CLINICAL NURSING

CLINICAL NURSING

June M. Thompson, R.N., M.S.

Assistant Professor, School of Nursing,
University of Texas Health Science Center,
Houston, Texas

Gertrude K. McFarland, R.N., D.N.Sc.

Nurse Consultant, Division of Nursing,
Health Resources and Services Administration,
U.S. Department of Health and Human Services,
Rockville, Maryland

Jane E. Hirsch, R.N., M.S.

Associate Director of Nursing,
University of California, San Francisco,
San Francisco, California

Susan M. Tucker, R.N., B.S.N., P.H.N.

Assistant Director of Nursing,
Kaiser Permanente Medical Center,
Panorama City, California

Arden C. Bowers, R.N., M.S.

Associate Professor,
Department of Nursing, College of Santa Fe,
Santa Fe, New Mexico

with 655 illustrations, including 132 in two colors
and 108 in full color

Original illustrations by **George Wassilchenko**

The C. V. Mosby Company

ST. LOUIS • TORONTO • PRINCETON   1986

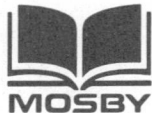

A TRADITION OF PUBLISHING EXCELLENCE

Editor: Barbara Ellen Norwitz
Developmental editor: Sally Adkisson
Editing Supervisor: Lin Dempsey
Manuscript editors: Patricia Tannian, Mary Wright, Idelle Winer,
Marjorie Sanson
Designer: Jeanne Genz
Cover designer: Diane M. Beasley
Production: Kathleen L. Teal, Mary G. Stueck, Suzanne C. Glazer

The authors and publisher have made a conscientious effort to ensure that the drug information and recommended dosages in this book are accurate and in accord with accepted standards at the time of publication. However, pharmacology is a rapidly changing science, so readers are advised to check the package insert provided by the manufacturer before administering any drug.

Printed in the United States of America

The C.V. Mosby Company
11830 Westline Industrial Drive, St. Louis, Missouri 63146

Library of Congress Cataloging in Publication Data

Main entry under title:

Clinical nursing.

   Includes bibliographies and index.
   1. Nursing. 2. Medicine, Clinical. I. Thompson,
June M., 1946-   . [DNLM: 1. Nursing Care.
2. Nursing Process.   WY 100 C6405]
RT41.C65 1986   610.73   85-21612
ISBN 0-8016-4953-6

GW/D/D 9 8 7 6 5 4 3 2 1   02/C/281

Contributors

LINDA D. ANDERSON, R.N., B.S.N.*

Clinical Nurse,
The National Institutes of Health,
Clinical Center, Nursing Department,
Bethesda, Maryland

ANNE ELIZABETH BELCHER, R.N., Ph.D.

Director of Nursing Staff Development,
University of Alabama Hospitals,
University of Alabama at Birmingham,
Birmingham, Alabama

CHARLOTTE ANNE BOSMAAS, R.N., A.A.N., P.N.A.*

Clinical Nurse,
The National Institutes of Health,
Clinical Center, Nursing Department,
Bethesda, Maryland

ARDEN C. BOWERS, R.N., M.S.

Associate Professor,
Department of Nursing,
College of Santa Fe,
Santa Fe, New Mexico

PRISCILLA C. BOYKIN, R.N., B.S.N., M.S.N.*

Educator,
The National Institutes of Health,
Clinical Center, Nursing Department,
Bethesda, Maryland

DEBRA C. BROADWELL, Ph.D., R.N.

Associate Professor,
Nell Hodgson Woodruff School of Nursing,
Emory University,
Atlanta, Georgia

DOROTHY BRUNDAGE, R.N., Ph.D., F.A.A.N.

Associate Professor of Nursing,
Duke University School of Nursing,
Durham, North Carolina

ANN WOLBERT BURGESS, R.N., D.N.Sc., C.S., F.A.A.N.

van Ameringen Professor of Psychiatric Mental Health Nursing,
University of Pennsylvania School of Nursing, Philadelphia;
Associate Director of Nursing Research,
Boston City Hospital,
Boston, Massachusetts

VICTOR G. CAMPBELL, M.S., R.N.

Ph.D. Student in Nursing,
Case Western Reserve University,
Cleveland, Ohio;
Formerly Instructor,
The Ohio State University College of Nursing,
Columbus, Ohio

MARY M. CANOBBIO, R.N., M.N.

Assistant Clinical Professor,
School of Nursing;
Cardiovascular Clinical Specialist,
Division of Cardiology,
University of California,
Los Angeles, California

*The opinions expressed herein are those of the author and do not necessarily reflect those of the U.S. Department of Health and Human Services or any of its component parts.

DEBORAH CESTARO-SEIFER, M.S., R.N.

Practitioner-Teacher,
Department of Pediatric Nursing,
Rush-Presbyterian-St. Luke's Medical Center,
Chicago, Illinois

TERESA M. CHOATE, R.N., B.S.N.*

Clinical Nurse,
The National Institutes of Health,
Clinical Center, Nursing Department,
Bethesda, Maryland

MARYANN COLLETTI, M.S., R.N.

Practitioner-Teacher,
Instructor, Rush University College of Nursing,
Department of Medical Nursing,
Rush-Presbyterian-St. Luke's Medical Center,
Chicago, Illinois

JOYCE E. DAINS, R.N., M.S.N.

Assistant Professor,
School of Nursing,
University of Texas Health Science Center,
Houston, Texas

JACQUELINE A. DIENEMANN, R.N., Ph.D.

Assistant Professor,
School of Nursing,
George Mason University,
Fairfax, Virginia

DIANE DIGIORGI, R.N., B.S.N.*

Clinical Nurse,
The National Institutes of Health,
Clinical Center, Nursing Department,
Bethesda, Maryland

JANICE ANN DRASS, R.N., B.S.N.*

Clinical Nurse,
The National Institutes of Health,
Clinical Center, Nursing Department,
Bethesda, Maryland

RICHARD J. FEHRING, D.N.Sc., R.N.

Assistant Professor,
Marquette University,
College of Nursing,
Milwaukee, Wisconsin

KAY FISCHER, R.N., M.N.

Clinical Nurse Specialist,
Private Practice,
Children's Health Care, Inc.,
Delafield, Wisconsin

MAGGIE GERMAN, M.S.N., R.N.

Nurse-Practitioner, Allergy/Clinical Immunology,
Instructor, Department of Immunology/Microbiology,
Rush University-College of Health Sciences,
Rush-Presbyterian-St. Luke's Medical Center,
Chicago, Illinois

MIKEL GRAY, R.N., M.S.N.

Clinical Nurse Specialist,
Section of Urology,
Emory University Clinic,
Atlanta, Georgia

DEANNA E. GRIMES, R.N., M.P.H.

Assistant Professor,
School of Nursing,
University of Texas Health Science Center,
Houston, Texas

KATHLEEN E. GUNTA, M.S.N., R.N.

Clinical Nurse Specialist-Orthopedics,
St. Luke's Samaritan Health Care Inc.,
Milwaukee, Wisconsin

JANICE C. HALLAL, R.N., D.N.Sc.

Assistant Professor, School of Nursing,
The Catholic University of America,
Washington, D.C.

CAROL R. HARTMAN, R.N., D.N.Sc.

Coordinator-Associate Professor,
Graduate Psychiatric/Mental Health Nursing Program,
School of Nursing,
Boston College,
Chestnut Hill, Massachusetts

KAREN D. HENCH, R.N., B.S.N.*

Clinical Nurse,
The National Institutes of Health,
Clinical Center, Nursing Department,
Bethesda, Maryland

JANE E. HIRSCH, R.N., M.S.

Associate Director of Nursing,
University of California, San Francisco,
San Francisco, California

LOIS M. HOSKINS, R.N., Ph.D.

Associate Professor, School of Nursing,
The Catholic University of America,
Washington, D.C.

RAE W. LANGFORD, R.N., Ed.D.

Associate Professor,
School of Nursing,
University of Texas Health Science Center,
Houston, Texas

LAUREN MEYERSON LONG, R.N., B.S.N.*

Clinical Nurse,
The National Institutes of Health,
Clinical Center, Nursing Department,
Bethesda, Maryland

NANETTE STEGMAN McATEE, R.N., B.S.N.*

Clinical Nurse,
The National Institutes of Health,
Clinical Center, Nursing Department,
Bethesda, Maryland

JAMES McCANN, R.N., D.N.Sc.*

Psychiatric Nurse Consultant,
Office of Survey and Certification,
Health Standards and Quality Bureau,
Health Care Financing Administration,
Baltimore, Maryland

ANN MARIE K. McDONNELL-KEENAN, M.S., R.N.

Practitioner-Teacher,
Instructor, Rush University, College of Nursing,
Department of Medical Nursing,
Rush-Presbyterian-St. Luke's Medical Center,
Chicago, Illinois

GERTRUDE K. McFARLAND, R.N., D.N.Sc.*

Nurse Consultant,
Division of Nursing,
Health Resources and Services Administration,
U.S. Department of Health and Human Services,
Rockville, Maryland

ELIZABETH A. McFARLANE, R.N., D.N.Sc.

Assistant Professor, School of Nursing,
The Catholic University of America,
Washington, D.C.

AUDREY M. McLANE, Ph.D., R.N.

Professor,
Marquette University,
College of Nursing,
Milwaukee, Wisconsin

RUTH E. McSHANE, M.S., R.N.

University of Wisconsin-Milwaukee,
Milwaukee, Wisconsin;
Doctoral Candidate,
University of Wisconsin-Madison,
Madison, Wisconsin

VIOLA MOROFKA, Ph.D., R.N.

Associate Professor of Nursing,
Kent State University,
School of Nursing,
Kent, Ohio

LEONA A. MOURAD, M.S.N., R.N.

Associate Professor, Emeritus,
The Ohio State University College of Nursing,
Columbus, Ohio

CHARLOTTE E. NASCHINSKI, R.N., M.S.*

Nurse Educator,
Saint Elizabeths Hospital,
National Institute of Mental Health,
U.S. Department of Health and Human Services,
Washington, D.C.

BARBARA K. REDMAN, R.N., Ph.D.

Executive Director,
American Association of Colleges of Nursing,
Washington, D.C.

PATRICE A. ROBINS, R.N., B.S.N.*

Clinical Nurse,
The National Institutes of Health,
Clinical Center, Nursing Department,
Bethesda, Maryland

M. GAIE RUBENFELD, R.N., M.S.

Assistant Professor, School of Nursing,
The Catholic University of America,
Washington, D.C.

POLLY RYAN, R.N., M.S.N.

Cardiovascular Clinical Nurse Specialist,
St. Luke's Samaritan Health Care Inc.,
Milwaukee, Wisconsin

ANN M. SCHREIER, R.N., Ph.D.

Adjunct Assistant Professor, School of Nursing,
The Catholic University of America,
Washington, D.C.

PAMELA M. SCHROEDER, M.S.N., R.N.

Clinical Nurse Specialist-Rheumatology,
St. Luke's Samaritan Health Care Inc.,
Milwaukee, Wisconsin

MARLENE F. SCHWARTZ, R.N., M.S.N.

Clinical Nurse Specialist, Psychotherapist,
Private Practice,
Psychiatric Associates,
Comprehensive Services,
Milwaukee, Wisconsin

BARBARA LEE BARRAT SOLOMON, D.N.Sc., R.N.*

ANA Certified Clinical Nurse Specialist,
The National Institutes of Health,
Clinical Center, Nursing Department,
Bethesda, Maryland

JUNE M. THOMPSON, R.N., M.S.

Assistant Professor,
School of Nursing,
University of Texas Health Science Center,
Houston, Texas

JEAN O. TROTTER, R.N., M.S.N.

Assistant Professor,
School of Nursing,
University of Maryland,
Baltimore, Maryland;
Case Manager, Inservice Instructor,
Home Call Incorporated,
Catonsville, Maryland

SUSAN M. TUCKER, R.N., B.S.N., P.H.N.

Assistant Director of Nursing,
Kaiser Permanente Medical Center,
Panorama City, California

EVELYN L. WASLI, R.N., D.N.Sc.*

Associate Chief Nurse, Saint Elizabeths Hospital,
National Institute of Mental Health,
U.S. Department of Health and Human Services,
Washington, D.C.

MARY WELLS, R.N., B.A.*

Clinical Nurse,
The National Institutes of Health,
Clinical Center, Nursing Department,
Bethesda, Maryland

SUSAN FICKERTT WILSON, R.N., Ph.D.

Assistant Professor,
School of Nursing,
University of Texas Health Science Center,
Houston, Texas

JANICE M. ZELLER, Ph.D., R.N.

Assistant Professor,
Departments of Medical Nursing
and Immunology/Microbiology,
Rush-Presbyterian-St. Luke's Medical Center,
Chicago, Illinois

Consultants

SANDRA S. BAUER, R.N., M.S.

Nurse Educator,
Saint Elizabeths Hospital,
National Institute of Mental Health,
U.S. Department of Health and Human Services,
Washington, D.C.

JACQUELINE A. DIENEMANN, R.N., Ph.D.

Assistant Professor,
School of Nursing,
George Mason University,
Fairfax, Virginia

LOIS K. EVANS, R.N., D.N.Sc.

Assistant Professor,
School of Nursing,
University of Pennsylvania,
Philadelphia, Pennsylvania

EDNA M. FORDYCE, R.N., M.N., Ed.D.

Associate Professor,
Department of Nursing,
Towson State University,
Baltimore, Maryland

ZERITA J. HAGERMAN, R.N., D.N.Sc.

Professor and Director,
Graduate Nursing,
Andrews University,
Berrien Springs, Michigan

MARY M. HALL, R.N., M.S.N.

Instructor, Emergency Medical Services Program,
School of Allied Health,
University of Texas Health Science Center,
Houston, Texas

MAXINE HARRIS, Ph.D.

Clinical Psychologist,
Co-Director, Community Connections,
Washington, D.C.

JOANNE D. JOYNER-McNEAL, M.S.N.

Clinical Nurse Specialist for Psychiatric Mental Health Nursing,
Veterans Administration Medical Center,
Washington, D.C.

MARIE E. KOENINGS, R.N.C.S., M.S.N.

Psychiatric Clinical Specialist,
Area D. Outpatient Department,
Saint Elizabeths Hospital,
Washington, D.C.

LORNA LARSON, R.N., M.S.N., D.N.Sc.

Research Nurse,
Saint Elizabeths Hospital,
National Institute of Mental Health,
Washington, D.C.

VALLORY G. LATHROP, D.N.Sc., F.A.A.N.

Deputy Director for Nursing,
Saint Elizabeths Hospital,
Washington, D.C.

GARLAND K. LEWIS, R.N., M.S.N.

Formerly Associate Professor of Psychiatric Nursing,
Catholic University of America,
Washington, D.C.

ELEANOR LOUIE, R.N.

Head Nurse,
University of California at San Francisco,
Medical Center,
San Francisco, California

MARY E. MARKERT, R.N., M.N.

Clinical Administrator,
Saint Elizabeths Hospital,
National Institute of Mental Health,
U.S. Department of Health and Human Services,
Washington, D.C.

KATHLEEN K. McCANN, R.N., M.S.N., C.S.

Clinical Specialist,
Montgomery General Hospital,
Olney, Maryland

ELAINE McKENNA, R.N., M.S.

Head Nurse,
University of California at San Francisco,
Medical Center,
San Francisco, California

GLORIA ODEN, R.N., M.S.

Psychiatric Coordinator,
Morristown Memorial Hospital,
Morristown, New Jersey

CYNTHIA A. RECTOR, R.N., M.S.

Director of Nursing,
Charter Glade Hospital,
Ft. Myers, Florida

SUZANNE S. RESNER, D.N.Sc.

Nurse Consultant,
Division of Nursing,
Health Resources and Services Administration,
U.S. Department of Health and Human Services;
Clinical Faculty, School of Nursing,
American University,
Washington, D.C.

KAREN V. SCIPIO-SKINNER, M.S.N.

Director of Staff Development,
Washington Psychiatric Institute,
Washington, D.C.

KATHERINE STEFOS, Ph.D.

Adjunct Associate Professor,
School of Nursing,
University of Texas Health Science Center,
Houston, Texas

KATHLEEN STONE, R.N., Ph.D.

Associate Professor,
College of Nursing,
The Ohio State University,
Columbus, Ohio

SUZANNE SUMMERHILL, R.N.

Clinical Practitioner-Teacher,
Pulmonary Department,
The Methodist Hospital,
Houston, Texas

SHEILA ZERR, R.N., M.Ed.

Assistant Professor,
School of Nursing,
University of Ottawa,
Ottawa, Ontario

Preface

We have developed what we believe to be the definitive reference source for the clinical nursing practice. No longer will you need to rely on the six or seven reference texts that you currently use. It's all here at last, a single text. A text that stands alone.

The Publisher

We didn't invent this text, you did. This text has evolved as a result of the demand by professional nurses from across the United States and Canada and in many parts of the world. Nurses said there was a need to clarify nursing practice—to "put it all together" in one book. They said, "Put together the nursing theories, nursing process including nursing diagnoses, and physiology and pathophysiology. Use those theory bases and an interdisciplinary health care approach to develop a contemporary and comprehensive text that reflects the potential scope and responsibilities of professional nursing practice."

So, here it is. We have written what we believe to be a succinct reference and text that is broad in scope and intensive in content. This text will permit nurses to easily relate nursing diagnosis to medical diagnosis and medical treatment to nursing process. *Clinical Nursing* is more than just "clinical nursing." It provides a strong foundation in nursing science, integrating the nursing process with nursing diagnoses throughout the text while at the same time providing thorough coverage in anatomy, physiology, pathophysiology, and the social sciences. The intent is to provide a single practical text that is also high level, theory based, interdisciplinary, contemporary, and comprehensive.

The framework for the text is *Nursing: A Social Policy Statement*, which was published by the American Nurses'

Association Congress for Nursing Practice in 1980. This document defines nursing as "the diagnosis and treatment of human responses to actual or potential health problems."* According to definition, practice is built upon phenomena (observable manifestations), theory application, nursing actions, and evaluation of effects of action in relation to the phenomena. Therefore these are the underlying principles of the text.

Clinical Nursing is designed for convenient use by both students and practitioners. Theoretical content provides the solid background required for the implementation of sound clinical practice, and the ready-reference format permits easy access to the detailed information needed to assess and provide care for individuals with actual or potential health care problems. The systematic design, layout, and two-color format make it easy to find information or extract specific data. Whether the reader wants to develop a nursing care plan, look up the details of a particular chemotherapeutic agent, read about the pathophysiology of a disease, or review the theory base and clinical application of a specific nursing diagnosis, the information is readily accessible and richly detailed.

Many steps were taken throughout the development of this text to ensure its quality. Authors and contributors were selected because of their clinical, educational, and research expertise. Thus they represent both theory and practice. Each chapter was carefully reviewed by clinical and educational experts in nursing, medicine, physiology, pharmacology, and related fields. We also consulted many others in nursing regarding the content and design of the text. Ideas and prototypes were circulated among

*American Nurses' Association: Nursing: a social policy statement, Kansas City, 1980, p. 9.

practicing nurses, students, and nursing educators to verify that this was the book they wanted. Laboratory and chemotherapeutic data were standardized where appropriate.*

*Laboratory values were taken from Jacobs, D., et al.: Laboratory test handbook, St. Louis, 1984, The C.V. Mosby Co. Chemotherapeutic data were taken from U.S. and Canadian sources: McEvoy, T.K., editor: American hospital formulary system: drug information 1985, Bethesda, Md., 1985, American Society of Hospital Pharmacists; and Canadian Pharmaceutical Association: Compendium of pharmaceuticals and specialties, ed. 20, Ottawa, Canada, 1985.

This text is based on the complex foundation of nursing theory and nursing science. We believe that it is unique, in-depth, comprehensive, precise, contemporary, and interdisciplinary.

June M. Thompson
Gertrude K. McFarland
Jane E. Hirsch
Susan M. Tucker
Arden C. Bowers

Acknowledgments

An undertaking of this magnitude is not the result of a single mind. It attests to the contributions, support, and encouragement of many. We owe a special debt and heartfelt thanks to Barbara Ellen Norwitz, Editor, for her vision, project initiation, and unstinting support; Sally Adkisson, Developmental Editor, for her forbearance, extensive assistance, and sound editorial sense; Lin Dempsey, Book Editing Manager, for careful reading, unending editing, and fruitful suggestions; George Wassilchenko for the beautiful artwork; all of the authors, consultants, and reviewers for their expertise and perseverance; and all of The C.V. Mosby Company staff involved in this project for their unending support and standard of excellence. This project was overwhelming. Without the kind support and expertise of all of the above it could not have been achieved.

JMT
GKM
JEH
SMT
ACB

Overview of Text

Clinical Nursing was designed to blend the traditional body system–disease approach with contemporary theory-based nursing practice. The text is divided into two major parts. The first part, "Clinical Nursing Practice," consists of 17 chapters. The second part, "Nursing Diagnoses," includes 13 functional patterns comprising all of the currently accepted nursing diagnoses.

Part One: Clinical Nursing Practice

Part One is organized by body systems for easy reference. The description of each body system is divided into three sections:

Overview. The overview presents the systems in terms of its importance and functioning. Presented in detail are:
Normal anatomy and physiology of the system
Normal clinical findings for the system
Normal laboratory values
Relevant diagnostic studies with nursing care

Conditions, Diseases, and Disorders. Health problems related to the specific body system are presented using a systematic format:
Definition of the condition, disease, or disorder
Pathophysiology of the problem
Diagnostic studies with anticipated findings
Treatment plan, including surgical, chemotherapeutic, electromechanical, and supportive interventions
Assessment criteria
Nursing diagnoses
Nursing interventions specifically related to the nursing diagnoses
Patient education
Evaluation based on patient outcome criteria

Medical Interventions. Major therapeutic interventions are presented and discussed thoroughly:
Overview of intervention including description and rationale
Contraindications and cautions
Preprocedural nursing care
Treatment plan
Assessment
Nursing interventions
Evaluation

Part Two: Nursing Diagnoses

Part Two is organized into the 13 functional patterns of the unitary person. It contains all of the nursing diagnoses accepted by the North American Nursing Diagnoses Association (NANDA). Each diagnosis includes the following information:
"Theory and Etiology" presents a discussion of the theories and research related to the development of the diagnosis and a list of etiologies.
"Defining Characteristics" includes the defining characteristics accepted by NANDA, as well as other research-based characteristics determined by the authors.
"Nursing Interventions" relates actions to goal statements.
"Evaluation" is based on the anticipated patient outcome and the data that indicate the outcome has been reached.

In addition to the two major parts of the text, three appendices provide supplemental content.

Appendix A: Current Status and Historical Evolution of the North American Nursing Diagnoses Association (NANDA)
Appendix A provides a brief overview of the evolution of nursing diagnoses and the North American Nursing Diagnoses Association. Also included is a list of the currently accepted nursing diagnoses.

Appendix B: Conversion Factors to International System of Units (SI Units)
In May 1977, the 30th World Health Assembly recommended that SI units be used in medicine. Although health care agencies in the United States continue to

use the metric system, many health care systems throughout the world have adopted SI units.

Appendix C: Chemotherapeutic Agents

Appendix C is a compilation of the chemotherapeutic agents discussed throughout the text. The agents presented are organized according to the format and description outlined by the American Hospital Formulary Service (1985). Each category of agents is presented as follows:

Category and class
    Generic and trade names (U.S. and Canadian)
    Actions
    Uses
    General side effects
    Adverse reactions
    Contraindications
    Nursing considerations

Parts One and Two of this text can be used independently or interdependently. The nurse can look up a particular disease in Part One and find virtually all the information needed to provide optimal care for the patient. The nurse can consult Part Two for a specific nursing diagnosis and can use the defining characteristics, interventions, and evaluation sections presented to implement a plan of care.

Although the nurse is concerned with medical diagnoses and nursing diagnoses as separate entities, the two should be integrated to deliver high-quality nursing care. The two separate component parts of this book will facilitate this integration. The nurse can look up a particular disorder in Part One. Within that discussion, in the section "Nursing Diagnoses and Nursing Interventions," are the details the nurse will need to provide nursing care for a patient with the disorder. In addition, many times cross-references are provided to specific nursing diagnoses discussed in Part Two. The expanded discussion in Part Two will help the nurse consider additional strategies of care.

The interrelationship of the two parts of the text will provide the nurse with complete information that can be used to develop an effective plan of care for patients. This book offers all the information the nurse needs to determine, implement, and evaluate an individualized plan of nursing care.

Contents

Appendixes

Detailed Contents

PART ONE

Clinical Nursing Practice

PART TWO

Nursing Diagnoses

Appendixes

CLINICAL NURSING

Plate 1. Integumentary system.

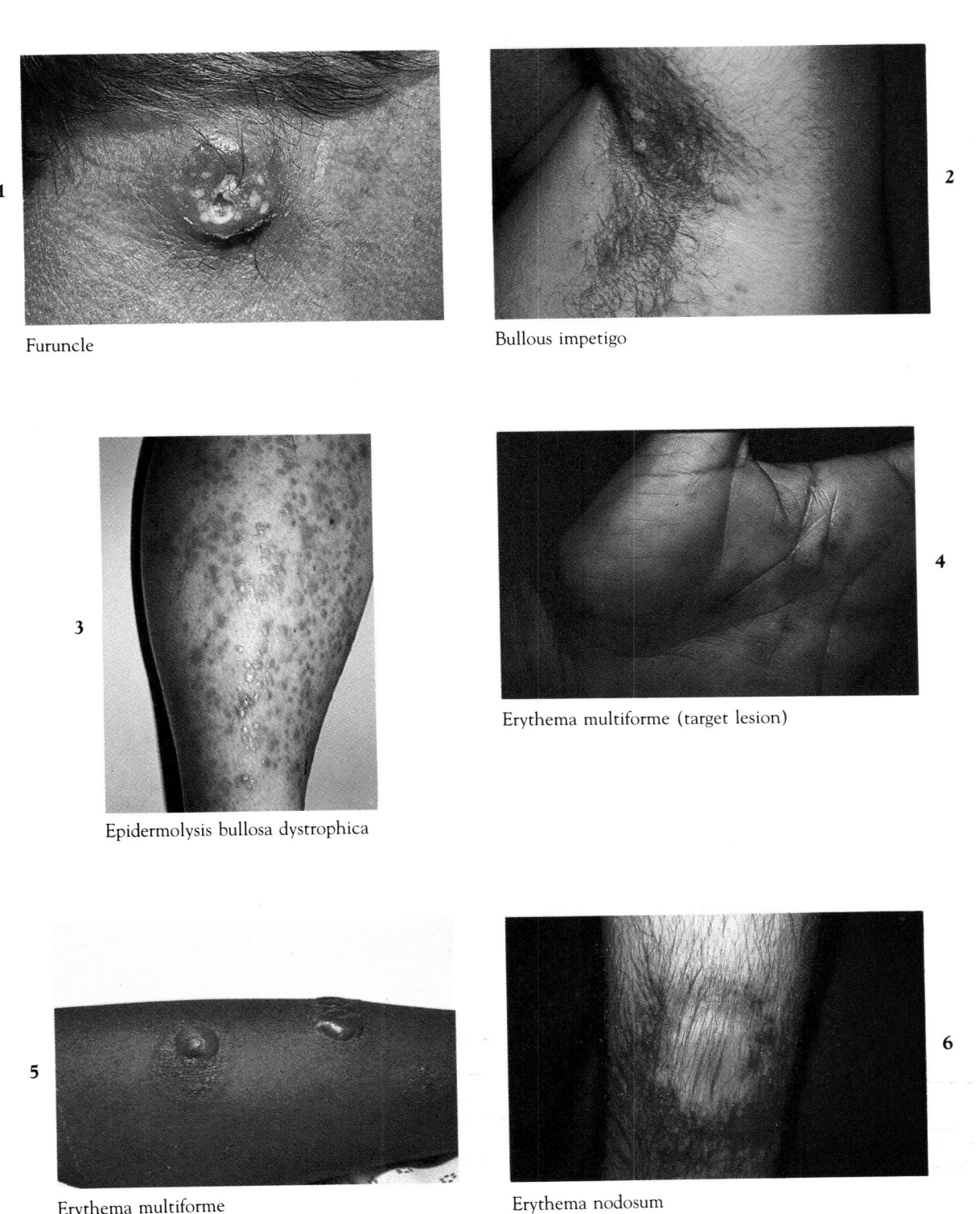

1   Furuncle

2   Bullous impetigo

3   Epidermolysis bullosa dystrophica

4   Erythema multiforme (target lesion)

5   Erythema multiforme

6   Erythema nodosum

Continued.

1 and **2,** Courtesy Jaime A. Tschen, M.D., Baylor College of Medicine, Department of Dermatology, Baylor College of Medicine, Houston; **3-6,** courtesy Stephen B. Tucker, M.D., Department of Dermatology, University of Texas Health Science Center at Houston.

7

Scabies

8

Fire ant bites

9

Contact dermatitis

10

Acute contact dermatitis

11

Seborrheic dermatitis

12

Ichthyosis vulgaris

7-12, Courtesy Stephen B. Tucker, M.D., Department of Dermatology, University of Texas Health Science Center at Houston.

Plate 1, cont'd. Integumentary system.

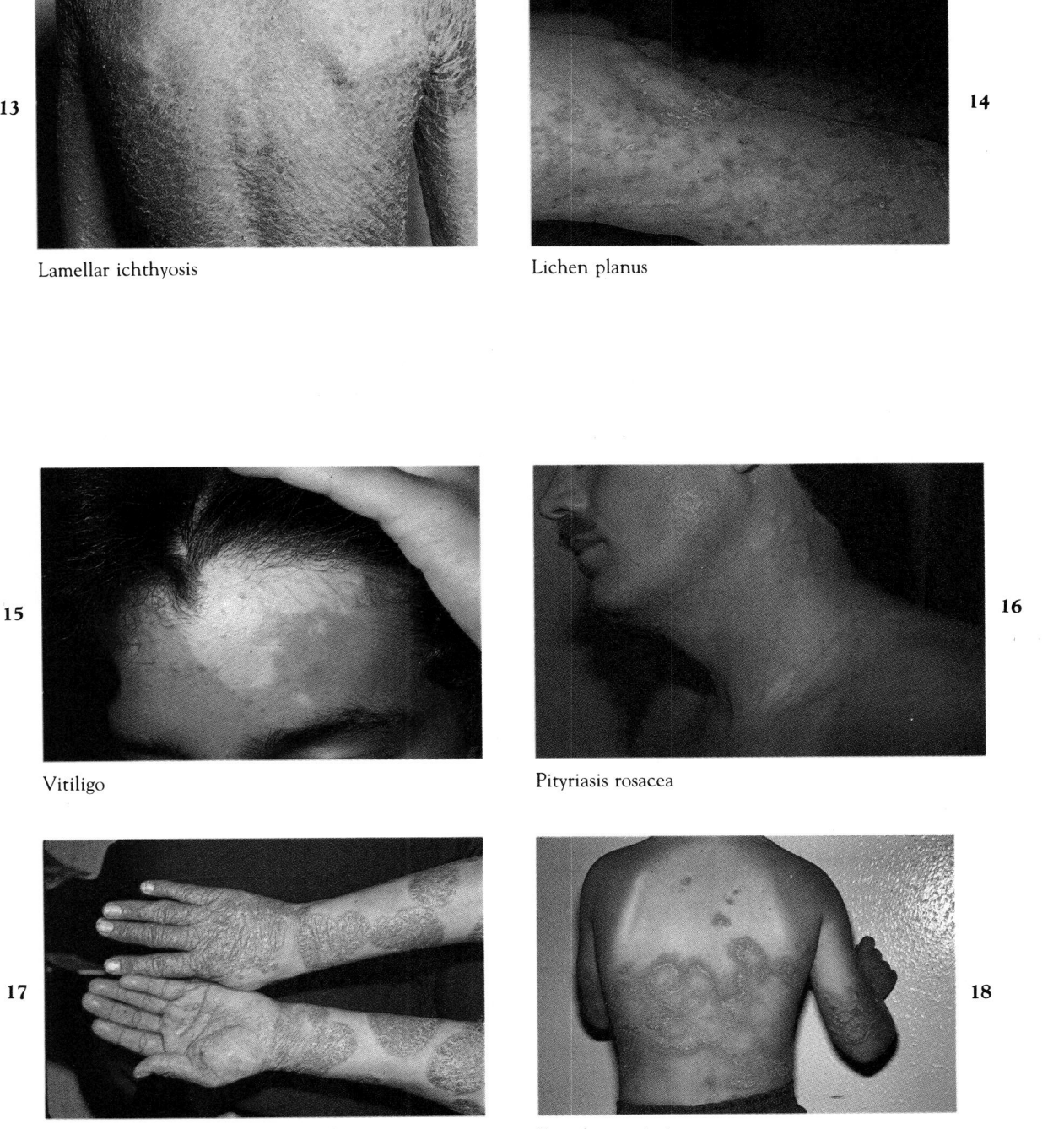

13 Lamellar ichthyosis

14 Lichen planus

15 Vitiligo

16 Pityriasis rosacea

17 Psoriasis vulgaris

18 Pustular psoriasis

Continued.

13, 14, and **18,** Courtesy Stephen B. Tucker, M.D., Department of Dermatology, University of Texas Health Science Center at Houston; **15, 16,** and **17,** courtesy Jaime A. Tschen, M.D., Baylor College of Medicine, Department of Dermatology, Houston.

Plate 1, cont'd. Integumentary system.

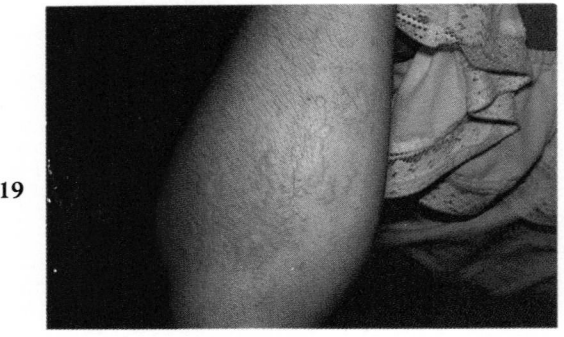

19

Urticaria

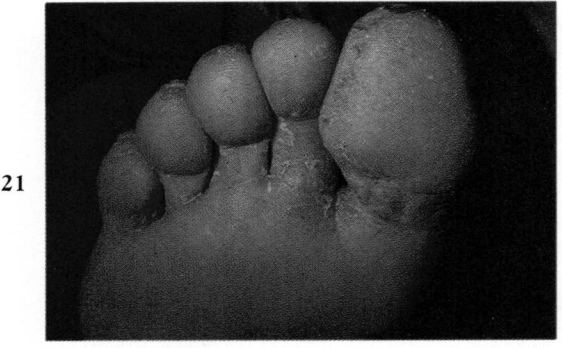

20

Tinea corporis

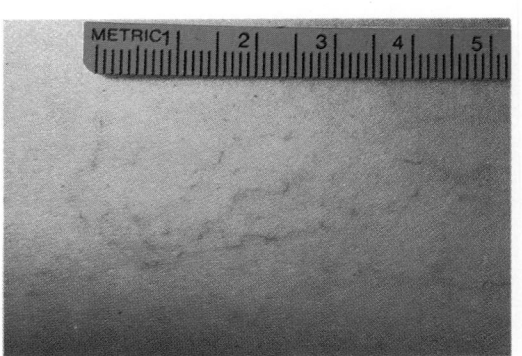

21

Tinea pedis

22

Telangiectasia

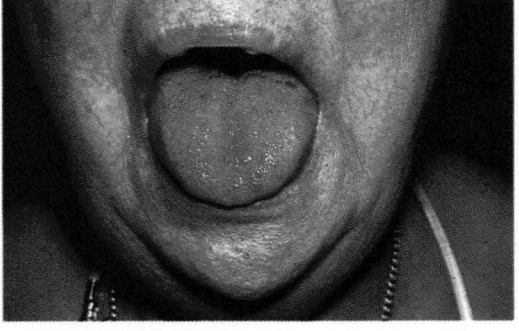

23

Hereditary hemorrhagic telangiectasia (Osler-Weber-Rendu disease)

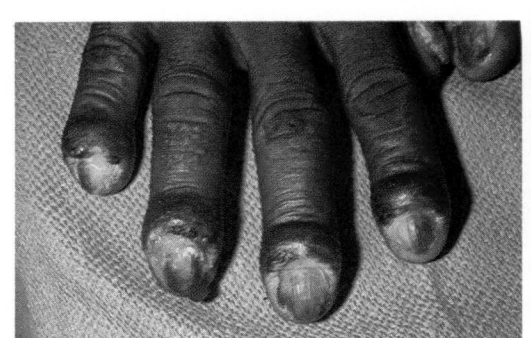

24

Chronic paronychia with nail dystrophy

19, 20, and 23, Courtesy Stephen B. Tucker, M.D., Department of Dermatology, University of Texas Health Science Center at Houston; 21, 22, and 24, courtesy Jaime A. Tschen, M.D., Baylor College of Medicine, Department of Dermatology, Houston.

Plate 2. Eye.

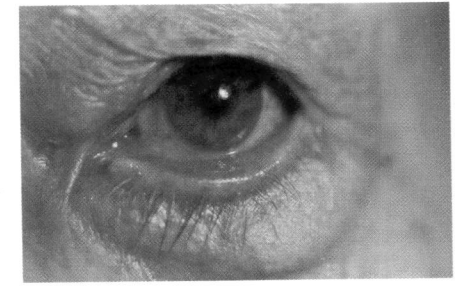

1

Ectropion. An outward turning of the lower eyelid from laxity of the eyelid muscle.

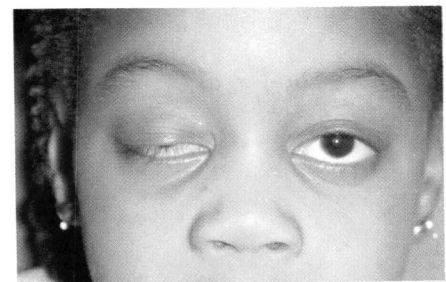

2

Ptosis. A drooping of the upper eyelid.

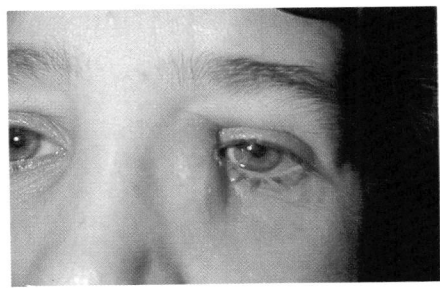

3

Acute dacryocystitis. Blockage of the lacrimal outflow system resulting in large swelling of the lacrimal sac.

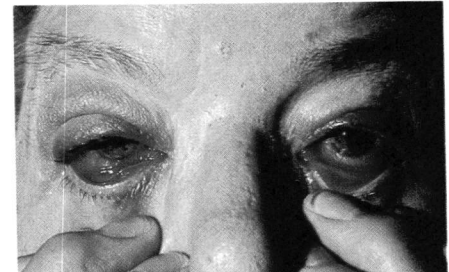

4

Acute bacterial conjunctivitis. Inflammation of the conjunctival lining caused by *Streptococcus.*

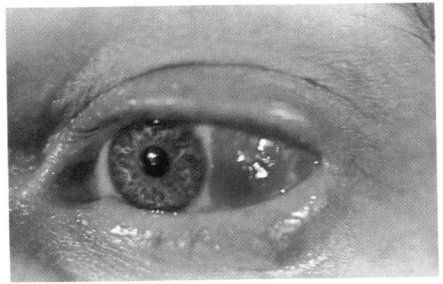

5

Subconjunctival hemorrhage. A spontaneous hemorrhage occurring under the conjunctiva and spreading over the globe.

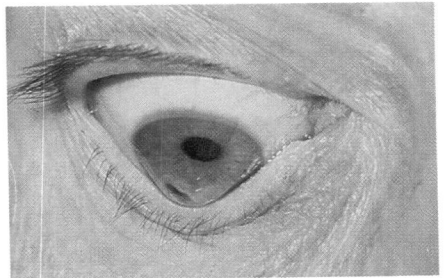

6

Advanced keratoconus. A cone-shaped deformity of the cornea with thinning of the cornea.

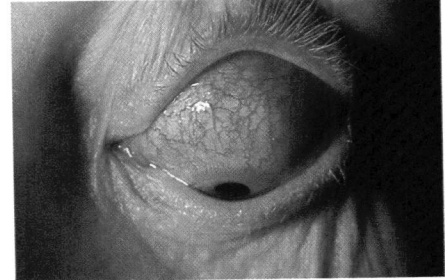

7

Scleritis. Nonbacterial inflammation of the sclera.

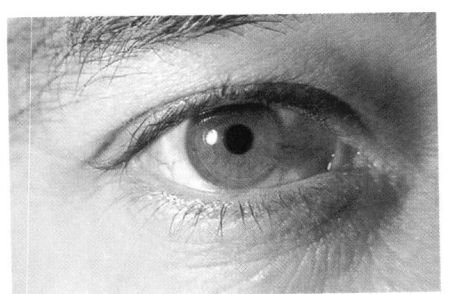

8

Pterygium. A triangular membrane extending from the conjunctiva over the cornea.

Continued.

1-8, From Stein, H.A., and Slatt, B.J.: The ophthalmic assistant: fundamentals and clinical practice, ed. 4, St. Louis, 1983, The C.V. Mosby Co.; **1,** courtesy Dr. Ira Abrahamson, Jr., Cincinnati; **6,** courtesy Dr. Dean Butcher, Australia.

Plate 2, cont'd. Eye.

9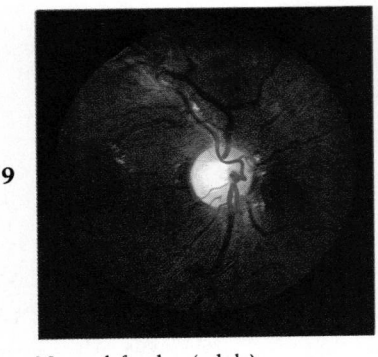

Normal fundus (adult)

10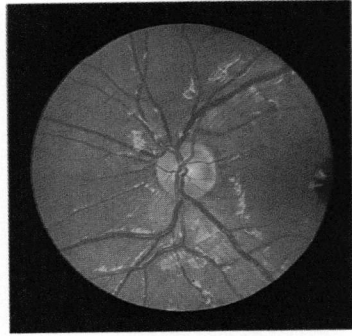

Normal fundus (child). Shows highlights reflected from the inner surface of the retina.

11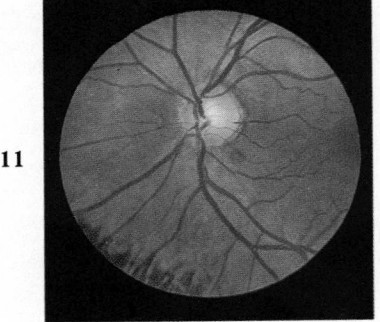

Normal negroid fundus. Shows uniform pigmentation that forms beneath and shows through the retina.

12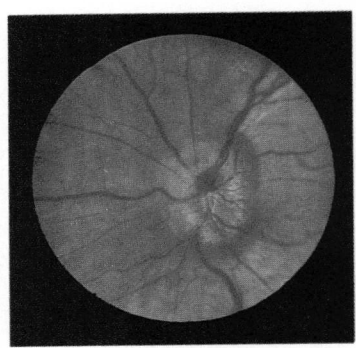

Papilledema. Disc is elevated. Disc border is obscured and hyperemic.

13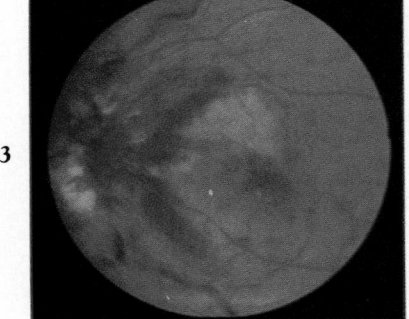

Central retinal artery occlusion.

14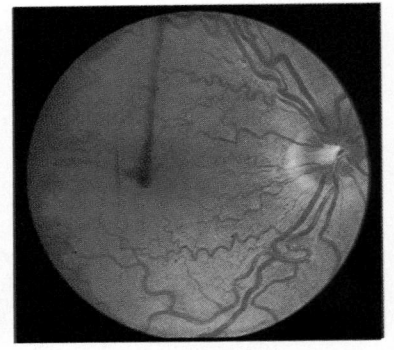

Arterial and venous tortuosity.

9-12, From MEDCOM: Selected topics in ophthalmology, Medcom Clinical Lecture Guides, Garden Grove, California, 1973, Medcom, Inc.; **13** and **14,** courtesy George Wassilchenko, Tulsa, Oklahoma.

Plate 2, cont'd. Eye.

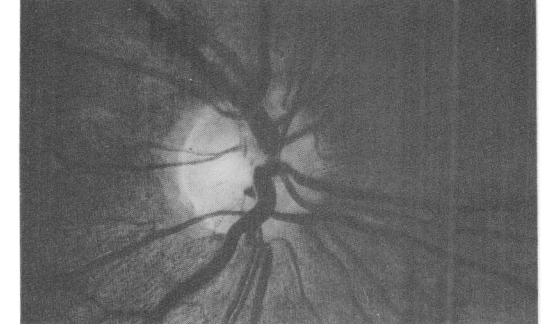

15

Diabetic retinopathy, proliferative.
Neovascularization appears above the disc.

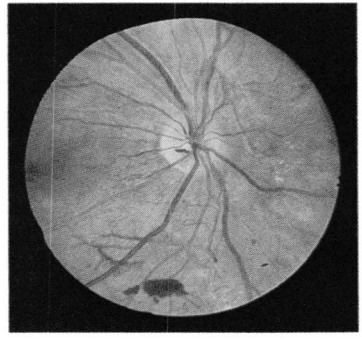

16

Diabetic retinopathy, proliferative.
A surface hemorrhage resulting
from neovascularization is in lower
right.

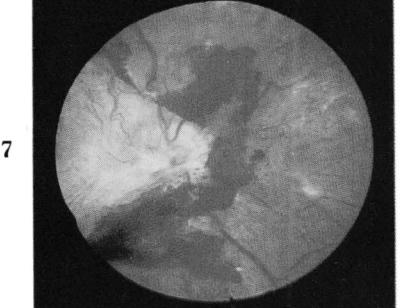

17

Diabetic retinopathy. Preretinal
hemorrhages surround the disc.
Older hemorrhages are darker, and
new ones are bright red.

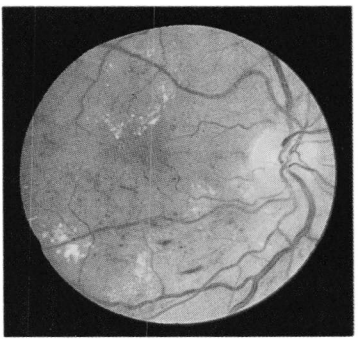

18

Diabetic retinopathy. Microaneurysms are temporal to macula.
Hard, yellow exudates are scattered
and flame hemorrhages.

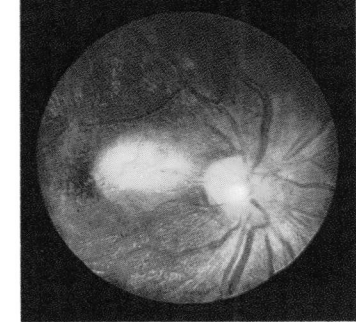

19

Chorioretinitis. Acute lesion with
opacification between disc and
macula.

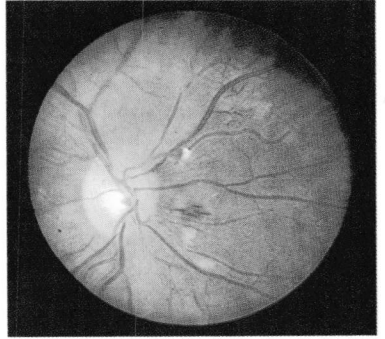

20

Retinal changes with hypertension.
Irregular caliber of major arterial
branches, cotton wool spots, and
splinter and punctate hemorrhages.

15-20, From MEDCOM: Selected topics in ophthalmology, Medcom Clinical Lecture Guides, Garden
Grove, California, 1973, Medcom, Inc.

Plate 3. Ear, nose, and throat.

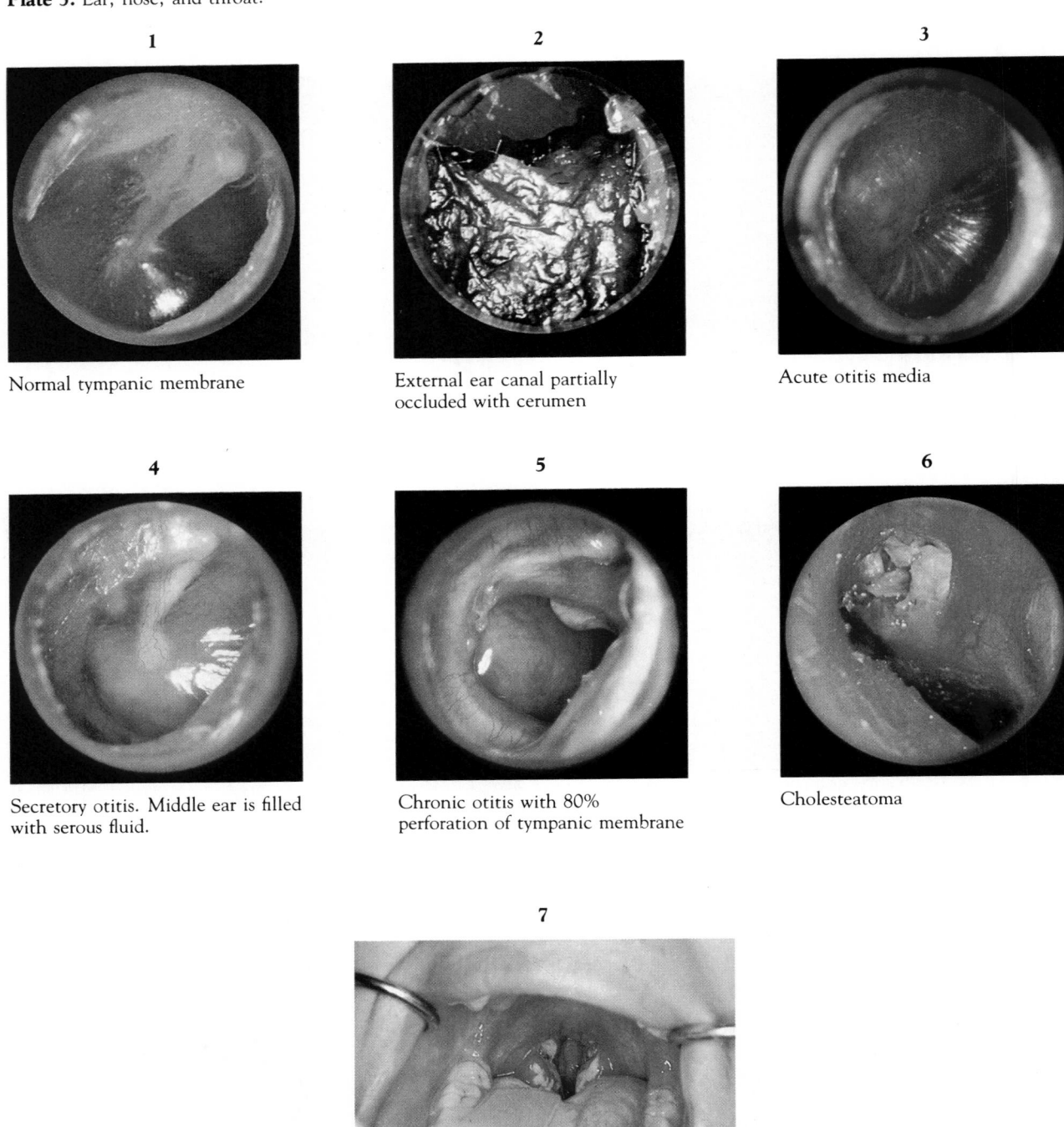

1

Normal tympanic membrane

2

External ear canal partially
occluded with cerumen

3

Acute otitis media

4

Secretory otitis. Middle ear is filled
with serous fluid.

5

Chronic otitis with 80%
perforation of tympanic membrane

6

Cholesteatoma

7

Tonsillitis and pharyngitis

From Malasanos, L., et al.: Health assessment, ed. 2, St. Louis, 1981, The C.V. Mosby Co.; **1-6,** Courtesy
Dr. Richard A. Buckingham, Clinical Professor, Otolaryngology, Abraham Lincoln School of Medicine,
University of Illinois, Chicago.

Plate 4. Hematolymphatic system.

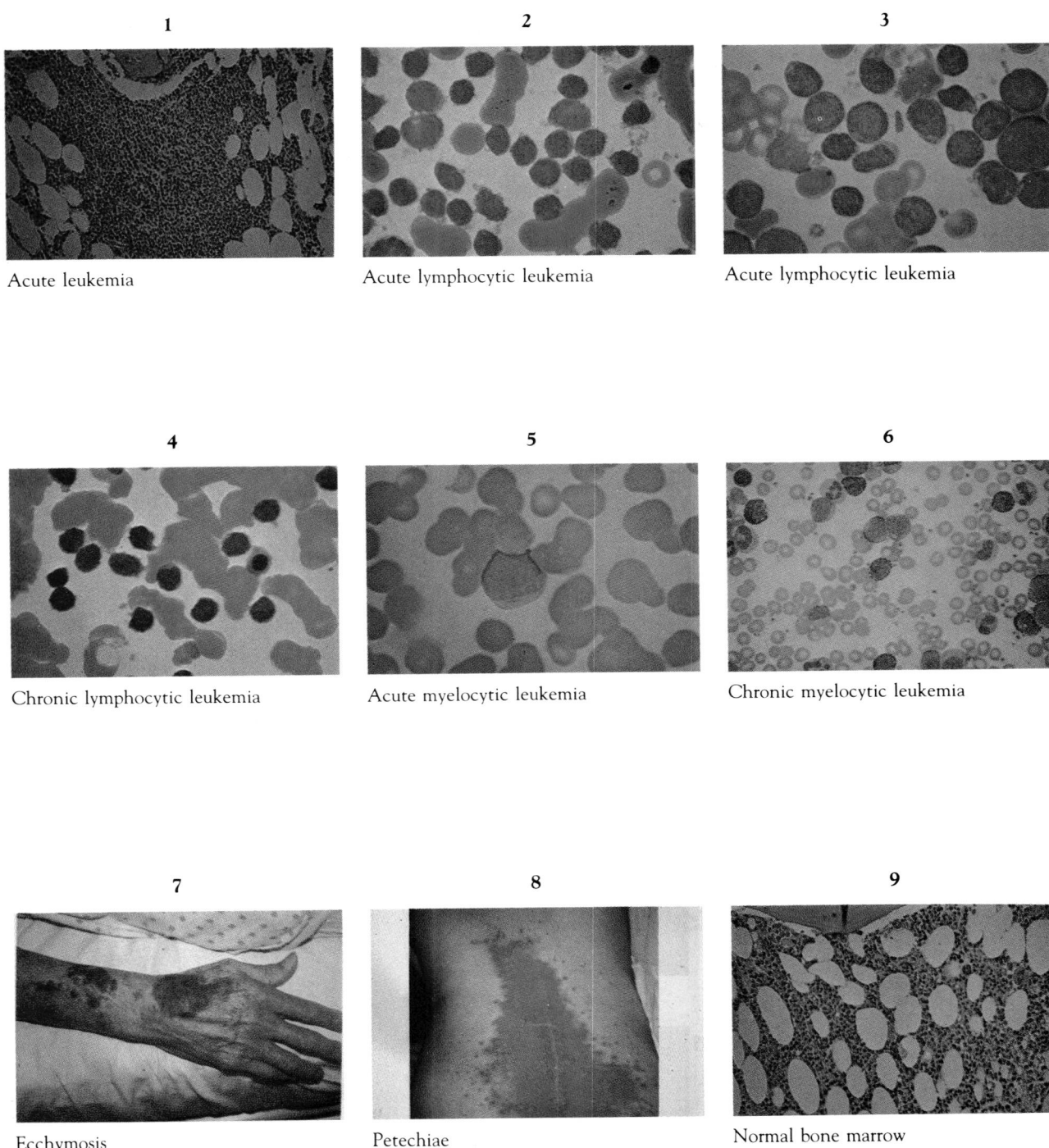

1

Acute leukemia

2

Acute lymphocytic leukemia

3

Acute lymphocytic leukemia

4

Chronic lymphocytic leukemia

5

Acute myelocytic leukemia

6

Chronic myelocytic leukemia

7

Ecchymosis

8

Petechiae

9

Normal bone marrow

Plate 5. Neoplasia.

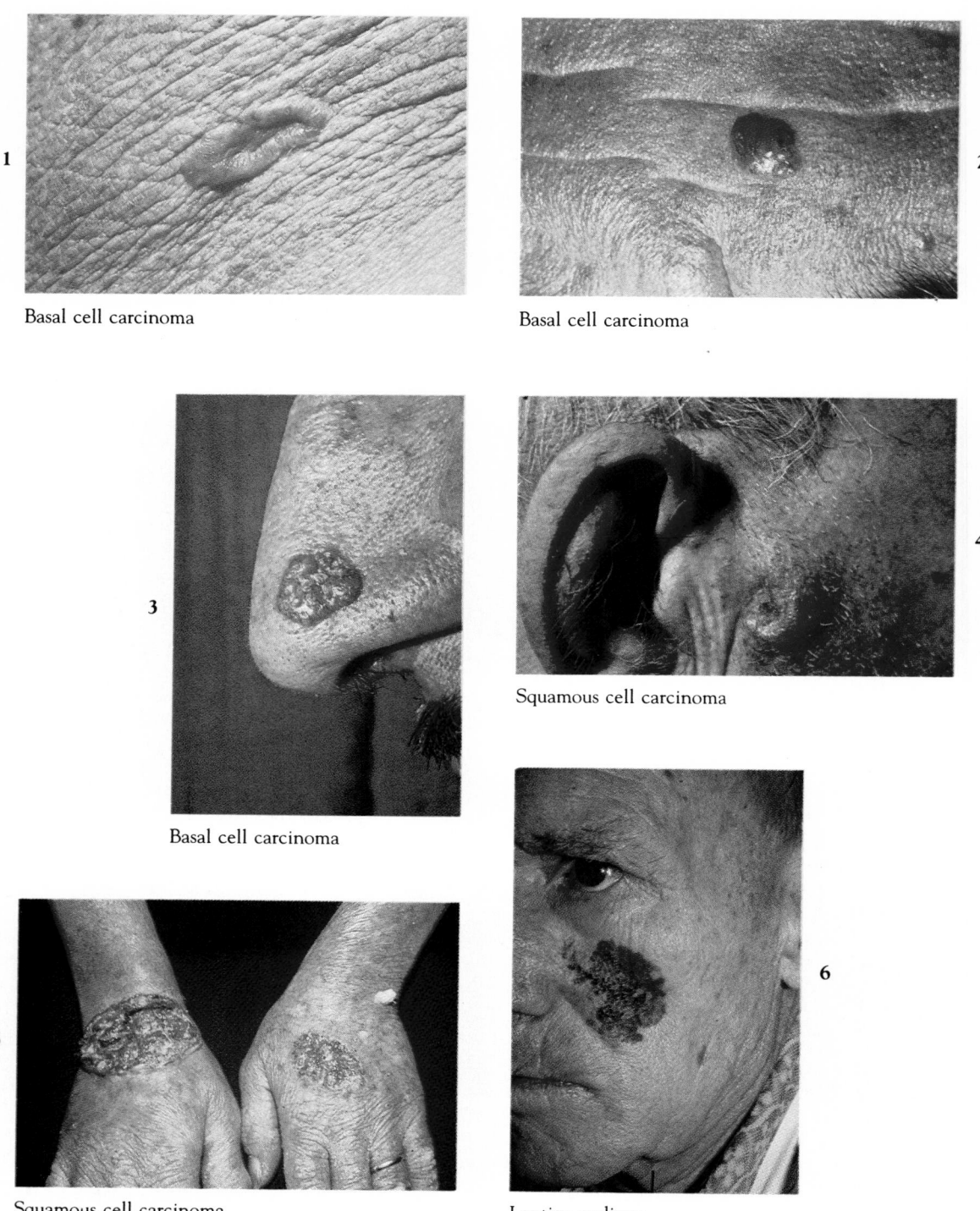

1 Basal cell carcinoma

2 Basal cell carcinoma

3 Basal cell carcinoma

4 Squamous cell carcinoma

5 Squamous cell carcinoma

6 Lentigo maligna

Courtesy Dr. Gary Monheit, University of Alabama at Birmingham School of Medicine.

Plate 5, cont'd. Neoplasia.

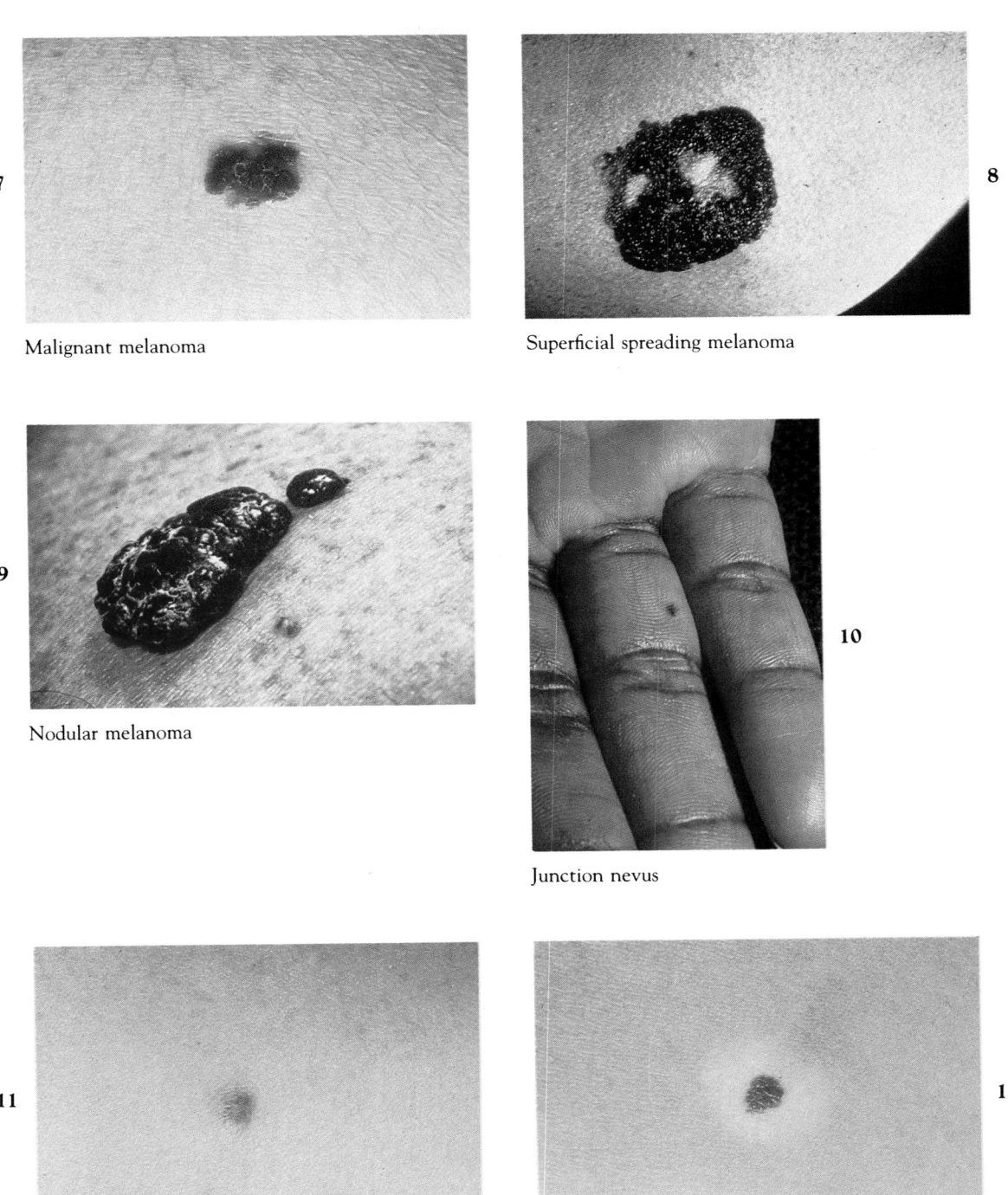

7   Malignant melanoma

8   Superficial spreading melanoma

9   Nodular melanoma

10   Junction nevus

11   Compound nevus

12   Halo nevus

Courtesy Dr. Gary Monheit, University of Alabama at Birmingham School of Medicine.

Plate 6. Infectious diseases.

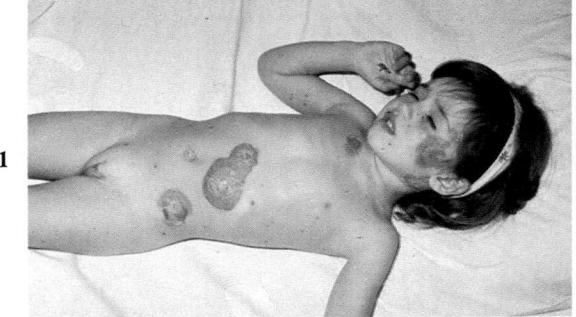

Combined infection of chickenpox with live measles vaccine virus produced bizarre bullae (ruptured) in addition to ordinary chickenpox lesions.

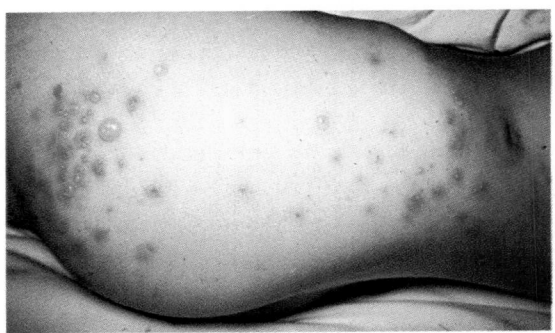

Staphylococcal bullous impetigo may produce lesions similar to chickenpox, but the distribution is in clusters rather than in a symmetric pattern.

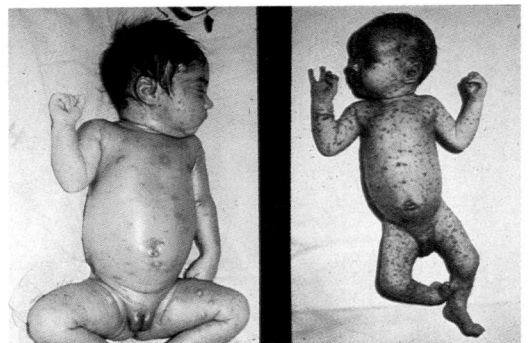

Left, Mild neonatal smallpox with atypical distribution. *Right,* Severe neonatal chickenpox with characteristic pleomorphic rash.

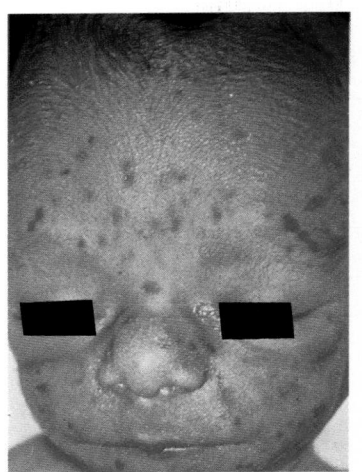

Congenital rubella

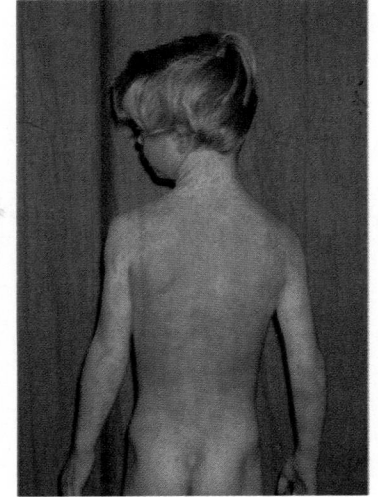

Rubeola

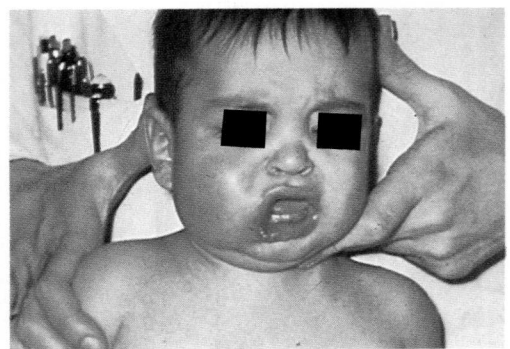

Facial cellulitis

1, 2, and **3,** Reproduced with permission of Burroughs Wellcome Co.; **4** and **5,** courtesy Donald C. Anderson, M.D., Baylor College of Medicine, Houston; **6,** courtesy Lisa M. Dunkle, M.D., St. Louis University School of Medicine, St. Louis.

Plate 6, cont'd. Infectious diseases.

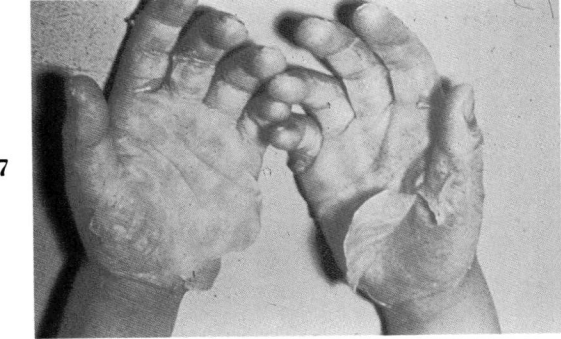

Palm desquamation (scarlet fever)

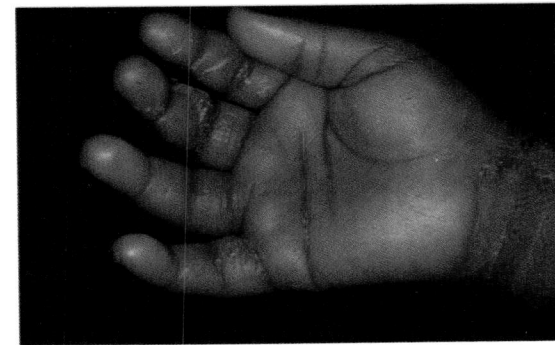

Palm desquamation (staphylococcal infection)

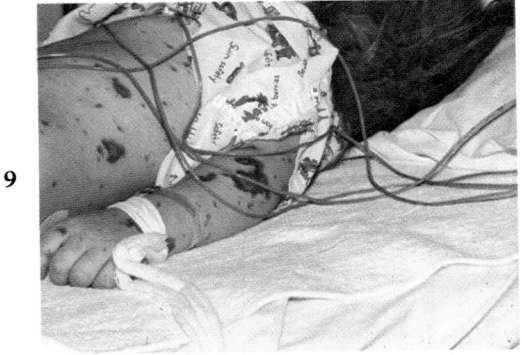

Meningococcemia

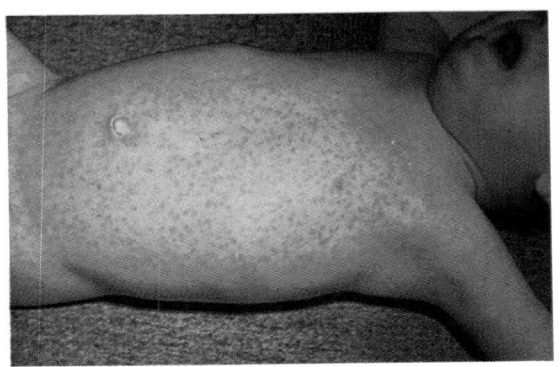

Echo virus can cause infectious viral encephalitis.

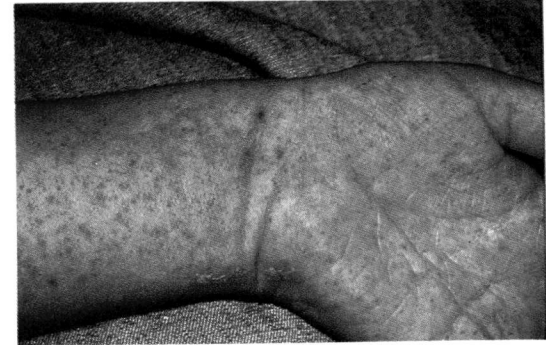

Rocky Mountain spotted fever

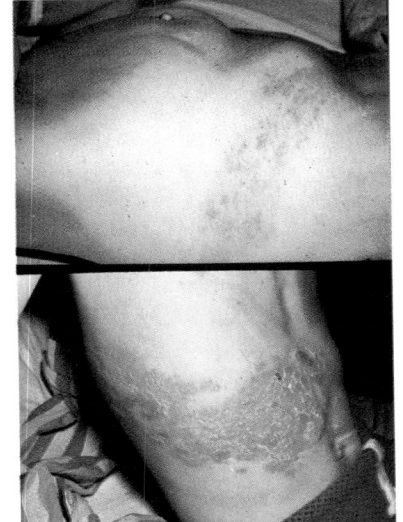

Uncomplicated shingles of the trunk. *Top,* Second day of rash. *Bottom,* Sixth day of rash.

Continued.

7, 9, and **10,** Courtesy Lisa M. Dunkle, M.D., St. Louis School of Medicine, St. Louis; **8,** courtesy Steven Buescher, M.D., University of Texas Health Science Center, Houston; **11,** courtesy Donald C. Anderson, M.D., Baylor College of Medicine, Houston; **12,** reproduced with permission of Burroughs Wellcome Co.

Plate 6, cont'd. Infectious diseases.

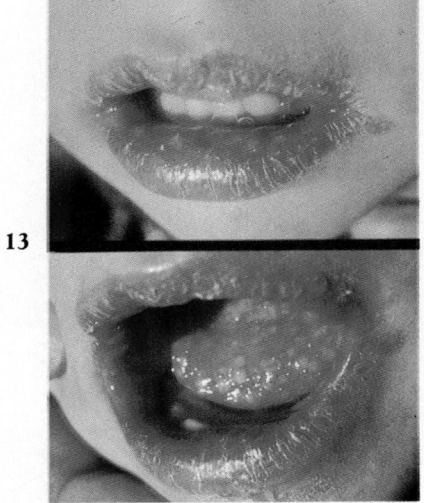

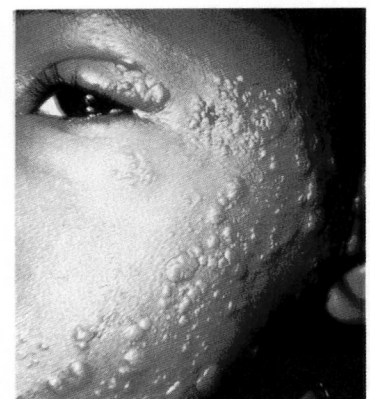

Herpes zoster

Primary gingivostomatitis showing
lesions on the lips and lesions on
the tongue and gums.

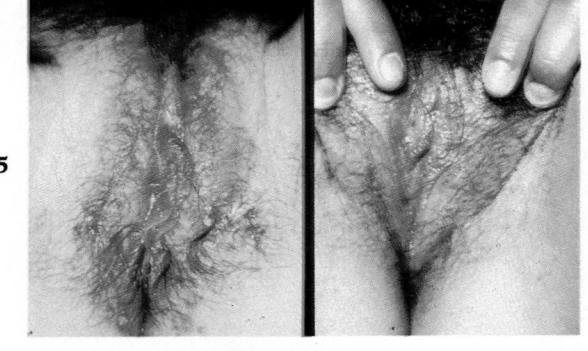

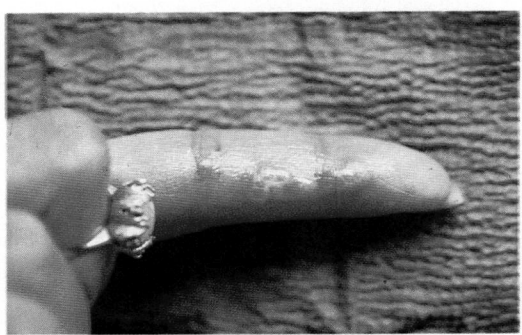

Left, Initial attack of genital herpes in a woman
with lesions extending onto the skin and
extending posteriorly. *Right,* A recurrent infection.
The attack is more limited and most of the lesions
have ruptured.

Herpetic whitlow on hand of health care provider
who did not wear gloves while caring for patient
with herpetic lesions.

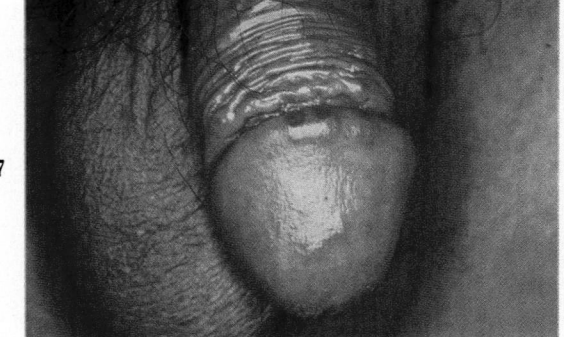

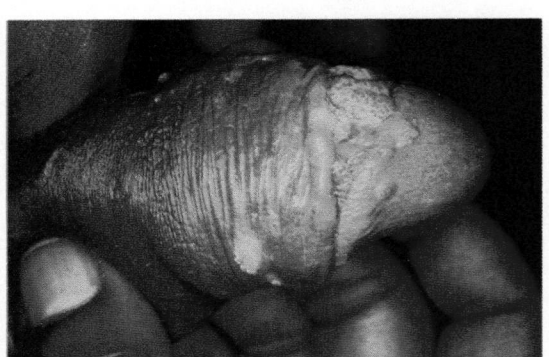

Lymphogranuloma venereum

Molluscum contagiosum (genital warts)

13 and **15,** Reproduced with permission of Burroughs Wellcome Co.; **14,** courtesy Donald C. Anderson,
M.D., Baylor College of Medicine, Houston; **16,** courtesy Steve Kohl, M.D., University of Texas Health
Science Center, Houston; **17** and **18,** courtesy Upjohn Co., Kalamazoo, Michigan.

Plate 7. Immunologic system.

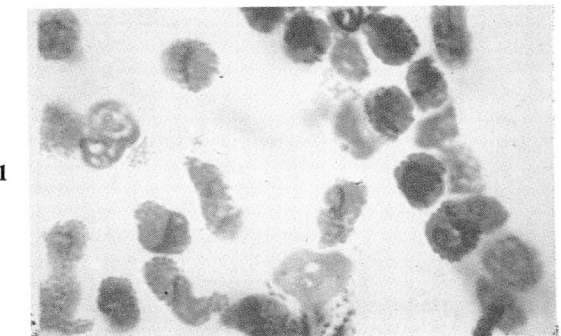

Eosinophil

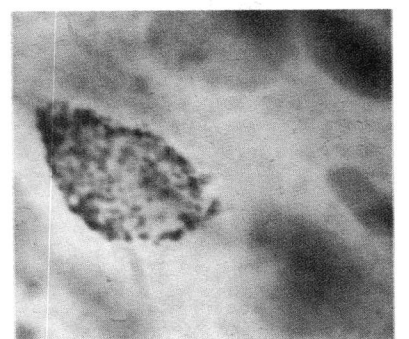

Mast cell

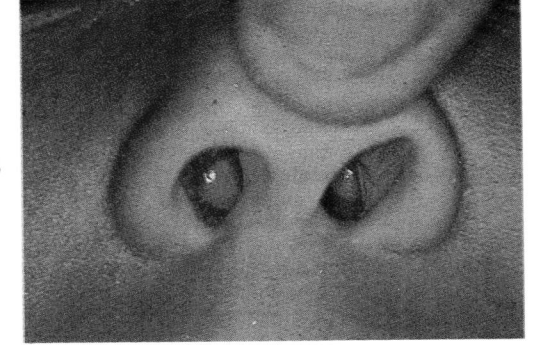

Allergic nose

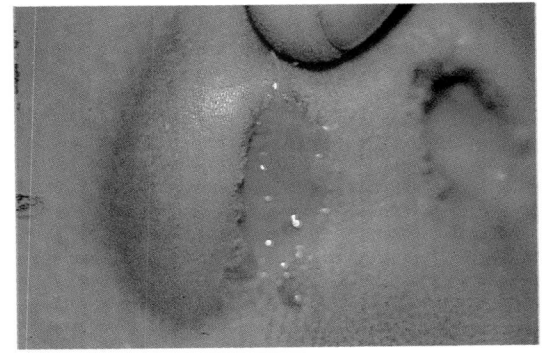

Allergic nasal polyp

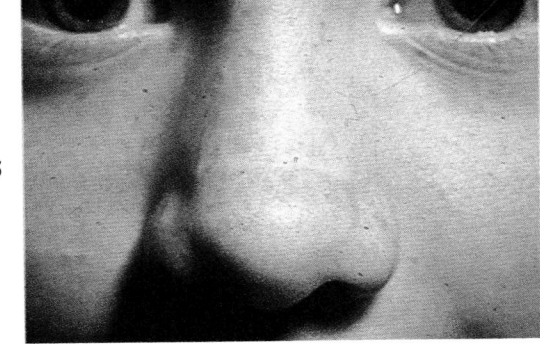

Allergic transverse nasal crease

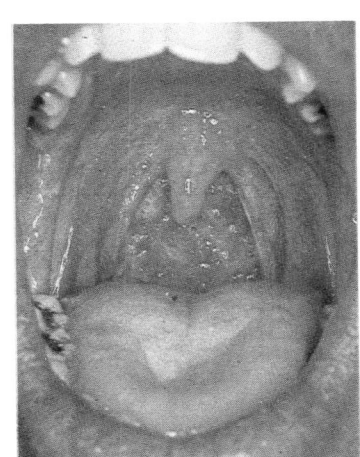

Postnasal drip

Continued.

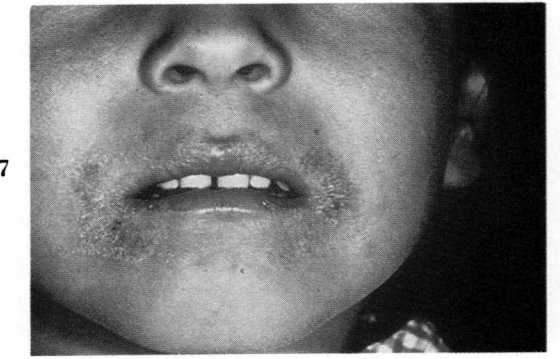

7

Allergic reaction caused by bubble gum

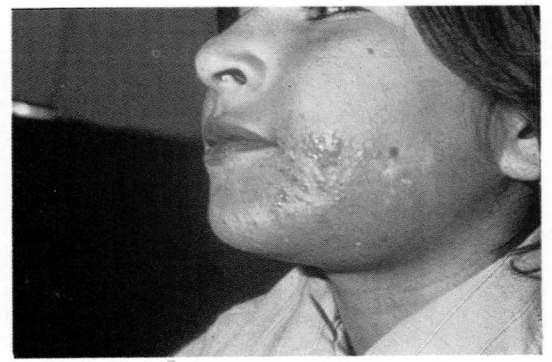

8

Drug eruption

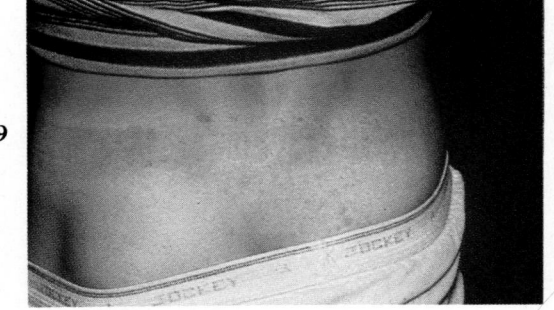

9

Allergic reaction caused by rubber and elastic

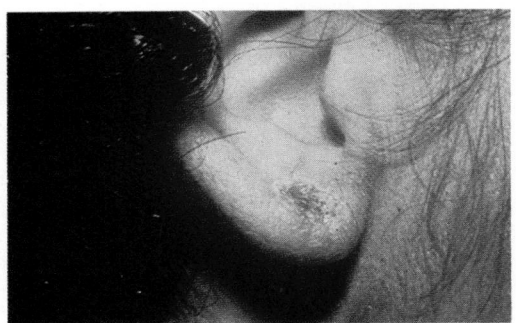

10

Allergic reaction caused by pierced earring

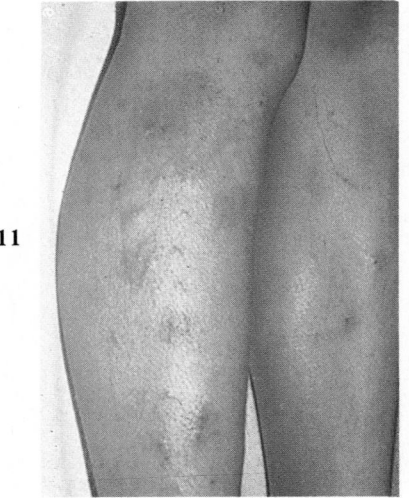

11

Allergic reaction caused by poison ivy

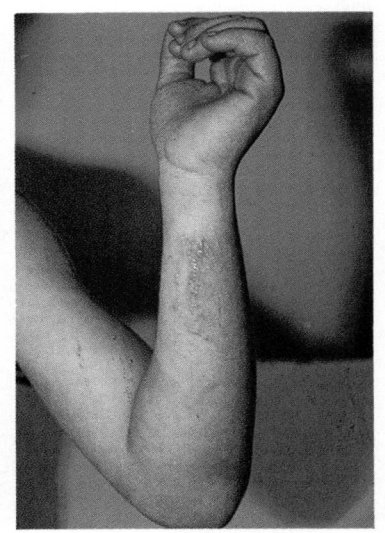

12

Allergic reaction caused by bird bite

PART ONE

Clinical Nursing Practice

Cardiovascular System

Overview

Despite recent advances in both medicine and surgery, cardiovascular disorders continue to be a principal cause of morbidity and mortality in the United States. In the day-to-day care of patients, nurses deal with cardiovascular disorders in terms of their physiologic signs and symptoms and appropriate therapeutic interventions. They must also consider the emotional impact of these disorders on the individual patient and family.

During the past 30 years progress has been made in prevention, diagnosis, treatment, and rehabilitation. Yet despite a demonstrated decrease in cardiac mortality, cardiovascular disease continues to claim more lives than all other causes of death combined. Over 40 million Americans have some form of cardiovascular disease, at an estimated annual cost of 40 billion dollars.[2] Additional costs incurred through production losses, labor turnover, and personnel training are difficult to determine.

In terms of morbidity and mortality, cardiac diseases can be divided into those acquired during life and those that are congenital defects.

Major acquired cardiovascular disorders, which are responsible for approximately 1 million deaths per year, include hypertension, myocardial infarction, congestive heart failure, cerebrovascular accident (stroke), and rheumatic heart disease.

High blood pressure, known as the silent killer, is a major contributing factor to heart attacks and cerebrovascular accidents. Studies have estimated that one in four adults has elevated blood pressure.[57] Among black Americans the prevalence is 50% or greater. Research is now focusing on early detection, particularly in light of studies that have identified hypertension in children as young as 4 years of age.[57]

Heart attacks remain the number one cause of death.[2] An estimated 4 million Americans are treated for heart attacks or angina pectoris each year. Major collaborative research has been undertaken to identify factors, such as occupation, sex, age, dietary habits, serum lipoprotein levels, and activity levels, that may be associated with the progression of underlying diseases that contribute to death by heart attack.[36] In recent years health professionals and community organizations have made major efforts to increase public awareness of risk factors and early warning signals of heart attack and cerebrovascular accident. Because less than half of cardiac deaths occur in hospitals, organizations such as the American Heart Association and the American Red Cross have initiated programs to teach laypersons the basic techniques of cardiopulmonary resuscitation.

Congestive heart failure is a consequence of myocardial dysfunction. Although often controllable with medication, it remains the major form of chronic cardiac disability. It is also one of the most expensive in terms of medical and nursing services, repeated hospital and nursing home services, medication costs, and lost production owing to disability.

3

Cerebrovascular accident is most commonly the result of high blood pressure. An estimated 2 million Americans have had cerebrovascular accidents despite the fact that they can usually be prevented.[2]

Rheumatic heart disease occurs in both children and adults. It is the result of rheumatic fever, a preventable disease. Although the incidence of rheumatic fever has declined, it continues to be a problem in urban populations where preventive measures are inadequate. An estimated 1.3% of deaths in the United States can be attributed to rheumatic heart disease.[2]

Congenital cardiovascular malformations are the major cause of death of children 5 years and younger. Since the advent of cardiac surgery, death from congenital heart disease has been on the decline. Approximately 1 in 300 live-born infants has some form of congenital heart defect. Although the severity and therefore the medical and surgical management of these disorders vary, most such children survive to adulthood. The growing number of adults with congenital heart disease presents a challenge to care givers, particularly because these adults have a greater risk for acquired cardiovascular disorders.

ANATOMY AND PHYSIOLOGY

The heart is a hollow muscular organ weighing between 250 to 350 g. It is located within the thoracic cavity in the mediastinal space, with two thirds extending to the left of the midline. It is flanked by the lungs and protected anteriorly by the sternum and ribs and posteriorly by the vertebral column.

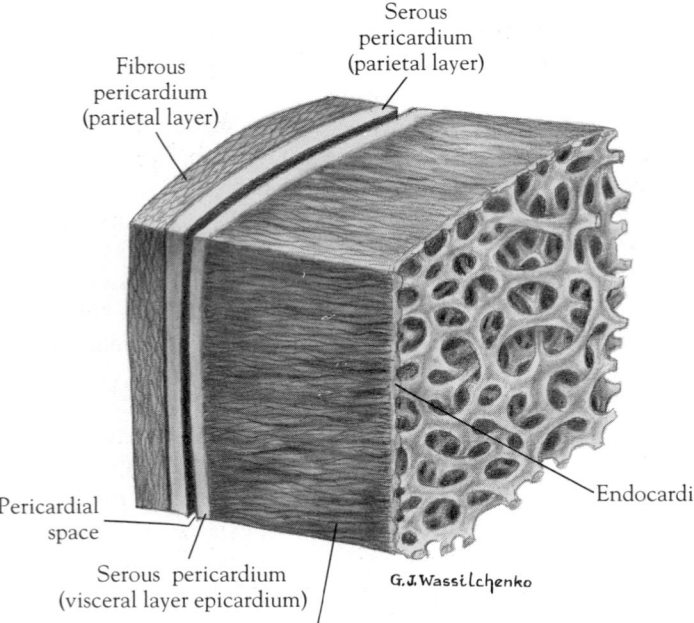

Serous pericardium (parietal layer)

Fibrous pericardium (parietal layer)

Pericardial space

Serous pericardium (visceral layer epicardium)

G. J. Wassilchenko

Myocardium

Endocardium

Layers of the Heart

Cardiac muscle is made up of three layers (Fig. 1-1). The epicardium, the outer layer, covers the surface of the heart and extends to the great vessels. The myocardium, the center layer of thick muscular tissue, is responsible for the major pumping action of the ventricles. Cardiac muscle cells are composed of striated muscle fibrils consisting of contractile elements known as myofibrils. The fibrils are grouped together in a band and are arranged in parallel rows extending from one end of a cell to the other (Fig. 1-2). A membrane junction, the intercalated disc, connects cell to cell. The endocardium, the innermost layer, is made up of a thin layer of endothelium and a thin layer of underlying connective tissue. The endocardium lines the inner chambers of the heart, valves, chordae tendineae, and papillary muscles. It is continuous with the blood vessels that enter and leave the heart.

Pericardium

The heart is enclosed in a double-walled fibroserous sac, the pericardium. The inner layer (visceral pericardium), composed of fibrous elastic connective tissue, covers the entire surface of the heart and constitutes the outermost layer of the heart wall (epicardium) (Fig. 1-1).

The outer layer (parietal pericardium) consists of strong, elastic, fibrous connective tissue lined with smooth, translucent serous membrane, attached inferiorly to the diaphragm and laterally to the pleura of the lung. Superiorly the pericardium attaches to the larger blood vessels (aorta, pulmonary artery, and superior vena cava) but not to the heart itself, thus giving rise to a potential space known as the pericardial cavity.

The space between the visceral and parietal layers contains 10 to 30 ml of clear lymphlike fluid that contributes to the smooth, easy motion of the heart during contraction and expansion. The pericardial cavity is capable of holding 300 ml of fluid without interference in cardiac function, and up to a liter in certain chronic disease states. The degree to which pericardial fluid compromises cardiac function depends largely on the rate of rise in intrapericardial volume rather than the amount. During rapid filling, as little as 100 ml may precipitate acute tamponade,[11] but patients who have slowly developing pericardial effusions have been shown to hold up to a liter of fluid without hampering heart function. The rate

Fig. 1-1
Cross section of cardiac muscle showing its three layers (endocardium, myocardium, and epicardium) and pericardium.

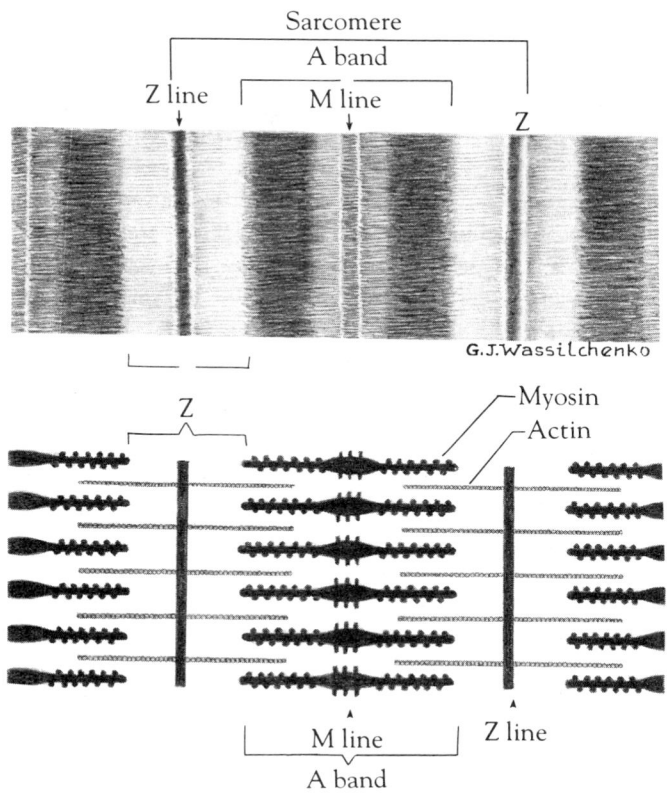

Fig. 1-2
Histologic representation of myocardial tissue, showing arrangement of myofibrils in relaxed state.

of filling is also more important than the amount in the relationship between intrapericardial fluid volume and intrapericardial pressure. Normal intrapericardial pressure is −2 to −5 mm Hg. A sudden increase in intrapericardial pressure may occur with rapid filling of fluid in the pericardial space, regardless of the amount of fluid.

The pericardium is a protective shield against infection and trauma and aids in efficiency of cardiac function by contributing to the free pumping motion of the heart.

Chambers of the Heart

The heart is a four-chambered organ but may be viewed functionally as a two-sided pump (Fig. 1-3). The right side is a low-pressure system pumping venous or deoxygenated blood to the lungs, whereas the left is a higher-pressure system pumping arterial or oxygenated blood to the systemic circulation.

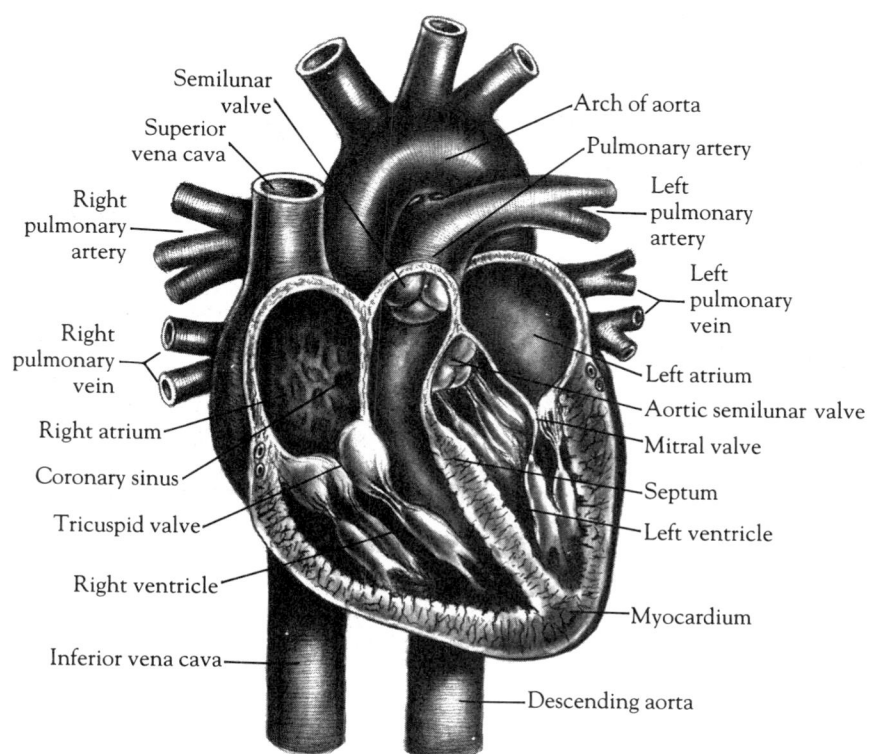

Fig. 1-3
Frontal schematic view of heart.

Right atrium. The right atrium (RA) is a thin-walled muscle that serves as a reservoir or receiving chamber. It receives systemic venous blood from the superior vena cava (SVC), which drains the upper portion of the body, and from the inferior vena cava (IVC), which drains blood from the lower extremities.

The coronary sinus, which drains venous blood from myocardial circulation, also empties into the RA just above the tricuspid valve. The pressure exerted during normal filling of the RA is 0 to 7 mm Hg and varies with respiration. During inspiration, RA pressure drops below the pressure in veins outside the chest cavity. Because blood flows from an area of high pressure to an area of lower pressure, blood flow to the RA occurs primarily during inspiration.

Oxygen saturations vary depending on the portal of entry (IVC, 80%; SVC, 70%; coronary sinus, 30%), but the combined oxygen saturation of RA mixed venous blood is about 75% or 40 mm Hg.

Right ventricle. The right ventricle (RV) is normally the most anterior chamber of the heart, lying directly beneath the sternum. Functionally the RV can be divided into an inflow and an outflow tract. The inflow tract includes the tricuspid area and the crisscross muscular bands called trabeculations, which make up the inner surface of the ventricle. The outflow tract is commonly referred to as the infundibulum.

During diastole blood enters the RV through the tricuspid valve and is ejected into the pulmonary circulation through the pulmonic valve. Because of low pulmonary resistance, systolic or ejection pressures of the RV are also low. RV pressures are 20-25/0-5 mm Hg with an oxygen saturation similar to that in the RA.

Left atrium. The left atrium (LA), the most posterior cardiac structure, receives oxygenated blood from the lungs via the right and left pulmonary veins. The wall of the LA is slightly thicker than that of the RA and exerts a filling pressure of 5 to 10 mm Hg with little respiratory variation. The arterial oxygen saturation is 98% (95 mm Hg).

Left ventricle. The left ventricle (LV) lies posterior to and to the left of the RV. It is ellipsoid in shape, with a wall composed of thick muscular tissue measuring 8 to 16 mm, two to three times thicker than that of the RV. This increased muscle mass is necessary to generate sufficient pressure to propel blood into the systemic circulation. LV pressure is normally 100-120/0-10 mm Hg with oxygen saturation of 95%. The inflow tract is funnel shaped, formed by the mitral anulus, the two mitral leaflets, and the chordae tendineae. The outflow tract is surrounded by the anterior mitral leaflet, the interventricular septum, and the left ventricular free wall. During systole, blood is propelled superiorly and to the right across the aortic valve.

Cardiac Valves

The heart's efficiency as a pump depends on the integrity of the cardiac valves (Fig. 1-4). Their sole purpose is to ensure one-way forward blood flow.

Atrioventricular valves. The two atrioventricular (A-V) valves are functionally similar but differ in several

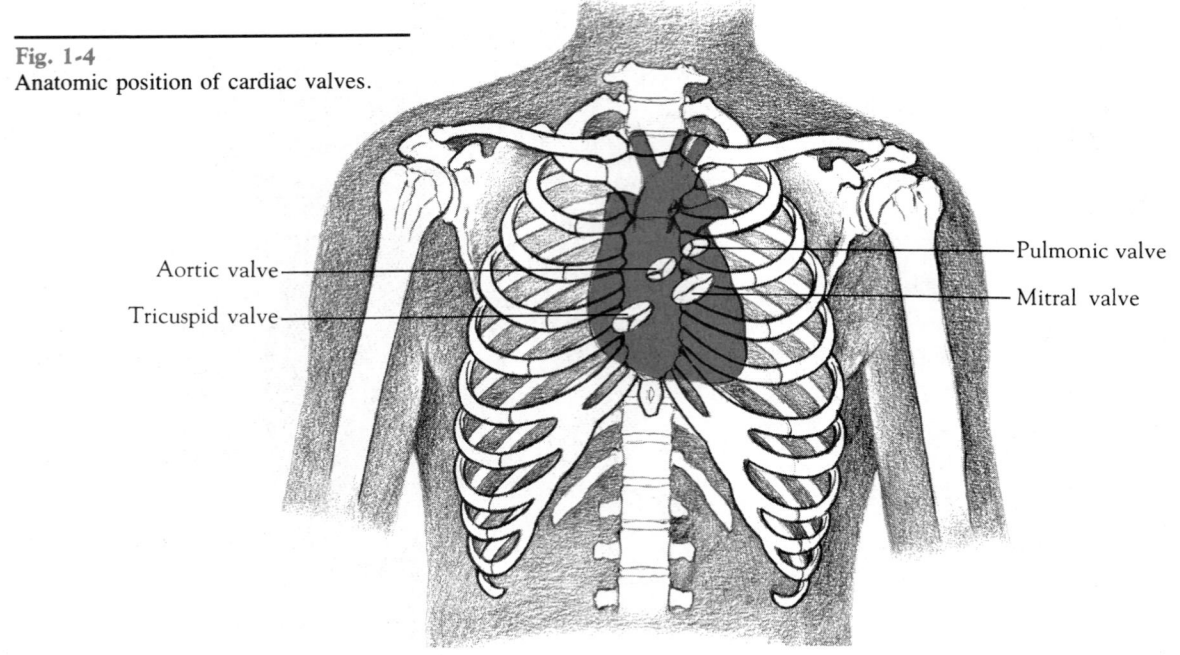

Fig. 1-4
Anatomic position of cardiac valves.

Aortic valve

Tricuspid valve

Pulmonic valve

Mitral valve

anatomic details. They are positioned along the atrio-ventricular groove, which separates the atria from the ventricles.

The anatomic elements that make up the tricuspid (right side) and mitral (left side) apparatus include the anulus fibrosus, the valvular tissue (leaflets) to which the chordae tendineae are attached, and the papillary muscles connecting the chordae to the floor of the ventricular wall. This arrangement allows the leaflets to balloon upward during ventricular systole but prevents eversion of the cusps into the atria. These components should be considered as a single unit, since disruption of any one element can result in serious hemodynamic dysfunction.

The tricuspid valve is larger and thinner than the mitral and has three separate leaflets: anterior, posterior, and septal. Competence of the anterior and posterior leaflets depends on RV lateral wall function. The septal leaflet attaches to portions of the interventricular septum and sits in close proximity to the A-V node.

The mitral valve is composed of two cusps: anterior and posterior. The anterior leaflet has a wide range of motion. It descends deep into the LV during diastole and rises quickly in systole to meet the posterior leaflet. The posterior leaflet is smaller and more restricted in its motion. The orifice is normally 4 to 6 cm² in adults.

Semilunar valves. The two semilunar valves are the aortic and pulmonic. They are smaller than the A-V valves and are similar to each other except that the aortic cusps tend to be thicker. The semilunar valves sit above the outflow tracts of their respective ventricles. Each is composed of a fibrous supporting ring called the anulus and three fibrous valve leaflet cusps. The normal valve orifice is 2.6 to 3.5 cm².

Coronary Circulation

Coronary circulation is described in terms of the two principal coronary arteries, which arise from the aorta just above and behind the aortic valve. These vessels supply blood to the myocardium.

Right coronary artery. The right coronary artery (RCA) arises from the right aortic sinus of Valsalva and branches out along the atrioventricular groove to supply the anterior portion of the right ventricle. In 90% of persons the RCA curves posteriorly within the interventricular groove and supplies the posterior septum, the posterior left papillary muscle, and the sinus and A-V nodes.

Left coronary artery. The left coronary artery (LCA) arises from the left aortic sinus of Valsalva, beginning as a common artery referred to as the left main and then dividing into the left anterior descending (LAD) artery and the circumflex artery. The LAD descends along the anterior intraventricular groove to nourish a large portion of the anterior left ventricular wall, including the anterior

septum, the anterior papillary muscle, and the apical portion of the myocardium.

The circumflex artery extends from the left main coronary artery along a groove between the LA and LV. In some persons the circumflex artery supplies the inferior and posterior portions of the LV. This is known as left coronary dominance.

Cardiac veins. Three main divisions of cardiac veins comprise the venous circulation and closely parallel the coronary arteries. These include the thebesian veins, most of which empty into the atria; the anterior cardiac veins, which empty into the RA; and the coronary sinus, a short vein lying on the posterior side of the heart. Most venous circulation drains into the coronary sinus, which receives blood from the deeper myocardium and empties into the RA at the coronary sinus ostium between the tricuspid valve and the opening of the inferior vena cava.

Conduction

A special system is concerned with the transmission and coordination of electrical impulses throughout the heart. It consists of atypical muscle fibers and has the following characteristics.

Impulse formation. The sinoatrial (S-A) or sinus node gives rise to a self-generating impulse known as the heart beat. The S-A node is located at the border of the superior vena cava and the right atrium. It is the primary pacemaker of the heart and has the inherent capacity to generate electrical impulses at a rate of 60 to 100 beats/minute (Fig. 1-5, A).

Stimulation of the S-A node causes a series of sequential ionic changes leading to the impulse, or action potential, which spreads rapidly throughout the heart muscle via the conduction system.

The S-A node is supplied primarily by the proximal RCA (60%) and the left circumflex artery and is innervated by sympathetic and parasympathetic nerve fibers. If the sinus node is depressed, escape ectopic beats from other inherent pacemakers in the A-V node or ventricle appear and can assume pacemaker function. In addition, rapid impulses in other areas of the heart may produce atrial, junctional, or ventricular tachycardias. These can occur when an ischemic myocardium causes an alteration in the heart's conductivity, producing what are called reentry pathways.

Conduction pathways. Once initiated the normal sinus impulse is transmitted through the heart via a highly specialized network of fibers known as the conduction system. When the impulse reaches the ventricles, stimulation of the myocardium causes depolarization of the cells, and contraction occurs.

The conduction system is made up of the A-V node, bundle of His, and right and left bundle branches. The A-V node filters atrial impulses as they pass through to

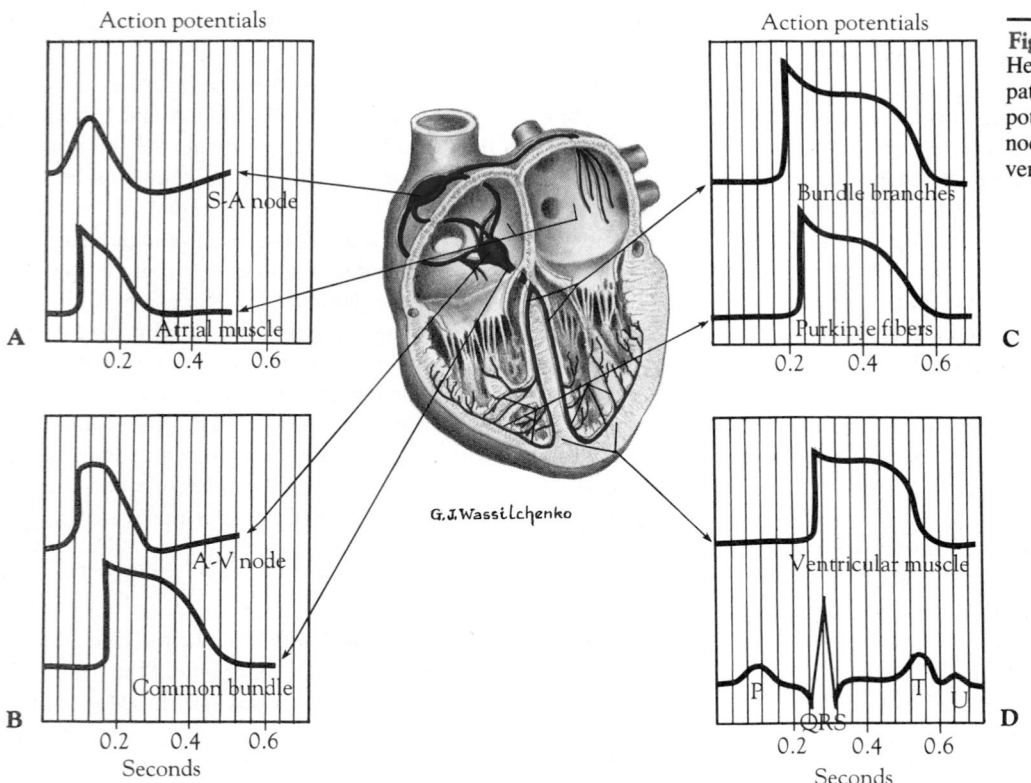

Fig. 1-5
Heart with normal conduction pathways and transmembrane action potential of, **A**, S-A node, **B**, A-V node, **C**, bundle branches, and **D**, ventricular muscle.

the ventricles. It can initiate its own impulse, but usually at lower rates (40 to 60 beats/minute). It is generally supplied by the RCA and is also innervated by the autonomic nervous system (Fig. 1-5, *B*).

The bundle of His provides infranodal conduction traversing the two sides of the intraventricular system, where it divides into the right and left bundle branches. The bundle branches terminate in a fine network of conductive tissue, the Purkinje fibers, which extend to the papillary muscles and lateral walls of the ventricles. The His bundle and its branches are supplied by the proximal branches of the LAD coronary artery (Fig. 1-5, *C*).

Electrophysiology. Transmission of the electrical impulse or action potential of the myocardium is preceded by a series of sequential ionic changes across the cardiac cell membrane, which results in depolarization and subsequent contraction of the myocardium. These events correspond in time to the mechanical events described on p.10. After depolarization the cells return for recovery to a resting state called repolarization, diastole, or relaxation.

A resting (polarized) cell has a net charge of -90 mV. Potassium is the predominant intracellular cation, and sodium the predominant extracellular cation. The difference in concentrations of these ions results in a resting state of electrical potential commonly referred to as the resting membrane potential (RMP).

On initiation of an electrical stimulus, sodium ions move across the cell membrane, converting the net electrical force within the cell to a positive charge. The cell is then depolarized, resulting in shortening of the cell.

The electrical potential created by this ionic movement progresses through adjacent regions of the cell membrane and is referred to as the action potential. Fig. 1-6 illustrates the five phases of the cardiac action potential and its relationship to the electrocardiogram.

Phase 0 represents the depolarization of the cell with the rapid influx of sodium causing a reversal of ionic changes (the inner surface of the cell becomes positive). This is depicted by the upstroke of the action potential curve (Fig. 1-6, *A*).

Phase 1 is the brief rapid change toward the repolarization process, during which the membrane potential returns to 0 mV.

Phase 2 is a plateau or stabilization period caused by the slow influx of sodium and the slow exit of potassium. During this period, calcium ions enter the cell through slow calcium channels, triggering the release of large quantities of calcium. Calcium functions in the process of cellular contraction.

Phase 3 represents sudden acceleration in repolarization as potassium leaves rapidly, causing the inside of the cell to move toward a more negative state.

Fig. 1-6
Cardiac action potentials. **A,** Action potential phases 0 to 4 of nonpacemaker cardiac cells. **B,** Action potential of pacemaker cell.

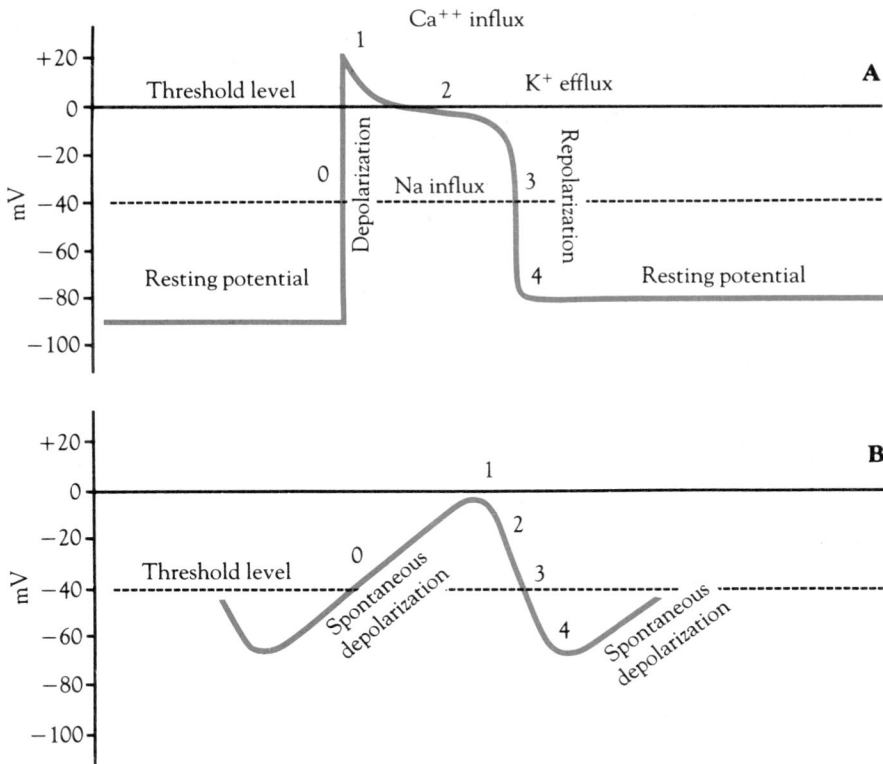

Phase 4 represents the return to the resting phase during which the intracellular charge is once again electronegative, leading to the initiation of the action potential (phase 0). Any excess sodium is eliminated from the cell in exchange for potassium that left the cell during phases 2 and 3.

Throughout these phases the cardiac cell goes through a series of refractory periods during which the cell is incapable of accepting another stimulus and responding with a full action potential. An *absolute refractory period* occurs during depolarization and at the beginning of repolarization (phases 0, 1, and 2). During this period, excitation of the cardiac cell will not result in another impulse no matter how strong the stimulus. The *relative refractory period* represents the time when the cell is once again electronegative. A stronger than threshold stimulus can initiate another impulse. A *vulnerable or supernormal period* occurs as phase 4 begins and the cell is returning to its resting potential. During this time a weaker than threshold stimulus can initiate an action potential.

Electrocardiogram. The electromechanical events of the heart can be recorded and interpreted on the electrocardiogram (ECG). The various waveforms in Fig. 1-7 have been correlated with the normal conduction sequence. Any deviation from normal is the basis for detection of arrhythmias.

Fig. 1-7
Normal electrocardiographic waveform.

From Tucker, S.M., et al.: Patient care standards, ed. 3, St. Louis, 1984, The C.V. Mosby Co.

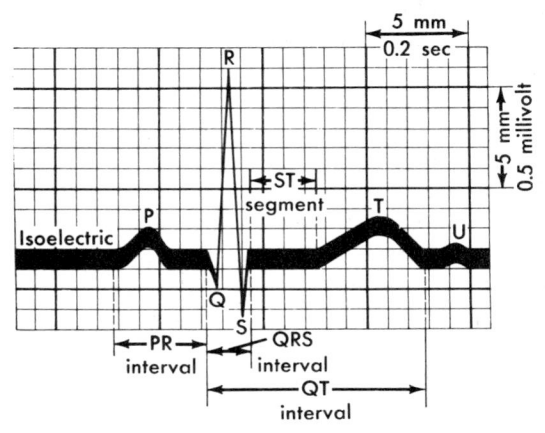

SYSTEMATIC APPROACH TO ECG INTERPRETATION

1. Calculate the heart rate. Calculate atrial (P waves) rate. Calculate ventricular (QRS complexes) rate.
2. Determine rhythm regularity.
3. Determine whether P waves are present. Determine the position of P waves with relation to the QRS complex.
4. Measure the PR interval.
5. Measure the QRS interval.
6. Identify and examine the ST segment and T wave.
7. Determine the origin of the rhythm. Is it of sinus, atrial, junctional, or ventricular origin?

The cardiac cycle includes the following waveforms and time intervals:

P wave—the electrical activity associated with the sinus node impulse and its depolarization of the atria

PR interval—the time the impulse takes to travel through the atria to the A-V node, the bundle of His and bundle branches, and the ventricles; normal duration is 0.12 to 0.20 second

QRS complex—electrical depolarization and contraction of the ventricles

ST segment—the period between the completion of depolarization and the repolarization of the ventricles

T wave—the recovery or repolarization phase of the ventricles

Intervals between these waveforms reflect the time an impulse takes to travel through the heart.

Identification of rhythms, normal or otherwise, requires a careful systematic approach to interpretation. One method is described in the box above.

Cardiac Cycle

The cardiac cycle is divided into two phases, systole and diastole. Systole is the time interval during which blood is ejected from the ventricles. Diastole is the time interval during which the ventricles are relaxed and filling with blood from the atria. Diastolic events are discussed first because filling pressures often predict the effectiveness of systolic ejection.

As described previously, the atria serve as reservoirs for blood entering the heart. During diastole the semilunar valves are closed, the ventricles are at rest, and the A-V valves are forced opened, allowing blood to flow from the atria into the ventricles. During the initial phase of diastole, approximately 70% of the blood flows rapidly into the ventricles. In the second half of diastole, blood flow slows until atrial contraction is accelerated, forcing the remainder of the blood into the ventricles. This added atrial thrust completes diastolic filling of the ventricle and is reflected as the a wave on the atrial pressure tracing

(Fig. 1-8). The blood present in the ventricles at the end of diastole is the end-diastolic volume.

With filling of the ventricles complete, isovolumetric contraction begins. During this initial phase, systolic pressures begin to rise, forcing the closure of the A-V valves. The deceleration of blood associated with the closure of the A-V valves is the source of the first heart sound (S_1) (Fig. 1-8). Isovolumetric contraction continues until ventricular pressure exceeds aortic pressure, forcing open the semilunar valves. Blood is ejected rapidly into the pulmonary artery and aorta on the left side.

As the ejection phase ends, the ventricular muscle relaxes, decreasing intraventricular pressures and causing reversal of blood flow in the aorta, which forces the semilunar valves to close. The onset of ventricular relaxation with the closure of the semilunar valves is the source of the second heart sound (S_2), reflected by a dicrotic notch on the pressure waveform of the aorta (Fig. 1-8).

After the semilunar valves close, ventricular wall tension or pressure falls rapidly. On the atrial pressure tracing the v wave reflects this period in which the ventricles are relaxing and blood is entering the atrium. The downsloping following the v wave is the signal that ventricular relaxation is complete. As ventricular pressure falls below atrial pressure, the A-V valves once again open and the cycle is repeated.

Factors Affecting Cardiac Function

A basic function of the heart is to transport oxygen and other nutrients to various portions of the body via the circulation and to return carbon dioxide and waste products of metabolism to the lungs for excretion.

The circulating volume varies according to the need of tissue cells. Any increase in the work of the cells causes an increase in blood flow and a subsequent increase in the work of the heart and myocardial oxygen consumption (MVO_2).

The heart's function is governed by the closely integrated working of three major factors: intrinsic properties

Fig. 1-8
Left ventricular pressure pulses
correlated in time with ventricular
volume, heart sounds, and
electrocardiogram.

From Guzzetta, C.E., and Dossey, B.M.:
Cardiovascular nursing: bodymind tapestry,
St. Louis, 1984, The C.V. Mosby Co.

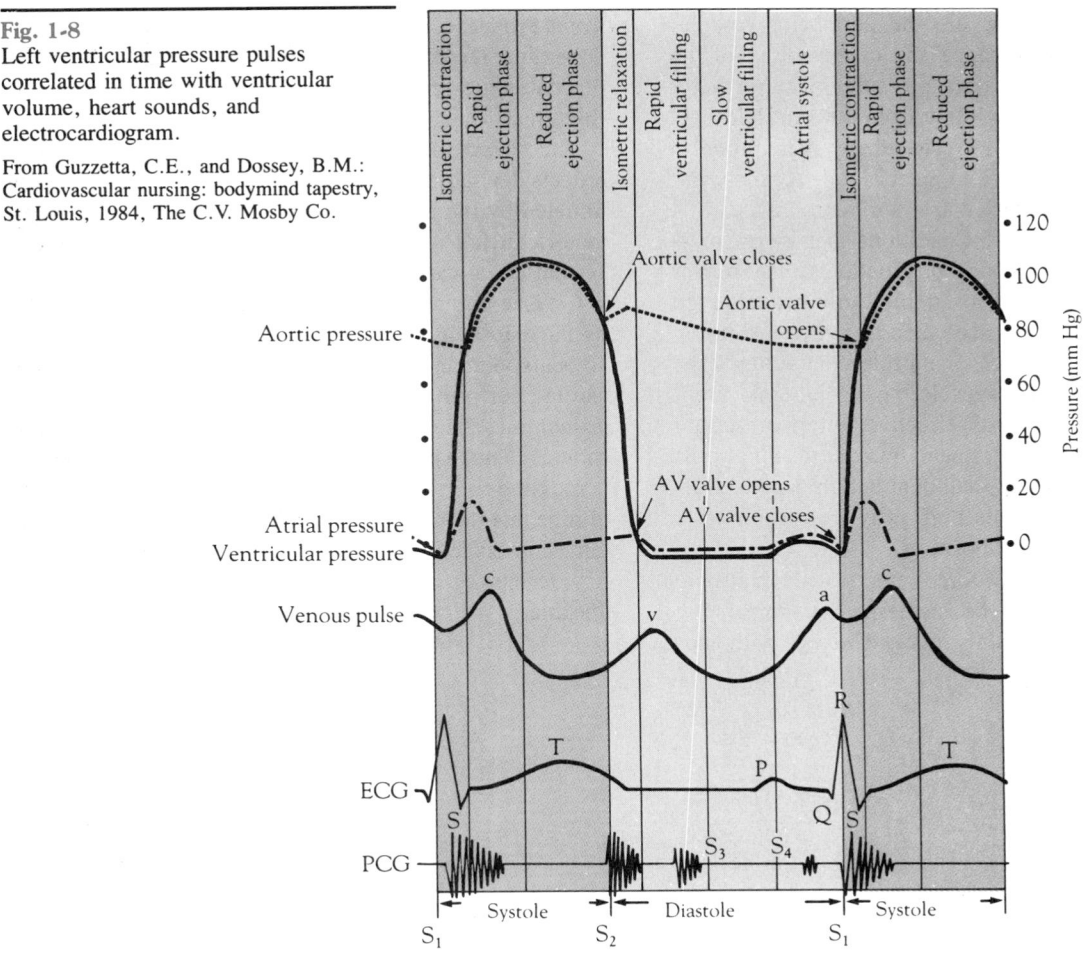

of the heart; extrinsic factors including nervous system, blood volume, and venous return; and peripheral circulation.

Cardiac function is based on the adequacy of the cardiac output (CO), which is the amount of blood pumped from the left ventricle per minute. CO is calculated by multiplying the amount of blood ejected from one ventricle with one heart beat (stroke volume, or SV) by the heart rate (HR): CO = SV × HR. In a normal 70 kg (150-pound) adult at rest, the CO is 5 L/minute. The primary factors affecting CO include preload (filling of the heart during diastole), afterload (the resistance against which the heart must pump), contractility of the heart muscle, and heart rate.

Preload is the degree of fiber stretch that occurs as a result of load or tension placed on the muscle before contraction. In discussing the heart the term ''load'' refers to the quantity of blood and the term ''tension'' to the pressure it exerts in the left ventricle at the end of diastole (filling) just before systole (ejection). This is

commonly referred to as left ventricular end-diastolic pressure (LVEDP).

The intrinsic ability of the muscle fibers to stretch in response to increasing loads of incoming blood (venous return) is related to the Frank-Starling principle. This principle is based on the length–active tension relationship curve and states that the greater the presystolic fiber stretch (within physiologic limits), the stronger the ventricular contraction. In other words, the more the ventricle fills with blood during diastole, the greater the quantity of blood it will pump during systole. Preload is a major determinant of myocardial oxygen consumption.

Afterload is the resistance to blood flow as it leaves the ventricles. Afterload is a function of both arterial pressure and left ventricular size. Any increase in vascular resistance (pressure against which the heart is forced to pump) will cause ventricular contractility to increase in an attempt to maintain stroke volume and cardiac output.

The principal factors causing impedance or resistance

to left ventricular outflow are the peripheral vascular resistance and the compliance and distensibility of the aorta and large arteries. Arterial pressure is a major factor offering resistance to blood flow from the ventricles. As arterial pressure increases, greater energy is required to generate sufficient pressure to eject blood. As more energy is required for ventricular systole, the myocardial oxygen demand increases. Conditions that increase afterload include those causing obstruction to ventricular outflow (such as aortic stenosis) and those causing high peripheral vascular resistance (such as hypertension).

Contractility is the force of muscle contraction. The myocardium is a unique muscle having intrinsic properties that contribute to its effective pumping action. When a stimulus is applied to heart muscle, the myofibrils slide together and overlap, and contraction occurs. During relaxation the filaments pull away from each other and return to their former positions.

The rate (chronotropic force) and force (inotropic force) of contraction can be increased by sympathetic nerve stimulation or administration of drugs with inotropic properties, such as isoproterenol, epinephrine, and dopamine. Depressed contractility is generally due to loss of contractile muscle mass through injury, disease, arrhythmias, or drugs.

The normal heart rate is 60 to 100 beats/minute and reflects depolarization of the ventricles. It is intrinsically initiated by the S-A node within the heart, but extrinsic factors such as stimulation of the autonomic nervous system can greatly influence heart rate and rhythm.

Cardiac output can be depressed or increased directly by fluctuation in heart rate. With a heart rate of less than 40 beats/minute, the cardiac output often falls, impairing cardiac performance. With low rates the tendency for arrhythmias increases because inherent automaticity contributes to uncoordinated myocardial contraction, further depressing contractility. With rapid pulse rates the length of time that the heart is in diastole is reduced. As a result, left ventricular filling is decreased as is coronary blood flow to the myocardium, which occurs primarily during diastole.

Fig. 1-9
Cross section of artery and vein showing the three layers: tunica intima, tunica media, and tunica adventitia. Note difference in wall thickness between artery and vein.

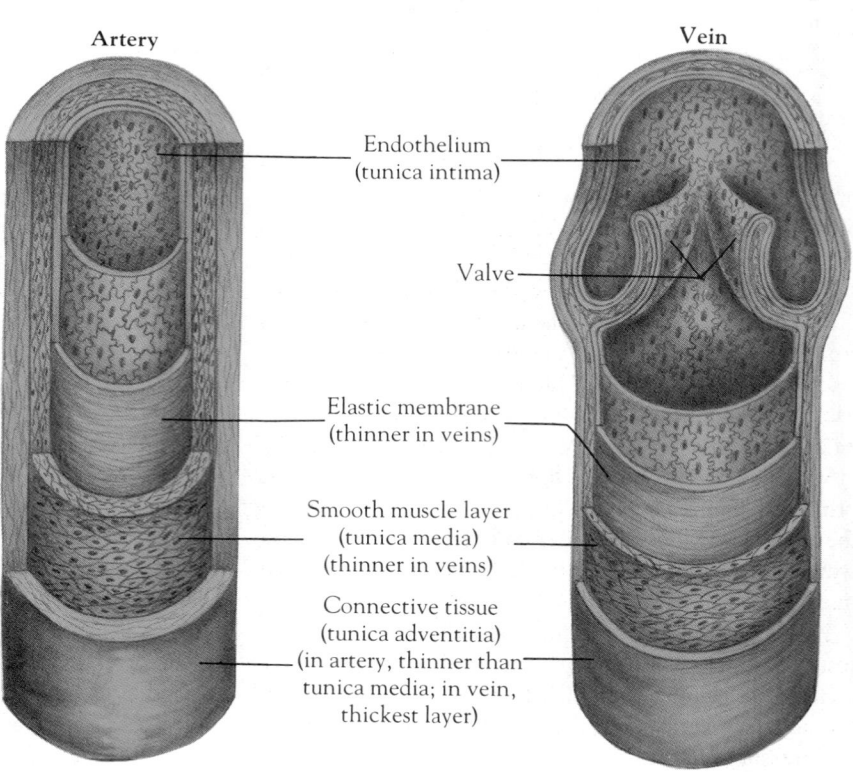

Artery

Vein

Endothelium (tunica intima)

Valve

Elastic membrane (thinner in veins)

Smooth muscle layer (tunica media) (thinner in veins)

Connective tissue (tunica adventitia) (in artery, thinner than tunica media; in vein, thickest layer)

Peripheral Vascular System

The components of the vascular system are the arteries, capillaries, and veins. The principal function of the systemic vascular system is to distribute blood to various body organs and tissues.

The arterial tree, which carries oxygenated blood to all body tissues, is comprised of arteries, arterioles, and capillaries. Arteries are distensible high-pressure conduits (Fig. 1-9). These vessels, known as resistance vessels, have a high elastic fiber content that can support high pressure and accommodate large volumes of blood. About 20% of the total circulating blood is contained within the arteries. Arterioles are smaller branches whose walls contain less elastic tissue and more smooth muscle. Constriction or dilation of the lumens of the arterioles is the major control of pressure and blood flow. By changing the diameter of the blood vessels, the volume of blood supplied to the tissues may be increased or decreased.

Arteries and arterioles respond to autonomic nervous system control and to chemical stimulation. Nervous impulses from reflex centers in the brain may constrict or dilate the vessels. Chemical substances may alter the size of a blood vessel by acting directly on the vessel or by stimulating sensory receptors, thus initiating reflex control. Physical factors such as temperature can also influence the size of the blood vessels.

Capillaries are microscopic (1 mm) endothelial vessels with no elastic properties. The extensive capillary bed is permeable to the molecules that are exchanged between blood cells and tissue cells (Fig. 1-10). Thus it is here that the vital exchange of oxygen, nutrients, and meta-bolic waste products between blood and interstitial fluid occurs. Blood flow through the capillaries is regulated by cellular oxygen demand. The precapillary sphincter assists in the regulation of blood flow through the capillary bed. As oxygen demand increases, the precapillary sphincter dilates and the capillaries open up, increasing blood flow to the tissue.

The capillaries are also responsive to nervous control such as sympathetic stimulation, which induces constriction. However, local capillary response is due primarily to humoral factors, that is, chemical substances resulting from tissue metabolism or the presence of chemical substances in the blood. Such substances include histamine (a powerful capillary dilator) and hormones such as epinephrine, which have a constricting effect. Oxygen and pH can also influence local blood flow.

The venous system, comprised of venules and veins, is responsible for returning blood to the heart. Venules, the exchange vessels, are small, thin tubules that converge to form veins. They collect blood from the capillary bed. Veins are thin, highly distensible vessels that can store large amounts of blood. Thus they are referred to as capacitance vessels (Fig. 1-9). This venous reservoir holds 60% to 70% of total blood volume and changes as tissue needs change. Veins contain valves at varying intervals to maintain forward blood flow to the heart (venous return) and prevent reflux. Venous blood flow is influenced by a variety of factors including arterial flow, skeletal muscle contractions, changes in thoracic and abdominal pressure, and right atrial pressure.

Fig. 1-10
Microcirculation involving blood, interstitial fluid, oxygen, and nutrients.

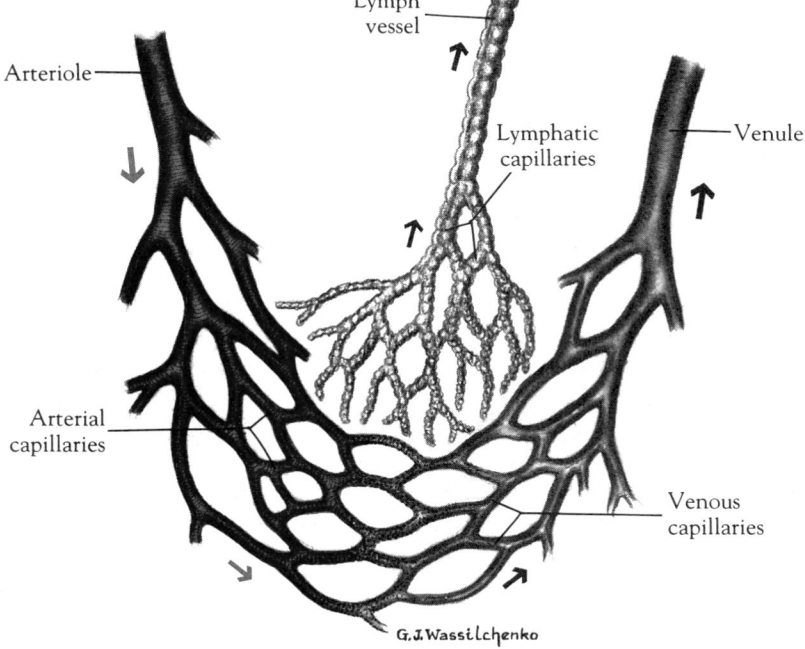

Neural Control of the Cardiovascular System

The heart and blood vessels are innervated by divisions of the autonomic nervous system.

Heart. The heart has the inherent ability to initiate its own impulse through the S-A node. This is known as automaticity and is influenced by both divisions of the autonomic nervous system. Sympathetic fibers innervate the heart through nerves arising from the cervical and upper thoracic ganglia of the sympathetic trunks and by the parasympathetic fibers arising in the vagal branches. Combined, they form the cardiac plexuses located close to the arch of the aorta.[4] From these plexuses, nerve fibers accompany the right and left coronary arteries to enter the heart. The fibers then extend to the S-A node, A-V node, and atrial myocardium.

Sympathetic cardiac nerves, or accelerator nerves, cause an increase in heart rate when activated. Parasympathetic nerves, or vagus fibers, serve as inhibitors, slowing the heart rate by decreasing conduction through the A-V node. The action of the sympathetic system is mediated through the release of epinephrine, whereas the parasympathetic effects are mediated by the vagal release of acetylcholine. Other factors such as pain, exercise, temperature, emotions, and drugs may also activate this autonomic receptor system.

Blood vessels. Arteries and arterioles are also under the control of the sympathetic division of the autonomic nervous system. Contraction and relaxation of the muscle fibers of the blood vessels determine the diameter of the vessels. The muscles are supplied by two sets of fibers: vasoconstrictors, which cause constriction of the vascular smooth muscle, and vasodilators, which relax it. Through a coordinated mechanism involving vascular reflexes, supplemented by the action of chemical substances in the blood, the diameter of vessels is regulated to bring about proper distribution of blood to various tissues in response to their physiologic needs.

Baroreceptors. Baroreceptor cells are located in the carotid sinus and aortic arch. Stimulation of these cells by stretch or pressure leads to inhibition of the vasomotor center, resulting in vasodilation. As more impulses go to the heart, stimulating parasympathetic fibers, the heart beat slows and the arterioles and venules dilate.

Chemoreceptors. Vasomotor chemoreceptors are located in the aortic arch and carotid bodies. They are particularly sensitive to decreased PaO_2, increased PcO_2, and decreased pH. When stimulated, the chemoreceptors send impulses to the vasoconstrictor centers in the medulla, causing vasoconstriction of arterioles and the venous reservoir.

Arterial Blood Pressure

Arterial blood pressure is a measure of the pressure blood exerts within the blood vessels. This pressure depends largely on work of the heart (cardiac output), blood volume, and peripheral resistance, including the elasticity of arterial walls.

Peripheral resistance is the resistance to blood flow imposed by the force created by the aorta, arteries, and arterioles. The amount of pressure exerted on the blood is highest in the aorta (120 mm Hg) and becomes progressively lower in arteries (80 mm Hg), arterioles (55 mm Hg), capillaries (30 mm Hg), and veins (20 mm Hg).[28] This pressure difference (gradient) is one of the determinants of blood flow, since blood flows naturally from high pressure to low. Other factors include the size and patency of the vessel lumen and blood viscosity.

The vascular tone of the arteries and arterioles allows them to constrict or dilate, influencing the resistance to flow. For example, the greater the resistance in the arteriole, the less the blood flow to capillaries. Therefore more blood remains in the arteries, creating a higher arterial pressure.

Blood viscosity depends on red blood cells and protein molecules in the blood. Greater pressure is required to propel viscous or thick fluid. Alteration in blood proteins or reduction in red cells as in anemia or hemorrhage reduces peripheral resistance and arterial pressure.

Measurement of arterial pressure. Arterial pressure may be measured by direct and indirect methods. Direct measurement is done by placing a catheter, attached to a recording monitor, into the artery.

Fetal Development

From the onset of gestation the developing embryo undergoes rapid cellular diffusion, forming tissues that will later become the heart. By the third week a primitive single tubular structure made up of two layers of germ cells is formed. The mesoderm contributes to the pericardial wall (epicardium) and myocardium, and within this layer a single longitudinal tube is formed that will eventually become the endocardium (Fig. 1-11, *A*).

The tube's position permits it to accommodate rapid growth. During the first 28 days the primitive cardiac tube grows and bends to the side, twisting into a loop. At this stage the cardiac structures are developing and identifiable: the sinuatrium, which connects the atria with the primitive ventricle, the conus cordis, which will later become the outflow tract for the ventricles; and the truncus arteriosus, which later divides into the aorta and pulmonary artery (Fig. 1-11, *B*).

From the fourth through the eighth weeks, transition to a four-chambered heart occurs. A midline groove forms at the apex of the ventricular loop, beginning the division between the right and left sides. Blood flow remains undivided and continuously enters the atria and sinus venosus and leaves via the truncus arteriosus (Fig. 1-11, *C*).

Fig. 1-11
Fetal development.

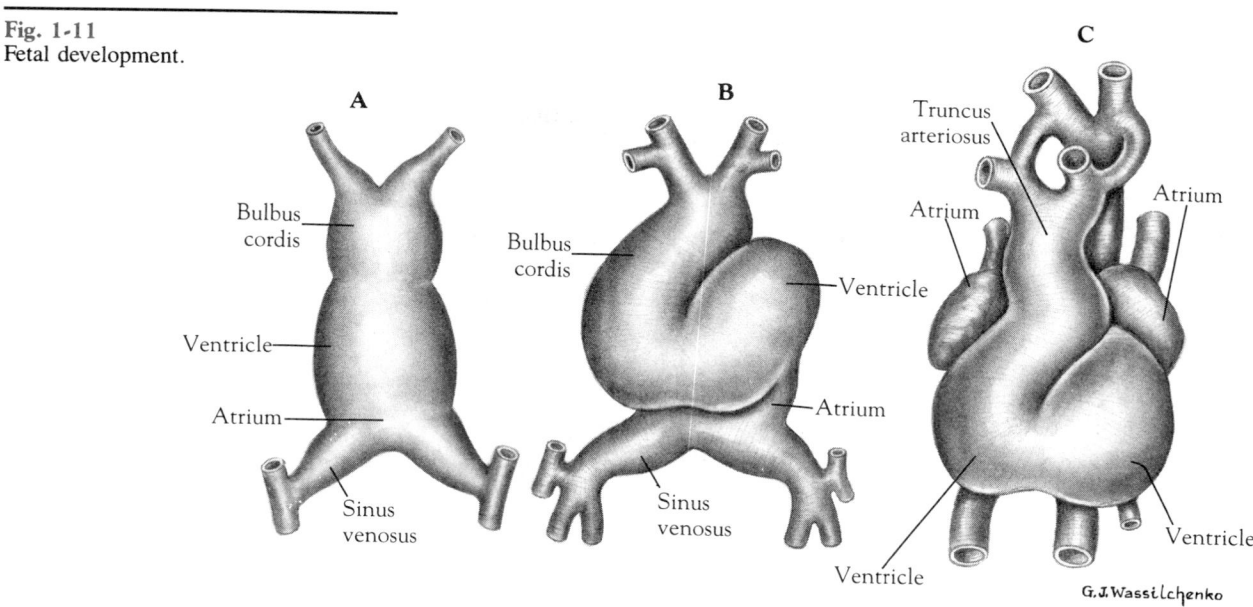

Fig. 1-12
Chamber development showing atrial
and ventricular septation.

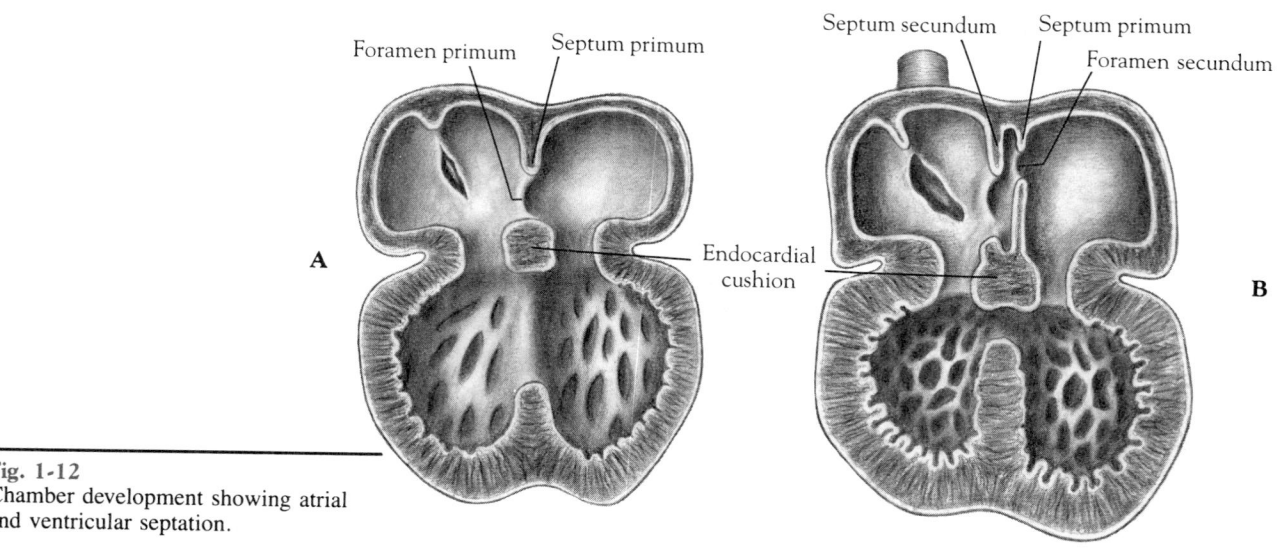

Atria. Atrial development begins from the common atrioventricular (A-V) canal. Two tissue bundles, the endocardial cushions, arise from the A-V canal, forming a dorsal (back) and ventral side. By the sixth week these tissues merge in the center of the heart, dividing the A-V canal into left and right channels and developing what will later be the tricuspid and mitral valves.

Atrial septation develops from the septum primum, which grows toward the A-V canal and endocardial cushions. An intercommunication between the left and right atria called the foramen primum remains (Fig. 1-12, *A*). As atrial division continues, a second atrial septum (septum secundum) is established in the center and to the

right of the septum primum. The septum primum continues to fuse with the endocardial cushions, obliterating the foramen primum. However, the lower portion remains as a flap valve that prevents blood flow from reversing to left to right. Throughout fetal life, blood flow is directed right to left through the foramen ovale, supplying oxygen to the left side of the heart and fetal structures (Fig. 1-13). The foramen ovale closes shortly after birth.

Ventricles. Septation of the ventricles takes place during the second month of fetal development. Rapid growth occurs from the apex of the common ventricle upward toward the expanding endocardial cushions and A-V canal. This upward-growing muscular tissue does

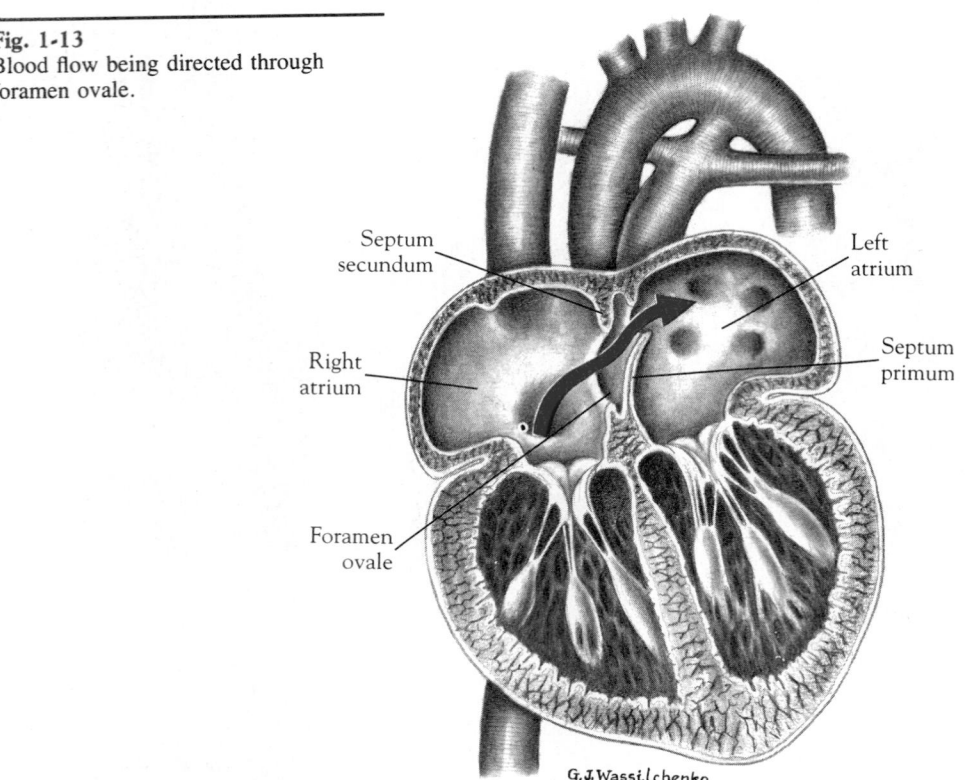

Fig. 1-13
Blood flow being directed through foramen ovale.

Septum secundum

Left atrium

Right atrium

Septum primum

Foramen ovale

G.J.Wassilchenko

not merge with the cushions. Thus an interventricular communication is created that exists until the tissues from the endocardial cushion and conus ridges of the truncus arteriosus grow downward and eventually obliterate it. The upper portion of the septum thins out into a fibrous sheet referred to as the membranous portion of the septum, while the lower portion remains muscular.

Great vessels and cardiac valves. The truncus arteriosus, which is initially a single undivided tubular structure, undergoes its own partitioning process. The conus ridges in the ventricular septum fuse and divide the truncus into a left and a right side, forming the aorta and pulmonary artery. These vessels continue to develop in a spiral fashion, so that the aorta receives blood from the left ventricle and the pulmonary artery receives blood from the right ventricle.

Embryonic connective tissue grows outward from the endocardial tissue of each conus ridge to form the three cusps of the aortic and pulmonic valves. Meanwhile the mitral and tricuspid valves are being formed by the proliferation and thinning of the tissues that project from the endocardial tissues and outer walls of the A-V canal. The papillary muscles and chordae tendineae arise from alteration of the muscular tissues of the inner sources of the ventricles.

Fetal circulation. Fetal circulation differs dramatically from that after birth. The developing fetus secures

oxygen and nutrients through the placenta, where an interchange of gases, foods, and wastes occurs between fetal and maternal blood. The fetal blood receives oxygen and nutritive substances by diffusion and gives up waste products. The fetus is connected to the placenta by the umbilical cord, which contains two umbilical arteries and one umbilical vein (Fig. 1-14).

Because the lungs are nonfunctional during fetal life, their blood supply is limited. However, three structures exist during the fetal life to ensure circulation within the heart. These are the foramen ovale in the interatrial septum, which allows the blood in the right atrium to pass directly into the left atrium; the ductus arteriosus, which connects the pulmonary artery directly with the aorta; and the ductus venosus, which allows blood to pass directly to the inferior vena cava.

The heart begins to beat in about the fourth week of fetal life. Fetal circulation of blood is similar to that in adults with the exception of the heart, lungs, and placenta. Blood reaches the placenta via the umbilical arteries. Within the placenta, blood passes through the capillaries of the villi and then returns to the fetus by way of the umbilical vein to the liver. Most of the blood is shunted directly to the inferior vena cava by way of the ductus venosus; the remainder is directed into the liver.

Circulation within the heart is a mixture of oxygenated

Fig. 1-14
Fetal circulation.

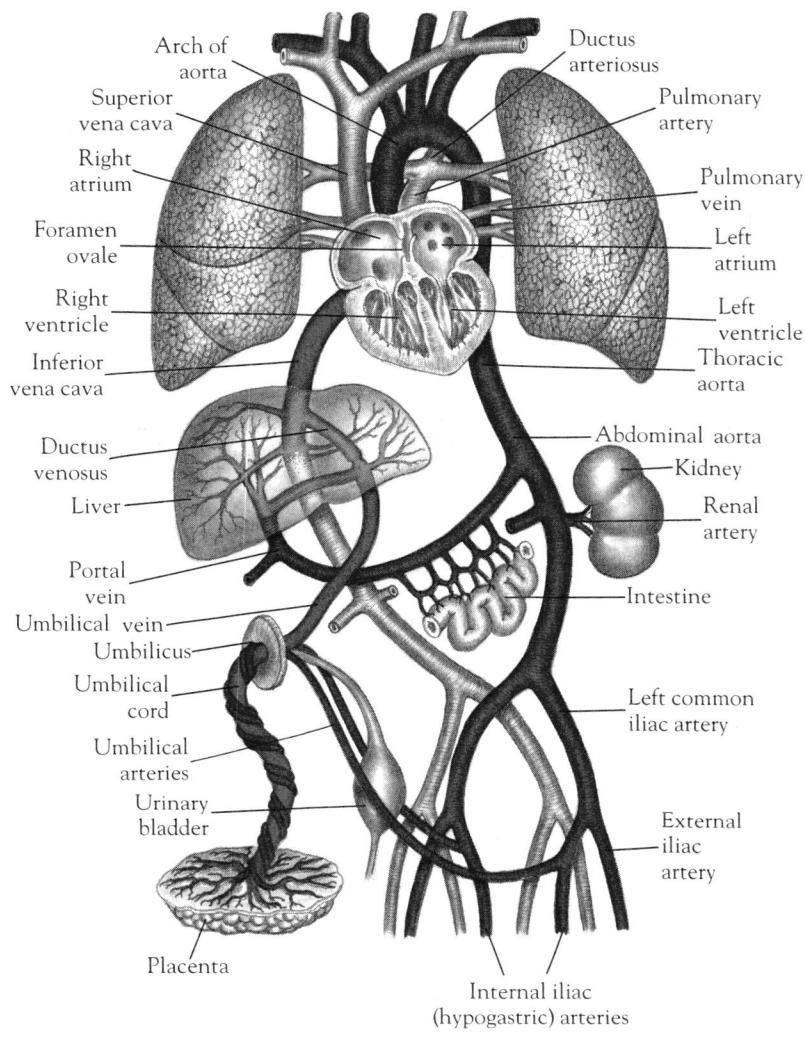

Arch of aorta
Superior vena cava
Right atrium
Foramen ovale
Right ventricle
Inferior vena cava
Ductus venosus
Liver
Portal vein
Umbilical vein
Umbilicus
Umbilical cord
Umbilical arteries
Urinary bladder
Placenta

Ductus arteriosus
Pulmonary artery
Pulmonary vein
Left atrium
Left ventricle
Thoracic aorta
Abdominal aorta
Kidney
Renal artery
Intestine
Left common iliac artery
External iliac artery
Internal iliac (hypogastric) arteries

blood received from the ductus venosus and deoxygenated blood returning from the alimentary canal, liver, and lower extremities, as well as from the coronary arteries, upper extremities, and superior vena cava. Blood enters the right atrium via the inferior vena cava and is shunted directly to the left atrium through the foramen ovale, bypassing most of the right ventricle and lungs. Blood that does enter the right ventricle is pumped to the pulmonary artery where it divides. A portion goes directly to the lung, and the remainder is shunted through the narrow ductus arteriosus to the descending aorta. Blood entering the left atrium mixes with a small amount of blood received from the pulmonary veins and passes into the left ventricle. From there it is pumped through the aorta and into the general circulation.

Circulatory changes at birth. With the first inspiration at birth, the lungs expand and begin functioning.

Placental circulation ceases, and the connection with the placenta ends with the cutting of the umbilical cord, causing several major changes. During fetal life the lungs have a high vascular resistance. As a result, the blood ejected from the right ventricle into the pulmonary artery is shunted via the ductus arteriosus into the descending aorta. With the first breath the alveoli expand, the pulmonary vascular resistance drops rapidly, and pulmonary blood flow increases. Simultaneously, the loss of placental blood flow causes the right atrial pressure to drop. The combination of decreased pulmonary vascular resistance, increased pulmonary blood flow, and decreased right atrial pressure causes the left atrial pressure to rise above right atrial pressure. The foramen ovale then closes, and the increase in oxygen saturation following the changes in pulmonary vascular resistance stimulates constriction and eventual closure of the ductus arteriosus.

NORMAL FINDINGS

The assessment of any patient begins with careful attention to the patient's chief complaint. The problem, whether chest pain, palpitations, or shortness of breath, should guide the direction of questioning. Questions regarding the problem may be organized into seven categories: location, quality, quantity, precipitating or aggravating factors, duration, and associated symptoms.

Area of Concern	Normal Adult Findings	Variations in Child	Variations in Older Adult
History			
Past medical history and general health status	Congenital heart disease; childhood disease (rheumatic fever, scarlet fever); coronary artery disease; vascular disorders; bleeding disorders; hypertension; kidney disease; diabetes; hyperlipidemia; heart murmurs; allergies		
Family history	Age, sex, and health of parents, siblings, and children and cause of death for deceased members; data regarding history of hypertension, heart disease, diabetes, elevated lipid levels		
Cardiovascular risk factor profile			
Sociocultural	Culture; occupation; smoking; alcohol consumption; economic situation		
Activity level	Normal activity level; sports		
Sleep	Number of pillows used; presence of paroxysmal nocturnal dyspnea; number of times up to urinate		
Nutrition	Fluid and dietary restriction; any recent weight increases or decreases		
Dental history	Major problems; last dental visit; knowledge regarding antibiotic prophylaxis if pertinent		
Medications	Prescription and nonprescription drugs; contraceptives		
Psychosocial	Perception of illness; response to health problems; patterns of coping or adaptation; understanding of current and past health problems		
Support system	Marital status; primary support system		
General appearance	Level of consciousness (alert, oriented); respiratory rate and pattern (passive breathing 12-20/minute, respiratory/pulse rate ratio 1:4, no shortness of breath [SOB] or dyspnea); nutritional state (well nourished); weight and height normal	Facial expression; nutritional state; height, weight based on percentile growth chart; motor development; posture assumed (squatting; knee-chest); quality of cry; color at rest and during crying episodes; activity level; respiration (nasal during infancy; 6-7 yr: thoracic or abdominal breathing) *Age* *Respirations/minute* Newborn 30-50 6 mo 20-40 1 yr 20-40 3 yr 20-30 6 yr 16-22 10 yr 16-20 17 yr 14-20	

Area of Concern	Normal Adult Findings	Variations in Child			Variations in Older Adult
Blood pressure	Systolic 100-140 mm Hg (tends to be 5-15 mm Hg higher in right arm); diastolic 60-90 mm Hg; pulse pressure 30-40 mm Hg	*Age*	*Systolic (mm Hg)*	*Diastolic (mm Hg)*	Maximum systolic pressure 160 mm Hg; with standing, there may be systolic drop of 10-15 mm Hg and diastolic drop of 5 mm Hg
		Newborn	80 ± 16	46 ± 16	
		2 mo to 1 yr	89 ± 29	60 ± 10	
		1 yr	96 ± 30	66 ± 25	
		2 yr	99 ± 25	64 ± 25	
		3 yr	100 ± 25	67 ± 23	
		4 yr	99 ± 20	65 ± 20	
		5-6 yr	94 ± 14	55 ± 9	
		6-7 yr	100 ± 15	56 ± 8	
		7-8 yr	102 ± 15	56 ± 8	
		8-9 yr	105 ± 16	57 ± 9	
		9-10 yr	107 ± 17	57 ± 9	
		10-11 yr	111 ± 17	58 ± 10	
		11-12 yr	113 ± 18	59 ± 10	
		12-13 yr	115 ± 19	59 ± 10	
		13-14 yr	118 ± 19	60 ± 10	
Arterial pulse (heart rate)	60-90 beats/minute	*Age*	*Average rate*		Slows with age due to increase in vagal tone
		Newborn	120-170		
		1 yr	80-160		
		2 yr	80-130		
		3 yr	80-120		
		4 yr	80-120		
		6 yr	75-115		
		over 6	70-110		

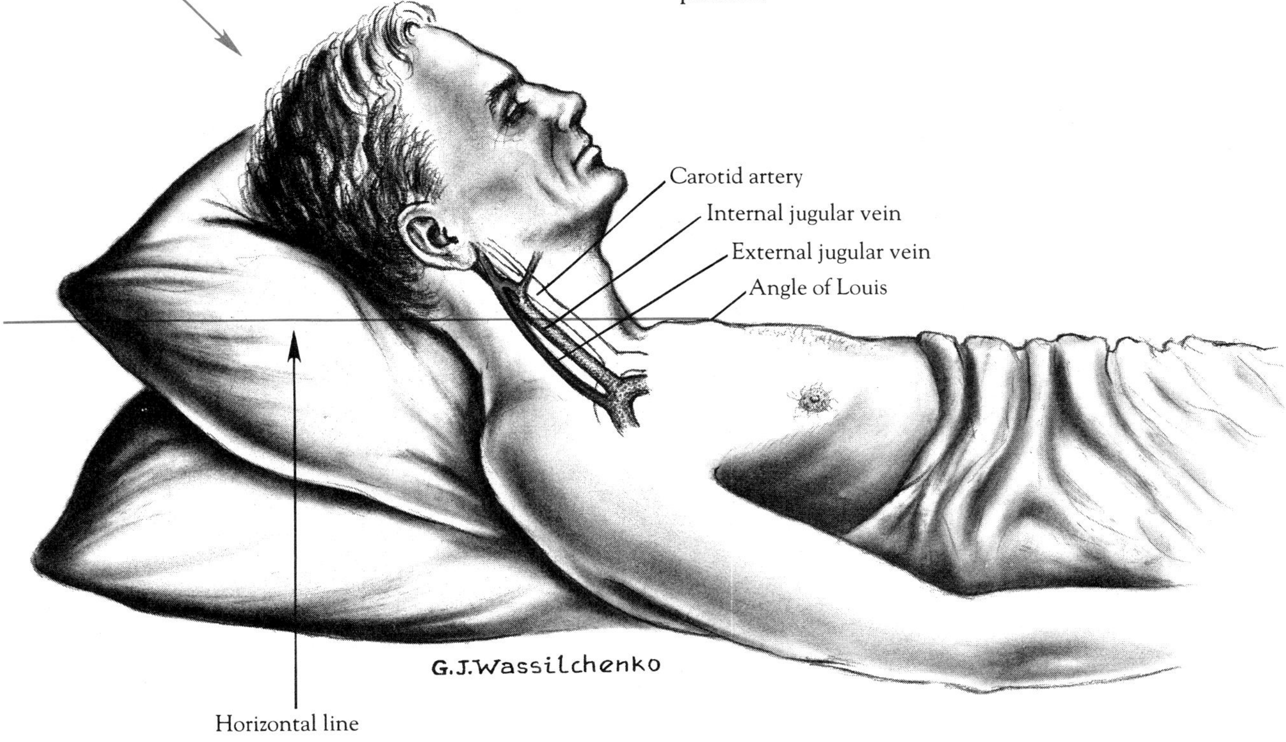

Fig. 1-15
Inspection of external jugular venous pressure.

45° angle
Carotid artery
Internal jugular vein
External jugular vein
Angle of Louis
Horizontal line
G.J.Wassilchenko

Area of Concern	Normal Adult Findings	Variations in Child	Variations in Older Adult
	Rhythm (regular); amplitude and contour (upstroke full, strong, rounded, brisk); symmetric response (equal on right and left); timing (equal for all arterial pulsations, e.g., brachial, femoral); auscultation (no murmurs or bruits)	Rhythm (irregular, varying with respiration); amplitude (upstroke smooth, rounded, full); auscultation (innocent supraclavicular murmur)	Amplitude and contour (upstroke more rapid, smooth)
Jugular venous pressure (JVP) (Fig. 1-15)	Should not exceed 3 cm (1 inch) above level of sternal angle (Fig. 1-15) with head of client elevated to 30-45 degrees	May be visible but does not usually pulsate or appear engorged	
Jugular pulsations	Undulations; movement with inspiration; increase or decrease with change in body position	Not routinely examined in children	
Wave pulsations			
a wave	First positive wave visualized; coincides with S_1		
X descent	First negative "trough" undulation; occurs between S_1 and S_2		
V wave	Third positive wave; coincides with S_2		
Precordium (Fig. 1-16)	Point of maximum impulse (PMI) 5-7 cm left of midsternal border at fifth intercostal space (ICS) and 1-2 cm (⅓-½ inch) in diameter; palpable areas: aortic area—at second ICS to right of sternal border, pulmonic area—at second ICS to left of sternal border, apex—at fifth ICS 5-7 cm to left of sternal border; precordial motion symmetric, even with respiration	PMI at fourth ICS to left of midsternal border; after age 7, similar to adults; 1-1.5 cm (⅓ inch) in diameter; palpable areas: aortic area—second ICS to right of sternal border, pulmonic area—second ICS to left of sternal border (may feel slight pulsations after exercise), apex (infants and small children)—fourth ICS to left of midsternal border; after age 7 similar to adults	

Fig. 1-16
Chest wall landmarks for inspection, percussion, and palpation.

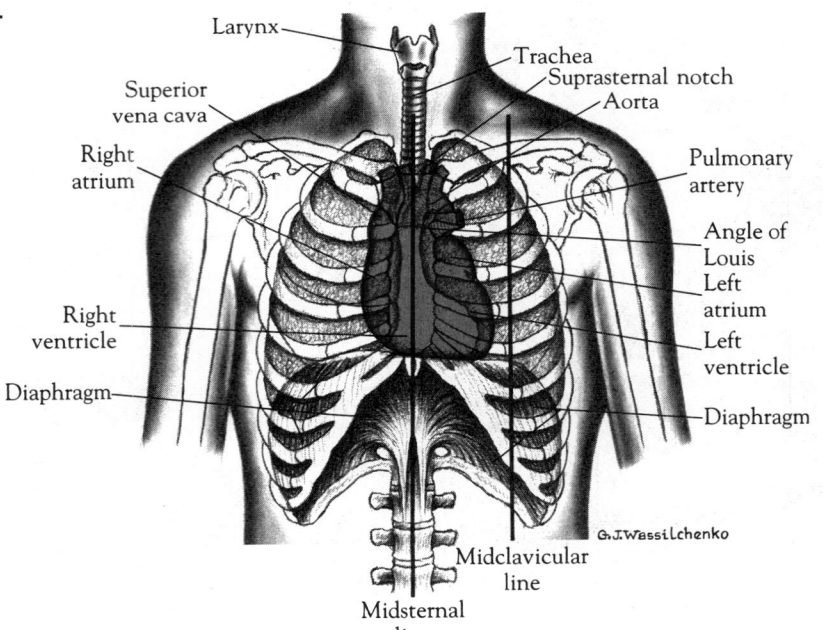

Larynx

Trachea
Suprasternal notch
Aorta

Superior vena cava

Pulmonary artery

Right atrium

Angle of Louis
Left atrium
Left ventricle

Right ventricle

Diaphragm

Diaphragm

G.J.Wassilchenko

Midclavicular line

Midsternal line

Area of Concern	Normal Adult Findings	Variations in Child	Variations in Older Adult
Heart sounds	First heart sound (S₁) closing of A-V valves; components are tricuspid (T₁), located at fifth intercostal space (ICS) and left lower sternal border (LLSB), and mitral (M₁), located in apical area at fifth ICS and 5-7 cm left of sternal border; loudest at apical area; normal splitting heard LLSB at fifth ICS Second heart sound (S₂) closure of semilunar valves; components are aortic (A₂), located at second ICS to right of sternal border, and pulmonic (P₂), located at second ICS to left of sternal border; loudest at base; normal splitting heard at P₂	Loudest at apex, rapid rate will accentuate; normal splitting heard in right ventricular area	

NORMAL LABORATORY DATA

Laboratory Test	Values	Laboratory Test	Values
Complete blood count (CBC)		Lactate dehydrogenase (LDH) isoenzymes (method dependent)	
Glycosylated hemoglobin	5.7%-8.8%	LDH₁	22%-36%
Plasma hemoglobin	1-5 mg/dl	LDH₂	35%-46%
Whole-blood hemoglobin		LDH₃	13%-26%
Birth (cord blood)	17.1 ± 1.8 g/dl	LDH₄	3%-10%
11-13.5 mo	11.9 ± 0.6 g/dl	LDH₅	2%-9%
1.5-3 yr	11.8 ± 0.5 g/dl	LDH (specific for heart, kidney, blood cells)	0.17-0.27 of total LDH
5 yr	12.7 ± 1.0 g/dl	Lipid profile	
10 yr	13.2 ± 1.2 g/dl	Total	400-800 mg/dl
Men	15.5 ± 1.1 g/dl	Cholesterol	100-210 mg/dl
Women	13.7 ± 1.0 g/dl	In cord blood	<100 mg/dl
Hematocrit		Birth–1 mo	45-100 mg/dl
First postnatal day		Triglycerides (at 95th percentile)	
24-25 wk gestational age	63%	White men	
26-27 wk gestational age	62%	25-29 yr	Up to 250 mg/dl
28-29 wk gestational age	60%	35-54 yr	Up to 320 mg/dl
30-31 wk gestational age	60%	55-64 yr	Up to 290 mg/dl
Newborn	54%-68%	65 and older	Up to 260 mg/dl
Males		White women	
2 yr	35%-44%	35-39 yr	Up to 195 mg/dl
6 yr	31%-43%	55-64 yr	Up to 250 mg/dl
Adult	42%-52%	Lipoproteins	
Females		High density (HDL)	
2 yr	35%-44%	Men 15-34 yr	30-65 mg/dl
6 yr	31%-43%	Women	35-80 mg/dl
Adult	35%-47%	Low density (LDL)	
Cardiac enzymes		White men 35-39 yr	Up to 190 mg/dl
Creatine phosphokinase (CPK)		Phospholipids	150-380 mg/dl
Males	55-70 units/L	Fatty acids	9-15 mmol/L
Females	15-57 units/L	Drug levels	
CPK-MB (isoenzyme)	0-7 IU/L	Digoxin	
SGOT	8-42 units/L	Therapeutic	1-2 ng/ml
	For infants, 2-3 times adult values; ranges decrease during childhood	Toxic	3 ng/ml
		Underdigitalization	<0.5 ng/ml
		Digitoxin	
		Therapeutic	10-30 ng/ml
		Toxic	>35 ng/ml

DIAGNOSTIC STUDIES

Electrocardiogram (ECG)

Electrical representation of myocardial activity; used to determine presence of abnormal transmission of heart impulse through conduction tissue of heart muscle (see p. 20 for normal findings)

Nursing care:

Explain procedure; ensure electrical safety measures

Exercise stress test (EST)

Examines cardiovascular response to exercise; used in detection and quantitation of ischemic heart disease, for patients considered at risk, and to determine cardiovascular fitness preceding exercise programs

Indications:

Differential diagnosis of chest pain; determining level of workload (exercise) when symptoms of ischemia occur; evaluation of therapy for angina; evaluation of patients who have multiple risk factors for coronary artery disease; evaluation of exercise-induced arrhythmias

Contraindications:

Recent myocardial infarction (4-6 weeks) (but such patients may perform submaximal EST before discharge from hospital); rapid ventricular or atrial arrhythmia; heart failure; severe aortic stenosis; blood pressure greater than 170/100 mm Hg before onset of exercise; complete A-V block

Nursing care:

Explain procedure, stressing need for patient to report any symptoms during and after procedure; instruct patient to dress comfortably in shorts or gym clothes and tennis shoes; instruct patient not to eat for 1 hour before test; during procedure, monitor blood pressure, heart rate, ECG changes such as ST elevation or depression and arrhythmias; observe for symptoms such as chest pain or pressure, shortness of breath, fatigue

Echocardiogram

Noninvasive method of evaluating internal structures and motion of heart; ultrasound beam penetrates cardiac structures, which reflect "echo" waves that travel back to transducer to form images; used to determine internal dimensions of ventricles, size and motion of intraventicular septum and posterior wall of left ventricle, valve motion and anatomy, presence of pericardial fluid, direction of blood flow, and presence of blood clots and myomatous tumors

Modes:

M-mode or one-dimensional (Fig. 1-17); two-dimensional, cross-sectional, real-time motion (Fig. 1-18); Doppler in which continuous wave combined with pulse ultrasound gives image of heart pulse and indicates direction of blood flow

Nursing care:

Explain procedure and that patient may sense discomfort from pressure of transducer across chest

Ambulatory electrocardiography (Holter monitor)

Used to detect ECG rhythm disturbances that may occur over extended period of time, to evaluate effectiveness of antiarrhythmic drug therapy, and to evaluate chest pain episodes; capable of recording ECG over 24- or 48-hour period

Nursing care:

Explain procedure; instruct patient in care of electrodes at home and about importance of keeping diary of symptoms or activities at times designated by physician

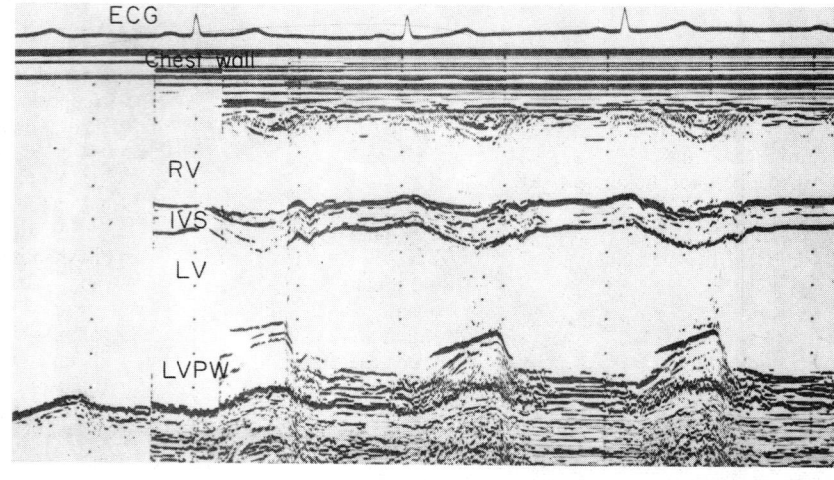

Fig. 1-17

Landmarks used to identify echo tracings: *ECG,* electrocardiography; chest wall; *RV,* right ventricle; *IVS,* intraventricular septum; *LV,* left ventricle; *LVPW,* left ventricular posterior wall.

Courtesy Non Invasive Labs, Division of Cardiology, UCLA School of Medicine, Los Angeles, Calif.; from Canobbio, M.M.: Noninvasive studies and diagnostic adjuncts for heart failure. In Michaelson, C.R.: Congestive heart failure, St. Louis, 1983, The C.V. Mosby Co.

Fig. 1-18
Two-dimensional echocardiography.
Apical, four-chamber view of heart.
A, Diagram of normal
echocardiogram. *CW,* Chest wall; *RV,*
right ventricle; *TV,* triscuspid valve;
AS, atrial septum; *RV,* right ventricle;
LV, left ventricle; *VS,* ventricular
septum; *MV,* mitral valve; *LA,* left
atrium; *PV,* pulmonary valve. **B,**
Two-dimensional echocardiogram,
apical view from patient with dilated
left atrium.

From Goldberger, E.: Textbook of clinical
cardiology, St. Louis, 1981, The C.V.
Mosby Co. **B** modified from Kotler, M.N.,
et al.: Am. J. Cardiol. **45:**1061, 1980.
Courtesy Dr. Joel Strom, Bronx, N.Y.

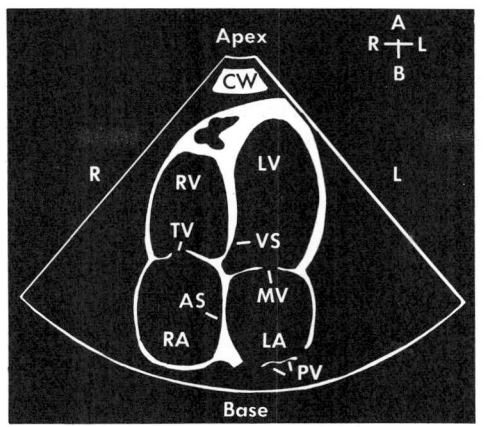

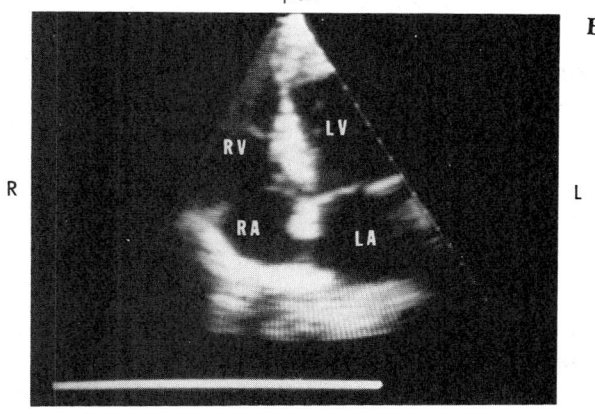

Chest roentgenogram

Gives information regarding anatomic location and abnormalities of heart, great vessels, and lungs; routine views in cardiac series: posterior-anterior (PA),
lateral, right anterior oblique (RAO), left anterior
oblique (LAO); used to determine position of heart
(normal is situs soltis: left thoracic heart), cardiothoracic size (normal is <50% of internal dimensions of thorax), cardiac silhouette (thorax, aorta,
ventricular chambers, atrial chambers, pulmonary
artery), presence of calcifications (visualized in
great vessels and on valves); lung fields used to
determine normal distribution of pulmonary blood
flow, increase of pulmonary congestion, presence
of pulmonary hypertension, presence of pleural effusions

Nursing care:
Explain procedure; inquire if patient is pregnant

Scintigraphy

Gives information regarding myocardial perfusion and
contractility through use of radionuclide imaging

Nursing care:
Explain procedure; obtain informed consent; instruct
patient that procedure involves injecting radioisotope and passing scanning camera over patient repeatedly; reassure patient that radiation exposure
involved is less than with chest roentgenogram; caution patient to remain quiet and still during study

Technetium 99m pyrophosphate myocardial imaging
Used to detect recent MI and extent of damage; "hot
spots" appear within 12 hours of infarct and dis-
appear after 1 week
Nursing care:
Explain to patient that tracer isotope will be injected

2-3 hours before procedure and that scanning will
take 30-60 minutes
Thallium 201 imaging
"Cold spot" myocardial imaging; used to assess
myocardial perfusion (myocardial blood flow), to
evaluate patency of grafts after bypass surgery,
and in conjunction with EST in diagnosis of coronary artery disease (stress imaging)

Nursing care:
If done in conjunction with EST instruct patient to
avoid tobacco, alcohol, or unprescribed medication for 24 hours before study and to take nothing by mouth for 3 hours before test; NOTE: if
chest pain, SOB, or drop in blood pressure develops, stress imaging is halted

Blood pool imaging (BPI)
Used to evaluate regional and global ventricular performance and to detect aneurysms of left ventricle
and areas of hypokinesis and dyskinesis; involves
injection of human serum albumin or RBCs
tagged with isotope technetium 99m pertechne-

tate; scintillation camera records several pass images of isotope as it passes through ventricle; imaging can be "gated" to systolic and diastolic events of cardiac cycle; normal left ventricular ejection fraction is 55% to 65%; procedure contraindicated in pregnancy

Electrophysiologic studies (bundle of His)

Invasive procedure involving insertion of catheter via peripheral vein into right atrium and right ventricle to detect A-V conduction disturbances, diagnose syncope, and assist in selection of antiarrhythmic agents; normal conduction intervals: H-V 35-55 msec, A-V 45-150 msec, P-A 20-40 msec

Complications:

Arrhythmias, phlebitis, pulmonary emboli, hemorrhage

Nursing care:

Obtain informed consent; explain that procedure will last 1-3 hours and that patient will be awake and may feel slight pressure; instruct patient to report any discomfort; permit nothing by mouth for 6 hours before procedure; after procedure check vital signs every 15 minutes for 1 hour, then every 4 hours; check insertion site for bleeding every 30 minutes to 1 hour for 8 hours

Cardiac catheterization

Invasive procedure involving insertion of radiopaque catheter via peripheral artery or vein into the heart; used to determine anatomy of heart chambers, valves, great vessels, and coronary arteries; ventricular wall thickness and motion; hemodynamic functions of the heart by pressure recordings of heart chambers and great vessels and pressure gradients across the valves; ventricular function and cardiac output; degree of valve competence; and intracardiac oxygen saturations; and to selectively visualize heart, coronary arteries, and great vessels by recording serial x-rays (angiograms)

Complications:

Myocardial infarction, arrhythmias, hematoma or hemorrhage at insertion site, reaction to contrast medium, infection, pulmonary edema, cardiac tamponade

Nursing care:

Obtain informed consent; explain that procedure will last 2-4 hours, that patient may feel pressure with insertion of catheter and hot flushing sensation or nausea with injection of contrast medium, that patient should cough when instructed by physician, and that patient will receive medication if chest pain occurs and may be given nitroglycerin to dilate coronary vessels; determine any allergies or hypersensitivity to shellfish, iodine, or other contrast media; after procedure check vital signs every 15 minutes, decreasing in frequency; keep patient flat in bed for 6-8 hours with pressurized dressing over puncture site; check dressing and surrounding area for bleeding, pain, and swelling; check peripheral pulses, color, warmth, and feeling of extremities distal to insertion site; give pain medication as indicated; encourage fluid intake for first 6-8 hours to assist in elimination of contrast medium

Digital vascular imaging (DVI) (digital subtraction angiography)

New invasive procedure using computer system and fluoroscopy with image intensifier to permit complete visualization of arterial supply to specific area

Indications:

Carotid and renal artery disease, aneurysms, thrombotic and embolic disease of great vessels, coarctation of aorta

Complications:

Arrhythmias, reaction to contrast medium, infection, bleeding at site

Nursing care:

Obtain informed consent; explain that procedure will last 1-2 hours, can be done on outpatient basis, and may cause certain sensations (similar to those with catheterization); after procedure check vital signs immediately and as ordered; check site for bleeding; instruct patient to observe site for infection and/or bleeding and to drink minimum of 1 L of fluid on day of procedure

Plethysmography

Measures venous flow in limbs by recording changes in volume and vascular resistance; used to detect deep vein thrombosis in leg and to screen patients at high risk for thrombophlebitis; two types: digital phethysmography to evaluate digital pulse volume and venous occlusion plethysmography to evaluate arterial responses to temporary block of venous system

Nursing care:
Explain procedure

Ultrasonography

Used to measure systolic blood pressure in distal arteries, to amplify audible sounds of peripheral pulses, and to measure blood flow velocity along course of an artery; ankle systolic pressure should be equal to or greater than brachial systolic pressure—0.45-0.75 mm Hg (ankle/brachial index)

Nursing care:

Explain procedure and that patient may sense discomfort from pressure of transducer

Conditions, Diseases, and Disorders

CARDIAC ARRHYTHMIAS

An arrhythmia is a disorder of the heart rate and rhythm caused by a disturbance of the conduction system.

The most serious consequence of cardiac arrhythmias is sudden death resulting from electromechanical failure (as in ventricular fibrillation) or from impaired cardiac function.

Early recognition and treatment are needed because various arrhythmias such as premature ventricular ectopic beats may spontaneously become frequent or multifocal. For example, in a patient with myocardial ischemia the ectopic beat may convert to ventricular tachycardia or ventricular fibrillation without warning. Approximately 40% to 70% of deaths from acute myocardial infarction occur within the first hour, generally before the victim can reach a hospital.

Careful continuous ECG monitoring now enables early detection and prompt treatment of potentially serious arrhythmias. However, proper treatment involves not only diagnosis but also a thorough understanding of the underlying etiologic factors.

PATHOPHYSIOLOGY

The pathogenesis of cardiac arrhythmias may be classified into abnormalities of impulse formation (sinus, atrial, ventricular) or impulse conduction or a combination of both.[31] Arrhythmias may also be described on the basis of rate (bradyarrhythmia, tachyarrhythmia) or clinical significance (minor, life threatening). Arrhythmias may occur as result of a primary cardiac disorder, as a secondary response to a systemic problem, or as a complication of drug toxicity or electrolyte imbalance.

Each of the major arrhythmias is described in the section on assessment.

DIAGNOSTIC STUDIES

Electrocardiogram (ECG)
See "Assessment: Areas of Concern" for ECG characteristics and findings for specific arrhythmias

24-Hour ambulatory electrocardiogram

Electrophysiologic studies

TREATMENT PLAN

Surgical
Electrophysiologic mapping—specialized procedure performed in catheterization laboratory or by direct visualization in operating room; performed only on patients with highly refractory tachyarrhythmias and to identify accessory A-V bundles in patients with Wolff-Parkinson-White syndrome, since tracts can be excised surgically once irritable focus is located; can also be performed on patients with recurrent ventricular tachycardia through use of programmed stimulation, which allows cardiologist or surgeon to induce ventricular tachycardia, identify arrhythmogenic site, and excise ectopic focus

Chemotherapeutic
Antiarrhythmic drugs: group I—potent local anesthetic drugs that affect nerves as well as myocardial fibers; decrease conduction velocity by retarding influx of sodium and reduce maximal rate of depolarizing action potential
Quinidine
Indications: Suppresses atrial, junctional, or ventricular ectopy, ventricular tachycardia, and paroxysmal atrial tachycardia; may be used to convert atrial fibrillation or flutter to sinus rhythm or to maintain sinus rhythm after cardioversion
Usual dosage: 200-400 mg po q4-6h
Onset of action: 15 min with peak activity in 2-4 h
Therapeutic blood levels: 2-6 mg/ml
Toxic signs: Widened QRS, prolonged QT bundle branch block, complete heart block, ventricular tachycardia, asystole
Sustained-release preparations: Quinidex, 300 mg q8-12h; Quinaglute, 324 mg q8-12h; Cardioquin, 275 mg q6h
Procainamide (Pronestyl)
Indications: Similar to quinidine; suppresses ventricular ectopy; may be less effective in controlling atrial arrhythmias
Usual dosage: 250-750 mg po q4-6h; 100 mg q5-15 min for total of 1 g IV
Peak action: Within 30 min
Therapeutic blood levels: 4-8 mg/ml
Sustained-release preparations: Procan SR, 500-1000 mg q6h

Disopyramide phosphate (Norpace)
  Indications: Suppresses or prevents ventricular arrhythmias; not particularly effective in treating atrial arrhythmias
  Usual dosage: 400-800 mg/day PO in four doses with loading dose of 200 mg
  Peak action: 2-4 h
  Therapeutic blood levels: 2-4 mg/ml
Lidocaine (Xylocaine)
  Indications and actions: Controls ventricular arrhythmias by depressing automaticity in Purkinje network and increasing excitability threshold of ventricles
  Usual dosage: 50-100 mg (1-2 mg/kg) by IV bolus followed by 1.5-4 mg/min
  Onset of action: 45-90 sec
  Duration of action: 20 min
  Therapeutic blood levels: 1.5-5 mg/ml
Phenytoin (Dilantin)
  Indications and actions: Depresses automaticity
  Usual dosage: 100 mg q6h po with loading dose of 200 mg or 50-100 mg IV over 5-10 min up to 1 g
  Onset of action: Slow and variable
  Therapeutic blood levels: 10-15 mg/ml
Mexiletine
  Indications: Investigational local anesthetic whose electrophysiologic properties closely resemble those of lidocaine; used in management of ventricular arrhythmias
  Usual dosage: IV loading 10-15 mg/min (200-300 mg over 30 min), maintenance 250-500 mg/12 h; po loading 100-400 mg, maintenance 200-300 mg q8h
  Onset of action: IV <5 min; po 1-2 h
  Therapeutic blood levels: 0.5-2 μg/ml
Tocainide
  Indications: Investigational drug given for control of ventricular arrhythmias
  Usual dosage: Loading 400-600 mg po, maintenance 400-800 mg q8h
  Onset of action: 1½ h
  Therapeutic blood levels: 6-12 μg/ml
Aprindine
  Indications: Investigational drug used in control of supraventricular and ventricular arrhythmias resistant to traditional agents
  Usual dosage: Loading 200-300 mg po, maintenance 100-150 mg/day
  Onset of action: 2 h
  Therapeutic blood levels: 1-2 μg/ml
Antiarrhythmic drugs: group II—control arrhythmias by blocking sympathetic stimulation, which shortens phase 4 depolarization of action potential
Propranolol (Inderal)

Indications and actions: Controls supraventricular tachycardia resulting from reentry mechanism; used to control ventricular response to atrial fibrillation and flutter by depressing A-V nodal conduction
  Usual dosage: 10-80 mg po qid; 0.5-1 mg IV push slowly to control heart rate
  Onset of action: 1-1½ h (po)
  Therapeutic blood levels: Not determined
Atenolol
  Usual dosage: 50-100 mg qd
Pindolol
  Usual dosage: 10-60 mg bid
Antiarrhythmic drugs: group III—act directly on myocardium, prolonging action potential
  Bretylium tosylate (Bretylol)
    Indications: Life-threatening ventricular arrhythmias; not recommended to treat asymptomatic ventricular ectopic beats
    Usual dosage: 5-10 mg/kg IV push up to total of 30 mg/kg; may repeat in 15-30 min; slow continuous infusion 5-10 mg/kg q6-8h
  Amiodarone
    Indications: Effective in treatment and prevention of wide variety of atrial and ventricular arrhythmias
    Usual dosage: 200-800 mg qd; loading dose 800-1200 mg qd for 1 wk
    Onset of action: 4-8 h
Antiarrhythmic drugs: group IV—inhibit calcium transport into cells, depress activity of the S-A and A-V nodes, prolong conduction in A-V node, and increase A-V node refractoriness
  Verapamil (Calan, Isoptin)
    Indications: Reentrant paroxysmal supraventricular tachyarrhythmias; suppresses A-V junctional tachycardia and controls ventricular response to atrial fibrillation and flutter
    Usual dosage: 5-10 mg (0.1 mg/kg) IV or 40-80 mg po q6-8h
    Peak action: IV 3-5 min; po 3-4 h

Electromechanical
Cardiac monitoring—continuous electrocardiographic monitoring provides most efficient and reliable method of detection of arrhythmias
Electrical countershock—often treatment of choice for tachyarrhythmias that are life threatening or producing a decrease in cardiac output and are resistant to pharmacologic interventions (see p. 97 for further discussion and nursing care)
Cardioversion—synchronized discharge of electrical impulse used to convert atrial fibrillation, atrial flutter, or supraventricular tachycardia to sinus rhythm

Defibrillation—emergency procedure that is unsynchronized; used in treatment of ventricular defibrillation

Cardiac pacemakers—battery-operated electrical devices used to initiate and control heart rate; system is composed of battery pack and electrodes through which electrical stimulation is delivered to myocardium; may be used as temporary assistive devices or implanted permanently; have variety of modalities that are selected on basis of rhythm disturbance; most common indication for pacemaker implantation is bradyarrhythmias, but recent advances in technology have broadened their use to treatment of suppressing supraventricular arrhythmias otherwise resistant to drug therapy (see p. 105 for further discussion)

Supportive

Diet—restrictions usually directed to underlying disease process; patients with diagnosed supraventricular tachyarrhythmias instructed to avoid using stimulants such as caffeine, which is found in coffee, certain teas, soft drinks, and chocolate

Smoking—use of nicotine contraindicated because of its effect on ventricular threshold, which may be basis for dysrhythmias that could precipitate fatal rhythms

ASSESSMENT: AREAS OF CONCERN

Rhythm	Characteristics	Etiology	Clinical Significance	Management
Sinus origin				
Sinus tachycardia (Fig. 1-19)	Regular rhythm; rate 100-180 beats/minute (higher in infants); normal P wave; normal QRS complex	Rate increase may be normal response to exercise, emotion, or abnormal stressors such as pain, fever, pump failure, hyperthyroidism, and certain pharmacologic agents, including caffeine, nitrates, atropine, epinephrine, isoproterenol, and nicotine	May have hemodynamic consequence in patient with damaged heart that is unable to sustain increased workloads brought on by persistent increases in heart rate	Correcting underlying factors; removing offending drugs

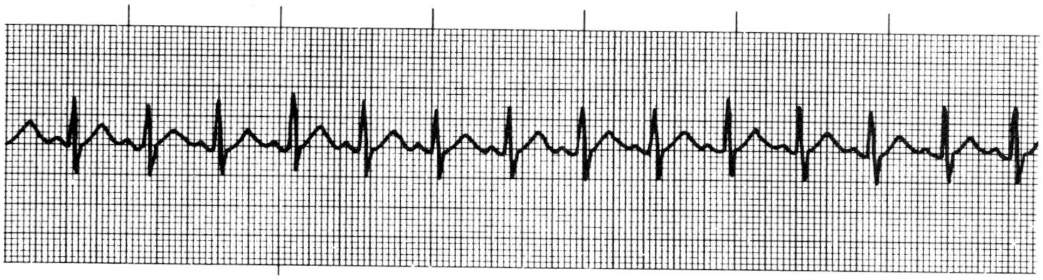

Fig. 1-19

From Andreoli, K., et al.: Comprehensive cardiac care: a text for nurses, physicians, and other health practitioners, ed. 5, St. Louis, 1983, The C.V. Mosby Co.

Rhythm	Characteristics	Etiology	Clinical Significance	Management
Sinus bradycardia (Fig. 1-20)	Regular rhythm; rate less than 60 beats/minute; normal P wave; normal PR interval; normal QRS complex	Rate decrease may be normal response to sleep or in well-conditioned athlete; abnormal drops in rate may be caused by diminished blood flow to S-A node, vagal stimulation, hypothyroidism, increased intracranial pressure, or pharmacologic agents such as digoxin, propranolol, quinidine, or procainamide	None unless associated with signs of impaired cardiac output; symptoms: dizziness, syncope, chest pain	Correcting underlying cause; atropine 0.5-1 mg IV; transvenous pacemaker

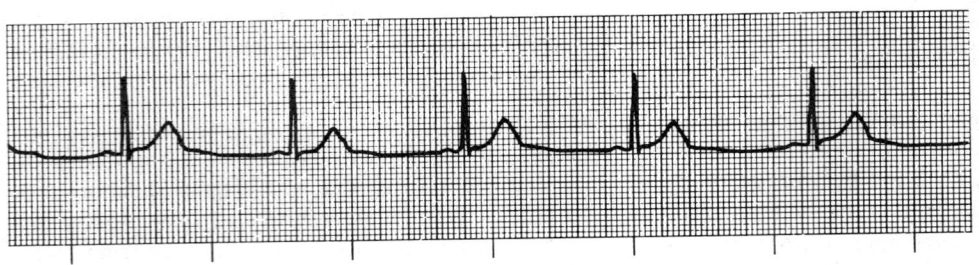

Fig. 1-20

From Andreoli, K., et al.: Comprehensive cardiac care: a text for nurses, physicians, and other health practitioners, ed. 5, St. Louis, 1983, The C.V. Mosby Co.

Rhythm	Characteristics	Etiology	Clinical Significance	Management
Sinus arrhythmia (Fig. 1-21)	Irregular rhythm; may be phasic with respiration, slowing during inspiration and increasing with expiration; rate 60-100 beats/minute; normal PR interval; normal QRS complex	Sinus rhythm with cyclic variation caused by vagal impulses that influence rhythm during respiration; occurs commonly in children, young adults, and the elderly; usually disappears as heart rate increases	None unless heart rate decreases; symptoms: dizziness with decreased rate	None indicated unless heart rate decreases and symptoms occur

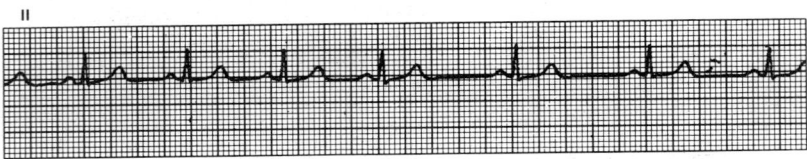

Fig. 1-21

From Conover, M.B.: Cardiac arrhythmias: exercises in pattern interpretation, ed. 2, St. Louis, 1978, The C.V. Mosby Co.

Rhythm	Characteristics	Etiology	Clinical Significance	Management
Atrial origin Atrial premature contractions (APCs, PACs) (Fig. 1-22)	Irregular rhythm owing to ectopic beats followed by incomplete compensatory pause; rate normal or increased depending on number of ectopic beats; P wave present but different from normal underlying sinus beat; PR interval may be shorter or longer than normal sinus beat; normal QRS complex	May be precipitated in healthy persons by anxiety, fatigue, caffeine, smoking, and alcohol; observed in patients with ischemia or organic heart disease and those receiving digoxin	May indicate atrial strain or hypoxia; frequent PACs (more than 6/minute) reflect atrial irritability and often mark onset of atrial fibrillation	Correcting underlying cause; for frequent PACs, quinidine or pronestyl

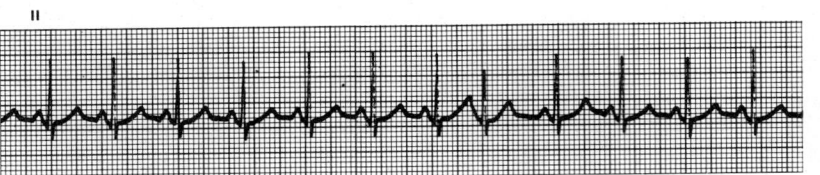

Fig. 1-22

From Conover, M.B.: Exercises in diagnosing ECG tracings, ed. 3, St. Louis, 1984, The C.V. Mosby Co.

Rhythm	Characteristics	Etiology	Clinical Significance	Management
Paroxysmal supraventricular tachycardia (PSVT) (Fig. 1-23)	Sudden, rapid onset of tachycardia with stimulus originating above A-V node; regular rhythm; rate 150-250 beats/minute; P wave uniform, may or may not be buried in preceding T wave; PR interval may vary, often difficult to measure; normal QRS complex	May begin and end spontaneously or be precipitated by excitement, fatigue, caffeine, smoking, or alcohol	Usually no significant impairment; patient complains of palpitations and shortness of breath; if persistent or occurring in patient with preexisting organic heart disease, may cause decrease in cardiac output and/or blood pressure resulting in pump failure or shock	Performing vagal stimulation with carotid sinus massage; using Valsalva maneuver to stimulate baroreceptors (may be used in conjunction with carotid sinus massage); decreasing ventricular response with medication to block A-V conduction; sedation to reduce sympathetic stimulation; verapamil 5-10 mg IV push; propranolol (Inderal) slowly IV in 1 mg increments up to 4 mg (contraindicated in patients with heart failure); edrophonium (Tensilon), test dose 1 mg followed by 10 mg IV; cardioversion if resistant to preceding

Fig. 1-23

From Andreoli, K., et al.: Comprehensive cardiac care: a text for nurses, physicians, and other health practitioners, ed. 5, St. Louis, 1983, The C.V. Mosby Co.

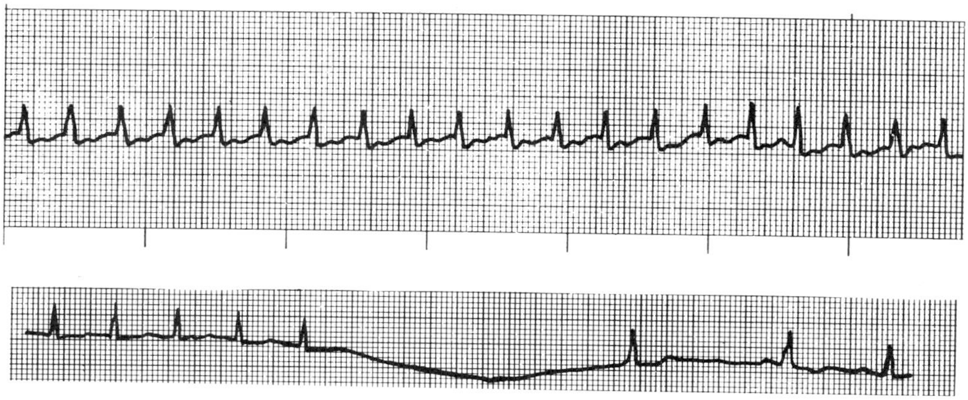

Rhythm	Characteristics	Etiology	Clinical Significance	Management
Atrial flutter (Fig. 1-24)	Rhythm may be regular or irregular; rate: atrial 250-350 beats/minute, characterized by sawtooth flutter waves; ventricular depends on A-V conduction, may occur at 2:1, 3:1, or 4:1 ratio; PR interval not measurable; normal QRS complex	Results from rapidly firing ectopic atrial focus; most likely underlying mechanism is localized atrial reentry phenomenon; seen in patients with organic heart disorders such as coronary artery disease and valvular heart disease	Patient complains of palpitations, which may be associated with heart failure, and chest pain, particularly in presence of rapid ventricular rates	Cardioversion; digoxin if cardioversion is not used or is unsuccessful; quinidine or procainamide

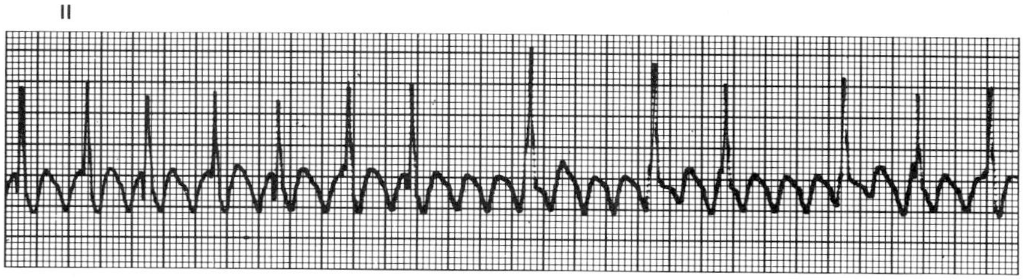

II

Fig. 1-24

From Conover, M.B.: Exercises in diagnosing ECG tracings, ed. 3, St. Louis, 1984, The C.V. Mosby Co.

Rhythm	Characteristics	Etiology	Clinical Significance	Management
Atrial fibrillation (Fig. 1-25)	Rhythm irregular; rate: atrial more than 350 beats/minute; absence of uniform atrial depolarization produces undulations (f waves); ventricular varies according to A-V conduction but may range between 50 and 150 beats/minute	Results from multiple atrial foci discharging almost simultaneously; atria never uniformly depolarize; reflects organic heart disease; may also occur with digitalis toxicity	With rapid ventricular rates, cardiac output may be impaired, resulting in heart failure, angina, and shock	Determination of underlying cause and whether acute or chronic; cardioversion for rapid ventricular response; digoxin if cardioversion is not used; quinidine; procainamide; verapamil

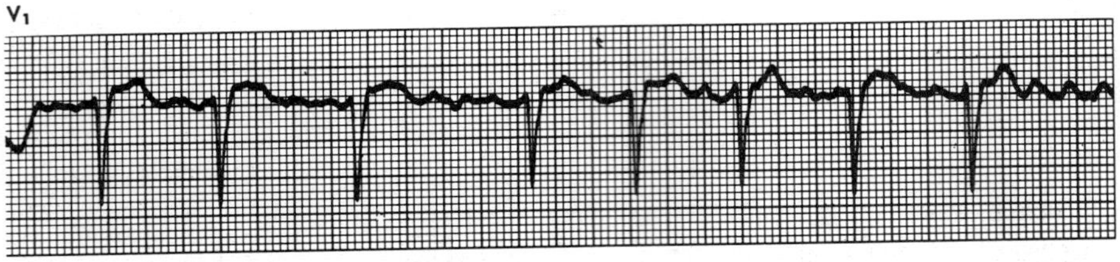

V₁

Fig. 1-25

From Conover, M.B.: Exercises in diagnosing ECG tracings, ed. 3, St. Louis, 1984, The C.V. Mosby Co.

Rhythm	Characteristics	Etiology	Clinical Significance	Management
Junctional rhythms Junctional escape rhythm (nodal) (Fig. 1-26)	Rhythm regular; rate 40-60 beats/minute; P wave abnormal, may occur before, during, or after QRS complex, may be inverted in leads II, III, and aVF; QRS complex usually normal	Occurs when sinus node is suppressed and atria fail to depolarize A-V junction; may be due to digitalis toxicity, vagal stimulation, or ischemic damage to S-A node	Usually none; transient; if condition persists, slow rates may allow foci with rapid rates to take over; may also produce symptoms of diminished cardiac output	Treatment or correction of underlying cause if persistent or if symptoms occur; atropine IV; pacemaker may be indicated

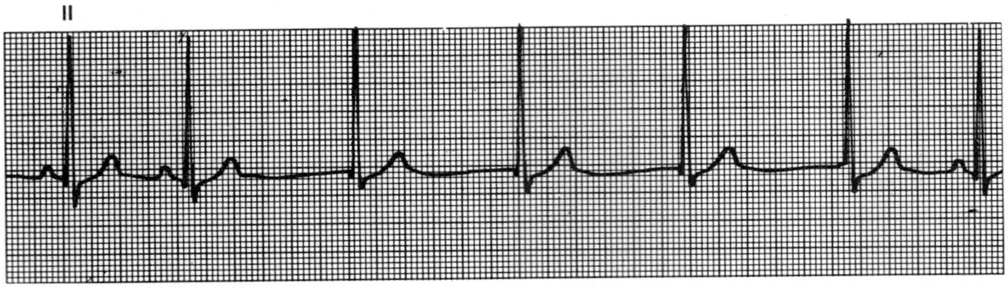

II

Fig. 1-26

From Conover, M.B.: Exercises in diagnosing ECG tracings, ed. 3, St. Louis, 1984, The C.V. Mosby Co.

Rhythm	Characteristics	Etiology	Clinical Significance	Management
Premature junctional contractions (Fig. 1-27)	Rhythm regular except for junctional beat; rate normal; P wave as described for junctional escape rhythm; PR interval shortened when P wave precedes QRS complex; QRS complex usually normal	Result from increased automaticity of A-V junction, causing ectopic focus in A-V node to discharge before onset of impulse from sinus node; these ectopic beats usually due to ischemia or digitalis toxicity	Usually none; frequency reflects junctional irritability	None indicated if infrequent; if frequent, quinidine

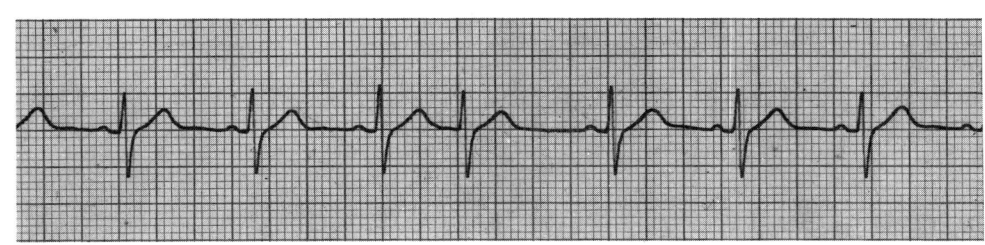

Fig. 1-27

From Conover, M.B.: Understanding electrocardiography, ed. 4, St. Louis, 1984, The C.V. Mosby Co.

Rhythm	Characteristics	Etiology	Clinical Significance	Management
Ventricular arrhythmias Premature ventricular contractions (PVCs) (Fig. 1-28)	Rhythm irregular owing to ectopic beats followed by full compensatory pause; rate normal or increased depending on number of ectopic beats; P wave absent in ectopic beat; PR interval absent; QRS complex widened and distorted; T wave is in opposition to R wave	Caused by irritable focus within ventricle, commonly associated with myocardial infarction; other causes include hypoxia, hypocalcemia, and acidosis	PVCs occurring frequently (more than 6/minute) or in pairs indicate increased ventricular irritability	Aimed at suppression of PVCs; if frequent, IV bolus of lidocaine (50-100 mg) followed by continuous IV infusion; additional antiarrhythmic agents in classes I and II may be given

II

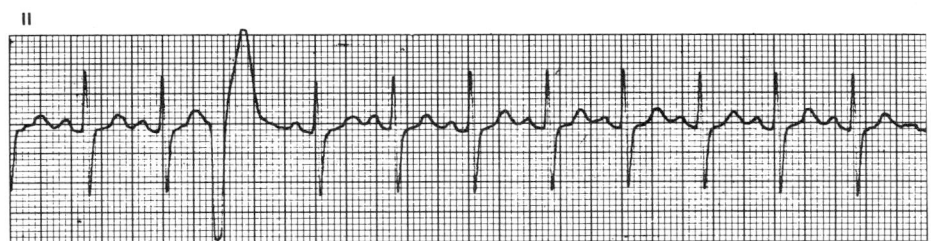

Fig. 1-28

From Conover, M.B.: Exercises in diagnosing ECG tracings, ed. 3, St. Louis, 1984, The C.V. Mosby Co.

Rhythm	Characteristics	Etiology	Clinical Significance	Management
Ventricular tachycardia (Fig. 1-29)	Rhythm slightly irregular; rate 100-200 beats/minute; P wave absent; PR interval absent; QRS complex wide and bizarre, greater than 0.12 second	Caused by irritable ventricular foci firing repetitively; commonly caused by myocardial infarction	Often a forerunner of ventricular fibrillation; if persistent and rapid, causes decreased cardiac output owing to decreased ventricular filling time	Most episodes terminate abruptly without treatment; lidocaine bolus 75-100 mg IV followed by continuous intravenous drip; defibrillation

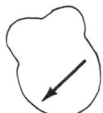

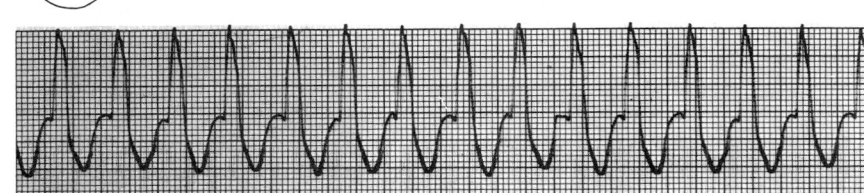

Fig. 1-29

From Conover, M.B.: Understanding electrocardiography, ed. 4, St. Louis, 1984, The C.V. Mosby Co.

Rhythm	Characteristics	Etiology	Clinical Significance	Management
Ventricular fibrillation (Fig. 1-30)	Rhythm irregular; rate: rapid repetitive waves or undulations that have no uniformity and are coarse or fine; P wave, QRS complex, and T wave cannot be identified	Lethal arrhythmia resulting from electrical stimulation of ventricular muscle, which leads to abrupt cessation of effective blood flow; occurs in severely damaged hearts as with ischemia, drug toxicity, trauma, or contact with high-voltage electricity	Loss of consciousness; decreases in blood pressure and peripheral pulse owing to loss of cardiac output	Cardiopulmonary resuscitation; defibrillation

Fig. 1-30
From Conover, M. B.: Understanding electrocardiography, ed. 4, St. Louis, 1984, The C.V. Mosby Co.

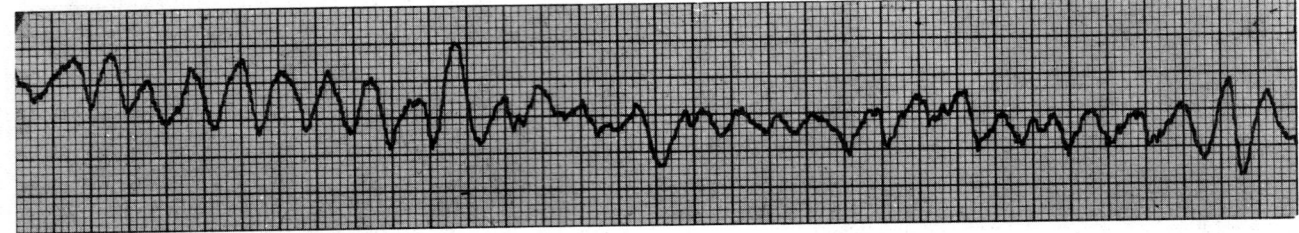

Rhythm	Characteristics	Etiology	Clinical Significance	Management
Conduction disturbances First-degree A-V heart block (Fig. 1-31)	Rhythm regular; rate normal; P wave normal; PR interval prolonged to greater than 0.20 second; QRS complex normal	Represents delay in impulse conduction through A-V node; occurs as result of increased vagal tone, digoxin administration, or congenital anomalies	No associated symptoms	None indicated; digitalis discontinued if causative factor; observation for development of further A-V block

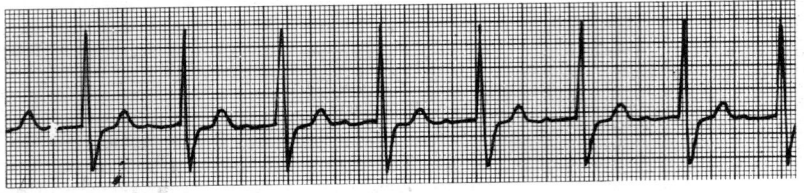

Fig. 1-31
From Conover, M.B.: Understanding electrocardiology: physiological and interpretive concepts, ed. 4, St. Louis, 1984, The C.V. Mosby Co.

Rhythm	Characteristics	Etiology	Clinical Significance	Management
Second-degree A-V heart block Mobitz type I (Wenckebach phenomenon) (Fig. 1-32, A)	Rhythm: atrial regular, ventricular irregular; rate: atrial greater than ventricular; P wave: multiple P waves before QRS complex; PR interval: progressive prolongation of PR interval until one impulse is completely blocked; QRS complex normal; RR interval becomes progressively shortened until one QRS complex is dropped	Represents progressive decrease in conduction velocity involving A-V node and proximal bundle of His; occurs as result of coronary artery disease, digitalis toxicity, rheumatic fever, viral infections, or inferior wall myocardial infarction	No associated symptoms if ventricular rate is adequately maintained	None usually indicated; elimination or correction of underlying cause; observation for progression to higher degree of block

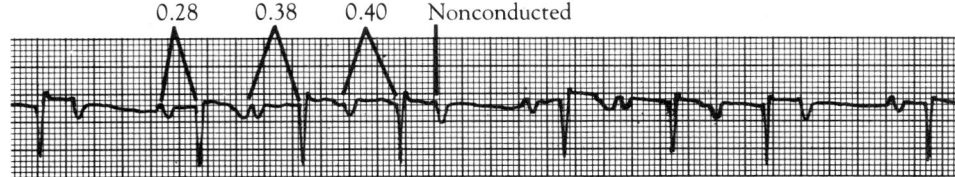

0.28   0.38   0.40   Nonconducted

Fig. 1-32, A

From Conover, M.B.: Understanding electrocardiology: physiological and interpretive concepts, ed. 3, St. Louis, 1980, The C.V. Mosby Co.

Rhythm	Characteristics	Etiology	Clinical Significance	Management
Mobitz type II (Fig. 1-32, *B*)	Rhythm: atrial regular, ventricular varies; rate: atrial slow to normal, ventricular may be slow, usually half or one-third atrial rate; P wave normal, occurring in multiples before QRS complex; PR interval normal or slightly prolonged, always constant; QRS complex normal or slightly prolonged	Represents block of impulse below level of A-V node and within His-Purkinje system; occurs as result of ischemia, digitalis or quinidine toxicity, anterior wall myocardial infarction	No associated symptoms if ventricular rate is adequately maintained; if rate is slow, cardiac output may be impaired, causing dizziness and weakness	Correction or elimination of underlying cause; tends to be recurrent, may progress to complete heart block; transvenous demand pacing may be required

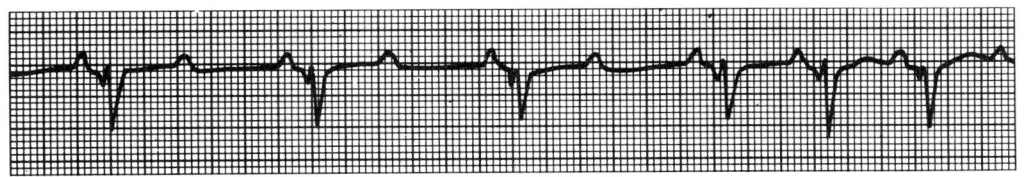

Fig. 1-32, B

From Conover, M.B.: Exercises in diagnosing ECG tracings, ed. 3, St. Louis, 1984, The C.V. Mosby Co.

Rhythm	Characteristics	Etiology	Clinical Significance	Management
Third-degree A-V block (complete heart block) (Fig. 1-33)	Rhythm: atrial and ventricular regular but act independent of each other; rate: atrial 60-90 beats/minute, ventricular 30-40 beats/minute; P wave normal but occurs in greater frequency than QRS complex; PR interval: no relationship with QRS complex, therefore never constant; QRS complex normal if ventricular depolarization initiated by junctional escape pacemaker, widened if depolarization initiated by ventricular pacemaker low in conduction system	Represents failure of A-V node to conduct impulse to ventricles; block may occur at any point in conduction system at or below level of A-V node; occurs as result of coronary artery disease, degenerative fibrosis of conduction system, congenital anomalies, myocarditis, drug toxicity (digitalis, quinidine, procainamide, verapamil), trauma	Symptoms associated with low cardiac output owing to slow ventricular rates; include syncope and signs of ventricular failure	Transvenous demand pacing; while awaiting pacemaker insertion, isoproterenol infusion to accelerate ventricular rate

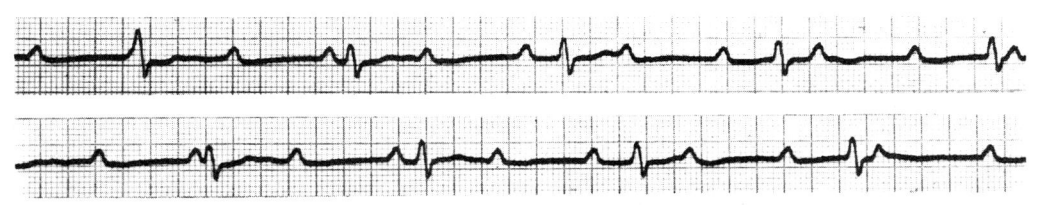

Fig. 1-33

From Andreoli, K., et al.: Comprehensive cardiac care: a text for nurses, physicians, and other health practitioners, ed. 5, St. Louis, 1983, The C.V. Mosby Co.

NURSING DIAGNOSES and NURSING INTERVENTIONS

Nursing Diagnosis	Nursing Intervention
Anxiety (related to altered heart action)	Provide continuous explanation for the various monitoring devices in use. Promote physical rest to reduce cardiac workload by maintaining bed rest, scheduled naptimes, and assistance with activities of daily living. Administer oxygen therapy as ordered to increase cardiac oxygenation. Administer sedatives as ordered to further reduce anxiety and promote rest.
Cardiac output, alteration in: decreased	Monitor patient continuously to determine cardiac rhythm. Monitor vital signs frequently, according to policy and patient's condition. Initiate prompt treatment of life-threatening arrhythmias per protocol: cardiopulmonary resuscitation (CPR), appropriate drug therapy, and preparation for pacemaker insertion. Continue to monitor and record changes in ECG tracings. Notify physician promptly if any decrease occurs in cardiac output as evidenced by disturbance in rate, respirations, blood pressure, or mental activity. Maintain patent IV as ordered.
Knowledge deficit	Provide explanation of disease etiology; medications, including purpose of drug, dosage, method of administration, and any untoward effects; and other therapies in use.

Patient Education

Instruction for a patient with a cardiac arrhythmia begins with the initial phase of care, whether in a coronary care unit or in an outpatient setting. The following points should be included:

1. Brief description of the rhythm disturbances and associated symptoms
2. Explanation of any diagnostic procedures that are planned
3. Explanation of monitoring equipment that may be used
4. Dietary restrictions that may be prescribed
5. Instructions regarding drug therapy, its purpose, desired effects, dosage, and side effects to report to the physician

EVALUATION

Patient Outcome	Data Indicating That Outcome is Reached
Heart returns to baseline rhythm.	ECG tracing reflects baseline rhythm. Blood pressure and heart rate are within normal limits. There is no ectopy.
Cardiac output is adequate to maintain cerebral perfusion.	Patient is alert and has no dizziness, syncopal episodes, or chest pains. Vital signs are stable. Peripheral perfusion is good.

CORONARY ARTERY DISEASE

Coronary artery disease is a disorder of the coronary arteries that ultimately leads to an interference in blood supply to the myocardium. Permanent disruption of blood flow causes myocardial dysfunction, including sudden death.

The incidence, mortality, and morbidity of coronary artery disease vary considerably among world populations. Serious study of the natural history of coronary artery disease began in 1950 with the Framingham study and other projects.[36] The data collected in these early studies have established certain factors related to the in-

cidence and progression of coronary atherosclerotic heart disease. These include age, sex, hypertension, lipid levels, obesity, smoking, sedentary life-style, and psychosocial factors.

Age and sex. Coronary artery disease is more prevalent in older men. Deaths from coronary artery disease are reported to be five times as frequent for men as for women in the 35- to 40-year-old group and two to three times as frequent in those 60 years and older. In recent years, however, these ratios appear to have changed, probably because of increased social and economic pressures on women and changes in their life-styles, including an increased incidence of smoking. The occurrence of coronary artery disease in persons less than 30 years of age is usually associated with hyperlipidemia, hypertension, and smoking.[2]

Hypertension. Although systolic hypertension is better correlated with cardiovascular disease, elevations in both systolic and diastolic pressure correlate with the development of ischemic heart disease. Systolic pressures greater than 160 mm Hg or diastolic pressures greater than 95 mm Hg are considered a significant risk factor for heart attacks, particularly when present in younger persons.[57]

Lipid levels. Of the various types of circulating lipoproteins, cholesterol and triglycerides are most commonly associated with coronary artery disease. Hyperlipidemia may be a primary disorder or may occur as a result of diabetes, myxedema, or alcoholism. Lipoproteins can now be fractioned and measured separately to determine levels of those that are atherogenic. Low-density lipids (LDLs) carry a high percentage of cholesterol in plasma and in high levels promote the production of atheromas. Conversely, high-density lipids (HDLs) are mostly protein and carry a smaller percentage of cholesterol, thereby assisting in the removal of lipids from the cell, primarily through liver metabolism. Recent studies show that the ratio of HDLs to LDLs is lower in patients with coronary artery disease and that a high ratio of HDLs helps reduce vascular disease. The formation of HDLs is stimulated through exercise, fat-controlled diets, and estrogens.[11]

Obesity. Studies have demonstrated that an increased food intake is associated with elevations in LDLs. Obese people also have a tendency toward hypertension and glucose intolerance.

Smoking. Cigarette smoking is now clearly associated with heart disease. Primarily through adrenergic stimulation, nicotine contributes to hemodynamic changes including increases in heart rate, stroke volume, cardiac output, and blood pressure. Nicotine also causes peripheral vasoconstriction and, in persons with decreased blood flow, enhances ischemic changes. Furthermore, smoking decreases the threshold for ventricular fibrillation through its interference with oxygen binding with hemoglobin, thus impairing oxygen diffusion into mitochondria.

Sedentary life-style. Although precise documentation of the positive effects of exercise on the risk of coronary artery disease is difficult, studies do support a decreased risk of coronary artery disease among well-conditioned persons such as joggers and marathon runners. Inactivity is associated with decreases in HDLs.

Psychosocial factors. The coronary-prone or type A personality has been demonstrated to be more characteristic of persons in whom coronary artery disease will develop. The characteristics of this personality include aggressiveness, competitiveness, and an urgent sense of time. When the type A personality is combined with other risk factors such as age, high lipid levels, and smoking, the risk of heart disease increases.

Other risk factors. Apart from the preceding factors that have been studied and strongly implicated in coronary artery disease, other factors have also been identified, including diabetes, genetic factors, and oral contraceptives.

Although the association is not clear, patients with diabetes have a high risk of coronary artery disease. The role of heredity beyond the predisposition to coronary artery disease is also unclear. Apparently a tendency toward hypertension, hyperlipidemia, and diabetes exists in some families. However, whether the tendency is inherited or simply the result of life-style patterns that are passed down from generation to generation is unknown. If the latter is true, these major risk factors may be altered favorably. Oral contraceptives have been demonstrated to be associated with coronary artery disease when taken by women 45 years or younger. This finding results from studies that show high serum cholesterol and triglyceride levels in women taking oral contraceptives.[2]

PATHOPHYSIOLOGY

Atherosclerosis, the basic underlying disease affecting coronary lumen size, is characterized by changes in the intimal lining of the arteries. It begins as an irregular thickening process producing fatty streaks. This advances to a more severe form involving the combination of large amounts of lipids with collagen to produce fibroblasts that ultimately lead to fibrous atherosclerotic plaques.

The severity of the disease is measured by the degree of obstruction within each artery, as well as the number of vessels involved. Obstructions exceeding 75% of the lumen of one or more of the three coronary arteries increase the risk of death. The annual mortality of persons with one-vessel disease is 1% to 3%. Three-vessel disease increases the risk to 10% to 15%. Among individuals with 75% obstruction of the left main artery, however, the annual mortality is 30% to 40%.

Myocardial Perfusion

The basic physiologic changes occurring as a result of the atherosclerotic process are problems of myocardial oxygen supply and demand. When myocardial oxygen demand exceeds the supply delivered by the coronary arteries, ischemia results. Myocardial metabolism is oxygen dependent (aerobic), extracting up to 80% of the oxygen from the coronary blood supply. Coronary blood flow to the myocardium occurs primarily during diastole.

The factors influencing supply include cardiac output, intramyocardial tension, aortic pressure, and coronary artery resistance. Coronary blood flow can be increased by increasing the cardiac output and aortic pressure and decreasing coronary artery resistance and intramyocardial tension.

The factors determining myocardial oxygen demand are heart rate, myocardial wall tension, and contractile state of the myocardium. As the heart rate increases, so does the demand for oxygen to the myocardial cells. Myocardial wall tension occurs during contraction and is influenced by ventricular and systolic (arterial) pressure. Myocardial contractility is stimulated through the release of catecholamines or sympathetic stimulation. Combined, these increase wall tension and thereby increase energy or oxygen demands.

Myocardial ischemia is the result of impaired myocardial perfusion. In the setting of coronary artery disease, it is the consequence of coronary atherosclerotic heart disease. The narrowing or obstruction varies in degree and may be well tolerated as long as the myocardial oxygen demand is minimal. As the demand increases and the obstruction persists or advances, ischemic changes result. Coronary blood vessel distribution is also important in providing oxygen to the myocardium. The coronary arteries sit on the epicardial surface of the heart. Blood travels inward toward the endocardium. The inner subendocardial layers of the myocardium therefore are particularly susceptible to ischemia. Increases in heart rate and wall tension can reduce flow to the endocardium.

In addition to ventricular perfusion, the coronary arteries supply major conduction structures within the myocardium. The right coronary artery (RCA) supplies the sinus node in 55% to 60% of persons, whereas in the remainder it is supplied by a branch of the circumflex artery. The RCA also supplies the A-V node in 85% of persons, whereas in the remaining 15% the left coronary artery does. The septum is supplied primarily by the left anterior descending (LAD) artery, although a portion of the posterior wall is supplied by the RCA. An obstruction or impedance to flow of any of the major arteries or their branches results in ischemia to the portion of myocardium nourished by that vessel. Obstruction of the LAD results in ischemic changes of the anterior wall of the ventricle. RCA obstruction results in infarction and ischemia of the right ventricle. The degree of obstruction and number of coronaries involved dictate the severity of the disease. Coronary artery disease is commonly described as single-, double-, or triple-vessel disease, the last referring to three major arteries. When a major obstruction occurs in the initial branch of the left coronary artery or the left main artery before bifurcation, the risk for a major infarction and death rises. This is referred to as left main disease.

The major clinical manifestations of ischemia are chest pain and ECG changes. The associated symptoms occur as a result of secondary effects brought on by compromised cardiac function.

Angina Pectoris

The term "angina pectoris," which means chest pain, is used to describe pain as a symptom of myocardial ischemia. Myocardial ischemia is the result of an imbalance between myocardial oxygen supply and demand. It occurs most commonly in the setting of coronary atherosclerosis but can also occur in patients with normal coronary arteries. For example, patients with aortic stenosis, hypertension, and hypertrophic cardiomyopathy may have clinical symptoms of angina pectoris. In these patients, myocardial work is increased but perfusion of the hypertrophied muscle is inadequate, resulting in myocardial ischemia despite normal coronary arteries.

Various terms have been used to describe the clinical syndromes associated with myocardial ischemia. The following are commonly used to describe chest pain that is transient and associated with myocardial ischemia.

Stable angina pectoris is characterized by effort-induced chest discomfort, with or without radiation, that lasts from a few seconds to 15 minutes. It is generally relieved by rest, removal of provoking factors, or sublingual vasodilators.

Unstable angina pectoris is characterized by pain that lasts longer, occurs more frequently, and may be precipitated by factors other than effort or activities. Various names are used to describe this syndrome, such as crescendo angina, preinfarction angina, angina decubitus, and nocturnal angina.

Variant (Prinzmetal's) angina is characterized by chest pain that occurs at rest and is often associated with ST elevations on the ECG. The underlying cause is thought to be coronary artery spasm. Unlike angina pectoris, variant angina is due to a sudden reduction in coronary blood flow brought on by the spasm and not by an increase in myocardial oxygen demand. It has been suggested that the decrease in myocardial consumption occurring during sleep or rest may lead to coronary artery vasoconstriction and is responsible for the spasm.[86]

The etiology of spasm is not clearly understood, but researchers have postulated a correlation with stimulation of α (vasoconstriction) and β (vasodilation) adrenergic receptors.[86] Other studies have suggested various mechanisms involved in the genesis of spasm, including parasympathetic nervous system activity[86] and possibly local abnormalities of vascular smooth muscle.[9]

Myocardial Infarction

Myocardial infarction is the development of ischemia and necrosis of myocardial tissue. It results from a sudden decrease in coronary perfusion or an increase in myocardial oxygen demand without adequate coronary perfusion.

Two types of infarction have been described. Subendocardial infarction is generally confined to small areas of myocardium, particularly within the subendocardial wall of the left ventricle, the ventricular septum, and papillary muscles. Transmural or full-thickness infarction is widespread myocardial necrosis extending from the endocardium through to the epicardium.

Myocardial tissue death is usually preceded by a sudden occlusion of one of the major coronary arteries. Coronary thrombosis is the most common cause of infarction, but multiple interrelated factors may be responsible. These include coronary artery spasm, platelet aggregation and embolism from a mural thrombus, a thrombus on a prosthetic mitral or aortic valve, or a dislodged calcium plaque from a calcified aortic or mitral valve.

Persistent cellular ischemia interferes with myocardial tissue metabolism, causing a rapid development of irreversible cellular damage. In the initial phases of the infarction there are three zones of tissue damage. The first is a central area consisting of necrotic myocardial cells, capillaries, and connective tissue. Surrounding this necrotic tissue is a second zone of "injured" myocardial cells that are potentially viable if adequate circulation is quickly restored. The third zone, called ischemia, is also viable and can be expected to recover unless the ischemia persists or worsens. The severity or extension of a myocardial infarction often depends on the fate of the injured and ischemic zones. Without appropriate interventions, ischemia may progress to necrosis. Since the infarction process may take up to 6 hours to complete, restoration of adequate myocardial perfusion is important if significant necrosis is to be limited.

DIAGNOSTIC STUDIES

Study	Stable Angina Pectoris	Variant (Prinzmetal's) Angina	Unstable Angina Pectoris	Myocardial Infarction
Electrocardiogram (ECG)	Changes usually seen during anginal episodes; 50%-70% of patients have normal ECG during pain-free episodes; ischemia determined by horizontal ST segment or downsloping with depression of 1 mm; T wave inversion represents impaired repolarization caused by ischemia	Ischemia appears as ST elevation during anginal attack but regresses as pain subsides; ECG changes may be seen before patient complains of chest pain or may be recorded in absence of pain; A-V conduction defects may occur, particularly when right coronary artery is involved, and include Mobitz type II and complete A-V block; ventricular irritability such as premature ventricular contractions, ventricular tachycardia, or fibrillation can occur, particularly during ischemic attack	Ischemia determined by horizontal ST segment or downsloping with depression of 1 mm; T wave inversion represents impaired repolarization caused by ischemia; ventricular irritability such as premature ventricular contractions, ventricular tachycardia, or fibrillation	Changes are evolutionary and indicate progression of infarction; in acute stage, ST elevations with subsequent T wave inversion and Q wave formation; Q waves indicate necrosis and are considered pathologic if they are 0.04 second or greater in duration, 0.4 mm or greater in depth, or present in leads that do not normally have Q waves; ST elevations reflect myocardial injury that interferes with polarization of cells, are seen in leads facing injured area, and return to normal (isoelectric) within days; ST elevations beyond 4-6 weeks should raise suspicion of ventricular aneurysm; infarction location determined by identifying leads that demonstrate characteristic ECG changes; such leads are those with positive terminals that face injured site of heart; reciprocal changes, seen in leads that face *opposite* surface of damaged heart, are absence of Q wave, increase in R wave amplitude, depressed ST segment, upright tall T wave

Laboratory tests				
Enzymes	No elevation; checked to rule out myocardial infarction	No elevation; checked to rule out myocardial infarction	No elevation; checked to rule out myocardial infarction	

	Onset	*Peak*	*Return to normal*
SGOT	6-12 hours	36 hours	5-7 days
CPK-MB	4-12 hours	24 hours	3-4 days
LDH (isoenzyme)	24-48 hours	3-6 days	8-14 days

Study	Stable Angina Pectoris	Variant (Prinzmetal's) Angina	Unstable Angina Pectoris	Myocardial Infarction
Complete blood count (CBC)	No elevation; checked to rule out anemia-induced angina	No elevation; checked to rule out anemia-induced angina	No elevation; checked to rule out anemia-induced angina	Elevated white count (WBC) and erythrocyte sedimentation rate (ESR) reflect myocardial damage

Glucose	No elevation	No elevation	No elevation	Transiently elevated owing to adrenergic response
Lipid levels (triglycerides, cholesterol, high- and low-density lipids)	Checked to determine any lipoprotein abnormalities	Checked to rule out presence of atherosclerotic process	Checked to determine any lipoprotein abnormalities	Checked to determine any lipoprotein abnormalities
Exercise stress test (EST)	Chest pain; horizontal ST segment or downsloping of 1 mm or more; failure of systolic blood pressure to rise or drop; ST elevations	Normal stress test done to differentiate between variant and classic angina; ST elevation with or without associated chest pain occasionally develops	As in stable angina pectoris; should not be done until patient has been stable and pain free for 24 hours	Not done in presence of documented myocardial infarction; low-level test may be performed before discharge from hospital
Thallium 201 scintigraphy	Ischemic areas appear as "cold" areas, reflecting reduced thallium uptake; when ischemia relieved, "cold" areas show normal thallium uptake		Similar to stable angina pectoris	Similar to stable angina pectoris
Radionuclide blood pool imaging with technetium 99m				Confirms myocardial damage by localizing and permitting estimation of size of transmural infarction; must be done within 2-6 days after acute infarction; determines wall motion abnormalities; permits estimation of ventricular function by determining ejection fractions
Cardiac catheterization and coronary angiography	Determines number and location of obstructive lesions, "graftability" of artery distal to obstructive lesion, and ventricular function	Distinguishes spasm in normal coronary arteries from those with severe obstructive lesions; intravenous injection of ergonovine maleate provokes coronary artery spasm in patients with variant angina	As in stable angina pectoris	Generally not performed as diagnostic procedure during acute period

TREATMENT PLAN

Surgical

Coronary artery bypass grafting (CABG)—only direct method of increasing myocardial coronary blood flow; provides symptomatic relief in 80% of patients with significant angina and has low operative mortality

Indications: Disabling angina that is refractory to medical therapy, significantly abnormal ECG response to exercise, 50% or greater obstruction of left main coronary artery, and significant obstructive lesions in all three coronary arteries (see p. 94 for care of patients undergoing open heart surgery)

Percutaneous transluminal coronary angioplasty—alternative approach to coronary artery bypass surgery in selected patients; attempts to restore luminal patency by compressing atheromatous plaques

Indications: Single-vessel disease in which there are high degree of stenosis, good left ventricular function, and recent onset of angina refractory to medical therapy

Chemotherapeutic

Vasodilators

Nitrates

Short-acting nitrates: Sublingual nitroglycerin (0.4-0.6 mg); isosorbide dinitrate (5 mg)

Duration of action: ½-2 h

Long-acting oral nitrates: Isosorbide dinitrate (10-20 mg qid)

Topical 2% nitroglycerin ointment (1-2 inches q4-6h)

Duration of action: Up to 6 h or longer

β-Adrenergic blocking agents

Propranolol (Inderal)

Usual dosage: 10-20 mg po tid or qid; IV 1 mg/min not exceeding 3-5 mg

Nadolol (Corgard)

Indications: Treatment of angina and hypertension

Usual dosage: 40-80 mg po up to 240 mg/day as necessary

Duration of action: About 20-24 h

Timolol

Indications: Reduction of mortality and reinfarction after myocardial infarctions; hypertension

Usual dosage: 20-60 mg bid

Atenolol

Indications: Approved for use of hypertension but may have potential use in treating angina and reducing infarct size

Usual dosage: 50-100 mg/day

Calcium antagonists

Nifedipine (Procardia)

Indications: Angina pectoris caused by coronary artery spasm

Usual dosage: 10 mg po; sublingual 10-40 mg q8h (not to exceed 180 mg); IV 5-15 mg/kg

Verapamil (Calan, Isoptin)

Usual dosage: 80-160 mg q8h (not to exceed 480 mg/day); IV 0.075-0.15 mg/kg (not to exceed 15 mg/30 min)

Diltiazem (Cardizem)

Indications: Treatment of variant angina

Usual dosage: Initially 30 mg po qid, increasing gradually to 80 mg tid (total 240 mg/day)

Antihyperlipidemic agents—interfere with reabsorption of cholesterol and lower triglyceride levels

Cholestyramine (Questran)

Usual dosage: 8-12 g bid

Neomycin sulfate

Usual dosage: 0.5-2 g/day

Clofibrate (Atromid-S)

Usual dosage: 0.5 g tid

Gemfibrozil (Lopid)

Usual dosage: 0.6 g bid

Niacin (nicotinic acid)

Usual dosage: 0.5-1 g tid

Intracoronary streptokinase infusion—still controversial and under investigation; used in early myocardial infarction (within 4-6 h of onset) to restore myocardial oxygen supply, thereby preserving myocardium and, ideally, limiting infarct size

Electromechanical

Monitoring—used to detect life-threatening complications of myocardial infarction, especially arrhythmias and pump failure; complications occur within first 5 days in half of patients with acute myocardial infarction; early detection depends on careful and often continuous monitoring of electrocardiogram, arterial and venous pressures, and clinical picture reflecting hemodynamic status of left ventricle (see p. 25 for description of arrhythmias)

Intra-aortic balloon counterpulsation (IABP)—used mainly in patients with acute myocardial infarction to protect ischemic myocardium by decreasing preload, afterload, and myocardial oxygen demand; diastolic pressure is supported, thus improving coronary perfusion and cardiac output; most successful in patients who are treated less than 6 hours after infarction, are undergoing their first myocardial infarction, and have no aortic insufficiency (see p. 102 for specific care)

Supportive

Oxygenation—patients evaluated early for hypoxemia, which may result from ventilation-perfusion abnormalities; providing additional inspired oxygen to patient in absence of hypoxemia does not ensure increased oxygen delivery to myocardium and may rarely increase systemic vascular resistance and arterial pressure, with subsequent decrease in cardiac output and oxygen delivery to tissues; arterial oxygen tension (PaO$_2$) should be measured on admission

to coronary care unit; if normal, oxygen therapy may be omitted; hypoxemic patients should receive oxygen therapy as required; serial arterial blood gas determinations to monitor effectiveness of therapy

ASSESSMENT: AREAS OF CONCERN

Area of Concern	Stable Angina Pectoris	Variant (Prinzmetal's) Angina	Unstable Angina Pectoris	Myocardial Infarction
Chest pain Quality	Aching, sharp, tingling, or burning sensation or pressure	Similar to stable angina pectoris	Similar to stable angina pectoris but may be more severe	Crushing, squeezing, stabbing, oppressive sensation or as if a heavy object is sitting on chest
Location and radiation	Substernal with radiation to left shoulder, down inner aspect of left arm or both arms; neck, jaw, and scapula may be additional sites of radiation	Similar to stable angina pectoris	Similar to stable angina pectoris	Retrosternal and left precordial radiating down left arm and to neck, jaws, teeth, epigastric area, and back
Precipitating factors	Onset classically associated with exercise or activities that increase myocardial oxygen demand, e.g., physical exercise, heavy lifting, emotional stress, cold temperatures	Onset at rest; pain is cyclic, often occurring during sleep	Pain may be brought on with less than usual exertion; may occur at rest	May occur at rest or during exertion
Duration and alleviating factors	3-15 minutes; relieved by rest, stopping pain-inducing activities; taking sublingual nitroglycerin (NTG) tablet	Characteristically, pain intensifies quickly, tends to last longer than angina, and subsides with exercise	Prolonged and not usually as quickly relieved by rest or taking NTG	Described as continuous, lasting more than 30 minutes, unrelieved by rest, position change, or taking NTG tablets
Associated signs and symptoms	During anginal attack, dyspnea, anxiety, diaphoresis, cool clammy skin	Similar to stable angina pectoris	Similar to stable angina pectoris but symptoms may be more prominent and may persist; may be associated with nausea	Anxiety, restlessness, weakness, associated profuse diaphoresis, dyspnea, dizziness; signs of vasomotor response including nausea, vomiting, faintness, and cold clammy skin; hiccough and other gastrointestinal distress may be present; low-grade temperature elevations common for first 24-48 hours but may last several days (this is inflammatory response to myocardial tissue damage)
Physical examination	Normal during asymptomatic periods; during anginal attacks, increased heart rate, pulsus alternans, and transient abnormal findings including precordial bulge and atrial and ventricular gallops (S$_3$, S$_4$)	Similar to stable angina pectoris	Similar to stable angina pectoris; may also demonstrate irregular pulse, hypotension, or signs of left ventricular dysfunction	May be unremarkable unless signs of ventricular failure or cardiogenic shock are present; blood pressure normal, elevated, or decreased—initially elevated when pain is present but usually decreases for first few days; respirations:

Area of Concern	Stable Angina Pectoris	Variant (Prinzmetal's) Angina	Unstable Angina Pectoris	Myocardial Infarction
				Cheyne-Stokes respiration owing to central nervous system hypoperfusion or opiate therapy; initial tachypnea returns to normal once pain subsides; heart sounds: S_3, S_4 gallops indicative of ventricular dysfunction; systolic murmurs reflecting papillary muscle dysfunction; diminished heart sounds and pericardial friction rub may occur; with left ventricular dysfunction: pulmonary rales, decreased urine output, increased amplitude of ''a'' wave in jugular vein; with right ventricular dysfunction: increased jugular venous distention, peripheral edema, liver tenderness; pulse often within normal limits; bradycardia present with inferior wall myocardial infarction; tachycardia with rates greater than 100 beats/minute may reflect compromised ventricle

NURSING DIAGNOSES and NURSING INTERVENTIONS

Nursing Diagnosis	Nursing Intervention
Comfort, alteration in: pain	*Acute care:* Stop angina-inducing activity. Encourage bed rest. Administer drug therapy as ordered to relieve pain. Administer oxygen therapy as ordered. Obtain 12-lead ECG to document ischemia during chest pain episode. Monitor vital signs frequently throughout episode of chest pain. *Convalescent care:* Administer long-acting nitrates as ordered. Encourage limitation of activities as needed to prevent pain.
Cardiac output, alteration in: decreased	*Acute care:* Evaluate vital signs every 5 to 15 minutes. Maintain bed rest. Monitor ECG for dysrhythmias and alterations. Maintain IV as ordered with 5% glucose in water for drug administration. Auscultate breath sounds and heart tones every 1 to 4 hours. Administer drug therapy as ordered. Prepare for insertion of Swan-Ganz catheter and/or central venous pressure line as needed. *Convalescent care:* Monitor for early complications: hypotension, arrhythmias, heart failure, and heart rupture. Begin armchair therapy as patient's condition stabilizes.
Gas exchange: impaired	*Acute care:* Administer oxygen therapy as ordered. Monitor arterial blood gases and report. Enforce safety precautions such as low oxygen concentrations for chronic respiratory patients.

Nursing Diagnosis	Nursing Intervention
	Prepare for possible intubation and assisted ventilation rehabilitation as ordered.
	Convalescent care:
	Begin respiratory exercises, especially for patients with chronic respiratory disease.
Nutrition: alteration in	Promote proper nutrition with liquid or soft diet as ordered.
	Avoid offering carbonated, very hot, or cold beverages and those with caffeine.
	Restrict sodium intake as ordered.
	Monitor intake and output closely to detect or prevent circulatory overload.
	Provide IV fluids as ordered if patient is unable to eat because of nausea or vomiting.
Anxiety	Continue to support patient and family.
	Offer reassurance during episodes of pain.
	Employ relaxation techniques as necessary.
	Administer drug therapy as ordered.
	Stay with patient as much as possible.
	Allow family members to assist patient if possible.
	Explain all procedures and routine care as they occur.
Bowel elimination: alteration in	Administer stool softeners as ordered.
	Caution patient not to strain with bowel movements.
	Avoid enemas and rectal insertions to prevent causing vagal stimulations.
	Monitor output to ensure normal bowel movements.
Urinary elimination: alteration in patterns	Monitor output to ensure adequate urine production.
	Administer diuretics as ordered to maintain urine output.
Activity intolerance	*Acute care:*
	Encourage bed rest.
	Allow patient to sit at bedside as ordered, for short intervals.
	Assist with activities of daily living as needed.
	Perform passive range of motion exercises to prevent thromboembolism, and encourage the patient to perform active range of motion exercises as soon as possible.
	Convalescent care:
	Begin phase I rehabilitation (see box below).
	Teach necessity to increase activity gradually at home while continuing periods of rest.
Knowledge deficit	Offer simple explanations of disease and treatment in the coronary care unit.
	Later, teach the patient and family about disease etiology, risk factors, exercise program, proper diet, drug therapy, and complications.

PHASES OF CARDIAC REHABILITATION

Phase I: Inpatient activities; anywhere from 4 to 16 stages; patient should be at 3 to 5 metabolic equivalents of tasks (METs) at discharge

Phase II: Begins with discharge and continues until healing has been completed; patient is evaluated with a stress test that is symptom limited

Phase III: Begins 4 to 6 weeks after myocardial infarction or surgery; training phase; patient exercises two to five times a week under supervision for usually 12 weeks; patient should be able to perform at 10 METs or greater at the end of this phase

Phase IV: Begins at the end of the training phase and continues for another 3 to 6 months (some believe it continues for the patient's lifetime); patient maintains his level of training by exercising two or three times a week; stress tests usually done at yearly intervals to measure effectiveness and amend the exercise prescription

Modified from Guzzetta, C.E., and Dossey, B.M.: Cardiovascular nursing: bodymind tapestry, St. Louis, 1984, The C.V. Mosby Co.

Patient Education

1. Explain the disease process, associated symptoms, and actions to take when the symptoms occur.
2. Explain the name, purpose, side effects, and method of administration of all drugs.
3. Explain activity allowances and limitations, including the patient's return to work and resumption of sexual activity.
4. Refer the patient to a rehabilitation program to assist with progressive increase in activity levels.
5. Teach the patient to avoid foods high in sodium, saturated fats, and triglycerides. Teach good nutritional habits and alternative ways of seasoning food to avoid cooking with salt and salt products.

EVALUATION

Patient Outcome	Data Indicating That Outcome is Reached
Cardiac output is improved.	ECG, vital signs, and electrolytes are within normal limits.
Gas exchange is improved.	P_{O_2} and P_{CO_2} are within normal limits. Patient has no complaints about shortness of breath.
Patient is free from chest pain.	Patient verbalizes absence of pain. Blood pressure and heart rate are within normal limits. Patient engages in hospital routines and activities without pain. Patient appears relaxed and verbalizes a sense of calm.

CONGESTIVE HEART FAILURE

Congestive heart failure is a complex clinical syndrome that results from the heart's inability to increase cardiac output sufficiently to meet the body's metabolic demands.

PATHOPHYSIOLOGY

The underlying causes of congestive heart failure vary, but the disorder ultimately results in the heart's inability to act as an effective pump.

Decreased myocardial contractility may result from a primary disorder or an excessive workload placed on the heart such as systemic hypertension or a valvular disorder. Causes of primary myocardial disorders and disorders that increase the heart's workload are summarized below.

Causes of decreased myocardial contractility
  Coronary artery disease
  Myocarditis
  Cardiomyopathies
    Congestive
    Restrictive
    Hypertrophic
  Infiltrative diseases
    Amyloidosis
    Tumors
    Sarcoidosis
  Collagen-vascular diseases
    Systemic lupus erythematosus
    Scleroderma
  Iatrogenic factors
    Drugs such as β-blockers; calcium antagonists
Causes of increased myocardial workload
  Hypertension
  Pulmonary hypertension
  Valvular heart disease
    Aortic or pulmonic stenosis
    Mitral, tricuspid, or aortic insufficiency
  Hypertrophic cardiomyopathy
  Intracardiac shunting
  High-output states
    Anemia
    Hyperthyroidism
    Beri-beri
    Arteriovenous fistula

Disorders that interfere with the normal stretch of the ventricle, thereby decreasing ventricular filling, cause a drop in cardiac output. Pericardial tamponade and constrictive pericarditis are examples.

Persistent tachyarrhythmias reduce ventricular filling time, and marked bradyarrhythmias significantly reduce cardiac output because the ventricles cannot augment the stroke volume.

Loss of coordinated atrial contraction, as occurs in atrial fibrillation, can decrease cardiac output, presumably because of loss of the atrial "booster pump" that contributes to normal ventricular filling.

The primary dysfunction in congestive heart failure is decreased myocardial contractility. However, secondary changes in preload and afterload contribute to the pathophysiologic state of heart failure.

Clinical manifestation of heart failure can be divided into left- and right-sided failure; they can occur independently or in combination.

Left-Sided Heart Failure

Any sustained elevation in left ventricular end-diastolic pressure (LVEDP) increases left atrial pressure, which is transmitted to the pulmonary vascular bed. Clinically, this is reflected by an increase in pulmonary capillary wedge pressure (PCWP). Should this pressure exceed the colloid osmotic pressure of the pulmonary capillaries, transudation of fluid into the interstitial spaces and eventually into alveolar spaces will occur. This leads to hypoxia resulting from poor oxygen exchange and clinically to dyspnea, cough orthopnea, and paroxysmal nocturnal dyspnea.

Right-Sided Heart Failure

Persistent elevation of LVEDP eventually leads to right-sided failure characterized by venous congestion in the systemic circulation. Right-sided heart failure may also occur as a primary disorder of the right ventricle as seen in tricuspid regurgitation, in right ventricular infarction, or as a result of pulmonary disease such as cor pulmonale. Clinically, distended neck veins, hepatomegaly, and dependent edema occur.

DIAGNOSTIC STUDIES

Laboratory tests
  Electrolytes
    Hyponatremia owing to water retention; urinary sodium loss in response to diuretics; hypokalemia as consequence of excessive use of diuretics or as secondary manifestation of aldosteronism; hypochloremia as result of diuretic therapy; metabolic acidosis or alkalosis
  Blood chemistry
    BUN, creatinine rise with decreased glomerular filtration; liver function values (SGOT, bilirubin, alkaline phosphatase) mildly increased; prothrombin time prolonged; glucose level elevated

  Arterial blood gases
    Hypoxemia; decreased oxygen saturation; (early) mild respiratory alkalosis; (late) hypercarbia, hypoxia
  Urine studies
    Urine output decreased; metabolic acidosis or alkalosis; specific gravity >1.010: excessive fluid intake, <1.035: decreased fluid intake; proteinuria; glucosuria
  Pulmonary function tests
    Reduced vital capacity; reduced total lung capacity; increased residual volume

Chest roentgenogram (Figs. 1-34 and 1-35)
  Increased pulmonary congestion: redistribution of pulmonary blood flow, interstitial edema (intraseptal edema—Kerley-B lines; perivascular edema), alveolar edema, pleural effusion; (early) little or no change in size or contour of cardiac silhouette; (late) increased cardiothoracic ratio

Electrocardiogram (ECG)
  Changes reflect primary disorders as well as chronic secondary effects of heart failure: left ventricular hypertrophy (LVH), right ventricular hypertrophy (RVH), atrial hypertrophy, tachycardia, arrhythmias

Echocardiogram (Fig. 1-36)
  Increased or decreased ventricular chambers or structures reflect primary disorder; left ventricular failure: increased LVEDP (>5.6 cm), decreased wall motion

Hemodynamic monitoring (right heart catheterization)
  Left ventricular failure: elevated pulmonary capillary wedge pressure and pulmonary artery diastolic pressure, decreased cardiac output, decreased ejection fractions; right ventricular failure: elevated pulmonary artery pressure, right ventricular pressure, and right atrial pressure

TREATMENT PLAN

Surgical
  Directed by underlying condition; mortality is greater among patients with left ventricular dysfunction

Chemotherapeutic
  Diuretics—potent loop diuretics that decrease tubular reabsorption and decrease total body sodium and water
    Furosemide (Lasix)
      Usual dosage: 20-300 mg/day
    Ethacrynic acid (Edecrin)
      Usual dosage: 25-200 mg/day

Fig. 1-34
Pulmonary congestion. Upper lobe distention *(arrows)*. Enlarged cardiac silhouette.

Courtesy P. Batra, M.D., Department of Radiology, UCLA School of Medicine, Los Angeles, Calif.; from Canobbio, M.M.: Noninvasive studies and diagnostic adjuncts for heart failure. In Michaelson, C.R.: Congestive heart failure, St. Louis, 1983, The C.V. Mosby Co.

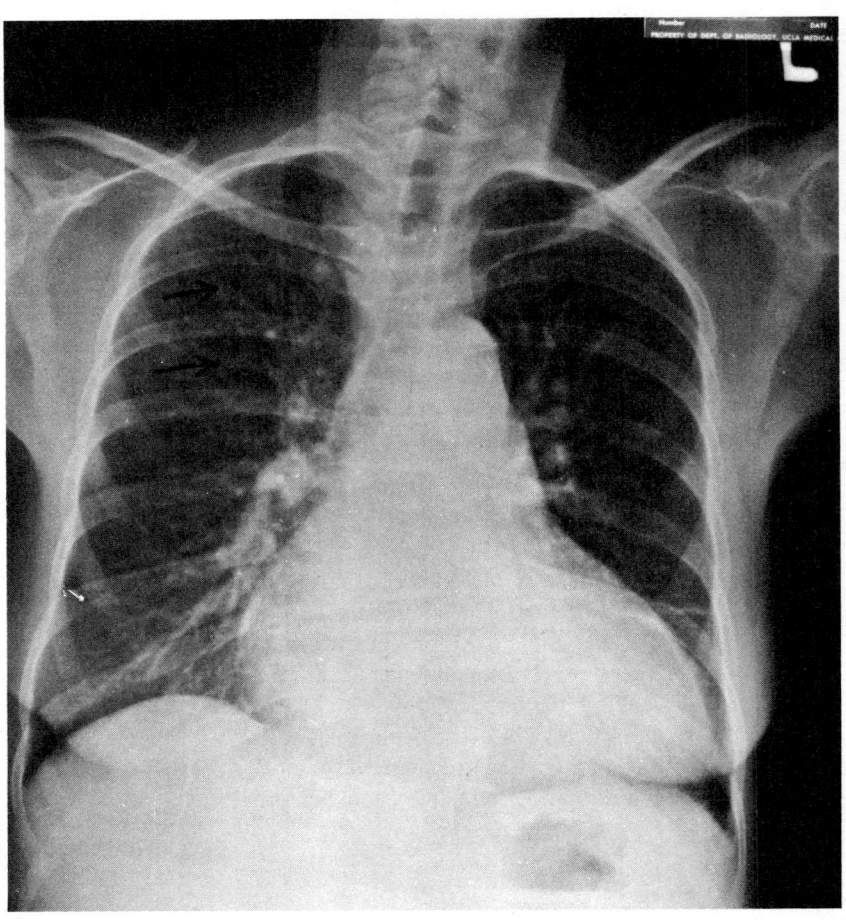

Thiazides
  Indications: Oral agents used in chronic management of congestive heart failure
Vasodilators—used therapeutically to dilate arterioles and veins, thereby achieving the following hemodynamic effects: (1) improving ejection fraction, which decreases LVEDP (preload) and pulmonary congestion; (2) reducing wall tension, which reduces myocardial oxygen demand; (3) decreasing pressure work of a failing ventricle
  Nitrates—act directly on smooth muscle, causing dilation of arterial and venous beds; used to decrease preload in acute left ventricular failure and to decrease pulmonary and venous pressure
Nitroprusside sodium (Nipride)
  Indications: Decreases preload and afterload
  Precautions: Excreted by kidney; requires careful monitoring of kidney function
  Half-life: 2-5 min; light sensitive
  Side effects: Hypotension, tachycardia, palpitations, dizziness, headache, nausea, and vomiting

  Usual dosage: 3 μg/kg/min IV; average dose 200 μg/min; should not exceed 800 μg/min
Isosorbide dinitrate (Isordil)
  Indications: Relaxes vascular smooth muscle
  Excretion: By liver
  Onset of action: Sublingual 2-3 min; po 20-40 min; chewable 3-4 min
  Side effects: Headache, flushing, dizziness
  Usual dosage: 10-30 mg sublingually; 20-80 mg po; 10-30 mg chewable
Antihypertensives (for vasodilator effect)
  Hydralazine (Apresoline)
    Indications: Arteriolar vasodilator, decreases afterload
    Excretion: Through liver and kidney
    Duration of action: 2-8 h (average 3 h)
    Side effects: Tachycardia, lupus syndrome, hypotension
    Usual dosage: IV 10-20 mg q4-6h; po 25-100 mg (not to exceed 400 mg/day)
α-Adrenergic blocking agents
  Prazosin (Minipress)

Fig. 1-35

Interstitial edema. Hilar areas are blurred and hazy. Cardiac silhouette is enlarged. Fluid collected within intralobular septa of lungs is visible as Kerley-B lines *(arrows)*.

Courtesy P. Batra, M.D., Department of Radiology, UCLA School of Medicine, Los Angeles, Calif.; from Canobbio, M.M.: Noninvasive studies and diagnostic adjuncts for heart failure. In Michaelson, C.R.: Congestive heart failure, St. Louis, 1983, The C.V. Mosby Co.

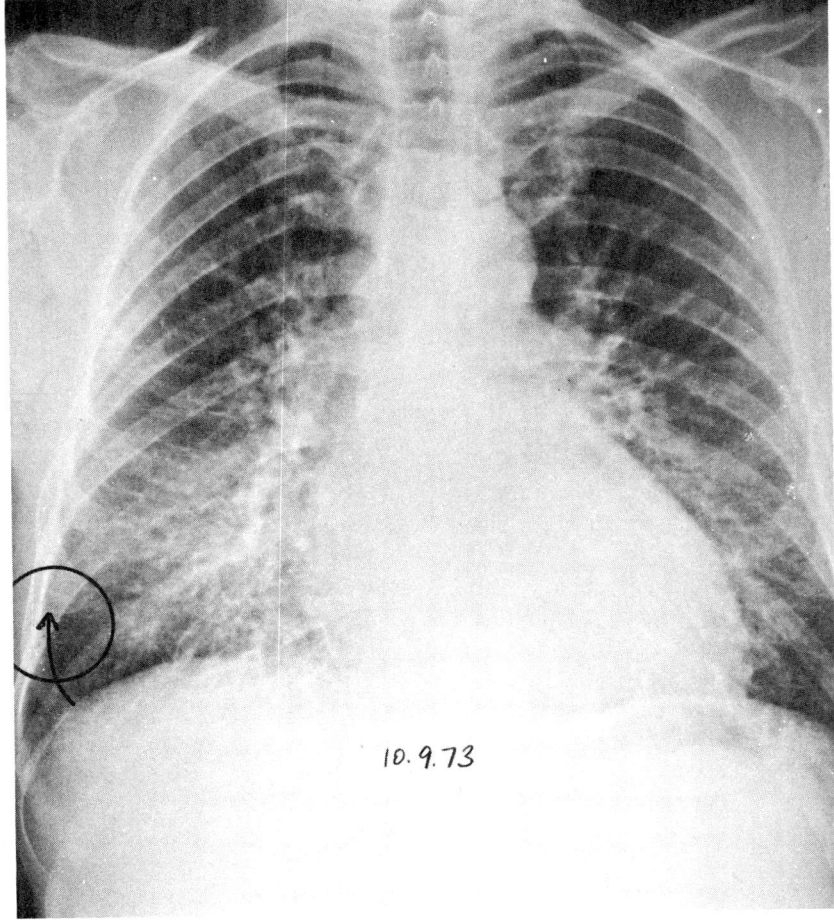

Fig. 1-36

Patient with dilated left ventricle (6.7 cm) and normal intraventricular septum (1 cm).

Courtesy Non Invasive Labs, Division of Cardiology, UCLA School of Medicine, Los Angeles, Calif.; from Canobbio, M.M.: Noninvasive studies and diagnostic adjuncts for heart failure. In Michaelson, C.R.: Congestive heart failure, St. Louis, 1983, The C.V. Mosby Co.

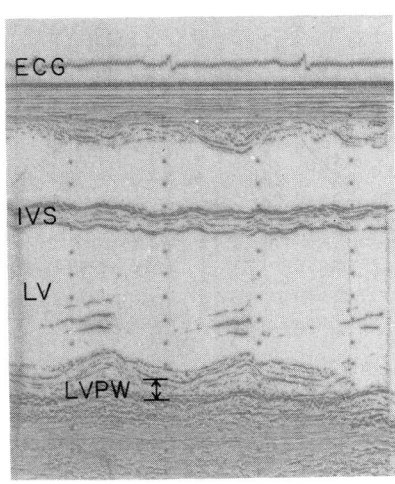

Indications: Relaxes vascular smooth muscle, decreases peripheral vascular resistance
Excretion: Through liver
Half-life: 3 h
Side effects: Syncope, dizziness, headache, drowsiness, nausea
Usual dosage: Initially 1-2 mg, increasing slowly to total of 20 mg bid or tid
Phentolamine (Regitine)
  Indications: Acts directly on vascular smooth muscle
  Excretion: Unknown
  Duration of action: IV 5-15 min; po 2-4 h
  Side effects: Hypotension
  Usual dosage: IV 0.2-2 mg/min; po 50-100 mg in four to six doses/day
Angiotensin-converting enzyme inhibitors
  Antihypertensive: Captopril (Capoten)
    Indications: Patients who have failed to respond to conventional drug therapy; inhibit formation

of angiotensin II, one of the most potent vasoconstrictors; decrease aldosterone secretion and renal-mediated vasoconstriction

Excretion: By kidney

Duration of action: 4-8 h

Side effects: Hypotension; metallic taste in mouth

Usual dosage: Initially 25 mg po tid, increasing to maximum dose of 150 mg

Morphine sulfate

Indications: Venous dilation rapidly decreases preload; sedative effect relieves anxiety; decreases hyperventilation by depressing respiratory center

Usual dosage: Slow IV push, 3-5 mg

Inotropic agents—increase contractile state of ventricle, thereby improving ejection fraction

Cardiac glycosides: Digitalis

Commonly used but use is limited because toxic effects occur when blood levels exceed 2 ng/ml

Excretion: By kidney; therefore daily dose should be reduced if renal function is impaired

Half-life: 30 h

Usual dosage: 0.25 mg/day

Precautions: May have toxic effects when blood levels exceed 2 ng/ml; toxicity more likely to occur in patients who are small or elderly or have chronic obstructive pulmonary disease; hypokalemia and digitalis in combination with quinidine can also cause toxicity; common symptoms are arrhythmias, nausea, anorexia

Adrenergic drugs: Dopamine (Intropin)

Indications: Directly stimulates myocardial contractility through β-receptors; produces positive inotropic effects through release of norepinephrine; like other inotropic agents, increases force of contraction, resulting in improved ejection fraction

Usual dosage: 5 to 20 μg/kg/min IV

Side effects: Tachycardia, headache, nausea, vomiting

Dobutamine (Dobutrex)

Indications: Synthetic cardioactive derivative of dopamine that stimulates α- and β_1-adrenergic receptors; increases contractility and possesses slight chronotropic effects

Usual dosage: 2.5-10 μg/kg/min

Side effects: Tachycardia, palpitations, nausea, headache

Electromechanical

Intra-aortic balloon pump (IABP)—counterpulsation device that assists failing heart by decreasing afterload and increasing coronary artery perfusion (see p. 102 for further discussion)

Hemodynamic monitoring—initiated as direct means of assessing hemodynamic status of heart and effectiveness of treatment; also assists in direction of therapy

Cardiac monitoring—used to assess for drug-induced arrhythmias and for arrhythmias induced by an underlying disorder

Supportive

Bed rest with head of bed elevated to 45 degrees to reduce myocardial oxygen demand and decrease circulating volume returning to heart

Restriction of sodium and water; weighing daily to monitor fluid retention

Oxygen therapy initiated if patient is hypoxic

Rotating tourniquets used for rapid reduction of circulating blood volume; however, effectiveness is questionable

ASSESSMENT: AREAS OF CONCERN

General complaints

Dyspnea owing to increased pulmonary venous and interstitial pressures; variations: dyspnea on exertion (DOE), orthopnea, paroxysmal nocturnal dyspnea (PND)

Fatigue moderate to severe owing to diminished cardiac output

Gastrointestinal symptoms as result of splanchnic congestion: anorexia, nausea, vomiting, abdominal distention, right upper quadrant pain

Physical examination

Decreased cardiac output: tachycardia, pulsus alternans, weak thready pulse, hypotension, narrowed pulse pressure, pallor, diaphoresis, cool skin, altered mental status, dizziness, syncope, decreased urine output

Increased pulmonary capillary pressure: rapid labored respiration, cough, frothy or blood-tinged sputum, moist rales on pulmonary auscultation, left ventricular S_3 and systolic murmur at apex on cardiac auscultation, precordial movement—displaced apical impulse and palpable thrills

Increased right atrial pressure: weight gain, elevated jugular venous pressure (rise in a and v waves), hepatojugular reflex, precordial movement (right ventricular impulse along lower left sternal border or subxiphoid), on auscultation right ventricular S_3 heard best at lower left sternal border; presence of systolic murmur, hepatomegaly, splenomegaly, peripheral edema, dilation of peripheral veins

NURSING DIAGNOSES and NURSING INTERVENTIONS

Nursing Diagnosis	Nursing Intervention
Cardiac output, alteration in: decreased (related to left ventricular dysfunction)	Maintain strict bed rest. Limit self-care activities, permitting progress as patient is able to increase activity level. Monitor vital signs frequently to prevent hypotension, arrhythmias, respiratory embarrassment, and loss of mental acuity. Perform hemodynamic monitoring, per institution policy, in pulmonary artery pressure catheters, central venous pressure lines, arterial lines, cardiac output, and intra-aortic balloon pumping. Administer drug therapy as ordered. Monitor ECG carefully to detect early arrhythmias and rate changes. Limit IV intake as ordered.
Gas exchange, impaired (related to elevated pulmonary capillary pressure)	Monitor arterial blood gases frequently. Administer oxygen therapy as ordered, via nasal prongs, mask, or positive-pressure device. Administer morphine sulfate IV per protocol to reduce hyperventilation. Elevate head of bed. Auscultate breath sounds every hour to detect increases in congestion and determine adequacy of ventilatory effort. Prepare for intubation and assisted ventilation if required. Explain all procedures and modalities briefly to patient to prevent hyperventilation resulting from fear or anxiety.
Fluid volume, alteration in: excess	Maintain patent IV for drug administration. Administer rapid-acting diuretics as ordered to decrease circulating volume. Restrict sodium and fluid intake. Weigh patient daily (same time of day, same amount of clothing) to determine fluid loss or retention. Monitor intake and output. Monitor serum electrolytes, especially sodium and potassium. Inspect for increased or decreased jugular venous distention. Auscultate heart sounds and breath sounds every 1 to 2 hours to detect increased congestion.
Nutrition, alteration in	Maintain fluid and sodium restrictions. Teach good nutritional habits and use of seasonings to make low-sodium diet more palatable.
Comfort, alteration in: pain	Administer morphine sulfate as ordered. Stay with patient as much as possible. Explain all procedures and routines to patient. Provide over-bed table and pillows as needed to maintain position of comfort. Allow family to stay with patient and assist with patient care.
Knowledge deficit	Begin teaching patient about disease condition as soon as possible, including lifelong dietary restrictions, medications, exercise limitations and potentials, and complications.

Patient Education

Instruction is directed toward long-term maintenance of the therapeutic program.

1. Instruct the patient to limit physical activity and avoid fatigue.
2. Instruct the patient to limit the intake of salt in the diet and avoid foods that have a high sodium content; instruct the patient in label reading. Provide information about alternative ways to season food.
3. Teach the patient to weigh daily in the morning before the first meal with the same scale and wearing the same clothing.
4. Teach the patient the name and method of administration of drugs and their potential side effects.
5. Describe the disease process, the underlying cause, and any precipitating factors.

EVALUATION

Patient Outcome	Data Indicating That Outcome is Reached
Ventricular function is improved.	Heart rate and PWP are decreased. Cardiac output is increased. Mental status is improved. Urine output is increased.
Fluid overload is decreased.	Patient loses weight. Jugular venous distention is decreased. Breath sounds are improved. Peripheral edema is decreased.
Gas exchange is improved.	Lung sounds are clear. Anxiety level is diminished. Orthopnea and dyspnea are reduced. Hypoxemia and hypercarbia are absent. Respirations are improved.
Knowledge level is increased.	Patient verbalizes knowledge regarding importance of daily weight, taking prescribed medication, activity allowances and limitation, and dietary restriction.
Anxiety level is decreased.	Patient appears relaxed. Patient demonstrates ability to rest and sleep without complaints. Patient verbalizes fears regarding disease process, asking appropriate questions.

SHOCK

Shock is an abnormal physiologic state that is the first phase of the body's alarm reaction to a stress situation.

Most commonly shock occurs as an extreme pathophysiologic syndrome associated with abnormal cellular metabolism, which in most cases is due to inadequate tissue perfusion. If shock is untreated, progressive circulatory collapse and impaired cellular metabolism develop, leading eventually to death.

PATHOPHYSIOLOGY

Various methods of identifying or classifying shock have been used. The following four categories based on etiology are commonly used in the clinical setting:
  Hypovolemic
    Loss of blood volume (hemorrhage)
    Loss of plasma volume (dehydration)
  Vasogenic
    Sepsis
    Immune-mediated (anaphylaxis)
    Deep anesthesia effects
  Cardiogenic
    Acute myocardial infarction
    Other causes (pulmonary emboli, cardiac surgery, tamponade)
  Neurogenic

Hypovolemic Shock

Hypovolemic or "cold" shock results from a decrease in intravascular volume and generally occurs when there is an associated deficit of at least 15% to 20% of the total blood volume. Hypovolemia is the most common cause of hypotension in critically ill patients, particularly in the postoperative phase.

Hypovolemic shock may be caused by excessive loss of plasma volume as occurs in burns or pancreatitis when extracellular fluid is sequestered in injured or inflamed tissue cells. Severe dehydration and hypovolemia may also be induced by diabetic ketoacidosis, excessive vomiting, or diarrhea. The most common cause of hypovolemic shock, however, is excessive loss of blood through trauma of a major blood vessel or vascular organ such as the kidney, spleen, or liver; through injury or disease of the gastrointestinal system such as rupture of esophageal varices; or through defects in vascular structures that lead to rupture as with aneurysms.

The severity of hypovolemic shock is related to the amount and rate of volume loss. If volume is replaced quickly, the shock state can be easily reversed, but if low aortic pressures persist longer than 60 minutes, the process may be irreversible.

The major hemodynamic changes initially associated with uncompensated fluid loss are low cardiac output, increased systemic vascular resistance, and decreased central venous pressure. Clinically the patient presents the classic textbook picture of shock: cool clammy skin, increased heart and respiratory rates, and decreased urine output owing to compensatory vasoconstriction. The blood pressure may be normal or low, particularly in the early phase of "cold shock."

Vasogenic Shock

Unlike hypovolemic shock, which leads to vasoconstriction, vasogenic shock results in massive vasodilation from an increase in total vascular capacity. Circulating volume is lost because of venous pooling, increased capillary permeability, and third spacing of fluid. If intravascular volume is not replaced, hypovolemia will occur. Whereas a patient with hypovolemia has cold extremities as a result of vasoconstriction, a patient with vasogenic shock has warm extremities, giving rise to the term "warm shock." Warm shock is present in 30% to 50% of patients in the early phase of septic shock.

The most common form of vasogenic shock is sepsis, but it may also occur as a result of other factors, including anaphylactic reactions from drugs, insect stings, and food allergies.

Septic shock is commonly related to the release of bacterial endotoxins following a gram-negative bacterial infection. The organisms most frequently found in septic shock are the gram-negative bacteria *Escherichia coli, Klebsiella, Enterobacter, Pseudomonas, Serratia, Proteus,* and *Bacteroides fragilis;* the gram-positive bacteria *Staphylococcus, Pneumococcus,* and α- or β-*Streptococcus;* and the fungus *Candida.* Many are part of the natural body flora or are common in the hospital environment. The microbes associated with the highest mortality are *Proteus, Pseudomonas, Candida,* and *B. fragilis.* Although patients in critical care units are the most vulnerable to hospital-acquired infections, a large subset of patients in general hospital units is also vulnerable. Patients particularly susceptible to septic shock are the elderly, immunosuppressed patients, patients who have indwelling catheters (urinary, intravenous, or intracardiac) or urinary tract infection, and patients who have undergone manipulative instrumentation or gastrointestinal or genitourinary surgical procedures.

Although deaths from septic shock have decreased since the 1960s, the mortality continues to be as high as 50%. This is due to several factors, the most striking of which are the changing pattern of microbial resistance to antimicrobial agents[3,10] and the rapidly changing microbial profile.

Although the exact mechanism by which toxins produce septic shock is unclear, certain hemodynamic changes have been recognized. In early phases a hyperdynamic state exists in which the cardiac output, stroke volume, and heart rate are increased and the systemic vascular resistance and central venous pressure are decreased. The patient appears warm, dry, and flushed because of generalized vasodilation and venous pooling. This hyperdynamic state is probably due to the effects of various vasoactive substances released by the exotoxins or from the injured or infected tissue.

The circulatory changes combined with the decreased systemic vascular resistance may stimulate sympathetic response, causing the increased heart rate and maintenance of normal blood pressure that occur during this "warm" shock phase.

If hyperdynamic shock is allowed to persist, the continued increase in capillary leaking will potentiate hypovolemia to the point that the process will convert to a hypodynamic phase known as the "cold" phase of septic shock. In this state the systemic vascular resistance increases, cardiac output drops, and the patient appears cold, pale, and clammy. The cause of this change is related to ineffective circulating blood volume, sympathetic vasoconstriction, and pump failure.[41]

In *anaphylactic reactions* from drugs, insect stings, or food allergies, the mechanism involved is an antibody-antigen interaction that provokes the release of chemical mediators such as histamine. These mediators act primarily on the vascular membranes and smooth muscles. Histamine release causes veins and arterioles to dilate, decreasing cardiac output and arterial pressure. In addition, histamine increases capillary permeability, causing fluid to escape from the intravascular compartment into the interstitial space. The result is volume depletion; however, while plasma water is removed from the capillaries, the red cells remain and the hemoglobin levels and hematocrit values rise. The immediate clinical reactions in anaphylaxis are pharyngeal and laryngeal edema, probably stemming from effects of histamines, and bronchoconstriction with the immediate threat of death from asphyxiation.

Deep anesthesia can cause severe depression of the vasomotor centers of the brain, which may result in vasomotor collapse and venous pooling. These in turn decrease venous return to the heart and diminish cardiac output.

Cardiogenic Shock

Cardiogenic shock occurs when the heart cannot maintain an adequate cardiac output to meet the body's metabolic demands.

The most common cause of cardiogenic shock is myocardial infarction, but it may be the result of a variety of cardiac disorders: acute myocardial infarction, endstage cardiomyopathy (congestive, hypertrophic, or restrictive), valvular heart disease, cardiopulmonary bypass, and cardiac tamponade. The cardinal feature of cardiogenic shock is inadequate tissue perfusion and oxygen delivery resulting from a severely impaired ventricle.

Despite advances in pharmacology and hemodynamic monitoring, the incidence of cardiogenic shock resulting from myocardial infarction remains at 10% to 15%, with a mortality greater than 60%. Since the prognosis depends largely on the extent of myocardial damage, current therapies focus on early intervention to reduce ischemia and limit permanent myocardial damage.

In patients with myocardial infarction, shock develops as a result of abnormal reflexes arising from the ischemic myocardium. The consequent inability to increase systemic vascular resistance makes it difficult to maintain an adequate arterial pressure. This leads to hypoperfusion of an already ischemic myocardium, producing further damage and further insufficiency of the pumping action of the left ventricle. Failure of the left ventricle to generate sufficient energy to pump blood into the systemic circulation further contributes to decreased coronary perfusion and decreased myocardial oxygen supply.

Cardiogenic shock has been correlated with destruction of 40% or more of left ventricular muscle mass. The mechanism of cardiogenic shock is complex, with a vicious cycle of metabolic and hemodynamic changes that lead rapidly to further deterioration of cardiac function. If left untreated, the reduction in tissue blood flow and oxygen delivery to the myocardium results in progressive circulatory collapse, impaired cellular metabolism, and eventual death.

The basic pathophysiologic defect associated with severe myocardial ischemia or necrosis is severely depressed ventricular function, which results in reduced cardiac output and inadequate tissue perfusion. The magnitude of impairment in ventricular function is related to total myocardial damage and the balance between oxygen supply and demand.

Neurogenic Shock

Neurogenic shock is produced by damage to or pharmacologic block of the sympathetic nervous system, resulting in vasodilation and increased vascular capacity. This leads to a relative hypovolemia brought on by a decrease in systemic vascular resistance with peripheral pooling and decrease in venous return. The result is a drop in cardiac output leading to tissue hypoperfusion.

Neurogenic shock is relatively rare and most commonly results from spinal anesthesia or damage or disease of the upper spinal cord. Brain trauma or injury rarely if ever causes shock.

Compensatory Mechanisms of Shock

A number of compensatory mechanisms are activated to maintain cardiovascular dynamics when arterial pressure and tissue perfusion are reduced. These compensatory mechanisms are mediated by the sympathetic nervous system and the release of endogenous vasoconstrictor and hormonal substances.[20]

Fig. 1-37
Different types of feedback that can lead to progression of shock.

Modified from Guyton, A.C.: Textbook of medical physiology, ed. 8, Philadelphia, 1980, W.B. Saunders Co.

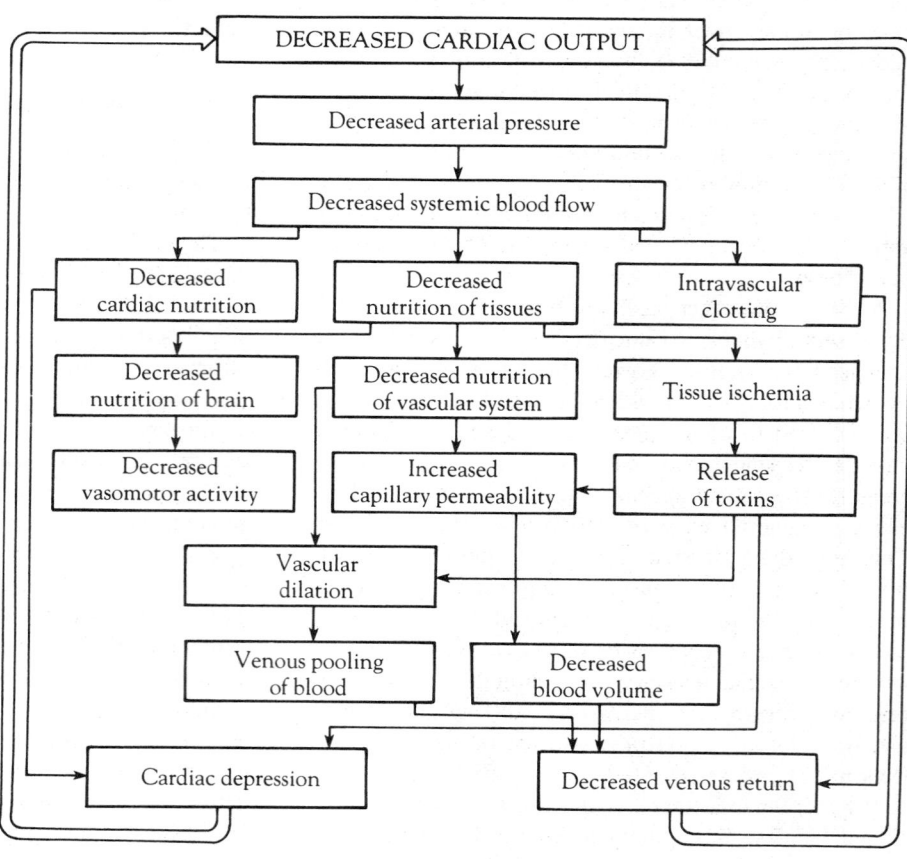

Baroreceptors. A reduction in mean arterial pressure and pulse pressure is sensed by baroreceptors in the carotid sinus and aortic arch, and they produce a generalized sympathetic stimulation with secretion of epinephrine and norepinephrine. The result is increases in peripheral vascular resistance, arterial pressure, and myocardial contractility.

Fluid shifts. The major endogenous vasoactive substances released during shock are catecholamines and vasopressin, which augment sympathetic activity when activated further. The release of these vasoactive substances also causes a reduction in vascular capacitance, which facilitates the osmotic movement of interstitial fluid into the vascular compartments to restore blood volume.

Renin-angiotensin-aldosterone system. When renal ischemia occurs, the renin-angiotensin-aldosterone system is activated to help maintain blood pressure and intravascular volume. The reduction of renal perfusion pressure results in release of renin, which in time is converted to angiotensin II, a powerful vasoconstrictor. Angiotensin II stimulates the release of aldosterone, which enhances sodium and water reabsorption by the renal tubules to help maintain intravascular volume.

Antidiuretic hormone. The release of antidiuretic hormone (ADH) from the posterior pituitary gland in response to hypotension is another hormonal system that plays a role in volume regulation during circulatory shock. ADH enhances reabsorption of sodium and water by increasing permeability of the renal tubules.

Progressive Shock

If the compensatory mechanisms are insufficient to restore effective perfusion to vital organs, circulatory function deteriorates further, perpetuating a cycle of progressive, irreversible changes that decrease cardiac output. Fig. 1-37 illustrates some of the changes that contribute to decreased cardiac output and circulatory collapse.

Cellular deterioration. As shock becomes severe, local changes in cellular metabolism occur. Prolonged tissue ischemia results in incomplete oxidation at the cellular level, diminishing mitochondrial activity. Cellular adenosine triphosphate (ATP) stores consequently begin to be used, and the cells resort to anaerobic metabolism of glucose to provide energy. This anaerobic process of glycolysis leads to the production of lactic acid, which builds up in the blood. The effects of an acidic pH include depressed myocardial function and a decreased vascular response to epinephrine and norepinephrine, thus potentiating the vasomotor collapse seen late in shock.[3]

Another significant cellular change resulting from continued cellular ischemia is the release of vasoactive metabolites into the systemic circulation. Substances such as bradykinin, histamine, serotonin, and prostaglandins, along with decreased vascular tone, lead to increases in venous pooling and capillary permeability. Excessive vasodilation then decreases venous return and cardiac filling. The increased permeability of the capillaries allows large quantities of fluid to escape into the interstitial spaces.

Organ and Tissue Changes

As the shock syndrome becomes severe, generalized organ deterioration begins.

Renal function. Although diminished renal perfusion activates certain compensatory mechanisms, in the early phase of shock prolonged decreased renal blood flow leads to renal ischemia and acute tubular necrosis. Clinically this is evidenced by fluid, electrolyte, and metabolic disturbances.

Pulmonary function. Ischemia to the pulmonary circulation in the early phases of shock can sufficiently damage pulmonary function to cause adult respiratory distress syndrome. Damage to the pulmonary capillary endothelial cells causes increased capillary permeability, which leads to interstitial and alveolar edema that impairs gas exchange. The resulting hypoxemia and respiratory acidosis further reduce tissue oxygen delivery and organ function.

Gastrointestinal function. Ischemic damage to the gastrointestinal tract causes a loss of the protective mucosal covering in the intestine. This can lead to intestinal damage and necrosis by digestive enzymes. It may also account for the release of bacteria and bacterial toxins into the bloodstream, causing sepsis and further circulatory dysfunction.

The reticuloendothelial system may also be damaged during shock, impairing the patient's ability to withstand infection.

Intravascular clotting. As the products of cellular deterioration begin to accumulate in the capillaries and vascular dilation occurs, blood flow becomes extremely sluggish. The stagnation, along with local chemical changes in the capillaries, leads to blood aggregation and intravascular clotting. The formation of microemboli enhances tissue ischemia by further decreasing blood flow through the capillaries. This hypercoagulability response may occur as an early compensatory mechanism, particularly with hemorrhage. In the late stages of shock, however, a reversal in coagulation occurs, leading to a hypocoagulability state. This results from loss in clotting factors through bleeding or decreased production owing to poor tissue perfusion. It may also be the result of a consumption of clotting factors that is seen in disseminated intravascular coagulation.

Myocardial depression. Except with cardiogenic shock, the major cardiac effects of shock occur in the late stage and are by far the most important factor in the progressive deterioration caused by shock. As arterial pressure continues to drop, so does coronary blood flow. This leads to depressed myocardial function and a further reduction of cardiac output. Myocardial contractility is depressed further by the combined effects of toxins, acidosis, and tissue hypoxia that result from cellular deterioration. Thus circulatory failure is a syndrome that involves all systems, and it is usually the deterioration of heart function that makes shock irreversible.[9]

DIAGNOSTIC STUDIES

Laboratory tests
Hematocrit
Increased in volume deficits
Hemoglobin
Decreased in hemorrhage
White blood count with differential
Increased; leukopenia in gram-negative sepsis; leukocytosis with increased neutrophils in all forms of shock
Erythrocyte sedimentation rate
Increased in response to tissue injury
Cultures (blood [obtain two to four cultures before initiation of antibiotic therapy], urine, sputum)
Positive growth of an organism
Serum electrolytes
Sodium
Increased during diuretic phase of acute tubular necrosis; decreased with administration of hypotonic fluid following fluid loss
Potassium
Increased with cellular death during oliguric phase, in acidosis, and after transfusion reactions
Serum chemistry
BUN, creatinine
Increased, reflecting impaired renal function
Lactate levels
Increased
Glucose levels
Increased in early shock, reflecting release of liver glycogen stores in response to catecholamines
Prothrombin time
Increased
Arterial blood gases
Respiratory alkalosis; metabolic acidosis
Urine studies
Specific gravity
Increased in response to action of ADH and during oliguric phase

Osmolality
High during oliguric phase

Electrocardiogram (ECG) (12-lead continuous monitoring)
To determine changes in heart rate and rhythm and ischemic changes

Chest roentgenogram
To determine pulmonary status and rule out other causes of shock state

Hemodynamic monitoring (pulmonary artery pressure, pulmonary capillary wedge pressure, cardiac output)
To provide information regarding serial changes in left ventricular function in response to specific treatments, such as fluid replacement

TREATMENT PLAN

Chemotherapeutic

Fluid-volume regulation. Except with patients in cardiogenic shock, restoration of intravascular volume is the most significant therapeutic intervention, particularly in the early phases of therapy.

Volume replacement should be initiated rapidly with 3 to 5 L of saline or other volume expanders over a 30- to 60-minute period. Ringer's lactate provides effective intravascular expansion and is the usual fluid of choice; however, a buffered solution with lactate may be used for severe shock.

Regulation of fluids should be based on hemodynamic response to the rapid fluid infusion. Careful monitoring of mean arterial pressure, pulmonary capillary wedge pressure (PCWP) or central venous pressure (CVP), and urine output is used to guide fluid replacement.

Blood plasma expanders should be given after the initial volume deficit is corrected. In cases of massive hemorrhage, replacement should be with whole blood if the hematocrit value is less than 30%. If the hematocrit value is greater than 30%, plasma expanders may be given. Packed cells are used if the right atrial pressure or PCWP is elevated and in cases such as cardiogenic shock in which myocardial dysfunction limits the amount and speed of fluid replacement.

In a patient in shock after acute myocardial infarction, volume deficits may occur and fluid replacement may be necessary to restore a depressed cardiac output to normal. Continuous monitoring of the PCWP is the most precise method of determining volume deficits. If the PCWP is below the desired level of 15 to 18 mm Hg, fluid replacement may be given to increase cardiac output (Starling's law). The PCWP should be kept below 18 mm Hg to avoid pulmonary congestion.

If the PCWP of a patient in shock is elevated, fluid replacement is contraindicated and diuretics may be necessary to return the PCWP to therapeutic range. Diuretics are generally given only to patients in cardiogenic shock with an elevated PCWP. They reduce preload through their effect on venous capacitance and decrease total circulating fluid.

Maintenance of adequate hemodynamic state. In shock, myocardial dysfunction develops as a result of workload, limited coronary blood flow, and decreased myocardial oxygenation. Sympathomimetic agents are used to maintain an adequate hemodynamic state. The effects of these agents are mediated through the action of α- and β-adrenergic receptors. α-Receptors located in the smooth muscle of the vascular bed cause vasoconstriction, thereby increasing peripheral resistance and venous return. By contrast, β_1-receptors are located in the myocardium, arteries, and lungs. Myocardial β_1-receptors act to increase heart rate and contractility, whereas activation of β_2-receptors causes vasodilation.

The various adrenergic drugs differ with respect to their relative α (peripheral) and β (peripheral, myocardial) effects. The rationale for selecting any drug depends on the specific vascular bed on which the drug acts and the desired cardiovascular effect. In cardiogenic shock, for example, drugs with positive inotropic and vasoconstrictor properties are used to increase cardiac output by augmenting myocardial contractility and to improve blood flow to vital organs by increasing total vascular resistance. Dopamine, norepinephrine, and epinephrine, which have both constrictor and inotropic properties, are commonly used in treatment of cardiogenic shock.

The following agents are most commonly used in the treatment of patients with shock.

Adrenergic drugs. Dopamine (Intropin) is one of the most widely used drugs in the treatment of shock. Its effects depend on the dose used. In low doses (2 to 5 μg/kg/min) it produces dilation of renal, mesenteric, coronary, and cerebral blood vessels. In higher doses (6 to 15 μg/kg/min) it improves cardiac output by increasing contractility (β effect) but has no effect on blood pressure. At therapeutic levels (10 to 15 μg/kg/min) dopamine increases cardiac output and blood pressure with little change or reduction in pulmonary vascular resistance. The increase in blood pressure is due primarily to an enhanced cardiac output. In addition, the vasodilator effect on renal blood vessels increases renal blood flow, which improves urine output. In very high doses (>20 μg/kg/min) dopamine causes generalized vasoconstriction (α effect), which opposes the desired vasodilator effect obtained with lower doses. Infusions should be started with low doses (3 to 5 μg/kg/min), increasing slowly until optimum arterial pressure is achieved.

Dobutamine (Dobutrex) is used primarily for its inotropic effect. It stimulates β_1-receptors to increase myocardial contractility and stroke volume, resulting in improved cardiac output. Since dobutamine has minimal β_2 and α effects, it produces little change in blood pressure and heart rate; however, systolic blood pressure may be increased because of increased cardiac output. Coronary blood flow and myocardial oxygen consumption (MVO_2) are also increased because of increased myocardial contractility. Infusions begin at 2 to 4 μg/kg/min, with therapeutic doses between 2.5 and 10 μg/kg/min.

Epinephrine is a potent β- and α-catecholamine causing vasoconstriction of the splanchnic and renal beds. Although it does increase cardiac output, its effects on peripheral resistance do not favor redistribution of blood flow to vital organs. It is also considered less advantageous than other adrenergic drugs because it increases automaticity, which can initiate serious arrhythmias.

Norepinephrine has both α and β actions. It increases myocardial contractility by stimulating β_1-receptors and causes arteriovenous constriction by stimulating α-receptors. Thus norephineprine increases systemic arterial pressure by increasing the cardiac output and peripheral vascular resistance. Once again the actual hemodynamic effects depend on the dose employed. With small doses a β effect predominates, causing slight increases in blood pressure and cardiac output. With very high doses norepinephrine produces significant vasoconstriction, causing an increased systemic resistance and blood pressure. However, the cardiac output may fall despite the positive inotropic effect. The usual starting dose is 2 to 8 μg/minute. Norepinephrine should be administered through an indwelling catheter placed in a large vein, since it is known to cause tissue necrosis with extravasation. The disadvantage of this drug is its vasconstricting effect on the kidneys, which can result in impaired renal perfusion and oliguria.

Isoproterenol (Isuprel) acts as a peripheral dilator through β_2 stimulation. More important is the β_1 effect, which augments myocardial contractility and heart rate, thereby improving cardiac output. However, it may cause a substantial increase in myocardial oxygen demand, which can exacerbate myocardial ischemia in a patient with cardiogenic shock.

Cardiac glycosides. The role of digitalis in the treatment of shock is now being questioned. It has been noted that inotropic drugs such as digoxin become less effective as the degree of left ventricular failure increases. As an inotropic agent for treatment of severe or cardiogenic shock, digitalis is relatively weak when compared with the sympathomimetic drugs. In addition, it could be hemodynamically detrimental because of the increased MVO_2 produced by the increased contractility, as well as by the decrease in afterload associated with it. Furthermore, because of the impaired renal function, acidosis, and hypoxia occurring in shock states, the patient is predisposed to digitalis-induced arrhythmias.[20]

Vasodilators. Vasodilator therapy is generally limited to patients with failing ventricular function and is still debated in the routine treatment of cardiogenic shock. However, it may be of use in patients with severe hypotension whose severe vasoconstriction continues despite volume replacement. Excessive vasoconstriction, which occurs initially as a compensatory response to hypoperfusion, can reduce blood flow and oxygen delivery, as well as cause such a loss of intravascular volume that it leads to further reduction of cardiac output. The rationale for using vasodilator therapy in shock is to break this progressive positive-feedback cycle.

Vasodilator agents improve left ventricular function by decreasing myocardial oxygen demand through the reduction of preload and afterload. These drugs have no direct inotropic action on the heart. The increased cardiac output produced by vasodilators is caused by the changes in preload and afterload.

Arterial vasodilators are used to decrease peripheral vascular resistance, which then decreases resistance to left ventricular ejection and therefore afterload. Venodilators are used to increase venous capacitance, causing a decrease in venous return that will decrease PCWP and preload.

The potential role of vasodilator therapy in cardiogenic shock merits further study. Although inappropriate as a single form of therapy, the use of vasodilators combined with external counterpulsation and other inotropic agents appears to be effective in providing efficient ventricular function. Nitroprusside and phentolamine are the vasodilator agents most commonly used in the treatment of cardiogenic shock.

Antihypertensive agents. Nitroprusside (Nipride, Nitropress) causes both arterial and venous dilation, thereby decreasing venous return and left ventricular filling (decreased preload), as well as resistance to left ventricular ejection (decreased afterload). The drug is administered intravenously with an initial dose of 0.5 to 10 μg/kg/min, which is increased in increments of 5 to 10 μg/kg/min every 5 minutes or until an improvement in hemodynamics is observed. Fluid replacement may be required if filling pressures drop excessively. Fluid volumes should be determined before administration of these agents. In hypovolemic patients, massive vasodilation will only worsen the clinical picture by further decreasing venous return.

α-Adrenergic blocking agents. Phentolamine mesylate (Regitine) inhibits vasoconstriction by blocking α-adrenergic receptors. It lowers arterial pressure, thereby decreasing afterload. The drug is given intravenously at a dosage of 0.1 to 2 mg/minute.

Electromechanical

Counterpulsation. Counterpulsation is the most frequently used method of mechanically assisting circulation to profound cardiovascular collapse. Counterpulsation augments aortic pressure during diastole with subsequent reduction of afterload, thus effectively reducing the work of the myocardium and improving coronary blood flow (see p. 102).

The intra-aortic balloon pump (IABP) is the most widely used counterpulsation technique. A catheter with a 10 to 50 cc balloon is inserted into the femoral artery and positioned in the thoracic aorta just distal to the left subclavian artery. With the ECG used for synchronization, the balloon is inflated during diastole and deflated during systole.

Oxygenation. Ventilation/perfusion ratios should be determined early to ensure adequate ventilation. Oxygen exchange may be impaired in patients with shock, especially if cardiac output is decreased. Oxygen therapy should be given from the onset of treatment to maintain an arterial PO_2 of at least 80 mm Hg. Intubation may be indicated if arterial blood gases show worsening hypoxemia despite high oxygen concentrations. The indications for mechanical ventilation are a PaO_2 of less than 50 mm Hg while the patient is receiving oxygen concentrations of 50%, a vital capacity of less than 15 ml/kg body weight, a PCO_2 of greater than 45 mm Hg, and an arterial pH of less than 7.25.

Hemodynamic monitoring. For diagnostic information and evaluation of ongoing therapy, arterial pressures, pulmonary artery pressure (PAP), and PCWP should be monitored initially every 5 to 10 minutes. A cardiac index of less than 2 L/minute is reflective of a shock state.

Supportive

Nutrition. Shock patients should receive nothing by mouth, but care must be taken to provide nutrition, preferably with hyperalimentation.

Acid-base balance. Frequent monitoring of acid-base balance is necessary to avert profound acidosis. Intravenous administration of sodium bicarbonate may be necessary to maintain or correct the pH to 7.35.

Renal function. Hourly urine output measurements with frequent checks are necessary to determine adequate kidney perfusion. Urine output of less than 30 ml/hour reflects inadequate renal perfusion. Elevated serum BUN and creatinine levels reflect renal dysfunction.

Activity. Efforts should be made to minimize energy expenditure. The patient should be maintained on complete bed rest in a supine position, with legs elevated to 45 degrees.

ASSESSMENT: AREAS OF CONCERN

Area of Concern	Hypovolemic Shock	Cardiogenic Shock	Vasogenic Shock	Neurogenic Shock
General appearance	Anxiety, restlessness	Anxiety, restlessness	Anxiety, restlessness	Anxiety, restlessness
Level of consciousness	Lethargy, stupor, or coma	Lethargy, stupor, or coma	Lethargy, stupor, or coma	Lethargy, stupor, or coma
Temperature	Increased or decreased	Increased	Increased or decreased	Increased or decreased
Heart rate	Increased, pulse thready	Increased, pulse thready	Increased, pulse thready	Normal or slow
Blood pressure				
Early	Pulse pressure decreased; diastolic pressure increased	Pulse pressure decreased; diastolic pressure increased	Normal; pulse pressure decreased	Normal; pulse pressure decreased
Late	Systolic pressure decreased	Systolic pressure decreased	Systolic pressure decreased	Systolic pressure decreased
Skin temperature and texture	Cool, moist, clammy, pale	Cool, moist, clammy, pale, cyanosis	Early: warm, dry; late: cool, moist, clammy; color: pale, cyanosis (late)	Early: warm, dry; late: cyanosis
Capillary refill time	Decreased	Decreased	Decreased	Decreased
Peripheral pulses	Absent or diminished	Absent or diminished	Absent or diminished (late)	Absent or diminished
Urine output				
Early	Decreased (less than 20 ml/mm)	Decreased (less than 20 ml/mm)	Decreased (less than 20 ml/mm)	Decreased (less than 20 ml/mm)
Late	Anuria	Anuria	Anuria	Anuria
Urine sodium concentration	Decreased	Decreased	Decreased	Decreased
Urine osmolality	Increased	Increased	Increased	Increased
Pulmonary function				
Respiratory rate	Increased	Increased; late: Cheyne-Stokes respirations, apnea	Increased; late: Cheyne-Stokes respirations	Varies
Auscultation	Early: clear; late: rales	Rales	Early: clear; late: rales	Early: clear; late: rales
Acid-base changes				
Early	Respiratory alkalosis	Respiratory alkalosis	Respiratory alkalosis	Respiratory alkalosis
Late	Metabolic acidosis	Metabolic acidosis	Metabolic acidosis	Metabolic acidosis
Hemodynamic findings				
Central venous pressure	Decreased			
Pulmonary capillary wedge pressure	Decreased	Increased	Decreased	Decreased
Cardiac output	Decreased	Decreased	Increased or decreased	Decreased
Peripheral vascular resistance	Decreased	Increased	Decreased	Decreased

NURSING DIAGNOSES and NURSING INTERVENTIONS

Nursing Diagnosis	Nursing Intervention
Cardiac output, alteration in: decreased	Maintain strict bed rest with patient in supine position and head of bed elevated slightly. (NOTE: Trendelenburg position is contraindicated.) Limit all activities. Monitor vital signs every 5 to 15 minutes and be alert for increasing pulse or thready pulse, decreasing blood pressure, and respiratory ineffectiveness. Monitor all hemodynamic parameters. Administer sympathomimetic drugs as ordered to maintain blood pressure at acceptable reading. Frequently assess cardiovascular response to drug therapy. Administer vasodilator drugs as ordered to increase cardiac output by decreasing peripheral vascular resistance. Maintain patent IV for drug administration. Initiate intra-aortic balloon pump as indicated by clinical state. Administer antiarrhythmic drugs as ordered for arrhythmias.
Fluid volume deficit, actual	Administer fluids as ordered. Assess patient for immediate response. Monitor hemodynamic parameters, including pulmonary capillary wedge pressure, heart rate, urine output, and central venous pressure. Assess skin for temperature, color, and elasticity. Maintain patient's core temperature by covering patient with blankets as needed. Maintain accurate intake and output record.
Gas exchange: impaired	Monitor arterial blood gases. Administer oxygen as ordered, via mask or through endotracheal tube. Auscultate breath sounds every hour for increasing pulmonary congestion and atelectasis. Ensure that chest roentgenograms are obtained as ordered. Monitor for signs of impairment in respiratory pattern by assessing skin color, respiratory rate, and breathing pattern. Suction as needed to ensure patent airway.
Injury, potential for	Implement safety precautions for patients who are restless or confused, including use of soft restraints and side rails.
Skin integrity, impairment of: potential	Perform skin care every 1 to 2 hours, carefully observing bony prominences for pressure points and evidence of breakdown. Provide egg-crate mattress, sheepskin mattress, or air-pressure mattress as ordered. Turn patient every 1 to 2 hours as condition permits. Begin passive range of motion exercises as condition permits.
Nutrition, alteration in: less than body requirements	Weigh daily. Begin tube feedings, intralipids, and/or hyperalimentation as ordered.
Anxiety	Explain all procedures and treatments. Remain with patient to offer reassurance. Maintain as quiet and calm an atmosphere as possible. Allow family to be with patient as condition permits. Provide alternative means of communication if patient is intubated or unable to verbalize fears and needs. Administer medications as ordered for persistent chest pain or discomfort. Maintain calm and reassuring manner.
Potential patient problem: infection	Maintain strict asepsis of all invasive lines. Administer antibiotics as ordered. Turn patient every 1 to 2 hours as condition permits.

Patient Education

1. Explain all procedures and treatments as they occur. Refer to primary disorder for specific teaching protocol.

EVALUATION

Patient Outcome	Data Indicating That Outcome is Reached
Cardiac output is improved.	Patient is normotensive. Cardiac output is 4 to 5 L/minute. PCWP is 10 to 15 mm Hg. Skin is warm and dry. Patient is resting quietly.
Fluid volume is restored.	Patient is normotensive. PCWP is 10 to 15 mm Hg. Urine output is increased.
Gas exchange is improved.	Pao_2 is 80 to 100 mm Hg. Pco_2 is 35 to 45 mm Hg. Lungs are clear. Patient verbalizes breathing easier.
Acid-base balance is normal.	CO_2 is 35 to 45 mm Hg. pH is 7.35 to 7.45.
Anxiety is decreased.	Patient verbalizes fears and asks questions. Patient appears relaxed and is resting quietly.

CARDIOMYOPATHY

The term ''cardiomyopathy'' is applied to diseases that diffusely affect the myocardium, resulting in enlargement or ventricular dysfunction.

In the past three decades, great advances in the understanding of this complex disorder have been made, particularly with regard to pathophysiology, diagnosis, and treatment. In an attempt to distinguish the various forms and causes of the myopathies, several classifications have been proposed. In *classifications according to cause,* terms such as idiopathic cardiomyopathy and myocardiomyopathy have been used to describe primary myocardial disease not caused by coronary artery, valvular, or congenital heart disease. Types of idiopathic cardiomyopathy include the following:

Endocardial fibroelastosis
Hypertrophic obstructive cardiomyopathy
Primary myocardial disease
Familial cardiomyopathies
   Metabolic storage diseases
      Pompe's disease (glycogen)
      Fabry's disease (glycolipid)
   Muscular dystrophies
   Friederich's ataxia
   Sickle cell anemia

Secondary cardiomyopathies occur as a result of a generalized disease process that affects other parts of the body before or after the myocardium is involved. The following are some examples of such conditions:

Inflammatory
   Infectious
      Viral (such as coxsackievirus, rubella)
      Rickettsial (typhus, Q fever)
      Bacterial (streptococcal)
      Spirochetal (leptospirosis, syphilis)
      Fungal (histoplasmosis, coccidioidomycosis)
      Parasitic (Chagas' disease, schistosomiasis)
   Noninfectious (collagen)
      Rheumatic heart disease
      Scleroderma
      Systemic lupus erythematosus
      Polyarteritis
      Löffler's disease
      Dermatomyositis
   Infiltrative
      Sarcoidosis
      Amyloidosis
      Neoplastic
   Metabolic
      Endocrine disorders
         Thyrotoxicosis
         Myxedema
      Nutritional
         Starvation, malnutrition
         Beri-beri
   Toxic
      Alcohol
      Carbon monoxide
      Arsenic
      Immunosuppressive drugs (doxorubicin)
      Emetine
   Miscellaneous
      Postpartum
      Radiation

In *functional classifications* three types exist: hypertrophic, dilated, and restricted.

PATHOPHYSIOLOGY
Hypertrophic Cardiomyopathy

Hypertrophic cardiomyopathy is the form of myocardial disease whose pathophysiologic, etiologic, and clinical features continue to receive the widest attention. As a result it has acquired an extensive list of identifying terms that generally describe features of the disease not present in all cases. These include idiopathic hypertrophic sub-

Fig. 1-38
Heart with hypertrophic
cardiomyopathy. Interventricular
septum, *IVS,* is thicker than posterior
wall, *PW.* Histologic section on right
shows marked disorganization of
myocardium that is especially
prominent in septum. (Hematoxylin
and eosin, ×50.)

From Bulkley, B.H.: Advances in cardiac
pathology, In The heart, update I, by J.
Willis Hurst, editor. Copyright © 1979,
McGraw-Hill Book Co. Used with the
permission of McGraw-Hill Book Co.

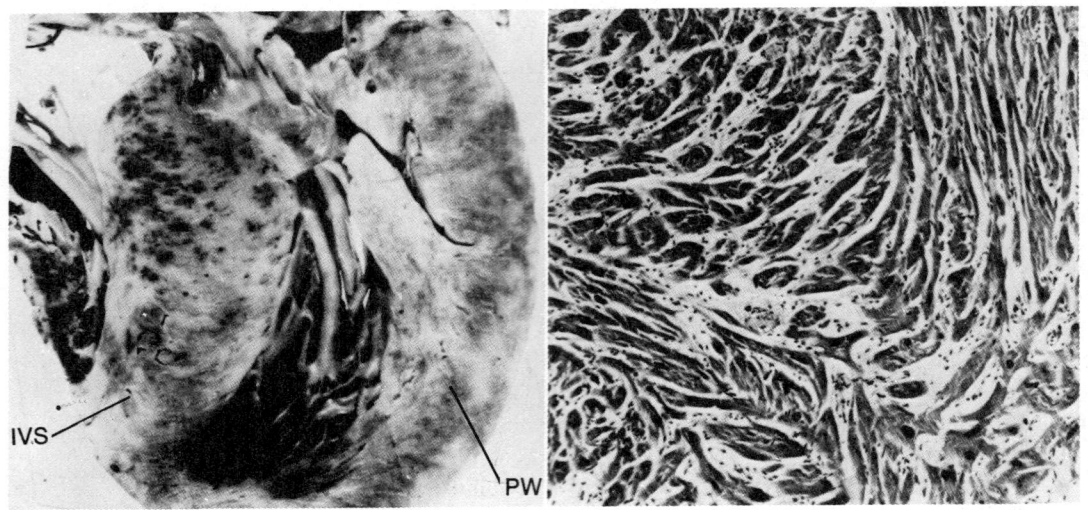

aortic stenosis (IHSS), asymmetric septal hypertrophy (ASH), and hypertrophic obstructive cardiomyopathy (HOCM).

Hypertrophic cardiomyopathy is characterized by a distinctive pattern of hypertrophy, with disproportionate thickening of the interventricular septum when compared with the free wall of the left ventricle (Fig. 1-38). The overgrowth of muscle mass renders the ventricular walls rigid, increasing resistance as blood enters from the left atrium. Obstruction to left ventricular outflow is another characteristic of hypertrophic cardiomyopathy. Consequently, left ventricular ejection is impeded throughout systole. Contributing to outflow obstruction is the obstruction produced by opposition of the anterior mitral leaflet against the hypertrophied septum during midsystole. Systolic motion of the anterior mitral leaflet has been used to determine the severity of outflow obstruction.[47] Elevated systolic pressure gradients occur in the range of 70% to 90% of left ventricular volumes.[12] Failure occurs as resistance to diastolic filling increases as the result of a stiff, noncompliant left ventricle.

On gross examination of these hearts, there is massive overgrowth of myocardial tissue with small ventricular cavities. The atria are also hypertrophied and dilated, reflecting the high resistance to ventricular filling.

Histologically the heart muscle may show myocardial fiber disarray. First described in 1958 by Donald Teare, this form of hypertrophic cardiomyopathy is thought to reflect an underlying genetic defect that manifests itself in abnormal cardiac structure. This feature of disorganized cellular architecture is not considered to be pathognomonic of hypertrophic cardiomyopathy. Similar disorganization has been seen in some cases of acquired or congenital heart disease.

Dilated Cardiomyopathy

The second and most common form of cardiomyopathy is characterized by gross dilation of the heart, interference with systolic function, and damage to myofibrils. Unlike hypertrophic cardiomyopathy, in which ventricular filling is impaired, dilated cardiomyopathy is characterized by impaired systolic ejection function with both the end-diastolic and end-systolic volumes increased.

On gross examination the heart has a globular shape with enlargement and dilation of all four chambers (Fig. 1-39). Although the heart may weigh up to 700 g (normal 350 g), the wall thickness may be normal or decreased. Left ventricular filling pressures are generally elevated as a consequence of poor contractile function. The cardiac valves are intrinsically normal, as are the coronary arteries. Endocardial thrombi are common, particularly in the ventricular apex.

Histologic examination reveals nonspecific changes including cellular hypertrophy and extensive interstitial and perivascular fibrosis.

Fig. 1-39
Heart with idiopathic dilated congestive cardiomyopathy. Opened left ventricle, *LV,* has dilated and globular configuration. Aortic valves, *AV,* and mitral valves, *MV,* are normal.

From Kaye, D., and Rose, L.F.: Fundamentals of internal medicine, St. Louis, 1983, The C.V. Mosby Co.

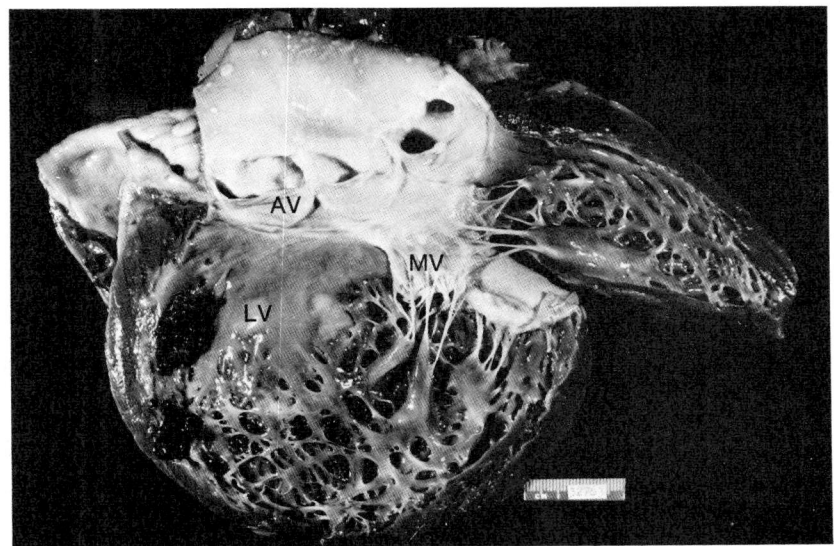

The cause of this disorder is not clear, but it has been linked etiologically to various factors that predispose to the development of cardiomyopathy, including alcohol, pregnancy, infections, and toxic agents.

Restrictive Cardiomyopathy

A less common form of cardiomyopathy, restrictive cardiomyopathy is characterized by abnormal diastolic (filling) function and excessively rigid ventricular walls. Contractility, however, is relatively unimpaired with normal systolic emptying of the ventricles. Hemodynamically, this group of cardiomyopathies resembles constrictive pericarditis.

The abnormal diastolic filling occurs as a result of infiltration of the endocardium or myocardium with fibroelastic tissue similar to that seen in Löffler's endocarditis, endomyocardial fibrosis, and amyloidosis.

DIAGNOSTIC STUDIES

Study	Hypertrophic Cardiomyopathy	Dilated Cardiomyopathy	Restrictive Cardiomyopathy
Chest roentgenogram	Enlarged cardiac silhouette (mild to moderate)	Enlarged cardiac silhouette; prominence of left ventricle (LV) (moderate to marked)	Cardiac enlargement (mild)
Electrocardiogram (ECG) (24-hour ambulatory monitor)	LV hypertrophy; ST segment and T wave changes; Q waves may be seen in precordial leads; atrial arrhythmias	LV hypertrophy; sinus tachycardia; atrial and ventricular arrhythmias; ST segment and T wave changes; conduction disturbances	Low-voltage; conduction disturbances
Echocardiogram	Asymmetric septal hypertrophy (ASH); narrow LV outflow tract; systolic anterior motion of mitral valve; decreased internal dimension of LV	LV dilation; abnormal diastolic mitral valve motion; enlarged atria	Increased LV wall thickness and mass; small or normal LV cavity; normal systolic function; pericardial effusion
Radionuclide studies	ASH; hyperdynamic systolic function; LV size small or normal	LV dilation and dysfunction	Myocardial infiltration; small or normal LV cavity; normal systolic function
Cardiac catheterization	Decreased LV compliance; mitral regurgitation; hyperdynamic systolic function; LV outflow obstruction	LV enlargement and dysfunction; mitral and tricuspid regurgitation; elevated diastolic filling pressures; decreased cardiac output	Decreased LV compliance; normal systolic function; elevated diastolic filling process

TREATMENT PLAN

Surgical

Myotomy-myectomy—for patient with hypertrophic cardiomyopathy who has intractable symptoms and severe obstruction; hypertrophied septum is excised, which diminishes left ventricular gradient and mitral regurgitation; procedure improves symptoms but has not been reported to prolong life

Excision of fibrotic endocardium—successful in limited number of cases of restrictive cardiomyopathy; procedure apparently decreases ventricular filling pressures and increases cardiac output

Other surgical interventions—essentially nonexistent; valve replacement considered in individual cases but generally not favored; cardiac transplantation may soon be favorable alternative for many patients but at present remains experimental treatment requiring enormous financial investment

Chemotherapeutic

Hypertrophic cardiomyopathy—goals of drug therapy are to decrease ventricular contractility and increase ventricular volume and left ventricular outflow

Cardiac glycosides: digitalis

Indications: Not favored in management of hypertrophic cardiomyopathy because it increases contractility and therefore degree of obstruction; used in presence of atrial fibrillation with rapid ventricular rates or left ventricular dysfunction without obstruction

β-Adrenergic blocking agents: propranolol (Inderal)

Indications: Principal mode of therapy; has negative inotropic effects on myocardial contractility and thus is believed to prevent increase in outflow obstruction, decrease myocardial oxygen consumption, and exert antiarrhythmic actions

Antiarrhythmic drugs: verapamil (Calan)

Indications: calcium channel blocking agent that has given best results in management of these patients; has been shown to decrease left ventricular outflow obstruction and increase exercise tolerance[13]

Usual dosage: 80-160 mg q8h (not to exceed 480 mg/day)

Dilated cardiomyopathy—cannot be halted or reversed by any pharmacologic agent; pharmacologic interventions directed largely by symptoms; as with any patient in congestive heart failure, digitalis, diuretic, and vasodilator therapy used (see p. 46); antiarrhythmics such as quinidine and procainamide used to treat arrhythmias

Restrictive cardiomyopathy—pharmacologic agents directed by underlying disorder; digitalis and diuretics often employed to treat arrhythmias and signs of failure, but their effectiveness is limited

Electromechanical

Hemodynamic monitoring—initiated as means of assessing left ventricular function and cardiac output

Intra-aortic balloon counterpulsation—used to sustain severely depressed ventricular function

Cardiac monitoring—used to determine presence of atrial or ventricular arrhythmias or conduction defects and to assess effectiveness of antiarrhythmic agents

Cardioversion—used in treatment of atrial fibrillation with rapid ventricular response

Supportive

Restriction of sodium and fluid intake
Oxygen therapy

ASSESSMENT: AREAS OF CONCERN

Area of Concern	Hypertrophic Cardiomyopathy	Dilated Cardiomyopathy	Restrictive Cardiomyopathy
General complaints	Dyspnea; shortness of breath; angina pectoris; fatigue; palpitations; syncope (may be exertional)	Dyspnea; fatigue; complaints associated with biventricular failure	Dyspnea; fatigue; complaints associated with right ventricular failure
Arterial pressure		Normal or low systolic; narrowed pulse pressure	
Arterial pulse	Brisk carotid upstroke	Low amplitude and volume; pulsus alternans	
Jugular venous pressure		Distended; prominent a and v waves	Distended
Palpation	Apical systolic thrill and heave	Apical impulse displaced laterally; parasternal impulses and heaves; pulsatile liver	Apical impulse difficult to palpate
Auscultation	Systolic murmur at lower left sternal border increasing in intensity with Valsalva maneuver; S_4 gallop	Murmurs of mitral and tricuspid regurgitation; S_3 and S_4 gallops; pulmonary rales	Murmurs of mitral regurgitation; S_3 and S_4 gallops; heart sounds distant

NURSING DIAGNOSES and NURSING INTERVENTIONS

Nursing Diagnosis	Nursing Intervention
Cardiac output, alteration in: decreased	Encourage bed rest. Limit self-care activities. Monitor arterial pressure, pulmonary capillary wedge pressure, cardiac output, and ECG every 1 to 2 hours. Observe for signs and symptoms of decreased left ventricular functioning, including chest pain, syncope, peripheral constriction, and cyanosis. Administer drugs as ordered. *Convalescent care:* Progressively increase activity level as indicated by improvement in patient status. Monitor vital signs and report any changes in heart rate or blood pressure. Teach patient and family the importance of monitoring vital signs and how to check blood pressure and pulse accurately.
Coping, ineffective individual	Determine baseline knowledge of disease. Answer all questions about disease and future health. Encourage discussion of feelings of hopelessness and fears. Assist patient to participate in decision-making process with regard to any adjustments in life-style. Provide patient education. Include family and/or significant other in care. Encourage family to learn cardiopulmonary resuscitation.
Gas exchange: impaired (related to elevated pulmonary capillary pressure)	Monitor arterial blood gases frequently. Administer oxygen therapy as ordered via nasal prongs, mask, or positive-pressure device. Administer morphine sulfate intravenously to reduce hyperventilation per protocol. Elevate head of bed. Auscultate breath sounds every hour to determine increases in congestion and adequacy of ventilatory effort. Prepare for intubation and assisted ventilation if required. Explain all procedures and modalities briefly to patient to prevent hyperventilation resulting from fear or anxiety.
Fluid volume: alteration in, excess	Maintain patent intravenous line for drug administration. Administer diuretics as ordered to decrease circulating volume. Restrict sodium and fluid intake. Weigh patient daily (same time of day, same amount of clothing) to determine fluid loss or retention. Monitor intake and output. Monitor serum electrolytes, especially sodium and potassium. Inspect for increased or decreased jugular venous distention. Auscultate heart tones and breath sounds every 1 to 2 hours for increased congestion.
Nutrition: alteration in	Maintain fluid and sodium restrictions. Teach good nutritional habits and alternative seasonings to make low-sodium diet more palatable.
Comfort, alteration in: pain	Administer morphine sulfate as ordered. Stay with patient as much as possible. Explain all procedures and routines to patient. Provide over-bed table and pillows as needed to maintain position of comfort. Allow family to stay with patient and assist with patient care.
Knowledge deficit	Begin teaching patient about disease as soon as possible, including lifelong dietary restrictions, medications, exercise limitations and potentials, and complications.

Patient Education

1. Describe the nature and type of cardiomyopathy.
2. Explain the limitations of the disease on life-style and the prognosis.
3. Explain the signs and symptoms to report to the physician.
4. Describe activity allowances and limitations; explain the importance of avoiding isometric exercises.
5. Explain dietary and fluid restrictions.
6. Explain the name, purpose, dosage, and side effects of prescribed medications; warn against the effects of abruptly stopping propranolol.
7. Explain the need for daily weights when ordered.

EVALUATION

Patient Outcome	Data Indicating That Outcome is Reached
Ventricular volume is increased; outflow obstruction is decreased.	Cardiac output and left ventricular end-diastolic pressure (LVEDP) are increased. Fatigue, dyspnea, and angina are relieved.
LV diastolic volume is decreased; ventricular contractility is improved.	LVEDP is decreased. Stroke volume is improved. Patient loses weight. Dyspnea and shortness of breath are relieved.
Patient copes effectively with diagnosis.	Patient follows up with medical therapy. Patient reports taking medications. Patient verbalizes feeling less anxious and fearful.

VALVULAR HEART DISEASE

Valvular heart disease is an acquired or congenital disorder of a cardiac valve, characterized by stenosis and obstructed blood flow or by valvular degeneration and regurgitation of blood.

With the introduction of antibiotic therapy and with improved diagnostic procedures, the incidence of valvular heart disease (VHD) has declined over the past three decades. It is most commonly a chronic illness, and symptoms requiring therapy may take years to develop. Valvular heart disease may also occur as an acute illness following trauma or myocardial infarction.

PATHOPHYSIOLOGY

The etiology of valvular heart disease can be classified into congenital and acquired disorders.

Congenital disorders include bicuspid aortic valve and pulmonary stenosis. Although not usually classified as valvular heart disease, tricuspid and pulmonary atresia and Ebstein's anomaly are all defects involving valve function. Mitral valve prolapse may also fall into this category.

Rheumatic fever and endocarditis account for the greatest number of cases of acquired valvular heart disease,[11,78] but other disorders such as Marfan's syndrome, cardiomyopathy, myocardial infarction, and myxomatous degeneration of the mitral valve, as well as trauma, can also lead to valve dysfunction.

Cardiac valves are unidirectional, ensuring efficient flow of blood throughout the heart, the pulmonary circulation, and the systemic circulation. Valve abnormalities occur when the integrity of the valve leaflets or the surrounding structures is disrupted.

Two basic valve abnormalities exist: stenosis and regurgitation. In stenosis, narrowing of the valve orifice occurs as a result of thickening and rigidity of the valve leaflets. Stenosis produces an obstruction to flow across the valve, increasing the pressure gradient. In regurgitation (insufficiency, incompetency), calcification, scarring, and retraction of the leaflets or adjacent structures lead to an incomplete valve closure that results in retrograde blood flow.

Mixed lesions can occur and produce both stenosis and regurgitation. In addition, more than one valve may be affected. The four major valve disorders are considered in the following sections.

Mitral Stenosis

The most common cause of mitral stenosis is rheumatic valvulitis that leads to fibrotic thickening and fusion of the valve commissures. In addition, scarring of the free margins of the anterior and posterior leaflets occurs with shortening and thickening of the chordae tendineae, which may contribute to the mitral regurgitation often seen with mitral stenosis.

The normal mitral valve orifice is 4 to 6 cm². When

this opening is reduced, flow across the valve is obstructed, increasing the pressure gradient necessary to eject blood from the left atrium to the left ventricle. The pressure gradient rises to ensure maintenance of cardiac output. When the mitral orifice is decreased to 1.5 cm^2, cardiac output drops and symptoms appear with exertion. As the disease progresses, the mean left atrial pressure rises, causing left atrial chamber enlargement. The increased left atrial pressure is reflected in the pulmonary capillaries and pulmonary artery. As pulmonary capillary pressure rises, fluid flows back across the alveolar membrane, eventually exceeding oncotic pressure of the plasma proteins in the blood and forcing fluid out of the capillaries into the lung. If this fluid cannot be removed by lymphatic drainage, pulmonary edema develops.

Mitral Regurgitation

Rheumatic fever, the usual cause of mitral regurgitation, produces thickening, scarring, rigidity, and calcification of the valve leaflets. The commissures become fused with the chordae tendineae, causing shortening and retraction of the leaflets, which prevents them from complete closure during systole. A nonrheumatic cause of mitral regurgitation is myocardial infarction, which causes dilation of the left ventricle and displacement of the papillary muscles. Papillary muscle dysfunction may also occur as a result of rupture or fibrosis caused by ischemia, infarction, and ventricular aneurysm at the base of a papillary muscle. In addition, annular dilation may lead to an incompetent mitral apparatus. The most common cause is left ventricular dilation resulting from coronary artery disease or congestive cardiomyopathy.

As mitral valve incompetence progresses, the retrograde flow to the left atrium causes left atrial pressure to rise. This pressure is reflected in the pulmonary veins, leading to transudation of fluid into the lungs.

The progressive increase in backward flow causes atrial dilation and enlargement. The left ventricle becomes hypertrophied, since it must deal with the larger volume of blood that is lost to the left atrium during systole.

Aortic Stenosis

Although rheumatic heart disease can lead to aortic stenosis, the most common cause is a congenital bicuspid valve. This defect occurs in 1% of the population, with a preponderance in males (3:1).

The normal aortic valve orifice measures 2.6 to 3.5 cm^2. Valve narrowing results from calcification of the leaflets. Calcification may extend into the aortic wall or onto the anterior leaflet of the mitral valve, which accounts for the mitral disease commonly occurring with aortic stenosis. Calcification may also extend into the conduction system, leading to conduction defects. As the disease progresses, calcification makes the valve inflexible, reducing the opening to a small slit.

As the aortic valve orifice decreases, left ventricular pressure rises to generate pressures sufficient to eject a normal stroke volume and propel flow across the valve into the aorta. This obstruction to left ventricular outflow leads to a pressure gradient between the aorta and left ventricle during systole. To maintain flow across the narrowed valve orifice, wall thickness gradually increases in the pressure-overloaded left ventricle, leading eventually to hypertrophy. In time the flow across the valve becomes fixed and cardiac output does not increase in response to demand. During exercise the increased flow to extremities in the setting of fixed cardiac output causes a decreased cerebral blood flow, resulting in dizziness or syncope.

Left atrial hypertrophy occurs in a compensatory attempt to increase cardiac output. To produce a forceful atrial contraction, left ventricular end-diastolic pressure (LVEDP) rises, which in turn increases the myocardial fiber stretch and leads to increased contraction and improvement in stroke volume.

The clinical course of aortic stenosis depends on the size of the valve orifice and the compensated left ventricle. When myocardial contractility falls, the left ventricle dilates, causing diastolic and left atrial pressures to increase further.

The onset of symptoms of heart failure indicates moderate to severe disease, and death often occurs less than 5 years after symptoms appear. Sudden death is associated with severe aortic stenosis (0.5 to 0.7 cm^2).

Aortic Regurgitation

Incompetency of the aortic valve is attributed to numerous causes. Rheumatic fever, syphilis, and infective endocarditis are common causes. Connective tissue disorders such as Marfan's syndrome are also implicated in this disease.

The basic hemodynamic problem in aortic regurgitation is a volume-overloaded left ventricle. Blood ejected during normal systole reenters the left ventricle in diastole. To compensate for this regurgitant volume, the left ventricle must produce a higher stroke volume by increasing the systolic pressure, resulting in eventual hypertrophy of the left ventricle.

With time, LVEDP and left atrial pressure increase. As myocardial contractility diminishes and failure takes place, mitral regurgitation may occur as a result of malposition of papillary muscles.

DIAGNOSTIC STUDIES

Study	Mitral Stenosis	Mitral Regurgitation	Aortic Stenosis	Aortic Regurgitation
Radionuclide studies	To determine resting and exercise ejection fraction	To determine resting and exercise ejection fraction	To determine resting and exercise ejection fraction	To determine resting and exercise ejection fraction
Cardiac catheterization	Pressure across mitral valve increased; left atrial (LA) pressure increased; PCWP increased; low cardiac output	Left ventricular end-diastolic pressure (LVEDP) increased; left atrial pressure (LAP) increased; angiography with contrast media performed to quantify regurgitation	Pressure gradient in systole across aortic valve; LVEDP increased	Pulse pressure increased; LVEDP increased; LAP increased; angiography with contrast media performed to quantify regurgitation
Electrocardiogram (ECG)	LA enlargement; notched P wave (P mitrale); right ventricular (RV) hypertrophy	LA enlargement; LV hypertrophy; atrial fibrillation	LV hypertrophy; conduction defects: first-degree A-V block, left bundle branch block	LV hypertrophy
Chest roentgenogram	LA and RV enlargement; pulmonary venous congestion; interstitial pulmonary edema	LA and LV enlargement; pulmonary vascular congestion	Poststenotic aortic dilation; aortic valve calcification	Aortic valve calcification; LV enlargement; dilation of ascending aorta
Echocardiogram	Decreased excursion of leaflets; diminished E to F slope	LA enlargement; hyperdynamic LV	Nonrestricted movement of aortic valve; thickening of LV wall	LV dilation; diastolic fluttering of anterior leaflet

TREATMENT PLAN

Surgical

Indicated when medical therapy no longer alleviates clinical symptoms or when there is diagnostic evidence of progressive myocardial failure (such as progressive enlargement of heart)

Open mitral commissurotomy (valvulotomy)—surgical splitting of fused valve leaflet by inserting expandable dilator through apex of ventricle and, with guidance provided by surgeon's finger, placing it in mitral orifice and separating fused commissures; palliative procedure performed only for pure mitral stenosis that involves leaflets and not chordae; contraindicated in patients with history of emboli

Valvular annuloplasty—reparative procedure of valve ring, chordae, or papillary muscle performed primarily for mitral and tricuspid regurgitation

Valve replacement—replacement of stenotic or incompetent valve with bioprosthetic or mechanical valve; commonly used valves include pynolite tilting disks, porcine heterografts, pericardial valves, and ball-in-cage valves

Chemotherapeutic

Guided by patient's clinical signs and symptoms

Digitalis and diuretics for heart failure (see pp. 45 and 48)

Quinidine, procainamide, propranolol for arrhythmias (see pp. 25 and 26)

Anticoagulants for patients in atrial fibrillation who are at risk for systemic or pulmonary embolization; warfarin sodium (Coumadin) in doses titrated to maintain prothrombin time at two times control

Antibiotic prophylaxis before any procedure that increases risk of endocarditis

Electromechanical

Cardioversion—indicated for patients with mitral stenosis in atrial fibrillation to decrease risk of emboli

Supportive

Dictated by severity of valvular disorder (see pp. 24 and 48 for supportive care of patients in heart failure or with arrhythmias)

Diet therapy—sodium restriction for patients with mild to moderate signs of pulmonary congestion

ASSESSMENT: AREAS OF CONCERN

Area of Concern	Mitral Stenosis	Mitral Regurgitation	Aortic Stenosis	Aortic Regurgitation
General complaints	Fatigue; dyspnea on exertion; palpitations; hemoptysis; hoarseness; orthopnea; paroxysmal nocturnal dyspnea	Dyspnea; fatigue; exercise intolerance; orthopnea; palpitations	Fatigue; dyspnea; orthopnea; angina pectoris; dizziness; syncope	Dyspnea on exertion; palpitations; orthopnea; exertional chest pain
Physical examination	Resting tachycardia; irregular pulse; jugular venous distention increased in presence of right ventricular (RV) failure; prominent "a" wave in presence of pulmonary hypertension (absent in atrial fibrillation)	Irregular pulse; sharp upstroke of arterial pulse; jugular venous distention increased in presence of RV failure; prominent "a" wave in presence of increased RV pressure	Early: normal blood pressure; late: systolic pressure decreased; narrow pulse pressure; carotid pulse slow with small pulse volume	Arterial pulsations: bounding pulse with rapid rise and fall (water-hammer pulse); widened pulse pressure; head bobbing (Musset's sign); skin warm, damp, and flushed
Palpation	Diastolic thrill at apex	Apical impulse forceful and displaced downward and to left	Systolic thrill palpable at base of heart; apical pulse strong and sustained throughout systole	Diastolic thrill along left sternal border; laterally displaced apical impulse; systolic thrill in jugular notch and along carotid arteries
Auscultation (Fig. 1-40)	Loud S_1; opening snap; low snap; low-pitched, rumbling diastolic murmur	Diminished or absent S_1; wide splitting of S_2; S_3, S_4 heard in severe regurgitation; holosystolic murmur heard best at apex	Diminished or absent A_2; crescendo-decrescendo harsh systolic murmur heard best at base (second intercostal space to right of sternum); aortic ejection sound	Decrescendo diastolic murmur (blowing), high pitched and heard best at base (second intercostal space to right of sternum); systolic ejection murmur heard best at base

Fig. 1-40

Auscultation of valvular heart disease murmurs. **A,** Mitral stenosis. **B,** Mitral regurgitation. **C,** Aortic stenosis. **D,** Aortic regurgitation.

From Guzzetta, C.E., and Dossey, B.M.: Cardiovascular nursing: bodymind tapestry, St. Louis, 1984, The C.V. Mosby Co.

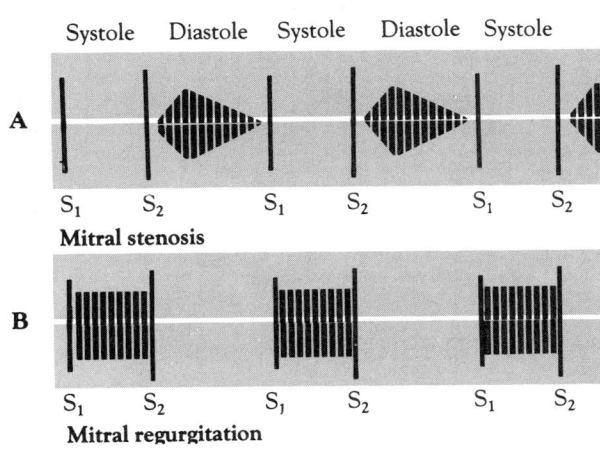
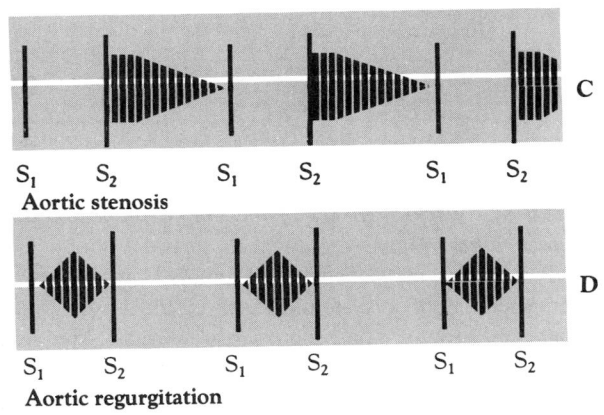

NURSING DIAGNOSES and NURSING INTERVENTIONS

Nursing Diagnosis	Nursing Intervention
Cardiac output, alteration in: decreased	Establish baseline assessment of cardiovascular status and evaluate response to therapy. Monitor vital signs every 2 to 4 hours. Administer medications as ordered to maintain blood pressure. Limit activities.
Fluid volume, alteration in: excess	Auscultate breath and heart sounds. Assess for increase or decrease in jugular venous distention. Administer diuretic and vasodilator therapy as ordered. Monitor nutrition within dietary sodium and fluid restrictions. Weigh patient daily (same time of day, same amount of clothing). Monitor intake and output. Assess level of comfort, determining irritating factors and means of eliminating them.
Comfort, alteration in: pain	For chest pain and shortness of breath, promote rest and relaxation by assisting with care during pain episodes. Administer medications as ordered. Instruct patient to limit activities during pain episodes. Provide oxygen therapy as ordered.
Knowledge deficit	Assess patient's level of knowledge and teach patient about disease, including etiology, medications, diet restrictions, exercise levels, and possible complications. Assist patient during diagnostic workup and assist with decision for medical or surgical treatment. Include patient's family in teaching and decision-making process.

Patient Education

1. Instruct the patient in the name, dose, and purpose of medications.
2. Instruct the patient in the disease process and associated symptoms to report to the physician.
3. Explain activity allowances and limitations.
4. Explain diet and fluid restrictions.
5. Instruct the patient about antibiotic prophylaxis to prevent infectious endocarditis (see p. 77).

EVALUATION

Patient Outcome	Data Indicating That Outcome is Reached
Cardiac output is adequate.	Lungs are clear. Patient reports improvement of symptoms. Heart rate is within acceptable limits.

PERICARDITIS

Pericarditis is an inflammatory process involving the parietal and visceral layers of the pericardium and outer myocardium.

Pericarditis may occur as an isolated process or as a complication of a systemic disease. Its designation as acute or chronic is based primarily on onset, frequency of occurrence, and symptoms. Acute pericarditis, which can occur within 2 weeks of the offending condition, lasts up to 6 weeks. It may be accompanied by effusion or tamponade. Chronic pericarditis may follow acute pericarditis and may last up to 6 months.

PATHOPHYSIOLOGY

Because of the close proximity of the pericardium to structures such as the pleura, lung, sternum, diaphragm, and myocardium, pericarditis may be the consequence

Table 1-1
Characteristics of Pericardial Fluid

Characteristic	Normal Fluid	Exudate Effusion
Appearance	Clear	Clear or turbid with fibrin sheds; straw or amber color; may appear hemorrhagic because of RBCs; may be purulent
Volume	50 ml	>100 ml (up to 3 L)
Specific gravity	<1.015	>1.015 (usually >1.017)
Total protein	<2 g/dl	>3 g/dl
Seromucin clot	Negative	Positive
Coagulation	Uncommon	Usual
Cells	Few	Few
Glucose	Nearly equal to plasma glucose	Nearly equal to plasma glucose
Culture	Negative	Negative

of a number of inflammatory or infectious processes. The most common cause is idiopathic, probably viral; this generally has a favorable prognosis. The causes of pericarditis can be summarized as follows:

Viral (idiopathic)—organism may never be isolated

Infectious—bacterial, tuberculous, fungal

Following myocardial infarction (Dressler's syndrome or postmyocardial infarction syndrome)

Following cardiac surgery (postpericardiotomy syndrome)

Neoplastic diseases

Chemotherapy

Radiotherapy

Uremia

Trauma, blunt or penetrating

Connective tissue diseases—systemic lupus erythematosus, rheumatoid arthritis, scleroderma, dermatomyositis

Agents or processes causing pericardial inflammation do so by direct extension or by irritation. Under normal conditions the pericardial sac contains up to 50 ml of clear, serouslike fluid. When an acute injury occurs, an exudate of fibrin, white blood cells, and endothelial cells is released, covering the parietal and visceral layers of pericardium. Resultant friction between the pericardial layers causes irritation and inflammation of the surrounding pleura and tissues. This fibrinous exudate may localize to one region of the heart or be generalized. Acute pericarditis may be "dry" and fibrinous or obstruct the heart's venous and lymphatic drainage, causing seepage of fibrin exudate and serous fluid into the pericardial sac, which creates pericardial effusion.[74]

Serofibrinous exudates occur in varying amounts from 100 ml to 3 L and may appear straw colored or turbid with fibrin strands. The exudate of pyrogenic pericarditis is purulent. The characteristics of pericardial exudate fluid are summarized in Table 1-1.

A slowly developing effusion of moderate amount (350 to 500 ml) may not alter cardiovascular dynamics. However, a rapidly accumulating effusion, regardless of amount, can interfere with diastolic filling and lead to cardiac tamponade.

The clinical syndrome of chronic pericarditis can occur in a variety of forms, including chronic pericardial effusion and constrictive or adhesive pericarditis. Chronic effusion may lead eventually to constrictive effusion, as described in the following paragraphs.

Constrictive pericarditis is characterized by pericardial thickening and scarring of the parietal or visceral pericardium. The layers become densely adherent to each other, obliterating the pericardial space. This adherence eventually involves the epicardial surface of the myocardium, causing the pericardium to become a totally noncompliant structure. In some cases the pericardium becomes calcified.

As the pericardium becomes scarred and rigid, normal diastolic filling of the heart is impeded. In severe cases, left ventricular end-diastolic volume may be less than stroke volume, causing the stroke volume to be reduced with a subsequent drop in cardiac output. The normal compensatory tachycardia is unable to improve the cardiac output because of the constriction of the myocardium.

Constrictive pericarditis is usually generalized to all four chambers but may be localized to areas such as the right ventricle, pulmonary artery, or aortic root. When the chambers are uniformly involved, left and right ventricular diastolic pressure and atrial pressures equalize. As stroke volume diminishes, left and right filling pressures rise. When this is combined with reduced cardiac output, systemic and pulmonary congestion results.

DIAGNOSTIC STUDIES

Laboratory tests

Complete blood count and differential

To determine infectious processes and inflammatory response

Fig. 1-41

In acute pericarditis, ST segment elevation is typically upward and concave in leads I, II, aV$_f$, and V$_4$ to V$_6$.

From Guzzetta, C.E., and Dossey, B.M.: Cardiovascular nursing: bodymind tapestry, St. Louis, 1984, The C.V. Mosby Co.

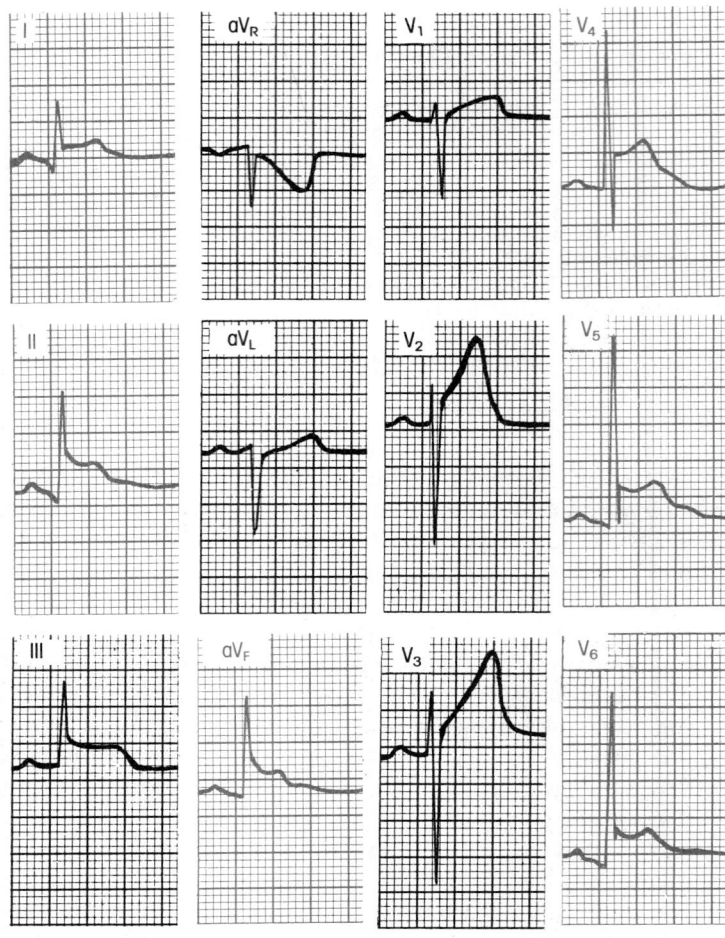

Sedimentation rate
  Usually elevated
Viral serology studies
  Performed during acute and convalescent periods
Blood and urine cultures
  Identification of organism in infectious process

Electrocardiogram (ECG)
Acute pericarditis
  Stage I (Fig. 1-41)
    ST-T segment elevation in left ventricular leads V$_5$, V$_6$, I, II, aV$_L$, and aV$_F$ during first few days; PR interval depression
  Stage II
    Return of ST segment to baseline; PR interval depression may persist
  Stage III
    T wave inversions
  Stage IV
    Normalization of T waves
  Low-voltage QRS complexes in presence of pericardial effusion
  Atrial arrhythmias

Constrictive pericarditis
  Wide P wave in leads I, II, and V$_6$; Q waves deep and wide; T waves flattened or inverted; low QRS voltage

Chest roentgenogram
Cardiac silhouette
  Enlargement depends on underlying disease or amount of pericardial effusion (enlarges with 250 ml or more of accumulated fluid) (Fig. 1-42)
Acute pericarditis
  Normal if pericardial fluid less than 250 ml
Constrictive pericarditis
  Normal or small; enlargement occurs as result of pericardial thickening or effusion; calcification of pericardium; pleural effusion

Echocardiogram
Confirms accumulation of free fluid in pericardial sac
  As fluid accumulates, separation of pericardial and epicardial echoes occurs, resulting in echo-free space; minimum of 20 ml detected

Fig. 1-42
A, Normal chest roentgenogram.
B, With pericardial effusion, cardiac silhouette is enlarged and has globular shape *(arrows)*.

From Guzzetta, C.E., and Dossey, B.M.: Cardiovascular nursing: bodymind tapestry, St. Louis, 1984, The C.V. Mosby Co.

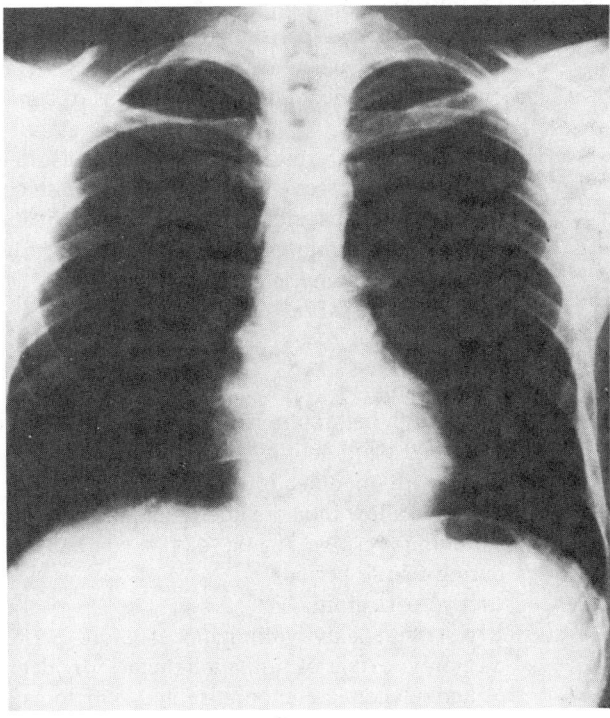
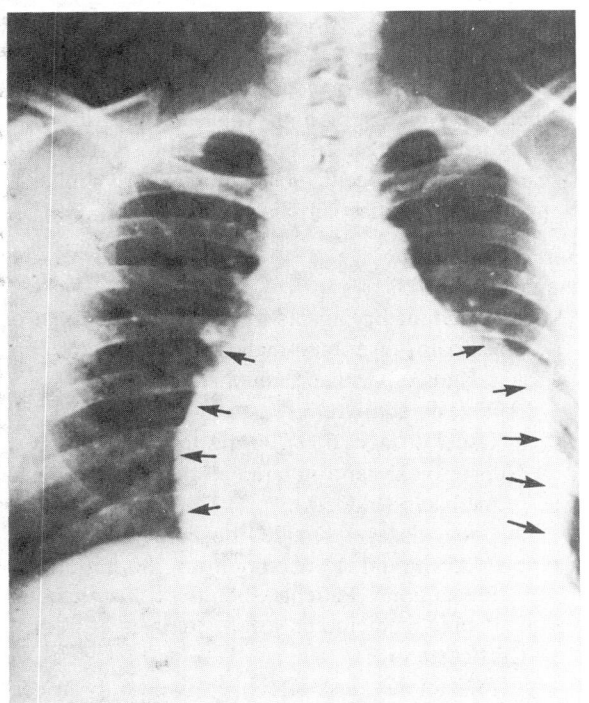

Evaluates ventricular function

In constrictive pericarditis demonstrates reduced motion of posterior wall of left ventricle (LV); abnormal movement of the interventricular septum characterized by flattening in systole and paradoxic movement in diastole; two separate echoes representing visceral and parietal pericardium separated by clear space of 1 mm throughout cardiac cycle

Radionuclide blood pool scanning (technetium-labeled macroaggregated albumin and thallium)

Demonstrates shadow of pericardial effusion outside of cardiac chambers; seen as abnormal space between heart and liver or heart and lungs

Cardiac catheterization

Demonstrates characteristic pericardial shadow outside opacified cardiac chambers, which are increased by pericardial thickening or fluid accumulation

Constrictive pericarditis

Increased left and right atrial (LA, RA) pressures; loss of respiratory variation of the RA pressure curve; elevated pulmonary artery (PA) systolic pressure (35 to 40 mm Hg); elevated diastolic pressures equal in all four chambers, rarely differing by more than 5 mm Hg at rest or during exercise; cardiac output normal in early stages, later decreased (<2.3 L/min/m^2); ejection fraction normal or decreased

TREATMENT PLAN

Surgical

Pericardiocentesis—removal of pericardial fluid or blood by aspiration through needle or catheter inserted into parietal pericardium; indicated when persistent or large effusions are compromising left ventricular function (see p. 108 for care)

Pericardial window—open pericardial drainage implemented for acute suppurative and chronic effusions: has certain advantages over pericardiocentesis: multiple aspirations can be avoided, pericardial tissue can be obtained for culture, pericardium can be visualized, and clots and fibrin deposits can be removed

Pericardiectomy—surgical removal of visceral and parietal pericardium; has excellent long-term benefits; operative mortality of about 10%; best results when myocardial fibrosis and ventricular atrophy are not far advanced and when total or near-total pericardiectomy is performed; if hemodynamic improvement not seen immediately, elevated pressures and abnormal waveforms continue for several weeks owing to atrophy of ventricles that have been immobilized for long periods—thus early pericardiectomy is encouraged before dense fibrosis and myocardial atrophy occur; postoperative care similar to that of any cardiac surgical patient (see p. 94)

Chemotherapeutic

Acute pericarditis

Anti-inflammatory agents for symptomatic relief of chest pain, fever, and malaise in absence of clinical signs of cardiac tamponade

Analgesic-antipyretics: aspirin

Usual dosage: 600-900 mg to qid

Nonsteroidal anti-inflammatory agents: indomethacin (Indocin)

Usual dosage: Divided doses beginning with 25 mg qid, to maximum of 200 mg/day

Precautions: Patients should be instructed to take medicine on a full stomach

Corticosteroids

Indications: Less effective; given only in persistent recurring pericarditis and effusion

Constrictive pericarditis

Chemotherapeutic agents aimed at specific cause; for example, patients with known or suspected tuberculosis should receive antituberculous therapy before and after pericardiectomy

Electromechanical

Electrocardiography—performed to rule out myocardial infarction, when cardiac tamponade is suspected, and if patient demonstrates signs of cardiac decompensation

Hemodynamic monitoring—indicated if cardiac tamponade is evident (see p. 73); for patients with constrictive pericarditis, closer monitoring of right atrial and pulmonary arterial pressures and cardiac output; after pericardiectomy, elevated pressures may continue for several weeks or months

Supportive

Acute pericarditis

Bed rest with bathroom privileges during period of fever and pain; activity limited during acute period, with modification of all activities for 2 weeks to allow inflammatory reaction of the pericardium to resolve; regular diet; encourage fluids during febrile period

Constrictive pericarditis

Bed rest with activity limitations before pericardiectomy; extent of limitation dictated by degree of hemodynamic compromise and symptoms

ASSESSMENT: AREAS OF CONCERN

Area of Concern	Acute Pericarditis	Constrictive Pericarditis
General complaints	Chest pain: location retrosternal or precordial radiating to neck and back, sudden pleuritic-like pain that worsens with deep inspiration, movement, or lying down and is relieved by sitting up or leaning forward; sharp, deep, persistent ache; tachypnea; shallow breathing; dyspnea in presence of pleural effusion or owing to impaired cardiac filling from compression of heart; restlessness; anxiety; malaise; dysphagia	Exertional dyspnea; fatigue; orthopnea; palpitations; paroxysmal nocturnal dyspnea; cough; peripheral edema
Physical examination	Low-grade temperature (39° C [102° F]); may be associated with diaphoresis and chills; auscultation: pericardial friction rub—best heard with patient leaning forward, heard in second, third, or fourth intercostal space to left of sternal border or at apex, loudest during inspiration, varies in intensity (grade 4 to 5), may be transient, triphasic consisting of presystolic, systolic, and diastolic components, scratchy, grating	Afebrile; elevated jugular venous pressure with presence of Kussmaul sign (increased distention during inspiration); arterial pressure normal or slightly reduced; diffuse precordial movement; decreased amplitude; absence of localized apical impulse; parodoxic pulse (rarely exceeds 15 mm Hg); auscultation: quiet, distant heart sounds, pericardial knock—early diastolic sound, accentuated with inspiration and heard best along lower left sternal border; clinical signs of elevated venous pressure: peripheral edema, hepatomegaly, ascites

NURSING DIAGNOSES and NURSING INTERVENTIONS

Nursing Diagnosis	Nursing Intervention
Anxiety	Provide supportive care. Explain disease process and procedures as they are implemented. Ensure quiet environment; reduce external stimuli as much as possible. Maintain family contact.
Comfort, alteration in: pain	Assess quality of chest pain. Administer pain medication as ordered for pericardial chest pain. Encourage bed rest with head of bed elevated or position of comfort; have patient lean forward on over-bed table.
Cardiac output, alteration in: decreased	Assess for signs of cardiac tamponade (see p. 74), including narrowing pulse pressure and pulsus paradoxus. Monitor vital signs for ventricular decompensation. Prepare for pericardiocentesis or pericardiectomy as indicated by clinical status.
Fluid volume, alteration in: excess	Auscultate heart and breath sounds every 1 to 2 hours during inflammatory period. Observe for increase in jugular venous pressure. Maintain accurate intake and output record. Maintain patent IV.

Patient Education

1. Explain the underlying cause and disease process.
2. Instruct the patient in signs and symptoms of recurring inflammation and tell the patient to notify the physician if they occur.
3. Explain the purpose, method of administration, and side effects of medications.

EVALUATION

Patient Outcome	Data Indicating That Outcome is Reached
Patient demonstrates decreased anxiety.	Patient verbalizes relief of pain. Patient demonstrates ability to rest and sleep without complaint. Patient appears relaxed. Patient tolerates routine activities and procedures without complaining of pain or shortness of breath.
There is no pericardial irritation.	ECG is normal. There is no friction rub or chest pain. White blood cell count and sedimentation rate are normal.
Patient shows an increased level of understanding.	Patient identifies signs and symptoms to report to physician. Patient verbalizes knowledge regarding disease, activity allowances and limitations, and medications.

CARDIAC TAMPONADE

Cardiac tamponade is acute cardiac compression caused when fluid accumulation within the pericardial sac exerts increased pressure around the heart. The result is restriction of flow in and out of the ventricles.

PATHOPHYSIOLOGY

Tamponade is most commonly caused by acute pericarditis but is quite common in patients with malignant and uremic pericardial effusions. A hemopericardium, bleeding into the pericardial spaces, may occur as a result of chest trauma, cardiac surgery, myocardial rupture, aortic dissection, or anticoagulant therapy.

As noted previously, the pericardial sac normally holds 30 to 50 ml of fluid, creating subatmospheric intrapericardial pressures of approximately -1 to -3 mm Hg during expiration and -5 mm Hg with inspiration. An increase in pericardial fluid can cause a rise in intrapericardial pressure, first to 0 mm Hg and eventually to a positive value. However, it is the rate of accumulation, not the volume, that determines the degree to which ventricular filling becomes restricted and whether cardiac tamponade will ensue.

When pericardial fluid accumulates slowly, large volumes (1 to 2 L) can be readily accommodated because of the stretching of pericardial fibers. During rapid filling, however, the pericardium fails to stretch, causing intrapericardial pressure to rise to a level exceeding normal filling pressure of the ventricles. When this occurs, filling of the ventricles is restricted, stroke volume decreases, and cardiac output falls. These hemodynamic alterations are followed by hypotension and shock. Pulsus paradoxus, an important hemodynamic feature of tamponade, is an abnormally large inspiratory fall in arterial pressure. When left ventricular filling and stroke volume are decreased, with inspiration blood pools in the lung and right side of the heart, increasing intrapericardial pressure. Therefore, during inspiration a greater negative intrathoracic pressure occurs, resulting in a dramatic fall in systolic blood pressure and pulse volume. The arterial blood pressure may normally fall 4 to 5 mm Hg during inspiration, but a decrease of 10 mm Hg or more is considered abnormal.

DIAGNOSTIC STUDIES

Chest roentgenogram
Enlarged cardiac silhouette (globular configuration depending on degree of effusion); lung fields clear

Electrocardiogram
Nonspecific ST and T wave changes; diminished voltage with specific alteration (electrical alternans) in QRS complex; peaked T waves in precordial leads associated with hemopericardium; changes associated with acute pericarditis (see p. 70)

Echocardiogram
Increased pericardial fluid; paradoxic septal motion; septum moves toward left ventricle during inspiration as right ventricle fills; may be possible to estimate fluid volume

Radionuclear scan
May be possible to identify presence of pericardial fluid by demonstrating increased space between inferior border of the heart and liver

Cardiac catheterization
Documents hemodynamic parameters associated with tamponade: decreased ventricular filling pressures, elevated right atrial pressure, alteration (equalization) of pressures during inspiration

TREATMENT PLAN

Surgical
Pericardiocentesis (see p. 108) or pericardial window (subxiphoid incision and placement of tube for continuous drainage) to remove pericardial fluid and relieve cardiac compression

Chemotherapeutic
Temporary supportive therapy—volume expansion with normal saline and infusion of inotropic agents to increase cardiac output and blood pressure

Electromechanical
Careful, continuous monitoring of clinical signs and symptoms, as well as changes in hemodynamic parameters, to support patient until definitive treatment is initiated; arterial pressure monitored for pulsus paradoxus and hypotension; right atrial pressure lines and electrocardiogram monitored for sudden changes.

Supportive
Bed rest with head of bed elevated to position of comfort; nothing by mouth (NPO) in anticipation of pericardiocentesis; parenteral therapy as ordered to maintain adequate blood pressure

ASSESSMENT: AREAS OF CONCERN

General complaints
Clinical presentation may vary from asymptomatic to dramatic and severe and is often nonspecific; anxiety; tachypnea; mild dyspnea to marked respiratory distress; lightheadedness; fatigue; chest discomfort (fullness, heaviness)

Physical examination
Tachycardia; peripheral cyanosis
Arterial pressure
Decreased systolic blood pressure; narrowing pulse pressure; pulsus paradoxus greater than 10 mm Hg; soft or absent pulse during inspiration
Venous pressure
Elevated venous pressure; distended neck veins on inspiration (positive Kussmaul's sign)
Auscultation
Distant, often inaudible heart sounds

NURSING DIAGNOSES and NURSING INTERVENTIONS

Nursing Diagnosis	Nursing Intervention
Cardiac output, alteration in: decreased (related to restricted ventricular filling pressure)	Determine degree of pulsus paradoxus. Assess jugular venous distention. Monitor arterial pressure, pulse pressure, pulse volume, ECG voltage, and level of consciousness every 5 to 15 minutes. Assist with pericardiocentesis or prepare patient for emergency surgery (pericardiectomy or pericardial window) as ordered. Administer inotropic medications as ordered. Administer fluids as ordered.
Activity intolerance	Encourage bed rest with head of bed elevated. Limit self-care activities.
Comfort, alteration in: pain	Assess quality and characteristics of chest pain. Provide bed rest in position of comfort. Provide medication as ordered to alleviate chest pain.

Patient Education

1. Provide an explanation of the condition.
2. Explain the need for and procedures regarding pericardiocentesis (see p. 108 for further detail) or for pericardiectomy as ordered.

EVALUATION

Patient Outcome	Data Indicating That Outcome is Reached
Improved ventricular compliance is shown by absence of tamponade.	Pulsus paradoxus decreases. Jugular venous distention decreases. Ventilation is improved. Pulse pressure and arterial pressure are normalized. Kussmaul's sign is absent.
Patient shows increased comfort.	Patient verbalizes relief of pain and dyspnea. Patient demonstrates ability to rest and sleep without complaint. Patient tolerates routine activities and procedures without complaint.

ENDOCARDITIS

Endocarditis is an inflammatory process involving the endothelial layer of the heart, including the cardiac valves and septal defects if present.

The designation of acute or subacute endocarditis describes the virulence of the infecting organism and the rapidity of destruction. Acute bacterial endocarditis (ABE) is considered fulminant, whereas subacute bacterial endocarditis (SBE) may be indolent for up to 8 weeks.

Statistically accurate information regarding the incidence of endocarditis is not available. In one report the frequency was estimated to be 0.16 to 5.4 cases per 1000 hospital admissions.[78] Reports do show a change in age distribution during the past 30 years. Considered a disease of young adults in the preantibiotic era, endocarditis now primarily involves older adults, with a mean age of 55 years. Men are affected more frequently by a ratio of 2:1 to 5:1 in several series.[11,57]

Persons at risk for endocarditis include patients with a history of rheumatic heart disease, valvular heart disease, or congenital heart defects or who have prosthetic heart valves, conduits, or pacemaker wires. Immunosuppressed patients are susceptible to transient bacteremia.

PATHOPHYSIOLOGY

Endocarditis can be attributed to a number of organisms. Diagnosis and treatment depend on isolation of the offending organism.

Streptococcal strains account for 40% to 80% of all SBE cases. These low-virulence bacteria generally affect already damaged valves. *S. viridans*, the most commonly implicated α-hemolytic organism, is found in the mouth and upper respiratory tract.

Staphylococcus aureus, which affects normal valves, is responsible for 50% of cases of acute endocarditis. A highly virulent organism, it is associated with a mortality ranging from 45% to 73%.[56] Less common enterococcal strains *(S. faecalis)* have increasingly been implicated in both acute and subacute endocarditis. *Enterococcus* is found in the gastrointestinal and genitourinary tracts and the oral cavity. It occurs frequently in elderly patients, particularly men undergoing urologic procedures, and has been reported in women of childbearing age. *S. epidermidis* is the pathogen commonly implicated in endocarditis following prosthetic valve replacement.

Other known pathogens associated with endocarditis include gram-negative organisms, fungi, and yeast. En-

docarditis caused by gram-negative cocci and bacilli *(Serratia marcescens, Klebsiella, Pseudomonas)* occurs in the elderly and "mainline" drug abusers. The increase in incidence of endocarditis caused by fungi *(Candida, Aspergillus)* may be attributed to the increase in intravenous drug abuse and the widespread use of antimicrobial and corticosteroid therapy. Fungal vegetations tend to be large and to embolize to major blood vessels, particularly in the lower extremities.

Endocarditis generally begins as a transient bacteremia (or fungemia) introduced into the circulation through several portals of entry (Table 1-2). For reasons not clearly understood, bacteria more commonly settle on cardiac structures that have preexisting damage. The valves, especially the mitral and aortic, are susceptible. Ventricular septal defects, coarctation of aorta, patent ductus arteriosus, and tetralogy of Fallot are predisposed to turbulent blood flow and therefore susceptible. Infected structures are often those in which turbulent blood flow is forced across an area of high pressure to low pressure. Trauma to the endothelial surface of the low-pressure side of the damaged site causes localized activation of clotting mechanisms. As a result, an aggregation of platelets and fibrin thrombi forms on the injured structure. During the active phase of the infection these thrombi can permit seeding and proliferation of microorganisms.

The pathogenesis of endocarditis is related to the adherence of infected thrombi to cardiac structures, which in the case of the valves can lead to scarring and retraction of the leaflets. The destruction may be sufficient to cause erosion of the leaflets and perforation leading to valvular insufficiency. The infectious process may also spread to the anulus, creating abscesses, or rupture the chordae tendineae. Mycotic aneurysms may result from septic embolization, which develops in the aorta, cerebral arteries, sinus of Valsalva, ligated ductus arteriosus, and smaller arterial vessels (of the lung, kidney, or spleen).

Table 1-2

Possible Ports of Entry and Factors Predisposing to Bacteremia

Port of Entry	Infecting Organism
Oral cavity Extractions, teeth cleaning, periodontal disease (abscesses), periodontal operations, use of unwaxed dental floss, oral irrigation, bridgework	*Streptococcus, Staphylococcus epidermidis*
Upper respiratory tract Tonsilloadenoidectomy, orotracheal intubation, bronchoscopy (rigid tubes), pneumonia	*Staphylococcus aureus, Streptococcus, Haemophilus* species, *Streptococcus pneumoniae, S. epidermidis*
Gastrointestinal tract Barium enema, sigmoidoscopy, colonoscopy, percutaneous biopsy of liver	Gram-negative rods, *Enterobacter, Escherichia coli, Klebsiella*
Genitourinary system Catheterization, urethrotomy, transurethral prostatectomy, retropubic prostatectomy, cystoscopy	*E. coli,* gram-negative bacilli, *Enterococcus*
Female reproductive system Delivery, abortion (therapeutic, illegal), intrauterine devices	*E. coli*
Skin Furuncles, acne (infected, squeezed)	*S. aureus, S. epidermidis*
Other sources of infection Pacemaker (transvenous), prolonged use of polyethylene catheter (arterial), hemodialysis (arteriovenous cannulas), infection (hematogenous osteomyelitis, Q fever, meningococcemia)	

DIAGNOSTIC STUDIES

Laboratory tests
   Complete blood count (CBC)
      Anemia; elevated sedimentation rate; leukocytosis
   Blood cultures (four to six cultures within 6 to 72 hours before therapy started)
      Identification of causative organism
   Urine
      Proteinuria; casts
   Rhuematoid factor
      Positive
   Blood chemistry
      Elevated BUN and creatinine values in patients with renal complications

Echocardiogram
Presence of vegetations or abscesses; involvement of cardiac valves; ventricular function

Electrocardiogram (ECG)
Conduction defects; atrial fibrillation, flutter

TREATMENT PLAN

Surgical
Surgical removal of vegetations and thrombi—not indicated unless uncontrollable sepsis occurs, and then combined with long-term antimicrobial therapy; if infectious process is fulminant and resistant to antimicrobial therapy, excision of vegetations, unroofing of abscesses, and valve replacement recommended[56]

Chemotherapeutic
Antibiotics—long-term IV antibiotic therapy inhibits bacterial growth; since appropriate therapy depends on isolation of infecting organism, serial blood cultures required *before* initiation of therapy; initiation of antibiotic therapy is guided by patient's clinical state: for subacute infection, delaying therapy until culture results are available will not endanger patient, but treatment for acutely ill patient should begin immediately; therapy usually continues 4-6 wk with parenteral administration as recommended route; in approximately 10%-20% of cases, primarily subacute bacterial endocarditis, culture findings are negative and therapy is directed at enterococcal infections, using combination of penicillin and streptomycin; blood cultures are obtained periodically to determine adequacy of regimen and sensitivity to antibiotics
Analgesic-antipyretics (salicylates) given for elevated temperature
Anticoagulants given prophylactically if large thrombus is visualized on echocardiogram or if atrial fibrillation develops
Other agents dictated by presence of complications
Cardiac
Abscesses
Valvular dysfunction (see p. 64)
Heart failure (see p. 44)
Myocarditis
Embolization
Cerebral
Renal
Splenic
Coronary
Mycotic aneurysms

Supportive
Rest—encouraged during acute phase; patient often requires prolonged hospitalization (2 to 6 weeks)
Vital signs—checked every 4 to 8 hours, decreasing frequency as indicated by improved clinical condition
Diet—regular; patient may require high-calorie supplemental feedings; force fluids during periods of elevated temperature provided there is no ventricular failure
Monitor parenteral therapy for rate and amount of infusion; check regularly for localized signs of inflammation, phlebitis

ASSESSMENT: AREAS OF CONCERN

General complaints
Acute: high-grade fever (39° to 40° C [102° to 104° F])
Subacute: low-grade fever (less than 39.4° C [103° F]), weakness, malaise, weight loss, anorexia, arthralgia, sweats, headache, dyspnea

Signs of embolization (peripheral, cerebral, systemic)
Petechiae in conjunctivae, palate, buccal mucosa, and extremities; splinter hemorrhages (linear, dark-red streaks on nail beds); Osler's nodes (small, tender, raised nodules frequently found on finger and toe pads); Janeway lesions (nontender, flat, erythematous macules on palms and soles); splenomegaly; Roth's spots (retinal hemorrhages with white centers); neurologic changes (behavioral changes, aphasia, paralysis)

Auscultation
Murmurs not usually present in early phase of infection but become apparent if valvular damage occurs (see discussion of valvular heart disease, p. 64); ventricular gallop (S_3) occurs in setting of ventricular failure (see p. 45)

NURSING DIAGNOSES and NURSING INTERVENTIONS

Nursing Diagnosis	Nursing Intervention
Nutrition, alteration in: less than body requirements	Weigh patient daily; decrease frequency of weighing as weight stabilizes. Offer high-calorie supplemental feedings. Restrict sodium if heart failure is present.
Fluid volume, alteration in: excess	Auscultate heart and lung sounds for increasing pulmonary congestion or presence of new murmurs. Monitor vital signs frequently. Assess peripheral extremities for evidence of edema. Weigh patient daily to detect increasing weight. Monitor for jugular venous distention.
Knowledge deficit	Provide instruction regarding disease process, precipitating factors, purpose and method of treatment, and need for lifelong antibiotic prophylaxis. Teach family member(s) with patient.
Diversional activity, deficit	Provide diversional activities such as occupational therapy, reading, television, radio, and out-of-hospital passes.
Thought processes, alteration in	Administer anticoagulant therapy as ordered. Instruct patient about need to continue with anticoagulants, if ordered, to prevent future embolic episodes.
Cardiac output, alteration in: decreased	Assess for signs and symptoms of impending heart failure, and initiate nursing care if they are present.

Patient Education

1. Instruct the patient about the nature of the disorder and the need for prolonged antibiotic therapy.
2. Explain precipitating factors that can lead to bacteremia and reinfection: dental work (gum cleaning or treatment, extractions), gastrointestinal or genitourinary procedures, vaginal deliveries, furuncles, staphylococcal infections, surgical procedures.
3. Encourage regular follow-up care with a medical physician.
4. Instruct the patient on the need for good oral hygiene and regular dental care.
5. Explain and reinforce the need for antibiotic prophylaxis before procedures that predispose to bacteremia.

EVALUATION

Patient Outcome	Data Indicating That Outcome is Reached
There are no inflammatory processes.	Temperature, blood cultures, white cell count, and other laboratory findings are normal. Patient's sense of well-being is improved. Patient reports feeling less fatigued, improved appetite, weight gain, and absence of sweats and headache.
Knowledge level is increased.	Patient verbalizes knowledge regarding factors that contribute to endocarditis, need for antibiotic prophylaxis, nature of disease, and signs and symptoms of recurrence.

SYSTEMIC HYPERTENSION

An intermittent or sustained elevation in systolic or diastolic blood pressure, hypertension is a major cause of cerebrovascular accident (stroke), cardiac disease, and renal failure.

Nearly one sixth of all Americans or 35 million persons have hypertension, and an additional 25 million have borderline hypertension. Half of those affected are unaware of their hypertension.

Hypertension may be defined as a blood pressure greater than 160/95 mm Hg. Persons with blood pressures less than 140/90 mm Hg are normotensive; those with blood pressure between 140/90 and 160/95 mm Hg are considered borderline hypertensive.[57]

Although there is no way of predicting in whom high blood pressure will develop, hypertension can be detected easily. Therefore the major emphasis in the control of hypertension should be on early detection and effective treatment.

PATHOPHYSIOLOGY

Primary (essential) hypertension is the most common form, accounting for 90% of all hypertension. It is an abnormal state in which excessive neurohumoral stimulation results in increased arterial tone. The etiology is unknown, but certain risk factors have been identified, including familial history, age group, race, obesity, stress, cigarette smoking, and high dietary intake of sodium and saturated fats.

Secondary hypertension occurs as a result of many factors:

Renal parenchymal disorders
  Pyelonephritis
  Glomerulonephritis
  Hydronephrosis
  Polycystic kidney
  Juxtaglomerular (renin-producing) tumors
  Following renal transplant
Renal artery disease
  Atherosclerosis
  Arthritis
  Embolism
  Aneurysm
  Diabetic nephrosclerosis
Endocrine and metabolic disorders
  Pheochromocytoma
  Cushing's syndrome
  Aldosteronism (primary)
  Hypercalcemia
  Neuroblastoma (in children)
  Acromegaly
  Myxedema
  Oral contraceptives
  Chronic licorice use
Central nervous system disorders
  Increased intracranial pressure
  Brain tumor
  Neurogenic; psychogenic
  Polyneuritis (porphyria)
Coarctation of aorta

Accelerated (malignant) hypertension is a state in which the blood pressure is extremely high (diastolic pressure greater than 120 mm Hg). It is accompanied by acute hypertensive retinopathy, nephrosclerosis, and encephalopathy.

The pathogenesis of hypertension is complex because various homeostatic mechanisms contribute to the maintenance of normal arterial pressure.

Cardiac output (stroke volume × heart rate) and peripheral vascular resistance are the hemodynamic determinants of arterial pressure. Increases in blood volume (high-output states), heart rate, or arterial vasoconstriction that cause an increase in peripheral resistance can lead to a hypertensive state.

Stimulation of stretch receptors (baroreceptors) in the wall of the carotid sinus and the aortic arch increases vagal activity (parasympathetic component) and decreases sympathetic activity. The result is a decrease in peripheral resistance and a reduction in blood pressure. Researchers currently believe that increased sympathetic activity with reduced vagal activity causes an autonomic dysregulation in persons with primary hypertension.[71]

Stimulation and production of high plasma levels of renin (a proteolytic enzyme produced by juxtaglomerular cells) contribute to a complex relationship between extracellular fluid and pressure, leading to sympathetic activation and elevated arterial pressure. Fig. 1-43 outlines the conversion of renin to angiotensin I and II.

DIAGNOSTIC STUDIES

Laboratory tests
  Urine studies including microscopic examination
    Proteinuria, hematuria
  Blood chemistry
    BUN >20 mg/dl
    Creatinine >1.5 mg/dl
    Potassium >5 mEq/L in renal failure; <3.5 mEq/L in primary aldosteronism and with diuretic administration
    Cholesterol and lipid levels elevated in hyperlipidemia
    Uric acid level may increase with diuretic therapy
    Calcium level may increase with diuretic therapy

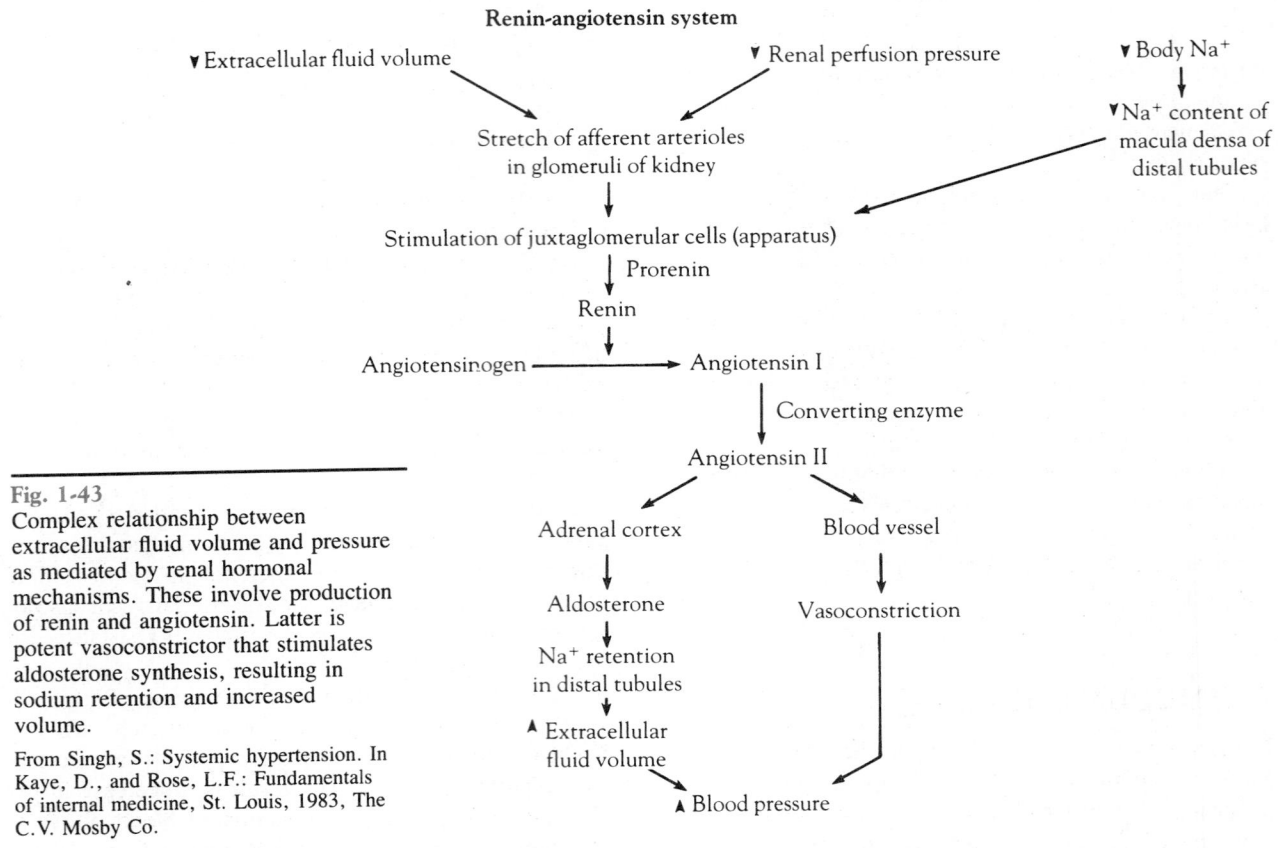

Renin-angiotensin system

Fig. 1-43

Complex relationship between extracellular fluid volume and pressure as mediated by renal hormonal mechanisms. These involve production of renin and angiotensin. Latter is potent vasoconstrictor that stimulates aldosterone synthesis, resulting in sodium retention and increased volume.

From Singh, S.: Systemic hypertension. In Kaye, D., and Rose, L.F.: Fundamentals of internal medicine, St. Louis, 1983, The C.V. Mosby Co.

Electrocardiogram (ECG)
   Evaluates presence of left ventricular hypertrophy and myocardial ischemia

Chest roentgenogram
   Cardiomegaly; aortic atherosclerosis

TREATMENT PLAN

Surgical
   None for primary hypertension (see Chapter 10 for surgical interventions for renal disorders)

Chemotherapeutic
   Diuretics
      Thiazides
         Chlorothiazide (Diuril) (0.5-1 g/day)
         Hydrochlorothiazide (Esidrex, HydroDIURIL) (50-100 mg/day)
         Bendroflumethiazide (Naturetin) (2.5-10 mg/day)
      Loop diuretics
         Furosemide (Lasix) (40-80 mg bid or qid)
         Ethacrynic acid (Edecrin) (initial dose 25-50 mg)

   Potassium-sparing diuretics
      Spironolactone (Aldactone) (100-400 mg bid or tid)
      Triamterene (Dyrenium) (100-300 mg bid)
      Amiloride (Midamor) (5-20 mg/day or bid)
   β-Adrenergic blocking agents
      Propranolol (Inderal) (10-80 mg po bid or qid)
      Metoprolol tartrate (Lopressor) (50-200 mg po qd or bid)
      Pindolol (Visken) (15-60 mg/day)
      Atenolol (Tenormin) (50-100 mg/day)
      Timolol maleate (Blocadren) (20-40 mg/day)
      Nadolol (Corgard) (80-320 mg/day)
   Antihypertensive agents
      Methyldopa (Aldomet) (up to 2 g/day po bid, tid, or qid)
      Guanethidine (Ismelin) (5-200 mg/day po)
      Clonidine (Catapres) (0.1-1.2 mg bid po)
      Captopril (Capoten) (24-150 mg tid)
      Hydrazaline (Apresoline) (10-50 mg po qid)
      Sodium nitroprusside (Nipride) (0.5-10 μg/kg/min IV)
      Diazoxide (Hyperstat) (300 mg by rapid IV bolus)

α-Adrenergic blocking agents
    Phentolamine (Regitine) (1-5 mg IV intermittently)
    Prazosin (Minipress) (initial dose 1 mg po, slowly increased to 10-15 mg/day)

Electromechanical
None for systemic hypertension
Cardiac monitoring for hypertensive crisis

Supportive
Dietary management
    Sodium restriction—may range from mild to rigid restriction depending on degree of hypertension; recommended dietary restriction 2 to 6 g/day
    Alcohol—limit intake to less than 3 drinks/day
    Caffeine—restrict intake
    Cholesterol, lipids, saturated fats—reduce intake
Weight control—recommend weight loss of 5% or more in obese patient
Exercise
    Aerobic exercise appropriate for age and health status
    Refer to cardiac rehabilitation for prescribed exercise program
    Avoid isometric exercises
Stress reduction and management
Monitoring of blood pressure on regular basis; frequency determined by blood pressure elevations

ASSESSMENT: AREAS OF CONCERN

Symptoms
Mild to moderate hypertension
    Asymptomatic

Moderate to severe hypertension
    Headaches, dizziness, fatigue, vertigo, palpitations
Severe hypertension
    Throbbing suboccipital headache (may be present when patient awakens in morning, disappearing spontaneously after several hours); epistaxis

Physical examination
Mild to moderate hypertension
    Normal with exception of blood pressure
Moderate hypertension
    Blood pressure (in both arms; sitting, standing, and supine; determined over at least two visits)
    160/90 mm Hg or higher
    Pulse
        Tachycardia; bounding; femoral delay as compared with radial or brachial pulsation
    Precordium
        Displaced but forceful apical impulse; ventricular heave (apical lift)
    Auscultation
        Bruits over carotid and femoral areas; accentuated S_2 at base; apical systolic murmur; audible S_4; early diastolic blowing murmur (right and left sternal borders and intercostal spaces)
    Optic fundi
        Retinal changes: grade I—minimal arterial narrowing or irregularity; grade II—marked arteriolar narrowing and irregularity with focal tortuosity or spasm; grade III—marked arteriolar narrowing and irregularity with generalized tortuosity, flame-shaped hemorrhages, cotton-wool exudates; grade IV—same as III plus papilledema

NURSING DIAGNOSES and NURSING INTERVENTIONS

Nursing Diagnosis	Nursing Intervention
Health maintenance, alteration in	Provide periodic monitoring of blood pressure. Identify risk factors and help patient modify risks. Administer antihypertensive agents as ordered. Initiate patient education program with patient and family.
Noncompliance	Assess factors that will influence patient's ability to adhere to therapeutic plan: financial status, age, culture, health status, occupation. Identify and clarify any misconceptions patient may have regarding disease state. Design program that is compatible with habits, life-style, and personality of patient; include patient in program design.
Powerlessness	Identify any misconceptions and fears patient may have regarding this chronic illness, such as forced dependence on health care system. Encourage patient to participate in determining therapeutic plan. Teach patient and family members to monitor blood pressure at home and interpret results.

Patient Education

1. Instruct the patient and family in blood pressure monitoring, procedure for taking blood pressure at home, frequency of monitoring, influencing factors, interpretation of results, and actions to take if significant change occurs.
2. Explain diet therapy including sodium, calorie, and lipid restrictions as ordered; include the rationale in explanation.
3. Explain the role of exercise in blood pressure regulation and weight control.
4. Explain the relationship between stress and hypertension, factors that produce stress, and methods to modify stress.
5. Explain antihypertensive therapy, including name, rationale, dosage, and side effects of all medications.

EVALUATION

Patient Outcome	Data Indicating That Outcome is Reached
Blood pressure is within acceptable limits.	Blood pressure is 140/90 mm Hg or less. Patient has no complaints of headache, dizziness, etc. Laboratory values are within normal limits.
Patient complies with therapeutic plan.	Patient is normotensive, reports taking medication, loses weight, and has no symptoms.

ACUTE ARTERIAL INSUFFICIENCY

Arterial insufficiency is a sudden decrease in the arterial supply to an extremity.

Classified as an acute disorder, obstruction of any major artery precipitates symptoms.

PATHOPHYSIOLOGY

The most common causes of acute arterial insufficiency are embolism, thrombosis, and trauma. Cardiac disorders such as mitral valve disease, rheumatic heart disease, atrial fibrillation, left atrial myxoma, or prosthetic valves are the primary source of thrombi on the left side of the heart. Once dislodged, an embolus may travel throughout the systemic circulation, lodging in an arterial branch and stagnating flow in the distal circulation. This sets up a condition of distal clotting or the formation of another thrombus. In the presence of inadequate collateral circulation, the clinical picture of acute arterial insufficiency occurs.

The lower extremities are most commonly involved in arterial occlusions. The femoral artery is most frequently affected (46%), followed by the popliteal tibial tree (11%) and the iliac arteries (8%).[73]

Acute arterial obstruction may also occur as a result of traumatic injury produced by compression, shearing, or laceration of a vessel. Furthermore, severe hypothermia may produce sudden severe vasoconstriction.

DIAGNOSTIC STUDIES

Doppler ultrasonography
Abnormal blood flow pattern proximal to occlusion; "pistol shot" sound characterizes absence of diastolic flow component; ankle/brachial index <0.25 reflects severe ischemia and impending gangrene

Arteriography
Determines location of obstruction and character of arterial circulation proximal and distal to obstruction

TREATMENT PLAN

Surgical
Embolectomy—embolus can be removed directly via femoral arteriotomy using soft balloon-tipped catheter known as Fogarty catheter; catheter is passed distal to occlusion, carefully inflated, and withdrawn

Chemotherapeutic
Anticoagulants
Heparin sodium (Lipo-Hepin and others)
Indications: Initiated once diagnosis of embolization is made and before operative treatment is performed

Usual dosage: Loading, 5000-10,000 units IV; maintenance, dose given to keep partial thromboplastin time to two times normal

Fibrinolytic agents

Streptokinase (Streptase), urokinase (Abbokinase)

Indications: Thrombolytic agents instilled by intra-arterial infusion into site of occlusion; method of action is fibrinolysis causing fibrin dissolution

Electromechanical

Percutaneous transluminal angioplasty—nonsurgical procedure involving mechanical dilation of occluded artery performed under local anesthesia with fluoroscopy; lesions considered suitable are stenotic vessels with intraluminal diameter of 2.5 mm and length of not more than 10 cm

ASSESSMENT: AREAS OF CONCERN

Peripheral extremity

Pain, sudden in onset; numbness; "embolic syndrome" characterized by five Ps: pain, pallor, paresthesia, pulselessness, and paralysis

NURSING DIAGNOSES and NURSING INTERVENTIONS

Nursing Diagnosis	Nursing Intervention
Tissue perfusion, alteration in: peripheral	Provide bed rest during acute period. Administer anticoagulants as ordered. Assess arterial pulses distal to occlusion every 1 to 2 hours. Assess skin color and temperature. Do not raise leg above level of heart.
Comfort, alteration in: pain	Provide for position of most comfort. Do not raise knee gatch. Administer analgesics as ordered. Protect affected extremity by using a bed cradle, cotton blankets, or sheepskin. Do active and passive range of motion exercises unless contraindicated.
Anxiety	Assess level of anxiety. Offer brief, accurate explanation of disease and therapeutic modalities. Correct any misconception about diagnosis and outcomes. Encourage verbalization, since patient may fear loss of extremity.

Patient Education

1. Instruct patient and family about the disease process, possible causes, and therapeutic modalities.
2. At discharge explain anticoagulant therapy and the need for follow-up monitoring with clotting studies.

EVALUATION

Patient Outcome	Data Indicating That Outcome is Reached
Peripheral perfusion is improved.	Pain is relieved. Distal and proximal pulses are present. Extremity has normal color. Normal motor function returns in affected extremity.

CHRONIC ARTERIAL INSUFFICIENCY

Chronic arterial insufficiency is inadequate blood flow in arteries, caused by occlusive atherosclerotic plaques or emboli, damaged or diseased vessels, aneurysms, hypercoagulability states, or heavy use of tobacco.

Arteriosclerosis obliterans is the primary cause of chronic arterial insufficiency. Other causes, although rare, may lead to arterial insufficiency of the lower extremities. These include thromboangiitis obliterans

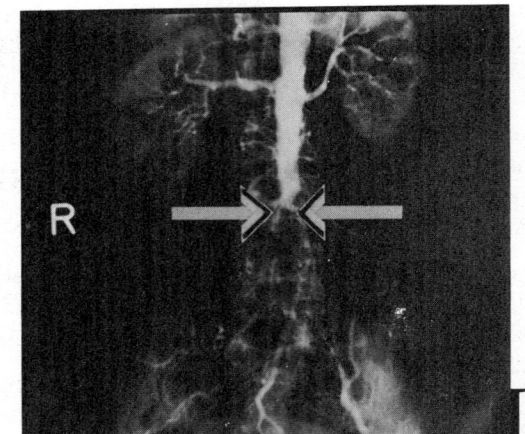

Fig. 1-44
A, Arteriogram depicting complete occlusion of distal abdominal aorta *(arrows)*. **B,** Aortobifemoral bypass graft using synthetic conduit.

From Guzzetta, C.E., and Dossey, B.M.: Cardiovascular nursing: bodymind tapestry, St. Louis, 1984, The C.V. Mosby Co.

(Buerger's disease), cystic degeneration of the popliteal artery, popliteal entrapment, and some connective tissue disorders.

Arteriosclerosis obliterans is a progressive ischemic syndrome. It is more prevalent in men, and the incidence rises with age. It is a diffuse process but is generally confined to short segments of arteries near bifurcations and origins. The aortoiliac and femoropopliteal areas are common sites.

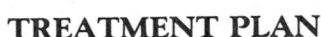

PATHOPHYSIOLOGY

Progressive narrowing of the arterial tree by atherosclerotic plaques gives rise to collateral vessels that tend to ensure adequate blood supply and prevent peripheral ischemia. However, the effectiveness of these collateral pathways is limited by their small size and high resistance, as well as by the extent of occlusive disease. Clinically, progressive occlusion leads to hypoperfusion and ischemia, which are related directly to the number of occlusions and the adequacy of collateral vessels. The distal extremities are the most vulnerable to ischemia.

DIAGNOSTIC STUDIES

Doppler ultrasonography
  Quantitates degree of ischemia; ankle/brachial index: arterial pressure less than pressure in brachial artery

Plethysmography
  Determines degree to which peripheral circulation is decreased

Angiography
  Provides visualization of arterial tree with exact localization of obstruction

TREATMENT PLAN

Surgical
  Arterial reconstruction—performed to restore unimpeded pulsatile blood flow, usually beginning with proximal segments (aortoiliac-femoral)
    Endarterectomy—removal of atheromatous intima from artery
    Bypass graft surgery—use of Dacron conduit to deliver blood from aorta to femoral vessels, bypassing diseased segments (Fig. 1-44)
  Femoropopliteal reconstruction
    Femoropopliteal bypass
    Profundoplasty—local endarterectomy of proximal profunda femoris artery
  Lumbar sympathectomy—removal of second and third lumbar ganglia; performed to improve blood flow to skin
  Amputation of limb—for severe, irreversible ischemia (gangrene)

Chemotherapeutic
  Several drugs such as anticoagulants, vasodilators, and antiplatelets have been used but are not part of standard care

Supportive

Weight reduction for obese patients

Daily foot care—inspection, cleaning, use of cotton socks; attention to nails, corns, calluses

Low-cholesterol diet as ordered

Education about atherosclerosis-producing factors (see pp. 34 and 35)

ASSESSMENT: AREAS OF CONCERN

Peripheral tissue perfusion

Intermittent claudication

Calf pain, fatigue induced by walking and relieved by rest, pain in thigh and buttocks (foot rarely involved)

Ischemic rest pain

Continuous burning pain confined to toes, aggravated by elevation and improved by dependence; occurs at rest and improved with walking

Arterial pulses

Palpation

Ranges from slightly reduced to absent

Auscultation

Presence of bruits at rest and after exercise; sites are abdominal aorta, and iliac and femoral arteries

Skin, nails, hair

Ulcerations, cold skin, pallor—increasing with elevation of extremity, atrophic nails, hair loss

NURSING DIAGNOSES and NURSING INTERVENTIONS

Nursing Diagnosis	Nursing Intervention
Tissue perfusion, alteration in: peripheral	Assess arterial pulses, determine pulse volume, and auscultate for bruits. Assess skin color, temperature, and elasticity. Avoid elevating affected extremity. Instruct patient to avoid use of nicotine. Avoid use of knee gatch. Instruct patient to avoid crossing legs and long periods of sitting or standing.
Comfort, alteration in: pain	Administer analgesics as ordered. Provide position of most comfort. Begin slow, progressive exercise program.
Skin integrity, impairment of: actual	Provide daily skin care and ensure that skin is thoroughly dried. Treat ulcerations as they occur. Avoid using adhesive tapes directly on skin. Avoid use of tight constricting socks or hose; use cotton socks. Observe for signs of necrosis. Avoid use of slipper socks; encourage patient to wear well-fitting, hard-soled shoes.

Patient Education

1. Provide information regarding disease and associated risk factors.
2. Explain the need to avoid use of nicotine.
3. Instruct the patient in a daily progressive walking program.
4. Explain skin care.
5. Provide weight counseling for obese patients.
6. Explain dietary limitations of a low-cholesterol, low-fat diet.

EVALUATION

Patient Outcome	Data Indicating That Outcome is Reached
Peripheral perfusion is improved.	Patient reports relief of pain (claudication). Pulses are present, equal, and bilateral. Skin color is normal; skin is warm to touch.
Skin integrity is maintained.	Skin shows no signs of ulcerations. Skin color and temperature are normal.

RAYNAUD'S DISEASE

Raynaud's disease is a disorder of small cutaneous arteries, most frequently involving the fingers; it is characterized by episodic vasospasm.

Raynaud's disease may occur as an idiopathic primary form or may follow other systemic disorders. As a primary disorder it occurs more commonly in young women, is often triggered by emotional stress and cold, and involves both hands.

PATHOPHYSIOLOGY

Raynaud's phenomenon involves three phases. Initially, severe constriction of cutaneous vessels results in blanching of the fingers. The digital vessels then dilate, slowing blood flow, which allows hemoglobin to release more oxygen into the tissues. During this ischemic phase the fingers are first white and then cyanotic, numb, and cold. The vasoconstriction phase is followed by a reactive hyperemic phase during which the fingers become red and the patient experiences throbbing pain. Because attacks are often triggered by stress and cold, it is believed that the disease may be related to vasoconstriction caused by release of catecholamines. The attacks may last a few minutes or, in severe cases, several hours.

In severe cases, progressive ischemia with trophic skin changes may lead to recurring infection and gangrene. Raynaud's phenomenon is a rare disorder, however, and generally occurs in mild form.

DIAGNOSTIC STUDIES

Digital plethysmography
Abnormal perfusion pressure and pulsatile contour

Peripheral arteriography
Visualization of distal arteries of hands

TREATMENT PLAN

Surgical
Sympathectomy
Lumbar ganglionectomy for relief of symptoms involving feet
Ganglionectomy for relief of symptoms involving hands
Amputation of terminal phalanges (very rare)

Chemotherapeutic
Antihypertensive agents
Reserpine (Serpasil, others)
Indications: Rauwolfia alkaloids that decrease vasoconstriction
Usual dosage: 0.25-0.5 mg/day po
α-Adrenergic blocking agents
Phenoxybenzamine (Dibenzyline)
Dosage is variable
Tolazoline (Prescoline)
Usual dosage: 25-50 mg po tid; 10-50 mg parenterally qid
Vasodilators
Nicotinyl alcohol (Roniacol)
Usual dosage: 50-100 mg po tid or 150 mg bid

Supportive
Avoidance of exposure to irritants such as cold, mechanical or chemical injury, and stressful situations

ASSESSMENT: AREAS OF CONCERN

Hands and fingers
Initially blanched and numb after exposure to cold or stress; then fingers become cyanotic; this is followed by change in color to red; trophic changes (ulcerations, chronic paronychia) may occur in long-standing disease

NURSING DIAGNOSES and NURSING INTERVENTIONS

Nursing Diagnosis	Nursing Intervention
Comfort, alteration in: pain	Assess for aggravating factors leading to vasospasm. Remove aggravating factors when possible; for example, provide warmth to fingers, have patient stop smoking. Assist patient to modify stressful periods that may aggravate vasospasm. Instruct patient as to cause of pain.
Skin integrity, alteration in	Perform daily assessment for color changes and ulcerations. Treat ulcerations if they occur. Avoid exposure to cold, mechanical and chemical irritants, or other stressful factors.

Patient Education

1. Instruct patient to avoid exposure to cold temperatures and to wear gloves or mittens when handling cold items and in cold weather.
2. Instruct patient to avoid smoking.
3. Explain the need to avoid stressful situations; teach ways to deal with stress, such as relaxation techniques.
4. Explain the purpose, side effects, and dosage of medications.

EVALUATION

Patient Outcome	Data Indicating That Outcome is Reached
Circulation in hands and fingers is improved.	There is no pain. Color is normal and skin is warm. Skin integrity is maintained.

VENOUS THROMBOSIS

Venous thrombosis is an abnormal vascular condition in which a thrombus develops within a blood vessel.

Venous thrombosis is the most common venous disorder. The greatest morbidity and mortality occur in the surgical population (30% to 60%) and in patients receiving intravenous therapy, because of the associated embolization of a thrombus to the lungs. The incidence of pulmonary embolism in surgical patients has been estimated to be between 7.3% and 54%, with the estimated number of deaths 200,000 per year.[70] The following terms are commonly used to describe venous disorders that reflect thrombus formation or inflammation:

phlebitis inflammation of vein.
phlebothrombosis (venous thrombosis) intraluminal thrombus with minimal or no inflammatory component; these have greater tendency to embolize.
thromboembolism the phenomenon of thrombus dislodgment and migration.
thrombophlebitis an acute condition characterized by thrombus and inflammation in deep or superficial veins.

intravenous therapy are common offenders. Endothelial damage leads to exposure of the subintimal collagen membrane, which promotes platelet adherence, and activation of intrinsic coagulation factors, which contribute to thrombus formation.

Hypercoagulability reflects an alteration in blood coagulability, which occurs in some patients with hematologic disorders (such as polycythemias and anemias), excessive estrogen or steroid use, or malignancies.

Once formed the thrombus initiates an inflammatory process leading to fibrosis. The enlarging thrombus eventually occludes the lumen of the vein or detaches and embolizes to the systemic circulation.

Frequent sites for venous thrombus formation are the soleal and gastrocnemius venous sinus and the larger veins such as the venae cavae and the femoral, iliac, and subclavian veins. Thrombosis of these veins is associated with increased risk of embolization. Thrombosis in superficial (subcutaneous) veins rarely leads to pulmonary embolism.

PATHOPHYSIOLOGY

The triad of stasis, intimal damage, and hypercoagulability is responsible for most venous thrombosis.

Venous stasis occurs in persons who are inactive for a time because of bed rest or immobilization of the lower extremities. Thrombus formation results from a reduction of flow-induced dilution and a decrease in natural circulating anticoagulants (antithrombin III, platelet factor IV, and some prostaglandins).[70] Stasis caused by reduced flow increases the contact between platelets and coagulation factors that enhance platelet aggregation.

Intimal damage may occur as a result of internal or external trauma. Venipuncture and traumatic or long-term

DIAGNOSTIC STUDIES

Plethysmography
Shows decreased circulation distal to affected area

Doppler ultrasonography
Identifies reduced blood flow to specific area; shows obstruction to venous flow

Phlebography
Confirms diagnosis; shows filling defects

^{125}I fibrinogen scan
Defines location of clot and any emboli that may have dislodged

TREATMENT PLAN

Surgical
Rarely indicated

Techniques used for deep vein thrombophlebitis necessitating venous interruption—ligation, vein plication, or clipping

Iliofemoral thrombectomy—may be considered for patients with acute iliofemoral thrombosis and compromised arterial perfusion that fail to respond to conventional therapy

Chemotherapeutic
Anticoagulants

Heparin sodium

Indications: Initially administered IV to augment fibrinolytic activity and aid in thrombolysis

Usual dosage: 300-500 units/kg followed by infusion of 1000 units/h

Warfarin

Indications: Given later to maintain prothrombin time to twice control level; usually for 3 mo

Fibrinolytic agents

Streptokinase (Streptase)

Indications: Produces total clot lysis and restores normal venous valve function

Usual dosage: IV initially 250,000 IU/30 min; maintenance 100,000 IU/h for 24-72 h

Antiplatelet agents (used in prevention of thrombus

Antiplatelet agents (to prevent thrombus formation)

Dipyridamole (Persantine)

Usual dosage: 800 mg/day; 400 mg/day if used with anticoagulants

Supportive
Bed rest with elevation of affected extremity above level of right atrium

Warm, moist heat

Custom-fitted elastic stockings when ambulatory

Monitoring of partial thromboplastin time and/or prothrombin time while patient is receiving anticoagulant therapy

ASSESSMENT: AREAS OF CONCERN

Lower extremity (deep veins)
Calf pain and tenderness; Homan's sign (calf pain on dorsiflexion of foot); dilated superficial veins; edema of involved extremity (30% to 50% of deep vein thromboses may be clinically silent); pain and tenderness over involved vein (for example, groin)

Upper extremity (superficial veins)
Redness, warmth, and tenderness over affected vein; veins visible and palpable

NURSING DIAGNOSES and NURSING INTERVENTIONS

Nursing Diagnosis	Nursing Intervention
Comfort, alteration in: pain	Provide bed rest; limit self-care activities. Elevate affected limb above level of right atrium. Do not use knee gatch. Administer analgesics as ordered. Apply warm moist compresses as ordered. Measure calf or thigh or both daily and record. Use elastic stockings as ordered. Maintain low elevation of affected extremity when patient is sitting in chair.
Gas exchange, impaired	Observe for signs of pulmonary embolism: chest pain, dyspnea, tachypnea. Monitor vital signs every 4 to 8 hours. Maintain bed rest during acute period. Administer anticoagulant therapy as ordered. Use elastic stockings during periods of ambulation.
Potential patient problem: hemorrhage	Monitor anticoagulant therapy, including dosage, sites of administration, and bleeding (epistaxis, bleeding gums, petechiae). Obtain daily coagulation laboratory values before administering medication. Teach patient and family need for medication, proper administration, and need for frequent laboratory evaluation.

Patient Education

1. Instruct the patient and family about the nature of the disorder and methods of preventing recurrence.
2. Instruct the patient to avoid constrictive clothing and crossing legs when sitting.
3. Explain the value of rest periods with legs raised.
4. Explain the need to lose weight if the patient is obese.
5. Instruct the patient to avoid use of oral contraceptives.
6. Explain the need for a regular or moderate exercise program.
7. Explain anticoagulant therapy.

EVALUATION

Patient Outcome	Data Indicating That Outcome is Reached
Inflammation is decreased, and venous blood flow is improved.	Patient has relief of pain, swelling, and redness.

CONGENITAL HEART DISEASE

A congenital cardiac anomaly is any structural or functional abnormality or defect of the heart or great vessels existing from birth.

Congenital heart disease is considered a specialty of pediatrics. With advances in surgical techniques, however, persons with congenital defects are living longer, presenting a new challenge to practitioners who treat adults. Although the incidence of congenital cardiac malformations has decreased over the decades, they continue to occur at a rate of 5 to 8 per 1000 live births.[52] Five of the most common of this large group of defects are presented here.

PATHOPHYSIOLOGY

In the majority of cases the cause for the congenital defect cannot be determined. However, various factors are believed to contribute to malformation of the human heart.

Genetics. Several studies have demonstrated prevalence rates among siblings and blood relatives to be 1.5% to 5%,[52] suggesting a genetic link in the etiology of cardiac malformations. Also, certain chromosomal abnormalities, including Turner's syndrome and Down's syndrome, have been found to be associated with cardiac defects.

Environmental factors. Although difficult to prove as isolated etiologic factors, environmental factors in combination with genetic factors have been implicated in cardiac anomalies. Factors implicated include pollution and smoking and alcohol use by the mother.

Teratogens. Use of certain drugs such as warfarin and exposure to viruses such as rubella during fetal development have been shown to cause not only cardiac malformations but also widespread injury to the embryo.

Altitude. Altitude has been implicated in the failure of the ductus arteriosus to close after birth.

Common Defects in Which Prolonged Survival Occurs

Patent ductus arteriosus (Fig. 1-45). The ductus arteriosus is a vascular connection that during fetal life directs blood flow from the pulmonary artery to the aorta, bypassing the lungs. Functional closure of the ductus occurs after birth. In some cases it takes 6 months to several years before complete obliteration occurs. If the

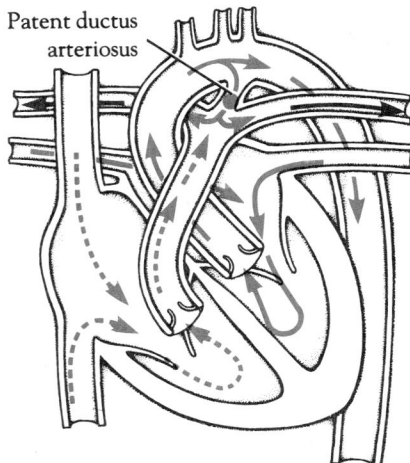

Fig. 1-45
Patent ductus arteriosus.

From Whaley, L.F., and Wong, D.L.: Nursing care of infants and children, ed. 2, St. Louis, 1983, The C.V. Mosby Co.

Patent ductus arteriosus

ductus remains patent, the direction of blood flow is reversed to left to right because of high systemic pressure in the aorta. Blood is shunted through the ductus to the pulmonary artery during both systole and diastole, raising pressure in the pulmonary circulation and increasing the pressure against which the right ventricle must work.

Survival into adulthood is possible. Patent ductus arteriosus occurs more frequently in girls and can be associated with other anomalies such as ventricular septal defect and coarctation of the aorta.

Atrial septal defect (Fig. 1-46). An atrial septal defect is an abnormal communication or opening between the right and left atria causing blood to be shunted from left to right. There are two common forms. In ostium secundum, the more common, the defect is in the middle of the septal wall near the fossa ovalis. Ostium primum results from failure of fusion of the left portions of the endocardial cushions occurring low in the atrial septum. An associated cleft (separation) is present in the anterior mitral valve leaflet, which can lead to mitral regurgitation.

Ventricular septal defect (Fig. 1-47). A ventricular septal defect is an abnormal communication or opening between the right and left ventricles. It varies in size (7 mm to 3 cm in diameter) and occurs in either the membranous (upper) or muscular (lower) portion of the ventricular septum. The size of the defect determines the clinical findings and the extent of the shunt from left to right ventricle. The larger the shunt, the greater the volume of blood ejected into the right ventricle and lungs. Therefore large defects cause a volume overload for both ventricles. Large defects can also lead to an increase in pulmonary vascular resistance, producing pulmonary hypertension. If this occurs, the shunt may be reversed to right to left, causing systemic cyanosis and producing the Eisenmenger syndrome, which renders the patient inoperable.

Tetralogy of Fallot (Fig. 1-48). Tetralogy of Fallot

Fig. 1-46
Atrial septal defect.

From Whaley, L.F., and Wong, D.L.:
Nursing care of infants and children, ed. 2,
St. Louis, 1983, The C.V. Mosby Co.

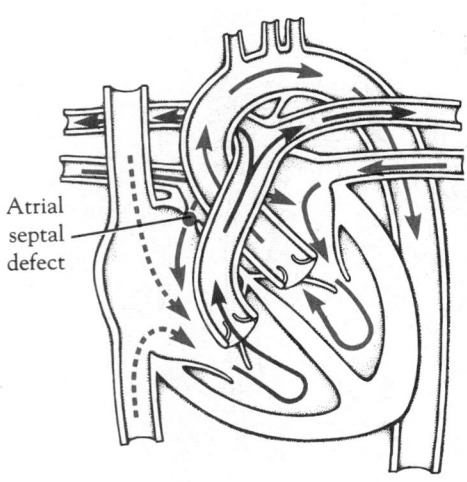

Atrial septal defect

Fig. 1-47
Ventricular septal defect.

From Whaley, L.F., and Wong, D.L.:
Nursing care of infants and children, ed. 2,
St. Louis, 1983, The C.V. Mosby Co.

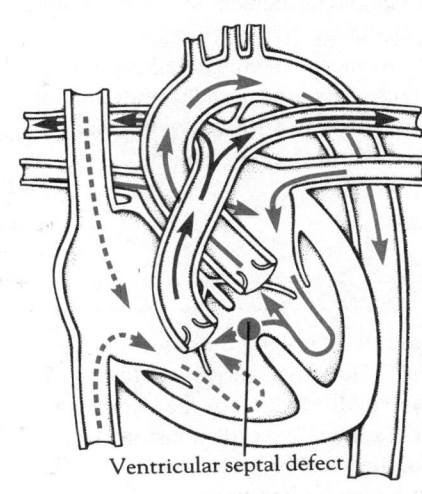

Ventricular septal defect

Fig. 1-48
Tetralogy of Fallot.

From Whaley, L.F., and Wong, D.L.:
Nursing care of infants and children, ed. 2,
St. Louis, 1983, The C.V. Mosby Co.

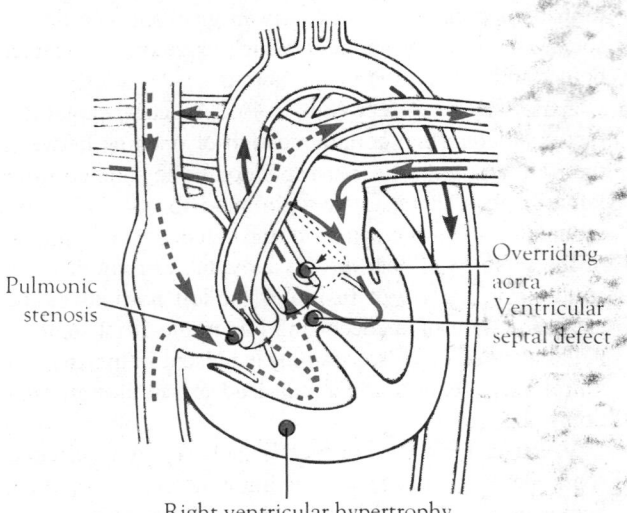

Pulmonic stenosis

Overriding aorta
Ventricular septal defect

Right ventricular hypertrophy

Fig. 1-49
Pulmonic stenosis.

From Whaley, L.F., and Wong, D.L.:
Nursing care of infants and children, ed. 2,
St. Louis, 1983, The C.V. Mosby Co.

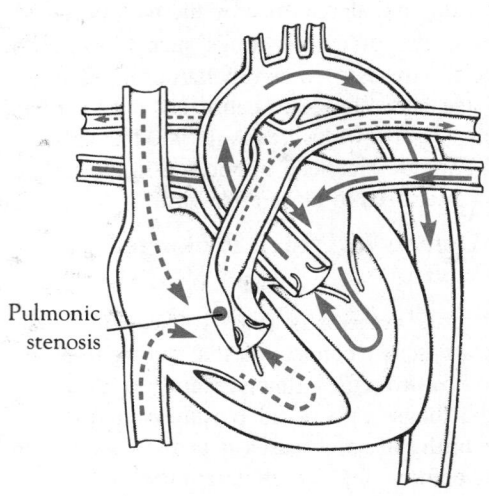

Pulmonic stenosis

is an anomaly characterized by four defects: ventricular septal defect, right ventricular outflow obstruction (pulmonic stenosis), deviation (dextroposition) of the aorta so it overrides the ventricular septum, and right ventricular hypertrophy. It is the most common cyanotic lesion in which survival to adulthood is expected. The severity of symptoms depends on the size of the ventricular septal defect, degree of pulmonic stenosis, and position of the aorta. Right ventricular outflow is obstructed, resulting in hypertrophy of the right ventricle and a right-to-left shunt. This produces a decrease in systemic arterial oxygen saturation, cyanosis, reduced pulmonary blood flow, and in some cases a hypoplastic pulmonary artery.

Pulmonic valvular stenosis (Fig. 1-49). Congenital pulmonic valvular stenosis may occur as an isolated anomaly, in conjunction with other defects such as atrial or ventricular septal defect, or as part of tetralogy of Fallot. If it is an isolated anomaly, the chance of survival to adulthood is good. Pulmonic stenosis may occur as one of three types: valvular, subvalvular (infundibular), or supravalvular. The degree of right ventricular hypertrophy varies with the degree of obstruction.

DIAGNOSTIC STUDIES

Study	Patent Ductus Arteriosus	Atrial Septal Defect	Ventricuiar Septal Defect	Tetralogy of Fallot	Pulmonic Stenosis
Electrocardiogram (ECG)	Normal (small ductus); left ventricular hypertrophy (LVH); PR interval may be prolonged; atrial fibrillation in adults	Normal; right ventricular hypertrophy (RVH); right bundle branch block; PR interval may be prolonged; left axis deviation (ostium primum); normal or right axis (ostium secundum)	Normal if defect is small; if moderate to large, LVH; LVH/RVH in presence of pulmonary hypertension	RVH	Normal if stenosis is mild; if moderate to severe, RVH and right axis deviation; if severe, right atrial hypertrophy (RAH)
Chest roentgenogram	Normal; with moderate to large shunt, enlarged cardiac silhouette with enlarged LA, LV, and pulmonary artery (PA); enlarged aorta; enlarged pulmonary trunk and increased pulmonary flow	Enlarged RA, RV, PA; increased pulmonary vascular markings; LA, LV, and aortic knob may be small	Mild LVH with small shunt; with large shunt, increased LV, dilation of PA, increased pulmonary vascular markings, enlarged LA	Small cardiac silhouette; small PA; prominent aorta (may arch to right in 25% of cases)	Enlarged RV and PA; if severe, decreased peripheral pulmonary vascular markings
Echocardiogram	Ductus not visualized; enlarged LA and LV owing to left-to-right shunt	With ostium secundum, enlarged RV, paradoxic movement of septum during systole; with ostium primum, mitral valve displaced inferiorly and anteriorly	Defect not visualized; large shunt; enlarged LA	Overriding aorta visualized; pulmonary stenosis visualized with degree of obstruction; enlarged ventricular septum (septal motion remains normal)	Normal if stenosis is mild; if moderate to severe, enlarged RA and RV
Laboratory tests	No specific findings	No specific findings	No specific findings unless patient is cyanotic, then increased hematocrit value, decreased hemoglobin level and arterial oxygen saturation	Increased hematocrit value; degree depends on amount of deoxygenated systemic blood	No specific findings

Study	Patent Ductus Arteriosus	Atrial Septal Defect	Ventricular Septal Defect	Tetralogy of Fallot	Pulmonic Stenosis
Cardiac catheterization	Increased pulmonary blood flow; increased oxygen saturation in PA; intracardiac pressures normal; RV and PA pressures may be slightly elevated	Left-to-right shunt at atrial level; increased oxygen saturation in RA; RA pressure usually normal; mitral regurgitation	Left-to-right shunt (LV to RV); study determines degree of shunt; increased pulmonary blood flow, oxygen saturation in RV, and systolic pressure in RV and PA	RV outflow obstruction; increased RV pressure RV to LV shunt; decreased PA pressure as catheter crosses obstruction	Increased RA pressure, which determines systolic pressure gradient between RV and PA

TREATMENT PLAN

Surgical

Patent ductus arteriosus
  Ligation of ductus
Atrial septal defect
  Direct closure by suturing or placement of Dacron patch across defect
  Correction of mitral regurgitation by valvuloplasty or replacement (depends on degree of regurgitation)
Ventricular septal defect
  Direct closure by suturing or with placement of Dacron patch across defect
Tetralogy of Fallot
  Palliative procedures performed on infants to enhance blood flow to lungs, thereby reducing hypoxia
    Blalock-Taussig procedure—anastomosis between subclavian artery and pulmonary artery
    Potts' anastomosis—side-to-side anastomosis of left pulmonary artery to descending aorta
    Waterston-Cooley procedure—anastomosis of right pulmonary artery to ascending aorta
Pulmonic stenosis
  Valvotomy; resection of excess infundibular muscle; valve replacement
Corrective surgery—intracardiac repair of ventricular septal defect and pulmonic stenosis; contraindicated if pulmonary artery is hypoplastic

Chemotherapeutic

Dictated by patient's clinical picture and presence of ventricular failure and arrhythmias

Electromechanical

Dictated by patient's clinical picture

Supportive

None specific unless indicated by complications such as heart failure, arrhythmias, or effects of polycythemia in cyanotic patient

ASSESSMENT: AREAS OF CONCERN

Area of Concern	Patent Ductus Arteriosus	Atrial Septal Defect	Ventricular Septal Defect	Tetralogy of Fallot	Pulmonic Stenosis
Physical examination	Small shunt: asymptomatic, increased respiratory infections, small for age; large shunt: exertional dyspnea, decreased exercise tolerance	Small shunt: asymptomatic; moderate to large shunt: exertional dyspnea, decreased exercise tolerance, palpitations	Small to moderate shunt: asymptomatic, exertional dyspnea; large shunt: failure in infancy, growth failure, feeding difficulties	In infancy: paroxysmal attacks of dyspnea with loss of consciousness ("blue" spells), small for age; in later childhood: cyanosis with clubbing of fingers and toes; in adulthood (following palliation): exertional dyspnea, cyanosis with clubbing	Asymptomatic during childhood; exertional dyspnea; decreased exercise tolerance

Area of Concern	Patent Ductus Arteriosus	Atrial Septal Defect	Ventricular Septal Defect	Tetralogy of Fallot	Pulmonic Stenosis
Palpation	Neck vessels dilated and pulsating	Left parasternal lift	Large shunt: left parasternal lift	Precordial prominence; parasternal heave	Left parasternal heave; subxiphoid pulsation
Auscultation	Systolic pressure normal; diastolic pressure low; wide pulse pressure; harsh, loud, continuous murmur in first, second, and third intercostal spaces (ICS) at lower sternal border (LSB); machinery-like murmur best heard when patient is lying, becoming fainter when patient is standing	Soft blowing systolic murmur at second ICS at LSB	Small shunt: holosystolic at third, fourth, and fifth ICS, systolic thrill; large shunt: holosystolic murmur at third, fourth, and fifth ICS, splitting of S_2 during expiration, widening during inspiration, systolic ejection sound at second ICS at LSB	Single S_2; systolic ejection murmur at third ICS, may radiate upward to left side of neck	S_1 normal; early systolic ejection click heard at base; midsystolic murmur at second and third ICS at LSB, radiates to suprasternal notch and to left side of neck; S_2 widely split

NURSING DIAGNOSES and NURSING INTERVENTIONS

Nursing Diagnosis	Nursing Intervention
Knowledge deficit	Instruct parents on type of defect and how to manage at home, and provide referral services for assistance with home care. For adult patients, provide detailed explanation of defect and treatments as dictated by defect.
Anxiety	Assess level of anxiety. Determine primary cause of anxiety. Encourage verbalization of feelings. Elicit questions and concerns of patient. Assist patient to deal realistically with anxiety, providing alternative methods for dealing with anxiety. Refer patient to long-term counseling if necessary.

Patient Education

1. Instruct the patient and family about the primary defect, explaining the associated signs and symptoms and describing what is normal and abnormal.
2. Explain activity allowances and limitations, including schooling, sports, and occupation.
3. For adolescents and adults provide counseling on issues concerning genetics, marriage, contraception, and childbearing.
4. Explain dietary restrictions.
5. Explain the need to prevent endocarditis (see p. 75).

EVALUATION

Patient Outcome	Data Indicating That Outcome is Reached
Level of knowledge is increased.	Patient and family verbalize knowledge regarding defect, prescribed care, medication, need for return visits, and endocarditis prophylaxis.
Anxiety is decreased.	Patient and family verbalize reeducation in anxiety level, and patient and family demonstrate appropriate behavior in self-care management.

Medical Interventions

CARE OF PATIENTS UNDERGOING CARDIAC SURGERY

Description and Rationale

Surgical interventions for cardiac disorders may be employed as a corrective measure in congenital heart disease or as an alternative treatment modality when a patient's clinical course becomes refractory to medical management.

Cardiac surgery may be broadly classified as an open or a closed procedure. Open heart techniques were made possible with the development of the cardiopulmonary bypass machine (extracorporeal circulation) in the early 1950s. Since that time, advances in myocardial preservation, in preoperative and postoperative support devices, and in pharmacology have contributed to improved mortality and morbidity and to increases in the number of operative procedures for cardiac disorders.

Procedures for acquired disorders include the following:

    Coronary artery bypass graft (CABG) surgery—myocardial revascularization for coronary artery disease; aimed at relief of unstable angina pectoris

    Valve surgery—valvulotomy (commissurotomy), valvuloplasty (repair of valve), and replacement with prosthetic valve

    Resection of ventricular aneurysm—resection of nonviable myocardium

    Septal defects—Closure of atrial or ventricular septal defect by direct suturing or placement of Dacron patch across defect

Procedures for congenital defects include these:

    Closure of patent ductus arteriosus

    Closure of atrial or ventricular septal defect

    Repair of coarctation of aorta

    Repair of tetralogy of Fallot

    Fontan or modified Fontan procedure for tricuspid atresia and single ventricle

    Mustard procedure for transposition of great vessels

Contraindications

Contraindications to cardiac surgery include bleeding disorders and acute (recent) cerebrovascular accident (stroke).

Cautions

Streptokinase should be administered within 24 hours before a cardiac surgical procedure. Cardiac surgery may be performed without added risk in the presence of pulmonary hypertension, in patients with an active infectious process, or in refractory ventricular failure.

Preprocedural Care

1. Determine the type of lesion and associated risks.
2. Initiate preoperative instruction for the patient and family, including information about the operative procedure and postoperative care: routine procedures of the intensive care unit (suctioning, coughing, turning, monitoring of vital signs); various tubes (endotracheal, chest, gastrointestinal, urinary catheter, intravenous); equipment (respirators, monitors); pain management; level of consciousness and emotional response; and visitor policies.
3. Obtain written informed consent.
4. Obtain baseline data: chest roentgenogram; ECG; laboratory work: complete blood count, blood type and cross-match, electrolytes, serum chemistries, and urinalysis; weight; height; and vital signs.
5. Perform skin preparation: chest; legs for vein harvesting.
6. Hold or modify preoperative medications:
   Digoxin—discontinued 24 to 36 hours before surgery
   Antiplatelets—instruct patient not to take these up to 1 week before surgery
   Anticoagulants—discontinue warfarin; initiate heparin therapy
   Antiarrhythmics, antihypertensives—in most cases continue until hours before surgery
7. Initiate pulmonary preparation by instructing the patient to stop smoking, teaching the patient methods for coughing and deep breathing, and using an incentive spirometer.
8. Deal with preoperative anxiety, offering reassurance and support.
9. Assist with insertion of balloon flotation catheter, if ordered, before surgery.
10. Administer preoperative sedation.

TREATMENT PLAN

Surgical

    Cardiopulmonary bypass machine (extracorporeal circulation; heart-lung machine)—assumes function of heart and lungs, providing quite bloodless operative field; procedure involves cannulation of great vessels, allowing drainage of unoxygenated blood that is emptied into venous reservoir; blood is then passed to oxygenator where it is fully saturated; to reduce tissue oxygen requirements, temperature of blood circulating in extracorporeal unit is lowered; cold blood is returned to patient, reducing total body temperature and slowing metabolic processes; myocardial preservation is required while the heart is arrested and includes coronary perfusion, topical cooling (profound hypothermia), and cold cardioplegia arrest

Chemotherapeutic
Preoperative management
  Cardiac glycosides
    Digoxin (Lanoxin)
      Indications: Atrial fibrillation and flutter
      Usual dosage: 0.25 mg or 0.5 mg (to control rate)
  Antiarrhythmics
    Lidocaine (Xylocaine)
      Indications: Ventricular ectopy, tachycardia
      Usual dosage: IV bolus 50-100 mg followed by continuous IV drip
    Quinidine sulfate (Quinora, others)
      Indications: Ventricular ectopy, tachycardia
      Dosage varies
    Procainamide (Pronestyl)
      Indications: Ventricular ectopy, tachycardia
      Usual dosage: 0.5-1 g IM; 0.2-1 g IV
  Potassium replacement
      Usual dosage: IV or po to maintain serum levels at 4 to 5 mEq/L
Postoperative management (based on clinical symptoms, complications, and progress of patient)
  Parenteral fluids
      Usual dosage: Calculated on basis of procedure performed and patient's body surface area: CABG, 50 ml/h; valve replacement, 1000-1500 ml/24 h; pediatric dosage, 60 ml/kg for first 10 kg body weight, 30 ml/kg for next 10 kg, 15 ml/kg for remainder of weight

Electromechanical
Intra-aortic balloon pump—used when severe ventricular dysfunction occurs as patient is removed from bypass; provides circulatory support to failing myocardium
Hemodynamic monitoring—arterial, left atrial, pulmonary artery, and pulmonary capillary wedge pressures; cardiac output measurements may be required
ECG monitoring—continuous evaluation of heart rate, rhythm
Pacemakers

Immediate postoperative
  Assisted ventilation
  Suctioning
  Chest tubes

Supportive
Diet therapy—sodium and fluid restrictions on basis of patient's clinical status
Pulmonary toilet—encourage coughing, deep breathing, and use of incentive spirometry

ASSESSMENT: AREAS OF CONCERN

Level of consciousness
Early
  Arousable
Late
  Alert and oriented

Pupils
May be small, but reactive to light

Motor function
As patient awakens, moves all extremities

Respiratory function
Early
  Atelectasis; diminished breath sounds at base
Late
  Clear with full aeration; arterial blood gases normal

Cardiovascular system
Low cardiac output
  Narrow pulse pressure; thready, rapid pulse; decreased urine output; labored respiration; disorientation
Arrhythmias
  Atrial fibrillation and flutter; junctional rhythms; heart block; ventricular rhythms: premature ventricular contractions, tachycardia, fibrillation
Cardiac tamponade
  Hypotension; narrowed pulse pressure (10 mm Hg); pulsus paradoxus; widened mediastinal shadow on chest roentgenogram; increased venous pressure
Bleeding
  Chest tube drainage at least 250 ml/hour; hypotension; disorientation; prolonged prothrombin time and partial thromboplastin time; decreased platelet levels
Infection
  Elevated temperature; purulent drainage from suture sites; chills; diaphoresis; malaise
Pericarditis; postpericardiotomy syndrome
  Pericardial friction rub; low-grade fever; chills; diaphoresis; malaise; chest pain

NURSING DIAGNOSES and NURSING INTERVENTIONS

Nursing Diagnosis	Nursing Intervention
Cardiac output, alteration in: decreased	Monitor pulmonary artery, pulmonary capillary wedge, and arterial pressures every 15 minutes during immediate postoperative period, decreasing frequency as clinical status stabilizes. Then monitor vital signs every 2 to 4 hours. Measure output every hour; report output of less than 30 ml/hour in an adult patient. Check peripheral perfusion: pulses, skin temperature, and color. Administer fluids and medications as ordered.
Gas exchange, impaired (related to ineffective airway clearance)	Administer oxygen therapy with assisted ventilation. Check respirations, observing rate and quality as patient is weaned from respirator. Obtain and monitor arterial blood gases per protocol. Auscultate lung sounds every 1 to 2 hours. Suction every 1 to 2 hours; oxygenate before suctioning procedure per institutional policy. Observe for signs of progressive atelectasis. *Convalescent care:* Encourage coughing and deep breathing. Encourage use of incentive spirometer. Auscultate lung sounds every 4 to 8 hours.
Fluid volume deficit, actual and potential	During rewarming check right atrial pressure, left atrial pressure, and pulmonary artery pressure every 5 minutes until stable, then every 30 to 60 minutes. Titrate parenteral fluids according to hemodynamic parameters per protocol. Measure output every hour; check specific gravity as ordered. Limit fluid intake as ordered. Monitor for signs of hypovolemia, including decreased blood pressure, increased heart rate, decreased central venous pressure, decreased pulmonary artery pressure, and oliguria. Monitor electrolytes, hemoglobin, and hematocrit. Measure chest tube drainage every 30 to 60 minutes. Weigh daily as indicated by clinical picture.
Potential patient problem: infection	Observe suture sites for local redness, drainage, and swelling. Check temperature every 2 hours for 48 hours, then every 4 hours for 48 hours, then every 8 hours. Observe for signs of generalized sepsis: elevated temperature, chills, and diaphoresis. Obtain blood cultures as ordered. Obtain complete blood count with differential as ordered.
Potential patient problem: hemorrhage	Observe for signs of hemorrhage: decreased blood pressure, disorientation, and falling hemoglobin level. Observe for signs of coagulopathy: blood oozing from incision, bloody secretions from endotracheal tube, and hematuria. Observe and measure chest tube drainage every 30 to 60 minutes. Report output in excess of 150 ml/hour for an adult or 5 ml/kg/hour for a child. Check hemoglobin, hematocrit, and clotting studies on patient's arrival to intensive care unit and every 2 to 4 hours as indicated. Administer blood and blood products as ordered.
Anxiety	*Preoperative:* Provide adequate instruction, allowing for questions and offering reassurance. Explain method of communication to be used after operation while patient is intubated. *Postoperative:* Orient patient to time, situation, and location. Inform patient that surgery is over. Assist with communication. Anticipate needs if possible. Allow family support and participation. Provide reassurance of daily progress. Encourage verbalization of fears and questions regarding operation, recovery, and discharge. Begin postoperative instruction.

Patient Education

1. Review the surgical procedure, emphasizing any precautions or complications that may be associated with the procedure.
2. Clarify what action(s) should be taken if symptoms of infection, bleeding, ventricular failure, or arrhythmias develop.
3. Review diet and fluid restrictions.
4. Review discharge medication, including purpose, dosages, side effects, and need for specific follow-up laboratory studies as indicated.
5. Discuss activity allowances or limitations. Refer patient to cardiac rehabilitation for progressive ambulation.
6. Discuss the importance of avoiding fatigue and sitting for prolonged periods of time.
7. Discuss care of incisions and symptoms of wound infection to report to the physician.

EVALUATION

Patient Outcome	Data Indicating That Outcome is Reached
Hemodynamic and electromechanical stability is achieved. Cardiac output is adequate.	Blood pressure, pulmonary artery pressure, and cardiac output are within acceptable range. There is no arrhythmia. ECG findings are within acceptable limits.
There is no infection.	Patient is afebrile.
Oxygenation, ventilation, and lung perfusion are adequate.	Pao_2 and Pco_2 are within normal limits. There is no dyspnea or tachypnea. Lungs are clear on auscultation and radiography.
Anxiety is reduced.	There is no pain. Anxiety is absent or decreased. Patient demonstrates appropriate behavior patterns: asking questions and participating in self-care.
Patient has knowledge and understanding of primary cardiac disorder, surgical procedure performed, and discharge instructions.	Patient is able to describe specific action to take regarding diet, medications, and care of incision(s). Patient is able to describe activity allowances and limitations.

CARDIOVERSION AND DEFIBRILLATION

Description and Rationale

Synchronous cardioversion is the electrical conversion of a tachyarrhythmia, such as atrial fibrillation, atrial flutter, or supraventricular tachycardia, to a normal sinus rhythm. A synchronized electrical shock is released through the chest wall, depolarizing the myocardium and simultaneously making it refractory, thereby enabling the S-A node to resume its function as primary pacemaker.

Defibrillation is the use of direct-current electrical countershock for the treatment of ventricular tachycardia and ventricular fibrillation. An emergency procedure, it is often performed in conjunction with basic life support measures.

Cautions

When cardioversion is performed, the electrical current must be timed so the discharge occurs at the apex of the R wave of the ECG pattern. Caution must be taken to avoid zones of vulnerability during which electrical current can produce ventricular fibrillation. The most vulnerable zone is the peak of the T wave on the ECG pattern.

Contraindications

Contraindications to cardioversion include atrial fibrillation of long standing or with slow ventricular rate, sick sinus syndrome with tachycardia, digitalis toxicity, and third-degree heart block.

Preprocedural Care

1. Explain the procedure to the patient and family, including rationale and associated risks.
2. Obtain written informed consent unless used in life-threatening situations.
3. Permit nothing by mouth for 6 to 8 hours before the procedure.
4. Withhold digitalis for 24 to 72 hours before the procedure.
5. Check digitalis and potassium levels.

6. Maintain an emergency cart at the bedside.
7. Attach the patient to an ECG and obtain baseline rhythm.
8. Insert an intravenous line.
9. Administer sedation as ordered (an anesthetist is usually in attendance).

TREATMENT PLAN

Chemotherapeutic
Antiarrhythmic drugs
  Quinidine sulfate (Quinora, others)
    Indications: Atrial fibrillation or flutter
    Usual dosage: 200-400 mg po q6h beginning 24-48 h before procedure
    For ventricular tachycardia or fibrillation, lidocaine (Xylocaine) bolus (50-100 mg) may be given
  Lidocaine (Xylocaine)
    Indications: Ventricular tachycardia or fibrillation
    Usual dosage: Bolus of 50-100 mg
Anesthesia during elective procedure—light intravenous anesthesia may be given by anesthetist
Tranquilizers
  Diazepam (Valium)
    Usual dosage: IV in 5 mg increments

Electromechanical
Cardiac monitoring—rhythm strip obtained before, during, and after procedure

Supportive
Oxygen therapy as ordered; intubation equipment on standby
Cardiopulmonary resuscitation in absence of breathing and pulse
Vital signs before, during, and after procedure

ASSESSMENT: AREAS OF CONCERN

During procedure
Cardioverter electrical voltage
  Synchronous cardioversion: 50-400 watt-seconds; defibrillation: 400 watt-seconds for person weighing 50 kg

After procedure
Mental status
  Awake, alert
Vital signs
  Within normal limits
ECG
  Normal sinus rhythm
Precordial chest
  Observe for skin burns

Complications
Ventricular fibrillation, cardiac arrest, pulmonary embolism, myocardial injury, hypotension, transient heart block

NURSING DIAGNOSES and NURSING INTERVENTIONS

Nursing Diagnosis	Nursing Intervention
Skin integrity, impairment of: actual	Check area where electrode paddles were placed. Wash area of electrode paddle placement with water and apply lanolin-based lotions as indicated.
Cardiac output, alteration in: decreased	Monitor blood pressure, pulse, and respirations every 5 to 10 minutes after procedure. Assess level of consciousness. Monitor ECG every 2 to 4 hours as ordered after procedure. Initiate hemodynamic monitoring as ordered.

EVALUATION

Patient Outcome	Data Indicating That Outcome is Reached
Sinus rhythm is reestablished.	ECG monitor shows normal sinus rhythm. Pulse rate is regular.

HEMODYNAMIC MONITORING

Description and Rationale

Monitoring to assess a patient's circulatory status may be done by indirect (noninvasive) or direct (invasive) methods. Indirect methods include arterial pressure monitoring by sphygmomanometer and stethoscope, heart rate monitoring by chest electrode placement, and cardiac monitoring. Direct methods are indicated by the term "hemodynamic monitoring."

Hemodynamic monitoring is a technique that permits close examination of cardiac function in acutely ill patients. Used primarily in critical care units, hemodynamic monitoring permits rapid identification of complications of myocardial infarction, guides the diagnosis and man-

agement of patients in shock, and helps to differentiate pulmonary disease from left ventricular failure.[29]

With use of a balloon-tipped, flow-directed catheter to provide continuous monitoring of the pulmonary artery pressure and pulmonary capillary wedge pressure, myocardial function can be evaluated in terms of preload, afterload, and contractility. From these parameters the left ventricular end-diastolic pressure (LVEDP) can be estimated. Other possible measurements include cardiac output by the thermodilution method and sampling of arteriovenous oxygen differences. Hemodynamic monitoring also provides a direct means of assessing the patient's progress and response to fluid and drug management.

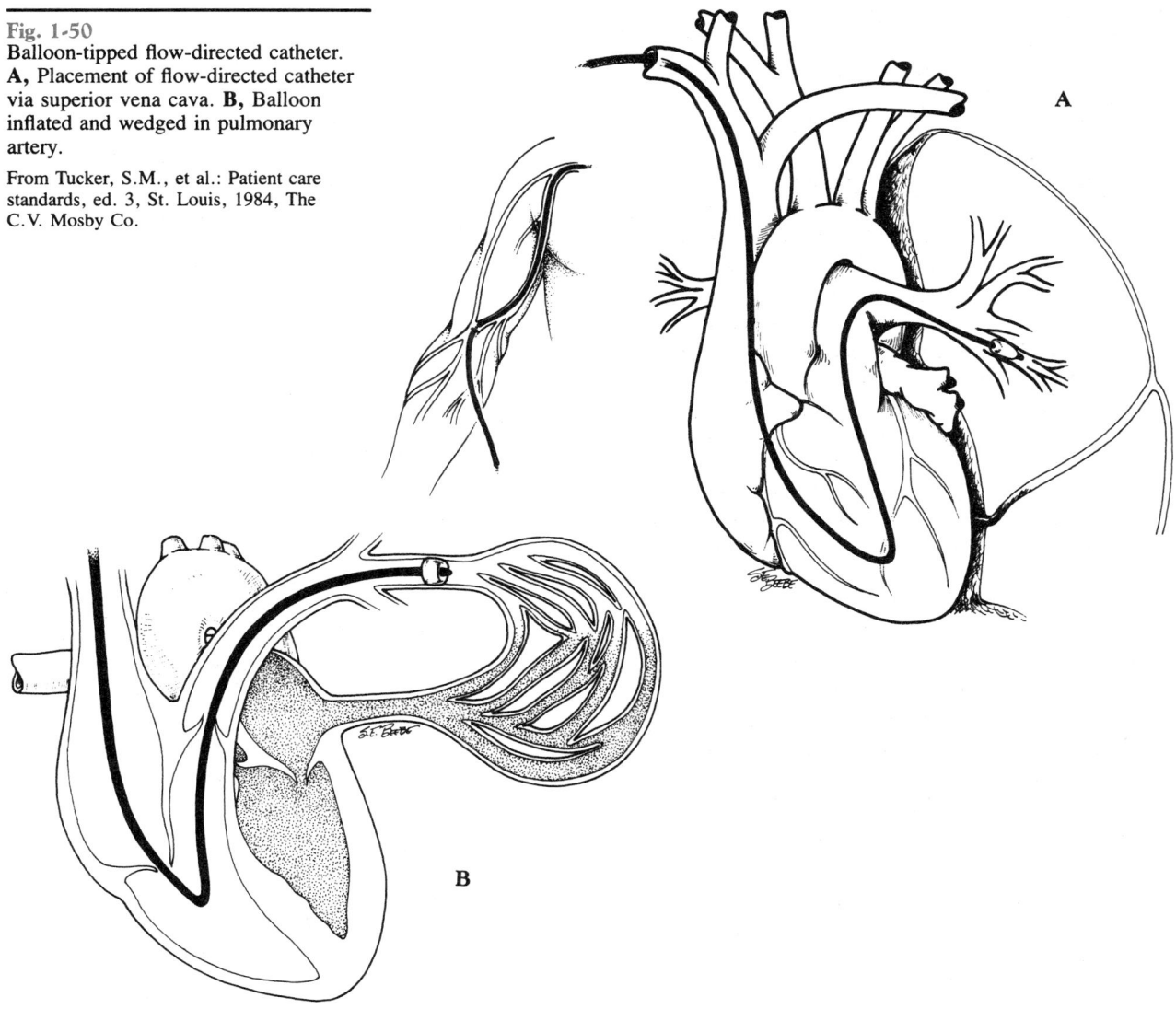

Fig. 1-50
Balloon-tipped flow-directed catheter. **A,** Placement of flow-directed catheter via superior vena cava. **B,** Balloon inflated and wedged in pulmonary artery.

From Tucker, S.M., et al.: Patient care standards, ed. 3, St. Louis, 1984, The C.V. Mosby Co.

Pulmonary artery pressure and pulmonary capillary wedge pressure. Although the LVEDP is the major determinant of left ventricular function, it cannot be measured at the bedside. However, the LVEDP can be reflected by the pressure in the pulmonary capillaries and by the pulmonary artery pressure (PAP) at the end of diastole. The catheter, which is introduced via the subclavian vein or by cutdown, is passed through the right heart into the pulmonary artery (Fig. 1-50). There the balloon is inflated, occluding the artery. With the balloon inflated, the catheter is wedged in a distal branch of the capillaries (Fig. 1-50). The pressure recorded reflects left atrial pressure, which corresponds to the LVEDP and is called the pulmonary capillary wedge pressure (PCWP).

Intra-arterial pressure (arterial line). Continuous monitoring of systemic arterial pressure is made possible by placement of an indwelling catheter, connected to a transducer and monitor, into a major artery. Central artery pressures, although more accurate, are used less frequently. The radial artery is the most common site for placement. The line also facilitates obtaining blood samples to measure arterial blood gases.

Cardiac output. The cardiac output, the volume of blood the heart pumps per minute, can be measured using a calibrated thermistor located near the tip of the pressure catheter. Based on the Fick principle, a thermodilution technique using blood temperature changes is used to produce cardiac output determinations. A known volume of iced solution is injected at a specific rate into the right atrium via the proximal port of a three- or four-lumen pulmonary pressure catheter. The temperature-sensitive thermistor records the temperature of the blood as it passes through the catheter. The difference in temperature between the iced injectate and the blood is calculated, and the cardiac output is then digitally displayed by a special computer.

Contraindications and Cautions

Patients with left bundle-branch block should be observed for development of right bundle-branch block during insertion and while the flotation catheter is in place. Insertion of the flotation catheter in a patient with right-sided endocarditis may cause dislodgment of septic emboli to the lung. Use of the radial artery for monitoring is contraindicated in the presence of inadequate circulation.

Preprocedural Care

1. The catheter can be inserted at the bedside, or the patient may be transferred to a special procedure room for insertion under fluoroscopy.

2. Explain the purpose, risks involved, and techniques of insertion.
3. Obtain written, informed consent.
4. Measure blood pressure, pulse, and respiration. If the cardiac output is to be measured, take the patient's temperature.
5. Connect the patient to a cardiac monitor; obtain a baseline rhythm strip.
6. Place the patient in a supine or slight Trendelenburg position.
7. Assemble the necessary equipment and supplies according to routine hospital policies:
   Monitoring equipment
     Pressure catheter with flush solution, related closed tubing, stopcocks, and a low-flush pressurized system
     Transducer with oscilloscope
   Insertion equipment
     Local anesthetic
     Skin preparation solution
     Sterile gloves
     Dressing supplies
8. Calibrate the pressure monitor according to the manufacturer's directions; for PAP readings, calibrate the transducer to the level of the right atrium.

TREATMENT PLAN

Surgical
Pulmonary pressure catheter (balloon flotation)—inserted via jugular, subclavian, brachial, or right femoral vein by cutdown or percutaneous puncture under local anesthesia
Arterial catheter—inserted via radial, brachial, or femoral artery by percutaneous method

Chemotherapeutic
Flushing system—continuous microdrip of heparinized solution (5% dextrose), kept in closed system under pressure greater than patient's systolic pressure (usually 300 mm Hg) by pressurized bag

Electromechanical
Continuous ECG monitoring

Supportive
Monitoring and recording of pressures every 1 to 2 hours or as ordered
Calibration of transducer and monitor every 4 hours or as specified by manufacturer
Maintaining patency of catheters with continuous pressurized flushing device

Table 1-3
Problems Observed in Pressure Waveforms

Observation	Etiologic Factors	Interventions
Loss of waveform on oscilloscope Loss of PAP; PCWP is displayed on monitor	Displacement of catheter Self-wedging	Reposition patient: notify physician Instruct patient to cough Obtain x-ray examination
Loss of PWP	Displaced into PAP; balloon rupture	Use diastolic of PAP
Decreased amplitude of waveform	Damping due to Clot in catheter	Flush lines: *Do not force if resistance is met*
	Air bubbles	Check all connections for air leaks: flush air bubbles
	Kinking of catheter	Notify physician
	Occluded catheter	Reposition patient; have patient cough
	Tip against artery wall	
Loss of PCWP; no resistance with inflation	Rupture of balloon	Seal off balloon lumen: *Do not allow any injection of air*
Air bubbles in pressure lines Damping of waveform Inaccurate reading	Air leak in system	Check all connections and secure
Artifacts and inadequate pressure readings	Respiratory interference from handling of pressure equipment during readings	Remove patient from respirator; instruct patient to hold his breath during reading
	Inaccurate calibration of equipment	Check for possible interference with tubing during readings
	Faulty equipment	Check electrical system for grounding Check calibration of and level to RA of transducer Check all equipment for proper functioning

From Tucker, S., et al.: Patient care standards, ed. 3, St. Louis, 1984, The C.V. Mosby Co.

ASSESSMENT: AREAS OF CONCERN

Pulmonary artery pressure catheters (Table 1-3)
Pneumothorax and arrhythmias during insertion; pulmonary and air embolism; pulmonary infarction; pulmonary perforation; sepsis or infection; thrombophlebitis at insertion site

Arterial lines
Hemorrhage; clot formation; diminished or absent pulse distal to insertion site; hematoma at insertion site; infection

NURSING DIAGNOSES and NURSING INTERVENTIONS

Nursing Diagnosis	Nursing Intervention
Gas exchange, impaired (potential for)	Observe for signs of pneumothorax and pulmonary air embolism. Observe for and prevent balloon rupture by (1) inflating balloon for few seconds only; (2) ensuring balloon is deflated following wedge pressure measurement; (3) observing waveform for signs of self wedge or damped tracing; (4) securing and labeling catheter and injection ports to avoid confusion of lines. Auscultate chest sounds every 4 hours. Monitor arterial blood gases as ordered. Administer oxygen therapy as ordered.

Nursing Diagnosis	Nursing Intervention
	Maintain aseptic technique during insertion. Change flushing solution and tubing to catheter every day. Change dressing every day, cleaning insertion site with antiseptic agents. Observe for signs of local inflammation or infection.
Anxiety	Provide continuous explanation of procedure. Offer frequent reassurance, encouraging verbalization and questions regarding progress. Allow family and significant others to visit patient when feasible.
Cardiac output, alteration in: decreased (potential for)	Monitor ECG rhythm during and after insertion. Keep lidocaine available at bedside during insertion. Monitor vital signs every 30 to 60 minutes as ordered.

Patient Education

1. Instruct the patient and family in the purpose of the procedure, as cited in preprocedure care.
2. Instruct the patient not to move the insertion area.

EVALUATION

Patient Outcome	Data Indicating That Outcome is Reached
Pressure lines are patent.	Waveform is normal.
There is no infection.	Patient is afebrile.
Anxiety is reduced.	Patient verbalizes absence of anxiety or decrease in anxiety level.
Lung aeration and perfusion are normal.	Lung sounds are clear to bases. There is bilateral aeration. Chest roentgenogram is normal.

INTRA-AORTIC BALLOON PUMPING

Description and Rationale

An intra-aortic balloon pump (IABP) is a mechanical device that provides circulatory assistance to the failing myocardium. Using the principles of counterpulsation, the balloon inflates with diastole and deflates during systole.

A sausage-shaped balloon is inserted through the common femoral artery and passed upward into the aorta. It lies in the descending aorta just distal to the left subclavian artery (Fig. 1-51). Externally the catheter is connected to a power console that has ECG input. Helium or carbon dioxide gas is used to inflate the balloon.

The IABP is used in the treatment of cardiogenic shock in low–cardiac output states, following cardiopulmonary bypass, in drug-resistant arrhythmias caused by ischemia, and in unstable angina. The effect of counterpulsation on left ventricular function is produced by diastolic augmentation and afterload reduction.

The first phase of balloon pumping (Fig. 1-52), with diastolic augmentations, occurs when the balloon inflates during diastole. This displaces the blood remaining in the aorta after ventricular ejection back into the aortic root. The increased blood in the aortic root results in an elevation of diastolic pressure, increasing coronary blood flow and perfusion.

Afterload reduction, the second phase of balloon pumping, occurs when the balloon deflates during systole. With balloon deflation blood flow is encouraged forward out of the left ventricle. This produces decreased myocardial wall tension during diastole (decreased resistance), decreased myocardial oxygen consumption, and improved left ventricular output.

Contraindications

Contraindications to IABP include severe aortic regurgitation, aortic dissection, abdominal aortic aneurysm, and terminal illness.

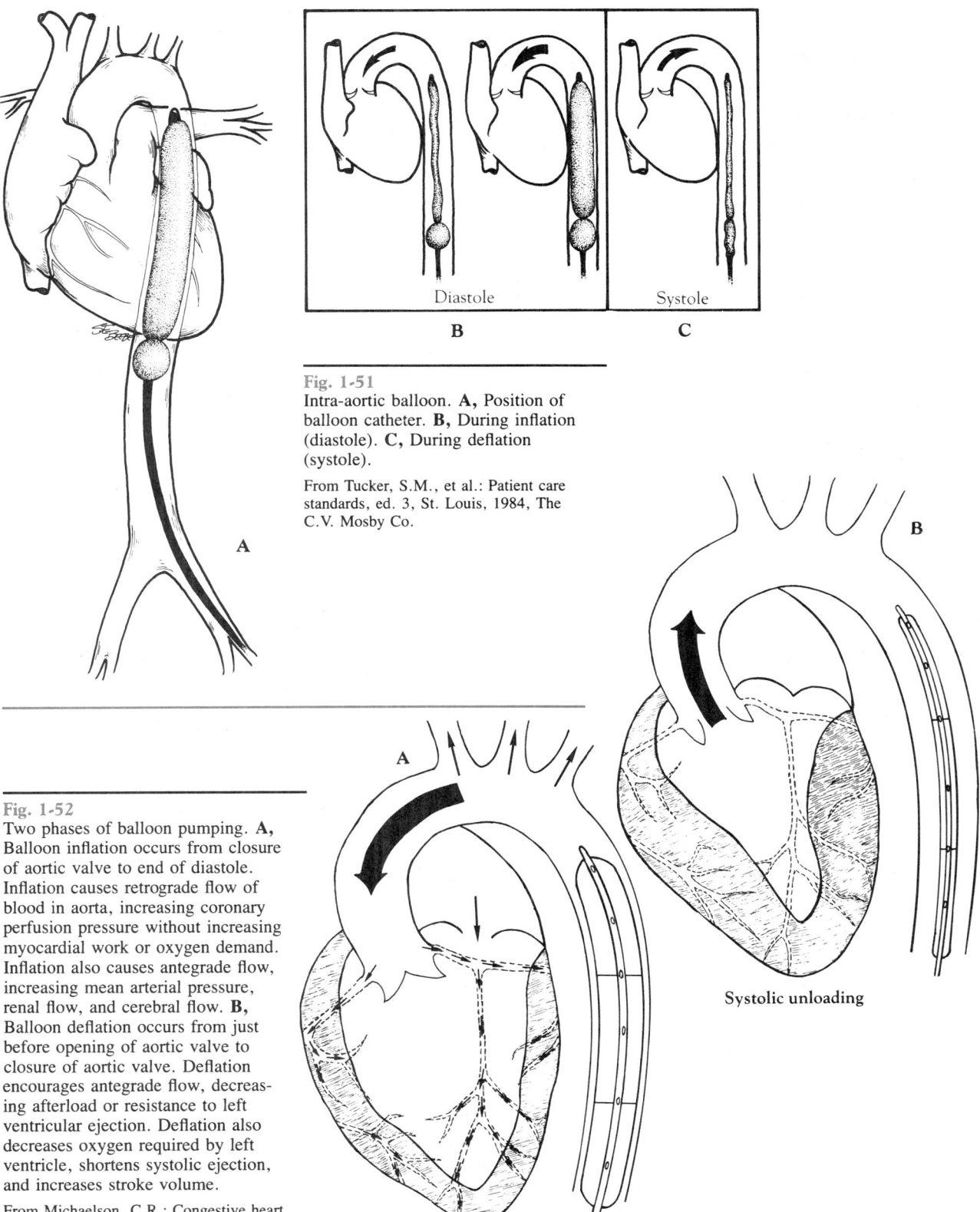

Fig. 1-51
Intra-aortic balloon. **A,** Position of balloon catheter. **B,** During inflation (diastole). **C,** During deflation (systole).

From Tucker, S.M., et al.: Patient care standards, ed. 3, St. Louis, 1984, The C.V. Mosby Co.

Fig. 1-52
Two phases of balloon pumping. **A,** Balloon inflation occurs from closure of aortic valve to end of diastole. Inflation causes retrograde flow of blood in aorta, increasing coronary perfusion pressure without increasing myocardial work or oxygen demand. Inflation also causes antegrade flow, increasing mean arterial pressure, renal flow, and cerebral flow. **B,** Balloon deflation occurs from just before opening of aortic valve to closure of aortic valve. Deflation encourages antegrade flow, decreasing afterload or resistance to left ventricular ejection. Deflation also decreases oxygen required by left ventricle, shortens systolic ejection, and increases stroke volume.

From Michaelson, C.R.: Congestive heart failure, St. Louis, 1983, The C.V. Mosby Co.

Diastole   Systole
B   C

Systolic unloading

Diastolic augmentation

Cautions

The cannulated extremity should not be flexed or bent.

Preprocedural care

1. Explain procedure, insertion technique, equipment to be used, and sensations that may be felt.
2. Obtain written informed consent from the patient or family.
3. Prepare the patient:
   a. Assess and record peripheral circulation, checking pulses and noting color and warmth of extremities; vital signs, including heart and breath sounds; hemodynamic status (arterial pressure, PAP, PCWP, cardiac output); and level of awareness (mentation).
   b. Obtain baseline laboratory data (clotting studies, hemoglobin, hematocrit, white blood cell count, and platelets).
   c. Obtain baseline ECG rate and rhythm.
   d. Prepare groin area.

TREATMENT PLAN

Chemotherapeutic
Local anesthetic agents
   Lidocaine (Xylocaine)

Electromechanical
Continuous monitoring during and after insertion, including ECG, arterial pressure, PAP, cardiac output

Supportive
Diet as ordered
Intravenous therapy as ordered
Oxygen therapy as indicated
Bed rest; turning every 2 hours with assistance

ASSESSMENT: AREAS OF CONCERN

Cannulated extremity
Normal
   Decreased pulse volume and contour
Complications at insertion site
   Infection
      Fever, local tenderness, swelling, purulent drainage
   Bleeding, hematoma
      Ecchymosis, swelling
   Ischemia
      Diminished or absent pulses, numbness, pallor, pain
   Arterial thrombus formation
      Diminished or absent pulses, numbness, pallor, pain

General complications
Aortic dissection, perforation
   Sudden, severe, sharp pain in abdomen and back; hypotension; tachycardia; decreased hematocrit value
Thrombocytopenia
   Bleeding; decreased platelet count (fewer than 150,000/ml)
Progressive myocardial failure
   Decreased cardiac output, arterial pressure, and urine output; increased PCWP; rales; rhonchi
Arrhythmias
   Ventricular ectopy: pulmonary ventricular contractions and ventricular tachycardia; atrial fibrillation

Machine console and equipment
Balloon synchronization
   Inflation (augmentation) at dicrotic notch of aortic waveform; deflation at end of diastole
Complications
   Catheter kinking; malposition; balloon rupture

NURSING DIAGNOSES and NURSING INTERVENTIONS

Nursing Diagnosis	Nursing Intervention
Tissue perfusion, alteration in: peripheral	Monitor peripheral extremities for decreased perfusion every 1 to 2 hours. Provide protection to extremity with sheepskin, lamb's wool, or foot cradle. Perform passive range of motion exercises every 4 hours. Avoid bending extremity. Check dressings every hour.
Cardiac output, alteration: decreased	Monitor arterial pressure, PAP, and PWCP every hour. Assess cardiac output as ordered. Monitor ECG rhythm every hour.
Tissue perfusion, alteration in: cerebral, renal, pulmonary	Assess level of consciousness. Auscultate breath sounds. Monitor arterial blood gases as ordered.

Nursing Diagnosis	Nursing Intervention
	Maintain oxygen therapy as ordered.
	Measure intake and output every hour.
	Ensure that ordered chest roentgenogram is done.
Skin integrity, impairment of: actual and potential	Assess for skin breakdown and decubitus formation.
	Turn and position every 2 hours.
	Provide skin care every 2 to 4 hours.
Anxiety	Provide continued explanation of procedure and treatments.
	Offer frequent reassurance, encouraging verbalization and questions regarding progress.
	Allow family and significant others to visit patient when feasible.

EVALUATION

Patient Outcome	Data Indicating That Outcome is Reached
Perfusion of cannulated extremity is adequate.	Extremity is warm. Capillary filling time is normal. Pulses are palpable. Color is normal. Mobility of extremity is normal.
Myocardial function is restored.	Arterial pressure, cardiac output, and PCWP are within normal limits. Urine output is restored to normal. Lungs are clear. S_3 and S_4 are absent.

PACEMAKERS

Description and Rationale

Pacemakers are battery-operated generators that initiate and control the heart rate by delivering an electrical impulse via an electrode to the myocardium. Implantation of myocardial electrodes is initiated when a patient has symptomatic atrioventricular block. However, since the development of pacemakers in 1960, their use has expanded to include treatment of symptomatic brachyarrhythmias from other causes and refractory tachyarrhythmias.

Pacemaker implantation may be performed for temporary or long-term pacing. In addition to control of the heart rate, temporary pacing is used to evaluate electrophysiologic responses to increased heart rates.

Pacemakers are described using a three-letter designation for the mode of pacing and the chambers to be sensed and paced. The first letter describes the chamber that will be paced: the atrium (A), ventricle (V), or both (dual) chambers (D). The second letter represents the chamber that will be sensed: atrium (A), ventricle (V), dual (D), or none (O). The third letter reflects the mode that will be used: triggered (T), inhibited (I), or both (D). For example:

VVI

V The pacemaker will pace the ventricle.

V The pacemaker will sense the ventricle.

I The pacemaker will inhibit pacing when the patient's own impulse is sensed.

There are three types of pacemakers:

Asynchronous or fixed rate, in which rate and rhythm of pacemaker beats are unaffected by spontaneous beats

Demand pacing or standby pacing, which discharges (fires) only when spontaneous beats drop below a preset minimum rate

Synchronous pacemakers, in which a sensing circuit is used to detect atrial and ventricular activity

Cautions

Safety from electrical hazards should be ensured.

Preprocedural Care

1. Initiate preoperative instruction for the patient and family.
2. Obtain written informed consent.
3. Perform skin preparation.
4. Obtain baseline assessment data: underlying ECG rhythm, heart rate, pulse, respirations, blood pressure, and level of consciousness.
5. Permit nothing by mouth.
6. Initiate intravenous line.
7. Check functioning of external generator (for a temporary unit).

TREATMENT PLAN

Surgical

Method of implantation depends on whether pacing will be temporary or permanent

Transvenous approach—most commonly used technique for temporary pacing; catheter passed into right ventricle via peripheral vein (brachial, femoral, subclavian, or internal jugular); electrode is connected to external battery-operated device that can be set manually for direct or demand pacing mode (Fig. 1-53)

Transthoracic approach—used primarily after open heart surgery; catheter is passed directly into heart through chest wall

Long-term transvenous pacing—catheter electrode is passed into right ventricle and attached to small, sealed, battery-operated pulse generator that is planted subcutaneously in shoulder or upper left quadrant (Fig. 1-54)

Epicardial pacing—performed less frequently; electrode is sutured to epicardial surface of right ventricle; procedure requires a thoracotomy

Chemotherapeutic

Preoperative

Local anesthesia, used for temporary and long-term transvenous pacing

General anesthesia, used for transthoracic approach

Electromechanical

Cardiac monitoring—ECG pattern observed for rate, pacemaker response, signs of pacemaker failure, and arrhythmias

Supportive

Bed rest for 8 hours after implantation, keeping arm below level of shoulder

Range of motion exercises to affected extremity when ordered after third postoperative day

Fig. 1-53
A, Temporary external pacemaker.
B, Temporary pacemaker unit, transvenous approach.

From Tucker, S.M., et al.: Patient care standards, ed. 3, St. Louis, 1984, The C.V. Mosby Co.

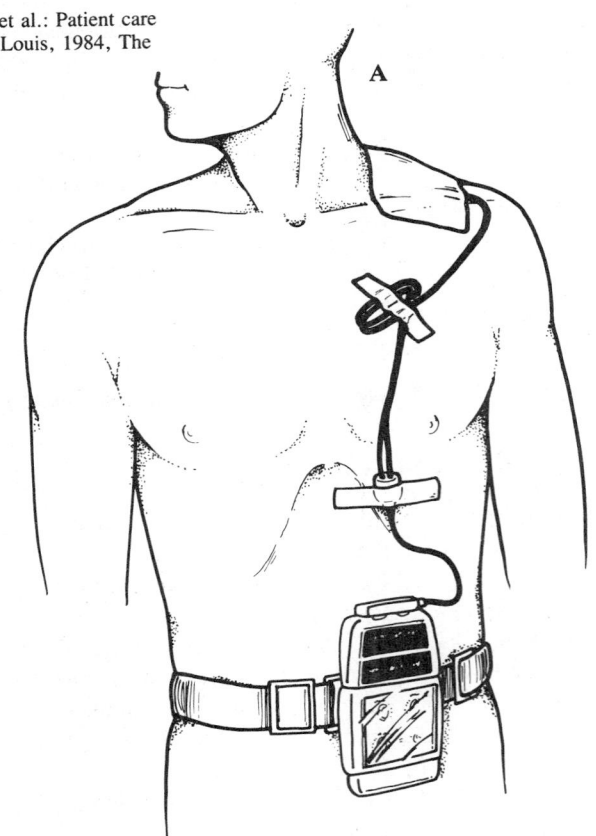
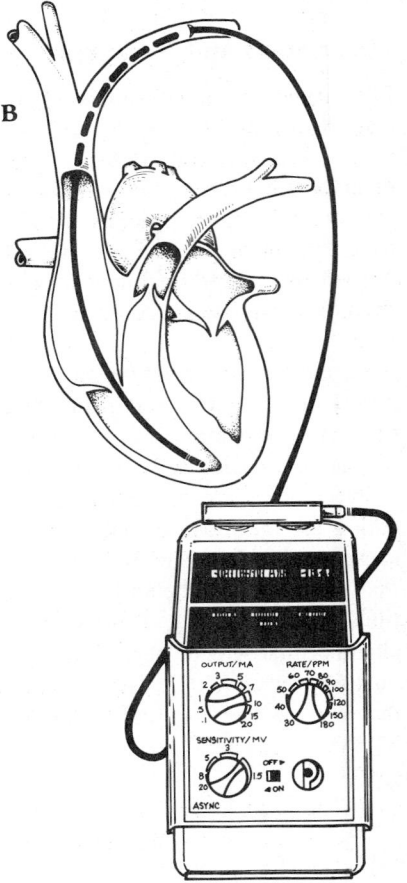

ASSESSMENT: AREAS OF CONCERN

Pacemaker failure
  Clinical symptoms
    Syncope; hypotension; brachycardia; pallor; shortness of breath; chest muscle spasm; hiccoughs
  ECG rhythm
    Loss of pacemaker artifact; change in paced QRS complex; decreased amplitude of pacemaker artifact; competition between patient's underlying rhythm and paced beats; arrhythmias

Infection at incisional site
  Redness; swelling; heat; fluid collection; skin breakdown

Arrhythmias
  Premature ventricular beats; ventricular tachycardia; patient complaints of palpitations

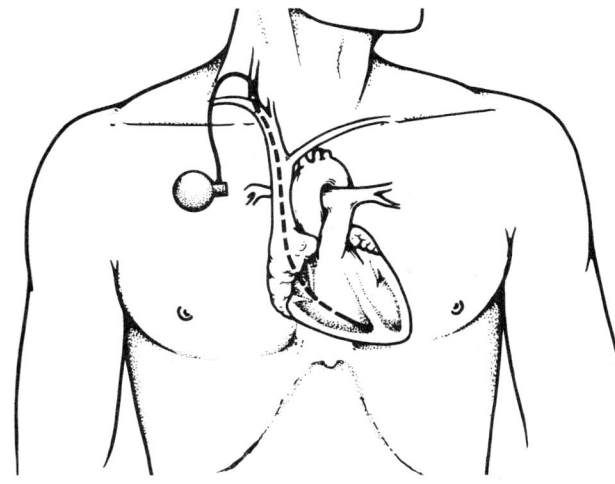

Fig. 1-54
Permanent pacemaker.

From Tucker, S.M., et al.: Patient care standards, ed. 3, St. Louis, 1984, The C.V. Mosby Co.

NURSING DIAGNOSES and NURSING INTERVENTIONS

Nursing Diagnosis	Nursing Intervention
Anxiety	Assess level of anxiety and contributing factors. Provide explanation and rationale for pacemaker, gauging reactions of patient. Anticipate and allow questions from patient regarding changes in life-style, cautions, and concerns over pacemaker management.
Comfort, alteration in: pain	Assess quality and source of pain. Administer pain medication as ordered. Encourage range of motion exercises to affected shoulder as ordered.
Cardiac output, alteration in: decreased	Assess patient and pacemaker unit for signs of pacemaker failure. Monitor vital signs every 4 hours after insertion. Monitor ECG rhythm strip every 4 hours after insertion for 24 hours.
Knowledge deficit	Assess level of knowledge. Correct any misconceptions regarding pacemaker function. Initiate patient education program, providing audiovisual presentations and pamphlets. Provide continued follow-up.

Patient Education

1. Instruct the patient and family about the purpose and rationale for a permanent pacemaker.
2. Describe the type of pacemaker and rate, and teach pulse taking.
3. Describe the signs and symptoms of pacemaker failure.
4. Explain the need for continued medical follow-up and the need for periodic battery replacements; refer the patient to a pacemaker clinic if available.
5. Describe the use of telephone transmitters if available.
6. Explain the signs and symptoms of infection over the incision site, and instruct the patient or family to report to the physician if fever or drainage develops.
7. Instruct in the need to protect the pacemaker site: avoid constricting clothing and direct contact or blows to the site; contact sports are usually contraindicated.
8. Explain avoidance of and protection against electrical hazards from high-output electrical generators.
9. Describe activity allowances and limitations.
10. Explain the need to carry an identification card.

EVALUATION

Patient Outcome	Data Indicating That Outcome is Reached
Pacemaker functions properly.	Patient is normotensive and without dizziness, syncope, palpitations, chest pain, shortness of breath, or fatigue. Heart rate is acceptable. A temporary pacemaker fires at preset rate, sensing mechanism is visualized, and pacemaker artifact is visualized on ECG. A permanent pacemaker fires at preset rate, and pacemaker artifact is visualized on ECG.
Patient is free of infection and pain.	Patient is afebrile. Incisional site is clean with no swelling or redness. Patient verbalizes comfort.

PERICARDIOCENTESIS

Description and Rationale

Pericardiocentesis (Fig. 1-55) is an invasive procedure performed by inserting a needle into the pericardial space (sac) to aspirate fluid. It may be done as a diagnostic procedure for analysis of pericardial fluid or as an emergency measure to relieve cardiac compression and drain the pericardial space.

Contraindications

The procedure is contraindicated in any patient who has been taking anticoagulants.

Fig. 1-55
Pericardiocentesis.

From Sheehy, S.B., and Barber, J.M.: Emergency nursing: principles and practice, ed. 2, St. Louis, 1985, The C.V. Mosby Co.

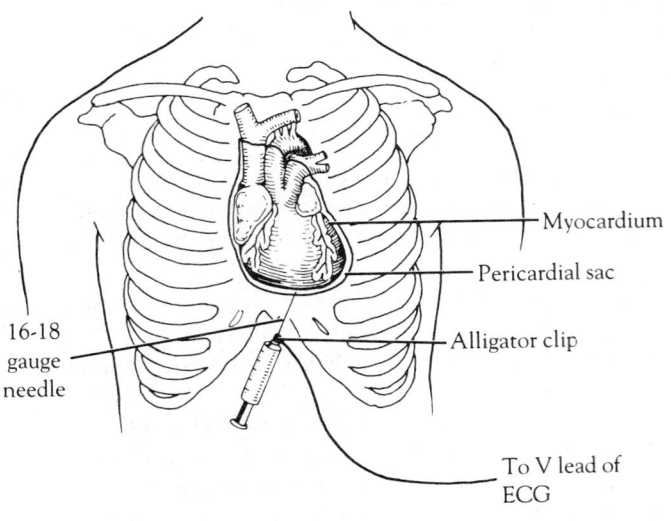

16-18 gauge needle — Myocardium — Pericardial sac — Alligator clip — To V lead of ECG

Cautions

All equipment must be secured and properly grounded to avoid delivering current to the myocardium, which would cause ventricular fibrillation.

Preprocedural Care

1. Explain the procedure, its purpose, and associated risks to the patient and family.
2. Obtain written informed consent.
3. Initiate and maintain the intravenous line.
4. Have an emergency crash cart close by.
5. Assemble equipment:
   Pericardiocentesis tray with 50 ml syringe
   Local anesthetic agents (lidocaine) and equipment (needles, syringes)
   Sterile test tubes and container
   Three-way stopcock
   Standard 12-lead ECG machine
   Kelly clamp
   Alligator clips
6. Perform skin preparation from the left costal margin to the xiphoid process.

TREATMENT PLAN

Surgical
Pericardial window if pericardiocentesis is unsuccessful

Chemotherapeutic
Tranquilizers
Diazepam (Valium)
Usual dosage: 5 mg IV

Electromechanical
Cardiac monitoring during and after procedure

Supportive
Oxygen therapy as ordered

Monitoring blood pressure, pulse, and respiration before and immediately after procedure

ASSESSMENT: AREAS OF CONCERN

ECG changes
Ventricular irritation: premature ventricular contractions, ventricular tachycardia; ischemia: ST elevation

Cardiac tamponade (hemopericardium)
Distended neck veins; paradoxic pulse; narrowed pulse pressure; dyspnea; cyanosis; distant heart sounds

Other complications
Respiratory distress; myocardial injury; shock

NURSING DIAGNOSES and NURSING INTERVENTIONS

Nursing Diagnosis	Nursing Intervention
Cardiac output, alteration in: decreased	After procedure, monitor blood pressure, pulse, respirations, and heart sounds every 15 minutes until stable, then every 30 minutes for 2 hours, then every hour for 4 hours, then every 4 hours. Check for pulsus paradoxus. Assess for improvement of symptoms.
Potential patient problem: infection	Ensure asepsis during procedure. Check temperature every 4 hours after procedure.

EVALUATION

Patient Outcome	Data Indicating That Outcome is Reached
Cardiac compression is relieved.	Pulse pressure is normal and pulsus paradoxus, if present, is less than 10 mm Hg. Symptoms of cardiac tamponade are relieved.

References

1. Akhtar, M.: Practical considerations in the treatment of ventricular arrhythmias with Mexiletine, Am. Heart J. **107**:1086, 1984.
2. American Heart Association: Heart facts—1980, Dallas, 1980, National Center.
3. Anderson, C.S.: The pathophysiology of shock: an overview. In Guthrie, M.M., editor: Shock, New York, 1982, Churchill Livingston, Inc.
4. Anthony, C.P., and Thibodeau, G.A.: Anatomy and physiology, ed. 11, St. Louis, 1983, The C.V. Mosby Co.
5. Arnsdorf, M.F.: Electrophysiologic properties of antiarrhythmic drugs as a rational basis for therapy, Med. Clin. North Am. **60**:213, 1976.
6. Barry, J., and Dieter, W.G.: Endocarditis: an overview, Heart Lung **11**:138, 1982.
7. Belloni, F.L.: The local control of coronary blood flow, Cardiovasc. Res. **13**:63, 1979.
8. Blake, S.: The clinical diagnosis of constrictive pericarditis, Am. Heart J. **106**:432, 1983.
9. Breu, C.S., Lindenmuth, J.E., and Tillisch, J.H.: Treatment of patients with congestive cardiomyopathy during hospitalization: a case study, Heart Lung **11**:229, 1982.
10. Brown, W.J.: A classification of microorganisms frequently causing sepsis, Heart Lung **5**:397, 1976.
11. Brunwald, E.: Heart disease: a textbook of cardiovascular medicine, Philadelphia, 1980, W.B. Saunders Co.
12. Bulkley, B.H.: Primary muscle disease of the heart. In Kaye, D., and Rose, L.F., editors: Fundamentals of internal medicine, St. Louis, 1983, The C.V. Mosby Co.
13. Bulkley, B.H., Weisfeldt, M.L., and Hutchins, G.M.: Asymmetric septal hypertrophy and myocardial fiber disarray, Circulation **56**:292, 1977.
14. Cain, R., Ferguson, R.M., and Tillisch, J.: Variant angina: a nursing approach, Heart Lung **8**:1122, 1979.
15. Canobbio, M.: Noninvasive studies and diagnostic adjuncts for heart failure. In Michaelson, C.R.: Congestive heart failure, St. Louis, 1983, The C.V. Mosby Co.
16. Conolly, M.E., Kersting, F., and Dollery, C.T.: The clinical pharmacology of beta-adrenoceptor-blocking drugs, Prog. Cardiovasc. Dis. **19**:203, 1976.
17. Craven, R.F., and Curry, T.D.: When the diagnosis is Raynaud's, Am. J. Nurs. **8**:1007, 1981.
18. Dalen, J.E., and Alpert, J.S.: Natural history of pulmonary embolism, Prog. Cardiovasc. Dis. **17**:259, 1975.
19. da Luz, P.L., Weil, M.H., and Shubin, H.: Current concepts and mechanisms and treatment of cardiogenic shock, Am. Heart J. **92**:103, 1976.
20. Dole, W.P., and O'Rourke, R.A.: Pathophysiology and management of cardiogenic shock, Curr. Probl. Cardiol. **8**:1, 1983.
21. Fenster, P.E.: Verapamil: new therapy for supraventricular arrhythmias, J. Cardiovasc. Med. **7**:410, 1982.
22. Ginzton, L.E., and Laks, M.M.: Acute pericarditis: recognition by ECG, Primary Cardiol. **10**:73, 1984.
23. Goldberger, E.: Textbook of clinical cardiology, St. Louis, 1982, The C.V. Mosby Co.
24. Goodwin, J.F.: Hypertrophic cardiomyopathy: a disease in search of its own identify, Am. J. Cardiol. **45**:177, 1980.

25. Gregoratos, G., and Karliner, J.S.: Infective endocarditis: diagnosis and management, Med. Clin. North Am. **63**:173, 1979.

26. Groër, M.W., and Shekleton, M.E.: Basic pathophysiology: a conceptual approach, St. Louis, 1983, The C.V. Mosby Co.

27. Guazzi, M., et al.: Repetitive myocardial ischemia of Prinzmetal type with angina pectoris, Am. J. Cardiol. **37**:923, 1976.

28. Guyton, A.C.: Textbook of medical physiology, ed. 8, Philadelphia, 1980, W.B. Saunders Co.

29. Guzzetta, C.E., and Dossey, B.M.: Cardiovascular nursing: body-mind tapestry, St. Louis, 1984, The C.V. Mosby Co.

30. Hardaway, R.M., et al.: The danger of hemolysis in shock, Ann. Surg. **189**:743, 1979.

31. Hoffman, B.F., and Cranefield, P.F.: The physiological basis of cardiac arrhythmias, Am. J. Med. **37**:670, 1964.

32. Hummelgard, A., and Esrig, B.: Calcium and calcium slow channel blockers: an overview, Crit. Care Q. **4**:17, 1981.

33. Johanson, B.C., et al.: Standards for critical care, St. Louis, 1981, The C.V. Mosby Co.

34. Josephson, M., Harken, A., and Horowitz, L.: Endocardial excision: a new surgical technique for the treatment of recurrent ventricular tachycardia, Circulation **60**:1430, 1979.

35. Josephson, M., and Horowitz, L.: Electrophysiologic approach to therapy of recurrent sustained ventricular tachycardia, Am. J. Cardiol. **43**:631, 1979.

36. Kannel, W.B., McGee, D., and Gordon, T.: A general cardiovascular risk profile: the Framingham study, Am. J. Cardiol. **38**:46, 1976.

37. Kaye, D., and Rose, L.F.: Fundamentals of internal medicine, St. Louis, 1983, The C.V. Mosby Co.

38. Kern, L.: Mechanical support of failing heart in congestive heart failure. In Michaelson, C.R.: Congestive heart failure, St. Louis, 1983, The C.V. Mosby Co.

39. King, S.L.: Patient care in vascular surgery, AORN J. **33**:843, 1981.

40. Kistner, R.L., et al.: Incidence of pulmonary embolism and thrombophlebitis of lower extremities, Am. J. Surg. **124**:169, 1972.

41. Lee, N.W.: The diagnosis and treatment of endotoxin shock, Anesthesia **31**:897, 1976.

42. Lees, R.S., and Lees, A.M.: Lipid lowering drugs: renewed enthusiasm, Drug Ther., p. 57, 1984.

43. LeFrock, J.L., et al.: Transient bacteremia associated with sigmoidoscopy, N. Engl. J. Med. **289**:469, 1973.

44. LeFrock, J.L., et al.: Transient bacteremia associated with nasotracheal suctioning, JAMA **236**:1610, 1977.

45. Lerner, P.I., and Weinstein, L.: Infective endocarditis in the antibiotic era, N. Engl. J. Med. **274**:199, 1966.

46. Lewis, S.M., and Collier, I.C.: Medical surgical nursing: assessment and management of clinical problems, New York, 1983, McGraw-Hill Book Co.

47. Maron, B., and Epstein, S.E.: Hypertrophic cardiomyopathy, Am. J. Cardiol. **45**:141, 1980.

48. McAnulty, J.H., and Rahimtoola, S.H.: Surgery for infective endocarditis, JAMA **242**:77, 1979.

49. Miller, D.C., and Roon, A.J.: Diagnosis and management of peripheral vascular disease, Menlo Park, Calif., 1982, Addison-Wesley Publishing Co.

50. Moore, S.: Pericarditis after acute myocardial infarction: manifestations and nursing implications, Heart Lung **8**:551, 1979.

51. Moore, W.S.: What's new in peripheral vascular surgery, J. Cardiovasc. Surg. **24**:49, 1983.

52. Neill, C.A.: Etiology of congenital heart disease, Cardiovasc. Clin. **4**:138, 1972.

53. O'Rourke, M.F.: Cardiogenic shock following myocardial infarction, Heart Lung **3**:353, 1974.

54. Perez, M.M., and Pintos Diaz, G.: Arteriosclerosis obliterans of the lower limbs, Cardiovasc. Rev. **4**:1357, 1983.

55. Perloff, J.K.: Clinical recognition of congenital heart disease, Philadelphia, 1980, W.B. Saunders Co.

56. Rahimtoola, S.: Surgery for infective endocarditis, Crit. Care Q. **4**:51, 1981.

57. Richardson, J.V., et al.: Treatment of infective endocarditis: a 10 year comparative analysis, Circulation **58**:589, 1978.

58. Roberts, B.: Balloon angioplasty in the treatment of peripheral vascular disease, J. Cardiovasc. Surg. **23**:225, 1982.

59. Romhilt, D.W., and Fowler, N.O.: Physical signs in acute myocardial infarction, Heart Lung **2**:74, 1973.

60. Rosenbaum, M.B., et al.: Clinical efficacy of amiodarone as an antiarrhythmic agent, Am. J. Cardiol. **38**:934, 1976.

61. Sacksteder, S., Gildea, J.H., and Dassy, C.: Common congenital cardiac defects, Am. J. Nurs. **78**:266, 1978.

62. Saunderson, R.G., and Kurth, C.L.: The cardiac patient, ed. 2, Philadelphia, 1983, W.B. Saunders Co.

63. Sawaya, J., Muyais, S., and Armenian, H.: Early diagnosis of pericarditis in acute myocardial infarction, Am. Heart J. **100**:144, 1980.

64. Schnittger, I., et al.: Echocardiography: pericardial thickening and constrictive pericarditis, Am. J. Cardiol. **42**:388, 1978.

65. Schomerus, M., et al.: Physiological disposition of verapamil in man, Cardiovasc. Res. **10**:605, 1976.

66. Shabetai, R.: Cardiomyopathy: how far have we come in 25 years, how far yet to go? J. Am. Coll. Cardiol. **1**:252, 1983.

67. Shine, K.I., et al.: Aspects of the management of shock, Ann. Intern. Med. **93**:723, 1980.

68. Silva, J.: Anaerobic infections, Heart Lung **5**:406, 1976.

69. Silver, D., and Stubbs, D.H.: Venous thrombosis, pulmonary embolism and the post phlebitis syndrome. In Miller, D.C., and Roon, A.J.: Diagnosis and management of peripheral vascular disease, Menlo Park, Calif., 1982, Addison-Wesley Publishing Co.

70. Singh, B.N., Collett, J.T., and Chew, C.: New perspectives in the pharmacologic therapy of cardiac arrhythmias, Prog. Cardiovasc. Dis. **22**:243, 1980.

71. Singh, S.: Systemic hypertension. In Kaye, D., and Rose, L.F., editors: Fundamentals of internal medicine, St. Louis, 1983, The C.V. Mosby Co.

72. Spittell, J.A.: Office and bedside diagnosis of occlusive arterial disease, Curr. Probl. Cardiol. **7**, May, 1983.

73. Spodick, D.H.: Acute pericarditis and pericardial effusion: guide to diagnosis and management, Hosp. Med. 72, 1979.

74. Stoddart, J.C.: Gram-negative infections in the ICU, Crit. Care Med. **2**:17, 1974.

75. The 1980 report of the Joint National Committee on Detection: evaluation and treatment of high blood pressure, Arch. Intern. Med. **140**:1280, 1980.

76. Tilkian, S.M., Conover, M.B., and Tilkian, A.: Clinical implications of laboratory tests, St. Louis, 1983, The C.V. Mosby Co.

77. Tucker, S., et al.: Patient care standards, ed. 3, St. Louis, 1984, The C.V. Mosby Co.

78. Watanakunakorn, C.: Changing epidemiology and newer aspects of infective endocarditis, Adv. Intern. Med. **22**:21, 1977.

79. Weil, M.H., and Shubin, H.: Anaphylactic shock in man. In Weil, M.H., and Shubin, H.: Critical care handbook, New York, 1974, John N. Kolen, Inc.

80. Weinstein, L., and Rubin, R.H.: Infective endocarditis—1973, Prog. Cardiovasc. Dis. **16**:239, 1973.

81. Wilson, R.F., and Wilson, F.A.: Sepsis. In Kinney, M.R., et al., editors: AACN's clinical reference for critical care nurses, New York, 1981, McGraw-Hill Book Co.

82. Winston, T.R., Henly, W.S., and Geis, R.C.: Surgery for peripheral vascular disease, AORN J. **33**:849, 1981.

83. Wirsing, P., Andriopoulous, A., and Botticher, R.: Arterial embolectomies in the upper extremity after acute occlusion, J. Cardiovasc. Surg. **24**:40, 1983.

84. Wit, A.L., and Rosen, M.R.: Pathophysiologic mechanisms of cardiac arrhythmias, Am. Heart J. **106**:798, 1983.

85. Wynne, J., and Braunwald, E.: The cardiomyopathies and myocarditis. In Braunwald, E., editor: Heart disease: a textbook of cardiovascular medicine, Philadelphia, 1980, W.B. Saunders Co.

86. Yasue, H., et al.: Prinzmetal's variant form of angina as a manifestation of alpha adrenergic receptor-mediated coronary artery spasm: documentation of coronary arteriography, Am. Heart J. **91**:148, 1976.

87. Zipis, D.P., and Troup, P.J.: New antiarrhythmic agents, Am. J. Cardiol. **41**:100, 1978.

88. Zsoter, T.T.: Calcium antagonist, Am. Heart J. **99**:805, 1980.

CHAPTER 2

Respiratory System

Overview

The primary function of the respiratory system is to supply oxygen to the body cells and to remove carbon dioxide from the cells. Oxygen is used at the cellular level, combining with adenosine diphosphate (ADP) and simple sugar (CHO) to produce energy in the form of adenosine triphosphate (ATP). Carbon dioxide and water are by-products of this cellular metabolism.

The success of the intended respiratory process involves factors external to the body as well as internal factors. The single most common cause of respiratory problems from an external source is, of course, smoking. It is considered to be the major cause of chronic bronchitis, emphysema, and lung cancer in the United States. Environmental respiratory factors have taken on increasing importance over the past 3 decades as by-products of industrialization and urbanization have polluted atmospheric conditions. Minute particles from air pollution inhaled into the respiratory tract frequently cause inflammatory and disease states. Major air pollutants of increasing concern include sulfur dioxide and sulfur trioxide, nitrogen dioxide, carbon monoxide, chlorine, ammonia, hydrocarbons, silica, cobalt, asbestos, and coal dust.[69] These chemicals, in addition to causing respiratory problems, are also responsible for atmospheric smog and haze, which in turn affects crop and vegetation growth and thus photosynthesis. The transportation and petrochemical industries are implicated in much of this pollution.

The internal respiratory factors that become operational once the ambient air reaches the nose and is available for inhalation include ventilation, diffusion and perfusion, blood flow, and control of breathing. All these internal factors must function effectively for adequate respiration to occur.

ANATOMY AND PHYSIOLOGY

The anatomy of the respiratory system is discussed from a functional perspective within each of the four respiratory factor levels:

1. *Ventilation:* the movement of air from outside to inside the body and its distribution within the tracheobronchial system to the gas exchange units of the lungs.
2. *Diffusion and perfusion:* the movement of oxygen and carbon dioxide across the alveolar-capillary membrane to the blood in the pulmonary capillaries.
3. *Blood flow:* the transportation of respiratory gases through the pulmonary and arterial circulation, the distribution and exchange of oxygen and carbon dioxide at the peripheral tissues, and the return of respiratory gases to the lungs.
4. *Control of breathing:* the regulation of ventilation

111

to maintain adequate gas exchange, usually in accord with changing metabolic demands or other special needs.

Ventilation

Ventilation is the process that moves air from outside the body to the gas exchange units of the lungs. To perform this function the muscles of respiration must exert sufficient force to move the chest wall and expand the lungs. There must be enough force to overcome the resistance in the respiratory system so that air will be drawn into the tracheobronchial tree. The volume of air that enters is determined by the mechanical properties of the lung parenchyma, the airways, and the chest wall.

Chest wall. The sternum, manubrium, and xiphoid process form the anterior border of the thorax. The posterior portion is formed by 12 thoracic vertebrae. The lateral boundaries are formed by 12 pairs of ribs, which have a posterior connection directly to the thoracic vertebrae. The first seven ribs also connect anteriorly to the sternum by the costal cartilages (Fig. 2-1).

The major muscle groups used in the ventilatory process are the diaphragm, and the intercostal muscles (Fig. 2-2).

The diaphragm is the principal muscle of inspiration.

Fig. 2-1
Ventilatory structures of the chest wall. **A,** Anterior view. **B,** Posterior view.

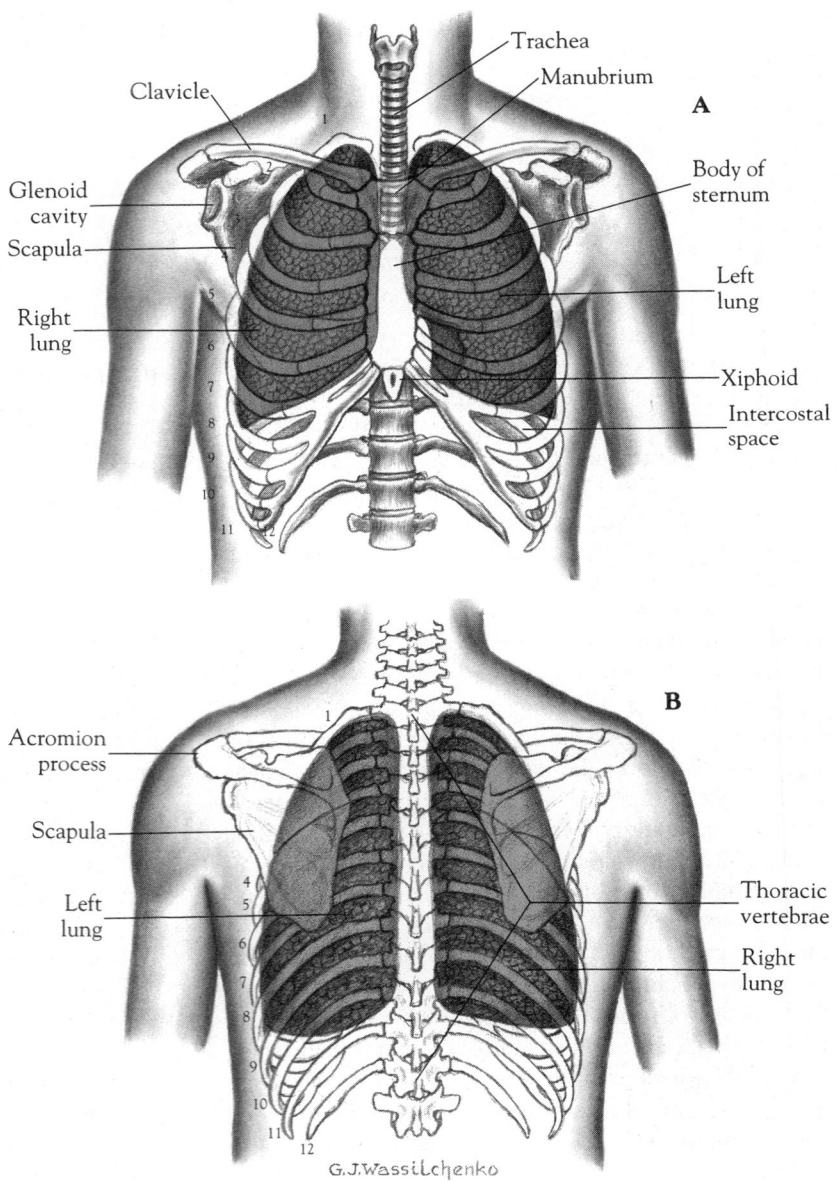

G.J.Wassilchenko

During a deep inspiration the diaphragm contracts and moves downward. This contraction, which occurs because of stimulation by the phrenic nerve, forces two major movements that facilitate ventilation. The first raises the lower ribs upward and laterally, increasing both the transverse and lateral intrathoracic space. The second action of diaphragmatic contraction forces the abdominal contents downward. Both actions facilitate ventilation.

The intercostal muscles are divided into the external and internal muscles. The external intercostal muscles contract to increase the anterior-posterior diameter of the thoracic cavity during inspiration. With deep and purposeful breathing the internal intercostal muscles contract to decrease the transverse diameter during expiration.

Three muscles function in an accessory capacity during

Fig. 2-2
Muscles of ventilation. **A,** Anterior view. **B,** Posterior view.

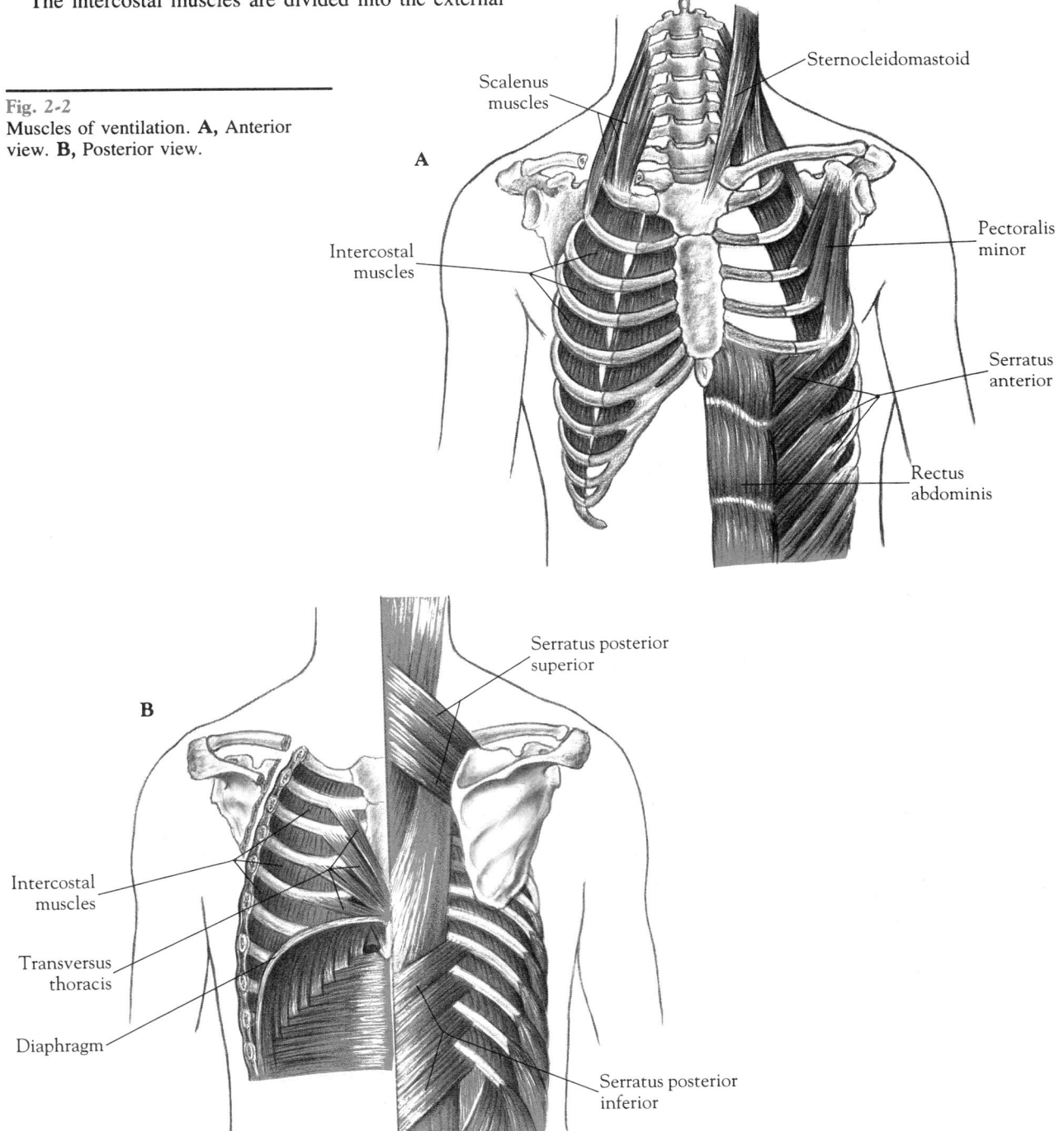

increased-effort ventilation: the scalene, sternocleido-mastoid, and abdominal muscles. During inspiration the scalene muscles contract to elevate the first two ribs and to stabilize the upper chest wall. The sternocleidomastoid muscle contracts during inspiration to elevate the sternum. During expiration these muscles relax and the abdominal wall muscles contract. During quiet ventilation the abdominal wall muscles are not used. If expiration is forced, as during exercise or ventilatory difficulties, the abdominal muscles may be used to depress the lower ribs of the chest wall. This in turn will assist with forced expiration.

Thoracic cavity. The primary structures of the thoracic cavity include the pleura, the pleural space, the mediastinum, and lungs. Fig. 2-3 details this anatomy.

The pleura is a two-layered protective membrane: the parietal pleura, which lines the thoracic cavity within the lung chambers, and the visceral or pulmonary pleura, which covers each lung. Although each is given a separate name, the pleurae are continuous with one another and form one closed sac. Between the two pleurae is a potential space, the pleural space, which contains a serous lubricant film that allows one pleura to slip over the other and thus facilitates movement of the lungs. In addition the intrapleural space maintains a subatmospheric pressure. At rest the pressure is 755 mm Hg; immediately prior to inspiration this pressure drops to 751 mm Hg.

The mediastinum is the region between the right and left parietal pleurae. It is bordered by the sternum anteriorly and the thoracic vertebrae posteriorly. The heart, contained within its own pericardial sac, is situated in

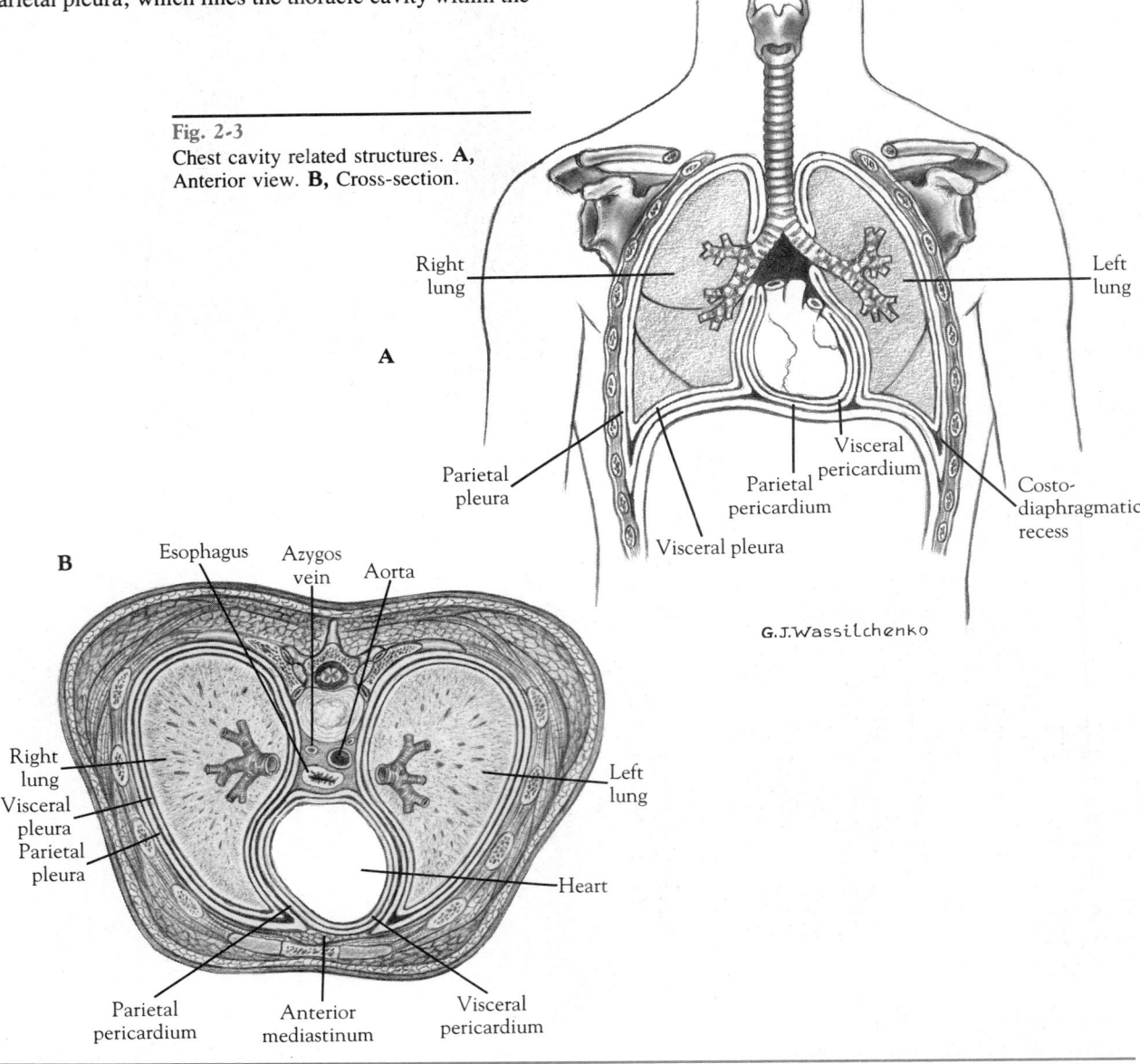

Fig. 2-3
Chest cavity related structures. **A,** Anterior view. **B,** Cross-section.

Fig. 2-4
Structures of the upper airway.

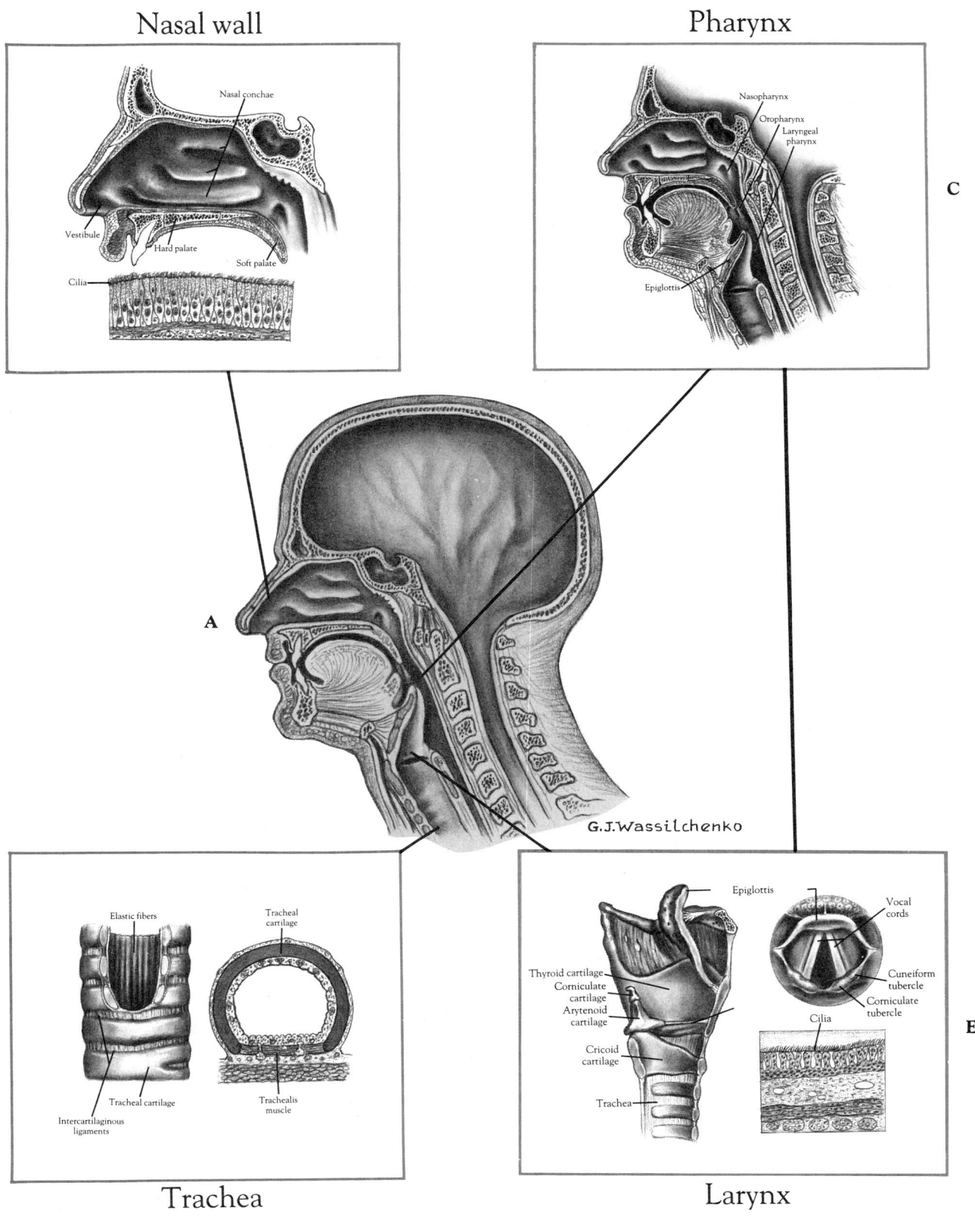

Nasal wall

Nasal conchae

Vestibule

Hard palate

Soft palate

Cilia

B

Pharynx

Nasopharynx

Oropharynx

Laryngeal pharynx

Epiglottis

C

A

G.J.Wassilchenko

Trachea

Elastic fibers

Tracheal cartilage

Tracheal cartilage

Trachealis muscle

Intercartilaginous ligaments

D

Larynx

Epiglottis

Vocal cords

Thyroid cartilage

Corniculate cartilage

Arytenoid cartilage

Cuneiform tubercle

Corniculate tubercle

Cilia

Cricoid cartilage

Trachea

E

the middle of the mediastinum. Also in the mediastinum are (1) the great vessels that enter and leave the heart, (2) the bifurcation of the trachea, (3) the large bronchi, (4) part of the esophagus, (5) the thymus gland, (6) lymph nodes, and (7) various nerves including the phrenic nerve, cardiac and splanchnic branches of the sympathetic system, and recurrent laryngeal and vagus branches of the parasympathetic system.

The hilum is located at the center of the mediastinal surface. This area contains the root of the lung and is the place where the visceral and parietal pleurae join and form a sheath around the bronchi. It is also the place where blood vessels and nerves connect with the lungs.

The right lung contains three lobes, has 10 bronchopulmonary segments, and is responsible for 55% of all normal lung activity.

The left lung has eight bronchopulmonary segments and is responsible for 45% of all normal lung functioning. Blood is supplied to the tissue of both lungs by the bronchial arteries.

Upper airway. The upper airway, consisting of the nose, pharynx, larynx, and extrathoracic trachea (Fig. 2-4), has three major functions:

1. To conduct air to the lower airway
2. To protect the lower airway from foreign matter
3. To warm, filter, and humidify inspired air

In addition to its olfactory function, the nose serves to warm, moisten, and filter inspired air. Temperature adjustment and proper humidification begin as soon as air hits the anterior nasal cavity. The structure of the nose, with its two nasal cavities, turbinates, and rich vasculature, provides maximum contact between inspired air and the nasal mucosa. By the time inspired air reaches the alveoli it is 100% water-vapor saturated.

Another function of the nose is to clear debris from the inspired air. The nasal cilia, hair, and moisture cluster small airborne particles. Sneezing is another means of clearing the inspired air: When a mechanical or chemical irritation occurs, sensory receptors in the nasal mucosa send impulses to the brain via the trigeminal and olfactory nerves, thus initiating a deep inhalation and an explosive exhalation—a sneeze.

Air passes from the nasal cavity into the three divisions of the pharynx: the nasopharynx, the oropharynx, and the laryngeal pharynx. The pharynx, which is covered with ciliated epithelium, filters and humidifies inspired air.

Fig. 2-5

Structures of the lower airway.

Adapted from Weilbrel, E.R.: Morphometry of human lung, New York, 1963, Academic Press.

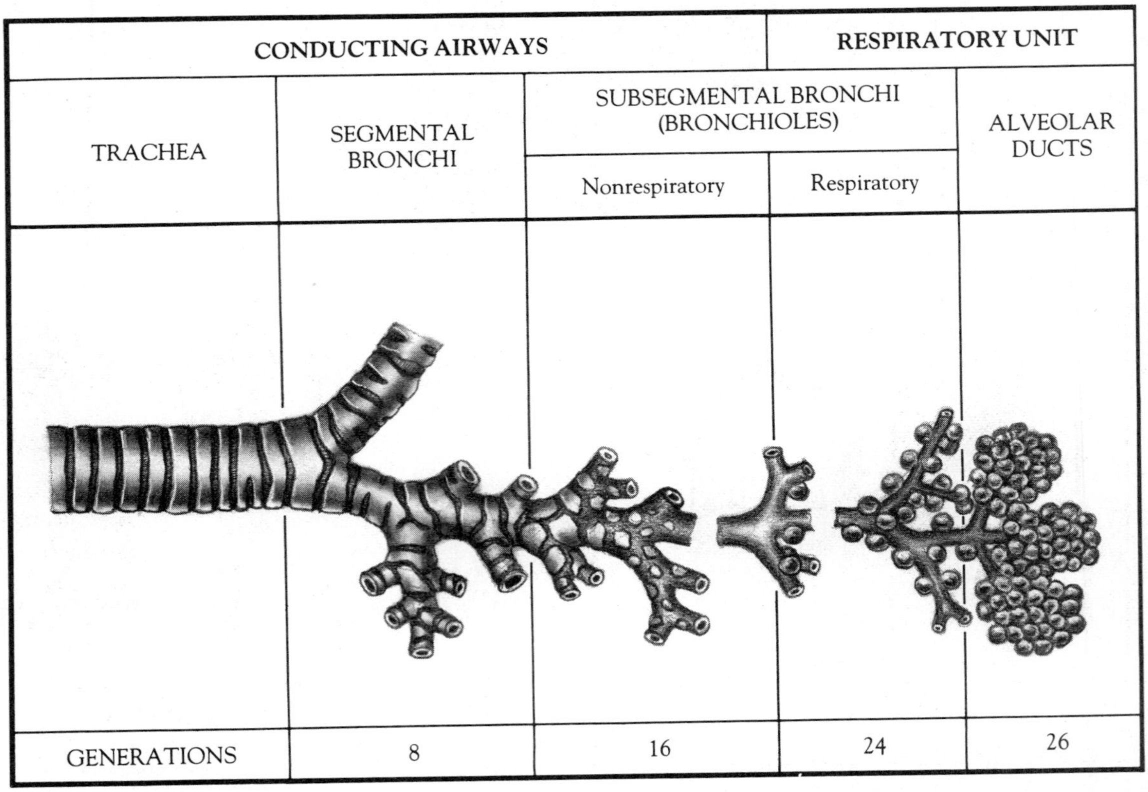

	CONDUCTING AIRWAYS			RESPIRATORY UNIT
TRACHEA	SEGMENTAL BRONCHI	SUBSEGMENTAL BRONCHI (BRONCHIOLES)		ALVEOLAR DUCTS
		Nonrespiratory	Respiratory	
GENERATIONS	8	16	24	26

The next major section of the upper respiratory tract, the larynx, contains the vocal cords for phonation, prevents aspiration of food into the trachea, and helps to initiate coughing. It extends vertically to the level of the sixth cervical vertebra (C-6) and is covered with the same pseudostratified ciliated columnar epithelium found in the nose and the pharynx.

The principal cartilages of the larynx are the thyroid, arytenoid, and cricoid. Attached to the anterior surface of the thyroid cartilage is the epiglottis. The cricoid cartilage, located beneath the thyroid cartilage, forms the narrowest part of the airway for infants and children. Innervation for the larynx comes from two separate branches of the vagus nerve. The recurrent laryngeal nerve provides motor innervation for the larynx, and the superior laryngeal nerve provides some motor and all sensory innervation. It is the sensory fibers of the superior laryngeal nerve that are responsible for the cough reflex.

Lower airway. The lower airway, consisting of the trachea, mainstem bronchi, segmental bronchi, subsegmental bronchioles, terminal bronchioles, and gas exchange units (Fig. 2-5), has three main functions:

1. Air conduction to the alveolar level of the lungs
2. Mucociliary clearance
3. Pulmonary surfactant production by the type II cells of the alveoli

There is a range of 23 to 26 levels of branches of conducting airways and terminal respiratory units involved. These branch levels, called generations, are divided into two categories and five types (Fig. 2-5).

The trachea, which is 4 to 5 cm wide and 11 to 12 cm long and which consists of C-shaped rings of cartilage, extends from the larynx and cricoid cartilage to the division of right and left mainstem bronchi at the level of the fifth thoracic vertebra (T5) in the chest.

The lining of the trachea consists of a pseudostratified, ciliated columnar epithelium interspersed with mucus-producing goblet cells.

The right and left mainstem bronchi conduct air between the trachea and the segmental bronchi. The right mainstem bronchus, which is approximately 5 cm shorter than the left bronchus, is positioned fairly vertically. Its vertical position results in aspiration of material into the bronchus. The bronchus subsequently divides into three branches, each of which supplies one of the three lobes of the right lung. The left mainstem bronchus lies more horizontal and divides into two branches, which supply the two lobes of the left lung.

The mainstem bronchi are composed of cartilaginous rings covered with the same fibroelastic membrane that covers the trachea. The inner mucosa of the bronchi consists of pseudostratified columnar epithelium with goblet and ciliated cells. Submucosal glands are present.

The segmental bronchi conduct the air between the main bronchi and the subsegmental bronchioles. There are 18 of these bronchi, which are divided into 10 in the right lung and 8 in the left lung. These bronchi, like the mainstem bronchi, are lined with mucosa consisting of pseudostratified, ciliated columnar epithelium and goblet cells. Submucosal glands are present.

The subsegmental bronchi (bronchioles) conduct air from the segmental bronchi to the alveoli via the terminal bronchioles. These airways have no cartilage, no goblet cells, and no submucosal glands. The bronchioles have a complete concentric ring of smooth muscle with two sets of smooth muscle fibers. When these muscle rings constrict as in asthma, the airways narrow.

The distal portion of the bronchioles consists of units, called the terminal bronchi, that conduct air from the subsegmental bronchi to the alveolar ducts. There are approximately 35,000 of these small bronchioles throughout both lungs. They are clustered so that three to five of them form a pulmonary lobule. Their mucosal lining consists of cuboidal epithelium and Clara cells. They contain no goblet cells. There are no submucosal glands.

The most distal section of the lower respiratory tract consists of the terminal respiratory units (acini), which include the respiratory bronchioles, the alveolar ducts, the alveolar sacs, and the terminal air sacs themselves, called the alveoli. An acinus is the site of gas exchange. Fig. 2-6 shows the cluster arrangement of these terminal respiratory units.

The membrane surface of the terminal respiratory unit is a flattened, one-cell-thick epithelial surface. It is the type II cell of the alveolar epithelium that secretes the lipoprotein substance called *surfactant*. Surfactant forms a thin layer between the surface of the alveoli and the air. Surfactant decreases the surface tension of the air-liquid interface in the alveoli. Without adequate surfactant, as occurs in hyaline membrane disease or respiratory distress syndrome, it becomes extremely difficult for the alveoli to inflate with inspiration because of the high pressure gradients required to overcome the high surface tension.

The alveolar membrane is composed of five layers. This membrane, as shown in Fig. 2-7, forms the division between the alveolar space and the pulmonary capillary.

Histology of the respiratory tract. Mucosa lines most of the structures of the upper respiratory tract. As seen in Fig. 2-8, this mucosa consists of an epithelial layer, a basement membrane, and lamina propria. The lamina propria, which has an elastic tissue layer boundary, contains lymphocytes, plasma cells, occasional polymorphonuclear leukocytes, and numerous mast cells. It is the mast cells that release histamine in the antigen-antibody reactions seen in asthma or allergic reactions. The lamina propria also contains lymphoid nodules at

Fig. 2-6
The terminal respiratory units.

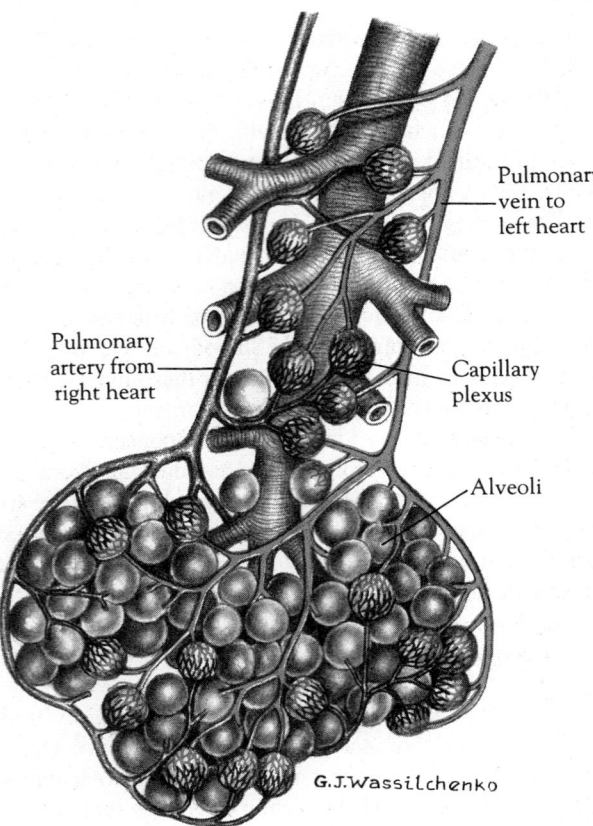

Pulmonary
vein to
left heart

Pulmonary
artery from
right heart

Capillary
plexus

Alveoli

G.J.Wassilchenko

various sites along the tracheobronchial tree. These nodules are thought to be important in a variety of immune responses occurring in the lungs. It is also involved in the production of immunoglobulin A (IgA).

The epithelial layer of the mucosa contains numerous cell types. Following are three significant types of cells:

1. Ciliated, pseudostratified epithelial cells: Found in the columnar epithelium of the larger airways and the cuboidal epithelium of the smaller airways. The main purpose of the cilia is to propel airway secretions toward the upper airway.
2. Goblet cells: Found among the columnar epithelial cells of the larger airways. Their function is synthesis and secretion of mucus.
3. Clara cells: Found in the cuboidal epithelium of the distal small airways. Although their exact function is unknown, it is thought that they are at least one of the sources of the fluid lining of the smallest airways.

The mucociliary system functions to trap and transport airborne particles (between 2 and 10 μm in diameter) not filtered in the nose and larger airways. Particles that make it to the smaller airways are trapped on the mucous blanket that coats the surface of the airways. This blanket consists of ciliated mucosal cells, which propel the debris upward at a velocity of 10 to 20 mm per minute.

Fig. 2-7
Alveolar wall and space.

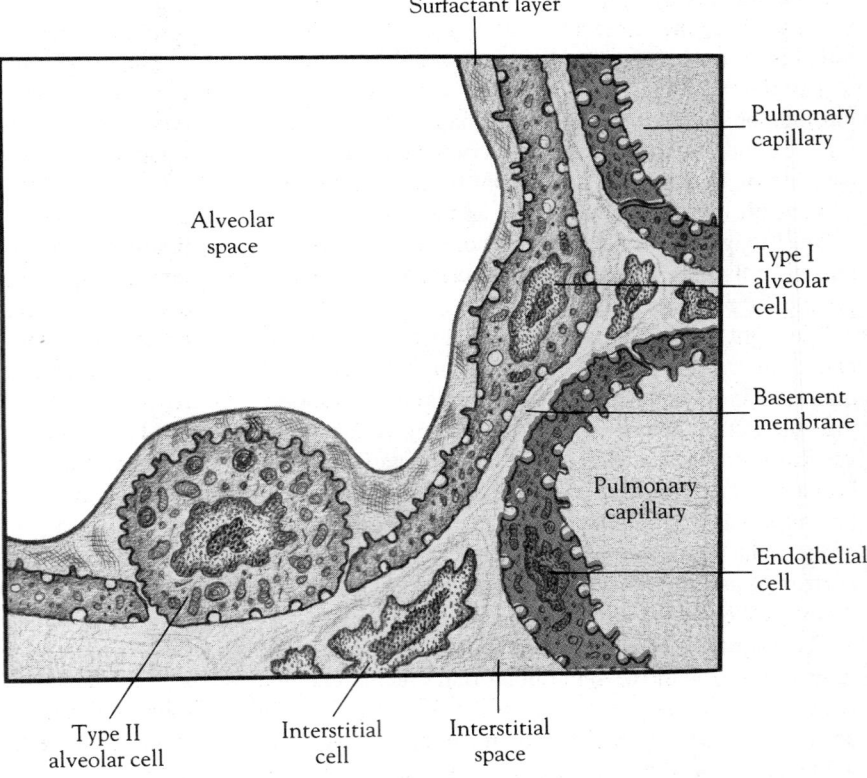

Surfactant layer

Pulmonary
capillary

Alveolar
space

Type I
alveolar
cell

Basement
membrane

Pulmonary
capillary

Endothelial
cell

Type II
alveolar cell

Interstitial
cell

Interstitial
space

The mucous blanket is approximately 95% water and consists of two layers. The bottom, watery layer cleans the cilia and is in direct contact with the epithelium. The top layer is the gel layer, which consists of streams of mucus that trap the particles.

Two immunoglobulins are found in the airway secretions:

1. Immunoglobulin G (IgG): This immunoglobulin plays an important part in the body's response to bacterial infections.
2. Immunoglobulin A (IgA): While its exact function is not known, IgA is thought to play an important part in protection from viral infections.

Process of ventilation. Ventilation is the movement of air in and out of the lungs. The numerous lung volumes and capacities are discussed in detail later in the chapter under Pulmonary Function Tests.

In addition to the air movement, two other processes affect the success of the ventilatory attempt: (1) respiratory pressures and surface tension and (2) lung compliance, or pulmonary elasticity.

Respiratory pressures and surface tension. Thoracic expansion occurs normally and quietly secondary to muscle contraction and rib cage elevation. When the rib cage expands, the intrapleural pressure drops from approximately 755 to 751 mm Hg. This slightly negative at-mospheric pressure is enough to draw air into the lungs.

The alveoli's surface tension augments the normal tendency of the lungs to collapse and pull away from the chest wall.

The presence of a lipoprotein substance called surfactant, at the interface between the lining of the alveoli and the air in the alveoli, plays an important part in decreasing the surface tension so that the lungs inflate easily. Surfactant decreases the surface tension within the alveoli and assists the gas to be distributed evenly over all the alveoli. In conditions such as hyaline membrane disease and adult respiratory distress syndrome (ARDS) surfactant is absent or decreased. Thus lung inflation becomes much more difficult.

Lung compliance. Compliance is a measure of the expansibility or elasticity of the lungs and the thorax. It is determined by plethysmography. The inspired or expired gas volume (ΔV) and the intrapleural pressure (ΔP) are measured, and ΔV is divided by ΔP (see Pulmonary Function Tests). Generally, when the intrapleural pressure is increased by 1 cm water, the lung volume increases 130 ml. Any condition that destroys lung tissue or causes it to become fibrotic or edematous, that blocks the alveoli, or that in any other way impedes lung expansion and contraction causes a decrease in lung compliance.

Fig. 2-8
Structures of the ventilatory mucosa.

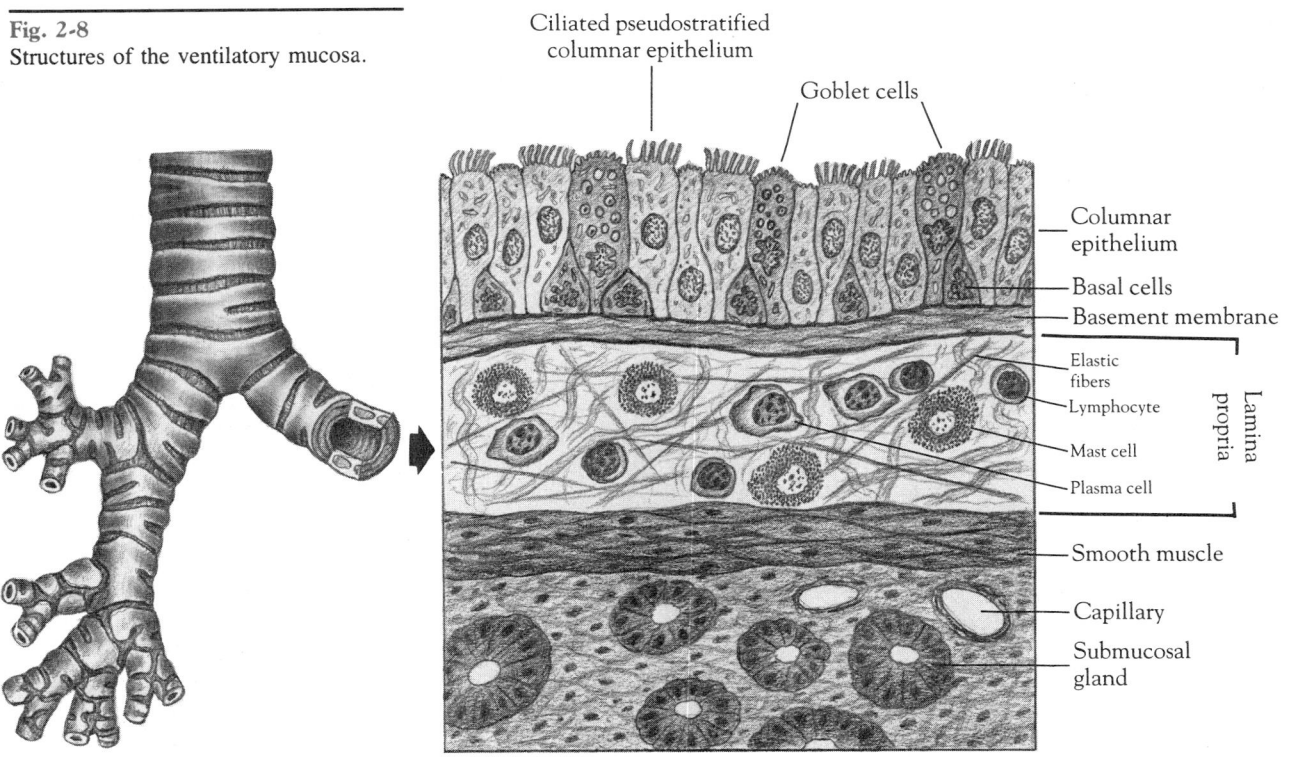

Ciliated pseudostratified columnar epithelium

Goblet cells

Columnar epithelium
Basal cells
Basement membrane
Elastic fibers
Lymphocyte
Mast cell
Plasma cell
Lamina propria
Smooth muscle
Capillary
Submucosal gland

Table 2-1

Relative Diffusion Coefficients for Respiratory Gases

Gas	Coefficient
Oxygen	1.0*
Carbon dioxide	20.3
Nitrogen	0.53

*1 is an assigned value against which to evaluate the diffusion rate of the other gases.

Diffusion and Perfusion

Once the oxygenated ambient air reaches the surface of the alveoli, the oxygen must cross the alveolar-capillary membrane and enter the pulmonary arterial system (contains venous blood). Likewise the carbon dioxide in the unoxygenated venous blood in the pulmonary system must cross the alveolar-capillary membrane to be expired from the lungs. Diffusion of the gases and perfusion of the alveoli are the two components that must be considered.

Diffusion. Diffusion of gases is dependent upon pressure gradients for exchange to occur. The diffusing capacity of the alveolar-capillary membrane is determined by the volume of gas that diffuses through the membrane each minute, for each millimeter of mercury difference in the pressure gradient across the membrane. The process of diffusion is dependent upon the thickness of the respiratory membrane, the surface area of the respiratory membrane, the diffusion coefficients of the involved gases, and the partial pressure differences of the gases being diffused. Each of these will be discussed separately.

Any changes in the alveolar membrane or the interstitial spaces between the alveoli and the capillary can affect the rate of gas diffusion. The rate of diffusion is inversely proportional to the thickness of the membrane.

The total alveolar surface for a normal adult is approximately 80 m². Pulmonary capillaries cover 85% to 90% of this surface. Therefore the total surface for gas diffusion is approximately 70 m². Any alteration such as the removal of a lung or emphysema will decrease the total surface area available for gas exchange. The pressure that gases exert against a surface is proportional to their individual concentrations. The diffusion coefficients for the respiratory gases are seen in Table 2-1. Note that carbon dioxide is 20 times more diffusible than oxygen.

The process of gas exchange between the air in the alveoli and the blood in the pulmonary capillaries occurs because of a difference in the partial pressures of the gases. Fig. 2-9 shows the partial pressures of respiratory gases. Each gas will diffuse from an area of high partial pressure to an area of low partial pressure.

By altering the concentration of oxygen, as is done with oxygen therapy, the diffusion partial pressures of the gases will also be altered (Fig. 2-10).

Perfusion. The major purpose of the pulmonary circulation is to deliver blood in a thin film to the alveoli so that oxygen uptake and carbon dioxide elimination can occur. The pulmonary vascular system is characterized as a high volume–low pressure system. This means that there is a large amount of blood flowing through the pulmonary circulation and that there is very low capillary resistance to that blood as it flows.

Pulmonary circulation begins when carbon dioxide–saturated blood from the right ventricle of the heart drains into the right and left pulmonary arteries, which branch into the 6 billion alveolar capillaries—the sites of gas exchange. After the blood is oxygenated, it flows into the four pulmonary veins, which return it to the left atrium of the heart.

The vascular pressure in the pulmonary system is very low. The pulmonary arterial pressure is approximately one fifth of that within the systemic system. The mean pressure is approximately 15 mm Hg.

Under normal resting conditions only about 25% of the pulmonary capillaries are actively perfused. As cardiac output increases, the pulmonary arterial pressure remains fairly constant. This is possible because of two mechanisms:

1. Recruitment: A mechanism that decreases pulmonary vascular resistance and thus permits increased blood flow through the vessels
2. Capillary dilation: A mechanism that directly increases the capillary size

Both these mechanisms accommodate an increase in cardiac output. Should there be malfunctioning of either of these compensatory mechanisms, pulmonary hypertension may occur. The Swan-Ganz catheter is now commonly used to measure the pulmonary arterial pressure.

Common alterations in perfusion

1. *Alveolar dead space:* Alveolar dead space occurs when the ventilation is normal but the perfusion of a variable number of alveoli is reduced or absent. Either there is not enough blood, or the blood is blocked from reaching the alveoli. This can have a variety of causes including gravitational shifts in pulmonary blood flow in the normal subject or impaired blood flow in the ill patient.[61]
2. *Physiologic shunting:* Physiologic shunting occurs when the pulmonary circulation is adequate but the air available in the alveoli is inadequate for normal diffusion. Thus a portion of the blood passing through the pulmonary system does not become oxygenated. There are three types of shunting that tend to occur:
   a. *Anatomic shunting:* This is the 2% to 5% of the cardiac output that normally bypasses the pul-

Fig. 2-9
Partial pressure of respiratory gases in
normal respiration.

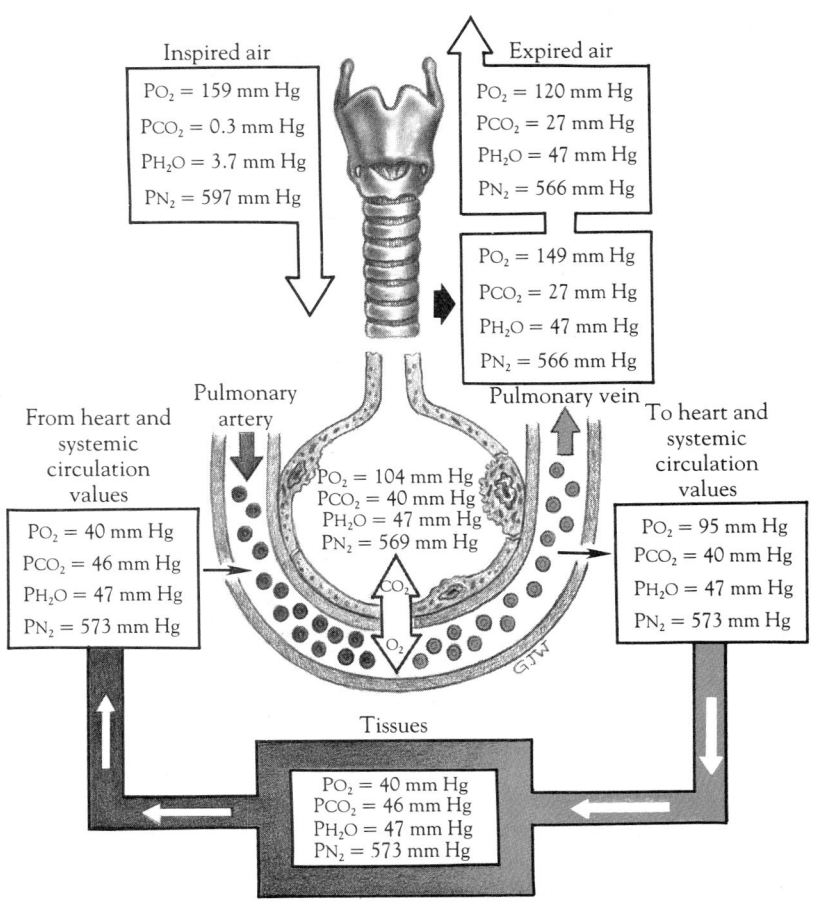

Inspired air

P_{O_2} = 159 mm Hg
P_{CO_2} = 0.3 mm Hg
P_{H_2O} = 3.7 mm Hg
P_{N_2} = 597 mm Hg

Expired air

P_{O_2} = 120 mm Hg
P_{CO_2} = 27 mm Hg
P_{H_2O} = 47 mm Hg
P_{N_2} = 566 mm Hg

P_{O_2} = 149 mm Hg
P_{CO_2} = 27 mm Hg
P_{H_2O} = 47 mm Hg
P_{N_2} = 566 mm Hg

Pulmonary artery

Pulmonary vein

From heart and
systemic
circulation
values

P_{O_2} = 40 mm Hg
P_{CO_2} = 46 mm Hg
P_{H_2O} = 47 mm Hg
P_{N_2} = 573 mm Hg

P_{O_2} = 104 mm Hg
P_{CO_2} = 40 mm Hg
P_{H_2O} = 47 mm Hg
P_{N_2} = 569 mm Hg

To heart and
systemic
circulation
values

P_{O_2} = 95 mm Hg
P_{CO_2} = 40 mm Hg
P_{H_2O} = 47 mm Hg
P_{N_2} = 573 mm Hg

Tissues

P_{O_2} = 40 mm Hg
P_{CO_2} = 46 mm Hg
P_{H_2O} = 47 mm Hg
P_{N_2} = 573 mm Hg

Fig. 2-10
Alteration of gas diffusion by varying
oxygen concentration.

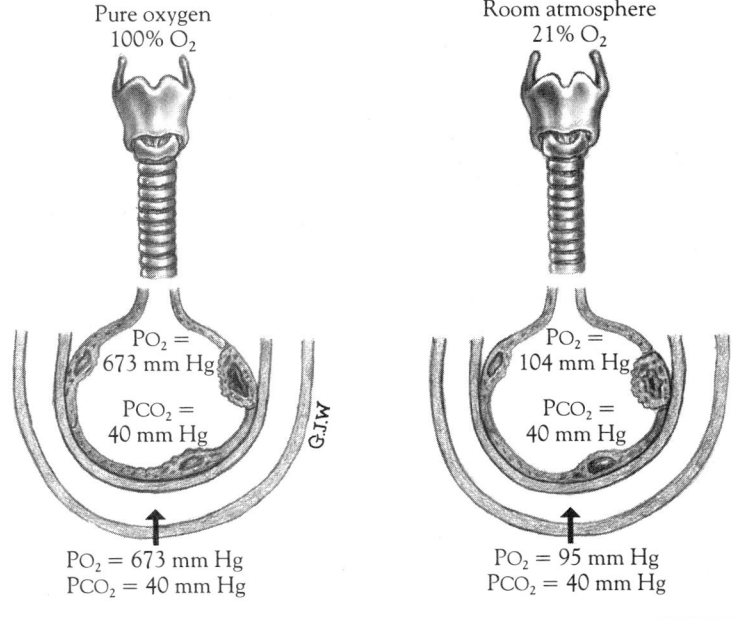

Pure oxygen
100% O_2

P_{O_2} = 673 mm Hg
P_{CO_2} = 40 mm Hg

P_{O_2} = 673 mm Hg
P_{CO_2} = 40 mm Hg

Room atmosphere
21% O_2

P_{O_2} = 104 mm Hg
P_{CO_2} = 40 mm Hg

P_{O_2} = 95 mm Hg
P_{CO_2} = 40 mm Hg

Fig. 2-11

Measurements of the distribution of blood flow in the lungs of an individual sitting in an upright position.

Adapted from West, J.: Respiratory physiology: the essentials, Baltimore, 1979, The Williams & Wilkins Co.

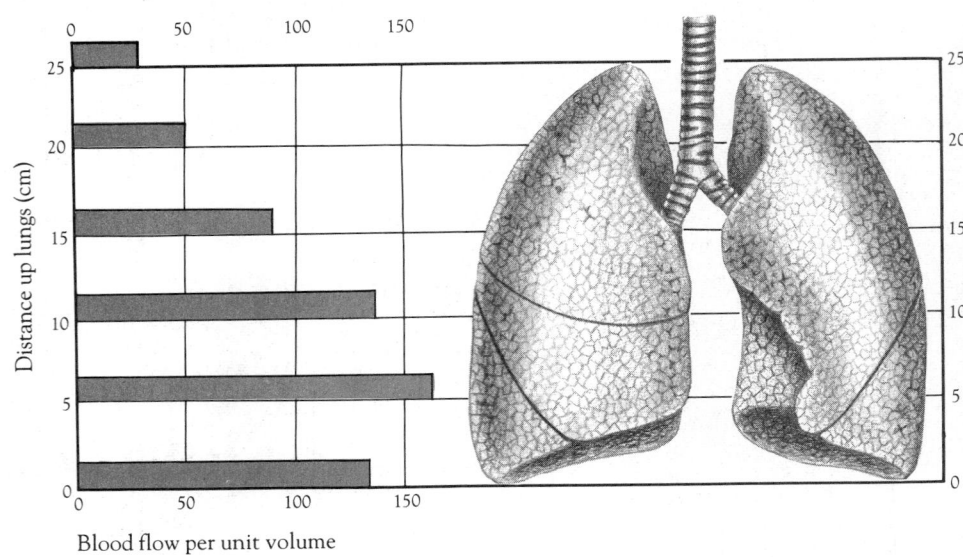

Blood flow per unit volume

monary arterial system. This blood is part of the bronchial, pleural, and coronary circulation.

b. *True shunt:* The blood perfuses the alveoli, but for one reason or another the alveoli are totally unventilated. Thus little or no diffusion occurs. Mechanical ventilation with oxygenation may be necessary to overcome this type of shunting.

c. *Shunt effect:* This occurs when the alveoli are underventilated or when the blood flows through the pulmonary system at an excessive rate. Oxygen and perhaps the use of a mechanical ventilator will help this type of shunting.

The distribution of blood flow throughout the pulmonary system is not uniform. The greatest amount of blood flow occurs in the lower segments of the lungs, and the least flow is in the apex. When the individual is supine, the blood flow distribution becomes more even. The distribution of pulmonary blood flow is easily measured by radioisotopes. Fig. 2-11 details the measurement of the distribution of blood in an upright individual.

The arterial blood gases (Table 2-2) indicate the effectiveness of the ventilation, diffusion, and perfusion processes. These are discussed in more detail in the blood gas section.

Blood Flow: Transportation of the Respiratory Gases

Following the diffusion of the gases at the alveolar level, they must be transported to the tissues for use. The fol-

lowing discussion includes the analysis of oxygen and carbon dioxide transport and a discussion of blood gases that can be used to evaluate gas exchange.

Oxygen. Oxygen in the blood is carried two ways: (1) dissolved in the liquid portion of the blood plasma and (2) in chemical combination with hemoglobin. Most oxygen is transported in the second manner.

The amount of dissolved oxygen carried in the plasma is directly proportional to the partial pressure of oxygen (Henry's law). There is 0.003 ml of oxygen dissolved in each 100 ml of blood for each 1 mm Hg partial pressure of oxygen. Thus at an ideal PaO_2 of 100 mm Hg, only 0.3 ml of oxygen would be carried per 100 ml of plasma. The individual's normal resting cardiac output is approximately 5 L per minute. If oxygen throughout the body were only carried in this dissolved state, the body's cardiac output would need to be increased to at least 120 L per minute.

Most oxygen in the body is transported to the cells in combination with hemoglobin. Oxygen combines loosely and reversibly with the heme portion of hemoglobin.

Table 2-2

Normal Values for Arterial Blood Gases

PO_2	90 ± 10 mm Hg
O_2 saturation	96% ± 1%
PCO_2	40 ± 3 mm Hg
pH	7.4 ± 0.03
Bicarbonate	22-26 mEq/L

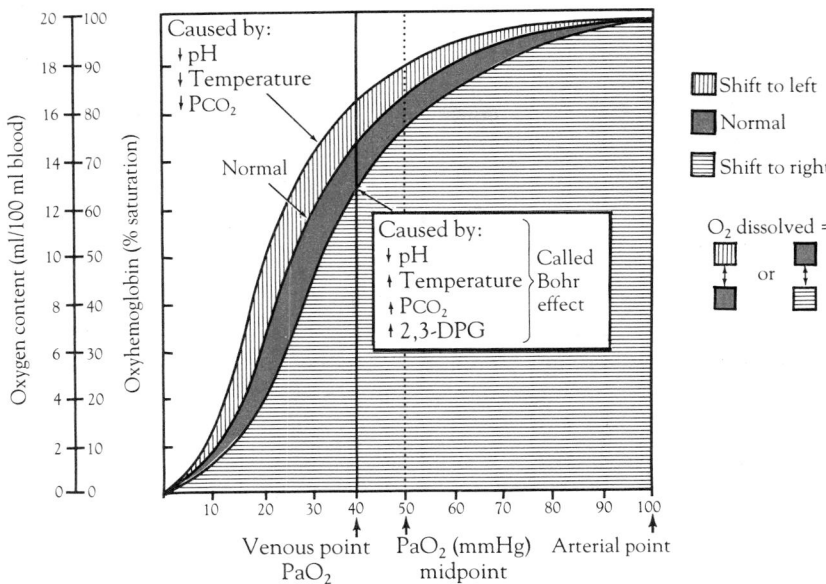

Fig. 2-12
Oxyhemoglobin dissociation curve
with pH 7.4 and temperature 98.6° F
(37° C).

Modified from Guenter, C.A., and Welch,
M.H.: Pulmonary medicine, Philadelphia,
1977, J.B. Lippincott Co.

When the PO_2 is high, as in the pulmonary capillaries, the oxygen readily combines with the hemoglobin. When the PO_2 is low, as in the tissue capillaries, the oxygen is released from the hemoglobin.

The amount of oxygen carried in the blood by hemoglobin is directly dependent on the concentration of hemoglobin. The average individual has approximately 15 g of hemoglobin in each 100 ml of blood. Each gram of hemoglobin has the maximum capability to combine with 1.34 ml of oxygen. Therefore a hemoglobin of 15 g/100 ml would result in 20.1 ml of oxygen combined with hemoglobin and 100% saturation.

$$\frac{15 \text{ g Hb}}{100 \text{ ml blood}} \times \frac{1.34 \text{ ml O}_2}{1 \text{ g Hb}} = \frac{20.1 \text{ ml O}_2}{100 \text{ ml blood}}$$

Tisi[64] discusses three terms that must be differentiated:
1. Oxygen content is the total amount of oxygen carried in both a dissolved and combined state per 100 ml of blood.
2. Oxygen capacity is the maximal amount of oxygen that can be carried in both states per 100 ml of blood.
3. Percent saturation is the relationship between the amount of oxygen that is carried and the amount of oxygen that can be carried.

$$\text{Saturation} = \frac{\text{Content (amount dissolved)}}{\text{Capacity (amount dissolved)}} = \frac{\text{``Is''}}{\text{``Can''}}$$

The amount of oxygen combined with hemoglobin depends on the partial pressure of oxygen dissolved in the arterial blood (PaO_2). The oxygen content at different partial pressures that combines with the hemoglobin is shown in the oxyhemoglobin dissociation curve (Fig. 2-12). When the blood leaves the lungs, the PaO_2 is approximately 100 mm Hg and the percent saturation is 97.5. In normal mixed venous blood the $P\bar{v}O_2$ is about 40 mm Hg with a 75% saturation. Tisi points out three important areas along the curve: (1) at a $P\bar{v}O_2$ of 40 mm Hg the percent saturation is 75, (2) at a PaO_2 of 50 mm Hg the percent saturation is approximately 84, and (3) at a PaO_2 of 100 mm Hg the percent saturation is 97.5.[64] On the steep portion of the curve, between points 1 and 2, there is almost a linear relationship in that for every 10 mm Hg PO_2 change there is a 10% saturation change. Note that between points 2 and 3 there is a 50 mm Hg change in the PO_2 but only a 13% change in saturation.

Various shifts in body functioning such as differences in pH, $PaCO_2$, or body temperature can also cause changes in the oxyhemoglobin dissociation curve. Fig. 2-12 also details this shift potential. Shifts to the right are produced by a decrease in pH, a rise in $PaCO_2$, and an increase in temperature. The curve can also be shifted to the right by an increase in 2,3-diphosphoglycerate (DPG) inside the red blood cells, which occurs as a result of prolonged hypoxia. A dissociation curve that shifts to the right tells us that something has weakened the hemoglobin's intrinsic ability to hold on to oxygen and that higher gas pressure is needed for binding. Oxygen escapes hemoglobin more easily and is more available to the tissues.

Shifts to the left are produced by an increase in pH, a decrease in $PaCO_2$, and a decrease in body temperature. This shift component may be a significant variable in explaining the difference between a patient's clinical appearance and the arterial blood gas results. When there is a shift to the left, something has happened to increase the affinity of hemoglobin for oxygen. The hemoglobin holds the oxygen more firmly than normal, and although less pressure is needed to bind the two, it is more difficult to separate the two at the cellular level.

Carbon dioxide. Carbon dioxide transportation is more complicated than that of oxygen but must be understood clearly, for the amount of carbon dioxide in transit is one of the major determinants of the acid-base balance of the body.[61] Most carbon dioxide is carried in three plasma and three erythrocyte compartments: *in plasma*—bound to protein to form carbamino compounds, as a bicarbonate (HCO_3^-), and in physical solution dissolved in plasma; *in erythrocytes*—dissolved in erythrocyte water, combined with the amino group of carbaminohemoglobin, and as carbonic acid (H_2CO_3). The carbonic acid further dissociates to form hydrogen and bicarbonate ions ($[H^+]$ and $[HCO_3^-]$). Fig. 2-13 summarizes the transport of carbon dioxide in the blood.

Just as the relationship between blood PaO_2 and oxygen saturation of hemoglobin was expressed by the oxygen saturation curve, so there is a relationship between blood $PaCO_2$ and the whole blood content of carbon dioxide, which is calculated in volume percent. The carbon dioxide dissociation curves as seen in Fig. 2-14 show this relationship. The purpose of the curves is to show how

Fig. 2-13

Transport of carbon dioxide and other gases in the blood.

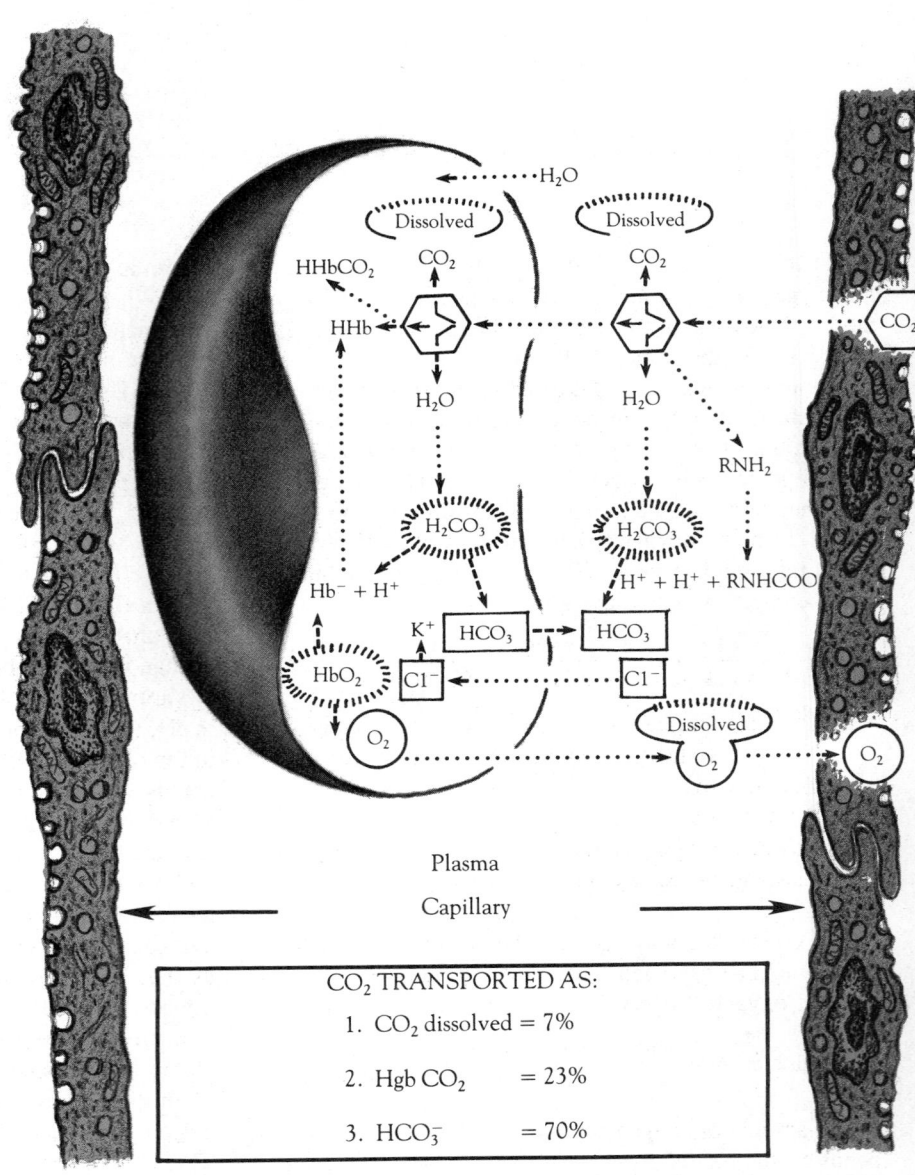

CO₂ TRANSPORTED AS:

1. CO₂ dissolved = 7%
2. Hgb CO₂   = 23%
3. HCO_3^- = 70%

carbon dioxide dissociates from, or leaves, the blood as its partial pressure drops. The curves also show that as the amount of carbon dioxide in the blood increases, so does the tension. When examining these curves note the influence of oxygen saturation (SO_2) on the $Paco_2$ content ratio. This influence, referred to as the Haldane effect, demonstrates that So_2 determines the course of carbon dioxide dissociation.[61] Fig. 2-14 shows selected segments of the curves to include the physiologic range of $Paco_2$ from the arterial point, with a $Paco_2$ of 40 mm Hg, So_2 of 97.5%, and carbon dioxide content of 48 vol%, to the venous point, with a Pco_2 of 46 mm Hg, So_2 of 70%, and carbon dioxide content of 53 vol%.[61] Since oxygen saturation changes from arterial to venous blood, the true

physiologic carbon dioxide dissociation curve must lie somewhere between these two curves.

Acid-Base Balance and Blood Gases

The term *acid-base balance* refers to the ratio between carbonic acid and its salt, sodium bicarbonate. For body cells to function optimally, body fluids and blood must remain within a specific, narrow acid-base balance (pH). Deviations of body pH outside this narrow range interfere with cellular metabolism and can cause cell death. Interactions of substances in the body should produce a hydrogen ion concentration sufficient to maintain a blood pH of 7.35 to 7.45. This normal acid-base balance is

Fig. 2-14
Carbon dioxide dissociation curve.

Adapted from Tisi, G.M.: Pulmonary physiology in clinical medicine, Baltimore, 1980, The Williams & Wilkins Co.

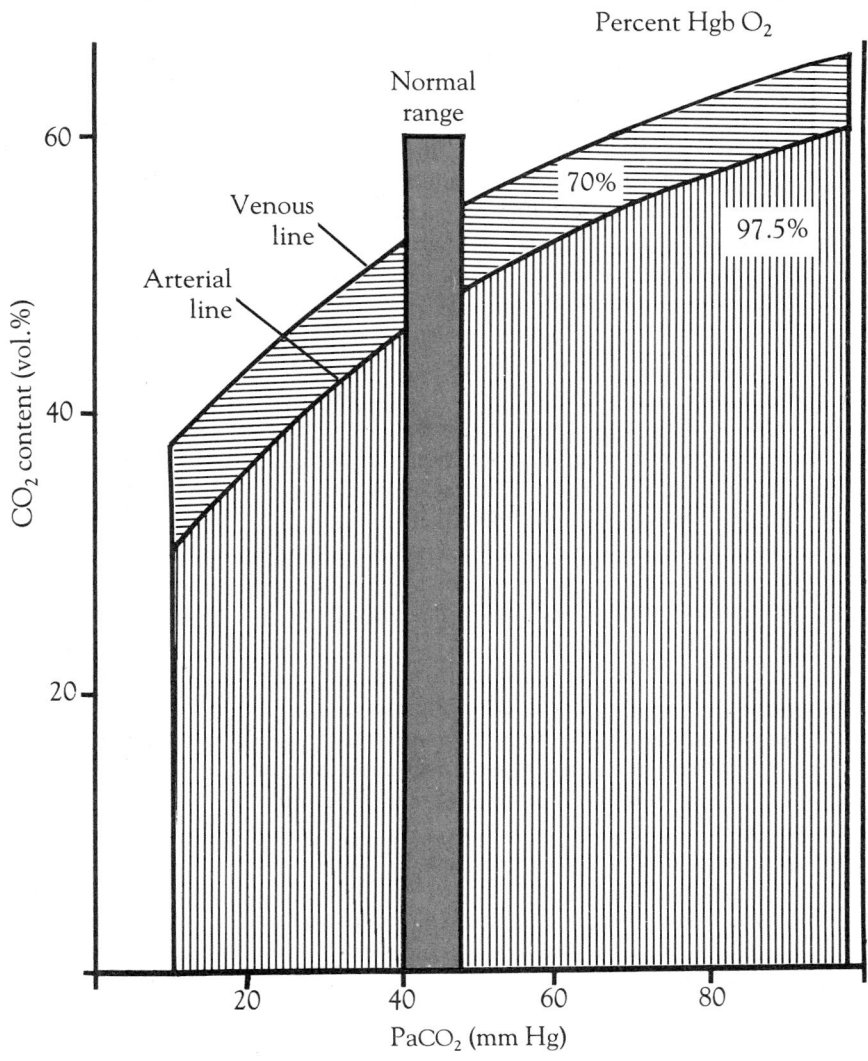

maintained by respiration and kidney function. The respiratory system determines the carbon dioxide concentration, thereby regulating the hydrogen ion concentration. The renal system uses buffering mechanisms to regulate bicarbonate concentration. Following is the Henderson-Hasselbach equation for the calculation of blood pH:

$$pH = pK^* + \log \frac{Base}{Acid}$$

$$(1)\ \frac{HCO_3^-}{H_2CO_3} = \frac{25.4\ mEq/L}{1.27\ mEq/L} = \frac{20}{1}$$

$$(2)\ Blood\ pK = 6.1$$

$$pH = 6.1 + \log \frac{20}{1}$$

$$pH = 6.1 + 1.3 = 7.4$$

Blood pH depends upon the ratio of bicarbonate to dissolved carbon dioxide. As long as that ratio is 20:1, the pH will be 7.4. If the blood pH falls below the normal range, becoming less alkaline, acidemia occurs, and if the pH is above normal, becoming more alkaline, alkalemia occurs.[1]

The body also has a buffer system that buffers or modifies large hydrogen ion concentrations to prevent wide swings in the pH. The buffering occurs primarily in the plasma and the erythrocytes. The carbonic acid–sodium bicarbonate buffer in the plasma is by far the most important of the buffers.[61]

Two types of disorders can cause an acid-base imbalance: respiratory disorders and metabolic disorders. Clinically an acid-base imbalance is referred to as acidosis or alkalosis. Acidosis caused by a respiratory disease is characterized by an elevated arterial carbon dioxide tension. When acidosis has a metabolic cause, arterial bicarbonate concentration is lowered. Alkalosis is characterized by lowered arterial carbon dioxide tension when it is the result of a respiratory disease, and by an elevated arterial bicarbonate concentration when it is caused by a metabolic problem.

Disorders of the respiratory system upset the denominator of the acid-base ratio because ventilation disrupts the blood carbon dioxide concentration, and the body compensates by attempting to adjust the numerator. Metabolic disorders upset the numerator of the ratio because the bicarbonate is either increased or decreased, and compensation attempts to adjust the denominator.[61]

Acid states

Respiratory acidosis ($\downarrow$ pH, $\uparrow$ Paco$_2$). Respiratory acidosis is the result of alveolar hypoventilation. The hypoventilation may occur secondary to cardiopulmonary, neuromuscular, skeletal, or obstructive lung dis-

ease, to acute infections, or to the action of drugs, such as narcotics or sedatives. Regardless of the cause, there is an increase in the partial pressure of arterial carbon dioxide and a drop in pH.

The body attempts to compensate for the elevated Paco$_2$ in two ways: (1) by immediately trying to chemically buffer the excess hydrogen ions as they are produced and (2) by excreting in the urine excess hydrogen ion in exchange for bicarbonate ions. The bicarbonate ions are concentrated in the plasma of the blood, where they help to restore the acid-base ratio and thus return the pH to a normal level. It is important to realize that through the process of compensation the patient may still have an elevated Paco$_2$ even though the pH may have returned to normal.[29]

Metabolic acidosis ($\downarrow$ pH, $\downarrow$ HCO$_3^-$). Metabolic acidosis is caused in one of two ways: (1) through the increase of fixed metabolic acids or (2) through the loss of bicarbonate in the body fluids. Examples of the first cause include salicylate poisoning, renal failure, diabetic ketoacidosis, and circulatory failure that produces a build-up of lactic acid. Persistent diarrhea, for example, will cause bicarbonate loss. In all situations of acidosis the body responds to the increase in body acids by using bicarbonate ions as a buffer. As a result the bicarbonate levels will be low. To compensate the respiratory system increases ventilation and the kidneys retain bicarbonate. Table 2-3 summarizes this process.

Alkalosis states

Respiratory alkalosis ($\uparrow$ pH, $\downarrow$ Paco$_2$). Respiratory alkalosis occurs when excess amounts of CO$_2$ are exhaled. Alveolar hyperventilation removes carbon dioxide from the blood, dropping the Paco$_2$ and elevating the pH. Hyperventilation due to anxiety is perhaps the best example. Other causes of alkalosis include brain injury or brain tumors, gram-negative sepsis, and improper management of the patient on a ventilator.

The body attempts to compensate by increasing renal excretion of bicarbonate, retaining chloride, and reducing the formation of ammonia and excretion of acid salts. These mechanisms lower the blood bicarbonate level and thus bring the acid-base ratio back into balance.[61]

Metabolic alkalosis ($\uparrow$ pH, $\uparrow$ HCO$_3^-$). Metabolic alkalosis is caused by an increase in the level of bicarbonate in the body. This occurs primarily when the patient ingests too much base or receives too much bicarbonate during cardiopulmonary resuscitation, and it occurs secondarily as a result of vomiting or gastric suctioning. In all cases the base-to-acid ratio is altered, and the pH rises. The respiratory system compensates by decreasing ventilation. This conserves CO$_2$ and raises the Paco$_2$. The kidneys respond to metabolic alkalosis by increasing the excretion of bicarbonate ions, thereby conserving hydrogen ions. The result is that the pH decreases to normal levels. Table 2-4 summarizes these processes.

*The pK is the pH at which the substance is half dissociated and half undissociated.

Table 2-3
Summary of the Acidosis Process

		$CO_2 + H_2O = H_2CO_3 = H^+ + HCO_3^-$	
	Initial Cause	Buffering	Compensation

Respiratory acidosis	↑ P_{CO_2}	Reaction moves to right to handle excess CO_2*
		 ↑ HCO_3^-
			Lungs
			   Elimination of CO_2
			 Kidneys
			   Elimination of H^+
			   HCO_3^- conserved (the higher the P_{CO_2}, the more HCO_3^- reabsorbed)

Metabolic acidosis	↓ Base
	 ↑ Fixed acids
		Reaction moves to the left to handle excess H^+
		 ↓ HCO_3^-
			Lungs
			   Elimination of CO_2
			 Kidneys
			   Conserve HCO_3^- (the lower the HCO_3^-, the more HCO_3^- conserved)

From Harper, R.: A guide to respiratory care, Philadelphia, 1981, J.B. Lippincott Co.
*Note movement to the right refers to moving from the left side of the equation above to the right side, therefore decreasing CO_2 production.

Table 2-4
Summary of Alkalosis Process

		$CO_2 + H_2O = H_2CO_3 = H^+ + HCO_3^-$	
	Initial Cause	Buffering	Compensation

Respiratory alkalosis	↓ P_{CO_2}	Movement to left to form more CO_2*
		 ↓ HCO_3^-
			Kidneys
			   Conservation of H^+
			   HCO_3^- excretion (the lower the P_{CO_2}, the less HCO_3^- reabsorbed)

Metabolic alkalosis	↑ Base
	 ↓ Fixed acids
		Movement to right to form more H^+ to offset increased base HCO_3^- ↑	Lungs
			   ↓ Ventilation to ↑ P_{CO_2}
			 Kidneys
			   Conserve H^+ by excreting HCO_3^- (the higher the plasma HCO_3^-, the greater the HCO_3^- excretion)

From Harper, R.: A guide to respiratory care, Philadelphia, 1981, J.B. Lippincott Co.
*Note, movement to the left refers to moving from the right side of the equation above to the left side, therefore increasing CO_2 production.

Control of Breathing

Until fairly recently the control of ventilation was believed to rest in a single respiratory center located in the medulla of the brain. Contemporary studies, however, more clearly indicate that the control mechanisms of breathing are exceedingly complex and that our knowledge of ventilatory control is incomplete and often speculative. The following discussion represents those factors thought by Spearman and others[61] to be generally accepted as the prime determinants of ventilation.

There are at least three respiratory centers. One is located in the medulla and two in the pons. In addition, there is a less well located area in the medulla containing chemoreceptors. Similar chemoreceptors are found among the peripheral stimulators, along with reflexes from the lung and a variety of other organs and tissues.

The medullary center is the final determinant of breathing patterns, as it responds to the autonomic stimuli as well as the voluntary stimuli of the higher centers of the cerebral cortex. The medullary center has two major functions: First it acts as the coordinator of data continuously received from sensory, gas exchange, and chemical units throughout the body, matching these needs and influences to determine the ventilatory pattern. The second function of the medullary center is to send nerve impulses to the two subcenters responsible for the muscles that control the inspiratory and expiratory phases of breathing.

The chemoreceptors in the medulla as seen in Fig. 2-15 are groups of specialized nerve cells that can differentiate between concentrations of hydrogen ions and oxygen. The medulla chemoreceptors, also called central

Fig. 2-15
Respiratory control system.

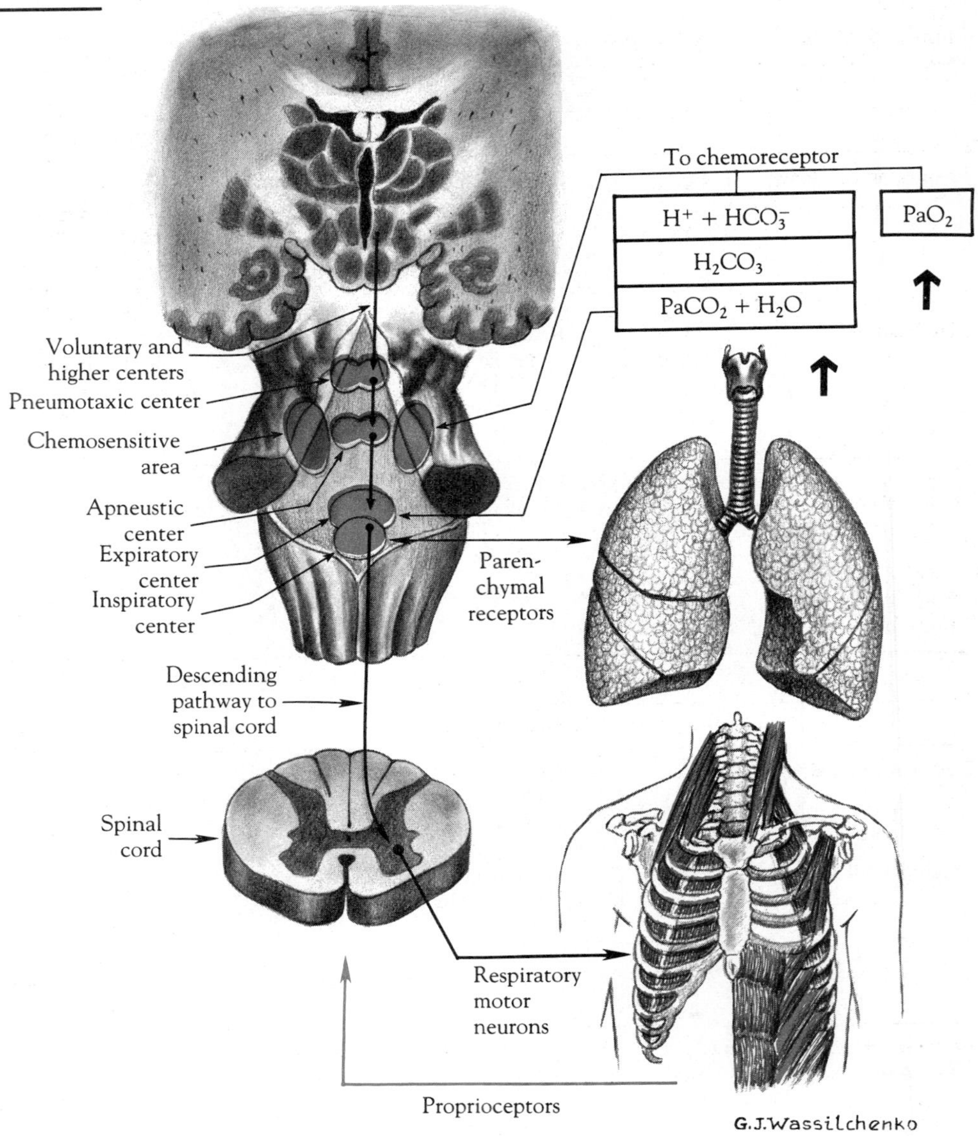

To chemoreceptor

$$H^+ + HCO_3^-$$
$$H_2CO_3$$
$$PaCO_2 + H_2O$$

PaO_2

Voluntary and higher centers

Pneumotaxic center

Chemosensitive area

Apneustic center

Expiratory center

Inspiratory center

Parenchymal receptors

Descending pathway to spinal cord

Spinal cord

Respiratory motor neurons

Proprioceptors

G.J.Wassilchenko

chemoreceptors, are the primary receptors. Other chemoreceptors, called peripheral chemoreceptors, are located at numerous body locations including the carotid arteries and the arch of the aorta. All chemoreceptors function basically the same way, responding to the concentration of either oxygen or hydrogen ions crossing their membranes to send ventilatory stimulus impulses to the medullary center.

The two respiratory centers located in the pons are the apneustic center and the pneumotaxic center. The apneustic center is located in the lower portion of the pons and is referred to as the pontine center. Apneusis is a condition in which ventilation stops in the inspiratory

position. The apneustic center is controlled by the pneumotaxic center and the inflation reflexes. Diseases of the pons may lead to abnormal stimulation of the apneustic center and apneustic breathing.

The pneumotaxic center, also in the pons, controls the effect of the apneustic center and encourages rhythmic ventilation. It is thought that the pneumotaxic center receives impulses from the medullary inspiratory subcenter and sends impulses to the medullary expiratory subcenter, thus limiting inspiration.

An inflation reflex, commonly called the Hering-Breuer reflex, carries impulses from the lung to the brain through the vagus nerve. This stretch reflex, originating in the bronchiolar or alveolar walls, modifies the apneustic center's action by limiting inhalation and by helping the medullary center establish a smooth and easy combination of tidal volume and rate.

In addition to these major areas, there are numerous miscellaneous reflexes that respond to pain, temperature, tissue pressure and stretch, and circulatory dynamics.

In summary, the greatest influences on the autonomic nervous system's ventilation control comes from the blood's hydrogen ion concentration and oxygen content stimulation of the medullary center's chemoreceptors. These help correlate ventilation with acid-base balance and with gas exchange needs. Finally the entire autonomic ventilatory control system is subject to voluntary override by higher areas of the cerebral cortex.

NORMAL FINDINGS

Area of Concern	Normal Adult Findings	Variations in Child	Variations in Older Adult
General appearance	Appears relaxed Breathing is quiet and easy without apparent effort Facial expressions and limb movements are relaxed		
Breathing pattern	Diaphragmatic-thoracic pattern is smooth and regular May have occasional sighing respirations Breathing is quiet and passive	Abdominal and nasal breathing during childhood until 6 to 7 years of age, then change to adult pattern Newborns may demonstrate Cheyne-Stokes breathing until 3 to 4 weeks of age	Pattern is same as for adults, but calcification at rib articulation points may decrease chest expansion
Respiratory rate	12-20 resp/min Ratio of pulse to respirations is 4:1	Newborn: 30-50 resp/min 1 yr: 20-40 resp/min 3 yr: 20-30 resp/min 6 yr: 16-22 resp/min 10 yr: 16-20 resp/min 17 yr: 14-20 resp/min	
Skin	Appears well oxygenated; no cyanosis or pallor present Palpation of skin and chest wall reveals smooth skin and a stable chest wall; there are no crepitations, bulging, or painful spots	Babies may become mottled if left uncovered	
Nail bed, nail configuration	Minimal angulation between base of nail and finger No thickening of distal finger width		
Chest wall configuration (Fig. 2-16)	Symmetric, bilateral muscle development A:P to transverse ratio is 1:2 to 5:7; larger than these ratios is considered to be barrel chest Straight spinal processes Downward and equal slope of ribs; costal angle 90 degrees or less Deviation of chest wall configuration discussed in Chapter 4 (Fig. 2-16)	Newborns have rounded chest wall configuration; by 6 years of age, A:P ratio should be 1:2	Kyphosis is a common finding in elderly persons; there is dorsal scoliosis with slight tracheal deviation; this may also cause a slight increase in A:P to transverse ratio
Tracheal position	Midline and straight directly above the suprasternal notch		May be slightly deviated if kyphosis is present

Fig. 2-16
Landmarks and structures of chest
wall. **A,** Anterior view. **B,** Posterior
view.

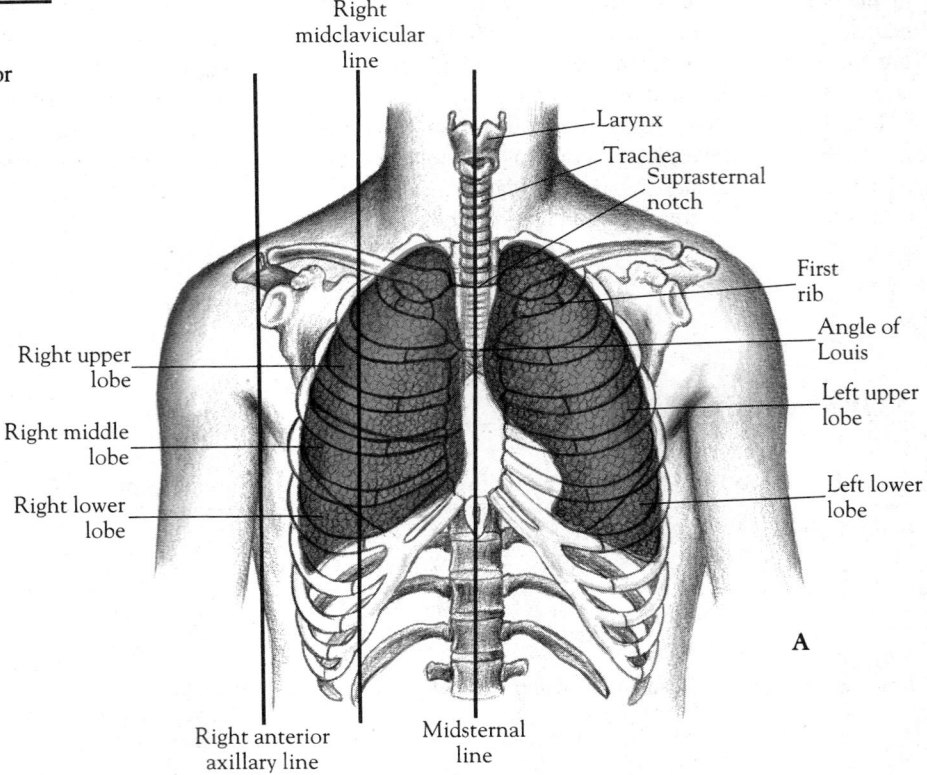

Right
midclavicular
line

Larynx

Trachea

Suprasternal
notch

First
rib

Angle of
Louis

Left upper
lobe

Left lower
lobe

Right upper
lobe

Right middle
lobe

Right lower
lobe

Right anterior
axillary line

Midsternal
line

A

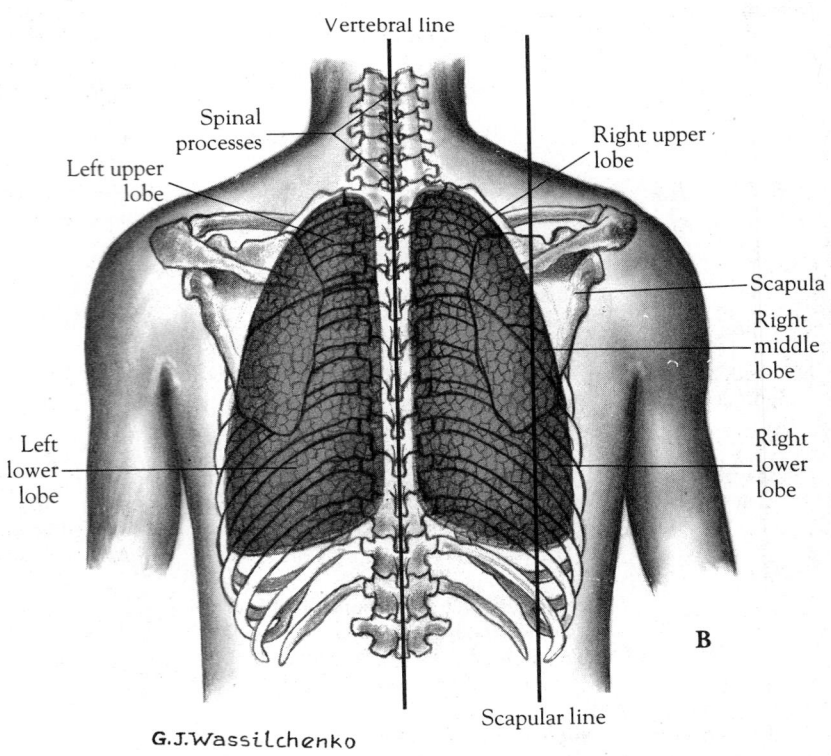

Vertebral line

Spinal
processes

Left upper
lobe

Right upper
lobe

Scapula

Right
middle
lobe

Right
lower
lobe

Left
lower
lobe

Scapular line

B

G.J.Wassilchenko

Fig. 2-17
Percussion tones. **A,** Anterior view.
B, Posterior view.

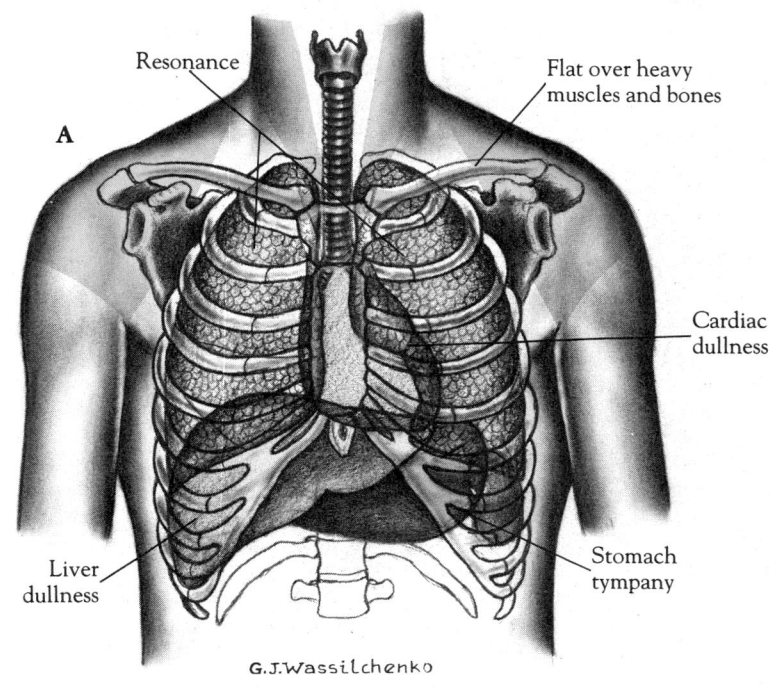

Resonance

Flat over heavy
muscles and bones

A

Cardiac
dullness

Liver
dullness

Stomach
tympany

G.J.Wassilchenko

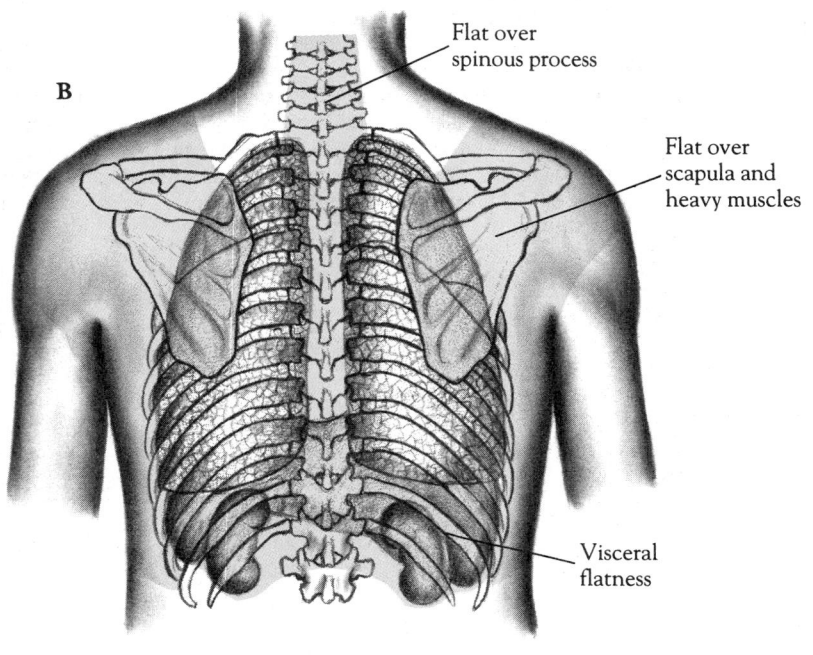

Flat over
spinous process

B

Flat over
scapula and
heavy muscles

Visceral
flatness

Area of Concern	Normal Adult Findings	Variations in Child	Variations in Older Adult
Vocal fremitus	Bilaterally equal mild sensation More intense vibratory feeling in upper posterior wall medial to scapula See box below		
Respiratory excursion	Bilaterally equal expansion of ribs during deep inspiration		Depth of breath may be less than in younger adult, but response should be the same
Percussion	Resonance heard throughout lung fields; see Fig. 2-17 and Table 2-5 for percussion tone characteristics Percussion of diaphragmatic excursion should measure 4 to 6 cm; inhaled position is approximately at tenth posterior rib level	Hyperresonance may be normally heard in young children	
Auscultation	Quiet breathing heard throughout all lung fields; Fig. 2-18 shows normal sounds heard in each lung field, and Table 2-6 describes the normal and abnormal breath and voice sounds	Bronchovesicular breath sounds are heard throughout the chest until child assumes adult breathing characteristics	

OVERVIEW OF VOCAL FREMITUS

Vocal fremitus is the sensation of sound vibrations produced when the patient speaks.

The examiner may feel for these vibrations by placing the extended hand gently on the chest wall. The spoken voice produces low-frequency vibrations through the vocal cords, the airways, and the pleura. These vibrations are felt and compared bilaterally.

The examiner instructs the patient to say "one-two-three" or "how-now-brown cow." As these words are spoken, the examiner feels for the vibrations.

Abnormal Responses

Increased fremitus. An increase in the vibratory sensation is felt when there is consolidation of the lung caused by fluid-filled or solid structures, which would transmit the vibrations better than air-filled lungs. This occurs, for example, with pneumonia or a tumor of the lung.

Decreased fremitus. A decrease in the vibratory sensation is felt when more air than normal is blocked or trapped in the lungs or pleural space; vibrations of the spoken voice are decreased. This occurs, for example, with emphysema or a pneumothorax.

Table 2-5
Percussion Tones Heard over Chest

Type of Tone	Intensity	Pitch	Duration	Quality
Resonant	Loud	Low	Long	Hollow
Flat	Soft	High	Short	Extremely dull
Dull	Medium	Medium-high	Medium	Thudlike
Tympanic	Loud	High	Medium	Drumlike
Hyperresonant*	Very loud	Very low	Longer	Booming

*Hyperresonance is abnormal sound heard during percussion in adults. It represents air trapping such as occurs in obstructive lung diseases.

Fig. 2-18
Normal auscultatory sounds. **A,**
Anterior view. **B,** Posterior view.

KEY:

Bronchovesicular
over main bronchi

Vesicular over lesser
bronchi, bronchioles, and lobes

Bronchial over trachea

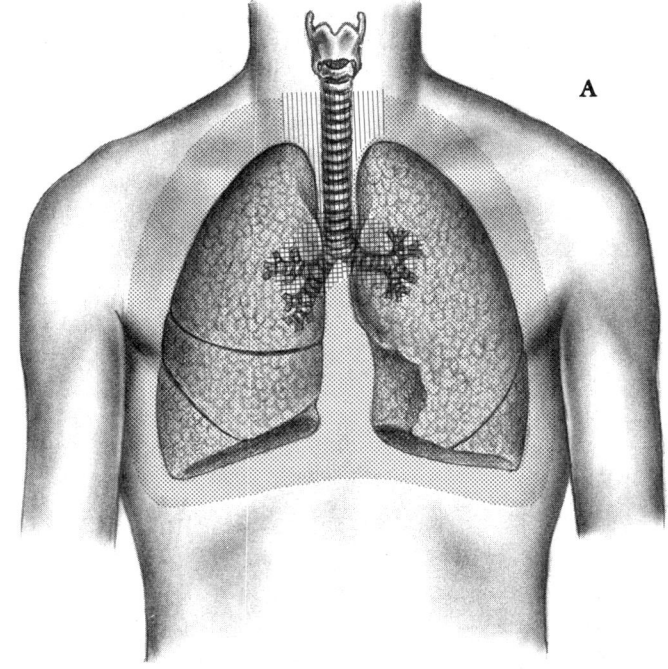

A

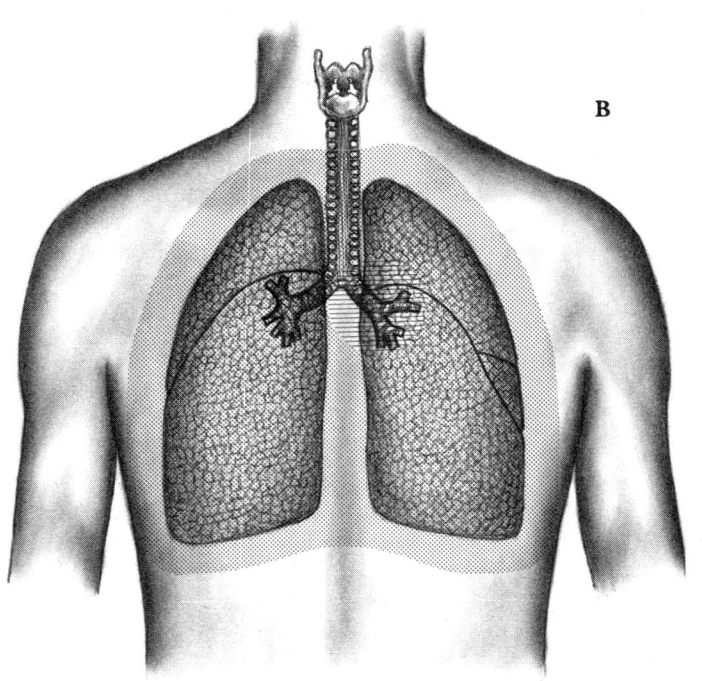

B

G.J.Wassilchenko

Table 2-6
Breath and Voice Sounds: Normal and Abnormal

Breath and Voice Sounds	Characteristics	Findings
Normal		
Vesicular	Heard over most of lung fields; low pitch; soft and short expirations (Fig. 2-18)	Low pitch, soft expirations
Bronchovesicular	Heard over main bronchus area and over upper right posterior lung field; medium pitch; expiration equals inspiration	Medium pitch, medium expirations
Bronchial	Heard only over trachea; high pitch; loud and long expirations	High pitch, loud expirations
Abnormal		
Bronchial when heard over peripheral lung fields	High pitch; loud and long expirations	
Bronchovesicular sounds when heard over peripheral lung fields	Medium pitch with inspirations equal to expirations	
Adventitious	Crackles: discrete, noncontinuous sounds	
	Fine crackles (rales): high-pitched, discrete, noncontinuous crackling sounds heard during the end of inspiration (indicates inflammation or congestion)	
	Medium crackles (rales): lower, more moist sound heard during the midstage of inspiration; not cleared by a cough	
	Coarse crackles (rales): loud, bubbly noise heard during inspiration; not cleared by a cough	
	Wheezes: continuous musical sounds; if low pitched, may be called rhonchi	
	Sibilant wheeze: musical noise sounding like a squeak; may be heard during inspiration or expiration; usually louder during expiration	
	Sonorous wheeze (rhonchi): loud, low, coarse sound like a snore heard at any point of inspiration or expiration; coughing may clear sound (usually means mucus accumulation in trachea or large bronchi)	

Breath and Voice Sounds	Characteristics	Findings
	Pleural friction rub: dry, rubbing, or grating sound, usually due to the inflammation of pleural surfaces; heard during inspiration or expiration; loudest over lower lateral anterior surface	
Resonance of spoken voice	*Bronchophony:* using diaphragm of stethoscope, listen to posterior chest as patient says "ninety-nine"	Negative response: muffled "nin-nin" sound heard Positive response: clear, loud "ninety-nine" response heard because the lung tissue is consolidated
	Whispered pectoriloquy: listen to posterior chest as patient whispers "one, two, three"	Negative response: muffled sounds heard Positive response: clear "one, two, three" is heard because of lung consolidation
	Egophony: listen to posterior chest as the patient says "e-e-e"	Negative response: muffled "e-e-e" sound heard Positive response: sound of *e* changes to an a-a-a sound because of consolidation

Common Abnormal Assessment Findings

Following are common abnormal findings that require in-depth subjective and objective assessment:

Finding	Subjective Assessment	Objective Assessment
Cough	Duration of coughing problem? Frequency of cough? Circumstances related to cough such as activity or position? Does activity make cough worse? Sputum production with cough? Currently smoking? If so, what and how much?	Frequency of cough? Characteristics of cough: hacky, dry, congested, barky, hoarse? Patient's position during coughing? Does coughing exhaust patient?
Sputum production	How long has sputum production occurred? Is sputum produced at certain times of the day or with certain activities or positions? Characteristics of sputum?	Characteristics of sputum: color, odor, consistency?
Shortness of breath	Describe onset of problem. History of breathing problem? If so, describe. What makes symptom better or worse? How does activity affect problem? How does different positioning affect problem? What seems to bring on episode? What does patient do for the problem?	Posturing during episode? Respiratory and pulse rates during episode? Circulatory response, i.e., pallor or cyanosis? Noisy breathing or wheezing noted?

NORMAL LABORATORY DATA

Laboratory Test	Normal Adult Values	Variations in Child
Whole Blood		
pH		Premature: 7.35-7.50
Arterial range	7.35-7.45 (average 7.4)	Newborn (arterialized capillary blood [heel, finger, big toe] or arterial blood): 7.32-7.49
Venous range	7.32-7.43	2 mo to 2 yr (arterialized capillary or arterial blood): 7.34-7.46
Pco_2		Newborn: 27-40 mm Hg
Arterial range	35-45 mm Hg (average 40 mm Hg)	Infant: 27-41 mm Hg
Venous range	35-50 mm Hg	Thereafter: 32-45 mm Hg
Po_2		Newborn: 60-70 mm Hg
Arterial range	80-95 mm Hg (average 95 mm Hg)	Thereafter: 83-108 mm Hg
		Average: 93.2 mm Hg
HCO_3^-		Infant: 16-24 mEq/L
Arterial range	21-28 mEq/L	
Venous range	22-29 mEq/L	
So_2		Newborn: 40%-90%
Arterial range	95%-99% (average 97%)	Thereafter: 95%-99%
Venous range	60%-85% (average 75%)	Newborn: 30%-80%
		Thereafter: 55%-85%
Pulmonary artery	75%-80%	
O_2 content		15-23 ml/100 ml or 15-23 vol%
Arterial range	17-21 ml/100 ml or 17-21 vol%	
Venous range	10-16 ml/100 ml or 10-16 vol%	
CO_2 content		Infants to 2 yr: 18-27 mEq/L
Arterial range	22-29 mEq/L	
Venous range	23-30 mEq/L	
Plasma		
CO_2 content		
Arterial range	21-30 mEq/L	
Venous range	24-34 mEq/L	
Hemoglobin		
CO saturation (carboxyhemoglobin)		Newborn: up to 10%-12%
Nonsmoker	0-2%	
Smoker	3%-5%	
Heavy smoker	9%-10%	

PULMONARY FUNCTION TESTS*

Test	Description	Significance
Lung Volume Tests†		
VC = Vital capacity (VC = ERV + V_T + IRV)	This capacity test combining more than one lung volume is the maximum amount of air that can be expired slowly and completely following a maximum inspiration. Response values of this test, as well as all other pulmonary function tests, are directly dependent on patient's effort. From VC other pulmonary function values may be calculated, including ERV, IRV, V_T, and IC.	A decrease in VC may be caused by a loss of distensible lung tissue, as seen in bronchiolar obstruction, pulmonary edema, pneumonia, atelectasis, pulmonary restriction, surgery, pulmonary congestion, or by depression of the respiratory center in the brain.
FRC = Functional residual capacity (FRC = ERV + RV)	This capacity test combining more than one lung volume is the volume of air remaining in the lungs at the end of normal expiration. Open- or closed-circuit techniques of body plethysmography are used to measure concentrations of a gas (either helium or nitrogen); from this the FRC can be calculated. This is actually calculated measurement of airway resistance.	The values help to differentiate obstructive from restrictive diseases. An increased FRC represents hyperinflation, which is seen with bronchiolar obstruction, emphysema, or asthma. An increased FRC results in muscular and mechanical inefficiency. A decreased FRC may be seen in diseases that occlude the alveoli such as pneumonia, and in fibrosis, asbestosis, or silicosis.
ERV = Expiratory reserve volume	This single-volume calculation is the maximum amount of air that can be exhaled following a resting expiratory level.	Although the ERV (approximately 25% of VC) has no diagnostic value, it must be calculated so that the RV can be calculated.
IRV = Inspiratory reserve volume	This single-volume calculation is the maximum amount of air that can be inspired following a normal inspiration.	
RV = Residual volume (RV = FRC − ERV)	This single-volume measurement is the volume of air remaining in the lungs at the end of maximal expiration. This is measured indirectly by subtracting the ERV from the FRC.	This value helps to differentiate restrictive from obstructive diseases. An increased RV indicates that despite maximal expiratory effort the lungs still contain an abnormally large amount of air. This may be seen in patients with emphysema or chronic bronchial obstruction. The RV usually decreases with restrictive lung disease.
IC = Inspiratory capacity (IC = V_T + IRV)	This calculated measurement is a capacity test involving more than one lung volume. It is the largest volume of air that can be inspired in one breath from the resting expiratory level.	IC normally composes approximately 75% of the VC. Changes in the IC usually parallel increases or decreases in VC. Other than its use in postoperative care, this value is not commonly measured.
TLC = Total lung capacity (TLC = FRC + IC) or (TLC = VC + RV)	This capacity test combining more than one lung volume is the volume of air contained in the lung at the end of a maximal inspiration. The TLC is a derived calculation.	TLC differentiates obstructive from restrictive diseases. It may be decreased in pulmonary edema, atelectasis, neoplasms, pulmonary congestion, pneumothorax, or thoracic restriction. TLC may be increased in bronchiolar obstruction with hyperinflation and in emphysema.

*Normal values for pulmonary tests vary depending on the patient's age, sex, weight, and race.
†To best interpret these tests see Figs. 2-19 and 2-20.

PULMONARY FUNCTION TESTS

Test	Description	Significance
RV/TLC Ratio = Residual volume/Total lung capacity ratio (RV/TLC × 100)	This is a statement of the fraction of the TLC that can be defined as RV, expressed as a percentage.	Values greater than 35% are seen in patients with emphysema or chronic air trapping.
Ventilation Tests		
V_T = Tidal volume	This single-volume measurement is the volume of air inspired or expired during each respiratory cycle. This is measured at the bedside by simple spirometer for 1 minute. The total is then divided by the rate (the number of breaths per minute) to determine the average V_T.	Decreased or increased V_T may occur in various pulmonary disorders. V_T should only be considered in relation to arterial blood gases and respiratory rate and minute volume.
V_E = Minute volume	This is the total volume of air inspired or expired in 1 minute. It is determined by measuring the inspired or expired air over several minutes and dividing by the number of minutes. It may also be measured easily at the bedside by simple spirometry.	This value must be considered in conjunction with arterial blood gases. V_E increases in response to hypoxia, hypercapnia, acidosis, and exercise. It is most commonly used in exercise testing.
V_D = Respiratory dead space	This is the volume of the lungs that is ventilated but not perfused by pulmonary capillary blood flow. This includes the conducting airways, or anatomic dead space, and the nonfunctioning alveoli, or alveolar dead space.	The measurement of V_D provides important information regarding the status of the functional lung capacity. It is used primarily for exercise testing.

Fig. 2-19

Lung volume measurements. All values are approximately 25% less in women. *TLC*, Total lung capacity; V_T, tidal volume; *FRC*, functional residual capacity; *IC*, inspiratory capacity; *IRV*, inspiratory reserve volume; *ERV*, expiratory reserve volume; *RV*, residual volume; *VC*, vital capacity.

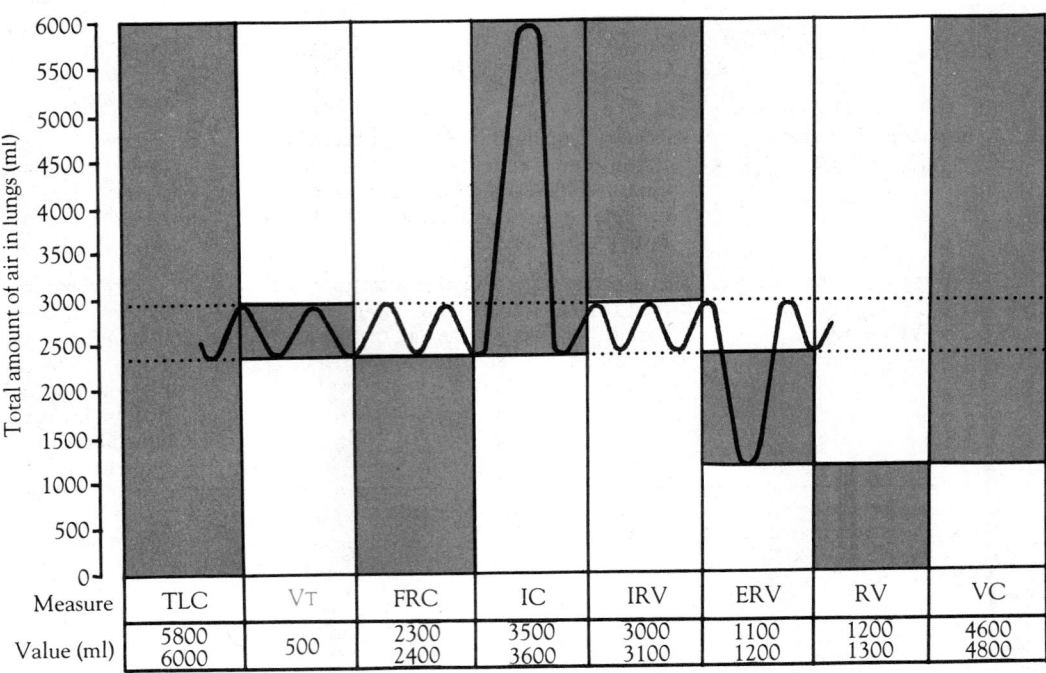

Measure	TLC	V_T	FRC	IC	IRV	ERV	RV	VC
Value (ml)	5800 6000	500	2300 2400	3500 3600	3000 3100	1100 1200	1200 1300	4600 4800

Test	Description	Significance
$\dot{V}_A$ = Alveolar ventilation $\dot{V}_A$ = $(V_T - V_D)$ f f = respiratory rate	This is the volume of air that participates in gas exchange in the lungs.	The adequacy of $\dot{V}_A$ can be determined only by arterial blood gas studies. It is used primarily for exercise testing.

Pulmonary Spirometry Tests

Test	Description	Significance
FVC = Forced vital capacity	This is the volume of air that can be expired forcefully and rapidly after maximal inspiration. The measurement is made directly by spirometer.	The FVC is normally equal to the VC. FVC may be reduced in chronic obstructive diseases, whereas the VC may appear close to normal. The FVC is decreased in restrictive diseases also. The test's validity depends largely on the individual's effort and cooperation.
FEV_T = Forced expiratory volume timed	This is the volume of air expired over a given interval during the performance of an FVC. The interval (T) is stated as a subscript to FEV. For example, $FEV_{0.5}$ indicates the interval is 0.5 second, and in FEV_1 the interval is 1 second. FEV_T is a calculated measurement by spirometer. After 3 seconds, FEV should equal FVC.	FEV_T is the most common screening test for detection of obstructive airways disease, in which the finding is a reduced response.
FEV% = FEV_T/FVC ratio $\times$ 100 (usually FEV_1/FVC%)	This is the percent of the measured FVC that a given FEV_T represents.	By measuring the expiratory flow over time the severity of obstruction can be assessed. FEV% or a reduced ratio is decreased in obstructive lung disease. It will usually remain within normal limits for persons with restrictive disease unless there is some type of secondary problem.
$FEF_{25\%-75\%}$ = Forced expiratory flow, 25%-75% or MMEF = Maximum midexpiratory flow rate	This is the average flow during the middle 50% of an FEV. It was previously known as the maximum midexpiratory flow rate (MMEF or MMF). Its reported value provides a picture of peripheral airways resistance. This value is then compared to the VC.	This measures the average flow rate over a given interval. It is an index of the status of the medium-sized airways. Decreased flow rates, when compared to the VC, are seen in early stages of obstructive diseases such as emphysema.
PEFR = Peak flow	This is the maximum flow rate attainable at any time during an FEV.	This measurement is of questionable diagnostic value. Children with asthma have a decreased PEFR.
F-V loop = Flow-volume loop	This is a graphic analysis of the maximum forced expiratory flow volume (MEFV) followed by a maximum inspiratory flow volume (MIFV). This technique uses a forced expiratory vital capacity followed by a forced inspiratory vital capacity. It is actually another way to display the forced vital capacity. Curves, reported as continuous loops on spirometric graphs, have distinctive sizes and shapes. The spirometry report of this technique is seen in Fig. 2-21.	The inspiratory flow may show evidence of upper airway obstruction. With obstructive disease the flow is reduced out of proportion to the volume. In restrictive disease the flow and volume are proportionally decreased, or the flow may be better than would be expected for the volume. As the flow-volume loop is examined, the shapes of the inspiratory and expiratory sides are analyzed.
MVV = Maximum voluntary ventilation	This is the largest volume of air that can be breathed per minute by voluntary effort. Actual testing period lasts 10 to 15 seconds.	The MVV measures the status of the respiratory muscles, the resistance offered by airways and tissues, and the compliance of the lung and thorax. This measurement depends greatly on the individual's effort.

Fig. 2-20

Spirometric standards for males and females.

From Morris, J.F., Roski, W.A., and Johnson, L.C.: Am. Rev. Respir. Dis. **103:**57, 1971.

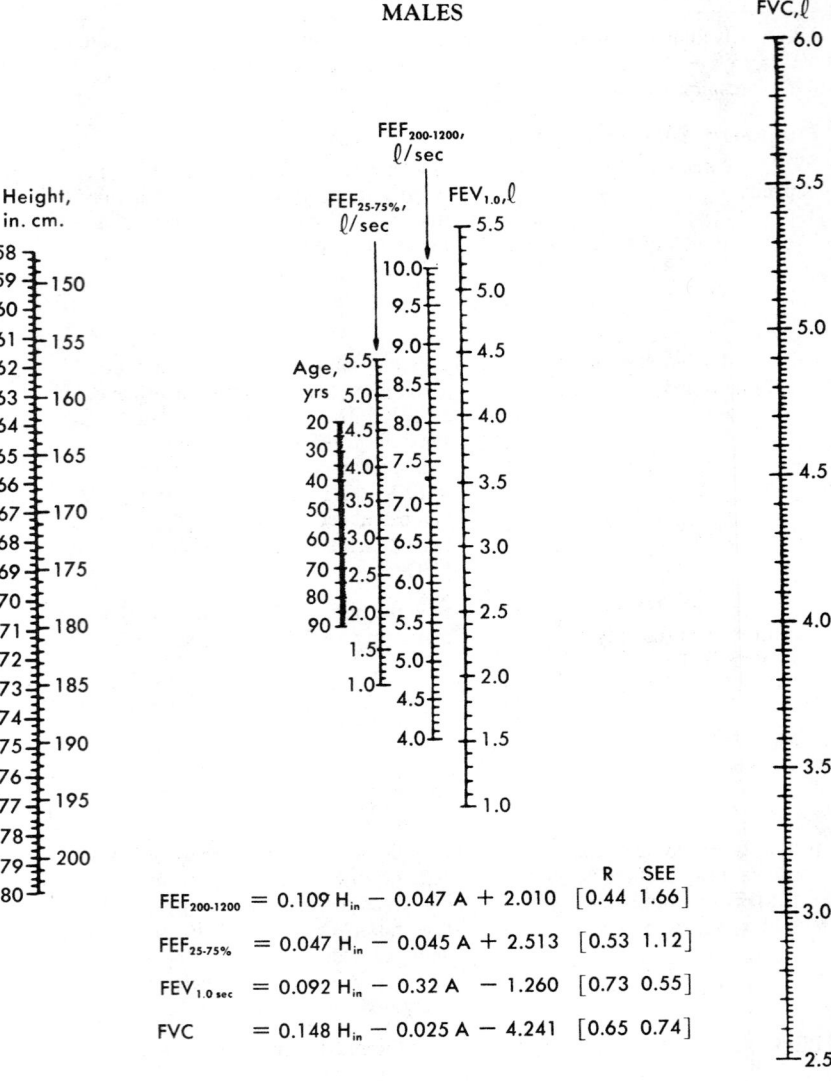

$$FEF_{200-1200} = 0.109\, H_{in} - 0.047\, A + 2.010 \quad [0.44 \quad 1.66]$$

$$FEF_{25-75\%} = 0.047\, H_{in} - 0.045\, A + 2.513 \quad [0.53 \quad 1.12]$$

$$FEV_{1.0\,sec} = 0.092\, H_{in} - 0.32\, A - 1.260 \quad [0.73 \quad 0.55]$$

$$FVC = 0.148\, H_{in} - 0.025\, A - 4.241 \quad [0.65 \quad 0.74]$$

PULMONARY FUNCTION TESTS

Test	Description	Significance
Gas Exchange DL_{CO} = Diffusing capacity of CO	The diffusing capacity rate of the lung provides a measure of the lung's gas exchange mechanism. It assesses the amount of functioning pulmonary capillary bed in contact with functioning alveoli. A common way to measure this is the *single-breath Krogh method:* the patient deeply inhales (from the residual volume level) a mixture of air containing 0.3% carbon monoxide and 10% helium gas, holds his breath for 10 seconds, and then exhales. The carbon monoxide levels are then remeasured.	The test is used primarily to differentiate various disease processes and for patient care monitoring.

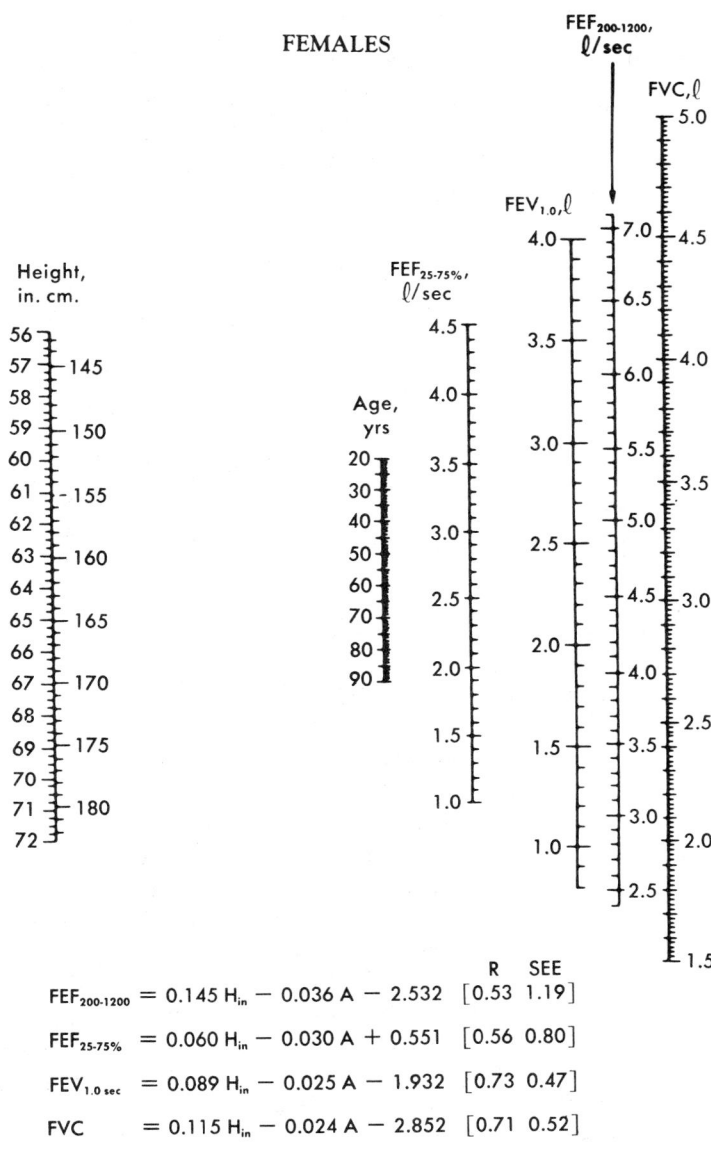

FEMALES

$$FEF_{200\text{-}1200} = 0.145\,H_{in} - 0.036\,A - 2.532 \quad [0.53 \quad 1.19]$$

$$FEF_{25\text{-}75\%} = 0.060\,H_{in} - 0.030\,A + 0.551 \quad [0.56 \quad 0.80]$$

$$FEV_{1.0\,sec} = 0.089\,H_{in} - 0.025\,A - 1.932 \quad [0.73 \quad 0.47]$$

$$FVC = 0.115\,H_{in} - 0.024\,A - 2.852 \quad [0.71 \quad 0.52]$$

R   SEE

PULMONARY FUNCTION TESTS

Test	Description	Significance
Raw = Airway resistance Gaw = Airway conductance	Raw is the pressure difference required for a unit flow change. Gaw is the flow generated per unit of pressure drop in the airway. It is the reciprocal of Raw. Measurements are made with a body plethysmograph. They are taken at the same time as FRC.	Raw increases in an acute asthmatic attack, emphysema, or other obstructive diseases. The calculations are most useful in evaluation of the qualitative response to various bronchodilators.

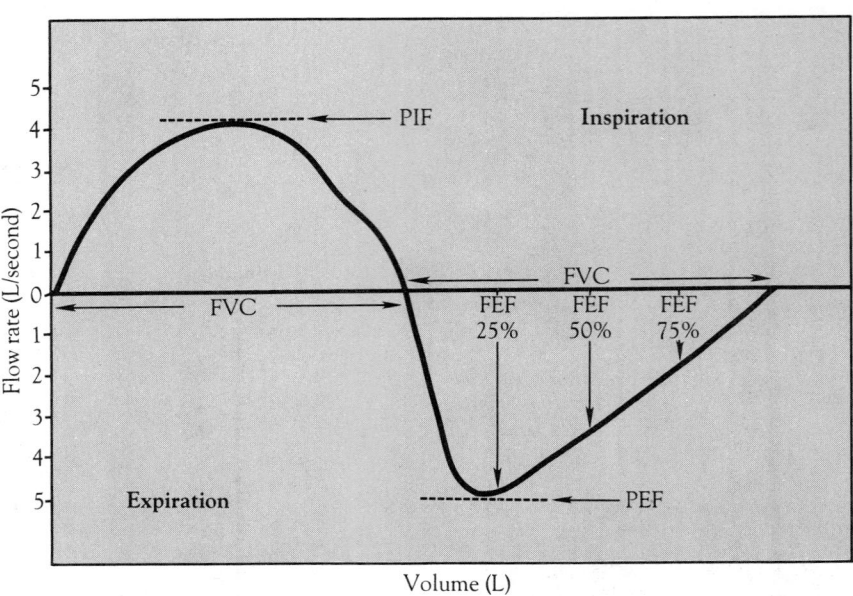

Fig. 2-21
Flow-volume loop. *PIF,* Peak inspiratory flow; *PEF,* peak expiratory flow; *FEF,* forced expiratory flow at *x*% FVC; *FVC,* forced vital capacity.

DIAGNOSTIC STUDIES

Pulmonary function testing
Simple spirometer

The simple spirometer is a basic office tool used to measure the presence and severity of disease in large and small airways and to distinguish between obstructive and restrictive patterns. It is most commonly used to measure VC, IC, ERV, T_v, IRV, $FEF_{200-1200}$, and $FEF_{25\%-75\%}$. There are two types of spirometers: volume and flow. Both of these types are commonly computerized. Two of the most common are the water seal and dry rolling seal spirometers (Fig. 2-22). The volume measurement spirometer is most common. This type works so that as the individual exhales or inhales into the mouthpiece, water or air already in the spirometer is displaced, causing the pen to touch the rotating drum and record the pattern. The presence and severity of respiratory dysfunction are determined by comparing observed values with those predicted for a normal person considering age, sex, height, weight, and race.

Spirometer with gas dilution

The spirometer with gas dilution is used to measure the following:
FRC
RV
RV/TLC ratio
D_LCO
The purpose of the technique is to measure the rate of diffusion. The measurement of lung volumes is by either the helium dilution technique or the nitrogen washout technique. In the *helium dilution technique* the patient rebreathes a known concentration of diluted helium through the spirometer mouthpiece until the helium concentration in the spirometer and the patient's lungs are equal. The helium concentration in the spirometer and the volume of gas can then be used to calculate the patient's FRC. In the *nitrogen washout technique* the patient breathes 100% O_2 from one source and exhales the expired gas into the spirometer.

Body plethysmography

Plethysmography is used to measure the following:
Raw
Gaw
FRC (V_{TG} = FRC shutter is closed at end of expiration)
The plethysmograph is an air-tight chamber in which the patient sits. The patient is seated in the air-tight chamber, is fitted with nose clips, and is instructed to breathe through the mouthpiece, which is connected to a transducer. To calculate V_{TG} the patient is instructed to pant into the mouthpiece while keeping the cheeks rigid and glottis open. This provides the pressure readings for the V_{TG} calculator. The Raw and Gaw may be mathematically calculated as the patient breathes rapidly and shallowly.

Arterial blood gases

Blood gas analysis is done for several reasons: (1)

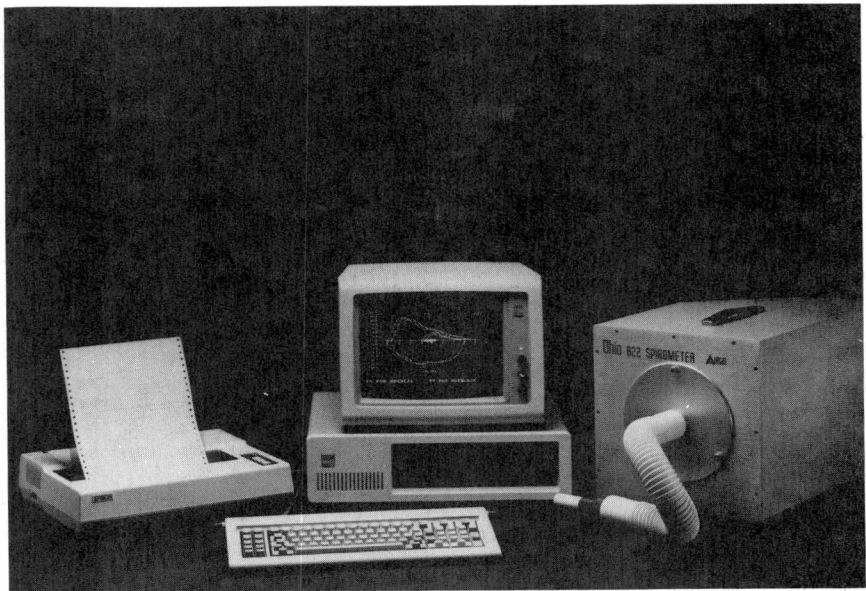

Fig. 2-22
Spirometer.

Courtesy Ohio Medical Products, Madison, Wisc.

assessment of adequacy of tissue oxygenation, (2) assessment of adequacy of ventilation, and (3) assessment of the body's acid-base status. Measurement of respiratory and nonrespiratory components is necessary to interpret arterial blood gas results.

Nursing care:

See pp. 233-235 for the procedure for obtaining arterial blood gas samples. The patient's vital signs including T, P, R should be evaluated prior to beginning the blood gas collection procedure. If patient is receiving O_2, record flow. If patient is on ventilator, record settings and oxygen flow.

If repeated or serial arterial blood gases are desired, an arterial catheter may be inserted.

Radiography: chest roentgenograms

The normal chest x-ray examination includes posterior-anterior (PA) and lateral views (as shown in Fig. 2-23). In young, healthy individuals or in asymptomatic persons only the PA view is used for screening. A lateral view should be obtained if disease is suspected or if the individual is over 40 years old. Chest x-ray films in the upright position are preferred so that the abdominal viscera is not pushing up on the diaphragm.

Chest x-ray films are evaluated for normal structure, position, and outlines, presence of fluid lines, foreign bodies, infiltration, abnormal shadows.

Nursing care:

All neck jewelry or garments containing metal closures, buttons, or ornaments must be removed. The patient should be wearing a hospital gown.

Tomography
Conventional tomography

This procedure produces films of multiple, sharply focused or plane "cuts" through the thorax with other planes blurred out.[26] It is most helpful when the exact morphologic characteristics of a lesion need to be identified.

Computerized axial tomography (CAT scan)

This technique produces x-ray absorption profiles at different angles in the same cross-sectional plane. This sensitive and highly accurate technique reconstructs internal structures into a picture format. (See Fig. 2-24.)

Contrast examinations
Barium swallow

This procedure, in which the patient swallows barium, outlines the esophageal lumen, thereby permitting detection of esophageal deviation by any of the adjacent mediastinal structures.

Bronchography

Radiopaque contrast medium is inserted into the lumina of the trachea and bronchial tree. Bronchography is being used more and more infrequently.[26] The advent of fiberoptic bronchoscopy has rendered fewer lesions inaccessible to direct vision. More precise methods for diagnosing a pulmonary lesion include bronchoscopic brush, forcep biopsy, and transthoracic needle puncture.

Nursing care:

1. Patient NPO for 8 hours before procedure.

Fig. 2-23

Normal PA and lateral chest roentgenogram. Note no abnormal bony prominences, heart of normal size, sharp costophrenic angles, lung fields clear, diaphragms visible throughout except against heart border, mediastinum midline with bronchial structures visible, and breast shadows.

Courtesy R. Keith Wilson, M.D., Baylor College of Medicine, Houston, Texas.

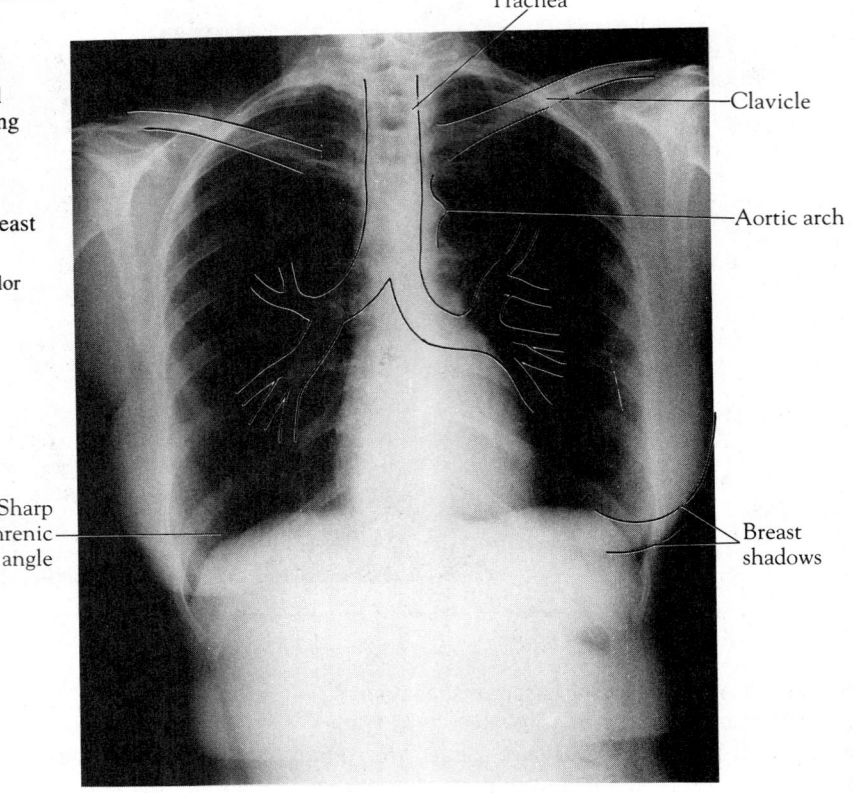

Trachea

Clavicle

Aortic arch

Sharp costophrenic angle

Breast shadows

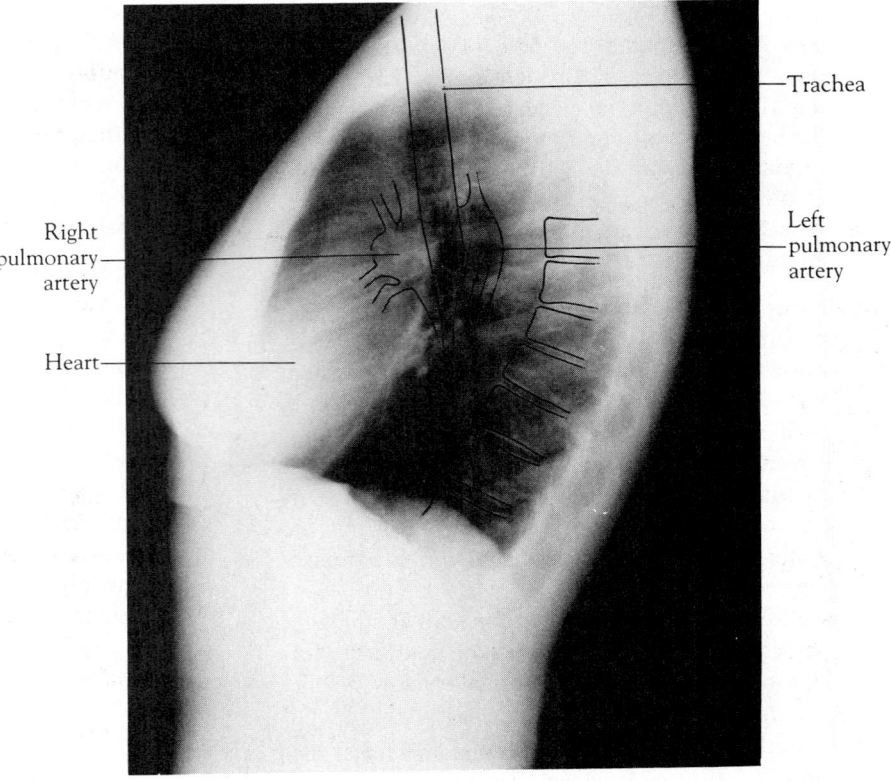

Trachea

Right pulmonary artery

Heart

Left pulmonary artery

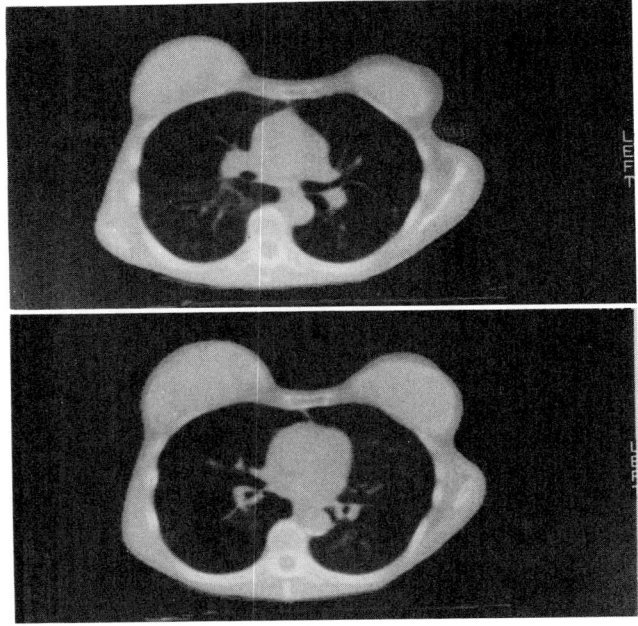

Fig. 2-24
CT scan of female patient. On this transverse scan through upper chest, bilateral breast shadows are evident. Heart, pulmonary arteries, and main bronchi are also visible.

Courtesy R. Keith Wilson, M.D., Baylor College of Medicine, Houston, Texas.

2. Assess allergies to anesthesia agent or contrast media.
3. Assess for dental prosthesis.
4. Approximately 1 hour before procedure administer barbiturate medication with atropine to decrease anxiety and secretions.
5. To lessen the patient's discomfort during the procedure, the throat may be sprayed with 0.5% tetracaine or similar substance.
6. Oxygen and suction should be available during process.
7. Following the procedure the patient should be evaluated for gag and cough reflex and tissue oxygenation.
8. Food and water should be withheld until the gag reflex returns.
9. Following the procedure the patient should be encouraged to cough. If cough is inadequate, postural drainage may be needed.

Pulmonary angiography

A radiopaque dye is injected rapidly into the pulmonary circulation by various routes: one or more systemic veins or the chambers of the heart or directly into the pulmonary arteries. Following the rapid injection a series of x-ray films is taken. The purpose of the examination is to detect pulmonary emboli and a variety of congenital and acquired thromboembolic lesions.

Nursing care
Prior to procedure assess allergies to radiopaque dye.
Following the procedure the patient must be observed for hematomas or inflammation around injection site, absence of peripheral pulses, or complaints of numbness or pain.

Ventilation/perfusion lung scanning

A scanning device records the pattern of pulmonary radioactivity after the inhalation or intravenous injection of gamma ray–emitting radionuclides (such as xenon 133), thus providing visual images of the distribution of blood flow in the lungs. The major indications for this procedure are the evaluation of a pulmonary thromboembolism and preoperative lung function studies.

Ultrasound

Ultrasound has limited usefulness in evaluation of the lungs because sound beams are not transmitted well by air-containing tissue. Ultrasound examination is useful to detect pericardial effusion and fluid-containing or solid tissue lesions.

Endoscopy procedures
Fiberoptic bronchoscope

This procedure, done under local anesthesia, permits the direct inspection of the larynx, trachea, and bronchi. The flexible fiberoptic bronchoscope

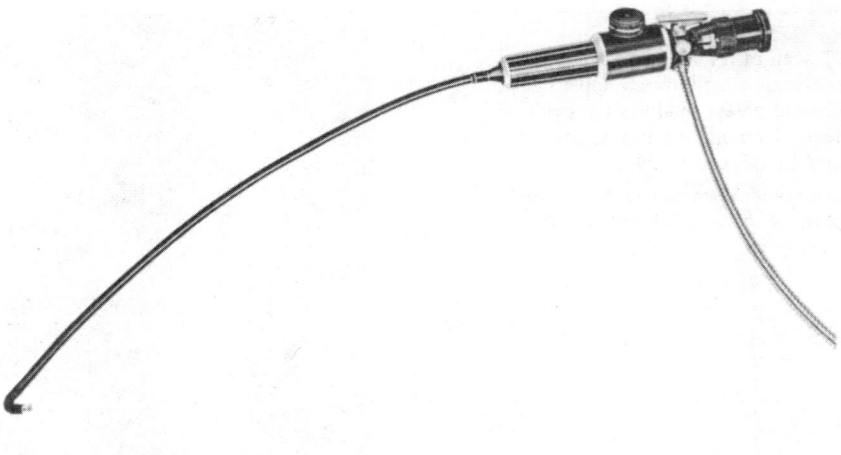

Fig. 2-25

Flexible fiberoptic bronchoscope.

Courtesy American Cystoscope Makers, Inc., Pelham, N.Y.

(Fig. 2-25) is the preferred instrument because it is better tolerated by patients and permits improved visualization of distal subsegmental airways. There are numerous purposes for bronchoscope:

1. To collect secretions for cytologic or bacterologic examination.
2. To collect tissue biopsy for examination.
3. To collect cells and secretions via a brush biopsy technique. This procedure involves using a small brush inserted through the bronchoscope to actually brush the tissue walls.
4. To locate and biopsy tumors.
5. To locate bleeding locations.
6. To remove foreign bodies or heavy blocking mucous plug secretions.
7. To implant radioactive gold seeds for tumor treatment.

The fiberoptic bronchoscope, which has an external diameter between 3 and 6 mm, is inserted either through the patient's nose or mouth.

General anesthesia may be used for this procedure if necessary.

Nursing care:

1. The patient should be NPO for 8 hours prior to the procedure.
2. A preprocedure sedative medication with atropine should be given.
3. Remove any dental prostheses.
4. When he is in the examination area, the patient's mouth, throat, and tongue will be sprayed with a topical anesthesia.
5. An oxygen catheter should be placed in one nostril and should remain there throughout the procedure.

6. Lidocaine jelly is generally used as the bronchoscope lubricant. This suppresses the patient's cough and gag reflexes.
7. Following the procedure the patient should be carefully watched and positioned until the full gag and swallowing reflexes return.
8. Increased sputum, productive mild bronchitis, a sore throat, and hoarseness are common complications of this procedure.
9. Patency of the patient's airway and the swallowing reflex should be evaluated as well as severe complications such as bronchospasms.

Mediastinoscopy, mediastinotomy, thoracoscopy

These are surgical endoscopy procedures in which a biopsy is taken from a tumor in the upper mediastinum, the pleura, or the lung. It is also used to determine if metastasis has occurred.

Mediastinoscopy: The incision is made in the suprasternal notch, and the scope is passed through that incision to biopsy tissue from the upper mediastinum.

Mediastinotomy: The incision is made above the third rib along the sternal border. Lung biopsy may also be done by this second technique.

Thoracoscopy: This is indicated to obtain a biopsy from a peripheral lesion of the lung or pleura. The incision site, along the lateral or anterior chest wall, is dependent upon the location of the lesion.

Nursing care:

For all procedures the patient receives a general

anesthetic. Therefore all preoperative procedures apply.

Postoperatively the patient should be observed for pneumothorax, cardiac arrhythmias, and bleeding.

A drainage chest tube is frequently used following the thoracoscopy procedure.

Biopsy

Scalene node biopsy

This procedure, done under local anesthesia, is to biopsy a palpable scalene node. The incision and biopsy are done in the supraclavicular scalene region.

Lung biopsy

Lung biopsy may be done in one of four ways. The purpose of all techniques is to obtain a tissue sample for histologic evaluation.

Transbronchial biopsy: This biopsy is taken with the fiberoptic bronchoscope from the bronchial area of concern.

Nursing care:

See fiberoptic bronchoscope above.

Percutaneous needle biopsy with aspiration: In this procedure, fluid and cells are aspirated into the syringe through a long, 18- to 20-gauge needle inserted percutaneously under fluoroscopic control into the suspected lesion. When the needle is in the lesion, the syringe is generally rotated to obtain a tissue specimen.

This procedure is used most often if malignancy is suspected.

A contraindication to needle aspiration is an uncooperative patient.

Nursing care:

The procedure is done under local anesthesia after the skin has been disinfected and a sterile field has been prepared.

The patient is instructed to hold his breath for 15 to 30 seconds during the procedure.

The aspirated material is sent for cytologic examination and for stains and cultures of microorganisms.

The major postprocedure complication is pneumothorax. Therefore careful respiratory assessment is indicated.

Percutaneous biopsy with a cutting needle: Three procedure options are possible:
1. Punch biopsy with Vim-Silvermann needle
2. High-speed drill biopsy with trephine lung biopsy drill
3. Suction excision biopsy with Abrams needle or a modification of the Abrams needle

The cutting needle procedure is indicated when the patient has diffuse pulmonary infiltrates. These techniques have significant complications and therefore are not usually done until other diagnostic procedures have failed to identify the problem.

Nursing care:

These procedures are also done under local anesthesia and a sterile field.

Major complications include hemorrhage and pneumothorax. Careful postprocedure assessment is indicated.

Open lung biopsy or exploratory thoracotomy: This is an invasive procedure used to confirm suspected diagnosis of lung or chest disease by obtaining lung specimens. The chest is opened through a standard thoracotomy incision, and the lung is inspected and biopsied. Open lung biopsy is indicated only after other investigative procedures have not clearly identified the patient's problem.

Nursing care:

For detailed nursing care see operative procedures, under Medical Interventions. General anesthesia is used.

A chest tube connected to water-seal drainage is used for 1 to 2 days after surgery because of the surgically induced pneumothorax.

Several days of postprocedural chest x-ray films are normally ordered.

The procedure may have several major complications including postoperative respiratory failure, emphysema, and chronic bronchopleural fistula.

Pleural fluid examination

Diagnostic thoracentesis

A needle is inserted through the chest wall into the pleural space for the purpose of removing pleural fluid. While it may be done therapeutically to drain off and relieve lung congestion, it is discussed here as a diagnostic procedure to collect pleural fluid for examination.

Nursing care:

Following the procedure follow-up chest x-ray films should be made, and the patient should be monitored for complications such as hemothorax, pneumothorax, air embolism, and subcutaneous emphysema.

Pleural biopsy

A small tissue sample is taken by special biopsy needle from the parietal pleura. It may be necessary to collect tissue samples from several different spots.

While some authorities advocate pleural biopsy every time a thoracentesis is done, others claim that it should only be done when granulomatous disease or malignancy is expected.

Nursing care:

This is generally done under local anesthesia before a thoracentesis.

The positioning of the patient is similar to that for a thoracentesis. Complications are rare but include pneumothorax, hemothorax, and intercostal nerve injury.

A postprocedure chest x-ray examination may be indicated if the patient has any complaints.

Sputum examination

The microbiologic evaluation of sputum is vitally important in the evaluation of the respiratory system. The two laboratory procedures commonly performed with sputum include microscopic Gram stain and culture and sensitivity.

Direct method

Voluntary coughing to produce sputum specimen. With this procedure, early morning specimens are sent on 3 consecutive days. It is most important to assure that a sputum and not a saliva specimen has been obtained.

Sputum induction

This technique may be used if voluntary coughing does not produce a specimen. With this technique the patient is instructed to breathe for several minutes using a heated, nebulized mist of distilled water or a sodium chloride (NaCl) solution. Following this nebulization the sputum collection technique as described is performed.

Nursing care:

Most important in the collection of sputum for laboratory analysis is ensuring that sputum, not saliva or postnasal drip, has been collected.

The sputum should be collected in a wide-mouth, sterile container with a tight fitting lid and should be transported immediately to the laboratory.

1. Instruct patient to brush teeth and gargle prior to collection of specimen.
2. Instruct patient to "hawk-up" any postnasal secretions and spit them out.
3. Instruct patient to take a deep breath to full capacity of lungs and then to exhale the air with an expulsive deep cough.
4. Specimen should be coughed directly into the sterile, wide-mouthed container.
5. Note color, consistency, odor, and amount. Serial number the specimens for each of the 3 days.

Indirect methods

One of 2 indirect methods may be used.

Nasotracheal suctioning

This technique is used to obtain specimens from the trachea via a catheter that has been passed transnasally.

Nursing care:

1. Assist the patient to a sitting position.
2. The nurse or physician passes a catheter through the patient's nose into the trachea to suction tracheobronchial secretions.
3. Oxygen should be administered during the procedure.
4. Cardiac response and the patient's oxygenation should be monitored.

Transtracheal aspiration

This technique may be preferred over nasotracheal suctioning. The specimens are better, but the patient may have discomfort. The technique involves puncture and needle aspiration. The needle is inserted through the criocothyroid membrane and the mucosal layer of the trachea. Procedural complications include subcutaneous or mediastinal emphysema and cervical infections at the site of the aspiration.

Nursing care:

1. Set up sterile procedural equipment including gloves, gauze sponges, large-bore intracath needle, 10 cc syringe, sterile specimen cup, local anesthetic with needles and syringe, and iodophor for skin cleansing.
2. Prepare patient for high-flow supplemental oxygen during the procedure.
3. Position the patient supine and hyperextend the patient's neck by placing a pillow under the shoulders.
4. Administer oxygen, assist the physician, and monitor the patient's cardiovascular and respiratory status during the procedure.
5. Following the procedure, light pressure should be placed over the site for at least 3 to 5 minutes.
6. Continue to assess the patient for postprocedural complications.
7. Anaerobic culture specimens are best sent to the laboratory in the aspirating syringe after all excess air has been expelled.

Gastric lavage

This technique, although not frequently used, may be helpful in the diagnosis of patients with suspected tuberculosis or lung cancer.

It is perhaps most valuable in those patients who may not be able to cooperate, such as young children and the acutely ill.

The procedure includes an early morning suctioning of gastric contents once a nasogastric tube has been properly placed. The timing of the procedure is early morning because it is assumed that the patient swallows sputum at night while sleeping and in the early morning with morning coughing.

The gastric contents are sent to the laboratory for sputum analysis.

Nursing care:
1. The patient is NPO since midnight.
2. A nasogastric (NG) tube is inserted through the patient's nose.
3. Suction by a large syringe is applied to the NG tube, and the gastric contents are removed.
4. The contents are placed in a specimen container and are sent immediately to the laboratory.
5. The NG tube is removed.

Skin tests

Tuberculin skin testing (Mantoux test)

This provides evidence of whether the tested individual has been infected, either past or present, with *Mycobacterium tuberculosis*.

Contraindications for testing include any rash, allergic dermatitis, scabies, current reactions to smallpox vaccinations, previous BCG vaccine.

Two types of tuberculin are currently being used for testing: old tubercu- (OT) and purified protein derivative (PPD). The PPD is the preferred tuberculin preparation because its strength is standardized and tests with the same dose are comparable.

Nursing care:
1. Each type of multiple puncture unit is slightly different.
2. Carefully read the manufacturers instructions regarding the administration of the test.
3. A positive reaction for all brands consists of the formation of separate papules at each of the puncture sites or a large papule over the entire area.
4. Refer to the manufacturer's instructions regarding specific interpretation.

Schick test (for susceptibility to diphtheria):

This is a test to determine the presence or absence of a significant quantity of diphtheria antitoxins in the blood. The presence of these antitoxins indicates immunity to diphtheria.

Nursing care:
1. Draw 0.1 ml of purified diphtheria toxin dissolved in human serum albumin into a tuberculin syringe.
2. In a second syringe draw up 0.1 ml of inactivated diphtheria toxoid to be used as control in the other arm to rule out sensitivity to culture proteins.
3. Attach 26- or 27-gauge, 1.25 cm (½ inch) needles to both syringes.
4. Clean the volar surfaces of both forearms.
5. Intradermally inject the toxin in one forearm, the toxoid in the other forearm.
6. Carefully record which was injected in each arm.
7. The areas are examined at 24 and 36 hours.
8. Evaluating the results:
   a. Positive reaction: the site of the toxin injection begins to redden in 24 hours. The redness, swelling, and tenderness continue until it reaches maximum size—usually 3 cm in diameter at the end of 1 week. The skin at the injection site may flake and in the center may appear as a dark pigmented spot. The area of the toxoid injection should show no reaction.
   b. Negative result: there is no flaking or erythema at either injection site.

Skin tests for fungal diseases

For patients suspected of having coccidioidomycosis, skin tests are available from lysates of both the mycelial (coccidioidin) and the spherule (spherulin) forms. Skin tests with either are highly specific and become positive 3 to 4 weeks after infection and 12 to 20 days after the onset of clinical illness.

Serologic tests

Serologic tests are frequently used to help determine the causative pathogens in fungal diseases and atypical pneumonia. The outcome of the test is dependent upon the development of antibodies to the organism in the patient's serum that can be detected by agglutination, complement fixation, or precipitation reactions when the serum is exposed to specific antigen. Examples are the fungal antibody tests for detection of coccidioidomycosis, blastomycosis, and histoplasmosis.

Conditions, Diseases, and Disorders

RESPIRATORY FAILURE, RESPIRATORY INSUFFICIENCY

The precise definition of respiratory insufficiency leading to respiratory failure is a condition in which the arterial PCO_2 is above 50 mm Hg when the patient is at rest and breathing room air or in which the PaO_2 is less than 55 mm Hg.[26]

Respiratory insufficiency refers to the inability of the lungs to maintain adequate gas exchange. That is, insufficient oxygen is taken up through ventilation to eliminate enough carbon dioxide to maintain normal partial pressures of these gases in the arterial blood. Respiratory insufficiency left untreated will result in respiratory failure and thus physiologic decompensation.

Respiratory insufficiency and respiratory failure are not diseases but more correctly are disorders of ventilation that may be caused by a variety of conditions either directly or indirectly.

Respiratory insufficiency and failure may be conveniently divided into three types:

Type I: Causes of severe hypoxemia with an abnormally low $PaCO_2$ include the following:
1. Increased pulmonary capillary pressure resulting from such conditions as:
   a. Left ventricular heart failure
   b. Pulmonary edema or fluid overload
2. Increased pulmonary capillary permeability from such conditions as:
   a. Pneumonia
   b. Tuberculosis
   c. Fungal infections
   d. Near drowning
   e. Chemical or smoke inhalation
   f. Liquid aspiration

In its most severe state, acute respiratory failure is referred to as adult respiratory distress syndrome (ARDS).

Type II: In type II respiratory failure the diseased lung is unable to normally excrete CO_2. Usually this is manifested by some type of chronic breathing problem accompanying such conditions as the following:
1. Chronic bronchitis
2. Emphysema
3. Massive obesity
4. Severe kyphoscoliosis
5. Asthma

Type III: The third type of respiratory failure is due to the inability of the neuromuscular system to ventilate normal or nearly normal lungs. There are two basic causes for this:
1. Respiratory center depression due to a malfunctioning central nervous system. This can be caused by:
   a. Drug overdoses
   b. Central nervous system lesions or infections
2. Inability of a normally functioning central nervous system to generate respiratory muscle power. Examples of disorders of neuromuscular transmission include the following:
   a. Guillain-Barré syndrome
   b. Multiple sclerosis
   c. Spinal cord injury
   d. Myasthenia gravis
   e. Muscular dystrophies
   f. Poliomyelitis
   g. Tetanus

PATHOPHYSIOLOGY

Each of the three types of respiratory insufficiency and respiratory failure has a specific pathophysiology, which is discussed below.

Type I

The most important factor in type I respiratory failure is increased extravascular lung fluid. The cause of this increased lung fluid may be (1) increased pulmonary capillary pressure or (2) increased pulmonary-capillary permeability. Patients who have diffuse pulmonary edema and respiratory failure secondary to increased pulmonary-capillary permeability are said to have ARDS. This is discussed below as a separate condition.

The process of hemodynamic pulmonary edema can be divided into three stages:

Initial stage: Pulmonary congestion and distended pulmonary vessels occur secondary to some specific condition. This leads to peripheral airway resistance and eventually to decreased compliance of the lungs.

Second stage: Peripheral airway resistance increases as additional fluid collects in the interstitial spaces, compressing the peripheral airways.

Third stage: As the alveoli become filled with fluid, total lung capacity is decreased, producing intrapulmonary shunting and hypoxia. The alveolar edema also suppresses the formation and effectiveness of surfactant. The surfactant problem leads to microatelectasis and a further reduction in the functional residual capacity.

The severe hypoxemia that occurs in patients with ARDS and respiratory failure is primarily due to the shunting of blood through fluid-filled alveoli and atelectatic alveoli. Because the small airways close and remain closed, distal atelectasis and loss of lung volume occur. Secondary to decreased compliance, a greater than normal inspiratory pressure is necessary to deliver the same tidal volume. As compliance decreases, there is also a decreasing overall lung volume.

Hypoxia is a cardinal feature of type I respiratory failure and ARDS. Even though the alveoli receive an adequate supply of blood, there is intrapulmonary shunting with little gas exchange. If uncorrected, acidosis results. In an attempt to compensate, cardiac output and alveolar minute ventilation increase.

Diagnostic studies for type I respiratory failure include evaluation of the $PaCO_2$ (significant finding is initially low when the body is still trying to compensate but then increases to greater than 50 mm Hg when compensation is no longer possible), of the pulmonary capillary wedge pressure (PCWP) (significant below 12 mm Hg), and of the protein concentration of fluid aspirated from the lung (significant finding is greater than 0.60).

Type II

The primary problem in type II respiratory failure is the inability to generate adequate alveolar ventilation. This results in an increased $PaCO_2$ and a decreased PaO_2.

The patient may have difficulty performing forced expiratory testing because of shortness of breath. In addition, because of the retention of carbon dioxide the kidneys tend to retain bicarbonate so that the arterial pH remains above 7.3.

Type III

The pathophysiologic discussion of type III respiratory failure needs to be subdivided into the two core divisions for the disorder.

Central nervous system (CNS) depression: Respiratory failure from CNS depression is most commonly seen following an overdose of opiates, alcohol, tricyclic antidepressants, barbiturates, or other sedative drugs. Following ingestion of significant quantities of any of these drugs, stimulation of the respiratory center is depressed, and there is a decreased rate of respiration with little change in the tidal volume. The respiratory center does not appear to respond to the rising $PaCO_2$.

Neuromuscular transmission difficulties: The main difficulty for patients with a neuromuscular disease is their inability to generate sufficient force for deep breathing or for coughing. Thus, although the individual is able to breathe easily with quiet respiration, exercise or a need for deep ventilation may cause difficulty. Chronically poor breathing will lead to secretion buildup and eventual airway obstruction. Because of the patient's inability to cough and thus clear the small airways, hypoventilation and an increase in $PaCO_2$ occur.

• • •

The diagnostic evaluation and nursing care of the patient with respiratory insufficiency and respiratory failure are cause specific. The reader is referred to the specific causes for a detailed discussion.

ADULT RESPIRATORY DISTRESS SYNDROME (ARDS)

In adult respiratory distress syndrome (ARDS) capillary permeability is increased, precipitating a clinical condition in which the lungs are wet and heavy, congested, hemorrhagic, stiff, and unable to diffuse oxygen.

ARDS left untreated leads to respiratory failure and death. The following are many of the disorders that may cause ARDS:

Trauma
    Hypovolemic shock
    Lung or cardiac contusion

Fat embolism
Head injury
Inhaled toxins
    Smoke
    Chemicals
    Oxygen toxicity
Liquid aspiration
    Gastric contents
    Near drowning
Hematologic disorders

Disseminated intravascular coagulation (DIC)
Blood transfusions
Infections
Gram-negative sepsis
Pneumonia
Drug overdose
Toxic metabolic disorders
Pancreatitis
Uremia
Eclampsia

This type of respiratory failure has been recognized for a long time. During World War I it was described as posttraumatic pulmonary insufficiency. During World War II it was called wet lung, and during the Viet Nam war it was described as Da Nang lung. The following terms are among the many synonyms for ARDS:

Wet lung
Shock lung
Pump lung
Congestive atelectasis
Acute pulmonary insufficiency
Noncardiogenic pulmonary edema
Stiff lung
White lung
Da Nang lung
Respirator lung
Progressive pulmonary consolidation
Adult hyaline membrane disease
Posttraumatic pulmonary insufficiency
Acute ventilatory insufficiency

Because of the variability of its diagnosis, the incidence and survival rates of ARDS are difficult to state. Studies done since the early 1970s have shown survival rates to be between 30% and 50%.[41] Other authors suggest that with prompt and aggressive treatment the survival rate may be increased to 60% to 70%. In all cases, early detection and aggressive interventions have direct impact on the patient's probability of survival.

PATHOPHYSIOLOGY

Although the insults responsible for precipitating ARDS may vary, the tissue response of the lung and the metabolic response of the body are virtually identical. On gross examination of the lung at biopsy the lung is found to be congested and hemorrhagic and to have the appearance of a liver. The amount of secretions in the large airways is not significant, and there is no visible obstruction of the major vessels.

There is always a time sequence in the development of ARDS. For example, it may be seen 12 to 24 hours after a trauma resulting in hypovolemic shock or lung contusion, or it may appear 5 to 10 days following the development of sepsis. In either case the sequence of physiologic response and the identification of clinical symptoms remain the same. Fig. 2-26 outlines the physiologic process.

As a result of this process the patient's major problems are:

1. A reduction in the functional vital capacity
2. Bronchovascular edema, resulting in a decrease of the interstitial negative pressure, distal atelectasis, and decreased vital capacity
3. Decreased pulmonary compliance secondary to pulmonary congestion, resulting in a decreased functional residual capacity (FRC)
4. Hypoxia secondary to the intrapulmonary shunting
5. Increased oxygen consumption, increased airway resistance, and increased venous blood return to the heart secondary to the patient's attempt to increase minute ventilation

DIAGNOSTIC STUDIES

Pulmonary function

Alveolar-arterial oxygen gradient $P(A-a)O_2$ (also A-a DO_2): 300-500 mm Hg; reflects the difficulty with which oxygen crosses the alveolar-capillary membrane

Shunt fraction (Qs-Qt): May be greater than 15%-20%; measures the degree of intrapulmonary shunting
Normal value <6%

Functional residual capacity (FRC): below normal

Compliance (C): below normal

Pulmonary capillary wedge pressure (PCWP): Low to normal pressure seen in ARDS

Pulmonary capillary wedge pressure: 3-12 mm Hg

Arterial blood gases

PaO_2 < 70 mm Hg
$PaCO_2$ < 35 mm Hg
HCO_3 < 22 mEq/L
pH increased in beginning; as ARDS becomes worse, pH decreases

Lactic acid levels

Increased regardless of measurement technique
Normal values
80-100 Wacker units
120-340 IU/I
150-450 Wroblewski units

Chest x-ray films

There must be a large increase in lung fluid before abnormalities are observed on chest x-ray films; early diagnostic x-ray changes include thickened or blurred margins of the bronchi or vessels; Fig.

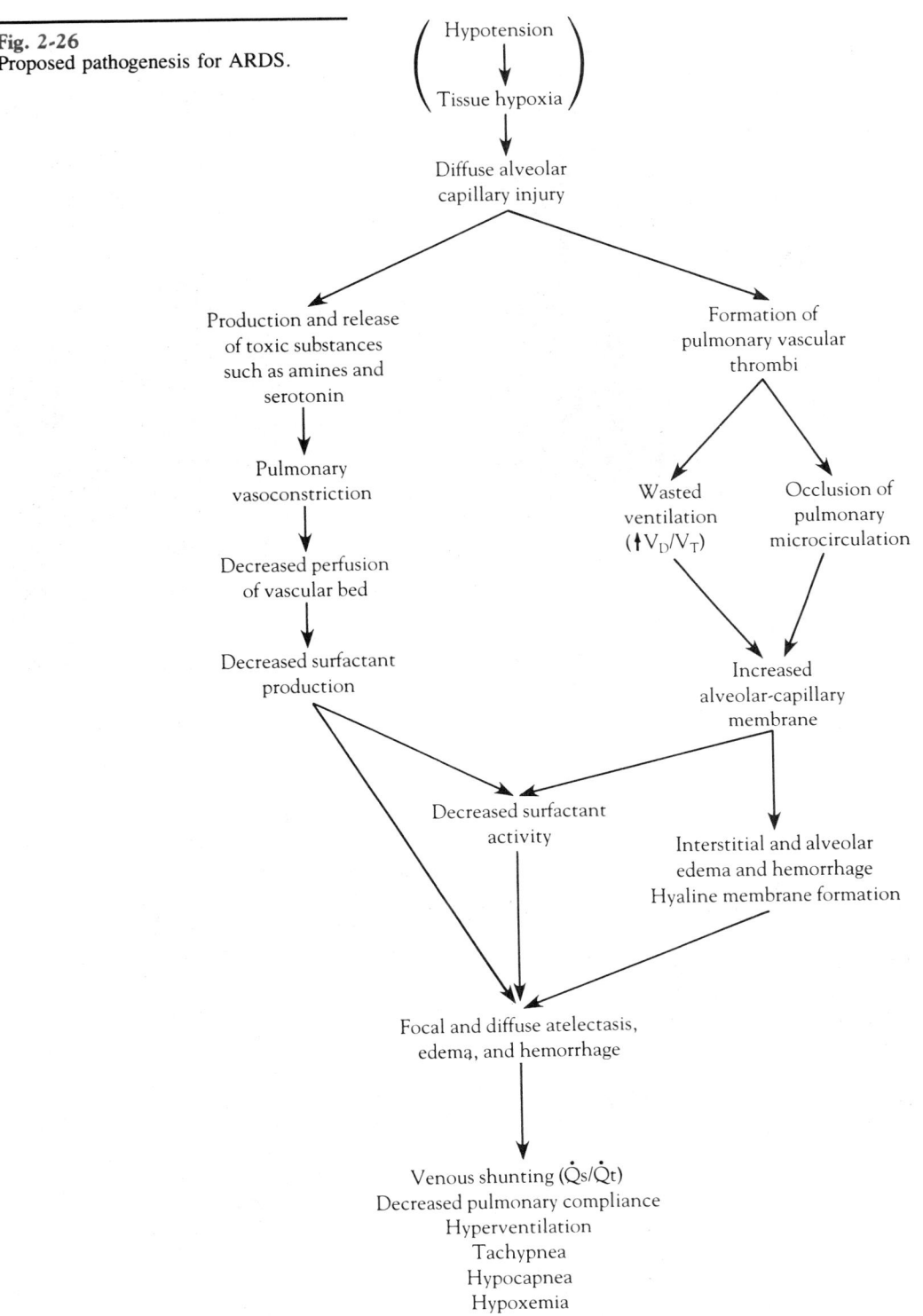

Fig. 2-26
Proposed pathogenesis for ARDS.

Hypotension

Tissue hypoxia

Diffuse alveolar
capillary injury

Production and release
of toxic substances
such as amines and
serotonin

Formation of
pulmonary vascular
thrombi

Pulmonary
vasoconstriction

Wasted
ventilation
($\uparrow V_D/V_T$)

Occlusion of
pulmonary
microcirculation

Decreased perfusion
of vascular bed

Decreased surfactant
production

Increased
alveolar-capillary
membrane

Decreased surfactant
activity

Interstitial and alveolar
edema and hemorrhage
Hyaline membrane formation

Focal and diffuse atelectasis,
edema, and hemorrhage

Venous shunting ($\dot{Q}s/\dot{Q}t$)
Decreased pulmonary compliance
Hyperventilation
Tachypnea
Hypocapnea
Hypoxemia

Fig. 2-27
Chest roentgenogram of patient with adult respiratory distress syndrome
(ARDS). Heart is normal size; note diffuse infiltrates in upper and middle
zones of lungs.

Courtesy R. Keith Wilson, M.D., Baylor College of Medicine, Houston, Texas.

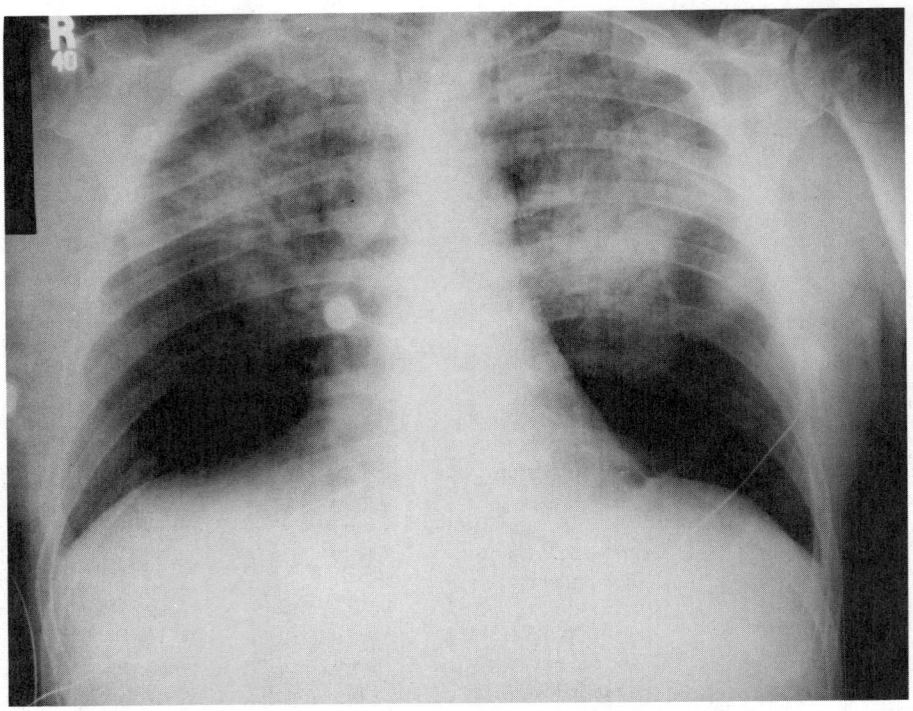

2-27 shows diffuse and hazy blurred appearance throughout the lung fields

TREATMENT PLAN

The major medical plan is focused in three areas:

1. Supportive: to provide adequate oxygenation and mechanical ventilation to reverse the hypoxemia and expand the distal gas exchange units so as to prevent further airway and alveolar collapse
2. Therapeutic: to treat the systemic responses caused by the alterations in pulmonary function
3. Curative: to locate and halt the causal insult

Chemotherapeutic

Fluid and electrolyte therapy: Fluids are monitored carefully. Excessive intravascular fluid administration may result in cardiogenic pulmonary edema. Patients with capillary damage from ARDS are especially susceptible to fluid leakage into the alveolar spaces.

Fluid types: There is some controversy regarding the use of colloids and crystalloids. It is most generally believed that colloidal fluids should be used in hypoalbuminemic patients. All other patients should receive crystalloid fluids.[61]

Quantity of fluids: The pulmonary capillary wedge pressure (PCWP) is much more reliable than the central venous pressure (CVP) when trying to determine the quantity of fluids to be administered. In most situations, maintenance of the PCWP at 10 to 15 mm Hg provides adequate, but not excessive, intravascular volumes. Certainly clinical parameters such as pulse, urinary output, and peripheral vasoconstriction should also be considered as assessment variables.

Pharmacologic: There are no specific drugs used to treat the syndrome. Drugs used are primarily supportive to other therapeutic measures such as mechanical ventilation.

Morphine (3 to 5 mg/h IV) may be given as sedation for mechanical ventilator patients who are restless and experiencing tachypnea.

Pavulon (pancuronium bromide) may be used as a neuroblocking agent to completely paralyze the voluntary respirations of the patient. Dosage must be carefully and individually calculated for each patient. The initial intravenous dosage range for an adult is 0.04 to 0.1 mg/kg.

Corticosteroid use is controversial. Evidence remains speculative that they are helpful in reducing pulmonary edema and stabilizing pulmonary membranes.

Heparin has been advocated by some sources as a drug to combat microvascular emboli. Most authorities, however, question the real benefits of heparin and warn that its risks outweigh any potential benefit for these critically ill individuals.

Electromechanical

Oxygenation: Oxygen support via mask may be used in the very early stages of ARDS but will not be sufficient as the syndrome becomes worse. The goal is to provide the lowest O_2 concentration to maintain the mixed venous O_2 at a level above 40 mm Hg (this may be measured by obtaining a blood sample from the distal lumen of the Swan-Ganz catheter). The $P\overline{v}O_2$ and PaO_2 must both be carefully monitored.

If oxygen concentrations of greater than 50% are required to maintain adequate blood gas oxygen levels, intubation and mechanical ventilation are indicated.

Mechanical ventilation: Early endotracheal intubation and mechanical ventilation should be considered as soon as subtle abnormalities in pulmonary function and laboratory and x-ray findings are observed. Unless the patient is to be maintained on the ventilator for longer than several weeks, tracheostomy is not usually required. See pp. 230-230 and 246-249 for discussion of endotracheal tubes and ventilatory maintenance.

The purpose of mechanical ventilation for ARDS is to produce a rapid inspiratory flow rate while also exerting a continuous positive end-expiratory pressure (PEEP). A pressure-cycled ventilator is therefore the ventilator of choice. Most commonly for the acute stages of ARDS a continuous positive pressure ventilator (CPPV) with PEEP is used. PEEP results in decreased shunt and an increase in PaO_2. The effects of PEEP in ARDS are[46]:

1. Pulmonary
   a. Increases mean airway pressure
   b. Increases functional residual capacity
   c. Increases compliance
   d. Decreases shunting
   e. Increases lung volumes
   f. Promotes clearing of lung fields
2. Circulatory
   a. Decreases venous return
   b. Increases pulmonary vascular resistance
3. Complications: may compromise circulation, resulting in:

   a. Peripheral vasoconstriction
   b. Hypotension
   c. Tachycardia
   d. Oliguria
   e. Increased pulmonary capillary wedge pressure (>15 mm Hg)
   f. Possible increased incidence of pneumothorax[2]

Guidelines for use of CPPV with PEEP for ARDS:
1. Tidal volume of 10 to 20 ml/kg body weight should be used. Tidal volumes greater than this used in conjunction with CPPV may cause alveolar hypertension.
2. PEEP should be regulated between 5 and 10 cm H_2O. Although a PEEP greater than 15 cm H_2O is generally contraindicated, many practitioners go much higher. The purpose of PEEP is to decrease the intrapulmonary shunting and to improve pulmonary compliance. Therefore, PEEP should be considered for use when an inspired oxygen concentration of >50% is required to maintain an adequate PaO_2 level.

   Optimal use of PEEP is to add it in small increments in an attempt to decrease the intrapulmonary shunt to the 15% to 20% range.
3. Physiologic respiratory rate should be between 10 and 20 per minute, although rates up to 30 per minute may be used.
4. The goal of mechanical ventilation is to keep the $PaCO_2$ in the range of 35 to 40 mm Hg. Below this will decrease cardiac output, increase airway resistance, and increase oxygen consumption.
5. If the patient fights the ventilator, sedation such as morphine or a neuroblocking agent such as pancuronium (Pavulon) may be necessary (see Chemotherapeutic discussion).
6. CPPV with PEEP should be used very cautiously in patients with low blood pressure. An increase in already high intrathoracic pressure may result. This in turn may compress thoracic vessels, leading to decreased venous return, decreased cardiac output, poor tissue perfusion, and a lactic acid buildup.

Other mechanical ventilation techniques used with ARDS:

Intermittent mandatory ventilation (IMV): This technique permits the patient to breathe spontaneously from a gas reservoir and still receive periodic mechanical hyperinflations. The patient's own spontaneous minute ventilation is thus augmented to a desired level by ventilator delivered breaths.

Continuous positive airway pressure (CPAP): For patients breathing on their own this technique provides a positive end-expiratory pressure to the end of each inhalation. It may be used in the patient who can maintain adequate $PaCO_2$ levels without mechanical ventilation but who cannot maintain adequate arterial oxygen.

Cardiovascular monitoring

Invasive cardiovascular monitoring as with the Swan-Ganz catheter should be used whenever cardiovascular compromise is anticipated. Once the catheter is in place, the pulmonary capillary wedge pressure (PCWP) should be optimized to 13 to 17 mm Hg.

Electrocardiogram: Monitor cardiac response.

Supportive

Tracheobronchial suctioning: To remove mucus secretions and to ensure patent airway.

Monitor ventilatory sufficiency: The patient's vital capacity, minute volume, and intrapulmonary shunting ($\dot{Q}s/\dot{Q}t$) should be monitored.

Monitor blood gases and pressure response: The patient's blood gases, pulmonary-capillary wedge pressure, and alveolar-arterial oxygen gradient ($P[A\text{-}a]O_2$) should be monitored.

Monitor sputum and bronchial secretions: Frequent laboratory analysis of bronchial secretions should be made to watch for signs of pulmonary system infection.

Monitor chest x-ray films: Frequent chest x-ray analysis is useful in monitoring the patient's response to the therapeutic treatment.

ASSESSMENT: AREAS OF CONCERN

One of the most important assessment rules in the care of the patient with ARDS or potential ARDS is to have good baseline data. Should the patient's condition deteriorate, subtle changes can be identified.

Respiratory status

Respiratory distress: nasal flaring, chest wall retractions, tachypnea or bradypnea, decreased chest wall movement, labored breathing

Breath sounds: rales, rhonchi, wheeze, decreased, bilaterally unequal

Breathing pattern: labored, irregular

Increased sputum, persistent cough, wet-sounding breathing

Pulmonary function: decreased vital capacity, minute volume, and functional residual capacity; increased intrapulmonary shunting

Hypercapnia: headache, dizziness, confusion, unconsciousness, twitching, hypertension, sweating, flushed face

Hypoxia: restlessness, confusion, impaired motor function, hypotension, cyanosis, tachycardia

Laboratory values

Blood gases: $PaCO_2$, PaO_2, PvO_2, $PA\text{-}aO_2$, pH, HCO_3^-, lactic acid levels

Cardiovascular status

Decreased cardiac output: restlessness, lethargy, tachycardia, hypotension, decreased urinary output

Pulmonary pressures: increased pulmonary wedge pressure (PWP), pulmonary artery pressure (PAP)

Fluid and electrolytes

Intake and output, cardiovascular response, potassium, and sodium bicarbonate

Bronchopulmonary infection

Temperature, sputum specimens for culture and sensitivity

Chest roentgenograms

Serial chest roentgenograms to monitor the clearing of thickened or blurred margins of the bronchi or vessels

Psychosocial

Fear of suffocation, fear of being out of control if on ventilator, fear of unknown, family understanding, support, ability to communicate

NURSING DIAGNOSES and NURSING INTERVENTIONS

Nursing Diagnosis	Nursing Intervention
Breathing pattern, ineffective	Assess ventilation to include evaluation of breathing rate, rhythm, and depth, chest expansion, presence of respiratory distress such as dyspnea, shortness of breath, nasal flaring, cyanosis, and changes in skin color including nail beds and mucous membranes.
	Assess tidal volume, vital capacity and minute volume, and intrapulmonary shunting.
	Identify contributing factors such as airway clearance or obstruction problem, pain, level of consciousness, or weakness.
	Maintain patient position to facilitate ventilation (that is, head of bed in semi-Fowler's position), cough, and deep breathing.

Nursing Diagnosis	Nursing Intervention
	Assess patient for tiring in relation to attempts to breathe; encourage pursed-lip breathing.
	Initiate techniques of pulmonary toileting to liquefy secretions and minimize pulmonary congestion, which may lead to secondary infections.
	Help to protect patient from known sources of secondary infection.
	In collaboration with physician, prepare for and administer mechanical ventilation when breathing pattern cannot maintain adequate blood gas levels or when patient demonstrates tiring with breathing efforts.
	When patient is receiving mechanical ventilation, provide care and monitoring consistent with the guidelines presented on pp. 246 to 249.
Gas exchange, impaired	Monitor arterial blood gases; report increases or decreases of $Paco_2$ and Pao_2 of more than 10 to 15 mm Hg.
	Assess pulmonary artery pressure and pulmonary capillary wedge pressure (PCWP).
	Monitor alveolar-arterial oxygen gradient.
	Assess patient to identify signs such as restlessness, confusion, and irritability, which may indicate the body's response to altered blood gas states.
	Prevent physiologic factors that promote restlessness or anxiety.
	Monitor for signs of cor pulmonale: pulmonary hypertension, gradually increasing edema of the legs, increasing central venous pressure and pulmonary-capillary wedge pressure, jugular venous distention, blood gas abnormalities, and hepatomegaly.
	Monitor electrocardiogram and cardiac status for arrhythmias secondary to alteration in blood gases.
	Monitor and record kidney functioning and urinary output, which may be affected secondary to chronic tissue hypoxia and alterations in metabolism.
	In collaboration with physician consultation, administer oxygen to maintain Pao_2 of at least 50 to 60 mm Hg; if blood gas levels cannot be maintained or if the concentration of oxygen exceeds 50%, mechanical ventilation must be considered.
	Monitor serum electrolytes, which may change because of alterations in oxygenation and metabolism.
	Carefully monitor body temperature, which may fluctuate because of alterations in metabolism or secondary infections.
	In collaboration with physician administer respiratory related medications and assess and document the patient's response.
Airway clearance, ineffective	Assess patient to identify inability to move secretions; if inability is identified, assist with appropriate measures (coughing, positioning, suctioning, liquefying secretions, etc.) on a regular and scheduled basis every 30 minutes to every 2 hours.
	Assist patient to maintain proper body positioning to ensure patent airway.
	Carefully monitor fluid intake and the corresponding pulmonary-capillary wedge pressure that may indicate fluid overload complicating pulmonary wetness.
Nutrition, alteration in: less than body requirements	Ensure intake of required fluids and nutrients.
	Maintain tube feedings or hyperalimentation in collaboration with physician.
	Monitor for signs and symptoms of malnutrition.
Fluid volume deficit, potential	Monitor for evidence of gastrointestinal bleeding secondary to physiologic stress; monitor serial hemoglobin and hematocrit; check all stools, emesis, and nasogastric aspirate for presence of blood; observe changes in vital signs or abdominal girth.
	Initiate prevention measures: for example, minimize activities for uninterrupted periods of time, maintain calm and restful environment, encourage patient to participate in care as tolerated, explain all therapy before administering.
Mobility, impaired physical	See p. 2106 of text for associated care.
Skin integrity, impairment of: potential	See p. 2020 of text for associated care.
Communication impaired: verbal (if patient is intubated or demonstrates significant dyspnea)	Provide alternative method of communication appropriate to the patient's comprehension ability.
	If patient is intubated, assure patient that speech will return as soon as endotracheal tube is removed.

Nursing Diagnosis	Nursing Intervention
	Observe for signs of frustration or patient withdrawal secondary to the inability to speak.
	Teach family members appropriate methods to communicate with patient.
Self-care deficit	See p. 2088 of text for associated care.
Coping, ineffective individual	See p. 1897 of text for associated care.
Coping, family: potential for growth	See p. 1899 for associated care.

Patient Education

1. Teach patient adaptive breathing techniques. Emphasize importance of periodic turning, coughing, and deep breathing.
2. Teach importance of not fighting the ventilator and relaxing instead to permit maximum ventilation. Assure patient that oxygen is being supplied.
3. Teach adaptive exercise and rest techniques.
4. Teach eating and food choice modifications.
5. Provide patient and family with information regarding all medications the patient is taking.

EVALUATION

Patient Outcome	Data Indicating That Outcome is Reached
Movement of air in and out of lungs is optimal. Airway is patent. Both lungs are fully aerated as visualized on chest x-ray films.	Vital capacity measurements including tidal and minute volumes are optimal for patient's status. Pulmonary capillary wedge pressure is within normal limits. Blood gas values are within normal limits. Airways are clear and breathing occurs without obstruction.
Breathing pattern occurs without tiring patient. Breath sounds are clear in all areas.	Patient demonstrates modified breathing techniques that facilitate ventilatory capacity. Behavior modified to conserve energy expenditure.
Physiologic function is stable.	Nutrition level is maintained. Kidney and bladder functioning is within normal limits. Gastrointestinal system is functioning adequately. Skin integrity is maintained. There are no secondary infections. Serum electrolytes are within normal limits.
Patient preserves pulmonary functioning by maintaining optimal activity level, preventing infection, and following prescribed treatments.	Patient demonstrates a variety of methods indicating ability to preserve and facilitate optimal respiratory functioning (e.g., breathing exercises, modified activities or exercise, taking medications as prescribed).
Patient and family have sufficient information to comply with discharge regimen.	Patient and family are able at time of discharge to discuss medications—purpose, side effects, route, and schedule—dietary therapy regimen, activity progression regimen, signs of infection or respiratory deterioration, and plan for follow-up visits.

CHRONIC OBSTRUCTIVE PULMONARY DISEASES

Chronic obstructive pulmonary disease (COPD) is a group of diseases that includes asthma, bronchitis, emphysema, and bronchiectasis.[26] Obstruction of airflow of a chronic irreversible or reversible recurrent nature is common to each of these diseases. At one end of the spectrum is periodic asthmatic attacks, and at the other end is pure emphysema.

COPD is a major cause of death and disability in the United States. It is estimated that up to 15% of the older population have some degree of COPD. The estimated economic costs for treatment are greater than $1 billion per year.[31] The actual incidence of COPD is difficult to determine because of the lack of agreement regarding diagnosis and because of the frequent coexistence of two or more obstructive diseases. In most patients with COPD two or more histopathologic elements aggravate the breathing process.[9]

Fig. 2-28 illustrates the interrelatedness of these obstructive diseases and the variety of host and environmental factors that tend to affect them. The degree of involvement and the physiologic response to therapy are individual.

The most important task for the health professional is to determine and maintain maximum ventilation and respiration for each patient. This means that the professional must be able to separate the reversible components of COPD from the irreversible components and to maximize each individual's potential.

Chronic Bronchitis and Emphysema

Obstructive airway disease refers to a continuum of pulmonary responses to various noxious stimuli. At one end of the spectrum is pure chronic bronchitis (e.g., congenital immune system dysfunction), and at the other end is pure emphysema (e.g., alpha-1-antitrypsin deficiency). It is because of this complexity that these two pure disease states are discussed in combination. Where possible, their differences are pointed out.

Chronic bronchitis refers to excessive mucus secretion in the bronchial tree. This mucus causes chronic and recurrent productive coughing.

Emphysema refers to anatomic alterations of the air spaces distal to the conducting airways. There is an abnormal enlargement of the air spaces. This causes physiologic destruction of the alveolar walls, which in turn causes increased lung compliance, decreased diffusing capacity, and increased airway resistance.

In present terminology, chronic bronchitis and emphysema represent a variety of respiratory disorders that all lead to a slowly progressive airway-obstructive disease. The airway obstruction is persistent and nonreversible.

The development of chronic bronchitis or emphysema is determined by evaluating the interrelatedness of the individual's susceptibility and genetic makeup with the structural and immunologic response to recurrent bronchial infections, environmental pollution, and chronic exposure to high concentrations of smoke, dust, or irritant gases.[26] The incidence of the diseases has increased dramatically in recent years. The American Lung Association attributes this increase to greater exposure to smoking and airborne irritants as well as to a better clinical understanding of the physiologic processes and diagnostic criteria.[2] Although changing in proportional relationships, the incidence of chronic bronchitis and emphysema remains greater in males than in females. This has most generally been thought to be due to smoking history and choice of occupation.

The course of the diseases prior to the development of symptoms is unclear. There is most likely a decrease in the FEV_1 before the signs of clinical illness appear. Once signs are evident, the FEV_1 (after bronchodilator administration) measurement may be the best indicator of prognosis and morbidity. Fig. 2-29 shows the survival curve of 200 patients after controlling for age.

In addition to predicting mortality, the FEV_1 may be a useful guide for evaluating morbidity. Table 2-7 summarizes the relationship between FEV_1 and activities of daily living.

Table 2-7
Relationship Between FEV_1 and the Activities of Daily Living

FEV_1 (L)	Activity Response
3.7-4	Normal value for the adult
2-1.5	Complaints of dyspnea on exertion such as carrying packages or climbing stairs
about 1	Breathlessness when trying to perform activities of daily living such as cooking, cleaning, bathing, dressing, walking
	Subject to complications of carbon dioxide retention and cor pulmonale
<0.75	Individual unable to work, usually housebound

Data from Dodge, R., and Burrows, B.: Chronic bronchitis and emphysema. In Fries, J., and Ehrlich, G.: Prognosis: contemporary outcomes of disease, Bowie, Md., 1981, The Charles Press Publishers, p. 230.

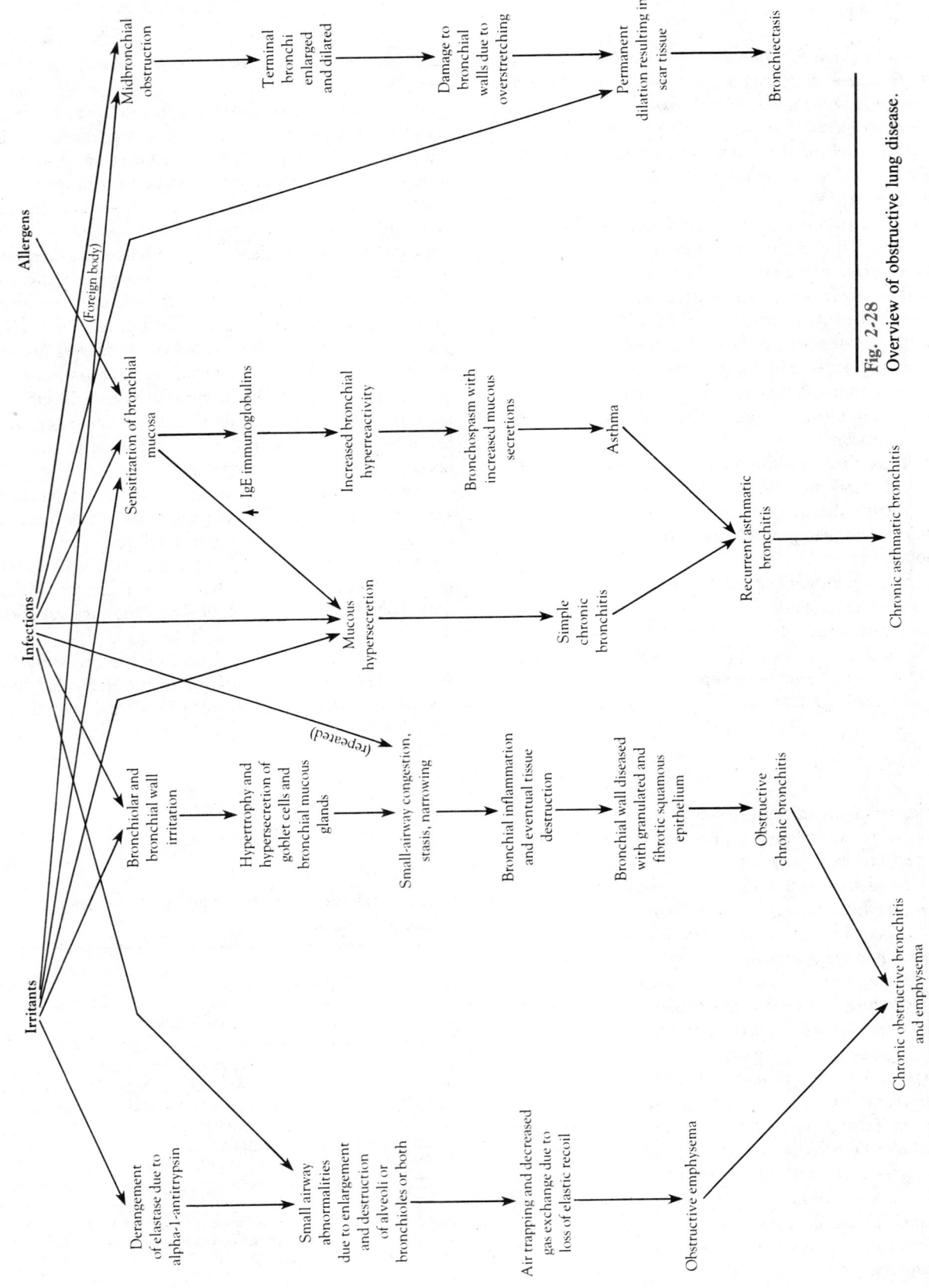

Fig. 2-28
Overview of obstructive lung disease.

Fig. 2-29
Cumulative survival rate for patients with chronic bronchitis and emphysema according to age and pulmonary function.

From Russell, D., and Burrows, B.: Chronic bronchitis and emphysema. In Fries, J.F., and Ehrlich, G.E.: Prognosis: contemporary outcomes of disease, Bowie, Md., 1981, The Charles Press Publishers.

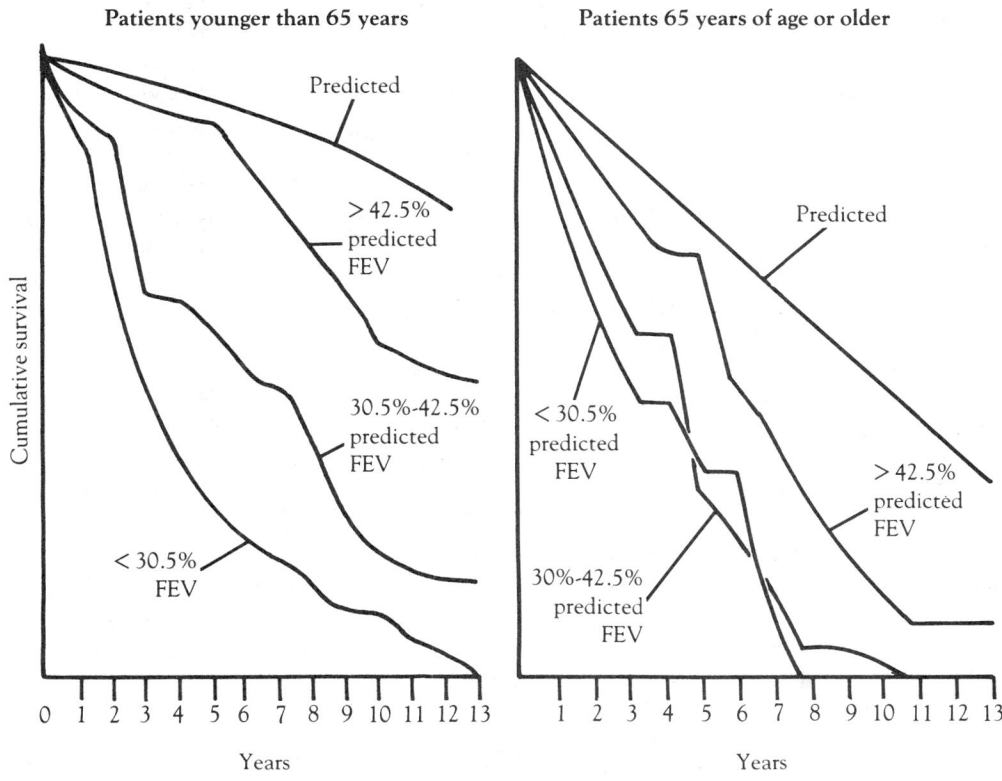

PATHOPHYSIOLOGY

Chronic Bronchitis

One of the earliest changes in chronic bronchitis appears in the secretory glands. There is hypertrophy and hypersecretion of the goblet cells and bronchial mucous glands. Both the goblet cells and the cells in the mucous glands increase in size and then in number. The goblet cells extend distally into the terminal bronchioles, where they are not normally found. The net result is increased quantities of sputum, bronchial congestion, and narrowing of bronchioles and small bronchi. With time the normally sterile lower respiratory tract becomes colonized by bacteria, and an increased number of polymorphonuclear neutrophil (PMN) leukocytes are found in the secretions.[26] It is felt that these leukocytes play a role in stimulating further bronchial inflammation and eventual tissue destruction.[60] As the bronchial wall becomes diseased, granulated and fibrotic squamous epithelium re-

places the normal ciliated epithelium. This scarring leads to stenosis and airway obstruction.

Emphysema

The primary defect underlying emphysema is the derangement of lung elastin by the neutral proteases, the most important of which is elastase. Elastase is produced and released by PMN leukocytes and alveolar macrophages. Under normal conditions, proteases become fused with bacteria that find their way to the alveolar level. A fraction of the total protease produced is liberated in the lung in response to particulate inhalation and following cell death; normally there is a counterbalancing supply of the protease inhibitor alpha-1-antitrypsin. It is thought that recurrent infections, environmental irritants, and cigarette smoking, along with an alpha-1-antitrypsin deficiency, yield a situation in which elastin in the distal airways and alveoli is degraded.[26] In addition, there is evidence that cigarette smoking alone depresses the activity of alpha-1-antitrypsin.[51] The resultant imbalance in this elastase-antielastase system allows for the destruction of the basic elastin structure of the distal airways and alveoli. As septal walls are lost, blood vessel density is also reduced, and emphysema results.[26]

NOTE: alpha-1-antitrypsin deficiency is estimated to be present in only 0.06% of the population[18] and is probably responsible for less than 10% of the clinically identified cases of emphysema.[26]

The lungs of an emphysematous patient appear large, overinflated, and pale. The walls of the bronchioles undergo destructive changes, and large bullae tend to form. If changes occur diffusely throughout the lobule and pulmonary acinus, the disease is referred to as panlobular emphysema (PLE). PLE, which is frequently found in elderly persons with no evidence of chronic bronchitis, shows a uniform enlargement and destruction of the alveoli throughout the acinus. Individuals with true alpha-1-antitrypsin deficiency are most likely to have PLE. In emphysema the normal architecture of the lung is destroyed. Lobule septal damage produces air sacs of various sizes, which leads to ventilation and perfusion abnormalities.

Two important consequences of emphysema are air trapping and decreased gas exchange. The air trapping is caused by a loss of elastic recoil. Ventilation is regionally decreased not only because of the elastic recoil problems but also because of poor support of terminal airways, which increases collapsibility of the noncartilaginous peripheral bronchioles. The decreased gas exchange causes both pulmonary diffusion and perfusion abnormalities. Pulmonary diffusion is reduced because of a loss of alveolar surface area and pulmonary vasoconstriction. The resulting hypoxemia causes a more generalized pulmonary artery constriction, shunting blood away from even the normal areas of the lung.[27] The clinically measurable result of these two processes is an increase in the functional residual capacity (FRC), increased compliance, and hypoxia.

DIAGNOSTIC STUDIES

Chronic bronchitis and emphysema are typically "silent" for years before the patient is even minimally symptomatic. It is at the time of symptoms that diagnostic studies evaluating the shortness of breath and cough are generally done.

Pulmonary function

FEV_1 (forced expiratory volume in 1 second): decreased, may fall as much as 50 to 75 ml per year

FVC (forced vital capacity): decreased

FEV_1/FVC ratio: decreased

TLC (total lung capacity): increased in emphysema because of decreased elastic recoil

RV (residual volume): increased
  In emphysema because of decreased elastic recoil
  In chronic bronchitis because of air trapping

FRC (functional residual capacity): increased
  In emphysema because of decreased elastic recoil
  In pure chronic bronchitis may be normal

C (compliance): increased in emphysema

R_{aw} (airway resistance): increased in both chronic bronchitis and emphysema

Ventilatory response: decreased with hypoxia and hypercapnia

Arterial blood gases

Alveolar-arterial (A-a) oxygen gradient: widened

PaO_2: decreased

$PaCO_2$: increased; patients with pure chronic bronchitis are more prone to CO_2 retention than are those patients with emphysema of comparable severity

Chest roentgenogram

May have flattened diaphragm and increased anterior-posterior (A-P) diameter

In emphysema, vascular markings may be decreased and intercostal spaces widened, and bullae may be present

TREATMENT PLAN

The medical plan for both of these diseases is to stop the progress of the disease and to maximize breathing by reducing airway secretions and inflammation and halting bronchospasms.

Chemotherapeutic

Acute exacerbation management

Bronchodilators (adrenergic and xanthine derivatives)
  The drugs used and dosages vary based upon patient response.
    Theophylline (Aerolate, Theo-Dur, Theolair), po 16 mg/kg in single or divided doses, or rectally 250-500 mg q8-12h
    Aminophylline (Aminophyl), IV loading dose 5.6-6 mg/kg in 100 ml normal saline; IV maintenance 0.2-1 mg/kg/hr; po 3.5 mg/kg q6h; rectally 300 mg tid
    Methylprednisolone (Solu-Medrol), 8.5 mg/kg IV q6h for 2-3 d

Anti-infective agents (for secondary infection)
  When the sputum is purulent and evidence of pneumonia is absent, the following antibiotics may be given:

Ampicillin (Amcill, Omnipen, others) 250-500 mg PO q6h for 10 d

Tetracycline (Achromycin, others) 250-500 mg PO q6h for 10 d

Long-term management

Bronchodilators:

Therapeutic theophylline levels should be maintained between 10 and 20 mEq/ml.

Corticosteroids:

If pulmonary function tests are improved after 3 to 4 weeks by corticosteroids, they may be continued at low doses. The goal is complete removal of the medication.

Influenza and pneumococcal vaccines:

These vaccines are recommended for patients with chronic bronchitis and emphysema.

Electromechanical

Acute exacerbations

Oxygenation: Administered at rates sufficient to maintain a PaO_2 between 50 and 60 mm Hg, usually by nasal cannula at a flow rate of 1 to 3 L per minute. Because patients with chronic bronchitis and emphysema may have chronic hypercapnia, they are considered to be sensitive to increased alveolar oxygen. This means that their borderline or diminished ventilatory drive may be further suppressed by increasing the PaO_2. Care must be taken to closely monitor oxygen administration and to increase the flow very slowly and carefully. Use of the Venturi mask allows more precise oxygen administration.

Mechanical ventilation: Intubation and mechanical ventilation may be necessary if supplemental oxygen cannot maintain the PaO_2 above 40 mm Hg with a pH greater than 7.25. If mechanical ventilation becomes necessary, the intermittent mandatory ventilation (IMV) technique becomes useful. The IMV allows the patient to breathe spontaneously with the exact amount of additional minute ventilation required to be delivered by the machine.

Long-term management

Oxygenation: Intermittent (at least 18 hours per day) oxygen therapy via nasal prongs may be indicated for patients who are unable to maintain a PaO_2 of at least 50 to 55 mm Hg while at rest and breathing room air. The flow rate should be adjusted to maintain a resting PaO_2 close to 60 mm Hg.

Supportive

Chest physiotherapy: Percussion and postural drainage may be administered at regular intervals for patients with large amounts of sputum production. See pp. 239 to 242 for techniques.

Physical training program: Physical training programs are based on the premise that improved ventilatory and cardiac muscle function might compensate for nonreversible lung disease. Bicycle and treadmill training appear to lead to decreased oxygen consumption with exercise and increased work capacity. These physical training techniques are currently used as methods of rehabilitation.[46]

ASSESSMENT: AREAS OF CONCERN

History

Smoking history and history of known respiratory irritants including duration of exposure of each; history of previous respiratory diseases, infections, allergies, etc.; history of chronic cough and characteristics; family history of respiratory diseases; description of activity tolerance including fatigue and dyspnea precipitation

Current medications

Careful and complete history of current respiratory-related medications as well as use of over-the-counter medications

Use of oxygen

History of use of oxygen, IPPB, or other related respiratory assistive devices; history to include amount, frequency, duration, and therapeutic response

Respiratory status

Respiratory distress as evidenced by dyspnea, cough, prolonged expiration; audible expiratory wheeze; diminished breath sounds over the diseased area; anxiety, bronchospasm; sputum-producing cough; hyperresonance due to overinflation of lungs; barrel chest; cyanosis of finger beds and mucous membranes; posturing and use of accessory muscles during breathing; respiratory failure signs (see discussion of respiratory failure at beginning of this chapter)

Hypoxia

Restlessness; tachycardia; confusion; hypotension; cyanosis; premature ventricular contractions and right bundle branch block if hypoxia becomes severe; somnolence; loss of memory; pulsus paradoxus

Laboratory values

Decreased chloride (from salt restriction and diuretics); decreased potassium (from diuretics)

ECG

May show atrial arrhythmias; tall, symmetric P waves in leads II, III, and aV_F; vertical QRS axis; and signs of right ventricular hypertrophy late in the disease

Pulmonary function

FEV_1; residual volume; forced vital capacity; total lung capacity; functional residual capacity; compliance; R_{aw}

Infection signs

Elevated temperature; purulent sputum; foul mouth odor or taste

GI response

Malaise and anorexia due to chronic hypoxic state; weight loss; constipation

Major complications

Cor pulmonale and pneumothorax

NURSING DIAGNOSES and NURSING INTERVENTIONS

Nursing Diagnosis	Nursing Intervention
Airway clearance, ineffective	Assess patient to identify inability to move secretions; if inability is identified, assist with appropriate measures (coughing, positioning, suctioning, liquefying secretions, etc.). Administer bronchodilators, mucolytics, and expectorants as ordered; observe for therapeutic response; monitor theophylline level if appropriate. Assist patient to maintain proper body positioning to assure maximal airway availability (e.g., semi-Fowler's position or sitting upright and leaning on overbed table). Provide hydration to liquefy secretions and replace fluids. Administer vaporization therapy and perform postural drainage with percussion as ordered; at least 1 hour prior to meals; provide oral hygiene after treatment. Carefully and frequently auscultate chest for quality of breath sounds and adventitious sounds; note cough and sputum characteristics.
Breathing pattern, ineffective	Assess ventilation to include evaluation of breathing rate, rhythm, and depth, chest expansion, presence of respiratory distress such as dyspnea, shortness of breath, nasal flaring, pursed-lip breathing or prolonged expiratory phase, use of accessory muscles. Assist to assess total lung capacity (TLC), residual volume (RV), functional residual capacity (FRC), forced expiratory volumes (FEV), and forced vital capacity (FVC) as ordered. Identify contributing factors such as airway clearance or obstruction problem, or weakness. Instruct patient in proper pulmonary routines, such as coughing, deep breathing, pursed-lip breathing, and diaphragmatic breathing. Suction as necessary to remove secretions. Assess patient for tiring in relation to attempts to breathe. Assist to protect patient from known sources of secondary infection or breathing irritation such as smoking. Should mechanical ventilation become necessary, provide care and monitoring consistent with the guidelines given in medical intervention section of this chapter (pp. 246 to 249).
Gas exchange, impaired	In collaboration with physician order, monitor arterial blood gases; report increases or decreases of Pa_{CO_2} and Pa_{O_2} of more than 10 to 15 mm Hg. Administer oxygen as ordered to maintain Pa_{O_2} of no less than 55 mm Hg; this usually may be maintained by administration of oxygen by nasal cannula at a flow rate of 1 to 3 L/min; if needed, a Venturi tube may be used; if blood gas levels cannot be maintained, mechanical ventilation must be considered. *Extreme caution must be exercised to maintain a low oxygen flow not to exceed 3 L/min.* Assess patient to identify signs such as restlessness, confusion, and irritability, which may indicate the body's response to altered blood gas states. Monitor electrocardiogram and cardiac status for arrhythmias secondary to alterations in blood gases. If patient is seriously ill, monitor for signs of cor pulmonale such as pulmonary hypertension, gradually increasing edema of the legs, increasing central venous pressure, jugular venous distention, blood gas abnormalities, and hepatomegaly.

Nursing Diagnosis	**Nursing Intervention**
	Monitor and record kidney function and urinary output, which may be affected secondary to chronic tissue hypoxia and alterations in metabolism.
	Monitor serum electrolytes, which may change because of alterations in oxygenation and metabolism.
	Carefully monitor body temperature, which may fluctuate because of alterations in metabolism or secondary infections.
Oral mucous membrane, alteration in	Instruct patients using aerosolized corticosteroids to perform thorough mouth washing after each use to prevent secondary infections of oral candidiasis.
	Observe oral mucosa for presence of mouth irritation; consult physician if noted.
Nutrition alteration in: less than body requirement	Assist patient to choose foods that are easy to chew and swallow; assist by cutting and feeding if patient tires easily.
	Diet should consist of high-protein and high-carbohydrate foods and fluids.
	Avoid gas-producing foods.
	Encourage smaller, more frequent meals.
	Encourage fluid intake of at least 2 L per day to facilitate liquefying secretions and promoting urinary output. (If patient has compromised cardiac or renal condition, fluid intake must be determined in collaboration with physician.)
	If indicated and in consultation with physician, administer stool softeners to relieve constipation.
	Monitor for signs and symptoms of malnutrition.
Fluid volume deficit, potential	In the seriously ill patient, monitor for evidence of gastrointestinal bleeding secondary to physiologic stress; monitor serial hemoglobin and hematocrit; check all stools, emesis, and nasogastric aspirate for presence of blood; observe changes in vital signs or abdominal girth.
Mobility, impaired physical	Encourage patient to use adaptive breathing techniques to decrease the work of breathing.
	Assist patient to space activities to provide periods of rest in between.
	Encourage gradual increase of activities as tolerated to prevent "pulmonary crippling."
	Problem solve with patient to determine methods of conserving energy while still performing activities of daily living (e.g., using stool to sit while in the bathroom shaving).
	Assess and document those activities that cause patient to tire easily and become short of breath.
	If patient is seriously ill and maintained on bed rest, encourage or provide active or passive range of motion exercises to maintain adequate muscle tone.
Fear	Observe for signs of frustration or fear secondary to hypoxia.
Self-care deficit	See p. 2088 for nursing care.
Health maintenance, alteration in	Assess with patient and family home and personally used irritants (smoking, fumes, vapors) that may exacerbate the chronic respiratory condition.
	Provide education regarding need to avoid irritants in home, work, and community environments.
	Provide education regarding need to identify early signs of complications and need for medical consultation.
Coping, ineffective individual	Determine patient's ability to cooperate with health care providers regarding intervention strategies such as breathing techniques, exercise progression, and alterations in the activities of daily living.
	Listen carefully to collect information significant to the current health care problem and the patient's perception of his ability to deal with alterations it is causing.
	Assist patient to develop appropriate coping strategies based upon his personal strengths and past experience.
Coping, family	See p. 1899 for associated nursing care.

Patient Education

1. Teach patient adaptive breathing techniques, and work with family to teach postural drainage techniques.
2. Teach importance of avoiding contact with persons with upper respiratory infections and influenza and pneumococcal vaccines.
3. Teach facts about and importance of prescribed medications such as bronchodilators and corticosteroids.
4. Provide patient and family with information regarding chronic lung diseases, how to assess individual capabilities and responses, and what to do during an acute episode of difficult breathing.
5. Teach change in health status that must be reported to the patient's health care providers; indicators of change may include change in sputum characteristics or color, decreased activity tolerance, increased use of IPPB or oxygen, decreased appetite, and fever.
6. Teach importance of consuming large quantities of fluid.
7. Teach importance of not smoking and of avoiding dust-producing articles (feathers, animal dander, cleaning equipment) and strong cooking odors, which may irritate the respiratory tract.
8. Teach eating and food choice modifications.
9. Provide patient and family with information regarding the care, cleaning, and maintenance of inhalation or oxygen equipment being used in the hospital or to be used at home, as signs of oxygen toxicity.
10. Provide patient and family with respiratory-related health information such as pollution indexes, secondary infection exposure, and community support groups.
11. Advise patient to avoid using powders and aerosol products, which may cause bronchospasm.

EVALUATION

Patient Outcome	Data Indicating That Outcome is Reached
Air moves optimally in and out of lungs	Vital capacity measurements including FEV_1, FVC, TLC, RV, and FRC are optimal for patient's status. Blood gas values are within acceptable limits for patient.
Airway is patent.	Airway clearance and breathing occur without obstruction and are optimal for patient.
Breathing pattern occurs without tiring patient.	Patient demonstrates modified breathing techniques that facilitate ventilatory capacity. Behavior is modified to conserve energy expenditure.
Physiologic function is stable.	Nutrition level is maintained. Kidney and bladder are functioning adequately. There are no secondary infections. Serum electrolytes are within normal limits.
Patient understands importance of daily pulmonary exercises.	Patient demonstrates pulmonary exercises and states rationale and importance of maintaining daily exercise routine.
Patient preserves pulmonary functioning by maintaining optimal activity level, preventing infection, and following prescribed treatments.	Patient demonstrates a variety of methods indicating ability to preserve and facilitate optimal respiratory functioning (e.g., breathing exercises, modified exercises, modified activities or exercise, taking medications as prescribed).
Patient and family have sufficient information to comply with discharge regimen.	Patient and family are able at time of discharge to discuss medications—purpose, side effects, route, and schedule; dietary therapy regimen; activity progression regimen; signs of infection or respiratory deterioration; and plan for follow-up visits.

Bronchial Asthma

Asthma, a disease characterized by increased responsiveness of the trachea and bronchi to various stimuli, is manifested by widespread narrowing of the airways that improves either spontaneously or as a result of therapy.[4]

Status asthmaticus is an intense, unrelenting attack that does not respond to the usual modes of therapy.

Bronchial asthma is actually a broad clinical syndrome rather than a specific disease. There is bronchial hypersensitivity characterized by a reversible airway bronchospasm. The bronchospasm causes increased mucosal edema, constriction of the bronchial muscles, production of viscous mucus, which eventually leads to increased mucus plugs, bronchial airway obstruction, and overdistention of the lungs.

Asthma affects approximately 2% to 3% of the U.S. population and has a mortality rate of 1 per 100,000 persons.[45] Approximately 50% of the cases begin prior to age 10 years, and another 30% occur prior to age 40. During childhood there is a 2:1 male to female ratio of prevalence. This ratio equalizes during adolescence and thereafter.[16]

Asthma is considered the most common chronic disease for children and adults. It is responsible for approximately 150,000 hospital admissions and 1,275,000 hospital days a year. Asthma accounts for at least 85 million days of restricted work and 5 million days of work lost each year.[21]

Asthma may be divided into two types: (1) extrinsic or atopic asthma and (2) intrinsic or nonatopic asthma.

Extrinsic or atopic asthma is caused by external agents such as dust, lint, insecticides, mold spores, or foods. This type is best understood as a reaction to specific allergens. It results from sensitization of an atopic person to specific allergens, so that exposure can precipitate an attack.

Intrinsic or nonatopic asthma indicates that the specific causes cannot be identified. It may be precipitated by a variety of situations such as a common cold, upper respiratory infection, or even exercise. This type usually begins in persons over 35 years of age and develops into a life-long condition, with episodes of increasing frequency and severity.

Table 2-8 differentiates characteristics of intrinsic and extrinsic asthma.

PATHOPHYSIOLOGY

While the trigger mechanism and physiologic response for intrinsic and extrinsic asthma are different, the clinical response appears the same. Fig. 2-30 provides a summary of the proposed pathogenesis for the two causes of an asthmatic response.

DIAGNOSTIC STUDIES

Arterial blood gases
  PaO_2: normal or slightly decreased secondary to decreased $\dot{V}/\dot{Q}$; has direct linear relationship with FEV_1 (as FEV_1 decreases, so does PaO_2)
  $PaCO_2$: will increase only when FEV_1 is decreased by at least 20%
  pH: normal or decreased
  HCO_3^-: normal or decreased

Pulmonary function
  FEV_1 (young healthy adult individual):
    Asthma before treatment: abnormally low
    After treatment: at least 2 L
  PEFR (young healthy adult individual):
    Asthma before treatment: as low as 100 L/min
    After treatment: at least 300 L/min
  TLC: increases during acute episode because of air trapping
  RV: increases during acute episode
  VC: abnormally low

Sputum examination
  Gross examination of sputum indicates sputum with increased viscosity and plugs

Table 2-8
Intrinsic Versus Extrinsic Asthma

Characteristic	Extrinsic	Intrinsic
Allergens as precipitants	Yes	No
Immediate skin test	Positive	Negative
Elevated IgE	Common	Uncommon
Eosinophilia	Yes	Yes
Childhood onset	Common	Uncommon
Other allergies	Common	Uncommon
Family history of multiple allergies	Common	Uncommon
Hyposensitization therapy	Helpful	Equivocal
Typical attack	Acute and self-limiting	Often fulminant and severe
Relationship of attack to infection	May be present	Common
Aspirin sensitivity	Uncommon	Uncommon

Data from Miller L.G., and Kazemi, H.: Manual of clinical pulmonary medicine, New York, 1983, McGraw-Hill Book Co., p. 45, and Weiss, E.B.: Bronchial asthma, Clin. Symp. **27:**39, 1975.

Fig. 2-30
Proposed pathogenesis of bronchial asthma.

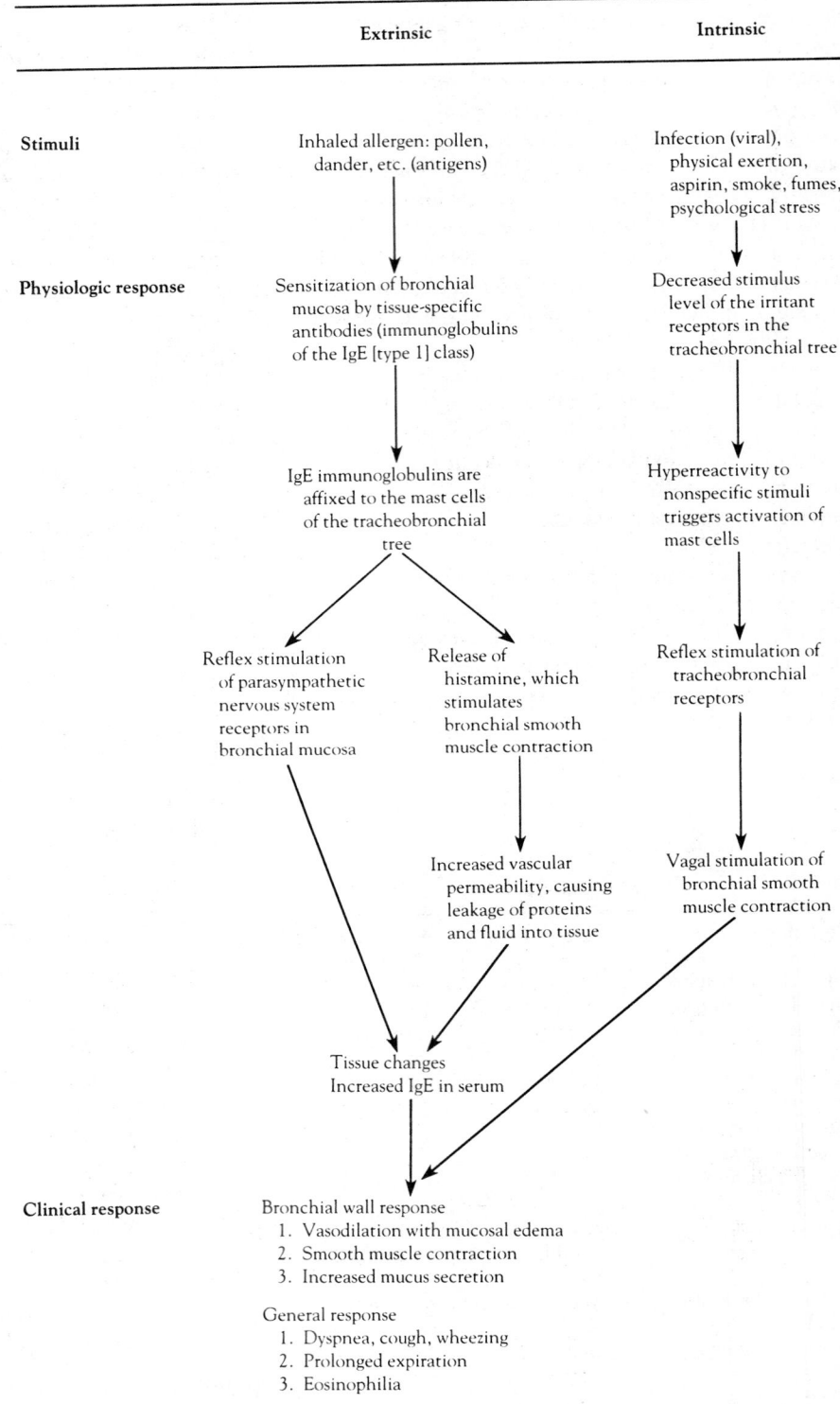

	Extrinsic	Intrinsic
Stimuli	Inhaled allergen: pollen, dander, etc. (antigens)	Infection (viral), physical exertion, aspirin, smoke, fumes, psychological stress
Physiologic response	Sensitization of bronchial mucosa by tissue-specific antibodies (immunoglobulins of the IgE [type 1] class)	Decreased stimulus level of the irritant receptors in the tracheobronchial tree
	IgE immunoglobulins are affixed to the mast cells of the tracheobronchial tree	Hyperreactivity to nonspecific stimuli triggers activation of mast cells
	Reflex stimulation of parasympathetic nervous system receptors in bronchial mucosa / Release of histamine, which stimulates bronchial smooth muscle contraction	Reflex stimulation of tracheobronchial receptors
	Increased vascular permeability, causing leakage of proteins and fluid into tissue	Vagal stimulation of bronchial smooth muscle contraction
	Tissue changes Increased IgE in serum	

Clinical response

Bronchial wall response
1. Vasodilation with mucosal edema
2. Smooth muscle contraction
3. Increased mucus secretion

General response
1. Dyspnea, cough, wheezing
2. Prolonged expiration
3. Eosinophilia

CBC
Eosinophilia usually seen, which is indicative of an allergic response

Chest roentgenogram
Roentgenogram usually clear; hyperinflation secondary to air trapping may be seen in persistent and long standing cases; transient migratory pulmonary infiltrations may also be seen

Electrocardiogram
Sinus tachycardia may be seen in acute episodes; prominent P waves occur in chronic asthma

Theophylline level
Any asthmatic patient taking theophylline should have baseline monitoring of theophylline levels; therapeutic level of theophylline in the blood is 10 to 20 μg/ml

TREATMENT PLAN

The intent of the immediate medical plan is to decrease the amount of bronchospasm and to increase pulmonary ventilation.

After the acute event is passed, the medical plan is to identify precipitating stimuli and to promote maximum health with this potentially degenerative chronic disease.

Surgical
Bronchoscopy: On the rare occasions when conventional therapy fails to obtain an improvement, a bronchoscopy for aspiration and saline lavage of secretions may be done.

Chemotherapeutic
Drug therapy for asthma can be divided into three categories: category I, acute phase therapy; category II, status asthmaticus therapy; and category III, interim therapy. For each of these treatment categories there are two types of pharmacologic agents used. Bronchodilators are used to increase the airway diameter, and corticosteroids are used to reduce the inflammatory response.

Category I: acute phase
Bronchodilators
  Parenteral
    Epinephrine 1:1000, 0.2 to 0.5 ml subcutaneously q15-30 min
    Terbutaline (Brethine, Bricanyl) 0.2 to 0.3 ml subcutaneously q30 min for 3 doses
    Aminophylline 250 mg in 20-30 ml normal saline IV (or 5.6-6 mg/kg in 100 ml normal saline) maximum rate = 25 mg/min
    Aerosols: 1 or 2 inhalations from hand nebulizer q3-4h or 0.5 ml in 2.5 or 3 ml normal saline by nebulization
      Isoproterenol (Isuprel) 1:200
      Isoetharine (Bronkosol) 1:200
Corticosteroids
  Parenteral
    Hydrocortisone sodium succinate (Solu-Cortef) 100-250 mg may be given with the first oral dose
  Oral
    Prednisone (Deltasone, others) 40-60 mg/d in divided doses; tapered rapidly over 3 wk period if possible

Category II: status asthmaticus
Bronchodilators
  Epinephrine: same as for category I
  Aminophylline (loading dose): 5.6-6 mg/kg in 100 ml normal saline for 20-30 min; maximum rate = 25 mg/min
  Continued therapy dose
    Children and young adult smokers: 1 mg/kg/h for 12h, then reduce to 0.8 mg/kg/h
    Healthy, nonsmoking adults: 0.7-0.9 mg/kg/h for 12h; then reduce to 0.5 mg/kg/h
    Older adults with cor pulmonale: 0.6 mg/kg/h for 12h; then reduce to 0.3 mg/kg/h
    Adults with congestive heart failure and liver failure: 0.5 mg/kg/h for 12h; then reduce to 0.1-0.2 mg/kg/h
  Subsequent doses should be determined by therapeutic serum level of aminophylline of 10-20 μg/ml
Corticosteroids
  Parenteral
    Hydrocortisone sodium succinate (Solu-Cortef) 4 mg/kg IV q4h
    Methylprednisolone sodium succinate (Solu-Medrol) 2 mg/kg IV q4h
  Oral: may also start on oral medications then reduce IV medications
    Hydrocortisone sodium succinate (Solu-Cortef) 300 mg/d divided into four doses
    Prednisone (Deltasone, others) 20 mg/d divided into four doses
    Methylprednisolone (Medrol) 16 mg/d divided into four doses

Category III: interim phase
Bronchodilator: Maintenance doses to keep serum level at 10-20 μg/ml
  Oral
    Theophylline (Aerolate, Elixophyllin, Quibron, Tedral, Theo-Dur, Theolair) 16 mg/kg/d in single dose or divided doses
    Aminophylline (Aminodur, Aminophyl, Somophyllin) 3.5-5 mg/kg q6h

Aerosol

    Albuterol (Proventil Inhaler, Ventolin Inhaler) 1-2 inhalations q4-6h

Corticosteroids

Aerosol

    Beclomethasone dipropionate (Vanceril Inhaler, others) 2 inhalations qid; long acting and not systematically absorbed

Fluid and electrolyte therapy: The purpose of fluid therapy is to liquefy secretions and to have a method by which to administer intravenous drugs. Providing that the patient has no cardiovascular dysfunction, fluid therapy should be aggressive. Dextrose 5% in water or 5% dextrose in 0.02 normal saline are adequate intravenous solutions. Electrolytes must be monitored frequently and replaced as indicated.

Electromechanical

Oxygenation: Humidified oxygen should be administered by nasal cannula or mask to counteract clinical and laboratory signs of hypoxemia.

Volume-cycled ventilator: Should the patient's condition continue to deteriorate despite aggressive therapy (1% to 3% of hospitalized asthmatics), endotracheal intubation and mechanical ventilation may become necessary.

The goal of ventilation by this method is to ensure adequate alveolar ventilation without hypercapnia or hypocapnia. To do this the practitioner should

1. Decrease tidal volume as tolerated to allow lower cycling pressures
2. Decrease respiratory rate as tolerated to allow adequate duration of expiration
3. Supply heated, humidified oxygen to maintain PaO_2
4. Sedate patient as required and ordered
5. Continue to administer medications as listed under the chemotherapeutic section
6. Administer chest physiotherapy and continue to encourage coughing[46]

Supportive

Chest physiotherapy: Postural drainage with chest percussion should be administered at least every 2 to 4 hours as long as the patient has congestion. See pp. 239 to 246 for techniques.

Environment: Provide an atmosphere void of known allergens.

Table 2-9
Assessment of Severity of Asthma

	Mild	Moderate	Severe
Episode Severity Analysis*			
Acute phase	Mild dyspnea Diffuse wheezes Adequate air exchange	Respiratory distress at rest Hyperpnea Marked wheezes Air exchange normal or ↓	Marked respiratory distress Marked wheezes or absent breath sounds Pulsus paradoxus >10 mm Chest wall retractions
	FEV_1 = 80% normal pH = Normal or ↑ PaO_2 = Normal or ↓ $PaCO_2$ = Normal or ↓	FEV_1 = 50% normal pH = Generally ↑ PaO_2 = ↓ $PaCO_2$ = Generally ↓	FEV_1 = 25% normal pH = Normal or ↓ PaO_2 = ↓ $PaCO_2$ = Normal or ↑
Disease Severity Analysis†			
General assessment	Attacks no more than once per week Responds to bronchodilators in 24 hours No signs of asthma between episodes No sleep interruption due to asthma No hyperventilation Normal chest x-ray Minimal evidence of airway obstruction No to minimal degree of increase in lung volume	Cough and wheeze episodes more than once per week Cough and low-grade wheeze between acute episodes Exercise tolerance diminished May be up at night because of cough and wheeze Hyperinflation seen on chest x-ray Lung volumes increased	Daily wheezing Frequent severe episodes Hospitalization frequently required to break cycle Poor exercise tolerance Much sleep interruption Chest deformity due to chronic hyperinflation Airway obstruction not completely reversible by bronchodilators Lung volumes markedly increased

*Adapted from The Merck manual of diagnosis and therapy, edition 14, p. 620, edited by Robert Berkow. Copyright 1982 by Merck & Co., Inc. Used with permission.
†From Ellis, E.F.: Asthma in childhood, J. Allergy Clin. Immunol. **72:**531, 1983.

ASSESSMENT: AREAS OF CONCERN

History
Known family or personal history of allergy, infantile eczema, or previous episodes of asthma

Current medications
Careful and complete history of current respiratory related medications as well as most recent dose and time prior to hospital arrival

Respiratory status
Respiratory distress: dyspnea, tachypnea, cough, prolonged expiration, use of accessory muscles during breathing, retractions

Breath sounds: inspiratory and expiratory wheeze, coarse rhonchi; in severe cases only coarse bronchial sounds heard; bilateral sounds heard throughout chest

Skin
Increases diaphoresis as respiratory distress increases

Hypoxia
Restlessness, tachycardia, confusion, hypotension, cyanosis, premature ventricular contractions and right bundle branch block if hypoxia becomes severe, pulsus paradoxus increase >10 mm Hg

Pulmonary function
FEV_1 decreased, peak expiratory flow rate decreased, total lung capacity increased, residual volume increased

Laboratory values
Blood gases: decreased Pao_2, increased $Paco_2$, decreased pH
CBC: eosinophilia, increased Hct

Chest roentgenogram
Unilateral obstruction or infiltration

Hydration
Intake and output to monitor hydration

Psychosocial
Fear of suffocation

Asthma not only must be assessed in the areas of concern as listed but also must be assessed as to its overall severity on both a short-term and long-term basis. Table 2-9 summarizes this assessment.

NURSING DIAGNOSES and NURSING INTERVENTIONS

Nursing Diagnosis	Nursing Intervention
Breathing pattern, ineffective	Assess ventilation to include evaluation of breathing rate, rhythm, and depth, chest expansion, presence of respiratory distress such as dyspnea, shortness of breath, nasal flaring, pursed-lip breathing or prolonged expiratory phase, and use of accessory muscles.
	Assess peak expiratory flow rate or forced expiratory volume as ordered.
	Identify contributing factors such as allergens in immediate environment or other irritants that may exacerbate condition.
	Maintain patient positioning to facilitate ventilation (that is, sitting upright and leaning forward on overbed table).
	Instruct patient in pulmonary hygiene routines that will facilitate effective breathing and minimize pulmonary congestion that could lead to secondary infections.
	Assess patient for tiring in relation to attempts to breathe.
	Initiate prevention measures such as uninterrupted periods of quiet time; maintain calm and restful environment; encourage patient to participate in care as tolerated; explain all therapy before administering.
	Encourage patient to use adaptive breathing techniques to decrease the work of breathing.
	Assist patient to space activities so as to provide periods of rest in between.
	Cover pillows with allergen-proof covers; eliminate dust factors and other irritants.
	Problem solve with patient to determine methods of conserving energy while still performing activities of daily living.
	Assist to protect patient from known sources of secondary infection.
	If mechanical ventilation is required, provide care and monitoring consistent with the guidelines presented on pp. 246-249.

Nursing Diagnosis	Nursing Intervention
Gas exchange, impaired	Monitor arterial blood gases; report increases or decreases of $Paco_2$ and Pao_2 of more than 10 mm Hg.
	Assess patient to identify signs such as restlessness, confusion, and irritability, which may indicate the body's response to altered blood gas states.
	Monitor electrocardiogram and cardiac status for arrhythmias secondary to alterations in blood gases.
	In collaboration with physician consultation, administer humidified oxygen to maintain Pao_2 of at least 50 mm Hg; if blood gas levels cannot be maintained or if the patient demonstrates exhaustion with breathing attempt, mechanical ventilation must be considered.
	Monitor serum electrolytes, which may change because of alterations in oxygenation and metabolism.
	Carefully monitor body temperature, which may fluctuate because of alterations in metabolism or secondary infections.
Airway clearance, ineffective	Promptly administer bronchodilator and corticosteroids as ordered; observe for therapeutic response and signs of side effects such as tachycardia, arrhythmia, nausea, and vomiting; monitor serum theophylline level if appropriate.
	Provide adequate hydration (up to 4000 ml/d) to ensure the liquefaction of secretions.
	Assess patient to identify inability to move secretions; if inability is identified, assist with appropriate measures (coughing, positioning, suctioning, etc.).
	Assist patient to maintain proper body positioning to assure patent airway.
	Carefully and frequently auscultate chest for quality of breath sounds and adventitious sounds; note cough and sputum characteristics.
Oral mucous membrane, alterations in	To prevent possible infections, instruct patients using aerated corticosteroids to perform thorough mouth washing after each use to prevent secondary infection of oral candidiasis.
	Observe oral mucosa for presence of mouth irritation; consult physician if noted.
Communication, impaired: verbal	Observe for signs of frustration or fear secondary to hypoxia that is causing fatigue when patient attempts to talk.
Self-care deficit	Assess the level of self-care deficit secondary to the patient's current condition.
	Provide assistive interventions for such activities of daily living as toileting, bathing, and feeding so as to minimize the patient's energy expenditures.
Health maintenance, alteration in	Assess with patient or family home and environmental stimulants (allergens) that may exacerbate asthma episode.
	Provide education regarding need to avoid contact with irritant allergens.
	Assist with allergy testing and desensitization if indicated.
	Assess for adverse systemic allergic response during allergy testing or desensitization process.
Coping, ineffective individual	Assess patient's response and perception related to the present breathing difficulties.
	Determine patient's ability to cooperate with health care providers regarding intervention strategies such as breathing techniques, exercise progression, and alterations in the activities of daily living.
	Listen carefully to collect information regarding the significance of asthma and the patient's perception of his ability to deal with alterations it is causing.
Coping, family	Assess family's anxiety related to limited understanding of diagnostic procedures, disease process and prognosis, and therapies employed.
	Provide information in areas needed.
	Explain relationship of disease process and rationale for various therapeutic interventions at a level appropriate for comprehension and degree of anxiety
	Involve family in care as appropriate.
	Encourage family to verbalize questions and concerns.

Patient Education

1. Teach facts about and importance of prescribed medications such as bronchodilators, cromolyn, and corticosteroids.
2. Provide patient and family with information about asthma as a disease, how to assess an asthmatic response, what to do during the process of care, criteria for requesting professional assistance, and acute emergency care.
3. Assist patient and family to examine secondary factors that may precipitate asthmatic episodes such as emotional stress, fatigue, or environmental changes or specific allergen contacts such as dust, animal dander, feathers, and pollen.

4. Teach patient adaptive breathing techniques and breathing exercises such as pursed-lip breathing and positioning.
5. Teach importance of consuming large quantities of fluid to maintain secretion liquefaction.
6. Teach adaptive exercise and rest techniques.
7. Provide patient and family with information regarding the care, cleaning, and maintenance of inhalation equipment being used in the hospital or to be used at home.
8. Provide patient and family with respiratory related health information such as pollution indexes, secondary infection exposure, and community support groups.

EVALUATION

Patient Outcome	Data Indicating That Outcome is Reached
Air moves optimally in and out of lungs. Airway is patent. Lungs are fully aerated as visualized on chest x-ray film.	Vital capacity measurements including FEV, TLC, and RV are optimal for patient's status. Serum level of IgE is normal for patient. WBC is within normal limits. Blood gas values are within normal limits. Airways are clear, breath sounds are clear, and breathing occurs without obstruction.
Breathing pattern occurs without tiring patient. Clear breath sounds are heard in all areas.	Patient demonstrates modified breathing techniques that facilitate ventilatory capacity. Behavior is modified to conserve energy expenditure.
Physiologic function is stable.	Hydration level is maintained within normal limits. Gastrointestinal system is functioning adequately. There are no secondary infections. Serum electrolytes are within normal limits.
Patient relates importance of pulmonary exercises.	Patient demonstrates pulmonary exercises and states rationale and importance of maintaining daily exercise routine.
Patient preserves pulmonary functioning by maintaining optimal activity level, preventing infection, and following prescribed treatments.	Patient demonstrates a variety of methods indicating ability to preserve and facilitate optimal respiratory functioning (e.g., breathing exercises, modified activities or exercise, taking medications as prescribed).
Patient and family have sufficient information to comply with discharge regimen.	Patient and family are able at time of discharge to discuss medications—purpose, side effects, route, and schedule—activity regimen, signs of infection or respiratory deterioration, and plan for long-term follow-up maintenance.
Patient and family have sufficient information to assist with preventing further asthma episodes or reduce severity of episodes.	Patient and family discuss pathophysiology of asthma, precipitating factors, and factor avoidance techniques, as well as treatment interventions should episode occur.

Bronchiectasis

Bronchiectasis is the chronic dilation of the medium size bronchi with eventual destruction of the bronchial elastic and muscular elements. The chronic dilation, usually secondary to repeated pulmonary infections or bronchial obstruction, leads to the eventual malfunctioning of bronchial muscle tone and elasticity.

The incidence of this acquired disorder has been much reduced since the development of antibiotics and aggressive management of pulmonary infections. Prior to the time of antibiotics, pulmonary infections would linger and secondary pulmonary obstruction would occur distal to the buildup of sputum and bronchial secretions. It is the chronic obstruction and tissue stretching that eventually lead to the destruction of bronchial elasticity and actual malfunctioning of bronchial muscle tone.

Children are at high risk for the development of bronchiectasis because their bronchi are small and soft and easily damaged by prolonged overinflation due to infection or bronchial foreign body obstruction. While the prevalence of childhood bronchiectasis is decreasing because of the use of antibiotics, it is still seen in children with cystic fibrosis and immune deficiency diseases.

While disease onset, especially in children, may follow a single episode of pulmonary disease, most adults relay a history of numerous pulmonary infections such as pneumonia and a chronic bronchitis type of cough. Delayed resolution of any type of pulmonary disease should raise suspicion of bronchiectasis.

PATHOPHYSIOLOGY

Initially there is a midbronchial obstruction due either to a foreign body or to pus or mucus secondary to a disease process. This obstruction causes impairment of normal bronchial functioning such as the movement of air and the loss of ciliary action responsible for moving secretions. As a result, the terminal bronchi become enlarged and dilated and secretions accumulate in the dilated distal segments. Unless the obstruction is cleared and the secretions drained, damage to the bronchial elasticity occurs and scar tissue develops, resulting in permanent dilation of the bronchial walls.

The development of bronchiectasis usually occurs over a period of time where there is a recurrence of an inflammatory and infectious process that slowly alters the structure of the bronchial walls and their elastic and muscular response. Once the alterations have occurred, however, it is irreversible.

DIAGNOSTIC STUDIES

Clinical examination
Severe and chronic sputum-producing cough, hemoptysis, moist rales and rhonchi heard over the lower lobes, dyspnea, fatigue, and general signs of pulmonary insufficiency

Sputum examination
Gross examination shows that the sputum divides into three layers (sediment, fluid, and foam); a sputum smear is done to rule out tuberculosis and to identify secondary bacterial infections such as those caused by pneumococci, *Pseudomonas*, and *Enterobacter*

CBC
With severe hypoxia may show polycythemia secondary to pulmonary insufficiency

Pulmonary function
Spirometry reveals a decreased forced expiratory volume (FEV_1) and a decreased forced vital capacity (FVC).

Chest roentgenogram
Clear but may show patches of inflammation with increased pulmonary markings at the lung bases

TREATMENT PLAN

The goals of the medical plan are to maintain maximum ventilation by controlling infections and removing secretions.

Surgical
Rarely bronchial resection may be done for patients with isolated areas of bronchiectasis that will not respond to conservative treatment. To consider this the disease must be localized enough to permit complete resection without inadvertently compromising pulmonary function.

Chemotherapeutic
Mucolytic agents
  Acetylcysteine (Mucomyst): Nebulization q2-6h with 20% solution (1-10 ml) or 10% solution (2-20 ml)
Anti-infective agents
  Antibiotic therapy should be specific to the organism identified in the sputum evaluation

Electromechanical
Warm or cool mist via vaporizer may be used to assist in the liquefying of secretions.

Supportive

1. Physiotherapy with postural drainage for at least 10 minutes 3 or 4 times a day.
2. Warm, dry climate void of smoke, fumes, and air pollution.
3. Patient should be encouraged not to smoke.
4. Encourage fluid increase to liquefy secretions and maintain hydration.
5. Culture sputum periodically to identify presence of secondary infections.

ASSESSMENT: AREAS OF CONCERN

Respiratory status

Breath sounds: rales and rhonchi over lower lobes

Breathing patterns: may be labored with prolonged expiration

Cough: chronic with production of large quantities of purulent sputum (coughing and sputum production may become worse with changes in posture and activity)

Hemoptysis in 50% of cases

Chest wall may have retractions during breathing and decreased expiratory excursion

Chest roentgenogram

Clear but may show some areas of inflammation with increased markings at the base

Mediastinal shift may be seen secondary to overinflation of specific lobes of the lung

Cardiovascular response

In advanced cases, cyanosis and clubbing of the fingers may be seen

Generalized response

Weight loss, night sweats, fever, gradual emaciation may be indications of disease progression with possible secondary infections

NURSING DIAGNOSES and NURSING INTERVENTIONS

Nursing Diagnosis	Nursing Intervention
Airway clearance, ineffective	Assess patient to identify inability to move secretions; promote aggressive techniques such as positioning, postural drainage, coughing, suctioning, and fluid promotion, to liquefy and drain excessive secretions. (See pp. 239-242 for techniques of postural drainage.) Assist patient to maintain proper body positioning and frequent alteration of body position to assure patent airway and secretion drainage. Suction if necessary to remove secretions. In collaboration with physician administer mucolytic drugs and antibiotics; assess and document patient response. Provide oral hygiene before and after respiratory therapy because of medication taste and increased sputum production.
Breathing pattern, ineffective	Assess ventilation to include evaluation of breathing rate, rhythm, and depth, chest expansion, presence of respiratory distress such as dyspnea, shortness of breath, nasal flaring, pursed-lip breathing or prolonged expiratory phase, use of abdominal muscles. Periodically assess forced expiratory volume (FEV_1) and forced vital capacity (FVC) to evaluate pulmonary function. Hygiene routines that will facilitate easy and effective breathing. Assess patient for tiring in relation to attempts to breathe.
Gas exchange, impaired	Assess patient to identify signs such as restlessness, confusion, and irritability, which may indicate the body's response to altered blood gas states. Carefully monitor body temperature, sputum characteristics, and cough characteristics, which may indicate the presence of secondary infection and which may lead to respiratory insufficiency if not properly treated. Assist to protect the patient from environmental situations that may put him at risk for secondary pulmonary infections. Assist patient to avoid environmental irritants such as smoke, fumes, and air pullution; patient should also be instructed not to smoke. Monitor and record kidney function and urinary output, which may be affected secondary to chronic tissue hypoxia and alterations in metabolism. Monitor serum electrolytes, which may change because of alterations in oxygenation and metabolism.

Nursing Diagnosis	Nursing Intervention
Nutrition alteration in: less than body requirement	Assist patient to choose foods that are easy to chew and swallow; assist by cutting and feeding if patient tires easily. Encourage smaller more frequent meals. Encourage fluid intake of at least 2 L per day to facilitate liquefying of secretions and promote urinary output. (If patient has compromised cardiac or renal condition, fluid intake must be determined in collaboration with physician.) Monitor for signs and symptoms of malnutrition.
Mobility, impaired physical	Encourage patient to use adaptive breathing techniques to decrease the work of breathing. Assist patient to space activities to provide periods of rest in between. Encourage gradual increase of activities as tolerated to prevent "pulmonary crippling." Problem solve with patient to determine methods of conserving energy while still performing activities of daily living. Assess and document those activities which cause patient to tire easily and become short of breath. If patient is seriously ill and maintained on bed rest, encourage or provide active or passive range of motion exercises to maintain adequate muscle tone.
Self-care deficit	See p. 2088 for associated care.
Anxiety	Assess patient's level of anxiety related to the present health state. Assess patient's level of anxiety related to chronic cough and sputum production.
Coping, ineffective individual	Determine patient's ability to cooperate with health care providers regarding intervention strategies such as breathing techniques, exercise progression, and alterations in the activities of daily living. See p. 1897 for additional strategies.
Coping, family	See p. 1899 for additional nursing care.

Patient Education

1. Teach patient adaptive breathing techniques such as pursed-lip and abdominal breathing.
2. Teach patient to prevent secondary infections by coughing and deep breathing, which will prevent the accumulation of secretion buildup in the lungs.
3. Teach importance of not smoking and avoiding fumes or smoke during active disease state.
4. Teach adaptive exercise and rest techniques.
5. Teach eating and food choice modifications.
6. Teach facts about and importance of prescribed medications.
7. Provide patient and family with respiratory related health information such as pollution indexes, home humidification techniques, and climate changes.
8. Teach importance of avoidance of contact with other persons who may expose patient to a secondary infection.
9. Teach signs of secondary infection such as change in characteristics of sputum or prolonged fever.

EVALUATION

Patient Outcome	Data Indicating That Outcome is Reached
Air moves optimally in and out of lungs.	Coughing if present is productive of sputum.
Airway is patent.	Airways are clear and breathing occurs without obstruction.
Chest x-ray film is clear.	No evidence of overinflation or infiltration is seen.
Patient is free of secondary respiratory infection.	Sputum evaluation shows no evidence of a secondary respiratory infection.
Breathing pattern occurs without tiring patient.	Patient demonstrates modified breathing techniques that facilitate ventilatory capacity. Behavior is modified to conserve energy expenditure.

Patient Outcome	Data Indicating That Outcome is Reached
Physiologic function is stable.	Nutrition level is maintained.
Patient relates importance of daily pulmonary exercises.	Patient demonstrates pulmonary exercises and states rationale and importance of maintaining daily exercise routine.
Patient preserves pulmonary functioning by maintaining optimal activity level, preventing infection, and following prescribed treatments.	Patient demonstrates a variety of methods indicating ability to preserve and facilitate optimal respiratory functioning (e.g., breathing exercises, modified activities or exercise, taking medications as prescribed).
Patient and family have sufficient information to comply with discharge regimen.	Patient and family are able at time of discharge to discuss medications—purpose, side effects, route, and schedule—activity progression regimen, signs of infection or respiratory deterioration, and plan for follow-up visits.

CYSTIC FIBROSIS

Cystic fibrosis is an autosomal recessive disorder of the exocrine glands that causes those glands to produce abnormally thick secretions of mucus. The glands most affected are those of the respiratory system, the pancreas, and the sweat glands.

In the United States, cystic fibrosis is the most common cause of life-threatening pulmonary disease of whites during childhood and adolescence. The disease incidence is 1 in 1500 to 2000 live births. Cystic fibrosis is most prevalent in blacks, American Indians, and persons of Asian ancestry. Boys and girls are equally affected.

Cystic fibrosis is the primary cause of pancreatic deficiency and chronic malabsorption in children and is responsible for many cases of intestinal obstruction in newborns. Although cystic fibrosis is a widespread multisystem disease, the progressive pulmonary infections are the most important clinical problem and are responsible for most of the morbidity and mortality.[66] Advances in the treatment of the respiratory components of the disease have played a primary role in improving the prognosis, but maximum success cannot be realized unless gastrointestinal, hepatic, and psychologic components and sweat abnormalities are also managed in the therapeutic plan.

The disease was first noted by Fanconi in 1936, and its pathophysiology was first discussed by Anderson in 1938. Since these early discoveries, much has been done to lengthen the survival of patients. At present, approximately 50% of patients with cystic fibrosis survive until their eighteenth birthdays.

Therapy for patients with cystic fibrosis is aimed at improving the nutritional status and minimizing pulmonary involvement. Respiratory and cardiac complications such as hemoptysis, pneumothorax, pulmonary insufficiency, cor pulmonale, and cardiac failure are additive and tend to become more severe with increasing age.

Death is most commonly due to cardiac and respiratory insufficiency.

Cystic fibrosis may be an extremely expensive disease. Dolan[15] estimates that average costs for just medications, laboratory tests, and clinic visits are at least $2000 annually. The costs are estimated to be much higher for patients requiring hospitalization, home oxygenation, or home nursing care.

PATHOPHYSIOLOGY

Cystic fibrosis (mucoviscidosis) is a pancreatic enzyme deficiency affecting the exocrine glands throughout the body, both mucus producing and other. Despite intensive research the exact defect in cystic fibrosis remains unknown.

Physiologically, the goblet cells of the mucus-producing (exocrine) glands of the body produce abnormal secretions. These secretions, instead of being thin and free flowing, are thick mucoproteins that precipitate or coagulate to form eosinophilic concentrations in the glands or ducts. Thus the glands and ducts clog and dilate, causing pathologic changes and consequent physical symptoms. The changes are thought to be secondary to the obstruction and not due directly to the abnormality of the secretions. Abnormalities of the non-mucus-producing glands are primarily evidenced in saliva and sweat.

Cystic fibrosis has significant and predictable physiologic impact throughout the body.

Pancreas. Thick secretions block the pancreatic ducts, causing cystic dilations of the small lobes of the acini. Degenerative and fibrotic changes in the pancreas result, and the essential pancreatic enzymes (trypsin, amylase, and lipase) are unable to participate in food absorption and digestion. Thus digestion of fats, proteins, and carbohydrates is disturbed. This altered digestive process is evidenced by increased stool fat and protein. Generalized pancreatic dysfunction also places patients with cystic fibrosis at higher risk for diabetes mellitus.

Pulmonary system. The thick, tenacious mucus causes bronchial and bronchiolar obstruction. Obstruction initially leads to areas of atelectasis and hyperinflation. As lung involvement progresses, reduced oxygen and retained oxygen and carbon dioxide result in hypoxia, hypercapnia, and acidosis. In addition, the heavy mucous secretions decrease ciliary activity and thus contribute to mucous obstruction. Mucous stasis provides an excellent medium for bacterial growth and resulting infection. With severe pulmonary involvement, compression of pulmonary blood vessels and progressive lung dysfunction frequently lead to pulmonary hypertension and cor pulmonale.

Cardiac system. Cardiac changes such as right ventricular hypertrophy occur as a result of obstructive bronchial disease, cor pulmonale, and pulmonary hypertension.

Biliary system. Foci of biliary obstruction and fibrosis are common and become progressively worse, resulting in a type of multilobular biliary cirrhosis. If liver involvement is extensive, portal hypertension and splenomegaly may also occur. Jaundice may be evidence of gallbladder obstruction.

Reproductive organs. In girls the cervical mucous glands may be dilated. Boys may have abnormal development and function of the epididymis, vas deferens, and seminal vesicles as a result of abnormal secretions during fetal development.

Non-mucus-producing glands. Although there are no histologic abnormalities, sweat and salivary gland secretions have abnormally high levels of sodium and chloride.

DIAGNOSTIC STUDIES

Diagnosis of cystic fibrosis requires a cluster of positive findings. Although not every evaluation may be significant, evidence such as elevated sweat chlorides in the presence of pulmonary disease or pancreatic insufficiency is considered to be diagnostic.

Family history
History of siblings or other family members with cystic fibrosis

Fig. 2-31
Chest roentgenogram of patient with cystic fibrosis. Note bronchial thickening and ill-defined shadows.

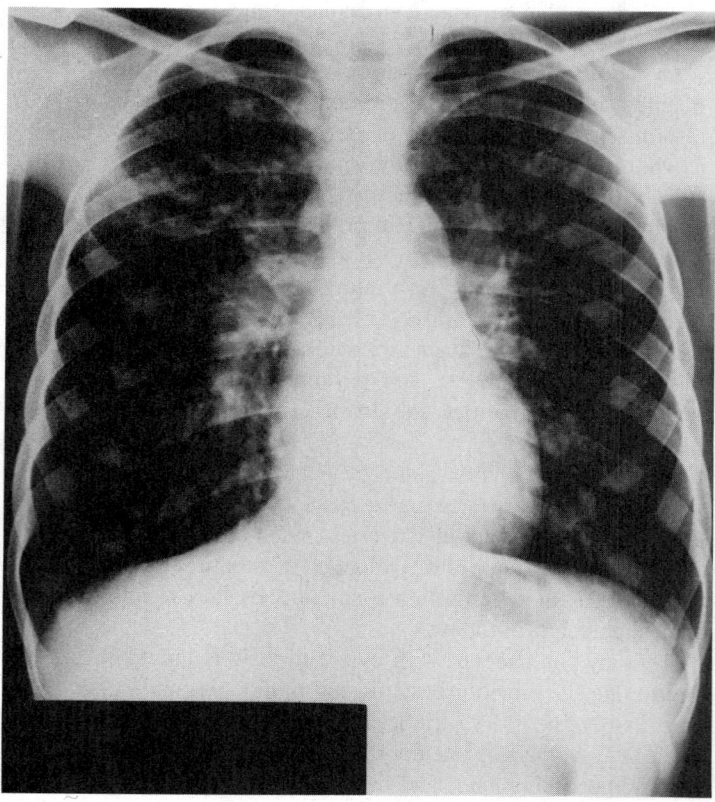

Sweat electrolytes

Normal mean value approximately 18 mEq/L (varies with age); sweat chloride 40-60 mEq/L suggestive of cystic fibrosis; sweat chloride over 60 mEq/L diagnostic of cystic fibrosis

Pancreatic enzymes

Examination of duodenal secretions or stool for presence of trypsin and chymotrypsin; absence of enzymes suggestive of potential cystic fibrosis

Stool examination for fat

Fat absorption tests conducted for 5 days to calculate ratio of fat in oral intake to fat in stool; impaired fat absorption in intestine, resulting in large volumes excreted in the stool (steatorrhea), suggestive of cystic fibrosis

Chest roentgenogram

Evidence of generalized obstructive emphysema suggestive of cystic fibrosis (Fig. 2-31); in advanced disease patchy atelectasis and disseminated infiltration pattern may be seen

TREATMENT PLAN

Surgical

Pulmonary lavage or bronchial washing—may be used for seriously ill patients whose bronchial airways cannot be cleared by other means

Resection of blebs and pleural scars—may be attempted if pulmonary disease is localized; purpose is resection of blebs and pleural scars by pleural stripping

Tracheostomy or endotracheal intubation—may be carried out for seriously ill patients; permits mechanical ventilation and facilitates mechanical pulmonary toileting

Chemotherapeutic

Mucolytic agents

Acetylcysteine (Mucomyst)

Nebulization q8-12h with 10% solution (2-3 ml)

Anti-infective agents

May be prescribed only at time of illness and infection or prophylactically; if prescribed for infection, antibiotic of choice depends on organism

Expectorants

Iodinated glycerol (Organidin), 60 mg q6h taken with liquid for adults, 15-30 mg q6h taken with liquid for children

Potassium iodide (Ki-N, Pima), 300-600 mg q4-6h for adults, 150-300 mg q4-6h for children

Digestive agents

Rationale: Provide enzymatic activity necessary to assist in digestion of carbohydrates, fats, and proteins

Pancreatin (Elzyme, Viokase), 325-1000 mg with meals or snacks

Pancrelipase (Cotazym, Ilozyme, Ku-Zyme HP, Pancrease), 1-3 tablets or capsules, 0.43-1.29 g powder, or 1-2 powder packets before or with meals or snacks; has 12 times the lipase and four times the amylase and protease activity of pancreatin

Contraindication: Hypersensitivity to pork or beef

Common side effects: Nausea, diarrhea, vomiting, anorexia

Immunizations

Routine immunizations against diphtheria, tetanus, pertussis, poliomyelitis, measles, mumps, and influenza recommended as preventive measures

Electromechanical

Oxygenation—may be indicated for persons unable to maintain adequate oxygen levels; oxygen concentrations should be as low as possible while maintaining adequate PaO_2 level; oxygen concentration should not exceed 24% to 40%; therapy may be initiated during times of infection or disease exacerbation

Aerosol therapy—may be used intermittently in conjunction with physiotherapy

Supportive

Diet—sufficient calories to promote normal growth (exceeding daily requirements by at least 25%); high-protein (at least 1.5 to 2 g/lb/day for infants and 1.25 g/lb/day for adults); low-fat (no more than 50% of normal); multivitamins with addition of vitamins A, D, and E; vitamin K if hypoprothrombinemia present; supplemental salt in hot weather

ASSESSMENT: AREAS OF CONCERN

Respiratory status

Respiratory distress: cough; congestion; tachypnea; retractions; decreased chest wall movement; labored breathing; dyspnea

Examination: barrel chest; tympanic percussion tone over consolidation or areas of atelectasis; clubbing of fingers and toes

Breath sounds: moist rales and rhonchi; decreased or unequal breath sounds

Sputum: productive cough with thick sputum; hemoptysis

Pulmonary function: decreased vital capacity; decreased FEV_1, decreased tidal volume; increased airway resistance

Acute respiratory complications: lobar atelectasis; lung abscess; spontaneous pneumothorax; cor pulmonale; congestive heart failure

Hypercapnia

Headache; dizziness; confusion; unconsciousness; twitching; sweating

Hypoxia

Restlessness; confusion; impaired motor function; cyanosis; tachycardia

Laboratory values

Blood gases: pH; $PaCO_2$; PaO_2

Serum levels: bicarbonate; sodium; chloride; potassium

Hematology: hematocrit; hemoglobin level

Sweat test: chloride concentrations greater than 50 mEq/L

Stool: no presence of pancreatic enzymes trypsin and chymotrypsin; increased fat in stool

Nutritional status

Appetite; percentages of carbohydrate, fat, and protein in diet; salt supplementation; evidence of malnutrition

Hepatic and biliary function

Jaundice; enlarged liver; ascites; abnormal liver function findings

Gastrointestinal function

Insufficient digestion producing bulky, foul-smelling, pale, watery stools; evidence of intestinal obstruction, fecal impaction, or rectal prolapse; evidence of gastrointestinal bleeding: tarry stools, positive guaiac findings

Cardiovascular status

Decreased cardiac output: restlessness, lethargy, tachycardia

Bronchopulmonary infection

Temperature; sputum specimens for culture and sensitivity; chest roentgenogram

Psychosocial

Support systems; networking with cystic fibrosis resource groups; activities of daily living; self-esteem; interaction with peers; sexuality

NURSING DIAGNOSES and NURSING INTERVENTIONS

Nursing Diagnosis	Nursing Intervention
Airway clearance, ineffective	Assess patient to identify inability to move secretions. If inability is identified, assist with appropriate measures (such as coughing, positioning, suctioning, and liquefying secretions).
	Promptly administer mucolytics and expectorants as ordered. Observe for therapeutic response and side effects.
	Assist patient to maintain body position that ensures maximum airway availability (semi-Fowler's position or sitting upright).
	Provide hydration to liquefy secretions and replace fluids.
	Administer aerosol and perform postural drainage with percussion at least 1 hour before meals; provide oral hygiene after treatment.
	Carefully and frequently auscultate chest for quality of breath sounds and adventitious sounds. Note cough and sputum characteristics.
Breathing pattern, ineffective	Assess ventilation to include evaluation of breathing rate, rhythm, and depth; chest expansion; presence of respiratory distress such as dyspnea, shortness of breath, nasal flaring, pursed-lip breathing, or prolonged expiratory phase; and use of accessory muscles.
	Identify contributing factors such as airway clearance or obstruction problem or weakness.
	Maintain patient positioning to facilitate easy ventilation (head of bed in semi-Fowler's position).
	Instruct patient in pulmonary hygiene routines that will promote easy and effective breathing, facilitate removal of secretions from the tracheobronchial tree, and minimize pulmonary congestion that could lead to secondary infections (see pp. 246-249).
	Suction if necessary to remove secretions.
	Assess patient for tiring in relation to attempts to breathe.

Nursing Diagnosis	Nursing Intervention
	Encourage patient to use adaptive breathing techniques to decrease work of breathing and to alternate activities with periods of rest. Protect patient from known sources of secondary infection or breathing irritation such as smoking. If mechanical ventilation is necessary, provide care and monitoring consistent with guidelines provided on pp. 246-249.
Gas exchange, impaired	If patient is very ill, monitor arterial blood gases. Report increases or decreases of more than 10 to 15 mm Hg in $PaCO_2$ and PaO_2. Administer oxygen as ordered and monitor to maintain PaO_2 between 45 and 60 mm Hg. This may usually be maintained by administering oxygen by nasal cannula at flow of 1 to 3 L/minute. Venturi mask may be used if needed. If adequate blood gas levels cannot be maintained, mechanical ventilation must be considered. Assess patient to identify signs, such as restlessness, confusion, and irritability, that may indicate body's response to altered blood gas states. If patient is very ill, monitor electrocardiogram and cardiac status for arrhythmias resulting from alterations in blood gases. Monitor and record kidney functioning and urinary output, which may be affected by chronic tissue hypoxia and alterations in metabolism. Monitor serum electrolytes, which may change owing to alterations in oxygenation and metabolism. Carefully monitor body temperature, which may fluctuate owing to alterations in metabolism or secondary infections.
Nutrition, alteration in: less than body requirements	Provide small, frequent feedings of high-calorie, high-protein, low-fat foods with supplemental vitamins. Assist by cutting food and feeding if patient tires easily. Administer pancreatic enzyme medications at mealtime. Assess nutritional status by daily weighing, monitoring intake and output, and observing skin turgor and muscle tone. Monitor serum levels of sodium and chloride. Observe for lethargy and signs of dehydration. Consult physician to administer sodium chloride should deficits occur. If indicated and in consultation with physician, administer stool softeners to relieve constipation. Monitor for signs and symptoms of malnutrition.
Fluid volume deficit, potential	If patient is seriously ill, monitor for evidence of gastrointestinal bleeding related to physiologic stress; monitor serial hemoglobin levels and hematocrit; check all stools, emesis, and nasogastric secretions for presence of blood; and observe changes in vital signs or abdominal girth.
Mobility, impaired physical	Encourage patient to use adaptive breathing techniques to decrease work of breathing. Assist patient to alternate activities with periods of rest. See p. 2104 for additional strategies.
Communication, impaired: verbal	Observe for signs of frustration or fear, fatigue, and tiring with attempts to communicate as result of hypoxia.
Self-care deficit	Assist with activities of daily living such as toileting, bathing, and feeding to minimize patient's energy expenditures. See p. 2086 for additional strategies.
Health maintenance, alteration in	With patient and family, assess home and personally used irritants (smoking, fumes, vapors) that may exacerbate chronic respiratory condition. Provide education regarding need to avoid irritants in home, work, and community environments.
Bowel elimination, alteration in: constipation	Observe stool; note odor, color, amount, frequency, and consistency. Observe for signs of intestinal obstruction or prolapse of rectum. Administer stool softener as ordered and report results. Observe for presence of blood in stool.

Nursing Diagnosis	Nursing Intervention
Coping, ineffective individual	Assess patient's perception of present and chronic disease state.
	Assess patient's level of frustration related to feeling of air hunger.
	Determine patient's ability to cooperate with health care providers in interventions such as breathing techniques, exercise progression, and alterations in activities of daily living.
	Listen carefully to collect information regarding significance of current health care problem and patient's perception of ability to deal with alterations caused by cystic fibrosis.
	Assist patient to develop appropriate coping strategies based on personal strengths and past experience.
	Explain all treatments and procedures in manner appropriate for patient's age and comprehension.
	Assist patient to participate in care.
	Encourage patient to maintain usual activities, especially school activities if patient is child.
	Arrange for continued schooling and peer contacts when patient is in hospital.
Coping, family: potential for growth	Assess family's understanding of diagnostic procedures, disease process and prognosis, and therapies employed.
	Explain relationship of disease processes and rationale for various therapeutic interventions at level appropriate for family members' comprehension and emotional state.
	Involve family in care as appropriate.

Patient Education

1. Teach the patient adaptive breathing techniques and work with the family to teach postural drainage techniques.
2. Teach the importance of avoiding contact with persons who have respiratory infections.
3. Teach the importance of obtaining appropriate immunizations and vaccinations to prevent as many childhood and communicable diseases as possible.
4. Teach the facts about and importance of prescribed medications and diet modifications.
5. Provide the patient and family with information regarding cystic fibrosis, assessment of individual capabilities and responses, and actions to take during an acute episode of difficult breathing.
6. Inform the patient and family that a change in health status must be reported to the patient's health care providers. Indicators of change may include change in sputum characteristics or color, decreased activity tolerance, nutrition or gastrointestinal changes, weight loss, fever, or stress symptoms indicating an inability to tolerate the disease state.
7. Teach adaptive exercise and rest techniques.
8. Provide the patient and family with information regarding the care, cleaning, and maintenance of inhalation or oxygen equipment used in the hospital or at home, as well as signs of oxygen toxicity.
9. Provide the patient and family with information related to respiratory health, such as pollution indexes, secondary infection exposure, and community support groups.

EVALUATION

Patient Outcome	Data Indicating That Outcome is Reached
Movement of air in and out of lungs is optimum.	Vital capacity measurements are optional for patient's health status.
Airway is patent.	Airways are clear and breathing is as optimum as possible for patient.
Breathing occurs without tiring patient. Breath sounds are clear in all areas.	Patient demonstrates modified breathing techniques that facilitate ventilatory capacity. Patient's behavior is modified to conserve energy expenditure.
	Patient's behavior is modified to conserve energy expenditure.
Physiologic stability is achieved.	Nutrition level is maintained. Kidney and bladder functioning is within normal limits. Gastrointestinal system is functioning

Patient Outcome	Data Indicating That Outcome is Reached
	adequately. There are no secondary infections. Serum electrolyte levels are within normal limits. Stool enzymes are present in normal levels. Stool fat content is within normal concentration.
Patient understands importance of daily pulmonary exercises.	Patient demonstrates pulmonary exercises and states rationale and importance of maintaining daily exercise routine.
Patient preserves pulmonary functioning by maintaining optimum activity level, avoiding infection, and following prescribed treatments.	Patient demonstrates variety of methods indicating ability to preserve and facilitate respiratory functioning (breathing exercise, taking medications as prescribed).
Patient and family have sufficient information to comply with discharge regimen.	Patient and family at time of discharge are able to discuss medications (purpose, side effects, route, and schedule), dietary therapy regimen, activity progression regimen, signs of infection or respiratory deterioration, and plan for follow-up visits.
Patient and family understand disease process and complications.	Patient and family discuss cystic fibrosis as disease: its consequences, outcome, and support strategies.

ATELECTASIS

Atelectasis is failure of the lung to expand.

In the pure sense atelectasis refers to atelectasis neonatorum, a condition occurring in premature infants. When used for adults, atelectasis refers to an acquired condition in which all or part of the normally aerated and expanded lung collapses. Atelectasis may be prevented by comprehensive nursing care of postoperative patients and injured patients with pneumothorax or hemothorax.

Atelectasis is a common complication of thoracic or upper abdominal surgery. The postoperative problem is due mostly to hypoventilation, which commonly leads to a bronchial obstruction with mucus. It may also be caused by compression of the lung tissue from hemothorax, pneumothorax, emphysema, oxygen therapy, or tumor.

PATHOPHYSIOLOGY

Atelectasis may occur suddenly and be extensive, or it may occur slowly and cause minor pulmonary dysfunction. The extent of the atelectasis depends on the site and rapidity of the blockage. If the mainstem bronchus to one lung is blocked, the entire lung becomes atelectatic and respiratory compromise is great. If only a small bronchiole becomes slowly blocked owing to buildup of secretions, symptoms may be minor and the respiratory system is able to compensate. In both cases, however, infection and lung tissue damage are possible.

The collapse of lung tissue results in hypoxia. Once obstruction has occurred, the gas distal to the obstruction is absorbed into the circulation because the oxygen tension in the pulmonary arteries is lower than in the alveoli. The higher the concentration (FIO_2) of the inspired gas at the time of the obstruction, the faster the alveolar collapse.

Surfactant levels may be an important factor in atelectasis. Decreased surfactant levels are thought to be a cause of the collapse of alveoli. Decreased blood flow postoperatively may play some part in causing decreased surfactant levels. The actual cause is yet to be determined.

DIAGNOSTIC STUDIES

Arterial blood gases
PaO_2 less than 80 mm Hg initially, often improving during first 24 hours; $PaCO_2$ often normal or low owing to hyperventilation

Chest roentgenogram
Airless area over region of atelectasis; trachea, heart, and mediastinum deviated toward atelectatic area; diaphragm elevated on affected side; rib spaces narrowed

Clinical examination
Rapid occlusion with massive collapse: hyperventilation, dyspnea, cyanosis, tachycardia, elevated temperature, diminished breath sounds over affected area, dull or flat percussion tones, restlessness, rales on auscultation
Slow occlusion with minor collapse: may be asymptomatic or have minor pulmonary symptoms

Bronchoscopy

May show bronchial obstruction

TREATMENT PLAN

The ultimate treatment plan for atelectasis is removal of the underlying cause.

Surgical

Surgical excision or insertion of drainage tube—performed to relieve atelectasis caused by compression component such as tumor, hemothorax, or pneumothorax

Bronchoscopy—may be performed when atelectasis not relieved by suction, coughing and deep breathing, or postural drainage

Chemotherapeutic

Bronchodilators

Isoetharine (Bronkosol), 2-4 ml of 0.125%-0.25% solution q4h

Metaproterenol sulfate (Alupent), 2-3 inhalations q3-4h

Anti-infective agents (use is controversial)

Broad-spectrum antibiotic (such as penicillin or ampicillin) given as soon as symptoms are noted; drug may be modified appropriately if specific pathogen is isolated from bronchial secretions

Electromechanical

High tidal volumes and/or positive end-expiratory pressure (PEEP)—used to maintain open alveoli if patient is intubated

Saline irrigation with suctioning—may help loosen secretions and enhance removal

Supportive

Positioning—patient placed with uninvolved side in dependent position to promote drainage of affected area; patient repositioned at least every hour

Chest physiotherapy with coughing and deep breathing

Ambulation as quickly as possible

ASSESSMENT: AREAS OF CONCERN

Respiratory status

Tachypnea; retractions; labored breathing; dyspnea; nasal flaring; retractions; rales, bilaterally unequal, diminished over affected area; labored or irregular breathing; hyperventilation; percussion tones dull or flat over affected area

Hypoxia

Restlessness; confusion; hypertension early; hypotension late; cyanosis; tachycardia

Laboratory values

Blood gases: pH; PaO_2; $PaCO_2$

Serum electrolyte levels: bicarbonate; sodium; potassium; chloride

Hematology: hematocrit; hemoglobin level

Bronchopulmonary infection

Temperature; characteristics of sputum; sputum specimens for culture and sensitivity

Chest roentgenogram

Periodic evaluation to monitor atelectasis region

Psychosocial

Fear of air hunger; fear of complications such as atelectasis

NURSING DIAGNOSES and NURSING INTERVENTIONS

Nursing Diagnosis	Nursing Intervention
Airway clearance, ineffective: potential	Prevent buildup of respiratory secretions after surgery by encouraging deep breathing and coughing; repositioning patient every hour; ambulating patient as soon as possible; not administering large doses of sedatives, which depress cough reflex and respirations; liquefying secretions by administering aerosol or intermittent positive-pressure breathing treatments, humidifying inspired air, and maintaining body hydration; and using incentive spirometer to encourage deep breathing. After surgery, position patient with pillow along incision site to function as splint. Administer analgesic medications before initiating deep breathing and coughing exercises.
Airway clearance, ineffective: actual	Assess patient to identify inability to move secretions. If inability is identified, assist with appropriate measures (such as coughing, positioning, suctioning, and liquefying secretions).

Nursing Diagnosis	Nursing Intervention
	Promptly administer bronchodilators, mucolytics, and expectorants per protocol to dilate bronchioles and remove secretions. Observe for therapeutic response and side effects.
	Assist patient to maintain body position that ensures maximum airway availability and draining of affected side (uninvolved side is in dependent position).
	Provide hydration to liquefy secretions and replace fluids.
	Administer IPPB and perform postural drainage with percussion.
	Carefully and frequently auscultate chest for quality of breath sounds and adventitious sounds. Note cough and sputum characteristics.
Breathing pattern, ineffective	Assess ventilation to include evaluation of breathing rate, rhythm, and depth; chest expansion; presence of respiratory distress such as dyspnea, shortness of breath, nasal flaring, pursed-lip breathing or prolonged expiratory phase; and use of accessory muscles.
	If possible, maintain patient in position that facilitates easy ventilation (head of bed in semi-Fowler's position or patient sitting and leaning forward on overbed table).
	Instruct patient in pulmonary hygiene routines that will promote easy and effective breathing, facilitate removal of secretions from tracheobronchial tree, and minimize pulmonary congestion that may lead to secondary infections.
	Suction if necessary to remove secretions.
	Assess patient for tiredness in relation to attempts to breathe.
	Protect patient from known sources of secondary infection or breathing irritation such as smoking.
Gas exchange, impaired	In collaboration with physician's order, monitor arterial blood gases. Report increases or decreases of more than 10 to 15 mm Hg in $Paco_2$ and Pao_2.
	Assess patient to identify signs, such as restlessness, confusion, and irritability, that may indicate body's response to altered blood gas states.
	Monitor electrocardiogram and cardiac status for arrhythmias resulting from alterations in blood gases.
	Monitor serum electrolyte levels, which may change owing to alterations in oxygenation and metabolism.
	Carefully monitor body temperature, which may fluctuate owing to alterations in metabolism or secondary infections.
Mobility, impaired physical	Encourage ambulation of patient as quickly as possible to encourage deeper breathing and lung expansion.
	Closely monitor amount of deep breathing and activity patient with altered respiratory state can tolerate before dyspnea occurs.
Fear	Observe for signs of frustration or fear, fatigue, and tiring with attempts to communicate that result from hypoxia.
	Assess patient's level of fear related to current health state.
	Assess patient's level of fear related to feeling of air hunger.
Self-care deficit	Assess level of self-care deficit resulting from patient's current condition.
	Assist with activities of daily living, such as toileting, bathing, and feeding, to minimize patient's energy expenditures.
Coping, ineffective individual	Determine patient's ability to cooperate with health care providers regarding intervention strategies such as deep breathing and coughing techniques and exercise progression.

Patient Education

1. Teach the patient deep breathing and coughing techniques, as well as increased movement and splinting when coughing.
2. Teach the patient facts about and the importance of prescribed medications such as bronchodilators and antibiotics.
3. If the patient has undergone surgery and does not have atelectasis, provide the patient and

family with information about techniques such as movement, deep breathing, and coughing and use of an incentive spirometer to facilitate aeration of the lungs.

4. Provide the patient and family with information regarding the care, cleaning, and maintenance of inhalation or oxygen equipment in the hospital or at home.

EVALUATION

Patient Outcome	Data Indicating That Outcome is Reached
Movement of air in and out of lungs is optimum.	Chest roentgenogram shows bilaterally equal and aerated lung fields.
Airway is patent.	Blood-gas findings are within normal range for patient. No signs of respiratory distress are noted. Airways are clear and breathing occurs without obstruction. Breath sounds are clear throughout.

PLEURISY (PLEURITIS)

Pleurisy is an inflammation of the visceral and parietal pleura. It is also referred to as dry pleurisy or fibrinous pleurisy.

Pleurisy often occurs as a result of pulmonary bacterial infections such as pneumonia or pulmonary infarction; viral infections of the intercostal muscles; transport of an infectious agent or neoplastic cells directly to the pleura by the bloodstream or lymphatics as occurs in collagen-vascular disease or uremic pleurisy; pleural trauma; asbestos-related pleural diseases; or early stages of tuberculosis or lung tumor. The size of the affected area may range from a very small space to most of the pleural surface. The disease onset is usually sudden, and the diagnosis is easily made based on the characteristic pleuritic pain and pleural friction rub heard by auscultation.

PATHOPHYSIOLOGY

The visceral pleura adheres to the lung's surface, whereas the parietal pleura lines the costal, diaphragmatic, mediastinal, and cervical regions of the thoracic cavity. Under normal circumstances these membranes slide easily over each other to reduce friction during respirations. When pleurisy develops, the pleural surfaces rub together in an irritating way as a result of the buildup of fibrinous exudate. It is the rough rubbing of the surfaces that causes the audible pleural friction rub.

During the development of pleurisy the pleura becomes edematous and congested, an exudate collects on the pleural surface, and cellular infiltration occurs. The exudate develops from plasma proteins leaking from damaged vessels. The exudate may be reabsorbed into the fibrous tissue, causing pleural adhesions.

The pain felt in pleurisy is due to stretching of the inflamed pleura. The pain is generally referred to the chest wall and occasionally to the abdominal wall. If the pleuritic area is along the diaphragm border, pain is referred to the shoulder.

DIAGNOSTIC STUDIES

Clinical examination
Auscultation during late inspiration and early expiration reveals dry rubbing sound (may not occur until 24 to 36 hours after onset of pain); history of pain with deep breath or coughing; with diaphragmatic pleurisy, pain referred to shoulder; respirations rapid and shallow; breath sounds diminished; if pleural effusion develops, pain subsides and fever and dry cough occur

Chest roentgenogram
Limited value in diagnosing pleurisy; diagnostic if fluid accumulates as in pleural effusion

TREATMENT PLAN

Chemotherapeutic
Local anesthetics
Paravertebral infiltration of anesthetic to block intercostal nerves
Narcotic analgesics
Analgesics to relieve discomfort; narcotics such as meperidine (Demerol), 50-75 mg q4-6h, or morphine, 15 mg q4-6h, to decrease pain while patient takes deep breaths and coughs

Analgesic-antipyretics
   Acetaminophen (Tylenol), 600 mg q4-6h

Supportive
   Treatment of underlying disease or problem
   Positioning patient on affected side to splint chest
   Deep breathing and coughing to prevent atelectasis and
      pneumonia
   Heat to affected area

ASSESSMENT: AREAS OF CONCERN

Respiratory status
   Pleural friction rub heard during late inspiration and
      early expiration

Pleural effusion
   Purulent sputum; fluid accumulation on chest roent-
      genogram; subsidence of pleural pain; dyspnea; dull
      percussion tone over chest

Pain
   Relationship between patient's level of pain and ability
      to cough and deep breathe; ability of analgesic or
      narcotic to relieve patient's pain

Bronchopulmonary infection
   Presence of fever; altered hematologic findings; spu-
      tum characteristics that might indicate secondary
      infection

NURSING DIAGNOSES and NURSING INTERVENTIONS

Nursing Diagnosis	Nursing Intervention
Comfort, alteration in: pain	Position patient on affected side to splint chest and minimize pain. In collaboration with physician, administer analgesic or narcotic medication as needed to minimize discomfort. Splint chest with pillow or other object during deep breathing and coughing.
Gas exchange, impaired	Monitor for signs of restlessness, confusion, and irritability, which may indicate altered blood gas levels resulting from shallow breathing. Monitor for signs of atelectasis (see pp. 183-184). Monitor for signs of pleural effusion (see pp. 188-190). Protect patient from known sources of secondary infection. Turn patient frequently to prevent pooling of secretions and promote expansion of all lung lobes. Position patient to facilitate maximum ventilation.

Patient Education

1. Teach the patient the importance of deep breathing and coughing to keep the lungs aerated.
2. Teach the patient splinting during deep breathing and coughing.

EVALUATION

Patient Outcome	Data Indicating That Outcome is Reached
Movement of air in and out of the lungs is optimum.	Breath sounds are clear with no evidence of pleural friction rub during inspiration and expiration.
There is no pain with breathing.	Patient is able to take deep breaths and cough without discomfort.
Disease state is corrected without atelectasis or secondary infection.	Patient recovers without development of atelectasis or secondary infection such as pneumonia.

PLEURAL EFFUSION (PLEURISY WITH EFFUSION)

A pleural effusion develops when excessive nonpurulent fluid accumulates in the pleural space between the visceral and parietal pleurae.

Pleural effusion is rarely a primary disease. It generally occurs as a secondary problem when the physiologic processes of capillary fluids, lymphatic drainage, membrane hydrostatic pressures, and colloidal osmotic pressures of the pleurae are disturbed.

Pleural effusions may be broken down into two categories, transudates and exudates, determined by the presence and amount of protein in the aspirated fluid (see below). Following are the common causes of pleural effusions:

Exudates
Viral infections
Tuberculosis
Bacterial infections
Chest trauma
Pancreatitis
Rheumatic fever
Collagen-vascular diseases
Metastic diseases
Uremia
Subphrenic abscess
Pulmonary infarction
Transudates
Peritoneal dialysis
Pericarditis
Cirrhosis
Congestive heart failure
Myxedema
Kidney disease
Sarcoidosis
Hypoproteinemia

PATHOPHYSIOLOGY

The visceral and parietal pleurae form a continuous sac between the lung and the chest wall. Normally, only a potential space containing less than 10 ml of fluid separates these surfaces. The fluid is continuously moving in and out of this space because of a balance between hydrostatic pressures, colloidal osmotic pressures, and the surface characteristics of capillaries and the pleurae. Any alteration in pressure gradients or surface characteristics can lead to the formation of an effusion. For example, inflammation may increase capillary permeability and thus allow the flow of fluid and protein into the pleural space.

As discussed previously, effusions may be categorized into transudate or exudate. The distinction is based on protein content. Transudates (also called hydrothorax) are produced when the flow of protein-free fluid into the pleural space is disturbed. Aspirated fluid is clear or pale yellow, has a specific gravity of 1.015 or less, and has a protein content that is either normal or less than 3 g/dl. Exudates result from either a disease of the pleural surface or an obstruction in the lymphatic system that inhibits drainage of proteins. The exudate fluid is often dark yellow or amber and has a specific gravity greater than 1.016 and a protein content greater than 3 g/dl.

DIAGNOSTIC STUDIES

Clinical examination
Dullness to percussion, which shifts with change in position; decreased or absent breath sounds over affected area; egophony above effusion site; dyspnea if effusion has occurred rapidly; if effusion is large, intercostal bulging or decreased chest wall movement during breathing

Chest roentgenogram
Effusions typically located at base of pleural space; moderate amount of fluid (250 to 300 ml) must accumulate to be seen on upright posteroanterior, decubitus, or lateral chest roentgenogram; effusion seen as dense opacity (Fig. 2-32); large effusions may obliterate hemothorax, simulating lung collapse; distinction between effusion and collapse based on shift of mediastinum away from effusion, but toward lung collapse.[46]

Thoracentesis
For pleural fluid analysis; submit several hundred milliliters if possible (see Table 2-10)

Stain, culture, and sensitivity of pleural fluid
Identification of causative agent (bacterial, fungal, or viral)

Cytologic examination of pleural fluid
Evaluation of potential neoplastic involvement

Pleural biopsy with tissue analysis
Indicated when fluid analysis fails to establish cause

TREATMENT PLAN

The treatment of pleural effusion depends on the etiology and clinical consequences. The following discussion refers to the general treatment of effusion. The reader is referred to the section of the text dealing with the cause of the effusion.

Fig. *2-32*
Chest roentgenogram of patient with
pleural effusion. **A,** PA view: note
obliteration of costophrenic angles
bilaterally; pulmonary vasculature
appears normal. **B,** Lateral view: note
lack of costophrenic angles.

Courtesy R. Keith Wilson, M.D., Baylor
College of Medicine, Houston, Texas.

A

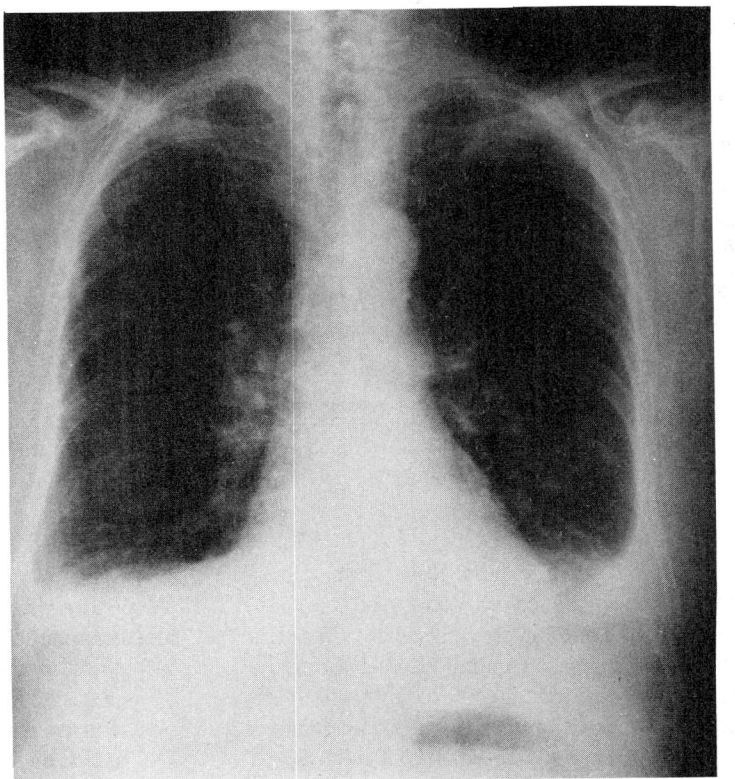

B

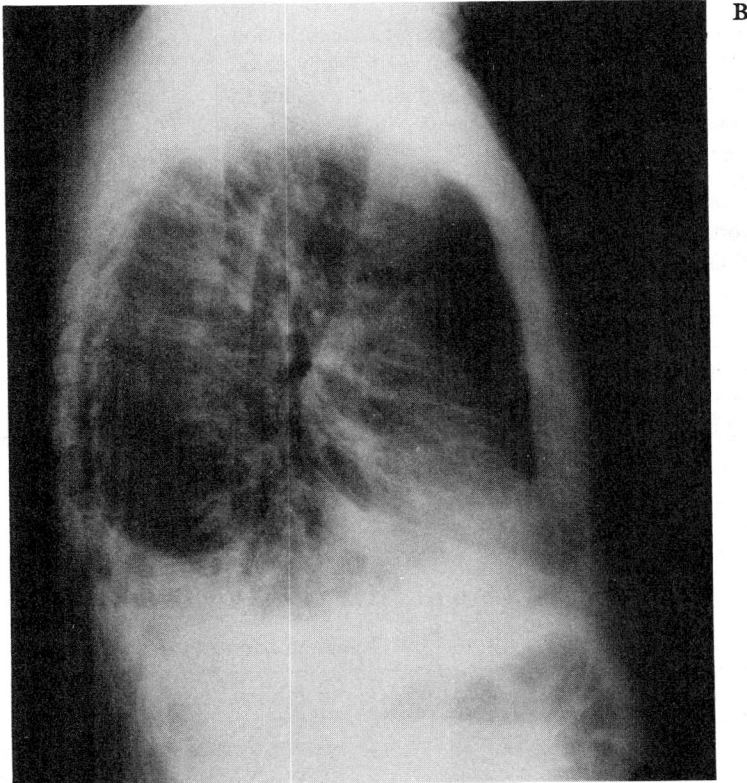

Table 2-10
Pleural Fluid Analysis

Measurement	Transudate	Exudate
Color	Pale yellow	Dark amber, blood or pus
Red blood cells (RBCs)	May increase	>5000 RBCs/mm³; may increase
Protein	<3 g/dl	>3 g/dl
Specific gravity	<1.016	>1.016
Lactic dehydrogenase (LDH)	<200 U/dl	>200 U/dl
Pleural LDH/serum LDH	<0.6	>0.6
White blood cells (WBCs)	Increase indicates empyema or infected effusion	
Amylase	Exceeds serum amylase level	
Glucose	Less than serum glucose level	
Triglyceride	May be increased	
pH	<7.3	>7.3

Modified from Miller, L.G., and Kazemi, H.: Manual of clinical pulmonary medicine, New York, 1983, McGraw-Hill Book Co.

Surgical

Thoracentesis—to drain excess fluid from pleural space and relieve dyspnea or hypoxemia (see p. 147 for procedure and nursing care); because of potential cardiovascular response to rapid removal of pleural fluids, removal limited to 1200 to 1500 ml at any one time; another complication of thoracentesis is pneumothorax (see pp. 223-228)

Insertion of small chest tube

Tube may be connected to underwater seal drainage system and left in place if accumulation of fluids is large and compromising respiratory function

If pleural effusion is caused by malignancy, tube may be inserted to drain fluid and left in place to provide insertion point for medications and therapeutic techniques

Chemotherapeutic

Antibiotics

Antibiotics specific to cause administered if effusion is thought to be caused by infectious process

Supportive

Treatment of underlying disease or problem

Deep breathing and coughing to encourage maximal ventilation; incentive spirometer may be used

Bed rest, which causes most effusions tend to absorb spontaneously

ASSESSMENT: AREAS OF CONCERN

Respiratory insufficiency resulting from fluid in pleural space

Respiratory distress: nasal flaring; tachypnea; decreased chest wall movement; dyspnea; restlessness; tachycardia; decreased breath sounds; paradoxic breathing; dull percussion tone

Pulmonary function studies: decreased vital capacity and minute volume

Reaccumulation of fluid in pleural space after drainage by thoracentesis

Assessment of potential respiratory distress as discussed above

Cardiovascular response to removal of large quantity of pleural fluid during thoracentesis

Hypotension; tachycardia; cardiac arrhythmias; syncopy; clammy skin; paleness

Bronchopulmonary infection

Temperature; sputum specimen for culture and sensitivity

Psychosocial

Fear of dyspnea or not being able to get enough air; potential fear of unknown cause of pleural effusion

NURSING DIAGNOSES and NURSING INTERVENTIONS

Nursing Diagnosis	Nursing Intervention
Fluid volume, alteration in: excess	Position patient so maximum ventilation can occur (semi-Fowler's or upright position). Assess for signs of respiratory distress caused by fluid buildup in pleural space. Assist with thoracentesis procedure and monitor patient's response after procedure.

Nursing Diagnosis	Nursing Intervention
	Assess for signs of secondary infection in pleural area or in lungs themselves. If chest tube is in place, assess and provide care as indicated on pp. 242-246.
Gas exchange, impaired	Monitor for signs of restlessness, confusion, change in respiratory pattern, or irritability that may indicate altered blood gas levels resulting from compromised breathing. Monitor for signs of atelectasis resulting from decreased ventilation. Turn patient frequently to prevent pooling of secretions within lungs and pleural space.

Patient Education

1. Teach the patient the importance of positioning to facilitate ventilatory effort.
2. Teach the patient the importance of deep breathing and coughing to keep the lungs aerated and to prevent complications.
3. If pleural effusion is a recurrent problem, ensure that the patient is able to identify signs of accumulating fluid so care can be sought early.
4. Prepare the patient for thoracentesis.

EVALUATION

Patient Outcome	Data Indicating That Outcome is Reached
Minimal fluid remains in pleural space.	Chest roentgenogram shows no evidence of fluid accumulation.
Movement of air in and out of lungs is optimum.	Breath sounds are clear and bilaterally equal; percussion tone is resonant over all lung fields.
Cause of pleural effusion is identified and treated.	There is no recurrence of disease.

EMPYEMA

Empyema is the accumulation or presence of infected fluid or pus in the pleural space.

The accumulation of purulent exudate in the pleural cavity may occur in several ways. The most common cause is direct extension from adjacent structures as occurs in pneumonia, tuberculosis, pulmonary abscess, bronchiectasis, or esophageal rupture. Exudate accumulation may also occur from direct contamination such as that induced by penetrating chest wounds or by chest surgery or other penetrating therapeutic procedures. Empyema is an uncommon but serious disorder that is seen most often in debilitated patients. If identified early and treated promptly with antibiotics, the condition can usually be controlled.

area appears inflamed and has a thin layer of exudate with a low leukocyte count. If untreated, the exudate thickens and frank pus may be aspirated. The pleura may thicken, and adhesions may occur. Chronic empyema develops when there are recurrent infections or when treatment of a previous infection was incomplete. Treatment of chronic empyema is difficult because the pleura often becomes thickened and fibrous and the lung may adhere to the chest wall. If the lung does adhere to the chest wall, ventilation is decreased. Pleural fibrosis with secondary limited ventilatory capacity may result. In addition to the changes and restrictions of the lungs and chest wall, the multiloculated cavities within the pleural space fill with pus and are difficult to drain.

PATHOPHYSIOLOGY

There are two kinds of empyema, acute and chronic. Either may affect a small area of pleura or may involve the entire pleural cavity. In the acute stage the affected

DIAGNOSTIC STUDIES

History

Recent thoracic or abdominal surgery; blunt or penetrating chest trauma; esophageal fistula; lung infections; aspiration; recent thoracentesis; persistent fever despite administration of antibiotics

Physical examination

Foul-smelling sputum; pleural friction rub; localized chest pain; dullness to percussion; decreased breath sounds at bases of lungs; decreased vocal fremitus

Chest roentgenogram

Pleural fluid, usually unilateral, with associated lung lesion

Thoracentesis

Evidence of pus in pleural exudate (because pus is difficult to aspirate, large-bore needle [18 gauge or larger] must be used)

Laboratory examination of pleural exudate

Odor and general appearance; specific gravity; cell count; Gram stains; aerobic and anaerobic cultures (NOTE: When materials are sent for culture, all air must be expressed from syringe and sample must be quickly transported to laboratory for anaerobic evaluation)

pH

Of special diagnostic value; fluid collected and analyzed in same manner as for arterial blood gases (using capped, 5 to 10 cc heparinized syringe); pH less than 7.20 suggestive of empyema that necessitates chest tube drainage

TREATMENT PLAN

Surgical

Thoracentesis—may be done to drain purulent drainage if area is small and localized

Thoracic drainage—either closed or open drainage system for large areas or quantities of collected pus; if intrapleural fluid and pus are thin and localized, large-diameter thoracotomy tube may be inserted and connected to closed system under waterseal drainage; open drainage possible only if there is no danger of lung collapse when atmospheric pressure enters pleural space; for open drainage, thoracotomy tube exits to room air and is covered with large, absorbent, sterile dressing (see pp. 242-246 for detailed discussion of thoracic drainage systems)

Intrapleural aspiration and instillation of medications—chest tube may be used to aspirate pleural drainage and as vehicle for instillation of antibiotics and fibrinolytic enzymes

Thoracotomy—may be necessary for patients not effectively treated by tube drainage system; area with empyema is resected and thickened membrane is stripped by process called decortication to permit reexpansion of lung

Chemotherapeutic

Anti-infective agents

Antibiotic therapy based initially on results of Gram's stain; alterations made if necessary when culture results are available

Fibrinolytic agents

Controversial; recommended by several researchers as method to decrease viscosity of pus and dissolve fibrin clots

Trypsin (Granulex) as aerosol, 0.1 mg/0.82 ml with balsam of Peru and castor oil; spray bid to debride necrotic areas

Streptokinase (Kabikinase, Streptase), 100,000 units/h IV over 24-72 h for adults; converts plasminogen to proteolytic enzyme fibrinolysin, which breaks down fibrin clots

Electromechanical

Oxygen support—may be necessary if signs of hypoxia are present

Irrigation of pleural cavity with sterile solution—periodically for patient with thoracotomy tube in place to flush out purulent and necrotic materials

Supportive

Bed rest while patient is febrile and has drainage mechanism in process

Deep breathing and coughing to encourage maximal ventilation and decrease congestion resulting from pulmonary problem and bed rest; incentive spirometer may be used

ASSESSMENT: AREAS OF CONCERN

Respiratory insufficiency resulting from presence of pus in pleural space

Nasal flaring; tachypnea; decreased chest wall movement; dyspnea; restlessness; tachycardia; decreased breath sounds; paradoxic breathing; dull percussion tone; decreased vital capacity and minute volume; arterial blood gases must be assessed if signs of hypoxia are present

Characteristics and amount of purulent drainage from pleural cavity and physiologic response to accumulation

Amount, odor, and color of drainage; specimens sent periodically to laboratory for analysis and culture; response to purulent accumulation, including fever, respiratory distress, and pain

Bronchopulmonary infection
Temperature; sputum specimen for culture and sensitivity

Common complications (pericarditis, endocarditis, meningitis, brain abscess)
Signs that patient is becoming more ill; for specific signs refer to appropriate sections in text

NURSING DIAGNOSES and NURSING INTERVENTIONS

Nursing Diagnosis	Nursing Intervention
Breathing pattern, ineffective	Assess ventilation, including evaluation of breathing rate, rhythm, and depth; chest expansion; and presence of respiratory distress such as dyspnea, shortness of breath, nasal flaring, or prolonged expiratory phase.
	Assess potential of purulent collection to interfere with ventilation and vital capacity.
	Identify contributing factors such as airway clearance or obstruction, pain, level of consciousness, or weakness.
	Maintain patient in position that facilitates easy ventilation (head of bed in semi-Fowler's position).
	Encourage deep breathing, coughing, and use of incentive spirometer.
Gas exchange, impaired	Monitor for signs of restlessness, confusion, and irritability, which may indicate altered blood gas levels resulting from compromised breathing.
	Assess blood gases if hypoxia is anticipated.
	Monitor for signs of atelectasis resulting from decreased ventilation.
	Encourage deep breathing and coughing to loosen secretions and facilitate expectoration. Incentive spirometry may be used.
	Turn patient frequently to prevent pooling of secretions within lungs and pleural space.
Self-care deficit	Assess level of self-care deficit resulting from empyema and associated chest tubes (if used).
	Assist with activities of daily living as needed.
	Encourage progressive activity after fever and acute stage are over.
Fluid volume deficit, potential	If patient is febrile because of empyema, monitor hydration and maintain at adequate level.
Potential patient problem: secondary infection	Carefully observe for signs that could indicate a secondary infection; report observations to physician.
	Protect patient from known sources of secondary infection.

Patient Education

1. Teach the patient the importance of positioning to facilitate the ventilatory effort.
2. Teach the patient the importance of deep breathing and coughing to keep the lungs aerated and prevent complications.
3. If empyema is a recurrent problem, teach the patient to identify signs of the problem so care can be sought early.
4. Prepare the patient for thoracentesis or the insertion of chest tubes (see pp. 242 to 246).
5. If the patient is to go home with an open chest tube left in place for drainage, teach care techniques (such as aseptic dressing change).
6. Teach the patient and family about empyema; inform them that the healing process may be slow and that repeated treatments, drainage, irrigation, and chest roentgenograms may be necessary.

EVALUATION

Patient Outcome	Data Indicating That Outcome is Reached
No purulent material remains in pleural space.	Chest roentgenogram shows no evidence of pus accumulation.
Movement of air in and out of lungs is optimum.	Breath sounds are clear and bilaterally equal; percussion tone is resonant over all lung fields.

ACUTE BRONCHITIS

Acute bronchitis is an inflammation of the bronchi or trachea or both that results from irritation or infection. It is usually self-limiting. It may occur as a primary disorder and is also a prominent finding in many chronic diseases such as bronchiectasis, emphysema, or tuberculosis.

Acute bronchitis is most prevalent in winter. It may also be seen as a secondary problem associated with systemic illnesses such as chickenpox, measles, and influenza. Once the disease is in process, exposure to air pollutants or physical disabilities such as malnutrition or fatigue may exacerbate it. If the patient already has a chronic disease such as chronic pulmonary or cardiovascular disease, acute bronchitis may become serious. Pneumonia is perhaps the most common complication.

Most cases of infective acute bronchitis are viral in origin, but bacterial causes (for example, *Streptococcus pneumoniae, Haemophilus influenzae*) are also common. Irritative bronchitis may be caused by fumes or dust, such as from strong acids, ammonia, chlorine, bromide, or smoke.

PATHOPHYSIOLOGY

Hyperemia or congestion of the bronchial mucous membranes is the earliest physiologic change. This is followed by desquamation or shedding of the submucosa. The congestion and shedding process causes submucosal edema with leukocyte infiltration. This process interferes with the normal function of the ciliated bronchial epithelium and the phagocytes. The result is the production of a sticky or mucopurulent exudate that stays in the bronchi until coughed out. The coughing mechanism is stimulated to remove the debris.

Because of the removal of the normally protective sterile environment of the bronchi, bacteria may invade and cause a secondary bacterial infection. At the beginning of the disease process the sputum of a patient with acute bronchitis is normally mucoid. If the sputum becomes mucopurulent or purulent, a superimposed bacterial infection can be suspected.

If the patient already has impaired cough, lung, or bronchial functioning, acute bronchitis may lead to respiratory failure.

DIAGNOSTIC STUDIES

Clinical examination
Cough initially dry and nonproductive but may produce mucoid sputum within few days; fever (38.3° to 38.9° C [101° to 102° F]); if cause is bacterial, midsternal chest pain, malaise, sore throat, diffuse rales and rhonchi throughout chest; if patient already has chronic lung disease, sputum may change from clear and thin to thick and tenacious or purulent

Chest roentgenogram
Clear; no evidence of lung consolidation

Sputum
Mucoid; may be thick; purulent sputum suggestive of superimposed infection

TREATMENT PLAN

The goals of the treatment plan are to provide supportive therapy during the course of the self-limiting disease and to prevent secondary infections.

Chemotherapeutic
Antitussive agents
  Cough suppressants (use with extreme caution in patients with chronic lung diseases)
    Hydrocodone bitartrate (Codone, Dicodid, Hycodan), 5-10 mg tid or qid for adults and children over 12
    Codeine phosphate (tablets and in mixture form in numerous syrups), 10-20 mg q4-6h for adults, 2.5-5 mg q4-6h for children 2-6 years, 5-10 mg q4-6h for children 6-12 years
Nonnarcotic analgesic agents
  Many agents available; following is incomplete list
    Dextromethorphan (Romilar, Benylin CM, Pertussin, Congespirin), 10-20 mg q4h or 30 mg q6-8 h for adults, 2.5-5 mg q4h or 7.5 mg q6-8h for children 2-6 years; 5-10 mg q4h or 15 mg q6-8h for children 6-12 years
    Noscapine (Tusscapine, Narcotine), 15-30 mg tid or qid for adults, 7.5-15 mg tid or qid for children 2-6 years, 15 mg tid or qid for children 6-12 years
    Levopropoxyphene napsylate (Novrad), 50-100 mg q4-6h for adults, 1.1 mg/kg q4h for children
Bronchodilators
  Terbutaline (Brethine, Bricanyl), 2.5-5 mg tid for adults, 2.5 mg tid for children over 12
  Theophylline (Aerolate, Theolair, Slo-Phyllin, Theo-Dur, Bronkodyl, Elixophyllin, others); *dosage highly individualized based on serum theophylline levels;* therapeutic level 10-20 μg/ml; 200-250 mg q6h or 1-2 timed-release preparations q8-12h (3.5-5 mg/kg) for adults; 80-100 mg q6h (1-1.2 mg/kg/h) for children

Anti-infective agents

Antibiotics when superimposed respiratory infection is suspected on basis of clinical evidence such as purulent sputum, high fever, and ill-appearing patient; antibiotics also indicated for patients with chronic obstructive lung disease

Doxycyclin (Vibramycin), oxytetracycline (Terramycin), others, 250-500 mg po qid for adults, 6.25-12.5 mg/kg qid for children over 8; should not be used for children under 8

Ampicillin (Amcill, Omnipen, others), 250-500 mg po qid for adults and children over 20 kg, 12.5-25 mg/kg q6h for children under 20 kg

Antipyretic-analgesics

To reduce fever and relieve malaise

Supportive

Increase in fluid intake—up to 4000 ml/day to liquefy secretions and maintain hydration

Steam or mist vaporizer to humidify air surrounding patient

Rest to conserve energy

Culture of sputum if sputum becomes purulent or patient's illness becomes progressively worse

ASSESSMENT: AREAS OF CONCERN

Because acute bronchitis is generally a self-limiting disease, assessment is important to identify complications, superimposed infections, or adverse effects of therapy.

Respiratory status

Sibilant and sonorous rhonchi; wet rales at base; labored or irregular breathing; dyspnea; substernal tightness with breathing; back pain; cough characteristics and duration

Chest roentgenogram

No evidence of lung consolidation

Bronchopulmonary infection

If bacterial, fever (38.3° to 38.9° C [101° to 102° F]) lasting several days; mucopurulent or purulent sputum; send sputum specimen for culture and sensitivity

NURSING DIAGNOSES and NURSING INTERVENTIONS

Nursing Diagnosis	Nursing Intervention
Breathing pattern, ineffective	Assess ventilation to include evaluation of breathing rate, rhythm, and depth; chest expansion; presence of respiratory distress such as dyspnea, shortness of breath, nasal flaring, pursed-lip breathing, or prolonged expiratory phase; and use of accessory muscles. Maintain patient in position that facilitates easy ventilation (patient sitting upright and leaning on overbed table). See p. 2030 for additional strategies.
Gas exchange, impaired	Assess patient to identify signs, such as restlessness, confusion, and irritability, that may indicate body's response to altered blood gas states. Assist patient to avoid smoking, fumes, smoke, or other inhaled irritants that may aggravate current disease state. See p. 2035 for additional strategies.
Airway clearance, ineffective	Assess patient to identify inability to move secretions. If inability is identified, assist with appropriate measures (coughing, positioning, suctioning, liquefying secretions, and so on). Provide adequate hydration to ensure liquefaction of secretions. Avoid offering dairy products, which tend to increase viscosity of mucus.
Self-care deficit	See p. 2086 for associated nursing care.
Coping, family: potential for growth	Assess family's level of understanding of diagnostic procedures, disease process and prognosis, and therapies employed. See p. 1899 for associated nursing care.

Patient Education

1. Teach the patient the importance of consuming large quantities of fluid.
2. Teach the patient the importance of not smoking and of avoiding fumes or smoke when the disease is active.
3. Teach the patient the importance of rest during the course of the disease.
4. Teach the patient facts about and the importance of prescribed medications.
5. Teach the patient how to use antipyretic-analgesics to reduce fever and relieve malaise.
6. Teach the patient the importance of avoiding contact with others, who may transmit infection.
7. Teach the patient signs of secondary infection such as a change in sputum characteristics or prolonged fever that may be suggestive of secondary infection.

EVALUATION

Patient Outcome	Data Indicating That Outcome is Reached
Movement of air in and out of lungs is optimum.	Breath sounds are clear with no evidence of adventitious sounds.
Airways are patent.	Breathing occurs without cough or substernal tightness. Chest roentgenogram is clear.
Tracheobronchial tree returns to noninflamed, predisease state.	Cough is decreased. Sputum if present is mucoid.

BRONCHIOLITIS

Bronchiolitis is an acute viral infection of the lower respiratory tract that affects primarily infants and young children. It is characterized by lower airway obstruction causing respiratory distress, expiratory prolongation, and wheezing.

Acute bronchiolitis is common among infants and small children, especially those under 1 year of age. The incidence peaks at about 6 months of age.

The causative agent in approximately 50% of cases is the respiratory syncytial virus. The remaining cases are caused by the parainfluenza 3 virus, *Mycoplasma,* and the adenoviruses. Cases caused by adenoviruses may be associated with long-term complications, including bronchiolitis obliterans and unilateral hyperlucent lung disease.[62]

The source of infection is usually a family member with an apparently minor respiratory illness. Clinical symptoms of bronchiolitis do not develop in an adult or older child because the larger airways tolerate the bronchial edema.

The disease is generally noncomplicated and self-limiting. Recovery is usually complete in a few days. The death rate is less than 1%, and death is usually a result of prolonged periods of apnea, severe uncompensated respiratory acidosis, or profound dehydration because of tachypnea and inability to drink fluids.

This disease must be differentiated clinically from bronchial asthma and other entities. Factors indicating asthma are family history, patient age over 18 months, and history of repeated episodes not preceded by cold symptoms. Other entities that must be considered during differential diagnosis include a foreign body in the trachea, congestive heart failure, pertussis, and cystic fibrosis.

PATHOPHYSIOLOGY

The virus spreads from the upper airway to the small bronchi and bronchioles of the lower respiratory tract. As it affects the tissue, edema and exudate of mucus and cellular debris develop and partially obstruct the small airways. Airway resistance is increased, especially during the expiratory phase of ventilation. This leads to eventual air trapping and overinflation. Atelectasis may occur if the obstruction becomes complete and the trapped air is absorbed. Hypoxemia is the result of these physiologic changes. Carbon dioxide retention usually does not occur except in severely affected patients. Stern[62] states that carbon dioxide retention is seldom seen until respirations exceed 60 per minute.

DIAGNOSTIC STUDIES

History

Recent exposure to adult or older child with minor respiratory illness

Clinical examination

Initially, serous nasal discharge, sneezing, diminished appetite, and sometimes low-grade fever; in mild cases symptoms may not progress beyond hacking cough; in serious cases respiratory distress with tachypnea (60 to 80 breaths/minute), tachycardia, hacking cough, nasal flaring, subcostal and intercostal retractions, circumoral cyanosis, and eventual lethargy; on chest auscultation, wheezing, fine moist rales, prolonged expiration; percussion tones hyperresonant as result of air trapping

Chest roentgenogram

Hyperinflation of lungs; increased anteroposterior diameter; depressed diaphragm; scattered areas of consolidation caused by atelectasis or obstruction or inflammation of alveoli

Laboratory studies

White blood cells usually within normal limits; 50% to 75% lymphocytes in most cases (common with viral illness); electrolytes show amount of dehydration

TREATMENT PLAN

Bronchiolitis is generally self-limiting, and only supportive therapy is indicated. The child is kept at home unless severe signs of respiratory distress or secondary infection are noted.

Chemotherapeutic
Intravenous fluids
  Should be administered if signs of dehydration are present
Anti-infective agents
  Not indicated unless secondary infection has been identified
Corticosteroids

Not proved to be of benefit; under certain conditions have proved to be harmful
Bronchodilators
  Ineffective

Electromechanical
Oxygenation—to relieve hypoxemia; specifically if PaO_2 drops below 55 mm Hg; may be given by tent, hood, face mask, or endotracheal tube

Supportive
Head positioned at 30- to 40-degree angle to ease breathing
Clear fluids to prevent dehydration

ASSESSMENT: AREAS OF CONCERN

Respiratory status
Respiratory distress: dyspnea; tachypnea; hacking cough; prolonged expiration; retractions; nasal flaring

Hypoxia
Restlessness; circumoral cyanosis; tachycardia

Laboratory values
Decreased PaO_2; increased $PaCO_2$; decreased pH; increased eosinophils; increased hematocrit

Chest roentgenogram
Observe for foreign body, unilateral obstruction, or infiltration

Hydration
Intake and output measurement to monitor for dehydration

Psychosocial
In child, fear of oxygen therapy technique (need to stay in tent), fear related to hypoxia; in parent, fear related to child's condition and necessary treatment

NURSING DIAGNOSES and NURSING INTERVENTIONS

Nursing Diagnosis	Nursing Intervention
Breathing pattern, ineffective	Assess ventilation to include evaluation of breathing rate, rhythm, and depth; chest expansion; presence of respiratory distress such as dyspnea, shortness of breath, nasal flaring, or prolonged expiratory phase; and use of accessory muscles.
	Identify contributing factors such as airway clearance or obstruction problem or weakness.
	Maintain patient in position that facilitates easy ventilation (head elevated to 30- to 40-degree angle).
	Assess patient for tiring in relation to attempts to breathe.
	Protect patient from known sources of secondary infection.
	Should mechanical ventilation become necessary, provide care and monitoring consistent with guidelines on pp. 246-249.

Nursing Diagnosis	Nursing Intervention
Gas exchange, impaired	Monitor arterial blood gases as ordered. Report increases or decreases of more than 10 to 15 mm Hg in $Paco_2$ and Pao_2.
	Administer oxygen as ordered to maintain Pao_2 over 80 mm Hg. This may usually be maintained by administering oxygen via tent, hood, or mask or if necessary by endotracheal intubation with ventilatory support.
	Assess patient to identify signs, such as restlessness, confusion, and irritability, that may indicate body's response to altered blood gas states.
	If patient is seriously ill, monitor electrocardiogram and cardiac status for arrhythmias resulting from alterations in blood gases.
	Carefully monitor body temperature, which may fluctuate owing to alterations in metabolism or secondary infections.
Fluid volume deficit, potential	Monitor intake and output, which may be altered owing to patient's inability to take fluids because of sucking difficulty and hypoxia.
	Encourage fluids in small amounts at frequent intervals to prevent dehydration.
	Monitor electrolytes, which show indications of dehydration.
	Administer intravenous fluids as ordered to correct or prevent dehydration.
Coping, ineffective individual	If a child, patient may experience difficulty in coping with environment or separation from family. Involve family in care as much as possible.
	Encourage parents to stay with child.
	Encourage uninterrupted periods of rest.
Coping, ineffective family: compromised	Assess family's level of fear related to patient's present health state.
	Determine family's ability to cooperate with health care providers regarding intervention strategies for patient.
	Listen carefully to collect information regarding significance of current health care problem and family's perception of patient's condition.
	Involve family as much as possible in caring for patient.

Patient Education

Because most patients with bronchiolitis are under 2 years of age, the following patient education strategies are directed toward the parents.
1. Teach the parents the importance of encouraging fluid intake.
2. Teach the parents the importance of keeping the child in an oxygen tent or maintaining the source of oxygen if needed.
3. Teach the parents the importance of keeping the child away from persons with upper respiratory infections and influenza.

EVALUATION

Patient Outcome	Data Indicating That Outcome is Reached
Movement of air in and out of lungs is optimum.	Blood gases are within normal limits. Airways are clear, and breathing occurs without obstruction.
Breathing occurs without tiring patient.	There are no signs of respiratory distress or restlessness. Breath sounds are clear in all lung fields.
Physiologic stability is achieved after respiratory insult.	Nutrition level is maintained. Kidney and bladder functioning is within normal limits. There are no secondary infections. Serum electrolytes are within normal limits.

CROUP AND EPIGLOTTITIS

Croup is a generalized term used to describe a hetero-geneous group of relatively acute infectious conditions characterized by a brassy "croupy" cough, which may or may not be accompanied by inspiratory stridor, hoarseness, and respiratory distress resulting from laryngeal obstruction.

Several types of infections are responsible for causing the symptoms of croup. Of the following list, epiglottitis is the most serious and must always be ruled out first.

Acute epiglottitis—life-threatening, rapidly progressive, inflammatory infection of epiglottis and surrounding areas; may result in severe respiratory distress and dysphagia

Acute infectious laryngitis—common viral illness causing inflammation and swelling of larynx; usually mild and produces no respiratory distress

Acute laryngotracheobronchitis—most common form of croup; caused primarily by virus; respiratory difficulty and expiratory prolongation may occur

Acute spasmodic laryngitis—periodic episodes of coryza, hoarseness, barking cough, noisy respirations, and respiratory distress; viral in most cases, but allergic and psychologic factors sometimes important

Croup is caused primarily by the parainfluenza viruses and to a lesser extent by the respiratory syncytial virus (RSV). Epiglottitis-type croup is caused by *Haemophilus influenzae* type B. Croup caused by the parainfluenza

viruses tends to occur in the fall. Croup caused by RSV and *H. influenzae* is more likely to occur in the winter and spring. The viruses are commonly transmitted by airborne secretions.

Persons affected most frequently by croup are children between the ages of 6 months and 3 years. Epiglottitis-type croup occurs most frequently in children between 3 and 7 years of age.

For most children croup is relatively mild and gradually improves with home treatment and rest. Recovery time is 3 to 7 days.

Table 2-11 summarizes the four types of croup.

PATHOPHYSIOLOGY

Croup symptoms occur most commonly in young children. Their airways are smaller and thus predisposed to greater narrowing with swelling. The infection of the respiratory system is rarely limited to a single section of the respiratory tract. As the disease progresses, areas of the larynx, trachea, and bronchi may be affected. Thus, with the exception of the "bark"-type cough, the symptoms vary.

With all types of croup the infecting agent causes the tissue to become inflamed and swollen. As a result, secretions and airway resistance are increased. In epiglottitis, the most serious type, the epiglottis becomes swol-

Table 2-11
Causes and Characteristics of Croup

	Acute Epiglottitis	Acute Infectious Laryngitis	Acute Laryngotracheobronchitis	Acute Spasmodic Laryngitis
Description	Severe, rapid onset; progressive infection of epiglottis	Preceded by upper respiratory infection with cough and sore throat; mild symptoms	Most common type; preceded by upper respiratory infection and sore throat; mild symptoms	Sudden onset; preceded by coryza and hoarseness
Initial manifestation	Respiratory distress; high fever (over 38.8° C [102° F]); aphonia; drooling; stridor; child appears ill	Croup cough followed by air hunger and fatigue of varying degree; may have low-grade fever	Croup cough; restlessness and fear; symptoms worse at night and may last for several days; fever below 39.4° C (103° F); bilateral diminished breath sounds; rhonchi; scattered rales	Croup cough; respiratory distress; noisy respirations; restlessness and fear; usually afebrile; episodes may last only several hours and may recur several times
Age affected	3 to 7 years; may occur in younger child	3 months to 3 years	Infants and small children	1 to 3 years
Causative agent	*Haemophilus influenzae* type B	Viral agents	Viral agents	Viral agents; allergy; psychogenic factors

len and cherry red and causes mechanical obstruction of the airway. The obstruction leads to hoarseness, drooling, dysphagia, and respiratory distress. Unless it is corrected, fatal asphyxia may result. Other types of croup cause inflammation of the larynx, trachea, bronchi, bronchioles, and lung parenchyma. Because the swelling and inflammation occur in the subglottic region, the symptoms and condition may be serious but generally are not life threatening. The obstruction, if not corrected, results in pulmonary compromise leading to hypoxemia, hypercapnia, and atelectasis.

DIAGNOSTIC STUDIES

	Acute Epiglottitis	Acute Infectious Laryngitis	Acute Laryngotracheo-bronchitis	Acute Spasmodic Laryngitis
Clinical Examination				
Cough	Bark-type cough	Bark-type cough	Bark-type cough	Bark-type cough
Fever	High	Low	May be low or high	Afebrile
Drooling, aphonia	Present	Absent	Absent	Absent
Respiratory distress with stridor	Present	May be present	May be present	May be present
Pharynx	Inflamed	Inflamed	Inflamed	May be inflamed
Epiglottis	Swollen, cherry red	Appears normal	Appears normal	Appears normal
Chest roentgenogram	Lateral neck view shows upper airway narrowing and edema in subglottic folds (Fig. 2-33)	—	—	—
Complete blood count	Leukocytosis initially, later shifting to leukopenia and lymphocytosis	—	—	—
Throat culture	Presence of *Haemophilus influenzae* type B	—	—	—

TREATMENT PLAN

Chemotherapeutic
  Epiglottitis—broad-spectrum antibiotics while waiting for culture reports
    Anti-infective agents
      Ampicillin (Amcill, Omnipen, others), 50-200 mg/kg in equal doses over 24 h (generally given by IV q6h)
      Chloramphenicol (Chloromycetin), 50 mg/kg in equal doses over 24 h (generally given by IV q6h)
  Acute spasmodic croup—caused by allergic reaction
    Bronchodilators
      Epinephrine 1:1000, 0.01 mg/kg to maximum of 0.5 ml/dose subcutaneously
      Isoproterenol (Isuprel) 1:200, 0.01-0.5 ml/dose by aerosol
    Corticosteroids
      Hydrocortisone, 50-100 mg q6h

Electromechanical
  Oxygenation—may be indicated if respiratory distress becomes severe and results in PaO$_2$ less than 60 mm Hg; may be administered by oxygen mask or less efficiently by placing child in croup tent with supplemental oxygen
  Artificial airway—for epiglottitis; usually nasotracheal intubation or tracheotomy

Supportive
  Humidification—nebulizer of ''cold steam'' (safety advantage) or hot steam vaporizer, or steam of hot shower or bath in closed bathroom, to stop laryngeal spasm; cool humidification with croup tent or cold steam nebulizer placed near child's bed may help to prevent further laryngeal spasms

Fig. 2-33
Roentgenogram of patient with epiglottitis. Note closing off of tracheal airway at approximate CS4 location.

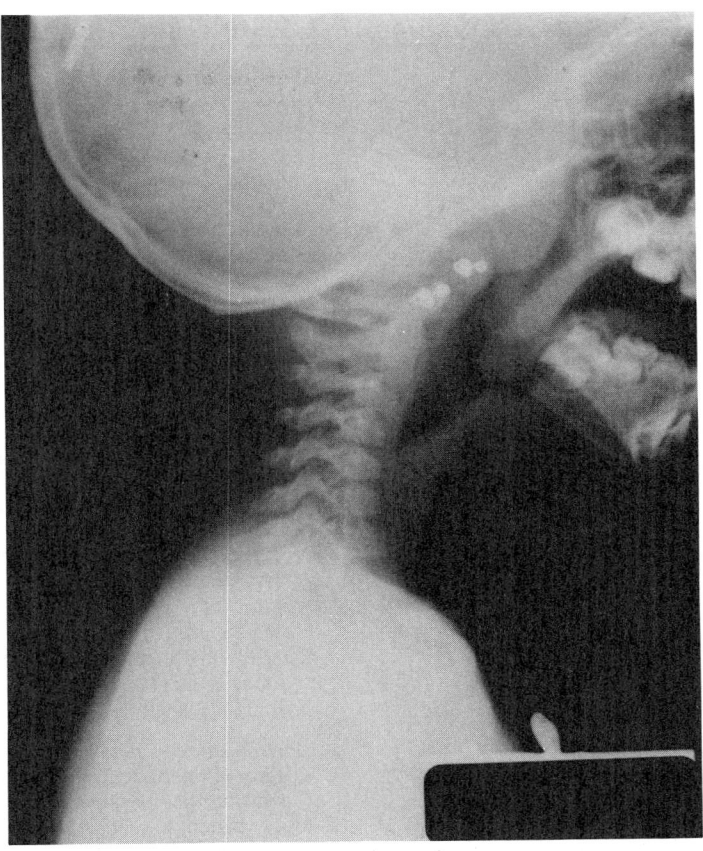

ASSESSMENT: AREAS OF CONCERN

History
Onset and previous symptoms important, especially in differentiating croup from possible foreign body aspiration

Respiratory distress
Dyspnea; cough; prolonged respirations; bronchospasm; diminished breath sounds over part of lung fields

Airway obstruction
Presence of or change in hoarseness, stridor, and cough

Hypoxia
Extreme restlessness; tachycardia; Pa_{CO_2} over 45 mm Hg; evidence of child tiring (indications for supportive oxygenation and ventilation)

Fever
Temperature monitored as indication of body's response to disease process

Fluid and electrolyte balance
Evidence of dehydration including skin turgor, urinary output, and alterations of electrolyte levels

Specific evidence of epiglottitis
Symptoms of croup with fever over 38.8° C (102° F); progressive stridor; respiratory distress; restlessness; hypoxia; cyanosis; pallor; depressed sensorium; ill appearance

NURSING DIAGNOSES and NURSING INTERVENTIONS

Nursing Diagnosis	Nursing Intervention
Breathing pattern, ineffective	Assess ventilation, including breathing rate, rhythm, and depth; chest expansion; presence of respiratory distress such as dyspnea, shortness of breath, nasal flaring, pursed-lip breathing, and prolonged expiratory phase; and use of accessory muscles.
	Identify contributing factors such as airway clearance or obstruction problem or weakness.
	Maintain patient in position that facilitates easy ventilation.
	Assess patient for tiring in relation to attempts to breathe.
	Provide rest and discourage activity as much as possible to decrease work of breathing.
	Protect patient from known sources of secondary infection.
	Should mechanical ventilation become necessary, provide care and monitoring consistent with guidelines on pp. 246-249.
Airway clearance, ineffective	Assess patient to identify inability to move secretions. If inability is identified, assist with appropriate measures (coughing, positioning, suctioning, liquefying secretions, and so on).
	Assess to detect airway clearance and impending airway obstruction resulting from tissue swelling.
	Provide humidification by croup tent or vaporizer.
	Provide hydration to liquefy secretions and replace fluids.
	Carefully and frequently auscultate chest for quality of breath sounds and adventitious sounds.
	Have tracheostomy tray at bedside as long as child is in acute distress.
Gas exchange, impaired	Monitor arterial blood gases as ordered. If unable to maintain PaO_2 above 60 mm Hg or if $PaCO_2$ is above 45 mm Hg, supplemental oxygen or ventilatory support must be considered.
	Assess patient to identify signs, such as restlessness, confusion, and irritability, that may indicate body's response to altered blood gas states.
	Monitor electrocardiogram and cardiac status for arrhythmias resulting from alterations in blood gases.
	Monitor serum electrolytes that may change owing to alterations in oxygenation and metabolism.
	Carefully monitor body temperature, which may fluctuate owing to alterations in metabolism during infection process.
Nutrition, alteration in: less than body requirement	As long as congestion and active signs of croup are present, encourage high-calorie liquids or administer fluids intravenously as ordered.
Fluid volume deficit, potential	Keep accurate records of intake and output.
	Administer advanced diet as tolerated.
	Encourage smaller, more frequent meals when fluids and food are tolerated.
	Monitor for signs and symptoms of dehydration.
Fear	Observe for signs of frustration or fear, fatigue, and tiring with attempts to communicate that result from hypoxia.
	Involve parents in care as much as possible to reduce child's fear.
	Avoid disturbances when child is resting.
Coping, family: potential for growth	Assess family's perception of and reaction to diagnostic procedures, disease process and prognosis, and therapies employed.
	See p. 1899 for additional strategies.

Patient Education

Because most patients with croup are under 7 years of age, the following patient education strategies are directed toward the parents.

1. Assess the parents' current knowledge and skills regarding croup and the care of croup.
2. Teach the parents techniques for providing vaporized cool or warm steam at home.
3. Teach the parents the importance of recognizing signs that might indicate worsening of the child's condition or the presence of epiglottitis.
4. Teach the parents the importance of increasing fluid intake and maintaining nutrition while the child is ill.
5. Teach the parents the importance of keeping the child in a croup tent or close to an oxygen source as long as necessary.
6. Teach the parents facts about and the importance of prescribed medications.

EVALUATION

Patient Outcome	Data Indicating That Outcome is Reached
Movement of air in and out of lungs is optimum. Airway is patent.	Child shows no signs of croup, such as ''bark''-type cough, or other signs of respiratory distress. Blood gas values are within normal limits. Airways are clear, and breathing occurs without obstruction. Breath sounds are clear in all lung fields.
Breathing occurs without tiring patient.	There are no signs of respiratory distress or restlessness.
Physiologic stability is achieved after respiratory insult.	Nutrition level is maintained. Kidney and bladder functioning is within normal limits. There is no secondary infection. Serum electrolytes are within normal limits.

LUNG ABSCESS

Lung abscess is an inflammatory lesion in the lung accompanied by necrosis. The abscess, which usually has well-defined borders, may be putrid (containing anaerobic bacteria) or nonputrid (containing aerobic bacteria).

The incidence of lung abscess has dropped significantly owing to the availability of effective antibiotics and the increased willingness of individuals to seek medical care. Lung abscesses are generally caused by the aspiration of infected material, which may occur during unconsciousness, general anesthesia, alcoholism, near-drowning, diabetic coma, or drug sedation or as a result of poor oral hygiene, gingival disease, infected tonsils, or aspiration of food. Bronchial carcinoma (squamous cell type) is also considered to be a common cause of lung abscess for male smokers over 55 years of age. Other, less common causes of lung abscess include septic pulmonary emboli from a pulmonary infarct and abscess transfers from the liver. Following are the common causes of lung abscess:

Alcoholism*

Coma*
Laryngeal palsy*
Septic emboli
Necrotic lesions
Infected tonsils*
Anesthesia*
Oral infection*
Carcinoma of esophagus
Pneumonia
Pyogenic bacteria
Infected cysts
Oversedation*
Food or foreign body*
Pulmonary infarct
Open chest wounds

PATHOPHYSIOLOGY

The site of the abscess is determined by the body's position at the time of aspiration. The aspirate gravitates to the most dependent position in the lung. Once the aspirate has settled, a fibrous granulation tissue forms

*May lead to aspiration or secretions and therefore to lung abscess.

around it and it embeds itself in the parenchyma.

As the abscess develops, it fills with pus. Pressure develops, and the granulated portion ruptures into the bronchus. Drainage of foul-smelling, purulent or bloody sputum results. The expectoration of purulent sputum may lead to partial healing and cavity formation. However, if the cavity does not drain adequately, small abscesses may form within the lung.

DIAGNOSTIC STUDIES

Clinical examination
Initial signs resembling pneumonia; cough producing bloody, purulent, foul-smelling sputum; general malaise; sporadic fever; pleuritic pain; dyspnea if abscess is large; dull percussion tone; rales; decreased or absent breath sounds over abscess area; pleural friction rub; if abscess left untreated and becomes chronic, auscultation may detect only fine rales or rhonchi; may be weight loss, anemia, and hypertrophic pulmonary osteoarthropathy

Chest roentgenogram
Initially, lobar consolidation, which becomes globular as disease progresses; rupture of consolidation causes fluid level, which indicates communication with bronchus; when fluid level is apparent, diagnosis can be narrowed down to either empyema with a bronchopleural fistula or a lung abscess

Laboratory examination of pleural exudate
Odor and general appearance; specific gravity; cell count; Gram stains; aerobic and anaerobic cultures to determine infective organisms; therapeutic intervention based on agent identification (NOTE: When material is sent for culture, all air must be expressed from syringe and sample must be quickly transported to laboratory for anaerobic evaluation)

White blood cell count
Leukocytosis common

Bronchoscopy
Unnecessary if roentgenography shows rapid resolution of abscess, but may be needed to verify presence of abscess or determine its severity if patient's condition does not improve

TREATMENT PLAN

The ability of the lung abscess to heal depends primarily on its ability to drain adequately through the bronchus. With free drainage, resolution occurs. Without free drainage, and without prompt antibiotic therapy, the abscess may become chronic.

Surgical
Bronchoscopy—occasionally necessary to remove thick, tenacious sputum

Pulmonary resection—necessary in rare cases if lung abscess does not respond to antibiotic therapy; single lesions removed by lobectomy and multiple lesions removed by pneumonectomy

Chemotherapeutic
Anti-infective agents
Antibiotic therapy directed at causative agent; should be monitored and perhaps changed depending on patient's clinical response; should begin as soon as the initial sputum specimens have been collected; drug of choice while awaiting test results is penicillin G, 1.2 million units po qid, or 300,000-600,000 units IM q6-8h; if after 4-7 d patient is not improved and specific organism is still not identified, medication may be changed to tetracycline (Achromycin, others), 500 mg po qid; antibiotic therapy continued until all signs of abscess are resolved on serial chest roentgenograms

Supportive
Postural drainage—extremely important to drain abscess (see pp. 239-242 for techniques)

Percussion—to loosen secretions and enhance their removal

Daily measurement of sputum volume output and assessment of sputum characteristics

ASSESSMENT: AREAS OF CONCERN

Characteristics and amount of purulent drainage from pleural cavity and physiologic response to infection
Amount, odor, and color of drainage; periodic specimens to laboratory for analysis and culture; body response to infectious process, including fever, respiratory distress, pleuritic chest pain, chills, diaphoresis, and weight loss; evidence that abscess continues to drain freely

Respiratory insufficiency resulting from presence of abscess in pleural cavity
Dyspnea; restlessness; tachycardia; decreased breath sounds; evidence of pleural friction rub; rales; rhonchi; dull percussion tones

Chest roentgenogram
Serial chest roentgenograms to monitor healing process of lung abscess

Response to antibiotic therapy
Monitoring of response to treatment process; if not improved, assessment for additional underlying cause of abscess such as tumor, or foreign body

Psychosocial
Concern that there is infection that must be treated for extended period of time

NURSING DIAGNOSES and NURSING INTERVENTIONS

Nursing Diagnosis	Nursing Intervention
Airway clearance, ineffective	Assess patient to identify inability to move secretions. If inability is identified, assist with appropriate measures (such as coughing, positioning, suctioning, and liquefying secretions). Assist patient to maintain proper body positioning to ensure maximum airway availability and to promote drainage position that will facilitate drainage of lobe. Provide hydration to liquefy secretions and replace fluids. Perform postural drainage with percussion at least 1 hour before meals; provide oral hygiene after treatment. Carefully and frequently auscultate chest for quality of breath sounds and adventitious sounds. Assess potential of purulent collection to interfere with ventilation. If necessary provide suctioning to remove sputum drainage. Note color, odor, and amount of sputum daily. Administer antibiotics as ordered.
Breathing pattern, ineffective	Assess ventilation, including evaluation of breathing rate, rhythm, and depth, chest expansion, breathing difficulty, or dyspnea. Identify contributing factors such as airway clearance or obstruction problem or weakness. Assess patient for tiring in relation to attempts to breathe. Protect patient from known sources of secondary infection or breathing irritation such as smoking.
Gas exchange, impaired	Monitor for signs of restlessness, confusion, and irritability, which may indicate altered blood gas levels resulting from compromised breathing. Assess blood gases if hypoxia is anticipated. Monitor for signs of atelectasis resulting from decreased ventilation. Encourage deep breathing and coughing to loosen secretions and facilitate expectoration. Assist patient to turn frequently to prevent pooling of secretions within lungs. Monitor white blood cells and electrolytes to evaluate changes that may be due to alterations in oxygenation, metabolism, and infection. Carefully monitor body temperature, which may fluctuate owing to alterations in metabolism or infectious process.
Self-care deficit: hygiene	Provide mouth care and toothbrushing after postural drainage and chest physiotherapy, as well as every several hours as long as abscess is draining. Encourage use of mouthwash to remove tastes associated with drainage.
Anxiety	Assess patient's level of anxiety related to present health state. See p. 1839 for additional strategies.
Coping, ineffective individual	Determine patient's ability to cooperate with health care providers regarding intervention strategies, such as frequent postural drainage sessions and need to sleep in positions that will facilitate abscess drainage. See p. 1897 for additional strategies.

Patient Education

1. Teach the patient the importance of positioning to facilitate abscess drainage.
2. Teach the patient the importance of deep breathing and coughing to keep the lung aerated and to prevent secondary complications.
3. Teach the patient facts about and the importance of prescribed medications such as antibiotics.
4. Provide the patient and family with information re- garding lung abscess and the treatment protocol, which may last as long as 6 to 8 weeks.
5. Teach the patient the importance of good oral hygiene, especially as long as there is active lung drainage.
6. Teach the patient methods to reduce the chances of a lung abscess in the future, such as good oral hygiene, avoidance of aspiration, and prompt medical attention for potential bacterial infection of the mouth or re- spiratory tract.

EVALUATION

Patient Outcome	Data Indicating That Outcome is Reached
No purulent material remains in lungs, and there is no evidence of lung abscess.	Serial chest roentgenograms show progressive improvement and healing. Temperature and laboratory values return to normal.
Movement of air in and out of lung is optimum.	Airways are clear and breathing occurs without obstruction. Breath sounds are clear and bilaterally equal; percussion tone is resonant over all lung fields.
Cause of lung abscess has been identified and treated.	Disease state does not recur.
Patient and family have sufficient information to comply with discharge regimen.	Patient and family at time of discharge are able to discuss med- ications (purpose, side effects, and route) and signs of ad- ditional infection or respiratory deterioration.

PNEUMONIA AND PNEUMONITIS

Pneumonia is an inflammatory process of the respiratory bronchioles and the alveolar spaces that is caused by infection. Pneumonitis is bronchial and alveolar inflam- mation of a noninfectious nature. Together, these terms are used to refer to inflammatory processes of the pa- renchyma of the lung.

Pneumonia is the most common cause of death from infectious disease in North America. It is also considered to be the major source of morbidity and mortality in critically ill patients.[38] Despite the use of antibiotics, pneumonia still accounts for 27.7 of every 100,000 deaths.[47]

Pneumonia may be caused by bacteria, viruses, *My- coplasma*, fungi, and parasites. Currently, approximately 50% of pneumonia is caused by bacteria and 50% is caused by virus. Up to 96% of bacterial pneumonia is caused by three organisms. Most of the organisms require specific therapy. It is therefore important to identify the specific causative agent.

Pneumonia is seen most frequently during the winter and early spring and in persons 60 years or older. The disease usually resolves within 2 to 3 weeks.

Bacterial Pneumonia

Streptococcus pneumoniae (pneumococcal) pneumonia. *S. pneumoniae* (hemolytic streptococcus type A), a gram-positive diplococcus, is by far the most common and important cause of bacterial pneumonia, accounting for 90% of cases. The infection usually results in extensive consolidation of part or all of the parenchyma of the lobe. *S. pneumoniae* pneumonia is frequently seen in infants, the elderly, and patients with sickle cell dis- ease, congestive heart failure, alcoholism, or diabetes mellitus. A vaccine is now available and is 80% to 90% effective against this type of pneumonia in adults.

Straphylococcus aureus pneumonia. *S. aureus*, a gram-positive coccus, may cause pneumonia as a primary disease in infants and the elderly and commonly causes pneumonia as a complication of influenza or in hospi- talized patients as a secondary infection after surgery, tracheostomy, coma, or immunosuppressive therapy. It accounts for 3% to 5% of bacterial pneumonia.

Haemophilus influenzae (type B) pneumonia. *H. influenzae*, a gram-negative bacillus, causes primary dis- ease in adults such as lobar-type pneumonia, broncho- pneumonia, or bronchiolitis. It accounts for 1% of bac- terial pneumonia.

Nonbacterial Pneumonia

Atypical pneumonia

Mycoplasma pneumoniae pneumonia. Infection with *M. pneumoniae*, which is seen most frequently among school-aged children and young adults, spreads among family members. Transmission is believed to be by contact with infected respiratory secretions. *M. pneumoniae* pneumonia is a type of bronchopneumonia.

Legionella pneumophila. *L. pneumophila*, a weakly organized gram-negative organism, is identified with a special fluorescent antibody stain. The disease, commonly called Legionnaires' disease, occurs most commonly in older adults and in persons who smoke or have predisposing chronic disease such as diabetes, renal disease, cancer, chronic bronchitis, or emphysema. It is three times more common in men than in women.

Aspiration Pneumonia Syndrome

Aspiration pneumonia syndrome occurs most commonly as a result of aspiration when the patient is in an altered state of consciousness owing to a seizure, drugs, alcohol, anesthesia, acute infection, or shock. It may also occur when the anatomy is altered by esophageal stricture, tracheal fistula, a nasogastric tube, or a tracheotomy. Aspiration pneumonia may be acquired through foreign body aspiration. Nonbacterial aspiration pneumonia may follow aspiration of toxic materials such as toxic fluids and inert substances; bacterial aspiration pneumonia may occur as a secondary problem.

The causative agents of bacterial pneumonia include the gram-positive coccus *Staphylococcus aureus*, the gram-negative coccus *Escherichia coli*, and the gram-negative bacilli *Klebsiella pneumoniae*, *Pseudomonas aeruginosa*, *Proteus*, and *Enterobacter*.

All of these bacterial aspiration pneumonias have a poor prognosis even with antibiotic therapy. They may cause extensive lung damage resulting in lung abscess or empyema. Mortality is 70% with *P. aeruginosa*, 45% with *E. coli*, 25% to 50% with *K. pneumoniae*, and 15% to 50% with *S. aureus*.[50]

PATHOPHYSIOLOGY

The pathophysiology depends on the etiologic agent. Bacterial pneumonia is characterized by an intra-alveolar suppurative exudate with consolidation. Lobar pneumonia causes consolidation of the entire lobe (see Fig. 2-34). Bronchopneumonia causes a patchy distribution of infectious areas around and involving the bronchi. A chest roentgenogram of bronchopneumonia shows patchy segmental or subsegmental infiltration in one or more dependent lobes.

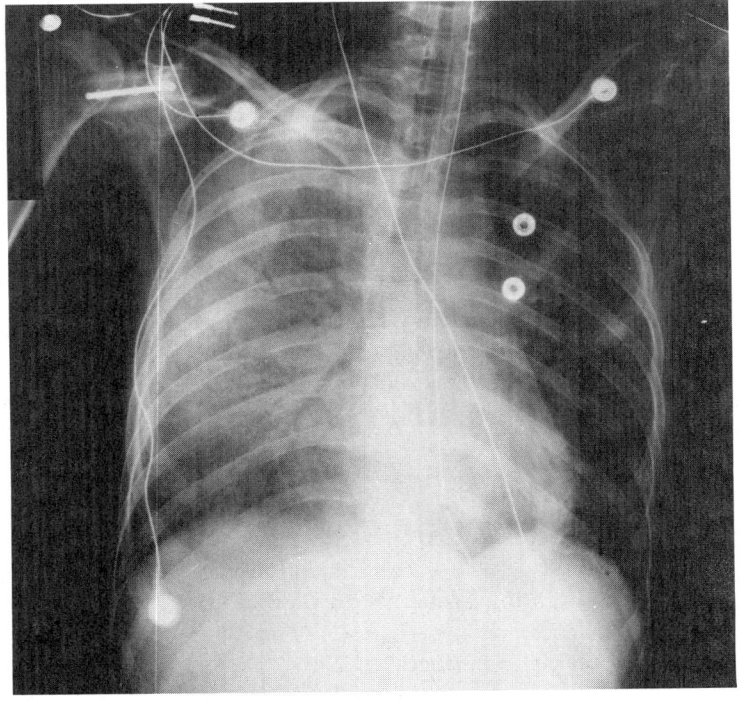

Fig. 2-34
Chest roentgenogram of patient with pneumonia. Note infiltrate of right middle and lower zones with air bronchogram seen; right heart border not obliterated. Also note monitor electrodes, gown snaps, endotracheal tube, and ventilator tubing.

Courtesy R. Keith Wilson, M.D., Baylor College of Medicine, Houston, Texas.

Mycoplasmal and viral pneumonia produces interstitial inflammation with accumulation of an infiltrate in the alveolar walls. There is no consolidation or exudate.

Fungal and mycobacterial pneumonia is characterized by patchy distribution of granulomas that may undergo necrosis with the development of cavities.

The most extensively studied type of pneumonia is pneumococcal or streptococcal pneumonia. The bacteria are thought to reach the alveoli in mucus or saliva. In the alveoli they undergo four predictable phases[50]:

1. *Engorgement (first 4 to 12 hours).* Serous exudate pours into alveoli from the dilated, leaking blood vessels.
2. *Red hepatization (next 48 hours).* The lung assumes a red granular appearance as red blood cells, fibrin, and polymorphonuclear leukocytes fill the alveoli.
3. *Gray hepatization (3 to 8 days).* The lung assumes a grayish appearance as the leukocytes and fibrin consolidate in the involved alveoli.
4. *Resolution (7 to 11 days).* Exudate is lysed and resorbed by macrophages, restoring the tissue to its original structure.

These stages represent the course of untreated pneumococcal pneumonia. With the use of antibiotics the course should run 3 to 5 days.

Viral pneumonia affects the tissues differently. The inflammatory response in the bronchi damages the ciliated epithelium. The lungs are congested and in some cases hemorrhagic. The inflammatory response is composed of mononuclear cells, lymphocytes, and plasma cells in proportions that vary with the type of virus causing the disease. In severe types of viral pneumonia the alveoli contain hyaline membranes. Characteristic intracellular viral inclusions may be seen in adenovirus, cytomegalovirus, respiratory syncytial virus, or varicella virus infections.

Aspiration pneumonia presents a still different physiologic response, which is based on the pH of the aspirated substance. If the pH is 2.5 or above, little necrosis results. If, however, the pH is below 2.5, atelectasis occurs, followed by pulmonary edema, hemorrhage, and type II cell necrosis. The alveolar-capillary "membrane" may be damaged, leading to exudation and in severe cases adult respiratory distress syndrome.[46]

DIAGNOSTIC STUDIES

Clinical examination (depends on type of pneumonia)

Streptococcal, pneumococcal
  Sudden onset; chest pain; chills; fever; headache; cough; rust-colored sputum; rales and possibly friction rub; hypoxemia as blood is shunted away from area of consolidation; cyanosis; area of consolidation visible on chest roentgenogram; sputum culture needed to determine causative agent

Staphylococcal
  Many of same signs as streptococcal; sputum copious and salmon colored

Klebsiella
  Many of same signs as streptococcal; onset more gradual; more bronchopneumonia visible on chest roentgenogram; if treatment delayed beyond second day after onset, patient will become critically ill; mortality high

Haemophilus
  Commonly follows upper respiratory infection; low-grade fever; croupy cough; malaise; arthralgias; yellow or green sputum

Mycoplasmal
  Gradual onset; headache; fever; malaise; chills; cough severe and nonproductive; decreased breath sounds and rales; chest roentgenogram clear; white blood cell count normal

Viral
  Symptoms generally mild; cold symptoms; headache; anorexia; fever; myalgia; irritating cough that produces mucopurulent or bloody sputum; bronchopneumonic type of infiltration on chest roentgenogram; white blood cell count usually normal; rise in antibody titers

Sputum examination

Sputum from lower respiratory tract needed for assessment; if necessary, may be obtained by needle aspiration, transtracheal aspiration, fiberoptic bronchoscopy, or open lung biopsy; sputum *must* be examined before initiation of antibiotic therapy

Macroexamination for odor, consistency, amount, color (see above for anticipated color)

Microexamination including Gram stain for etiologic agent, neutrophilia, increased epithelial cells, presence of other organisms

Sputum culture for organism identification; although routinely done, culture thought to be only 50% sensitive for pneumococcal disease and only 35% to 50% sensitive for pneumonia caused by *Haemophilus influenzae*[46]

Blood cultures

May be transient bacteremia in pneumococcal pneumonia

Acid-fast stains and cultures

To rule out tuberculosis

Serum specimen for cold agglutinins

10 ml of clotted blood needed for test; used for dif-

ferential diagnosis of viral or mycoplasmal infections; cold agglutinins present in about 50% of diseases caused by these two agents

White blood cell count

Leukocytosis (15,000 to 25,000/mm^3); neutrophilia (normal or low white blood cell count in mycoplasmal or viral infection)

Chest roentgenogram

Presence of density changes involving primarily lower lobes (Fig. 2-34)

Lung function studies

Volumes—congestion and collapse of alveoli; decreased lung volumes

Pressures—in increased airway resistance and decreased compliance

Gas exchange—shunting as a result of hypoxemia

TREATMENT PLAN

Surgical

Thoracentesis with chest tube insertion—may be necessary if secondary problem such as empyema occurs

Chemotherapeutic

Anti-infective agents

The main therapy for pneumonia is etiology specific; the following are drugs of first choice for specific organisms

Streptococcus pneumoniae—penicillin G, 1.2-2.4 million units IV or IM

Staphylococcus aureus—semisynthetic penicillin such as nafcillin or oxacillin, 4-12 g IV

Haemophilus influenzae—ampicillin, 4-8 g IV

Mycoplasma pneumoniae—erythromycin or tetracycline, 2 g/d po

Klebsiella pneumoniae—gentamicin, 3-5 mg/kg IM or IV, and cephalothin, 4-12 g IV

Pseudomonas aeruginosa—carbenicillin, 300-400 mg/kg IV, and tobramycin, 3-5 mg/kg IV or IM

Escherichia coli—gentamicin, 3-5 mg/kg IV, and cephalothin, 4-12 g IV, or ampicillin, 4-8 g IV

Proteus—ampicillin, 4-8 g IV

Enterobacter—tobramycin, 3-5 mg/kg IV or IM

Bronchodilators

May be indicated if patient has bronchospasm or secondary condition such as chronic obstructive pulmonary disease or asthma

Electromechanical

Humidification—Humidifier or nebulizer if secretions are thick and copious

Oxygenation—if patient has PaO_2 less than 60 mm Hg; Venturi mask or nasal prongs commonly used

Supportive

Physiotherapy—role in hastening resolution of pneumonia uncertain; patient should be encouraged at least to cough and deep breathe to maximize ventilatory capabilities[46]

Hydration—monitoring of intake and output; supplemental fluids to maintain hydration and liquefy secretions

ASSESSMENT: AREAS OF CONCERN

Respiratory status

Tachypnea; retractions; labored breathing; dyspnea; nasal flaring; rales; pleural friction rub; diminished breath sounds over area of consolidation; hypoventilation; labored or irregular breathing; breathing tiring for patient; percussion tone dull over area of consolidation

Hypoxia

Restlessness; confusion; tachycardia; cyanosis

Laboratory values

If patient seriously ill, monitor for decreased pH and PaO_2 and increased $PaCO_2$; evidence of elevated leukocyte count

Temperature

Must be carefully monitored and controlled because of nature of infection

Cough and sputum

Amount and productivity of coughing; color, consistency, odor, and amount of sputum; fatigue related to coughing; periodic laboratory evaluation of sputum needed to evaluate patient's response to treatment

Hydration state

Intake and output; tissue turgor; liquidity of sputum; electrolytes

Chest roentgenogram

Periodic evaluation to monitor improvement

Potential complications

Complications most common with pneumonia caused by gram-negative bacteria

Pleurisy

Pleuritic pain; fever; shallow, rapid breathing; dull

percussion tones; occasional hemoptysis with coughing; pleural friction rub

Atelectasis

Pleuritic pain; tachypnea; dyspnea; absence of breath sounds over affected area; anxiety; cyanosis; flat percussion tone over area; mediastinal shift toward affected side

Empyema

Persistent fever despite antibiotics; foul-smelling sputum; pleural friction rub; localized chest pain; dullness to percussion; decreased breath sounds at bases of lung; decreased vocal fremitus

Lung abscess

Usually foul-smelling and purulent sputum (unless abscess is walled off); high fever; chest pain; persistent fever despite antibiotics

Pulmonary edema

Acute respiratory distress; frothy, red-tinged sputum; coarse rales or rhonchi; tachycardia and tachypnea; diaphoresis; moist noisy breathing

Superinfection pericarditis

Sharp, sudden chest pain that radiates to neck, shoulders, and back; pericardial friction rub; tachycardia; fever; dyspnea; possible pulsus paradoxus; elevated ST segment on electrocardiogram; elevated white blood cell count; widened space between pericardial layers on echocardiogram; erythrocyte sedimentation rate elevated

Meningitis

Nuchal rigidity; altered neurologic signs; fever; papilledema; positive Kernig's sign; projectile vomiting

NURSING DIAGNOSES and NURSING INTERVENTIONS

Nursing Diagnosis	Nursing Intervention
Airway clearance, ineffective	Assess patient to identify inability to move secretions. If inability is identified, assist with appropriate measures (such as coughing, positioning, suctioning, and liquefying secretions). Promptly administer bronchodilators, mucolytics, and expectorants per protocol to dilate bronchioles and remove secretions. Observe for therapeutic response and side effects. Assist patient to maintain body position that ensures maximum airway availability (semi-Fowler's position or sitting upright and leaning on overbed table). Provide hydration to liquefy secretions and replace fluids. Carefully and frequently auscultate chest for quality of breath sounds and adventitious sounds. Note cough and sputum characteristics.
Breathing pattern, ineffective	Assess ventilation to include evaluation of breathing rate, rhythm, and depth; chest expansion; presence of respiratory distress such as dyspnea, shortness of breath, nasal flaring, pursed-lip breathing, or prolonged expiratory phase; and use of accessory muscles. Identify contributing factors such as airway clearance or obstruction problem or weakness. Maintain patient in position that facilitates ventilation (head of bed in semi-Fowler's position or patient sitting and leaning forward on overbed table). Instruct patient in proper pulmonary hygiene routines that will promote easy and effective breathing, facilitate removal of secretions from tracheobronchial tree, and minimize pulmonary congestion, which could lead to superinfections. Assess patient for tiring in relation to attempts to breathe. Protect patient from known sources of secondary infection.
Gas exchange, impaired	If necessary and with physician consultation, administer oxygen by nasal cannula or Venturi mask to maintain Pao_2 above 60 mm Hg. Assess patient to identify signs, such as restlessness, confusion, and irritability, that may indicate body's response to altered blood gas states. Monitor serum electrolytes that may change owing to alterations in oxygenation and metabolism. Carefully monitor body temperature, which may fluctuate owing to alterations in metabolism or infection.
Health maintenance, alteration in	Provide strict isolation for patient with pneumonia caused by *Staphylococcus* (see Chapter 15 for techniques). Adhere to strict handwashing to prevent spread of disease.

Nursing Diagnosis	Nursing Intervention
Nutrition, alteration in: less than body requirements	Help patient choose foods that are easy to chew and swallow. Assist by cutting and feeding if patient tires easily. See p. 2042 for additional strategies.
Fluid volume deficit, potential	If patient is seriously ill, monitor for evidence of dehydration resulting from fever and lack of fluid intake. Carefully monitor intake and output. Encourage fluid intake if needed.
Mobility, impaired physical	Encourage patient to use adaptive breathing techniques to decrease work of breathing. Assist patient to alternate activities with periods of rest. Encourage gradual increase of activities as tolerated. If patient is seriously ill and maintained on bed rest, encourage or provide active or passive range of motion to maintain adequate muscle tone.
Self-care deficit	Assess level of self-care deficit resulting from patient's current condition.
Anxiety	Assess patient's level of anxiety related to present health state.
Coping, ineffective individual	Assess patient's emotional response to feeling of air hunger or pulmonary congestion. Determine patient's ability to cooperate with health care providers in intervention strategies such as breathing techniques and coughing exercises. See p. 1897 for additional strategies.
Coping, family: potential for growth	Assess family's understanding of diagnostic procedures, disease process and prognosis, and therapies employed. Involve family in care as appropriate. Teach family about strict handwashing to prevent spread of pneumonia.

Patient Education

1. Teach the patient deep breathing and coughing techniques.
2. Teach the family the importance of handwashing when working with the patient to prevent the spread of the disease.
3. Teach the patient and family facts about and the importance of prescribed medications such as antibiotics.
4. Provide the patient and family with information regarding the specific type of pneumonia the patient has, treatment, anticipated response, possible complications, and probable disease duration.
5. Inform the patient and family that a change in health status must be reported to the patient's health care providers. Indicators of change may include a change in sputum characteristics or color, decreased activity tolerance, fever despite the antibiotics, increasing chest pain, or a feeling that things are not getting better.
6. Teach the patient the importance of consuming large quantities of fluid.
7. Teach the patient adaptive exercise and rest techniques.

EVALUATION

Patient Outcome	Data Indicating That Outcome is Reached
Movement of air in and out of lungs is optimum.	Airways are clear, and breathing occurs without obstruction.
Airway is patent.	There is no cough or pulmonary congestion and no sputum production.
Breath sounds are clear in all areas.	Bronchovesicular breath sounds are heard throughout lungs. There are no areas of decreased breath sounds or consolidation.
Physiologic stability is achieved after pneumonia.	Nutrition level is maintained. Kidney and bladder functioning is within normal limits. There is no secondary infection. Serum electrolytes are within normal limits.

Patient Outcome	Data Indicating That Outcome is Reached
Patient and family have sufficient information to comply with discharge regimen.	Patient and family at time of discharge are able to discuss medications (purpose, side effects, route, and schedule), dietary therapy regimen, activity progression regimen, and signs of secondary infection.

COR PULMONALE AND PULMONARY HYPERTENSION

Cor pulmonale is a condition of hypertrophy and dilation of the right ventricle of the heart resulting from a disease process that affects the function or structure of the lung or its vasculature. This may occur with or without heart failure. Pulmonary hypertension is an increase in the main pulmonary artery pressure at rest or during exercise. This means that the systolic/diastolic pressure in the pulmonary artery exceeds 30/15 mm Hg at rest.

Cor pulmonale occurs as a secondary process following a primary pulmonary disease. The four most common disorders leading to cor pulmonale are restrictive lung diseases, obstructive lung diseases, chest wall disorders, and vascular diseases:

Obstructive lung diseases
    Chronic bronchitis
    Emphysema
    Asthma
    Cystic fibrosis
    Bronchiectasis
Vascular disease
    Thromboembolism
Restrictive lung diseases
    Atelectasis
    Pneumonia
    Interstitial fibrosis
    Sarcoidosis
Chest wall disorders
    Kyphoscoliosis

Chronic obstructive pulmonary disease accounts for approximately 75% of cases of cor pulmonale in the United States.

There are four primary factors in the development of cor pulmonale and right-sided failure: (1) reduction in the size of the pulmonary vascular bed as a result of destruction of pulmonary capillaries or loss of large amounts of lung tissue; (2) increased resistance in the pulmonary vascular bed; (3) shunting of nonaerated blood; and (4) the effect of reduced blood oxygen in causing pulmonary vasoconstriction and elevation of pressure in the pulmonary artery.[44] The most common direct cause of cor pulmonale is pulmonary hypertension. Right-sided heart failure is most frequently the terminal event in the disease process.

PATHOPHYSIOLOGY

The pulmonary circulation is normally a low-pressure, low-resistance system that may increase output, without increasing pulmonary pressure, to increase cardiac output. As pulmonary vascular resistance of the small arterioles and arteries increases in some types of disease, pulmonary hypertension results. Pulmonary hypertension, in turn, increases the workload of the right side of the heart, causing it to hypertrophy and eventually fail.[50]

A second major process causing pulmonary hypertension is an alteration in pulmonary arteriolar vasoconstriction. Chronic vasoconstriction, resulting from hypoxemia, and acidosis may lead to pulmonary hypertension. Fig. 2-35 shows the pathogenesis of cor pulmonale.

DIAGNOSTIC STUDIES

Clinical examination
    Evidence of other chronic lung diseases; dyspnea; cough; cyanosis; wheezing; distended neck veins; loud pulmonic secondary sound on cardiac auscultation; gallop rhythm and occasional murmur resulting from functional insufficiency of tricuspid and pulmonic valves

Chest roentgenogram
    Right ventricular hypertrophy

Echocardiogram
    Right ventricular enlargement

Arterial blood gases
    Decreased PaO_2 in range of 40 to 60 mm Hg; $PaCO_2$ in range of 40 to 70 mm Hg

Electrocardiogram
    Arrhythmias resulting from hypoxia; right bundle-branch block; right axis deviation; right ventricular hypertrophy

Complete blood count
    Elevated hemoglobin level and hematocrit value and polycythemia resulting from chronic hypoxia

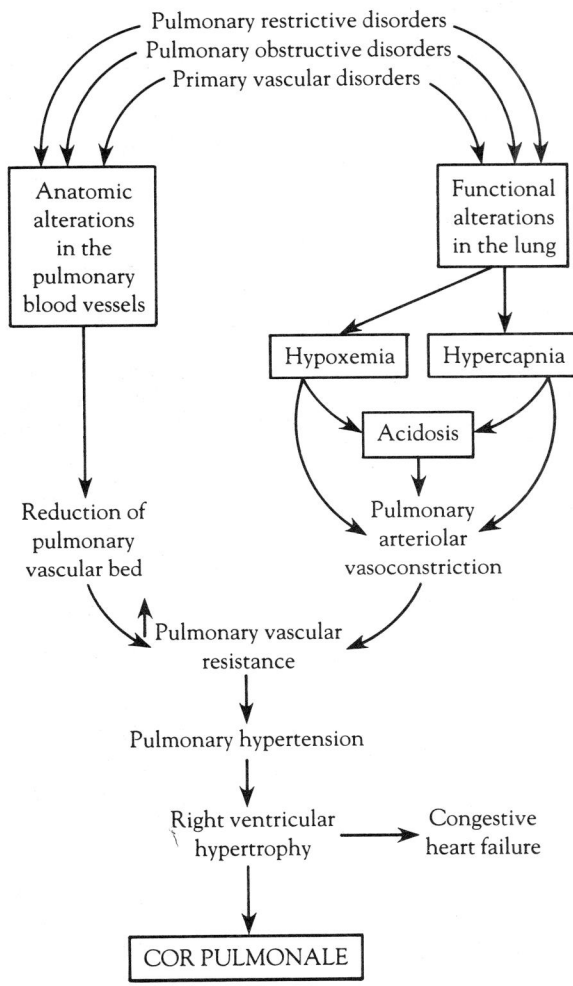

Fig. 2-35
Etiology and pathogenesis of cor pulmonale.

From Price, S.A., and Wilson, L.M.: Pathophysiology: clinical concepts of disease processes, ed. 2, New York, 1982, McGraw-Hill Book Co.

Pulmonary arterial pressure
  Systolic pressure above 30 mm Hg; diastolic pressure above 15 mm Hg; pulmonary function findings consistent with underlying pulmonary disease

TREATMENT PLAN

The underlying pulmonary and cardiac diseases must be treated first. (See Chapter 1 for cardiac disease guidelines.)

Chemotherapeutic
  Diuretics
    Initial diuresis can lower pulmonary artery pressure by decreasing total blood volume; careful monitoring of serum electrolytes needed when administering diuretics
    Furosemide (Lasix), 20-80 mg/d to maximum of 600 mg/d for adults, 1-2 mg/kg/d to maximum of 6 mg/kg/d for children
  Bronchodilators
    Concomitant administration of theophylline and terbutaline recommended to improve airway obstruction and reduce afterload on right and left sides of heart, thereby improving cardiac output[26]
    Theophylline (Theo-Dur, Theolair, Elixophyllin, others), 16 mg/kg divided into 3 or 4 doses
    Terbutaline (Brethine, Bricanyl), 2.5-5 mg po tid
  Anti-infective agents
    Antibiotics administered after Gram stain analysis of sputum specimens

Electromechanical
  Oxygenation—administered in concentrations ranging from 24% to 40% unless contraindicated by underlying pulmonary disease; 85% to 95% arterial oxygen saturation or arterial oxygen tension greater than 55 mm Hg[26]

Supportive
  Sodium-restricted test
  Bed rest during acute episodes to conserve energy and pulmonary effort

ASSESSMENT: AREAS OF CONCERN

Primary disease state
  See assessment for specific primary disease state

Pulmonary artery pressure
  Carefully monitored

Arterial blood gases
  PaO_2; $PaCO_2$; pH

Laboratory values
  Hemoglobin; hematocrit; serum electrolytes

Sputum characteristics
  Periodic laboratory analysis of sputum specimens

Fluid retention
  Careful monitoring of intake and output

Presence of complications
  Ankle edema; distended neck veins; abdominal pain; hepatomegaly; cardiac ventricular gallop (S_3); tachycardia; tachypnea

NURSING DIAGNOSES and NURSING INTERVENTIONS

The primary nursing diagnoses and nursing care should be directed toward the primary disease state. In addition, the following diagnoses and care strategies are specific for cor pulmonale.

Nursing Diagnosis	Nursing Intervention
Gas exchange, impaired	In collaboration with physician, order and monitor arterial blood gas studies.
	In collaboration with physician, administer oxygen to maintain oxygen saturation between 85% to 95%. *If patient has chronic obstructive lung disease, administer oxygen at low flow and with extreme caution.*
	Administer and monitor bronchodilators as ordered. Monitor patient response.
	Assess patient to identify signs, such as restlessness, confusion, and irritability, that may indicate body's response to altered blood gases.
	Monitor electrocardiogram and cardiac status for arrhythmias resulting from alterations in blood gases.
	Monitor for signs of increasing cor pulmonale such as increased pulmonary artery pressure, increased edema in extremities, jugular venous distention, and hepatomegaly.
	Monitor body temperature, which may fluctuate owing to alterations in metabolism or secondary infection.
	Evaluate for need to continue low-flow oxygen use at home to maintain arterial blood gas level. Indicators include continued reduced Pao_2 (50 to 55 mm Hg while patient is at rest), continuing pulmonary artery hypertension, and clinically apparent right ventricular failure.[26]
Fluid volume, alteration in: excess	Monitor and record weight daily.
	Carefully monitor and record intake and output.
	In collaboration with physician, administer diuretic medications.
	Assist patient to maintain sodium-restricted diet.
	Assist patient to limit fluid intake.
	Monitor serum electrolytes, which may change owing to administration of diuretics or alterations in metabolism.

Patient Education

The primary education is directed toward the patient's primary disease state; refer to patient education for specific primary disease.

1. Teach the patient the importance of restricting salt intake and limiting fluid intake.
2. Teach the patient to weigh self daily.
3. Provide the patient and family with information regarding chronic lung diseases, assessment of the patient's capabilities and responses, and actions to take during an acute episode.
4. Teach the patient the importance of avoiding environmental pollutants and not smoking.
5. Teach the patient facts about and the importance of prescribed medications.
6. Provide the patient and family with information regarding the care, cleaning, and maintenance of inhalation or oxygen equipment being used in the hospital or to be used at home, as well as the signs of oxygen toxicity.

EVALUATION

Also see the patient outcomes for the underlying disease state.

Patient Outcome	Data Indicating That Outcome is Reached
Breathing pattern occurs without tiring patient.	Modified breathing technique is maintained.
Optimal gas exchange occurs throughout lungs.	Blood gas values are within normal limits for patient's condition.
Fluid and electrolyte balance is restored.	There is no evidence of fluid retention; serum electrolytes are within normal limits.
Patient and family have sufficient information to comply with discharge regimen.	Patient and family at time of discharge are able to discuss medications, dietary therapy, activity progression, evidence of respiratory infection or compromise, and plan for follow-up visit.

PULMONARY EDEMA

Pulmonary edema is the accumulation of serous fluid in the interstitial tissue of the lung.

Pulmonary edema may result from many causes:

Heart failure owing to arteriosclerosis, mitral valve disease, or hypertension

Near-drowning

Pulmonary embolism

Overdose from heroin, barbiturates, or opiates

Overload or rapid infusion of intravenous fluids, plasma, or blood products

Renal disease

Pulmonary disease

Diffuse infections

Hemorrhagic pancreatitis

Pulmonary edema is acute and extensive and may lead to death unless treated rapidly. As may be inferred from the preceding list of causes, pulmonary edema results from one of three conditions: damage to the capillary walls, a decrease in colloid osmotic pressure as occurs in nephritis, or an increase in hydrostatic pressure within the pulmonary capillary walls. Pulmonary edema has therefore been conveniently divided into cardiogenic and noncardiogenic types. The remainder of this section is devoted to the cardiogenic type. For discussion of the noncardiogenic type, see the discussion of adult respiratory distress syndrome (pp. 151-158). The most common cause of cardiogenic pulmonary edema is left ventricular failure resulting from heart disease.

PATHOPHYSIOLOGY

Pulmonary edema occurs when left ventricular failure or fluid overload causes fluid to leave the vascular space and collect in the interstitial tissue of the lungs, increasing hydrostatic pressure and altering pulmonary capillary dynamics.

The formation of pulmonary edema has two stages: engorgement and fluid movement. In the first stage, interstitial edema causes engorgement of the perivascular and peribronchial spaces. The body has three safety mechanisms to protect against alveolar flooding.[26] First, lung lymph flow increases to help clear the edema fluid from the lung. Second, the concentration of protein in the interstitial space falls because of an increase of water and solutes entering the interstitial space around the alveolar vessels. This leads to an oncotic pressure difference between the plasma and the interstitial fluid, resulting in resorption of fluid into the circulation. The third safety factor is the capacity of the interstitial spaces in the lung, which can contain up to 500 ml of edema fluid in the bronchovascular cuffs before edema symptoms become severe.

Once engorgement reaches its limits and the safety factors are overwhelmed, alveolar edema occurs and fluid moves into the alveolar spaces. Blood plasma pours into the alveoli faster than coughing or the safety factors can clear it.[50] The result of this process is acute pulmonary edema, which causes interference with the diffusion of oxygen, tissue hypoxia, and asphyxia. Unless emergency procedures are implemented, respiratory failure occurs.

DIAGNOSTIC STUDIES

Clinical examination

Severe dyspnea; grunting and labored respirations; tachypnea; cyanosis; tachycardia; cough; rales; frothy, blood-tinged sputum; distended neck veins; restlessness; vague uneasiness; agitation or confusion resulting from hypoxia; diaphoresis

Chest roentgenogram

Prominent interlobular septa (Kerley-B lines) (Fig. 2-36)

Pulmonary capillary wedge pressure

Left atrial pressure increased: 14 to 20 mm Hg in mild cases, 25 to 30 mm Hg in severe cases[26]

Arterial blood gases

PaO_2 and $PaCO_2$ variable; respiratory alkalosis or acidosis may occur

TREATMENT PLAN

Chemotherapeutic

D5W IV with microdrip tubing running at keep-open rate for medication infusion

Narcotic analgesics

Morphine sulfate, 10-15 mg IV, to reduce anxiety, slow respirations, and reduce venous return

Diuretics

Furosemide (Lasix), loading dose of 40 mg IV over 1-2 min, increasing to 80 mg IV after 1 h for adults; loading dose of 1 mg/kg IV or IM, increasing by 1 mg/kg no sooner than 2 h after previous dose for children; maximum dose is 6 mg/kg for children; monitor serum potassium level

Ethacrynic acid (Edecrin), loading dose of 50 mg slow IV push (may be repeated once if needed) for adults; loading dose of 0.5 mg/kg for children; monitor serum potassium level

Fig. 2-36
Chest roentgenogram of patient with pulmonary edema. Note cardiomegaly, increased pulmonary vascularity, and obliteration of costophrenic angles indicating increase of pleural space fluid. Note infiltration of fluid indicating alveolar edema.

Courtesy R. Keith Wilson, M.D., Baylor College of Medicine, Houston, Texas.

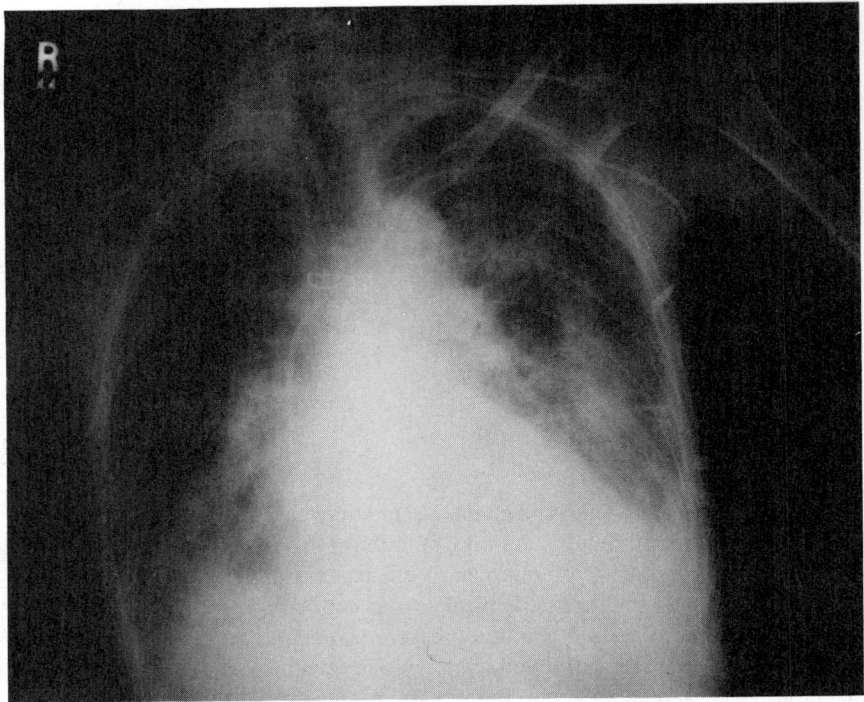

Bronchodilators
  Aminophylline, 250-500 mg (diluted in 50 mg IV solution) IV over 15-20 min
  Other drugs to treat underlying cause of pulmonary edema, e.g., cardiac drugs for cardiac-related problem

Electromechanical
  Rotation of tourniquets—manually or by machine; pressure applied to three limbs at a time; cuff inflation slightly above patient's diastolic blood pressure; cuff inflated for 45 minutes followed by 15 minutes free of compression
  Oxygenation—high flow by Venturi mask at 50% concentration or intermittent positive-pressure breathing tolerated; short-term intubation with mechanical ventilatory support if patient unable to maintain adequate arterial blood gas levels and adequate tidal volume
  Foley catheter attached to closed system drainage—for careful monitoring of intake and output
  Cardiac monitoring
  Pulmonary capillary wedge pressure monitoring

Supportive
  High Fowler's position or patient permitted to sit on edge of bed and dangle legs

ASSESSMENT: AREAS OF CONCERN

Respiratory status
  Nasal flaring; retractions; tachypnea; retractions; labored noisy breathing; diaphoresis; rales; wheezing; noisy wet breathing; cough productive of sputum; frothy, blood-tinged sputum; persistent cough; decreased vital capacity; decreased minute volume; increased intrapulmonary shunting

Tourniquets
  Careful monitoring and systematic rotation of tourniquets; patient's response; tissue oxygenation and pulses distal to tourniquets

Hypoxia
  Restlessness; confusion; hypotension, anxiety; tachycardia

Laboratory values
  $PaCO_2$; PaO_2; pH; HCO_3; alveolar-arterial oxygen gradient; potassium; sodium

Cardiovascular status
  Decreased cardiac output; restlessness; lethargy; tachycardia; hypotension

Intake and output
  Careful monitoring of intake and urinary output

Pulmonary pressures
Pulmonary capillary wedge pressure; pulmonary artery pressure

Bronchopulmonary infection
Temperature; sputum specimens for periodic culture and sensitivity

Chest roentgenogram
Serial chest roentgenograms to monitor clearing of edema

Psychosocial
Fear of suffocation

Associated complications or indications that condition is worsening
Sudden weight gain; swollen feet or ankles; chest pain; decreased urinary output; persistent cough

NURSING DIAGNOSES and NURSING INTERVENTIONS

Nursing Diagnosis	Nursing Intervention
Fluid volume, alteration in: excess	In collaboration with physician apply and monitor tourniquets. Rotate tourniquets, with 45 minutes on and 15 minutes off. Keep pressure slightly above patient's diastolic pressure. Carefully observe color and temperature of limb distal to each tourniquet. To discontinue tourniquets, remove one at a time, waiting at least 15 minutes before removing another. Carefully monitor cardiovascular and respiratory system response. Carefully monitor intake and output. Monitor pulmonary capillary wedge pressure as ordered (may indicate fluid overload complicating pulmonary wetness). Administer diuretics, and monitor and record patient response as ordered. Monitor serum electrolytes as ordered (may change owing to diuretics and alterations in oxygenation and metabolism). Weigh patient at same time each day.
Breathing pattern, ineffective	Assess ventilation to include evaluation of breathing rate, rhythm, and depth; chest expansion; presence of respiratory distress such as dyspnea, shortness of breath, nasal flaring, pursed-lip breathing or prolonged expiratory phase; and use of accessory muscles. Assess tidal volume, vital capacity, minute volume, functional residual capacity, and intrapulmonary shunting. Identify contributing factors such as airway clearance or obstruction problem or weakness. Position patient in high Fowler's position or sitting and leaning forward on overbed table to facilitate ventilation. Suction if necessary to remove secretions. Assess patient for tiring in relation to attempts to breath. Collaborate with physician to prepare for and administer mechanical ventilation when breathing pattern is unable to maintain adequate blood gas levels or when patient demonstrates tiring with breathing efforts.
Airway clearance, ineffective	Assess patient to identify inability to move secretions. If inability is identified, assist with appropriate measures (such as coughing, positioning, suctioning, and liquefying secretions). Promptly administer bronchodilators as ordered to dilate bronchioles and remove secretions. Monitor serum theophylline level. Assist patient to maintain body position that ensures maximum airway availability. Carefully and frequently auscultate chest for quality of breath sounds and adventitious sounds. Note cough and sputum characteristics.
Gas exchange, impaired	In collaboration with physician, monitor arterial blood gases. Report increases or decreases of more than 10 to 15 mm Hg in $Paco_2$ and Pao_2. In collaboration with physician, administer oxygen and intermittent positive-pressure breathing. Assess patient to identify signs, such as restlessness, confusion, and irritability, that may indicate body's response to altered blood gas states.

Nursing Diagnosis	Nursing Intervention
	Monitor electrocardiogram and cardiac status for arrhythmias resulting from alterations in blood gases.
	Monitor for signs of cor pulmonale such as pulmonary hypertension, gradual increasing edema of legs, increasing central venous pressure and pulmonary capillary wedge pressure, jugular venous distention, blood gas abnormalities, and hepatomegaly.
	Carefully monitor body temperature, which may fluctuate owing to alterations in metabolism or secondary infections.
	In collaboration with physician, administer respiratory and cardiac medications and assess and document patient response.
Mobility, impaired physical	Encourage patient to use adaptive breathing techniques to decrease work of breathing.
	Assist patient to alternate activities with periods of rest.
	Provide active or passive range of motion exercises to maintain adequate muscle tone.
Skin integrity, impairment of: potential	Provide meticulous skin care and observe skin for hygiene and potential for skin breakdown.
	Reposition patient at least every 2 hours to prevent extended periods of lying on known pressure points.
Fear	Observe for signs of frustration, fear, fatigue, and tiring with attempts to communicate resulting from hypoxia.
Self-care deficit	Assess patient's level of fear related to present health state.
	Assess patient's level of fear related to feeling of air hunger.
	Assess level of self-care deficit resulting from patient's current condition.
	Assist with activities of daily living such as toileting, bathing, and feeding to minimize patient's energy expenditures.
Coping, ineffective individual	Determine patient's ability to cooperate with health care providers in intervention strategies.
Coping, family: potential for growth	Assess family's understanding of diagnostic procedures, disease process and prognosis, and therapies employed.
	Provide information in areas needed.
	See p. 1899 for additional strategies.

Patient Education

1. Teach the patient adaptive breathing techniques.
2. Teach the patient the importance of avoiding contact with persons who have upper respiratory infections.
3. Teach the patient facts about and the importance of prescribed medications such as bronchodilators and diuretics.
4. Teach the patient the importance of maintaining a low-sodium diet.
5. Inform the patient that a change in health status must be reported to the patient's health care providers. Indicators of change may include change in sputum characteristics or color, decreased activity tolerance, increased cough or chest fullness, noisy wet breathing, or leg or ankle edema.
6. Teach the patient adaptive exercises and rest techniques.

EVALUATION

Patient Outcome	Data Indicating That Outcome is Reached
Movement of air in and out of lungs is optimum. Airway is patent.	Vital capacity measurements including tidal and minute volumes are normal for patient.
Both lungs are fully aerated as visualized chest roentgenogram.	Blood gas values are within normal limits. Airways are clear, and breathing occurs without obstruction.

Patient Outcome	Data Indicating That Outcome is Reached
Breathing pattern occurs without tiring patient.	Patient demonstrates modified breathing techniques that facilitate ventilator capacity. Behavior is modified to conserve energy expenditure.
Physiologic stability is achieved after respiratory insult.	Nutrition level is maintained. Kidney and bladder functioning is within normal limits. Gastrointestinal system functions adequately. There is no secondary infection. Serum electrolytes are within normal limits.
Patient understands importance of daily pulmonary exercises.	Patient demonstrates pulmonary exercises and states rationale and importance of maintaining daily exercise routine.
Patient preserves pulmonary functioning by maintaining optimum activity level, preventing infection, and following prescribed treatments.	Patient demonstrates variety of methods indicating ability to preserve and facilitate optimum respiration (for example, breathing exercises, modified activities or exercise, taking medications as prescribed).
Patient and family have sufficient information to comply with discharge regimen.	Patient and family at time of discharge are able to discuss medications (purpose, side effects, route, and schedule), dietary therapy regimen, activity progression regimen, signs of infection or respiratory deterioration, plan for follow-up visits.

PULMONARY EMBOLISM AND PULMONARY INFARCTION

Pulmonary embolism is the blockage of a pulmonary artery by foreign matter such as a thrombus that usually arises from a peripheral vein, fat, air, or tumor tissue. Subsequent to the blockage is obstruction of blood supply to the lung tissue.

Pulmonary infarction is an uncommon complication of pulmonary embolism resulting in a localized area of lung tissue ischemic necrosis distal to the area of embolus.

The formation of a pulmonary embolism usually occurs in patients with well-defined risk factors. Following are the most common predisposing factors:

Thrombophlebitis	Chronic illness
Major surgery	Congestive heart
Use of estrogens	failure
Pregnancy	Obesity
Recent childbirth	Venous insufficiency
Leg trauma	Immobilization from
Myocardial infarction	fracture
Elderly	Polycythemia vera

Perhaps at the base of many of these predisposing factors is the factor of immobilization. Horwitz suggests that up to 5% of all hospital deaths may be due to pulmonary embolism secondary in part to immobilization.[34]

Death from pulmonary embolism usually occurs within the first 24 hours. After that time and with proper treatment the mortality rate drops significantly. Resolution of the embolus occurs within 7 to 10 days.

PATHOPHYSIOLOGY

Three factors are related to the development of a venous thrombus: (1) venous stasis, (2) injury to the vein wall, and (3) increased blood coagulability. Together these factors are called Virchow's triad.

The most common sites for the thrombus to form are the deep veins of the legs (90%); the second most common sites are the pelvic veins. At some given point the thrombus breaks loose and travels to and lodges in one of the pulmonary arteries.

The effect of a pulmonary embolism is to produce an area of the lung that is ventilated but underperfused. There is therefore an increase in physiologic dead-space ventilation. Reflex bronchoconstriction occurs in the affected area and is thought to result from the release of histamine or serotonin from the clot.[50] If the embolism is large and sufficiently reduces the pulmonary perfusion, pulmonary hypertension may result.

If the embolism lodges in a large or medium size artery, there may be insufficient collateral bronchial blood circulation. If this occurs, there may be significant tissue underperfusion, and pulmonary infarction may result.

DIAGNOSTIC STUDIES

Clinical examination

Dyspnea, pleuritic pain, apprehension, cough, unexplained hemoptysis, sweats, tachypnea, localized rales, pleural friction rub, tachycardia, cyanosis, low grade fever, thrombophlebitis

Blood gases

PaO_2 less than 60 mm Hg in association with hyperventilation leads to $PaCO_2$ less than 40 mm Hg; alveolar arterial oxygen tension gradient ($PA\text{-}aO_2$) increased

Electrocardiogram

The following classic signs help to differentiate pulmonary embolism from myocardial infarction: right axis deviation, incomplete or complete right bundle branch block, tall peaked P waves, S wave in lead I, a Q wave in lead III, T wave inversion, ST and T wave changes in the right precordial leads

Chest roentgenogram

Unilateral diaphragm elevation, enlarged main pulmonary artery associated with decreased vascular markings on one side, unilateral pulmonary effusion, occasional wedge-shaped area of consolidation

Lung scans

Rapid, relatively safe and easy screening tests for establishing the diagnosis (Fig. 2-37); if the patient has a chronic lung disease, asthma, or congestive heart failure, the lung scan is of little diagnostic value; two scans are commonly used sequentially: perfusion lung scan and ventilation lung scan; comparison of scans may be diagnostic of pulmonary embolism

Perfusion lung scan

This study involves the intravenous injection of serum albumin tagged with tracer amounts of a radioisotope; the radioactive particles pass through the right side of the heart and lodge in the pulmonary capillary bed; significant diagnostic findings reveal an area deficient in radioactivity

Ventilation lung scan

The patient initially breathes a radioactive gas through a carefully sealed system for several minutes; during this time the lungs are scanned by a gamma camera

Pulmonary angiography

Although it is the most specific diagnostic procedure, pulmonary angiography also has the most risk; the two diagnostic criteria of this technique are intra-arterial filling defects and complete obstruction of a pulmonary artery branch

Laboratory tests

Serum assays (looking for the triad of elevated lactate dehydrogenase [LDH] and bilirubin with a normal serum glutamic-oxaloacetic transaminase [SGOT] and white blood cell count [WBC] [less than 15,000], and elevated fibrin split products [FSP]).

TREATMENT PLAN

Surgical

Surgical therapy of pulmonary embolism is infrequently indicated. When there are multiple emboli, an umbrella filter (Mobin-Uddin umbrella) may be surgically placed in the inferior vena cava. Other techniques are surgical removal of the embolus, which requires cardiopulmonary bypass, and interruption of blood flow through the inferior vena cava via ligation.

Chemotherapeutic

Anticoagulants: The main purpose of this therapy is supportive.

Fig. 2-37
Lung scan showing pulmonary embolism. Note decreased perfusion of right upper lobe indicative of pulmonary embolism.

Courtesy R. Keith Wilson, M.D., Baylor College of Medicine, Houston, Texas.

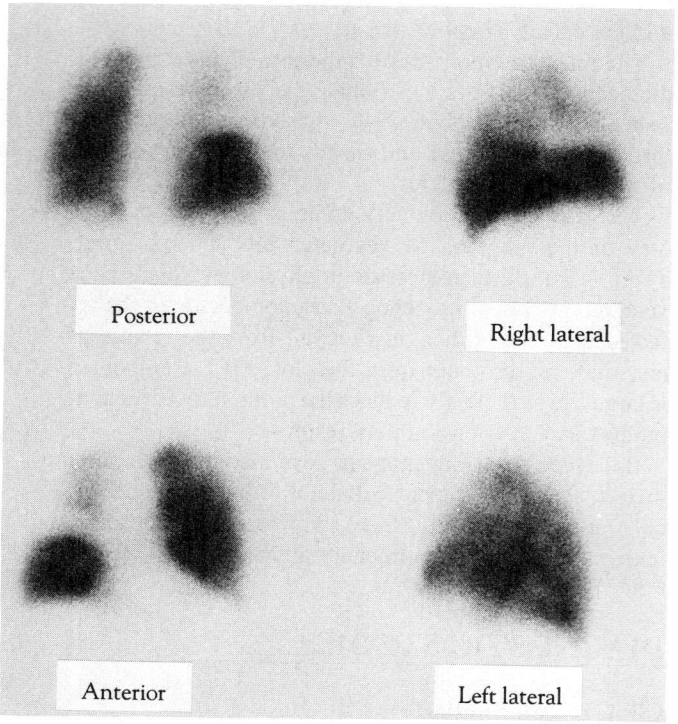

Posterior

Right lateral

Anterior

Left lateral

Heparin: does not directly lead to clot lysis; instead, heparin halts clot propagation, enabling endogenous fibrinolytic mechanisms to remove the clot.[46] Heparin may be administered by continuous intravenous infusion or by intermittent intravenous injections.
Initial bolus loading dose: 5000-10,000 units
Continuous infusion: 20 units/kg/h or 800-1500 units/h
Intermittent bolus doses: 70-100 units/kg q4h using a heparin lock
The dose of heparin is best monitored and regulated by obtaining serial venous samples for partial thromboplastin time (PTT) coagulation studies. The dose should be adjusted to maintain clotting times in the range of 1.5 to 2.5 times the control values. The drug is generally continued from 7 to 14 days.
Should a severe bleeding event occur secondary to the use of heparin, protamine sulfate may be given intravenously. In such a case, 1 mg of protamine is given for every 100 units of heparin received in the dose prior to the bleeding episode. The drug should be administered slowly over 3 to 5 minutes in 20 ml saline. The total amount of protamine should not exceed 100 mg.
Long-term anticoagulation: necessary when the patient is predisposed to another pulmonary embolus.
Warfarin: should be started before the heparin is terminated.
Oral dose: 5-10 mg daily
Warfarin may be used for 6 months up to life in some cases. Clotting time should be monitored by the prothrombin time (PT).
Fibrinolytic enzymes: some authors believe fibrinolytic therapy to be superior to heparin therapy.[46] The two drugs of choice are:
Urokinase (Abbokinase, Breokinase): 4400 units/kg IV over 10 min, followed by 4400 units/kg/h for 12 h
Thrombin time (TT) or PTT should be monitored after 2 hours.
Streptokinase (Kabikinase, Streptase): 250,000 units IV over 20-30 min followed by 100,000 units/h over 24-72 h
TT or PTT should be monitored after 2 hours.
The main side effects of these two drugs include bleeding and allergic reactions.

Electromechanical
Oxygen therapy: administer oxygen by mask or cannula to maintain blood gas levels.

Supportive
Bed rest should be maintained for the first 2 or 3 days. Following that, mobilization should be gradually increased.

ASSESSMENT: AREAS OF CONCERN

Respiratory status
Respiratory distress: tachypnea, labored breathing, dyspnea, coughing, shallow breathing
Breath sounds: rales or pleural friction rub

Hypoxia
Restlessness, confusion, tachycardia, cyanosis

Laboratory values
Blood gases: monitor pH, PaO_2, $PaCO_2$
As long as patient is on anticoagulants, daily monitor clotting time, hematocrit, urinalysis, and stool for occult blood
Platelet count should be monitored at least twice weekly for thrombocytopenia

Cough sputum
Characteristics of cough and sputum should be monitored daily

Chest roentgenogram
Should be monitored periodically for changes

Potential complications
Cardiac arrhythmias, cor pulmonale, hypotension, severe hypoxemia, pulmonary hypertension, atelectasis, chest congestion

Psychosocial
Fear, air hunger, pain, confusion

Potential risk for developing pulmonary embolism
Identification of persons at risk for development of pulmonary embolism
Preoperative teaching and postoperative care to maximize early ambulation of surgical patients
Leg exercises to maintain peripheral circulation and antiembolism stockings

NURSING DIAGNOSES and NURSING INTERVENTIONS

Nursing Diagnosis	Nursing Intervention
Gas exchange, impaired	In collaboration with physician order, monitor arterial blood gases; report increases or decreases of $Paco_2$ and Pao_2 of more than 10 mm Hg.
	In collaboration with physician consultation, administer oxygen to maintain adequate blood gas levels.
	Assess patient to identify signs such as restlessness, confusion, and irritability, which may indicate the body's response to altered blood gas states.
	Monitor electrocardiogram and cardiac status for arrhythmias secondary to alterations in blood gases.
	If patient is seriously ill, monitor for signs of cor pulmonale such as pulmonary hypertension, cardiac compromise, jugular venous distention, blood gas abnormalities, and hepatomegaly.
	Monitor and record kidney functioning and urinary output, which may be affected secondary to tissue hypoxia and alterations in metabolism.
	Monitor serum electrolytes that may change because of alterations in oxygenation and metabolism.
	Carefully monitor body temperature, which may fluctuate because of alterations in metabolism or secondary infections.
	As long as patient has an active pulmonary embolism, maintain bed rest; proceed with ambulation as quickly as possible.
Fluid volume deficit, potential	As long as patient is on anticoagulants, monitor PTT, PT, or TT as indicated.
	Carefully evaluate urine and stool samples for occult blood.
	Avoid use of any drug that may potentiate heparin action such as aspirin.
Breathing pattern, ineffective	Assess ventilation to include evaluation of breathing rate, rhythm, and depth, chest expansion, presence of respiratory distress such as dyspnea, shortness of breath, tachypnea, shallow breathing, ineffective breathing, and use of accessory muscles.
	Carefully and frequently auscultate chest for quality of breath sounds and adventitious sounds; note cough and sputum characteristics.
	Help to assess total lung capacity (TLC), residual volume (RV), functional residual capacity (FEV_1), and forced vital capacity (FVC) as ordered.
	Identify contributing factors such as airway clearance or obstruction problem, or weakness.
	Maintain patient positioning to facilitate easy ventilation (i.e., head of bed in semi-Fowler's position).
	Assess patient for tiring in relation to attempts to breathe.
	Encourage patient to use adaptive breathing techniques to decrease the work of breathing and to space activities so as to provide periods of rest in between.
Mobility, impaired physical	Encourage patient to use adaptive breathing techniques to decrease the work of breathing.
	Provide range of motion exercises for legs as soon as ordered.
	Provide antiembolism stockings.
	See p. 2106 for additional strategies.
Anxiety	Assess patient's level of anxiety related to feeling of air hunger.
Coping, ineffective individual	Listen carefully to collect information regarding the significance of the current health care problem and the patient's perception of his ability to deal with alterations it is causing.
Coping, family	See p. 1897 for associated nursing care.

Patient Education

1. Teach patient about medications as well as side effects that are currently being used to treat the pulmonary embolism.
2. Teach preventive measures to all high-risk patients preoperatively and initiate interventions postoperatively that will help to prevent pulmonary embolism.

3. Teach strategies for persons of high risk to prevent venous pooling, which may lead to thrombophlebitis.
4. Changes in the health status of individuals recovering from pulmonary embolism must be reported immediately to the patient's health care provider. Changes include chest pain, shortness of breath, tachypnea, blood-tinged sputum, blood in the stool or urine.

EVALUATION

Patient Outcome	Data Indicating That Outcome is Reached
Optimal movement of air in and out of lungs occurs.	Vital capacity measurements are optimal for patient's status.
Airway is patent.	Blood gas values are within normal limits for patient. Airways are clear and breathing occurs without obstruction. Chest x-ray film or lung scan shows no evidence of pulmonary embolism.
Breathing pattern is adequate.	There is no shortness of breath, dyspnea, tachypnea, or shallow breathing. Clear breath sounds are heard in all areas.
Physiologic stability occurs secondary to respiratory insult.	Nutrition level is maintained. Kidney and bladder functioning is within normal limits. Gastrointestinal system functioning is adequate. Secondary infections do not occur. Serum electrolytes are within normal limits.
Patient and family have sufficient information to comply with discharge regimen.	Patient and family are able at time of discharge to discuss medications—purpose, side effects, route, and schedule; dietary therapy regimen; activity progression regimen; signs of infection or respiratory deterioration; and plan for follow-up visits.

PNEUMOTHORAX AND HEMOTHORAX

The presence of air in the pleural space between the parietal and visceral pleurae is a pneumothorax.

The presence of blood in the pleural space is a hemothorax.

Many times, especially with trauma, victims have a combination of pneumothorax and hemothorax. In these cases the term hemopneumothorax is used.

A pneumothorax may be caused by trauma or by surgery, or it may occur spontaneously. Historically a pneumothorax may have been therapeutically caused as a common treatment for tuberculosis. Today, however, that treatment mode is no longer used.

Trauma may cause a penetrating injury to the chest wall and thus permit air to directly enter the pleural space. It may also result in a fractured rib, which from the inside tears the lung surface. In either case, air may accumulate in the pleural space, and a pneumothorax results.

A spontaneous pneumothorax occurs suddenly without injury and may or may not be the result of underlying pulmonary disease. Specifically, there is a rupture of the bronchus or alveolus. Pulmonary diseases such as em-physema, pneumonia, and neoplasms may provide weak tissue where a spontaneous pneumothorax may occur. A spontaneous pneumothorax may occur in apparently healthy young persons usually between 20 and 40 years of age. For these persons there may be rupture of a subpleural bleb secondary to a hard cough or sneeze. The rupture again permits air from the lungs to leak into the pleural space.

A pneumothorax occurs secondary to chest surgery such as thoracotomy or a thoracentesis.

In addition to cause, a pneumothorax may be classified by its type: open pneumothorax, closed pneumothorax, or tension pneumothorax.

An open pneumothorax is one that is communicating with the outside air (also called a sucking chest wound). The cause of this type of pneumothorax is almost always a penetrating trauma.

A closed pneumothorax is noncommunicating with the outside air (also called a simple pneumothorax). The cause may be a needle puncture or stab wound from the outside or a fractured rib or simple hard cough or sneeze from the inside. If the insult came from outside the body, the chest wall has again become airtight after penetration. Thus there is no air transfer into or out of the chest wall.

A tension pneumothorax occurs secondary to a traumatic event when a check-valve mechanism in a bronchiole permits air to continue to leak into the pleural space. The air continues to collect with each breath, causing a pressure within the space to rise above the atmospheric pressure. The result is collapse of the lung, shift of the mediastinum to the opposite side, and impairment of venous return.

A hemothorax may be the result of a blunt or penetrating chest trauma. The bleeding is generally self-limiting. If not, however, a thoracotomy may be indicated to ligate the bleeding vessels.

PATHOPHYSIOLOGY

The pleural space normally maintains a negative pressure between -10 to -12 mm Hg. This negative pressure as explained at the beginning of this chapter facilitates lung expansion during ventilation. When there is penetration into the pleural space by an object external to the chest wall such as a knife or needle or when there is penetration into the pleural space by an internal mechanism such as a broken rib or bleb rupture of the lung, air enters the pleural space and the negative pressure is decreased. Depending on the amount of air that enters initially and the amount that continues to enter, such as with a tension pneumothorax, the lung is no longer able to remain inflated to its full extent.

As the pleural space pressure increases and as the lung collapses, there is a mediastinal shift toward the direction of the unaffected side. This shift causes pressure on the great vessels returning to the heart and thus causes a decreased venous return. If pneumothorax is left untreated, cardiac output is compromised, and a shut-down systemic response may occur.

DIAGNOSTIC STUDIES

The types of pneumothorax and hemothorax have both similarities and differences. The following diagnostic studies discuss the differences where they exist.

Spontaneous, simple, or noncommunicating pneumothorax

History

Patient generally is male between the ages of 20 and 40 years and is in good health

Patient is older and has a chronic obstructive pulmonary disease, pneumonia, or a neoplasm

Patient usually awakens to note shortness of breath and chest pain

Clinical examination

Shortness of breath and chest pain in only 50% of all cases; patient may appear acutely ill with cyanosis and tachypnea or may appear to be healthy; the difference in the clinical signs is dependent on the size of the pneumothorax; breath sounds are generally diminished; percussion tones are hyperresonant over involved area; approximately 25% of patients may have subcutaneous emphysema[68]; in addition the patient demonstrates syncope and Hamman's sign (a crunching sound with each heartbeat due to mediastinal air accumulation)

Open, communicating, penetrating-trauma pneumothorax

History

Some event that has caused a penetration of the chest wall

Clinical examination

Penetration of the chest wall, a sucking sound on inspiration as the chest wall rises, and varying signs of respiratory distress depending on the size of the pneumothorax

Tension pneumothorax

History

Blunt trauma to the chest that may have resulted in fractured ribs or penetrating injury to the chest that permits air to enter the chest wall but then seals off as the air tries to escape

Clinical examination

As the positive pressure on the affected side increases, the clinical signs will become more severe; these include neck vein enlargement due to pressure on the superior vena cava, dyspnea, cardiogenic shock because of the lack of oxygenated blood, paradoxical movement of the chest, deviated trachea toward the unaffected side, cyanosis, distant heart sounds, absence of breath sounds on the affected side, and hyperresonance on percussion of the affected side

Hemothorax

History

Same as that for open pneumothorax or tension pneumothorax

Clinical examination

Same as above with the addition of tachycardia, hypotension, dullness on chest percussion, and signs of hypovolemic shock such as pallor and anxiety; the severity of the hemothorax may be determined by the amount of blood accumulation: less than 300 ml is considered minor and may not cause significant clinical signs; 300 to 1400 ml is moderate; and over 1400 ml is severe, indicating that most clinical signs will also be present

Chest roentgenogram

Simple and open pneumothorax

The characteristic finding shows air in the pleural cavity without the lateral markings of the lungs; instead there is a sharp pleural margin seen medially, indicating that the lung has collapsed; if the lung is not entirely collapsed, this margin may not be as obvious; it is, therefore, desirable to take an expiratory film with the patient sitting in an upright position; because intrapleural air first collects in the apex, partial pneumothorax identification may be made; Fig. 2-38 shows a classic picture of a pneumothorax

Tension pneumothorax

The chest x-ray film of an individual with a tension pneumothorax shows complete lung collapse and a shift of mediastinal structures toward the unaffected side.

Hemothorax

A minimum of 250 ml of intrapleural fluid is required to show a blunting of the costophrenic angle on an upright chest roentgenogram[40]; it is therefore desirable to obtain an upright chest roentgenogram if possible; findings are decreased lung expansion as in Fig. 2-38.

Blood gases

$\downarrow$ pH; $\downarrow$ Pao_2; $\uparrow$ $Paco_2$

TREATMENT PLAN

Surgical

Closed-tube thoracostomy (chest tube): this technique is used to treat most types of pneumothorax. The exception is a small, spontaneous pneumothorax in an otherwise healthy individual. The indications for closed-tube thoracostomy* include the following:

*Data from Vukich, D.J., and Markovchick, V.J.: Pneumothorax. In Rosen, P., Baker, F.J., Braen, G.R., et al., editors: Emergency medicine: concepts and clinical practice, St. Louis, 1983, The C.V. Mosby Co., p. 339.

Fig. 2-38
Chest roentgenogram of patient with pneumothorax. Note narrowing of pleural edge at arrow point and lack of lung markings beyond pleural line.

Courtesy R. Keith Wilson, M.D., Baylor College of Medicine, Houston, Texas.

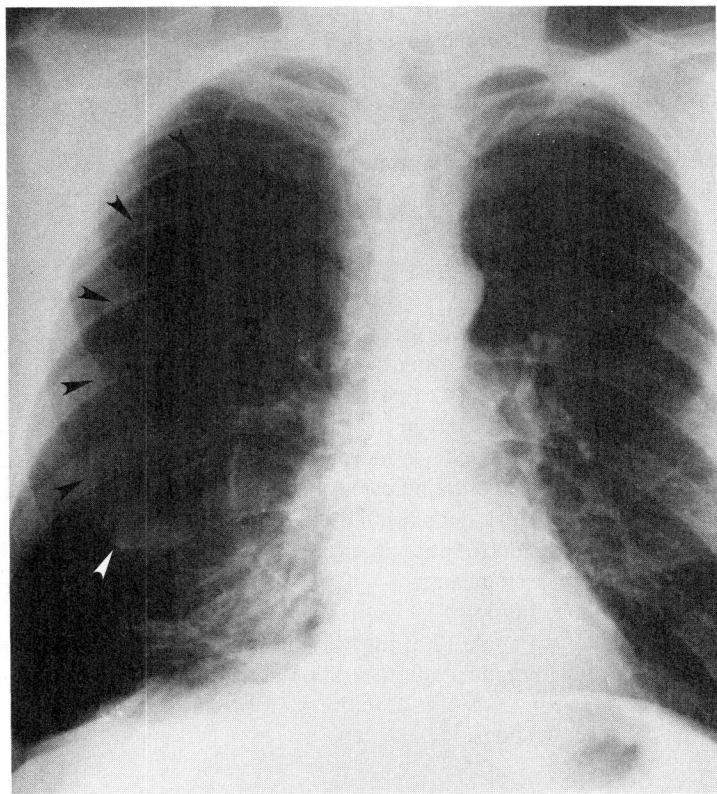

Traumatic causes
Pneumothorax with respiratory distress
Recurrent pneumothorax
Patient requires ventilatory support
Moderate to large pneumothorax
Pneumothorax that continues to get larger despite treatment
Patient requires anesthesia
Associated hemothorax
Tension pneumothorax

The chest tube should be inserted in the fifth or sixth intercostal space at the midaxillary line. If the tube is positioned posteriorly and toward the apex of the lung, it can effectively remove air and fluid. The lateral placement is preferred not only because it is most efficient but also because it does not produce a cosmetic defect, as does the anterior site of the second intercostal space at the midclavicular line.[68] See pp. 242-246 for discussion of chest tubes and their care.

Tension pneumothorax requires immediate and specific medical intervention. The building pressure in the pleural space must be reversed. A mechanism must be provided to release the pressure. The most effective way to release the pressure is to insert a large-bore needle (16 to 18 gauge) either anteriorly at the midclavicle line between the second and third intercostal space or at the midlateral line between the fifth and sixth intercostal space. Once the needle is inserted, the patient's condition should improve remarkably.

Thoracotomy: A hemothorax may require a thoracotomy for correction. Indications for this procedure include initial thoracostomy tube drainage greater than 1500 ml of blood; persistent bleeding rate greater than 500 m/h; increasing hemothorax seen on chest x-ray film; patient remains in an unstable and hypotensive state despite adequate blood replacement.[68]

Chemotherapeutic

Hemothorax requires aggressive intravenous therapy to restore the circulating blood volume.

Narcotic analgesics: Analgesics such as meperidine (Demerol) may be given for pain if respirations are adequate. Drugs such as morphine and barbiturates are generally contraindicated because they may cause respiratory depression.

Adrenergic agents: Antihypotensives such as dopamine may be indicated.

Dopamine (Intropin)

Dilute 1 ampule (200 mg) in 250 ml D5W; use with microdrip administration set; usual dose is 2-5 mg/kg/min initially; then titrate to desired response.

Electromechanical

Airway maintenance: done by positioning, a simple airway, or endotracheal intubation, depending on the patient's condition.

Oxygenation: provide oxygen to maintain adequate blood gas levels.

If the patient shows evidence of respiratory failure, mechanical ventilation with PEEP may be initiated after the chest tubes have been inserted and determined to be functioning adequately. See p. 246 for discussion of technique.

Supportive

If the patient has an active and communicating pneumothorax, the entrance wound into the chest wall should be immediately covered by a petroleum jelly gauze. Three sides of the gauze pad should be taped. The fourth is left open to permit exhale ventilation. If the gauze is placed on too tightly, a tension pneumothorax may result.

ASSESSMENT: AREAS OF CONCERN

Respiratory status

Respiratory distress to include dyspnea, tachypnea, retractions, labored breathing, nasal flaring

Breath sounds are distant, bilaterally unequal, diminished; vocal fremitus on the affected side; hyperresonance to percussion on affected side

Breathing pattern; presence of splinting or hypoventilation that may lead to atelectasis; breathing seems inadequate, causing patient to tire but still be "air hungry"

Evaluate chest wall for stability and movement

Tracheal deviation is noted with palpation

Evaluate for presence of crepitation

Cough, characteristics and amount; sputum, amount and characteristics

Hypoxia

Restlessness, confusion, tachycardia, cyanosis; note mucous membranes, nail beds

Cardiovascular status

Blood pressure, heart rate, auscultation quality, tissue perfusion, and urinary output

Laboratory values

Blood gases; electrolytes; CBC

Chest roentgenogram

For presence of pneumothorax and change since the last chest roentgenogram

Chest-tube drainage

Assess intact drainage system and amount and characteristics of drainage

Anxiety
Fear, air hunger, pain, confusion

Secondary complications
Atelectasis, ARDS, chest congestion, infection, pulmonary edema, pulmonary embolus

NURSING DIAGNOSES and NURSING INTERVENTIONS

Nursing Diagnosis	Nursing Intervention
Breathing pattern, ineffective	Assess ventilation to include evaluation of breathing rate, rhythm, and depth, chest expansion, presence of respiratory distress such as dyspnea, shortness of breath, nasal flaring, anxiety, retractions, prolonged expiratory phase, use of accessory muscles. Assist to insert chest tubes as indicated. Provide chest tube care consistent with the guidelines presented on pp. 242 to 246; carefully maintain to avoid interruption in the airtight system via dislodgment of the tubing or breaking of the bottles. Identify contributing factors such as airway clearance or obstruction problem, or weakness that may contribute to the patient's respiratory distress. Maintain patient positioning to facilitate easy ventilation (i.e., head of bed in semi-Fowler's position). Suction if necessary to remove secretions. Assess patient for tiring in relation to attempts to breathe. Encourage patient to breathe deeply but also to use adaptive breathing techniques to decrease the work of breathing and to space activities so as to provide periods of rest in between. Assist to protect patient from known sources of secondary infection. Should mechanical ventilation become necessary, provide care and monitoring consistent with the guidelines on pp. 246 to 249.
Gas exchange, impaired	In collaboration with physician order, monitor arterial blood gases; report increases or decreases of $Paco_2$ and Pao_2 of more than 10 to 15 mm Hg. Administer oxygen to maintain the arterial blood gases as ordered. Assess patient to identify signs such as restlessness, confusion, and irritability, which may indicate the body's response to altered blood gas states. Monitor electrocardiogram and cardiac status for arrhythmias secondary to alterations in blood gases. Monitor and record kidney functioning and urinary output, which may be affected secondary to chronic tissue hypoxia and alterations in metabolism. Monitor serum electrolytes, which may change because of alterations in oxygenation and metabolism. Carefully monitor body temperature, which may fluctuate because of alterations in metabolism or secondary infections.
Airway clearance, ineffective	Assess patient to identify inability to move secretions; if inability is identified, assist with appropriate measures (coughing, positioning, suctioning, liquefying secretions, etc.). Assist patient to maintain proper body positioning to assure maximal airway availability (e.g., semi-Fowler's position). Carefully and frequently auscultate chest for quality of breath sounds and adventitious sounds; note cough and sputum characteristics.
Nutrition alteration in: less than body requirements	See p. 2042 for associated nursing care.
Fluid volume deficit, potential	In the seriously ill patient, monitor for evidence of gastrointestinal bleeding secondary to physiologic stress; monitor serial hemoglobin and hematocrit; check all stools, emesis, and nasogastric aspirate for presence of blood; observe changes in vital signs or abdominal girth.
Mobility, impaired physical	Encourage patient to use adaptive breathing techniques to decrease the work of breathing. See p. 2106 for additional strategies.

Nursing Diagnosis	**Nursing Intervention**
Fear	Assess patient's level of fear related to the present health state. Assess patient's level of fear related to feeling of air hunger.
Self-care deficit	Assess the level of self-care deficit secondary to the patient's current condition. See p. 2088 for additional strategies.
Coping, ineffective individual	Listen carefully to collect information regarding the significance of the current health care problem and the patient's perception of his ability to deal with alterations it is causing.
Coping, family: potential for growth	Assess family's understanding of diagnostic procedures, disease process and prognosis, and therapies employed. See p. 1899 for additional strategies.

Patient Education

1. Teach patient and family about the chest tubes, their purpose, function, and care that must be taken during their use.
2. Teach patient adaptive breathing techniques so as to maximize potential lung reexpansion and prevent complications.
3. Teach importance of contact avoidance with persons with upper respiratory infections and influenza.
4. Teach importance of regular medical reevaluations for an extended period following the pneumothorax.

EVALUATION

Patient Outcome	Data Indicating That Outcome is Reached
Full expansion of lungs is achieved.	Chest x-ray films show full lung expansion with no evidence of pneumothorax or hemothorax.
Optimal movement of air in and out of lungs occurs.	Vital capacity measurements are optimal for patient. Blood gas values are within normal limits. Airways are clear, and breathing occurs without obstruction. Clear breath sounds are heard in all areas. Behavior is modified to conserve energy expenditure.
Physiologic stability occurs secondary to respiratory insult.	Nutrition level is maintained. Kidney and bladder functioning is within normal limits. Gastrointestinal system functioning is adequate. Secondary infections do not occur. Serum electrolytes are within normal limits.
Patient can relate importance of daily pulmonary exercises until pneumothorax is completely healed.	Patient demonstrates pulmonary exercises and states rationale and importance of maintaining daily exercise routine.
Patient and family have sufficient information to comply with discharge regimen.	Patient and family are able at time of discharge to discuss medications—purpose, side effects, route, and schedule; dietary therapy regimen; activity progression regimen; signs of infection or respiratory deterioration; and plan for follow-up visits.

Medical Interventions

AIRWAY MAINTENANCE

Airway maintenance may occur in many forms including the following:

Suctioning
Oropharyngeal airway
Nasopharyngeal airway
Endotracheal intubation
Tracheostomy (see Chapter 7 for procedures)

Regardless of technique, the purpose of maintaining a patent airway is so that ventilation may occur. Certain airway maintenance methods such as endotracheal intubation are usually connected to oxygen sources or mechanical ventilators.

Preprocedural Care

Clinical assessment indicating airway obstruction

Restlessness
Wheezing
Noisy respirations
Difficulty breathing
Tachycardia
Rhonchi over large airways
Decreased breath sounds
Retractions: intercostal, suprasternal, supraclavicular, nasal flaring
Stridor
Mouth breathing
Low tidal volume

Preprocedural teaching. Because of the patient's situation requiring airway maintenance procedures, preprocedural teaching may seem inappropriate. The care provider is still required to anticipate teaching opportunities and to provide the following information as appropriate:

Explain procedure to patient and family members
Discuss with patient and family what procedure will be like for the patient
Demonstrate equipment and its purpose

PROCEDURAL TECHNIQUES AND ASSOCIATED CARE[29,32,37,49,65]

Orotracheal or nasotracheal suctioning

Indications:
Signs of respiratory distress
Noisy wet breathing

Contraindications:
Tight wheeze at bronchospasm or croup

Procedural guidelines:
1. If possible, position patient in semi-Fowler's position.
2. Use sterile, gloved technique.
3. Use smallest catheter size possible to remove secretions.
4. Hyperoxygenate patient prior to suctioning procedure if patient is on respiratory assistance ventilator.
5. Encourage patient to breath slowly during procedure.
6. Lubricate catheter tip with sterile saline or water prior to procedure.
7. Insert vented catheter for suctioning.
8. Insert and advance catheter as patient slowly breathes.
9. Do not apply suction until catheter is fully inserted.
10. Once catheter is in place, apply suction for 5- to 10-second interval; rotate and slowly withdraw catheter during suctioning.
11. At least 3 minutes should be allowed between suctioning periods; during this time, administer oxygen.
12. Note and record amount and characteristics of sputum.
13. Note and record patient's response to suctioning procedure.
14. Discard catheter after each treatment.
15. Change vacuum container and tubing every day.

Complications:
Wheezing or crowing respiratory sounds after or during procedure indicating potential bronchospasm or laryngospasm (if noted, administer oxygen and contact physician)
Bloody drainage due to trauma or respiratory secretions
Prolonged spasmodic coughing
Traumatic ulceration of the airways
Infection
Atelectasis if catheter greater than two thirds the size of bronchus is used
Hypoxemia
Cardiac rhythm and rate disturbance

Oropharyngeal or nasopharyngeal airways

Indications:

Potential or actual upper airway obstruction due to altered levels of consciousness resulting in relaxation of the tongue against the hypopharynx

Trauma-induced upper airway obstruction

Procedural guidelines:

1. Determine type of airway according to individual patient needs:
   a. Oropharyngeal airway: length should be from teeth to the mandibular end of jaw.
   b. Nasopharyngeal airway: may be indicated if patient has associated mouth injury; the length should be slightly narrower than the nares diameter.
2. Insertion techniques:
   a. Oropharyngeal airway: insert airway upside down to prevent tongue from being pushed posteriorly; as the airway passes the uvula, rotate the airway 180 degrees; the flange of the airway should be securely positioned outside the lips.
   b. Nasopharyngeal airway: should be inserted in anatomic line with the nasal passage.
3. Position patient on side to facilitate drainage.
4. Remove and change airway at least every 6 to 8 hours; observe for ulcerations of mucous membranes.
5. Remove and change nasal airway at least every 72 hours; rotate to other nares; observe for ulcerations of mucous membranes.
6. Carefully observe position of airway at least every hour; suction if needed.
7. Provide mouth and nose care at least every 2 hours.
8. Airway removal: observe patient's level of consciousness and presence of gag and swallow reflexes; when patient is awake, instruct him to push airway out with tongue; carefully observe patient for adequate airway maintenance after removal.

Complications:

Will not prevent aspiration of secretions; suction must be available

May cause patient to gag

May become clogged

May become dislodged if not secured in place

Bleeding secondary to trauma of insertion

Potential infection secondary to airway

Ulceration of nares or of pharynx secondary to prolonged insertion

Observe for mucus plugs or other signs of noisy breathing, restlessness, or malpositioning of airway, which indicate blockage of airway or malpositioning

Endotracheal intubation

Indications:

Intubation:

Airway obstruction that occurs despite the use of an oral airway

To prevent possible aspiration in an unconscious patient

To remove secretions from the tracheobronchial tree

To provide controlled ventilation, which may or may not be accomplished by face masks

To provide high concentrations of oxygen

Extubation:

Should only be attempted in a planned and controlled environment

Procedural guidelines:

1. Assemble all equipment prior to attempting intubation procedure.
2. Check the cuff on endotracheal tubes for leakage.
3. Assist to position patient so that the neck is flexed and the head is extended; this should bring the mouth, larynx, and trachea in line.
4. If patient is awake or combative, succinylcholine may be given to block voluntary ventilation; prior to administering this drug, ventilatory assistance equipment must be available for immediate use.
5. Prior to intubation the nurse should explain the procedure and ensure that any false teeth or bridges have been removed.
6. Prior to intubation, hyperventilate patient using an Ambu bag with supplemental 100% oxygen.
7. If intubation is prolonged, the procedure should be interrupted and the patient should be oxygenated.
8. Once the endotracheal tube is in place, the nurse must assist to determine proper endotracheal tube placement; this is done by considering the following:
9. Correct placement: bilateral lung inflation, breath sounds heard equally throughout all lobes.
10. Incorrect placement:
    a. Esophagus: absence of breath sounds, respiratory distress and cyanosis; if these are noted, the endotracheal tube should be removed and reinserted.
    b. Right mainstem bronchus or carina: the endotracheal tube has been inserted too far; clinical signs include unilateral breath

sounds, lung inflation, and coughing; if this is noted and confirmed by x-ray examination, the endotracheal tube should be retracted slightly and resecured; reassessment should indicate proper placement.

11. Once in correct position, the endotracheal tube should be taped securely so that movement of the tube is impossible.
12. Tube placement and patency should be monitored at least every hour; this assessment should include:
    a. Tube position.
    b. Tube patency.
    c. Select lung inflation.
    d. Absence of respiratory distress.
    e. Generalized respiratory response.
    f. Monitoring of arterial blood gases.
13. Ongoing care for patients with endotracheal tube in place:
    a. Provide mouth care every 2 hours.
    b. Clean nares and around endotracheal tube at least every 6 to 8 hours.
    c. Reposition and retape endotracheal tube at least every 6 to 8 hours.
    d. Take precaution not to dislodge tube position.
14. If tube has cuff, use minimal leak technique or deflate cuff every 4 to 5 hours for at least 20 minutes (prolonged cuff deflation will not work if patient is attached to ventilator); this should follow careful and thorough suctioning of oral secretions; the cuff should then be reinflated until no air leakage is noted; record the amount of air inserted to inflate the cuff.
15. Bite block should be used if the patient bites the endotracheal tube.
16. Mucus plugs may be removed by instillation of saline into the endotracheal tube:
    a. Children less than 5 kg = 0.5 ml saline.
    b. Children over 5 kg = 1 to 2 ml saline.
    c. Adults = 8 to 10 ml saline.
17. Chest physiotherapy should be performed at least every 4 hours.
18. Patient should receive humidified oxygen while intubated.
19. If patient is awake, provide writing materials so that patient has method of communicating.
20. Extubation:
    a. Assess patient's ability to breathe on own prior to extubation.
    b. Determine that patient is able to maintain spontaneous respiratory rate sufficient to maintain stable blood gas values.
    c. Carefully suction endotracheal tube and mouth prior to extubation.
    d. Immediately following extubation, assess for signs of respiratory distress or laryngeal spasm such as dyspnea, noisy breathing, use of abdominal or accessory muscles, restlessness, irritability, tachycardia, tachypnea, ↓ PaO_2, ↑ $PaCO_2$; if these are noted, consult physician immediately and prepare for reinsertion of endotracheal tube.

Complications:
Delay of oxygenation or ventilation during intubation procedure
Placement of endotracheal tube into right mainstem bronchi, resulting in unilateral and thus diminished lung aeration
Endotracheal tube cuff inflated for more than 8 hours may cause ulceration of trachea, or tracheoesophageal fistula
Mucus plugs or other blockage of endotracheal tube may lead to hypoxia and respiratory distress
Unplanned extubation by combative patient or secondary to poor securement of tube will require immediate airway and ventilatory assessment by the nurse as well as potential need for oral airway, patient positioning, and ventilation by Ambu bag with supplemental oxygen
Aspiration of secretions secondary to poorly inflated cuff; inadequate suctioning prior to cuff deflation; or too small noncuffed endotracheal tube used
Potential laryngospasm or edema following intubation

ASSESSMENT: AREAS OF CONCERN

Inability to maintain patent airway
Despite the selected technique, patent airway is not obtained; patient continues to have same or different airway obstruction signs as noted during preprocedural assessment (see above)
Carefully observe patent condition of tubing; clean or reposition as necessary to maximize airway potential
For tracheostomy and endotracheal intubation, obtain a chest x-ray film after insertion to ascertain exact positioning of tube

Positioning to maximize airway potential
Carefully assess for patent airway, presence of bilaterally equal breath sounds, and bilateral expansion of chest wall

Bleeding or trauma caused by the airway maintenance technique

Observe for presence of bleeding and for wet breath sounds; bleeding is usually self-limiting, unless the patient is receiving anticoagulants or has a bleeding disorder

Potential dental damage secondary to insertion

Observe condition of patient's teeth

Ulcerations of nasal tissue or pharynx

Carefully observe tissue around the airway mechanism; when possible, change position of the mechanism or its taped location

Secondary infection due to airway maintenance mechanism

Observe for signs of infection such as increased temperature, change in secretions, or foul odor

NURSING DIAGNOSES and NURSING INTERVENTIONS

Nursing Diagnosis	Nursing Intervention
Airway clearance, ineffective	Position patient to maximize airway potential. Using sterile technique, suction as needed to maintain airway. At least hourly, auscultate chest for presence and quality of bilateral breath sounds and adventitious sounds. Observe patient for other signs of hypoxia or airway blockage as indicated in the preprocedural assessment section. If patient has endotracheal tube in place, provide oropharyngeal airway or bite-block to prevent biting on the endotracheal tube.
Anxiety	Observe for signs of anxiety secondary to airway blockage or hypoxia. Observe for signs of anxiety secondary to the airway maintenance procedure.
Breathing pattern, ineffective	Observe breathing pattern secondary to airway maintenance procedure or which remains ineffective despite the airway maintenance procedure; in collaboration with physician prepare to administer supportive ventilation.
Gas exchange, impaired	Monitor arterial blood gases secondary to airway maintenance procedure; in collaboration with physician prepare to administer oxygen therapy secondary to airway maintenance procedure.
Oral mucous membrane, alterations in	Provide mouth care at least every 2 hours for those patients with an airway maintenance device left in place.
Skin integrity, impairment of: potential	Provide careful skin care around the airway maintenance device at least every 4 hours. If taping is involved, rotate the taping site often.
Communication, impaired: verbal	Provide patient with note paper and pencil or Magic Slate for easy communication. Place call-light cord in easy reach.
Injury, potential for	Should patient demonstrate restlessness and confusion secondary to hypoxia or systemic condition, provide soft restraints for the patient's wrists so that airway does not become dislodged.

EVALUATION

Patient Outcome	Data Indicating That Outcome is Reached
Airway is patent.	Breath sounds are clear and bilaterally equal. There are adventitious sounds. Breathing occurs easily and seems to be adequate for patient's attempt.
Gas exchange is adequate.	Blood gas values are within normal limits.

ARTERIAL BLOOD GAS ANALYSIS

Description and Rationale

Arterial blood gas analysis is the most direct method to assess the patient's oxygen and blood-gas status. The procedure is indicated for any patient who is seriously ill or injured whose respiratory status and metabolic balance are in question. Most commonly, arterial blood gases are required for those patients with hypoxemia or desaturation secondary to altered ventilatory patterns due to any cause.

Cautions[58]

1. Potential inadequate collateral circulation (See Allen test below to test for collateral circulation.)
2. Potential hematoma from multiple unsuccessful attempts at injection at any one site or from inadequate pressure (less than 5 minutes) to puncture site following artery stick
3. Potential ischemia secondary to thrombus following the procedure
4. Adjunct nerve damage secondary to incorrect technique

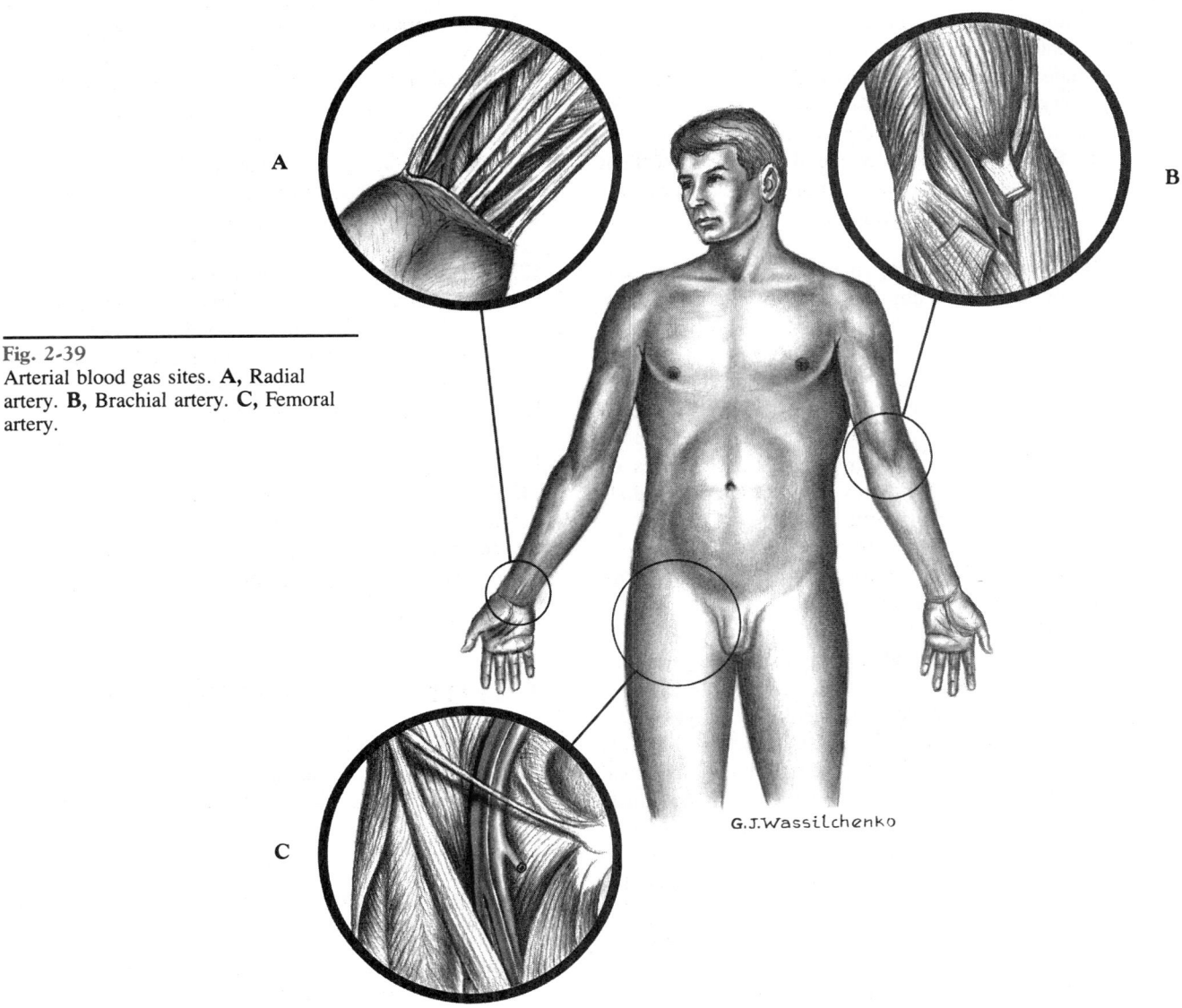

Fig. 2-39
Arterial blood gas sites. **A,** Radial artery. **B,** Brachial artery. **C,** Femoral artery.

G.J.Wassilchenko

ARTERIAL BLOOD GAS COLLECTION PROCEDURE

1. Gather equipment: 2 or 3 ml syringe with 25-gauge needle; 10 ml glass or disposable syringe with 20-21-gauge needle (21-23-gauge for children); rubber stopper or Luer-Lok cap, 1 ml sodium heparin (1:1000), lidocaine (Xylocaine) or procaine, alcohol swab or iodophor prep, gauze pads, and basin with crushed ice and water.

2. Heparinize the 10 ml glass syringe by using the 20-21-gauge needle and drawing up 0.5 ml heparin into the syringe to wet the cylinder and plunger; then discard the heparin as much as possible by holding the syringe upright and expelling the heparin and air bubbles. Recover the needle and lay aside.

3. Position the patient in either a sitting or supine position and explain procedure.

4. Locate the arterial puncture site: possible sites include the radial artery, brachial artery, and femoral artery (Fig. 2-39). Vessel criteria include the following:

   a. Collateral blood flow: radial artery has excellent collateral flow; brachial artery has reasonable collateral flow; and femoral artery has no collateral blood flow.

   b. Vessel accessibility: it is easier to palpate, stabilize, and puncture superficial vessels than deep ones. The more distal an artery, the more superficial it is.

   c. Periarterial tissue: muscles, tendon, and fat are reasonably insensitive to pain. Bone periosteum and nerves are very sensitive. Therefore, choose a site that avoids close sensitive structures or parallel veins. The sites of choice are first, radial; second, brachial; third, femoral.

5. When using the radial artery, perform the Allen test. This will evaluate the collateral blood supply. The technique is as follows:

   a. Instruct patient to close fist tightly.

   b. Obliterate both radial and ulnar nerves simultaneously.

   c. Instruct patient to relax hand (not fully); watch for blanching of palm and fingers.

   d. Remove obstructing pressure from only the ulnar artery and observe for capillary refill and flush of hand (within 15 seconds). This refill response, which is a positive Allen test, verifies that the ulnar artery alone is capable of supplying the entire hand.

   e. If there is a negative Allen test, do not use the radial artery for arterial puncture.

   f. If the patient is unconscious or uncooperative, a similar response to the closed fist can be obtained by placing the patient's hand up in the air until blanching occurs; obliterate the arteries, lower the hand, and release pressure over the ulnar artery.

NOTE: The remaining procedure assumes that the radial artery has been chosen for arterial puncture:

6. Palpate the radial artery to locate a spot where maximum pulsation is felt.

7. Clean the area with iodophor prep, then with alcohol swab.

8. The skin may then be injected with an anesthetic agent using the small syringe with 25-gauge needle.

9. With one hand locate the radial pulse proximal to the area cleaned. This will provide landmark information. Keeping the fingers of the one hand on the pulse, insert the heparinized needle and syringe into the radial artery distal to the palpating fingers. The angle between the needle and the artery should be approximately 45 degrees (Fig. 2-40). This makes the hole through the arterial wall oblique so that the muscle fiber will seal the hole as soon as the needle is removed.

10. When the artery is punctured, the pulsating blood will push up the hub of the syringe. Do not make more than two attempts at any one site.

11. Obtain a sample of approximately 3 to 5 ml.

12. After the blood is obtained, remove the needle, apply gauze, and use firm and continuous pressure over the site for a minimum of 5 minutes. If the patient is on anticoagulants, pressure must be maintained for a much longer period of time.

13. Remove all air bubbles from syringe (will affect blood gas results) and apply rubber stopper to the needle tip.

14. Place capped syringe in the basin of crushed ice and water and send it to the laboratory. The ice will decrease the alterations of the true pH, oxygen, and carbon dioxide levels of the specimen.

ASSESSMENT: AREAS OF CONCERN

Peripheral circulation
Distal limb color bilaterally equal
Pulses distal to puncture site strong and bilaterally equal

Intact nerves
Bilaterally equal sensation and motor function distal to puncture site

Hematoma or bleeding around puncture site
Assess for signs of swelling, discoloration, pain, or free bleeding

Fig. 2-40

Arterial blood gas drawing technique.
A, Palpate artery chosen to draw
arterial blood. **B,** Penetrate skin,
holding syringe at 45-degree angle
with needle bevel up. **C,** Gently and
slowly advance syringe until arterial
vessel is punctured. Pulsating bright
blood should fill heparinized syringe.

From Hirsch, J., and Hannock, L.:
Mosby's manual of clinical nursing
procedures, St. Louis, 1981, The C.V.
Mosby Co.

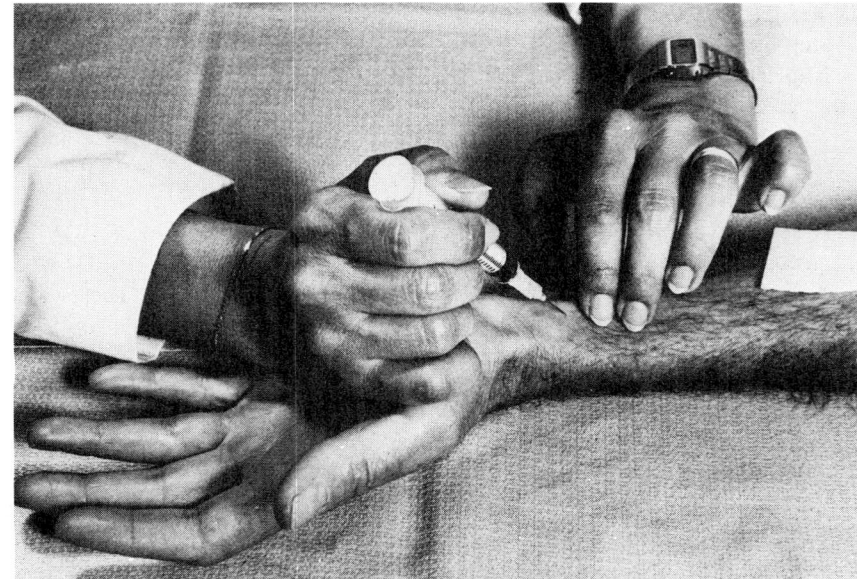

A

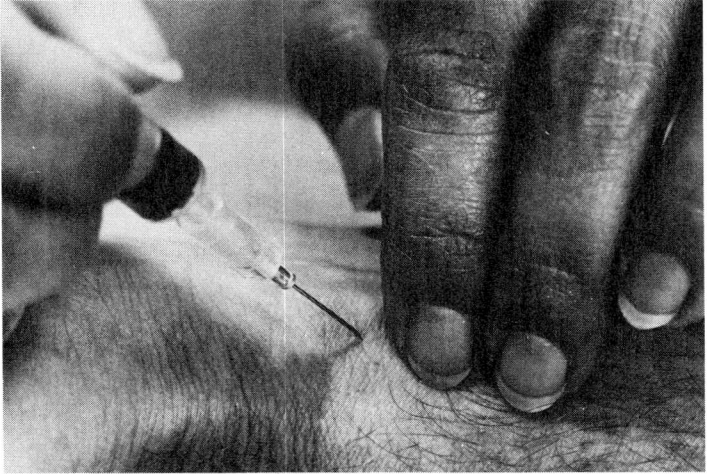

B

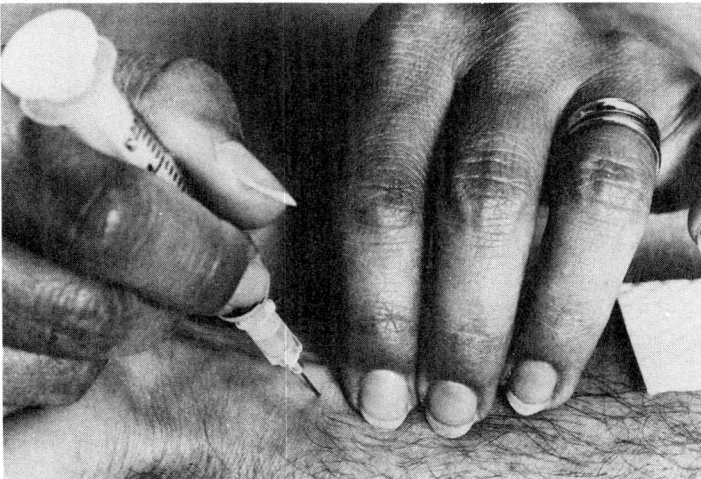

C

Blood gas analysis[46,55]

Step by step analysis

1. pH (hydrogen ion concentration): assess patient's acid-base status

   Normal = 7.35 to 7.45

   Acidosis = Less than 7.35

   Alkalosis = Greater than 7.43 (when pH is normal, but when $PaCO_2$ and HCO_3^- are both abnormal, compensation is probably occurring)

2. $PaCO_2$ (carbon dioxide tension): evaluates the patient's ventilation

   Normal = 35 to 45 mm Hg

   Hyperventilation (hypocarbia) = Less than 34 mm Hg; this means that there is excessive loss of carbon dioxide

   Abnormal value indicates there is no respiratory compensation for a metabolic problem

   Decreased values may be due to hyperventilation or ventilation-perfusion inequality

   To evaluate for respiratory acidosis and alkalosis and for compensation due to metabolic acidosis and alkalosis

3. $PaCO_2$ in relation to pH

   $\uparrow PaCO_2 + \downarrow$ pH = Acidemia of respiratory origin

   $\uparrow PaCO_2 + \uparrow$ pH = Respiratory retention of carbon dioxide to compensate for metabolic alkalosis

   $\downarrow PaCO_2 + \uparrow$ pH = Alkalosis of respiratory origin

   $\downarrow PaCO_2 + \downarrow$ pH = Respiratory elimination of carbon dioxide to compensate for metabolic acidosis

4. Bicarbonate (HCO_3^-): This is the metabolic component

   Normal = 16 to 24 mEq/L (infant), 21 to 28 mEq/L (arterial children and adults), 22 to 27 mEq/L (venous children and adults)

   Alkalosis = Greater than 26 mEq/L

   Acidosis = Less than 22 mEq/L

   A normal value indicates that there are no primary metabolic problems and that there is no metabolic compensation for a respiratory problem

5. HCO_3^- in relation to pH: To evaluate for metabolic acidosis and alkalosis and for compensation due to respiratory acidosis and alkalosis

   $\downarrow HCO_3^- + \downarrow$ pH = Acidemia of metabolic origin

   $\downarrow HCO_3^- + \uparrow$ pH = Renal retention of hydrogen ion or elimination of HCO_3^- to compensate for respiratory alkalosis

   $\uparrow HCO_3^- + \uparrow$ pH = Alkalosis of metabolic origin

   $\uparrow HCO_3^- + \downarrow$ pH = Renal retention of HCO_3^- or elimination of hydrogen ion

6. PaO_2 and O_2 saturation

   PaO_2 saturation: Normal = 80 to 95 mm Hg
   60 to 70 mm Hg (newborn)

   O_2 saturation: Normal = 95% to 99%

   These values may be due to hypoventilation, shunting, ventilation-perfusion inequality, or a reduction of inspired oxygen

Acid-base imbalance[54]

Alkalosis

  Respiratory

   $\downarrow PaCO_2 + \downarrow HCO_3^- =$ Patient attempting to compensate

   $\downarrow PaCO_2 +$ Normal $HCO_3^- =$ No patient compensation

  Metabolic

   $\uparrow HCO_3^- + \uparrow PaCO_2 =$ Patient attempting to compensate

   $\uparrow HCO_4^- +$ Normal $PaCO_2 =$ No patient compensation

  Clinical signs of alkalosis: dizziness, tingling of fingers and toes, muscle weakness or muscle spasm, muscle twitching, sweating, cardiac arrhythmia, shallow respirations, nausea or vomiting, tachypnea, tremor, or convulsion

  Fluid and electrolyte imbalances

   $\downarrow$ Serum sodium

   $\uparrow$ Serum chloride

   $\downarrow$ Serum chloride (if alkalosis is due to gastric suctioning)

   $\downarrow$ Potassium

Acidosis

  Respiratory

   $\uparrow PaCO_2 + \uparrow HCO_3^- =$ Patient attempting to compensate

   $\uparrow PaCO_2 +$ Normal $HCO_3^- =$ No patient compensation

  Metabolic

   $\downarrow HCO_3^- + \downarrow PaCO_2 =$ Patient attempting to compensate

   $\downarrow HCO_3^- +$ Normal $PaCO_2 =$ No patient compensation

  Clinical signs of acidosis: headache, slow to respond to questions, hand tremor when patient instructed to extend arms, confusion, drowsiness, Kussmaul respirations, nausea or vomiting, tremor, confusion, tachycardia, coma

  Fluid and electrolyte imbalances

   $\downarrow$ Serum sodium

   $\downarrow$ Serum chloride

   $\uparrow$ Serum potassium

NURSING DIAGNOSES and NURSING INTERVENTIONS

Nursing Diagnosis	Nursing Intervention
Fear	Explain procedure fully before attempting technique.
Comfort, alteration in: pain	Carefully assess potential pain response for patient. Assist physician to use local anesthesia if indicated prior to obtaining arterial blood gases.
Skin integrity, impairment of: actual	Following technique, apply direct pressure over puncture site for at least 5 minutes to prevent hematoma, or bleeding into the tissues.
Gas exchange, impaired	Carefully and systematically analyze the blood gas results according to the assessment guidelines. Monitor patient response to actual or potential blood-gas acid-base imbalances to include the following: Mental state: depression or stimulation of the central nervous system Respiratory status: monitor breathing pattern and depth and quality of respiration Cardiovascular response: pulse rate, rhythm, and quality Fluid and electrolyte status: monitor disorders such as vomiting and diarrhea that could cause the imbalance as well as monitor patient responses secondary to fluid and electrolyte imbalances

EVALUATION

Patient Outcome	Data Indicating That Outcome is Reached
Blood gas values are within normal limits.	Pao_2 80 to 95 mm Hg 60 to 70 mm Hg (newborn) O_2 saturation 95% to 98% $Paco_2$ 35 to 45 mm Hg pH 7.35 to 7.45 HCO_3^- 16 to 24 mEq/L (infant) 21 to 28 mEq/L (arterial children and adult) 22 to 29 mEq/L (venous children and adult)

BREATHING TECHNIQUES

Following are some breathing techniques that may be taught to the patient that will facilitate effective ventilation:

- Abdominal or diaphragmatic breathing
- Pursed-lip breathing
- Deep breathing: coughing and splinting
- Incentive spirometer

These are useful and specific measures to increase the volume of air entering the lungs as well as being expelled from the lungs. These techniques are discussed according to indications and procedural techniques.

Abdominal or diaphragmatic breathing

Indications:

Patients with chronic and acute respiratory dysfunction may be taught to use the abdominal muscles and diaphragm as the primary structures for facilitating and maximizing the ventilatory attempts of the lungs.

Procedural guidelines[35,44]:

1. Nasal passage and trachea should be free of secretions and congestion. If necessary, suction, use aerosol, encourage coughing, or perform postural drainage prior to teaching diaphragmatic breathing.
2. Assist patient to attain position of comfort, either sitting or in semi-Fowler's position in bed. Abdominal muscles should be relaxed and knees and hips flexed.
3. Instruct patient to inhale deeply through nose (keep mouth shut). As patient inhales, the focus should be to pull the diaphragm down and to force the abdominal wall outward. If a hand is placed on the patient's abdomen, the hand should rise.
4. Following a deep and even inspiration the patient should be instructed to pause slightly and then, using a pursed-lip technique, to quietly and naturally exhale.

5. The patient should be encouraged to use the abdominal muscles during exhalation to remove all air from the lungs.
6. Expiration should last 2 to 3 times longer than inspiration.
7. After the technique is mastered, a 5-pound (2.25 kg) weight may be placed on the patient's abdomen to further strengthen the abdominal muscles.
8. The diaphragmatic breathing technique must be practiced 10 to 20 minutes at least every 4 hours until the patient adequately demonstrates ability and willingness to implement the technique alone.

Pursed-lip breathing

Indications:

This technique is used to control expiration and to facilitate the maximal emptying of the alveoli. It functions to maintain a positive pressure in the airways and thus keep them open longer. In this way more air may be exhaled.

Procedural guidelines:
1. Assist patient to a position of comfort.
2. Instruct patient to inhale deeply through the nose (keep mouth shut). At end of inspiration pause slightly.
3. Then instruct patient to slowly exhale through "pursed" lips so that a blowing effect occurs.
4. Exhalation should be slow and purposeful.
5. As the technique is practiced and used on a continual basis, patient anxiety and anxiety-related dyspnea should decrease.

Deep breathing, coughing, and splinting

Indications:

This technique is most frequently used during the first 48 hours after surgery to loosen secretions and force them to be expelled. The deep breathing dilates the airways, stimulates surfactant production, and expands the lung tissue surface, thereby increasing the area for respiratory gas exchange.[44] Coughing is used to force collected and consolidated secretions to be expelled. Splinting of the chest wall is used to produce stabilization, which in turn will decrease discomfort.

Procedural guidelines:
1. Position patient so that deep inspiration and coughing may be facilitated.
2. The incision area may be splinted with a pillow and hand pressure from the nurse. As the patient coughs, the nurse should firmly assist the patient to stabilize the incisional area.
3. Instruct patient to take a slow, deep inspiration. If patient is postoperative pain medications may need to be administered 20 to 30 minutes prior to initiating procedure.
4. Instruct patient to quickly close glottis and forcefully expel an explosive current of air.
5. Provide patient with tissues to collect expelled sputum.

Incentive spirometers

Indications:

The incentive spirometer may be used postoperatively to encourage deep breathing. While it may provide assistive deep breathing exercises, it should not replace other deep breathing and coughing interventions.

Procedural guidelines:
1. Position patient in seated or semi-Fowler's position.
2. Instruct patient to seal mouth around mouthpiece and to inhale or exhale so as to activate the spirometer. Each brand of spirometer functions slightly differently. Some are operated by exhalation into the system; others are activated by inspiration. In either case the deeper the ventilatory effort, the more successful the use of the spirometer. The nurse must carefully inspect the operation of a specific unit prior to instructing the patient.
3. It is advantageous for the patient to hold a deep breath for a few seconds prior to exhaling. This will assist to prevent pulmonary complications.
4. After the spirometer is used, the mouthpiece and tubing should be washed and not used for any other patient.
5. The incentive spirometer should be used at least every 3 or 4 hours during the postoperative period until the patient is ambulatory and initiates effective deep breathing and coughing on his own.

EVALUATION

All of the breathing techniques have similar evaluation criteria.

Patient Outcome	Data Indicating That Outcome is Reached
Optimal movement of air in and out of the lungs occurs.	Airway is clear and breathing occurs without obstruction. Patient is able to inhale deeply and exhale effectively. There is no evidence of dyspnea or hypoxia.
Airway is patent.	There is no evidence of pulmonary congestion, or condition is optimal for patient; if sputum is present, patient is able to demonstrate productive sputum cough.
Clear breath sounds are heard in all areas.	Bronchovesicular breath sounds are heard throughout, or optimal breath sounds for patient. No areas of decreased breath sounds or consolidation are heard.
Patient is comfortable during coughing and deep breathing.	Patient is able to ask for splinting assistance or splints self during deep breathing and coughing exercises.

CHEST PHYSIOTHERAPY AND POSTURAL DRAINAGE

Postural drainage, chest percussion, and vibration are effective methods by which to loosen and move secretions for patients who are unable to loosen and cough up secretions on their own. The nursing diagnosis most frequently indicated is airway clearance, ineffective.

Specifically, these techniques are helpful for preoperative or postoperative patients who have large amounts of sputum, patients with cystic fibrosis or other types of lung diseases in which copious secretions are produced, and for any patient who has difficulty coughing up sputum.

Contraindications:
1. Cyanosis or dyspnea caused by the techniques
2. Increased pain or discomfort with the techniques
3. Suction equipment not available for:
   a. Patients with copious sputum
   b. Patients with prolonged bleeding and clotting times
   c. Extremely obese patients
   d. Patients with history of predisposition to pathologic fractures

Procedural guidelines:
Postural drainage consists of positioning the patient in specific and controlled positions so as to drain and remove secretions from particular segments of the lungs.

The various positions for postural drainage differ based upon the lobes being drained. Fig. 2-41 details the various positions, lobes drained, and special instructions. Many times chest physiotherapy is combined with postural drainage.

The patient should maintain each postural drainage position for a minimum of 5 minutes. At the end of each positioned period the patient should cough and deep breathe before moving to the next position. Should one position cause the patient dyspnea or discomfort, move on to the next position. Do not terminate the techniques completely.

Chest physiotherapy consists of chest percussion and vibration. Each indicated lung lobe area may be percussed and vibrated as indicated in Fig. 2-41.

To *percuss,* cup hands and lightly and rhythmically strike the chest wall. A hollow, deep sound indicates that the technique is being performed correctly. Each area should be percussed for 1 to 2 minutes. Do not percuss over soft tissue or areas where the technique causes increased pain. To vibrate the area, gently but firmly vibrate hand against the thoracic wall directly over the area that was percussed. This technique should be done at least 5 to 7 times during the patient's expiration.

Chest physiotherapy and postural drainage techniques take on a therapeutic treatment when they are performed systematically and routinely as ordered by the physician. The therapy most frequently involves the following:
1. Patient assumes a specific postural drainage position for 5 minutes.
2. The area is percussed for 1 to 2 minutes.
3. The area is vibrated.

Fig. 2-41
Positions for postural drainage. **A,** Anterior apical segment; sitting. **B,** Posterior apical segment; sitting. **C,** Anterior segment; lying flat on back. **D,** Right posterior segment; lying on left side. **E,** Left posterior segment; lying on right side. **F,** Right middle lobe; lying on left side. **G,** Left lingula; lying on right side. **H,** Anterior segments; lying on back. **I,** Right lateral segment; lying on left side. **J,** Left lateral segment; lying on right side. **K,** Posterior segments; lying on stomach. **L,** Superior segments; lying on stomach.

From Hirsch, J., and Hannock, L.: Mosby's manual of clinical nursing procedures, St. Louis, 1981, The C.V. Mosby Co.

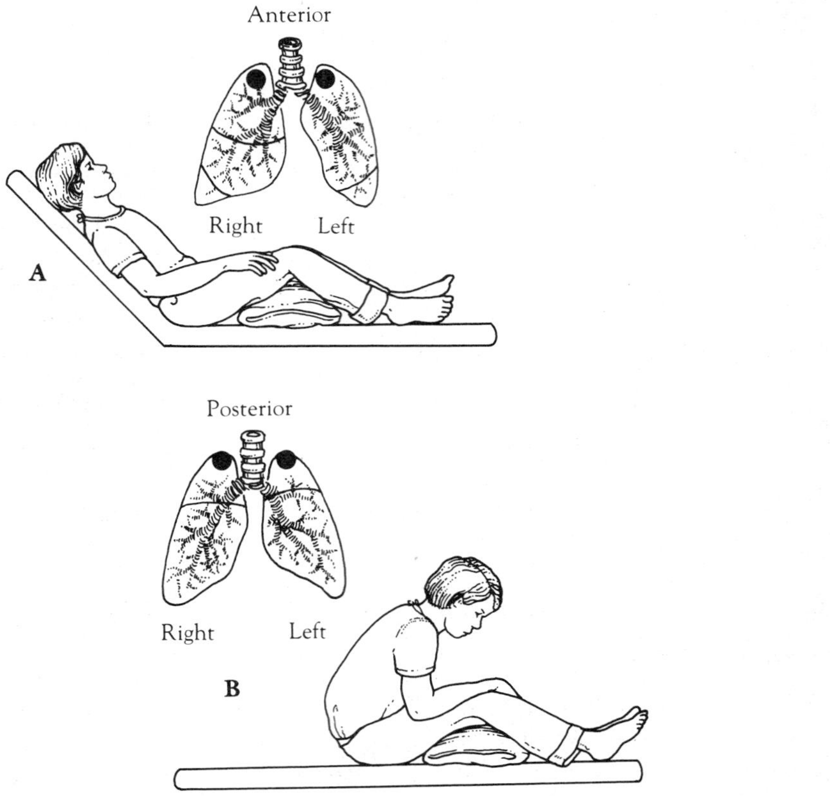

Anterior
Right   Left
A

Posterior
Right   Left
B

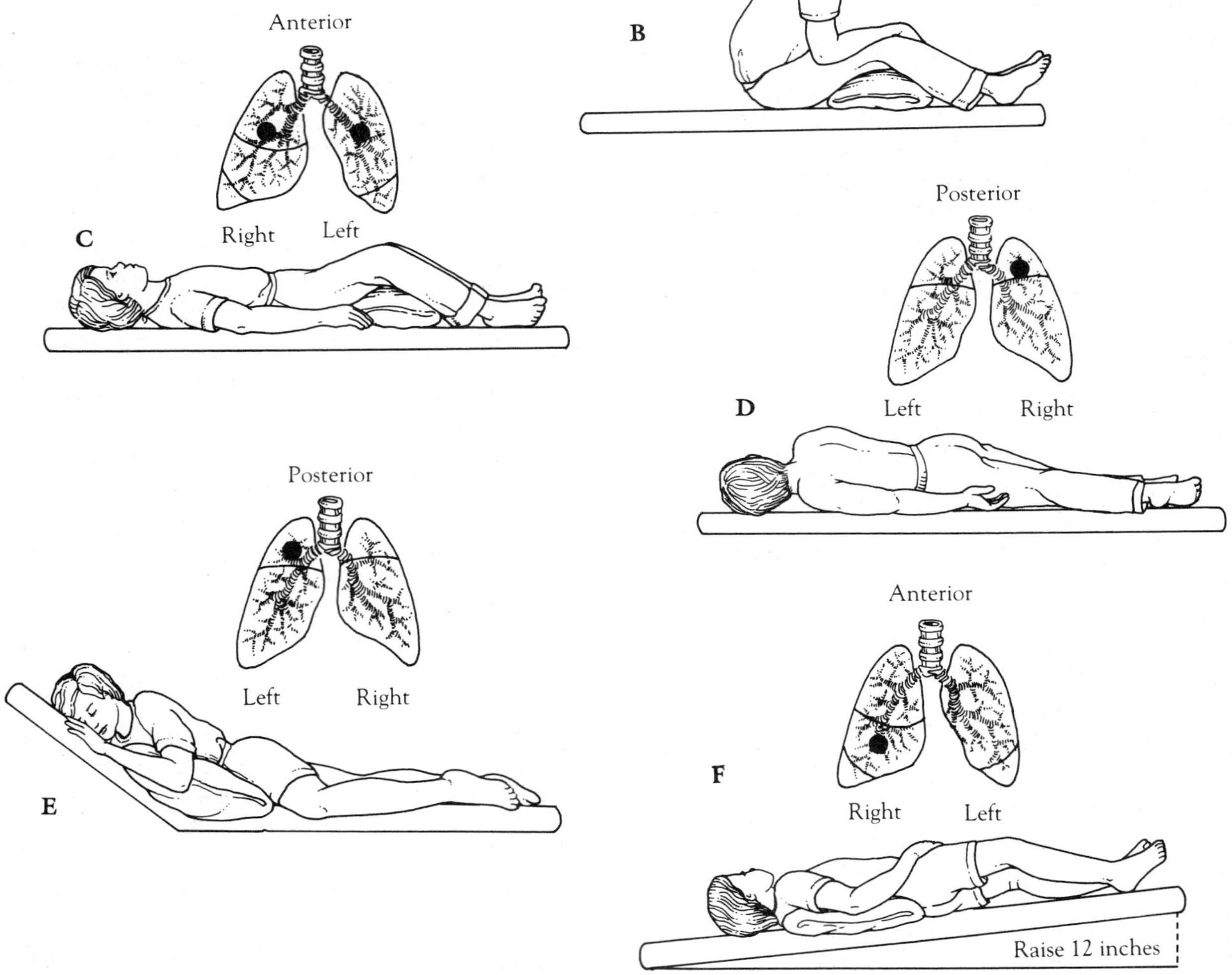

Anterior
C   Right   Left

Posterior
D   Left   Right

Posterior
Left   Right
E

Anterior
F   Right   Left

Raise 12 inches

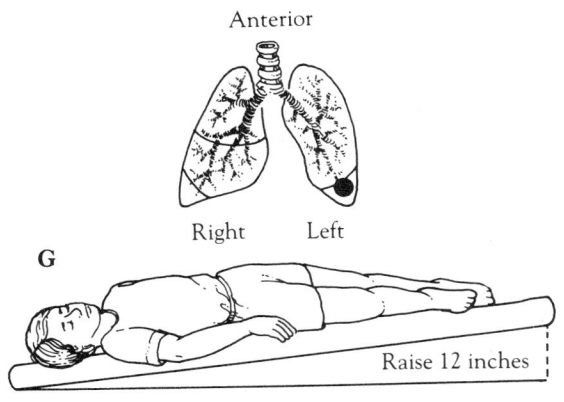

Anterior

Right Left

G

Raise 12 inches

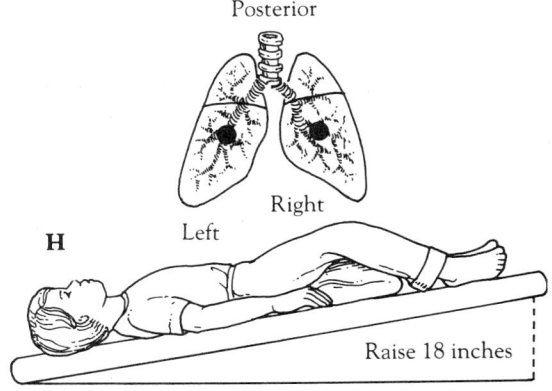

Posterior

Left Right

H

Raise 18 inches

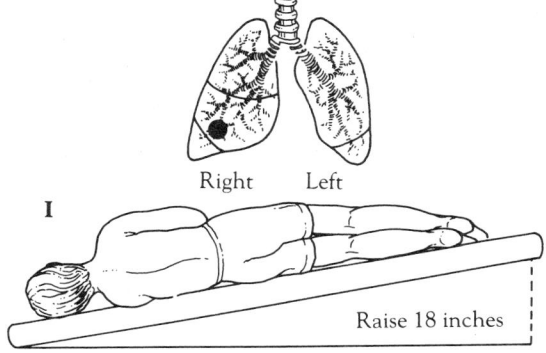

Anterior

Right Left

I

Raise 18 inches

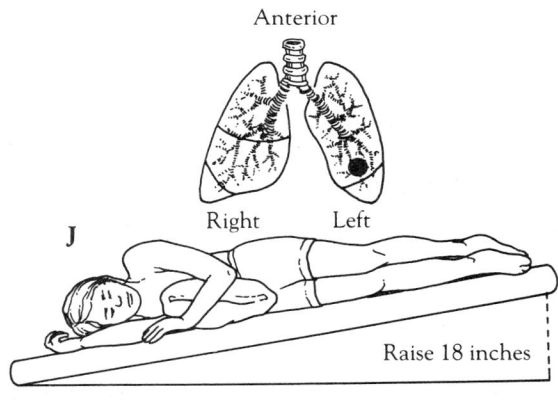

Anterior

Right Left

J

Raise 18 inches

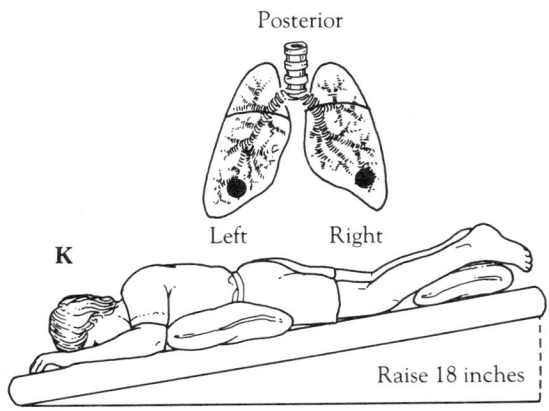

Posterior

Left Right

K

Raise 18 inches

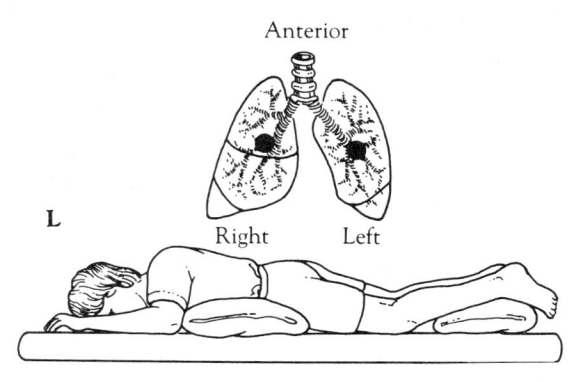

Anterior

Right Left

L

4. Patient is encouraged to cough up and spit out sputum.
5. A different postural drainage position is attained, and the percussion and vibration techniques are repeated.

Patient Education

1. Patients may be taught to perform postural drainage at home; a specific routine should be encouraged.
2. Although it is impossible for patients to perform chest physiotherapy on themselves, they may perform "tapping" movements on the chest wall by using the fingertips of both hands. This may assist to loosen secretions.
3. Family members may be taught vibratory and percussion techniques.
4. Patients should be encouraged to perform oral hygiene after procedure.
5. Procedure should be completed at least 30 minutes prior to meals, or at least 2 hours following the last meal.
6. Encourage patient to use tissues during coughing and to inspect characteristics of sputum.

EVALUATION

Patient Outcome	Data Indicating That Outcome is Reached
Airways are clear.	Breath sounds are clear bilaterally following techniques.
Chest physiotherapy and postural drainage are maintained at a therapeutic level.	Patient tolerates procedures, and procedures appear to be beneficial to patient.
Productive sputum specimen is produced.	Patient is able to expectorate sputum following each postural drainage position.

CHEST TUBES AND CHEST DRAINAGE SYSTEMS

Description and Rationale

Chest tubes with attached drainage systems are placed in the pleural cavity to drain fluid, blood, or air from the pleural cavity and to reestablish a negative pressure that will facilitate expansion of the lung. Chest tubes may be inserted postoperatively, as an emergency procedure following chest trauma, or therapeutically as a disease treatment modality. Following are chest tube insertion sites:

- Pneumothorax: usually in second and third intercostal space—anterior
- Hemothorax: usually in seventh, eighth, or ninth intercostal space—posterior
- Thoracotomy: one tube generally inserted in second or third intercostal space anterior chest and another in lower-posterior axillary line

Chest tubes may be terminated when x-ray examination determines that the lung is reexpanded and when the drainage has slowed to less than 75 ml per day.[29]

Cautions

Chest tubes are inserted by a physician and sutured into place. Cautions specific to chest tubes and drainage systems include the following:

- Sterility must be maintained so as not to introduce infection into pleural cavity.
- The system must remain patent: the tubing must not become blocked; if this occurs, a tension pneumothorax may result.
- Should the drainage tubing become dislodged from the patient or should a drainage bottle break, cross-clamps should be quickly applied to the tube(s) nearest the patient until the system's integrity can be reestablished.
- Should the chest tube become dislodged from the patient's chest, the patient should forcefully exhale, and the chest wall incision should be quickly covered with a petroleum jelly gauze.

Preprocedural Nursing Care

Carefully assess patient's preprocedural condition including respiratory rate and quality. Note evidence of dyspnea, labored breathing, tachypnea, tachycardia, quality and distribution of breath sounds, mediastinal shift, subcutaneous emphysema, and crepitus.

Set up drainage equipment appropriately for the type of system being used.

Fig. 2-42
Bottle chest drainage systems. **A,** Single-bottle system. **B,** Double-bottle system. **C,** Triple-bottle system.

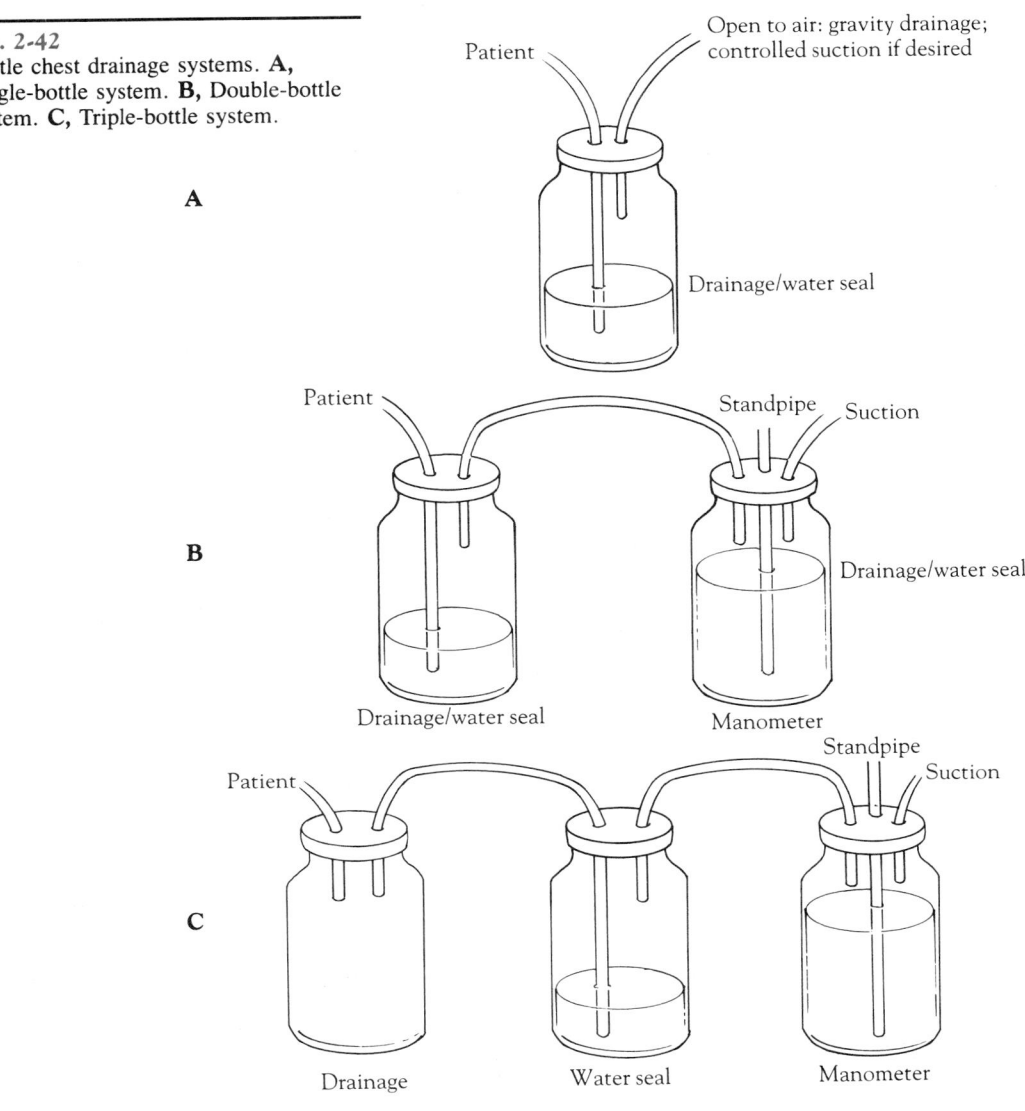

A

Patient

Open to air: gravity drainage; controlled suction if desired

Drainage/water seal

B

Patient

Standpipe   Suction

Drainage/water seal

Drainage/water seal   Manometer

C

Patient

Standpipe   Suction

Drainage   Water seal   Manometer

Single-bottle system (Fig. 2-42, *A*)
1. Unwrap bottles and tubing; maintain sterility.
2. Fill bottle with sterile water until the long glass tubing is submerged 2 cm. This bottle is called the water-seal bottle.
3. The short glass tubing, air vent, should never be covered with water.
4. The long glass tubing is connected to the patient's chest tube, and the short tubing air vent may be open to the air or connected to gravity drainage.

Double-bottle system (Fig. 2-42, *B*)
1. Prepare first bottle as described for the single-bottle system.

2. Prepare the second bottle (the suction control or manometer bottle) by running a tube from the air vent of the first bottle to an air vent in the second bottle. This is the bottle that regulates the amount of vacuum in the system.
3. Fill the second bottle with sterile water to the designated depth.
4. The second bottle contains a long glass middle tube that acts as the air vent. The length of the large tube submerged under water determines the amount of negative pressure required to drain the chest. A common depth of water is 10 to 20 cm.

Fig. 2-43
Commercial chest drainage system.

From Budassi, S.A., and Barber, J.M.:
Mosby's manual of emergency care, ed. 2,
St. Louis, 1984, The C.V. Mosby Co.

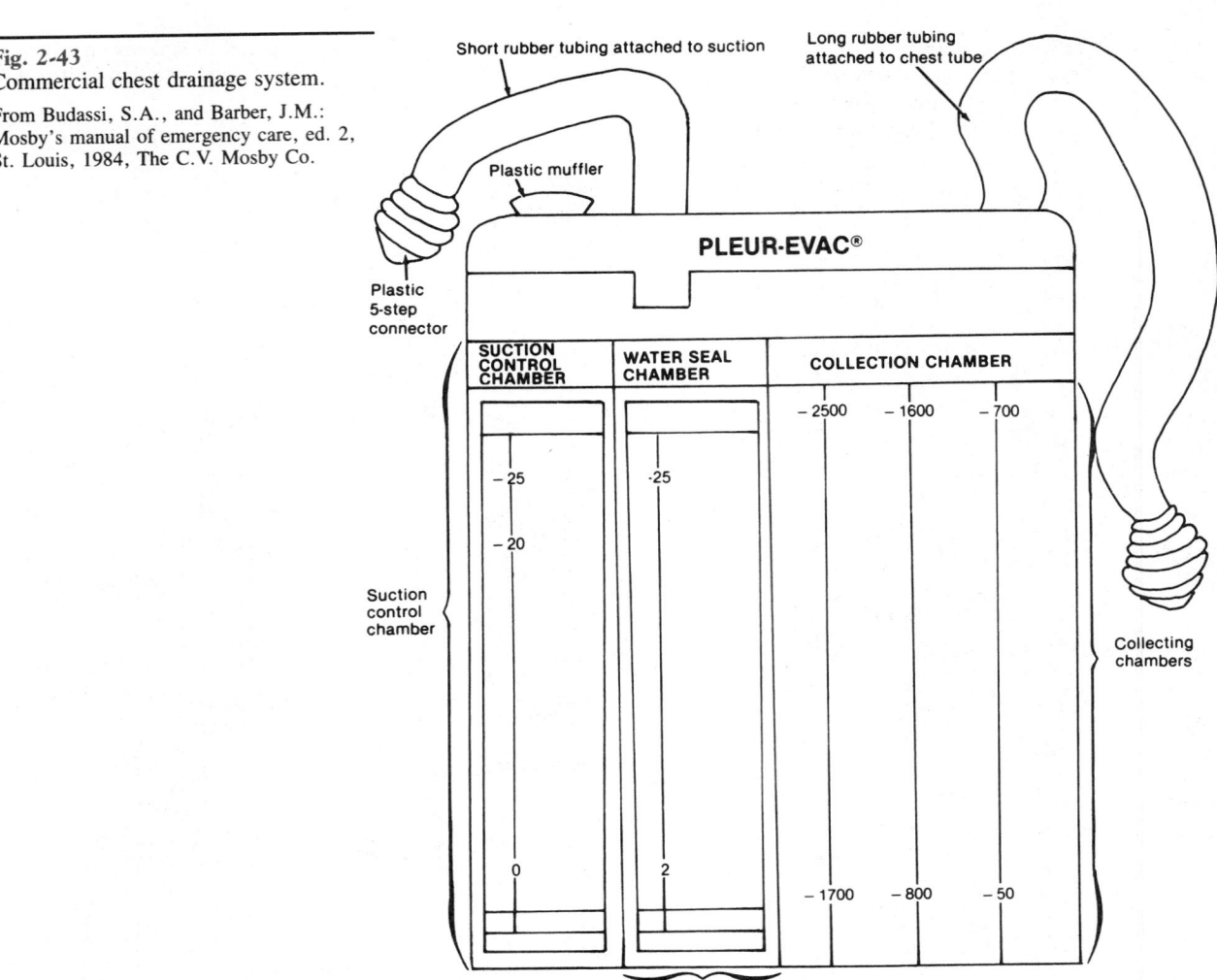

5. The suction control or manometer bottle is generally connected to a suction device such as an Emerson or Stedman pump.

Triple-bottle system (Fig. 2-42, *C*)
1. Prepare first two bottles as previously described.
2. A third bottle is prepared for a position closest to the patient. This bottle acts entirely as a drainage collection bottle.

Commercial disposable three-chamber units (Fig. 2-43)
1. Pleur-Evac and Thoraseal are two common brands.
2. These systems function like the three-bottle systems.
3. Set-up and operation directions are provided with the sterile units.

ASSESSMENT: AREAS OF CONCERN

System functioning properly[29]
Water in the water-seal bottle should fluctuate slightly when suction is applied to the patient's chest
There should be no bubbling in the water-seal bottle with expiration; *continuous bubbling suggests an air leak*

Potential atelectasis due to hypoventilation
Dyspnea, evidence of consolidation on chest x-ray film

Increased accumulation of air in the pleural space
Check for air leaks in the system
Assess to make sure chest tubes are securely placed and patent

Clinical signs include increased evidence of dyspnea, tachypnea, tachycardia, anxiety, restlessness, and shortness of breath

Infection

↑ WBC, ↑ temperature, evidence of purulent drainage

NURSING DIAGNOSES and NURSING INTERVENTIONS

Nursing Diagnosis	Nursing Intervention
Breathing pattern, ineffective	Assess and assure patency of chest tubes by stripping and milking chest tubes every hour to keep them clear of clots; observe for tube kinking. Observe for signs of intrapleural fluid accumulation such as decreased breath sounds on affected side, increased dyspnea, and mediastinal shift. Always keep chest tube drainage system lower than patient's chest. Observe volume, shade, color, and consistency of drainage from lung and record findings regularly. Observe for "tidaling" or fluctuation of fluid in the water-seal bottle; this should rise and fall with breathing; if fluctuation is not seen, carefully evaluate the patency of the tubing. Assure that all tubing connections are securely attached and taped. Have at the bedside two rubber-shod clamps to cross clamp the chest tube near the patient should the water-seal drainage system become disconnected or break. Assist patient to cough, deep breathe, and move position at least every 2 hours. Observe special positioning if indicated due to special technique or surgery. Auscultate breath sounds at least every 2 to 4 hours to assess quality of breath sounds.
Comfort, alteration in: pain	Provide splinting to chest tube area when encouraging patient to cough or deep breathe; if necessary, administer medications as ordered to relieve pain associated with chest tubes; monitor and report patient response. Place padding around chest tube when assisting patient to turn or move. Make sure chest tubes are adequately taped to patient's chest so that they may not be pulled with moving or turning.
Skin integrity, impairment of: actual	Provide wound care around chest tube site; use sterile technique to clean area at least daily. Change dressing around chest tube daily. Observe for signs of infection, including increased temperature, purulent drainage, odor, or increased WBC.
Mobility, impaired physical	Provide passive and active range of motion to arm and shoulder of affected side. Encourage patient to exercise lower legs to prevent venous stasis. Ambulate patient as ordered.
Fear	Carefully and completely explain all procedures to patient. Assure patient that splinting and support will be provided to decrease discomfort. Provide patient with opportunities to participate in own care.

Removal of Chest Tubes

Chest tubes may be removed after the lung has been reinflated for 24 hours to several days. Indications for removal are usually confirmed by chest x-ray examination. Removal procedures include the following:

1. Place patient in semi-Fowler's position or on side.
2. Physician instructs patient to take a deep breath and hold it.
3. The chest tube suture is clipped and the tube is quickly removed.
4. A pressure dressing with antibiotic ointment or petroleum jelly gauze is placed over chest wall wound.
5. The patient is instructed to breathe normally, and the pressure dressing is taped securely.
6. Careful patient assessment should follow on a continuing basis, including rate of respirations, quality of breath sounds, and drainage from chest tube dressing, sudden chest pains, or shortness of breath.

EVALUATION

Patient Outcome	Data Indicating That Outcome is Reached
Chest tube drainage system is intact and operational.	System remains intact. Water fluctuates in water-seal container. Drainage accumulates in drainage bottle.
Lungs reexpand.	X-ray films confirm lung reexpansion. Breath sounds are bilaterally equal and clear. Blood gases are within normal limits for patient. There is no atelectasis, consolidation, or associated infection.

MECHANICAL VENTILATION[29,35,44,54]

Mechanical ventilation is indicated for patients who are unable to maintain adequate ventilation on their own. The ventilator does not cure; it is simply a temporary support that merely "buys time" for correction of the underlying situation that precipitated its use in the first place.

There are currently three categories of ventilators in use: volume-cycled ventilators, pressure-cycled ventilators, and external body ventilators. Each of these is discussed separately.

Volume-Cycled Ventilators

These volume-cycled (volume-preset) ventilators terminate inspiration after delivering a preset volume of gas. The desired volume of gas is delivered regardless of the required pressure to do so. The ventilator will continue to deliver a constant tidal volume regardless of the changes in the airway resistance or in compliance of the lungs and thorax.

The volume remains the same unless excessively high peak airway pressures are reached, in which case, safety release valves stop the flow. The safety release pressure is usually set about 10 cm H_2O above the peak inspiratory pressure.

Inspiratory time is determined by adjusting the flow rate of gas to be delivered (more rapid the flow, shorter the inspiratory time; slower the flow, longer the inspiratory time).

Expiratory time is most commonly determined by setting the respiratory rate. The operator must preset the following:

1. Tidal volume
2. Inspiratory pressure
3. Rate of breaks per minute
4. Peak flow
5. Degree of sensitivity required by patient to trigger inspiration
6. Frequency of sighs per hour
7. Sigh volume—or amount of gas to be delivered during a sigh
8. Sigh pressure limit during a sigh inspiration
9. Oxygen percent concentration to be delivered

Pressure-Cycled Ventilators

These pressure-cycled (pressure preset) ventilators terminate inspiration when a preset pressure is achieved. When the pressure is reached, the gas flow stops and the patient passively exhales. The largest patient variable is that varying degrees of resistance interfere with gas flow. Thus the delivered volume may vary as the degree of resistance varies.

These ventilators are most commonly used for patients whose ventilatory resistance has not changed (i.e., drug overdose). They are not appropriately used in patients whose resistance may have changed (i.e., postoperative status or patients with severe respiratory infections). These respirators have only a low peak pressure capability (i.e., 30 to 40 cm).

External Body Ventilator

External body ventilators function by applying intermittent subatmospheric pressure to the thorax and trunk of the body, thus assisting the patient to breathe.

ASSESSMENT: AREAS OF CONCERN

Preprocedural

Alveolar-arterial difference $(P(A-a)_{O_2})$ >400 mm Hg when patient is on 100% oxygen
$PaCO_2$ >55 mm Hg
PaO_2 <60 mm Hg
pH <7.35
Dead space to total volume (V_D/V_T) >0.60

Inspiratory force (IF) <25 cm H_2O
Tidal volume (V_T) <5 ml/kg
Vital capacity (VC) <10 ml/kg
Expiratory force <60 cm H_2O

Procedural problems[32]
Pa_{O_2} >110 mm Hg
Determine $F_{I_{O_2}}$; report $F_{I_{O_2}}$ setting and Pa_{O_2} to physician (make sure $F_{I_{O_2}}$ was not left on 100% oxygen)
Note patient's position; diaphragm movement and blood flow and ventilation ($\dot{V}/\dot{Q}$) relationships are affected by gravity and position
Pa_{O_2} <50 to 90 mm Hg depending on patient's underlying disease
If patient shows signs of cyanosis, tachycardia, arrhythmias, restlessness, or decreased sensorium, remove patient from ventilator and bag breathe patient with 100% oxygen until physician help and further assessment are possible
Assessment of problem should include:

Machine or tubing malfunction
Patient's need for suctioning
Diminished patient lung functioning due to pneumothorax or atelectasis
Malplaced endotracheal tube
Pa_{CO_2} >45 mm Hg or the patient's baseline if the patient has COPD
Verify that patient is connected to ventilator and that ventilator tubing is clear of obstruction or water accumulation
Suction patient if necessary and determine position and patency of endotracheal tube
Evaluate patient for metabolic acidosis
If patient is on low, intermittent mandatory ventilation, determine whether patient has recently received respiratory depressing sedation, which would affect respiratory status
Pa_{CO_2} <35 mm Hg (unless desired for control of cerebral blood flow)
Assess patient's respiratory rate and depth
Assess for metabolic acidosis

NURSING DIAGNOSES and NURSING INTERVENTIONS

Nursing Diagnosis	Nursing Intervention
Airway clearance, ineffective	Endotracheal tube should be secured in place (see associated procedure in airway maintenance section). Assure 100% humidification and warming (between 32° and 36° C) of inspired gases as ordered. Suction and clean tube as indicated to maintain patency. Because patient is disconnected from ventilator prior to suctioning, the nurse must: • Warn patient • Deliver high concentrations of oxygen for several minutes prior to and following suctioning so that hypoxia and cardiac arrhythmias may be avoided Wait 20 minutes after suctioning to obtain arterial blood gases. Monitor airway pressure (should remain constant or <20 cm H_2O) frequently; empty water from tubing.
Breathing pattern, ineffective	Consistently evaluate ventilatory pattern for rate, quality, signs of respiratory distress, or inappropriate inspiratory to expiratory ratio (should be at least 1:1). Monitor patient signs of fighting the ventilator, which indicate that the patient's respiratory cycle is inconsistent with the mechanical cycle; may be due to pain, hypoxemia, secretions, fear, and anxiety; to correct, clear airways as indicated or give sedatives as ordered. PEEP (positive end expiratory pressure breathing) may be used to prevent alveolar collapse and thereby increase tidal volume. The major goal of PEEP is to enhance oxygen transport. CPAP (continuous positive airway pressure) functions similar to PEEP but is intended to be used with patients who are breathing spontaneously.
Gas exchange, impaired	Position patient so that all lobes of lungs are adequately ventilated and perfused. Reposition patient every 30 to 60 minutes; rotate positioning from right and left lateral positions to a semi-Fowler's position. Carefully monitor ventilator pressure readings and the patient's breath sounds for presence and quality; pneumothorax, pneumomediastinum, and subcutaneous emphysema may be signs of barotrauma secondary to a high mechanical ventilator pressure.

Nursing Diagnosis	Nursing Intervention
	Pneumothorax may be anticipated by seeing an abrupt rise in the peak inspiratory pressure for a constant tidal volume. Carefully monitor all ventilator settings as well as patient's arterial blood gas response.
Breathing pattern, ineffective	Ensure that the alarm on the ventilator is turned to the ON position whenever the patient is left alone. Carefully check all connections of the ventilator tubing regularly to assure that they are tightly secured.
Cardiac output, alteration in: decreased	May be due to hyperventilation or hypoventilation; therefore carefully assess ventilatory rate, rhythm, and quality; $Paco_2$ may cause a transient alkalosis.
Potential patient problem: susceptibility to infection	Because of warm moist nature of the ventilator equipment, the patient is prone to nosocomial infections. Change all parts of the ventilator equipment that come in contact with the patient every 24 hours. Send sputum specimens to the laboratory for analysis as ordered. Carefully monitor patient's temperature and characteristics of sputum.
Fear	Assure patient that he will not be left alone. Provide call-bell button for immediate access. Assure patient that adequate ventilation is being provided.
Communication, impaired: verbal	Provide Magic Slate or other mechanism by which patient may communicate.

Weaning from the Ventilator

Physiologic guidelines:
1. Vital capacity (at least 10 to 15 ml/kg body weight)
2. Alveolar-arterial oxygen tension difference ($PA\text{-}a_{O_2}$) measured with patient receiving 100% oxygen (should be less than 300 to 500 mm Hg)
3. Maximum inspiratory force (greater than 20 cm H_2O)
4. Tidal volume (greater than 5 ml/kg)
5. Resting minute ventilation greater than 101 per minute
6. $Paco_2$ within stable range
7. Pao_2 greater than 70 to 80 mm Hg on 0.5 Fi_{O_2}
8. Pao_2 on 100% oxygen greater than 300 mm Hg
9. Shunt fraction less than 15%

If patient is not completely ready to be weaned from ventilator, he may be changed to intermittent mandatory ventilation (IMV) or intermittent demand ventilation (IDV):

IMV allows patient's own reasonable breathing pattern to be maintained with positive-pressure breaths intermittently delivered by the ventilator. The positive pressure breaths are completely independent of the patient's own breathing pattern.

Because mechanical ventilatory assistance leaves the patient's respiratory muscles weakened, it may be helpful to transfer the patient to IMV for gradual transition weaning.

IDV allows the patient to breathe a controlled atmosphere at a reasonable, spontaneous pattern, with intermittent positive augmentation in phase with the patient's own breathing pattern (on demand).

When the patient is disconnected from the ventilator, he should be in a sitting position, and humidified oxygen should be readily available by mask.

EVALUATION

Patient Outcome	Data Indicating That Outcome is Reached
Pulmonary system with assistance of mechanical ventilator has the power to maintain physiologic ventilation.	Breath sounds are heard in all lobes of lungs. Bilaterally equal lung expansion occurs. Tidal volume >5 ml/kg Vital capacity >10 ml/kg Inspiratory force >25 cm H_2O Dead space to tidal volume ratio <0.60

Patient Outcome	Data Indicating That Outcome is Reached
Effectiveness of ventilation or oxygenation is maintained.	$Paco_2$ 35 to 45 mm Hg Pao_2 >80 mm Hg with Fi_{O_2} 0.4 or above pH >7.35 There are no clinical signs of dyspnea, restlessness, or cyanosis.
Myocardial work is decreased by diminishing ventilatory effort and improving ventilatory efficiency.	Blood pressure and pulse are within normal limits for patient. Patient appears restful without signs of agitation or hypoxia.

THORACIC SURGERY

Description and Rationale[44]

Thoracotomy. Thoracotomy refers to a surgical incision of the chest wall. Many times an exploratory thoracotomy is performed to biopsy a specimen or to locate a source of bleeding. During the procedure the ribs are spread and the pleura is opened. Closed chest drainage is generally required postoperatively.

Pneumonectomy. Pneumonectomy refers to surgical removal of an entire lung. The surgeon severs and sutures off the main arteries, veins, and the mainstem bronchus at the bifurcation. The major indication for pneumonectomy is lung cancer. Closed chest drainage is generally not done postoperatively. It is desirable for the thoracic cavity on the affected side to fill with serous exudate. The exudate eventually consolidates. The phrenic nerve on the affected side may be severed by the surgeon. This permits the diaphragm to assume an elevated position, which also assists to fill the empty thoracic space.

Lobectomy. Lobectomy refers to removal of a lobe of the lung. Major indications for this procedure include isolated tumors, cysts, tuberculosis, abscess, or localized injury. Closed chest drainage is used following a lobectomy.

Segmental resection. Segmental resection refers to the removal of one or more segments of the lung lobe. Indications for the procedure include tuberculosis, bleb, localized abscess, or bronchiectasis. Closed chest drainage is used following this procedure.

Wedge resection. Wedge resection refers to the removal of a small, wedge-shaped localized area near the lung surface. Indications for the procedure include biopsy and removal of a small area of tuberculosis. The resected area is sutured off prior to removal. There is generally little disruption of overall lung function. Closed chest drainage is used following the procedure.

Decortication. Decortication refers to the stripping off of a thick fibrous membrane that may develop over the visceral pleura secondary to empyema or the prolonged presence of blood or fluid in the pleural space. Closed chest drainage is required postoperatively.

Thoracoplasty. Thoracoplasty refers to a surgical procedure intended to remove select portions of the ribs with the intent of reducing the overall size of the thoracic cavity.

Contraindications and Cautions

The following complications of surgery should be anticipated:
  Respiratory insufficiency
  Tension pneumothorax
  Cardiac failure or myocardial infarction
  Thrombosis or pulmonary embolism
  Atelectasis
  Bronchopleural fistula
  Pulmonary edema
  Subcutaneous emphysema
  Infection

Preprocedural Nursing Care

Carefully determine preoperative status of patient including the following:
  Baseline pulmonary function studies
  Electrocardiogram
  Arterial blood gases
  Electrolytes
  Other existing medical problems
  Current respiratory status: amount and extent of dyspnea, cough, and respiratory distress
  General nutrition and hydration state
  Provide preoperative teaching to include the following:
  Need to stop smoking preoperatively
  Coughing and deep breathing techniques
  Need for and technique of suctioning and closed chest drainage postoperatively
  Overview of equipment and procedures that will most likely occur postoperatively
  Listen preoperatively to patient and family questions and concerns; provide information and clarification when indicated

Assure patient that pain medication will be available postoperatively to assist with discomfort

Teach patient the need for postoperative range of motion and leg exercises

ASSESSMENT: AREAS OF CONCERN

Blood gases

pH, PaO_2, $PaCO_2$, HCO_3^- to monitor ventilator assistance or patient's ability to ventilate self

Chest tube drainage

Amount of drainage, characteristics of drainage, patency of closed drainage system

Incision status

Suture line characteristics; lack of signs of infection

Respiratory status

Lung expansion status, lack of signs of atelectasis, consolidation, infection, pulmonary edema, pulmonary embolus, mediastinal shift, paradoxical motion

Cardiovascular status

Electrocardiogram changes, hypovolemia, pulmonary edema, venous stasis, cardiac arrhythmias, central venous pressure within normal limits for patient

Pain

Pain management that facilitates patient's activities of turning, coughing, deep breathing, and range of motion

Fluid and electrolyte balance

Fluid intake managed in manner to facilitate adequate nutritional and electrolyte requirements

Adequate urinary output

Electrolytes remain within normal limits

Infection

↑ WBC, fever, purulent drainage, redness around incision area

NURSING DIAGNOSES and NURSING INTERVENTIONS

Nursing Diagnosis	Nursing Intervention
Airway clearance, ineffective	Maintain patent airway by suctioning and adequate position; if patient has endotracheal tube, see p. 230 for additional strategies. Observe for signs of airway obstruction including restlessness, inadequate chest expansion, stridor, noisy respirations, cyanosis, or dyspnea (*atelectasis may be preventable with proper nursing care*). Evaluate for signs of atelectasis that may result secondary to airway obstruction; signs include increased respiratory rate, rapid pulse, increased temperature, cyanosis, and diaphoresis.
Breathing pattern, ineffective	Carefully monitor status of closed chest drainage system; note fluctuation or tidaling in the water-seal chamber and the drainage tubing near the patient; see closed-chest drainage system for additional strategies. If patient is on mechanical ventilator, see pp. 246-249 for specific nursing strategies. When patient is ventilating on his own, carefully assess respiratory rate, depth, and quality; note signs of dyspnea and respiratory distress, hemoptysis. Administer intermittent positive pressure breathing (IPPB) as ordered; evaluate and record response. Encourage coughing and deep breathing on a regular basis until patient is able to maintain procedure by self; observe and record response. Carefully auscultate lungs at least every 2 hours; note quality of breath sounds, rate and depth of respirations, presence of adventitious sounds, presence of paradoxical respirations, mediastinal shift. Observe for chest wall movement and potential splinting secondary to pain. Observe for signs of pulmonary embolism, which include dyspnea, fear, hemoptysis, symptoms of right-sided heart failure, hypoxia, engorgement of neck veins, tachycardia, hypotension, apprehension, sense of impending doom, nausea, sweating. Observe for signs of gastric distention that may occur secondary to swallowing air and anesthesia; if this occurs, it may cause ventilatory compromise, which will further complicate the postoperative period; if gastric distention is noted and confirmed by x-ray examination, the physician may elect to insert a nasogastric tube until gastrointestinal mobility returns.

Nursing Diagnosis	Nursing Intervention
Comfort, alteration in: pain	Administer pain medications approximately 30 minutes prior to deep breathing and coughing and ambulation. Provide adequate splinting prior to coughing and deep breathing.
Gas exchange, impaired	Monitor arterial blood gases as ordered; report alterations. Maintain oxygenation as ordered; monitor patient response. Reposition patient frequently so as to facilitate aeration of the lung. Lobectomy patients should be moved from supine to side-lying positions (a rolled towel should be placed around the chest tubes to protect them from collapse).
Fluid volume deficit	Monitor for signs of circulatory insufficiency secondary to hypovolemia; this circulatory insufficiency may cause clinical signs such as hypotension, tachycardia, tachypnea, hypoxia, acidosis, and ischemia to vital organs. Maintain accurate intake and output records. Provide intravenous fluids as ordered and monitor patient's cardiovascular and urinary output response. Observe for signs of fluid overload such as pulmonary congestion.
Mobility, impaired physical	Initiate passive and encourage active range of motion throughout the postoperative period. The patient is at risk for developing stiffness and ankylosis of the shoulder on the side with the chest tubes; specify range of motion should be encouraged for that shoulder on a regular schedule. Passive and active range of motion of the legs will decrease the potential for thrombosis. Ambulate patient as soon as possible and in accord with patient's ability to tolerate ambulation.
Skin integrity, impairment of: actual	Provide sterile technique wound care of incision according to physician's orders. Observe and record condition of suture line. Observe and record amount and characteristics of drainage including color, odor, and amount. Observe for raised temperature or fever, which may be an indication of infection; report observations to physician.
Fear	Assure patient that nursing assistance is constantly available. Provide reassurance and explain all procedures before they are performed. Assist patient to see progress being made from one day to the next.
Communication, impaired: verbal	If patient is unable to communicate verbally because of mechanical ventilation, endotracheal tube, or tracheostomy, provide a Magic Slate or similar writing material to facilitate communication. Make sure call button is conveniently placed for patient's use.

EVALUATION

Evaluation criteria are based on the individual procedure performed as well as the underlying disease state.

OXYGEN THERAPY

Description and Rationale

The goal of oxygen therapy is to provide sufficient amounts of oxygen to the tissues so that normal metabolism can occur. Clinically this means to provide oxygen at the lowest fractional inspired oxygen (F_{IO_2}) to maintain a Pa_{O_2} of at least 55 mm Hg. Therapy is indicated when the patient is unable to maintain an adequate Pa_{O_2} by his own ventilatory efforts.

Spearman, Sheldon, and Egan[61] give the following clinical objectives for oxygen therapy:

1. To reduce or correct arterial hypoxemia and tissue hypoxia
2. To reduce or correct the need for physiologic compensatory mechanisms to hypoxemia

Hypoxemia may be caused by a variety of factors. Following are the most common:

1. Reduced alveolar oxygen: results from either low ambient PaO_2 or hypoventilation
2. Impaired alveolar-capillary diffusion: occurs secondary to pathologic changes such as fibrosis, increased connective tissue, interstitial edema, or tumors
3. Hemoglobin deficiencies: may be either absolute due to anemia, or relative as is seen in patients with carbon monoxide ingestion
4. Ventilation/perfusion ratio imbalance: anatomic shunting that occurs secondary to congenital defects, disease or trauma, or physiologic shunting
5. Circulatory failure: occurs secondary to decreased cardiac output or hypovolemia

Contraindications and Cautions

The following discussion of precautions regarding oxygen therapy is based primarily on Spearman, Sheldon, and Egan[61] and Holloway.[33] Following are risks and precautions regarding the use of therapeutic oxygen:

1. Oxygen-induced hypoventilation: when the arterial carbon dioxide tension is greater than 50 mm Hg, the risk of oxygen-induced hypoventilation increases. It is therefore advised, especially for patients with chronic lung diseases, to maintain oxygen therapy so that the arterial oxygen tension remains about 50 to 60 mm Hg.

    To prevent this problem use low concentrations of oxygen if the patient is not mechanically ventilated. Observe ventilatory pattern and quality.
2. Atelectasis: the collapse of alveoli may occur secondary to high concentrations of oxygen in inspired air, which causes malfunctioning pulmonary surfactant

    To prevent this complication, if possible limit the duration of 100% inspired oxygen to no more than 15 to 20 minutes; maintain patent airway; sigh the patient if on a ventilator; and provide high tidal volumes
3. Oxygen toxicity: the lungs can normally handle oxygen concentrations of 21%. Although it is not clear exactly what fractional inspired oxygen percent (FIO_2) causes oxygen toxicity, it is most probable that an FIO_2 of over 50% administered for longer than 24 hours increases the risk (see assessment section for additional guidelines).

Preprocedural Nursing Care: Assessment of Need for Supplemental Oxygen

Hypoxia
  Hypotension
  Cyanosis
  Dyspnea
  Disorientation
  Anxiety
  Nausea
Nasal flaring
Retractions
Atelectasis
Pulmonary edema
Central nervous system
  depression
Muscle weakness

Altered blood gas states
  PaO_2 below 55 mm Hg
  $PaCO_2$ above 42 mm Hg
  Bradycardia
  Cardiac arrhythmias
  Tachypnea
  Drowsiness
  Headache
  Poor judgment
  Shortness of breath
Pneumonia
Emphysema
Airway obstruction

TREATMENT PLAN

Oxygen therapy equipment may be divided into two major types:

Low-flow systems: systems that do not apply all of the inspired gases that the patient breathes. This means that the patient breathes some room air along with the oxygen. For the system to be effective, the patient must be able to maintain a normal tidal volume, have a regular ventilatory pattern, and be able to cooperate. As the patient's ventilatory pattern changes, so does the concentration of inspired oxygen. Examples of low-flow systems include nasal cannula, simple oxygen mask, partial rebreathing mask with reservoir bag, and nonrebreathing mask with reservoir bag.

High-flow systems: systems that supply all gases at a preset FIO_2. These systems are generally not affected by changes in ventilatory pattern. The most common example of the high-flow system is the Venturi mask.

In addition to these two main types of systems there are blended-type systems that may use either high-flow or low-flow techniques. Examples of this type include oxygen hoods, Isolettes, T-tubes, and oxygen tents.

Table 2-13 summarizes the major types of oxygen therapy systems, their benefits, problems, and precautions.

Table 2-13
Oxygen Therapy Systems

Type System	Description	Flow Rate (L/min)*	Approximate Oxygen Concentration Delivered	Benefits	Problems	Nursing Care
Low-Flow Systems						
Nasal cannula		1	22%-24%	Comfortable, convenient method of delivering concentration of oxygen ranging from 25%-45%	Unable to deliver oxygen concentration over 44%	Clean equipment
		2	26%-28%		Assumes an adequate breathing pattern	Evaluate for pressure sores over ears and cheek areas
		3	28%-30%	If minute ventilation is relatively low and constant, then FIO_2 delivered approaches the percentages presented	Equipment may not be used if patient has nasal problem or if unable to tolerate nasal prongs	Lubricate nasal prongs before inserting into nose
		4	32%-36%		Patient must be able to cooperate to keep prongs in place	Liter flow above 6 L/min will *not* increase the FIO_2
		5	36%-40%	Major advantages of this method are low cost of equipment, allowance for patient mobility, the ability to deliver oxygen and still permit patient to eat and talk, and the lack of necessity for humidification of inspired gas mixture	Requires tight face seal similar to regular mask	
		6	40%-44%		Must be removed for eating and talking	Must maintain flow sufficient to keep reservoir bag from completely deflating during inspiration
				Practical system for long-term therapy	If liter flow is maintained below 4 L/min, CO_2 may build up in the reservoir bag	All other functions as with simple mask
				Mouth breathing will not affect the concentration of delivered oxygen	Bag may kink or twist	To initially fill bag apply mask as the patient exhales
Partial rebreathing mask with reservoir bag	Masks similar to simple face mask with addition of a reservoir oxygen bag; the purpose of the rebreathing mask is to conserve oxygen by permitting it to be rebreathed from the reservoir bag	8	40%-50%	The bag makes possible the delivery of oxygen concentration between 40% and 60% provided that the reservoir is kept full by a continuous flow of oxygen	Requires tight face seal	Arterial blood gases should be monitored
		10-12	60%		Impractical for long-term therapy	Check mask for leaks around face; FIO_2 may decrease if mask is not tight fitting
					Must be removed for eating and talking	All other functions as with simple mask
					May lead to signs of oxygen toxicity	

*Normal breathing patterns are assumed.

Table 2-13, cont'd
Oxygen Therapy Systems

Type System	Description	Flow Rate (L/min)	Approximate Oxygen Concentration Delivered	Benefits	Problems	Nursing Care
Nonbreathing mask with reservoir bag	Similar to rebreathing bag, but this mask has one-way expiratory valve that prevents rebreathing of expired gases	6 8 10 12-15	55%-60% 60%-80% 80%-90% 90%	Effective as short-term therapy May deliver oxygen concentration up to 90%	Requires tight face seal Impractical for long-term therapy Must be removed for eating and talking May lead to signs of oxygen toxicity	Arterial blood gases should be monitored Check mask for leaks around face; FiO_2 may decrease if mask is not tight fitting All other functions as with simple mask
Simple face mask		5-6 6-7 7-8	40% 50% 60%	If patient's ventilatory needs exceed the flow of gas, the holes on the sides of the mask allow for entry of room air Permits higher oxygen delivery than nasal cannula System does not tend to dry out mucous membranes of nose or mouth	Mask must be removed prior to patient's eating May not be operated at flow less than 5 L/min A tight face mask seal may cause facial irritation Face mask may increase anxiety in some patients, especially children Not practical for long-term therapy May feel hot and confining for some patients	Do not operate at flow less than 5 L/min (will not flush out accumulated CO_2) If FiO_2 above 60% is desired, patient must be switched to rebreathing mask with reservoir bag Should not be used for patients with chronic lung diseases Powdering may be necessary along bony prominence of face Equipment should be removed and cleaned several times each day

High-Flow Systems

Type	Flow (L)	%	Description		Considerations	Nursing actions
Venturi mask	3	24% 24% 28%	Works on the Bernoulli principle of air entrainment: for each liter of oxygen that passes through a fixed orifice, a fixed proportion of room air will be entrained; by varying the size of the orifice and the flow of oxygen, the precise FiO_2 is maintained	Delivers exact concentration If greater than 40% concentration is desired, must switch to different oxygen delivery system The FiO_2 remains constant regardless of the patient's ventilatory pattern	May irritate face skin Interferes with eating and drinking Tight face seal must be maintained Condensation may collect within system	Arterial blood gases should be monitored Check mask for leaks around face; FiO_2 may be altered if system not properly fitting All other functions as with simple face mask
	6	30% 35%		FiO_2 may be measured directly by an oxygen analyzer The FiO_2 dial may be changed and set to deliver a calculated oxygen concentration		
	8	40% 50%	The system operates by actually setting the FiO_2			
Oxygen hood	10-12		Most convenient method to provide oxygen therapy to infants	Hood covers head only, leaving rest of the body available for patient care May be used in conjunction with high-flow Venturi system May be used in conjunction with Isolettes, which provide temperature and humidity regulation Oxygen analyzer should be used to determine level of concentration	Oxygen between 10 and 12 L may be necessary to keep oxygen concentrations steady (dependent on size of oxygen hood)	Make sure oxygen is warmed and humidified Active infants must be carefully observed; they may dislodge hood Pad edges of hood with towels or foam Condensation in tubing will build and must be emptied frequently Heat nebulizer should be maintained between 94° F (34.4° C) and 96° F (35.6 C)

ASSESSMENT: AREAS OF CONCERN

Respiratory status
Ventilatory pattern
Tachypnea
Retractions
Work of breathing
Accessory muscle use
Posturing

Tissue oxygenation
Restlessness
Irritability
Disorientation
Confusion

Cardiovascular
Hypotension
Sudden hypertension
Tachycardia
Cardiac arrhythmia

Predicting effects of oxygen therapy
When the $P(A\text{-}a)O_2$ gradient is known, the FiO_2 may be calculated

$$FiO_2 = \frac{P(A\text{-}a)_{O_2} : \text{Desired } PaO_2}{760} \times 100 \%$$

Oxygen analyzer may be used to monitor concentrations given (especially useful when oxygen hood is used)

Mucosa hydration
Nasal and mucous membranes

Skin integrity
Protect bony prominences against pressure sores
Dry skin from oxygen contact

Absorption atelectasis
This can occur when oxygen washes out nitrogen in the alveoli; without nitrogen the residual volume decreases and the alveoli collapse

Patients at risk for developing:
Low tidal volume
Normal tidal volume without sighing
Airway trapping such as in chronic lung disease
Problem may be prevented by:
Limiting 100% oxygen delivery to no more than 30 minutes at a time
Patent airway
Mobilizing secretions
Encouraging sighing
Providing continuous high tidal volume

Oxygen toxicity
Clinical signs that may occur after:
6 hours of 100% oxygen therapy:
Sharp chest pain
Dry cough
18 hours: decreased pulmonary function studies
24-48 hours: ARDS occurs
Guidelines to prevent oxygen toxicity:
1. Limit use of 100% oxygen to brief periods
2. As early as possible reduce FiO_2 to lowest possible level to maintain oxygenation
3. Up to 70% oxygen may be used safely for 24 hours
4. Up to 50% oxygen may be used safely for 2 days
5. After 2 days an FiO_2 above 40% is potentially toxic
6. Prolonged use of FiO_2 below 40% rarely causes oxygen toxicity[33]

Equipment
Patency of tubing and bags
Cleanliness
Humidification
Correct size for the patient

Safety
While oxygen is in use, prohibit smoking in the area

NURSING DIAGNOSES and NURSING INTERVENTIONS

Nursing Diagnosis	Nursing Intervention
Airway clearance, ineffective	Assess patient to identify inability to move secretions, which would interfere with oxygenation. Assist patient to maintain proper body positioning to ensure maximal airway availability. Carefully and frequently auscultate chest for quality of breath sounds and adventitious sounds that could indicate complications of oxygen therapy.
Breathing pattern, ineffective	Assess ventilation to include evaluation of breathing rate, rhythm, and depth, chest expansion, presence of respiratory distress such as dyspnea, shortness of breath, nasal flaring, pursed-lip breathing and prolonged expiratory phase, use of accessory muscles.

Nursing Diagnosis	Nursing Intervention
	Observe for signs of oxygen-induced hypoventilation.
	Suction if necessary to remove secretions.
	Assess patient for tiring in relation to attempts to breathe.
	Assess to make sure that oxygen therapy equipment is not interfering with patient's attempts to breathe.
Gas exchange, impaired	In collaboration with physician order, monitor arterial blood gases; report increases or decreases of $Paco_2$ of more than 10 to 15 mm Hg.
	In collaboration with physician consultation, administer oxygen to maintain Pao_2 above 55 mm Hg.
	Assess patient to determine which oxygen therapy system is best to maintain the required Pao_2 level.
	Assess patient to identify signs such as restlessness, confusion, and irritability, which may indicate the body's response to altered blood gas states.
	Assess for signs of oxygen toxicity and absorption atelectasis.
	Monitor electrocardiogram and cardiac status for arrhythmias secondary to alterations in blood gases.
	Monitor serum electrolytes that may change due to alterations in oxygenation and metabolism.
	Carefully observe effectiveness of selected oxygen equipment to maintain determined F_{IO_2} levels.
	Clean equipment several times daily.
Oral mucous membrane, alteration in:	Assess and care for drying of mucous membranes of the nose and mouth secondary to oxygen therapy.
Nutrition, alteration in: less than body requirement	Assess patient's ability to remove oxygen equipment during periods of eating and respiratory response.
	If mask system is being used for oxygen therapy, assess need for nasal cannula therapy during meal time.
Communication, impaired: verbal	Observe for signs of frustration secondary to hypoxia that are causing fatigue as patient attempts to communicate; provide alternative communication techniques
	Observe for signs of frustration secondary to wearing oxygen mask; provide alternative communication techniques
Anxiety	Assess patient's level of anxiety related to the need to have oxygen therapy
	Assess patient's level of anxiety related to feeling of air hunger
Coping, ineffective individual	Determine patient's ability to cooperate with health care providers regarding intervention strategies

Patient Education

1. Assess patient's current knowledge and skills regarding the use of oxygen equipment.
2. Teach patient the purpose and process of the selected type of oxygen equipment.
3. Teach importance of not smoking (or having others in the area smoke) during administration of oxygen.
4. Provide patient and family with information regarding the care, cleaning, and maintenance of oxygen equipment being used in the hospital or to be used at home.

EVALUATION

Patient Outcome	Data Indicating That Outcome is Reached
Optimal movement of air in and out of lungs occurs.	Vital capacity measurements including FEV_1, FVC, TLC, RV, and FRC are optimal for patient's status.
Airway is patent.	Blood gas values are within normal limits.
	Airways are clear and breathing occurs without obstruction.
Patient and family have sufficient information to comply with oxygen therapy plan.	Therapy plan is maintained.

References

1. A.C.C.P.-A.T.S. Joint Committee on Pulmonary Terms and Symbols: Chest **67:**583, 1975.
2. American Lung Association: Chronic obstructive pulmonary disease, New York, 1981, The Association.
3. American Lung Association: Occupational lung diseases: an introduction, New York, 1983, The Association.
4. American Thoracic Society: A statement by the Committee on Diagnostic Standards for Nontuberculosis Respiratory Diseases, Am. Rev. Respir. Dis. **85:**762, 1962.
5. American Thoracic Society: Surveillance for respiratory hazards in the occupational setting, Am. Rev. Respir. Dis. **126**(5), 1982.
6. American Trauma Society: Definitions and classifications of chronic bronchitis, asthma, and pulmonary emphysema, Am. Rev. Respir. Dis. **85:**762, 1962.
7. Brown, M., and Andrews, J.: How to manage adult respiratory distress syndrome, Geriatrics **34:**39, April, 1979.
8. Burkhart, C.: After pneumonectomy, Am. J. Nurs. **83:**1563, 1983.
9. Burrows, B.: An overview of obstructive lung diseases, Med. Clin. North Am. **65:**455, 1981.
10. Canobbio, M.: Chest x-ray film interpretation, Focus Crit. Care **11**(2):18, 1984.
11. Carrieri, V., Murdaugh, C., and Jason-Bjerklie, S.: A framework for assessing pulmonary disease categories, Focus Crit. Care **11**(2):10, 1984.
12. Chin, R., and Pesce, R.: Practical aspects in management of respiratory failure in chronic obstructive pulmonary disease, Crit. Care Q. **6**(2):1, 1983.
13. Cronin, L.R., and Carrizosa, A.: The computer as a communication device for ventilator and tracheostomy patients in the intensive care unit, Crit. Care Nurse **4:**72, 1984.
14. D'Agostino, J.S.: Teaching tips for lung with COPD at home, Nurs. '84 **14**(2):57, 1984.
15. Dolan, T.F.: Cystic fibrosis. In Fries, J.F., and Ehrlick, G.E., editors: Prognosis: contemporary outcomes of disease, Bowie, Md., 1981, The Charles Press Publishers, p. 242.
16. Ellis, E.F.: Asthma. In Vaughn, V.C., McKay, R.J., and Behrman, R.E., editors: Nelson's textbook of pediatrics, ed. 11, Philadelphia, 1979, W.B. Saunders Co., p. 627.
17. Ellis, E.F.: Asthma in childhood, J. Allergy Clin. Immunol. **72:**526, 1983.
18. Erikkson, S.: Pulmonary emphysema and alpha-1-antitrypsin deficiency, Acta Med. Scand. **175:**197, 1964.
19. Ferris, B.G.: Epidemiology standardization project respiratory questionnaires, Am. Rev. Respir. Dis. **118:**7, 1978.
20. Fletcher, C.M., et al.: The significance of respiratory symptoms and the diagnosis of chronic bronchitis in a working population, Br. Med. J. **2:**257, 1959.
21. Fries, J.F., and Ehrlich, G.E.: Prognosis: contemporary outcomes of disease, Bowie, Md., 1981, The Charles Press Publishers.
22. Fuchs, P.: Streamlining your suctioning techniques. I: Nasotracheal suctioning, Nurs. '84 **14**(5):55, 1984.
23. Fuchs, P.: Streamlining your suctioning techniques. II: Endotracheal suctioning, Nurs. '84 **14**(6):46, 1984.
24. Fuchs, P.: Streamlining your suctioning technique. III: Tracheostomy suctioning, Nurs. '84 **14**(7):39, 1984.
25. Gaensler, E.A., et al.: Epidemiology standardization project III. Recommended standardized procedures for pulmonary function testing, Am. Rev. Respir. Dis. **118**(suppl.):55, 1978.
26. George, R.B., Light, R.W., and Matthay, R.A., editors: Chest physiology, New York, 1983, Churchill Livingstone.
27. Glennon, S., Matus, V., and Bryan-Brown, C.: Respiratory disorders. In Kinney, M.R., et al., editors: AACN's clinical reference for critical care nursing, New York, 1981, McGraw-Hill Book Co., p. 516.
28. Grossbach-Landis, I.: Successful weaning of ventilator dependent patients. In Topics in clinical nursing: breathing and breathlessness, Germantown, Md., 1980, Aspen Systems Corp.
29. Harper, R.W.: A guide to respiratory care: physiology and clinical approaches, Philadelphia, 1981, J.B. Lippincott Co.
30. Hess, D.: Bedside monitoring of the patient on a ventilator, Crit. Care Q. **6**(2):23, 1983.
31. Higgins, T.T.: Epidemiology of bronchitis and emphysema. In Fishman, A.P., editor: Pulmonary diseases and disorders, New York, 1980, McGraw-Hill Book Co.
32. Hirsh, J., and Hannock, L., editors: Mosby's manual of clinical nursing practice, St. Louis, 1981, The C.V. Mosby Co.
33. Holloway, N.M.: Nursing the critically ill adult, ed. 2, Menlo Park, Calif., 1984, Addison-Wesley Publishing Co.
34. Horwitz, O.: Pulmonary embolus. In Fries, J.F., and Ehrlich, G.E.: Prognosis: contemporary outcomes of disease, Bowie, Md., 1981, The Charles Press Publishers.
35. Jacob, J.: Performance of chest physiotherapy. In Hirsch, J., and Hannock, L., editors: Mosby's manual of clinical nursing procedures, St. Louis, 1981, The C.V. Mosby Co., p. 59.
36. Janson-Bjerklie, S.: Defense mechanisms: protecting the healthy lung, Heart Lung **12:**643, 1983.
37. Johanson, B.C., et al.: Standards for critical care, St. Louis, 1981, The C.V. Mosby Co.
38. Kinney, M.R., et al., editors: AACN's clinical reference for critical-care nursing, New York, 1981, McGraw-Hill Book Co.
39. Kirilloff, L.H., and Tibbals, S.C.: Drugs for asthma: a complete guide, Am. J. Nurs. **83:**55, 1983.
40. Kirsh, M.M., and Shoan, H.: Blunt chest trauma: general principles of management, Boston, 1977, Little, Brown & Co.
41. Lakshminarayan, S., and Hudson, L.D.: Pulmonary function following the adult respiratory distress syndrome, Chest **74:**489, 1978.
42. Landis, K., and Smith, S.: The mechanically ventilated patient: a comprehensive nursing care plan, Crit. Care Q. **6**(2):43, 1983.
43. Loopstra, S., and Martin, K.: Care of the patient with a tracheostomy. In Hirsch, J., and Hannock, L., editors: Mosby's manual of clinical nursing procedures, St. Louis, 1981, The C.V. Mosby Co.
44. Luckmann, J., and Sorenson, K.: Medical-surgical nursing: a psychophysiological approach, ed. 2, Philadelphia, 1980, W.B. Saunders Co.
45. McFadden, E.R., and Austin, K.F.: Asthma. In Thorn, G.W., et al., editors: Harrison's principles of internal medicine, ed. 8, New York, 1977, McGraw-Hill Book Co.
46. Miller, L.G., and Kazemi, H.: Manual of clinical pulmonary medicine, New York, 1983, McGraw-Hill Book Co.
47. Morbidity and Mortality Weekly Report **32:**463, September 9, 1983.
48. Nowak, R.: Acute bronchial asthma. In Rosen, P., editor: Emergency medicine: concepts and clinical practice, St. Louis, 1983, The C.V. Mosby Co., pp. 774-789.
49. Phipps, W., Long, B., and Woods, N.: Medical-surgical nursing: concepts and clinical practice, St. Louis, 1983, The C.V. Mosby Co.
50. Price, S.A., and Wilson, L.M.: Pathophysiology: clinical concepts of disease processes, ed. 2, New York, 1982, McGraw-Hill Book Co.
51. Reynolds, H.Y., and Merrill, W.W.: Airway changes in young smokers that may antedate chronic obstructive disease, Med. Clin. North Am. **65:**667, 1981.
52. Rhodes, M.: Update on chest trauma, Crit. Care Q. **6**(2):59, 1983.
53. Rifas, E.: Teaching patients to manage acute asthma: the future is now, Nurs. '83 **13**(4):77, 1983.
54. Robinson, S., and Russo, P., editors: Providing respiratory care: nursing photobook, Springhouse, Pa., 1979, Intermed Communications.
55. Rokosky, J.S.: Assessment of altered respiratory function, Nurs. Clin. North Am. **16**(2):198, 1981.
56. Sexton, D.: The supporting cast: wives of COPD patients, J. Gerontol. Nurs. **10**(2):82, 1984.
57. Shapiro, B.: Clinical application of blood gases, Chicago, 1979, Year Book Medical Publishers.
58. Shelley, R.: Performance of radial artery puncture. In Hirsch, J., and Hannock, L.: Mosby's manual of clinical nursing procedures, St. Louis, 1981, The C.V. Mosby Co.

59. Smith, L., and Thier, S.: Pathophysiology: the biological principles of disease, Philadelphia, 1981, W.B. Saunders Co.
60. Snider, G.L.: Pathogenesis of emphysema and chronic bronchitis, Med. Clin. North Am. **65:**647, 1981.
61. Spearman, C., Sheldon, R., and Egan, D.: Egan's fundamentals of respiratory therapy, ed. 4, St. Louis, 1982, The C.V. Mosby Co.
62. Stern, R.: Lower respiratory tract. In Vaughn, V.C., McKay, R.J., and Behrman, R.E.: Nelson's textbook of pediatrics, ed. 11, Philadelphia, 1979, W.B. Saunders Co., p. 1203.
63. Tinits, P.: Oxygen therapy and oxygen toxicity, Ann. Emerg. Med. **12:**89, 1983.
64. Tisi, G.M.: Pulmonary physiology in clinical medicine, Baltimore, 1980, The Williams & Wilkins Co.
65. Tucker, S.M., et al.: Patient care standards, ed. 3, St. Louis, 1984, The C.V. Mosby Co.
66. Vaughn, V.C., McKay, R.J., and Behrman, R.E., editors: Nelson's textbook of pediatrics, ed. 11, Philadelphia, 1979, W.B. Saunders Co.
67. Vincent, J.E.: Medical problems in the patient on a ventilator, Crit. Care Q. **6**(2):33, 1983.
68. Vukich, D.J., and Markovchick, V.J.: Pneumothorax. In Rosen, P., et al., editors: Emergency medicine: concepts and clinical practice, St. Louis, 1983, The C.V. Mosby Co., vol. 1.
69. Waldbott, G.: Health effects of environmental pollutants, ed. 2, St. Louis, 1978, The C.V. Mosby Co.
70. Weiss, E.B.: Bronchial asthma, Clin. Symp. **27:**39, 1975.
71. Weiss, E.B., and Segal, M.S., editors: Bronchial asthma, Boston, 1976, Little, Brown & Co.
72. West, J.: Respiratory physiology: the essentials, Baltimore, 1979, The Williams & Wilkins Co.

CHAPTER 3

Neurologic System

Overview

The human nervous system consists of complex structures and processes that coordinate one's ability to perceive and respond to the internal and external environments. In basic terms the nervous system provides an intricate "circuit board" through which the functions of various body subsystems are integrated. Because these functions are integrative, the physiologic and psychologic ramifications of a neurologic dysfunction can be devastating for both the patient and the family.

Estimates from The National Committee for Research in Neurological Disorders indicate the prevalence of neurologic disorders as follows:

1. Each year, several hundred thousand deaths occur from sensory and neurologic disorders—almost 190,000 from strokes alone.
2. Cerebrovascular accidents rank third as the major cause of death.
3. Over 8 million individuals are disabled by diseases affecting the brain and spinal cord.
4. In the United States, 1 in every 16 infants born suffers from some type of neurologic disability.[29]

Nervous system trauma affects a tremendous number of individuals, particularly older adolescents and young adults. In developed countries of the Western world, craniocerebral trauma is now the most important cause of death. These traumatic injuries appear to be the unwanted by-product of modern technology; their incidence increases as an area becomes more technologically developed.[47]

ANATOMY AND PHYSIOLOGY

The nervous system is divided into two fairly distinct structural categories. The central nervous system (CNS) consists of the brain and spinal cord. The peripheral nervous system (PNS) is made up of 12 pairs of cranial nerves, 31 pairs of spinal nerves, and the sympathetic and parasympathetic subdivisions of the autonomic nervous system. Functionally, the central and peripheral nervous systems are interdependent in that each is composed of millions of neurons and neuroglia cells. These microscopic cells are derived from the inner ependymal layer of the neuronal tube during embryonic development. The neuron is the basic structural and functional unit of the nervous system, with the neuroglia cells functioning in a supportive capacity for the neuron.

Neuroglia Cells

Approximately 40% of the microscopic structures of the brain and spinal cord consist of neuroglia cells. The purpose of these cells is to provide protection, structural support, and nourishment for the cell bodies and processes of the neurons. There are four distinct types of neuroglia cells: (1) astrocyte, (2) ependyma, (3) microglia, and (4) oligodendroglia (Fig. 3-1). All of these cells, except the microglia, are derived from the embryonic ectoderm. Unlike neurons, neuroglia cells can divide and multiply by mitosis. Therefore these cells are a primary source for nervous system tumors.

Fig. 3-1
Types of neuroglia cells.

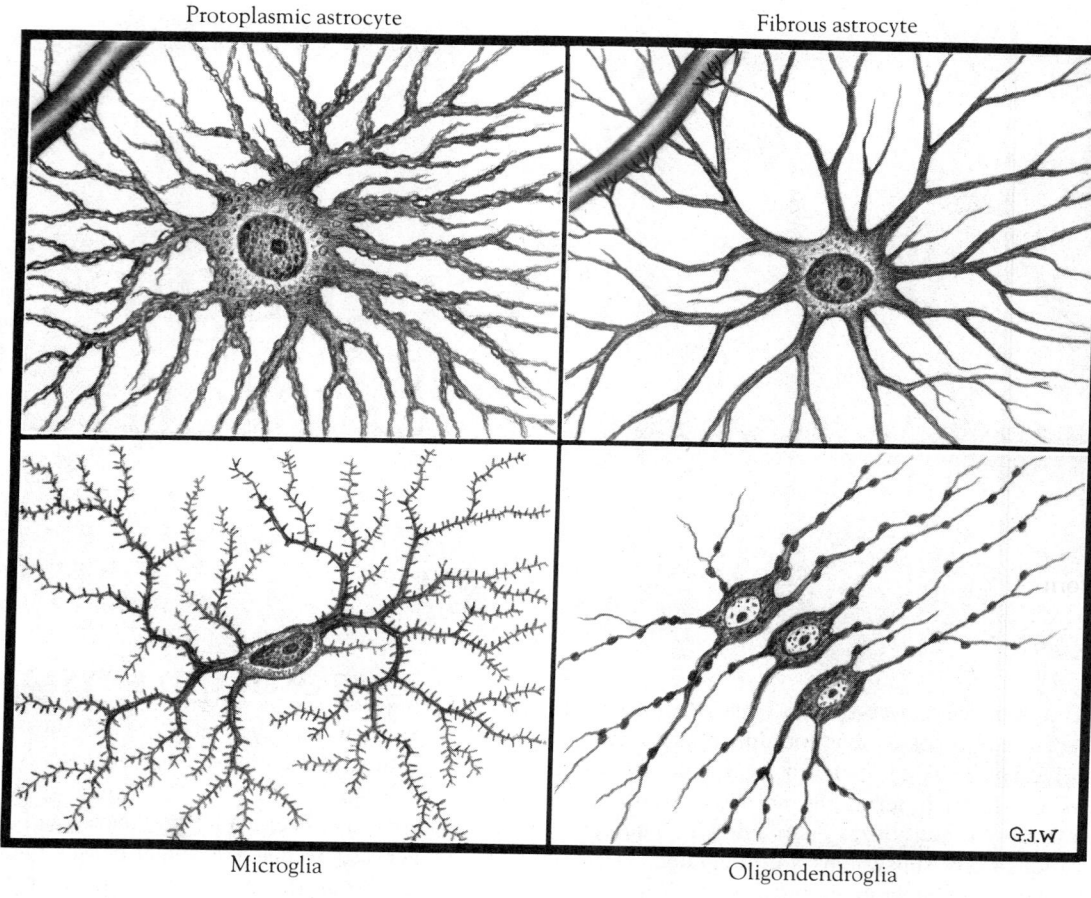

Protoplasmic astrocyte

Fibrous astrocyte

Microglia

Oligondendroglia

Astrocytes (astroglia) cells are starlike in appearance because of the many processes extending from the cell body. Their functions include (1) maintenance of the neuron's chemical environment for impulse conduction and synaptic transmission, (2) maintenance of neuronal nutritional needs, (3) information storage, (4) neuronal structural support, and (5) participation in the blood-brain barrier via the proliferation process of gliosis. Further, astrocytes are divided into fibrillary astrocytes, found chiefly in white matter, and protoplasmic astrocytes, located chiefly in gray matter.

Ependyma cells are distributed within the epithelial lining of the cerebral ventricles, the choroid plexuses, and the spinal cord's central canal. The main function of the ependyma cells is in the production of cerebrospinal fluid.

Microglia are usually stationary cells scattered throughout the central nervous system, mainly in the white matter. These cells are derived from the embryonic mesoderm. The function of microglia is phagocytosis, during which the microglia become mobile, ingesting and digesting tissue debris. These properties of microglia are similar to those of histocytes found in the peripheral connective tissue.

Oligodendroglia cells synthesize a lipid-protein complex that forms myelin sheaths around the axonal projections of neurons in the central nervous system. (Myelin is formed in the peripheral nervous system by Schwann cells.) The functions of the myelin sheath include (1) holding nerve fibers together, (2) providing insulation along the nerve processes, (3) promoting ionic flow across the neuronal cell membrane, and (4) transmission of nerve impulses (saltatory conduction). Oligodendroglia begin forming at approximately the fourth fetal month and continue until approximately 20 years of age. Unlike the Schwann cells in the peripheral nervous system, the oligodendroglia cannot regenerate because the cells of the central nervous system lack

Fig. 3-2
Diagram of neuron with composite parts.

From Rudy, E.B.: Advanced neurological and neurosurgical nursing, St. Louis, 1984, The C.V. Mosby Co.

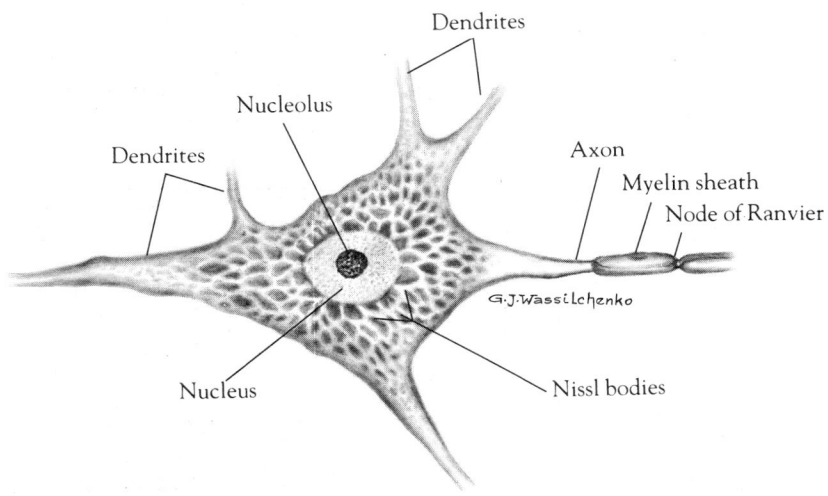

the neurilemma membrane. Instead, damaged neuronal structures are replaced primarily with astrocytes, which form a gliotic scar that can disrupt the surrounding neuronal tissue.

The Neuron

The neuron (Fig. 3-2) is a specialized cell that comes in a variety of sizes and shapes; each cell has the function of transmitting specific nervous stimuli. The neurons have the specialized properties of (1) excitation and (2) electrical-chemical conductivity. In the central nervous system, groups of neurons are called nuclei; in the peripheral nervous system they are termed ganglia.

Cytologic features. The neuron is composed of a *cell body*, or perikaryon, and *prosections*, called dendrites, which carry information to the neuron (afferent fibers), and an axon, which carries information away from the nerve cell body (efferent fibers). The nerve cell body is referred to as the gray matter of the nervous system.

Each neuron typically contains only one centrally located *nucleus*. The nucleus is a large double-membraned structure containing deoxyribonucleic acid (DNA). Inside the nucleus is a single prominent nucleolus containing ribonucleic acid (RNA), which is crucial for protein synthesis and maintenance in the long cellular projections.

Surrounding the nucleus is the granular *cytoplasm* containing many organelles including Nissl bodies, mitochondria, the Golgi complex, neurofilaments, and microtubules. Nissl bodies are highly ordered masses of granular endoplasmic reticulum. These organelles function as the protein-synthesizing machinery of the neuron cell. *Mitochondria* are rod-shaped structures that regulate the cell's respiratory metabolism. Metabolic energy is stored as adenosine triphosphate (ATP). The *Golgi complex*, located in the cellular cytoplasm, condenses and stores secretory substances necessary for impulse transmission. Dense neurofilaments are found throughout the cytoplasm as well as in the axonal and dendritic processes. Individual neurofilaments are made up of structures called neurotubules or microtubules. The neurofilaments and microtubules together form the neurofibril, which is involved in the intracellular axoplasmic transport system.

Processes. Extending from the cell body is a long, smooth projection termed the *axon*, or *axis cylinder* (Fig. 3-2). The axon generally originates from the neuron's cell body at a point called the axon hillock. Surrounding the axon is the myelin that provides protection and insulation for the axonal structure. The axon carries efferent impulses away from the cell body. The axons form the white matter of the central nervous system. Terminal branches of the axon are called terminal filaments or buttons (axon telodendria).

Extending from the cell body to the immediate surrounding areas are short receptive processes, or *dendrites*. The branchlike dendrites are unmyelinated and lie with the cell body in the gray matter. The purpose of the dendritic branches is to increase the surface area from which neuronal impulses may be picked up. Dendrites transmit afferent impulses toward the cell body. Rootlike terminal endings of the dendrite, or dendritic spines, provide for synaptic transmission.

Classification. The neuron cell can be classified by structure and function. Structurally, the neuron can be subdivided according to the number of processes and the axon length (Fig. 3-3).

Unipolar neurons have only one process or pole, which divides close to the cell body. One branch of this division,

Fig. 3-3
Structural and functional neuron
classification.

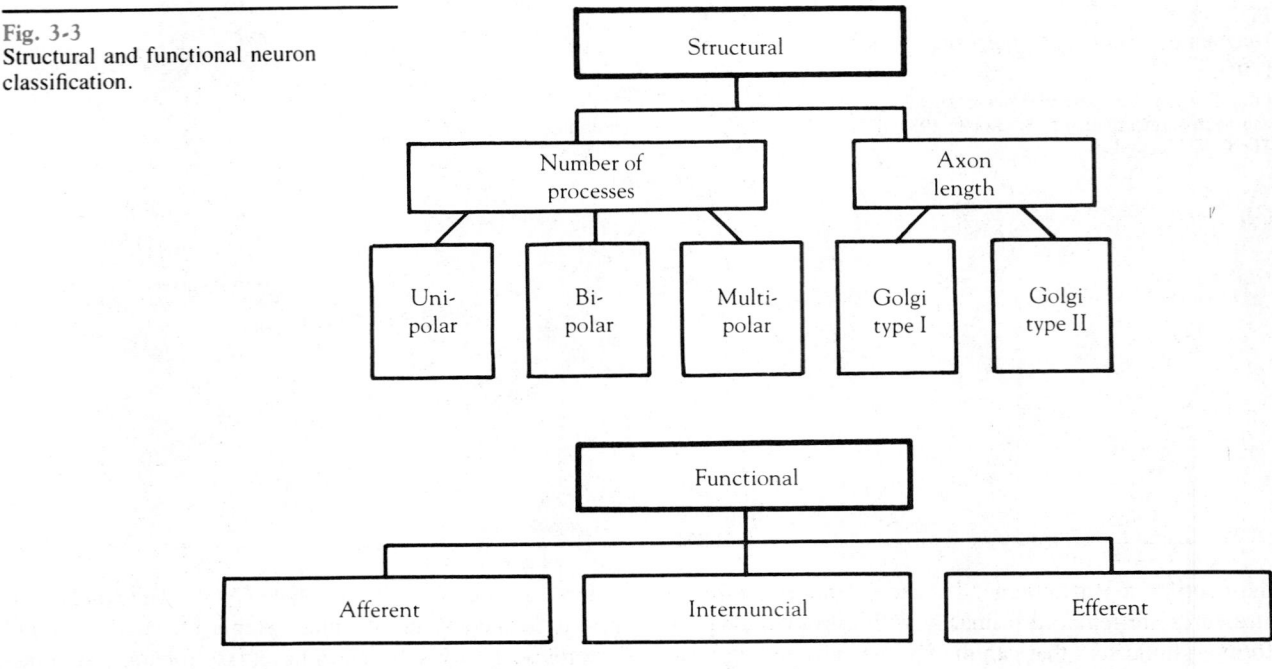

Fig. 3-4
Types of neurons. **A,** Multipolar.
B, Unipolar.

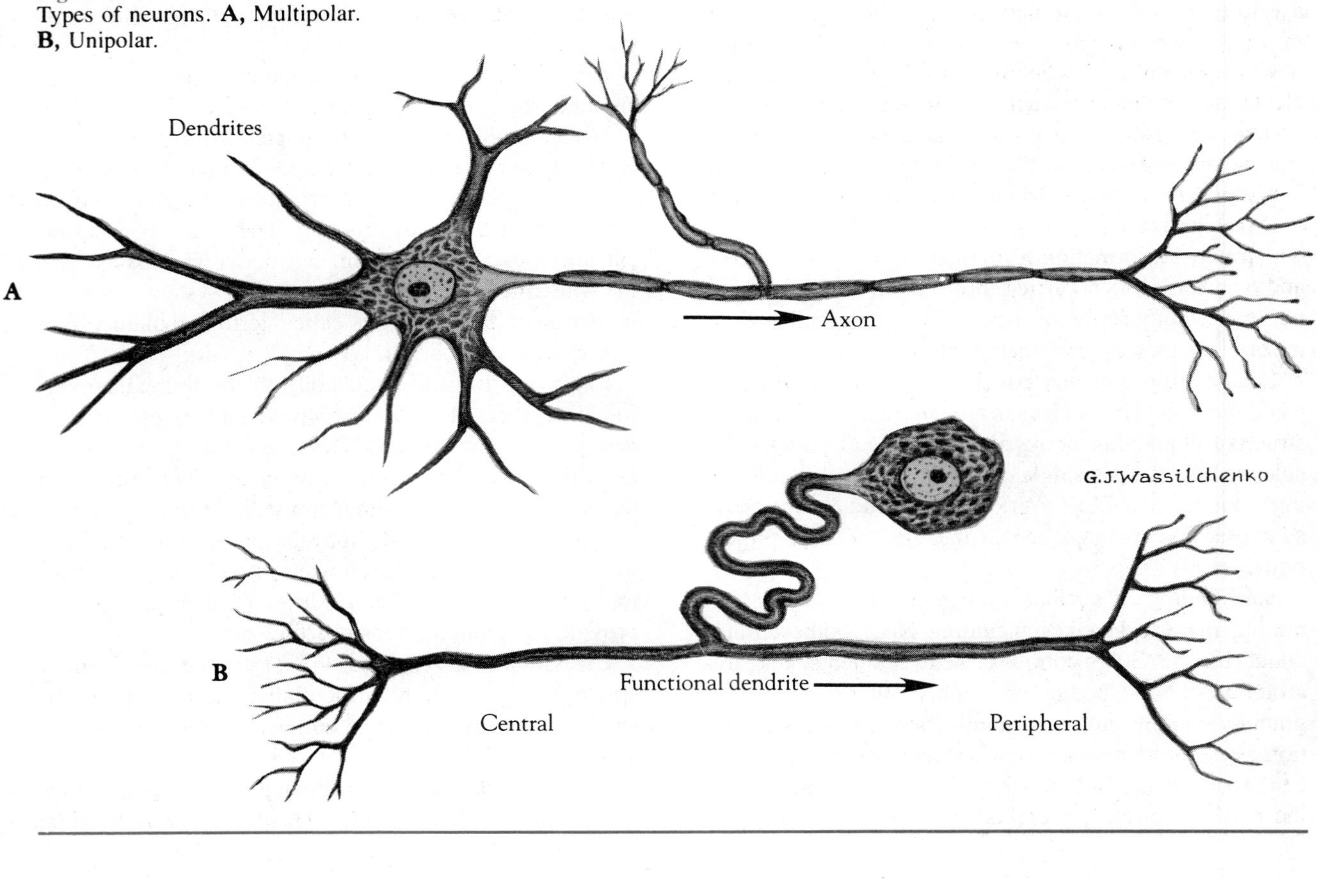

Dendrites

A

Axon

G.J.Wassilchenko

B

Functional dendrite

Central   Peripheral

Fig. 3-5
Peripheral nerve.

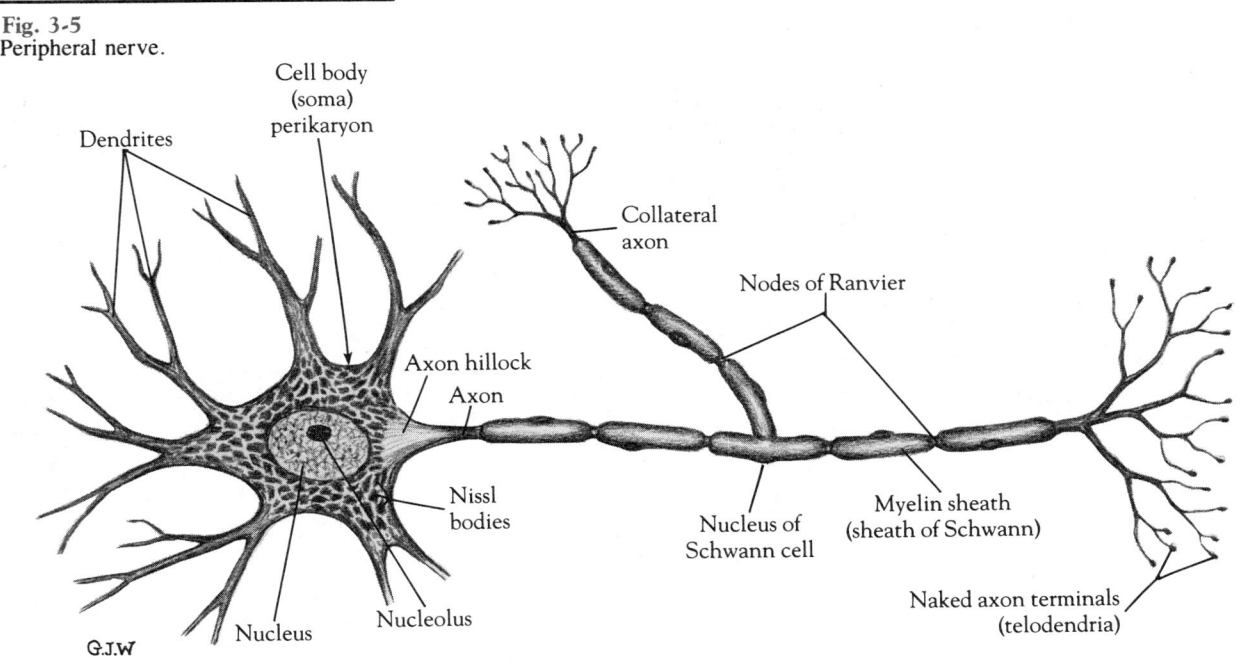

the peripheral process, carries afferent impulses from the periphery toward the cell body. The other branch, the central process, conducts efferent impulses away from the cell body toward the spinal cord or brainstem. The general sensory neuron is unipolar and has its nerve cell body in the dorsal root ganglia.[10] *Bipolar* neurons have two processes: one axon and one dendrite. Bipolar neurons are found in special sensory areas such as the spinal ganglia, the olfactory mucous membrane, and the rod and cone cells of the retina. *Multipolar* neurons make up most of the central nervous system, including all internuncial (association) and motor neurons. Multipolar neurons consist of a cell body, one long projection (axon), and one or more shorter branches (dendrites).

Fig. 3-4 illustrates the anatomic structures of the unipolar, bipolar, and multipolar neurons.

Neurons can also be classified by the axon length. Subdivisions within this classification are Golgi type I and Golgi type II (Fig. 3-3). *Golgi type I* neurons are large and have long axons. They are found in the long fiber tracts located in the cerebral cortex, the cerebellum, and the spinal cord. *Golgi type II* neurons are small cells, interposed between larger neurons, that establish complex circuits in the nervous system. These neurons are found throughout the brain and spinal cord. Golgi type II neurons characteristically have short axons that branch repeatedly and terminate near the cell body.

Functionally, the neurons are classified as (1) afferent, (2) internuncial (association), or (3) efferent (Fig. 3-3).

Afferent (sensory) neurons conduct impulses from peripheral nerve endings to the central nervous system. *Internuncial* (association) neurons are located in the central nervous system and assist in afferent and efferent impulse conduction. *Efferent* (motor) neurons transmit impulses from the central nervous system to effector organs and tissue.

The Nerve

In the peripheral nervous system the neuron has the function of carrying impulses to and from the central nervous system. This function is accomplished via the chainlike grouping of neuron cell fibers into *nerves* (Fig. 3-5). (The term *nerve* applies only to cell fibers found in the peripheral nervous system. In the central nervous system these are referred to as *fiber tracts*.)

The axon is the impulse-conducting component of the nerve. Surrounding the axon is the discontinuous layer of the myelin sheath. This sheath insulates, protects, and nourishes the axon. In peripheral myelinated nerve fibers, there are periodic interruptions of the myelin sheath called *nodes of Ranvier*. These nodes allow action potentials to skip from node to node, resulting in increased impulse conduction. *Neurilemma* is a thin cytoplasmic membrane formed by the Schwann cells. The neurilemma membrane wraps spirally around the segmented myelin sheaths of myelinated nerve fibers or the axons of unmyelinated nerves in the peripheral nervous system.

Fig. 3-6
Peripheral nerve trunk and coverings.

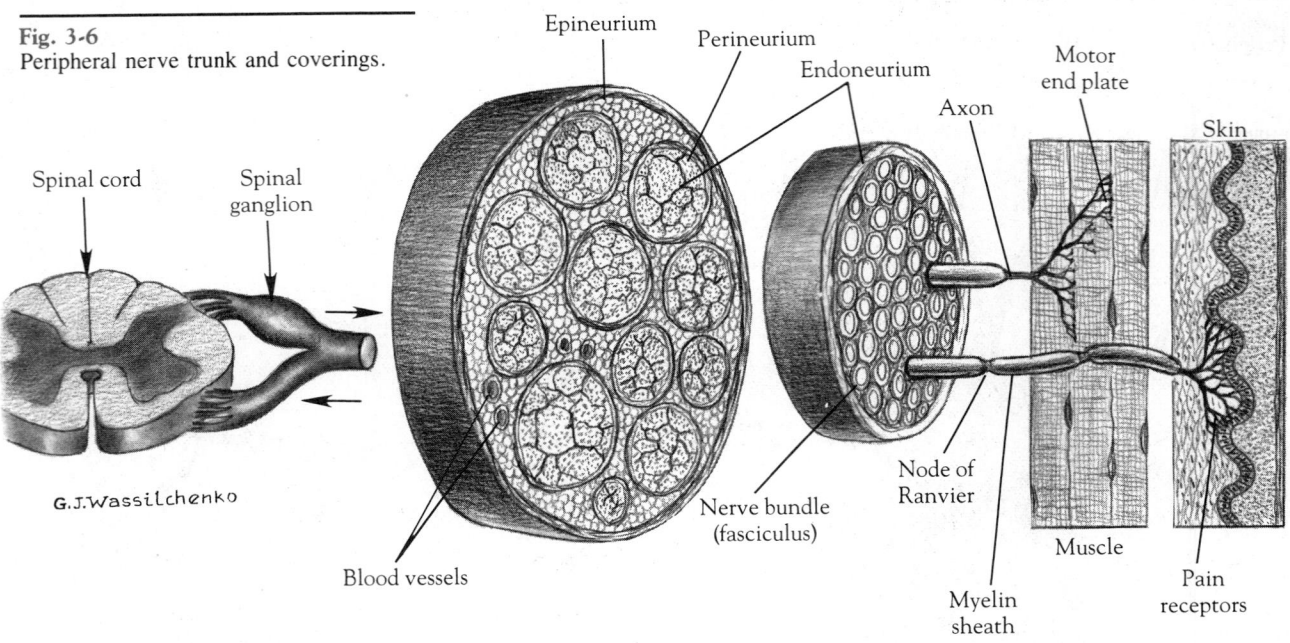

G.J.Wassilchenko

Functions of the neurilemma membrane include protection and support of the nerve processes. This membrane provides a basic structure for regeneration of peripheral nerve processes following injury or destruction. The myelin, nodes of Ranvier, and neurilemma are sometimes referred to collectively as the neurilemma cells.

Surrounding the nerve fibers are three layers of connective tissue coverings (Fig. 3-6). The *endoneurium* is a delicate covering that ensheathes the neurilemma cells. Adjacent to the endoneurium is the *perineurium,* which surrounds groups of nerve fibers (fascicles). The *epineurium* is the outer fibrous covering that binds the groups of fascicles together.

The nerve fibers in the peripheral nervous system, like the neuron, are classified according to their function: afferent, internuncial (association), or efferent.

The nerve impulse. As with other cells in the body, nerve fibers are polarized, or charged, in their resting state. In this state, the cells have a resting membrane potential of -70 mV, which means the inside of the cell membrane is negatively charged in relation to the outside. Specifically, there is a high concentration of sodium (Na^+) extracellularly and a high concentration of potassium (K^+) intracellularly, resulting in unequal electrical charges across the cell membrane. This difference in electrical polarity is the result of the relative impermeability of the cell to sodium and the sodium-potassium pump mechanism whereby sodium is continuously pumped out of the cell and potassium is pumped in.

When a chemical, mechanical, or electrical stimulus of sufficient strength and magnitude (referred to as threshold intensity) is initiated, there is a rapid, marked change in the permeability of the cell membrane. This change in permeability results in an influx of sodium and a loss (via diffusion) of intracellular potassium. With the influx of sodium, the cell becomes positive, relative to the interstitial space, and an action potential or depolarization results. At the cell membrane the depolarization stimulus excites one local area, which in turn excites adjacent portions of the cell membrane (conduction) until the entire membrane is stimulated at the same intensity. As a result, the wave of depolarization is propagated in a cyclic manner along the entire length of the nerve process. Following depolarization, there is a reversal of the ionic flow. Sodium is pumped out as potassium is pumped back into the cell. Reversal of ionic flow constitutes the repolarization process whereby the membrane is returned to its resting potential. During depolarization and one third of the repolarization process, the neuron cell cannot be restimulated with another action potential. This time interval, termed the *absolute refractory period,* prevents repeated excitation of the neuron. Fig. 3-7 illustrates the depolarization-repolarization process.

The speed of impulse conduction depends on whether the nerve is myelinated or unmyelinated. In the unmyelinated nerve the action potential must travel the entire length of the nerve fiber. In myelinated nerves the axolemma is exposed only at the nodes of Ranvier; therefore

Fig. 3-7
Stages in impulse propagation.

From Schottelius, B.A., and Schottelius, D.D.: Textbook of physiology, ed. 18, St. Louis, 1978, The C.V. Mosby Co.

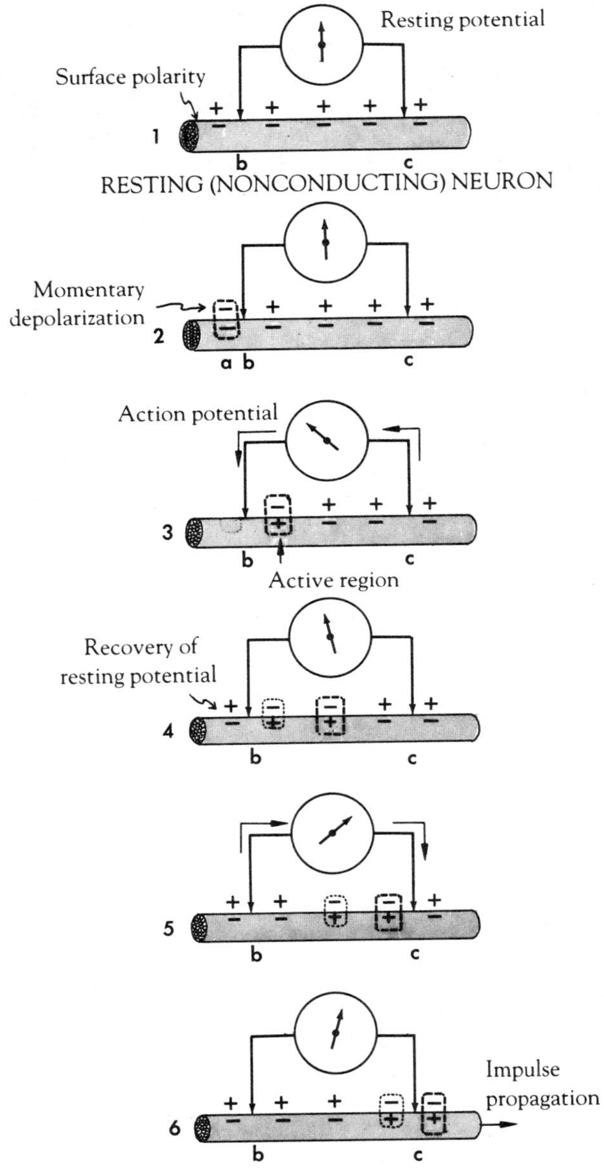

Resting potential

Surface polarity

1
RESTING (NONCONDUCTING) NEURON

Momentary depolarization
2

Action potential
3
Active region

Recovery of resting potential
4

5

Impulse propagation
6

the action potential is not transmitted by way of the entire axon membrane. Instead, the action potential "skips," in a discontinuous fashion, from one node of Ranvier to the next. With this node-to-node conduction (termed *saltatory transmission*) the action potential travels faster, thereby increasing the velocity of impulse transmission and decreasing energy demands.

Synapse. Because neurons occur in chainlike pathways, impulses must travel from one cell to another via functional junctions called *synapses*. Actual synaptic transmission is a chemical process accomplished through the release of neurotransmitters. Additionally, synapses are polarized so the impulse flow is unidirectional (e.g., axon of one neuron to the axon, dendrites, or cell body of another neuron in a pathway).

The anatomic structures of the synapse consist of (1) presynaptic terminals, (2) the synaptic cleft, and (3) the postsynaptic membrane (Fig. 3-8). The presynaptic terminals (also referred to as presynaptic knobs) contain hundreds of minute circular vesicles that store excitatory or inhibitory neurotransmitters. When an impulse stimulates the presynaptic terminals, a specific type of neurotransmitter is secreted into the microscopic extracellular space, the synaptic cleft. The release of the neurotransmitter into the synaptic cleft then stimulates receptor sites, on the postsynaptic membranes, of the next neuron in the pathway. To prevent overstimulation of the postsynaptic receptor membrane, the neurotransmitter is chemically inactivated following the synaptic transmission.

There are three types of interneuronal synapses: *axosomatic*, in which the axon of one neuron synapses with the cell body of another neuron; *axodendritic*, in which the axon of one neuron transmits to the dendrites of another nerve cell; and *axoaxonic*, in which one axon comes into contact with another axon.

Neurotransmitters. At least 30 different substances, the neurotransmitters, can affect chemical transmission of an impulse at the synapse. Presynaptic terminals secrete neurotransmitters into the synaptic cleft, causing a change in the permeability of the postsynaptic membrane. Neurotransmitters cause either excitation or inhibition activity in the postsynaptic cell.

Excitatory neurotransmitters react with receptor sites on the postsynaptic membrane to cause an enhanced permeability to sodium, potassium, and choride ions. The influx of sodium lowers the membrane potential (depolarization), developing an excitatory postsynaptic potential (EPSP) and facilitating the postsynaptic neuron toward an action potential. The principal excitatory neurotransmitter of the voluntary nervous system and the parasympathetic division of the autonomic nervous system is acetylcholine. Other central excitatory neurotransmitters include norepinephrine, dopamine, serotonin, L-asparate, and glutamic acid. The major postsynaptic excitatory neurotransmitter in the sympathetic division of the autonomic nervous system is norepinephrine.[10]

Inhibitory neurotransmitters decrease the permeability of the postsynaptic membrane to sodium, while increasing permeability to potassium and choride ions. The potassium ion flows out and chloride flows in, hyperpolarizing (less toward depolarization) the postsynaptic cell membrane and forming an inhibitory postsynaptic potential (IPSP). The formation of the IPSP is known as direct inhibition and moves the neuron farther away from depolarization. Another type of inhibitory action results from stimulation of the excitatory presynaptic terminals by an inhibitory neuron. In presynaptic inhibition there is partial depolarization of the excitatory presynaptic terminals so that less excitatory neurotransmitters are released from these endings. Consequently, the amplitude of the action potential as it arrives at the presynaptic terminals is reduced and end-excitation of the neuron decreases. Inhibitory neurotransmitters include gamma-aminobutyric acid (presynaptic) and glycine (postsynaptic).

The quantity of neurotransmitters released does not follow the all-or-none principle but rather depends on the rate and amount of impulses stimulating the presynaptic terminals. Therefore, eliciting an action potential on the postsynaptic membranes may require that one presynaptic terminal depolarize repeatedly (referred to as temporal summation) or that many presynaptic terminals depolarize and release neurotransmitters (spatial summation).

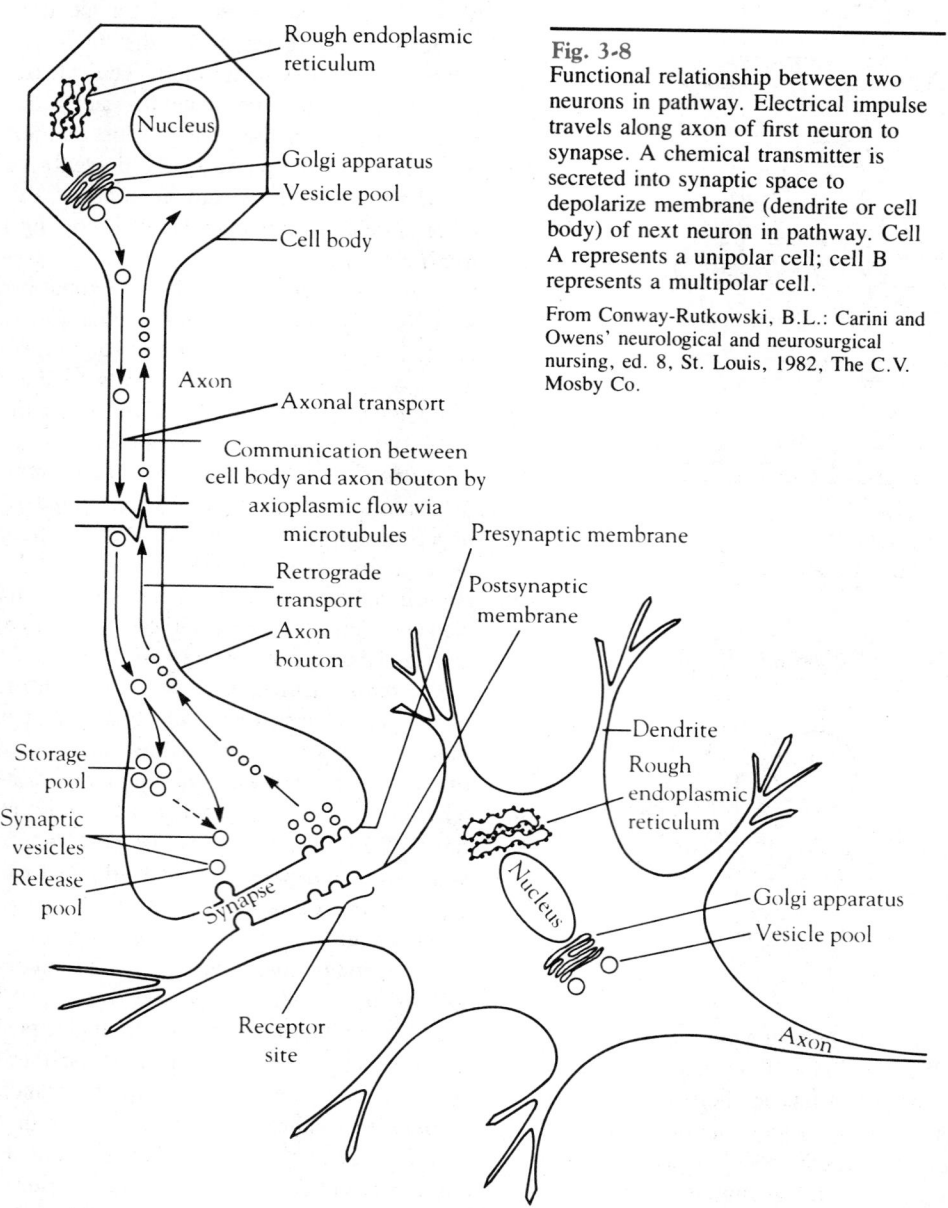

Fig. 3-8
Functional relationship between two neurons in pathway. Electrical impulse travels along axon of first neuron to synapse. A chemical transmitter is secreted into synaptic space to depolarize membrane (dendrite or cell body) of next neuron in pathway. Cell A represents a unipolar cell; cell B represents a multipolar cell.

From Conway-Rutkowski, B.L.: Carini and Owens' neurological and neurosurgical nursing, ed. 8, St. Louis, 1982, The C.V. Mosby Co.

Following synaptic transmission, the chemical neurotransmitter continues to bind with the postsynaptic membrane until it is (1) inactivated by enzyme degradation (i.e., acetylcholine is inactivated by acetylcholinesterase), (2) retaken up by presynaptic terminals (i.e., dopamine, serotonin, and GABA), or (3) diffused away from the postsynaptic membrane.

Central Nervous System

Skull. The brain is enclosed and protected by the bony structure of the skull (Fig. 3-9). The skull itself is divided into two primary sections, the cranium and the skeleton of the face. Since it is the cranial portion of the skull that most directly protects the vulnerable brain tissue, only this portion will be addressed. It is made up of eight relatively flat and irregular bones joined together by a series of fixed joints called sutures. These bones are composed of three layers: the solid *outer table*, the spongy middle *diploë*, and the solid *inner table*. The inner table of the skull forms a cavity filled with ridges and convolutions that are "custom designed" for holding the brain. This internal cavity is anatomically divided into three major regions: (1) the anterior fossa, (2) the middle fossa, and (3) the posterior fossa. The anterior fossa contains the frontal lobes; the middle fossa contains the temporal, parietal, and occipital lobes; and the posterior fossa contains the brainstem and cerebellum.[10]

At the base of the skull in the inferior-anterior portion of the occipital bone is a large oval opening called the foramen magnum. It is at the level of the foramen magnum that the brain and spinal cord become continuous. Also located at the base of the skull is a series of foramina that provide openings for the entrance and exit of paired cranial nerves, as well as cerebral blood vessels.

Cranial meninges. Between the skull and the brain are three connective tissue layers collectively referred to as the meninges. Each meningeal layer is a continuous separate sheet that, like the skull, protects the soft brain tissue (Fig. 3-10).

Fig. 3-9
Lateral view of skull.

From Anthony, C.P., and Kolthoff, N.J.: Textbook of anatomy and physiology, ed. 9, St. Louis, 1975, The C.V. Mosby Co.

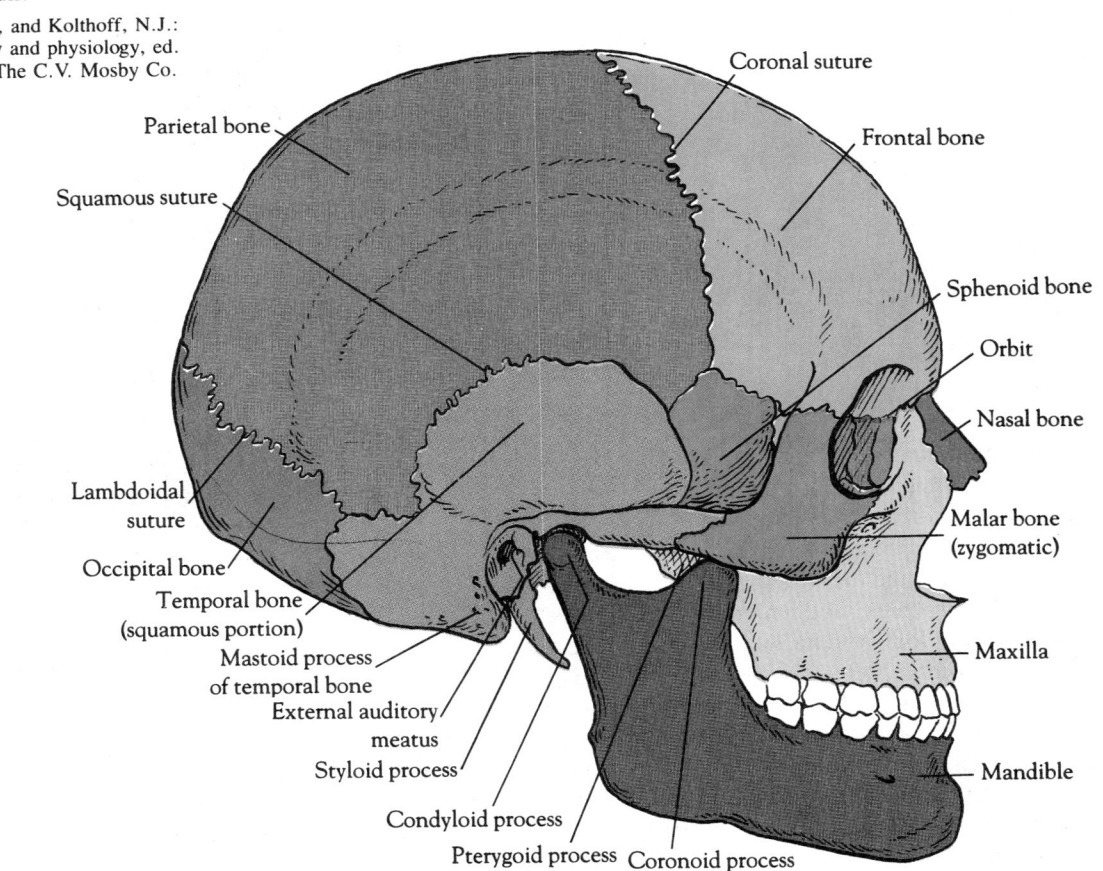

Fig. 3-10
Schematic drawing of sagittal section
of head.

From Rudy, E.B.: Advanced neurological
and neurosurgical nursing, St. Louis, 1984,
The C.V. Mosby Co.

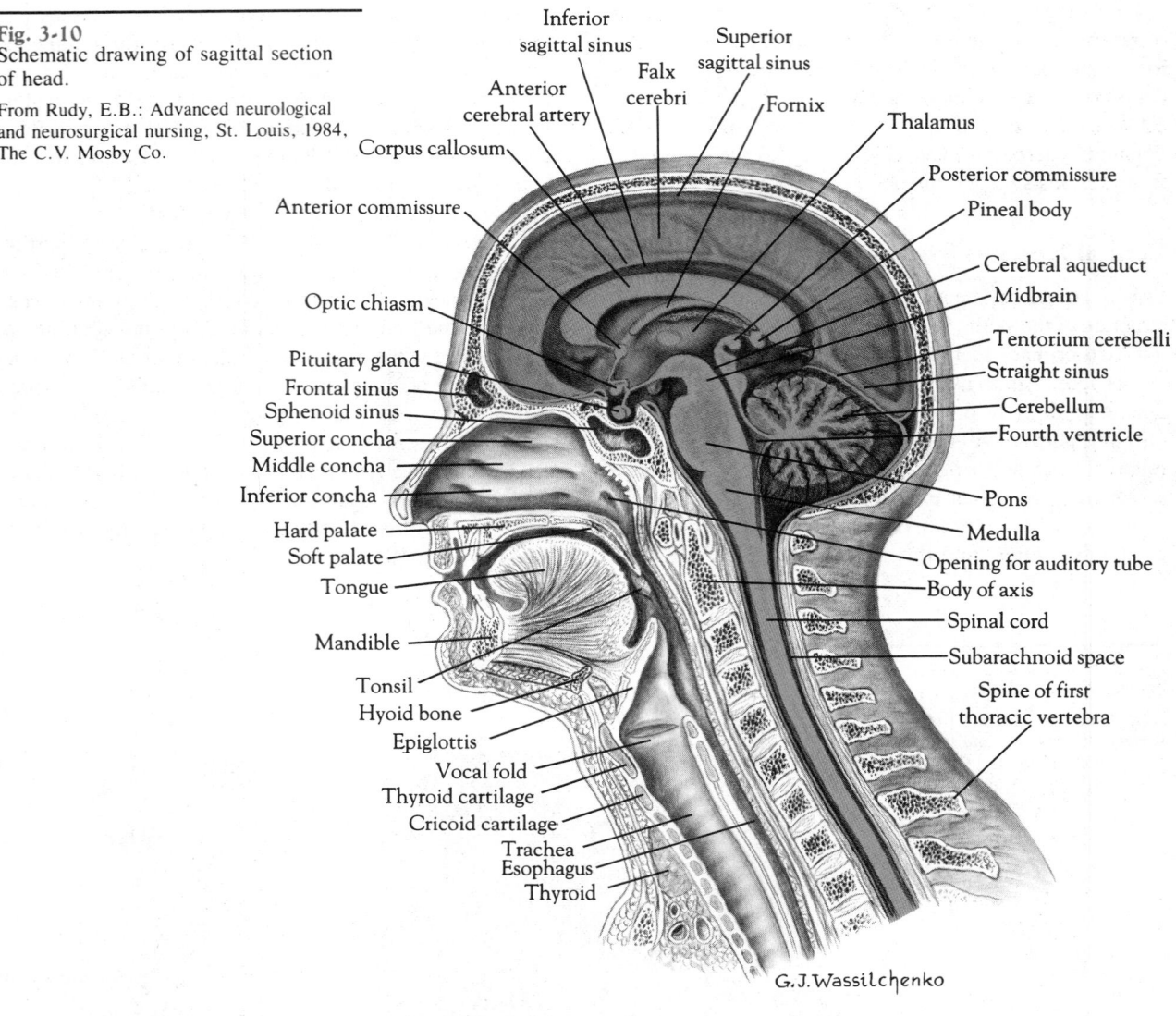

G.J.Wassilchenko

The fibrous outermost meninx is the double-layered *dura mater,* which envelops the brain and separates the skull into compartments by its various folds or processes. The falx cerebri process is formed by a vertical fold of the dura mater at the midsagittal line, separating the two cerebral hemispheres. The tentorium cerebelli is a horizontal double fold of dura that supports the temporal and occipital lobes, separating the cerebral hemispheres from the brainstem and the cerebellum. (The tentorium provides an important line of demarcation. Structures above the tentorium are termed supratentorial, and those below it are termed infratentorial.) The falx cerebelli process separates the two hemispheres of the cerebellum.

The dura mater in the skull significantly differs from spinal dura mater in the following ways: (1) the cranial dura is firmly attached, but the spinal dura is not attached to the vertebrae; (2) cranial dura consists of two layers, periosteal and meningeal, whereas the spinal dura consists of one meningeal layer; and (3) the cranial dura separates in places and forms venous sinuses, whereas this is not possible in the one-layer spinal dura.[10] These differences are important to understand when dealing with craniocerebral injuries or disorders causing increased intracranial pressure.

Between the dura mater and the middle meningeal layer is a narrow serous cavity called the subdural space. Vessels located within the subdural space have minimal support structures and therefore are quite vulnerable to injury.

The middle layer of the meninges is the arachnoid. It

Fig. 3-11
Lateral view of cerebral hemisphere (showing lobes and principal fissures), cerebellum, pons, and medulla oblongata.

From Rudy, E.B.: Advanced neurological and neurosurgical nursing, St. Louis, 1984, The C.V. Mosby Co.

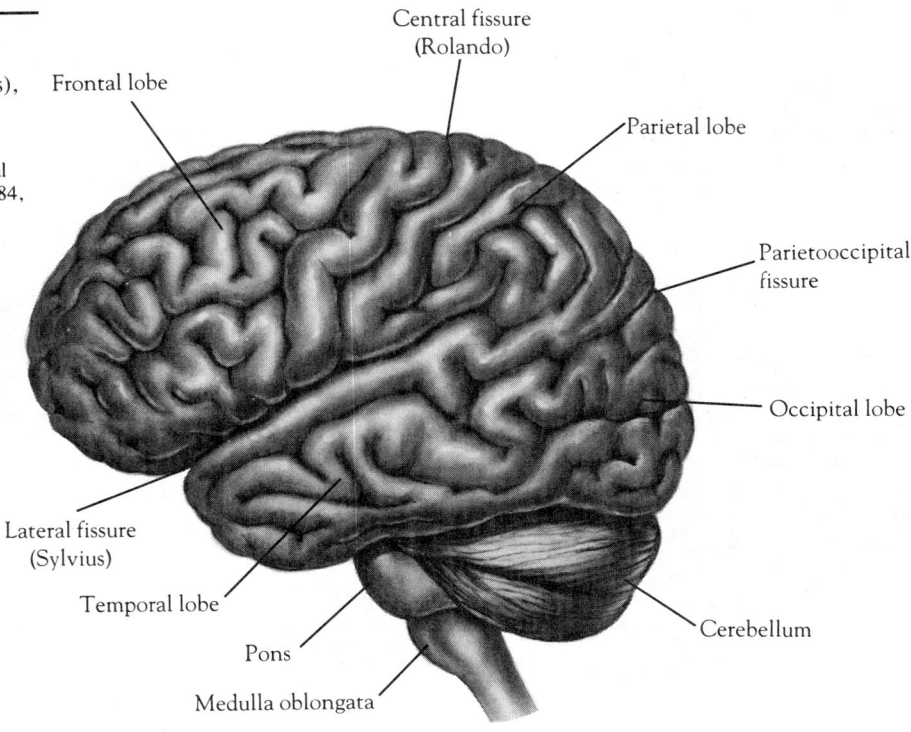

Central fissure (Rolando)

Frontal lobe

Parietal lobe

Parietooccipital fissure

Occipital lobe

Lateral fissure (Sylvius)

Temporal lobe

Pons

Medulla oblongata

Cerebellum

consists of a two-layered, fibrous, elastic membrane that crosses over the folds and fissures of the brain, creating the spongy subarachnoid space. Within the subarachnoid space are various-sized cerebral arteries and veins. At the base of the brain, dilations in the subarachnoid space form cisterns. The largest of these cisterns is the cisterna magna, which forms a direct communication with the fourth ventricle. It is in the subarachnoid space that cerebrospinal fluid circulates over the surfaces of the brain.

The innermost layer of meninges, the *pia mater,* is rich in small blood vessels, which supply the brain with a large volume of blood. The pia mater is directly continuous to the external structure of the brain tissue. The arachnoid and pia membranes are collectively referred to as the leptomeninges.

The brain. Adjacent to the pia mater is the brain, which is pinkish gray in color. The brain, which constitutes approximately 2% (about 3 pounds) of the total body weight of an adult, receives about 20% of the cardiac output and requires 20% of the body's oxygen utilization.[39]

The surface of the brain has numerous convolutions, which are separated by shallow folds. Sulci and fissures are the deeper grooves that divide the brain into lobes and hemispheres.

The brain (encephalon) can be divided into three major anatomic areas: the cerebrum, the cerebellum, and the brainstem. The cerebrum consists of cerebral hemispheres, the rhinencephalon, the internal capsule and basal ganglia, and the diencephalon (i.e., thalamus, hypothalamus). The brainstem is composed of the mesencephalon (midbrain), the metencephalon (pons), and the myelencephalon (medulla oblongata).

Cerebrum. The cerebrum is the largest anatomic portion of the brain and is covered on the outside with multiple layers of gray cells, the cerebral cortex. The internal white matter of the cerebrum consists of a large number of myelinated nerve fibers and neuroglia cells. The cerebrum is divided lengthwise into right and left sides by the longitudinal fissure. Each of these symmetric halves is referred to as a lateral cerebral hemisphere. The hemispheres are joined longitudinally by the large tract of white commissural fibers, the corpus callosum, that serves as the communication link between the hemispheres. The major folds of the cortex divide each lateral hemisphere into four lobes, or cerebral hemispheres, which are named for the overlying cranial bones: frontal, parietal, occipital, and temporal (Fig. 3-11).

Specific functions of the cerebrum have been localized to certain areas of the cerebral cortex. Probably the best-

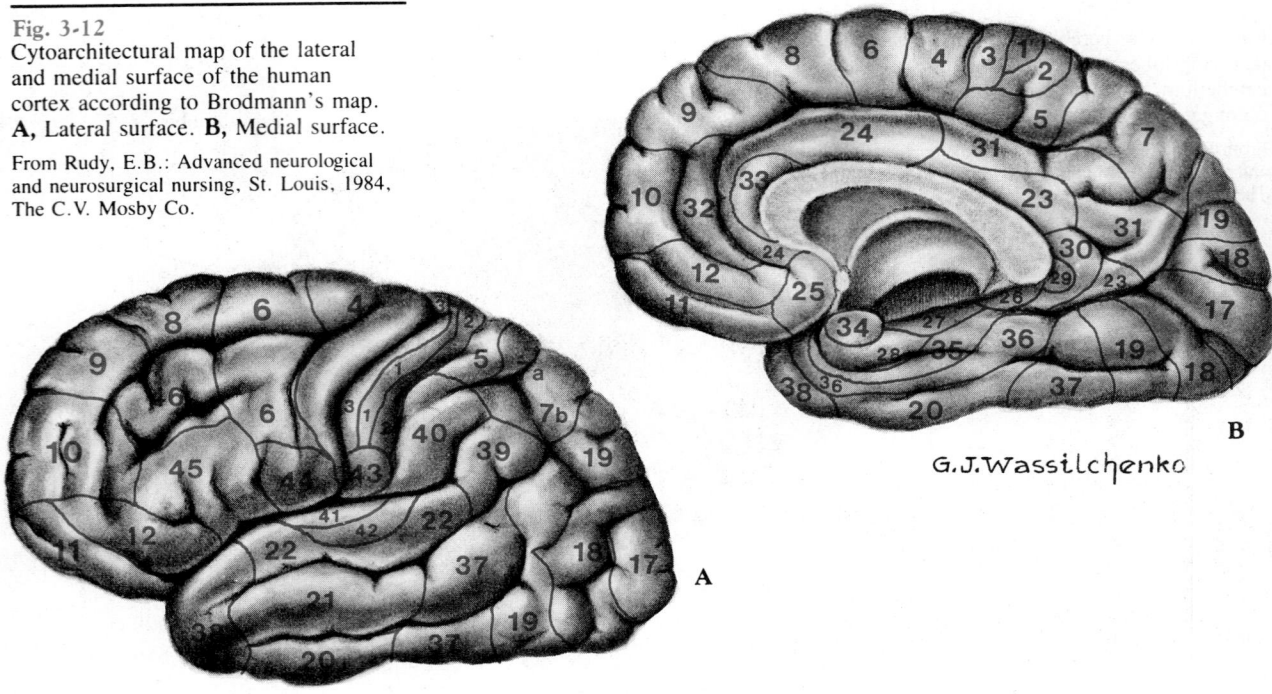

Fig. 3-12
Cytoarchitectural map of the lateral
and medial surface of the human
cortex according to Brodmann's map.
A, Lateral surface. **B,** Medial surface.

From Rudy, E.B.: Advanced neurological
and neurosurgical nursing, St. Louis, 1984,
The C.V. Mosby Co.

known classification of these areas is *Brodmann's map*. On the basis of histologic studies performed in 1909, Brodmann developed a map of 47 different areas of the cerebral cortex (Fig. 3-12) and classified them as primary function areas or association areas.

Primary function areas are those in which the movement or perception of movement occurs. Brodmann's area 4, located at the precentral gyrus, is the primary motor area. At the postcentral gyrus are Brodmann's areas 1, 2, and 3, which are the primary somatic sensory areas. Brodmann's areas 41 and 42 are the primary auditory cortex and are located in the temporal lobe. The occipital lobe contains the primary visual cortex, Brodmann's area 17.

Association areas are areas 1 to 5 cm in diameter surrounding the primary function areas. The function of the association areas is to provide a higher level of integration (i.e., memory, learning) for sensory experiences. Brodmann's association areas include 9, 10, 11, and 12 (frontal); 5 and 7 (sensory); 42 (auditory); 18 and 19 (visual); and areas 20, 21, 38, and 40. Other association areas worth noting include 44 and 45 of the frontal lobe (Broca's area) and area 22 of the temporal lobe (Wernicke's area).

The *frontal lobe* is located in the anterior fossa and extends from the anterior portion of each hemisphere to the central sulcus (fissure of Rolando) posteriorly. The inferior border is the lateral cerebral fissure (fissure of Sylvius). The overall function of the frontal lobe is concerned with psychic and higher intellectual functions. The frontal lobe also contains higher level centers for autonomic functioning, such as cardiovascular responses, and gastrointestinal activity. Additionally, Broca's area, which assists in the formation of words, is located in the frontal lobe.

The *parietal lobe* is located in the middle fossa. Specifically, it lies in the area between the central sulcus (fissure of Rolando) and the parieto-occipital fissure. The major functions of the parietal lobe deal with position sense, touch, and motor movement.

The *occipital lobe* is a pyramid-shaped structure situated in the middle fossa, posterior to the parieto-occipital fissure and just above the cerebellum. The occipital lobe contains the primary vision centers (primary vision cortex).

The *temporal lobe* is also located in the middle fossa. It lies inferior to the lateral cerebral fissure (fissure of Sylvius) and extends posteriorly to the parieto-occipital fissure. Primary functions of the temporal lobe are memory storage and hearing. Wernicke's area, the auditory association area, is found in the temporal lobe.

The *rhinencephalon* (limbic lobe) is anatomically part of the temporal lobe but is separate in its functions. Specifically, the rhinencephalon consists of cortical and subcortical structures that form the border of the lateral ventricles of each cerebral hemisphere. The functions of

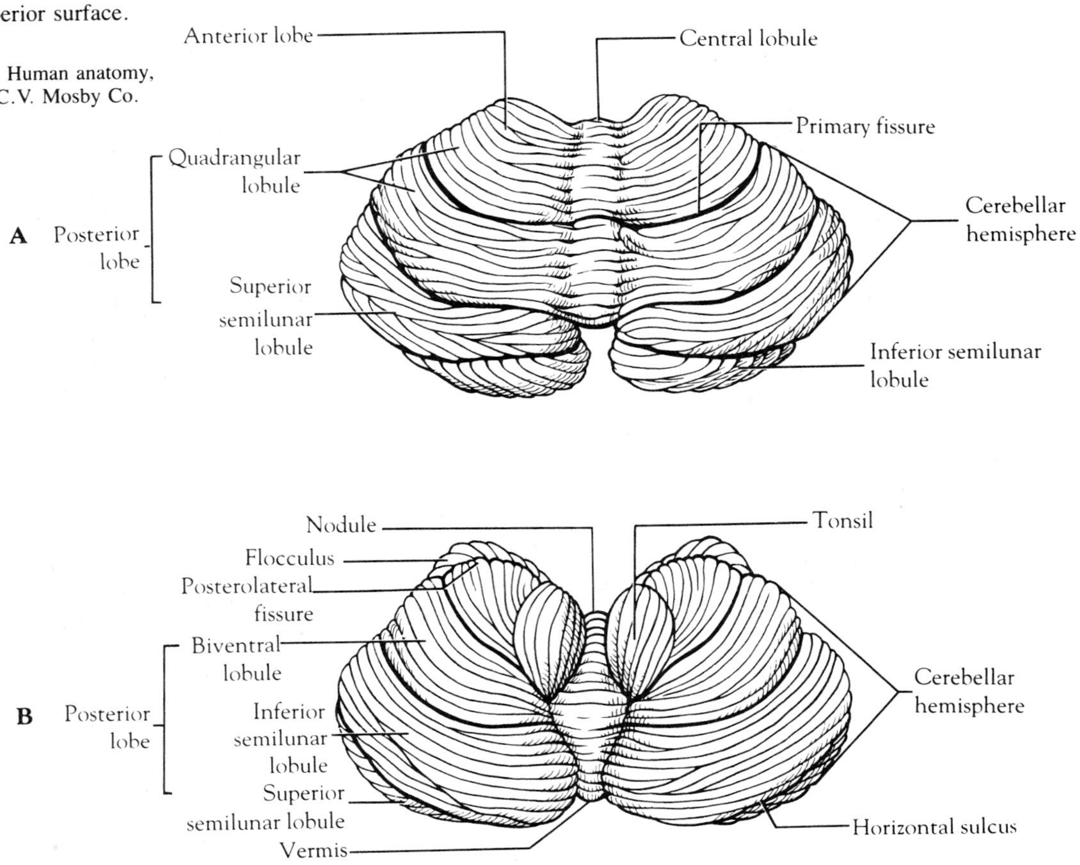

Fig. 3-13
Cerebellum. **A,** Superior surface.
B, Inferior surface.

From McClintic, J.R.: Human anatomy,
St. Louis, 1982, The C.V. Mosby Co.

the rhinencephalon are relative to self-preservation, visceral activities, instincts, feeling states, and moods.

The *basal ganglia* are gray nuclei located deep within the white matter of each cerebral hemisphere. The basal ganglia consist of the paired anatomic structures of the lenticular nucleus, caudate nucleus, amygdaloid body, and claustrum. The lenticular and caudate nuclei are collectively referred to as the corpus striatum. Functions include motor control of fine body movements, particularly in the hands and lower extremities.

The internal capsule, located in the thalamic-hypothalamic area, is a massive bundle of white matter. It consists of afferent and efferent fiber tracts that transmit impulses from the cerebrum to the brainstem and spinal cord.

Diencephalon. The oval-shaped diencephalon forms the rostral (toward the head) end of the brainstem and consists of gray matter.[25] Functionally the diencephalon contains pathways for visceral, sensory, somatic, and motor impulses. Structurally it consists of the epithalamus, thalamus, hypothalamus, and subthalamus. The epithalamus, located in the most dorsal aspect of the dien-

cephalon, consists of the pineal body, habenula, habenular commissure, posterior commissure, and striae medullares. The pineal body, the most important structure of the epithalamus, is composed primarily of neuroglia cells and plays a role in growth and sexual development. The thalamus consists of two connected ovoid masses of gray matter in the dorsal portion of the diencephalon. Each half of the thalamus is located deep within the corresponding cerebral hemisphere.[25] The thalamus functions as a relay and integration station for cerebral, cerebellar, and brainstem activity. The hypothalamus lies inferior to the thalamus, forming the floor and portions of the walls of the third ventricle. Functions of the hypothalamus are indicated in Table 3-1. The subthalamus is anatomically situated between the tegmentum of the midbrain and the dorsal aspect of the thalamus. The subthalamus is functionally integrated with the extrapyramidal system of the autonomic nervous system.

Cerebellum. Separated from the cerebrum by the tentorium cerebelli is the cerebellum (Fig. 3-13), which is approximately one fifth the size of the cerebrum and

Table 3-1
Principal Thalamic Nuclei

Neuroanatomic Classification	Functional Classification	Principal Connections		General Functions
		Afferent Fibers	Efferent Fibers	
Anterior nuclei				
Anteromedial	Nonspecific projection			
Anterodorsal	Nonspecific projection			
Anteroventral	Nonspecific projection	From hypothalamus via mammillothalamic tract (of Vicq d'Azyr); higher order olfactory neurons	To cingulate gyrus of cerebral cortex	Part of circuit involved in limbic system, convey olfactory impulses
Midline nuclei				
Cell groups beneath lining of wall, third ventricle	Nonspecific projection	From spinothalamic, trigeminothalamic tracts, medial lemniscus, reticular formation, other thalamic nuclei, hypothalamus	To hypothalamus and cortex (few to anterior rhinencephalon (?); basal ganglia (?); other thalamic nuclei	Center for integrating crude visceral and somatic sensations
Massa intermedia	Nonspecific projection			
Medial nuclei				
Scattered cells in internal medullary lamina (intralaminar nuclei)	Nonspecific projection	From prefrontal cortex, septal areas, basal ganglia, and other thalamic nuclei	To prefrontal cortex	Integrate somatic and visceral sensory impulses before projecting this information to cortex; association center for synthesis of crude somatic sensations
Dorsomedial	Nonspecific projection	From thalamic nuclei, prefrontal cortex, basal ganglia	To prefrontal cortex	
Centromedian	Nonspecific projection	From putamen, caudate nucleus, other thalamic nuclei	To basal ganglia, other thalamic nuclei (?)	Intrathalamic integrating center (?)
Lateral nuclei				
Anterior ventral	Nonspecific projection	From globus pallidus via thalamic fasciculus	To corpus striatum; cortex (frontal lobe)	
Lateral ventral	Specific projection	From cerebellum via superior cerebellar peduncle; globus pallidus via thalamic fasciculus	To cerebral cortex (premotor areas) via posterior limb of internal capsule	Part of circuit involved in voluntary motor functions
Posterolateral ventral	Specific projection	Termination of spinothalamic tracts, medial lemniscus	To sensory areas of cortex (postcentral gyrus) via posterior limb of internal capsule	Relays sensory impulses from trunk and limbs*
Posteromedial ventral	Specific projection	Termination of secondary trigeminal and taste fibers		Relays sensory impulses from face†
Dorsal lateral	Specific projection	From other thalamic nuclei; parietal lobe of cerebral cortex	To cerebral cortex (parietal lobe)	Primary sensory relay nuclei
Posterior lateral	Specific projection			
Reticular	Nonspecific projection	From entire cerebral cortex, other thalamic nuclei, reticular formation of brainstem	To other thalamic nuclei; tegmentum of midbrain	Functions controversial
Posterior nuclei				
Pulvinar	Specific projection	From other thalamic nuclei, cerebral cortex (parietal, temporal, occipital lobes)	To cerebral cortex (parietal, temporal, occipital lobes)	Integrates auditory, visual, somatic impulses (?)

Medial geniculate†	Specific projection	From brachium of inferior colliculus	To auditory cortex via sublenticular portion of internal capsule (bilateral projection)	Audition
Lateral geniculate†	Specific projection	From optic tract (cranial nerve II)	To ipsilateral striate cortex via retrolenticular portion of internal capsule	Vision

From Jensen, D.: The principles of physiology, ed. 2, New York, 1982, Appleton-Century-Crofts.

*The posterolateral ventral and posteromedial ventral nuclei of the thalamus are of major physiologic significance, since these structures provide the principal thalamic relay system for somesthetic afferent fibers.

†The medial and lateral geniculate bodies sometimes are classed together as the *metathalamus*.

comprises two lateral hemispheres and a medial portion, the *vermis*. The cerebellum consists of an outer cortex of gray matter and an internal medulla of white matter. Embedded deep within the white matter are four pairs of nuclei: dentate, emboliform, globose, and fastigial. The cerebellum is connected, via the midbrain, to the cerebral cortex and attaches on each side of the brainstem by means of three large bundles of nerve fibers, the *cerebellar peduncles*. Additionally, the cerebellum connects with the semicircular canals, or organs of balance. The cerebellum is primarily involved in coordinating movement, equilibrium, muscle tone, and position sense. Each of the cerebellar hemispheres controls movement coordination for the same side of the body (ipsilateral).

Brainstem. The brainstem (Fig. 3-14) consists of the midbrain (mesencephalon), the pons, and the medulla oblongata. The overall functions of the brainstem deal with maintaining involuntary reflexes for vital functioning of the body.

The *midbrain* (mesencephalon) forms a junction between the diencephalon and the pons. The lower surface contains two bundles of fibers, crura cerebri, which are made of the corticospinal, corticopontine, and corticobulbar tracts of the voluntary nervous system carrying descending motor fiber tracts from the cerebral cortex to the pons. The oculomotor nerves (cranial nerve III) originate from each side of the fossae separating the peduncles of the crura cerebri. The superior cerebral peduncles contain the point of decussation where fibers from the dentate nucleus of one side cross over to the red nuclei of the opposite side. The dorsal surface of the midbrain consists of four rounded elevations, collectively called the corpora quadrigemina. The rostral pair of elevations is the superior colliculi (eye tracking), and the caudal pair is the inferior colliculi (auditory reflexes). The trochlear nerves (cranial nerve IV) exit the brain posterior to the inferior colliculi. Additionally, the tectospinal and rubrospinal tracts of the nonpyramidal motor pathway originate in the midbrain. Both of these tracts decussate near their respective points of origin. The tectospinal tract mediates reflex movements in response to visual and auditory stimuli. The rubrospinal tract controls tone of flexor muscles. The major function of the midbrain is the relay of stimuli dealing with muscle movement, visual reflexes, and auditory reflexes from the spinal cord, medulla oblongata, and the cerebellum to the cerebrum.

The *pons* (metencephalon; Fig. 3-14) connects the midbrain to the medulla oblongata and relays impulses to the brain centers as well as to the lower spinal centers of the nervous system. Sensory and motor nuclei of the trigeminal (cranial V), abducens (cranial VI), facial (cranial VII), and acoustic (cranial VIII) nerves originate in the pons. The corticobulbar and corticospinal tracts make up the white matter of the pons.

Fig. 3-14
Brainstem. **A,** Posterior view.
B, Lateral view.

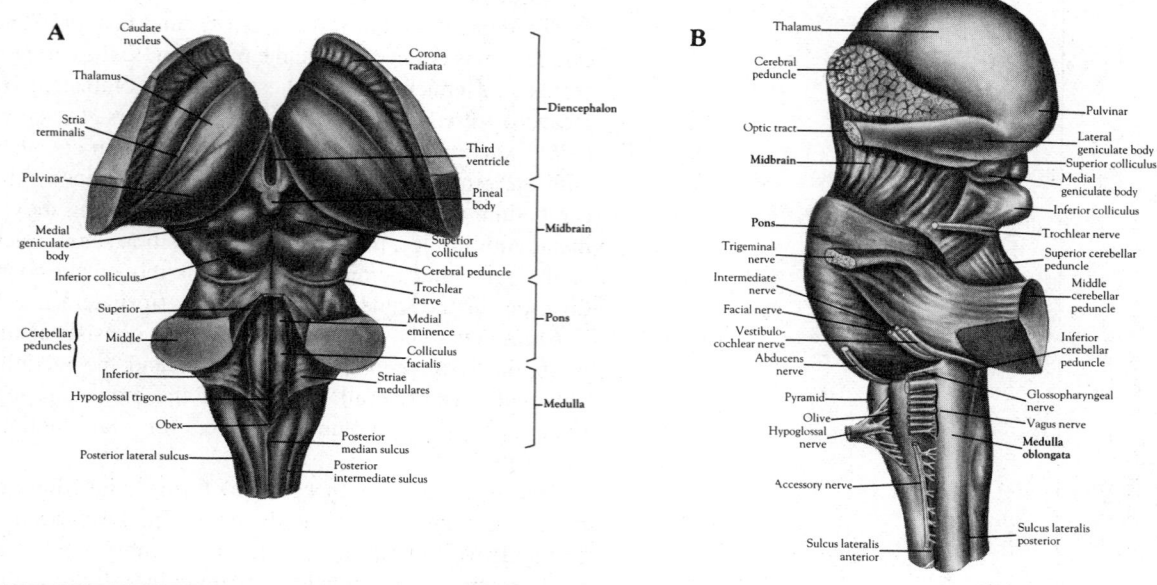

Fig. 3-15
Reticular activating system.

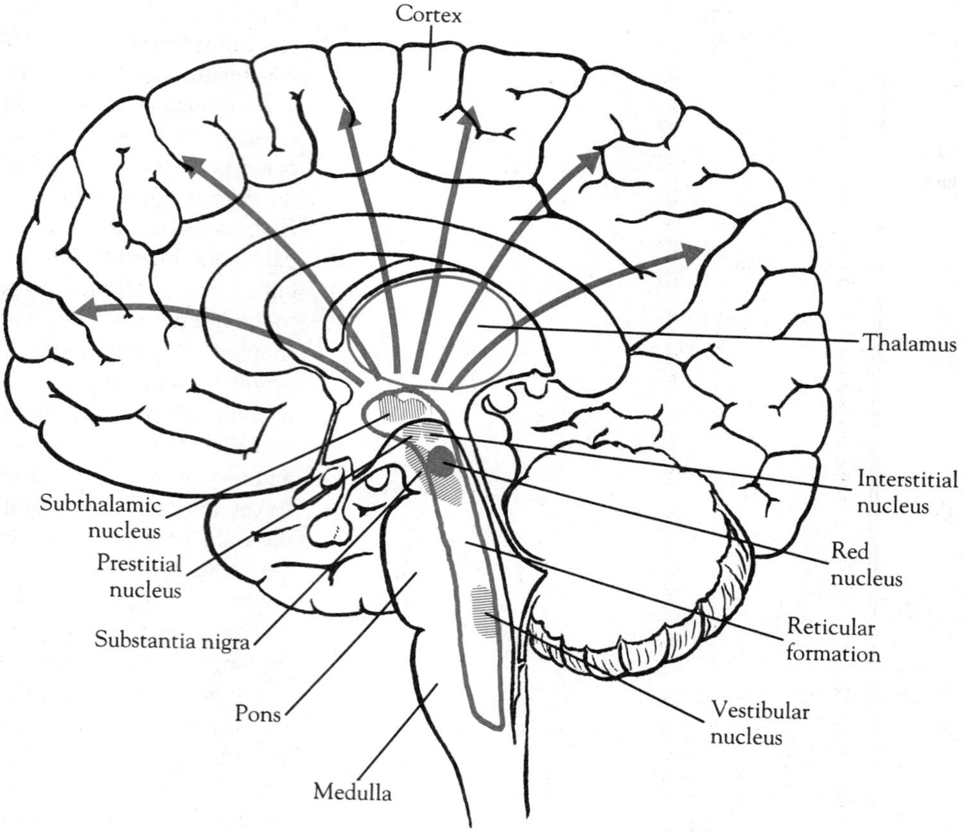

The *medulla oblongata* (myelencephalon; Fig. 3-14) contains the reflex centers for controlling involuntary functions such as breathing, sneezing, swallowing, coughing, salivation, vomiting, and vasoconstriction. Additionally, the medulla provides points of origin for the glossopharyngeal (cranial IX), vagus (cranial X), spinal accessory (cranial XI), and hypoglossal (cranial XII) nerves.

Reticular formation. Extending from the upper spinal cord through the midventral portion of the medulla, pons, midbrain, and diencephalon are extensions of gray matter intermeshed with filaments of nuclei and fibers called the reticular formation. The reticular formation is a scattered and interconnected complex of sensory nerve fibers. Located in the reticular formation are centers that regulate respiration, blood pressure, heart rate (medulla), and vegetative functions (Fig. 3-15).

Reticular activating system. The reticular activating system (RAS) is a polysynaptic, nonspecific sensory pathway considered to be an integral regulatory center of the central nervous system. It extends from the superior level of the brainstem to the cerebral cortex. Functionally, most of the RAS is excitatory and is involved in the following processes: maintaining attention; the sleep-wake cycle; regulation of visceral functions such as respiration and vasomotor tone; consciousness; perception of sensory input; regulation of temperature; emotional states; learning; conditioned reflexes; and regulation of skeletal muscle tone and activity.[25]

Spinal vertebrae. The vertebral column (Fig. 3-16) is made up of 33 vertebrae divided into five anatomic and functional regions: cervical, thoracic, lumbar, sacral, and coccygeal. Vertebrae are joined together by numerous ligaments and intervertebral discs that provide strength and flexibility.

There are seven *cervical* vertebrae. C1 is a highly developed vertebra referred to as the atlas because it supports the head. The atlas is modified from other cervical vertebrae in that it does not have a vertebral body or spinous process. C2, termed the axis, forms a pivot on which the skull and atlas rotate. The axis is also modified in that the vertebral body has a perpendicular toothlike projection, the odontoid process, on which the atlas articulates.

The 12 *thoracic* vertebrae progressively enlarge as they descend. The thoracic vertebrae body is characterized by four costal facets. The costal facets, two inferior and two superior, provide articulation for the heads of the ribs. Due to rib articulation, the vertebral column is least free for movement and rotation in the thoracic region.

Fig. 3-16

Vertebral column and anatomic structure of vertebrae.

From Rudy, E.B.: Advanced neurological and neurosurgical nursing, St. Louis, 1984, The C.V. Mosby Co.

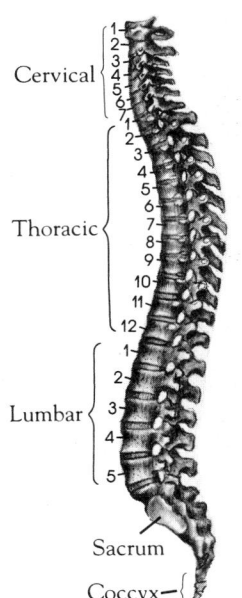

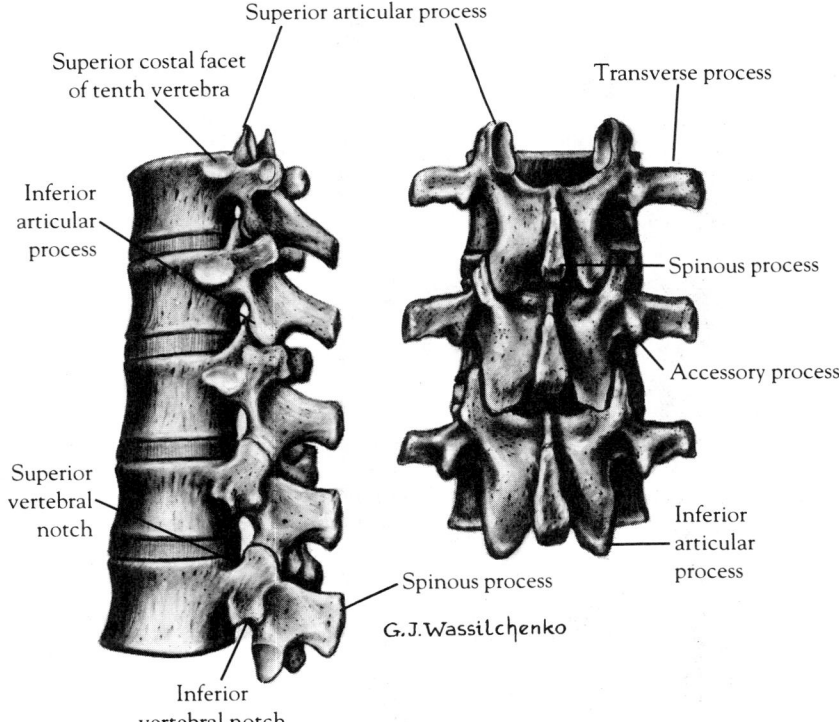

G.J. Wassilchenko

The five *lumbar* vertebrae allow for great freedom of movement. L5 and the base of the sacrum together form the lumbosacral angle.

The *sacrum* in the adult is a single wedge-shaped bone formed by the fusion of the five sacral vertebrae. The sacral canal, which contains the cauda equina and filium terminale, originates in this region.

The *coccyx* in the adult is also a fused bone consisting of from three to five coccygeal vertebrae.

The typical *vertebra* (Fig. 3-16) found in the cervical, thoracic, lumbar, or sacral regions listed above consists of several important anatomic characteristics. The vertebral body is the cylindric ventral portion that assumes the responsibility of weight bearing. It is separated from the vertebral bodies above and below it by cartilage and fibrous tissue called intervertebral discs. The dorsal portion of the vertebra is the vertebral arch, which is formed by two laminae and two pedicles. In the center of the vertebra is the vertebral foramen, which, in conjunction with other vertebrae, forms the vertebral canal containing the spinal cord and spinal meninges. The vertebral notch forms a part of the vertebral foramen from which spinal nerves and blood vessels exit the spinal cord. Finally, the vertebral processes (one spinous, two transverse, two superior articular, and two inferior articular) provide sites for attachment of muscles and ligaments as well as for articulation with adjacent vertebrae.

Protective structures: meninges. The spinal cord, like the brain, is enveloped by the three layers of meninges: dura mater, arachnoid, and pia mater. Between the lining of the vertebral canal and the spinal dura mater is the epidural space. The epidural space contains areolar

Fig. 3-17

Spinal cord within vertebral canal and exiting spinal nerves. **A,** Posterior view of brainstem and spinal cord in situ with spinal nerves and plexuses. **B,** Anterior view of brainstem and spinal cord. **C,** Lateral view showing relationship of spinal cord to vertebrae. **D,** Enlargement of caudal area showing termination of spinal cord (conus medullaris) and group of nerve fibers constituting the cauda equina.

From Rudy, E.B.: Advanced neurological and neurosurgical nursing, St. Louis, 1984, The C.V. Mosby Co.

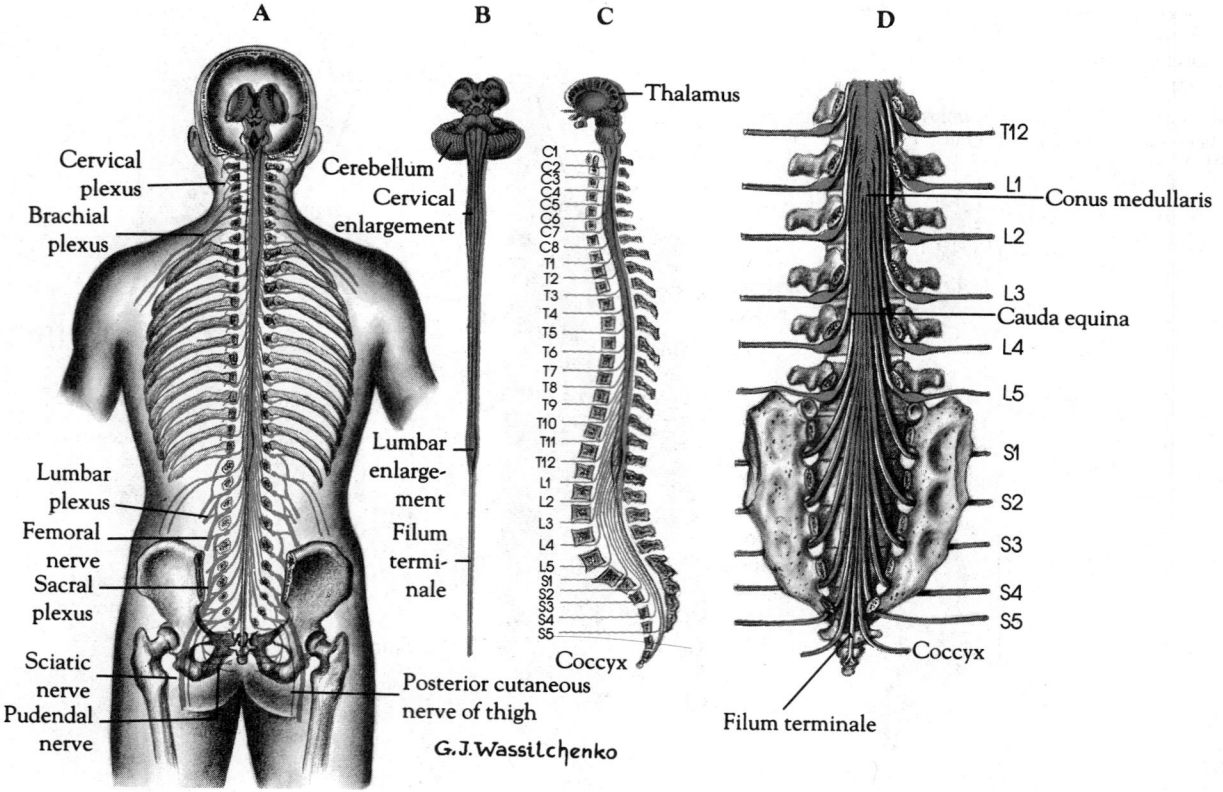

tissue, fat, and a number of venous plexuses. Adjacent to the epidural space is the spinal dura mater. The spinal dura mater extends from the foramen magnum, where it is continuous with the cranial dura, to the second sacral vertebra, where it blends with the filium terminale. Laterally, the dura continues over the roots of the spinal nerves forming dural root sleeves. Between the dura mater and the intermediate meningeal layer is the subdural space. The subdural space contains a small amount of fluid, which decreases friction between opposing surfaces. The second meningeal layer, the spinal arachnoid, extends superiorly from the foramen magnum, to inferior surfaces of the cauda equina and the filum terminale. Laterally, the spinal arachnoid encloses the spinal nerve roots to the point of exit from the vertebral canal. The space between the arachnoid and the pia mater is the subarachnoid space, which contains cerebrospinal fluid. The innermost layer, the spinal pia mater, also envelops the spinal nerves. The pia mater extends downward to the filum terminale, where it is connected by the denticulate ligaments to the spinal dura mater between the ventral and dorsal spinal nerve roots.

Spinal cord. The spinal cord (Fig. 3-17) is a downward continuation from the medulla oblongata, originating at the foramen magnum and ending at the superior border of L2. The cord tapers in the lower thoracic area into a cone-shaped structure called the *conus medullaris.*

Extending inferiorly from the conus medullaris is a thin prolongation, the *filum terminale,* that anchors the spinal cord to the coccyx. The spinal cord consists of 31 segments, each giving rise to a pair of spinal nerves.

Microscopically, the spinal cord consists of gray (unmyelinated) and white (myelinated) matter. The *gray matter* integrates the cord reflexes and is concentrated into an internal core. When this internal core is viewed in cross section, it resembles a butterfly (Fig. 3-18). The pair of gray matter projections forming the front ''wings'' of the butterfly are the anterior, or ventral, horns. The pair of projections forming the back ''wings'' are called the posterior, or dorsal, horns. The ventral horn consists of multipolar neuron structures (e.g., cell bodies, dendrites) that together form the motor efferent neurons of the ventral roots and spinal nerves. The dorsal horn contains cell bodies and dendrites of sensory (afferent) neurons and sensory receptors from the periphery. Additionally, the gray matter contains internuncial (association) neurons. The internuncial neurons transmit impulses from one lateral half of the cord to the other, from dorsal to ventral, and to other levels of the central nervous system.

Surrounding the gray matter of the spinal cord is the *white matter* (Fig. 3-18), which comprises long ascending and descending tracts that serve as pathways between the spinal cord and brain for afferent and efferent im-

Fig. 3-18
Cross section of spinal cord illustrating subdivisions of white and gray matter.

From Rudy, E.B.: Advanced neurological and neurosurgical nursing, St. Louis, 1984, The C.V. Mosby Co.

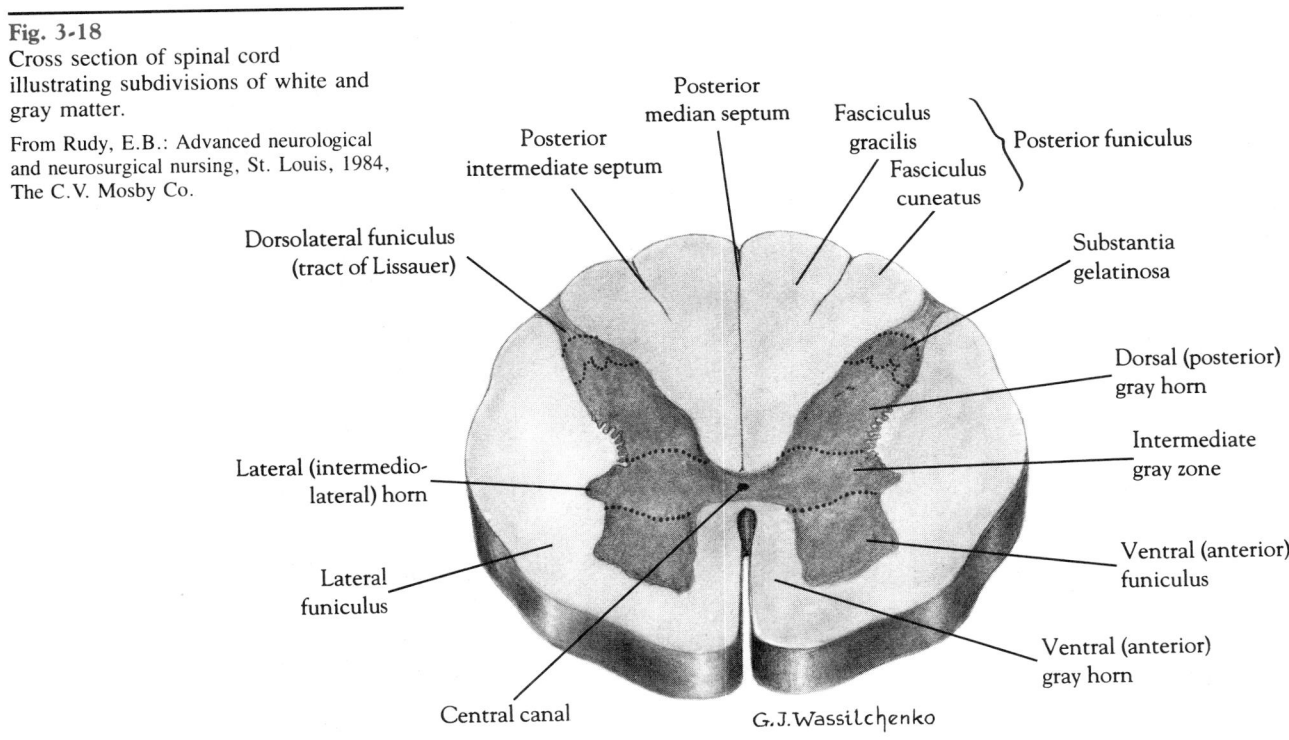

Posterior median septum

Posterior intermediate septum

Posterior intermediate septum

Fasciculus gracilis

Fasciculus cuneatus

Posterior funiculus

Dorsolateral funiculus (tract of Lissauer)

Substantia gelatinosa

Dorsal (posterior) gray horn

Intermediate gray zone

Lateral (intermediolateral) horn

Ventral (anterior) funiculus

Lateral funiculus

Ventral (anterior) gray horn

Central canal

G.J.Wassilchenko

pulses. The white matter is grouped into anatomic and functional bundles called fasciculi.

The spinal cord is divided into lateral halves by the *anterior fissure* and the *posterior sulcus*. Each lateral half is connected to the other half by commissures of gray and white matter. Each lateral half of the spinal cord is divided into three sections that run the length of the spinal cord: dorsal, lateral, and ventral. Within each of these divisions are distinct fiber tracts: (1) ascending fibers, which bring sensory information to the central nervous system; (2) descending fibers, which carry impulses from the brain to motor neurons of the brainstem and the spinal cord; and (3) internuncial (association) neurons, which form short ascending and descending tracts that travel between spinal segments. These short tracts are referred to as intersegmental tracts. Both ascending and descending tracts are detailed further below.

The neurons in the *ascending* pathways transmit sensory information from peripheral receptors to the spinal cord and brain. The sensory chain consists of a three-neuron pathway. The first-order neuron's cell body originates in the dorsal root ganglion and conducts impulses from peripheral receptors to the spinal cord. The second-order neuron's cell body is found at various levels of the gray matter of the spinal cord and the brainstem. These neurons conduct impulses, in the white matter, to the thalamus. The third-order neuron's cell body lies in the thalamus and conducts impulses from the thalamus to the cerebral cortex.

The pathways are organized according to body surface areas and cross in the brain so that sensory information enters the cerebral cortex from the opposite side of the body. This crossing over is usually done by the second-order neuron.

The *descending* pathways involve two principal types of neurons. The first type is the upper motor neuron, which has its cell body in the cerebral motor areas or subcortical areas (i.e., brainstem) of the central nervous system. The upper motor neuron transmits impulses from the brain to motor neurons in the anterior (ventral) horn of the spinal cord as well as to motor neurons in the cranial nerves. The second type of neuron, the lower motor neuron, begins in the central nervous system and terminates in the peripheral nervous system. The lower

Fig. 3-19
Schematic drawing to show decussation of pyramids at level of medulla.

From Rudy, E.B.: Advanced neurological and neurosurgical nursing, St. Louis, 1984, The C.V. Mosby Co.

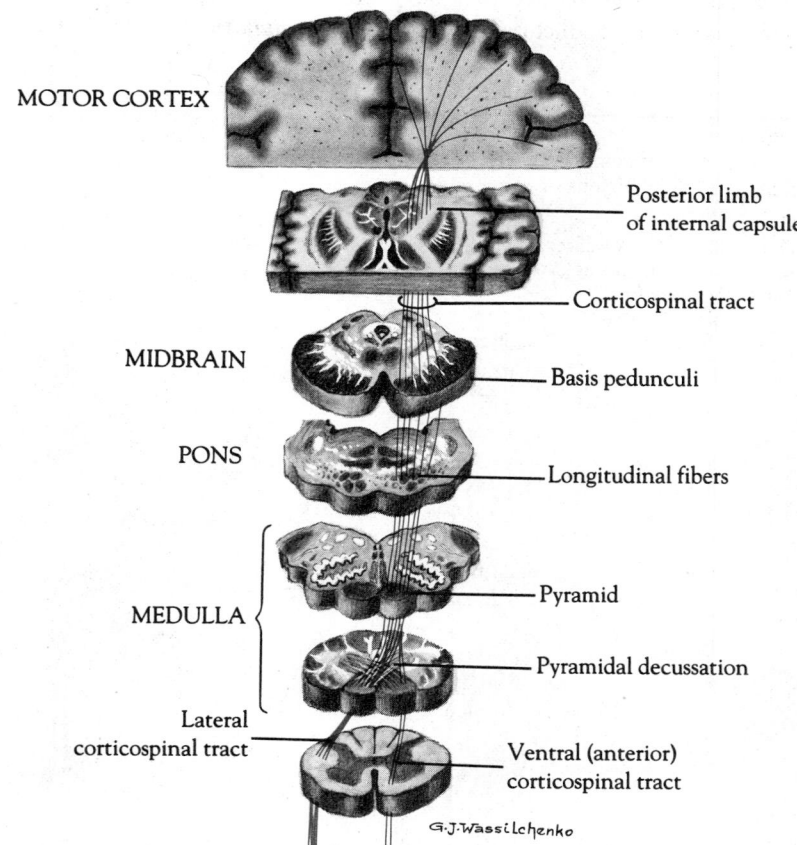

MOTOR CORTEX

Posterior limb of internal capsule

Corticospinal tract

MIDBRAIN

Basis pedunculi

PONS

Longitudinal fibers

Pyramid

MEDULLA

Pyramidal decussation

Lateral corticospinal tract

Ventral (anterior) corticospinal tract

G.J.Wassilchenko

motor neurons consist of motor nuclei of the cranial nerves, and the motor cells in the anterior horn of the spinal cord. The two major subdivisions of the descending pathways originating from the cerebral cortex are the pyramidal and extrapyramidal tracts.

The pyramidal tracts (corticospinal tracts) originate from the large pyramid-shaped motor neurons in the cerebral precentral cortex of the parietal lobe and descend through the diencephalon, midbrain, pons, medulla, and the white matter of the spinal cord to the motor cells in the anterior horns of the gray matter. In the medulla the pyramidal tracts form the medullary pyramids where the majority of fibers decussate (cross over) to the other side, forming the larger of the two corticospinal tracts, the *lateral corticospinal tract*. Fibers that do not decussate at the medulla form the *anterior corticospinal tract*, which descends (on the same side of origin) in the spinal cord in the anterior white matter to the cervical and upper thoracic regions. Many fibers of the anterior corticospinal tract decussate at respective levels of the anterior white commissure before synapsing with the lower motor neurons. The pyramidal tracts conduct voluntary impulses and reflex muscle contractions (Fig. 3-19).

The extrapyramidal tracts (Fig. 3-20) originate in the

Fig. 3-20

Extrapyramidal descending tracts. Upper motor neurons originate below level of cortex and converge on lower motor neurons (final common pathway) along with upper motor neurons of pyramidal tracts. Rubrospinal tract *(A)* originates in the red area.

From Conway-Rutkowski, B.L.: Carini and Owens' neurological and neurosurgical nursing, ed. 8, St. Louis, 1982, The C.V. Mosby Co.

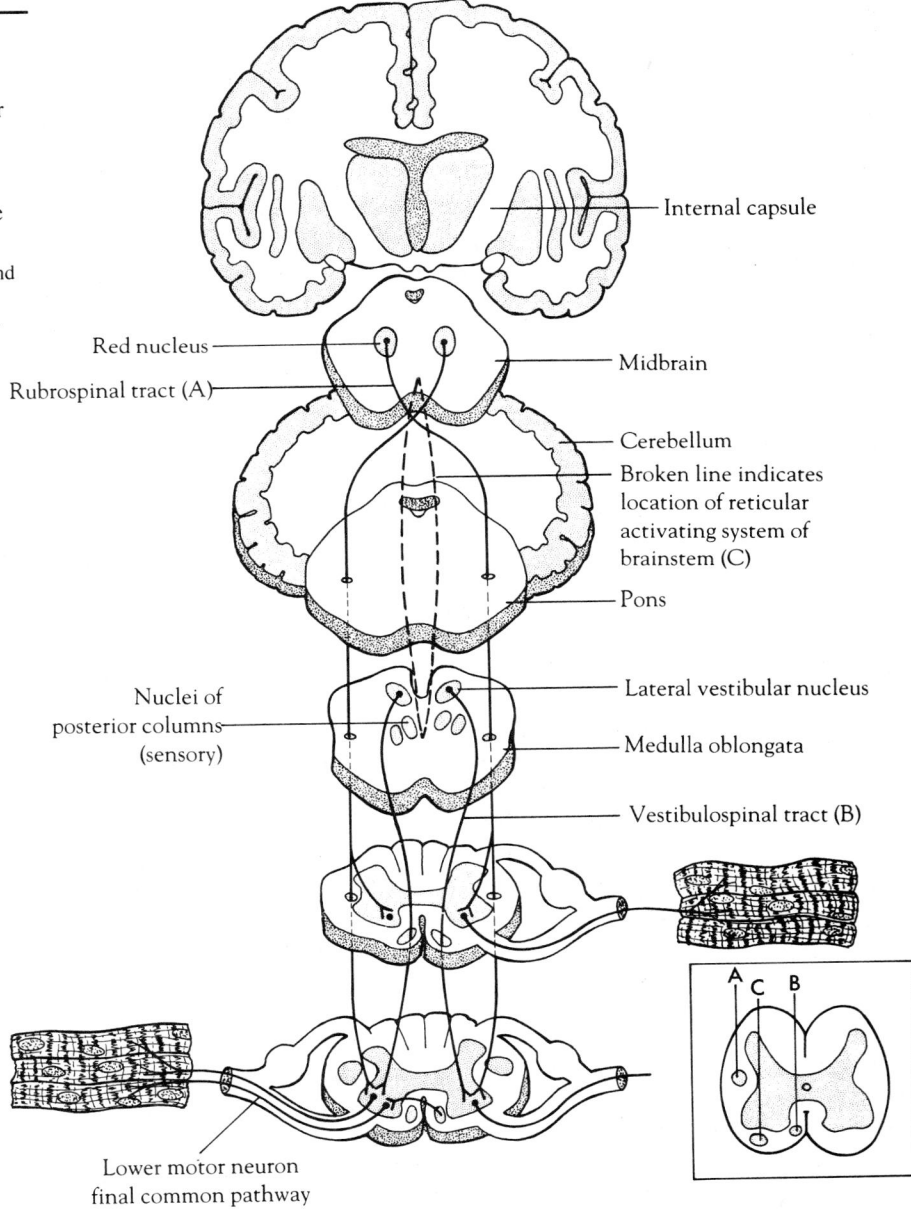

Table 3-2
Major Ascending and Descending Spinal Cord Tracts

Name	Function	Location	Origin*	Termination†
Ascending				
Lateral spinothalamic	Pain, temperature, and crude touch opposite side	Lateral white columns	Posterior gray column opposite side	Thalamus
Ventral spinothalamic	Crude touch, pain, and temperature	Anterior white columns	Posterior gray column opposite side	Thalamus
Fasciculi gracilis and cuneatus	Discriminating touch and pressure sensations, including vibration, stereognosis, and two-point discrimination; also conscious kinesthesia	Posterior white columns	Spinal ganglia same side	Medulla
Spinocerebellar	Unconscious kinesthesia	Lateral white columns	Posterior gray column	Cerebellum
Descending				
Lateral corticospinal (or crossed pyramidal)	Voluntary movement, contraction of individual or small groups of muscles, particularly those moving hands, fingers, feet, and toes of opposite side	Lateral white columns	Motor areas of cerebral cortex (mainly areas 4 and 6) opposite side from tract location in cord	Intermediate or anterior gray columns
Ventral corticospinal (direct pyramidal)	Same as lateral corticospinal except mainly muscles of same side	Lateral white columns	Motor cortex but on same side as tract location in cord	Intermediate or anterior gray columns
Lateral reticulospinal	Mainly facilitatory influence on motorneurons to skeletal muscles	Lateral white columns	Reticular formation, midbrain, pons, and medulla	Intermediate or anterior gray columns
Medial reticulospinal	Mainly inhibitory influence on motorneurons to skeletal muscles	Anterior white columns	Reticular formation, medulla mainly	Intermediate or anterior gray columns

From Anthony, C.P., and Thibodeau, G.M.: Textbook of anatomy and physiology, ed. 11, St. Louis, 1983, The C.V. Mosby Co.
*Location of cell bodies of neurons from which axons of tract arise.
†Structure in which axons of tract terminate.

brainstem, basal ganglia, and cerebellum. These pathways are motor systems coordinating muscular activity. The *rubrospinal* tract originates in the red nucleus of the brainstem where it immediately decussates and transmits impulses for tonus in flexor muscles. The *medial reticulospinal* tract originates in the reticular formation of the brainstem and descends uncrossed. The medial reticulospinal tract stimulates flexor and inhibits extensor responses. The *lateral reticulospinal* tract also originates from the brainstem and is primarily uncrossed. The lateral tract stimulates extensor and inhibits flexor responses, maintaining posture. The *medial vestibulospinal* and the *lateral vestibulospinal* tracts originate in the medulla. The lateral tract descends uncrossed, while some fibers in the medial tract decussate (cross over). Both the lateral and medial vestibulospinal tracts conduct impulses that provide muscle tone and aid in maintaining equilibrium. The *olivospinal* tract is mainly crossed and descends only to the cervical region. The specific functions

of the olivospinal tract are unknown, but it may mediate thalamospinal reflexes. Finally, the *tectospinal* tract arises from the superior colliculus of the midbrain where they decussate. This tract primarily innervates the upper four cervical segments and mediates head and neck muscle positions in response to visual and auditory stimuli. Table 3-2 summarizes the principal ascending and descending tracts of the spinal cord, with their respective functions.

The *extrapyramidal system* is a functional rather than an anatomic unit and depends on an intact pyramidal system. This system consists of extrapyramidal areas of the cerebral cortex, the corpus striatum, thalamic nuclei connected to the corpus striatum, the subthalamus, and rubral and reticular systems. The extrapyramidal system coordinates associated movements and changes in posture and integrates functions of the autonomic nervous system.[25] The system has fibers that originate from the cerebral cortex and project to the basal ganglia. The basal

Fig. 3-21
Three-neuron reflex arc.

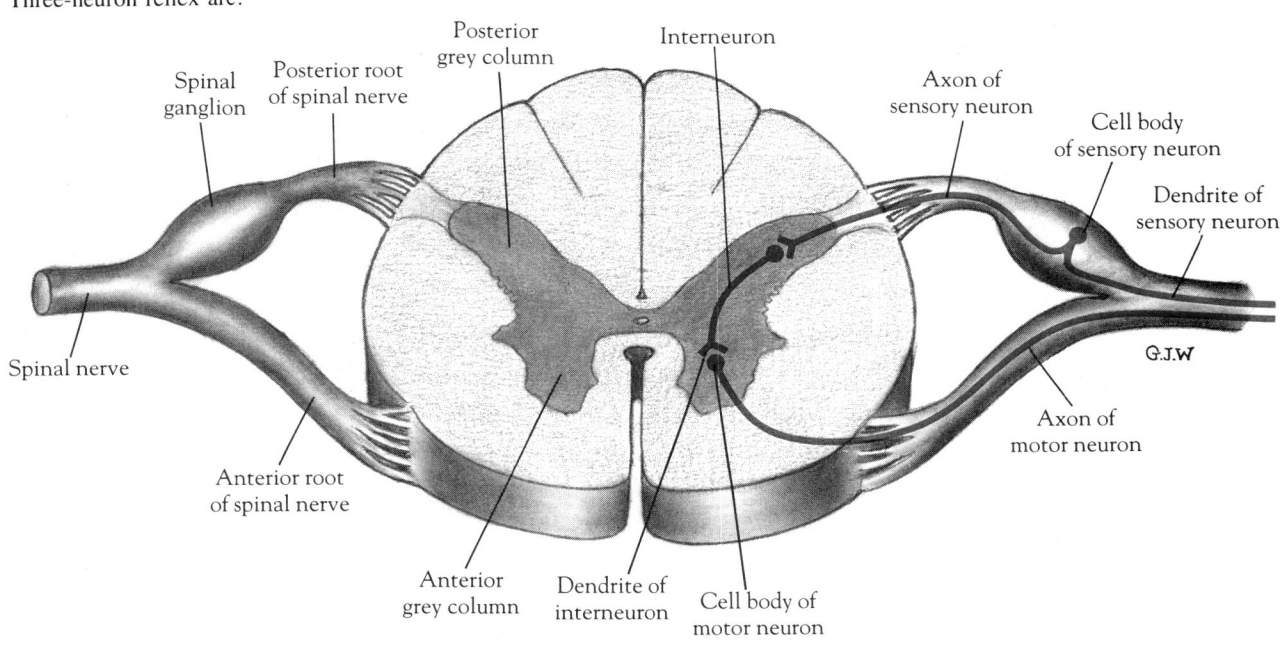

ganglia with respect to the extrapyramidal system act to coordinate movement.

Reflexes

The reflex arc (Fig. 3-21) is the basic functional unit responsible for maintaining body integrity by automatic conduction of impulses from sensory receptors (afferent) to efferent neurons. Specifically, the reflex arc or loop consists of stimulation of a sensory nerve ending, which then conveys the impulse via sensory (afferent) neurons to gray matter nuclei in the spinal cord. In the gray matter the afferent neuron may synapse directly with lower motor neurons, or it may synapse with one or more internuncial (association) neurons, which transfer the impulse to the lower motor neuron. The lower motor neurons (efferent) carry the impulse via the ventral roots of the spinal cord to the neuroeffector junction. Stimulation of the neuroeffector junction then results in a response of the effector organ (e.g., muscle contraction or glandular secretion). An example of a simple reflex involving only two neurons and one synapse is the knee-jerk (patellar) reflex. When the knee is tapped, afferent receptors are stimulated and send the impulse to the spinal cord. In the spinal cord the impulse is directly relayed to the lower motor neurons. These series of events result in contraction of the quadriceps muscles, which jerk the leg. Unlike this example, which is the only monosynaptic reflex in

the body, most reflex pathways involve numerous synaptic connections (polysynaptic). Reflex response time increases proportionately with the number of synapses. Some reflexes involve only one half of the body (e.g., flexor reflex) and are termed ipsilateral. There are other reflexes that cross over, eliciting responses on the opposite side of the body (e.g., crossed extensor reflex), and these are called contralateral reflexes. For example, when one steps on a tack, there is a reflex flexion in the one leg to move away from the tack, while in the opposite leg there is extension to maintain body balance.

Finally, both the brain and the spinal cord contain reflex centers that provide important data regarding level of functioning. Examples of brain reflexes include pupillary response, cardioregulatory mechanisms, and the medullary vasomotor centers. Examples of reflexes controlled predominantly by the spinal cord include emptying of the bowel and bladder, withdrawal from painful stimuli (known as a nociceptive reflex), increased blood flow to the skin, and stretch reflexes that maintain normal posture and position. Specific reflexes as well as responses elicited are discussed in the section on normal findings of the neurologic system.

Peripheral Nervous System

Cranial nerves. The 12 pairs of cranial nerves (Fig. 3-22) form the peripheral nerves of the brain. Some have

Table 3-3
Cranial Nerves

Nerve*	Sensory Fibers†			Motor Fibers†		Functions‡
	Receptors	Cell Bodies	Termination	Cell Bodies	Termination	
I Olfactory	Nasal mucosa	Nasal mucosa	Olfactory bulbs (new relay of neurons of olfactory cortex)			Sense of smell
II Optic	Retina	Retina	Nucleus in thalamus (lateral geniculate body); some fibers terminate in superior colliculus of midbrain			Vision
III Oculomotor	External eye muscles except superior oblique and lateral rectus	?	?	Midbrain (oculomotor nucleus and Edinger-Westphal nucleus)	External eye muscles except superior oblique and lateral rectus; fibers from Edinger-Westphal nucleus terminate in ciliary ganglion and then to ciliary and iris muscles	Eye movements, regulation of size of pupil, accommodation, proprioception (muscle sense)
IV Trochlear	Superior oblique	?	?	Midbrain	Superior oblique muscle of eye	Eye movements, proprioception
V Trigeminal	Skin and mucosa of head, teeth	Gasserian ganglion	Pons (sensory nucleus)	Pons (motor nucleus)	Muscles of mastication	Sensations of head and face, chewing movements, muscle sense
VI Abducens	Lateral rectus			Pons	Lateral rectus muscle of eye	Abduction of eye, proprioception
VII Facial	Taste buds of anterior two thirds of tongue	Geniculate ganglion	Medulla (nucleus solitarius)	Pons	Superficial muscles of face and scalp	Facial expressions, secretion of saliva, taste
VIII Acoustic						
1 Vestibular branch	Semicircular canals and vestibule (utricle and saccule)	Vestibular ganglion	Pons and medulla (vestibular nuclei)			Balance or equilibrium sense
2 Cochlear or auditory branch	Organ of Corti in cochlear duct	Spiral ganglion	Pons and medulla (cochlear nuclei)			Hearing

Cranial nerve	Receptors	Cell bodies (ganglia)	Termination	Origin	Termination (muscle/gland)	General functions
IX Glossopharyngeal	*Pharynx; taste buds and other receptors of posterior one third of tongue*	*Jugular and petrous ganglia*	*Medulla (nucleus solitarius)*	**Medulla (nucleus ambiguus)**	**Muscles of pharynx**	*Taste and other sensations of tongue,* **swallowing movements, secretion of saliva,** *aid in reflex control of blood pressure and respiration*
	Carotid sinus and carotid body	Jugular and petrous ganglia	Medulla (respiratory and vasomotor centers)	**Medulla at junction of pons (nucleus salivatorius)**	**Otic ganglion and then to parotid gland**	
X Vagus	*Pharynx, larynx, carotid body, and thoracic and abdominal viscera*	*Jugular and nodose ganglia*	*Medulla (nucleus solitarius), pons (nucleus of fifth cranial nerve)*	**Medulla (dorsal motor nucleus)**	**Ganglia of vagal plexus and then to muscles of pharynx, larynx, and thoracic and abdominal viscera**	*Sensations* **and movements** *or organs supplied; for example,* **slows heart, increases peristalsis, and contracts muscles for voice production**
XI Spinal accessory	?	?	?	**Medulla (dorsal motor nucleus of vagus and nucleus ambiguus)**	**Muscles of thoracic and abdominal viscera and pharynx and larynx**	**Shoulder movements, turning movements of head, movements of viscera, voice productions,** *proprioception?*
				Anterior gray column of first five or six cervical segments of spinal cord	**Trapezius and sternocleidomastoid muscle**	
XII Hypoglossal	?	?	?	**Medulla (hypoglossal nucleus)**	**Muscles of tongue**	**Tongue movements,** *proprioception?*

From Anthony, C.P., and Thibodeau, G.M.: Textbook of anatomy and physiology, ed. 11, St. Louis, 1983, The C.V. Mosby Co.

*The first letters of the words in the following sentence are the first letters of the names of the cranial nerves. Many generations of anatomy students have used this sentence as an aid to memorizing these names. It is "On Old Olympus Tiny Tops, A Finn and German Viewed Some Hops." (There are several slightly differing versions of this mnemonic.)

†Italics indicate sensory fibers and functions. Boldface type indicates motor fibers and functions.

‡An aid for remembering the general function of each cranial nerve is the following 12-word saying: "Some say marry money but my brothers say bad business marry money." Words beginning with S indicate sensory function. Words beginning with M indicate motor function. Words beginning with B indicate both sensory and motor functions. For example, the first, second, and eighth words in the saying start with S, which indicates that the first, second, and eighth cranial nerves perform sensory functions.

Fig. 3-22
Cranial nerves.

From Rudy, E.B.: Advanced neurological
and neurosurgical nursing, St. Louis, 1984,
The C.V. Mosby Co.

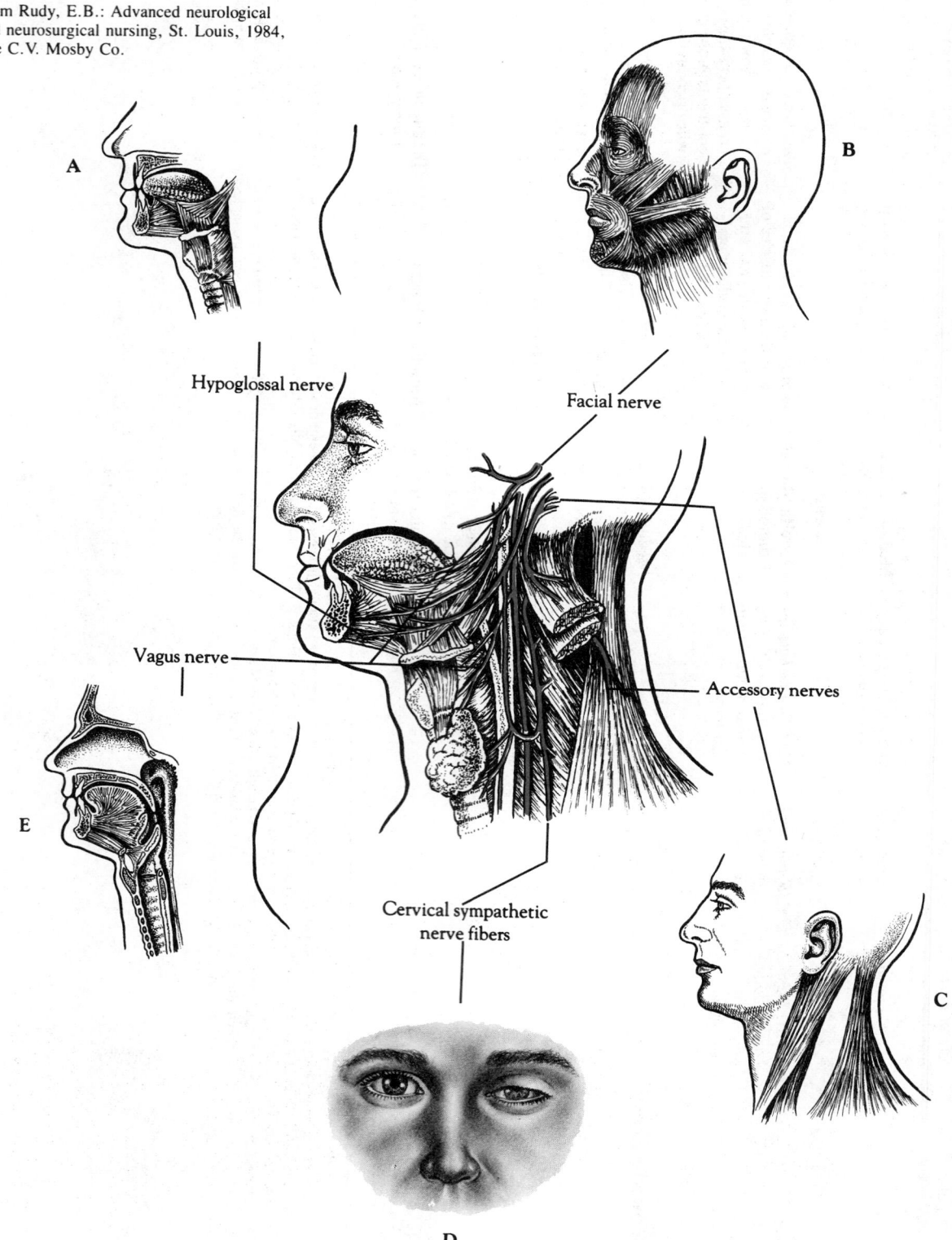

only motor fibers (five pairs), some have only sensory fibers (three pairs), and the rest (four pairs) have both sensory and motor fibers. The cranial nerves "correspond to the spinal nerves serving common sensation, voluntary control of muscles, and autonomic functions in the head; in addition, they include the mechanism for the special senses of vision, hearing, smell, and taste."[23]

Table 3-3 summarizes origin, functional class, and primary functions of the cranial nerves. Assessment of their functions is in the section on neurologic assessment.

Spinal nerves. The 31 pairs of spinal nerves arise from different segments of the spinal cord. Each pair of spinal nerves is formed by the union of anterior and posterior roots attached to the spinal cord. Each pair of spinal nerves and its corresponding part of the spinal

cord constitute a *spinal segment*. Individual spinal segments in turn innervate specific body segments. Some spinal nerves join at the anterior rami to form a complex network of nerve fibers called *plexuses*. The *cervical* and *brachial plexuses* provide peripheral nerves for innervation to the upper extremities. The lower extremities are innervated by peripheral nerves from the *lumbar* and *sacral plexuses*. Unlike the cervical and thoracic spinal nerves, the lumbar and sacral nerves do not exit from the intervertebral foramen at right angles. Instead, these nerves extend obliquely and inferiorly forming a large bundle of nerve fibers termed the *cauda equina*.

Table 3-4 summarizes the spinal nerves, corresponding plexuses, and peripheral innervation (see also Table 3-5).

Table 3-4
Spinal Nerves and Peripheral Branches

Spinal Nerves	Plexuses Formed from Anterior Rami	Spinal Nerve Branches from Plexuses	Parts Supplied
Cervical 1 2 3 4	Cervical plexus	Lesser occipital; Great auricular; Cutaneous nerve of neck; Anterior supraclavicular; Middle supraclavicular; Posterior supraclavicular; Branches to numerous neck muscles	Sensory to back of head, front of neck, and upper part of shoulder, motor to numerous neck muscles
		Phrenic (branches from cervical nerves before formation of plexus; most of its fibers from fourth cervical nerve)	Diaphragm
		Suprascapular and dorsoscapular	Superficial muscles* of scapula
		Thoracic nerves, medial and lateral branches	Pectoralis major and minor
Cervical 5 6 7 8 Thoracic (or dorsal) 1	Brachial plexus	Long thoracic nerve	Serratus anterior
		Thoracodorsal	Latissimus dorsi
		Subscapular	Subscapular and teres major muscles
		Axillary (circumflex)	Deltoid and teres minor muscles and skin over deltoid
		Musculocutaneous	Muscles of front of arm (biceps brachii, coracobrachialis, and brachialis) and skin on outer side of forearm
		Ulnar	Flexor carpi ulnaris and part of flexor digitorum profundus; some of muscles of hand; sensory to medial side of hand, little finger, and medial half of fourth finger
2 3 4 5 6 7 8 9 10 11 12	No plexus formed; branches run directly to intercostal muscles and skin of thorax	Median	Rest of muscles of front of forearm and hand; sensory to skin of palmar surface of thumb, index, and middle fingers
		Radial	Triceps muscle and muscles of back of forearm; sensory to skin of back of forearm and hand
		Medial cutaneous	Sensory to inner surface of arm and forearm

From Anthony, C.P., and Thibodeau, G.M.: Textbook of anatomy and physiology, ed. 11, St. Louis, 1983, The C.V. Mosby Co.
*Although nerves to muscles are considered motor, they do contain some sensory fibers that transmit proprioceptive impulses.   *Continued.*

Table 3-4, cont'd
Spinal Nerves and Peripheral Branches

Spinal Nerves	Plexuses Formed from Anterior Rami	Spinal Nerve Branches from Plexuses	Parts Supplied
Lumbar 1 2 3 4 5 Sacral 1 2 3 4 5 Coccygeal 1	Lumbosacral plexus	Iliohypogastric Ilioinguinal } Sometimes fused	Sensory to anterior abdominal wall Sensory to anterior abdominal wall and external genitalia; motor to muscles of abdominal wall
		Genitofemoral	Sensory to skin of external genitalia and inguinal region
		Lateral cutaneous of thigh	Sensory to outer side of thigh
		Femoral	Motor to quadriceps, sartorius, and iliacus muscles; sensory to front of thigh and medial side of lower leg (saphenous nerve)
		Obturator	Motor to adductor muscles of thigh
		Tibial† (medial popliteal)	Motor to muscles of calf of leg; sensory to skin of calf of leg and sole of foot
		Common peroneal (lateral popliteal)	Motor to evertors and dorsiflexors of foot; sensory to lateral surface of leg and dorsal surface of foot
		Nerves to hamstring muscles	Motor to muscles of back of thigh
		Gluteal nerves, superior and inferior	Motor to buttock muscles and tensor fasciae latae
		Posterior cutaneous nerve	Sensory to skin of buttocks, posterior surface of thigh, and leg
		Pudendal nerve	Motor to perineal muscles; sensory to skin of perineum

†Sensory fibers from the tibial and peroneal nerves unit to form the *medial cutaneous* (or sural) *nerve* that supplies the calf of the leg and the lateral surface of the foot. In the thigh the tibial and common peroneal nerves are usually enclosed in a single sheath to form the *sciatic nerve*, the largest nerve in the body with its width of approximately ¾ of an inch. About two thirds of the way down the posterior part of the thigh, it divides into its component parts. Branches of the sciatic nerve extend into the hamstring muscles.

Table 3-5
Cranial Nerves Contrasted with Spinal Nerves

	Cranial Nerves	Spinal Nerves
Origin	Base of brain	Spinal cord
Distribution	Mainly to head and neck	Skin, skeletal muscles, joints, blood vessels, sweat glands, and mucosa except of head and neck
Structure	Some composed of sensory fibers only; some of both motor axons and sensory dendrites; some motor fibers belong to somatic nervous system, some to autonomic	All of them composed of both sensory dendrites and motor axons; some of latter somatic, some autonomic
Function	Vision, hearing, sense of smell, sense of taste, eye movements	Sensations, movements, and sweat secretion

From Anthony, C.P., and Thibodeau, G.A.: Textbook of anatomy and physiology, ed. 10, St. Louis, 1979, The C.V. Mosby Co.

Dermatomes. Each spinal nerve root innervates a specific area of the body surface for superficial or cutaneous sensation; each area is known as a *dermatome.* Although there is a great deal of overlap in the spinal nerves, knowledge of the distribution of dermatomes (Fig. 3-23) is clinically useful for assessment and evaluation purposes.

Autonomic Nervous System

The autonomic nervous system (ANS), considered part of the peripheral nervous system, regulates the body's internal environment in close conjunction with the endocrine system. It is responsible for the unconscious moment-to-moment functioning of all internal systems including visceral organs (e.g., digestive, urogenital), involuntary muscle fibers (e.g., smooth muscle), and glandular functions (e.g., islets of Langerhans in the pancreas, and the adrenal medulla). The autonomic nervous system is activated by centers located in the hypothalamus, brainstem, and spinal cord and is characterized by a two-neuron chain consisting of a preganglionic neuron and a postganglionic neuron.

Preganglionic neurons have cell bodies in the central nervous system and efferent fibers that terminate in the autonomic ganglia. *Postganglionic* neurons have cell bodies outside the central nervous system in the autonomic ganglia and innervate the target, or effector, organ (e.g., cardiac muscle). The purpose of the postganglionic neuron is to relay impulses beyond the ganglia.

The autonomic nervous system has two major subdivisions (the sympathetic and the parasympathetic), each of which consists of autonomic ganglia and nerves. Generally each effector organ has both sympathetic and parasympathetic innervation. The subdivisions differ in the following ways: (1) type of neurotransmitters released, (2) distribution of nerve fibers, and (3) effects on organs innervated, in that the subdivisions produce antagonistic physiologic responses.

The *sympathetic* (thoracolumbar) subdivision is oriented to maintaining survival and is activated during internal and external stress situations (i.e., flight-fight phenomenon). During those stressful situations, sympathetic responses include increases in blood pressure and heart rate as well as vasoconstriction of peripheral blood vessels. The sympathetic division is also referred to as *adrenergic* since the transmitter substance, norepinephrine (noradrenalin), is secreted by its postganglionic nerve terminals.

Anatomically, the preganglionic fibers are located in the intermediolateral columns of the thoracic and first two lumbar segments in the spinal cord (i.e., T1 to L2); thus the term thoracolumbar. After leaving the spinal nerves, the small, myelinated, preganglionic, sympa-

thetic fibers enter, via the white ramus, the sympathetic trunk. The sympathetic trunk is a chain of ganglions extending from the base of the skull to the coccyx on either side of the spinal cord.

Most axons of sympathetic neurons synapse in the sympathetic trunk or travel up and down the trunk before synapsing. Some axons do not synapse within the sympathetic trunk and instead exit to synapse in collateral ganglia nearer to the organ of innervation. The neurotransmitter at all preganglionic nerve terminals of the sympathetic division is acetylcholine. The neurotransmitter at all postganglionic nerve terminals of the sympathetic system is norepinephrine (noradrenalin). Therefore the sympathetic division is adrenergic. Because of the sympathetic chain ganglia, the nerve fibers of the sympathetic system generally have short and long postganglionic fibers. Fibers terminate on two receptor sites (alpha or beta), which determine the effects of the neurotransmitters. Beta receptors are divided into beta and beta$_2$ receptors since some drugs affect some, but not all, beta receptors.

The adrenal medulla is a functional extension of the sympathetic nervous system whose postganglionic neurons are specialized secretory cells. The catecholamine hormones, epinephrine and norepinephrine, are secreted by the adrenal medulla at the same time the sympathetic nerves are stimulating afferent organs and have almost the same effect as direct sympathetic stimulation. As a result, body tissues are stimulated simultaneously, directly by the sympathetic nerves and indirectly by the hormones of the adrenal medulla. Following release, the hormones are rapidly metabolized, primarily by the liver. Approximately one half of the catecholamines are excreted in the urine as free or conjugated normetanephrine and metanephrine. Daily normal urinary output of the catecholamines equals approximately 6 mg of epinephrine and 30 mg of norepinephrine.[21,25] The reader is referred to Chapter 12 for further detail on the adrenal medulla and the catecholamines.

The *parasympathetic* (craniosacral) subdivision of the autonomic nervous system consists of preganglionic fibers arising from cell bodies in cranial nerves III, VII, IX, and X as well as sacral spinal nerves II through VII. This division is activated when an individual is at rest or relaxed, protecting and restoring the body's resources. It works slower than the sympathetic division, has a more discrete effect, and dominates control over the sympathetic subdivision during nonstressful conditions. Parasympathetic fibers in the cranial and sacral nerves form synaptic connections only with terminal ganglia located near the organs innervated. Therefore in the parasympathetic division, preganglionic fibers are long; postganglionic fibers are short. Both preganglionic and postganglionic fibers secrete the neurotransmitter *acetylcholine;*

Fig. 3-23
Dermatomes of the body. Each dorsal (sensory) spinal root innervates one dermatome. The first cervical nerve usually has no cutaneous distribution. The trigeminal nerve (fifth cranial nerve) supplies most of the general somatic sensory innervation to the anterior part of the head.

From Rudy, E.B.: Advanced neurological and neurosurgical nursing, St. Louis, 1984, The C.V. Mosby Co.

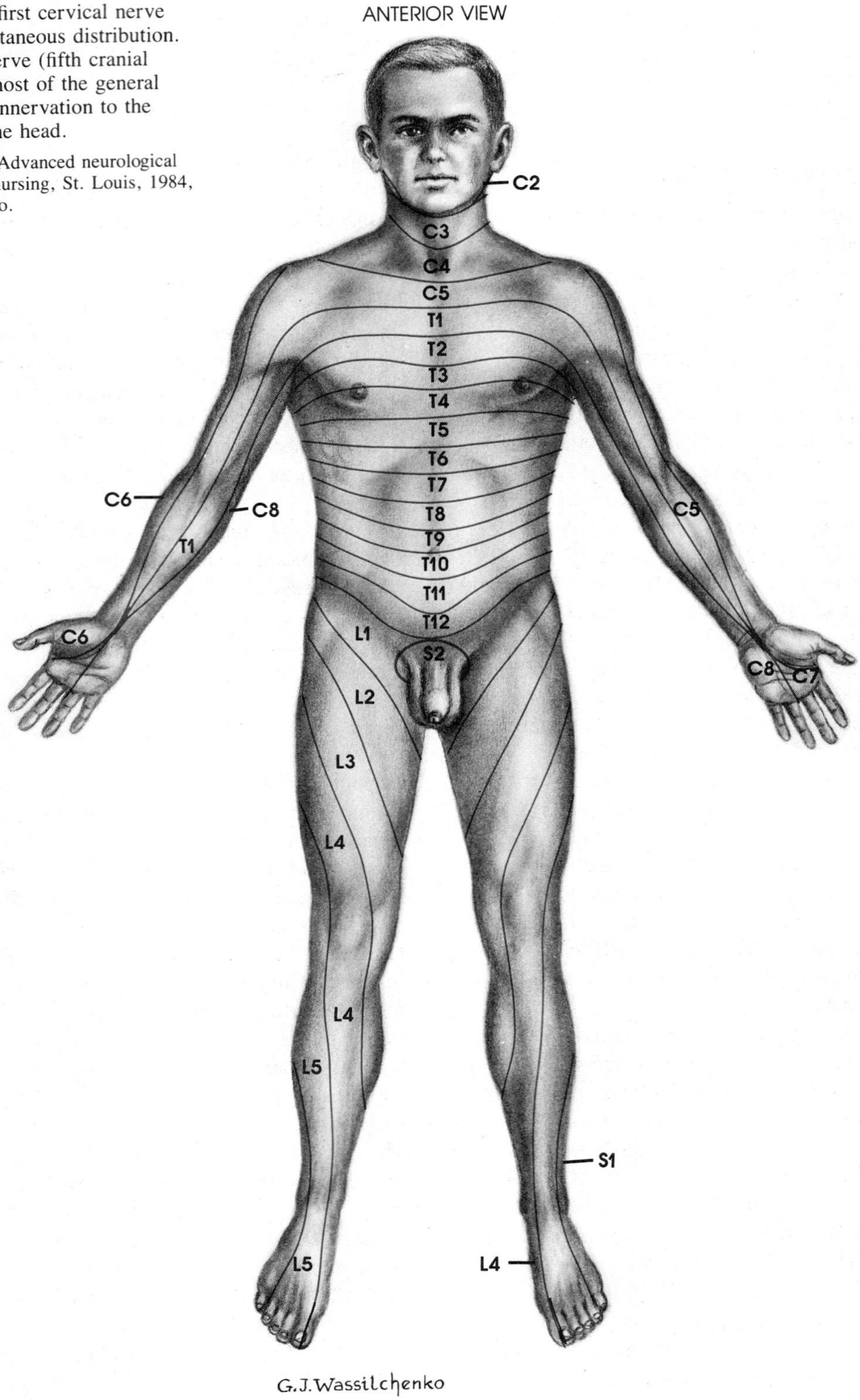

ANTERIOR VIEW

G.J. Wassilchenko

POSTERIOR VIEW

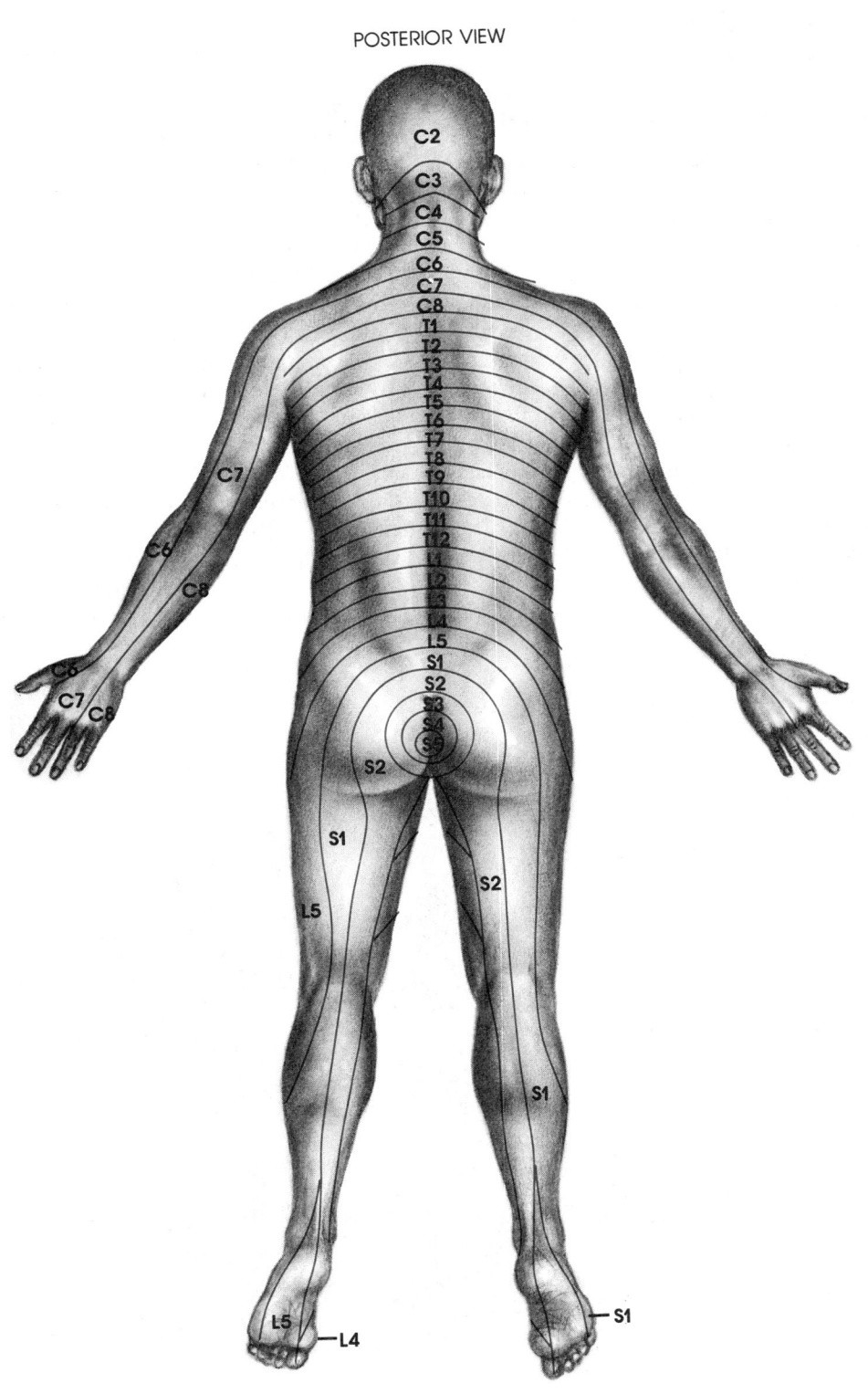

therefore the parasympathetic subdivision is called *cholinergic*.

The organs innervated and effects of stimulation by sympathetic and parasympathetic subdivisions are summarized in Tables 3-4 and 3-5.

Vascular Supply to Brain and Spinal Cord

Maintaining adequate blood supply to the brain and spinal cord is vital for proper functioning of the nervous system. The blood removes metabolic waste products and supplies the cells with nutrients.

Brain. The blood supply to the brain comes principally from two pairs of arteries, the internal carotids and the vertebral arteries. The *internal carotids*, which provide approximately 80% of the blood supply to the brain, arise from the common carotid artery at the level of the thyroid cartilage. The internal carotids then give rise to the anterior and middle cerebral arteries at about the level of the optic chiasm. The *anterior cerebral artery* supplies portions of the medial surfaces of the frontal and parietal lobes, nuclei of the basal ganglia, caudate putamen, and portions of the internal capsule and corpus callosum. The *middle cerebral artery* supplies lateral surfaces of the parietal, frontal, and temporal lobes. It is the major

source of blood supply to the precentral (motor) and postcentral (sensory) gyri. The vertebral arteries arise respectively from the right and left *subclavian arteries,* providing the remaining 20% of cerebral blood supply. The vertebral arteries anastomose at the base of the brain and form the basilar artery. The *basilar artery* enters the skull at the foramen magnum and ascends to the midbrain. Branches of the vertebral and basilar arteries supply the brainstem and cerebellum. In the midbrain the basilar artery bifurcates into the pair of *posterior cerebral arteries*. The posterior cerebral arteries supply portions of the temporal and occipital lobes of each hemisphere, the vestibular organs, and the cochlear apparatus. Fig. 3-24 illustrates the vessels supplying the brain tissue.

At the base of the brain the cerebral arteries are connected into an arterial circle, the *circle of Willis* (Fig. 3-25), by their communicating branches. More specifically, the posterior cerebral artery is connected to the middle cerebral artery by the posterior communicating branches. The anterior cerebral arteries are connected by the anterior communicating branches. The purpose of the circle of Willis is to ensure circulation should there be an interruption in one of the four main blood vessels.

Branches of cerebral arteries extend throughout the brain. These branches are called end arteries because

Fig. 3-24

Blood supply of the brain.

From Rudy, E.B.: Advanced neurological and neurosurgical nursing, St. Louis, 1984, The C.V. Mosby Co.

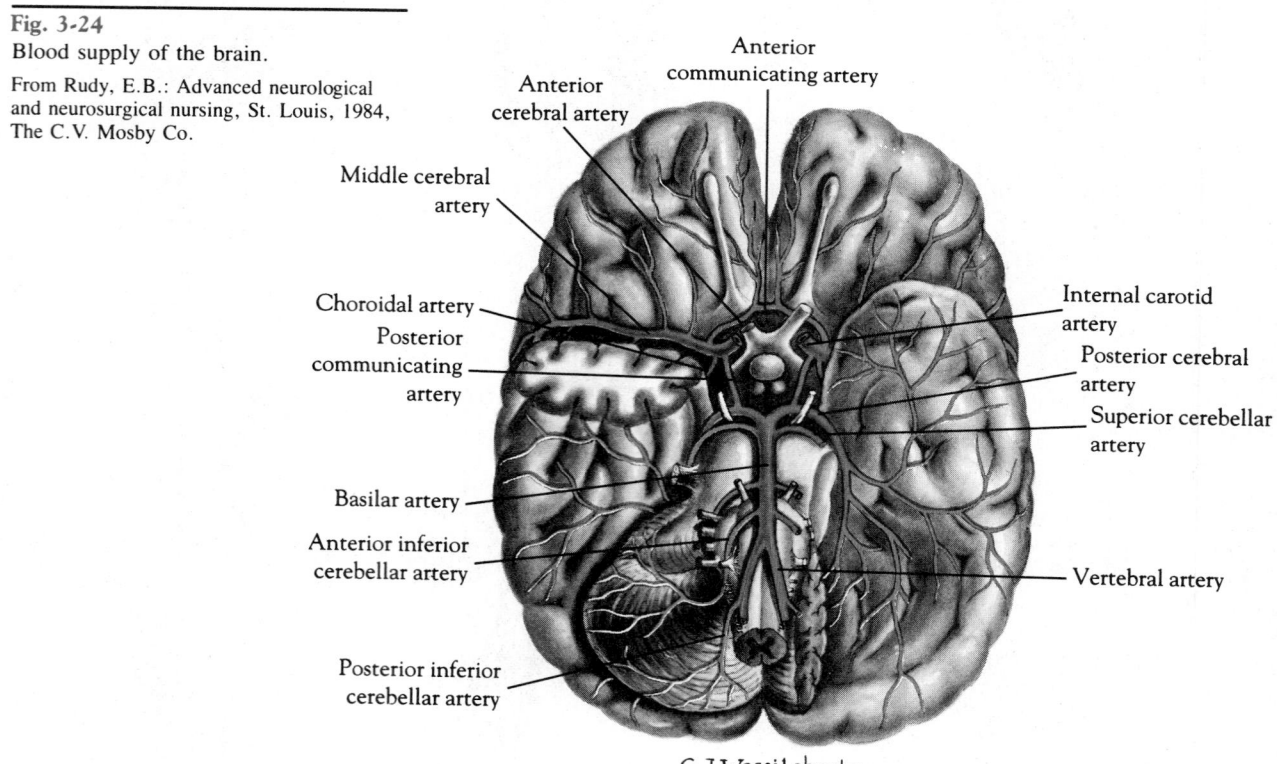

G.J. Wassilchenko

there are few branching connections. Since there is minimal branching, there is decreased potential for collateral circulation.

Dense networks of capillaries are found in the gray matter of the brain. These capillaries are surrounded by a protective membrane formed by the end-feet of *astrocyte cells*. The capillary blood enters the deep veins, which then empty into the superficial venous plexuses and dural sinuses (principally the superior longitudinal sinus). The venous blood is drained from these sinuses by the internal jugular veins, which return the blood to the general circulation (a small volume of blood drains via the *pterygoid* and ophthalmic venous sinuses).

The anterior, middle, and posterior meningeal arteries provide an abundant blood supply to the cranial meninges.

Spinal cord. The arterial blood supply to the spinal cord comes from three main vessels: the one spinal artery and the two radicular arteries. The *spinal artery* arises from branches of the vertebral arteries at the level of the foramen magnum. The spinal artery then divides into one anterior and two posterior branches. These branches then enter the vertebral canal with the dorsal and ventral nerve roots. The *radicular* artery arises from the thoracic and abdominal aorta. The vessel then divides into anterior and posterior branches that enter the spinal cord at the intervertebral foramina. At the spinal segments the radicular arteries connect with the spinal arteries to form an extensive vascular plexus around the entire spinal cord.

The spinal venous system is extensive, with many intradural veins exiting from the ventral median fissure. Additionally, there are numerous extradural veins that

Fig. 3-25
Anatomic diagram of the circle of Willis and its common variations. **A,** "Classic" circle of Willis. No component is hypoplastic or absent. **B,** Hypoplasia of one or both posterior communicating arteries. **C,** Absent or hypoplastic segment of the anterior cerebral artery. **D,** "Fetal" origin of the posterior cerebral artery with hypoplasia of the segment. **E,** Multichanneled or duplicated anterior communicating artery. In **B** to **E** the absent or hypoplastic segments are shaded *(arrows)*.

From Osborn, A.G., and Maack, J.G.: Introduction to cerebral angiography, Philadelphia, 1980, Harper & Row, Publishers, Inc.

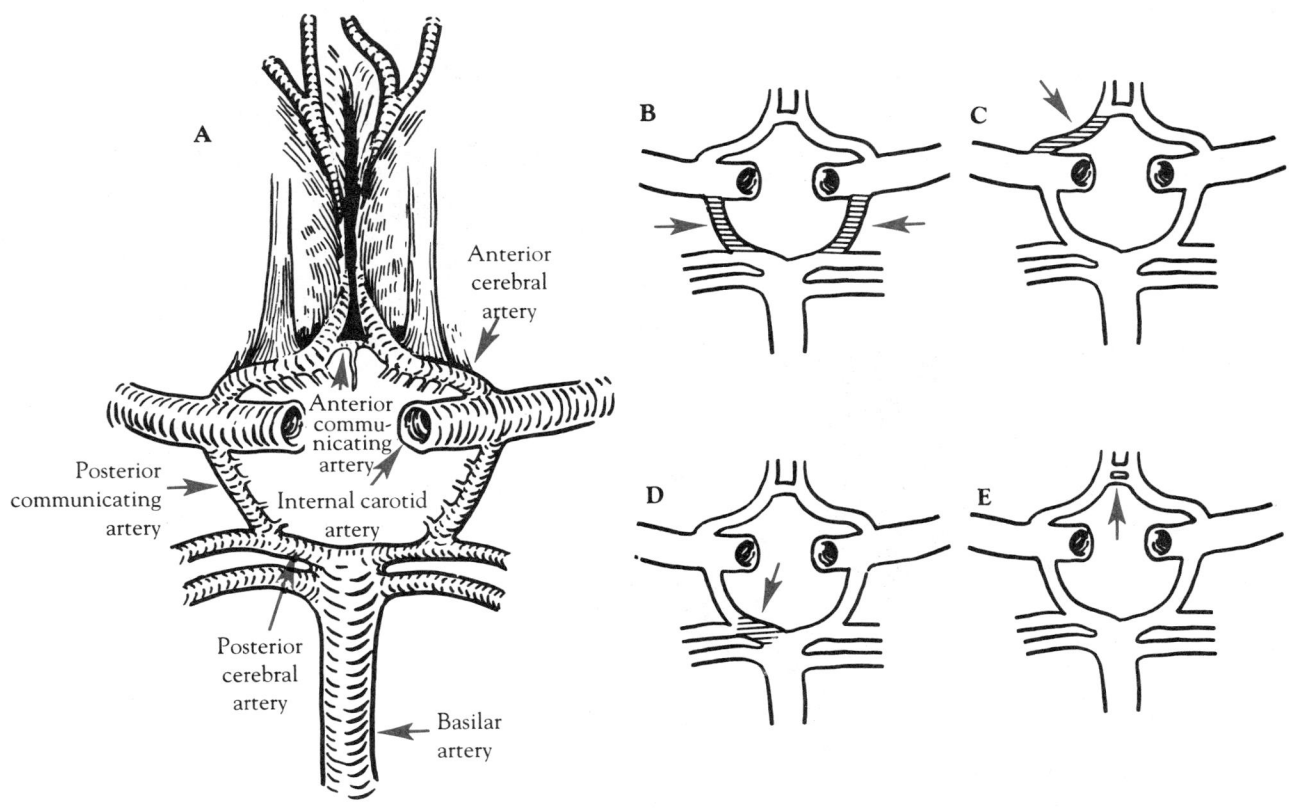

form a dense venous plexus in the pia mater. Venous blood is drained from the plexus by veins accompanying roots of the spinal nerves.

Brain barriers. The neuronal tissue of the brain is extremely sensitive to any quantitative changes in the ionic concentration of their environment. Therefore the composition of the brain's internal environment must be delicately balanced to ensure normal functioning. The *blood-brain barrier* is a physiologic mechanism that assists in maintaining and protecting this homeostatic balance by way of selective capillary permeability. Since substances from the blood enter the brain either by way of capillaries into the cerebrospinal fluid or by way of capillaries into the extracellular fluid, there are actually two barrier mechanisms. The blood-brain and blood-cerebrospinal barriers function together to protect the neuronal brain tissue from injury. The complex of inter-membranes that form these barriers is found in most regions of brain parenchyma, the choroid plexus, and the vasculature of the brain. Unlike most capillaries in the body, these capillaries are surrounded by astrocyte end-feet that form tight junctions of the endothelial cells. It is thought the tight junctions and glial end-feet affect capillary permeability. Both the blood-brain and blood-

cerebrospinal barriers are permeable to oxygen, carbon dioxide, and water. They are slightly permeable to electrolytes (e.g., Na^+, K^+, Cl^-) but are impermeable to fixed acids and bases as well as many pharmaceutical agents. Finally, these barriers develop in the postnatal period; therefore the cerebral capillaries of the newborn are far more permeable than those of the adult.

Cerebral Ventricular System

Fig. 3-26 depicts the cerebral ventricular system, which is a series of four ependymal-lined cavities. The non-nervous ventricles are interconnecting structures that originate from the single cavity of the embryonic neural tube. The two largest cavities, the lateral ventricles, are located within each cerebral hemisphere. Each lateral ventricle consists of a body and anterior (frontal), inferior (temporal), and posterior (occipital) horns. The lateral ventricles are separated from each other (in their respective hemispheres) by a thin layer called the septum pellucidum. Further, each of these ventricles communicates, via the interventricular foramen of Monro, with a central cavity. This central cavity constitutes the third ventricle, which is a small cleft space between the thalamic struc-

Fig. 3-26
Cerebral ventricles. **A,** Lateral view.
B, Superior view.

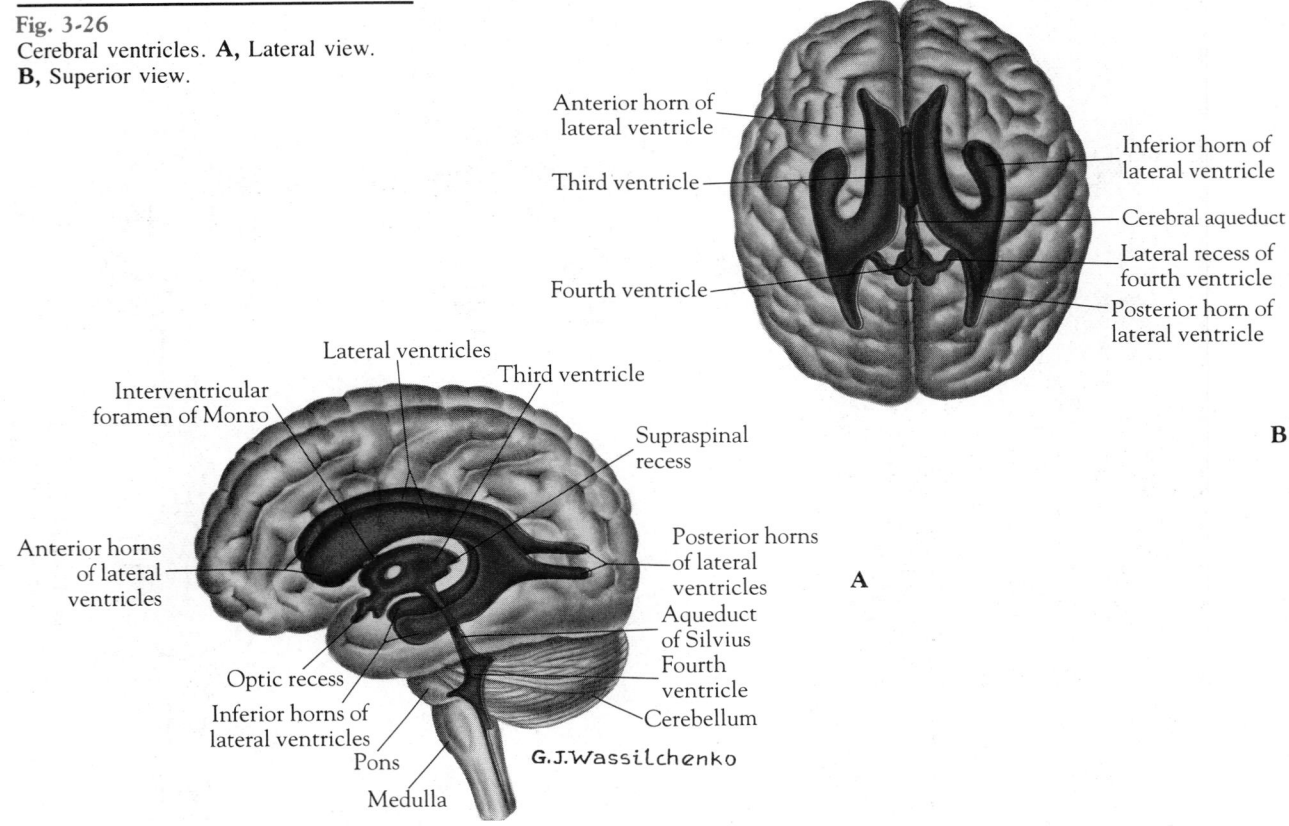

Anterior horn of lateral ventricle

Third ventricle

Fourth ventricle

Inferior horn of lateral ventricle

Cerebral aqueduct

Lateral recess of fourth ventricle

Posterior horn of lateral ventricle

B

Interventricular foramen of Monro

Lateral ventricles

Third ventricle

Supraspinal recess

Anterior horns of lateral ventricles

Posterior horns of lateral ventricles

A

Aqueduct of Silvius

Optic recess

Fourth ventricle

Inferior horns of lateral ventricles

Cerebellum

Pons

Medulla

G.J.Wassilchenko

tures of the diencephalon. In the midbrain the third ventricle communicates with the fourth ventricle via the aqueduct of Sylvius. The rhomboid fourth ventricle is located posterior to the pons and anterior to the cerebellum, extending down to the central canal of the upper cervical portion of the spinal cord. The fourth ventricle is connected by three foramina to the subarachnoid space.

Cerebrospinal Fluid

Parts of the lateral, third, and fourth ventricular structures are lined with dense networks of capillaries called the *choroid plexus* (tela choroidea). The choroid plexus secretes cerebrospinal fluid (CSF), which is a colorless, clear, and odorless fluid containing glucose, electrolytes, oxygen, water, carbon dioxide, small amounts of protein, and a few leukocytes. The purposes of the cerebrospinal fluid include removal of metabolic wastes, nutrition, mechanical function (i.e., shock absorber), and participation in the maintenance of normal intracranial pressure. In a 24-hour period the choroid plexuses secrete approximately 500 to 750 ml of cerebrospinal fluid; however, only about 125 to 150 ml is present in the system at any one time.

After the cerebrospinal fluid is secreted by the choroid plexuses in the lateral ventricles, it passes through the foramen of Monro to the third ventricle. From here, the cerebrospinal fluid slowly flows through the aqueduct of Sylvius to the fourth ventricle. The fluid then leaves the fourth ventricle by way of the single medial foramen of Magendie (located in the roof of the fourth ventricle) and the paired foramina of Luschka (located in the lateral portion of the fourth ventricle). After leaving the fourth ventricle, the cerebrospinal fluid enters the subarachnoid space, where it fills the spinal cisterns and slowly diffuses upward over the convexities of the brain. The fluid is slowly absorbed from the subarachnoid space by the arachnoid villi. The arachnoid villi are clusterlike protrusions extending into the superior sagittal sinus. The cerebrospinal fluid diffuses from the arachnoid villi into the intradural venous sinuses, where it is reabsorbed into the venous system.

Intracranial Pressure: Normal Dynamics

Approximately 88% of the contents of the cranial cavity consists of brain tissue, 2% is composed of the intravascular blood volume, and the final 10% consists of cerebrospinal fluid. These three components are the essential elements of intracranial pressure (ICP) dynamics. Specifically, intracranial pressure equals the volume of brain tissue (BTV) plus the volume of blood (BV) plus the volume of cerebrospinal fluid (CSFV).

$$ICP = BTV + BV + CSFV$$

The normal intracranial pressure in the recumbent position is about 0 to 15 mm Hg (110 to 140 mm H_2O). Standing decreases intracranial pressure while activities such as sitting, sneezing, coughing, isometric exercises, sexual intercourse, and the Valsalva maneuver result in a transient rise of intracranial pressure. Since expansion of the brain is limited by the skull, these activities are normally compensated for by a redistribution of cerebrospinal fluid to the spinal subarachnoid space or by partial collapse of the cisterns and cerebral ventricles. (In the young child, the skull is not rigid; therefore expansion is not so severely limited.)

Another very important determinant in the dynamics of intracranial pressure is the autoregulation of cerebral blood flow. This blood flow is generally expressed as cerebral perfusion pressure (CPP) and is accomplished by the regulation of resistance vessel diameters. The cerebral perfusion pressure equals the mean arterial blood pressure (MABP)* minus the intracranial pressure (ICP).

$$CPP = MABP - ICP$$

The normal range of cerebral perfusion pressure is 80 to 100 mm Hg. A cerebral perfusion pressure of at least 50 mm Hg is necessary for the brain to receive an adequate blood supply. To maintain normal cerebral perfusion, the blood vessels constrict or dilate and therefore directly affect intracranial pressure.

The third and final component in intracranial pressure is the actual brain tissue. The compensatory mechanism of brain tissue displacement or shifting is not usually considered a part of normal dynamics.

An important point to understand in relation to intracranial pressure is that any activity or condition causing a sustained increase in one of the essential elements listed above must be compensated for by a decrease in one or both of the other two essential elements. This principle is known as the Monro-Kellie doctrine and must be understood in relation to normal dynamics of intracranial pressure as well as pathologic states that lead to the condition of increased intracranial pressure.

Variations in Child

Development of the human neurologic system proceeds in an orderly manner starting at approximately the third week after conception. Throughout embryonic growth the rostral portion increases in size at a faster rate than the caudal portion. At birth the central nervous system, the peripheral nervous system, and their supporting structures are not fully developed.

Skull. The newborn's skull (Fig. 3-27) is large in

---

*MABP is calculated as follows: $\dfrac{\text{Systolic BP} + 2\,(\text{diastolic BP})}{3}$.

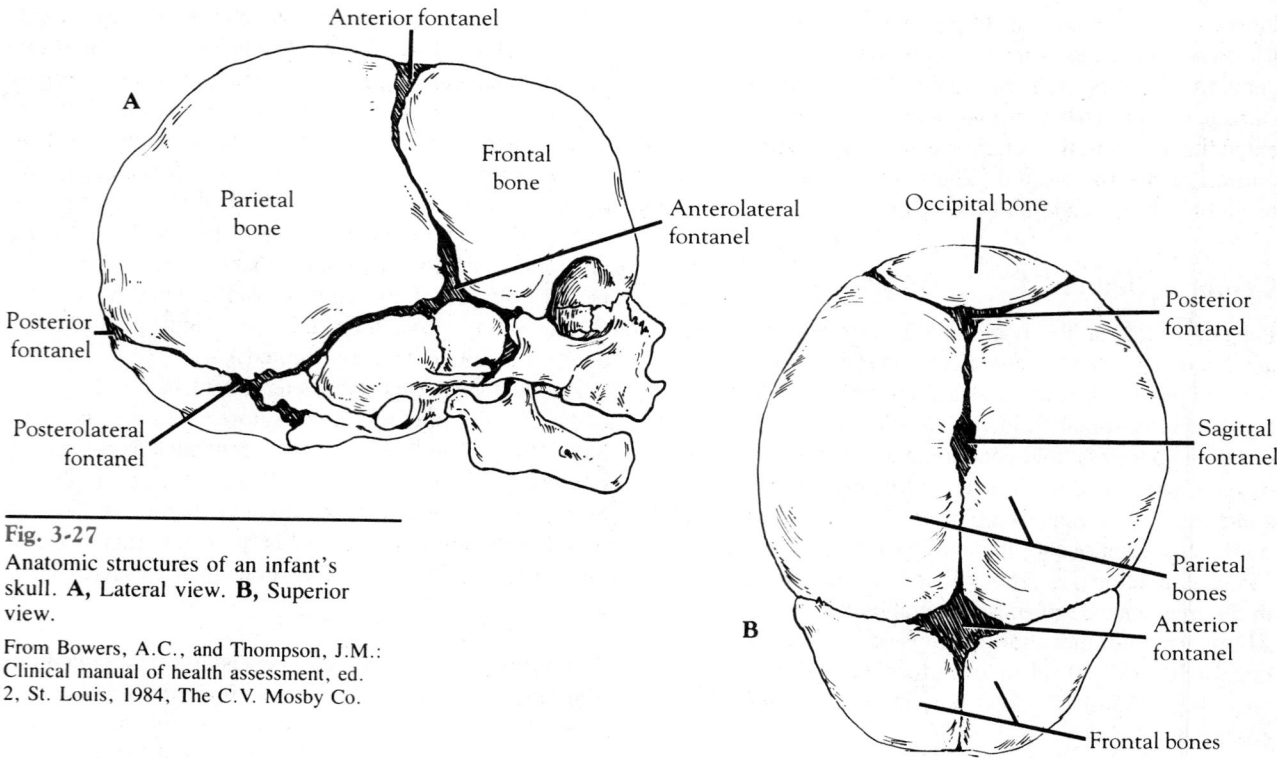

Fig. 3-27
Anatomic structures of an infant's skull. **A,** Lateral view. **B,** Superior view.

From Bowers, A.C., and Thompson, J.M.: Clinical manual of health assessment, ed. 2, St. Louis, 1984, The C.V. Mosby Co.

relation to the body, with the cranial portion constituting the largest part of the skull itself. The ossification process of the cranial bones is incomplete at birth so the newborn has six major membrane-filled spaces, the fontanels, where the suture lines of the bones intersect. The *anterior fontanel* is located between the two sections of the frontal bone and the angles of the parietal bones. Since it is superior to the sagittal dural venous sinus, the anterior fontanel shows a vascular pulsation. It measures approximately 4 to 6 cm in size and closes around the age of 18 months. The *posterior fontanel* is a triangular space between the occipital and two parietal bones. It measures 0.5 to 1 cm in size and usually closes around the age of 2 months. Two *anterolateral fontanels* are found at the intersections of the frontal, parietal, temporal, and sphenoid bones. The anterolateral fontanels close at about 2 months. The two *posterolateral fontanels* are located at the junction of the parietal, occipital, and temporal bones and close at about 2 years of age.

At birth the average head circumference is 34 to 35 cm. This circumference increases to 44 cm by the age of 6 months and to 47 cm by the age of 1 year because the rate of brain growth is rapid. Following the infancy period, the head circumference will slowly increase in size, reaching approximately 50 cm by the age of 5 years. At this time a tough fibrous tissue joint is evident at the cranial suture lines.

Brain. The brain is one fourth the adult size at birth. By the end of the first year, it is one half, and by the age of 3 years, the brain grows to four fifths of the adult size. Growth then slows down considerably, with actual adult size obtained around the age of 12 years. There are two distinct peaks of growth rate at the cellular level. During the first peak, occurring between 10 and 18 weeks of fetal life, there is a multiplication of neuroblasts. The second spurt of brain growth occurs between midgestation and about 1½ years of age, when there is multiplication of glial cells, production of myelin by the glial cells, and development of dendrites and synaptic connections.[20] The majority of neurons are present at birth; however, the gray and white matter of the cerebral hemispheres is not well differentiated. The newborn has sheaths of myelin around the axons of the brainstem, basal ganglia, and cerebellum; but the fibers connecting the cerebral cortex and the thalamus are unmyelinated. At 6 months of age, cortical development, which progresses in a cephalocaudal fashion, is about one half complete, and at 2 years it is three fourths complete. Cortical development is completed around the age of 4 years. It is important to note that since the cerebral cortex is not fully developed at birth, the brainstem and spinal cord dominate neurologic functioning and are responsible for the primitive infantile reflexes (i.e., Moro, palmar and plantar grasp, sucking, rooting, stepping, glabellar, and Babinski). These primitive reflexes begin to disappear between the ages of 6 weeks to 2 years as the higher cerebral centers dominate neurologic functioning.

Nerve conduction velocity of the newborn is quite slow (i.e., 30 m/s) compared to that of the adult. Conduction increases rapidly; by approximately 3 years of age almost all values are at the lower adult range; and by age 5 maximal adult levels are achieved.[7] Average nerve conduction velocity of the healthy adult is 60 m/s.

Vertebrae. Like the skull, the vertebral column has only partial ossification at birth. Only the primary curves (thoracic and pelvic) are present, giving the vertebral column a continuous convex curve from the top to the bottom. Secondary curves (cervical and lumbar) develop in the postnatal period. Specifically, the cervical curve is evident around 3 to 4 months, and the lumbar curve appears around 12 to 18 months of age. The sacrum is composed of five separate bones at birth that fuse into one large bone by 18 to 20 years of age. The coccyx is made of three to five small rudiments of vertebrae that begin to fuse between the ages of 1 to 4 years and become fused into one bone by 25 years of age.

Spinal cord. Initially, spinal cord growth is most rapid in the lumbar and cervical regions. The thoracic region develops most rapidly during the third trimester of pregnancy. Because of the rapid growth rate of the developing vertebral column during the third fetal month, the terminal end of the spinal cord moves cranially, with the conus medullaris moving from the level of the fourth vertebra in the fifth fetal month to the adult level of the first or second lumbar vertebra by the second postnatal month. Spinal cord myelination proceeds in a cephalocaudal direction.[20] The myelination process is completed by approximately 2 years of age.

Variations in Older Adult

As with other systems in the body, the neural structures undergo significant changes as a result of the aging process. Understanding these anatomic and physiologic changes assists the practitioner to establish realistic normative behaviors for the elderly population.

Brain. The neuronal cells of the central nervous system (brain and spinal cord) of all adults are postmitotic and therefore do not regenerate once destroyed. Studies indicate the aging process causes a loss of brain cells, and that cells not destroyed may undergo significant structural changes. More specifically, brain cells decrease in number at a rate of about 1% a year after 50 years of age. However, this rate of loss is not consistent throughout the brain, so that certain areas may lose cells at a faster (e.g., cortex) or slower (e.g., brainstem) rate than others. Other cells, such as the neurons of the prefrontal neocortex, undergo structural changes that result in a progressive decline of dendritic interconnections. Additionally, neuronal cells of the elderly contain the age pigment *lipofuscin* in the storage granules, as well as senile plaques and neurofibrillary tangles.

Cerebral blood flow studies indicate there is a change with age in cerebral blood flow and oxygen utilization. Cerebral blood flow showed a decline from 79.3 ml/min/100 g of brain tissue at the mean age of 17 to 46.0 ml/min/100 g at the mean age of 80, a net loss of 33.3 ml/min/100 g of brain. The rate of cerebral oxygen consumption declined from 3.6 ml/min/100 g of brain tissue at the mean age of 17 to 2.7 ml/min/100 g at the mean age of 80.[7]

Nerve conduction velocity of the individual over 50 years also differs from that of younger adults. By 80 to 90 years of age, conduction velocity equals about 50 m/s, whereas the young adult has a conduction velocity of approximately 60 m/s. This loss of conduction velocity appears to be slightly greater in the aging female. Nerve conduction velocity in the elderly is also affected by an increased synaptic delay and a change in neurotransmitters. Recent studies indicate that in the human brain, monoamine oxidase (MAO) and serotonin increase with age while norepinephrine decreases. This reciprocal increase may explain the depression and apathy often associated with aging.[7]

Vertebrae. The vertebral column may show advancing kyphosis in the thoracic region of the elderly patient. This degenerative change is the result of osteoporosis, vertebral collapse, or changes in vertebral cartilage. As the vertebral cartilage calcifies, there is decreased mobility of the vertebral column.

Spinal cord. The basic reflex arc does not change with the aging process. However, the spinal cord may show changes in sensory conduction because of decreased vascularity of the white matter in the cord. Therefore diminished reflexes in the distal portion of the lower extremities (i.e., ankle) are not uncommon. Degenerative changes in the peripheral nerves are responsible for the loss of vibratory sense at the ankles. Reflexes of the upper extremities should be intact in the healthy elderly individual.

NORMAL FINDINGS

The normal assessment findings for the neurologic system of the adult, geriatric, child, toddler, and infant are summarized in the following table. The reader is encouraged to review these findings for the appropriate age group before and after performing a neurologic examination.

"Normal" behaviors must be evaluated in terms of the patient's baseline pattern as well as significant variables (i.e., anxiety) affecting the assessment process. One way to establish the patient's baseline is through a careful and thorough health history. The health history component is equally as important in the assessment of the geriatric or pediatric patient. Whenever the health history or the physical examination provides data that indicate a deviation from normal, that symptom or complex of symptoms requires a comprehensive symptom analysis.

Normative behaviors of the geriatric patient may vary from source to source. With that fact in mind, it is recommended that the examiner cross reference the assessment findings with the patient's previous patterns of behavior. The examiner must also carefully consider the affect on behavior of such variables as physical illness, displacement, examiner approach, change in self-image, and physiologic changes (i.e., diminished sense of hearing or vision).

The evaluation of assessment findings for the pediatric patient requires similar consideration in that behaviors as well as the developmental milestones must be weighted against the child's overall pattern of development. It is recommended that all children between the ages of 1 month through 6 years be screened with the Denver Developmental Screening Test (DDST) to evaluate language, fine motor adaptive, gross motor, and personal-social functioning. The school-aged child should routinely be evaluated for "soft" neurologic signs. If the child demonstrates difficulty in performing any of these tasks, the responses should be clustered and the child referred for further evaluation.

Area of Concern	Normal Adult Findings	Variations in Child	Variations in Older Adult
General Cerebral Functions			
Appearance and behavior	Age, height, weight; body proportionate in size in terms of body parts; clean; groomed; dressed appropriate to age, sex, peers, and background	Infant: appears content and is quiet except for when hungry or tired; head larger in proportion to other body parts Toddler: appears happy and playful	Length of trunk decreased in relation to extremities
Posture	Shoulders back and relaxed; arms rest at sides; feet rest on floor (if applicable); stands with narrow base	Infant: limbs semiflexed; hips slightly abducted; symmetric posture predominates; sits alone without support at 7 mo Toddler: maintains balance most of time; stands with wide base	May assume posture with slight semiflexion at principal joints; stands with narrow to medium base; may exhibit kyphosis in thoracic spine region with accompanying backward tilt of head
Gestures	Smooth; coordinated; deliberate	Not assessed in infant Toddler: deliberate; not always coordinated	
Movements	Coordinated; smooth; deliberate; able to change positions with smooth, even movements	Infant: generalized and symmetric; predominance of flexor tone in extremities; movements somewhat hypertonic Toddler: deliberate; may fall if movements too hurried	Changes position with slow, even movements
Facial expression	Facial features symmetric; establishes eye contact; acknowledges examiner presence; uses eye contact throughout interview	Infant: facial features symmetric; eyes open; blinks at bright light; smiles responsively (after 2 mo) and spontaneously Toddler: facial features symmetric: eyes at same level, ears at same level; lips equidistant from midline on both sides; establishes eye contact with care giver	

Area of Concern	Normal Adult Findings	Variations in Child	Variations in Older Adult
Attention	Able to complete thought processes (i.e., able to repeat series of numbers forward and backward); has continuity of ideas	Not assessed in infant Toddler: short attention span	
Level of con-sciousness	Responds appropriately to visual, audito-ry, tactile, and painful stimuli; oriented to person, place, time; able to carry out simple and complex commands; opens eyes spontaneously; extraocular eye movement present	Infant: alert; eyes open sponta-neously; may coo or babble; re-sponds to visual, auditory, tactile stimuli Toddler: alert; recognizes and re-sponds to name; able to carry out simple commands; eyes open spontaneously; frequent move-ments	May respond slower, appropriately to vi-sual, auditory stimu-li; may demonstrate diminished response to tactile and painful stimuli; able to carry out simple and com-plex commands, with slower response time
Intellectual func-tions Memory Immediate	Able to repeat a series of numbers (e.g., 12, 9, 5, 1, 6)	Toddler: may be able to repeat 2-digit number; 4 yr: able to repeat 3-digit number; 5 yr: able to re-peat 4-digit number; 6 yr: able to repeat 5-digit number	
Recent	Able to repeat correct series of numbers after 5 min	Not assessed in infant Toddler: able to identify familiar object after 5 min	
Remote	Able to state correct birthplace; able to correctly state personal vocational history	Not assessed until age 7; then is able to state birthplace and par-ents' names	
Abstract rea-soning	Able to describe meaning of simple prov-erbs such as "a stitch in time saves nine," or "Rome wasn't built in a day"	Not assessed until about 10 yr	
Insight	Demonstrates consistent awareness of reality and perception of self	Not assessed	May demonstrate in-creased resistance to "new" ideas

Specific Cerebral Functions

Area of Concern	Normal Adult Findings	Variations in Child	Variations in Older Adult
Sensory interpre-tation Visual	Recognizes objects; differentiates between size and shape	Infant: will fix gaze on bright or shiny object brought into field of vision Toddler: able to recognize pictures and objects of different sizes and shapes	
Auditory	Able to identify sound made by ringing bell	Infant: will respond to moderate to loud noise with generalized movement or eye blink Toddler: able to respond to audito-ry stimuli by turning in direction of sound, fixing gaze on object, and reaching for object	
Tactile	Able to recognize familiar objects through use of touch (stereognosis)	Not assessed in infant and toddler	Longer response time

Area of Concern	Normal Adult Findings	Variations in Child	Variations in Older Adult
Cortical Motor integration	Able to carry out a skilled act such as protruding tongue, using a comb	Infant: able to reach for an object, grasp it, and bring it to mouth Toddler: able to carry out a skilled act such as feeding self or folding a piece of paper Able to carry out a skilled act such as putting folded paper in envelope	
Comprehension	Able to correctly answer questions throughout history, interview, and examination	Not assessed in infant 18 mo: able to point to body parts; comprehends "hot," "cold," "hungry" 5 yr: able to comprehend 3-stage command	
Judgment	Able to discuss plans for future	Not assessed	
Language and speech	Smooth, flowing; able to easily formulate words; varied inflections; demonstrates ability to read appropriate to educational level; able to write letters and numbers to dictation	Infant: cry loud with moderate pitch; coos after 3 mo; babbles after 4 mo; 1-2 words (e.g., da-da, ba-ba) after 9 mo Able to speak 1-3 words (nouns) by *12 mo;* 10-20 words (nouns) by *18 mo;* 200-300 words (nouns and verbs), 2-3 word sentences by *24 mo;* 900 words (all types), 3-4 word sentences by *36 mo* Able to speak 1500 words, 4-5 word sentences, uses plurals at *4 yr;* 2200 words, 5-6 word sentences, uses compound sentences at *5 yr;* 3000 words, sentences over 6 words in length at *6 yr;* able to read words appropriate to educational level; able to write letters or numbers to dictation after 6 yr of age	Flow may be slightly decreased
Emotional status Affect	Appropriate to verbalization; body behaviors indicative of mild to moderate anxiety	Infant: laughs, smiles spontaneously and in response to care giver Toddler: laughter, smiling appropriate to activity	
Mood	Consistent with conversation; cooperates with examiner	Infant: smiles and laughs when not tired or hungry Toddler: happy, playful	
Thought processes Content	Spontaneous, natural, logical, and free flowing	Not assessed in infant and toddler	Thought patterns become more concrete; thought patterns increase in orderliness

Area of Concern	Normal Adult Findings	Variations in Child	Variations in Older Adult
Cranial nerves			
Olfactory	Able to identify aromatic, volatile, nonirritating substances (e.g., lemon, peppermint) with each nostril	Infant: grimace to aromatic substances Toddler: able to identify changes in odors; not able to always identify specific odors (e.g., oranges, onions) Then able to identify pleasant, familiar substances, such as lemon or peppermint, with each nostril	May demonstrate diminished sense of smell; able to identify changes in aromatic substances with each nostril
Optic	See Chapter 6		
Oculomotor Trochlear Abducens	Eyelids symmetric and not drooping; pupils equal in size, regular in outline, with prompt and equal reaction (direct and consensual) to light stimulus; conjugate gaze; smooth conjugate eye movements intact through six cardinal positions of gaze; prompt accommodation to distant and near objects; bilaterally, equal corneal light reflex	Infant: eyelids symmetric and cover eye to limbus; smooth conjugate eye movements when tracking a bright object; constriction and convergence when bright shiny object brought midline to tip of nose	Eyelids appear less elastic; eye movements intact with some limitation of upward gaze; eyes unable to converge
Trigeminal Sensory	Bilateral blink when limbus of cornea touched with cotton wisp; symmetric tickling sensation when cotton wisp touched to anterior scalp, paranasal sinuses, and jaws; symmetric pressure and pain sensation when alternating blunt and sharp ends of a safety pin are touched to anterior scalp, paranasal sinuses, and jaws; symmetric warm and cold sensation felt when tested for temperature over anterior scalp, paranasal sinuses, and jaws	Infant: bilateral blink when limbus of cornea touched with cotton wisp; symmetric sucking and rooting response; other responses not assessed	
Motor	Bilaterally strong contractions of temporal and masseter muscles	Infant: swallowing coordinated	
Facial Sensory	Able to correctly identify sweet, sour, salty, and bitter substances placed on anterior tongue	Infant: likes sweet (smile); dislikes salty (grimace and perhaps cry) Toddler: able to respond to tastes of sweet, sour, and salty (bitter not tested) on anterior tongue	
Motor	Symmetry of facial movements such as smiling, frowning, closing eyes, raising eyebrows, showing teeth, and puffing out cheeks	Infant: facial movements symmetric when smiling, laughing (after 2 mo), or crying; symmetry of wrinkles, facial contours, and nasolabial fold; purses lips for sucking Toddler: symmetry of facial movements when playing "make face" game	
Acoustic Cochlear division	Bilateral ability to hear whispered voice (from distance of 1-2 ft); able to hear watch ticking (from distance of 1-2 in)	Newborn: responds to noises (e.g., ringing bell) by facial movements such as blinking, or startle reflex 3 mo: turns eyes toward sound or head toward source of noise	

Area of Concern	Normal Adult Findings	Variations in Child	Variations in Older Adult
		9-12 mo: able to determine specific location from which sound is coming Toddler: able to determine origin of sound and turn head toward it Air vs. bone conduction not assessed in infant and toddler	
Weber test	Sound heard equally in both ears		
Rinne test	Sound heard twice as long by air conduction as by bone conduction		
Vestibular division (tested only with history of vertigo)			
Bárány test	Demonstrates a feeling of nausea, slow horizontal nystagmus toward side irrigated, with past pointing and falling	Not assessed in infant and toddler	
Bárány chair rotation	Nystagmus, past pointing, and postural deviation in direction of chair movement; vertigo and sensation of continued movement in opposite direction of chair movement	Not assessed	
Electronystagmography	No displacement of corneal-retinal potential bilaterally	Not assessed	
Glossopharyngeal and vagus	Immediate contraction of pharyngeal muscles, with or without gagging, with lateral, upper, lower, and posterior stimulation; speech smooth, without hoarseness; able to identify tastes of sweet, salty, sour, and bitter on posterior third of tongue	Infant: coordinated, smooth swallow; gag reflex when pharyngeal muscles stimulated	
Spinal accessory	Able to turn head against resistance: sternocleidomastoid muscle bilaterally equal in strength and symmetry; able to shrug shoulders against resistance with bilaterally equal strength of upward movement	Infant: symmetric, coordinated swallow and suck reflex Head turn not easily assessed in toddler Shoulder shrug not assessed in infant nor easily assessed in toddler	
Hypoglossal	Able to protrude tongue in midline; able to move tongue in and out of mouth rapidly; able to wiggle tongue from side to side	Infant: reflex opening of mouth and raising of tip of tongue when nostrils pinched	
Proprioception; Cerebellar and Motor Function			
Gait	Maintains upright posture of trunk; walks unaided with narrow base, weight shifts from one extremity to another, pelvis approximately at right angle to weight-bearing extremity; maintains balance; opposing arm swing	9-12 mo: wide-base waddling 12-18 mo: unsteady, broad base; 18 mo: broad base; maintains balance; opposing arm swing	Maintains upright posture of trunk (if no kyphosis); walks with narrow to medium base
Romberg test	Slight swaying, but upright posture and narrow foot stance maintained	Not assessed in infant Toddler: minimal swaying	
Tandem walk	Able to walk heel to toe in straight line	Tested after 3 yr of age	

Area of Concern	Normal Adult Findings	Variations in Child	Variations in Older Adult
One-foot balance	Able to maintain position for at least 5 sec; bilaterally equal response with eyes open and eyes closed	Not assessed in infant 20-30 mo: 1 sec with eyes open; 36 mo: 5 sec with eyes open	
Hop in place	Able to maintain balance, hop on one foot, and stay in place: bilaterally equal response	Not assessed in infant 20-30 mo: able to jump in place (base of jump broad); 3-4½ yr: as adult	
Knee bends	Able to perform knee bends while maintaining balance	Not assessed in infant Toddler: usually not assessed; may be able to imitate examiner	
Upper extremity testing	Able to rapidly pronate and supinate hands with bilaterally equal timing, purposeful movement; able to repeatedly touch nose with alternate index finger in rhythmic fashion (eyes open and eyes closed); able to rapidly and purposefully touch each finger to thumb; able to move index finger from nose to examiner's finger in coordinated fashion (each hand tested)	Not assessed in infant Toddler: may be able to imitate examiner; tests done with eyes open and slower responses expected	
Lower extremity testing	Able to purposefully run heel down contralateral shin with bilaterally equal coordination	Not assessed in infant and toddler	
Muscle strength and tone	See Chapter 4		
Sensory Functions Primary Light touch	Able to perceive light or tickling sensation; able to correctly identify location touched	Infant: facial and motor response to stimulus	
Pain	Able to perceive pain sensation as sharp or dull; able to correctly identify area touched	Not assessed in infant and toddler	
Temperature	Able to perceive sensation as hot or cold	Not assessed in infant and toddler	
Vibration	Able to perceive sensation of vibration	Not assessed in infant and toddler	
Discriminating sensation Stereognosis	Able to identify common objects (e.g., key, pencil) by handling it	Not assessed in infant Toddler: may be able to identify objects such as coins or buttons by touch	
Two-point discrimination	Able to distinguish whether touched by one or two objects; palms, 8-12 mm; dorsum of hands, 20-30 mm; fingertips 2.8-5 mm; dorsa of fingers, 4-6 mm; chest and forearm, 40 mm; back, 40-70 mm; upper arms and thighs, 75 mm; shins, 30-40 mm	Not assessed in infant and toddler	May evidence diminishment from adult normal findings

Area of Concern	Normal Adult Findings	Variations in Child	Variations in Older Adult
Graphesthesia	Able to recognize traced letter or number on hand, back, etc.	Not assessed in infant Toddler: may be able to identify geometric shape, parallel lines, or crossed lines Child: able to recognize traced letter or number on hand, back, etc.; numbers best identified are 0, 7, 1, or 3	
Double simultaneous sensation	Able to distinguish if touched on one or two sides of body (at same level)	Not assessed in infant and toddler	May not be able to distinguish
Kinesthetic	Able to identify change in position of fingers as up or down	Not assessed in infant and toddler	
Reflexes Superficial Upper abdominal (T8, T9, T10)	Upward movement of umbilicus toward area of stimulus		May be diminished or absent
Lower abdominal (T10, T11, T12)	Downward movement of umbilicus toward area of stimulation		May be diminished or absent
Cremasteric (T12, L1)	Elevation of ipsilateral testicle as cremaster muscle contracts (males only)		
Gluteal (L4 to S3)	Contraction of anal sphincter		
Deep tendon Biceps (C5, C6)	Flexion of arm at elbow		
Triceps (C6, C7, C8)	Extension of arm at elbow and contraction of triceps muscles		
Finger flexion (C7 to T1)	Fingers flexed		
Brachioradialis (C5, C6)	Flexion at elbow and pronation of forearm		
Patellar (L2, L3, L4)	Extension of leg at knee and contraction of quadriceps		May be diminished
Achilles (S1, S2)	Plantar flexion of foot at ankle		May be absent
Pathologic Plantar (Babinski) (L4, L5, S1, S2)	Dorsal flexion of great toe with fanning of other toes	Up to 18 mo: fanning of toes	
Chaddock (L4, L5, S1, S2)	Dorsal flexion of great toe with fanning of other toes		
Clonus	No movement of foot		

Normal Infantile Reflexes

Reflex	Findings	Reflex	Findings
Moro's (startle reflex)	Symmetric abduction and extension of arms and legs; thumb and index finger assume C position; pulls legs and arms up against trunk; appears at birth; disappears at 1-4 mo	Clonus*	Clonus movement of foot (if present); appears at birth; disappears at 4 mo
Tonic neck	Extension of leg and arm on side to which head turned; flexion of contralateral arm and leg; assumes fencing position; appears at birth to 6 wk; disappears at 4-6 mo	Rooting	Turns head in direction of stimulus and opens mouth slightly; appears at birth; disappears at 3-4 mo
Plantar grasp	Toes flex tightly downward; appears at birth; disappears at 8-10 mo	Sucking	Sucking motion of lips and tongue; appears at birth; disappears at 10-12 mo
Palmar grasp	Tightly grasps object (i.e., finger) with fingers; appears at birth; disappears at 3-4 mo	Galant's	Lateral curvature of trunk; easiest to obtain at 5-6 d of age
Babinski's*	Positive response with fanning of toes; appears at birth. 12-18 mo: fanning of toes; 18 mo to 3 yr: flexion of great toe with fanning of other toes	Glabella	Eyes closed tightly
		Crossed-extensor	Extension and slight adduction of contralateral leg
		Landau's	Extension of spine and legs and lifting of head; appears at 6-8 mo; disappears at 3 yr
Step in place	Paces forward using alternating steps; appears at birth; disappears at 3 mo	Parachute	Extension of arms and legs; appears at 4-6 mo

*May occur in adults and older children as symptom of a pathologic condition.

NORMAL LABORATORY DATA

Indications for obtaining cerebrospinal fluid include all the following:
1. To measure or reduce pressure within the subarachnoid space (i.e., subarachnoid block from a neoplasm, vertebral fracture, or dislocation)
2. To assist in the diagnosis of bacterial or viral infections (e.g., meningitis)
3. To administer anticancer drugs
4. To administer antibiotics (not commonly used)
5. To assist in the diagnosis of demyelinating diseases, a subarachnoid hemorrhage, an intracranial hemorrhage, and brain abscesses

Samples of the cerebrospinal fluid are most commonly collected via the lumbar puncture. If the lumbar site is infected or deformed, the cerebrospinal fluid can be aspirated by a cisternal or ventricular puncture.

Laboratory Test	Normal Adult Values	Variations in Child
Appearance	Crystal clear, colorless	
Pressure (lateral recumbent)	50-180 mm H_2O	
Protein Lumbar	6 mo and up: approximately 15-50 mg/dl Ventricular CSF protein is generally lower	0-1 mo: 30-170 mg/dl
Cisternal	15-25 mg/dl	
Ventricular	6-15 mg/dl	
Cell count	No RBCs 0-5 WBCs 0-10 cells/cmm (all lymphocytes and monocytes)	<1 mo: <30 cells/cmm 1 yr: <10 cells/cmm 1-4 yr: <8 cells/cmm 5 yr to puberty: <5 cells/cmm
Glucose	50-80 mg/dl (60-70% of plasma glucose)	

Laboratory Test	Normal Adult Values	Variations in Child
A/G rates	8:1 (albumin to globulin)	
Serologic studies		
Complement fixation	Nonreactive	
Treponema pallidum immune adherence	Nonreactive	
Treponema immobilization test	Nonreactive	
Gram stain	Negative for organisms	
Culture and sensitivity	No growth of organisms	
Electrolytes		
Sodium	141 mEq/L	
Potassium	3.3 mEq/L	
Chloride	110-125 mEq/L	
Bilirubin	Negative	
Cholesterol	0.2-0.6/dl	
Creatinine	0.5-1.2 mg/dl	
Urea	7-15 mg/dl	
Urea nitrogen	10-15 mg/dl	
Uric acid	0.5-4.5 mg/dl	
pH	7.32-7.35	
Specific gravity	1.007	
Glutamine	6-15 mg/dl (enzymatic)	Infants: 24-193 mg/L
IgG index	0.3-0.7	
IgG	0-11% of total protein	
Lactic acid	Control group with no CNS disorder: 0.6-2.2 mEq/L (0.6-2.2 mmol/L; 10-20 mg/dl)	Increased in first 2 wk of life
LDH	Fluid LDH activity normally much less than plasma LDH activity; normal spinal fluid LDH levels are about 10% of serum levels	
Myelin basic protein	<4 ng/ml CSF is normal	
Oligoclonal bands	Normal CSF: no demonstrable oligoclonal bands	
Protein electrophoresis (normal range depends on methodology)		
Gamma	3.0-13.0%	
Beta	7.3-17.9%	
Alpha$_2$	3.0-12.6%	
Alpha$_1$	1.1-6.6%	
Albumin	56.8-76.9%	
Prealbumin	2.2-7.1%	
CSF Albumin	13.4-23.7 mg/dl	
Total protein	15-50 mg/dl	
Beta-gamma ratio	1.67-2.3	
Oligoclonal bands	Absent	
FTA-ABS	Nonreactive	
Cryptococcal antigen titer	Negative	
VDRL	Nonreactive	
Mycobacteria culture	No growth	
Counterimmunoelectrophoresis	Negative	
India ink preparation	No *Cryptococcus* identified	

DIAGNOSTIC STUDIES

Brain scan

Intravenous injection of a small amount of radioactive substance (e.g., technetium 99). Head is then scanned with a special sensing device to pick up areas of concentrated uptake.

Nursing care:

Obtain careful history regarding any existing allergies, particularly to iodine.

Assure patient that procedure is painless, radioactive substance is harmless, and there are no after effects.

Caloric tests
Caloric test for vestibular function

Injection of cold or hot water into external auditory canal; with patient lying down and head elevated at 30 degrees. Patient observed for nystagmus.

Hallpike caloric test

Injection of hot or cold water into external auditory canal. Time interval from beginning of water flow to end of visible nystagmus is recorded.

Nelson caloric test

Injection of small amounts of ice water into external aural canal while patient is in supine position with head tilted 30 degrees forward or in sitting position with head tilted 60 degrees backward. Patient observed for nystagmus.

Nursing care:

Maintain bed rest, with head of bed elevated at 20 to 30 degrees until subjective symptoms disappear.

Patient is given nothing by mouth 6 hours before procedure.

Cerebrospinal fluid studies
Lumbar puncture

Insertion of needle into lumbar subarachnoid space to obtain cerebrospinal fluid for examination and to detect spinal subarachnoid block. Needle is inserted between L3-L4 interspace.

Nursing care:

Position patient on firm surface and maintain spine in horizontal position.

Assist in obtaining manometer reading of cerebrospinal fluid pressure.

If subarachnoid block is suspected, a Queckenstedt test is performed.

Place blood pressure cuff around patient's neck and inflate to 20 mm Hg pressure (or compress jugular veins) for 10 seconds.

Obtain manometer pressure readings at 10-second intervals until pressure stabilizes.

Keep patient flat in bed (or on side) for 4 to 6 hours after procedure.

Force fluids, unless contraindicated.

Frequent monitoring of vital signs and neurologic signs. Procedure should be done with *extreme* caution when intracranial pressure is elevated.

Lateral cervical puncture

Insertion of a needle into C1-C2 interspace through to subarachnoid space to obtain cerebrospinal fluid. Needle is inserted perpendicular to neck with patient in supine position.

Nursing care:

Keep patient flat for 4 to 6 hours after procedure.
Force fluids, unless contraindicated.

Cisternal puncture

Insertion of short-beveled needle immediately below occipital bone into cisterna magna to obtain cerebrospinal fluid. Can be done simultaneously with lumbar puncture to demonstrate subarachnoid block.

Nursing care:

Assist patient to bend head slightly forward.
Monitor for cyanosis, dyspnea, or apnea.

Ventricular puncture

Insertion of ventricular needle (in adults and older children) through burr holes into lateral ventricle.

Insertion of short-beveled needle (in infant) through scalp and anterior fontanel into lateral ventricle.

Nursing care:

Infant usually must be sedated (i.e., Nembutal) and immobilized (i.e., wrap in draw sheet) for procedure.

Assist in obtaining manometer pressure readings.
Frequently monitor vital signs and neurologic signs.
Position patient on side with head of bed elevated 10 degrees.

Echoencephalogram

Rapid and simple diagnostic test that records echoes from deep structures in skull. Indicates position of midline structures and estimation of ventricular size. Echoes are converted to electrical impulses and recorded on screen.

Electrodiagnostic
Electroencephalogram (EEG)

Measurement and recording of brain's electrical impulses: alpha, beta, and delta waves.

Nursing care:

Stimulants such as coffee, tea, and cola not permitted for 8 hours before procedure.

Adult patient should have minimal sleep (i.e., 4 to 5 hours) night before procedure.

Young child should be put to bed later (i.e., 2 hours) than usual.

Electromyography (EMG)

Surface electrodes or monopolar electrodes measure and record electrical properties of skeletal muscle and nerve conduction. Electrical activity is picked up by a needle electrode inserted into muscle and displayed on a cathode-ray oscilloscope.

Nursing care:
Patient should be informed about temporary discomfort experienced during insertion of electrode needles.
Provide postprocedural pain relief, if indicated.

Electronystagmography

Graphic recording and measurement of electrical potentials of eye movements during spontaneous, positional, or calorically evoked nystagmus. Intensity, frequency, and speed of fast and slow component of nystagmus are recorded.

Nursing care:
Instruct patient to keep eyes open during procedure.

Lumbar venography

Injection of contrast medium to visualize epidural venous plexus. Catheter is inserted percutaneously into femoral vein and then guided into internal iliac vein or ascending lumbar vein.

Nursing care:
Monitor site for signs of hemorrhage or infection.
Immobilize affected extremity for 12 hours after procedure.

Neuroradiologic
Routine skull

Simple radiographic study of skull. Anteroposterior and lateral views most frequently ordered to detect configuration, density, and vascular markings of skull.

Routine spine

Simple radiographic study of different spinal regions: cervical, thoracic, lumbar, or sacral. Anterior, posterior, and lateral views most common.

Computerized tomography (CT scan)

Scanning of brain, in successive layers, by narrow beam of x rays. Provides scanning in two planes simultaneously and at various angles: distinguishes different densities of brain tissues and displays computer printout of tissues scanned.

Nursing care:
Monitor for signs of allergic reaction if contrast medium is utilized.

Positron emission tomography (PET)

Intravenous injection of deoxyglucose with radioactive fluorine. Head is scanned, and color composite picture is obtained. Various shades of colors indicate levels of glucose metabolism.

Nursing care:
As for CT scan.

Pneumoencephalography

Injection of gases (i.e., nitrogen, oxygen) into subarachnoid space, by lumbar or cisternal puncture, for visualization of ventricular system, and intraspinal, intracranial, subarachnoid spaces. Provides greater visualization of posterior fossae than does ventriculogram.

Fractional pneumoencephalography

Injection of small amounts of air to visualize ventricular system.

Nursing care:
Keep patient flat in bed for 12 to 24 hours after procedure.
Force fluids, unless contraindicated. Maintain accurate intake and output records.
Frequently monitor vital signs and neurologic signs. (Many patients will be febrile for as long as 36 to 48 hours after procedure.)
If indicated, administer analgesics as per order.

Ventriculography

Gas or a positive-contrast medium is directly introduced into lateral ventricles by ventricular puncture. In infants, puncture is through coronal sutures. In older children and adults, puncture is through a small trephine opening (burr holes) into frontal, posterior, parietal, or occipital region.

Nursing care:
General anesthesia may be required for young pediatric patient.
Observe for signs and symptoms of intracranial or subdural hematoma (especially in patients with noncommunicating hydrocephalus).
Frequently monitor vital signs and neurologic signs.
Keep patient flat in bed for 24 to 48 hours after procedure.
Encourage fluids. Keep accurate intake and output records.
Institute seizure precautions after procedure for 24 hours.

Myelography

Radiographic study of spinal cord by introduction of negative (air) or positive (Pantopaque) contrast medium into subarachnoid space by lumbar or cisternal puncture.

Nursing care:
As for lumbar puncture.

Cerebral arteriography

Injection of contrast medium into arterial bloodstream for roentgenographic visualization of brain's vascular system.

Injection into carotid system is made to visualize anterior, middle, and posterior cerebral arteries and returning venous circulation; injection into vertebral artery visualizes vertebral-basilar system in posterior fossae.

Nursing care:
Observe puncture site for hematoma or hemorrhage.
Frequently monitor vital signs and neurologic signs during and after procedure.
Observe for signs of allergic dye reactions.

Cisternography
Injection of radioisotope into subarachnoid space through cisternal or lumbar puncture. Head is then scanned at regular intervals to determine amount of time it takes for radioisotope to clear from circulating cerebrospinal fluid.

Nursing care:
As for cisternal or lumbar puncture.

Discography
Injection of contrast medium into intervertebral disc or discs for radiographic study. Anteroposterior and lateral spine films are taken. Procedure limited to L3, L4, L5 areas.

Nursing care:
Frequently monitor vital signs and neurologic signs.
Analgesics are indicated, as procedure is very painful.

Nerve conduction studies
Study of nerve conduction velocity calculated by division of distance between proximal and distal points by time required for stimulus (electrical) to travel between those two points.

Tissue sampling
Brain biopsy
Removal of a small brain tissue sample, usually done during intracranial surgery.

Nursing care:
Frequently monitor vital signs and neurologic signs.

Muscle biopsy
Removal of a small muscle tissue sample for histologic, histochemical, ultrastructural, or biochemical studies.

Nursing care:
Monitor site for signs of hemorrhage and infection.
Symptomatic pain relief, if indicated.
Sutures removed in 7 to 10 days.

Nerve biopsy
Removal of a small nerve tissue sample. Determines extent of damage to myelinated and unmyelinated nerve fibers.

Nursing care:
As for muscle biopsy.

Conditions, Diseases, and Disorders

BRAIN ABSCESS

A brain abscess is a suppurative infection consisting of a collection of pus within the parenchyma of the brain.

The frequency of abscesses in areas of the brain is site specific, depending on factors such as the size of the area and the amount of cerebral blood flow. As a result, 80% of the abscesses are found in the cerebrum, while the remaining 20% are found in the cerebellum. Statistics indicate that 5% to 20% of brain abscesses have multiple site frequency. The individual with a brain abscess presents a difficult clinical situation since there is a 30% to 60% mortality associated with the disorder. Surgical intervention may reduce the mortality, but this depends on accessibility of the abscess as well as the general condition of the patient. Morbidity following a brain abscess presents continued difficulties. Individuals surviving brain abscesses may experience different types of neurologic residue, including paralysis and seizures.

The majority of brain abscesses result from extension of chronic middle ear, sinus, or mastoid infections. The bacteria of these infections can invade the cranial vault directly through the bone, through spinal dura mater, across the subdural and subarachnoid spaces, or along venous channels as in the extension of a septic thrombophlebitis. Suppuration from the ear accounts for one third to one half of all brain abscesses, producing disease in either the ipsilateral cerebellar hemisphere or in the temporal lobe. Extended infections from the frontal sinuses primarily affect the anteroinferior parts of the frontal lobes. Sphenoidal sinusitis may extend to the frontal or temporal lobes, and ethmoid sinusitis may extend to the frontal lobes. Penetrating head injuries, compound skull fractures, and osteomyelitis of the skull may lead to the formation of a brain abscess. Patients with right-to-left cardiac shunts are susceptible to the formation of brain abscesses because of polycythemia, which causes cerebral ischemia and necrosis. Most abscesses disseminated through the bloodstream are multiple and found in the white matter, particularly in areas distal to those perfused by the middle cerebral artery.

Organisms commonly isolated as the cause of brain abscesses include streptococci, aerobic Enterobacteriaceae, and the staphylococci. Specifically, anaerobic bacteria (i.e., *Bacteroides fragilis*) and aerobic Enterobacteriaceae (i.e., *Escherichia coli*, *Klebsiella*) are found in suppurative ear infections. Anaerobic and microaerophilic streptococci, *Bacteroides*, *Fusobacterium*, and *Veillonella* species are found in suppurative lung infections. Staphylococci are frequently associated with penetrating head injuries and endocarditis. In patients with impaired host resistance, disseminated fungal infections (e.g., candidiasis) may also result in brain abscesses.

PATHOPHYSIOLOGY

Following the initial implantation of bacteria there is a localized inflammatory reaction (i.e., cerebritis or encephalitis), which is characterized by local edema, hyperemia, leukocyte infiltration, and parenchymal softening. Several days to weeks after invasion of the brain tissue by the bacteria, there is central liquefaction and necrosis of brain tissue resulting in a cystic mass of pus. The cystic mass is enclosed by an abscess wall from migration of fibroblasts. Continued fibroblastic activity and gliosis result in replacement of granulation tissue of the abscess wall by collagenous connective tissues. The encapsulation process is usually completed within about 3 weeks. The abscess wall is usually thinnest on the ventricular side, predisposing this side to rupture. Infiltration of the leptomeninges (subarachnoid and pia mater) may lead to low-grade cerebrospinal fluid pleocytosis

without abscess rupture. When the infection extends toward the cortex, meningitis results; when it extends toward the ventricles, ventriculitis results.

DIAGNOSTIC STUDIES

Lumbar puncture
Contraindication:
1. May precipitate brain herniation if intracranial pressure is severely elevated

Roentgenograms: skull, sinuses, mastoid processes, chest
Helpful in locating associated suppurative processes

CT scan
Locates well-formed and encapsulated abscesses
Visualizes ventricle size and midline displacement

Brain scan
Locates abscesses over 1 cm in size
Sensitive in early cerebritis when local alteration in permeability of blood-brain barrier can be visualized

CSF studies (if done)
Slight increase in pressure
Increase in WBC
Increased protein
Normal glucose levels
CSF cultures nonspecific unless abscess has ruptured

Carotid arteriography
Locates temporal lobe abscesses
Posterior circulatory arteriography used to locate cerebellar abscesses

Magnetic resonance imaging (MRI)
Same as CT scan without radiation

Electroencephalogram (EEG)
Marked slowing at sites of abscess

TREATMENT PLAN

Surgical
Aspiration or complete excision and evacuation of abscess (method depends on site and accessibility)

Chemotherapeutic
Anti-infective agents; course of therapy may be 6 wk
Penicillin G, 20 million units IV qd
Chloramphenicol (Chloromycetin), 50 mg/kg/d in divided doses q6h IV
Nafcillin (Unipen)

Adult: 500 mg IV q4h
Child: 50 mg/kg/d in 4 divided doses
Semisynthetic, resistant penicillin used if *Staphylococcus aureus* isolated
Metronidazole (Flagyl) (adults)
Loading: 15 mg/kg IV over 1 h
Maintenance: 7.5 mg/kg IV over 1 h q6h
Used if anaerobic bacteria such as *Bacteroides fragilis* are isolated

Electromechanical
Serial-order CT scans or brain scans
Support of vital functions (e.g., ventilator) if indicated

Supportive
Physical therapy
Nutritional services

ASSESSMENT: AREAS OF CONCERN

Pain
Activation
Headache (70% of patients)
Increased pulse
Increased blood pressure
Increased respiratory rate
Dilated pupils
Pallor
Increased muscle tension
Cold perspiration
Raised hairs on some parts of body
Rebound phase
Blood pressure lower than before pain experience
Pulse rate slower than before pain experience
Adaptation phase
Pain occurring frequently or for long duration: pulse rate and blood pressure not increased as much as in activation phase
Stress reaction
Pain persisting for many days
Increased production of 17-ketosteroids
Increased production of eosinophils
Increased susceptibility to other infections
Vocalizations
Grunt
Whimper
Groan
Sob
Cry
Gasp
Facial expressions
Clenched teeth

Eyes open wide or tightly shut lids
Wrinkled forehead
Biting lower lip
Other
May withdraw
May not initiate conversation

Level of consciousness
Lethargy
Irritability
Confusion or coma

Increased intracranial pressure
Nausea, vomiting
Changing level of consciousness (see p. 349 for additional signs and symptoms of increased intracranial pressure)
Papilledema (late sign)

Meningeal irritability
Nuchal rigidity (25% of patients)

Seizure activity
Generalized or focal (30% of patients)
Preconvulsive (preictal) stage
Aura: flash of light; sense of loss, fear; weakness; dizziness; peculiar taste, smell, and sounds
Cry or scream
Fall to floor
Loss of consciousness
Tachypnea
Convulsive stage
Tonic: rigid body; flexed jaws; clenched fists; extended legs; cyanosis; holding breath
Clonic: urinary and/or fecal incontinence; jerking of facial muscles and extremities; biting tongue; frothing at mouth
Postconvulsive (postictal) stage
Altered level of consciousness
Headache
Nausea and/or vomiting
Malaise
Muscle soreness
Aspiration
Breathing difficulty, choking, cyanosis, decreased breath sounds, tachycardia, tachypnea

Other
Selective aphasia (if temporal lobe involved)
Homonymous upper quadrantic or hemianopic defects in visual fields
Weakness of lower face
Ataxia, nystagmus, incoordination of extremities, and occasionally intention tremors (cerebellar abscess)
Impaired 2-point discrimination, altered position

sense, astereognosis, visual inattention, and impaired opticokinetic nystagmus (parietal lobe abscess)

Anxiety
Appearance
  Increased perspiration, clammy skin
  Fatigue
  Increased muscle tension (rigidity)
  Skin blanches; pale
  Increased small motor activity (i.e., tremors, restlessness)

Behavior
  Decreased attention span
  Increased immobility
  Decreased ability to follow directions
Other
  Increased rate or depth of respirations
  Increased heart rate
  Rapid shifts in body temperature, blood pressure
  Urinary urgency
  Diarrhea
  Dry mouth
  Decreased appetite
  Pupillary dilation

NURSING DIAGNOSES and NURSING INTERVENTIONS

Nursing Diagnosis	Nursing Intervention
Airway clearance, ineffective	Maintain patent airway; avoid flexion of neck if patient is comatose. Suction as needed. Assist ventilation as per protocol. Monitor vital signs and neurologic status every 1 to 2 hours. Keep emergency drugs and ventilator at bedside. Maintain nothing-by-mouth status to prevent risk of choking and aspiration.
Breathing pattern, ineffective	Maintain patent airway; intubation and assisted ventilation may be indicated. Monitor arterial blood gases as per protocol: Report decrease of Po_2 of 10 to 15 mm Hg. Report increase of Pco_2 greater than 10 to 15 mm Hg. Note respiratory rate, depth, and level of consciousness every 15 to 30 minutes and as needed. Check blood pressure, temperature, and pulse rate every 1 to 2 hours and as needed. Administer medications as per protocol. Measure and record vital capacity of 2 to 4 hours. Limit fluid intake as ordered; may include titrating according to pulmonary artery pressure, central venous pressure, or pulmonary capillary wedge pressure. Take and record ECG rhythm strips every 2 to 4 hours and as needed, noting rate and rhythm. Measure intake and output: report hourly output less than 30 ml. Monitor hemodynamics (central venous pressure, arterial pressure, pulmonary artery pressure, pulmonary capillary wedge pressure) as per protocol. Monitor intracranial pressure (if monitoring device is used) every 30 minutes to 1 hour. Monitor vital signs every 1 to 2 hours and as needed.
Tissue perfusion, alteration in: cerebral	Monitor arterial blood gases, blood chemistry, and electrolytes. Maintain head of bed at 20- to 45-degree elevation. Maintain body alignment. Monitor intake and output every 1 to 2 hours or as condition indicates. Monitor ECG rhythm and arterial pulses.
Comfort, alteration in: pain	See general intervention strategies listed on p. 1979.
Skin integrity, impairment of: potential	Administer skin care every 2 to 4 hours. Turn patient every 2 hours. Use air mattress or egg-crate mattress. Use sand bags or footboard. Keep skin dry.
Mobility, impaired physical	Perform passive range of motion (ROM) exercises to all extremities every 4 hours.

Nursing Diagnosis	Nursing Intervention
Sensory-perceptual alteration	Keep siderails up at all times when patient is alone. Maintain patient safety at all times. Maintain quiet environment, reducing external stimuli to a minimum. Reorient patient frequently to time, place, and person. Introduce self each time you reorient patient. Repeat explanations frequently and simply. Have family bring in familiar objects. Maintain planned rest periods, allowing sufficient time for REM sleep. Use day-night lighting appropriately. Stimulate senses of touch, taste, position.
Self-concept, disturbance in: body image, role performance, personal identity	See general intervention strategies listed on p. 1820. Avoid facial expressions that may indicate rejection. Perform care in a quiet, unhurried manner.
Injury, potential for: seizures Preconvulsive	Have oral airway at bedside. Have suction equipment available at bedside. Pad side rails, if indicated. Administer oxygen as per protocol. Establish means of communication. Identify auras if possible.
Convulsive	Maintain patent airway. Support and protect head; turn to side if possible. Prevent injury. Ease to floor if in chair. Place pillows along side rails if in bed. Remove surrounding furniture. Loosen constrictive clothing. Provide privacy as necessary. Stay with patient; remain calm. Note frequency, time, involved body parts, and length of seizure.
Postconvulsive	Maintain patent airway. Suction as needed and as indicated. Check vital signs and neurologic status every 15 minutes. Administer oxygen as per protocol. Reorient patient to environment. Provide emotional support. Place patient in position of comfort; turn head to side. Administer oral hygiene as necessary for secretions and bleeding. Prepare for diagnostic tests if ordered: CT scan, skull series, arteriogram, EEG.

Patient Education

1. Make certain the patient and family know and understand the following:
   a. Nature of a brain abscess, treatments, and procedures; explain as they occur.
   b. Need to ambulate as tolerated.
   c. Importance of maintaining planned rest periods.
   d. Names of medications, dosages, frequency of administration, purposes, and toxic or side effects.
   e. Need to avoid taking over-the-counter medications without consulting physician.
   f. Possible residual effects such as headaches, sensory or motor deficits, seizures.

2. Teach the patient and the family to recognize seizure activity and appropriate course of action:
   a. Sit or lie down.
   b. Avoid trying to stop seizure or restraining patient.
   c. Protect patient from injury.
   d. Observe and record body parts involved and duration of seizure activity.

3. Ensure that the patient and family understand importance of ongoing outpatient care (i.e., physician's visits and physical therapy).

4. Teach the patient and family the importance of maintaining a well-balanced diet.

EVALUATION

Patient Outcome	Data Indicating That Outcome is Reached
The patient demonstrates effective airway clearance.	Breath sounds are normal. Chest excursion is symmetric. Rate and depth of respirations are normal. Cough is effective. There are no subjective or objective findings of shortness of breath, air hunger, or dyspnea on exertion.
The patient demonstrates an effective breathing pattern.	Patent airway is maintained. Chest excursion is symmetric. Breath sounds are normal, or there is no increase in adventitious sounds. ABG values are within normal ranges or consistent with patient's baseline. Vital signs are within normal ranges or consistent with patient's baseline. Hemoglobin levels are 14 to 18 g/dl (male) and 12 to 16 g/dl (female). Intake and output are stable. There are no signs of respiratory distress. Resonance of all lobes is evident on percussion. Skin color is without cyanosis.
The patient maintains adequate cerebral and spinal tissue perfusion.	There is no change in level of consciousness. There is no evidence of neurologic deficits. Pattern of electrolytes is stable. There is no seizure activity.
The patient demonstrates an optimal level of mobility.	Skin integrity is maintained. The patient remains free of contractures and deformities. Level of mobility is appropriate to physiologic status. Intake and output pattern is stable. Nutritional status is adequate. The patient remains free of thrombophlebitis. The patient remains free of local infection.
The patient experiences minimal alterations in comfort.	The patient openly verbalizes feelings of discomfort when they occur. The patient is able to utilize measures to decrease discomfort. The patient verbalizes a decrease in subjective feelings of discomfort. There is a decrease in objective findings of pain.
The patient demonstrates minimal complications of sensory-perceptual alterations.	The patient maintains optimal level of mobility. The patient remains free of injury. Skin integrity is maintained. Nutritional status is adequate. The patient demonstrates minimal self-care deficits. The patient demonstrates social participation appropriate to physiologic status.
The patient demonstrates intact self-concepts.	The patient openly verbalizes feelings of grief, loss, etc. The patient verbalizes positive feelings about self. The patient acknowledges actual change in self-image. The patient focuses on present and future appearance and function. The patient verbalizes feelings of hopefulness and helpfulness.
The patient remains free of traumatic injury.	Safety measures appropriate to level of physiologic status are used. Skin integrity is maintained. Skin is free of bruises, burns, abrasions, redness, etc. Environment is safe. The patient is free of nosocomial infections.

HYDROCEPHALUS

Hydrocephalus is a condition in which there is an abnormal accumulation of cerebrospinal fluid within the cranial vault and subsequent dilation of the cerebral ventricles.[39]

Hydrocephalus has an incidence of 4 per 1000 births through the age of 3 months. However, hydrocephalus can occur at any age. In infants it is considered a primary disease, whereas in later life it occurs as a complication of other diseases.

Hydrocephalus has several known causes, which can be categorized as congenital or acquired. Obstructions to the flow of cerebrospinal fluid are attributable to congenital abnormalities, with 70% resulting from stenosis of the aqueduct of Sylvius. Other anomalies causing or associated with hydrocephalus are the Arnold-Chiari malformation, Dandy-Walker syndrome, and spina bifida cystica.[36] Flow and absorption of cerebrospinal fluid can also be affected by fibrosis of meninges and obstruction of the aqueduct and basal cisterns caused by inflammatory lesions.

The causative mechanisms of hydrocephalus have been classified as follows: (1) excessive secretion of cerebrospinal fluid as a result of a choroid plexus papilloma, (2) obstruction of cerebrospinal fluid flow in the ventricles or subarachnoid space, (3) obstruction by pacchionian granulations, and (4) hemodynamic production. Common sites for obstruction to the flow of cerebrospinal fluid include the third ventricle, the fourth ventricle, the foramina of Monro, and the aqueduct of Sylvius. Each site may be obstructed by a mass within or outside the lumen. Pacchionian granulations caused by inflammatory processes and fibrosis can occlude the arachnoid villi, preventing the escape of cerebrospinal fluid from the subarachnoid space and resulting in hydrocephalus.

Although most causes of hydrocephalus are associated with intraventricular hypertension, there are two types in which intraventricular pressure is not elevated. *Hydrocephalus ex vacuo* results in ventricular dilation to fill spaces caused by a decreasing neural mass (e.g., Alzheimer's disease and stroke). *Normal pressure hydrocephalus* is characterized by dilated ventricles, normal neural tissue mass, and normal intracranial pressure. The etiology and pathology of normal pressure hydrocephalus remain to be elucidated.

Communicating vs. Noncommunicating Hydrocephalus

A *communicating* or extraventricular hydrocephalus occurs when the obstruction is outside the ventricular system; therefore flow between the ventricles is not blocked.

An excessive amount of cerebrospinal fluid accumulates in the ventricles because the fluid is not adequately absorbed from the cerebral subarachnoid space. The *noncommunicating,* or intraventricular, hydrocephalus results in an accumulation of cerebrospinal fluid from a block of the normal flow at some point in the ventricular system. The cerebral ventricles proximal to the block then dilate.

PATHOPHYSIOLOGY

When there is an obstruction in the ventricular system or in the subarachnoid space, the cerebral ventricles dilate, causing the ventricular surface to stretch, disrupting its ependymal lining. The underlying white matter atrophies and may be reduced to a thin ribbon. There is selective preservation of the gray matter, even when the ventricles have obtained enormous size. The dilation process may be an insidious or acute process and may be selective, depending on the site of blockage. The acute process may represent a medical emergency. In the infant and young child, the cranial sutures split and widen in order to accommodate the increase of cranial mass. If the anterior fontanel is not closed, it will bulge and feel tense to palpation. Aqueductal stenosis, a sex-linked familial disease, causes a marked dilation of the lateral and third ventricles. This dilation gives the head a characteristic dominant frontal brow appearance. The Dandy-Walker syndrome occurs when there is an obstruction of the exit foramina of the fourth ventricle. Consequently the fourth ventricle dilates, with the posterior fossae becoming prominent and bossing below the tentorium. This type of hydrocephalus gives the patient generalized symmetric enlargement of the cerebrum, and the face appears disproportionately small.

In the older individual the cranial sutures have closed; therefore the space is fixed and limits expansion of the brain mass. As a result the older person usually exhibits the signs and symptoms of increased intracranial pressure before the cerebral ventricles become greatly enlarged.

Defects of cerebrospinal fluid absorption and circulation in hydrocephalus are not complete. Formation of cerebrospinal fluid exceeds the capacity of the normal ventricular system every 6 to 8 hours, and a total lack of absorption is incompatible with life. Ventricular dilation causes a disruption of the normal ependymal lining of the walls of the cavities, permitting increased absorption. If the collateral route is adequate to prevent progressive ventricular dilation, a state of compensation may exist.[6]

DIAGNOSTIC STUDIES

Angiography
Detection of vessel abnormalities caused by stretching
Vascular lesions

Computerized axial tomography
Detection of variations in tissue density
Presence of cysts or masses
Visualization of the ventricular system

Lumbar puncture
Diagnosis of communicating hydrocephalus
Contraindication:
Elevated intracranial pressure

Pneumoencephalography
Contraindication:
Presence of increased intracranial pressure

Subdural/ventricular tap
As for lumbar puncture

Ventriculography
Visualization of ventricular system configuration
Shows ventricular dilation with hydrocephalus

Magnetic resonance imaging (MRI)
Same as computerized axial tomography (CT scan)

TREATMENT PLAN

Surgical*
Correction of CSF obstruction such as resection of cyst, neoplasm, or hematoma
Ventricular bypass into normal intracranial channel (i.e., Torkildsen procedure where CSF is shunted from lateral to cisterna magna) in noncommunicating hydrocephalus
Ventricular bypass into extracranial compartment (i.e., ventriculoperitoneal or ventriculoatrial shunt)
Reduction of CSF production as in third or fourth ventriculostomy or endoscopic choroid plexus extirpation (plexectomy or electric coagulation)

Chemotherapeutic
Acetazolamide (Diamox), 8-30 mg/kg in divided doses, IV

*Therapy of choice.

Mannitol (Osmitrol), in initial management of severe increased intracranial pressure
Corticosteroids: Dexamethasone (Decadron), adults, 6-20 mg q6h IV

Electromechanical
Intracranial pressure monitoring
Cardiac monitoring
Respiratory monitoring

ASSESSMENT

Head circumference
Severely enlarged head
Bulging fontanels after pulsation
Fixed downward gaze of eyes with visible sclera above (sunset gaze)
Visible, distended scalp veins
Radiation of light throughout accumulated cerebrospinal fluid with translumination

Vomiting
More frequent in older patient
Likely to occur in morning (frequency may increase with increased intracranial pressure)

Seizures
Focal or general tonic-clonic seizures
May assume opisthotonic position

Behavioral changes
Feeds poorly
Lethargy
Irritability when stimulated

Alterations in vital signs (with increased intracranial pressure)
Decreased pulse
Increased systolic blood pressure
Irregular and decreased respirations

Muscle tone
Alteration of muscle tone in extremities

Later assessment findings
Physical and/or mental development lag
Prominence of forehead
Scalp shiny, with scalp veins prominent
Optic atrophy, strabismus, nystagmus, exposed sclera

NURSING DIAGNOSES and NURSING INTERVENTIONS

Nursing Diagnosis	Nursing Intervention

Breathing pattern, ineffective	Maintain patent airway. Have intubation and assisted ventilation equipment at bedside.
	Suction as needed. Ausculate breath sounds before and after suctioning.
	Position for maximal lung expansion; elevate head of bed slightly (10 to 20 degrees).
	Monitor arterial blood gases as ordered:
	    Report decrease of Po_2 of 10 to 15 mm Hg.
	    Report increase of Pco_2 greater than 10 to 15 mm Hg.
	Note respiratory rate and depth and level of consciousness every 15 to 30 minutes and as needed. Check pulse rate, temperature, and blood pressure every 1 to 2 hours and as needed.
	Administer medications as per protocol.
	Limit fluid intake as per protocol; include titrating according to intracranial pressure.
	Measure and record intake and output; report hourly output less than 30 ml.
	Administer tube feedings as per protocol.

Fluid volume, alteration in: excess	Do ongoing assessment of findings indicating increased intracranial pressure.
	Provide preoperative nursing care for patient who will have shunt implantation:
	    Monitor vital signs and neurologic status every 15 minutes to 1 hour and as needed.
	    Suction or aspirate mucus as needed.
	    Observe for signs and symptoms of shock.
	    Administer medications (i.e., antibiotics and anticonvulsants).
	    Turn every 2 hours and provide skin care every 2 hours.
	    Insert nasogastric tube for abdominal decompression, if indicated.
	    Avoid hyperthermia and hypothermia.
	Provide postoperative nursing care after shunt implantation:
	    Position patient and pump shunt per protocol.
	    Compress valve specified number of times at regular intervals.
	    Accurately measure intake and output and record on flow sheet.
	    Administer parenteral fluids as per protocol.
	    Administer feedings as per protocol.
	    Monitor for signs of complications, such as dehydration and infection.

Tissue perfusion, alteration in: cerebral	Intervene to monitor and/or prevent increased intracranial pressure:
	    Administer medications, treatments, and intravenous lines as per protocol.
	    Maintain elevation of head of bed as per protocol.
	    Accurately record intake and output.
	    Monitor serum electrolytes, blood count, and arterial blood gases for abnormalities.
	    Monitor values and wave forms of intracranial pressure line, if appropriate:
	        Maintain patency and sterility of system.
	        Monitor effects of treatments on intracranial pressure.
	        Correlate neurologic status with intracranial pressure values, and notify physician if inconsistent.
	        Assist with drainage of cerebrospinal fluid from system, if indicated.
	Intervene to monitor or prevent seizures:
	    Assess seizure history of patient.
	    Institute seizure precautions:
	        Padded tongue blade and airway at bedside
	        Bed height at lowest level
	        Side rails up at all times and padded
	        Oxygen and suction equipment at bedside
	        Emergency medications at bedside
	Administer anticonvulsants as per protocol:
	    Monitor effects and side effects.
	    Monitor serum for therapeutic levels of anticonvulsant.

Nursing Diagnosis	Nursing Intervention
Sensory-perceptual alteration	Have side rails up at all times when patient is alone. Maintain patient safety at all times. *Judiciously* use soft restraints; monitor patient's response. Involve family in aspects of care as appropriate. Frequently reorient patient to time, person, and place. Reintroduce yourself each time you reorient patient. Have family bring in familiar objects. Allow family to stay with patient. Maintain planned rest periods, allowing sufficient time for REM sleep. Use day-night lighting appropriately. Stimulate patient's sense of touch, taste, and position.

Skin integrity, impairment of: potential	See general intervention strategies listed on p. 2020.
	Prevent pressure sores and contractures:
	  Keep scalp dry and clean.
	  Reposition every 2 hours, and turn head frequently. Rotate head and body together to prevent strain on neck.
	  Provide passive ROM exercises every 4 hours and as needed, especially to lower extremities.

Nutrition, alteration in: less than body requirements	Offer small, frequent feedings. Complete nursing care before feeding times. Allow ample time for feeding. Position patient in a semisitting position. Support head. Encourage a high-protein diet. Accurately measure and record intake on a flow sheet. Administer parenteral fluids as per protocol. Administer tube feedings as per protocol. Position patient on his side to prevent aspiration after feeding. Elevate head.

Patient Education

1. Make certain the patient and family know and understand the following:
   a. Nature of hydrocephalus, treatments, and procedures; explain as they occur.
   b. Care of shunt devices if indicated.
   c. Need to ambulate as tolerated.
   d. Importance of maintaining planned rest periods.
   e. Names of medications, dosages, frequency of administration, purposes, and toxic or side effects.
   f. Need to avoid taking over-the-counter medications without consulting physician.
   g. Possible residual effects such as headaches, sensory or motor deficits, seizures.

2. Teach the patient and the family to recognize seizure activity and appropriate course of action:
   a. Sit or lie down.
   b. Avoid trying to stop seizure or restraining patient.
   c. Protect patient from injury.
   d. Observe and record body parts involved and duration of seizure activity.

3. Ensure that the patient and family understand importance of ongoing outpatient care (i.e., physician's visits and physical therapy).

4. Teach the patient and family the importance of maintaining a well-balanced diet.

EVALUATION

Patient Outcome	Data Indicating That Outcome is Reached
The patient demonstrates an effective breathing pattern.	Patent airway is maintained. Chest excursion is symmetric. Breath sounds are normal or there is no increase in adventitious sounds. Arterial blood gas values are within normal ranges or consistent with patient's baseline. Vital signs are within normal ranges or consistent with patient's baseline. Hemoglobin levels are 14 to 18 g/dl (male) and 12 to 16 g/dl (female). Intake and output are stable. There are no signs of respiratory distress. Resonance of all lobes is evident on percussion. Skin color is without cyanosis.
The patient maintains adequate cerebral tissue perfusion.	There is no change in level of consciousness. There is no evidence of neurologic deficits. Pattern of electrolytes is stable. There is no seizure activity.
The patient demonstrates minimal complications of sensory-perceptual alterations.	Optimal level of orientation is maintained. The patient remains free of injury. Skin integrity is maintained. Nutritional status is adequate. Self-care deficits are minimal. Social participation is appropriate to physiologic status.
The patient demonstrates skin integrity.	Skin is intact. Nutritional status is adequate. Electrolyte balance is maintained. The patient remains free of pressure sores and contractures.
The patient experiences minimal alterations in comfort.	The patient openly verbalizes feelings of discomfort when they occur. The patient is able to utilize measures to decrease discomfort. The patient verbally validates a decrease in subjective feelings of discomfort. Objective findings of pain are decreased.
The patient demonstrates intact self-concepts.	The patient openly verbalizes feelings of grief and loss. The patient verbalizes positive feelings about self. The patient acknowledges actual change in self-image. The patient focuses on present and future appearance and function. The patient verbalizes feelings of hopefulness, helpfulness, and powerfulness.

CRANIAL AND PERIPHERAL NERVE DISORDERS
Bell's Palsy

Bell's palsy is the paralysis of the facial nerve (cranial nerve VII), resulting in a sudden loss of ability to move the muscles of expression of the face.

Any or all of the three branches of the facial nerve may be affected. The disorder can be unilateral or bilateral, transient or permanent. Generally the disorder appears static for about 10 days to 2 weeks, at which time muscle tone begins to reappear. Voluntary movement of the muscles may appear within 3 or 4 weeks. However, some individuals manifest no recovery for almost 6 months, and maximal recovery (which may not be complete) may occur in approximately a year. More than 80% of the patients with Bell's palsy recover without residual neurologic deficits.[10]

PATHOPHYSIOLOGY

The pathogenesis and pathophysiology of Bell's palsy are yet to be elucidated. One theory proposes that a viral infection of the geniculate ganglion is responsible for the disorder. Other possible mechanisms may include local ischemia and edema or emotional trauma and the resulting vasoconstriction.[16]

The disorder can occur at any age but is most frequently found in individuals between 20 to 60 years. Men and women are affected about equally. The diagnosis of Bell's palsy is made by clinical features and a characteristic history.

TREATMENT PLAN

Chemotherapeutic
    Corticosteroids
        Prednisone (Deltasone), 20-60 mg po qid; dosage is gradually reduced

Electromechanical
    Electrical stimulation of nerve
    Warm, moist heat
    Massage
    Facial sling to prevent muscle stretching and to facilitate eating (by improving lip alignment)

Supportive
    Facial exercises (i.e., wrinkling brow, forcing eyes closed, puffing out cheeks) for 5 minutes three or four times daily, as muscle tone returns

ASSESSMENT: AREAS OF CONCERN

Pain
    Usually begins behind the ear
    May or may not be accompanied by herpetic vesicles in the external ear

Paralysis
    Drawing sensation on affected side, followed by complete paralysis of affected side of face: all muscles powerless and flaccid (i.e., cannot smile, wrinkle forehead, or close eye; drooling of saliva; constant eye tearing)

Taste
    Loss of taste sensation over anterior two thirds of tongue on affected side

Eating/drinking difficulties
    May see anorexia and weight loss

NURSING DIAGNOSES and NURSING INTERVENTIONS

Nursing Diagnosis	Nursing Intervention
Comfort, alteration in: pain	Establish baseline and ongoing assessment of patient's perception of level of discomfort. Provide gentle massage as needed. Provide warm moist heat as per protocol. Provide for electrical stimulation as per protocol. Apply facial sling as needed. Administer pain medications as per protocol. Provide eye care every 1 to 2 hours and as needed. Apply eye pads as indicated. Teach patient to perform facial exercises three or four times daily for 5 minutes, when facial tone returns: Wrinkling brow / Grimacing / Whistling / Puffing out cheeks / Forcing eyes closed. Provide patient with sunglasses to prevent eye strain as needed.
Nutrition, alteration in: less than body requirements	Offer the patient frequent, small feedings. Maintain soft diet as indicated. Avoid hot fluids and foods to prevent burns to insensitive areas. Provide patient with privacy at mealtimes. Provide patient with adequate time for eating meals. Teach patient to take foods on unaffected side.

Nursing Diagnosis	Nursing Intervention
	Apply facial sling to improve lip alignment. Teach patient to chew food on unaffected side. Provide meticulous mouth care before and after meals. Provide dietary supplements as indicated.
Communication, impaired: verbal	See general intervention strategies listed on p. 1870.
Anxiety	See general intervention strategies listed on p. 1839. Assist patient to deal with anxiety about the disorder, discomfort, changes in self-image, and fear of recurrence. Explain possible causes and treatments for the disorder: State simply and monitor reactions. Repeat explanations as indicated.
Self-concept, disturbance in: body image	See general intervention strategies listed on p. 1820.
Social isolation	See general intervention strategies listed on p. 1938.

Patient Education

1. Instruct regarding possible causes, involvement, symptoms, treatments, and usual course of Bell's palsy (explain procedures as they occur).
2. Instruct regarding signs of complications and progression of the disorder.
3. Teach special techniques such as the use of facial slings, massage, dietary adjustments, and exercise program to minimize discomfort.
4. Stress importance of continued eye care.
5. Instruct regarding safety measures for minimizing trauma to insensitive areas.
6. Instruct regarding name of medications, dosage, frequency of administration, purpose, and toxic or side effects of the medication.
7. Stress importance of ongoing outpatient care: physician's visits, physical therapy and exercise program, and support groups.

EVALUATION

Patient Outcome	Data Indicating That Outcome is Reached
The patient and family demonstrate adequate knowledge of Bell's palsy.	The patient is able to explain possible causes of Bell's palsy. The patient is able to explain treatment modalities for the disorder. The patient is able to explain the usual course of the disorder.
The patient demonstrates a low level of anxiety.	The patient openly verbalizes concerns and feelings of grief, loss, and discomfort. Open verbalization of feelings is supported by the health care professionals and family.
The patient demonstrates minimal discomfort.	The patient is able to utilize measures such as facial sling and warm massage as needed. The patient openly expresses feelings of discomfort when they occur. The patient is able to perform facial exercises as indicated.
The patient does not demonstrate the complications of impaired communication.	
The patient demonstrates adequate nutritional status.	Weight pattern is stable: normal for height, age, sex, and previous baseline. Intake and output are balanced and stable. Diet is appropriate to age. Skin turgor is good. There is fluid and electrolyte balance. Dietary supplements are used as appropriate.
The patient demonstrates an intact, realistic body image.	See p. 327.

Patient Outcome	Data Indicating That Outcome is Reached
The patient demonstrates social participation.	The patient can state the importance of interpersonal relationships. The patient can relate to self and others. The patient participates in unit or group activities. The patient participates in family activities as appropriate to his condition.

Guillain-Barré Syndrome

Guillain-Barré syndrome is an acute type of ascending or descending peripheral nerve syndrome resulting in widespread inflammation and demyelination of the peripheral nervous system.

Of those individuals affected by Guillain-Barré syndrome, 85% will experience complete functional recovery. The recovery period usually extends over several weeks, but it may last months or even years. The remaining 15% of affected individuals will experience some degree of permanent neurologic deficit.

Guillain-Barré syndrome is also known by the following names: acute idiopathic polyneuritis, acute polyradiculoneuropathy, postinfectious polyneuritis, Landry-Guillain-Barré-Strohl syndrome, infectious neuronitis, infectious polyneuritis, acute polyradiculitis, acute idiopathic polyradiculoneuritis, and acute inflammatory polyradiculoneuropathy.

PATHOPHYSIOLOGY

The pathogenesis of Guillain-Barré syndrome appears to be related to the sensitization of peripheral nerve myelin and is characterized by infiltration, at all levels of the peripheral nervous system, of mononuclear cells. Over half of individuals affected have had a nonspecific infection 10 to 14 days before the onset of Guillain-Barré symptoms, suggesting that sensitized lymphocytes may produce demyelination. A significant number of persons developed symptoms characteristic of Guillain-Barré syndrome after being inoculated for the swine flu. The syndrome occurs in both sexes and can affect persons of any age.

Morphologic alterations that characterize Guillain-Barré syndrome include (1) widespread monocytic inflammatory infiltrate around vessels (i.e., veins and capillaries) throughout the cranial and spinal nerves, including nerve roots, ganglia, and distal nerves; (2) segmental demyelination; and (3) in severe cases, axon destruction with resultant axonal reaction and wallerian degeneration. Anterior horn cells and neurons in dorsal root ganglia occasionally show central chromatolysis. If the axon loss is severe, denervation group atrophy can be seen in distal muscles. Electron microscopic studies have shown a breakthrough of the basement membrane of the Schwann cell by phagocytic cells, which insinuate themselves beneath the myelin layers, which are then stripped away.[41]

DIAGNOSTIC STUDIES

CSF sampling
Albuminocytologic dissociation: decreased protein normal initially (15 to 45 mg); then increases as high as 600 mg; followed by return to normal
Lymphocyte count normal

Electromyography (EMG)
Reduced nerve conduction velocity when tested near peak of illness (usually 4 to 8 weeks after onset)
Slow F wave conduction velocities
Low voltage potentials
Fibrillations and positive sharp waves (more common in late stages)

TREATMENT PLAN

Surgical
Tracheostomy

Chemotherapeutic
Pituitary hormones
Corticosporin (ACTH), 25-40 units IM or subq tid (possibly valuable if given early in course of the disorder; dosage and frequency individually determined)
Corticosteroids
Prednisone (Deltasone), 5-80 mg/d in divided doses
Anti-infective agents
Prophylactic antibotics

Electromechanical
Cardiac monitoring
Mechanical ventilation
Plasmapheresis

Supportive
Chest physiotherapy
Arterial blood gas monitoring
Nutritional maintenance (e.g., IV or nasogastric feedings)
Special eye care

ASSESSMENT: AREAS OF CONCERN

Autonomic function
Hypertension
Sinus tachycardia or bradycardia
Postural hypotension
Chest and abdominal tightness
Profuse diaphoresis

Urinary and rectal incontinence
Paroxysmal facial flushing

Cranial nerve function
Cranial nerve VII most commonly involved; abnormal testing response elicited

Motor function
Weakness following paresthesia
Most common type of weakness is ascending (i.e., lower to upper limbs to trunk)
Equal involvement of proximal and distal muscles
Atrophy possible

Reflex status
Deep tendon reflexes absent or diminished

Sensory function
Usually less severe than motor involvement
Superficial or deep sensory involvement: usually stocking-glove distribution

NURSING DIAGNOSES and NURSING INTERVENTIONS

Nursing Diagnosis	Nursing Intervention

Breathing pattern, ineffective	Maintain patent airway. Intubation, tracheostomy, and mechanical ventilation may be indicated.
	 Auscultate breath sounds every 1 to 2 hours; note quality and any increase in adventitious sounds.
	 Suction as needed. Hyperinflate lungs with 100% oxygen for 1 minute before and 1 minute after suction, unless contraindicated. Maintain aseptic technique.
	 Monitor mechanical ventilation, if used:
	   Ensure that tidal volume, rate, mode, and oxygen concentration are set as ordered.
	   Ensure that ventilator alarms are on and functional.
	 Monitor arterial blood gases, as per protocol.
	   Report decrease in Po_2 of 10 to 15 mm Hg.
	   Report increase in Pco_2 greater than 10 to 15 mm Hg.
	 Note respiratory rate, depth, and level of consciousness every 15 to 30 minutes and as needed.
	 Check blood pressure, temperature, and pulse rate every 1 to 2 hours and as needed based on patient's condition.
	 Assist and teach patient to cough and deep breath every 2 hours.
	 Administer medications per protocol.
	 Administer parenteral fluids as per protocol.
	 Limit fluid intake as per protocol; may include titrating fluids according to pulmonary artery, pulmonary capillary wedge, or central venous pressure.
	 Measure and record intake and output; report hourly output less than 30 ml.
	 Monitor hemodynamics (central venous pressure, arterial pressure, pulmonary artery pressure, pulmonary capillary wedge pressure) as per protocol.

Comfort, alteration in: pain	See general intervention strategies listed on p. 1979.
Mobility, impaired physical	See general intervention strategies listed on p. 2104.
Self-care deficit: feeding, bathing/hygiene, dressing/grooming, toileting	Avoid oral feedings; administer IV or nasogastric feedings as per protocol. Administer oral hygiene every 2 hours and as needed. Provide daily hygiene care.

Nursing Diagnosis	Nursing Intervention
	Provide eye care every 2 hours:
	Cleanse eyes and remove crust formation.
	Apply eye shields or tape eyes closed.
	Administer artificial tears or eye drops as per protocol.
	Maintain bowel function with regular evacuation.
Anxiety	Deal realistically and honestly with the patient's anxiety about the disorder, the discomfort, and the change in self-image.
	Explain potential treatments for the disorder:
	State simply and monitor patient's reactions.
	Repeat explanations, as indicated.
	Teach the patient basic relaxation techniques. Reinforce teaching, as indicated.
	Teach the patient the essential aspects of care, as indicated by the patient's condition.
	Assist the patient to participate in making decisions about care, as indicated by patient's condition.
	Alert staff to possible emotional changes; expect mood swings.
Self-concept, disturbance in: body image, self-esteem, role performance, personal identity	See general intervention strategies listed on p. 1820.

Patient Education

1. Stress need to encourage open verbalization.
2. Emphasize importance of dealing with fears of permanent disability, loss of function, and dying as well as with changes in body image.
3. Stress importance of avoiding individuals who have upper respiratory infections.
4. Emphasize importance of maintaining planned rest periods.
5. Stress need for independence and socialization:
   a. Encourage self-care.
   b. Encourage patient to eat meals with family.
6. Instruct regarding name of each medication, dosage, frequency of administration, purpose, and toxic or side effects.
7. Stress need to check with physician before taking any over-the-counter medication.
8. Emphasize need to exercise to tolerance level and avoid fatigue.
9. Stress need for high-caloric, high-protein diet; progress from soft to solid as tolerated.
10. Emphasize need to arrange utensils and food so they are easily managed by the patient.
11. Teach need to maintain fluid intake at 2000 ml daily, unless contraindicated.
12. Stress need to avoid constipation:
    a. Drink fluids.
    b. Use stool softeners.
    c. Eat foods and fruits high in roughage.
13. Emphasize need for diversional activities (e.g., watching television, reading, listening to radio).
14. Stress importance of ongoing outpatient care: physician's visits, physical therapy, and occupational therapy.
15. Ensure the patient or family demonstrates the following: speech exercises, active and/or passive ROM exercises with massage to all extremities, and exercises that increase strength and mobility of fingers (e.g., squeeze toys, balls, clay).
16. Stress importance of warm baths to alleviate pain and stiffness.

EVALUATION

Patient Outcome	Data Indicating That Outcome is Reached
The patient demonstrates a low level of anxiety.	The patient openly verbalizes concerns and feelings of grief, loss, and discomfort.
	The patient openly verbalizes feelings, supported by health care professionals and significant others.
	The patient verbalizes essential aspects of care.
	The patient is able to demonstrate relaxation techniques when feelings of anxiety begin.

Patient Outcome	Data Indicating That Outcome is Reached
The patient demonstrates an effective breathing pattern.	Airway remains patent. Chest excursion is symmetric. Vesicular, bronchial, and bronchovesicular breath sounds are normal with no adventitious sounds. Arterial blood gas values are within normal ranges or consistent with patient's baseline. Vital signs are within normal limits or consistent with patient's baseline. Hemoglobin levels are 14 to 18 g/dl (male) and 12 to 16 g/dl (female). Intake and output are stable. There are no signs of respiratory distress (i.e., nasal flaring, increased pulse rate, air hunger). All lobes are resonant on percussion. Skin color is not cyanotic.
The patient demonstrates a minimal level of discomfort.	The patient openly verbalizes feelings of discomfort when they occur. The patient is able to utilize measures to decrease discomfort. The patient is able to verbally validate a decrease in subjective feelings of discomfort. Objective findings of pain are decreased.
The patient demonstrates minimal complications of impaired physical mobility.	Skin integrity is maintained. Contractures and deformities do not form. Level of mobility is appropriate to physiologic status. Intake and output pattern is stable. Nutritional status is adequate. There are no signs or symptoms of thrombophlebitis. There are no signs or symptoms of local infection.
The patient demonstrates minimal self-care deficits.	Outcome criteria stated for impaired physical mobility are met. Level of self-care is appropriate to physiologic status. Diet is high in calories and protein. Physical and occupational therapy are given as indicated.
The patient demonstrates intact self-concept.	The patient openly verbalizes feelings of grief and loss. The patient verbalizes positive feelings about self. The patient acknowledges actual change in self-image. The patient focuses on present and future appearance and function. The patient verbalizes feelings of hopefulness, helpfulness, and powerfulness.

Trigeminal Neuralgia

Trigeminal neuralgia, or tic douloureux, is a neurologic condition that affects the sensory distribution of the trigeminal facial nerve (cranial nerve V) and is characterized by flashing, stablike paroxysms of pain radiating along the course of a branch of cranial nerve V from the angle of the jaw.[50]

Trigeminal neuralgia is caused by degeneration of the nerve or by pressure on it. Any of the three branches of the nerve may be affected. Attacks of lancinating pain, caused by trigeminal neuralgia, often will cause the person to wince with facial contractions, thus the term *tic douloureux*.

PATHOPHYSIOLOGY

The etiology of trigeminal neuralgia is unknown. The term *neuralgia* is applied because there is no demonstrable structural lesion along the course of the nerve. A similar syndrome can occur in cases of multiple sclerosis, gasserian ganglion tumor, cerebellopontine tumor, or brainstem infarction.[26]

The idiopathic form of trigeminal neuralgia affects 15,000 individuals each year in the middle adult to late adulthood phases. It is slightly more common in women. Although any of the nerve's three branches can be affected, the second and third divisions are most commonly involved. Neuralgia of the first division results in pain over the forehead and around the eyes; of the second division, pain in the nose, cheek, and upper lip. Neuralgia of the third division results in pain in the lower lip and on the side of the tongue. Episodes of the pain recur over weeks or months, although there may be spontaneous remissions. Tender areas (trigger zones) and any mechanical activity such as smiling, talking, or touching the face can set off an attack.[26] These trigger points are the part of mucous membrane or skin that is close to the appearance of the nerve involved. The following are common trigger points:

First division: supraorbital notch
Second division: infraorbital foramen close to the junction of the cheek and nose
Third division: side of the tongue or the mental foramen

The diagnosis of trigeminal neuralgia is based on the characteristic history of the disorder.

TREATMENT PLAN

Surgical
Microvascular decompression procedure for selective cutting of fibers within the trigeminal nerve
Radio frequency retrogasserian rhizotomy (surgical lesions, made at selected points on the trigeminal nerve, by radio frequency current)
Avulsion of the peripheral branches of the trigeminal nerve
Intracranial division of the sensory root of the trigeminal nerve

Chemotherapeutic
Carbamazepine (Tegretol), 400-1000 mg/d po or IV
Phenytoin (Dilantin), 200-400 mg/d po or IV
Absolute alcohol: injected into gasserian ganglion in very small amounts
Analgesics

Supportive
Semisolid, fluid diet
Psychosocial counseling

ASSESSMENT: AREAS OF CONCERN

Pain
Severe, shooting pain, starting at a particular point with a repetitive tic and increasing in severity to where it shoots violently and with explosive force through the face on the affected side

Apprehension
Protects face from any stimulation

Personal identity
Actual change in function of facial nerve
Protection of face from any form of stimulation
Change in social involvement
Verbalization of:
  Negative feelings about self
  Preoccupation with change or loss
  Focus on past appearance and function
  Change in life-style
  Fear of rejection by others
  Feelings of powerlessness, helplessness, hopelessness
  Refusal to acknowledge actual change

Social isolation
Preoccupation with own thoughts and meaningless, repetitive activities
Dull, sad affect
Hostility projected in voice and behavior
Seeks to be alone
Withdrawn, uncommunicative, no eye contact
Activities and interests inappropriate for developmental stage and age
Verbalizes feelings of rejection
Verbalizes interests inappropriate for developmental stage and age
Insecurity in public
Expresses feeling different from others
Inability to meet others' expectations
Absence of, or insecurity in, significant purpose in life

NURSING DIAGNOSES and NURSING INTERVENTIONS

Nursing Diagnosis	Nursing Intervention
Anxiety	See general strategies listed on p. 1839.
Comfort, alteration in: pain	Promote rest and relaxation. Decrease noxious stimuli by assessing what precipitates the pain and assist patient to avoid these factors.

Nursing Diagnosis	Nursing Intervention
	Modify anxiety associated with the pain experience.
	Provide other sensory input. Administer medications as per protocol.
	Remain with the patient.
	Improve effectiveness of pain relief measures by using them before the pain becomes intense.
Self-concept, disturbance in: body image, self-esteem, role performance, personal identity	See general intervention strategies listed on p. 1820.
	Assist the patient to become involved in self-care.
	Assist the patient to become involved in unit activities.
Social isolation	Allow the patient to express perceptions regarding the illness. Offer support and clarification.
	Foster a sense of relatedness to self.
	Foster a sense of relatedness to family:
	Provide for physical closeness of family member.
	Include family in care as appropriate to do so.
	Have patient teach family about the disorder.
	Encourage the patient to personalize the environment. Allow personal items to be brought from home.
	Use touch as therapeutic intervention.
	Encourage patient to verbalize needs met through interpersonal relationships.
	Encourage group activities.
	Encourage patient to maintain good grooming habits.

Patient Education

1. Instruct regarding involvement, symptoms, treatments, and usual course of trigeminal neuralgia (explain procedures as they occur).
2. Instruct regarding signs of complications and progression of the disorder.
3. Teach measures for minimizing stimulation of affected areas.

4. Instruct regarding name of medications, dosage, frequency of administration, purpose, and toxic or side effects of the medication.
5. Stress the importance of ongoing outpatient care and physician's visits.
6. Give referral to support groups.

EVALUATION

Patient Outcome	Data Indicating That Outcome is Reached
The patient and family demonstrate adequate knowledge of trigeminal neuralgia.	The patient is able to explain treatment modalities for the disorder.
	The patient is able to explain the usual course of the disorder.
The patient demonstrates a low level of anxiety.	The patient openly verbalizes concerns and feelings of grief, loss, and discomfort.
	The patient openly verbalizes feelings, supported by health care professionals and family.
	The patient verbalizes essential aspects of care.
The patient demonstrates minimal discomfort from the disorder.	The patient openly expresses feelings of discomfort when they occur.
	The patient is able to utilize measures to decrease discomfort such as decreasing stimuli to affected areas and judicious use of analgesics.
The patient demonstrates an intact, realistic body image.	The patient openly verbalizes feelings of grief and loss.
	The patient verbalizes positive feelings about self.
	The patient acknowledges actual changes in self-image.
	The patient focuses on present appearance and function.
	The patient verbalizes feelings of hopefulness, helpfulness, and powerfulness.

Patient Outcome	Data Indicating That Outcome is Reached
The patient demonstrates social participation.	The patient states the importance of interpersonal relationships. The patient experiences a sense of relatedness to self and to others. The patient participates in unit or group activities. The patient participates in family activities, as appropriate to the patient's condition.

DEGENERATIVE DISORDERS
Amyotrophic Lateral Sclerosis

Amyotrophic lateral sclerosis (ALS) is a degenerative neurologic disease of the motor neurons, which is characterized by atrophy of the muscles of the hands, forearms, and legs that eventually spreads to involve most of the body.[50]

Amyotrophic lateral sclerosis, also called Lou Gehrig's disease, is the most common variant of motor neuron disease. The cause and the cure of amyotrophic lateral sclerosis remain unknown.

The onset of amyotrophic lateral sclerosis usually occurs between the ages of 40 to 70 years, but it may also occur in the very aged. It has an incidence of 2 to 7 cases per 100,000 persons in the United States. In the United States, 95% of the cases are sporadic, and 5% are familial. Approximately two to three men are affected to each woman with amyotrophic lateral sclerosis. The disorder is usually fatal within 2 to 3 years after diagnosis, but one fifth of the patients may survive for between 5 and 20 years. A clustering of cases occurs in the western Pacific regions of Guam and Mariana Islands, where a form of amyotrophic lateral sclerosis is perhaps 50 to 100 times more common than in other regions.

As previously stated, the cause of amyotrophic lateral sclerosis has not been established. Virologic studies have not revealed any disease-specific abnormality, and most ultrastructural studies for virus material have been inconclusive or negative. Immunologic factors have been suggested by the finding of immune complex deposition in the glomeruli of some patients with the disease and the cytotoxicity of amyotrophic lateral sclerosis serum to anterior horn cells in tissue culture.[26] Epidemiologic studies in Guam support a genetic or external agent as a possible causative agent. Other proposed causes include metabolic disturbances (i.e., metal imbalances), inappropriate nutrition, and systemic stimuli responses (i.e., infection, trauma).

PATHOPHYSIOLOGY

The pathophysiology of amyotrophic lateral sclerosis is characterized by the deterioration of the anterior horn cells. Atrophy of the cortex, particularly of the precentral gyrus, may be grossly apparent in the cerebrum. Other pathologic changes include reduced numbers and size of the Betz cells of the motor cortex. In the brainstem there is loss of the motor neurons of the brainstem except for those serving the extraocular muscles. In the spinal cord there is a loss of large motor neurons and degeneration of the corticospinal tract.[26] The surviving motor neurons show pyknotic nuclei and are atrophic. The loss of the anterior horn cells results in denervation of the muscle fibers.

DIAGNOSTIC STUDIES

Serum
Creatinine phosphokinase may be twice normal value

CSF sampling
Mild elevation of total protein with a normal IgG concentration and normal cell count

Myelography
Normal or shrunken spinal cord

CT scan (brain)
Normal; shows cerebral atrophy

Muscle biopsy
Abnormalities and changes of denervation

Electromyogram
Remarkable abnormalities
Useful in confirming diffuse process in monoparetic or unilateral forms of the disease

TREATMENT PLAN

No specific treatment for amyotrophic lateral sclerosis has been established.

Surgical
Cricopharyngeal myotomy to alleviate dysphagia
Cervical esophagostomy
Transtympanic neurectomy to control neural supply to parotid glands

Chemotherapeutic
Antianxiety agents (used for muscle relaxant effect)
Diazepam (Valium), 5 mg po bid to tid
Muscle relaxants
Baclofen (Lioresal), 5 mg po tid; up to 15-25 mg po tid (therapy initiated at low dosage and increased gradually until optimal results are achieved)

Electromechanical
Cardiac monitoring
Mechanical ventilation
Prosthesis to support weakened muscles

Supportive
Physical therapy
Psychosocial counseling and support
Nutritional support: soft or liquid diet
Community referrals

ASSESSMENT: AREAS OF CONCERN

Symptoms of amyotrophic lateral sclerosis vary, depending on which motor neuron cells are affected.

Muscle functioning
Fasciculation of muscles; may be accompanied by weakness

Upper extremity (usually unilateral)
Atrophy evident in palms and both sides of thumbs
Loss of dexterity for fine hand movements
Lower extremities
Spasticity and progressive weakness until flaccidity and atrophy occur
Foot-drop

Bulbar palsy
Fasciculations and atrophy of the tongue
Dysphagia
Dysphonia
Dysarthria
Excessive drooling

Reflexes
Progressive decrease
Increase in pathologic reflexes

Mental faculties
Not affected

Fear
Subjective statements of feeling fearful about health status and future life-style

NURSING DIAGNOSES and NURSING INTERVENTIONS

Nursing Diagnosis	Nursing Intervention
Airway clearance, ineffective	Maintain patent airway; avoid flexion of the neck if patient is comatose. Auscultate for breath sounds every 1 to 2 hours; report any changes. Suction as needed. Assist ventilation as per protocol. Monitor vital signs every 1 to 2 hours; monitor neurologic status every 1 to 2 hours. Keep emergency drugs at the bedside. Maintain nothing-by-mouth status to prevent risk of choking or aspiration. Maintain quiet, nonstressful environment whenever possible.
Breathing pattern, ineffective	See general intervention strategies listed on p. 2030.
Nutrition, alteration in: less than body requirements	Offer the patient frequent, small feedings. Maintain soft or liquid diet as indicated. Have suction equipment at bedside at all times. Have patient eat and drink in an upright position with neck flexed. Apply soft cervical collar if patient is unable to hold head upright. Avoid mucus-producing foods such as milk. Institute IV, nasogastric, or gastric feedings as per protocol.
Mobility, impaired physical	Use braces (hand splint; ankle-foot braces) to maintain function. Teach family turning, positioning, and transfer techniques.
Self-care deficit: feeding, bathing/hygiene, dressing/grooming, toileting	See general intervention strategies listed on p. 2086.
Anxiety	See general intervention strategies listed on p. 1839.

Nursing Diagnosis	Nursing Intervention

Communication, impaired: verbal	Develop a means of communication with the patient:
	    When restricted to eye or eyelid movement, develop a code with the patient.
	    Reinforce the techniques established.
	Assist the patient and family to identify other outlets for communication.
	Continue to use sense of touch and nonverbal forms of communication.

Powerlessness	Assist patient to reestablish as much physiologic control as condition allows.
	    Share knowledge of physiologic functioning with the patient.
	Assist patient to reestablish some means of psychologic control:
	    Encourage patient to express feelings as long as possible.
	    Encourage patient to participate in care as long as able to do so.
	    Encourage patient to become an active decision maker about care and immediate environment.

Self-concept, disturbance in: body image, role performance, personal identity	See general intervention strategies listed on p. 1820.
Social isolation	See general intervention strategies listed on p. 1938.

Patient Education

1. Encourage open verbalization of feelings.
2. Stress importance of dealing with fears of loss of function, changes in body image, and dying.
3. Emphasize importance of maintaining planned rest periods.
4. Stress need for independence and socialization:
   a. Encourage self-care.
   b. Encourage family to eat meals together for as long as possible.
5. Emphasize need to exercise to tolerance levels.
   a. Tell patient to avoid fatigue.
   b. Teach patient and family active exercises and ROM exercises.
6. Instruct regarding name of each medication, dosage, frequency of administration, purpose, and toxic and side effects.
7. Stress need to check with physician before taking any over-the-counter medications.
8. Emphasize need to maintain fluid intake at 2000 ml daily, unless contraindicated.
9. Teach proper techniques for turning, positioning, and transfer.
10. Stress importance of ongoing outpatient care:
    a. Physician's visits
    b. Physical therapy
    c. Occupational therapy
    d. Home nursing care, if indicated
    e. ALS Foundation referral
11. Ensure the patient and family demonstrate application of hand splints and ankle-foot braces.

EVALUATION

Patient Outcome	Data Indicating That Outcome is Reached
The patient demonstrates adequate airway clearance.	Airway remains patent. Breath sounds can be auscultated in all lobes. All lobes move during respiratory cycle. There are no signs of respiratory distress.
The patient demonstrates a low level of anxiety.	The patient openly verbalizes, as possible, concerns and feelings of grief, loss, and discomfort. The patient openly verbalizes, as possible, of feeling supported by health professionals or significant others. The patient verbalizes, as possible, essential aspects of care.
The patient demonstrates an effective breathing pattern.	Airway remains patent. Chest excursion is symmetric. Vesicular, bronchial, and bronchovesicular breath sounds are normal.

Patient Outcome	Data Indicating That Outcome is Reached
	Arterial blood gas values are within normal limits or consistent with patient's baseline.
	Vital signs are within normal limits or consistent with patient's baseline.
	Hemoglobin levels are 14 to 18 g/dl (male) and 12 to 16 g/dl (female).
	Intake and output are stable.
	There are no signs of respiratory distress.
	Skin tone is appropriate to racial background.
	All lobes are resonant on palpation.
The patient demonstrates minimal impaired verbal communication.	The patient verbalizes feelings as long as physically able to do so.
	The patient develops alternate methods of communication.
The patient experiences a minimal level of impaired physical mobility.	Skin integrity is maintained.
	The patient remains free of contractures or deformities.
	The patient demonstrates a level of mobility appropriate to physiologic status.
	Intake and output are stable.
	Nutritional status is adequate.
	There are no signs or symptoms of local infection.
The patient demonstrates adequate nutritional status.	Weight pattern is stable.
	Intake and output pattern is stable.
	Diet is appropriate to physiologic status.
	Skin turgor is good.
	There is fluid and electrolyte balance.
	Dietary supplements are taken, as appropriate.
The patient demonstrates minimal feelings of powerlessness.	The patient maintains optimal level of physiologic control, as possible for current physiologic status.
	The patient maintains optimal level of psychologic control, as possible for current physiologic status.
	The patient participates, as possible, in decision making about care.
	The patient participates, as possible, in self-care.
The patient demonstrates minimal self-care deficits.	Outcome criteria listed for impaired physical mobility are met.
	Level of self-care is appropriate to physiologic status.
	The patient participates in physical and occupational therapy.
The patient demonstrates intact self-concepts.	The patient verbalizes, as possible, positive feelings about self.
	The patient acknowledges actual change in self-image.
	The patient verbalizes, as possible, feelings of grief, loss of functioning, and dying.
The patient demonstrates social participation, as possible.	The patient states importance of interpersonal relationships.
	The patient relates to self and others.
	The patient participates, as possible, in unit and group activities.
	The patient participates, as possible, in family activities.

Multiple Sclerosis

Multiple sclerosis, or disseminated sclerosis, is a progressive neurologic disease that is characterized by disseminating demyelination of nerve fibers of the brain and spinal cord.[50]

Multiple sclerosis is the most prevalent of the human demyelinating diseases, with an incidence of 40 to 60 per 10,000 persons in the United States and Canada. Women are affected with the disorder slightly less often than men. The onset of symptoms occurs between 20 and 40 years of age in 75% of the cases. Onset is rare in childhood, and the onset of symptoms rapidly decreases in frequency in old age. The course and prognosis of multiple sclerosis vary from person to person in severity and duration. The survival rate of individuals with multiple sclerosis is approximately 85% of that for the general population. It is important to note that multiple sclerosis is not contagious. The prerequisites for diagnosis of this disorder include the presence of multiple lesions in the central nervous system and dissemination over time.

Numerous studies have confirmed the well-known association between the prevalence of multiple sclerosis and distance from the equator. Geographically, multiple sclerosis is most prevalent in western Europe, southern Canada, southern Australia, and New Zealand.[26] Within the Unites States, the prevalence of multiple sclerosis is higher in the Great Lakes region, the northern Atlantic states, and the Pacific Northwest.

Etiology

The etiology of multiple sclerosis has not been clearly established. Etiologic hypotheses include genetic, virologic, epidemiologic, and immunologic features.

Genetic features. Studies indicate that first-degree relatives of a family member with multiple sclerosis have 15 times greater incidence of multiple sclerosis than the general population. A person who has an identical twin affected with multiple sclerosis has a 20% risk of the disease, 300 times greater than in the general population.

Virologic features. Individuals with multiple sclerosis have been found to have elevated (i.e., up to twofold) serum and cerebrospinal fluid titers of antibodies to many viruses including herpes simplex, type I; parainfluenza, rubella, mumps, measles, and Epstein-Barr virus.

Epidemiologic features. As previously stated, the prevalence of multiple sclerosis is very low in warm climates and increases in frequency in temperate and colder climates. Studies that have evaluated the effect of migrations of populations on the prevalence of multiple sclerosis have shown that persons who move from areas of higher prevalence to areas of lower prevalence after 15 years of age retain the risk of multiple sclerosis at the level of their previous environment. Individuals below 15 years of age acquire the risk prevalence of the new environment.[26]

Immunologic features. Research indicates that approximately 90% of individuals affected with multiple sclerosis have abnormalities of the cerebrospinal fluid. In particular are increased IgG and oligoclonal bands. Suppressor lymphocyte function is altered, and acute deteriorations are accompanied or perhaps preceded by defective immunoregulation allowing unimpeded damage to the myelin membrane and oligodendrocytes. Remission is accompanied by a rebound elevation in suppressor function.[26]

PATHOPHYSIOLOGY

The neuropathologic changes in multiple sclerosis include multifocal plaques of demyelinization distributed randomly within the white matter of the brainstem, spinal cord, optic nerve, and cerebrum. In acute stages, perivenular cuffs of inflammatory cells have been noted. The active changes occurring include three nearly concurrent processes: breakdown of myelin structure, lysis of oligodendrocytes, and activation of astroglial processes.[16] Within the cerebrum there is a predilection of plaques in the periventricular areas, particularly around the third and fourth ventricles. Accompanying the parenchymal changes may be a mild lymphocytic meningitis predominantly in deep sulcal recesses. The external surface of the brain appears normal. Brain weight may be diminished, and the ventricles may be enlarged. The most characteristic feature of the chronic lesions is a proliferation of astrocytic processes, which transform the lesion into a glial scar. As lesions age, the lipid products of myelin breakdown are phagocytosed.[16]

During the demyelination process (termed primary demyelination), the myelin sheath and the myelin sheath cells are destroyed. The demyelination process leads to four significant central disturbances: (1) a decrease in nerve conduction velocity, (2) nerve conduction block (frequency-related), (3) differential rate of transmission of impulses, and (4) complete failure of impulse transmission. These disturbances account for the variety of clinical signs and symptoms.

DIAGNOSTIC STUDIES

CSF sampling
  Elevated CSF gamma globulin
  Normal or low CSF protein
  Negative VDRL
  Increased WBC count
  Abnormal colloidal gold curve (in absence of neurosyphilis)
  Presence of myelin basic pattern

CT scan
  May show ventricular enlargement and cerebral atrophy (with long-term disease)
  Areas of low attenuation around cerebral ventricles

Evoked response
  Visual: may reveal optic atrophy; impaired in 85% of patients with multiple sclerosis
  Rolandic somatosensory: abnormal
  Brainstem evoked: often abnormal

TREATMENT PLAN

Surgical
Contralateral thalamotomy
Rhizotomy

Chemotherapeutic
Corticosteroids
   Prednisone, 40-60 mg po qd for 8 d
   Dexamethasone (Decadron), initial dose of 0.75-9 mg qd; maintenance dose individually adjusted to maintain an adequate clinical response
Pituitary hormones
   Corticotropin (ACTH, Athcar), 40-50 units bid for 7-10 d
Muscle relaxants
   Dantrolene sodium (Dantrium), initial dose of 25 mg po qid; maintenance dose up to 400 mg/d po
Psychotherapeutic agents
   Chlorpromazine (Thorazine), 10 mg po tid
Muscle relaxants
   Baclofen (Lioresal), 15-25 mg po tid
Beta-adrenergic blocking agents
   Propranolol (Inderal), 40-240 mg po qd

Electromechanical
Braces
Splints
Wheelchair, walker, cane

Supportive
Nutritional consultation
Physiotherapy
Occupational therapy
Home nursing services
Extended care facility referrals
Hydrotherapy
Speech therapy

ASSESSMENT: AREAS OF CONCERN

Sensory symptoms
Numbness and tingling of involved extremity or face
Loss of joint sensation and proprioception (generally accompanies extremity edema)
Loss of sense of position, shape, texture, and vibration (50% of patients)

Ocular symptoms
Optic neuritis (pain with eye movement, visual clouding, decrease in visual field)
Nystagmus (70% of patients)
Diplopia
Marcus-Gunn phenomenon (dilation of affected pupil when light is shone into eye)
"Swinging-flashlight sign" (dilation of affected pupil when light is moved from intact eye to eye with defect)

Motor symptoms
Weakness in lower extremities (initially)
Decline in motor function after hot bath or shower (Uhthoff's phenomenon)
Incoordination
Intentional tremors of upper extremities and ataxia of lower extremities
Staggering gait and spastic weakness of speech muscles
Facial palsy

Vestibular/auditory functions
Vertigo

Mental/behavioral symptoms
Irritability
Inattentiveness
Emotional lability
Mild depression
Poor judgment
Later: memory deficits; depression; confusion; disorientation

Other
Hyperactive reflexes
Positive Babinski's sign
Ankle clonus (50%)
Impotence
Loss or impairment of sphincter control
Loss of abdominal reflexes (80%)
Lhermitte's phenomenon
Charcot triad (intentional tremors, nystagmus, and staccato speech) with brainstem involvement
Urine and fecal incontinence
Respiratory failure

NURSING DIAGNOSES and NURSING INTERVENTIONS

Nursing Diagnosis	Nursing Intervention
Airway clearance, ineffective	Maintain patent airway, and avoid flexion of the neck if patient is immobile. Auscultate for breath sounds every 1 to 2 hours and as needed; report changes in breath sounds. Suction as needed. Assist ventilation as indicated. Monitor vital signs every 1 to 2 hours; monitor neurologic status every 1 to 2 hours. Keep emergency drugs at bedside. Maintain nothing-by-mouth status to prevent risk of choking or aspiration.
Breathing pattern, ineffective	See general intervention strategies listed on p. 2030.
Injury: potential for	See general intervention strategies listed on p. 1990.
Comfort, alteration in: pain	Decrease the noxious stimuli, whenever possible, by assessing precipitating factors and assisting patient to modify or avoid these factors. Assist patient to modify the anxiety associated with the pain experience. Provide other sensory input (e.g., gentle back rub). Administer medications as per protocol: analgesics and muscle relaxants.
Anxiety	Assist patient to deal realistically with anxiety about: 　Inability to predict course of the disorder 　Discomfort from spasticity 　Change in self-image and self-esteem Explain potential treatments for the symptoms of the disorder: 　State in basic terms and monitor patient's response. 　Repeat explanations as needed. Alert other health care professionals and family to potential emotional changes.
Self-care deficit	Assist with feeding, as indicated: 　Use of hand braces 　Use of IV or nasogastric feedings, as ordered Administer oral hygiene every 2 hours and as needed. Assist with daily hygiene care, as indicated. Administer eye care every 2 to 4 hours. Perform intermittent catheterization as per protocol. Maintain bowel function with regular evacuation.
Sensory-perceptual alteration	See general intervention strategies listed on p. 1967.
Nutrition, alteration in: less than body requirements	See general intervention strategies listed on p. 2042.
Urinary elimination, alteration in patterns	See general intervention strategies listed on p. 2077.
Bowel elimination, alteration in: incontinence	See general intervention strategies listed on p. 2074.
Communication, impaired: verbal	Develop means of communication with the patient: 　Pad and pencil 　Magic slate Teach patient to speak in a slow, unhurried manner. Obtain referral for speech therapy. Reinforce techniques established. Assist patient and family to identify other outlets for communication. Continue to use sense of touch and other nonverbal forms of communication.

Patient Education

1. Instruct regarding nature of multiple sclerosis and treatment modalities (explain procedures as they occur).
2. Stress importance of routines for activities of daily living.
3. Emphasize importance of avoiding fatigue, overwork, and emotional stress.
4. Stress importance of regular exercise and planned rest periods.
5. Emphasize importance of diversional activities.

6. Stress importance of speech therapy, physical therapy, and occupational therapy.
7. Encourage verbalization about feelings.
8. Emphasize need for socialization with significant others.
9. Stress need for independence and self-care to level of tolerance:
   a. Support patient when ambulating.
   b. Help patient to walk with a wide base.
10. Instruct regarding symptoms of disease progression and flu or cold to report to the physician.
11. Emphasize need to avoid persons with upper respiratory infections.
12. Stress need to avoid extremes of hot and cold.
13. Teach name of medication, dosage, frequency of administration, purpose, and toxic or side effects.
14. Emphasize importance of avoiding over-the-counter medications.

15. Stress importance of ongoing outpatient care:
    a. Physician's visits
    b. Physical therapy
    c. Speech therapy
    d. Occupational therapy
    e. Home nursing services
    f. MS Society referral
16. Ensure the patient and family demonstrate the following:
    a. Active and/or passive ROM exercises
    b. Proper techniques of ambulation
    c. Proper techniques for turning, positioning, and transfer
    d. Application of hand splints and braces
    e. Methods for maintaining patient safety

EVALUATION

Patient Outcome	Data Indicating That Outcome is Reached
The patient and family demonstrate adequate knowledge of multiple sclerosis.	The patient and family state that the disorder is not hereditary. The patient and family state the nature of the disease in basic terms. The patient and family can identify possible treatment modalities. The patient and family can identify symptoms of progression.
The patient demonstrates a patent airway.	Breath sounds are normal. Chest excursion is bilateral and symmetric. Rate and depth of respiration are normal. Cough is effective. There are no subjective or objective findings of shortness of breath, air hunger, or dyspnea on exertion.
The patient demonstrates a low level of anxiety.	The patient openly verbalizes concerns and feelings of grief, loss, and discomfort. The patient openly verbalizes feelings, supported by health care professionals and family. The patient verbalizes essential aspects of care. The patient identifies methods to effectively deal with anxious feelings.
The patient demonstrates minimal complications of bowel incontinence.	Skin in perineal area is clean and dry. Dietary intake is adequate. Fluid intake is adequate (2000 ml daily, unless contraindicated). Intake and output patterns are stable. There is no fecal impaction. Bowel evacuation pattern is regular.
The patient demonstrates an effective breathing pattern.	Airway is patent. Chest excursion is symmetric. Breath sounds are normal, or there is no increase in adventitious sounds. Arterial blood gas values are within normal ranges or consistent with patient's baseline. Hemoglobin levels are 14 to 18 g/dl (male) and 12 to 16 g/dl (female). Intake and output are stable.

Patient Outcome	Data Indicating That Outcome is Reached
	There are no signs of respiratory distress. All lobes are resonant on percussion. Skin color is not cyanotic.
The patient experiences minimal alterations in comfort.	The patient openly verbalizes feelings of discomfort when they occur. The patient can utilize measures to decrease comfort. The patient verbally validates a decrease in subjective feelings of discomfort. Objective findings of pain are decreased.
The patient remains free of traumatic injury.	Safety measures are appropriate to level of physiologic status. Skin integrity is maintained. Skin is free of bruises, burns, abrasions, and redness. Environment is safe. The patient is free of nosocomial infections.
The patient demonstrates minimal impaired verbal communication.	The patient verbalizes feelings for as long as physically able to do so. The patient develops alternate methods of communication.
The patient demonstrates social participation.	The patient states importance of interpersonal relationships. The patient relates to self and others. The patient participates, as possible, in unit and group activities. The patient participates, as possible, in family activities.
The patient demonstrates minimal complications from alterations in urinary elimination patterns.	Intake and output patterns are stable. Urine is clear, yellow to amber in color, and without sediment. Skin in perineal area is clean and dry. Urine is acetic (pH 6.0). The patient remains free of urinary tract infections. The patient remains free of bladder distention. The patient can describe symptoms of urinary tract infections that require medical intervention.
The patient demonstrates minimal complications of sensory-perceptual alterations.	Level of orientation is optimal. The patient remains free of injury. Skin integrity is maintained. Nutritional status is adequate. Self-care deficits are minimal. Social participation is appropriate to physiologic status.

Parkinson's Disease

Parkinson's disease is a slowly progressive degeneration of the brain's dopamine neuronal systems and is characterized by the clinical symptoms of masklike facies, trunk-forward flexion, muscle weakness and rigidity, shuffling gait, resting tremors, finger pill-rolling, and bradykinesia.

Parkinson's disease is also referred to as idiopathic Parkinson's and paralysis agitans. The progressive, degenerative course of Parkinson's disease varies from individual to individual. Of the patients affected with Parkinson's disease, approximately 30% will experience dementia.

The cause of Parkinson's disease includes known genetic, viral, vascular, and toxic etiologies as well as many unknown factors. Parkinson's disease occurs throughout the world in all racial and ethnic groups. Results of population surveys indicate an incidence of about 130 per 100,000 standard population. The disorder is uncommon in individuals under 40 years of age, with the mean age of onset at 60 years. The prevalence of Parkinson's disease increases with age, and statistics indicate that 1% of the population over 60 years of age are afflicted with the disorder. Family studies indicate that approximately 2% of the adult siblings of individuals with Parkinson's disease also have the disorder.

PATHOPHYSIOLOGY

Parkinson's can be divided into three major types in terms of pathophysiologic mechanisms: (1) parkinsonism-dementia complex, (2) Lewy body Parkinson's disease, and (3) neurofibrillary tangle Parkinson's disease. Parkinsonism-dementia complex is unique to certain Pacific islands and is often associated with amyotrophic lateral sclerosis. The pathologic characteristics of this complex include neurofibrillary tangles found throughout the neuraxis, atrophy of the thalamus and temporal and frontal lobes, and granulovascular degeneration in structures such as the hippocampus.

Lewy body Parkinson's disease involves the degeneration of the pigmented neurons of the substantia nigra and locus ceruleus. Other melanin-bearing neurons of the brainstem and spinal cord also degenerate, such as the dorsal motor nucleus of the vagal nerve, and paravertebral ganglia. The surviving melanin-bearing cells contain structures known as Lewy bodies. Lewy bodies are cytoplasmic inclusions consisting of a central core of filamentous proteins. Radiating from the central core is a less dense array of tubules that may represent excess axoplasmic transport material or degenerated storage granules.[30]

Neurofibrillary tangle parkinsonism demonstrates the following pathologic changes: (1) atrophy of the cerebral cortex with an increased subarachnoid space and narrow gyri, (2) depigmentation (usually) of the substantia nigra, and (3) the presence of neurofibrillary tangles in the surviving neuronal cells of the substantia nigra. These neurofibrillary tangles consist of helically twisted pairs of filaments and result from proliferation of the neurofilaments. Studies suggest a possible relationship between this form of Parkinson's disease and viral encephalitis.

Iatrogenic parkinsonism, which closely resembles Parkinson's disease, may be induced by different drugs, such as the major tranquilizers or, rarely, methyldopa, a-methyl-para-tyrosine, and reserpine. These agents interfere with the synthesis or the storage of dopamine or block the striatal dopamine receptors.[26] The effects of chemical-induced parkinsonism are reversible within 1 to 2 weeks after discontinuation of the offending agent.

DIAGNOSTIC STUDIES

Serum
Mild microcytic anemia

Chest roentgenograms
Slight scoliosis

CT scan, skull films
Normal results (CT scan may show cerebral atrophy, with history of chronic dementia.)

Electroencephalogram (EEG)
Normal results or shows minimal slowing and/or disorganization
With marked dementia and bradykinesia, may show moderate to marked slowing and diffuse disorganization

Cineradiographic study of swallowing
Abnormal pattern: delayed relaxation of cricopharyngeal muscles

Gastrointestinal studies
Hypomotility
Delayed emptying of stomach
Varying degrees of large bowel distention (frank megacolon in patients with severe constipation)

TREATMENT PLAN

Surgical
Stereotactic thalamotomy: produces small lesion in ventrolateral nucleus of thalamus to alleviate contralateral tremor and rigidity

Chemotherapeutic
Antiparkinsonism agents
Carbidopa (Sinemet), 10-25 mg po tid or qid
Trihexyphenidyl (Artane), 2-5 mg po tid or qid
Benztropine mesylate (Cogentin), 0.5-6.0 mg po qd
Amantadine hydrochloride (Symmetrel), 100 mg po qd q5-7d
Ethopropazine hydrochloride (Parsidol), 20-600 mg po qd
Bromocriptine mesylate (Parlodel), 2.5 mg po bid or tid
L-dihydroxyphenylalamine (L-dopa), 100-250 mg po tid or qid
Orphenadrine hydrochloride (Disipal), 50 mg po tid
Antidepressant agents
Amitriptyline hydrochloride (Elavil), 75-150 mg po qd
Antihistamine
Diphenhydramine hydrochloride (Benadryl), 10-50 mg po q6h prn

Electromechanical
Heat massage
Walkers, canes, wheelchairs

Supportive
Physiotherapy

Bowel and bladder program
Nutritional program
Occupational therapy
Extended care facility referral
Speech therapy
Resources available (National Parkinson Foundation)

ASSESSMENT: AREAS OF CONCERN

Initial symptoms
Weakness, tendency to tremble (usually in one hand)
Slowness or awkwardness of affected limb
Some loss of facial expression
Deliberate quality of speech
Tendency to posture arm flexed at elbow
May progress to other side of the body after 1 to 2 years

Autonomic dysfunction
Increased secretion of sebum resulting in scaly erythematous eruptions of skin (particularly by ears and eyebrows and in scalp and nasolabial folds)
Intermittent, profuse diaphoresis
Chronic constipation
Urgency and hesitancy in micturition
Orthostatic hypotension
Dysphagia

Equilibrium
Festination (leaning of the trunk farther and farther with each step):
Propulsion (forward stepping with leaning of trunk)
Retropulsion (backward stepping with leaning of trunk)
Lateropulsion (sidewise stepping with leaning of trunk)

Face
Masklike facies
Decreased eye blinking

Gradual dementia
Initial
Forgetfulness
Minor confusional episodes
Later
Irritability
Paranoia and visual hallucinations
Frank delirium

Hands
Fingers extended with metacarpophalangeal joints flexed approximately 30 degrees

Handwriting
Letters becoming progressively smaller (micrographia)
Tremulous writing

Nutrition
Impaired deglutition
Drooling
Weight loss
Failure of cricopharyngeal muscles to relax

Posture and rigidity
Shuffling gait without arm swing
Akathisia (most evident in spinal musculature)
Hypertonicity

Speech
Involuntary repetition of sentences
Decreased amplitude
Soft, rapid monotone

Toes
Toe flexion with dorsiflexion of proximal phalanges
Great toe may assume continuous dorsiflexion position

Tremors
Lips, jaws, tongue, facial muscles, axial muscles, and limb muscles
Usually resting tremors (most apparent when affected area is at rest)

NURSING DIAGNOSES and NURSING INTERVENTIONS

Nursing Diagnosis	Nursing Intervention
Airway clearance, ineffective	Maintain patent airway, and avoid flexion of the neck if patient is immobile. Auscultate for breath sounds every 1 to 2 hours and as needed. Suction as needed. Assist ventilation as indicated. Monitor vital signs every 1 to 2 hours; monitor neurologic status every 1 to 2 hours. Keep emergency drugs and ventilator at bedside. Maintain nothing-by-mouth status to prevent risk of choking or aspiration, if indicated.

Nursing Diagnosis	Nursing Intervention

Breathing pattern, ineffective	Maintain patent airway. Intubation/tracheostomy and mechanical ventilation may be indicated.
	Auscultate breath sounds every 1 to 2 hours; note quality and any increase in adventitious sounds:
	  Suction as needed. Hyperinflate lungs with 100% oxygen for 1 minute before and 1 minute after suctioning, unless contraindicated.
	Monitor mechanical ventilator, if used:
	  Ensure tidal volume, rate, mode, and oxygen concentration are set as ordered.
	  Ensure ventilator alarms are on and functional.
	Monitor arterial blood gases, as ordered:
	  Report decrease in Po_2 of 10 to 15 mm Hg.
	  Report increase in Pco_2 greater than 10 to 15 mm Hg.
	Note respiratory rate, depth, and level of consciousness every 15 to 30 minutes and as needed based on the patient's condition.
	Check blood pressure, temperature, and pulse rate every 1 to 2 hours and as needed based on the patient's condition.

Comfort, alteration in: pain	See general intervention strategies listed on p. 1979.

Bowel elimination, alteration in: constipation	Provide high-residue diet.
	Maintain activity level to tolerance.
	Maintain regular bowel evacuation:
	  Stool softeners
	  Rectal suppositories
	  Mild cathartics
	  Natural laxatives; prune juice

Injury: potential for	See general intervention strategies listed on p. 1990. Provide the patient with a call light within easy reach. Maintain side rails in up position at bedtime, after sedation, when patient is confused, and as needed. Pad side rails if patient is overactive. Assist patient to change positions slowly (helpful in preventing orthostatic hypotension). Keep walkways clear.
Sensory-perceptual alteration	See general intervention strategies listed on p. 1967.

Mobility, impaired physical	Institute gait-retaining program, if indicated.
	Apply splints and braces, as indicated.
	Continue with physiotherapy program.
	Encourage outdoor ambulation (avoid extremes of hot and cold).
	Encourage the patient to dress daily:
	  Avoid shoes with laces or snaps.
	  Avoid clothes with buttons; use zippers.
	  Place head of bed or chair on blocks to facilitate getting up.
	  Provide raised toilet seat and side rails to facilitate sitting and standing.

Self-care deficit	Assist with feeding, as indicated:
	  Use of hand braces
	  Use of IV or nasogastric feedings, as ordered
	Administer oral hygiene every 2 hours and as needed; control drooling.
	Assist with daily hygiene care, as indicated.
	Administer skin care every 2 to 4 hours and as needed.
	Administer eye care every 2 to 4 hours.
	Perform intermittent urinary catheterization as per protocol.

Anxiety	See general intervention strategies listed on p. 1839.
	Support the family:
	  Provide for ongoing contact.
	  Give appropriate referrals to support groups.
	Assist patient to deal realistically and honestly with anxiety about:
	  Inability to predict course of the disorder
	  Discomfort from spasticity
	  Change in self-image and self-esteem

Nursing Diagnosis	Nursing Intervention

	Explain potential treatments for the symptoms of the disorder:
	    State in basic terms and monitor patient's response.
	    Repeat explanations as needed.
	Alert other health care professionals and family to potential emotional changes.
	Instruct family that the patient is intellectually normal, despite physical disability.

Communication, impaired: verbal	Develop means of communication with the patient:
	    Pad and pencil
	    Magic slate
	    Call light
	Teach patient to speak in a slow, unhurried manner. Provide electronic amplifiers as needed.
	Obtain referral for speech therapy. Reinforce techniques established.
	Assist patient and family to identify other outlets for communication.
	Continue to use sense of touch and other nonverbal forms of communication.

Nutrition, alteration in: less than body requirements	Offer small, frequent feedings.
	Complete nursing care before mealtimes.
	Apply braces if severe tremors are present.
	Encourage a high-protein, high-bulk, high-roughage diet. Provide supplements as needed.
	Allow ample time for eating, and keep food warm:
	    Place utensils within easy reach.
	    Cut foods for patient.
	    Use blender for thick foods.
	Use bibs or straws as indicated.

Self-concept, disturbance in: body image, self-esteem, role performance, personal identity	Reorient to time, person, and place, as appropriate. Carefully explain what you are doing and why you are doing it. Answer questions simply and honestly. Correct misinformation. Protect the patient's privacy. Provide gentle physical care in a caring environment. Provide an ongoing assessment of the patient's interpersonal strengths. Focus on strengths and potential. Assist the patient to become involved in self-care. Assist the patient to become involved in unit activities.
Social isolation	See general intervention strategies listed on p. 1938.
Urinary elimination, alteration in patterns	Assess characteristics of the patient's voiding pattern (frequency, amount). Perform intermittent catheterization, as per protocol. Monitor intake and output. Maintain fluid intake at 2000 ml daily, unless contraindicated. Assess urine for sediment, concentration, color, and odor. Acidify urine with foods such as orange juice and cranberry juice. Administer urinary tract germicides (e.g., methenamine mandalate [Mandelamine]) as ordered.

Patient Education

1. Instruct regarding causes, symptoms, and treatment modalities for Parkinson's disease (explain procedures as they occur.)
2. Stress importance of verbalization about loss of self-esteem, sexuality, and body functions.
3. Emphasize importance of verbalization about feelings.
4. Encourage social participation.
5. Emphasize capabilities.
6. Encourage independence and self-care; avoid overprotection.
7. Stress need for daily exercise program.
8. Emphasize need for high-calorie, high-protein, soft diet; instruct patient to eat slowly and take small bites.
9. Stress need for diversional activities.
10. Teach safety measures to prevent injury.
11. Emphasize need for speech therapy.

12. Stress need for frequent skin care and oral hygiene.
13. Emphasize need for bowel and bladder programs.
14. Instruct regarding name of medication, dosage, frequency of administration, purpose, and toxic or side effects.

15. Stress importance of ongoing outpatient care:
    a. Physician's visits
    b. Physical therapy
    c. Home nursing care
    d. Parkinson's Disease Information Center; Parkinson's Foundation

EVALUATION

Patient Outcome	Data Indicating That Outcome is Reached
The patient and family demonstrate adequate knowledge of Parkinson's disease.	The patient and family state the nature of the disease in basic terms. The patient and family can identify possible treatment modalities. The patient and family can identify symptoms of progression.
The patient demonstrates a patent airway.	Breath sounds are normal. Chest excursion is bilateral and symmetric. Rate and depth of respiration are normal. Cough is effective. There are no subjective or objective findings of shortness of breath, air hunger, or dyspnea on exertion.
The patient demonstrates minimal complications of bowel incontinence.	Skin in perineal area is clean and dry. Dietary intake is adequate. Fluid intake is adequate (2000 ml daily, unless contraindicated). Intake and output patterns are stable. The patient remains free of fecal impaction. The patient demonstrates a regular bowel evacuation pattern.
The patient demonstrates a low level of anxiety.	The patient openly verbalizes concerns and feelings of grief, loss, and discomfort. The patient openly verbalizes feelings, supported by health care professionals and family. The patient verbalizes essential aspects of care. The patient can identify methods to effectively deal with anxious feelings.
The patient demonstrates an effective breathing pattern.	Airway is patent. Chest excursion is symmetric. Breath sounds are normal, or there is no increase in adventitious sounds. Arterial blood gas values are within normal ranges or consistent with patient's baseline. Vital signs are within normal ranges or consistent with patient's baseline. Hemoglobin levels are 14 to 18 g/dl (male) and 12 to 16 g/dl (female). Intake and output are stable. There are no signs of respiratory distress. All lobes are resonant on percussion. Skin is not cyanotic.
The patient experiences minimal alterations in comfort.	The patient openly verbalizes feelings of discomfort when they occur. The patient can utilize measures to increase comfort. The patient verbally validates a decrease in subjective feelings of discomfort. Objective findings of pain are decreased.
The patient demonstrates minimal impaired verbal communication.	The patient verbalizes feelings for as long as physically able to do so. The patient develops alternate methods of communication.

Patient Outcome	Data Indicating That Outcome is Reached
The patient remains free of traumatic injury.	The patient uses safety measures appropriate to level of physiologic status. Skin integrity is maintained. Skin is free of bruises, burns, abrasions, and redness. Environment is safe. The patient is free of nosocomial infections.
The patient demonstrates an optimal level of mobility.	Skin integrity is maintained. There are no contractures and deformities. The patient's level of mobility is appropriate to physiologic status. Intake and output pattern is stable. Nutritional status is adequate. There is no thrombophlebitis. There is no local infection. The patient participates in an ongoing physical therapy program.
The patient demonstrates adequate nutritional status.	Weight pattern is stable. Intake and output pattern is stable. Diet is appropriate to physiologic status. Skin turgor is good. Fluid and electrolyte balance is maintained. The patient takes dietary supplements, as appropriate.
The patient demonstrates minimal self-care deficits.	Outcome criteria listed for impaired physical mobility are met. Level of self-care activities is appropriate to physiologic status. The patient participates in physical and occupational therapy.
The patient demonstrates minimal complications of sensory-perceptual alterations.	Optimal level of orientation is maintained. The patient remains free of injury. Skin integrity is maintained. Nutritional status is adequate. Self-care deficits are minimal. Social participation is appropriate to physiologic status.
The patient demonstrates intact self-concepts.	The patient openly verbalizes feelings of grief and loss. The patient verbalizes positive feelings about self. The patient acknowledges actual change in self-image. The patient focuses on present and future appearance and function. The patient verbalizes feelings of hopefulness, helpfulness, and powerfulness.
The patient demonstrates social participation.	The patient states importance of interpersonal relationships. The patient relates to self and others. The patient participates, as possible, in unit and group activities. The patient participates, as possible, in family activities.
The patient demonstrates minimal complications from alterations in urinary elimination patterns.	Intake and output pattern is stable. Urine is clear, yellow to amber in color, and without sediment. Skin in perineal area is clean and dry. Urine is acetic (pH 6.0). The patient is free of urinary tract infections. The patient is free of bladder distention. The patient can describe symptoms of urinary tract infections that require medical intervention.

MYASTHENIA GRAVIS

Myasthenia gravis is a neuromuscular disease involving lower motor neurons and muscle fibers; it is characterized by abnormal fatigue and motor weakness of skeletal muscles that worsens with effort and improves with rest.

Voluntary muscles most commonly affected in myasthenia gravis include the oculomotor, facial, laryngeal, pharyngeal, and respiratory muscles.

The cause of myasthenia gravis is presently unknown, although there is considerable data that suggest it is a systemic autoimmune disease. Although myasthenia gravis is not a hereditary condition, 15% of infants born to myasthenic mothers manifest transitory symptoms lasting from 7 to 14 days after birth. The incidence of myasthenia gravis is 3 to 6 per 100,000 individuals. There are two characteristic ages of onset: (1) between the ages of 20 and 30 years and (2) in late middle age. When the disorder begins in the second or third decade, women are more commonly affected than men. When the disorder begins in late middle age, men are affected more often than women. Epidemiologic studies have not produced any specific socioeconomic or racial factors relevant to the development of the disease. Clinical studies have indicated that 80% of the patients with myasthenia gravis have thymic abnormalities (10% have a thymoma, and 70% have thymic hyperplasia). The role of the thymus in the pathogenesis is unclear. Mortality for individuals with myasthenia gravis is 15 times greater than for the general population.

PATHOPHYSIOLOGY

Regardless of the cause, the basic physiologic defect in myasthenia gravis is that nerve impulses do not pass onto the skeletal muscle at the myoneuronal junction. This defect appears to result either from a deficiency in release of acetylcholine from the presynaptic terminals or a deficiency (i.e., blockage or reduced numbers) in the postsynaptic membrane receptor sites. Biopsy studies of myasthenic patients have shown that small end-plate potentials are normal in frequency but have markedly decreased amplitudes. Postsynaptic potentials are slightly smaller than normal but contain the normal number of acetylcholine quanta.[16]

Research pursuing the prospect that myasthenia gravis is produced by an autoimmune mechanism has shown that a major feature in the pathogenesis is an attack on end-plate acetylcholine receptors by circulating antibodies.[16] The reasons why these antibodies to acetylcholine receptors develop remains to be elucidated.

There is no evidence in myasthenia gravis of central or peripheral nervous system disease. Involved skeletal muscles usually do not atrophy, and there is no loss of sensation. The primary manifestation is extreme fatigability and weakness of voluntary muscles.

DIAGNOSTIC STUDIES

Chest roentgenogram, CT scan of chest
May indicate presence of thymoma

Edrophonium (Tensilon) test
Marked improvement in 30 seconds to 1 minute, with improvement lasting only several minutes

Electromyogram (EMG)
Muscle fiber contraction with progressive decremental response

Single-fiber electromyogram
Time response variation of two fibers stimulated

Curare test
Myasthenia gravis patient will be curarized with 1/32 of the normal curare dose
Done by a neurologist with anesthesia at the bedside, ready to intubate
Done only if all the other tests are normal or questionable
Frequently seen as the ultimate diagnostic technique for myasthenia gravis

TREATMENT PLAN

Surgical
Tracheostomy
Thymectomy
Bronchoscopy

Chemotherapeutic
Cholinergic agents
Neostigmine (Prostigmin), 15-90 mg po qd
Pyridostigmine (Mestinon), individualized size and frequency of dosage
Ambenonium chloride (Mytelase), 10-25 mg po tid or qid
Corticosteroids
Prednisone, 100 mg po qd
Diphenoxylate hydrochloride (Lomotil), prn
Pituitary hormones
ACTH, 100-160 units qd for 10 d (rarely used)

Electromechanical
Mechanical ventilation, if indicated
Plasma exchange (plasmapheresis)

Supportive
    Physical therapy
    Occupational therapy

ASSESSMENT: AREAS OF CONCERN

Eye muscles
    Ocular palsy
    Ptosis
    Diplopia

Facial muscles
    Masklike expression and mobility (weakness) of face
    Weak voice
    Dysphagia
    Choking
    Aspiration
    Drooling
    Nasal speech

Neck muscles
    Head bobbing up and down

Respiratory muscles
    Breathlessness
    Respiratory weakness
    Respiratory failure, reduced tidal volume, and vital
       capacity

Other muscles
    Stress incontinence
    Anal sphincter weakness

Reflexes
    Normal or brisk

Myasthenia gravis crisis
    Respiratory distress
    Tachypnea
    Increased muscular weakness
    Extreme fatigue
    Anxiety
    Restlessness
    Irritability
    Facial weakness
    Dysphagia
    Inability to chew
    Elevated temperature
    Ptosis
    Speech impairment

Cholinergic crisis
    Respiratory distress
    Vertigo
    Blurred vision
    Sweating
    Lacrimation
    Salivation
    Anorexia
    Dysarthria
    Dysphagia
    Abdominal cramps
    Nausea and vomiting
    Muscular spasms or cramps
    Generalized weakness
    Dyspnea and wheezing

NURSING DIAGNOSES and NURSING INTERVENTIONS

Nursing Diagnosis	Nursing Intervention
Airway clearance, ineffective	Maintain patent airway, and avoid flexion of the neck if patient is comatose.
	Auscultate for breath sounds every 1 to 2 hours, and report any changes to the physician.
	Suction as needed.
	Assist ventilation as indicated.
	Monitor vital signs every 1 to 2 hours; monitor neurologic status every 1 to 2 hours.
	Keep emergency drugs and ventilator at the bedside.
	Maintain nothing-by-mouth status to prevent risk of choking or aspiration.
Breathing pattern, ineffective	See general intervention strategies listed on p. 2030.
	If patient has a thymectomy, observe for signs of pneumothorax:
	Restlessness
	Tachycardia
	Respiratory distress
	Cyanosis
	Diaphoresis
	Maintain patency of chest tubes.
	Provide chest physiotherapy.
	Monitor tidal volume and vital capacity every hour in acute stage.

Nursing Diagnosis	Nursing Intervention
Mobility, impaired physical	See general intervention strategies listed on p. 2106.
Self-care deficit: feeding, bathing/hygiene, dressing/grooming, toileting	See general intervention strategies listed on p. 2088.
Nutrition, alteration in: less than body requirements	Offer small, frequent feedings. Encourage a high-protein, high-bulk, high-roughage diet. Allow ample time for eating. Stay with patient. Accurately measure and record intake on a flow sheet. Administer parenteral fluids as per protocol. Monitor the patient's weight pattern, and report any significant changes. Obtain nutritional services consultation.
Bowel elimination, alteration in: constipation	See general intervention strategies listed on p. 2062. Check patient for impaction every 1 to 2 days.

Communication, impaired: verbal	Develop means of communication with the patient:
	    Pad and pencil
	    Magic slate
	    Call light
	Teach patient to speak in a slow, unhurried manner.
	Obtain referral for speech therapy. Reinforce technique established.
	Assist patient and family to identify other outlets for communication.
	Continue to use sense of touch and other nonverbal forms of communication.

Powerlessness	See general intervention strategies listed on p. 1830.

Patient Education[49]

1. Encourage verbalization.
2. Encourage independence and continued socialization.
3. Deal with fears and body image changes.
4. Instruct regarding name of medication, dosage, time of administration, purpose, and side effects. For anticholinesterase medications:
   a. Stress importance of dosage.
   b. Instruct patient to take at scheduled times.
   c. Instruct patient not to skip doses.
   d. Instruct patient to avoid taking with fruit, tomato juice, coffee, or other medications.
   e. Inform patient of toxic side effects (i.e., diarrhea, abdominal cramping, muscular weakness).
5. Stress need to avoid taking over-the-counter medications without notifying the physician.
6. Teach symptoms of progression or recurrence to report to physician.
7. Emphasize need to wear medical alert tag.
8. Stress importance of avoiding individuals with upper respiratory infection.
9. Teach symptoms of upper respiratory infection to report to physician (i.e., chills, cough, low-grade temperature).
10. Stress need to avoid alcohol, tobacco, and prolonged exposure to heat or cold.
11. Emphasize need for adequate nutritional status:
    a. Give diet as tolerated.
    b. Arrange food and utensils so they can be managed by patient.
    c. Instruct to chew thoroughly, and eat slowly and in small pieces.
12. Stress need for activity and exercise to tolerance:
    a. Plan activities of daily living.
    b. Maintain rest periods as planned.
    c. Do active and passive ROM exercises.
    d. Get at least 8 hours of sleep at night.
13. Emphasize need for diversional activities.
14. Stress importance of avoiding physical and emotional stress.
15. Emphasize need for speech therapy.
16. Stress importance of avoiding constipation.
17. Emphasize importance of ongoing outpatient care.
18. Give available agencies for reference (e.g., Myasthenia Gravis Foundation).
19. Give outpatient or home nursing care referrals.

EVALUATION

Patient Outcome	Data Indicating That Outcome is Reached
The patient and family demonstrate adequate knowledge of myasthenia gravis.	The patient states the nature of the disorder in basic terms. The patient can identify treatment modalities. The patient can state treatment regimen. The patient can identify symptoms of progression.
The patient demonstrates a patent airway.	Breath sounds are normal. Chest excursion is bilateral and symmetric. Rate and depth of respirations are normal. Cough is effective. There are no subjective or objective findings of shortness of breath, air hunger, or dyspnea on exertion.
The patient demonstrates an effective breathing pattern.	Airway is patent. Chest excursion is symmetric. Breath sounds are normal, or there is no increase in adventitious sounds. Arterial blood gas values are within normal ranges or consistent with patient's baseline. Vital signs are within normal ranges or consistent with patient's baseline. Hemoglobin levels are 14 to 18 g/dl (male) and 12 to 16 g/dl (female). Intake and output are stable. There are no signs of respiratory distress. All lobes are resonant on percussion. Skin is not cyanotic.
The patient demonstrates an optimal level of mobility.	Skin integrity is maintained. The patient is free of contractures and deformities. Level of mobility is appropriate to physiologic status. Intake and output pattern is stable. Nutritional status is adequate. The patient remains free of thrombophlebitis. The patient remains free of local infection.
The patient demonstrates minimal self-care deficits.	Outcome criteria stated for impaired physical mobility are met. Level of self-care is appropriate to physiologic status. Diet is high in calories and protein. The patient participates in physical and occupational therapy as indicated.
The patient demonstrates minimal impaired verbal communication.	The patient verbalizes feelings for as long as physically able to do so. The patient develops alternate methods of communication.
The patient experiences minimal feelings of fear.	The patient has no subjective feelings of fear. The patient has no objective findings of fear.
The patient demonstrates minimal feelings of powerlessness.	Optimal level of physiologic control, as possible for current health status, is maintained. Optimal level of psychologic control, as possible, is maintained. The patient participates, as possible, in decision making about care. The patient participates, as possible, in self-care.
The patient demonstrates minimal complications of bowel incontinence.	Skin in perineal area is clean and dry. Dietary intake is adequate. Fluid intake is adequate (2000 ml daily, unless contraindicated). Intake and output pattern is stable. The patient remains free of fecal impaction. The patient demonstrates a regular bowel evacuation pattern.

INTRACRANIAL TUMORS

Intracranial tumors include both benign space-occupying (primary) and malignant (metastatic) lesions. Every age group can be affected by intracranial tumors, and all brain structures and areas are vulnerable. Growth rates of intracranial tumors vary, ranging from the rapid growth of glioblastomas to the almost imperceptible changes of some meningiomas.[26] Brain tumors are named according to the tissues from which they arise. The types of primary brain tumors include oligodendrogliomas, ependymomas, astrocytomas and glioblastomas, medulloblastomas, and meningiomas. Secondary or metastatic tumors include metastatic carcinoma or sarcoma. (See Chapter 16 for a discussion of malignant brain tumors.)

Oligodendrogliomas originate from the oligodendroglia cells that are responsible for the formation of the central nervous system myelin sheaths. These tumors evolve slowly and may be detected on a routine skull roentgenogram because of intracranial calcification. Microscopically, an oligodendroglioma is composed of small, round cells with spheric nuclei.[26] The most common site for oligodendrogliomas is the temporal lobe. This type of tumor makes up only 5% or less of all intracranial tumors. There is a high incidence among young adults who have a childhood history of temporal lobe epilepsy.[30]

Ependymomas are fairly rare in the general adult population and make up only 5% of all intracranial tumors. They are more commonly found in young children and adolescents and account for 20% of brain tumors in this age group. Ependymomas originate from the ependymal cells and astrocytes that line the walls of the cerebral ventricular system and most commonly affect the fourth ventricle.

Astrocytomas originate from astrocyte cells at any level of the central nervous system. Astrocytomas in the adult are usually lateral and supratentorial, whereas astrocytes in children are in or near the midline.[30] Cerebellar astrocytomas, which constitute 30% of all pediatric brain tumors, are usually located just lateral to the midline in the cerebellar hemisphere. Simple surgical excision provides a long survival rate. Brainstem astrocytomas primarily affect school-aged children, for whom there is a high mortality because of destruction of the local cranial nerve nuclei and the long tracts.

Cerebral astrocytomas are classified according to grade (Table 3-6). Cerebral astrocytomas are common between 30 and 50 years of age, making up 30% of the brain tumors for this age group. These tumors have a growth rate that is proportional to their grade. For example, grades I and II grow slowly, whereas grades III and IV grow rapidly.[30]

Medulloblastomas constitute 20% of brain tumors in children and occur most frequently in children under 10 years of age. The tumor eventually will obstruct the flow of cerebrospinal fluid from the aqueduct, resulting in hydrocephalus and cerebellar signs. Without irradiation, the tumor is fatal; with irradiation there is a 30% survival rate.

Meningiomas are adult tumors arising from the cells of vessels, pia-arachnoid, and surrounding fibroblasts. Meningiomas make up 15% of all adult tumors of the central nervous system and its coverings. They occur more frequently in women than men and are found in approximately 40% to 50% of patients with von Recklinghausen's disease (neurofibromatosis).[30] The symptoms of a meningioma are manifested as the tumor indents a local area of the brain and raises the intracranial pressure.

PATHOPHYSIOLOGY

An *oligodendroglioma* is microscopically composed of small round cells with spheric nuclei. Many of these tumors have an astrocytic component; therefore recurrence of the tumor may have astrocytic characteristics.

An *ependymoma* has several variants. The *myxopapillary ependymoma* is a special variant occurring in adolescents, developing in the fifth ventricle (ventriculus terminalis), formed by the caudal opening of the central canal of the spinal cord.[30] Generally, symptoms of increased intracranial pressure are manifested when the ependymoma fills the fourth ventricle, blocking the flow of cerebrospinal fluid.

An *astrocytoma* of low grade (I or II) is gelatinous and frequently indistinguishable from cerebral gliosis. This type of tumor is slow growing and infiltrative. Astrocytomas commonly arise in the white matter. Their cellularity is almost normal.[30] Astrocytomas of grades III

Table 3-6

Grades of Astrocytoma

	Growth Rate	Prognosis
Astrocytoma		
Grade I	Slow	Good; 15-20 yr after surgery
Grade II	Slow	Good; 10-15 yr after surgery
Glioblastoma		
Grade III	Rapid, invasive	Poor; less than 2 yr without therapy
Grade IV (glioblastoma multiforme)	Rapid, invasive	Very poor; 6-9 mo without surgery

and IV are rapid-growing tumors that are characterized by a high degree of macroscopic necrosis. This grade of astrocytoma is not confined to white matter and may grow into areas of the subarchnoid space and the brainstem. These tumors are very cellular, pleomorphic, and necrotic and demonstrate marked endothelial proliferation.[30]

A *medulloblastoma* arises in the caudal cerebellar vermis and is markedly cellular. The cells in the tumor have very little cytoplasm and do not demonstrate differentiation. When they occur beyond the first decade of life, medulloblastomas arise more rostrally and laterally in the cerebellar hemispheres.[30]

A *meningioma* may be one of several cell types, and each may have a different prognosis depending on the cellular variety. The tumor cells are commonly uniform and may form characteristic whorls.[26] Frequent locations for these tumors include the ethmoid regions, parasagittal region, the sphenoid ridge, and the dorsal roots of the spinal cord.

Regardless of the pathologic type of intracranial tumor, signs and symptoms reflect progressive neurologic deficits caused by focal disturbances and increased intracranial pressure. Focal disturbances are caused by increasing compression of brain tissue and the infiltration or direct invasion of brain parenchyma resulting in destruction of neural tissue.[39] Cerebral blood supply may also be altered by the tumor's compression of blood vessels, resulting in necrotic cerebral tissue or seizures. Increased intracranial pressure may result from regional edema, alterations in cerebrospinal fluid circulation, and an increase in tissue within the skull. As previously presented, hydrocephalus results from disruption in the circulation of cerebrospinal fluid from the cerebral ventricles to the subarachnoid spaces.

The size and location of the specific tumor can effect shifts of brain tissue with associated brain herniation syndromes. If left untreated, herniation can lead to infarction and hemorrhage in the upper pons and the midbrain, resulting in pontomedullary decompensation.[16]

DIAGNOSTIC STUDIES

Skull roentgenograms
Erosion of posterior clinoid process or presence of intracranial calcifications

Chest roentgenograms
Detection of primary lung tumor or metastatic disease

CT scan
Identification of vascular tumors
Shifts in midline structures
Changes in cerebral ventricular sizes

Electroencephalogram (EEG)
Marked focal slowing (with rapidly developing tumors)
Rhythmic, periodic, and high-voltage slowing (with increased intracranial pressure)

Isotope scanning
Increased concentration of labeled substance (most useful with highly malignant tumors)

Dural sinus venography
May indicate narrowed sinuses and interference with cranial drainage

Echoencephalogram
Shifts in midline structures

Ophthalmoscopic examination
Papilledema

Brain scan
Increased uptake of isotope in the tumor

Pneumoencephalogram
Tumor localization

Cerebral angiography
Cerebral vascularity
Blood vessel deviations

Magnetic resonance imaging (MRI)
Same as CT scan, without radiation

TREATMENT PLAN

Surgical
Intracranial pressure monitoring
Tumor excision; craniotomy
Shunting procedure
Laser therapy

Chemotherapeutic
Corticosteroids
Dexamethasone (Decadron), 20-40 mg po qd
Anticonvulsants
Phenytoin (Dilantin), 100 mg po tid
Analgesic/antipyretics
Acetaminophen, gr X po q 4h prn
Laxatives
Docusate sodium (Colace), 100 mg po bid or tid
Histamine receptor antagonist
Cimetidine (Tagamet), 300 mg po qid
Antacids
Magnesium hydroxide, (Maalox), 30 ml po qid

Electromechanical
Radiation therapy

Mechanical ventilation, if indicated
Cardiac monitoring

Supportive
Nutritional consultation
Physical therapy

ASSESSMENT: AREAS OF CONCERN

Focal neurologic disturbance
Gradually increasing weakness
Subtle sensory loss
Adult-onset seizures not always relieved by medications

Mentation
Personality changes
Insidious decrease in mentation
Depression
Memory deficits
Judgment deficits

Pain
Headaches with steady, persistent, or intractable dull pain
Changes in character of headaches
Stress-induced headaches

Increased intracranial pressure
Restlessness, lethargy
Changes in level of consciousness
Changes in vital signs (i.e., Cushing response with increased systolic blood pressure, wide pulse pressure, and decreased pulse rate)

Pupillary changes (i.e., mydriasis)
Impaired pupillary reflex
Papilledema
Vomiting
Fluctuations in temperature
Seizures
Worsening of focal neurologic signs
Changes in respiratory patterns

Seizure activity
Preconvulsive (preictal stage)
Aura: flash of light; sense of loss; fear; weakness; dizziness; peculiar taste, smell, and sounds
Cry or scream
Fall to floor
Loss of consciousness
Tachypnea
Convulsive stage
Tonic: rigid body; fixed jaws; clenched fists; extended legs; cyanosis; holding breath
Clonic: urinary and/or fecal incontinence; jerking of facial muscles and extremities; biting tongue; frothing at mouth
Postconvulsive (postictal stage)
Altered level of consciousness
Headache
Nausea or vomiting
Malaise
Muscle soreness
Aspiration: breathing difficulty, choking, cyanosis, decreased breath sounds, tachycardia, tachypnea
Pneumonia

NURSING DIAGNOSES and NURSING INTERVENTIONS

Nursing Diagnosis	Nursing Intervention
Airway clearance, ineffective	See general intervention strategies listed on p. 2028.
Breathing pattern, ineffective	See general intervention strategies listed on p. 2030.
Tissue perfusion, alteration in: cerebral	Establish baseline and ongoing neurologic assessment every 1 to 2 hours and as needed as indicated by the patient's condition, level of consciousness, motor or sensory deficits, cranial nerve functioning, auditory functioning, nausea/vomiting, reflex status, pupillary size, reaction, behavior and personality changes, posturing spontaneously, or stimuli response. Intervene to monitor and prevent increased intracranial pressure: Administer medications, treatments, and IV lines as per protocol. Maintain elevation of head of bed as per protocol. Accurately record intake and output; monitor for imbalance. Monitor serum electrolytes, blood count, and arterial blood gases for abnormalities.
Tissue perfusion, alteration in: cerebral	Monitor values and wave forms of intracranial pressure line, if appropriate: Maintain patency and sterility of the system. Monitor effects of treatments of intracranial pressure.

Nursing Diagnosis	Nursing Intervention
	Correlate neurologic status with intracranial pressure values; notify physician if inconsistent.
	Assist with drainage of cerebrospinal fluid from the system.
	Intervene to monitor and prevent seizures:
	Assess seizure history of the client.
	Institute seizure precautions:
	Padded tongue blade and airway at bedside
	Bed height at lowest level
	Side rails up at all times and padded
	Oxygen and suction equipment at bedside
	Emergency medications at bedside
	Administer anticonvulsants as per protocol:
	Monitor effects and side effects.
	Monitor serum for therapeutic levels of the anticonvulsant.
	Maintain balance between hyperthermia and hypothermia.
Sensory-perceptual alteration	Maintain quiet environment, reducing external stimuli to a minimum.
	Reorient patient frequently to time, place, and person. Introduce self each time you reorient patient.
	Repeat explanations frequently and simply.
	Assist patient in judgments, perceptions, and reorientation as needed.
	Have family bring in familiar objects.
	Maintain planned rest periods, allowing sufficient time for REM sleep.
	Use day-night lighting appropriately.
	Stimulate senses of touch, taste, and position.
Injury, potential for: trauma	Maintain bed in low position at all times unless side rails are up or when nurse is with the patient.
	Provide the patient with a call light within easy reach.
	Maintain side rails in up position.
	Pad side rails if patient is overactive.
Preconvulsive	Have oral airway at bedside.
	Support and protect head; turn to side if possible.
	Prevent injury:
	Ease to floor if in chair.
	Place pillows along side rails if in bed.
	Remove surrounding furniture.
	Loosen constrictive clothing.
	Provide privacy as necessary. Stay with patient; stay calm.
	Note frequency, time, involved body parts, and length of seizure.
Postconvulsive	Maintain patent airway.
	Suction as needed, as indicated.
	Check vital signs and neurologic status.
	Administer oxygen as per protocol.
	Reorient patient to environment.
	Place patient in position of comfort; turn head to side.
	Administer oral hygiene as necessary for secretions and bleeding.
Mobility, impaired physical	See general intervention strategies listed on p. 2104.
Self-care deficit	Assist with feeding, as indicated. Use IV or nasogastric feedings, as per protocol.
	Assist with daily hygiene care, as indicated.
	Administer eye care every 2 to 4 hours, if indicated.
	Maintain bowel function with regular evacuation.
Skin integrity, impairment of: potential	See general intervention strategies listed on p. 2020.
Comfort, alteration in: pain	Modify anxiety associated with the pain experience.
	Provide other sensory input.
	For patients receiving radiation or chemotherapy:
	Explain procedure or medication before implementing.
	Administer antiemetics and antidiarrheal medications as needed.
	Provide frequent skin care.

Nursing Diagnosis	Nursing Intervention
	Provide frequent mouth care.
	Monitor the patient's laboratory values for depressed RBCs, WBCs, or platelets.
	Report to physician.
	Maintain planned rest periods.
	Offer frequent, small feedings to combat anorexia and discomfort of nausea.
Powerlessness	See general intervention strategies listed on p. 1830.

Patient Education

1. Involve family in care, as possible; teach essential aspects of care.
2. Reinforce physician's explanation of medical management.
3. Stress importance of ongoing outpatient care and follow-up visits.
4. Encourage independent activities, as possible:
   a. Alert patient to limitations.
   b. Avoid overprotection.
   c. Stress need for supportive devices as indicated.
5. Stress need for regular exercise program. Teach ROM exercises to family.
6. Stress importance of diet as ordered:
   a. Offer supplemental feedings.
   b. Offer small portions, and instruct patient to chew slowly.
7. Stress importance of safety measures: side rails, ramps, shower chairs, and walkers and canes.
8. Instruct patient regarding name of medication, dosage, time of administration, and toxic or side effects.
9. Instruct patient regarding need to avoid over-the-counter medications without first consulting physician.
10. Encourage socialization with friends and family.
11. Stress importance of verbalization of feelings about anxiety, fear, and body image changes.
12. Teach patient and family about seizures: safety measures and who to contact.

EVALUATION

Patient Outcome	Data Indicating That Outcome is Reached
The patient demonstrates a patent airway.	Breath sounds are normal. Chest excursion is bilateral and symmetric. Rate and depth of respirations are normal. Cough is effective. There are no subjective or objective findings of shortness of breath, air hunger, or dyspnea on exertion.
The patient demonstrates an effective breathing pattern.	Airway is patent. Chest excursion is symmetric. Breath sounds are normal, or there is no increase in adventitious sounds. Arterial blood gas values are within normal ranges or consistent with patient's baseline. Vital signs are within normal ranges or consistent with patient's baseline. Hemoglobin levels are 14 to 18 g/dl (male) and 12 to 16 g/dl (female). Intake and output are stable. There are no signs of respiratory distress. All lobes are resonant on percussion. Skin color is not cyanotic.
The patient maintains adequate cerebral tissue perfusion.	Level of consciousness is unchanged. There is no evidence of neurologic deficits. Pattern of electrolytes is stable. There is no seizure activity.

Patient Outcome	Data Indicating That Outcome is Reached
The patient demonstrates minimal complications of sensory-perceptual alterations.	Level of orientation is optimal. The patient is free of injury. The patient demonstrates skin integrity. Nutritional status is adequate. Self-care deficits are minimal. Social participation is appropriate to physiologic status.
The patient remains free of traumatic injury.	Safety measures are appropriate to physiologic status. Skin integrity is maintained. Skin is free of bruises, burns, abrasions, and redness. Environment is safe. The patient is free of nosocomial infections.
The patient demonstrates an optimal level of mobility.	Skin integrity is maintained. The patient remains free of contractures and deformities. Level of mobility is appropriate to physiologic status. Intake and output pattern is stable. Nutritional status is adequate. The patient is free of thrombophlebitis. The patient is free of local infection. The patient participates in an ongoing physical therapy program.
The patient demonstrates minimal self-care deficits.	Outcome criteria listed for impaired physical mobility are met. Level of self-care activities is appropriate to physiologic status. The patient participates in physical and occupational therapy.
The patient demonstrates skin integrity.	Skin is intact. Nutritional status is adequate. Electrolyte balance is maintained. The patient is free of pressure sores and contractures.
The patient experiences minimal alterations in comfort.	The patient openly verbalizes feelings of discomfort when they occur. The patient can utilize measures to decrease discomfort. The patient can verbally validate a decrease in subjective feelings of discomfort. There is a decrease in objective findings of pain.
The patient demonstrates minimal feelings of powerlessness.	Optimal level of physiologic control, as possible for current health status, is maintained. Optimal level of psychologic control, as possible, is maintained. The patient participates, as possible, in decision making about care. The patient participates, as possible, in self-care.

SPINAL TUMORS

Spinal tumors, although less common than intracranial tumors, are similar in pathologic types. They can arise from spinal nerve roots, the meninges, parenchyma of the cord, vertebral column, or the spinal vascular network. Spinal tumors frequently affect young and middle-aged adults, and most involve the thoracic (50%), cervical (30%), and lumbosacral (20%) areas. The tumors are relatively rare in children and elderly persons. Spinal tumors can be classified according to their location; those occurring within the spinal cord tissue are termed *intramedullary,* and those outside the spinal cord are termed *extramedullary.* Extramedullary tumors may be further divided into categories of intradural, extradural, or extravertebral. Spinal lesions constitute approximately 1% of all tumors in the general population. Men and women are affected about equally, except with meningiomas, which affect women more frequently. Approximately 85% of intraspinal tumors are benign.

PATHOPHYSIOLOGY

Intramedullary tumors, located within the tissue of the spinal cord, primarily arise from astrocyte or ependymal cells. Expanding intramedullary lesions may compress the spinal cord and nerve roots and destroy the parenchyma. Extramedullary tumors can be inside or outside the dural sac and produce spinal cord and spinal nerve root compression. Lesions outside the dural sac are termed *extradural* and include herniated vertebral discs, acute and chronic infectious processes, metastatic lesions, meningiomas (5% to 10%), schwannomas (25% to 30%), and epidural hemorrhages. Tumors located within the dural sac but outside the spinal cord and nerve roots are called *extramedullary intradural* and include the following: several types of glial tumors (e.g., ependymoma); most meningiomas and schwannomas; hemorrhages; and embryonic or congenital lesions. *Extramedullary extravertebral* tumors are commonly associated with bony destruction of vertebrae.[23]

Schwannomas are the most common spinal tumor arising from the nerve sheath and can be found in all portions of the spinal cord. These tumors appear as a firm, encapsulated, rounded mass that contains many small cysts. Microscopically, schwannomas consist of interlacing bands of cells with parallel intracellular fibrils and elongated nuclei that are usually arranged in parallel rows. There are also a number of star-shaped cells resembling astrocytes loosely arranged in the microscopic structure. Small foci of degeneration with cysts are common. Initially, the schwannoma will compress the spinal nerve root in the foramen of the canal, producing localized nerve root symptoms. As the lesion progresses, further compression of other nerve roots and the spinal cord occurs, producing neurologic findings of cord compression. Symptoms are usually asymmetric. Extradural schwannomas are often hourglass or dumbbell in shape with a portion in the spinal canal attached by a narrow band of tumor through the foramen to a part outside the spinal canal. This type of tumor can compress cervical, mediastinum, or abdominal tissue.[34]

Meningiomas constitute approximately 22% of all primary spinal tumors. Most meningiomas are extramedullary. Eighty percent of meningiomas affect women, usually in the fourth, fifth, or sixth decade of life. These tumors can appear anywhere in the spinal canal, but they are most common in the region of the nerve roots, particularly in the thoracic region (two thirds of meningiomas occur in this region). They appear as small, rounded, nodular masses that frequently attach to the insertion of the dendate ligament and extend dorsally or ventrally. Meningiomas consist of groups of elongated cells with round or oval nuclei. There is a tendency toward the formation of whorls, and frequently calcification is present in the center of the whorls. Symptoms are initially produced by traction or irritation of the nerve roots (i.e., radicular pain) and progress to long motor tract signs (i.e., spasticity) as a result of compression. Meningiomas can undergo malignant changes.[34]

Ependymomas make up approximately 13% of all spi-nal cord tumors. They arise from the lining of the internal spaces of the central nervous system and are usually intramedullary. Ependymomas can be found throughout the spinal cord but commonly are located caudally in the conus medullaris and the filum terminale (cauda equina ependymoma). There is a predilection for men, generally affecting them in the fourth or fifth decade of life. These tumors appear as loculated masses in the spinal canal, frequently with fusiform swelling. Microscopically, ependymomas appear as a crowded mass of polygonal-type cells. In the filum they appear as a central core of connective tissue and blood vessels that is surrounded by a single layer of ependymal cells. Ependymomas may extend to 10 vertebral spaces in length and produce symptoms resulting from cord compression.[34]

Astrocytomas and *oligodendrogliomas* are clinically similar and will therefore be discussed together. The oligodendroglioma is a rare type of spinal cord tumor. Astrocytomas, less common than ependymomas, are generally intramedullary, and there is a predilection for men. Astrocytomas appear as elongated, fusiform swellings of the spinal cord. (See Table 3-6 for grading of astrocytomas.) Symptoms are produced by compression of the long tracts of the spinal cord.

The pathologic processes occurring with any spinal tumors can result from spinal cord destruction and infiltration, spinal cord displacement and compression, spinal nerve root irritation and compression, disruption in spinal blood supply, or disruption of cerebrospinal fluid circulation.[23]

Most benign lesions produce neurologic symptoms by compression and displacement of the spinal cord and irritation and compression of the spinal nerve roots rather than by invasion and destruction of the spinal cord. The severity of neurologic symptoms depends on the degree of compression and the rapidity with which it develops. With slower-growing tumors, the spinal cord can accommodate the mass by compressing itself into a slender, ribbonlike tissue. This slow-growing tumor may produce minimal deficits. Fast-growing tumors can produce sudden cord compression, edema, and severe neurologic deficits.[20]

DIAGNOSTIC STUDIES

Roentgenograms
Determine presence of vertebral column lesions and bony destruction

Myelography (with contrast)
Identifies size, boundaries, and level of tumor (with incomplete blockage of subarachnoid space)

CSF sampling
Elevated protein levels

Electromyogram (EMG)
Assistive in differential diagnosis

Queckenstedt test
Positive

CT scan
Lesion location identified

Spinal angiograms
Differentiates vascular lesions from tumors

TREATMENT PLAN

Surgical
Tumor excision
Decompression laminectomy
Tracheostomy, if indicated
Spinal fusion
Lumbar puncture

Chemotherapeutic
Corticosteroids
Dexamethasone (Decadron), 10-40 mg IV qid
Antacids
Maalox, 15-30 ml po or ng q4h
Histamine antagonist
Cimetidine (Tagamet), 300 mg po or IV
Analgesic/antipyretics
Acetaminophen, gr X po q4h prn

Electromechanical
Radiation therapy
Mechanical ventilation, if indicated
CT scans
Soft cervical collar, if indicated
Spinal prostheses

Supportive
Physiotherapy
Nutritional consultation
Psychosocial counseling and support
Extended care facility referral, if appropriate

ASSESSMENT: AREAS OF CONCERN

General signs
Sensory impairment
Slow, progressive numbness or tingling, and coldness in an extremity
Hyperesthesia at level of lesion
Loss of touch, vibration, and position sense (later signs)
Motor impairment
Weakness, spasticity, and clumsiness: spreading contralaterally or homolaterally
Hyperactive reflexes
Hypotonia and ataxia (cerebellar signs)
Spasticity
Positive Babinski's reflex
Paresis
Pain
Intermittent nerve root (radicular) pain, aggravated by straining, movement, and coughing
Persistent back pain
Sphincter disturbances
Urinary urgency
Difficulty in initiating urination
Retention and overflow incontinence
Decreased sphincter control (later sign)
Other
Brown-Séquard's syndrome
Contralateral loss of temperature and pain
Ipsilateral motor loss
Ipsilateral loss of vibration, touch, and position sense

Cervical tumors
C4 and above
Sensory
Vertigo
Motor
Quadriparesis
Atrophy of sternocleidomastoid muscles
Dysphagia
Dysarthria
Tongue deviation
Respiratory insufficiency
Respiratory failure
Other
Occipital headaches
Nuchal rigidity
Down-beat nystagmus
Papilledema
C4 and below
Sensory
Paresthesia
Horner's syndrome (ipsilateral pupillary constriction, ptosis, and anhidrosis)
Motor
Weakness
Muscle fasciculations
Muscle atrophy
Other
Shoulder and arm pain

Thoracic tumors
Sensory
Hyperesthesia band immediately above level of lesion
Motor
Spastic paresis of lower extremities
Positive Babinski's sign
Lower motor neuron deficits
Other
Sphincter impairment

Lumbar tumors
Sensory
Localized loss in legs and saddle area
Motor
Foot-drop
Diminished or absent patellar and Achilles reflexes
Other
Severe low back pain with radiation down legs
Perineal and bladder discomfort
Decreased libido
Impotence
Bladder disturbances

NURSING DIAGNOSES and NURSING INTERVENTIONS

Nursing Diagnosis	Nursing Intervention
Airway clearance, ineffective	Maintain patent airway, and avoid flexion of the neck if patient is immobile. Auscultate for breath sounds every 1 to 2 hours and as needed. Assist ventilation as indicated. Keep "Ambu" bag at bedside. Monitor vital signs every 1 to 2 hours; monitor neurologic status every 1 to 2 hours. Keep emergency drugs and ventilator at bedside. Maintain nothing-by-mouth status to prevent risk of choking or aspiration, if indicated.
Breathing pattern, ineffective	Maintain patent airway. Intubation/tracheostomy and mechanical ventilation may be indicated. Auscultate for breath sounds every 1 to 2 hours; note quality and any increase in adventitious sounds: Suction as needed. Hyperinflate lungs with 100% oxygen for 1 minute before and 1 minute after suctioning, unless contraindicated. Monitor mechanical ventilator, if used: Ensure tidal volume, rate, mode, and oxygen concentration are set as ordered. Ensure ventilator alarms are on and functional. Monitor arterial blood gases, as per protocol: Report decrease in Po_2 of 10 to 15 mm Hg. Report increase in Pco_2 greater than 10 to 15 mm Hg. Check blood pressure, temperature, and pulse rate every 1 to 2 hours and as needed.
Tissue perfusion, alteration in: cerebral and/or spinal	Establish baseline and ongoing neurologic assessment every 1 to 2 hours and as needed. Intervene to monitor or prevent increased intracranial pressure: Administer medications, treatments, and IV lines as per protocol. Maintain elevation of head of bed as per protocol. Accurately record intake and output; monitor for imbalance. Monitor serum electrolytes, blood count, and arterial blood gases for abnormalities. Monitor values and wave forms of intracranial pressure line, if appropriate. Maintain patency and sterility of the system. Monitor effects of treatments on intracranial pressure. Correlate neurologic status with intracranial pressure values; notify physician if inconsistent. Assist with drainage of cerebrospinal fluid from the system. Intervene to monitor or prevent seizures. Institute seizure precautions: Padded tongue blade and airway at bedside Bed height at lowest level

Nursing Diagnosis	Nursing Intervention

	Side rails up at all times and padded
	Oxygen and suction equipment at bedside
	Emergency medications at bedside
	Administer anticonvulsants as per protocol:
	    Monitor effects and side effects.
	    Monitor serum for therapeutic levels of the anticonvulsant.
	Maintain balance between hyperthermia and hypothermia.

Sensory-perceptual alteration: kinesthetic, tactile	See general intervention strategies listed on p. 1967.
Injury, potential for: trauma	Maintain bed in low position at all times unless side rails are up or when nurse is with the patient. Provide the patient with a call light within easy reach. Maintain side rails in up position at bedtime, after sedation, when patient is confused, and as needed. Maintain wheelchairs and stretchers in locked position when transferring patient. Pad side rails if patient is overactive.

Preconvulsive	Have oral airway at bedside.
	Support and protect head; turn to side if possible.
	Prevent injury:
	    Ease to floor if in chair.
	    Place pillows along side rails if in bed.
	    Remove surrounding furniture.
	    Loosen constrictive clothing.
	Provide privacy as necessary. Stay with patient; stay calm.
	Note frequency, time, involved body parts, and length of seizure.

Postconvulsive	Maintain patent airway. Suction as needed, as indicated. Check vital signs and neurologic status. Administer oxygen as per protocol. Reorient patient to environment. Place patient in position of comfort; turn head to side. Administer oral hygiene as necessary for secretions and bleeding.

Mobility, impaired physical	Administer skin care every 2 hours.
	    Turn patient every 2 hours and as needed, unless contraindicated:
	        Change position slowly.
	        Position in proper body alignment.
	    Massage pressure points every 2 hours to stimulate circulation; give gentle back rubs every shift and as needed.
	Use firm mattress or bed board.
	Use footboard or Spence boots to prevent foot-drop.
	Apply antiembolus stockings to lower extremities.
	Administer anticoagulation therapy as per protocol.
	Encourage self-care activities to tolerance.
	Plan all activities to avoid fatigue. Maintain planned rest periods.
	Obtain physical therapy referral.

Self-care deficit: feeding, bathing/hygiene, dressing/grooming, toileting	Assist with feeding, as indicated; use IV or nasogastric feedings, as per protocol. Administer oral hygiene every 2 hours and as needed. Assist with daily hygiene care, as indicated. Administer eye care every 2 to 4 hours, if indicated. Perform intermittent urinary catheterization, as per protocol. Maintain bowel function with regular evacuation.

Skin integrity, impairment of: potential	Prevent pressure sores and contractures:
	    Keep skin dry and clean.
	    Reposition every 2 hours; massage pressure areas after turning.
	    Provide passive ROM exercises every 4 hours and as needed:
	        Perform ROM exercises gently, slowly, and rhythmically.
	        Repeat each ROM exercise three times, every 4 hours.
	    Use footboard or Spence boots to prevent foot-drop.
	Maintain high-protein, low-calcium diet.

Nursing Diagnosis	Nursing Intervention
Comfort, alteration in: pain	See general intervention strategies listed on p. 1979.
Self-concept, disturbance in: body image, self-esteem, role performance, personal identity	Provide for a safe, comfortable, secure environment. Reorient to time, person, and place, as appropriate. Carefully explain what you are doing and why you are doing it. Answer questions simply and honestly. Correct misinformation. Protect the patient's privacy. Provide gentle physical care in a caring environment.

Patient Education

1. Involve family in care, as possible; teach essential aspects of care.
2. Reinforce physician's explanation of medical management.
3. Stress importance of ongoing outpatient care and follow-up visits.
4. Encourage independent activities, as possible:
   a. Alert to limitations.
   b. Avoid overprotection.
   c. Stress need for supportive devices as indicated.
5. Stress need for regular exercise program; teach ROM exercises to family.
6. Stress importance of diet as ordered:
   a. Offer supplemental feedings.
   b. Give small portions, and instruct patient to chew slowly.
7. Stress importance of safety measures:
   a. Side rails
   b. Ramps
   c. Shower chairs
   d. Removal of scatter rugs
   e. Walker, canes
8. Instruct regarding name of medication, dosage, time of administration, and toxic or side effects.
9. Stress need to avoid over-the-counter medications without first consulting physician.
10. Encourage socialization with friends and family.
11. Stress importance of verbalization of feelings about anxiety, fear, and body image changes.
12. Teach patient and family about seizures (i.e., safety measures and who to contact).

EVALUATION

Patient Outcome	Data Indicating That Outcome is Reached
The patient demonstrates a patent airway.	Breath sounds are normal. Chest excursion is bilateral and symmetric. Rate and depth of respirations are normal. Cough is effective. There are no subjective or objective findings of shortness of breath, air hunger, or dyspnea on exertion.
The patient demonstrates an effective breathing pattern.	Airway is patent. Chest excursion is symmetric. Breath sounds are normal, or there is no increase in adventitious sounds. Arterial blood gas values are within normal ranges or consistent with patient's baseline. Vital signs are within normal ranges or consistent with patient's baseline. Hemoglobin levels are 14 to 18 g/dl (male) and 12 to 16 g/dl (female). Intake and output are stable. There are no signs of respiratory distress. All lobes are resonant on percussion. Skin color is not cyanotic.
The patient maintains adequate cerebral and spinal tissue perfusion.	Level of consciousness is unchanged. There is no evidence of neurologic deficits.

Patient Outcome	Data Indicating That Outcome is Reached
	Electrolyte pattern is stable. There is no seizure activity.
The patient demonstrates minimal complications of sensory-perceptual alterations.	Level of orientation is optimal. The patient remains free of injury. The patient demonstrates skin integrity. Nutritional status is adequate. Self-care deficits are minimal. Social participation is appropriate to physiologic status.
The patient remains free of traumatic injury.	Safety measures are appropriate to level of physiologic status. Skin integrity is maintained. Skin is free of bruises, burns, abrasions, and redness. Environment is safe. The patient is free of nosocomial infections.
The patient demonstrates an optimal level of mobility.	The patient exhibits skin integrity. The patient is free of contractures and deformities. Level of mobility is appropriate to physiologic status. Nutritional status is adequate. Intake and output pattern is stable. The patient is free of thrombophlebitis. The patient is free of local infection. The patient participates in an ongoing physical therapy program.
The patient demonstrates minimal self-care deficits.	Outcome criteria listed for impaired physical mobility are met. Level of self-care activities is appropriate to physiologic status. The patient participates in physical and occupational therapy.
The patient demonstrates skin integrity.	Skin is intact. Nutritional status is adequate. Electrolyte balance is maintained. The patient is free of pressure sores and contractures.
The patient experiences minimal alterations in comfort.	The patient openly verbalizes feelings of discomfort when they occur. The patient can utilize measures to decrease discomfort. The patient verbally validates a decrease in subjective feelings of discomfort. The patient verbally validates a decrease in objective findings of pain.
The patient demonstrates intact self-concepts.	The patient openly verbalizes feelings of grief and loss. The patient acknowledges actual change in self-image. The patient verbalizes positive feelings about self. The patient focuses on present and future appearance and function. The patient verbalizes feelings of hopefulness, helpfulness, and powerfulness.

NEUROFIBROMATOSIS (VON RECKLINGHAUSEN'S DISEASE)

Neurofibromatosis, also known as multiple neuroma, neuromatosis, and von Recklinghausen's disease, is a genetic disorder transmitted as an autosomal dominant trait by either parent.

The disorder is characterized by numerous fibromas of spinal or cranial nerves and skin, café au lait spots on the skin, and developmental anomalies of bone, muscles, and viscera. It has an estimated frequency of 1:2500 to 1:3000 live births and is sometimes associated with spina bifida, meningocele, or epilepsy. Approximately 50% of the cases of neurofibromatosis are sporadic and demonstrate no familial history. Men are more commonly affected than women. There is malignant degeneration in 2% to 5% of the cases of neurofibromatosis. Mental retardation occurs in 10% of the patients.

A method for classification of neurofibromatosis is according to central or peripheral involvement. The *central* form is characterized by various combinations of gliomas, meningiomas, neurofibromas, and schwannomas that affect the intraspinal and intracranial nervous systems.[30] *Peripheral* neurofibromatosis shows little evidence of central nervous system involvement, primarily affecting peripheral nerve. The *visceral* form is characterized by involvement of the viscera and autonomic nervous system. The clinical symptoms of neurofibromatosis usually appear in later childhood or adolescence and continue to develop with advancing age.

PATHOPHYSIOLOGY

In neurofibromatosis there is a proliferation of Schwann cells or fibroblasts, which results in a tortuous interlacing of tissue cords that is manifest as circumscribed or poorly defined tumors in multiple areas.[30] These tumors vary in size from minute lesions to those that are several centimeters in size. The majority of the lesions are soft or firm and smoothly rounded or lobulated and occur as nodules scattered along the course of involved peripheral, intracranial, or intraspinal nerves. Often the superficial dermal tumors (cutaneous neurofibromas) sink into the subcutaneous fat on gentle pressure ("buttonholing"). Most subcutaneous neurofibromas occur over the trunk and are asymptomatic. Along with neuromas, there may also be tumors of the meninges (meningiomas) and tumors of the glia cells (astrocytomas, ependymomas, glioblastomas, etc.), as well as small, gliotic or glial nodules within the central nervous system.[33]

The café au lait macule is composed of melanin located deep in the epidermis. Usually it is a uniformly pale brown macule, unevenly round to ovoid, ranging in size from 0.5 to 15 cm or more in diameter. Five or more of the café au lait macules of at least 1.5 cm diameter (Crowe's sign) are sufficient for establishment of a diagnosis even without the neurofibromas. The macules are most frequently found in the axilla (axillary freckles), over the trunk, and over the pelvis. Because of giant melanosomes in pigment epithelial cells, the pigmented areas become even more evident with age.

DIAGNOSTIC STUDIES

CSF sampling
Elevated protein levels

Myelography
Determination of presence of spinal cord tumors

CT scan
Determination of presence of intracranial tumors

Skull roentgenograms
Bone erosion from tumor growth

TREATMENT PLAN

Surgical
Tumor excision
Shunting procedures for hydrocephalus

Electromechanical
Intracranial pressure monitoring, if indicated

Supportive
Genetic counseling
Psychosocial counseling
Support groups

ASSESSMENT: AREAS OF CONCERN

Skin
Multiple cutaneous neurofibromas
Café au lait, pigmented skin lesions with regular, sharp borders in axilla, pelvis, and trunk
Skin bronzing
Sacral hypertrichosis
Nevus anemicus
Macroglossia
Cutis verticus gyrata
Large, hairy, pigmented nevi

Endocrine system
Hyperparathyroidism
Cretinism
Acromegaly
Myxedema
Precocious puberty
Pheochromocytoma

Skeletal system
Lordosis
Kyphosis
Scoliosis
Spina bifida
Pseudoarthrosis
Spontaneous fractures
Dislocations
Osteitis fibrosa cystica

Cranial nerves
Facial numbness or weakness
Visual loss
Deafness
Optic nerve atrophy

Hydrocephalus
Increased intracranial pressure
Vertigo
Atrophy of muscles of mastication

Pain
Paresthetic or neurologic discomfort
Tumors possibly painful to pressure

Spinal nerves and spinal cord
Paralyses
Brown-Séquard syndrome (with large fibromas in cervical or thoracic areas of the spinal cord)

Other
Ipsilateral cerebellar signs (with cerebellopontine angle meningiomas):
Elephantiasis neuromatosa (diffuse fibrosis and proliferation of affected part)
Mental retardation
Epilepsy
Visceral hypertrophy

NURSING DIAGNOSES and NURSING INTERVENTIONS

Nursing Diagnosis	Nursing Intervention
Skin integrity, impairment of: potential	Keep skin clean and dry. Assist with active and/or passive ROM exercises. Maintain adequate nutritional status. Monitor fluid and electrolyte balance: 　Monitor weights. 　Maintain intake and output. 　Monitor laboratory values (i.e., electrolytes).
Tissue perfusion, alteration in: peripheral	Monitor for signs of increased intracranial pressure or neurologic deficits every 2 to 4 hours and as needed. If tumors are surgically excised: 　Monitor vital signs and neurologic status. 　Maintain patent airway and effective breathing pattern. 　Check incision site frequently. 　Administer parenteral fluids as ordered. 　Administer medications as ordered. 　Maintain pain management. 　Keep patient warm and dry. 　Stay with patient, if restless.
Anxiety	See general intervention strategies listed on p. 1839.
Comfort, alteration in: pain	Establish a baseline and ongoing assessment of the patient's pain and response to the pain experience. Promote rest and relaxation. Decrease noxious stimuli, whenever possible. Assist patient to modify the anxiety associated with the pain experience. Provide other sensory input (e.g., gentle back rub). Utilize behavior modification, if indicated. Administer medications (analgesics), as per protocol. Teach the patient about his pain (i.e., ways to modify precipitating and environmental factors).
Self-concept, disturbance in: body image, self-esteem, role performance, personal identity	Reorient to time, person, and place, as appropriate. Carefully explain what you are doing and why you are doing it. Listen to the feelings the patient expresses. Answer questions simply and honestly. Correct misinformation. Protect the patient's privacy. Provide gentle physical care in a caring environment. Provide an ongoing assessment of the patient's interpersonal strengths. Focus on strengths and potential. Assist the patient to become involved in self-care.
Social isolation	See general intervention strategies listed on p. 1938.

Patient Education

1. Instruct regarding cause of the disorder, signs, and symptoms of progression.
2. Stress importance of genetic counseling.
3. Emphasize need for open expression of feelings of anxiety, fear, and changing body image.
4. Stress need for continued interactions with family and friends.
5. Teach methods of controlling physical discomfort.
6. Teach methods of controlling anxiety.
7. Instruct regarding name of medication, dosage, time of administration, purpose, and side effects.
8. Emphasize need to avoid over-the-counter medications without first consulting physician.
9. Stress importance of ongoing outpatient care.

EVALUATION

Patient Outcome	Data Indicating That Outcome is Reached
The patient demonstrates skin integrity.	Skin is intact. Nutritional status is adequate. Electrolyte balance is maintained. The patient is free of pressure sores and contractures.
The patient demonstrates adequate tissue perfusion.	Criteria listed for skin integrity are met. The patient is free of signs of increased intracranial pressure. Present neurologic status is maintained. The patient is free of infections and complications.
The patient demonstrates a low level of anxiety.	The patient openly verbalizes concerns and feelings of grief, loss, and discomfort. The patient openly verbalizes feelings supported by health care professionals and family. The patient verbalizes essential aspects of care. The patient can identify methods to effectively deal with anxious feelings.
The patient experiences minimal alterations in comfort.	The patient openly verbalizes feelings of discomfort when they occur. The patient can utilize measures to decrease discomfort. The patient can verbally validate a decrease in subjective feelings of discomfort. The patient can verbally validate a decrease in objective findings of pain.
The patient demonstrates intact self-concepts.	The patient openly verbalizes feelings of grief and loss. The patient verbalizes positive feelings about self. The patient acknowledges actual change in self-image. The patient focuses on present and future appearance and function. The patient verbalizes feelings of hopefulness, helpfulness, and powerfulness.
The patient demonstrates social participation.	The patient can state importance of interpersonal relationships. The patient relates to self and others. The patient participates, as possible, in unit and group activities. The patient participates, as possible, in family activities.

VASCULAR DISORDERS
Aneurysm

An intracranial aneurysm is a localized arterial wall dilation that develops secondary to a weakness of the arterial wall.

Cerebral aneurysm is the fourth most frequent cerebrovascular disorder. The prevalence of cerebral aneurysm is estimated to be 9.6 per 100,000 in the general population. The peak incidence is in the 35- to 60-year-old age group, and women are affected slightly more often than men. Cerebral aneurysms are rarely found in children and adolescents. Saccular aneurysms are associated with an increased incidence of congenital polycystic disease of the kidney and coarctation of the aorta.[37] Hypertension is found more frequently than in the average population; however, aneurysms occur in normotensive individuals as well.[37]

Ruptured cerebral aneurysm is the most common cause of nontraumatic subarachnoid hemorrhage. At least 28% of individuals with ruptured cerebral aneurysm die immediately. Of those individuals surviving the initial hemorrhage untreated, approximately 50% experience rebleeding within a year. Approximately one third of individuals who survive ruptured cerebral aneurysms demonstrate some residual paralysis, headaches and mental changes, or epilepsy. Aneurysmal rupture is often associated with physical exertion (i.e., sports or coitus), severe emotional excitement, and a sudden rise in blood pressure, but it can also occur during sleep.

PATHOPHYSIOLOGY

No single mechanism has been established in the pathogenesis of intracranial aneurysm. Possible causes include congenital structural defects in the media and elastica of the vessel wall, incomplete involution of embryonic vessels, and secondarily acquired factors such as arterial hypertension, atherosclerosis, and hemodynamic disturbances.

Aneurysms may be generally classified according to their predominant characteristics into (1) saccular, or berry; (2) fusiform, or atherosclerotic; and (3) mycotic. *Saccular* aneurysms constitute 95% of all ruptured aneurysms. They appear as small, thin-walled "berries" protruding from arteries primarily at points of bifurcations and branchings. Because of the local weakness in the vessel, the intima bulges outward, and the sac slowly enlarges, until finally wall dissolution and rupture occur.[16]

Fusiform aneurysms are spindle-shaped dilations of the entire circumference of an artery for several centimeters.

They are characterized by degenerative changes of the elastic fibers and deposits of cholesterol in the intima as well as a fibrous replacement of smooth muscle.[1] This type of aneurysm occurs most commonly along the trunk of the basilar artery. They infrequently rupture and generally produce symptoms by compression of adjacent cerebral tissue or cranial nerves. When rupture does occur, the atherosclerotic or fusiform aneurysm is more often fatal.

Mycotic aneurysms are rare and can result when a septic embolus from acute or subacute bacterial endocarditis or other infectious process produces arterial necrosis that may lead to thrombosis or aneurysm formation. Mycotic aneurysms usually arise in a characteristic location along the distal branches of the middle and anterior cerebral arteries.[54] They tend to be multiple.

Since the saccular, or berry, aneurysm constitutes the majority of ruptured aneurysms, its pathophysiology is further detailed. Saccular aneurysms characteristically occur at specific locations in the intracranial circulation. They primarily are situated on the vessels that form the circle of Willis, at sites of arterial bifurcation. Approximately 85% of berry aneurysms are found in the anterior portion of the circle of Willis and 15% are situated in the vertebral or basilar arteries. Within the anterior portion, there are three main sites of rupture: (1) termination of the internal carotid artery (25%), (2) the anterior communicating artery (23%), and (3) the middle cerebral artery bifurcation (16%).[41] Aneurysms of the internal carotid are frequently large and may be situated either in the angle formed by the internal carotid and the posterior communicating artery or at the site of bifurcation of the internal carotid into the anterior and middle cerebral arteries. Aneurysms of the middle cerebral artery are usually located approximately 2 to 3 cm from the vessel's origin, at the site of origin of the first main branches.[17] Multiple aneurysms, often bilateral and symmetric, may be found in 15% to 20% of cases.

Gross examination of saccular cerebral aneurysms indicates that most have a definable neck and many are multilobular. Thickening, thrombosis, and wall calcification are frequently seen.[11] The aneurysms may vary in size from 2 mm up to 2 to 5 cm in diameter. Most aneurysms have reached a size of at least 10 mm at the time of rupture. Larger aneurysms may result in erosion of the bones of the skull and compression of cerebral tissue and adjacent cranial nerves.[11] Histopathologic examination shows thinning of the arterial wall with fragmentation of internal elastica and degeneration or absence of its smooth muscle wall.

Aneurysmal rupture occurs when the pulse pressure

tears a very small hole in the fundus of the aneurysm, which results in direct hemorrhage into the leptomeningeal compartment (subarachnoid hemorrhage) under arterial pressure. Such a hemorrhage spreads rapidly, producing localized changes in the underlying cortex and focal irritation of the cranial nerves and arteries.[17] The bleeding is commonly stopped by the formation of a fibrin-platelet plug at the point of rupture and by tissue compression. Within approximately 3 weeks the hemorrhage undergoes *resorption*. Resorption occurs by the arachnoidal villi after the leukocytes and macrophages have begun their scavenging.[17] There is a serious risk of recurrent rupture 7 to 10 days after the original hemorrhage.

Massive hemorrhage (i.e., 30 to 50 ml) may produce rapid filling of the ventricular system and basal cisterns or produce a hematoma that locally distorts the subarachnoid space and brain tissue. Aneurysms of the anterior communicating artery lying next to the medial surfaces of the frontal lobes and aneurysms of the middle cerebral artery within the sylvian fissure next to the frontal and temporal lobes are particularly prone to rupture into the parenchyma of the brain. Aneurysms of the anterior communicating artery may rupture into the frontal lobes. Aneurysms of the basilar artery may rupture into the midbrain or diencephalon. Secondary rupture into the cerebral ventricles can occur because these intracerebral hemorrhages commonly extend through the brain tissue.[11] Aneurysmal rupture may include bleeding in nearby cranial nerves. The most commonly affected cranial nerve is the oculomotor, or cranial nerve III, due to the rupture of an aneurysm at the origin of the posterior communicating artery from the internal carotid. The optic nerve is frequently involved with ophthalmic artery aneurysms, and carotid aneurysms in the cavernous sinus involve cranial nerves III, IV, and VI, which act on the muscles and the first division of the trigeminal nerve. Increased intracranial pressure commonly results in distortions that can produce unilateral or bilateral sixth nerve palsies. Most of the cranial nerve palsies that develop in individuals with aneurysm result from hemorrhage in the nerve and not from compression of the nerve by the aneurysm.[11]

Increased intracranial pressure is frequently a sequel of acute subarachnoid hemorrhage and occurs because of several mechanisms. First, an expanding hematoma acts as a rapidly enlarging space-occupying lesion that compresses or displaces adjacent brain tissue. Second, blood in the basal cistern may impede or interrupt the flow of cerebrospinal fluid. Last, if the pacchionian granulations become distended with blood, the spinal fluid reabsorption is impeded.[16] The presence of the increased intracranial pressure may retard subsequent hemorrhage. Cerebral vasospasms are a frequent complication of subarachnoid hemorrhage, occurring in 35% to 40% of individuals with ruptured intracranial aneurysms. The pathophysiology of vasospasms is not clearly understood, but it is believed that certain substances, such as prostaglandins, serotonin, catecholamines, and methemoglobin, are released by the blood into the subarachnoid space. These vasoactive substances are thought to precipitate the vasospasms.[16] Edema, media necrosis, and proliferation of the intima have been described as sequelae to the initial vasospasms. Cerebral vasospasms usually appear 4 to 10 days after the hemorrhage and are characterized by measurable constriction or reactive narrowing of the cerebral arteries. The vasospasms are most evident in arteries adjacent to the site of hemorrhage and tend to be lessened when bleeding is minimal. Vasospasms can produce focal neurologic deterioration, cerebral ischemia, and infarction. The diagnosis of cerebral vasospasms is made by angiographic confirmation of severely constricted cerebral vessels.

Subarachnoid hemorrhages can be graded according to their severity and clinical status. In one method for grading hemorrhages, individuals in grades 1 and 2 are managed medically for an average of 10 days and then surgically treated to prevent recurrent bleeding. Individuals in grades 3 and 4 are medically managed for 3 to 4 weeks in order to stabilize for surgery. Those individuals in grade 5 are not surgical candidates except for life-threatening complications.

DIAGNOSTIC STUDIES

Lumbar puncture
NOTE: Should be done with caution
Increased opening pressures
Elevated protein content (80 to 130 mg/dl)
Increased WBC count
Slightly decreased glucose
Bloody cerebrospinal fluid with xanthochromia (hemolyzed RBCs)

CT scan (serial)
Demonstration of blood in the subarachnoid space
Displaced midline structures
Localized blood clots

Magnetic resonance imaging (MRI)
Same as CT scan

Cerebral arteriogram (four-vessel)
Identification of local or general vasospasm
Outlining of cerebral vasculature

Skull roentgenograms
May reveal calcified wall of aneurysm and areas of bone erosion

Echoencephalogram
Shifts in midline structure

Brain scan
May indicate the presence of local diminution of flow

Serum tests
Electrolyte imbalances
Changes in bleeding parameters (i.e., prothrombin time, partial thromboplastin time, and platelet count)

Plethysmography
Screen for deep vein thrombosis

Regional cerebral blood flow (rCBF)
Mean flow values for both hemispheres and determination of status of cerebral vasospasm

TREATMENT PLAN

Surgical
Tracheostomy or endotracheal intubation
Intracranial pressure monitoring
Ventriculoatrial shunting (hydrocephalus)
Clipping of aneurysm
Ligating of aneurysm
Wrapping of aneurysmal sac
Trapping of aneurysm with bypass grafting
Embolization of aneurysm
Evacuation of intracerebral clot

Chemotherapeutic
Anticonvulsants
Phenytoin (Dilantin), 100 mg po or IV tid or qid (do not exceed 50 mg/min IV)
Phenobarbital, adult, 50-100 mg po in two or three divided doses
Antihypertensive agents
Hydralazine hydrochloride (Apresoline) as ordered
Methyldopa (Aldomet), 250-500 mg IV q6h
Hemostatic agents
Aminocaproic acid (Amicar), 24-36 g IV qd for 3 wk (not given with coagulopathies)
Corticosteroids
Dexamethasone (Decadron), 6-10 mg IV q6h
Analgesic/antipyretics
Acetaminophen (Tylenol), grain X po or rectal suppository q4h prn
Pituitary hormone
Vasopressin injection (Pitressin), 5-10 units IM or subq tid or qid (treatment of diabetes insipidus)
Antihistamine (antiserotinin effect)
Methysergide (Sansert), 4-8 mg, po
Serotonin antagonist (Debenzyline), 10-40 mg

Narcotic analgesic
Acetaminophen with codeine, 30 mg po or IV q4-6h prn
Laxative
Docusate sodium (Colace), 100 mg po or NG bid
Psychotherapeutic agents
Chlorpromazine (Thorazine), dosage individualized (for shivering)

Electromechanical
Ventilatory support
Hypothermia blanket
ECG; cardiac monitoring
Arterial blood pressure monitoring

Supportive
Elevation of head of bed
Serial arterial blood gases
Subarachnoid precautions
Strict intake and output
Intermittent catheterization
Seizure precautions

ASSESSMENT: AREAS OF CONCERN

Assessment findings dependent on the location of the hemorrhage.

Level of consciousness
Varies from brief loss of consciousness to persistent coma

Meningeal irritation
Nuchal rigidity
Positive Kernig's sign
Positive Brudzinski's sign
Fever
Irritability
Restlessness
Later stages: seizures and blurred vision

Visual disturbances
Blurred vision
Double vision
Visual field defects: unilateral blindness

Cranial nerve involvement
Ptosis and dilation of pupil
Inability to move eye upward or inward
Papilledema
Photophobia

Autonomic function
Diaphoresis
Chills
Heart rate changes

Changes in blood pressure
Slight temperature elevation (100° to 102° F)
Altered respiratory rhythm

Motor function
Onset and worsening of hemiparesis
Aphasia
Dysphagia
Hemiplegia
Transient paresis of one or both lower extremities

Increased intracranial pressure
Restlessness and lethargy
Changes in level of consciousness
Changes in vital signs (i.e., Cushing response with increased systolic blood pressure, wide pulse pressure, and decreased pulse rate)
Pupillary changes (i.e., mydriasis)
Impaired pupillary reflex
Papilledema
Vomiting
Fluctuations in temperature
Seizures
Worsening of focal neurologic signs
Changes in respiratory patterns

Seizure activity
Preconvulsive (preictal stage)
Aura: flash of light; sense of loss; fear; weakness; dizziness; peculiar taste, smell, and sounds
Cry or scream
Fall to floor
Loss of consciousness
Tachypnea

Convulsive state
Tonic: rigid body; fixed jaws; clenched fists; extended legs; cyanosis; holding breath
Clonic: urinary and/or fecal incontinence; jerking of facial muscles and extremities; biting tongue; frothing at the mouth
Postconvulsive (postictal) stage
Altered level of consciousness
Headache
Nausea or vomiting
Malaise
Muscle soreness
Aspiration: breathing difficulty, choking, cyanosis, decreased breath sounds, tachycardia, and tachypnea
Pneumonia

Pain
Sudden onset of a violent headache usually beginning as localized frontally or temporally and then generalizing to involve entire head

Vasospasms
Drowsiness followed by hemiplegia or hemiparesis
Aphasia
Focal neurologic deficits

ECG abnormalities
Q waves
Elevated ST segments
ST and T wave changes

Other
Dizziness, nausea, and vomiting are frequent
Cranial bruits may sometimes be auscultated on affected side
Babinski's sign

NURSING DIAGNOSES and NURSING INTERVENTIONS

Nursing Diagnosis	Nursing Intervention
Airway clearance, ineffective	See general intervention strategies listed on p. 2028.
Breathing pattern, ineffective	See general intervention strategies listed on p. 2030.

Tissue perfusion, alteration in: cerebral	Perform neurologic checks every hour and as needed.
	Report any changes to physician.
	Monitor closely for signs of increased incranial pressure.
	Maintain patency and sterility of intracranial pressure monitoring device, if used:
	    Use surgical asepsis for all dressing changes.
	    Monitor intracranial pressure responses to care and treatments.
	Administer medications, as per protocol: anticonvulsants, steroids, antibiotics, antifibrinolytics (monitor prothrombin time, partial thromboplastin time, and platelet count), analgesics, control of vasospasms.
	Elevate head of bed 30 to 40 degrees, unless contraindicated.
	Maintain strict intake and output (1500 to 1800 ml/24 h).
	Observe for signs of dehydration or overhydration.
	Maintain balance between hyperthermia and hypothermia, as per protocol.

Nursing Diagnosis	Nursing Intervention

	Maintain safe, quiet environment (subarachnoid hemorrhage precautions, if appropriate):
	    Private room with lights dimmed
	    Absolute bed rest
	 Elevate head of bed.
	 Provide all care for the patient.
	 Instruct patient to avoid coughing and straining. Administer mild laxatives or stool softeners.
	 Maintain dietary restrictions (no stimulants such as coffee or tea).
	 Limit visitors.
	 Instruct patient not to watch television, listen to radio, or read.

Sensory-perceptual alteration: kinesthetic, tactile	See general intervention strategies listed on p. 1967.
Injury, potential for: trauma	Maintain bed in low position at all times unless side rails are up or when nurse is with patient. Provide the patient with a call light within easy reach. Maintain side rails in up position at bedtime, after sedation, when patient is confused, and as needed. Maintain wheelchairs and stretchers in locked position when transferring patient.

Preconvulsive	Maintain seizure precautions:
	    Have oral airway at bedside.
	    Have suction equipment available at bedside.
	    Pad side rails, if indicated.
	 Administer oxygen as per protocol.
	 Establish means of communication. Identify auras if possible.

Convulsive	Maintain patent airway.
	 Support and protect head; turn to side if possible.
	 Prevent injury:
	    Ease to floor if in chair.
	    Place pillows along side rails if in bed.
	    Remove surrounding furniture.
	    Loosen constrictive clothing.
	 Provide privacy as necessary; stay with patient.
	 Note frequency, time, involved body parts, and length of seizure.

Postconvulsive	Maintain patent airway. Suction as needed, as indicated. Check vital signs and neurologic status. Administer oxygen as per protocol. Reorient patient to environment. Place patient in position of comfort, and turn head to side. Administer oral hygiene as necessary for secretions and bleeding.
Mobility, impaired physical	See general intervention strategies listed on p. 2106. Encourage mobility to tolerance, unless contraindicated with subarachnoid hemorrhage precautions. Encourage self-care activities to tolerance unless contraindicated with subarachnoid hemorrhage precautions. Plan all activities to avoid fatigue; maintain planned rest periods. Obtain physical therapy referral.
Skin integrity, impairment of: potential	See general intervention strategies listed on p. 2020.
Bowel elimination, alteration in: incontinence	See general intervention strategies listed on p. 2074.
Urinary elimination, alteration in patterns	See general intervention strategies listed on p. 2079.
Anxiety	See general intervention strategies listed on p. 1839.
Communication, impaired: verbal	Develop a means of communication with the patient: pencil, magic slate, or call light within easy reach. Reinforce the techniques established. Assist patient and family to identify other outlets for communication. Continue to use sense of touch and nonverbal forms of communication.

Patient Education[49]

1. Involve family in care, as possible; teach essential aspects of care.
2. Reinforce physician's explanation of medical management.
3. Stress importance of ongoing outpatient care and follow-up visits.
4. Stress need for regular exercise program:
   a. Teach ROM exercises to family.
   b. Instruct person to perform ROM exercises to all body joints every 2 to 4 hours.
5. Encourage independent activities, as possible:
   a. Be alert to limitations.
   b. Avoid overprotection.
   c. Instruct regarding need for supportive devices as indicated (wheelchair, braces, walker, canes, overhead trapeze).
6. Stress importance of diet as ordered:
   a. Offer supplemental feedings.
   b. Offer small portions, and instruct patient to chew slowly.
   c. Arrange food and utensils within easy reach.
   d. Avoid foods such as soft breads, mashed potatoes, semicooked vegetables and large pieces of meat that can cause choking.
7. Stress importance of safety measures:
   a. Side rails
   b. Ramps
   c. Shower chains
   d. Removal of scatter rugs
   e. Walker, canes, flat shoes
8. Instruct patient regarding name of medication, dosage, time of administration and toxic or side effects
9. Instruct patient regarding need to avoid over-the-counter medications without first consulting physician.
10. Encourage socialization with friends and family.
11. Stress importance of communication:
    a. Speak slowly and distinctly.
    b. Use one-word commands and short sentences. Repeat as needed.
    c. Use gestures and touch when giving directions. Maintain eye contact.
    d. Implement speech exercises twice a day.
12. Stress importance of verbalization of feelings about anxiety, fear, and body image changes.
13. Teach patient and family about seizures (i.e., safety measures and who to contact).

EVALUATION

Patient Outcome	Data Indicating That Outcome is Reached
The patient demonstrates a patent airway.	Breath sounds are normal. Chest excursion is bilateral and symmetric. Rate and depth of respirations are normal. Cough is effective. There are no subjective or objective findings of shortness of breath, air hunger, or dyspnea on exertion.
The patient demonstrates an effective breathing pattern.	Airway is patent. Chest excursion is symmetric. Breath sounds are normal, or there is no increase in adventitious sounds. Arterial blood gas values are within normal ranges or consistent with patient's baseline. Vital signs are within normal ranges or consistent with patient's baseline. Hemoglobin levels are 14 to 18 g/dl (male) and 12 to 16 g/dl (female). Intake and output are stable. There are no signs of respiratory distress. All lobes are resonant on percussion. Skin color is not cyanotic.
The patient maintains adequate cerebral tissue perfusion.	Level of consciousness is unchanged. There is no evidence of neurologic deficits. Pattern of electrolytes is stable. There is no seizure activity.
The patient demonstrates skin integrity.	Skin is intact. Nutritional status is adequate.

Patient Outcome	Data Indicating That Outcome is Reached
	Electrolyte balance is maintained. The patient remains free of pressure sores and contractures.
The patient demonstrates a low level of anxiety.	The patient openly verbalizes concerns and feelings of grief, loss, and discomfort. The patient openly verbalizes feelings, supported by health care professionals and family. The patient verbalizes essential aspects of care. The patient can identify methods to effectively deal with anxious feelings.
The patient demonstrates minimal impaired verbal communication.	The patient verbalizes feelings for as long as physically able to do so. The patient develops alternate methods of communication.
The patient demonstrates minimal complications of bowel incontinence.	Skin in perineal area is clean and dry. Dietary intake is adequate. Fluid intake is adequate (2000 ml daily unless contraindicated). Intake and output pattern is stable. The patient is free of fecal impaction. The patient demonstrates a regular bowel evacuation pattern.
The patient demonstrates minimal complications of sensory-perceptual alterations.	Level of orientation is optimal. The patient remains free of injury. Skin integrity is maintained. Nutritional status is adequate. Self-care deficits are minimal. Social participation is appropriate to physiologic status.
The patient remains free of traumatic injury.	Safety measures are appropriate to level of physiologic status. Skin integrity is maintained. Skin is free of bruises, burns, abrasions, and redness. Environment is safe. The patient is free of nosocomial infections.
The patient demonstrates an optimal level of mobility.	Skin integrity is maintained. The patient remains free of contractures and deformities. Level of mobility is appropriate to physiologic status. Nutritional status is adequate. Intake and output pattern is stable. The patient remains free of thrombophlebitis. The patient remains free of local infection. The patient participates in an ongoing physical therapy program.

Stroke

Stroke, or cerebrovascular accident, is a pathologic condition of the cerebral blood vessels in which the vessels are occluded by an embolus or cerebrovascular hemorrhage, resulting in ischemia of the area of the brain normally perfused by the damaged vessels.[50]

The sequelae of a stroke depend on the extent and the location of the ischemia. It is ranked as the third leading cause of death in the United States and accounts for approximately 200,000 deaths annually. Furthermore, stroke is the second cause of chronic disability and illness, with approximately 200,000 individuals experiencing some degree of disability from the residual effects. Statistics from 1980 indicate that stroke has an incidence of 196 per 100,000 general population. Individuals in the age range of 25 to 64 are affected, but incidence increases rapidly from age 35 upward. The greatest increase in frequency occurs between 75 and 85 years of age.[23] Epidemiologic studies indicate variations in incidence in different geographic areas in the United States and in other parts of the world.

Certain risk factors that may predispose an individual to a stroke have been identified through ongoing research. The major risk factor identified in the stroke syndrome is hypertension. Risk factors showing some familial tendencies include diabetes mellitus, hypertension, cardiac disease, and high serum cholesterol. The risk factors of obesity, sedentary life-style, cigarette smoking, stress, and high serum levels of cholesterol, lipoprotein, and triglycerides make the individual a high-risk candidate for stroke. In women the use of oral contraceptives and cigarette smoking increase the risk of stroke. Combinations of risk factors put the individual at a greater risk.[10]

PATHOPHYSIOLOGY

The pathologic mechanisms of stroke can be divided into three categories: hemorrhage, occlusion, and hypotension. The three categories are more commonly listed as hemorrhagic, thrombotic, and embolic in most recent vascular literature. The major types of stroke are (1) hemorrhage, which may be subarachnoid from rupture of the subarachnoid artery or intraparenchymal from rupture of an intraparenchymal artery; (2) embolic occlusion from tumors, valvular cardiac diseases, and most commonly, plaques released from cerebral vessels that produce infarctions; and (3) thrombotic arterial occlusion producing various ischemic or hypoxic insults.[30]

Cerebral Hemorrhage

Intraparenchymal or intracerebral hemorrhage is most commonly caused by hypertensive vascular disease.

The pathogenesis of hypertensive cerebral hemorrhage is not completely understood. Several facts about this type of hemorrhage are known: (1) the hemorrhage usually occurs in relation to some mild exertion; and (2) it occurs in individuals who have experienced significant increases in systolic-diastolic pressures for several years. Some researchers theorized that microaneurysms, known as *Charcot-Bouchard aneurysms*, in small arteries or arteriolar necrosis may precipitate the bleeding. The major sites of bleeding in hypertensive cerebral hemorrhage include the following: putamen (55%), cortex and subcortex (15%), thalamus (10%), pons (10%), and the cerebellar hemisphere (10%).[41]

Since hypertensive vascular disorders primarily affect the smaller arteries and arterioles, the following changes are seen: thickening of vessel walls, increase in cellularity of some vessels, and hyalinization, possibly with necrosis.[41]

Resolution of the hemorrhage occurs via resorption and begins when macrophages and reactive fibrillary astrocytes appear. After the tissue has been cleared of blood by the macrophages, there results a cavity that is surrounded by dense, fibrillary gliosis and hemosiderin-laden macrophages.[41]

Cerebral Infarction

Cerebral infarction results when a local area of brain tissue is deprived of blood supply because of some type of vascular occlusion. Several hypotheses regarding the pathogenesis of cerebral infarcts include the following: (1) abrupt vessel occlusion (i.e., embolus) will generally result in tissue infarction in the distribution supply of the occluded vessel; (2) gradual vessel occlusion (i.e., atheroma) may not necessarily result in an infarction if collateral blood supply is sufficient; and (3) vessels that are stenosed but not completely occluded may precipitate an infarction if the collateral blood supply to the hypoxic area becomes comprised.[41]

The most common causes of vascular occlusions are cerebral thrombi and cerebral emboli. Thrombi usually occur in larger vessels (i.e., internal carotids) and are associated with localized damage to the vessel wall at the point of occlusion. Atherosclerosis and hypotension are the most important underlying processes, but other types of vascular injury (i.e., arteritis) can initiate thrombosis. Emboli usually affect smaller vessels and are commonly found at points of narrowed vessel lumen and bifurcation. The sources of cerebral emboli vary, but the most common is a mural thrombus in the left atrium or ventricle. Septic emboli may originate from bacterial endocarditis. Cerebral infarcts from embolic occlusions are frequently hemorrhagic, whereas thrombotic infarcts are bland or ischemic. Emboli most frequently occur in the middle cerebral artery.

On examination a cerebral infarction may be ischemic or hemorrhagic. *Ischemic* infarctions are usually not demonstrable on gross examination for 6 to 12 hours. The initial change of the affected area is a slight discoloration and softening with the gray matter taking on a muddy color and the white matter losing its normal fine-grained appearance.[41] Forty-eight to seventy-two hours after the infarct, necrosis, circumlesional swelling, and mushy disintegration of the affected area are evident. Eventually there is liquefaction and cyst formation, which is surrounded by a firm glial tissue.

Histologic changes after an infarction include cell body changes, interruption and disintegration of the myelin sheath and axis cylinder, and loss of oligodendroglia and astrocytes. Approximately 48 hours after infarct, polymorphonuclear leukocytes begin to appear. At 78 to 96 hours, macrophages appear about blood vessels.

Hemorrhagic infarctions usually occur in the cerebral cortex and result from a reflow of blood into the infarcted area. This reperfusion is caused by a fragmentation or lysis of the embolus or a reduction of vascular compression and reestablishment of blood flow.[41] Hemorrhagic infarcts therefore are originally ischemic.

DIAGNOSTIC STUDIES

Computerized tomography (CT scan)

Infarct: appears initially (24 hours) as area of decreased density surrounded by area of intermediate density; shifts in midline structures and ventricular system

Older infarct: area of low density extending toward cortex or shift in ventricular system toward lesion

Magnetic resonance imaging (MRI)
Same as CT scan
Hemorrhage: rounded shape and uniformly high density

Cerebral arteriography
Vessel abnormalities

Lumbar puncture*
Increased pressure
Bloody spinal fluid

Electroencephalography
May show focal slowing around area of lesion

Brain scan
Diminished perfusion
Detection of infarction, encapsulated hemorrhage, hematoma, and arteriovenous malformations

*Perform with caution.

Digital subtraction angiography
Shows occlusion or narrowing of large vessels, particularly carotid artery occlusions

B mode ultrasound
Outlines with ultrasound the flow of blood through large neck vessels

Skull roentgenogram
Pineal position
Intracranial calcifications

Echoencephalography
Detection of shifts in midline structures
Displaced ventricles

Doppler ultrasonography
Measurement of direction and velocity of blood flow through vessels

OPG studies
Retinal artery pressures

ASSESSMENT: AREAS OF CONCERN

The following table summarizes assessment findings and diagnostic studies in seven types of strokes.

	Intracerebral Hemorrhage	Subarachnoid Hemorrhage	Subdural Hemorrhage
Onset	Rapid; minutes to 1-2h	Sudden; varied progression	Insidious; occasionally acute
Duration	Permanent if lesion is large; small lesions are potentially reversible	Variable; complete clearing may occur in days or weeks	Hours to months
Relation to activity	Usually occurs during activity	Most commonly related to head trauma	Usually related to head trauma
Contributing or associated factors	Hypertensive cardiovascular disease; coagulation defects	Intracerebral arterial aneurysm; trauma; vascular malformations	Chronic alcoholism
Sensorium	Coma common	Coma common	Generally clouded
Nuchal (neck) rigidity	Frequently present	Present	Rare
Location of cerebral deficit	Focal; arterial syndrome not common	Diffuse aneurysm may give focal sign before and after	Frontal lobe signs; ipsilateral pupil may dilate
Convulsions	Common	Common	Infrequent
Cerebrospinal fluid	Bloody unless hemorrhage entirely intracerebral	Grossly bloody; increased pressure	Normal to slightly elevated protein
Skull x-ray films	Pineal shift, edema, hemorrhage, or hematoma	Normal or calcified aneurysm	Frequent contralateral shift of pineal gland

TREATMENT PLAN

Surgical
Carotid endarterectomy
Anastomosis of superior temporal artery and middle cerebral artery
Intracranial pressure monitoring
Endotracheal intubation or tracheostomy
Evacuation of intracerebral clot or hematoma

Chemotherapeutic
Anticoagulants
    Warfarin sodium (Coumadin), loading doses: 40-60 mg (adult), 20-30 mg (elderly); maintenance dose: 5-10 mg
Antihypertensives
    Diazoxide (Hyperstat), 5 mg/kg IV
Diuretic
    Furosemide (Lasix), 40-80 mg IV, 30-60 min before each dose of diazoxide
Corticosteroids
    Dexamethasone (Decadron), 10 mg initially, then 4 mg q4-6h IV or IM

Anticonvulsants
    Phenytoin (Dilantin), 100-600 mg/d
Narcotic analgesic
    Codeine, 30-60 mg q3-4h
Analgesic/antipyretics
    Acetaminophen, gr X q4h po or rectal suppository
Antacids

Electromechanical
Mechanical ventilation
Hypothermia blanket
ECG and cardiac monitoring

Supportive
Subarachnoid precautions
Strict intake and output
Bed rest
Elevation of head of bed
Nasogastric tube
Foley or indwelling catheter
Elastic stockings
Serial arterial blood gases
Seizure precautions

Extradural Hemorrhage	Focal Cerebral Ischemia	Cerebral Thrombosis	Cerebral Embolism
Rapid; minutes to hours	Rapid; seconds to minutes	Minutes to hours	Sudden
Initially fluctuating; then steadily progressive	Seconds to minutes	Permanent if lesion is large; potentially reversible if lesion is small	Rapid improvement may occur depending on collateral flow
Almost always related to head trauma	Occurs during activity if related to decreased cardiac output	Usually occurs at rest	Unrelated to activity
Any condition that predisposes to trauma	Peripheral and coronary atherosclerosis; hypertension	Peripheral and coronary atherosclerosis; hypertension	Atrial fibrillation; aortic and mitral valve disease; myocardial infarct; atherosclerotic plaque
Rapidly advancing coma	Usually conscious	Usually conscious	Usually conscious
Rare	Absent	Absent	Absent
Temporal lobe signs; ipsilateral pupil may dilate; high intracranial pressure	Focal; or arterial syndrome	Focal; or arterial syndrome	Focal; or arterial syndrome
Common	Rare	Rare	Rare
Increased pressure; color and cells usually normal	Usually normal	Usually normal	Usually normal
Frequently fracture across middle meningeal artery groove	May show calcification of intracranial arteries	Possible arterial calcification and pineal shift from edema	Usually normal

NURSING DIAGNOSES and NURSING INTERVENTIONS

Nursing Diagnosis	Nursing Intervention
Airway clearance, ineffective	See general intervention strategies listed on p. 2028.
Breathing pattern, ineffective	See general intervention strategies listed on p. 2030.
Tissue perfusion, alteration in: cerebral	Perform neurologic checks every hour and as needed. Report any changes. Monitor closely for signs of increased intracranial pressure. Maintain patency and sterility of intracranial pressure monitoring device, if used: Use surgical asepsis for all dressing changes. Monitor intracranial pressure responses to care and treatments. Administer medications, as per protocol: anticonvulsants, steroids, antibiotics, antifibrinolytics (monitor prothrombin time, partial thromboplastin time, and platelets), analgesics, and agent for control of vasospasms. Elevate head of bed 30 to 40 degrees, unless contraindicated. Maintain strict intake and output (1500 to 1800 ml/24 h). Observe for signs of dehydration or overhydration. Maintain balance between hyperthermia and hypothermia, as per protocol. Maintain safe, quiet environment (subarachnoid hemorrhage precautions, if appropriate): Have patient in private room with lights dimmed. Use absolute bed rest. Elevate head of bed. Provide all care for the patient. Instruct patient to avoid coughing and straining. Administer mild laxatives or stool softeners. Maintain dietary restrictions (no stimulants such as coffee and tea). Limit visitors. Instruct patient not to watch television, listen to radio, or read.
Sensory-perceptual alteration: kinesthetic, tactile	See general intervention strategies listed on p. 1967.
Injury, potential for: trauma	Maintain bed in low position at all times unless side rails are up or when nurse is with patient. Provide patient with a call light within easy reach. Maintain side rails in up position at bedtime, after sedation, when patient is confused, and as needed. Maintain wheelchairs and stretchers in locked position when transferring patient.
Preconvulsive	Maintain seizure precautions: Have oral airway at bedside. Have suction equipment available at bedside. Pad side rails, if indicated. Administer oxygen as per protocol. Establish means of communication; identify auras if possible.
Convulsive	Maintain patent airway. Support and protect head; turn to side if possible. Prevent injury: Ease to floor if in chair. Place pillows along side rails if in bed. Remove surrounding furniture. Loosen constrictive clothing. Provide privacy as necessary. Stay with patient. Note frequency, time, involved body parts, and length of seizure.
Postconvulsive	Maintain patent airway. Suction as needed, as indicated. Check vital signs and neurologic status. Administer oxygen as per protocol. Reorient patient to environment. Place patient in position of comfort, and turn head to side. Administer oral hygiene as necessary for secretions and bleeding.

Nursing Diagnosis	Nursing Intervention

Mobility, impaired physical	Administer skin care every 2 hours:
	  Turn patient every 2 hours and as needed, unless contraindicated:
	    Change position slowly.
	    Position in proper body alignment.
	    Keep skin dry; administer perineal care as needed.
	    Massage pressure points every 2 hours to stimulate circulation; give gentle back rubs every shift and as needed.
	    Use air mattress.
	    Use firm mattress or bedboard.
	    Perform active or passive ROM exercises every 2 to 4 hours.
	Perform dorsiflexion of quadriceps and ankles every 2 to 4 hours.
	Assist out of bed to chair two or three times daily; unless contraindicated.
	Use footboard or Spence boots to prevent foot-drop.
	Administer anticoagulation therapy as per protocol.
	Monitor nutritional status.
	Encourage mobility to tolerance unless contraindicated with subarachnoid hemorrhage precautions.
	Encourage self-care activities to tolerance unless contraindicated with subarachnoid hemorrhage precautions.
	Plan all activities to avoid fatigue; maintain planned rest periods.
	Obtain physical therapy referral.
	Encourage diversional activities, if appropriate.

Self-care deficit: feeding, bathing/hygiene, dressing/grooming, toileting	Assist with feeding, if indicated; use IV or nasogastric feedings, as ordered. Administer oral hygiene every 2 hours and as needed. Assist with daily hygiene care, as indicated. Administer eye care every 2 to 4 hours, if indicated. Insert indwelling urinary catheter, or do intermittent urinary catheterizations as per protocol. Maintain bowel function with regular evacuation.
Skin integrity, impairment of: potential	See general intervention strategies listed on p. 2020.
Self-concept, disturbance in: body image, self-esteem, role performance, personal identity	See general intervention strategies listed on p. 1820.
Bowel elimination, alteration in: incontinence	See general intervention strategies listed on p. 2074.
Urinary elimination, alteration in patterns	See general intervention strategies listed on p. 2079.

Powerlessness	Assist patient to reestablish as much physiologic control as condition allows.
	  Share knowledge of physiologic functioning with patient and family.
	Assist patient to reestablish some means of psychologic control:
	  Encourage patient to express feelings.
	  Encourage patient and family to participate in care.
	  Encourage patient to become an active decision maker about care and immediate environment.

Communication, impaired: verbal	Develop a means of communication with patient: pencil, magic slate, or call light within easy reach. Reinforce the techniques established. Assist patient and family to identify other outlets for communication. Continue to use sense of touch and nonverbal forms of communication.

Patient Education

1. Involve family in care, as possible. Teach essential aspects of care.
2. Reinforce physician's explanation of medical management.
3. Stress importance of ongoing outpatient care and follow-up visits.
4. Stress need for regular exercise program:
   a. Teach ROM exercises to family.
   b. Perform ROM exercises to all body joints every 2 to 4 hours.
5. Encourage independent activities, as possible:
   a. Alert to limitations.

b. Avoid overprotection.

c. Emphasize need for supportive devices as indicated (wheelchair, braces, walker, canes, overhead trapeze).

6. Stress importance of diet as ordered:
   a. Offer supplemental findings.
   b. Offer small portions, and instruct patient to chew slowly.
   c. Arrange food and utensils within easy reach.
   d. Avoid foods such as soft breads, mashed potatoes, semicooked vegetables, and large pieces of meat that can cause choking.

7. Stress importance of safety measures: side rails; ramps; shower chains; removal of scatter rugs; and walker, canes, and flat shoes.

8. Instruct regarding name of medication, dosage, time of administration, and toxic or side effects.

9. Stress need to avoid over-the-counter medications without first consulting physician.

10. Encourage socialization with friends and family.

11. Stress importance of communication:
    a. Speak slowly and distinctly.
    b. Use one-word commands and short sentences. Repeat as needed.
    c. Use gestures and touch when giving directions. Maintain eye contact.
    d. Implement speech exercises twice a day.

12. Stress importance of verbalization of feelings about anxiety, fear, and body image changes.

13. Teach patient and family about seizures (i.e., safety measures and who to contact).

EVALUATION

Patient Outcome	Data Indicating That Outcome is Reached
The patient demonstrates a patent airway.	Breath sounds are normal. Chest excursion is bilateral and symmetric. Rate and depth of respirations are normal. Cough is effective. There are no subjective or objective findings of shortness of breath, air hunger, or dyspnea on exertion.
The patient demonstrates an effective breathing pattern.	Airway is patent. Chest excursion is symmetric. Breath sounds are normal, or there is no increase in adventitious sounds. Arterial blood gas values are within normal ranges or consistent with patient's baseline. Vital signs are within normal ranges or consistent with patient's baseline. Hemoglobin levels are 14 to 18 g/dl (male) and 12 to 16 g/dl (female). Intake and output are stable. There are no signs of respiratory distress. All lobes are resonant on percussion. Skin color is not cyanotic.
The patient maintains adequate cerebral tissue perfusion.	Level of consciousness is unchanged. There is no evidence of neurologic deficits. Electrolyte pattern is stable. There is no seizure activity.
The patient demonstrates minimal complications of sensory-perceptual alterations.	Optimal level of orientation is maintained. The patient remains free of injury. The patient demonstrates skin integrity. Nutritional status is adequate. Self-care deficits are minimal. Social participation is appropriate to physiologic status.
The patient remains free of traumatic injury.	Safety measures are appropriate to physiologic status. Skin integrity is maintained. Skin is free of bruises, burns, abrasions, and redness. Environment is safe. The patient is free of nosocomial infections.

Patient Outcome	Data Indicating That Outcome is Reached
The patient demonstrates an optimal level of mobility.	Skin integrity is maintained. The patient remains free of contractures and deformities. Level of mobility is appropriate to physiologic status. Intake and output pattern is stable. Nutritional status is adequate. The patient remains free of thrombophlebitis. The patient remains free of local infections. The patient participates in an ongoing physical therapy program. The patient demonstrates minimal self-care deficits. Outcome criteria listed for impaired physical mobility are met. Level of self-care activities is appropriate to physiologic status. The patient participates in physical and occupational therapy.
The patient demonstrates skin integrity.	Skin is intact. Nutritional status is adequate. Electrolyte balance is maintained. The patient remains free of pressure sores and contractures.
The patient demonstrates minimal complications of bowel incontinence.	Skin in perineal area is clean and dry. Dietary intake is adequate. Fluid intake is adequate (2000 ml daily unless contraindicated). Intake and output pattern is stable. The patient remains free of fecal impaction. The patient demonstrates a regular bowel evacuation pattern.
The patient demonstrates intact self-concepts.	The patient openly verbalizes feelings of grief and loss. The patient verbalizes positive feelings about self. The patient acknowledges actual change in self-image. The patient focuses on present and future appearance and function. The patient verbalizes feelings of hopefulness, helpfulness, and powerfulness.
The patient demonstrates minimal feelings of powerlessness.	Optimal level of physiologic control, as possible for current health status, is maintained. Optimal level of psychologic control, as possible, is maintained. The patient participates, as possible, in decision making about care. The patient participates, as possible, in self-care.
The patient demonstrates minimal impaired verbal communication.	The patient verbalizes feelings for as long as physically able to do so. The patient develops alternate methods of communication.
The patient demonstrates minimal complications from alterations in urinary elimination patterns.	Intake and output pattern are stable. Urine is clear, yellow to amber in color, and without sediment. Skin in perineal area is clean and dry. Urine is acidic (pH 6.0). The patient remains free of urinary tract infections. The patient remains free of bladder distention. The patient can describe symptoms of urinary tract infections that require medical intervention.

CRANIOCEREBRAL TRAUMA

Trauma, as an entity, is the leading cause of death for individuals between the ages of 1 and 35 years of age. Craniocerebral trauma is a major factor in half of the deaths resulting from physical injuries and is the second most common cause of neurologic deficits. In addition to the 77,000 individuals who die each year in the United States from traumatic brain injury, another 50,000 to 60,000 individuals survive head injuries with varying levels of permanent deficits. It is estimated that each year 3000 children in the United States are affected by head trauma. Actual injury to the brain represents the most serious complication of head trauma.

General effects of moderate to severe head injuries include cerebral edema, sensorimotor deficits, and increased intracranial pressure. Following the initial brain injury, secondary damage can result from brain herniation, cerebral ischemia, and hypoxemia. Leading causes of craniocerebral trauma include falls, industrial accidents, vehicular accidents (70% of victims sustain head injuries), assaults, sport accidents (i.e., football, boxing, diving), and intrauterine and birth injuries.

PATHOPHYSIOLOGY

Craniocerebral injuries can result from direct or indirect trauma to the head. Indirect trauma is caused by tension strains and shearing forces transmitted to the cranium by extreme torsion and stretching of the neck (i.e., hard fall on buttocks). Direct trauma occurs when traumatic forces directly impact the head, setting into action the mechanisms of injury. The mechanisms of direct trauma that produce actual brain deformation include acceleration-deceleration with cavitation, and rotation of the skull and its cranial contents. These forces can occur simultaneously or in succession and damage the brain by compression, shearing, or tension. Acceleration injuries result when the head is struck by a moving object and set in motion. The slower-moving brain tissue is damaged by sudden contact with the edges of the dural membrane or the boney prominences of the skull. As a result of acceleration forces, there may be bruising or contusion of the undersurfaces of the occipital lobes, the brainstem, the superior surface of the cerebellum at the edge of the tentorium, or the tips of the frontal and temporal lobes. Another factor in the acceleration mechanism is the effect of positive and negative pressure waves traversing the skull. At the point of impact, a high pressure wave (positive) occurs, while a low pressure wave (negative) occurs opposite the site of impact. If the negative pressure reaches vapor pressure, theoretically it may produce cavitation and a contrecoup injury.

Deceleration occurs when the moving head strikes a solid, immovable object (e.g., head hitting windshield). As a result there is rapid deceleration of the skull, but the brain decelerates slower (i.e., 20 ms), and the brain tissue may travel 2 to 3 cm in that time frame.

Acceleration-deceleration movements from lateral flexion, hyperflexion, hyperextension, and turning movements during the injury cause the cerebrum to rotate about the brainstem, resulting in shearing, straining, and distortion of neural tissue. Microscopically, the stretching or tension causes fracture of axons in the longitudinal bundles of the cerebrum and the long axons in the brainstem. This rotational mechanism is a major cause of contrecoup lesions (severe head injuries) and may ac-

count for most of the contusions to the brain tissue. Areas most frequently injured during rotation are the frontal and temporal lobes.

Head injuries can be classified as open or closed. *Open* head injuries result from skull fractures or penetrating (i.e., missile) wounds. The velocity, mass, shape, and direction of impact are the major determinants of brain injury. With an open head injury there is some type of skull fracture, such as linear, comminuted, depressed, or perforated.

A linear fracture is a simple break in bone continuity that results in an inbending of the bone at the point of impact and an outbending of the skull in the surrounding area. A comminuted skull fracture occurs when two or more communicating breaks divide the bone into more than two fragments. Depressed fractures result when the bone is forced below the line of normal contour from impact with a moving object. Compound fractures may be linear, comminuted, or depressed.

Another and serious type of break in the integrity of the skull is the basal fracture, which can be linear, comminuted, or depressed. Structures most commonly damaged with this type of fracture include the internal carotid artery and cranial nerves I, II, VII, and VIII. With basal skull fractures the fractures usually traverse the paranasal sinuses. The fragility of the bones and the close adherence of the dura account for the frequency of this type of fracture and the resulting leakage of cerebrospinal fluid through the dural tear.[23]

With open head injuries there can be high- or low-velocity impacts. The higher the velocity of impact, the greater the explosive effect within the cranium. For example, in high-velocity impacts, such as with gunshot wounds, there is entry site laceration, cerebral edema, hemorrhage into the destroyed area, and remote contusions (secondary to tissue displacement).[47] Lower-velocity impacts usually result in distortion and linear fractures of the skull.

A *closed*, blunt head injury can produce the pathologic signs of cerebral concussion, contusion, or laceration. A *concussion* is a transient neural dysfunction of paralysis and is the least serious type of brain injury. With a concussion there are immediate and transitory disturbances in equilibrium, consciousness, and vision. *Contusions* result in bruising of brain tissue, usually accompanied by hemorrhages of surface vessels. *Lacerations* are the actual tearing of the cortical surface. Contusions and lacerations result in microscopic hemorrhages around blood vessels with destruction of surrounding brain tissue.

A contusion or laceration directly beneath the site of cranial impact is termed a *coup* lesion; those occurring opposite the site of impact are *contrecoup* lesions. The two major factors that determine the distribution of coup and contrecoup lesions are the ability of cerebrospinal fluid to act as a shock dampener and shifts of the intracranial contents. With a coup lesion the impact causes greater displacement of the skull than the brain. At the site of impact, the cerebrospinal fluid is squeezed out from between the brain and skull, and the skull hits the brain at the point of impact.[30] Contrecoup lesions occur because of the following changes: (1) dissipation of the cerebrospinal fluid between the trailing edge of the brain and the trailing surface of the skull and (2) a compensatory increase in the volume of cerebrospinal fluid between the leading edge of the brain and the leading surface of the skull.[30] The coup or contrecoup lesion may be accompanied by cavitation, which is the release of dissolved gases from cerebrospinal fluid, blood, or brain tissue. The release of these gases produces microscopic bubbles that can extensively disrupt neural tissue, primarily in cerebrospinal pathways and near blood vessels.

Secondary responses to craniocerebral trauma may include the formation of an epidural, subdural, or intracerebral hematoma, a subarachnoid hemorrhage, cerebral edema, and brain herniation. An *epidural* hematoma usually occurs when there is a linear fracture of one of the skull's membranous bones, such as the temporal area near the meningeal artery and vein. Following rupture, the arterial blood forms a convex mass that indents the brain. If the hemorrhage continues, the hematoma may break periosteal attachments and the dural collagen.

A *subdural* hematoma may result from cerebral hemorrhage in the temporal, frontal, or midline region or in any region there is a laceration of brain tissue or its parenchymal vessels. Because the subdural hematoma is venous in origin, symptoms may appear much later than with the arterial epidural hematoma and can be classified as acute, subacute, or chronic. *Acute* subdural hematomas usually manifest symptoms within 24 to 48 hours after the severe trauma. Symptoms of a *subacute* subdural hematoma usually develop anywhere from 48 hours to 2 weeks following severe head injury. *Chronic* subdural hematomas develop over weeks, months, and possibly even years after an apparently minor head injury. The chronic type of subdural hematoma is most common for those individuals in the 60 to 70 year age group because brain atrophy permits more room for expansion.

An *intracerebral hematoma*, which is a collection of blood within the actual brain tissue, usually occurs in the temporal or frontal region. Extensive removal of the hematoma and surrounding necrotic brain tissue is usually necessary to prevent further brain injury.

Subarachnoid hemorrhage is a frequent complication of head trauma. The pathologic processes of subarachnoid hemorrhage are presented in the discussion of vascular lesions.

The pathologic findings with cerebral hematoma are similar to those of space-occupying intracerebral tumors. As the hematoma forms, localized, and later generalized, cerebral edema contributes to increased intracranial pressure and the possibility of brain herniation syndromes.

Cerebral edema following craniocerebral trauma can occur locally around the injury as well as throughout the brain. The peak of cerebral edema is usually around 72 hours after the traumatic injury. Responses to the cerebral edema include increased intracranial pressure as well as the cerebral herniation syndromes.

Brain herniation is a secondary complication that can develop as a result of a primary head injury. The main types of brain herniation syndromes include uncal, transtentorial, and cerebellar. *Uncal* (lateral transtentorial) herniation involves displacement of the medial portion of the temporal lobe across the tentorium into the posterior fossa, compressing the midbrain and brainstem. *Transtentorial* (central) herniation involves downward displacement of the cerebral ventricles through the tentorial incisura resulting in compression of the diencephalon against the midbrain. Cerebellar herniation results when the cerebellar tonsils move downward through the foramen magnum and compress the medulla.

Variations in Children

Craniocerebral injury in the child differs substantially from craniocerebral trauma in the adult. For example, in children the cerebral tissues are softer, thinner, and more flexible, which permits diffusion of the impact. However, the cerebral tissues of the child are fragile and may be easily damaged, resulting in many long-term effects.[52] Because the child's skull is more expansible than the adult's, a greater amount of posttraumatic edema and serious hemorrhage can occur without evidence of neurologic deficits. Compared with the adult blood volume, a greater portion of a child's blood volume flows to the head, thereby creating a potentially dangerous situation if the hemorrhage is undetected over a period of time. Unlike the adult with craniocerebral trauma, a child may experience hypovolemic shock from the intracranial bleeding.[52]

Perinatal trauma can result in the formation of a subdural hematoma, intracerebral and subarachnoid hemorrhage, cephalohematoma, or depressed skull fractures. The most common and most serious birth injury is the subdural hematoma; it may be precipitated by prenatal anoxia. Cephalohematomas occur in approximately 5% of all live births. Causes for cephalohematoma include delivery by forceps, primiparity, and cephalopelvic disproportion. This type of hematoma, which resolves spontaneously in 2 to 3 weeks, usually occurs in the parietal area and does not cross the midline.[52] Most depressed skull fractures in the newborn elevate spontaneously and cause little neurologic damage.

Hematomas following head injury in children include subdural, epidural, and intracerebral hematomas. The subdural hematoma is the most frequent complication, whereas the intracerebral hematoma is a rare finding.

The most frequent neurologic problem in infants and children is the closed head injury that results in concussion, contusion, or laceration to the brain tissue. Pathophysiologic processes detailed on p. 376 are applicable to the pediatric patient.

DIAGNOSTIC STUDIES

Skull roentgenogram
   Detection of calvaria fractures (i.e., simple, compound, depressed, or comminuted)

Cervical roentgenogram
   To confirm or rule out cervical spinal injury

Chest roentgenogram
   Indicates presence of aspiration and chest injuries

CT scan
   May indicate subdural hematoma, intracerebral hematoma, or shift and distortion of cerebral ventricles

Magnetic resonance imaging (MRI)
   Same as CT scan

CSF sampling
   May be contraindicated with increased intracranial pressure
   Normal in cerebral edema and brain concussion
   Increased pressure and blood with laceration and contusion

Cerebral angiography
   May indicate intracerebral or subdural hematoma by showing avascular areas with displacement of surrounding vessels

Pneumoencephalogram
   Demonstration of cerebral ventricular shift, distortion, or dilation

Electroencephalogram (EEG) (done serially)
   Appearance or development of pathologic waves
   Determination of brain death

Cisternogram
   Identification of dural tear site with basal skull fracture

Echoencephalogram
   Detects shifts in midline structures

Serum electrolytes
   Natriuresis
   Hypernatremia
   Elevated plasma cortisol
   Increased serum lactic dehydrogenase

TREATMENT PLAN

Surgical
   Suturing of head and scalp lacerations
   Debridement of wounds
   Ventricular catheter, subarachnoid bolt, and epidural sensor
   Ventriculostomy
   Cranioplasty
   Shunting procedures for hydrocephalus
   Craniectomy
   Craniotomy
   Tracheostomy
   Skull trephine

Chemotherapeutic
   Diuretics
      Mannitol 20%, 0.25 mg/kg IV q4-6h
      Furosemide (Lasix), 20-40 mg IV q6-8h
   Anticonvulsants
      Phenytoin sodium (Dilantin)
         Adult, 18 mg/kg; then maintenance dose of 5 mg/kg qd
         Child, initially 5 mg/kg/d in divided doses; then maintenance dose of 4-8 mg/kg/d in divided doses
      Phenobarbital sodium
         Adult, 30-120 mg qd in 2 or 3 individual doses
         Child, 6 mg/kg qd in 3 divided doses
      Carbamazepine (Tegretol)
         Adult, 200 mg bid initially; gradually increased up to 800-1 200 mg/qd in divided doses
         Child (6-12 yrs), 100 mg bid initially; gradually increased by 100 mg/d up to 1000 mg/qd in divided doses
   Corticosteroids
      Dexamethasone (Decadron), 4-10 mg IV q6h
   Histamine antagonist
      Cimetidine (Tagamet), adult, 300 mg IV q6h
   Analgesic/antipyretics
      Avoid morphone sulfate because of medullary depressant effects.
      Acetaminophen
         Adult, 325-650 mg prn
         Child (6-12 yr), 160-325 mg tid or qid
   Antacids
      Maalox, 30 ml po or NG q2h

Artificial tears, prn
Stool softeners
Muscle relaxants
  Pancuronium (Pavulon), 1-4 mg IV q4h

Electromechanical

Controlled mechanical ventilation
Cervical collars
Central venous pressure line
Arterial pressure line
Intracranial pressure monitoring
Hypothermia-hyperthermia balance
Incentive spirometry
Cardiac monitoring
Salem sump, nasogastric tube

Supportive

Nutritional support (i.e., enteral feedings, intravenous
  hyperalimentation)
Physical therapy program
Warm or cold compresses for periorbital edema and
  ecchymosis
Indwelling urinary catheter
Speech therapy, if indicated
Psychosocial counseling
Seizure precautions

ASSESSMENT: AREAS OF CONCERN

Cranial nerve palsies

Bilateral anosmia
Agnosia (less common)
Paralysis of ocular movements: diplopia, nystagmus
Partial or complete blindness
Vertigo
Deafness
Numbness, paresthesias, or neuralgia of areas supplied
  by trigeminal nerve
Strabismus

Level of consciousness

Mental changes
  Irritability
  Restlessness
  Confusion
  Delirium
  Stupor
  Coma
Posttraumatic amnesia (loss of day-to-day memory af-
  ter the injury)
Retrograde amnesia (loss of memory regarding events
  immediately preceding the injury)

Pain

Headache

Motor function

Concussion
  Transitory extensor spasms
Contusion
  Weakness
  Paresis
  Paralysis
  Decorticate (flexor) posturing: upper extremity flex-
    ion, lower extremity extension
  Decerebrate (extension) posturing: extension and in-
    ternal rotation of upper extremities, extension of
    lower extremities
  Areflexia

Meningeal irritability

Nuchal rigidity
Positive Kernig's sign
Positive Brudzinski's sign

Skull fracture

Linear
  No bone displacement
  Possible epidural hematoma
Depressed
  Focal neurologic deficits
  Cranial nerve injuries
Basilar
  CSF rhinorrhea
  Bilateral periorbital ecchymosis
  CSF otorrhea
  Mastoid bone ecchymosis (Battle's sign)
  Hearing impairments
  Positive halo sign

Cerebral edema/increased intracranial pressure

Changes in level of consciousness
Slow, labored respirations
Changes in arterial blood pressure and pulse pressure
Bradycardia
Anorexia
Papilledema
Changes in motor function (i.e., posturing)
Nausea and vomiting (may be projectile)
Positive Babinski's sign (usually contralateral to le-
  sion)

Brain herniation

Uncal
Decreased level of consciousness with almost simultaneous rapid motor function changes (decerebrate or decorticate posturing) and rapid changes
  in pupillary equality
Respiratory acidosis or alkalosis
Loss of oculocephalic reflex

Transentorial
  Decreased level of consciousness
  Nuchal rigidity
  Headache
  Unilateral or bilateral pupil dilation
  Elevated blood pressure
  Bradycardia
  Cheyne-Stokes respiration
  Cardiac arrhythmias
  Decerebrate or decorticate posturing
Cerebellar
  Pupils constricted and nonreactive
  Decreased level of consciousness
  Apnea or ataxis respiration
  Decreased ROM

Hemorrhage
Epidural hematoma
  Transient loss of consciousness
  Increasing intracranial pressure (rapid development)
  Ipsilateral dilated pupil
Subdural hematoma
  Increasing lethargy
  Headache
  Increasing intracranial pressure
  Seizures
  Minimal dilation of unilateral pupil
Intracerebral hematoma
  Increasing intracranial pressure
  Sensory and motor deficits

Reflexes
Pupils dilated

Loss of cutaneous and tendon reflexes (concussion)
Babinski's reflex positive (with increased intracranial pressure)

Vital signs
Decreased blood pressure
Pulse slow or rapid and feeble
Respirations shallow or temporary cessation (concussion)
Widening pulse pressure with hypertension
Hyperventilation
Cheyne-Stokes, apneustic, ataxic, or cluster respirations (dependent on level of function)
Temperature elevation

Other
Punch-drunk encephalopathy: memory impairment, dysarthria, ataxias, tremors, parkinsonian manifestations
Postconcussion syndrome: headache, insomnia, nervousness, fatigability, giddiness
Dehydration
Polyuria
Shock

Extracranial complications
Cervical fracture not diagnosed
Chest injuries
Fat emboli
Gastrointestinal hemorrhage
Hypoxia
Hypercapnia
Anemia
Hypotension

NURSING DIAGNOSES and NURSING INTERVENTIONS

Nursing Diagnosis	Nursing Intervention
Airway clearance, ineffective	Maintain patent airway; avoid flexion of the neck if patient is immobile. Auscultate for breath sounds every 1 to 2 hours and as needed. Suction as needed. Monitor vital signs every 1 to 2 hours; monitor neurologic status every 1 to 2 hours. Keep emergency drugs and ventilator at bedside. Maintain nothing-by-mouth status to prevent risk of choking or aspiration, if indicated.

Breathing pattern, ineffective	Maintain patent airway. Intubation/tracheostomy and mechanical ventilation may be indicated.
	Auscultate breath sounds every 1 to 2 hours; note quality and any increase in adventitious sounds:
	  Suction as needed. Hyperinflate lungs with 100% oxygen for 1 minute before and 1 minute after suctioning, unless contraindicated.
	Monitor mechanical ventilator, if used:
	  Ensure tidal volume, rate, mode, and oxygen concentration are set as ordered.
	  Ensure ventilator alarms are on and functional.

Nursing Diagnosis	Nursing Intervention

	Monitor arterial blood gases, as per protocol:
	  Report decrease in P_{O_2} of 10 to 15 mm Hg.
	  Report increase in P_{CO_2} greater than 10 to 15 mm Hg.
	Check blood pressure, respirations, and pulse rate every 1 to 2 hours and as needed based on patient's condition.

Tissue perfusion, alteration in: cerebral	Establish baseline and ongoing neurologic assessment every 1 to 2 hours and as needed as indicated by the patient's condition.
	Intervene to monitor or prevent increased intracranial pressure:
	  Administer medications, treatments, and IV lines as per protocol.
	  Maintain elevation of head of bed as per protocol.
	  Accurately record intake and output; monitor for imbalance.
	  Monitor serum electrolytes, blood count, and arterial blood gases for abnormalities.
	  Monitor values and wave forms of intracranial pressure line, if appropriate:
	    Maintain patency and sterility of the system.
	    Monitor effects of treatments on intracranial pressure.
	    Correlate neurologic status with intracranial pressure values; notify physician if inconsistent.
	    Assist with drainage of cerebrospinal fluid from the system.
	Intervene to monitor or prevent seizures:
	  Institute seizure precautions:
	    Padded tongue blade and airway at bedside
	    Bed height at lowest level
	    Side rails up at all times and padded
	    Oxygen and suction equipment at bedside
	    Emergency medications at bedside
	  Administer anticonvulsants as per protocol:
	    Monitor effects and side effects.
	    Monitor serum for therapeutic levels of the anticonvulsant.
	Maintain balance between hyperthermia and hypothermia.

Sensory-perceptual alteration: visual, auditory, gustatory, kinesthetic, tactile, olfactory	Keep side rails up at all times when patient is alone. Maintain patient safety at all times. Maintain quiet environment, reducing external stimuli to a minimum. Reorient patient frequently to time, place, and person. Introduce self each time you reorient the patient. Repeat explanations frequently and simply. Have family bring in familiar objects. Maintain planned rest periods, allowing sufficient time for REM sleep. Use day-night lighting appropriately. Stimulate senses of touch, taste, and position. Support family members to understand what is happening as a result of perceptual alterations.
Injury, potential for: trauma	Maintain bed in low position at all times unless side rails are up or when nurse is with the patient. Provide the patient with a call light within easy reach. Maintain side rails in up position at bedtime, after sedation, when patient is confused, and as needed. Maintain wheelchairs and stretchers in locked position when transferring patient.

Preconvulsive	Have oral airway at bedside.
	Support and protect head; turn to side if possible.
	Prevent injury:
	  Ease to floor if in chair.
	  Place pillows along side rails if in bed.
	  Remove surrounding furniture.
	  Loosen constrictive clothing.
	Provide privacy as necessary; stay with patient.
	Note frequency, time, involved body parts, and length of seizure.

Postconvulsive	Maintain patent airway. Suction as needed, as indicated. Check vital signs and neurologic status.

Nursing Diagnosis	Nursing Intervention
	Administer oxygen as per protocol.
	Reorient the patient to environment.
	Provide emotional support.
	Place patient in position of comfort; turn head to side.
	Administer oral hygiene as necessary for secretions and bleeding.
Mobility, impaired physical	Administer skin care every 1 to 2 hours:
	Turn patient every 2 hours and as needed, unless contraindicated.
	Change position slowly.
	Position in proper body alignment; may need to use "log-roll" technique when turning.
	Massage pressure points every 2 hours to stimulate circulation; give gentle back rubs every shift and as needed.
	Use firm mattress or bed board.
	Use footboard or Spence boots to prevent foot-drop.
	Apply antiembolus stockings to lower extremities.
	Administer anticoagulation therapy as per protocol.
	Monitor nutritional status.
	Encourage mobility to tolerance or as per protocol.
	Encourage self-care activities to tolerance.
	Plan all activities to avoid fatigue; maintain planned rest periods.
	Obtain physical therapy referral.
Self-care deficits: feeding, bathing/ hygiene, dressing/grooming, toileting	Assist with feeding, as indicated.
	Use IV or nasogastric feedings, as per protocol.
	Administer oral hygiene every 2 hours and as needed.
	Assist with daily hygiene care, as indicated.
	Administer eye care every 2 to 4 hours, if indicated.
	Maintain bowel function with regular evacuation.
Skin integrity, impairment of: potential	See general intervention strategies listed on p. 2020.
Comfort, alteration in: pain	See general intervention strategies listed on p. 1979.
Self-concept, disturbance in: body image, self-esteem, role performance, personal identity	Provide for a safe, comfortable, secure environment.
	Reorient the patient to time, person, and place, as appropriate.
	Carefully explain what you are doing and why you are doing it.
	Answer questions simply and honestly.
	Correct misinformation.
	Protect the patient's privacy.
Anxiety; powerlessness	See general intervention strategies listed on pp. 1830 and 1938.
	Assist patient to reestablish as much physiologic control as condition allows.
	Share knowledge of physiologic functioning with the patient and family.
	Assist patient to reestablish some means of psychologic control.
	Encourage the patient to express feelings.
	Encourage the patient and family to participate in care.
	Encourage the patient to become an active decision maker about care and immediate environment.
Communication, impaired: verbal	Develop a means of communication with the patient: pencil, magic slate, or call light within easy reach.
	Reinforce the techniques established.
	Assist patient and family to identify other outlets for communication.
	Continue to use sense of touch and nonverbal forms of communication.

Patient Education

1. Involve family in care, as possible; teach essential aspects of care.
2. Reinforce physician's explanation of medical management.
3. Stress importance of ongoing outpatient care and follow-up visits.
4. Encourage independent activities, as possible:
   a. Alert to limitations.
   b. Avoid overprotection.
   c. Stress need for supportive devices as indicated.
5. Emphasize need for regular exercise program. Teach ROM exercises to family.
6. Stress importance of diet as ordered:
   a. Offer supplemental feedings.
   b. Offer small portions; instruct patient to chew slowly.
7. Stress importance of safety measures: side rails; ramps; shower chairs; walker, canes.
8. Instruct patient regarding name of medication, dosage, time of administration, and toxic or side effects.
9. Stress need to avoid over-the-counter medications without first consulting physician.
10. Encourage socialization with friends and family.
11. Emphasize importance of verbalization of feelings about anxiety, fear, and body image changes.
12. Teach patient and family about seizures (i.e., safety measures and who to contact).

EVALUATION

Patient Outcome	Data Indicating That Outcome is Reached
The patient demonstrates a patent airway.	Breath sounds are normal. Chest excursion is bilateral and symmetric. Rate and depth of respirations are normal. Cough is effective. There are no subjective or objective findings of shortness of breath, air hunger, or dyspnea on exertion.
The patient demonstrates an effective breathing pattern.	Airway is patent. Chest excursion is symmetric. Breath sounds are normal, or there is no increase in adventitious sounds. Arterial blood gas values are within normal ranges or consistent with patient's baseline. Vital signs are within normal ranges or consistent with patient's baseline. Hemoglobin levels are 14 to 18 g/dl (male) and 12 to 16 g/dl (female). Intake and output are stable. There are no signs of respiratory distress. All lobes are resonant on percussion. Skin color is not cyanotic.
The patient maintains adequate cerebral and spinal tissue perfusion.	Level of consciousness is unchanged. There is no evidence of neurologic deficits. Electrolyte pattern is stable. There is no seizure activity.
The patient demonstrates minimal complications of sensory-perceptual alterations.	Optimal level of orientation is maintained. The patient remains free of injury. The patient demonstrates skin integrity. Nutritional status is adequate. Self-care deficits are minimal. Social participation is appropriate to physiologic status.
The patient remains free of traumatic injury.	Safety measures are appropriate to level of physiologic status. Skin integrity is maintained. Skin is free of bruises, burns, abrasions, and redness. Environment is safe. The patient is free of nosocomial infections.
The patient demonstrates an optimal level of mobility.	The patient exhibits skin integrity. The patient remains free of contractures and deformities.

Patient Outcome	Data Indicating That Outcome is Reached
	Level of mobility is appropriate to physiologic status.
	Intake and output pattern is stable.
	Nutritional status is adequate.
	The patient remains free of thrombophlebitis.
	The patient remains free of local infection.
	The patient participates in an ongoing physical therapy program.
The patient demonstrates minimal self-care deficits.	Outcome criteria listed for impaired physical mobility are met. Level of self-care activities is appropriate to physiologic status. The patient participates in physical and occupational therapy.
The patient demonstrates skin integrity.	Skin is intact. Nutritional status is adequate. Electrolyte balance is maintained. The patient remains free of pressure sores and contractures.
The patient experiences minimal alterations in comfort.	The patient openly verbalizes feelings of discomfort when they occur. The patient can utilize measures to decrease discomfort. The patient verbally validates a decrease in subjective feelings of discomfort. Objective findings of pain are decreased.
The patient demonstrates intact self-concepts.	The patient openly verbalizes feelings of grief and loss. The patient verbalizes positive feelings about self. The patient acknowledges actual change in self-image. The patient focuses on present and future appearance and function. The patient verbalizes feelings of hopefulness, helpfulness, and powerfulness.
The patient demonstrates a low level of anxiety.	The patient openly verbalizes concerns and feelings of grief, loss, and discomfort. The patient openly verbalizes feelings supported by health care professionals and family. The patient verbalizes essential aspects of care. The patient identifies methods to effectively deal with anxious feelings.
The patient demonstrates minimal feelings of powerlessness.	The patient maintains an optimal level of physiologic control, as possible for current health status. The patient maintains an optimal level of psychologic control, as possible. The patient participates, as possible, in decision making about care. The patient participates, as possible, in self-care.
The patient demonstrates minimal impaired verbal communication.	The patient verbalizes feelings for as long as physically able to do so. The patient develops alternate methods of communication.

SPINAL CORD TRAUMA

Injuries to the spinal cord constitute approximately 10% of traumatic injuries to the nervous system. Causes of spinal cord trauma include assaults (e.g., bullet wounds), falls, sport injuries (e.g., diving accidents), industrial accidents, birth injuries, degenerative changes (e.g., vertebral disk deterioration), and vehicular accidents. Approximately 10,000 spinal cord injuries occur each year in the United States, and spinal cord trauma from vehicular accidents accounts for one half to two thirds of that number. Approximately one third of the individuals sustaining spinal cord injuries die before reaching an acute-care facility. About 80% of individuals sustaining spinal cord injury are between the ages of 18 and 25 years and most are male. It is estimated that there are presently over 100,000 individuals in the United States who are paralyzed as a result of spinal cord trauma.

The most common sites of injury are the lower cervical region (C4-C7 and T1) and the thoracolumbar junction (T12, L1, and L2). Trauma to the spinal cord can result in concussion, contusion, laceration, hemorrhage, transection (partial or complete), or impairment in the spinal vascular supply.

PATHOPHYSIOLOGY

As with craniocerebral trauma, the spine (and spinal cord) can be injured by direct or indirect forces. Direct injuries such as falls on the head or seat can result in spinal cord lesions from fractured vertebrae or in direct compression of the cord by depressed bone fragments. Indirect injuries, which constitute the major type of spinal cord injuries, can occur when excessive forces accelerate the cranium in relation to the trunk (i.e., whiplash injury) or when the trunk is suddenly decelerated in regard to the lumbar spine. Whether the forces are direct or indirect, the subsequent fractures of vertebrae can seriously injure the neural elements of the spinal cord.

Vertebral Injuries

The vertebral column is a generally rigid structure that protects the soft tissue of the spinal cord. The major mechanisms of vertebral injury, occurring alone or in combination, include hyperextension, hyperflexion, vertical compression trauma, and rotation.[23]

Hyperextension injuries (commonly termed *whiplash*) are most common in the cervical region, and damage results from the forces of acceleration-deceleration and the sudden reduction in the anterior-posterior diameter of the spinal canal. Since the spinal canal is full of neural tissue in the cervical area, injury can produce profound disability. With a hyperextension injury the cord can be compressed between the body of one vertebra and the leading edge of the laminal arch of adjacent vertebrae, causing complete or partial transection. Additionally, the ligamentum flavum may be torn or bulge inward, and intervertebral disks may tear. Severe hyperextension injuries can result in complete transverse fracture of the vertebral body. With the compression and shearing forces of a hyperextension injury, there is destruction of gray matter of the cord and disruption in microcirculation at and around the level of the injury.

Hyperflexion injury results in an overstretching, compression, and deformation of the spinal cord from a sudden and excessive force that propels the neck forward or an exaggerated lateral movement of the neck to one side or another. Hyperflexion injuries can occur with wedge or compression fractures of the vertebral body with or without dislocation, fracture of the pedicle with

or without dislocation of intraspinal ligaments, or fracture of the vertebral body and rupture of the intervertebral discs.

Vertical compression trauma primarily occurs around the area of the thoracolumbar junction (T12 to L2) and results from a force applied along an axis from the top of the cranium through the vertebral bodies. With compression injuries the vertebral body bursts, compressing the spinal cord and damaging nerve roots with bony fragments.

Rotation injury can involve all portions of the vertebral body including pedicles, ligaments, and the articulation. Fracture of the pedicles or locked facets of the vertebrae can rupture ligaments and shear spinal cord tissue.

Vertebral injuries can be classified into four main groups: simple fractures, compressed or wedged fractures, comminuted fractures, and vertebral dislocation.[23] A *simple* fracture is a single break usually affecting transverse or spinous processes. Vertebral alignment usually remains intact, and compression of the spinal cord is not usually present.

Compressed, or *wedged*, vertebral fractures occur when the vertebral body is compressed anteriorly. Spinal cord compression may or may not be present with a wedged fracture.

Comminuted, or *burst*, fractures can cause serious injury to the spinal cord. With this type of fracture, the vertebral body shatters into multiple fragments, and these fragments may penetrate the spinal cord. Burst fractures occur at the cervical, thoracic, and lumbar regions.

Dislocation of a vertebra may rupture the ligamentum flavum, resulting in dislocation of the vertebral facets, which can be unilateral or bilateral. This dislocation disrupts alignment of the vertebral column, and injury to the spinal cord may or may not be present. Partial dislocation of the spinal cord is termed *subluxation*.

Spinal Cord Injuries

The neural elements of the spinal cord and spinal nerve roots are injured by the mechanisms of compression from bone, disc herniation, hematoma, and ligaments; edema following compression or concussion; overstretching or disruption of neural tissue; and disturbances in spinal circulation.[16]

Sequential pathologic processes following an impact injury to the spinal cord include localized hemorrhaging, which advances from the gray to the white matter; reduced vascular perfusion and production of ischemic areas and decreased oxygen tension in tissue at the site of injury; edema; cellular and subcellular alterations; and tissue necrosis. Several minutes after the traumatic injury, microscopic hemorrhages appear in the central gray matter and in the pia-arachnoid. The small hemorrhages increase in size until the entire gray matter is hemorrhagic and necrotic. Hemorrhaging and peritraumatic edema progress transversely and longitudinally to the white matter, forming vacuolation and wedge-shaped foci and thus impairing the microcirculation to the spinal cord. This impaired microcirculation produces ischemia or vascular stasis.

Circulation in the white matter returns to normal within approximately 24 hours, but circulation in the gray matter remains altered.

Changes in the chemistry and metabolism of the traumatized regions include a transitory increase in tissue lactate, a rapid decrease in tissue oxygen tension within 30 minutes of the injury, and an increased concentration of norepinephrine. It has been proposed that the increased concentration of norepinephrine released to the cord tissue may produce ischemia, vascular rupture, or necrosis of neuronal tissue.[2]

Localized ischemia of neural tissue may also occur as a result of compression on the vasculature of the cord or nerve roots by bony fragments or herniated disks. If the flow of blood from the vertebral artery to the anterior spinal artery or to the branches of the radicular arteries is impaired, severe cord ischemia results. Hemorrhage, other than that occurring with contusion and edema, usually does not produce significant neural impairment. Epidural and subdural hematomas rarely reach a sufficient size to result in serious compression. Although subarachnoid bleeding is usual, it is of little clinical significance. Larger intramedullary hematomas, on the other hand, may produce a tubular hematomyelia that can cause partial or complete interruption in spinal cord functioning.[16]

Following the immediate posttraumatic period, which is characterized by necrosis, a phase of resorption and organization begins. This state is characterized by the appearance of phagocytes, proliferation of microglial and mesenchymal cells, and changes in astroglias. The phagocytes appear around the necrotized area within 36 to 48 hours after injury. Blood is gradually removed from the tissue by disintegration of red cells and resorption of hemorrhages. Macrophages engulf degenerating axons in the first 10 days after injury.[2]

Beginning the third to fourth week after the injury, the traumatized section of the cord is removed and gradually replaced with connective scar tissue or glial fibers. Injured segments of the spinal cord are replaced with acellular collagenous tissue, which connects the meninges to the cord and central canal. Scarring, in the area of destruction, consists mainly of thickened meninges and connective tissue.

Spinal Shock

Following a complete (and sometimes an incomplete) cord transection, spinal shock occurs in the area at which the cord is severed, producing a complete loss of sensory, motor, autonomic, and reflex functioning below the level of the lesion. Spinal shock results from the loss of inhibition from descending tracts, continued inhibition of supraspinal impulses, and axonal degeneration of the interneurons.

Autonomic Hyperreflexia

A syndrome that may occur after spinal shock has been restored and reflex activity has returned is autonomic hyperreflexia. The syndrome is associated with a massive uncompensated cardiovascular response to stimulation of the sympathetic division of the autonomic nervous system.[10] Individuals most likely to be affected with autonomic hyperreflexia have lesions at the level of T6 or above. If symptoms of autonomic hyperreflexia are not treated, serious damage and possibly even death can result.

Cord Syndromes

Trauma to the spinal cord results in several types of neurologic syndromes that develop from the specific area of cord damaged and that vary in severity depending on the amount of cord compression or cord transection.

The *anterior* cord syndrome occurs after an acute flexion injury to the cervical area and is the most common type of cord syndrome. Damage to the anterior spinal artery, the ventral portion of the spinal cord, or both accounts for the loss of upper and lower motor function.

The *posterior* cord syndrome, although rare, is associated with cervical hyperextension trauma.

Central cord syndrome may result from hyperextension injuries or flexion injuries. Pathologic processes in the central cord syndrome are characterized by central edema of the spinal cord and compression on the anterior horn cells. Neurologic deficits include mixed upper and lower motor neuron loss (disproportionately more impairment in upper extremities) and spasticity below the level of injury.

The *Brown-Séquard* syndrome results from rotation-flexion injuries where subluxation or dislocation of the fracture fragments occurs by unilateral pedicle-laminar injuries.[10] Neurologic deficits include ipsilateral paresis, loss of proprioception, and contralateral loss of pain and temperature sensations.

The *herniated disc* syndrome is one of the most common spinal cord syndromes. Degenerative changes with the fraying and tears of the anulus fibrosus predispose the intervertebral discs to posterior displacement through a laceration of the anulus fibrosus and the posterior longitudinal ligament. The extrusion of fibrocartilaginous material may occur spontaneously or in response to activity (i.e., lifting) or slight injury. The severity of symptoms depends on (1) quantity of herniated disc tissue, (2) number of involved discs and amount of nerve root compression, and (3) the amount of spinal canal narrowing.[23] Herniated discs most frequently (90%) affect the lower lumbar and lumbosacral regions.

Motor Neurons

The motor neurons are the nerve cells that are responsible for transmitting impulses from the brain or spinal cord to muscular or glandular tissue. Spinal cord trauma can result in varying degrees of motor neuron impairment, and differentiation between the upper and lower motor neurons is important to understand. *Upper* motor neuron lesions result from damage in the corticobulbar or corticospinal tract. *Lower* motor neuron lesions result in the loss of reflex and voluntary responses of muscles because of destruction of anterior horn cells, peripheral nerves, or ventral nerve roots or motor fibers.[23]

DIAGNOSTIC STUDIES

Roentgenograms (anteroposterior and lateral)
Vertebral fractures

Serum chemistry
Hypoglycemia or hyperglycemia
Electrolyte imbalance
Possibly decreased hemoglobin and hematocrit

CT scan
Spinal cord edema

Magnetic resonance imaging (MRI)
Spinal cord edema and compression

Spinal puncture
Establishes presence or absence of spinal block

Myelography
Establishes presence of spinal block

TREATMENT PLAN

Surgical
Laminectomy
Tracheostomy or endotracheal intubation (nasal)
Spinal fusion
Wound débridement; suturing of lacerations
Cervical tongs (i.e., Cone, Vinke, Crutchfield, Gardner-Wells)
Halo traction
Halo with femoral traction
Body casts
Spinal cord cooling
Myotomies, tenotomies, neurectomies, rhizotomies, and muscle transplants (treatment for spasticity)
Harrington rod insertion

Chemotherapeutic
Antianxiety agents
Diazepam (Valium)
Adult, 2-10 mg tid or qid po
Child, 1-2.5 mg tid or qid po
Meprobamate (Equanil)
Adult, 1200-1600 mg/d po in divided doses
Child (6-12 yr), 100-200 mg po bid or tid
Corticosteroids
Dexamethasone (Decadron): 5-10 mg qid po
Anticoagulants
Heparin, 5000-7000 units subq q12h
Antihypertensive agents
Diazoxide (Hyperstat),* adult, 1-3 mg/kg, up to 150 mg, IV, repeated at intervals of 5-15 min until blood pressure reduced
Hydralazine (Apresoline),* adult, 20 mg in slow IV push
Muscle relaxants
Dantrolene sodium (Dantrium)
Adult, 25 mg tid to 200 mg qid
Child (5-12 yr), 0.5 mg/kg bid initially; then up to 3 mg/kg bid to qid (not to exceed 100 mg qid)
Anti-infective agents
Sulfisoxazole (Gantrisin)
Adult, 2-4 g initially, then 4-8 g/d in divided doses
Child, 75 mg/kg initially, then 150 mg/kg/d in divided doses
Methenamine mendelate (Mandelamine): adult, 1-2 g qid
Laxatives
Glycerin or bisacodyl (Dulcolax), as rectal suppository
Antacids
Magnesium hydroxide and aluminum hydroxide (Maalox T.C.): adult, 20 ml po q4h

Electromechanical
Mechanical ventilation
Stryker or Foster frame bed
Skeletal traction
Vital capacity and tidal volume measurements
Splints and braces

Supportive
Bed board and firm mattress
Shock blocks under head of bed

*Treatment for autonomic hyperreflexia.

Intermittent urinary catheterization
Intake and output recording
Dietary consultation
Sex counseling
Psychosocial counseling for individual and family
Cervical collar (soft or hard)
Immobilization of part with sandbags
Serial measurement of arterial blood gases
Urine sugar and acetone; guaiac
Antiembolus stockings
Nasogastric tube

ASSESSMENT: AREAS OF CONCERN

Spinal shock
Complete transection
  Flaccid paralysis below level of lesion
  Loss of proprioception, pain, temperature, touch, and pressure below level of lesion
  Loss of all spinal reflexes below level of lesion
  Loss of vasomotor tone
  Loss of visceral and somatic sensations below level of lesion
  Loss of ability to perspire below level of lesion
  Dysfunction of bowel and bladder
  Possible priapism[23]
Partial transection
  Asymmetric flaccid paralysis below level of lesion
  Asymmetric loss of reflexes below level of lesion
  Some senses of proprioception, pain, temperature, touch, and pressure intact below level of injury
  Some visceral and somatic sensations intact below level of lesion
  Less vasomotor instability
  Less bowel and bladder dysfunction
  Possible priapism

Autonomic hyperreflexia
Paroxysmal hypertension
Pounding headache
Diaphoresis above level of lesion
Flushing above level of lesion
Cutis anserina below level of lesion
Nasal stuffiness
Nausea
Bradycardia

Anterior cord syndrome
Loss of pain and temperature senses below level of lesion
Loss of motor function below level of lesion
Senses of vibration, touch, and proprioception intact

Posterior cord syndrome
Motor function of extremities intact
Loss of light touch and proprioception senses

Central cord syndrome
Disproportionate amount of upper extremity paresis or paralysis as compared to lower extremities
Various degrees of bladder dysfunction

Brown-Séquard syndrome
Paresis or paralysis on ipsilateral side
Contralateral loss of pain and temperature sensations
Ipsilateral loss of vibration, touch, pressure, and proprioception

Herniated disk syndrome
Lumbar
  Pain in lower back with radiation down back of one leg
  Restricted spinal mobility
  Walking painful
  Back appears straight with loss of lumbar curve
  Spastic paravertebral muscles
  Impaired sensation of affected leg and foot
  Less active ipsilateral ankle jerk may be present
  Pain aggravated by jugular compression
Cervical
  Stiffness of neck
  Pain radiating down arm to fingers

Pain
Hyperesthesia immediately above level of lesion
Intense tingling and burning pain below level of lesion (in paraplegia)

Spasticity
Partial or complete loss of voluntary control
Exaggerated deep tendon reflexes

Sexual function
Varies from normal function to complete impotence
Menstrual irregularities for short time after injury

Trophic skin changes
Trophic ulcers
Skin and nail changes

NURSING DIAGNOSES and NURSING INTERVENTIONS

Nursing Diagnosis	Nursing Intervention
Airway clearance, ineffective	Maintain patent airway, and avoid flexion of the neck.
	Auscultate for breath sounds every 1 to 2 hours and as needed.
	Suction as needed.
	Assist ventilation as indicated. Keep ''Ambu'' bag at bedside.
	Monitor vital signs every 1 to 2 hours; monitor neurologic status every 1 to 2 hours.
	Maintain nothing-by-mouth status to prevent risk of choking or aspiration, if indicated.
Breathing pattern, ineffective	Maintain patent airway. Intubation/tracheostomy and mechanical ventilation may be indicated.
	Auscultate for breath sounds every 1 to 2 hours; note quality and any increase in adventitious sounds:
	Suction as needed. Hyperinflate lungs with 100% oxygen for 1 minute before and 1 minute after suctioning, unless contraindicated.
	Monitor mechanical ventilator, if used:
	Ensure tidal volume, rate, mode, and oxygen concentration are set as ordered.
	Ensure ventilator alarms are on and functional.
	Monitor arterial blood gases, as ordered:
	Report decrease in Po_2 of 10 to 15 mm Hg.
	Report increase in Pco_2 greater than 10 to 15 mm Hg.
	Check blood pressure, temperature, and pulse rate every 1 to 2 hours and as needed based on the patient's condition.
Tissue perfusion, alteration in: cerebral	Perform neurologic assessment every 1 to 2 hours and as needed.
	Ensure immobilization vertebral column:
	Maintain skeletal traction.
	Maintain cervical skeletal traction:
	Crutchfield tongs:
	Check traction and orthopedic frame every 4 hours.
	Make sure tongs are secure.
	Ensure weights hang freely.
	Assess tong sites every 4 hours and as needed.
	Provide tong site skin care: clean with hydrogen peroxide, and then apply povidone-iodine solution. Cover with sterile dressing.
	Halo traction:
	Assess traction pins to ensure they are tight and secure.
	Assess fiberglass cast jacket for proper fit (should be able to insert index finger between cast and skin).
	Assess cast edges for roughness or crumbling; petal rough edges:
	Provide routine cast care.
	Provide pin site skin care: clean site with hydrogen peroxide, and then apply povidone-iodine solution.
	Cover with sterile dressing.
	Stryker frame:
	Inspect pressure points (face, chin, scapula, coccyx, and heels) every 2 to 4 hours.
	Administer skin care every 2 to 4 hours.
	Secure all bolts before turning patient.
	Assess pulse and respirations before and after turning.
	Check position of canvas under patient after turning.
	Use armrests to maintain alignment.
	Establish method of elimination.
	Maintain *strict* body alignment; keep body straight and head flat:
	Do not move head or spinal column.
	Utilize sandbags, if needed, to maintain alignment.
	Administer medications as ordered:
	Give steroids to control cord edema.
	Avoid injections below the level of the lesion.
	Maintain parenteral fluids, as per protocol.
	Measure intake and output every hour. Immediately report urine output of less than 30 ml/h.

Nursing Diagnosis	Nursing Intervention
Sensory-perceptual alteration: visual, auditory, kinesthetic, gustatory, tactile, olfactory	See general intervention strategies listed on p. 1967.
Injury, potential for: trauma	Maintain bed in low position at all times unless side rails are up or when nurse is with the patient. Provide the patient with a call light within easy reach. Maintain side rails in up position at bedtime, after sedation, and as needed. Maintain stretchers in locked position when transferring patient. Pad side rails if patient is overactive.

Mobility, impaired physical	Administer skin care every 2 hours:
	  Turn patient every 2 hours and as needed, unless contraindicated.
	  Change position slowly.
	  Position in straight body alignment; use "log-roll" technique when turning.
	Keep skin dry; give perineal care as needed.
	Massage pressure points every 2 hours to stimulate circulation; give gentle back-rubs every shift and as needed.
	Use heel and elbow guards as needed.
	Use firm mattress.
	Perform active or passive ROM exercises every 2 to 4 hours.
	Use footboard or Spence boots to prevent foot-drop.
	Apply antiembolus stockings to lower extremities.
	Administer anticoagulation therapy as per protocol.
	Encourage mobility to tolerance or as per protocol.
	Encourage self-care activities to tolerance.
	Plan all activities to avoid fatigue. Maintain planned rest periods.
	Obtain physical therapy referral.
	Encourage diversional activities.

Self-care deficit: feeding, bathing/hygiene, dressing/grooming, toileting	See general intervention strategies listed on p. 2088.

Bowel elimination, alteration in: incontinence	Maintain fluid intake of 2000 ml daily, unless contraindicated.
	Monitor intake and output.
	Provide patient with diet that is high in roughage, protein, and bulk.
	Monitor pattern of bowel elimination.
	Keep patient's skin clean and dry.
	Check patient for impaction every 1 to 2 days.
	Institute a regular bowel evacuation program:
	  Begin bowel retraining program.
	  Instruct patient to take 8 to 10 oz of prune juice 12 hours before time set for defecating; insert glycerin suppository high in rectum 15 to 20 minutes before set time; then place patient on bedpan, toilet, or commode.
	  Insert lubricated glycerin suppository 2 hours before set time, and position patient in sitting position or transfer to bedpan or commode at set time.
	  Instruct patient to drink 4 to 8 oz of prune juice each night.
	  Instruct patient to drink a warm drink (water, coffee, or milk) 30 minutes before set time.
	  Insert laxative suppository for 2 to 4 days, then glycerin suppository for 2 to 4 days; note length of time between insertion and defecation; place patient on bedside commode at appropriate time; if no bowel movement, give small tap water enema.[49]

Urinary elimination, alteration in patterns	Assess the characteristics of the patient's voiding pattern (frequency, amount).
	Observe for bladder distention every 2 to 4 hours.
	Perform intermittent catheterization, as per protocol.
	Perform catheter care every shift:
	  Maintain closed system.
	  Tape catheter to thigh to prevent pulling and tension.
	Monitor intake and output. Maintain fluid intake of 2000 ml daily unless contraindicated.
	Assess urine for sediment, concentration, color, and odor.
	Acidify urine with foods such as cranberry juice.
	Administer urinary tract germicides (e.g., Mandelamine) as ordered.

Nursing Diagnosis	Nursing Intervention

Begin bladder retraining program:

Upper motor neuron bladder:

Administer fluids between 7 AM and 7 PM.

Remove urinary catheter at 7 AM.

Force fluids (i.e., 240 ml) every hour.

After approximately 3 or 4 hours, trigger area (i.e., digital stimulation of rectum) until stimulated and attempt to void is made; if patient is able to void, residual urine is immediately checked:

Residual urine of less than 100 ml is needed to continue with training.

Residual urine of greater than 100 ml requires catheter reinsertion. Bladder retraining is then resumed on another day.

Lower motor neuron bladder:

Administer fluids between 7 AM and 7 PM.

Remove urinary catheter at 7 AM.

Force fluids (i.e., 240 ml) every hour.

After approximately 3 or 4 hours, patient attempts to void by Valsalva's maneuver, Credé's maneuver of bladder, or contraction of abdominal muscles.

If patient is able to void, residual urine is immediately checked:

Residual urine of less than 50 to 75 ml is needed to continue with training.

Residual urine of greater than 75 ml requires catheter reinsertion. Retraining is then resumed on another day.

Skin integrity, impairment of: potential

See general intervention strategies listed on p. 2020.

Self-concept, disturbance in: body image, self-esteem, role performance, personal identity

Provide for a safe, comfortable, secure environment.

Carefully explain what you are doing and why you are doing it.

Listen to the feelings the patient expresses (i.e., feelings of grief and loss).

Answer questions simply and honestly.

Correct misinformation.

Protect the patient's privacy.

Provide gentle physical care in a caring environment.

Provide an ongoing assessment of the patient's interpersonal strengths. Focus on strengths and potential.

Assist the patient to become involved in self-care.

Assist the patient to become involved in unit activities.

Anxiety

See general intervention strategies listed on p. 1839.

Powerlessness

See general intervention strategies listed on p. 1830.

Patient Education[49]

1. Stress importance of regular exercise program and need to exercise to tolerance.
2. Turn every 2 to 4 hours while in bed.
3. Inspect skin and bony prominences for breakdown.
4. Emphasize importance of skin care every 2 to 4 hours while in bed.
5. Encourage verbalization; deal with anxieties over body image changes and disabilities.
6. Instruct regarding name of medication, dosage, time of administration, purpose, and side effects.
7. Avoid over-the-counter medications without first checking with physicians.
8. Teach muscle-building exercises: rubber balls, clay, trapezes, pulleys, squeeze toys, and sit-ups.
9. Stress importance of bladder retraining:
   a. Avoid food low in calcium.
   b. Force fluids to 3000 ml daily unless contraindicated.
   c. Maintain an acidic urine by drinking cranberry juice and taking ascorbic acid if ordered.
   d. Avoid alcoholic beverages, coffee, and tea.
   e. Maintain mobility as tolerated.
   f. Stress that rehabilitation may be a long process.
   g. Instruct regarding signs of full bladder.
   h. Avoid use of penile clamp to control incontinence.
   i. Avoid persons with infections, especially upper respiratory infections.
   j. Instruct regarding care of indwelling catheter.
   k. List symptoms to report to physician: urinary tract infection, kidney stone, upper respiratory infection, or skin lesions.

10. Ensure that the patient or family demonstrates:
    a. Bladder exercises every 2 to 4 hours:
        (1) Tighten rectum or vaginal vault.
        (2) Hold contraction for 5 seconds; then relax.
        (3) Continue tightening and relaxing for 5-min period.
    b. Credé's maneuver for manual bladder stimulation:
        (1) Apply manual pressure over suprapubic region.
        (2) Contract abdominal muscles.
    c. Palpation of bladder distention
    d. Intake and output measurement
    e. Recording of time and amount of fluid intake
    f. Recording of time and amount of urine voided
    g. Testing of urine for pH
    h. Application of condom catheter if necessary
    i. Self-catheterization
11. Instruct regarding importance of bowel retraining program:
    a. Encourage patient participation in developing program.
    b. Evaluate previous bowel habits.
    c. Establish regular bowel habits: (1) time of day that will be convenient for patient once discharged (e.g., after breakfast) and (2) development of program to have bowel evacuation at same time of day or every 3 days.
    d. Teach exercises that will help develop abdominal muscles and tone: pushing up, bearing down, and contracting abdominal muscles.
    e. Ensure privacy.
    f. Provide bedside commode rather than bedpan when possible: encourage sitting position rather than lying position.
    g. Keep equipment easily available at bedside.
    h. Teach patient to recognize signals that may indicate full bowel: goose pimples, perspiration, rising of hair on arms or legs, and sense of fullness.
    i. Instruct patient to develop exercise or signals that may help to stimulate urge to defecate: (1) pressure on inner thigh, (2) stroking anus, (3) digital rectal stimulation, (4) drinking coffee, and (5) massaging abdomen downward or side to side.
    j. Instruct patient to respond to signals promptly.
    k. Discuss importance of establishing well-balanced diet that includes bulk and roughage.
    l. Discuss foods to avoid: bananas, beans, and cabbage.
    m. Instruct patient to recognize signs of impaction: (1) no formed stool for 3 days, (2) semiliquid stools, and (3) restlessness and increased feeling of discomfort.
    n. Discuss treatment for impaction: (1) laxative suppository, (2) tap water or oil retention enema, or (3) manual clearing of bowel followed by enema.
    o. Stress importance of reporting symptoms of autonomic hyperreflexia to physician immediately.
    p. Discuss possibility of accidental incontinence once program has been established.
    q. Instructing patient to relate incontinence to change in diet or daily routine.
13. Stress importance of ongoing outpatient care such as physician's visits and physical therapy.
14. Refer to Spinal Cord Injury Foundation.

EVALUATION

Patient Outcome	Data Indicating That Outcome is Reached
The patient demonstrates a patent airway.	Breath sounds are normal. Chest excursion is bilateral and symmetric. Rate and depth of respirations are normal. Cough is effective. There are no subjective or objective findings of shortness of breath, air hunger, or dyspnea on exertion.
The patient demonstrates an effective breathing pattern.	Airway is patent. Chest excursion is symmetric. Breath sounds are normal, or there is no increase in adventitious sounds. Arterial blood gas values are within normal ranges or consistent with patient's baseline. Vital signs are within normal ranges or consistent with patient's baseline. Hemoglobin levels are 14 to 18 g/dl (male) and 12 to 16 g/dl (female). Intake and output are stable. There are no signs of respiratory distress.

Patient Outcome	**Data Indicating That Outcome is Reached**
	All lobes are resonant on percussion. Skin color is not cyanotic.
The patient demonstrates adequate spinal tissue perfusion.	Neurologic and vital signs are stable. Spinal column is immobilized via appropriate method. Straight body alignment is maintained. Intake and output are adequate.
The patient demonstrates minimal complications of sensory-perceptual alterations.	Level of orientation is optimal. The patient remains free of injury. Nutritional status is adequate. Skin integrity is maintained. Self-care deficits are minimal. Social participation is appropriate to physiologic status.
The patient remains free of traumatic injury.	Safety measures are appropriate to level of physiologic status. Skin integrity is maintained. Skin is free of bruises, burns, abrasions, and redness. Environment is safe. The patient is free of nosocomial infections.
The patient demonstrates an optimal level of mobility.	Skin integrity is maintained. The patient remains free of contractures and deformities. Level of mobility is appropriate to physiologic status. Intake and output pattern is stable. Nutritional status is adequate. The patient remains free of thrombophlebitis. The patient remains free of local infection. The patient participates in an ongoing physical therapy program.
The patient demonstrates minimal self-care deficits.	Outcome criteria listed for impaired physical mobility are met. Level of self-care activities is appropriate to physiologic status. The patient participates in physical and occupational therapy.
The patient demonstrates skin integrity.	Skin is intact. Nutritional status is adequate. Electrolyte balance is maintained. The patient remains free of pressure sores and contractures.
The patient demonstrates minimal complications of bowel incontinence.	Skin in perineal area is clean and dry. Dietary intake is adequate. Fluid intake is adequate (2000 ml daily, unless contraindicated). Intake and output pattern is stable. The patient remains free of fecal impaction. The patient demonstrates a regular bowel evacuation pattern.
The patient demonstrates intact self-concepts.	The patient openly verbalizes feelings of grief and loss. The patient verbalizes positive feelings about self. The patient acknowledges actual change in self-image. The patient focuses on present and future appearance and function. The patient verbalizes feelings of hopefulness, helpfulness, and powerfulness.
The patient demonstrates a low level of anxiety.	The patient openly verbalizes concerns and feelings of grief, loss, and discomfort. The patient openly verbalizes feelings supported by health care professionals and family. The patient verbalizes essential aspects of care. The patient identifies methods to effectively deal with anxious feelings.
The patient demonstrates minimal feelings of powerlessness.	The patient maintains optimal level of physiologic control, as possible for current health status. The patient maintains optimal level of psychologic control, as possible. The patient participates, as possible, in decision making about care. The patient participates, as possible, in self-care.

HEADACHE

Headache, or cephalalgia, may be defined as any ache or pain in the head that results from the stimulation of pain-sensitive structures in the cranium or the extracranial tissues in the head and neck.

Approximately 30 million individuals in the United States seek health care for recent or recurring headaches. There are many different types of headaches ranging in severity from a relatively benign and transient discomfort to a severe, incapacitating pain. Headaches may be the symptom of some potentially destructive pathologic process such as cerebral hypoxia, head trauma, inflamed meninges, cerebral hemorrhage, or expanding cranial mass. Therefore headaches, and particularly *recurring* headaches, require thorough investigation including a complete history and neurologic examination.

Headaches may be classified into the major catagories of (1) vascular, (2) muscle contraction, and (3) traction-inflammatory. Vascular headaches include migraine, cluster, and hypertensive headaches, as well as headaches from secondary responses (e.g., to infectious process). Muscle contraction headaches may occur from psychogenic problems, such as response to trauma or as a result of medical disorders such as cervical arthritis. Traction-inflammatory headaches may result from infection, intracranial or extracranial lesions, occlusive vascular disorders, diseases of facial structures, and medical disorders such as arteritis.[10]

PATHOPHYSIOLOGY

Pain-sensitive extracranial structures include (1) skin of the scalp; (2) periosteum; (3) temporal, frontal, and occipital muscle groups; (4) arteries traversing the subcutaneous tissue; and (5) the delicate tissues of the eye, nasal cavity, and ear. Intracranial structures include (1) the venous sinuses and their tributary veins, (2) the meninges (in particular part of the basal dura mater), (3) the larger arteries within the pia-arachnoid and dura mater, and (4) the first three cervical nerves as well as the vagus, glossopharyngeal, and trigeminal cranial nerves. The cranial bones, most of the pia-arachnoid membranes and dura, the brain parenchyma, the choroid plexuses, and the ependymal lining of the cerebral ventricles are relatively insensitive to painful stimuli.

Afferent pain fibers carry sensory stimuli to the tissues of the central nervous system by the three divisions of the trigeminal nerve, the first three cervical nerves, and cranial nerves IX (glossopharyngeal) and X (vagus). Intracranially, the trigeminal nerve supplies structures in the anterior and middle fossae of the skull above the tentorium. Trigeminal innervation extracranially includes all or most of the nervous supply to the facial skin; the

subcutaneous tissues, and especially the blood vessels in this region; the eyes, nose, sinuses, and teeth; and most of the ear and external auditory canal.[2] The first three cervical nerves serve structures in the posterior fossae and the infradural region. Cranial nerves IX and X also supply portions of the posterior fossae and refer pain to the throat and ear.

Head pain can be caused by any of the following mechanisms: (1) distention, dilation, or traction of intracranial or extracranial arteries; (2) traction, compression, or disease states affecting sensory cranial or spinal nerves; (3) meningeal irritation and increased intracranial pressure; (4) displacement or traction of large intracranial veins or their dural envelopes; and (5) voluntary or involuntary spasms and possible interstitial inflammation or traction of cervical and cranial muscles.

Extracranial causes of headaches include emotional tension, disorders of extracranial arteries, sinusitis, and inflammatory lesions of the bone and its coverings. Pain results from chronic sustained contractions of skeletal muscles, changes in intracranial pressure, vessel dilation and stretching of surrounding tissue, or a combination of the preceding factors.

Intracranial causes of headaches, such as mass lesions, produce pain from the compression, inflammation, distortion, or traction of the pain-sensitive blood vessels and meninges at the base of the brain.

Headaches of diffuse meningeal irritation are most likely caused by the chemical irritation of nerve endings and the stretching of pain-sensitive structures by dilation and congestion of inflamed meningeal vessels. This type of headache is typically throbbing in nature because of the transmission of arterial pulsation to cerebral tissues already under increased tension.[43]

Vascular Headaches

Migraine headaches. Migraine headache generally begins in childhood, adolescence, or early adult life and is found in approximately 5% of the general population. It is frequently familial, and there appears to be some predilection for young women. These young women appear to be particularly susceptible just before or during the menstrual period. Migraine is characterized by a paroxysmal, throbbing, unilateral head pain that frequently is accompanied by autonomic symptoms such as nausea and vomiting. Attacks generally decrease in frequency and intensity with advancing years.

The precise pathogenesis of migraine remains to be elucidated. The initial physiologic change is that of vasospasm in the intracranial and extracranial arteries and their branches on one side of the head. Ten to thirty minutes later, dilation of the same vessels occurs. The constriction of the arteries is responsible for the symptoms of the aura, while vessel dilation produces the headache part of the syndrome. In headache-free intervals, the cranial vessels of the migraine patient are hypersensitive to inhalation of carbon dioxide and intravenous histamine.[37]

Recent studies indicate there is a rise in serotonin levels during the prodromal phase, and these levels drop during the headache phase. Also, the urinary excretion of 5-hydroxyindoleacetic acid (5-HIAA), a metabolite of serotonin, is increased during the migraine episodes. Platelet aggregability, which increases just before a migraine attack, is thought to be responsible for the release of serotonin.[26]

Agents and circumstances thought to precipitate migraine attacks include emotional stress and tension, menstruation, too much or too little sleep, and dietary agents such as tyramine, nitrate, and glutamate. However, none of these affect all individuals or consistently produce attacks in the same individual.[9] There is no evidence to support allergy or autonomic disorders as responsible for migraine attacks.

Cluster headaches. Cluster headaches (Horton's syndrome, histamine headache, migrainous neuralgia, or paroxysmal nocturnal cephalalgia) are intense repetitive vascular events. Cluster headaches are four times more common in men, generally occurring in the third and fourth decades of life.[26] Cluster headaches are characterized by a distinct episode of excruciating pain, usually unilateral, which lasts from ½ to 1 hour, and is accompanied by ipsilateral lacrimation, nasal stuffiness, and drainage.[9] Usually, the same side of the head is involved in the cluster of attacks. There is no prodrome and usually only slight nausea. The attack may occur at any time (usually they are nocturnal), and multiple attacks are common.

Headaches may occur in an episodic or chronic pattern. The episodic pattern of cluster headaches is characterized by occurrence of the headache event for several weeks to months, followed by months to years during which no headaches occur.

Chronic cluster headaches can be divided into a primary chronic type and a secondary chronic type. The primary chronic pattern is characterized by persistent, repetitive attacks for years at a time. The secondary chronic type occurs when the episodic attacks evolve into chronic, unremitting attacks.[9]

The exact mechanism of cluster headaches is unknown. Increased histamine with resultant vasodilation has been implicated.

Tension Headaches

Muscle contraction headaches. Muscle contraction headaches are the most common type of head pain. Research studies indicate a preponderance of muscle contraction headaches in women and a higher incidence in adults from 20 to 40 years of age. This type of headache is usually bilateral and may be diffuse or confined to the frontal, temporal, parietal, or occipital area. The onset of an attack is more gradual than with a migraine, and duration is highly variable, but it may last for several days up to several months or years.

Muscle contraction headaches are frequently accompanied by contraction of skeletal muscles of the face, jaw, and neck. Concurrent arterial vasodilation may contribute further to the discomfort. There are no structural changes in the involved muscle groups.

Traumatic headaches. The posttraumatic, or postconcussion, headache, which consists of a dull, generalized pain, may develop after head injury and may be coupled with other symptoms such as lack of concentration, giddiness, or dizziness. Symptoms are much the same whether the head injury is mild or severe. Traumatic headaches are usually nonfocal, appearing for at least part of every day and persisting over days, weeks, or months. The headache is made worse by coughing and straining, which raises the pressure in both intracranial and extracranial venous systems.

The pathogenesis of posttraumatic headaches is thought to be caused by vascular dilation, muscle contraction, or direct injury to the scalp.

Traction-Inflammatory Headaches

Traction headaches. Traction headaches may result from increased intracranial pressure, cerebral hemorrhage, decreased intracranial pressure (e.g., lumbar puncture), and inflammatory processes (e.g., encephalitis, meningitis). The discomfort produced with traction headaches results from referred pain when the pain-sensitive structures (i.e., cranial nerves, arteries, etc.) are stretched or displaced by a mass lesion.

Temporal arteritis. The headache produced in temporal arteritis, also termed cranial arteritis or giant cell arteritis, generally affects individuals over 60 years of age. This type of headache is usually located in the temporal area and may be accompanied by visual loss, which is caused by ophthalmic artery involvement.[26]

The pathogenesis of temporal arteritis is thought to result from an autoimmune mechanism and is included in the group of collagen-vascular diseases. The temporal arteries may be palpated as firm, tender cords or may be seen as tortuous, enlarged vessels.

Other clinical types of headaches include those from angioma and aneurysm, chronic subdural hematoma, brain tumor, and medical disorders such as hypothyroidism, Cushing's disease, fevers of any cause, chronic lung disease with hypercapnia, hypertension, acute anemia, chronic nitrate or ergot exposure, corticosteroid withdrawal, carbon monoxide exposure, adrenal tumors producing aldosterone, and sometimes Addison's disease.

DIAGNOSTIC STUDIES

Cervical and skull roentgenograms
Detection of abnormalities at base of brain

Funduscopic eye examination
Possible irritation of iris and ciliary body

Serum
Increased sedimentation rate
Anemia (lithium serum level *not* to exceed 1.0 mEq/L)

CT scan
Possible intracranial lesions

Magnetic resonance imaging (MRI)
Same as CT scan

Cerebral angiography
Detection of vascular abnormalities

Neurologic history and examination
Identification of precipitating influences
Effects on activities of daily living
Neurologic deficits

TREATMENT PLAN

Chemotherapeutic
Analgesic/anti-inflammatory agents
Ergot preparations (Table 3-7)

Table 3-7

Drugs Used in the Treatment of Vascular Migraine Headaches

Drug	Use	Dose	Action	Side Effects
Ergotamine tartrate (Gynergen)	Treatment of vascular migraine headaches A single dose of ergotamine (1 or 3 mg by injection at bedtime) is effective for *cluster headaches*	2 mg orally 2 mg sublingually, initially to be followed by 2 mg every 30 min until the headache subsides, or until 6 mg have been taken (Some texts suggest that up to a total of 9 mg may be taken.) 0.25-0.5 mg *subcutaneously* or *IM* at onset; dose may be repeated hourly up to 1.0 mg in 24 h 0.25 mg intravenously at onset; no more than 0.5 mg/24 h; rarely given IV 2-4 mg by *rectal suppository* at onset; 2 mg may be repeated hourly, up to 6-8 mg	Ergot alkaloids result in cerebral vasoconstriction, which decreases the amplitude of the pulsations of the cranial arteries. In addition to its powerful vasoconstrictive property, it also constricts the smooth muscles of the uterus. However, the major use of ergot alkaloids is for the treatment of migraine headaches.	Has a *cumulative action,* so that it must be taken sparingly and as ordered or ergotism will develop (*Ergotism:* numbness and tingling of fingers and toes, muscle pain and weakness, gangrene, and blindness) *Contraindications:* Diabetes mellitus, sepsis, hepatorenal disease, peripheral and coronary disease, hypertension, and pregnancy
Dihydroergotamine (DHE 45)	Treatment of migraine headaches which tend to be severe	1 mg IM or IV at onset; repeat in 1 h	Action is not clear, but a majority of patients receive relief in 15 min to 2 h after administration.	Less toxic and fewer side effects than ergotamine; less likely to cause vomiting than ergotamine

From Hickey, J.: The clinical practice of neurological and neurosurgical nursing, Philadelphia, 1981, J.B. Lippincott Co, p. 402.

Table 3-7, cont'd
Drugs Used in the Treatment of Vascular Migraine Headaches

Drug	Use	Dose	Action	Side Effects
Ergotamine with caffeine (Cafergot)	Same as ergotamine	Each tablet contains 1 mg of ergotamine tartrate and 100 mg of caffeine. Usual dose is 1-2 tablets at onset and another tablet in 30 min, not to exceed 6 tablets per attack (also available in suppositories if vomiting occurs).	The caffeine increases the effectiveness of the ergotamine by its vasoconstrictive action.	Same as ergotamine
Ergotamine tartrate, 0.3 mg Phenobarbital, 20 mg Belladonna alkaloid, 0.1 mg (Bellergal)	Reduces the number of attacks in patients who have one or more weekly	Give 2 or 3 times daily for a few weeks.	Vasoconstriction, sedation, and reduction of spasm	Same as ergotamine, along with dryness of mucous membrane and drowsiness *Contraindications:* In addition to those of ergotamine, do not give to patients with glaucoma.
Methysergide maleate (Sansert)	For prophylactic treatment of vascular headaches such as migraine, cluster, and others which have been difficult to control; not effective for an acute attack; a serotonin antagonist *Alert:* Patient must be under medical supervision because this drug has such serious side effects.	2 mg orally tid with meals; after taking drug for 5 mo, it should be discontinued for 3-4 wk to reduce the incidence of serious side effects; dosage should be reduced gradually to prevent rebound headache.	The action is not clear, but it decreases the frequency of headache in patients who have a few headaches weekly and are difficult to control with other drugs.	Fibrotic changes in the retroperitoneal and pleuropulmonary tissue and in the mitral and aortic valves are the most serious complications. Any of the following symptoms should be reported at once: urinary tract obstruction, dysuria, back pain, peripheral vascular insufficiency, cold, numb, or painful extremities and diminished pulse, dyspnea, and chest pain. *Contraindications:* Cardiac conditions, severe hypertension, pregnancy, peripheral vascular disease, and atherosclerosis

Others
  Analgesics
    Codeine sulfate, 30 mg
         or
    Meperidine (Demerol), 50 mg

Either drug may be given for severe pain once the headache has become full-blown. Narcotics are avoided unless the pain is very severe, and precautions should be taken to avoid addiction.

    Aspirin, 0.6 g
    Propoxyphene (Darvon), 65 mg
    Butalbital (Fiorinal), 2 tablets

These drugs may be tried for less severe pain.

  Diuretics
    Hydrochlorothiazide (Esidrix)
      or acetazolamide (Diamox)

These drugs are given 1 wk before menstruation if premenstrual tension predisposes the individual to headaches. In addition, mild tranquilizers and analgesics such as aspirin may be given.

  Antihistamines
    Diphenhydramine (Benadryl)
      and others

May be helpful in cluster headaches.

Adrenergic agents
Isometheptene mucate (Midrin, Octinum), 1-2 capsules at onset of headache; followed by 1-2 capsules 1 h later

Psychotherapeutic agents
Chlorpromazine (Thorazine), 25 mg IM, po, or rectal suppository
Promethazine (Phenergan), 25 mg IM or rectally; 50 mg po
Hydroxyzine (Vistaril), 75 mg IM or 50-100 mg po
Lithium carbonate (Lithane; others), initial dose of 300 mg po bid to qid; *must* be monitored by serum levels

Analgesic/antipyretics
Acetaminophen (Tylenol)

Narcotic analgesics
Meperidine (Demerol), 50-75 mg IM q4-6h prn

Corticosteroids
Dexamethasone (Decadron), 8-12 mg IM

Beta-adrenergic blocking agent
Propranolol (Inderal), initial dose 20 mg po bid or tid; titrated gradually up to 80-200 mg/d in divided doses

Antihistamines
Methysergide maleate (Sansert), 2 mg tid or qid; for up to 5-6 mo; followed by mandatory discontinuance for at least 1 mo
Cyproheptadine (Periactin), 4 mg po bid to qid

Antidepressants
Phenelzine (Nardil), 10-15 mg po bid to qid

Antihypertensive agents
Clonidine hydrochloride (Catapres), 0.2 mg po bid to tid

Antianginal agents
Dipyridamole (Persantine), 25-50 mg po tid or qid

Nonsteroidal anti-inflammatory agents
Sulfinpyrazone (Anturane), 200 mg po bid to qid

Antidepressants
Amitriptyline (Elavil), 25-100 mg po qid

Electromechanical
Application of heat or cold to affected areas

Supportive
Dietary counseling to eliminate food items that may provoke headaches:

vinegar	canned figs
chocolate	ripened cheeses
pork	herring
onions	doughnuts
excessive caffeine	cured sandwich meats
citrus fruits	chicken livers
bananas	broad bean pods
yogurt	fermented or marinated foods
sour cream	avocados
alcohol	MSG

Psychologic counseling for behavioral modification, stress management, and biofeedback

ASSESSMENT: AREAS OF CONCERN

Migraine
Classic migraine
Prodrome
Visual scotoma
Aphasia
Hemiparesis
Altered mood, hunger, and taste
Drowsiness
Pain
Throbbing, high-intensity, unilateral discomfort in temporal area, upper cranium, or lower hemicranium (rare)
Other
Photophobia
Nausea and vomiting
Ergotism: tingling and numbness of toes and fingers; muscle weakness and pain; gangrene; blindness
Common migraine
Prodrome
None
Pain
Throbbing intense pain progressing to generalized, nonthrobbing head pain
Other
Photophobia
Nausea and vomiting
Irritability

Cluster
Pain
Sudden, intense unilateral head pain beginning in area of nostril and spreading to area of adjacent eye and sometimes forehead
Other
Flushing of skin
Nose and eyes water
Homolateral Horner's syndrome with ptosis and pupillary constriction
Steady, nonpulsating, unilateral or bilateral head pain in temporal, frontal, parietal, or occipital areas

Posttraumatic
Pain
Generalized, dull, aching head pain
Other
Personality changes
Insomnia

Fatigue
Giddiness
Unsteadiness
Concentration difficulties
Nausea and vomiting

Hypertensive
Throbbing pain that is predominantly occipital

Traction
Deep, dull, steady ache usually worse in morning and aggravated by coughing or straining

Cerebral arteritis
Variable intensity of unilateral or bilateral head pain in temporal, occipital, or fronto-occipital regions; may be accompanied by tenderness of painful areas

Lumbar puncture headache
Dull, pulsating occipital-nuchal discomfort and frontal pain after rising from a recumbent position

NURSING DIAGNOSES and NURSING INTERVENTIONS

Nursing Diagnosis	Nursing Intervention
Anxiety	See general intervention strategies listed on p. 1839.
Comfort, alteration in: pain	Promote rest and relaxation. Decrease noxious stimuli. Modify anxiety associated with the pain experience. Provide other sensory input. Administer medication as per protocol. Remain with the patient. Utilize whatever measures the patient believes will alleviate the pain. Teach the patient about his discomfort. Utilize other professionals, as appropriate. Improve effectiveness of pain relief measures by using them before the pain becomes intense.

Patient Education

1. Reinforce physician's explanation of medical management.
2. Instruct regarding name of medication, dosage, time of administration, and toxic or side effects.
3. Instruct regarding proper use of ergot drugs:
   a. Take medication at earliest symptom of a headache.
   b. Dosages greater than 10 mg/wk can lead to ergotism and cumulative effects.
   c. Lie in quiet, dark room after taking the medication.
4. Stress need to avoid over-the-counter medications without first consulting physician.
5. Emphasize need for regular exercise program.
6. Instruct regarding possible food causes of headaches.

EVALUATION

Patient Outcome	Data Indicating That Outcome is Reached
The patient experiences minimal alterations in comfort.	The patient openly verbalizes feelings of discomfort when they occur. The patient can utilize measures to decrease discomfort. The patient verbally validates a decrease in subjective feelings of discomfort. Objective findings of pain are decreased.
The patient demonstrates a low level of anxiety.	The patient openly verbalizes concerns and feelings of grief, loss, and discomfort. The patient openly verbalizes feelings, supported by health care professionals and family. The patient verbalizes essential aspects of care. The patient identifies methods to effectively deal with anxious feelings.

SEIZURES

A seizure, or convulsion, is "a sudden, violent involuntary contraction of a group of muscles that may be paroxysmal and episodic, as in a seizure disorder, or transient and acute, as following a head concussion."[50]

Seizures may be tonic or clonic, focal, and unilateral or bilateral. The term *epilepsy* is used to denote a group of neurologic disorders characterized by the repeated occurrence of any of the various forms of seizures. Approximately 2 to 4 million Americans are affected with epilepsy, and many of this number are children. The social consequences of a seizure disorder are many, including possible loss of driving or educational privileges. Of all persons with epilepsy, 25% have recurrent seizures while on medication, 10% are institutionalized, and 5% are home-bound invalids.[30]

PATHOPHYSIOLOGY

Seizure disorders can be classified into five basic groups of causative factors: (1) pathologic processes, (2) endogenous or exogenous poisons, (3) metabolic disturbances, (4) fever, and (5) idiopathic. *Pathologic processes* include formation errors (e.g., vascular anomalies), space-occupying lesions (e.g., brain abscess, tumors, hematomas), craniocerebral trauma, acute cerebral edema (e.g., secondary to acute renal failure), infection (e.g., encephalitis), degenerative changes (e.g., leukodystrophies), vascular lesions (e.g., embolus, cerebrovascular accidents, and hemorrhages), and neuronal injury (e.g., anoxia from deficient oxygen supply.

Toxic endogenous substances (e.g., uremia) or *exogenous* substances such as certain medications (e.g., phenothiazines), lead ingestion, and alcohol intoxication or sudden withdrawal may precipitate seizures.

Metabolic disturbances (i.e., electrolyte imbalances) that cause an interference with crucial substances such as oxygen, glucose, or calcium being delivered to cerebral tissues can result in seizures.

Individuals with decreased neuronal thresholds may experience a seizure secondary to a *febrile* state.

Finally, *idiopathic* seizures may occur without any identifiable cause. The basis of idiopathic seizure disorders is thought to be some type of biochemical imbalance.

The factors listed above as causative agents can be grouped under the general headings of genetic factors and acquired factors. *Genetically*, epilepsy is rarely a predictable, inherited entity. The only well-defined inherited seizure pattern is that of the classic 2.5 to 3/s spike-and-wave pattern on the EEG.[26] Therefore, although inheritance may be a risk in developing seizures, environmental risk factors (e.g., trauma) play a significant role. *Acquired* factors listed above include pathologic processes (e.g., infection), trauma that produces epileptogenic lesions, toxic substances, metabolic disturbances, and febrile states.

Seizures have traditionally been classified into categories of grand mal, petit mal, psychomotor (temporal lobe), and focal motor (jacksonian). With advanced technology it became evident that many neurologic manifestations of seizures did not fit into these categories. In 1969 the International League Against Epilepsy formulated a revised classification that incorporated pathophysiologic principles of all types of seizure activity.

Partial seizures originate from a localized activation of neurons and generally do not involve the whole brain or significantly impair consciousness or memory. Partial seizures with simple symptoms produce symptoms of which the individual is aware, including autonomic, sensory, or focal motor symptoms. Simple partial seizures with focal motor symptoms (jacksonian seizures) generally originate from the contralateral precentral gyrus. Symptoms occur initially in the part of the body controlled by that brain area and can then spread to involve the entire limb and frequently the entire half of the body. The seizure ends with a gradual reduction of clonic, jerking movements. Seizure activity occurring usually in the hand or face which is continuous, clonic, and localized is termed *epilepsia partialis continua*. Simple sensory seizures are not common, but when present, they originate from hyperexcitable neurons in the postcentral gyrus. Symptoms of a partial sensory seizure include various degrees of numbness and paresthesias. Autonomic seizures result from hyperexcitable neurons of the frontal, temporal, mesial, orbital, or insular cortices. These seizures may begin with disturbances in gastric motility, which may progress to nausea and vomiting, tenesmus, or sudden bowel evacuation.[16] Partial seizures with only autonomic symptoms are rare.

Partial seizures with complex symptoms generally produce some type of episodic loss of consciousness. This type of seizure may include cognitive, affective, psychosensory, or psychomotor symptoms. Triggering events occur within the structures of the temporal lobe. The onset of complex partial seizures consists of various types of auras such as sensory illusions, déjà vu, or unusual smells. The individual may recognize these auras, or memory of them may be lost in postictal amnesia. In complex partial seizures, electroencephalographic abnormalities are localized in temporal or frontotemporal areas, including rhinencephalic structures. Complex partial seizures are characterized by purposeful behavior that is inappropriate for the time and place.[2] Automatisms such as lip smacking, walking aimlessly, or picking at one's clothing are common. The individual with this type of seizure is usually amnestic for events of the seizure, but consciousness is not lost totally.

Psychomotor seizures in children can be confused with absence attacks because of the relative paucity of memory patterns in the temporal lobe of the young child. Complex partial attacks in children may be differentiated from absence attacks by the fact that the psychomotor attacks occur much less frequently and are of longer duration.

Generalized seizures begin locally but almost immediately result in bilateral involvement of the corticoreticular and reticulocortical systems of the diencephalon. Generalized seizures are usually petit mal (absence seizures) or grand mal (tonic-clonic) in nature. Petit mal seizures usually affect children after the age of 4 years and before puberty,[23] and although rare, they can occur in adults up to 70 years of age. Petit mal seizures consist of a sudden cessation of conscious activity without loss of postural control or convulsive motor activity.[37] These absence attacks usually last for seconds or minutes. The brief lapses of consciousness may be accompanied by minor motor manifestations (e.g., eyelid flickering and isolated myoclonic jerks). Following a petit mal seizure the individual quickly regains consciousness or awareness and usually experiences no postictal confusion.

Grand mal seizures are one of the most common types of epileptic paroxysms and may be primarily generalized seizures or the result of secondary generalization of partial seizures. Grand mal seizures usually occur without warning and follow a common pattern: (1) *tonic* phase: forceful contraction of axial and appendicular muscles, loss of postural control, epileptic cry, cyanosis; tonic phase usually lasts 2 or 3 minutes; (2) *clonic* phase, characterized by gradual transition from tonic contractions to intermittent bilateral brisk clonic movements; this phase is representative of recurring inhibition phases interrupting the initial tonic phase; (3) *postictal* phase: amnesia of seizure and possibly even retrograde amnesia.

Generalized seizures can also result from secondary generalization of focal cortical discharges and are identical to primary generalized seizures, making it difficult to distinguish these from primarily generalized tonic-clonic seizures. With secondary generalized seizures, however, there are usually diffuse cerebral pathologic findings.[2]

Generalized seizures such as myoclonic seizures, tonic seizures, infantile spasms, and atonic seizures usually occur during childhood and are generally associated with some type of genetic, perinatal, or metabolic brain disease. *Myoclonic* seizures may occur alone or coexist with other types of seizures. Individuals with severe and generalized myoclonus demonstrate evidence of disturbances

in function of the reticular substance in relevant areas of the sensory cortex.

Tonic seizures are a less common type of primary generalized seizure and consist of sudden onset of rigid posturing of trunk and extremities, frequently with deviation to one side of the head and eyes. Tonic seizures are frequently of a shorter duration than tonic-clonic seizures and are not followed by a clonic phase. These seizures usually indicate a lesion in the area of the midbrain and are sometimes seen in individuals with severe cerebral palsy.

Infantile spasms (hypsarhythmia) are generalized seizures occurring between birth and approximately 12 months of age. They consist of brief synchronous contractions of the neck, torso, and arms.[37] Infantile spasms rarely occur in an apparently normal infant; rather, they usually occur in children with an underlying neurologic disorder (e.g., anoxic encephalopathy). Approximately 90% of children with infantile spasms develop mental retardation.

Atonic seizures consist of brief loss of consciousness and postural tone; these symptoms are not associated with tonic muscular contractions.[37] This type of seizure is frequently accompanied by other forms of seizure activity.

Unilateral seizure refers to a type of seizure activity in which clinical signs usually occur on one side of the body and the electroencephalographic discharges are recorded over the contralateral cerebral hemisphere.[2] Unilateral seizures may shift from one side to another but generally do not become symmetric.

Unclassified epileptic seizures consist of all the types that cannot be classified under any of the preceding headings because of insufficient data for classification or atypical characteristics of the seizure activity.

The microscopic changes leading to pathologic processes occurring during the different types of seizure activities are essentially the same. The major alteration in the physiologic state is a hypersynchronous discharge in a localized area of the brain.[37] This localized area of hypersynchronized discharge is termed the *epileptogenic focus*, producing a large, sharp EEG wave form known as the spike discharge.

Metabolic changes occurring within the cerebrum during the epileptic discharges include (1) release of unusually large amounts of neuropeptides and neurotransmitters during the seizure, (2) increased cerebral blood flow to primary involved areas, (3) increased extracellular concentrations of potassium and decreased extracellular concentrations of calcium, (4) changes in oxidative metabolism and local pH, and (5) increased utilization of glucose.

Termination of seizure activity appears to be related to the large and lasting hyperpolarization of the neuronal

402   Clinical Nursing Practice

cell membrane. This hyperpolarization is possibly generated by an electrogenic sodium pump. As the hyperpolarization is sustained, the neuronal cells cease firing and the surface potentials of the brain are suppressed.[16]

DIAGNOSTIC STUDIES

CT scan
Structural changes

Magnetic resonance imaging (MRI)
Structural changes

Skull roentgenogram
Evidence of fractures
Shift of calcified pineal gland
Bony erosion
Separated sutures

Echoencephalogram
Possible midline shifts of brain structures

Cerebral angiography
Possible vascular abnormalities
Evaluation of a subdural hematoma

Electroencephalogram (EEG)
Grand mal: high, fast voltage spiked in all leads
Petit mal: 3/s, rounded spike wave complexes in all leads
Psychomotor (temporal lobe): square-topped 4-6/s spike wave complexes over involved lobe
Delta waves: usually associated with destroyed brain tissue
Theta waves: not always abnormal

Urine screening
Indicates presence and levels of certain medications

Serum chemistry
Hypoglycemia
Electrolyte imbalance
Increased blood urea nitrogen
Blood alcohol levels

History and neurologic examination
Pattern of onset and characteristics of seizure activity
Precipitating factors

TREATMENT PLAN

Surgical
Excision of epileptogenic focus
Stereotactic lesions

Chemotherapeutic
Anticonvulsants
Grand mal, simple partial, and complex partial
Phenytoin (Dilantin), adult, 100 mg po or IV tid or qid; child, 5 mg/kg/d
Phenobarbital
Primidone (Mysoline)
Day 1-3: 100-125 mg po hs
Day 4-6: 100-125 mg po bid
Day 7-9: 100-125 mg po tid
Day 10 and maintenance: 250 mg po tid
Carbamazepine (Tegretol), adult, initially 200 mg po bid; increase dosage gradually until desired response is obtained (should not exceed 120 mg/d; child (6-12 yr), initially 100 mg po bid; increase by 100 mg/d until desired response is achieved (should not exceed 1000 mg/d)
Petit mal
Ethosuximide (Zarontin), initially at 3-6 yr of age, 250 mg po qd; 6 yr and older, 500 mg po qd; maintenance dose, individually determined according to patient's response

Electromechanical
Emergency equipment at bedside

Supportive
Serum chemistry monitoring (complete blood count, platelet count)
Routine urinalysis
Dietary therapy (i.e., ketogenic diet)
Serum drug levels (e.g., Dilantin, phenobarbital)
Seizure precautions

ASSESSMENT: AREAS OF CONCERN

Simple partial seizures
Motor signs
Involuntary recurrent contractions of muscles (e.g., face, hand, arm, finger) of one body part; may be confined to one body area or spread to contiguous ipsilateral body parts (Spread of activity such as left thumb to left hand to left arm to left side of face is known as *jacksonian march*.)
Behavioral manifestations
Sensory: auditory or visual hallucinations; paresthesias; vertigo
Autonomic and psychic: sensation of déjà vu; complex hallucinations; illusions; unwarranted feelings of anger or fear; pupillary dilation; sweating
Level of consciousness
No loss of consciousness

Complex partial seizures
Onset
May consist of variety of auras (e.g., sensory hallucinations, déjà vu, unusual smells)
Motor activity
Compulsive patting or rubbing of body parts, lip smacking, walking aimlessly, swallowing, picking at clothing (termed *automatisms*)
Unconscious performance of highly skilled acts
Level of consciousness
Episodic loss of conscious contact with environment
Postictal amnesia
Amnestic for seizure events
May be amnestic of auras

Generalized seizures
Petit mal
Transient loss of consciousness for few seconds to minutes
May be accompanied by flickering eyelids or intermittent jerking movements of hands
Grand mal
See findings listed on p. 311
Myoclonic
Sudden brief contraction of muscle groups producing rapid jerky movements in one or more extremities or entire body
May be accompanied by violent fall without loss of consciousness
Tonic
Sudden assumption of an abnormal dystonic posture for a few seconds to minutes
Consciousness usually retained
Head and eyes may deviate toward one side
Infantile spasms
Brief synchronous contractions (usually flexion) of both arms, neck, and trunk
Mental retardation (90% of cases)
Atonic "drop attacks"
Brief loss of consciousness and postural tone without associated tonic muscular contractions

Unilateral seizures
Clonic, tonic, or tonic-clonic seizures affecting only or predominantly one side of body
May be with or without impairment in level of consciousness
Seizures may shift from one side to another (usually not symmetric)

Unclassified seizures
Any atypical seizure activity

NURSING DIAGNOSES and NURSING INTERVENTIONS

Nursing Diagnosis	Nursing Intervention
Airway clearance, ineffective	See general intervention strategies listed on p. 2028.
Breathing pattern, ineffective	See general intervention strategies listed on p. 2030.
Sensory-perceptual alteration: visual, auditory, kinesthetic, gustatory, tactile, olfactory	See general intervention strategies listed on p. 1967.
Injury, potential for: trauma	Maintain bed in low position at all times unless side rails are up or when nurse is with patient. Provide the patient with a call light within easy reach. Maintain side rails in up position at bedtime, after sedation, when patient is confused, and as needed. Maintain wheelchairs and stretchers in locked position when transferring patient.

Preconvulsive	Maintain seizure precautions:
	  Have oral airway at bedside.
	  Have suction equipment available at bedside.
	  Pad side rails, if indicated.
	Administer oxygen as per protocol.
	Establish means of communication; identify auras if possible.
	Reorient the patient to environment.
	Provide emotional support
	Place head in position of comfort; turn head to side.
	Administer oral hygiene as necessary for secretions and bleeding.

Anxiety	See general intervention strategies listed on p. 1839.
Social isolation	See general intervention strategies listed on p. 1938.

Patient Education

1. Instruct regarding nature of the seizure disorder and need to adopt positive attitude.
2. Stress importance of verbalizing feelings of shame, humiliation, anxiety, and fears regarding seizure disorder. Assist in clarifying common fears and myths about epilepsy (i.e., not a form of insanity).
3. Emphasize need to avoid overprotection.
4. Stress need to continue with normal work and recreation routines. Assure patient that activity may inhibit seizure activity.
5. Emphasize need to avoid excessive stress or emotional excitement.
6. Teach importance of wearing a medical alert band or carrying a medical alert card at all times.
7. Stress importance of well-balanced diet and avoidance of excessive use of stimulants such as alcohol.
8. Emphasize importance of identifying aura and course of action to take.
9. Instruct regarding name of medication, action, side effects, dosage, and frequency of administration.
10. Stress need to avoid taking over-the-counter medications without first consulting physician.
11. Emphasize importance of ongoing outpatient care.

EVALUATION

Patient Outcome	Data Indicating That Outcome is Reached
The patient demonstrates a patent airway.	Breath sounds are normal. Chest excursion is bilateral and symmetric. Rate and depth of respirations are normal. Cough is effective. There are no subjective or objective findings of shortness of breath, air hunger, or dyspnea on exertion.
The patient demonstrates an effective breathing pattern.	Airway is patent. Chest excursion is symmetric. Breath sounds are normal, or there is no increase in adventitious sounds. Arterial blood gas values are within normal ranges or consistent with patient's baseline. Vital signs are within normal ranges or consistent with patient's baseline. Hemoglobin levels are 14 to 18 g/dl (male) and 12 to 16 g/dl (female). Intake and output are stable. There are no signs of respiratory distress. All lobes are resonant on percussion.
The patient remains free of traumatic injury.	Safety measures are appropriate to physiologic status. Skin integrity is maintained. Skin is free of bruises, burns, abrasions, and redness. Environment is safe. The patient is free of nosocomial infections.
The patient demonstrates a low level of anxiety.	The patient openly verbalizes concerns and feelings of grief, loss, and discomfort. The patient openly verbalizes feelings, supported by health care professionals and family. The patient verbalizes essential aspects of care. The patient can identify methods to effectively deal with anxious feelings.
The patient demonstrates social participation.	The patient can state importance of interpersonal relationships. The patient relates to self and others. The patient participates, as possible, in unit and group activities. The patient participates, as possible, in family activities.

Medical Interventions

ASSESSMENT PROCEDURES
Noninvasive Assessment Procedures

Noninvasive procedures for evaluating neurologic function consist of the following: (1) roentgenography, (2) echoencephalography, and (3) electroencephalography.

Roentgenography. Roentgenographic studies commonly include skull and spinal x-rays films to assist in identification of relationships between injured tissue or bone and the surrounding tissue. Skull films provide important data about vascular abnormalities, shape and size of the skull bones, presence of fractured skull bones, degenerative changes (i.e., bone erosion), unusual calcifications (e.g., tumors or chronic subdural hematomas), and the position of the pineal body. Spinal x-ray films are taken when there has been any trauma, pain, or sensory or motor impairment to the back or vertebral column. Radiographs of the spine usually include anterior, posterior, and lateral views in order to pinpoint fractures of the irregularly shaped vertebrae. Abnormal findings of spinal roentgenography include (1) vertebral dislocation or fracture, (2) bone erosion, (3) unusual calcification, (4) collapsed vertebrae and wedging, (5) spondylosis, and (6) spurs.

Echoencephalography. An echoencephalogram is a simple and noninvasive diagnostic technique that records the sonic pulses from cerebral structures by reflection of ultrasonic impulses directed through the patient's skull and back toward the source. These pulses are then recorded and projected on an oscilloscope screen.[3]

Echoencepholography is useful in determining ventricular size and cerebral midline shifts. The procedure is performed by placing an ultrasonic transducer on the skull's midaxis at the temporoparietal region. The waves produced are called M-echos, which are then recorded and projected on the oscilloscope screen to provide a graphic representation of the distance from the reflecting surface to the source of the ultrasonic beam.[42] Pictures of these M-echo waves may be recorded to become a permanent part of the client's record.

The procedure takes only several minutes, and the reliability of the results depends on the skill of the technician. Abnormal shifts of the midline structures are recorded in millimeters, and a shift of 3 mm or more in the adult client is considered abnormal.

Electroencephalography. An electroencephalogram (EEG) provides a graphic record of brain wave activity (Fig. 3-28). It is used to diagnose brainstem disorders, impaired level of consciousness, focal lesions, seizure disorders, drug overdose, and brain death.

Generally, between 17 and 21 electrodes are attached with collodion to the patient's head at corresponding areas over the prefrontal, frontal, temporal, parietal, and occipital lobes. After the electrodes are attached, the patient is instructed to remain quiet with eyes closed and is informed of the need to refrain from talking or moving unless otherwise requested (i.e., patient will be asked to hyperventilate for a short period during the test to accentuate abnormalities).

The brain waves recorded during an EEG are called alpha, beta, delta, and theta rhythms. *Alpha* rhythms occur in the adult at 8 to 13 cycles/s and are most prominent in the occipital leads. Apprehension and anxiety can decrease the frequency of the alpha waves. *Beta* wave forms are most prominent in the frontal and central areas and occur at a rate of 18 to 30 cycles/s. Beta rhythm indicates normal activity when an individual is alert and attentive with eyes open. *Delta* wave forms indicate serious brain dysfunction or deep sleep. This rhythm occurs at a rate of less than 4 cycles/s. *Theta* wave forms occur at a rate of 4 to 7 cycles/s and come primarily from the temporal and parietal areas. Theta rhythm indicates drowsiness or emotional stress in adults. They are common in children.

Preprocedural Nursing Care

1. Assisting physician in obtaining consent form from the patient
2. Establishing and maintaining an accurate neurologic baseline
3. Administration of a sedative, unless contraindicated
4. Administration of routine medications, unless otherwise ordered
5. Preprocedural education

ASSESSMENT: AREAS OF CONCERN

Knowledge deficit
Verbalization of deficiency in knowledge of diagnostic procedure

Fig. 3-28
Electroencephalograms. **A,** Normal record with regular, 10-per-second alpha waves dominant throughout. **B,** Irregular high-amplitude delta waves (one to two per second) prominent over the left side. This patient had intracranial tumor. **C,** Three-per-second, synchronous "spike and dome" waves present in all areas, as seen in minor epilepsy.

From Conway-Rutkowski, B.L.: Carini and Owens' neurological and neurosurgical nursing, ed. 8, St. Louis, 1982, The C.V. Mosby Co.

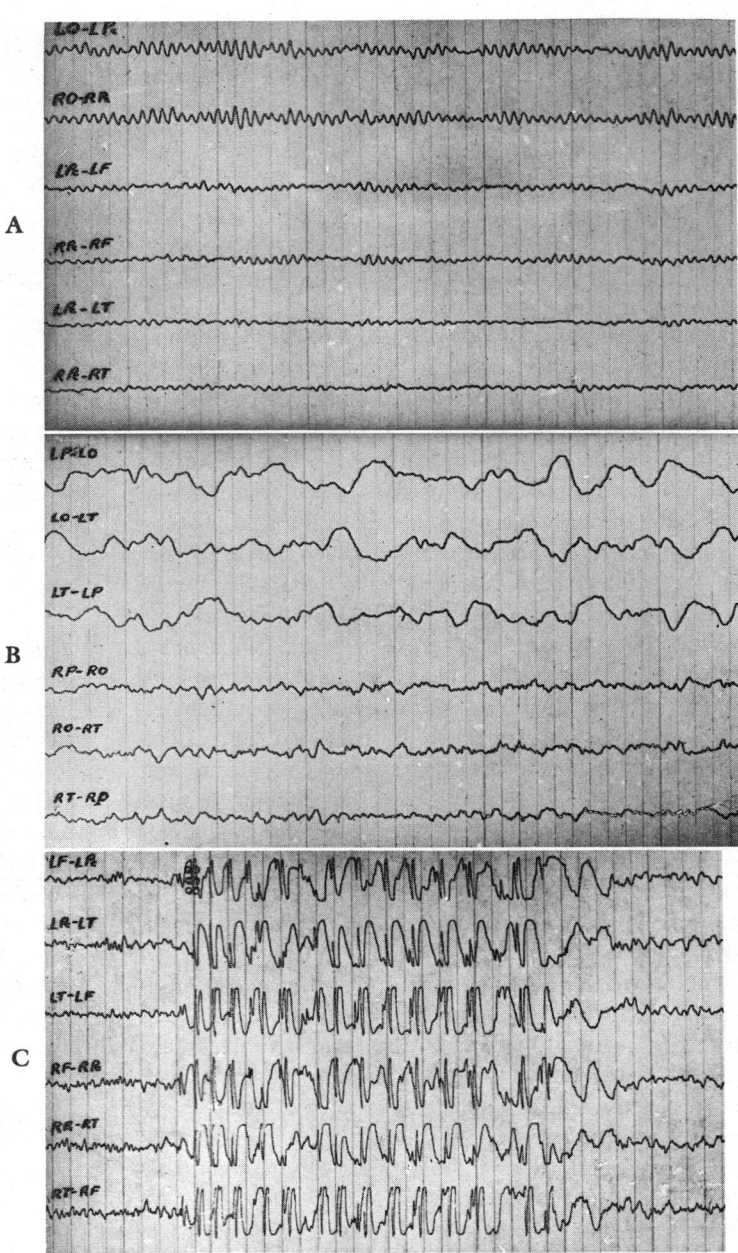

Anxiety
  Appearance
    Increased perspiration, clammy skin
    Fatigue
    Increased muscle tension (rigidity)
    Skin blanches; pale
    Increased small motor activity (i.e., tremors, restlessness)
  Behavior
    Decreased attention span
    Increased somatizing

    Increased immobility
    Decreased ability to follow directions
  Other
    Increased rate or depth of respirations
    Increased heart rate
    Rapid shifts in body temperature and blood pressure
    Urinary urgency
    Diarrhea
    Dry mouth
    Decreased appetite
    Pupillary dilation

NURSING DIAGNOSES and NURSING INTERVENTIONS

Nursing Diagnosis	Nursing Intervention
Knowledge deficit	Implement teaching plan: 　Reason that test was ordered 　Description of equipment used and the testing 　Description of possible sensations patient may experience Provide repetition of teaching plan to strengthen learning. Implement teaching plan in an environment free of distractions and other obstacles. Encourage questions and answer the questions simply and completely. Evaluate and revise teaching plan as necessary.
Anxiety	Establish baseline and ongoing assessment of the patient's anxiety and response to anxiety. Encourage the patient to openly verbalize feelings. Listen to the patient's concerns. Support the patient as he verbalizes feelings of anxiety and provide feedback as indicated. Assist patient in techniques that promote relaxation.

EVALUATION

Patient Outcome	Data Indicating That Outcome is Reached
The patient demonstrates adequate knowledge regarding the diagnostic procedure.	The patient can state why test was ordered. The patient can state what the testing procedure consists of and what equipment is used.

Cerebrospinal Fluid Sampling

Sampling of the cerebrospinal fluid can be obtained from the spinal canal (lumbar puncture), the cisterna magna (cisternal puncture), or the lateral ventricles (ventricular puncture).

Lumbar puncture. The lumbar puncture, or spinal tap, is one of the most common neurologic tests and is performed to (1) measure cerebrospinal fluid pressure, (2) remove cerebrospinal fluid for visualization and laboratory analysis, (3) inject medications or contrast media, and (4) determine degree of subarachnoid block by means of spinal dynamics. The procedure consists of the introduction of a hollow needle and stylet into the lumbar subarchnoid space of the spinal canal, using strict aseptic technique. The patient assumes the lateral recumbent position and curves his back with the head and shoulders bent toward the knees, the legs flexed, and thighs on the abdomen. This position affords maximal space between the vertebrae. The needle is then inserted through the interspace between the third and fourth lumbar vertebrae into the subarachnoid space and the stylet is withdrawn. (The site of insertion for infants and young children is usually lower.) After the stylet is removed, cerebrospinal fluid should begin to slowly drip out. A stopcock with manometer is connected to the needle for recording of opening and closing pressures and removal of cerebrospinal fluid (usually 8 to 10 ml) for visualization and laboratory analysis. The needle is then removed and the puncture site covered with a small dressing.

Contraindications to the lumbar puncture include the following:

1. Infection at the puncture site
2. Clinical evidence of significantly increased intracranial pressure
3. If the procedure does not contribute to diagnosis or treatment

Complications following the procedure include infection, leakage of cerebrospinal fluid, dysuria, signs of meningeal irritation, headaches, nausea, and vomiting.

Cisternal puncture. A cisternal puncture may be performed (1) if a subarachnoid block is present, (2) if a lumbar puncture is contraindicated, (3) to reduce intracranial pressure, (4) to perform encephalography, and (5) to introduce air or a contrast medium for myelography. The patient is positioned on his side with head bent slightly forward at the edge of the bed. After the skin is cleaned and anesthetized, a short, beveled needle with stylet is inserted between the atlas and the occipital bone to a depth of approximately 5 cm (adult) into the cisterna magna. The cerebrospinal fluid is then removed and a

Fig. 3-29
Patient position for lumbar puncture.

From Rudy, E.B.: Advanced neurological
and neurosurgical nursing, St. Louis, 1984,
The C.V. Mosby Co.

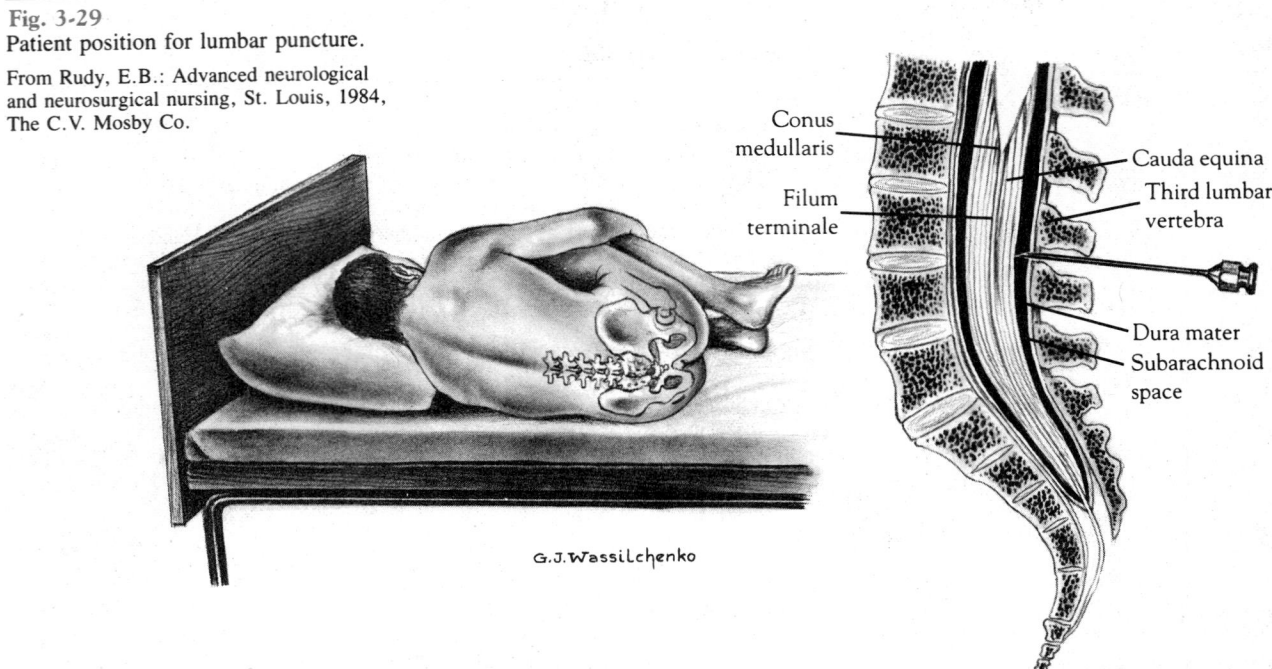

G.J.Wassilchenko

cisternogram may be performed. A *cisternogram* is done
by injecting a radioisotope material into the subarachnoid
space. Following injection, the patient is scanned at regular intervals (i.e., 6, 12, and 24 hours) to determine
the amount of time needed for the radioisotope to clear
from the circulating cerebrospinal fluid.

Ventricular puncture. A ventricular puncture is indicated (1) if lumbar or cisternal puncture is contraindicated, (2) for injection of contrast media into an infant's
ventricles to determine the type of hydrocephalus, (3)
for removal of cerebrospinal fluid, (4) for injection of
air or oxygen to localize a tumor, and (5) as a preliminary
to ventricular drainage. The procedure consists of the
insertion of a needle into the lateral ventricle. The patient
is placed on the side opposite the lateral ventricle to be
tapped and the head is immobilized. After the skin is
cleaned and anesthetized, the needle is inserted into the
ventricle; the sampling then proceeds as for the lumbar
puncture.

Complications following the procedure may include
headache, respiratory distress, increased intracranial
pressure, convulsions, infection, fever, hemorrhage, or
oozing of cerebrospinal fluid.

TREATMENT PLAN

Chemotherapeutic
Sedative hypnotic agents
Pentobarbital sodium (Nembutal), 30 mg po

Analgesic agents
Acetaminophen (Tylenol), 650 mg po q4h prn
Narcotic analgesic agents
Codeine phosphate, 30 mg po q4h prn
Antiemetic agents
Trimethobenzamide hydrochloride (Tigan), 100-
250 mg IM q4-6h prn
Prochlorperazine (Compazine), 10 mg IM q4-6h prn

Electromechanical
Emergency equipment at bedside: airway; Ambu bag

Supportive
Bed rest, as ordered (i.e., 12 to 24 hours after procedure)
Maintenance of input and output; encourage fluids as
ordered

ASSESSMENT: AREAS OF CONCERN

Pain
Headache or nuchal rigidity
Local pain at puncture site
Transient leg or back pain

Increased intracranial pressure
Restlessness; lethargy
Changes in level of consciousness
Changes in vital signs (i.e., Cushing response with
increased systolic blood pressure, wide pulse pres-
sure, and decreased pulse rate)

Pupillary changes (i.e., mydriasis)
Impaired pupillary reflex
Papilledema
Vomiting
Fluctuations in temperature
Seizures

Worsening of focal neurologic signs
Changes in respiratory patterns
Other
Dysuria
Temperature rise without preceding chill

NURSING DIAGNOSES and NURSING INTERVENTIONS

Nursing Diagnosis	Nursing Intervention
Tissue perfusion, alteration in: cerebrospinal	Check vital signs (pulse, respirations, and blood pressure) every 15 minutes for four times, then every hour for four times, then as per routine. Observe puncture site for redness, swelling, or drainage. Assist patient to cough and deep breathe every 2 to 4 hours and as needed. Force fluids, unless contraindicated. Maintain bed rest as per protocol; explain importance of keeping head and body flat in bed.
Comfort, alteration in	Administer pain medications as ordered.

EVALUATION

Patient Outcome	Data Indicating That Outcome is Reached
The patient remains free of postprocedural complications.	The patient does not have a headache. The patient takes fluids well. Vital signs are stable. There is no nausea and vomiting. There is no nuchal rigidity. Cerebral tissue perfusion is adequate.

Contrast Studies

Neurologic contrast studies are all invasive procedures and include cerebral angiography, pneumoencephalography, ventriculography, and brain scan myelography.

Cerebral angiography. Cerebral angiography consists of the infusion of a radiopaque substance into the cerebral arterial system. During infusion of the contrast medium, a series of x-ray films is taken for visualization of the extracranial and intracranial vessels. To outline the anterior, middle, and posterior cerebral arteries and returning venous circulation, the injection is made into the carotid system. If visualization of the vertebral-basilar system in the posterior fossa is needed, the injection is made into the vertebral artery.[3]

Indications for performing cerebral angiography include identification of cerebral circulatory anomalies (i.e., aneurysm, hematoma) and their site and size, and visualization of cerebral arteries and veins.

Contraindications include the following:
1. Anticoagulant therapy
2. Age
3. Recent embolic or thrombotic occurrences

4. Sensitivity to the contrast medium
5. Severe liver, thyroid, or kidney disease

There are two approaches (open or closed) to performing the angiography. The *open* method is performed in the operating room and involves the surgical exposure of the internal carotid before injection of the contrast substance. Following the procedure, the incision is sutured and dressed. The actual procedure and aftercare are the same as those for the closed method. The *closed* method involves injection of the contrast medium directly into the carotid or vertebral arteries or indirectly by injection of the carotid or vertebral vessels by way of the femoral, brachial, subclavian, or axillary artery.[10] Following injection, repeated radiographs are taken for visualization of arterial and venous circulations.

Complications generally occur during or shortly after the procedure and include seizures, stroke, allergic reactions (to dye), thrombosis, hemiparesis, visual disturbances, pulmonary emboli, and dysphasia.

Pneumoencephalography. A pneumoencephalogram (PEG) involves the injection of air, helium, or oxygen into the lumbar subarachnoid space after intermittent removal of the cerebrospinal fluid by lumbar puncture. This procedure allows for the radiologic visualization of the ventricular space, basal cisterns, and subarachnoid space overlying the cerebral hemispheres of the brain.[27]

Indications for a pneumoencephalogram include localization of intracranial lesions, demonstration of the ventricular system and subarachnoid space, and demonstration of cerebral atrophy.

Contraindications to the pneumoencephalogram include the following:

1. Infection at the puncture site
2. Clinical evidence of significantly increased intracranial pressure
3. If the procedure does not contribute to diagnosis or treatment

The procedure is performed with the patient in a sitting position. Following the lumbar puncture, a small amount of cerebrospinal fluid (about 5 ml) is withdrawn and then replaced with an equal amount of air, helium, or oxygen. Repeated radiographs are taken for visualization of the ventricular system.

Complications following the procedure can include nausea and vomiting, headache, increased intracranial pressure, respiratory distress, seizures, air embolus, and shock.

Ventriculography. A ventriculogram consists of the injection of air or positive contrast medium, via a ventricular puncture, directly into the lateral cerebral ventricles. Indications for a ventriculogram include determination of patency of the ventricular system, localization of a brain tumor, and detection of cerebral anomalies.

The procedure is performed in the operating room under strict aseptic technique. Following the ventricular puncture, cerebrospinal fluid is gradually removed and replaced with air or a positive contrast medium and radiographs are taken. Complications of a ventriculogram are as outlined for the pneumoencephalogram.

Myelography. A myelogram involves the injection of air or a positive contrast medium, via a lumbar or cisternal puncture, into the subarachnoid space. Following the puncture, approximately 10 ml of cerebrospinal fluid is removed and the contrast medium is injected. Repeated radiographs are then taken to detect distortions of the spinal cord, spinal nerve roots, and the subarachnoid space.[50]

TREATMENT PLAN

Surgical
Open method angiography
Burr holes or trephine

Chemotherapeutic
Sedative hypnotic agents
Secobarbital (Seconal), 10-100 mg IV (for severe apprehension)
Diphenhydramine (Benadryl), 20 mg IV (for allergic symptoms)
Adrenergic agents
Methoxamine hydrochloride (Vasoxyl), 5 mg IV (used in shock and acute hypotension)
Antiemetic agents
Trimethobenzamide hydrochloride (Tigan), 100-250 mg IM q4-6h prn, *or*
Prochlorperazine (Compazine), 10 mg IM q4-6h prn
Narcotic analgesic agents
Codeine, 30 mg po q4-6h prn

Electromechanical
Roentgenography

Supportive
Bed rest for 12 to 24 hours (flat for pneumoencephalogram; head of bed elevated 15 degrees for ventriculogram)
Maintenance of intake and output; encourage fluids
Neurologic checks every 15 minutes for 1 hour following procedure

ASSESSMENT: AREAS OF CONCERN

Pain
Headache
Nuchal rigidity
Puncture site discomfort

Complications
Anaphylactic shock
    Urticaria
    Diminished urine output
    Flushed skin
Arterial occlusion (angiogram)
    Pale, mottled, cool skin
    Absent peripheral pulses of affected extremity
Tracheal obstruction (carotid angiography)
    Tachypnea
    Cyanosis
    Crowing respirations
Shock
    Altered level of consciousness
    Decreased blood pressure
    Tachycardia
    Tachypnea
    Pallor
    Cool, clammy skin
    Diminished urine output
    Collapsed peripheral veins

Flat neck veins
Cyanosis
Hemorrhage
    Hematoma at puncture site
    Findings listed above for shock
Increased intracranial pressure
    Restlessness; lethargy
    Changes in level of consciousness
    Changes in vital signs (i.e., Cushing response with increased systolic blood pressure, wide pulse pressure, and decreased pulse rate)

Pupillary changes (i.e., mydriasis)
Impaired pupillary reflex
Papilledema
Vomiting
Fluctuations in temperature
Seizures
Worsening of focal neurologic signs
Changes in respiratory patterns

NURSING DIAGNOSES and NURSING INTERVENTIONS

Nursing Diagnosis	Nursing Intervention
Tissue perfusion, alteration in: cerebral	Perform neurologic checks every 15 minutes for four times, every 30 minutes for two times, and then every hour and as needed. Report any changes to physician.
	Monitor closely for signs of increased intracranial pressure.
	Maintain patency and sterility of intracranial pressure monitoring device, if used.
	Use surgical asepsis for all dressing changes.
	Monitor intracranial pressure responses to care and treatments.
	Administer medications as ordered:
	Anticonvulsants as ordered
	Antifibrinolytics (monitor prothrombin time, partial thromboplastin time, and platelets) as ordered
	Analgesics as ordered
	Antibiotics as ordered
	Control of vasospasm
	Steroids
	Elevate head of bed 30 to 45 degrees unless contraindicated.
	Maintain strict intake and output (1500 to 1800 ml/24 h). Observe for signs of dehydration or overhydration.
	Maintain balance between hyperthermia and hypothermia as ordered.
	Maintain safe, quiet environment.
	Institute subarachnoid hemorrhage precautions, if appropriate:
	Use private room with lights dimmed.
	Maintain absolute bed rest.
	Elevate head of bed.
	Provide all care for the patient.
	Instruct patient to avoid coughing and straining. Administer mild laxatives or stool softeners.
	Maintain dietary restrictions (no stimulants such as coffee or tea)
	Limit visitors.
	Instruct patient not to watch television, listen to radio, or read.
Injury: potential for (trauma)	See general intervention strategies listed on p. 1990.
Preconvulsive	Have oral airway at bedside.
	Have suction equipment available at bedside.
	Pad side rails, if indicated.
	Administer oxygen as ordered.
	Establish means of communications. Identify auras, if possible.
Convulsive	Maintain patent airway.
	Support and protect head; turn to side, if possible.
	Prevent injury:
	Ease to floor if in chair.
	Place pillows along side rails if in bed.
	Remove surrounding furniture.
	Loosen constrictive clothing.

Nursing Diagnosis	Nursing Intervention
	Provide privacy as necessary. Stay with patient; stay calm.
	Note frequency, time, involved body parts, and length of seizure.
Postconvulsive	Maintain patent airway.
	Suction as needed, as indicated.
	Check vital signs and neurologic status.
	Administer oxygen as ordered.
	Reorient patient to environment.
	Place patient in position of comfort; turn head to side.
	Administer oral hygiene as necessary for secretions and bleeding.
	Check injection sites (angiography) every 15 minutes for four times, then every 4 hours for 24 hours. Immediately report swelling or bleeding to physician.
Comfort, alteration in: pain	See general intervention strategies listed on p. 1979.
	Improve effectiveness of pain relief measures by using them before the pain becomes intense.
	Apply ice (i.e., collar or pack) to puncture sites.

EVALUATION

Patient Outcome	Data Indicating That Outcome is Reached
The patient remains free of complications after the procedure.	The patient has no nausea or vomiting.
	The patient has no pain.
	Peripheral pulses are palpable.
	Vital signs are stable.
	Motor and sensory status is normal.
	The patient voids without difficulty.
The patient maintains adequate cerebral tissue perfusion.	Level of consciousness is unchanged.
	There is no evidence of neurologic deficits.
	Pattern of electrolytes is stable.
	There is no seizure activity.
The patient remains free of traumatic injury.	Safety measures are appropriate to level of physiologic status.
	Skin integrity is maintained.
	Skin is free of bruises, burns, abrasions, and redness.
	Environment is safe.
	The patient is free of nosocomial infections.

Computerized Tomography

Computerized tomography (CT) scanning was introduced in the early 1970s. CT scans utilize an x-ray beam and a computer to provide very accurate images of thin cross sections (0.8 to 1.3 cm) of the brain and skull.[10] Indications for use of the CT scan include (1) head trauma, (2) cerebrovascular disturbances, (3) hydrocephalus, (4) abnormal brain development, (5) identification of space-occupying lesions, (6) metastatic tumors, and (7) brain abscesses. The CT scanner has many advantages including that it is safe and painless; there is a very small amount of radiation exposure; data can be collected in early stages of the dysfunction; and it reduces the need for more serious diagnostic procedures such as the ventriculogram. The disadvantages to the use of CT scanning are primarily related to the cost of the equipment and some lack of vessel and posterior fossa visualization.

The CT scan may be done with or without a contrast medium. When the contrast medium is used, the patient should be closely observed for any type of allergic reactions.

Before the procedure, the patient should be instructed regarding the need to remain quiet and perfectly still during the test. If a contrast medium is to be used, collect a comprehensive history about the patient's allergies, particularly shellfish and iodine. Inform the patient that during the test, he will hear clicking noises and these are normal.

During the CT scan procedure the patient lies on a table with his head inside the scanner's opening. The scanner is then moved to various angles and rotated slow-

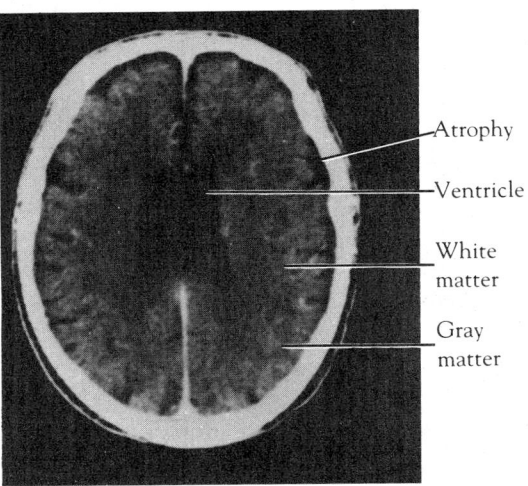

Fig. 3-30
CT scan printouts. CT brain scan differentiates between gray and white brain matter.

From Ballinger, P.W.: Merrill's atlas of radiographic positions and radiologic procedures, ed. 5, St. Louis, 1982, The C.V. Mosby Co.

—Atrophy

—Ventricle

White matter

Gray matter

ly around the patient's head as repeated x-ray films are taken. This information is recorded on a computer print-out, and film prints (i.e., hard copy) of these visual images are taken. The scan is usually completed in 10 to 45 minutes.

TREATMENT PLAN

Chemotherapeutic
Sedatives as ordered
Contrast medium
   Metrizamide (Amipaque)
Antihistamine agents

Diphenhydramine hydrochloride (Benadryl), 25-50 mg IV

Supportive
Withhold solid foods 2 hours before test (if contrast medium is used).

ASSESSMENT: AREAS OF CONCERN

Anxiety
Appearance
   Increased perspiration, clammy skin
   Fatigue
   Increased muscle tension (rigidity)
   Skin blanches, pale
   Increased small motor activity (i.e., tremors, rest-lessness)
Behavior
   Decreased attention span
   Increased somatizing
   Increased immobility
   Decreased ability to follow directions
Other
   Increased rate or depth of respirations
   Increased heart rate
   Rapid shifts in body temperature and blood pressure
   Urinary urgency
   Diarrhea
   Dry mouth
   Decreased appetite
   Pupillary dilation

Complications (with use of contrast medium)
Hemorrhage
Shock
Dye reaction: anaphylactic shock
   Urticaria
   Flushed skin
   Decreased urine output

NURSING DIAGNOSES and NURSING INTERVENTIONS

Nursing Diagnosis	Nursing Intervention

Knowledge deficit	Implement teaching plan:
	   Explain why the test was ordered.
	   Describe equipment used and the testing.
	   Describe possible sensations patient may experience.
	Provide repetition of teaching plan to strengthen learning.
	Implement teaching plan in an environment free of distractions and other obstacles.
	Encourage questions and answer the questions simply and completely.
	Evaluate and revise teaching plan as necessary.

EVALUATION

Patient Outcome	Data Indicating That Outcome is Reached
The patient remains free of postprocedural complications.	Vital signs are stable. Cerebral tissue perfusion is adequate. There is no reaction to dye.
The patient demonstrates adequate knowledge regarding the diagnostic procedure.	The patient can state why test was ordered. The patient can state what the testing procedure consists of and what equipment is used.

Electromyography

An electromyogram (EMG) consists of an evaluation of skeletal muscle electrical activity, which is detected by the application of surface electrodes or insertion of needle electrodes into the muscle. The electrical activity of the motor unit (action potential) is observed with an oscilloscope and a loudspeaker for abnormalities in amplitude, duration, frequency, wave formation, and sound. Indications for performing electromyography include (1) assessment of peripheral nerve reinnervation and (2) identification and localization of lower motor neuron disease that affects skeletal muscle fibers, neuromuscular junction, and voluntary and reflex muscle activity.

The procedure consists of application or insertion of the electrodes into the muscles. If needle electrodes are used, the patient should be forewarned regarding the discomfort on insertion. Length and extent of the testing procedure vary.

TREATMENT PLAN

Surgical
   Needle electrode insertion

Electromechanical
   Oscilloscope

ASSESSMENT: AREAS OF CONCERN

Pain
   Pain on insertion
   Discomfort during test
   Muscle tenderness after the procedure

NURSING DIAGNOSES and NURSING INTERVENTIONS

Nursing Diagnosis	Nursing Intervention
	Establish a baseline and ongoing assessment of the patient's pain and response to the pain experience. Promote rest and relaxation Decrease the noxious stimuli, whenever possible. Assist patient to modify the anxiety associated with the pain experience. Provide other sensory input (e.g., gentle back rub). Administer medications, as ordered: analgesics and muscle-relaxing drugs. Improve effectiveness of pain relief measures by using them before the pain becomes intense.
Anxiety	See general intervention strategies listed on p. 1839.

EVALUATION

Patient Outcome	Data Indicating That Outcome is Reached
The patient demonstrates minimal alterations in comfort.	There is no pain after the procedure is terminated.
The patient experiences minimal anxiety.	The patient openly verbalizes concerns and discomfort. The patient openly verbalizes feelings supported by health care professionals and family. The patient can identify methods to effectively deal with anxious feelings.

CRANIOTOMY

A craniotomy is a surgical procedure in which an opening is made into the cranium for removal of a tumor, control of bleeding, or relief of intracranial pressure. A flap is created by leaving the bone attached to the muscle so that the tissue can be turned down.[10] Next the dura is incised in the opposite direction so that its base is near the midline. After the surgery's purpose is accomplished, closure is done in layers (i.e., dura, muscles, fascial, galea, and scalp).[3] Craniotomies can be classified into two major categories: supratentorial and subtentorial.

Supratentorial craniotomy refers to a surgical procedure performed on the brain structures located above the tentorium for removal of space-occupying lesions in the frontal, temporal, parietal, and occipital lobes. The incision is usually made behind the hairline. *Subtentorial* craniotomy is performed to relieve the discomfort of trigeminal neuralgia and for tumor removal from the cerebellum or cerebellar-pontine angle.[25] The incision is usually made slightly above the nape of the neck.

Complications following a craniotomy can include any or all of the following: (1) increased intracranial pressure, (2) seizures, (3) meningitis, (4) respiratory distress, (5) cardiac arrhythmias, (6) wound infection, (7) diabetes insipidus, (8) thrombophlebitis, (9) visual disturbances, (10) personality changes, (11) bowel or bladder dysfunction, (12) periocular edema, (13) motor and sensory disturbances, (14) headache, and (15) postoperative hydrocephalus.

If part of the cranium is removed without replacement (i.e., to provide decompression from cerebral edema), the procedure is termed a *craniectomy*. *Cranioplasty* is the surgical repair of a cranial defect to reestablish the integrity and normal contour of the skull. The area of cranial defect is repaired through the use of substitute bone materials (i.e., tantalum, vitallium, or plastic).

TREATMENT PLAN

Surgical
Intracranial pressure monitoring

Chemotherapeutic
Corticosteroids
Dexamethasone (Decadron), 20-40 mg po qd
Anticonvulsants
Phenytoin (Dilantin), 100 mg po tid
Laxative agents
Docusate sodium (Colace), 100 mg po bid or tid
Antiemetic agents
Cimetidine (Tagamet), 300 mg po qid
Antacids
Magnesium hydroxide (Maalox), 30 ml po qid

Anti-infective agents
Organism specific

Electromechanical
Mechanical ventilation, if indicated
Cardiac monitoring

Supportive
Nutritional consultation
Physical therapy

ASSESSMENT: AREAS OF CONCERN

Focal neurologic disturbance
Gradually increasing weakness
Subtle sensory loss
Adult-onset seizures not always relieved by medications

Mentation
Personality changes
Insidious decrease in mentation
Depression
Memory deficits
Judgment deficits

Pain
Headaches with steady, persistent, or intractable dull pain
Changes in character of headaches
Stress-induced headaches

Increased intracranial pressure
Restlessness, lethargy
Changes in level of consciousness
Changes in vital signs (i.e., Cushing response with increased systolic blood pressure, wide pulse pressure, and decreased pulse rate)
Pupillary changes (i.e., mydriasis)
Impaired pupillary reflex
Papilledema
Vomiting
Fluctuations in temperature
Seizures
Worsening of focal neurologic signs
Changes in respiratory patterns

Seizure activity
Preconvulsive (preictal) stage
Aura: flash of light; sense of loss; fear; weakness; dizziness; peculiar taste, smell, and sounds
Cry or scream
Fall to floor
Loss of consciousness
Tachypnea

Convulsive stage
    Tonic: rigid body; fixed jaws; clenched fists; extended legs; cyanosis; holding breath
    Clonic: urinary or fecal incontinence; jerking of facial muscles and extremities; biting tongue; frothing at mouth
Postconvulsive (postictal) stage
    Altered level of consciousness
    Headache
    Nausea and/or vomiting
    Malaise
    Muscle soreness
    Aspiration
        Breathing difficulty
        Choking
        Cyanosis
        Decreased breath sounds
        Tachycardia
        Tachypnea
    Pneumonia

Diabetes insipidus
    Marked polyuria
    Marked polydipsia
    Anorexia
    Weight loss
    Dehydration
    Dry skin
    Poor turgor
    Headache
    General weakness
    Irritability
    Apathy
    Laboratory studies
        Urinary specific gravity of 1.001 to 1.005
        Electrolyte imbalance
        Increased plasma osmolality
Other
    Periocular edema
    Thrombophlebitis

NURSING DIAGNOSES and NURSING INTERVENTIONS

Nursing Diagnosis	Nursing Intervention
Airway clearance, ineffective	See general intervention strategies listed on p. 2028.
Breathing pattern, ineffective	See general intervention strategies listed on p. 2030.

Tissue perfusion, alteration in: cerebral	Establish baseline and ongoing neurologic assessment every 1 to 2 hours and as needed.
	Assess level of consciousness and motor or sensory deficits:
	  Cranial nerve functioning
	  Auditory functioning
	  Nausea and vomiting
	  Reflex status
	  Pupillary size and reaction
	  Behavior and personality changes
	  Posturing spontaneously or stimuli response
	Intervene to monitor and prevent increased intracranial pressure:
	  Administer medications, treatment, and IV lines as ordered.
	Maintain elevation of head of bed as ordered.
	Accurately record intake and output; monitor for imbalance.
	Monitor serum electrolytes, blood count, and arterial blood gases for abnormalities.
	Monitor values and wave forms of intracranial pressure line, if appropriate.
	  Maintain patency and sterility of the system.
	  Monitor effects of temperature on intracranial pressures
	  Correlate neurologic status with intracranial pressure values; notify physician if inconsistent.
	  Assist with drainage of cerebrospinal fluid from the system.
	Intervene to monitor and prevent seizures:
	  Assess seizure history of the client.
	  Institute seizure precautions:
	    Padded tongue blade and airway at bedside
	    Bed height at lowest level
	    Side rails up at all times and padded
	    Oxygen and suction equipment at bedside
	    Emergency medications at bedside

Nursing Diagnosis	**Nursing Intervention**
	Administer anticonvulsants as ordered:
	Monitor effects and side effects.
	Monitor serum for therapeutic levels of the anticonvulsant.
Skin integrity, impairment of: actual	Maintain head elevation at 30 to 45 degrees if supratentorial approach used.
	Keep head of bed flat with subtentorial approach; avoid neck flexion.
	Check head dressing every hour and as needed. Report any new or increased drainage. Measure and mark all drainage.
	Change head dressing as ordered.
	Maintain patency of ventricular drainage system is used.
	Provide wound care every shift and as needed when head dressing is removed.
	Monitor laboratory results for elevated white blood cell count.
Sensory-perceptual alteration	Keep side rails up at all times when patient is alone. Maintain patient safety at all times.
	Maintain quiet environment, reducing external stimuli to a minimum.
	Reorient patient frequently to time, place, and person. Introduce self each time you reorient the patient.
	Repeat explanations frequently and simply.
	Assist patient in judgments, perceptions, and reorientation as needed.
	Have family bring in familiar objects.
	Maintain planned rest periods, allowing sufficient time for REM sleep.
	Use day-night lighting appropriately.
	Stimulate senses of touch, taste, and position.
	Support family members to understand what is happening as a result of perceptual alterations.
Injury, potential for: trauma	Maintain bed in low position at all times unless side rails are up or when nurse is with the patient.
	Provide the patient with a call light within easy reach.
	Maintain side rails in up position at bedtime, after sedation, when patient is confused, and as needed.
	Maintain wheelchairs and stretchers in locked position when transferring patient.
	Pad side rails if patient is overactive.
Preconvulsive	Have oral airway at bedside.
	Support and protect head; turn to side if possible.
	Prevent injury:
	Ease to floor if in chair.
	Place pillows along side rails if in bed.
	Remove surrounding furniture.
	Loosen constrictive clothing.
	Provide privacy as necessary.
	Note frequency, time, involved body parts, and length of seizure.
Postconvulsive	Maintain patent airway.
	Suction as needed, as indicated.
	Check vital signs and neurologic status.
	Administer oxygen as ordered.
	Reorient patient to environment.
	Place patient in position of comfort; turn head to side.
	Administer oral hygiene as necessary for secretions and bleeding.
Mobility, impaired physical	See general intervention strategies listed on p. 2106.
Self-care deficit	Assist with feeding as indicated; use IV or nasogastric feedings as ordered.
	Administer oral hygiene every 2 hours and as needed.
	Assist with daily hygiene care as indicated.
	Administer eye care every 2 to 4 hours if indicated.
	Perform intermittent urinary catheterization as ordered.
Comfort, alteration in: pain	Promote rest and relaxation.
	Modify anxiety associated with the pain experience.
	Provide other sensory input.
	Remain with the patient.

Nursing Diagnosis	Nursing Intervention
	Improve effectiveness of pain relief measures by using them before the pain becomes intense.
	For patients receiving radiation or chemotherapy:
	Explain procedure or medication before implementing.
	Administer antiemetics and antidiarrheal medications as needed.
	Provide frequent skin care.
	Provide frequent mouth care.
	Monitor the patient's laboratory values for depressed red blood cells, white blood cells, or platelets. Report to physician.
	Maintain planned rest periods.
	Offer frequent, small feedings to combat anorexia and discomfort of nausea.
Self-concept, disturbance in: body image, self-esteem, role performance, personal identity	See general intervention strategies listed on p. 1820.

Patient Education

1. Involve family in care, as possible; teach essential aspects of care.
2. Reinforce physician's explanation of medical management.
3. Emphasize the importance of ongoing outpatient care and follow-up visits.
4. Encourage independent activities, as possible:
   a. Alert patient to limitations.
   b. Avoid overprotection.
   c. Stress need for supportive devices as indicated.
5. Explain the need for regular exercise program. Teach ROM exercises to family.
6. Teach the importance of diet as ordered:
   a. Offer supplemental feedings.
   b. Offer small portions; instruct patient to chew slowly.
7. Teach the importance of safety measures: side rails, ramps, shower chairs, removal of scatter rugs, walker, and canes.
8. Explain name of medication, dosage, time of administration, and toxic or side effects.
9. Explain need to avoid over-the-counter medications without first consulting physician.
10. Encourage socialization with friends and family.
11. Teach the importance of verbalization of feelings about anxiety, fear, and body image changes.
12. Teach patient and family about seizures (i.e., safety measures and who to contact).

EVALUATION

Patient Outcome	Data Indicating That Outcome is Reached
The patient's airway is patent.	Breath sounds are normal.
	Chest excursion is bilateral and symmetric.
	Rate and depth of respirations are normal.
	Cough is effective.
	There are no subjective or objective findings of shortness of breath, air hunger, or dyspnea on exertion.
The patient's breathing pattern is effective.	Airway remains patent.
	Chest excursion is symmetric.
	Breath sounds are normal, or there is no increase in adventitious sounds.
	Arterial blood gas values are within normal ranges or consistent with patient's baseline.
	Vital signs are within normal ranges or consistent with patient's baseline.
	Hemoglobin levels are 14 to 18 g/dl (male) and 12 to 16 g/dl (female).
	Intake and output are stable.
	There are no signs of respiratory distress.
	All lobes are resonant on percussion.
	Skin color is not cyanotic.

Patient Outcome	Data Indicating That Outcome is Reached
Cerebral tissue perfusion is adequate.	Level of consciousness is unchanged. There is no evidence of neurologic deficits. Pattern of electrolytes is stable. There is no seizure activity.
The patient experiences minimal complications of sensory-perceptual alterations.	The patient maintains an optimal level of orientation. The patient remains free of injury. Skin integrity is maintained. Nutritional status is adequate. Self-care deficits are minimal. Social participation is appropriate to physiologic status.
The patient remains free of traumatic injury.	Safety measures are appropriate to level of physiologic status. Skin integrity is maintained. Skin is free of bruises, burns, abrasions, and redness. Environment is safe. The patient is free of nosocomial infections.
The patient's level of mobility is optimal.	Skin integrity is maintained. The patient remains free of contractures and deformities. Level of mobility is appropriate to physiologic status. Intake and output pattern is stable. Nutritional status is adequate. The patient remains free of thrombophlebitis. The patient remains free of local infection. The patient participates in an ongoing physical therapy program.
Self-care deficits are minimal.	Criteria listed for impaired physical mobility are met. Level of self-care activities is appropriate to physiologic status. The patient participates in physical and occupational therapy.
Alterations in comfort are minimal.	The patient openly verbalizes feelings of discomfort when they occur. The patient can utilize measures to decrease discomfort. The patient verbally validates a decrease in subjective feelings of discomfort. There is a decrease in objective findings of pain.
The patient maintains intact self-concepts.	The patient openly verbalizes feelings of grief and loss. The patient verbalizes positive feelings about self. The patient acknowledges actual change in self-image. The patient focuses on present and future appearance and function. The patient verbalizes feelings of hopefulness, helpfulness, and powerfulness.

CHORDOTOMY

A chordotomy is a surgical procedure in which the lateral spinothalamic tract of the spinal cord is surgically divided to relieve pain. The lesion is created on the contralateral side, approximately two to three spinal segments above the desired level of anesthesia, which then severs the pain pathways. If the pain is midline, the lesions must be made bilaterally. Currently, the preferred surgical technique is the *percutaneous chordotomy*.

The procedure consists of stereotactic insertion of a spinal lumbar puncture needle laterally between C1 and C2 (at the cervical level). A wire electrode is then inserted into the anterior quadrant, and a lesion is made by use of a radio-frequency generator at a designated site in order to destroy ascending pain fibers. The percutaneous chordotomy may be repeated if pain perception recurs or the level of anesthesia falls. The other method for performing a chordotomy consists of a *surgical thoracic resection approach*. Following exposure of the spinal cord, the dendate ligament is divided at the level selected for the chordotomy.

Following a chordotomy, the patient may experience an interruption in respiratory reflex pathways causing periods of apnea or respiratory arrest, temporary paralysis, permanent loss of temperature sensation, and loss of bowel and bladder control.

TREATMENT PLAN

Surgical
Tracheostomy, if indicated

Chemotherapeutic
Local anesthesia (percutaneous chordotomy)
General anesthesia
Regional anesthetic blocks (preoperatively)

Electromechanical
Radio-frequency generator (percutaneous chordotomy)
Mechanical ventilator, if indicated (i.e., high cervical chordotomy)
Pulmonary function testing (preoperatively and post-operatively)

Supportive
Counseling and support regarding coping effectively with diffuse pain
Occupational therapy
Physical therapy

ASSESSMENT: AREAS OF CONCERN

Pain
Discomfort at puncture or incision site

Complications
Paralysis
  Leg weakness
  Temporary paralysis
Bowel/bladder control
  Temporary (i.e., several weeks) urine retention
  Incontinence
Respiratory function
  Periods of apnea
  Respiratory arrest (with cervical chordotomy)
Sensation
  Permanent loss of temperature sensation below level of interruption
  Paresthesias
  Decreased position sense
Other
  Postural hypotension

NURSING DIAGNOSES and NURSING INTERVENTIONS

Nursing Diagnosis	Nursing Intervention

Breathing pattern, ineffective	Maintain patent airway; intubation/tracheostomy and mechanical ventilation may be indicated:
	  Suction as needed. Hyperinflate lungs with 100% oxygen for 1 minute before and 1 minute after suctioning, unless contraindicated.
	  Maintain aseptic technique.
	Monitor mechanical ventilator, if used:
	  Ensure tidal volume, rate, mode, and oxygen concentration are set as ordered.
	  Ensure ventilator alarms are on and functional.
	Monitor arterial blood gases as ordered:
	  Report decrease in P_{O_2} of 10 to 15 mm Hg.
	  Report increase in P_{CO_2} greater than 10 to 15 mm Hg.
	Note respiratory rate, depth, and level of consciousness every 15 to 30 minutes and as needed.
	Stay with patient if he is in acute distress.

Tissue perfusion, alteration in: spinal	Perform neurologic assessment every 1 to 2 hours and as needed:
	  Check level of consciousness.
	  Assess pupillary size, reaction, and equality.
	  Check for extraocular eye movements.
	  Note motor and sensory deficits (i.e., color and strength of extremities). Report any increase in deficits immediately to the physician.
	Administer medications as ordered (i.e., steroids to control cord edema).
	Maintain parenteral fluids as ordered.
	Measure intake and output every hour. Immediately report urine output of less than 30 ml/h.

Sensory-perceptual alteration	See general intervention strategies listed on p. 1967.

Mobility, impaired physical	Administer skin care every 2 hours:
	  Turn patient every 2 hours and as needed unless contraindicated:
	    Change position slowly.
	    Position in straight body alignment.

Nursing Diagnosis	Nursing Intervention

Use "log-roll" technique when turning.
Keep skin dry; give perineal care as needed.
Massage pressure points every 2 hours to stimulate circulation; give gentle back rubs every shift and as needed.
Use heel and elbow guards as needed.
Use firm mattress or bed board.
Perform active or passive ROM exercises every 2 to 4 hours.
Apply antiembolus stockings to lower extremities.
Administer anticoagulation therapy as ordered.
Monitor nutritional status.
Encourage mobility to tolerance or as ordered.
Encourage self-care activities to tolerance.
Plan all activities to avoid fatigue. Maintain planned rest periods.
Obtain physical therapy referral.

Patient Education

1. Stress need to continue with physical and occupational therapy as ordered.
2. Teach methods of avoiding injury (e.g., burns) to lower trunk and legs.
3. Teach methods and routine for inspecting lower portion of the body and feet for infection and breaks in the skin.
4. Instruct regarding care of surgical incision (with thoracic approach chordotomy).
5. Emphasize importance of ongoing outpatient care by physician.

EVALUATION

Patient Outcome	Data Indicating That Outcome is Reached
The patient demonstrates a patent airway.	Breath sounds are normal. Chest excursion is bilateral and symmetric. Rate and depth of respirations are normal. Cough is effective. There are no subjective or objective findings of shortness of breath, air hunger, or dyspnea on exertion.
The patient demonstrates an effective breathing pattern.	Airway is patent. Chest excursion is symmetric. Breath sounds are normal or there is no increase in adventitious sounds. Arterial blood gas values are within normal ranges or consistent with patient's baseline. Vital signs are within normal ranges or consistent with patient's baseline. Hemoglobin levels are 14 to 18 g/dl (male) and 12 to 16 g/dl (female). Intake and output are stable. There are no signs of respiratory distress. All lobes are resonant on percussion. Skin color is not cyanotic.
The patient demonstrates adequate cerebral tissue perfusion.	Level of consciousness is unchanged. There is no evidence of further neurologic deficits. Pattern of electrolytes is stable. There is no seizure activity. Vital signs are stable.
The patient demonstrates minimal complications of sensory-perceptual alterations.	Level of orientation is optimal. The patient remains free of injury. Skin integrity is maintained.

Patient Outcome	Data Indicating That Outcome is Reached
	Nutritional status is adequate. Self-care deficits are minimal. Social participation is appropriate to physiologic status.
The patient remains free of traumatic injury.	Safety measures are appropriate to physiologic status. Skin integrity is maintained. Skin is free of bruises, burns, abrasions, and redness. Environment is safe. The patient is free of nosocomial infections.
The patient demonstrates an optimal level of mobility.	Skin integrity is maintained. The patient remains free of contractures and deformities. Level of mobility is appropriate to physiologic status. Intake and output pattern is stable. Nutritional status is adequate. The patient remains free of thrombophlebitis. The patient remains free of local infection. The patient participates in an ongoing physical therapy program.
The patient demonstrates minimal self-care deficits.	Outcome criteria listed for impaired physical mobility are met. Level of self-care activities is appropriate to physiologic status. The patient participates in physical and occupational therapy.
The patient demonstrates skin integrity.	Skin is intact. Nutritional status is adequate. Electrolyte balance is maintained. The patient remains free of pressure sores and contractures.
The patient experiences minimal alterations in comfort.	The patient openly verbalizes feelings of discomfort when they occur. The patient utilizes measures to decrease discomfort. The patient verbally validates a decrease in subjective feelings of discomfort. There is a decrease in objective findings of pain.
The patient demonstrates a low level of anxiety.	The patient openly verbalizes concerns and feelings of grief, loss, and discomfort. The patient openly verbalizes feelings, supported by health care professionals and family. The patient verbalizes essential aspects of care. The patient can identify methods to effectively deal with anxious feelings.

INTRACRANIAL PRESSURE MONITORING

Intracranial pressure monitoring devices now make it possible to reliably measure the parameters of intracranial dynamics such as volume-pressure relationships, pressure waves, and cerebral perfusion pressures. Indications for intracranial pressure monitoring include any of the following: (1) head trauma; (2) cerebral hemorrhage; (3) massive brain lesions; (4) encephalitis; (5) congenital hydrocephalus; (6) hydrocephalus resulting in an alteration of cerebrospinal fluid production or absorption; and (7) symptoms of increased intracranial pressure such as change in level of consciousness, headache, vomiting, or deterioration in respiratory status and motor function.[22] Intracranial pressure can be measured continuously via three basic monitoring systems: the ventricular catheter, the subarachnoid bolt, and the epidural sensor (Fig. 3-31).

The *ventricular* catheter consists of a cannula that is implanted, via burr holes, into the anterior horn of the lateral ventricle of the nondominant cerebral hemisphere. The catheter is then connected by pressure-resistant, fluid-filled tubing to a transducer and recording instrument.[10] (NOTE: Continuous flushing devices are not used for intracranial pressure measurement.) The transducer is positioned so the dome is at the level of the foramen of Monro. The external anatomic landmarks for this position are the tragus of the ear or the edge of the brow.

Fig. 3-31
Subarachnoid screw monitoring *(left)* and intraventricular *(right)* devices for measuring intracranial pressure. Both require attachment to transducer using a stopcock or pressure tubing.

From Budassi, S.A., and Barber, J.M.: Emergency nursing: principles and practice, St. Louis, 1981, The C.V. Mosby Co.

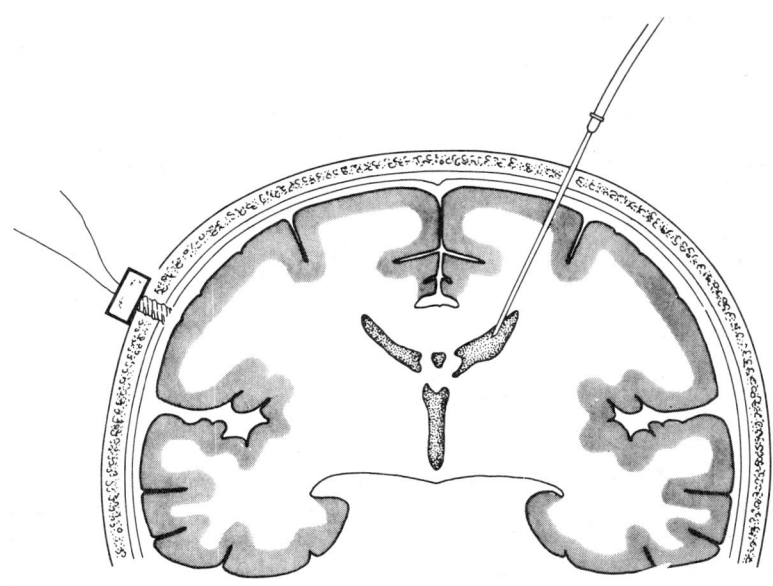

An error of approximately 2 torr exists for each inch of discrepancy between the level of the transducer and the pressure source.

Advantages to the use of the ventricular catheter include (1) accurate measurement of intracranial pressure; (2) instillation of a contrast medium; (3) evaluation of pressure/volume responses; and (4) ability to drain large amounts of cerebrospinal fluid, if needed.

Disadvantages to the ventricular catheter are (1) catheter placement may be difficult if the lateral ventricle is displaced, swollen, or collapsed; (2) the catheter is the most invasive type of monitoring and can provide another route for infection; (3) excessive cerebrospinal fluid drainage can occur if stopcock is not positioned properly; (4) brain tissue or blood may occlude the catheter; (5) false pressure readings may occur if the ventricle collapses and compresses the catheter; and (6) frequent recalibration of the transducer and monitor is necessary for accurate readings.

The *subarachnoid bolt* or screw method of intracranial pressure measurement was started in the early 1970s. The device consists of a metal screw with a sensory tip that is inserted through a twist drill hole into the subdural or subarachnoid space. Although the cerebrum is not penetrated, the intracranial pressure is measured directly from the cerebrospinal fluid. The bolt is connected to a transducer and recording device via pressure-resistant, fluid-filled tubing. Here, as with the intraventricular catheter, continuous flushing devices are contraindicated. Indications for use of the subarachnoid bolt are to provide a means to measure and monitor intracranial pressure and to provide access for sampling of the cerebrospinal fluid.

Advantages of the bolt include (1) intracranial pressure is measured directly and accurately from cerebrospinal fluid; (2) it provides access for cerebrospinal fluid sampling and drainage; (3) it provides access for volume-pressure responses; and (4) it can be quickly placed without penetrating the cerebrum.

Disadvantages to the bolt are (1) it may become occluded with tissue or blood; (2) the infection rate is comparable to that of the ventricular catheter; (3) it requires a closed skull; and (4) frequent recalibration of the transducer and monitor is necessary for accurate readings.

The *epidural sensor* consists of placement of a fiber-optic sensor, radio transmitter, or tiny balloon with radioisotopes in the epidural space through a burr hole in the skull. The sensor cable then plugs directly into the monitor. The indication for use of the epidural sensor is to measure intracranial pressure.

Advantages to the sensor include (1) it is less invasive; (2) it can be easily placed; and (3) it cannot become occluded.

The major disadvantage of the sensor is that its reliability remains questionable. Other disadvantages include (1) the system cannot be recalibrated if the sensor is affected by pressure or heat; (2) cerebrospinal fluid sampling and drainage are not possible; and (3) volume/pressure responses cannot be evaluated.

Pressure waves. Intracranial pressure's dynamic state is reflected by the pressure waves produced. These wave forms are most commonly known as A-waves, B-waves, and C-waves (Fig. 3-32).

A-waves (or plateau waves), which occur at variable intervals, are spontaneous, rapid increases in pressure

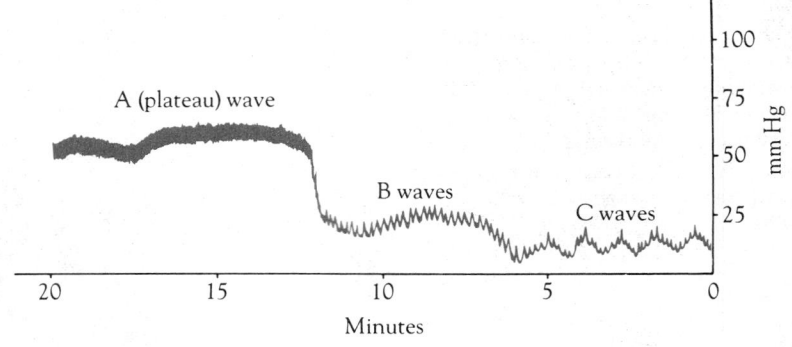

Fig. 3-32
Intracranial pressure waves.
Composite drawing of A (plateau)
waves, B waves, and C waves.

Reprinted by permission from Holloway,
N.M.: Nursing the critically ill adult, p.
521. Copyright © 1979 by Addison-
Wesley Publishing Co., Inc.

between 50 to 200 torr. Plateau waves usually occur in patients with moderate intracranial pressure elevations and last 5 to 20 minutes, falling spontaneously. Factors that can trigger plateau waves include the following: (1) REM sleep, (2) emotional stimuli, (3) isometric muscle contractions, (4) the rebound phase of the Valsalva maneuver, (5) hypercapnia, (6) hypoxemia, (7) sustained coughing and sneezing, (8) arousal from sleep, and (9) certain positions such as neck flexion or extreme hip flexion. A-waves are known to cause cerebral ischemia and brain damage and can produce paroxysmal or transient symptoms of (1) change in level of consciousness, (2) headache, (3) nausea and vomiting, (4) altered motor function, (5) abnormal pupillary reactions, (6) changes in vital signs (i.e., increased blood pressure, widened pulse pressure, and decreased pulse rate) and respiratory patterns (i.e., ataxic breathing and central neurogenic hyperventilation).[10] Due to the ischemia and previously stated symptoms, A-waves are the most clinically significant intracranial pressure wave forms and require immediate intervention to prevent further brain injury.

B-waves appear as sharp, rhythmic, and sawtooth waves that occur every ½ to 2 minutes and have pressures up to 50 torr. B-waves correlate to changes in respiration, such as Cheyne-Stokes respirations. B-waves can also occur in patients with normal intracranial pressure.

C-waves are small, rapid, and rhythmic waves that occur at a rate of approximately 4 to 8/min and increase pressures up to 20 torr. C-waves are also called Traube-Herring-Mayer waves. These wave forms correspond to normal changes in the systemic arterial pressure and are not clinically significant.

TREATMENT PLAN

Surgical
Intracranial pressure monitoring (pp. 422-425)
Tumor excision
Shunting procedure

Chemotherapeutic
Corticosteroid agents
   Dexamethasone (Decadron), 20-40 mg po qd
Anticonvulsant agents
   Phenytoin (Dilantin), 100 mg po tid
Laxative agents
   Docusate sodium (Colace), 100 mg po bid or tid
Antiemetic agents
   Cimetidine (Tagamet), 300 mg po qid
Antacids
   Magnesium hydroxide (Maalox), 30 ml po qid
Anti-infective agents
   Organism specific

Electromechanical
Radiation therapy
Mechanical ventilation, if indicated
Cardiac monitoring
Arterial blood pressure monitoring

Supportive
Nutritional consultation
Physical therapy

ASSESSMENT: AREAS OF CONCERN

The reader is referred to the appropriate disorder for specific physical assessment findings.

Loss of intracranial pressure wave form
Transducer may be incorrectly connected
Monitoring device could be occluded
Air may be between pressure source and transducer
   diaphragm

Low intracranial pressure
Cerebral ventricles may have collapsed
Transducer may have been incorrectly zeroed and calibrated

High intracranial pressure
Excessive activity

Body posture with neck or extreme hip flexion
Use of positive end-expiratory pressure (PEEP)
Hyperthermia
Respiratory distress
Fluid and electrolyte imbalances
Infection
Blood pressure changes

False high intracranial pressure
Transducer too low or incorrectly balanced
System incorrectly calibrated
Air in system

False low intracranial pressure
Transducer too high
Air in system

NURSING DIAGNOSES and NURSING INTERVENTIONS

Nursing Diagnosis	Nursing Intervention

Tissue perfusion, alteration in: cerebral	Maintain sterility of the intracranial pressure monitoring equipment:
	  Maintain strict sterile technique.
	  Change equipment (i.e., tubing) daily or as ordered.
	Maintain patency of intracranial pressure monitoring device:
	  Keep all stopcock ports capped.
	  Keep system free of air.
	  Never flush the system.
	  Observe for cerebrospinal fluid leaks and blood in the tubing.
	Obtain accurate pressure measurements:
	  Place patient in baseline position. Obtain measurements when patient is at rest—not when moving, coughing, sneezing, etc.
	  Level the transducer.
	  Recalibrate the transducer according to the manufacturer's instructions.
	  Obtain measurements and record. Report significant changes in intracranial pressure to physician immediately.

EVALUATION

Patient Outcome	Data Indicating That Outcome is Reached
The patient will maintain adequate cerebral tissue perfusion.	Level of consciousness is unchanged. There is no evidence of neurologic deficits. Pattern of electrolytes is stable. There is no seizure activity. Vital signs are stable.

References

1. Anthony, C.P., and Thibodeau, G.A.: Structure and function of the body, ed. 7, St. Louis, 1984, The C.V. Mosby Co.
2. Baker, A.B., editor: Clinical neurology, ed. 2, New York, 1983, Harper & Row, Publishers Inc.
3. Bates, B.: A guide to physical assessment, ed. 3, Philadelphia, 1983, J.B. Lippincott Co.
4. Burns, K.R., and Johnson, P.J.: Health assessment in clinical practice, Englewood Cliffs, N.J., 1980, Prentice-Hall, Inc.
5. Burrell, O., and Burrell, Jr., Z.L.: Critical care, ed. 4, St. Louis, 1982, The C.V. Mosby Co.
6. Caird, F.I., and Judge, T.G.: Assessment of the elderly patient, ed. 3, California, 1977, Pitman Medical Publishing Corp.
7. Carnevali, D.L., and Patrick, M.: Nursing management for the elderly, Philadelphia, 1979, J.B. Lippincott Co.
8. Carotenuto, R., and Bullock, J.: Physical assessment of the gerontologic client, Philadelphia, 1980, F.A. Davis Co.
9. Conn, H.F., and Conn, Jr., R.B.: Current diagnosis, Philadelphia, 1980, W.B. Saunders Co.
10. Conway-Rutkowski, B.L.: Carini and Owens' neurological and neurosurgical nursing, ed. 8, St. Louis, 1982, The C.V. Mosby Co.
11. Crowell, R.M., and Zervas, N.T.: Management of intracranial aneurysm, Med. Clin. North Am. **63**:695, 1979.
12. Davis, G.T., and Hill, P.M.: Cerebral palsy, Nurs. Clin. North Am. **15**:35, 1980.
13. Davis, J.E., and Mason, C.B.: Neurologic critical care, New York, 1979, Van Nostrand Reinhold Co.
14. Demyer, W.: Technique of the neurologic examination: a programmed text, ed. 3, New York, 1980, McGraw-Hill Book Co.
15. De Young, S.: The neurologic patient: a nursing perspective, Englewood Cliffs, N.J., 1983, Prentice-Hall, Inc.
16. Eliasson, S.G., et al., editors: Neurological pathophysiology, ed. 2, New York, 1978, Oxford University Press.
17. Escourolle, R., and Poirier, J.: Manual of basic neuropathology, ed. 2, Philadelphia, 1978, W.B. Saunders Co.
18. Geffner, E.S., editor: Compendium of drug therapy, New York, 1983, Biomedical Information Corp.

19. Groer, M.W., and Shekleton, M.E.: Basic pathophysiology: a conceptual approach, ed. 2, St. Louis, 1983, The C.V. Mosby Co.
20. Grundy, J.H.: Assessment of the child in primary health care, New York, 1981, McGraw-Hill Book Co.
21. Guyton, A.: Textbook of medical physiology, ed. 5, Philadelphia, 1976, W.B. Saunders Co.
22. Hazinski, M.F.: Nursing care of the critically ill child, St. Louis, 1984, The C.V. Mosby Co.
23. Hickey J.: The clinical practice of neurological and neurosurgical nursing, Philadelphia, 1981, J.B. Lippincott Co.
24. Hudak, C.M., et al.: Critical care nursing, ed. 3, Philadelphia, 1982, J.B. Lippincott Co.
25. Jensen, D.: The principles of physiology, ed. 2, New York, 1982, Appleton-Century-Crofts.
26. Kaye, D., and Rose, L.F.: Fundamentals of internal medicine, St. Louis, 1982, The C.V. Mosby Co.
27. Kim, M.J., McFarland, G.K., and McLane, A.M., editors: Pocket guide to nursing diagnosis, St. Louis, 1984, The C.V. Mosby Co.
28. Kinney, M.R., editor: AACN's clinical reference for critical-care nursing, New York, 1981, McGraw-Hill Book Co.
29. Kintzel, K., editor: Advanced concepts in clinical nursing, ed. 2, Philadelphia, 1977, J.B. Lippincott Co.
30. Leech, R.W., and Shuman, R.M.: Neuropathology: a summary for students, New York, 1982, Harper & Row, Publishers Inc.
31. Malasanos, L., et al.: Health assessment, ed. 2, St. Louis, 1981, The C.V. Mosby Co.
32. McElroy, D.B.: Hydrocephalus in children, Nurs. Clin. North Am. **15:**23, 1980.
33. Merrit, H.H.: A textbook of neurology, ed. 6, Philadelphia, 1979, Lea & Febiger.
34. Mulder, D.W., and Allen, J.D.: Spinal cord tumors and disks. In Clinical neurology, vol. 3, New York, 1983, Harper & Row, Publishers Inc.
35. Nikas, D.L., editor: The critically ill neurosurgical patient: contemporary issues in critical care nursing, vol. 3, New York, 1982, Churchill Livingstone, Inc.
36. Passo, S.: Malformations of the neural tube, Nurs. Clin. North Am. **15:**5, 1980.
37. Petersdorf, R.G., editor: Harrison's principles of internal medicine, ed. 10, New York, 1983, McGraw-Hill Book Co.
38. Phipps, W.J., Long, B.C., and Woods, N.F.: Shafer's medical-surgical nursing, ed. 7, St. Louis, 1980, The C.V. Mosby Co.
39. Price, S.A., and Wilson, L.M.: Pathophysiology: clinical concepts of disease processes, ed. 2, New York, 1982, McGraw-Hill Book Co.
40. Ramirez, B.: When your're faced with neuro patients, RN **42:**67, 1979.
41. Robbins, S.L., and Cotran, R.S.: Pathologic basis of disease, ed. 2, Philadelphia, 1977, W.B. Saunders Co.
42. Robinson, J., editor: Coping with neurologic problems proficiently. Nursing skillbook series, Springhouse, Pa., 1982, Intermed Communications, Inc.
43. Smith, L.H., and Thier, S.O.: Pathophysiology: the biological principles of disease, Philadelphia, 1981, W.B. Saunders Co.
44. Steinberg, F.U.: Cowdry's the care of the geriatric patient, ed. 5, St. Louis, 1976, The C.V. Mosby Co.
45. Stub, R.L., and Black, F.W.: The mental status examination in neurology, Philadelphia, 1977, F.A. Davis Co.
46. Swaiman, K.F., and Wright, F.S.: The practice of pediatric neurology, ed. 2, St. Louis, 1982, The C.V. Mosby Co.
47. Taylor, J.W., and Ballinger, S.: Neurological dysfunctions and nursing interventions, New York, 1980, McGraw-Hill Book Co.
48. Thompson, J.M., and Bowers, A.C.: Clinical manual of health assessment, St. Louis, 1980, The C.V. Mosby Co.
49. Tucker, S.M., et al.: Patient care standards, ed. 3, St. Louis, 1984, The C.V. Mosby Co.
50. Urdang, L., editor: Mosby's medical and nursing dictionary, St. Louis, 1983, The C.V. Mosby Co.
51. Urosevich, P.R.: Coping with neurologic disorders. Nursing photobook series, Springhouse, Pa., 1981, Intermed Communications, Inc.
52. Walleck, C.: Head trauma in children, Nurs. Clin. North Am. **15:**115, 1980.
53. Whaley, L.F., and Wong, D.L.: Nursing care of infants and children, ed. 2, St. Louis, 1983, The C.V. Mosby Co.
54. Wyngaarden, J.B., and Smith, L.H., editors: Cecil's textbook of medicine, Philadelphia, 1982, W.B. Saunders Co.

CHAPTER 4

Musculoskeletal System

Overview

The tissues of the musculoskeletal system make up the framework on, in, and around which the rest of the body is built and provide the means for easy, comfortable movements. Because of their vital and multiple structures and functions, they greatly influence the general health when they are inflamed, injured, or anomalous. Musculoskeletal anomalies and birth injuries affect newborns and lead to disability in growth, development, and productivity throughout the life span. Injuries from sports, jogging, or other physical fitness activities are major factors in the health of young to middle-aged adults. Formerly, men were the ones primarily affected with musculoskeletal injuries, but with the increasing participation of women in sports and physical fitness programs, the gender gap is narrowing. Trauma, primarily from automobile crashes, is the number one cause of death in persons aged 16 to 24 years. Inflammatory, rheumatic, and degenerative diseases of the musculoskeletal tissues not only exact a toll of young adult lives but also account for a large portion of the illness and disability of middle-aged and elderly adults. Billions of dollars are spent yearly for care and treatment of persons of all ages with musculoskeletal conditions. The economic costs are a major health care problem.

ANATOMY AND PHYSIOLOGY

Skeleton

According to Wolff's law, the 206 bones of the skeleton are shaped according to their function. They may be long (arm or leg), short (wrist or ankle bone), flat (sternum or scapula), irregular (vertebrae), or rounded (patella). The skull, face and auditory ossicles, vertebrae, ribs, sternum, and the hyoid bone make up the *axial* skeleton; the *appendicular* skeleton consists of the bones in the upper and lower extremities, shoulders, and pelvis.

Bones perform the following functions:
1. Support the body, enabling it to stand erect
2. Protect internal organs and other soft tissues
3. Assist in movements by leverage and in coordination with muscles
4. Make blood cells within the red bone marrow
5. Provide for storage of minerals, particularly calcium and phosphorus

Structure of bone tissue. Long bones of the extremities and thorax consist of a long shaft, the diaphysis, and two ends, the epiphyses, which are covered with articular cartilage and separated from the shaft by the growth plate and nutrient arteries of the metaphysis (Fig.

427

Fig. 4-1
Bone showing relationships of
compact and cancellous bone,
epiphysis, epiphyseal plate, and
diaphysis.

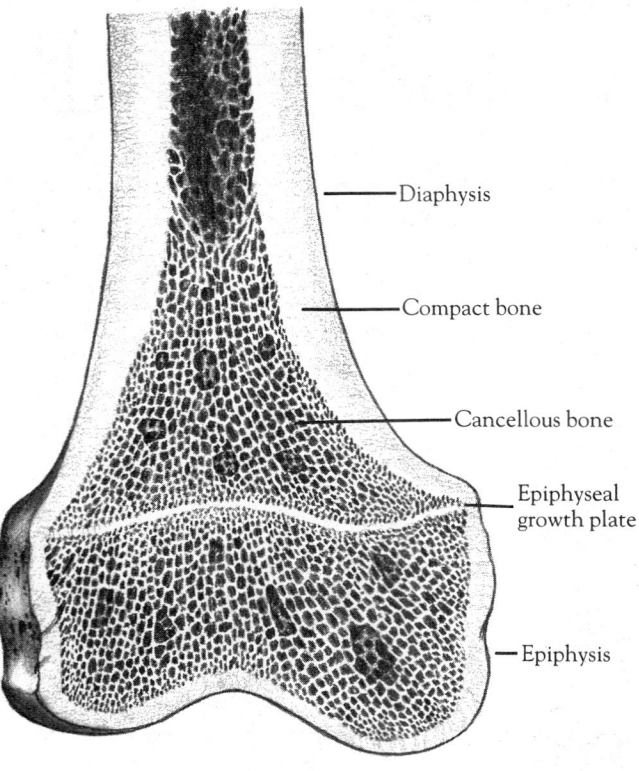

— Diaphysis

— Compact bone

— Cancellous bone

— Epiphyseal
   growth plate

— Epiphysis

nect to the blood vessels in the haversian canal by smaller canals, the canaliculi (Fig. 4-2). The haversian canal provides nutrients to osteocytes for bone building and removes wastes and debris from bone growth and resorption. Osteocytes, the major bone-forming cells, develop from osteoblasts, which are spindle-shaped cells found beneath the periosteum and in the inner region of bones, the endosteum. Osteoblasts remain dormant until needed for bone growth, when they mature into osteocytes. A third cell, the osteoclast, is also needed for shaping and remodeling bone and is used for resorption of unneeded or necrotic bone cells.

Bones are in a constant process of reabsorption counterbalanced by new bone formation. This process prevents bones from becoming excessively thick or heavy, as well as preventing them from becoming thinner or weakened from reabsorption. The formation and reabsorption processes are related to calcium and phosphate levels and metabolism in the body.

Approximately 99% of the total calcium of the body is contained in bone, with the remainder circulating in the blood plasma and in interstitial fluid.

Levels of extracellular calcium and phosphate concentrations are regulated by secretions of parathyroid hormone from the parathyroid glands, by absorption in the intestinal tract, and by retention or excretion by the kidneys so that relatively stable concentrations are maintained. Low calcium levels stimulate parathyroid hormone production, which stimulates osteoclasts to break down bone structure, freeing calcium phosphate crystals to be available to increase serum calcium concentrations. Additionally, the gastrointestinal ion-transport system absorbs calcium and moves the ion from the gut lumen to the blood. Thirdly, reabsorption of calcium is increased in the renal tubules to raise serum calcium levels, which concurrently reduce the reabsorption of phosphate. Through the processes just described, calcium levels remain relatively constant in healthy persons, and bone remains strong with relatively stable calcium concentration through formation and resorption.

Lastly, bone strength, formation, and resorption are affected by the amount and metabolism of vitamin D, which facilitates the absorption of calcium and phosphorus from the intestine. A deficiency of either vitamin D or sunshine (needed to activate sterol precursors in the skin to vitamin D) will cause changes in bones known as rickets in children and osteomalacia in adults. These two conditions are discussed on pp. 468-470.

The skeleton begins to develop from mesenchymal cells in the first prenatal month and is completely formed by the third month. Bones form through two basic processes: intramembranous and endochondral bone formation. Both involve the formation of a cancellous or spongy stage, which is later transformed into compact bone by deposition of bone matrix, which becomes cal-

4-1). The outer surface (cortex) of a bone is hard, dense tissue called compact bone, containing approximately 99% of the calcium in the body. The ends of long bones, the flat bones, and the ridges or crests of the ilium and tibia contain cancellous bone, which is soft and spongy with cavities containing the red bone marrow for hematopoiesis. Red bone marrow depletions are replaced by fat cells of the yellow bone marrow, which is found in the shafts of long bones.

The periosteum is the tough outer membrane of connective tissue covering each bone for protection and nutrition. Blood vessels in the inner layer of the periosteum bring nutrients and remove wastes. The periosteal blood vessels communicate with vessels in the central canal of the haversian system, which is the microscopic unit of compact bone.

The haversian system contains layers or plates of compact bone cells called lamellae surrounding the haversian canal, which contains two blood vessels and a nerve. The lamellae are aligned parallel to the shaft of the bone and encompass the lacunae, which are small cavities filled with bone cells and tissue fluids. The lacunae con-

Fig. 4-2

1, Three-dimensional view of compact bone; *2*, transverse section of compact bone depicting lamellae, lacunae, and canaliculi; *3*, longitudinal section of bone with lacunae and canaliculi; *4*, lacunae occupied by osteocyte.

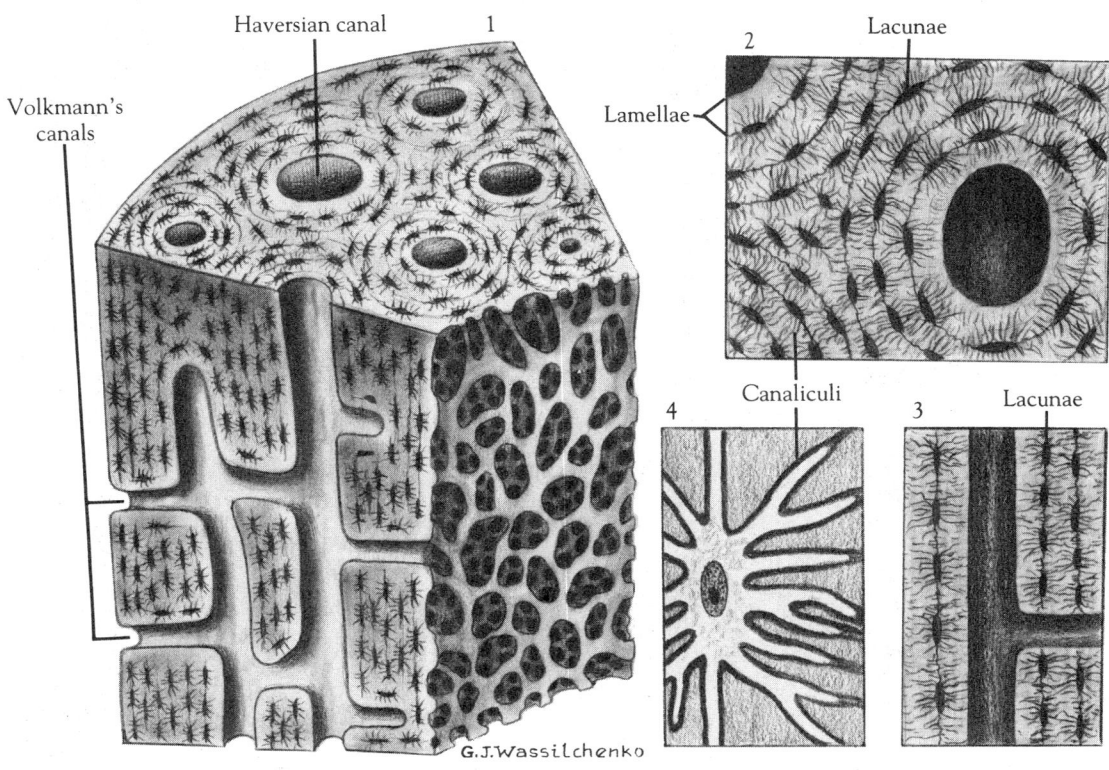

G.J.Wassilchenko

cified. Bone formation occurs where blood vessels supply minerals, oxygen, and nutrients. Where cancellous bone tissues predominate, the blood vessels are transformed into hemopoietic cells.[8]

Briefly, in intramembranous bone formation, mesenchymal cells differentiate into osteoblasts, which align themselves into a preliminary framework of osteoid tissue containing large endoplasmic reticulum. The well-differentiated osteoblasts are surrounded by a bone matrix and are then called osteocytes. Although the newly formed bones are derived from type I collagen (see p. 440 for collagen types), the major form of collagen that is eventually found in the bone matrix is type III. Calcification of the osteoid tissues depends on the supply of minerals and nutrients from the adjacent capillaries. Mineral deposits align into the bone trabeculae, which become surrounded by lamellae, which eventually replace the initial trabeculae by lamellar compact bone. The bones of the skull and other flat bones are formed through intramembranous pathways.

Bones formed endochondrally develop within a preformed cartilage framework. Gradually the cartilage is resorbed as the bones develop through the activity of osteoblasts. All long bones are formed from endochondral tissues. These bones begin to ossify from the center in the middle of the diaphysis. The chondrocytes align themselves in long, parallel columns, hypertrophy, and eventually die while initiating the synthesis of type I collagen laid down on the inner sides of their lacunae. As the lacunae enlarge, their intervening matrix decreases in quantity and becomes irregularly calcified. Simultaneously, intramembranous bone formation is begun at the periphery of the diaphysis, mediated through cells of type I and type III collagen molecules, which eventually transform this portion of the bone into the periosteum. The remaining cartilaginous mold cells are resorbed, and type III collagen molecules infiltrate the newly formed bone trabeculae and extend the mineralization and ossification toward both ends of the bone. After birth, secondary centers for ossification develop in the epiphyseal

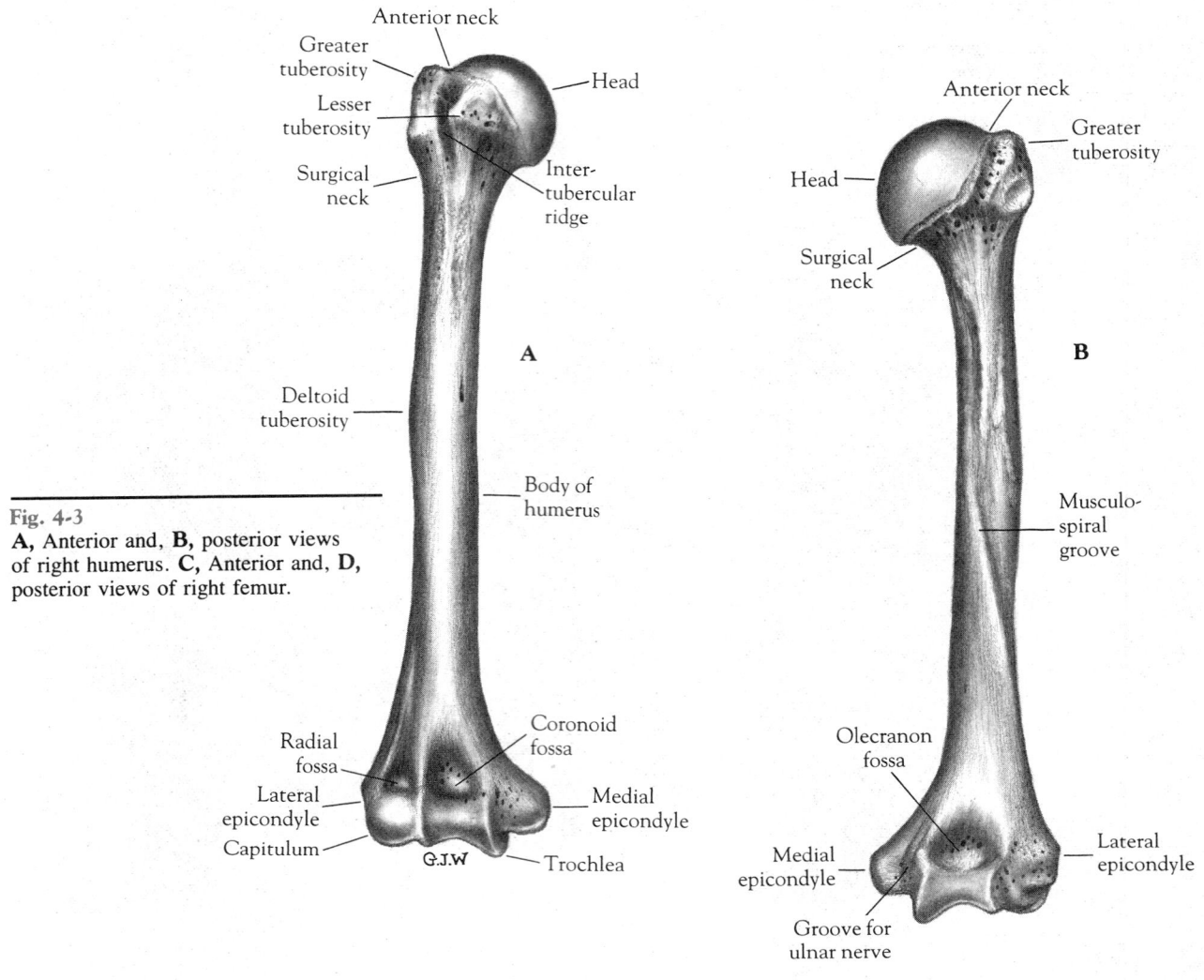

Fig. 4-3
A, Anterior and, **B**, posterior views of right humerus. **C**, Anterior and, **D**, posterior views of right femur.

regions with the cartilage that remains becoming the epiphyseal plate. The growth or proliferation of the columnar cartilage cells in this region results in the increased length of bones as the body grows. Eventually these growth zones are resorbed and replaced by bone when the bone has reached its final size. As the bone expands in length, its outer diameter is increased slightly accompanied by an increase in volume in the bone marrow cavity. New bone is continuously deposited on the outer surfaces with resorption from the inner surfaces, until the final bone shape is achieved. The shape is designed to maximize the specific bone's load-bearing capacities while minimizing its mass or weight. Bone growth and ossification generally continue longitudinally until 15 years of age in girls and 16 years of age in boys. Bone maturation and shaping, however, continue until 21 years

in both sexes with such regularity and accuracy that one's age can be closely approximated by x-ray examination of the bones.

As shown in Fig. 4-3, many processes (prominences) project outward from the surfaces of bones where tendons or ligaments attach themselves to the bones. Bony prominences may be rounded and knucklelike (condyles); small, rounded projections (tubercles); large processes (trochanters); or narrow ridges or crests (frontal bone and iliac crests). Projections may be transverse (transverse processes of vertebrae and ear), or they may project posteriorly (posterior spinous processes) or anteriorly (nasal cartilages). Bones also contain alveoli (sockets), fossae (depressions), fissures (narrow slits), foramina (openings for nerves, muscles, and blood vessels), sinuses (cavities), and sulci (grooves).

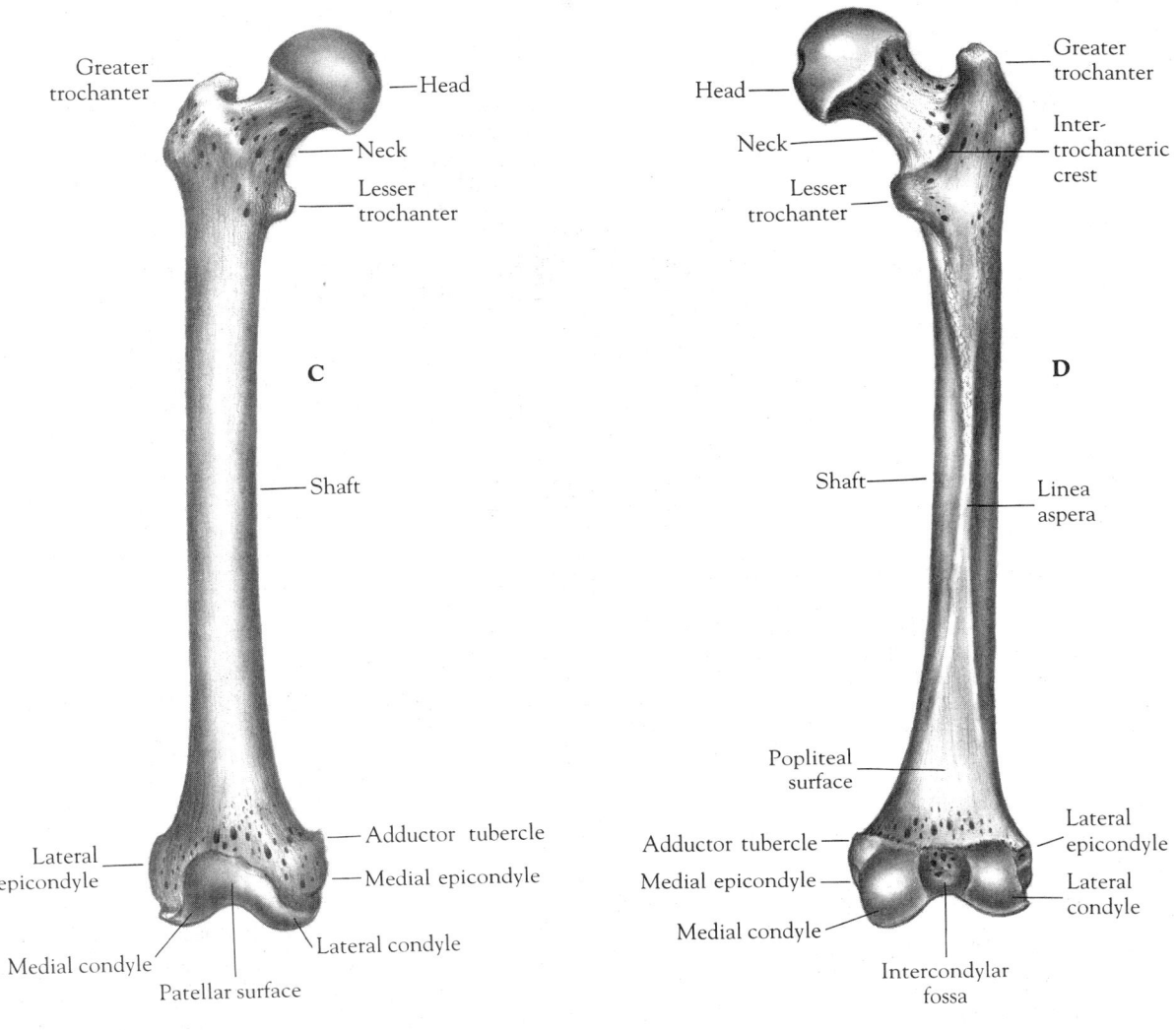

C

Greater trochanter — Head — Neck — Lesser trochanter — Shaft — Lateral epicondyle — Adductor tubercle — Medial epicondyle — Medial condyle — Patellar surface — Lateral condyle

D

Head — Greater trochanter — Neck — Intertrochanteric crest — Lesser trochanter — Shaft — Linea aspera — Popliteal surface — Adductor tubercle — Medial epicondyle — Medial condyle — Lateral epicondyle — Lateral condyle — Intercondylar fossa

Muscles

Muscles move the body through a tightening and shortening of the fibers (contraction) brought about through the *motor unit*. Each motor unit is composed of 100 to 200 muscle fibers innervated by a single motor nerve axon that stimulates the motor unit, sending the contraction through the muscle body. The muscle responds through the "all or none principle": it responds entirely or not at all to the stimulus. The strength of the muscle contraction is determined by the number of motor units contracting and by the number of times per second each motor unit is stimulated. A stimulus strong enough to bring about contraction is called a *liminal* stimulus; a stimulus of lesser intensity is called *subliminal*. A phenomenon known as *treppe* occurs from the additive effects of rapid subliminal stimuli. Treppe occurs when a second stimulus takes place at the apex of a preceding one resulting in a summation of stimuli and an increased strength of contraction (treppe) from the additive effects of the rapid subliminal stimuli.

Muscle *spasm* is an involuntary contraction of one or a group of muscles caused by repetitive activation of entire motor units from the repetitive firing of a motor nerve. *Tetanus* is a sustained summated contraction resulting from a repetitive series of stimuli conducted along the sarcolemmal membrane.

Muscle contraction. Muscle contraction results from a series of interactions at the myoneural junction in the muscle tissue. The stimulus travels along the motor nerve to the motor end-plate (myoneural junction) of the muscle fiber. Acetylcholine is produced at this synapse (junction) and released to bring about the muscle contraction by

Fig. 4-4
Motor end-plate and myoneural
junction involved in muscle
contraction (see text for content).

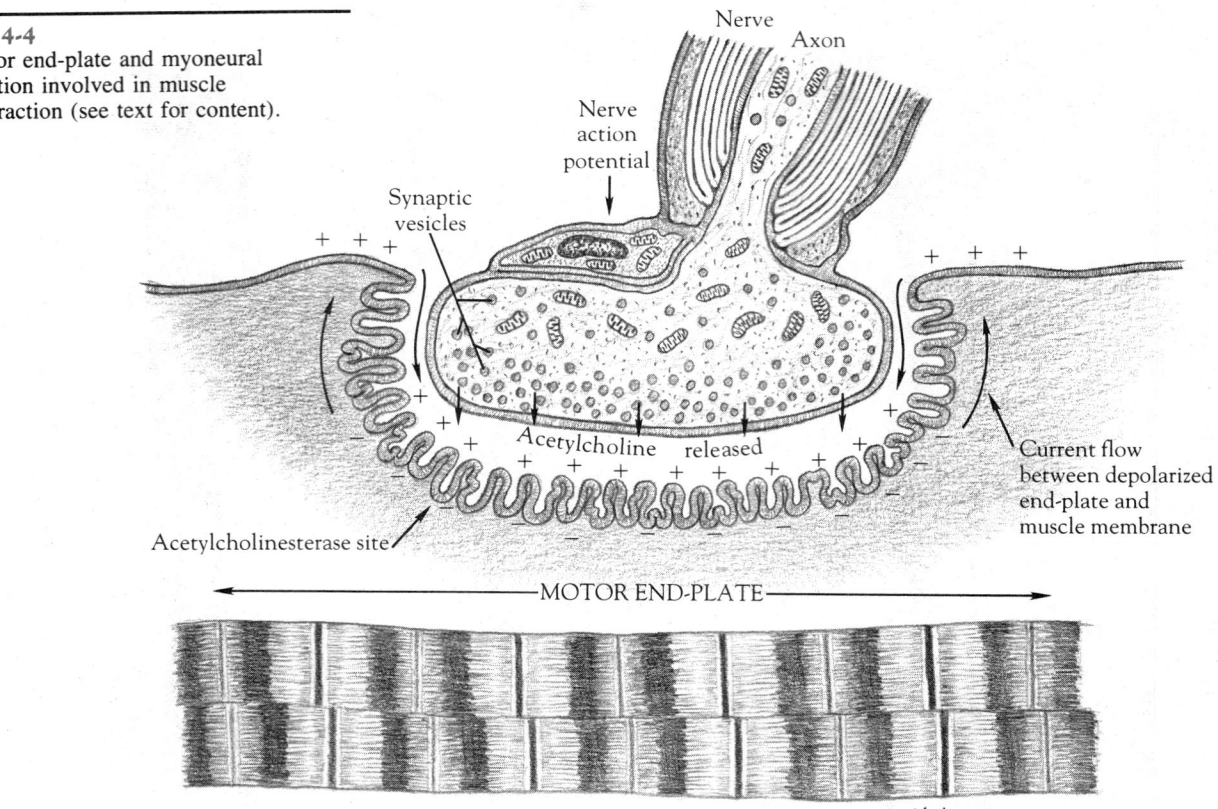

Nerve

Axon

Nerve
action
potential

Synaptic
vesicles

Acetylcholine released

Acetylcholinesterase site

Current flow
between depolarized
end-plate and
muscle membrane

MOTOR END-PLATE

G.J.Wassilchenko

depolarizing the sarcolemma. Depolarization permits interstitial calcium ions to enter the muscle membrane to aid the contraction. The wave of depolarization travels through the muscle fiber until it is deactivated by the enzyme acetylcholinesterase, after which the fiber is again ready for reactivation. The positive calcium ions catalyze an energy-releasing reaction to bring about the sliding of actin along the myosin, which results in contraction and shortening of the muscle (Fig. 4-4).

The energy for muscle contraction comes from the hydrolysis of ATP into ADP + phosphate + energy. The energy is used by the actin and myosin fibers to effect the intermeshing. Additional energy sources are from phosphocreatine, a protein-energy source found only in muscle tissues, and from oxygen, which facilitates contraction by oxidizing the lactic acid resulting from the anaerobic hydrolysis of the high-energy ATP bonds.

Along with contraction, muscles also have the ability to relax. A relaxing factor, as yet unnamed, acts by rendering ATP inactive until the next stimulus reaches a particular fiber, thereby keeping the muscle relaxed.

Muscle twitch. A muscle twitch occurs when a liminal stimulus is attained. All muscle fibers associated with the stimulated nerve contract and then relax.

Muscle twitches are classified as either isotonic or isometric. An *isotonic* twitch causes the muscle to change length when constant tension is applied throughout its contraction. An *isometric* twitch is one in which the muscle remains or retains a constant length even with a sudden increase in muscle tension.

Muscle tone. Muscle *tone* results from the steady state of readiness maintained within a muscle to ensure a rapid reaction to an external stimulus. Tone in muscles provides resistance to passive elongation or stretch and results from a continuous flow of stimuli from the spinal cord to each motor unit. Muscle tone can be increased or decreased depending on the activity within the nervous system. Tone is increased in anxiety states and decreased during restful periods.

Structure of skeletal muscles. Skeletal muscles make up 40% to 45% of the body's weight. They move the body as a whole or in part through their contractions. They cover the skeletal bones and help produce the contours of the body. Muscles are attached at each end to a bone, ligament, tendon, or fascia. One end of the muscle, the more fixed end, is referred to as the *origin* and the more movable end is the muscle *insertion*. Muscles of the skeletal system are voluntary muscles that are controlled by the will; in contrast, visceral muscles move

Fig. 4-5
Structure of muscle fibers and their coverings.

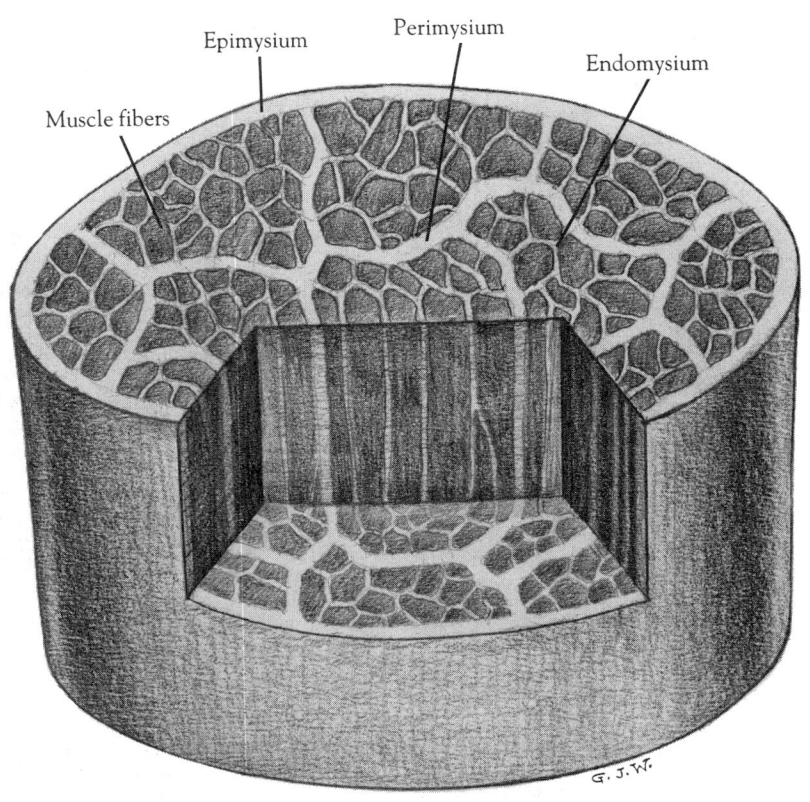

Epimysium   Perimysium   Endomysium

Muscle fibers

G.J.W.

involuntarily and are not initiated by conscious effort. Voluntary movement of muscle requires electrical stimulation as previously discussed.

Muscles of the skeletal system, or striated muscles, are generally long, slender bundles containing dark cross markings or lines called striations. Each muscle is made up of fibers enclosed in a sarcolemma and bound together in bundles (fasciculi) by a connective tissue sheath (perimysium). The fasciculi are further bound together by a stronger sheath (epimysium). These bundles of bound fibers make up the muscle belly, the fleshy part of the muscle. The epimysium extends beyond the belly of the muscle to form a *tendon*. All the muscles of the limbs are bound together by a layer of connective tissue called fascia, a tough, silvery-appearing covering.

Skeletal muscles vary in length, width, diameter, and color, being either red or white. Red muscle contains the pigment myoglobin, which gives it its color and, being closely related to hemoglobin, acts as a temporary oxygen store for the muscle. White muscle fibers contain less myoglobin and appear lighter colored. White muscles react more rapidly when stimulated, whereas red muscles carry out slower, sustained movements (Fig. 4-5).

The striations of skeletal muscles result from bands of muscle fibers composed of cylindric cytoplasmic ele-

ments called *myofibrils*. Myofibrils form the longitudinal striation of the muscle; transverse striations form the banding patterns in the myofibrils. Each myofibril consists of smaller *myofilaments*, which form a regular repeating pattern along the length of the fibril. One unit of this repeating pattern is called a *sarcomere*. The sarcomere is the functional unit of the contractile system in muscles.

Each sarcomere contains two types of myofilaments: thick and thin. The thick myofilaments are found in the central region of the sarcomere, where their orderly, parallel arrangement results in the dark bands, called A bands, that are seen in striated muscles. The thick filaments contain the protein myosin. The thin myofilaments contain the protein actin and are attached at either end of the sarcomere to a structure known as the Z line. Two successive Z lines define the limits of one sarcomere. The Z lines contain short elements that interconnect the thin filaments from two adjoining sarcomeres to provide an anchoring point for the thin filaments. The thin elements extend from the Z lines toward the center of the sarcomere where they overlap with the thick filaments (Fig. 4-6).

Two other bands have been identified as changing during contraction relative to the positions of the thick and

Fig. 4-6
A, Lines and bands in striated muscle.
B, Relationships of bands, actin, myosin, and lines in relaxed and contracted muscle fibers (see text for content).

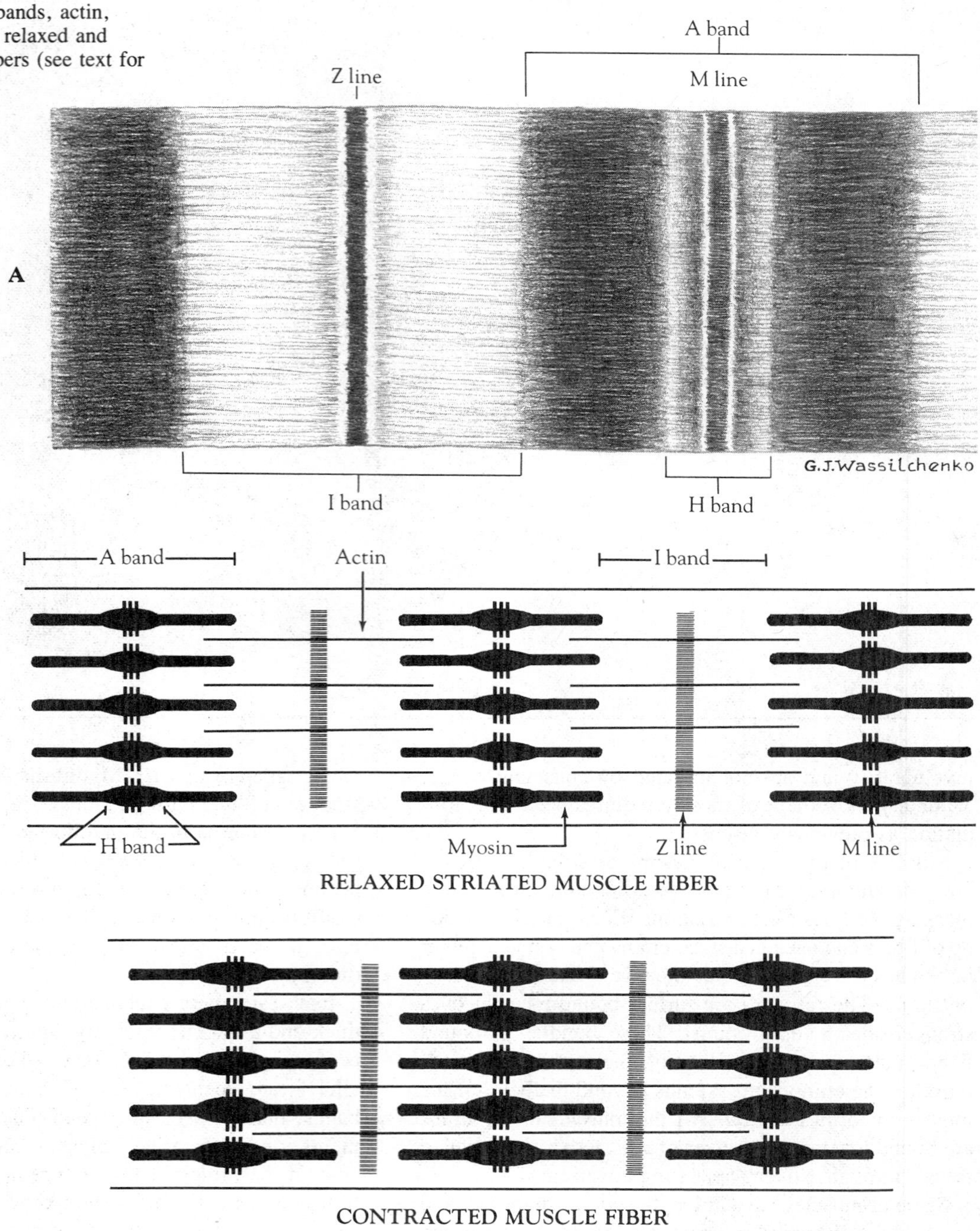

A

Z line

A band

M line

I band

H band

G.J.Wassilchenko

A band — Actin — I band

H band — Myosin — Z line — M line

B

RELAXED STRIATED MUSCLE FIBER

CONTRACTED MUSCLE FIBER

thin filaments in the sarcomere. One, the *I band,* is between the ends of the A bands in two adjoining sarcomeres. Because it contains only thin filaments, it usually appears as a light band separating the dark A bands. The other band, the *H zone,* is a thin, lighter band in the center of the A band that corresponds to the space be-

tween the ends of the thin filaments. Only thick filaments are found in the H zone region.

During contraction the thick and thin filaments slide past each other, but the lengths of the individual thick and thin filaments do not change. As the thin filaments move past the thick filaments, the width of the H zone

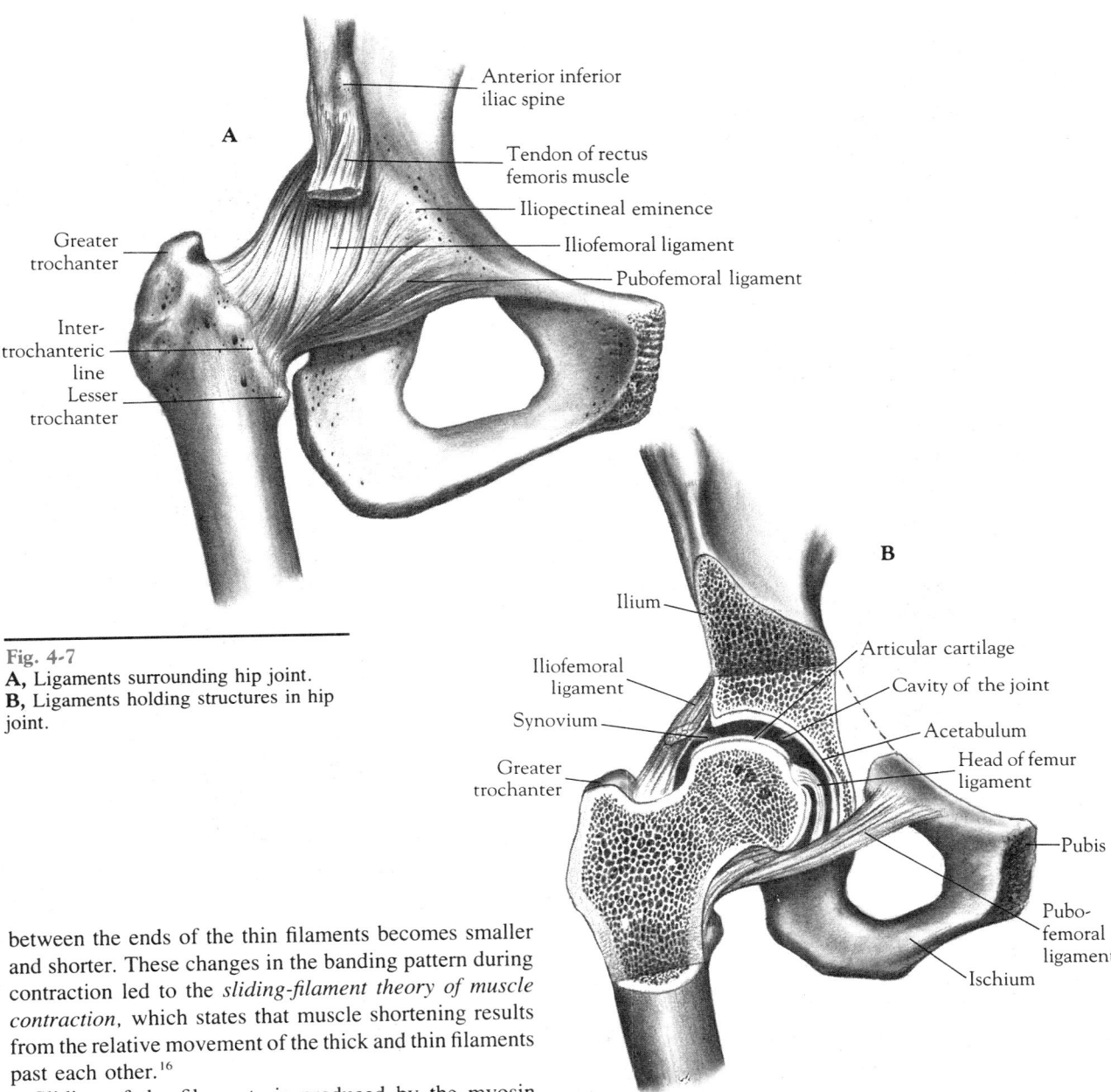

Fig. 4-7
A, Ligaments surrounding hip joint.
B, Ligaments holding structures in hip joint.

between the ends of the thin filaments becomes smaller and shorter. These changes in the banding pattern during contraction led to the *sliding-filament theory of muscle contraction*, which states that muscle shortening results from the relative movement of the thick and thin filaments past each other.[16]

Sliding of the filaments is produced by the myosin cross bridges, which swivel in an arc around their fixed positions on the surface of the thick filament. The movement of the cross bridges in contact with the actin thin filaments produces the sliding of the thick and thin filaments past each other. The cross bridges undergo many repeated cycles of movement during a contraction. The myosin bridges detach themselves from actin, rebind to new actin sites, and repeat these cycles of movements, brought about by the binding of a molecule to ATP to myosin.[16] The process of binding ATP appears to break the linkage between actin and myosin. The reaction returns the bridge to its initial state so that it can repeat the cycle of bridge movement.

Ligaments

Ligaments hold bones to bones. They may encircle a joint to add strength and stability as they do around the hip joint (Fig. 4-7), or they may hold obliquely or parallel to the ends of bones across the joint as they do in and around the knee joint (Fig. 4-8). Ligaments are relatively long bands in order to perform their functions; they are made up of tough bands of collagen fibers arranged in parallel bundles of fibers to add strength. The type of

Fig. 4-8
Ligaments of the knee joint.

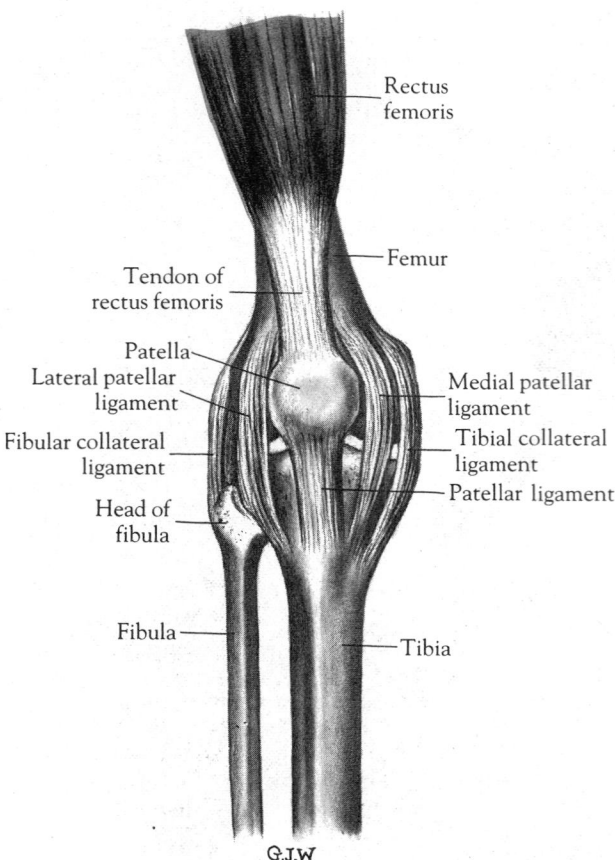

Fig. 4-9
Tendons and muscles around the knee joint (anterior view).

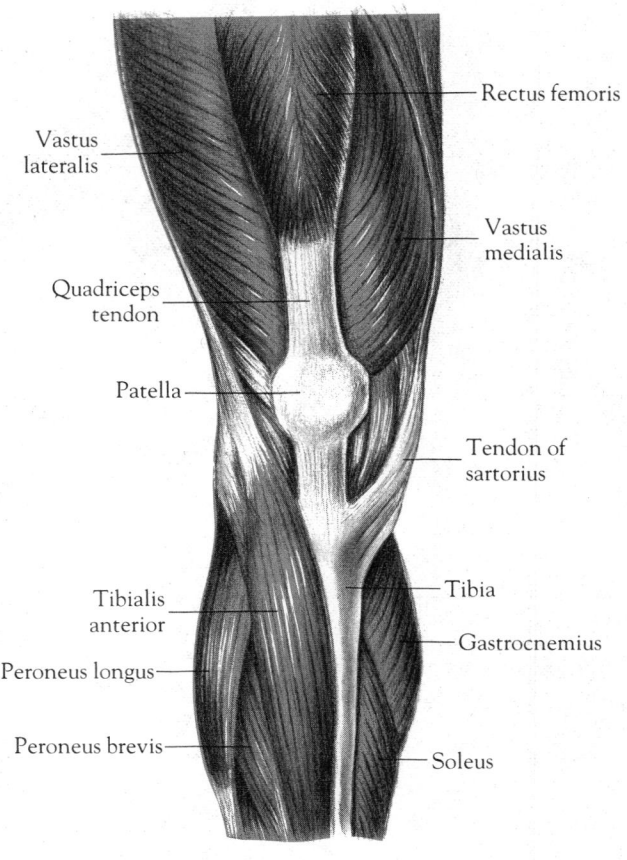

collagen producing these large, densely packed fibers is type I (see pp. 439-440 for discussion of collagen structure and types), which gives ligaments great tensile strength with limited extensibility. When ligaments are taut they provide the greatest stability to the specific joint. Ligaments allow movements in some directions while restricting movements in other directions.

Tendons

Tendons hold muscles to bones (Fig. 4-9). They form at the ends of muscles into strong, nonelastic cords of type I collagen, which gives them great strength as it does with ligaments. The cells of tendons are arranged in coarse, parallel bundles bound together into fascicles to provide the high tensile strength while allowing them to transmit forces from contractile muscle to bone or cartilage and still remain undamaged themselves. Tendons vary in length from 1 inch to approximately 1 foot,

the longest being the Achilles tendon of the heel (Fig. 4-10).

Joints

Joints are formed where two surfaces of bones come together and articulate. Classified by their degree of movement, joints are either immovable (synarthrotic), slightly movable (ampiarthrotic), or freely movable (diarthrotic). Synarthrotic joints are in the skull held together by fibrous tissues called sutures. Ampiarthrotic joints allow slight movement through their fibrocartilage disc such as in the symphysis pubis or by a fibroligament as in the radioulnar articulation.

The majority of joints are diarthrotic and freely movable. They are also called synovial joints because they are lined with synovial membranes. In addition to the synovium, other structures included in diarthrodial joints are bones, articular cartilage, synovial fluid, nerves, lym-

Fig. 4-10
Achilles tendon in leg.

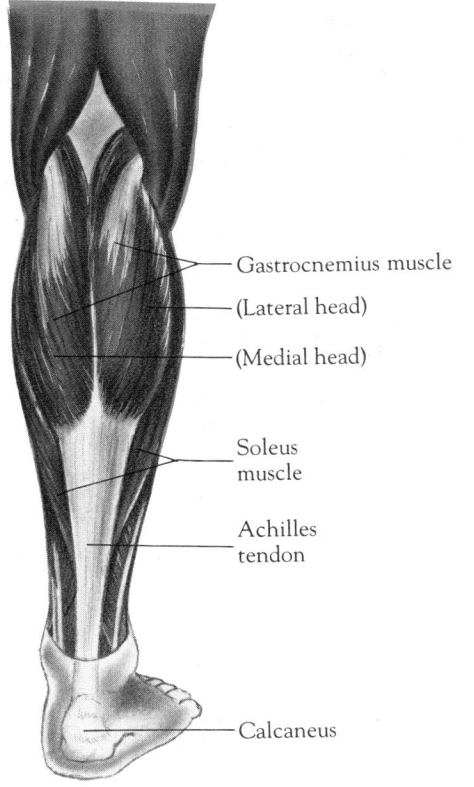

Gastrocnemius muscle

(Lateral head)

(Medial head)

Soleus muscle

Achilles tendon

Calcaneus

circumduction   Making a conical movement, exemplified by winding up to throw a ball.

supination   Turning the palm upward and forward.

pronation   Turning the palm downward and backward.

eversion   Turning the sole of the foot outward.

inversion   Turning the sole of the foot inward.

dorsiflexion   Pulling the foot and toes upward and forward.

plantar flexion   Pushing the foot and toes downward and backward.

elevation   Lifting upward.

depression   Lowering.

protraction   Moving a part forward.

retraction   Moving a part backward.

opposition   Moving the thumb toward the little finger to touch together.

When joints cannot or do not maintain their usual ranges of movements, they exert effects on all musculoskeletal tissues plus other body tissues as noted later. Table 4-1 gives ranges of motion of major joints.

Synovium

The synovium is a membrane that completely lines the inner surfaces of the joint. It forms from mesenchymal cells within the inner layer of the joint capsule. The membrane has villous folds that contain the blood vessels and lymphatics. The membrane is made of cells derived primarily from type I collagen molecules, although the blood vessels are derived from type III collagen (see pp. 439-440 for a discussion of collagens).

The villous folds of the synovial membrane are filled with fluid, called the synovial fluid, that bathes the articular cartilage to facilitate articulation as well as providing nutrients, phagocytes, and other immunologic functions within the joints.

Cartilage

Cartilage is a smooth, white or yellow, resilient supporting tissue made up of elastic fibers containing the protein chondrin. There are three types of cartilage:

hyaline   Bluish white, elastic cartilage covering the ends of bones making up synovial joints, the ends of the ribs, the nasal septum, and the walls of the trachea; made up of type II collagen molecules with some type I cells.

fibrous   White fibers that are particularly resistant to tension and are found in the symphysis pubis and the knee; made up of type I collagen molecules.

yellow   Elastic yellow fibers found in the epiglottis and the pinna (outer ear); made up of type I collagen molecules.

Cartilage serves as a smooth surface for articulating bones. It also absorbs weight and, through its elasticity and moldability, absorbs shock, stress, and strain to pre-

phatics, and blood vessels, all encased in the joint capsule made up of ligaments and tendons encircling or surrounding the joints.

Since diarthrodial joints are freely movable they are named for their major form of movement, such as ball and socket (hip, shoulder), hinge (elbow, knee), pivot (atlas, axis), condyloid (wrist), saddle (first metacarpal/trapezium), and gliding (intervertebral).

The degree of movement of a joint is referred to as its range of motion. Joints have one or more of the movements listed below:

flexion   Bending forward; shortening that decreases the angle between two bones.

extension   Bending backward or lengthening that increases the angle between two bones or straightens the joint.

abduction   Moving away from the midline of the body.

adduction   Moving toward the midline.

rotation   Moving around a central axis, perpendicular to the axis.

Table 4-1

Range of Motion of Major Joints

Joint	Movements	Average ranges (in degrees)* Adult	Older Adult
Cervical spine	Flexion	35-45	35
	Extension	35	May have pain and some stiffness
	Lateral bending	45	
	Rotation	45	
	Hyperextension	45	
Thoracic and lumbar spine	Flexion	80-90	
	Extension	30	
	Lateral bending	28-35	
	Rotation	35-38	30
	Hyperextension	30	
Shoulder	Flexion	90	Some stiffness
	Backward extension	45-55	
	Abduction	90	
	Adduction	45-50	
	Circumduction	360	May have crepitation
Elbow	Flexion	145-160	May only be able to flex 135 degrees
	Hyperextension	0	
Forearm	Pronation	70-90	
	Supination	85-90	
Wrist	Extension	70	May have soreness or stiffness
	Flexion	73-90	
	Ulnar deviation	33-55	
	Radial deviation	19	
Thumb	Abduction	58	
Fingers	Flexion		Decreased (may be caused by Heberden's or Bouchard's nodes)
	Distal joint	80	
	Middle joint	100	
	Proximal joint	90	
	Extension		
	Distal joint	0	
	Middle joint	0	
	Proximal joint	45	
Hip	Flexion	120-135	Decreased because of degenerative changes
	Extension	28	
	Abduction	45-48	
	Adduction	20-30	
	Rotation		
	In flexion		
	Internal rotation	45	
	External rotation	45	
	In extension		
	Internal rotation	35	
	External rotation	48	
	Abduction in 90-degree flexion	45-60	
Knee	Flexion	120-130	Same or decreased but with soreness and stiffness; may have crepitation
	Hyperextension	10	
Ankle	Flexion	48-50	
	Extension	18-20	
Forefoot	Inversion	30-33	Same or decreased because of hallux valgus or degenerative changes
	Eversion	18-20	
	Dorsiflexion	20	
	Plantar flexion	45-50	

*Zero degrees is the extended position; movement is measured by degrees in the specific directions in which the joint moves.

vent or lessen injury to bones within joints as well as other joint tissues (Fig. 4-25).

Cartilage contains no intrinsic blood vessels within its cells. It receives its nutrition from the synovial fluids that are forced into its porous cellular network by the movements and weight bearing of the joints. Therefore, when a particular joint ceases to bear weight or develops limitations of its usual range of movements, articular cartilage will begin to atrophy. Atrophy of the cartilage continues until joint motion and weight bearing are resumed.

Bursa

A bursa is a small sac or cavity found in the connective tissues (usually the tendons) surrounding or near a joint (Fig. 4-11). The bursa is lined with synovial membrane and contains synovial fluid. Normally the bursa is a part of the musculoskeletal tissues, but a bursa can also form as a result of pressure or friction over a prominent part. Just such a bursa forms to become a bunion in hallux valgus deformity.

The bursa reduces friction between tendons and bones or between tendons and ligaments by lubrication with synovial fluid from the bursal sac. New bursae can develop as a result of increased pressure or friction for the purpose, again, of providing lubrication to lessen the friction. Their formation may indeed increase the pressure and cause pain.

Collagen

Collagen is the principal supporting element in connective tissues. It is a protein that constitutes approximately one half the total body protein in fully developed adults. Along with its supporting function, collagen also plays an active role in developmental processes, cell attachment, chemotaxis, and the binding of antigen-antibody complexes. Thus collagen is more than an inert structural protein.

The collagen molecule is an asymmetric, rigid, rodlike structure made up of three individual polypeptide strands that are aligned colinearly throughout the molecule. At one end is an NH_2 radical, and it is at this terminal that the cross-links originate. The central region accounts for about 95% of the length of the molecule. The third portion of the molecule contains the COOH terminal, comprising about 3% of the molecule.

The three individual strands of collagen are tightly coiled together in the form of a left-handed helix (the minor helix). They are then coiled around a common central axis to form a right-handed helix (the major helix). This coiled-coil configuration is stabilized by interchain hydrogen bonds with the collagen chains containing the amino acid glycine at every third position.

Collagen strands are made up of many amino acid residues, approximately 23% of which are proline plus hydroxyproline and 33% of which are glycine. Other amino acids are glutamic acid, alanine, and hydroxylysine. Lesser amounts of amino acids such as methionine, isoleucine, tyrosine, and histidine are also present in the molecule.

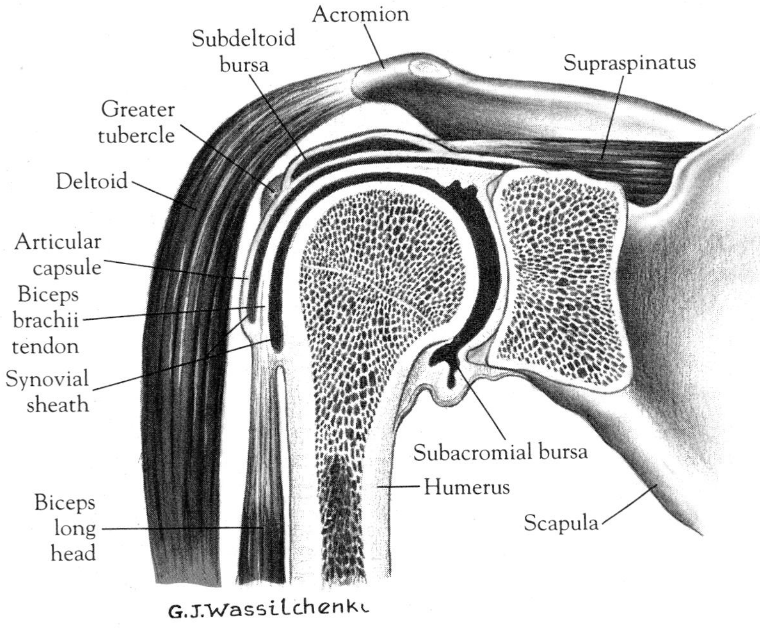

Fig. 4-11
Subdeltoid and subacromial bursae.

G.J.Wassilchenki

Collagen molecules presently are referred to as type I, II, or III; these types make up the most extensively occurring molecules. Fibers from these types are found predominantly in spaces between the cellular elements of a tissue or organ; thus they are called interstitial collagens.

Fibers from type I collagen molecules are found in all major connective tissues and in the stroma of several organs. Tissues such as bone, tendon, and dentin and fibrocartilage appear to be formed exclusively of type I collagen molecules. The distribution patterns of type I molecules indicate that they play a major role as supporting elements in tissues that normally exhibit very little distensibility under mechanical stress. Additionally, it appears that type I collagen molecules can be synthesized by the connective tissue cells in which they are found.

Type I collagen molecules are composed of two identical alpha-1 strands and a different but homologous alpha-2 chain. Type II is composed of three alpha-1 chains, found primarily in hyaline cartilage, where they lend their special properties to the mechanical strengths of the car-

tilage. Type III collagen molecules, also composed of three identical alpha-1 chains, are found in tissues that are the most distensible such as the skin, blood-vessel walls, and the uterine wall and in several organs. Type III fibers coexist as fine reticular networks with type I molecules with larger fibers in the same tissues.

Differences in the three chains can be discerned by electron microscopy. The alpha-2 chain contains more basic amino acid residues than the other chains. The alpha-chain of type II collagen contains significantly higher levels of threonine and glutamic acid compared to the other chains, and it has markedly increased levels of hydroxylysine and glycosylated hydroxylysine. The alpha-1 chain of type III collagen contains relatively high levels of 4-hydroxyproline, glycine, and cysteinyl residues.[8] Each chain yields a unique set of peptides when examined, and each type of collagen has been determined to develop from or under the control of separate and distinct structural genes. Thus the specific chain type and arrangement give the particular collagen the strength and distensibility most suited to its specific tissue and distribution within the connective tissues of the body.

NORMAL FINDINGS

The orthopedic examination should take into account both the history and the physical examination.

The history should include any past and present orthopedic problems as well as patterns of local and systemic signs and symptoms with review of all systems; social, marital, employment (occupational), and psychologic state; and habits or hobbies.

The physical examination includes an overall general inspection; observance of gait, posture, and movements while walking, sitting, and standing; assessment of *bilateral* symmetry, size and shape of musculoskeletal tissues, muscular development, generalized or localized edema, range of movements of each joint, condition of skin of body and of fingers and toes (with presence or complaints of Raynaud's phenomenon), lesions, rash (color and site), pain at rest or with movement in one or more joints, temperature of skin of and around joints, texture of skin and nails, nodules in or around joints, hair growth and distribution, and evidence of bruises, hemorrhage, bone or joint deformity, congenital defects or deformities, condition of blood vessels, peripheral pulses, color of tissues, lymph nodes, leg length equality, and "point" tenderness.

The following equipment is needed: goniometer to measure range of movements, percussion hammer, pin, cotton, sphygmomanometer, thermometer, tourniquet, tape measure, and stethoscope.

The following principles should be kept in mind in performing an orthopedic examination:
- Normal tissues are examined before injured, inflamed, or otherwise involved ones.
- Local signs and symptoms are assessed with systemic findings.
- Bilateral local and systemic observations are made.
- Palpation is gently performed while observing facial or other reactions to note tenderness or sensitivity within the tissues.
- Movements are assessed within norms for ranges of movements; differences between the right and left sides are noted.
- Physical examination is but one part of the orthopedic examination, along with the history and radiologic, serologic, surgical biopsy or exploratory, and consultative examinations.

Area of Concern	Normal Adult Findings	Variations in Child	Variations in Older Adult
Skeleton Posture	Stands upright; head perpendicular to shoulders and pelvis; shoulders and pelvis aligned; convex curve to thoracic spine; concave curve to lumbar spine; arms hang freely from shoulders; feet aligned with toes pointing straight ahead.	Newborn lies on back or sides; upper extremities held flexed and may appear to have exaggerated length in comparison to body trunk; bones seem very flexible. Body growth is rapid in first years; height is rapidly increased in first 1-3 years. Arms and hands carried at sides by 15 months of age. Sitting upright by 6-8 months while able to maintain balance.	Stance less upright with head and neck more forward; thoracic curvature more pronounced; lumbar curvature less pronounced; shoulders may be hunched or rolled forward; angle of head of femur into acetabulum changes, leading to varus planting or placement of thighs, legs, and feet.
Stature	Long, slender bones varying to short, thick bones. Bone maturation ceases approximately age 21.	Boys are slightly longer at birth than girls. With growth, extremities become more proportional to trunk. Bones become firmer and stronger. Child grows 2-3 inches per year until age 15-16 when longitudinal growth ceases.	Height may decrease because of curvature changes; upper extremities appear longer and out of proportion to rest of body. Calcium losses from bones also affect stature from osteoporosis.
Symmetry	Slight differences in upper extremities because of handedness. Hands may appear larger in larger persons.	Symmetric in contour and size.	
Gait	Smooth, coordinated, easy, rhythmic with push off and swing through; arms move freely at sides. Easy acceleration and deceleration. Can stand still without swaying or tilt.	Crawling initiated by 7-10 months; standing, assisted, by 8 months; standing, unassisted, by 12-14 months; walking assisted by 9-12 months, and unassisted, by 15 months; running by 18 months and walking up or down stairs by 24 months.	Gait slow to initiate and stop; gait may be shuffling at times with less knee and ankle lifts; more stiffness of hips, knees, and back; steps may be shorter and more rapid but cover less overall distance.
Muscles Shape and contour	"Full-bellied"; firm and supple; muscle mass in overall conformity with body build; tapered at either end of muscle mass.	Soft, less firm with less "belly" or mass; less shape and contour until weight bearing when firming increases.	Shape and contour decrease with less belly and mass common.
Strength	Peak of muscle strength is 25-30 years; able to perform work of movements on demand and to maintain work activity over time; very smooth and firm when contracted; loose when relaxed. Strong grip/push/pull strength.	Initially baby grips as part of reflex behavior, then grasp and grip become meaningful, differentiated, and controlled; can sustain some work (e.g., hold head up for brief time after 2-4 weeks).	Initial work energy strong, but strength lessens over time (gradual 10% loss in muscle strength between 30-60 years). Movements may be somewhat uncoordinated and jerky. Grip/push/pull strength weaker than young adult.

Area of Concern	Normal Adult Findings	Variations in Child	Variations in Older Adult
Muscles—cont'd			
Range of movements	Able to move bones and joints through movements required or permitted by the bone/joint structures. Movements are smooth and sustained if necessary; muscle action begins smoothly without jerking. Usual length is regained when muscle is relaxed. Paired opposing actions are smooth. There should be no limitation of movement (Table 4-1).	All muscles can be passively moved through range of movements at birth. Active range of movements proceeds as child matures and should be smooth and coordinated. Pot-bellied appearance is common in toddlers because of undeveloped abdominal muscles. Preschool boys surpass girls in muscle strength tasks whereas girls are superior in small muscle coordination.	All muscles can be put through passive range of movement slowly. Active range of movement may be slower or limited in one or more joints either symmetrically or asymmetrically. Slight to moderate tenderness or pain may accompany movement.
Joints			
Shape and contour	Depends on the specific type and position in body. Bones of joint should articulate without deformity on one another in alignment. Joint is firm and strong.	Joints appear larger than bones surrounding joint at birth, and size gradually becomes more in conformity as child grows; joints may appear "looser" or less firm at birth and gradually gain tightness as child grows.	Joints appear larger than surrounding tissues; contour may be irregular in one or more joints. Bones may glide over one another with slightly audible click or sound. Joint is stiffer than younger adult.
Movements	Bones should move quietly and freely over one another; no clicks, crepitation, or pain should occur. Movements should be smooth and coordinated according to particular type of joint. Active range of movements should be pain free.	Movements less coordinated with child initiating "locking" of joints to help with balance at times. As child gains muscle strength from preschool to adolescence, movements are smooth, strong, and coordinated.	Movements slower and more deliberate. Balance may be harder to maintain. Joints may be somewhat limited in range of movements. Movements may be jerky and slightly painful.
Temperature	Warmth around joint should be same as surrounding tissues.	Same.	Same.
Swelling/edema	None.	None.	May have slight edema.
Ligaments, Cartilage, and Tendons			
Shape and contour	Taut, elastic, and firm; permit weight bearing.	Same; easily stretched.	Taut but may be tighter and less elastic; may limit bone/joint contour.
Movements	Easily moves through range of motion and holds joints and muscles according to place or function. Movements of joints can be sustained without deformity or curvature. Weight bearing is pain free.	Same, with more "looseness" at birth. Tiring noted with sustained movements but full function regained with rest.	Less ease and range of movements. Joints are stiffer. May have some joint laxity and weakness. Weight bearing may cause some soreness or pain.

SPECIAL ASSESSMENT TECHNIQUES

Examination or Test	Site	Normal Findings	Abnormal Findings
Joint range of movements	Any or all joints	Specific range of motion (ROM) as per Table 4-1; no soreness or pain; no edema or elevated temperature in or around joint or joints.	Limitation of range of movements in one or more spheres; pain, soreness, muscle weakness, edema, elevated temperature in or around joint or joints.
Straight leg raising (Lasègue's)	Legs (one at a time)	No pain or soreness in back, buttocks when leg is raised while fully extended at knee; patient lies on back.	Pain, soreness, or radiation of pain from low back to buttocks; may spread down leg to toes.
McMurray's	Knee	No excessive or palpable pop or click in knee noted when ankle is grasped to turn knee medially and laterally, and while moving knee backward and forward from full flexion to extension.	Click or pop felt or heard; pain or local tenderness is positive for meniscal damage or tears.
Fabere-Patrick	Knee and hip	Knee can be flexed and brought to almost horizontal position to body with heel resting on opposite knee.	Knee cannot be brought to horizontal position; limitation may be in hip, knee, or back (usually hip disease prevents knee rotation to horizontal position).
Drawer	Knee	Knee has slight forward or backward movement while flexed on tibia and fibula.	Knee has more movement forward or backward (direction indicates tear of either anterior or posterior cruciate ligaments).
Trendelenburg's	Pelvis and gluteus muscles	With weight on one leg, pelvis on opposite side will be slightly elevated (observed posteriorly).	With weight on one leg, pelvis will drop (due to weakness or pain in hip joint or its muscles) on opposite side (Fig. 4-19).
Thomas'	Hip, knee, and lumbar spine	With patient on back, hip and knee are flexed to abdomen without flexion simultaneously occurring in lumbar spine.	When patient flexes knee and hip to abdomen, lumbar spine will flex if there is a pathologic condition of the hip, and opposite leg will rise from table.
Ortolani's	Hip joints of newborns	With hips in flexion, hips should abduct nearly to right angles.	With hips flexed, abduction will not be to full right angle but either hip may stop part way; if pressure is applied, it may abduct fully with a jerk or clunk as dislocation is reduced (sign of congenital hip dislocation) (Fig. 4-18).
Barlow's	Hip joints of newborns	Femur stays in hip joint bilaterally.	Femoral head can be "levered" in or out of hip joint in congenital dislocation of hip.

NORMAL LABORATORY DATA

Laboratory Test	Normal Adult Values	Variations in Child	Variations in Older Adult
Serum calcium	See pediatric values	Normal range slowly descends Up to 30 yr: 8.2-10.5 mg/dl	Decreases very slightly with age
Serum calcium (ionized)	4.75-5.2 mg/dl		
Serum calcium (ionized, calculated, blood)	3.9-4.8 mg/dl		
Serum phosphorus	2.5-4.5 mg/dl	At birth: 5.6-8.0 mg/dl Childhood: 4-7 mg/dl	
Alkaline phosphatase*	3-13 King-Armstrong units or 1.5-4.0 Bodansky units	15-25 King-Armstrong units	
Acid phosphatase	Method dependent; up to 0.8 IU/L, ACA		
Creatinine (24-h urine)	Adult male: 1-2 g/24 h Adult female: 0.8-1.8 g/24 h	2-3 yr: 6-22 mg/kg/24 h Child over 3 yr: 12-30 mg/kg/24 h	Creatinine excretion decreases with advanced age as muscle mass diminishes
Creatinine clearance	Adult male: 85-125 ml/min/1.73 m^2 Adult female: 75-115 ml/min/1.73 m^2	70-140 ml/min/1.73 m^2	
BUN/creatinine ratio	6-20; mean about 10:1		
Creatinine (serum)	Adult males: up to 1.2 mg/dl Adult females: up to 1.1 mg/dl There are slight differences between the sexes with males higher, since the range relates to the amount of muscle mass present.	1-5 yr: 0.30-0.50 mg/dl 5-10 yr: 0.50-0.80 mg/dl	
Uric acid (serum)	Adult males: 3.4-7.0 mg/dl or slightly more Adult females: 2.4-6.0 mg/dl or slightly more	An increase occurs during childhood.	
Uric acid (urine)	Approximately 250-750 mg/24 h		
Serum glutamic pyruvic transaminase (SGPT)	3-30 IU/L (method dependent)	Slightly increased ranges in infancy compared to adult normal range	
Serum glutamic oxaloacetic transaminase (SGOT)	8-42 IU/L	Infants: 2-3 times adult values Ranges decrease during childhood	
Creatine phosphokinase (CPK)	0-50 IU (method dependent)		
Aldolase	1.5-7.2 m/M/min/L		
Erythrocyte sedimentation rate (ESR): Westergren method	Males <50 yr: 0-15 mm/h Males >50 yr: 0-20 mm/h Females <50 yr: 0-25 mm/h Females >50 yr: 0-30 mm/h		
Zeta sedimentation ratio	<50 yr: <55% 50-80 yr: 40-60%		

*In nonpregnant subjects, percent residual activity >25% favors hepatic origin; <10% favors bone origin.

DIAGNOSTIC STUDIES

Electromyogram (EMG)

Studies electrical activity of skeletal muscle to determine strength and ability to respond to a stimulus (responses are decreased in myopathies)

Nursing care:

Explain to patient that examination is similar to an electrocardiogram except that a needle will be inserted into one or more muscles to be studied; can be done in patient's room; no preexamination or postexamination care needed

Nerve conduction velocity determination

Studies muscle response to nerve stimulation and velocity of conduction of stimulus

Uses same machine as for EMG; can be done in conjunction with EMG; no preexamination or postexamination care needed

Muscle biopsy

Removal of small section or sections of one or more muscles for analysis

Usually done in operating room for asepsis

Arthroscopy

Examination of a joint via arthroscope inserted following injection of a local anesthetic (may use more than one insertion "port")

Done in physician's office or operating room aseptically; may involve removal of "loose bodies" or small pieces of cartilage

Nursing care:

Dressing changes required postoperatively; checking for edema, pain, bleeding is needed; peripheral pulses checked

Arthrogram

Insertion of dye into a joint to outline structures; dye is flushed from joint when examination is completed, remainder will be absorbed

May be done before open surgery of a joint; usual preoperative care is given, in either case

Myelogram

Injection of dye (either water-soluble or oil based) into spinal canal to outline posterior spinal nerves and their coverings; shows obstruction if intervertebral disc is ruptured or rupturing

Nursing care:

Preoperative allergy to iodine determined

Postoperative care differs if water-based or oily dye used:

Water-soluble: observe for anaphylactic or circulatory complications; can have head of bed raised and can be up as desired

Oily dye: flat in bed 8-12 hours; observe for headache

For both: force fluids to restore cerebrospinal fluid; if patient complains of a headache, put on flat bed rest

Synovial biopsy

Removal of small section of synovium or synovial fluid for analysis; local anesthetic injected before examination

Nursing care:

Preoperatively, no special care required; biopsy done with strict asepsis; meperidine may be administered before biopsy to calm patient and relieve pain; after biopsy, analgesics are given and a compression bandage is applied for 24 hours; following its removal, patient is allowed to ambulate normally

X-ray examination

Done to determine injury to one or more bones or tissues in or around a joint, or for inflammatory, degenerative, or neoplastic conditions

Discogram

Injection of a dye into one or more intervertebral discs to determine their condition

Nursing care:

Postexamination analgesics required and laminectomy checks are done

Bone scan

Following injection of a radioisotope, entire skeleton (or a specific part) is "scanned"; injured or diseased tissues will show up as darker or "hot" areas on scan pictures

Computed tomography (CT) scan

Using special cameras, tables, and depths of exposure, pictures are obtained of all body tissues and organs as person moves through scanner lying on table

Nuclear magnetic resonance (available presently in only a few centers)

Sound waves used to "see" organs, tissues, and cells of parts or entire body

Conditions, Diseases, and Disorders

INFLAMMATORY CONDITIONS

Inflammatory conditions can affect one or more muscles, tendons, ligaments, bones, and structures in and around the joints. Because of the interaction of the structures with each other, diagnosis and treatment of specific tissue inflammations may be difficult; overlapping therapy may be needed to ensure relief of the condition. Treatment modalities for many specific musculoskeletal inflammatory conditions are identical, as will be noted in the following pages. Additionally, it will be noted that inflammatory or degenerative effects in one musculoskeletal tissue may have long-term effects on contiguous tissues. Therefore inflammatory conditions must be considered as serious alterations even if only one small area of localized inflammation is noted.

Ankylosing Spondylitis

Ankylosing spondylitis is a localized inflammatory condition that begins with low back (lumbar) pain, which progresses throughout the entire spinal column and eventually results in hardening (ankylosis) and severe deformity of the vertebral column and adjacent tissues.

Ankylosing spondylitis progressively inhibits the mobility of those persons affected. Formerly known as Marie-Strümpell disease, its present name more accurately reflects its changes. This disease affects men at a ratio of 8:1 or 9:1 over women; it occurs between 20 and 40 years of age and rarely occurs over 50 years of age. Also associated with ankylosing spondylitis is a marked hereditary factor, histocompatibility antigen HLA-B27.

PATHOPHYSIOLOGY

The exact pathologic condition in ankylosing spondylitis is unknown; the disease appears to begin in the sacroiliac bones and joints. The intervertebral discs become inflamed and are infiltrated by vascular connective tissue that then undergoes ossification. The peripheral portions of the anulus fibrosus are the major areas initially affected, but as the disease progresses the entire anulus, intervertebral ligaments, and the vertebrae themselves undergo similar inflammatory and ossifying changes. The disease gradually moves up the entire spinal column with the vertebral calcifications being referred to as "bamboo" spines because the x-ray signs look like bamboo canes.

DIAGNOSTIC STUDIES

Physical examination of back and all musculoskeletal tissues

Local or systemic limitations and pain

Reiter's syndrome of conjunctivitis with uveitis, urethritis, and arthritis may be the presenting complaint of patients with ankylosing spondylitis

X-ray examination

Inflammatory or degenerative changes referred to as "bamboo" spine

Serologic examination

Positive test for the histocompatibility antigen HLA-B27, present in over 90% of patients with ankylosing spondylitis but in less than 10% of the general population[6]

Erythrocyte sedimentation rate

Elevated during the disease activity (normal [male, 0 to 9 mm/h, and female, 0 to 20 mm/h] elevations increase to 10 to 15 and 20 to 25 mm/h respectively)

TREATMENT PLAN

Surgical

Total hip replacement to correct postinflammatory fixed flexion of the hip joints

Osteotomy of the midlumbar vertebrae, only if the patient cannot see straight ahead because of kyphosis

Cervical spinal fusion to aid in maintaining upright position in the neck

Chemotherapeutic

Analgesic-antipyretic agents

Salicylate analgesics (aspirin), 600 mg q4h

Nonsteroidal anti-inflammatory agents

Indomethacin (Indocin), 25 mg tid; may be increased to a maximum of 200 mg/d

Table 4-2
Syndromes Associated with Arthritic Diseases

Syndrome	Patterns	Associated Diseases
Reiter's	Triad of conjunctivitis, urethritis, and arthritis; oral, genital, and mucocutaneous lesions (stomatitis, ulcerations, papules)	Ankylosing spondylitis; rheumatoid arthritis
Behçet's	Triad of iritis, oral lesions, and genital lesions; cutaneous lesions; phlebitis; colitis; polyarthritis	Polyarthritis of unknown etiology
Sjögren's	"Sicca" patterns of dryness (sicca) of conjunctiva and salivary glands; arthritis; swelling of parotid gland; Raynaud's phenomenon in some patients	Connective tissue diseases such as systemic lupus erythematosus (SLE), progressive systemic sclerosis (PSS), polymyositis
Stevens-Johnson (variant of erythema multiforme)	Stomatitis with ulcerations of oral mucosa; high fever; genital ulcerations; erythematous skin eruptions; arthritis	Erythema multiforme; erythema nodosum; rheumatic fever; rheumatoid arthritis and juvenile rheumatoid arthritis; ulcerative colitis

Phenylbutazone (Butazolidin), 200-400 mg/d, given last because of multiple side effects, although it is very effective as an anti-inflammatory medication

Supportive
Occupational therapy for identification and learning of modifications in activities of daily living (ADL), employment, and changes in life-style necessary because of rigidity and curvature of spinal column
Consultations with social service and community nursing personnel to plan for long-term care and follow-up
Exercises to maintain mobility, including swimming and walking (rest is not beneficial in ankylosing spondylitis)
Physical therapy for exercises of the entire back, specific joint and muscle exercises, and deep-breathing exercises
A firm mattress and bed with only a small pillow
Occasionally, use of a back brace

ASSESSMENT: AREAS OF CONCERN

Lumbar area of back
Pain (may alternate side to side and is usually worse on getting up or when rising in the morning)
Stiffness
Limitation of motion
Radiation to buttocks

Systemic responses
Polyarthritis (asymmetric and of the large joints of the lower limbs)
Malaise, fatigue, weight loss, vague chest pains
Reiter's syndrome possible (Table 4-2)

Spread
Throughout entire spinal column as disease progresses

Psychosocial concerns
Self-concept and body image concerns from limitation of social interactions and loss of mobility and independence

NURSING DIAGNOSES and NURSING INTERVENTIONS

Nursing Diagnosis	Nursing Intervention
Mobility, impaired physical: actual and potential	Observe movements for signs of relief or progressive impairment. Assist with active ROM exercises as able. Encourage performance of prescribed exercises (swimming and walking). Massage back as needed.

Nursing Diagnosis	Nursing Intervention
Comfort, alteration in: pain	Administer analgesic and anti-inflammatory medications as ordered. Observe patient's movements for increasing ease and frequency. Listen for patient's verbalizations of pain relief or continuation. Observe all involved points for abatement or continuation of inflammation. Encourage proper pillow and mattress use. Observe for side effects of medications (e.g., gastric irritation or burning; changes in complete blood count [CBC] and erythrocyte sedimentation rate [ESR]; diarrhea or constipation).
Self-concept, disturbance in: body image, role performance	Encourage socialization with family and friends. Encourage team recreational activities and games, such as team swimming and walking with others. Encourage compliance with treatment regimen to prevent severe deformity. Encourage continuation of physician consultation for continuity of care and for current or recent developments in treatment of ankylosing spondylitis.

Patient Education

1. Reiterate explanations of inflammatory processes and rationale for medical care to ensure understanding by patient and family.
2. Explain rationale for exercise as opposed to rest of affected tissues: rest is harmful in ankylosing spondylitis.
3. Explain actions and side effects of salicylates and other anti-inflammatory medications. Patient should understand and be alert to the many side effects of ordered medications.
4. Explain skin reactions (reasons for and signs of) if radiotherapy is administered, to lessen patient's concern if skin reaction occurs.
5. Teach (or reiterate explanations for) deep breathing and ROM and joint mobility exercises to encourage the patient's compliance.
6. Include family members in evaluation, practice, and performance of ADL as necessary for home-care continuity.

EVALUATION

Patient Outcome	Data Indicating That Outcome is Reached
Patient retains adequate vertebral mobility and satisfactory curvature.	Patient's inflammation is abated without ankylosis or severe curvature.
Patient maintains independence, social interactions, and self-care activities.	Patient continues own ADL and usual employment activities, interactions, and recreation.
Patient complies with medical regimen.	Patient continues prescribed daily medication, rest, and exercise regimens.

Bursitis

Bursitis is the inflammation of a bursa.

Since the bursa is an enclosed sac situated between muscles or tendons and bony prominences, the inflammation may spread to certain structures or simply be an inflammation of the bursal fluid and sac.

One or more bursae can become inflamed, but the commonest sites are the subdeltoid and subacromial bursae of the shoulder, the olecranon (elbow) bursa, the greater trochanteric bursa lateral to the hip, and the anserine bursa in the medial aspect of the upper tibia.

Children may develop enlargement of the bursa between the semimembranosus and medial head of the gastrocnemius muscle behind the knee. The enlargement is a painless lump but must be differentiated from an acute bursitis.

PATHOPHYSIOLOGY

Bursitis may result from constant friction between the skin and musculoskeletal tissues around the joint. Bursitis from friction would be sterile or aseptic without pathogenic organisms. Rarely, bursitis may result from a foreign body or microorganism invasion. The area around the bursa becomes exquisitely tender (with ''point tenderness,'' the patient can point to the spot or area of greatest tenderness). Motion is either partially or greatly limited by the swollen, enlarged sac, which causes pressure and pain when the tissues are moved. The area may be reddened, hot, and edematous with only point tenderness or with soreness radiating to the tendons at the site; tendinitis may also occur, causing further limitation of motion and prolonging recovery. Calcium may be deposited in the sacs in long-standing or recurring bursitis.

DIAGNOSTIC STUDIES

Physical examination
  Localized inflammation
  Point tenderness
  Limitation of motion of one or more bursae

X-ray examination
  May or may not show calcified deposits

TREATMENT PLAN

Surgical
  Open removal of the calcified deposits
  Aspiration of fluid within the sac (infrequently) for persistent edema and pressure
  Removal of the bursal sac (rarely)

Chemotherapeutic
  Analgesic-antipyretic agents
    Salicylates (aspirin), 600-1000 mg q4h
  Nonsteroidal anti-inflammatory agents
    Indomethacin (Indocin), 25 mg bid, tid or qid
  If the bursa is infected, antibiotics specific for the offending organism following culture
  Injections of steroids into the sac to relieve the inflammation; dosage is individualized

Supportive
  Avoidance of activities (such as kneeling) that cause pressure
  Avoidance of constant friction movements (such as throwing or hitting a ball) that cause the inflammatory reaction
  Moist heat applications every 4 hours to the inflamed area
  ROM exercises to help regain or maintain motion
  Wrapping with elastic bandages, if bursa is accessible, to reduce edema

ASSESSMENT: AREAS OF CONCERN

Inflammatory process
  Heat
  Redness
  Swelling
  Tenderness
  Limitation of motion

Systemic response
  Similar responses in one or more joints/bursae
  Fever and malaise if pathogen is involved

Psychosocial concerns
  Limitation of use of muscles and joint possibly curtailing income or livelihood

NURSING DIAGNOSES and NURSING INTERVENTIONS

Nursing Diagnosis	Nursing Intervention
Mobility, impaired physical limitation of motion	Encourage exercise to maintain ROM as prescribed. Caution against continuing activities that may cause recurrence. Observe for edema, pain, and redness related to limiting or increasing motion. Apply compresses every 4 hours as ordered. Remove bandages, observe site, and rewrap bandages (if used) to prevent disarrangement or tightening.
Comfort, alteration in: pain	Administer medications as ordered. Note continuation or relief of pain, tenderness, or inflammation. Observe for side effects of medications. Handle inflamed tissues gently.

Patient Education

1. Instruct the patient in ROM exercises he can perform correctly to lessen possibility of bursa inflammation.
2. Instruct the patient about side effects of medications.
3. Alert the patient to the possibility that pain may be temporarily increased after injection of steroids (1 to 24 hours), followed by noticeable pain relief and increasing ROM.
4. Caution the patient to avoid activities that could cause exacerbation until inflammation is resolved (4 to 6 weeks).

EVALUATION

Patient Outcome	Data Indicating That Outcome is Reached
Patient experiences relief of pain in joint.	Patient states pain, soreness, and stiffness are no longer present.
Patient regains ROM of affected joint.	Patient can again engage in usual activities with affected joint.
Patient no longer needs medication.	Patient has no pain with ROM or use of joint for usual activities.

Epicondylitis and Tendonitis (Tenosynovitis)

Epicondylitis is an inflammation of the tendons of the medial or lateral epicondyles of the radius or ulna. Tendonitis (tenosynovitis) is an inflammation of the tendons and their sheaths.

Epicondylitis and tendonitis will be considered together because they may occur together and, with some variations, the treatments are similar for both. The local sites of inflammation are contiguous, which adds to the diagnostic challenge.

Epicondylitis, commonly called "tennis elbow," occurs as a result of repetitive twisting and swinging movements of the elbow that accompany, among other activities, swinging a tennis racket or golf club and use of a hammer or other tools. The specific inflammation is of the tendons that originate in the medial or lateral epicondyles of the radius or ulna. The tendons and their sheaths may both become inflamed (tendonitis and tenosynovitis, respectively).

lateral epicondylar pain may be elicited by pronation or supination of the hand when the elbow is in 45 degrees of flexion.

DIAGNOSTIC STUDIES

History
> Elbow flexion and rotation and repetitive ROM actions from occupational or sports activities resulting in localized elbow pain, tenderness, and limitation of motion

Physical examination
> Point tenderness and increased pain with supination and pronation of hand
> Edema and tenderness radiating along the tendon and its sheath

PATHOPHYSIOLOGY

Fibers of the common extensor tendon are damaged and torn by repetitive trauma. Extravasation of tissue fluids sets up inflammatory reactions; healing produces scar tissue and adhesions, which limit the range of motion of the elbow joint and can become inflamed by the repetitive trauma to the scarred, inelastic fibers. The inflammation can spread to the tendon sheath, with fibrosis binding it to the tendon, further limiting joint movements. Classic symptoms of epicondylitis include tenderness (frequently point tenderness), pain, and edema. Severe medial and

TREATMENT PLAN

Surgical
> Removal of calcium deposits from the inflammatory processes occasionally required
> Removal of a degenerated (scarred and bound-down) tendon sheath for chronic, persistent synovitis of a shoulder, elbow, or heel because of calcium deposits from repeated trauma

Chemotherapeutic
> Corticosteroids

Injection of steroids into the inflamed area to produce pain relief; may need to be repeated at intervals for complete pain relief; dosage and type individualized

Analgesic-antipyretic agents

Salicylates (aspirin), 600 mg q4h for mild conditions

Supportive

Moist heat applications to area every 4 hours

Rest to the part or parts

Splint to the forearm and elbow applied occasionally

ASSESSMENT: AREAS OF CONCERN

Inflammatory process

Localized pain

Tenderness

Edema in elbow area

Range of motion

Pain increased with supination and pronation of hand

Psychosocial concerns

Concern for ability to earn a living if in an occupation requiring full elbow ROM (such as carpenter or sports professional)

NURSING DIAGNOSES and NURSING INTERVENTIONS

Nursing Diagnosis	Nursing Intervention
Mobility, impaired physical	Encourage exercises to maintain ROM as prescribed. Caution against continuing activities that may cause recurrence. Observe for edema, pain, and redness related to limiting or increasing motion. Apply compresses every 4 hours as ordered.
Comfort, alteration in: pain	Administer medications as ordered. Note continuation or relief of pain, tenderness, or inflammation. Observe for side effects of medications. Handle inflamed tissues gently.
Self-concept, alteration in: role performance	Encourage expression of concerns; seek guidance to resolve concerns regarding employment or recurrence of condition. Encourage patient's continued compliance with treatment regimen and continued medical care to note recovery.

Patient Education

1. Explain inflammatory processes and effects of repetitive trauma to lessen painful episodes and inflammation.
2. Instruct the patient about side effects of medications.
3. Alert the patient to the possibility that pain may be temporarily increased after injection of steroids (1 to 24 hours), followed by noticeable pain relief and increasing ROM.
4. Caution the patient to avoid activities that could cause exacerbation until inflammation is resolved (4 to 6 weeks).

EVALUATION

Patient Outcome	Data Indicating That Outcome is Reached
Patient's inflammation is resolved.	Patient has normal temperature and no pain or edema in elbow area.
Patient regains joint mobility without limitation.	Patient can put joint through normal ROM without pain or limitation.
Patient returns to employment as before.	No restrictions are necessary during employment activities.

Gouty Arthritis

Gout is a metabolic condition of improper production of uric acid (hyperuricemia), which must be excreted through the kidneys. Some of the uric acid crystals may precipitate in joints, setting up an inflammation, or gouty arthritis.

Gout is actually a metabolic disease, but because of the hyperuricemia, the urate crystals frequently are deposited in joints. Thus gouty arthritis must be included in inflammatory conditions of musculoskeletal tissues. Men constitute nearly 95% of the patients with gout.

PATHOPHYSIOLOGY

Arthritis associated with gout results from the deposition of sodium biurate crystals within the joint cartilage. The crystals are very irritating and initiate an inflammatory response producing painful arthritis. The skin overlying the joint becomes red and hot; the joint is swollen and very tender, forcing the patient to attempt to hold it still. The biurate crystals can also be deposited in bone resulting in cystlike, punched-out, translucent areas under the cartilage noted on x-ray examination.

Severe, excruciating pain results from the inflammatory responses to the crystallization in the joint tissues. Acute attacks usually last 3 to 5 days. Although any joint can be affected, the one most commonly affected is the metatarsophalangeal joint of the great toe. Also commonly affected are the ankle and knee joints.

When biurate crystals are deposited in other tissues, such as the ear cartilage or fingers, these deposits are referred to as tophi, a physical diagnostic feature of gout.

DIAGNOSTIC STUDIES

History
Severe pain localizing in joint of great toe or other joint
History of gout

Physical examination
Inflamed joint or joints
Tophi possible

Serum uric acid
Elevated (normal levels: men, 3.9 to 7.8 mg/dl; women, 2.5 to 6.8 mg/dl)

Microscopic examination of aspirated fluid
Characteristic biurate crystallizations

TREATMENT PLAN

Chemotherapeutic
Antigout agents
  Colchicine (Colsalide), 0.5-1 mg every hour during acute pain episode; continue administration of 1 mg/h until patient experiences nausea, vomiting, or diarrhea (stop administration because therapeutic blood level has been achieved [administer a maximum of 8-10 tablets])[12]
  Probenecid (Benemid), 0.5 g/d, with gradual increases to total dose of 2-3 g/d; decreases incidence of acute attacks and controls serum uric acid levels
Nonsteroidal anti-inflammatory agents
  Indomethacin (Indocin); dosages vary for acute attacks to maximum of 200 mg/d
  Phenylbutazone (Butazolidin), 400-600 mg/d; given in divided doses for several days during acute attacks, with gradually decreasing doses over 6-8 days
  Allopurinol (Zyloprim), 50-100 mg bid; reduces serum uric acid levels by reducing uric acid formation; dosage gradually increased in increments of 100 mg every 2-4 wk until total daily dose is 300-600 mg[12] and serum uric acid is at normal level
Analgesic-antipyretic agents
  Mild analgesics such as aspirin (for pain relief) in 600-1000 mg doses q4h

Supportive
Application of cold via ice bags to decrease inflammatory processes; allow affected joint to rest on ice bag so pain is not increased
Gentle ROM exercises when the acute pain has subsided

ASSESSMENT: AREAS OF CONCERN

Inflammatory processes
Exquisite pain in joint
Tenderness
Swelling
Heat

Systemic processes
Tophi (deposits of monosodium urate): may be found in ear cartilages, small joints of fingers
Serum uric acid levels: may be elevated

Psychosocial concerns
Loss of social interactions from pain and enforced immobility

NURSING DIAGNOSES and NURSING INTERVENTIONS

Nursing Diagnosis	Nursing Intervention
Comfort, alteration in: pain	Do not allow patient to bear weight on involved joints. Apply ice bags to decrease inflammation, if tolerated due to pain. Administer ordered medications to relieve pain. Observe for side effects of medications (particularly colchicine) and for therapeutic blood levels and then discontinue (for acute attacks). Apply splint to affected joint if ordered. Keep bedding and pressure off affected joint or joints.
Mobility, impaired physical	Perform gentle ROM exercises after acute pain has subsided. Encourage ambulation when pain relief has been achieved. Encourage return to normal activities.

Patient Education

1. Explain rationale for hourly administration of medications during acute attacks to achieve desired blood levels.
2. Explain side effects of each medication used during acute attacks and as maintenance medications; have the patient list them for reference.
3. Encourage the patient to maintain physician visits for medication or dosage change to control systemic aspects of gout.

EVALUATION

Patient Outcome	Data Indicating That Outcome is Reached
Patient's gout is controlled with medications.	Patient is able to maintain usual activities with absent or infrequent acute attacks of pain relieved with intensified medication dosages.
Patient experiences no side effects of maintenance medications.	Patient has no nausea, vomiting, leukopenia, or pruritus.

Rheumatoid Arthritis

Rheumatoid arthritis is a chronic systemic disease characterized by inflammation of the connective tissues throughout the body.

This severely disabling chronic disease is one of the major rheumatic diseases. Although it is a systemic disease, the major focus of this discussion will be on the local effects on the tissues in and around joints.

Rheumatoid arthritis is thought to be an autoimmune disease (see Chapter 16 for discussion of autoimmune diseases), but the exact etiology has not been established. Women are affected three times as often as men, and there is a marked familial tendency. The majority of patients develop rheumatoid arthritis between 25 and 55 years of age, although the disease also occurs in children between 8 and 15 years old, when it is referred to as juvenile rheumatoid arthritis or Still's disease.

PATHOPHYSIOLOGY

The disease begins in the synovial membrane within the joint, usually in one of the smaller joints of the wrist, fingers, or hand, but symmetric joint involvement is a characteristic finding. The synovial membrane becomes inflamed from the autoimmune antigen-antibody effects, and the membrane becomes swollen, irritated, and painful. Fibrotic changes and hypertrophy of the synovial membrane occur, referred to as pannus formation. The inflammatory reaction spreads to other joint tissues, including the cartilage, and eventually the bones. Ligaments and tendons also are involved, leading to scarring and shortening and eventually bringing about deformities, subluxations (partial dislocations), and contractures. Cartilage degeneration results in pain and grating with weight bearing and movements. As the cartilage erodes and degeneration continues, the bone ends are exposed and also develop erosions, bone cysts, or fissures; eventually bone spurs and osteophytes develop, further limiting joint mobility and use. The entire joint and its structures remain inflamed, edematous, and painful. Additionally, collections of fibroblasts in collagen tissues near joints enlarge into rheumatoid nodules, a classic feature of rheumatoid arthritis.

Characteristically, rheumatoid arthritis affects smaller joints symmetrically before involving the larger weight-bearing joints. Bouchard's nodes are the classic enlargements of the proximal phalangeal and metacarpophalangeal joints.

Eventually the local disease in the joints involves major organ systems in the remainder of the body including the heart, kidneys, lungs, and skin.

DIAGNOSTIC STUDIES

History
Monoarticular or polyarticular inflammation

Physical examination
Criteria for the diagnosis of rheumatoid arthritis have been established by the American Rheumatism Association (ARA); presence of 10 of the following confirms the diagnosis:
Morning stiffness on arising; pain and tenderness in at least one joint
Swelling in at least one and possibly two joints
Symmetric joint swelling
Fatigue, malaise, and weight loss
Paresthesias of hands or feet
Raynaud's phenomenon of fingers and toes
Development of subcutaneous nodules
Involvement of major organs such as heart and kidney
Pericarditis; valvular lesions; vasculitis
Pneumonitis; fibrosis
Tenosynovitis; ankylosis of joints
Felty's syndrome (splenomegaly and leukopenia)

Serologic examination
Rheumatoid factor (a large immune globulin)
Positive in 95% of patients with rheumatoid arthritis
Erythrocyte sedimentation rate (ESR)
Elevated (moderate to severe elevation [to 15 mm/h in males and 25 mm/h in females]); normal: 0-9 mm/h in males and 0-20 mm/h in females
C-reactive protein
Present during acute phases
Red cell count
Anemia, primarily hypochromic (normocytic is common)
White cell count
Elevated over all cell types

Synovial fluid aspiration and analysis
May reveal immune complexes and elevated white cell counts

Synovial membrane biopsy
Positive for pannus formation and inflammatory changes

X-ray examination
Rarefaction of bones, plus erosions of involved bone, as disease progresses

TREATMENT PLAN

Surgical
Synovectomy of inflamed synovial membranes to relieve pain and maintain muscle and joint balance
Repair of ruptured or fibrotic tendon sheaths to prevent deformity and subluxations
Total joint replacement to increase mobility
Arthrodesis (fusion of a joint): may be done to decrease deformity and joint instability; spinal fusion may be required to treat subluxation
Osteotomy to change weight-bearing surfaces and relieve pain

Table 4-3
Levels of Treatment in Management of Rheumatoid Arthritis*

First	Second	Third	Fourth	Fifth
Education for patient and family	Occupational and physical therapy	Gold	High-dose glucocorticoids	Immunosuppressive drugs, penicillamine
Heat	Orthotic devices	Low-dose glucocorticoids	Hospitalization	
Therapeutic exercises	Nonsteroidal anti-inflammatory drugs	Hydroxychloroquine	Reconstructive surgery	
Rest	Analgesic drugs	Intra-articular glucocorticoids		
Salicylates at therapeutic doses				

*Treatment of rheumatoid arthritis generally includes each of the above modalities during the course of the disease process.

Chemotherapeutic
Analgesic-antipyretic agents
   Aspirin, divided doses up to 5 g/d
Nonsteroidal anti-inflammatory agents
   Ibuprofen (Motrin), single oral dose of 400 mg
   Fenoprofen (Nalfon), single oral dose of 200 mg
   Tolmetin (Tolectin), initially 400 mg tid to reach
      optimal daily dose of 600-1800 mg/d
   Naproxen (Naprosyn), 250-375 mg bid for chronic
      state; 250 mg tid for acute inflammatory attack
Antirheumatic agents
   Gold thiomaleate (Myochrysine), 20-50 mg/wk IM
      to decrease inflammation
   Penicillamine (Cuprimine, Depen), 125-250 mg/d
      increased to 500-750 mg/d; may be used as a
      substitute for patients sensitive to gold
Antineoplastic agents
   Azathioprine (Imuran), 3-5 mg/kg/d initially; then
      1-2 mg/kg/d maintenance dose
Corticosteroids
   Primarily prednisone (Deltasone, others) or pred-
      nisolone (Delta-Cortef, others) in titrated doses
      of 2-10 mg/d, used after other medications for
      anti-inflammatory effects
   Hydrocortisone (Cortef, others), 100 mg, injected
      into the joint to reduce inflammation

Electromechanical
Immersion in paraffin ''glove''
Immersion in whirlpool
Application of splints to inflamed joints to maintain
   proper position

Supportive
Moist warm applications to joints
Applications of cold alternating with heat

ROM exercises to maintain motion
Prescribed rest periods in morning and afternoon
Well-balanced diet; avoidance of obesity because of
   increased joint stress
Providing knowledge about the disease to ease patient's fears and increase compliance with treatment
   regimen

ASSESSMENT: AREAS OF CONCERN

Local inflammatory processes in joint
Edema
Pain
Heat
Redness
Limitation of motion

Systemic processes
Malaise
Fever
Elevated erythrocyte sedimentation rate
Multiple joint involvement
Subcutaneous rheumatoid nodules
Weight loss
Later, inflammatory changes within major organs

Psychosocial concerns
Concerns with self-concept, body image disturbances,
   loss of mobility because of chronicity
Eventual death from major organ involvement

Economic concerns
Major costs for treatments over extended periods of
   time

NURSING DIAGNOSES and NURSING INTERVENTIONS

Nursing Diagnosis	Nursing Intervention
Activity intolerance	Provide rest periods in morning and afternoon. Provide 8 to 10 hours for uninterrupted nighttime sleep. Alternate activities with rest periods to prevent fatigue.
Comfort, alteration in: pain	Administer medications as ordered to relieve pain. Have patient sleep and rest on a firm mattress with a small pillow to prevent deformities. Provide back massage to ease tightness and pressure. Encourage patient to be active during periods when pain relief is experienced. Encourage expression of patient's thoughts and feelings about pain, disease, and loss of independence. Encourage diversionary activities to decrease focus on pain. Encourage patient's active and positive participation in each treatment modality to increase comfort.
Home maintenance management, impaired	Use occupational therapists to teach modifications in home environment to lessen joint stress.

Nursing Diagnosis	Nursing Intervention
	Use community health nurses for home evaluation and continuity of care.
	Have patient practice and use implements and utensils to gain skill and independence.
	Encourage self-care and modify with utensils and learning experiences for skill.
Mobility, impaired physical	Assist with treatment regimen (such as heat, cold, paraffin) to maintain joint mobility.
	Provide ROM exercises as able to prevent stiffening.
	Provide splints and ambulatory aids such as cane or crutch to lessen joint stress.
	Turn and position the patient every 2 to 4 hours to prevent joint deformity.
Sleep pattern disturbance	Prepare patient for rest with massage and bed straightening of linens.
	Position to prevent contractures.
	Administer medications to relieve pain and inflammation as ordered.
	Give warm milk or snack to induce sleep.
	Maintain a quiet environment to promote and maintain sleep periods.
Self-concept, disturbance in: body image, role performance	Encourage active participation in usual roles as able.
	Allow patient to ventilate feelings about deformities and limitation of movements.
	Offer support and encouragement to the patient to help maintain a positive attitude about the disease and its treatment.
	Encourage family members to maintain open communications with the patient to help maintain usual roles.
	Employ team concept (occupational therapy, physical therapy, medicine, and nursing) to discuss plan of care, to provide continuity of care, and to build trust relationships with patient and family.

Patient Education

1. Reiterate explanations of chronicity and controllability of rheumatoid arthritis and its symptoms to aid understanding.
2. Reiterate necessity for patient compliance with treatment regimen for maximal benefits.
3. Teach patient and family members about each medication and common side effects to be aware of and to report to the physician.
4. Encourage patient's active and full participation in each aspect of the disease, its treatments, and alternatives for long-term care.
5. Explain the necessity for cooperative family relationships in the patient's care and treatments to maintain self-worth and role relationships.
6. Teach foods needed for a balanced diet.

EVALUATION

Patient Outcome	Data Indicating That Outcome is Reached
Patient continues with localized disease for long periods.	Patient can maintain ADL with mild restrictions of mobility and strength and minimal deformity of tissues.
Systemic organ involvement responds to medical regimen.	Patient has symptoms of cardiac or renal involvement controlled with minimal arrhythmias, no signs of congestive failure, mild edema, and no proteinuria or fever.
Surgical corrective procedures restore joint mobility and relieve pain and deformity.	Patient regains joint strength and structure and has tolerable pain and relief of deviation or deformity.
Patient retains or returns to social interactions over long periods of time.	Patient maintains roles in family and society.
Patient adheres to medication regimen over time without undue side effects.	Patient has minimal nausea, vomiting, bleeding disorders, gastrointestinal burning or pain, and anemia.
Patient engages in prescribed programs of physical therapy.	Patient participates actively in rest and activity periods, exercises, and joint mobility programs as prescribed.

Paget's Disease

Paget's disease is a chronic inflammatory disease of bones that results in thickening, softening, and eventual bowing of the bones.

Paget's disease (osteitis deformans) is a fairly common disease affecting 3% of persons over 40 years of age. It is inflammatory because of the increased warmth over the rapidly changing bone, although it is also a metabolic condition because of the high rates of bone formation and resorption.

PATHOPHYSIOLOGY

The cause of Paget's disease is unknown. It is very rare in Norway and Japan for unknown reasons. This disease is characterized by high rates of bone resorption and bone formation occurring in several stages. In the so-called vascular stage[6] spaces left by bone absorption fill with vascular fibrous tissue. New osteoid bone tissue forms on both sides of the cortex, but it is not completely converted to mature bone. Thus even though it is thick, the bone is soft and bendable. Additionally, the newly formed lamellae are not regularly layered as in correctly formed bones. During the later, so-called sclerotic, stage even though the lamellae calcify and become thick and sclerosed, the bone is easily broken. The disease may begin in one bone only and remain localized for years. The most common sites for Paget's disease are the pelvis and tibia followed by the femur, skull, spine, and clavicle.[6] When only a single bone is involved, it becomes painful and deformed from bending. The pain is a dull ache that is worse at night. As the disease becomes more generalized, other signs, in addition to the pain, become more evident, including deafness, deformities, stiffness, limb pain, fractures, headaches, and possibly even heart failure.[6] Deafness results from otosclerosis; enlargement of the skull bones increases the head size, and pressure on the optic nerve may produce blindness. Kyphosis may be pronounced with the patient becoming shorter and appearing apelike with bent legs and arms hanging in front of the trunk.[6] The legs become bowed, and the patient experiences backache with nerve root pressure pain. Fractures become more common as the disease becomes systemic.

DIAGNOSTIC STUDIES

History and physical examination
Tenderness and increased warmth over involved sites
Pain worse at night
Involvement of special senses
Signs of heart failure
Bones easily bendable
Possibility of fracture

X-ray films
Thickened, bent bone, its density possibly decreased in the vascular stage and increased in the sclerotic stage
Coarse and widened trabeculae of bone, with a honeycomb appearance
Fine periosteal cracks as a result of stress

Serum alkaline phosphatase and hydroxyproline
High; urinary excretion of hydroxyproline increased

TREATMENT PLAN

Surgical
Fracture reduction by closed or open manipulation
External casts or splints to maintain reduction and to help straighten bone

Chemotherapeutic
Thyroid hormones
Calcitonin (Calcimar), 50-100 IU, injected qd for 3-6 mo; then given 3 times weekly for 6 more mo
Diphosphonates, po; dosages not fully established to date
Glucagon and mithramycin may also be used during high disease activity; dosage according to need

ASSESSMENT: AREAS OF CONCERN

Inflammatory processes
Increased warmth over affected bone site or sites
Dull pain
Stiffness and limitation of motion (although bone may be easily manipulated and bent)

Systemic processes
Headache
Back and limb pain
Heart failure signs
Hearing loss or deficit and visual changes possible

Psychosocial concerns
Body image
Progressive nature of disease (possibility of development of sarcoma and easy fracturing of bones)

NURSING DIAGNOSES and NURSING INTERVENTIONS

Nursing Diagnosis	Nursing Intervention
Comfort, alteration in: pain	Note complaints of bone pain, headache, joint pain and stiffness, dyspnea and edema from congestive heart failure. Encourage active exercise and range of motion to unaffected musculoskeletal tissues. Administer medications as ordered: calcitonin lowers osteoclastic (bone reabsorption) activity and serum alkaline phosphatase, thereby strengthening bones and lessening pain and deformity. Note patient's responses to medication: pain relief, increased bone and joint strength, less edema and dyspnea.
Injury, potential for	Record and report patient's complaints of sudden increase in pain, hearing or sensing bone crack, experiencing inability to bear weight or use bone normally. If fracture occurs and is treated with manipulation, do necessary nursing care (see p. 514 for care of persons in a cast or having open reduction with internal fixation) to facilitate patient's recovery.
Mobility, impaired physical	Secure physical therapy for proper joint and muscle use and exercises.
Self-concept, disturbance in: body image, role performance	Encourage patient to ventilate feelings about bone "brittleness," deformity and loss of bone, joint strength, and mobility as desired. Secure consultation with occupational therapist to maintain customary roles with necessary modifications. Secure consultation with hearing and vision specialists to maintain or regain adequate functions of these senses when possible. Instruct family members of possible role changes necessitated by the progressive nature of this disease.

Patient Education

1. Reiterate explanations of bone formation and reabsorption for patient understanding.
2. Explain purposes of drug therapy and side effects of medication.
3. Caution the patient to use care when moving to lessen probability of fracture.
4. Encourage patient and family activities to maintain independence and social roles.

EVALUATION

Patient Outcome	Data Indicating That Outcome is Reached
Patient's disease is controlled over long periods without systemic effects.	Patient experiences no progression of pain, deformity, fracture, or loss of bone strength and no joint or other organ involvement.
Patient's pain is relieved with medications without side effects.	Patient is able to have long pain-free periods, and if pain occurs, it is controlled with medications. Patient experiences no nausea, vomiting, or constipation.

BACTERIAL INFECTIONS
Osteomyelitis

Osteomyelitis is an infection of bones.

Osteomyelitis is of great concern in any patient with an open wound, sore throat, or pneumonia because it may "smolder" undiagnosed for extensive periods. Its long-term effects on bones and their contiguous tissues necessitate constant vigilance to prevent recurrence, bone damage, and eventually, even amputation. Although the incidence of osteomyelitis may not be high, even one occurrence is to be prevented or avoided whenever possible because of the destructive nature of this infection.

Osteomyelitis occurs as a direct invasion into bone tissues from an open wound or bone fracture or secondary to an infection in distant organs in the body, such as following streptococcal sore throat or bacterial pneumonia. The major pathogens are staphylococci and streptococci, but *Escherichia coli* and tubercle bacilli may also be involved. Children develop osteomyelitis from throat infections, and hematogenous spread is a major factor in childhood osteomyelitis. Adults experience more infection from direct invasion following trauma. No sex or age group is immune.

PATHOPHYSIOLOGY

The invading organisms travel to the site within the metaphysis (part of the bone between the shaft and epiphyseal area), either by direct invasion or indirectly by hematogenous spread. The metaphysis provides a secluded, warm, well-nourished area for the organisms to grow and multiply. The pathogens produce pus, which initially remains localized and confined. As greater quantities of purulent matter are produced, the enlarging mass eventually spreads out of the confined area, through the cortex of the bone, into contiguous tissues, and eventually, if undetected or untreated, to the surface of the skin through a sinus tract. The purulent matter also continues to spread around and along the bone shaft and into more soft tissues. Bone cells are destroyed, and the dead bone, called sequestrum, becomes dense and walled off. New bone begins to form from the deeper layers of periosteal cells; this new bone is referred to as involucrum. As the infection progresses, the affected bone becomes weakened and may fracture, giving the first evidence of the existence of the infection. If the soft tissues around the infected bone become tense from accumulated purulent matter, the patient may experience soreness, tenderness, increased warmth at the site, and occasionally edema. Occasionally the patient may experience severe pain that is not relieved by rest and may stop using the extremity (most commonly the lower extremity around the knee). With the soft tissue spread the patient may experience high, spiking temperatures and appear toxic and ill.

DIAGNOSTIC STUDIES

History
Antecedent infection or open trauma in previous 3 to 4 weeks

Physical examination
Area of tenderness, edema, warmth, redness, and possibly mass or drainage in ends of long bones
Increased pain with movement
Spiking fevers in 103° to 104° range intermittently noted

Culture of mass or drainage
Infecting pathogenic organisms

White cell count
Elevated with increased levels of polymorphonuclear neutrophils (PMNs) indicative of bacterial infection

Erythrocyte sedimentation rate
Increased

X-ray films
Initially may not reveal the destructive processes but will later show rarefaction of the involved bone with evidence of formation of sequestrum and involucrum

Serum cultures
Pathogenic organism

TREATMENT PLAN

Surgical
Aspiration of abscess for culture purposes only
Following "sterilization" of abscess, sequestrum is removed and replaced by bone grafts
Saucerization is performed: involved bone is scraped to remove all necrotic cells, following which bone regenerates; if the defect is pronounced, bone grafts may be applied or metallic fixation may be applied (never used in infected areas or if uncertainty exists about the possibility of lingering pathogens remaining)
External fixation devices such as Hoffman apparatus (pp. 517-519) may be used to hold bones weakened from the initial infection or saucerization
Amputation of limb (done less frequently now because of improved treatment modalities)

Chemotherapeutic
Anti-infective agents: according to culture and sensitivity results and patient sensitivity or allergy
  Adults
    Aqueous penicillin, 500,000 to 1 million U, IV q6h continuously for 30 d or longer, up to 6 wk
    Erythromycin (Erythrocin), 1-2 g, IV q6h (for penicillin-sensitive patients)
    Ampicillin (Omnipen), 1 g IV q6h
    Cephalosporin (cephalothin or Keflin), 1 g q6h IV for penicillin-resistant organisms
  Children: Erythromycin (Erythrocin), 30 mg/kg IV q6h

Supportive
Splints to decrease joint pain
Bed rest to conserve energy

Sling for the arm

Cast to prevent a fracture of weakened bones; should have "windows" for dressing changes, if needed

ASSESSMENT: AREAS OF CONCERN

Inflammatory processes
Increased warmth at site
Edema
Tenderness
Mild to severe pain
Affected part may not be used

Systemic processes
Fever
Malaise
Weakness

Spread
Local tissues
Distant sites, where infection continues

Psychosocial concerns
Body image
Disability from long-term disease processes

NURSING DIAGNOSES and NURSING INTERVENTIONS

Nursing Diagnosis	Nursing Intervention
Comfort, alteration in: pain	Maintain bed rest or limited activity to lessen stress on involved tissues. Administer analgesics, if ordered, for relief of pain. Aspirin, 300 to 600 mg, is usually the medication ordered. Handle affected limb gently to lessen pressure and pain. Use sling when appropriate. Administer intravenous antibiotics in collaboration with physician to clear infection and thereby lessen pain. Monitor patient's response. Encourage diversionary activities to divert attention from condition; take child to playroom, outside, etc. Use care and caution when initiating intravenous therapy per physician order and during therapy to preserve venous integrity for long-term need. Use caution to maintain asepsis of all equipment.
Mobility, impaired physical	Encourage ROM to unaffected joints to decrease tiredness and prevent weakening. Encourage self-care to maintain muscle strength. Encourage hobby and diversionary activities to maintain motion and strength in all uninvolved joints. Use wheelchair or crutches to aid patient's ambulation and increase socialization.
Tissue perfusion, alteration in	Perform postoperative neurovascular checks to determine tissue perfusion.
Skin integrity, impairment of: actual	Remove splint for care and to check skin condition. Change dressings as needed to remove drainage and to lessen odor and skin maceration. If surgical procedures are performed, perform thorough skin preparation and "scrub" to lessen postoperative wound infections.
Self-concept, disturbance in: body image	Explain rationale for long-term therapy to clear disease. Assess equipment (splint, Hoffman apparatus, etc.) for proper functioning and patient responses. If amputation is required, do preoperative preparation allowing patient to verbalize concerns over loss of body part. Following amputation do necessary care to promote wound healing and prevent complications. Encourage patient and family interactions to maintain relationships and usual roles.

Patient Education

1. Reiterate need for prompt medical attention to local or systemic infections to prevent recurrence.
2. Explain rationale, purposes, and expected outcomes for long-term antibiotic therapy to increase understanding and compliance.
3. Explain side effects of long-term antibiotic therapy.
4. Explain purposes for continuing ROM exercises to maintain strength and mobility.

EVALUATION

Patient Outcome	Data Indicating That Outcome is Reached
Patient's infection is cleared without local or systemic extension or recurrence.	Patient's temperature is normal; patient has no pain, tenderness, or edema at site and no limitation of mobility; bone heals without loss of length, sequestrum, or involucrum.
Patient regains social interactions and returns to employment activities.	Patient returns to family and social roles and employment as before illness.

CONNECTIVE TISSUE DISORDERS

Formerly known as collagen diseases, connective tissue diseases affect the musculoskeletal tissues either directly or indirectly from the effects on tissues common to both groups such as muscles, arteries, skin, and joints, all of which contain collagen tissues.

Collagen is the most prevalent protein in the body, constituting approximately one half the total protein in adults. Collagen is the principal supporting element in the connective tissues. Also, collagen functions in active roles in developmental processes, cell attachment, chemotaxis, and the binding of antigen-antibody complexes.

Collagen is made of three polypeptide strands aligned colinearly (in the same straight line) throughout the molecule. Sites for cross linking occur in one of the three strands. The strands form coils around a central region with the coils stabilized by interchain hydrogen bands.

Another characteristic of collagen tissues is that interstitial collagens as well as their biosynthetic precursors (procollagens) are "now recognized as distinct antigens capable of eliciting significant humoral and cellular immune responses."[8] Some of the major arthritides are also thought to be of autoimmune origins, thus another correlation of connective and musculoskeletal tissues. Indeed, rheumatoid arthritis and ankylosing spondylitis are diseases of specific connective tissues.

Specific types of collagen make up the connective tissues of bones, tendons, cartilage, and other connective tissues including skin, muscles, uterine wall, and blood vessel walls, among others.

For our purposes, discussion will be limited to progressive systemic sclerosis as a prototypical connective tissue disease.

NOTE: With all connective tissue diseases compliance with medication regimens over extended periods is a basic necessity and requirement for control of these disabling chronic diseases. It is understood that a major goal would be to achieve maximal patient compliance not only with the intake of all the requisite medications, but also with every part of the therapeutic regimen. Patient compliance is a nursing and medical concern with the connective tissue diseases because treatments are symptomatic, noncurative, and multiple in modalities.

Progressive Systemic Sclerosis

Progressive systemic sclerosis is a chronic inflammatory disease of the collagen (connective) tissues.

The name *progressive systemic sclerosis* has replaced the term *scleroderma* because it accurately reflects the inexorable effects of this disease on multiple organs and other connective tissues throughout the body. Although progressive systemic sclerosis is a very rare disease, it merits discussion because of its multiple connective tissue involvements.

PATHOPHYSIOLOGY

In the early stages of progressive systemic sclerosis the skin may be edematous and of a "doughy" consistency.

As the inflammation proceeds through its stages to fibrous tissue formation, large amounts of collagen are deposited and the skin becomes thickened, leathery, and bound to the subcutaneous connective tissues. In the later stages, atrophic changes are noted in the dermis and fat tissues, with thin, translucent skin stretched tightly over the subcutaneous structures. The face is pinched, nonexpressive, and stiff. The sclerosis (hardening) and fibrosis also occur in the gastrointestinal tract, heart, lungs, and kidneys. Arterial walls develop thickened intima and thickened basement membranes leading to ischemic changes characterized as Raynaud's phenomenon, a classic accompaniment of progressive systemic sclerosis. The disease proceeds slowly with complications arising in specific tissues, such as bowel obstruction, congestive heart failure, nephrosclerosis, esophageal thickening leading to dysphagia, and lung fibrosis causing respiratory problems.

DIAGNOSTIC STUDIES

Physical examination
CREST syndrome
C = calcinosis, hardening
R = Raynaud's phenomenon
E = esophageal dysfunction; dysphagia
S = sclerodactyly (hardening, thinning of fingers and skin)
T = telangiectasis (dilation of superficial capillaries, commonly called spider nevi)

Biopsy and angiography
Capillaries
Large dilated capillary loops with loss of capillaries from adjacent areas leading to marked avascularity (seen in over 80% of patients with progressive systemic sclerosis)
Skin, subcutaneous tissues, fascia, and muscle
Collagen hypertrophy with cellular infiltrates and inflammatory changes

TREATMENT PLAN

Surgical
Joint arthroplasty for ankylosis
Bowel resection for bowel obstruction; occasionally, colostomy may be required

Chemotherapeutic
Corticosteroids
Prednisone (Deltasone, others), 40-60 mg/d in divided doses for 8-12 wk
Nutritional supplements
Potassium para-aminobenzoate (Potaba), 12 g/d in divided doses, for cutaneous changes; dose reduced as response is noted
Cholinergic agents
Bethanechol (Urecholine), 5-10 mg 30 min ac for dysphagia
Analgesic-antipyretic agents
Aspirin, 600-1000 mg qd for joint symptoms
Refer to chapters 1 and 9 for chemotherapeutic treatment of associated hypertension and renal dysfunction.

Supportive
Individualized exercise programs to maintain ROM of joints affected are vital to prevent contractures
Planned rest programs in morning and afternoon to prevent overtiring
Wearing warm clothing and gloves and, in extreme cases, moving to a warmer climate for patients with pronounced Raynaud's phenomenon
Avoidance of exposure to cold
Forcing fluids lessens bowel and renal concerns
Diet nutritious, well balanced, and high in bulk-forming foods

ASSESSMENT: AREAS OF CONCERN

Inflammatory processes (localized to skin and joints)
Edema
Tenderness
Weakness and limitation of movements
Raynaud's phenomenon in fingers and hands
Tough and hardened feeling to skin
Skin rash (may be localized to hands and feet)
Taut and shiny appearance to skin as disease progresses with loss of skin folds

Systemic responses to inflammation (vary with particular patient)
Esophageal: dysphagia
Respiratory
Dyspnea
Repeated respiratory infections
Intestinal
Bowel distention
Constipation
Obstruction
Renal
Hematuria
Decreased urinary output (late pattern)
Hypertension
Musculoskeletal: multiple joint involvements with deformity and ankylosis

Psychosocial concerns
Body image changes and disturbances

NURSING DIAGNOSES and NURSING INTERVENTIONS

Nursing Diagnosis	Nursing Intervention
Mobility, impaired physical	Perform ROM exercises to joints. Assist patient to ambulate four times daily. Provide rest periods.
Mobility, impaired physical (etiology related to other involved organs/tissues)	Assess swallowing to note dysphagia. Check for bowel movement; note characteristics of stool. Check for peripheral edema; hypertension or cardiac involvement. Assist with ADL as requested while maintaining patient's independence as desired. Provide nutritious diet, high in bulk.
Urinary elimination, alteration in patterns	Check urine and urinary output with renal involvement. Force fluids if feasible and required.
Tissue perfusion, alteration in	Observe fingers, hands, and toes, particularly for evidence of Raynaud's phenomenon: blanching, cyanosis, then redness (pattern is white to blue to red). Assess for tingling and paresthesia in fingers and toes. Observe for unusual reactions to cold. Note thinning, tightness, and shininess of skin (patient has a ''pinched,'' expressionless facies); fingers appear more pointed and tips are thin and fragile looking; tips may develop ulcers.
Self-concept, disturbance in: body image	Encourage social interactions to maintain self-esteem.

Patient Education

1. Reiterate progressive nature of progressive systemic sclerosis.
2. Encourage patient to maintain ADL and social roles to prevent or lessen complications.
3. Explain patterns indicative of specific organ involvement: signs of congestive heart failure, hypertension, dysphagia, bowel obstruction and urinary/renal hematuria, and oliguria, if pertinent.
4. Explain side effects of medications.
5. Encourage patient and family interactions for clarifications as needed.

EVALUATION

Patient Outcome	Data Indicating That Outcome is Reached
Patient maintains mobility for extended periods.	Patient is able to do self-care and ADL and to move about adequately without undue limitations.
Patient experiences no skin breakdown or circulatory deficits.	Patient has no ulcers, numbness, tingling, or Raynaud's phenomenon; skin thickening or hardening is minimal.

DEGENERATIVE CONDITIONS

As people age they experience some musculoskeletal conditions resulting from degeneration. Even though such conditions may begin in a specific tissue such as the cartilage or bone, they affect not only that specific tissue but also other musculoskeletal tissues because of their contiguous and interrelated anatomic and physiologic arrangements. Therefore these conditions have local and systemic effects as do the conditions previously discussed.

Hallux Valgus

Hallux valgus is deviation of the great toe toward the other toes.

Hallux (great toe) valgus is either a congenital or acquired deformity. The great toe deviates toward the other toes either from congenital abnormality or from degeneration caused by increasing weight and weight-bearing activities. The forefoot becomes splayed, allowing the first metatarsal bone to deviate into a more varus position (Fig. 4-12).

Fig. 4-12
Hallux valgus (bunion). **A,** External
view. **B,** Anatomic view.

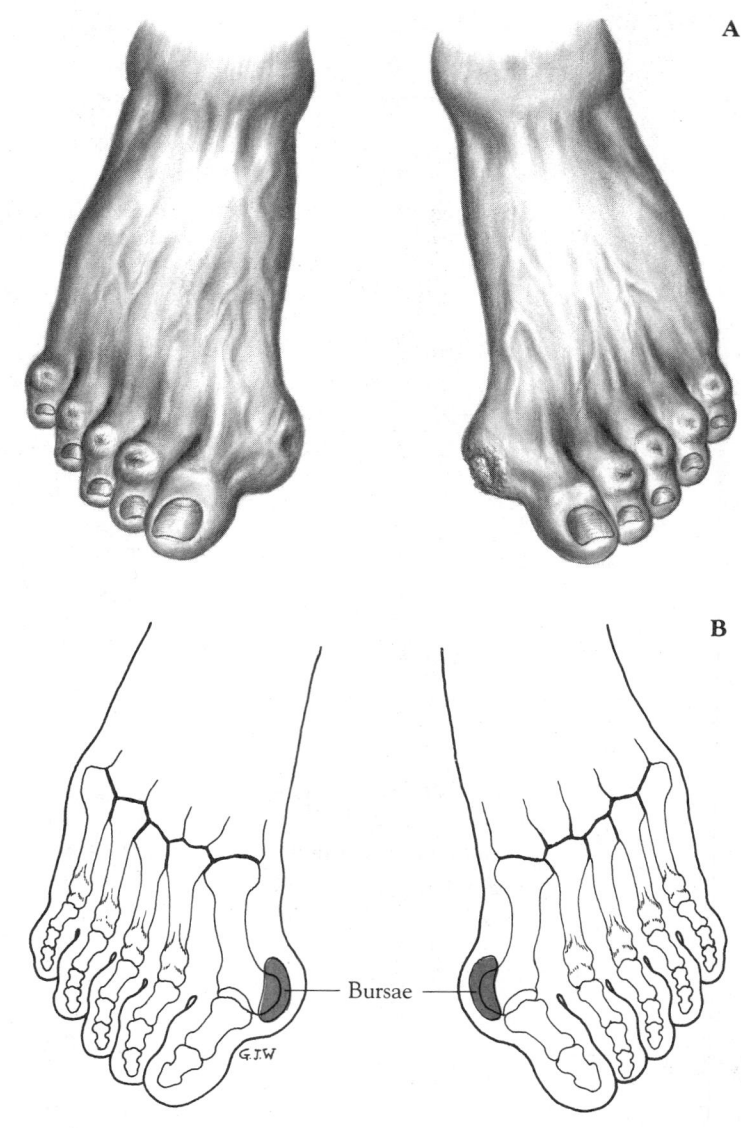

Bursae

PATHOPHYSIOLOGY

Hallux valgus is most obvious from the increasing prominence and deformity of the first metatarsal bone, with this bone's shaft deviated medially away from the second metatarsal. The head of the first metatarsal bone develops a protective bursa (bunion) wherever it rubs against a shoe. As the valgus deformity of the proximal phalanx of the great toe increases, the second toe is crowded and may also become deformed.

Usually hallux valgus is bilateral with one side more prominent and symptomatic than the other. It is most commonly noted in women during the sixth decade with a strong familial tendency. Adolescents also may have hallux valgus.

DIAGNOSTIC STUDIES

Physical examination
  Valgus deformity of great toe, with or without bursa development (bunion), hammer toe, corns, calluses, and bilaterality

X-ray films
  Deformities described above

History
  Familial occurrence

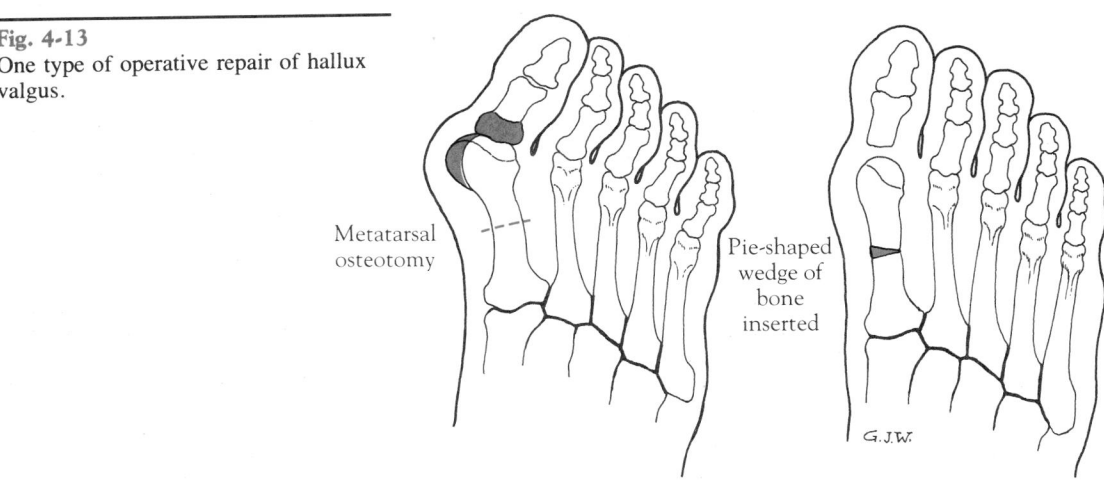

Fig. 4-13
One type of operative repair of hallux valgus.

Metatarsal osteotomy

Pie-shaped wedge of bone inserted

G.J.W.

TREATMENT PLAN

Surgical
Osteotomy to realign bones
Arthroplasty: Keller operation; Mayo procedure (Fig. 4-13)
Arthrodesis
Bunionectomy

Chemotherapeutic
Analgesic-antipyretics
Aspirin, 600-1000 mg qid
Acetaminophen, 600-1000 mg qid

Supportive
Placing and taping pad under metatarsal heads to change weight-bearing pressure
Changing shoe style to wider, open-toed shoe with soft upper portions
Foot exercises to lessen splayfoot
Application of ice bag to site

ASSESSMENT: AREAS OF CONCERN

Signs of degeneration
Valgus (away from midline) deformity of great toe and first metatarsal bone
Presence of bunion
Corn development from pressure
Deformity or crowding of second toe
Hammer toe possible
Callus possible under metatarsal head

Other accompanying signs
Presence of inflamed bursa producing tenderness and often exquisite pain in and around joint
Condition usually bilateral

Psychosocial concerns
Concern with body image from deformity and pain

NURSING DIAGNOSES and NURSING INTERVENTIONS

Nursing Diagnosis	Nursing Intervention
Self-concept, alteration in: body image	Encourage wearing of well-fitting footwear. Encourage consulting with physician for possible surgical removal. Encourage exercises to lessen progressive deformity.
Comfort, alteration in: pain	Administer ordered medication. Apply ice bag to inflamed bursa. Encourage temporary cessation of weight bearing when pain is acute.
Mobility, impaired physical	Encourage use of padding in shoes to change weight-bearing sites. Encourage usual activities when pain is relieved. Encourage consulting with physician to remove bursa if necessary.

Patient Education

1. Clarify bunion as accompanying hallux valgus, not being only condition.
2. Instruct about preventive measures with proper footwear and exercises.
3. Explain surgical options previously discussed with physician if necessary for clarity.

EVALUATION

Patient Outcome	Data Indicating That Outcome is Reached
Patient walks without pain or deformity of toe joint.	Patient uses orthotic devices as ordered, wears well-fitted shoes, applies ice during acute inflammation, and rests the joint. Patient undergoes surgical correction if necessary to relieve deformity and regain joint mobility.

Osteoarthrosis (Osteoarthritis)

The term *osteoarthritis* has been replaced by the term *osteoarthrosis* because the condition is degenerative rather than inflammatory.

Osteoarthrosis is a degenerative condition of the articular cartilage primarily within the major weight-bearing joints, although other joints are also affected.

Osteoarthrosis is a disease of older adults, becoming manifest after middle age. It is the major cause of loss of joint mobility and increasing pain episodes in those persons affected. Although biochemical changes occur in the joints with age, aging alone does not account for the degeneration of the cartilage. The essential feature is a discrepancy between the strength of the cartilage and the force to which it is subjected. If the load to which the cartilage is subjected is too great, the cartilage gives way. It will also give way with normal loads if it has been weakened by damage or disease or if it is unsupported by normal bone.[6] Osteoarthrosis is slightly more common in women than men.

PATHOPHYSIOLOGY

Early changes in the normal, whitish smooth hyaline cartilage are an increase in its water content and a decrease in the amount of proteoglycan (complex protein-carbohydrate molecules). The cartilage looks irregular, pitted, and softer. It undergoes fibrillation, and cartilage flakes (detritus) are shed into the joint. This shedding process rubs away the cartilage primarily from sites where the maximal load is greatest. Repeated wear and erosion cause the cartilage to become thin.

Even in nonstress areas the cartilage, although not rubbed away or thinned, is unhealthy from undernourishment. Cartilage is nourished by imbibition of synovial fluid and of transudates from subchondral vessels, a process facilitated by compression; this pumping action is lacking in nonstress areas; hence, there is undernourishment. The subchondral vessels hypertrophy and invade the cartilage, which calcifies and later ossifies, forming osteophytes. The hyperemia spreads into the bone beneath the stress area, but in this area pressure prevents the vessels from penetrating into the cartilage. The cartilage continues to be rubbed away, exposing the underlying bone, which becomes dense and hard. Stress (fatigue) fractures occur in the subchondral trabeculae, and cysts develop where pressure is greatest.[6]

In the process of cartilage erosion, detritus is deposited on the synovial lining, which then hypertrophies; flakes of cartilage also penetrate into the subsynovial layer, where they induce fibrosis, extending into the capsule. The capsule becomes thickened and inelastic. As the fibrous tissue matures, it shrinks, thereby limiting joint movement.

This restriction of movement resulting from fibrosis is a cardinal feature of osteoarthrosis. Symptoms appear early in joints such as the hip where full extension is required for walking. Since the hip joint capsule is well supplied with pain fibers, slight restriction is noted by pain with attempts at full extension. Thus major weight-bearing joints show earlier symptoms. Weight bearing continues as an aggravation in osteoarthrosis.

Joints other than the hip and knee are also involved in osteoarthrosis, including the carpometacarpal joint at the base of the thumb, the vertebrae, and the distal joints of the fingers.

Limitation of movements and pain are the major symptoms. Pain frequently occurs after a night's rest. Usually there are no systemic signs, just the local signs confined to the joints and their contiguous tissues.

DIAGNOSTIC STUDIES

Physical examination

Enlarged edematous joint with some stiffness and deformity

Usually only one joint has most pronounced signs, although more than one can be involved

If hip is involved, patient may hold it flexed, adducted, and externally rotated

Joint may be tender but rarely feels hot

Movements of joint limited

Crepitus common

Heberden's nodes may be present in distal interphalangeal joints of fingers

X-ray films

Decreased or diminished joint space

Sclerotic bone

Bone cysts

Osteophytes and lipping in some joints

TREATMENT PLAN

Surgical

Arthroplasty to repair the joint

Total joint replacement to replace diseased tissues

Osteotomy to change weight-bearing surfaces

Arthrodesis to limit joint movements (done to abolish pain)

Chemotherapeutic

Analgesic-antipyretic agents

Aspirin, 600-1000 mg 3-4 times daily

Nonsteroidal anti-inflammatory agents

Ibuprofen (Motrin), 300-400 mg 3-4 times daily

Naproxen (Naprosyn) 250-375 mg bid

Tolmetin (Tolectin), 200-400 mg 3-4 times daily

Indomethacin (Indocin), 25-50 mg 3-4 times daily

Sulindac (Clinoril), 150-200 mg bid

Phenylbutazone (Butazolidin), 300-400 mg/d, for short-term use only

Electromechanical

Moist heat applications with diathermy, hot water bottles, and radiant heat

Rest and modified weight-bearing activities beneficial

Canes, crutches, or walkers to aid walking and decrease joint stress

Soft collar and cervical traction to lessen pain

ASSESSMENT: AREAS OF CONCERN

Local (joint) signs of degeneration

Limitation of full extension, pain on arising and on weight bearing in joint

Pain disturbing sleep as disease progresses

Joint stiffness and deformity from fibrosis, shrinkage, and muscle imbalance

Limp

Joint feels unstable and may give way

Edema in superficial joints

Systemic signs

None

Psychosocial concerns

Body image changes

Pain

Limitation of movement

NURSING DIAGNOSES and NURSING INTERVENTIONS

Nursing Diagnosis	Nursing Intervention
Mobility, impaired physical	Encourage and assist with ambulation as needed. Assist with ADL is needed. Use ambulatory aid as ordered to facilitate walking. Assist patient to ambulate after pain is relieved with heat or medication.
Comfort, alteration in: pain	Administer ordered analgesic or anti-inflammatory medications. Assess effects of medications for pain relief. Use heat and diathermy as ordered to relieve pain. Stress proper posture when walking, standing, or sitting. Encourage weight loss to decrease joint stress if needed. Apply traction or collar if necessary and ordered.
Self-concept, alteration in: body image, role performance	Encourage patient to perform usual activities and ADL for self-esteem. Encourage compliance with plan of medical care to lessen joint deformity and decrease pain. Encourage planned rest to maintain strength. If surgery is contemplated, review and clarify options previously discussed by physician with patient.

Patient Education

1. Clarify understandings of degenerative nature of this disease and effects on mobility.
2. Explain side effects of medications.
3. Caution of effects of heat on less sensitive tissues.

EVALUATION

Patient Outcome	Data Indicating That Outcome is Reached
Patient walks with minimal limitation of motion or pain.	Patient maintains self-care, ADL, and employment for as long as desired without experiencing uncontrollable pain or joint movement limitations or deformity.
Patient will comply with medication regimen without distressing side effects.	Patient takes medications as ordered without nausea, vomiting, gastrointestinal burning, bleeding, or pain, and no hematologic changes. Pain is relieved with medications, and joint mobility is enhanced.
Patient returns to social interactions.	Patient returns to usual family, social, and employment roles.

DEFICIENCY DISEASES
Osteomalacia and Rickets

Osteomalacia is a disease of adults characterized by increasing softening, brittleness, flexibility, and deformity of bones.

Rickets is a disease of children characterized by inadequate calcification of developing bones, resulting in deformity in the shape and structure of bones.

Osteomalacia is the adult equivalent of rickets in children; both result from a deficiency of vitamin D, which leads to reduced absorption of calcium and phosphorus. The vitamin D deficiency may be from inadequate dietary intake, insufficient sunshine, malabsorption in the intestines, or defective metabolism of vitamin D. Although rare, this disease can cause severe illness in children; adults are less seriously affected.

PATHOPHYSIOLOGY

Without vitamin D, the amount of calcium and phosphorus available for bone calcification is inadequate to maintain strong bones. Defective growth and replacement of rigid bones are noted first in immature skeletal bones at sites of growth and in mature bones at points of stress, where turnover is most rapid: the physiologic balance of bone growth and reabsorption is hereby disrupted. Defective replacement at the sites mentioned is noticed first because of the increased demand for new bone formation. Failure of mineralization and its resultant inability of the bone to resist stress because of lack of rigidity are then evident through the patient's symptoms and x-ray evidence.

DIAGNOSTIC STUDIES

History

Decreased intake or absorption of vitamin D, from unfortified milk, following gastrectomy, or other cause

Physical examination

Fretful baby with obvious deformities in skull, ribs, or long bones with abnormal curvatures

Adult: bone pain, muscle weakness, and general malaise

Serum calcium levels

Lower than normal (4.5 to 5.5 mEq/L)

Serum alkaline phosphatase

Elevated above 13 King-Armstrong units

Sedimentation rate

May be slightly elevated

X-ray films

General decalcification

Pseudofractures (Looser's zones): incomplete fractures in various stages of healing

Children with rickets: epiphyses that appear late, growth discs that are too deep, and metaphyses that are too wide[6]

Biopsy of iliac crest
Excessive uncalcified bones

Renal osteodystrophy (chronic renal failure)
From lack of completion of vitamin D metabolism

TREATMENT PLAN

Surgical
Osteotomy may be done for children with severe bone deformities to permit proper weight bearing.

Chemotherapeutic
Nutritional supplements: vitamin D, 400-600 USP units, po or IV, daily, until deficiency is removed

Supportive
Supplying well-balanced diet with fortified milk, and sources of vitamin D (egg yolks, tuna, cod liver oil, and salmon)

ASSESSMENT: AREAS OF CONCERN

Skeleton: bone growth, maturation
Children with rickets
Lack of bone mineralization leading to softening of skeleton
Abnormal curvature of bones
Enlargement of bone ends
Skull changes giving a "hot-cross bun" appearance
Enlargement of the costochondral junctions of the ribs referred to as rosary
Bone possibly tender
Adults with osteomalacia
Bone pain present
Strength of bone less
May have backache and muscle weakness

Systemic processes
Children with rickets
Dentition (eruption of teeth) delayed
Flabby muscles
Prone to bronchitis, diarrhea, convulsions, and tetany
May be fretful and restless
Adults with osteomalacia
General feeling throughout body; may have malaise and fatigue

Psychosocial concerns
Body image disturbances

NURSING DIAGNOSES and NURSING INTERVENTIONS

Nursing Diagnosis	Nursing Intervention
Mobility, impaired physical	Handle baby gently and carefully to avoid further trauma. Position to support affected tissues; use pillows appropriately. For adults, assist with ambulation if no fracture is present. Prevent additional injury through maintenance of a safe environment: side rails, nonskid surfaces, and clean, dry areas. Observe baby for signs of tetany or convulsions.
Nutrition, alteration in: less than body requirements	Administer medications (vitamin D) per physician order to remove deficiency. Explain how this therapy will improve patient's condition. Supply well-balanced diet high in vitamin D foods. Inform patient how this therapy will affect condition.
Self-concept, disturbance in: body image	Listen to parents/patients ventilate feelings of deformity. Discuss surgical purposes, if contemplated, to remove deformity and prevent later degenerative changes.

Patient Education
1. Instruct about sources of vitamin D and need for adequate intake.
2. Explain surgical treatment and recovery processes.

EVALUATION

Patient Outcome	Data Indicating That Outcome is Reached
Patient regains and maintains adequate vitamin D levels.	Patient has normal serum levels of vitamin D.
Patient regains and maintains normal calcium levels and strength of bones without deformity.	Patient has normal serum calcium levels. Bones regain proper calcification and x-ray films show increased density and minimal or no deformity.

Osteoporosis

Osteoporosis is a condition of overall reduction in bone mass or density in which bone resorption has outstripped bone formation, thereby upsetting the normal balance.

Characteristically, persons with osteoporosis have reduced amount or quantity of bone per unit volume, but the bones themselves are otherwise normal.[6] The disease is most common in postmenopausal women probably because of endocrine involution and inactivity. Younger persons may develop osteoporosis following injuries leading to paralysis and long periods of immobility. Persons with rheumatoid arthritis and liver disease may also develop osteoporosis.

PATHOPHYSIOLOGY

Even though patients with osteoporosis have normal bones, they do have less overall bone quantity. The remaining bone becomes weakened from the demands of weight bearing. Fractures can occur with little force, especially in the lower radius, femoral neck, and vertebrae. The vertebral column's overall mass is diminished, leading to increasing kyphosis (dowager's hump) and loss of height. Backache is common.

DIAGNOSTIC STUDIES

History
Prolonged immobility
Menopause
Decreased activity

Physical examination
Increased kyphosis
Backache or neck ache
Few other symptoms

X-ray films
Soft vertebral bodies that are indented by the discs and become biconcave
Vertebrae possibly wedged from fractures
Thoracic vertebral curvature increased

TREATMENT PLAN

Chemotherapeutic
Nutritional supplements
Calcium carbonate (Os-Cal or Os-Cal-Fluor), 1 g qd
Vitamin D, 50,000 IU once or twice weekly
Estrogens for postmenopausal women who have undergone hysterectomy; because of increased risk of endometrial cancer and cardiovascular complications, use of estrogens is controversial for osteoporosis

Electromechanical
Application of back corset or support to prevent stress fractures
Ambulation and maintaining activity to hold calcium in bones

ASSESSMENT: AREAS OF CONCERN

Skeletal tissues
Degree of strength
Presence of increased kyphosis
Loss of height
Fracture

Other tissues
Backache
Neck pain

Psychosocial concerns
Self-concept: disturbances in self-esteem and body image
Alteration in physical mobility

NURSING DIAGNOSES and NURSING INTERVENTIONS

Nursing Diagnosis	Nursing Intervention
Self-concept, disturbance in: self-esteem, performance role	Explain or clarify the processes accompanying menopause as normal and natural. Encourage usual ADL and other activities to maintain bone mass. Encourage fashion consultation for clothing to lessen effects of increased kyphosis.
Mobility, impaired physical	Administer medications, if ordered; monitor patient's response. Perform ROM exercises actively and passively if necessary to maintain muscle and joint strength. Use ambulatory aid (cane or crutch) if needed to lessen stress on bones. Apply back corset to lessen pain and increase mobility.

Patient Education

1. Refute lay perception of osteoporosis as "thin" bones; bone mass is decreased, but bones are not thinner in this disease.
2. Instruct patient and family of advantages of activity to maintain bone mass and calcium in bones.
3. Clarify effects of increased calcium intake and reiterate need for serial examinations of serum calcium levels.

EVALUATION

Patient Outcome	Data Indicating That Outcome is Reached
Patient maintains or regains bone calcification.	Patient has normal serum calcium levels; x-ray films show normal bone densities.
Patient maintains pain-free ambulation and joint mobility.	Patient maintains self-care, ADL, and mobility as desired without pain.
Patient's osteoporosis is not progressively debilitating.	Patient's disease is controlled by medication, calcium intake, or activity. Patient does not experience major loss of bone density.

TRAUMA

Trauma accounts for a significant portion of medical care associated with the musculoskeletal tissues with injuries occurring in all age groups. One in five emergency department visits is associated with musculoskeletal trauma, and one in four patient visits to physicians correlates with musculoskeletal conditions. Older persons are admitted to hospitals for musculoskeletal conditions and trauma second only to admissions for respiratory conditions. Additionally because of our high-paced lifestyles, the injured person may suffer multiple injuries affecting not only the musculoskeletal tissues but other tissues as well, which, if not life ending or life threatening, may require long hospitalization and recovery periods without assurance of future lack of disability or pain and probable periods of decreased mobility.

Contusions, Strains, and Sprains

A contusion is a bruise without an external break in the skin.

A strain is a "pull" in a muscle, ligament, or tendon caused by excessive stretch.

A sprain is a tear in a muscle, ligament, or tendon; it may be mild to severe.

Trauma to the musculoskeletal tissues may involve one specific tissue, such as one ligament, one tendon, or a single muscle mass, although injury to single tissues alone is very rare. The more common occurrence is multiple tissues injured in the traumatic incident such as multiple fractures of bones with many fracture fragments associated with skin, nerve, and blood vessel trauma. Such injuries may be and frequently are life threatening.

Injuries of a lesser nature involve bruises or contusions of the skin, strain (stretch) of tendon or ligament fibers, or sprains (tearing) of some, many, or all tendons, ligaments, or even bones in and around a joint. Since these three conditions (contusion, strain, and sprain) have similar initial signs (with some differences), require similar assessments, and have similar treatment modalities (again, with some differences), they will be considered together, with the differences compared and contrasted.

PATHOPHYSIOLOGY

Contusions are bruises that occur from sudden external pressure causing tears in the subcutaneous circulatory veins and capillaries. Bleeding occurs in the injured subcutaneous tissues, noted by bluish discoloration of the injured tissues with edema or swelling accompanying the vessel or tissue injury. Depending on the extent or severity of the contusion, the edema and discoloration begin to abate in 48 to 72 hours.

A *strain* is an undue force applied to muscles, ligaments, or tendons; it stretches the fibers causing a temporary weakness, numbness, and some bleeding if the veins or capillaries within the injured tissues are excessively stretched. The weakness may last 24 to 72 hours, but the numbness usually disappears within hours. Bleeding may continue for 30 minutes or longer unless pressure or cold is applied to stop it. A strained muscle, ligament, or tendon can regain its full function following conservative treatments, discussed later.

A *sprain* is a different matter altogether from a contusion or strain. A sprain is a partial or full tearing off or away (avulsion) of one or more ligaments or tendons or portions of the bone in and around a joint caused by undue force, twisting, or pull exerted during sports or work activities. Most sprains occur in the ankles, wrists, fingers, and toes. Other joints can also be sprained if undue force, pressure, or pull is applied without relief.

DIAGNOSTIC STUDIES

History
   Pressure
   Undue force
   Pull without relief (if strain or sprain)

Physical examination
   Skin, circulatory, and musculoskeletal signs as described on pp. 440-443

TREATMENT PLAN

	Contusion	Strain	Sprain
Surgical			
Open reduction and repair of torn or avulsed tissues	None	None	May be needed for full joint function; ligament or tendon may be reattached or may need to be removed
Chemotherapeutic			
Analgesics	None	Aspirin, 300-600 mg qid prn; or acetaminophen, 300-600 mg qid prn	Aspirin, 300-1000 mg q4h to relieve pain and inflammation
Narcotics	None	None	Codeine, 30-60 mg po q4-6h for severe pain
Electromechanical			
Cold application	Ice bag for 24°	Ice bag for 24°	Ice bag for 24°
External wrap	None	Ace wrap or sling	Ace wrap or cast; sling
Elevation	None	Elevate if extremity	Elevate if extremity
Exercises (ROM)	Gentle exercises after 48 h	Gentle exercises and use as able after 48 h	No exercises while severe edema and bleeding present; gentle exercises may be begun after 7-10 d, depending on tissue injured

	Contusion	Strain	Sprain
Weight bearing	Full use	As able; full use	Cessation of weight bearing with crutch use for 7 d or more depending on tissues involved

ASSESSMENT: AREAS OF CONCERN

	Contusion	Strain	Sprain
Specific tissue or tissues	Skin and subcutaneous tissue	Tendon, ligament, bone, and entire joint	Same as with strain
Local processes	Bluish discoloration and edema; skin openings; pain; soreness	Weakness, numbness, bleeding noted by discoloration; skin opening?; joint mobility, stability, or laxness; pain; edema; ability to bear weight or use joint normally	Same as with strain only more pronounced: more edema, bleeding, and discoloration; inability to use joint, muscles, or tendons normally; can not bear weight; pain more severe and constant
Systemic processes	Other bruises or contusions possibly present	Distant joints possibly sore from initial injury	Same as with strain
Psychosocial concerns	Minor discomfort; no major concerns	Temporary (24-72 hours) impairment of mobility	Mobility impaired for varying periods (10 days to 3 or more weeks)

NURSING DIAGNOSES and NURSING INTERVENTIONS

Nursing Diagnosis	Nursing Intervention
Mobility, impaired physical	Handle injured tissues gently to avoid further trauma. Apply ice bag to aid healing to regain mobility. Elevate injured part or parts to decrease edema. Assist with ROM exercises when allowed; perform as able. Use sling for upper extremity injury to lessen pain. Perform neurovascular checks as ordered. Assist with crutch walking as needed; assess crutches for proper length. Administer analgesics to lessen pain and aid in relief of inflammation. Assist with personal hygiene as needed.
Self-concept, disturbance in: role performance	Assure patient that full function should be regained. Encourage resumption of ADL and usual activities as able. Caution about possibility of reinjury if care not taken.

EVALUATION

Patient Outcome	Data Indicating That Outcome is Reached
Patient recovers ROM of affected joints and tissues without limitations.	Patient experiences no pain, tenderness, limitation of motion, edema, or loss of function of tissues.
Patient returns to social interactions.	Patient returns to usual family, social, and employment roles.

Dislocation

A dislocation is displacement of a part, usually a bone, from its normal anatomic position within a joint.

Dislocations may be complete or partial (called subluxations). Dislocations usually result from a blow, force, or pull of sufficient magnitude to cause the bone to be forced or pulled from the joint. Repeated dislocations are common for some persons from repetitive or chronic trauma to a joint, which weakens ligaments, tendons, or muscles. Some joints, such as the shoulder, elbow, and knee, are more commonly dislocated than others.

Subluxations are more common in persons with long-standing rheumatoid arthritis because fibrosis shortens the tendons, forcing the bones to subluxate; this is referred to as a swan neck or boutonniere deformity.

PATHOPHYSIOLOGY

The major signs of dislocation are deformity and inability to use the part or joint normally. Tendons or ligaments can become interposed, making reduction and replacement of the dislocated part into the joint difficult or impossible without open surgical reduction. The latter situation is more common with subluxations associated with rheumatoid arthritis because of the tendon shortening.

DIAGNOSTIC STUDIES

History
Repetitive trauma, such as throwing or hitting a ball

Physical examination
Head or other part of bone out of the normal anatomic position

Deformity
Inability to use joint normally

X-ray film
Dislocated parts

TREATMENT PLAN

Surgical
Open reduction of the dislocated bone
Tendon transplant for swan neck and boutonniere deformities

Mechanical
Manual closed reduction of the dislocated bone into the joint
Application of a sling for the upper extremity to lessen stress
Adhesive or Ace wrap of lower extremity joint

ASSESSMENT: AREAS OF CONCERN

Joint and bones of joint
Palpation of dislocated part out of usual position
Deformity
Inability to use joint normally
Tenderness, soreness, or pain

Psychosocial concerns
Self-concept
Disturbances of role expectations
Impaired mobility

NURSING DIAGNOSES and NURSING INTERVENTIONS

Nursing Diagnosis	Nursing Intervention
Self-concept, disturbance in: role performance	Assure patient that full ROM should be regained after reduction and healing. Assist with hygiene and ADL as needed. Provide postoperative care as needed.
Mobility, impaired physical	Apply sling or Ace wrap to maintain reduction. Perform ROM to all unaffected joints to maintain strength. Assist patient to ambulate four times daily to maintain strength.

Patient Education
1. Explain how repetitive trauma weakens joint supports and predisposes to repeated dislocations.
2. Explain that prompt treatment lessens long-term effects of repetitive dislocations.

EVALUATION

Patient Outcome	Data Indicating That Outcome is Reached
Patient has reduction of dislocation without recurrence.	Patient's bones are in normal anatomic positions.
Patient has normal ROM of affected joint.	Patient performs ADL and ROM without pain, limitation, or recurrence of dislocation.

Fractures

A fracture is a discontinuity or break in a bone.

Major trauma of musculoskeletal tissues occurs when bones are fractured. Not only is the most vital part (bone) unable to perform its normal functions, but all other surrounding tissues also cannot carry out their activities from the domino effect of the bone trauma. The cumu- lative effects may or may not be in direct relationship to the severity of the injury because of the ripples experienced in these interrelated tissues.

The type of fracture is usually related to the source or force of the blow (Table 4-4; Fig. 4-14). Only minor force may be needed for a greenstick fracture of one bone

Table 4-4
Classification of Fractures

Type of Fracture	Age of Persons Affected	Description	Force or Power Causing Fracture
Greenstick	Children and older adults	Break in one cortex (covering) of bone	Minor direct or indirect force
Transverse	All ages	Horizontal break across both cortices	Direct or indirect moderate force with angulation toward bone
Spiral	Young and older adults	Fracture curves around both cortices, which may twist out of place (become displaced)	Twisting force, direct or indirect
Oblique	All ages	Fracture at oblique angle across both cortices with or without displacement	Force is twisting and angulating, with axial compression
Comminuted	Young and older adults	Fracture has more than two pieces with much soft tissue trauma	Crushing force directly to tissues
Compression	All ages	Bone squeezed or wedged together at one cortex	Axial compressive force, directly applied to superior skeleton
Pathologic	Older adults	Transverse, oblique, or spiral fracture	Minor direct or indirect force through bone weakened by tumor
Open	All ages	Bones fractured, skin is opened, and there may be much soft tissue trauma	Moderate to severe force suddenly applied without relief; exceeds tissue tolerances
Avulsed	Children and young adults	Fracture pulls bone away from its normal attachments and place (occurs frequently at knee and elbow with patella or olecranon being avulsed from joints)	Force is direct or indirect with resisted extension of knee or elbow muscles causing pulling away of bone involved; muscles may also avulse from bones or tendons from resisted actions
Stress	Young and older adults	Crack in one cortex of a bone (scaphoid, lunate, or hamate in wrist) and others	Repetitive application of force (as striking a lever); also may result from steroids causing osteoporosis
Closed	All ages	Bone fractured, but skin over site remains intact	Minor, as with greenstick or pathologic fractures

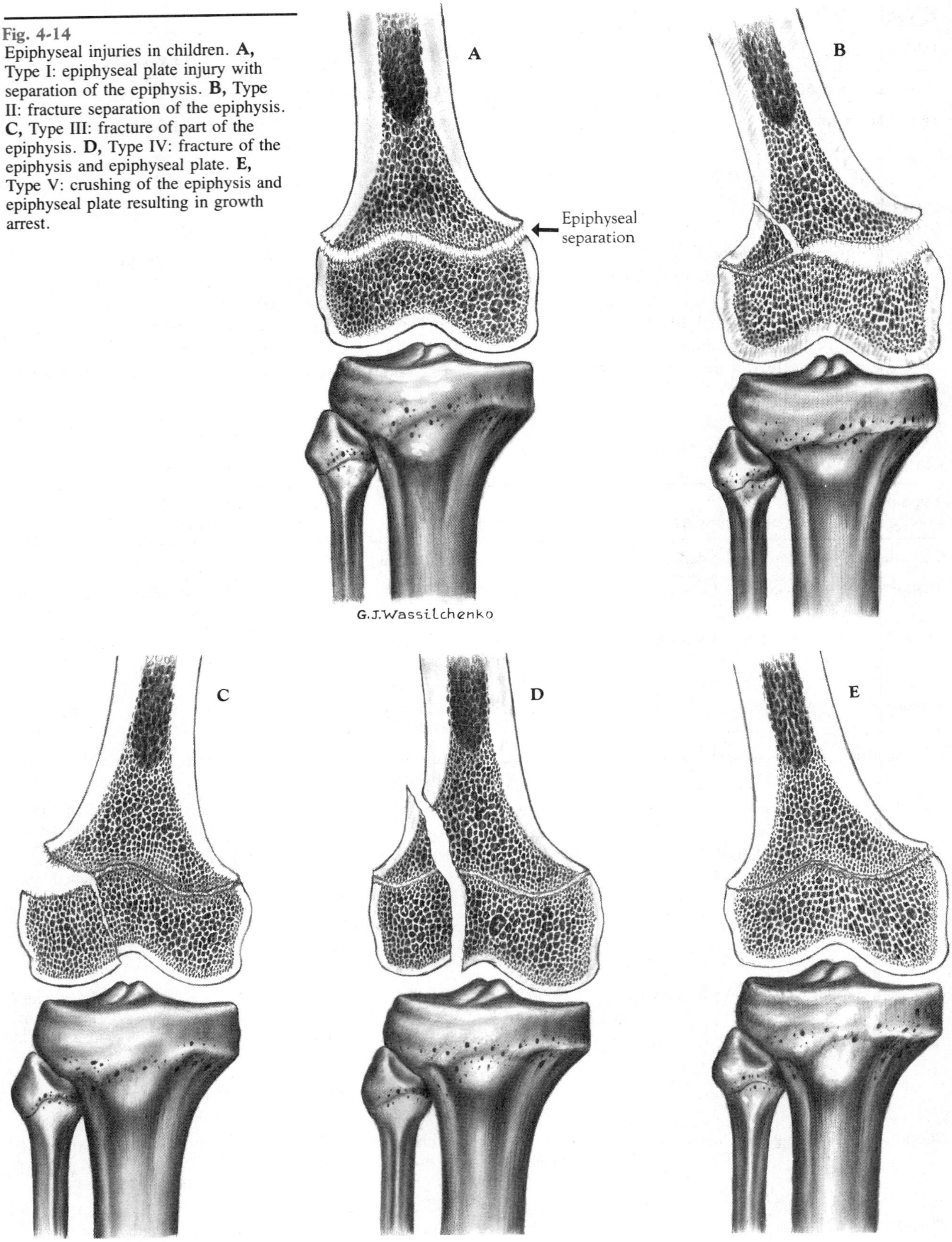

Fig. 4-14
Epiphyseal injuries in children. **A,**
Type I: epiphyseal plate injury with
separation of the epiphysis. **B,** Type
II: fracture separation of the epiphysis.
C, Type III: fracture of part of the
epiphysis. **D,** Type IV: fracture of the
epiphysis and epiphyseal plate. **E,**
Type V: crushing of the epiphysis and
epiphyseal plate resulting in growth
arrest.

Epiphyseal
separation

G.J.Wassilchenko

cortex, whereas more powerful forces cause comminuted fractures with associated soft tissue trauma. All ages of persons are susceptible to fractures; however, younger children and aged persons may experience fractures from minor forces. Young and middle-aged adults, because of their stronger musculoskeletal tissues, require greater forces to fracture a bone, and there is more associated soft tissue trauma.

PATHOPHYSIOLOGY

Bones are held relatively firmly in their normal anatomic positions by their shape, bony projections and processes, and the strong ligaments and tendons that hold them in their joints. Muscles surrounding the bones along their shafts also provide protection. However, when forces are applied either directly or indirectly to the bone that are superior to the strength of the bone, muscles, tendons, or ligaments, they cause the tissues to resist or "give in." Bones break when they cannot continue to resist the strength, duration, or repetitive nature of the applied forces.

A fractured bone can no longer maintain its normal length unless the two fragments impact into each other at the time of the fracture. Usually there will be shortening of the tissues around the fractured bone brought about from muscle contraction and spasms as the muscles respond to the stimulus of trauma. As the muscles contract and shorten, they move the distal fragment cephalad (toward the head or upward). The distal fragment is less stable and more movable than the proximal fragment, which is held more firmly from the muscles' originations (the origins of muscles are less movable than their insertions). The shortening of the muscles and the displacement of the distal fragment result in deformity, a characteristic sign of a fracture. The deformity can generally be noted on gross examination as a deviation from the normal appearance of the tissues. Displacement of the distal fragment is diagnostically and therapeutically significant, because the distal fragment must be replaced in continuity with the proximal fragment for healing and bone union to transpire. The amount of displacement and the angulation and rotation of the distal fragment are caused by the loss of the bone's continuity and the severity or strength of the muscle spasms and contraction. Force must be applied to the distal fragment and to the muscles to overcome the muscle contraction so that the two or more fracture fragments can again become aligned. Terms used to describe the position of the distal fragment include varus or valgus displacement, rotation, and medial, lateral, anterior, or posterior displacement.

When a bone is fractured, many or all of the following events occur sequentially from the trauma. These events begin immediately with the injury, but they continue for weeks, months, and even years in some situations before they are completed:

1. Hematoma formation: blood and blood cells extravasate into the injured tissues from vessels broken or bruised at the time of injury and from the inflammatory response to release of histamine, bradykinins, and serotonin into the injury site. Bleeding into the tissues causes a hematoma to form. Blood cells, especially thrombocytes, begin to work with fibroblasts to form a fibrin (clot) meshwork within the hematoma. Usually, the hematoma is well formed in 24 to 48 hours, and frank or continued bleeding slows or ceases completely. There appears to be an optimal-size hematoma to facilitate bone union. Healing is delayed or prevented by hematomas that are too small or too large, although the exact favorable size is still undetermined.

2. Consolidation: fibroblasts continue to invade the hematoma, firming up the fibrin meshwork. Mucopolysaccharides brought to the area aid adherence of the fibrils to each other. Additionally, white cells brought to and circulating in the injured tissues "wall off" and surround the hematoma, adding strength while also localizing and removing wastes from the inflammatory responses. The fibrin meshwork is very fragile at this stage, and therefore it is very important to maintain relative immobility of the fractured bones. This period of consolidation lasts 10 days to 3 weeks.

3. Granulation: osteoblasts (bone-forming cells) move into the meshwork, firming it and intertwining it with collagen connective tissue fibers to form strong scar tissues and to form new bone to bridge the gap between the fractured ends. Capillary buds develop into new blood vessels, which bring more nutrients and calcium molecules into the area to form bone callus. The granulation period lasts 3 to 6 weeks or longer.

4. Callus formation: this is probably the most vital period for bone healing for two reasons: (1) Sufficient nutrients must be present and in continuous supply to carry bone formation to completion. A major nutrient is oxygen, along with sufficient amounts of vitamins A, B, C, and D, carbohydrates, proteins, minerals, and water. (2) Callus formation is enhanced by the "right" amount of compression of the fractured fragments. Too little compression may result in pseudobone (false bone), and too much compression may decrease oxygen supply and tension, resulting in bone-end absorption and creating too large a gap for the collagen fibers to bridge, thus decreasing or preventing

formation of strong callus. Osteoclast activity is greater when compressive forces are too great, because osteoclasts act to absorb or resorb bone cells, while osteoblasts aid formation. The balance is disrupted between the two cells, decreasing the callus or new bone formation. This period lasts for varying periods of 3 to 6 months or more, depending on the type of fracture and the above conditions.

5. Remodeling: if present, excess is resorbed during this period. The collagen fibers and fibrous tissues are aligned to form trabeculae along the lines of stress according to Wolff's law, which states that bone will respond to stress by becoming thicker and stronger and that the structure of a bone depends on its function. Osteoclasts resorb the excess callus or poorly aligned trabeculae until they are firm and strong.

Bone healing, then, depends on multiple *local* factors, including the severity of the injury, nutrient supply, amount of bone bridge or gap, degree of immobilization, infection or necrosis of bone cells, and type of bone fractured. Cancellous bone fractures heal more quickly than fractures of compact bone because of the presence of blood and blood cells in greater quantities than in compact bone. *Systemic* factors influencing bone healing include the patient's age (children heal more quickly), concomitant diseases such as diabetes, hormonal balances (growth hormones aid healing while excess corticosteroids delay healing), and stress, immobility, or mobility at the fracture site. Application of electric current aids bone healing and has become a valuable adjunct in recent years.

DIAGNOSTIC STUDIES

History
Sudden, unexpected trauma; chronic, repetitive forces rather than sudden force usually cause stress fractures

Physical examination
Local deformity
Edema or a mass
Distal tissues held at abnormal angles or positions
Limitation of use of part
Crepitation
Pain or tenderness at or around the site
Subjective signs of numbness, tingling, weakness, or inability to use part normally
Distal tissues cooler than proximal
Peripheral pulses
Skin over injury site open or intact

X-ray films
Complete break in bone continuity or in one cortex
Rarely, may fail to reveal fracture initially
Repeat in 10 days for certainty[6] since bone absorption at fracture site makes diagnosis easier

TREATMENT PLAN

Surgical
Open reduction of the fracture with internal fixation of the fracture fragments with pins, nails, screws, staples, plates, intramedullary nails, or wire
Arthroplasty with replacement with prosthesis
Total joint replacement for crush injuries
Amputation for severe crush injuries
Application of external apparatus such as the Hoffman or Ace-Fischer device

Chemotherapeutic
Narcotic analgesics
Meperidine (Demerol, others), 50-100 mg q3h IM for acute pain
Morphine, 5-20 mg q4h, subq, or hydromorphone (Dilaudid), 2-4 mg q4h subq, for acute pain
Analgesic-antipyretics
Aspirin, 600-1000 mg q4h between narcotic administration times
Acetaminophen, 600-1000 mg q4h between narcotic administration
Tranquilizers
Hydroxyzine (Vistaril), 25-50 mg IM, with narcotic as a narcotic potentiator (This drug is the *only* one that potentiates narcotic activity for pain relief.)
Diazepam (Valium), 2-10 mg q4-6h po, for muscle relaxant effects
Anti-infective agents specific to the invading organisms (noted by culture) if the skin is open; commonly prescribed antibiotics include the following:
Ampicillin (Amcill, others), 1-2 g q6h IV and later, po
Cefamandole (Mandol), 500-1000 mg q4-8h IM or IV
Cephalexin (Keflex), 500-1000 mg po
Sedative-hypnotics, barbiturate
Phenobarbitol (Luminal), 15-30 mg 2-3 times daily
Flurazepam (Dalmane), 15-30 mg hs
Glutethimide (Doriden), 250-500 mg hs

Fig. 4-15
Examples of casts for upper extremity injuries.

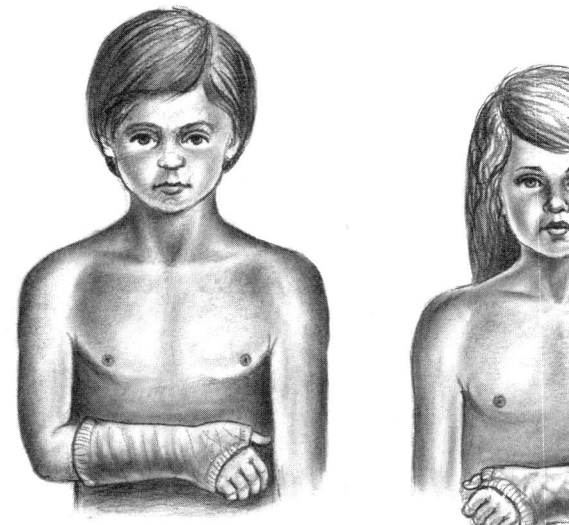
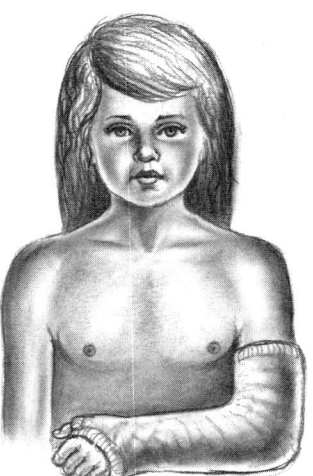
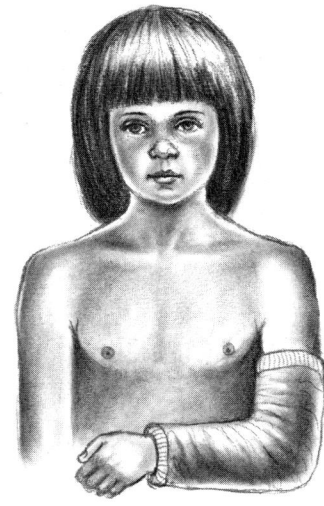

Short arm cast   Long arm cast   Arm cylinder cast

Fig. 4-16
A, Plaster body jacket cast. **B,** Body jacket with halo apparatus attached.

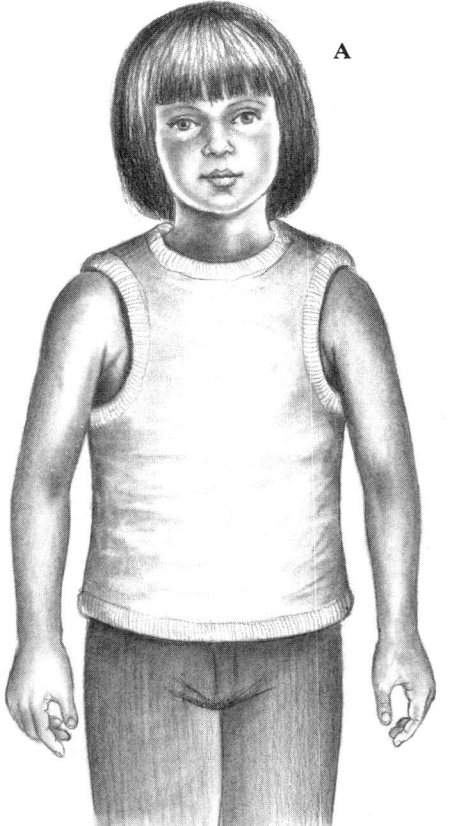

A

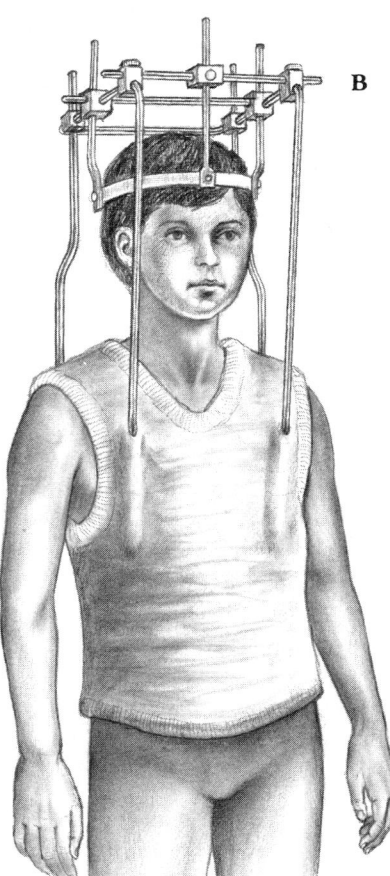

B

G.J.Wassilchenko

Electromechanical

Reduction of the fracture through closed, manual manipulation or open, direct manipulation of the fractured bones if fragments are displaced; if no displacement is present, reduction is not done

Application of an anterior and posterior splint for undisplaced or well-reduced, stable fractures of the radius, ulna, or wrist bones

Application of circular cast (see Figs. 4-15 to 4-17 for types of casts and p. 514 for nursing concerns)

Wrapping injured tissues with elastic wraps for temporary immobilization (primarily for undisplaced stress fractures of wrist bones)

Placing patient in one or another type of traction (see Table 4-6 for traction forms and p. 519 for specific care)

Supportive

Application of ice bags to decrease bleeding and edema formation and relieve pain

Elevation of injured tissues if extremity

Application of a sling or splint to lessen stress on contiguous tissues

Placing on bed rest, if feasible

Making patient "non-weight-bearing" to affected bone and joints

Use of cane, crutches, or walker when not bearing weight

Well-balanced diet high in vitamins, proteins, carbohydrates, and minerals

Forcing fluids

Concurrent treatment of systemic diseases if present

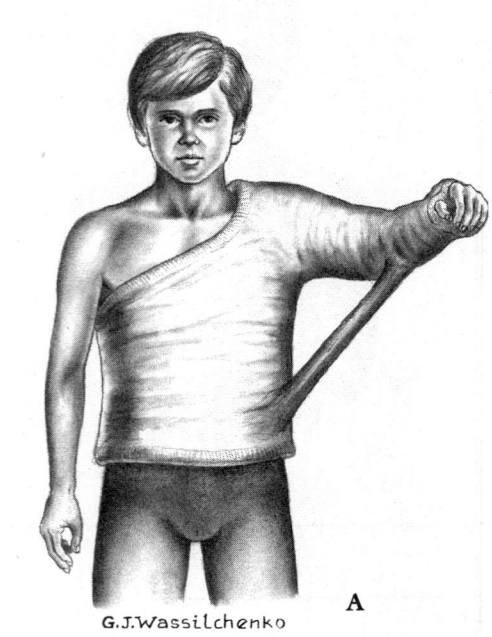

Fig. 4-17
Spica casts. **A,** Shoulder spica (bivalved). **B,** Unilateral hip spica. **C,** One and one-half hip spica. **D,** Bilateral long leg hip spica.

G.J.Wassilchenko

A

ASSESSMENT: AREAS OF CONCERN

Fracture site and surrounding tissues

Edema

Color changes

Deformity

Paresthesia with numbness and tingling

Pain

Limitation of movement or inability to use part

Skin closed or open

Crepitation (movement of parts normally not movable)

Bruising

Bleeding or hematoma (noted by mass)

Presence or absence of pulses distal to injury

Systemic concerns

Pallor

Confusion

Dyspnea

Shock

Changes in blood pressure

Sweating or perspiring

Fear and anxiety

Concomitant diseases or other injuries to distant organs

Psychosocial concerns

Self-concept

Disturbances in body image and impairment of physical mobility

Alteration in comfort, acute pain

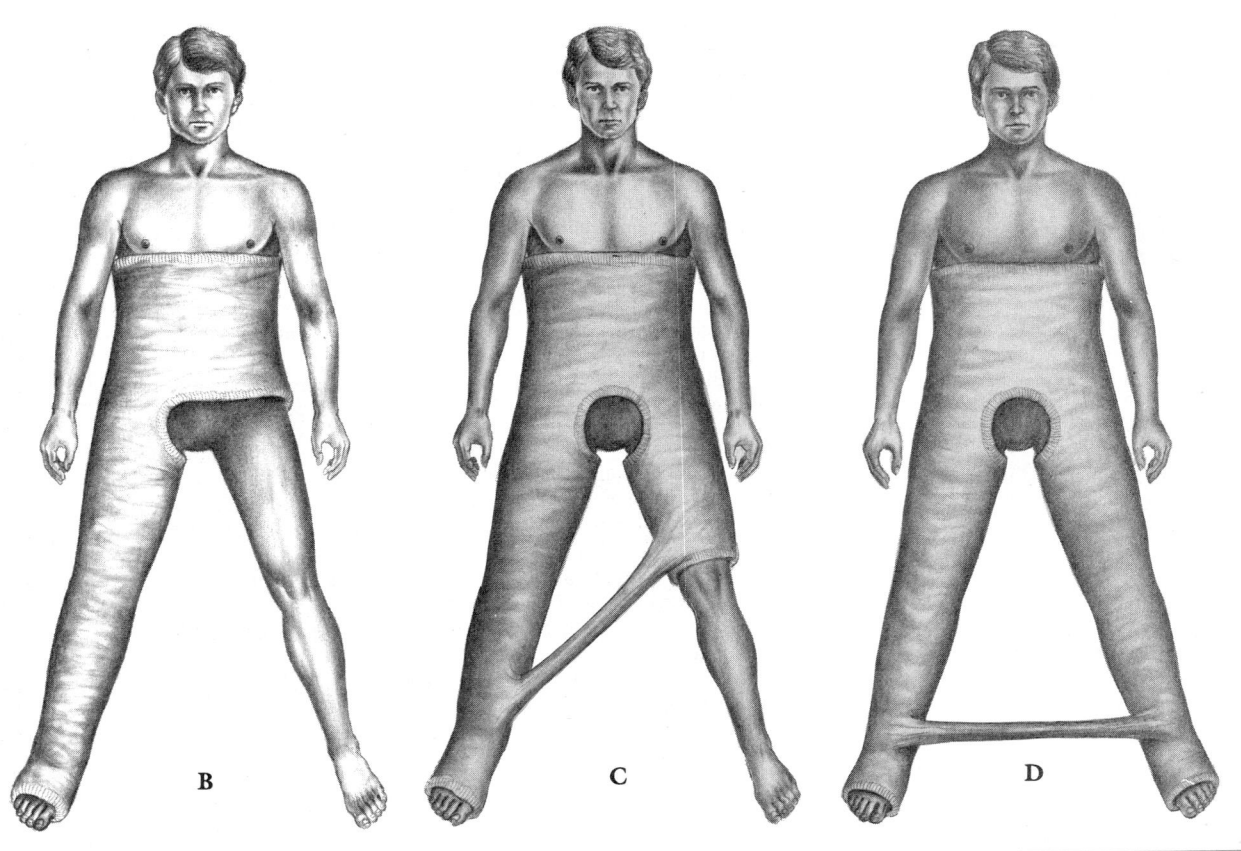

B   C   D

NURSING DIAGNOSES and NURSING INTERVENTIONS

Nursing Diagnosis	Nursing Intervention
Mobility, impaired physical	Gently handle injured tissues by supporting joint above and below site to prevent additional injury and lessen pain.
	Apply ice bags to site.
	Elevate extremity as ordered; support with pillows.
	Put patient on bed rest if ordered.
	Explain purposes for rest and not bearing weight.
	Perform neurovascular checks.
	Assess integrity of cast, function of traction or wrapping every 1 to 2 hours initially, then every 4 hours.
	Explain position required for maximal healing.
	Assist patient to proper position; change position every 2 hours or assist patient to position self correctly.
	Teach patient the ''post position'' to lift self (patient plants [posts] unaffected foot flat on bed with knee bent at right angle; lifts self using trapeze while pushing down with foot and leg). Assist with lifting patient's buttocks if needed.
	Teach patient exercises to maintain strength and facilitate resolution of inflammation: quadriceps, buttocks, and triceps setting exercises done every 4 hours when allowed.

Nursing Diagnosis	Nursing Intervention
Comfort, alteration in: pain	Assist patient to assume a position of comfort, if possible. Administer ordered narcotic analgesics: every 3 hours for meperidine (action is lost after 3 hours) or every 4 hours for opiate narcotics. Administer narcotics around the clock for 3 to 5 days or longer as ordered to maintain adequate blood levels to relieve pain. Periods between narcotics may be increased after the acute muscle spasms are relieved. Administer nonnarcotic analgesics as ordered every 4 hours between narcotic administrations to enhance pain relief. Aspirin has the additional anti-inflammatory effect to aid its resolution. Change position every 2 hours to lessen muscle fatigue. Do back and buttocks massage to remove waste products of pressure and fatigue and to increase circulation to those areas. Administer muscle relaxant or sedatives as ordered to aid reduction of muscle spasms to lessen pain.
Self-concept, disturbance in: body image, role performance	Maintain privacy while assisting patient to perform ADL and hygienic care for personal cleanliness and esteem. Offer oral hygiene and back care frequently to maintain healthy tissues. Explain the purposes for proper positioning and prolonged immobility required to facilitate bone healing. Encourage ventilation of patient's feelings regarding enforced immobility and displacement from familiar surroundings. Secure physical therapy and occupational therapy consultations to maintain muscle strength and self-esteem. Encourage family members to interact with patient to maintain customary roles and esteem. Assist patient to take high-nutrient diet to lessen weight loss (a patient in skeletal traction may lose 20 to 30 pounds) and maintain positive body image.

Patient Education

1. Reiterate explanations of purposes of immobility and not bearing weight (anxiety may preclude patient's hearing or understanding initial explanations).
2. Explain reasons for weight loss and how patient can lessen by active exercises and diet.
3. Explain pain relief measures for dealing with acute pain and changes in medication administration patterns as pain decreases.
4. Explain bone healing processes for patient's maximal cooperation.

EVALUATION

Patient Outcome	Data Indicating That Outcome is Reached
Patient experiences bone union in anatomic position.	X-ray films reveal union of bones. Patient can use part without limitation or pain.
Patient resumes ambulation with full weight bearing without limitation or discomfort.	Patient experiences no discomfort or pain with ambulation and weight bearing.
Patient resumes social interactions and roles.	Patient returns to family, social, and employment roles.

CONGENITAL ANOMALIES

Anomalies are abnormalities in the structure or function of specific tissues; they may be congenital or acquired. Musculoskeletal congenital anomalies most frequently involve the lower extremities, feet, hips, and vertebrae. Such anomalies may be caused by the fetus's remaining for prolonged periods in one unchanging position (e.g., breech position), from a shallower than normal maternal pelvic structure, or from the side effects of maternal ingestion of drugs. Drugs known to cause musculoskeletal anomalies include thalidomide (withdrawn from the market), corticosteroids, chlorpropamide (Diabinese), tolbutamide (Orinase), tetracyclines, alcohol and tobacco, and other drugs. Musculoskeletal anomalies caused by these medications occur in the limbs and facial and palatal structures. Structures may be absent, malformed, fused together, or *not* fused when they should be, such as in spina bifida. Curvatures may be exaggerated or maldirected, and the relationships may be altered between neighboring structures, as in clubfoot or congenital hip dysplasia.

Clubfoot

Clubfoot is deformity of the foot. The foot may turn in (varus), outward (valgus), downward (equinus), or upward (calcaneus), or in a combination of several positions (e.g., equinovarus and adduction of the forefoot).

Clubfoot is one of the most common congenital anomalies of musculoskeletal tissues, as well as being one of the oldest known. It may be unilateral or bilateral, with the foot turned in (varus) or out (valgus), forefoot down (equinus), forefoot up (calcaneus), or forefoot adducted or abducted. The most common clubfoot combines three factors: forefoot adduction, hindfoot varus, and equinus of the foot and ankle.

PATHOPHYSIOLOGY

Normal growth and development of all the musculoskeletal tissues in and around the foot are prevented by the abnormal positions of the foot and ankle. Abnormal stress is put on the immature bones, ligaments, tendons, and muscles; unless the position is corrected, they grow and develop in flexed, contracted, or abnormal positions. Because of the requirement of proper alignment of the foot and ankle and the maintenance of proper muscle balances for walking, clubfoot corrective procedures are begun within days of the baby's birth.

DIAGNOSTIC STUDIES

Physical examination
Abnormal positions of parts or all of foot in relation to the ankles (Baby cannot maintain normal position of one or both feet.)

X-ray films
Abnormal positions of one or more bones of foot or ankle
Useful to determine treatment

TREATMENT PLAN

Electromechanical
Application of plaster cast to one or both feet with casts changed every week, 10 days, or 2 weeks as correction is achieved
Immobilization in Denis Browne splint at bedtime or nap time

ASSESSMENT: AREAS OF CONCERN

Both feet and ankles
Position of feet in relation to ankles
Unusual rotation or turning
Unusual bending up or down of forefoot or heel
Inability of baby to maintain foot and ankle in normal positions
Lax or weak muscles or joints
Legs turning in or out
Thin calves

Systemic processes
Fingers anomalous in number or structure
Hips easily dislocated (dysplastic)

Psychosocial concerns
Self-concept and body image disturbances
Impaired physical mobility

NURSING DIAGNOSES and NURSING INTERVENTIONS

Nursing Diagnosis	Nursing Intervention
Mobility, impaired physical	Teach parents care of the cast (p. 514). Instruct parents about necessity for frequent cast changes as child grows and correction is proceeding. Teach parents about maintaining correction through use of Denis Browne splint, if ordered. Instruct parents about skin care under and around the cast or splint.
Self-concept, disturbances in: body image (if uncorrected)	Allow child to verbalize feelings about walking "funny" and about being teased by peers. Encourage parents to seek medical guidance for proper care or treatment of their child's anomaly. Encourage ventilation of feelings about changed body image. Teach exercises (if prescribed) to strengthen weak muscles and improve feelings about body image.

Patient Education

1. Teach parents about need for frequent cast changes.
2. Teach parents use of Denis Browne splint.
3. Encourage parents to continue pediatric follow-up care.
4. If condition is uncorrected until age 3 or 4, surgical correction may be needed; parents should understand that early corrective procedures usually negate need for surgery. Surgery may involve tendon lengthening or osteotomy.

EVALUATION

Patient Outcome	Data Indicating That Outcome is Reached
Baby's feet and ankles will be anatomically aligned and can be maintained as aligned.	Inspection or x-ray films indicate proper anatomic positions and alignment. Alignment can be maintained with ROM.
Baby ambulates without limitation.	Baby walks easily and with no evidence of pain or rotation of feet or ankles.

Congenital Hip Dysplasia

Congenital hip dysplasia is the abnormal placement (location) and development of the head of the femur and the acetabulum resulting in dysfunction of the hip.

Congenital hip dysplasia is more commonly noted in female babies (6:1 ratio) and those born in breech position. Possibly from prolonged intrauterine breech positioning, the acetabulum is shallower and the head of the femur is dislocated from the acetabular socket. This anomaly also has a genetic link, being more common in areas where intermarriage of close relatives is common. The left hip is more commonly affected than the right.

PATHOPHYSIOLOGY

Because the head of the femur and the acetabulum are not in their normal anatomic positions either from joint laxity or malformation, one or both of the bones develop abnormally. The acetabular roof is too steep while the socket is too shallow. The bony femoral head is smaller than normal, and the cartilaginous head is larger. The femoral neck is usually short and is often excessively anteverted. The head of the femur is dislocated posteriorly, with the slope of the pelvis pushing the femoral head laterally as it rides upward and back.[6]

The capsule of the hip joint remains intact but over time becomes more hourglass in shape,[6] and the ligamentum teres, through which the femoral head receives its blood supply through the acetabulum, becomes thicker. In time, also, muscles arising from the pelvis become adaptively shortened.

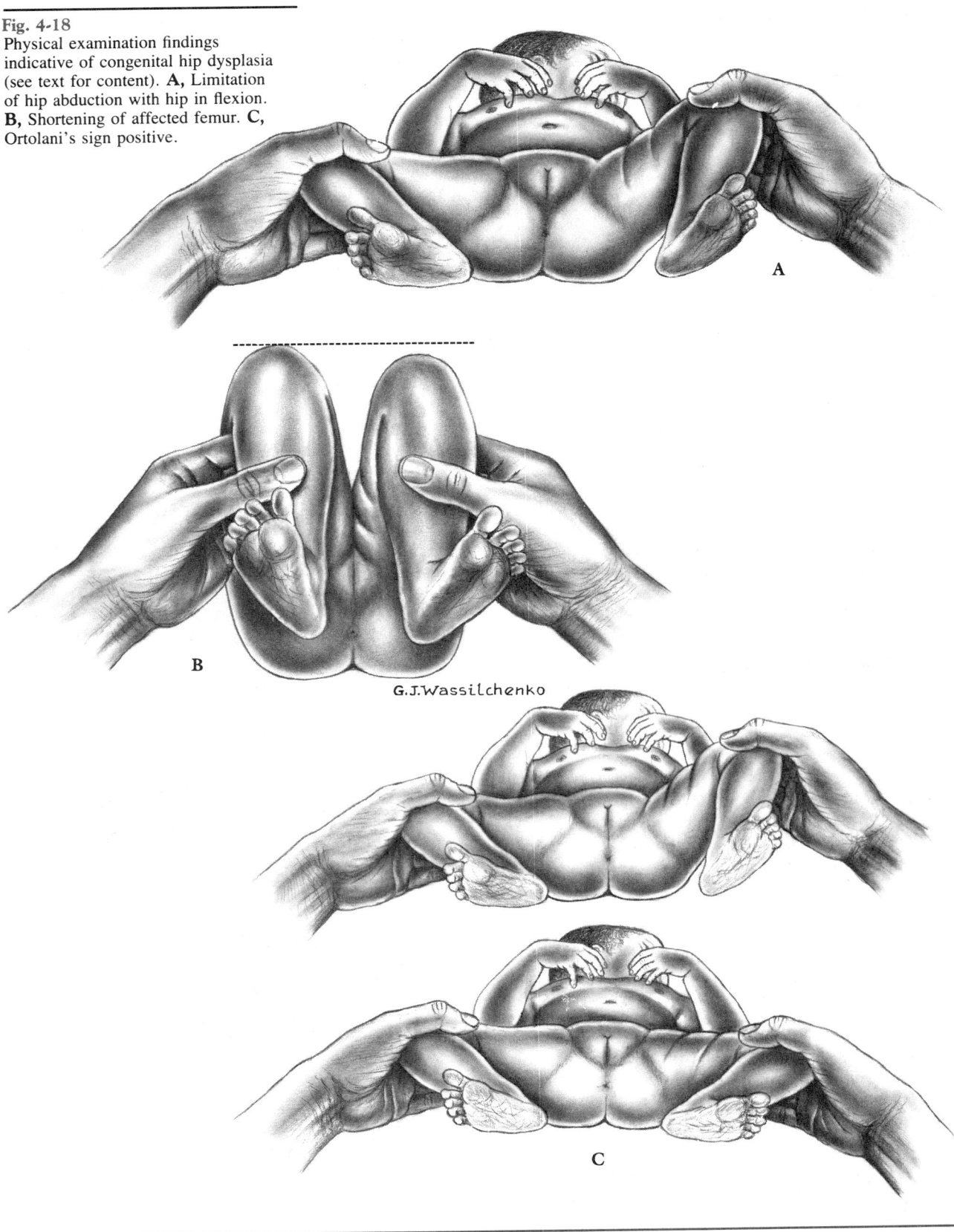

Fig. 4-18
Physical examination findings
indicative of congenital hip dysplasia
(see text for content). **A,** Limitation
of hip abduction with hip in flexion.
B, Shortening of affected femur. **C,**
Ortolani's sign positive.

G.J.Wassilchenko

DIAGNOSTIC STUDIES

Physical examination
Asymmetric skin folds or creases
Limited hip abduction
Click
Unilateral wider pelvis
Shorter limb on affected side (Fig. 4-18)

X-ray film
Dislocated femoral head

TREATMENT PLAN

Surgical
For hips that repeatedly dislocate:
Open reduction followed by plaster cast for 6 weeks
Subtrochanteric osteotomy, which rotates the femur to hold the head into the acetabulum (Internal fixation holds the osteotomized bones, and a cast may also be applied.)

Electromechanical
Use of double diapers or folded diapers (wider than necessary) to separate legs
Use of foam or stuffed pillow between legs to separate legs
Use of lightweight plastic or aluminum splint applied so legs are abducted when in the splint
Application of a plaster cast encasing the hips, thighs, and legs with the hips flexed to 90 degrees with moderate abduction (less used currently since it may cause ischemia of head of femur)
Application of skin traction after reduction of femoral head into acetabulum (Traction is usually bilateral for immobility purposes.)
Application of Denis Browne congenital hip dislocation splint (holds thighs abducted, but permits movement for the child)

ASSESSMENT: AREAS OF CONCERN

Hip joint, acetabulum, and head of femur (bilateral examination)
Asymmetric skin folds of gluteus and thigh
Limited hip abduction
Shortened femur
Click when affected limb is moved from a flexed adducted position
Pelvis appears wider on affected side, and abduction decreased (normal hip in newborn should abduct almost to a right angle)

Manipulation may bring about dislocation from acetabulum
Examination of older child: gait changes and positive Trendelenburg's sign (Figs. 4-18 and 4-19)

Systemic processes
Assessment for other congenital anomalies, especially clubfoot

Psychosocial concerns
Impaired physical mobility

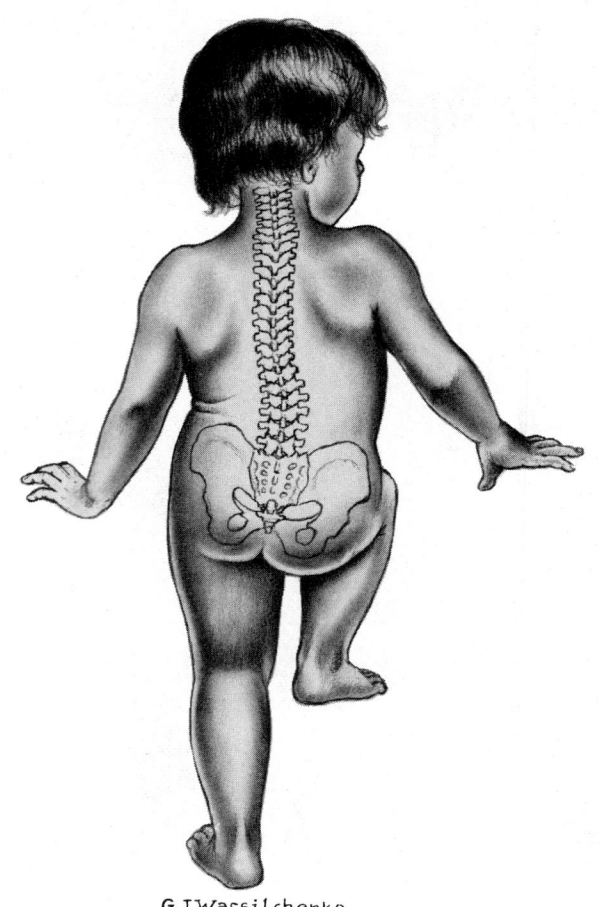

Fig. 4-19
Trendelenburg's sign (see text).

G.J.Wassilchenko

NURSING DIAGNOSES and NURSING INTERVENTIONS

Nursing Diagnosis	Nursing Intervention
Mobility, impaired physical	Explain purposes of double diapering and abduction position, *or* explain purpose of foam pillow, brace, or cast.
	Clarify skin care needed to maintain skin integrity with each form of cast or splint, with traction, or following surgery: bathing, drying, inspecting skin surfaces and folds, massaging pressure areas and prominences, changing damp linens and dressings, using powders sparingly to prevent caking, removing wrinkled pads or linens, turning and repositioning patient frequently.
	Stress wearing of double diapers, pillow, or brace at all times for molding and shaping joint structures to prevent dislocations.
	Stress continuing pediatric medical care until condition is corrected.

Patient Education

1. Instruct parents about purposes of positions of flexion and abduction of hip.
2. Reiterate purposes for long-term follow-up care.

EVALUATION

Patient Outcome	Data Indicating That Outcome is Reached
Patient regains normal joint configuration and mobility.	Patient has equal limb length, no unequal folds or joint limitation of motion, and no limp or unequal hip heights.
Patient experiences no recurrence of hip disabilities.	Patient experiences no long-term disabilities, limp or avascular necrosis, or other hip problems.

CURVATURES OF THE SPINAL COLUMN

The spine develops its characteristic curves during fetal growth (Fig. 4-20). Both prenatally and postnatally the curves may become abnormal because of defective bone, muscle, nerve, or other growth factors. The abnormal curves are called kyphosis (excessive curvature of thoracic spine), scoliosis (lateral or rotary curvature of thoracic spine), and lordosis (excessive curvature of lumbar spine) (Fig. 4-21).

Kyphosis

Kyphosis is excessive curvature of the thoracic vertebrae.

Kyphosis can occur in various age groups. When it occurs in young children, it is usually congenital in origin. It may become apparent in the adolescent years, when it is referred to as juvenile kyphosis, or Scheuermann's disease. Occasionally, kyphosis may be compensatory for lumbar lordosis. Kyphosis is also a classic symptom of ankylosing spondylitis, discussed previously. And kyphosis occurs in postmenopausal women, when it is referred to as senile kyphosis.

PATHOPHYSIOLOGY

Since the thoracic vertebrae have a physiologic posterior curve normally, the curvature becomes pathologic only when it becomes excessive or exaggerated.

In young children the abnormal curvature may be the only pathologic sign without a specific etiology. As children become adolescents, the curvature may become quite pronounced especially in Scheuermann's disease, in which there is irregular epiphyseal plate growth and ossification placing undue strain on the anterior portion of the vertebral bodies. This irregular growth and the additional strain lead to the excessive curvature.

In older persons with kyphosis, there usually are some degenerative changes in the intervertebral cartilages leading to the excessive curvature. In postmenopausal women kyphosis is commonly associated with osteoporosis and degeneration in the anulus fibrosus rings between the vertebrae.

Fig. 4-20
Normal spinal alignment and abnormal spinal curvatures associated with scoliosis. **A,** Normal. **B,** Mild. **C,** Severe. **D,** Rotation and curvature of scoliosis.

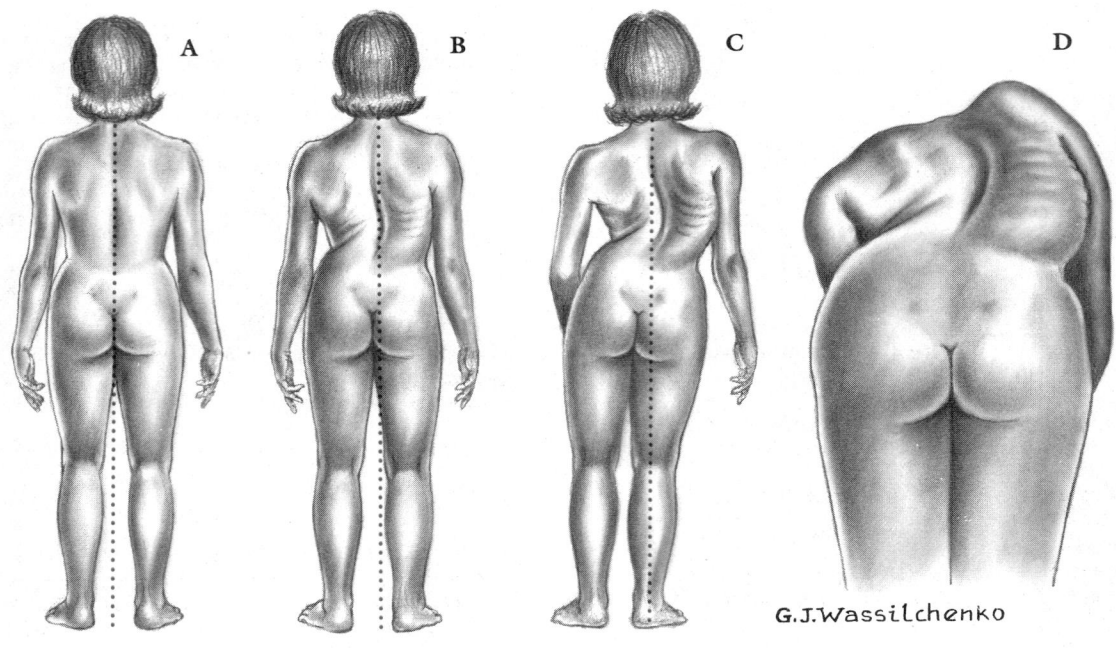

G.J.Wassilchenko

Fig. 4-21
A, Normal spinal alignment and curvatures. **B,** Kyphosis. **C,** Lordosis.

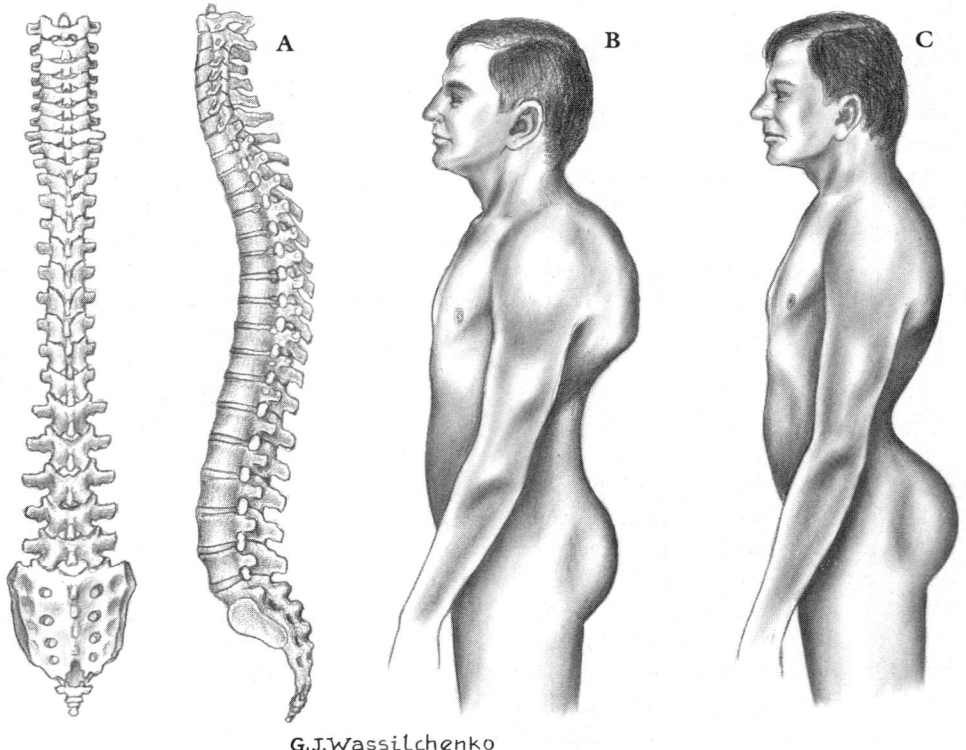

G.J.Wassilchenko

DIAGNOSTIC STUDIES

Physical examination
Excessive thoracic spinal curvature
Rounded shoulders
Occasional low back pain

X-ray film
Forward curvature of thoracic spine
Geriatric patients: possible osteoporosis
Wedging and narrowing of anterior portions of thoracic
  vertebral bodies (6 to 10)

Histocompatibility testing
Serum HLA-B27 antigen present in young adults with
  ankylosing spondylitis

TREATMENT PLAN

Chemotherapeutic
Older adults may have hormonal treatment or mineral
  administration
Young adults with ankylosing spondylitis receive several agents (p. 446) for treatment of their disease
  process

Electromechanical
Milwaukee brace for adolescents
Back corset for older adults

Supportive
Teach patient to stand up as straight as possible

ASSESSMENT: AREAS OF CONCERN

Thoracic spine
Child
  Excessive posterior convexity of thoracic spine
Adolescent
  Rounded shoulders
  Backache
  Excessive curvature of thoracic spine
  Lumbar lordosis increased
Young adult
  Stiffness and soreness of back when rising
  Low back pain
  Increasing curvature of thoracic spine
Older adult
  Female
  Postmenopause
  Loss of height
  Excessive curvature of thoracic spine

Systemic processes
Young adult
  Positive HLA-B27 histocompatibility antigen
  Reiter's syndrome (conjunctivitis, uveitis, genital
    lesions, low back pain)

Psychosocial concerns
Self-concept
Disturbances in self-esteem, body image, and role ex-
  pectations

NURSING DIAGNOSES and NURSING INTERVENTIONS

Nursing Diagnosis	Nursing Intervention
Self-concept, disturbance in: self-esteem, body image, role performance	Discuss principles of proper posture. Discuss non-life-threatening nature of condition. Assist with application of brace, if used, until patient can self-apply. Discuss clothing and other apparel to "cover" brace's presence. Discuss exercises to strengthen back muscles. Discuss patient's life goals and review need for possible alteration (patient should be able to do what he desires without many limitations; see p. 447, for limitations with ankylosing spondylitis).
Mobility, impaired physical	Nursing care measures have been discussed under ankylosing spondylitis.

Patient Education

1. Reiterate patient's means to help self through exercises and posture changes.
2. Reiterate that the patient should be able to achieve life's goals even with kyphosis.

EVALUATION

Patient Outcome	Data Indicating That Outcome is Reached
Patient's posture has improved and curvature is lessened after treatment.	Patient stands straighter with less curvature and/or rotation; hips and shoulders are more normally aligned; respiratory functions are regained; and mobility is improved.
Patient returns to social interactions and roles.	Patient has improved self-concept and body image, is more able to regain family and social roles, and is positive about self and the future.

Scoliosis

Scoliosis is the lateral curvature of the vertebral column.
Scoliosis may be noted in babies, young children, and adolescents. Infants experience two types of scoliosis, referred to as resolving and progressive, both of which are idiopathic. There is a familial genetic factor associated with scoliosis, but the exact factor or factors have not yet been determined. Some hormonal and metabolic factors may be involved, affecting general skeletal growth of the trunk and upper limbs and leading to an abnormal skeletal symmetry in the upper body, although these factors as causes of idiopathic scoliosis have not yet been proven. The curvature may be minimal and barely noticeable in infants and young children.

As the child grows toward adolescence, the curvature becomes more pronounced and noticeable because of the laterality, rotation of the spine, and uneven shoulder and hip levels. Generally treatment is required for curvatures beyond 20 degrees.

PATHOPHYSIOLOGY

The curvatures of scoliosis may be mild to severe and may also be associated with rotation of the spinal column. The curve is convex and the vertebral bodies usually rotate toward the convexity of the curve, although the spinous processes and neural arches rotate toward the concave part of the curve. Both the curves and rotation are likely to increase with growth and stop as spinal growth ceases with maturity.

Scoliosis affects more females, although the exact ratio is difficult to determine with accuracy.

DIAGNOSTIC STUDIES

History
Asymmetry of shoulders or hips
Uneven hemlines, pant length, or waistline

Physical examination
Lateral deviation with or without rotation of vertebrae
Curvature may become more pronounced when patient bends forward
Rotation may also be more noticeable when patient bends forward
When hands of examiner are placed on hips, one hand is higher than other when patient is standing upright
Examination of leg length reveals one leg shorter, and when patient sits, the curvature disappears
Rib angles may protrude and one hip may stick out

X-ray films
Curvature and angle of curvature, plus rotation

Fig. 4-22
Types of casts for correcting scoliosis.
A, Risser localizer cast.
B, Turnbuckle cast.

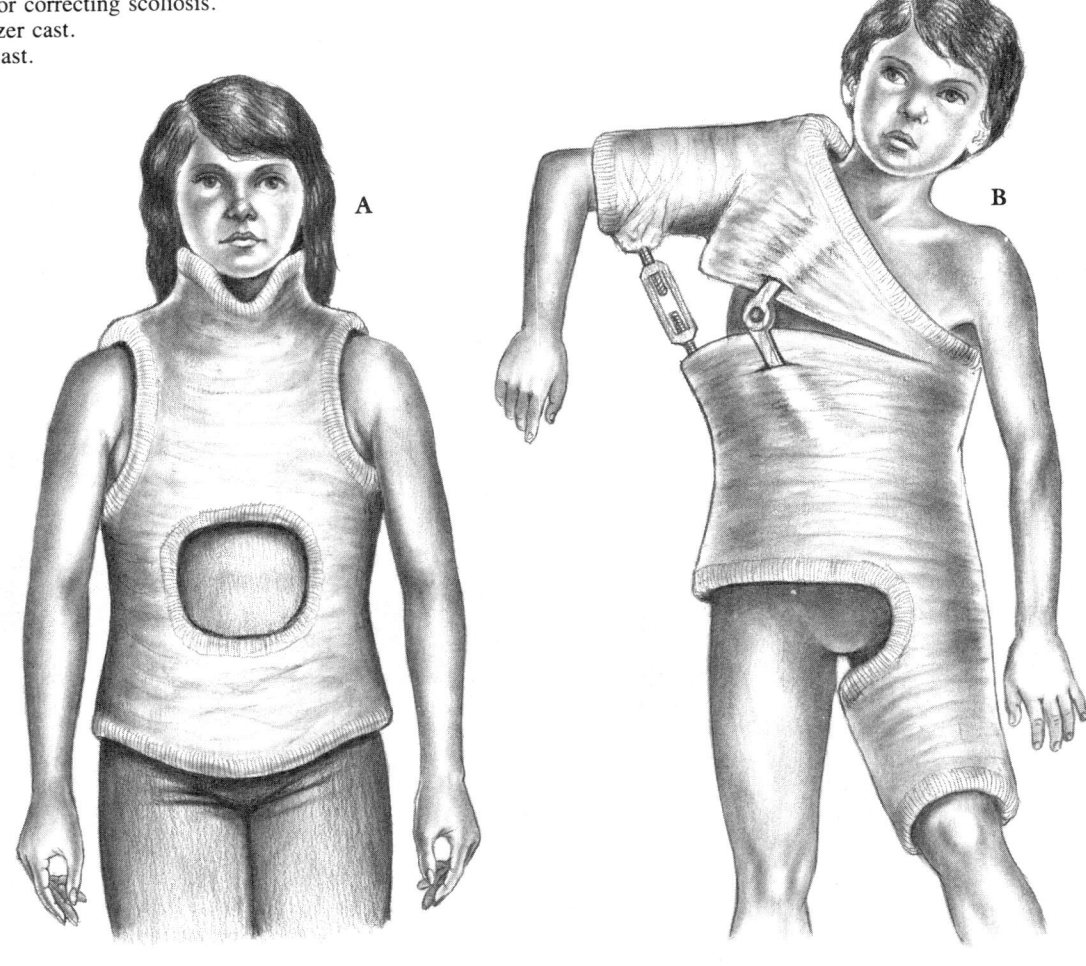

TREATMENT PLAN

Surgical

Straightening of curve with Harrington rod internal fixation with bone grafts to fuse spine

Dwyer procedure involves removal of wedges of vertebral bodies containing intervertebral discs and their adjoining end-plates; staples and screws are fixed to the vertebral bodies, and a cable is inserted through the screw heads; tightening the cable closes the vertebral wedges and straightens the curve

Electromechanical

Use of Milwaukee (or similar) brace

Application of distraction plaster cast to permit gradual straightening of curve (Fig. 4-22)

Application of Cotrel's traction (Fig. 4-23) or halo-femoral traction

ASSESSMENT: AREAS OF CONCERN

Entire spinal column

Spinal column will curve away from the midline

One shoulder or hip will be a different height than the other

Spine will have a noticeable hump when patient bends over

Spine will rotate when patient bends over

Systemic concerns

Patient may have muscle weakness through body

Cardiac or respiratory signs such as pulse rate or rhythm changes, dyspnea, or shortness of breath may be noted in more severe scoliosis

Psychosocial concerns

Self-concept

Alteration in body image and role expectations

Impaired physical mobility

Fig. 4-23
Cotrel's traction for scoliosis.

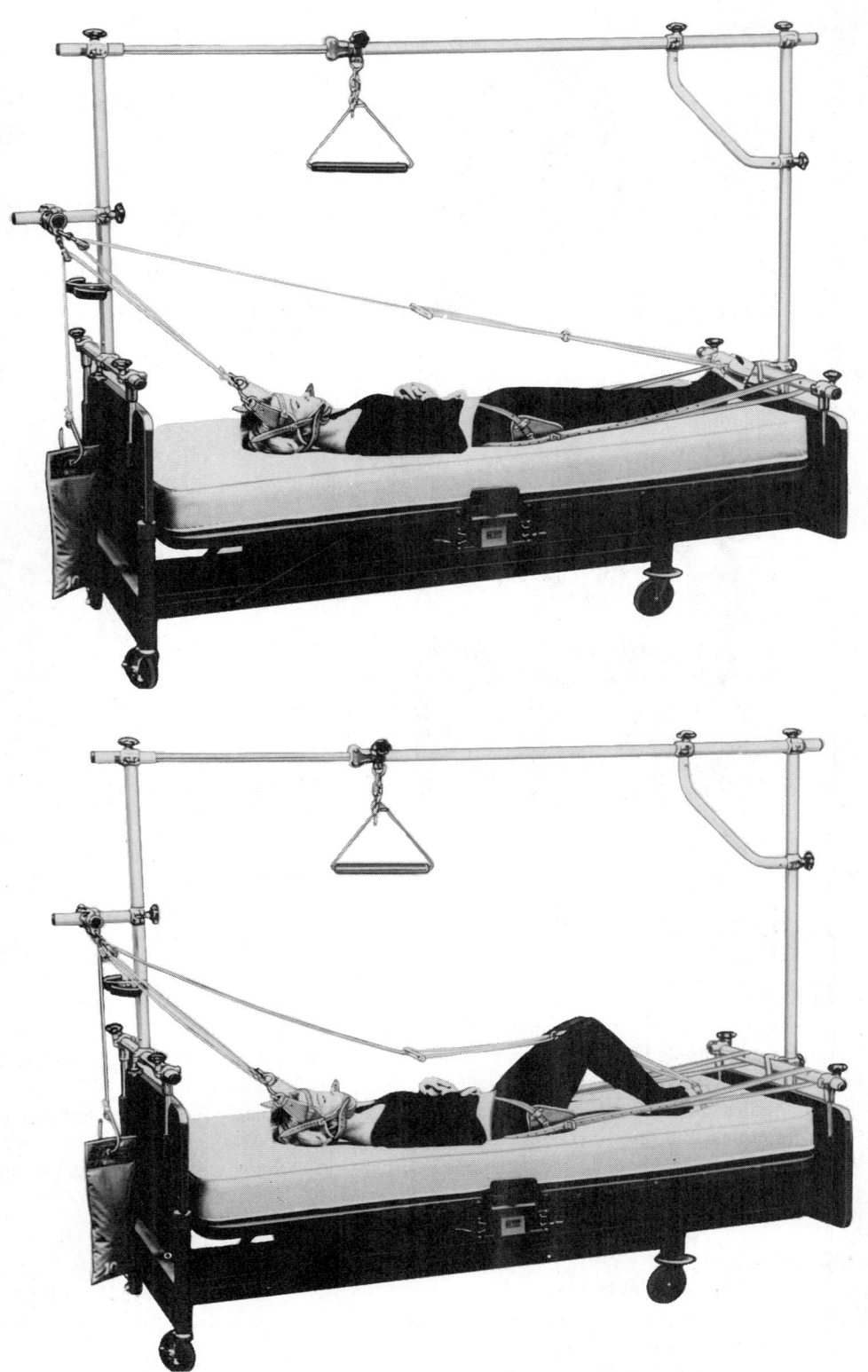

NURSING DIAGNOSES and NURSING INTERVENTIONS

Nursing Diagnosis	Nursing Intervention
Self-concept, disturbance in: body image, role performance	Discuss patient's feelings of inadequacy because of deformity. Discuss clothing to make brace less noticeable. Discuss need to continue wearing brace to prevent increase in rotation or lateralization. Discuss adjustments to clothing hemlines and so on to negate effects of scoliosis. Encourage usual peer relationships and activities.
Activity intolerance, potential	Teach proper posture and back-strengthening exercises to prevent progression.
Mobility, impaired physical	Discuss purposes of bed rest and Cotrel's or halo-femoral traction (Fig. 4-23). Change patient's position every 2 to 3 hours to maintain tissue integrity when necessary. Discuss need to limit activities to maintain traction or brace use. Discuss possibilities of brace; stress positive activities that patient can do. If surgery performed, discuss need for bed rest to permit healing (see p. 553 for spinal fusion nursing care). Encourage maintaining peer visits and interactions while on restricted movements to foster personal growth and esteem. Seek educational tutoring to maintain learning processes. Seek occupational therapy and physical therapy consultations to maintain muscle strength and spirits of patient. Provide well-balanced diet to promote healing after surgery.

Patient Education

1. Clarify inexorable progression of lateralization without treatment.
2. Encourage continuity of medical care to monitor status of scoliosis.
3. Reiterate need to wear brace at all times to prevent progression of scoliosis.

EVALUATION

Patient Outcome	Data Indicating That Outcome is Reached
Patient's posture has improved and curvature is lessened after treatment.	Patient stands straighter with less curvature and rotation; hips and shoulders are more normally aligned; respiratory functions are regained; and mobility is improved.
Patient returns to social interactions and roles.	Patient has improved self-concept and body image, is more able to regain family and social roles, and is positive about self and future.

Lordosis

Lordosis is a normal curvature of the lumbar spine.

Lordosis may become exaggerated during pregnancy or with large abdominal tumors or obesity that necessitates overcorrection to maintain balance when upright. Structural changes do not occur, and the condition is relieved with delivery, tumor removal, or weight loss.

Permanent hyperlordosis, although very rare, can occur from degenerative conditions of the lumbosacral discs or vertebral bodies such as osteoporosis, discussed previously. Treatments for hyperlordosis include use of a brace, lumbar belt, spinal fusion, or osteotomy.

ACQUIRED ANOMALIES

Acquired anomalies of musculoskeletal tissues usually result from trauma, including birth injuries, causing disruption of blood flow, inadequate oxygen supply, disruption of nerve stimulus transmission, or lack of proper muscle function. Examples of acquired anomalies are Erb's palsy, Klumpke's paralysis, Legg-Perthes disease, and Osgood-Schlatter disease.

Legg-Perthes Disease

Legg-Perthes disease is a disease of the femoral head in which either the cartilage or the femoral head itself develops avascular necrosis.

Legg-Perthes disease becomes evident between 3 and 10 years of age and is predominantly found in boys. The exact etiology is unknown although it may be associated with joint effusion from inflammatory processes, from repeated trauma, or from alterations in the blood supply during growth periods, resulting in ischemic changes.

PATHOPHYSIOLOGY

The femoral head becomes partly or wholly avascular. The avascular head does not grow; but the cartilage envelope surrounding the head does continue to enlarge (cartilage receives its nourishment from the synovial fluid). The growing cartilage is not occupied by growing bone so there is an increase in joint space. Blood vessels grow into the avascular head from the femoral neck. The metaphyseal area below the epiphysis becomes hyperemic and soft, compresses, and bends easily. The new blood vessels in the femoral head bring about some bone absorption in piecemeal fashion, distorting the roundness of the head. Even though new bone is formed with normal density, the femoral head remains permanently flat.

DIAGNOSTIC STUDIES

Physical examination
Irritable hip and joint with slightly diminished range of movements in all directions

Painless but diminished movements when disease is not active

X-ray films
Increased joint space with femoral head standing too far laterally

Increased density in avascular areas of head with flattening and patchy fragmentation

Variation in findings with degree of progression of pathologic condition

TREATMENT PLAN

Surgical
Osteotomy to change femur and acetabulum "fit," followed by plaster cast until union is achieved (2 to 3 months)

Electromechanical
Skin traction, applied to affected leg

Modified weight bearing with use of crutches

Maintenance of abduction of hip with plaster cast or brace to contain head within acetabulum

Supportive
Bed rest when hip is irritated

ASSESSMENT: AREAS OF CONCERN

Hip joint (one or both)
Range of movements

Soreness

Tenderness or pain

Limp

Systemic concerns
Urogenital anomaly (in about 4% of patients)

No other systemic signs

Psychosocial concerns
Mobility impaired

Self-concept: disturbance in body image and role expectations

NURSING DIAGNOSES and NURSING INTERVENTIONS

Nursing Diagnosis	Nursing Intervention
Mobility, impaired physical	Explain to child and parents purposes of bed rest. Assist with application of traction. Explain traction to child and parents. Change patient's position as traction allows every 3 to 4 hours. Encourage play activities to maintain child's strength and interest. Encourage parents to stay and participate in patient's care as able. Move child to play with other patients or bring them to child. Encourage activities appropriate to age to use and maximize interests and strength. Observe traction for proper and safe functioning. Assist or provide hygienic care as needed. Encourage intake of well-balanced diet. Teach child and parents crutch-walking techniques.
Self-concept, disturbance in: body image	Discuss need for cast, brace, or surgery with child and parents. Discuss self-limiting nature of disease and stress return to usual activities with some limitations depending on specific pathologic condition. Build on child's strengths during interactions for esteem.

Patient Education

1. Clarify purposes for various treatments.
2. Clarify bone healing after surgery.
3. Instruct about crutch walking.

EVALUATION

Patient Outcome	Data Indicating That Outcome is Reached
Patient's condition is arrested or relieved by treatments.	Patient has x-ray evidence of no continuation of disease processes and improved hip alignment, has no pain or joint limitation of movement, no limp, and increased ROM.
Patient resumes age-related social interactions and roles.	Patient returns to family, social, and educational activities and roles as related to age.

Osgood-Schlatter Disease

Osgood-Schlatter disease is a usually self-limiting condition of the patellar apophysis characterized by pain and tenderness below the knee and thought to be caused by injury to the apophysis or patellar tendon.

Osgood-Schlatter disease is a fairly common condition in young adolescents. Since it is a localized, self-limiting condition without sequelae, it will only be summarized here.

Osgood-Schlatter disease is centered around the knee and tibial plateau. It consists of a traction (pull) injury of the apophysis, the bony projection in the center of the tibia just below the knee, into which part of the patellar tendon is inserted (the remainder of the tendon is inserted on each side of the apophysis and prevents complete separation). The injury may be caused by, for example, repeated knee bends onto a hard surface, as by a baseball catcher. It can also result from the twisting motion of the knee with the leg extended while kicking a ball "soc-cer style." Although sports activities are major interests of young adolescents, they do experience aches and pains in their maturing tissues, even without significant injury, and Osgood-Schlatter condition is a prime example. The youngster complains of pain below the knee, and there is usually a noticeable lump. The lump is on the bony apophysis and is tender. Extension of the knee against resistance is also painful since it stretches the tendon. The two signs (i.e., a tender lump below the knee and an adolescent patient) are diagnostic of Osgood-Schlatter disease. An x-ray film may show fragmentation of the apophysis.[6] Treatments are few; the symptoms resolve spontaneously with the restriction of repetitive activities such as soccer and cycling. If symptoms persist after a period of time, the knee may be wrapped with elastic bandages, and for more severe involvement, the leg and knee may be placed in a cast or brace. Recovery is usually complete.

MISCELLANEOUS CONDITIONS ASSOCIATED WITH THE MUSCULOSKELETAL SYSTEM

During a difficult delivery, the baby may be injured about the neck and shoulder from the force required to deliver the baby through a snug or tight pelvis and vagina. The injuries that result may be traction injuries to the nerves of the brachial plexus, but the end results of such injuries are musculoskeletal from weakness and atrophy. Table 4-5 shows several injuries that can occur at birth but also can be experienced later in life from trauma. Nerve damage at any time of life causes significant musculoskeletal defects.

Without stimuli, muscles will become weakened and flaccid and will eventually shrink and atrophy. As muscles atrophy, they pull other tissues with them, namely, the tendons, ligaments, bones, and skin. Since the flexor muscles are generally stronger than the extensors, flexion contractures will usually result. Also, adduction is frequently more noted than abduction, although either may be present. Rotation and pronation of the muscles and joints are also commonly seen. Changes may also accompany the motor losses, with the affected tissues being either markedly more sensitive or entirely insensitive with variations between the extremes.

Table 4-5
Musculoskeletal Effects of Nerve Injuries

Brachial plexus nerves	Cervical roots of C5-7	Traction to arm or shoulder during delivery; gun shot wound; avulsion of nerves from excess traction accidentally applied	Erb's palsy: affected arm, forearm, and hand internally rotated and pronated. Injury may cause temporary weakness and palsy or if severe, will cause permanent paralysis with contracture of lower forearm, wrist, and fingers; sensory loss to outer arm.
Brachial, axillary, and musculocutaneous nerves	Cervical roots of C8 and T1	Breech delivery with arm above head; gun shot wound	Klumpke's palsy: intrinsic muscles of hand and flexor muscles of fingers are paralyzed; some sensory loss may be present in ulnar forearm and hand. Permanent effects: a claw hand develops in a flaccid, weak limb.
Radial nerve	Shoulder or elbow	Leaning on crutches in axillae; elbow: fracture; other: cutting of nerve	Radial weakness from leaning on crutches with axillary pressure is fully reversible. Elbow lesions: may have paralysis of wrist extensor and supinator muscles; eventually may need tendon transplants to wrist and fingers.
Ulnar nerve	Shoulder to elbow and to forearm	Open wounds (cut); fracture of medial epicondyle or lateral condyle; osteoarthritic changes	Ring and little fingers may be temporarily or permanently held in hyperextended positions while rest of the hand is clawed. Sensation is lost over ringer and little fingers. There is muscle wasting of intrinsic muscles of hand.
Median nerve	Wrist under transverse carpal ligament	Trauma; pregnancy; rheumatoid arthritis; postmenopausal state	Wasting of palmar thenar prominence (base of thumb; edema of hand; heavy, "clumsy" hand; sensory loss over radial 3½ fingers. If median nerve is severed without repair, paralysis of middle finger or index finger causes it to point ahead while other fingers are held in flexion; muscle wasting of hand (see pp. 497-499 for carpal tunnel syndrome).
Peroneal nerve	Neck of fibula	Pressure of splint; traction with leg in external rotation	Patient cannot dorsiflex or evert foot and toes; outer side of leg is wasted; foot-drop is present; sensation is lost over front and outer half of leg and dorsum of foot and toes. Posterior tibial nerve injuries may cause tarsal tunnel syndrome (p. 498).

Carpal Tunnel Syndrome

Carpal tunnel syndrome is a cluster of symptoms affecting the functions of the wrist, hand, and fingers, caused by compression of the median nerve.

Carpal tunnel syndrome is secondary to compression of the median nerve in the tendon sheath under the transverse ligament on the ventral surface of the wrist (Fig. 4-24). The syndrome usually follows trauma with subsequent fibrosis and scarring of the tendon sheath. However, no previous trauma may be noted, and curiously, pregnant women may experience carpal tunnel syndrome during their last trimester for as yet undetermined reasons, although fluid retention and edema may be contributing factors.

Overall, more women than men experience carpal tunnel syndrome. Menopausal women and patients with rheumatoid arthritis also have an increased incidence of this condition.

PATHOPHYSIOLOGY

The syndrome follows compression of the median nerve beneath the anterior carpal ligament. Because the tissues

in this part of the wrist normally fit closely together, any swelling will usually bring on the compressive symptoms.

Pain is one of the first symptoms, often occurring at night and waking the person with burning, tingling, and numbness. The fingers feel swollen, and the hand feels heavy. The person must usually hang the arm over the bed or get up and walk around to relieve the pain.

During the day the patient has few symptoms except when performing activities requiring turning of the wrist, such as knitting and crocheting. The hand is weaker and feels clumsy to the person. At times pain may also radiate up the arm.

Either one or both hands may be involved.

NOTE: A condition similar to carpal tunnel syndrome can occur in one or more other peripheral nerves, including the radial and ulnar tunnels in the upper extremity; and tarsal tunnel syndrome may occur in the lower extremity. Radial nerve weakness can temporarily occur from improper use of crutches; this clears when the person ceases resting the axillae on the shoulder supports of the crutches. Ulnar nerve injuries frequently accompany elbow trauma, which, when severe, can cause claw-

Fig. 4-24
A, Wrist structures affected in carpal tunnel syndrome. **B,** Decompression of the median nerve.

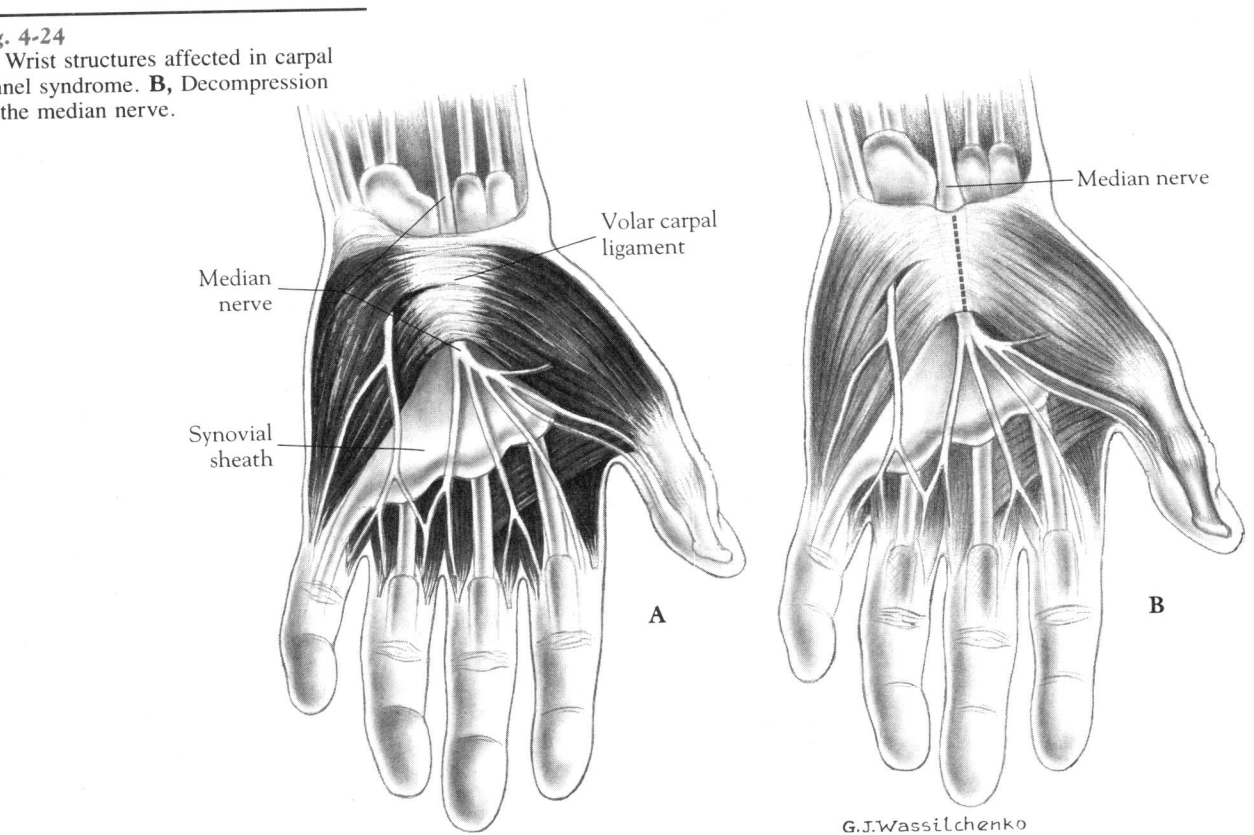

G.J.Wassilchenko

ing of the ring and little fingers plus loss of sensation over those fingers.

Trauma to the posterior tibial nerve or entrapment in the transverse tunnel over the Achilles tendon can give rise to the tarsal tunnel syndrome. The symptom patterns are the same as those of the carpal tunnel with the foot and ankle having the symptoms instead of the hand and wrist. Treatments for tarsal tunnel are the same as for other entrapment syndromes, being specific to the particular nerve, ligament, and tendon sheath involved.

DIAGNOSTIC STUDIES

History
Sensory changes
Paresthesia and numbness
Pain waking patient at night
Motor changes with clumsiness, heaviness of hand, and edema
Pain possibly radiating up arm
Similar symptoms in lower extremity with tarsal tunnel syndrome
Correlation with pregnancy, rheumatoid arthritis, or postmenopausal state

Physical examination
Deficits in sensory mapping along median nerve innervation pathways
Positive Tinel's sign: increased tingling with gentle tap over tendon sheath on ventral surface of central wrist
Edema of fingers noted
Thenar surfaces of palm thinner than normal (wasting)
Holding wrist in forced palmar flexion for 1 minute can elicit sensory changes

Electromyogram
Weakened muscle response

TREATMENT PLAN

Surgical
Release of carpal ligament and tendon to relieve compression (Fig. 4-24)

Chemotherapeutic
Injection of hydrocortisone (dosage varies) into tendon sheath to relieve inflammation

Electromechanical
Use of a cock-up splint to relieve pressure
Elevation to relieve edema
ROM exercises to lessen sense of clumsiness
Restriction of twisting and turning activities of wrist

Supportive
Continuation of usual medical care for systemic illness (rheumatoid arthritis) if present

ASSESSMENT: AREAS OF CONCERN

Wrist, hand, and fingers (both extremities)
Inability to use hands and fingers through normal ranges of motion
Movements limited
Presence or absence of edema, numbness, tingling, pain
Assessment of time when pain is present, severity, and activities that increase or decrease pain
Assessment of palmar thenar (base of thumb) surfaces for atrophy
Assessment of distribution of paresthesia (if present) into fingers or up arm

Systemic concerns
Rheumatoid arthritis
Postmenopausal state
Pregnancy in last trimester

Psychosocial concerns
Self-concept: disturbances in body image and role expectations
Impaired physical mobility

NURSING DIAGNOSES and NURSING INTERVENTIONS

Nursing Diagnosis	Nursing Intervention
Tissue perfusion, alteration in	Assess circulatory status of limb.
Mobility, impaired physical	Explain inflammatory processes to correlate need to limit activities of wrist and hand.
	Assist with and teach patient proper splint application; assist with hygienic care if necessary.

Nursing Diagnosis	Nursing Intervention
	Elevate hand and wrist if edema present. Assist with ROM exercises if ordered. Continue care for concomitant illnesses. Observe and assess site for relief of symptoms following injection of hydrocortisone, if used, or after surgical release. Encourage continuing follow-up medical care until recovery is complete.
Comfort, alteration in: pain	Administer pain medication as ordered; monitor and report patient response.

Patient Education

1. Reiterate explanations of inflammatory processes as bases for symptoms.
2. Teach about activities to lessen stress on inflamed tissues.
3. Reassure about relief of symptoms after surgical release or injection of steroids that follows reduction of edema and healing of involved tissues.
4. If patient is pregnant, discuss probable relief of symptoms following delivery.

EVALUATION

Patient Outcome	Data Indicating That Outcome is Reached
Patient regains joint ROM and muscle strength over time.	Patient performs self-care and regains strength after incisional healing.
Patient experiences pain-free wrist and hand functions.	Patient has no pain, edema, numbness, or tingling with use of wrist and hand.

Sciatic Nerve Injury

Sciatic nerve injury is a pathologic condition caused by some external trauma to the nerve.

Injury to the sciatic nerve may be primary from a gunshot wound, stabbing, fall, or other cause, or it may be secondary to pressure from a rupture of an intervertebral nucleus pulposus, which exerts pressure on the spinal nerves as they exit the spinal cord and traverse the sciatic nerve. The intervertebral discs that suffer the most frequent ruptures are at L5-S1 (95%) and L4-L5 interspaces. Cervical intervertebral discs rupture less frequently.

The following discussion is focused on the sciatic nerve pathologic findings secondary to herniation (rupture) of one or more lumbar intervertebral nuclei pulposi.

PATHOPHYSIOLOGY

The nucleus pulposus is a semigelatinous mass inside the cartilaginous anulus (disc) between the bodies of each vertebra. When the cartilage of the anulus cracks or degenerates, it allows the nucleus pulposus to herniate or rupture out through the cracks. A ruptured disc, then, is a two-fold process of degeneration of the anulus with herniation of the nucleus pulposus material.

Rupture of the anulus is generally caused by degenerative changes in the cartilaginous structures of the anulus. As the disc (anulus) ages, it loses elasticity, partly from changes in its collagen fibers and partly from decreases in its fluid content. These changes weaken the disc, making it unable to tolerate even usual body weight. It flattens or bulges, and additional pressure from lifting, straining, increased weight, or a sudden twist, turn, or sharp bending of the back may cause the anulus to bulge backward or to tear, allowing the nucleus pulposus to extrude through the crack. The mass can extrude anteriorly toward the cord, laterally toward the lamina and facets, or posteriorly toward the posterior spinous processes. The extruded mass presses on the dura mater or on the nerve roots or both, causing pain in the back with radiation to the sciatic nerve. The presence of the extruded mass plus the pressure cause edema to develop, which also increases pain. At times, if the entire nucleus mass has not extruded, it may move back inside the disc when the edema subsides. If the mass stays extruded, it can adhere to the nerve roots or their dural sheaths, adding to the scarring and pain. In time the prolapsed material can also disturb the functioning of the facets of the vertebrae, leading to further degeneration of these joints.

The incident that causes the acute rupture can be as trivial as a sneeze or cough while the person is bent forward. Usually it is brought about by lifting something while the body is not in optimal lift position or if the load is unexpectedly heavy. Excessive pressure is referred from tensed abdominal and back muscles to the anulus and then to the nucleus, which ruptures through the weakened, cracked anulus. Signs of sciatic nerve pressure follow the rupture.

DIAGNOSTIC STUDIES

History
Sudden acute pain in low back

Physical examination
Loss of normal lordotic curve
"List" or tilt to side
Tense, tight back muscles
Tenderness in low back that may radiate to buttocks
ROM movements limited in forward flexion, in lateral flexion, and sometimes in extension
Pain radiating down (usually) one leg to foot and toes
Straight leg raising limited by pain
Pain increased with foot dorsiflexion
Sensations impaired on outer thigh, calf, and foot
Paresthesia with numbness and tingling
Knee and ankle reflexes possibly diminished or absent (knee reflex rarely lost)

X-ray film of back
Tilt
Diminished disc space (not necessarily diagnostic)

Myelogram
Location of rupture revealed by impaired dye flow (see p. 445 for myelography)

CT scan
Ruptured disc

TREATMENT PLAN

Surgical
Hemilaminectomy with removal of extruded nucleus and degenerated anulus
Spinal fusion
Fenestration to open nerve root exit sites

Chemotherapeutic
Analgesic-antipyretics
Aspirin, 600-1000 mg q4h
Acetaminophen, 600-1000 mg q4h
Antianxiety agents
Diazepam (Valium), 2-10 mg po q4-6h
Narcotic analgesics
Oxycodone (Percodan), 30-60 mg q4h for severe pain uncontrolled by aspirin
Meperidine (Demerol), 50-150 mg IM q3h

Electromechanical
Application of skin traction (pelvic belt)
Williams (head of bed and knee gatch each elevated 45 degrees) position in bed
Diathermy to low back three or four times daily; ice massage
Application of canvas back support or metal back brace
Physical therapy with specific exercises to strengthen back and abdominal muscles

Supportive
Bed rest on firm mattress
Cessation of lifting and stooping
Back massage after diathermy

ASSESSMENT: AREAS OF CONCERN

Vertebral column, lumbar back, and sciatic nerve dermatomes
Degree of lumbar lordotic curve
Range of movements of back (forward, backward, lateral to each side)
"List" or tilt to either side
Tenderness
Pain in back or buttocks, radiating down posterior thighs and legs to feet and toes
Assessment of muscles for spasm, tenseness, or tightness
Leg-raising assessments
Sensory functions "around" thigh, leg, and foot (bilaterally)
Strength or absence of knee and ankle reflexes
Bowel or bladder function changes

Systemic concerns
  Concomitant systemic diseases
    Rheumatoid arthritis
    Ankylosing spondylitis
    Osteoarthrosis

Psychosocial concerns
  Self-concept, disturbance in: body image, role performance
  Mobility, impaired physical
  Comfort, alteration in: acute pain in lower back with radiation

NURSING DIAGNOSES and NURSING INTERVENTIONS

Nursing Diagnosis	Nursing Intervention
Mobility, impaired physical	Explain purposes of hospitalization, bed rest, and traction. Explain use of firm mattress and bed position (Williams position) to relax spasm of back muscles. Prepare patient for physical therapy, diathermy, and massage; assist with hygienic care to have patient ready and to lessen strain to back. Assist patient to apply back support, brace, or belt; teach self-application. Place in skin traction belt; observe patient's responses; remove traction while sleeping to lessen muscle spasms.
Self-concept, disturbance in: body image, role performance	Encourage patient to discuss usual roles and temporary adjustments needed with family members.
Comfort, alteration in: pain	Keep patient on bed rest to relieve inflammation with acute low back pain. Administer analgesics around the clock as ordered to maintain an adequate blood level for first 2 or 3 days. Administer muscle relaxants as ordered to relieve spasms. Assess effects of Williams position to relieve spasms and pain. Offer back massage to relax muscles and relieve inflammation. Assess relief of pressure signs on sciatic nerve by determining relief of paresthesia, numbness, etc. Perform "laminectomy checks." Report continued presence of pain, paresthesia, and muscle spasms to physician. Use dietary measures, high fluid intake, and medication to prevent constipation (straining increases pain).

Patient Education

1. Teach patient bed positions to relieve pain and inflammation.
2. Teach patient proper lifting postures, when feasible.
3. Teach exercises to strengthen muscles.

EVALUATION

Patient Outcome	Data Indicating That Outcome is Reached
Patient experiences relief of back pain and muscle spasms.	Patient uses back for ADL without pain, numbness, radiation to legs, or muscle spasms. Patient has no limitations in ROM.
Patient resumes social interactions and roles.	Patient returns to usual family, social, and employment roles and activities.

Medical Interventions

AMPUTATION

Description and Rationale

An amputation is the removal of all or part of a specific tissue or organ. Musculoskeletal tissues are frequently amputated because of crush injuries, severe sepsis, malignant tumors, or gangrene resulting from loss of arterial or venous circulatory integrity. Less frequently a limb may be amputated because of intractable pain from paralysis or multiple recurrent flare-ups of osteomyelitis threatening not only the limb but also the individual's life.

The following terms are used to refer to amputations involving the extremities:

forequarter Removal of entire arm, forearm, and hand; extremity disarticulated at shoulder joint

arm Amputation above elbow or along forearm

hemipelvectomy Removal of thigh, leg, and foot; also referred to as hindquarter amputation

thigh Amputation above the knee (AKA)

lower leg Amputation below the knee (BKA)

foot Amputation of toes and part of foot at metatarsal joints

finger or toe Amputation of part or all of one or more fingers or toes

The varieties of amputations are referred to as (1) *provisional,* which is done when primary healing is unlikely, (2) *definitive end-bearing,* which is done when weight bearing is to be borne through the end of the stump, and (3) *definitive non-end-bearing,* which is done when weight will not be borne at the end of the stump. When weight is to be borne through the end of the stump, the incision is not made at the end but is cut through or near a joint; if weight will not be borne at the end of the stump, the incision can be terminal (at the end of the stump). Also, the incision may be cut perpendicularly to the bone through all the tissues, called a guillotine incision, with little or no incisional closure and only loosely applied dressings. The guillotine incision is used in grossly infected tissues. The more frequently used incision is closed and snugly dressed after the tissues are amputated; it is commonly done in noninfected tissues.

During the surgical procedure, bleeding is controlled through application of a tourniquet unless there is arterial insufficiency. Skin flaps are made, usually of equal length for upper limb or above-knee amputations and with a longer posterior flap for below-knee amputations. The muscles are divided distal to the intended site of bone resection, and later opposing muscle groups are sutured over the bone end to each other and to the periosteum to provide better muscle control and circulation. Nerves are divided proximal to the bone end. After the bone is cut, all vessels and bleeders are ligated carefully and the skin flaps are sutured closed (unless tissues are infected), drains are inserted, and the stump is firmly dressed.

Contraindications and Cautions

1. If the amputation is to be done to remove a malignant tumor, metastasis to distant sites is a contraindication.
2. Lack of arterial circulation requires that the amputation be proximal to the gangrenous or necrotic tissues.
3. Sufficient tissues must be left on and over the stump for fitting of a prosthesis when possible.

Preprocedural Nursing Care

1. Meticulous skin cleansing with antiseptic solutions removes transient and some resident bacteria.
2. Presence of peripheral pulses (may be absent in "dry" gangrene) is determined.
3. Edema, color, temperature, skin condition, and pain (when present) are compared with tissues on the opposite side of body. Edema may be pronounced in venous obstruction associated with "wet" gangrene.
4. The skin is observed for open or draining areas.
5. Vital signs are checked for evidence of systemic infection and to monitor the patient's general condition.
6. The patient is observed for hemorrhage and possible shock with crush injuries.

7. If the patient is a child or older adult, factors related to age and developmental or educational level that could affect recovery and self-care after the amputation are determined.

8. A rehabilitated person with a similar amputation may visit the patient preoperatively when feasible.

TREATMENT PLAN

Surgical
Wound suction continuously
Change of dressings as needed

Chemotherapeutic
Anti-infective agents
    Cephalothin sodium (Keflin), 500-1000 mg IV q4-6h for 48-72 h (or longer, if ordered)
Narcotic analgesic agents
    Meperidine (Demerol), 50-100 mg IM q3h for pain
Intravenous fluid replacement with 5% dextrose in 0.45 normal saline, 2000-3000 ml for 24 h

Electromechanical
Stump elevated for 24 hours, then kept flat and extended (Order for elevation depends on presence or amount of edema in stump.)
Adduction exercises of amputated extremity, 10 times per hour after 24 hours
For lower extremity amputation, turning to prone position four times daily
Thigh (hamstring) tightening exercises in prone position begun after 24 hours (10 times every 4 hours)
Up with crutches three times daily on second postoperative day

Supportive
Physical therapy consultation for exercise regimen and to assist with ambulation
Regular diet as desired
Stump wrapping after fifth postoperative day (or after sutures are removed)
Orthotic technician (prosthetist) to measure stump for prosthesis
Stump check every hour for first 24 hours to note color, drainage, edema, bleeding, sutures (wound), and pulses proximal to incision site

Tourniquet present at bedside continuously
Up in chair after 12 to 24 hours
Pulmonary deep breathing and coughing every 4 hours
NOTE: Some patients may return from surgery with a prosthesis already in place, held to the stump with plaster (an immediate postsurgical fitting). It is usually left in place up to 10 days, after which it is removed, the sutures are removed, and a new cast is applied. This fitting lessens edema and pain, although the rigidity of the plaster delays the shaping of the stump into a conical shape. However, the immediate postsurgical prosthesis does permit earlier ambulation and discharge, particularly in younger patients.

ASSESSMENT: AREAS OF CONCERN

Site of amputation (stump)
Drainage or bleeding scant and serosanguineous
Edema slight
Dressing intact without constriction
Pain may be sharp and acute in incisional area
If Penrose drain is present, drainage may be scant to moderate amount, although still serosanguineous
Tourniquet should be at bedside

Entire extremity
Extremity should remain extended
Range of motion of muscles and joints may be slightly limited by pain or stiffness
Only incisional area edema or erythema unless infection develops

Psychosocial concerns
Concern with alteration in body image and appearance
Presence of phantom pain
Alteration in mobility and ability to maintain livelihood and income

Other complications
Hemorrhage, wound infection, or dehiscence
Development of contractures
Persistence of phantom pain
Development of neuromas
Excessive scar formation

NURSING DIAGNOSES and NURSING INTERVENTIONS

Nursing Diagnosis	Nursing Intervention
Self-concept, alteration in: body image	Allow and encourage patient to ventilate feelings of mutilation, grief, and loss; avoidance of looking at stump; anger; and such.
	Encourage patient to assist with dressing changes and wrapping of stump as able. Teach family member wrapping techniques if necessary.
	Encourage family members to walk with patient to maintain strength and social contacts.
	Encourage wearing of personal clothing and grooming to maintain individuality and personality.
Mobility, impaired physical	Turn and position on side, back, and abdomen (after 24 hours) to maintain muscle and joint ROM.
	Teach adduction and extension exercises and assist patient to perform them every 4 hours.
	Assist with sitting in chair and ambulation with aid as able.
	Prepare patient for physical therapy, transportation for exercises, and stump wrapping if appropriate. Encourage family members to learn wrapping.
	Encourage family members to walk with patient during initial ambulation periods, accompanied by health professionals.
	Teach patient purposes of prone and extension positions to prevent contractures.
	Assist prosthetist with prosthesis measurements and fitting as needed.
Comfort, alteration in: pain (nerve trauma following surgery)	Administer narcotics as ordered every 3 hours for first 24 to 48 hours until surgical trauma is lessened; then administer as needed.
	Explain causes for phantom pain sensations and methods to overcome them.
	Administer antibiotics as ordered to prevent infection, thereby lessening pain and scarring.
	Encourage activities for self-care and ambulation to maintain positive outlook and maximal strength.
	Encourage or secure social service consultation for economic and employment aid.
	Secure continuity of care referral for follow-up care.

Patient Education

1. Teach patient and family proper positions, exercises, and ambulation techniques.
2. Teach patient and family stump-wrapping techniques.
3. Teach patient and family that prolonged phantom pain experiences are unusual and should receive medical attention.
4. Teach patient and family skin care to prevent stump irritation or breakdown.
5. Teach patient and family signs of a wound infection.

EVALUATION

Patient Outcome	Data Indicating That Outcome is Reached
Skin and incision heal.	Scar is well approximated with no excess scarring.
Patient and family demonstrate ability to perform care.	Patient can wrap stump correctly and can ambulate with crutches or prosthesis.
Alteration in body image and self-concept is achieved.	Patient has positive outlook toward condition and is able to return to usual personal and employment/economic position following convalescence.

ARTHROSCOPY

Description and Rationale

With the advent and development of the arthroscope, startling changes have occurred in operative examination and treatment of pathologic joint conditions. Although the knee joint is still a major focus, nearly all joints including the spinal canal (experimentally in Japan) can be examined with the arthroscope. The multiple benefits of early arthroscopic treatment with specialized techniques and instruments in the hands of a skilled practitioner include lessened inflammation, degeneration, and posttraumatic arthrosis. Patients can usually return to their daily activities sooner with full use of the involved joint following arthroscopic examination and repair.

Arthroscopy is most frequently done for diagnosis and treatment of knee injuries, primarily torn or damaged menisci. The menisci, C-shaped rings of cartilage covering the ends of the tibia within the knee joint, are subject to degeneration, tears, and wear. Cartilage has no intrinsic blood supply, and if torn, worn, or degenerated it rarely heals without development of unsatisfactory fibrocartilage. Trauma to the meniscus is greatest among athletes who experience tears from external forces such as a tackle or from internal forces when a load exceeds the compressibility and resiliency of the cartilage; this may occur in a single incident or over time from repeated stressors. The meniscal tear may cause slight, partial, or complete avulsion from adjoining bone tissues.

The discussion that follows will focus on the knee because it is the joint most commonly examined and treated arthroscopically.

Loose or torn pieces of menisci up to 1 inch in size can be removed arthroscopically. One or more small incisions may be required for full visualization of the joint. Incisions or "ports" for arthroscopic procedures are on the mediolateral or posterolateral surfaces of the knee joint superior to the patella.

Contraindications and Cautions

1. Arthroscopy requires skilled practitioners and more specialized techniques than with more extensive arthrotomy procedures.
2. The use of more than one port for visualization of the joint may lead to infection.
3. Small pieces of torn or loose cartilage may be missed if hidden under other joint tissues.
4. Hemorrhage must be prevented to lessen posttraumatic arthrosis.
5. Scar formation may predispose to future tears of ligaments or cartilage.

6. Postoperative physical therapy and individualized programs of exercises must be prescribed and performed to maintain or regain the joint's mobility, stability, and strength.

TREATMENT PLAN

Chemotherapeutic

Finish IV fluids; then attach IV needle to heparin well

Narcotic analgesics

Meperidine (Demerol), 50-100 mg IM q3h as needed for 3 d

Oxycodone (Percodan), 30-60 mg po q4h prn after 3 d

Anti-infective agents

Cephazolin (Ancef), 250-1000 mg q6-8h IM

Cephalexin (Keflex), 500 mg po q6h

Supportive

Bed rest until patient is fully alert; then can be up with crutches four times daily

Check of vital signs every 2 hours for 6 hours; then every 4 hours

Neurovascular checks every hour for 24 hours

Ice bags to knee continuously

Change dressing as needed

Advancement to regular diet as tolerated

Physical therapy consultation for knee exercises

ASSESSMENT: AREAS OF CONCERN

Neurovascular status of knee joint and lower extremity

Color: may be slightly paler, but perfusion should be within 2 to 4 seconds

Temperature: slightly cooler

Peripheral pulses: should be present

Movement: should be normal in ankle; knee should be able to be flexed with moderate discomfort

Sensations: should be normal

Psychosocial concerns

Concern with regaining knee mobility to return to usual ADL and activities without deficit

Complications

Hemorrhage

Thrombus formation

Posttraumatic degeneration and arthrosis

NURSING DIAGNOSES and NURSING INTERVENTIONS

Nursing Diagnosis	Nursing Intervention
Tissue perfusion, alteration in	Assess neurovascular status as ordered. Apply ice bags to knee continuously.
Mobility, impaired physical	Assist to positions of comfort; assist to ambulate as needed. Assess drainage and change dressing as needed (drainage should be scant, serosanguineous). Assist with physical therapy exercises as needed. Teach walking up and down stairs to regain joint motion.
Comfort, alteration in: pain	Administer medications as ordered for pain. Assist to stand to void. Assist and prepare tray for dietary intake.

EVALUATION

Patient Outcome	Data Indicating That Outcome is Reached
Patient regains joint motion.	Patient has full ROM without pain or limitation, has returned to usual activities, and does not have degenerative changes.

MENISCECTOMY

Description and Rationale

Traditional meniscectomy for removal of larger portions of damaged or degenerated cartilage from the knee joint is still required at times although the incidence of this more extensive procedure will surely lessen as arthroscopic techniques and skilled practitioners become more available. The techniques and equipment have only been in use in the United States since 1974, but in these past 10 years the knowledge and understanding gained are revolutionizing the thinking and surgical treatment of meniscal lesions. Open meniscectomy is still required for many patients, however, and some nursing care differs from that of closed arthroscopy (Fig. 4-25).

Contraindications and Cautions

1. Small pieces of torn or loose cartilage may be missed if hidden under other joint tissues.
2. Hemorrhage must be prevented to lessen posttraumatic arthrosis.
3. Scar formation may predispose to future tears of ligament or cartilage.
4. Postoperative physical therapy and individualized programs of exercises must be prescribed and performed to maintain or regain the joint's mobility, stability, and strength.

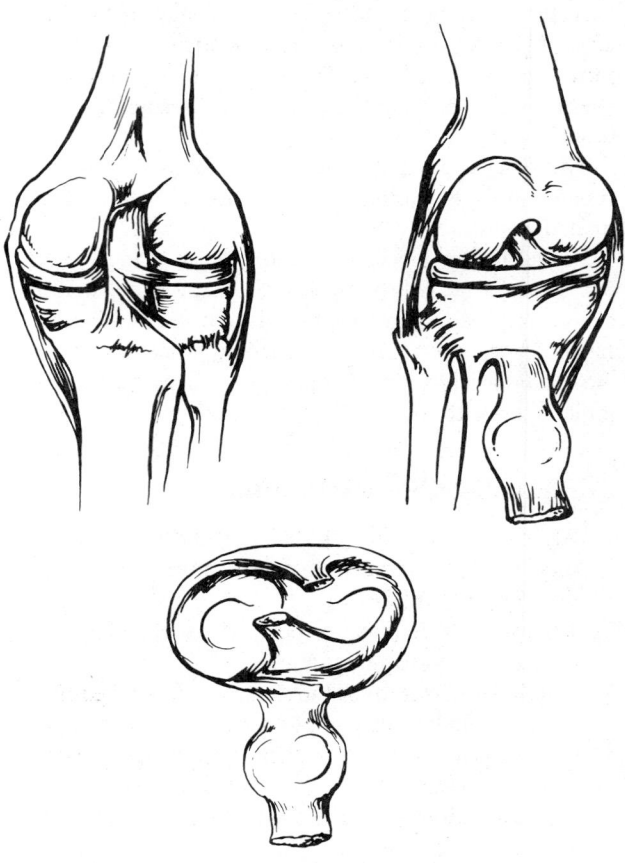

Fig. 4-25
Meniscus of knee joint.

TREATMENT PLAN

Chemotherapeutic

Narcotic analgesic agents

Meperidine (Demerol), 75-100 mg IM q3h for severe pain

Antianxiety agents

Hydroxyzine (Vistaril), 25-50 mg IM q3h with meperidine

Analgesic-antipyretic agents

Aspirin, 600-1000 mg po q4h prn

Anti-infective agents

Cefazolin sodium (Ancef) or cephalothin sodium (Keflin) (or other cephalosporin), 500-1000 mg q6-8 h for 48-72 h, or longer as individually required

Cephalexin (Keflex), 250-500 mg q6h po, after IV antibiotic is discontinued

Electromechanical

Crutch walking with partial weight bearing; varies with specific procedure but may begin as early as 24 to 48 hours postoperatively

Apply knee immobilizer splint between exercise periods

Supportive

Maintain postoperative dressing and immobilization as ordered (varies with specific procedure; for meniscectomy, 24 hours and then up with crutches four times daily)

Check peripheral pulses every 2 hours with neurovascular checks

Elevate leg and foot of bed

Apply ice bags to incisional area

On third postoperative day, begin straight leg–raising (SLR) exercises

Begin active and passive ROM knee exercises in physical therapy on third to fifth postoperative day (varies with procedure and patient need, but specific program will be prescribed)

ASSESSMENT: AREAS OF CONCERN

Knee joint and incisional area

Presence, amount, and type of drainage (usually is scant, serosanguineous)

Skin color (paler than unoperative knee)

Edema and pain (increasing edema and pain are untoward signs of excessive bleeding)

Ability or inability to move leg with knee extended

Psychosocial concerns

Alteration in or concerns with body image and ability to return to usual activities and sports (if an athlete)

Limitation of mobility over time

Other complications

Development of hematoma or thrombus in or distal to knee or calf

Instability of knee joint

Recurrence of pain with or without degeneration or reinjury of tissues of knee joint

Compartment syndrome also possible (ischemia of muscles leading to necrosis of tissues)

NURSING DIAGNOSES and NURSING INTERVENTIONS

Nursing Diagnosis	Nursing Intervention
Tissue perfusion, alteration in: peripheral	Perform *neurovascular (circulation) checks* every 2 hours including check of color, edema, temperature, pain, sensory or motor changes, ability to use or lift leg, peripheral pulses, extension of inflammation to contiguous tissues above or below knee, and comparison of operative leg characteristics with unoperative leg. Report changes in findings; may require removal of constricting dressings or additional surgery if pulses absent. Elevate leg and foot of bed. Apply ice bags to site. Continue checks every 4 to 6 hours to note changes early.
Mobility, impaired physical	Maintain bed rest as ordered. Begin SLR exercises on second or third postoperative day as ordered. Encourage performing quadriceps setting exercises every 2 hours. Encourage setting of gluteus muscles every 2 hours when ordered. Assist to be up in a chair without weight bearing initially. Then progress as ordered to assist with crutch walking as needed. Monitor patient's response. Teach patient necessity to continue exercise program at home. Teach patient application of knee immobilizer, splint, or brace if required.

Nursing Diagnosis	Nursing Intervention
	Assist with ADL as required.
	Encourage weight lifting of operative leg as ordered.
Urinary elimination, alteration in patterns	Assist to stand to void. Check adequacy of voiding three times.
	Monitor intake and output.
Skin integrity, impairment of: actual	Change dressings of wound as needed.
	Observe drainage characteristics and amount; report findings to physician.
Comfort, alteration in: pain	Administer narcotics per order every 3 hours with potentiator. Increase time periods between administration of narcotics or analgesics as acute pain abates.
	Administer aspirin between narcotics (enhances pain relief and relief of inflammation). Encourage use of aspirin as anti-inflammatory drug if ordered (patients are usually discharged with either aspirin or acetaminophen ''prescription'' for over the counter securing).
	Encourage position changes to lessen pressure and fatigue.
	Report continuing severe pain, change in peripheral pulses, or increasing edema as signs indicative of ischemia, thrombus formation, or developing compartment syndrome.

Patient Education

1. Clarify recovery program and exercise and leg-raising activities to aid recovery.
2. Clarify rationale for each part of neurovascular check to gather thorough information about tissues.
3. Reiterate the need for continuing the exercise and ambulation programs prescribed for long-term recovery.
4. Encourage return to social contacts to regain mobility and comfort even though using crutches and having partial weight bearing only.
5. Stress need to refrain from sports activities that could retraumatize unhealed tissues until physician permits resumption.

EVALUATION

Patient Outcome	Data Indicating That Outcome is Reached
ROM of knee joint is regained.	Patient has 90 degree flexion and full extension of knee without pain.
Patient engages in usual ADL as desired.	Patient returns to sports activities or usual ADL with protective knee covering, if required. Patient does not experience post-traumatic arthrosis.

ARTHROPLASTY

Arthroplasty refers to repair or refashioning of one or both sides, parts, or specific tissues within a joint. Parts of a joint repaired during an arthroplasty include bones, cartilage, synovium, ligaments, and tendons. Bursae are outside a joint, but they may be removed during an arthroplastic procedure.

Arthroplasties are described as (1) *interpositional arthroplasty,* in which a metal barrier is interposed between the bones after reshaping one or both bone ends (e.g., cup arthroplasty done currently to preserve as much bone as possible, particularly the head of the femur); (2) *gap arthroplasty,* in which one of the bones in the joint is excised (e.g., Girdlestone arthroplasty performed mainly now to remove infected bones); (3) *partial joint replacement arthroplasty,* in which one joint bone end is replaced with a prosthesis (e.g., Moore prosthesis of head of femur), and (4) *total joint replacement arthroplasty,* in which both bone ends are replaced (e.g., total hip or knee replacement). Synovectomy is an example of an excisional arthroplasty, as is a meniscectomy with removal of the meniscus within the knee joint.

Refashioning or repairing a joint usually follows trauma, degeneration, or inflammation of one or more tissues within the joint. The surgery may be performed within hours after a traumatic injury, such as a hip fracture or meniscus tear, or it may be done after years of inflammatory processes in a joint, such as occurs with rheumatoid arthritis or after degenerative erosions accompanying osteoarthrosis from restrictive joint movements.

An arthroplasty, therefore, is usually performed to relieve restrictive movements of a joint, to relieve pain, to remove loose or torn tissues (ligaments, cartilage, or calcium), to reshape one or both bone ends to make a joint perform more smoothly, or to remove overgrown, hypertrophied tissue (synovium) or atrophic, avascular tissue (avascular head of femur).

Contraindications and Cautions

The age of a specific patient may be a contraindication to a particular arthroplasty. Arthroplasties are performed infrequently in children because they may damage the growth epiphyses and the immature cartilage and bones. Surgical repair of childhood conditions such as Legg-Perthes disease (p. 494) is undertaken only after more conservative medical treatments fail to resolve the condition. Adolescents with large, unsightly bunions may have an arthroplasty to correct them, but often surgical correction is required again in later years. Older adults with rheumatoid arthritis or degenerative osteoarthrosis may have their surgical procedures delayed to correct a concurrent endocrine, cardiac, or respiratory condition, as also will those patients having arthroplastic surgery following trauma.

Bunionectomy: Keller or Mayo Arthroplasty
Description and Rationale

Keller arthroplasty is the most commonly performed one for hallux valgus and bunions. It involves excision of the proximal part of the proximal phalanx plus trimming of the prominent portion of the metatarsal head. Mayo procedure involves excision of the first metatarsal head and trimming of the prominent portion of the proximal phalanx. Both procedures are examples of gap arthroplasty; the gap is usually filled with a Silastic implant. Removal of the bunion (enlarged bursa and knob of bone) is also done during the arthroplasty. A plaster toe cap or splint is applied to some patients.

Contraindications and Cautions

1. Hallux valgus in an adolescent is primarily unsightly and deforming; surgical correction may be delayed until the patient is older since osteotomy is a fairly radical procedure at this age.
2. Surgery may be delayed or avoided in some patients through careful attention to properly fitting footwear. Padding may protect the bunion to lessen pain. Exercises and use of a metatarsal arch support may lessen splayfoot.
3. Surgery may not be entirely successful or satisfactory. Bunions can recur, and surgery may weaken the foot slightly.

TREATMENT PLAN

Surgical
Arthroplasty
Bunionectomy

Chemotherapeutic
Narcotic analgesics
Meperidine (Demerol), 75-100 mg IM q3h for 24-48 h for severe pain
Codeine (codeine sulfate or phosphate), 30-60 mg
Oxycodone (Percodan), 5-10 mg po
Analgesic-antipyretic agents
Aspirin, 600-1000 mg po q4h for minor pain

Electromechanical
Up with crutches when edema lessens, usually in 2 days (depends on whether surgery is bilateral)

Supportive
Check cast or splint for tightness, intactness, and drainage
Assess wound for edema, pain, and drainage
Elevate foot (feet) on pillows
Elevate foot of bed
Keep patient on bed rest for 24 to 48 hours and then up in chair without weight bearing
Apply ice bags to operative site continuously

ASSESSMENT: AREAS OF CONCERN

Preoperative
Area of great toe (bilateral)
Presence of deformity
Swelling over first metatarsal head (bursa)
Pain
Limitation of movement of joint with or without pain
Presence of hallux valgus deviation

Hammer toe
Crowding of second toe
Splayfoot
Calluses or corns
Foot
   Varus or valgus deviation of one or both feet usually
     noted
Shoes
   Condition
   Type
   Evidence of wear
   Softness
   Data indicative of footwear contributing to hallux
     condition
Systemic
   Evidence of gout
     Tophi
     Elevated serum uric acid levels
     Pattern of acute pain

Postoperative
   Great toe or toes and incisional site
     Assessment of plaster cast or splint for intactness
     Visible portions of toe
       Color
       Edema
       Pain
       Pulses proximal or distal to incision (if able to
         locate in toe)
       Drainage
       Bleeding
     Dressing
       Tightness
       Drainage
     Amount of sensation and motion in operative area
       (cast may limit movement)
   Psychosocial concerns
     Alteration in body image, comfort, and mobility
     Possibility of recurrence or lack of wound healing
   Other complications
     Excessive scarring or recurrence of bursa
     Weakening of foot joint or joints of or near one or
       more toes

NURSING DIAGNOSES and NURSING INTERVENTIONS

Nursing Diagnosis	Nursing Intervention
Comfort, alteration in: pain	Put bed cradles on bed to cover feet without pressure of linens. Keep foot of bed and feet elevated. Administer narcotics as ordered for acute pain. Administer analgesics after acute pain is relieved. Apply ice bags as ordered. Assist with position changes and skin care; do back massage as needed. Instruct patient about analgesic and anti-inflammatory effects of aspirin and ice.
Mobility, impaired physical	Assist to be up in chair when able. Assist with use of crutches when able. Encourage activities as strength and cast or splints permit. Encourage return to social activities "in spite of" cast, splint, or crutches. Assist with application or fitting of soft shoes if or when cast is removed (to lessen pressure or rubbing on tender tissues).

Patient Education

1. Explain wound healing and signs of wound dehiscence to report to physician.
2. Teach patient principles and examples of proper footwear. Explain that friction and pressure of snug footwear can precipitate recurrence.
3. Teach patient bone and wound healing for long-term follow-up.

EVALUATION

Patient Outcome	Data Indicating That Outcome is Reached
Incisional area and operated bones and joints have regained healing and functions.	Deformity has been removed; ROM is normal; scar formation is not excessive; pain is gone in and around joint.
Self-concept is positive and enhanced.	Patient returns to usual activities with unassisted, pain-free mobility. Footwear is comfortable.

Total Joint Replacement Arthroplasty

Work done since the late 1950s and early 1960s has made it possible to repair and replace both bone surfaces of many joints. Initially, work with total replacement of hip joints has led to the ability to totally replace many joints including ankles, knees, shoulders, elbows, wrists, and joints of the fingers and toes. Not all prosthetic materials or arthroplastic procedures work entirely satisfactorily in the joints with more and varied movements, such as the elbow, wrist, knee, and ankle. To date, more successful replacements have been in the ball and socket joints, primarily the hip. Research and design changes continue in efforts to perfect the prostheses and the techniques for all total arthroplastic procedures.

Replacement of both joint surfaces is required primarily in inflammatory or degenerative conditions within the joint, such as those accompanying rheumatoid arthritis or osteoarthrosis from degeneration of the synovium or cartilage. As one or more of the normal joint tissues deteriorate or degenerate, the bone ends are exposed, leading to pain and limitation of joint movements. Joint stiffness and muscle atrophy follow, further increasing pain and limiting movement and mobility, both locally in the involved joint and systemically as other joints become involved. Exposed bone surfaces will lead to bone growth that may eventually adhere to the opposing bone ends, causing bony ankylosis and loss of joint movements. Therefore replacement of the deteriorated or degenerated tissues and bones can and does restore movement and relieve pain.

Total joint replacements involve removal of some or all of the synovium, cartilage, and bone in both sides of the joint. One of the joint bone surfaces is then replaced with a metallic prosthesis while the other surface is replaced with a plastic, silicone-lined prosthesis. This metallic-plastic approximation is necessary to prevent metal-to-metal wear, friction, and possible electrolytic reactions from the interactions and intermingling of joint fluids. Individual physicians prefer specific combinations of prostheses for particular joints according to the individual patient's condition. Also, the timing for total joint replacement varies with physician and patient, since this procedure is usually elective except in situations of trauma.

Presently, each prosthetic replacement on both sides of the joint is secured in place with methyl methacrylate, a pliable polymer that hardens to hold the prosthesis firmly. Through research and development, ceramic and metallic components have been designed that are self-adhering and immovable and do not require methacrylate adherence. Use of the self-adhering replacements is occurring in selected centers at the present time but should become more widespread as the technique for their insertion is learned and the differences in postoperative recovery and rehabilitation are accepted. Ambulation is slower and use of crutches or other aids is more prolonged with the self-adhering replacements because of the need for the bone particles used as the natural interfacing material to granulate and ossify for solid adherence to the prosthetic replacements. Obviously use of the patient's own bone for the interface with the prostheses is more desirable since methyl methacrylate sets up an inflammatory response that may eventually lead to loosening or instability within the joint.

Total joint replacement involves special operative tables, instruments, and positions of patient and physicians. Expert anesthesic administration is required to prevent hypotension as the methyl methacrylate and prostheses are inserted; the temperature of and the methyl methacrylate itself may cause a temporary and sudden drop in blood pressure as it is inserted, and communication between the surgeon and anesthesiologist prevents the hypotension from being prolonged or sufficient to lead to other complications. Total joint replacements require careful ongoing physician-patient contact and consultation before and after surgery. When successful, as the great majority of joint replacements are, this surgery provides the patient with a welcome relief of pain, increased mobility, and freedom not available with more conservative procedures.

Contraindications and Cautions

1. Joint infection with or without an associated systemic infection is the major deterrent to total replacement. Infection loosens components, prevents healing, and may eventually lead to osteomyelitis.

2. Active flare-up of a chronic rheumatic or other inflammatory disease is another deterrent. Flare-ups of rheumatoid arthritis, ulcerative colitis, systemic lupus, and such preclude surgery until the condition is controlled or becomes quiescent.
3. Respiratory diseases and limitations from chronic conditions may preclude surgery. Methyl methacrylate is excreted through the lungs; this may set up a pneumonitis that could severely limit respiratory reserves.
4. Chronic renal conditions or mild failure may also preclude replacement since hypotension could lead to acute renal shutdown.
5. Bleeding or clotting disorders would usually preclude surgery unless special care is provided to prevent hemorrhage.
6. Insertion of the femoral component into the femoral shaft during total hip replacement causes pressure changes in the venous system, which can lead to thrombophlebitis and pulmonary or fat embolization.
7. Limb length inequality can occur from inadequate muscle strength or improper operative fit. If limbs are unequal in length preoperatively, the inequality can possibly be corrected with the surgical procedure.

Preprocedural Nursing Care

1. Skin cleansing procedures are begun 1 to 5 days preoperatively; these include shampoo, shower, and local scrub of operative site with antiseptic antibacterial soaps and thorough flushing with water.
2. X-ray films are taken, and the limbs are measured bilaterally to assure use of the best-fitting prostheses.
3. If total hip replacement is to be done, the patient is taught the proper position for postoperative lifting.
4. Respiratory care is begun preoperatively, including deep breathing and coughing exercises, respiratory therapy (intermittent positive pressure breathing [IPPB]), and use of respiratory aids such as Triflow or Respirex apparatus.
5. Antibiotics are begun intravenously 12 to 24 hours preoperatively to establish a therapeutic blood level.
6. Occasionally, skin traction may be applied preoperatively to relieve muscle spasms.

TREATMENT PLAN

Chemotherapeutic
Anti-infective agents
    Cefamandole (Mandol), 500-1000 mg q4-8h IM or IV
    Cefazolin (Ancef), 250-1000 mg q4-6h IV for 7 d

    Cephalexin (Keflex), 250-500 mg q6h po when IV antibiotics are discontinued
Narcotic analgesic agents
    Meperidine (Demerol), 50-100 mg IM q3h for pain
Antianxiety agents
    Hydroxyzine (Vistaril), 25-50 mg IM with meperidine
Anticoagulants
    Heparin, 2000-3000 units subq q12h
Sedative-hypnotics
    Flurazepam (Dalmane), 15-30 mg at bedtime
Cathartic or laxative agents
    Bisacodyl (Dulcolax), 1-2 tablets or rectal suppository prn
Analgesic-antipyretic agents
    Acetaminophen (Tylenol), 600 mg q4h prn for elevated temperature
If rheumatic or inflammatory disease is present, antirheumatic or anti-inflammatory medications are begun postoperatively as soon as patient can tolerate oral intake

Electromechanical
Empty and record suction drainage every 4 hours, if ordered; otherwise, empty as needed
Give oxygen at 2 to 3 L per nasal cannula for 24 hours, then as needed
Perform respiratory therapy with IPPB every 4 hours, or instruct patient in use of incentive spirometer every 2 to 4 hours
Assist patient to do deep breathing and coughing every 2 hours
Record intake and output

Supportive
Maintain bed rest for 24 to 72 hours (varies with specific joint replaced, the security of the replacement prostheses, and physician's choice)
Change dressing after 24 to 48 hours; may reinforce dressing if necessary
Give nothing by mouth for 24 hours; then clear liquids and advance to regular diet as tolerated
Perform neurovascular checks every hour for 24 hours, then every 2 hours for 24 hours, and then every 4 hours
Check vital signs every 4 hours
Maintain position of operative area with sling, splint, abduction pillow, immobilizer, brace, or Ace wrappings (varies with specific joint replaced)
Patient should be up with no weight bearing to operative limb after bed rest order expires (may be after 24, 48, or 72 hours, depending on joint replaced and whether or not cemented or noncemented replacement was done)
Begin physical therapy exercises on second postop-

erative day; exercises and schedule vary with joint replaced; exercises are either active or passive to all joints with exclusion of the operated joint and include quadriceps setting, straight leg raising, flexion and extension, or other individually prescribed exercises for the particular joint replaced

Patient should be up with walker or crutches four times daily; ambulation should increase as patient is able with up to 25 pounds weight to operative limb, gradually increasing to full weight bearing with crutches

Patient should sit in chair for 10 to 15 minutes only (after hip replacement), two or three times daily for first week; then may sit in chair 20 or 30 minutes four times daily

Patient should wear antiembolism hose

Encourage fluid intake and high-fiber foods (if tolerated) to prevent constipation; administer rectal suppository if needed to empty rectum

Patient should use toilet riser for toilet (prevents hyperflexion of hip after total replacement)

ASSESSMENT: AREAS OF CONCERN

Joint and incisional area
Presence, amount, and type of drainage
Edema
Color of tissues
Presence, type, and tightness of dressing or bandages
Presence of peripheral pulses
Pain in incision or distal to operative site
Presence of immobilizing device, splint, or pillow to maintain proper position of prosthesis within joint

Systemic concerns
Respiratory functions
Excursion
Dyspnea
Orthopnea
Pain in chest or lung areas
Cough
Decreased lung sounds

Psychosocial concerns
Concern with body image
Acute pain
Regaining mobility and weight bearing

Other complications
Pneumonitis
Pneumonia
Wound infection (superficial or deep)
Limb inequality or limp

NURSING DIAGNOSES and NURSING INTERVENTIONS

Nursing Diagnosis	Nursing Intervention
Mobility, impaired physical	Maintain bed rest as ordered. Begin ambulation with ambulatory aid and weight-bearing restrictions as ordered. Encourage performance of active and passive ROM exercises, isometric exercises, and other specific ordered exercises. Encourage use of trapeze to assist with lifting, turning, and positioning.
Skin integrity, impairment of: actual	Reinforce and then change dressing with strict aseptic technique: note wound edge approximation, redness, edema, hematoma, or unusual tenderness of wound.
Tissue perfusion, alteration in	Apply ice bags to operative site. Do circulation checks and record findings; note presence or absence of pain in calf and positive Homans' sign. Check drainage in suction apparatus and record. Report unusual amounts. Remove antiembolism hose twice daily; check color, presence of pulses, and skin condition; replace hose after 1 hour off. Check vital signs; note presence of hypotension and elevated pulse or temperature; record and report. Maintain proper and ordered flexion, extension, and/or abduction of operative tissues according to specific joint replaced.

Nursing Diagnosis	Nursing Intervention
Comfort, alteration in: pain	Administer narcotics with potentiator as ordered every 3 hours for first 24 hours; then use as needed for pain relief. Turn, raise, or adjust position to prevent pressure and lessen fatigue Administer medications for concomitant disease as ordered to relieve symptoms and pain. Administer sedative at bedtime as ordered. Assess bowel and bladder output; may need laxative, suppository, or enema. Convalescent care: encourage self-care and return to ADL as able. Stress alternatives to medication for restful sleep (activity to become tired, reading, warm milk, snack).
Mobility, impaired physical	Encourage ambulation as feasible and able. Assist with ROM exercises. Monitor use of crutches or walker to ascertain proper amount of weight bearing. Complete continuity of care referral for home care follow-up. Stress compliance with prescribed rehabilitation program after discharge. Encourage continued contact with physician for follow-up care.

Patient Education

1. Stress that rehabilitation of muscles and joint tissues, locally and systemically, will require daily practice over time.
2. Stress compliance with medication regimen for chronic disease if present.
3. Stress that joint ROM and mobility should be regained after recovery and rehabilitation are accomplished.

EVALUATION

Patient Outcome	Data Indicating That Outcome is Reached
Incision is well healed.	Wound edges are well approximated; there is no edema or drainage.
Patient regains joint mobility and ROM.	Patient ambulates with crutches (if lower extremity) and performs prescribed exercises with comfort and assistance if required; discomfort is eased with analgesics only.
Self-concept is positive.	Patient returns to family and social roles when able.

EXTERNAL FIXATION FOR IMMOBILIZATION OF BONES
Casts

Description and Rationale

Casts are hard structures of plaster, fiberglass, or plastic materials used to immobilize musculoskeletal tissues following injuries. Although plaster (gypsum) is still the most frequently used material for casts, newer fiberglass, plastic, and cast-tape casts are also becoming more commonly used. Each of the particular materials requires specific application techniques and has advantages and disadvantages, such as being heavy, cumbersome, or expensive or requiring special drying procedures and care to prevent skin breakdown. The use of a particular material is determined by the patient's injury, length of time needed for immobilization, and the physician's preference (Figs. 4-15 to 4-17).

Preparation for encasement in a cast varies from simply explaining its impending application and purpose for use to complete physical preparation including an enema, bath, and skin cleansing with antiseptic solutions. Explanations and care should be geared to the patient's level of comprehension and need to prevent undue fear or anxiety. Gentle handling of the entire patient and specifically the parts to be encased in a cast alleviates tension and facilitates application without additional trauma.

Depending on the type of cast and the materials used, assembling all supplies together and securing assistance for positioning and holding are prerequisites. Privacy is required when the skin is exposed and breast and genital areas should be covered for respect of the patient. Padding may be used over bony prominences before the cast is applied.

Once a cast is applied, drying times vary with the material used, the amount of plaster used, the areas of the body to be put into a cast, and the weather conditions. Plaster casts dry more slowly in damp, high-humidity conditions and can take 3 or 4 days to dry thoroughly. While drying, the areas in a cast must remain uncovered for drying to proceed from inside out. Drying is also facilitated with fans (except with open reductions) and use of heat lights with low-voltage bulbs.

During the drying periods, care must be taken to avoid making finger indentations in the cast, which would be reflected inward and cause a pressure area on the skin under the indented area. Pressure is also eased by turning the patient every 2 hours while the cast is drying to prevent molding and deformation. Propping or elevating with pillows helps maintain proper positioning. Pillows used should not have a plastic or rubber covering since the heat given off by the cast material will be trapped by the rubber or plastic and reflected back to the tissues in the cast causing injury or even a burn.

Contraindications and Cautions

1. Open fractures may not be treated with casts initially because of the need to observe the injury site over an extended period.
2. Plaster casts must be kept dry to prevent disintegration and weakening of the cast.
3. Fiberglass, plastic, and cast-tape casts can become wet without weakening; however, the skin under the cast must be dried if it becomes very wet to prevent maceration under the cast.

Preprocedural Nursing Care

1. The skin areas to be encased must be clean, dry, and free of open lesions.
2. X-ray films are taken to ascertain the extent of trauma.
3. All equipment and supplies must be assembled before the procedure is begun for ease and safety of application without unnecessary delay.
4. Sufficient skilled personnel should be present to assist with the application; two or three persons may be needed to assist the physician with a spica or body cast.
5. A sedative, narcotic, or anesthetic may be given before cast application.

TREATMENT PLAN

Chemotherapeutic
    Narcotic analgesics
        Meperidine (Demerol), 25-100 mg IM q3h (exact dosage varies with age and trauma)
    Analgesic-antipyretic agents
        Aspirin, 300-600 mg po or rectally (if NPO) for moderate pain q4h prn
    Sedative-hypnotics, nonbarbiturate
        Flurazepam (Dalmane), 30 mg po at hs, prn

Electromechanical
    Ice bags to site (would be ordered to a specific site)

Supportive
    Bed rest until cast is dry
    Elevation of cast (extremity) on pillows
    Neurovascular checks every hour for 24 hours, then every 2 hours for 24 hours, and then every 4 hours
    For open reduction, recording and report of amount of drainage or hemorrhage
    Forcing of fluids

ASSESSMENT: AREAS OF CONCERN

Cast and contiguous tissues
    Neurovascular condition of tissues around cast
    Position of tissues in cast (e.g., in flexed or extended position)
    Condition of cast (damp or dry)
    Temperature of cast and tissues around cast
    Ice bags to area

NURSING DIAGNOSES and NURSING INTERVENTIONS

Nursing Diagnosis	Nursing Intervention
Mobility, impaired physical	Teach isometric exercises as feasible, such as quadriceps and buttocks setting exercises. If fracture is below knee, quadriceps setting exercises of affected leg are vital to retain muscle strength and prevent atrophy. Assist with ambulation as needed. Teach techniques for crutch walking. Apply sling to hold cast snugly; teach patient to allow cast to lie in sling with shoulder loose to prevent shoulder pain or "freeze" of muscles.
Mobility, impaired physical (edema and muscle weakness after cast removal)	Explain that affected tissues may develop edema and tenderness with reuse. Caution patient to begin usual activities slowly to lessen edema and soreness.
Comfort, alteration in: pain	Assess presence of and degree of pain. Stress that return of pain after pain-free period should be reported to physician (may indicate loss of reduction or other complication). Administer narcotic or analgesic as necessary and ordered. Note increase in pain, numbness, or tingling and decrease or absence of pulses as indicative of compartment syndrome or that cast may be too tight; report promptly to physician since cast may need to be cut (bivalved). Stress need to elevate extremity if edema recurs after discharge. Note signs of increasing anxiety, dyspnea, nausea or vomiting, eructation or complaints of abdominal distention; may be caused by "cast syndrome" from excessive aerophagia (air swallowing) leading to gastric or intestinal distention and ileus; cast may need to be bivalved, and a nasogastric tube may be inserted to relieve ileus. Consult occupational therapist and physical therapist for activities to relieve boredom and maintain muscle strength.
Bowel elimination, alteration in: constipation (potential)	Stress intake of well-balanced, nourishing meals, high in residue and bulk to prevent bowel problems (after on full diet).
Urinary elimination, alteration in patterns (potential)	Force fluids to maintain urinary functions.

Patient Education

1. Explain techniques to keep cast clean and dry.
2. Explain need to have intake of well-balanced meals, foods, and adequate fluids.
3. Explain proper crutch use and ambulation techniques.
4. Explain skin care after cast removal: gently cleanse skin with cold-water wash containing enzymes; allow to soak in skin for 20 or 30 minutes; then flush with clear water; dry carefully and apply a lubricating lotion to prevent cracking or drying of the skin.
5. Explain that the patient should report persistent pain, weakness, and edema to the physician (usually all symptoms are relieved in 3 or 4 days after cast removal, although muscle weakness may persist longer); at times special exercises may be prescribed.

EVALUATION

Patient Outcome	Data Indicating That Outcome is Reached
Patient regains mobility and ROM.	Patient uses muscles and joints normally and without limitation, edema, and minimal initial postremoval pain and discomfort.

Immobilization with Hoffman or Other Apparatus

Description and Rationale

Several types of externally applied fixation devices are currently used for immobilization of bones including the Wagner, Roger Anderson, Murray, Hoffman, and Ace-Fischer apparatuses. The Hoffman apparatus consists of pins placed at right angles to the long axis of a bone and held by the clamps and screws of the device. The Ace-Fischer device has pins placed in oblique and vertical angles to the long axis of the bone and then attached to the retaining device. The latter device has only recently become available, whereas the former (Hoffman) one has been in use for approximately 15 years. The use of one or another device depends on the patient's condition and physician choice as with any medical treatment (Fig. 4-26).

Externally applied fixation is used in many sites and for many conditions. Sites where such fixation may be applied include bones of the face, jaw, upper and lower arm or leg, pelvis, ribs, and fingers or toes. Pins used vary in number, length, and thickness according to the bones or area to be treated. The major reasons for use of these devices are that they allow increased use of contiguous joints while maintaining the local immobility, they permit the patient's discharge to home, they hold unstable fractures or reductions and weakened muscles while allowing ambulation, and they hold bones with tissue or bone infection (pins are above and below the infected areas).

Contraindications and Cautions

1. Severely comminuted bone fractures may be a contraindication for use of these devices because the multiple pins needed may cause more fractures or weakening. Comminution with good alignment may be an indication for use.

Fig. 4-26
External fixation apparatuses. **A,** Hoffman. **B,** Roger Anderson.

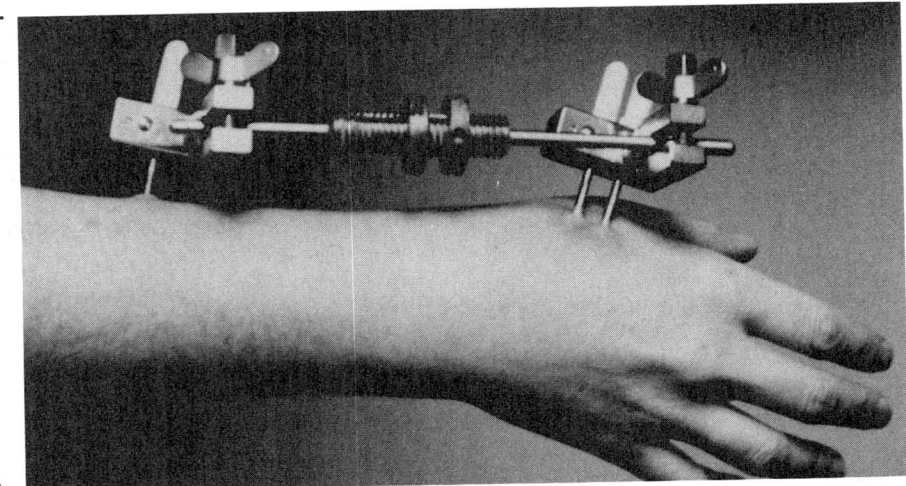

A

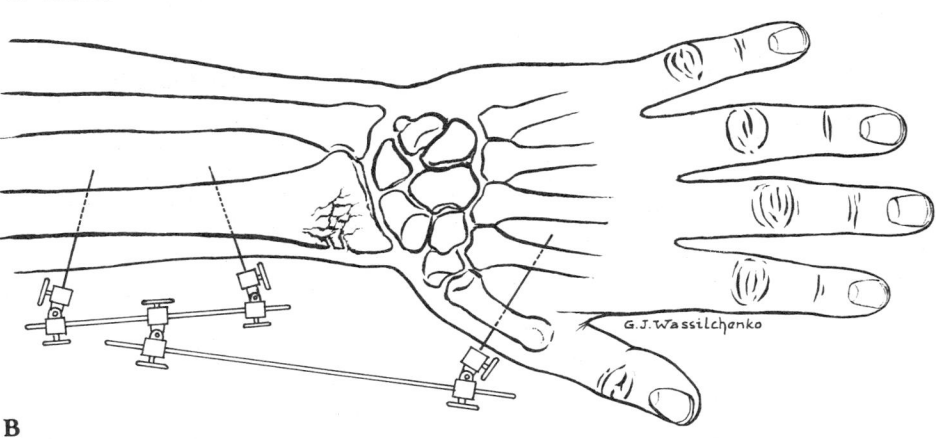

G.J.Wassilchenko

B

2. Severe or spreading osteomyelitis may be another contraindication since the multiple sites can be sources for progressive infection.
3. Overuse or excessive muscular movements may cause loosening or pin movements.
4. The multiple pin entrance and exit sites can be sources of skin and bone infections.
5. Following removal of the pins, bones can be refractured because of the multiple tracts through the bones; patients must be cautioned to increase activities slowly to prevent reinjury.

Preprocedural Nursing Care

1. Meticulous skin cleansing and preparation are required.
2. X-ray films must be taken.
3. Antibiotics are given intravenously.

TREATMENT PLAN

Surgical
Pin care every 4 hours and as needed

Chemotherapeutic
Narcotic analgesic agents
  Meperidine (Demerol), 50-100 mg IM q3h (dosage varies with age and trauma)
Anti-infective agents
  Cefamandole (Mandol) or cefazolin (Ancef), 250-1000 mg IV q6h for 7 d
  Cephalexin (Keflex), 500 mg q6h po after IV antibiotic is discontinued
Analgesic-antipyretic agents
  Aspirin, 600 mg q4h po, for moderate pain or temperature above 101° F

Supportive
Neurovascular checks every hour for 24 hours, then every 2 hours for 24 hours, and then every 4 hours
Ice bags to site continuously
Elevation of extremity on pillows
Up with sling (if upper extremity) or with crutches and no weight bearing (if lower extremity; after recovery from anesthetic)
ROM to unaffected joints and muscles

ASSESSMENT: AREAS OF CONCERN

Site of injury and external apparatus
Assessment of each pin entrance and exit site
  Color
  Temperature and edema of tissues
  Drainage
  Peripheral pulses
  Ability to move contiguous muscles and joints (unless ordered to be held immobilized)
  Pain, numbness, or tingling

Systemic concerns
Temperature and other vital signs
Nausea
Headache or other pain

Psychosocial concerns
Concern with body image
Degree of mobility/immobility
Acute pain
Possibility of infection

Other complications
Nonunion or malunion
Infection
Muscle or nerve damage or injury
Compartment syndrome

NURSING DIAGNOSES and NURSING INTERVENTIONS

Nursing Diagnosis	Nursing Intervention
Mobility, impaired physical	Maintain bed rest until recovered from anesthesia. Ambulate as ordered with sling or crutches. Turn and alter bed position as needed.
Self-concept, disturbance in: body image (related to external apparatus)	Clarify purposes of multiple pins and external device. Stress positive aspects of use of external devices to increase self-concept and body image. Explain that pins can be removed in physician's office when union has been achieved as determined by x-ray films.
Skin integrity, impairment of: actual	Wound care as needed. Pin care: clean each site with hydrogen peroxide–soaked swabs; remove drainage with normal saline; then dry. Topical antibiotic ointment may or may not then be lightly applied, depending on physician or insti-

Nursing Diagnosis	**Nursing Intervention**
	tutional policy. (Pin care may be stopped if sites are clean, dry, and without drainage).
	Clean all sutures if present with antiseptic and redress if drainage is present. Sutures may be left open to air if unit policy.
Comfort, alteration in: pain	Assess site and amount of pain (may initially be acute, sharp pain at pin insertion sites on skin).
	Administer narcotics and analgesics as needed and ordered.
	Stress that recurrence of pain at site is sign to be reported to physician.
	Stress that acute pain experiences will lessen in 24 to 48 hours and that all pain will be relieved in approximately 7 to 10 days.
	Note localization of pain to one site (may be sign of infection or inflammation); continue hourly neurovascular checks to note early changes.
	Note change in sensations, numbness, and tingling as signs of circulatory pressure; report increases in either sign.
	Apply ice bags as ordered to lessen edema and pain.

Patient Education

1. Teach patient and family member pin care techniques to continue at home if needed.
2. Stress the need to increase movements and weight bearing slowly after the pins are removed to lessen tenderness and to permit the muscles to regain strength.

EVALUATION

Patient Outcome	Data Indicating That Outcome is Reached
Patient regains mobility and ROM.	Patient uses muscles and joints normally and without limitation or edema and with minimal initial postremoval pain and discomfort.
Wound sites remain infection-free.	No drainage, redness, or erythema is noted at pin sites.

Traction

Description and Rationale

Traction is the application of force to the skin, muscles, and bones to aid in reduction of fractures, hold the reduced bones in alignment for healing, relieve muscle spasms and pain, and exert sufficient pull on muscles and bones to relieve pressure on peripheral spinal nerves. Traction can be applied to the skin and thus indirectly to the bones and muscles, or it can be applied directly to the bones through skeletal pins inserted through the skin and bones with the pins then being attached to ropes, pulleys, and weights. The particular type of skin or skeletal traction applied is determined by the physician with regard to the patient's injury or condition, the purpose of the traction, the age of the patient, the weight of the patient, the condition of the skin tissues to be placed in traction, and the length of time the patient will need to be kept in traction. Table 4-6 summarizes the various types of skin and skeletal traction and the specific points pertinent to each type of traction (Figs. 4-27 to 4-29).

Because time is required to overcome muscle spasms, bone overriding, angulation, and shortening, patients may be in traction for as short a time as 24 to 48 hours or as long a time as 10 or more weeks. Generally, patients in traction must remain hospitalized for the entire time because of the specialized care and equipment required (except for patients being treated with home cervical traction with a head halter). Since hospitalization in traction is extensive and also expensive, patients may be placed in traction for periods only to achieve relief of muscle spasms and to correct fracture overriding or angulation; once alignment is regained, the patient may be taken to surgery to have internal metallic fixation. Therefore although traction is still frequently required for specific treatment of an individual patient's injuries, the traction may be removed sooner than in the past because of use of metallic implants to maintain the reduction.

Table 4-6
Traction

Type	Patient's Age	Amount of Weight	Purposes and Principles	Considerations for Care
Skin Traction				
Bryant's (both legs) (Fig. 4-28)	1-3 year old child; weight under 40 lb	2-5 lb/leg	Applied for femoral fractures; realigns fracture fragments; overcomes muscle spasm. Legs should be at right angles to buttocks; buttocks should be held off the bed slightly.	Child remains on back at all times; must have supervision to maintain back-lying position; traction remains on for 7-10 days. If permitted, traction may be removed for skin care by two persons; one maintains gentle manual traction while second does care. Traction is removed from unaffected leg first, then from injured leg. Bilateral checks of color, edema, and peripheral pulses are performed as ordered.
Buck's extension (one or both legs) (Fig. 4-27, *A*)	Any age; most commonly used in adults	5-8 lb/leg	Applied preoperatively for hip fractures; for "pulling" contracted muscles; for relieving muscle spasms of legs or back. Patient usually lies in recumbent position; may be turned to either side if no fracture is present; if there is a fracture, patient is turned to unaffected side.	Skin of older patients is more "friable" and subject to loosening because of less subcutaneous fat. Patient's complaints of burning under tape, moleskin, or traction boot should be assessed. Traction may be removed for skin care even in presence of fracture.
Russell's (one or both legs) (Fig. 4-27, *B*)	Children 5 years or more to older adults	2-5 lb/leg	Applied for "pulling" contracted muscles; preoperatively for hip fractures. Uses principle that "for every force in one direction, there is an equal force in the opposite direction" for the pulley placement and amount of weights used, because weight pull is doubled.	Patient is positioned on back for most effective pull. Knee sling can be loosened for skin care and checking pulses in popliteal area.
Pelvic belt or girdle (abdomen and pelvis are enclosed) (Fig. 4-27, *C*)	Adults or older adolescents	20-35 lb	Relieve muscle spasms and pain associated with "disc" conditions. Pull is from iliac crests to relieve spasm.	Patient may be positioned in Williams position, which permits 45 degrees of flexion of the knees and hips to relax the lumbosacral muscles. Orders usually state to be "in traction 2 hours, out 2 hours" and out of traction at night. Traction straps should not put pressure over sciatic nerves.
Pelvic sling (under pelvis and buttocks like a hammock)	Adults	20-35 lb	For holding fractured pelvic bones. Buttocks must be slightly off the bed.	Patients are very comfortable in the sling even with extensive pelvic bruising. They may become quite dependent on being in the sling, and gradual "weaning" may be required. The sling should be kept clean and dry, and the patient can be removed from the sling for care and toileting, if institutional policies permit.

Table 4-6, cont'd
Traction

Type	Patient's Age	Amount of Weight	Purposes of Principles	Considerations for Care
Cervical head halter (under chin, around face, head, and back of head) (Fig. 4-27, *D*)	Adults	5-15 lb	For relieving muscle spasms caused by degenerative or arthritic conditions in or of the cervical vertebrae. Halter should be applied so pull comes from occipital area not through chin portion.	Patients may be in low or high Fowler's position depending on the purpose of the traction. Halter is usually incorrectly positioned if the patient complains of pain of chin, teeth, or temperomandibular joint; the side straps usually should be adjusted to relieve these complaints. Patients should be removed from the traction for sleeping. Patients may also use this type of traction at home for cervical arthritic conditions.
Cotrel's (cervical head halter and pelvic belt to pelvis)	Adolescents	5-7 lb to head halter and 10-20 lb to pelvic belt	For stretching muscles preoperatively for scoliosis. Principle is to pull muscles and joints apart.	Patient is put in this traction to relax muscles and curvature; should be in traction except for sleeping. Rarely, patient may be placed in Cotrel's postoperatively, too, although less frequently because of newer operative techniques such as Harrington rod insertion.
Dunlop's (lower humerus and forearm)	Children to adults	5-7 lb to humerus; 3-5 lb to forearm	For realigning fractures of the humerus. Body is used for countertraction by slightly elevating side of bed of arm in traction. Forearm is merely held at right angles to the humerus for comfort, by using Buck's extension to the forearm.	Dunlop's can be totally skin traction by Buck's extension to the humerus or can be skeletal with a Steinmann pin inserted through the distal humerus; use of either depends on the patient's injury. The traction to the *forearm* should be removed daily for skin care, pulse checks, and ROM exercises since the forearm traction is merely a means to keep the forearm vertically at a right angle to the humerus. Patients must have assistance during ADL because they are held flat on their backs. They can turn enough for back care only.
Cervical via skull tongs (skull bones bilaterally)	Any age (most commonly young adults)	20-30 lb (depends on weight of patient)	To realign fractures of cervical vertebrae and to relieve pressure on cervical nerves. Patient must be on a special bed or frame such as a Circ-Olectric bed or Stryker frame to facilitate care. Traction weights must never be "lifted"; traction must always be continuous.	Patients with this traction may be severely injured, having either upper or lower spinal cord injury or complete transection, making them quadriplegics or paraplegics. Neurovascular checks and "craniotomy" checks are required hourly to assess progression or relief of symptoms. Patients also may develop paralytic ileus (therefore are given nothing by mouth), may have a nasogastric tube inserted to suction, and have an indwelling urinary catheter. Pin care is done every 4 hr: soak sterile applicators in a half-strength solution of hydrogen peroxide and normal saline; apply to each pin site; allow to stand 5-10 min; use soaked applicators to remove drainage; dry sites; apply antibiotic or antiseptic ointment to pin sites if ordered.

Continued.

Table 4-6, cont'd
Traction

Type	Patient's Age	Amount of Weight	Purposes and Principles	Considerations for Care
Halo-pelvic (pins inserted into skull in four areas to hold halo part and pins inserted through iliac pelvic bones for pelvic part)	Adolescents and adults	None; bars extending between skull and pelvic portions hold body in desired positions	For preoperative straightening of scoliosis curvature. Straightening is accomplished by overcoming muscle contractions through tightening the bars.	This traction is "comfortable" after a few days to recover from the insertional trauma; however, dressing is very complicated because of the vertical bar placements that interfere with most clothing. Children with this traction are usually hospitalized. The traction may remain in place postoperatively to be replaced by a brace or cast. Halo-pelvic traction is a variant of halo-femoral traction, in which the pins are inserted through the distal femurs instead of the pelvic bones and the skull pins pull away from the femoral pins, thereby bringing about straightening.
Balanced suspension to femur (Steinmann pin or Kirschner wire inserted through upper tibia; thigh and leg are suspended in a splint and leg attachment) (Fig. 4-29)	Any age from 3 yr	20-35 lb	For realignment of fractures of the femur; to overcome muscle spasms associated with fractures of the femur. Suspension of the thigh and leg is "balanced" by countertraction to the top of the thigh splint (Fig. 4-29).	Patients in this traction should be recumbent for best effects. They can turn approximately 30 degrees to either side briefly for back care or can lift themselves using the trapeze and by using the uninjured leg and foot. Neurovascular checks are vital to assess circulatory status and to prevent compartment syndrome. Tissue pressure monitoring is done (Table 4-7).

Table 4-7
Tissue Pressure—Monitoring Procedures for Detection of Compartment Syndrome

Steps	Purpose and Interpretation
1. Cleanse skin over site with antiseptic.	To lessen chance of infection.
2. Insert needle-tipped catheter into muscle to be assessed; attach catheter to stopcock and syringe filled with normal saline; attach to tubing of mercury manometer.	
3. Open stopcock; depress plunger of syringe to inject saline.	
4. Observe pressure readings on manometer.	Normal tissue pressures are 0-30 mm Hg; rising pressures that approach patient's diastolic blood pressure readings may indicate compartment syndrome. Patient may need fasciotomy.
5. Remove saline; close stopcock.	
6. Record findings; report increasing pressures to physician.	
7. Check distal peripheral pulses bilaterally; compare.	
8. Measure site (usually thigh, calf, arm, or forearm) *bilaterally* to assess presence of, amount of, or increase in edema formation.	Rising venous pressures may exceed arterial tissue perfusion; peripheral pulses may be weak or nonpalpable; edema may be pronounced.

Fig. 4-27

Types of skin traction. **A,** Buck's extension. **B,** Russell's. **C,** Pelvic belt. **D,** Cervical head halter. Bryant's traction, a type of skin traction used for small children, is shown in Fig. 4-28.

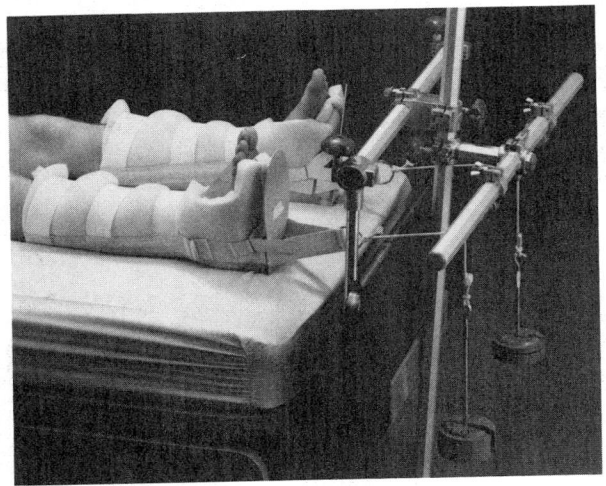

A

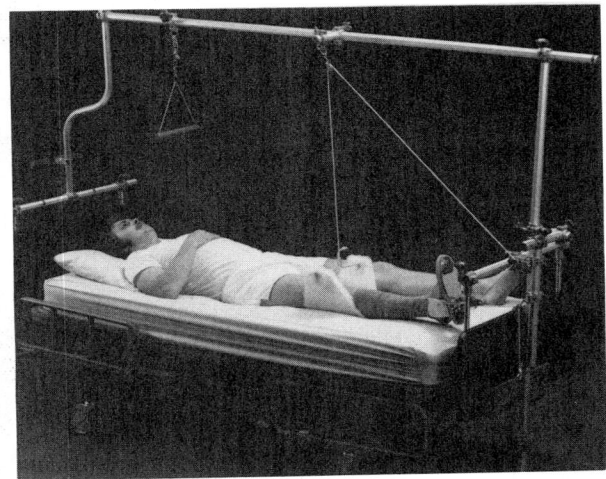

B

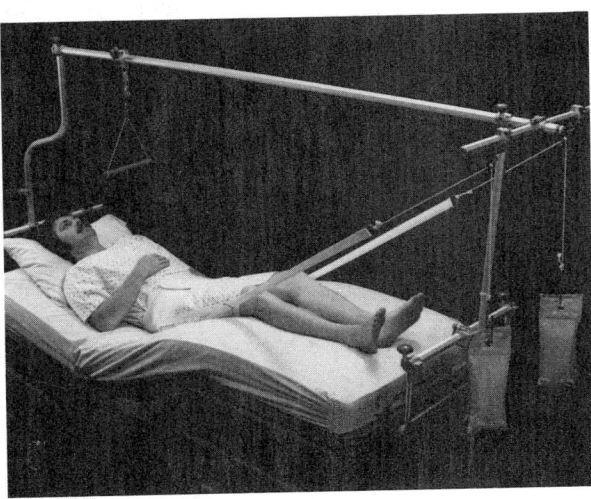

C

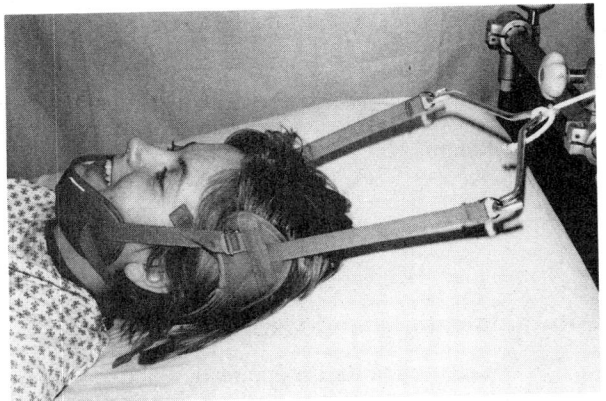

D

Fig. 4-28
Child in Bryant's traction, buttocks off bed properly.

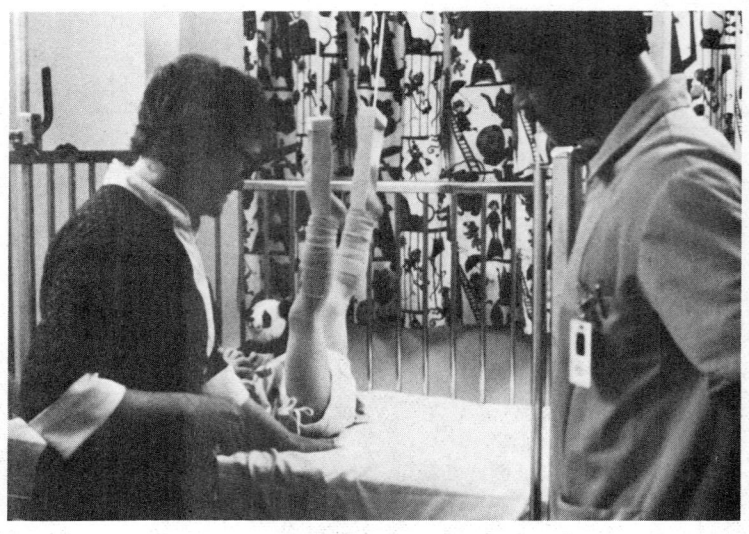

Fig. 4-29
Balanced suspension skeletal traction to the femur.

From Brashear, R.H., Jr., and Raney, R.B., Sr.: Shands' handbook of orthopaedic surgery, ed. 9, St. Louis, 1978, The C.V. Mosby Co.

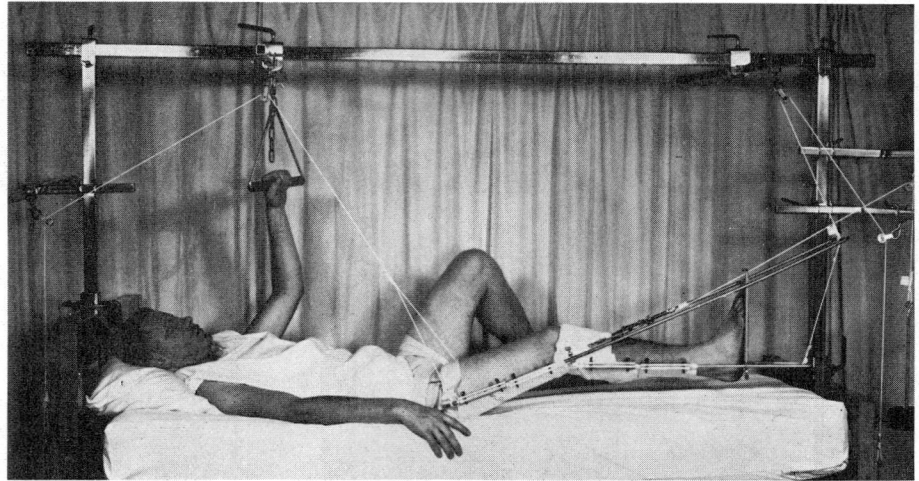

Contraindications and Cautions

1. Age is a restriction for the application of one or more types of skin or skeletal traction (Table 4-6). Because of lack of muscle mass or strength, a newborn baby or an elderly adult may not benefit from traction.
2. Open draining wounds or lesions are also contraindications to the use of either skin or skeletal traction since such wounds predispose to infection.
3. The amount of weight applied must be determined by the physician considering the amount of muscle spasm, the degree of overriding and angulation, and the specific purposes of the treatment. The weight may be increased or decreased as x-ray films indicate the need for weight changes.

Preprocedural nursing care

1. Reiterate or clarify upcoming events for patient's traction.
2. Assess local and systemic physical condition for indications or contraindications to placement in traction (such as open lesions, drainage, deep calf pain).
3. Assist with hygienic self-care for clean, dry skin surfaces.
4. Assist with positioning for x-ray films.
5. Administer preprocedural medication if ordered.
6. Assemble all equipment for application of specific traction.

TREATMENT PLAN

Chemotherapeutic
Narcotic analgesics
  Meperidine (Demerol), 50-100 mg IM q3h for
  72 h
  Morphine, 10-15 mg IM q4h
Analgesic-antipyretic agents
  Aspirin, 600-1000 mg q4h prn for moderate pain
Tranquilizers
  Diazepam (Valium), 2-10 mg po q4-6h

Electromechanical
Application of skin or skeletal traction (Table 4-6)
Diathermy to back (lumbar area) twice daily

Supportive
Bed rest: specific position or positions as per Table
  4-6
Neurovascular checks every hour for 24 hours, then
  every 2 hours, and then every 4 hours
Monitoring of tissue pressure if ordered
Ice bags to affected tissues (site always ordered for
  application)
Diet: high protein, high vitamin, low fat; force fluids
Physical therapy for ROM and isometric exercises
Pin care twice daily for skeletal traction

ASSESSMENT: AREAS OF CONCERN

Area of body in traction*
Tissues
  Color

*See Table 4-6 for specific tissues.

Edema
Signs of pressure around traction
Pain
Amount of weight
Direction of pull

Systemic concerns
Patient
  Pressure areas over bony prominences
  Muscle strength or weakness
  Weight loss
  Position in bed
Traction (entire traction setup)
  Ropes
  Pulleys
  Weights
  Knots
  Pins
  Slings
  Belts
  Each part of setup (Table 4-6)

Psychosocial concerns
Concern with changes in body image
Immobility and loss of livelihood
Acute pain

Other complications
Nonunion
Malunion
Embolic phenomena
Pin necrosis
Skin lesions or pressure areas

NURSING DIAGNOSES and NURSING INTERVENTIONS

Nursing Diagnosis	Nursing Intervention
Comfort, alteration in: pain	Assess pain experiences to determine extent, etiology, and patient's reactions.
	Monitor tissue pressures every hour (Table 4-7).
	Assist with and alter patient's position within traction limitations to relieve muscle/joint stiffness or soreness.
	Administer narcotic analgesics as ordered to relieve acute pain and nonnarcotic analgesic (aspirin) to relieve inflammation.
	Assess patient's entire pain experiences: *local* pain at site of injury and *systemic* spread (e.g., chest pain, dyspnea, calf pain, headache, confusion); may be indications of pulmonary, circulatory, neurologic, or other complications.
	Assess for evidence of fat embolism with symptoms of mental confusion, dyspnea, chest pain, and vital sign changes. A petechial rash may also develop over upper chest and neck with fat emboli.
	Assess and perform Homans' procedure to determine possible cause of calf pain; could indicate thrombophlebitis if positive Homans' sign.
	Assess degree of muscle spasms in injury site; clarify causes of and measures to relieve spasms through traction and muscle-relaxant medications.

Nursing Diagnosis	Nursing Intervention
	Clarify use of ice bags and apply ice bags to assist with relief of muscle spasms. Assist with ROM exercises to maintain strength in unaffected muscles. Assess effects of diathermy to relieve pain and muscle spasms if pertinent to injury. Perform pin care (Table 4-6).
Self-concept, disturbance in: body image (related to weight loss and weakness)	Explain purposes of traction repeatedly since patient's anxiety and pain may preclude hearing or full understanding. Explain reasons for bed rest, weakness, and anorexia. Encourage increasing intake as appetite returns to help regain weight. Patients can lose up to 30 pounds in skeletal traction because of decreased muscle activities. Explain purposes of position changes to maintain healthy tissues. Assess appetite and intake and output.
Mobility, impaired physical (related to traction, hospitalization, and loss of livelihood)	Clarify use of traction as one part of treatment regimen for this patient's specific injury. Encourage patient and family communications with physician for "timetable" of plans for overall treatment. Seek consultations (per physician's order) for occupational therapy and physical therapy to assist patient's recovery and adjustment to treatment regimen and hospitalization. Seek consultation with social service personnel to assist patient and family to plan and prepare for possible economic needs to regain livelihood (may lose employment while hospitalized). Encourage patient's self-care activities to maintain mobility within traction limits. If surgical repair follows traction use, assist to ambulate as ordered to regain mobility.

Patient Education

1. Ensure that patient and family can apply traction correctly if it is to be used in the home.
2. Instruct patient and family in use of muscle relaxants and pain medications if prescribed for home use.
3. Ensure that patient and family recognize when to contact physician if symptoms recur.

EVALUATION

Patient Outcome	Data Indicating That Outcome is Reached
Patient regains mobility and ROM.	Patient uses muscles and joints normally and without limitation or edema, and with minimal initial postremoval pain and discomfort.

NOTE: One or another form of skin or skeletal traction may be applied as the major treatment for a specific musculoskeletal condition, as has been indicated throughout this chapter. Traction also can be used before surgical repair or placement within a cast. Other nursing care concerns are discussed in those areas of the chapter and in Table 4-6.

INTERNAL FIXATION FOR IMMOBILIZATION OF BONES

Description and Rationale

Surgical implantation of metallic pins, nails, screws, plates, and other devices for immobilizing or repairing traumatized or damaged bones and joints is a major orthopedic treatment modality. With the development in the early 1930s of nonreactive metal alloys, surgical repair has provided markedly decreased hospitalization periods, a more rapid return to home and social and employment opportunities, and a more rapid regaining of mobility. Surgical repair requires the concurrent administration of antibiotics to prevent infection, the major hazard and deterrent to use of more orthopedic surgical and metallic implants for a wider range of injuries. However, in most instances, the advantages of internal metallic fixation far exceed the disadvantages; therefore surgery is a major viable modality for orthopedic trauma.

Fractures of bones may be immobilized by (1) screws attached to a compression plate, (2) nails or pins as in a hip nailing, (3) a rod or nail placed within the intrame-dullary canal (intramedullary rod) or placed parallel to the bones (Harrington rod), (4) screws or staples to hold fracture fragments together, or (5) natural bone grafts to fill in gaps in bones or to fuse two bone surfaces together as in a spinal fusion (Fig. 4-30).

This section will focus on three procedures representative of internal fixation procedures: hip nailing or pinning, spinal fusion by Harrington rods, and spinal fusion by natural bone grafts.

Internal Fixation with Hip Nails or Pins

Contraindications and Cautions

The patient's specific injury, general physical and mental condition, and the physician's choice from the many available metallic nails and pins determine which type will be used for the particular patient. The injury may

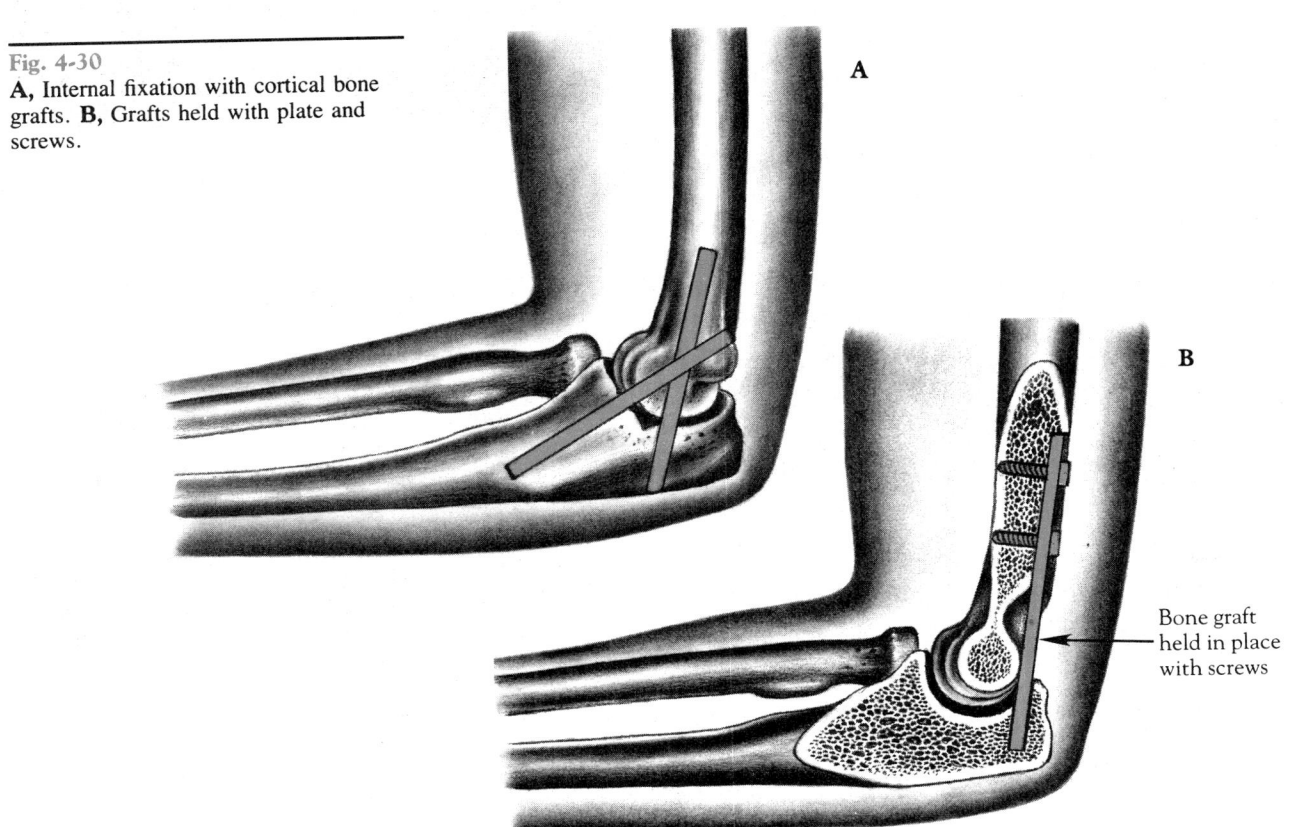

Fig. 4-30

A, Internal fixation with cortical bone grafts. **B,** Grafts held with plate and screws.

Bone graft held in place with screws

be a fairly stable fracture that requires only a single nail such as a compression screw or a sliding compression nail. Unstable fractures may require multiple pins, such as Knowles pins, or use of a nail with a side plate.

The type of internal fixation used is also determined by the particular fracture type and site. Hip fractures are referred to as intracapsular or extracapsular. Intracapsular fractures are those of the femoral head or neck that are contained within the hip capsule (Fig. 4-7). Intracapsular fractures may disrupt the blood supply to the head of the femur with subsequent development of avascular necrosis of the head of the femur. Therefore fractures of the head or proximal femoral neck may be treated with insertion of a femoral prosthesis. Subcapital or distal neck fractures may heal without avascular necrosis; thus these latter fractures may be nailed or pinned.

Extracapsular fractures are those around or through the trochanters and are referred to as intertrochanteric or subtrochanteric fractures. These fractures heal well with the use of compression screws or nails because the blood supply to the fracture site comes from the surrounding vessels outside the capsule. Side plates attached to the nails help maintain a stable reduction while healing progresses (Fig. 4-31).

Finally, the patient's physical and mental condition may also help determine which type of internal fixation is performed. The weak or confused patient would benefit from a compression interlocking nail, which can withstand some weight bearing; a single nail with or without a side plate would be appropriate for a stable fracture in a mentally clear patient who could be cautioned and expected to ambulate with only minimal or touch-down weight bearing.

Thus the specific internal fixation and repair require careful evaluation and assessment by the surgeon and other health professionals for the patient's greatest benefit.

Preprocedural Nursing Care

1. The patient is placed in traction, usually Buck's extension or Russell's, while preparations for surgery are completed.
2. Chest and injury site x-ray films are evaluated.
3. An enema is given, if needed, and an indwelling catheter may be inserted.
4. An electrocardiogram is done to determine cardiovascular status.
5. Serologic studies are done for chemistry analysis; urinalysis is done.
6. Skin cleansing is done to decrease organisms in the operative site.
7. Preoperative medication is administered.
8. Intravenous therapy is initiated for fluid intake.

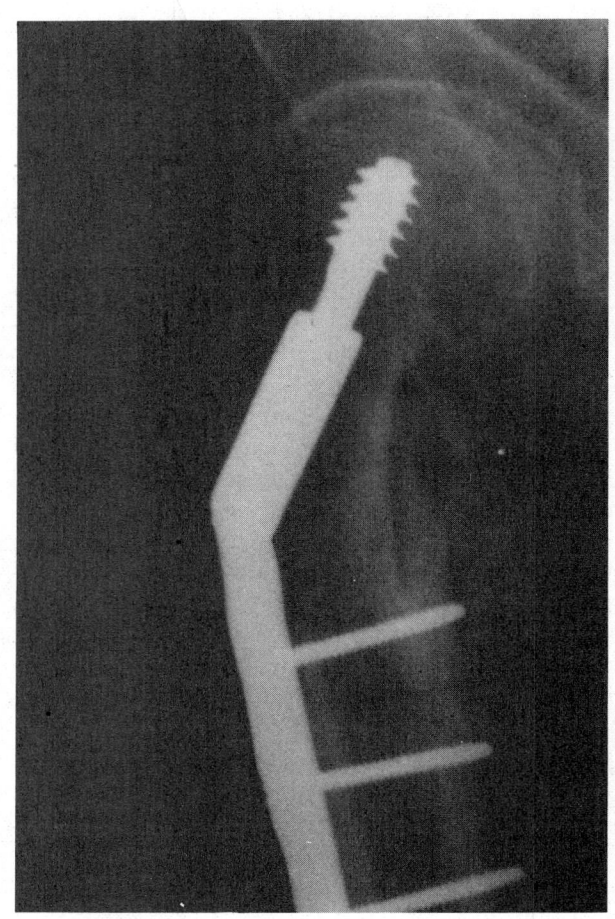

A

TREATMENT PLAN

Chemotherapeutic
Anti-infective agents
    Cefazolin (Ancef), 250-1000 mg IV q6h
Narcotic analgesic agents
    Meperidine (Demerol), 50-75 mg q3h for 24 h, then q3h prn
Analgesic-antipyretic agents
    Aspirin, 600 mg R suppository q4h for temperature elevation above 101° F and for moderate pain
Intravenous 1000 ml 5% D/.2N/S at 125 ml/h; add 20 mEq KCl to each liter

Electromechanical
Pulmonary IPPB every 4 hours

Supportive
Bed rest with operative leg in neutral position
Turning to unoperative side and back every 2 hours
Change of dressing as needed; reinforce as needed

Fig. 4-31
A, Type of hip nail. **B,** Prosthesis replacing head of humerus. **C,** Femoral head prosthesis.

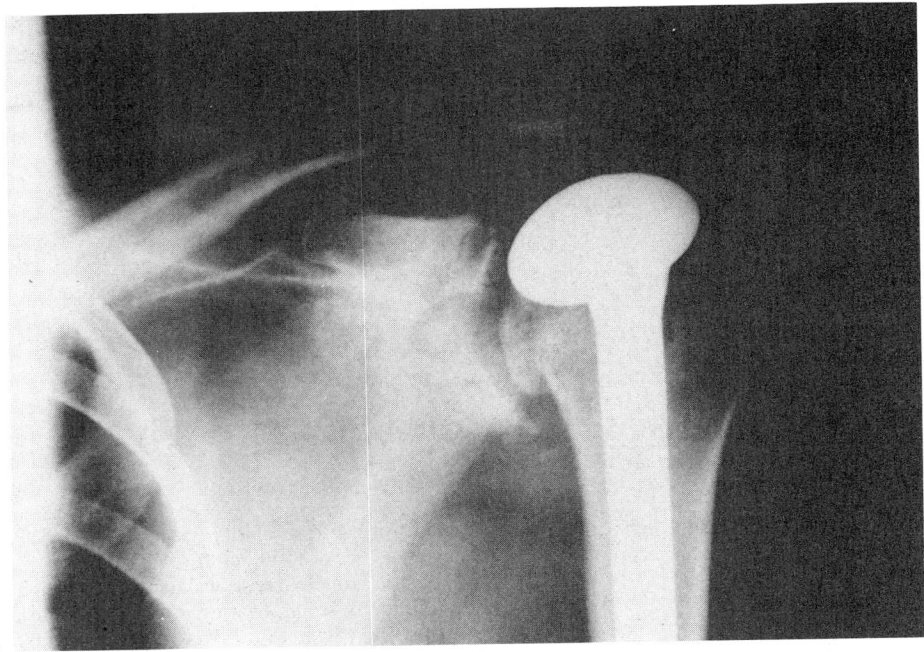

B

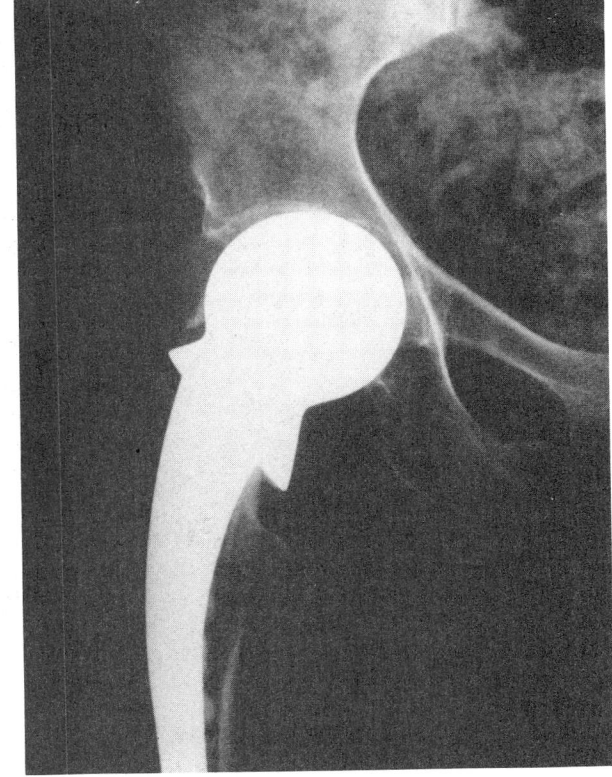

C

Record of input and output; separate record of suction drainage

Deep breathing and coughing every 2 hours; Respirex (or Triflow) 10 times every hour

Vital signs every 15 minutes for four times, every 30 minutes for four times, every hour for four times, then every 4 hours

Up in chair three times on first postoperative day with no weight bearing

Up with walker on second postoperative day; no weight bearing on operated leg

Clear liquids after nausea has subsided; advance to regular diet as tolerated

CBC, electrolytes, and CO_2 in morning and daily for 4 days

Physical therapy to assist with ambulation

ASSESSMENT: AREAS OF CONCERN

Hip and upper thigh incisional and wound area
  Assessment
    Dressing
    Drainage
    Wound suction equipment
    Drainage in container
  Presence of edema at wound site
  Position of thigh and leg
  Complaints of pain
  Color of tissues

Systemic concerns
Respiratory and circulatory status
Vital signs
Mental state and recovery from anesthesia
Muscle strength or weakness
Urinary output and catheter-drainage setup
Intravenous fluid type, amount, and rate

Psychosocial concerns
Concern with body image
Immobility

Confusion
Acute pain

Other complications
Loss of reduction and/or dislocation
Thrombophlebitis
Avascular necrosis of femoral head
Pneumonia
Cardiac arrhythmias

NURSING DIAGNOSES and NURSING INTERVENTIONS

Nursing Diagnosis	Nursing Intervention
Self-concept, disturbance in: body image	Maintain bed rest; clarify need for, if needed.
	Massage back to aid comfort and circulation.
	Assist to ambulate with walker and no weight bearing as ordered (may continue either no weight bearing or partial weight bearing for up to 3 months, gradually increasing to full weight by 5 months).
Mobility, impaired physical (related to modification in weight bearing)	Assist to dangle at bedside on first postoperative day, then to pivot to chair with no weight on operative leg.
	Stress that operative foot should be placed on floor but all weight should be borne on unoperative leg (refer to limb as either left or right leg so patient has a clear understanding).
	Turn every 2 hours; prop with pillows between legs or back to maintain position.
	Assist with ROM exercises to maintain muscle strength.
	Assist physical therapist to ambulate patient with walker and no weight to operative limb (if assistance is needed).
	Encourage patient and family members to ambulate together to aid patient's security. Instruct family about non-weight-bearing techniques for clarity and safety.
Comfort, alteration in: pain	Assess wound for evidence of resolution of surgical trauma and inflammation.
	Assess patient's complaints of pain; clarify site, type, and amount of pain.
	Administer analgesics judiciously because of patient's age; dosage should be sufficient to relieve pain without causing confusion (may need to vary dosage within ordered ranges).
	Turn or reposition patient and massage back to increase comfort.
	Perform Homans' test to determine development of thrombophlebitis, which could lead to pulmonary embolism. Observe for chest pain, dyspnea, and changes in vital signs, which could indicate pulmonary embolism, atelectasis, or pneumonia.
	Assist with meal and food selections to aid in healing, resolution of inflammation, and enhancement of bone calcification.
	Force fluids to aid digestion and bowel and bladder elimination.

Patient Education

1. Clarify need for weight-bearing restrictions for bone union.
2. Clarify signs to report to the physician: increased soreness or pain at operative site, fever, decreased urine output or burning with urination.
3. Reiterate techniques for use of walker.
4. Teach patient and family necessity to continue intake of well-balanced diet and good fluid intake for healing, circulation, and elimination.

EVALUATION

Patient Outcome	Data Indicating That Outcome is Reached
Patient regains mobility.	Patient ambulates with progressive weight bearing as healing occurs, with minimal discomfort and satisfactory ROM.
Fracture has united.	Patient has no pain in fracture site. Muscle and joint strength is regained.

Internal Fixation with Harrington or Other Rods

Description and Rationale

Harrington rods are long metallic implants attached posteriorly to the vertebral column following corrective repair and fusion as treatment for scoliosis. The rod or rods (they may be bilaterally used) hold the vertebrae in the corrected alignment to permit the bone grafts to heal and fuse the vertebrae solidly. The rods may remain in the site for extended periods or may be removed (rarely done) after x-ray films indicate there is sound, solid fusion. In the early postoperative period some patients may wear a fitted brace to assist the rods to maintain spinal immobility if the curvature was marked preoperatively and multiple grafts were implanted during surgery. The brace is worn during the waking hours and is removed for sleep.

Luque rods are another kind of metallic implant used for corrective spinal surgery. Luque rods are used on both sides of the spinal column with multiple attachments to each spinal segment to add corrective forces throughout the deformity. Additionally, Luque rods are contoured to aid in correcting the deformation.

Contraindications and Cautions

1. Harrington and other rods are foreign bodies, as are all metallic implants; thus they may cause a severe inflammatory reaction, which may necessitate their removal.
2. Open surgery may predispose to local wound infection or may lead to meningeal infections.
3. One or more bone grafts may be needed to maintain the correction of the curvature; parts or whole grafts may not unite firmly, which may necessitate prolonged wearing of a brace, encasement in a plaster cast, or even reoperation.
4. The spinal attachments holding the rods may loosen, allowing the rods to move. Major movement of either end of the attachments would necessitate reoperation.

Preprocedural Nursing Care

1. The patient may be placed in Cotrel's or halo-femoral traction (Table 4-6) or a Risser cast (Fig. 4-22) before surgery to stretch contracted muscles.
2. Meticulous skin cleansing is done to remove organisms to prevent infections.
3. X-ray films determine respiratory and spinal conditions; respiratory therapy with IPPB and a respiratory aid is done every 4 hours.
4. Serologic and urologic studies are done.
5. An enema is administered to clear the lower bowel.
6. An indwelling catheter is inserted into the urinary bladder.

TREATMENT PLAN

Chemotherapeutic

Narcotic analgesics
  Meperidine (Demerol), 50-100 mg IM q3h
  Morphine, 10-15 mg IM q4h
Analgesic-antipyretic agents
  Aspirin, 600 mg R suppository for moderate pain q4h prn; or for temperature over 101° F (38.3° C)
Anti-infective agents
  Cefazolin (Ancef) or cefamandole (Mandol), 250-500 mg q6h IV (children's dosage is 50-100 mg/kg/day in divided doses)
  Intravenous 1000 ml 5% D/.45N/S at 75 ml/h with 10 mEq KCl in every other liter

Electromechanical

IPPB every 4 hours

Supportive

Maintain patient flat in bed
Do log roll every 2 hours
Assist patient to deep breathe and cough every 2 hours; use respiratory aid 10 times every hour
Do not change dressing; reinforce if needed
Do laminectomy checks every hour
Give clear liquids after patient has had nothing by mouth for 24 hours; advance to regular diet as tolerated
Force fluids after intravenous line is discontinued
Do ROM exercises to arms and legs every 4 hours

Keep cast uncovered until dry or keep brace on at all times (if ordered and used)

Consult physical therapist for ROM and isometric exercises

ASSESSMENT: AREAS OF CONCERN

Vertebral column, incisional wound site
Check of alignment and position of back and entire patient

Check of wound

  Drainage (may have suction drainage)

  Edema

  Dressing

  Presence of brace or plaster cast with open window in back portion

Skin condition of formerly contracted tissues

Respiratory excursions; depth, rate, and character of respirations

Site and amount of pain

Systemic concerns
Assessment of motor and sensory functions by "laminectomy checks"

Catheter drainage

Intravenous fluid infusion site, solution, and rate

Presense of nausea or vomiting

Abdominal distention/ileus

Psychosocial concerns
Self-concept and body image

Immobility

Acute pain

Length of convalescence

Other complications
Shock

Hemorrhage

Wound infection

Nonunion

Loss of reduction

Pneumonia

Urinary tract infection

Meningitis

NURSING DIAGNOSES and NURSING INTERVENTIONS

Nursing Diagnosis	Nursing Intervention
Self-concept, disturbance in: body image (related to deformity and dependence because of bed rest and surgery)	Stress patient's improved appearance following fusion. Encourage self-care as able; assist with placement and removal of supplies to maintain an esthetic atmosphere.
Mobility, impaired physical (related to prolonged convalescence and muscle weakness and spasms)	Turn, with assistance of another health professional, by log rolling every 2 hours. (Teach family log-rolling technique if feasible and utilize their assistance.) Do not let patient turn self since log rolling cannot be self-accomplished safely because patient would twist. Twisting could disrupt fibrin meshwork (see pp. 477-478 for bone healing), thereby delaying or preventing bone union and fusion. Brace will hold back sufficiently rigid after discharge so patient can safely turn or get up unassisted.
	Encourage deep breathing and leg exercises to increase self-activities and independence and promote healing and circulation.
	Perform laminectomy checks every hour: observe and compare in all four extremities: color, temperature, edema; ROM in each extremity; grip, push, and pull strength; sharp and dull discrimination; presence of and type of pain, radiation, numbness, and tingling.
	Place full-length bed pad or alternating-pressure mattress on bed.
	Provide massage to exposed areas of shoulders, neck, back, and buttocks to relieve tiredness and muscle spasms.
	Assist with stretching exercises if needed to relieve skin restrictions from preoperative curvature limitations.
Comfort, alteration in: pain	Assess patient's complaints of pain; clarify site, type, and amount of pain.
	Administer age-adjusted (if younger child or adolescent) and pain severity–adjusted medication dosage as ordered.
	Assess wound as pain source; note signs of resolution of inflammation and surgical trauma. Report continued edema, redness, and increased drainage as untoward signs.

Nursing Diagnosis	Nursing Intervention
	Assist to increase amount and time of ambulation (when allowed up) to help resolve muscle soreness and weakness and to lessen soreness and pain in operative site.
	Change dressings over incision (after initial dressing change by physician) as needed; note lessening of soreness and acute pain as healing proceeds.
	Check bowel sounds, abdominal distention, passage of flatus (ileus may be source of pain).

Patient Education

1. Teach application of brace to patient and family.
2. Clarify that muscle stiffness, weakness, and soreness may increase with increase in activities but will last for brief periods only.
3. Reiterate stages of bone healing for strong union; stress need for caution against sudden position changes and need to continue wearing the brace.
4. Stress need for intake of well-balanced diet for regaining muscle strength and for healthy bone growth.
5. Explain that sudden or gradually increasing amounts of pain should be reported to physician.

EVALUATION

Patient Outcome	Data Indicating That Outcome is Reached
Patient has regained satisfactory spinal curves.	Patient has satisfactory posture and curvatures without spinal rotation.
Patient regains independence, mobility, and spinal motion with limited flexion.	Patient moves freely without muscle weakness, discomfort, or pain and has learned to use muscles of lower extremities and hips to assist lumbar muscles when stooping or bending (must kneel or bend from hips rather than from lumbar area).
Self-concept is positive.	Patient resumes social contacts.

Skeletal Traction

Skeletal traction is a modified form of internal fixation that combines internal with external immobilization. The uses, purposes, and care of patients in skeletal traction have been discussed on pp. 519–526 and in Table 4-6.

Spinal Fusion with Bone Grafts

Spinal fusion with natural autogenous bone grafts is done as treatment of a herniated nucleus pulposus. Nursing care of patients following spinal fusion for treatment of a ruptured disc is very similar to that discussed above with the addition of assessing relief of sensory pressure signs, numbness, and tingling as surgical wound healing progresses. Use of autogenous bone grafts usually provides solid union without the problems associated with metallic implants, including foreign body reactions, loosening, or infections.

Nursing care for spinal fusion is the same as for internal fixation with Harrington rods.

HEMILAMINECTOMY

Description and Discussion

Hemilaminectomy is the partial removal of the lamina to gain access to the intervertebral space to remove a ruptured disc. The pathophysiology leading to disc degeneration and rupture is discussed on p. 463.

Contraindications and Cautions

1. Determination of the cause and location of one or more degenerated or ruptured discs requires physiologic and psychologic diagnostic profiles before surgery.

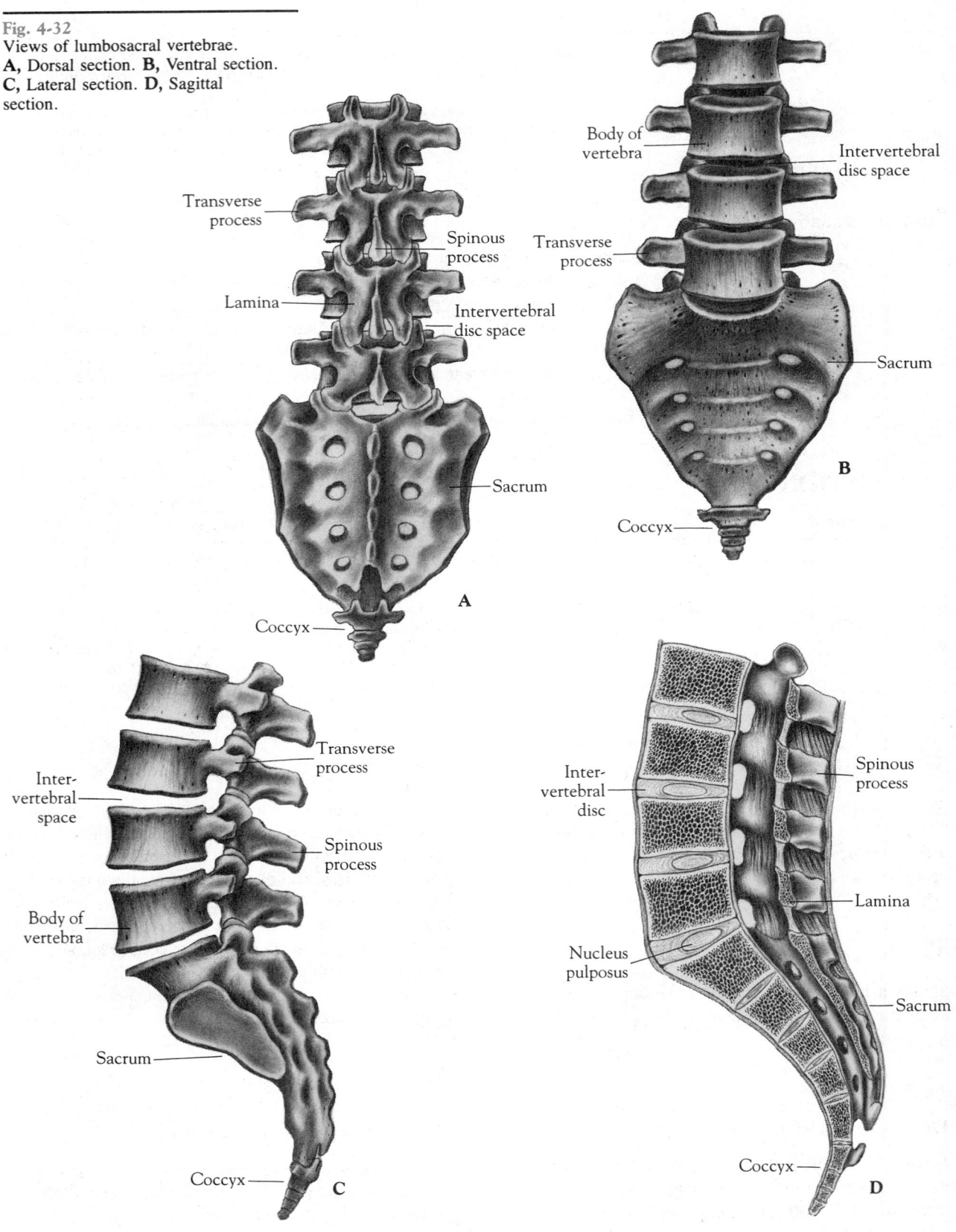

Fig. 4-32
Views of lumbosacral vertebrae.
A, Dorsal section. **B,** Ventral section.
C, Lateral section. **D,** Sagittal
section.

A
- Transverse process
- Spinous process
- Lamina
- Intervertebral disc space
- Sacrum
- Coccyx

B
- Body of vertebra
- Intervertebral disc space
- Transverse process
- Sacrum
- Coccyx

C
- Transverse process
- Intervertebral space
- Spinous process
- Body of vertebra
- Sacrum
- Coccyx

D
- Intervertebral disc
- Spinous process
- Lamina
- Nucleus pulposus
- Sacrum
- Coccyx

Fig. 4-33
A, Spinal nerves exiting from cord.
B, Herniated nucleus pulposus; note
pressure on nerve.

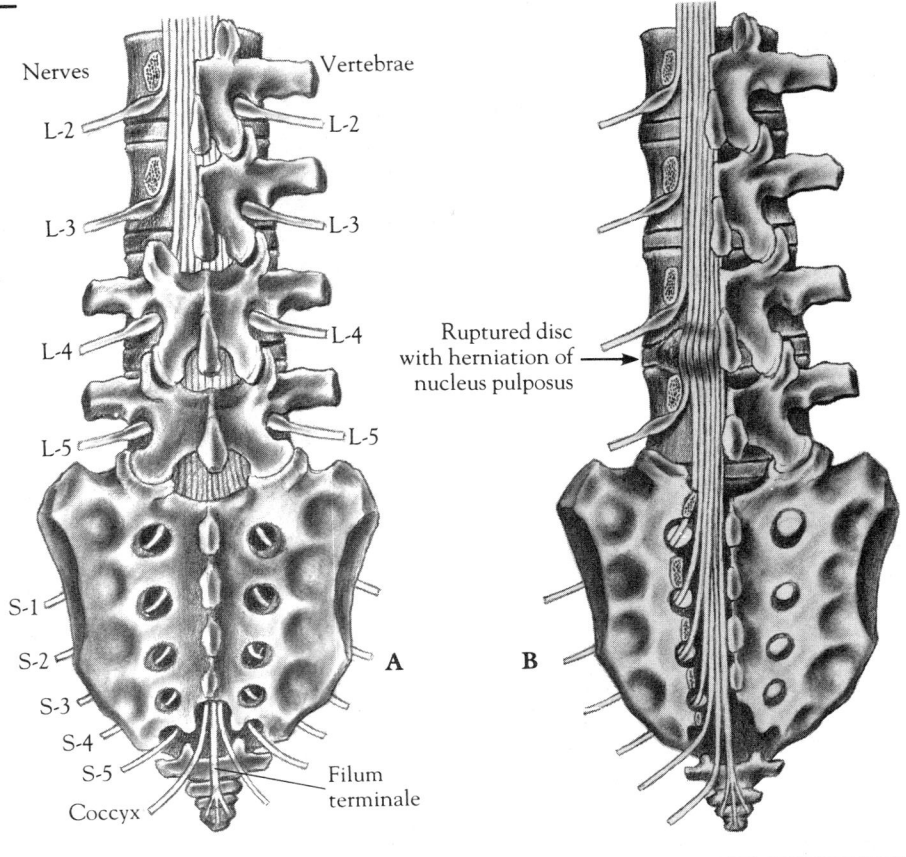

Nerves

Vertebrae

L-2   L-2

L-3   L-3

L-4   L-4

L-5   L-5

Ruptured disc
with herniation of
nucleus pulposus

S-1

S-2

S-3

S-4

S-5

Coccyx

Filum
terminale

A   B

Fig. 4-34
Mechanisms that can cause
degeneration of the anulus leading to
herniation of the nucleus pulposus. **A,**
Axial pressure. **B,** Lateral pressure.
C, Posterior pressure.

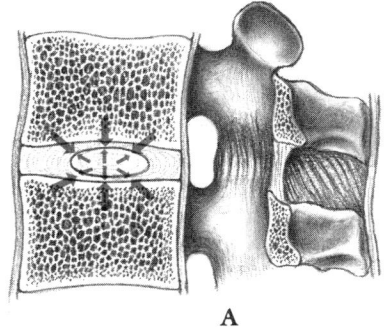

A

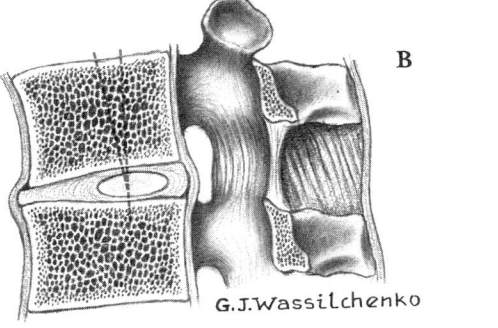

B

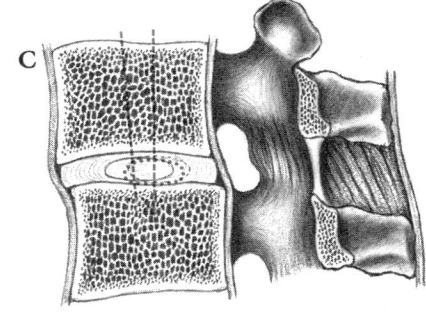

C

G.J.Wassilchenko

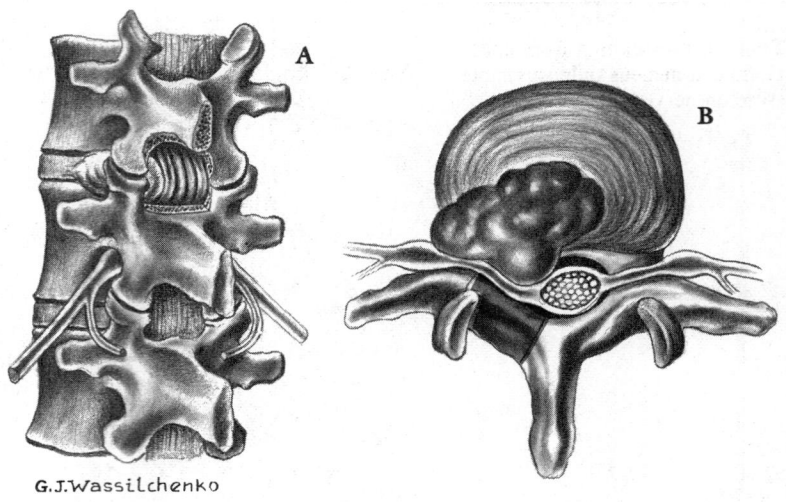

Fig. 4-35
Laminectomy for herniation of nucleus pulposus. **A,** Area of lamina removed during a hemilaminectomy. **B,** Herniated nucleus pulposus.

G.J.Wassilchenko

2. Removal of a degenerated or ruptured disc may not relieve the patient's complaints of pain.
3. Postoperative rehabilitation requires the patient's cooperation and performance of daily exercises to strengthen the spinal and abdominal muscles.

TREATMENT PLAN

Chemotherapeutic
Narcotic analgesic agents
    Meperidine (Demerol) 50-100 mg q3-4h for pain
Anti-infective agents
    Cefazolin (Ancef) or cefamandole (Mandol), 250-500 mg q6h IV
Intravenous, 1000 ml 5% D/.45 N/S at 75-100 ml/h

Supportive
Nothing by mouth until morning; then clear liquids and advance to regular diet
Bed rest until evening of surgery
Turn side to side every 2 hours
Patient up at bedside evening of surgery and up three times daily thereafter
Laminectomy checks every hour for 4 hours, then every 2 hours for four times, and then every 4 hours
Patient may stand to void
Reinforce dressing if needed; change dressing after 24 hours
Check vital signs every hour for 4 hours, then every 2 hours for four times, and then every 4 hours
Have patient deep breathe and cough every 2 hours; use Respirex 10 times every hour
Physical therapy consultation for exercise regimen and program

ASSESSMENT: AREAS OF CONCERN

Incisional area of lumbar back or cervical area
Assessment of motor strengths and sensory condition of feet and legs or arms and hands bilaterally (usually are within normal limits for push, pull strength; may have some remaining sensory changes such as lingering numbness or decreased sensitivity to sharp pinpricks)
All peripheral pulses palpable
Skin temperature of feet, legs, arms, and hands: may be slightly cool and pale
Drainage on dressing scant to moderate amount and serosanguineous
Pain mild to moderate in operative area with some radiation to shoulders and occipital area (if cervical) and to hips and buttocks (if lumbar)

Systemic concerns
Headache
Nausea
Abdominal distention
Urinary retention (may need to stand to void)

Psychosocial concerns
Acute pain
Lingering chronic pain
Limitation of neck or back muscle and joint mobility and strength

Other complications
Hemorrhage
Motor and sensory weakness
Continued pain

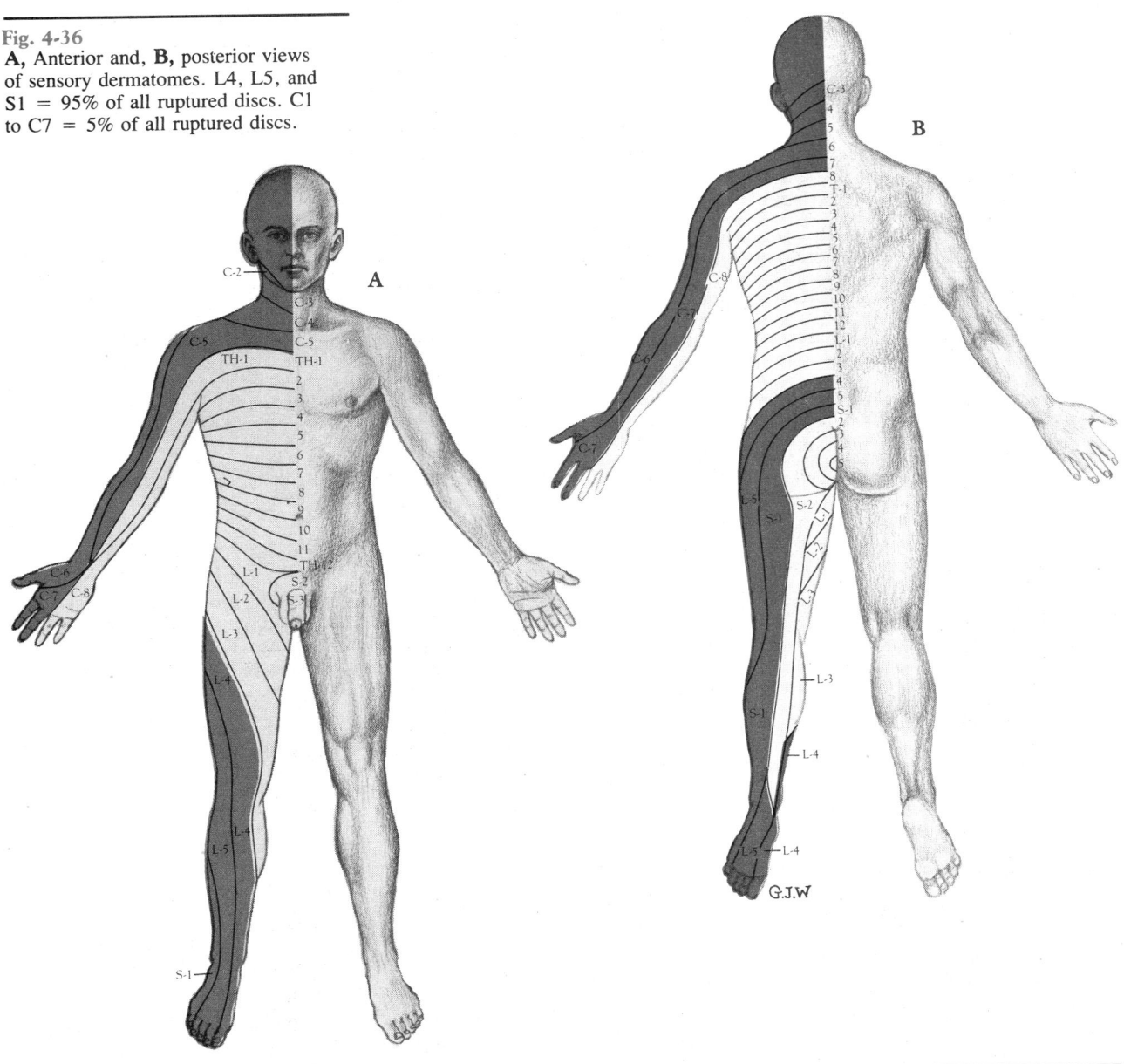

Fig. 4-36
A, Anterior and, **B,** posterior views of sensory dermatomes. L4, L5, and S1 = 95% of all ruptured discs. C1 to C7 = 5% of all ruptured discs.

NURSING DIAGNOSES and NURSING INTERVENTIONS

Nursing Diagnosis	Nursing Intervention
Comfort, alteration in: pain	Assess degree, site, type, and amount of pain. Medicate as necessary. Turn or adjust position to relieve fatigue and discomfort.
	Get patient up to change position and ease pain. Instruct on proper techniques to turn, sit up, and walk.
	Increase up time as able.
	Perform laminectomy checks. Report any decreases in motor or sensory functions.
Mobility, impaired physical	Encourage physical therapy as ordered and prescribed.
	Note and assess muscle spasms or limitation of movements when moving and doing wound care or hygienic care.

Nursing Diagnosis	Nursing Intervention
	Assess incisional area for relief of inflammation and wound healing evidence (approximation of wound edges, no drainage and, later, removal of sutures or staples).
	Assess vital signs for fluctuations that could indicate inflammation or infection.
	Encourage fluid and food intake of regular diet.

Patient Education

1. Reiterate need to do exercises to regain muscle strength following surgery.
2. Clarify and stress normal motor and sensory functions as evidence of regaining full functions with relief of inflammation.
3. Explain lingering numbness as sign of former nerve pressure that may or may not completely abate.
4. Clarify physician's home care limitations in lifting and driving for 3 to 6 weeks or longer (individualized based on specific condition). Stress follow-up visit to physician to determine recovery.
5. Explain signs of fever, continued pain, and wound drainage as reportable to physician.

EVALUATION

Patient Outcome	Data Indicating That Outcome is Reached
Patient has relief of neck or back pain.	Patient has little residual motor or sensory deficit and little or no pain, locally or systemically.
Patient has satisfactory ROM without muscle spasms or weakness.	Patient can move about comfortably and easily, can do prescribed exercises well, and returns to family, social, and employment activities.

CHEMONUCLEOLYSIS

Description and Discussion

Chemonucleolysis is the chemical reduction by an enzyme of a ruptured or herniating disc. The enzyme used is chymopapain, obtained from the papaya plant. It acts similarly to a meat tenderizer to alter the fluid content of collagen fibers by "breaking" the disc into its biochemical constituents of sugars, amino acids, and water; this softens the disc and lessens its pressure. Scar tissue then replaces the disc tissues as the inflammatory processes resolve.

Chymopapain was first used in 1964; it was approved by the U.S. Food and Drug Administration (FDA) in 1975, but the approval was withdrawn because statistics showed it offered no statistical differences in patients' symptom relief following its injection when compared to those persons treated with a placebo. Researchers disputed these data because it was found the placebo contained an enzyme. In November 1982 the FDA reapproved the use of chymopapain for relief of pain associated with disc herniations.

Contraindications and Cautions

1. Allergic history, reactions to meat tenderizers, and other allergens are contraindications.
2. Pregnancy and prior injection with chymopapain are also contraindications.
3. Chymopapain is also not used in progressive nerve deficits, whether motor or sensory, or bowel or bladder dysfunction.
4. Postoperative muscle spasms are a common occurrence.
5. Some patients may still require operative disc removal; surgery is more difficult following chemonucleolysis because of scar tissue formation.
6. Discs treated with chymopapain age more rapidly because they lose water.
7. If the sedimentation rate is elevated above 20 mm in women, chemonucleolysis is contraindicated, because anaphylactic reactions may occur.
8. Some physicians order preoperative diphenhydramine (Benadryl) and cimetidine (Tagamet) to lower histamine receptors.

Preprocedural Nursing Care

1. Obtain a detailed history of allergies.
2. Perform meticulous skin care.

TREATMENT PLAN

Chemotherapeutic
Adrenergic agents
   Epinephrine (Adrenalin), 1:100,000, on hand
Antihistamines
   Diphenhydramine (Benadryl), 50 mg on hand
Narcotic analgesic agents
   Meperidine (Demerol), 50-100 mg q3h for severe pain
Tranquilizers
   Diazepam (Valium), 2-5 mg IM q4-6h for muscle spasms
Intravenous, 1000 ml 5% D/.45 N/S at 75-100 ml/h for 12 h; then to "keep open" rate

Supportive
Check vital signs every hour for 4 hours, then every 2 hours for four times, and then every 4 hours
Observe for development of signs of anaphylaxis: wheezing, dyspnea, anxiety, rash, vital sign changes, flushed skin
Give nothing by mouth until patient is fully awake; then give clear liquids and advance to regular diet as tolerated
Patient should be up in morning and then three times daily
Help patient to deep breathe and cough every 2 hours
Do laminectomy checks every hour for 4 hours, then every 2 hours for four times, and then every 4 hours
Monitor voiding and input and output
Discharge in morning after physician visits (varies per physician and patient's progress)

NURSING DIAGNOSES and NURSING INTERVENTIONS

Nursing Diagnosis	Nursing Intervention
Comfort, alteration in: pain	Observe for presence and amount of muscle spasms (some physicians order ice applications; others order heat). Administer analgesics and/or muscle relaxants as ordered; see that patient has prescriptions for home medications. Perform laminectomy checks every 2 to 4 hours. Assist to stand to void. Assist with ambulation as needed. Change bed position as desired (lying prone is contraindicated).
Potential patient problem: anaphylactic reaction	Monitor vital signs as ordered, observe for rash, changes in pulse, blood pressure drop, dyspnea, or wheezing, anxiety (most commonly occur in first 2 to 4 hours).

Patient Education

1. Discuss anaphylaxis signs to report to physician (can occur as late as 1 week after procedure).
2. Stress that relief of symptoms may not occur for several weeks or longer.
3. Instruct patient to comply with physician's follow-up visit in 1 week.

EVALUATION

Since the use of and experience with chymopapain are so new, data are not available to fully evaluate this treatment.

Patient Outcome	Data Indicating That Outcome is Reached
Patient experiences no anaphylaxis.	Patient has no rash, blood pressure or pulse changes, wheezing, or dyspnea.
Patient is relieved of neurologic deficits.	Patient experiences tolerable muscle spasms initially with easing over time; motor and sensory changes are reversed: peripheral pulses are present; color is pink; temperature is warm; patient is able to move with normal ROM, void easily, and walk with upright posture with ease.

References

1. Adams, J.C.: Standard orthopaedic operations, ed 2, New York, 1980, Churchill Livingstone.
2. American Academy of Orthopaedic Surgeons: Joint motion method of measuring and recording, Chicago, 1965, American Academy of Orthopaedic Surgeons.
3. American Academy of Orthopaedic Surgeons: Symposium on osteoarthritis, St. Louis, 1976, The C.V. Mosby Co.
4. American Academy of Orthopaedic Surgeons: Reconstructive surgery of the knee, St. Louis, 1978, The C.V. Mosby Co.
5. American Academy of Orthopaedic Surgeons: Symposium on idiopathic low back pain, St. Louis, 1982, The C.V. Mosby Co.
6. Apley, A.G.: System of orthopaedics and fractures, ed. 5, Boston, 1977, Butterworth Publishers Inc.
7. Eftekhar, M.S.: Principles of total hip arthroplasty, St. Louis, 1978, The C.V. Mosby Co.
8. Gay, S., and Miller, E.J.: Collagen in the physiology and pathology of connective tissue, New York, 1978, Gustav Fischer Verlag.
9. Hall, D.: The aging of connective tissue, New York, 1976, Academic Press.
10. Johnson, L.: Diagnostic and surgical arthroscopy, ed. 2, St. Louis, 1981, The C.V. Mosby Co.
11. Marmor, L.: Arthritis surgery, Philadelphia, 1976, Lea & Febiger.
12. Moskowitz, R.W.: Clinical rheumatology, ed. 2, Philadelphia, 1982, Lea & Febiger.
13. Riseborough, E.J., and Herndon, J.H.: Scoliosis and other deformities of the axial skeleton, Boston, 1975, Little, Brown & Co.
14. Seligson, D., and Pope, M.: Concepts in external fixation. New York, 1982, Grune & Stratton.
15. Swanson, S.A.V., and Freeman, M.A.R.: The scientific basis of joint replacement, London, 1977, Pitman Medical.
16. Vander, A.J., Sherman, J.S., and Luciano, D.S.: Human physiology, ed. 2, New York, 1975, McGraw-Hill, Inc.
17. Widmann, F.K.: Clinical interpretation of laboratory tests, ed. 8, Philadelphia, 1979, F.A. Davis Co.

Suggested Readings

BOOKS

Aegerter, E., and Kirkpatrick, J.A.: Orthopedic diseases, ed. 4, Philadelphia, 1975, W.B. Saunders Co.

American Academy of Orthopaedic Surgeons: Symposium on microsurgery, St. Louis, 1979, The C.V. Mosby Co.

Bonica, J.J.: Sympathetic nerve blocks for pain diagnosis and therapy, vol. 1, New York, 1980, Breon Laboratories, Inc.

Burns, K.R., and Johnson, P.J.: Health assessment in clinical practice, Englewood Cliffs, N.J., 1980, Prentice-Hall, Inc.

Burny, F., et al., editors: Electric stimulation of bone growth and repair, New York, 1978, Springer-Verlag.

Carini, G.K., and Birmingham, J.J.: Traction made manageable, New York, 1980, McGraw-Hill Book Co.

Coleman, S.S.: Congenital dysplasia and dislocation of the hip, St. Louis, 1978, The C.V. Mosby Co.

Delagi, E.F., and Perotto, A.: Anatomic guide for the electromyographer, Springfield, Ill., 1980, Charles C Thomas, Publisher.

Dudrick, S., et al.: Manual of preoperative and postoperative care, Philadelphia, 1983, W.B. Saunders Co.

Farrell, J.: Illustrated guide to orthopedic nursing, ed. 2, Philadelphia, 1982, J.B. Lippincott Co.

Hanak, M., and Scott, A.: Spinal cord injury, New York, 1983, Springer Publishing Co.

Hilt, N., and Schmitt, E.W.: Pediatric orthopedic nursing, St. Louis, 1975, The C.V. Mosby Co.

Jones, D., et al.: Medical-surgical nursing, ed. 2, New York, 1982, McGraw-Hill Book Co.

Kerr, A.: Orthopedic nursing procedures, ed. 3, New York, 1980, Springer Publishing Co.

Kessel, L., and Boundy, U.: Color atlas of clinical orthopaedics, Chicago, 1980, Year Book Medical Publishers, Inc.

LaMaitre, G.D., and Finnegan, J.A.: The patient in surgery: a guide for nurses, ed. 4, Philadelphia, 1980, W.B. Saunders Co.

Lenman, J.A.R., and Ritchie, A.E.: Clinical electromyography, Philadelphia, 1977, J.B. Lippincott Co.

Loebl, S., and Spratto, G.: The nurse's drug handbook, ed. 2, New York, 1980, John Wiley & Sons.

Louis, R.: Chirurgie durachis, New York, 1982, Springer-Verlag.

Martin, M., et al., editors: Comprehensive rehabilitation nursing, New York, 1981, McGraw-Hill Book Co.

McWilliams, N.: Manual of orthopaedic surgery for nurses, Bowie, Md., 1982, Robert J. Brady Co.

Meinhart, N.T., and McCaffery, M.: Pain: a nursing approach to assessment and analysis, Norwalk, Conn., 1983, Appleton-Century-Crofts.

Mourad, L.: Nursing care of adults with orthopedic conditions, New York, 1980, John Wiley & Sons.

Price, S., and Wilson, L.: Pathophysiology clinical concepts of disease processes, New York, 1982, McGraw-Hill Book Co.

Rand, R.W.: Microneurosurgery, ed. 2, St. Louis, 1978, The C.V. Mosby Co.

Rowe, J.W., and Wheble, V.H.: A concise textbook of anatomy and physiology, ed. 3, Baltimore, 1972, The Williams & Wilkins Co.

Schneider, F.R.: Handbook for the orthopaedic assistant, ed. 2, St. Louis, 1976, The C.V. Mosby Co.

Silber, S., editor: Microsurgery, Baltimore, 1979, The Williams & Wilkins Co.

Thompson, J., and Bowers, A.C.: Clinical manual of health assessment, St. Louis, 1980, The C.V. Mosby Co.

Torbert, M.P., and Budesheim, G.C.: Arthritis. In Community health nursing, Philadelphia, 1981, F.A. Davis Co.

Urdang, L., and Swallow, H., editors: Mosby's medical and surgical nursing dictionary, St. Louis, 1983, The C.V. Mosby Co.

JOURNALS

Allen, B.L., and Ferguson, R.L.: A pictorial guide to the Galveston LRI pelvic fixation technique, Contemp. Orthop. **7:**51, 1983.

Arem, A.J.: The stiff hand: an approach to prevention and treatment, Contemp. Orthop. **3:**501, 1981.

Aviole, L.V.: Osteoporosis: diagnosis and treatment, Myology **4:**3, 1979.

Beckenbaugh, R.D.: Preliminary experience with a noncemented nonconstrained total joint arthroplasty for the metacarpophalangeal joints, Orthopedics **6:**962, 1983.

Brown, R.: Electrical bone growth stimulation, J. Operating Room Research Institute **4:**27, 1982.

Brumfield, R.H.: Carpal tunnel syndrome in rheumatoid arthritis, Orthop. Rev. **12:**69, 1983.

Carron, H.: Case study: postlaminectomy syndrome, Curr. Concepts Pain, **1:**16, 1983.

Cox, J.S.: Chondromalacia of the patella: a review and update. Part II, Contemp. Orthop. **7:**35, 1983.

Clancy, W.G., and Graf, B.K.: Arthroscopic meniscal repair, Orthopedics **6:**1125, 1983.

Crowninshield, R.D., et al.: An engineering analysis of total hip component design, Orthop. Rev. **12:**33, 1983.

DeLisa, J.A., et al.: Clinical electromyography and nerve conduction studies, Orthop. Rev. **12:**75, 1978.

Deyo, R.A.: Conservative therapy for low back pain, J.A.M.A. **250:**1057, 1983.

DiNubile, N.A., and Joyce, J.: Arthroscopy of the postmenisectomy knee, Orthopedics **6:**1301, 1983.

DiStefano, V.J.: A technique of arthroscopic meniscoplasty, Orthopedics **6:**1135, 1983.

Duncan, B.F.: Rehabilitation of the tennis elbow syndrome, Contemp. Orthop. **7:**61, 1983.

Eftekhar, N.S.: Hip surgery: then and now, The Bulletin **31:**16, 1983.

Farrell, J.: Caring for the laminectomy patient: how to strengthen your support, Nursing '78, **6:**65, 1978.

Fischer, D.A., et al.: Symposium: external fixation of fractures, Contemp. Orthop. **6:**113, 1983.

Frame, B.: Aspects of osteoporosis, Transition Med. Aging Process, **1:**16, 1983.

Garcia, A.: The ankle, Orthop. Rev. **12:**21, 1983.

Geelhoed, G.W., and Sharpe, K.: The rationale and ritual of preoperative skin preparation, Contemp. Orthop. **7**:29, 1983.

Graham, R.A.: Carpal tunnel syndrome: statistical analysis of 214 cases, Orthopedics **6**:1283, 1983.

Guhl, J.F.: Evolution and development of operative arthroscopy; 1974 to present, Orthopedics **6**:1104, 1983.

Hawkins, R.J., and Hobeika, P.: Physical examination of the shoulder, Orthopedics **6**:1270, 1983.

Hench, P.K.: Myofascial pain syndromes, Myology **5**:3, 1980.

Henning, C.: Arthroscopic repair of meniscus tears, Orthopedics **6**:1130, 1983.

Henry, J.H.: Lateral ligament tears of the ankle, Orthop. Rev. **12**:31, 1983.

Herndon, J.: Long-term results of silicone arthroplasty, Surg. Rounds **6**:94, 1983.

Joyce, J.J.: Arthroscopic anatomy, Orthopedics **6**:1115, 1983.

Kalisman, M., and Millendorf, J.B.: Managing osteomyelitic wounds of the lower extremity, Infect. Surg. **2**:321, 1983.

Kaplan, J.: Electromyography and nerve conduction velocities, Curr. Concepts Pain **1**:11, 1983.

Kasdon, D.L.: The neurosurgical approach to pain, Surg. Rounds **6**:28, 1983.

Kasdon, D.L.: The perception of pain, Surg. Rounds **6**:22, 1983.

Khan, M.A., and Khan, N.K.: Diagnostic value of HLA-B27 testing in ankylosing spondylitis and Reiter's syndrome, Ann. Intern. Med. **96**:70, 1982.

Klein, K.: Developmental asymmetries and knee injury, Physician Sport Medicine **11**:67, 1983.

Kornberg, M., and Eismont, F.J.: Discitis: an elusive infection, Infect. Surg. **2**:818, 1983.

Kreigsman, J.: Horizontal cleavage tears of menisci presenting with oblique tears: a computer assisted statistical analysis, Contemp. Orthop. **7**:43, 1983.

Kumar, P., et al.: Metal hypersensitivity in total joint replacement: review of the literature and practical guidelines for evaluating prospective recipients, Orthopedics **6**:1455, 1983.

Kunec, P.: Total hip replacement in patients under thirty-five years of age, Orthopedics **6**:1426, 1983.

Lee, M.H.M., and Ernst, M.: The sympatholytic effect of acupuncture as evidenced by thermography, Orthop. Rev. **12**:67, 1983.

London, J.T., moderator: Total elbow arthroplasty symposium, Contemp. Orthop. **3**:541, 1981.

Macnab, I.: Chemonucleolysis, Clin. Neurosurg. **20**:183, 1973.

Marmor, L.: Hematogenous infection of total joint replacement, Orthop. Rev. **12**:99, 1983.

Marmor, L.: Hip disease presenting as knee pain, Contemp. Orthop. **7**:19, 1983.

Marshall, J.L., et al.: Anterior cruciate ligament, the diagnosis and treatment of its injuries, Orthop. Rev. **12**:35, 1983.

Mooney, V., et al.: Symposium: back disease, Contemp. Orthop. **7**:71, 1983.

Munson, M.: Operative treatment for subtrochanteric fractures, Orthopedics **6**:874, 1983.

Navarro, A.H.: Physical therapy in the management of rheumatoid arthritis, Clin. Rheum. Pract. **1**:125, 1983.

Nisonson, B.: A guide to portal selection for diagnosis and surgery, Field of View Orthopaedics/Arthroscopy, **2**:1, 1983.

Pope, M.: Understanding and rehabilitation of low back disease, The Spinal Column **1**:9, 1983.

Rand, J.A., and Sim, F.H.: Evaluation and management of unicompartmental osteoarthritis: role of arthroscopy in upper tibial osteotomy, Orthopedics **6**:1288, 1983.

Reddy, M.P.: Ulnar nerve entrapment syndrome at the elbow, Orthop. Rev. **12**:69, 1983.

Reichman, H., et al.: The influence of immobilization of the wrist joint on the development of osteoporosis, Contemp. Orthop. **7**:55, 1983.

Rezaian, S.M., et al.: Spinal fixator for surgical treatment of spinal injury, Orthop. Rev. **12**:31, 1983.

Ritter, M.A.: Ambulatory care of medial collateral ligament tears, Physician Sports Medicine **11**:47, 1983.

Ritter, M.A., and Misamore, G.W.: Incidence of infection in total joint replacement arthroplasty, Contemp. Orthop. **7**:29, 1983.

Ritter, M.A., et al.: Cephalosporin prophylaxis for total hip replacement, Orthopedics **6**:850, 1983.

Rodts, M.F.: An orthopedic assessment you can do in 15 minutes, Nursing '83 **13**:65, 1983.

Roth, S.H., and April, P.A.: A preliminary reappraisal of salicylates as hypouricemic agents, Orthop. Rev. **12**:49, 1983.

Sakellarides, H.T.: The management of carpal tunnel syndrome, Orthop. Rev. **12**:77, 1983.

Schilling, J.: Wound healing, Surg. Rounds **6**:46, 1983.

Schwartz, D.P., and DeGood, D.E.: An approach to the psychosocial assessment of the chronic pain patient, Curr. Concept Pain **1**:3, 1983.

Shamberger, R.C., et al.: Progressive systemic sclerosis resulting in megacolon, J.A.M.A. **250**:1063, 1983.

Sherman, O., et al.: Peroneal nerve compression secondary to posterior osteophyte, Orthopedics **6**:1317, 1983.

Simmons, J.W.: Chemonucleolysis: an alternative to back surgery, The Spinal Column **1**:3, 1983.

Smith, M.J.: Electrical stimulation for relief of musculoskeletal pain, Physician Sports Medicine **11**:46, 1983.

Waldron, V.D.: Technique of hip nailing, Orthop. Rev. **12**:45, 1983.

Waldron, V.D.: Test for chondromalacia patellae, Orthop. Rev. **12**:103, 1983.

Ward, J.R.: Tertiary therapy of rheumatoid arthritis: suggested guidelines, Arthron **2**:2, 1983.

Weiss, A.B., et al.: Surgical protocols for PLA: carbon ligament implants, Contemp. Orthop. **7**:39, 1983.

Wexler, C.E.: Diagnosing spinal problems with thermography, Diagnostic Imaging, 1981.

Whipple, T.L., et al.: Laser energy in arthroscopic meniscectomy, Orthopedics **6**:1165, 1983.

Zarins, B.: Technique of arthroscopic medial meniscectomy, Contemp. Orthop. **6**:19, 1983.

CHAPTER 5

Integumentary System

The integument, or the skin, is the largest organ of the body. It serves as the protective barrier between the internal structure and the external environment. It is tough, resilient, and virtually impermeable, and yet at the same time it is affected by changes in the internal environment. Assessment of the integument provides data about how an individual is affected by and coping with both the internal and external environments.

According to the National Health and Nutrition Examination Survey, almost one third of all persons in the United States have a skin disease requiring treatment. However, the true extent of skin disorders is difficult to determine, since many persons with skin disorders treat themselves rather than seek medical care. An estimated 60.6 million persons between the ages of 1 and 74 years have one or more significant skin diseases. Of these, approximately 3.4% have a skin disorder severe enough to be a handicap to gainful employment or housework. The economic cost of skin diseases is substantial.[64]

ANATOMY AND PHYSIOLOGY

Structure

Anatomically the skin is made up of two principal layers, the outermost layer, the epidermis, and an underlying connective tissue layer, the dermis. Beneath the dermis is the hypodermis (subcutaneous tissue), which is technically not part of the skin but is composed of loose connective tissue and fat cells that provide a layer of insulation. Specialized structures of the epidermis include glands, hair, and nails.

The anatomy of the skin varies from one part of the body to another, and therefore the diagram of the skin in Fig. 5-1 shows only the main parts and their approximate spatial relationships. The pathologic conditions that arise in skin disorders occur in one or more of the various layers. The variation in anatomy often accounts for the distribution of skin diseases.

Epidermis. The epidermis is composed of stratified squamous epithelium. Two cell types, keratinocytes and melanocytes, make up most of the epidermal cells. The epidermis is composed of two major sublayers, the stratum corneum, which protects the body against harmful environmental substances and restricts water loss, and the cellular stratum, where keratin cells are synthesized. The basement membrane lies beneath the cellular stratum and connects the epidermis to the dermis. The epidermis is devoid of blood and lymph channels and depends on the underlying dermis for its nutrition.

The *stratum corneum* is the outer horny layer of closely packed dead squamous cells that contain the waterproofing protein keratin and form the protective barrier of the skin. The variation in skin thickness (0.5 mm in

543

Fig. 5-1
Structures of the skin.

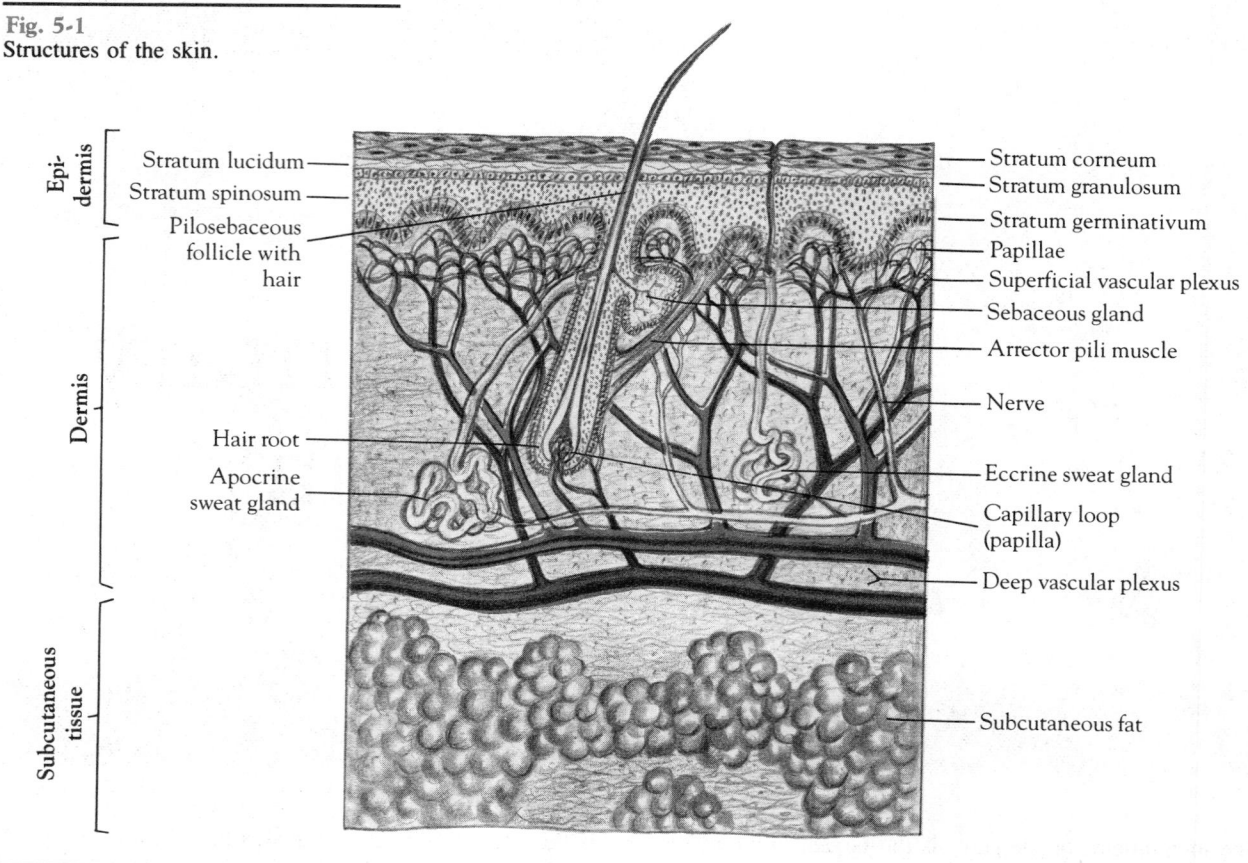

the eyelids to 4 mm in the palms and soles) is due mostly to differences in the thickness of the stratum corneum.

The *cellular stratum* is composed of three or four layers; from the most superficial to the deepest they can be identified as follows:

1. *Stratum lucidum.* This is a thin translucent layer of protein-filled cells found only in the thicker skin of the palms and in the soles. The cells of this layer are filled with a transparent substance that appears to be a precursor of keratin.
2. *Stratum granulosum.* This granular layer is composed of cells containing granules of keratohyalin, which is an intermediate in keratin formation.
3. *Stratum spinosum.* This is the prickle cell layer where cells begin to flatten and precursors of keratin appear.
4. *Stratum germinativum.* This is the basal cell layer where mitotic activity occurs to replace the cells in the upper epidermal layer. The basal layer also contains the melanocytes, which synthesize the melanin that gives the skin its color.

The keratinocytes in the basal layer evolve into cells of the stratum corneum as they mature (keratinize) and make their way to the surface, where they are eventually desquamated. The transit time of basal layer cells to the final stage of desquamation is approximately 28 days.

Appendages. The epidermis invaginates into the dermis and forms the following appendages: eccrine sweat glands, apocrine sweat glands, sebaceous glands, hair, and nails.

The *eccrine sweat glands* are small, convoluted secretory coils that transverse the dermis and open directly on the surface of the skin. Eccrine glands are peculiar to humans and are distributed throughout the body except for the lip margins, eardrums, nail beds, inner surface of the prepuce, and glans penis. The main function of the sweat glands is regulation of body temperature through water secretion. The eccrine sweat glands are innervated by sympathetic cholinergic nerve fibers, with heat the primary stimulus for their secretion. Muscle exertion and emotional stress also act as stimuli for secretion of water, chlorides and other electrolytes, and waste products such as lactate and urea.

Fig. 5-2
Structures of the nail.

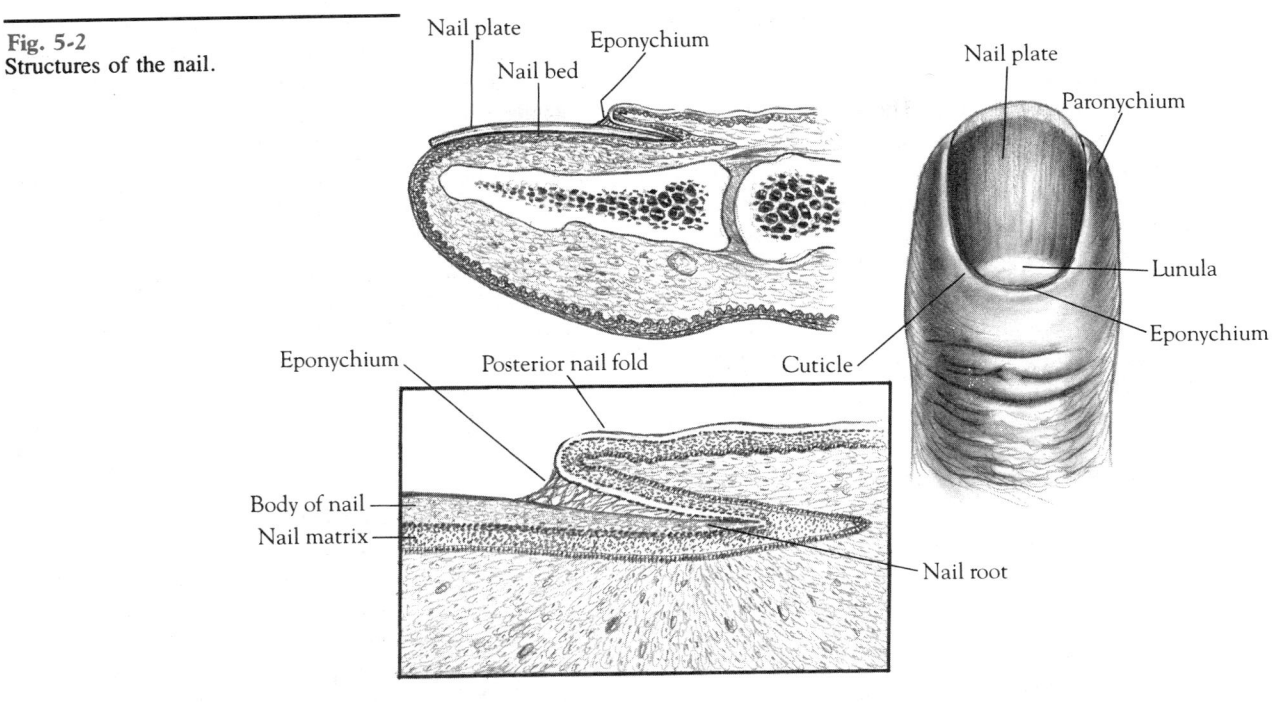

The *apocrine sweat glands* are specialized structures found only in the axilla, nipple and areola, anogenital area, eyelids, and external ear. They do not develop fully until puberty. These glands are much larger and are located more deeply than the eccrine glands. The secretory duct of an apocrine sweat gland enters the hair follicle above the entrance of the sebaceous duct. The apocrine glands are adrenergic and secrete a white fluid containing water, salt, protein, carbohydrate, and other substances in response to emotional stimulation. Secretions from these glands are initially odorless. The action of bacteria on the skin surface decomposes the organic components of sweat, resulting in distinctive body odors.

The *sebaceous glands* are distributed throughout the body except for the palms and soles. They are continuous with and secrete into a pilosebaceous follicle, which may or may not contain a hair. They occasionally open directly onto the skin. They secrete sebum, a lipid-rich substance that functions to help keep the skin and hair from drying out. The activity of sebaceous glands, which is stimulated by sex hormones, primarily testosterone, varies according to hormonal levels throughout the life span.

Hair is formed by epidermal cells that invaginate into the underlying dermal layers. Hair consists of keratin that is synthesized by cells in the papilla at the base of the hair shaft. The papilla provides nourishment for mitosis, which causes the hair to grow. The hair shaft projects above the skin surface and at an acute angle with the hair root. Hair goes through cyclic changes: growth (anagen), atrophy (catagen), and rest (telogen), after which the hair is shed. The normal loss of hair is not noticeable because neighboring follicles have differently timed cycles. Hair grows on most of the body except for the palms, soles, and parts of the genitalia. Men and women have about the same number of hair follicles, which are stimulated to differential growth by hormones. Melanocytes in the hair shaft give the hair its color. Hair follicle muscles, arrectores pilorum, are immediately beneath the sebaceous glands. When innervated by adrenergic fibers, they elevate the hair to a more vertical position and indent the surrounding skin, producing "goose bumps."

The *nails* (Fig. 5-2) are epidermal cells converted to hard plates of keratin. The nail root lies beneath the skin; the nail body (plate) is the visible part lying on the nail bed, which is a highly vascular area giving the transparent nail body a pink color. The white crescent-shaped area extending beyond the proximal nail fold (lunula) marks the end of the matrix, the site of mitosis and nail growth. The stratum corneum of the skin covering the nail root is the cuticle, or eponychium, which pushes up and over the lower part of the nail body. The paronychium is the soft tissue surrounding the nail border. Nails function to protect the toes and fingers.

Dermis. The dermis is the connective tissue layer of the skin that supports the epidermis and separates it from the cutaneous adipose tissue. The dermis is highly vascular and serves as the source of nutrition for the epidermis. The vascular structure also acts to control body temperature and blood pressure. The appendages of the epidermis are located in the dermis.

The dermis is composed of two parts, the papillary layer and the reticular layer. The *papillary layer* contains blood vessels and some nerve elements that respond to stimuli applied to the skin. This layer is folded into ridges, or papillae, that extend into the upper epidermal layer producing ridges on the surface of the skin, most notably on the palmar surface of the hands. The papillae also provide nourishment for the living epidermal cells and maintain a strong attachment between the dermis and epidermis.

The *reticular layer* contains elastin fibers for resilience, collagen fibers for strength, and reticulin fibers for stability. This connective tissue portion also contains blood vessels, lymphatics, nerves, matrix, and various cells. Collagen forms the greatest part of the substance of the dermis.

The major part of the body's sensory apparatus is the skin. The sensory fibers located in the dermis form a complex network to provide the sensations of pain, touch, and temperature. The dermis also contains autonomic motor nerves that innervate blood vessels, glands, and the arrectores pilorum muscles.

Hypodermis (subcutaneous tissue). The dermis is connected to underlying organs by a layer of subcutaneous tissue that is composed mainly of loose connective tissue filled with fatty cells. This layer of adipose tissue provides heat, insulation, shock absorption, and a reserve of calories. Both sensory and autonomic motor nerve fibers are also located in the subcutaneous tissue.

Function

The integument provides several functions that are integral to the functioning of the entire body.

Protection. An intact stratum corneum creates a physical barrier against invasion by bacteria and foreign substances and minor physical trauma. Glandular secretions wash microorganisms from the pores, and colonies of nonpathogenic bacteria present on the skin retard the growth of pathogens. Hairs in the nose, ears, anogenital areas, eyebrows, and eyelids act as a barrier against the entry of foreign materials. Sebaceous gland secretions along with the skin prevent absorption of water during immersion. The skin reduces potential damage to de-

oxyribonucleic acid (DNA) from ultraviolet radiation through thickening of the stratum corneum that disperses radiation and through melanin production that forms a protective cap over the nucleus of the cell.

Retardation of body fluid loss. The skin acts as a barrier to minimize loss of internal content and to prevent the internal fluid environment from leaking out.

Excretion. The skin acts as a minor organ of excretion. Some urea and lactic acid are lost through the skin along with sweat and sodium chloride.

Regulation of body temperature. The skin controls body temperature by four processes: *radiation* of heat energy from the body surface; *conduction* of heat from the skin to other objects or the air; *convection* or removal of heat by air currents; and *evaporation* of perspiration that is stimulated by the sympathetic nervous system when the body is overheated.

Blood vessels of the skin assist in control of body temperature by dilation in warm environments to promote heat loss through radiation and by constriction in cold environments to promote conservation of heat. If the skin is directly exposed to temperatures below 15° C (59° F), blood vessels begin to dilate to prevent the tissues from freezing.

Blood pressure regulation. During strenuous exercise, anxiety, or hemorrhage, constriction of skin blood vessels through sympathetic stimulation reduces blood flow to the skin, promotes increased venous return, increases cardiac output, and thereby increases blood pressure.

Tissue repair. The skin maintains itself and repairs its own wounds through exaggeration of the normal process of replacement of desquamated stratum corneum along with scar tissue formation.

Vitamin D production. The skin provides an area for irradiation of vitamin D precursors. Through catalytic action, ultraviolet light converts the precursor found in the skin to vitamin D_3, which is reabsorbed into blood vessels. Vitamin D is necessary in the metabolism of calcium and phosphorus.

Sensory perception. Free nerve endings and specialized receptors in the skin function alone or in conjunction to permit detection of environmental stimuli including pain, touch, heat, cold, pressure, vibration, tickle, itch, wetness, oiliness, and stickiness.

Expression. Feelings such as anxiety, fear, and anger may be visible on the skin through sweating, pallor, or flushing. Because of its visibility, skin is also closely connected with an individual's body image.

NORMAL FINDINGS

Area of Concern	Normal Adult Findings	Variations in Child	Variations in Older Adult
Skin			
Color			
Tone	Deep to light brown in blacks; whitish pink to ruddy with olive or yellow overtones in whites	Newborn reddish first 8 to 24 hours, then pale pink with transparent tone; slight jaundice starting second or third day of life, may last up to a month; mottled appearance of hands and feet in newborns, disappears with warming; in black newborns melanotic pigmentation not intense with exception of nail beds and scrotum	Skin of white persons tends to look paler and more opaque
Uniformity	Sun-darkened areas; areas of lighter pigmentation in dark-skinned persons (palms, lips, nail beds); labile pigmented areas associated with use of hormones or pregnancy; callused areas appear yellow; crinkled skin areas darker (knees and elbows); dark-skinned (Mediterranean origin) persons may have lips with bluish hue; vascular flush areas (cheeks, neck, upper chest, or genital area) may appear red, especially with excitement or anxiety; skin color masked through use of cosmetics or tanning agents	Upper and lower extremities similar in color	More freckles; uneven tanning; pigment deposits; hypopigmented patches
Moisture	Minimum perspiration or oiliness felt; dampness in skin folds; increased perspiration associated with warm environment or activity; wet palms, scalp, forehead, and axilla associated with anxiety	Perspiration present in all children over 1 month of age	Increased dryness, especially of extremities; decreased perspiration
Surface temperature	Cool to warm		
Texture	Smooth, even, soft; some roughness on exposed areas (elbows and soles of feet)	Smooth; soft; flexible; dryness and flakiness of skin in infants less than 1 month of age (shedding of vernix caseosa), may appear as white cheesy skin; presence of milia; small white papules over nose and cheeks (plugged sebaceous glands) may remain for 2 months	Flaking and scaling associated with dry skin, especially on lower extremities
Thickness	Wide body variation; increased thickness in areas of pressure or rubbing (hands and feet)	Varying degrees of adipose tissue; dimpling of skin over joint areas	Thinner skin, especially over dorsal surface of hands and feet, forearms, lower legs, and bony prominences

*Modified from Bowers, A., and Thompson, J.: Clinical manual of health assessment, St. Louis, 1984, The C.V. Mosby Co.

Area of Concern	Normal Adult Findings	Variations in Child	Variations in Older Adult
Turgor	Skin moves easily when lifted and returns to place immediately when released	Skin moves easily when lifted but falls quickly when released; skin over extremities taut	General loss of elasticity; skin moves easily when lifted but does not return to place immediately when released; skin appears lax; increased wrinkle pattern more marked in sun-exposed areas, in fair skin, and in expressive areas of face; pendulous parts sag or droop (under chin, earlobes, breasts, and scrotum)
Hygiene	Clean, free of odor		
Alterations	Striae (stretch marks) usually silver or pinkish; freckles (prominent in sun-exposed areas); some birthmarks	Café au lait spots (light, cream-colored spots on darkened background); some nevi; stork bites (small red or pink spots on back of neck, upper lip, or upper eyelid; usually disappear by 5 years of age)	Nevi often become lighter or disappear; seborrheic keratoses (pigmented, raised, warty, slightly greasy lesions most often found on trunk or face); senile (actinic) keratoses on exposed surfaces, first seen as small reddened areas and then as raised, rough, yellow to brown lesions; senile sebaceous adenomas (yellowish flattened papules with central depressions); cherry adenomas (tiny, bright, ruby red, round; may become brown with age)

Nails

Configuration	Nail edges smooth and rounded; nail base angle 160 degrees; nail surface flat or slightly curved	Nails generally longer than wide	Toenails may be thickened and distorted
Consistency	Smooth, hard surface; uniform thickness	Soft nails in infants and small children; become hardened with age; vernix may be found under nails of newborns	Fingernails may be more brittle or may peel
Color	Variations of pink; pigment deposits in nail beds of dark-skinned individuals	Postmature infants may show yellow staining	Toenails may lose translucence and luster and may become yellow
Adherence to nail bed	Nail base feels firm when palpated		

Area of Concern	Normal Adult Findings	Variations in Child	Variations in Older Adult
Hair			
Surface characteristics	Scalp smooth; hair shiny; vellus hair short, fine, inconspicuous, and unpigmented; terminal hair coarser, thicker, more conspicuous, and usually pigmented	Scalp smooth and soft	Sebaceous hyperplasia may extend into scalp
Distribution and configuration	''Normal'' varies with individual; hair present on scalp, lower face, nares, ears, axillae, anterior chest around nipples, arms, legs, back, buttocks; female pubic configuration forms inverted triangle; hairline may extend up linea alba; male pubic configuration is upright triangle with hair extending up linea alba to umbilicus	Newborn displays lanugo (fine hair over body, mostly over shoulders and back; will disappear during first 3 months of life); pubic hair begins to develop between 8 and 12 years old; smooth hair at first, changing to coarse, curly hair; followed approximately 6 months later by facial hair in boys	Increased facial hair (especially in women), bristly quality; men may have coarse hair in ears, nose, and eyebrows; decreased scalp hair; symmetric balding in men (most often frontal or occipital); decreased pubic and axillary hair
Texture	Scalp hair may be fine or coarse; fine vellus hair over body; coarse terminal hair in pubic and axillary areas	Scalp hair soft and fine; as child grows, hair takes on adult characteristics	Facial hair coarse; body hair fine
Color	Wide variation from pale to black; color may be masked or changed with rinses or dyes	Irregularity of pigmentation	Graying; whitening; hairs that do not lose pigment often become darker
Quantity	''Normal'' varies with individuals; gradual symmetric balding of scalp hair in some men		General decrease of body and scalp hair

DESCRIPTIONS AND CHARACTERISTICS OF SKIN LESIONS

Primary Skin Lesions

Primary skin lesions occur as initial spontaneous manifestations of an underlying pathologic process.

Lesion		Description	Examples
Macule		Flat; nonpalpable; circumscribed; less than 1 cm in diameter; brown, red, purple, white, or tan in color	Freckles; flat moles; rubella; rubeola

Lesion		Description	Examples
Patch		Flat; nonpalpable; irregular in shape; macule that is greater than 1 cm in diameter	Vitiligo; port-wine marks
Papule		Elevated; palpable; firm; circumscribed; less than 1 cm in diameter; brown, red, pink, tan, or bluish red in color	Warts; drug-related eruptions; pigmented nevi
Plaque		Elevated; flat topped; firm; rough; superficial papule greater than 1 cm in diameter; may be coalesced papules	Psoriasis; seborrheic and actinic keratoses
Wheal		Elevated, irregular-shaped area of cutaneous edema; solid, transient, changing; variable diameter; pale pink in color	Urticaria; insect bites
Nodule		Elevated; firm; circumscribed; palpable; deeper in dermis than papule; 1 to 2 cm in diameter	Erythema nodosum; lipomas

Lesion		Description	Examples
Tumor		Elevated; solid; may or may not be clearly demarcated; greater than 2 cm in diameter; may or may not vary from skin color	Neoplasms
Vesicle		Elevated; circumscribed; superficial; filled with serous fluid; less than 1 cm in diameter	Blister; varicella
Bulla		Vesicle greater than 1 cm in diameter	Blister; pemphigus vulgaris
Pustule		Elevated; superficial; similar to vesicle but filled with purulent fluid	Impetigo; acne; variola
Cyst		Elevated; circumscribed; palpable; encapsulated; filled with liquid or semisolid material	Sebaceous cyst

Lesion		Description	Examples
Telangiectasia		Fine, irregular red line produced by dilation of capillary	Telangiectasia in rosacea

Secondary Skin Lesions

Secondary lesions are a result of later evolution of a primary lesion or are induced by external trauma to the primary lesion.

Lesion		Description	Examples
Scale		Heaped-up keratinized cells; flaky exfoliation; irregular; thick or thin; dry or oily; varied size; silver, white, or tan in color	Psoriasis; exfoliative dermatitis
Crust		Dried serum, blood, or purulent exudate; slightly elevated; size varies; brown, red, black, tan, or straw in color	Scab on abrasion; eczema
Lichenification		Rough, thickened epidermis; accentuated skin markings due to rubbing or irritation; often involves flexor aspect of extremity	Chronic dermatitis

Lesion		Description	Examples
Scar		Thin to thick fibrous tissue replacing injured dermis; irregular; pink, red, or white in color; may be atrophic or hypertrophic	Healed wound or surgical incision
Keloid		Irregularly shaped, elevated, progressively enlarging scar; grows beyond boundaries of wound; due to excessive collagen formation during healing	Keloid from ear piercing or burn scar
Excoriation		Loss of epidermis; linear or hollowed-out crusted area; dermis exposed	Abrasion; scratch
Fissure		Linear crack or break from epidermis to dermis; small; deep; red	Athlete's foot; cheilois

Lesion		Description	Examples
Erosion		Loss of all or part of epidermis; depressed; moist; glistening; follows rupture of vesicle or bulla; larger than fissure	Varicella; variola following rupture
Ulcer		Loss of epidermis and dermis; concave; varies in size; exudative; red or reddish blue	Decubiti; stasis ulcers
Atrophy		Thinning of skin surface and loss of skin markings; skin translucent and paperlike	Striae; aged skin

Patterns of Arrangement and Distribution

The patterns of arrangement of skin lesions have diagnostic value in many cases. The patterns can sometimes be explained by their pathogenesis. There are three common patterns of arrangement:

1. *Annular*. The formation of rings indicates a process of extension of the lesions from the initial location to the periphery with clearing in the center. The skin may revert to normal appearance or may be scarred. Annular configuration can also be from an allergic process in which the central area becomes refractory. Annular patterns are commonly seen in pityriasis rosea, tinea corporis, tinea cruris, urticaria, and erythema annulare.

2. *Grouped*. This pattern is the localization of numerous small primary lesions in one area. It may be from mechanical factors (as in insect bites) or from a predisposition of a particular body area to a specific lesion as in herpes simplex.

3. *Linear*. This arrangement may be from external factors such as trauma or occur in contact dermatitis. It may also be determined by developmental origins of the lesions as in herpes zoster.

Skin disorders may present either generalized or localized lesions. The distribution of lesions may provide diagnostic clues. Generalized lesions may be indicative of an underlying systemic disorder as in erythema multiforme, an allergic response as with drug reactions, or a genetic disorder as with lamellar ichthyosis. Localized lesions occur frequently as the result of a primary irritant or allergic eczematous dermatitis. Many disorders produce lesions in specific regions of the body. For example, erythema nodosum produces nodules that are limited to the legs and thighs. Acne vulgaris produces lesions on the face, chest, back, and shoulders. Candidal infections usually manifest in intertriginous areas. Tinea cruris produces lesions in the perineal region. Pityriasis rosea may be distinguished from tinea corporis by the absence of lesions on the face and scalp. Pediculosis corporis is characterized by lesions along clothing lines, while scabies lesions are found in interdigital webs along the fingers and on the wrist and penis. In contrast, lesions from flea bites are limited to the ankles and lower legs.

In assessing skin lesions the following characteristics should be considered and described:

Characteristics of the lesion
  Size
  Shape or configuration
  Color
  Elevation or depression
Pattern of arrangement
  Annular
  Grouped
  Linear
Location and distribution
  Generalized or localized
  Region of the body
  Discrete or confluent

DIAGNOSTIC STUDIES

Many skin diseases can be diagnosed by physical examination alone through observation of changes in normal findings (see pp. 547-549) and through identification of primary or secondary lesions and their arrangement and usual distribution (see pp. 549-555).

The patient should undress and be examined completely to determine the presence of lesions on clothed areas of the body. The oral mucosa, anogenital area, scalp, and nails also frequently provide clues to the diagnosis. Good lighting, preferably daylight, is essential. A thorough history is also important in assessing physical findings.

The following areas should be included in a dermatologic history:

Usual care of skin, hair, and nails
  Products used
  Sun exposure patterns
  Cleaning regimens
  Home remedies or preparations
Dermatologic history
  Skin sensitivities
  Allergic skin reactions
  Tolerance to sunlight
  Increased or decreased sensitivity to stimuli

Family history
  Dermatologic diseases or disorders (acute, chronic, intermittent, and allergic)
  Genetic-related allergic conditions such as asthma or hayfever
Present dermatologic problem
  Temporal sequence: date of onset, sequence of lesion occurrence and development, and date of recurrence
  Symptoms
  Apparent cause
  Seasonal or climate variations
  Exposure to drugs, environmental toxins, or chemicals
  Relationship to stress or leisure activity
  What makes the condition worse or better
  How the patient is adjusting to the problem
Medications
  Topical or systemic
  Prescribed or over-the-counter
Travel history
  Where, when, length of stay
  Exposure to diseases
  Contact with travelers

The following studies are commonly used for diagnostic purposes.

Biopsy

Lesion marked and area infiltrated with lidocaine; small circular punch or scalpel used to obtain tissue to determine cell histology

Nursing care:
  Cleanse site with antibacterial solution; give patient information regarding procedure; apply direct pressure over area to stop bleeding (sutures may be used for areas larger than 3 cm); bandage

Scrapings

Area cleansed with alcohol and air dried so superficial fine dry scale is apparent; scale scraped with sharp scalpel and gathered on glass slide or in blood collection tube; nail and hair clippings also used; scrapings are covered with 10% KOH (potassium hydroxide) and viewed microscopically for presence of mycelia in fungal infections; fungus appears as branching, threadlike elements

Culture

For pustular lesions, swab sample placed in broth culture media; for chronic bacterial and fungal infections, biopsy specimen used for culturing; cultures incubated or refrigerated and observed for fungal or bacterial growth

Wood's light

Skin viewed in darkened room under ultraviolet light with wavelength of 360 nm ("black light"); certain disease-producing fungi and bacteria show characteristic color

Gram stain

Exudate from lesion smeared onto glass slide and stained with gentian or crystal violet; violet is washed off and smear flooded with iodine solution, which is then washed off; smear flooded with 95% alcohol and counterstained with safranin red dye; stain will differentiate gram-negative from gram-positive bacteria based on their ability to pick up one or both of the two stains

Cytology

Cellular material scraped from base of vesicle and stained with Wright's or Giemsa stain, or clean glass slide touched to surface of lesion so cells can adhere to it; cells sprayed with fixative and viewed microscopically after staining; multinucleated giant cells present in herpes simplex, herpes zoster, and varicella; pemphigus diagnosed by presence of typical acantholytic cells

Immunofluorescence (IF)

Serum or tissue specimen viewed microscopically; indirect IF test demonstrates that serum of patient with pemphigus or bullous pemphigoid contains specific antibodies that bind to different areas of epithelium; in direct IF test skin sample shows characteristic patterns for specific diseases

Electron microscopy

Glass slide smear of vesicular fluid or crusted tissue viewed under electron microscope to determine presence of virus

Patch test

Suspected allergen applied to skin under nonabsorbent adhesive patch and left for 48 hours; positive test consists of erythema with some induration and occasional vesicle formation; some reactions do not occur until after patch is removed from site

Nursing care:

Instruct patient to leave patch on, to keep area dry, and to return for inspection of the site in 48 hours; instruct patient to remove patch if itching or burning develops before 48 hours and to return for inspection of the site; reinspect site at 72 hours

Diascopy

Lesion covered with glass slide or piece of clear plastic to determine whether dilated capillaries or extravasated blood is causing redness of lesion

Side lighting

Beam of light directed from side over lesion to reveal minor elevations or depressions in lesion; helps determine configuration and degree of eruption

Conditions, Diseases, and Disorders

BACTERIAL CONDITIONS
Furuncles and Carbuncles

A furuncle is an acute localized staphylococcal infection that is initially limited to a hair follicle but spreads rapidly to the surrounding dermis and subcutaneous tissue. A carbuncle is a group of furuncles confluent into one larger lesion and involving adjoining hair follicles.

Furuncles and carbuncles usually occur in areas exposed to friction, pressure, or plugging, such as sweat glands in the axilla. These skin lesions tend to develop in persons who are debilitated, malnourished, fatigued, or obese. They also develop in persons who have altered immune mechanisms, diabetes mellitus, severe acne, or seborrheic dermatitis. Poor personal hygiene is a further predisposing factor.

Furuncles occur most frequently on the neck, breasts, face, and buttocks. The condition may be recurrent and troublesome (furunculosis) and often occurs in healthy young adults.

Carbuncles develop more slowly than single furuncles. They occur most frequently on the nape of the neck in men.

PATHOPHYSIOLOGY

A furuncle develops as a small perifollicular abscess that ordinarily destroys the hair and follicle during its early stages. A carbuncle involves more than one pilosebaceous unit and may involve many.

The invading organism, *Staphylococcus aureus,* which is found anywhere on the body, usually gains entry after trauma causes a break in the skin. The organism produces an acute inflammatory process around the hair follicle. The initial nodule becomes a pustule that is 5 to 20 mm in diameter at the base of the hair follicle. The surrounding skin becomes red, hot, and tender, with local edema occurring in 3 to 5 days. The center of the lesion becomes filled with yellow pus and forms a core that may rupture spontaneously or require surgical incision (Plate 1, *1*). The initial drainage is purulent and progresses to a serosanguineous discharge. Healing occurs gradually, usually with residual scarring.

The infection is usually walled off by local defense mechanisms. However, if the inflammatory process spreads to the deeper structures of the dermis and subcutaneous tissue (cellulitis), the bacteria may reach the dermal vascular plexus and cause septicemia. This complication is more likely to occur in persons with altered immune status and in infants whose defense mechanisms are less efficient.

DIAGNOSTIC STUDIES

Physical examination
   Characteristic lesion

Culture of lesion discharge
   Presence of infecting organism *(Staphylococcus aureus)*

TREATMENT PLAN

Surgical
   Incision to promote drainage after lesion has become localized and filled with pus

Chemotherapeutic
   Anti-infective agents
      Systemic antibiotics even for cutaneous lesions only
         Penicillinase-resistant penicillin for 4-6 wk to prevent subsequent development of new lesions
         Cloxacillin (Cloxapen, Tegopen), 250-500 mg po q8h for adults, 20-40 mg/kg/d po in divided doses q8h for children
         Dicloxacillin (Dycill, Dynapen, Pathocil, Veracillin), 125-250 mg po q6h for adults, 12.5-25 mg/kg/d in divided doses q6h for children
         Nafcillin (Nafcil, Unipen), 250-1000 mg po q4-6h for adults, 50 mg/kg/d po q4h for children
         Cephalexin (Keflex) for patients allergic to penicillin, 250-500 mg po q6h for adults, 25-50 mg/kg/d in 4 divided doses for children
      Topical antibiotics once the lesions begin to drain, bacitracin or Neosporin applied locally tid or qid
      Analgesics if lesions are extensive or if pain is severe

Supportive
   Warm, moist compresses to promote suppuration
   Nutritional therapy for underlying malnourishment, obesity, or debilitation
   Appropriate therapies for underlying disease

ASSESSMENT: AREAS OF CONCERN

Inflammatory process
   Tenderness; pain; swelling; redness around infected follicle

Systemic response to infection
   Malaise; fever; regional lymphadenopathy; increased white blood count; increased eosinophils; decreased neutrophils; increased lymphocytes; increased erythrocyte sedimentation rate

Spread of infection
   Personal hygiene; family hygiene

Psychosocial concerns
   Concern with body image

NURSING DIAGNOSES and NURSING INTERVENTIONS

Nursing Diagnosis	Nursing Intervention
Skin integrity, impairment of: actual	Use meticulous handwashing. Apply hot, moist compresses to promote suppuration. Change sterile dressings frequently after spontaneous drainage or surgical incision; properly dispose of contaminated articles.

Nursing Diagnosis	Nursing Intervention
	Teach the importance of not picking or squeezing lesions, since this may spread infection and increase the risk of scarring.
	Observe for signs of systemic infection (see p. 557).
	Instruct patient in correct use of antibiotic therapies.
Skin integrity, impairment of: potential	When drainage begins, eliminate compresses to prevent skin maceration and infection.
	Teach meticulous handwashing and proper hygiene practices to prevent autoinoculation.
	To reduce risk of recurrence, instruct patient to bathe daily with bacteriostatic soap and to avoid use of oily preparations.
	Address predisposing factors such as altered nutritional status and obesity; patient should modify intake of fats and sugars.
Self-concept, disturbance in: body image	Assess for presence of defining characteristics.
	Recognize importance of body image in growth and development.
	Teach importance of not picking or squeezing lesion, which may increase the risk of scarring.
	See p. 1820 for additional strategies.
Comfort, alteration in: pain	Apply warm, moist compresses.
	Instruct patient in use of analgesics.

Patient Education

1. Instruct the patient or family members to make sure that:
   a. The patient bathes daily with a bacteriostatic soap
   b. The patient uses towels, linens, and clothing separate from the rest of the family
   c. The patient's clothing, linen, and towels are changed and washed daily
   d. A clean washcloth is used each time lesions are cleaned or soaked; lesions should be washed gently, not scrubbed
2. Teach the patient and family to apply warm compresses and to change dressings using aseptic technique.
3. Teach the patient and family the need to maintain the correct regimen of antibiotic therapy.

EVALUATION

Patient Outcome	Data Indicating That Outcome is Reached
Therapeutic effect is achieved.	Existing lesions heal. Integument is intact and free of infection. Scarring is minimal. Pain is alleviated.
Hygiene measures to prevent spread or recurrence are instituted.	Lesions do not recur. Infection does not spread to family members.
Appearance is evaluated by patient in realistic manner.	Patient engages in usual activities and relationships.

Folliculitis

Folliculitis is a superficial or deep bacterial infection and irritation of the hair follicle usually caused by Staphylococcus aureus.

The bacterial infection can be limited to the hair follicle, resulting in its destruction, or the process can extend deeper to involve all of the hair follicle and the surrounding dermis.

Newborn infants may demonstrate multiple lesions of the forehead, face, and neck. In adults the lesions are found in hairy areas such as the thigh, face, scalp, groin, or axilla.

Folliculitis may become chronic where the hair follicles are deep in the skin, as in the bearded area. Stiff hairs in the bearded area may emerge from the follicle, curve, and reenter the skin, producing a chronic low-grade irritation without significant infection (pseudofolliculitis). Pseudofolliculitis occurs most often in black men.

PATHOPHYSIOLOGY

Folliculitis is a variable condition, with lesions ranging from minute, white-topped pustules in newborns to large, yellow, tender, pus-containing lesions in adults.

The primary lesion is a small pustule 1 to 2 mm in diameter, which is located over the pilosebaceous orifice and is sometimes perforated by a hair. The pustule may be surrounded by inflammation or nodular lesions. A crust develops after rupture of the pustule.

Predisposing factors include superficial damage to the skin, exposure to certain chemicals, solvents, and greases, and the presence of staphylococci. Other bacteria can also cause folliculitis, especially after antibiotic therapy. Gram-negative folliculitis occurs in patients who receive long-term tetracycline or erythromycin therapy for acne.

DIAGNOSTIC STUDIES

Physical examination
  Characteristic lesions

Culture of lesion
  Presence of infecting organism: gram-positive *Staphylococcus aureus* or gram-negative organisms

TREATMENT PLAN

Chemotherapeutic
  Anti-infective agents
    Systemic antibiotics
      Erythromycin (Delta-E, E-Mycin, Ery-Tab, Eryc, others), 250 mg po q6h for 10 d for adults, 30-50 mg/kg/d po in 3 or 4 divided doses for 10-14 d for children
      Penicillin V (Pen-Vee-K, V-Cillin K), 125-500 mg po q6h for 10 d for adults, 15-50 mg/kg/d in 3-6 divided doses for 10 d for children
    Penicillinase-resistant penicillins
      Cloxacillin (Cloxapen, Tegopen), 250-500 mg po q6h for adults, 50-100 mg/kg/d po in divided doses q6h for children
      Dicloxacillin (Dycill, Dynapen, Pathocil, Veracillin), 125-250 mg po q6h for adults, 12.5-25 mg/kg/d po in divided doses q6h for children
      Cephalexin (Keflex), 250-500 mg po q6h for adults, 25-50 mg/kg/d in 4 divided doses for children
  Topical antibiotics
    Bacitracin or Neosporin, applied locally tid or qid

ASSESSMENT: AREAS OF CONCERN

Inflammatory process
  Tenderness; pain; swelling; redness around infected follicle

Spread of infection
  Personal hygiene; presence of precipitating factors such as exposure to oils, greases, and solvents

NURSING DIAGNOSES and NURSING INTERVENTIONS

Nursing Diagnosis	Nursing Intervention
Skin integrity, impairment of: actual	Use meticulous handwashing. Apply hot, moist compresses to promote suppuration. Prevent maceration of skin, which delays healing. Instruct patient to use antibacterial soap. Instruct patient in correct use of antibiotic therapies.
Skin integrity, impairment of: potential	Teach meticulous handwashing and proper hygiene practices. Assist patient in identification and elimination of precipitating factors such as skin maceration and exposure to oils, greases, and solvents. Encourage growth of beard for men with chronic folliculitis or pseudofolliculitis in bearded area.
Self-concept, disturbance in: body image	Assess for presence of defining characteristics. Recognize importance of body image in growth and development. Assist in verbalization of feelings about body and body appearance. See p. 1820 for additional strategies.

Patient Education

1. Instruct the patient or family members to make sure that:
   a. The patient bathes daily with a bacteriostatic soap
   b. The patient uses towels, linens, and clothing separate from the rest of the family
   c. The patient's clothing, linen, and towels are changed and washed daily

EVALUATION

Patient Outcome	Data Indicating That Outcome is Reached
Lesions heal.	Integument is intact and free of infection.
Hygienic measures to prevent spread or recurrence are instituted.	Lesions do not spread; no new lesions develop. Lesions do not spread to family members.
Precipitating factors are avoided.	No new lesions develop.
Appearance is evaluated by patient in realistic manner.	Patient engages in usual activities and relationships.

Impetigo and Ecthyma

Impetigo (impetigo contagiosa) is a superficial vesiculopustular infection. Ecthyma is an ulcerative form of impetigo.

Impetigo and ecthyma occur primarily in infants, children, and the elderly. They are highly contagious among the newborn in nurseries and in young children and less contagious in older persons.

The arms, legs, and face are more susceptible to impetigo and ecthyma than are unexposed areas, although lesions may occur at any site. Impetigo occurs most commonly on the face. It usually appears first on the central facial area adjacent to the nose and mouth. Ecthyma occurs most often on the legs, the posterior aspect of the thighs, and the buttocks.

Outbreaks of impetigo occur most frequently during the late summer and early fall. Biting insects, mosquitoes, and flies appear to be important in the transmission of these infections. Predisposing factors include poor hygiene, anemia, and malnutrition. The infection spreads easily among family members and from one child to another in a classroom or playgroup.

PATHOPHYSIOLOGY

Impetigo is produced by coagulase-positive staphylococci and β-hemolytic streptococci. The bacteria may be found alone or in combination. Staphylococci are usually seen in very early lesions, but streptococci predominate in chronic lesions.

The infectious process is located subcorneally. The initial lesion is a small erythematous macule that changes into a vesicle or bulla with a thin roof. In streptococcal impetigo the vesicle becomes pustular in a matter of hours. A characteristic thick, honey-colored crust forms on rupture. In staphylococcal impetigo the thin-walled bulla breaks and a thin clear crust forms from the exudate (Plate 1, 2). Both forms usually produce pruritus, burning, and regional lymphadenopathy. Autoinoculation from scratching may cause satellite lesions to form. Since the process is very superficial, healing can occur spontaneously in the center of the lesion, resulting in the formation of annular or circinate patterns.

A serious complication that develops in 2% to 5% of patients is acute glomerulonephritis from a nephritogenic strain of β-hemolytic streptococci. In adults impetigo may have a more serious prognosis than impetigo occurring during childhood.

Ecthyma, a deeper infection than impetigo, often develops in neglected superficial abrasions or from the scratching of insect bites. The inflammatory process is deeper and involves both the dermis and epidermis with resultant scarring.

Ecthyma is characterized by localized thick, adherent crusted plaques with underlying ulceration and purulent exudate. The early lesions may appear as a vesicle or pustule surrounded by an area of erythema. Itching is common, and autoinoculation from scratching can transmit ecthyma to other parts of the body.

DIAGNOSTIC STUDIES

Physical examination
Characteristic lesion

Gram stain
Identification of infecting organism (gram-positive or gram-negative)

Culture

Identification of infecting organism (coagulase-positive staphylococci; β-hemolytic streptococci)

TREATMENT PLAN

Chemotherapeutic

Anti-infective agents

Systemic antibiotics

Penicillin V (Pen-Vee-K, V-Cillin K), 125-500 mg po q6-8 h for 10-14 d for adults, 15-50 mg/kg/d po in 3-6 divided doses for 10-14 d for children

Benzathine penicillin G (Bicillin, Permapen), 1.2 million units IM as single injection for adults, 600,000 units IM as single injection for children

Erythromycin (Delta-E, E-Mycin, Ery-Tab, Eryc, others), 250 mg po q6h for 10-14 d for adults, 30-50 mg/kg/d po in 3-4 divided doses for 10-14 d for children

Cloxacillin (Cloxapen, Tegopen) if initial treatment fails, 250-500 mg po q6h for adults, 50-100 mg/kg/d po in divided doses q6h for children

Cephalexin (Keflex) if initial treatment fails, 250-500 mg po q6h for adults, 25-50 mg/kg/d po in 4 divided doses for children

Topical antibiotics

Bacitracin or Neosporin applied locally tid or qid

Antihistamines for itching

Supportive

Crust removal through soap and water washing and cool, moist compresses

Nutritional therapy for underlying malnourishment or debilitation

Appropriate therapies for underlying disease

ASSESSMENT: AREAS OF CONCERN

Lesion

Vesicle, bulla, exudate, crust, or ulceration; satellite lesions; itching

Spread of infection

Personal hygiene, particularly fingernails; family hygiene; contact with others; presence of lesions in other family members

Glomerulonephritis

Oliguria; periorbital edema; hypertension; abnormal urinalysis with presence of red blood cells, white blood cells, protein, or casts

Psychosocial concerns

Concern that others may react to highly contagious disease; concern with body image

NURSING DIAGNOSES and NURSING INTERVENTIONS

Nursing Diagnosis	Nursing Intervention
Skin integrity, impairment of: actual	Use meticulous handwashing. Remove crusts: clean lesion with bactericidal soap and water; apply compresses of Burow's solution and cool water to soften crust; gently scrub crust; dispose of contaminated articles properly. Apply topical antibiotics to area of lesion for 2 days after lesion disappears Cut patient's fingernails short to minimize damage to lesion and to prevent autoinoculation from scratching.
Skin integrity, impairment of: potential	Cut patient's fingernails short to prevent autoinoculation and new skin breaks. Teach patient and family meticulous handwashing to prevent autoinoculation and spread to family members. Have patient and family bathe daily with bactericidal soap to reduce recurrences and prevent spread to family members. Check family members for lesions. Address predisposing factors such as insect control and nutrition.
Self-concept, disturbance in: body image	Assess for presence of defining characteristics. Recognize importance of body image in growth and development. Encourage patient to verbalize feelings about own or child's body appearance and fear of reaction or rejection by others. Prepare parents that they may encounter negative reaction from others because of child's contagious disease. See p. 1820 for additional strategies.

Patient Education

1. Instruct the patient or family members to make sure that:
   a. The patient and all family members bathe daily with bacteriostatic soap
   b. The patient or any family member with lesions uses towels, linens, and clothing separate from the rest of the family
   c. The patient's clothing, linen, and towels are changed and washed daily
   d. A clean washcloth is used each time lesions are cleaned or soaked
2. Teach the patient and family how to remove the crust from the lesions: apply cool compresses of water and Burow's solution to soften the crust and then scrub the crust gently.
3. Instruct parents to check other family members, particularly other children, for lesions; have infected family members treated.
4. Instruct the parents to notify the school nurse if infection is present in a school-age child.
5. Instruct the parents to isolate the child from other children until oral antibiotics have been given for 2 days.
6. Instruct the parents to watch the child for signs of glomerulonephritis for 5 days to 5 weeks after the onset of a streptococcal infection: dark urine, puffy eyes, decreased urinary output, headaches, and visual disturbances.
7. Teach the patient and family the need to maintain the correct regimen of antibiotic therapy even though the skin lesions have healed.

EVALUATION

Patient Outcome	Data Indicating That Outcome is Reached
Lesions resolve.	Integument is intact and free of infection.
Hygienic measures are instituted.	Lesions do not spread to other areas of the body. Lesions do not recur.
Measures to prevent spread of infection are instituted.	Infected family members are treated. Infection does not spread to noninfected family members or to child's classmates or playmates.
Glomerulonephritis, if it occurs, is promptly recognized and treated.	Medical treatment is sought for following symptoms: dark urine, puffy eyes, decreased urinary output, headaches, and visual disturbances.

Cellulitis and Erysipelas

Cellulitis is a diffuse, acute streptococcal or staphylococcal infection of the skin and subcutaneous tissue. Erysipelas is a rarer form of streptococcal cellulitis.

Cellulitis occurs most frequently in the lower extremities, usually from bacterial invasion through a wound in the skin or an open lesion. The infection may also spread through the lymphatic system from an existing infection site. Often, however, no predisposing condition or site of entry is evident.

Erysipelas occurs on the face (bilaterally), ears, arms, and legs. Recurrences in the same area are not uncommon.

PATHOPHYSIOLOGY

Cellulitis is most commonly caused by group A β-hemolytic *Streptococcus* or *Staphylococcus aureus*. Diffuse spread of infection occurs because enzymes produced by the organism break down cellular components that would otherwise localize the inflammatory process. Areas of skin trauma, ulceration, or lymphedema are especially susceptible to developing cellulitis.

The area of infection is diffuse and involves all layers of the skin and subcutaneous tissue, with ill-defined borders. The skin is red, hot, indurated, and tender. Sometimes pitting is evident with pressure. Irregular lymphangitic streaks (seen as red streaks) may extend from the periphery, and regional lymphadenopathy may be present. The skin frequently has an infiltrated surface resembling the skin of an orange (peau d'orange). Breakdown of the infected area can occur with purulent discharge. Local abscesses form occasionally and require surgical incision.

Erysipelas occurs at the dermal level of the skin and is caused specifically by group A β-hemolytic streptococci. The inflammatory process is acute with sudden onset. The area of infection is characterized by an erythematous, hot, and tender raised plaque with well-defined, sharply demarcated margins. Burning and pain, which may be severe, are common at the lesion site. Vesicles and bullae may develop and rupture, occasionally with necrosis of the involved skin. There is a pronounced exfoliation of the overlying skin as erysipelas heals.

Both cellulitis and erysipelas may be accompanied by systemic manifestations.

DIAGNOSTIC STUDIES

Physical examination
Characteristic lesion

Culture of lesion
For infecting organisms (group A β-hemolytic *Streptococcus* or *Staphylococcus aureus*); organism difficult to isolate unless drainage is present

Blood culture
For infecting organism: only occasionally positive

TREATMENT PLAN

Surgical
Incision and drainage of localized abscess

Chemotherapeutic
Anti-infective agents
Systemic antibiotics
Should be continued for 1 wk after infection has cleared; may need to be prolonged for several wks for erysipelas
Penicillin V (Pen-Vee-K, V-Cillin K), 125-500 mg po q6h for 10 d for adults, 15-50 mg/kg/d in 3-6 divided doses for 10 d for children
Penicillin G or benzathine (Bicillin, Permapen), 1.2 million units IM in single dose for adults, 600,000 units IM in single dose for children
Erythromycin (Delta-E, E-Mycin, Ery-Tab, Eryc, others), 250-500 mg po q6h for 10-14 d for adults, 30-50 mg/kg/d po in 3 or 4 divided doses for 10-14 d for children
For severe infections requiring hospitalization: penicillin G aqueous, 400,000-1.2 million units IV q6h followed by oral therapy after 36-48 h
Analgesics
Aspirin (ASA) or acetaminophen (Tylenol), alone or combined with codeine

Supportive
Immobilization and elevation of affected limb to reduce edema
Hospitalization for patients with severe infections or with systemic symptoms
Cool compresses for discomfort alternated with warm compresses or soaks to increase circulation
Appropriate therapies for underlying disease

ASSESSMENT: AREAS OF CONCERN

Inflammatory process
Cellulitis: tenderness; pain; redness; heat; swelling; lymphangitic streaks; peau d'orange skin; purulent discharge; abscesses
Erysipelas: tenderness; pain; redness; heat; swelling; raised plaque; vesicles; bullae; purulent exudate

Systemic response to infection
Regional lymphadenopathy; fever; chills; tachycardia; headache; hypotension; malaise; increased white blood count; decreased neutrophils; increased eosinophils; increased lymphocytes; increased erythrocyte sedimentation rate

NURSING DIAGNOSES and NURSING INTERVENTIONS

Nursing Diagnosis	Nursing Intervention
Skin integrity, impairment of: actual	Elevate and immobilize affected area for 2 to 3 days to decrease edema and increase circulation for healing. Use meticulous handwashing. Use sterile dressing changes for ulcers and open or draining lesions. Observe for signs of systemic infection (see assessment section above). Instruct patient in correct use of antibiotic therapies.
Comfort, alteration in: pain	Elevate and immobilize affected area. Apply cool wet compresses alternated with warm compresses or soaks. Instruct patient in use of analgesics.

Nursing Diagnosis	Nursing Intervention
Mobility, impaired physical	Elevated affected area to decrease edema and pain. Explain to patient need to maintain elevation and immobility for at least 2 to 3 days. Explore with patient options to maximize elevation and immobility depending on patient's situation and severity of infection: bed rest, sling, crutches, or leg propped above heart level.

Patient Education

1. Explain the need to elevate and immobilize the affected area for at least 2 to 3 days or until redness and edema decrease.
2. Instruct the patient to wash an open or draining wound gently with clean washcloth and soap and water and to change dressings using aseptic technique.
3. Instruct the patient to apply a cool compress for discomfort alternated with a warm compress or warm soak to increase circulation.

EVALUATION

Patient Outcome	Data Indicating That Outcome is Reached
Infection resolves.	Lesions heal. Integument is intact and free of infection.
Pain relief is obtained.	Symptoms of pain, burning, and discomfort are alleviated.
Mobility is regained.	Patient engages in usual activities.
Systemic infection does not occur or is quickly resolved.	Laboratory values are normal; temperature is normal.

Acne Vulgaris

Acne vulgaris is an inflammatory disease of the pilosebaceous follicles characterized by comedones, pustules, papules, or nodular lesions.

Acne is a pubertal onset disease, although lesions may occur as early as 8 years of age and continue through the 20s and 30s. The peak incidence appears to be around 14 years of age for girls and 16 years for boys. Acne occurs more frequently in boys but tends to be more severe and prolonged in girls. Almost all adolescents experience some degree of acne; about 80% have substantial lesions that range from superficial noninflammatory comedones to cysts and scars. Only a small percentage of these persons seek medical attention; most treat themselves with over-the-counter preparations that may be ineffective.

Acne lesions occur most frequently on the face, neck, upper back, and chest. The precise etiology of acne is unknown. Research now centers on hormonal dysfunction and oversecretion of sebum as primary causes.[71,83] The course and severity of the disease seem to be genetically determined. Dietary factors have little or no influence on the development of the disease, although certain foods may aggravate the condition in some patients.[11,90] Predisposing factors include the use of cosmetics, steroids, oral contraceptives, and certain drugs (iodides, bromides, phenytoin, phenobarbital, trimethadione, isoniazid, ethionamide, rifampin, and lithium); exposure to heavy oils, greases, and tars; friction or occlusion from clothing such as sweatbands, shoulder straps, and football shoulder pads; emotional stress; hyperalimentation; or an unfavorable climate. Acne seems to improve during the summer and to become worse in the fall and winter, probably because of the favorable effects of exposure to sunlight during the summer months. However, a hot, humid climate can produce severe acne in some persons.

PATHOPHYSIOLOGY

The sebaceous gland increases in size and produces more sebum because of androgenic activity. This is accompanied by abnormal keratinization of the middle third of the hair follicle, which results in obstruction of the pilosebaceous unit. This blockage prevents the normal flow of sebum to the skin surface, causing retention of cells, lipids, fatty acids, hair, and focal masses of *Corynebacterium acnes (Propionibacterium acnes)*. Subsequent comedones form either as open comedones (blackheads) or closed comedones (whiteheads). Open comedones have a distended orifice that allows the contents to escape to the skin surface. The black appearance is due to oxidation of the keratinous material or to melanin granules. Closed comedones have a skin covering that prevents extrusion of the contents and promotes further retention of keratin and sebum. The open or closed comedones can remain free from inflammation, despite the presence of bacteria. As the contents of the structure continue to accumulate, the enlarging comedone becomes visible. This process may take weeks, months, or a year. If the wall of the upper third of the hair follicle becomes disrupted, its contents are discharged onto the epidermis and a pustule develops.

An enlarged follicle can eventually rupture, discharging its contents into the surrounding dermis with the resulting development of the inflammatory papule, nodule, or cyst. There is usually a combination of acute inflammation and foreign body reaction induced by keratin and hair in the dermis. Rupture of the follicle can occur spontaneously because of the inflammatory effects of the bacteria or can be caused by trauma such as squeezing the comedone. The deeper the lesions, the more severe the potential and degree of scarring.

The regeneration of the ruptured follicular wall is accomplished by proliferating keratinizing epidermis, but cystic structures with surrounding fibrosis can form in the process. These can progress to deep cystic processes with interconnecting channels, gross inflammation, and abscess formation. Chronic, recurring lesions produce distinctive acne scars.

DIAGNOSTIC STUDIES

Physical examination
Characteristic lesions and scarring

TREATMENT PLAN

Surgical
Surgical removal of fibrotic cysts that have not responded to intralesional injections or liquid nitrogen therapy; excision should not be performed on actively inflamed acne cysts[56]
Intralesional injections of corticosteroids (triamcinolone [Aristocort, Kenalog]) into cysts, 2.5-5 mg/ml of injectable steroid in saline or lidocaine, 0.1-0.3 ml in each cyst

Chemotherapeutic
Vitamins
Oral retinoids[55,72,74]
Isoretinoin (Accutane), 1-2 mg/kg/d po in 2 divided doses for 15-20 wk; initial dose individualized for patient's weight and severity of disease, with dosage adjusted after 2 wk according to response of disease; second course may be initiated for persistent acne after 2 mo without therapy
Topical
Vitamin A acid (retinoic acid) gel or cream, 0.05%-0.1% applied nightly 30 min after washing face and 1 h before bedtime
Anti-infective agents
Systemic antibiotics (for severe acne)
Tetracycline, 250-500 mg po qid for 4 wk then decreased to lowest maintenance dose that gives good response
Erythromycin (Delta-E, E-Mycin, Ery-Tab, Eryc, others), 250-500 mg po qid; same regimen as with tetracycline, if response to tetracycline is poor
Topical antibiotics
Clindamycin 1%, apply tid or qid to lesions
Erythromycin 2%, apply tid or qid to lesions
Tetracycline, apply tid or qid to lesions
Keratolytic agents
Salicylic acid gel, apply nightly to affected areas
Benzoyl peroxide 2.5%-20%, 3-4 h/d for 4 d, then overnight if tolerated; patient establishes own level of tolerance for strength and time
Estrogens (for women)
Mestranol, 0.075-0.1 mg or equivalent po in cyclic monthly routine

Electromechanical
Cryotherapy—liquid nitrogen applied with cotton-tipped applicator or fine spray onto cysts
Expression of comedones by means of Schamberg or other extractor
Ultraviolet light in increasing doses at least once a week

Supportive
Well-balanced diet to eliminate foods known to aggravate condition; foods will be specific to each individual

ASSESSMENT: AREAS OF CONCERN

Lesion

Presence of comedones (open or closed), pustules, papules, nodules, cysts, pitting scars on face, neck, shoulders, upper back, or chest; seasonal or monthly pattern and history of past inflammatory lesions; evidence of picking or squeezing lesions

Inflammatory process

Tenderness; pain; swelling; redness around infected follicle

Psychosocial concerns

Concern with body image and social relationships

NURSING DIAGNOSES and NURSING INTERVENTIONS

Nursing Diagnosis	Nursing Intervention
Skin integrity, impairment of: actual	Encourage patient to seek medical attention when acne develops. Stress importance of adhering to therapeutic regimen; assist in setting up overall schedule for managing regimen on daily basis. Plan schedule for facial hygiene: clean skin with acne soap or mild soap once or twice a day, keep skin clean and dry, and avoid abrasive soaps. Give written instructions for use of peeling agents such as benzoyl peroxide or retinoic acid. Alternating the creams can give better results. Never apply the two together. Discourage squeezing, picking, and rubbing of lesions. Teach patient how to use comedone extractor. Set up criteria for which comedones can be removed. Establish limited schedule for removal. Apply hot packs to cystic lesions. Encourage frequent shampooing and hairstyle that keeps hair off face. Analyze dietary intake and help patient identify foods that cause flare-ups. Help patient deal with stress. Help patient label feelings, identify alternative courses of action, and set reachable goals. Identify and eliminate predisposing factors. Dispel myths that sexual activity or abstinence causes or affects acne. Instruct patient in correct use of antibiotic therapies.
Self-concept, disturbance in: body image	Recognize importance of body image in growth and development. Assess patient's perception of own appearance. Teach importance of not picking or squeezing lesions, which may increase risk of scarring. Encourage patient to verbalize feelings about body, body appearance, or fear of reaction or rejection by others. Encourage patient to develop interests and other attributes to support positive self-image, feelings of self-worth, and self-confidence. Help patient evaluate facial scarring in realistic perspective so it does not become focal point of existence. Advise patient of availability of tinted acne lotions that can mask lesions and scars. Arrange for individual or group therapy if patient is unable to adjust to appearance.

Patient Education

1. Provide written instructions regarding:
   a. Side effects of systemic antibiotics and oral retinoids
   b. Need for and schedule of follow-up laboratory work for long-term antibiotic therapy or with oral retinoids
   c. Untoward effects of topical preparations:
      (1) For increased redness and peeling reduce time and strength of preparation until symptoms subside, then increase slowly
      (2) Photosensitizing properties of retinoic acid: use only at bedtime; do not go out into sunlight with it on
   d. Safe use of ultraviolet lamp: eyes covered, timed exposure with backup timer, and measured distance

2. Teach good hygiene practices to prevent secondary infection.
3. Instruct the patient how to maintain a well-balanced diet and to get adequate rest.
4. Instruct the patient to go out into the sunlight unless contraindicated.

5. Discuss with the patient and family that successful therapy requires the patient's full cooperation and patience and that therapy is long-term and results may not be immediate.
6. Instruct the patient to continue local lesion care even after the lesions have resolved.

EVALUATION

Patient Outcome	Data Indicating That Outcome is Reached
Disease condition improves.	There are fewer comedones, pustules, papules, nodules, or cysts.
Acne lesions improve.	Lesions heal with as little scarring as possible. There is no secondary infection.
Inflammatory process recedes.	There is no pain, tenderness, swelling, or redness around affected follicle.
Side effects or untoward effects of medications are recognized and treated quickly.	Patient seeks medical attention for untoward or side effects.
Patient has realistic self-concept.	Acne disorder is not used as excuse for unsuccessful interpersonal relationships. Patient's perception of own appearance is realistic.

Rosacea

Rosacea is a chronic inflammatory disorder involving the central area of the face, which is characterized by erythema, telangiectasia, papules, and pustules.

Rosacea tends to occur in two types of persons: those who blush easily and those who become red easily from brief exposure to the sun. It appears most often in white women in their 40s and 50s. When it occurs in men, it is usually more severe and is often associated with rhinophyma. Rhinophyma is characterized by thickened red skin on the nose that can be disfiguring.

The etiology of rosacea is unknown, although alcohol, coffee, spicy foods, stress, and sun exposure may precipitate or exacerbate it in some persons. Physical activity, infection, endocrine abnormalities, use of tobacco, and extreme heat or cold—anything that produces flushing—can also aggravate rosacea. The use of fluorinated steroid creams can lead to the development of rosacea.

The onset of rosacea is gradual, beginning with periodic flushing across the forehead, nose, chin, and cheeks. The redness is intermittent initially but later becomes permanent. Telangiectasia develops along with pustules and papules. The inflammatory process causing the papules is granulomatous, differentiating it from the papules of acne. The pustules of rosacea appear similar to those of acne but do not have the characteristic comedones of acne. Rhinophyma is seen in advanced cases where there is marked hyperplasia of the sebaceous glands of the nose. Rhinophyma develops on the lower half of the nose and produces red, thickened, bulbous skin with dilated follicles.

Rosacea is sometimes associated with ocular symptoms of keratitis, corneal vascularization and blepharitis, and uveitis.

Rosacea usually spreads slowly and does not subside spontaneously.

PATHOPHYSIOLOGY

The main pathologic processes of rosacea are instability of the superficial blood vessels, which result in persistent erythema and telangiectasia; overgrowth of normal bacteria, which results in pustules; and a granulomatous inflammation, which results in papular localization.

DIAGNOSTIC STUDIES

Physical examination

Characteristic vascular flushing and acneform lesions without comedones of acne vulgaris; rhinophyma

TREATMENT PLAN

See Chapter 6 for treatment of eye symptoms.

Surgical
Excision of excess tissue in rhinophyma

Chemotherapeutic
Anti-infective agents
  Systemic antibiotics
    Tetracycline, 250-500 mg po qid initially for 1-
    to 2-wk periods to prevent pustules; decrease
    doses as symptoms subside
    Topical erythromycin 2% or clindamycin 2% alter-
    nated with hydocortisone cream
Corticosteroids (topical preparations)
  Sulfur 20% in hydrocortisone cream 1% applied bid
  Hydrocortisone cream 1% applied bid

Electromechanical
Electrolysis for large dilated blood vessels
Cryotherapy for rhinophyma

ASSESSMENT: AREAS OF CONCERN

Inflammatory process
Erythema, telangiectasia, papules, and pustules across
forehead, nose, chin, and cheeks; rhinophyma

Extension of inflammation
Ocular symptoms of keratitis, conjunctivitis, uveitis,
and vascular dilation

Precipitating factors
Erythema in response to sunlight, hot beverages, spicy
foods, vegetables, vinegar, alcohol, physical activity, and stress

Psychosocial concerns
Concern with body image

NURSING DIAGNOSES and NURSING INTERVENTIONS

Nursing Diagnosis	Nursing Intervention
Skin integrity, impairment of: actual	Instruct patient not to squeeze or pick pustules. Instruct patient to keep skin clean and oil free, but to avoid excessive dryness and irritation. Instruct patient to shampoo hair often to avoid oiliness. Instruct patient in correct use of antibiotic and medication therapies.
Skin integrity, impairment of: potential	Assist patient in identifying factors that cause exacerbations, and work with patient to eliminate them.
Self-concept, disturbance in: body image	Assess patient's perception of own appearance. Encourage patient to verbalize feelings about body, body appearance, and fear of reaction or rejection by others. Assist patient to evaluate own appearance in realistic manner.

Patient Education

1. Instruct the patient to eliminate factors leading to facial hyperemia: injection of hot beverages, spicy foods, alcohol, exposure to external irritants, and extremes of environmental heat or cold.
2. Instruct the patient to avoid excessive sun exposure.
3. Teach the patient about the effects of long-term antibiotic therapy and to report untoward reactions.

EVALUATION

Patient Outcome	Data Indicating That Outcome is Reached
Pustular lesions resolve.	Integument is intact with no papules or pustules.
Exacerbations are not triggered by avoidable factors.	Patient avoids factors leading to facial hyperemia.
Side effects or untoward reactions from long-term antibiotic therapy are recognized and treated.	Patient seeks medical attention for untoward or side effects.
Patient evaluates own appearance in realistic manner.	Patient engages in usual activities and relationships.

BENIGN SKIN CHANGES
Corns and Calluses

A corn (clavus) is a painful circumscribed area of hyperkeratosis caused by external pressure. A callus is a superficial area of hyperkeratosis that forms at the site of repeated pressure or friction.

A corn is a flat to slightly elevated circumscribed lesion with a smooth hard surface. "Soft" corns are caused by the pressure of a bony prominence. They appear as whitish thickenings and are most commonly found between the fourth and fifth toes. "Hard" corns are sharply delineated with a conical appearance. They appear most frequently over bony prominences, such as the interphalangeal joints of the toes at the site of pressure from footwear, and are usually quite painful. The pain may be dull and constant or sharp when pressure is applied, giving the sensation of stepping on a pebble.

Calluses are not well demarcated and may be quite large. They are elevated with a normal pattern of skin ridges running over the surface. Calluses usually occur on the weight-bearing areas of the feet, overlying bony prominences. Calluses may form over plantar warts and must be differentiated from them. They are also very common on the palmar surface of the hands, often indicating occupational acquisition. Calluses are usually not tender, but pressure may produce dull pain.

PATHOPHYSIOLOGY

A corn contains a localized pinpoint accumulation of keratin that forms an elongated hard plug in the horny layer of the epidermis with thinning of the underlying epidermis. The plug presses downward on the dermal structures.

In callus formation the epidermis reacts to repeated friction with an increased mitotic rate that results in hyperkeratosis and thickening of the stratum corneum.

The severity of a corn or callus depends on the degree and duration of the trauma that caused it to form.

DIAGNOSTIC STUDIES

Physical examination
Characteristic lesion consistent with history of chronic pressure or friction

TREATMENT PLAN

Surgical
Excision of superficial cornified layer of corn

Chemotherapeutic
Keratolytics
40% salicylic acid plaster or ointment
Corticosteroids
Injection of triamcinolone (Kenalog, Aristocort), 10 mg/ml at base of corn to relieve pain

Supportive
Orthopedic correction of weight-bearing mechanics through use of bars and support devices
Corn pads to redistribute weight and relieve pressure

ASSESSMENT: AREAS OF CONCERN

Lesion
Thickened skin; may be tender to touch

Pain
Location, duration, and intensity

NURSING DIAGNOSES and NURSING INTERVENTIONS

Nursing Diagnosis	Nursing Intervention
Skin integrity, impairment of: actual	Instruct patient how to apply keratolytic substance and to avoid normal skin. Demonstrate to patient proper application of corn pads.
Comfort, alteration in: pain	Instruct patient in use of corn pads to relieve pressure.
Knowledge deficit, cause and prevention	Teach patient that most corns and calluses on feet are caused by tight, ill-fitting shoes and that new lesions can be avoided by wearing properly fitting shoes. Show patient potential areas of pressure and how shoes should fit.

Patient Education

1. Instruct the patient not to pare away existing corns and calluses.
2. Give the patient instructions for the use of keratolytic plaster: Apply sticky side to skin making sure the plaster is large enough to cover the affected area. Cover the plaster with adhesive tape and leave in place for the designated period of time (overnight to 7 days). After the plaster is removed, soak the area in warm water and rub the soft macerated skin with a rough towel or pumice stone. Reapply the plaster and repeat the process until all hyperkeratotic skin is removed.

EVALUATION

Patient Outcome	Data Indicating That Outcome is Reached
Source of pressure is relieved.	Shoes fit properly. Orthopedic correction is used. Corn pads redistribute weight. New lesions do not form.
Existing lesions resolve.	Symptoms of pain are alleviated. Thickened areas disappear.

Sebaceous, Epidermal, and Dermoid Cysts

Sebaceous, epidermal, and dermoid cysts are slow growing, benign, cystic, intradermal, or subcutaneous tumors.

Cysts are classified into three basic types depending on their histopathology: (1) epidermal cysts, (2) pilar or trichilemmal cysts (sebaceous cysts), and (3) dermoid cysts.

Epidermal cysts are usually found on the face, scalp, neck, and back. Epidermal cysts include milia, acne cysts, and traumatic inclusion cysts. Only a few lesions are usually present unless the patient has had severe acne, in which case multiple lesions may be present.

Pilar or trichilemmal cysts (wens) occur most frequently on the scalp but may also occur elsewhere. These cysts have conventionally been referred to as sebaceous cysts. However, this is a misnomer. True sebaceous cysts are seen only in steatocystoma multiplex, a relatively rare inherited condition.

Dermoid cysts are usually found at birth. They are located deep in the subcutaneous tissue and may be adherent to the periosteum.

Cystic lesions vary in size from 1 mm to several centimeters. Most cysts are less than 3 cm in diameter but can enlarge to the size of an orange. On palpation the mass is firm, movable, round, globular, and nontender unless infected.

PATHOPHYSIOLOGY

The wall of the epidermal cyst is composed of keratinizing epidermis. The cyst contains keratin in laminated layers. The wall of the pilar cyst is made up of epidermal cells derived from the central part of the hair follicle. The contents of the pilar cyst are homogeneous rather than in laminated layers. The walls of the dermoid cyst are composed of keratinizing epidermis containing hair follicles, sebaceous glands, and sweat glands.

Cyst formation may occur after inflammation, trauma, or rupture of closed comedones. A person may also have a genetic predisposition to cyst formation. The contents of the cyst are the result of the obstructed hair follicle, and the exact nature depends on the level of the obstruction. The contents are soft and yellow-white and have a rancid odor.

DIAGNOSTIC STUDIES

Physical examination
Characteristic lesion

TREATMENT PLAN

Surgical
Excision of cyst, including wall, to prevent recurrence
Incision and drainage of infected cysts

Chemotherapeutic
Corticosteroids
Triamcinolone (Aristocort, Kenalog) by intralesional injection

ASSESSMENT: AREAS OF CONCERN

Lesion
Size; location; number; presence of tenderness, inflammation, or infection; on palpation, firm, movable, round, globular, and nontender

Psychosocial concerns
Concern about body image

NURSING DIAGNOSES and NURSING INTERVENTIONS

Nursing Diagnosis	Nursing Intervention
Skin integrity, impairment of: actual	Teach importance of not picking or squeezing lesions, since this may lead to infection of cyst. Instruct patient in dressing changes and suture care after surgical excision.
Self-concept, disturbance in: body image	Assess for presence of defining characteristics. Recognize importance of body image in growth and development. Teach importance of not picking or squeezing lesions, which may lead to infection and result in scarring. Assist in verbalization of feelings about body, body appearance, and fear of reaction or rejection by others.

Patient Education

1. Instruct the patient in dressing changes and suture care after excision of the cyst.

EVALUATION

Patient Outcome	Data Indicating That Outcome is Reached
Nonexcised lesions do not become infected.	There is no redness, swelling, tenderness, pus, or fever; scarring is minimal.
Excised lesions heal.	Integument is intact and smooth.
Patient evaluates own appearance realistically.	Patient engages in usual activities and relationships.

Cutaneous Tag (Acrochordon)

Cutaneous tags are common, small, flesh-colored or pigmented pedunculated lesions.

Acrochordons are found most often in middle-aged and elderly people. The number increases with pregnancy and menopause. The lesion occurs most frequently around the neck, upper chest, axilla, groin, and in association with seborrheic keratoses. They may occur singularly or in the hundreds. Although the lesion is benign, it may cause concern because of cosmetic embarrassment or irritation by clothing.

PATHOPHYSIOLOGY

The cutaneous tag consists of an outpouched core of loose connective tissue and dilated capillaries covered by normal epidermis. The papilloma is pedunculated and varies in size from 12 mm in diameter to considerably larger, soft, baglike, fibrous lesions.

DIAGNOSTIC STUDIES

Physical examination
  Characteristic lesion

TREATMENT PLAN

Surgical
  Removal with scalpel or scissors, with electrocoagulation of central vessel if needed

Electromechanical
  Removal through electrodesiccation or cryotherapy

ASSESSMENT: AREAS OF CONCERN

Lesion
  Location; number; size; presence of irritation, tenderness, and inflammation

Psychosocial concerns
  Concern about body image

NURSING DIAGNOSES and NURSING INTERVENTIONS

Nursing Diagnosis	Nursing Intervention
Skin integrity, impairment of: potential	Evaluate with patient the potential for irritation of tags through friction from clothing or rubbing against other body parts.
Self-concept, disturbance in: body image	Assess for presence of defining characteristics. Encourage patient to verbalize feelings about body, body appearance, or fear of reaction or rejection by others.

Patient Education

1. Instruct the patient in the benign nature of the lesions.
2. Instruct the patient that removal of the lesions can be accomplished relatively easily for cosmetic purposes or if tags become irritated.

EVALUATION

Patient Outcome	Data Indicating That Outcome is Reached
Patient evaluates lesions in realistic manner.	Patient seeks treatment for lesions that are irritated or inflamed. Lesions are removed if they become irritated or if patient is embarrassed.

Keloid

A keloid is an overgrowth of fibroelastic tissue that arises spontaneously or at the site of dermal trauma.

The factors that trigger keloid formation are unknown. There appears to be a genetic predisposition and a regional susceptibility in that keloids commonly occur on the sternum, chest, upper back, and earlobes and where an injury crosses normal flexion creases. Keloids occur predominantly in children or young adults, particularly in dark-skinned persons (Fig. 5-3).

PATHOPHYSIOLOGY

In susceptible persons keloids form after any dermal trauma or may arise spontaneously. Keloids represent abnormal progressive deposition of collagen that exceeds the requirements for wound repair. This may be the result of immune activity. The lesions are soft and pink in the early stages and then become firm and white. Keloids are raised, smooth, or ridged, extend beyond the edges of the initial wound, and may continue to grow for many months or years to form large irregular lesions. Keloid scars are frequently tender and pruritic.

DIAGNOSTIC STUDIES

Physical examination
  Characteristic lesion; clinical differentiation from hypertrophic scar not possible in first 3 months of lesion, but thereafter any continued increase in size and sensitivity of firm, indurated scar is indicative of keloid formation

TREATMENT PLAN

Keloids may become worse as the result of treatment; therefore the need for intervention must first be carefully assessed. Small keloids are often best left untreated. Many keloids gradually soften and flatten out over a period of years even without treatment.

Surgical
  Surgical excision combined with radiation therapy or intralesional injection of steroids for large keloids—surgical excision alone will result in the formation of new and larger keloids

Chemotherapeutic
  Corticosteroids
    Triamcinolone (Aristocort, Kenalog), 20-40 mg/ml by intralesional injection; may require repeated injections at monthly intervals until keloid remains flattened and asymptomatic

Supportive
  Solid carbon dioxide or liquid nitrogen applied toically at 2-week intervals

ASSESSMENT: AREAS OF CONCERN

Lesion
  Size; location; color; tenderness; pruritus

Psychosocial concerns
  Concern about body image

Fig. 5-3
Keloid.
Courtesy of Stephen B. Tucker, M.D., Department of Dermatology, University of Texas Health Science Center at Houston.

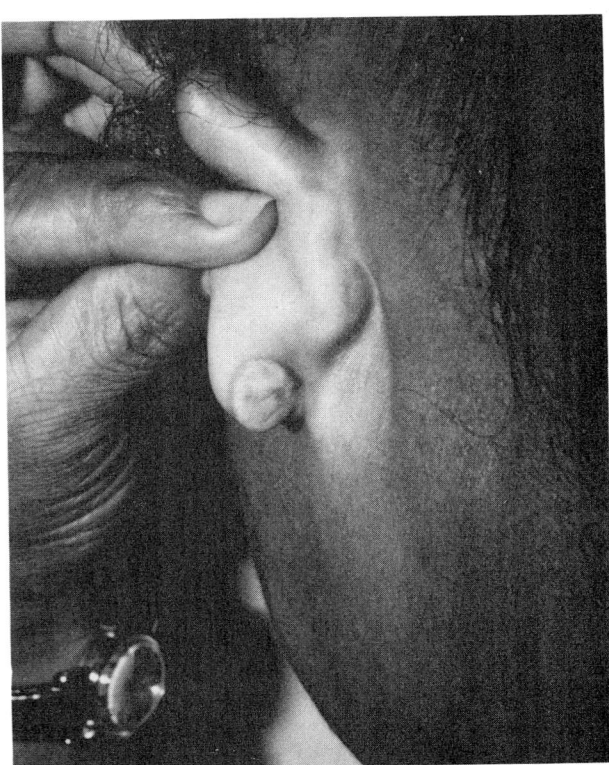

NURSING DIAGNOSES and NURSING INTERVENTIONS

Nursing Diagnosis	Nursing Intervention
Skin integrity, impairment of: actual	Discuss with patient the nature of keloid formation and assist patient in seeking skilled practitioners for therapeutic intervention. Inform patient that optimum time for treatment is within first few months of scar formation while lesions are still vascular and growing and that older keloids may be resistant to treatment. Instruct patient not to scratch keloid that itches to avoid dermal trauma that could cause further keloid formation.
Skin integrity, impairment of: potential	Discuss with patient safety habits to avoid injury that leads to keloid formation: protective clothing, proper equipment, and so on.
Self-concept, disturbance in: body image	Assess patient's perception of own appearance. Assist in verbalization of feelings about body, body appearance, and fear of reaction or rejection by others. Assist patient to evaluate own appearance in realistic manner.

Patient Education

1. Discuss with the patient the nature of keloid behavior and the need to evaluate therapeutic intervention carefully with practitioners who are familiar with and skilled in treating keloids.
2. Inform the patient that many keloids gradually soften and flatten out over a period of years even without treatment.

EVALUATION

Patient Outcome	Data Indicating That Outcome is Reached
Patient is knowledgeable about keloid therapies and risks.	Patient seeks intervention early and from practitioners who are familiar with and skilled in keloid treatment. Patient avoids surgical excision of keloids.
Patient takes measures to prevent injury that would result in keloid formation.	Patient uses safety measures, such as protective clothing and use of proper equipment, to avoid injury. Patient refrains from scratching or irritating scar tissue.
Patient evaluates appearance in realistic manner.	Patient engages in usual activities and relationships.

Seborrheic Keratoses

Seborrheic keratoses are common, benign, superficial, epithelial, pigmented tumors.

The cause of seborrheic keratoses is not known. They occur most frequently after 40 years of age. The most common sites of occurrence are the back, central chest, face, and scalp. In blacks the lesions tend to be more numerous and smaller and to occur earlier. The lesions are inherited as a dominant trait.

Seborrheic keratoses vary in color from yellow to brownish black. They are elevated plaques with sharply circumscribed borders and give the appearance of being stuck on the skin. The size of the lesion varies from a few millimeters to several centimeters. They almost always occur in multiples rather than singly. These lesions do not become malignant, although a sudden increase in the number and degree of itching of the lesions can occur in association with an internal malignancy.

PATHOPHYSIOLOGY

Immature keratinocytes accumulate, causing formation of seborrheic keratoses. Keratinization eventually occurs, causing the lesions to become warty, dry, and fissured. The surface of the lesions often have a greasy appearance, with pits filled with keratotic material. These represent invaginations of the epidermis. There is also a papular variant of the lesion that has a smooth surface. Epidermal thickening is associated with an increase of dermal papillae and the formation of the verrucous surface. The lesions grow slowly and are round or oval in shape.

Seborrheic keratoses are usually asymptomatic unless they become irritated. They may itch occasionally. Irritation of the lesions by physical or chemical trauma results in tenderness, itching, erythema, and an increase in the size of the lesion.

DIAGNOSTIC STUDIES

Physical examination
Characteristic lesion

Biopsy
Done if squamous cell carcinoma is suspected

TREATMENT PLAN

In most instances small, asymptomatic seborrheic keratoses require no treatment. Treatment is instituted for lesions that itch, are irritated, or are cosmetically embarrassing.

Surgical
Shave ablation or curettage using local anesthesia

Supportive
Liquid nitrogen cryotherapy at 2- to 3-week intervals
Carbon dioxide pencil applied with light to moderate pressure for 12 to 20 seconds.

ASSESSMENT: AREAS OF CONCERN

Lesion
Location; size; number; appearance; color; surface characteristics; borders; pruritus; changes in characteristics

Irritation of lesion
Erythema; tenderness; increased pruritus

Psychosocial concerns
Concern with body image

NURSING DIAGNOSES and NURSING INTERVENTIONS

Nursing Diagnosis	Nursing Intervention
Skin integrity, impairment of: actual	Reassure patient that this lesion has no potential for malignancy. Have patient identify lesions that itch, are irritated, or are cosmetically embarrassing. Evaluate with patient lesions that are likely to become irritated from clothing or rubbing against other body parts.
Self-concept, disturbance in: body image	Assess patient's perception of own appearance. Encourage patient's verbalization of feelings about body, body appearance, or fear of reaction or rejection by others. Inform patient that bothersome lesions can be removed, usually with minimal or no scarring.

Patient Education

1. Inform the patient that the lesion has no potential for malignancy.
2. Instruct the patient to seek medical therapy for lesions that become irritated or bothersome or that are cosmetically embarrassing.

EVALUATION

Patient Outcome	Data Indicating That Outcome is Reached
Patient evaluates lesions realistically.	Patient seeks treatment for lesions that itch, are irritated, or are cosmetically embarrassing.
Patient evaluates appearance realistically.	Patient engages in usual activities and relationships.
Treated lesions heal.	Integument is intact with minimal scarring and is free of infection.

BULLOUS DISEASES
Pemphigus

Pemphigus is an uncommon, chronic, and potentially fatal skin disease that is characterized by the formation of intraepidermal bullae on apparently healthy skin and mucous membrane.

Pemphigus occurs most often in middle-aged persons of Jewish descent and Mediterranean extraction. It often affects debilitated individuals and occurs equally in men and women. Pemphigus may occur at any age, although it is rare in children.

Mortality from untreated pemphigus is high. The disease may be fatal even with treatment; 50% of patients die within 6 months to 10 years of onset of the disease. Corticosteroid therapy has decreased mortality by two thirds.

In *pemphigus vulgaris and pemphigus vegetans* erosion of the buccal mucosa is the first indicator of disease in approximately 50% of cases. The erosions are painful and persistent. Other cutaneous membranes such as the conjunctiva, esophagus, vulva, and rectal mucosa may be involved.

Cutaneous lesions can occur anywhere on the body as tense, fluid-filled bullae that become flaccid and rupture easily, leading to painful denuded erosions that bleed, ooze, and crust. Large areas of denuded skin result in substantial body fluid, protein, and electrolyte loss and predispose the patient to secondary bacterial infection. Intact skin surfaces are easily damaged and separated from the dermis by light rubbing or friction (Nikolsky's sign). The lesions heal slowly, but when healing does occur, there is no scar because the lesion is intraepidermal.

Lesions are common in pressure areas, axillae, groin, face, and scalp. Generalized eruptions develop in 6 to 12 months from the onset of early lesions.

Pemphigus foliaceus is characterized by extensive generalized eruptions with a moist, red, edematous, exfoliating appearance. The buccal mucosa is rarely involved. In *pemphigus erythematosus* the lesions are localized to the face and chest and are red, moist, and crusted over. Both are benign forms of pemphigus.

PATHOPHYSIOLOGY

The basic mechanism of pemphigus is an antigen-antibody reaction or an autoimmune response that causes destruction of the mucopolysaccharide protein complex of the intercellular cement. The epidermal cells lose their cohesion, which results in splitting and separation of the normal intercellular contact between epidermal cells (acantholysis) and the formation of bullae. The basal cells remain attached to the basement membrane, and the bullae that form contain detached, rounded, epidermal cells.

The clinical appearance of pemphigus depends on the level and type of acantholysis. Thin-walled bullae and eruptions develop in pemphigus vulgaris and pemphigus vegetans, in which the acantholysis is predominantly suprabasal. Erythema and scaling occur in pemphigus foliaceus and pemphigus erythematosus, in which the acantholysis occurs higher in the epidermis.

DIAGNOSTIC STUDIES

Physical examination
   Characteristic lesion; positive Nikolsky's sign: lateral pressure on skin separates epidermis from dermis

Complete blood count
   Eosinophilia

Immunofluorescence (IF)
   Presence of IgG antibodies in serum (direct IF) or on epidermal or epithelial cell surfaces (indirect IF)

Biopsy
   Suprabasal cell separation

Cytology
   Tzanck smear: acantholytic cells stain blue with Wright's or Giemsa stain

TREATMENT PLAN

Chemotherapeutic
   Corticosteroids
      Systemic
         Prednisone, 150-300 mg/d po for 6-8 wk, then decreasing doses when no new lesions appear for 7-10 d
      Topical
         Fluocinonide (Lidex, Topsyn) 0.05% tid or qid; triamcinolone (Aristocort, Kenalog) 0.025%-0.1%, tid or qid
   Antineoplastic agents (used for immunosuppressive effect)
      Methotrexate, azathioprine, and cyclophosphamide in individualized doses
   Analgesics if lesions are extensive or pain is severe

Supportive
   Cool compresses or soaks

Wet Dakin's dressings
Potassium permanganate baths (see p. 638)
Intravenous therapy for fluid and electrolyte balance
Blood and plasma transfusions for fluid and protein loss
Nutrition—high-protein, high-calorie diet to support healing and reepithelization and to replace protein loss through extensive bullae

ASSESSMENT: AREAS OF CONCERN

Lesion
Raw, round, weeping lesions; pruritus; burning; odor; bullae with little or no inflammation; location and number of lesions; extent of body covered

Systemic involvement
Anorexia; weight loss; weakness; fever; eosinophilia

Fluid and electrolyte balance
Weight loss; weakness; dry mucous membrane; hydration status; lowered serum sodium, chloride, and potassium levels

Secondary infection
Inflammation; pus; odor; increased white blood count; increased eosinophils; increased lymphocytes; increased erythrocyte sedimentation rate; decreased neutrophils

Nutrition
Inability to eat because of mouth sores

Psychosocial concerns
Concern with body image; concern about dying

NURSING DIAGNOSES and NURSING INTERVENTIONS

Nursing Diagnosis	Nursing Intervention
Skin integrity, impairment of: actual	In collaboration with physician, provide cool baths and soaks, Dakin's dressings, and potassium permanganate baths using aseptic technique. In collaboration with physician, use Stryker frame or CircOlectric bed to relieve pressure and decrease painful movement on raw surfaces. Use meticulous hygiene. Observe for signs of septicemia. Assess for and prevent secondary infection; reverse isolation as needed. Use room deodorizer. Test urine for glucose and albumin when patient is receiving high doses of corticosteroids.
Oral mucous membrane, alteration in	Provide mouth care with saline or alkaline mouthwash. Provide soft, bland diet. Avoid acidic and astringent fluids. Have patient use viscous lidocaine mouthwash.
Body fluid, alteration in composition: fluid volume deficit, potential for	Provide adequate hydration by mouth and intravenously. Monitor intake and output. Weigh daily. Monitor vital signs and hydration status. Observe for adverse reaction after administration of blood or blood components.
Nutrition, alteration in: less than body requirements	Provide high-protein, high-calorie diet. Provide small, frequent feedings. Provide snacks between meals.
Comfort, alteration in: pain	Apply cool compresses or soaks. Use Stryker frame or CircOlectric bed. Use talcum powder liberally on bedsheets. Provide soft, bland foods. Offer nonacidic, nonastringent fluids.
Self-concept, disturbance in: body image	Assist patient in verbalization of feelings about body, body appearance, or fear of reaction or rejection by others. Spend time with patient. Prepare visitors for patient's appearance. Encourage positive self-esteem by continued interest in patient and attentiveness to patient's needs.

Nursing Diagnosis	Nursing Intervention
Powerlessness	Assess for presence of defining characteristics. Observe for signs of depression and apathy. Involve patient in decision making. Encourage patient to express dissatisfaction and frustration. Accept feelings of anger. Provide support for patient who is dying.
Grieving, anticipatory	Assess for presence of defining characteristics. Encourage patient's verbalization of distress, anger, sorrow, and fear. Assist in movement through stages of grief.

Patient Education

1. Instruct the patient in the effects of long-term, high-dose corticosteroid therapy.
2. Teach the patient who is at home to apply cool compress and Dakin's dressings and to prepare potassium permanganate baths (see p. 638).
3. Instruct the patient in aseptic technique.
4. Teach the patient the signs and symptoms of secondary infection and to seek medical attention if they occur.
5. Teach the patient the importance of a high-calorie, high-protein diet and provide specific diet instructions.

EVALUATION

Patient Outcome	Data Indicating That Outcome is Reached
Disease condition improves.	Bulla formation decreases. Denuded areas are reepithelized. Integument and mucosa heal. Pain is alleviated.
Fluid and electrolyte balance is maintained.	Mucous membrane is moist. There is no dry skin or weight loss. Blood values are normal: pH 7.35 to 7.45, sodium 136-145 mEq/L, potassium 3.5-5 mEq/L, and chloride 100-106 mEq/L.
Nutritional requirements are satisfied.	Weight is maintained. Patient eats diet high in protein and calories. Lesions heal.
Secondary infection does not develop.	There is no pus, redness, swelling, or fever.
Patient works through psychosocial concerns.	Patient verbalizes dissatisfaction, frustration, anger, distress, sorrow, and fear. Patient moves through stages of grief.

Epidermolysis Bullosa

Epidermolysis bullosa is a group of hereditary bullous disorders caused by abnormalities of the epidermis and dermoepidermal junction.

PATHOPHYSIOLOGY

The six disorders of epidermolysis bullosa have varying characteristics and degrees of severity. They are classified as (1) simple, (2) recurrent, (3) lethal, (4) dystrophic dominant, (5) dystrophic recessive, and (6) dystrophic acquired.

Simple and recurrent epidermolysis bullosa. These two forms are inherited dominant disorders that are relatively mild. The blisters are caused by disintegration of the intraepidermal cells in the basal and subbasal layers. The clinical features are tense clear bullae that first appear in infancy with the normal trauma from bedsheets or crawling. Lesions occur on the feet, on the extensor aspects of the extremities, and over joints. Bullae are more numerous during the summer months because of exposed skin surfaces. The lesions heal without scarring.

Recurrent epidermolysis bullosa may not become apparent until early adulthood. Lesions are superficial and are precipitated by trauma from footwear and warm weather exposure. These lesions also heal without scarring.

Lethal epidermolysis bullosa. This is an inherited recessive disorder. Blistering occurs at the basement membrane. It is extensive and nonscarring, with the mucous membrane affected. Death usually occurs shortly after birth because of involvement of the mucous membrane in the gastrointestinal and respiratory tracts.

Dystrophic dominant, recessive, and acquired epidermolysis bullosa (Plate 1, 3). These are the deepest forms of the disorder and produce scars and chronic mucocutaneous erosions.

In the dominant form the abnormality is within the basal lamina of the dermoepidermal junction; bullae are subepidermal. The blisters leave atrophic or hypertrophic scars.

In the recessive form bullae occur within the upper dermis rather than in the immediate subepidermis. Large areas of erosion and scarring develop. The oral and esophageal mucosa may also be involved. The condition progresses to gross hypertrophic scarring of the fingers and toes with adhesions between the digits. All nails are dystrophic. One feature of this form is the presence of milia within the epidermis.

The acquired variant is not hereditary. The mechanism of acquisition is not known. The disease follows the course of the hereditary dystrophic forms of epidermolysis bullosa.

DIAGNOSTIC STUDIES

Physical examination
Characteristic lesions that occur spontaneously or as result of trauma

Biopsy
Bulla formation in basal layer, basement membrane zone, and dermis

TREATMENT PLAN

Chemotherapeutic
Corticosteroids
Systemic glucocorticoids such as prednisone; dosage determined by type and severity of disease
Vitamin derivatives
Vitamin E, 200-3200 IU po qd; use controversial; effect at best limited to selected cases[6]
Anti-infective agents
Systemic antibiotics for secondary infection; specific drug and dosage dependent on infecting organism

Supportive
Permanent or long-term hospitalization for disabilities

ASSESSMENT: AREAS OF CONCERN

Lesion
Bullae or scars on extremities, hands, feet, and mucous membranes; number, size, and location of bullae; degree of involvement

Secondary infection
Redness; swelling; tenderness; pus or purulent exudate; odor

Systemic response to infection
Regional lymphadenopathy; fever; chills; tachycardia; headache; hypotension; malaise; increased white blood count; increased eosinophils; increased lymphocytes; decreased neutrophils; increased erythrocyte sedimentation rate

Psychosocial concerns
Concern with body image; loss of family member; fear of having other children with disease

NURSING DIAGNOSES and NURSING INTERVENTIONS

Nursing Diagnosis	Nursing Intervention
Skin integrity, impairment of: actual	Use meticulous hygiene and handwashing to prevent secondary infection. Use antibacterial soap. Assess for and prevent secondary infection; provide reverse isolation if required. In collaboration with physician, provide Stryker frame or CircOlectric bed to relieve pressure and decrease painful movement in eroded areas.
Oral mucous membrane, alteration in	Assess for presence of defining characteristics.

Nursing Diagnosis	Nursing Intervention
	Provide mouth care with saline or alkaline mouthwash. Avoid astringent or acidic fluids. Provide soft, bland diet.
Self-concept, disturbance in: body image	Assess for presence of defining characteristics. Encourage patient to verbalize feelings about body, body appearance, or fear of reaction or rejection by others.
Mobility, impaired from scarring and disabilities	Assess for presence of defining characteristics. Maintain skin integrity and circulation. Implement passive and active range of motion exercises. In collaboration with physician, provide Stryker frame or CircOlectric bed. Refer patient to physical therapy.
Powerlessness	Assess for presence of defining characteristics. Observe for signs of depression and apathy. Involve patient in decision making. Assist patient in expressing dissatisfaction and frustration. Assist family in expressing fear and anxiety regarding future children; assist in seeking genetic counseling.
Grieving, anticipatory	Assess for presence of defining characteristics. Assist in expression of distress, anger, sorrow, and fear. Assist in movement through grief process.

Patient Education

1. Instruct the patient and family in meticulous hygiene and handwashing to prevent secondary infection.
2. Instruct the patient and family in aseptic technique for dressing changes required for oozing or infected lesions.
3. Instruct the patient and family in signs and symptoms of secondary infection and to seek medical attention if they occur.
4. Instruct the patient and family in the importance of preventing trauma that can cause blister formation.
5. Assist in identifying ways to eliminate potential trauma, such as protective footwear, long sleeves, and long pant legs.
6. Instruct patients with dystrophic forms who are at home to perform range of motion exercises to minimize disability from scarring at the joints.

EVALUATION

Patient Outcome	Data Indicating That Outcome is Reached
Existing lesions heal.	Bullae resolve. Integument and mucous membranes heal.
Secondary infection is absent.	There is no redness, swelling, or pus in healing lesions.
Systemic response to infection resolves.	There are no systemic indicators: lymphadenopathy, fever, tachycardia, hypotension, or malaise. Laboratory values are normal: white blood count, 5000-10,000/mm^3; eosinophils, 50-400/mm^3; lymphocytes, 1000-4000/mm^3; neutrophils, 3000-7000/mm^3; and erythrocyte sedimentation rate normal (depends on method).
External trauma to integument is minimized.	Patient wears protective clothing and footwear. Patient avoids activities that are conducive to integumentary trauma.
Disability from scarring is minimized.	Patient performs active and passive range of motion exercises. Range of motion of joints is preserved.
Psychosocial needs are recognized and addressed.	Patient is involved in decision making. Patient and family express dissatisfaction, frustration, fear, anger, and sorrow. Patient and family move through grief process. Parents seek genetic counseling.

ERYTHEMA MULTIFORME

Erythema multiforme is an acute inflammatory eruption characterized by symmetric erythematous, edematous, or bullous lesions precipitated by numerous factors.

The etiology and pathogenesis of erythema multiforme are unknown. The mechanism of response seems to be an allergic hypersensitivity.

The disease is associated with herpes simplex, bacterial and other infections, endocrine changes, and internal malignancies. Almost any drug can cause erythema multiforme; penicillin, sulfonamides, salicylates, and barbiturates are the most commonly implicated drugs. Bacterial and viral infections are often implicated in children and young adults, whereas association with drugs and malignancy is more common in adults. Attacks sometimes last for 2 to 4 weeks and recur in the fall.

PATHOPHYSIOLOGY

In mild cases of erythema multiforme, eruption is limited to cutaneous lesions of erythematous macules, papules, and plaques that are localized predominantly in the distal portion of the extremities and face and are symmetrically distributed. The classic lesion (target or iris lesion) is a dark, urticarial plaque with elevated circular borders and a depressed inner ring (Plate 1, *4*). After a few days the central area of erythema develops a dusky purplish discoloration that can become bullous (Plate 1, *5*).

In more severe cases systemic symptoms of fever, coryza, malaise, and arthralgia may also occur. In these more severe cases the lesions are predominantly vesiculobullous and involve mucous membranes as well as skin. In children and young adults a severe and sometimes fatal form of erythema multiforme known as Stevens-Johnson syndrome can develop. In this syndrome mucous membrane lesions are present and may or may not be accompanied by cutaneous lesions. Vesicles and ulcerations develop on the mucous membrane of the lips, mouth, nasal passages, eyes, and genitalia. Conjunctival and corneal lesions are present in 90% of the cases.

Genitourinary lesions in erythema multiforme can compromise bladder function, and the inflammatory process can involve the kidneys with consequent hematuria and renal tubular necrosis. Mucous membrane ulceration can extend into the pharynx, esophagus, larynx, trachea, and bronchi.

The spectrum of histologic changes in erythema multiforme depends on the site of involvement and the degree of the inflammatory process. The blood vessels are dilated and are surrounded by lymphohistiocytic infiltrate with substantial edema of the papillary dermis. Edema of the upper dermis leads to the formation of bullae that are subepidermal without acantholysis. Epidermal necrosis occurs primarily in the center of the lesion, the site of the dusky iris (target) lesion.

DIAGNOSTIC STUDIES

Physical examination
   Characteristic lesion, particularly iris or target lesion; lesions fixed and do not fade or change location; absence of itching

Complete blood count
   Increased white blood count, increased erythrocyte sedimentation rate

Urinalysis
   Red blood cells and albumin in urine if genitourinary lesions are present

Antistreptolysin titer
   Elevated if disease occurs after streptococcal infection

TREATMENT PLAN

Mild erythema multiforme clears spontaneously and may require no treatment other than elimination of the precipitating factor. For treatment of eye symptoms see Chapter 6.

Chemotherapeutic
   Anti-infective agents
      Systemic antibiotics for underlying infection or to control secondary infection; specific drug and dosage depends on infection, its severity, and age of patient
   Corticosteroids
      Systemic glucocorticoids (controversial)[86,87]
         Prednisone, 60-80 mg po qd in divided doses, then decreased, for adults; 1-2 mg/kg/d in 3 or 4 divided doses, then decreased, for children
   Local anesthetic agents
      Viscous lidocaine (Xylocaine) swish for mouth lesions
   Analgesics
      Aspirin (ASA), 300 mg po q4-6h

Supportive
   Wet dressings to debride crusted lesions
   Bed rest; hospitalization for severe cases
   Bland diet for mouth lesions
   Intravenous fluids for hydration in severe cases

ASSESSMENT: AREAS OF CONCERN

Lesion
Erythematous macules, papules, vesicles, or bullae at distal aspect of extremities and face; target or iris lesion; vesicles or ulcerations of mucous membranes

Systemic involvement
Fever; coryza; arthralgia; malaise; chest pain; vomiting; diarrhea; hematuria; albuminuria; increased erythrocyte sedimentation rate; increased white blood count; radiologic changes in lungs

Nutrition
Inability to eat because of mouth ulcerations

Psychosocial concerns
Concern about body image

NURSING DIAGNOSES and NURSING INTERVENTIONS

Nursing Diagnosis	Nursing Intervention
Skin integrity, impairment of: actual	In collaboration with physician, apply wet dressings to debride lesions (see p. 639). Scrub crusted lesions gently with antibacterial soap. Teach meticulous handwashing and good hygiene to prevent secondary infection.
Oral mucous membrane, alteration in	Provide soft, bland diet. Avoid astringent or acidic liquids. Provide mouth care with alkaline or saline mouthwash. Instruct patient in use of viscous lidocaine mouth swish.
Comfort, alteration in: pain	Apply cool compresses or soaks. Encourage bed rest. Instruct patient in use of analgesics.
Nutrition, alteration in: less than body requirements	Provide soft, bland diet. In collaboration with physician, offer viscous lidocaine mouth swish 15 minutes before eating.
Self-concept, disturbance in: body image	Assist patient in verbalization of feelings about body, body appearance, or fear of reaction or rejection by others.

Patient Education

1. Instruct the patient and family in the application of cool compresses or soaks using aseptic technique.
2. Instruct the patient and family in the need for follow-up urinalysis to detect the presence of renal tubular necrosis.
3. Instruct the patient and family in signs and symptoms of secondary infection and to seek medical attention if they occur.
4. Assist the patient in identifying potential precipitating factors and to eliminate those factors when possible.

EVALUATION

Patient Outcome	Data Indicating That Outcome is Reached
Existing lesions heal.	Lesions resolve. Ulcerations and erosions reepithelize. Integument and mucous membrane heal. Discomfort is alleviated.
Secondary infection is avoided.	There is no swelling, redness, or pus in healing lesions.
Nutritional status is adequate.	Weight is maintained. Lesions heal.

Patient Outcome	Data Indicating That Outcome is Reached
Systemic involvement resolves.	There are no red blood cells or protein in urine. White blood count is 5000-10,000/mm^3. Erythrocyte sedimentation rate is normal (depends on method).
Complications are recognized early.	Patient has follow-up urinalysis. Patient seeds medical attention for vision changes.
Patient evaluates appearance in realistic manner.	Patient engages in usual activities and relationships.

ERYTHEMA NODOSUM

Erythema nodosum is an acute inflammatory nodular eruption that involves primarily the lower extremities and is precipitated by various factors.

Erythema nodosum is found equally in boys and girls but is more common in adults, particularly young women. It occurs more commonly from January to June.

Numerous precipitating factors have been identified, including various infections, drugs, diseases, and pregnancy. Erythema nodosum frequently follows an infection of the upper respiratory tract, especially from streptococci. In adults streptococcal infections and sarcoidosis are the most common causes. An underlying systemic cause is identifiable in more than 50% of cases. The remainder of the cases occur in apparently healthy young adults.

The prodromal symptoms may be fever, chills, malaise, and arthralgia, which occur a few days or several weeks before the onset of the eruption. Some of the prodromal symptoms may be from the underlying condition.

PATHOPHYSIOLOGY

Erythema nodosum is a vascular reaction pattern, most likely a hypersensitivity response involving both cellular and humoral mechanisms (see Chapter 16).

The eruption is sudden with discrete, erythematous, hot, and very tender nodules on the shins, knees, ankles, thighs, buttocks, and sometimes lower arms (Plate 1, 6). The nodules are bright red initially, changing to a purplish color, and finally becoming a flat brown pigmentation that slowly fades completely. The total evolution of lesions takes 3 to 4 weeks.

The nodules vary in size from 6 to 8 mm and are usually bilaterally symmetric. There may be only a few lesions or numerous nodules appearing in crops. New crops may occur periodically. Edema of the ankles and general aching of the legs are common and are aggravated by ambulation.

Cellular changes are probably due to the immunologic processes. Deep dermal inflammation extends down into subcutaneous tissue. Small blood vessels experience mild vasculitis and inflammatory infiltrate with partial obstruction of blood flow.

DIAGNOSTIC STUDIES

Physical examination
Characteristic lesion; history consistent with possible precipitating factors

Complete blood count
Increased erythrocyte sedimentation rate; platelet estimate

Biopsy
Deep excision biopsy including subcutaneous tissue; shows histologic changes described previously

Diagnostic studies to isolate underlying disorders
Antistreptolysin titer; throat culture; tuberculosis test; rheumatoid factor; antinuclear factor

TREATMENT PLAN

Management of the disease is aimed at identifying and treating the precipitating factor or underlying disorder.

Chemotherapeutic
Analgesics
Aspirin (ASA), 300 mg po q4-6h
Anti-infective agents
Systemic antibiotics for underlying infection; may require long-term therapy; specific antibiotic depends on the underlying infection
Corticosteroids
Intralesional injection of triamcinolone (Aristocort, Kenalog), 5 mg/ml

Supportive
Bed rest

Cool compresses applied to nodules
Support stockings or elastic bandages

ASSESSMENT: AREAS OF CONCERN

Lesions
Red, hot, tender nodules (initially) on anterior aspect of lower extremities

Systemic involvement
Fever; chills; malaise; arthralgia; ankle edema; aching legs

Underlying disorder
Complete blood count; urinalysis; antistreptolysin titer; tuberculosis test; rheumatoid factor; throat culture; antinuclear factor

Psychosocial concerns
Concern about body image

NURSING DIAGNOSES and NURSING INTERVENTIONS

Nursing Diagnosis	Nursing Intervention
Comfort, alteration in: pain	Encourage bed rest and elevation of legs. Have patient use support hose and elastic bandages.
Skin integrity, impairment of: actual	Apply cool compresses.
Self-concept, disturbance in: body image	Encourage patient to verbalize feelings about body, body appearance, or fear of reaction or rejection by others. Assure patient that lesions heal without scarring.

Patient Education

1. Assist the patient in identifying potential precipitating factors and eliminating them when possible (such as with drugs).
2. Instruct the patient in the effects of long-term antibiotic therapy if indicated.
3. Instruct the patient in management of symptoms: elevation of legs, rest, use of support hose or elastic bandages, and application of cool compresses.

EVALUATION

Patient Outcome	Data Indicating That Outcome is Reached
Nodules resolve.	Discomfort is alleviated. Skin integrity is restored.
Underlying condition is identified and treated.	Symptoms of underlying disorder improve and resolve.
Precipitating factors are eliminated when possible.	Condition does not recur.
Patient evaluates appearance in realistic manner.	Patient engages in usual activities when possible and in usual relationships.

INFESTATIONS AND PARASITIC DISORDERS
Pediculosis

Pediculosis is an infestation by lice of the head (pediculosis capitis), the body (pediculosis corporis), or the genital area (pediculosis pubis).

Pediculosis is a highly pruritic and often secondarily infected disorder that results from two species of lice: (1) *Pediculus humanus,* which affects the head and body, and (2) *Phthirus pubis,* which infests the pubic area, the lower abdomen, and sometimes the eyebrows, eyelashes, and scalp.

Pediculosis capitis occurs most frequently in schoolchildren and is easily transmitted by personal contact and by objects such as combs and hats. Itching and excoriation are present. The posterior aspect of the scalp commonly shows the greatest degree of involvement. The posterior occipital nodes may be enlarged and tender.

Pediculosis corporis is characterized by pruritus and parallel linear excoriations that are frequently secondarily infected. The infesting lice live in the seams of clothing and move onto the skin to feed at frequent intervals. Lesions are most common on the shoulders, buttocks, and abdomen. Infestation is associated with unhygienic living conditions ("vagabond's disease").

Pediculosis pubis is transmitted by close personal contact, usually through sexual contact. Infestation is usually in the pubic hair but may occur in the chest or axillary hair, eyebrows, or eyelashes. A sign of infestation is the presence of reddish brown specks on undergarments as a result of the excreta of lice.

PATHOPHYSIOLOGY

In pediculosis capitis, injection of saliva from the lice during feeding produces severe pruritus. Scratching causes excoriation, and secondary infection is common. Each day the female louse lays seven to 10 eggs that hatch in 8 days. The eggs (nits) are cemented to the hair shaft and cannot be dislodged.

In pediculosis corporis the primary lesion is an urticarial papule, which is often obscured by secondary excoriation and infection. With prolonged infestation the skin becomes dry, scaly, and hyperpigmented.

Pediculosis pubis is manifested primarily by itching. The lice ova are commonly attached to the skin at the base of the hair follicle. Discrete, small, 1 to 3 cm, gray-blue macules can be seen on the trunk, thighs, and axillae. These lesions are due to a reaction of the lice's saliva with bilirubin, converting it to biliverdin. Excoriation and secondary infection are uncommon.

DIAGNOSTIC STUDIES

Physical examination
Presence of lice or eggs; presence of nonspecific lesion with characteristic distribution

Wood's light
Fluorescence of adult louse

Microscopic examination
Examination of hair shaft for eggs

TREATMENT PLAN

Chemotherapeutic
Anti-infective agents
Lindane (Kwell) shampoo, cream, or lotion, applied qd for 2 d; application repeated in 10 d; used with caution with young children because of neurotoxicity
Ophthalmic preparation of yellow mercury oxide qd for infested eyelashes
Cholinergic agents
Physostigmine (Eserine) 0.25% ophthalmic ointment qd for infested eyelashes

Supportive
Rinsing with white vinegar diluted with equal amounts of water followed by washing to remove residual nits from hair
Lice removed from eyelashes with forceps
Body lice eliminated from clothing and bedding by thorough washing, hot ironing, boiling, and steaming

ASSESSMENT: AREAS OF CONCERN

Local response to infestation
Pruritus; excoriation; secondary infection

Infestation
Location and distribution of lesions or local responses

Psychosocial concerns
Concern that others may react to transmissible infestation

NURSING DIAGNOSES and NURSING INTERVENTIONS

Nursing Diagnosis	Nursing Intervention
Skin integrity, impairment of: actual	Isolate patient until treatment is complete. Instruct patient in use of lindane. Instruct patient to comb hair with fine-toothed comb to remove eggs after preparation is used. Instruct patient to remove lice from eyelashes with cotton-tipped applicator. Instruct patient in good hygiene, meticulous handwashing, and need for short fingernails to avoid secondary infection.
Skin integrity, impairment of: potential	Teach patient how to decontaminate sources of infestation. Treat all family members and sexual partners. Advise patient that recurrence is common. Notify contacts and school nurse if child is infested. Teach patient importance of not borrowing personal items such as combs.

Patient Education

1. See the patient education interventions above.
2. Instruct the patient that prolonged use of lindane may result in dermatitis.

EVALUATION

Patient Outcome	Data Indicating That Outcome is Reached
Infestation is cleared in patient and affected family members and partners.	Pruritus subsides. No new areas of itching or excoriation develop. There are no lice or eggs on examination.
Lesions heal.	Excoriations resolve. Integument is intact.
Secondary infection is resolved or avoided.	Lesions heal without redness, swelling, or pus.
Infestation does not spread to unaffected family members, partners, schoolmates, and playmates.	Associates of patient do not develop symptoms. Hair and skin are free of lice or eggs. All family members and sexual partners receive treatment.

Scabies

Scabies is a transmissible parasitic infestation characterized by burrows, pruritus, and excoriations with secondary infection.

Scabies is caused by the *Sarcoptes scabiei* mite. The infestation and lesions occur most commonly on the finger webs, the flexor surfaces of the wrist, and the elbows and axillary folds, along the belt line, and on the lower buttocks (Plate 1, 7). The areolae in women and the genitals in men are particularly susceptible. Lesions do not extend to the face in adults but may do so in infants.

Scabies is transmitted readily by personal contact. It characteristically spreads to other family members, to intimate contacts, and between schoolchildren. It is not transmitted by clothing, bedding, or inanimate objects. Infestation can occur from cats, dogs, and other small animals, but the animal scabies mite does not burrow, only feeds.

PATHOPHYSIOLOGY

The impregnated female mite burrows into the stratum corneum forming a small tunnel that is seen as a fine, wavy, dark line. The burrow is a few millimeters to 1 cm long with a minute papule at the open end. The mite extends the burrow daily and deposits eggs and feces in it (Fig. 5-4).

The lesions are initially asymptomatic. After several weeks, a state of sensitization to the mite develops and itching becomes noticeable. The itching is intense and is characterized by increased severity at night. The itching intensifies over a period of several weeks. The burrows and papules are often obscured by secondary excoriation, bacterial infection, crusting, and lichenification. A fine rash is present that consists of papules of various sizes.

Fig. 5-4
Scabies burrow.
Courtesy of Stephen B. Tucker, M.D.,
Department of Dermatology, University of
Texas Health Science Center at Houston.

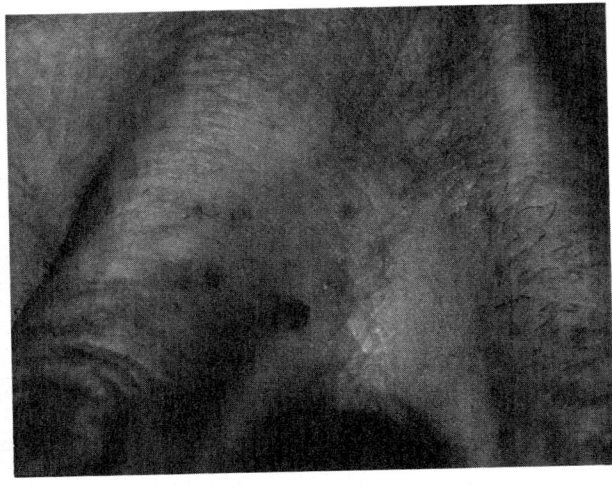

DIAGNOSTIC STUDIES

Physical examination
 Burrows; nonspecific excoriations; papules with characteristic distribution; intense itching that worsens at night

Scrapings
 Taken from burrow and placed in oil; presence of mite on microscopic examination

TREATMENT PLAN

Chemotherapeutic
 Anti-infective agents
  Benzyl benzoate topical emulsion 20%-25%; applied to entire cutaneous surface from neck down; left on 12-24h for adults, less time with children, and then washed off; procedure repeated after 2 d; third treatment may be necessary in 2 wk
  Lindane (Kwell) 1% cream or lotion applied according to above instructions; not used for young children because of neurotoxicity; not recommended during pregnancy
  Sulfur ointment 5%-10% applied as above; used for infants
  Crotamiton (Eurax) applied with benzyl benzoate; less irritating than benzyl benzoate
 Corticosteroids
  Fluorinated corticosteroid ointment 1% applied topically bid, tid, or qid for persistent itching

ASSESSMENT: AREAS OF CONCERN

Lesion
 Linear gray-brown burrows a few millimeters in length; excoriation; secondary infection; crusting; papules; vesicles; lichenification

Local response to infestation
 Intense itching out of proportion to visible signs; itching worse at night

Psychosocial concerns
 Concern that others may react to transmissible infestation

NURSING DIAGNOSES and NURSING INTERVENTIONS

Nursing Diagnosis	Nursing Intervention
Skin integrity, impairment of: actual	Isolate patient until treatment is completed. Instruct patient in meticulous handwashing and good hygiene to avoid secondary infection. Have patient's fingernails cut short to avoid excoriation from scratching. Instruct patient in use of treatment lotion; all skin surfaces except face must be covered.
Skin integrity, impairment of: potential	Have all family members and sexual partners treated.[67] Have patient notify sexual contacts; if child is infested, have parents notify school nurse. Instruct patient and family in modes of infestation and transmission.
Social isolation	Prepare patient and family for potential reaction of others to transmissible infestation. Assure patient and family that infestation can be treated successfully.

Patient Education

1. Tell the patient and family that treatment irritates the skin and does not quickly reduce the pruritus; discomfort may persist for a few weeks.
2. Instruct the patient in the use of cool soaks and compresses to reduce itching after treatment is complete.
3. Stress the importance of the correct use of treatment lotion to avoid neurotoxicity and undue irritation.
4. Advise that all family members and sexual partners be treated.

EVALUATION

Patient Outcome	Data Indicating That Outcome is Reached
Infestation is cleared in patient and affected family members and partners.	No new papules, burrows, or areas of itching develop.
Lesions heal.	Excoriations resolve. Integument is intact.
Secondary infection is resolved or avoided.	Lesions heal without redness, swelling, crusts, or pus.
Spread of infestation to child's schoolmates or playmates is minimized.	These persons do not develop symptoms of infestation, or they seek treatment if symptoms develop.
Infestation does not spread to seemingly unaffected family members or sexual partners.	

Arachnid and Hymenoptera Bites

Arachnids are ticks, spiders, and scorpions; their bites cause toxic and allergic reactions as a result of the injection of a venom or toxin. Hymenoptera are bees, wasps, yellow jackets, and ants; their bites cause toxic and allergic reactions as a result of the injection of a venom or toxin.

Tick bites. Tick bites are common in woods and fields throughout the United States. The tick attaches itself to a passing animal or person and after biting remains attached to the skin for several days or longer. Ticks transmit Rocky Mountain spotted fever, Q fever, relapsing fever, and Lyme disease. The tick bite is initially painless but begins to itch after several days. Infiltration and erythema develop around the bite with formation of firm, discrete, intensely pruritic nodules that may be present for several months or longer.

Systemic symptoms attributed to a toxin include fever, malaise, headache, and abdominal pain. Several species of ticks inject a salivary neurotoxin that causes paralysis. Paresthesia and pain in the lower extremities, weakness, and incoordination develop. The condition may progress to respiratory failure and death from bulbar involvement. Symptoms clear dramatically with tick removal.

Spider bites. The most important spider bites are caused by the black widow and brown recluse spiders. The black widow is common throughout the United States and southern Canada. It lives in old lumber, unused sheds, and outdoor toilets and may be found in attics, drawers, and closets. Only the female bites and only in self-defense. The female is recognized by her coal black coloring with a red or orange marking on the ventral side.

The black widow bite results from the injection of a neurotoxic venom through a clawlike appendage. The bite, which may go unnoticed, is felt as a pinprick sensation followed by a dull numbing pain. Local necrosis may cause a small ulcer at the site. Within 10 to 60 minutes muscle spasms occur locally and then spread to include all extremities and the trunk. Excruciating pain is felt in waves. The attack subsides after several hours.

Systemic symptoms may include restlessness, vertigo, sweating, chills, pallor, hyperactive reflexes, hypertension, tachycardia, thready pulse, nausea and vomiting, headache, eyelid edema, urticaria, pruritus, and fever. Ascending paralysis, severe hypotension, circulatory collapse, convulsions, and death may result. Mortality is less than 1%.

The brown recluse spider is common in the south-central United States and is usually found in dark areas such as drawers and closets. It commonly bites people when they are asleep. The spider is small, and fawn to dark brown, with a light violin-shaped mark on its head. The female is more dangerous than the male. Most bites occur between April and October.

Brown recluse venom is coagulotoxic. Pain and local symptoms develop 2 to 8 hours after the bite. Localized vasoconstriction causes ischemic necrosis at the site. The area is red with blisters and blebs surrounded by ischemia. After several days the center becomes dark and hard. After 2 weeks it becomes depressed, demarcated, and necrotic, and a large open ulcer forms. The ulcer may take several weeks to heal and may require grafting.

Systemic symptoms include fever, chills, malaise, weakness, arthralgia, nausea, vomiting, petechiae, hemolysis, and thrombocytopenia.

Scorpion bites. Scorpions are found throughout the United States but are most common in the southern United States and Mexico. The two deadly species are found in the southwest United States.

Scorpions are nocturnal and photophobic. They sting by means of a hooked caudal stinger that discharges venom. Most stings occur during the warmer months. Nonlethal bites cause local swelling, tenderness, pain, a sharp burning sensation, skin discoloration, paresthesia, regional lymphadenopathy, and rarely anaphylaxis. Lethal bites are neurotoxic and result in pain, hyperesthesia followed by hypoesthesia, drowsiness, itching of the nose, mouth, and throat, slurred speech, incontinence, vomiting, and convulsions. Symptoms last 24 to 48 hours. Death may follow cardiovascular or respiratory failure. Mortality is less than 1%.

Bee, wasp, hornet, yellow jacket, and ant stings. All female Hymenoptera have an egg-laying organ (stinger) that can be used for defense or offense. The venom of bees, hornets, wasps, and yellow jackets contains four to six distinct chemical compounds, each of which can produce an allergic reaction. The venoms of all stinging Hymenoptera are closely related and therefore cross-sensitizing.

Local reactions include swelling, pain, erythema, urticaria, and pruritus (Plate 1, 8). Generalized allergic reactions include nausea, vomiting, diarrhea, urticaria, pruritus, and anaphylaxis, with shortness of breath, tightness in the chest, difficulty swallowing, anxiety, convulsions, or unconsciousness. Delayed reaction (serum sickness) occurs 1 to 4 weeks after the sting and is characterized by fever, malaise, lymphadenopathy, rash, urticaria, and arthralgia.

PATHOPHYSIOLOGY

The local or systemic response to injection of a venom occurs as a result of: (1) direct action of the venom on susceptible cells; (2) IgE-mediated humoral immune response (type I), and (3) immune complex humoral response (type III).

The arthropod or Hymenoptera venom is toxic to all humans. The biologically active venom exerts its effect directly on susceptible cells (such as nerve cells and blood cells). The protein component of the venom may contain enzymes that cause cell lysis, histamine release, anticoagulation, or interference with neuromuscular transmission.

The IgE-mediated immune response occurs in persons who are sensitive to the protein component of the venom, which acts as an antigen. These persons have come in contact with the allergen in the past and have become sensitized rather than immunized. Sensitization triggers the synthesis of specific antiallergenic IgE antibodies. On subsequent contact with the allergen, the person responds with a type I immune reaction.

IgE immunoglobulins are bound to mast cells and basophils. Mast cells are found in all body tissues, in close proximity to blood vessels, and in abundance in the skin. Basophils circulate as leukocytes in the blood. Both mast cells and basophils contain potent pharmacologically active substances such as histamine, bradykinin, serotonin, and other vasoactive amines. The venom (antigen) becomes bound to the IgE on the surface of the cell, creating degranulation of the cell that releases the active agents. These mediators cause increased vascular permeability and smooth muscle contraction. Histamine seems to be the most important agent. Its release causes (1) peripheral vasodilation, (2) increased permeability of capillaries with subsequent loss of plasma from the circulation, (3) smooth muscle constriction (as in the bronchi), and (4) increased mucous gland secretion. If the agents remain confined to the area of the bite, the tissue reaction remains localized (local anaphylaxis) with tissue swelling, wheal formation, and itching. If the mediators are released systemically, systemic anaphylaxis (anaphylactic shock) may result. The widespread response to histamine release causes profound bronchoconstriction and vasodilation with subsequent circulatory collapse. The severity of the reaction depends on the amount of the sensitizing dose, the amount and distribution of the IgE antibodies, and the dose of toxin that causes the reaction.

A type III (immune complex) reaction, or serum sickness, can develop 1 to 3 weeks after the antigen is injected. The antigen initiates an immune response, and antibodies are formed. The response is mediated by IgG or IgM and complement. The immune complexes are deposited in joints, blood vessels, kidneys, and the heart. Platelet aggregation is caused by the collection of immune complexes and complement along blood vessel walls. Anaphylatoxins are released during activation of the complement system, causing a severe inflammatory response.

DIAGNOSTIC STUDIES

Physical examination
Puncture wound with characteristic symptoms

Complete blood count
Eosinophilia in type I reaction

Direct immunofluorescence
Presence of antigen, immunoglobulin, or complement in type III reaction

TREATMENT PLAN

Surgical
Skin grafting—split-thickness graft to close brown recluse spider bite

Chemotherapeutic
For anaphylaxis
Bronchodilators
Epinephrine (Adrenalin), 1:1000 for allergic reactions, 0.3-0.5 ml subcutaneously or IM for mild or severe reactions repeated q5-20 min as needed; 0.1-0.2 ml subcutaneously injected into site to decrease absorption of antigen; 0.25-0.5 ml IV in 10 ml saline repeated in 5-10 min for severe anaphylaxis with cardiovascular involvement
Epinephrine 1:200 aqueous suspension, 0.3 ml subcutaneously; long-acting for severe reactions without cardiovascular involvement after edema has subsided
Aminophylline (Aminodur, Lixaminol, Phyllacontin, Somophyllin) for bronchospasm, 6 mg/kg IV over 10-20 min followed by 0.5 mg/kg/h IV
Antihistamines
Diphenhydramine (Benadryl), 50-100 mg IV
Adrenergic agents
Isoproterenol (Isuprel, Proterenol), 1 mg diluted in 500 ml D5W infused at rate of 0.5-1 ml/min for myocardial insufficiency
Vasoconstrictors for prolonged hypotension
Norepinephrine (Levophed, Levarterenol), 8-12 μg/min IV of 4 μg/ml dilution, titrated
Metaraminol (Aramine), 15-100 mg/500 ml D5W IV, titrated, for adults; 0.4 mg/kg IV for children
Corticosteroids
Hydrocortisone, 100 mg IV for prolonged symptoms

Oral antihistamines
Diphenhydramine (Benadryl), 25-50 mg po qid for mild reaction
For toxins
Antivenin, 1 ampule IV in 10-50 ml saline for black widow and scorpion bites
Anticonvulsant muscle relaxants
Calcium gluconate 10% 10 ml IV slowly q4h
Methocarbamol (Delaxin, Forbaxin, Metho-500, Robaxin, others), 300 mg/min IV to total of 3 g qd
Orphenadrine (Flexon, Flexoject, Norflex, others), 60 mg IV q12h
For convulsions from scorpion bites
Phenobarbital, 30-60 mg/min IV up to 600 mg
Corticosteroids
Dexamethasone (Decadron, Hexadrol), 4 mg IM q6h for brown recluse spider bites during acute phase, then in decremental doses
Antihistamines
Diphenhydramine (Benadryl), 25-50 mg po qid
Anti-infective agents
Bacitracin or Neosporin applied tid or qid as topical antibiotic for brown recluse spider bite
Immunologic agents
Tetanus prophylaxis as indicated with tetanus toxoid, 0.5 ml IM
Intravenous infusion with D5W or lactated Ringer's solution

Supportive
Scraping to remove stinger is present by scraping; do not squeeze or pinch, since retained venom sacs discharge residual venom
Application of meat tenderizer paste (containing proteolytic enzyme) to sting site
Hospitalization for observation or ventilator support

ASSESSMENT: AREAS OF CONCERN

Local response
Presence or absence of stinger; pain; itching; edema; blister; ulceration; tissue necrosis

Systemic response
Anxiety; feeling of doom; fever; malaise

Cardiovascular
Respiratory distress; tightness in chest; shortness of breath; wheezing; dyspnea

Neurologic
Tachycardia; bradycardia; hypotension; imperceptible pulse; pallor

Musculoskeletal
Cramping; pain; rigidity; weakness

Gastrointestinal
Nausea; vomiting; diarrhea; cramping; constipation

Skin
Flushing; diffuse erythema; urticaria; pruritus

Delayed response
One to 4 weeks after sting: fever; malaise; lymphadenopathy; arthralgia; rash; urticaria

Psychosocial concerns
Concern about body image as result of disfigurement, depending on severity of tissue damage; fear of insects, spiders, bees, and scorpions

NURSING DIAGNOSES and NURSING INTERVENTIONS

Nursing Diagnosis	Nursing Intervention
Breathing pattern, ineffective	Maintain airway. In collaboration with physician, perform oropharyngeal suctioning as needed. Provide oxygen by cannula or mask. Position for ease of respiration. Administer drugs as indicated.
Cardiac output, alteration in: decreased, and fluid volume deficit, actual	Monitor vital signs. Initiate intravenous line in collaboration with physician. Administer drugs as indicated.
Skin integrity, impairment of: actual	Apply meat tenderizer or paste to neutralize venom. Apply ice packs to decrease pain and swelling and to limit venom absorption. Keep patient quiet. Remove stinger by scraping. Remove tick; do not pull since head and mouth may remain embedded; apply heat to body and tick will back out, or cover with oil, which blocks its breathing and causes it to withdraw. Clean bite with antiseptic. Clean brown recluse bite with 1:20 Burow's solution.
Comfort, alteration in: pain	Apply ice packs to area. Apply meat tenderizer paste to neutralize venom.
Fear (of arachnids and hymenoptera)	Encourage patient to verbalize fears. Assist patient in developing preventive measures (see below).
Self-concept, alteration in: body image	Assess for presence of defining characteristics. Assist patient in verbalization of feelings about body, body appearance, or fear of reaction or rejection by others. Reassure patient with disfiguring ulcer that skin grafting can improve appearance.

Patient Education

1. Instruct patients who are sensitive to stings to carry an emergency kit that has an antihistamine and epinephrine. Teach the patient or a family member or friend how to inject epinephrine.
2. Instruct patients who are sensitive to wear or carry medical alert information and identification.
3. Refer the patient to an allergist for desensitization.
4. Instruct the patient in the removal of ticks and stingers.
5. Instruct the patient and family in general preventive measures such as wearing protective clothing when outdoors, spraying areas of spider infestation with creosote every 2 months, inspecting clothing before putting it on in infested areas, and not wearing bright colors or scents that attract bees when outdoors.
6. Instruct the patient and family to keep the site of the bite clean by washing two or three times daily with warm soapy water or water with hydrogen peroxide; apply antibiotic ointment as needed.
7. Instruct the patient in changing the dressing if needed.

EVALUATION

Patient Outcome	Data Indicating That Outcome is Reached
Local toxic reaction is minimized.	Stinger or tick is removed correctly and treatment is initiated immediately. Areas of ulceration and necrosis are limited. Pain is alleviated.
Systemic response is avoided or resolved.	Cardiovascular, neurologic, musculoskeletal, or gastrointestinal symptoms are avoided or resolved. Respirations are regular and easy. Pulse rate is 60 to 100 and regular. Blood pressure is within patient's usual limits. Reflexes, sensation, and motion are intact. Patient has urinary continence and bowel function. There is no malaise, fever, lymphadenopathy, arthralgia, rash, or urticaria after delayed response.
Lesions heal.	Areas of necrosis, ulceration, and blistering reepithelize. Integument is intact and free of infection.
Sensitized patients institute precautionary measures.	Patient carries medical alert information and identification. Patient carries emergency kit. Patient, family member, or friend demonstrates injection of epinephrine. Patient seeks allergist for desensitization.
Psychosocial concerns are addressed.	Patient expresses feelings about body appearance. Patient with disfiguring ulcer has opportunity to seek surgical interventions.

Beetles and Caterpillars

Toxic reactions to beetles and caterpillars occur from contact with the toxin on the skin.

Blister beetles produce local irritation and blistering if they are crushed while on the skin surface. Damage to the beetle causes release of a toxic substance in the insect's body fluids.

More than 50 species of caterpillars possess spines that contain a venom capable of producing dermatitis on human skin. These caterpillars are widely distributed throughout the United States and Canada. Contact with the venom occurs from direct contact with the insect or its nest or from windblown hairs. Papular lesions or urticaria may develop at the site or elsewhere on the body. The venom produces a stinging sensation followed by swelling and erythema. Symptoms can occur systemically depending on the species and amount of venom received by the person. Painful and persistent nodules are formed if the toxin comes in contact with the conjunctiva.

PATHOPHYSIOLOGY

The venom produces a direct toxic response to human tissue. The caterpillar's venom is biologically very active and causes histamine release, anticoagulation, fibrinolysis, and plasminogen activity. The toxins are capable of producing impaired cellular activity or cellular destruction.

DIAGNOSTIC STUDIES

Physical examination
Lesion consistent with history of beetle or caterpillar contact

TREATMENT PLAN

Chemotherapeutic
Corticosteroids
Topical corticosteroid for skin inflammation: hydrocortisone 1% applied tid
Ophthalmic corticosteroid and analgesic for eye injury: cortisporin ophthalmic solution, 1-2 gtt qid

ASSESSMENT: AREAS OF CONCERN

Local reaction
Pain; swelling; blister; papule; urticaria; necrosis

Systemic reaction
Widespread papular lesions; urticaria

NURSING DIAGNOSES and NURSING INTERVENTIONS

Nursing Diagnosis	Nursing Intervention
Skin integrity, impairment of: actual	Flush skin with copious amounts of water and scrub gently with soap and water. Irrigate eye with copious amounts of normal saline.

Patient Education

1. Instruct the patient to avoid crushing beetles.
2. Teach the patient how to flush the skin and eye.
3. Teach the patient to keep the site clean by washing two or three times a day with soap and water.
4. Instruct the patient in the use of eye drops.

EVALUATION

Patient Outcome	Data Indicating That Outcome is Reached
Lesions heal.	Urticaria, blisters, or papules resolve. Necrotic areas reepithelize; Pain is alleviated. Integument is intact and free of infection. Eye symptoms or visual disturbances resolve.

Lesions Caused by Fleas, Flies, and Mosquitoes

Toxic reactions to fleas, flies, and mosquitoes occur as a result of saliva that is injected during feeding.

Fleas. Any of the human or domestic animal fleas will attack humans. Adult fleas are attracted to moving objects and leap to attain them. Thus flea bites are often found on the ankles or lower legs. The bites are characteristically found in groups of three on the ankles, legs, or waist. The flea penetrates the skin, feeds, and then crawls to a higher location until stopped by constrictive clothing.

A flea bite usually results in a small wheal with a hemorrhagic puncture at the center. In susceptible persons the flea bite produces larger wheals, urticaria, intensely pruritic papules, bullae, and small necrotic ulcers. Flea bites are usually innocuous but can produce a severe reaction in sensitive persons.

Flies. There are innumerable biting flies in the United States. Most common are the blackflies, houseflies, deer flies, gadflies, and dog or stable flies. Most flies feed during the day or at dusk and attack in swarms on exposed parts of the body such as the face, neck, and arms. Fly-transmitted tularemia occurs in the central and western United States.

Fly bites are painful and pruritic for several days. Urticaria may occur as a result of a protein in the fly's saliva.

Mosquitoes. Mosquitoes are important because of their role in transmitting viral encephalitis, dengue fever, yellow fever, malaria, and filariasis. Cutaneous lesions are produced when the mosquito feeds and deposits droplets of saliva. These lesions commonly occur on exposed areas of the hands, arms, face, and legs.

Mosquitoes are attracted by lights, dark clothing, and the presence of warm-blooded creatures. In most species the female mosquito is the bloodsucking biter.

The usual mosquito bite produces transient local irritation and pruritic erythematous papules. Large numbers of bites can produce intense pruritus. Urticaria and serum sickness can develop in sensitive persons.

PATHOPHYSIOLOGY

For an explanation of toxic reactions and antigen-antibody reactions see p. 589.

DIAGNOSTIC STUDIES

Physical examination
Puncture wound with characteristic symptoms

TREATMENT PLAN

For treatment of systemic reactions see p. 590.

Chemotherapeutic

Corticosteroids

Glucocorticoid ointment (e.g., hydrocortisone 1%) with 0.5% menthol and 0.5% phenol applied topically to lesions q1-2h

Anti-infective agents

Topical antibiotics

Bacitracin or Neosporin applied qd or bid

ASSESSMENT: AREAS OF CONCERN

Local response

Puncture wound with any of the following: pain, pruritus, wheal, urticaria, erythematous papule, bullae, or small necrotic ulcer; secondary infection: pain, swelling, tenderness, exudate

Systemic response

See pp. 590 and 591

Serum sickness

Fever; malaise; lymphadenopathy; arthralgia; rash; urticaria

NURSING DIAGNOSES and NURSING INTERVENTIONS

For care of systemic reactions see p. 591.

Nursing Diagnosis	Nursing Intervention
Skin integrity, impairment of: actual	Apply ice to puncture wound to decrease pain and swelling. Trim fingernails to decrease damage and secondary infection from scratching. Instruct patient in good hygiene and handwashing to prevent secondary infection.
Skin integrity, impairment of: potential	Instruct patient in personal and prophylactic environmental control; see below.

Patient Education

1. Teach the patient how to keep the lesion clean by washing two or three times a day with soap and water.
2. Teach the patient how to change the dressing for infected lesions.
3. Instruct the patient in the correct use of appropriate insect repellents:
   a. For flies: Repellent should contain at least 20% N,N-diethyl-m-toluamide; reapply every 1 to 2 hours or after swimming.
   b. For mosquitoes: Repellent should contain at least 20% N,N-diethyl-m-toluamide, indalone, or dimethyl pthalate; reapply every 1 to 2 hours or after swimming.

4. Instruct the patient in controlling fleas in the environment and animals.
   a. Environment: apply chlordane 1%, dimpylate 1%, lindane 1%, malathion 3%, methoxychlor 5%, ronnel 1%, or trichlorfon 1% in kerosene; use according to instructions on container.
   b. Animals and furniture: dust with malathion 4% powder, rotenone 1% powder, or methoxychlor 10%; use according to instructions on container. Repeat procedure at 2-week intervals to eliminate newly hatching fleas.

EVALUATION

Patient Outcome	Data Indicating That Outcome is Reached
Lesions heal.	Puncture wound resolves. Pain disappears. Integument is intact and free of infection.
Systemic responses resolve.	There is no fever, malaise, lymphadenopathy, arthralgia, rash, or urticaria. Cardiovascular, neurologic, gastrointestinal, and musculoskeletal symptoms are also resolved.
Patient takes precautionary measures and uses environmental control.	No new lesions occur.

DERMATITIS
Eczematous Dermatitis (Eczema)

Eczematous dermatitis is a superficial inflammation of the skin that is characterized by vesicles, redness, edema, oozing, crusting, scaling, and itching.

Eczematous dermatitis is a reaction pattern of the skin. Several forms of dermatitis occur, including primary contact dermatitis, allergic contact dermatitis, atopic dermatitis, diaper dermatitis, and seborrheic dermatitis. The common denominator of the various forms is the breakdown of the epidermis, usually as a result of intracellular vesiculation. Eczematous dermatitis is the model for understanding the other forms of dermatitis.[42,87] The treatment modalities are similar, and the nursing care is virtually the same. Individual differences are identified in the following discussion when appropriate.

PATHOPHYSIOLOGY

Eczematous dermatitis can be classified as acute, subacute, or chronic. The skin responds to a wide variety of noxious stimuli with a limited number of changes, including vasodilation, edema of the upper dermis, inflammatory cell infiltration of the upper dermis and epidermis, and breakdown of epidermal cells. Vesicles or bullae form when fluid accumulates between epidermal cells (spongiosis) or when there are changes within the cell itself.

The result of this inflammatory process is a skin surface that is erythematous (from vasodilation), edematous, exudative, or eroded (from vesicle formation), and crusted or scabbed (from infection or an accumulation of serous exudate). Thickening and scaling occur as a result of attempted or exaggerated reparative efforts (hyperkeratosis or parakeratosis).

Table 5-1 summarizes the clinical features and changes occurring in eczematous dermatitis. Acute dermatitis becomes subacute as it heals, as a result of either treatment or natural reparative processes. Subacute eczematous dermatitis can resolve or can become chronic if exposure to noxious stimuli persists. Acute, subacute, and chronic eczematous dermatitis may occur simultaneously.

DIAGNOSTIC STUDIES

See discussions of contact dermatitis, atopic dermatitis, diaper dermatitis and seborrheic dermatitis.

Physical examination
Characteristic eruption; history congruent with specific forms of eczematous dermatitis

TREATMENT PLAN

Table 5-2 summarizes the specific treatment measures used for the different classes of eczematous dermatitis.

Chemotherapeutic
Antipruritic agents
  Antihistamines
    Cyproheptadine (Cyproheptadine, Periactin), 12-16 mg qd po in divided doses for adults, 6 mg qd po in divided doses for children under 6 yr, 12 mg qd po in divided doses for children over 6 yr
    Trimeprazine (Temaril), 2.5 mg po qid for adults, 1.25 mg po tid for children under 3 yr, 2.5 mg po tid for children over 3 yr
  Antianxiety agents
    Hydroxyzine (Atarax, Vistaril), 25-100 mg po tid or qid for adults, 50 mg qd po in divided doses for children under 6 yr, 50-100 mg qd po in divided doses for children over 6 yr

Table 5-1
Clinical Features and Changes in Eczematous Dermatitis

	Acute	Subacute	Chronic
Clinical features	Erythema; exudate; weeping vesicles; crusts; pruritus	Less erythema; involuting vesicles; excoriation; some scaling; pruritus	Dryness; scaling; lichenification; pruritus
Microscopic changes	Vasodilation; edema; inflammatory infiltrates; spongiotic vesicles	Less vasodilation, inflammatory infiltrates, and vesiculation; parakeratosis; hyperkeratosis; acanthosis	Hyperkeratosis; no frank vesicles; acanthosis

Table 5-2
Summary of Treatment Modalities for Eczematous Dermatitis

	Acute	Subacute	Chronic
Chemotherapeutic	Antihistamines; systemic corticosteroids; topical corticosteroids (water miscible); topical antibacterials; topical antifungals	Topical corticosteroids in emollient base	Keratolytic agents; tars; topical corticosteroids
Supportive	Wet dressings (Burow's, saline, or tap water)	Oil-in-water compresses; emollient creams	Oil soaks or compresses; occlusive dressings; hydration

Corticosteroids
  Systemic
    Prednisone, 40-80 mg po in divided doses; dosage depends on severity of condition
  Topical
    Hydrocortisone (Cort-Dome, others) 1% tid or qid
    Betamethasone valerate (Valisone) 0.1% tid or qid
Anti-infective agents
  Systemic—for secondary infection; specific drug and dosage depends on infecting organism and severity of condition
  Topical antibacterials
    Bacitracin or Neosporin applied tid or qid
  Topical antifungals
    Nystatin (Mycostatin, Nilstat, others), miconazole (Monistat-Derm), or clotrimazole (Lotrimin, Mycelex), applied bid
Keratolytics
  Salicylic acid, 3%-5% added to topical corticosteroid
  Urea 10%-20% added to topical corticosteroids

Supportive (see pp. 637 and 638)
  Wet Burow's dressings, saline, and plain water dressings
  Occlusive dressings
  Oil-in-water compresses
  Hydration

ASSESSMENT: AREAS OF CONCERN

Eruption
  Clinical features as described in Table 5-1

Secondary infection
  Purulent drainage; fever; tenderness; regional lymphadenopathy

Psychosocial concerns
  Concern with body image; inability to sleep because of pruritus

NURSING DIAGNOSES and NURSING INTERVENTIONS

Nursing Diagnosis	Nursing Intervention
Skin integrity, impairment of: actual	Instruct patient in handwashing and good hygiene to prevent secondary infection. Instruct patient to cut fingernails short to decrease trauma and secondary infection. Apply dressings: wet, oil, or occlusive, as indicated (see pp. 637 and 638). Scrub crusted lesions gently with antibacterial soap to debride. Establish realistic therapeutic regimen with patient. Instruct patient in use of medications.
Comfort: alteration in, and sleep pattern disturbance	Apply cool compresses for wet skin or oil compresses for dry skin. Instruct patient in use of antipruritics.
Self-concept, disturbance in: body image	Assess patient's perception of personal appearance. Encourage patient to verbalize feelings about body, body appearance, or fear of reaction or rejection by others. Encourage development of other interests so skin condition does not become focal point of patient's existence.

Patient Education

1. Instruct the patient in the application of compresses, soaks, and scrubs using aseptic technique.
2. Instruct the patient in the use and side effects of medications.
3. Inform the patient and family that successful therapy requires patience, that therapy may be long-term, and that results may not be immediate.
4. Teach the patient the signs and symptoms of secondary infection and to seek medical treatment if they occur.

EVALUATION

Patient Outcome	Data Indicating That Outcome is Reached
Eruption improves.	Erythema, exudate, crusts, dryness, scaling, and pruritus are decreased. Excoriated areas reepithelize.
Pruritus is alleviated.	There are fewer areas of excoriation. Patient is able to sleep.
Secondary infection is avoided.	Lesions heal without purulent exudate. Temperature is normal.
Patient evaluates appearance in realistic manner.	Patient engages in usual activities and relationships.

Contact Dermatitis

Contact dermatitis is an acute or chronic inflammation of the skin that is due to external factors (primary irritant dermatitis) or specific sensitizers (allergic contact dermatitis).

Contact dermatitis is a form of eczematous dermatitis (see p. 595). Primary irritant dermatitis is caused by irritation from various chemical and biologic substances, including acids, alkalies, solvents, detergents, oils, salts, secretions, and excretions (Plate 1, 9). Chronic hand dermatitis ("housewife's eczema") and industrial dermatoses are common primary irritant dermatoses. The degree of irritation depends on the physical and chemical characteristics of the substance and the degree and time of exposure. The amount of consequent inflammation varies from person to person and depends on factors such as race, degree and pH of perspiration, type of skin, preexisting disease, and family history. Persons with little skin pigmentation are more susceptible to the effects of irritants.

Allergic contact dermatitis is a manifestation of delayed hypersensitivity. The allergen is an environmental substance to which the person has become sensitized. Genetically predisposed persons and those who have had a previous episode of allergic contact dermatitis are more likely to experience episodes of the disorder. The most common causes of allergic contact dermatitis are chemicals that have a high sensitizing index, including certain plants (tulips and chrysanthemums), plant oils (poison ivy, oak, and sumac), nickel, chrome, rubber, and paraphenylenediamine (an ingredient in many dyes).

The severity of the reaction depends on the duration and frequency of the contact. Since allergic contact dermatitis is enhanced by friction and pressure, the addition of these factors to simple exposure produces a more severe reaction.

PATHOPHYSIOLOGY

The irritating substances of primary irritant dermatitis cause damage to the stratum corneum, alter its elasticity, and change the physical features of the skin's lipid film. This impairs the barrier function of the skin and allows absorption of the irritating substance and the subsequent changes of eczematous dermatitis. The basic features of primary irritant dermatitis are the same as those of eczematous dermatitis (see p. 595). The condition can be acute, subacute, or chronic (Plate 1, 10). Primary irritant dermatitis is frequently complicated by secondary bacterial infection.

Allergic contact dermatitis is a cell-mediated, type IV immune response (see Chapter 16). The sensitizing chemical (hapten) enters the epidermis through the stratum corneum and combines with epidermal proteins to form a new molecule (hapten-protein or hapten-carrier complex) that has antigenic potential. This molecule enters the local cutaneous lymphoid tissue where specific committed lymphocytes are developed and are selectively directed against the antigen. Subsequent exposure to the hapten results in release of the committed lymphocytes around the capillary endothelial cells with the development of inflammation and eczematous dermatitis.

DIAGNOSTIC STUDIES

Physical examination
Characteristic history of contact with irritating or sensitizing substance; detailed history essential

Patch test (see p. 556)
Usually positive to allergen in allergic contact dermatitis; should not be performed if patient has active acute dermatitis

TREATMENT PLAN

Management is directed toward identification and elimination of the precipitating factor (see also p. 595).

ASSESSMENT: AREAS OF CONCERN

Eruption
Erythema; exudate; vesicles; crusts; scaling; dryness; lichenification; pruritus; location and distribution of eruption; history of eruption; site of initial eruption; history of contact with irritating or sensitizing substances; pattern of flare-ups

Secondary infection
Purulent drainage; fever; tenderness; regional lymphadenopathy

Psychosocial concerns
Concern with body image; inability to sleep

NURSING DIAGNOSES and NURSING INTERVENTIONS
See p. 596.

Patient Education
1. Instruct the patient to eliminate or avoid the precipitating factors (also see p. 597).

EVALUATION

Patient Outcome	Data Indicating That Outcome is Reached
Precipitating factor is identified and avoided.	No recurrent episodes of dermatitis appear.

Atopic Dermatitis

Atopic dermatitis is a chronic, superficial, pruritic, inflammatory response of the skin that is often associated with other atopic diseases (asthma, hay fever, and allergic rhinitis).

Atopy refers to a type I immunologic response that is hereditary (see Chapter 16). Patients with atopic dermatitis usually have high serum levels of IgE. A patient with atopic dermatitis manifests vasomotor changes, great susceptibility to environmental irritants, and susceptibility to bacterial and viral infections. Atopic dermatitis is associated with ichthyosis and xerosis and with numerous abnormalities of humoral and cell-mediated immunity.

Patients with atopic dermatitis have dry, highly sensitive skin with a lowered threshold to pruritus so that a minor stimulus causes exaggerated itching. Scratching leads to epidermal breakdown and damage to nerve endings, which in turn increase the itch sensation. This itch-scratch cycle is characteristic of atopic dermatitis.

Atopic dermatitis can begin at any time. There are usually three phases: (1) an infantile phase (3 or 4 months to 2 years of age), (2) the childhood phase (4 to 10 or 12 years), and (3) the adolescent and young adult phase. The condition gradually improves.

PATHOPHYSIOLOGY

The disease is the result of a type I immunologic response. The findings are clinically and microscopically the same as those of eczematous dermatitis and may be acute, subacute, or chronic (see discussion of eczematous dermatitis).

There is a marked tendency toward vasoconstriction of superficial blood vessels, decreased response to cooling and warmth, increased sweat production in flexor areas, and a blanch phenomenon on stroking (white dermographism). Cold and low humidity are poorly tolerated. Heat and high humidity are also poorly tolerated; vasodilation increases the inflammatory response, thereby aggravating the dermatitis and causing increased itching. Psychologic and emotional factors do not play an etiologic role but do modify symptoms. Food allergies may exacerbate the skin disease in some patients, and a good history is extremely important.

DIAGNOSTIC STUDIES

Physical examination
Characteristic eruption with typical distribution; personal or family history of allergies

Immunofluorescence
Serum IgE may be elevated

TREATMENT PLAN

Atopic dermatitis presents the whole range of the eczematous process from acute to chronic, and treatment must be directed accordingly. The focus of therapy is to interrupt the itch-scratch cycle.

Chemotherapeutic
Infantile phase
Corticosteroids
Topical hydrocortisone cream 0.1% (Cort-Dome, others) applied bid or tid

Anti-infective agents
Topical antifungals
Clotrimazole (Lotrimin, Mycelex), 0.1% applied bid
Miconazole (Monistat-Derm), 0.2% applied bid
Nystatin (Candex, Mycostatin, Nilstat, others), 100,000 units/g applied bid
Systemic or topical antibiotics for secondary infection; drug and dosage dependent on causative organism and severity of infection
Childhood and adolescent and young adult phases
Corticosteroids
Topical steroids with menthol or camphor 0.25%-0.5% applied bid or tid
Systemic
Prednisone (Deltasone, Orasone, others), 60-80 mg/qd as single morning dose for 1-2 wk; smaller dose for children
Keratolytics
Coal tar 2% (Alphosyl, Tar-Doak) applied topically at bedtime
Antihistamines
Diphenhydramine (Benadryl), 25-50 mg po tid or qid; smaller doses for children
Tripelennamine (Pyribenzamine, PBZ), 100 mg po bid or tid; smaller doses for children
Anti-infective agents
Systemic antibiotics for secondary infection; drug and dosage dependent on causative organism and severity of infection

Supportive
Burow's dressings and saline compresses (see pp. 637 and 638)
Oatmeal and oil baths (see pp. 637 and 638)
Occlusive dressings (see pp. 637 and 638)
Allergy diet (controversial)[27,87]
House humidified
Light, cotton clothing

ASSESSMENT: AREAS OF CONCERN

Infantile Phase (3 mo-2 yr)	Childhood Phase (4-12 yr)	Adolescent and Young Adult Phase (12 yr and older)
Eruption Acute eczematous eruption; erythema; vesicles; crusts; oozing; excoriation; pruritus	Subacute papular eruptions; dusky erythema; dryness; scaling; lichenification; pruritus	Lichenification; excoriation; subacute papular eruptions; generalized erythema; pruritus

Infantile Phase (3 mo-2 yr)	Childhood Phase (4-12 yr)	Adolescent and Young Adult Phase (12 yr and older)
Location		
Scalp; face; neck; intertriginous areas	Flexor surfaces; foot; lip and perioral surface	Face; neck; upper chest; flexor surfaces; wrists, feet; upper back; generalized
Special disease manifestations		
Diaper dermatitis; cradle cap	Foot dermatitis; pityriasis alba	Chronic hand eczema; nummular eczema

Secondary infection

Purulent drainage; fever; tenderness; regional lymphadenopathy

Psychosocial concerns

Concern with body image; inability to sleep because of pruritus; exacerbations caused by stress

NURSING DIAGNOSES and NURSING INTERVENTIONS

See p. 596.

Patient Education

1. Teach the patient and family that the patient should avoid:
   a. Heat, high humidity, and rapid changes of temperature
   b. Sweating
   c. Excessive bathing
   d. Strong soaps and detergents that can irritate skin
   e. Emotional stress
   f. Wools, coarse synthetic fabrics, and tight-fitting clothing
   g. Primary irritants

2. Teach the patient and family that the patient should:
   a. Keep skin well lubricated
   b. Wear light, loose, cotton clothing that "breathes"
   c. Bathe in lukewarm, not hot, water
3. Teach the patient and family the signs and symptoms of secondary infection and to seek medical attention if they occur.
4. Explain to the patient and family that therapy requires patience and that results may not be immediate.
5. Teach the child to manage the skin condition as soon as possible.
6. Counsel the family not to allow a child to use manipulative behavior through scratching.

EVALUATION

Patient Outcome	Data Indicating That Outcome is Reached
Known causative agents are avoided.	Eruption subsides. Exacerbations are limited.
Pruritus is relieved.	Scratching decreases. Excoriations heal. Patient is able to sleep.
Secondary infection is avoided.	Eruption is free from tenderness and purulent exudate. There is no fever or lymphadenopathy.
Patient assesses appearance in realistic manner.	Patient engages in usual relationships and activities when possible.

Seborrheic Dermatitis

Seborrheic dermatitis is a chronic, recurrent, erythematous scaling eruption that is localized in areas where sebaceous glands are concentrated.

In infants seborrheic dermatitis may develop on the scalp, back, and intertriginous and diaper areas. The scalp lesions are scaling, adherent, thick, yellow, and crusted. Lesions elsewhere are erythematous, scaling, and fissured.

After puberty lesions tend to occur in the scalp, eyebrows, eyelids, nasolabial areas, postauricular areas, and presternal and intertriginous areas (Plate 1, *11*). Lesions may be mild or severe and vary from dry, greasy scales to erythema, excoriation, and crusting. Secondary bacterial or fungal infection may occur. Genetic factors seem to affect the incidence and severity of the disease. The disorder is worse during the winter months.

PATHOPHYSIOLOGY

The etiology of seborrheic dermatitis is unknown. Histologic changes include vasodilation and discharge of inflammatory cells into the epidermis from the capillary loops. Epidermal inflammation and eczema may be present. Scales are produced as a result of an increased mitotic rate and an accumulation of corneocytes. Despite the name, the composition, production, and flow of sebum are normal.

DIAGNOSTIC STUDIES

Physical examination
Characteristic lesions and distribution

TREATMENT PLAN

Chemotherapeutic
  Corticosteroids
    Topical
      Hydrocortisone (Cort-Dome, others) 0.1% bid or tid in nonhairy areas
      Betamethasone (Valisone) 0.05% bid in hairy areas
  Antiseborrheic shampoos
    Zinc pyrithione 1%-2% (Head & Shoulders) qd
    Selenium sulfide (Selsun suspension) qd
  Anti-infective agents
    Topical antibiotics for secondary infection
      Neomycin 0.1% bid or tid
      Chloramphenicol (Chloromycetin cream) 0.1% bid or tid
  Keratolytics
    Salicylic acid 1%-3% topically bid
    Precipitated sulfur 1%-5% topically bid
    Tar cream 4% topically bid

Supportive
  Oils—castor, mineral, and olive, rubbed into scalp lesions and left overnight
  Frequent shampooing
  Burow's solution for weeping lesions

ASSESSMENT: AREAS OF CONCERN

Eruption
  Erythema; scaling; fissures; inflammation; pruritus

Secondary infection
  Purulent discharge; fever; tenderness; increased inflammation; regional lymphadenopathy

Psychosocial concerns
  Concern about body image

NURSING DIAGNOSES and NURSING INTERVENTIONS

Nursing Diagnosis	Nursing Intervention
Skin integrity, impairment of: actual	Instruct patient in use of medications and topical preparations. Instruct patient to shampoo daily. Instruct patient not to scratch or rub lesions, since that will prolong course of disease.
Self-concept, disturbance in: body image	Encourage patient to verbalize feelings about body, body appearance, or fear of reaction or rejection by others. Assure patient that treatment can be successful.

Patient Education

1. Instruct the patient in the use of medications and preparations.
2. Explain the care regimen to the patient.
3. Instruct the patient in the signs and symptoms of secondary infection and to seek medical care if they occur.
4. Instruct the patient to avoid external irritants, excessive heat, and excessive perspiration.

EVALUATION

Patient Outcome	Data Indicating That Outcome is Reached
Eruption resolves.	Erythema and inflammation disappear. Scaling decreases. Fissures heal. Pruritus is relieved. Integument is intact.
Secondary infection is resolved or prevented.	There is no purulent discharge, fever, or lymphadenopathy.
Patient evaluates appearance in realistic manner.	Patient engages in usual activities and relationships.

ICHTHYOSIS

Ichthyosis is a common inherited keratinization disorder that is characterized by varying degrees of dryness, scaling, and exfoliation.

Several genetic keratinization abnormalities result in dry, scaly skin. The most common condition is ichthyosis vulgaris, an autosomal dominant inherited disease that occurs in 1 in 1000 persons (Plate 1, *12*). The other forms of ichthyosis are rarer.

PATHOPHYSIOLOGY

In ichthyosis vulgaris the mitotic rate is decreased and the stratum corneum fails to desquamate normally. The granular layer is reduced or absent, and sweat and sebaceous glands may be reduced. The follicular orifices are hyperkeratotic and are often plugged with keratin. The ability of the stratum corneum to retain water is decreased. Aggravation during the winter months and improvement during the summer are common. The other forms of ichthyosis show similar pathologic changes.

Table 5-3 summarizes the clinical, pathologic, and genetic features of the four patterns of inherited ichthyosis (Plate 1, *13*).

DIAGNOSTIC STUDIES

Physical examination
Characteristic lesion

TREATMENT PLAN

Chemotherapeutic
Emollients (apply to moist skin bid after bathing)
Propylene glycol 40%-50%
Propylene glycol 60%, ethanol 2%, and salicylic acid 6% in gel base under occlusive dressing for 1-4 d and then every third night
Hydrophilic petrolatum
Water-miscible bath oil
Keratolytics (apply after bathing to moist skin or 3-7 times/wk)
Salicylic acid 5% in emollient base
Urea 10% in water-miscible base
Sodium chloride 10% and salicylic acid 5%
Vitamins
Tretinoin (Retin-A) 0.1% (vitamin A, retinoic acid), applied topically for lamellar ichthyosis
Oral synthetic retinoids, still under testing[19,85,86]

ASSESSMENT: AREAS OF CONCERN

Lesions
Type of scale and distribution as in Table 5-3; severity

Secondary infection
Redness; tenderness; swelling; exudate; odor

Comfort and mobility
Discomfort from dry cracked skin; limitation on mobility

Psychosocial concerns
Concern about body image

Table 5-3
Summary of Ichthyosis Disorders

Disorder	Inheritance Pattern	Age of Onset	Prognosis	Histopathology	Type Scale	Distribution
Vulgaris	Dominant	Childhood (1 to 4 years)	Improves during adult years	Increased mitotic rate; retained stratum corneum; decreased granular layer; plugged follicular orifices	Fine, small, thin, light	Back and extensor surfaces; flexures spared; increased markings on palms and soles
Male, sex-linked	Recessive X-linked	Birth	Persistent	As above; increased plugging	Large, brown	Neck and trunk; total extremities; flexures spared; normal markings
Lamellar non-bullous	Recessive	Birth	Persistent	Increased mitotic rate; granular layer present; acanthosis; hyperkeratosis; plugged follicular orifices	Large, coarse, yellow, raised corners	Generalized; thick palms and soles
Bullous epidermolytic hyperkaratoses	Dominant	Birth	Persistent; very severe forms may cause death in early infancy from secondary infection	As above; vacuolation of epidermal cells	Thick, gray-brown, coarse, warty, vesicular, and bullous lesions	Patchy or generalized; flexures affected

NURSING DIAGNOSES and NURSING INTERVENTIONS

Nursing Diagnosis	Nursing Intervention
Skin integrity, impairment of: actual	Instruct patient and parent in use of topical preparations. Stress importance of good hygiene to prevent secondary infection.
Comfort, alteration in and mobility, impaired physical	Instruct patient in use of emollients to decrease dryness. Instruct patient not to use soap or to use it sparingly while bathing. Instruct patient to maintain humidity in living environment.
Self-concept, disturbance in: body image	Assess patient's or parents' perception of patient's appearance. Encourage patient to verbalize feelings about body, body appearance, and fear of reaction or rejection by others. Encourage patient to develop interests and other attributes to support positive self-image, feelings of self-worth, and self-confidence. Help patient evaluate appearance in realistic manner so it does not become focal point of existence. Inform parents that condition may improve as child matures.

Patient Education

1. Instruct the patient and family in the use of emollients and keratolytics.
2. Instruct the patient in the signs and symptoms of secondary infection and to seek medical care if they occur.
3. Inform the patient and family that successful therapy requires the patient's full cooperation and patience, that therapy is long-term, and that results may not be immediate.

EVALUATION

Patient Outcome	Data Indicating That Outcome is Reached
Dryness is decreased.	Discomfort is relieved. Cracks and fissures improve. Limitations on mobility lessen.
Secondary infection is avoided.	There is no redness, tenderness, swelling, or purulent exudate.
Patient makes successful adaptations in self-concept.	Patient develops interests and participates in activities compatible with degree of mobility. Patient engages in satisfying relationships. Patient does not use disorder as excuse for unsuccessful relationships.

LICHEN PLANUS

Lichen planus is a chronic pruritic inflammatory eruption of the skin and mucous membrane. It is characterized by small angular papules that may coalesce into larger plaques.

Lichen planus occurs most frequently in adults. The onset may be gradual or abrupt. The average duration of the disease is 15 to 24 months, but it may persist or recur for years. Healing is followed by residual pigmentation that eventually fades.

PATHOPHYSIOLOGY

The etiology of lichen planus is unknown. It can be represented as an immunologic process with cytotoxic damage to the basal cells. Certain drugs and chemicals used in developing color photographs can cause an eruption.

Inflammation occurs primarily at the dermal level with lymphocytic infiltrate. There are hyperkeratosis and prominence of the granular layer. Vacuolation, degeneration, and inflammatory changes occur in the basal layer. Fibrin and IgM are deposited in the papillary dermis.

Cutaneous lesions are pruritic, flat-topped, reddish violet, angular papules that are 0.5 to 5 mm in diameter. The papules have a sheen on cross-lighting (Plate 1, *14*). Whitish gray lines (Wickham's striae) are seen on the skin. The individual papules can coalesce to larger plaques, becoming more scaly and verrucous. The lesions are usually symmetrically distributed and occur most commonly on the flexor surfaces of the wrist, forearm, and ankles and on the abdomen and sacrum. The face, palms, and soles are rarely affected. Eruption can occur at the site of minor trauma (Köbner's phenomenon).

Lesions of the buccal mucosa are present in 50% to 60% of the cases. These gray lacy lesions may ulcerate and be painful. Malignant degeneration occurs in about 1 in 100 cases.

Clinical variants include annular, bullous, hypertrophic, and atrophic lesions. Nails can be involved, with pitting, thinning, and increase in longitudinal ridging. In severe cases the nail may be shed completely.

DIAGNOSTIC STUDIES

Physical examination
Characteristic lesion

Biopsy
Characteristic histologic changes

Immunofluorescence
IgG deposits in papillary dermis

TREATMENT PLAN

Chemotherapeutic
Corticosteroids
Topical
Hydrocortisone (Cort-Dome, others) 0.1% or triamcinolone (Aristocort, Kenalog, others) 0.1% in occlusive dressing at bedtime; must be maintained until all signs of lesions disappear
Triamcinolone 0.1% in dental paste (Kenalog in Orabase) applied q3-5h for mouth lesions
Intralesional injection
Triamcinolone (Aristocort, Kenalog) 5 mg/ml (see p. 640)
Systemic corticosteroids for very severe or generalized lesions
Prednisone, 40-60 mg po qd, then decreasing doses
Vitamins
Tretinoin (Retin-A) 0.1% applied with cotton-tipped applicator at night followed by triamcinolone 0.1% tid

Local anesthetics
  Viscous lidocaine (Xylocaine) mouth swish before
    meals
Antipruritics
  Anti-anxiety agents
    Hydroxyzine (Atarax, Orgatrax, Vistaril), 25-100
      mg po tid or qid
  Antihistamines
    Cyproheptadine (Cyproheptadine, Periactin), 4
      mg po tid

Supportive
Withdrawal of all current medications and replacement
  with substitutes

ASSESSMENT: AREAS OF CONCERN

Lesion
Angular papules; bullous, hypertrophic, and atrophic
  lesions; coalesced plaques, mucosal plaques, or ulceration; distribution of lesions

Discomfort
Pruritus; pain from buccal ulceration

Nutrition
Inability to eat because of buccal ulceration

Psychosocial concerns
Concern with body image

NURSING DIAGNOSES and NURSING INTERVENTIONS

Nursing Diagnosis	Nursing Intervention
Skin integrity, impairment of: actual	Instruct patient in good hygiene and need for short fingernails to prevent secondary infection. Apply cool compresses to relieve itching. Instruct patient in use of occlusive dressing (see p. 637).
Oral mucous membrane, alteration in	Instruct patient in use of viscous lidocaine (Xylocaine): 15 minutes before eating, swish in mouth. Instruct patient to avoid astringent and acidic fluids. Provide mouth care with alkaline or saline mouthwash.
Comfort, alteration in: pain	Provide soft diet. Provide bland foods.
Self-concept, disturbance in: body image	Assess patient's perception of own appearance. Encourage patient to verbalize feelings about body, body appearance, or fear of reaction or rejection by others.

Patient Education
1. Instruct the patient in the treatment regimen, medications, and dressings.
2. Instruct the patient in the side effects of medications.
3. Teach the patient the signs and symptoms of secondary infection and to seek medical treatment if they occur.
4. Discuss the long-term nature of the disorder and the fact that treatment requires persistence and patience.
5. Instruct the patient to avoid precipitating drugs and chemicals.

EVALUATION

Patient Outcome	Data Indicating That Outcome is Reached
Eruption improves.	Papules, bullae, and plaques resolve. Ulcerations reepithelize. Pruritus resolves. Secondary infection does not occur.
Discomfort from buccal lesions is alleviated.	Patient is able to eat and does not lose weight.
Pruritus is alleviated.	Areas of excoriation resolve or do not recur.
Patient evaluates appearance in realistic manner.	Patient engages in usual activities and relationships.

PIGMENTED DISORDERS
Pigmented Nevi, Blue Nevi, and Mongolian Spots

Pigmented nevi, blue nevi, and mongolian spots are benign skin lesions that are caused by accumulation of pigment in the dermis.

Pigmented nevi occur in various forms that vary in size and degree of pigmentation. Nevi are present on most persons and may occur anywhere on the body. They vary in appearance and may be flat, slightly raised, dome shaped, smooth, rough, or hairy. Their color ranges from tan, gray, and shades of brown to black.

The blue nevus usually occurs as a single nodular lesion on the dorsal surface of the hands, face, or buttocks. The nevus is present at birth and remains unchanged through life.

Mongolian spots have a dusky blue color and blend into the surrounding normal skin. The spots occur primarily in Oriental and dark-skinned infants, usually in the lumbosacral area. The spots vary in diameter from 1 cm to several centimeters. They cause no symptoms and usually disappear during childhood.

PATHOPHYSIOLOGY

The lesions occur as the result of nevus cells that migrate to the dermis during embryonic development. The nevus cells have the same origin as melanocytes and are closely associated with them. The nevus cells contain melanin pigment, which gives the lesions their color. The blue color of the blue nevus and the mongolian spots is due to the concentration of melanin and its depth below the epidermis.

Table 5-4 summarizes the features of the various types of pigmented nevi.

DIAGNOSTIC STUDIES

Physical examination
  Characteristic lesion

Biopsy
  Shows histologic configuration

TREATMENT PLAN

Most nevi do not require any treatment. Surgical removal may be indicated for cosmetic purposes or if changes occur in the nevus. Mongolian spots require no treatment.

Surgical
  Shave ablation with electrodesiccation of base for intradermal nevus
  Excisional or punch biopsy removal of junction nevus
  Excision of hairy nevus with full-thickness skin grafting (see pp. 640-641)

Table 5-4

Features and Occurrence of Various Types of Pigmented Nevi

Type	Features	Occurrence	Comments
Halo nevus	Sharp, oval, or circular; depigmented halo around mole; may undergo many morphologic changes; usually disappears and halo repigments (may take years)	Usually on back in young adult	Usually benign; biopsy indicated because same process can occur around melanoma
Intradermal nevus	Dome shaped; raised; flesh to black color; may be pedunculated or hair bearing	Cells limited to dermis	No indication for removal other than cosmetic
Junction nevus	Flat or slightly elevated; dark brown	Nevus cells lining dermoepidermal junction	Should be removed if exposed to repeated trauma
Compound nevus	Slightly elevated brownish papule; indistinct border	Nevus cells in dermis and lining dermoepidermal junction	Should be removed if exposed to repeated trauma
Hairy nevus	May be present at birth; may cover large area; hair growth occurring after several years		Should be removed if changes occur

ASSESSMENT: AREAS OF CONCERN

Lesion
Location; size; color; shape

Lesion changes
Enlargement; darkening; crusting; bleeding; inflammation; ulceration; appearance of satellite lesions

Psychosocial concerns
Concern about body image

NURSING DIAGNOSES and NURSING INTERVENTIONS

Nursing Diagnosis	Nursing Intervention
Self-concept, disturbance in: body image	Assess for presence of defining characteristics. Assist in verbalization of feelings about body, body image, or fear of reaction or rejection by others.

Patient Education

1. Instruct the patient regarding the benign nature of the lesions.
2. Instruct the patient regarding changes that might indicate malignancy and to seek medical attention if they occur.

EVALUATION

Patient Outcome	Data Indicating That Outcome is Reached
Patient seeks treatment for changes in lesions.	Patient seeks medical attention if color or size of nevus changes, if it bleeds, or if it is exposed to repeated trauma.
Patient evaluates appearance in realistic manner.	Patient seeks removal if lesion is cosmetically embarrassing.

Chloasma

Chloasma is a diffuse, mottled brown pigmentation that appears over areas of the face and forehead.

PATHOPHYSIOLOGY

Chloasma is a blotchy brown pigmentation that involves the forehead, malar prominences, and preauricular areas. The distribution is usually symmetric. Chloasma occurs primarily in women during and after childbearing years. Increased activity of melanocytes with a resultant increase in melanin deposits in the basal cells of the epidermis can occur secondary to pregnancy or from the use of anovulatory hormones. Exposure to sunlight exaggerates the pigmentation. It fades somewhat after childbirth or after the hormones are discontinued. Chloasma rarely occurs idiopathically in dark-skinned men.

DIAGNOSTIC STUDIES

Physical examination
Characteristic pigmentation and distribution; in women history congruent with pregnancy or anovulatory hormones

TREATMENT PLAN

Chemotherapeutic
Topical depigmenting agents
Hydroquinone (Eldopaque, Eldoquin), 2%-4% applied sparingly bid
Compound of retinoic acid 0.1%, hydroquinone 5%, and dexamethasone 0.1% applied sparingly bid[86]

Sunscreen—para-aminobenzoic acid (PABA) 5% (Pabanol, Sunbrella) in ethyl alcohol 95%, applied twice a day and after swimming and bathing

Supportive

Discontinuation of anovulatory hormones

ASSESSMENT: AREAS OF CONCERN

Pigmentation

Severity and extent of pigmentation; questioning to determine if woman is pregnant or taking anovulatory hormones

Psychosocial concerns

Concern about body image

NURSING DIAGNOSES and NURSING INTERVENTIONS

Nursing Diagnosis	Nursing Intervention
Self-concept, disturbance in: body image	Assess patient's self-perception. Encourage patient to verbalize feelings about body, body image, or fear of reaction or rejection by others. Inform patient that pigmentation fades in time. Instruct patient in use of medications.

Patient Education

1. Instruct the patient to avoid sun exposure, which will worsen the condition.
2. Instruct the patient to use sunscreens.
3. Instruct the patient in the side effects of depigmenting agents.

EVALUATION

Patient Outcome	Data Indicating That Outcome is Reached
Existing pigmentation fades.	Blotchy brown areas become less noticeable.
Patient avoids sunlight and use of anovulatory hormones.	New areas of pigmentation do not occur.
Patient evaluates appearance in realistic manner.	Patient seeks treatment for areas that are cosmetically embarrassing. Patient engages in usual activities and relationships.

Depigmentation: Albinism and Vitiligo

Albinism and vitiligo are depigmentation that results from a congenital or acquired decrease in melanin production.

Albinism is a rare inherited disease that may be complete or partial. Partial albinism is autosomal dominant. The affected areas are usually linear and unilateral. The same area may be affected in more than one family member. A small area on the scalp with a white streak of hair is frequently seen.

Complete or universal albinism is autosomal recessive or irregularly dominant. There is no pigmentation in the skin, hair, and eyes. (Some pigmentation may occur with increasing age.) The skin is pale, the hair white, and the iris pink or red. Nystagmus and errors of refraction are common. Skin cancer and premature actinic keratosis are common.

Vitiligo is localized areas of depigmentation that are caused by the disappearance of previously active melanocytes. Vitiligo is fairly common, occurring in 1% of the world's population. It is a familial trait and can occur at any age. Initial lesions frequently develop in areas exposed to the sun. The process may remain stable for years and involve only small areas, or it may progress to affect more extensive areas or the entire skin surface and hair. The eyes do not lose their pigment.

The lesions are completely depigmented and have well-demarcated borders that may be hyperpigmented (Plate 1, *15*). Vitiligo usually develops symmetrically and may follow trauma to the area. Common areas of involvement are the hands, axillae, perineum, and periorbital areas. The surface of the depigmented skin is normal except for the absence of pigmentation. There is no scaling. Some spontaneous repigmentation occurs in about 10% of patients, but complete repigmentation is rare.

Vitiligo is associated with thyroid dysfunction, diabetes mellitus, Addison's disease, and pernicious anemia.

PATHOPHYSIOLOGY

In partial albinism melanocytes are not present in the depigmented area because they failed to migrate to the skin during embryonic development. In complete albinism melanocytes are present in the dermis, but they are unable to synthesize pigment because of a block in the formation of melanin from its precursor.

The etiology of vitiligo is unknown. It is considered an autoimmune process that causes destruction of preexisting melanocytes. The melanocytes are abnormal and in various stages of cell death at the periphery of the lesions. Repigmentation is thought to result from the migration of melanocytes from residual areas of melanocytic activity within hair follicles.

DIAGNOSTIC STUDIES

Physical examination
  Distinctive lesions with characteristic configuration and distribution

TREATMENT PLAN

There is no treatment for albinism other than protection from sun exposure and actinic damage. The treatment for vitiligo is protracted and has mixed results.

Chemotherapeutic
  Photosensitizers
    Psoralen therapy with 8-methoxypsoralen or methoxsalen (Oxsoralen, Trisoralen) to repigment
    Psoralen, 40-50 mg po 2h before sun exposure; sun exposure time initially 20 min then gradually increased
    Psoralen, 40-50 mg po with long-wave ultraviolet light (PUVA), exposure time gradually increased[30,86] (see p. 641)
  Sunscreens
    Para-aminobenzoic acid (PABA) 5% (Pabanol, Sunbrella) as protection against sunburn, applied topically q3h and after swimming
  Skin dyes containing dihydroxyacetone (Vitadye); stain stratum corneum; applied topically several times a week
  Corticosteroids
    Oral glucocorticoids or topical glucocorticoids used in occlusive dressings to repigment
  Depigmenting agents
    For surrounding area in extensive vitiligo
      20% monobenzyl ether or hydroquinone

ASSESSMENT: AREAS OF CONCERN

Lesions
  Location and distribution; extent of involvement

Psychosocial concerns
  Concern about body image

NURSING DIAGNOSES and NURSING INTERVENTIONS

Nursing Diagnosis	Nursing Intervention
Skin integrity, impairment of: potential	Instruct patient to protect against skin exposure to sun through use of protective clothing and hats. Instruct patient to use PABA as sunscreen.
Self-concept, disturbance in: body image	Assess patient's perception of own appearance. Encourage patient to verbalize feelings about body, body image, or fear of reaction or rejection by others. Encourage development of interests and other attributes to support positive self-image and feelings of worth and self-confidence. Help patient evaluate appearance in realistic way so it does not become focal point of patient's existence. Advise patient of cosmetic products (Covermark) available for use on small areas. Facilitate initiation of counseling if patient is unable to adjust to appearance.

Patient Education

1. Instruct the patient to protect against exposure to the sun to prevent premature actinic damage.
2. Instruct in the use and side effects of medications and preparations.
3. Inform the patient that treatment for vitiligo is protracted and that results vary.

EVALUATION

Patient Outcome	Data Indicating That Outcome is Reached
Actinic damage is avoided.	Epidermis is not dry or fissured. There are no actinic keratoses. Skin remains smooth and elastic.
Patient evaluates appearance in realistic manner.	Disorder is not used as excuse for unsuccessful interpersonal relationships. Patient develops interests and relationships so appearance is not focal point of existence.

PITYRIASIS ROSEA

Pityriasis rosea is a self-limiting inflammation of unknown etiology.

The disease peaks in spring and fall. It is less likely to occur on tanned skin, and sunlight apparently hastens the course. Onset is sudden with occurrence of a herald patch followed 1 to 3 weeks later by a generalized eruption. New lesions continue to appear for about a week after onset of the generalized eruption. A gradual involution follows. Total duration is 4 to 12 weeks with rare recurrence. The disease is not infectious or contagious.

PATHOPHYSIOLOGY

The etiology of pityriasis rosea is unknown. The herald patch is a single oval or round plaque with fine superficial scaling (Plate 1, *16*). The remainder of the lesions are smaller but are similar in configuration to the primary lesion. The lesions develop on the trunk and extremities. The palms and soles are not involved, and facial involvement is rare. The lesions are characteristically distributed in parallel alignment following the direction of the ribs in a Christmas tree–like pattern. An inverse pattern can occur, with concentration of the lesions on the extremities and relative sparing of the trunk. The lesions are usually pale, erythematous, and macular with fine scaling, but they may be papular or vesicular. Pruritus may be present.

Microscopic examination reveals nonspecific inflammation of the dermis, perivascular infiltrates, and localized epidermal changes with spongiosis and focal parakeratosis.

DIAGNOSTIC STUDIES

Physical examination
  Characteristic lesion with distinct distribution and congruent history

VDRL or rapid plasma reagin (RPR) test
  Done to rule out secondary syphilis

TREATMENT PLAN

Treatment is usually unnecessary.

Chemotherapeutic
  Antipruritic effects
    Antipruritic agents
      Menthol 0.25% in cream base applied topically bid or tid
    Antihistamines
      Cyproheptadine (Cyproheptadine, Periactin), 4 mg po tid
    Antianxiety agents
      Hydroxyzine (Atarax, Orgatrax, Vistaril), 25-100 mg po tid or qid
  Corticosteroids
    Prednisone, 10 mg po qid for severe pruritus til itching subsides, then in decremental doses over 14 d

ASSESSMENT: AREAS OF CONCERN

Lesion

Pale, erythematous macules with fine scaling or papules and vesicles; herald patch larger than new lesions; characteristic distribution

Psychosocial concerns

Concern with body image

NURSING DIAGNOSES and NURSING INTERVENTIONS

Nursing Diagnosis	Nursing Intervention
Skin integrity, impairment of: actual	Lubricate skin with emollient and water-miscible bath oil. Stress importance of good hygiene to avoid secondary infection. Have patient cut fingernails short to avoid tissue trauma from scratching.
Self-concept, disturbance in: body image	Reassure patient that lesions will clear in 4 to 12 weeks. Assist in verbalization of feelings about body, body appearance, or fear of reaction or rejection by others.

Patient Education

1. Instruct the patient that the disease is self-limiting and will resolve.
2. Instruct the patient that exposure to sunlight may hasten the course of the disease.
3. Teach the patient the signs and symptoms of secondary infection and to seek medical attention if they occur.
4. Instruct the patient in the use and side effects of medications.

EVALUATION

Patient Outcome	Data Indicating That Outcome is Reached
Lesions resolve.	Macules, papules, vesicles, and scaling disappear. Pruritus is relieved. Integument is intact.
Secondary infection is resolved or avoided.	There is no tenderness, swelling, purulent discharge, or fever.
Patient evaluates appearance in realistic manner.	Patient engages in usual activities and relationships.

PSORIASIS

Psoriasis is a chronic and recurrent disease of keratin synthesis that is characterized by dry, well-circumscribed, silvery, scaling papules and plaques.

Psoriasis occurs in 3% to 5% of the population. Onset is usually between the ages of 10 and 40 years. A family history of psoriasis is common.

The onset of the disease is insidious, and the course is characterized by periods of inactivity and exacerbation. Emotional stress may precipitate exacerbations. Spontaneous remission may occur. Psoriasis characteristically involves the back, buttocks, and extensor surfaces of the extremities, particularly the knees and elbows, and the scalp. The nails, axillae, umbilicus, eyebrows, and anogenital areas may be affected. Generalized eruptions can occur. Approximately 5% of persons with psoriasis have an associated arthritis. Lesions may develop at sites of recent epidermal injury.

The characteristic lesions of psoriasis are raised, erythematous, sharply demarcated papules covered with overlapping, silvery or shiny scales. The papules may coalesce, forming large plaques. When the scales are removed, a deep red base, covered with a thin membrane that bleeds, is revealed.

Table 5-5
Clinical Features and Distribution of the Various Forms of Psoriasis

Clinical Pattern	Clinical Features	Distribution
Localized plaques	Erythematous plaques with silver scales; nails pitted, thickened, discolored, and crumbling beneath free edge	Extensor aspect of extremities; elbows; knees; scalp; nails
Generalized plaques	As above	Disseminated
Guttate	Tiny plaques (0.5-2 cm); sudden onset usually after streptococcal infection; may progress to other types; may itch	Disseminated
Pustular	Pustular lesions covered by thin scale	Palms and soles only or generalized
Erythrodermic exfoliative	More inflammatory; skin red and hot; deep erythema with massive shedding of scales; usually follows overly aggressive therapy; can cause temperature and fluid imbalances	Generalized

PATHOPHYSIOLOGY

The basic defect in psoriasis is in the control of the growth of epidermal cells. This defect may be genetic, biochemical, or immunologic. The three main components of the psoritic process are: (1) increased mitotic rate that results in rapid cellular turnover and shortened transit time of the epidermal cell from the basal layer to the epidermis (4 to 7 days versus the normal 28 days); (2) faulty keratinization of the horny layer, which desquamates readily and affords little protection to the underlying skin; and (3) dilation of upper dermal vessels and intermittent discharge of polymorphonuclear leukocytes into the dermis.

The three processes occur in different degrees that result in varying forms of psoriasis with differing clinical features. If the increased mitotic rate predominates, the result is a thick silvery scale because of the separation of corneocytes and the presence of air between them. If vasodilation predominates, the result is diffusely red, hot, slightly scaling skin (Plate 1, 17 and 18).

The forms of psoriasis and their clinical features are summarized in Table 5-5.

DIAGNOSTIC STUDIES

Physical examination
  Characteristic lesions

TREATMENT PLAN

Chemotherapeutic
  Corticosteroids
    Topical nonfluorinated corticosteroids for lesions on face and intertriginous areas
      Hydrocortisone (Cort-Dome, others) 2%-3% applied sparingly bid

Topical fluorinated corticosteroids for lesions on scalp, body, and extremities
  Fluocinolone (Fluonid, Synalar) 0.025%-0.01% applied sparingly bid, tid, or qid
  Betamethasone (Valisone) 0.05%-0.1% applied sparingly bid, tid, or qid
  Triamcinolone (Aristocort, Kenalog) 0.05%-0.1% applied sparingly bid, tid, or qid
Topical corticosteroids in conjunction with tar preparations or in occlusive therapy (see p. 637)
Intralesional injections of corticosteroids
  Triamcinolone (Kenalog) 10 mg/ml
Systemic corticosteroids—individualized treatment regimen; rarely used[28,86,97]
Keratolytics
  Coal tar preparations (Alphosyl, Psorigel, Balnetar) added to bath oil or shampoo or applied sparingly to lesions
  Dianthrol compounds[53,93]
    Anthralin (Anthra-Derm) 0.1%-1% applied sparingly at bedtime or bid; very irritating and stains clothing permanently; cannot be used simultaneously with corticosteroids
  Phenol-saline mixture (P & S liquid) massaged into scalp and left for 3-4h for scalp lesions, followed by tar shampoo
Photosensitizing agents
  Psoralen (Trisoralen, Oxysoralen), 0.6 mg/kg, 2-4h before exposure to ultraviolet light; used as photoactivator in combination with long-wave ultraviolet light therapy (see p. 641)
Vitamins
  Oral retinoids
    Etretinate, 25 mg/kg; still under testing[25,43,85,94]
Antineoplastic agents (used for antimetabolite effect)
  Methotrexate in individualized treatment regimen for very severe disease; use is controversial[27,86,92]

Anti-infective agents
 Penicillin (Pen Vee-K, V-Cillin, others), 250 mg po qid for 10 days for underlying streptococcal infection in guttate psoriasis

Electromechanical

See pp. 641 and 642

Exposure to short-wave ultraviolet light (UV-B)—one to three times weekly with increasing UV-B exposure; kept below level that would cause erythema

Goeckerman therapy—UV-B therapy in combination with coal tar applications that are photosensitizing; coal tar ointment applied and left on for several hours and then washed off; UV-B therapy then administered in doses to account for photosensitization; Tar finally reapplied[54,60]

Long-wave ultraviolet light (UV-A) in combination with psoralen as a photosensitizer (PUVA therapy)—psoralen administered in initial dose of 0.6 mg/kg; UV-A irradiation delivered 2 to 4 hours after psoralen administration; dosage and exposure determined by individual response; special equipment and careful monitoring required, so therapy usually provided in special treatment centers; long-term effects remain controversial; treatment usually reserved for chronic, severe, refractory psoriasis[23,27,30,36]

X-ray therapy and Grenz-ray therapy—used to provide temporary clearing of stubborn plaques; of limited value as therapeutic tools in psoriasis therapy[27,86]

Peritoneal dialysis—mechanism for antipsoriasis effect unknown; therapy experimental[2,91]

Supportive

Occlusive dressings with topical corticosteroids or tar preparations or both (see p. 637)

Day care treatment centers for psoriasis—patients with severe psoriasis can undergo treatment regimens that are intensive or that require special equipment and supervision[60]

ASSESSMENT: AREAS OF CONCERN

Lesions
Characteristics and distribution as in Table 5-5

Psoritic arthritis
Pain; tenderness; stiffness in small distal joints (early); larger joints involved later

Environment
Presence of mechanical injury that can exacerbate lesions; stress factors

NURSING DIAGNOSES and NURSING INTERVENTIONS

Nursing Diagnosis	Nursing Intervention
Skin integrity, impairment of: actual	Explain disease process regarding exacerbations and remissions. Stress importance of adhering to therapeutic regimen; assist patient in setting up overall schedule for managing regimen on daily basis. Give written instructions for use of topical preparations, tar baths, and shampoos. Instruct patient in application of occlusive dressings. Instruct patient to scrub scales gently during daily bath with soft brush and to apply medications after removing scales. Instruct patient not to apply keratolytics and tar to nonaffected areas, since they may precipitate new lesions. Explore stress factors affecting patient and alternatives for dealing with stress.
Self-concept, disturbance in: body image	Recognize importance of body image in growth and development. Assess patient's perception of own appearance. Assist in verbalization of feelings about body, body appearance, or fear of reaction or rejection by others. Encourage patient to develop interests and other attributes to support positive self-image, feelings of worth, and self-confidence. Facilitate initiation of individual or group therapy if patient is unable to adjust to appearance.
Social isolation	Involve family members in treatment regimen. Stress that psoriasis is not communicable. Refer patient for counseling if patient is socially disabled by disease.
Powerlessness	Assess for presence of defining characteristics. Observe for signs of depression and apathy. Involve patient in decision making. Encourage patient to express dissatisfaction and frustration.

Patient Education

1. Instruct the patient in the treatment regimen and the use of medications.
2. Instruct the patient in the side effects of medications.
3. Inform the patient that anthralin (Dithranol) stains skin, sheets, and clothing. Skin discoloration resolves in a few weeks as the stratum corneum is shed.
4. Evaluate the patient's ability to carry out home care and reteach procedures as necessary.
5. Instruct the patient in good hygiene to avoid secondary infection.

EVALUATION

Patient Outcome	Data Indicating That Outcome is Reached
Lesions improve.	Scaling, pustules, erythema, and size of plaques decrease.
Exacerbating factors are avoided.	Patient takes precautions against integumentary trauma. Patient avoids or tries alternative strategies for reducing stress factors.
Untoward effects from therapies are minimized.	Patient seeks medical attention for untoward or side effects from medications or therapies.
Patient copes with disorder in an effective manner.	Patient engages in satisfying relationships. Patient seeks counseling when feeling overwhelmed by disease. Patient does not use disorder as excuse for failures in life or in relationships. Patient participates actively in treatment regimen.

PRURITUS

Pruritus is a localized or generalized itching sensation that elicits the desire to scratch.

Pruritus may occur as a primary disorder or may be a symptom of a systemic disorder. Pruritus may result from inflammations caused by various factors including irritation, infection, infestations, and allergic reactions. It may be the result of systemic disease, malignancy, and altered physiologic states.

Three areas of the body are most frequently affected by pruritus: the anus (pruritus ani), vulva (pruritus vulvae), and ear (otitis externa). These are body orifices that have an abundance of sensory nerve endings.

Pruritus ani occurs primarily in men. It is caused by many factors and is associated with various diseases. Perianal erythema and scratches or gross excoriation are evident. Lichenification or fissures occur in long-term cases. The entire gluteal fold may be involved. Aggravating factors include contact dermatitis, anatomic abnormalities, infection, and systemic disorders. Common irritating factors include feces, irritation from toilet tissue, tight clothing, sweating, and long periods of sitting. The itching is often associated with tension, irritability, and depression.

Pruritus vulvae is caused by many factors and is associated with various diseases. Pruritus vulvae begins with intermittent episodes that can develop into unremitting pruritus. Erythema develops in the labia majora, with lichenification in long-standing disease. The perianal region may also be affected. Tight clothing, heat, perspiration, motion, sitting, and lying aggravate the condition.

Otitis externa occurs in the external ear usually as a result of trauma, moisture, and bacterial colonization. The distal third of the external canal and the meatal skin develop a scaling erythema that becomes moist and oozing as the condition worsens. Itching is the main complaint. Otitis externa is aggravated by heat, humidity, moisture, and overzealous cleansing.

Generalized pruritus can signify a systemic disorder. Diabetes mellitus, drug reactions, biliary obstruction, renal disease, malignancy, and pregnancy are common causes of generalized pruritus.

PATHOPHYSIOLOGY

The exact mechanism of pruritus is undetermined. The itch sensation seems to arise from nerve endings that are just below the epidermis and in the dermis. Itching may be a result of repetitive, low-frequency stimulation of C fibers that are similar to but distinct from those that transmit pain.[38]

Persistent scratching may produce erythema, urticarial papules, excoriation, and fissures (Plate 1, *19*). Prolonged scratching and rubbing may produce lichenification and pigmentation. Many factors, including personality, determine whether itching will be ignored, rubbed, or scratched and excoriated.

DIAGNOSTIC STUDIES

Physical examination and history
To determine underlying cause or systemic disorder

Laboratory studies with generalized pruritus
To determine possible systemic cause: complete blood count, blood urea nitrogen, serum bilirubin, serum iron, blood glucose, sulfobromophthalein retention, stool for occult blood, and parasites

Biopsy
To determine histopathologic changes

TREATMENT PLAN

Treatment is aimed at the specific underlying cause (see specific diseases for treatment modalities) and at eliminating aggravating factors (see ''Patient Education'').

Chemotherapeutic
Topical preparation: combination of menthol 0.5%, phenol 0.5%, and betamethasone 0.1% applied sparingly tid

Anti-infective agents
Topical antibiotics if pruritus has bacterial etiology; gentamicin (Garamycin) or polymycin, applied tid
Antianxiety agents (used for antipruritic effect)
Hydroxyzine (Atarax, Orgatrax, Vistaril), 25 mg po at bedtime or q6h for localized itching
Antihistamines (used for antipruritic effect)
Trimeprazine (Temaril), 5 mg po at bedtime or q6h for localized itching
Psychotherapeutic agents (used for antipruritic effect)
Chlorpromazine (Thorazine), 10-25 mg po q6-8h for severe generalized itching

Supportive
Sitz baths
Burow's compresses
Emollients for dry skin

ASSESSMENT: AREAS OF CONCERN

Pruritus
Severity; localization; diurnal or seasonal patterns; distribution

Lesion
Erythema; scaling; excoriation; fissures

Environment
Aggravating factors; stress, tension; depression; irritability

NURSING DIAGNOSES and NURSING INTERVENTIONS

Nursing Diagnosis	Nursing Intervention
Skin integrity, impairment of: actual	Instruct patient in good hygiene to prevent secondary infection. Instruct patient to cut fingernails short to avoid tissue damage from scratching.
Comfort, alteration in	Assist patient in identifying and eliminating potentially aggravating factors (see ''Patient Education''). Assist patient in identifying stress factors and alternative approaches to stress. Apply cool compresses and Burow's compresses. Offer sitz baths. Apply emollients. Instruct patient in use of medications.

Patient Education

1. Instruct the patient to avoid aggravating factors:
   a. Heat and humidity
   b. Rubbing and friction from clothing
   c. Tight clothing
   d. Wool and rough fabrics
   e. Fabrics that do not allow ventilation
   f. Excessive perspiration
   g. External irritants (such as soap)
   h. Dry skin
   i. Temperature changes
2. Instruct the patient in the use and side effects of medications.
3. Instruct the patient in the use of compresses (see p. 637).
4. Instruct the patient in the signs and symptoms of secondary infection.

EVALUATION

Patient Outcome	Data Indicating That Outcome is Reached
Aggravating factors are avoided.	Pruritus decreases. Exacerbations do not occur.
Underlying disease is identified and treated.	Erythema, scaling, excoriation, and fissures resolve. Pruritus is alleviated.
Secondary infection is resolved or avoided.	There is no tenderness, swelling, or purulent exudate in resolving lesions.
Discomfort is alleviated.	Scratching and excoriations decrease. Patient is able to sleep.

TINEA (DERMATOPHYTOSIS)

Tinea is a group of superficial fungal infections.

Dermatophytes (ringworm fungi) cause various superficial fungal infections through invasion of the stratum corneum, nails, or hair. The disorders are usually classified according to the anatomic location, since treatment of most superficial fungal disorders is the same and the clinical appearance of the eruption is not always related to the species of fungus. The disorder varies from mild inflammation to acute vesicular infection. Remissions and exacerbations may occur. Itching is usually present.

The condition is transmissible from other persons or from animals.

PATHOPHYSIOLOGY

The local response to fungal invasion is inflammation, scaling, erythema, and pruritus. A cell-mediated immunologic response may develop with the production of further erythema, spongiosis, vesicles, and oozing (Plate 1, *20* and *21*). Table 5-6 summarizes the features of tinea.

Table 5-6
Summary of Tinea

Type	Distribution	Occurrence	Clinical Features
Tinea corporis	Nonhairy parts of body; face; neck; extremities	More common in hot and humid climates; more common in rural than in urban settings; occurs in both adults and children	Pruritus; papulosquamous annular lesions with raised borders; lesions expand peripherally with central clearing
Tinea cruris	Groin; inner thigh; scrotum or labia not involved	More common in adult men; tends to recur; flare-ups common in summer; aggravated by tight clothes, perspiration and physical activity	Pruritus; hypopigmented; well-demarcated lesions; dryness and scaling; pustules present at margins; central clearing sometimes present; secondary bacterial or candidal infection and maceration common
Tinea capitis	Scalp	More common in children; contagious	Lesions vary: small, gray scaly patches with short broken hairs; mild erythematous papules; raised, boggy, inflamed nodules dotted with perifollicular abscesses; thick, yellow, suppurative lesions; lesions may be small, coalesced, or cover entire scalp; hairless patches
Tinea pedis	Feet; begins in third and fourth interdigital spaces and spreads to involve plantar surface; may involve nails	Rare in children; not transmitted by simple exposure	Lesions vary: maceration, scaling, fissuring of interdigital space; vesicular scaling, erythema of plantar surface; chronic, noninflamed, diffuse scaling; nails brittle, discolored; pruritus
Tinea unguium	Toenails and (less commonly) fingernails	—	Nails thickened, lusterless, and discolored; subungual debris; nail plate crumbling or absent

DIAGNOSTIC STUDIES

Physical examination
Characteristic lesion and distribution

KOH (potassium hydroxide) scraping
Presence of branching mycelia or spores

Fungal culture
Infecting organism

Wood's light
Affected hairs fluoresce

TREATMENT PLAN

Chemotherapeutic
Anti-infective agents
Griseofulvin (Fulvicin, Grifulvin, Grisactin, Gris Owen, Gris-Peg) for tinea capitis and severe cases of other tineas, 1 g po in divided doses with meals for adults; 0.5 g/day po in divided doses with meals for children 30-50 lb, 0.75 g/day po in divided doses with meals for children over 50 lb;
may require more than 4 mo therapy; continue therapy for 2 wk after last sign of clinical activity
Topical antifungals rubbed in bid for 3 wk
Tolnaftate 1% (Aftate, Tinactin)
Miconazole 2% (Monistat-Derm)
Clotrimazole 1% (Lotrimin, Mycelex)
Ketoconazole, under investigation in United States[55]
Keratolytic agents (for noninflammatory scaling)
Salicylic acid 3% and benzane acid 6% in ointment or alcohol

ASSESSMENT: AREAS OF CONCERN

Lesion
For description and distribution see Table 5-6

Secondary infection (bacterial or candidal)
Itching; exudate; inflammation; odor; tenderness; maceration

Environment
Aggravating factors; hygiene; contacts

NURSING DIAGNOSES and NURSING INTERVENTIONS

Nursing Diagnosis	Nursing Intervention
Skin integrity, impairment of: actual	Decrease moisture in affected areas. Stress importance of good hygiene and handwashing to prevent secondary infection. Have patient's fingernails cut short to avoid tissue trauma from scratching. Shave head in affected area for tinea capitis. For tinea capitis remove scales with shampoo and gently scrub before medication is applied. Instruct in use of medications and preparations.
Skin integrity, impairment of: potential for	Inform patient that contacts should be screened and referred for treatment if symptoms appear. Instruct patient that pets should be checked and treated for fungal infection. Instruct patient and family members to protect themselves and others by not sharing towels or personal articles and by wearing protective footwear in public showers.
Comfort, alteration in	Instruct patient to avoid tight clothing. Instruct patient to wear cotton next to skin. Instruct patient to stay in areas of decreased humidity. Instruct patient in use of medications and preparations as prescribed.

Patient Education

1. Teach the patient and family about the transmission, recurrence, and reinfection of the disease.
2. Instruct the patient to avoid aggravating factors: tight clothing, moist skin, and excessive humidity.
3. Stress the importance of following the therapeutic regimen to avoid recurrence and reinfection.
4. Instruct the patient and family in the side effects of medications.
5. Instruct the patient and family in the signs and symptoms of secondary infection and to seek medical attention if they occur.

EVALUATION

Patient Outcome	Data Indicating That Outcome is Reached
Eruption clears up.	Papules, scaling, pustules, erythema, vesicles, and pruritus resolve. Nails resume smooth texture.
Secondary infection is avoided or resolved.	There is no tenderness, swelling, or purulent exudate.
Spread of infection is contained.	Contacts are notified and treated if symptoms appear. Personal articles and items are not shared.
Aggravating environmental factors are avoided.	Eruption clears. Exacerbations do not recur. Pruritus is alleviated.

VASCULAR DISORDERS OF CUTANEOUS BLOOD VESSELS
Hemangiomas

Hemangiomas are congenital vascular lesions of the skin and subcutaneous tissue.

PATHOPHYSIOLOGY

There are three common types of hemangiomas: (1) nevus flammeus, (2) capillary hemangiomas, and (3) cavernous hemangioma.

Nevus flammeus (port-wine stain) is a flat purple-red lesion that is present at birth and is due to a mass of mature, dilated, congested capillaries in the dermis. The color depends on whether the superficial, middle, or deep dermal vessels are involved. The lesion does not disappear or fade over time, does not enlarge, and may develop a thickened nodular surface.

The occipital area of the scalp is the most common site of occurrence. The lesion may occur elsewhere and is frequently seen on the face. The lesions are usually unilateral and tend to follow the course of a cutaneous nerve. There is no satisfactory treatment for hemangiomas.

Capillary hemangioma (strawberry mark) is a very common raised, bright red lesion that usually appears in the third to fifth week of life. It consists of a proliferation of endothelial cells arranged in strawberry-like lobules. It may occur anywhere on the body. It may enlarge for the first several months but rarely enlarges after the first year. It involutes spontaneously and is usually completely regressed by 3 to 5 years of age. Involution begins with an area of fibrosis in the center. The lesion may leave a brownish pigmentation or scarring and wrinkling of the skin as it involutes. No treatment is required unless the lesion is massively disfiguring or is near the eye or a body orifice where it might interfere with body functioning.

Cavernous hemangioma is a large vascular pool lined with mature epithelial cells that are located in the subcutaneous tissue of the dermis. It is deeper than the other types of hemangiomas and may contain numerous arteriovenous shunts and vascular formations.

The lesion, which is present at birth, is reddish blue and round and may be elevated and compressible. It can occur on any part of the body. Most lesions eventually involute at least partially.

DIAGNOSTIC STUDIES

Physical examination
Characteristic lesion and congruent history

TREATMENT PLAN

No treatment for nevus flammeus currently exists. Laser techniques are under development.[3,4,15,17] For capillary or cavernous hemangiomas treatment is as follows.

Surgical
Used for capillary or cavernous hemangiomas only if lesion does not involute; may leave more scarring than spontaneous resolution

Excision with grafting

Cryosurgery (see p. 639)

Chemotherapeutic
Corticosteroids
Prednisone, 10 mg po bid or tid with decremental doses until lesion resolves
Intralesional injection of triamcinolone (Kenalog, Aristocort); may cause scar formation

Supportive
Electrocoagulation for small lesions; may leave scars

ASSESSMENT: AREAS OF CONCERN

Lesion history
Present or absent at birth; rate of growth or involution

Lesion
Size; color; texture; elevation; location; secondary trauma or bleeding

NURSING DIAGNOSES and NURSING INTERVENTIONS

Nursing Diagnosis	Nursing Intervention
Skin integrity, impairment of: potential	Instruct patient in ways to protect lesions from scratching (cut nails short) and trauma to avoid tissue damage and secondary bleeding. Stress importance of good hygiene to avoid secondary infection. Advise that it is better to wait for involution of capillary and cavernous hemangiomas than to cause complications and scarring through early treatment.
Self-concept, disturbance in: body image	Advise patients of excellent prognosis for involution of capillary and cavernous hemangiomas but warn them that lesion may grow before it involutes. Use accurate measurements or photographs to show progress of involution. Assess patient's self-perception or parents' perception of child's appearance. Encourage verbalization of feelings about body, body image, and fear of reaction or rejection by others. As child matures, encourage development of other interests and attributes to support feelings of self-worth and self-esteem. Assist patient or parent in evaluating appearance in realistic manner so lesion does not become focal point of existence.

Patient Education
1. Inform the patient and family of the likelihood of involution.
2. Advise the patient and family of the hazards of unnecessary treatment.

EVALUATION

Patient Outcome	Data Indicating That Outcome is Reached
Secondary trauma and infection are minimized.	Lesion remains intact and free of bleeding, crusting, excoriation, and purulent exudate.
Unnecessary scarring is avoided.	Family waits for spontaneous involution in capillary and cavernous hemangiomas before seeking treatment.
Patient and parents evaluate appearance in realistic manner.	Patient develops interests and attributes and engages in activities so hemangioma is not focal point of existence. Lesion is not used as excuse for unsuccessful interpersonal relationships.

Telangiectasia and Hereditary Hemorrhagic Telangiectasia

Telangiectasia is a network of dilated superficial dermal capillaries and venules.

PATHOPHYSIOLOGY

Essential telangiectasia is a disorder that is characterized by a network of small dilated veins on the thighs and calves of adult women (Plate 1, *22*). The condition is localized and often symmetric. The vessels involved are the superficial venous plexuses. The condition has cosmetic significance only.

Telangiectasia is also a component of certain systemic diseases such as lupus erythematosus and scleroderma and certain hereditary disorders. Hereditary hemorrhagic telangiectasia (Rendu-Osler-Weber disease) is a rare, autosomal dominant, inherited disorder. Telangiectatic lesions of the skin, mucous membranes, and internal organs are present in this disease (Plate 1, *23*). Lesions occur most commonly after puberty and increase throughout adult life. The small, red to violet lesions consist of thin, dilated vessels that blanch with pressure and tend to bleed spontaneously or with minor trauma. Bleeding may also occur from lesions in the mouth, pharynx, and gastrointestinal and genitourinary tracts. Anemia may result from continued oozing. Bleeding tends to become more severe with age. Systemic problems may arise from associated pulmonary arteriovenous fistulas and cerebrovascular malformations.

DIAGNOSTIC STUDIES

Physical examination
   Characteristic lesions

Complete blood count
   Iron deficiency anemia

TREATMENT PLAN

For treatment of anemia see Chapter 13. For treatment of underlying systemic disorders see the specific diseases.

Chemotherapeutic (for Rendu-Osler-Weber disease)
   Estrogens
      Cyclic therapy to decrease bleeding tendency
   Corticosteroids
      Nasal spray to control bleeding
   Hematinic agents
      Iron po for iron loss through repeated bleeding

Electromechanical (for localized lesions)
   Electrolysis—free hydrogen via electric current to obliterate vessels

Supportive
   Blood transfusions for acute hemorrhage

ASSESSMENT: AREAS OF CONCERN

Lesion
   Number, location and bleeding tendency; symptoms of anemia (see Chapter 13)

NURSING DIAGNOSES and NURSING INTERVENTIONS

For nursing care of patients with anemia see Chapter 13.

Nursing Diagnosis	Nursing Intervention
Skin integrity, impairment of: actual	Instruct patient to avoid trauma to lesions; wear protective clothing and cut fingernails short.
Oral mucous membrane, alteration in	Instruct patient to eat soft foods. Instruct patient to use soft toothbrush.
Self-concept, disturbance in: body image	Encourage patient to verbalize feelings about body, body image, or fear of reaction or rejection by others. Advise patient of availability of covering makeup (Covermark).

Patient Education

1. Instruct the patient in protective measures to avoid trauma that may cause bleeding (see Nursing Interventions).
2. Instruct the patient in the use and side effects of medications.
3. Instruct the patient to seek medical attention if unable to stop a bleeding episode.

EVALUATION

Patient Outcome	Data Indicating That Outcome is Reached
Trauma is minimized.	Bleeding episodes are less frequent.
Patient assesses self-concept in realistic manner.	Patient engages in activities compatible with limitations of disorder. Patient engages in interpersonal relationships. Patient employs protective measures and seeks medical attention as needed.

Vasculitis

Vasculitis is a range of cutaneous lesions associated with inflammation of the wall of blood vessels of the skin and subcutaneous tissue.

Vasculitis is a comprehensive term for a large number of disorders that manifest skin lesions as a result of inflammation of the walls of cutaneous blood vessels. The diseases range in severity from mild to fatal. The cutaneous lesions appear as erythematous papules and plaques, nodules, urticaria, purpuric or hemorrhagic papules and vesicles, and pustular and necrotic lesions.

Lesions, which tend to develop in crops, occur most commonly on the legs, thighs, and buttocks. Some lesions begin as erythematous papules or plaques and progress to ulcerations that heal slowly. In severe ulcerative forms, lesions are progressive and involve other body organs. There is currently no universal or satisfactory classification system for the vasculitis disorders.

PATHOPHYSIOLOGY

Vasculitis involves intravascular and extravascular changes. The sequence of events occurs as a result of damage to the vessel that is precipitated by numerous factors and modified by the body's response to noxious stimuli.

The inflammatory process of the vessel includes increased permeability; epithelial shedding; increased deposition of fibrin, platelets, and leukocytes; changes in endothelial cells during repair; and thrombosis. The cutaneous changes that occur as a result of the inflammation processes depend on the degree of inflammation and the size of the involved vessel.

The pathogenesis of vasculitis can be summarized as follows:

Intravascular component
  Deposition of circulating antigen-antibody complexes with chemotaxis of leukocytes and release of mediators of inflammation
  Direct toxic effect of circulating chemicals, drugs, and bacterial antigens
  Bacterial emboli and reaction to products of bacterial breakdown
Vascular wall component
  Endothelial proliferation in reparative attempt
  Infiltration by lymphocytes and polymorphonuclear leukocytes
  Fibrinoid necrosis and scarring from fibrin deposits
  Granulomatous infiltrates
Extravascular component
  Leakage of red blood cells and fibrin into surrounding tissue
  Deposition of inflammatory infiltrates
  Thrombosis of small vessels with secondary tissue; ischemia
  Increased fibrosis
  Venous stasis

DIAGNOSTIC STUDIES

Physical examination
  Lesions and history as described in "Assessment: Areas of Concern"

Biopsy of blood vessel

Immunofluorescence shows cellular changes as described above; will determine type and severity of vasculitis

Further studies to determine systemic involvement and underlying conditions

Complete blood count

Antinuclear factor, serum protein, and rheumatoid factor

Serum fibrinolytic activity

VDRL test or rapid plasma reagin test

Culture and antistreptolysin titer

Urinalysis for red blood cells and casts

Serum complement and cryoglobulin

Roentgenograms of chest, sinuses, and teeth

Roentgenograms of gastrointestinal tract if symptoms indicate

TREATMENT PLAN

Specific treatment is aimed at the particular clinical condition or underlying disease process.

Chemotherapeutic

Antihypertensive agents

If needed to minimize small vessel damage

Anti-infective agents

Agent-specific to clear infection

Corticosteroids

Systemic glucocorticoids for deep tender nodular lesions

Nonsteroidal anti-inflammatory agents

Aspirin, potassium iodide, indomethacin (Indocin), ibuprofen (Motrin), phenylbutazone (Butazolidin, Azolid)

ASSESSMENT: AREAS OF CONCERN

Lesion

Erythematous papules, plaques, or nodules; persistent urticaria; purpuric papules and vesicles; pustules; necrotic lesions

Surrounding tissue

Abnormal vascular patterns; abnormal reactions to cold

History

Precipitating factors; infection; food and drug allergies or sensitivity

General medical problems

Diabetes mellitus; arthritis; cardiovascular diseases; respiratory diseases; connective tissue diseases

NURSING DIAGNOSES and NURSING INTERVENTIONS

Nursing Diagnosis	Nursing Intervention
Skin integrity, impairment of: actual	Instruct patient in good hygiene and handwashing to prevent secondary infection. Apply dressings on open or draining lesions.
Skin integrity, impairment of: potential	Encourage rest and elevation of affected part. Initiate range of motion exercises to maintain blood flow. Protect affected area from cold.
Comfort, alteration in: pain	Encourage patient to rest affected area. Apply cool compresses to hot, nodular lesions.

Other nursing interventions depend on the symptoms produced by the particular clinical condition and disorder.

Patient Education

1. Teach the patient how to change dressings, if indicated, using aseptic technique.
2. Teach the patient how to use cool compresses as needed.
3. Instruct the patient in the use of medications and their side effects.
4. Instruct the patient in the signs and symptoms of secondary infection and to seek medical attention if they occur.

EVALUATION

Patient Outcome	Data Indicating That Outcome is Reached
Clinical disorder is identified and treated.	Inflammatory response is not exacerbated or does not recur.
Cutaneous lesions improve.	Erythema and lesions resolve. Necrotic areas reepithelize. Discomfort is alleviated. Integument is intact.
Secondary infection is resolved or avoided.	There is no swelling, purulent exudate, fever, or lymphadenopathy.

BURNS (THERMAL, CHEMICAL, AND ELECTRICAL)

Thermal burns are injuries caused by exposure to flames, hot liquids, and radiation. Chemical burns are caused by contact, ingestion, inhalation, or injection of acids, alkalies, or vesicants. True electrical burns occur when current passes through the body to the ground. Electrical current can also cause secondary flash or flame burns.

More than 2 million persons in the United States are burned each year. Although most of these burn injuries are minor, approximately 3% to 5% are life threatening. Burn injury is the second leading cause of death among young children and is the fourth overall cause of accidental death for persons of all ages.[65]

PATHOPHYSIOLOGY

Burns occur when excessive thermal or chemical energy is transferred to the body. Thermal and chemical injury disrupts the normal protective barrier function of the skin, causing a wide range of sequelae. In electrical injury heat is generated as the electricity passes through tissues. The thermal energy released is the cause of clinical injury.

The extent and depth of the burn injury determine the extent and severity of burn sequelae. Injury to the stratum corneum results in evaporative heat and water loss as a result of the loss or disruption of the lipid-water barrier of that layer. Injury to the stratum germinativum results in delayed or absent reepithelization and healing. Injury to the deeper structures results in scarring and tissue damage that may require skin grafting.

Vascular changes are caused by direct cellular damage or inflammatory processes. During the first few hours after the burn, vasoactive substances are released from the injured cells and vasoconstriction occurs. Vasodilation then occurs as a result of kinin release. During this period histamine causes increased capillary permeability, which allows plasma to leak into the burn area.

There are three zones of associated tissue damage[14]:

1. *Zone of coagulation.* This is the area of greatest destruction where coagulation and irreversible cellular death occur. The area remains white because all viable tissue has been destroyed. Leukocytosis is inhibited or totally blocked. The zone can extend deeply into the tissue structures, causing full-thickness skin destruction.

2. *Zone of stasis.* This area surrounds the zone of coagulation and involves the vasculative dermis. Shortly after the burn, leukocytes and platelets aggregate in underlying capillaries, causing thrombosis. This, combined with the vasoconstriction, causes decreased circulation and transient ischemia to the area. With appropriate protection and treatment, circulation to the area can be restored, thereby salvaging the tissue. However, the tissue in this area is very fragile, and any further trauma because of rough handling or infection can convert this zone to one resembling the zone of coagulation.

3. *Zone of hyperemia.* This area, which is the least affected, forms the border of the burn wound. Vascular integrity is maintained with no cellular death. The area is bright red and blanches with pressure. The inflammatory processes are present.

In electrical injury, vessel wall changes occur that are characterized by cellular disintegration of the media of the arteries and arterioles and by severe arterial spasm.

Vascular changes and tissue loss cause fluid shifts. The first of these shifts, the hypovolemic stage, occurs during the first 24 to 48 hours and is characterized by a rapid shift of fluid and protein from the vascular compartment into the interstitial spaces, causing blisters, edema, and fluid escape. Deep in the wound sodium is translocated into skeletal muscle and other tissues and pulls water with it, which results in hyponatremia and hyperkalemia. This fluid shift, along with evaporative fluid loss from the surface of the wound, causes an abrupt decrease in the circulating blood volume resulting in hypovolemic shock. In turn hypovolemic shock causes decreased cardiac stroke volume, decreased blood pressure, increased peripheral resistance, decreased tissue perfusion, and circulatory collapse. Anuria, renal failure, and death result if treatment is delayed or inadequate.

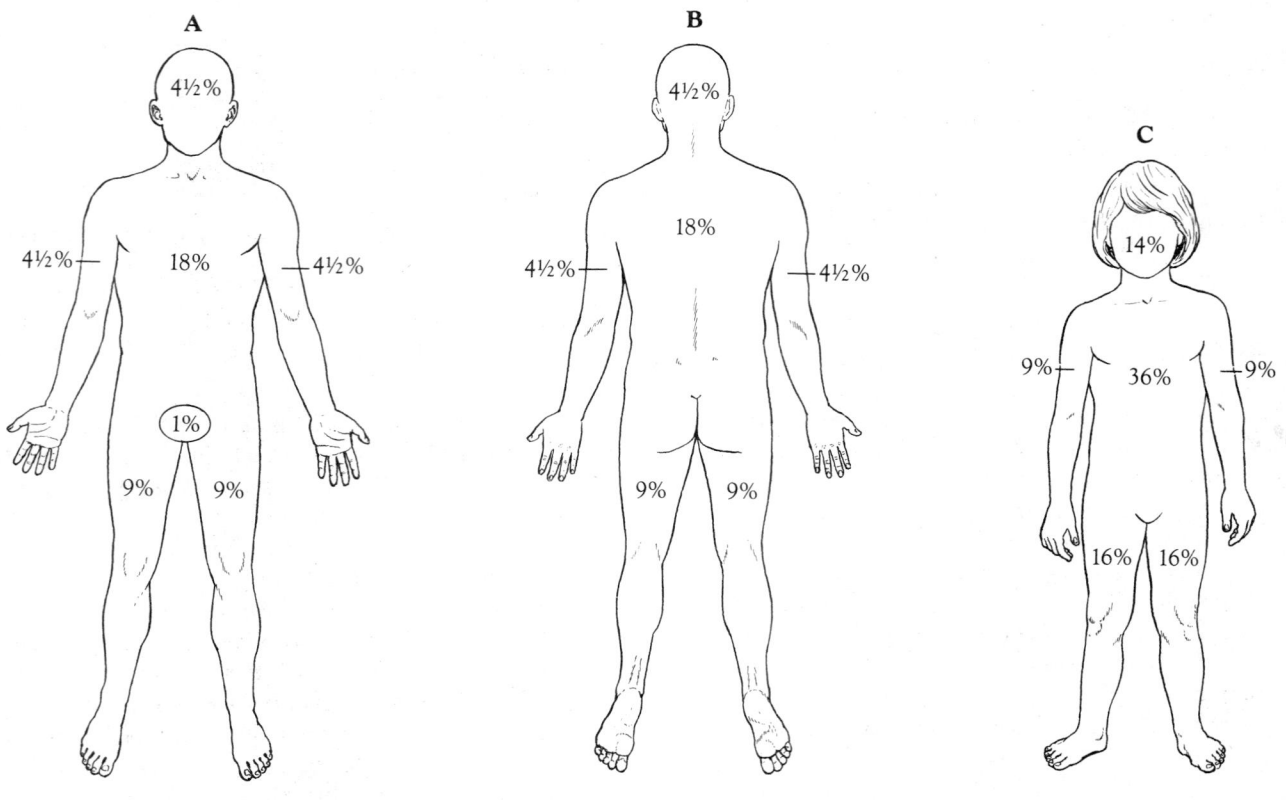

Uninjured cells may become dehydrated as a result of this fluid shift. Hypoproteinemia develops from continued loss of protein as a result of increased capillary permeability. Nitrogen is lost through renal catabolism, and a negative nitrogen balance develops. Metabolic acidosis can occur as a result of decreased tissue perfusion, anaerobic metabolism, and retained acid end products.

Within 18 hours of the burn injury, the sodium and water shunting reverse, and within 48 to 72 hours of the burn, a second fluid shift occurs in the opposite direction that causes fluid to return to the vascular compartment. In this phase the rapidly increasing blood volume causes diuresis and hemodilution that may result in dehydration, hyponatremia, and hypokalemia. Metabolic acidosis may occur because of bicarbonate loss in the urine and the catabolic state. Protein continues to be lost through the burn wound. Hypovitaminosis and weight loss also occur.

The evaporative fluid loss that occurs after the burn may be five to 19 times the normal loss. Associated with this fluid loss are tremendous heat loss and hypermetabolism that cause enormous caloric expenditure and hypothermia.

Erythrocyte hemolysis and a decrease in red cell mass occur as a result of direct damage and a decreased half-life of damaged red cells. Platelet function and half-life are also diminished. Hemoconcentration occurs as a result of fluid loss from the vascular system, which causes hematocrit values to rise.

Patients who have been injured in a fire may also have carbon monoxide poisoning from inhaling the gas that results from incomplete combustion of some materials. Poisoning occurs because carbon monoxide has 200 times the affinity of oxygen to combine with hemoglobin.

DIAGNOSTIC STUDIES

Physical examination

Determination of extent of injury using rule of nines (Fig. 5-5); Lund and Browder charts (Fig. 5-6); determination of degree of injury (Tables 5-7 and 5-8)

Determination of mechanism of injury

Thermal, chemical, or electrical

Fig. 5-5
Estimation of burn injury: rule of
nines. **A,** Adults (anterior view). **B,**
Adults (posterior view). **C,** Children.
D, Infants.

D

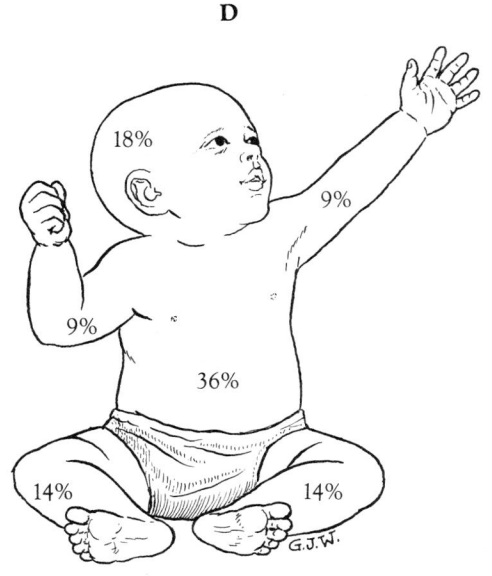

Baseline laboratory studies
Complete blood count
Serum electrolytes
Blood urea nitrogen
Creatinine
Arterial carboxyhemoglobin
Arterial blood gases
Bilirubin
Phosphorus
Alkaline phosphatase
Urine for myoglobin and hemoglobin levels

Fiberoptic bronchoscopy
Inspection of major and proximal airways to determine
upper airway injury

Xenon lung scan
Determination of small airway and parenchymal burns;
bolus of xenon is injected; as xenon gas is expired
from lungs, injured areas trap gas and show high-
density levels

Fig. 5-6
Estimation of burn injury: Lund and
Browder chart. Areas designated by
letters (*A, B,* and *C*) represent
percentages of body surface area that
vary according to age. The
accompanying table indicates the
relative percentages of these areas at
various stages in life.

From Artz, C.P., and Yarbrough, D.R. III:
Burns: including cold, chemical, and
electrical injuries. In Sabiston, D.C., Jr.,
editor: Textbook of surgery: the biological
basis of modern surgical practice, ed. 11,
Philadelphia, 1977, W.B. Saunders Co.

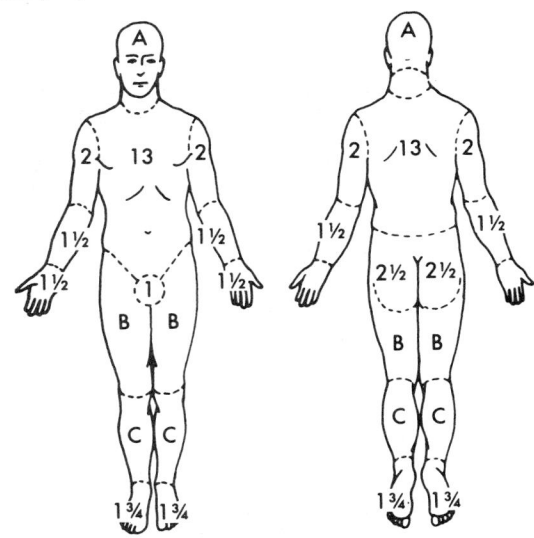

Relative percentages of areas affected by growth
(age in years)

	0	1	5	10	15	Adult
A: half of head	9½	8½	6½	5½	4½	3½
B: half of thigh	2¾	3¼	4	4¼	4½	4¾
C: half of leg	2½	2½	2¾	3	3¼	3½

Second degree _____ and
Third degree _____ =
Total percent burned _____

Table 5-7

Assessment of Burn Injury

Degree	Depth	Characteristics
Superficial (first degree)	Epidermis only; devitalization of epidermis and dilation of intradermal vessels	Pain; erythema; blanching with pressure; normal texture
Partial-thickness (second degree)	Destruction of epidermis and part of dermis	Erythema; blisters; pain; blanching with pressure; firm texture
Full-thickness (third and fourth degree)	Destruction of all layers of skin extending into subcutaneous tissue, muscle, nerves, and bone	Dryness; pale, white, brown, or red color; charring; no capillary refill; no pain; firm and leathery texture

Table 5-8

American Burn Association Classification of Burn Injury

Class	Description
Major	Full-thickness burns over 10% or more of body surface area (BSA)
	Partial-thickness burns over 25% of BSA for adults and 20% of BSA for children
	All burns on face, hands, eyes, ears, feet, or perineum
	All inhalation and electrical burns
	All burns complicated by trauma
	All burns in poor-risk patients
Moderate	Full-thickness burns over 2%-10% of BSA
	Partial-thickness burns over 15%-25% of BSA for adults and 10%-20% of BSA for children
Minor	Full-thickness burns over less than 2% of BSA
	Partial-thickness burns over less than 15% of BSA for adults and less than 10% of BSA for children

TREATMENT PLAN

Short-term Care of Major Burns

Surgical

Escharotomy—may be needed for circumferentially burned extremities or chest

Fasciotomy—may be needed for electrical injuries

Chemotherapeutic

Narcotic analgesics

　Meperidine (Demerol) for pain, 20-25 mg IV for adults; 0.5 mg/kg for children

Immunologic agents

　Tetanus immunization

　　0.5 ml IM for immunized patients

　　0.5 ml IM plus 250 units tetanus immune globulin (Hyper-tet) for nonimmunized patients

Anti-infective agents

　Aqueous penicillin G for prophylaxis against gram-positive organisms, 1.2-2 million units IV in divided doses for adults and 0.6-1.2 million units IV in divided doses for children

Supportive

Airway maintenance; intubation if needed

Humidification with 100% oxygen for inhalation injuries

Emergency treatment of musculoskeletal injuries or hemorrhage

Fluid replacement

　Parkland (Baxter formula)—2-4 ml lactated Ringer's solution/kg/% of BSA burned/24 hr; give one half of total amount in first 8 hours and one half during next 16 hours

　Brooke formula (after first 24 hours)—colloids (plasma, plasmanate, or dextran) 0.5 ml/kg/% of BSA burned plus 2000 ml of dextrose in water for adults (less for children)

　Electrical and inhalation injuries require more fluids

Uretheral catheterization

Nasogastric tube insertion

Wound cleansing with povidone-iodine (Betadine), saline, or hydrogen peroxide

Central venous line insertion

Swan-Ganz catheter to monitor pulmonary arterial and capillary wedge pressures

Long-term Care of Major Burns

Surgical

Skin grafts (see p. 640)

　Split-thickness—autograft from unburned area; postage stamp or strip application

　Mesh graft—split-thickness graft meshed with special instrument to cover large areas; held in place by dressing or sutures

　Homograft—skin from deceased person; used as

Table 5-9
Comparison of Topical Burn Agents

Agent	Advantages	Disadvantages
Mafenide acetate (Sulfamylon)	Penetrates rapidly; not inactivated by pus or body fluids; softens wound, allowing better mobility; more effective in established infection	Painful; sulfa sensitivities; acidosis with renal or pulmonary impairment; antibacterial activity lasts 4-6 hours
Silver sulfadiazine (Silvadene)	Penetrates slowly; not inactivated by pus or body fluids; minimum systemic absorption; painless; antibacterial activity lasts up to 48 hours	Sulfa sensitivities; not as effective in established infection
Silver nitrate	Wet dressings retain heat, moisture, and reduce evaporation; no sensitivities	Painful; staining

temporary cover for about 10 days; may survive 4 to 5 weeks

Heterograft—pigskin or synthetic substitute; acts as biologic dressing

Autologous cultured human epithelium—epidermal cells from unburned area cultured into sheets in flask; cultured sheets then attached to petrolatum gauze squares and sutured in place in wound; petrolatum gauze removed 7 to 10 days later[33]

Amputation of limb severely injured from electrical injury

Chemotherapeutic

Anti-infective agents

Topical (Table 5-9)

Mafenide acetate 10% (Sulfamylon); sterile application of amounts sufficient to just cover wound; wound left open to air; reapplied bid after washing off previous application and debriding wound

Silver sulfadiazine 1% (Silvadene) cream applied tid or qid; left open or covered with mesh gauze dressing; washed off before application, but no wound debridement done

Silver nitrate solution 0.5%; saturated thick gauze pads replaced q12-24h

Narcotic analgesics

Codeine, meperidine (Demerol), methadone (Dolophine); dosage determined on individual basis

Supportive

Wound debridement (see p. 639)

Hydrotherapy (see p. 637) once or twice daily for 20 to 30 minutes for dressing removal and debridement

Dressings, wet or dry (see p. 637 for wet dressings)

Dry dressing—single layer of nonadherent fine mesh gauze held in place by coarse gauze wrap

Nutrition

2 to 4 mg protein/kg/day

3500 to 5000 calories daily for adults; 90 to 100 calories/kg/day for children 3 years or under; 70 calories/kg/day for children 4 to 12 years

Vitamin and iron replacement

Total parenteral nutrition (hyperalimentation) if needed

Physiotherapy

Care of Minor Burns

Chemotherapeutic

Immunologic agents

Tetanus immunization, 0.5 ml IM for immunized patients, 0.5 ml IM plus 250 units tetanus immune globulin (Hyper-tet) for nonimmunized patients

Anti-infective agents

Topical (applied with sterile tongue blade to completely cover wound with ⅛-inch thickness)

Mafenide acetate (Sulfamylon) 5%

Silver sulfadiazine (Silvadene) 1%

Povidone-iodine (Betadine)

Polymyxin B, Bacitracin, Neosporin

Narcotic analgesics

Codeine, 30-60 mg po or subcutaneously q4-6h

Morphine, 8-10 mg subcutaneously

Meperidine (Demerol), 50-100 mg po q4-6h

Analgesic-antipyretics

Aspirin, 650 mg po q4-6h

Supportive

Wound cleansed with one-half strength Betadine solution

Wound debridement (see p. 639)

Dressing—innermost layer of nonadherent, porous, fine mesh gauze (fine enough to prevent epithelization into gauze); second layer of bulky, fluffed coarse mesh gauze to absorb exudate; outer layer of semielastic coarse mesh to apply even pressure and hold dressing in place; change once or twice daily

ASSESSMENT: AREAS OF CONCERN

Wound
Degree and extent of injury; see Tables 5-7 and 5-8 and Figs. 5-25 through 5-29; mechanism of injury (thermal, chemical, or mechanical)

First fluid shift and hypovolemic shock
Vital signs: decreased blood pressure, increased pulse; urinary output (desirable: 50 ml/hour for adults; 1 ml/kg/hour for children); monitoring of central venous pressure; potassium levels increased

Second fluid shift
Hyperpnea; blood pH less than 7.35; CO_2 combining power less than 21 mEq/L; $PaCO_2$ less than 40 mm Hg

Airway
Pulmonary edema (see Chapter 2); singed nasal hair; soot in mouth or nose; darkened septum; rales, cough, or cyanosis; dyspnea or stridor

Carbon monoxide poisoning
Vomiting; chest pain; tachycardia; confusion; agitation; decreased coordination

Neurologic
Changes in level of consciousness

Cardiovascular
Vital signs; dysrhythmias; fluid shifts; cyanosis; capillary refill; pulses

Musculoskeletal
Fractures; decreased mobility; deformities; exposed bone or muscle

Hypermetabolism and heat loss
Body temperature; weight loss

Hemopoietic
Increased hematocrit; hemoglobinuria

Gastrointestinal
Mouth injuries; nausea and vomiting; blood in gastric contents; bowel sounds; paralytic ileus; stress ulcer

Renal
Renal failure resulting from hypovolemic shock; oliguria; anuria; desirable output 50 ml/hour for adults, 1 ml/kg/hour for children; myoglobinuria; hemoglobinuria; diuresis (second phase)

Pain
Presence or absence; location; intensity; severity

Psychosocial
Body image

Infection
Inflammation; exudate; odor

NURSING DIAGNOSES and NURSING INTERVENTIONS

Nursing Diagnosis	Nursing Intervention
Skin integrity, impairment of: actual	Handle wound gently to avoid converting zone of stasis to zone of coagulation. Implement isolation precautions. Use sterile technique in wound care: debridement, topical preparations, and dressing changes. Provide hydrotherapy. Provide wound care to graft donor site. Use sterile linen. Use bed cradles. Keep patient warm through control of environmental temperature.
Fluid volume deficit, actual	Observe patency of urinary catheter. Monitor input and output. Replace fluids to achieve output of 50 ml/hour for adults; 1 ml/kg/hour for children per physician order. Monitor vital signs. Monitor urine specific gravity. Monitor central venous pressure.
Tissue perfusion, alteration in	Maintain adequate fluid replacement. Maintain optimum mobility. Provide adequate nutrition.

Nursing Diagnosis	**Nursing Intervention**
Mobility, impaired physical	Provide active and passive range of motion exercises. Use circOlectric bed per physician order. Refer patient for physiotherapy. Apply splints to prevent contractures. Have patient participate in water exercises.
Nutrition, alteration in: changes related to body requirements	Monitor protein intake: 2 to 4 g/kg/day. Monitor caloric intake: adults, 3000 to 3500 calories daily; children under age 3 years, 90 to 100 calories/kg/day; children over age 3 years, 70 calories/kg/day. Monitor vitamin replacement. In collaboration with physician institute total parenteral nutrition. Provide high-protein powdered milk preparations. Encourage self-feeding. Offer favorite foods. Avoid performing painful procedures near mealtime. Offer snacks.
Bowel elimination, alteration in: constipation	Give nothing by mouth until bowel sounds return. Provide bulk foods. Provide fruit juices. Administer stool softeners.
Comfort, alteration in:	Administer analgesics as ordered. Position patient for comfort. Provide or refer patient for hydrotherapy. Instruct in relaxation techniques. Refer patient for biofeedback training.
Self-concept, disturbance in: body image	Encourage patient to verbalize feelings about body, body appearance, or fear of reaction or rejection by others. Spend time with patient. Prepare visitors for patient's appearance. Encourage positive self-esteem by continued interest in patient and attentiveness to patient's needs.
Grieving, anticipatory	Encourage patient to verbalize distress, anger, sorrow, guilt, and fear. Assist patient in movement through stages of grieving.
Powerlessness	Observe for signs of depression or apathy. Involve patient in decision making. Encourage patient to express dissatisfaction and frustration. Accept patient's feelings of anger.

Patient Education

1. Instruct the patient in the care of minor burns:
   a. Cleanse wound with one-half strength Betadine using sterile gauze; rub gently to remove existing topical agent.
   b. Apply topical agent thick enough to cover wound with ⅛ inch of agent to provide healing and prevent bandage from adhering.
   c. Apply nonadherent fine mesh gauze (fine enough not to be epithelized), then fluffed bulky coarse gauze to trap exudate; hold in place with semi-elastic net to exert even pressure.

2. Instruct the patient in the care of healed burns:
   a. Wash skin gently, rinse well, dry thoroughly, and apply cream.
   b. Avoid exposure to sunlight, harsh detergents, fabric softeners, and irritation by rubbing of clothing.
3. Instruct the patient to watch for signs of infection and to seek early treatment to avoid further complications.
4. Instruct the patient that increased calories and protein may be required until healing is complete.
5. Advise the patient of available support groups and community resources to assist in the resumption of usual activities and relationships.

EVALUATION

Patient Outcome	Data Indicating That Outcome is Reached
State of homeostasis exists.	Normal blood values include the following: pH of 7.35-7.45; $Paco_2$ of 40-43; CO_2 combining power of 21-28 mEq/L; sodium 136-145 mEq/L; potassium 3.5-5 mEq/L; chloride 100-106 mEq/L. Nitrogen is in balance. Fluids are in balance.
Burn area heals.	Reepithelization occurs. Integument is intact and free of infection.
Nutrition is adequate.	Patient eats diet high in protein, calories, minerals, and vitamins. Patient does not lose weight. Wounds heal.
Patient is free of contractures.	Patient has full extremity flexion and extension.
Patient resocializes and evaluates appearance in realistic manner.	Patient returns or plans to return to former activities if possible. Patient develops interests and activities compatible with degree of limitation. Patient engages in satisfactory interpersonal relationships.
Home care is satisfactory.	Healing remains uninterrupted. New tissue is free from irritation or infection. Scar tissue remains soft and pliable.
Complications are recognized and treatment is sought.	Patient seeks medical attention for infection, weight loss, contractures, or changes in scar tissue.

COLD INJURY (FROSTBITE)

Frostbite is a localized cold injury caused by exposure to freezing temperatures.

Several predisposing factors are associated with the occurrence of frostbite. Persons who are not acclimated to the cold and those from warmer climates have more vasospasm and less heat production in their extremities when exposed to cold temperatures; thus their risk of cold injury is increased. A racial predisposition of blacks to cold injury has been noted.[81] Fatigue, hunger, young or old age, circulatory disorders, fear, alcohol, and hypoxia increase the risk of cold injury. Factors that promote heat loss such as contact with metal, wet skin, and wind velocity contribute to the occurrence and severity of frostbite injuries.

PATHOPHYSIOLOGY

Cellular injury in frostbite is caused by direct freezing of cells at the time of injury or by inadequate tissue perfusion resulting from vascular spasm and occlusion of small vessels in the injured area.

With direct freezing of cells (crystallization), ice crystals form in extracellular fluids and osmotically draw intracellular fluid, thereby causing cell dehydration. Vascular changes include vasoconstriction, decreased cap-

illary perfusion, and increased viscosity of the blood with sludging and thrombus formation.

After thawing, vascular stasis occurs in the injured area as a result of obstruction in the vascular bed. Edema occurs in the injured area and is maximal 2 to 3 days after thawing. Thrombi, interstitial hemorrhaging, and leukocyte infiltration are present. Tissue necrosis occurs and becomes more prominent as the edema resolves. It may take 60 to 90 days before the necrotic tissue becomes fully evident.

The extent of the injury is determined by the magnitude and rate of heat loss from the skin. Frostbite is classified as superficial or deep. Superficial injury involves the skin and subcutaneous tissue. The injured area is white, waxy, soft, and anesthetic. Capillary refill is absent. On thawing the area becomes flushed, edematous, and painful and then may turn mottled or purplish. Large blisters may develop within 24 hours and resolve in about 10 days, leaving a hard dark eschar. After 3 to 4 weeks the eschar separates, leaving sensitive new epithelium. Throbbing and burning pain last for several weeks. The area is sensitive to heat and cold for months, and the frostbitten part may perspire excessively.

Deep frostbite causes injury to the skin, subcutaneous tissue, muscle, tendon, and neurovascular structures. The injured part is hard and solid and remains cold, mottled, and blue or gray after thawing. Blisters may be absent or form after several weeks at the juncture of viable and nonviable tissue. Edema occurs in the entire limb and may take months to resolve. When the blisters dry, blacken, and slough off, a line of demarcation remains where the viable tissue separates and retracts from the dead tissue.

DIAGNOSTIC STUDIES

Physical examination
Characteristic findings with congruent history

TREATMENT PLAN

Surgical
Escharotomy
Sympathectomy for severe vasospasm and pain
Debridement after retraction of viable tissue (13 weeks to 4 months after injury)
Amputation of nonviable extremity after retraction of viable tissue and medical intervention; may be several months after injury

Chemotherapeutic
Immunologic agents
Tetanus immunization, 0.5 ml IM for immunized patients, 0.5 ml IM plus 250 units tetanus immune globulin (Hyper-tet) for nonimmunized patients
Plasma expanders
Low–molecular weight dextran 40, 20 ml/kg IV q24h to decrease sludging; this therapy controversial[81]

Anti-infective agents
Tetracycline or ampicillin (Amcill, Omnipen, others) for prophylaxis, 250 mg po q6h
Narcotic analgesics
Morphine, up to 15 mg IM q3h
Analgesic-antipyretics
Aspirin, 650 po q3h

Supportive
Rapid rewarming by immersion for 20 minutes in water at 38° to 45° C (100° to 112° F)
Protective isolation of patient or extremity
Whirlpool baths three times a day at 32° to 37° C (90° to 98° F)

ASSESSMENT: AREAS OF CONCERN

Injured area
Color of skin; resilience of tissue; extent of limb involvement; duration of contact with cold; superficial injury: white, waxy, soft, no capillary refill; deep injury: hard, solid, mottled, blue or gray

Healing process
Pain; edema; color; blister formation; eschar formation; line of demarcation between viable and nonviable tissue

Infection
Pus; odor; redness; heat; fever

Complications
Vasospasm; pain; hyperesthesia; increased perspiration spiration

NURSING DIAGNOSES and NURSING INTERVENTIONS

Nursing Diagnosis	Nursing Intervention
Tissue perfusion, alteration in	In collaboration with physician, initiate rapid rewarming in water at 38° to 45° C (100° to 112° F) for 20 minutes. Completely immerse affected area in water, avoiding contact of skin with container. Instruct patient not to smoke to avoid vasoconstriction.
Skin integrity, impairment of: actual	Use sterile sheets. Isolate patient or extremity if necessary to prevent infection. Use bed cradle. Keep blisters intact. Keep extremity exposed to air circulation. Avoid debridement.
Mobility, impaired physical	Elevate extremities periodically. Initiate range of motion exercises.

Nursing Diagnosis	Nursing Intervention
Comfort, alteration in: pain	Keep sheets off extremity. Administer analgesics as ordered. Instruct patient in relaxation techniques. Refer patient for biofeedback training.
Self-concept, disturbance in: body image	Encourage patient to verbalize feelings about body, body appearance, or fear of reaction or rejection by others.
Grieving, anticipatory	Encourage patient to verbalize distress, anger, sorrow, guilt, and fear about potential loss of extremity part or function. Assist in movement through stages of grieving.
Powerlessness	Observe for signs of depression and apathy. Inform patient that healing process is long-term, slow, and uncertain; provide accurate information regarding healing. Encourage patient to express dissatisfaction and frustration. Involve patient in decision making. Accept patient's feelings of anger.

Patient Education

1. Instruct the patient to protect the extremity from temperature extremes and rapid changes in temperature, since the tissue is sensitive to temperature changes and refreezing will cause tissue loss.
2. Instruct the patient to avoid tight, constrictive clothing or pressure to an area that might decrease circulation.
3. Instruct the patient in the application of dry, sterile dressing to small, open areas.
4. Instruct the patient to avoid smoking to reduce vasoconstriction.
5. Instruct the patient in preventive measures to avoid future episodes or reinjury of the frostbitten part: protective, multilayered, warm, nonconstrictive clothing; avoidance of fatigue, hunger, and alcohol when exposed to the cold.

EVALUATION

Patient Outcome	Data Indicating That Outcome is Reached
Maximum tissue is preserved.	Initial rapid thawing with no refreezing of tissue occurs. Tissue is free of infection. Healing is allowed to occur without premature surgical intervention.
Joints are functional.	Patient has full extension and flexion of joints.
Patient evaluates self in realistic manner.	Patient resumes former activities if possible. Patient develops interests and activities compatible with degree of limitation. Patient engages in satisfactory interpersonal relationships.
Patient prevents further injury to area.	Patient avoids tight, constrictive clothing or pressure to area. Patient does not smoke.
Patient prevents further episodes of cold injury.	Patient wears protective clothing. Patient avoids hunger, fatigue, and alcohol when exposed to cold.

DISEASES OF THE NAILS
Fungal Infections

See "Tinea."

Paronychia

Paronychia is an acute or chronic inflammation of the proximal nail fold.

Erythema, induration, and swelling of the nail folds and consequent pain and tenderness are the primary features of paronychia. Staphylococci, streptococci, and sometimes *Candida* are the organisms usually responsible for the infection. One or more fingers or toes may be involved. Paronychia may be acute or chronic (Plate 1, *24*). Acute paronychia usually results from minor trauma or a hangnail. Chronic paronychia occurs in persons whose hands are exposed to chronic irritation and moisture.

PATHOPHYSIOLOGY

In acute paronychia organisms enter through a break in the epidermis. The infection may follow the nail margin or extend beneath the nail and suppurate. Purulent exudate may drain from beneath the nail fold. The eponychium remains attached to the nail plate. This separation creates a space in which foreign material and inflammatory exudate accumulate, an environment that is conducive to bacterial and yeast growth. Chronic paroncyhia usually leads to nail ridging, distortion, and discoloration.

DIAGNOSTIC STUDIES

Physical examination
Characteristic lesion

Culture
Growth of infecting organism

TREATMENT PLAN

Surgical
Incision and drainage of purulent pocket

Chemotherapeutic
Anti-infective agents
Systemic antibiotics; depending on infecting organism
Anticandidal solutions or lotions applied topically tid, clotrimazole (Lotrimin, Mycelex), miconazole (Monistat-Derm)
Thymol 4% in chloroform solution, 1 drop tid to affected area

ASSESSMENT: AREAS OF CONCERN

Inflammatory and infectious processes
Erythema; swelling; heat; tenderness; pain; purulent exudate; nails ridged, distorted, and discolored

Environmental factors
Constant moisture and trauma to hands or feet; history of previous infections

NURSING DIAGNOSES and NURSING INTERVENTIONS

Nursing Diagnosis	Nursing Intervention
Skin integrity, impairment of: actual	Apply hot soaks. Instruct patient in proper handwashing. Instruct patient to scrupulously dry hands and feet, especially around nails, and to use hot air drying rather than towel when possible.
Skin integrity, impairment of: potential	Instruct patient to protect hands and feet from moisture by wearing cotton socks and rubber gloves with cotton liners when hands are in water. Discuss with patient role of environmental factors such as moisture and trauma, and explore ways to eliminate them.
Comfort, alteration in: pain	Offer hot soaks to decrease swelling. Elevate affected limb.

Patient Education

1. Instruct the patient regarding handwashing, drying, protection from moisture, and trauma (see "Nursing Care").
2. Instruct the patient in the use of medications and side effects.
3. Instruct the patient in aseptic dressing changes if needed for draining lesions or after incision and drainage.

EVALUATION

Patient Outcome	Data Indicating That Outcome is Reached
Inflammation subsides and infection resolves.	There is no erythema, swelling, heat, tenderness, pain, or purulent exudate.
Chronic moisture and trauma are avoided.	Paronychia does not recur.

DISEASES OF THE HAIR
Alopecia

Alopecia is a partial or complete loss of hair.

Alopecia may occur as a result of genetic factors, the aging process, or local or systemic disease. Alopecia can be scarring or nonscarring and localized, patterned, or diffuse. The biologic dysfunctions of hair have little clinical importance, but the psychologic and social importance is substantial.

Fig. 5-7

Alopecia areata.

Courtesy of Stephen B. Tucker, M.D., Department of Dermatology, University of Texas Health Science Center at Houston.

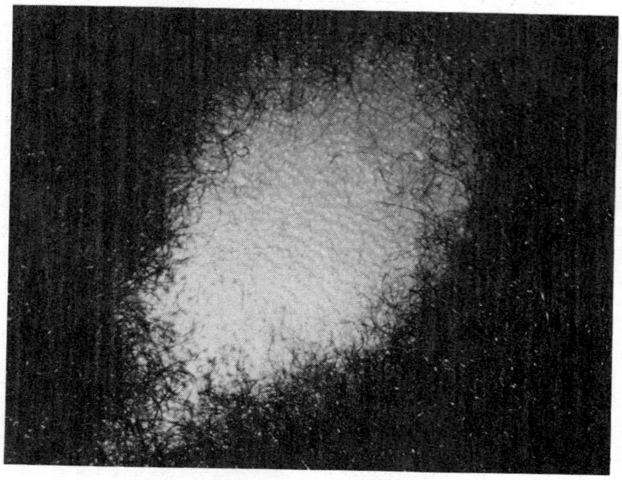

PATHOPHYSIOLOGY

Table 5-10 summarizes the clinical features and pathophysiology of the various types of hair loss.

DIAGNOSTIC STUDIES

Physical examination
Hair loss distribution, characteristics, and history

Biopsy
Reveals hair phase and structural damage

Culture
Infecting bacteria or fungus

TREATMENT PLAN

Surgical
Hair transplant for androgenic hair loss

Chemotherapeutic
Corticosteroids
Intralesional injection of 1-2 ml of triamcinolone (Kenalog), 10 mg/ml
Topical glucocorticoids under occlusive dressing (see pp. 637-639)
Betamethasone (Valisone) 0.1%
Fluocinolone (Fluonid, Synalar, Fluosyn, Synemol) 0.025%
For scarring alopecia, treatment directed at eliminating cause

Table 5-10
Clinical Features and Pathology of Various Forms of Alopecia

Disease	Type	Features	Pathology
Areata	Nonscarring; localized or general	Occurs on any part of body; associated with family incidence; skin soft, smooth, not inflamed; one or several patches of loss; loss sudden; regrowth may occur with fine, light hair; hair pigments eventually	Inflammatory infiltrate around hair bulb; retraction in anagen hair; abnormal keratinization; loss of melanin and melanocytes; increased number of hair follicles in telogen phase
Androgenic	Nonscarring; patterned	Occurs on scalp; in men frontal and temporal loss; thinning over vertex in women; mild, severe, or complete loss; familial trait	Androgens cause hair follicles to become smaller in size; terminal hair no longer formed; most hair follicles eventually disappear
Mechanical and chemical	Nonscarring; localized	Acute or chronic; attributable to hairdressing procedures or habitual hair pulling; skin may show trauma from tight braids or curlers	Trauma to hair shaft; localized breakage of hair
Telogen effluvium	Nonscarring; diffuse	Occurs 6 to 16 weeks after precipitating episode; hair loss seen on shampooing or brushing; occurs as diffuse thining; common precipitating factors are pregnancy, hormone therapy, stress, surgery, fever, and illness	Increased percentage of hairs in resting phase and subsequently in normal process of shedding
Drug related	Nonscarring Diffuse	Caused by antimitotic drugs (anagen hair loss) or by oral contraceptives, anticoagulants, propanolol (telogen hair loss); usually temporary	Antimitotic drugs cause decreased mitosis and decreased number of anagen hairs; hair shaft constricted; cause increase in percentage of hairs in telogen phase and subsequently in normal process of shedding
Scarring	Scarring	Due to systemic diseases such as lupus erythematosus, scleroderma, lichen planus, folliculitis decalvans; regrowth does not occur	Follicle destroyed by infection or scarring

ASSESSMENT: AREAS OF CONCERN

Lesion
As described in Table 5-10; location; distribution; scarring

Precipitating factors
Trauma; drugs; family history; systemic diseases

Psychosocial concerns
Concern about body image

NURSING DIAGNOSES and NURSING INTERVENTIONS

Nursing Diagnosis	Nursing Intervention
Self-concept, disturbance in: body image	Assess patient's self-perception. Encourage patient to verbalize feelings about body, body appearance, or fear of reaction or rejection by others. Advise patient that regrowth will occur in certain temporary conditions. Discuss use of wigs and hairpieces.

Patient Education

1. Advise the patient that commercial preparations will not restore hair or encourage hair growth.
2. Instruct the patient in the cause and course of the disease.
3. Instruct the patient in the use of glucocorticoids under an occlusive dressing when indicated (see pp. 637-639).

EVALUATION

Patient Outcome	Data Indicating That Outcome is Reached
Underlying cause of hair loss is diagnosed and treated.	There is no new hair loss. Hair regrowth occurs in some conditions.
Patient evaluates appearance in realistic manner.	Patient does not use commercial hair restorative preparation. Patient uses wigs or hairpieces. Patient engages in satisfactory interpersonal relationships.

Hypertrichosis and Hirsutism

Hypertrichosis refers to nonspecific hair growth of all types. Hirsutism is excessive hair growth induced by androgens in women.

PATHOPHYSIOLOGY

Hypertrichosis occurs as a result of increased activity of the hair follicle with the production of a coarse terminal hair. Localized hypertrichosis can be the result of persistent trauma that causes chronic hyperemia and inflammation of the dermis. Hypertrichosis can also be caused by systemic disorders, including severe infection, gross malnutrition, and gluten enteropathy.

Hirsutism occurs as a result of increased androgen activity and simulates the male pattern of hair distribution with increased coarse terminal hair on the face, areolae, midline of the abdomen, and extremities. Hirsutism may be familial. Onset usually occurs slowly with no other symptoms of virilization. It may occur after menarche. Sudden onset of hirsutism may be from increased androgen production from adrenal, ovarian, or pituitary sources or by certain drugs such as systemic steroids, androgens, testosterone, progesterone, norethindrone, and phenytoin.

DIAGNOSTIC STUDIES

Physical examination
Distribution of hair with congruent history

Screening for adrenal, ovarian, and pituitary disorders

TREATMENT PLAN

For treatment of adrenal, ovarian, or pituitary disorders see the specific diseases. Generally, tumors are removed surgically; glucocorticoids are used for adrenal hyperplasia.

Electromechanical
Electrolysis—hair follicle destroyed by passage of galvanic electric current
Diathermy—tissue destroyed through electrocoagulation; not recommended, since it may cause scarring[27]

Supportive
Depilatories (wax or chemical)—chemicals can be irritating
Shaving
Bleaching with hydrogen peroxide and ammonia to depigment hair

ASSESSMENT: AREAS OF CONCERN

History
Onset; menstrual history; drug history; family history of hirsutism

Hair characteristics
Description of hair; type; distribution and pattern

Systemic features
Signs of virilization; size of ovaries and clitoris; uterine development

Psychosocial concerns
Concern about body image

NURSING DIAGNOSES and NURSING INTERVENTIONS

Nursing Diagnosis	Nursing Intervention
Self-concept, disturbance in: body image	Assess patient's self-perception. Assist in verbalization of feelings about body, body image, and fear of reaction or rejection by others. Advise of treatment modalities available for hair removal or bleaching.

Patient Education

1. Advise the patient of the advantages and disadvantages of the methods to remove or bleach the hair.
2. Instruct the patient in the cause and course of the disorder.

EVALUATION

Patient Outcome	Data Indicating That Outcome is Reached
Underlying or systemic disorders are diagnosed and treated.	Hair growth diminishes or ceases.
Patient chooses acceptable method for removing or bleaching hair.	Patient is satisfied with method and appearance.
Patient evaluates appearance in realistic manner.	Patient engages in usual activities and relationships.

Medical Interventions

Common Therapeutic Interventions

Intervention	Therapeutic Effect	Nursing Care/Patient Education
Balneotherapy Tap water Colloid, oatmeal, 1 cup Colloid, cornstarch, 2 cups Tar, commercial preparations, 2 teaspoons Carbonis detergens liquor, 1 ounce Oil (Alpha-Keri, Domol, Lubath, Jeri-Bath, etc.)	Treat large areas of body or widely disseminated lesions Antipruritic cooling; anti-inflammatory Antipruritic; nondrying Antipruritic; drying Antipruritic; nondrying Antipruritic; nondrying Lubrication	Fill tub half full (20 to 25 gallons) at room temperature. Keep water from cooling. Bathe for 10 to 15 minutes. Use safety mat, since medications make tub slippery. Keep room warm. Remove loose skin and crusts after bath. Apply medications while skin is still moist. Blot dry. Have patient dress in light, loose clothing.
Burn hydrotherapy: May add prescribed amounts sodium chloride, potassium chloride, calcium hypochlorite, or detergent	Facilitate dressing change and debridement	Immerse in water at temperature of 100° F (37.8° C) for 20 to 30 minutes. Stay with patient. Administer pain medications. Plug catheter. Shave and debride as needed. Use aseptic technique.
Occlusive dressings	Increased absorption and penetration of topical preparations; produces moisture retention, skin maceration, and decreased evaporation to increase effect of topical preparations	Apply airtight plastic film over medicated skin. Remove for 12 of 24 hours to prevent complications. Watch for complications: bacterial and candidal infections, sweat retention, folliculitis, and side effects of medications.
Shampoos Selenium sulfide Betadine Zinc pyrithione 2% Carbonis detergens liquor, 5% Triethanolamine sulfate 40%	Antiseborrheic Antibacterial Antiseborrheic Antiseborrheic Antipruritic Bland (can add medications)	Lather sufficiently. Gently work into scalp. Avoid contact with eyes.

Interventions	Therapeutic Effect	Nursing Care/Patient Education
Wet Dressings and Compresses Tap water or normal saline Aluminum acetate (Burow's) Potassium permanganate 1:10,000 solution; 5 grains/3 quarts water	Cool and dry acute inflammation through evaporation Antipruritic; antiinflammatory; used in acute oozing dermatoses As above; also antibacterial As above; also antifungal and antibacterial	Soak compress to point of dripping. Keep at room temperature. Remoisten every few minutes. Apply for 15 minutes every 2 to 3 hours. Do not rub or blot. Do not treat more than one third of the body at one time. Keep patient warm and covered. Advise patient that potassium permanganate stains skin, clothing, and tub. Instruct patient to use soft towels or cotton sheeting for home care to avoid irritating skin. Instruct patient to use clean towel or sheet each time compress is used, to keep them separate from rest of family linens, and to launder between each use.
Dry Burn Dressing Nonadherent, porous, fine mesh gauze Bulky, fluffed, coarse, mesh gauze Semielastic coarse mesh	First layer; nonadherent; fine enough to prevent epithelization into gauze Second layer; absorbs exudate Outer layer; applies even pressure; holds dressing in place	Cleanse wound with one-half strength Betadine using sterile gauze; rub gently to remove existing topical agent. Apply topical agent thick enough to cover wound with ⅛ inch of agent to provide healing and prevent bandage from adhering. Apply layers of dressing: fine gauze, bulky coarse gauze; semielastic mesh. Change dressing one or two times daily.

Topical Preparations

Preparation	Therapeutic Effect	Nursing Care/Patient Education
Creams and Ointments Petrolatum, mineral oil, lanolin, Eurin, Qualatum, Unibase, Dermabase	Lubrication; protection; vehicle for medications; decrease water loss; ointments greasy with oil base; creams lighter and water washable	Rub into skin by hand. Cover ointments with light dressing to protect clothing. Apply frequently. Wash off before reapplication.
Gels Contain propylene glycol and carboxymethylene	Like creams and ointments; clear and non-greasy; may be used on hairy areas	Apply with fingers. Avoid rubbing, since they are thixotropic agents (become thinner with rubbing). Apply frequently.
Lotions With 0.5% menthol and 0.25% phenol	Liquid vehicles for medications; lubrication; cooling through evaporation Antipruritic; drying	Apply with cotton gauze. Lotions are usually not washed off between applications.
Pastes	Stiff vehicle of powder and ointment; porous and less occlusive than ointments; protective	Apply with tongue depressor. Wash off between applications. Scrub gently if paste is difficult to remove.
Powders Talc, zinc, oxide, cornstarch	Absorbent; hygroscopic (take up water); reduce friction	Apply with shaker. Avoid accumulation in intertriginous areas.

Topical Medications

Medication	Therapeutic Effect	Nursing Care/Patient Education
Antiseptic Agents Chlorhexidine, povidone-iodine, hexachlorophene	Treat carriers of pathogens; reduce overall skin bacterial count	Observe for sensitivities. Do not use hexachlorophene for infants and children.

Medication	Therapeutic Effect	Nursing Care/Patient Education
Antibacterial Agents Neomycin Bacitracin Silver sulfadiazine (Silvadene) Sulfamylon	Like antiseptic agents For gram-negative and gram-positive organisms For gram-negative organisms and *Pseudomonas* For burns; for gram-negative and gram-positive organisms and yeast For burns; bacteriostatic only; for gram-negative and gram-positive organisms	Observe for sensitivities. Cover with light dressing to protect clothing. Apply two to four times a day. Wash off before reapplication. With sulfamylon debride wound before reapplication.
Precipitated Sulfur 3%	Antiseborrheic	Observe for irritation.
Salicylic Acid 3%-5%; **Urea 10%-20%**	Keratolytic; increases absorption of other medications	Observe for irritation.
Corticosteroids Hydrocortisone 1%; fluocinolone 0.01%; triamcinolone 0.025%-0.1%; betamethasone	Decrease inflammation through vasoconstriction and direct action on leukocytes; decrease prostaglandin synthesis; decrease mitotic rate of epidermal cells	Apply sparingly to skin or apply in occlusive dressing. When used for prolonged periods, especially under occlusive dressings, watch for thinning of skin, striae formation, telangiectasia, and follicular hyperkeratosis.

CRYOSURGERY

In cryosurgery tissue is frozen to remove hyperkerolytic growths (such as warts) or to cause involution of cysts.

Contraindications and Cautions

1. Overfreezing can cause scarring and hyperpigmentation.
2. Application of liquid nitrogen can be painful and is not well tolerated by children.

Procedure

1. Liquid nitrogen is applied with a cotton-tipped applicator and is held in place for 10 to 20 seconds.
2. Carbon dioxide is applied via CO_2 pencil, which is held in place with moderate pressure for 20 to 30 seconds.

NURSING INTERVENTIONS

1. Inform the patient before treatment of the possibility of scarring or hyperpigmentation, and help the patient evaluate the benefit/risk trade-off.
2. Instruct the patient in the procedure.
3. Observe for blister formation immediately with CO_2 or in 5 to 10 hours with liquid nitrogen.
4. Instruct the patient to prevent infection by keeping the area clean and dry, not puncturing the blister, and not picking at the scab.
5. Instruct the patient to observe for signs of infection and to seek medical attention if they occur.

DEBRIDEMENT

In debridement dead tissue or eschar is removed to facilitate healing or in preparation for skin grafting.

Procedure

Surgical
Surgical excision—large areas removed down to fascia
Tangential excision—layers of eschar removed with dermatome or scalpel to point of capillary bleeding; edge of tissue picked up with forceps and necrotic tissue cut with scissors; margin of 0.5 cm left to avoid cutting viable tissue; debridement limited to area of 10 cm; bleeding controlled by direct pressure; topical agent applied

Chemotherapeutic
Proteolytic enzymes applied with saline to erode and consume eschar

Mechanical
Removal through mechanical action in dressing changes, hydrotherapy, and showers

NURSING INTERVENTIONS

1. Describe the procedure to the patient.
2. Administer analgesics 20 minutes before debridement.
3. After the procedure, assess the area for exudate, color, sensation, bleeding, and size of area debrided.
4. Assess the patient's response: pain, stress, or fear.

INTRALESIONAL INJECTIONS

Intralesional injections are injections of a corticosteroid into a lesion. The anti-inflammatory action helps clear lesions and reduce the size of cysts.

Contraindications and Cautions

1. Injection into subcutaneous tissue can result in transient or permanent atrophy and local tissue depression.

Procedure

1. Aqueous suspension (usually triamcinolone, 5-10 mg/2 ml) is injected intracutaneously into the lesion or cyst with a fine-gauge needle. The more superficial the injection, the better the result.

NURSING INTERVENTIONS

1. Inform the patient before treatment of the possibility of atrophy and help the patient evaluate the benefit/risk trade-off.
2. Instruct the patient to observe for side effects of treatment: bleeding, hemorrhaging, pigmentation, and atrophy; adrenal suppression may occur with multiple injections.
3. Instruct the patient to observe for desired effects: cyst decreases in size and lesion clears.
4. Instruct the patient to keep the area clean to avoid secondary infection.

SKIN GRAFT

In a skin graft a section of skin tissue that is separated from its blood supply is transferred to a recipient site to provide tissue for epithelization.

split-thickness graft   Composed of epidermis and superficial layers of dermis.
full-thickness graft   Composed of epidermis and all layers of dermis.
homograft (allograft)   Skin from a deceased person that is used as temporary cover for about 10 days, and may survive for 4 to 5 weeks.
heterograft (xenograft)   Pigskin or synthetic substitute that acts as biologic dressing.
autograft   Skin from another part of the patient's own body.
mesh graft   Split-thickness graft meshed with a special instrument to cover large areas and is held in place by a dressing or by sutures.

autologous cultured human epithelium   Unburned epidermal cells cultured into sheets in a flask. The cultured sheets are then attached to petrolatum gauze squares and sutured in place in the wound. The petrolatum gauze is removed 7 to 10 days later.[33]

Procedure

1. The donor site is prepared by surgical scrub. The recipient site is debrided and cleansed.
2. A split- or full-thickness graft is taken from the donor site with a dermatome. The graft is cut as "postage stamps" or strips or is meshed and is placed on recipient sites.
3. The graft is held in place by a pressure dressing or by sutures.
4. The donor site is covered with nonadherent gauze that is held in place by a gauze dressing.

NURSING INTERVENTIONS

Donor site
1. Remove the outer dressing in 24 hours.
2. Inspect the site daily.
3. Assess for bleeding, pain, and infection.
4. Leave nonadherent gauze in place until it separates spontaneously.
5. If infection occurs, treat it with medicated wet dressing.

Recipient (graft) site
1. Inspect the site daily.
2. Assess for edema, hematoma formation, fluid collection, infection, and viability of graft tissue.
3. Immobilize the affected part to avoid disrupting the graft.
4. Elevate the grafted extremity for 7 to 10 days.
5. Protect the graft from scratching by the patient.
6. If infection occurs, treat it with a medicated wet dressing.
7. The heterograft acts as a biologic dressing; expect it to slough off in 10 days to 5 weeks.

Healing phase
1. Inform the patient about the changing hues of graft scar tissue: pale, then pink, then red, then fading to resemble surrounding skin; a full-thickness graft may remain deeply red for several months.
2. Anticipate skin scaling with a full-thickness graft.
3. Lubricate the donor site with lanolin or cocoa butter to keep the tissue soft and pliable.
4. Apply mineral oil or lanolin to the graft site after the second or third week to remove superficial crusts, moisten the graft, and stimulate circulation.

5. Instruct the patient who will be at home to avoid overexposure of the graft site to the sun, since the site is sensitive to the sun and can burn easily.
6. Encourage the patient to verbalize feelings about body, body appearance, or fear of reaction or rejection by others.

4. Advise the patient not to suddenly stop taking the medication, which could precipitate adrenal crisis.
5. Advise the patient to have routine checkups while receiving steroid therapy to evaluate the response to medication and to monitor side effects.

SYSTEMIC STEROID THERAPY

In systemic steroid therapy parenteral or oral glucocorticoids are used for their anti-inflammatory action.

Contraindications and Cautions

1. Hypertension and diabetes mellitus can be exacerbated.
2. Concurrent infections can be masked.
3. Therapy is used with caution in patients who are predisposed to peptic ulceration, thrombophlebitis, adrenal suppression, and mood swings.

Procedure

The dose and duration of treatment depend on the severity of the disease and the patient's response. The patient should receive a dose sufficient to produce a therapeutic response and then be maintained with the minimum effective dose; the dose should be tapered slowly after the lesions have cleared.

Approximate equivalent doses of various steroids are:
Betamethasone, 0.5 mg
Dexamethasone, 0.75 mg
Fludrocortisone, 2 mg
Hydrocortisone, 20 mg
Methylprednisolone, 4 mg
Prednisolone, 5 mg
Prednisone, 5 mg
Triamcinolone, 4 mg

NURSING INTERVENTIONS

1. Inform the patient about the side effects to watch for and to seek medical attention if they occur: euphoria, gastrointestinal pain or bleeding, bruising, thrombophlebitis, hypertension, moon face, cushingoid features, acne, hirsutism, osteoporosis, and mood swings.
2. Instruct the patient to take medication with milk or antacids to decrease gastric irritation.
3. Instruct the patient to increase protein intake to combat osteoporosis.

ULTRAVIOLET LIGHT THERAPY

SHORT-WAVE ULTRAVIOLET LIGHT

Short-wave ultraviolet light (UV-B) is used for the treatment of psoriasis and acne.

Procedure

1. The patient is exposed one to three times per week.
2. The exposure time is increased to keep skin just below erythema level.

GOECKERMAN THERAPY

In Goeckerman therapy ultraviolet light therapy is used in combination with coal tar applications that are photosensitizing; it is used for the treatment of psoriasis.

Procedure

1. Coal tar ointment is applied, left on for several hours, and then washed off.
2. UV-B therapy is given in doses to account for photosensitization.
3. The skin is kept just below erythema level.
4. Coal tar ointment is reapplied after UV-B exposure.

PUVA THERAPY

In PUVA therapy long-wave ultraviolet light (UV-A) is used in combination with psoralen, which is a photosensitizer (P + UV-A = PUVA); it is used for treating psoriasis.

Contraindications and Cautions

1. Long-term effects of PUVA therapy remain controversial, and treatment is usually reserved for chronic, severe, refractory psoriasis.[27,36,86]

Procedure

1. Psoralen is administered in an initial dose of 0.6 mg/kg.
2. UV-A irradiation is delivered 2 to 4 hours after psoralen administration.
3. Dosage and exposure are determined by individual response.
4. Therapy is usually provided in specific treatment centers, since specialized equipment, careful calibration, and close monitoring are required.

NURSING INTERVENTIONS

1. Instruct the patient in the procedure.
2. Assist the patient in setting up a schedule to maintain the therapeutic regimen.
3. Instruct a patient who is using short-wave ultraviolet light therapy at home to:
   a. Use a lamp with an automatic timer to shut off
   b. Use a backup timer
   c. Measure the distance from the lamp carefully and maintain the correct distance
   d. Increase exposure time slowly and keep the skin below erythema level
   e. Wear an occlusive protective eye covering
4. Advise a patient who is using concomitant photosensitizing agents to avoid lengthy exposure to sunlight.
5. Advise a patient who is receiving PUVA therapy of the undetermined long-term effects, and assist the patient in evaluating the risk/benefit trade-off.

References

1. Abel, E., and Farber, E.: Hazards of PUVA therapy. In Epstein, E., editor: Controversies in dermatology, Philadelphia, 1984, W.B. Saunders Co.
2. Anderson, P.: Peritoneal dialysis. In Epstein, E., editor: Controversies in dermatology, Philadelphia, 1984, W.B. Saunders Co.
3. Apfelberg, D., et al.: The role of the argon laser in the management of hemangiomas, Int. J. Dermatol. 21:579, 1982.
4. Arndt, K.: Treatment technics in argon laser therapy, J. Am. Acad. Dermatol. 11:90, 1984.
5. Ashton, R., et al.: Anthralin: historical and current perspectives, J. Am. Acad. Dermatol. 9:173, 1983.
6. Ayres, S.: Vitamin E: an effective therapeutic agent in dermatology. In Epstein, E., editor: Controversies in dermatology, Philadelphia, 1984, W.B. Saunders Co.
7. Barkin, R., and Rosen, P., editors: Emergency pediatrics, St. Louis, 1984, The C.V. Mosby Co.
8. Baron, M.: The skin and wound healing, Top. Clin. Nurs. 5:11, 1983.
9. Bates, B.: A guide to physical examination, ed. 3, Philadelphia, 1983, J.B. Lippincott Co.
10. Bickers, D.: Position paper: PUVA therapy, J. Am. Acad. Dermatol. 8:265, 1983.
11. Bickers, D.: The etiologic irrelevance of diet in acne vulgaris. In Epstein, E., editor: Controversies in dermatology, Philadelphia, 1984, W.B. Saunders Co.
12. Bowers, A., and Thompson, J.: Clinical manual of health assessment, ed. 2, St. Louis, 1984, The C.V. Mosby Co.
13. Braen, G.R.: Burns. In Kravis, T., and Warner, C.G., editors: Emergency medicine: a comprehensive review, St. Louis, 1983, The C.V. Mosby Co.
14. Braen, G.R., and Jelenko III, C.: Thermal injuries (burns). In Rosen, P., et al.: Emergency medicine: concepts and clinical practice, St. Louis, 1983, The C.V. Mosby Co.
15. Buecker, J., Ratz, J., and Richfield, D.: Histology of port-wine stain treated with carbon dioxide laser, J. Am. Acad. Dermatol. 10:1014, 1984.
16. Camp, R.: Generalized pruritus and its management, Clin. Exper. Dermatol. 7:557, 1982.
17. Carruth, J., and McKenzie, J.: The argon laser in dermatology: safety aspects, Clin. Exp. Dermatol. 7:247, 1982.
18. Clayton, B.: Mosby's handbook of pharmacology in nursing, ed. 3, St. Louis, 1984, The C.V. Mosby Co.
19. Coskey, R.: Dermatologic therapy: December, 1982, through November, 1983, J. Am. Acad. Dermatol. 11:25, 1984.
20. Cronin, E.: The management of allergic contact dermatitis, Clin. Exp. Dermatol. 7:281, 1982.
21. Dawber, R.: Alopecia and hirsutism, Clin. Exp. Dermatol. 7:177, 1982.
22. Delancy, V., and North, C.: Skin assessment, Top. Clin. Nurs. 5:5, 1983.
23. Diette, K., et al.: Role of ultraviolet A in phototherapy for psoriasis, J. Am. Acad. Dermatol. 11:441, 1984.
24. Dimick, A.: The burn at first sight, Emerg. Med. 15:130, 1983.
25. Ellis, C., et al.: Isotretinoin therapy is associated with early skeletal radiographic changes, J. Am. Acad. Dermatol. 10:1024, 1984.
26. Elton, R.: Complications of cutaneous cryosurgery, J. Am. Acad. Dermatol. 8:513, 1983.
27. Epstein, E.: Common skin disorders: a physician's illustrated manual, ed. 2, Oradell, N.J., 1983, Medical Economics Books.
28. Farber, E., Abel, E., and Charuworn, A.: Recent advances in the treatment of psoriasis, J. Am. Acad. Dermatol. 8:311, 1983.
29. Fischbach, F.T.: A manual of laboratory diagnostic tests, Philadelphia, 1980, J.B. Lippincott Co.
30. Fitzpatrick, T., and Parrish, J.: PUVA in perspective. In Epstein, E., editor: Controversies in dermatology, Philadelphia, 1984, W.B. Saunders Co.
31. Fry, L.: The treatment of dermatitis herpetiformis, Clin. Exp. Dermatol. 7:633, 1982.
32. Galles, E.: Identifying dermatological conditions in blacks, J. Emerg. Nurs. 4:56, 1978.

33. Gallico, G., et al.: Permanent coverage of large burn wounds with autologous cultured human epithelium, N. Engl. J. Med. **311:**448, 1984.

34. Graham, J., and Jouhar, A.: The importance of cosmetics in the psychology of appearance, Int. J. Dermatol. **22:**153, 1983.

35. Grice, K.: Treatment of hyperhidrosis, Clin. Exp. Dermatol. **7:**183, 1982.

36. Grupper, C., and Berretti, B.: Psoriasis: PUVA therapy. In Epstein, E., editor: Controversies in dermatology, Philadelphia, 1984, W.B. Saunders Co.

37. Gurevitch, A.: Dermatologic disorders. In Steinberg, F., editor: Care of the geriatric patient, ed. 6, St. Louis, 1983, The C.V. Mosby Co.

38. Guyton, A.: Human physiology and mechanisms of disease, Philadelphia, 1982, W.B. Saunders Co.

39. Heng, M., Kloss, S., and Haberfelde, G.: Pathogenesis of papular urticaria, J. Am. Acad. Dermatol. **10:**1030, 1984.

40. Henwood, B., and MacDonald, D.: Caterpillar dermatitis, Clin. Exp. Dermatol. **8:**77, 1983.

41. Huff, J.C., Weston, W., and Tonnesen, M.: Erythema multiforme: a critical review of characteristics, diagnostic criteria, and causes, J. Am. Acad. Dermatol. **8:**763, 1983.

42. Jones, R.R.: The histogenesis of eczema, Clin. Exp. Dermatol. **8:**213, 1983.

43. Kaplan, R., Russell, D., and Lowe, N.: Etretinate therapy for psoriasis: clinical responses, remission times, epidermal DNA and polyamine responses, J. Am. Acad. Dermatol. **8:**95, 1983.

44. Kim, M.J., McFarland, G., and McLane, A.: Pocket guide to nursing diagnosis, St. Louis, 1984, The C.V. Mosby Co.

45. Korting, G.: Geriatric dermatology, Philadelphia, 1980, W.B. Saunders Co.

46. Lane, A., Wachs, G., and Weston, W.: Once-daily treatment of psoriasis with topical glucocorticosteroid ointments, J. Am. Acad. Dermatol. **8:**523, 1983.

47. Lawlis, G., and Achterberg, J.: Acne: the disease and stress, Top. Clin. Nurs. **5:**23, 1983.

48. Lever, R., and Mackie, R.: The use of oral sodium cromoglycate in young adults with severe chronic atopic dermatitis, Clin. Exp. Dermatol. **9:**143, 1984.

49. Leverne, G.: The treatment of pemphigus and pemphigoid, Clin. Exp. Dermatol. **7:**643, 1982.

50. Long, B.: Assessment of the integument and immune status. In Phipps, W., Long, B., and Woods, N., editors: Medical-surgical nursing, ed. 2, St. Louis, 1983, The C.V. Mosby Co.

51. Long, B.: Intervention in the person with a dermatologic problem. In Phipps, W., Long, B., and Woods, N., editors: Medical-surgical nursing, ed. 2, St. Louis, 1983, The C.V. Mosby Co.

52. Long, B., Wright, E.R., and Phipps, W.: Problems associated with impaired immune response. In Phipps, W., Long, B., and Woods, N., editors: Medical-surgical nursing, ed. 2, St. Louis, 1983, The C.V. Mosby Co.

53. Lowe, N., et al.: Coal tar phototherapy for psoriasis reevaluated: erythemagenic versus suberythemagenic ultraviolet with a tar extract in oil and crude coal tar, J. Am. Acad. Dermatol. **8:**781, 1983.

54. Lowe, N., et al.: Anthralin for psoriasis: short-contact anthralin therapy compared with topical steroid and conventional anthralin, J. Am. Acad. Dermatol. **10:**9, 1984.

55. Lyell, A.: Review of significant progress in clinical dermatology since 1977, J. Am. Acad. Dermatol. **6:**195, 1982.

56. Maddin, S.: Acne surgery. In Epstein, E., editor: Controversies in dermatology, Philadelphia, 1984, W.B. Saunders Co.

57. Malasanos, L., et al.: Health assessment, ed. 2, St. Louis, 1981, The C.V. Mosby Co.

58. Malseed, R.: Quick reference to drug therapy and nursing considerations, Philadelphia, 1983, J.B. Lippincott Co.

59. Marks, R.: Chronic idiopathic urticaria, Int. J. Dermatol. **21:**19, 1982.

60. Menter, A., and Cram, D.: The Goeckerman regimen in two psoriasis day care centers, J. Am. Acad. Dermatol. **9:**59, 1983.

61. Monroe, E.: Urticaria, Int. J. Dermatol. **20:**32, 1981.

62. Moynahan, E.: The treatment and management of epidermolysis bullosa, Clin. Exp. Dermatol. **7:**665, 1982.

63. Nater, J., and DeGroot, A.: Unwanted effects of cosmetics and drugs used in dermatology, Princeton, N.J., 1983, Excerpta Medica.

64. National Center for Health Statistics: Prevalence of dermatological disease among persons 1-74 years of age: United States, Advance Data from Vital and Health Statistics 572(4), Public Health Service, Washington, D.C., Jan. 26, 1977, U.S. Government Printing Office.

65. National Safety Council: Accident facts: 1983 edition, Chicago, 1983, The Council.

66. O'Malley, C.: Intervention in the person with burns. In Phipps, W., Long, B., and Woods, N., editors: Medical-surgical nursing, ed. 2, St. Louis, 1983, The C.V. Mosby Co.

67. Orkin, M., Juranek, D., and Maibach, H.: Treatment of household and sexual contacts of patients with scabies. In Epstein, E., editor: Controversies in dermatology, Philadelphia, 1984, W.B. Saunders Co.

68. Perry, H.: Psoriasis: the Goeckerman treatment. In Epstein, E., editor: Controversies in dermatology, Philadelphia, 1984, W.B. Saunders Co.

69. Pillsbury, D.M., and Heaton, C.L.: A manual of dermatology, ed. 2, Philadelphia, 1980, W.B. Saunders Co.

70. Pittman, R.: Disorders of the skin and its appendages. In Luckmann, J., and Sorensen, K.: Medical-surgical nursing: a psychophysiologic approach, ed. 2, Philadelphia, 1980, W.B. Saunders Co.

71. Ponchi, P.: Pathogenesis of acne: importance of follicular epithelial changes. In Epstein, E., editor: Controversies in dermatology, Philadelphia, 1984, W.B. Saunders Co.

72. Pye, R.: Prospects for the treatment of acne vulgaris and rosacea, Clin. Exp. Dermatol. **7:**195, 1982.

73. Rand, R., and Baden, H.: The ichthyoses: a review, J. Am. Acad. Dermatol. **8:**285, 1983.

74. Reisner, R.: 13–cis–retinoic acid in the treatment of acne. In Epstein, E., editor: Controversies in dermatology, Philadelphia, 1984, W.B. Saunders Co.

75. Reisner, R.: Some controversial areas in the topical treatment of acne. In Epstein, E., editor: Controversies in dermatology, Philadelphia, 1984, W.B. Saunders Co.

76. Rentoul, J.: Management of the hirsute woman, Int. J. Dermatol. **22:**265, 1983.

77. Roberts, H.: The vitamin E enigma: perspectives for physicians. In Epstein, E., editor: Controversies in dermatology, Philadelphia, 1984, W.B. Saunders Co.

78. Robertson, D., and Maibach, H.: Topical corticosteroids, Int. J. Dermatol. **21:**59, 1982.

79. Samman, P.: Management of disorders of the nails, Clin. Exp. Dermatol. **7:**189, 1982.

80. Sauer, G.: Manual of skin diseases, ed. 3, Philadelphia, 1973, J.B. Lippincott Co.

81. Shaw, J.: Frostbite. In Rosen, P., et al.: editors: Emergency medicine: concepts and clinical practice, St. Louis, 1983, The C.V. Mosby Co.

82. Sheddon, I., and Church, R.: Skin disorders in clinical practice, Reading, Mass., 1976, Addison-Wesley Publishing Co.

83. Shuster, S.: Acne: the ashes of a burnt-out controversy. In Epstein, E., editor: Controversies in dermatology, Philadelphia, 1984, W.B. Saunders Co.

84. Stawiski, M., and Callen, J.: Dermatology. In Price, S., and Wilson, L.: Pathophysiology: clinical concepts of disease processes, New York, 1982, McGraw-Hill Book Co.

85. Stewart, W.: An appraisal of the retinoids in the treatment of psoriasis. In Epstein, E., editor: Controversies in dermatology, Philadelphia, 1984, W.B. Saunders Co.

86. Stewart, W., Danto, J., and Maddin, S.: Dermatology: diagnosis and treatment of cutaneous disorders, St. Louis, 1978, The C.V. Mosby Co.

87. Vasarinsh, P.: Clinical dermatology: diagnosis and therapy of common skin diseases, Woburn, Mass., 1982, Butterworth Publishers.

88. Verbov, J.: Pruritus ani and its management: a study and reappraisal, Clin. Exp. Dermatol. **9:**46, 1984.

89. Verbov, J., and Morley, N.: Color atlas of pediatric dermatology, Philadelphia, 1983, J.B. Lippincott Co.

90. Waisman, M.: Diet in acne. In Epstein, E., editor: Controversies in dermatology, Philadelphia, 1984, W.B. Saunders Co.

91. Ward, R., and Wathen, R.: Principles of dialysis: utilization in nonuremic psoriatic subjects, Int. J. Dermatol. **21:**154, 1982.

92. Weinstein, G.: Psoriasis and the selection of methotrexate for therapy. In Epstein, E., editor: Controversies in dermatology, Philadelphia, 1984, W.B. Saunders Co.

93. Williamson, D.: Treatment of chronic psoriasis by Psoradrate (0.1% dithranol in a 17% urea base) applied under occlusion, Clin. Exp. Dermatol. **8:**287, 1983.

94. Wolska, H., Jablonska, S., and Bounameaux, Y.: Etretinate in severe psoriasis, J. Am. Acad. Dermatol. **9:**883, 1983.

95. Wright, E.R.: Biologic defense mechanisms. In Phipps, W., Long, B., and Woods, N., editors: Medical-surgical nursing, ed. 2, St. Louis, 1983, The C.V. Mosby Co.

96. Yeganef, R., and Long, B.: Management of the person with a dermatologic problem. In Phipps, W., Long, B., and Woods, N., editors: Medical-surgical nursing, St. Louis, 1979, The C.V. Mosby Co.

97. Zackheim, H.: Treatment of psoriasis: use of corticosteroids. In Epstein, E., editor: Controversies in dermatology, Philadelphia, 1984, W.B. Saunders Co.

CHAPTER 6

The Eye

ANATOMY AND PHYSIOLOGY

External Structures

Orbit and its contents. The human eye is a spheric organ that is approximately 24 mm in diameter and rests within a fatty cushion in a bony orbit of the skull.[17] The orbit is composed of six bones forming a cavity that converges into two major posterior openings, the optic foramen and the superior orbital fissure (Fig. 6-1). These openings admit blood vessels and nerves that connect the eyeball to the brain and the body's blood supply. The ophthalmic artery, the optic nerve, and sympathetic nerves from the carotid plexus enter the orbit through the optic foramen. The oculomotor nerve (CN III), trochlear nerve (CN IV), abducent nerve (CN VI), and ophthalmic branch of the trigeminal nerve (CN V) pass through the superior orbital fissure.[28]

Some of the pertinent eye measurements are as follows:

Orbit volume 29 to 30 ml
Height at entrance 35 mm
Width at entrance 40 mm
Extraorbital width (anterior margin to anterior margin) 100 mm
Intraorbital width (medial margin to medial margin) 25 mm

The orbit contains the eyeball, which is cradled in the anterior portion; six oculomotor muscles, which surround and insert into the eyeball; a muscle for elevating the eyelid; and fat, ligaments, and connective tissue in the posterior section, which cushion and support the sphere and the extrinsic muscles. The anterior orbital walls are relatively thick and provide good protection for the eye. The medial wall, which separates the orbit from the ethmoid sinus, is extremely thin and vulnerable to ethmoid sinus infection.[28] The medial wall also contains a fossa for the lacrimal sac, which extends downward through the nasal lacrimal duct into the nose. The lateral posterior wall is also very thin and separates the orbit from the temporal lobe.

The anterior roof of the orbit contains the fossa for the lacrimal gland. The floor of the orbit is supported primarily by the orbital plate of the maxilla, which contains the infraorbital fissure. The maxillary branch of the trigeminal nerve (CN V) passes through this opening. The posterior wall of the orbit contains a fibrous sheet that encircles the optic foramen and serves as the origin for the extrinsic muscles, which stretch forward to encircle and insert in the anterior and medial aspects of the eyeball (Fig. 6-2). The orbital contents are supported and separated from the bone by a periosteal lining and fascial tissue that form the eye socket upon which the eyeball rests.

Eyelid. The exposed part of the eye is protected with a lid that serves as a shield from external assault and a barrier to excessive light. As the upper lid blinks, it distributes tears over the surface to maintain moisture. When the lids are open, they form the palpebral fissure (the elliptical opening), which results in the upper lid covering a portion of the iris (Fig. 6-3). The lids meet

Fig. 6-1
Right bony orbit.

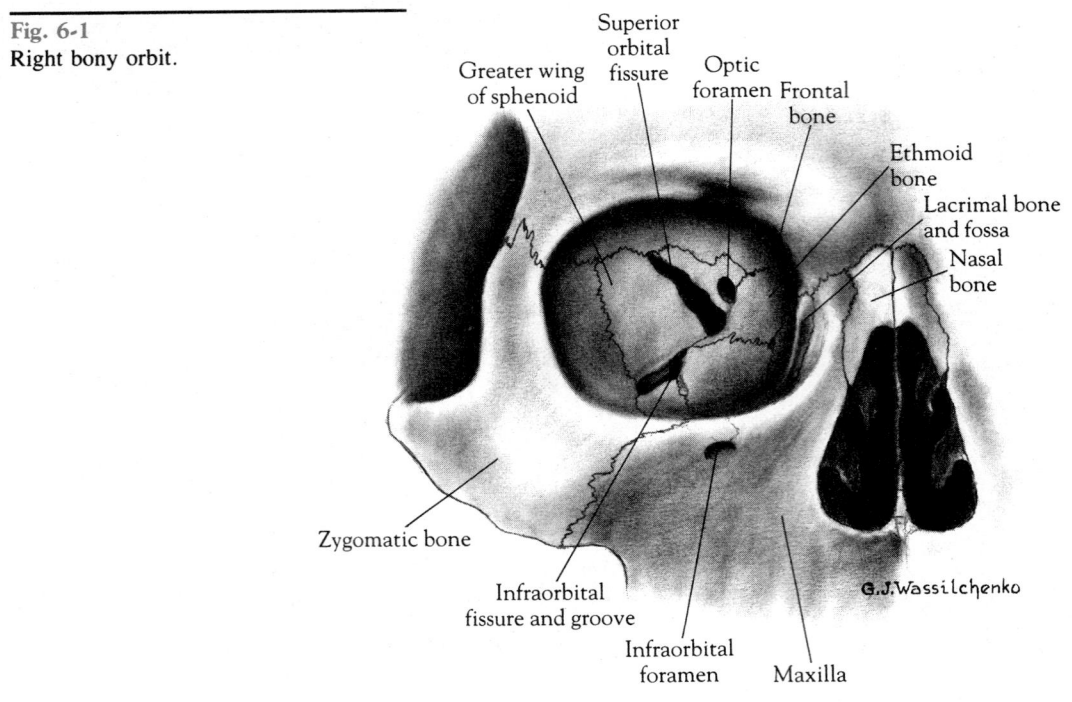

Superior orbital fissure
Greater wing of sphenoid
Optic foramen
Frontal bone
Ethmoid bone
Lacrimal bone and fossa
Nasal bone
Zygomatic bone
Infraorbital fissure and groove
Infraorbital foramen
Maxilla
G.J.Wassilchenko

Fig. 6-2
Diagrammatic section of orbit.

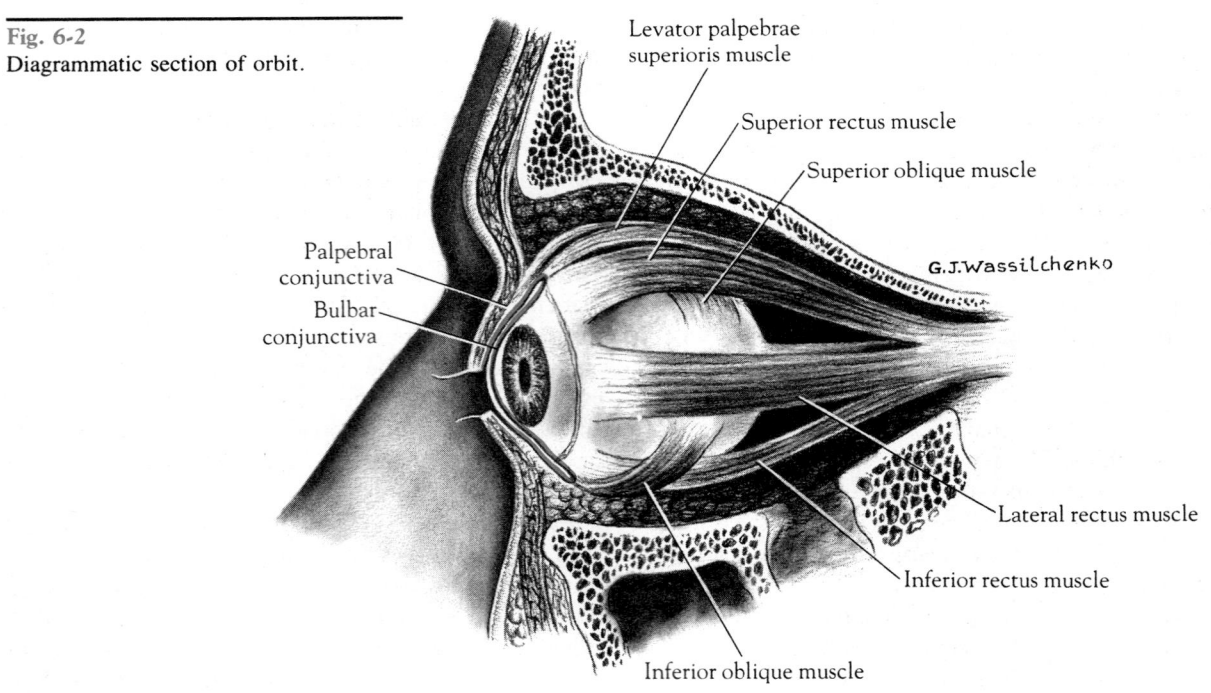

Levator palpebrae superioris muscle
Superior rectus muscle
Superior oblique muscle
G.J.Wassilchenko
Palpebral conjunctiva
Bulbar conjunctiva
Lateral rectus muscle
Inferior rectus muscle
Inferior oblique muscle

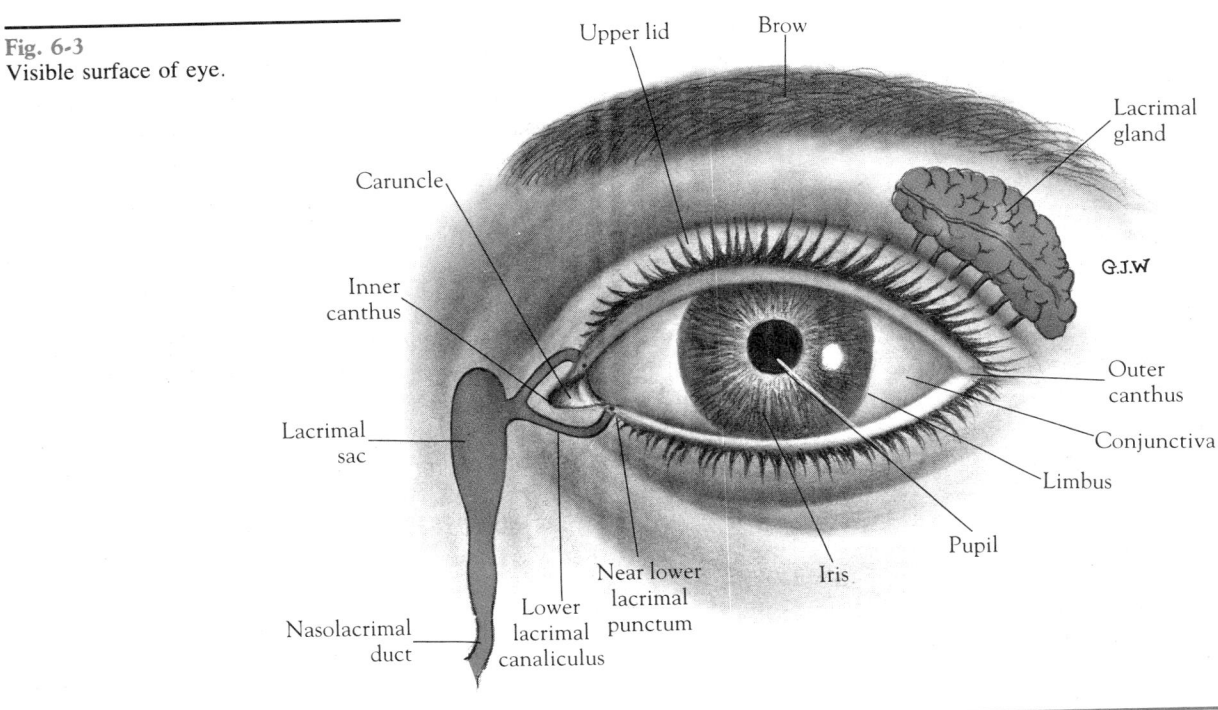

Fig. 6-3
Visible surface of eye.

Labels: Upper lid, Brow, Lacrimal gland, Caruncle, Inner canthus, Lacrimal sac, Nasolacrimal duct, Lower lacrimal canaliculus, Near lower lacrimal punctum, Iris, Pupil, Limbus, Conjunctiva, Outer canthus. G.J.W

at the medial (inner) canthus and enfold a small elevation, the lacrimal caruncle, which contains large sebaceous glands. The inner canthus is sometimes obscured by a vertical skin fold (epicanthus) in Oriental people and young children.[4] The central portion of the upper and lower lid is thickened with a firm connective tissue (tarsal plate) that protects the eye and maintains the shape of the lid. The eyelids are lined with a thin, transparent mucous membrane (palpebral conjunctiva) that continues as an outer cover for the sclera of the eyeball (bulbar conjunctiva) (Fig. 6-2). The conjunctiva contains blood vessels, nerves, hair follicles, and sebaceous glands (meibomian glands). The meibomian glands are situated along the margin of the lids; their secretions prevent rapid evaporation and overflow of tears and create an airtight lid closure.[1] Lid movement is supplied from the superior division of the oculomotor nerve (CN III), which activates the superior palpebral levator muscle for upper lid elevation and the inferior rectus muscle for lower lid retraction. The facial nerve (CN VII) activates the orbicularis oculi muscle, an oval sheet of fibers that surround the palpebral fissure, for lid closure. Superior and inferior palpebral smooth muscles and a central portion of the orbicularis oculi muscle respond to sympathetic innervation for involuntary blinking. The upper lid receives its sensory innervation from the ophthalmic division of the trigeminal nerve (CN V), and the lower lid is innervated by the maxillary branch of the trigeminal nerve. The eyelids are the only portion of the eye that

has a lymphatic system. The medial portions of the upper and lower lids drain into the submaxillary nodes, and the lateral aspects drain into the preauricular nodes.[28]

Lacrimal apparatus. The lacrimal apparatus secretes and drains a fluid that moistens and lubricates the anterior surface of the eye. Tears are produced in the lacrimal gland, which is located in the anterior lateral fossa of the orbit. Smaller accessory glands scattered throughout the palpebral conjunctiva also secrete fluid. Lacrimal fluid is normally clear and does not overflow unless reflex or psychic stimuli produce excessive tearing. Sebaceous gland secretions and a thin mucin layer combine with the aqueous portion of tears to maintain a constant film over the cornea. Lacrimal fluid contains immunoglobins, lymphocytes, phagocytes, and lysozyme as protective substances.[28]

Lid blinking assists in the distribution of tears over the eye and draws the tears inward to the puncta, small openings in the margins of the upper and lower lids at the inner canthus (Fig. 6-3). The puncta empty into the lacrimal canaliculi, which join to form the nasolacrimal sac (Fig. 6-3). The adjacent lacrimal duct empties into the nasal cavity in the inferior nasal meatus.[1]

Eyeball

Layers of the eye
Outer layer: cornea and sclera. The eyeball is surrounded by the sclera, a tough fibrous layer that covers the

posterior five sixths of the eye. The sclera merges with the cornea, which covers the anterior one sixth of the eye, at a junction called the limbus (Fig. 6-3).

The cornea is transparent, avascular, and richly innervated with sensory nerves (trigeminal [CN V]). The anterior surface of the cornea is convex, and irregularities of the curvature cause astigmatism. The anterior portion is bathed in lacrimal fluids, and the posterior surface is washed with aqueous humor in the anterior chamber. Since the cornea is avascular, it depends on the atmosphere, tears, and aqueous humor for oxygenation and nourishment. The cornea has three layers: the superficial epithelial layer, which is continuous with the bulbar conjunctiva; the substantia propria, which constitutes 90% of corneal thickness; and an endothelial layer.[1,40]

The epithelial layer is a regenerative multilayered barrier. If its cells are injured, uninjured cells migrate to the traumatized area and form a new barrier one cell thick within an hour of the injury.[28] Total repair of the corneal epithelium takes approximately 6 weeks. Because of its dependence on exposure to tears, corneal epithelium is subject to edema if deprived of oxygen. The implications for contact lenses are discussed later. The substantia propria is lined anteriorly with a collagenous membrane (Bowman's membrane) that resists infection and trauma.

If Bowman's membrane is destroyed, it reforms with scarring and irregular cell formation that contribute to astigmatism. The endothelial layer pumps fluid from the other corneal layers into the aqueous humor. A relatively diminished fluid volume is necessary for corneal transparency.[1] If the endothelium is destroyed, it does not regenerate and the remaining corneal layers become edematous.

The corneoscleral limbus has a rich vascular supply that encircles and nourishes the periphery of the cornea. The limbus is a transition area where corneal cells are mixed with conjunctival and scleral layers. Bowman's membrane ends abruptly at this junction. The posterior inner surface of the limbus adjoins the trabecular meshwork and the canal of Schlemm, which drain aqueous fluid from the anterior chamber.[40]

The sclera, the ''white'' of the eye, is the outer layer that surrounds most of the eye. It is adjacent to the second layer, the uveal tract, which includes the choroid layer, the ciliary body, and the iris (Fig. 6-4). The sclera has three layers. The outermost is the episclera, which merges with fascial tissue at the limbus; it is vascular and dense, and the minute vessels can be seen through the conjunctiva. The middle layer, the scleral stroma, is composed of tough collagenous fibers that create the

Fig. 6-4
Cross section of eye.

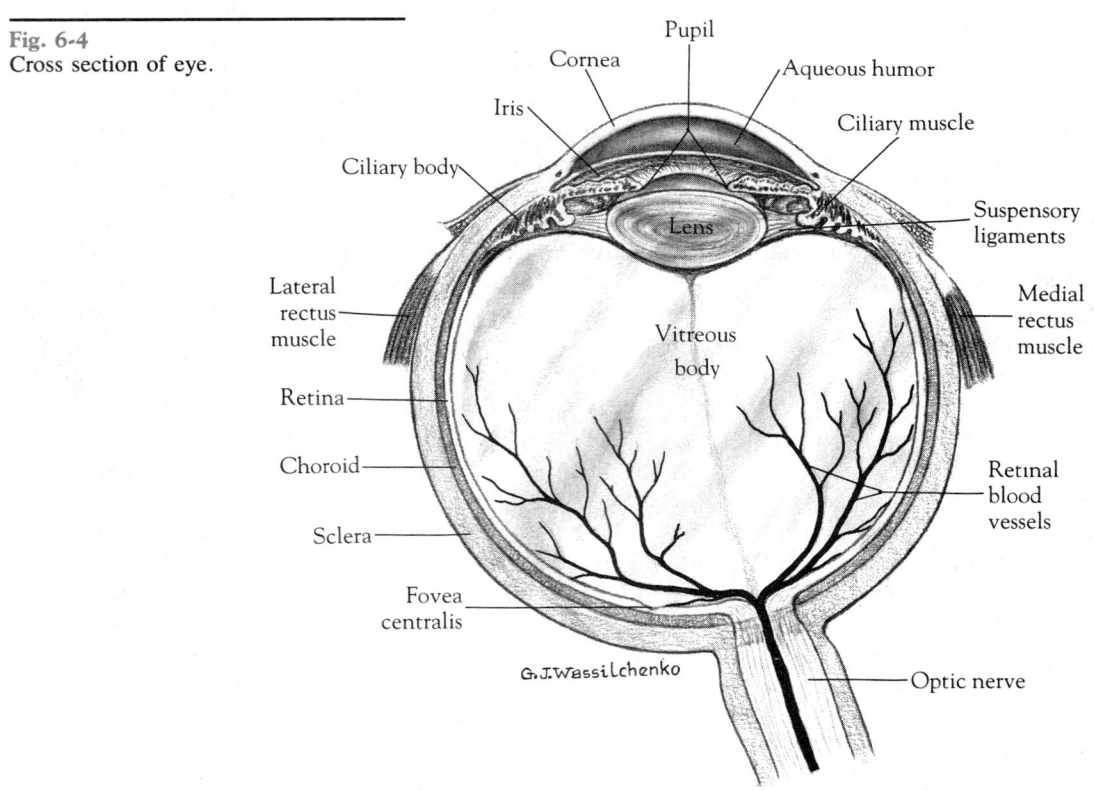

white appearance of the sclera. The innermost layer, the lamina fusca, contains melanocytes that may contribute to a yellow-brown scleral hue in dark-skinned persons. The lamina fusca contains collagenous fibers that filter into the choroid layer for adherence. The oculomotor muscles attach to the sclera at various points near the midsection of the eyeball (Fig. 6-2). The sclera also has numerous openings through which nerves and blood vessels pass. The two major openings are the posterior foramen, which admits the optic nerve into the eye, and the anterior foramen, where the ciliary muscle adjoins at the limbus in the anterior chamber.

Middle layer: choroid, ciliary body, and iris. The middle layer of the eyeball (the uveal tract) is comprised of the choroid, a vascular layer; the ciliary body, which contains smooth muscles attached to the lens and an epithelial portion for secreting aqueous humor; and the iris, which surrounds the pupil (Fig. 6-4).

The choroid adheres to the sclera at the entrance point of the optic nerve and extends anteriorly to the ciliary body. It has five layers. The outer layer, the suprachoroid, contains melanocytes, smooth muscle fibers, and ciliary arteries that nourish a portion of the choroid. The three middle layers contain veins and arterioles that feed into the ciliary body, the iris, and the outer portion of the retina. The inner layer of the choroid, Bruch's membrane, is multilayered and collagenous and contains cells from the adjacent retinal and choroid layers.

The ciliary body has both a muscular and a secretory function. The ciliary muscles expand from the choroid and extend anteriorly and medially toward the lens (Fig. 6-5). The body forms a ring of smooth muscle that surrounds the lens and parallels the overlying sclera. There are three groups of ciliary muscles. Muscles in the outer division are longitudinal and are parallel and adjacent to the sclera. Contraction of these fibers opens the canal of Schlemm, a thin-walled vessel that encircles the eye and drains aqueous fluid from the anterior chamber. The canal of Schlemm is located at the inner aspect of the sclerocorneal junction (limbus) (Fig. 6-5). The middle layer of ciliary muscles is a meshwork of fibers that connect the longitudinal muscles to the inner circular fibers. The circular fibers are directed medially toward the lens. A series of delicate ligaments (the lens zonule) attach the ciliary muscles to the equator of the lens (Fig. 6-5). The tension of the zonular fibers suspends the lens and stabilizes its position. The zonular tension relaxes with ciliary circular muscle contraction to increase the convexity of the lens for accommodation.[28]

Aqueous humor is secreted from the epithelial portion of the ciliary body. The ciliary body culminates in ciliary processes behind the peripheral portion of the iris. The processes are lined with nonpigmented epithelium that secretes aqueous humor. The nonpigmented epithelial cells extend into the sensory portion of the retina. The retina also joins the inner lining of the ciliary epithelium (the pars plana) at a serrated structure called the ora serrata, which corresponds in shape to the ciliary processes (Fig. 6-6).[17]

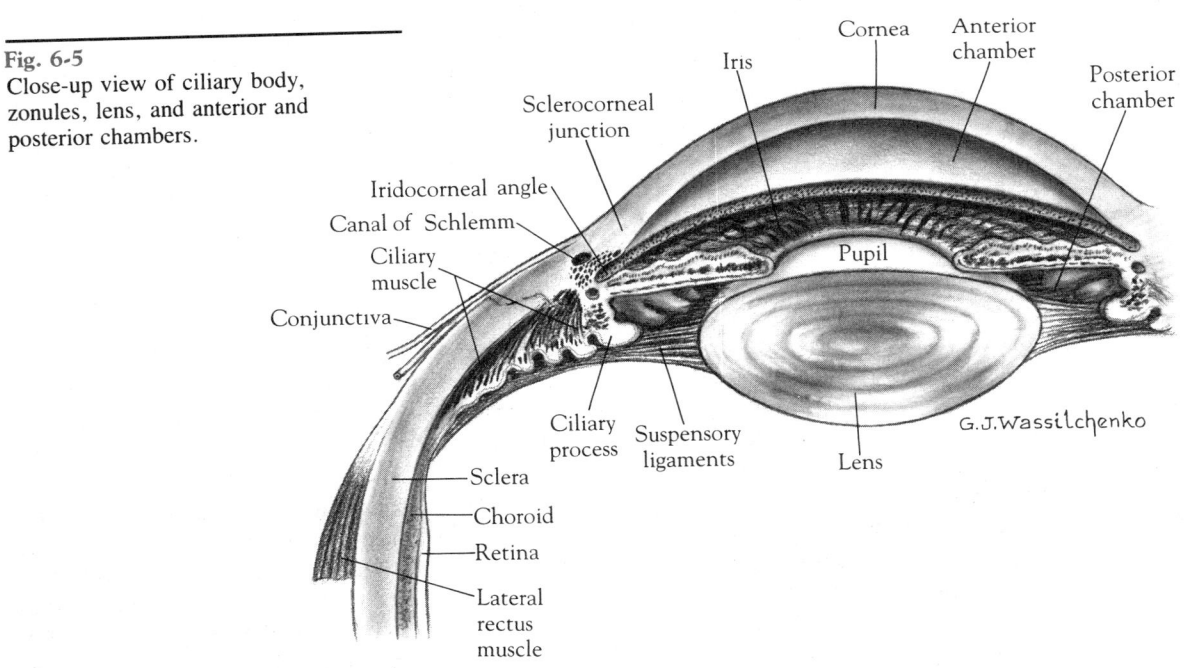

Fig. 6-5
Close-up view of ciliary body, zonules, lens, and anterior and posterior chambers.

Fig. 6-6
Posterior view of ciliary body and
surrounding structures. (Retina and
ciliary body join at ora serrata.)

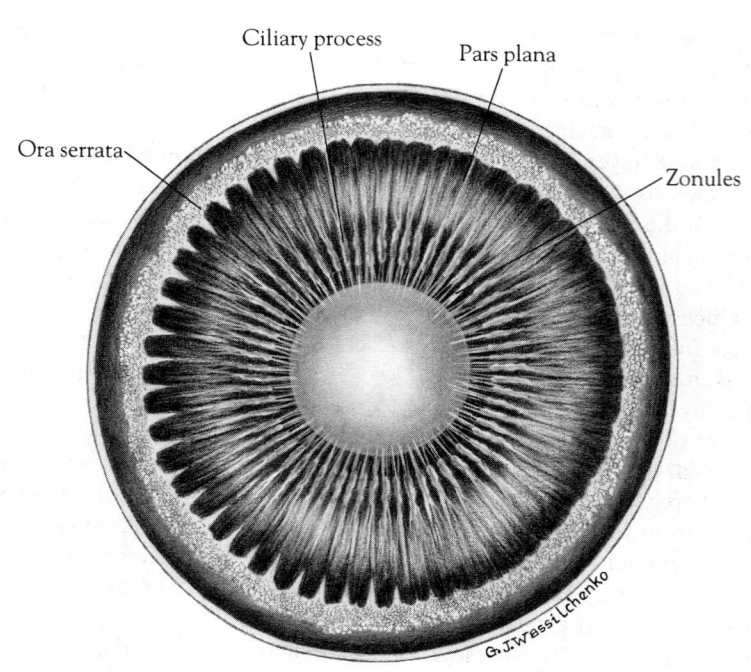

The iris is a circular muscular membrane that surrounds the pupil. The pupil is an aperture (hole) that
appears black because light cannot be seen behind it. The
iris separates the anterior and posterior eye chambers and
is positioned in front of the lens (Fig. 6-5). The iris has
two layers; the stroma, which is the anterior surface, and
the pigmented epithelium. The amount of melanin in the
stroma determines the color of the eyes. If a small amount
of melanin exists, the reflection from the pigment in the
underlying pigmented epithelium appears to be blue. The
more melanin in the stroma, the darker the iris. The
sphincter pupillae muscle is in the posterior aspect of the
stroma. It is innervated by parasympathetic fibers from
the oculomotor nerve. The iris sphincter surrounds the
pupil, and its contraction decreases pupil size. The pigmented epithelium layer contains the dilator pupillae
muscle, which dilates the pupil when contracted and is
sympathetically innervated. Pupillary response is described further in the discussion of the nervous system
of the eye.

The iris is located at the medial portion of the iridocorneal angle (Fig. 6-5), which separates the canal of
Schlemm and the underlying trabecular meshwork from
the iris. If the iris inserts at the anterior edge of the ciliary
body, the angle may become narrow. Pupillary dilation
also thickens the iris, which may affect the status of the
angle. The implications for iris location and shape in
relation to the iridocorneal angle are discussed in the
section on glaucoma.

Inner layer: retina. The retina is an extension of the
central nervous system. This inner layer begins posteriorly at the optic nerve, coats the inside of the sphere,
and ends at the ora serrata where it joins the ciliary body
(Figs. 6-4 and 6-6). The retina is normally transparent.
Ophthalmoscopic viewing shows arterioles and veins that
nourish the retina, as well as the underlying choroid layer,
which appears fluorescent and pale orange. The retina
has 10 layers and contains rods and cones (photoreceptor
cells), connecting cells that synapse with ganglion cells
in a peripheral layer, and optic nerve fibers (axons) that
pass into the optic nerve (Fig. 6-7). The pigmented epithelium (adjacent to the choroid surface) contains enzymes and protein binding sites for vitamin A, which
are necessary for the photochemical visual process. The
rods and cones, elongated cells that respond to light and
convert it into electrical energy, pass through the next
four layers. Both types of cells contain light-sensitive
pigments that undergo chemical changes necessary for
neural transmission of light. Rods are light sensitive in
low illumination (scotopic vision). Cones perceive images and color in higher levels of illumination (photopic
vision). Rods and cones are so named because of their
microscopic appearance; rods are more cylindric and generally more elongated. Rods and cones connect with each
other in the plexiform layer and synapse with a variety
of cells that ultimately reach the ganglion cells. The
ganglion cells transmit electrical discharges through their
axons to the midbrain.[17]

Fig. 6-7
Layers of retina.

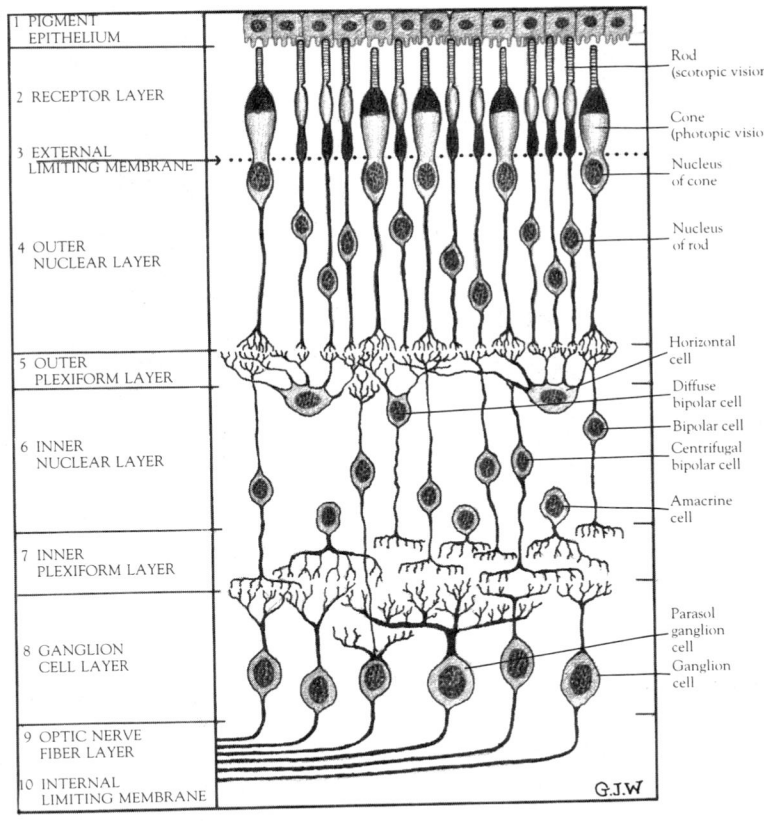

1 PIGMENT EPITHELIUM

2 RECEPTOR LAYER

3 EXTERNAL LIMITING MEMBRANE

4 OUTER NUCLEAR LAYER

5 OUTER PLEXIFORM LAYER

6 INNER NUCLEAR LAYER

7 INNER PLEXIFORM LAYER

8 GANGLION CELL LAYER

9 OPTIC NERVE FIBER LAYER

10 INTERNAL LIMITING MEMBRANE

Rod (scotopic vision)

Cone (photopic vision)

Nucleus of cone

Nucleus of rod

Horizontal cell

Diffuse bipolar cell

Bipolar cell

Centrifugal bipolar cell

Amacrine cell

Parasol ganglion cell

Ganglion cell

G.J.W

Rods and cones are dispersed irregularly in the various regions of the retinal surface. If the retina were laid out on a flat surface, its center would be the fovea centralis, a small depression containing a concentration of cones but no rods. The fovea contains about 150,000 cones/mm², each of which synapses with more than one foveal photoreceptor and ganglion cell but with fewer of these cells than elsewhere in the retina. Visual acuity is sharpest in this area if enough light is available for photopic vision. The fovea is surrounded by the macula lutea, a pigmented area about 4.5 mm in diameter. Rods are densely packed in the periphery of this region (approximately 150,000 rods/mm²) and become less dense as they extend toward the periphery. Cones average about 4500/mm² and also become sparse in the periphery.[28] The optic disc (the head of the optic nerve) perforates the retina about 3 mm toward the nose from the fovea. The disc is approximately 1.5 mm in diameter and contains no rods or cones. This results in a small physiologic blind spot for each eye located about 15 degrees laterally from the center of vision. The viewer is not aware of this because the other eye compensates for the loss. The periphery of the retina contains primarily rods. When viewed through the ophthalmoscope, the fovea appears as a small pinpoint of light surrounded by a yellow-brown pigmented area (the macula) approximately 3 mm temporally from the optic disc. The head of the optic nerve appears as a pink or cream-colored circle with a white depression in the center where the central retinal artery and central vein bifurcate, emerge, and feed into smaller branches throughout the retinal surface.

Chambers, fluids, and inner structures of the eye

Aqueous fluid and intraocular pressure. The eye contains three chambers: the anterior, the posterior, and the vitreous body. The anterior chamber is bounded anteriorly by the cornea and posteriorly by the iris. It maintains a depth of approximately 3 mm between the central portion of the cornea and the pupil.[4] It is filled with approximately 0.2 ml of aqueous humor, which flows from the posterior chamber and empties at the canal of Schlemm (Fig. 6-5). The canal of Schlemm is an oval channel that encircles the anterior chamber. The canal is a highly permeable vessel adjacent to the trabecular meshwork, which filters the fluid en route to the canal (Fig. 6-8). The meshwork also encircles the anterior chamber and lies at the apex of the iridocorneal angle. The posterior chamber is a narrow passage behind the

Fig. 6-8
Close view of trabecular meshwork
and flow of aqueous humor.

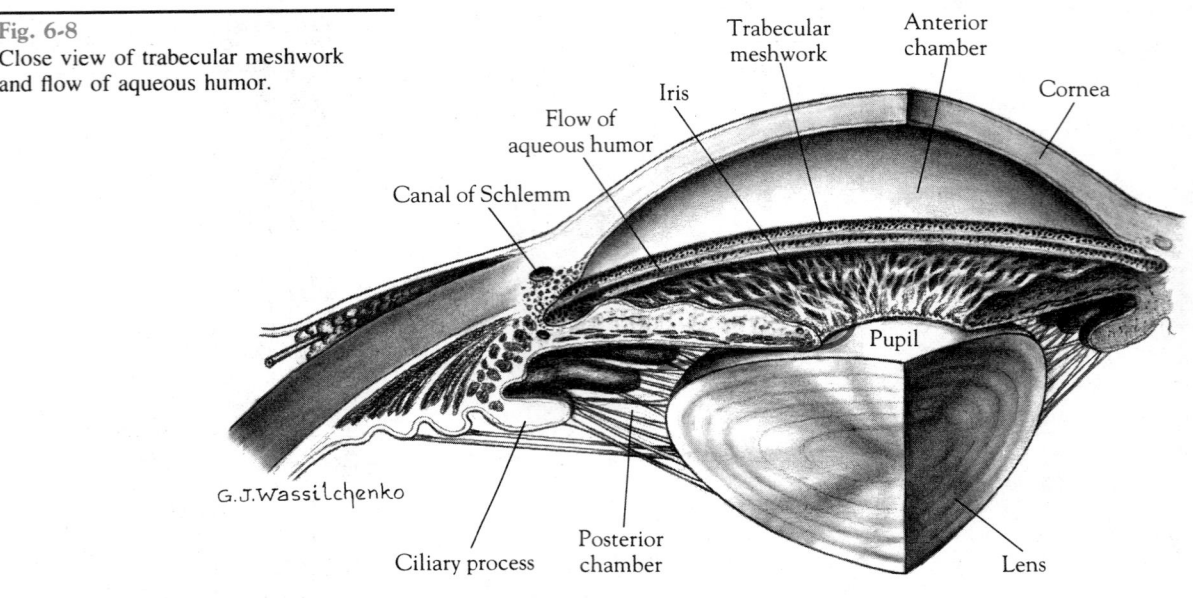

iris and in front of the lens and the ciliary body. Aqueous humor is secreted by the ciliary processes and flows into the anterior chamber through the pupil (Fig. 6-8).

Aqueous humor maintains intraocular pressure (normally within a range of 10 to 22 mm Hg), contributes to metabolism of the lens, and nourishes the cornea. Intraocular pressure is maintained by the rate of fluid secretion and the resistance to outflow by the trabecular meshwork. Eyeball pressure must exceed atmospheric pressure to maintain the contour of the sphere. Intraocular pressure fluctuates 1 to 2 mm Hg with each heartbeat. Pressure fluctuations are based on the pressure within the episcleral veins, which connect to the canal of Schlemm, and the osmotic pressure of the blood. Normal pressure changes (up to 5 mm Hg) are usually quickly compensated for by trabecular meshwork distention, which lowers outflow resistance.[28] The Valsalva maneuver (bearing down to complete a bowel movement) increases venous pressure and thus causes a marked intraocular pressure increase, which quickly returns to normal when the maneuver ceases. Drinking large quantities of water or receiving saline intravenous fluids causes a slight increase in intraocular pressure.

Lens. The lens separates the posterior chamber from the vitreous body. It is a biconvex, transparent structure that is stabilized in its position by suspensory ligaments attached to the ciliary body. The lens is composed of a capsule that encases it, a cortex (the peripheral portion), and a central core. It is transparent because its cells are predominantly anuclear. Newly formed cells, with nuclei, originate at the periphery and move toward the center where mature fibers have lost their nuclei. New fibers

are formed throughout the life span of the lens and continue to migrate and become compressed in the center core. Therefore an older lens is larger, denser, less elastic, and less able to contract to accommodate for near vision. The lens also maintains transparency by its ability to avoid excessive hydration. The lens is surrounded by media that are high in sodium. The lens membrane is relatively impermeable to sodium and lens metabolism pumps out sodium, which decreases osmotic activity. The lens becomes yellow in middle age, which diminishes the intensity of blue-toned light on the retina.[17]

Vitreous body. The vitreous cavity contains approximately 4.5 ml of vitreous humor, a gelatinous substance that adheres firmly to its adjacent structures: the retina, the ciliary epithelium (at the base of the lens), and the margin of the optic nerve. If the vitreous humor diminishes in volume or degenerates, retinal tears may occur because of traction on the retina.

Image Formation

Light reception and refraction. The receptors of the eye are sensitive to only a small portion of the electromagnetic spectrum. Massless particles called photons, which travel in wavelengths between 400 and 700 nm, stimulate retinal photoreceptors and become visible light to the human observer. Light in wavelengths less than 400 nm or greater than 700 nm is not absorbed by rods and cones and therefore not seen.[23]

To reach the retina, light must pass through the clear media of the cornea, aqueous fluid, the lens, and the vitreous body. Light rays are emitted in all directions

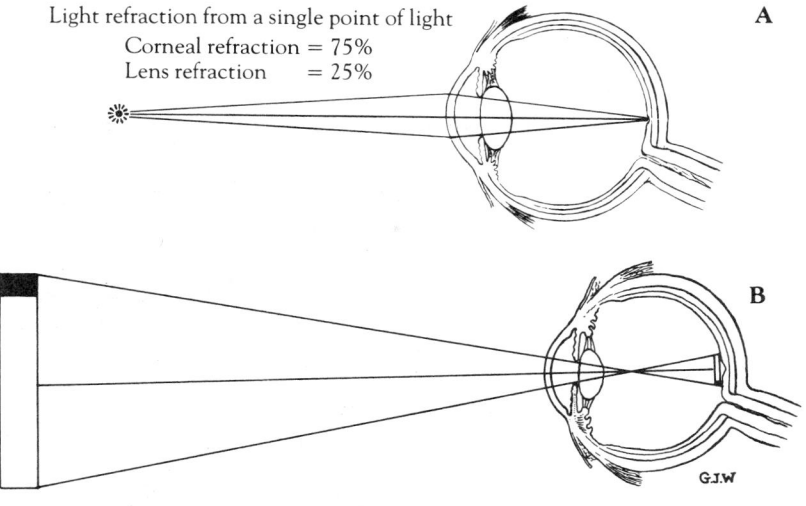

Fig. 6-9
A, Light refraction from single point of light. **B,** Light refraction from object with more than one point of light.

Light refraction from a single point of light
Corneal refraction = 75%
Lens refraction   = 25%

A

B

from any single source. These divergent waves pass through the optic system, which focuses them at a specific point to achieve image accuracy.

When a ray of light passes from one clear medium into another, its velocity is affected by the density of the medium. The density of the cornea slows the light ray, and the curvature of the cornea bends it. This process is known as refraction. The surface of the cornea is curved so light rays emitted from a single source hit the surface at different angles but are bent to redirect them to the lens, which further bends and directs them to a single point on the retina (Fig. 6-9, *A*). When a person focuses on an object, the light waves from that object are directed to the fovea centralis for image identification and clarity (called focal vision). Most objects have more than one point of focus. As different points of focus from an object reach the retina, they form an image that is upside down and reversed (Fig. 6-9, *B*). Light waves also enter the eye from a wide visual field (approximately 170-degree arc for each eye) that surrounds the object of focus. These peripheral sources focus on the periphery of the retina (ambient vision) and assist with spatial sense.[28]

The anterior surface of the cornea is the primary refractive area of the eye. The more a surface bends light rays, the greater the refractive power. The shift in the direction of light from air to corneal surface is greater than the second shift at the lens surface.

Accommodation. Accommodation is the process by which the lens alters its shape for visual clarity when the eye is viewing an object at close range. In other words, the lens surface increases its refractive power (becomes thicker and more convex) to accommodate near objects. Normally the lens is somewhat flattened and held taut by the ligaments that attach to the circular ciliary muscle.

When these muscles contract, the ligaments relax and release their tension on the lens. The lens contracts and becomes more spheric. The lens is constantly adjusting to stimuli at different distances. Ciliary branches of the oculomotor nerve respond to brain signals for this automatic response.

Binocular vision and vergence. Normal eyes are aligned in their respective orbits in such a way that they can direct light rays from an outer object to the fovea centralis of each eye. The visual axis is an imaginary line that is drawn from each fovea centralis to a fixation point. When a three-dimensional object is focused on the back of both eyes, a slight disparity occurs in the horizontal placement of the two retinal images. This slight difference sets up two images in the brain, which permits the binocular viewer to experience the visual sensation of depth (stereopsis).

Vergence is a visual reflex of simultaneous eye movements. When distant objects are viewed, the visual axes of the eyes become more parallel and the eyes are rotated outward (divergence). As the fixation point draws nearer, the medius rectus muscles contract and pull the eyes inward (convergence).[1] This reflex is necessary to prevent diplopia (double vision). If a person holds a finger about 10 inches in front of his nose and focuses on the finger, he sees one finger. If he suddenly shifts his focus to a distant object, he sees two fingers because the parallel visual axes do not meet at the finger.

Image Interpretation

Visual pathway. Vision occurs when refracted light rays stimulate retinal photoreceptors, are converted into electrical energy, and are transmitted to different cerebral

Fig. 6-10
Visual pathway.

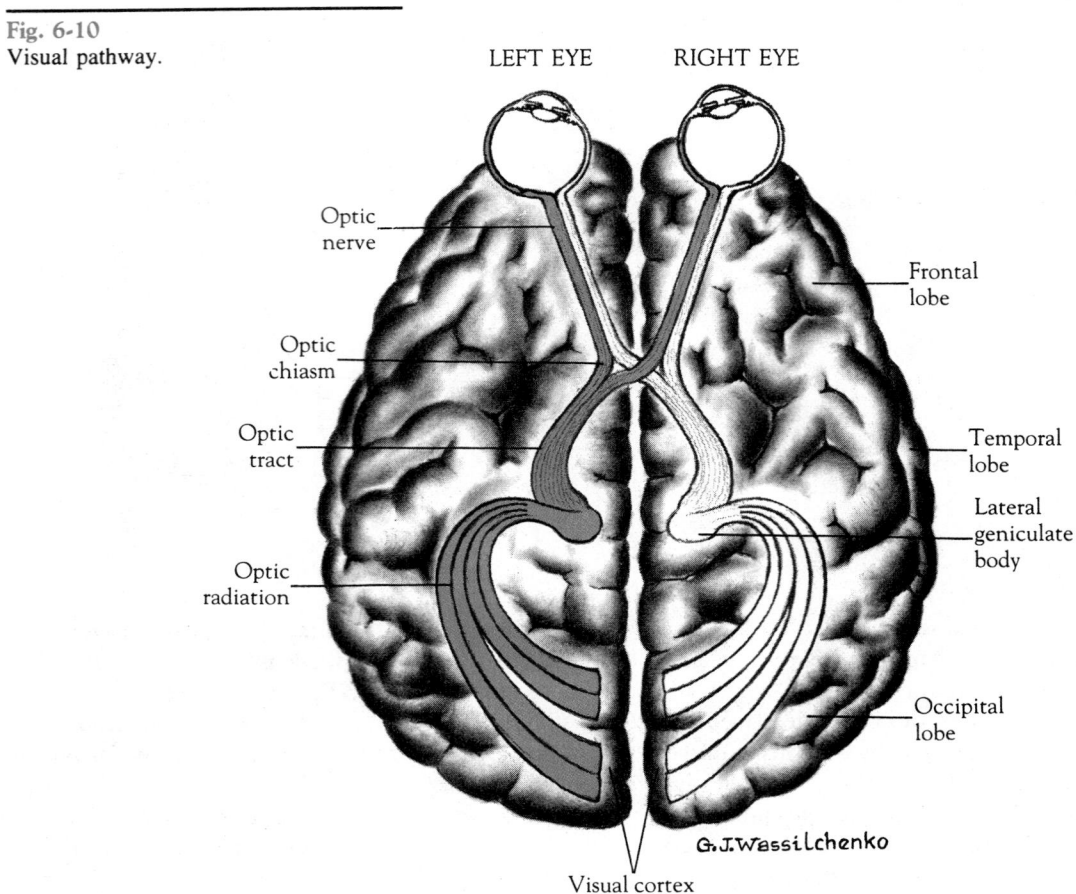

LEFT EYE   RIGHT EYE

Optic nerve

Optic chiasm

Optic tract

Optic radiation

Frontal lobe

Temporal lobe

Lateral geniculate body

Occipital lobe

G.J.Wassilchenko

Visual cortex

cortical areas for interpretation. Light rays constantly bombard and stimulate photoreceptors. Rods and cones contain specific pigments (opsins) that combine with a form of vitamin A to absorb light and convert it to a graded electrical potential. These photoreceptors synapse with second- and third-order neurons within the retina, which converge into fibers that enter the optic nerve. The optic nerve forms the optic disc and exits the eyeball at the posterior region. The choroid and all the retinal layers except the nerve fiber layer end at the edge of the disc.

The optic nerve contains over 1 million fibers (axons of ganglion cells), which control vision, eye movement, and pupillary reflexes. As the optic nerve exits from the sphere, it is encased in dura mater, an arachnoid sheath, and pia mater and forms an S-shaped curve to allow for stretching with eye movement. The orbital portion of the nerve is about 30 mm long. The optic nerve also contains the central retinal artery and vein, which bifurcate and branch into the eyeball near the head of the nerve (the disc). The central artery and vein exit from the optic nerve about 12 mm behind the eyeball.[28]

The optic nerves from each eye pass through the optic foramen and meet at the optic chiasm, which lies above and in front of the pituitary gland. Optic tracts emerge from the chiasm and are directed laterally to encircle the hypothalamus and terminate in the lateral geniculate bodies in the temporal lobes (Fig. 6-10). Cells in the lateral geniculate bodies send fibers (optic radiation) to the occipital lobe of each cerebral hemisphere. The visual cortex in the posterior aspect of the occipital lobe receives a majority of visual fibers representing central vision (stimuli from the fovea centralis and the surrounding macula). Adjacent occipital lobe areas receive fibers representing the more peripheral portions of the retina. Reversed images are righted when perceived in the cortex.

Objects in the visual field stimulate the opposite side of the retina. In other words, a fixation point on a person's right (temporal) side would stimulate the nasal aspect of the right eye (Fig. 6-11). A superiorly located object would stimulate the inferior aspect of the retina, and an inferior object would be directed superiorly. When nerve fibers pass into the optic nerve, the nasal and temporal fibers are separate within the sheath. Temporal fibers pass on the temporal side of the nerve, nasal fibers are on the nasal side, and central (foveal) fibers are in the center of the nerve. When the nerves merge at the chiasm, nasal fibers cross (decussate) to the opposite optic tract. Temporal fibers do not cross but continue in the optic tract on the same side as the nerve that conveys them to the chiasm (Fig. 6-10). Therefore the pathway of vision for an object seen on a person's right side would be through nasal receptors in the right eye and then through the nasal side of the optic nerve to the chiasm, where it would cross to the left optic tract and proceed to the left cerebral occipital lobe. Visual field defects can often be traced to disorders in specific anatomic locations because of the arrangement of nerve fibers. A left or right optic nerve lesion would cause a corresponding defect in the left or right eye. Chiasm lesions can cause a variety of defects depending on the location of the lesion; a common defect is bitemporal hemianopia, which results from a pituitary tumor. A left optic tract lesion would result in a bilateral right visual field deficit. These defects are depicted in Fig. 6-12.

Light and dark adaptation. The concentration of pigment in the photoreceptor cells of the retina determines the sensitivity of these cells to light. Photoreceptive pigments are constantly being used and replaced through chemical changes in the retina. When the eyes

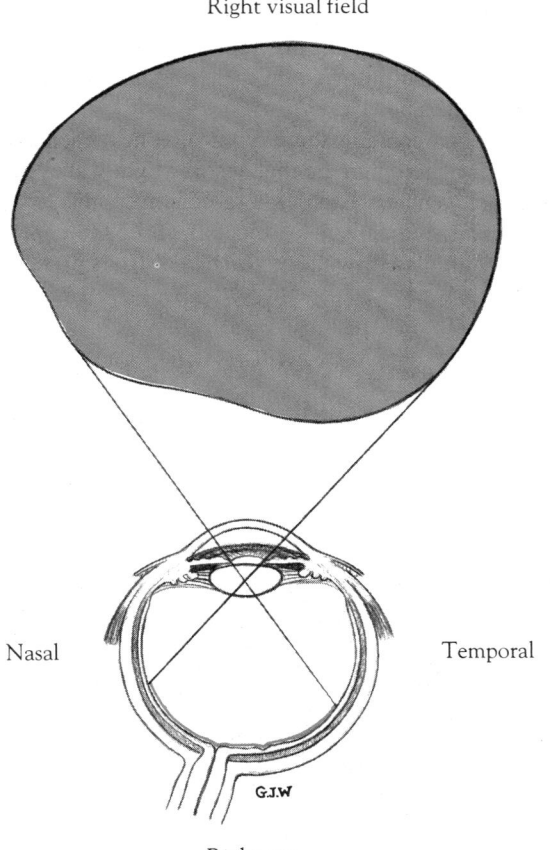

Fig. 6-11
Image placement on retina.

Right visual field

Nasal

Temporal

G.J.W

Right eye

Fig. 6-12
Visual pathway defects.

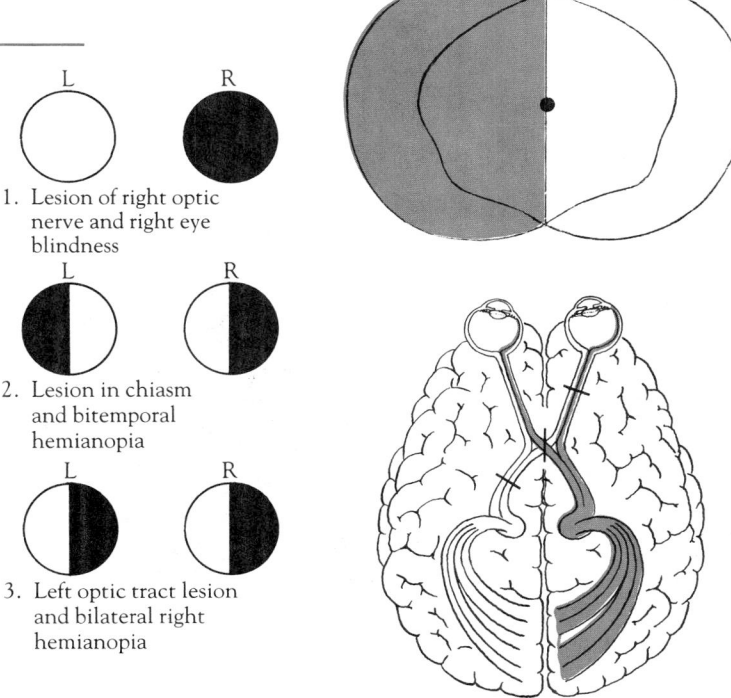

1. Lesion of right optic nerve and right eye blindness

2. Lesion in chiasm and bitemporal hemianopia

3. Left optic tract lesion and bilateral right hemianopia

LEFT   RIGHT

are exposed to bright light, the pigments become bleached (used) and the sensitivity of the photoreceptors diminishes. Bright light causes discomfort for several minutes until breakdown of the photopigments produces a gradual rise of the visual threshold. Coupled with pupillary constriction, decreased rod and cone sensitivity to light protects the retinal cells in bright light. This is called light adaptation.[17]

Exposure to darkness tends to stimulate an increase of photopigment regeneration to increase sensitivity to light. Rhodopsin, the photopigment in rods, is particularly sensitive to dim light and enables a person to visualize dim forms and shapes in near darkness. Since rhodopsin does not absorb color wavelengths, color is not perceived in dim light. Dark adaptation involves pupillary dilation and regeneration of rhodopsin to increase sensitivity to light.

Color perception. Light waves do not contain color. Color is perceived by humans according to the wavelength (frequency) of a light ray. Colors are determined by hue, or the standard recognition of a particular shade, and saturation, or the intensity of a color. A less intense color contains larger amounts of white and appears relatively pale. Any object that reflects all visible light rays evokes a sensation of white. The absence of light rays is perceived as black.

The retina contains three types of cones, each having a different photopigment that absorbs light waves of different frequencies. Each type of cone responds to a primary color: red, green, or blue. If all of the cones are equally stimulated, white is perceived. Rods do not perceive color.[17]

Eye Movement

The movement of each eye is controlled by six muscles. Four of these (the recti) originate posterior to the eyeball,

Fig. 6-13
Extraocular muscles.

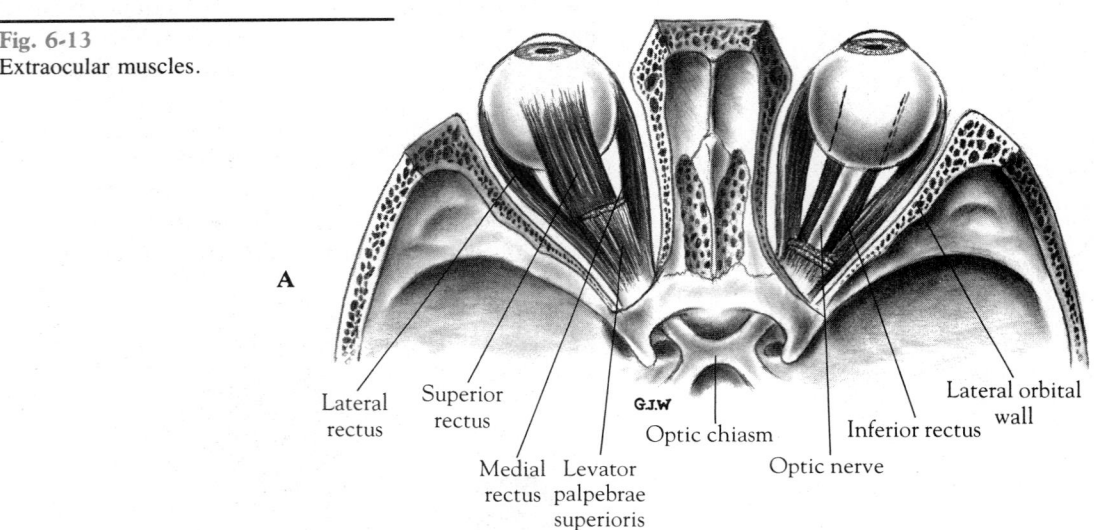

A

Lateral rectus Superior rectus G.J.W Optic chiasm Inferior rectus Lateral orbital wall

Medial rectus Levator palpebrae superioris Optic nerve

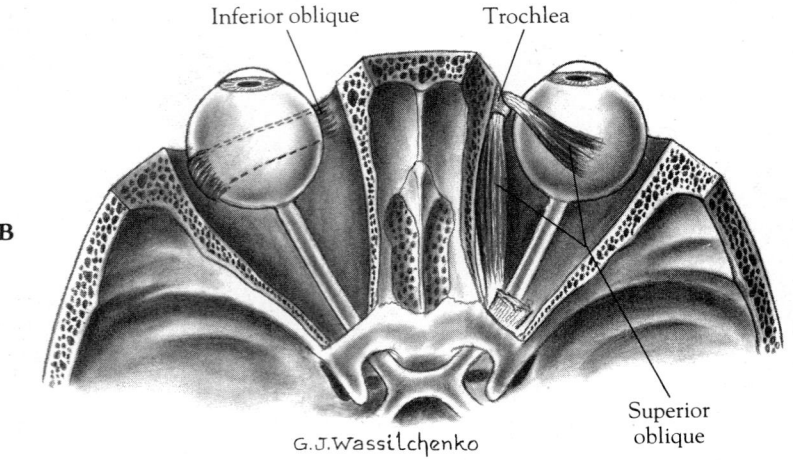

B

Inferior oblique Trochlea

Superior oblique

G.J.Wassilchenko

project forward around the sphere, and insert into the sclera about 7 mm behind the limbus (Fig. 6-13, *A*). The superior oblique muscle arises at the posterior orbit, passes forward to the anterior orbital rim, loops through the trochlea (a fibrocartilaginous structure) to return to the eyeball, and inserts into the sclera under the belly of the superior rectus muscle (Fig. 6-13, *B*). The sixth muscle, the inferior oblique, originates at the nasal side of the orbit and passes under the eyeball to attach at its lateral surface (Fig. 6-13, *B*). The oculomotor nerve (CN III) supplies the medial, inferior, and superior rectus muscles and the inferior oblique muscle. The trochlear nerve (CN IV) supplies the superior oblique muscle, and the abducens nerve (CN VI) supplies the lateral rectus muscle (Fig. 6-14).[1]

Contraction of an eye muscle turns the eye toward that muscle. For example, medial rectus contraction rotates the eye toward the nose. The antagonist muscle stretches or relaxes to permit eyeball rotation. If the eye rotates inward (nasally), the medial rectus contracts and the lateral rectus relaxes. All six muscles are constantly coordinating stretch and contraction functions to permit full and continuous eye movement.

Both eyes must move together to maintain a clear focus. When a person looks to the right, the right lateral rectus muscle and the left medial rectus muscle contract. The innervation stimulus to both muscles is equal, so the speed and destination of the two eyeball movements are equal. Muscles that produce equal movement of each eye in the same direction are called yoke muscles. Conjugate ocular movements are simultaneous, equal, and coordinated eye movements.[1]

The fibers within the extraocular muscles are highly differentiated. Eye muscles are capable of slow graded contractions and very rapid contractions. Rapid eye movements may be voluntary or involuntary. One type of rapid reflex movement is called saccade. Saccadic movements are small rapid jerks that alternate with steady

Table 6-1

Summary of Major Nervous System Mechanisms of the Eye

Function	Mechanism
Lid movement	
Oculomotor (CN III)	Innervates levator palpebrae superioris and inferior rectus
Facial (CN VII)	Innervates orbicularis oculi
Sensation (trigeminal [CN V])	Ophthalmic division for upper lid; maxillary division for lower lid
Reflex response	Sympathetic fibers from superior cervical ganglion innervate palpebral muscles
Tears	Normal moisture maintained by secretory function of palpebral accessory glands; excess tears mediated through stimulation of facial nerve (CN VII) and trigeminal nerve (CN V)
Corneal sensation	Trigeminal nerve (CN V)
Pupil	
Constriction	Light stimulates retina and afferent fibers that pass through optic nerve (CN II) and chiasm and then deviate from tract to area of midbrain (superior colliculus); axons leave this area and connect to nucleus of oculomotor nerve (CN III), which sends efferent fibers to ciliary ganglion (between optic chiasm and posterior orbit); parasympathetic fibers leave ciliary ganglion and enter eye to stimulate iris sphincter
Consensual response	Both pupils constrict when only one is stimulated; oculomotor nucleus responds to afferent fibers from one eye and sends signals through its fibers and parasympathetic fibers to both iris muscles
Dilation	Reduction of parasympathetic tonic flow to iris sphincters in dim light; sympathetic stimulation of fibers from carotid plexus occurs with startle or pleasure responses
Lens accommodation	Oculomotor nerve (CN III) mediates parasympathetic stimulation for ciliary muscle contraction and resultant lens convexity
Vision	Light focuses on retinal receptors; axons pass into optic nerve (CN II), chiasm, optic tracts, lateral geniculate bodies, and optic radiation to occipital lobe and visual cortex
Eye movement	Conjugate movements occur because nuclei of CN III, IV, and VI connect in fiber tract in midbrain
Oculomotor nerve (CN III)	Innervates superior rectus, medial rectus, inferior rectus, and inferior oblique muscles
Trochlear nerve (CN IV)	Innervates superior oblique muscle
Abducent nerve (CN VI)	Innervates lateral rectus muscle

Data from Jensen, D.: The principles of physiology, ed. 2, New York, 1980, Appleton-Century-Crofts; Newell, F.W.: Ophthalmology: principles and concepts, ed. 5, St. Louis, 1982, The C.V. Mosby Co.; and Vaughn, D., and Asbury, T.: General ophthalmology, ed. 10, Los Altos, Calif., 1983, Lange Medical Publications.

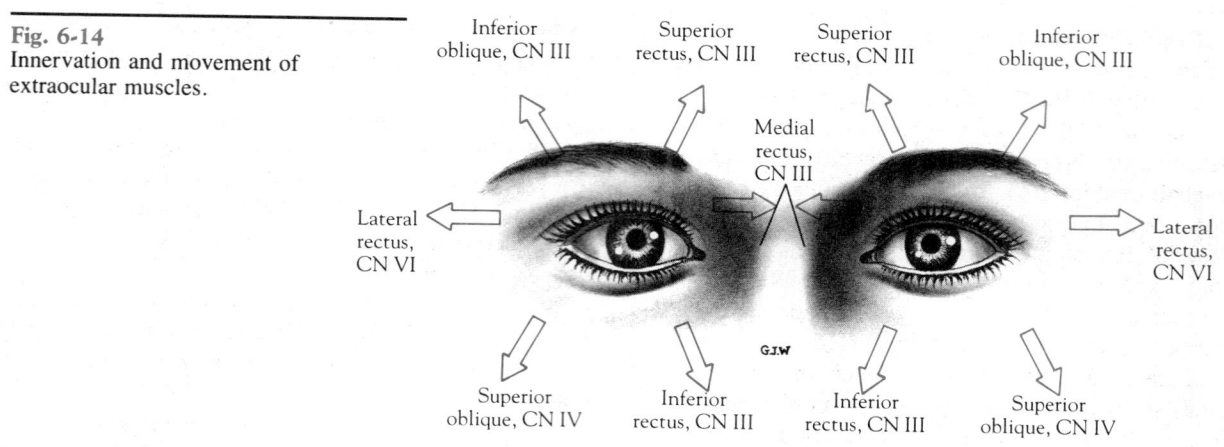

Fig. 6-14
Innervation and movement of extraocular muscles.

fixation (particularly when the eye is focusing on a near object). Saccadic movements bring peripheral retinal images to the fovea centralis for clarity. These movements also sweep images over retinal receptors to prevent light adaptation. If one continued to focus an image in one retinal area, color and detail would fade in a few seconds. Saccade also occurs during sleep as rapid eye movement (REM).[23]

Reflexes from the vestibular apparatus permit the eyes to maintain a steady gaze of fixation in spite of head movements. If the head turns to the right, the eyes can

shift an equal rotation to the left. Upward head movement causes downward rotation of the eyes.

In summary, eye movements can be classified as (1) tracking (slow, smooth, coordinated rotations for maintaining the image of an object on the fovea centralis); (2) vergence (slow, smooth movements that rotate the eyes inward or outward to track an object in depth); (3) saccadic movements (rapid reflexes that alternate with fixation for clarity and image maintenance); and (4) compensatory movements (reflexes that coordinate head movement with object fixation and steady gaze).

NORMAL FINDINGS[4,34,37,38,43]

Area of Concern	Normal Adult Findings	Variations in Child	Variations in Older Adult
Eyelids	Blink response to light or corneal touch; frequent involuntary bilateral blinks (average 15-20/minute); lid margins rest over inferior and superior borders of cornea	Eyes usually closed at birth, blink response to light or corneal touch; voluntary blink intact at 28 weeks	
Eyeball	Anteroposterior diameter 22-27 mm Caucasian: Eyeball does not protrude beyond supraorbital bridge of frontal bone Negroid: Eyeball may protrude slightly beyond ridge	Birth: Relatively short anteroposterior diameter (average 17.3 mm) and less spheric than adult 8 years: Globe is adult sized	
Lacrimal function	Eyeball surface moist; excess tears in response to emotion or noxious atmospheric stimuli; puncta nontender and without discharge on palpation	Birth-2 weeks: Tear glands begin to secrete; nasolacrimal duct opens 6-12 weeks: Tears produced with emotion	Over 50 years: Diminished reflex response for excess tearing
Conjunctivae	Palpebral: Pink with uniform small vessels showing no discharge Bulbar: Clear, tiny, red vessels may be visible		Bulbar: May lack luster of young adult

Area of Concern	Normal Adult Findings	Variations in Child	Variations in Older Adult
Sclera	White; slight overall yellowish cast or black dots (pigmentation) in dark skinned-individuals		
Cornea	Transparent; smooth surface; convex curvature	Birth: Flatter surface than adult 2 years: Adult curvature	Arcus senilis (gray ring of lipid deposit around limbus)
Iris	Rounded; consistent, bilateral coloration	Birth: Dark blue appearance 20-28 weeks: Permanent color established	Bilateral irregularity of pigment density (color may appear paler)
Pupil	Equal; round; reacts to light and accommodation; consensual response	Birth: Miotic; equal; round; reacts to light Twelve months: Diameter nearing adult size	Often miotic with slower dilation reaction to dark
Anterior chamber	Clear; approximately 3.3 mm between cornea and iris		Becomes slightly shallower with aging
Internal eye Retina	Full, round, bilateral red reflex Uniform pink and granular texture (negroid surface uniformly more pigmented); choroid layer may be visible showing linear light orange vessels	Periphery mature at birth; many movable light reflections on surface	May appear slightly paler
Vessels	Central vein and artery emerge on nasal side of physiologic cup within disc, and each immediately breaks into two branches; arteries light red and 25% narrower than dark red veins; narrow band of light may appear at center of arteries; vessel caliber regular and uniformly decreases as vessel branches toward periphery; venous pulsations more prominent in young adults		Arteries slightly narrower; arterial light reflex may be widened; arterial caliber may be slightly irregular
Disc, cup	Whitish, cream, or pink; vertically oval or round with distinct border (nasal side may be slightly less demarcated and temporal border may appear as grayish crescent); approximately 1.5 mm diameter (magnified 15 times through ophthalmoscope); cup is small, white or pale depression in center of disc and occupies approximately half of disc diameter		Disc may appear slightly smaller and more opaque
Macula, fovea	Macula is darker area two disc diameters temporally from disc; fovea is pinpoint bright light in center of macula	Birth: Macula absent 1 year: Macula fully mature	
Visual acuity Distant vision	20/20 (able to read designated size letter on standardized chart at 20 feet distance)	Birth: 20/300 20 weeks: 20/200 1 year: 20/200 2 years: 20/100 3 years: 20/50 4-5 years: 20/20	20/20-20/30
Near vision	Able to read newsprint at 14 inches	Birth: Hyperopic (owing to shape of eyeball) 1-2 years: Can increasingly fixate on small objects 3-5 years: Approaching reading readiness	Presbyopic owing to loss of lens refractive power (average person over 60 years cannot focus more closely than 3 feet without corrective lenses)

Area of Concern	Normal Adult Findings	Variations in Child	Variations in Older Adult
Peripheral vision	Temporal vision 90 degrees from central visual axis Upward: 50 degrees Nasalward: 60 degress Downward: 70 degrees		May be slightly diminished but usually not measurable with confrontation testing
Eye movement, co-ordination, and interpretation	Both eyes demonstrate coordinated, parallel movements in six cardinal fields of gaze; physiologic nystagmus (mild rhythmic twitching if eye held in extreme gaze); eyes converge and diverge in smooth coordinated fashion as person focuses on near and far objects; tracking, saccadic, and compensatory movements enable person to perceive objects clearly in depth and accurately in terms of distance and surrounding space	Birth: Poor coordination but able to fixate briefly on moving object at 8-10 inches; doll's head reflex (when head is turned, eyes lag behind) 4 weeks: Able to watch speaking parent intently when face is held close 6 weeks: Brief binocular fixation 8 weeks: Vergence still jerky and inexact 12 weeks: Doll's head reflex disappears; convergence on near vision intact 16-20 weeks: Binocular vision established; interest in stimuli more than 3 feet away; able to fixate on ½-inch block and inspect hands 1 year: Depth perception developing; visual loss may develop if binocular vision not intact; eye muscles fully functional 18 months: Interpretation of distance and space improving 2-3 years: Able to recall visual images; convergence is smoother 3-5 years: Able to copy geometric figures; approaching reading readiness 6 years: Depth perception fully developed	
Color perception	Able to identify all colors accurately when tested with series of pictures or cards that present multicolored field for color differentiation	20-28 weeks: Development of color preference for red and yellow	Brightness of colors may be dimmed; yellow overcast to hues owing to aging lens

DIAGNOSTIC STUDIES[28,36,40]

Mydriatic medication

Short-acting, topical medication used for pupil dilation during direct ophthalmoscopy; sympathomimetic (adrenergic) drugs such as phenylephrine (2.5% to 10%) or parasympatholytic (anticholinergic) drugs such as eucatropine (2% to 5%) used; drug should dilate pupil but not inhibit accommodation; cycloplegic drugs (which inhibit accommodation) used for indirect ophthalmoscopy to maintain pupil dilation in very bright light

Nursing care:

May be contraindicated with shallow anterior chamber, certain intraocular lens implants, or vascular hypertension; remove contact lenses before instilling drops

Direct ophthalmoscopy

Examiner uses ophthalmoscope to view retinal surface and inner structures of eye; pupils usually *dilated*, and examination takes place in dark room; retinal structures and vessels magnified 15 times

Nursing care:
Indicate length of effect of medication used to dilate pupil and limitation in vision

Indirect ophthalmoscopy
Examiner wears head-mounted binocular instrument; patient is supine; examiner stands 30 inches away and holds convex lens over patient's eye for focusing; image is magnified four to five times; greater visual field can be viewed than with direct ophthalmoscopy; scleral depressor (blunt rod) may be used to compress eyeball so ora serrata (tissue behind iris) can be viewed

Nursing care:
Assure client that mild or no discomfort will be experienced if scleral depressor is used

Fluorescein angiography
10% solution of sodium fluorescein injected into antecubital vein is relayed to retinal arteries in 10 to 16 seconds and to veins in 25 seconds; pupils are dilated with short-acting cycloplegics in combination with mydriatic; ophthalmoscope with blue filter can show entire diameter of vessel, whereas ordinary ophthalmoscopy provides only surface view

Nursing care:
Inquire about previous allergy to fluorescein (allergic response usually hives and itching); subcutaneous leakage of dye causes local burning; patient may experience brief hot flash or nausea; temporary yellowish discoloration of sclera may occur until dye is excreted in urine (within 48 hours); inform patient what to expect in terms of effect on vision

Photography
Black and white film with appropriate filters used in camera that takes rapid sequence photographs from 9 to 30 seconds after injection of fluorescein; patient and examiner are seated at table opposite each other, each looking into camera

Ultrasonography (diagnostic ultrasound)
Ultrasound machine uses high-frequency waves (5000 to 20,000 Hz) to detect vibrations reflected from soft tissues of varying density; vibrations (echoes) are converted into electrical potential and displayed on oscillograph; A-scan machine registers varying acoustic densities as spikes on linear tracing; B-scan registers two-dimensional "picture" of eye and its contents; useful for diagnosing intraocular tumors, retinal detachment, and fibrous tissue proliferation; examiner holds probe (attached to machine) over patient's eyelid

Computed tomography
X-ray beam scans transverse axial slices of head and gives off light that is reconstructed as image by computer; image is much more accurate than conventional roentgenograms and is useful for contrasting orbital contents and tumors because of differences in tissue density; procedure is noninvasive and has become primary procedure for x-ray diagnosis of eye disorders

Tonometry
Several types of instruments (tonometers) measure intraocular pressure; all of them indent globe and measure force (or weight) necessary to cause indentation

Nursing care:
Sterilize tonometer daily and clean before each use; inquire about corneal injuries or abrasions; assure patient that no discomfort will be experienced

Schiötz
Hand-held instrument with curved footplate that is rested on cornea; local anesthetic is instilled in each eye; patient lies supine and is asked to stare straight ahead; examiner holds lids open; as tonometer is placed on corneal surface, scale reading is taken from instrument and converted with chart to pressure in mm Hg

Applanation
Machine that measures force required to flatten rather than indent central cornea; more accurate than Schiötz tonometry; spring tension knob records pressure; local anesthetic is used

Noncontact
Machine that uses rapid puff of air to exert and register pressure; does not require anesthetic and is very accurate except in higher pressure ranges; cannot be used for patients with corneal edema or those with irregular optic interface

Conditions, Diseases, and Disorders

DISORDERS OF THE EYELID

Lid disorders are extremely common and varied. Since the lids are responsible for tear maintenance and dispersion, structure and position defects can result in excess tears or drying of the eyeball surface. Deformities and movement abnormalities interfere with the lid's vital protective function and with vision. Structure and movement malfunctions alter facial expression and appearance and create cosmetic concerns. Many pain receptors are near the lid margin, and stretching and inflammation of the tissue result in acute discomfort. Since the palpebral conjunctiva is adjacent to the lid margin, disorders in this area can produce acute and diffuse redness of the eye.

Two types of lid disorders are covered: those involving position, structure, and movement and inflammatory disorders. Most disorders of lid structure and function require surgical intervention if localized nerve or muscle malfunction is diagnosed as the causative factor. Inflammatory disorders can affect the glands in the eyelids, the eyelid margins, and the meibomian glands. The skin of the eyelids may also be involved in a variety of inflammations because of the skin's looseness, its exposed position, and the secondary involvement of the eye. Contact dermatitis is common in the eye area because of use of cosmetics and frequent rubbing of the eyes.

Entropion

Entropion is an abnormal turning inward of the margin of the eyelid.

PATHOPHYSIOLOGY

The lower lid is most commonly involved.[40] Involution of the lid can be caused by atrophy of the lower lid retractor muscle (atonia), spasms of the orbicularis oculi muscle, or scarring and deformity of the tarsal plate resulting from trauma or chemical or inflammatory assaults. Atonia is relatively common in the elderly and can occur in varying degrees of severity. If the lashes are turned inward, corneal and conjunctival inflammation may occur. Spastic entropion results from chronic or acute irritation of the horizontal muscle. Corneal inflammation, conjunctivitis, and ocular surgery are common causes of spasm. Congenital entropion occurs with a deformity of the tarsal plate.

TREATMENT PLAN

Surgical
  Orbicularis procedure—small section of orbicularis oculi muscle is resected to tighten remaining muscle farthest from lid margin, which results in peripheral lid eversion
  Tarsal resection—wedge of tarsal plate is removed, which prevents lid margin from rotating inward
  Mucosal graft—scarred, atrophied conjunctiva may be replaced with section of mucous membrane from mouth[28,40]

Supportive
  For entropion (spasm from irritation), remove irritation (such as eye dressing) to reduce or relieve spasms; stabilize lower lid with pressure patch or tape lower lid to cheek for temporary relief

ASSESSMENT: AREAS OF CONCERN

Eyelid and lashes
  Lashes turned inward; possible tear spillage

Cornea and conjunctiva
  Possible conjunctivitis; secondary corneal infection

NURSING DIAGNOSES and NURSING INTERVENTIONS

Nursing Diagnosis	Nursing Intervention
Injury, potential for: cornea and conjunctiva (related to entropion spasms or inverted eyelashes)	Monitor eye for inflammatory signs. Remove irritation if possible (for example, by removing eye dressing). Splint or stabilize everted lid by taping to cheek. Place pressure patch over eye.
Injury, potential for: cornea and conjunctiva (related to inadequate tearing)	Monitor eye for symptoms of dryness. Administer artificial tears, sustained-release tear insert, or lubricating ointment as ordered. Be certain that lid is closed when applying dressing.
Anxiety	Assess level of anxiety. Listen to patient's concerns. Provide supportive counseling.
Sensory-perceptual alteration: visual (related to use of unilateral eye patch)	*Before surgery:* Warn patient that depth perception will be lost and that 50% of peripheral vision will be lost on affected side. *After surgery:* Assist patient with activities of daily living. Caution patient to bring hand forward slowly to touch objects (especially containers of hot liquid and containers receiving poured liquids). Explain that patient should turn head fully toward affected side to view objects or obstacles. Teach patient to use up and down head movements to judge stair dimensions and oncoming objects when walking and to proceed slowly.[24]

Sensory-perceptual alteration: visual (related to use of bilateral eye patches)	*Before surgery:*
	Warn patient that eyes will be patched.
	Orient patient to bedside equipment and room arrangement.
	Arrange for placement of personal belongings in advance and review plan with patient.
	Warn patient that side rails will be raised for safety.
	
	After surgery:
	Raise side rails.
	Address patient by name from doorway and identify self.
	Complement voice stimulation with touch to notify patient of your proximity.
	Reorient patient to equipment (such as call light) and personal belongings at bedside by directing patient's hand.
	Encourage patient to perform self-care with personal hygiene.
	Ensure patient's privacy, and assure patient that he will have privacy.
	Provide patient with television set or radio to encourage mental and memory stimulation.
	Engage patient in discussions about news or other items heard.
	Provide patient with clock that can be felt and remind patient of date.
	Discourage napping, which patient may want to do as he loses track of time.
	Assist patient with meals.
	  Read menu selections.
	  Guide hand to utensils and food on tray.
	  Describe food on tray in clock terms (for example, coffee is at 2 o'clock, knife and spoon are at 3 o'clock).
	  Assist with cutting meats, removing lids from containers, buttering bread, and so on.
	Assist with walking.
	  Walk slowly and slightly ahead of patient; his hand should rest on your arm at elbow.
	  If possible, allow patient to trace his progress by running the dorsal aspect of his free hand along a wall.
	  Describe surroundings as you proceed.
	  Warn of steps, turns, and narrow passageways in advance.
	  Allow patient to feel chair, toilet, or bed before he turns to sit.[24]

Nursing Diagnosis	Nursing Intervention
Comfort, alteration in: pain (related to postoperative eyelid surgery)	Inquire about discomfort. Give pain medication as ordered.
Injury: potential for (to surgically repaired lid, related to nausea or vomiting)	Monitor patient's feelings of nausea. Request order for antiemetic and administer if needed.

Patient Education

1. Teach the patient to avoid rubbing or picking at the eyes.

EVALUATION

Patient Outcome	Data Indicating That Outcome is Reached
Cornea and conjunctiva are healthy.	Cornea is transparent, smooth, glossy, and moist. Palpebral conjunctiva is homogeneous pink color and bulbar conjunctiva is clear. There is no burning or itching.
Surgically repaired eyelid maintains proper position and movement.	Lid margins are flush against eyeball surface. Eyelids close completely. Lid margins rest over inferior and superior borders of cornea. There is no tear spillage.
Patient is able to care for abnormally positioned lid that is not surgically repaired.	Patient administers prescribed medications successfully. Patient is able to monitor condition of eye and to report conjunctival or corneal irritation in early stage.[4]

Ectropion

Ectropion is an abnormal outward turning of the margin of the eyelid.[39]

PATHOPHYSIOLOGY

Ectropion occurs in two main forms, atonic and cicatricial. Only the lower eyelid is involved in the atonic type, which is the more common. Older adults are frequently subject to the atonic type from the bulbar conjunctiva owing to relaxation of the orbicularis oculi muscle. This condition can occur in all degrees of severity and may cause corneal drying and irritation and conjunctivitis. Paralysis of the orbicularis oculi muscle (CN VII) also results in atonic ectropion. Cicatricial entropion can affect either the upper or lower eyelid and follows burns, lacerations, and infections of the eyelid skin.

TREATMENT PLAN

Surgical
Ectropion repair—wedge of skin, muscle, and tarsal plate removed to tighten lower lid(s)[39]
Skin grafting—replacement of scar tissue that relieves constriction of inferior part of lower lid

Supportive
Monitoring of exposed conjunctiva for infection and drying
Lubricating ointment as needed

ASSESSMENT: AREAS OF CONCERN

Eyelid
Possible tear spillage

Cornea and conjunctiva
Corneal drying; conjunctivitis

NURSING DIAGNOSES and NURSING INTERVENTIONS

Nursing Diagnosis	Nursing Intervention
Injury, potential for: cornea and conjunctiva (related to inadequate tearing)	Monitor eye for symptoms of dryness. Administer artificial tears, sustained-release tear insert, or lubricating ointment as ordered. Be certain that lid is closed when applying dressing.
Self-concept, disturbance in: body image (related to eyelid deformities)	Listen to patient's concerns. Assist family members with being supportive. See p. 1820.
Knowledge deficit	Educate patient about disorder. Discuss alternative care plans, rationale, and consequences.
Anxiety	Assess level of anxiety. Listen to patient's concerns. Provide supportive counseling.
Sensory-perceptual alteration: visual (related to use of unilateral eye patch)	*Before surgery:* Warn patient that depth perception will be lost and that 50% of peripheral vision will be lost on affected side. *After surgery:* Assist patient with activities of daily living. Caution patient to bring hand forward slowly to touch objects (especially containers of hot liquid and containers receiving poured liquids). Explain that patient should turn head fully toward affected side to view objects or obstacles. Teach patient to use up and down head movements to judge stair dimensions and oncoming objects when walking and to proceed slowly.[24]

Sensory-perceptual alteration: visual (related to use of bilateral eye patches)	*Before surgery:*
	Warn patient that eyes will be patched.
	Orient patient to bedside equipment and room arrangement.
	Arrange for placement of personal belongings in advance and review plan with patient.
	Warn patient that side rails will be raised for safety.
	
	After surgery:
	Raise side rails.
	Address patient by name from doorway and identify self.
	Complement voice stimulation with touch to notify patient of your proximity.
	Reorient patient to equipment (such as call light) and personal belongings at bedside by directing patient's hand.
	Encourage patient to perform self-care with personal hygiene.
	Ensure patient's privacy, and assure patient that he will have privacy.
	Provide patient with television set or radio to encourage mental and memory stimulation.
	Engage patient in discussions about news or other items heard.
	Provide patient with clock that can be felt and remind patient of date.
	Discourage napping, which patient may want to do as he loses track of time.
	Assist patient with meals.
	  Read menu selections.
	  Guide hand to utensils and food on tray.
	  Describe food on tray in clock terms (for example, coffee is at 2 o'clock, knife and spoon are at 3 o'clock).
	  Assist with cutting meats, removing lids from containers, buttering bread, and so on.
	Assist with walking.
	  Walk slowly and slightly ahead of patient; his hand should rest on your arm at elbow.
	  If possible, allow patient to trace his progress by running the dorsal aspect of his free hand along a wall.
	  Describe surroundings as you proceed.
	  Warn of steps, turns, and narrow passageways in advance.
	  Allow patient to feel chair, toilet, or bed before he turns to sit.[24]

Nursing Diagnosis	Nursing Intervention
Comfort, alteration in: pain (related to postoperative eyelid surgery)	Inquire about discomfort. Give pain medication as ordered.
Injury: potential for (to surgically repaired lid, related to nausea or vomiting)	Monitor patient's feelings of nausea. Request order for antiemetic and administer if needed.

Patient Education

1. Teach the patient to avoid rubbing or picking at the eyes.

EVALUATION

Patient Outcome	Data Indicating That Outcome is Reached
Cornea and conjunctiva are healthy.	Cornea is transparent, smooth, glossy, and moist. Palpebral conjunctiva is homogeneous pink color and bulbar conjunctiva is clear. There is no burning or itching.
Surgically repaired eyelid maintains proper position and movement.	Lid margins are flush against eyeball surface. Eyelids close completely. Lid margins rest over inferior and superior borders of cornea. There is no tear spillage.
Patient is able to care for abnormally positioned lid that is not surgically repaired.	Patient administers prescribed medications successfully. Patient is able to monitor condition of eye and to report conjunctival or corneal irritation in early stage.[4]

Ptosis

Ptosis is a drooping of the upper eyelid.

PATHOPHYSIOLOGY

Ptosis can be bilateral or unilateral, constant or intermittent, and congenital or acquired.[40] Congenital deformity usually involves malfunction of the levator muscle and is often accompanied by limited eye movement associated with superior rectus muscle failure. Acquired ptosis is mechanical, neurogenic, or myogenic in origin. Mechanical factors usually stem from abnormal weight of the eyelid imposed by such conditions as chronic edema, tumor, or excess tissue. Malfunction of the oculomotor nerve (CN III) interferes with lid elevation, eye movement, and pupillary constriction. Carotid aneurysms and diabetic neuropathy are common causes of CN III degeneration. Interruption of the sympathetic innervation of the smooth muscle that maintains lid tone and dilates the pupil causes ptosis. Horner's syndrome (a miotic pupil and drooping lid) occurs with sympathetic pathway lesions such as goiter, cervical lymph node enlargement, or apical bronchogenic carcinoma.[28] Unilateral ptosis is frequently the first sign of myasthenia gravis, which is characterized by fatigability of striated muscles. Bilateral involvement with progressive diminished eye movement may ensue. Aging eyes lose muscle tone of the lid elevator and the smooth muscle within the lid, and a general mild lid sag may occur.

TREATMENT PLAN

Surgical

Resection of levator palpebrae superioris muscle—if functioning, muscle is reattached to tarsus at shorter length to increase muscle strength and lid-raising capacity

Upper eyelid suspension—when levator muscle is not functioning, supportive band of material is threaded within lid and attached to frontalis muscle to provide sling effect; lid movement is not affected, but cosmetic effect is improved[28,40]

Supportive

Glasses with "crutch" can be worn to suspend inoperable lid

Treatment of systemic disorder (such as treatment of myasthenia gravis or removal of sympathetic pathway lesion) may relieve lid drooping[28]

ASSESSMENT: AREAS OF CONCERN

Ptosis
If both lids involved, head may be thrown back and
forehead constantly furrowed

NURSING DIAGNOSES and NURSING INTERVENTIONS

Nursing Diagnosis	Nursing Intervention
Self-concept, disturbance in: body image (related to eyelid deformities)	Listen to patient's concerns. Assist family members with being supportive. See p. 1820.
Knowledge deficit	Educate patient about disorder. Discuss alternative care plans, rationale, and consequences.
Anxiety	Assess level of anxiety. Listen to patient's concerns. Provide supportive counseling.
Comfort, alteration in: pain (related to postoperative eyelid surgery)	Inquire about discomfort. Give pain medication as ordered.

EVALUATION

Patient Outcome	Data Indicating That Outcome is Reached
Cornea and conjunctiva are healthy.	Cornea is transparent, smooth, glossy, and moist. Palpebral conjunctiva is homogeneous pink color and bulbar conjunctiva is clear. There is no burning or itching.
Surgically repaired eyelid maintains proper position and movement.	Lid margins are flush against eyeball surface. Eyelids close completely. Lid margins rest over inferior and superior borders of cornea. There is no tear spillage.
Patient is able to care for abnormally positioned lid that is not surgically repaired.	Patient administers prescribed medications successfully. Patient is able to monitor condition of eye and to report conjunctival or corneal irritation in early stage.[4]

Lagophthalmos

Lagophthalmos is inadequate closure of the eyelids.
Lagophthalmos may result from facial nerve (CN VII) weakness or enlargement or protrusion of the eyeball.[28]

TREATMENT PLAN

Surgical
Immediate surgical closure of lids may be necessary to prevent corneal drying and trauma; upper and lower eyelid adhesions can be temporarily or permanently created[36]

Supportive
When only small portion of central cornea is exposed
Lubricating ointment instilled at bedtime for protection during sleep
Soft contact lens worn or artificial tears administered several times a day
Sustained-release tear insert in each eye once a day[28]

ASSESSMENT: AREAS OF CONCERN

Cornea
Corneal drying; secondary keratitis

NURSING DIAGNOSES and NURSING INTERVENTIONS

Nursing Diagnosis	Nursing Intervention
Injury, potential for: cornea and conjunctiva (related to inadequate tearing)	Monitor eye for symptoms of dryness. Administer artificial tears, sustained-release tear insert, or lubricating ointment as ordered. Be certain that lid is closed when applying dressing.
Self-concept, disturbance in: body image (related to eyelid deformities)	Listen to patient's concerns. Assist family members with being supportive. See p. 1820.
Knowledge deficit	Educate patient about disorder. Discuss alternative care plans, rationale, and consequences.
Anxiety	Assess level of anxiety. Listen to patient's concerns. Provide supportive counseling.
Sensory-perceptual alteration: visual (related to use of unilateral eye patch)	*Before surgery:* Warn patient that depth perception will be lost and that 50% of peripheral vision will be lost on affected side. *After surgery:* Assist patient with activities of daily living. Caution patient to bring hand forward slowly to touch objects (especially containers of hot liquid and containers receiving poured liquids). Teach patient to turn head fully toward affected side to view objects or obstacles. Tell patient to use up and down head movements to judge stair dimensions and oncoming objects when walking and to proceed slowly.[24]

Sensory-perceptual alteration: visual (related to use of bilateral eye patches)	*Before surgery:*
	Warn patient that eyes will be patched.
	Orient patient to bedside equipment and room arrangement.
	Arrange for placement of personal belongings in advance and review plan with patient.
	Warn patient that side rails will be raised for safety.
	
	After surgery:
	Raise side rails.
	Address patient by name from doorway and identify self.
	Complement voice stimulation with touch to notify patient of your proximity.
	Reorient patient to equipment (such as call light) and personal belongings at bedside by directing patient's hand.
	Encourage patient to perform self-care with personal hygiene.
	Ensure patient's privacy, and notify patient that he will have privacy.
	Provide patient with television set or radio to encourage mental and memory stimulation.
	Engage patient in discussions about news or other items heard.
	Provide patient with clock that can be felt and remind patient of date.
	Discourage napping, which patient may want to do as he loses track of time.
	Assist patient with meals.
	  Read menu selections.
	  Guide hand to utensils and food on tray.
	  Describe food on tray in clock terms (for example, coffee is at 2 o'clock, knife and spoon are at 3 o'clock).
	  Assist with cutting meats, removing lids from containers, buttering bread, and so on.
	Assist with walking.
	  Walk slowly and slightly ahead of patient; his hand should rest on your arm at elbow.
	  If possible, allow patient to trace his progress by running the dorsal aspect of his free hand along a wall.
	  Describe surroundings as you proceed.
	  Warn of steps, turns, and narrow passageways in advance.
	  Allow patient to feel chair, toilet, or bed before he turns to sit.[24]

Nursing Diagnosis	Nursing Intervention
Comfort, alteration in: pain (related to postoperative eyelid surgery)	Inquire about discomfort. Give pain medication as ordered.
Injury: potential for (to surgically repaired lid, related to nausea or vomiting)	Monitor patient's feelings of nausea. Request order for antiemetic and administer if needed.

Patient Education

1. Teach the patient to administer eye drops, lubricant, or tear insert if ordered; tell the patient to wash hands before and after the procedure.
2. Caution the patient to avoid rubbing or picking at the eyes.
3. Tell the patient to avoid noxious odors or fumes such as cigarette smoke.
4. Suggest that the patient use a humidifier in the home if the atmosphere is dry.
5. Show the patient how to monitor the eye for signs and symptoms of dryness or irritation.

EVALUATION

Patient Outcome	Data Indicating That Outcome is Reached
Cornea and conjunctiva are healthy.	Cornea is transparent, smooth, glossy, and moist. Palpebral conjunctiva is homogeneous pink color and bulbar conjunctiva is clear. There is no burning or itching.
Surgically repaired eyelid maintains proper position and movement.	Lid margins are flush against eyeball surface. Eyelids close completely. Lid margins rest over inferior and superior borders of cornea. There is no tear spillage.
Patient is able to care for abnormally positioned lid that is not surgically repaired.	Patient administers prescribed medications successfully. Patient is able to monitor condition of eye and to report conjunctival or corneal irritation in early stage.[4]

Epicanthus

Epicanthus is a vertical fold of skin in the medial canthus of the eye.

This extra fold occurs normally in Orientals and sometimes in newborns. The configuration and extent of the fold vary widely. The fold may extend over the eye and cover the medial angle so the eye (or eyes) appears to turn inward. Cover-uncover testing can rule out strabismus. As the infant's face and nose develop, the epicanthus disappears. Deformities of eye and lid shape and symmetry are commonly associated with chromosomal disorders and should be carefully evaluated. For example, epicanthal folds, upward slanted eyes, and widely spaced eyes are characteristically associated with Down's syndrome.[43] Epicanthal folds are generally not treated and become less prominent or disappear as facial features mature.

Blinking Disorders

Blinking disorders may occur as excessive blinking or a diminished rate of blinking.

PATHOPHYSIOLOGY

Blinking is both a voluntary and an involuntary action. The rate of involuntary blinking varies among individuals, but blinking occurs frequently enough to spread tears over the surface of the eye. Reflex blinking increases in response to conjunctival or corneal irritation or pain in the eye. Chronic irritation may result in a continuous clonic response that is sustained until the stimulus is removed. Rapid blinking also accompanies anxiety and may become a prolonged pattern with chronic stress. Spasms of the orbicularis oculi muscle (blepharospasm) sometimes occur in elderly persons.[40] These spasms are involuntary, tonic, spasmodic, usually bilateral contractions. They range from an annoying tic to a dangerous level during which the person cannot see. They are also unattractive. Causative factors include irritation of the eyes, facial nerve lesions, fatigue, and anxiety. Absence or diminishment of blinking may accompany parkinsonism or hyperthyroidism.

TREATMENT PLAN

Blinking disorders are usually relieved when the cause (systemic origin, anxiety, or local irritation) is treated or removed.

ASSESSMENT: AREA OF CONCERN

Blinking disorder
Rapid bilateral blinking
Multiple anxiety behaviors
Tics
Anxiety; statements of stress

Cornea and conjunctiva
Diminished blinking
Conjunctival drying and irritation or corneal drying; keratitis

NURSING DIAGNOSES and NURSING INTERVENTIONS

Nursing Diagnosis	Nursing Intervention
Injury: potential for (cornea and conjunctiva, related to inadequate tearing)	Monitor eye for symptoms of dryness. Administer artificial tears, sustained-release tear insert, or lubricating ointment as ordered. Be certain that lid is closed when applying dressing.
Knowledge deficit	Educate patient about disorder. Discuss alternative care plans, rationale, and consequences.
Anxiety	Assess level of anxiety. Listen to patient's concerns. Provide supportive counseling.

Patient Education

1. Teach the patient to administer eye drops, lubricant, or tear insert if ordered; tell the patient to wash hands before and after the procedure.
2. Caution the patient avoid rubbing or picking at the eyes.
3. Tell the patient to avoid noxious odors or fumes such as cigarette smoke.
4. Suggest that the patient use a humidifier in the home if the atmosphere is dry.
5. Teach the patient to monitor the eye for signs and symptoms of dryness or irritation.

EVALUATION

Patient Outcome	Data Indicating That Outcome is Reached
Cornea and conjunctiva are healthy.	Cornea is transparent, smooth, glossy, and moist. Palpebral conjunctiva is homogeneous pink color, and bulbar conjunctiva is clear. There is no burning or itching.
Lid movement is normal.	Open and closure movement of lid is not excessive. Vision is not obscured. Source for nervous mannerisms or local irritant has been removed.

Blepharitis

Blepharitis is an inflammation of the eyelid margins.

PATHOPHYSIOLOGY

Blepharitis is a chronic condition that can be caused by organisms (chiefly *Staphylococcus*), associated with seborrheic dermatitis, or aggravated by allergies. Often the causative factors are inseparable. Other conditions commonly associated with chronic blepharitis are diabetes, gout, anemia, and rosacea.[28] Infections of the nose and mouth can be transferred to the eyes and lids by frequent eye rubbing. Staphylococcal lesions usually ulcerate and often involve the conjunctiva and meibomian glands. Chalazions and hordeola (styes) may develop and recur. Seborrheic blepharitis is frequently accompanied by dermatitis of the scalp, eyebrows, and external ears. Some persons first have this chronic condition in childhood and continue to have intermittent exacerbations throughout life.[36]

TREATMENT PLAN

Chemotherapeutic[28,36,40]
  Anti-infective agents
    Ointment applied locally qd or bid, usually at bedtime
    Sulfacetamide sodium (Sulamyd, others), 10%-30% solution or 10% ointment
    Bacitracin (Baciguent), 500 units/1 g ointment
    Neomycin sulfate (Myciguent), 0.5% ointment
    Selenium sulfide shampoo and soak for brows, eyelids[36]

Supportive
  Warm compresses to soften and remove crusts and scaling twice a day for 10 to 20 minutes
  Oil to soften crusts
  Mild baby shampoo to clean lids

ASSESSMENT: AREAS OF CONCERN

Eyelid and lashes
  Red lid margins; flaking and scaling around lashes; localized discomfort; loss of lashes; ingrown lashes; thickening and eversion of lid margins; tear spillage; in ulcerative staphylococcal blepharitis, pus, multiple lesions and crusting at lid margins, development of ulcers, lids glued shut by dried drainage

Cornea and conjunctiva
  Light sensitivity; possible chronic conjunctivitis; possible corneal inflammation

NURSING DIAGNOSES and NURSING INTERVENTIONS

Nursing Diagnosis	Nursing Intervention
Skin integrity, impairment of: actual and potential	Demonstrate and instruct patient in self-care. Use oil to soften crusts. Apply warm compresses with clean cloth for 10 to 20 minutes two or three times a day. Soften crusts and clean lids lightly, stroking toward lid margin with cotton applicator.[36]

EVALUATION

Patient Outcome	Data Indicating That Outcome is Reached
Eyelids are normal.	Lid margins are smooth and without scaling.
Conjunctiva is normal.	Palpebral conjunctiva is homogeneous pink color and bulbar conjunctiva is clear. There is no excessive tearing.

Meibomianitis

Meibomianitis is excessive secretion and inflammation of the meibomian glands.

PATHOPHYSIOLOGY

Meibomianitis most often occurs in middle adulthood. It may accompany acute blepharitis or may recur periodically without infection.[40] Mild compression over the lid margins expresses an oily, yellowish discharge that contains no organisms.

TREATMENT PLAN

Chemotherapeutic[28,36,40]
  Anti-infective agents
    Ointment applied locally qd or bid, usually at bedtime if infection is present

  Sulfacetamide sodium (Sulamyd, others), 10%-30% solution or 10% ointment
  Bacitracin (Baciguent), 500 units/1 g ointment
  Neomycin sulfate (Myciguent), 0.5% ointment

Supportive
  Warm compresses with clean cloth two or three times a day
  Tarsal massage—mild compression at lid margin to express gland contents twice a day

ASSESSMENT: AREAS OF CONCERN

Eyelids
  Red-rimmed eyes; localized burning and discomfort; prominent meibomian glands; continuous frothy, yellowish discharge

Conjunctiva
  Possible chronic conjunctivitis

NURSING DIAGNOSES and NURSING INTERVENTIONS

Nursing Diagnosis	Nursing Intervention
Skin integrity, impairment of: actual and potential	Demonstrate tarsal massage (light compression over lid margin to express gland contents) and instruct patient to perform it twice a day. (This is difficult to do to oneself because the lid must be elevated to massage it well.[28]) Demonstrate and instruct patient in application of warm compresses.

Patient Education

1. Instruct the patient in the application of warm compresses and antibiotic ointment if ordered.
2. Instruct the patient in hygiene practices related to self-care of the eye, such as washing hands before and after self-care and avoiding fumes and smoke.
3. If the patient is a woman, tell her to avoid using eye makeup during the acute phase of lid infection, since makeup is a common allergen.

EVALUATION

Patient Outcome	Data Indicating That Outcome is Reached
Eyelids are normal.	Lid margins are smooth, without crusting.
Conjunctiva is normal.	Palpebral conjunctiva is homogeneous pink color, and bulbar conjunctiva is clear. There is no excessive tearing.[4]

Chalazion

Chalazion is a granulomatous inflammation of a meibomian gland.

PATHOPHYSIOLOGY

A chalazion forms on the conjunctival aspect of the upper or lower eyelid as glands in both are affected. It begins as a nontender swelling and may take several weeks to develop. It does not appear inflamed unless a secondary infection occurs. If large enough, the nodule can compress the eyeball and cause an astigmatism. A large nodule also produces discomfort as the upper lid closes, causing pressure on the cornea. Some chalazia disappear in a few months without ever causing symptoms. Chronic chalazia tend to subside partially and reactivate periodically.

TREATMENT PLAN

Surgical
 Localized excision of chronic chalazion with patient under local anesthesia; antibiotic eye drops administered three or four times a day before and after surgery

Chemotherapeutic
 Anti-infective agents
  Ointment applied locally once or twice daily, usually at bedtime if infected
   Sulfacetamide sodium (Sulamyd, others), 10%-30% solution or 10% ointment
   Bacitracin (Baciguent), 500 units/1 g ointment
   Neomycin sulfate (Myciguent), 0.5% ointment

ASSESSMENT: AREAS OF CONCERN

Eyelids
 Small, nontender, noninflamed lump on outer lid; lid eversion reveals nodule that points toward conjunctiva; secondary infection produces redness, pain, and suppuration; sensitivity to light

NURSING DIAGNOSES and NURSING INTERVENTIONS

Nursing Diagnosis	Nursing Intervention
Skin integrity, impairment of: actual and potential	Demonstrate and instruct patient in self-care. Apply warm compresses with clean cloth for 10 to 20 minutes two or three times a day after excision of chalazion.

Patient Education

1. Instruct the patient in hygiene practices related to self-care of the eye, such as washing hands before and after self-care and avoiding fumes and smoke.
2. If the patient is a woman, tell her to avoid using eye makeup during the acute phase of lid infection, since makeup is a common allergen.

EVALUATION

Patient Outcome	Data Indicating That Outcome is Reached
Eyelids are normal.	Lid margins are smooth, without lesions.
Conjunctiva is normal.	Palpebral conjunctiva is homogeneous pink color, and bulbar conjunctiva is clear. There is no excessive tearing.[4]

Hordeolum

A hordeolum (sty) is an acute infection of an eyelash follicle or the glands of Moll or Zeis (sebaceous glands).

PATHOPHYSIOLOGY

The offending organism is usually *Staphylococcus*. The lesion becomes a pustule that eventually points and may rupture. Multiple pustules may occur along adjacent lash follicles because of reinfection.[40]

TREATMENT PLAN

Chemotherapeutic
Anti-infective agents (ointment applied locally once or twice daily, usually at bedtime)

Sulfacetamide sodium (Sulamyd, others), 10%-30% solution or 10% ointment
Bacitracin (Baciguent), 500 units/1 g ointment
Neomycin sulfate (Myciguent), 0.5% ointment

Supportive
Warm compresses with clean cloth for 10 to 20 minutes two or three times a day
Local incision of pustule if rupture is not spontaneous

ASSESSMENT: AREAS OF CONCERN

Eyelids
Initial tenderness with localized redness and swelling that forms pustule at lid margin; may be multiple pustules; generalized lid edema; pain that increases as pustule enlarges and ceases with rupture

NURSING DIAGNOSES and NURSING INTERVENTIONS

Nursing Diagnosis	Nursing Intervention
Skin integrity, impairment of: actual and potential	Demonstrate and instruct patient in self-care. Apply warm compresses with clean cloth for 10 to 20 minutes two or three times a day.

Patient Education

1. Instruct the patient in the application of warm compresses and antibiotic ointment if ordered.
2. Instruct the patient in hygiene practices related to self-care of the eye, such as washing hands before and after self-care and avoiding fumes and smoke.
3. If the patient is a woman, tell her to avoid using eye makeup during the acute phase of lid infection, since makeup is a common allergen.

EVALUATION

Patient Outcome	Data Indicating That Outcome is Reached
Eyelids are normal.	Lid margins are smooth, without lesions.
Conjunctiva is normal.	Palpebral conjunctiva is homogeneous pink color, and bulbar conjunctiva is clear. There is no excessive tearing.[4]

LACRIMAL APPARATUS DISORDERS

Patients with lacrimal disorders usually complain of "dry eyes," excessive tearing, or pain and swelling of the lacrimal duct. Inadequate tearing can result in drying and severe damage to the cornea. Excessive tearing can be caused by overproduction of tears by the lacrimal gland or a faulty drainage system that results in tear spillage. Tear accumulation can interfere with vision and irritate the eyeball. Inflammation of the lacrimal sac and adjacent canaliculi can be associated with conjunctivitis, nasal disease, or drainage obstruction.

Dry Eye Syndrome

Dry eye syndrome is a condition in which tear production is inadequate.

PATHOPHYSIOLOGY

Dry eye syndrome occurs for three primary reasons: lacrimal gland malfunction, mucin deficiency, and mechanical abnormalities that interfere with the spread or maintenance of tears over the eyeball surface. Lacrimal gland malfunctions can be congenital or acquired. The most common congenital disorders are lacrimal gland aplasia, ectodermal dysplasia, and trigeminal nerve (CN V) malfunction, which disrupts sensory stimulation to the upper lid. Acquired disorders that affect lacrimal gland function can be systemic, infectious, or related to trauma. Common systemic disorders that may be associated with diminished tear production are rheumatoid arthritis (Sjögren's syndrome), leukemia, lymphoma, sarcoidosis, and systemic sclerosis.[28] Facial nerve (CN VII) palsy inhibits tearing. Mumps and some forms of conjunctivitis may obstruct tear flow. Chemical burns and irradiation may reduce lacrimal gland function. Some medications such as antihistamines, atropine, and β-adrenergic blockers decrease tear production. Even if the lacrimal gland is not functioning, accessory glands in the palpebral conjunctiva may secrete sufficient tears to prevent severe corneal damage.

A layer of mucin, produced by goblet cells in the lid, maintains a homogeneous tear spread over the eyeball surface. The absence of mucin causes the tear film to break up, leaving "dry holes" over the cornea. Mucin deficiency is commonly associated with some forms of chronic conjunctivitis, vitamin A deficiency, and medications such as antihistamines and β-adrenergic blockers.[28]

Mechanical defects that contribute to dry eyes include abnormalities of eyelid structure and function (see p. 662), protrusion of the eyeball (proptosis), and misuse of contact lenses (see p. 725).

DIAGNOSTIC STUDIES[28,36,40]

Rose bengal staining
Drop of 1% or 2% solution placed in conjunctival sac; 2% solution demonstrates loss of corneal and conjunctival epithelium in keratoconjunctivitis sicca; 1% solution valuable in demonstrating conjunctival and corneal epithelial cell loss and degeneration; patients with deficiency of aqueous portion of tears have punctate staining of lower two thirds of cornea and bright red staining of bulbar conjunctiva in area corresponding to palpable aperture

Schirmer's test
Strip of filter paper, 3.5 × 0.05 cm, placed in conjunctival cul-de-sac of lower lid for 5 minutes; 10 mm length of paper wetted with tears considered normal; more than 25 mm moistened paper indicates excessive tearing

Basic secretion test
Topical anesthesia administered to eyeball before filter paper inserted; anesthesia reduces lacrimal output to allow measurement of tear production of accessory glands in eyelid

TREATMENT PLAN

Surgical
Occlusion of puncta to conserve tears
Surgical repair of lid position or movement abnormalities

Supportive
Treatment varies depending on severity of condition
Artificial tears as needed
Lubricating ointment at bedtime
Humidifier in environment
Sustained-release tear insert once a day

ASSESSMENT: AREAS OF CONCERN

Dry eyes
Burning; itching; sensitivity to light; blurred vision; lack of tears; loss of glossy appearance of cornea; tear film interspersed with mucus strands

NURSING DIAGNOSES and NURSING INTERVENTIONS

Nursing Diagnosis	Nursing Intervention
Injury: potential for (cornea and conjunctiva, related to lack of tears)	Monitor eye for signs and symptoms of irritation (itching, burning, and loss of glossy appearance of eyeball surface). Administer artificial tears, sustained-release tear insert, or lubricating ointments as ordered.
Sensory-perceptual alteration: visual (related to bilateral eye patches or lid closure)	Raise side rails. Address patient by name from doorway and identify self. Complement voice stimulation with touch to notify patient of your proximity. Orient patient to bedside equipment (such as call light, bed control, and side rails) and personal belongings at bedside by directing his hand over objects. Encourage patient to perform self-care with personal hygiene. Provide support and supervision. Provide patient privacy and assure patient that privacy is provided. Assist with meals. (Patients may become so frustrated at mealtime that they may not eat without this assistance.) Read menu selections. Guide hand to utensils and food on tray. Describe food on tray in clock terms. Teach patient to "trail," that is, to use dorsal aspect of index and middle fingers to find objects on food tray. Fill glasses only half full, since patient may spill easily. Assist patient with cutting meat, removing lids from cartons, buttering bread, and so on. Assist with walking. Walk slowly and slightly ahead of patient. Patient's hand should rest on your arm at your elbow. If possible, allow patient to trace his progress by running the dorsal aspect of his free hand along a wall. Describe surroundings as you proceed. Allow patient to feel chair, toilet, or bed before he turns to sit.[24]
Comfort, alteration in: pain (related to localized inflammation)	Assess patient's degree of discomfort. Provide analgesics as ordered.

Patient Education

1. Teach the patient how to administer eye drops, lubricant, or a tear insert; stress the importance of washing hands before and after the procedure.
2. Instruct the patient to avoid rubbing or picking at the eyes.
3. Instruct the patient to avoid noxious odors or fumes and to use a humidifier in the home if the atmosphere is dry.
4. Teach the patient how to monitor the eye for signs and symptoms of dryness or irritation.

EVALUATION

Patient Outcome	Data Indicating That Outcome is Reached
Cornea and conjunctiva are healthy.	Cornea is transparent, smooth, glossy, and moist. Palpebral conjunctiva is homogeneous pink color, and bulbar conjunctiva is clear. There is no burning or itching.[4]

Excessive Tears

Excessive tears can occur from overproduction or in-adequate drainage of tears.

PATHOPHYSIOLOGY

Tear spillage most commonly occurs because the drainage system is faulty (epiphora). The puncta can be occluded because of congenital absence of an opening or because of infection in the lacrimal sac. Lid abnormalities, such as ectropion, cause abnormal alignment of the lacrimal tear pool and the puncta. An accumulation of tears in the inner canthus is an irritant that stimulates more tear production. Obstructions may also occur in the lacrimal duct or the meatus in the nasal cavity.

Lacrimation (excessive tear production) occurs most commonly with reflex stimulation of the lacrimal gland. Corneal injury, eye pain, noxious odors, eyestrain, bright light, and allergies are examples of sensory stimuli affecting the trigeminal nerve (CN V). Glaucoma often stimulates tear production because of trigeminal irritation. Facial nerve (CN VII) irritation during vomiting or laughter also stimulates tear production. Abnormal regeneration of the facial nerve following Bell's palsy causes "crocodile tears," a phenomenon of excess tearing that occurs during eating. Parasympathetic stimulants (cholinergic drugs) and some endocrine disorders (such as hyperthyroidism) can also increase tearing.[28]

DIAGNOSTIC STUDIES

Dye disappearance
Cul-de-sac of lower lid flooded with 2% fluorescein solution; fluorescein normally disappears from cul-de-sac in 1 minute

Dacryocystography
Radiopaque medium injected into lacrimal sac before roentgenography; shows patent lacrimal passage

Dacryoscintography
Isotope instilled in cul-de-sac and traced with gamma camera; irrigation of lacrimal sac before dacryo-scintography will stain mucosal lining a readily identifiable blue color; shows patent lacrimal passage

TREATMENT PLAN

Surgical
Repair of lid structure abnormalities to enhance punctal access to tear pool
Probing of obstructed punctum
Construction of tube connecting conjunctival cul-de-sac to nasal cavity

Supportive
Related to removal of cause of lacrimation

ASSESSMENT: AREAS OF CONCERN

Excessive tears
Tear spillage; blurred vision; puncta red and swollen; puncta may exude purulent material on mild compression over lacrimal sac; conjunctivitis (reddened conjunctiva)

NURSING DIAGNOSES and NURSING INTERVENTIONS

Nursing Diagnosis	Nursing Intervention
Sensory-perceptual alteration: visual (blurred vision caused by excessive tears)	Monitor eye for amount of lacrimation or increased symptoms of irritation or infection. Encourage patient to maintain excellent hygiene.

Patient Education

1. Instruct the patient in hygiene practices related to self-care of the eyes, such as washing hands before and after self-care and keeping hands away from the eyes.

EVALUATION

Patient Outcome	Data Indicating That Outcome is Reached
Lacrimal drainage system is patent.	There is no excess tearing. Inner canthus of eye is homogeneous pink color. When eye is compressed at medial infraorbital rim, punctum does not exude any material.[4]
Underlying endocrine cause, if any, is corrected.	Amount of tears produced is not excessive.

Dacryocystitis

Dacryocystitis is an inflammation of the lacrimal sac.

PATHOPHYSIOLOGY

Dacryocystitis can be acute or chronic and is usually caused by obstruction of tear drainage from the punctum or lacrimal sac.

Normal newborns often do not have patent nasolacrimal ducts. The duct usually opens about the third week of life. If the duct fails to open, tearing occurs and eventually purulent material exudes from the punctum. The condition often corrects itself by 3 to 6 months of age. Lacrimal probing may be performed if spontaneous patency does not occur. Surgical construction of a duct is rarely needed, but if necessary it is performed when the child reaches 3 or 4 years of age.[28]

Chronic dacrocystitis most often occurs in middle-aged adults. Spontaneous punctum obstruction is followed by bacterial infection with a mucopurulent discharge. The nasolacrimal duct can also be obstructed by injury or nasal lesions, which causes an inflammatory response. Acute dacrocystitis has a rapid onset with marked swelling and tenderness of surrounding tissue.[40]

TREATMENT PLAN[28,40]

Surgical
Incision and drainage of abscess
Dacryocystorhinostomy for construction of passage between lacrimal sac and nasal cavity

Chemotherapeutic
Anti-infective agents
Systemic antibiotics for acute, severe infection
Instillation of antibiotic or sulfonamide eye drops 4-5 times/d until infection subsides

Supportive
Daily massage of lacrimal sac to rid it of purulent material
Warm compresses over affected eye during acute phase
Lacrimal probing with graduated sizes of probe while patient is under local anesthesia
Temporary lacrimal drainage splint

ASSESSMENT: AREAS OF CONCERN

Lacrimal inflammation
Tear spillage; purulent material exuding from punctum on compression; punctum swollen and surrounding tissue may be reddened; localized pain

NURSING DIAGNOSES and NURSING INTERVENTIONS

Nursing Diagnosis	Nursing Intervention
Injury: potential for (infection of surrounding tissue related to dysfunction in lacrimal drainage)	Apply warm compresses over affected eye for 10 to 20 minutes three or four times a day. Lightly massage lacrimal sac at medial infraorbital rim to rid sac of accumulated purulent material. Administer antibiotic or sulfonamide eye drops or ointment as ordered. Wash hands thoroughly before and after care of affected eye.

Patient Education

1. Instruct the patient in hygiene practices related to self-care of the eyes, such as washing hands before and after self-care and keeping hands away from the eyes.

EVALUATION

Patient Outcome	Data Indicating That Outcome is Reached
Cornea and conjunctiva are healthy.	Cornea is transparent, smooth, glossy, and moist. Palpebral conjunctiva is homogeneous pink color. Bulbar conjunctiva is clear. There is no burning or itching.[4]
Lacrimal drainage system is patent.	There is no excess tearing. Inner canthus of eye is homogeneous pink color. Punctum does not exude any material when eye is compressed at medial infraorbital rim.[4]

CONJUNCTIVAL DISORDERS

The bulbar conjunctiva serves as a protective coating for the scleral portion of the eyeball and is subject to numerous environmental assaults. It adjoins the palpebral conjunctiva in the lid cul-de-sac and is susceptible to infection because of its proximity to the eyelid. The conjunctiva also responds to internal infections or diseases such as measles, diabetes mellitus, or riboflavin deficiency. This outer layer contains blood vessels that dilate rapidly and pain receptors that register mild to moderate discomfort in response to inflammation. The conjunctiva is adjacent to the cornea and can be an avenue for spread of infection to this vital area.

Conjunctivitis

Conjunctivitis is an inflammation or infection of the conjunctiva.

Conjunctival tissue can show inflammatory responses to such stimuli as dust, smog, tobacco smoke, noxious fumes, wind, sun, and airborne allergens. Conjunctivitis is common and easily spread, particularly in crowded environments such as schools and nursing homes.

PATHOPHYSIOLOGY

Conjunctivitis occurs in varying degrees of severity. Vascular dilation and engorgement can be a response to external irritants such as smog, hair sprays, or fumes. Lacrimation and a foreign body sensation may be experienced, but no discharge or progressive infectious process appears. Generalized hyperemia and burning are an initial response to insufficient tearing, and a secondary infection can rapidly follow. Allergic responses may be seasonal and include vascular injection, moderate tearing, and severe itching. Viral conjunctivitis is characterized by generalized hyperemia, profuse tearing, and a minimal showing of exudate. Preauricular nodes are commonly associated with a viral infection. Bacterial conjunctivitis,

the most common type, is frequently called "pinkeye." Almost any bacterium can be involved, but *Pneumococcus*, *Staphylococcus*, and *Streptococcus* organisms are common. The infection usually begins in one eye and is transferred to the other eye through contamination. The onset is acute, with a mucopurulent exudate, tearing, generalized hyperemia, and moderate discomfort. This form of conjunctivitis is highly contagious.[40]

Some organisms rapidly invade the cornea, as well as the conjunctiva, and lead to corneal ulceration and perforation. Two of the most virulent organisms are *Neisseria gonorrhoeae* and *Chlamydia trachomatis*. Ophthalmia neonatorum, a conjunctivitis that occurs in newborns, is commonly transmitted from the mother with acute gonorrheal urethritis during birth. Ophthalmia neonatorum occurs within the first 10 days of life and is characterized by a rapid progression of signs from mild inflammation to marked redness, swelling, and purulent exudate. Corneal involvement is common and severe. *Chlamydia trachomatis* organisms can also be transmitted during a newborn's passage through the vagina. The early symptoms are similar to those of gonococcal conjunctivitis, but the incubation period is slightly longer (5 to 14 days). *Chlamydia* organisms do not respond to silver nitrate, which has been traditionally administered prophylactically to newborns. Since 1980, erythromycin has been more commonly used because it is effective against both *N. gonorrhoeae* and *Chlamydia*. Both gonococcal and chlamydial organisms (which are transmitted venereally) can invade adult conjunctivae and cause severe, acute, purulent infection.[28]

The conjunctival infections that have been described are generally acute in nature and can be successfully treated. Some persons have a chronic recurrent conjunctivitis characterized by periodic exacerbations of eye discomfort, redness, and discharge. Repeated inflammatory episodes can result in a thickening of the conjunctiva and lid margins. The causes are numerous, but the most common are contact allergens (such as cosmetics or chlorine), airborne allergens, excessive meibomian gland secretions, and chronic blepharitis. Trachoma (a chronic *Chlamydia trachomatis* conjunctivitis) has been described as the leading cause of blindness in the world. It is prevalent in warm climates where living conditions are crowded and hygienic practices are poor. Insects may participate in disease transmission. In some cases the disease heals spontaneously, but in others, untreated, it leads to conjunctival scarring and loss of vision.[40]

DIAGNOSTIC STUDIES[40]

Microscopic examination of stained conjunctival scrapings
Numerous polymorphonuclear neutrophils in bacterial infections; monocytes in viral infections or trachoma; eosinophils and basophils in allergies

Culture of exudate or conjunctival scrapings
Organism identification

TREATMENT PLAN

Chemotherapeutic
Anti-infective agents (medication varies with causative organism)
Sulfacetamide sodium (Sulamid, others), 10%-30% solution; 10% ointment for 3-7 d
Erythromycin (Ilotycin), topical 0.5% ointment for 3-7 d
Gentamicin sulfate (Garamycin, others), topical, 3 mg/ml solution or 3 mg/g ointment, use for 3-7 d
For gonococcal or chlamydial conjunctivitis or severe purulent conjunctivitis
Tetracycline (Achromycin), 250-500 mg qid for 21 d

Erythromycin (E-Mycin, others), 250 mg qid for 21 d
Prophylactic dose within first hour of life for newborns
Erythromycin ophthalmic ointment, 0.5%, in each eye
Tetracycline ophthalmic ointment, 1%, in each eye[28,40]

Supportive
Saline irrigations for purulent discharge
Warm compresses for discomfort and inflammation, 10 to 15 minutes two or three times a day
Cold compresses for allergic itching, 10 to 15 minutes two or three times a day
Oil or shampoo swabbing for softening, loosening, and removing crusts on eyelids[28,36]

ASSESSMENT: AREAS OF CONCERN

Allergic and general irritant responses
Lacrimation; generalized hyperemia; gritty, sandy sensation; severe itching (with allergies)

Viral inflammation
Lacrimation; minimum mucopurulent discharge; generalized hyperemia; possible preauricular nodes; some lid swelling; moderate discomfort; possible photophobia

Bacterial inflammation
Purulent discharge; lid swelling; generalized hyperemia; moderate discomfort; possible photophobia; complaints of blurred vision (owing to excess exudate over eye surface); blurring may disappear with blinking

Severe (corneal) involvement
Moderate discomfort that becomes severe

NURSING DIAGNOSES and NURSING INTERVENTIONS

Nursing Diagnosis	Nursing Intervention
Injury: potential for (corneal or conjunctival damage related to conjunctival infection)	Isolate patient from others (in institutional setting) and use isolation precautions. Administer prescribed topical ointments or systemic antibiotics. Administer saline irrigations for excessive discharge. Apply warm compresses for discomfort 10 to 15 minutes two or three times a day. Cleanse lids with mild shampoo and applicators for crusting.[36]

Patient Education

1. Teach the patient to perform saline irrigation of the eye.
2. Teach the patient to apply warm compresses with a clean cloth or cold compresses (ice should not be applied directly to eyelids).
3. Instruct the patient to wash hands thoroughly before and after treating each eye.
4. Tell the patient to keep the hands away from the face.
5. Instruct the patient to avoid crowded environments when possible.
6. Instruct family members to avoid touching their faces and to wash hands thoroughly when contact has occurred.[40]
7. Tell the patient to avoid noxious fumes and smoke.
8. Instruct the patient not to wear contact lens during the suppuration period.

EVALUATION

Patient Outcome	Data Indicating That Outcome is Reached
Conjunctiva and cornea are healthy.	Palpebral conjunctiva is homogeneous pink color. Bulbar conjunctiva is clear and glossy. Cornea is clear and glossy. There is no eye discomfort, lacrimation, or discharge.[4]

Subconjunctival Hemorrhage

Subconjunctival hemorrhage is a common phenomenon caused by the rupture of a blood vessel. It appears suddenly as a well-defined, bright red area on the surface of the eyeball and gradually disappears in 2 to 3 weeks. A large hemorrhage may be darker in color and expand for the first few days. The patient feels no discomfort but is usually quite alarmed. The ruptured vessel is usually the result of localized increased pressure (following a severe coughing, vomiting, or sneezing episode) or minor trauma. Often a cause cannot be found, and no treatment exists to hasten resolution. In rare instances blood dyscrasias, hypertension, or viral conjunctivitis is associated with this hemorrhage.

Conjunctival Discolorations and Growths

The conjunctiva is subject to a large variety of growths, tumors, and discolorations. Bilirubin is absorbed in the conjunctiva with jaundice and gives the underlying sclera a yellow hue. This discoloration must be differentiated from the normal yellowish pigmentation that occurs with increased melanin deposits in dark-skinned persons.

Two of the most common benign growths are pterygium and pinguecula. A pterygium is a triangular growth of connective tissue that usually advances from the nasal side of the conjunctiva and encroaches on the cornea. It occurs more commonly among people who are frequently exposed to the sun and wind. It is not surgically removed unless it creates a cosmetic concern or threatens to involve the central cornea. A pinguecula is very common in older adults and appears as a yellow nodule on either side of the cornea at the limbus. It usually involves both eyes. It may be subject to periodic inflammation but does not invade the cornea and is usually not treated unless the patient expresses cosmetic concerns.

DISORDERS OF THE CORNEA AND SCLERA

The cornea is the primary exterior guardian of vision. Visual clarity depends on uniformity, smoothness, and transparency throughout the corneal layers. The avascular central cornea depends on its periphery (the limbus) for nourishment and on its epithelial (outer layer) and endothelial (inner layer) activity for hydration stability. Exposure of the cornea to the external environment increases its vulnerability to trauma and infection. Injury to the outer epithelial layer exposes Bowman's membrane and the substantia propria (stromal layer) to infection. If untreated infection perforates the cornea, the eye may be lost. The epithelial layer regenerates rapidly without scarring, but the deeper layers form opacities that may cause astigmatism or mild to severe visual loss.

In recent years, surgical techniques for corneal transplantation involving new microscopic and illuminating systems have greatly improved the prognosis for patients needing new corneas.[15] Corneal transplant and implications for nursing are covered in the last section of this chapter (p. 732).

Keratitis (Corneal Inflammation)

Keratitis is an inflammation of the cornea.

PATHOPHYSIOLOGY

The cornea is subject to injury through exposure (drying), ischemia, nutritional deficiency, microbe invasion, anesthesia (sensory interruption), and trauma. Keratitis (corneal inflammation) may be superficial (epithelial), invade the stroma (subepithelial), or eventually break through the inner layer (Descemet's membrane) to the endothelium. Most organisms require a break in the epithelium for entrance into the cornea. The epithelium can be jeopardized by hypersensitivity to conjunctival inflammation, corneal drying, mechanical injury, or chemical irritants. Since the epithelium is richly innervated, superficial inflammation causes moderate to severe pain. Epithelial erosions may appear in the form of tiny pits or small or coarse lesions scattered over the surface. Some of the medical treatments prescribed for therapy or relief of discomfort may facilitate bacterial invasion. Immunosuppressed persons are more vulnerable to infection; the misuse of local corticosteroid therapy increases the tissue destruction activity of collagenase, which is produced when epithelial cells are injured. Immunosuppressed persons are also more vulnerable to invasion by fungi, which have an affinity for penetrating Descemet's membrane. Fluorescein solution, which is used to stain and detect epithelial damage, is easily contaminated and can inoculate the epithelium with organisms. A patient who is given local anesthetics (particularly for use at home) can further abrade the cornea without knowing it. In addition to inhibiting the protective corneal reflex, anesthesia of the eye interrupts epithelial regeneration.[40]

Almost any bacterium can invade the cornea. *Pneumococcus*, *Staphylococcus*, *Streptococcus*, and *Pseudomonas* organisms are the most common. Fungal infections have become much more common since the introduction of topical corticosteroids and antibiotics. Chronic debilitating disease increases vulnerability to fungal infections. Viral infections, most commonly caused by herpes simplex, are also prevalent.

The sclera surrounds the eyeball and is adjacent to the uveal tract (including the choroid layer). It opens posteriorly to admit the optic nerve and other nerves and vessels into the eye. Scleral inflammation and disease are often associated with systemic connective tissue disorders.

The severity of corneal destruction depends on the virulence of the organism, the degree of corneal destruction (with trauma), the accuracy and promptness of therapy, and the immunocompetence of the host. *Pneumococcus* and *Pseudomonas* organisms tend to spread rapidly and form ulcers that penetrate deep into the stroma. Herpes keratitis can be recurrent, is triggered by stress, exposure to ultraviolet light (sun), or other illness, and is relatively asymptomatic because it attacks the trigeminal nerve (CN V) and diminishes pain. Corneal ulceration and optic atrophy develop rapidly in neonates contaminated with herpesvirus at birth. Adults with recurrent herpes keratitis may heal with or without scarring.[28] Herpesvirus is also activated with the use of topical steroids. Some virus forms are highly contagious and cause outbreaks, especially in schools, institutions, and eye clinics. Chronic disabling illness increases vulnerability to corneal damage, as do certain diseases such as diabetes mellitus, leukemia, chronic alcoholism, severe vitamin A deficiency, and autoimmune diseases.[28]

DIAGNOSTIC STUDIES[28,40]

Fluorescein stain (2%)
Sterile paper strips most commonly used; breaks in epithelium are stained green

Ulcer scrapings for microscopic viewing (Gram or Giemsa stain)
Organism identification

Ulcer scrapings for culture
Organism identification

TREATMENT PLAN

Surgical
Corneal transplantation (see p. 732)
Enucleation (or evisceration) (see p. 729)

Chemotherapeutic
Mode, frequency, and duration of therapy depend on identified organism and degree of corneal penetration[28,40]
Anti-infective agents
Topical
Erythromycin, 5 mg/g
Gentamicin, 3-8 mg/ml
Penicillin G, 10,000-20,000 units/ml
Bacitracin, 10,000 units/ml
Sodium sulfacetamide, 10% solution
Natamycin (Pimaricin), 4%-5%
Amphotericin B, 1.5-3 mg/ml
Idoxuridine, 0.1% solution or 0.5% ointment
Subconjunctival injections of antibiotics for acute, severe central ulcerations
Systemic antibiotics (IV or po) for acute severe central ulcerations, if sclera is involved, or if perforation threatens
Mydriatic-cycloplegic agents
Atropine, 1% solution bid or tid for painful inflammation of iris and inflammatory constriction of pupil
Mucolytics
Acetylcysteine, 10%-20% solution for inhibiting collagenase
Analgesics (for severe pain)
Acetaminophen (Tylenol), 650 mg po q4h prn
Acetaminophen (Tylenol 650 mg) with codeine (30 mg), 1-2 tablets po q4h prn
Codeine, 30-60 mg po q4h prn

Supportive
Supportive therapy according to cause and severity of condition
Hospitalization for extensive central ulcer (over 3 mm diameter or penetrating deep into stroma)[28]

Pressure dressings (often over both eyes) for discomfort
Loose epithelium mechanically removed with applicator and local anesthetic for viral keratitis
Warm compresses for 10 to 15 minutes two or three times a day for discomfort and inflammation
Cool compresses for 10 to 15 minutes two or three times a day for burns (ultraviolet exposure), allergic response relief, or epithelial abrasions
Therapeutic soft contact lenses for recurrent corneal erosion or other chronic keratopathy[28,40]

ASSESSMENT: AREAS OF CONCERN

Corneal epithelium
Moderate to severe pain; blurred vision; haloes seen around lights; lacrimation; generalized hyperemia; fluorescein stains green on corneal surface; possible photophobia; possible purulent exudate, especially with accompanying conjunctivitis

Scarring
Opacity or irregular light reflection may be visible on corneal surface; diminished vision if opacity in visual axis

Edema
Cornea appears dull and uneven; visual loss (blurring)

Ulceration
Ulcers vary in appearance and size; whitish gray opacity with overhanging margins; fungous ulcer may be white, fluffy, and elevated; severe pain with epithelial damage or iritis; lacrimation and possible purulent discharge; generalized hyperemia

NURSING DIAGNOSES and NURSING INTERVENTIONS

Nursing Diagnosis	Nursing Intervention
Injury, potential for (related to foreign body)	Remove foreign body or irritant, if possible, by mechanical removal or saline or water rinse. Identify epithelial breaks with fluorescein (2%) stain. Instill prescribed medications such as topical antibiotics and cycloplegic agents for pain.
Comfort, alteration in: pain (related to corneal epithelial damage)	Apply pressure bandage to eye for discomfort; be certain covered eye is closed. Apply warm compress for 10 to 15 minutes for inflammation and discomfort. Apply cool compress for 10 to 15 minutes for burn or allergic response. Provide systemic analgesic as ordered. Administer topical and systemic medications as ordered for infection and iritis (cycloplegic). Ensure comfort and safety of hospitalized patient.

Nursing Diagnosis	Nursing Intervention
	Apply pressure dressings to one or both eyes as needed. Both eyes may need to be covered to limit movement of affected eye. Provide comfort and support.[36,40]

Sensory perception, alteration in: visual (related to bilateral eye patches)	Raise side rails.
	 Address patient by name from doorway and identify self.
	 Complement voice stimulation with touch to notify patient of your proximity.
	 Orient patient to bedside equipment (such as call light, bed control, and side rails) and personal belongings at bedside by directing his hand over objects.
	 Encourage patient to perform self-care with personal hygiene.
	 Provide patient's privacy and assure patient that privacy is provided.
	 Assist with meals.
	  Read menu selections.
	  Guide hand to utensils and food on tray.
	  Describe food on tray in clock terms.
	  Assist with cutting meat, removing lids from cartons, buttering bread, and so on.
	 Assist with walking.
	  Walk slowly and slightly ahead of patient.
	  Place patient's hand on your arm at your elbow.
	  If possible, allow patient to trace progress by running the dorsal aspect of his free hand along a wall.
	  Describe surroundings as you proceed.
	  Allow patient to feel chair, toilet, or bed before he turns to sit.[24]

Patient Education

1. Teach the patient self-care of corneal abrasion.
2. Teach the patient how to apply eye drops or ointments as ordered.
3. Teach the patient the application of warm or cold compresses.
4. Instruct the patient to wear dark glasses if a cycloplegic drug is ordered.
5. Tell the patient to wash hands before and after treating each eye.
6. Instruct the patient to keep hands away from the face and eyes except when treating self.
7. Instruct the patient not to use a soiled handkerchief or tissue on the eyes.
8. Instruct the patient to avoid noxious fumes and smoke.
9. Teach the patient to monitor the eye for increased pain or change in discharge.
10. Explain visual changes (increased blurring) or visual blockage.

EVALUATION

Patient Outcome	Data Indicating That Outcome is Reached
Cornea is healthy.	Cornea is clear and glossy. There is no eye discomfort, lacrimation, or discharge.[4]

Scleritis

Scleritis is an inflammation of the sclera.

Scleral inflammations are uncommon. The sclera has a poor blood supply and a low metabolism that does not encourage infection. Deep-seated aching and tenderness to touch without loss of vision are early indicators of disease. An ocular muscle may contract and turn the eye if the inflammation is near its insertion. Because of the proximity of the sclera to the uveal tract, a secondary choroiditis or retinal detachment may occur.

The episclera (located anteriorly) is more vascular than the rest of the sclera, and infections in this area may be worse. Infection is usually unilateral, has a sudden onset, and is accompanied by marked generalized hyperemia and pain. The cause is not always apparent, and the inflammation often subsides spontaneously.

Chronic or recurrent scleritis may result in scleral thinning with a localized outward bulging of the choroid layer. Perforation may occur.

DISORDERS OF THE UVEAL TRACT AND PUPIL

The uveal tract is composed of the iris, ciliary body, and choroid layer. The iris surrounds the pupil and controls its size; the ciliary body secretes aqueous humor and controls accommodation; and the vascular choroid nourishes the anterior uveal tract and part of the retina. The location and extent of uveal lesions determine the variety and severity of signs, symptoms, and visual alterations. Deep corneal inflammation often spreads to the iris and results in a painful contraction of the iris and ciliary body.

Iris abnormalities or inflammation can alter the shape of the pupil, disrupt the pupillary light reflex, or form adhesions to the cornea or lens to cause glaucoma. Ciliary body lesions can interfere with accommodation or cause anterior chamber or vitreous clouding with exudates, which diminishes visual acuity. Choroidal inflammation can spread to the sensory retinal layer and destroy central or peripheral vision. Retinal detachment may occur because of vitreous pull on the retina.[28]

Uveitis

Uveitis is an inflammation or infection of the uveal tract.

Uveitis is the most common uveal lesion. Organisms can be identified if the inflammation is peripheral enough to give the examiner access to infected tissue for staining or culture. Often the cause is unknown and the inflammation is treated on the basis of the presumed cause. Some inflammatory processes are associated with endogenous causes or chronic conditions that can be diagnosed and treated systemically. Acute inflammations vary in severity and may subside without residual alterations. The uveal tract is also subject to congenital or developmental lesions that may or may not affect vision.[28]

PATHOPHYSIOLOGY

Inflammation of the uveal tract can be acute or chronic and mild or severe and can involve primarily the anterior tract (iris, ciliary body, and anterior choroid), the posterior choroid, or the entire eye. The most common form of uveitis is acute anterior inflammation. The onset is sudden, and the symptoms of pain and visual loss appear abruptly and are sometimes severe. The arteries of the anterior ciliary body become engorged and dilated, which creates a purplish discoloration around the limbus (circumcorneal flush).[40] The iris and the ciliary body release an exudate that results in an increase of protein and inflammatory cells in the anterior chamber. The protein causes clouding of the chamber (aqueous flare), and the cells form in clumps that adhere to the posterior cornea (keratic precipitates). Keratic precipitates, a diagnostic determinant, can be viewed with a slit lamp and occasionally with the ophthalmoscope if the deposits are large enough.[28] A massive production of cells forms pus in the anterior chamber (hypopyon). The ciliary body also releases exudate into the vitreous to cause clouding and cell production. The iris is usually constricted (miotic

pupil) and does not respond to light. The constriction is painful, and pain intensity increases with light stimulation. If the pain is severe, it is difficult to open the lid for examination. If the iris remains constricted, it quickly forms adhesions to the underlying lens (posterior synechiae) that may obstruct aqueous flow and cause a pupillary block glaucoma. With anterior inflammation the iris, ciliary body, and anterior choroid are usually all involved because of a common blood supply.[28]

Posterior uveitis is usually confined to the posterior choroid and quickly spreads to the sensory retina. The vitreous becomes clouded with cells and exudate that can be viewed with an ophthalmoscope. Chorioretinal lesions can also be seen as irregular gray-white areas on the retinal surface. Vision impairment is the chief symptom of posterior choroiditis. Often there is no pain, redness, or photophobia. The degree of visual impairment depends on the extent of vitreous clouding and the location of retinal sensory layer inflammation. If the macula is involved, central vision is severely impaired. Retinal inflammations often leave scars that permanently impair vision.[40]

Acute uveitis results from external infection, trauma (laceration, puncture, or contusion), or chemical burns. Herpes simplex, herpes zoster, and fungal infections are common causes of iritis. There are many endogenous sources. Rubella, rubeola, or mumps may cause a mild, transient uveitis. A hypermature cataract may release exudate into the anterior chamber and cause severe inflammation. Systemic diseases such as rheumatoid arthritis, regional enteritis, ankylosing spondylitis, and collagen disorders may contribute to uveitis. Many uveitis exacerbations are idiopathic and are treated symptomatically. Acute uveitis can recur, particularly if the cause is endogenous and chronic.

Chronic uveitis is usually a continuous and progressive inflammation that involves cell production in the anterior and posterior chambers, frequent posterior synechia formation, retinal involvement, minimal exterior inflammatory signs or pain, and residual scarring of inflammatory sites. Some organisms invade and remain in the uveal tract. Tuberculosis, herpes zoster, and some forms of fungi are common causes of chronic inflammation. Systemic diseases such as sarcoidosis, rheumatoid arthritis (Still's disease), and histoplasmosis may be implicated. Some of the chronic syndromes are caused by local eye degenerative reactions. Chronic infections resulting from the degenerative changes in blind eyes may force a decision to perform enucleation for relief. Pars planitis is a chronic inflammation of the posterior choroid that involves vitreous opacities with a chief complaint of "floaters," retinal inflammation, and scarring. The cause is unknown, and the disease extends over 5 to 10 years.[28]

In severe infections the entire inner eyeball may become inflamed (panophthalmitis). Pyogenic bacteria may penetrate to the uvea with trauma, through rupture of a corneal ulcer, or through endogenous sources such as septicemia, meningitis, or bacterial endocarditis. *Staphylococcus aureus, Pseudomonas,* and *Proteus* are commonly involved organisms. Suppurative panophthalmitis is acute and severe. Severe pain, visual loss, and necrosis of the sclera may be followed by rupture of the globe. Sometimes the infection does not invade the sclera but remains confined to the inner eyeball (endophthalmitis). In this case the onset and course are less severe and the infection is more responsive to treatment.[28]

DIAGNOSTIC STUDIES[28,40]

Staining and culture of scrapings
Performed if uveitis is associated with peripheral inflammation or ulceration; organism is identified through culture and Gram stain

Slit-lamp (binocular microscope) examination
Patient's head is stabilized on chin rest; examiner sits opposite patient and views anterior parts of eye through movable microscope that magnifies objects five to 40 times (depending on design of instrument); beam of light is narrowed to slit that focuses on thin sections of cornea, anterior chamber, lens, or anterior vitreous; presence and extent of inflammatory cells or pus in anterior chamber and anterior vitreous can be viewed

Gonioscopy
Corneal contact lens (goniolens) is placed over anesthetized cornea to permit viewing of anterior chamber angles with microscopic lens; cellular debris and adhesions are seen in anterior chamber; angles can be viewed

Ophthalmoscopy
Vitreous opacities and chorioretinal lesions can be viewed

Diagnostic studies to rule out or identify systemic disease
Syphilis; primary tuberculosis; sarcoidosis; histoplasmosis; toxoplasmosis; ankylosing spondylitis; genitourinary infections; connective tissue disorders

TREATMENT PLAN[28,40]

Acute uveitis is often treated symptomatically because the etiology cannot be identified.

Surgical
Enucleation for ruptured globe or marked eye degeneration (see p. 729)
Lens extraction for lens-induced uveitis

Chemotherapeutic
Topical medications
  Anti-infective agents
    Erythromycin, 5 mg/g
    Gentamicin, 3-8 mg/ml
    Penicillin G, 10,000-20,000 units/ml
    Bacitracin, 10,000 units/ml
    Sodium sulfacetamide, 10% solution
    Natamycin (Pimaricin) 5% suspension
    Amphotericin B, 1.5-3 mg/ml
    Idoxuridine, 0.1% solution or 0.5% ointment
  Mydriatic-cycloplegic agents
    Atropine sulfate, 1% solution bid or tid to maintain full pupillary dilation
  Corticosteroids
    Instilled as frequently as q1-2h initially for severe inflammation, or bid or tid; to reduce inflammation and prevent iritic adhesions; patient response must be carefully supervised; herpes simplex and fungal organisms increase in activity and growth with steroid therapy; immunosuppression may increase host susceptibility to secondary infection; since open-angle glaucoma is common complication of topical steroid treatment, ocular tension must be carefully monitored
    Prednisolone suspension (Metimyd, others) (0.2%) or solution (0.125% or 1%)
    Dexamethasone suspension (Decadron phosphate), 0.1% solution or 0.05% ointment
    Hydrocortisone acetate suspension (Cortef, others), 0.5%, 1%, or 2.5%
    Fluorometholone suspension (FML Liquifilm), 0.1%

Medrysone suspension (HMS Liquifilm), 1%
Systemic medications
  Analgesics
    Acetaminophen (Tylenol), 650 mg po q4h prn
    Acetaminophen (Tylenol 650 mg) with codeine (30 mg), po q4h prn
  Corticosteroids
    For posterior uveitis and inflammations that do not respond to local treatment

ASSESSMENT: AREAS OF CONCERN

Anterior uveitis

Moderate pain; severe pain if associated with keratitis; intense photophobia; no visual change, possible blurred vision if eye chambers clouded with exudate, or possible blurred distant vision with ciliary spasm; circumcorneal flush (purplish coloration); pupillary constriction

Posterior uveitis

Minimal or no pain; blurred vision from vitreous opacities or sensory retina inflammation (may be central [macular] or peripheral depending on extent and location of inflammation); ophthalmoscopy may reveal vitreous opacities as black dots

NURSING DIAGNOSES and NURSING INTERVENTIONS

Nursing Diagnosis	Nursing Intervention
Comfort, alteration in: pain (related to acute anterior iridocyclitis)	Administer cycloplegics as ordered. Apply warm compresses for 10 to 15 minutes two or three times a day. Administer systemic analgesics as ordered. Instruct patient to wear dark glasses or avoid light.
Injury, potential for (adhesions and increased ocular pressure related to iridocyclitis)	Administer cycloplegics as ordered. Monitor patient for signs of increased ocular pressure, increased hazy vision (corneal edema), extreme pain, nausea, vomiting, or onset of conjunctival injection.[28]
Injury, potential for (retinal damage related to posterior chorioretinitis)	Administer topical and systemic medications (such as steroids) as ordered.[36]

Patient Education

1. Teach the patient self-care of uveitis in the home setting.
2. Teach the patient how to apply eye drops and ointments.
3. Teach the patient to apply warm compresses.
4. Instruct the patient to wear dark glasses.
5. Teach the patient to monitor the eye for increased pain, visual changes (increased blurring), and inflammatory signs.
6. Warn the patient that vision will be blurred because the pupil will be dilated.[36]

EVALUATION

Patient Outcome	Data Indicating That Outcome is Reached
Uveal tissue is healthy.	Cornea is clear and glossy. There is no photophobia, eye discomfort, inflammation (corneal, circumcorneal, or conjunctival), or discharge.
Vision is restored.	There is no blurring at close or distant range.[4]

Uveal Tract Deformities

Uveal tract deformities range from minor defects to severe impediments to visual functioning.

A coloboma is a localized absence of uveal tissue. An absence of a portion of the iris may cause a pupil shape defect (see p. 690) with no visual defects. If the choroidal coloboma is large, the overlying retina is deprived of blood supply in that area, which affects sensory vision. Aniridia is absence or diminishment of the iris. The pupil appears greatly enlarged, and no iris is showing. Photophobia and severe reduction of visual acuity follow. Aniridia may be inherited or associated with other chromosomal disorders such as mental retardation, Wilms' tumor, and urogenital abnormalities. The iris can atrophy over a period of years leaving a misshapen pupil or holes (looking like additional pupils) over the visible surface of the iris. The presence of holes can cause diplopia. Atrophy can follow severe eye inflammation or trauma or occur as a primary disease. Choroid atrophy can be a benign disorder or result in marked retinal degeneration. Some forms of choroid atrophy cause progressive night blindness and diminished visual acuity.[28]

The size of the pupil is controlled by dilator and constrictor muscles in the iris. There are no disorders of the pupil, but its size, response to light (accommodation), uniformity of shape, and symmetric responses with the corresponding eye are indicators of iris, eye, or systemic disorders.[25,28,29]

Table 6-2
Pupil Abnormalities

Abnormality	Contributing Factors	Appearance
Bilateral		
Miosis (pupillary constriction; usually less than 2 mm in diameter)	Iridocyclitis; miotic eye drops (such as pilocarpine given for glaucoma)	
Mydriasis (pupillary dilation; usually more than 6 mm in diameter)	Iridocyclitis; mydriatic or cycloplegic drops (such as atropine); midbrain (reflex arc) lesions or hypoxia; oculomotor (CN III) damage; acute-angle glaucoma (slight dilation)	
Failure to respond (constrict) with increased light stimulus	Iridocyclitis; corneal or lens opacity (light does not reach retina); retinal degeneration; optic nerve (CN II) destruction; midbrain synapses involving afferent pupillary fibers or oculomotor nerve (CN III) (consensual response is also lost); impairment of efferent fibers (parasympathetic) that innervate sphincter pupillae muscle	
Argyll Robertson pupil	Bilateral, miotic, irregular-shaped pupils that fail to constrict with light but retain constriction with convergence; pupils may or may not be equal in size; commonly caused by neurosyphilis or lesions in midbrain where afferent pupillary fibers synapse	
Oval pupil	Sometimes occurs with head injury or intracranial hemorrhage; transitional stage between normal pupil and dilated, fixed pupil with increased intracranial pressure (ICP); in most instances returns to normal when ICP is returned to normal	

Table 6-2, cont'd
Pupil Abnormalities

Abnormality	Contributing Factors	Appearance
Unilateral Anisocoria (unequal size of pupils)	Congenital (approximately 20% of normal people have minor or noticeable differences in pupil size, but reflexes are normal) or caused by local eye medications (constrictors or dilators), amblyopia, or unilateral sympathetic or parasympathetic pupillary pathway destruction (NOTE: Examiner should test whether pupils react equally to light; if response is unequal, examiner should note whether larger or smaller eye reacts more slowly [or not at all], since either pupil could be abnormal size)	
Iritis constrictive response	Acute uveitis is frequently unilateral; constriction of pupil accompanied by pain and circumcorneal flush (redness)	Normal eye Affected eye
Oculomotor nerve (CN III) damage	Pupil dilated and fixed; eye deviated laterally and downward; ptosis	Normal eye Affected eye
Horner's syndrome	Miotic pupil; ptosis; interruption of sympathetic nerve supply to dilator pupillae muscle; may be due to goiter, cervical lymph enlargement, apical bronchogenic carcinoma, or surgical injury to neck	Normal eye Affected eye
Adie's pupil (tonic pupil)	Affected pupil dilated and reacts slowly or fails to react to light; response to convergence normal; caused by impairment of postganglionic parasympathetic innervation to sphincter pupillae muscle or ciliary malfunction; often accompanied by diminished tendon reflexes (as with diabetic neuropathy or alcoholism)	Normal eye Affected eye
Other Irregularities Iridectomy	Sector iridectomy	

Table 6-2, cont'd
Pupil Abnormalities

Abnormality	Contributing Factors	Appearance
	Peripheral iridectomy Surgical excision of portion of iris usually done in superior area so upper lid will cover additional exposure	
Coloboma (localized absence of portion of iris)	Congenital absence of area of iris; remaining iris shows normal light response	
Iridodialysis (circumferential tearing of iris from scleral spur)	Blunt trauma; more than one "pupil" in eye can cause diplopia	

GLAUCOMA

Glaucoma incorporates a variety of diseases that exhibit all or at least one of the following abnormalities: increase in intraocular pressure, degeneration of the optic nerve (disc), and visual field losses that may lead to total loss of vision.

Glaucoma is detected in a variety of ways. Simple tonometry testing reveals intraocular pressure (IOP) that exceeds the normal range of 10 to 22 mm Hg. Only 5% to 10% of persons with IOP over 21 mm Hg have visual defects or optic nerve changes.[20] A variety of variables (discussed later) determine whether an unaffected person with a high IOP will only be monitored or will be treated for glaucoma. When screening methods include ophthalmoscopy or perimetry testing for visual field defects, some patients with a normal IOP exhibit optic nerve degeneration or visual field losses. Approximately one third of the visual defect population have a normal IOP when first examined.[20] The prevalence of glaucoma is difficult to determine because of the different screening methods and criteria for diagnosis among physicians and regions of the world. An estimated 1.5% of persons over 40 years of age have glaucoma, and approximately 50,000 persons in the United States are blind as a result of this disease.[40] Tonometry alone is not an adequate screening method for detecting glaucoma, and higher incidences are reported when persons are more thoroughly examined.

Glaucoma occurs because aqueous fluid cannot be drained adequately from the anterior chamber to maintain a normal IOP. Excessive pressure results in optic nerve degeneration. Primary glaucomas include open-angle and angle-closure disorder. Open-angle glaucoma is the more common and generally affects adults over 40 years of age. The onset is insidious and asymptomatic, and the disease progresses slowly. Many elderly persons with glaucoma are successfully treated with medications and retain vision. Closed-angle glaucoma occurs because of eye structure defects or changes and results in a mechanically blocked drainage system. The onset is usually acute and dramatic. Secondary glaucomas can be caused by inflammation, trauma, systemic disorders, or local eye changes. In addition, a number of congenital syndromes include glaucoma.

Glaucoma can be classified as follows*:

I. Primary
   A. Open-angle
      1. Chronic open-angle glaucoma and ocular hypotension
      2. Low-tension glaucoma
   B. Angle-closure
      1. Pupillary block
      2. Ciliary body block
      3. Peripheral iris block
II. Secondary
   A. Open-angle (aqueous humor has access to uveal trabecular meshwork)
      1. Uveal tract-related
         a. Inflammation
         b. Pigment dispersion
         c. Heterochromia iridis (Fuchs)
         d. Glaucomatocyclitic crisis
         e. Primary and secondary ocular tumors
         f. Anterior chamber epithelization
         g. Exfoliation syndrome
         h. Trabecular inflammation
         i. Phacolytic (hypermature lens)
         j. Phacoanaphylactic uveitis
      2. Trauma
         a. Recessed angle after contusion
         b. Hyphema
            (1) Erythrocytes, free or clotted, obstructing pupil or angle
            (2) Hemosiderin free or in macrophages
            (3) Ghost cells
         c. Siderosis from iron foreign bodies
      3. Miscellaneous
         a. Corticosteroid-induced
         b. Increased episcleral venous pressure
         c. Thyrotropic exophthalmos
         d. Alpha-chymotrypsin glaucoma
         e. Fuchs dystrophy
   B. Angle-closure (aqueous humor does not have access to uveal trabecular meshwork)
      1. Intumescent cataract
      2. Anterior displacement of iris lens diaphragm (malignant glaucoma)
      3. Ciliary body tumors
      4. Dislocated lens
      5. Rubeosis iridis
      6. Flat anterior chamber after accidental or surgical trauma
      7. Iridocorneoendothelial syndrome
         a. Chandler's syndrome
         b. Iris-nevus syndrome
         c. Iris atrophy
      8. Retrolental fibroplasia
      9. Persistent hyperplastic primary vitreous
   C. Pupillary block
      1. Inflammatory adhesions of iris to lens or vitreous face (in aphakia)
      2. Vitreous block (in aphakia)
      3. Intraocular lens block
      4. Anterior dislocation of lens
III. Congenital and hereditary
   A. Autosomal recessive congenital glaucoma
   B. Associated systemic disorders
      1. Phacomatosis
         a. Neurofibromatosis
         b. Sturge-Weber syndomre
      2. Lens dislocation
         a. Marfan's syndrome
         b. Homocystinuria
      3. Congenital infections
         a. Maternal rubella
         b. Syphilis
   C. Associated ocular disorders
      1. Mesodermal dysgenesis
      2. Posterior polymorphous dystrophy cornea
      3. Nanophthalmos and microcornea
      4. Aniridia

*From Newell, F.W.: Ophthalmology: principles and concepts, ed. 5, St. Louis, 1982, The C.V. Mosby Co.

PATHOPHYSIOLOGY

Open-Angle Glaucoma

Approximately 90% of cases of primary glaucoma are of the open-angle type. The incidence of this disease increases with age. Population studies have shown that less than 1% of persons under 65 years of age have glaucoma and that approximately 3% of the population over 75 years of age have this disorder.[20] Other risk factors for open-angle glaucoma have been identified. Nonwhite persons have a much higher incidence and frequently exhibit an earlier onset and a more rapid eye degeneration. Hypertension has been linked to glaucoma, as have the hypotensive episodes associated with treatment for hypertension. Approximately 20% to 25% of glaucoma patients have a family history of this disease. Myopic and diabetic persons are reported to have a higher incidence of glaucoma.[20]

Increased IOP occurs because of degenerative changes of unknown cause in the trabecular meshwork and the canal of Schlemm. Excess fluid cannot be emptied from the anterior chamber.

IOP is not static but normally varies 2 to 5 mm Hg with increased heart rate, activity, or excitement. One high reading does not constitute a basis for diagnosis. Some persons exhibit visual field defects and optic nerve changes with normal or near-normal IOP, whereas others are able to tolerate elevated IOP without eye damage. Elevated IOP without ocular damage is called ocular hypertension. Some physicians believe that this elevation is a precursor of glaucoma, but others think that a mildly elevated IOP (20 to 24 mm Hg) is a normal state. The risk for eye damage increases with age, a family history of glaucoma, diabetes, and systemic vascular disorders.

Early open-angle glaucoma may be difficult to diagnose because it is asymptomatic. Even persons with visual field defects do not usually perceive them until they become extensive. There is no pain or blurred vision, and the outer eye does not appear inflamed or abnormal to the examiner. Tonometry usually shows an elevated IOP. The Schiötz tonometer is less accurate in higher pressure ranges and consistently shows lower pressures than applanation or noncontact tonometers. Direct ophthalmoscopy may reveal the earliest finding if the examiner is sufficiently skilled. The physiologic cup (a depression in the center of the disc) may be larger in one eye than the other. As the disease progresses, the cup widens and extends toward the disc temporal margin. The temporal vessels appear to drop (or bend) abruptly into the cup. The large vessels become displaced and crowded toward the nasal side of the disc. The temporal disc border atrophies and loses its pink coloration to appear a flat white. The cup widens and deepens (excavation) as the surrounding optic nerve margin diminishes and atrophies.

Visual field testing often shows the most tangible alterations. Visual field testing by confrontation does not measure early or limited defects. The Goldmann perimeter measures both central and peripheral losses. Characteristic defects (blind areas or scotomas) appear and enlarge as the disease progresses. Nerve fiber bundles originating from the optic nerve cease to function as the nerve head atrophies. The nasal visual field is often first affected, and eventually the periphery is diminished. The person may retain only a small portion of central vision with acuity of the unaffected area.[40]

Many older adults are treated successfully with medication. Parasympathomimetic agents (miotic eye drops) increase the outflow of fluid by enlarging the area around the trabecular meshwork. β-Adrenergic blocking agents (eye drops) and orally administered carbonic anhydrase inhibitors decrease aqueous production. These drugs are given in various combinations. Miotic drops disturb vision because of pupillary constriction and may cause ciliary spasms. β-Blockers must be administered cautiously to asthmatic patients. Epinephrine drops are sometimes prescribed to increase outflow, but their use should be evaluated carefully because of potential systemic effects (tachycardia) and occasional local effects (macular edema). Diuretics deplete potassium and may cause thirst and drinking of large amounts of fluids, which could increase pressure. Patient receiving medication need careful and continuous supervision.[33]

If IOP cannot be controlled through medication, laser trabeculoplasty (creating openings in the trabecular meshwork with laser beams), laser iridotomy, or surgery

---

Fig. 6-15
A, Normal anterior chamber. **B,** Shallow anterior chamber. Shallow chamber shows forward displacement of iris and narrow anterior angle.

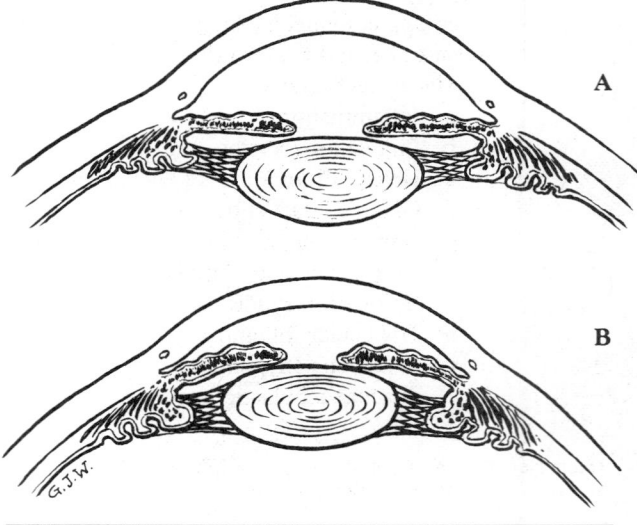

may be performed. Surgery usually involves the creation of an opening between the anterior chamber and the subconjunctival space. Many physicians prefer laser therapy because it is less damaging to the eye (see p. 734). Success rates for laser and surgical therapies are variable.[33] The openings or filter systems may not remain patent. Invasive therapy for open-angle glaucoma is a last resort for eyes that do not respond to chemotherapeutic regimens.

Angle-Closure Glaucoma

Angle-closure glaucoma occurs because mechanical blockage of the anterior chamber angle results in accumulation of aqueous fluid and increased IOP. Most persons with angle-closure glaucoma have shallow anterior chambers (less than 3 mm depth between the iris and the posterior corneal surface), which is often a familial trait.[1,28] These persons do not exhibit IOP elevations unless the angle is closed and obscures the trabecular meshwork, which ordinarily drains fluid from the anterior chamber. The shallow chamber is often accompanied by narrowed anterior angles (Fig. 6-15). Narrow angles are more vulnerable to other physiologic events that cause further crowding of the angles.

Angle closure occurs because of pupillary dilation or forward displacement of the iris. In some instances pupillary dilation (physiologic or induced) causes the iris to crowd into the anterior angle, resulting in obstruction. Forward displacement of the iris occurs with enlargement of the lens, which normally thickens with aging. The iris can also be pushed forward with physiologic pupillary block. In a shallow anterior chamber the iris may press against the lens and obstruct aqueous flow from the posterior chamber to the anterior chamber. As fluid accumulates posteriorly, it bulges forward against the iris. A bulging iris can be viewed by an examiner with a penlight aimed obliquely at the cornea. The bulge casts a shadow on the opposite side of the light source. If the examiner views the iris laterally, the normally flat iris can sometimes be seen as a convex curve that parallels the overlying cornea.

Angle closure can occur in a subacute, acute, or chronic form. Subacute episodes often precede an acute attack. These episodes may involve transient angle obstruction with symptoms of blurred vision, mild to severe pain, and haloes seen around lights. Persons with subacute angle closure may not exhibit increased IOP during an examination, but provocative testing with rapid drinking of water, sitting in a dark room to cause pupil dilation, or induced mydriasis may elicit an increased IOP (see descriptions of methods on p. 694).

Acute angle closure causes a dramatic response. A sudden onset of blurred vision, severe ocular pain, and haloes seen around lights is followed by a progression of symptoms as the pressure increases. Ciliary injection (a purplish red coloration around the limbus), profuse lacrimation, a mildly dilated, nonreactive pupil (5 to 6 mm in diameter), and nausea and vomiting may occur. Corneal edema causes the cornea to appear hazy. An acute episode constitutes a medical emergency. If the pressure is not relieved within several hours, eye damage occurs. Adhesions (anterior synechiae) begin to form between the iris and the cornea, which eventually closes the angle. Within a few days the iris and ciliary body begin to atrophy, the cornea shows permanent changes because of chronic edema, and optic atrophy and deterioration of nerve fibers occur. Total loss of vision is the result.[40]

Emergency medical treatment consists of (1) oral or intravenous administration of carbonic anhydrase inhibitors or osmotics to reduce pressure, (2) miotic eye drops to pull the iris away from the inner angle, and (3) systemic analgesics to reduce pain. Surgical treatment (usually iridotomy) follows as soon as ocular pressure is stabilized. Although usually only one eye is affected at a time, surgery is eventually performed on the other eye as a preventive measure.[28,40]

Chronic episodes of increased IOP can occur when anterior angles are sufficiently narrowed to partially obstruct outflow. The patient may have minimal symptoms (hazy vision, mild pain) or none, and the IOP is usually elevated when measured. Subacute and chronic forms of angle closure are often treated medically or surgically to prevent insidious eye damage such as slow formation of anterior adhesions.

Secondary Glaucomas

Trabecular meshwork obstruction or closed-angle glaucoma can occur because of eye deformities, inflammation, or trauma (surgical or accidental). Corticosteroid therapy increases IOP; this may be transient or may cause permanent eye damage.[28]

A displaced, enlarged, hypermature, or ruptured lens can result in a crowding of the angle, an associated trabecular meshwork obstruction, or uveitis. Uveitis may cause a pupillary block with ciliary spasms or posterior synechiae (adhesions of the iris to the lens), which ultimately obstructs angle drainage. Trabeculitis with resultant scarring and damage may follow iridocyclitis when inflammatory cells and fibrous material are deposited in the anterior angles. Eye contusions elevate IOP, usually temporarily. If hemorrhage or edema of the iris or ciliary body ensues, the IOP increase is sustained and the angle flow may be compromised. If the anterior eye is traumatized through surgery or laceration, the iris root may reform or adhere to the ciliary body to obstruct the anterior angle.[40]

Congenital Glaucoma

Primary congenital glaucoma is a hereditary disease. It occurs when the structures of the anterior chamber angle do not fully develop at about the fifth month of fetal life. A thin remnant of iris tissue inserts into the trabecular meshwork and partially or fully covers it. The IOP increases, and corneal and optic nerve destruction ensues. Boys are affected more often than girls, and the disease is most commonly diagnosed at birth or within the first 2 years of life. The disease is most often bilateral. The earlier the symptoms, the less favorable the prognosis because earlier onset indicates a greater anatomic abnormality. Other systemic congenital defects may accompany primary congenital glaucoma. Early symptoms are excessive tearing and photophobia. A hazy cornea eventually becomes opaque because of edema and stretching with breaks in Descemet's membrane, which allows fluid into the cornea. The eye enlarges because the tissue is elastic, and the diameter of the cornea increases. Optic nerve deterioration occurs rapidly, resulting in total loss of vision. If the symptoms are diagnosed early, goniotomy (cutting away the tissue covering the meshwork) is performed. In some instances the goniotomy must be repeated a number of times to ensure adequate drainage. Approximately 80% of these surgeries are successful.[40]

Secondary congenital glaucomas are associated with a variety of systemic and eye disorders. Aniridia, the absence of an iris, may be associated with other anterior eye deformities to cause glaucoma. A dystrophic cornea or a congenital cataract may be associated with glaucoma. Neurofibromatosis and Sturge-Weber syndrome (hemangioma of the face) are two of the more common systemic disorders that accompany congenital glaucoma. Usually filtering or trabeculoplasty procedures are performed with varying success depending on the severity of the anatomic abnormality.[28]

DIAGNOSTIC STUDIES[28,40]

Tonometry (Schiötz, applanation, or contact methods)
Test for intraocular pressure; normal range 10 to 22 mm Hg

Visual field studies
Central field tangent screen
Central vision covers approximately 50 degrees of patient's central vision, 25 degrees in each direction from central fixation point; black screen 1 m² is placed 1 m from eye; blind spots are outlined by using 1 to 3 mm white target placed

on board; normal blind spot is 13 to 18 degrees temporal from central fixation; abnormal isolated spots (scotomas) or confluent areas can be identified; nasal areas are usually lost first
Automated perimetry
Various automatic machines (such as Goldmann perimeter) measure both central and peripheral fields

Gonioscopy
Corneal contact lens (goniolens) placed over anesthetized cornea to permit viewing of anterior chamber angles with microscopic lens; cellular debris and adhesions in anterior chamber angles can also be viewed

Ophthalmoscopy
See pp. 660-661

Provocative tests
Used for patients with mildly elevated IOP, those who have optic nerve changes or field defects without elevated IOP, and those with shallow anterior chambers and compromised anterior angles; results not definitive but may distinguish potentially glaucomatous persons from others
Water drinking test
In morning, fasting patient drinks approximately 1 L of water as fast as possible (within 2 to 4 minutes); IOP is measured before and at 15-minute intervals for 45 minutes; normal eyes show IOP increase of 3 to 5 mm Hg; increase of 8 mm Hg is indicative of glaucoma
Dark room test (for narrow-angle glaucoma)
Patient sits in dark room for 60 minutes to dilate pupils; IOP increase of 7 to 8 mm Hg is indicative of iris bunching into and blocking anterior angle flow
Mydriatic testing
One eye is dilated at a time (under careful supervision), and pupil is constricted when test is ended; IOP increase of 8 mm Hg is indicative of glaucoma

TREATMENT PLAN

Open-Angle Glaucoma[28,36,40]

Surgical
Surgery performed if medications do not control pressure
Laser trabeculoplasty—may be done on outpatient basis; 100 to 120 laser impacts aimed evenly spaced around anterior portion of trabecular meshwork

through goniolens; resultant scarring thought to increase tension within meshwork to maintain openings; success rate not fully determined[33]; see p. 736

External trabeculectomy—favored over other filter device procedures because it does not disrupt anterior chamber and adhesions do not form between iris and posterior canal; portion of meshwork is removed through scleral flap incision; flap is replaced over surgical site to keep anterior chamber intact; procedure performed in hospital with patient under general anesthesia[28]

Chemotherapeutic

Adrenergic-blocking agents

Timolol maleate (Timoptic) to reduce aqueous production, 1 drop of 0.25%-0.5% eye drops in each eye, usually bid

Miotics

Pilocarpine, 1 or 2 drops of 0.25%-4% eye drops, 2-6 times/d

Anticholinesterase drops (long-acting, strong miotics) for aphakic glaucoma; miotic response is strong, and these agents should not be used for narrow-angle glaucoma because pupillary block may occur

Echothiophate iodide (Phospholine), 1 drop of 0.03%-0.25% solution qd or bid

Physostigmine salicylate (Eserine), 0.1 ml of 0.25%-1% solution several times/d

Adrenergic agents

Epinephrine drops (Epifrin), to decrease aqueous secretion, 1 or 2 drops of 0.25%-2% solution qd

Diuretics

Acetazolamide (Diamox) to suppress aqueous production, 125-250 mg po qid

Angle-Closure Glaucoma[28,36,40]

Surgical

Laser iridotomy—lens placed over anesthetized cornea; argon laser aimed at iris for approximately 50 deliveries to penetrate iris and create opening for aqueous flow; laser sessions repeated several times if necessary; ultimately both eyes usually treated; see p. 736

Peripheral iridectomy—3 to 4 mm incision made at limbus or parallel to limbus over cornea; iris prolapses through limbus, or forceps is inserted into anterior chamber to pull portion of iris outward so small wedge or piece of iris can be excised; remaining iris is massaged back into chamber, and pupil is constricted to assure therapist that it is intact and round surrounding excised wedge; incision is then closed; pupil is dilated postoperatively, and

steroid eye medication is given for few days so inflamed iris will not form adhesions; iridectomy opens channel between anterior and posterior chambers and creates opening in anterior angle for aqueous flow

Chemotherapeutic

In acute attacks, medications given to lower and control IOP so surgery can be performed

Hyperosmotic agents

Glycerin (Glycerol) to draw fluid from eye, 1.5 g/kg body weight po

Mannitol (Osmitrol), usually IV, 2 g/kg body weight

Carbonic anhydrase inhibitors

Acetazolamide (Diamox), 250 mg po bid or qid, or 500 mg followed by 250 mg IV q4h; should be given immediately to abort acute attack

Narcotic analgesics

Meperidine, 100 mg IM q4-6h prn

Congenital Glaucoma[28,36,40]

Surgical

Goniotomy—knife inserted near limbus to penetrate anterior chamber and reach area of trabecular meshwork in anterior angle; special goniolens used to scrutinize angle while knife tears away tissue covering meshwork; procedure may be repeated a number of times to ensure patency of drainage system

Chemotherapeutic

Medications not usually given; surgery necessary for alleviation; miotics sometimes given in preparation for surgery

ASSESSMENT: AREAS OF CONCERN

Open-angle glaucoma

Asymptomatic (no blurring, pain, or inflammatory signs, early visual defects not perceived by patient); outer eye appears normal

Tonometry

IOP usually elevated (more than 24 mm Hg) but may be within normal limits (under 22 mm Hg)

Optic disc

Cupping and disc atrophy

Initial one cup larger than other; enlarged cup occupies more than half of disc diameter; cup widens and extends toward temporal disc border; temporal disc border loses translucence and appears flat white; crowding of disc vessels toward nasal border

Visual fields (perimetry)
  Typical central blind spots (scotomas) identifiable; nasal vision usually lost before peripheral vision

Angle-closure glaucoma
  Excessive lacrimation; acute, severe ocular pain (usually bilateral; blurred vision; haloes seen around lights; pupil in mild dilation (5 to 6 mm diameter); corneoscleral flush (purplish red coloration at limbus); cornea may appear hazy; possible nausea and vomiting

Tonometry
  IOP usually markedly elevated (more than 24 mm Hg)

Congenital glaucoma
  Excessive lacrimation; photophobia; hazy opaque cornea; affected eye enlarged (both eyes may be affected); affected cornea enlarged in diameter
Tonometry
  IOP usually elevated but elastic eye tissue may stretch and give false low reading

NURSING DIAGNOSES and NURSING INTERVENTIONS

Nursing Diagnosis	Nursing Intervention
Open-Angle Glaucoma	
Noncompliance (related to side effects of eye medications)	Educate patient about disease and its insidious progress without treatment. Be certain that patient can read medication labels. Explain that number of medications and number of administrations can be confusing, inconvenient, and easy to forget. Enlist patient's assistance and understanding in devising medication schedule that patient can meet. Discuss with patient that medications do not relieve any symptoms and may cause unpleasant side effects. Ensure that patient is aware of possible side effects: Miotics—blurred vision for 1 to 2 hours after administration, diarrhea; Timolol—fatigue, weakness, depression; Diamox—numbness, tingling of extremities and lips, decreased appetite or nausea, impotence. Assess patient's needs and response to medications regularly to see if negative responses are occurring and that medication schedule is being followed. Physician may be able to change medication if side effects are severe.
Injury: potential for	Instruct patient with new prescription that frequent checkups by physician are needed to detect side effects and other symptoms such as increased IOP, sudden blurred vision, and inflammation of eyes. Teach patient about possible side effects: Miotics—pupillary block, myopia from excessive accommodation; Timolol—keratitis, asthma, bradycardia; Epinephrine—eye irritation, periorbital edema, tachycardia; Diamox—hypokalemia, confusion, urinary calculi. Inform patient that examination (tonometry, health history, ophthalmoscopy, gonioscopy, and perimetry) will be needed every 2 to 3 months until physician determines that IOP is stable and there is no further optic nerve damage or visual field loss. Examination should be annually performed thereafter. Demonstrate correct method for administration and storage of eye drops. Have patient repeat demonstration to ensure proper technique.
Sensory-perceptual alteration: visual	Review patient's life-style and suggest adjustments to blurred vision associated with miotics. Assess and review patient's family and support system for assistance in dealing with visual loss. Assess patient's feelings about visual loss or changes. Offer support for feelings of loss and helplessness. Inform patient that peripheral vision is a great safety hazard and may be markedly reduced with advanced glaucoma. Explain that patient must learn to turn head to visualize either side. Ask patient to reduce clutter in home (such as electrical cords, loose rugs, and items on floor) that could cause fall. Inform patient that home should be well lighted (especially stairways) and that night light in bathroom is helpful.

Nursing Diagnosis	Nursing Intervention
	Warn patient that seeing at night, at dusk, or in dim lighting will be difficult because miotic pupils do not dilate to admit more light to retina in subdued lighting or darkness.[4,36]
Laser Trabeculoplasty Knowledge deficit	Describe procedure carefully to patient and family members, including discussion of equipment, length of procedure, nature of procedure, and postoperative events.
Anxiety (related to uncertainty about discomfort and outcome of laser procedure)	Offer support and comfort. Administer anesthetic eye drops immediately before procedure. Inform patient that headache and blurred vision may occur for first 24 hours after procedure. Administer medications as ordered. Educate patient about administering eye medications and necessity for maintaining prescribed therapy, since iris may become inflamed postoperatively and IOP may be increased: 　Glaucoma medications—resumed until inflammatory process subsides and then discontinued or adjusted 　Topical steroid drops—often prescribed for approximately 1 week after surgery; reduce inflammation but may raise IOP Inform patient that IOP may rise postoperatively and needs to be carefully monitored. Educate patient about necessity for keeping appointments for monitoring IOP. Educate patient about self-monitoring for symptoms (especially sudden onset): 　Excessive lacrimation 　Photophobia 　Severe ocular pain Advise patient that vision will be blurred for first day or two after procedure.[33]
Comfort, alteration in: pain	Administer systemic analgesics as ordered for headache that may occur a day or two after procedure. Apply eye patch for few hours postoperatively to avoid discomfort associated with light exposure.
Peripheral Trabeculectomy Knowledge deficit (related to lack of information needed about the procedure)	Describe procedure carefully to patient and family members, including discussion of equipment used, length of procedure, nature of procedure, and postoperative events.
Anxiety	Offer support and comfort. Orient patient to surroundings and inform him that affected eye will be patched postoperatively. Explain to patient that already damaged vision cannot be restored but that there is likelihood that further damage will be stopped.[36]
Injury: potential for	Maintain vital signs until stable. Observe eye dressing for excessive bleeding (small amount of serosanguineous drainage may be present). Inform patient that periodic tonometry measurements are usually performed because IOP may temporarily increase postoperatively. Administer antiemetics as ordered for nausea. Administer mydriatics as ordered; pupil of affected eye is dilated immediately or within 2 or 3 days postoperatively to prevent formation of iris adhesion. Administer glaucoma medications as ordered for unoperated eye.
Sensory-perceptual alteration: visual	*Before surgery:* Warn patient that depth perception will be lost and that 50% of peripheral vision will be lost on affected side. *After surgery:* Assist patient with activities of daily living. Caution patient to bring hand forward slowly to touch objects (especially containers of hot liquid and containers receiving poured liquids).

Nursing Diagnosis	Nursing Intervention
	Teach patient to turn head fully toward affected side to view objects or obstacles.
	Tell patient to use up and down head movements to judge stairs and oncoming objects and to go slowly.[24]
	See p. 1967.
Comfort, alteration in: pain	Monitor patient for postoperative discomfort and give systemic analgesics as ordered.
Angle-Closure Glaucoma	
Comfort, alteration in: pain	Offer comfort and support to patient and family.
	Give medications as ordered (meperidine may not be ordered for some patients because it tends to cause nausea and vomiting).
	Administer osmotics or carbonic anhydrase inhibitors as ordered to reduce aqueous production, and document response.
Anxiety	Offer comfort and support.
	Give realistic assurance about maintenance of vision if IOP is brought under control quickly.
	Keep patient informed of progress and planned medical and surgical interventions.
	Describe impending surgical procedures, including equipment, length of procedure, nature of procedure, and postoperative events.
Laser Iridotomy	
Comfort, alteration in: pain	During procedure, assist patient to hold still (head is stabilized on chin rest).
	Offer reassurance and support.
	Administer topical anesthetic as ordered.
	Administer postoperative medications as ordered.
	Educate patient about necessity of maintaining prescribed therapy.
	Educate patient about necessity of keeping appointments for monitoring IOP. (This procedure may be done on outpatient basis, and patient compliance is vital factor.)
	Educate patient about self-monitoring for symptoms (especially sudden onset): Excessive lacrimation / Photophobia / Severe ocular pain
	Advise patient that vision will be blurred for first day or two after procedure.
	Advise patient that procedure may have to be repeated several times to ensure patency of angle.
	Administer systemic analgesics as ordered if headache and mild eye pain continue for day or two.
	Eye patch is usually applied for a few hours postoperatively to avoid discomfort associated with light exposure.[33,36]
	Maintain vital signs until stable.
	Observe eye dressing for excessive bleeding.
	Observe patient for sudden onset of severe pain in operated eye and administer medications as ordered.
	Inform patient that tonometry measurements will probably be performed periodically.
	Administer antiemetics as ordered for nausea.
	Administer mydriatics and steroid drops for operated eye as ordered. (Unoperated eye may need to be maintained with glaucoma medications if patient has previously received them.)
Sensory-perceptual alteration: visual	*Before surgery:*
	Warn patient that depth perception will be lost and that 50% of peripheral vision will be lost on affected side.
	After surgery:
	Assist patient with activities of daily living.
	Caution patient to bring hand forward slowly to touch objects (especially containers of hot liquid and containers receiving poured liquids).

Nursing Diagnosis	Nursing Intervention
	Teach patient to turn head fully toward affected side to view objects or obstacles.[24]
	Tell patient to use up and down head movements to judge stairs and oncoming objects and to go slowly.
	See p. 1967.
Comfort, alteration in: pain	Monitor patient for postoperative discomfort and give systemic analgesics as ordered.

Patient Education

Specific knowledge needs are described in "Nursing Diagnosis and Nursing Interventions" because glaucoma is commonly managed on an outpatient basis.

1. Inform the patient that glaucoma is not curable but can be controlled.
2. Explain to the patient that medications *must* be taken regularly.
3. Instruct the patient to visit the physician regularly as prescribed.
4. Explain that the patient must monitor self for side effects (see p. 696) and report any to the therapist, since therapy may be changed according to the patient's response to medications (either undesirable side effects or ineffective therapy).
5. Tell the patient to watch for sudden changes, including severe eye pain, inflamed eye, excessive lacrimation, marked photophobia, and visual field losses (inability to use peripheral vision), which may be noted because of bumping into obstacles from the side or at the patient's feet.
6. Remind the patient of any existing limited vision and related safety concerns (see p. 696).
7. Warn the patient of factors that may increase IOP, such as constrictive clothing around the neck or torso, constipation (straining), heavy exertion or lifting, and sneezing or coughing (upper respiratory infection).
8. Explain that family members should be examined regularly because glaucoma and shallow interior chambers are often familial.

EVALUATION

Patient Outcome	Data Indicating That Outcome is Reached
IOP is under control.	Tonometry shows IOP of less than 24 mm Hg.
Eye damage is not present or not increasing.	There are no visual field defects, or existing field defects are not increasing. Eye examination shows normal findings. Eyeball surface is moist without excessive tearing. Conjunctiva is clear without injection. Cornea is clear, and no redness appears at limbus. Pupil may be constricted because of medication. Red reflex is full and round. Retinal surface is pink, granular, and uniform in color and consistency. Optic disc is pinkish white and translucent with physiologic cup that occupies no more than half of disc diameter. Both optic cups are same size. Central vessels emerge evenly from optic disc and are not crowded toward nasal side.[4]

DISORDERS OF THE LENS

The lens is a 4 mm (sagittal diameter) by 9 mm (equatorial diameter), transparent structure between the anterior chamber and the vitreous body.[17] Its transparency and biconvex shape enable it to focus light rays on the retina through refraction. The lens is suspended by fibers (zonule) that attach to the ciliary muscles, and it is stabilized behind the iris. The elasticity of the lens enables it to increase its spheric shape in response to ciliary contraction for near vision (accommodation). Loss of elasticity with aging results in diminished refractive power for near vision (presbyopia).

Diseases of the lens result in either opacity or dislocation of the lens. Because the lens contains no pain fibers or blood vessels, usually the only symptom is blurred vision without discomfort.

Lens Dislocation

The lens can be dislocated by trauma (a blow to the eye), systemic congenital disorders, or deformities of the lens itself.

In most instances the lens loses the full support of the zonular fibers and is either partially dislocated or fully detached and floating in the vitreous. Iritis and glaucoma are common complications of a lens in the vitreous. Surgical removal of the detached lens may be performed to prevent further eye damage, although complications may ensue because of disruption and loss of vitreous. Partially dislocated lenses are often successfully treated with glasses to correct blurred vision.[28]

Cataract

Cataract is an opacity of the lens.

No one has perfectly transparent lenses. Minor imperfections do not impair vision and are not apparent with gross examination. Gradual opacification of the lens is a physiologic process; if all humans lived long enough, they would develop cataracts. The diagnosis of cataract is usually confirmed when a patient reports visual impairment.[9] Considerable opacification may occur before the patient notices visual changes. The prevalence of the disease is difficult to determine because in some studies cataracts are defined as lens changes, whereas in others the disease is reported when vision is altered or the lens must be surgically removed. A summary of available data states that visible lens changes occur in 42% of the 52- to 64-year-old population and that 5% of these persons demonstrate some visual impairment. Between 60% and 91% of the 65- to 85-year-old group show senile lens opacities, and approximately 25% to 46% of these persons demonstrate visual impairment.[21] Cataracts are the third leading cause of blindness.

Congenital cataracts are relatively rare and occur in all degrees of severity. Newborns can exhibit total or minimum opacification. Surgery may be performed in infancy, or the eyes may be observed and surgically treated at a later time. In many instances opacification does not impair vision sufficiently to warrant surgical removal.

The only therapy for lens opacities that impair vision is surgical removal of the lens. Surgical procedures for the eye have changed dramatically in the last 20 years. Fine suture materials, the operating microscope, microsurgical instruments, improved general anesthetic procedures, and ultrasonic probes for lens emulsification and lens suction have all contributed to an improved prognosis and rapid recovery from surgery.[10,42] In the past, patients had to wait for the cataract to become "ripe" (develop marked edema and liquefaction) before surgery was possible. Newer techniques permit the decision to be made jointly by the patient and physician on the basis of visual impairment and the patient's need for visual clarity.[2] Extended-wear soft contact lenses and, in some instances, surgically implanted lenses allow monophakic persons (those with one lens removed) to enjoy binocular vision. Over 95% of surgically treated cataract patients can now look forward to restored useful vision.[9]

PATHOPHYSIOLOGY

Acquired cataracts can occur because of trauma, heat, toxins, intraocular inflammation, systemic disease, or aging. Aging is considered the primary risk factor for cataract formation. Senile cataracts occur because of protein alterations, accumulation of water, increasing edema, and migration and disruption of normal fibers within the lens. The exact cause for these changes is unknown.[26] Cataracts are usually bilateral but progress more rapidly in one eye than the other.

Opacities occur in different formations and in different areas of the lens (Fig. 6-16). The central part of the lens (nucleus) is harder and denser than the periphery (cortex) because newly formed fibers continuously migrate toward and pack together in the central nucleus. The lens is surrounded by the capsule, a semipermeable membrane. The most common type of senile cataract occurs in the posterior subcapsular area. These opacities tend to obscure central vision relatively early. Cortical (or peripheral) cataracts, called soft cataracts, may cause marked opacification without interfering with vision. Eventually the opacities encroach on the visual axis and decrease visual acuity. Nuclear (or hard) cataracts occur in the central area of the lens.[40] As the central lens changes, it enlarges and increases its spheric shape, which permits some persons to enjoy "second sight," an increase in near vision. This diminished presbyopia is a temporary improvement and is followed by increased opacities that ultimately reduce vision. Opacities may develop very slowly and form different configurations. An early symptom may be glare (especially at night) because the opacities reflect light rays inefficiently. In some instances central opacities split light rays and cause a monocular diplopia. This symptom disappears as the

Fig. 6-16
Various types of senile cataracts. **A,** Nuclear sclerosis. **B,** Nuclear sclerosis and posterior subcapsular cataract. **C,** Nuclear sclerosis and anterior and posterior cortical cataracts.

From Newell, F.W.: Ophthalmology: principles and concepts, ed. 5, St. Louis, 1982, The C.V. Mosby Co.

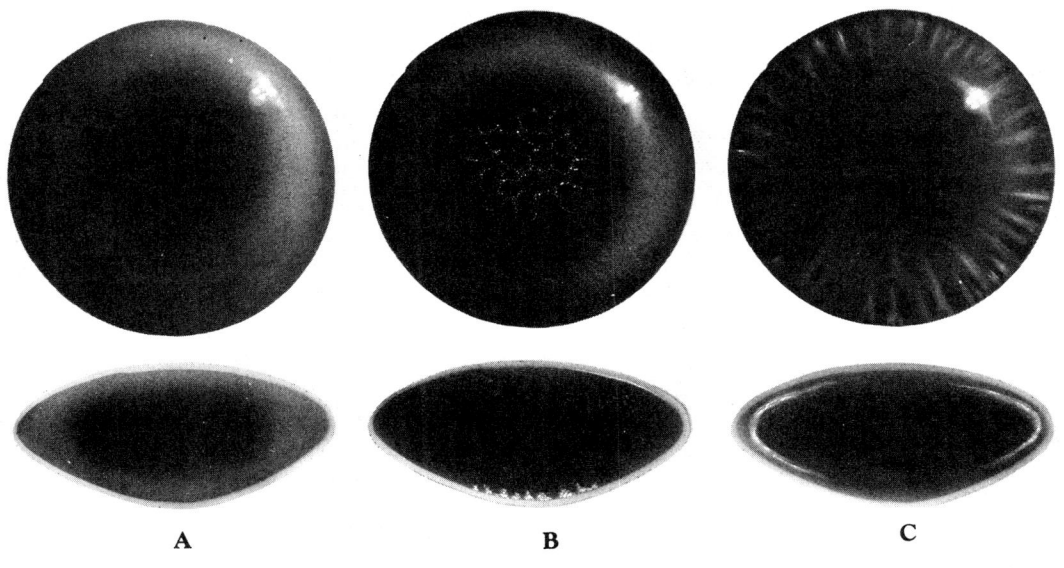

A   B   C

opacity increases. Vision may improve in dim light (or with pupil dilation) because the person has more pupil available to see around the opacity. Some patients are able to "see" the dark spots, which remain fixed in the visual field, unlike floaters (debris in the vitreous) that move around.

If the cataract is not removed, it may eventually cause the entire lens to be opaque. This can be seen with casual observation as a whitish discoloration of the entire pupil. Less advanced opacities may be seen through the ophthalmoscope as dark spots, patches, or networks of lines that disrupt the red reflex.

Decision for removal of the lens is usually based on the patient's need to see. Vision is evaluated by examining both eyes. If one eye enables the patient to maintain adequate vision, the failing eye is often not surgically treated. In some instances the lens swells and encroaches on the anterior chamber angle to cause glaucoma. Hypermature cataracts may release toxic products that cause a secondary uveitis or glaucoma or both. Surgical intervention is sometimes undertaken to prevent eye damage regardless of visual acuity.[28]

Risk factors other than age have been identified as possible sources for cataract formation. Women over 65 years of age are reported to have a higher rate of cataract formation than men. Some studies have shown that persons living in warm, sunny climates have a significantly higher incidence of cataracts. The correlation between cataract formation and ultraviolet light exposure is under further investigation. The lens is susceptible to heat because its avascular tissue does not transfer heat efficiently.[21]

High-dose radiation has been proved to cause cataracts. Survivors of atomic bomb explosions have exhibited a high prevalence of this disease. Study findings of the effects of exposure to low doses of radiation over a prolonged period are not conclusive. Some concern has been raised about computed tomography scans of the skull as a direct source of radiation to the eyes.[21]

Some drugs are reported to be associated with early cataract formation. Corticosteroids, phenothiazines, and some cancer chemotherapy agents are commonly used medications cited in clinical and animal studies.[21]

Diabetes is associated with an earlier onset of cataracts. Young adults with poorly controlled diabetes may rarely exhibit fulminating bilateral cataracts. Sorbitol, a by-product of excessive glucose, is known to accumulate in and damage the lens. Hypertensive patients also have a higher incidence of cataracts.

Blunt trauma (contusion) to the eye may result in opacification of the lens that occurs several months after the injury. If the trauma is invasive, localized opacification occurs as a response to rupture of the lens capsule.

Congenital cataracts may be associated with multiple

systemic disorders or other eye deformities, or they may occur in the absence of other signs or symptoms. Maternal rubella in the first trimester often results in infant cataracts that may be accompanied with other signs of deformity. Down's syndrome is commonly associated with cataracts, which usually do not progress sufficiently to impair vision. Infants with identifiable cataracts should be examined and monitored for other physical abnormalities, developmental delay, impaired hearing, and mental retardation.[43]

Most infants and children with cataracts do not exhibit enough opacification to interfere with normal vision. If a newborn has dense opacities, surgery is often performed shortly after birth to prevent permanent sensory loss from disuse of the eye. Foveal stimulation must occur in both eyes in the first 4 months of life to allow normal visual development. Long-wearing contact lenses may be prescribed for monophakic infants if the parents are able to manage the care involved. Children with slowly progressive cataracts have a better prognosis for normal binocular vision if surgery can be delayed until 10 to 12 years of age.[40]

Congenital cataracts can be detected at birth if severe opacification is present. Marked density can be seen with casual observation. The newborn normally manifests a full round red reflex when examined with an ophthalmoscope. Lens opacities interrupt the red reflex and require further examination with a gonioscope. In some instances the parent may notice that the infant is not responding visually at home.[36] The family of the affected child should be examined for cataracts.

DIAGNOSTIC STUDIES

Cataracts are identified through ophthalmoscopy or slit-lamp examination. Visual acuity is measured periodically to assess visual function in both the impaired eye and the less impaired eye.

TREATMENT PLAN

Surgical

Surgical removal of the lens. Indications for surgical intervention include diminished visual acuity (by definition of the patient's life-style needs), hypermature cataracts that threaten to cause eye damage (glaucoma, uveitis), and the necessity to treat or view the structure behind the lens.[9,28,40]

Two procedures are used for extraction: intracapsular and extracapsular. Intracapsular extraction is removal of the entire lens, including its surrounding capsule. An 18

to 20 mm incision is made at the superior limbus arc, and the entire lens is extracted through the incision. A peripheral iridectomy may be performed at the same time. The lens is extracted by forceps or a cryoprobe (which has a low temperature tip that freezes and adheres to the lens surface so that it can be easily extracted). Chymotrypsin, a proteolytic enzyme, is sometimes briefly instilled in the anterior chamber to dissolve resistant zonular fibers in younger patients. Total lens extraction has traditionally been performed on elderly patients.

Extracapsular extraction is removal of the anterior portion of the capsule and the lens, leaving the posterior capsule intact. An incision at the limbus provides access to the anterior capsule, which is mechanically disrupted so the lens nucleus can be removed. The remaining lens cortex is irrigated and suctioned out, leaving the posterior capsule in place. This procedure is often used with younger adults and children because the posterior lens capsule adheres to the vitreous until about 20 years of age. Leaving the capsule in place avoids disruption and loss of vitreous. This method is also favored by some surgeons to accommodate placement of a lens implant. Occasionally the posterior capsule becomes opaque and has to be removed at a later date.

With younger adults, ultrasonic fragmentation (phacoemulsification) is used to disintegrate the lens so it can be aspirated. A rapidly vibrating needle powered by ultrasonic energy breaks up the lens tissue. This method is not used with older adults because the lens nucleus is hardened and resistant to emulsification. The incision for this procedure is only 3 mm, and the patient is usually able to leave the hospital the following day.

The lens can be removed with either general or local anesthesia. General anesthesia is usually used if a lens is implanted. Postoperative care is usually uncomplicated, and the patient is ambulatory on the first or second day. An eye patch may be applied to the operative eye for a brief period, or longer if the physician prefers. An eye patch is not worn after phacoemulsification. A metal eye shield is applied to the eye at night for several weeks to prevent accidental rubbing or injury. The postoperative phase requires patient precautions to avoid increased intraocular pressure, as well as adjustments to distorted vision (see p. 705) unless a lens is implanted in the eye.[36]

Lens implantation. Indications for lens implantation include the following[26]:

1. Persons who cannot manage the care and insertion or removal of extended-wear or regular contact lenses (for example, because of mental impairment or limited manual dexterity)
2. Other eye conditions that contraindicate contact lens wear (such as dry eyes, severe allergies, or severe astigmatism)
3. Adverse work environment (such as presence of

dust or fumes) that does not permit tolerance of contact lenses

4. Only one eye affected

Polymethylmethacrylate (Plexiglas), the lens material originally discovered to be nonirritating to the eyes, is still used today. A wide variety of sizes, shapes, and lens placements have been devised and are selected according to the surgeon's preference, the overall condition of the patient's eye, and the cataract extraction method used. The implant is usually placed at the time of the cataract removal, and the limbus incision may have to be enlarged to allow implantation. Common types of implant lenses include the following:

1. Anterior chamber lens that rests over the pupillary opening and lodges in the anterior angle (Fig. 6-17, *A*)
2. Iris plane lens suspended in the pupil that clips in front of and behind the iris (Fig. 6-17, *B*)
3. Iridocapsular lens supported by the posterior capsule that has been left in place (Fig. 6-17, *C*)

4. Posterior chamber lens held in position either in the capsule of the lens or sutured to the iris

Miotic drops are usually prescribed for iris plane lenses to avoid the risk of lens displacement. Mydriatic drops are usually prescribed for anterior chamber lenses to avoid the development of adhesions and secondary glaucoma. The lens may be sutured in place or may be stabilized with clips or hooks.[26,28,36]

Lens implantation offers many advantages over the use of spectacles and is particularly useful for patients with good vision in the unoperated eye. Binocular vision is rapidly restored, with improved depth perception and good distant and near visual acuity. The lens implant provides accurate distant vision, and glasses are often prescribed to correct near vision difficulties. However, many patients are not good candidates for implantation because of potential postoperative complications. Patients with severe myopia, a history of chronic iritis, retinal detachment, diabetic retinopathy and glaucoma, congenital cataracts, or complications during surgery

Fig. 6-17

Common types and configurations of lens implants. **A,** Anterior chamber lens. **B,** Iris plane lens. **C,** Lens supported by remaining posterior capsule.

From Newell, F.W.: Ophthalmology: principles and concepts, ed. 5, St. Louis, 1982, The C.V. Mosby Co.

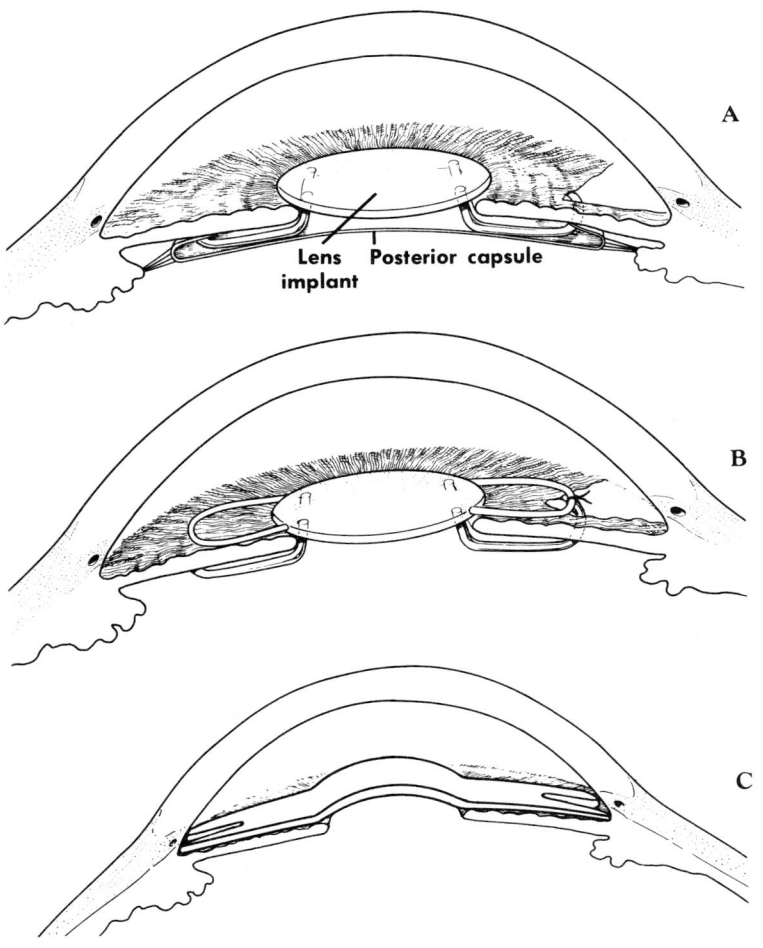

would not be advised to receive an implant. The rate of surgical complications is reported to be 2% to 5% of implantations performed, and complications include corneal edema, secondary glaucoma, iritis, hemorrhage, retinal detachment, and lens displacement.[19,26,44]

Some surgeons believe that implants should be used only if the patient cannot tolerate contact lenses. The long-range durability of the lenses is uncertain, and in most instances they are used only for patients over 65 years of age. Some surgeons believe that extended-wear lenses will eventually replace lens implants as methods for the manufacture and use of contact lenses improve.

Chemotherapeutic

A wide variety of preoperative and postoperative medications are ordered according to the surgeon's preference, the patient's condition, and the nature of the procedure.[28,38,40]

Preoperative

Topical anti-infective agents (usually prescribed 1 wk before surgery)
    Gentamicin, 1-2 drops bid or tid
    Chloramphenicol ointment 1%, small amount q3h
Mydriatic-cycloplegic agents
    Atropine sulfate 1%, 1 drop q5
    Cyclopentolate (Cyclogyl), 1 drop of 1% solution or 2 drops of 0.5% solution q5 min for 15 min
Hyperosmotic agents
    Glycerine, po 1-2 g/kg mixed with equal amount of water
    Mannitol, IV 500 mg by slow drip
Sedative-hypnotics
    Secobarbitol (Seconal), 100 mg po
Antiemetics
    Promethazine (Phenergan), 25 mg IM
Narcotic analgesics
    Meperidine (Demerol), 50-100 mg IM

Postoperative

Mydriatic-cycloplegic agents
    Atropine sulfate 1%, 1 drop bid for 2-6 wk after surgery
Miotic agents (pupil constrictors) prescribed to keep certain types of lens implants in place
    Pilocarpine, 0.1 ml of 0.5%-4% solution 1-6 times/d
Corticosteroids
    Prednisolone suspension (Metimyd, others), 1 drop of 0.2%-0.5% suspension qid
    Hydrocortisone acetate (Cortef, others), 1 drop of 0.5%-2.5% suspension qid
Analgesics

    Acetylsalicylic acid with codeine (Empirin #3), po q4h prn
    Acetaminophen (Tylenol), 650 mg po q4h prn

Supportive

Corrective lenses may be prescribed for aphakic patients. The removal of the lens causes a severe hyperopia because of loss of accommodative powers and a marked magnification of visual objects. Adults must receive some type of corrective lens to maintain visual function. Based on the patient's overall condition, the physician prescribes spectacles or contact lenses or performs lens implantation. Aphakic infants must have corrective lenses to permit development of vision in the first 6 months of life.[28]

Spectacles are still commonly prescribed for elderly patients who cannot tolerate contact or implanted lenses. Adjusting to spectacles is difficult because image magnification of approximately 30% is still present and peripheral vision and depth perception are obscured. Binocular vision is not possible with a unilateral cataract removal unless contact lenses are prescribed. Corrective lenses are usually trifocal or bifocal, and the prescription may have to be changed several times over a period of months until the most effective visual correction is attained.[26]

Contact lenses are usually the prescription of choice for adults and infants if the wearer can tolerate them. Increased depth perception, less image magnification (approximately 7%), and binocular vision are attained with unilateral or bilateral cataracts. Many elderly patients who cannot remove and insert lenses visit a physician weekly and later monthly or quarterly for removal and cleansing of extended-wear lenses and examination of the eyes. Parents of infants receiving contact lenses must be capable of removing, inserting, and cleansing the lenses and monitoring the eyes for complications. For further discussion of contact lens care and precautions see p. 724. A permanent corrective lens can usually be prescribed within 4 to 6 weeks after surgery.[9]

Many patients are good candidates for lens implantation. An implantation offers the advantage of rapid recovery of accurate binocular vision. The complication rate is slightly higher than that of cataract surgery without implantation.[26]

ASSESSMENT: AREAS OF CONCERN

Cataract

Opacities usually not visible on gross examination but may be seen as dark spots, clusters, or linear networks against retinal background with ophthalmoscope; glare at night and in bright light; blurred vision; peripheral vision may diminish before central vision; near vision may improve temporarily (with nuclear cataract); monocular diplopia if central opacity splits visual axis

Advanced cataract
Pupil cloudy and white on gross examination; total blindness

Aphakia with spectacle correction
Thick lenses; 30% magnification of images; clear vision perceived only when looking through center of lens; diminished and distorted peripheral vision; good near vision; monocular aphakic patient unable to use binocular vision (diminished depth perception)

Aphakia with contact lens correction
7% to 10% magnification of images; peripheral vision intact; monocular aphakic patient able to experience binocular vision (improved depth perception); improved near and far visual acuity; reading glasses may be needed

Aphakia with implanted lens correction
Most often used for monocular aphakia and useful in unoperated eye; full binocular vision restored; minimum magnification; peripheral vision intact; improved near and far visual acuity; reading glasses may be needed[9]

NURSING DIAGNOSES and NURSING INTERVENTIONS

Nursing Diagnosis	Nursing Intervention
Sensory-perceptual alteration: visual (related to cataract formation)	Review patient's life-style needs and suggest possible alterations for adjustment to blurred vision or reduced peripheral vision. Assess patient's family and support system for assistance in dealing with visual loss. Review with patient and family safety measures in home and community, necessary life-style changes and resultant feelings, and factors contributing to decisions about surgery to remove cataract(s).[26,36]
Fear (related to anticipation of eye surgery)	Assess patient for fears regarding blindness, pain, and hospitalization. Discuss with patient concerns about cataract surgery and correct any misconceptions, such as that the remaining eye will deteriorate faster after surgery or that total immobilization is necessary postoperatively for a prolonged period. Assess patient for visual acuity, other physical problems, frailty, knowledge about condition, and available support system. Offer support and comfort. Orient patient to room and surroundings. Describe procedure carefully to patient and family members, including equipment, length of procedure, nature of procedure, and postoperative events.
Injury, potential for (eye infection or trauma related to lack of preoperative measures)	Educate patient to refrain from squeezing eyelids shut or touching eyes postoperatively. Encourage older patient to wear glasses during day as reminder not to rub eye. Teach patient to avoid heavy lifting, straining, or bending over at waist, since this might cause dizziness and precipitate fall. Administer preoperative medications as ordered (antibiotic drops or ointments, mydriatic or cycloplegic drops, ocular hypotensive agents, and preanesthetic medications).
Injury, potential for (postoperative complications related to cataract surgery)	Position head of bed at 30-degree elevation. Observe dressing for excessive drainage or bleeding. Assess patient for increased intraocular pressure and report immediately. Observe patient for marked temperature elevation or sudden onset of severe pain. Assist patient to avoid nausea, vomiting, sneezing, coughing, straining with elimination, and touching operated eye. Assist patient to turn to unoperated side. Approach patient from unoperated side. Assist patient with ambulation the night of surgery. Maintain eye patch in place (usually for first or second day). Apply eye shield at night.

Nursing Diagnosis	Nursing Intervention
	Give postoperative medications as ordered (mydriatic drops, miotic medication lens implant, antibiotic or steroid drops to prevent infection, laxative as needed, and antiemetic as needed).[6,26,36]
Sensory-perceptual alteration: visual (related to unilateral eye patch)	*Before surgery:* Assist in measuring visual acuity of unoperated eye preoperatively. Have patient's glasses available for immediate use postoperatively. Warn patient that depth perception will be lost and that 50% of peripheral vision will be lost on affected side.
	After surgery: Assist patient with activities of daily living. Caution patient to bring hand forward slowly to touch objects (especially containers of hot liquids and containers receiving poured liquids). Teach patient to turn head fully toward affected side to view objects or obstacles. Tell patient to use up and down head movements to judge stairs and oncoming objects and to go slowly.[24]
Comfort, alteration in: pain (related to surgery)	Monitor patient for postoperative discomfort (which is usually mild) and itching, and administer analgesics as ordered to prevent patient from inadvertently rubbing eye.

Patient Education

1. Instruct the patient to avoid heavy lifting, straining with elimination, and strenuous exercise for 6 weeks, since increased intraocular pressure should be avoided until the eye is healed.
2. Teach the patient to wear an eye shield at night for 2 to 6 weeks to avoid injury to the eye.[36]
3. Inform the patient that dark glasses may be worn during the day to avoid pupil constriction and glare associated with mydriatic medication. The eye is sensitive to light after surgery, and tearing or squinting may occur in bright natural or artificial light.
4. Teach the patient the correct procedures for instilling eye drops and ointments and applying an eye shield (without touching or applying pressure on the eyeball) to avoid self-inflicted injury.
5. Instruct the patient and family that the patient's life-style must be altered to deal with continued diminished vision in one or both eyes, since final prescription spectacles or contact lenses take 4 to 8 weeks to attain.
6. Explain to a patient receiving spectacles that images will be magnified 30%, peripheral vision will be obscured and distorted, and the lenses will probably be bifocal or trifocal. Therefore life-style changes and safety concerns will need to be assessed; for example, the patient must learn to judge distances when descending stairs or viewing oncoming objects and must turn the head from side to side to see the peripheral environment.
7. Explain to a patient receiving contact lenses that images will be magnified 7% to 10%, peripheral vision will be intact, and reading glasses may also be prescribed. Therefore the patient must learn to care for, insert, and remove lenses (see p. 728) or arrange to visit a physician routinely for removal, cleansing, and reinsertion of extended-wear lenses (see p. 728).
8. Warn the patient that it will be necessary to adjust to mild magnification when performing daily activities.[26,36]
9. Alert the patient and family to signs and symptoms of complications to watch for and report: sudden onset of eye pain, redness and watering of eyes, photophobia, and sudden onset of visual changes.

EVALUATION

Patient Outcome	Data Indicating That Outcome is Reached
Patient with cataracts has adjusted to visual changes.	Life-style needs are not hampered by diminished vision. Patient is able to participate in activities requiring near and far vision. Patient understands cause of visual changes and recognizes that further changes will ensue. Patient expresses feeling of self-control in terms of participating in future decisions about

Patient Outcome	Data Indicating That Outcome is Reached
	cataract surgery. Patient is not endangering self with activities requiring more vision than patient has, such as driving, venturing into community without assistance, home maintenance, self-care activities (self-administering medication), or working at a job.
Patient with cataract removal has adjusted to visual correction with spectacles.	Patient recognizes and avoids safety hazards, does not trip or fall, and does not feel physically insecure. There is no eye pain, further marked visual change, eye redness, lacrimation, or photophobia.
Patient with cataract removal has adjusted to visual correction with contact lenses.	Patient can demonstrate insertion, removal, and cleansing of lens or reports regular visits to practitioner for lens care. Peripheral vision is intact. Binocular vision is intact. There is no eye pain, further marked visual change, eye redness, lacrimation, or photophobia.
Patient with cataract removal has adjusted to visual correction with lens implant.	Peripheral vision is intact. Binocular vision is intact. There is no eye pain, marked visual change, eye redness, lacrimation, or photophobia.[26,36]

DISORDERS OF THE RETINA

The retina, the inner lining of the eyeball, is a multilayered extension of the central nervous system that receives images and transmits them to the brain. Lesions or disorders affecting this surface result in altered vision without pain because sensory fibers do not exist in this area. The degree and type of diminished vision depend on the extent and location of the lesions. Central retinal lesions encroach on the macula and the fovea centralis, severely reducing central vision, near vision, and color differentiation. Peripheral (rod) lesions affect peripheral vision, causing isolated blind spots, night blindness, or gradual peripheral loss until the person is reduced to tunnel (or tubular) vision. Retinal diseases can be congenital or acquired through inflammation, trauma, vascular insufficiency, or aging. The diseases vary in severity from total blindness at birth or a slowly deteriorating condition to minor defects that are unnoticed by the person. The cause and cure for many of these diseases are unknown. Photocoagulation can sometimes arrest the pathologic process, but treatment is difficult if the lesion is in the macular area because photocoagulation causes scarring and further vision reduction. Alterations in the configuration of the retina can cause traction, hole formation, and tearing that are surgically treatable.

Retinal Vascular Occlusion

Occlusion of the retinal artery or vein can cause loss of vision.

PATHOPHYSIOLOGY

Retinal arterial occlusion causes a sudden, unilateral, painless loss of vision. The severity of vision diminishment ranges from total loss with an occluded central artery to a visual field defect that corresponds to blockage of a branch. Emboli associated with atherosclerosis, valvular heart disease, and blood hyperviscosity are among the most common causes. Emboli sometimes form in elderly patients with carotid plaques. Retinal arterial spasms cause transient vision losses that often progress to a permanent loss. Treatment for occlusion must be swift (within 2 hours) to restore vision. Massage of the eyeball (intermittent moderate pressure on the globe) may dislodge an embolus and send it to a more peripheral branch.[28,40] Evaluation and treatment of the systemic disorder that led to the retinal artery occlusion follow emergency treatment.

Retinal vein occlusion results in a more gradual loss of vision, occurring over several hours in contrast to the abrupt loss with arterial blockage. Venous blockage usually occurs in only one eye, and the degree of vision interruption depends on whether the central vein or one of its branches is occluded. Vein occlusion is associated with systemic vascular disease, venous stasis, arterial hypertension, and blood hyperviscosity.[40] Branch occlusion is more common than central blockage and is sometimes successfully treated with photocoagulation.

Photocoagulation does not cure the vascular or systemic disease but deters localized hemorrhage and neovascularization (formation of new vessels). When retinal veins are obstructed, they become engorged and tortuous, and neovascularization occurs in the retina and iris and may extend into the vitreous. The new vessels leak protein and blood. Hemorrhage from dilated veins, retinal edema, and neovascularization may result in anterior synechia formation (adhesions at the anterior angle) and acute glaucoma. Some patients recover from venous stasis retinopathy without treatment. Others respond to photocoagulation. Some patients are left with irreversible visual defects.[40]

DIAGNOSTIC STUDIES[28,38,40]

Direct ophthalmoscopy
Venous dilation and tortuosity; arterial narrowing or obliteration; opacities; hemorrhage; microaneurysms; neovascularization; retinal pallor, detachment, breaks, and folds

Fluorescein angiography
Abnormal placement of vessels (crowding, shunts, obliteration); vessel leakage; microaneurysms; neovascularization

TREATMENT PLAN[28,40]

Retinal Artery Occlusion

Surgical
Anterior chamber paracentesis—with patient under local anesthesia, needle is injected through limbus into anterior chamber; 1 or 2 drops of aqueous fluid is removed to cause sudden lowering of intraocular pressure, which might dislodge embolus[40]

Chemotherapeutic
Anticoagulant agents (may be prescribed in early phases of occlusion[28])
Heparin, IV loading dose of 5000-10,000 units followed by 5000-10,000 units q4-6h for adult[11]

Supportive
Intermittent massage of eyeball—physician applies moderate pressure to globe for 5 seconds, releases pressure for another 5 seconds, and then repeats maneuver in attempt to dislodge embolus to more peripheral branch
Oxygenation—95% oxygen for 10 minutes each hour over period of hours[28]
Evaluation and treatment of systemic cardiovascular dysfunction

Retinal Vein Occlusion

Recovery may be spontaneous, and no curative therapy exists. Therapy is given to prevent further retinopathy in the affected eye and occlusive responses to the other eye.

Surgical
Photocoagulation (see p. 738) to burn small or new vessels

Chemotherapeutic
Anticoagulant agents[28]
Heparin, for adult, IV loading dose of 5000-10,000 units followed by 5000-10,000 units q4-6h, followed by bishydroxycoumarin (Dicumarol), 25-150 mg qd as maintenance dose[11]
Analgesics
Acetylsalicyclic acid (aspirin), for adult, 200 mg every third day[28]; may be given for antithrombotic effect as preventive measure for remaining eye
Corticosteroids
Prednisone (Deltasone, others), 30 mg qd in divided doses for retinal edema[11]

Supportive
Monitoring of eye for increased intraocular pressure

ASSESSMENT: AREAS OF CONCERN

Central retinal artery occlusion
Monocular event; sudden (within seconds), painless loss of vision; pale posterior retina; opaque posterior retina; fovea cherry red in contrast to surrounding whiteness; narrowed arteriole columns; no pupil constriction response; consensual response present

Central retinal vein occlusion
Usually monocular event; gradual (within hours), painless loss of vision; retinal veins dilated and tortuous; optic disc swollen; neovascularization; cotton wool patches; visible hemorrhages

NURSING DIAGNOSES and NURSING INTERVENTIONS

Nursing Diagnosis	Nursing Intervention
Sensory-perceptual alteration: visual (related to sudden unilateral loss)	Offer support and comfort. Keep patient informed of status, progress, and events during emergency care.
Anxiety (related to threat of further visual loss)	Inform patient of related systemic disease and its effect on present and future visual dysfunction. Be realistic in describing health status assessment and prognosis to patient. Offer continuing support and comfort to patient and family.
Potential patient problem: bleeding (related to anticoagulant therapy)	Observe patient for spontaneous bleeding such as hematuria, tarry stools, bleeding gums, or bruising. Observe patient for allergic responses (pruritus, rash, or wheals). If medication is continued at home, educate patient concerning dosage, frequency, signs of bleeding, necessity for keeping appointments with physician, drug interactions, and necessity for keeping laboratory appointments for prothrombin time monitoring.

Patient Education

1. Teach the patient about the systemic disease that contributes to the vascular problem.
2. Explain the degree of visual loss (usually unilateral) and its effect on the patient's life-style.

EVALUATION

Outcomes vary from a fully restored healthy retina with fully functional vision to total loss of central or peripheral vision, or both, with marked retinal destruction.

Patient Outcome	Data Indicating That Outcome is Reached
Vision returns.	Vision returns to or approaches previous acuity.
Condition of retina is normal for patient.	Appearance of retina returns to normal or shows improvement.
Patient has adjusted to partial or complete loss of vision.	Patient is fully informed about present visual status and prognosis. Patient is able to draw on effective support system to supplement self-care. Patient is aware of safety measures to use at home or in community related to visual changes or loss.

Retrolental Fibroplasia

Retrolental fibroplasia is a retinopathy caused by oxygen administered to premature infants.

Retrolental fibroplasia was the leading cause of blindness in infants until the 1940s, when it was discovered that the concentrated oxygen administered for survival to premature infants was related to visual defects in infancy. Even though oxygen administration methods have been altered and oxygenation is now carefully monitored, premature infants are still at risk for retinal damage.

PATHOPHYSIOLOGY

Premature infants who receive supplemental oxygen are vulnerable to retinopathy and consequent total loss of vision. Some of the peripheral retina vessels are not fully mature at birth and respond to excessive oxygen by constricting and eventually disappearing. The corresponding retina (initially the temporal area) is deprived of nourishment, and eventually the remaining vessels dilate and neovascularization occurs. Retinal hemorrhage and edema follow with eventual fibrosis and contraction of the entire area behind the lens. Iritis, cataracts, glaucoma, and retinal traction or tears are common complications of severe retinopathy.[28]

Some infants experience partial or full recovery in the first or second month of life. Myopia, strabismus, and retinal detachment are common complications later in life (often in adolescence). Infants receiving high concentrations of oxygen should be carefully monitored for retinal vascular changes at birth and throughout childhood.[43]

DIAGNOSTIC STUDIES[28,38,40]

Indirect ophthalmoscopy
Performed on discharge from nursery or at 3 months of age, whichever is earlier; venous dilation and tortuosity; arterial narrowing or obliteration; opacities; hemorrhage; microaneurysms; neovascularization

TREATMENT PLAN

No curative therapy exists. Therapy is aimed at preventing further retinopathy and is controversial.

ASSESSMENT: AREAS OF CONCERN

General factors
Low-birth-weight infant requiring supplemental oxygen; retinal changes in first few weeks of life; bilateral event

Visible retinal changes (occur in stages)
Lack of blood vessels in peripheral retina; dilated vessels in central retina; neovascularization; hemorrhage

Advanced stage
Eyes appear sunken; white mass seen through pupil; total blindness

NURSING DIAGNOSES and NURSING INTERVENTIONS

Nursing Diagnosis	Nursing Intervention
Grieving, anticipatory (related to parent's perceived potential loss of child's vision)	Inform parents of infant's visual status and prognosis for visual functioning. Offer comfort and support (encourage expressions of fear, anger, and conflict). Offer alternatives to visual bonding mechanisms (for example, touch, vocalizing, and changes in level of infant activity as response to parent).[43]
Sensory-perceptual alteration	See p. 1967.

Patient Education

Education is affected by the degree of visual loss that can be expected. Visual changes range from minimal loss to total blindness for the child.

1. If the infant's prognosis is uncertain, instruct the parents to assess the child's visual responses carefully for the first 2 to 3 months of life (when recovery may occur):
   a. A newborn normally demonstrates a blink reflex and is able to follow a moving object at an 8- to 10-inch distance within 45-degree range.
   b. At 4 weeks the visual range increases to 90 degrees and the infant is able to watch a speaking parent's face intently.
   c. At 6 weeks the infant shows brief binocular fixation, but vergence and coordinated eye movements are inexact until 3 months of age.
   d. Eye movements may not be fully coordinated until 6 months of age.[40]
2. Instruct the parents to keep in close touch with the nurse or physician and report their observations.
3. Inform the parents of the child's visual potential after each examination. Review the child's prognosis with the parents frequently if their anxiety, grief, or guilt interferes with realistic perceptions.
4. Inform the parents that the child will need regular visual examinations throughout life, since visual complications such as myopia, strabismus, and retinal detachment may occur in later years.

EVALUATION

Outcomes vary from a fully restored healthy retina with fully functional vision to total loss of central and/or peripheral vision with marked retinal destruction.

Patient Outcome	Data Indicating That Outcome is Reached
Vision is fully functional.	Patient's vision develops normally as described under "Patient Education."
Condition of retina is optimum for patient.	Appearance of retina is nearly normal or improved.
Patient has adjusted to partial or complete loss of vision.	Patient or family is fully informed about present visual status and prognosis. Patient or family is able to draw on effective support system to supplement patient's care. Patient or family is aware of safety measures to use in home or in community related to visual changes or loss.

Diabetic Retinopathy

Diabetic retinopathy is a vascular disorder that occurs in patients with diabetes.

Diabetic retinopathy is one of the leading causes of blindness in the Western world.[38] The prevalence of retinal pathology is directly related to the length of time that diabetes has been present. Newell[28] states that 7% of diabetics who have had the disease less than 10 years have retinopathy, as do 26% of those with diabetes of 10 to 14 years' duration and 63% of those with diabetes for 15 years or more. These figures are estimates because the onset of non-insulin-dependent diabetes is not easily determined. The incidence of retinopathy is increasing as diabetics receive better treatment and live longer. Retinopathy is also related to the degree of control of diabetes in the early years of the disease.[38]

PATHOPHYSIOLOGY

Diabetic retinopathy exists in all degrees of severity, and the loss of visual acuity depends on the location of the lesion rather than its extent. An early lesion in the central retina (macular area) can obliterate central vision. Multiple scattered lesions throughout the periphery may not affect visual acuity. Clinicians divide retinopathy into background retinopathy and proliferative retinopathy on the basis of severity. Both conditions involve the same lesions of deterioration, but proliferation is marked by the onset of neovascularization and greater tissue destruction.

Initially the venous capillaries lose vascular tone, dilate, and develop permeable microaneurysms that contribute to ischemia and edema of the surrounding retinal tissue. Hard yellow exudates (lipid deposits) form in the edematous tissue as the fluid is being reabsorbed. The remaining retinal veins become dilated, tortuous, and irregular in caliber. Soft deposits (cotton wool patches) also form in response to vascular insufficiency. These patches, which are small, white, and fluffy in appear-

ance, indicate microinfarction in the nerve fiber area of the retina.[38] Hemorrhages within the layers of the retina appear as small red dots that eventually are reabsorbed and disappear. Larger hemorrhages also occur between the vitreous and the retina. Opacities and hemorrhages obscure vision to the extent that they occur in the visual axis. A preretinal hemorrhage might suddenly obliterate vision as it spills into the vitreous.

The formation of new vessels (neovascularization) marks the onset of proliferative retinopathy.[28] A network of fine, permeable vessels, venous in origin, leaks protein and blood into the surrounding tissue, which becomes edematous and opaque in appearance. More hard and soft deposits form in the retina in response to edema and vascular insufficiency. The tiny vessels spread out over the inner surface of the retina and contribute to further hemorrhage and vitreous detachment from the retina. Eventually the vessels and surrounding tissue become fibrous and the vitreous contracts and fully detaches.

The course of retinopathy varies greatly. The pathologic changes may take many years to develop, and the patient may or may not lose functional vision.

Photocoagulation of the vascular abnormalities frequently slows the progress of microaneurysm formation and neovascularization. However, photocoagulation cannot be used in the macular area. Control of diabetes after retinopathy has begun is less effective in reducing retinal damage than careful control at the onset of diabetes.[38]

DIAGNOSTIC STUDIES[28,38,40]

Indirect ophthalmoscopy
Venous dilation and tortuosity; arterial narrowing or obliteration; opacities; hemorrhage; microaneurysms; neovascularization

Slit-lamp examination (biomicroscopy)
Magnification of lesions

TREATMENT PLAN

Surgical

Photocoagulation (see p. 738) to destroy neovascular-ization sites, prevent retinal edema, and seal small leaking vessels

Vitrectomy—if portion of vitreous is clouded with blood or fibrous membrane, opacities can be re-moved with fine probe passed through anterior scler-al incision; fiberoptic light attached to probe permits direct viewing of vitreous and retina with micro-scope and special contact lens; cannulated probe cuts and removes vitreous fragments; removed vitreous is replaced with fortified Ringer's solution; simul-taneous infusion and aspiration maintain intraocular pressure during surgery[10]

Supportive

Assessment and careful control of diabetes; some think this is more effective in preventing or delaying ret-inopathy during first 5 years of disease, although this is controversial[28]

ASSESSMENT: AREAS OF CONCERN

Background Retinopathy

General factors

Visual loss may be total, partial, or absent; may not correspond to number or severity of lesions seen; possible complaints of glare; absence of pain; visible retinal changes

Microaneurysms

Small, round, red dots; usually located away from visible vessels; may turn white (hyalinized)

Hard yellow exudates

Yellow, waxy, confluent deposits that surround micro-aneurysm area

Cotton wool patches

Fluffy, white soft deposits scattered over retinal sur-face

Subretinal hemorrhages

Small, round, red spots, less circumscribed and usually larger than microaneurysms

Preretinal hemorrhages

Larger, blotchy, red spots

Dilated retinal veins

Enlarged and tortuous; may appear "beaded" (irreg-ular in caliber)

Proliferative Retinopathy

General factors

Visual loss still may not correspond to number or se-verity of lesions seen; visible retinal changes

Neovascularization

Minute network of fine vessels (often at arteriovenous crossing)

Retinal opacification

Increased clouding or whitening of area surrounding neovascularization

Vitreous hemorrhage

Large, red blotches (may obscure much of retina); patient may "see" vitreous hemorrhage as red shower over eyes or multiple floaters, or vision may suddenly be obscured; lesions described in back-ground retinopathy may also be present

NURSING DIAGNOSES and NURSING INTERVENTIONS

Nursing Diagnosis	Nursing Intervention
Sensory-perceptual alteration: visual (related to bilateral gradual loss of vision)	Offer comfort and support. Assess visual acuity and review activities of daily living that are affected or di-minished because of loss of vision. Devise strategies for carrying out activities of daily living with patient (see p. 1967). Assess patient's support system at home and encourage full use of it. Give realistic encouragement for maintenance of independent functioning.
Knowledge deficit (related to self-care and monitoring of diabetes mellitus)	Review patient's knowledge of disease status and self-care practices. Be alert for patient feelings of guilt about lack of self-care. (Patient may express misconceptions and blame self for present condition.[36])
Injury: potential for (related to self-care and safety threatened by diminished vision)	Assist patient to adopt self-care practices to visual handicaps. Review activities that require close vision and color differentiation (such as urine testing, reading medication labels [use large print], and administering insulin injections).

Nursing Diagnosis	Nursing Intervention
	Review patient's support system and encourage full use of it. Assist patient in identifying resources available in community for other assistance as needed.
Anxiety (related to hospitalization and uncertainty about outcome of vitrectomy)	Assess level of anxiety, which may be increased because of patient's poor vision. Assess patient for present visual acuity, other physical problems, frailty, knowledge about condition, and available support system. Offer support and comfort. Orient patient to room and surroundings. Ensure that small personal items are within easy reach. Describe procedure and warn patient that one or both eyes may be patched after surgery and that operative eye will be swollen and bruised for a period of time. Explain that patient will not be totally immobilized for a long period. Bathroom privileges are usually permitted by second day. Inform patient that outcome for functional vision depends on condition of retina. Patient should be able to learn his visual status from physician (to the extent that physician can offer prognosis). Inform patient that decision for using general or local anesthetic will be made by physician.[28,36,40]
Injury: potential for (related to postoperative vitrectomy)	*Before surgery:* Administer antibiotic, mydriatic, and cycloplegic eye drops as ordered. *After surgery:* Monitor vital signs until stable. Be alert for fever. If position of head is not stipulated, semi-Fowler's position or side-lying position with operated eye upward is favored. Check dressing for excessive bleeding (swelling and serous drainage will exist for first 24 to 48 hours). Give postoperative eye drops as ordered (mydriatic, cycloplegic, antibiotic, and anti-inflammatory). Assess patient for nausea, coughing, excessive restlessness, and disorientation. Give narcotics and antiemetics as ordered to prevent excessive restlessness, bumping head, sneezing, coughing, and vomiting.[36] (Avoidance of vomiting is especially important.) Report any signs of upper respiratory infection to physician. Encourage patient to do periodic deep breathing.
Sensory-perceptual alteration: visual (related to monocular vision with postoperative eye patch)	*Before surgery:* Be sure patient's glasses are available for immediate use postoperatively. Warn patient that depth perception will be lost and that 50% of peripheral vision will be lost on affected side. Notify patient that no reading will be permitted while operative eye is patched (to prevent eye movement) but that watching television may be permitted. *After surgery:* Assist patient with activities of daily living. Caution patient to bring hand forward slowly to touch objects (especially containers of hot liquids and containers receiving poured liquids). Teach patient to turn head fully toward affected side to view objects or obstacles. Tell patient to use up and down head movements to judge stairs and oncoming objects and to go slowly.[24]
Sensory-perceptual alteration (related to binocular patches postoperatively)	Keep side rails up at all times. Identify self when entering room; touch patient as you approach and identify self and what you are doing. Put note at door instructing all who enter to identify self and explain reason for being there, for example, cleaning staff. Assist with feeding and hygienic measures as needed. (Patient may have entered hospital with severely diminished vision and may have some self-care skills.) Place call bell and all personal articles within reach; have patient locate them with hand.

Nursing Diagnosis	Nursing Intervention
	Maintain patient's independence as much as possible. Describe events and nursing activities as they occur. Visit patient frequently and offer backrubs, deep breathing, range of motion exercises, and conversation to provide stimulation. Assess patient for depression, anxiety, restlessness, or disorientation.[24]

Patient Education

1. Maintain the patient's awareness of the diabetic state and self-care needs.
2. Inform the patient of the need for regular visual examinations.
3. Teach the patient to monitor visual responses and changes at home and to report any sudden changes to the physician:
   a. Sudden loss of vision (usually unilateral; loss may be within seconds or persist over a day or two)
   b. Increase in floaters or persistent floaters
   c. Flashes of light
   d. Sharp pain in or around eyes
4. Tell the patient to be aware of any changes in visual status, especially changes in peripheral vision (as evidenced by running into large objects, "blind" spots on either side of central vision, or changes in ability to differentiate colors).
5. Inform the patient that visual changes may be very gradual (over many years). Give the patient realistic reassurance to help him continue an independent lifestyle to the fullest extent and develop ways to adapt to diminishing vision.
6. If the patient has had a vitrectomy:
   a. Cycloplegic, antibiotic, and anti-inflammatory eye drops will be continued at home. Review the procedure for administering eye drops and emphasize the importance of maintaining the prescribed dosage. Tell the patient to wash hands before administering drops.
   b. Tell the patient to avoid constipation (straining), sneezing, coughing, heavy lifting (more than 5 pounds), rapid or jarring head movements, and heavy exercise the first week or two at home.
   c. Watching television or reading is acceptable.
   d. Have the patient make an appointment with the physician for a week after discharge.
   e. Visual function should be restored to the extent that the retina is intact. Tell the patient to review visual prognosis with the physician.[36]

EVALUATION

Outcomes vary from a healthy retina with fully functional vision to total loss of central and or peripheral vision with marked retinal destruction.

Patient Outcome	Data Indicating That Outcome is Reached
Condition of retina is optimal for patient.	Changes in retinal appearance are slowed or stopped.
Patient has adjusted to partial or complete loss of vision.	Patient is fully informed about present visual status and prognosis. Patient is able to draw on effective support system to supplement self-care. Patient is aware of safety measures to use in home or in community related to visual changes or loss.

Retinal Degeneration

Degenerative changes in the retina cause a partial or complete loss of vision.

PATHOPHYSIOLOGY

Retinal degeneration may occur because of genetic defects, inflammation, vascular insufficiency, or aging. In many instances the cause of the disorder is unknown; the defect is often familial. Some defects occur at birth with total blindness, whereas others develop insidiously and lead to severe visual loss. Some degenerative changes only minimally affect vision or are considered harmless. The extent, spread, and location of the deterioration and ensuing lesions determine the effect on visual acuity. Lesions that encroach on the macula often diminish vision dramatically.

Senile macular degeneration occurs because layers of the choroid thicken and the capillaries of the choroid are sclerosed and deprive the fovea centralis of nourishment. The onset is slow, involving both eyes, but deterioration may progress faster in one eye than the other. Near and central vision diminishes over a period of years, but some of the peripheral vision remains intact. No treatment is available for this condition.[36,38]

DIAGNOSTIC STUDIES[28,38,40]

Indirect ophthalmoscopy
Opacities; hemorrhage; microaneurysms; neovascularization; retinal pallor, detachment, breaks, and folds

Slit-lamp examination (biomicroscopy)
Magnification of lesions

ASSESSMENT: AREAS OF CONCERN

Senile macular degeneration
Bilateral event (pathologic progress usually not the same in both eyes); gradual diminishment of vision over months or years

Drusen
Hyaline bodies associated with choriocapillaris sclerotic changes; ophthalmoscopy may show cluster (or coalescence) of yellowish dots in macular area[30]; retinal field may show minimum changes in contrast to visual changes

NURSING DIAGNOSES and NURSING INTERVENTIONS

Nursing Diagnosis	Nursing Intervention
Sensory-perceptual alteration: visual (related to bilateral gradual loss)	Offer comfort and support. Assess visual acuity and review activities of daily living that are affected or diminished because of loss. Devise strategies for carrying out activities of daily living. Assess patient's support system at home and encourage full use of it. Give realistic encouragement for maintenance of independent functioning. See p. 1967.

Patient Education

Education depends on the extent of visual changes (usually bilateral) and whether the prognosis indicates that further changes will occur.
1. Inform the patient or parents that the patient should have regular visual examinations.
2. Provide full information to the patient or parents about visual status and prognosis (realistic reassurance about a gradual loss may help the patient to maintain an independent life-style).

EVALUATION

Outcomes vary from mild to severe loss of vision.

Patient Outcome	Data Indicating That Outcome is Reached
Patient has adjusted to loss of vision.	Patient is fully informed about present visual status and prognosis. Patient is able to draw on effective support system to supplement self-care. Patient is aware of safety measures to use in the home or community.

Retinal Holes, Tears, and Detachment

Retinal holes and tears are breaks in the continuity of the retina. Detachment is a separation of the sensory layers of the retina from the pigmented epithelium.

PATHOPHYSIOLOGY

The retina is a smooth, unbroken, multilayered surface that attaches to the hyaloid membrane of the vitreous on its inner aspect. The posterior retinal lining (pigmented epithelium) attaches to Bruch's membrane of the choroid layer on its outer aspect. Breaks in the continuity of the retina can occur in the form of small holes caused by degeneration or tearing (tears are U shaped with flaps over the holes).

Degenerative holes usually occur in the retinal periphery and are the result of retinal thinning that often parallels the ora serrata. Multiple holes form a row of latticework that is fluid filled and covered by vitreous that adheres to either side of the series of holes. Latticework degeneration occurs in about 8% of the population in all age groups and contributes to about 30% of hole-formation retinal separations.[40] The holes are often missed during general ophthalmoscopic inspection and can be seen only with scleral depression and an indirect ophthalmoscope. Many of these patients are asymptomatic, and retinal detachment does not occur. They are carefully monitored for further degeneration or tearing throughout their lifetimes.

Retinal tears occur most often because of vitreous traction. The vitreous degenerates with age and falls forward, resulting in fluid-filled cavities and collagenous areas that tug on the inner lining of the retina. The vitreous also contracts with fibrous band formations associated with retinal degeneration or diabetic retinopathy. Aphakic and myopic persons are at a higher risk for separation because the posterior chamber space is enlarged, which increases vitreous pull. A tear may be small or large, and underlying tissue bulges through it. Holes and tears may lead to detachment, a pulling away of the sensory retinal layers from the pigmented epithelium. The inner layers buckle or fold into the vitreous.[40]

Holes and tears in the retina do not cause pain. Visual diminishment does not occur unless the retinal break is in the macular area. Vitreous pull often stimulates a sensation of lightning flashes or bright streaks of light that are momentary and unilateral. The light sensation may be a harmless phenomenon or may signal potential retinal damage. If the retina breaks or tears with vitreous pull, the patient may experience a shower of floaters (black spots or dots) because minute capillary hemorrhages send particles floating within the visual axis.[40]

Retinal detachment occurs because of traction holes or breaks in the retina (rhegmatogenous) or because fluid, blood, or a mass separates the sensory portion from the pigmented epithelium (exudative). Inflammation, hemorrhage, and tumors are common contributors to retinal separation.

Detachment often begins in the periphery and continues to spread posteriorly. The circumferential spread may occur over a few hours or may continue for several years. A relatively rapid separation gives the sensation that a curtain is being pulled over the eyes. A slow separation may offer no symptoms until the macular area is invaded or the person closes the unaffected eye and notes decreased vision in the affected eye.

Examination with an ophthalmoscope shows the detached portion of the retina as a gray bulge, ripple, or fold in contrast to the pink attached retina. If holes or tears are within the examiner's visual range, the choroid layer shows through as a contrasting cherry red spot.[28]

DIAGNOSTIC STUDIES[28,38,40]

Indirect ophthalmoscopy
Retinal pallor, detachment, breaks, and folds

Slit-lamp examination (biomicroscopy)
Magnification of lesions

Three-mirror gonioscopy
Magnified view of retinal lesions

TREATMENT PLAN

The use and type of surgical therapy depend on the extent and location of the retinal detachment.

Surgical
Photocoagulation (see p. 738)—used to burn and eventually seal localized tears or breaks in posterior portion of eyeball
Cryothermy—frozen-tipped probe placed on sclera directly over area of retinal hole; borders of hole are "frozen," inflammatory response ensues, and eventual scarring seals hole
Diathermy—heat applied by means of ultrasonic probe to scleral surface directly over site of retinal break; resultant burn causes inflammatory response with eventual scarring and sealing
Scleral buckle—sclera indented by means of local implant or encircling strap so it is flattened against retinal tissue that has fallen away from inner surface;

conjunctiva pulled back to expose scleral surface; indirect ophthalmoscopy and diathermy probe used to identify areas of detachment; partial thickness of sclera is incised and pulled back to form flaps that eventually hold implant in place; rectus muscles tied with sutures so eyeball can be rotated to expose equator; detached area may be treated with diathermy before implant is put in place; encircling rod or strap often used if multiple retinal holes exist; implant sutured in place, and subretinal fluid drained from site of detachment; air, other gases such as sulfur hexafluoride, or liquids such as silicone oil may be injected into vitreous to flatten detached retina against choroid surface; air or liquid is absorbed and eventually replaced with vitreous fluid[10,36]

Chemotherapeutic
Adrenergic-mydriatic agents
Phenylephrine (Neo-Synephrine) 2.5%-10%, 1-2 drops instilled for preoperative pupil dilation
Mydriatic-cycloplegic agents
Cyclopentolate (Cyclogyl), 1 drop of 1% solution or 2 drops of 0.5% solution preoperatively and postoperatively, frequency and duration of postoperative dosage vary with degree of inflammation
Anti-infective agents (postoperative eye drops to prevent uveitis complications)
Gentamicin sulfate (Garamycin), 3 mg/ml topical solution, 1-2 drops qid
Neomycin sulfate and prednisolone sodium phosphate, neomycin 3.5 mg/ml and prednisolone 5 mg/ml, frequency and duration of prescription vary according to physician's order, usually 1 drop tid or qid for 4-6 wk

Supportive
Postoperative monocular or binocular eye patches (according to physician's preference) to rest eyes for day or two (usually bilateral patches because operated eye may move when unoperated eye moves)
If air is injected into vitreous cavity, head positioned so air bubble will rise and remain flush against detached retinal segment; physician specifies optimum head position and duration for positioning (usually 4 to 5 days); usual position is face down or angled to side; pillows or rubber or plastic ring used to support head; pillows under abdomen for support[36]

ASSESSMENT: AREAS OF CONCERN

Visual symptoms reported by patient
Flashing lights (unilateral, may be repeated over a period of days, months, or years); shower of floaters (black dots within visual field); sensation of curtain folding over eyes

Appearance of retina
Detached portion grayish and less transparent than surrounding retina; retinal folds may be visible; vessels over detached portion dark red in color; holes or breaks within detached area cherry red, in contrast to the grayish area

NURSING DIAGNOSES and NURSING INTERVENTIONS

Nursing Diagnosis	Nursing Intervention
Anxiety (related to sudden loss of unilateral vision)	Offer comfort, support, and realistic reassurance (about 90% of retinal detachment repairs are successful).[10] Inform patient that both eyes may be patched postoperatively.
Injury, potential for (related to preoperative status: detached retina)	Supervise limited activities or bed rest as ordered. Maintain bilateral eye patches if ordered. Keep room dark. Keep patient supine. Keep side rails up if patient is bedfast. Assist with ambulation and avoid jarring, bumps, or falls. Administer mydriatic and cycloplegic drops as ordered.
Sensory-perceptual alteration: visual (related to preoperative or postoperative binocular patching)	Keep patient quiet preoperatively. Identify self when entering room; touch patient as you approach and identify self. Instruct others to identify themselves and state purpose of entering room. Assist with feeding, hygienic measures, and ambulation as needed. Provide frequent sensory stimulation with visits and conversation postoperatively. Monitor patient for disorientation and agitation.

Nursing Diagnosis	Nursing Intervention
Injury, potential for (related to postoperative status)	Monitor vital signs until stable. Position patient as ordered. (If gas or air has been injected into vitreous, head position may need to be maintained for 4 to 5 days.) Supervise bed rest or limited activities as ordered (bathroom privileges are usually ordered on second day). Keep patient's head parallel to floor when patient is out of bed for brief periods. Check dressing for excessive bleeding. Report sudden severe pain. Assess and document marked swelling and serous drainage, which is present for first 24 to 48 hours. Initiate deep breathing exercises four times a day. Administer cycloplegic, mydriatic, antibiotic, and anti-inflammatory eye drops as ordered. Assess patient for nausea, coughing, excessive restlessness, and disorientation. Administer antiemetics as ordered. Avoid excessive restlessness, jarring or bumping head, sneezing, coughing, and vomiting.[36]
Comfort, alteration in: pain (related to postoperative status)	Monitor patient's pain (which is usually moderate) and administer narcotics according to physician's orders.

Patient Education

1. Inform the patient that cycloplegic and antibiotic eye drops will be continued at home. Review the procedure for administering eye drops and emphasize the importance of maintaining the prescribed dosage and washing the hands thoroughly before administration.
2. Tell the patient to avoid constipation (straining), sneezing, jarring head movements, and heavy exercise for the first 4 to 6 weeks at home.
3. Inform the patient that television watching is permitted but reading should generally be avoided for the first week (physician will specify).
4. If the patient's occupation is sedentary, work may be resumed after the second week at home (physician will specify).

5. Tell the patient to be aware of visual changes or sensation and to report sudden loss of vision, severe pain in the eyeball, a heavy shower of floaters, or flashing lights to the physician. (Usually some floaters are seen for a period of weeks postoperatively, but they should be reported.)
6. Have the patient schedule an appointment with the physician a week after hospital discharge.[36]
7. With the patient and physician review and ensure that the patient understands his visual status, including the possibility of recurrence of detachment in the affected eye, ultimate visual acuity and macular damage, and potential for retinal detachment or holes in the other eye.

EVALUATION

Outcomes vary from a fully restored healthy retina with fully functional vision to total loss of central or peripheral vision, or both, with marked retinal destruction.

Patient Outcome	Data Indicating That Outcome is Reached
Vision returns.	Vision returns to or approaches previous acuity.
Condition of retina is optimal for patient.	Appearance of retina returns to normal or shows improvement.
Patient adjusts to partial or complete loss of vision.	Patient is fully informed about present visual status and prognosis. Patient is able to draw on effective support system to supplement self-care. Patient is aware of safety measures to use in home or community.

STRABISMUS AND AMBLYOPIA

Strabismus is a deviation of one or both eyes so one fovea fails to receive the same visual image as the fovea of the nondeviated eye. Amblyopia is a unilateral or bilateral reduction of vision without evidence of disease in the eyes or brain; it is often caused by strabismus.

Strabismus, a misalignment of one or both eyes, occurs in approximately 3% of infants and children. Because of the immaturity of the visual and neurologic systems, strabismus often causes a loss of vision (suppression amblyopia) in the deviated eye. If uncorrected the visual loss can become permanent.

Although strabismus more commonly occurs in children, eye deviation can also occur in adults, usually in association with a systemic disorder. If the deviating eye has adequate vision, defective eye alignment in an adult usually causes diplopia (double vision) rather than a loss of vision.

This discussion concentrates on the common strabismus that affects children and threatens loss of vision.

PATHOPHYSIOLOGY

The development of normal binocular vision requires full bilateral visual acuity with coordinated movements that enable the foveas of both eyes to receive the same image simultaneously. The two images are transmitted to the occipital cortex and interpreted as a single image, a process called fusion. If one or both eyes are deviated so they are unable to direct their gaze at a single object, double vision (diplopia) results.

The mind is able to suppress a double image. When looking through an ophthalmoscope, a person may keep both eyes open and suppress the images perceived by the eye not being used. This phenomenon, called suppression scotoma, quickly occurs in many persons with diplopia resulting from a deviated eye. In a mature vision system, suppression scotoma occurs only when both eyes are being used. If the less dominant eye is tested alone, it transmits a full image to the cortex. In an immature vision system (before 7 years of age) the suppression may evolve into amblyopia with atrophied cells in the visual cortex.[28] Amblyopia may be fully or partially reversible if it is treated before 7 years of age. Experts disagree about the age limits for reversing amblyopia. It is generally stated that the prognosis improves if suppression or amblyopia occurs in the later years of early childhood.

Congenital strabismus (occurring at birth) and congenital cataracts, which also deprive the eye of form vision, are treated in early infancy to prevent permanent visual loss. Congenital cataracts must be treated before 4 months of age.[28] In the first 4 weeks of life the infant develops the ability to follow a moving object 8 to 10 inches from the face within a range of approximately 45 degrees. As the infant matures, conjugate fixation skills improve, and binocular vision is established by 4 months of age.[43] Since the eyes may still exhibit occasional erratic movements up to the age of 6 months,[40] early strabismus may be difficult to diagnose. However, the condition can usually be diagnosed by 4 months of age, and early surgical correction can occur between 8 and 12 months of age.[13]

Strabismus occurs in many forms. One or both eyes may be fixed in one position, or the eye(s) may deviate intermittently or alternately. Deviations can take the form of the eye(s) turning inward (esotropia), outward (exotropia), upward (hypertropia), or downward (hypotropia). Some deviations occur only when one eye is covered. The fusion mechanism of binocular vision controls the latent deviation (phoria). Esophoria is an inward deviation that occurs only when one eye is covered. Esotropia is a medial deviation that is apparent when both eyes are uncovered.

Strabismus is traditionally divided into two categories: paralytic and nonparalytic. Paralytic strabismus is caused by one or more weakened eye muscles. Nonparalytic strabismus does not initially involve weakened muscles; for reasons not fully understood the fusion mechanism is faulty and causes eye deviations.

Nonparalytic strabismus is further divided into three categories: accommodative, nonaccommodative, and combined accommodative and nonaccommodative. Accommodative strabismus occurs when a person is making an effort to adjust from far to near vision or from near to far vision. Esotropia may occur in hyperopic (farsighted) persons attempting to focus on near objects, and exotropia may develop in myopic (nearsighted) persons. The eye deviations may occur only at the time of refocusing, or the deviation may be fixed. Optical correction can often control accommodative strabismus.

The most common type of strabismus (approximately 40%) is infantile esotropia. It is frequently inherited and is usually diagnosed before 1 year of age.[14] It is nonparalytic and nonaccommodative. The angle of eye deviation is the same in all directions of gaze and is not affected by accommodation. The deviation may involve one or both eyes. Visual acuity is usually not affected if both eyes alternate in deviation, but a monocular deviation often develops into amblyopia. In early infancy the newborn is carefully observed by the physician and parents. The infant should be able to follow a large moving object with both eyes by 4 to 6 weeks of age. If one eye fails to fixate consistently, strabismus and amblyopia should be suspected. An older infant or toddler may object to having the dominant eye covered for testing, which is another indication. Toddlers who have markedly different test results between each eye with picture cards are also suspected of having amblyopia.[13]

As soon as amblyopia is suspected, it may be treated by patching the dominant eye. Eye patching of infants must be carefully supervised because amblyopia from disuse can develop in the dominant eye within 1 to 3 days. Parents are asked to observe the child's eye preference when fixating on an object and to switch the patch to the other eye if the fixation preference has shifted from one eye to the other. Patching supervision is lessened somewhat after the child reaches 1 year of age. Parents are still asked to observe for fixation preference daily, but patching periods may be extended to 4 days.[13]

As soon as maximum visual acuity is achieved or the defective eye is showing no further improvement, the eye is surgically repaired by shortening a muscle (resection) or reattaching a muscle insertion at a new site (recession). Surgical repair satisfies cosmetic concerns but does not improve visual acuity. Intermittent patching may continue after surgical therapy. Parents should be told that surgical correction may not be exact and that surgery may have to be repeated at a later date.

In some children, amblyopia develops without apparent strabismus (anismetropic amblyopia). The reduced visual acuity is often first discovered in preschool visual examinations (at 3 or 4 years of age).[14] The eye with reduced acuity may receive correction with eyeglasses for a brief period. An eye patching program may also be used to correct the amblyopia.

Some amblyopic problems involve both refractive errors (hyperopia or myopia) and defects in the fusion mechanism. Visual refraction (eyeglasses) alone or coupled with a patching program may correct the problem.

DIAGNOSTIC STUDIES

Cover-uncover test
Patient is asked to stare straight ahead at fixed point; examiner covers one eye with card and observes uncovered eye for movement to focus on designated point; examiner then removes card from eye and observes eye for movement to focus; same process of covering and uncovering is repeated with other eye; normal eyes do not move in process of covering or uncovering; procedure can also be employed with infants to observe for fixation preference[4]

Prism tests
Variety of visual tests in which prisms are used as eye covers; prisms deflect light rays, forcing covered eye to turn in direction of prism light path to focus light on fovea; prism is held in front of one eye and then the other, and degree of eye movement is noted for each eye; prisms of different strengths are used to cover each eye until eyes no longer have to move to fix on object; angle of eye deviation is measured in prism strengths or diopters[32] (prism diopter is prism strength required to bend light ray by 1 cm from light source 1 m from prism)

Corneal reflection
Patient fixes on light held at distance of 13 inches (33 cm); light reflex normally appears as pinpoint of light near center of each pupil; esotropic eye reflects light temporally to pupil; exotropic eye reflects light from pupil toward nose; prisms are also used to center corneal light reflex; strength of prism required to bend light ray so it appears at pupil center of deviated eye measure angle of deviation in prism diopters; average medial deviation in infantile esotropia is 50^Δ (diopters)[13]

Visual acuity tests
Allen cards
Toddlers asked to identify familiar objects on series of cards with one eye at a time; cards usually held at 10 feet, and standardized figures reported in 10/30 measurements; normal visual acuity 10/30 in right eye (OD), left eye (OS), and both eyes (OU) at 2½ to 3½ years of age; decreased acuity measured by moving cards closer to child until figures are identified; therefore top number (which registers distance from patient) becomes smaller as examiner moves closer (for example, 6/30, 4/30); marked discrepancy in test results between eyes suggestive of amblyopia or refractive error or both[13] (NOTE: test is subjective and depends on child's ability to cooperate and identify such figures as telephone and house)

E chart
Young children (3 to 5 years of age) and illiterate persons stand 20 feet from chart with series of standard-sized E's; with one eye covered, patient identifies direction legs of E are pointing (up, down, right, or left); 20/20 OD, OS, and OU indicates that vision is normal because patient identified at 20 feet the same-size letter that persons with normal vision would identify at 20 feet; 3- to 5-year-old with normal vision should be able to identify letters in 20/30 line; marked discrepancy between eyes suggests amblyopia, refractive error, or both

Amblyoscope
Used with older children who are able to sit at machine and identify objects presented separately to each

eye; machine measures grades of fusion, stability of fusion with convergence, suppression, and retinal correspondence; child looks into machine through tubes that present different images to each eye; tubes can be moved to measure stability of fusion as images are pulled closer together[36,40]; if two images are perceived as superimposed, both eyes are being used; if only one image is reported, suppression exists; as images are pulled closer together, degree of eye movement (convergence) is measured before diplopia occurs; other images are used to record diplopia, indicating that light source is falling at different points on each retina

Eye movement tests

Six cardinal fields of gaze

Patient stabilizes head and looks directly at examiner; patient is asked to follow object in examiner's hand with eyes only; examiner slowly moves object from center position to outer extremes and back to center in six cardinal fields of gaze[4]; normal eyes show coordinated parallel movements in all directions; fixed deviated eye may maintain same angle of deviation regardless of direction of gaze; if muscle is weakened or nerve supply to muscle is faulty, eye may fail to move in given direction with other eye

Accommodation

Patient fixes gaze at distant object; examiner holds up vertical object, centered with patient's nose, about 10 to 12 cm (4 to 5 inches) from nose; patient is asked to redirect distant gaze to near object in front of nose; normal eyes converge easily, smoothly, and in coordinated fashion; accommodative esotropic patient may demonstrate normal alignment with straight-on gaze, but when eyes converge, one eye deviates medially more than the other

TREATMENT PLAN

Surgical

Surgical correction is not performed until the amblyopia is either reversed or maximally improved through occlusion (eye patching). The purpose of surgical correction is to straighten the deviated eye. Surgery does not correct amblyopia. An eye occlusion program may be continued after the surgery if needed.

The angle of eye deviation is interpreted through prism diopters and converted into the prescribed millimeter measurement for moving a muscle from its insertion point to a new location (muscle recession) or shortening a muscle (resection). The procedures may be performed simultaneously on a number of muscles, or only one muscle may be surgically altered.

Since the surgery is based on an estimation, full or cosmetically satisfactory correction is not always achieved. Ten per cent of congenitally esotropic patients must have further surgery because of overcorrection or undercorrection.[13]

Recession for infantile esotropia weakens the medial rectus muscle. The patient is given a general asesthestic. An incision is made through the conjunctiva at the nasal limbus. The medial rectus muscle is isolated and exposed at its insertion. It is severed and reattached to the sclera at a prescribed new distance from the limbus. Weakening of this muscle frees the eye to rotate temporally.

Sometimes medial rectus muscle recession is sufficient to produce the desired effect. In other instances the lateral rectus muscle is strengthened in the same operation. The choice of surgery and the number of muscles altered depend on surgeon preference, the severity of deviation, and other variables.

Resection for infantile esotropia strengthens the lateral rectus muscle. A temporal incision is made at the limbus. The lateral rectus muscle is isolated at its insertion. The muscle is clamped and severed from its insertion. The muscle is measured and resewn beyond the insertion point of the muscle, and the excess muscle is cut off. Strengthening of the lateral rectus muscle assists the eye with temporal rotation.

The child is usually ambulatory on the day of surgery. Recovery is rapid, and the child is able to return to normal activities with 2 to 3 days after surgery.

Chemotherapeutic

Miotics

In accommodative esotropia, anticholinesterase eye medication used as substitute for eyeglasses if child is too young to wear spectacles or is uncooperative; eye drops inhibit accommodation and relieve convergence esotropia

Echothiophate iodide (Phospholine), 1 or 2 drops of 0.03%-0.06% solution for children qd or bid

Isoflurophate (Floropryl) ointment, 0.025% applied qd[40]

Supportive

Eye patching programs vary somewhat according to physician preference. Patching is begun in infancy as soon as amblyopia is suspected. The patch remains on the dominant eye during all the waking hours. The parents are asked to make daily observations of the child's fixation preference (that is, which eye is fixed on a moving object). If the fixation has shifted from the patched eye to the nonpatched eye, the patch is placed over the other eye to prevent disuse amblyopia of the dominant eye. A suggested routine is to patch the dominant eye for 3 days and then switch the patch to the amblyopic eye on the fourth day. Initially the child visits the physician within 1 week's time. Thereafter, frequent appointments are made to measure visual acuity and examine the fusion mechanism.[13]

In children over 1 year of age the patching of the dominant eye may be extended to 4 days, after which the patch is switched to the other eye for 1 day. Visits to the doctor are still frequent (every 2 weeks) until children reach 3 years of age. After 3 years of age, dominant eye patching is further extended with continued visual acuity checks.[41] The patching program continues until the amblyopic eye fails to improve with visual acuity tests for a 3-month period. In some instances amblyopia recurs and patching is resumed either full time or intermittently. Patching may continue until the child is 9 or 10 years of age.[28]

ASSESSMENT: AREAS OF CONCERN

Nonaccommodative infantile esotropia

Family history of strabismus; onset at birth or usually under 1 year of age; both eyes may deviate medially; often deviation is monocular; angle of deviation remains the same regardless of direction of gaze; infant may show fixation preference—one eye tends to follow slowly moving object at close range (8 to 10 inches); infant may object (push examiner's hand away) when dominant eye is covered; diagnosis often confirmed by 4 months of age; monocular strabismus usually evolves into amblyopia

Accommodative esotropia

Family history of strabismus; onset at 2 to 3 years of age (when accommodative powers are being used); onset often abrupt; child usually hyperopic (farsighted) when vision is tested; eyes often appear aligned with distant vision; one or both eyes exhibit medial deviation during accommodation (use of near vision); amblyopia may develop in weakened eye

Amblyopia

Usually monocular event; visual acuity tests show one eye testing at least two lines below the other on the Snellen E chart, for example, dominant eye 20/20, weakened eye 20/40; defective eye may show severe loss (for example, 20/200)

Anisometropic amblyopia

Child's eyes usually not deviated; usually not discovered until preschool vision tests 3½ to 4½ years of age; when vision is tested, one eye manifests refractive error that does not exist in other eye

NURSING DIAGNOSES and NURSING INTERVENTIONS

Nursing Diagnosis	Nursing Intervention
Parenting, alteration in	Assess family members' ability to cope with ordinary care of infant coupled with anxiety of having to monitor infant's visual responses at home. Instruct family in normal visual responses of infant and specific behaviors to look for (see "Patient Education"). Offer support and reassurance. Encourage family to communicate with nurse and to keep appointments with physician. Inform family members fully about methods for monitoring eye responses and rationale for switching patch from one eye to the other (see "Patient Education").
Injury: potential for (related to side effects of anticholinesterase drops or ointment)	Inform parents fully about medication and administration (see "Patient Education").
Anxiety (related to need for surgical correction of strabismus)	Offer emotional support geared to child's developmental status. (Children are frequently admitted to the hospital the morning of surgery or are admitted and sent home the day of surgery to avoid trauma of hospital stay.[32]) Note that child beyond 9 months will become fearful of mother's absence. Offer support and reassurance of parents. Fully inform parents about procedure. Address any questions or concerns. Warn parents that operative eye will appear reddened with little drainage after surgery. The eye may or may not be patched according to surgeon's preference.

Nursing Diagnosis	Nursing Intervention
Injury: potential for (related to postoperative status)	Administer antibiotic eye drops preoperatively as ordered. Administer preoperative injection as ordered. Keep side rails up at all times. Take vital signs until patient is stable. Provide close supervision of child until fully alert (operative eye may or may not be patched). Observe eye or dressing for drainage (usually little or none apparent). Conjunctiva will be red.
Sensory-perceptual alteration: visual (related to monocular patching)	Observe whether child is accustomed to patching and able to function without difficulty. Assist child with getting in and out of bed or caution parent to supervise child closely.

Patient Education

1. Explain normal development of vision and how to observe an infant for strabismus.[4,40,43]
   a. Between birth and 4 weeks of age the infant should be able to *briefly* follow (with both eyes) a large, slowly moving target held 8 to 10 inches from the face within a 45-degree range.
   b. As the infant matures, the duration of bilateral fixation and the range for following the target should increase.
   c. By 3 months of age, convergence with near vision should be intact (exhibiting smooth coordinated movement).
   d. By 4 months of age, binocular vision is usually established. The infant is able to fix on smaller objects 3 feet away.
   e. Erratic, uncoordinated eye movements may still be exhibited until the child is 6 months of age.
   f. All infants develop at their own rate. The ages related to developmental accomplishments are only estimates.
   g. Infants respond to sound with their eyes. Be careful to differentiate eye fixation as a response to sound from visual stimulation. (For example, a mother who holds her face close to the infant and talks to him is stimulating with sound as well as sight.)
   h. Observe the child daily for fixation patterns. Note whether one eye tends to fix and follow an object more than the other.
   i. Observe eyes turning inward for near vision. Note whether one eye consistently turns in farther than the other.
   j. Report concerns and questions to the nurse or physician.
2. Explain the patching program.
   a. Patching the dominant eye enables the visual system in the defective eye to develop and prevents further or total loss of vision.
   b. The physician prescribes a specific patching schedule based on the child's age and other factors related to the deviation. The schedule must be followed carefully.
   c. The patch must be applied during all waking hours.
   d. Initially the child may object to having the dominant eye patched and will have to be closely supervised until adjusted.
   e. The young child should be observed daily for eye preference when fixating. If fixation shifts from one eye to the other, either switch the patch (if the physician has ordered this) or report to the physician.
   f. Regular appointments must be kept with the physician for eye examination.
   g. The patch will be prescribed until the defective eye either is restored to normal or ceases to improve for a period of 3 to 6 months.
   h. The prognosis for restored vision may not be known.
3. Explain hyperopia correction.
   a. The parents and physician determine whether the child is mature enough to wear eyeglasses (usually a question if child is between 2 and 4 years of age).
   b. If anticholinesterose medication is prescribed instead of glasses (to inhibit accommodation), the parents must learn to administer eye drops or ointment, carefully following the prescription for amount and frequency of dosage.
   c. If eyeglasses are prescribed, straps are available to help the young child keep the glasses in place.
   d. Parents should examine the glasses regularly for scratches or other damage.
   e. If amblyopia is diagnosed, a patching program is prescribed along with the eyeglasses or medication.

f. The eyeglasses (or medication) may not correct the amblyopia or eye deviation. Stress that child needs regular examinations to determine visual progress.

4. Explain surgical correction of strabismus.

   a. The physician may prescribe an eye patch to be worn at home for 2 to 7 days.
   b. The operative eye is reddened for about a week after surgery. A small amount of clear pinkish discharge may appear at the eye for a day or so.
   c. Warm compresses three times a day may be prescribed for inflammation.

d. The child's hands and fingernails should be kept clean, and the child's hands should be kept away from the eyes.
e. An antibiotic or anti-inflammatory eye drop is prescribed for administration three times a day for a week. Parents must know how to administer eye drops.
f. The child can resume normal activities in 2 to 3 days.
g. Continued visits for eye examinations will be necessary. (Occasionally, eye patching is continued or resumed after strabismus repair.)

EVALUATION

Patient Outcome	Data Indicating That Outcome is Reached
Binocular vision is restored.	Child has 20/20 vision OD, OS, and OU (20/30 vision may be appropriate for 3-year-old). (Full restoration of vision in defective eye may not be possible.) Although depth perception (stereopsis) is usually not fully recovered, child has learned to gauge depth by contrasting sizes of images and colors at different distances. Both eyes fixate and follow image consistently.
Strabismus is corrected.	Eyes are in good alignment when looking straight on. Eyes remain in good alignment when one eye is covered. Eyes move in smooth, coordinated fashion in six cardinal fields of gaze. Bilateral eye movements are smooth and coordinated with convergence and divergence.[4]

Medical Interventions

CONTACT LENSES

Description and Rationale

Contact lenses are rounded plastic disks that are curved and shaped to fit over the cornea and beneath the eyelid. As methods for producing them improve, they are being used increasingly as a substitute for eyeglasses to correct refractive errors.

Contact lenses, introduced in the 1940s, are available in many forms and serve a multitude of purposes. Hard lenses were originally used to correct refractive errors and high astigmatism associated with corneal irregularities.[40] The introduction of soft lenses in 1971 and extended-wear lenses in 1981 has expanded the benefits of

contact lenses and the indications for their use.[27] Some of the major indications for contact lenses are (1) cosmetic preference over eyeglasses, (2) monocular aphakia, (3) marked difference in refractive error between eyes (anisometropia), (4) active occupation or sports participation, and (5) severe corneal irregularities.

A major concern with all types of lenses is to maintain an adequate oxygen supply to the corneal surface. The cornea receives most of its oxygen from precorneal tears. Contact lenses float on the precorneal tear film and act as foreign bodies that interrupt normal tear flow.

Hard or rigid lenses often cover only the corneal surface (7 to 9 mm in diameter).[28,36] Blinking action pumps tear fluid under the lens to keep the corneal surface moist. The corneal lens is small enough to shift during blinking so tears can be pumped under the lens and debris can be carried away from the cornea. Some hard lenses are fashioned to cover the cornea and part of the sclera. A buffer solution is then required to keep the chamber between the cornea and the lens full of fluid.[36] Scleral lenses are less comfortable than corneal lenses and more difficult to wear. Hard lenses are still prescribed for correction of marked corneal irregularities because their shape does not conform to the corneal surface as readily as soft lenses and they provide better peripheral vision. Hard lenses can be worn only for a limited time (10 to 14 hours) and are not worn during sleep. They eventually change the shape of the corneal surface and therefore cannot be worn alternately with eyeglasses.

Soft lenses are made of hydrophilic plastics that increase access of fluid to the cornea. They are usually larger in diameter and more easily tolerated than hard lenses and can be worn longer. They are regarded as a medical device and are regulated by the Food and Drug Administration. Soft lenses absorb medications, cleansing solutions, and chlorinated water from swimming pools and gradually release them into the tear film.[28] This can cause local irritation and systemic side effects. Soft lenses are removed every day for cleansing and are not worn during sleeping hours to allow the cornea to recover.

Extended-wear lenses are designed to provide continuous oxygen to the cornea. One type of lens is ultrathin and permits absorption of oxygen through it. The other type is thicker but has a higher concentration of water (70% to 80%), which continuously bathes the corneal surface.[7] Extended-wear lenses can be worn for periods ranging from a few days to several months depending on patient tolerance, self-care habits, and the patient's eye condition. The effects of extended wear and the development of new materials are receiving considerable research.[3]

Contact lenses are successfully worn by many people but are definitely contraindicated in some instances. Corneal infection and damage can occur if lenses are not handled appropriately. Persons who wear lenses must have a clear understanding of how to insert, remove, and care for them. Misuse can result in severe eye damage and the loss of vision.

Contraindications

Chaotic or disorganized life-style
Lack of motivation to monitor eye responses and care for lenses
Manual dexterity problems or any condition that inter-feres with daily removal and insertion and lens care (Daily wear lenses can sometimes be replaced with extended-wear lenses that are monitored, removed, and cleaned by a professional.)
Poor blinking or lid function
Diminished corneal sensation
Chronic blepharitis or conjunctivitis
Occupation or life-style that involves heavy fumes or dust in the environment
High astigmatism (contraindicated for soft and extended-wear lenses)[4,5]

TREATMENT PLAN[27,40]

The patient is evaluated for indications and contraindications for lens wearing and the appropriate type of lens. After the lenses are prescribed and fitted, the patient is closely followed for signs of complications. The major complications are corneal abrasion, corneal edema, infection, ulceration, tight lens syndrome, and giant papillary syndrome.

Corneal Abrasions

Corneal abrasions occur when hard lenses are left in too long (overwear syndrome) and drying of the corneal surface results in minute epithelial breaks. Abrasions also form if foreign bodies lie between the lens and the cornea or if the corneal surface is scraped during insertion or removal. A fluorescein stain can be used to identify epithelial breaks. The patient experiences severe pain and usually seeks care immediately. Epithelial abrasions can heal in 24 to 48 hours.

Chemotherapeutic
Anti-infective agents
Sulfisoxazole (Gantrisan) 4% ointment applied to each eye before 24-h patching
Sulfacetamide sodium (Sulamyd) 10% ointment applied to each eye before 24-h patching
Anesthetics
Proparacaine (Ophthaine) 0.5% solution, 1-2 drops in each eye, gives relief for 10-15 min
Mydriatic-cycloplegic agents
Tropicamide (Mydriacyl) 0.5%-1% solution, 1-2 drops bid or tid for 24 h

Supportive
Binocular tight patches for 24 hours (if patient has someone to care for him) or monocular patch on more painful eye and mydriatic drops in open eye to reduce ciliary spasm and pain (see above for dosage); reexamination of patient in 24 hours[27]

Corneal Edema

Corneal edema most commonly occurs with soft or extended-wear lenses because of a more gradual oxygen deprivation to the cornea. The epithelium becomes edematous, and vision becomes blurred. There is usually no pain, but slight redness of the eye may be evident.

Supportive

Removal of contact lens reverses condition; lens prescription may have to be changed

Corneal Ulceration and Infection

Corneal ulceration and infection occur if corneal abrasions or edema are not successfully treated. A secondary uveitis may ensue and require intensive emergency care to prevent loss of vision (see p. 685 for pathophysiology and interventions). Infection also occurs if insertion, removal, and lens care are not managed hygienically by the patient.

Chemotherapeutic

Anti-infective agents
Sulfacetamide sodium (Sulamyd) 10% or 30% solution, 1-2 drops several times/d for 3-7 d (varies with severity of infection)
Sulfisoxazole (Gantrisan) 4% solution, 1-2 drops several times/d (varies with severity of infection)

Supportive

Warm compresses for discomfort and inflammation for 10 to 15 minutes two or three times a day

Tight Lens Syndrome

Tight lens syndrome occurs in soft lens wearers. The lens tends to change in shape and become more curved and less mobile over the cornea. The change may take place within hours after the fitting or within several days (with extended-wear lenses). The wearer experiences decreased visual acuity and conjunctival congestion.[8]

Supportive

Removal of lens reverses process; wearer may have to be refitted with new prescription

Giant Papillary Syndrome

Giant papillary syndrome occurs after several months or years of lens wearing and manifests itself as a cobblestone-appearing inflammation of the inner lining of the upper lid. Redness, tearing, and discharge accompany the tissue inflammation. The cause is unknown, and the treatment is removal of the lens.[40]

ASSESSMENT: AREAS OF CONCERN[3,27,28,40]

Corneal abrasion (epithelial)

Moderate to severe pain; blurred vision; halo seen around lights; generalized hyperemia; lacrimation; fluorescein stains (green) on corneal surface; patient unable to open eyes (owing to pain)

Corneal edema

Blurred vision; absence of pain; dull appearance of cornea; slightly reddened conjunctiva

Corneal ulceration

Ulcers varying in appearance and size; whitish gray opacity with overhanging margins; severe pain associated with epithelial damage; iritis; lacrimation and possible purulent discharge; generalized hyperemia

Localized infection

Purulent discharge; generalized hyperemia; moderate discomfort; possible photophobia; crusting around lids; eyes may be "stuck together" in morning (or on awakening); complaints of blurred vision (owing to excessive exudate over eye surface), which disappears with blinking

Tight lens syndrome

Eye discomfort; decreased visual acuity (onset may be sudden [within hours] or more gradual); patient unable to remove lens; conjunctival congestion with some redness

Giant papillary syndrome

Bilateral cobblestone appearance of inner lining of upper eyelids; slow onset over months or years; lacrimation; conjunctival redness; discharge may be present

NURSING DIAGNOSES and NURSING INTERVENTIONS

Nursing Diagnosis	Nursing Intervention
Knowledge deficit (care of contact lenses)	See "Patient Education" for specific instructions. Deficit exists with new prescription or if medical problems arise after lenses are fitted.
Injury: potential for (related to epithelial damage to cornea with potential for stroma injury)	Assist with identification of epithelial breaks with flourescein stain as ordered. Instill medications as ordered, such as topical antibiotics and cycloplegic drops.
Comfort, alteration in: pain (related to corneal epithelial damage)	Apply pressure bandage to eye(s) as ordered, being certain that covered eye is closed. Apply topical anesthetic as ordered. Apply warm compress as ordered for 10 to 15 minutes for inflammation or discomfort. Administer systemic analgesic as ordered and document response. Discourage patient from reading.
Sensory-perceptual alteration: visual (related to total loss of vision with binocular patches)	Raise side rails. Address patient by name from doorway and identify yourself and reason for presence. Complement voice stimulation with touch to notify patient of your proximity. Orient patient to bedside equipment (such as call light, bed control, and side rails) and personal belongings at bedside by directing his hand over objects. Encourage patient to perform self-care with personal hygiene. Provide support and supervision. Provide privacy and ensure patient that privacy is provided. Assist with meals. Read menu selections. Guide hand to utensils and food on tray. Describe food on tray in clock terms. Assist with cutting meat, removing lids from cartons, and so on. Assist with walking. Walk slowly and slightly ahead of patient with his hand resting on your arm at your elbow or on your shoulders. If possible, allow patient to trace his progress by running the dorsal aspect of his free hand along the wall. Describe surroundings as you proceed. Allow patient to feel chair, toilet, or bed as he turns to sit. Visit patient frequently to be certain that he is sufficiently stimulated. Be certain that someone will be at home to supervise patient's activity after discharge. Review above safety and comfort measures with caretaker.[24]
Sensory-perceptual alteration: visual (related to blurred vision with corneal edema or tight lens)	Assure patient that condition is temporary. Review activities of daily living (such as driving, preparing food, housekeeping, personal hygiene, toileting, and maneuvering around house) and responsibilities at work to be certain that they can be performed safely by patient or with assistance from someone else.

Patient Education[3,27,28,40]

1. Caution the patient to wash hands and dry well before inserting and removing lenses.
2. Tell the patient that eyelashes and face should be thoroughly cleaned before lenses are inserted.
3. Inform the patient that instructions for care and follow-up should be carried out meticulously.
4. Explain the care of hard contact lenses.

a. Encourage the patient to monitor self for sudden onset of pain, excessive eye redness, sudden decrease in vision, mucus discharge, or foreign body sensation. Tell the patient to remove the lenses and report to the physician.
b. Inform the patient that adjustment to new lenses may take 2 to 3 weeks and that mild photophobia, tearing, and lid edema may occur.

c. Inform the patient that hard lenses are not recommended for wearing alternately with glasses or on a part-time basis after initial adjustment and that wearing time will increase to 10 to 14 hours after the adjustment period.

d. Inform the patient that hard lenses should not be worn when engaging in contact sports.

e. Tell the patient that lenses must be removed at night or before sleeping.

f. Explain that lenses must be cleaned after each removal according to the manufacturer's directions and stored in their case.

g. Explain that the lens is wetted with an approved wetting solution before being placed over the cornea.

h. Review the insertion and removal procedure with the patient and have the patient demonstrate it to ensure competence.

i. Inform the patient of the importance of consistently applying one lens before the other to avoid mixing the lenses. If vision is blurred immediately after application, the lenses may be reversed.

j. Tell the patient to check the lenses daily for scratches, tears, loose debris, or clouding. Tell the patient to report to the physician if unable to wash the lenses clear.

k. Emphasize the need to keep appointments with the physician. Eyes may change shape, or refractory error may cause changes. Lenses should be replaced regularly (usually every 1 to 2 years).

5. Explain the care of soft and extended-wear lenses.

a. Encourage the patient to monitor self for sudden onset of pain, excessive eye redness, sudden decrease in vision, mucus discharge, or foreign body sensation. Tell the patient to remove the lenses and report to the physician.

b. Inform the patient that the adjustment time for soft lenses is usually shorter and involves less eye irritation than with hard lenses.

c. Inform the patient that soft lenses are less likely to pop out.

d. Tell the patient that soft lenses can be alternated with glasses.

e. Caution the patient not to wear soft lenses while swimming, applying eye medications, or using hair or body sprays because soft lenses absorb chemicals easily.

f. Explain that soft lenses are usually removed at night and that the wearing time will increase to 12 to 14 hours after adjustment time.

g. Tell the patient that lenses must be cleaned after each removal according to the manufacturer's instructions and stored in a specified solution. Soft lenses should not be permitted to dry out.

h. Explain that the storage solution must be changed as directed.

i. Inform the patient soft lenses are fragile and can be damaged by exposure to makeup, creams, or mascara or nicked by fingernails.

j. Tell the patient that lenses should be checked daily for scratches, tears, loose debris, or clouding. Tell the patient to report to the physician if unable to wash the lenses clear.

k. Explain that the lens must be wetted with an approved wetting solution before being placed in the eye.

l. Review the insertion and removal procedure with the patient and have the patient demonstrate it to ensure competence.

m. Inform the patient of the importance of consistently applying one lens before the other to avoid mixing the lenses. If vision is blurred immediately after application, the lenses may be reversed.

n. Stress the need to keep appointments with the physician, since the eyes and lenses should be checked regularly.

EVALUATION

Patient Outcome	Data Indicating That Outcome is Reached
Cornea is healthy.	Cornea is clear and glossy without eye discomfort, redness, or discharge.
Contact lenses are successfully worn.	Visual acuity is 20/20 OD, OS, and OU. Near vision is clear at 14 inches.[4]

ENUCLEATION

Description and Rationale

Enucleation, or surgical removal of the eyeball, is performed when other treatment of the eyeball is insufficient to prevent pain, disfigurement, or spread of malignant disease. Indications include severe infections, malignancies such as melanoma and retinoblastoma, large and infiltrating tumors, extensive trauma to the eye, blindness when severe eye pain is also present, and end-stage glaucoma when the patient is blind with no light perception and has increased intraocular pressure. Enucleation may also be performed for cosmetic improvement of a blind eye and as a prophylactic measure when sympathetic ophthalmia is likely to occur. Sympathetic ophthalmia is a rare granulomatous inflammation that usually develops within 3 months of an injury to one eye and involves the entire area. The injured eye is called the exciting eye, and the other eye (the sympathizing eye) can also become inflamed with uveitis unless the exciting eye is enucleated before the inflammation spreads.

Enucleation can be performed with the patient under local or general anesthetic. During surgery a 360-degree peritomy is performed at the limbus (Fig. 6-18), opening the conjunctiva and allowing Tenon's fascia to be separated between the rectus muscles. The rectus muscles are separated, hooked, and cut with scissors near their insertion into the sclera. The inferior oblique muscle and superior oblique tendons are hooked and cut, the medius rectus muscle is clamped, and enucleation scissors are placed between the sclera and Tenon's capsule. The optic nerve is then cut as far behind the globe as possible, and the eye is removed.[35] After adequate hemostasis is obtained at the socket, the muscles may be sutured to each other around a plastic or Teflon sphere to build up the eye and provide a more acceptable cosmetic appearance.

After the enucleation a "conformer" is placed in the socket until postoperative edema subsides and an artificial eye can be placed, usually 10 to 14 days after enucleation.

Two relevant surgical procedures are evisceration and exenteration. In evisceration the entire contents of the eyeball and sometimes the cornea are removed but the sclera remains. This procedure may be used when panophthalmitis, an inflammation of the entire inner eye including the sclera, is present. Exenteration is a more radical procedure in which the eyelids, eyeball, and orbital contents are removed, usually in cases of malignancies of the lacrimal gland, extension of eyelid malignancies in the orbit, malignant melanoma of the conjunctiva, or melanoma or retinoblastoma that has invaded the orbit.

Contraindications and Cautions

Panophthalmitis is a contraindication to enucleation because the risk of postoperative meningitis is increased after removal of an actively infected eyeball.

TREATMENT PLAN

Surgical
Removal of the eyeball as described previously

Chemotherapeutic
Narcotic-analgesic agents
   Meperidine (Demerol), 50-75 mg IM q4-6h prn for severe pain
   Acetaminophen with codeine (Tylenol with Codeine), 30-60 mg po q4-6h prn for less severe pain

Supportive
Firm pressure dressing applied to operative site for 24 to 48 hours
Activity progression without restrictions as tolerated
Progressive diet as tolerated

ASSESSMENT: AREAS OF CONCERN

Eye socket
Pain at enucleation site; headache on side of enucleation; no fever or bleeding

NURSING DIAGNOSES and NURSING INTERVENTIONS

Nursing Diagnosis	Nursing Intervention
Comfort, alteration in: pain	Administer pain medications as ordered by physician and document response. Notify physician if pain or headache persists, since this may indicate infection. Notify physician if temperature is elevated.
Potential patient problem: potential hemorrhage	Maintain firm pressure dressing at operative site until removal is ordered by physician.

Fig. 6-18

Technique of standard enucleation. **A,** Peritomy is performed. **B,** Tenon's fascia is separated. **C,** Rectus muscles are hooked. **D,** Rectus muscles are cut near their insertions. **E,** Inferior oblique muscle and, **F,** superior oblique tendon are hooked and cut. **G,** Enucleation scissors are placed nasally. **H,** After optic nerve has been cut, globe removed, and ball implant inserted, rectus muscles and Tenon's capsule are closed with interrupted 4-0 chromic catgut sutures. **I,** Tenon's capsule is closed more superficially with interrupted 4-0 chromic catgut sutures. **J,** Conjunctiva is closed with running 6-0 plain catgut sutures. **K,** Conformer is placed between eyelids and conjunctiva.

From Shields, J.A.: Diagnosis and management of intraocular tumors, St. Louis, 1983, The C.V. Mosby Co.

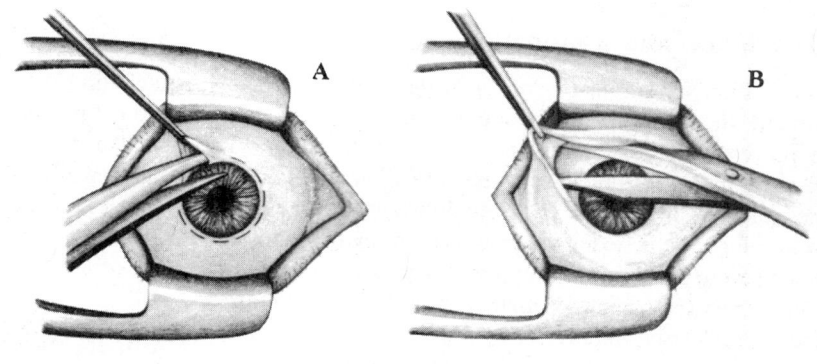

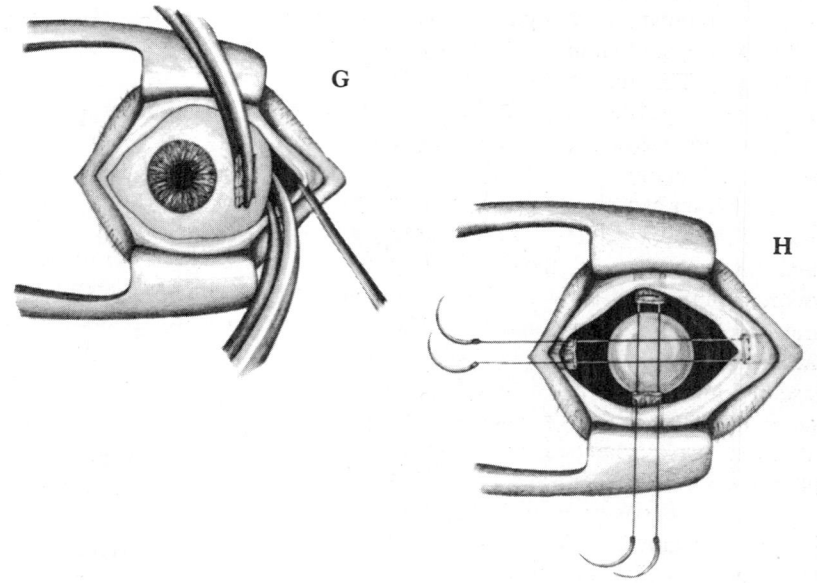

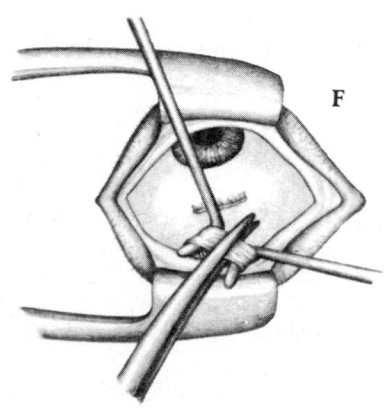

Nursing Diagnosis	Nursing Intervention
	Observe dressing at operative site frequently for signs of oozing or frank bleeding.
	Document absence of blood or amount if present.
	Monitor and document vital signs according to protocol, and report any change in pulse and blood pressure.
Sensory-perceptual alteration: visual	Assist patient with ambulation as tolerated.
	Ensure that patient's call light and personal belongings are close by on unaffected side.
	Assist patient with meals as needed.
Self-concept, disturbance in: body image	Assure patient that appearance will be quite normal when patient is fitted with artificial eye and that satisfactory visual adjustment usually occurs.
	Listen to patient's fears and concerns in comforting, supportive manner.
	Assure patient that period of depression is normal after procedure such as removal of eye.

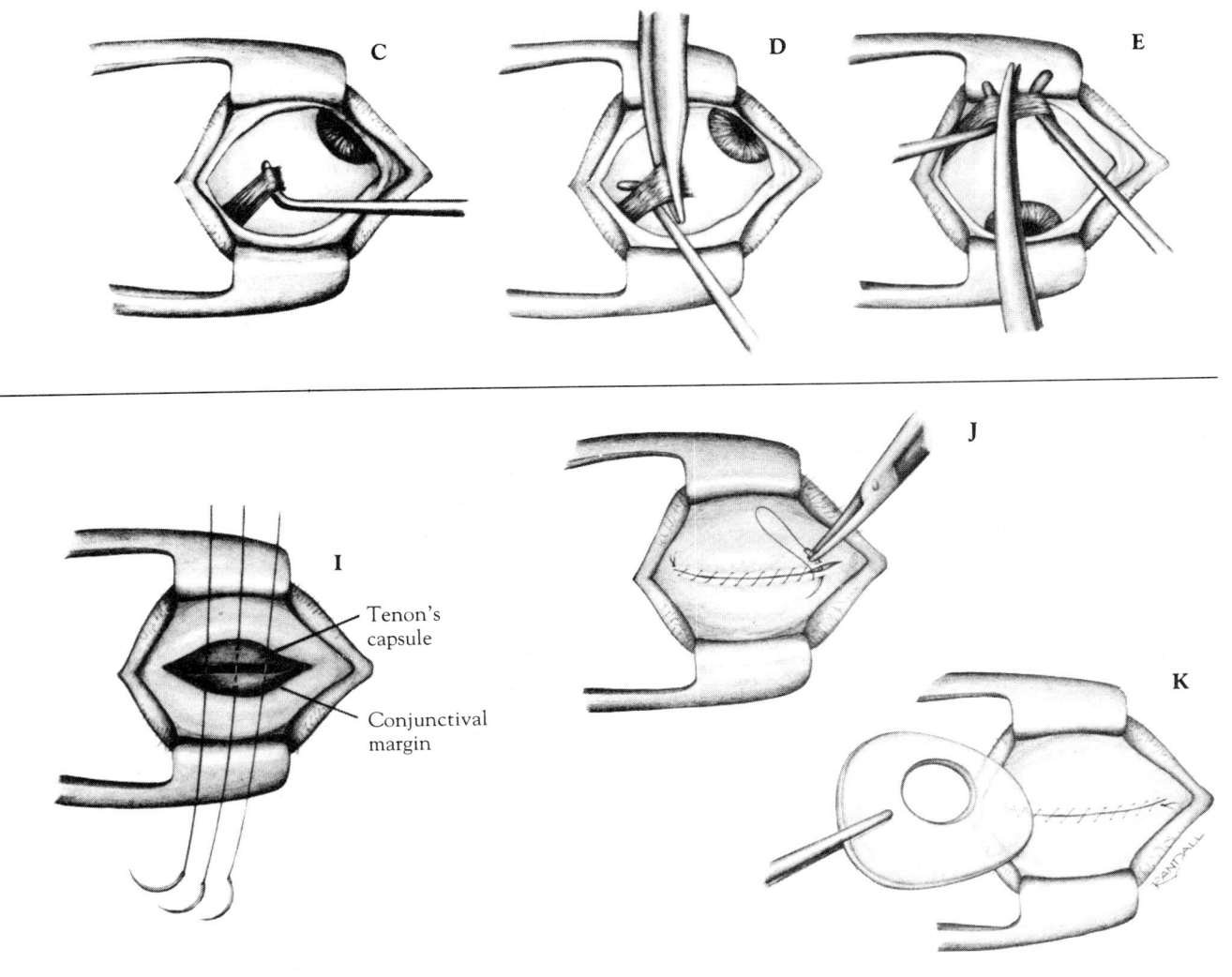

Tenon's
capsule

Conjunctival
margin

Patient Education

1. Teach the patient how to care for the eye socket. These instructions are usually given on an outpatient basis.
2. Teach the paient and family how to care for, insert, and remove an artificial eye if one is used. The artificial eye is fitted after the patient leaves the hospital and the wound has healed.
3. Ensure that the patient is aware of the need to protect the vision in the remaining eye. Some physicians recommend that a patient wear safety glasses for protection.
4. Educate the patient regarding the signs and symptoms of infection, abscess, and meningitis.
5. Discuss the limited field of vision and the need to exaggerate head movement to achieve a full visual field, for example, when driving. Discuss the changes in depth perception.

EVALUATION

Patient Outcome	Data Indicating That Outcome is Reached
There is no infection.	Patient and family demonstrate ability to care for eye socket and artificial eye after discharge from hospital. Patient verbalizes signs and symptoms of possible infection: pain, headache, drainage, and elevated temperature.
Body image is adequate.	Patient is fitted with and wears artificial eye, if appropriate, to improve appearance after discharge from hospital. Patient verbalizes understanding of need for eye removal and expresses concerns and frustrations regarding disease process and body image.

KERATOPLASTY

Description and Rationale

Keratoplasty, or corneal transplant, is the excision of corneal tissue and its replacement by a cornea from a human donor.[28] This procedure may be performed to replace a corneal opacity, which is a lack of corneal transparency resulting from injury or inflammation, or to correct a variety of corneal abnormalities called corneal dystrophies. Certain bilateral hereditary disorders may be present at birth but usually develop during adolescence and progress through adulthood. Some do not affect vision, but many do. The success of corneal transplantation as a treatment for these dystrophies depends on the type and extent of the corneal abnormality. The dystrophy may possibly recur in the donor graft. One of the dystrophies for which keratoplasty is particularly successful is keratoconus, a condition in which the symmetric curvature of the cornea is distorted by an abnormal thinning and forward bulging of the central portion of the cornea (Fig. 6-19). A penetrating corneal transplant restores useful vision with a 95% success rate.[28] Corneal perforation, which is usually a complication of a corneal ulcer, is a serious condition that may destroy vision if not treated rapidly. Keratoplasty may be performed if there is imminent danger of perforation of a corneal ulcer.

There are two types of keratoplasty: lamellar and penetrating. Lamellar or nonpenetrating keratoplasty is a partial-thickness graft in which the surgeon removes and replaces a superficial layer of cornea without entering the anterior chamber. In a penetrating keratoplasty the entire thickness of cornea is removed and replaced by donor corneal tissue. This is the traditional type of keratoplasty and can be either complete or partial, depending on whether the entire cornea is excised.

Donor eyes are obtained from cadavers of noninfected persons who have died as a result of injury or acute disease or from patients whose eyes have been surgically removed for some reason but whose corneas are normal.

Ideally the donor is between 25 and 35 years of age. Corneas should not be used from patients who were ill for a long time before death or who had such diseases as leukemia, sepsis, hepatitis, or certain tumors of the eye.

If it is known when a patient dies that the eyes are to be donated, the lids should be closed and covered with small ice bags. Nothing should touch the corneas themselves. The donor eyes should be enucleated within an hour after death, but up to 5 hours is acceptable if ice bags have been placed on the eyes at death. Ideally cor-

Fig. 6-19
Abnormal corneal profile in keratoconus.

From Newell, F.W.: Ophthalmology: principles and concepts, ed. 5, St. Louis, 1982, The C.V. Mosby Co.

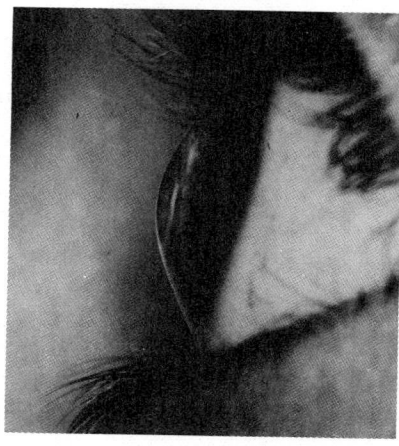

neas are transplanted into the recipient immediately after removal, but many eye banks can now safely store corneas for longer periods. Whole eyes can be stored from 24 to 48 hours if refrigerated; corneal tissue can be kept longer if removed with a 3 mm rim of scleral tissue attached. Corneas must not be folded during storage because this damages the endothelium. They must be stored at a temperature of 4° C (39° F) in a modified tissue culture medium.[28]

Transplantation is usually performed with the patient under topical and retrobulbar anesthesia. The surgeon removes the cornea from the donor's eye with a trephine and then removes the impaired areas from the recipient eye using another trephine the same size or slightly larger. The donor cornea, called the donor button, is sutured into place with continuous or interrupted sutures to align and graft and ensure a watertight wound (Fig. 6-20).

Contraindications and Cautions

Light perception and projection must be normal before surgery will be considered.

There is the possibility that some corneal dystrophy will recur in the transplanted cornea.

Corneal graft rejection may occur. This starts 3 weeks or more after keratoplasty and is limited to the donor cornea, since there are no blood vessels or lymphatics to sensitize the recipient. The inflammatory process begins at the graft margin and spreads to involve the entire graft.

TREATMENT PLAN

Surgical
Lamellar or penetrating keratoplasty as described previously

Chemotherapeutic
Narcotic analgesic agents
Meperidine (Demerol), 50-100 mg IM q4h prn for pain
Antiemetic agents
Prochlorperazine (Compazine), 25 mg by rectum bid or 5-10 mg IM q4-6h for nausea
Corticosteroids
Pred-Forte eye drops, 1 drop qid
Laxatives
Docusate sodium (Colace), 240 mg po to prevent straining during bowel movement

Supportive
Unilateral eye patch for 24 hours
Activity and diet progress as tolerated

ASSESSMENT: AREAS OF CONCERN

Cornea
Wound edema; inflammation; photophobia; decreased vision; clouding caused by vascularization as result of graft rejection

Fig. 6-20
Keratoplasty. Excised central portion of cornea is being replaced with clear donor cornea.

From Newell, F.W.: Ophthalmology: principles and concepts, ed. 5, St. Louis, 1982, The C.V. Mosby Co.

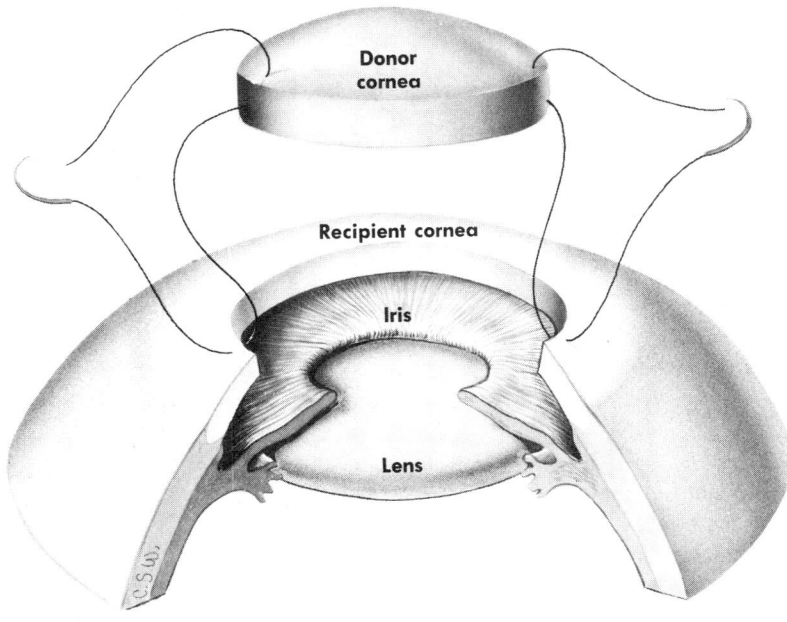

NURSING DIAGNOSES and NURSING INTERVENTIONS

Nursing Diagnosis	Nursing Intervention
Sensory-perceptual alteration: visual	Ensure that eye patch remains securely in place for at least 24 hours. Assist patient with ambulation postoperatively, since patient may be unsteady and must be prevented from falling and injuring eye. Ensure that call light is in place, side rails are up, and items at bedside are in familiar place for patient. Administer eye drops as ordered by physician.
Comfort, alteration in: pain	Administer pain medication as ordered, particularly on first postoperative night, to decrease discomfort and promote rest and healing of eye.
Injury: potential for	Institute measures designed to prevent increases in intraocular pressure that might push healing graft forward. Administer antiemetics as ordered to prevent vomiting. Encourage patient not to cough but to breathe deeply often to increase lung expansion. Avoid using any material that may cause sneezing: talcum powder, perfumes, room sprays, or pepper on meal trays. Instruct patient not to lean over, lift, or push heavy objects and to avoid straining when having a bowel movement.

Patient Education

1. Instruct the patient regarding the need to prevent increases in intraocular pressure, since eye tissue requires more time to heal than other tissue. Warn the patient to avoid extreme exertion or emotion, sudden jerky movements, lifting or pushing heavy objects, or straining at stool.
2. Inform the patient that the sutures will remain in the eye for as long as a year to ensure adequate healing.
3. Inform the patient that the photophobia experienced after surgery will gradually decrease, that vision will slowly improve, that dark glasses may be worn if needed, and that further correction with eyeglasses may be necessary.
4. If the patient is discharged with eye drops, ensure that the patient or family can demonstrate the appropriate technique of instillation.
5. Instruct the patient and family in the signs and symptoms of graft rejection (inflammation, clouding, drainage, and pain at graft site), and tell them to notify the physician immediately so treatment can begin promptly.

EVALUATION

Patient Outcome	Data Indicating That Outcome is Reached
Corneal graft heals adequately.	Wound edema and inflammation dissipate. Photophobia decreases. Vision improves slowly. No evidence of graft rejection occurs. No injury is caused to the graft from increase in intraocular pressure.

LASER THERAPY

Description and Rationale

The word "laser" is an acronym for *l*ight *a*mplification by *s*timulated *e*mission of *r*adiation. Experimentation with the effect of light on the retina began in the 1800s after the invention of the ophthalmoscope, when ophthalmologists began noticing solar burns in patients' eyes after solar eclipses. Early investigators used the effects of the sun or the carbon arc to produce a lesion in the retina.[22] Since that time, research with laser therapy has refined and broadened its use, and lasers are now the treatment of choice for a wide variety of ophthalmic disorders. Laser therapy produces excellent results (Table

Table 6-3

Results of Treatment of Various Ocular Abnormalities by Argon, Xenon Arc, Ruby, Dye, Carbon Dioxide, and Krypton Lasers

Disease	Argon Laser	Xenon Arc	Ruby Laser	Dye Laser	Carbon Dioxide Laser	Krypton Laser Red	Krypton Laser Green-Yellow
Peripheral Retinal Structural Abnormalities							
Retinal tears	Excellent*	Excellent	Excellent	Excellent	None	Excellent	Excellent
Retinal degenerations	Excellent*	Excellent	Excellent	Excellent	None	Excellent	Excellent
Retinal detachments	Excellent—requires absorbent pigment*	Excellent—effective with slightly elevated retinas, meridional folds, tears	Good—effective if retina attached	Excellent	None	Good—effective if retina attached	Excellent
Retinoschisis	Good—use limited to delimiting bulla,* possibly barrage	Good—used to barrage* or delimit bulla; with encircling element*	Fair—to delimit bulla after collapse by surgery	Good	None	Fair—to delimit bulla after collapse by surgery	Excellent
Peripheral Retinal Vascular Abnormalities							
Eales' disease	Excellent*	Excellent	Poor	Excellent	None	Poor	Excellent
Leber's disease	Excellent—especially for macular lesions*	Excellent	Poor	Excellent	None	Poor	Excellent
Coats' disease	Excellent	Excellent*	Poor	Excellent	None	Poor	Excellent
Proliferative sickle retinopathy	Excellent*	Excellent	Poor	Excellent	None	Poor	Excellent
Retrolental fibroplasia	Equivocal*	Equivocal	Poor	Equivocal	None	Poor	Excellent
Diabetic Retinopathy							
Nonproliferative	Excellent*	Excellent	Poor	Excellent	None	Good	Excellent
Proliferative	Excellent—especially for epipapillary, peripapillary, papillovitreal, and retinovitreal neovascularization*	Excellent—especially for surface neovascularization*	Fair—ablation technique only	Excellent	None	Good—ablation technique only	Excellent
Peripheral Chorioretinal Tumors							
Retinoblastoma	Fair	Good*	Poor	Excellent*	None	Poor	Poor
Malignant melanoma	Good—6 disc diameters	Good*—<6 disc diameters	Poor	Excellent*	None	Poor	Poor
Angiomatosis retinae	Excellent	Excellent*	Poor	Excellent*	None	Poor	Excellent

From L'Esperance, F.A., Jr.: Ophthalmic lasers: photocoagulation, photoradiation, and surgery, ed. 2, St. Louis, 1982, The C.V. Mosby Co.
*Preferred method of treatment.

Continued.

Table 6-3, cont'd
Results of Treatment of Various Ocular Abnormalities by Argon, Xenon Arc, Ruby, Dye, Carbon Dioxide, and Krypton Lasers

Disease	Argon Laser	Xenon Arc	Ruby Laser	Dye Laser	Carbon Dioxide Laser	Krypton Laser Red	Krypton Laser Green-Yellow
Macular Serous Abnormalities							
Serous detachment of pigment epithelium	Excellent*	Excellent	Good	Excellent	None	Good	Excellent
Central serous choroidopathy	Excellent*	Excellent	Excellent	Excellent	None	Excellent*	Excellent
Macular Hemorrhagic Abnormalities							
Hemorrhagic detachment of the pigment epithelium	Excellent	Excellent	Poor	Excellent	None	Excellent*—especially in foveolar avascular zone	Excellent—especially in foveolar avascular zone
Hemorrhagic detachment of the sensory retina	Good*	Good	Poor	Excellent	None	Excellent*	Excellent
Choroidal neovascularization and secondary exudative maculopathy	Excellent	Excellent	Poor	Excellent	None	Excellent—especially for perifoveal and macular area*	Excellent
Macular Intraretinal Abnormalities							
Branch retinal vein occlusion	Excellent*	Excellent	Good—ablation technique only	Excellent	None	Excellent*	Excellent
Central retinal vein occlusion	Excellent*	Good	Good—ablation technique only	Excellent	None	Excellent*	Excellent
Miscellaneous Macular Diseases							
Macular hole, penetrating	Fair*	Fair	Good	Excellent	None	Excellent	Excellent
Preretinal fibrosis	Equivocal* Good(?)*	Equivocal Good(?)	Equivocal Good(?)	Equivocal Good	None None	Equivocal Equivocal	Equivocal Equivocal
Toxoplasmic retinochoroiditis							
Toxocara canis infestation	Equivocal(?)	Equivocal(?)*	Poor	Equivocal	None	Equivocal	Equivocal
Pigment epitheliopathy	Good	Good	Fair	Excellent	None	Excellent*	Excellent
Angioid streaks	Good	Good	Poor	Excellent	None	Excellent*	Excellent

Anterior Segment Abnormalities

Iris defects							
Deformed pupils	Excellent*	Good	Poor	Excellent	None	Good	Excellent
Iris cyst	Excellent*	Excellent	Poor	Excellent	None	Good	Good
Iridocyclitic membrane	Excellent*	Good	Poor	Excellent	None	Poor	Excellent
Glaucoma							
Laser photomydriasis	Excellent—especially if lens present*	Good	Poor	Excellent	None	Excellent	Excellent
Laser iridotomy	Excellent*	Good	Excellent—Q-switched only	Excellent	None	Good	Good
Laser trabeculoplasty	Excellent*	Poor	Good—Q-switched	Good	None	Good	Excellent
Laser gonioplasty	Excellent*	Good	Poor	Excellent	None	Excellent	Excellent
Laser goniophotocoagulation	Excellent*	Poor	Poor	Excellent	None	Poor	Excellent
Laser trabeculostomy	Good(?)	Poor	Poor	Poor	Excellent*	Poor	Poor
Laser trabeculosclerostomy							
Internal	Good*	Poor	Poor	Excellent	None	Poor	Good
External	Poor	Poor	Poor	Poor	Excellent*	Poor	Poor
Laser cyclocautery							
Transpupillary	Excellent*	Excellent	Poor	Excellent	None	Poor	Good
Transscleral	Poor(?)	Poor	Good—Q-switched only*	Poor	None	Poor	Poor

*Preferred method of treatment.

6-3). Types of laser used today include argon, xenon arc, ruby, dye, carbon dioxide, and krypton.

A basic principle of laser therapy is that the light absorbed by pigment is converted to heat energy. When enough heat is generated to coagulate the protein in the tissue, a thermal burn, called photocoagulation, ensues. The retinal pigment epithelium and the uveal pigment within the eye are ideal for this absorption of light.[35] Two other types of laser therapy, less widely used than photocoagulation, are photoradiation therapy and photovaporization therapy. Photoradiation therapy is the use of photosensitizing drugs and a dye laser to treat malignant tumors such as melanomas of the eye, and photovaporization therapy is the use of carbon dioxide laser radiation to vaporize malignant intraocular and extraocular tumors in a very precise manner. When repeated surface impacts are made with the carbon dioxide laser, carbon dioxide radiation is highly absorbed by ocular tissue, with almost complete absorption and conversion to heat within a tissue depth of 100 μm.[22]

Photocoagulation provides a nonsurgical approach to many ophthalmic disorders and can usually be performed on an outpatient basis. The goal of photocoagulation therapy is to maintain the hemodynamics, fluid dynamics, and physiologic structure of the macular region. In cases of anatomic barrier breakdown, photocoagulation is used to destroy the offending tissue elements or retinal vessels in an effort to seal the abnormal area and prevent leakage from a retinal or choroidal vascular system into the sensitive sensory retina. In cases of neovascularization, photocoagulation is used to obliterate the newly vascularized areas to prevent further deterioration of the

TREATMENT PLAN*

	Argon Laser	Xenon Arc	Ruby Laser
Energy source	Electrically pumped gaseous discharge tube	High-pressure xenon arc bulb	Ruby crystal pumped by xenon flash
Tissue reaction	Absorption primarily at pigmented areas, such as melanin, xanthophyll, and hemoglobin; heat production and coagulum formed, resulting in eventual pigment and glial proliferation	Coagulation with sufficient absorption of any wavelength (400 to 1600 nm); edema, exudation, pigment proliferation, gliosis, and atrophy	Absorption primarily at pigmented areas, with production of heat; late result similar to light coagulation
Anesthesia	Topical anesthesia required; occasionally retrobulbar akinesia and anesthesia necessary	Occasionally preoperative sedation, retrobulbar and lid akinesia and anesthesia; topical anesthesia necessary	None required
Ancillary equipment	Low vacuum or three-mirror contact lens for retinal photocoagulation; occasionally cooling contact lens for anterior segment therapy	Contact lens for correcting high ametropia, lid speculum, and constant saline corneal lavage; forceps manipulation of eye may be necessary	None required
Hospitalization and aftercare	None required	Monocular patch for 12 hours	None required
Hazards	No danger to operator; overall hazards to patient minimal because of minute total energy transmitted through refractive media	Accidental retinal burn of operator; overheating of anterior chamber, thermal cataract, vitreous hemorrhages, secondary retinal necrosis and tears, secondary excudative retinal detachment, and macular deterioration	Accidental retinal burn of operator more probable because of coherence and energy density of stray laser beam; similar ocular complications; less total energy transmitted through media

*Modified from L'Esperance, F.A., Jr.: Ophthalmic lasers, ed. 2, 1983, St. Louis, The C.V. Mosby Co.

involved regions.[22] It has offered new hope to patients with diabetic retinopathy. Although photocoagulation does not increase vision, it can prevent further loss of vision by cauterization of the newly formed, fragile vessels of the retina with an intense minuscule light beam, thereby diverting blood to the already established sturdy vessels on the retina and eliminating the most likely areas of stress and hemorrhage.[31]

Photocoagulation has also become useful in the treatment of glaucoma to control intraocular pressure. A procedure called laser goniophotocoagulation can control pressure successfully in about 85% of cases, especially in eyes with wide angles and slight pigmentation of the trabecular meshwork.

Laser therapy is also useful in treating chronic primary angle-closure glaucoma. The aim of therapy is to prevent the pressure in the posterior chamber from exceeding that of the anterior chamber by creating an opening that eliminates the accumulation of aqueous humor in the posterior chamber. The surgeon performs a laser iridotomy in which a localized area of the midperipheral iris is caused to bulge forward by means of mild laser burns. The central portion of this area is then perforated by a laser beam of much higher energy. Many applications of the beam may be necessary.[28]

Dye Laser	Carbon Dioxide Laser	Krypton Laser
Dye pumped by argon laser	Gaseous discharge tube pumped electrically	Gaseous discharge tube pumped electrically
Absorption in various portions of ocular tissues depending on dye used and wavelength generated; heat production and coagulum formed, resulting in pigment and glial proliferation; certain wavelengths useful in phototherapy and photosensitization of tumors	100% absorption by all ocular and extraocular tissues within 100 μm of surface impact; solid tissue vaporized to water vapor and smoke instantaneously; absorption independent of pigmented material; beam hemostatic, bacteriostatic, lymphostatic; tissue response, slight char and minimal injury; healing excellent	Absorption primarily at pigmented areas such as melanin (red, yellow, and green beams), xanthophyll (violet and blue beams), and hemoglobin (blue, green, and yellow beams); heat production and coagulum formed, resulting in eventual pigment and glial proliferation
Topical anesthesia required; occasionally retrobulbar akinesia and anesthesia necessary	Topical anesthesia required as well as local infiltration anesthesia for external lesions; retrobulbar akinesia and anesthesia necessary for intraocular therapy; occasionally general anesthesia required	Topical anesthesia required; occasionally retrobulbar akinesia and anesthesia necessary
Low-vacuum or three-mirror contact lens for retinal photocoagulation; stereotaxic manipulator for delivery and distribution of laser beam by fiberoptic cables	Low reflective instruments necessary; positive pressure nitrogen flow and/or vacuum apparatus for smoke and vapor; glasses for operating room personnel	Plano–low-vacuum or three-mirror contact lens for retinal photocoagulation; occasionally other specialized lenses for anterior segment therapy
None usually required; phototherapy and photosensitization procedures may require brief hospitalization	May be required for intraocular and extraocular dissections	None required
No danger to operator; minimal hazards to patient possible with phototherapy procedures	Mild danger to operator and operating room personnel; ordinary glasses should be worn; nonreflective instruments and noninflammable draperies should be used; constant monitoring by technician of instrumentation and personnel necessary	No danger to operator; overall hazards to patient minimal because of minute total energy transmitted through refractive media

Table 6-4
Factors That Affect Photocoagulation

Eye Segment	Consideration	Caution
Cornea	Defects in epithelium; embedded foreign bodies; disruptions of Bowman's membrane; stromal haze, maculas, or opacities	Could cause scatter, deflection, or absorption of laser beam
Corneal endothelium	Increase in guttata; pigment deposition; breaks, doubling, or rolling of Descemet's membrane; accumulations of red or white cells or keratotic precipitates on posterior surfaces	Could decrease effectiveness of laser beam and could introduce complications
Anterior chamber	Presence of cells; protein accumulation; blood, pigment flecks, or other unusual particles	Could decrease effectiveness of photocoagulation and visualization of posterior segment
Iris	Should dilate to at least 4 mm in diameter	To permit adequate visualization of areas of retina
Lens	Wedgelike cortical opacities	Could decrease impact power of beam by occlusion of segment as beam passes through opacity
	Presence of nuclear or posterior subcapsular cataracts	Could refract beam in various directions and diminish or negate effectiveness of procedure
	Presence of anterior and posterior polar cataracts	Presents problem if pupil cannot be dilated; beam must be channeled eccentrically through outer portion of pupillary sphere to avoid central opacification
Vitreous	Blood clots; opacities; pigment accumulation; collagen condensations and membranes	Could decrease effectiveness of beam and cause further deterioration or damage
Retina	Areas of hemorrhagic activity; edema or exudate; retinoschisis; serous accumulations beneath sensory retina; increase in sensory retinal edema	Would require change in laser approach or increase in energy to ensure adequate coagulation of underlying neovascularization

Modified from L'Esperance, F.A.: Ophthalmic lasers, ed. 2, 1981, The C.V. Mosby Co.

Contraindications and Cautions

Before photocoagulation therapy each segment of the eye must be closely examined for factors that would diminish the effectiveness of therapy, as described in Table 6-4.

ASSESSMENT: AREAS OF CONCERN

Vision
Constriction of peripheral fields; temporary decrease in central vision; slight decrease in night vision; headache from bright laser light

NURSING DIAGNOSES and NURSING INTERVENTIONS

Nursing Diagnosis	Nursing Intervention
Knowledge deficit	Explain purpose of laser therapy.
	Assure patient that procedure causes little pain and that topical anesthetic (eye drops) will be administered.
	Describe procedure to patient and family. Explain that patient will be awake and sitting up in a chair and may have special contact lens placed on eye.
	Describe bright lights caused by laser beam that patient will see during procedure.
	Explain that procedure may take 15 to 40 minutes.
	Tell patient that family member or friend should accompany patient and drive home, since patient's eyes will be dilated and vision may be temporarily blurred.

Nursing Diagnosis	**Nursing Intervention**
Comfort, alteration in: pain	Explain to patient that headache may develop after treatment because of bright laser light. Suggest acetaminophen to relieve discomfort. Advise patient not to use aspirin because of its anticoagulant effect.

Patient Education

1. Emphasize the importance of not increasing the venous pressure in the head, neck, and eyes, particularly with the Valsalva maneuver. Instruct the patient to keep the head up and to move slowly and not to bend over or make sudden movements.
2. Caution the patient not to lift anything heavier than 5 pounds and not to strain for any reason, as when having a bowel movement. Encourage the patient to take a stool softener to avoid constipation.
3. Instruct the patient to avoid strenuous activities such as athletics and sexual intercourse for approximately 3 weeks, but encourage the patient to participate in mild forms of exercise such as walking.
4. Explain that spots may be seen before the eyes for 24 to 48 hours after treatment. Inform the patient that there may be some discomfort around the eye for about 3 weeks; the lid may be black and blue, the eye may be bloodshot, the vision may be somewhat blurred temporarily, and night vision may be temporarily decreased.
5. Instruct the patient to sleep with the head of the bed elevated 15 to 20 degrees to decrease the pressure in the eyes.
6. Advise the patient to avoid coughing and sneezing and not to blow the nose vigorously. (However, sneezes should not be stifled, since this raises the pressure in the eyes.)
7. Teach the patient not to rub the eyes.
8. Caution the patient to avoid altitudes above 8000 feet. The patient may fly on commercial airlines, however, since the cabins are pressurized.
9. Instruct the patient to avoid medications that contain epinephrine, such as nose drops or sprays, since these may raise the blood pressure.

EVALUATION

Patient Outcome	Data Indicating That Outcome is Reached
Vision is restored or improved.	Blurred vision decreases after about 3 weeks, and normal vision returns.

References

1. Adler, F.H.: Physiology of the eye: clinical application, St. Louis, 1965, The C.V. Mosby Co.
2. Bernth-Petersen, P.: A change in indications for cataract surgery? A 10 year comparative epidemiological study, Acta Ophthalmol. **59**:206, 1981.
3. Binder, P.S.: The physiologic effects of extended wear soft contact lenses, Am. Acad. Ophthalmol. **87**:745, 1980.
4. Bowers, A.C., and Thompson, J.: Clinical manual of health assessment, St. Louis, 1984, The C.V. Mosby Co.
5. Boyd-Monk, H.: Taking a closer look at contact lenses, Nursing 78 **8**:38, 1978.
6. Cataract surgery: providing total patient care, Nursing 83 **13**:65, 1983.
7. Cavanagh, H.D., Bodner, B.I., and Wilson, L.A.: Extended wear hydrogel lenses, Am. Acad. Ophthalmol. **87**:871, 1980.
8. Eichenbaum, J.W., Feldstein, M., and Podos, S.M.: Extended-wear aphakic soft contact lenses and corneal ulcers, Br. J. Ophthalmol. **66**:663, 1982.
9. Ellis, R.A.: Advances in cataract surgery, Occupational Health Nurs. **29**:34, 1981.
10. Foulds, W.S.: The changing pattern of eye surgery, Br. J. Anaesth. **52**:643, 1980.
11. Gilman, A.G., Goodman, L.S., and Gilman, A., editors: The pharmacological basis of therapeutics, ed. 6, New York, 1980, MacMillan Publishing Co., Inc.
12. Groër, M.W., and Shekleton, M.E.: Basic pathophysiology: a conceptual approach, St. Louis, 1983, The C.V. Mosby Co.
13. Helveston, E.M., and Ellis, F.D.: Pediatric ophthalmology practice, St. Louis, 1980, The C.V. Mosby Co.
14. Hillis, A., Flynn, J.T., and Hawkins, B.S.: The evolving concept of amblyopia: a challenge to epidemiologists, Am. J. Epidemiol. **118**:192, 1983.
15. Hirst, L.W., Smiddy, W.E., and Stark, W.J.: Corneal perforations: changing methods of treatment, 1960-1980, Ophthalmology **89**:630, 1982.
16. Reference deleted in proofs.
17. Jensen, D.: The principles of physiology, ed. 2, New York, 1980, Appleton-Century-Crofts.
18. Kim, M., McFarland, G., and McLane, A.: Pocket guide to nursing diagnoses, St. Louis, 1984, The C.V. Mosby Co.
19. Kornzweig, A.L.: New ideas for old eyes, J. Geriatr. Soc. **28**:145, 1980.
20. Leske, M.C.: The epidemiology of open-angle glaucoma: a review, Am. J. Epidemiol. **118**:166, 1983.
21. Leske, M.C., and Sperduto, R.D.: The epidemiology of senile cataracts: a review, Am. J. Epidemiol. **118**:152, 1983.
22. L'Esperance, F.A.: Ophthalmic lasers, ed. 2, St. Louis, 1983, The C.V. Mosby Co.
23. Luciano, D.S., Vander, A.J., and Sherman, J.H.: Human function and structure, New York, 1978, McGraw-Hill Book.

24. Luckmann, J., and Sorensen, K.C.: Medical-surgical nursing: a psychophysiologic approach, Philadelphia, 1980, W.B. Saunders Co.

25. Marshall, L.F.: The oval pupil: clinical significance and relationship to intracranial hypertension, J. Neurosurg. **58:**566, 1983.

26. McCoy, K.: Cataracts and intraocular lenses: from cloudy to clear, Nurs. Clin. North Am. **16:**405, 1981.

27. Melamed, M.: Complications of contact lenses, Emergency Med. **12:**218, 1982.

28. Newell, F.W.: Ophthalmology: principles and concepts, ed. 5, St. Louis, 1982, The C.V. Mosby Co.

29. Norman, S.: The pupil check, Am. J. Nurs. **82:**588, 1982.

30. Pearson, L.J., and Kotthoff, M.E.: Geriatric clinical protocols, Philadelphia, 1979, J.B. Lippincott Co.

31. Perrin, E.D.: Laser therapy for diabetic retinopathy, Am. J. Nurs. **80:**664, 1980.

32. Price, S.A., and Wilson, L.M.: Pathophysiology: clinical concepts of disease processes, ed. 2, New York, 1982, McGraw-Hill Book Co.

33. Resler, M., and Tumulty, G.: Glaucoma update, Am. J. Nurs. **83:**752, 1983.

34. Saunders, W.H., et al.: Nursing care in eye, ear, nose and throat disorders, St. Louis, 1979, The C.V. Mosby Co.

35. Shields, J.A.: Diagnosis and management of intraocular tumors, St. Louis, 1983, The C.V. Mosby Co.

36. Smith, J.F., and Nachazel, D.P.: Ophthalmologic nursing, Boston, 1980, Little, Brown & Co.

37. Steinberg, F.U., editor: Care of the geriatric patient, ed. 6, St. Louis, 1983, The C.V. Mosby Co.

38. Straatsma, B.R.: The aging eye, Transition p. 18, 1984.

39. Tyers, A.G.: Aging and the ocular adnexa: a review, J. R. Soc. Med. **75:**900.

40. Vaughan, D., and Asbury, T.: General ophthalmology, ed. 10, Los Altos, Calif., 1983, Lange Medical Publications.

41. Von Noorden, G.K.: Practical management of amblyopia, Int. Ophthalmol. **6:**7, 1983.

42. Waring, G.O., editor: Pars plana lensectomy by ultrasonic fragmentation, Surv. Ophthalmol. **27:**96, 1982.

43. Whaley, L.F., and Wong, D.L.: Nursing care of infants and children, ed. 2, St. Louis, 1983, The C.V. Mosby Co.

44. Yanoff, M.: Cataract surgery—when and how, Geriatrics **37:**71, 1982.

CHAPTER 7

Ear, Nose, and Throat

Overview

The ear, nose, and throat (ENT) are responsible for many of the body's senses: sound, smell, and taste, as well as equilibrium and speaking. These are obviously important in human functioning; health professionals who care for patients with disorders affecting these areas must be highly sensitive and skilled in assessing the symptoms of disorders that may have a great impact on a patient's life or self-perception.

Although few ENT disorders prove fatal (with the exception of neoplastic diseases, which are discussed in Chapter 14), they nevertheless can cause painful, incapacitating illnesses and major disruptions in communication, personal appearance, eating, swallowing, and air intake.

Since many ENT disorders are treated on an outpatient basis, patient education is a focus of this chapter.

The advent of antibiotics and recent surgical advances have greatly minimized the impact of ENT diseases. Hearing loss, once a common occurrence after severe or repeated ear infections, has almost been eliminated in the United States, and other diseases that once were life threatening are now considered minor if treated early. Surgical techniques such as microsurgery, stapedectomy, cochlear implant, and tympanoplasty have brought great progress to the treatment of hearing loss.

ANATOMY AND PHYSIOLOGY

Ear

The ears are a pair of sensory organs that participate in both *hearing* and *equilibrium*. The ear can be divided into three anatomic sections: external, middle, and inner (Fig. 7-1).

External ear. The external ear includes the outer projection, or the auricle, and a passageway called the external auditory meatus or external auditory canal. The function of the external ear is to receive sound waves and direct them to the tympanic membrane. The auricle, or pinna, is attached to the head by muscles innervated by the facial nerve, is composed of cartilage, and is covered by skin, except for the dependent lobe, which contains no cartilage (Fig. 7-2). The auricle is highly susceptible to frostbite because it has little subcutaneous fat to protect it and only one layer of blood vessels. The sensory nerve supply of the auricle is provided by the great auricular nerve, the lesser occipital nerve, the auricular branch of the vagus nerve, the auriculotemporal nerve, and the fifth, seventh, and tenth cranial nerves.

The external auditory meatus or canal, which is about 1 inch deep and has a slight downward curve, ends blindly at the tympanic membrane. The outer half is cartilaginous and the inner half is bony except in infants in whom ossification has not yet occurred. The skin that lines the

743

Fig. 7-1
Relationship of external, middle, and
inner ear.

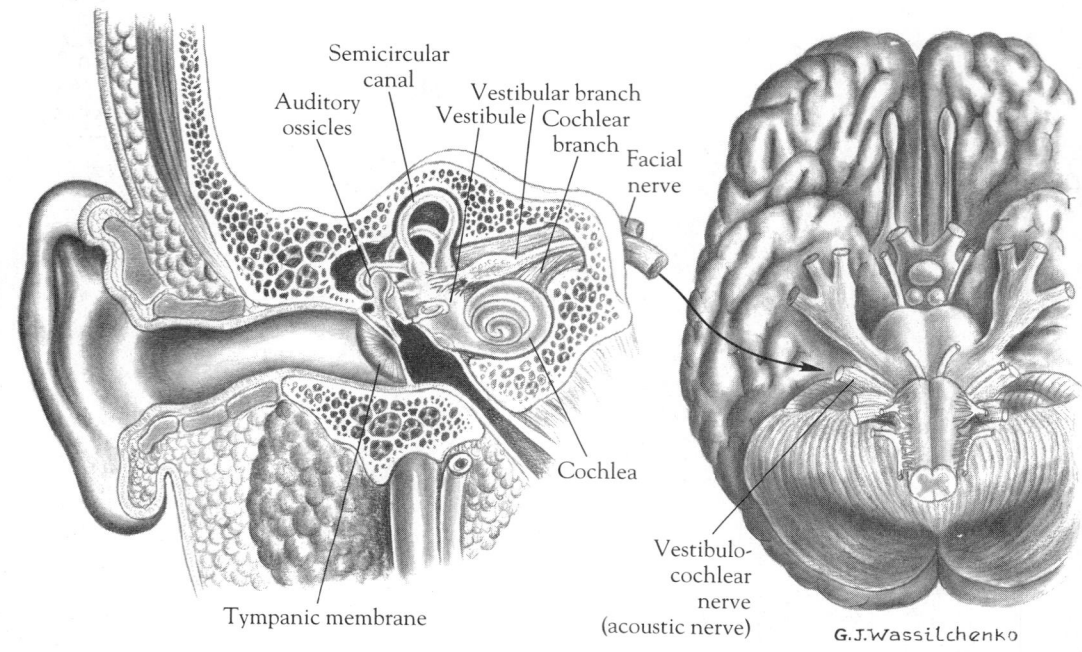

cartilaginous portion of the canal is thick and contains
fine hairs, large sebaceous glands, and ceruminous
glands. Cerumen, the combined secretion of the sebaceous and ceruminous glands, may accumulate to the
point of obstructing sound transmission. The epithelium
that lines the bony half of the external canal is very thin

and contains no hair or glands. In adults the external
canal is approximately 24 mm long and the bony portion
is slightly longer than the cartilaginous (Fig. 7-3).

Anterior to the ear canal is the temporomandibular
joint. Diseases of this joint can cause referred pain to
the ear.

Middle ear. The tympanic membrane separates the
external ear from the middle ear. The tympanic membrane is made up of two layers of epithelium—the outer
layer squamous and the inner cuboidal—and a middle
layer of fibrous collagen tissue. New cells of the tympanic
membrane are produced in the periphery and migrate
toward the center of the drum. The drum is slightly cone
shaped and slightly inclined; the concavity of the drumhead and its position relative to the ear canal vary and
may be greatly altered during disease.

The fibers of the tympanic membrane condense into a
ring called the anulus, which fits into the tympanic sulcus. The anulus is an incomplete ring that contains a
superior break between the anterior and posterior malleolar ligaments; this break is known as the notch of
Rivinus. The portion of the tympanic membrane closing
this area is the pars flaccida, so named because it does
not contain a fibrous collagen layer.

The tympanic membrane is described as a translucent
window through which the middle ear may be viewed.
The color is usually a pearl gray, although this may vary
slightly in normal membranes (Fig. 7-4).

Fig. 7-2
External ear.

From Whaley, L.F., and Wong, D.L.:
Nursing care of infants and children, ed. 2,
St. Louis, 1983, The C.V. Mosby Co.

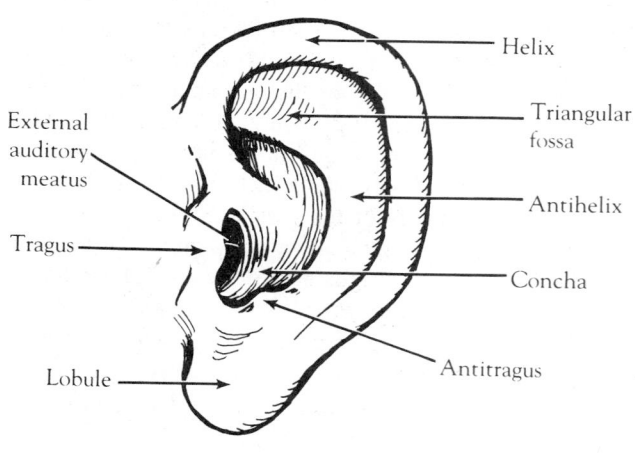

Fig. 7-3
External auditory canal. **A,**
Cartilaginous ear canal showing hair
follicles, sebaceous glands, and
ceruminous glands. **B,** Bony ear canal
with thin epithelial lining, containing
no hair or glands.

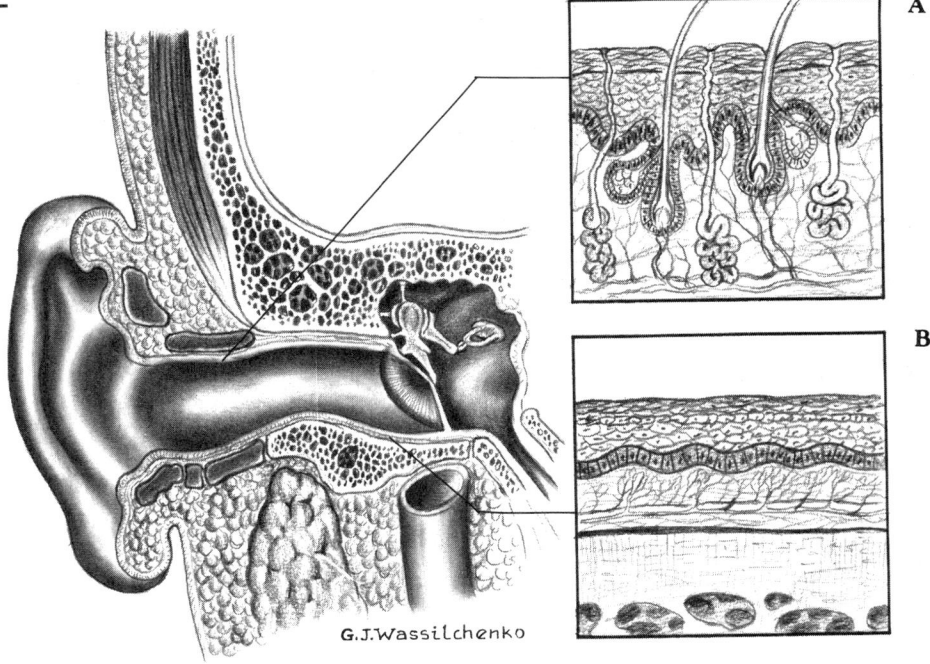

G.J.Wassilchenko

A

B

Fig. 7-4
Normal tympanic membrane.

From Whaley, L.F., and Wong, D.L.:
Nursing care of infants and children, ed. 2,
St. Louis, 1983, The C.V. Mosby Co.

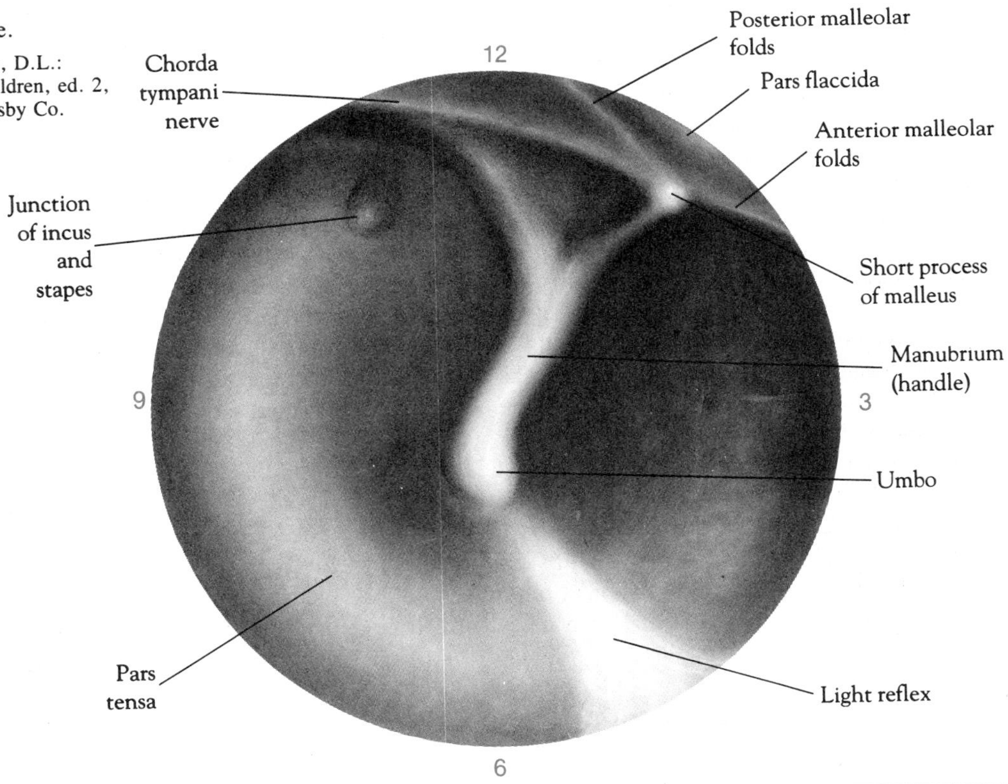

Chorda
tympani
nerve

Junction
of incus
and
stapes

Pars
tensa

12

9

6

3

Posterior malleolar
folds

Pars flaccida

Anterior malleolar
folds

Short process
of malleus

Manubrium
(handle)

Umbo

Light reflex

Fig. 7-5
Ossicles of right middle ear.

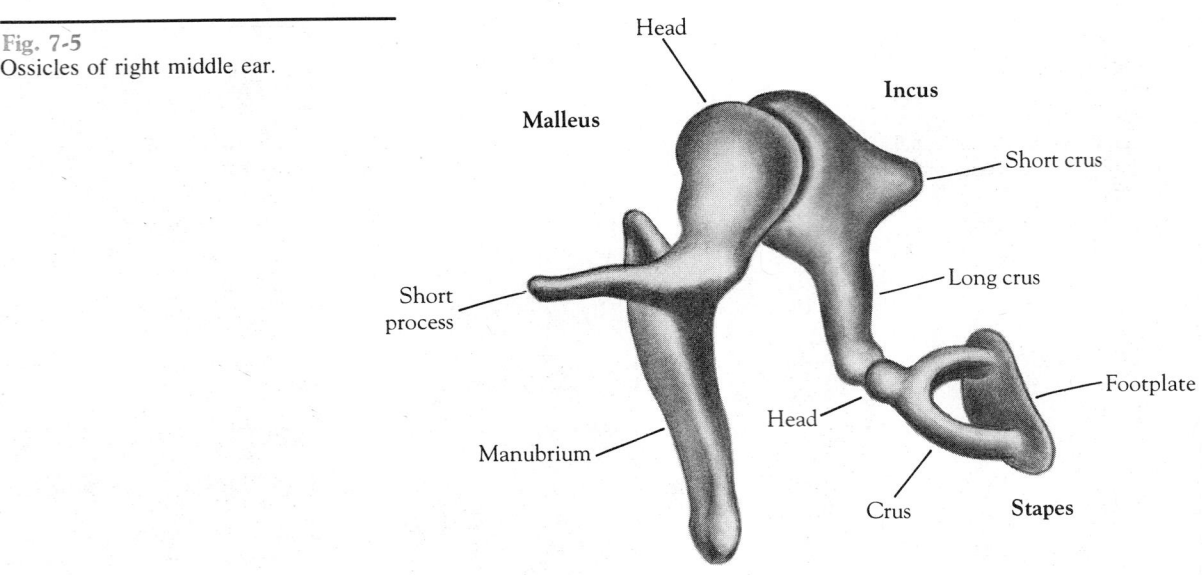

The middle ear, or tympanic cavity, is covered by the tightly stretched tympanic membrane. It is a small, roughly oblong, flattened space that is lined with non-ciliated, single-layered mucous membrane and contains bony walls. During an infection the membrane becomes ciliated and multilayered. This area holds air and three small bones, or ossicles: the malleus, the incus, and the stapes (Fig. 7-5).

The ossicles are three bones that connect the tympanic membrane with the oval window and represent the normal pathway of sound transmission across the middle ear space. The first bone is the malleus or hammer; it has a head, neck, handle, and short process. The manubrium (the handle) and the short process attach to the tympanic membrane, and the headlike portion is connected to the second bone, the incus or anvil, forming a true joint. The incus connects to the third bone, the stapes or stirrup. The footplate of the stapes fits into the oval or vestibular window, which is a small opening in the wall between the middle and inner ear.

The major function of the middle ear is to transfer sound waves from the outer ear to the fluid-filled inner ear. Since the fluid in the inner ear is more difficult to move than air, the pressure waves must be increased. The bony ossicles are joined so they amplify sound waves received by the tympanic membrane and transmit these waves to the inner ear by a lever action of their freely movable joints. The oval window's membrane vibrates and conducts sound waves to the fluid in the inner ear. In otosclerosis the joints of the ossicles are no longer freely movable, resulting in decreased sound transmission. Two small skeletal muscles attached to the ossicles affect the transmission of sound waves. The tensor tympani muscle pulls the malleus inward to tense the tympanic membrane, which attenuates high-pitched sounds. The stapedius muscle pulls the footplate of the stapes outward, possibly making low-frequency sounds more audible.

The middle ear communicates directly with the nasopharynx by means of the eustachian tube. This tube, which leads downward and medially to the nasopharynx, carries air into the middle ear to equalize pressure on both sides of the tympanic membrane. The mucosal lining of the middle ear is continuous with that of the nasopharynx via the eustachian tube. Normally the eustachian tube is passively closed; it opens by action of the tensor and levator muscles of the palate, usually, although not always, during swallowing. The eustachian tube offers a direct route for infection to reach the middle ear from the upper respiratory tract.

A third structure of the middle ear is the collection of mastoid air cells. These are air-filled spaces in a portion of the temporal bone in the skull. They communicate posteriorly with the middle ear. They are present at birth but are small and filled with diploic bone and loose osseous tissue between the two tables of cranial bones. Between the ages of 2 and 6 years the diploic bone is gradually replaced by air cells that bud off from the mastoid antrum, which is the first and largest air cell and connects directly to the middle ear.

Inner ear. The functions of the ear are hearing and equilibrium. The end organs supplying these two functions are housed in the inner ear. The inner ear, or labyrinth, is composed of two portions, one inside the other

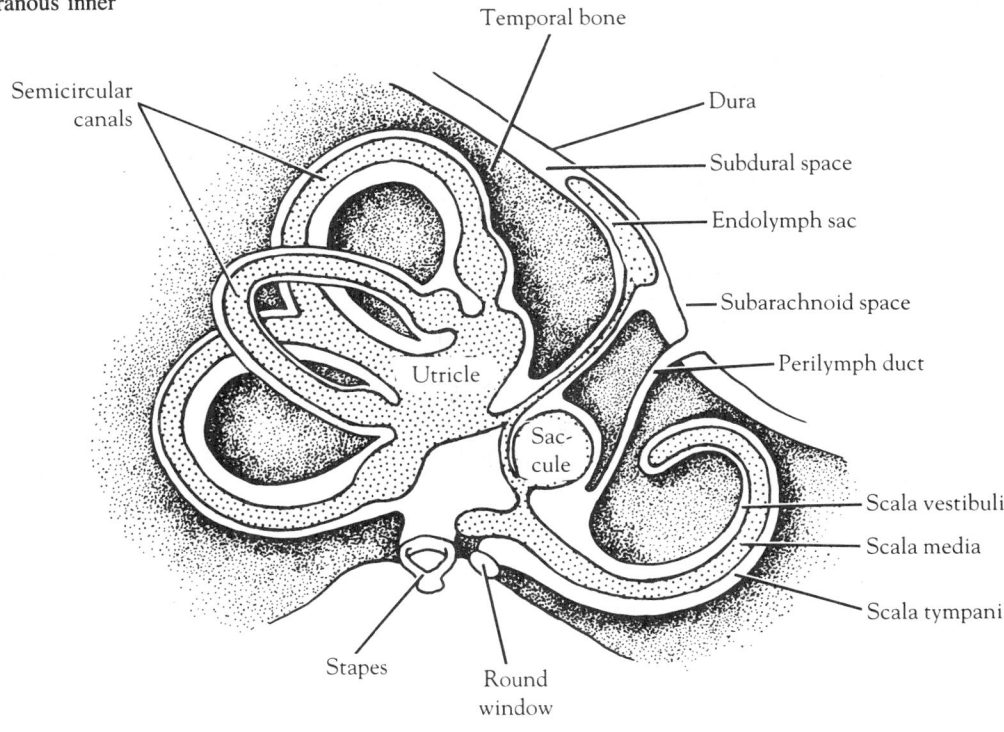

Fig. 7-6
Bony labyrinth and membranous inner labyrinth.

From Ganong, W.F.: Review of medical physiology, ed. 11, Los Altos, Calif., 1983, Lange Medical Publications.

Semicircular canals

Temporal bone

Dura

Subdural space

Endolymph sac

Subarachnoid space

Perilymph duct

Utricle

Sac-cule

Scala vestibuli

Scala media

Scala tympani

Stapes

Round window

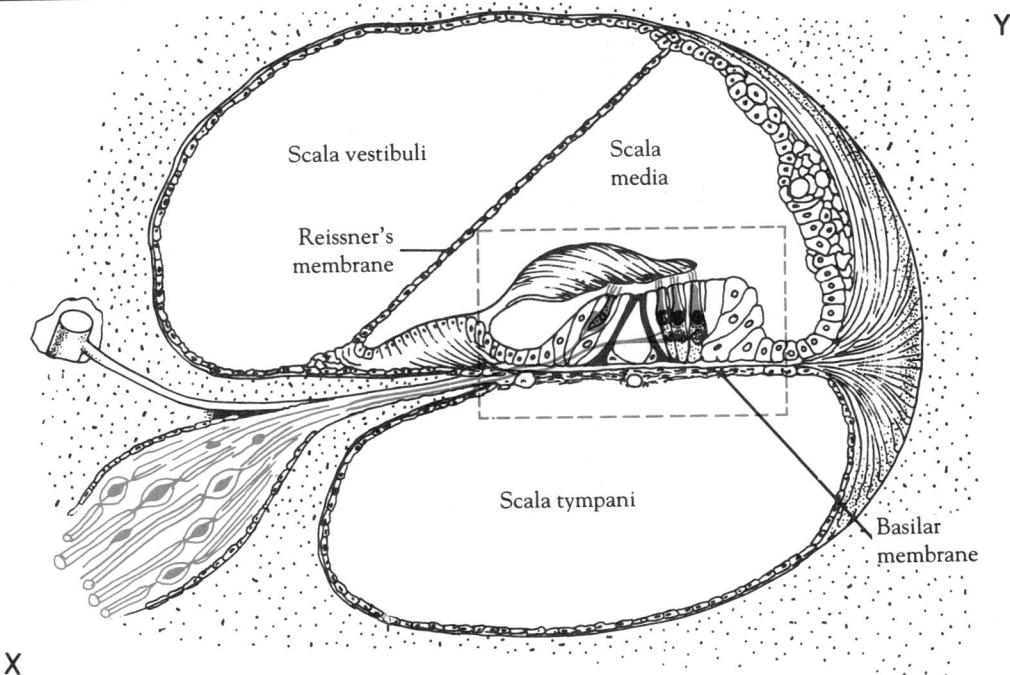

Fig. 7-7
Scalae of the cochlea, separated by Reissner's membrane and basilar membrane. *X* and *Y* indicate orientation vis-a-vis drawing on right in Fig. 7-9.

From Berne, R.M., and Levy, M.: Physiology, St. Louis, 1983, The C.V. Mosby Co.

Y

Scala vestibuli

Scala media

Reissner's membrane

Scala tympani

Basilar membrane

X

Fig. 7-8
Middle ear, showing relationship of ossicles and cochlea. Communication between scala vestibuli and scala tympani is shown. Arrows indicate displacement of liquid inside bony cochlea and round window from movement of stapedial footplate and displacement of oval window.

From Berne, R.M., and Levy, M.: Physiology, St. Louis, 1983, The C.V. Mosby Co.

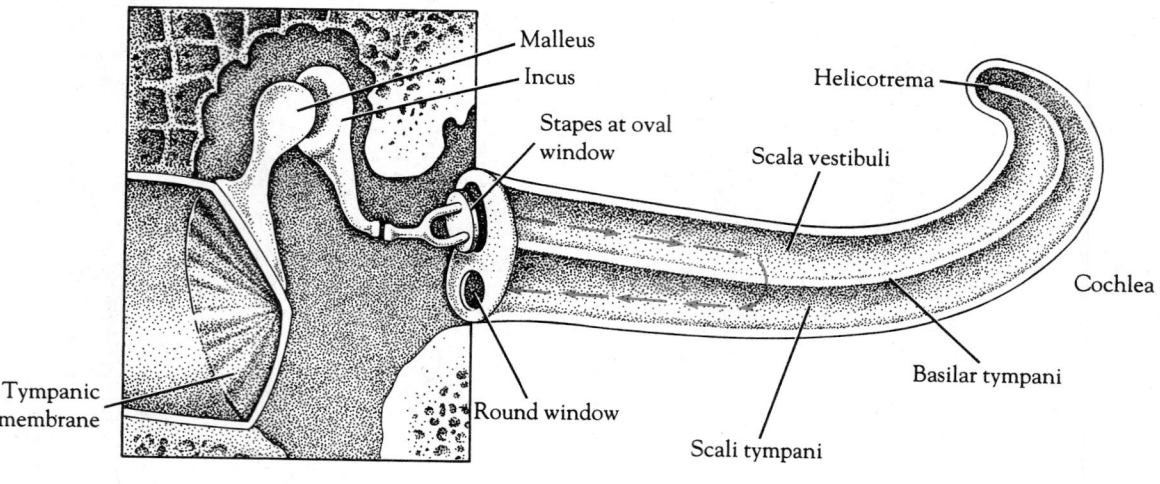

Fig. 7-9
Coiled structure of cochlea showing relationships of oval window, scala vestibuli, scala media, and scala tympani. Arrows indicate path of continuous flow from scala vestibuli through helicotrema to scala tympani.

From Berne, R.M., and Levy, M.: Physiology, St. Louis, 1983, The C.V. Mosby Co.

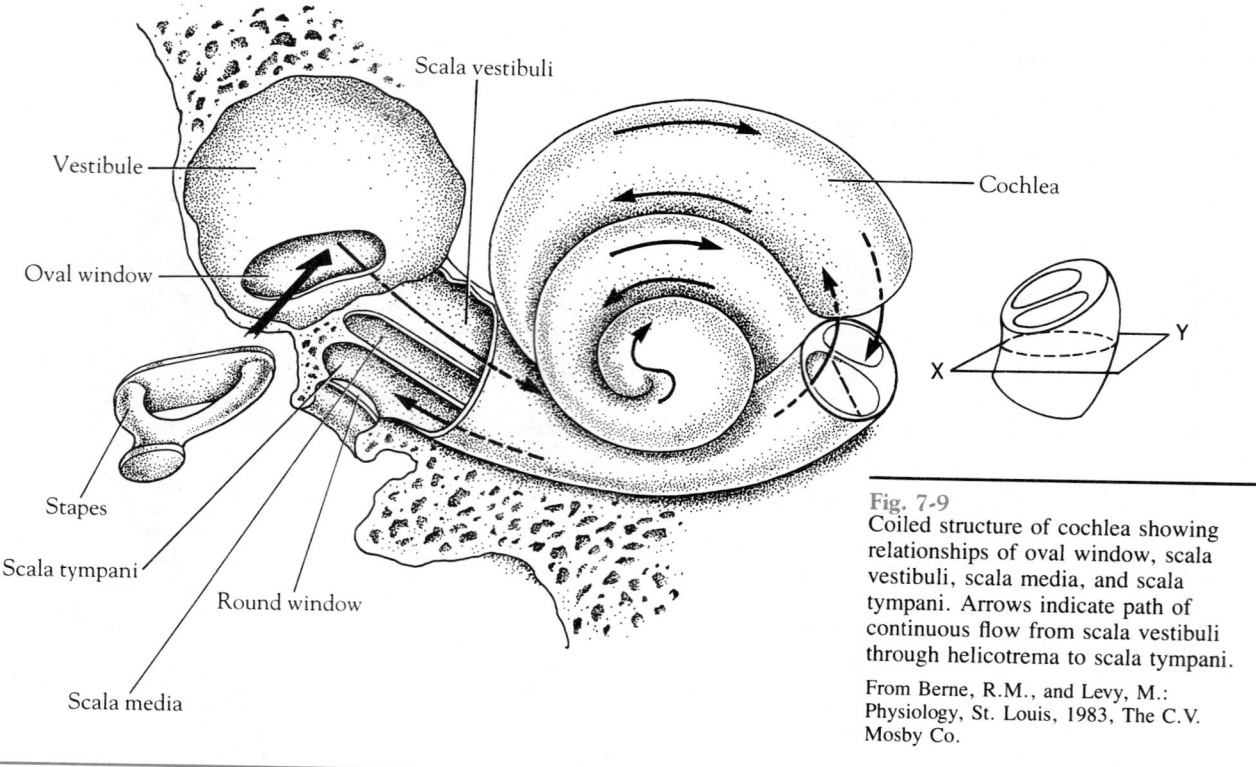

(Fig. 7-6). The bony labyrinth is a series of tubes or channels within the petrous portion of the temporal bone. Lining the bony labyrinth is the membranous labyrinth, which duplicates the shape of the bony channels. Inside the bony channels is fluid called perilymph, which surrounds the membranous labyrinth. The membranous labyrinth is filled with endolymph, and there is no communication between the fluid-filled spaces.[10]

Components of the inner ear include the cochlea for hearing, the semicircular canals for equilibrium, that is, rotational and angular acceleration, and the vestibule, which houses the utricle and saccule responsible for sensing changes in gravity and linear and angular acceleration. The vestibule is a space that opens onto the oval window and serves as the entrance into the inner ear. It communicates anteriorly with the cochlea and posteriorly with the semicircular canals and utricle.

Cochlea. The cochlea is a snail-shaped bony tube that contains the organ of Corti, which is the neural end organ for hearing. The cochlea is about 3.5 cm long with about 2¾ spiral turns. If the cochlea were internally uncoiled,

one would see that it could be divided into three independent tubes lying side by side. Throughout its length, the basilar and Reissner membranes separate it into three tubes or chambers called scalae (Fig. 7-7).[3]

The upper scala vestibuli and the lower scala tympani contain perilymph and communicate with each other through the helicotrema, a small opening at the apex of the cochlea. The scala vestibuli at the base of the cochlea ends at the oval window, where the footplate of the stapes is attached. The scala tympani ends at the base of the cochlea into or at the round window, which is an opening enclosed by a secondary tympanic membrane. The round window bulges outward to dissipate the pressure waves that are set up in the inner ear fluid during sound transmission. The scala media, or the middle cochlear chamber, contains endolymph and does not communicate with the other two scalae (Figs. 7-8 and 7-9).[3]

Located on the basilar membrane is the organ of Corti, which contains the receptors for hearing (Fig. 7-10). It extends from the base of the cochlea to the apex and therefore has a spiral shape. The receptors for hearing

Fig. 7-10
A, Organ of Corti on basilar membrane. **B,** Hair cells embedded in tectorial membrane.

From Berne, R.M., and Levy, M.: Physiology, St. Louis, 1983, The C.V. Mosby Co.

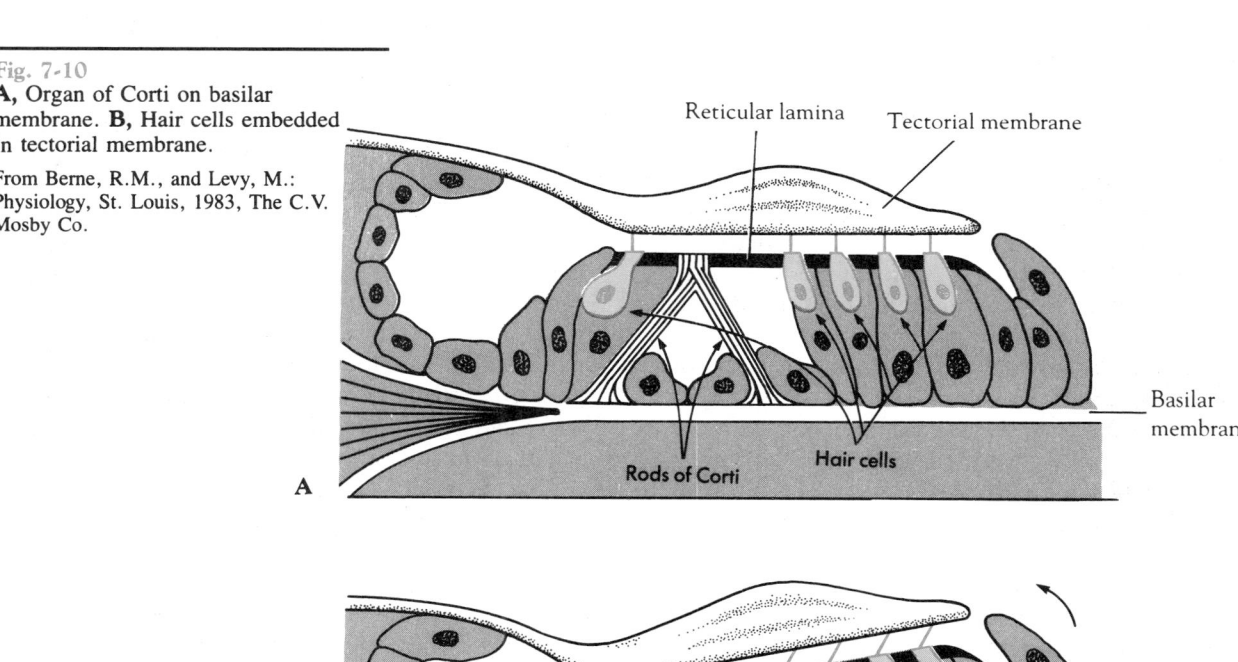

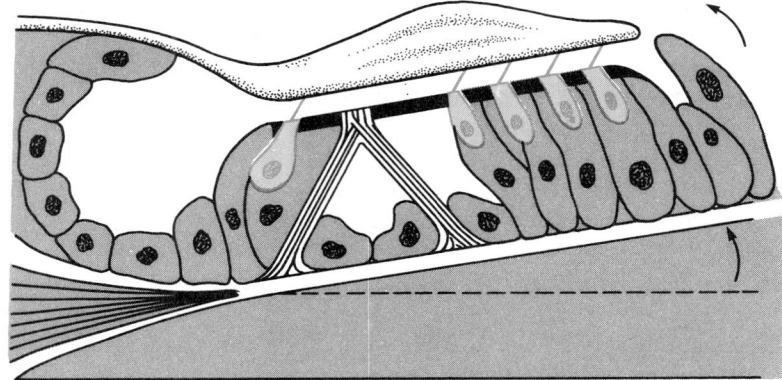

are hair cells arranged in two rows. There are 3500 inner and 20,000 outer hair cells, whose tips are embedded in the tectorial membrane (Fig. 7-10).[3] When these hair cells are bent or distorted by pressure waves, sound is converted (transduced) into an electromechanical impulse. This impulse is carried over the afferent neuron to the spiral ganglion in the bony core of the cochlea. The axons of these nerves form the auditory division of the eighth cranial nerve (vestibulocochlear nerve) and terminate in the dorsal and ventral cochlear nuclei of the medulla oblongata. From the cochlear nuclei, axons carry auditory information to the inferior canaliculi for reflexes associated with audition, such as turning the head to locate a sound. The fibers then pass to the medial geniculate body in the thalamus and to the primary auditory cortex, Brodmann areas 41 and 42, which are located in the superior portion of the temporal lobe.[31]

Semicircular canals. The semicircular canals are perpendicular to each other on each side of the head. Three canals are on each side: a superior, posterior, and horizontal canal; they are so oriented to sense changes in the three planes of space. Inside the bony canals are the membranous canals suspended in the perilymph. Near the end of each canal is an enlargement called the ampulla, which houses the crista ampullaris, or the vestibular receptors. The hair cells of the crista ampullaris are stimulated with rotation. The pattern of stimulation varies with the direction and plane of rotation. Nerve fiber tracts compose the vestibular portion of the vestibulocochlear nerve, or cranial nerve VIII, to the vestibular nuclei and terminate the four vestibular nuclei at the level of the pons and medulla in the brainstem. Tracts that descend from the vestibular nuclei into the spinal cord are responsible for head-righting reflexes and changes with muscle tone associated with rotation. Ascending fibers from the vestibular nuclei are concerned with eye movements, that is, nystagmus associated with rotation.

Utricle and saccule. Housed within the vestibule are the utricle and saccule, which are responsible for sensing changes in gravity and linear acceleration. Hair cells in the macula of the utricle and saccule are stimulated by head tilting and by jumping or falling, respectively. Both macular structures are sensitive to linear acceleration in the horizontal plane. Fibers from the utricle and saccule compose portions of the vestibular division of cranial nerve VIII, which is the vestibulocochlear nerve. The vestibular division is important for the control of posture and the maintenance of balance, while the cochlear division is responsible for hearing.

Hearing loss. Hearing loss can be partial or total and can occur in low, medium, or high frequencies or in combination. Hearing is measured in decibels (dB), which is a ratio that compares the relationship between two sound intensities.

The American Medical Association's formula for hearing loss is that hearing is impaired 1.5% for every decibel that the pure tone average exceeds 25 dB. A hearing loss of 40 dB in both ears, or a 22.5% hearing impairment, usually impairs a person's ability to function normally in social situations and requires the use of a hearing aid unless it can be medically or surgically treated. True deafness, however, is defined as 85 to 90 dB below normal. Hearing losses can occur in one or both ears, depending on the etiology, and may imply only a partial loss of function, depending on the severity. The following are six types of hearing losses.

Sensorineural hearing loss. Sensorineural hearing loss is the result of disease within the cochlea, the cochlear nerve, or the brain. It usually results from trauma; an infectious process; a degenerative process such as presbycusis, a senile degenerative change in the hair cells in the organ of Corti; a congenital abnormality; or exposure to ototoxic substances such as certain drugs. Intense noise may also cause destruction of cochlear hair cells, thereby causing a sensorineural hearing loss, as may injury to the organ of Corti. This may also be called perceptive or ''nerve-type'' hearing loss. Patients with sensorineural hearing losses are often unable to use hearing aids satisfactorily.

Conductive hearing loss. This is also called transmission hearing loss. It occurs in disorders of the external or middle ear such as otitis media, otosclerosis, or a perforated eardrum. These patients have a normal inner ear, but sound waves are prevented from reaching the inner ear normally. If sound is amplified, these patients may be able to hear very well and thus can usually benefit greatly from the use of a hearing aid. With the exception of otosclerosis in which the drumhead usually appears normal, disorders that cause conductive hearing loss also cause changes in the normal appearance of the drumhead, such as thickening or retraction.

Mixed hearing loss. Some patients have both conductive and sensorineural hearing losses.

Congenital hearing loss. This type of hearing loss is present from birth or early infancy. ''Neonatal'' causes may be from anoxia or trauma during delivery or from Rh incompatibility. Other causes may include maternal exposure to syphilis or rubella during pregnancy or the use of ototoxic drugs during pregnancy. Infants with serum bilirubin levels above 20 mg/dl may also incur hearing losses from the toxic effect of high bilirubin levels on the brain.

Simulated hearing loss. This is also called functional, psychogenic, or nonorganic hearing loss. It means that an apparent hearing loss is not the result of an organic cause and may represent malingering or a functional disorder.

Central hearing loss. This is caused by damage to the brain's auditory pathways, such as occurs in a cerebrovascular accident.

Nose

The nose is an external organ comprised of two nares or nostrils through which air enters and passes posteriorly to the nasopharynx; it is separated in the middle by the septum, which is composed of both cartilage and bone (Fig. 7-11). The septum is usually straight at birth but becomes deformed or deviated from the midline in almost every adult; it can appear dislocated into one nasal vestibule. The nasal cavity is an irregularly shaped space extending from the bony palate that separates the nose and mouth cavities upward to the frontal ethmoid and sphenoid bones of the cranial cavity. The walls of the nasal cavity are bone covered with mucous membrane.

The vestibule of the nostril is lined with skin containing vibrissae, or nasal hairs, and some sebaceous and sweat glands. The nose is lined with respiratory mucosa except for the skin in the vestibule and the olfactory epithelium. Mucus secreted by the mucosa is carried back to the nasopharynx by the cilia of the mucosa. The nasal mucosa is extremely vascular, which makes it appear redder than the oral mucosa.

The lateral wall of the nose has four nasal turbinates or conchae: the inferior, middle, superior, and supreme (Fig. 7-12). The supreme turbinate is quite small and cannot be seen during examination. The inferior turbinate is a separate bone, but the other three are part of the ethmoid bone. The turbinates greatly increase the surface area of the mucous membrane over which air travels as it passes through the nasal passages and into the nasopharynx. The nasolacrimal duct communicates indirectly with the lacrimal gland and opens onto the lateral surface of the inferior meatus of the nose. Tears drain continuously into the nose. If any part of the system becomes blocked or if tears are formed at an unusual rate, the fluid runs out onto the face.

The blood supply to the nose is from the external and internal carotid arteries. The external carotid artery supplies blood primarily through one of its terminal divisions, the internal maxillary artery. This artery and its terminal branch, the sphenopalatine artery, supply blood to most of the posterior nasal septum and the lateral wall of the nose. The second largest vessel that supplies blood to the internal nose is the anterior ethmoidal artery, which derives its blood from the internal carotid system. The ethmoidal artery supplies blood to the anterosuperior part of the septum and the lateral wall of the nose. The external nose receives blood mostly from the same arteries as the internal nose; however, venous drainage differs in that part of it is through the angular vein, which leads

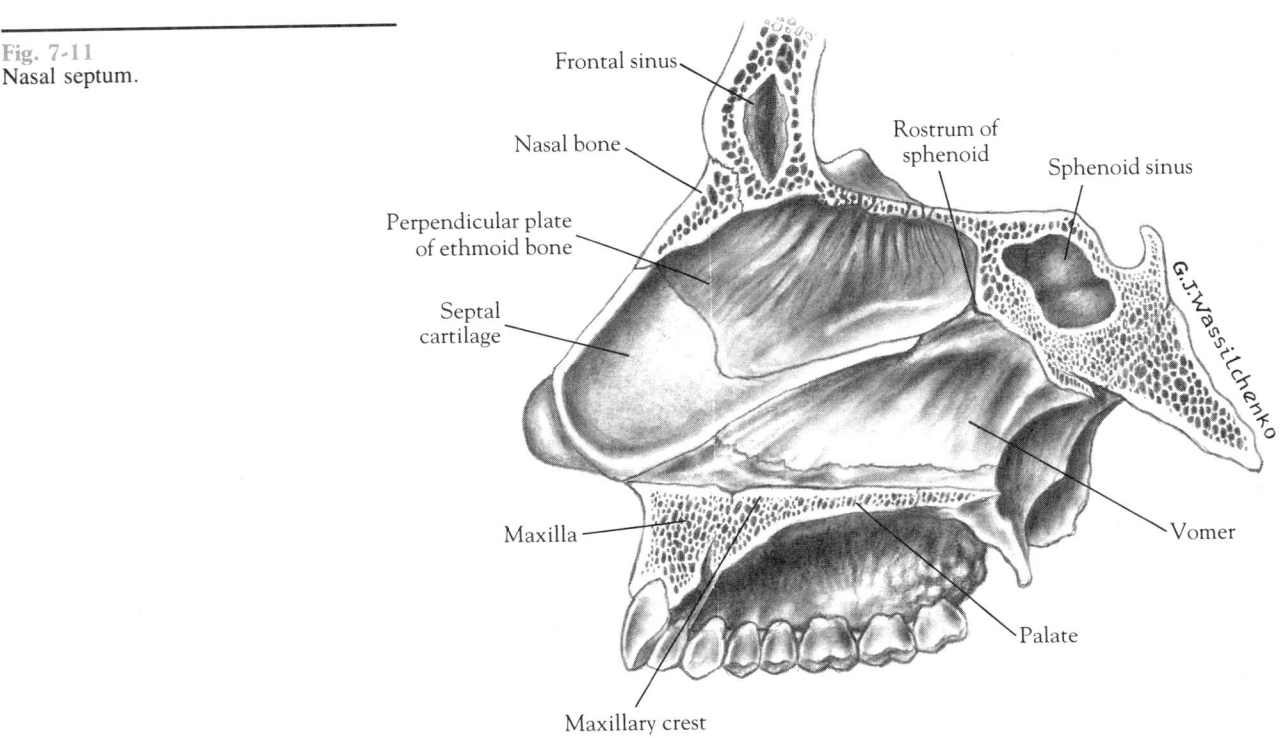

Fig. 7-11
Nasal septum.

Fig. 7-12
Lateral wall of nose.

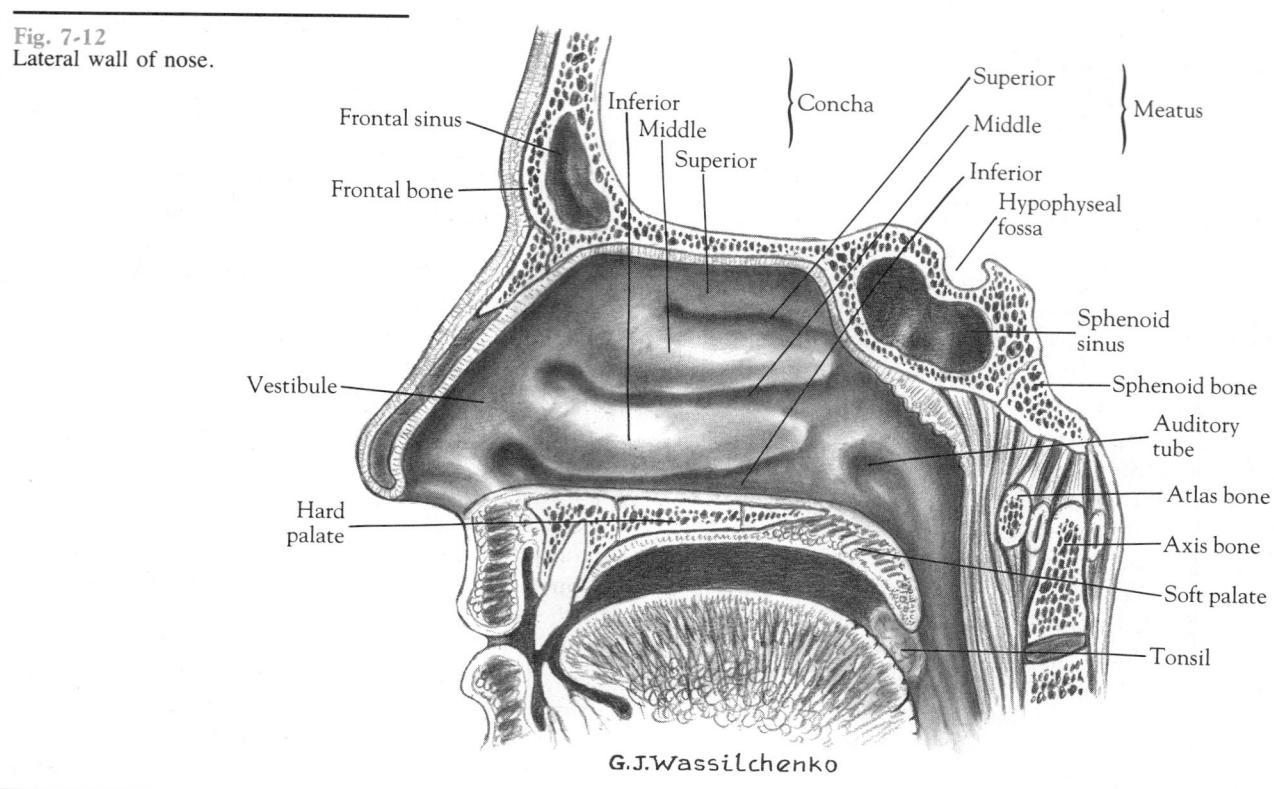

G.J.Wassilchenko

into the inferior ophthalmic vein and the cavernous sinus. Most venous drainage is through the anterior facial vein.

The muscles of the external nose receive their nerve supply from the seventh cranial nerve, and the external skin is innervated by the first and second divisions of the fifth cranial nerve. The nerve supply to the internal nose is provided by the olfactory nerve and also from the first and second divisions of the fifth cranial nerve.

The sinuses, which serve to lighten the weight of the skull and give resonance and timbre to the voice, are mucous membrane–lined cavities in the facial bones surrounding the nasal cavities. They drain into the nasal cavities through openings in grooves between the turbinates. The sinuses are in the frontal, sphenoid, ethmoid, and maxillary bones. The maxillary sinuses (or antrum of Highmore) are the largest and most accessible if treatment is required. They are within the maxillary bones on either side of the nose. The frontal sinuses are between and above the eyes, the ethmoid sinuses are between the eyes and nose, and the sphenoid sinuses lie at the rear of the nasal cavity. The sphenoid sinuses, which are the most deeply placed of the sinuses, are directly below the sella turcica, from which pituitary tumors can erode downward to fill them. Only the maxillary and ethmoid sinuses are present at birth; the frontal sinuses begin to pneumatize the frontal bone during the

second year of life, and the sphenoid sinuses form during the third year.

Functions of the nose. The major functions of the nose are air conditioning and olfaction; the former refers to temperature and humidity control, as well as to filtration of particulate matter and bacteria in inspired air before it reaches the trachea, bronchi, and lungs. Inspired air reaches the nasopharynx in about ¼ second; during this short period, the temperature of the air reaches 97° to 98° F and the humidity becomes a constant 75% to 80%.

Serum and mucus cover the surface of the nasal mucosa and can provide large amounts of water to be absorbed by cold, dry air. As much as 1 L of moisture can evaporate from the nose during 24 hours of normal breathing; the submucosal glands replenish this moisture as the water evaporates. The turbinates are covered with erectile tissue that is capable of becoming rapidly filled with blood, which allows greater control of temperature and humidification. The nose, sinuses, pharynx, trachea, bronchi, and bronchioles are covered by a continuous mucous blanket to which airborne particles cling on contact. The blanket contains lysozyme, an enzyme that causes most bacteria to disintegrate on contact. Cilia carry the mucous blanket with its trapped particulate matter back toward the pharynx where it is swallowed. Residual bacteria are then destroyed by hydrochloric acid and gastric juices.

The olfactory sense organs are located in the olfactory membrane that covers the roof of the nose and is reflected medially downward over the superior turbinate. The olfactory receptors are hair cells or chemoreceptors that are stimulated by molecules dissolved in the fluids of the nasal mucosa when air is inspired through the nose.

Pharynx

The pharynx, which is the Greek word for throat, is the muscular tube behind the oral cavity that extends downward from the base of the skull to the larynx. The pharynx is a somewhat conical chamber that serves as the common passageway for the respiratory and digestive systems. It conducts air between the nasal cavities, eustachian tubes, and larynx and food from the mouth to the esophagus.

The pharynx is divided into three sections: the nasopharynx, oropharynx, and laryngopharynx. The nasopharynx is above the margin of the soft palate posterior to the nose; the oropharynx is the area that is visible when the tongue is depressed with a tongue blade behind the mouth; and the laryngopharynx is dorsal to the larynx. The structures of the pharynx include the uvula, epiglottis, tonsils, and anterior and posterior tonsillar pillars (Fig. 7-13). The nasopharynx lies behind the nasal cavities and communicates with them through the posterior nasal apertures. The nasopharynx also communicates with the middle ear through the eustachian tube about 1 cm behind the posterior end of the inferior turbinate. Near these openings are patches of lymphoid tissue called the pharyngeal tonsils, which lie in the mucous membrane at the junction of the posterior wall and roof. (Hypertrophied pharyngeal tonsils are adenoids.) The nasopharyngeal space opens inferiorly into the oropharynx so the floor is formed by the dorsal aspect of the soft palate, which is its only movable boundary. At birth the mucosal lining of the nasopharyngeal cavity is columnar ciliated epithelium, but this changes to patchy squamous epithelium between the ages of 10 and 80 years. Squamous epithelium covers about 80% of the posterior wall, and surface mucosa is stratified squamous after about the

Fig. 7-13
Structures of pharynx. **A,** Uvula, epiglottis, and tonsils. **B,** Hypopharynx (posterior view).

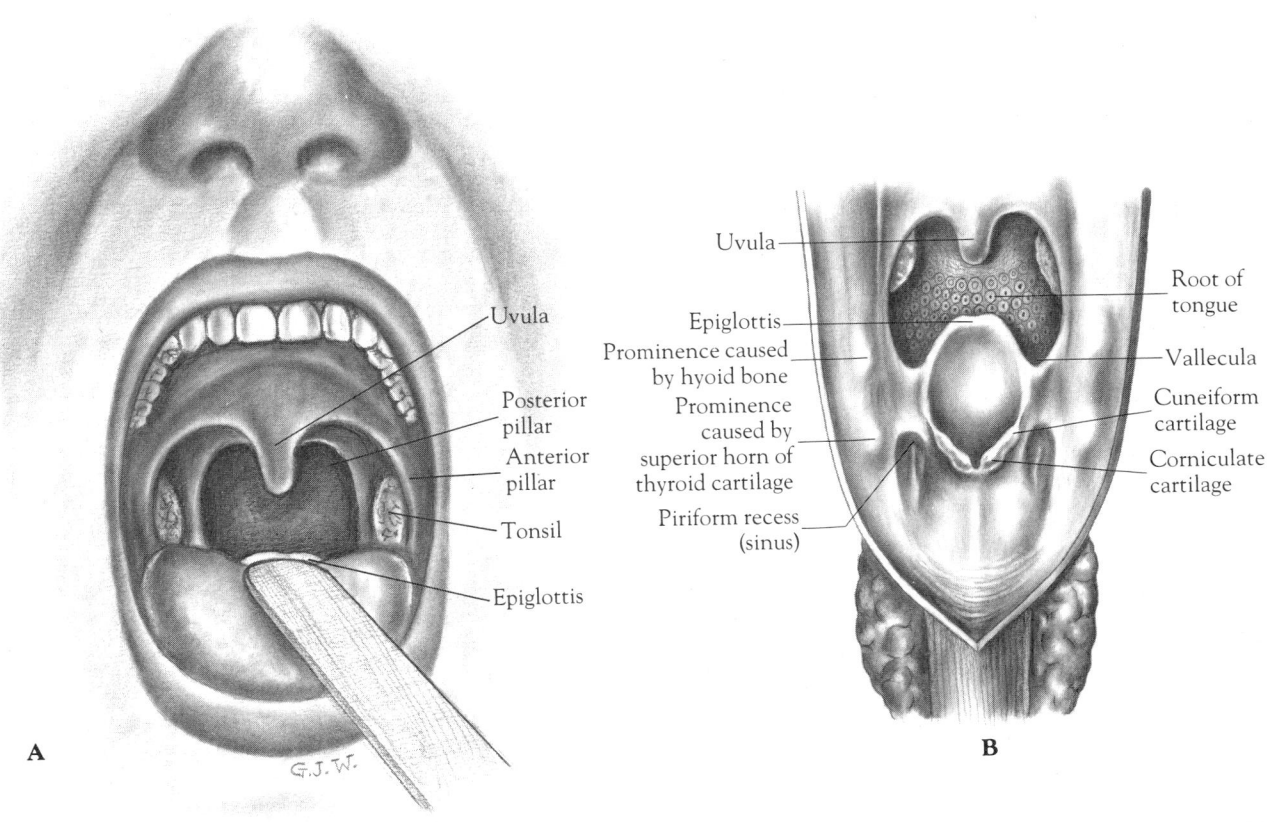

A

Uvula
Posterior pillar
Anterior pillar
Tonsil
Epiglottis

G.J.W.

B

Uvula
Epiglottis
Prominence caused by hyoid bone
Prominence caused by superior horn of thyroid cartilage
Piriform recess (sinus)
Root of tongue
Vallecula
Cuneiform cartilage
Corniculate cartilage

Table 7-1
Tonsils

Structure	Description
Pharyngeal tonsil or adenoid	Mass of lymphoid tissue in nasopharynx; extends from its roof almost to free end of soft palate; present in all infants and children; starts to regress just before puberty; normally absent in adults
Lateral pharyngeal bands	Extend down lateral wall of pharynx from adenoids; located behind posterior tonsillar pillar; gradually become thinner until they disappear below level of faucial tonsil
Faucial (palatine) tonsil	Located laterally at junction of oropharynx and oral cavity; composed of large lymphoid follicles; contains numerous crypts lined with squamous epithelium; supplied by tonsillar and palatine arteries, which come from external carotid artery
Lingual tonsils	Two masses of lymphoid tissue located on dorsum of tongue; extend from circumvallate papillae of tongue to epiglottis

age of 10 years. Glands secreting mucus and serous fluid are scattered throughout the mucous membrane.

The oropharynx communicates with the nasopharynx above and the laryngopharynx below to the level of the epiglottis. The oropharynx contains the palatine tonsils, which with the pharyngeal and lingual tonsils (on the dorsum of the tongue) comprise Waldeyer's ring, a protective barrier of lymphoid tissue between the mouth and throat and the respiratory and digestive tracts. This lymphoid tissue is considered important in the development of immune bodies, which, if stimulated by bacterial infection, promote the production of additional immune factors that provide future protection from bacterial infection.[7]

The laryngopharynx boundaries are the superior constrictor muscle and vertebrae posteriorly, the larynx and piriform fossa below, and the hyoid bone, base of the tongue, and constrictor muscle above. The upper end of the epiglottis projects into the laryngopharynx.

The oropharynx and laryngopharynx are spaces surrounded by muscles that provide support to the surrounding tissue and a passageway through which air, food, and fluids can be ingested. Swallowing is accomplished by the action of the constrictor muscles in the pharynx, as well as by the suprahyoid and infrahyoid muscles. Action of these muscles and their nerves is also responsible for the gag reflex, which protects the air and food passages from the entrance of any unwanted material. Two cranial nerves are responsible for the gag reflex: the glossopharyngeal nerve (cranial nerve IX) and the vagus nerve (cranial nerve X). The glossopharyngeal nerve has sensory and motor divisions. The sensory division supplies sensation to the pharynx, and the motor division innervates the posterior wall of the pharynx. The vagus nerve innervates all of the thoracic and abdominal viscera

A

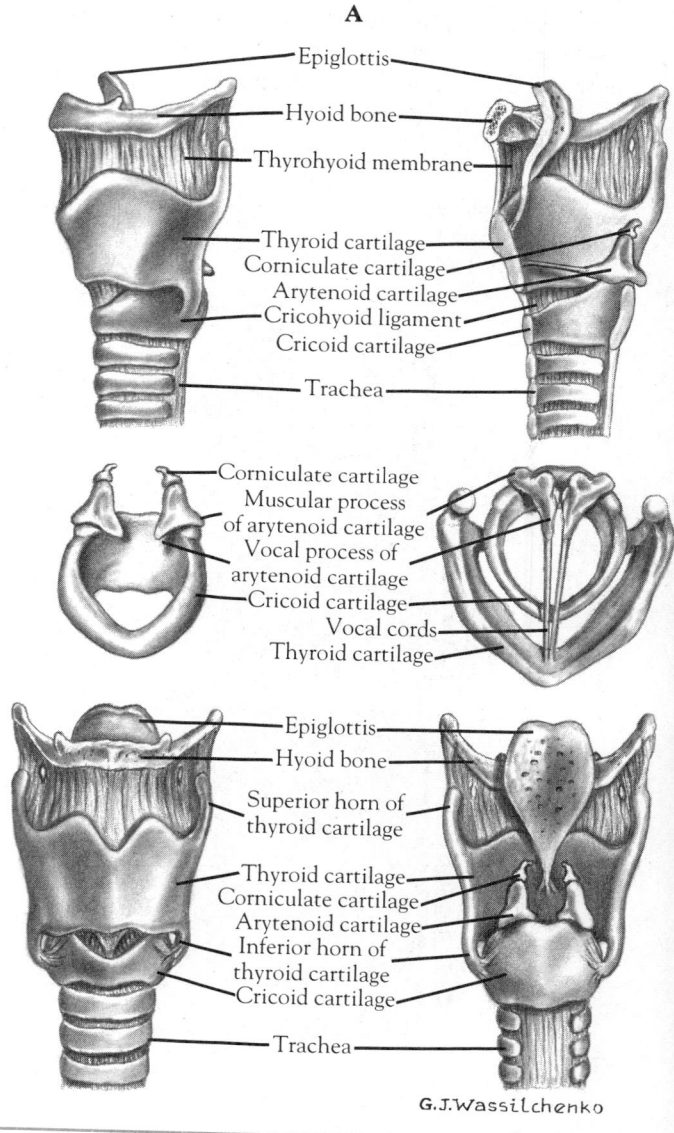

Epiglottis
Hyoid bone
Thyrohyoid membrane
Thyroid cartilage
Corniculate cartilage
Arytenoid cartilage
Cricohyoid ligament
Cricoid cartilage
Trachea

Corniculate cartilage
Muscular process of arytenoid cartilage
Vocal process of arytenoid cartilage
Cricoid cartilage
Vocal cords
Thyroid cartilage

Epiglottis
Hyoid bone
Superior horn of thyroid cartilage
Thyroid cartilage
Corniculate cartilage
Arytenoid cartilage
Inferior horn of thyroid cartilage
Cricoid cartilage
Trachea

G.J.Wassilchenko

and conveys impulses from the walls of the intestines, the heart, and the lungs.[31]

Tonsils. The tonsils, which are small masses of primarily lymphoid tissue, are covered by mucous membrane and contain small openings that deliver phagocytes to the mouth and pharynx.

In the past, removal of the tonsils and adenoids was commonplace, but it is now known that the lymphoid tissue of the pharynx plays an important role in the immune system of the body, and they are not removed as frequently (Table 7-1).

The lymphatic tissues of Waldeyer's ring drain into the lymph nodes of the neck. The adenoids in the nasopharynx drain into the posterior cervical lymph glands, and the palatine and lingual tonsils drain into the anterior cervical lymph nodes.

Larynx

The larynx has several functions: (1) it is the air passageway between the pharynx and the lungs; (2) it prevents food and fluid from entering the lungs; and (3) it is involved in sound production or phonation.

The larynx is a roughly tubular structure with an irregular shape. It is somewhat wider at the top where it is attached to the pharynx and narrower below where it attaches to the trachea. The larynx is composed of cartilages, ligaments, and muscles that keep its walls from collapsing on inspiration (Fig. 7-14). Three of the cartilages are paired and three are unpaired, for a total of nine cartilages (Table 7-2).

Cartilages and muscles of the larynx. The larynx is protected on its front and sides by thyroid cartilage (thyroid means shieldlike) and from behind by vertebrae,

Fig. 7-14
Larynx. **A,** Cartilages and ligaments.
B, Neck muscles.

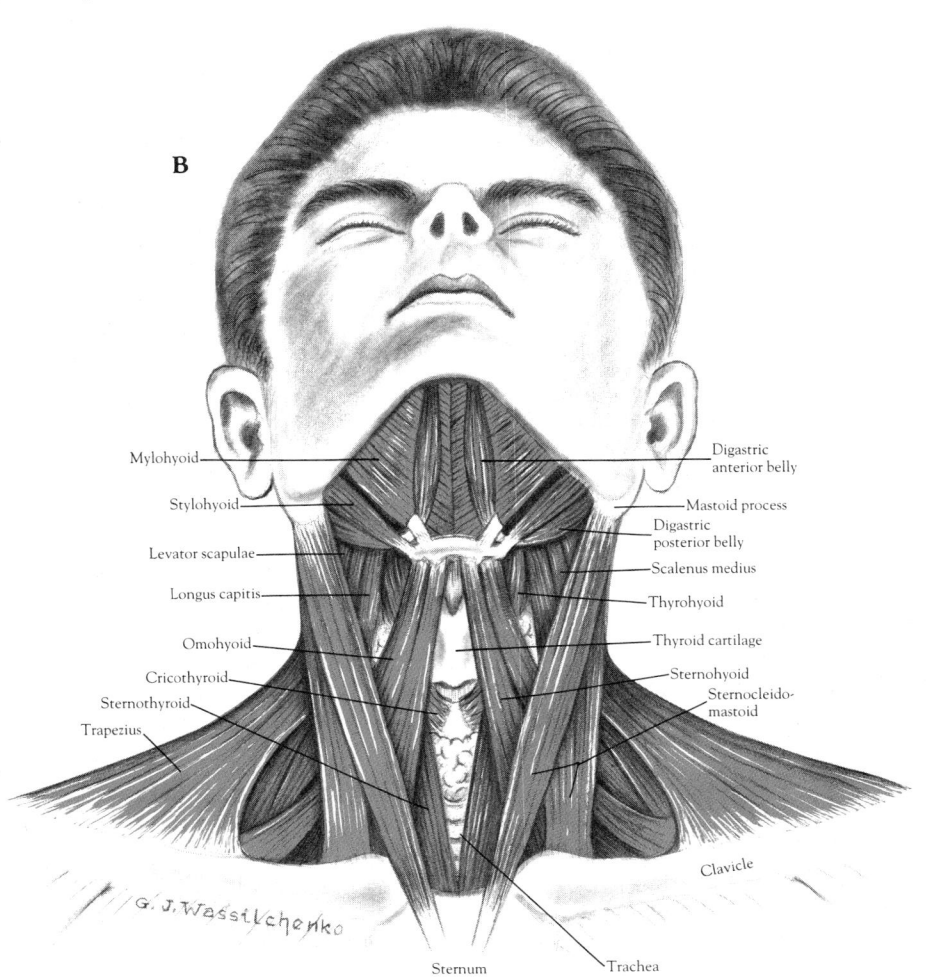

B

Mylohyoid
Stylohyoid
Levator scapulae
Longus capitis
Omohyoid
Cricothyroid
Sternothyroid
Trapezius

Digastric anterior belly
Mastoid process
Digastric posterior belly
Scalenus medius
Thyrohyoid
Thyroid cartilage
Sternohyoid
Sternocleidomastoid

Clavicle

G. J. Wassilchenko

Sternum   Trachea

Table 7-2

Cartilages and Muscles of the Larynx

Structure	Description
Unpaired Cartilages	
Thyroid	Largest cartilage of larynx; forms anterior midline shield called laryngeal prominence or Adam's apple
Cricoid	Only complete cartilaginous ring in respiratory tract; located just below thyroid cartilage
Epiglottis	Leaf shaped; projects upward at base of tongue and guards opening of larynx
Paired Cartilages	
Arytenoid, corniculate, and cuneiform	Serve as attachment for vocal ligaments; movement of cartilages controls tension of vocal ligaments
Intrinsic Muscles	
Thyroarytenoideus	Tilts arytenoid cartilages toward thyroid; results in shortening and relaxation of vocal cords
Arytenoideus	Approximates arytenoid cartilages and closes glottis
Cricothyroideus	Lifts anterior section of cricoid cartilage; results in increased tension on vocal cords
Posterior	
Cricoarytenoideus	Produces lateral rotation of arytenoid cartilages; results in separation of vocal cords and opening of glottis
Lateral	
Cricoarytenoideus	Produces medial rotation of arytenoid cartilages; results in approximation of vocal cords and closing of glottis

since the thyroid cartilage is incomplete posteriorly. The thyroid cartilage is the largest cartilage of the larynx. Its midline prominence forms the hard bump in the front of the neck called the laryngeal prominence, or "Adam's apple." This prominence is hardly visible in children or women but is noticeable in men.

Just below the thyroid cartilage lies the cricoid cartilage, which can be palpated in normal necks and can usually be seen in people with thin necks. The cricoid (ring-shaped) cartilage is the only complete ring of cartilage in the respiratory tract. It structurally resembles a signet ring, with the signet portion located posteriorly. The cricoid cartilage articulates with the thyroid and ar-

ytenoid cartilages. The cricoid and thyroid cartilages are attached by the cricothyroid membrane.

The arytenoid, corniculate, and cuneiform cartilages are the paired cartilages of the larynx and serve as attachments for the vocal ligaments. The arytenoid cartilages swing in and out as though rotating around a fixed central point. This action opens or closes the space between the vocal cords, since the posterior end of each vocal cord is attached to an arytenoid cartilage and thus must move with it.

The epiglottis is a leaf-shaped cartilaginous structure that is attached to the thyroid cartilage by ligaments and projects upward and posterior to the base of the tongue to guard the opening of the larynx.

The larynx contains extrinsic and intrinsic striated muscles. The extrinsic muscles connect the larynx to adjacent structures of the neck (the hyoid and sternum) and assist in swallowing. The five intrinsic muscles (Table 7-2) connect the laryngeal cartilages and alter the shape of the laryngeal cavity by contracting. The intrinsic muscles act as constrictors, dilators, and tensors and hence have an important role in sound production or phonation. A branch of the vagus nerve, the recurrent laryngeal nerve, supplies the intrinsic muscles except for the cricothyroid muscle, which is supplied by the superior laryngeal nerve. This innervation becomes particularly significant during endotracheal intubation; mechanical manipulation of the vocal cords and musculature may result in bradycardia from vagal stimulation.

Internal structures of the larynx. The internal structures lie behind the protective shield of the thyroid cartilage in front and include the vestibule, the false vocal cords, the true vocal cords, the laryngeal ventricle, and the glottis.

The inlet to the larynx lies in the anterior wall of the pharynx and is bounded by the epiglottis and arytenoid cartilages. From the inlet the larynx expands into a wide vestibule that ends below at the level of the true vocal folds.

Inside the larynx are two pairs of shelflike folds that project inward from the lateral walls of the larynx. The superior folds, or false vocal cords, are attached to the cartilage anteriorly and the arytenoid cartilage posteriorly, making them immobile or stationary. Immediately beneath the false vocal cords are the true vocal cords. The true vocal cords are joined anteriorly where they attach to the inner surface of the thyroid cartilage. This is a fixed point at which the cords are held immobile, but they attach posteriorly to the movable arytenoid cartilages, which allow them to adduct and abduct.

The laryngeal ventricle, a fold of mucous membrane between the true and false cords, extends up under the thyroid cartilage. Glands in the upper portion of the ventricle secrete mucus that lubricates the vocal cords.

The narrowest portion of the larynx is the glottis; this is the space between the vocal cords. Somewhat larger in men than in women, the glottis is very small in infants, thereby causing much greater danger when the airway becomes edematous as with laryngitis.

Additional structures of the larynx. The larynx is lined with mucous membrane that is continuous with the pharynx above and the trachea below. The mucosa folds over the false cords beneath the epiglottis, invaginates into the laryngeal ventricle, and comes out again to cover the true vocal cords before descending into the trachea.

Most of the blood supply to the larynx is provided by the superior and inferior thyroid arteries through their branches, the superior and inferior laryngeal arteries.

Lymphatic drainage is provided by lymph nodes in the middle and upper cervical chains along the internal jugular vein. All parts of the extrinsic larynx and the arytenoid area contain a somewhat rich lymphatic network, while the true vocal cords have a sparse supply. Most carcinomas of the larynx develop in the true vocal cords.

Functions of the larynx. The most important function of the larynx is to form an airway between the pharynx and the trachea. The larynx is not merely a tube, as is the trachea, but rather an organ with sphincter functions that help prevent aspiration and assist in coughing. During swallowing the aryepiglottic folds, the arytenoids, and the tubercle of the epiglottis fold inward, close the larynx, and prevent food from entering the trachea. Other actions close the glottis when a foreign body enters the throat and assist in expelling it by increasing intrathoracic pressure when coughing. The cough reflex is an important protective mechanism. This reflex is set off whenever the highly sensitive laryngeal mucosa is touched by a foreign body.

Phonation, or the formation of speech sounds, is also an important function of the larynx, although not its chief purpose, even though the larynx is sometimes called the "voice box." During phonation, tracheal air pressure increases and decreases; as the edges of the cords firm and relax, the larynx moves up and down so the air columns above and below are lengthened and shortened. The larynx creates sounds (humming or buzzing) as a result of vocal cord vibrations, but words are formed when the vibrating column of air comes up from the larynx to the tongue, lips, palate, and teeth (Fig. 7-15). Movements of the oral structure (articulation) actually form the words.

Fig. 7-15

Larynx. **A,** In quiet respiration. **B,** In phonation.

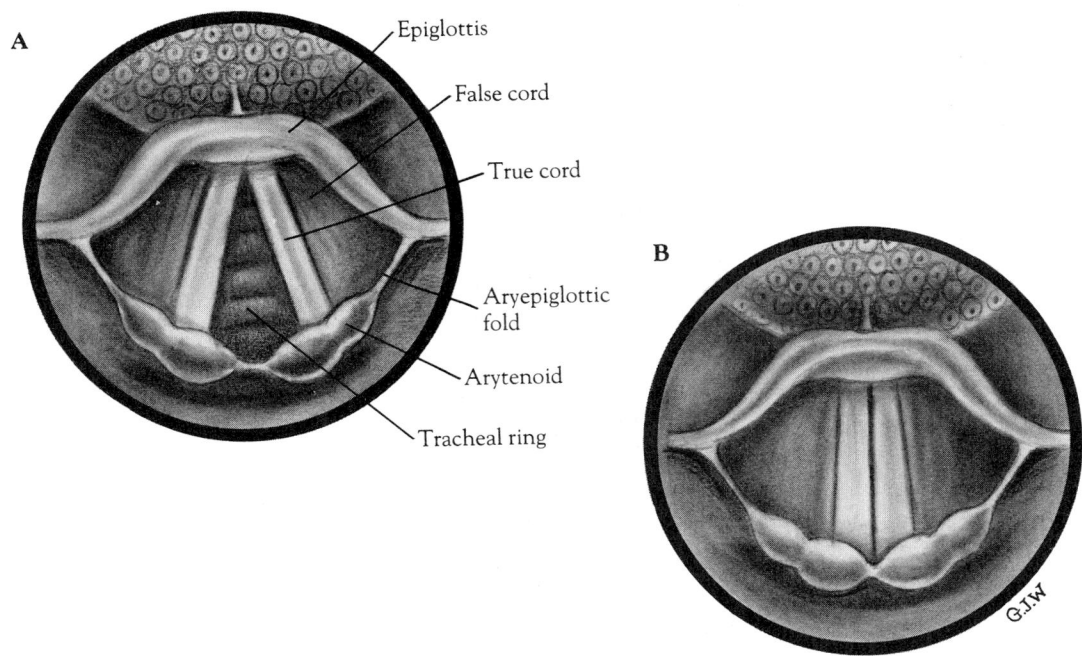

NORMAL FINDINGS

Area of Concern	Normal Adult Findings	Variations in Child	Variations in Older Adult
Ear			
External ear	Height and size equal; skin clean; no evidence of injury or trauma		Earlobes may appear pendulous
Auricle	Moves freely without causing pain		
Tympanic membrane	Drumhead slightly conical, quite shiny, and pearl gray in color; oblique position when viewed with otoscope; cerumen color varying from black to brown to creamy pink; cerumen waxy or flaky; depending on translucency, should be possible to visualize following in normal drumhead: malleus, anterior and posterior malleolar folds, anulus (whiter and denser than rest of drumhead), long process of incus (frequently seen posterior to manubrium of malleus), occasionally chorda tympani nerve seen crossing transversely behind drumhead at about level of short process of malleus		Some landmarks may appear more pronounced because of atrophied or sclerotic tympanic changes
Eustachian tube	Eardrum moves with Valsalva maneuver if tube is patent		
Vestibulocochlear nerve (cranial nerve VIII)	Patient able to hear whisper from distance of 2 feet; tuning fork placed in middle of head heard equally well in both ears	May not be tested	Presbycusis (hearing loss from senile degenerative changes) may be present
Nose			
Mucosa	Nose mostly lined with respiratory mucosa that is dark red		May be somewhat drier
Septum	Septum usually not straight but deviates from midline	Usually straight from midline	Usually deviates
Turbinates	Turbinates deep pink and similar in color to rest of nasal mucosa		
Sinuses	No tenderness, swelling, or purulent secretions from sinuses		
Olfactory nerve (cranial nerve I)	Patient able to identify odor of substances such as lemon or coffee	Not usually tested	Sense of smell may be somewhat depressed
Pharynx			
Oropharynx	Soft palate pink, showing fine vessels under mucosa; hard palate white, more irregular, showing rugae running transversely; ducts of mucous glands may be seen in back of hard palate; uvula may vary greatly in size and may be bifid or "split"; tonsils same color as rest of oral mucosa, with crypts of whitish epithelium showing; small irregular red or pink spots of lymphoid tissue commonly seen in mucosa of posterior pharyngeal wall; gag reflex induced by touching posterior wall of pharynx	Tonsils vary in size from barely visible to very large	
Nasopharynx	Superior, middle, and inferior turbinates can be seen and may vary greatly in appearance; orifice of eustachian tube seen, usually pale, yellowish, and small; orifice normally closed but	Adenoids may occlude eustachian tube	

Area of Concern	Normal Adult Findings	Variations in Child	Variations in Older Adult
Hypopharynx	opens during yawning and swallowing; adenoids seen growing from roof and posterior wall if not surgically removed, usually small Circumvallate papillae in inverted V, may vary greatly in size; lingual tonsils on either side of tongue, may vary in size; small white spots that are debris in tonsillar crypts frequently seen; valleculae seen as cup-shaped spaces between tongue and epiglottis, may have large veins; epiglottis varies in size, shape, and color, free edge thin and slightly curved	Lingual tonsils may not be visible; epiglottis furled in infants, called ''omega shaped''	
Larynx External (by visual examination)	Thyroid cartilage (Adam's apple) protrudes, more obvious in men; laryngeal crepitation should occur when thyroid cartilage is grasped between thumb and forefinger and is moved from side to side; cricoid cartilage can be seen in thin persons with head extended and can be easily palpated; hyoid bone palpable above thyroid cartilage; cricoid cartilage drawn upward when patient says high-pitched E-E-E as normal cricothyroid muscle contracts	Thyroid and cricoid cartilages not usually visible	Thyroid cartilage may be very noticeable
Internal (via indirect laryngoscopy)	Cords move only slightly during normal respiration; phonation causes adduction of cords, which should approximate perfectly; true vocal cords appear white and sharp edged, although they are actually pink with rounded edges; a few tracheal rings sometimes seen all the way to carina; false vocal cords appear dull pink and thicker than true vocal cords; arytenoids dull red, mobile, and swing in and out with phonation; they appear as small mounds at posterior end of glottis	Small glottic area	Musculature control decreases, producing characteristic hoarseness and quavering voice; atrophy of muscles and mucosa in trachea; fatty infiltration of trachea

DIAGNOSTIC STUDIES

Mastoid films

Roentgenograms of temporal bone; if mastoiditis present, characteristic findings are clouding of mastoid air cells and decalcification of bony walls between cells

Sinus films

Roentgenograms taken to diagnose sinusitis by determining clouding or possible fluid levels in sinuses; usual views include:

Waters' view—orbits, frontal and maxillary sinuses, and nasal septum

Caldwell view—frontal sinuses, ethmoid air cells between each orbit, nasal septum, and petrous portion of temporal bone

Lateral view—sphenoid sinus and posterior wall of frontal sinuses

Direct laryngoscopy

Direct examination of larynx under local or general anesthesia; done by introducing laryngoscope into patient's mouth over tongue; tongue is raised, patient's neck is slowly extended, and laryngoscope is passed over posterior portion of epiglottis and raised to expose vocal cords

Nursing care:

Patient may return from study with intravenous line, which can be discontinued as soon as patient can take fluids; observe patient for respiratory distress for first 2 to 4 hours; if patient had local anesthesia before procedure, be aware that gag reflex may be absent until anesthesia wears off; humidified oxygen to provide additional moisture to patient's airway

Indirect laryngoscopy

Most common way to examine larynx; usually performed in physician's office; patient sits upright in chair, and laryngeal mirror is used to visualize larynx; method can be used for biopsy or excision of polyp

Suspension laryngoscopy

Essentially the same as direct laryngoscopy, but attachment holds laryngoscope and examiner then can use both hands; usually used in conjunction with microscope that provides magnification and binocular vision

Specific audiometric and hearing tests. The following are some of the tests used to determine hearing losses:

1. *Rinne.* The normal ear hears a tuning fork about twice as long by air conduction as by bone conduction.
2. *Weber.* The handle of a lightly vibrating tuning fork is placed in the middle of the forehead. Tones should normally be heard equally in both ears.
3. *Schwabach.* The examiner and patient hear tones equally when a tuning fork is alternately placed on the patient's and the examiner's mastoid processes.
4. *Pure tone.* Pure tone is a series of tones at calibrated volume at different frequencies (400 to 3000 Hz). The speech threshold represents the loudness at which a person with normal hearing can perceive tone. Both air and bone conduction are measured for each ear and the results are graphed. With normal hearing, the line is plotted at 0 dB.
5. *Speech audiometry.* A person with normal hearing hears and correctly repeats 95% of the words transmitted by the examiner.
6. *Impedance audiometry.* This detects disorders of the middle ear, thereby determining the degree of tympanic membrane and middle ear mobility. An impedance audiometer is used; one end is a probe with three small tubes inserted into the external canal and the other end attaches to an oscillator. One tube delivers a low tone of varying intensity, the second contains a microphone, and the third has an air pump. A normal tympanic membrane reflects minimal sound waves and produces a low-voltage curve on the graph.
7. *Tympanometry.* This uses the impedance audiometer, measures tympanic membrane compliance with air pressure variations in the external canal, and determines the degree of negative pressure in the middle ear.

In addition to these tests, patients may be tested to differentiate sensory (cochlear) hearing losses from neural (acoustic nerve) hearing losses. These tests include recruitment, sensitivity to small increases in intensity, and pathologic adaptation.

Recruitment is the ability to hear loud sounds normally despite a hearing loss or an abnormal increase in the perception of loudness. This is absent in neural hearing losses and present in sensory hearing losses. It can be demonstrated by having the patient compare the loudness of sounds in the affected ear with the loudness of sounds in the normal ear. In sensory hearing losses, the sensation of loudness in the affected ear increases more with each increment in intensity than it does in the normal ear. In neural hearing losses, the sensation of loudness in the affected ear increases less with each increment in intensity than it does in the normal ear. This is called decruitment.[1]

Sensitivity to small increments in intensity can be determined by having a patient listen to a continuous tone of 20 dB and then briefly and intermittently increasing the intensity. Patients with neural hearing losses, as well as those with normal hearing, cannot detect small changes in intensity. On the other hand, a patient with a sensory hearing loss can easily perceive these changes.

Pathologic adaptation, or tone decay, is found when a person cannot continue to hear a constant tone above the hearing threshold. The findings are mildly abnormal with sensory losses and severely abnormal with neural losses.

Conditions, Diseases, and Disorders

BENIGN TUMORS

Benign tumors affecting the ear are nonmalignant growths such as keloids, nodules, sebaceous cysts, polyps, and exostoses.

Nonmalignant tumors may develop on the external ear or anywhere in the ear canal. They rarely become malignant, but they may occlude the ear canal and cause retention of cerumen and a conductive hearing loss. The prognosis is excellent with proper diagnosis and treatment.

PATHOPHYSIOLOGY

Keloids are large overgrowths of hypertrophied scar tissue that result from surgery or trauma. They are much more common in blacks than in whites. In the ear keloids commonly form as a result of ear piercing, but other trauma to the auricle can cause them as well. The treatment is excision followed by repeated injections of a long-lasting steroid.

Nodules may form along the superior rim of the auricle and become indurated or painful. The cause is unknown, and treatment is excision or injection of a long-lasting steroid such as methylprednisolone or triamcinolone (Kenalog).

Sebaceous cysts are sebaceous glands that become obstructed with sebum, a soft, cheesy material. These cysts may occur in the meatus of the canal or just behind the earlobe. Normally painless, they can enlarge quickly and become painful if infected. Acute sebaceous cysts are incised and drained, and hot, moist compresses are applied.

Exostoses are small, hard, bony lumps, covered with normal epithelium, that arise from the osseous ear canal near the tympanic membrane and are attached to the posterior wall. The bases of these exostoses are close to the facial nerve. Exostoses are usually bilateral and frequently occur in multiples. They rarely occur during childhood and are more common in men than in women. They are usually asymptomatic and rarely cause an obstruction of the canal. It is believed that they form from an irritation of the periosteum as a result of swimming in cold water. Treatment is usually unnecessary, although removal may be indicated if they grow to a large size.

EXTERNAL OTITIS

External otitis is a general term used to describe inflammatory diseases of the auricle and the external auditory canal.

External otitis may be acute or chronic and may be localized as with furunculosis or diffuse, involving the entire canal. The disorder may be caused by either infections or dermatosis or by a combination of the two. It is more common in summer and is sometimes called swimmer's ear. External otitis varies in severity; there is occasionally no infection and it may be from either contact or seborrheic dermatitis. Either bacteria or fungi may produce infectious external otitis. Bacterial causes are usually attributed to *Pseudomonas*, *Proteus*, *Streptococcus*, and *Staphylococcus*. Fungi, which are most common in the tropics, are usually *Aspergillus* and *Candida*. Predisposing factors include: (1) allergies that may increase the likelihood of external otitis; (2) irritants such as hair sprays, hair dyes, or dust that cause the person to scratch the ear canal, resulting in excoriation; (3) attempts at cleaning or scratching the ear canal with a foreign object, such as a cotton swab, bobby pin, or finger, which causes irritation and possible introduction of infectious organisms; (4) continual use of earphones, earplugs, or earmuffs, which trap moisture in the ear, thereby creating a medium for infection; and (5) swimming in contaminated water, which is absorbed by the wax in the ear, macerates the skin of the canal, and allows the introduction of organisms.

PATHOPHYSIOLOGY

Acute external otitis can range from mild to severe. In the mild stage, pain is moderate to severe and is aggravated by traction on the auricle or pressure on the tragus. The patient may experience a low-grade fever and may have a sticky, yellow discharge from the ear canal. There may be a partial loss of hearing or the feeling of a blocked ear if the ear canal is swollen or obstructed with debris.

Pain is more intense during the severe stage of external otitis. The entire side of the head often aches, and the patient cannot tolerate examination of the auricle. There is usually a sticky, yellow discharge from the ear canal, hearing may be diminished, and the ear feels blocked. The patient's temperature may be as high as 40° C (104° F). The external auditory canal is swollen or entirely closed, and the tragus and external meatus are also swollen. The epithelium of the canal is usually soggy and pale. Desquamated epithelium and wax are often present in the canal. However, the canal may be reddened rather than pale, or the epithelium may be dry instead of wet. Patients may also have lymphadenopathy anterior to the tragus, behind the ear, or in the upper neck. If the auricle is involved, the skin is crusted and oozing. Pustules may be present and the ear swollen and tender. If the infection did not originate on the face or scalp, it may spread to these areas. The eardrum frequently cannot be seen well in acute external otitis because the ear canal is so swollen. An infected canal usually causes much more pain than if the auricle alone is affected because the epithelium of the ear canal cannot stretch much without causing pain.

With chronic external otitis, itching rather than pain is the usual complaint. There is no pain even with manipulation of the auricle or tragus. An examination reveals that the epithelium is thickened and red, and the canal and drumhead are insensitive to pressure from cotton applicators. A discharge is usually present.

A rare, lethal type of external otitis, which is called malignant external otitis, is caused by *Pseudomonas;* it is a fulminant bone-destroying infection. Principally seen in patients with diabetes, it quickly involves all contiguous structures and has a mortality of 50% to 75% unless recognized early and treated with potent parenteral antibiotics.[23]

In fungally caused external otitis, a characteristic mass (black or grayish with *Aspergillus niger*) forms in the ear canal, and its removal reveals a hyperemic, edematous epithelium that may be denuded. Fungal infections may be asymptomatic, since frequently the growth is found only on wax or other debris in the ear and has not invaded the tissue.

Furunculosis is a localized type of external otitis in the outer half of the ear canal. Glands and hair follicles in this area may become infected and form boils or furuncles. The onset of a furuncle may be acute; the patient may notice a feeling of fullness in the ear, loss of hearing, adenopathy, and swelling behind the ear. The area is reddened, may be very swollen, and may obstruct the entire canal. Pain is intense; even a small furuncle causes severe pain until it is surgically drained or breaks spontaneously. Movement of the auricle and tragus causes pain, as does chewing if the furuncle is on the canal floor or anterior wall.

DIAGNOSTIC STUDIES

Culture of discharge
Identification of causative organisms; usual organisms are *Pseudomonas, Proteus, Streptococcus, Staphylococcus, Aspergillus,* and *Candida*

TREATMENT PLAN

Surgical
Surgery not performed unless furuncle needs incision and drainage

Chemotherapeutic
Narcotic analgesics
  Analgesic for pain is codeine, 30 mg po q4h
Corticosteroids
  A wick is inserted into the ear canal; 1% hydrocortisone is sometimes used to reduce swelling and to allow penetration of antibiotics
Anti-infective agents
  Antibiotic or antifungal ear drops may be prescribed, which usually contain 0.5% neomycin or 10,000 U/ml of polymyxin
  Systemic antibiotics may be prescribed if infection is severe; specific drug depends on causative organism

Supportive
Careful cleansing of ear canal to remove debris and impacted cerumen
Heat therapy to external ear for pain relief

ASSESSMENT: AREAS OF CONCERN

Infection of external ear
Acute
  Moderate to severe pain in the ear, which is exacerbated by chewing and manipulation of the auricle or tragus; headache; fever; feeling of fullness or blockage in ear; foul-smelling, yellow, sticky discharge from ear (black if from fungal infection); hearing normal or decreased; tinnitus; localized swelling; erythema; lymphadenopathy behind ear and in upper neck

General ear
Chronic
  Chief complaint itching rather than pain; discharge usually present; thickened, red epithelium; canal and drumhead insensitive to pressure

NURSING DIAGNOSES and NURSING INTERVENTIONS

Nursing Diagnosis	Nursing Intervention
Comfort, alteration in: pain	In collaboration with physician, provide medication as required for pain relief; assess and document effectiveness. Monitor vital signs, especially temperature. If chewing is painful, arrange for soft or full-liquid diet.
Skin integrity, impairment of: actual	Keep ear canal clean: Cleanse gently with cotton swab soaked with Burow's solution and also apply directly to auricle. Dry gentle and completely. Administer antibiotics as ordered. Instill medicated ear drops as ordered. Observe and record amount of aural drainage.
Sensory-perceptual alteration: auditory	If patient's hearing is diminished, be sure that adequate method of communication is used. Speak slowly and clearly and stand directly in front of patient when speaking. Instruct patient and family about factors contributing to development of external otitis and encourage patient to keep foreign objects such as bobby pins out of ears. Encourage patient to use earplugs when swimming and to minimize amount of water that gets into ears when showering and shampooing.

Patient Education

1. Inform the patient and family of the necessity of completing the prescribed course of medication, whether antibiotics or ear drops, to avoid inadequate treatment or possible recurrence.
2. Teach the patient and family the proper way to instill ear drops.
3. If Burow's soaks are done, give instructions in the proper method.

EVALUATION

Patient Outcome	Data Indicating That Outcome is Reached
Inflammation of external ear and canal is cleared.	There is no pain in the ear. Patient's temperature is within normal limits. There is no discharge from ear canal. Hearing is within normal limits for patient. There is no cervical lymphadenopathy.
Patient and family verbalize increased knowledge of disease and its treatment.	Patient and family verbalize understanding of cause of, contributing factors to, and ways to prevent recurrence of disease. Patient and family verbalize understanding of necessity of completing prescribed course of antibiotics.

OBSTRUCTION

Obstruction of the ear canal is usually caused by excessive secretion or impaction of cerumen or by foreign bodies, including insects.

Young children put various objects, such as beads, pebbles, beans, and small toys, into their ears. An obstruction of the ear canal can lead to infection and to conductive hearing loss if auditory function is disrupted.

PATHOPHYSIOLOGY

Cerumen is normally produced in small amounts and dries in the ear, where it is forced out bit by bit during chewing and talking. Some people, however, have overactive glands, producing excessive amounts of cerumen that can completely occlude the ear canal. Others have narrow or tortuous ear canals that can become impacted with cerumen.

Insects occasionally fly into the ear, which causes an unpleasant sensation as they beat their wings.

Foreign objects, which children frequently put into their ears, may not cause symptoms or may cause intense pain if deep in the canal. Physicians occasionally find foreign objects in children's ears during a routine examination.

DIAGNOSTIC STUDIES

Examination of ear with an otoscope
Visualization of obstructing object

TREATMENT PLAN

Surgical
Surgical removal of foreign object with patient under anesthesia may be necessary if patient, who is often a child, is unable to remain still during removal

Chemotherapeutic
Carbamide peroxide 6.5% (Debrox drops), 5-10 gtts in ear canal to soften cerumen

Electromechanical
Removal of cerumen by irrigation or with cerumen spoon
If insect is cause of obstruction, it is smothered with drops of oily substance and removed with forceps
Other foreign objects removed with forceps if possible

ASSESSMENT: AREAS OF CONCERN

Auditory function
Ear feels occluded; some tinnitus or "buzzing" may be present; pain in ear; slight hearing loss; canal may be completely occluded by cerumen; may be insect or foreign body in canal

NURSING DIAGNOSES and NURSING INTERVENTIONS

Nursing Diagnosis	Nursing Intervention
Sensory-perceptual alteration: auditory	Instill ear drops or perform irrigation if ordered. Use solution at room temperature to avoid stimulating a caloric response. Warn patient and family not to put foreign objects in ears.
Comfort, alteration in: pain	Provide instruction about safe analgesic medications.

Patient Education

1. For patients who produce excessive cerumen, suggest a method for preventing impaction or obstruction.
2. Once a week put 1 or 2 drops of an oily substance in the ears at night. In the morning put 1 or 2 drops of hydrogen peroxide in the ears and clean gently with a soft cotton wick.

EVALUATION

Patient Outcome	Data Indicating That Outcome is Reached
Obstruction is removed.	There is no feeling of occlusion, tinnitus, or pain in ear. Hearing is normal for patient.

PERICHONDRITIS

Perichondritis is an inflammation of the auricular cartilage.

Perichondritis may follow a skin infection, but it more usually follows exposure of the cartilage from infection or trauma, which allows bacteria to enter.

PATHOPHYSIOLOGY

Perichondritis may be initiated by trauma, insect bites, or incision of superficial infections of the pinna, which causes pus to accumulate between the cartilage and the perichondrium. The causative organism is usually a gram-negative rod, frequently *Pseudomonas*. Perichondritis can cause a loss of blood supply to the cartilage, resulting in breakdown and necrosis of the cartilage. The pinna appears enlarged, inflamed, and shiny. Pain is usually severe, and localized fluctuant areas may be present on the auricle. Perichondritis must be treated early and aggressively to prevent a lengthy, destructive course.

DIAGNOSTIC STUDIES

Culture of purulent material
Identification of causative organism

TREATMENT PLAN

Surgical
Incision and drainage of any purulent material; removal of any necrotic cartilage

Chemotherapeutic
Anti-infective agents

Systemic parenteral antibiotic therapy, depending on cultured organism; local irrigations with antibiotic solutions (usually polymyxin B [10,000 units/ml], bacitracin, neomycin 0.5%, or a combination)
Narcotic analgesics or analgesic/antipyretic agents
Analgesia for pain relief; aspirin or acetaminophen (Tylenol), 650 mg, with codeine, 30 mg po q4h

Electromechanical
Small polyethylene tube inserted into area beneath nonpressure dressing to facilitate irrigation

Supportive
Local heat applications for relief

ASSESSMENT: AREAS OF CONCERN

Auricular cartilage
Inflammation and swelling of the cartilage, usually with pus; fluctuant areas on auricle; severe pain; history of trauma, insect bite, or incision of superficial infection on pinna

NURSING DIAGNOSES and NURSING INTERVENTIONS

Nursing Diagnosis	Nursing Intervention
Comfort, alteration in: pain	Provide analgesic medications for pain relief as ordered. Assess and document effectiveness.
Sensory-perceptual alteration: auditory	Administer antibiotics as ordered. Perform irrigations as ordered with room-temperature antibiotic solution. Be aware that irrigating solution contains potentially ototoxic drugs. Monitor vital signs, especially temperature.
Skin integrity, impairment of	Perform wound care of affected area if incision and drainage have been done. Apply local heat for comfort. Assess area for increased signs of infection.

Patient Education

1. Instruct the patient and family in the necessity of completing the prescribed course of antibiotics to avoid recurrence or complications.
2. If wound care is being done, be sure that the patient and family know the procedures to change the dressing and aseptic techniques to avoid wound contamination.

EVALUATION

Patient Outcome	Data Indicating That Outcome is Reached
Inflammation of auricular cartilage is absent.	There is no pain or drainage from affected ear. Temperature is within normal limits for patient. There are no fluctuant areas on auricle. Patient and family demonstrate ability to change dressing properly using aseptic technique.
Patient and family verbalize and demonstrate knowledge of treatment.	Patient and family verbalize understanding of necessity of completing prescribed course of antibiotics.

INFECTIOUS MYRINGITIS

Infectious or bullous myringitis is an inflammation of the tympanic membrane.

Vesicles in the tympanic membrane and at the end of the external auditory canal appear hemorrhagic and rupture spontaneously, which is revealed by serosanguineous fluid in the external ear. The cause is either viral or bacterial, and the disorder sometimes occurs after acute otitis media. It is common in children.

The patient experiences severe ear pain and some tenderness over the mastoid area. Occasionally fever and mild hearing loss are present. Treatment consists of pain management with aspirin or other analgesics, local heat for comfort, and either local or systemic antibiotic therapy to prevent secondary infection. Infectious myringitis usually resolves spontaneously within 3 days to 2 weeks.

OTITIS MEDIA

Otitis media is an inflammation of the middle ear and can be classified as acute or chronic and suppurative or secretory (serous).

Acute Otitis Media

Acute suppurative otitis media is very common in young children and is usually the result of a bacterial or viral infection of the upper respiratory tract. Organisms travel from the nasopharynx to the middle ear via the eustachian tube. Infants and children have shorter, straighter eustachian tubes than do adults; this easier access to the middle ear is probably the reason otitis media is common in children. Another contributing factor is that children have not developed immunities to the causative organisms. Furthermore, children have a very large mass of adenoid tissue that usually disappears during adolescence. This lymphoid tissue, if swollen, can obstruct the orifice of the eustachian tube and contribute to the development of otitis media by preventing equalization of the atmospheric pressure in the ear, thereby causing a vacuum and effusion of the middle ear.

PATHOPHYSIOLOGY

The usual pathogens of acute otitis media are grampositive cocci, but *Haemophilus influenzae* is also frequently found. Generally resulting from an infection that ascends via the eustachian tube, the inflammation usually involves the lining of the whole middle ear. This has

several effects. Exudate and edema interfere with ciliary action in the eustachian tube so its efficiency as a barrier to infection is lost. The opening of the tube is also abnormal, since edema has decreased the size of the lumen, and inflammation has caused hyperemia of the mucosal lining of the middle ear, which results in increased oxygen absorption. This leads to decreased aeration, development of a partial vacuum, retraction of the tympanic membrane, and serous exudation. This stage is common in viral infections of the upper respiratory tract, but does not progress if the middle ear is reaerated. If there is bacterial superinfection, however, the exudate becomes purulent and causes bulging of the tympanic membrane as the pus collects behind it. This is called purulent otitis media.

DIAGNOSTIC STUDIES

Culture of purulent organism
Identification of causative organisms

TREATMENT PLAN

Surgical
Myringotomy—to drain pus and fluid from middle ear (see p. 808)

Chemotherapeutic
Anti-infective agents
Penicillin G or V, 250 mg po q6h for 10 d for patients older than 8 yr
Ampicillin (Amcil, others), 50-100 mg/kg/d for 10 d for children under 8 yr because of frequency of *H. influenzae* infections in this age group
If patient is allergic to penicillin, erythromycin (E-Mycin, others), 250 mg po for adults and older children; combination of erythromycin and sulfisoxazole for children younger than 8 yr
Analgesic/antipyretic or narcotic analgesics
Codeine, 30 mg po q4h (for severe pain); sedatives sometimes given to small children
Antihistamines
Chlorpheniramine (Chlor-Trimeton), 4 mg po q4-6h for 7-10 d for adults; 0.35 mg/kg qid for children
Bronchodilators
Pseudoephedrine (Sudafed), 30 mg po q4-6h for adults

ASSESSMENT: AREAS OF CONCERN

Tympanic membrane

Severe, deep, throbbing pain behind tympanic membrane; pain may disappear if eardrum ruptures; feeling of fullness in ears; partial loss of hearing

Infectious process

Fever that may be as high as 104° F; chills; malaise, weakness and dizziness; nausea and vomiting; tympanic membrane appears red, inflamed, and bulging; if it is perforated, pulsating purulent material can be seen coming through it after ear is cleaned of pus and debris

NURSING DIAGNOSES and NURSING INTERVENTIONS

Nursing Diagnosis	Nursing Intervention
Comfort, alteration in: pain	Provide analgesia as ordered and assess and document effectiveness. Administer sedatives, if ordered, to young children as needed. Instruct parents in appropriate dosages of medication to give child at home.
Skin integrity, impairment of	If patient has had myringotomy, keep ear clean and dry. Place sterile cotton in outer ear to absorb drainage and prevent possible contamination of outer ear, which leads to development of external otitis media. Encourage bed rest if patient is weak, complains of malaise, or has nausea and vomiting. Monitor vital signs, especially temperature, and report any changes.
Sensory-perceptual alteration: auditory	Observe patient for symptoms of hearing deficit. If patient is child, ask parents if they have noticed any signs of hearing loss: inattentiveness, blank stares, lack of response to questions, or pulling at affected ear. (Ear pain is frequently so severe that hearing loss is not noticed.) Administer antibiotics as ordered and instruct patient and family about appropriate dosages. Instruct patient or family to monitor level of hearing (it should return to normal with appropriate antibiotic therapy).

Patient Education

1. Instruct the patient and family of the necessity for completing the entire course of antibiotics to prevent a recurrence or complications.
2. Instruct the parents to feed children in an upright position and not lying down to prevent reflux of nasopharyngeal flora through the eustachian tube into the middle ear.
3. Instruct the patient not to blow the nose forcefully, which forces contaminated material into the eustachian tube.
4. If the patient has had a myringotomy, instruct the patient and family how to change the cotton in the outer ear at least twice a day.

EVALUATION

Patient Outcome	Data Indicating That Outcome is Reached
Otitis media is resolved.	There is no purulent drainage from tympanic membrane. Tympanic membrane appears normal with no bulging, redness, retraction, or inflammation. Hearing is normal for patient. Patient is afebrile. Patient's activity level is normal.
Patient and family have increased knowledge of treatment.	Patient and family verbalize understanding of necessity for completing prescribed course of antibiotics.

Secretory Otitis Media

Secretory (serous) otitis media is an effusion in the middle ear that results from incomplete resolution or inadequate treatment of acute otitis media. Effusions can also be caused by an obstruction of the eustachian tube, resulting in an increase in negative pressure in the middle ear that produces transudation of fluid from the blood vessels in the membranes of the middle ear. This fluid is usually sterile but may contain pathogens. Secretory (serous) otitis media can also be caused by allergies that produce edema in the lumen of the eustachian tube or by barotrauma that results from the external pressure markedly exceeding lowered pressure of the middle ear, as during diving or the descent of an airplane. It is common in children.

Patients feel a fullness in their ears but have no pain or fever. A conductive hearing loss may occur, especially in chronic secretory otitis media. Otoscopic examination reveals mild retraction of the tympanic membrane with a clear transudate from the blood vessels. The tympanic membrane is immobile and amber colored, and a fluid level or air bubbles may be seen through the tympanic membrane. The meniscus of the fluid may appear as a thin black hair or line across the tympanic membrane. If blood is present, as with barotrauma, the fluid may appear blue-black.

Treatment consists of inflation of the eustachian tube, a Valsalva maneuver (in which the patient inspires, holds the breath, and bears down as though having a bowel movement) several times a day, myringotomy to drain fluid from the middle ear, or antihistamine therapy to improve eustachian tube function. A small plastic tube may be left in place for several weeks to promote drainage and equalize air pressure; this is most commonly done in children but occasionally in adults.

Chronic secretory otitis media resulting from inadequate treatment of acute otitis media or from overgrowth of the lymphoid tissue in the nasopharynx caused by nasal sinus infections or allergies poses a serious threat to the patient's hearing. Symptoms are minimal; a fluctuating hearing loss or a feeling of heaviness on one side of the head is most common. Treatment is directed at the underlying cause and the removal of fluid by myringotomy. A small tube is frequently inserted during myringotomy to equalize pressure on both sides of the eardrum and is left in place for 8 to 9 months, when it usually falls out spontaneously. These tubes may need to be replaced. Patients should be instructed not to swim while a tube is in place.

Not to be overlooked as a cause of chronic secretory otitis media in adults is carcinoma of the nasopharynx; if the effusion is unilateral, a thorough workup must be done to eliminate carcinoma.[7]

Chronic Otitis Media

Chronic otitis media is usually caused by repeated attacks of acute otitis media and acute mastoiditis; it generally results in a permanent perforation of the tympanic membrane. Chronic changes such as thickening and scarring of the mucosa eventually occur in the middle ear, and the ossicles may be destroyed. These permanent tympanic perforations result in a slight conductive hearing loss. If the ossicles are involved, the hearing loss may be greater.

There are two types of perforations: central, in which the margin of the eardrum is not involved, and marginal, in which the anulus or margin of the drum is destroyed. Central perforations are more benign than marginal ones, and less likely to result in cholesteatomas. Cholesteatomas occur when the marginal perforation of the eardrum allows squamous epithelium of the external auditory canal to grow into the middle ear, which then becomes lined with squamous epithelium. As the epithelium grows, it desquamates and the debris collects inside the middle ear. Cholesteatomas enlarge slowly, expand into the mastoid antrum, and destroy adjacent structures.

The most common symptom of chronic otitis media is a constant, painless, serous discharge from the ear, which varies from foul smelling to nearly odorless. The discharge becomes much worse when the patient has an infection of the upper respiratory tract, and it occasionally causes slight discomfort in the ear.

Treatment during exacerbations consists of thoroughly cleaning the ear and instilling a solution of 0.5% acetic acid with 1.0% hydrocortisone three times a day for 5 to 7 days. Severe exacerbations require systemic antibiotic therapy. Tympanoplasty can also be performed to restore and reconstruct the mechanisms of the middle ear (see p. 817).

MASTOIDITIS

Mastoiditis is an inflammation of the air cells of the antrum.

Usually of bacterial origin, mastoiditis is the result of the extension of a middle ear infection. It was quite common before the discovery of antibiotics but is now found only in patients whose otitis media was untreated or inadequately treated.

PATHOPHYSIOLOGY

Mastoiditis occurs when pus is left in the middle ear from otitis media, and infection progresses into the bony portion of the mastoid antrum and cells. This can cause bony necrosis of the mastoid process and breakdown of its bony structure. If untreated, the infection can lead to formation of subperiosteal abscesses and other complications, including meningitis, facial paralysis, brain abscesses, and sigmoid sinus thrombosis.

With mastoiditis, large amounts of thick purulent material usually fill the external auditory canal, which indicates perforation of the tympanum, and the soft tissue that is next to the eardrum may be ruptured and sagging. Roentgenograms of the mastoid are needed to determine the extent of involvement. Findings vary from clouding of the air cells and some decalcification of the bony walls to complete coalescence of the air cells. If early decalcification is present, intense antibiotic therapy and myringotomy can usually cure mastoiditis; if it has progressed to further destruction, simple mastoidectomy is necessary.[7]

DIAGNOSTIC STUDIES

Mastoid films
   May show cloudy air cells and decalcification of cell walls

TREATMENT PLAN

Surgical
   Mastoidectomy if necessary; involves removing involved bone and cleansing area; can be performed through postaural or endaural incision
   Myringotomy to drain fluid and pus from middle ear (see p. 808)

Chemotherapeutic
   Anti-infective agents
      Penicillin G procaine suspension (Wycillin, Duracillin), 600,000-1,200,000 units IM
      Penicillin G aqueous, 1.5 million units q4-6h for severe infections
   Other agents specific to organism

ASSESSMENT: AREAS OF CONCERN

Tympanic membrane
   Thick purulent discharge; membrane appears dull, thickened, and edematous, and otoscopic examination reveals that it is ruptured; dull aching behind ear; low-grade fever; auricle may be pushed out from head by erythema or edema; conductive hearing loss

NURSING DIAGNOSES and NURSING INTERVENTIONS

Nursing Diagnosis	Nursing Intervention
Comfort, alteration in: pain	Administer analgesics as ordered. Assess and record effectiveness of pain relief. Administer antibiotics as ordered.
Skin integrity, impairment of	After mastoidectomy, check dressings and reinforce as necessary. Place gauze between ear and head to avoid crushing ear against head and to promote adequate circulation. Record amount and color of wound drainage and patient's temperature.
Sensory-perceptual alteration: auditory	Monitor patient's hearing before and after mastoidectomy and myringotomy. If patient experiences hearing loss, speak slowly and clearly when talking with patient. Ensure that family and other staff members are aware of hearing loss and use appropriate methods of communication. Assist patient with standing and ambulation initially, since patient may experience some vertigo.

Patient Education

1. Inform the patient and family of the necessity of completing the prescribed course of antibiotics to prevent recurrence or complications.

EVALUATION

Patient Outcome	Data Indicating That Outcome is Reached
Inflammation of mastoid is cleared.	There is no pain in ear. There is no drainage in external canal. If mastoidectomy was performed, wound is well healed. Temperature is within normal limits for patient. Hearing is normal for patient.
Patient and family verbalize knowledge of treatment of mastoiditis.	Patient and family verbalize understanding of necessity for completing the prescribed course of medication.

OTOSCLEROSIS

Otosclerosis is a disease of the bone in the bony labyrinth, or the otic capsule, in which normal bone is replaced by the formation of highly vascular, "spongy" otosclerotic bone.

Otosclerosis most commonly occurs (85%) at the oval window and eventually causes a conductive hearing loss. Most patients have the disease in both ears, although not to the same degree. It is unilateral in about 10% to 15% of patients.

Otosclerosis is present to some degree in about 10% of the white population. It is not found as frequently in Orientals and blacks but is reported as common in southern India. About half of patients with otosclerosis have a family history of the disease. Women are apparently affected more often than men, and although the etiology is unclear, pregnancy frequently triggers a rapid onset of this condition. It is usually noticed first in the late teens or early twenties.

PATHOPHYSIOLOGY

The cause of otosclerosis is unknown; it is thought to have no relationship to previous ear infections. However, normal bone in the otic capsule is gradually replaced by otosclerotic bone that is highly vascular and described as spongy. As this bone advances, it impedes the normal mobility of the stapes and causes progressive fixation of the footplate of the stapes, which virtually immobilizes the footplate in the oval window. This produces a conductive hearing loss, since sound pressure vibrations can no longer be transmitted to the fluid media. Patients may also experience a mixed or sensorineural hearing loss if the cochlea is involved.

In otosclerosis the eardrum usually appears normal, although a pink blush called Schwartz's sign can occasionally be seen through the eardrum. This indicates a high degree of vascularity in active otosclerotic bone.

DIAGNOSTIC STUDIES

Rinne test
Bone conduction lasting longer than air conduction in affected ear

Weber test
Reverse is true in normal hearing

Audiometric tests
Hearing loss ranges from 60 dB in early stages to total loss in later stages; sound lateralizes more to affected ear

TREATMENT PLAN

Surgical
Stapedectomy (see p. 810)

Chemotherapeutic
Anti-infective agents
Tetracycline (Achromycin), 250 mg po q6h for 10 d (before and after surgery)

Electromechanical
Air conduction hearing aid if stapedectomy is not indicated

ASSESSMENT: AREAS OF CONCERN

Auditory function
Slowly progressive conductive hearing loss; low- to medium-pitched tinnitus; tympanic membrane normal on examination with otoscope

NURSING DIAGNOSES and NURSING INTERVENTIONS

Nursing Diagnosis	Nursing Intervention
Sensory-perceptual alteration: auditory	Encourage activity level within physician's protocol. (Some patients will be up the day of surgery, others will require bed rest for at least a day.)
	Instruct the patient to lie flat with head turned to side and operated ear facing upward so position of inserted prosthesis is maintained.
	Point out to the patient that vertigo, pain, nausea, and vomiting may occur.
	Administer pain medication as needed.
	Keep side rails up.
	Convalescent care: Assist patient to begin ambulation gradually to minimize vertigo.

Patient Education

1. Instruct the patient not to cough, sneeze, or blow his nose for at least 1 week to prevent bacteria from entering the eustachian tube and to prevent dislodging the prosthesis and graft over the oval window.
2. Instruct the patient to avoid loud noises, although there is no evidence that any damage is caused.
3. Inform the patient that a decrease in hearing may occur after surgery because of increased fluid in the middle ear.
4. Tell the patient to ask the physician when flying will be permitted, since pressure changes may cause injury to the prosthesis and graft. This varies greatly from physician to physician and can range from 2 to 3 days after surgery to 1 to 2 months after surgery.

EVALUATION

Patient Outcome	Data Indicating That Outcome is Reached
Patient recovers uneventfully from stapedectomy.	Patient experiences no vertigo. Patient experiences no pain. Hearing is improved to normal (remember that patient may experience decrease in hearing after surgery until blood in middle ear is reabsorbed).
Patient and family verbalize understanding of stapedectomy.	Patient verbalizes understanding of importance of completing antibiotic regimen and knowledge of convalescent care.

ACOUSTIC NEUROMA

Neuromas are tumors that arise from the neurilemma or Schwann cell sheath in the covering of the axon of a neuron.

Acoustic neuromas actually arise from the vestibular portion rather than from the cochlear portion of the eighth cranial nerve; the origin is only occasionally found to be the acoustic nerve. Thus these tumors are also called vestibular schwannomas, tumors of the eighth cranial nerve, or cerebellopontine angle tumors. Since most of these neuromas arise within the internal auditory meatus, early effects may be from pressure on the meatus, the cochlear division of the eighth cranial nerve, and the vestibular nerve. Patients usually have tinnitus, hearing loss, dizziness, and unsteadiness. Although these tumors can affect people at any age, most patients are 40 to 50 years of age, with women affected slightly more frequently (60%) than men. Acoustic neuromas comprise approximately 5% to 10% of all intracranial tumors.[4]

During the past 20 years, advances in diagnosis and techniques for removal of these tumors, such as the use of lasers and microsurgery, have greatly reduced morbidity and mortality.

PATHOPHYSIOLOGY

The neuroma is a well-defined, fleshy, lobulated mass that is soft and cystic in some areas; it has a variegated appearance that may be caused by areas of old hemorrhage, although the tumor itself is quite avascular. Small, white, patchy areas of calcification may also be present.

As previously mentioned, the tumor usually arises in the internal auditory meatus. It is called an intracanalicular tumor if it lies entirely within the auditory canal and is considered an ear tumor. Small tumors measure between 2 and 5 cm, and large tumors have a minimum diameter of 5 cm.[42] As the tumor increases in size, it grows into the cerebellopontine angle and may begin to erode the wall of the internal meatus above and below. After the tumor grows out of the bony canal, it can expand medially, anterosuperiorly, and posteroinferiorly. As it grows medially, the tumor encroaches on the brainstem in the region of the pons. By this time the neuroma is usually about 2.5 cm in diameter and may be in contact with the anterior inferior cerebellar artery, which is responsible for the blood supply to the side of the pons and medulla. Continued enlargement medially compresses and distorts the pons and aqueduct, thereby producing brainstem signs and causing an obstructing hydrocephalus.

As the tumor expands anterosuperiorly, it displaces the facial nerve and stretches it over the surface of the tumor. Although it may adhere to the facial nerve, the tumor can usually be separated from the nerve at surgery because the tumor does not normally wrap itself around the nerve. As the tumor extends farther, it usually involves the trigeminal nerve, lifting it up from below, thereby causing facial numbness, pain, and decreased corneal sensation.

If the tumor extends inferiorly and posteriorly, it may cause compression of the middle cerebellar peduncle and the cerebellum. It also stretches the ninth, tenth, and eleventh cranial nerves as it approaches the foramen magnum.

Most acoustic neuromas grow within the subarachnoid space. They are usually considered slow growing, although this can vary from patient to patient. Tumors seem to grow fairly rapidly in young adults and more slowly in the elderly.

Substantial cochlear and labyrinthine changes occur with these space-occupying lesions of the internal meatus (Fig. 7-16), causing abnormalities of the cochlear and eighth cranial nerves. There may be chemical alterations, such as high concentrations of protein in the perilymph, and the sense organs themselves may be destroyed, although the hair cells of the organ of Corti often remain quite normal.

Von Recklinghausen's disease, or neurofibromatosis, can also cause acoustic neuromas that are usually bilateral and expand within the nerve rather than against the nerve such as in isolated neuromas.[42]

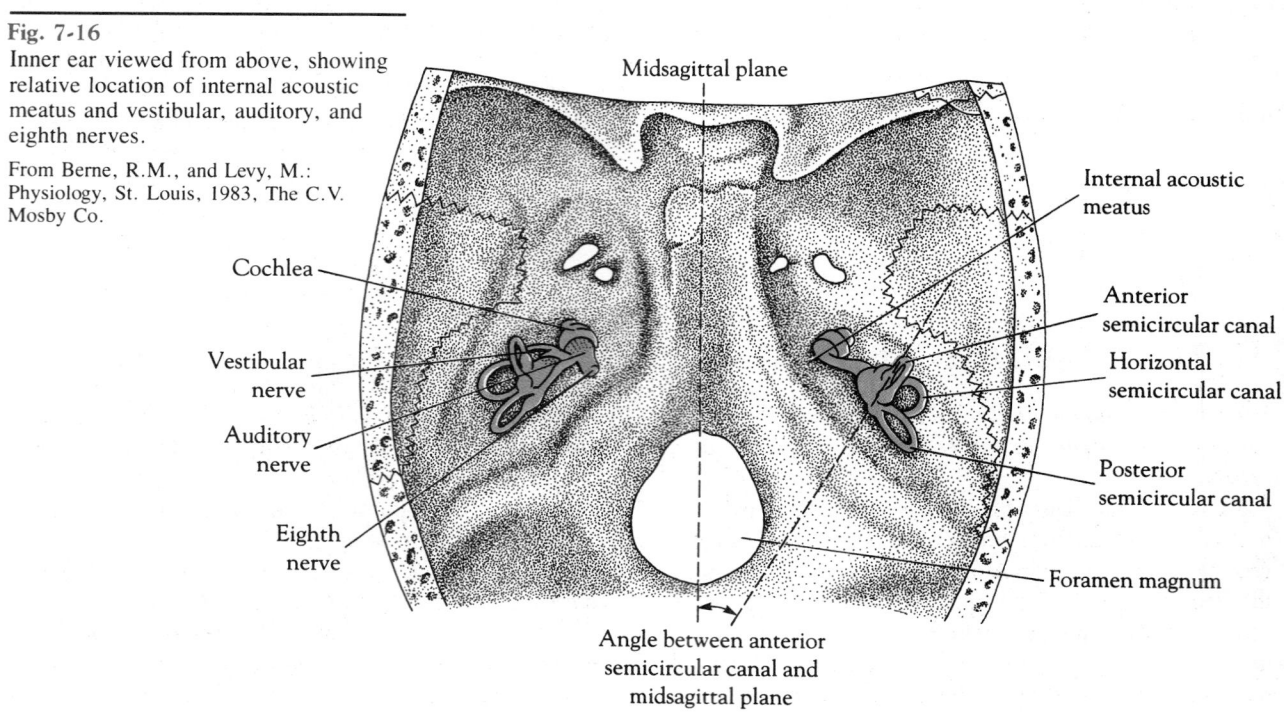

Fig. 7-16
Inner ear viewed from above, showing relative location of internal acoustic meatus and vestibular, auditory, and eighth nerves.

From Berne, R.M., and Levy, M.: Physiology, St. Louis, 1983, The C.V. Mosby Co.

Midsagittal plane

Internal acoustic meatus

Anterior semicircular canal

Horizontal semicircular canal

Posterior semicircular canal

Foramen magnum

Cochlea

Vestibular nerve

Auditory nerve

Eighth nerve

Angle between anterior semicircular canal and midsagittal plane

DIAGNOSTIC STUDIES

Audiology, electrocochleography, and brainstem response to audiometry
Performed to evaluate degree of hearing loss and to differentiate between conductive and sensorineural hearing losses

Cerebral arteriography
Used less frequently in recent years but may be performed to diagnose aneurysms, to outline size and location of tumors, and to determine location and deviation of major vessels

Computerized axial tomography and magnetic resonance imaging (MRI) scan
Can indicate presence of tumor, pinpoint location, and show evidence of enlarged ventricles

Lumbar puncture
Cerebrospinal fluid examined for increased protein; should not be performed if increased intracranial pressure is suspected to prevent herniation of cerebellar tonsils through foramen magnum or uncal herniation through tentorial notch[42]

Tomograms
Can show flaring of internal acoustic canal along medial aspect and erosion of posterior wall of canal[38]

Roentgenograms of petrous pyramid of temporal bone
May show erosion of petrous portion of temporal bone or internal acoustic meatus by tumor[38]

TREATMENT PLAN

Surgical
Surgery is treatment of choice, since these tumors do not respond well to chemotherapy or radiation; objective is to remove tumor completely while saving facial nerve; surgery can last from 9 to 14 hours and is done with patient in sitting position; either suboccipital or translabyrinthine approach used; for suboccipital approach, small portion of hair at base of neck is shaved; some surgeons prefer translabyrinthine approach: one institution reports that all acoustic neuromas, regardless of size, can be removed with this approach, although there may be technical problems with very large tumors; translabyrinthine approach associated with lower mortality, better facial nerve function, less postoperative ataxia, and much less postoperative hydrocephalus than with suboccipital approach; advantage is avoidance of pressure on cerebellum[39]
If tumor is large and adheres to facial nerve, total removal of tumor may necessitate sacrifice of facial nerve; if possible, end-to-end anastomosis of nerve stumps is done at time of surgery and should result in return of nerve function[42]
Ventriculostomy—sometimes performed during surgery so intracranial pressure can be monitored after surgery

Chemotherapeutic
Corticosteroids
Dexamethasone (Decadron), 4-6 mg IV q4h to decrease cerebral edema

Electromechanical
Cardiac and intracranial pressure monitoring; mechanical ventilation immediately after surgery

Supportive
Nothing by mouth and intravenous feedings until patient is able to eat; tube feedings necessary in some patients until gag reflex or ability to chew returns
Physical therapy and possibly speech therapy after surgery

ASSESSMENT: AREAS OF CONCERN

Symptoms are dependent on size and location of tumor.

Auditory function
Sensorineural hearing loss, usually unilateral and slowly progressive; tinnitus; dizziness and transient unsteadiness; true vertigo (sense of rotation, nausea, and vomiting) in some patients; otalgia (ache within ear or mastoid); tension or neck pain on same side as otalgia; occasional facial numbness; occasional tic douloureux

Visual function
Depression of corneal reflex; delayed blink reflex; decreased tear production; eyes feel dry and gritty

Gustatory function
Diminished sense of taste on anterior two thirds of tongue; with large tumors, diplopia, nystagmus, ataxia, headaches, papilledema, loss of vision, and difficulty chewing

Motor function
Poor coordination and gait disturbances

NURSING DIAGNOSES and NURSING INTERVENTIONS

Nursing Diagnosis	Nursing Intervention
Tissue perfusion, alteration in: cerebral	Establish neurologic baseline and monitor neurologic status and vital signs every 15 minutes until stable, and then every 4 hours. Be alert for hypertension, which could be significant after surgery. Monitor amount of and describe ventricular drainage if used. Observe for signs of increasing intracranial pressure: widening pulse pressures, decreased level of consciousness, papilledema, seizures, and hyperactive deep tendon reflexes. Administer dexamethasone as ordered. Administer antacids to decrease increased gastric acidity and prevent stress ulcers. Observe for symptoms of hydrocephalus from edema or bleeding into ventricles, which is possible after surgery. Observe cardiac monitor for any arrhythmias, which could be result of cerebral edema or vagal stimulation during surgery. Keep head of bed elevated 30 degrees to promote venous drainage and limit cerebral edema.
Respiratory function, alteration in	Patient will be mechanically ventilated for 1 or 2 days after surgery: maintain ventilator settings; suction patient as needed; and observe patient after extubation for return of gag reflex and ability to cough effectively. Patient may need continued suctioning or physical therapy of the chest.
Fluid volume excess	Monitor and record intravenous infusions. Patient will initially take nothing by mouth. Maintain strict intake and output records. Assess skin turgor. Be alert for fluid retention as result of decreased sodium. Monitor electrolyte levels, since patients are given diuretics to decrease brain bulk during surgery. Patient will have Foley catheter until able to void normally; perform catheter care to prevent urinary tract infection.
Comfort, alteration in: pain	Assess for pain and give medication as needed to minimize pain, nausea, and vomiting.
Nutrition, alteration in: less than body requirements	Maintain nothing by mouth until gag reflex has returned. Begin offering patient soft or pureed foods, feeding on unaffected side if patient experiences difficulty or facial numbness. Evaluate need for dietary consultation. Provide tube feedings in collaboration with physician until gag reflex returns. Provide excellent mouth care.
Skin integrity, impairment of	Observe dressing for drainage and bleeding and reinforce or change as needed. Remove dressing 3 to 5 days after surgery. Observe for redness, inflammation, drainage, or puffiness near operative site. Puffiness may be from accumulation of subgaleal fluid, since dura was entered; fluid should be reabsorbed in few days. To prevent skin breakdown, position patient comfortably and change position frequently until patient is mobile. Since neck muscles will be weakened, provide adequate support to head and back when positioning. Provide artifical tears to patient's eyes as needed to maintain normal lubrication because of loss of corneal reflex and decreased secretions.
Sensory-perceptual alteration: auditory	Assess and record level of hearing. If hearing is decreased, face patient when speaking and speak clearly and loudly if necessary.
Mobility, impaired physical	Assist patient with ambulation and consult with physical therapy department for continued exercise, strengthening, and gait training.
Self-concept, disturbance in	Be sensitive to body image problems if patient experiences continued weakness, especially facial weakness, drooping, or ptosis.

Patient Education

1. Instruct the patient and family regarding signs and symptoms of wound infection.
2. Instruct the patient and family regarding signs and symptoms of hydrocephalus, which in rare cases occurs several weeks after surgery.
3. Instruct the patient and family regarding the need for continued physical therapy and rehabilitation and possible speech therapy.
4. Instruct the patient and family regarding maintenance of nutrition, especially if a chewing or swallowing deficit remains. If the patient is discharged but will continue tube feedings, be sure that the patient or a family member can perform the procedure safely.
5. Ensure that the patient and family understand that deficits may take several months to resolve or may not resolve at all; assess the family's coping mechanisms and the possible need for assistance in dealing with these deficits.

EVALUATION

Patient Outcome	Data Indicating That Outcome is Reached
Preoperative symptoms are improved or absent.	Hearing is improved or normal. Tinnitus is absent. Dizziness or unsteadiness has improved or disappeared. Facial numbness, tickling, and pain have improved or disappeared (this may take 3 to 6 months). Headaches and vomiting are absent. Gait and coordination difficulties are improved.

LABYRINTHITIS

Labyrinthitis is an inflammation of the labyrinth of the inner ear.

Labyrinthitis is quite rare, and it is usually classified into four types: (1) paralabyrinthitis, (2) serous, (3) purulent, and (4) viral. Because the membranous labyrinth is protected by bone, it is difficult for microorganisms to enter the area unless the bony labyrinth is eroded, as with cholesteatoma formation in chronic otitis media. However, organisms can gain entry through the oval and round windows during acute otitis media or through the cochlear aqueduct during meningitis. Symptoms are usually severe vertigo and nystagmus, followed by total sensorineural hearing loss on the affected side.

Paralabyrinthitis causes the least serious symptoms of the four types of labyrinthitis. A fistula between the bony and membranous labyrinths is caused by erosion of the bone from granulation or cholesteatoma formation, but no inflammation or infection is present. There is no spontaneous nystagmus, and vertigo may be present only because the membranous labyrinth is exposed when exogenous stimulation occurs. A diagnosis is usually made when alternating positive and negative pressures are applied to the external meatus: applying positive pressure may induce nystagmus toward the affected ear, and negative pressure has the opposite effect. Nystagmus is not always produced, however, and the presence of vertigo usually assists in making the diagnosis. Treatment consists of surgically exteriorizing the fistula.

In *serous labyrinthitis* the membranous labyrinth is inflamed and direct labyrinthine stimulation occurs, probably by a direct effect on the nerve endings, producing nystagmus on the affected side. Nystagmus may also result from the caloric effect caused by the hyperemia. The patient experiences severe vertigo and nausea and vomiting, characteristically lies quietly with the affected side down, and looks up in an attempt to decrease the nystagmus. The patient may experience some deafness. Any type of movement may worsen the vertigo, and an attempt to stand results in a fall. Heavy sedation, bed rest, and systemic antibiotics in high doses are indicated. If the patient's hearing returns, the labyrinthitis was serous rather than purulent.

Purulent labyrinthitis results in the destruction of the labyrinth and cochlea, causing permanent deafness in the affected ear. Symptoms and treatment are the same as for serous labyrinthitis; massive doses of antibiotics are administered to prevent the spread of infection and pus and resultant meningitis. Drugs such as ampicillin are usually prescribed because penicillin does not easily cross into the labyrinth. Patients may require intravenous hydration and administration of antivertigo drugs such as meclizine.

Viral labyrinthitis may be suspected after infections of the upper respiratory tract or if sudden unilateral deafness occurs in a young patient with no concomitant infection of the middle ear. The mumps virus is commonly associated with sudden deafness in young children. Rubella during the first trimester of gestation may cause congenital deafness. Infants born of these mothers have elevated rubella titers. The best prevention is prophylactic vaccination of young women during their childbearing years.

As mentioned previously, patients with labyrinthitis have severe vertigo, nystagmus, nausea, and vomiting. Nursing care is aimed at preventing falls. Bed rails are kept up, and the patient is instructed to lie quietly and not to get out of bed without assistance. Antiemetic and antivertigo medications are administered for patient comfort. Antibiotics are given if ordered. The patient's intake and output are monitored for symptoms of dehydration, and intravenous fluids are given if ordered.

If not hospitalized, the patient should maintain bed rest at home and request assistance from a family member before getting up.

The patient and family should be informed that recovery from the symptoms may take up to 6 weeks, and the patient is cautioned about activities that may result in vertigo, such as climbing or working in high places.

MÉNIÈRE'S DISEASE

Ménière's disease, also called endolymphatic hydrops, is a labyrinthine dysfunction associated with dilation of the membranous labyrinth.

The dilation causes three typical symptoms: severe vertigo, tinnitus, and a sensorineural hearing loss, which is usually initially of low tones. Although never fatal, this disorder is nonetheless quite incapacitating during attacks, which occur episodically with intervals of remission. As hearing decreases, the attacks become less frequent, and they may stop altogether when the patient's hearing loss is almost total. The acute attacks usually last for several hours, but between attacks the patient may have no symptoms except for tinnitus and a gradually progressive hearing loss. In severe or untreated cases, however, the patient may have daily attacks, although with periods of complete relief from vertigo between attacks.

Adults between the ages of 30 and 60 years are usually affected. Although it can occur at any age, Ménière's disease is rare in children and the elderly. Men are perhaps affected slightly more often than women, and the condition is more often unilateral than bilateral.

Some researchers believe that the incidence of Ménière's disease may have increased since World War II, possibly because of a correlation between the disease, current living habits, and environmental conditions, such as increased stress and increased salt intake.

PATHOPHYSIOLOGY

The most widely accepted theories regarding the cause of Ménière's disease fall into two categories: (1) an overproduction of endolymph from some disturbance in the formation of fluid in the inner ear and (2) decreased absorption of endolymph from a disturbance in the sac, which leads to an accumulation of endolymph.

Many other theories have been postulated, but few have gained wide acceptance. Endolymphatic hydrops, however, is thought to cause degeneration of the neural end organ of the labyrinth and cochlea. Some researchers believe that fluid disturbances are caused by sodium retention, allergies, or vascular spasm. Small vesicles may form in the walls of the endolymphatic system, and the sudden rupture of these vesicles may cause acute attacks of vertigo. The cause of the formation of these vesicles is unclear. Premenstrual edema precipitates attacks in some women.

Reissner's membrane and the saccular wall (Fig. 7-7) frequently undergo enormous stretching and rupture. This causes the membranes to lose their ability to maintain normal electrolyte gradients between the endolymph and the perilymph; potassium contamination of the scala vestibuli may occur as a result. The contaminated perilymph could pass through the helicotrema to the scala tympani to alter the electrolyte environment of the nerve fibers and the organ of Corti. There is conjecture that fluctuating low-tone hearing losses are caused by the repeated loss of control of the electrolyte gradients or by ruptures of Reissner's membrane or the saccular wall with consequent potassium intoxication.[4] In some cases the membranous labyrinth may collapse completely, possibly as a result of rupture, which causes the utricle to come in direct contact with the footplate of the stapes.

DIAGNOSTIC STUDIES

Audiology
Tuning fork test
  Shows sensorineural deficit
Rinne test
  May be false-positive if there is severe unilateral hearing loss
Pure tone test
  Shows sensorineural loss involving low tones

Electrocochleography
Used frequently to aid in differential diagnosis of auditory diseases

Caloric tests
5 ml ice water instilled into each ear with patient's head elevated 30 degrees to cause acute attack with

nausea, vomiting, vertigo, and nystagmus; response is occasionally hypoactive in involved ear and sometimes in both ears

Roentgenograms of petrous bones

Internal auditory meatus examined carefully; patients with Ménière's disease usually have shorter, straighter vestibular aqueducts than do patients without Ménière's disease

Injection of intravenous acetazolamide

Causes temporary increase in pure tone and speech audiometric thresholds, which suggest temporary increase in preexisting hydrops, possibly from transient reduction in plasma osmolality (many patients with Ménière's disease have moderately elevated serum osmolality[42])

TREATMENT PLAN

Goals are preservation of hearing and control of vertigo.

Surgical

Recent increased interest in surgical therapies because medical therapy has failed to halt hearing losses; if medical therapy has failed, two surgical procedures may be performed

Decompression of endolymphatic sac—done by inserting Teflon endolymphatic subarachnoid shunt or by incision in sac kept patent by muscle flap or Teflon sheet; has some benefit in about two thirds of patients

Destruction of end organ and neural connections by labyrinthectomy or vestibular neurectomy; labyrinthectomy performed only as last resort when vertigo is persistent and little or no hearing is left, since cochlear function is destroyed; vertigo disappears in almost every case but tinnitus may remain; vestibular neurectomy may be regarded as operation of choice; middle cranial fossa approach is used; 90% of patients have relief from vertigo, some with improvement in hearing; in one study 16% of 52 patients had improvement in hearing and 64% had stabilization of hearing loss; in another study 32% of 78 patients had improvement in hearing at least 2 years after neurectomy[38]

Chemotherapeutic

Vasodilators (used for histamine effect)

Histamine (Diphosphate), 2.75 mg given in 200-500 ml of 5% glucose; drip over 1 h (in remission); based on theory that labyrinthine ischemia is cause of disease; most have not been found to be effective, but β-histamine may improve vertigo, hearing, and tinnitus[1]

Antiemetics (used for symptomatic vestibular suppressant effect)

Prochlorperazine (Compazine), 10 mg po q6h

Antianxiety agents (used for symptomatic vestibular suppressant effect)

Diazepam (Valium), 2.5-5 mg po q6h

Diuretics (used as vestibular decompressant)

Furosemide (Lasix), 40-80 mg/d

Hydrochlorothiazide (Hydrodiuril), 25-200 mg/d

Cholinergic blocking agents

Atropine, 0.01 mg/kg to maximum of 0.04 mg/kg subcutaneously or IM

Adrenergic agents

Epinephrine, 0.2-0.5 mg IV may be administered to stop an attack; sedatives and antiemetics such as meclizine (Antivert), 25 mg po qid, and prochlorperazine (Compazine), 10 mg po q6h may be used

Supportive

Bed rest maintained during acute attack

To prevent attacks, Furstenberg diet (neutral ash and salt free)

Restriction of salt and water intake

ASSESSMENT: AREAS OF CONCERN

During acute attack

Balance

Sudden onset of acute vertigo

Auditory function

Tinnitus described by patient as a persistent background hum

Visual function

Nystagmus

General

Nausea and vomiting; sweating; abdominal pain; diarrhea; and bradycardia

Between attacks

Auditory function

Gradually progressive sensorineural hearing loss; tinnitus; some patients describe a fullness, pressure, or dull ache in ear; normal tympanic membranes

NURSING DIAGNOSES and NURSING INTERVENTIONS

Nursing Diagnosis	Nursing Intervention
Injury: potential for (trauma)	Keep side rails of bed up.
	Encourage patient to lie quietly and *not* to get up without assistance during attack.
	Instruct patient to avoid sudden head movements or position changes, since attacks may begin without warning.
	Administer antiemetics and sedatives to help prevent vomiting and promote rest.
Sensory-perceptual alteration: auditory	See p. 1967.

Patient Education

1. Instruct the patient in theories about the etiology of the disease and acute attacks.
2. Ensure that the patient is aware that there may be a progressive hearing loss unless treatment is successful.
3. Inform the patient of ways to minimize tinnitus if the patient is bothered by it.
4. Inform the patient that the attacks will last a few hours and will stop on their own, but that treatment is available to diminish or stop them if necessary.
5. Ensure that the patient understands the danger of trying to walk unassisted during an attack because of vertigo.
6. Instruct the patient and family in dietary or medical regimen if used or inform them about surgical interventions if used.

EVALUATION

Patient Outcome	Data Indicating That Outcome is Reached
Patient has increased knowledge of Ménière's disease.	Patient verbalizes understanding that attacks will eventually stop of their own accord. Patient verbalizes understanding that sudden movements and hazardous tasks should be avoided because of sudden onset of vertigo. Patient expresses knowledge of side effects of medical regimen if ordered or of surgical intervention if used. Patient expresses understanding of possibility of hearing loss.

TINNITUS

Tinnitus is the perception of sound in the absence of an acoustic stimulus.

Tinnitus is usually described as a ringing in the ears, although it may also be perceived by the patient as roaring, sizzling, whistling, or humming. Although usually a subjective experience, tinnitus is occasionally objective and can be heard as a blowing sound or bruit by the examiner.

The intensity of tinnitus varies greatly from patient to patient. It is often slight and is noticed by the patient only at night when other sounds are minimal. At other times it can be loud and continuous to the point that some patients may even consider suicide. It can be intermittent or continuous and may be accompanied by a hearing loss. It may also be unilateral or bilateral.

Although the mechanism that produces tinnitus is not thoroughly understood, it can be a symptom of nearly all ear disorders. In many cases it is the first or only symptom of disease, and any patient complaining of tinnitus must have a thorough examination to determine the cause.

PATHOPHYSIOLOGY

As mentioned previously, the exact mechanism that causes tinnitus is obscure. However, it is known that tinnitus can be caused by a disturbance anywhere in the ear, as well as in the acoustic nerve, brainstem, or cortex (Fig. 7-17). Two disorders with tinnitus as a major symptom, Ménière's disease and acoustic neuroma, are discussed separately in this section.

External ear causes include obstruction of the canal by foreign bodies or cerumen; patients usually describe the sound as low pitched, muffled, and intermittent. These patients may perceive their own voices as having a hollow sound.

Most middle ear disorders can also cause tinnitus. Otosclerosis is usually accompanied by tinnitus, which is described by patients as a ringing or whistling. It is constant, and some patients may experience more than one sound. Infectious or inflammatory processes usually produce tinnitus, which is described as pulsating. This type of tinnitus usually ends when the infection is cleared.

Acoustic trauma caused by very loud noises frequently produces tinnitus of a high-pitched nature and may be associated with a temporary hearing loss. These symptoms should serve as a warning to the patient that the ears should be protected before future exposure to loud noises or a permanent hearing loss may result. The pitch of tinnitus in these patients is usually near the frequency where their hearing loss is the greatest.

Tinnitus is commonly caused by certain drugs. Quinine, salicylates, some diuretics, and aminoglycoside antibiotics frequently cause tinnitus and can also cause a hearing loss. These drugs damage the cochlea and the eighth cranial nerve; the tinnitus is usually high pitched and may or may not continue after the drug is stopped.

Other causes of tinnitus include anemia and hypotension. This tinnitus usually resolves when the underlying condition is corrected. Cardiovascular diseases, such as arteriosclerosis and hypertension, may also produce a tinnitus that may fluctuate with the patient's blood pressure.

Audible or objective tinnitus can also be heard by another person. Objective tinnitus is better understood, and the cause usually is easily diagnosed. If a patient complains of a blowing sound that coincides with respirations or complains of clicking sounds, the physician should suspect audible tinnitus, and may be able to hear

Fig. 7-17
Areas where tinnitus may occur.

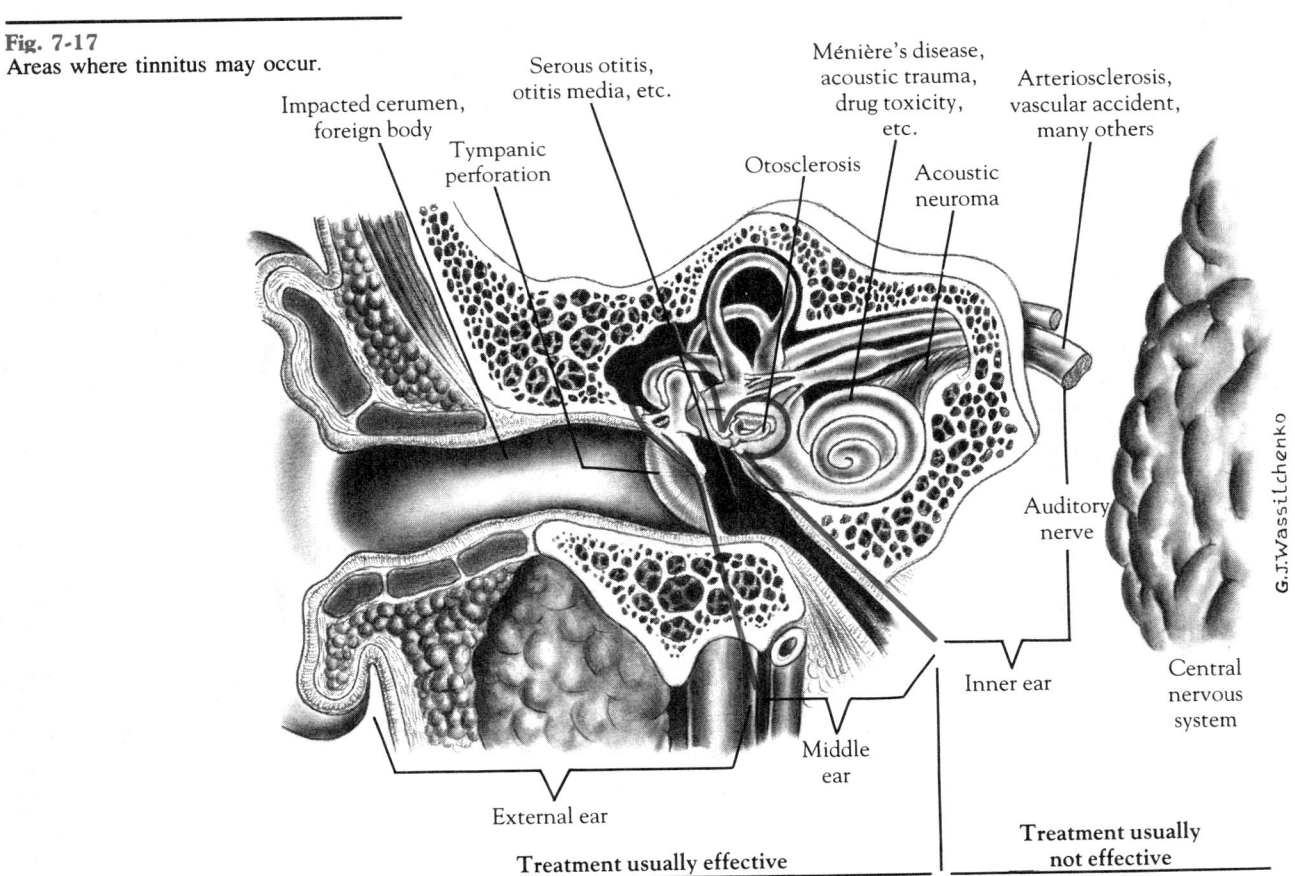

Impacted cerumen, foreign body

Serous otitis, otitis media, etc.

Ménière's disease, acoustic trauma, drug toxicity, etc.

Arteriosclerosis, vascular accident, many others

Tympanic perforation

Otosclerosis

Acoustic neuroma

Auditory nerve

Inner ear

Central nervous system

Middle ear

External ear

G.J.Wassilchenko

Treatment usually effective

Treatment usually not effective

it by placing an ear over the patient's ear or by placing a stethoscope over the patient's external auditory canal. An abnormally patent eustachian tube is usually the cause of blowing tinnitus, and this is quite annoying to patients. Luckily it may be of short duration, and patients can improve the condition somewhat by performing repeated Valsalva maneuvers to increase the negative pressure in the nasopharynx or equalize the pressure in the middle ear with the atmosphere. The clicking noises are fairly rare, are usually intermittent, and are produced by tetanic contractions of the muscles of the soft palate. The cause of this condition is unknown, but it is a reflex action, and the palate can be seen to contract, sometimes 175 to 200 times a minute. This is usually treated with injections of lidocaine on the involved side to disrupt the activity.

DIAGNOSTIC STUDIES

Audiology

Presence or absence of concurrent hearing loss; any diagnostic study may be performed to rule out the presence of systemic or ear diseases known to produce tinnitus

TREATMENT PLAN

Surgical

None, unless surgery is indicated for particular disorder that is found to be cause of tinnitus

Chemotherapeutic

Hypocholesterolemic agents
Nicotinic acid (Niacin), 50-200 mg po qd, to vasodilate blood vessels that supply inner ear; its efficacy is questionable
Antianxiety agents (used for sedative effect)
Diazepam (Valium), 5 mg po q4-6h
Anticonvulsants (used for sedative effect)
Carbamazepine (Tegretol), 200 mg po bid for 1 d, then maintenance dose of 800 mg-1.2 g qd
Phenytoin (Dilantin), 100 mg po tid
Primidone (Mysoline), 100-125 mg qd at bedtime for 3 d, then 250 mg tid or qid, and carbamazapine in combination; have helped in some cases, but exact mechanism is unknown

Supportive

Feedback helpful in some cases; radios or masking units to drown out tinnitus or to make it less noticeable to patient

ASSESSMENT: AREAS OF CONCERN

Auditory function

Patient describes sound in one or both ears as ringing, sizzling, whistling, roaring, humming, or hissing; may be intermittent or continuous; may be high pitched; history of acoustic trauma, that is, exposure to loud noise; history of ototoxic drugs; hearing may be normal to decreased

NURSING DIAGNOSES and NURSING INTERVENTIONS

Nursing Diagnosis	Nursing Intervention
Sensory-perceptual alteration: auditory	Encourage use of background noise, that is, radios or masking units to present a more pleasant noise. Ensure that use of any ototoxic substances is discontinued. Assist with any procedures necessary for diagnosis or treatment.

Patient Education

1. Inform the patient that tinnitus is usually a symptom of a systemic or ear disease and that a thorough examination should be performed.
2. Warn the patient against exposure to loud noises that may cause acoustic trauma.
3. Inform the patient about the ototoxic effects of some drugs. If the patient must take an ototoxic drug, be sure that periodic audiologic testing is performed to detect any hearing loss.

EVALUATION

Patient Outcome	Data Indicating That Outcome is Reached
Patient's understanding of cause of tinnitus is increased.	Patient verbalizes understanding of cause of tinnitus if known. Patient verbalizes understanding that tinnitus can be side effect of certain drugs. Patient understands that loud noises may be damaging and cause tinnitus and hearing loss. Patient verbalizes knowledge of various ways to diminish or minimize the tinnitus, that is, radios or masking units.

CHOANAL ATRESIA

Choanal atresia, which may be unilateral or bilateral, is an obstruction at the posterior end of the nose that blocks the passage to the pharynx.

Choanal atresia occurs in about 1 in 5000 births, is more common in boys than in girls, and occurs more often on the right side. There is thought to be some correlation with the presence of thyroid disease in the mother, which may cause interference with chromosomal separation during cell division.[39]

Other multiple anomalies may be present if a child is born with choanal atresia. Abnormalities may be present in 45% of the unilateral cases and in 60% of the bilateral cases, with the head, heart, and digestive system particularly affected.

PATHOPHYSIOLOGY

Choanal atresia is caused by failure of the embryologic "temporary" bucconasal membrane at the posterior end of each nasal sac to rupture when it should at about 40 days of fetal life. The obstruction may be bony or membranous and may be complete or incomplete.

If the atresia is unilateral, the infant may have almost no symptoms at birth, and the condition may remain undiagnosed for years. However, it usually causes a continuous, thick, viscid nasal discharge that occasionally becomes purulent. The child usually has a normal middle ear, eustachian tube function, and mastoid aeration.

Bilateral atresia is obvious at birth, since the infant has cyanosis and difficulty with respirations. The child cannot feed normally and chokes, although the symptoms are temporarily relieved when the infant cries. Some babies quickly begin oral breathing, but most do not and require the assistance of an oral airway.

DIAGNOSTIC STUDIES

Nasal roentgenograms
Will demonstrate a posterior blockage after radiopaque dye is injected

TREATMENT PLAN

Surgical
Operative removal of obstruction, usually through transpalatal approach

Electromechanical
Airway placed immediately after birth if atresia is bilateral and if infant is cyanotic and has respiratory difficulty

Supportive
Nutritional supplements provided by tube feedings if infant cannot feed normally

ASSESSMENT: AREAS OF CONCERN

Nasal obstruction
Unilateral
  Continuous, thick rhinorrhea; failure of catheter to enter pharynx when passed through obstructed side of nose

Respiratory function
Bilateral
  Cyanosis and respiratory difficulty at birth; child aspirates and cannot feed; no aeration or bubbling through nose

NURSING DIAGNOSES and NURSING INTERVENTIONS

Nursing Diagnosis	Nursing Intervention
Breathing pattern, ineffective	Observe infant at birth for presence of thick nasal discharge. If infant obviously has respiratory distress and is cyanotic, immediately place oral airway and continue to monitor child's respiratory status until obstruction can be removed surgically.
Injury, potential for	Tape oral airway in place so child can breathe orally until surgery is performed. Watch infant closely when feeding, since child will probably aspirate. Explain all procedures and rationale to baby's parents.
Nutrition, alteration in: less than body requirements	Ensure that infant receives adequate nutrition. Since baby cannot feed normally, be sure feeding tube is placed so infant can receive required number of calories.

Patient Education

1. Ensure that the parents learn about the child's disorder and the surgical procedure to correct it. Although the problem will be corrected before the baby is discharged, the parents must be aware of the potential problems with feedings and breathing, since they may assist in caring for the child before surgery.

EVALUATION

Patient Outcome	Data Indicating That Outcome is Reached
Respiratory function and feedings are normal.	Child breathes and feeds normally without distress. Child's weight is normal for age. There is no abnormal mucoid discharge.

EPISTAXIS

Epistaxis is bleeding from the nose caused by irritation, trauma, coagulation disorders, hypertension, or chronic infection.

Epistaxis is thought to have occurred at least once in over 10% of the normal population. It is either a primary disorder or secondary to another condition such as hemophilia or leukemia.

In children, who are twice as likely to have epistaxis as adults, the bleeding is usually mild and tends to originate from the anterior nasal septum. In adults bleeding is more likely to originate from the posterior septum so that the bleeding point is more difficult to locate and the bleeding may be profuse.[31] Epistaxis is more common in men than in women and occurs more frequently in winter, probably because of the dryness of the air.

Epistaxis is a frightening experience for the patient but generally looks and feels worse than it actually is. The blood is usually bright red and the patient may swallow some of it, producing an unpleasant sensation. Although adults can lose up to 1 L per hour during severe bleeding, the mortality is extremely low. When the patient bleeds enough to show signs of shock, the nosebleed usually stops because of low blood pressure. Some deaths are thought to have been caused by coronary ischemia from blood loss.[31]

PATHOPHYSIOLOGY

The most common cause of epistaxis is trauma to the nasal mucosa from damage by a foreign object, picking crusts from the nasal septum, or dryness of the nasal mucosa. Nosebleeds are fairly common in hypertensive patients and occur in patients with coagulation defects such as hemophilia, leukemia, and purpura. Infection, tumors, and some drugs and toxins may cause nosebleeds; in many instances, however, the cause is simply not identified or is considered idiopathic.

Children experience frequent nosebleeds from the anteroinferior part of the septum known as Little's area or Kiesselbach's plexus (Fig. 7-18). The etiology is not clear, but the area is richly vascular, and children have

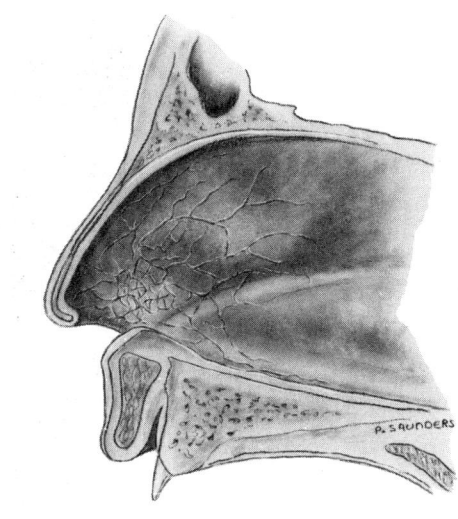

Fig. 7-18
Kiesselbach's plexus.

From DeWeese, D.D., and Saunders,
W.H.: Textbook of otolaryngology, ed. 6,
St. Louis, 1982, The C.V. Mosby Co.

hyperemic and congested upper respiratory tracts. Children also pick and rub their noses in the area where the mucosa is stretched over cartilage and bone.

Intractable nose picking is another cause of anterior nosebleeds. Some patients cannot stop picking their noses, either because of a nervous habit or because crusts are present from an earlier ulceration or perforation. Constant nose picking can cause septal ulceration or even a perforation, which leads to epistaxis.

A hereditary disease that is an unusual cause of epistaxis is Rendu-Osler-Weber disease or hemorrhagic hereditary telangiectasia. This disease is gene dominant and may be passed from either parent to a child of either sex. Epistaxis is usually the initial symptom, but telangiectasis is commonly found in other mucous membranes or anywhere on the external surface of the body. Bleeding usually occurs from the nose and gastrointestinal tract because mucosa in those areas is very fragile, whereas other areas have protective layers of squamous epithelium.

Most nosebleeds in the anterior part of the nose originate from Kiesselbach's plexus, the highly vascular network in the anterior nasal septum. Since the vessels are fairly small and easily accessible, these nosebleeds are the easiest to treat. If bleeding is from the posterior part of the nose, the exact source of bleeding is more difficult to locate, since it is sometimes impossible to see and bleeding is more profuse. Usually just one source on one side of the nose bleeds, although bleeding frequently originates from both sides in patients with blood dyscrasias.

DIAGNOSTIC STUDIES

Hematocrit, hemoglobin, platelets, prothrombin time, partial thromboplastin time, reticulocyte count, and differential
    Done to rule out coagulation defect; results usually normal; bleeding from other parts of body likely in patients with hematologic disorders

TREATMENT PLAN

Surgical
    Arterial ligation if proper packing fails to control nosebleed
    Septal dermoplasty for Rendu-Osler-Weber disease—skin graft is placed in nose to cover anterior parts of septum and floor and walls of nose anteriorly to provide protective covering over fragile mucosa

Chemotherapeutic
    Fibrinolytics
        Vitamin K (Aquamephyton), 10 mg po or IM qd; useful in some cases of epistaxis, but packing remains therapy of choice
    Anti-infective agents
        Penicillin, 1-5 million units IV q6h recommended for infection prevention because packing obstructs drainage of paranasal sinuses

Electromechanical
    Nosebleed from anterior part of nose
        Easiest to treat; source of bleeding located, and clots and fresh blood aspirated with suction; cotton ball saturated with 1:1000 epinephrine inserted into bleeding nostril, and strong pressure applied to compress cotton ball against septum for several minutes; after cotton ball is removed, cauterization performed by means of silver nitrate or electric cautery; packing unnecessary if bleeding is controlled with cauterization; pressure alone may control bleeding
    Intractable nose picking
        Both sides of nose packed with antibiotic-saturated cotton ball and nose taped completely shut for 7 to 10 days to facilitate healing of mucous membranes
    Epistaxis from posterior part of nose
        Postnasal packing: with patient sitting to prevent aspiration of blood, bleeding site located by ad-

Fig. 7-19
Postnasal packing for epistaxis.

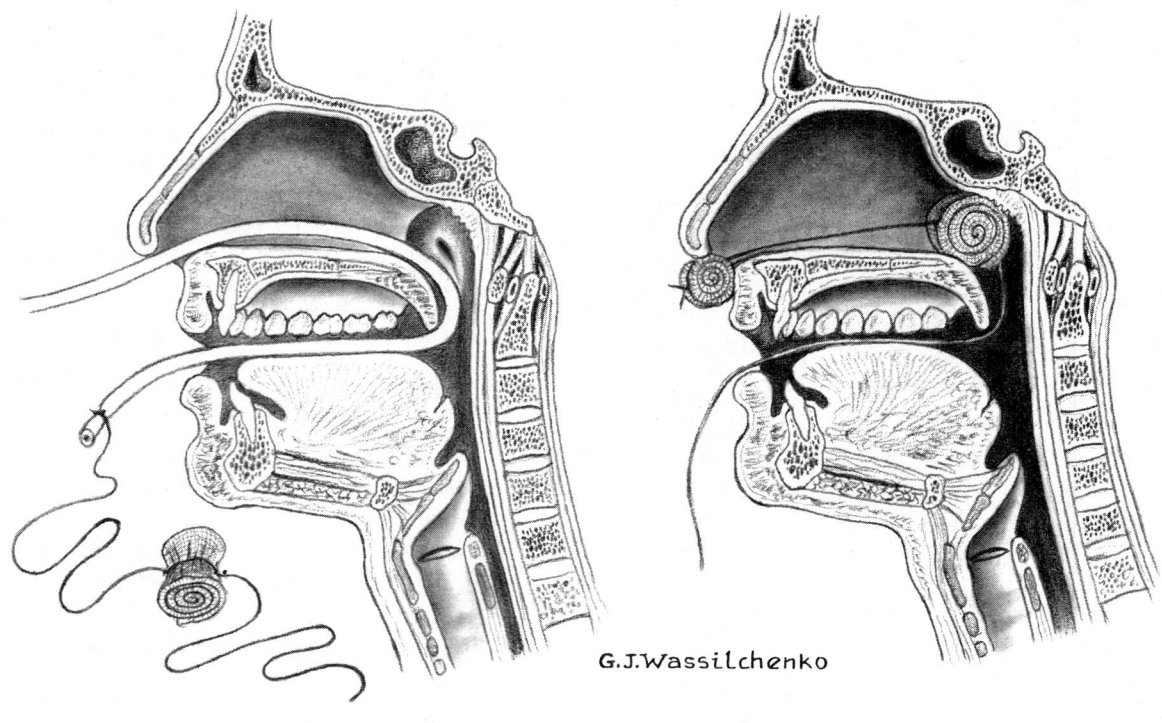

G.J.Wassilchenko

vancing strong suction tip until nose fills with blood when suction tip has passed; large postnasal pack introduced through mouth by attaching it to catheter that is inserted into nostril and out mouth (Fig. 7-19); catheter pulled through nose, lodging pack in posterior part of nose and providing compression to bleeding site; packing remains in place 48 to 96 hours; if both choanae occluded because of large size of pack, patient must be checked daily for ear or eustachian tube symptoms; patient will have some difficulty swallowing

ASSESSMENT: AREAS OF CONCERN

Nasal bleeding
Bright red blood comes from the nares; patient may also swallow or expectorate blood; history of trauma, nose picking, hypertension, or other known cause; inspection of anterior part of nose with the patient seated and using bright light (if bleeding spot seen, treatment may begin; if patient continues to swallow blood and no source is located, bleeding may be from posterior source); examination of patient's body for bruises or petechiae that may indicate underlying hematologic disorder

NURSING DIAGNOSES and NURSING INTERVENTIONS

Nursing Diagnosis	Nursing Intervention
Fear	Reassure patient that amount of blood lost looks worse than it probably is. Encourage patient not to swallow blood. Have patient breathe through mouth. Have basin nearby for patient to expectorate blood.

Nursing Diagnosis	Nursing Intervention
Airway clearance, ineffective: potential	Elevate head of bed or have patient sit to prevent aspiration of blood. Pinch patient's nostrils together for 5 to 10 minutes to compress soft portion of nostril against septum. Apply ice or cold compress to nose to help stop bleeding. Notify patient's physician. Assist with packing if necessary. If nasal packing is in place, encourage fluids and provide frequent oral hygiene to decrease mucosal dryness, since patient will be breathing through mouth. Inspect oropharynx for presence of blood.
Tissue perfusion, alteration in: cerebral, cardiopulmonary	Monitor patient's vital signs and level of consciousness. Record color and amount of blood loss.

Patient Education

1. Inform the patient of the inherent dangers in nose picking.
2. Inform the patient and family of the dangers of inserting foreign objects into the nose.
3. Encourage the patient and family to seek medical assistance immediately if nasal infection or epistaxis occurs.
4. If epistaxis is from dryness of mucous membranes, inform the patient about possible benefits of using a humidifier or vaporizer to provide additional humidity in the home, especially during the winter months.

EVALUATION

Patient Outcome	Data Indicating That Outcome is Reached
Epistaxis is well controlled.	Bleeding is absent. Patient's hematocrit value and hemoglobin level are normal. Mucous membranes are healed if bleeding is from picking or ulceration. Patient verbalizes understanding of cause of epistaxis, if known, and ways to prevent bleeding in future.

NASAL FRACTURES

A nasal fracture is a traumatic injury to the nasal bones, resulting in discontinuity of the tissues of the bone.

Nasal fractures occur quite commonly and more often than fractures of the other facial bones. However, when nasal fractures are diagnosed, it is essential to rule out fractures of associated facial bones such as zygomatic or mandibular fractures, since facial injuries or trauma may also damage these bones.

Even a nasal fracture that appears simple usually has associated damage to the mucosal lining of the nose. If a patient has suffered a facial trauma that causes epistaxis, damage to the bone-cartilage structures of the nose is likely.

PATHOPHYSIOLOGY

A nasal fracture occasionally occurs in the birth canal during delivery. These are usually of the "greenstick" type, and the baby's nose inclines slightly to one side. The nose can be grasped at the tip and pulled toward the midline to realign it in these cases.

Nasal fractures can be classified as unilateral, bilateral, or complex. A unilateral fracture may produce little or no displacement and may appear as a simple crack on a roentgenogram. Bilateral fractures, which are the most common, may be caused by a "right cross" blow that pushes both nasal bones to one side or by a frontal blow that depresses the nasal bones and gives a flattened look to the nose. The entire nose may be deviated, and the nose may have a C or S deformity.

Complex fractures are usually a result of powerful frontal blows that may shatter the nasal pyramid and frequently the frontal bones as well, causing a marked depression of the nasal and facial bones.

The usual findings are epistaxis, a noticeable facial deformity, and a history of trauma. Edema occurs quickly at the injury site and depending on the severity may include periorbital swelling. Ecchymosis is common, the nose is exquisitely tender, and nasal obstruction occasionally occurs. Complex fractures of the nose and face may result in diplopia or subscleral hemorrhage.

DIAGNOSTIC STUDIES

Roentgenograms of face and nose
Show fractures and depressed areas of facial and nasal bones

TREATMENT PLAN

Surgical
Reduction and fixation of the fractures as quickly as possible after injury (within first 3 to 4 days) because fragments tend to stabilize quickly; bilateral nasal packing usually done during surgery to maintain stability and position of nasal structure; wiring or splinting may be required for complex fractures

Chemotherapeutic
Narcotic analgesics or analgesic/antipyretics
Acetaminophen (Tylenol), 325-650 mg q4-6h
Acetylsalicylic acid (aspirin) with codeine, po q4h prn

Electromechanical
Simple thumb pressure on convex side of the nose occasionally enough to push bones back together

ASSESSMENT: AREAS OF CONCERN

Facial swelling
Deformity; ecchymosis; epistaxis; nose very tender; history of trauma to face and nose; possible accompanying lacerations; possible bony crepitus; if leak of cerebrospinal fluid is present, clear fluid dripping from nose and ears

Respiratory status
Difficulty in breathing; mouth breathing

NURSING DIAGNOSES and NURSING INTERVENTIONS

Nursing Diagnosis	Nursing Intervention
Comfort, alteration in: pain	Provide adequate analgesia for pain relief; assess and document effectiveness.
Breathing pattern, ineffective	Observe for shortness of breath, dyspnea from nasal obstruction, or difficulty in swallowing.
	Apply ice to face and nose to minimize swelling and bleeding without pressure to nose.
	Monitor amount and color of epistaxis and record.
	Keep head of bed elevated.
	Prevent patient from swallowing blood or aspirating; encourage patient to breathe through mouth.
	Have basin nearby for patient to expectorate blood.
	Provide frequent oral hygiene and encourage intake of oral fluids.
	Monitor vital signs and level of consciousness.
Sensory-perceptual alteration: visual	Observe for eye swelling; apply ice to minimize edema.
	Observe for scleral hemorrhage and periorbital edema.
	If eyes are not completely closed, assess patient's ability to see.

EVALUATION

Patient Outcome	Data Indicating That Outcome is Reached
Nasal fracture is well healed.	There is no facial deformity. There is no nasal obstruction; patient can breathe normally through nose. Sclera is clear without redness or swelling.

NASAL POLYPS

Polyps are benign growths that appear as soft, pale gray, nontender masses and gradually form from recurrent localized swelling of the sinuses or nasal mucosa (Fig. 7-20).

Polyps are seen in about 90% of patients with chronic maxillary sinusitis. Polyps may become quite large, are usually bilateral, occur in multiples, and may cause actual distention and enlargement of the bony structures of the nose. Even after surgical removal, nasal polyps tend to recur. Although rare in children, polyps are occasionally found in children with cystic fibrosis and allergies and in those with Peutz-Jeghers syndrome, the symptoms of which include pigmented spots on the skin, especially around the mouth, and polyposis of the gastrointestinal tract.

PATHOPHYSIOLOGY

The etiology of nasal polyps is not totally clear. It is accepted that they are a common consequence of aller-gies, and they are thought to be produced by pressure resulting from prolonged edema of the nasal and sinus mucous membranes. One theory is that this pressure causes the epithelium to rupture, forming a small polyp. Mucous glands then grow from the epithelium that forms the polyp. The volume of the polyp increases, from gravity as well as from congestion of its vascular stalk. In a 1973 study,[39] a large number of patients with nasal polyps were studied. Only 28% of the patients had allergies; the rest probably had chronic infection as the cause of their polyps.

Polyps are usually found in the middle meatus near the openings of the sinuses and occasionally in the roof of the nose. They are never found on the septum or in the lower meatus; the reason for this is not known.

Patients with bronchial asthma frequently have nasal polyps that may be part of a disorder of the entire respiratory tract. An interesting phenomenon that occurs in some patients with asthma and nasal polyposis is an intolerance to aspirin, indomethacin, and some coal tar dyes. This intolerance is severe and can cause respiratory

Fig. 7-20
Nasal polyps.

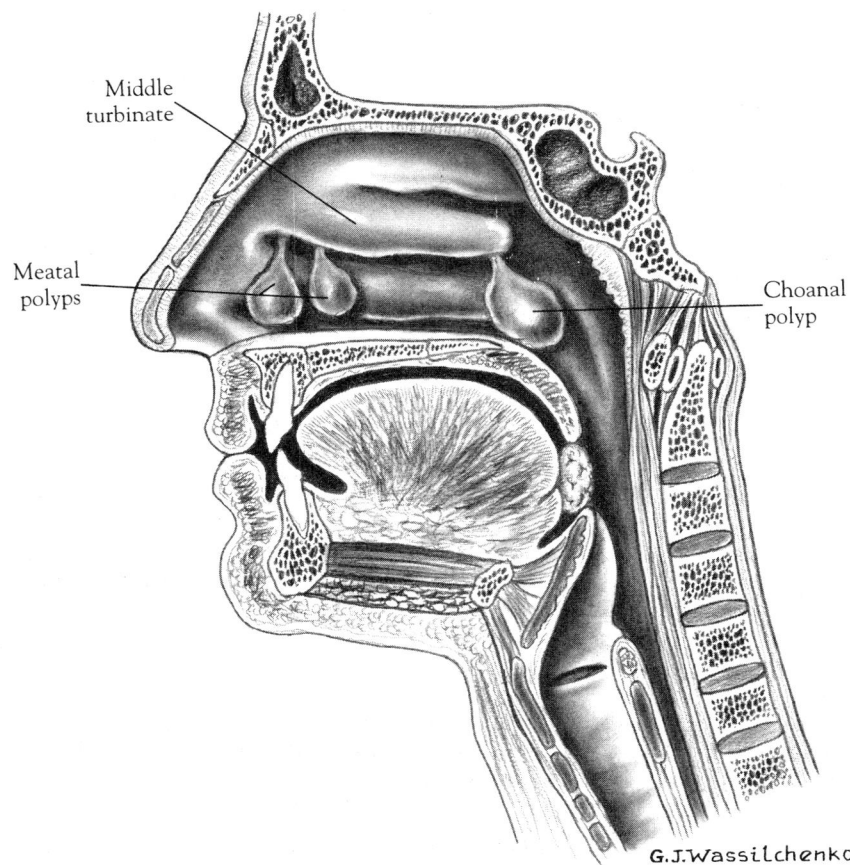

Middle turbinate

Meatal polyps

Choanal polyp

G.J.Wassilchenko

arrest if these substances are ingested. The reason for this is unclear but is thought to be related to the inhibitory action of these substances on prostaglandin synthesis.[39]

DIAGNOSTIC STUDIES

Roentgenograms of sinuses
  Shadows over affected areas

TREATMENT PLAN

Surgical
  Polypectomy—each polyp avulsed with wire snare
  Caldwell-Luc procedure—may be performed if polyps are caused by chronic maxillary sinusitis

Chemotherapeutic
  Corticosteroids
    Betamethasone (Celestone), 0.6-4.8 mg qd, will cause polyps to disappear
    Cortisone not recommended for long-term use; local sprays such as beclomethasone (Vanceril Inhaler) may be useful, since they are effective in treating asthma (0.1 mg/spray, 2 sprays in each nostril bid or tid)
  Antihistamines (to treat allergy symptoms)
    Chlorpheniramine (Chlor-Trimetron), 4 mg po q4-6h as needed for adults; 0.35 mg/kg qd in divided doses for children
  Adrenergic agents (for antihistamine effect)
    Pseudoephedrine (Sudafed), 30 mg po q4-6h prn for adults
  Anti-infective agents
    Agent-specific antibiotics if infection is present

ASSESSMENT: AREAS OF CONCERN

Nasal obstruction
  Feeling of fullness in face or nose; shortness of breath; nasal discharge; anosmia; other symptoms of allergic rhinitis, such as sneezing, watery eyes, eczema, and asthma; grayish growths visible on examination with nasal speculum

NURSING DIAGNOSES and NURSING INTERVENTIONS

Nursing Diagnosis	Nursing Intervention
Breathing pattern, ineffective	After polypectomy, prevent bleeding, elevate head of bed, and apply ice compresses to nose to minimize swelling and bleeding.
	Change nasal drip pad as indicated and record amount and consistency of drainage.
	Encourage patient not to swallow blood or secretions but to expectorate into basin.
	Monitor patient's vital signs.
	Instruct patient not to blow nose.
	Convalescent care: Observe for bleeding, especially after packing has been removed (1 to 2 days after surgery).
	If patient is still hospitalized, notify physician, elevate head of bed, check vital signs, and compress outside of nose against septum.
	If bleeding persists, pack if necessary.
Sensory-perceptual alteration: olfactory	Assure patient that sense of smell should return postoperatively after packing is removed and swelling is decreased.

Patient Education

1. Ensure that the patient knows how to reach the physician immediately if bleeding begins after the patient has been discharged.
2. Instruct the patient with allergies to avoid known allergens if possible and to take antihistamines early to minimize allergic reactions.
3. Instruct the patient to use nose drops and sprays cautiously because of the rebound effect on the mucous membranes.

EVALUATION

Patient Outcome	Data Indicating That Outcome is Reached
Patient's knowledge of polyps is increased.	Patient verbalizes understanding of possible causes and ways to prevent recurrence of nasal polyps. Patient seeks early treatment for sinusitis or minimizes severity of allergies by taking antihistamines.
Patient's recovery from polypectomy is unremarkable.	There is no bleeding, nasal obstruction, shortness of breath, or anosmia after surgery.

SEPTAL DEVIATION AND PERFORATION

A deviated septum is a shift of the septum from the midline, which is common in many adults.

Although the septum is usually straight at birth, it may shift from one side to another as a result of trauma or injury.

A septal perforation is a hole in the nasal septum between the nostrils, which is usually in the anterior or cartilaginous septum but may occasionally occur in the bony septum. A small perforation, which can be caused by infections, nasal crusting, or nose picking, is often asymptomatic, although a slight whistle may be heard as the patient breathes. Larger perforations may produce rhinitis, nasal crusting, or epistaxis.

PATHOPHYSIOLOGY

As previously mentioned, the nasal septum is usually straight. The septum is occasionally bent during the trauma of birth, and the infant may have a twisted-appearing nose. This can usually be corrected when first noticed by placing light pressure on the convex side of the nose. There is no need for packing or a splint.

With aging, the septum has a tendency to become deviated or to form a hump. There is frequently no history of injury to account for the deviation. As a result, few adults have a totally straight septum. Trauma during the growth years may also contribute to septal deviation.

Although there are frequently no symptoms associated with a deviated septum, some patients experience moderate to severe degrees of nasal obstruction. Other, less well-defined symptoms include headaches, which are found in some patients who have a septal spur impinging on the inferior turbinate; epistaxis; and symptoms of sinusitis, which are rare but may be influenced by a deviated septum that obstructs a sinus opening.

Septal perforations may be small or large; they may be asymptomatic or cause annoying symptoms such as crusting, a watery discharge, or a whistling noise as the patient breathes. Small perforations are usually caused by repeated irritation of the nose, such as picking it. Less frequent causes are repeated cauterizations because of epistaxis, snorting cocaine, and chronic nasal infections. Although once quite common, perforations resulting from syphilis and tuberculosis are now infrequently found.

DIAGNOSTIC STUDIES

Facial roentgenograms, examination with otoscope
Show a shift of the septum

TREATMENT PLAN

Surgical
For deviation
Submucous resection—may be performed to reposition septum and relieve nasal obstruction
Rhinoplasty—may be done to correct nasal structure deformity
Septoplasty to replace septum in midline—may be done to relieve nasal obstruction and to enhance external appearance of nose
For perforation
Bilateral nasal packs—used for 24 to 48 hours to hold mucosa and septum in place
Surgical closure—possible but not always successful; a Silastic "button" prosthesis may be inserted to close perforation[9]

Chemotherapeutic
Analgesic/antipyretics
Acetylsalicylic acid (aspirin), 600 mg po q4-6h to relieve headache if present (for deviation)
Antihistamines (to decrease secretions and congestion)
Chlorpheniramine (Chlor-Trimeton), 4 mg po q4-

6h for adults; 0.35 mg/kg qd in divided doses for children

Adrenergic agents

Pseudoephedrine (Sudafed), 30 mg po q4-6h for adults (for perforation)

Anti-infective agents

Antibiotics topically applied to prevent infection; bacitracin (Baciquent), 500 units/g in petrolatum base

Supportive

Local application of lanolin or petrolatum to prevent crusting (for perforation)

Packing to control bleeding if present (for deviation)

ASSESSMENT: AREAS OF CONCERN

Nasal obstruction

Irregularities or deformity of external nose; examination with bright light and nasal speculum shows septal deviation from midline, which is sometimes S shaped with a greatly reduced airway; feeling of facial fullness, headaches, epistaxis, or sinusitis

NURSING DIAGNOSES and NURSING INTERVENTIONS

Nursing Diagnosis	Nursing Intervention
Breathing pattern, ineffective	Postoperative care includes explanation to patient that facial and periorbital edema will be present and that nasal packing will be in place for 24 to 48 hours. Instruct patient to breathe through mouth during this time.
Skin integrity, impairment of	To prevent edema and promote drainage, keep head of bed slightly elevated. Use ice packs on face to decrease edema, pain, and bleeding. Use cool vaporizer to assist in liquifying secretions. Point out that patient will experience difficulty swallowing while nasal packs are in place. Change drip pad as necessary, recording color, consistency, and amount of drainage. Provide meticulous mouth care, since the patient is breathing through mouth.
Injury: potential for	Assess and report presence of excessive bleeding, swallowing, or purulent drainage. Caution patient against blowing nose, which may cause bruising and edema. Caution patient not to smoke for at least 2 days and to limit physical activity for 2 to 3 days.

Patient Education

1. To prevent tissue trauma, remind the patient not to smoke or blow the nose.
2. Remind the patient to avoid overexertion at home for several days.

EVALUATION

Patient Outcome	Data Indicating That Outcome is Reached
Nasal obstruction is lessened.	The patient breathes comfortably. There is no epistaxis, headache, or infection. If the septum was perforated, the area is well healed without evidence of infection.

SINUSITIS

Sinusitis is an inflammatory process producing changes in the mucosa of a sinus that are caused by bacterial, viral, or allergic conditions.

Frequently blamed for symptoms such as headaches or nasal problems, sinusitis is actually present in fewer than 10 of every 100 patients who consult an otolaryngologist. The types of sinusitis are acute, subacute, and chronic suppurative; allergic; and hyperplastic.

The changes in the sinus mucosa caused by sinusitis produce definite signs and symptoms, most of which can be assessed during physical examination or on roentgenograms.

An attack of sinusitis frequently follows a common cold as infection spreads from the nasal passages to the sinuses; excessive or forceful nose blowing may also force infected material into the sinuses. Since the sinuses normally drain secretions through their normal routes into the meatus, any condition that obstructs these openings and forces the secretions to back up into the sinuses may cause an infection to occur there. These conditions may include the presence of nasal polyps, a deviated nasal septum, or edema of the turbinates resulting from an allergic disorder.

The maxillary sinus (antrum) is the one most frequently affected with acute sinusitis, although the entire anterior group of sinuses may be involved. These are the maxillary, frontal, and anterior and middle ethmoid, all of which drain into the middle meatus of the nose. The posterior group of sinuses, the posterior ethmoid and sphenoid, are usually affected with chronic sinusitis only when the anterior group is also involved.

The prognosis for sinusitis is usually good with identification and treatment if necessary, but some complications may result from sinusitis if the infection spreads. These include septicemia, periorbital abscesses, brain abscesses, and osteomyelitis.

Regardless of the type of sinusitis, patients should avoid cold, damp conditions and maintain a constant room temperature and humidity. Air conditioning aggravates sinusitis as does smoking, since smoke irritates the mucous membranes and inhibits their normal self-cleansing ciliary action.

PATHOPHYSIOLOGY

Acute suppurative sinusitis follows a common cold or may be caused endemically by a specific organism after a sudden drop in temperature. In addition, during swimming or diving, infected water may be forced into the nose and cause a bacterial infection.

Bacteria that are commonly responsible include gram-positive cocci, such as *Streptococcus*, *Staphylococcus*, and *Pneumococcus*, and *H. influenzae*. Others are less commonly responsible.

Swimming and diving may cause an acute onset of sinusitis; otherwise there is a gradual onset of symptoms as the involved sinus becomes more inflamed. The nasal mucosa appears red and swollen, and purulent discharge is obvious in the middle meatus. The discharge becomes more copious, may be blood tinged in the first 24 to 48 hours, and may cause an inflamed, sore throat from the postnasal discharge. As fluid fills the sinuses, they become opaque to transillumination and an actual fluid level may be seen on roentgenograms of the sinus.

Pain varies from low-grade to intense as the oxygen in the sinus is absorbed into the blood vessels. This creates negative pressure in the sinus and allows it to be filled with transudate, which produces a painful positive pressure. Tenderness is also present over the involved sinus.

Most cases of acute sinusitis are cured with conservative treatment; antibiotics are unnecessary. Purulent secretions are present for 3 to 4 days and then slowly resolve over the next 10 days to 2 weeks. In a few cases, however, a purulent nasal discharge persists, and the patient may continue to complain of nasal congestion and vague discomfort over the sinuses or face. This is classified as subacute sinusitis. These patients may have persistent pus in the nose for more than 3 weeks after the acute infection. Since antibiotic therapy may be needed, a culture of the exudate should be done and roentgenograms taken to determine if more than one sinus is involved.

Patients with persistent subacute sinus infections may have an allergy; recognition of this will obviously aid in treatment.

If sinus infections are neglected or if a patient has repeated attacks, the mucosal lining of the sinus may become permanently damaged. This is known as chronic suppurative sinusitis. Often the only symptom is continued purulent nasal discharge. If a patient seems unable to overcome the infection, the physician must evaluate the patient for systemic conditions that may lower resistance to infection, such as anemia, malnutrition, or hypometabolism.

Allergic sinusitis occurs only in conjunction with allergic rhinitis. The symptoms are the same, and the sinus mucosa undergoes the same changes as the nasal mucosa. Patients with allergic rhinitis probably also have allergic sinusitis; polyps, which are common with allergic rhinitis, also occur with regularity in the mucosal lining of the sinuses.

Purulent sinusitis superimposed on allergic rhinitis and sinusitis is called hyperplastic sinusitis. The lining of the mucosa and submucosa becomes chronically thickened, and nasal polyps tend to form and recur even after surgical removal. These polyps may block the natural openings to the meatus and obstruct drainage of purulent material. Tissue swelling remains severe, and the nasal tissue does not respond to the usual shrinking solutions. The nose feels plugged most of the time, and a frontal headache is common.

DIAGNOSTIC STUDIES

Transillumination

Examiner shines bright light in patient's mouth with lips closed around bulb; involved sinus appears dark whereas normal sinus transilluminates

Sinus roentgenograms

Involved sinuses appear clouded or actual fluid level may be seen (Fig. 7-21)

TREATMENT PLAN

Surgical

For maxillary sinusitis

Creation of nasal window—to open sinus and allow pus and secretions to drain through nose

Caldwell-Luc procedure (radical antrum operation) through incision under upper lip to remove diseased mucosa and periosteum

For chronic ethmoid sinusitis

Ethmoidectomy—to remove infected tissue through incision into ethmoid sinus

For chronic frontal sinusitis

Creation of osteoplastic flap—involves incision across skull and behind hairline to drain sinuses

Frontoethmoidectomy—allows removal of infected frontal sinus tissue through external ethmoidectomy

For sphenoid sinusitis

External ethmoidectomy—performed through incision that begins under eyebrow and extends along side of nose, allowing removal of infected sinus tissue

Chemotherapeutic

Narcotic analgesics (used to relieve headache from acute sinusitis)

Codeine, 30-60 mg po q4-6h

Meperidine (Demerol), 50 mg po q4-6h

Antihistamines (used to decrease secretions and congestion)

Fig. 7-21
Sinus films showing clouding and fluid level from sinusitis.

From DeWeese, D.D., and Saunders, W.H.: Textbook of otolaryngology, ed. 6, St. Louis, 1982, The C.V. Mosby Co.

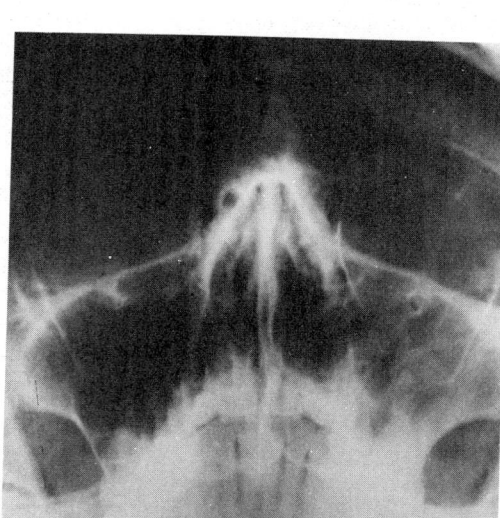

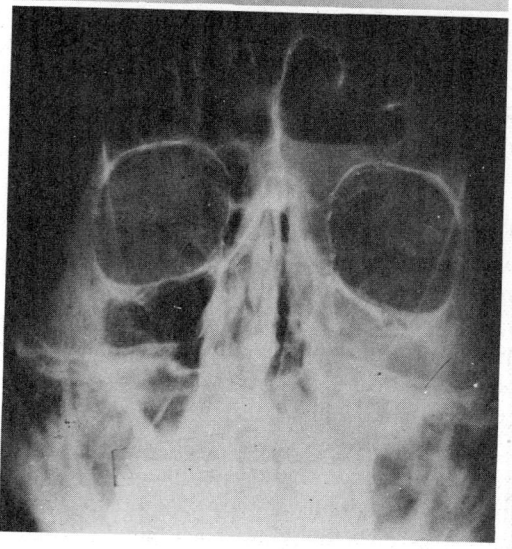

Azatadine (Optimine), 1 or 2 mg po q12h

Adrenergic agents

Pseudoephedrine (Sudafed), 30 mg po q4-6h prn for adults

Anti-infective agents

Penicillin G or V, 250 mg po q6h

Erythromycin (E-Mycin), 250 mg po q6h

Ampicillin, 250 mg po q6h (for chronic sinusitis)

Tetracycline, 250 mg po q6h (for chronic sinusitis)

Aerosol bacitracin (for chronic sinusitis)

Vasoconstrictors

Nose drops or nasal spray containing vasoconstrictor to keep the nose open; Afrin (1 spray in each nostril q12h) is commonly prescribed

Electromechanical

Drainage of involved sinus if usual therapy fails

Antral puncture (puncture of medial wall of maxillary sinus) to provide means of irrigation (may also be done to collect specimen for diagnosis)

Proetz displacement method—used infrequently now; was more common before antibiotics; with one side of nose occluded, physician creates and releases vacuum and replaces pus in sinus with thin fluid

Supportive

Steam inhalation to encourage drainage and promote vasoconstriction

Hot, wet packs applied locally for relief of pain and congestion at least four times a day

ASSESSMENT: AREAS OF CONCERN

Acute sinusitis

Malaise; anorexia; nasal congestion; purulent nasal discharge; cough; sore throat; fever, usually low-grade; pain over sinus areas that worsens as patient lowers head; pressure over involved areas and upper teeth; orbital or facial edema; constant, severe headaches; enlarged turbinates; pus apparent in nasal cavity and nasopharynx when examined with nasopharyngeal mirror

Subacute sinusitis

Stuffy nose; vague intermittent discomfort in involved areas; fatigue; pus in nose more than 3 weeks after acute infection; nonproductive cough

Chronic sinusitis

Continued purulent nasal discharge; occasional slight headache (from edema of nasal tissue or allergic rhinitis, and not from sinuses) that is worse in the morning and relieved slightly during the day

Allergic sinusitis

Nasal stuffiness; symptoms of allergic rhinitis: watery eyes, eczema, and asthma; itching and burning of nose; sneezing; frontal headache; thin nasal discharge; presence of nasal polyps

Hyperplastic sinusitis

Severe tissue edema; mucosal polyps; thickened mucosal lining of sinuses; poor response of nasal tissue to shrinking solutions; low-grade frontal headache

NURSING DIAGNOSES and NURSING INTERVENTIONS

Nursing Diagnosis	Nursing Intervention
Comfort, alteration in: pain	Encourage bed rest with head of bed slightly elevated to promote drainage of secretions. In collaboration with physician, give analgesics and antihistamines as needed for relief. Assess and document effectiveness. Administer antibiotics if ordered. Apply warm, moist compresses locally at least four times a day for pain relief and promotion of drainage. Monitor vital signs, especially temperature. Watch for and report increase in headaches, blurred vision, periorbital edema, chills, or vomiting.
Sensory-perceptual alteration: olfactory	Administer antihistamines and nose drops or spray to relieve nasal congestion in collaboration with physician. Reassure patient that condition is temporary.
Sleep pattern disturbance	To minimize headaches, give analgesic medications per physician's orders before patient goes to bed; administer antihistamines or nose drops at bedtime to clear nasal passages. Make sure that patient understands importance of using nose drops as prescribed because of rebound effect on mucous membranes if they are used over long period of time.
Breathing pattern, ineffective (potential)	Inform patient before surgery that nasal packing will be in place for 12 to 48 hours and that breathing through the mouth will be necessary and nose blowing cannot be performed postoperatively.

Nursing Diagnosis	Nursing Intervention
Potential patient problem: bleeding after surgery	Observe patient for bleeding after surgery. Monitor vital signs and watch for frequent swallowing, which may indicate hemorrhaging and swallowing of blood.
Skin integrity, impairment of	Place patient in semi-Fowler's position to prevent edema and promote drainage. Use iced compresses to minimize swelling and bleeding for first 24 hours. Apply cool or warm vapor inhalations as ordered. Provide meticulous mouth care, since patient will be breathing through mouth and may have copious bloody secretions. Change dressing or nasal drip pad and record amount and color of drainage. (There will normally be small amounts of bright red blood with some clots.) Inform patient that some numbness of upper lip and teeth may be present after Caldwell-Luc procedure and that black eye and some swelling of operative area are not uncommon for about a week after sinus surgery. Instruct patient not to brush teeth in this area during this time.

Patient Education

1. Instruct the patient not to smoke for 2 to 3 days after surgery to minimize irritation of the mucous membranes.
2. Tell the patient to watch for bleeding after the nasal packing is removed and to notify the physician immediately if it occurs.
3. Instruct the patient about the early signs and symptoms of sinusitis so prompt treatment can be sought.

EVALUATION

Patient Outcome	Data Indicating That Outcome is Reached
There are no signs or symptoms of sinusitis.	There is no headache, nasal congestion, or purulent discharge.
There are no surgical complications if a procedure was performed.	There is no excessive bleeding or postoperative infection; the wound is completely healed.
Patient's knowledge of sinusitis is increased.	Patient verbalizes understanding of causative factors of sinusitis, signs and symptoms of infection, and when to seek medical assistance.

ABSCESSES

Throat abscesses are infections in the fascial spaces.

The most common throat abscesses are peritonsillar (quinsy), retropharyngeal, and pharyngomaxillary. These abscesses form after tonsillitis or an infection of the upper respiratory tract. A peritonsillar abscess forms in the space between the tonsil and the fascia that covers the superior constrictor muscle; a retropharyngeal abscess forms between the posterior pharyngeal wall and the prevertebral fascia; and a pharyngomaxillary abscess forms in the deep space between the fascia of the parotid gland, the internal pterygoid muscle, and the superior constrictor muscle (Fig. 7-22).

PATHOPHYSIOLOGY

A peritonsillar abscess usually forms after a patient has had tonsillitis for a few days and appears to improve. Usually caused by group A β-hemolytic streptococci or occasionally anaerobic organisms, peritonsillar abscesses are rare in children but fairly common in young adults.

Retropharyngeal abscesses are found almost exclusively in infants and young children because the lymph nodes in the retropharyngeal space have usually disappeared by young adulthood. These are usually found as complications of infections in the pharynx, sinuses, adenoids, or ears that have spread to the retropharyngeal lymph nodes.

Fig. 7-22
A, Retropharyngeal abscess. **B,**
Pharyngomaxillary space infection.

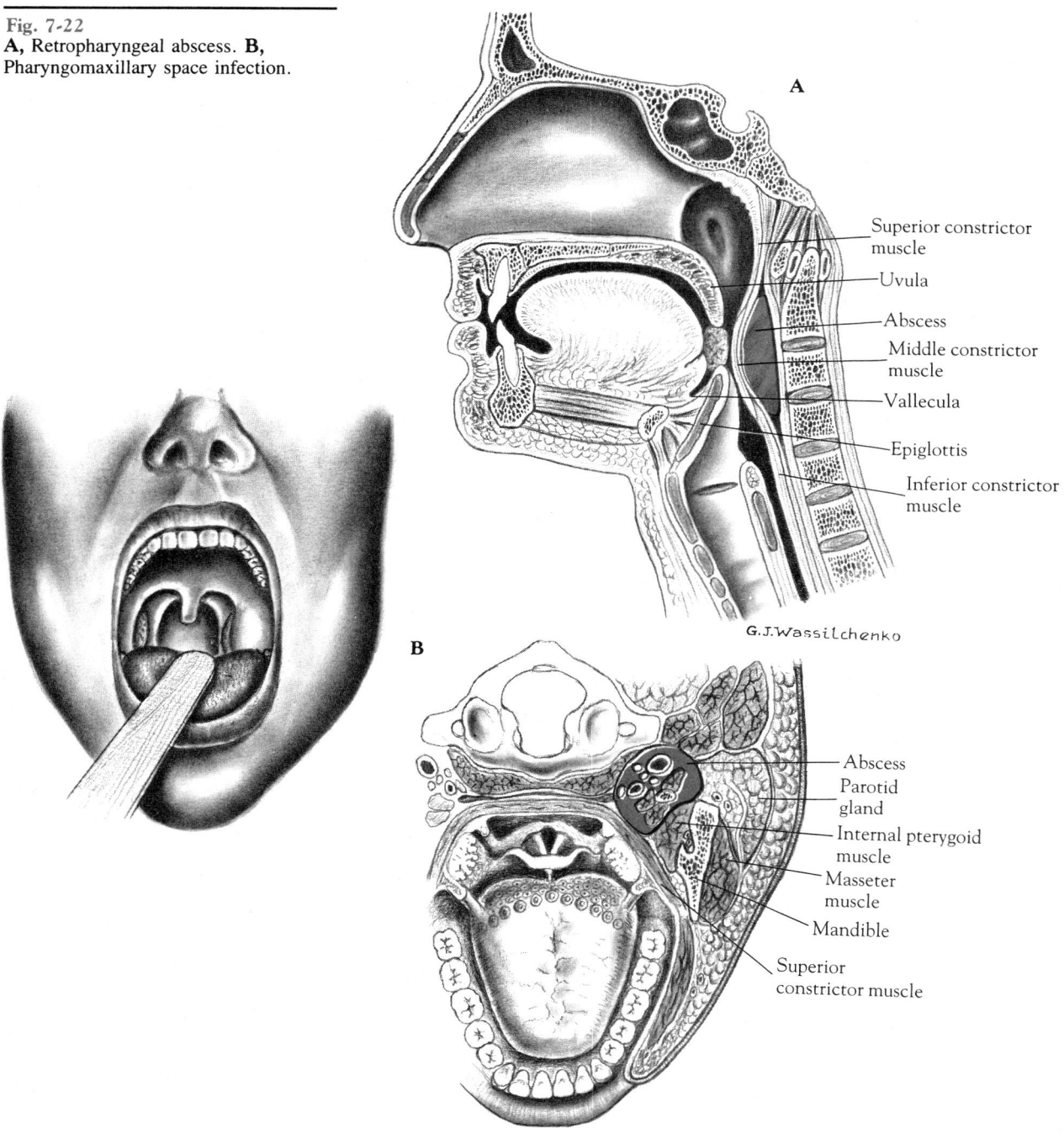

A

Superior constrictor
muscle

Uvula

Abscess

Middle constrictor
muscle

Vallecula

Epiglottis

Inferior constrictor
muscle

G.J.Wassilchenko

B

Abscess
Parotid
gland

Internal pterygoid
muscle

Masseter
muscle

Mandible

Superior
constrictor muscle

Pott's disease, or tuberculosis of the cervical spine, can also cause a ''cold'' retropharyngeal abscess that may appear at any age.

Pharyngomaxillary abscesses are less common than peritonsillar abscesses, but more common than retropharyngeal, and usually occur as a result of direct contamination with a needle or by the spread of an adjacent infection.

DIAGNOSTIC STUDIES

Roentgenograms of neck area

Larynx appears pushed forward; mass shows in posterior pharynx with retropharyngeal abscesses

TREATMENT PLAN

Surgical
Incision and drainage of abscess with or without local anesthetic

Tonsillectomy about 1 month after peritonsillar abscess has healed to prevent recurrence

Chemotherapeutic
Anti-infective agents

Penicillin G aqueous, 1-5 million units q4h IV or another broad-spectrum antibiotic for 7-10 d

ASSESSMENT: AREAS OF CONCERN

Peritonsillar area
Severe sore throat; difficulty in swallowing; trismus; drooling; muffled voice; thick secretions; fever, chills, nausea, and malaise; tonsil appears pushed towards midline, forward, and downward; uvula may rest against the tonsil or palate

Retropharyngeal area
Stridor and nasal obstruction; muffled cry; child lies with head extended; fever; posterior pharyngeal wall soft, red, and bulging

Pharyngomaxillary area
Fullness behind jaw; Trismus

NURSING DIAGNOSES and NURSING INTERVENTIONS

Nursing Diagnosis	Nursing Intervention
Comfort, alteration in: pain	Administer analgesics and antipyretics as ordered. Assess and document effectiveness. Administer hot saline gargles or irrigation for comfort.
Breathing pattern, ineffective	In particular, observe children with retropharyngeal abscesses, since they are most at risk because of laryngeal obstruction and edema. Observe airway until abscess has been drained. Monitor for dyspnea, restlessness, stridor, and cyanosis.
Airway clearance, ineffective: potential	Before abscess is drained, watch patient closely for signs of spontaneous rupture of abscess and possible asphyxiation from pus. (When abscesses are drained, it is not unusual for pus to pour out.) Keep patient upright with strong suction applied continuously through mouth to prevent aspiration of pus that would result in suffocation. After incision and drainage, administer antibiotics as ordered. Monitor and document vital signs, skin color, and presence of bleeding. Ensure adequate fluid intake; intravenous therapy will probably be ordered.

Patient Education

1. Instruct the patient or family about the necessity of continuing antibiotic therapy for the entire prescribed course to prevent recurrence or complications.
2. Inform the patient that peritonsillar abscesses are likely to recur and that a tonsillectomy will probably be performed about a month after the abscess has healed to prevent recurrence.

EVALUATION

Patient Outcome	Data Indicating That Outcome is Reached
Throat abscess is well healed.	There is no pain in throat. Temperature is within normal limits for patient. Trismus and drooling are absent. Incised area is healing well.
The patient and family understand course of treatment for abscess.	Patient and family verbalize understanding about completing prescribed course of antibiotic therapy.

ADENOID HYPERTROPHY

Adenoid hypertrophy is the enlargement of adenoidal tissue in the nasopharynx resulting from lymphoid hyperplasia.

Adenoid hypertrophy occurs exclusively in children, since adenoidal tissue normally reaches its maximum growth by about the age of 5 years and atrophies during puberty. However, the adenoids eventually hypertrophy if a child suffers repeated attacks of acute adenoid inflammation.

PATHOPHYSIOLOGY

There are several characteristic complications of adenoid hypertrophy. Some degree of nasal obstruction is usually present. The child's voice has a slightly nasal quality, since the nasal cavities are not used for resonance because of the enlarged adenoids. Other complications include mouth breathing, snoring at night, and frequent head colds and stuffiness. These children also have what is known as adenoid facies, that is, a broadened nose, a staring expression in the eyes, shortening of the upper lip, and a high arch of the hard palate that results in a slight elongation of the face (Fig. 7-23). This may be caused by chronic mouth breathing during the formative years when the facial bones are changing, but some researchers believe that the anatomic development of the maxilla may predispose certain children to nasal obstruction.

Changes in the ears and eustachian tubes are also found with adenoid hyperplasia. There is usually partial blockage of the eustachian tube, which leads to retraction of the eardrum, hearing loss, and fluid behind the eardrum. These children may also have recurrent acute or chronic otitis media.

The children occasionally do not breathe effectively through the mouth and may develop symptoms of nocturnal respiratory insufficiency, that is, nasal flaring and intercostal retractions; on rare occasions this has led to pulmonary hypertension and cor pulmonale.

DIAGNOSTIC STUDIES

Nasopharyngoscopy
Abnormal adenoid tissue

Rhinoscopy
Light reflected on hand mirror shows abnormally large adenoid mass

Fig. 7-23
Adenoid facies.

From DeWeese, D.D., and Saunders, W.H.: Textbook of otolaryngology, ed. 6, St. Louis, 1982, The C.V. Mosby Co.

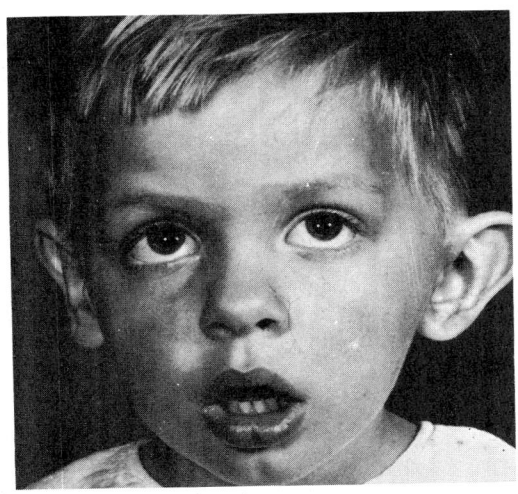

TREATMENT PLAN

Surgical
Adenoidectomy for child with persistent mouth breathing, nasal quality of voice, adenoid facies, and recurrent otitis media

ASSESSMENT: AREAS OF CONCERN

Facial appearance
Adenoid facies

Respiratory function
Child breathes through mouth and snores at night; history of frequent head colds

Auditory function
Nasal quality of voice; eustachian tube partially blocked; fluid present behind eardrum

NURSING DIAGNOSES and NURSING INTERVENTIONS

Nursing Diagnosis	Nursing Intervention
Breathing pattern, ineffective	After adenoidectomy, maintain patent airway. Keep child in side-lying position to prevent aspiration of secretions.
Airway clearance, ineffective: potential	Check throat frequently for bleeding using flashlight to visualize back of throat. Encourage child to avoid clearing throat for 8 to 10 hours. Monitor child's vital signs frequently during first night after surgery. Document and report changes in blood pressure, pulse, respiratory rate, and skin color or presence of bleeding. Examine any emesis (not uncommon after surgery) for "coffee-ground" material.
Sleep pattern disturbance	Inform parents that symptoms of adenoid hypertrophy (mouth breathing, restlessness, snoring, and poor sleep) should disappear after adenoidectomy.
Sensory-perceptual alteration: auditory	Reassure parents that any hearing loss child may have experienced is reversible with treatment.

Patient Education

1. Warn the child and parents that the child's voice will temporarily have a nasal quality after adenoidectomy. It usually takes several weeks for the palate to adjust to the absence of the large adenoid and to approximate the posterior pharyngeal wall. Speech therapy may be necessary if voice quality does not improve.
2. Inform the child and parents to watch for delayed postoperative bleeding, which can occur around the fifth postoperative day. Instruct them to immediately report any symptoms such as spitting up of blood or a nosebleed.
3. Instruct the parents to encourage large amounts of cool oral fluids and soft foods for several days.
4. The child should remain in bed for 1 or 2 days and then gradually resume normal activities.

EVALUATION

Patient Outcome	Data Indicating That Outcome is Reached
Child recovers uneventfully from adenoidectomy.	There is no undue blood loss. Weight remains normal. Fluid intake is normal.
Child and parents verbalize knowledge of postoperative care.	Parents are given list of postoperative suggestions for food and fluids. Child and parents verbalize understanding of importance of observing for delayed postoperative bleeding (around fifth postoperative day) and know that voice will temporarily have nasal quality. Parents verbalize understanding that preoperative symptoms of adenoid hypertrophy should disappear.

LARYNGITIS

Laryngitis, or inflammation of the larynx, is a common disorder that may be either acute or chronic.

Acute laryngitis may be found as part of a viral or bacterial infection of the upper respiratory tract, or it may be an isolated infection limited to the vocal cords.

Trauma such as abuse of the voice may also cause acute laryngitis.

Chronic laryngitis implies inflammatory changes in the laryngeal mucosa. It can be progressive and may lead to a serious voice disability.

PATHOPHYSIOLOGY

Acute laryngitis is often found in combination with viral or bacterial infections of the upper respiratory tract. Viral infections are the most common, but organisms such as β-hemolytic streptococci and *Streptococcus pneumoniae* are also causative agents. Laryngitis may occur in conjunction with colds, bronchitis, pneumonia, or influenza.

Noninfectious causes include excessive use of the voice, such as by public speakers or singers, inhalation of toxic or irritating fumes, or occasional aspiration of caustic chemicals.

Chronic laryngitis can be caused by frequent attacks of acute laryngitis, chronic abuse of the voice, and smoking; chronic tonsillitis and adenoiditis, allergies, or hypermetabolic states may occasionally be causative factors.

DIAGNOSTIC STUDIES

Laryngoscopy, either direct or indirect
Shows abnormalities in true cords, reddened mucosa, and secretions on vocal cords

TREATMENT PLAN

Surgical
None unless tracheotomy is required because of severe laryngeal edema

Chemotherapeutic
Anti-infective agents
Penicillin G; 250 mg po q6h for 10-12 d
Analgesic/antipyretics

Acetaminophen (Tylenol), 600 mg po q4-6h prn
Analgesics
Throat lozenges (Chloraseptic or Cepacol) if necessary for throat pain
Antitussive agents
Guaifenesin (Robitussin), 100-400 mg q4h for adults, 50-100 mg q4h for children to relieve cough

Supportive
Voice rest
Steam inhalation

ASSESSMENT: AREAS OF CONCERN

Laryngeal function
Acute
Hoarseness to aphonia; nonproductive cough; rough, scratchy throat; edema, stridor, and dyspnea in very severe cases; fever or malaise; true vocal cords appear red rather than white with rounded rather than sharp edges as determined by indirect laryngoscopy; entire laryngeal area erythematous; bilateral swelling of cords; drops of secretions in trachea or on vocal cords
Chronic
Progressive hoarseness, if present, is worse in morning because of dried secretions in larynx; voice improves during day and deteriorates again toward evening; usually no throat pain; nonproductive cough; laryngeal mucosa uniformly reddened but smooth; usually no swelling; in some cases polypoid growths, which are called chronic polypoid laryngitis

NURSING DIAGNOSES and NURSING INTERVENTIONS

Nursing Diagnosis	Nursing Intervention
Comfort, alteration in: pain	Administer analgesics, throat lozenges, or antitussives for comfort. Administer antibiotics as ordered. Provide for inhalation of warm steam for symptomatic relief.
Communication, impaired: verbal	Encourage complete voice rest. Provide magic slate or paper and pencil to facilitate communication. Anticipate patient's needs as much as possible to eliminate need for patient to talk. Encourage family and friends to assist patient by asking questions patient can answer by nodding. If patient is hospitalized, mark on intercom that patient cannot respond and notify patient that someone will come to room when light is turned on.

Patient Education

1. Ensure that the patient understands possible sequelae of constant voice abuse and smoking and encourage improvement of these habits.

EVALUATION

Patient Outcome	Data Indicating That Outcome is Reached
There is no inflammation of larynx.	There is no hoarseness, and voice is normal for patient. Raw, tickling feeling in throat is gone. Cough and throat pain are absent. Temperature is within normal limits for patient. There is no inflammation or swelling in laryngeal mucosa or vocal cords.
Patient's understanding of laryngitis is increased.	Patient verbalizes understanding of causes of laryngitis and preventive measures: no smoking, no voice abuse, early treatment of colds, and recognition of symptoms of bronchitis.

LUDWIG'S ANGINA

Ludwig's angina is a virulent, rapidly spreading cellulitis of the floor of the mouth that occurs in both the sublingual and submaxillary spaces (Fig. 7-24).

Ludwig's angina is actually not an abscess, although it resembles one, and there is no lymphatic involvement. Over 80% of cases develop in patients with dental disease such as gingivitis, tooth extraction, or trauma (fractures of the mandible, peritonsillar abscess, or lacerations of the floor of the mouth).[5]

PATHOPHYSIOLOGY

As stated previously, patients in whom Ludwig's angina develops usually have dental disease or poor dental hygiene. These patients' lower molars oddly have the roots closer to the inner than to the outer side of the jaw, and the tips of the roots may extend below the mylohyoid line. The infection usually begins around a tooth root that drains into the submaxillary space rather than into the sublingual space because of root placement. The usual causative organisms are *Streptococcus viridans* and *Escherichia coli*.

The infection spreads rapidly to the sublingual space, which causes the floor of the mouth to become very swollen; it may involve all the tissues under the mandible and usually one or both submaxillary spaces. The swelling may extend all the way down to the clavicle. The tongue is elevated in the back of the mouth, and airway obstruction is a danger. The patient has a fever and systemic signs of illness.

Pus is seldom found if an incision and drainage are performed, although they must occasionally be done to drain the fluid present and to relieve the pressure on the swollen tissues.

Tracheostomy must often be performed, since the patient's airway is greatly compromised from both swelling and excessive secretions.

DIAGNOSTIC STUDIES

Identification of causative organism
Culture of exudate; visual examination

TREATMENT PLAN

Surgical
Incision and drainage—to relieve pressure
Tracheotomy if airway is impaired

Chemotherapeutic
Anti-infective agents
Penicillin G aqueous, 1-5 million units q4h IV
Cefotaxime (Claforan), 1-2 g q6-8h IM or IV (given if patient is allergic to penicillin)

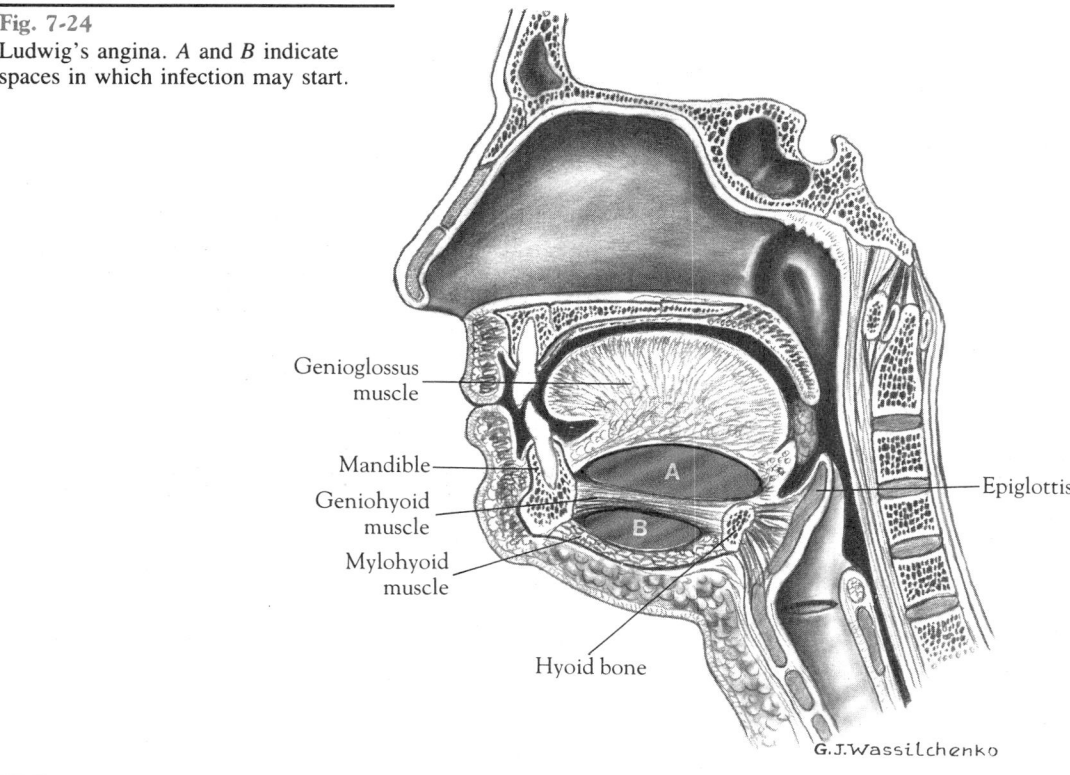

Fig. 7-24
Ludwig's angina. *A* and *B* indicate
spaces in which infection may start.

Genioglossus muscle

Mandible

Geniohyoid muscle

Mylohyoid muscle

Hyoid bone

Epiglottis

G.J.Wassilchenko

ASSESSMENT: AREAS OF CONCERN

Infectious process in mouth
Severe pain in involved tooth area; trismus (difficulty opening mouth); dysphonia; patient unable to eat; excessive secretions and drooling; tongue elevation from swelling of the floor of the mouth

Respiratory function
Dyspnea and stridor from laryngeal edema

NURSING DIAGNOSES and NURSING INTERVENTIONS

Nursing Diagnosis	Nursing Intervention
Airway clearance, ineffective	Do usual tracheostomy care and frequent suctioning; assist patient in handling secretions. Observe patient for signs of airway obstruction. Observe vital signs and signs and symptoms of dyspnea and stridor.
Comfort, alteration in: pain	Provide adequate analgesia for pain relief; assess and document effectiveness. Perform wound care gently but thoroughly if incision and drainage were performed.
Fear	Provide reassurance that patient is being closely monitored. Explain tracheostomy procedure and suctioning and assure patient that it will assist with breathing.
Nutrition, alteration in: less than body requirements	Ensure adequate fluid intake. Monitor intravenous line closely. As soon as patient can take food and fluids orally, have nutritionist visit patient to plan diet that will provide needed caloric intake.

Patient Education

1. Stress the importance of good dental hygiene to prevent recurrence of Ludwig's angina or other oral or dental problems.

EVALUATION

Patient Outcome	Data Indicating That Outcome is Reached
Abscess is well healed.	Airway is patent without respiratory difficulty.
	Tracheostomy stoma is healing well. There is no swelling in floor of mouth. Tongue is not elevated. Temperature is within normal limits. There is no pain. Wound is healed if incision and drainage were performed. Nutritional status is adequate for patient.
Patient's knowledge base is increased.	Patient verbalizes understanding of importance of prophylactic dental care and early treatment of any oral inflammation.

PHARYNGITIS

Pharyngitis is an acute or chronic inflammation of the pharynx.

PATHOPHYSIOLOGY

Pharyngitis is the most common of the throat disorders. It frequently precedes or accompanies the common cold and is characterized by a mild sore throat, difficulty and pain in swallowing, and a low-grade fever. In 90% of cases pharyngitis is viral in origin; the bacterial cause is usually *Streptococcus,* especially in children. Unless complicated by other bacteria, pharyngitis usually resolves in 4 to 6 days. It is communicable for 2 or 3 days after the initial symptoms appear.

If follicular pharyngitis develops, usually from infection by β-hemolytic streptococci, the mucous membrane becomes severely inflamed and studded with white or yellow follicles. If these follicles are present, most are on the tonsils; if the tonsils have been removed, the follicles appear on the lymph areas in the posterior pharynx and also on the lingual tonsil and in the nasopharynx.

DIAGNOSTIC STUDIES

Throat culture
Taken to rule out streptococcal infection

TREATMENT PLAN

Chemotherapeutic
Anti-infective agents
Penicillin G or V, 250 mg po q6h for 10 d (if pharyngitis has bacterial cause)
Analgesic/antipyretics
Acetylsalicylic acid (aspirin), 300-600 mg po q4-6h

Supportive
Bed rest
Humidification
Warm saline throat irrigations
Adequate fluid intake; if throat is so painful and swollen that adequate fluids cannot be taken orally, the patient is often hospitalized for intravenous fluid intake for 24 to 72 hours or until inflammation subsides

ASSESSMENT: AREAS OF CONCERN

Infectious process in throat
Sore throat, with slight difficulty swallowing, especially saliva; mild fever; headaches, malaise, and joint pain; cervical lymphadenopathy; pharynx reddened and inflamed; blisters or follicles on tonsils or lymph areas

NURSING DIAGNOSES and NURSING INTERVENTIONS

Nursing Diagnosis	Nursing Intervention
Comfort, alteration in: pain	Administer antibiotics and analgesics as ordered. Assess and document effectiveness. Provide warm saline throat irrigations for comfort. Encourage bed rest.
Fluid volume deficit, potential	Encourage a fluid intake of at least 2500 ml per day. Monitor intake and output, observe for signs of dehydration (dry skin, cracked lips, and decreased urine output). If intravenous fluid is ordered, maintain adequate flow rate. Assist patient with frequent oral hygiene; patient may be mouth breathing, which adds to discomfort. Monitor patient's temperature and report abnormalities.

Patient Education

1. Instruct the patient and family about the necessity of completing the prescribed course of antibiotics to prevent complications or recurrence of infection.
2. Inform the patient and family of possible irritants (smoking and lack of humidity) and ways to prevent inflammation.

EVALUATION

Patient Outcome	Data Indicating That Outcome is Reached
Pharyngitis is resolved.	Sore throat is gone. Patient is afebrile. Activity level is normal for patient. Fluid and nutritional status are adequate for patient. There is no swelling or infection in throat. Cervical lymphadenopathy is absent.
Patient verbalizes knowledge of treatment.	Patient verbalizes understanding of necessity of completing prescribed course of antibiotics.

TONSILLITIS

Tonsillitis is an inflammation of the palatine tonsil.

Tonsillitis may be acute or chronic. It usually remains localized in the tonsillar tissue and is considered mildly contagious. It is characterized by a sore throat, but the patient may experience referred pain to the ears.

Usually an airborne or foodborne bacterial infection, tonsillitis can occur at any age but is most frequently found in children between the ages of 5 and 10 years. If uncomplicated, it usually resolves after 5 to 7 days. Treatment makes the patient more comfortable and may prevent serious complications such as arthritis, glomerulonephritis, or chronic tonsillitis. A less common cause of tonsillitis is viral infection; epidemics of viral tonsillitis have occurred among military recruits.[5]

Several years ago the role of the tonsils and adenoids in the immune system was not as well known as it is today, and surgical removal of the tonsils and adenoids was common. These procedures are performed less today because the importance of this lymphoid tissue to the body's immune system is known.

PATHOPHYSIOLOGY

Tonsillitis begins as a sore throat accompanied by fever, chills, headache, myalgia, joint pain, and anorexia. The patient may also have enlarged and tender anterior cervical lymph nodes. The tonsils appear enlarged, reddened, and inflamed with pus or exudate projecting from between the pillars of the fauces or in the crypts. Some of the exudate can be pulled away from the tonsil, which causes bleeding. The white blood cell count is frequently increased to 10,000 to 20,000/mm^3.

A throat culture should be done to identify the infecting organism. *Streptococcus* (β-hemolytic streptococci group A) is the most common organism. If this is the cause, the tonsils appear studded with yellow follicles. Other causative agents are *Pneumococcus* and gram-negative organisms (*Proteus, Pseudomonas,* or coliforms), which have steadily increased as infective agents over the past 10 years.

DIAGNOSTIC STUDIES

Throat culture
Identification of causative organism

TREATMENT PLAN

Surgical
Tonsillectomy, if indicated, after acute infection has subsided (see p. 812)

Chemotherapeutic
Analgesic/antipyretics
Acetylsalicylic acid (aspirin) or acetaminophen (Tylenol), 600 mg po q4-6h for adults
Anti-infective agents
Penicillin V (PenVee), 125 mg po q6h
Penicillin G (Bicillin), 600,000-1,200,000 units IM

ASSESSMENT: AREAS OF CONCERN

Infectious process in throat
Moderate to severe sore throat; pain referred to ears; anterior cervical lymphadenopathy; fever and chills; headache; muscle and joint pain; anorexia; increased secretions from throat; enlarged, reddened, inflamed tonsils; pus or exudate on tonsils; edematous or inflamed uvula; white blood count of 10,000 to 20,000/mm^3

NURSING DIAGNOSES and NURSING INTERVENTIONS

Nursing Diagnosis	Nursing Intervention
Comfort, alteration in: pain	Provide adequate analgesia for relief of throat pain; assess and document effectiveness. Administer antibiotics as ordered. Perform throat irrigations; provide hot saline gargles or ice collar as comfort measures. Maintain bed rest during acute phase and emphasize importance of rest while convalescing.
Fluid volume deficit, potential	Encourage increased fluid intake keeping in mind that children can become dehydrated very quickly. Note that the child may like ice cream, sherbet, or flavored drinks; avoid juices, since they may burn throat. If child is hospitalized, monitor intravenous intake to ensure adequate intake of fluid.
Nutrition, alteration in: less than body requirements	Ensure that patient has adequate intake of soft, nourishing foods. Encourage patient to eat foods that are minimally irritating to throat and provide adequate caloric intake, that is, soups and milkshakes.

Patient Education

1. Stress to the patient and family the importance of completing the prescribed course of antibiotics to prevent complications or recurrence.

EVALUATION

Patient Outcome	Data Indicating That Outcome is Reached
Patient recovers uneventfully from attack of tonsillitis.	Patient is afebrile. Tonsils are normal in size and free of pus and exudate. There is no pain in throat. Lymph nodes are not enlarged, although this might persist after other symptoms have disappeared. White blood count is within normal limits. Patient and family verbalize understanding of necessity of completing the required course of medication.

VOCAL CORD PARALYSIS

Vocal cord paralysis is the loss of nerve and motor supply to the vocal cords resulting in fixation and abnormal position of one or both cords.

Paralysis of the vocal cords is the result of either disease or injury to the superior laryngeal nerve or the recurrent laryngeal nerve, which is the branch of the vagus nerve that provides the entire motor supply to the larynx.

Vocal cord paralysis may be unilateral or bilateral; the quality of the voice depends on whether one or both cords are affected, as well as the position and tenseness of the affected cords. Paralysis of the vocal cords may also be described as complete or incomplete or abductor or adductor.

PATHOPHYSIOLOGY

Vocal cord paralysis can have central, peripheral, or idiopathic causes. The causes are usually peripheral, but lesions of the central nervous system such as multiple sclerosis, syringomyelia, brain tumors, and vascular accidents do produce paralysis of the vocal cords.

The left recurrent laryngeal nerve, which follows a longer path, is paralyzed in over 70% of cases in contrast to about 15% for the right recurrent laryngeal nerve. Men are affected about 10 times more commonly than women, and the most common age is in the seventies. The most common cause is malignant disease, possibly from an increased incidence of smoking and cancers of the lung and larynx. One in four recurrent laryngeal nerve paralyses is caused by cancer.

Peripheral causes are the most common. These include stretching of the nerve, as with aortic aneurysms and mitral stenosis, which causes enlargement of the left auricle and also stretches the left recurrent laryngeal nerve. The nerve can be infiltrated or stretched by lung or bronchial tumors. Thyroid carcinomas may cause paralysis, and tumors of the larynx itself eventually cause fixation of one or both cords.

Probably 10% of the cases of vocal cord paralysis are unexplained and are called idiopathic. These cases may be from viral infections that remain undiagnosed. In many of these cases the function of the vocal cord recovers spontaneously; this is probably true in 80% of the patients with vocal cord paralysis if recovery has begun before 6 months has passed. The high incidence of infections of the upper respiratory tract suggests a viral etiology in many cases; improved methods of diagnosis should decrease the frequency of the idiopathic label.[6]

The most common form of paralysis is unilateral: one cord is paralyzed and the other remains normal. If the affected cord is paralyzed in the midline, the normal cord can usually approximate it and the patient may have a normal voice. However, if the paralyzed cord is abducted, the normal cord cannot meet it and the patient has a husky, "breathy" voice.

Dyspnea is not associated with unilateral cord paralysis because the laryngeal airway is adequate; the good cord abducts enough for the airway. However, bilateral cord paralysis affects the airway more seriously. The cords are usually paralyzed in the adducted position. The cords may be within 2 to 3 mm of the midline, and the patient suffers both stridor and dyspnea on exertion.

DIAGNOSTIC STUDIES

Laryngoscopy
Shows paralyzed condition of cords

Bronchoscopy and esophagoscopy
Done as part of malignancy workup

Skull roentgenograms, thyroid scan, upper gastrointestinal series, and complete neurologic examination
Performed to rule out other causes

TREATMENT PLAN

Surgical
For unilateral paralysis
  Injection of measured amounts of Teflon into paralyzed cord under direct laryngoscopy; enlarges or swells cord and brings it closer to midline so normal cord can better approximate it; strengthens voice and prevents aspiration
For bilateral paralysis
  Tracheotomy may be needed because of inadequate airway
  Alternative therapy is arytenoidectomy in which one arytenoid cartilage is removed and glottis is opened posteriorly
  King procedure is another alternative in which suture is passed around arytenoid cartilage and through adjacent cricoid cartilage; arytenoid is rotated and fixed laterally; improves airway patency but may adversely affect quality of voice; many patients decide to conserve their voices and keep tracheotomy tube
  Lateralization of vocal cords; used in 22 patients with paralysis of bilateral abductor cord; consists of segmental removal of thyroarytenoid muscle fibers that are adjacent to vocal ligament down to

conus elasticus medially and thyroid cartilage laterally; excision made by microcautery, and surgical defect closed after vocal cord is lateralized with two sutures, one into endolarynx superiorly and other into vocal ligament inferiorly; voice becomes whispery and coarse, but procedure negates need for tracheotomy[26]

ASSESSMENT: AREAS OF CONCERN

Voice
   Vocal weakness; hoarse, breathy quality

Respiratory function
   Stridor and dyspnea on exertion if paralysis is bilateral

NURSING DIAGNOSES and NURSING INTERVENTIONS

Nursing Diagnosis	Nursing Intervention
Communication, impaired: verbal	Ensure that patient understands Teflon procedure. Indicate to patient that voice will be improved but may not be completely normal.
Breathing pattern, ineffective	Provide usual postoperative care after tracheotomy is performed. Observe patient closely for excessive secretions and need for suctioning. After assessing patient's readiness, teach patient to care for tracheotomy tube: suctioning, cleaning, and changing tube.

Patient Education

1. Remind the patient that speaking can be accomplished normally by using a tracheotomy plug or by occluding the lumen of the tracheotomy with a finger.
2. Advise the patient to wear a Medic-Alert bracelet indicating that a tracheotomy is present.

EVALUATION

Patient Outcome	Data Indicating That Outcome is Reached
Vocal cord paralysis has resolved.	Airway is patent. Voice maintains good quality.
Patient demonstrates ability to care for tracheotomy tube.	Patient demonstrates ability to suction, clean, and humidify tracheotomy tube.

VOCAL CORD POLYPS AND NODULES

Polyps usually develop on the vocal cords from chronic abuse of the voice, allergies, or chronic inhalation of irritants, which frequently starts during an acute infection of the upper respiratory tract. Polyps are edematous masses of mucous membrane that attach to the vocal cords by either broad or narrow bases. Most have a broad base so there is permanent interference with voice production; however, some polyps are pedunculated, hang under the vocal cord, and cause only intermittent symptoms. Polyps are usually unilateral and may appear anywhere on the cord. They are common in adults who smoke, have allergies, or live in very dry climates. Rarely found in children, polyps are far more common in men. Since the cords are inhibited from approximation, painless hoarseness is the only symptom.

Polyps are gelatinous and telangiectatic, but mainly transitional types of polyps can be discriminated. Examination may show an alteration in the permeability of blood vessels, allowing extravasation of fluid, fibrin, or erythrocytes. After this, reactive processes develop with the formation of labyrinthine vascular spaces. This process is similar to the formation of a thrombus. The polyps develop at the site of maximum muscular and aerodynamic forces exerted during phonation and are considered a sequela of phonotrauma.[29]

Vocal cord nodules, also called singer's, teacher's, or screamer's nodules, are caused by chronic voice abuse, such as singing, screaming, or constantly speaking outside the natural voice range. Nodules occur at any age and usually in girls and women, although they are some-

Fig. 7-25
Vocal cord nodules. **A,** During
respiration. **B,** During phonation.

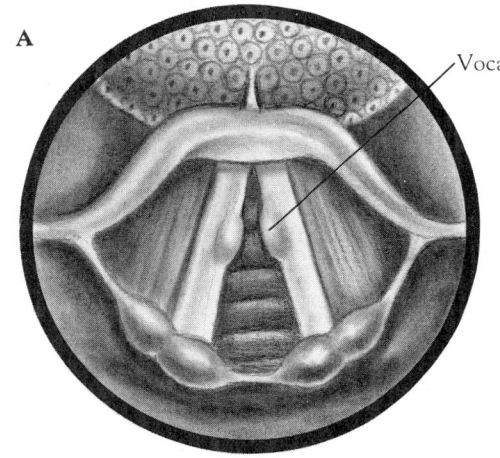

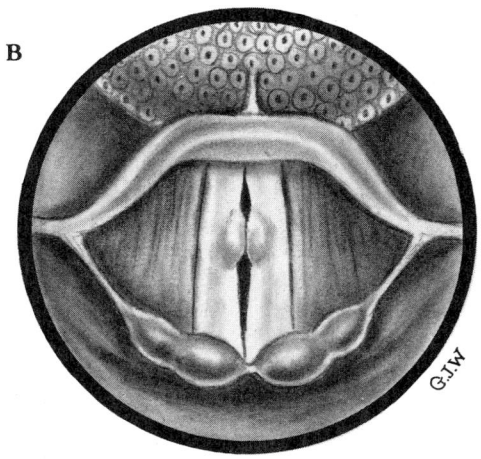

times found in young boys who scream and shout excessively.

The nodules are benign growths that first appear red and raised above the vocal cord surface, later changing into small white lumps that touch when the cords approximate. Since they are raised, the cords are kept apart and produce a characteristic hoarse, breathy voice (Fig. 7-25).

Conservative treatment of nodules and complete voice rest often cause even large nodules to disappear. After voice rest, speech therapy may be indicated to prevent recurrence of the nodules and restore a normal voice. In contrast polyps usually require surgical removal; they do not disappear with voice rest. Direct laryngoscopy is performed, and the polyps are excised. If a patient has bilateral polyps, the excision should be done in two stages, since doing both sides at the same time may cause a laryngeal web to form between the two raw surfaces.

NURSING DIAGNOSES and NURSING INTERVENTIONS

Nursing Diagnosis	Nursing Intervention
Communication, impaired: verbal	Ensure that patient does not speak during period of voice rest; provide patient with magic slate or paper and pencil.
	Remind visitors and staff members that patient is not to speak; attempt to anticipate patient's needs to eliminate need to speak.
	Use humidifier in room to provide adequate moisture in air and decrease throat irritation.
	Discourage patient from smoking during recovery from polyp removal.

Patient Education

1. Refer the patient to a speech therapist after discharge to prevent recurrence of nodules or polyps.
2. Discourage the patient from smoking, since exposure to irritants such as smoke predisposes patients to polyp formation.
3. Instruct the patient about the importance of adequate humidification in the home to prevent throat irritation.

EVALUATION

Patient Outcome	Data Indicating That Outcome is Reached
Patient recovers uneventfully from removal of nodules or polyps.	There are no nodules or polyps on vocal cords. Patient is able to speak in a normal voice. Patient verbalizes understanding of stresses on voice and how to minimize these: no smoking, avoidance of allergens, and no excessive shouting or screaming.

Medical Interventions

MYRINGOTOMY

Description and Rationale

Myringotomy is an incision of the tympanic membrane, usually to drain pus or fluid from the middle ear. Myringotomy was once performed routinely for ear infections such as otitis media, but the advent of antibiotics has greatly decreased the need for it.

A local or general anesthetic may be used, although the procedure is relatively painless. A curved incision is made in the posteroinferior portion of the drumhead (Fig. 7-26) with a very sharp myringotomy knife. The physician wears a head mirror and uses an aural speculum to visualize the drumhead to avoid injuring the ossicles.

Myringotomy may also be performed by touching a heated wire loop to the drumhead for 1 second to produce a 2 mm hole. This small opening stays open for about 3 to 4 weeks and heals without scarring.[2]

After the drumhead is incised, pus may pour out or suction may be used to remove fluid. Cotton is then placed in the ear to absorb the drainage, which may continue for several days.

A myringotomy incision heals quickly with only minimal scarring and causes no disruption in hearing.

Contraindications and Cautions

When making the incision the physician must be careful to avoid injuring the ossicles and cutting too deep. A deep incision may cut the mucous membrane covering the promontory, causing bleeding and pain. If it is cut, however, the injury is not serious. The drumhead can be easily visualized posteriorly and inferiorly, which is where the incision should be made to avoid injury to the medial wall of the middle ear and the ossicles.

There are no apparent contraindications to myringotomy if the disease process requires its performance.

TREATMENT PLAN

Surgical
Incision of eardrum with sharp myringotomy knife for evacuation of pus and fluid

Chemotherapeutic
Anti-infective agents
Tetracycline (Achromycin), 250 mg po q6h
Polmyxin B sulfate (Neosporin) ear drops
Narcotic analgesics
Acetaminophen (Tylenol), 600 mg with codeine q4-6h prn

Electromechanical
Cotton in ear to absorb drainage

ASSESSMENT: AREAS OF CONCERN

Tympanic membrane
Drainage from eardrum; bleeding and pain at incision site; no impairment of hearing

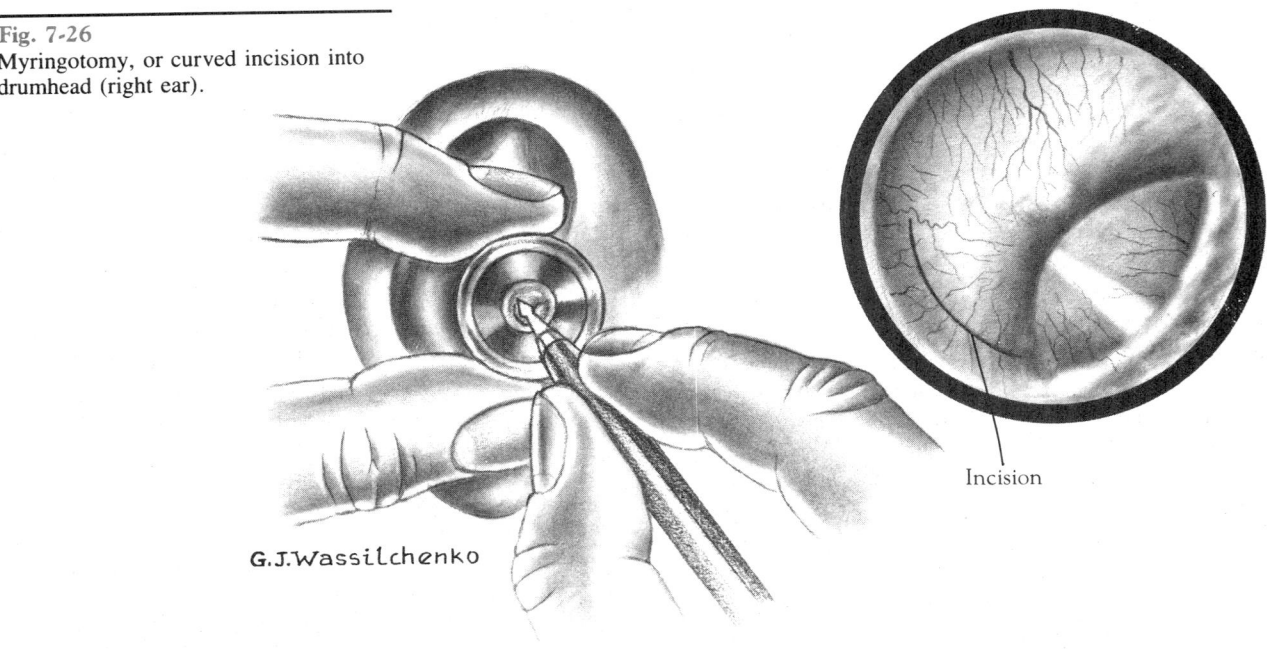

Fig. 7-26
Myringotomy, or curved incision into drumhead (right ear).

Incision

G.J.Wassilchenko

NURSING DIAGNOSES and NURSING INTERVENTIONS

Nursing Diagnosis	Nursing Intervention
Comfort, alteration in: pain	Provide analgesia as needed for pain relief; assess and document effectiveness. Administer antibiotics and ear drops as ordered. If patient is child, instruct parents in treatment regimen and proper instillation technique for ear drops. Observe amount of drainage from ear. Change cotton as needed. Teach technique to patient or to parent. Since drainage is usually infected, wash hands well after handling drainage and teach patient or parents to do same to prevent contamination. Keep external ear dry and clean. Assess for and report symptoms such as headache, nausea, fever, or increased ear pain.

Patient Education

1. Instruct the patient and family of the necessity for completing the prescribed course of antibiotics to prevent recurrence or complications.
2. Instruct the patient or family to monitor for hearing loss or increased ear pain. Myringotomies occasionally need to be performed again for reaccumulation of fluid.

EVALUATION

Patient Outcome	Data Indicating That Outcome is Reached
Patient recovers uneventfully from myringotomy.	Myringotomy incision is healed well with no evidence of pus or fluid behind eardrum. There is no drainage from eardrum. Patient is afebrile. Patient experiences no hearing loss.

STAPEDECTOMY

Description and Rationale

Attempts to improve hearing losses that result from otosclerosis have been made for almost 100 years. Stapedectomy is the result of refinement of these various attempts and is now the operation of choice in many patients with hearing losses from otosclerosis. One author states that the conductive component of stapedectomy is better understood than the sensorineural component.[34] Preliminary results of studies indicate that the sensorineural component of otosclerosis may be an autoimmune response to the primitive cartilage in the fissula ante fenestrum and otic capsule in which the otosclerotic process begins.[34] During stapedectomy the surgeon partially or completely removes the footplate and the stapes and replaces them with a prosthesis that allows the reestablishment of normal sound pathways. The prostheses are usually made of tissue or of plastic materials.

If patients are appropriately selected for the procedure and the surgeon has the appropriate skills, 90% of patients experience an improvement in the level of hearing and in many instances hearing is almost normal.

Patients who may benefit from stapedectomy include those with a negative Rinne test of at least 572 Hz with a vibrating tuning fork and an air-bone gap of at least 20 dB for speech frequencies. Patients with otosclerosis and accompanying tinnitus may experience relief from tinnitus after stapedectomy.

Since the ''worst'' ear is the one operated on, patients selected for this surgery must have one ear functioning at a fairly adequate level. The operative ear must have a mobile malleus and a normally situated tympanic membrane.

Contraindications and Cautions

Active external otitis or otitis media must be well healed before stapedectomy will be considered

Severe vertigo from Ménière's disease

Occupation that requires frequent or large changes in barometric pressure, that is, divers, pilots, and those who work at heights

''Dead'' or nonfunctioning ear on one side, unless patient has reached stage at which hearing aid can no longer be satisfactorily used

Patients younger than 25 years of age, since otosclerosis may still be in an active stage

Older patients assessed carefully for general health status and adequate sensorineural reserve and for evidence of vestibular damage; caution exercised in patients with any vestibular damage and poor sensorineural reserve because results may not be satisfactory

TREATMENT PLAN

Surgical

With patient under local anesthetic surgeon turns eardrum back on itself like omelette; microscope used to magnify bones of middle ear; stapes and footplate removed by means of various picks and sometimes electric drill; when footplate is removed, open oval window sealed with fascial graft from temporal muscle, and prosthesis connected to incus to restore normal sound conduction; several types of prostheses used; one end attached to the incus and other to graft or plug in oval window; external ear canal packed to ensure healing of tympanum; packing left in place 5 or 6 days

Chemotherapeutic

Narcotic analgesics
  Meperidine (Demerol), 50-100 mg IM q4h prn
Antiemetic agents
  Prochlorperazine (Compazine), 10 mg IM q6h prn
  Meclizine (Antivert) for vertigo effect, 25 mg po ½h ac and hs
Sedative agents
  Sedation, such as pentobarbital (Nembutal), 60-100 mg po before surgery
  Phenobarbital, 60-100 mg po before surgery
Anti-infective agents
  Tetracycline (Achromycin), 250 mg po q6h for 10 d

Supportive

Bed rest for 24 hours (may vary with physician) with operative side facing upward to maintain position of prosthesis and graft

ASSESSMENT: AREAS OF CONCERN

Infectious process
  Fever or other symptoms of infection; pain in operated ear

Auditory function
  Hearing ability; vertigo

Gustatory function
  Ability to taste with anterior tongue

Complications

Reparative granuloma occurs in about 1% of stapedectomies; the cause is unknown, but it may be related to contamination of the implant or trauma to the tissue. Granuloma can be recognized if the flap and tympanic membrane still appear reddened and inflamed and there has been no hearing improvement 1 week after surgery. A granuloma can fill much of the middle ear and must be completely removed along with the prosthesis. A different type of prosthesis must then be inserted.

NURSING DIAGNOSES and NURSING INTERVENTIONS

Nursing Diagnosis	Nursing Intervention
Mobility, impaired physical	Enforce bed rest as ordered; patient should lie flat with operative side up. Do not turn patient. Keep side rails up. When patient is allowed to be up, assist patient, since vertigo may be present. Begin movement and ambulation gradually and provide medication for pain or dizziness as needed.
Sensory-perceptual alteration: auditory	Improvement in hearing may not be noticeable immediately because of packing in ear and bleeding. Make sure that patient is aware of this fact to avoid disappointment immediately after surgery.
Skin integrity, impairment of: potential	Inform patient that after usual 5- to 6-day packing a piece of cotton may be placed in ear for few days for protection. Instruct patient in appropriate technique of changing cotton and tell patient to do it once or twice a day. While patient is hospitalized, monitor for excessive bleeding, drainage, fever, and ear pain and report any symptoms immediately.
Comfort, alteration in: pain	Administer pain medication and antiemetics as needed; assess and document effectiveness. Report excessive ear pain immediately. Encourage patient to move gradually, avoiding sudden movement.

Patient Education

1. Inform the patient to avoid sneezing or nose blowing for at least 1 week to protect the eustachian tube from contaminated material and to prevent dislodgment of prosthesis and graft.
2. Ensure that the patient is aware of the necessity of careful ear care both immediately before surgery and on an ongoing basis.
3. The patient must avoid getting the ear wet (as by shampooing) while deep external packing remains in place.
4. Inform the patient that smoking is contraindicated after stapedectomy.

EVALUATION

Patient Outcome	Data Indicating That Outcome is Reached
Patient recovers uneventfully from stapedectomy.	Activity level is normal for patient; no weakness or vertigo is present. There is no pain or excessive drainage from operated ear. Hearing is improved to normal. Patient verbalizes understanding of ear care regimen and symptoms to report to physician.

TONSILLECTOMY

Description and Rationale

Tonsillectomy is the surgical removal of the tonsils and usually the adenoids (adenoidectomy). The rationale for this procedure is usually the removal of chronically infected tissue. A general anesthetic is used; the most common method for removal of the tonsils is dissection and snare, since it can be used for all sizes of tonsils whether they are in shallow or deep fossae. Although it has disadvantages, the guillotine method is chosen by some physicians. Injury to the tonsillar pillar is more common with this method, and it is not suitable for deeply recessed tonsils. It may also not reach the base of the tonsils and will leave a tonsil tag. Adenoids are removed with an adenotome; a curette may also be used to remove residual adenoid tissue.

Contraindications and Cautions

Presence of any acute infection, especially tonsillitis
Active tuberculosis
Presence of hematologic disorders, such as hemophilia, leukemia, or aplastic anemia

TREATMENT PLAN

Surgical

Tonsil and adenoidal tissue removed to secure all bleeding points

Chemotherapeutic

Narcotic analgesics
Acetaminophen (Tylenol), 600 mg with codeine, po q4-6h prn (avoid aspirin because of possibility of bleeding)

Supportive

Intravenous fluids, until nausea has subsided and patient is drinking well
Soft or liquid diet
Bed rest

ASSESSMENT: AREAS OF CONCERN

Postoperative status

Vital signs stable; patient afebrile with pulse and blood pressure normal for patient; skin warm and dry; level of consciousness appropriate for recovery from anesthesia; no bleeding at operative site; if adenoidectomy is done, there may be some nasopharyngeal trickling down back of throat

Complications

Bleeding from failure to secure bleeding points during surgery
Airway obstruction from blood or secretions
Aspiration of blood or secretions

NURSING DIAGNOSES and NURSING INTERVENTIONS

Nursing Diagnosis	Nursing Intervention
Comfort, alteration in: pain	Provide adequate pain relief; assess and document effectiveness. Provide hot saline gargles for comfort. Ensure adequate fluid intake. Monitor intravenous intake at prescribed rate until discontinued and then provide soothing fluids to prevent dehydration. Do not offer juices, since they may burn the throat. Provide ice chips to suck. Monitor vital signs, level of consciousness, and presence of bleeding and report any change immediately. Maintain patent airway; keep patient on bed rest lying on side as much as possible. Observe for vomiting of dark brown fluid because of "swallowed" blood during surgery. Watch for frequent swallowing, which may indicate bleeding; check frequently with flashlight to see if blood is trickling down back of throat if adenoidectomy was done.

POSTOPERATIVE INSTRUCTIONS FOR TONSILLECTOMY AND ADENOIDECTOMY

1. For the next 7 to 10 days, there may be pain and soreness in the throat and ears.
2. Small amounts of bleeding will occur during this period. If bleeding persists, call the physician immediately.
3. If signs and symptoms of infection occur, such as purulent exudate or increase in pain or fever, call the physician immediately.
4. Keep the fluid intake high for the first few days after surgery, which will help keep the temperature down.
5. The diet should consist of soft bland foods, gelatin, cooked cereals, ice cream, soft-boiled eggs, custard, broth, mashed potatoes, and noncitrus juices for about 1 week. Apple and grape juice are the best liquids. Carbonated beverages may be taken if the patient tolerates them. Well-ground hamburger and well-cooked meats should be added as soon as tolerated.
6. Activity should not cause overexertion for the next 7 to 10 days. If the weather is good, the patient may go outside after the second day. Persons with acute infections should be kept away. Bathing may be carried out in the usual manner.
7. Acetaminophen (Tylenol) (if not allergic) may be taken by mouth, 650 mg every 4 hours for pain, especially ½ hour before meals. If the patient is given medications to take home from the hospital, they may be substituted for Tylenol.
8. The patient should not gargle but only gently rinse mouth.
9. If you have any questions or concerns, call your physician to discuss these areas.

Courtesy Ruth Weddle, RN, and Eden Rivera, RN, University of California, San Francisco.

Patient Education

1. Instruct the patient not to clear the throat, to watch for bleeding, and to call the physician immediately if any symptoms occur. They may occur on about the fifth day after surgery when the scab sloughs from the operative area.
2. Since most patients are hospitalized for only a short time, give the patient a preprinted list of instructions for postoperative care at home (see box above).

EVALUATION

Patient Outcome	Data Indicating That Outcome is Reached
Patient recovers uneventfully from tonsillectomy.	There is no bleeding from operative site. Patient is afebrile and takes fluids and food well. Activity level is normal for patient. Patient verbalizes understanding of necessity of watching for late postoperative bleeding and calling physician immediately. Patient verbalizes knowledge of when to return to physician for postoperative visit.

TRACHEOSTOMY

Description and Rationale

A tracheotomy is an incision into the trachea to form a temporary or permanent opening, which is called a tracheostomy. The incision is made through the second, third, or fourth tracheal ring, and a tube is usually inserted through the opening to allow passage of air and the removal of tracheobronchial secretions.

Except in cases of head, neck, and face trauma, a tracheotomy is rarely performed as an emergency procedure. If immediate airway control is needed and the patient is hospitalized, endotracheal intubation is usually performed; a tracheotomy is performed as an elective procedure if an artificial airway is necessary longer than an endotracheal tube should be left in place.

Aside from tracheotomy performed to reduce anatomic dead space (by approximately 150 cc) in patients with chronic pulmonary disease or to aid in mechanical ventilation of an unconscious patient, most patients fall into one of two categories. Patients in the first group have an obstruction at or above the level of the larynx, such as foreign body obstruction, carcinoma of the larynx, severe infection (such as Ludwig's angina), or trauma to the tongue or mandible. Patients in the second group have no actual obstruction but are unable to raise their own secretions and are in danger of anoxia if secretions accumulate and are not removed from the chest. These patients include those with paralysis of the chest muscles and diaphragm (as in Guillain-Barré syndrome), patients who are unconscious or semiconscious with head injuries, and patients with fractured ribs or other chest injuries causing severe pain that inhibits them from coughing. Tracheotomy is an excellent way to provide access to the trachea when a patient needs frequent suctioning. Other indications include patients with smoke inhalation or severe burns around the head and neck and patients who are at risk of bleeding from thyroidectomy or radical neck dissection.

Contraindications and Cautions

Caution exercised in infants because of extremely small size of their tracheas and small size of tube that must be used[19,21]

Caution exercised if surgical incision in neck would increase risk of infection

TREATMENT PLAN

Surgical

Vertical incision in midline of neck from lower border of thyroid cartilage to slightly above suprasternal notch; soft tissue and muscle layers divided and isthmus of thyroid exposed and divided between clamps or retracted upward, which exposes rings of trachea; vertical incision made, usually between third and fourth rings, secretions thoroughly aspirated, and tracheostomy tube of correct size for patient inserted; first tracheal ring should not be cut (Fig. 7-27); complete hemostasis ensured after pro-

Fig. 7-27
Correct area of trachea for incision and insertion of tracheotomy tube.

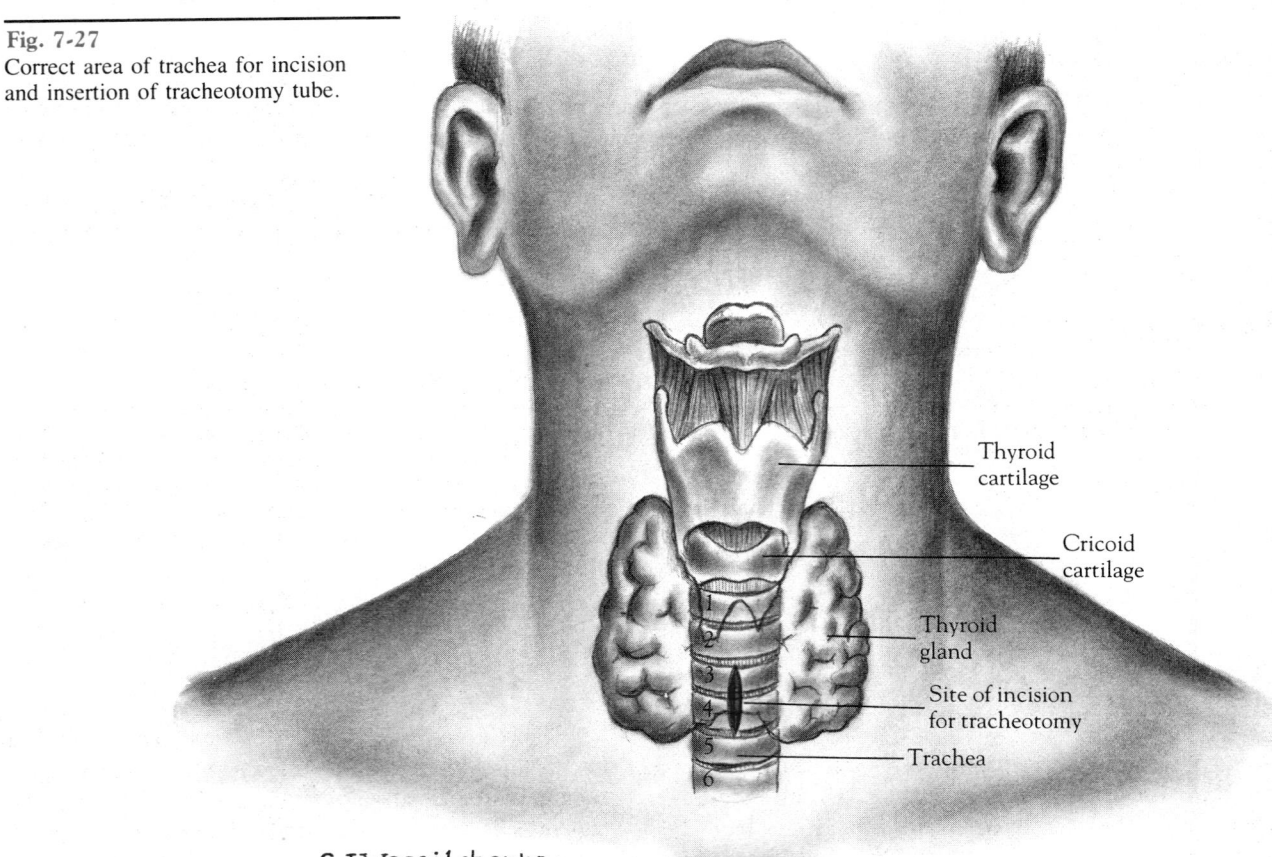

Thyroid cartilage

Cricoid cartilage

Thyroid gland

Site of incision for tracheotomy

Trachea

G.J.Wassilchenko

cedure; if procedure is elective, endotracheal tube left in place and tracheotomy performed over tube; endotracheal tube can be removed after airway is secured

Chemotherapeutic

Drugs prescribed depending on reason for tracheotomy, that is, infection or laryngeal edema

Electromechanical

Tracheobronchial suctioning

Supportive

Humidification of inspired air

ASSESSMENT: AREAS OF CONCERN

Respiratory function

Respiratory rate; amount and color of tracheal secretions; need for frequency of suctioning; anxiety level; arterial blood gases; presence of bleeding at tracheostomy site (should be absent); no excessive coughing after suctioning; adequate humidification provided to tracheostomy (mucus is thin and without thick plugs); breath sounds audible in all lobes after suctioning; tracheostomy ties securely fastened

Pneumomediastinum

No dyspnea, crepitus, or edema of face and neck

Pneumothorax

No cough, anxiety, sharp chest pain, or tachycardia

Cardiac tamponade

No increase in central venous pressure, narrowed pulse pressure, paradoxic pulse, decreased blood pressure, dyspnea, or decreased level of consciousness

NURSING DIAGNOSES and NURSING INTERVENTIONS

Nursing Diagnosis	Nursing Intervention
Airway clearance, ineffective; breathing pattern, ineffective; and gas exchange, impaired	Observe for and report any symptoms suggesting: (1) pneumomediastinum; (2) pneumothorax; (3) cardiac tamponade; (4) hemorrhage; or (5) subcutaneous emphysema.
	Suction airway as often as necessary to maintain patent airway and remove secretions. This can be done as frequently as every 5 to 10 minutes immediately after surgery to every 3 to 4 hours after tracheostomy has been in place awhile. Use catheter that is no greater than half diameter of tracheostomy tube. Preoxygenate and hyperinflate patient using Ambu bag before suctioning. Give patient five sigh breaths. Do not suction for more than 5 to 10 seconds, since suctioning decreases alveolar oxygen pressure by 30 mm Hg. Keep bypass port open on catheter while inserting it to minimize oxygen removal. Gentle twisting motion of catheter should be used while suctioning.
	Stop suctioning immediately if any signs of respiratory distress occur, since there may be mucus blockage and patient may quickly become hypoxic. Postoxygenate patient after suctioning by giving five sigh breaths with Ambu bag to reopen small airways. Maintain adequate humidification to keep secretions loose and minimize difficulty in secretion removal. (Sputum is 95% water and mucous membranes dry out easily without proper hydration.) If necessary, 1 to 5 ml of sterile saline can be instilled into tracheostomy tube before suctioning to facilitate removal of secretions.
	Clean inner cannula (if present) of tracheostomy tube every 4 hours or as necessary using sterile technique.
	If appropriate, ensure that patient receives chest physiotherapy depending on condition and reason for tracheotomy.
	Document suctioning, patient response, result of chest assessment, and all treatments.
	If tracheostomy tube is Portex, inflate cuff when patient eats or receives ventilation assistance or intermittent positive-positive breathing treatments. At these times cuff pressure should be maintained at level that just occludes trachea. Pressure should be less than 20 mm Hg.
	Convalescent care: Observe for any frank bleeding from tracheostomy or pulsation of cannula. (Innominate artery is in close proximity, and tracheostomy tube may erode through the artery wall.)

Nursing Diagnosis	Nursing Intervention
	Ensure that tracheostomy ties are secured at all times so tube does not fall out or become dislocated.
	When tracheotomy has just been performed, change ties with assistance so tracheostomy tube is held in place while ties are replaced. Institutional policy may vary regarding whether nurses may change tracheostomy ties within first 48 hours after surgery.
	To prevent patient from inhaling foreign particles, avoid using aerosol sprays, talcum powder, or tissue or gauze containing cotton.
	Use precut tracheostomy gauze or unlined gauze opened full-length and folded into U shape.
Anxiety	Carefully explain suctioning procedure to patient.
	Provide assurance that patient will be closely observed for respiratory distress or need for suctioning and that call light will be answered promptly.
Communication, impaired: verbal	Provide patient with magic slate or pen and paper to facilitate communication.
	Use word cards with commonly used phrases to decrease patient frustration.
	Convalescent care: Instruct patient to occlude tracheostomy opening with finger or plug to allow verbal communication.
Skin integrity, impairment of	Assess stoma during every shift and note any bleeding, purulent drainage, and condition of surrounding tissue.
	Check skin under tracheostomy dressing and note areas of breakdown.
	Wear gloves to change dressing when soiled or on every shift.
	Clean wound thoroughly when changing dressing.
	Clean inner cannula of tracheostomy tube during every shift or as necessary.
	Ensure that sterile technique is maintained while suctioning.
	Make sure that patient is turned at least hourly if condition warrants and that areas of breakdown are noted and treatment begun promptly.
Nutrition, alteration in: less than body requirements	Monitor intravenous or tube feedings as necessary and document appropriately.
	Weigh patient daily.
	Watch closely for signs of dehydration and malnutrition and report immediately.
	Convalescent care: Evaluate patient's ability to swallow.
	If patient is eating and has a cuffed tracheostomy tube, inflate cuff while patient eats and deflate after meals.
	Consult nutritionist to plan attractive, nourishing meals.
	Provide high-calorie snacks if needed.
	Provide attractive, clean environment at meals and meticulous mouth care before meals, since patient may experience loss of taste because of decreased sense of smell.
	Weigh patient daily and maintain accurate record of intake and output.
	If the patient is receiving tube feedings, ensure that they are of sufficient caloric value to maintain weight and promote wound healing.
	Monitor patient's hydration and nutritional status.
	Follow established guidelines for tube feedings, that is, check for placement in stomach and residual before next tube feeding.
	Replace residual, and hold feeding if greater than 100 ml.
	Feed patient with head of bed elevated.
	Assess patient's bowel activity.
Home maintenance management, impaired	*Convalescent care:* If patient will be discharged with tracheostomy, ensure that patient and family have been instructed in and understand management of tracheostomy at home, including suctioning, cleaning, wound care, humidification, changing tracheostomy tapes, and tube feeding if necessary.
	Ensure that family and patient know where to purchase supplies and when to return to see physician.[12]
	To prepare tracheostomy tube for decannulation:
	Evaluate patient's ability to breathe and cough effectively, gag reflex, and swallowing reflexes.
	Report any symptoms of distress to physician immediately.
	"Plug" tracheostomy tube intermittently and increase length of time for occlusion as patient tolerates.

Nursing Diagnosis	Nursing Intervention
	Remove tracheostomy tube or assist physician with removal of tube when patient tolerates occlusion well.
	Apply Steri-Strips or tape to approximate wound edges.
	Check and cleanse wound site daily.
	Observe for signs of infection; opening should heal within few days.
	Make referral to visiting nurse or public health nurse.

Patient Education

1. Inform the patient that there will be frequent suctioning, a loss of speech, and decreased ability to smell and that he will not be breathing through the nose or mouth while the tracheostomy is present.
2. Refer the patient to a speech therapist, if appropriate, to learn esophageal or alternative method of speech.

EVALUATION

Patient Outcome	Data Indicating That Outcome is Reached
If short-term tracheostomy, respiratory status is within normal limits.	Patient has no excess secretions and tracheostomy stoma is healed without signs of infection. Patient experiences no dyspnea or shortness of breath.
Nutritional status is maintained.	Weight is normal and patient eats regularly.
If long-term tracheostomy, patient and family demonstrate ability to care for all aspects of tracheostomy at home.	Patient or family demonstrates suctioning and cleaning techniques, wound care, changing tapes, and methods for humidification. Visiting or public health nurse assists patient or family if necessary.
Nutritional status is maintained.	Weight and caloric intake are normal for patient. Patient and family demonstrate ability to administer tube feedings as necessary.

TYMPANOPLASTY

Description and Rationale

Tympanoplasty is a reconstructive or reparative procedure of the middle ear that is usually performed to correct conductive hearing loss caused by chronic suppurative otitis media. The procedure involves rebuilding the structures of the middle ear or replacing them with prostheses. Tympanoplasty may also be occasionally performed to close a perforation of the tympanic membrane (myringoplasty or type I tympanoplasty) or to assist with clearing infections in patients with chronic suppurative otitis media and a sensorineural (rather than conductive) hearing loss. There is no chance of correcting the hearing loss in these patients. Tympanoplasty may also be indicated in patients with ossicular problems such as dislocation of the incus from trauma, congenital middle ear problems, or tympanosclerosis, in which the malleus is

fused to the incus. In these cases metal or plastic prostheses, autogenous material, or cadaveric ossicles are commonly used. Since these patients have no concomitant infection, the results are often good.[7]

The principal rationale for tympanoplasty is to improve hearing in patients with conductive hearing loss but intact nerve function or cochlear reserve. The greatest improvement is seen in patients with bilateral disease and a large difference between air and bone measurements. In chronic otitis media the tympanic membrane, malleus, and incus are frequently damaged or destroyed. If this occurs, sound waves can enter the oval and round window with equal intensity and cancel each other, since the tympanic membrane is not there to protect the round window from sound pressure. Chronic otitis media also disrupts the areal ratio, or the tympanic membrane–foot-

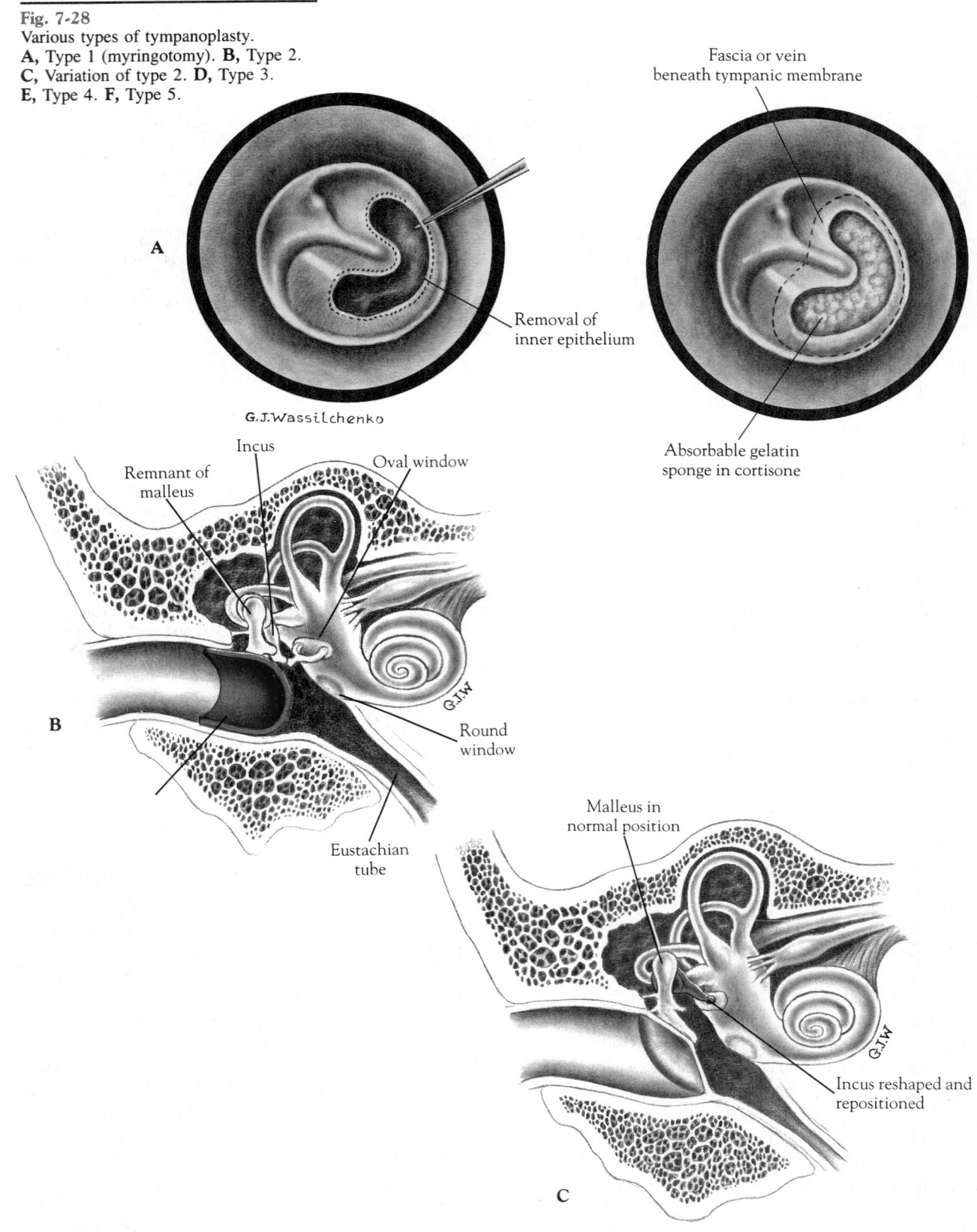

Fig. 7-28
Various types of tympanoplasty.
A, Type 1 (myringotomy). **B,** Type 2.
C, Variation of type 2. **D,** Type 3.
E, Type 4. **F,** Type 5.

A

Removal of inner epithelium

G.J.Wassilchenko

Fascia or vein beneath tympanic membrane

Absorbable gelatin sponge in cortisone

B

Remnant of malleus

Incus

Oval window

Round window

Eustachian tube

C

Malleus in normal position

Incus reshaped and repositioned

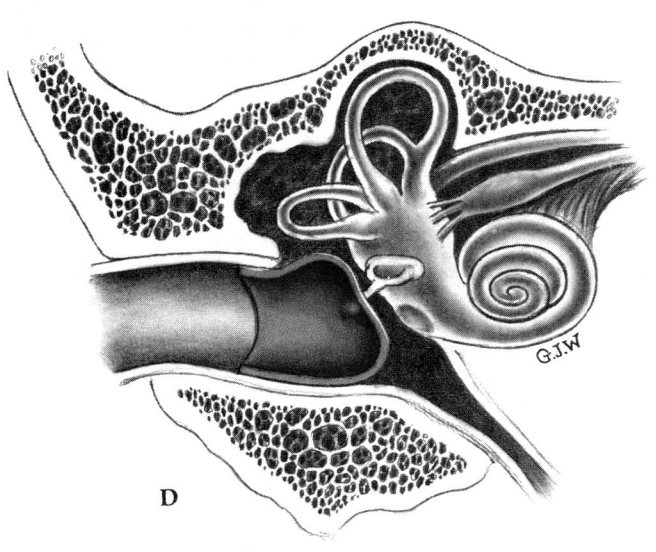

D

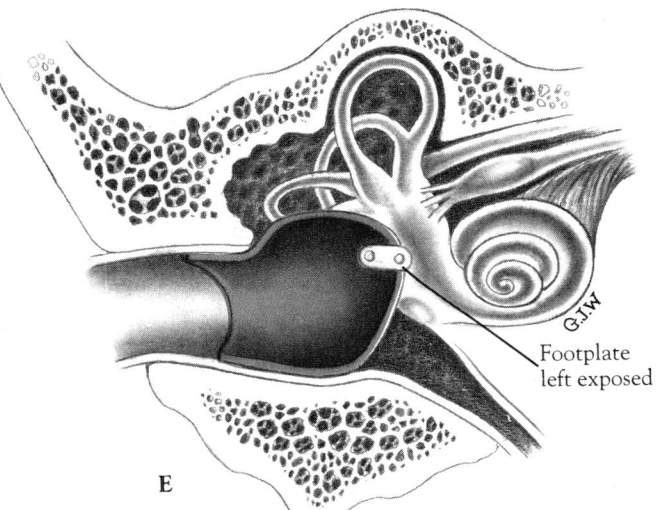

Footplate
left exposed

E

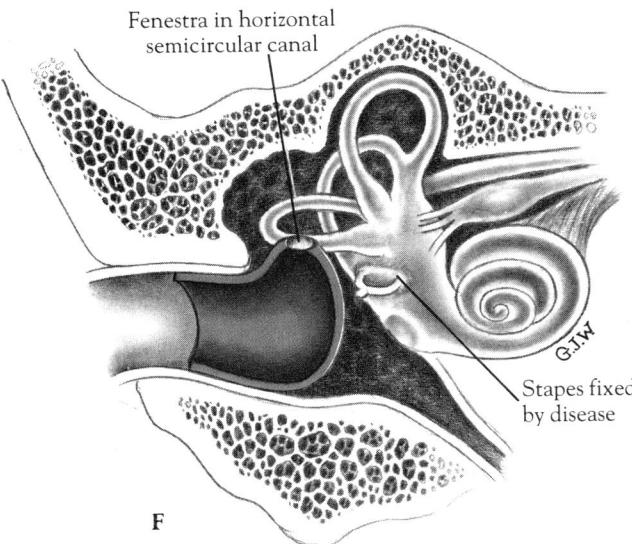

Fenestra in horizontal
semicircular canal

Stapes fixed
by disease

F

plate ratio, thereby negating the transformer action of the middle ear.

Tympanoplasty, of which there are five types described below, improves hearing by reestablishing two important middle ear functions: restoring the areal ratio and creating sound protection for the round window.

Contraindications and Cautions

Presence of infection; procedure to clear infection must be performed before tympanoplasty

Patients with poor nerve function as determined by bone conduction tests

Hearing loss from otosclerosis or serous otitis media rather than chronic suppurative otitis media

TREATMENT PLAN

Surgical (See Fig. 7-28)

Postaural or endaural approach; with operating microscope at high magnification, surgeon performs one of five types of tympanoplasty, using either temporal fascia or tissue from nearby vein as graft; tympanic membranes from human cadavers sometimes used as graft, although this technique is still being evaluated; Teflon or stainless steel wires also used occasionally

Type I (myringoplasty)—performed for closure and perforation; epithelium removed from edge of perforation and graft of autogenous tissue, usually fascia or vein placed under tympanic membrane; areal ratio and round window sound protection restored

Type II—performed when malleus is eroded; perforation closed with graft against incus or what remains of malleus; enough ossicular chain must remain to create new areal ratio

Type III—also restores both areal ratio and sound protection of round window by means of autogenous graft; performed when tympanic membrane and ossicular chain are destroyed but normal stapes remains; graft is placed in contact with stapes

Type IV—areal ratio cannot be restored, but round window sound protection is provided; only footplate remains intact, and air pocket is placed between round window and graft to provide sound protection

Type V—only round window sound protection provided; footplate is fixed and fenestration into inner ear must be performed

Chemotherapeutic

Narcotic analgesics

Meperidine (Demerol), 50 mg IM q4h prn

Acetaminophen (Tylenol), 600 mg with codeine q4-6h prn

Anti-infective agents

Tetracycline (Achromycin), 250 mg po q6h, or penicillin G, 250-500 mg po q6h

Antiemetics (for antivertigo effect)

Meclizine (Antivert), 250 mg po ½ h ac and hs

Supportive

Bed rest until next morning with head of bed elevated 40 degrees and operative side facing upward

ASSESSMENT: AREAS OF CONCERN

Middle ear function

Bleeding; amount, color, and consistency of drainage; temperature and dizziness when getting out of bed or with sudden movement; nausea; vertigo

NURSING DIAGNOSES and NURSING INTERVENTIONS

Nursing Diagnosis	Nursing Intervention
Injury: potential for	Encourage patient to maintain bed rest until first morning after surgery. Keep patient from lying on operative side. Elevate head of bed 40 degrees. Assess, record, and report unusual bleeding or drainage from operative side. Assist with ambulation when patient is allowed to get up.
Sensory-perceptual alteration: auditory	Reassure patient that hearing improvement, if expected, will not be noticed until edema and drainage at operative site have decreased.

Patient Education

1. Instruct the patient to avoid showering or shampooing until permitted by the physician in order to prevent contamination of the ear canal.
2. Instruct the patient to notify the physician immediately if there is evidence of fever, bleeding, increased drainage, or dizziness after discharge.
3. Instruct the patient to use Antivert for about 1 month after surgery to minimize dizziness.
4. Instruct the patient to avoid blowing the nose with force.

EVALUATION

Patient Outcome	Data Indicating That Outcome is Reached
Graft heals well.	There is no fever, excessive drainage, or dizziness.
Hearing is improved if this was reason for procedure.	Increased hearing is verified by audiometric testing.

References

1. Baugh, R., and Baker, S.: Epiglottitis in children: review of 24 cases, Otolaryngol. Head Neck Surg. **90**:157, 1982.
2. Berkow, R., editor-in-chief: The Merck manual of diagnosis and therapy, ed. 14, Rahway, N.J., 1982, Merck Sharp & Dohme Laboratories.
3. Berne, R.M., and Levy, M.: Physiology, St. Louis, 1983, The C.V. Mosby Co.
4. Blanco, K.M.: Acoustic neuroma: postoperative nursing care and rehabilitation, J. Neurosurg. Nurs. **13**:153, 1981.
5. Brooks, G.B., et al.: Acetazolamide in Ménière's disease: evaluation of a new diagnostic test for reversible endolymphatic hydrops, Otolaryngol. Head Neck Surg. **90**:358, 1982.
6. Chiu, R.T.K., et al.: Ménière's disease at the University of Iowa, 1973-1980, Otolaryngol. Head Neck Surg. **90**:482, 1982.
7. DeWeese, D.D., and Saunders, W.H.: Textbook of otolaryngology, ed. 6, St. Louis, 1982, The C.V. Mosby Co.
8. Diseases—the nurses reference library, Nursing 82 Books, Springhouse, Pa., 1982, Intermed Communications, Inc.
9. Dohlmann, G.F.: Mechanism of the Ménière attack, ORL J. Otorhinolaryngology Relat. Spec. **42**:10, 1980.
10. Ganong, W.F.: Review of medical physiology, ed. 11, Los Altos, Calif., 1983, Lange Medical Publications.
11. Gerson, C.R., and Tucker, G.F.: Infant tracheotomy, Ann. Otol. Rhinol. Laryngol. **91**:413, 1982.
12. Goode, R.L., and Schulz, W.: Heat myringotomy for the treatment of serous otitis media, Otolaryngol. Head Neck Surg. **90**:764, 1982.
13. Havener, W.H., et al.: Nursing care in eye, ear, nose and throat disorders, ed. 4, St. Louis, 1979, The C.V. Mosby Co.
14. Hirsch, J.E., and Hannock, L.A., editors: Mosby's manual of clinical nursing procedures, St. Louis, 1981, The C.V. Mosby Co.
15. Hughes, G.B., et al.: Cerebrospinal fluid leaks and meningitis following acoustic tumor surgery, Otolaryngol. Head Neck Surg. **90**:117, 1982.
16. Jazbi, B.: Subluxation of the nasal septum in the newborn: etiology, diagnosis and treatment, Otolaryngol. Clin. North Am., Philadelphia, 1977, W.B. Saunders Co.
17. Jongkees, L.B.W.: Some remarks on Ménière's disease, ORL J. Otorhinolaryngology Relat. Spec. **42**:1, 1980.
18. Kim, M.J., and Moritz, D.A.: Classification of nursing diagnoses, Proceedings from third and fourth national conferences, New York, 1982, McGraw-Hill Book Co.
19. Kirchner, F.R.: Endoscopic rehabilitation of the airway in laryngeal paralysis, Ann. Otol. Rhinol. Laryngol. **91**:382, 1982.
20. Kitahara, M., et al.: Experimental study on Ménière's disease, Otolaryngol. Head Neck Surg. **90**:470, 1982.
21. Kleinsasser, O.: Pathogenesis of vocal cord polyps, Ann. Otol. Rhinol. Laryngol. **91**:378, 1982.
22. Leonidas, J.D.: Radiologic diagnosis in pediatric otorhinolaryngology, Otolaryngol. Clin. North Am. **10**:1, 1977.
23. Lucente, F.E., et al.: Malignant external otitis: a dangerous misnomer, Otolaryngol. Head Neck Surg. **90**:266, 1982.
24. Luckmann, J., and Sorensen, K.: Medical-surgical nursing: a psychophysiologic approach, ed. 2, Philadelphia, 1980, W.B. Saunders Co.
25. Malasanos, L., et al.: Health assessment, ed. 2, St. Louis, 1981, The C.V. Mosby Co.
26. Maran, A.G.D., and Stell, P.M., editors: Clinical otolaryngology, Oxford, Eng., 1979, Blackwell Scientific Publications.
27. Moran, W.B.: Nasal trauma in children, Otolaryngol. Clin. North Am. **10**:95, 1977.
28. Nordmark, M.T., and Rohweder, A.W.: Scientific foundations of nursing, ed. 3, Philadelphia, 1975, J.B. Lippincott Co.
29. Pallanch, J.F.: Prosthetic closure of nasal septal perforations, Otolaryngol. Head Neck Surg. **90**:448, 1982.
30. Parisier, S.C.: Surgical therapy of chronic mastoiditis with cholesteatoma, Otolaryngol. Head Neck Surg. **90**:767, 1982.
31. Price, S., and Wilson, L.: Pathophysiology: clinical concepts of disease processes, New York, 1982, McGraw-Hill Book Co.
32. Rejowski, J., et al.: Nasal polyps causing bone destruction and blindness, Otolaryngol. Head Neck Surg. **90**:505, 1982.
33. Saxton, D.F., et al.: The Addison-Wesley manual of nursing practice, Menlo Park, Calif., 1983, Addison-Wesley Publishing Co.
34. Shea, J.J.: Stapedectomy—a long term report, Ann. Otol. Rhinol. Laryngol. **91**:516, 1982.
35. Sheehy, J.L.: Diffuse exostoses and osteomata of the external auditory canal: a report of 100 operations, Otolaryngol. Head Neck Surg. **90**:337, 1982.
36. Silverstein, H., and Norrell, H.: Retrolabyrinthine vestibular neurectomy, Otolaryngol. Head Neck Surg. **90**:778, 1982.
37. Thompson, J.M., and Bowers, A.C.: Clinical manual of health assessment, St. Louis, 1980, The C.V. Mosby Co.
38. Tortorelli, B.A.: Acoustic neuroma: an overview of the disorder and nursing care for these patients, J. Neurosurg. Nurs. **13**:170, 1981.
39. Tos, M., and Thomsen, J.: The price of preservation of hearing in acoustic neuroma surgery, Ann. Otol. Rhinol. Laryngol. **91**:240, 1982.

40. Tucker, S.M., et al.: Patient care standards, St. Louis, 1980, The C.V. Mosby Co.
41. Ward, P., and Berci, G.: Observations on so-called idiopathic vocal cord paralysis, Ann. Otol. Rhinol. Laryngol. **91:**558, 1982.
42. Wehrmaker, S.L., and Wintermute, J.R.: Case studies in neurological nursing, Boston, 1978, Little, Brown & Co.

Suggested Readings

Black, F.O., et al.: Diagnosis and management of drop attacks of vestibular origin: Tumarkin's otolithic crisis, Otolaryngol. Head Neck Surg. **90:**256, 1982.
Geurkink, N.: Nasal anatomy, physiology and function, J. Allergy Clin. Immunol. **72:**123, 1983.

Hough, J. Van Doren: Tympanoplasty. In Gibb, A.G., and Mansfield, F.W.S., editors: Otolaryngology 1, London, 1982, Butterworth's International Medical Reviews.
Merzenich, M., et al.: Cochlear implant prostheses: strategies and progress, Ann. Biomed. Eng. **8:**361, 1980.
Rybak, L.P.: Medical treatment of chronic sinusitis in the immunocompetent and immunosuppressed patient: a review, Otolaryngol. Head Neck Surg. **90:**534, 1982.
Saunders, W.H., and Gardner, R.W.: Pharmacotherapy in otolaryngology, St. Louis, 1976, The C.V. Mosby Co.
Saunders, W.H., et al.: Atlas of ear surgery, ed. 3, St. Louis, 1980, The C.V. Mosby Co.

CHAPTER 8

Endocrine and Metabolic Systems

Overview

The endocrine system is a widely diversified system of glands, hormones, intermediate metabolites, and cellular responses. The functional responsibilities of this system include growth, development, reproduction, production of energy, fluid and electrolyte balance, and a response to stress. A single gland may hold primary responsibility for a particular function, but the interrelationships between and among glandular functions are called the endocrine and metabolic systems.

The hypothalamus and anterior pituitary gland work together to regulate the endocrine system. These two very small organs mediate essential functions such as growth, thyroid balance, and fertility. The hypothalamus coordinates central nervous system input with hormone release. It regulates the anterior lobe of the pituitary gland, which in turn directs target organ release of specific hormones (e.g., release of cortisol from the adrenal glands).

The posterior lobe of the pituitary gland is known as the neurohypophysis. It secretes two hormones, vasopressin (antidiuretic hormone) and oxytocin. These hormones are responsible for the control of water balance and the milk letdown reflex, respectively.[73]

The thyroid gland is one of the largest endocrine glands. A well-functioning and healthy thyroid gland is essential for normal growth and development and maintenance of metabolic stability in the adult.[25] Thyroid disease is relatively common.[25] Special diagnostic problems may occur because a multiplicity of metabolic processes are affected by the thyroid hormones. Thyroid hormones, for example, influence the concentration and activity of numerous enzymes as well as the metabolism of substrates, vitamins, and minerals.[73] The secretion and degradation rates of all other hormones as well as their target tissue responses are also affected by the thyroid hormones. For these reasons, thyroid hormones affect all tissues and organ systems.[73]

Parathyroid glands regulate calcium exchange through three major hormones: parathyroid hormone, calcitonin, and $1,25(OH)_2D_3$ (vitamin D). Calcium is regulated by a negative-feedback mechanism involving the intestines, kidneys, bones, and mammary glands during lactation. Homeostasis of calcium ion concentration is essential for bone formation, transmission of nerve impulses, maintenance of cardiac and skeletal muscle contractility, and

823

efficient blood clotting. Calcium levels are maintained in equilibrium with phosphate levels for storage and release of energy, metabolism of carbohydrates and lipids, and regulation of serum pH.

The adrenal glands are two of the major endocrine organs in the body. Although small in size, their impact on the body system is significant and, in fact, vital to human life.[20] The condition of the adrenal cortex will determine how effectively the body can respond to stress, trauma, and infections as well as perform carbohydrate, fat, and protein metabolism. The adrenal medulla is part of the sympathetic nervous system. Homeostasis is maintained during physical and emotional stress in part by the release of catecholamines from the chromaffin cells of the adrenal medulla. Catecholamines are hormones that evoke an adrenergic, metabolic, and glycemic response from the body systems. The central nervous system also secretes catecholamines, making survival possible without adrenal medullary activity.[32]

The pancreas functions primarily as an exocrine gland, secreting enzymes for the digestion of food. Twenty percent of the gland (islets of Langerhans) has an endocrine function, secreting glucagon, insulin, gastrin, and somatostatin. The endocrine role of the pancreas was first demonstrated in 1886 when Minkowski and Von Mering produced diabetes in a dog by total pancreatectomy.

The gonads are the endocrine glands responsible for production of the reproductive (sex) cells. They are also the body's major contributor of the sex hormones. The male gonads, the testes, secrete testosterone in utero, which is necessary for sex differentiation of the fetus. The female gonads, the ovaries, primarily secrete estrogen. Through direct stimulation by the pituitary gland, gonadal hormones initiate pubertal development. Likewise, they take the child through puberty into adulthood, sustaining the development of secondary sexual characteristics and fertility.[35]

Genetic disorders may result in a direct alteration in the formation of a gland or the release and effect of a hormone. More often, however, genetic alterations result in problems of intermediary metabolism.

ANATOMY AND PHYSIOLOGY
Hypothalamus and Anterior Pituitary Gland

The hypothalamus is part of the cerebrum of the brain and is located beneath the cerebral hemisphere on each side of the third ventricle. It is connected to the thalamus above by neural tissue and to the pituitary gland below by the pituitary stalk[52] (Fig. 8-1). The hypothalamus is approximately 6 cm in diameter.[43a]

The pituitary gland is located in an indentation of the sphenoid bone, the sella turcica, at the base of the brain. The gland is oval shaped and approximately 1 cm in diameter. It consists of two distinct parts: 75% of the gland is the anterior lobe, and 25% is the posterior lobe. Phylogenetically, the anterior pituitary gland (the adenohypophysis) originates from an outpouching of the roof of the mouth.[52] It is the anterior pituitary gland that is involved in the regulation of the majority of endocrine functions.

The hypothalamus has the dual function of regulating autonomic nervous system and endocrine functions.[52] With neural regulation, it affects multiple diverse functions such as body temperature, sweating, gastrointestinal secretion and motility, blood pressure, sleep, and response to pleasure and pain. The hypothalamus influences fluid and electrolyte balance as well as cell metabolism by the production and release of hypothalamic hormones, which directly affect the pituitary gland. These hormones are known as releasing hormones (if a chemical structure has been identified) or as releasing factors (if the chemical structure is unknown).[71] The hypothalamic-stimulating hormones are corticotropin-releasing hormone (CRH), growth hormone–releasing factor (GRF), thyrotropin-releasing hormone (TRH), and gonadotropin-releasing hormone (GnRH, LHRH). The hypothalamic-inhibiting factors and hormones are melanocyte-inhibiting factor (MIF), prolactin-inhibiting factor (PIF), and somatostatin (also known as growth hormone–inhibiting hormone).[29]

The hypothalamic hormones travel down the pituitary stalk through the portal blood supply to their target, the anterior pituitary gland. They cause the pituitary gland to release specific hormones: luteinizing hormone (LH), follicle-stimulating hormone (FSH), growth hormone (GH), prolactin (PRL), adrenocorticotropic hormone (ACTH), thyroid-stimulating hormone (TSH), and melanocyte-stimulating hormone (MSH). These hormones travel through the bloodstream to their target tissues.

The physiologic effects of GH are multiple and diverse, whereas PRL, MSH, LH, and FSH cause more specific tissue responses. GH influences the body in two general areas: growth and metabolism. It promotes bone growth, "stimulates protein anabolism, promotes lipolysis, enhances absorption of dietary calcium, and antagonizes the action of insulin."[31] PRL is responsible for breast development and lactation. MSH stimulates pigmentation activity in the skin. LH and FSH are responsible for the development of secondary sexual characteristics as well as fertility. LH and FSH are released in a cyclic, pulsatile fashion in both sexes; this release is necessary for normal gonadal function.

The three tropic hormones directly affecting gonadal function are FSH, LH, and PRL. In males, LH and FSH bind to specific receptors in the testes, Leydig's cells and

Fig. 8-1
Anatomy of the hypothalamus and pituitary.

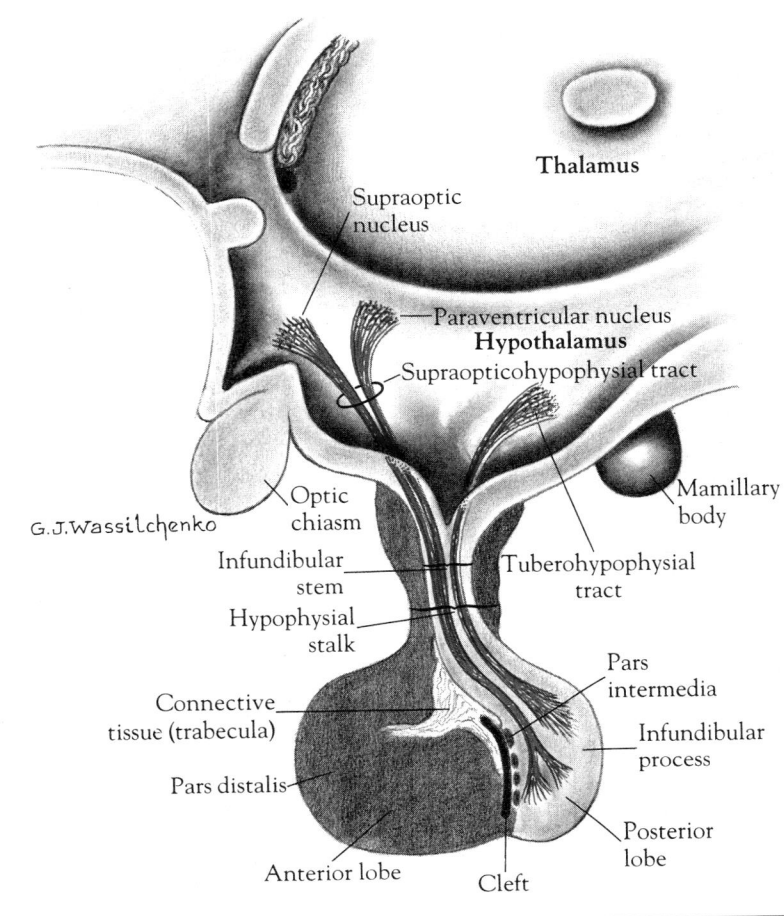

Sertoli cells, respectively. LH stimulates maturation of Leydig's cells and stimulates synthesis and secretion of the gonadal steroid, testosterone. Testosterone and FSH facilitate LH effects by helping develop LH receptors in Leydig's cells. Studies suggest that PRL and FSH may also help androgen synthesis in Leydig's cells.[25]

FSH was originally thought to be the hormone responsible for spermatogenesis. However, LH and testosterone both are needed for full spermatogenesis.[25] FSH is necessary for the conversion of spermatogonia into sperm and testosterone is postulated to be necessary for final maturation.[41]

The gonadotropin release is regulated by a negative-feedback system from testicular secretions. Testosterone has a negative feedback on LH secretion. Estradiol, produced through testosterone, has also been found to inhibit LH secretion.[25] A testicular hormone, inhibin, produced in the Sertoli cells, has been identified as the negative feedback for FSH. These negative feedbacks appear not only at the pituitary level but at the hypothalamic level as well. Tissues in the hypothalamus have a high affinity for testosterone and estradiol, and these both inhibit GnRH secretion.[3]

Communication along the hypothalamus–pituitary–target tissue axis is maintained through feedback mechanisms to control the fluctuating hormone levels. The feedback system between the hypothalamus and pituitary gland is known as a short-loop, negative-feedback mechanism.[20] With this mechanism, high levels of pituitary hormones cause the hypothalamus to decrease the release of its hormones, which in turn causes levels of pituitary hormones to decrease. The target organs also communicate by a long-loop, negative-feedback mechanism to regulate hormone release from the pituitary gland and the hypothalamus (Fig. 8-2).

Another factor that affects circulating hormone levels is an intrinsic rhythm of the release of pituitary hormones. This is probably controlled by the central nervous system through the hypothalamus.[73] One example of this rhythmicity is the sharp release of GH, LH (during puberty), and PRL from the pituitary gland 1 hour after the onset of deep sleep.[73] Another example is the diurnal variation

Fig. 8-2
Negative-feedback mechanism.

Adapted from information in Muthe, M.C.:
Endocrinology: a nursing approach,
Boston, 1981, Little, Brown & Co.; and
Williams, R., editor: Textbook of
endocrinology, Philadelphia, 1981, W.B.
Saunders Co.

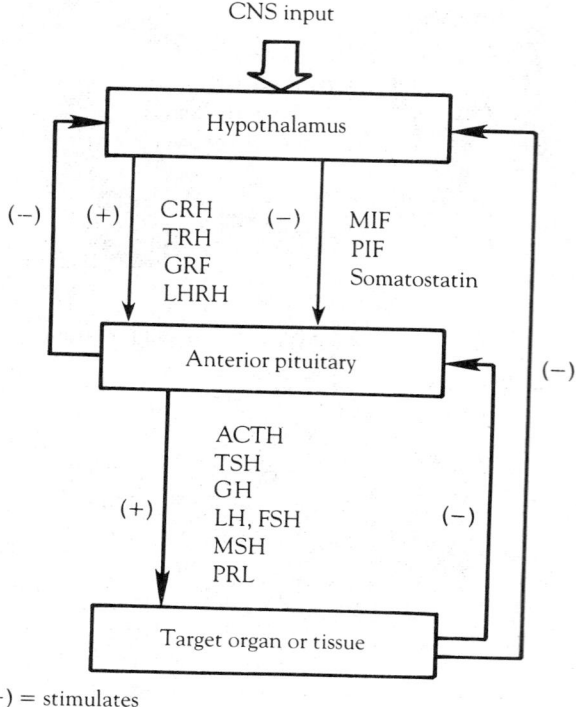

(+) = stimulates
(−) = inhibits

may be inhibited by emotional stress, pain, or fright. Oxytocin release is stimulated by a crying baby, sexual excitement, and orgasm. Although oxytocin may be used to induce labor and control obstetric hemorrhage, its physiologic role in initiating and maintaining normal labor is still unclear. Patients with complete hypophysectomy seem to progress through labor normally.[20,73]

Vasopressin acts to conserve water in the renal collecting duct; thus it is also known as the antidiuretic hormone (ADH). ADH causes an increase in the permeability of the renal collecting ducts to water, thereby increasing water retention and decreasing urine output. The production of ADH in the hypothalamus and the release of ADH from the posterior pituitary gland are determined by plasma osmolality and extracellular fluid volume. The secretion of ADH is regulated by three factors:

1. Osmoreceptors in the median eminence of the hypothalamus respond to changes in plasma osmolality. Increases in osmolality stimulate the release of ADH; decreases in osmolality inhibit ADH release.
2. Volume receptors in the left atrium and great vessels inhibit ADH release when vascular volume is increased.
3. Baroreceptors in the carotid sinus and aortic arch stimulate ADH release when blood pressure is decreased.[73]

ADH secretion is stimulated by factors such as hemorrhage, a reduction in cardiac output, dehydration, and hypoalbuminemic states. The limbic system also plays a role in the stimulation of ADH during stress, trauma, heat, fear, and pain. Certain drugs may also promote ADH secretion, such as morphine, nicotine, barbiturates, beta-adrenergic agents, general anesthetics, vincristine, cyclophosphamide (Cytoxan), carbamazepine, and chlorpropamide. Inhibition of ADH occurs during states of hypervolemia and hypo-osmolality. Total body immersion in water and a sensation of cold also inhibit ADH secretion. Pharmacologic agents inhibiting ADH include morphine antagonists, alpha-adrenergic agents, and ethyl alcohol.[20]

Free water loss leads to concentration of the blood, and plasma osmolality rises. When plasma osmolality reaches about 288 mOsm/kg, two things occur. First, the osmoreceptors in the hypothalamus are stimulated and promote synthesis of ADH in the hypothalamic nuclei and release of ADH from the posterior pituitary gland. Second, a perception of thirst occurs, leading to the ingestion of water. ADH causes the kidney to increase water reabsorption, resulting in antidiuresis. As plasma osmolality returns toward normal, stimulation of osmoreceptors is reduced, and ADH secretion decreases. The sensation of thirst is reduced. Overhydration dilutes the

of ACTH secretion. The secretion of hypothalamic hormones is also affected by psychoneurologic components, such as stress.

The neurohypophysis secretes two hormones: vasopressin and oxytocin. Vasopressin is the primary regulator of water metabolism in human beings. Oxytocin is responsible for the milk letdown phenomenon and stimulates the contraction of uterine muscles in labor. Neurogenic reflexes from the nipple travel through the spinal cord and midbrain to the hypothalamus. The neurohypophysis then releases oxytocin, which stimulates contractions of mammary myoepithelium; this results in the ejection of milk. Both of these hormones are synthesized in the supraoptic and paraventricular nuclei of the hypothalamus. They are transported along the neurohypophyseal tract to the posterior lobe of the pituitary gland, where they are stored. Rapid release of these hormones occurs in response to a variety of stimuli.[73] Oxytocin

Fig. 8-3
Thyroid anatomy.

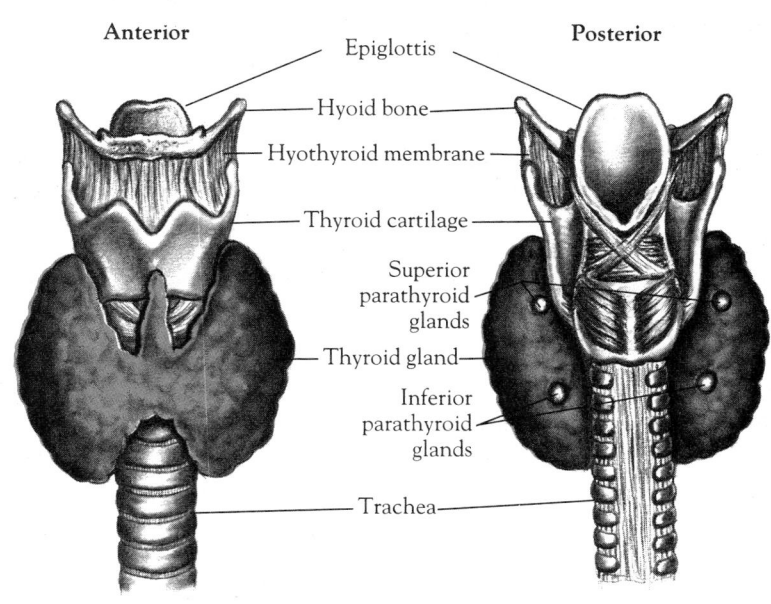

Thyroid Gland

The thyroid gland weighs approximately 20 g in the healthy adult. It is composed of two lobes positioned on either side of the trachea and joined by the isthmus. The right lobe is larger and more vascular than the left lobe. The recurrent laryngeal nerves run in the grooves beside the trachea and behind the lobes of the thyroid gland. The thyroid gland is located anteriorly just below the cricoid cartilage (Fig. 8-3).

Embryologically, the thyroid gland begins as epithelial tissue in the pharyngeal floor. Deviations in normal embryonic development may consist of (1) failure of lobe development, (2) development of a lingual thyroid gland from remnants of the thyroglossal duct, (3) thyroglossal cyst formation from duct remnants, or (4) substernal goiter formation from resultant descent of the thyroid gland along the developmental path of the thymus into the thorax.[25,73]

Thyroid blood supply is well in excess of the kidney blood supply. This blood supply is furnished by two major pairs of arteries that account for the rich vascularity of the gland and for the increased risk of hemorrhage that may occur postoperatively. The presence of a palpable thrill or audible bruit over the gland or surrounding area is indicative of an increased blood flow.[73]

The thyroid gland is innervated by (1) the adrenergic nervous system, from the cervical ganglia; (2) the cholinergic nervous system, from the vagus nerve; and (3) a network of adrenergic fibers that terminate near the basement membrane of the follicular walls.[73] Thyroid blood flow is regulated by neurogenic stimuli.

The thyroid is composed of follicular and parafollicular cells. The follicles are filled with proteinaceous colloid.[25] Colloid is the major constituent of total thyroid mass.

The function of the follicular cells is to secrete the two major thyroid hormones, thyroxine (T_4) and triiodothyronine (T_3). The parafollicular cells or C cells secrete a third hormone, thyrocalcitonin (calcitonin), a calcium-lowering substance. Parafollicular cells are located in the interfollicular connective tissue.[73]

The major component of thyroid hormones is iodine. Normal iodine balance depends on sufficient dietary intake. Seafoods are the major natural sources. Medications, diagnostic agents, dietary supplements, and the use of iodine by the food-processing industry and in the food given to animals have increased iodine ingestion in the more highly developed countries.[73] Normal daily dietary intake of iodine varies widely throughout the world primarily because of the varying iodine content of soil and water and because of cultural food preferences.[73] The minimum daily requirement of iodide is about 80

blood, and plasma osmolality decreases. When it reaches about 282 mOsm/kg, the synthesis and release of ADH are inhibited. The kidneys decrease water reabsorption, and diuresis ensues. Serum osmolality returns toward normal.[25,42]

μg.[25] However, dietary intake of iodine ranges as high as 500 μg or more daily in most areas of the United States.[25]

Iodine is rapidly absorbed from the gastrointestinal tract, primarily as iodide, the form in which it is carried in the blood, and is largely confined to the extracellular fluid (ECF) compartment.[73] When absorbed in organic form, iodine is converted to iodide in the liver.[25] Small quantities of iodine are lost in the stool, in expired air, and through the skin.[73] During lactation, more notable losses occur.[73] Primary removal from the ECF pool occurs by (1) excretion of iodine into the urine and (2) transport of iodine into the thyroid gland.

Renal clearance of iodide is important because it determines the availability of iodide to the thyroid gland.[73] The kidneys are considered passive participants in iodide metabolism and are not a part of the body's defense mechanism for maintenance of thyroidal homeostasis.

Biosynthesis of the thyroid hormones occurs in sequential stages: (1) iodide trapping; (2) oxidation of the

Fig. 8-4
Biosynthesis of thyroid hormones.

From Clark, J.F., Queener, S.F., and Karb, V.B.: Pharmacological basis of nursing practice, ed. 2, St. Louis, 1986, The C.V. Mosby Co.

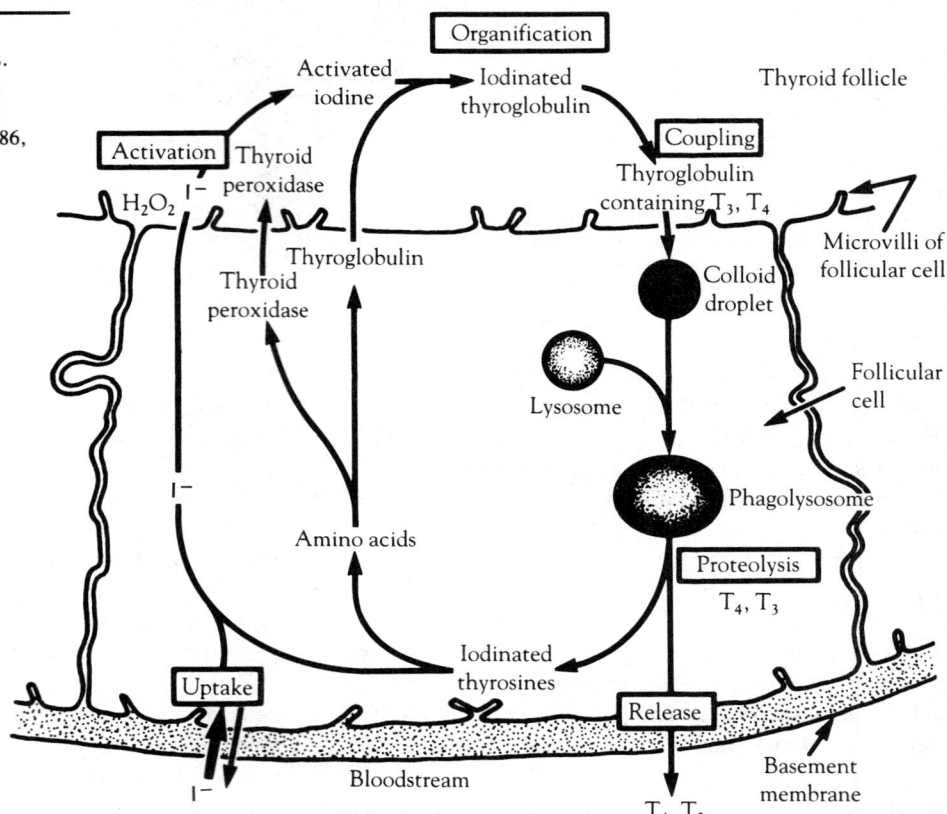

Sequential steps in release of T_4 and T_3 into the general circulation:

1. Stimulation of the thyroid by TSH.
2. Formation of pseudopodia occurs at the apical surface of the follicular cells.
3. Endocytosis of thyroglobulin in colloid to yield multiple vesicles termed colloid droplets.
4. Movement of colloid droplet into the cell and fusion with lysosomes to form phagolysosomes.
5. Migration of phagolysosomes toward base of the cell.
6. Proteolysis of the thyroglobulin molecule (proteinases for digestion are located within phagolysosomes) with the resultant disappearance of colloid and release of T_3 and T_4, MIT, and DIT into the cell.
7. Diffusion of T_3 and T_4 out of cell into the circulation.

iodide ion; (3) organification of thyroglobulin; and (4) coupling of iodotyrosines to form the active hormones, T_4 and T_3 (Fig. 8-4).

The first step in synthesis is iodide uptake by the follicular cells. This step is referred to as iodide transport or the iodide pump. Iodide is transported from the ECF into the thyroid glandular cells and follicles. TSH stimulates iodide transport activity.[73] In addition, iodide transport is depressed by excess iodide administration and increased by iodide deficiency.[25]

During the second phase of biosynthesis, the iodide ions are converted to an oxidized form of iodine capable of combining directly with tyrosine amino acids located within thyroglobulin. Thyroglobulin is a large glycoprotein molecule synthesized and secreted into the follicles.

The binding of iodine with the thyroglobulin molecule is called organification. Oxidized iodine combines with tyrosine to form the hormonally *inactive* iodotyrosines, monoiodotyrosine (MIT) and diiodotyrosine (DIT). The coupling phase continues and results in the formation of the hormonally *active* iodothyronines. T_4 is formed when

two molecules of DIT combine. T_3 results when one molecule of MIT couples with one molecule of DIT.

Thyroglobulin serves as a storage depot for the thyroid hormones and the precursors MIT and DIT. A 30-day supply of T_3 and T_4 and a 2-day supply of iodine stored as MIT or DIT are normally contained within the thyroglobulin.[15] The thyroid gland is therefore unique among the endocrine glands because of its large storage of hormones.

T_4 and T_3 enter the bloodstream directly after being cleaved from the thyroglobulin molecule. This process occurs in sequential steps as outlined in Fig. 8-4. The inactive iodotyrosines do not reach the circulation. Instead, their iodine is cleaved from them and reutilized in the thyroid gland.[25] This process is an important salvage mechanism for maintenance of iodothyronine synthesis.

T_4 is solely produced by the thyroid gland with a total daily production rate of 80 to 100 μg.[25] T_3 is secreted from the thyroid gland, but most of it is produced by extrathyroidal deiodination of T_4. Approximately 80% of the daily T_3 production (20 to 30 μg) is produced in this manner.[25] The half-life of T_4 in the circulation is 6 to 7 days.[25] T_3 has a half-life of 30 hours in the circulation.[25]

Upon entering the bloodstream, T_4 and T_3 are bound to circulating plasma proteins.[25] These proteins are (1) thyroxine-binding globulin (TBG), a glycoprotein synthesized in the liver; (2) thyroxine-binding prealbumin; and (3) albumin. Any disorders producing changes in the serum-binding protein concentrations have major effects on serum T_4 and T_3 concentrations. Unbound T_4 and T_3 levels are reflected in measurements of serum *free* T_4 and T_3.

Regulation of thyroid function is achieved through (1) the hypothalamic-pituitary-thyroid axis (Fig. 8-5) and (2) an autoregulatory mechanism within the gland. Thyrotropin-releasing hormone (TRH) is synthesized by neurons in the hypothalamus and is transported to cells of the anterior pituitary gland that contain specific cell membrane receptors for TRH binding. Thyroid-stimulating hormone (TSH) in the anterior pituitary gland is stimulated by the secretion of TRH. Most of the thyroid gland's metabolic processes are regulated by TSH. However, the primary action of TSH is the production and secretion of the thyroid hormones. The thyroid hormones, on the other hand, inhibit TSH secretion at the level of the anterior pituitary gland. Small alterations in serum T_4 and T_3 concentrations result in reciprocal changes in both TSH secretion and TSH response to exogenous TRH. Serum thyroid hormone levels will override the pituitary gland's response to TRH if the T_4 and T_3 levels are high.[25]

Blockage or removal of TSH stimulation results in hypovascularity and atrophy of the thyroid gland.[73] The

Fig. 8-5
Thyroid negative-feedback mechanism.

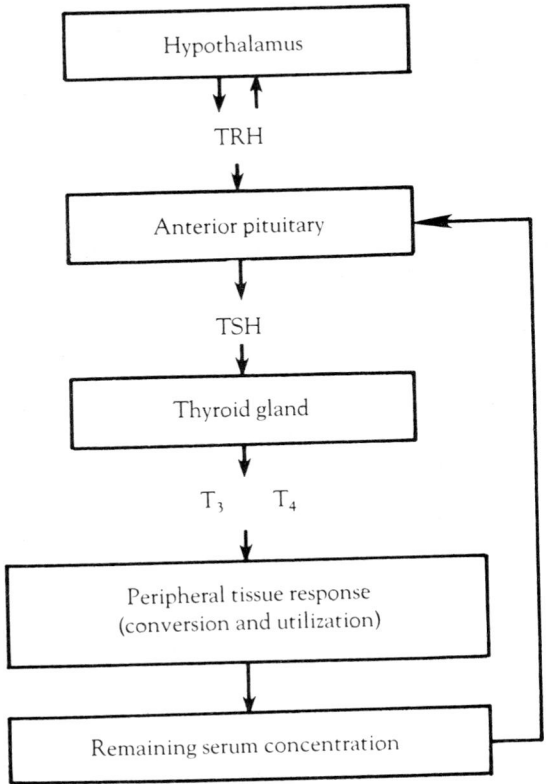

reverse effects occurs when stimulatory doses of TSH are produced. Secretion of TSH in serum is pulsatile in nature and is subject to a circadian rhythm. TSH secretion is characterized by fluctuations at 1- to 2-hour intervals and by a nocturnal surge before the onset of sleep.[73] The circadian variation does not appear to be determined by the cortisol rhythm or by fluctuations in serum T_4 and T_3 levels. If TSH secretion is completely destroyed (i.e., by hypophysectomy or suppression), there is a decreased activity of the thyroid iodide transport mechanism and organic binding is inhibited. The reverse effect occurs with administration of TSH.[73]

Many factors influence thyroid hormone function. For example, TSH secretion is affected by somatostatin, dopamine, and the catecholamines. Other factors that influence thyroid hormone functioning include (1) sex and sex hormones; (2) pregnancy; (3) the newborn state; (4) age; (5) the glucocorticoids; (6) environmental temperatures, especially exposure to extreme cold; (7) alterations in nutritional states (i.e., starvation or overfeeding); and (8) other nonthyroid illnesses such as cirrhosis and chronic renal failure.

Parathyroid Glands

There are usually two pairs of parathyroid glands located near the posterior surface of the thyroid gland. However, there may be as few as three glands or as many as six, and their location may vary. These glands are sometimes found in the mediastinum, within the thyroid gland, or behind the esophagus. The usual size of a gland is $5 \times 5 \times 3$ mm.

The parathyroid glands are made up of three types of cells: (1) chief cells, which are the main source of parathyroid hormone (PTH); (2) water clear cells, which increase in number as hormone secretion increases; and (3) oxyphil cells, which may be involved in the synthesis and secretion of PTH. PTH is a polypeptide that regulates calcium and phosphate metabolism. Its functions include the regulation of bone metabolism, maintenance of calcium concentration, and regulation of vitamin D synthesis.

PTH has three target areas, which are affected by the amount of hormone secreted. The first of these areas is bone. PTH increases the activity of osteoclasts, which form a pool to inhibit osteoblasts from forming bone when serum calcium levels are low. This mechanism allows calcium resorption into the ECF. Increased serum calcium levels cause a decrease in PTH secretion, which causes the reverse effect (i.e., osteoblasts are stimulated to form bone and calcium resorption is decreased).

The second target area affected by PTH is the kidney. As PTH secretion is increased there is an increase in renal tubular resorption of calcium and increased excre-

tion of phosphate. This mechanism keeps calcium levels in equilibrium with phosphate.

The third target area is the gastrointestinal tract, where PTH stimulates $1,25(OH)_2D_3$ (vitamin D) to increase absorption of calcium in the small intestine. Vitamin D allows calcium to transfer from the intestinal lumen into the intestinal wall. There is evidence that vitamin D is also essential for PTH to act effectively on bone synthesis.

Adrenal Glands

The adrenal glands are located at the level of the eleventh thoracic rib, lateral to the first lumbar vertebra. Positioned suprarenally, the adult adrenal glands are one-thirtieth the size of the kidney. The left adrenal gland is larger than the right and weighs 4 to 6 g.[20] There are two structures making up the adrenal gland: the adrenal cortex and the adrenal medulla.

Embryonically, the *adrenal cortex* is of mesodermic origin and arises from the coelomic epithelium.[56] The cortex has three distinct zones containing specific cell types responsible for the production of the glucocorticoids, mineralocorticoids, and androgen. The zona glomerulosa is the chief producer of aldosterone (the major mineralocorticoid), while the glucocorticoids and androgens are produced by the zona fasciculata and zona reticularis.[20,56]

The mineralocorticoids are responsible for sodium conservation and potassium excretion via the renal tubules, and maintenance of adequate extracellular volume.[73] The secretion of aldosterone is regulated by potassium ion concentration, the renin-angiotensin system, and ACTH (although this is a weak regulator).[50] The renin-angiotensin system influences ECF volume by regulating aldosterone secretion.[66] When fluid volume or intra-arterial volume is decreased, renin is released from the renal juxtaglomerular cells. This results in the formation of angiotensin I, which then converts to angiotensin II. The cells of the zona glomerulosa produce aldosterone in response to angiotensin II. Sodium is reabsorbed, extracellular volume increases, and renin secretion is decreased.[50,66] Aldosterone secretion increases as serum potassium increases.[66] When ACTH is administered, a rise in aldosterone secretion is documented.

Cortisol is the principal glucocorticoid secreted in humans.[66] Cortisol is secreted in a circadian rhythm. The level is higher in the morning than the evening.[43] Carbohydrate, protein, and fat metabolism are regulated by cortisol. Gluconeogenesis is potentiated by cortisol.[66] Glucocorticoids exert a catabolic effect on protein cells except in the liver, where there is an anabolic effect.[43] The excretion of digestive enzymes, maintenance of emotional well-being, maintenance of normal excitability of

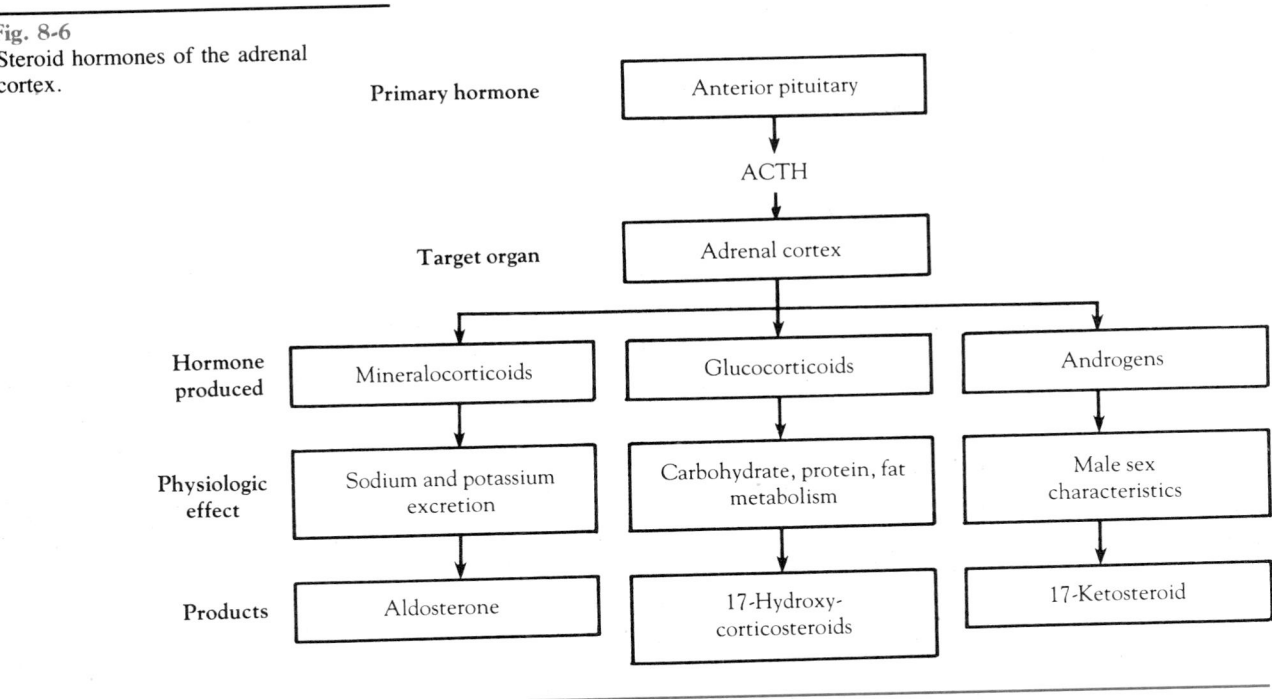

Fig. 8-6
Steroid hormones of the adrenal cortex.

the myocardium, and catecholamine action depend on the presence of glucocorticoids.[66] Studies have shown that without the existence of increased glucocorticoids in response to increased stress, death will occur.[66] The term *stress* is defined by Nelson to be "anything that exerts an effect upon the cell that disturbs its homeostatic balance beyond the cell's ability to compensate for that disturbance."[56] Glucocorticoids also exhibit an anti-inflammatory effect. Leukocytes are produced and neutrophils are increased along with a corresponding decrease in lymphocytes and eosinophils.[66] Capillary permeability is decreased.[27] The regulation of glucocorticoid release is via a negative-feedback system. The release of corticotropin-releasing hormone and ACTH does not depend on the source of cortisol. Exogenous forms of cortisol will influence the negative-feedback system.

ACTH secretion regulates the release of androgens. Androgens are responsible for the masculinization present in females (axillary and pubic hair) and supplement the major source of androgens in males (the testes)[66] (Fig. 8-6).

The adrenal medulla is the middle portion of each adrenal gland; it is made up of chromaffin cells and arises from the neural crest in the embryo. The chromaffin cells, or pheochromocytes, are functional at birth. The medulla is normally dark red-brown in color and is 8% to 10% of total adrenal weight. Central nervous system stimulation of the medulla is provided by the splanchnic nerve.

The medulla receives its vascular supply from blood that has flowed through the adrenal cortex, thus exposing the medulla to high levels of corticosteroids.[20]

The sympathetic nervous system innervates the adrenal medulla and on stimulation causes release of catecholamines. Catecholamines are both hormones (chemical substances that are released into the circulation and elicit a response from a target organ) and neurotransmitters (chemical substances released from nerve endings that have local effects).[25] Catecholamines are biosynthesized from tyrosine, an amino acid that comes from dietary sources, or from conversion of phenylalanine to tyrosine in the liver. Tyrosine is acted on by enzymes to initiate the catecholamine pathway (Fig. 8-7).

Norepinephrine and *epinephrine* are the main products of the pathway. Medullary catecholamine secretions are approximately 15% norepinephrine and 85% epinephrine. It is thought that the steroid-rich blood supply of the adrenal medulla maintains the enzyme phenylethanolamine N-methyl transferase (PNMT) and thus promotes the conversion of norepinephrine to epinephrine (Fig. 8-7). The medulla is the primary source of epinephrine production, while the central nervous system secretes norepinephrine almost exclusively. Epinephrine is 5 to 10 times more potent than norepinephrine, although norepinephrine has a longer duration of action.[25,52]

Norepinephrine and epinephrine are both alpha- and beta-adrenergic agonists, but norepinephrine primarily

Fig. 8-7
Catecholamine biosynthesis in the adrenal medulla.

From Felig, P., et al.: Endocrinology and metabolism, New York, 1981, McGraw-Hill Book Co.

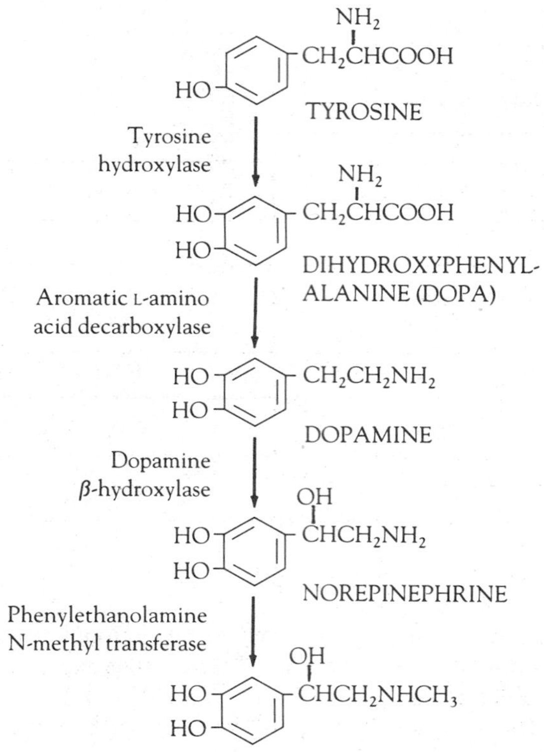
NH2
CH2CHCOOH
HO
TYROSINE
Tyrosine hydroxylase
NH2
HO
CH2CHCOOH
HO
DIHYDROXYPHENYL-ALANINE (DOPA)
Aromatic L-amino acid decarboxylase
HO
CH2CH2NH2
HO
DOPAMINE
Dopamine β-hydroxylase
OH
HO
CHCH2NH2
HO
NOREPINEPHRINE
Phenylethanolamine N-methyl transferase
OH
HO
CHCH2NHCH3
HO

stimulates the alpha-adrenergic receptors, and epinephrine stimulates the beta-adrenergic receptors. The actions of these catecholamines are briefly summarized in Table 8-1.

Catecholamines are excreted in the urine as urinary epinephrine and norepinephrine and are metabolized by enzymes and excreted as urinary metanephrine and urinary vanillylmandelic acid (VMA) (Fig. 8-8).

Pancreas

The pancreas lies behind the stomach to the left of the liver and is attached to the duodenum by ducts from the head and body section of the pancreas. It is through this duct that the pancreatic digestive enzymes enter the small intestine.

Each islet of Langerhans consists of a grouping of two to several hundred cells. The islets are scattered over the entire gland but are mainly concentrated in the tail section of the pancreas. The islets contain at least four different types of cells. About 10% to 20% of islet cells are alpha (A) cells, which secrete glucagon; 60% to 70% of the cells are beta (B) cells, which produce and secrete insulin.[9] The delta (D) and gamma (G) cells, which make up 2% to 8% of the islet cells, secrete somatostatin and gastrin, respectively.

The islet cells have a large blood supply and many nerve fibers. The central nervous system is linked to the islets through the autonomic nervous system's adrenergic and cholinergic fibers.[24] Stimulation of the sympathetic fibers increases blood sugar through stimulation of glucagon and inhibition of insulin.[24] Parasympathetic stimulation causes the opposite effect.[24] It is thought that various neurotransmitters (somatostatin, serotonin, and prostaglandins) may also affect the activity of the islet cells.[24]

Glucagon is produced chiefly by the alpha cells of the pancreas and is also found in the mucosa of the stomach and small intestine. Like insulin, glucagon plays an important role in the body's metabolism of nutrients. Details regarding the synthesis and secretion of glucagon are not completely known. Secretion of glucagon is stimulated by low blood sugar. The chief effects of glucagon are to trap amino acids in the liver and to increase gluconeogenesis, glycogenolysis, and lipolysis. The primary tar-

Table 8-1
Catecholamine Functions

Class and Function	Alpha-Adrenergic	Beta-Adrenergic	Dopaminergic
Agonist	Norepinephrine	Epinephrine	Dopamine
Antagonist	Phentolamine	Propranolol	Haloperidol
Actions			
Heart		Inotropic and chronotropic	Inotropic
Smooth muscle	Contracts	Relaxes	Mixed
Metabolic		Lipolysis Glycogenolysis Gluconeogenesis	
Molecular	Decreases cAMP	Increases cAMP	Increases cAMP

From Karenman et al.: Practical diagnosis/endocrine disease, Boston, 1978, Houghton-Mifflin Professional Publishers.

Fig. 8-8
Catecholamine metabolism. *COMT*, catechol-O-methyl transferase; *MAO*, monoamine oxidase; *AO*, aldehyde oxidase; *AD*, alcohol dehydrogenase.

From Felig, P., et al.: Endocrinology and metabolism, New York, 1981, McGraw-Hill Book Co.

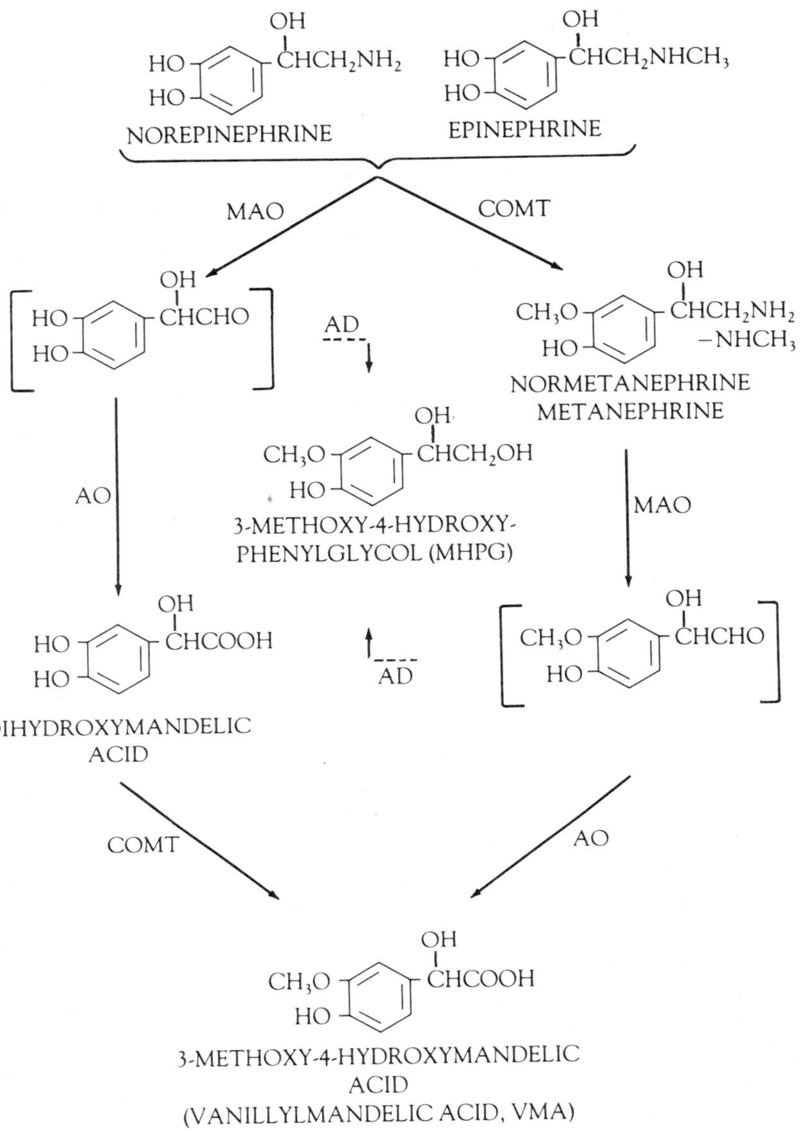

get organ of this hormone is the liver, where it attaches to a glucagon receptor on a liver cell.[39] Glucagon output from islet alpha cells varies inversely with blood glucose concentrations, in the presence of insulin. Stimulation of glucagon also stimulates release of insulin by either raising the blood sugar level or by directly stimulating beta cells to increase insulin secretion, or both.[52] Glucagon also stimulates release of epinephrine and norepinephrine from the adrenal medulla, causing conversion of glycogen to glucose, which further elevates blood sugar.

Insulin is synthesized in the endoplasmic reticulum of the beta cells, under the direction of messenger RNA. After the terminal connecting C-peptide fragment is re-moved (Fig. 8-9), the insulin molecule is folded and held together by disulfide bonds. Both insulin and C-peptide are secreted into the circulation. C-peptide has little, if any, insulin activity and can be measured in the circulation by radioimmunoassay as an indicator of pancreatic beta-cell function in persons receiving exogenous insulin.[24] The main stimulus for insulin secretion is glucose, although fats, proteins, and other carbohydrates also enhance secretion. Once secreted, insulin travels in the portal circulation to the liver and then into the general circulation. In order to be effective, insulin must first bind to cell membrane receptors on target tissues (liver, fat, and muscle cells).

Fig. 8-9

Formation of insulin and connecting peptide from proinsulin.

Reprinted with permission from Imagimedic Productions, Practical Diabetology 2(1):3, 1983.

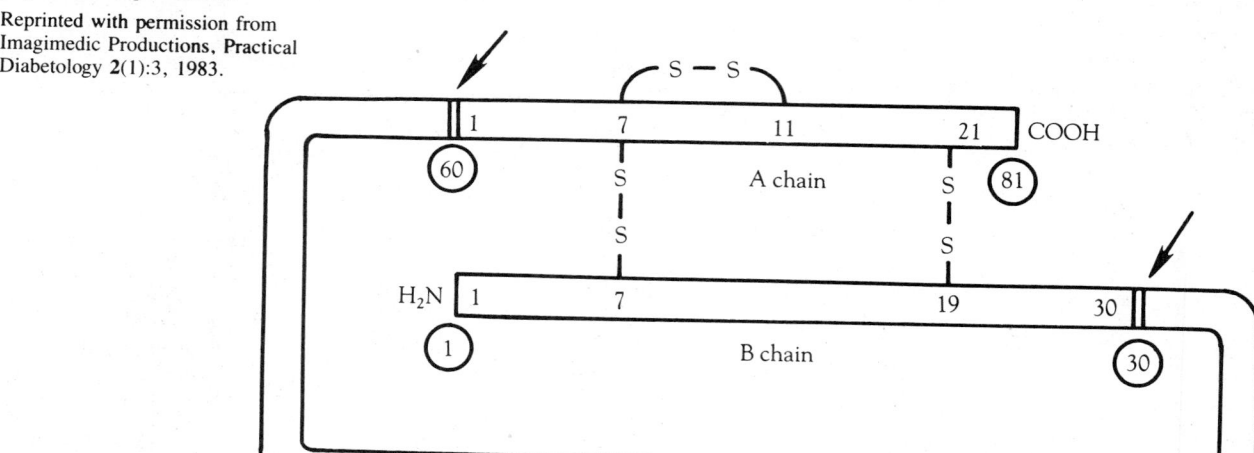

In the fasting state, low insulin levels (and high glucagon levels) allow glycogenolysis and gluconeogenesis by the liver to maintain blood glucose levels and adequate glucose supply to the cells for energy. In the fed state, insulin levels may rise to 30 to 80 μg/mg to prevent severe elevations in blood sugar by both suppressing liver production of glucose and stimulating glucose uptake by liver, fat, and muscle cells.[24] An estimated 25% of glucose ingested is used by non-insulin-dependent tissues (brain, eye, red blood cells) for energy.[25]

The net effects of insulin are growth promoting and are summarized in Table 8-2. In muscle tissues, insulin causes the uptake of glucose and amino acids, the formation of glycogen, and protein synthesis. In the liver, insulin increases fatty acid and glycogen synthesis through its effect on major enzyme systems. Gluconeogenesis is also inhibited. The action of insulin on fat metabolism involves increasing the uptake of fatty acids and inhibiting lipase activity within the fat cell. The end result is a stimulation of glucose uptake, fatty acid synthesis, enhanced triglyceride synthesis, and inhibition of fatty acid oxidation. Insulin also has a suppressive effect on circulating ketones.

While blood glucose regulation is mainly affected by insulin, at least four other counterregulatory hormones (including glucagon) interact with insulin to maintain a normal blood sugar at all times. Growth hormone, secreted from the anterior pituitary gland, has the effect of increasing blood sugar levels and accelerating anabolic processes in the body. Its secretion is enhanced by hypoglycemia, exercise, and amino acids; it is suppressed by hyperglycemia.[24] Insulin is secreted in response to hyperglycemia and has the effect of decreasing blood sugar, growth hormone, glucagon, and catecholamines.

Table 8-2
Action of Insulin

	Liver	Adipose Tissue	Muscle
Anticatabolic effects	Decreased glycogenolysis Decreased gluconeogenesis Decreased ketogenesis	Decreased lipolysis	Decreased protein catabolism Decreased amino acid output Decreased amino acid oxidation
Anabolic effects	Increased glycogen synthesis Increased fatty acid synthesis	Increased glycerol synthesis Increased fatty acid synthesis	Increased amino acid uptake Increased protein synthesis Increased glycogen synthesis

Reprinted with permission from Felig, P.: Physiologic action of insulin. In Ellenberg, M., and Rifkin, H., editors: Diabetes mellitus: theory and practice, ed. 3, New York, 1983, Medical Examination Publishing Co.

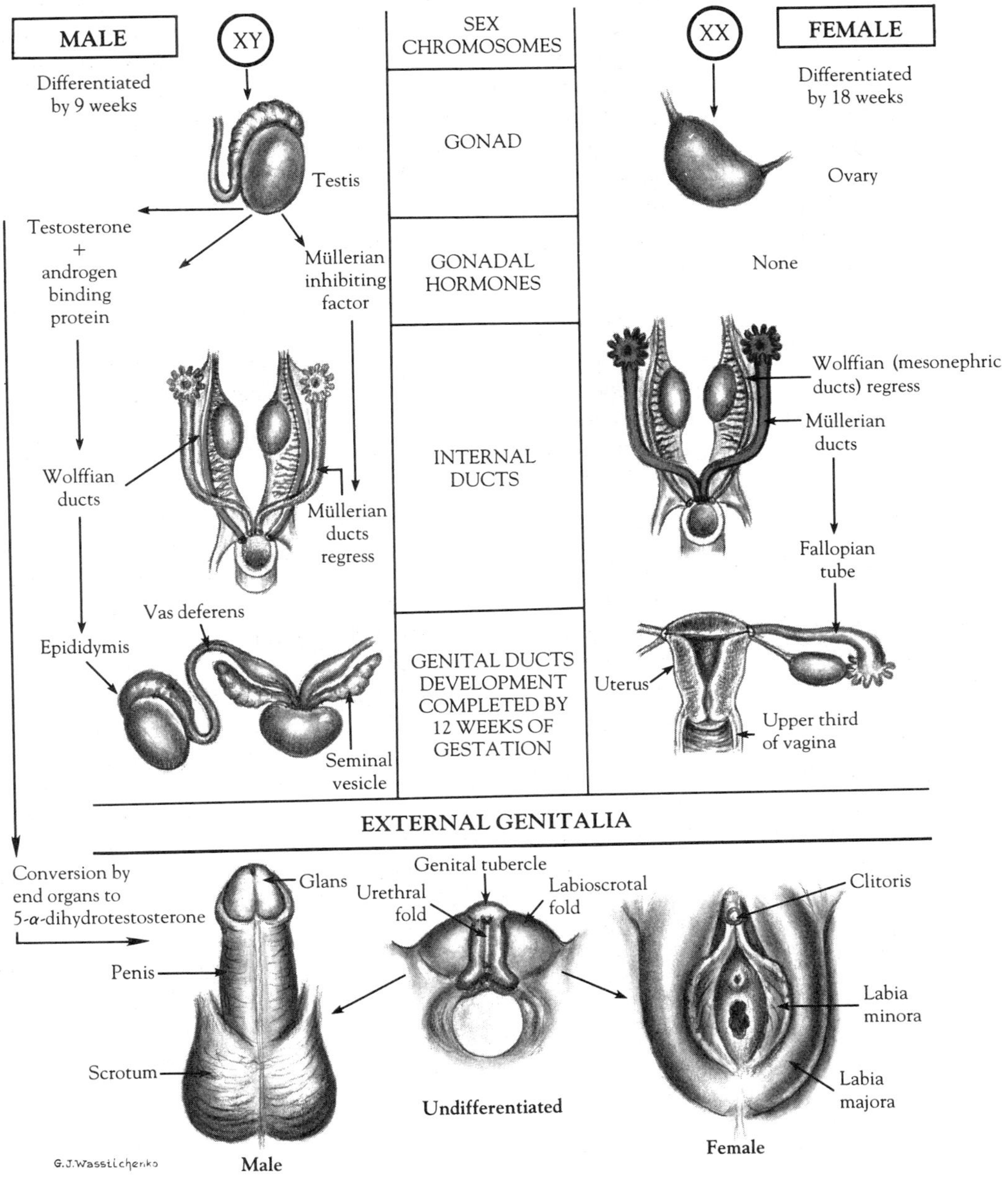

Fig. 8-10
Sexual differentiation in utero.

	SEX CHROMOSOMES	
MALE (XY)		(XX) FEMALE
Differentiated by 9 weeks	GONAD	Differentiated by 18 weeks
Testis		Ovary
Testosterone + androgen binding protein	GONADAL HORMONES	None
Müllerian inhibiting factor		
Wolffian ducts	INTERNAL DUCTS	Wolffian (mesonephric ducts) regress
Müllerian ducts regress		Müllerian ducts
Vas deferens		Fallopian tube
Epididymis	GENITAL DUCTS DEVELOPMENT COMPLETED BY 12 WEEKS OF GESTATION	Uterus
Seminal vesicle		Upper third of vagina

EXTERNAL GENITALIA

Conversion by end organs to 5-α-dihydrotestosterone

Glans — Penis — Scrotum

Male

Genital tubercle
Urethral fold
Labioscrotal fold

Undifferentiated

Clitoris
Labia minora
Labia majora

Female

G.J.Wasstichenko

Finally, insulin lowers serum potassium through stimulation of potassium uptake by liver and muscle cells.[24]

Gastrin is a polypeptide hormone secreted by pancreatic gamma-islet cells, as well as by the pyloric gland, proximal duodenum, and upper duodenum.[52] Release of gastrin may be stimulated by any of the following: (1) mechanical distention of the antrum of the stomach; (2) foods entering the stomach, especially those containing alcohol, amino acids, or calcium[52]; (3) increased stomach acid; (4) decreased blood sugar; and (5) vagal stimulation.[41]

Once gastrin is released, it is carried in the circulation to the target tissues, the parietal cells of the stomach. Its actions are as follows[52]: (1) increases gastrointestinal muscular tone (including stomach, large and small intestine, and gallbladder); (2) increases digestive secretions from the stomach and pancreas (including insulin); (3) promotes growth of the gastric mucosa by increasing the number of parietal cells, including their ability to secrete hydrochloric acid; and (4) activates secretin release from the intestinal mucosa.

Somatostatin is formed in the secretory granules of the

islet delta cells as preprosomatostatin, changed to prosomatostatin, and finally secreted as somatostatin in a calcium-dependent process. The secretory granules expel their contents (somatostatin) into the intercellular space. The main effects of somatostatin are inhibitory on (1) growth hormone, (2) thyrotropin, (3) insulin, (4) glucagon, and (5) various gastrointestinal hormones. Somatostatin secretion is stimulated by glucose, arginine, leucine, ketoisocaproic acid, and beta hydroxybutyrate. Increases in extracellular calcium and potassium increase somatostatin release.[24]

A negative-feedback system exists between the alpha and beta cells of the islets mediated by somatostatin. Glucagon release stimulates somatostatin release, which in turn decreases insulin secretion. Insulin does not appear to have any direct effect on somatostatin release.[24]

Gonads

Sexual differentiation of the fetus begins with the distribution of the sex chromosomes, X and Y, during cell division, or meiosis, and is completed at conception with the formation of the zygote. Initially, internal and external genitalia are identical. Shortly after conception primordial germ cells move from the endoderm of the yolk sac to the gonadal ridge. Here they await further instruction to form ovaries or testes. Sexual differentiation is further outlined in Fig. 8-10.

Formation of the male gonad is an active process primarily mediated by the presence of androgens. Determination is also thought to be made by the presence of the H-Y (histoincompatibility-Y) antigen located near the centromere of the Y chromosome.[35] It is thought that this

antigen directs the germ cell to proceed into the testes. By 6 to 9 weeks of gestation, the testes are secreting testosterone, which maintains the wolffian ducts (precursor of the male internal system) and converts to dihydrotestosterone to direct the external genitalia into forming the penis and scrotum.[35] The testes also secrete a müllerian-inhibiting factor (substance) (MIF), which causes the regression of the müllerian ducts (precursor of the female internal system), thereby preventing the formation of the female internal genitalia.

During the seventh to ninth month of gestation the testes descend from the posterior abdominal cavity to the scrotal sac. Because the scrotum temperature is approximately 2° C lower than the abdominal cavity, this descent is necessary to permit spermatogenesis during puberty. A tubelike structure projecting from the peritoneal cavity, the processus vaginalis, precedes the descending testis into the inguinal canal. Failure of the tube to shrink and close after proper positioning of the testis produces a congenital indirect inguinal hernia.[7] Varying degrees of cryptorchidism occur with incomplete or misdirected descent of the testis.

The testes are ovoid shaped; their size varies with age and degree of sexual maturity. Age-related testicular dimensions are found in Table 8-3. In adulthood the mature testes can weigh between 10 and 45 g. Clinically, testicular volume is measured by the Prader Orchiometer and is expressed in cubic centimeters. Approximately 95% of the testes is made up of convoluted seminiferous tubules that are contained in septa (septate testis) and separated by the tunica albuginea. Fig. 8-11 illustrates a crosscut view of the adult testis. In utero the tubule is lined with Sertoli cells (support cells that secrete MIF) and later by germinal epithelium that produces sperm. During ejaculation, sperm is emptied into the epididymis, to the vas deferens, passing finally into the urethra. The remaining 5% of the testis is interstitial tissue made up of Leydig's cells, lymphatic tissue, blood vessels, and connective tissue. Leydig's cells are responsible for the production of androgens, primarily testosterone.[26] Further information on gonadal hormones is given in Table 8-4.

In the absence of the Y chromosome and MIF, the female reproductive system begins to develop at 6 to 11 weeks of gestation and is recognizable by 18 weeks of gestation. Without circulating testosterone the wolffian ducts regress and the müllerian system progresses to form the internal fallopian tubes, uterus, and proximal one third of the vagina. Although development of the müllerian system is not maintained by ovarian function, further evolution of the ovary does depend on two normally structured X chromosomes.[35] At approximately the sixth month of pregnancy, primordial follicles are forming from meiotic oocytes. Here they will await further mat-

Table 8-3
Testicular Size from Birth to Maturity

Age (yr)	Length (cm)	Volume (cc)
Under 1	1.5	0.6
1-2	1.6	0.7
3-4	1.6	0.8
5-6	1.6	0.8
7-8	1.6	0.8
9-10	1.6	0.9
11	1.7	1.5
12	1.9	2.0
13	2.3	5.0
14	2.8	8.0
15	3.0	12.0
16	3.5	13.0
17	—	15.0
18-19	—	16.0-20.0
20-25	4.0-5.0	16.0-20.0

From Kaplan, S.A.: Clinical pediatric and adolescent endocrinology, Philadelphia, 1982, W.B. Saunders Co.

Fig. 8-11
Mature testis.

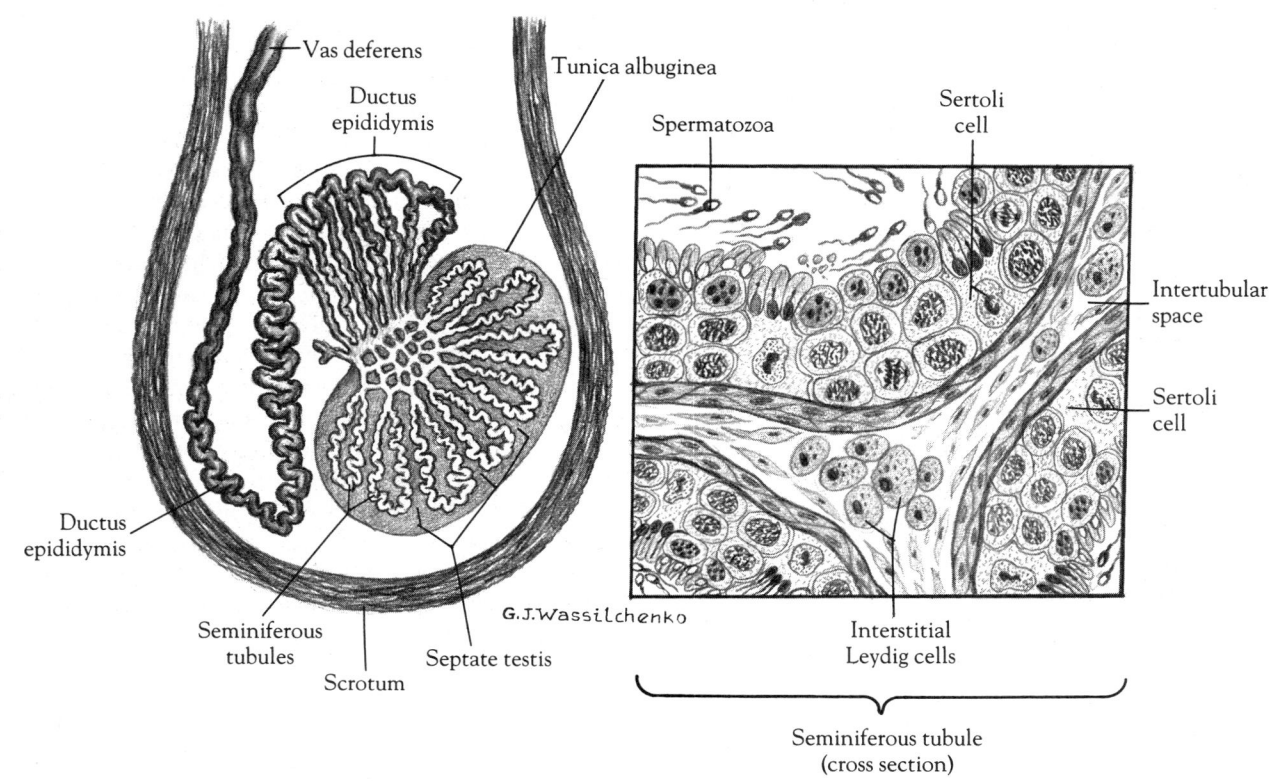

G.J.Wassilchenko

Seminiferous tubule
(cross section)

Table 8-4
Gonadal Hormones

	Origin	Location	Appearance	Function
Male				
Sertoli cells	Surface epithelium; development of gonad and testis	Line seminiferous tubules	Fetal	Secrete MIF Provide support for developing spermatids
Leydig's cells	Mesenchyme	Interstitial tissue of testes	Fetal and pubertal	Secrete testosterone
Female				
Granulosa/follicular	Surface epithelium; rete ovary	Cortex of ovary	Early fetal	Houses maturing ova Secretes small amounts of nonaromatized testosterone (theca cells)
Corpus luteum	Postovulatory follicle	Cortex of ovary	Postovulatory	Secretes progesterone for support of pregnancy Produces 17OH progesterone Produces small amounts of estrogen and androgen

Table 8-5
Summary of Hormonal Effects

Area of Concern	Hormonal Influence
Normal growth	Thyroid
	Insulin
	Growth hormone
	Gonadotropins
	Sex steroids
Metabolic rate	Thyroid
Protein, carbohydrate, and fat metabolism	Thyroid
	Glucagon
	Insulin
	Gastrin, glucocorticoids
Cardiac contractility	Calcium, epinephrine
Blood pressure; pulse rate	Glucocorticoids, mineralocorticoids
	Epinephrine, norepinephrine
Muscle mass and contractility	Glucocorticoids
	Insulin
	Growth hormone
	Androgens
Skin turgor	Mineralocortocoids, glucocorticoids
	Epinephrine, norepinephrine
Secondary sex characteristics	Gonadotropins
	Sex steroids
Lactation	Calcium
	Prolactin, oxytocin
Skin pigmentation	Melanocyte-stimulating hormone

uration during puberty. Generally each ovary is whitish, flat, and almond shaped, situated to either side of the uterus just posterior of the fallopian tube and held in place by the meso-ovarian ligament, a portion of the broad ligament. As in the male testes, size and weight depend on normal development and stage of maturation. Each ovary consists of a medulla and cortex similar to the adrenal gland, which shares a similar embryonic origin. Contained in the cortex are the maturing follicles, whereas the medulla supports tissues of the lymphatic, nervous, and circulatory systems. The entire unit is protected by the tunica albuginea and again by the germinal epithelium.[26] Fig. 8-12 gives a crosscut diagram of the ovary. In response to pituitary secretion of LH and FSH, graafian follicles, each housing an ovum, begin maturing. Normally, the two ovaries contain an average total of 400,000 ova.[26] Following an LH surge and fall in estrogen, a mature ovum is released to be swept up the fimbrae of the fallopian tubes. The two primary ovarian hormones are given in Table 8-4. The primary hormone of the follicle, or granulosa, is estrogen, whereas the corpus luteum secretes progesterone. In the mature ovary, interstitial cells seem to have androgenic properties that are unclear at this time.[26]

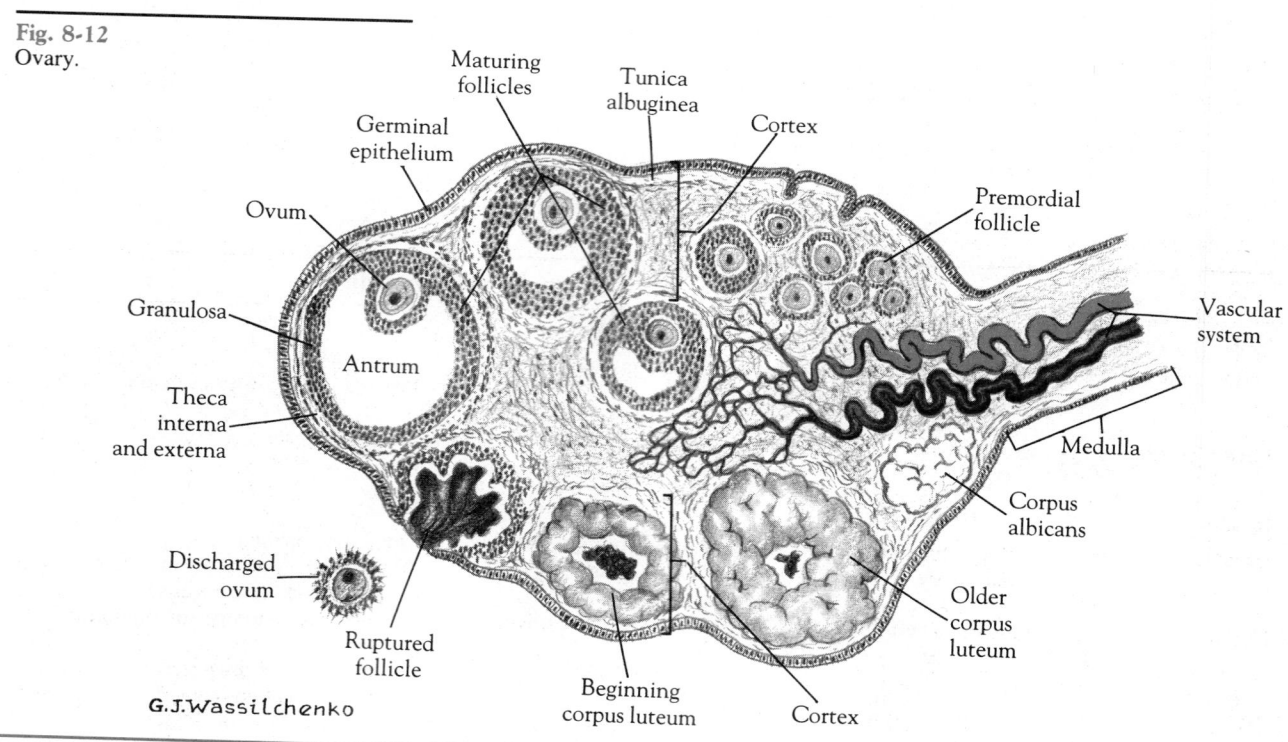

Fig. 8-12
Ovary.

Maturing follicles
Germinal epithelium
Tunica albuginea
Cortex
Ovum
Premordial follicle
Granulosa
Antrum
Vascular system
Theca interna and externa
Medulla
Discharged ovum
Corpus albicans
Older corpus luteum
Ruptured follicle
Beginning corpus luteum
Cortex
G.J.Wassilchenko

NORMAL FINDINGS*[35,46,47]

Tanner Stage and Mean Age	Normal Findings	

Male

Tanner I

Prepubertal; less than 10 yr of age
Nonmature genitalia; testes volume approximately
   3 ml
Vellus hairs over genitalia

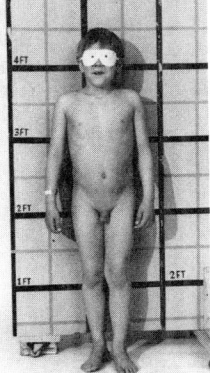

Tanner II (11.7 yr ± 1.3 [SD])

Increase in testicular size
Few sparse terminal (pigmented) straight pubic
   hairs (difficult to appreciate in illustration)
Testicular volume greater than 3 ml
Scrotum somewhat reddened and thinning with
   increased rugae

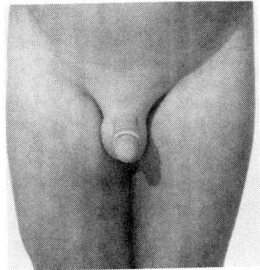

Tanner III (13.2 yr ± 0.8 [SD])

Further testicular growth
Penile enlargement in length and circumference
Increasing number of pubic hairs, at base of shaft
   (curled, coarse)
Increased muscle bulk, acne and oil production,
   body odor

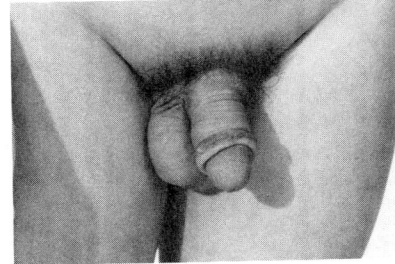

Tanner IV (14.7 yr ± 1.1 [SD])

Continued growth of testes, scrotum, and penis
Development of glans penis
Increased pigmentation of genital skin
Developing libido
Growth spurt at 13-14 yr
Pubic hair over symphysis pubis
Possible temporary gynecomastia (or earlier)

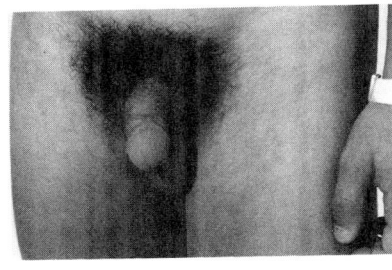

Tanner V (15.5 yr ± 0.7 [SD])

Pubic hair extends to medial surfaces of thighs
Mature genitalia
Facial and axillary hair
Adult height reached with epiphyseal closure
Reproductive capability
Libido

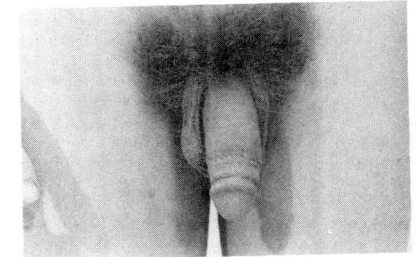

*Illustrations courtesy Dr. F. Comite, National Institutes of Health.

Continued.

Tanner Stage and Mean Age	Normal Findings

Female

Tanner I

Immature genitalia
Less than 9 yr of age
Vellus hairs present
No palpable breast tissue
Mean areolar diameter of 11.9 mm

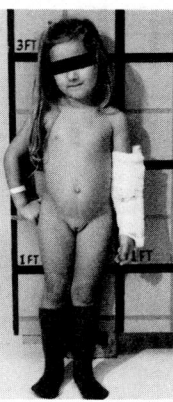

Tanner II (10.08 yr ± 1.1 [SD])

Few terminal hairs along labia
Beginning estrogen stimulation of breast tissue
Small buttonlike mound (breast bud) over nipple
Labia pinker and moist

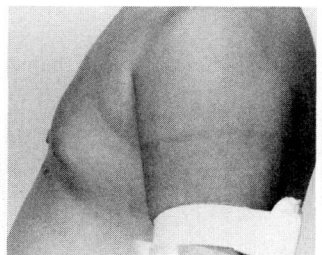

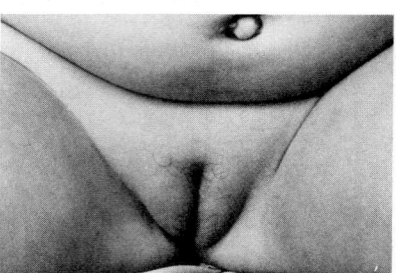

Tanner III (12.0 yr ± 1.1 [SD])

Pelvic widening
Pubic hair increased on mons
Breast tissue extends beyond areola to form
    doughnut-shaped mound
Asymmetry of breast development likely
Menarche (mean age of 12.7 yr ± 1.0)
Body odor, increased oil production, and acne

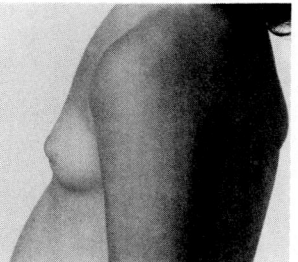

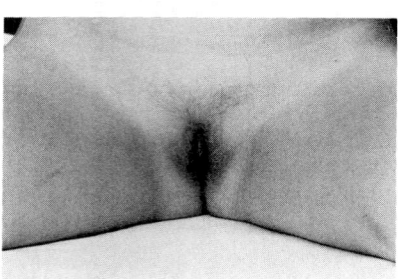

Tanner Stage and Mean Age	Normal Findings

Tanner IV (13.0 yr ± 2.2 [SD])   Pubic hair approaching feminine triangle
Contour separation of areolar mound from breast
Growth spurt at 11-13 yr
Moderate amount of axillary hair

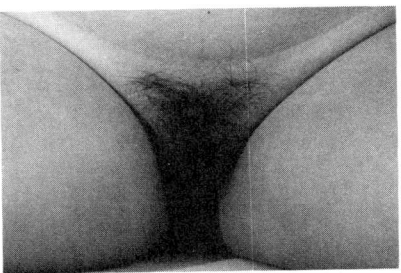
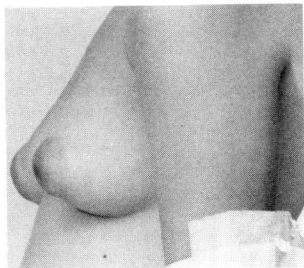

Tanner V (14.0 yr ± 1.2 [SD])   Pubic hair extending up on thighs and up linea
alba
Areola and breast as one; similar to Tanner stage
III
Asymmetry of breast development may persist
Cyclic moodiness with monthly menses
Conception possible with ovulation
Adult height reached with epiphyseal closure

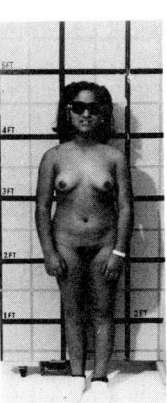

NORMAL LABORATORY DATA

Laboratory Test	Normal Adult Values	Variations in Child	Variations in Older Adult
Blood or Serum			
Adrenocorticotropic hormone (ACTH)	8 AM: <140 pg/ml 4 PM: 10-50 pg/ml		
Aldosterone			
Normal salt diet			
Supine	5.4-9.8 ng/dl	30-90 ng/dl	
Upright	8.9-58 ng/dl		
Low salt diet	2-4 times above values		
Androstenedione	<250 ng/dl	8-240 ng/dl	
Calcitonin	<150 pg/ml; usual basal fasting level is about 20-100 pg/ml, depending on assay		
Calcium			
Serum	Up to 30 yr: 8.2-10.5 mg/dl; decreases very slightly in older years	Infants up to 1 mo: 7-11.5 mg/dl Normal range slowly descends	
Ionized serum	4.75-5.0 mg/dl		
Calculated ionized	3.9-4.8 mg/dl		

Laboratory Test	Normal Adult Values	Variations in Child	Variations in Older Adult
Catecholamines			
Supine			
Epinephrine	20-97 pg/ml	20-115 pg/ml	
Norepi-nephrine	125-310 pg/ml	150-400 pg/ml	
Standing			
Epinephrine	20-109 pg/ml		
Norepi-nephrine	169-515 pg/ml		
Cortisol	8 AM: 8-18 μg/dl 4 PM: 4-10 μg/dl	3-21 μg/dl	
C-peptide			
Fasting	0.9-4.2 ng/ml	1-4 ng/ml	
Nonfasting	1.5-9.0 ng/ml		
Dehydroepian-dosterone (DHEA)	Adult male: 270-1400 ng/dl Adult female: 200-800 ng/dl	31-900 ng/dl; varies with Tanner stage	
DHEA sulfate (serum)	Adult male: 130-550 μg/dl Premenopausal female: 60-340 μg/dl Postmenopausal female: <130 μg/dl		
Estrogen			
Male	2-8 ng/ml	<2 ng/ml	
Female	6-40 ng/ml	<2 ng/ml	

Follicle-stimulating hormone	Male: <22 IU/L
	Female:
	  Midcycle: <40 IU/L
	  Preovulation or postovulation: <20 IU/L
		Prepubertal children: <10 IU/L	Postmenopausal women: 40-160 IU/L

Free thyroxine	Approximately 0.7-1.8 ng/dl (varies among laboratories)		
Gastrin	Fasting: 50-100 pg/ml (up to 300 pg/ml in some laboratories) Postprandial: 95-140 pg/ml; usually <250 pg/ml	<10-125 pg/ml	
Glucagon	20-100 pg/ml		
Glucose	Adult: 70-120 mg/dl	Birth to 1 wk: 30-80 mg/dl 2 yr to puberty: 60-100 mg/dl	
Growth hormone	<10 ng/ml	<20 ng/ml	
Hemoglobin$_{A1C}$	5.7-8.8%		
Human chorionic gonadotropin	<3 mIU/ml (nonpregnant)		
Insulin	Fasting level: up to 25 μU/ml with slight differences in upper limit of normal among laboratories	<2-13 μU/ml	
Luteinizing hormone			
Male	7-24 mIU/ml; normal ranges vary among laboratories	<1-4 mIU/ml	
Female	Follicular phase: 6-27 mIU/ml Midcycle: 35-154 mIU/ml Luteal: 5-17 mIU/ml		Postmenopausal: 29-96 mIU/ml
Parathyroid hormone	Dependent on individual laboratory, calcium result; the calcium value is related to the parathyroid hormone value by some laboratories on a two-dimensional graph or nomogram to ascertain abnormality		
Progesterone			
Male	13-97 ng/dl		7-33 ng/dl
Female	Follicular: 95 ng/dl Luteal: 1130 ng/dl		
Progesterone receptor assay	<5 fmol/mg protein is negative		

Laboratory Test	Normal Adult Values	Variations in Child	Variations in Older Adult
Prolactin	2-37 ng/ml	3-18 ng/ml	
Renin*			
Supine	20-160 ng/dl/h	50-330 ng/dl/h	
Upright	70-330 ng/dl/h		
Somatomedin C	0.4-2.0 U/ml	0.17-3 U/ml	
Somatostatin	10-25 pg/ml		
Testosterone	Male: 300-1100 ng/dl	<3-10 ng/dl; varies with Tanner stage	
	Female: 20-100 ng/dl		
Triiodothyronine	Approximately 80 to 200-230 ng/dl with some variation among laboratories; increase occurs in pregnancy	Values in infancy and childhood are higher than in adulthood	
Thyroglobulin	About 1-20 ng/ml; mean values of 5.1-9.5 ng/ml		
Thyroid stimulating hormone (TSH)	Upper limit of normal varies among laboratories from about 5.4 μU/ml to approximately 10 μU/ml	Neonates: less than 20 μIU by third day of life	
Thyroxine	5.5-11.5 μg/dl	Neonatal values are much higher	
	Pregnancy: approximately 5.5-16 μg/dl	10 yr and up: approximately 5.8-11.0 μg/dl	
Thyroxine binding globulin	Variability among laboratories exists; 10-28 μg/ml; increased in pregnancy	2.0-5.3 mg/dl	
Urine			
Aldosterone	3-19 μg/24 h	1-8 μg/24 h	
Calcium	Varies with diet; based on average calcium intake of 600-800 mg/24 h, excretion may be 100-250 mg/24 h		
	On a diet of 400-800 mg of calcium daily, others set the upper limit at 200 mg calcium in a 24-h urine collection		
Catecholamines			
Epinephrine	0-20 μg/24 h		
Norepinephrine	15-80 μg/24 h		
Metanephrine	0.2-0.8 g/24 h		
Dopamine	65-400 μg/24 h		
Creatinine clearance	Male: 85-125 ml/min/1.73 m²	70-140 ml/min/1.73 m²	
	Female: 75-115 ml/min/1.73 m²		
Free cortisol	Male: 11-84 μg/24 h	Lower in infants and children as a result of decreased cortisol production	
	Female: 10-34 μg/24 h		
FSH			
Male	3-11 IU/24 h	<1.0-3.3 IU/24 h	
Female	5-50 IU/24 h	<1.0-3.4 IU/24 h	Postmenopausal: 2-3 times adult values
HCG	<10 IU/24 h		
Hydroxyprolines	See individual laboratory reference ranges; excretion on meat-free, gelatin-free diet is approximately 10-50 mg/24 h	Normal range is higher in infancy, childhood, and adolescence, especially during growth spurts	
17-Ketosteroids	Male: 9-22 mg/24 h		Decrease in advancing years
	Female: 6-15 mg/24 h		
VMA	1.8-7 mg/24 h		
17-Hydroxysteroids	Male: 3-10 mg/24 h		
	Female: 2.5-10/24 h		
LH	Male: 5-25 IU/24 h		Postmenopausal: 2-3 times adult values
	Female: 8-90 IU/24 h		

*Varies between laboratories; depends on sodium intake, age, and posture and whether there has been stimulation (e.g., furosemide). Values from right and left renal veins should normally be equal. In arterial constriction, abnormal result is considered a ratio of greater than 1.5.

DIAGNOSTIC STUDIES

Provocative endocrine testing is classified as either stimulation or suppression studies. Evaluation of secretory reserve by a *stimulation* test is useful for diagnosing hypofunction and for detecting impaired secretory reserve. *Suppression* tests are useful for diagnosis of hyperfunction because the hyperfunctioning gland by definition is not operating under normal control mechanisms.

Below is a list of tests according to the hormone being evaluated. These tests are associated with specific procedures dependent on the laboratory capabilities of the institution. Injection of some hormones (e.g., TRH) may produce a warm, flushed feeling. The nursing care includes education of the patient about the purpose, procedure, and possible side effects and support of the patient during the procedure. The insulin tolerance test will cause profound and purposeful hypoglycemia, requiring a nurse in attendance at all times. When the physician terminates the test, intravenous glucose (10% D/W; 20% D/W; 50% D) is infused immediately and followed by a high-protein meal.

Hormone	Stimulation	Suppression
Antidiuretic hormone (ADH)	Water deprivation	Saline infusion
	Nicotine	Pitressin
Growth hormone (GH)	Insulin tolerance test	Glucose tolerance test
	Arginine tolerance test	
	Levodopa	
	Exercise stimulation test	
Thyroid-stimulating hormone (TSH)	Thyrotropin releasing hormone (TRH)	Triiodothyronine
		Thyroxine
Prolactin (PRL)	Insulin tolerance test	Levodopa
	Chlorpromazine	
	TRH	
Adrenocorticotropic hormone (ACTH)	Insulin tolerance test (hypoglycemia will occur)	Dexamethasone
	Corticotropin-releasing hormone (CRH)	Metyrapone
Luteinizing hormone (LH)	Luteinizing-releasing hormone (LRH)	Testosterone
		Estrogen
Follicle-stimulating hormone (FSH)	Clomiphene	
Triiodothyronine (T_3)	TSH	T_3
Thyroxine (T_4)		T_4
Cortisol	ACTH	Dexamethasone
	CRH	Metyrapone
	Insulin tolerance test	
	Arginine tolerance test	
Aldosterone	ACTH	Salt loading/volume expansion
		Spironolactone
Norepinephrine	Histamine	Phentolamine
	Tyramine	
	Glucagon	
Progesterone	Human menopausal gonadotropin (HMG)	Provera
	Human chorionic gonadotropin (HCG)	Progesterone
Testosterone	HMG	Testosterone
	HCG	
Parathyroid hormone (PTH; vitamin D)	PTH infusion	Calcium infusion
Glucose	Glucagon	Insulin tolerance test
		Tolbutamide
Insulin	Glucose tolerance test (GTT)	Prolonged fast
	Leucine	
	Fructose	
Gastrin	Pentagastrin	Cimetidine
	Calcium infusion	
	High-protein, high-carbohydrate meal	

The following outline gives diagnostic studies in endocrine testing.

X-ray films of sella turcica

CT scans of sella turcica, abdomen

Nursing care:
Varies with institution

Ultrasonograms of thyroid, pelvis, abdomen, testes

Mineral oil or other transmission jelly spread over region; ultrasonoscope transmits ultrasonic beams through tissues while a picture of findings is created on an oscilloscope

Nursing care:
Varies with institution

Thyroid uptake and scan

Amount of radioactive iodine taken up by the thyroid over a period of time (e.g., 6, 8, or 24 h)

Closed percutaneous thyroid biopsy

Sterile aspiration of thyroid tissue

Nursing care:
Support during procedure; assess for esophageal or tracheal puncture

Selective arteriography: parathyroid, adrenal, pancreatic

Injection of contrast media into selected blood vessels for visualization and localization of possible tumors in preparation for surgery

Nursing care:
Give nothing by mouth; assess for hematoma or hemorrhage

Venous sampling

Insertion of catheter similar to arteriography but for the purpose of serial sampling for hormone levels

Nursing care:
Same as for arteriography

Visual field and acuity tests

Conditions, Diseases, and Disorders

ADRENAL INSUFFICIENCY

Adrenal insufficiency can be defined as an abnormality of the adrenal glands with destruction of the adrenal cortex so that glucocorticoid production and mineralocorticoid production are impaired.

Primary adrenal insufficiency can be found in all age groups ranging from newborn to elderly. Men and women alike are affected, and there is no differentiation between races. Secondary adrenal insufficiency is most common among patients who have withdrawn from exogenous cortisol therapy.

In patients with idiopathic primary adrenal insufficiency the prognosis is favorable because of advances made in cortisol replacement therapy. Although the condition is lifelong, with appropriate management and an increased patient awareness, the disease is manageable.

Patients diagnosed with secondary adrenal insufficiency may have other causes for a reduction in ACTH secretion. These causes include pituitary tumors, hypophysectomy for pituitary tumors, postpartum pituitary necrosis, tumors of the third ventricle, trauma, and optic glioma.[31]

Adrenal crisis can occur in any patient deficient in adrenal steroids. Many times, the patient who is adrenally insufficient may not have the diagnosis made until a crisis occurs. Once the signs and symptoms are recognized and treatment initiated, response is encouraging.[20] Because of the life-threatening nature of adrenal crisis, response must be prompt.

Many factors can be the precipitating cause of adrenal crisis. Anything that causes additional stress in the adrenally insufficient patient may be significant, such as infection, surgery, or trauma (automobile accident). If the patient does not receive sufficient coverage with glucocorticoids, crisis ensues.

PATHOPHYSIOLOGY

Sixty-six to eighty percent of cases of primary adrenal insufficiency have an idiopathic cause (most likely autoimmune). Causes of primary adrenal insufficiency include fungal infections and vascular and metastatic disease.[9]

Secondary adrenal insufficiency results from an impairment of the hypothalamic-pituitary-adrenal axis. Insufficient ACTH stimulation is responsible for the hypofunction of the adrenal gland. If the cause of the decreased ACTH production is a pharmacologic source of cortisol, the axis may recover; however, it may take months or even years.[31]

Primary adrenal insufficiency reflects both mineralocorticoid and glucocorticoid deficiency. Patients with secondary adrenal insufficiency have only glucocorticoid deficiency[73] because the regulation of mineralocorticoid secretion by the renin-angiotensin system is independent of ACTH secretion.

Adrenal insufficiency affects the balance of metabolic regulators. Muscle work capacity is diminished. Cardiac contractility and output decrease, and this may lead to circulatory collapse. Decreased cardiac output results in reflex tachycardia and increased secretion of ADH, which leads to water retention. Free fatty acid mobilization is impaired, which reduces free fatty acid levels. This in turn leads to increased utilization of glucose resulting in hypoglycemia.[42] Decreased cortisol increases ACTH production causing hyperpigmentation,[13a] and there is a decrease in gastrointestinal enzymes. The loss of diurnal cortisol causes a loss of mental acuity and vitality.[65] Mineralocorticoid deficiency is reflected by hyperkalemia and hyponatremia, which may be manifested by hypotension.[66] Androgen deficiency results in loss of body hair.[31]

Adrenal insufficiency is manifested only after 90% of the adrenal gland is not working. The onset is usually gradual although one third of the cases diagnosed have a history of 3 months from wellness to insufficiency.[25] With the gradual onset, symptoms may not be readily apparent. Plasma steroids may, in fact, be within the normal range. With exposure to stress, however, the glands are unable to provide the appropriate response and adrenal crisis may occur.[25]

Adrenal crisis is characterized by a worsening of the symptoms associated with adrenal insufficiency. Hypovolemic shock may develop as sodium is depleted and ECF volume decreases. Vomiting and diarrhea contribute to volume depletion. Fever may be present, either as a result of a precipitating infection or as a result of hypoadrenalism. The presence of hyperpigmentation may be the only clue to the diagnosis. Therefore examination of scars, buccal mucosa, and palmar surfaces should be included in any patient in unexplained shock.[25]

DIAGNOSTIC STUDIES

ACTH stimulation
Primary adrenal insufficiency: little or no cortisol and 17-hydroxysteroid response

Secondary adrenal insufficiency: normal to intermediate cortisol and 17-hydroxysteroid response

Insulin tolerance test
Secondary adrenal insufficiency: abnormal response

Blood
Adrenal crisis: hyponatremia, hyperkalemia, lymphocytosis, and eosinophilia[25]; these findings are helpful for differentiating the diagnosis of a patient in shock

Urine collection (24-hour) for 17-hydroxysteroids and 17-ketosteroids
Decreased in both primary and secondary adrenal insufficiency

TREATMENT PLAN

Chemotherapeutic
Corticosteroids

Hydrocortisone, 20 mg in morning and 10 mg in evening

Hydrocortisone acetate, 25 mg in morning and 12.5 mg in evening

Prednisone, 5 mg in morning and 2.5 mg in evening

Dexamethasone, 0.5-0.75 mg/d

Fludrocortisone, 0.05-0.2 mg/d

These medications are considered life sustaining for the patient. This fact cannot be overemphasized.

Because of the ever-present potential of adrenal crisis, these patients need to be able to use the intramuscular injection of hydrocortisone (Hydrocortone Phosphate) for times when oral medication is not tolerated. This injection should be carried with the patient at all times, and a family member or significant other should be taught how to use the intramuscular injection along with the patient.

Special Medication Complications

Incorrect dosage. It may take time to determine correct replacement.

Overtreatment with glucocorticoids may result in short stature and symptoms of Cushing's syndrome. Excess mineralocorticoids may result in fluid overload and hypertension.

ASSESSMENT: AREAS OF CONCERN

Circulation
   Postural hypotension
   Lightheadedness
   Hypopyrexia or hyperpyrexia*
   Shock*

Food and fluid needs
   Salt craving
   Weight loss
   Nausea
   Vomiting
   Hyponatremia*
   Hyperkalemia*

Elimination
   Diarrhea
   Renal shutdown*

Neurosensory area
   Lassitude
   Coma*
   Confusion*

Sleep and rest
   Tires easily

Mobility
   Muscle aches
   Muscle wasting
   Muscle weakness

Comfort and pain
   Severe headache*
   Severe abdominal pain*
   Severe leg pain*
   Severe lower back pain*

Hygiene and skin care
   Hyperpigmentation
   Decreased body hair

Sexuality
   Amenorrhea
   Decreased libido

*Characteristic of adrenal crisis.

NURSING DIAGNOSES and NURSING INTERVENTIONS

Nursing Diagnosis	Nursing Intervention
Potential patient problem: susceptibility to infection	Keep patient in environment as free from stress as possible (lighting, warm temperature, noise level). Encourage frequent rest. Reinforce importance of medications to patient.
Potential patient problem: electrolyte balance, alteration	Encourage patient to choose foods high in sodium and low in potassium. Take apical pulse to detect cardiac arrhythmias. Employ means to combat nausea. Maintain intake and output records.
Tissue perfusion, alteration in: peripheral	Recognize early presyncopal signs (dizziness, lightheadedness, visual changes, etc.). Have patient change positions (from lying to sitting to standing) slowly. Take lying and standing blood pressures and pulses. Administer IV fluids as ordered. Monitor intake and output. Monitor vital signs frequently (every 15 to 30 minutes). Explain rationale for IV therapy to patient.
Sleep pattern disturbance	Do not disturb patient when sleeping. Encourage methods of achieving relaxation (back rub, warm milk, dark room, etc.). Allow for period of uninterrupted rest during the day. Decrease amount of external stimuli.
Fluid volume deficit, actual	Monitor intake and output. Observe for signs and symptoms of shock. Monitor vital signs frequently. Maintain IV line. Employ means to combat vomiting and diarrhea. Assess skin turgor.

Patient Education

1. Teach the patient the importance of avoiding obvious sources of infection such as persons with infections.
2. Teach the patient the importance of and how to take medication regularly and in emergency situations.
3. Teach the steps to follow when early symptoms of crises are noted.
4. Teach the importance of regular medical follow-up and wearing medical identification.

EVALUATION

Patient Outcome	Data Indicating That Outcome is Reached
The patient is free of infection.	Temperature is within normal range. The patient has no signs or symptoms of infection. Glucocorticoid and mineralocorticoid levels are within therapeutic range.
Electrolytes are within the normal range.	Sodium and potassium blood levels are within normal limits.
Tissue perfusion is adequate.	The patient makes no statements concerning syncope. Peripheral pulses are adequate. Output equals intake. The patient adheres to activity limitations.
The sleep pattern is undisturbed.	The patient verbalizes and demonstrates methods of achieving relaxation. The patient verbalizes receiving an increased amount of sleep.
Hydration is adequate.	Urine output is greater than 40 ml/h. Blood pressure is maintained within normal limits. Skin is intact, and turgor is normal.

PRIMARY ALDOSTERONISM

Primary aldosteronism is defined by Biglieri and Baxter as "a condition in which there is increased and inappropriate production of aldosterone by the adrenal gland leading to a mineralocorticoid excess state."[8]

Primary aldosteronism is not a common disease. When patients are first seen with hypertension, it is prudent to consider the diagnosis of primary aldosteronism since the incidence of this syndrome ranges from 0.5% to 2.0% of the hypertensive population.[20] It occurs in women more frequently than men in a ratio of 3:1 and is more prevalent between 30 and 50 years of age.[20]

PATHOPHYSIOLOGY

Primary aldosteronism is a disorder of the adrenal cortex. Causes include adrenal adenoma, idiopathic adrenocortical nodular hyperplasia, and adrenal carcinoma.[65] Sixty to seventy percent of patients diagnosed with primary aldosteronism have an adrenal adenoma.[20]

Excess aldosterone results in increased sodium reabsorption, increased total body sodium, and hypervolemia. Edema is rarely exhibited because of an "escape" mechanism, where proximal tubular sodium reabsorption is inhibited by the renal regulatory system.[20,31]

Arterial hypertension is present because of volume expansion, arteriolar sodium content, and vascular and sympathetic reactivity.[31] The degree of hypertension ranges from mild to severe.

Potassium depletion, both intracellular and extracellular, occurs because of increased renal tubular excretion of potassium.[31] Hypokalemia results in muscle weakness, fatigue, nocturnal polyuria (because of defective urinary concentration), altered electrical conductivity of the myocardium, and diminished glucose tolerance.[31]

Hydrogen ion secretion is increased with hyperaldosteronism, resulting in metabolic alkalosis. The alkalosis correlates to the degree of hypokalemia.[31] Marked alkalosis may be demonstrated by positive Chvostek's and positive Trousseau's signs.[50]

Plasma renin activity is suppressed. Laboratory values will reveal suppressed renin levels after the patient is exposed to conditions that will cause elevated levels in normal patients.[73] Simultaneous elevation of aldosterone secretion is also observed in these patients.

DIAGNOSTIC STUDIES

Diagnosis of primary aldosteronism is based on the following[73]:

1. The observation of hypertension
2. Presence of hypokalemia
3. Suppressed renin levels
4. Elevated aldosterone secretion

Renin and aldosterone levels

Measured after challenging the system with upright posture and restricted sodium or diuretic therapy. Normally, renin levels would increase under this challenge; with primary aldosteronism renin levels remain low.[31,50] Aldosterone levels can be measured after volume expansion through salt loading. This can be accomplished by diet, infusion of normal saline, or administration of a mineralocorticoid. The failure to suppress aldosterone secretion occurs with primary aldosteronism.[31]

CT scans of adrenal gland

Used to detect the presence and location of an adenoma. Because less radiation and time is involved than that with an iodocholesterol scan, it is a preferred diagnostic aid.[25]

Venous catheterization of adrenal glands with measurement of plasma cortisol and aldosterone

May be performed to distinguish between a unilateral and bilateral source of the hyperaldosteronism.[43]

TREATMENT PLAN

Surgical
Adrenalectomy

Chemotherapeutic
Receptor blockade: spironolactone (Aldactone), 400-600 mg qd

Supportive
Low-sodium diet

ASSESSMENT: AREAS OF CONCERN

Circulation
Mild to severe hypertension
Hypokalemia
U waves and widened QT intervals on ECG
Hypernatremia

Food and fluid
Polydipsia

Elimination
Polyuria
Nocturia

Neurosensory area
Positive Chvostek's sign
Trousseau's sign

Sleep and rest
Fatigue

Mobility
Muscle weakness

Comfort and pain
Muscle aches
Frontal headache

NURSING DIAGNOSES and NURSING INTERVENTIONS

Nursing Diagnosis	Nursing Intervention
Tissue perfusion, alteration in: cardiopulmonary	Obtain daily weight. Provide rest periods. Reinforce diet restrictions. Explain rationale for diet and mobility restrictions.
Fluid volume, alteration in: excess	Assess vital signs every 4 hours. Monitor intake and output. Check peripheral pulses. Observe for edematous tissue. Elevate any edematous area when possible.
Potential patient problem: acid-base imbalance	Assess respiratory status and quality of respirations. Reinforce low-sodium diet. Monitor laboratory data. Assess for Chvostek's and Trousseau's signs.

Patient Education

1. With surgical intervention, see p. 931.
2. With chemotherapeutic intervention, teach the patient the importance of and how to take medication regularly and the side and toxic effects to report.

EVALUATION

Patient Outcome	Data Indicating That Outcome is Reached
Cardiopulmonary tissue perfusion is adequate.	Blood pressure is within the normal range. No dysrhythmias are present. Electrolytes are within the normal range.
Excess fluid is decreased or absent.	There is no edema. Output equals intake. Skin turgor is normal. Peripheral pulses are within the normal range.
Acid-base balance is normal.	Respirations are within the normal range. Chvostek's and Trousseau's signs are absent. Potassium and sodium blood levels are within the normal range.

CONGENITAL ADRENAL HYPERPLASIA

Congenital adrenal hyperplasia is an inherited syndrome of adrenal insufficiency caused by an enzymatic alteration in steroid synthesis.

There are many classifications of congenital adrenal hyperplasia, which is caused by different enzyme deficiencies. Only the most common deficiencies (21-hydroxylase deficiency and 11-beta-hydroxylase deficiency) will be addressed here. In these deficiencies, the lack of enzyme compromises the biosynthesis of cortisol in the adrenal cortex. The two types of 21-hydroxylase deficiency are a simple type with decreased cortisol production and a salt-wasting type that includes decreased aldosterone production. 11-Beta-hydroxylase deficiency also includes a compromised biosynthesis of aldosterone.

The incidence of congenital adrenal hyperplasia is estimated at 1:15,000 births, but the incidence differs according to geographic location. It is transmitted as an autosomal recessive trait, meaning that paired carriers have a one in four chance with each pregnancy of producing an affected infant. Affected members in a family will always have the same type of enzyme deficiency.[33]

PATHOPHYSIOLOGY

Adrenal hyperplasia is brought about by excessive adrenocorticotropic hormone (ACTH) stimulation caused by lack of cortisol feedback inhibition. Normally, low serum cortisol sends signals through the hypothalamic-pituitary-adrenal feedback system, stimulating production of ACTH, which in turn acts on the adrenal cortex to synthesize steroids through a complex step-by-step enzyme system. In congenital adrenal hyperplasia the precursors to an enzymatic alteration build up and are shunted to the unaltered androgen pathway, resulting in excessive formation of sex steroids and their metabolites in blood and urine (Fig. 8-13). (See p. 845 for life-threatening nature of steroid deficiencies.)

The effects of virilizing hormones are progressive and cause pseudohermaphroditism in the female and precocious pseudopuberty in the male.

Because high androgen levels accelerate growth and maturation, the triggering of true precocious puberty can occur in both sexes. Cortisol levels either remain low or are normal depending on the adrenal gland's compensatory abilities.[73]

At birth, male infants appear to have normal genitalia. Diagnosis is often missed until outward signs of precocious pseudopuberty have appeared, such as penile enlargement and pubic hair. Because the testes do not mature, the diagnosis of precocious pseudopuberty can be distinguished from that of true precocious puberty. Affected female infants often have ambiguous genitalia and may receive wrong gender identification if not examined thoroughly. In these girls gonads will not be found in the "scrotal sac." The internal reproductive organs in both the male and female are normal, but if the female patient is not treated early enough, normal pubertal

Fig. 8-13
Alteration in adrenal steroid biosynthesis in congenital adrenal hyperplasia. The deficiency may occur in the cortisol pathway or in both the cortisol and aldosterone pathways.

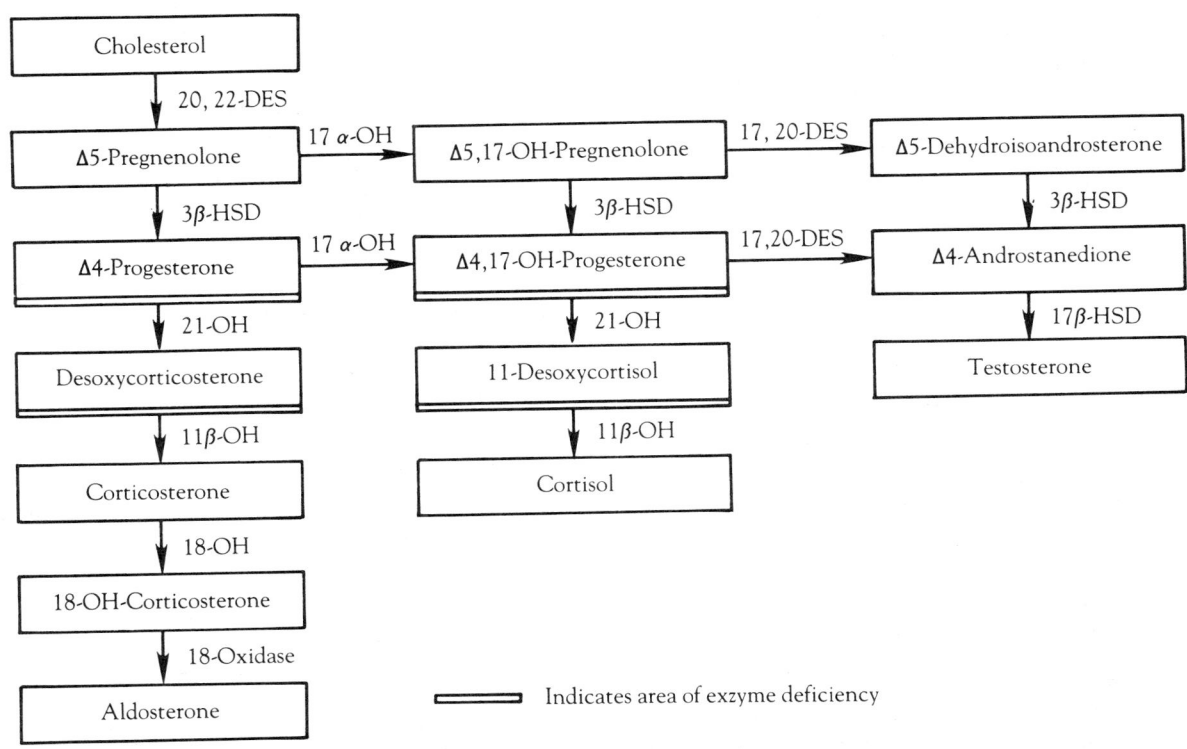

changes might not occur and there may be problems with fertility later in life. Untreated individuals are tall as children and short as adults. This phenomenon is caused by rapid bone growth and maturation, resulting in early epiphyseal closure.[7]

In the salt-wasting type of 21-hydroxylase deficiency, which has the added enzymatic alteration occurring in the biosynthesis of aldosterone, precursors are shunted to the same unaltered androgen pathway and the inadequate production of aldosterone results in salt loss through the urine.[38] Aldosterone levels can sometimes remain normal with the patient asymptomatic, if the adrenal gland has been able to compensate. The biosynthesis of aldosterone is thought to be activated by the renin-angiotensin feedback system or by an increase in serum potassium.

11-Beta-hydroxylase deficiency exhibits no salt wasting, but there may or may not be hypertension. High blood pressure is considered to be a consequence of the buildup of deoxycorticosterone, a precursor to aldosterone. The high levels of deoxycorticosterone seem to act as potent mineralocorticoids and protect against salt loss.[10]

Differences in expression of enzyme deficiencies in congenital adrenal hyperplasia and the adrenal gland's varying ability to compensate for those differences remain unexplained. The current hypothesis is that the adrenal cortex acts as two separate glands, one responding to ACTH stimulation and the other responding to angiotensin II stimulation.[72]

If treated early and continuously with replacement steroids, the patient with congenital adrenal hyperplasia can achieve normal growth and development with fertility possible. Increase in medication during times of stress aids in maintaining normal body homeostasis and prevention of adrenal crisis.

DIAGNOSTIC STUDIES

Prenatal
   17-Hydroxyprogesterone and Δ4-androstenedione
      Amniotic fluid levels

Human leukocyte antigen (HLA) genotyping
Amniotic cells compared with those of affected sibling (11-beta-hydroxylase deficiency not detected by this method)

11-Deoxycortisol and tetrahydrocortisol
Amniotic fluid levels increased in 11-beta-hydroxylase deficiency

Neonatal

17-Hydroxyprogesterone (capillary)
57 pg/disc or greater indicates need for further study[59]

Serum steroid levels
Elevated

ACTH stimulation test
Subnormal cortisol response

Dexamethasone suppression test
17-Ketosteroids reduced to normal

Urinary steroids and metabolites
Elevated (> 1 year of age)

TREATMENT PLAN

Surgical
Clitororecession for clitoral hypertrophy in females
Vaginoplasty for ambiguous genitalia in females
See discussion of surgical repair of ambiguous genitalia in females

Chemotherapeutic
Emergency steroid replacement; fluids and electrolytes (refer to Crisis Intervention for Adrenal Insufficiency)
After stabilization
Corticosteroids: treat infant with intramuscular cortisone acetate daily for 5 days; then every third day until 18 months; after 18 months, oral cortisone acetate or hydrocortisone daily in divided doses[20]; double dose of cortisone at times of major stress
Mineralocorticoids in salt wasters and in all with elevated plasma renin activity[72]: oral fludrocortisone daily or desoxycorticosterone (DOCA) in oil intramuscularly daily or desoxycorticosterone pellets subcutaneously every 6 to 9 months; oral salt supplements[20]

The patient with congenital adrenal hyperplasia must be carefully observed for growth curves, bone age, and steroid levels in blood and urine, all of which help determine the most beneficial dosage of medication.[20]

ASSESSMENT: AREAS OF CONCERN

Electrolyte balance
Nausea, vomiting, diarrhea
Output greater than intake
Weight loss

Cardiovascular concerns
Hypotension in 21-hydroxylase deficiency (salt-wasting type)
Hypertension in 11-beta-hydroxylase deficiency

Sexuality
Male
Early penile enlargement without maturation of testes

Female
Ambiguous genitalia
No gonads in "scrotal sac"
Mild clitoral hypertrophy to complete labioscrotal fusion with "phallus"
Progressive clitoral enlargement
Failure to develop female secondary sex characteristics (breasts, menses)
Infertility

Male and female
Early or excessive acne, facial hair, pubic hair, axillary hair, body hair, skin pigmentation, deepening of voice

Activity
Weakness
Fatigue
Frequent or prolonged illness

Psychosocial concerns
Taller than peers as child
Shorter than peers as adult
Alteration in genitalia

NURSING DIAGNOSES and NURSING INTERVENTIONS

Nursing Diagnosis	Nursing Intervention
Potential patient problem: electrolyte imbalance	Maintain IV lines as ordered. Administer medications as ordered. Record intake and output. Record weight every 8 hours (infants) to every day. Monitor vital signs every 30 minutes to every 8 hours. Check for signs and symptoms of dehydration. Assess level of consciousness.
Tissue perfusion, alteration in: cardiopulmonary	Administer replacement steroids as ordered. Monitor blood pressure every 30 minutes to every 8 hours.
Self-concept, disturbance in: body image, personal identity	Ask parent or patient to tell you what he or she knows about altered development; discuss and encourage questions. Encourage parent or patient to verbalize fears and anxieties about sexuality. Discourage discussion of altered development as a disease.

Patient Education

1. Teach about the disorder: the cause, implications, and treatments.
2. Teach the importance of regular medication and the role it plays in management of the disorder.
3. Teach the steps to be taken to prevent adrenal crisis.
4. Identify resource and support groups available.

EVALUATION

Patient Outcome	Data Indicating That Outcome is Reached
Electrolyte balance is normal.	Intake equals output. Weight is maintained for body requirements. Skin is warm and moist, with good turgor. Serum electrolyte levels are normal.
Tissue perfusion is normal.	Blood pressure is maintained within normal range.
Self-concept improves.	The patient verbalizes understanding of altered development, realistic expectations, and strengths. The patient accepts body changes. The patient maintains relationships with peers. The patient participates in age-related activities.

DELAYED ADOLESCENCE

The diagnosis of delayed puberty is assigned to adolescents whose pubertal changes begin after two standard deviations of the accepted mean age for that sex.

In the United States, girls who have not experienced breast budding (thelarche) by age 13 or menarche by age 15 are suspected of having delayed puberty. Comparatively, boys who do not show signs of pubertal development by age 14 or who have not completed puberty in a mean of 4.7 years after initiation have maturational delay.[63] Although the exact mechanism by which puberty is initiated remains unclear, standards have been set outlining the onset and progression of the physical signs of puberty.[46,47] The ages at which breast, sexual hair, and genital development begin differ in boys and girls. Aside from age, other endogenous and exogenous factors (nutrition, genetics, endocrine disorders) influence the onset and regulation of puberty. A careful balance of all factors must be maintained. When puberty does not occur as expected, each factor must be evaluated through a careful medical examination.

Constitutional delay in development is the most common form of delayed puberty. The slow but eventual beginning of puberty represents a delay in the mechanism that triggers the onset of puberty. Numerous other etiologies of delayed adolescence are outlined below:

I. Constitutional/familial
II. Endocrine disorders
  A. Chromosomal abnormalities
    1. Turner's syndrome (XO, XO/XX)
    2. Klinefelter's syndrome (XXY)
    3. Pure or mixed gonadal dysgenesis
  B. Hypogonadotropic hypogonadism (low gonadotropins)
    1. Hypothalamic/pituitary disorders (absent or incomplete stimulation of pituitary by LHRH)
      a. Infection or inflammation (e.g., encephalitis)
      b. Neoplasms (e.g., craniopharyngioma, gliomas)
      c. Trauma
      d. Syndromes (examples)
        (1) Kallmann's
        (2) Prader-Willi
        (3) Laurence-Moon-Bardet-Biedl
        (4) Fertile eunuch
        (5) Fröhlich's
        (6) Reifenstein's
      e. Suppression by exogenous hormones
      f. Receptor disorders (hypothalamic/pituitary)
    2. Systemic disorders or chronic illness affecting:
      a. Cardiovascular system
      b. Respiratory system
      c. Gastrointestinal system
      d. Renal system
      e. Endocrine system (hypothyroidism, hyperthyroidism, diabetes mellitus, hyperprolactinemia)
      f. Anemia
      g. Collagen vascular system (rheumatoid disorders)
  C. Hypergonadotropic hypogonadism (elevated gonadotropins)
    1. Disorders of the ovaries and testes
      a. Trauma
      b. Inflammation (polycystic ovarian disease)
      c. Iatrogenic; malfunction resulting from:
        (1) Surgery
        (2) Irradiation
        (3) Chemotherapy
      d. Neoplasms
      e. True hermaphroditism and pseudohermaphroditism
      f. Gonadotropin receptor disorders
    2. Defect in biosynthesis of androgens and estrogens
      a. 17-Alpha-hydroxylase deficiency
      b. Desmolase deficiency
    3. Malnutrition
      a. Anorexia nervosa
      b. Isolated vitamin or mineral deficiency (zinc)
      c. Deprivation related to socioeconomic status
      d. Inadequate percentage of body fat (related to athletics)
    4. Congenital anomalies
      a. Testicular feminization
      b. Absent uterus or vagina (müllerian abnormality)
      c. Imperforate hymen
      d. Del Castillo syndrome (Sertoli cell)

The more common disorders will be discussed in other sections of this chapter. This section will discuss constitutionally delayed adolescence.

It is estimated that 25 out of every 1000 children will not have entered puberty by the expected age.[63] Although this disorder is common to both boys and girls, the exact ratio of occurrence is unclear. Culturally, a delay in pubertal development is more acceptable for girls than boys. Frequently, it is the boy who seeks medical help because of concern for this problem. The parents' first indication of their child's delayed puberty may be his short stature. Further examination shows infantile or early maturing genitalia. If these findings are very disturbing to the adolescent, hormonal treatment may be considered, although psychologic support and reassurance are all that is usually needed. The adolescent who does not experience the same overt physical changes as peers may experience a disturbance in self-concept and well-being. Thus he may lack the confidence to establish successful peer relationships. In order to allay concerns, the patient and family need the assurance provided in understanding the diagnosis, treatment options, and prognosis.

PATHOPHYSIOLOGY

Constitutionally delayed puberty can usually be differentiated from other causes of delayed puberty by a few diagnostic tests. A careful family history including age of onset and characteristics of puberty in parents, siblings, and immediate relatives gives clues to familial influences. Physical examination shows sexual maturation delayed for chronologic age; bone age is also delayed. Growth of about 2 inches (5 cm) per year is usually present. The typical patient has early signs of development (breast buds, testes enlargement) and a growth

Fig. 8-14

Hypothalamic-pituitary-gonadal (H-P-G) axis diagrams illustrate gradual decreasing inhibition of the hypothalamus as the individual passes through puberty. The negative-feedback mechanism is enhanced by increased gonadal secretions (sex steroids) trying to overcome the decrease in hypothalamic sensitivity. The resulting increase in all H-P-G secretions maintains adult sexual development.

Redrawn from Grumbach, M.M., Grave, G.D., and Mayer, F.E., editors: Control of the onset of puberty, New York, 1974, John Wiley & Sons, Inc.

	Prepuberty	Initiation of puberty	Adult
Gonadal steroids	Low	Unchanged	Adult level
Feedback	Operative and sensitive	Decreasing in sensitivity	Operative at adult level
Gonadotropins	Low	Increasing	Adult level

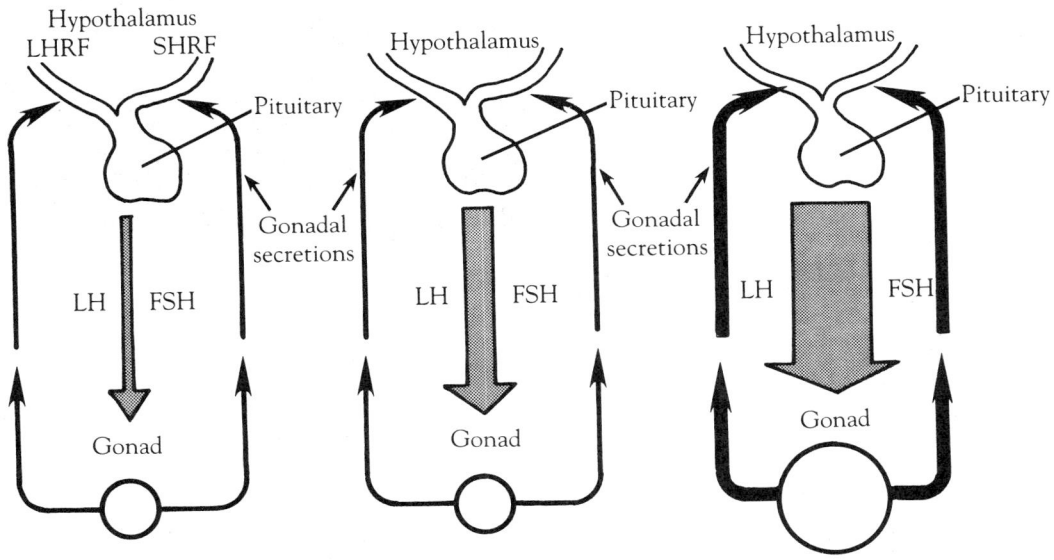

curve showing height below but parallel to the first percentile.[35]

Data suggest that a lag in maturation of the hypothalamic-pituitary-gonadal axis exists.[10] Pubertal progression depends on secretion of GnRH and then LH and FSH with negative feedback provided by sex steroids to maintain development (Fig. 8-14). In delayed puberty, pulsatile synchronization between secretion of GnRH and the gonadotropins with sustained sex steroid secretion by the gonads has not been achieved. Without this vital hormonal stimulation and feedback mechanism, puberty cannot be sustained. In time, this system does mature and puberty progresses to completion. This suggests that constitutionally delayed adolescence is not the result of genetic anomalies or nutritional, endocrinologic, or systemic diseases but of a delay in the hormonal regulation.

Differential diagnosis of delayed adolescence includes various diagnostic procedures (p. 856). Once an etiology has been determined, treatment is aimed at correcting the systemic or hormonal disorder. Hormonal treatment for constitutionally delayed puberty is considered only after age 14 in boys and age 13 in girls. After adequate nutritional status has been confirmed, hormonal treatment is indicated for the child who is suffering psychologically from short, immature stature. As depicted in Fig. 8-15, constitutionally delayed adolescence, left untreated, progresses naturally.

Fig. 8-15
Constitutional delay of puberty and
progression into puberty without
treatment.

From Prader, A.: Constitutional delay of
growth and puberty. In Chiumello, G., and
Laron, Z., editors: Recent progress in
pediatric endocrinology, New York, 1977,
Academic Press Inc.

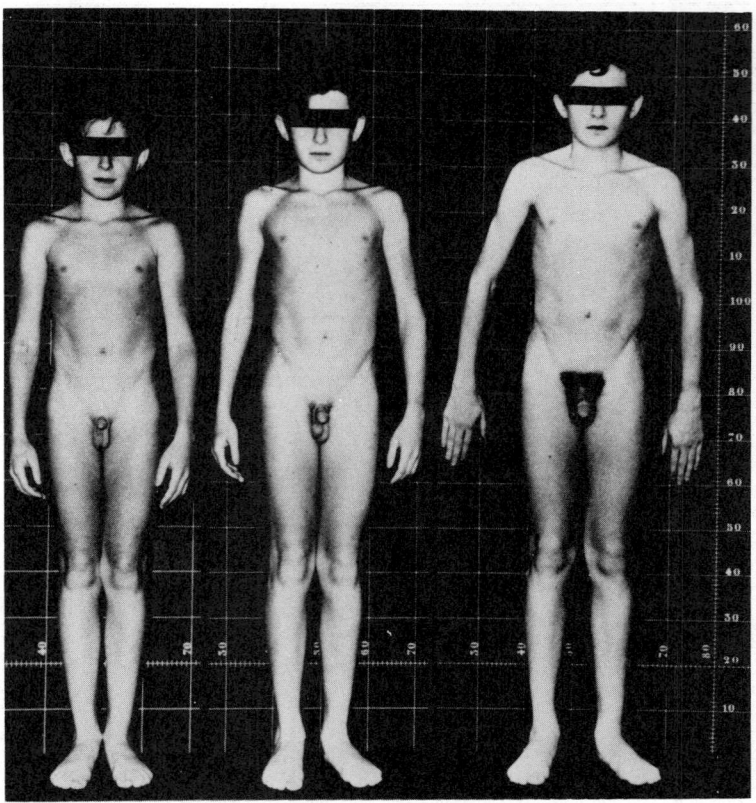

Age	14 ½₂ yr	15 ³⁄₁₂ yr	16 ²⁄₁₂ yr
Height	142.6 cm	146.6 cm	155.4 cm
Bone age		12 yr	13 yr

DIAGNOSTIC STUDIES

The following studies are most commonly used in the
differential diagnosis of delayed puberty. A child with
constitutionally delayed puberty will have normal findings.

Skull films
Free of abnormalities (i.e., masses)

Abdominal and genital ultrasonography
Normal internal structures free of masses and congenital anomalies

Buccal smear or karyotype
Chromosomal analysis appropriate for stated gender

**Baseline and stimulated gonadotropins, sex
hormones, and adrenal hormones**
Baseline and stimulated levels may be prepubertal or
appropriate for Tanner stage of development

Routine hematologic and blood/urine tests
Normal findings

Bone age
Delayed

TREATMENT PLAN

Chemotherapeutic
Only if indicated. Therapy is usually discontinued at
a bone age of 13 since the natural hypothalamic-
pituitary-gonadal axis should be activated.
Girls
Estrogens: rarely given and usually prescribed in
gradually increasing doses
Ethinyl estradiol, 0.02 mg/d for 21 d of a 28-d
cycle

Conjugated estrogens (Premarin), 0.6-2.5 mg/d until vaginal spotting and genital maturation begin

Cyclic estrogen therapy may be chosen at this point

Boys

Androgenic agents: treatment of choice is a long-acting intramuscular testosterone preparation in gradually increasing doses (50-300 mg/mo) q4-6 mo

Oral methyltestosterone, 25-50 mg/d

Fluoxymesterone (Halotestine), 2-10 mg/d po for 3-6 mo

Treatment usually lasts from 3 to 6 months and should be interrupted by an equal period of time off the treatment.

ASSESSMENT: AREAS OF CONCERN

Pubertal development

Delayed sexual development for age (Tanner stage)

Growth pattern below but parallel to first percentile

Child appears younger than stated age

Physical (congenital) anomalies may or may not be present

Psychosocial concerns

Note psychologic adjustment to delayed maturation (i.e., peer and school adjustments)

Parents note child is withdrawn, refrains from peer involvement (e.g., sports)

Teased by peers for short stature and immature (small) genitalia

Child treated inappropriately for chronologic age

NURSING DIAGNOSES and NURSING INTERVENTIONS

Nursing Diagnosis	Nursing Intervention
Self-concept, disturbance in: body image, personal identity	Assess understanding, correct misconceptions, and adjust explanations to learner level. Reassure that puberty will occur with or without treatment (diagnosis dependent). Give positive feedback. Provide illustrated literature where appropriate (contact local child health organization or see government publications). Aid patient and family to identify familial pattern of delayed sexual development. Assess ability to achieve successful interpersonal relationships with peers. Role play interactions with peers and family. See also p. 1820.

Patient Education

1. Ensure that understanding of process is adequate for treatment or nontreatment decision.
2. Teach effects and possible side effects of prescribed hormones.
3. Teach knowledge of medication dosage schedule and administration and duration of treatment.
4. Explain the importance of regular medical care.

EVALUATION

Patient Outcome	Data Indicating That Outcome is Reached
Self-concept improves.	Child and family accept altered development. Child and family verbalize realistic expectations of potential growth. Child maintains successful peer and family relationships. Child displays improved sense of self-worth. Child participates in age-related activities.

INSULIN-DEPENDENT AND NON-INSULIN-DEPENDENT DIABETES MELLITUS

Diabetes mellitus is a condition of relative or absolute lack of insulin, affecting carbohydrate, protein, and fat metabolism.

In 1982, 300,000 to 500,000 persons in the United States had insulin-dependent diabetes mellitus (IDDM).[54] In the same year, 5.5 to 5.7 million persons in the United States had non-insulin-dependent diabetes mellitus (NIDDM).[54]

The guidelines for classifying diabetes mellitus come from the NIH National Diabetes Data Group. Their classification of diabetes mellitus is as follows[53]:

1. Insulin-dependent
2. Non-insulin-dependent
3. Other types (diabetes mellitus associated with certain conditions or syndromes)
4. Impaired glucose tolerance
5. Gestational diabetes mellitus
6. Previous abnormality in glucose tolerance
7. Potential abnormality in glucose tolerance

(This discussion is limited to the first two types.)

PATHOPHYSIOLOGY

Insulin-dependent diabetes mellitus is a different disorder from non-insulin-dependent diabetes mellitus although both share a common defect: relative or absolute lack of insulin (Table 8-6). Genetic predisposition for insulin-dependent diabetes mellitus seems to be conferred by a certain histocompatibility antigen, human leukocyte antigen (HLA), coded on chromosome 6.[24] Environmental factors may have a role in the development of insulin-dependent diabetes in the genetically susceptible individual. Viruses (coxsackie, mumps, rubella) may either

Table 8-6

Types of Diabetes and Characteristics

	Type I: Insulin-Dependent Diabetes (Juvenile Onset [JOD])	Type II: Non-Insulin-Dependent Diabetes (Maturity Onset [MOD])
Age of onset	<30 yr	>40 yr
Body weight	Normal or underweight	Overweight (80%)
Prevalence	0.5%	5%
Etiology	Unknown	Unknown
	Heredity: associated with specific human leukocyte antigen (HLA) types but only 50% concordance in twins	Heredity: not associated with specific HLA types but 95% concordance in twins
	Autoimmune disease: 70% circulating islet cell antibodies	Autoimmune disease: 10% circulating islet cell antibodies
	Viral infections are possible trigger	No evidence for viral infections
Insulin	Early in disease, insulin secretion is impaired; late in disease, secretion may be totally absent	Insulin deficiency and/or insulin resistance
		Deficiency: insulin secretion insufficient to meet demands created by obese state; possible impairment in glucose receptor of the beta cell
		Resistance: in nonobese patients, there is hyperinsulinemia and a defect in tissue responsiveness to insulin; insulin resistance may be mediated by a decreased number of insulin receptors
Ketosis	Common	Rare
Complications	Frequent	Frequent
	Microangiopathies	Accelerated atherosclerosis
	Neuropathies	Microangiopathies
	Accelerated atherosclerosis	Neuropathies
Leading cause of death	Microangiopathies (i.e., renal failure secondary to diabetic nephropathy)	Accelerated atherosclerosis (i.e., myocardial infarction)
Treatment	Diet and insulin	Diet (reduction) *or*
		Diet and oral hypoglycemic agents *or*
		Diet and insulin

From Busick, E.J.: Natural history and diagnosis. In Kozak, G.P., editor: Clinical diabetes mellitus, Philadelphia, 1982, W.B. Saunders Co.

cause direct destruction of the beta cells or induce an immunologic reaction to the beta cells of the pancreas.[24]

Initially, insulin dependence appears as insulitis and mononuclear cell infiltration of the pancreas, progressing to actual destruction of the functioning beta cells.[24] Islet cell antibodies, cell-surface antibodies, and cell-mediated immunity are present, suggesting the possible role of autoimmunity in the development of insulin-dependent diabetes.

Once beta cells are destroyed, metabolic compensation and the ability to maintain blood sugar within normal limits deteriorate steadily. Symptoms are the direct result of the lack of insulin and subsequent deterioration of body processes and metabolism associated with or requiring insulin.

Insulin deficiency causes hyperglycemia by decreasing glucose uptake by peripheral adipose and muscle tissues. The lack of restraining effect on the liver processes of glycogenolysis and gluconeogenesis causes the liver to overproduce glucose.[39] Glucose and amino acid uptake by muscle and fat tissue is impaired; synthesis of protein, glycogen, fat, DNA, RNA, and ATP is decreased.[39] Protein and fat are actually broken down, freeing up more substrate for the liver to use in out-of-control gluconeogenesis. Elevated levels of triglyceride and cholesterol bind to proteins in the blood. Since these lipoproteins cannot be metabolized in the peripheral tissues, they deposit under the skin.

Individuals with non-insulin-dependent diabetes are usually over 30 years of age at the time of diagnosis, and 80% are obese. Environmental etiologic factors are related to the urban life-style and include obesity, decreased exercise, and possible dietary factors.[24] A possible genetic component has not yet been identified.

Obesity is associated with insulin resistance or diminished sensitivity to insulin or both.[24] The exact cause of the defect is unknown, but it could occur at any step in the sequence of insulin action, from receptor binding to intracellular metabolism. Down regulation of receptors in response to hyperinsulinism has been demonstrated.[24] Therefore insulin resistance may begin as an adaptive mechanism to protect the body from hypoglycemia in the face of sometimes severe hyperinsulinemia. Hyperglycemia causes overactivity of the polyol pathway, causing sorbitol to accumulate in Schwann cells. This process damages myelin nerve coverings, causing diabetic neuropathies.[39] Attachment of glucose to proteins (glycosylation) in the basement membranes of capillaries causes a thickening of the membranes and resultant diabetic microangiopathy. Microangiopathy is implicated in the development of retinopathy and nephropathy. Accelerated atherosclerosis in the heart and large arteries combined with decreased elasticity of arterial walls and the hypercoagulable state of diabetic blood result in high cardiac-related morbidity and mortality among the diabetic population.[24]

Other metabolic abnormalities associated with hyperglycemia, including elevated serum lipids, elevated plasma glucagon, and elevated growth hormone, may also have a contributory effect on the development of long-term complications. Although a number of these abnormalities return to normal with proper management of diabetes, none are causally related to the pathologic changes in the long-term complications of diabetes mellitus.

DIAGNOSTIC STUDIES

Fasting blood sugar
  Venous plasma: $\geq$140 mg/dl
  Venous whole blood: $\geq$200 mg/dl

Glucose tolerance test
  Two-hour oral glucose tolerance test sample and one other sample after 75 g glucose (adult) or 1.75 g/kg ideal body weight (children)
  Venous plasma: $\geq$200 mg/dl
  Venous whole blood: $\geq$180 mg/dl

Blood insulin levels
  Absent in insulin-dependent diabetes
  Normal to high in non-insulin-dependent diabetes

Plasma proinsulin
  Not applicable in insulin-dependent diabetes
  Normal to high in non-insulin-dependent diabetes mellitus

Plasma C-peptide
  Absent in insulin-dependent diabetes
  Normal to high in non-insulin-dependent diabetes

TREATMENT PLAN

Surgical
  Interventions for complications (i.e., bypass grafts, eye surgery)

Chemotherapeutic
  Insulin preparations—doses are individually adjusted
    Rapid-acting preparations
      Regular
        Iletin I, II (beef, pork)
        Velosulin or Quick (pork)
        Actrapid (pork)
      Semilente
        Iletin I (beef, pork)
        Semitard (pork)

Human
  Humulin R
  Actrapid Human
Intermediate-acting preparations
  NPH
    Iletin I, II (beef, pork)
    Insulatard NPH (pork)
    Lentard (beef, pork)
  Lente
    Iletin I, II (beef, pork)
    Monotard (pork)
    Lentard (beef, pork)
  Globin
  Human
    Humulin N
    Monotard Human
Long-acting preparations
  Utralente
    Ultratard (beef)
    Iletin I (beef, pork)
  Protamine Zinc
    Iletin I, II (beef, pork)
Hypoglycemic agents: sulfonylureas (first generation)
  Tolbutamide (Orinase), 500 mg to 2.0 g/d in divided
    doses
  Chlorpropamide (Diabinese), 100-250 mg/d
  Acetohexamide (Dymelor), 250 mg to 1.5 g/d in
    divided doses
  Tolazamide (Tolinase), 100 mg to 1 g/d

Electromechanical
Open-loop infusion pumps (listing not inclusive)
  Autosyringe: AS6C and AS6C-U100, AS6MP
    (Baxter-Travenol Laboratories, Inc.)
  Beta 1 (Orange Medical Instruments)
  Delta SP-250 (Delta Medical Industries)
  Medix 209-100 (Medix Corp.)
  Pacesetter Systems Inc. (Micromed)
  CPI (Eli Lilly Co.), model 9100
  Photocoagulation (see Chapter 6)
  Penile prosthesis (see Chapter 10)
  Kidney dialysis (see Chapter 9)

Supportive
ADA diet

ASSESSMENT: AREAS OF CONCERN

Food and fluid
  Hunger, thirst, nausea
  Weight loss or obesity

Elimination
  Frequent urination in large amounts
  Nocturia
  Diarrhea or constipation

Neurosensory concerns
  Decreased sensation to pain and temperature in feet
  Blurred vision
  Headaches, cataracts, halos around lights

Mobility
  Muscle weakness
  Tiredness
  Wrist-drop
  Ankle-drop

Skin
  Infection (frequent skin boils and ulceration)
  Rubeosis; dermopathy

Sexuality
  Impotence
  Vaginal discharge
  Increased susceptibility to vaginal infection

Circulation
  Cold extremities
  Loss of hair on toes; skin shiny, thin, and atrophic
  Orthostatic hypotension
  Painful calves when walking
  Numbness and tingling of lower extremities
  Weak pedal pulse

Psychosocial concerns
  Verbalization of inability to cope
  Verbalization of change in life-style
  Negative feeling about body

Teaching and learning
  Lack of exposure to diabetes if newly diagnosed
  Lack of recall
  Misinformation
  Inadequate demonstration of skills required (urine and/
    or blood testing, injection technique)
  Lack of interest
  Unfamiliarity with facts of management

NURSING DIAGNOSES and NURSING INTERVENTIONS

Nursing Diagnosis	Nursing Intervention
Tissue perfusion, alteration in: peripheral	Assess peripheral pulses and color, temperature, blanching, and tenderness of lower extremities. Avoid pressure at back of knees by crossing legs or sitting on a chair that is too high. Avoid constricting garments on lower trunk and extremities. Instruct patient regarding Buerger-Allen exercises to develop collateral circulation.
Fluid volume deficit, potential	Encourage noncaloric fluids for hyperglycemia. Assess skin turgor for dehydration.
Nutrition, alteration in: more than body requirements	Arrange a dietary consultation. Reinforce meal plan as ordered. Suggest support group such as Weight Watchers. Allow patient to verbalize feelings regarding weight. Positively reinforce patient's effort at weight loss. Assess for psychosocial concerns that may be related to overeating.
Nutrition, alteration in: less than body requirements	Arrange a dietary consultation. Reinforce meal plan as ordered. Assess for factors that may influence diet preferences. Encourage verbalization of feelings about weight, body size, and eating behavior.
Skin integrity, impairment of: potential	Assess feet every day for pressure areas and skin changes. Maintain good hydration and nutritional status. Instruct patient regarding proper foot care.
Coping, ineffective individual and family	Emphasize that daily management can become as routine as personal hygiene. Encourage self-care to maximal ability. Encourage participation in diabetic support groups through local American Diabetes Association (ADA) and Juvenile Diabetes Foundation (JDF). See pp. 1897 and 1899.

Patient Education

1. Teach importance of and how to administer insulin or oral hypoglycemics; teach side or toxic effects to report.
2. Teach method for monitoring blood sugar:
   a. Regular urine testing or home blood glucose monitoring
3. Teach need for maintenance of prescribed diet and regular, routine exercise and activity to maintain blood sugar control.
4. Teach early recognition and treatment of hypoglycemia and hyperglycemia.
5. Ensure knowledge of sick day management.
6. Teach personal hygiene stressing specifics related to dental, foot, and skin care.
7. Stress methods of care to prevent complications.
8. Teach importance of regular medical care.
9. Ensure adequate information about disease process to permit informed decision making (e.g., about pregnancy).

EVALUATION

Patient Outcome	Data Indicating That Outcome is Reached
Tissue perfusion is adequate.	Peripheral pulses are present. Skin is warm and moist. Turgor is normal. Capillary refill time is less than 3 seconds.
Nutrition is adequate.	Weight is within range for height and stature. Blood sugar is below 150 mg/d. Output equals intake.

Patient Outcome	Data Indicating That Outcome is Reached
Skin is intact.	There are no breaks, cracks, ulcers, or discoloration. There are no infections. Wound healing is normal.
The patient copes effectively.	The patient verbalizes coping with limitations imposed by required care. The patient expresses feelings of control. The patient accepts support from others as needed. The patient exhibits no destructive behavior. The patient functions independently in activities of daily living to maximal ability. The patient incorporates diabetic care into life-style.
Self-care is achieved.	The patient verbalizes understanding of and demonstrates the following: Insulin or oral hypoglycemic administration Urine or home blood glucose testing Procedures to follow for hypoglycemia, hyperglycemia, and other illnesses General personal hygiene and specific hygiene related to dental care, skin, and feet Prescribed diet, exercise, activity Disease process and related complications

DIABETIC KETOACIDOSIS AND HYPERGLYCEMIC HYPEROSMOLAR NONKETOTIC COMA

Diabetic ketoacidosis (DKA) is acute insulin deficiency that causes metabolic acidosis from ketone bodies (organic acids) as a result of fat breakdown.

Hyperglycemic hyperosmolar nonketotic coma (HHNC) is severe hyperglycemia and hypertonic dehydration without significant ketoacidosis.

DKA accounts for 14% of all diabetic hospital admissions.[24] It is estimated that 15% to 30% of all episodes of DKA occur during initial diagnosis; and 50% of all cases are related to the occurrence of a stressful event, such as an infection.[24] There are many predisposing factors possible in the development of DKA: (1) failure to take insulin, (2) insufficient amount of insulin taken, (3) infection, or (4) physiologic or emotional stress. Frequently the cause is not clear.

Currently, HHNC accounts for approximately 5% to 15% of all hospital admissions for diabetic coma.[24] Serious hyperosmolarity is not restricted to the diabetic individual. Severe hyperglycemic hyperosmolarity has been observed in association with diabetes insipidus; central nervous system damage; gastrointestinal hemorrhage; intravenous therapy with large amounts of glucose solutions; dialysis of hyperosmolar dialysate; concentration milk formula in feeding of infants; acromegaly; hypothermia; and drugs such as the thiazide diuretics, phenytoin, diazoxide, glucocorticoids, furosemide, propranolol, and cimetidine; and after the ingestion of large amounts of sugary beverages or high-protein gastric tube feedings.[24] About 80% of patients with HHNC have impaired renal function, a significant predisposing condition that contributes to the development of HHNC.[24]

Most victims are elderly and infirm, institutionalized, or mentally impaired.

Unfortunately, both hyperglycemia and hyperosmolarity are also present in the patient with DKA, making it very difficult to separate these entities entirely. Usually the precipitating factors are the same. Research is currently focused on explaining the exact biochemical basis for the nonketotic condition of HHNC and developing a recommendation on preferred rate of insulin and intravenous therapy.

PATHOPHYSIOLOGY

The contribution of counterregulatory (stress) hormones to the extreme hyperglycemia of insulin deficiency can quickly cause the development of diabetic ketoacidosis (DKA). During stress, the secretion of these hormones (glucagon, catecholamines, growth hormone, and cortisol) increases. In the insulin-deficient individual the effects of these hormones are magnified because of both an exaggerated release and an enhanced responsiveness when insulin levels are below normal.[24] Specifically, catecholamines increase liver glycogenolysis; cortisol increases hepatic gluconeogenesis and blocks peripheral use of glucose; growth hormone stimulates lipolysis, freeing up fatty acids and glycerol to be used in gluconeogenesis; and glucagon stimulates glycogenolysis, gluconeogenesis, and lipolysis. Thus deficiency of insulin itself permits an out-of-control secretion and response to the secretion of counterregulatory hormones, which only serve to accelerate the development of DKA. Since the stress that precipitates the occurrence of DKA is prolonged, the effects of all four stress hormones are also

prolonged. In addition, there appears to be a synergistic effect among all four stress hormones, which further increases blood sugar and causes a rapid deterioration of metabolic balance.[24]

The events of DKA are summarized in Fig. 8-16. In the absence of adequate insulin, peripheral fat, muscle, and liver cells are unable to utilize glucose. Breakdown of fat and protein is accelerated, freeing up more substrate (fatty acids and amino acids) for use in gluconeogenesis affected by the counterregulatory hormones.

Excessive amounts of fatty acids are used by the liver

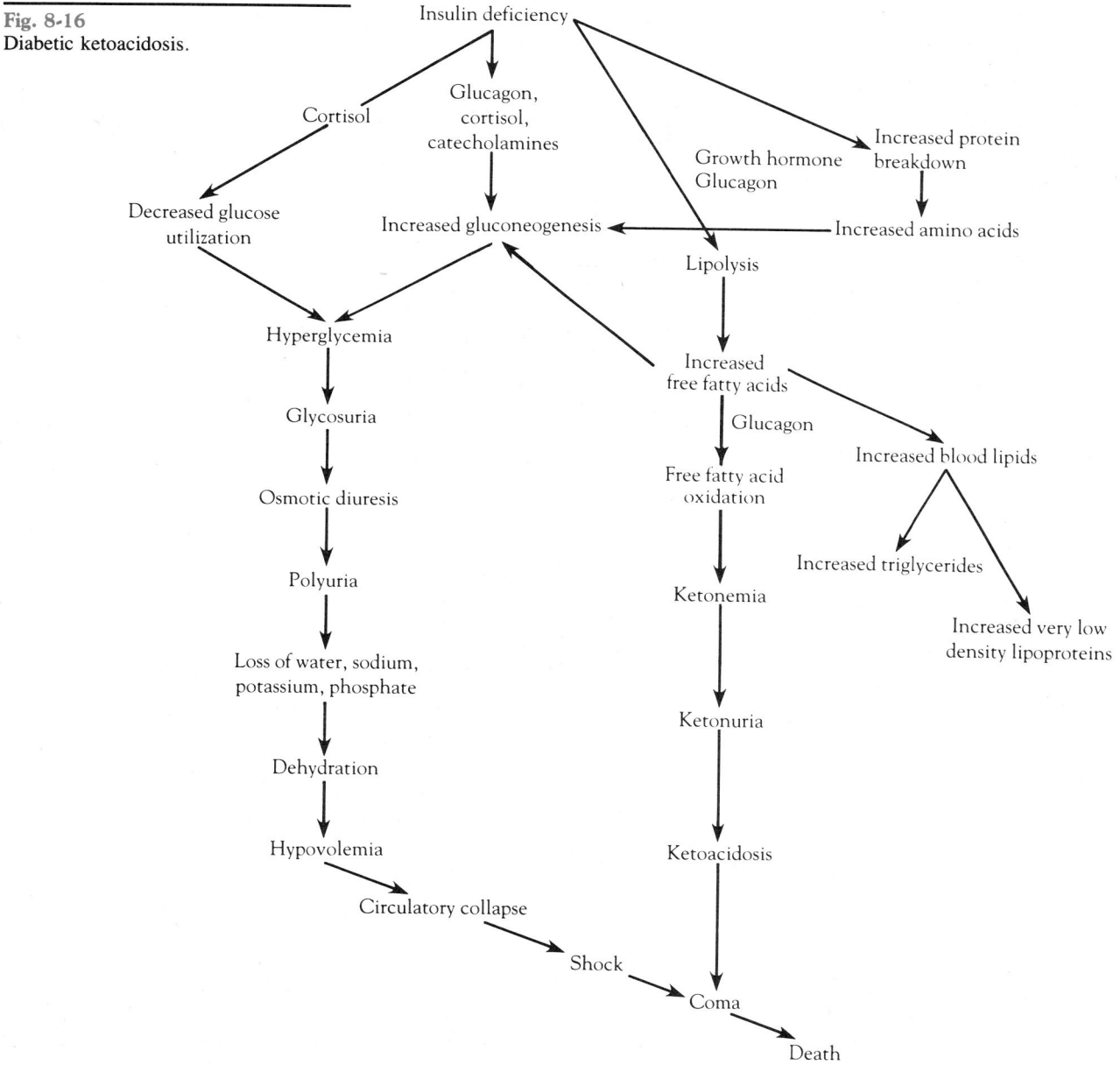

Fig. 8-16
Diabetic ketoacidosis.

(under the control of glucagon) for the formation of ke-tone bodies, beta-hydroxybutyric acid, and acetoacetic acid.[39] Acetone, responsible for the characteristic fruity breath in DKA, is formed from acetoacetic acid by a simple decarboxylation reaction.[39] The ketone bodies are produced faster than they can be metabolized or excreted. Acetoacetic acid and beta-hydroxybutyric acid cannot be metabolized in the absence of insulin; therefore their levels also increase in the plasma.[39] These strong organic acids dissociate at body pH and provide 1 mEq of H+ cation and a ketoacid anion. Metabolic acidosis occurs when the body's buffer system and respiratory compensatory mechanisms are unable to maintain normal pH.

Hyperglycemia results in glycosuria with a large os-motic water and electrolyte loss through the kidneys.[28] In addition, the organic acids are excreted through the kidneys as anions, significantly decreasing potassium and sodium in the body. The acidotic state also creates a shift in electrolytes; extracellular H+ is exchanged for intra-cellular K+. Therefore serum K+ may be elevated as H+ moves intracellularly. Hypovolemia may seem to increase the degree of hyperkalemia, but eventually the loss of potassium through the kidneys seriously depletes body potassium. There are many contributing factors to the changes in levels of consciousness in the DKA pa-tient, such as decreased oxygenation of tissues, increased

Fig. 8-17
Pathophysiology of hyperosmolar coma.

From Arieff, A.E., and Felts, P.W., editors: Current concepts: hyperosmolar coma, Upjohn, 1974, A Scope Publication, p. 23.

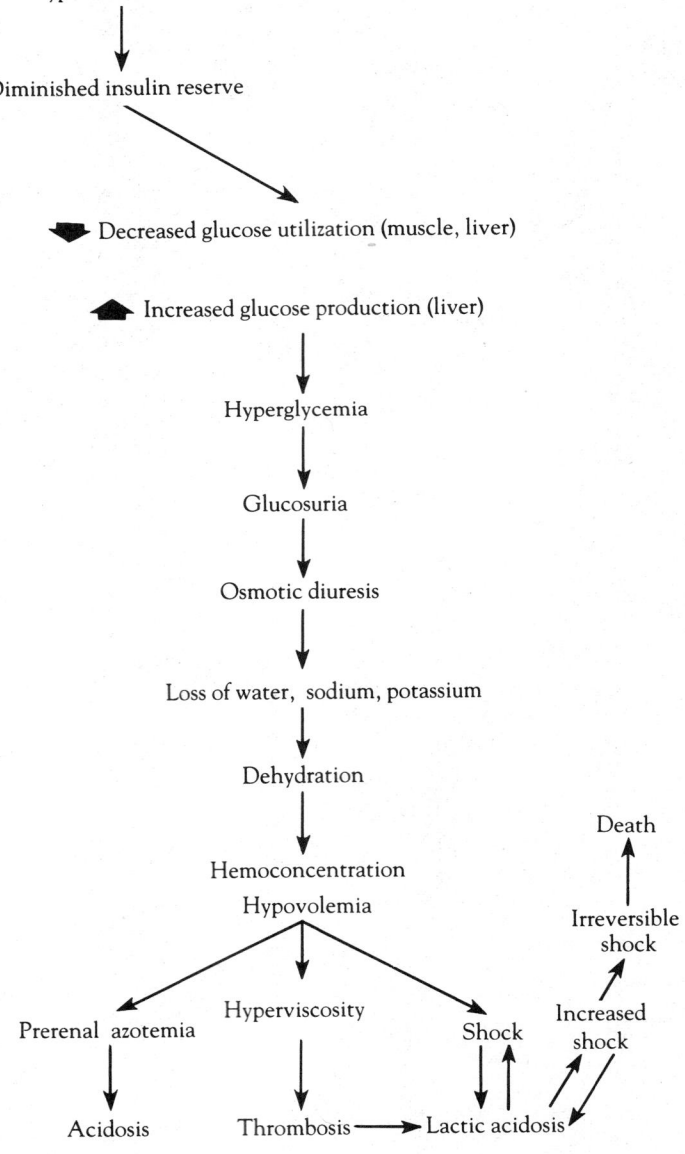

H +, hyperosmolarity, and increased acetoacetic acid.

Twenty to sixty-five percent of DKA patients experience an abnormality of plasma serum enzymes including serum amylase, creatine phosphokinase (CPK), transaminases (SGOT, SGPT), and lysosomal enzymes.[24] These changes may be directly related to the metabolic acidosis or to the underlying cause of the acidosis. Phosphorus deficiency is thought to be related to increased protein breakdown, impaired glucose use by the cells, and altered renal excretion of electrolytes in acidosis.[24] Magnesium is an intracellular cation lost in a manner parallel to potassium in DKA. Initially, serum magnesium may be normal or elevated, but a total body deficit may be recognizable only after insulin therapy has begun.

The initial step in the progression from non-insulin-dependent diabetes mellitus (NIDDM) to hyperglycemic hyperosmolar nonketotic coma (HHNC) begins with low serum insulin levels, which cause derangement in carbohydrate, fat, and protein metabolism (Fig. 8-17). Blood sugar rises in response to decreased glucose use by the cells and increased glucose production by the liver in the total or partial lack of insulin. Osmotic water and electrolyte loss begins in response to glycosuria. Amino acid uptake and protein synthesis are halted. Breakdown of protein furnishes the liver with more substrate for gluconeogenesis. Fat is also broken down, causing an excess of fatty acids.

The most significant aspect of the disease that differentiates HHNC from DKA is the serum level of free fatty acids, which are lower in HHNC than in DKA[39] (see Table 8-7 for a comprehensive comparison of the two conditions). This may be the most plausible explanation for the lack of ketosis in HHNC. There are a number of theories that attempt to explain why serum free fatty acids are lower in HHNC: (1) there is decreased release of fatty acids from adipose cells and a concomitant decrease in their use by the liver because of the presence of small amounts of insulin in the circulation[24]; (2) glucagon levels are higher in HHNC[24]; (3) hyperosmolarity or severe dehydration itself inhibits fatty acid release and production of ketones by the liver[39]; and (4) the excess fatty acids are instead utilized in other pathways, such as triglyceride synthesis.[34]

Serum concentrations of the counterregulatory hormones differ significantly from those in DKA: serum glucagon levels are higher and growth hormone and cor-

Table 8-7

Comparison of Hyperglycemic Hyperosmolar Nonketotic Coma (HHNC) and Diabetic Ketoacidosis (DKA)

Clinical Picture	HHNC	DKA
General	More dehydrated, not acidotic	More acidotic and less dehydrated
	Frequently comatose	Rarely comatose
	No hyperventilation	Hyperventilation
Age frequency	Usually elderly	Younger patients
Type of diabetes mellitus	Type II or non-insulin-dependent	Type I or insulin-dependent
Previous history of diabetes mellitus	In only 50%	Almost always
Prodromes	Several days duration	Less than 1 day
Neurologic symptoms and signs	Very common	Rare
Underlying renal or cardiovascular disease	About 85%	About 15%
Laboratory findings		
Blood sugar	Over 800 mg/dl	Usually less than 800 mg/dl
Plasma ketones	Less than large in undiluted specimen	Positive in several dilutions
Serum sodium	Normal, elevated, low	Usually low
Serum potassium	Normal or elevated	Elevated, normal, or low
Serum bicarbonate	Over 16 mEq	Less than 10 mEq
Anion gap	10-12 mEq	Over 12 mEq
Blood pH	Normal	Less than 7.35
Serum osmolality	Over 350 mOsm/L	Less than 330 mOsm/L
Serum BUN	Higher than DKA ($\uparrow\uparrow\uparrow$ to $\uparrow\uparrow\uparrow\uparrow$)	Not as high as in HHNC ($\uparrow\uparrow$)
Free fatty acids	Less than 1000 mEq/L	Over 1500 mEq/L
Complications		
Thrombosis	Frequent	Very rare
Mortality	20-50%	1-10%
Diabetes treatment postrecovery	Diet alone or oral agents sometimes	Always insulin

From Kozak, G.P., and Rolla, A.R.: Diabetic comas. In Kozak, G.P., editor: Clinical diabetes mellitus, Philadelphia, 1982, W.B. Saunders Co., p. 132.

tisol levels are lower in HHNC. The elevated glucagon levels appear to be primarily responsible for the severely elevated blood sugar values, a direct result of stimulation of liver gluconeogenesis by glucagon. The presence of renal impairment (80% of patients), either primary (kidney disease) or secondary to circulating volume depletion, also appears to play a significant role in elevating blood sugar levels in HHNC.[24] The kidneys are unable to rid the body of excess sugar or maintain water balance. Body water loss that is not replaced results in hyperosmolality and dehydration. Increased solutes increase osmotic pressure. The effective serum osmolarity (Eosm) is calculated as follows[24]:

$$Eosm = 2(Na + K \text{ [in mEq]}) + Glucose \frac{\text{(mg/dl)}}{18}$$

When this value exceeds 320 mOsm/L, severe hyperosmolarity is present.[24] The hyperosmolarity of HHNC is a direct result of excessive blood sugar and increasing sodium concentration in dehydration.

Insulin output continues at a level to prevent ketosis. The steady loss of sodium, potassium, and water with hyperglycemia and glycosuria exacerbates the hyperosmolar state and ultimately results in hypovolemia and increased blood viscosity.[5] These two factors are primarily responsible for decreasing the blood flow to vital organs and resultant tissue hypoxia. Decreased circulation to brain cells combined with intracellular fluid and electrolyte shifts are responsible for the abnormal and confusing neurologic findings in HHNC.[5] Since most abnormalities resolve after therapy, it is suggested that the neurologic examination be repeated 48 hours after fluids and insulin therapy have been effective in restoring homeostasis.

DIAGNOSTIC STUDIES

Diagnostic Study	Diabetic Ketoacidosis (DKA)	Hyperglycemic Hyperosmolar Nonketotic Coma (HHNC)
Blood sugar	High (300 to over 800 mg/dl)	Over 800 mg/dl
Plasma ketones	Positive	Less than large
Serum sodium	Low	Normal, elevated, or low
Serum potassium	Elevated, low, or normal	Normal or elevated
Serum bicarbonate	Less than 10 mEq/L	Greater than 16 mEq/L
Blood pH	Less than 7.35	Normal
Serum osmolarity	Less than 330 mOsm/L	Greater than 350 mOsm/L
Free fatty acids	Over 1500 mEq/L	Less than 1000 mEq/L

TREATMENT PLAN

Chemotherapeutic
IV fluids
  DKA
    Adult deficit is usually 6-12 L
  HHNC
    Rapid IV fluid replacement
    Plasma expanders:
      Dextran 70 (Macrodex; others), 500-1000 ml of 6% solution, IV
      Dextran 75 (Gentran 75; others), 500-1000 ml of 6% solution, IV
      Dextran 40 (LMD; others), 10-20 ml/kg of 10% solution, IV

Insulin: regular insulin, U-40 or U-100
  Given at same rate for both DKA and HHNC, although less needed totally in HHNC
  Given until blood sugar reaches about 250 mg/dl
Electrolytes
  Sodium chloride, IV as required
  Potassium chloride, IV up to 10 mEq/h or up to 100-200 mEq/d
  Phosphate, IV as required
  Magnesium sulfate, up to 2 mEq/kg q4h

ASSESSMENT: AREAS OF CONCERN

Area of Concern	Diabetic Ketoacidosis (DKA)	Hyperglycemic Hyperosmolar Nonketotic Coma (HHNC)
Air	Rapid, deep respirations Acetone breath	
Circulation	Hypotension Tachycardia Weak, thready pulse ECG changes: elevated P wave, flattened T wave or inverted prolonged Q-T interval	Rapid, thready pulse Cool extremities Normal to low blood pressure Orthostatic hypotension 30% in frank shock[39]
Food and fluid	Extreme thirst Nausea and vomiting	Extreme thirst Weight loss Nausea and vomiting
Elimination	Nocturia Polyuria	Polyuria
Neurosensory concerns	Twitching and tremors Muscle weakness Drowsiness; lethargy; coma Headache Decreased reflexes	50% have impaired consciousness[39] Visual changes Increased or decreased reflexes Positive Babinski's sign Various abnormal neurologic findings such as aphasia, hemisensory defects, seizures, hemiparesis
Mobility	Decreased muscle tone Muscle wasting Muscle weakness	Muscle weakness
Comfort and pain	Abdominal bloating Abdominal cramping	Abdominal pain and cramping Leg cramping
Hygiene and skin	Hyperthermia Dried mucous membranes Sunken eyeballs Hot, dry flushed skin Parched tongue	Hypothermia Parched, dry lips and tongue Poor skin turgor Soft, sunken eyeballs Flushed face
Psychosocial concerns	Frightened Crying; restlessness Unable to care for self because of high levels of anxiety or decreased consciousness	Unable to care for self because of change in levels of consciousness

NURSING DIAGNOSES and NURSING INTERVENTIONS

Nursing Diagnosis	Nursing Intervention
Fluid volume deficit, actual	Start and maintain patent peripheral IV line. Monitor intake and output every hour and urine specific gravity. Administer intravenous fluids at rate prescribed. Assess pulse, temperature, and blood pressure every 30 to 60 minutes. Report signs and symptoms of circulatory collapse immediately. Provide mouth care every hour. Assess skin turgor. Instruct patient and family about therapy ordered.
Potential patient problem: acid-base balance, alteration in	Administer insulin at times ordered. Monitor laboratory data. Assess respiratory status. Monitor and record changes in levels of consciousness.

Nursing Diagnosis	Nursing Intervention
	Check all voidings for sugar and acetone.
	Instruct patient and family about therapy ordered and results of laboratory tests.
Potential patient problem: electrolyte imbalance	Assess patient for development of signs and symptoms of decreased serum electrolytes.
	Administer electrolyte replacements as ordered.
Coping, ineffective individual	See p. 1897.
	Explain all procedures to patient and family.
	Encourage participation in self-care to maximum ability as soon as able.

Patient Education

1. Teach patient essential skills and concepts of diabetes mellitus education (p. 861), especially sick day rules.

EVALUATION

Patient Outcome	Data Indicating That Outcome is Reached
Fluid balance is achieved, and cardiac output is normal.	Blood pressure is within normal limits.
	Pulse is within normal limits.
	Shock is not present.
	Circulation to peripheral tissues is adequate.
	There is no dehydration.
	Output equals intake.
	Skin turgor is normal.
Acid-base balance is achieved.	Blood pH is normal.
	Blood sugar is within normal limits.
	The patient is conscious and alert.
	Respiratory rate and character are normal.
Electrolyte balance is achieved.	Electrolytes are within normal level.
	ECG is at baseline.
The patient copes effectively.	Family and patient participate in care.
	The patient verbalizes concerns and fears.
	Behavior is calm and appropriate.
	The patient discusses potential causes of condition.
	The patient verbalizes methods to prevent recurrence.
Self-care is achieved.	The patient verbalizes understanding and demonstrates knowledge and skills required to control disease process (see discussion of diabetes mellitus, p. 861).

DIABETES INSIPIDUS

Diabetes insipidus is a transient or permanent disturbance of water metabolism that results in the excretion of a large volume of dilute urine. It may be pituitary, nephrogenic, or psychogenic in nature.

Central (or pituitary) diabetes insipidus results from a failure of vasopressin synthesis or release. Nephrogenic diabetes insipidus results from a deficiency of vasopressin receptors in the renal collecting ducts. Psychogenic diabetes insipidus (polydipsia) occurs following a large intake of fluid that may suppress antidiuretic hormone (ADH). All these causes result in the excretion of large volumes of dilute urine. Current research centers on the development of more effective and specific analogues of vasopressin, such as DDAVP, a vasopressin analogue with prolonged action.

PATHOPHYSIOLOGY

The maintenance of water homeostasis is a function of the posterior pituitary gland and the kidney. The neurohypophysis secretes a polypeptide hormone with marked antidiuretic properties called antidiuretic hormone (ADH), or vasopressin. ADH acts on the collecting duct of the nephron and regulates its permeability to water. In the absence of ADH, an average adult will produce about 10 to 12 L of dilute (specific gravity = 1.001; osmolality = 100 mOsm/kg) urine daily. In the presence of maximal vasopressin concentrations, urine flow can be reduced to less than 0.5 L/d of very concentrated (specific gravity = 1.035; osmolality = 1000 mOsm/kg) urine.[42]

Central diabetes insipidus may be caused by head trauma, neurosurgery, hypothalamic tumors, or infiltrative diseases. Half of all cases are idiopathic. Diabetes insipidus is transient when the supraoptic hypophyseal tract is damaged below the median eminence, and it is permanent when damage is above the median eminence. Only 10% of the neurosecretory neurons need to be present to prevent diabetes insipidus. It may be corrected by vasopressin replacement therapy.[74]

Nephrogenic diabetes insipidus is inherited as an autosomal dominant trait and is therefore predominantly found in males. It may be acquired in association with disorders causing a decrease in glomerular filtration rate (chronic renal disease, electrolyte disturbances, pharmacologic agents, sickle cell disease, or dietary abnormalities). Treatment of nephrogenic diabetes insipidus is directed toward the primary disorder and may involve the use of diuretics to produce a paradoxical antidiuretic effect to enhance fluid reabsorption.

Psychogenic polydipsia results in the same clinical picture as central and nephrogenic diabetes insipidus. This disorder is only dangerous when intake exceeds renal capacity to excrete water. Treatment is directed at control of fluid intake.

DIAGNOSTIC STUDIES

Dehydration test

Administration of vasopressin

Hypertonic saline infusion

Visual field testing

CT scan and x-ray films of sella turcica

TREATMENT PLAN

Chemotherapeutic

Pituitary hormones

Vasopressin (Aqueous Pitressin), 2-5 units two to four times daily, IM, subq, or IV; duration of drug: 2-8 h; used in acute settings or for initial emergency treatment; for close monitoring during transient episodes; too short acting for chronic use; used for differential diagnosis of diabetes mellitus

Vasopressin (Pitressin Tannate in oil), 5-10 units q2-4d IM or subq; duration of drug: 48-72 h; longer duration, preferred for chronic therapy; used for differential diagnosis of diabetes insipidus

Lypressin nasal solution (Diapid Nasal Spray; synthetic lysine), one or two sprays in one or both nostrils qid; onset: 1 h; duration of drug: 3-8 h; may be used alone or in conjunction with vasopressin tannate; if patient has nasal congestion, there will be decreased absorption of drug

Desmopressin (DDAVP; synthetic arginine, vasopressin), 5-40 μg/d in one to three divided doses; administer by nasal insufflation (high in nose, not inhaled into throat); onset: 1 h; duration of drug: 8-20 h; drug of choice for chronic treatment because of its long duration and infrequent side effects

ASSESSMENT: AREAS OF CONCERN

Thirst
Polydipsia
Unquenchable thirst
Preference for cold or iced water

Urinary function
Polyuria (output greater than 4 L/d)
Frequency
Nocturia
Low specific gravity (1.001 to 1.005)

Hydration status
Poor skin turgor
Dry skin
Weight loss

Bowel function
Constipation

NURSING DIAGNOSES and NURSING INTERVENTIONS

Nursing Diagnosis	Nursing Intervention
Fluid volume deficit, actual	Measure and record intake and output.
	Measure urine specific gravity.
	Check patient's weight every day at same time with same clothing.
	Assess degree of dehydration.

Patient Education

1. Teach patient how to measure and record intake and output.
2. Teach patient to weigh self daily in the morning in same clothes.
3. Teach importance of why and how to administer vasopressin; side or toxic effects to report to physician; and parameters for as-needed administration based on output volume and characteristics.
4. Teach patient how to check urine specific gravity.
5. Teach importance of wearing medical alert bracelet to identify the disorder.

EVALUATION

Patient Outcome	Data Indicating That Outcome is Reached
Hydration is adequate.	Intake approximates output.
	Specific gravity is 1.005 to 1.015.
	Weight is stable.
	Skin is warm and dry with good turgor (no signs of dehydration).

GALACTOSEMIA, HEREDITARY FRUCTOSE INTOLERANCE, AND GLYCOGEN STORAGE DISEASES

Galactosemia, hereditary fructose intolerance, and glycogen storage diseases are metabolic disorders of carbohydrate metabolism.

Galactosemia, hereditary fructose intolerance, and glycogen storage diseases are rare inborn errors of metabolism that usually first appear within the neonatal period or early childhood. Early and precise diagnosis of specific genetic metabolic defects is essential in providing a level of functioning for the patient and family.

PATHOPHYSIOLOGY

Galactosemia is a disorder of galactose metabolism and may be classified into two types of enzyme deficiencies. Classic galactosemia is the result of the missing enzyme galactose-1-phosphate uridyl transferase. Galactokinase-deficiency galactosemia is a mild and rare form of the disorder. This form of galactosemia is the result of the deficient enzyme galactokinase. In both forms of the disorder, glyconeogenesis is impaired, and a toxic build-up of galactose-1-phosphate and galactitol accumulates in the enzyme-deficient cells. Toxicity may lead to cell death and impaired organ energy metabolism in the kidney, liver, brain, intestinal mucosa, and eyes. Symptoms of hypoglycemia occur as blood glucose decreases. Infants affected with classic galactosemia appear normal at birth and present signs and symptoms of genetic metabolic defect shortly after the ingestion of milk or other lactose products.[18] Lenticular cataracts may be the clinical finding for those individuals with galactokinase-deficiency galactosemia. Cataracts develop only after a prolonged period of lactose ingestion. Consequently, the patient may not be diagnosed until later in life. Diagnosis of galactosemia can be assumed by clinical presentation, the presence of reducing substances in the urine, lesions in the lens nucleus, elevated liver enzymes, acinar formation in liver biopsy, and absence of galactose-1-phosphate uridyl transferase or deficiency of galactokinase in the red blood cells.[73]

Hereditary fructose intolerance is apparent when fructose-1-phosphate aldolase is deficient in the cells. A toxic

Table 8-8
Types of Glycogen Storage Diseases

Type	Disease Name	Defective or Deficient Enzyme	Organ Involvement	Prognosis
I	von Gierke's	Glucose-6-phosphate	Hepatorenal with kidney, liver, and intestine as primary sites	Guarded in infancy; variable in later life depending on severity of signs and symptoms
II	Pompe's	2-Acid glucosidase (acid maltase)	Generalized with blood cells, heart, liver, and muscle as primary sites	Poor: death within first 1-2 yr of life
III	Cori's (debrancher's)	Amylo-1,6-glucosidase (debrancher enzyme)	Generalized with blood cells, kidney, and liver as primary sites	Good: high probability for reaching adulthood
IV	Andersen's	2-1,4-Glucan: 2-1,4-glucan 6-glycosol transferase (brancher enzyme)	Generalized with liver and blood cells as primary sites	Poor: death usually within first 6-24 mo of life
V	McArdle's	Muscle phosphorylase	Musculoskeletal with blood cell involvement	Good: high probability for reaching adulthood
VI	Liver phosphorylase defect	Phosphorylase	Hepatorenal with blood cell, kidney, and liver as primary sites	Guarded in infancy, with probability for reaching adulthood
VII	Muscle phosphofructokinase defect	Phosphofructokinase	Musculoskeletal with blood cell involvement	Variable, depending on severity of signs and symptoms
VIII	Spencer-Peet	Fructose isomerase	Hepatorenal with liver as primary site	Guarded in infancy; probability for reaching adulthood
IX	Type IX	Phosphorylase kinase	Generalized with liver muscle and blood cells as primary sites	Variable, depending on severity of signs and symptoms
O	Lewis'	Glycogen synthase	Hepatorenal with blood cell, kidney, and liver as primary sites	Variable, depending on severity of signs and symptoms

buildup of fructose-1-phosphate occurs directly after fructose ingestion. Glyconeogenesis is impaired, and the liver is unable to replenish glucose supplies. The liver is unable to properly metabolize fructose after ingestion of foods containing fructose. Hepatomegaly occurs secondary to lipid accumulation. Nausea, vomiting, and diarrhea occur with rapid onset of hypoglycemia after fructose ingestion and the accumulation of fructose-1-phosphate. Following the ingestion of fructose, blood glucose drops and blood fructose rises. Elimination of fructose from the diet leads to a marked reversal of symptoms. Signs and symptoms of metabolic disorder usually appear in the neonate. Clinical manifestations may vary with age, and less severely affected individuals may not develop symptomatology until later in childhood or early adulthood. The evaluation of fructose ingestion and fructose-1-phosphate leads to the diagnosis for this inborn error of metabolism.

The glycogen storage diseases may be broken down into hepatorenal, musculoskeletal, and generalized symptomatology directly related to the accumulation and deposits of glycogen and fat in the affected individual. The corresponding enzyme deficiency is responsible for impeding glycogen metabolism and synthesis. Blood sugar and lactate levels as well as clinical manifestations may vary with each specific enzyme deficiency. Life-threatening hypoglycemia is present after a prolonged period of fasting. Diagnosis can be confirmed with altered molecular structure or concentration of glycogen in body tissue, and the absence of a specific enzyme (Table 8-8).

TREATMENT PLAN

Supportive
Dietary management

ASSESSMENT: AREAS OF CONCERN

Air
Respiratory difficulty

Circulation
Hemorrhagic manifestations

Hepatomegaly
Splenomegaly

Food and fluids
Chronic vomiting and diarrhea
Failure to thrive
Hypoglycemia
Food intolerances

Neurosensory concerns
Decreased visual fields
Decreased intellectual functioning
Delayed developmental milestones

Neuromuscular concerns
Progressive muscular atrophy, myopathy, hypotonia,
pain

Psychosocial concerns
Unresolved feelings related to growth retardation,
short stature, degenerating disease, progressive
signs and symptoms
Death during childhood in severe cases

Body image concerns
Enlarged abdomen
Short stature

Comfort and pain
Frequent headaches

Family coping
Prognosis
Management of chronic illness
Diagnosis of genetic defect

NURSING DIAGNOSES and NURSING INTERVENTIONS

Nursing Diagnosis	Nursing Intervention
Fluid volume deficit: actual/potential	Monitor intake and output. Assess skin turgor and other signs of dehydration. Offer small frequent feedings every 1 to 3 hours. Monitor urine specific gravity. Monitor patient for signs and symptoms of hypoglycemia. Encourage fluid and electrolyte replacement.
Tissue perfusion, alteration in: cardiopulmonary	Monitor patient for epistaxis, hematomas, and abdominal distention. Monitor vital signs. Encourage rehabilitation and physical therapy. Provide comfort measures.
Nutrition, alteration in: less than body requirements	Encourage calorie count daily. Offer foods and fluids allowed every 1 to 3 hours. Weigh daily at same time with same scale. Assess physical developmental stage. Assess intellectual functioning.
Self-concept, disturbance in: body image, self-esteem	Encourage verbalization concerning delayed maturation. Explore strengths in intellectual and physical functioning; reinforce use of these strengths. Discuss and urge practice of alternate methods of mental and physical functioning.
Coping, ineffective family	Encourage verbalization concerning guilt related to genetic defect. Reinforce positive actions toward care giving and providing maximal functioning of patient. Promote discussions about disappointment in patient's ability to achieve and function to expectations. Support throughout grieving process.

Patient Education

1. Teach dietary plan for achieving maximal growth and development possible.
2. Teach how to assess hydration and calorie utilization.
3. Teach early recognition of signs and symptoms of exacerbation and plan to follow.
4. Stress methods of care to permit maximal independent functioning.
5. Teach importance of support groups and psychologic assistance.

EVALUATION

Patient Outcome	Data Indicating That Outcome is Reached
Hydration is adequate.	Intake equals output. There are no signs of dehydration. Episodes of vomiting and diarrhea decrease.
Tissue perfusion is normal.	Heart rate is within normal limits. Peripheral pulses are present. Hemorrhagic tendencies are absent.
Nutrition is adequate.	Weight is in proportion to height and stature. Blood sugar level is within normal limits. The patient verbalizes understanding of dietary restrictions.
Self-concept improves.	The patient participates in age-related activities. The patient maintains relationships with peers. The patient capitalizes on strong areas of functioning.
Coping improves.	The family verbalizes plans for maximizing independent functioning of patient, needed alterations in life-style consistent with required medical plan, and realistic developmental expectations.

GROWTH HORMONE DEFICIENCY AND SHORT STATURE

Short stature is a sign of diminished growth that may have one or more causes, including growth hormone deficiency.

Pathophysiologic causes of short stature are varied and often difficult to differentiate. Individuals affected with short stature may appear physically small, with normal body and limb proportions, or they may have obviously disproportionate features of the trunk, limbs, and face.

Current therapy consists of the identification and correction of the underlying cause of short stature. Present research involves more precise determination of growth patterns and the biochemical mechanisms of growth regulation as well as new forms of treatment, primarily synthesized growth hormone, utilizing recombinant DNA techniques, and the use of gonadotropin-releasing hormone (GnRH) analogues to delay puberty and prolong the active growth period.

PATHOPHYSIOLOGY

Growth Hormone Deficiencies

Growth hormone deficiencies are classified by specific deficit in release, synthesis, or utilization of growth hormone or by inappropriate response to somatomedin, the intermediary of growth hormone.

Isolated growth hormone deficiency is the result of impaired release or production of growth hormone from the body. This deficiency may be familial in origin, as an autosomal recessive gene. In such cases, pituitary functioning is normal. Isolated growth hormone deficiency may also be nonfamilial in origin with abnormal pituitary or hypothalamic functioning. Individuals with pituitary deficits, suprapituitary disorders, and hypothalamic disorders may exhibit any or all of the following hormonal effects: appropriate response of leuteinizing hormone (LH) and follicle-stimulating hormone (FSH) to gonadotropin-releasing hormone (GnRH) stimulation; excess somatostatin; growth hormone–releasing factor (GRF) deficiency; and delayed response of thyroid-stimulating hormone (TSH) to thyrotropin-releasing hormone (TRH). Untreated isolated growth hormone deficiency may result in subnormal amounts or lack of growth hormone in the bloodstream.[20]

Individuals with inappropriate response to somatomedin closely parallel those with isolated growth hormone deficiencies. The major difference is the high serum level of growth hormone found in the bloodstream. This serum level is ineffective in promoting normal growth and development because of the inappropriate response or generation of somatomedin. Individuals with somatomedin generation disorders will not respond to human growth hormone therapy. They are unable to utilize exogenous or endogenous growth hormone to generate somatomedin and subsequent growth and development.

Pathophysiology related to short stature is complex, with multiple causative factors (Table 8-9). A great variety of environmental, physiologic, and psychologic components must be combined to result in a child's normal growth and development. When one component or part of one component is lacking, short stature may result.

One of the most common types of short stature is constitutional short stature. These children show no abnormal biologic or endocrine function related to their physical size and usually have parents who are also short in stature. Thus constitutional short stature is genetic in origin. These children are usually mildly affected and do not have the body disproportions and facial and skin characteristics commonly associated with other forms of short stature or growth hormone deficiency.[13]

Table 8-9

Possible Causes of Short Stature

Possible Cause	Example of Disease State or Disorder	Pathophysiology	Medical Plans and Treatment
Chronic Disease (hepatorenal, metabolic, or cardiopulmonary disease)	Congenital heart disease; chronic liver diseases	Adequate growth; varied pathophysiology; related to chronic disease	Optimal treatment of chronic illness
Growth Abnormalities			
Congenital or chromosomal defects	Down's syndrome; Turner's syndrome	Adequate growth hormone; possible decreased estrogen	None; supportive, experimental treatment: LHRH and estrogen therapy
Inborn errors of metabolism	Phenylketonuria (PKU); galactosemia; hereditary fructose intolerance; glycogen storage diseases	Nutrition deficiency; adequate growth hormone	Optimal dietary management of disease and nutrition
Skeletal malformations	Osteogenesis imperfecta; spondyloepiphyseal dysplasia	Adequate growth hormone; impaired nutrition and absorption	None
Hormonal Imbalances			
Inappropriate hormone secretion	Hypopituitarism; hypothyroidism	Decreased growth hormone	Exogenous growth hormone
Inappropriate hormone action	Precocious puberty; adrenal cortical hyperplasia	Adequate growth hormone; other hormones unbalanced	Correction of hormonal action with medication
Hormone deficiency	Growth hormone deficiency; thyroid deficiencies; dwarfisms	Decreased growth hormone, decreased TSH	Exogenous growth hormone; thyroid replacement
Glucocorticoid	Cushing's syndrome	Increased cortisol; varied response of growth hormone	Medication or surgery
Normal Endocrine Functioning	Constitutional short stature; familial growth hormone deficiency	Adequate or decreased growth hormone	No treatment; experimental: delay puberty or use estrogen therapy
Nutritional Defects			
Prenatal period or infancy	Intrauterine growth retardation; failure to thrive; dehydration	Adequate growth hormone	Adequate nutrition
Childhood or adult onset	Gastrointestinal malabsorption syndromes; malnutrition	Adequate growth hormone	Correction of nutritional deficit
Psychosocial Deficits	Maternal deprivation syndrome; psychosocial dwarfism; anorexia nervosa	Adequate growth hormone	Psychologic intervention
Unknown Etiology (miscellaneous)	Noonan's syndrome; Prader-Willi syndrome	Unknown	None

DIAGNOSTIC STUDIES

	Isolated Growth Hormone Deficiency	Somatomedin Generation Disorders	Lack of Responsiveness to Somatomedin
Arginine/insulin tolerance test	No release of serum growth hormone; prolonged hypoglycemia	Release of serum growth hormone	Prolonged hypoglycemia; release of serum growth hormone
Levadopa tolerance test	No release of serum growth hormone	Release of serum growth hormone	Release of serum growth hormone
Exogenous growth hormone	Increased somatomedin and growth	No increase in somatomedin; no growth	Increased somatomedin; no growth

TREATMENT PLAN

Chemotherapeutic

For isolated growth hormone deficiency or short stature only

Exogenous growth hormone: human growth hormone (Somatotropin), 0.1-2.0 IU by IM injection

ASSESSMENT: AREAS OF CONCERN

Adult
Psychosocial concerns
Delayed puberty
Small genitalia
Men tend to be thin
Women tend to be overweight

Pediatric
Mobility
Short stature
Decreased arm and leg span
Small hands and feet

Psychosocial concerns
Physical size may limit abilities and activities of daily living (ADL)
Poor acceptance by peers
Treated as a child of lesser chronologic age
Difficulty obtaining size- and age-appropriate necessities for ADL
No mental or IQ deficits related to impaired growth
Feelings of hopelessness and powerlessness

Altered physical appearance
Childlike face
Small mandible
Prominent forehead
Sparse hair
High-pitched voice
Increased skin elasticity

Growth
Below fifth percentile for height
Distance below fifth percentile as age increases
Growth rate and age-appropriate norm (for at least 6 months)

Nutrition
Adequate or inadequate intake of calories, protein, and minerals for age or size

NURSING DIAGNOSES and NURSING INTERVENTIONS

Nursing Diagnosis	Nursing Intervention
Self-concept, disturbance in: body image, self-esteem, role performance, personal identity	Discuss alternate methods of maintaining ADL. Relate to patient in an age-appropriate manner. Encourage age-appropriate behaviors and needs. Adapt environment to suit limitations. Encourage independence. Encourage reality-based goals.
Coping, ineffective individual	Encourage support groups and psychologic counseling. Encourage family involvement in care. Encourage visit by well-adjusted individual or family with same diagnosis. Provide for appropriate role model for patient and family.

Patient Education

1. Teach alternate methods of maintaining ADL.
2. Instruct regarding environmental adaptations.
3. Teach parenting skills to encourage independence and appropriate behaviors.
4. Instruct regarding age-appropriate expectations, activities, and experiences.

EVALUATION

Patient Outcome	Data Indicating That Outcome is Reached
The patient's self-esteem and coping mechanisms improve.	Patient and family participate in support groups and psychologic counseling.
	Patient demonstrates independent and appropriate ADL for chronologic age.
	Patient verbalizes appropriate goals for chronologic age and abilities.
	Patient meets developmental milestones within age-appropriate time.
	Patient and family verbalize resolution of feelings of guilt, sorrow, anger, powerlessness, and resentment.
Home management is successful.	Siblings are involved in patient care.
	Appropriate parenting skills are provided by family members.
	Patient and family demonstrate maximal level of independent functioning.
	Patient and family demonstrate successful environmental adaptations.
	Patient and family verbalize acceptance of limitations at highest possible level.

HYPERCORTISOLISM (CUSHING'S SYNDROME)

Hypercortisolism is the overproduction of cortisol, the primary glucocorticoid, from the adrenal cortex. The numerous clinical features present in glucocorticoid excess are referred to as Cushing's syndrome.[43]

Cushing's syndrome is rare; approximately 10 cases per million population occur per year. Sex predominance and age predominance depend on the specific etiology of the disorder. Generally, there is a higher ratio of females to males affected (3:1). Hypercortisolism from adrenocorticotropic hormone (ACTH) secreting tumors of ectopic origin occurs more often in males. Cushing's syndrome in children is very unusual.[43]

Scientific developments have been ongoing in the diagnosis of hypercortisolism, the search for pathologic causes, and treatment. Investigations are now under way to develop more accurate and more reliable methods to diagnose and identify the source of the hypercortisolism. Interventions such as petrosal sinus sampling for steroids and the corticotropin-releasing hormone (CRH) stimulation test are being instituted and tested in hopes of improving the accuracy of diagnosis.[25a,67a] Current research also includes the role of beta endorphins in the hypothalamic-pituitary-adrenal axis, cortisol production in association with endogenous depression, and the use of antiglucocorticoids as a new approach to treatment of hypercortisolism.[26a]

PATHOPHYSIOLOGY

In adrenocortical hyperfunctioning, hypercortisolism occurs in association with mineralocorticoid excess and hyperandrogenism.[43]

The etiology of hypercortisolism (Cushing's syndrome) falls into two major classifications: ACTH dependent and ACTH independent.

Pituitary hypersecretion of ACTH is called Cushing's disease and occurs in 70% of patients with Cushing's syndrome. Extrapituitary sources of ACTH secretion are referred to as ectopic ACTH syndromes (e.g., oat cell carcinoma of the lung). The amount of cortisol produced in these disorders depends on the amount of ACTH secreted. Elevated ACTH levels result in adrenal hyperstimulation and hyperplasia.[43]

Fig. 8-18
Forty-six–year–old woman diagnosed with Cushing's disease. Note classic cushingoid habitus with prominent supraclavicular fat pads and muscle wasting in extremities.

Courtesy National Institutes of Child Health, Bethesda, Md.

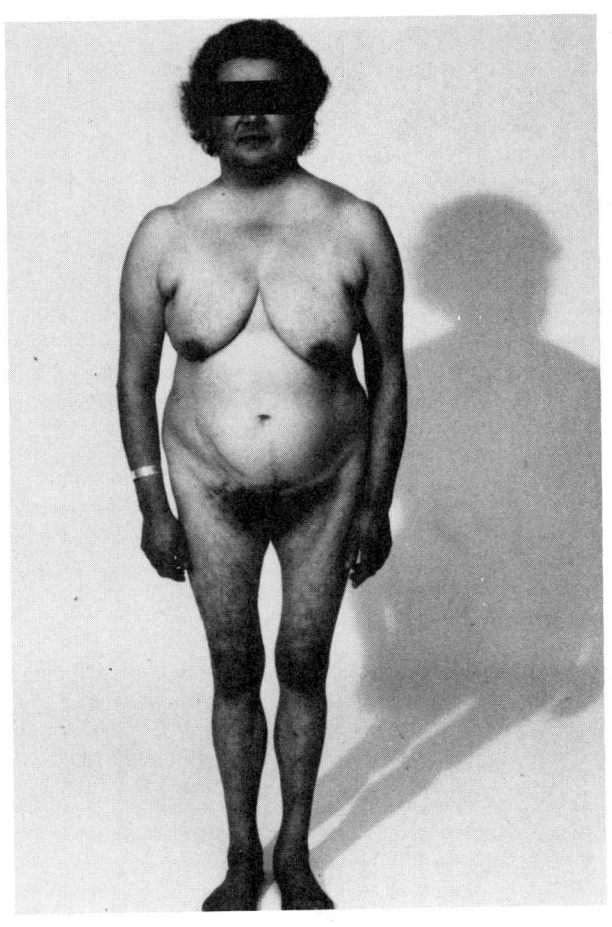

Adrenal adenomas (benign) and adrenal carcinomas (malignant) involve pathologic conditions in the gland itself. Normal tissue transforms into neoplastic tissue and produces cortisol independently of ACTH. Levels of ACTH are low, owing to the negative feedback within the axis.

Hypercortisolism can also be a result of other conditions such as chronic alcoholism, endogenous depression, and factitious use of corticosteroids.[43] Hypothalamic disease resulting in hypercortisolism has been postulated as a cause in some cases of Cushing's disease.

High levels of cortisol have profound effects on many tissue and organ systems. Cortisol possesses sodium-retaining properties, increasing extracellular fluid volume and causing mild to moderate hypertension.[20]

Carbohydrate metabolism is affected by the ability of cortisol to (1) increase glucose formation from circulating amino acids, (2) stimulate gluconeogenesis, and (3) render muscle and fat cells insulin resistant. The resulting state of hyperglycemia, glucose intolerance, and glycosuria has been labeled "steroid diabetes." The severity depends on the individual's own predisposition to diabetes.[20]

The mechanism for the fat deposition and distribution in hypercortisolism is yet unclear. It has been suggested that the increased secretion of insulin (resulting from the hyperglycemia) stimulates lipogenesis.[20] Some individuals with simple exogenous obesity present with fat distribution typical of Cushing's syndrome without classic biochemical findings.

Catabolic effects of cortisol cause muscle atrophy, especially in the extremities, and muscular weakness. A mild hypokalemia, present in hypercortisolism, contributes to debilitation (Fig. 8-18).

Atrophy of the epidermis and the inhibition of collagen formation are thought to be the result of excess cortisol. Increased susceptibility to infection is present, resulting in frequently observed fungal infections of the skin and nails. Hyperpigmentation is caused by the concomitant release of beta-lipotropic hormone (β-LPH) with ACTH from the pituitary or ectopic site. β-LPH has melanocyte-stimulating activity and results in darkening of the skin.[13a] Cortisol inhibits the protein matrix in bone; calcium is abnormally absorbed. Demineralization and hypercalciuria occur. Subsequent osteoporosis in hypercortisolism of long duration and renal calculi may develop.[20] Inhibition of growth hormone by cortisol, as well as cortisol's direct effect on growth cartilage, causes growth retardation and delayed skeletal development in children with this disorder. Psychiatric disturbances are recognized in some patients with hypercortisolism. Loss of the normal diurnal rhythm of cortisol release has been associated with insomnia.

Hyperandrogenism from adrenal hyperfunctioning in Cushing's syndrome causes menstrual irregularities (oligomenorrhea or amenorrhea). Mild to moderate hirsutism in females is seen depending on the amount of androgen secreted and the sensitivity of the hair follicle to androgen (Fig. 8-19).

DIAGNOSTIC STUDIES

Blood
Serum cortisol
Loss of diurnal rhythm
Elevated at night

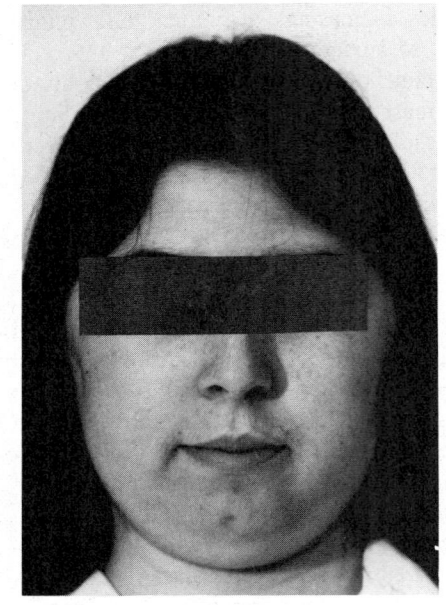

A

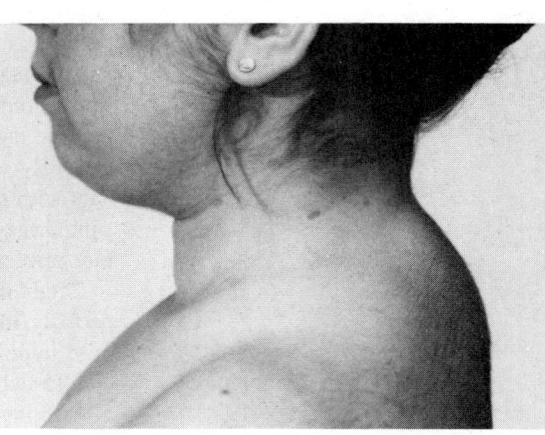

B

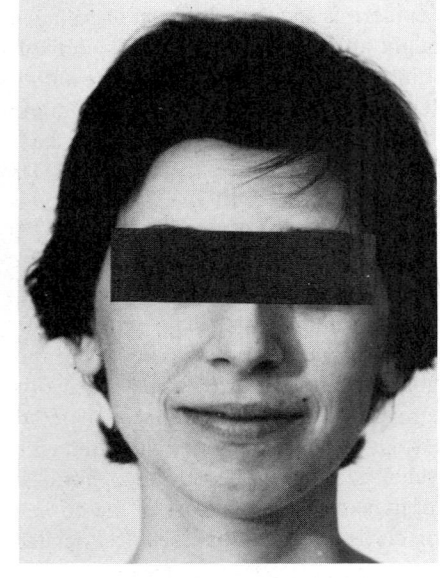

C

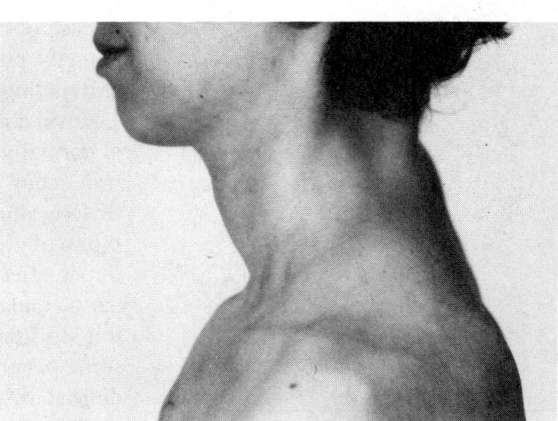

D

Fig. 8-19
Preoperative and postoperative appearance of 23-year-old woman with adrenal carcinoma. Note moon facies, buffalo hump, supraclavicular fat pads, and mild hirsutism. **A,** Preoperative adrenal carcinoma with moon facies and hirsutism. **B,** Preoperative adrenal carcinoma with buffalo hump. **C,** Postoperative adrenal carcinoma with loss of moon facies and hirsutism. **D,** Postoperative adrenal carcinoma with loss of buffalo hump.

Courtesy National Institutes of Child Health, Bethesda, Md.

Plasma ACTH
   Elevated (ectopic syndromes)
   Normal to slightly elevated (Cushing's disease)
   Low to immeasurable (adenoma or carcinoma)
   Loss of diurnal variation

Potassium
   Decreased concentration

Eosinophil
   Reduction in number

Urine
Urinary free cortisol (UFC): 24 hours
   Elevated; greater than 100g/24 h

Urinary 17-ketosteroids (17-KS): 24 hours
   Elevated (age dependent)

Urinary 17-hydroxysteroids (17-OH): 24 hours
   Elevated

Endocrine

Dexamethasone suppression test

Tests the state of negative feedback between the adrenal and the hypothalamic-pituitary unit; false positive readings may occur in depression, alcoholism, or patients receiving phenytoin and phenobarbital

Low dose (0.5 mg q6h for 2 d)

Normal response: suppression of ACTH; decreased production of urinary 17-OH

Cushing's disease: little or no effect

High dose (2.0 mg q6h)

Cushing's disease: urinary 17-OH less than 50% of baseline

Metyrapone test (750 mg q4h for six doses)

Tests hypothalamic-pituitary feedback response; altered response when patient has thyroid abnormalities or is taking estrogen or phenytoin

Normal response: increased ACTH and 11-deoxycortisol

Adrenal adenoma: no rise in ACTH or 11-deoxycortisol

Radiologic tests

Chest tomograms

CT scan of sella

Sellar x-ray film

CT scan of adrenal glands

Electromechanical

Pituitary irradiation (p. 928)

ASSESSMENT: AREAS OF CONCERN

Circulation

Mild to moderate hypertension

Nutrition

Moderate weight gain

Fat distribution: truncal obesity, supraclavicular fat pads, buffalo hump, moon facies

Hyperglycemia

Increased appetite

Elimination

Glycosuria

Proteinuria

Hypercalciuria

Neurologic concerns

Impaired memory

Impaired concentration

Musculoskeletal concerns

Fatigue

Muscle weakness

Inability to rise from squat position

Muscle wasting in extremities

Growth retardation (pediatrics)

Pain and discomfort

Back pain

Rib pain

Skin

Blood vessel fragility: plethora and easy bruisability

Thin, translucent skin

Hyperpigmentation

Poor wound healing

Psychosocial concerns

Irritability

Altered body image

TREATMENT PLAN

Surgical

Adrenalectomy

Hypophysectomy (p. 935)

Chemotherapeutic

Antineoplastic agents: mitotane (Lysodren), 8-10 g/d in divided doses; aminoglutethimide (Cytadren), 250 mg q6h; increase slowly to maximal daily dose of 2 g

NURSING DIAGNOSES and NURSING INTERVENTIONS

Nursing Diagnosis	Nursing Intervention
Nutrition, alteration in: less than body requirements	Observe compliance to prescribed caloric, high-protein diet. Record urine chemistry daily (i.e., sugar, acetone, and protein). Administer insulin as prescribed.
Activity intolerance	Plan activity and rest periods with patient daily. Discuss limitations with patient.

Nursing Diagnosis	Nursing Intervention

Skin integrity, impairment of: actual	Instruct patient concerning good skin hygiene:
	  Wash and dry thoroughly.
	  Use lotions as needed.
	  Use antifungal cream as needed.
	  Perform aseptic care to minor lacerations and abrasions.
	Provide adequate pressure to venipuncture sites.
	Instruct patient to avoid minor bumps and trauma.
	Keep patient's room clear of obstructions (excess furniture, etc.).

Coping, ineffective individual	Discuss with patient emotional factors related to disorder:
	  Give emotional support.
	  Identify sources of irritability and depression.
	  Assist patient with problem solving.
	  Collaborate with mental health nursing specialist or psychiatrist.

Self-concept, disturbance in: body image	Discuss with patient cushingoid features of the disorder; give emotional support. Discuss palliative treatment for hirsutism (i.e., shaving or depilatories).

Patient Education

1. Teach importance of and how to administer chemotherapeutic medication and side or toxic effects to report.
2. Stress importance of regular, lifelong medical follow-up.
3. Teach importance of wearing or carrying medical alert information.

EVALUATION

Patient Outcome	Data Indicating That Outcome is Reached
Nutrition is adequate.	Weight is proportionate to height and stature. Urine chemistry levels are within normal limits. Blood sugar is within normal limits. The patient verbalizes use of appropriate dietary regimen.
Activity tolerance increases.	The patient maintains maximal activity levels for physical limitations. The patient verbalizes realistic plan for alternating activities and rest based on limitations. The patient participates in recreational activities.
Skin is intact.	There are no breaks, cracks, ulcers, or ecchymosis. There is no infection. Wound healing is normal. The patient verbalizes a method for maintaining hygiene.
The patient copes effectively.	The patient verbalizes one or more sources of stress and a plan to prevent or decrease stress. The patient seeks assistance with coping when appropriate. The patient functions to maximal level of independence based on limitations.
The patient's self-concept improves.	The patient utilizes realistic self-care methods to enhance physical features. The patient is not preoccupied with negative aspects of physical appearance. The patient participates in age-related activities and groups. The patient maintains peer relationships. The patient expresses realistic expectations concerning physical abilities and appearance.

HYPERINSULINISM

Hyperinsulinism is a condition of excess serum insulin, which causes a reduction in blood sugar, producing symptoms of hypoglycemia.

One classification of hyperinsulinism is based on insulin levels in the (1) fasting, (2) postprandial, or (3) induced hypoglycemic state. Some of the most frequent causes of hyperinsulinism are outlined as follows:

Fasting
    Insulin-producing islet cell tumor
    Extrapancreatic neoplasm
    Nesidioblastosis
    Infants of diabetic mothers
    Leucine-induced
Postprandial
    Reactive hypoglycemia
    Early diabetes mellitus
    Rapid gastric emptying
Induced
    Exogenous insulin
    Miscellaneous drugs

The true prevalence of each entity is uncertain. However, insulin-producing islet cell tumors (arising from beta-cell tumors or insulinomas) are the most frequently occurring of the islet cell tumors, with 80% showing excessive insulin secretion with measurable hypoglycemia.[9] These tumors vary in size with no relationship between the size of the tumor and severity of symptoms.[9] Ninety percent of insulinomas are benign, and 90% occur in individuals over age 30.[25] Beta-cell tumors can be present with other endocrine abnormalities, such as in the MEN I (multiple endocrine neoplasias, type 1) syndrome associated with adenomas of the pituitary and parathyroid tissue and the occurrence of Zollinger-Ellison syndrome.

Induced hypoglycemia is a condition brought about by various agents, most commonly by insulin use in the insulin-dependent diabetic and alcohol abuse in the adult population.[31] The following discussion will be limited to hypoglycemia associated with hyperinsulinism.

Insulin abuse in the nondiabetic patient was first described in 1947, but it was not until the 1970s that C-peptide was recognized to be a marker of endogenous insulin production,[24] useful in determining whether the hyperinsulinemia was endogenous or exogenous in source. The possibility of self-injection of insulin in the nondiabetic patient, or surreptitious insulin use, should be considered in all cases of fasting hypoglycemia, particularly in health professionals and persons acquainted with or having contact with diabetes.[31] These persons often display no psychologic disorder and are very ingenious in concealing their use of insulin. Sulfonylurea abuse has also been reported as a cause of factitious hypoglycemia, and together with surreptitious insulin abuse, factitious hypoglycemia may occur as frequently as insulinoma.[24]

PATHOPHYSIOLOGY

Normally, varying concentrations of insulin are responsible for maintaining blood sugar in the normal range. In hyperinsulinemia, excess serum insulin disrupts this balance by increasing glucose use and inhibiting hepatic glycogenolysis, which results in a decreasing serum glucose level. The early subjective feelings associated with low blood sugar are associated with inhibition of glucose receptors in the ventromedial hypothalamic nucleus, which in turn stimulate the sympathetic fibers of the autonomic nervous system and epinephrine release in an attempt to restore blood glucose levels to normal. This adrenergic response is most noticeable when the blood sugar fall is rapid. A fall in blood sugar actually results in an increase in secretion of all four counterregulatory hormones (growth hormone, glucagon, cortisol, and catecholamines) although it appears that the catecholamines exert the major influence.[31]

The brain is most sensitive to disruption in normal blood sugar since brain cells cannot utilize free fatty acids as an energy source. With a continued decline in blood sugar, brain cells are deprived of glucose, with decreased cerebral oxygen consumption.[31] The neuroglycopenic symptoms predominate when blood sugar decline is gradual. They are more severe and occur at a higher blood sugar level in the elderly than in the young.[24] It has been suggested that some irreversible brain damage, including decrease in intellectual function, impaired nerve function, and personality changes, may occur as the result of frequent or prolonged hypoglycemia.[24]

Insulin-secreting pancreatic tumors as well as nesidioblastosis (in which exocrine cells are transformed to endocrine cells) produce absolute elevations of plasma insulin levels in the fasting state. Insulin levels are not responsive to changes in blood glucose levels, and the hypoglycemia results from elevated glucose uptake by insulin-dependent tissues and inhibition of glycogenolysis and gluconeogenesis mechanisms. Exercise intensifies hypoglycemic symptoms caused by increased use of glucose by muscle cells. Seventy-five to ninety percent of patients with insulinoma will develop symptoms of hypoglycemia during the first 24 hours of a fast.[67]

Immediately after birth, the neonate must produce the energy needed to maintain life and vital functions. The main source of energy supply in these early days of life is carbohydrates, mainly from glycogen stores in the liver. Therefore any interruption in the normal mechanism for glucose regulation (liver glycogen stores, glucagon, insulin, etc.) results in neonatal hypoglycemia. Infants at risk include (1) the premature infant with inadequate liver glycogen stores, (2) the small-for-gestational-age infant who has depleted liver glycogen stores in utero, (3) the infant with erythroblastosis fetalis and resultant hyperinsulinemia caused by glutathione destruction of insulin, and (4) the infant of the diabetic mother with beta-cell hyperplasia and hyperinsulinemia induced by maternal hyperglycemia.

The mean blood glucose value during the first 72 hours of life is about 30 mg/dl for the full-term infant and above 20 mg/dl for the premature infant. Any blood glucose value below these values indicates neonatal hypoglycemia. Certain infants will also develop hypoglycemia in response to the leucine in cow's milk, which stimulates excessive insulin secretion. Hypertrophy of the islet cells is present. Postprandial hypoglycemia and fasting hypoglycemia are present in about 75% of these cases, with onset of symptoms occurring before 6 months of age.[24]

In the patient with reactive hypoglycemia, adrenergic symptoms of hypoglycemia are usual, with neuroglycopenic symptoms only rarely occurring, because of the abrupt decline of blood sugar levels and shorter duration of symptoms.[25] These patients have no symptoms of hypoglycemia when fasting but experience hypoglycemic symptoms most commonly after a breakfast or lunch containing large amounts of carbohydrates.[31]

A similar pattern of postprandial hypoglycemia is seen in individuals with mildly impaired glucose tolerance or early non-insulin-dependent diabetes mellitus and obesity where the early rise in blood glucose related to inadequate insulin release is followed by a delayed but excessive insulin response resulting in a sudden drop of blood sugar and adrenergic symptoms of low blood sugar.

Rapid gastric emptying of carbohydrates into the small intestine following gastrectomy, gastrojejunostomy, or vagotomy with pyloroplasty or with hyperthyroidism causes an early hyperglycemia that stimulates excessive insulin secretion resulting in alimentary hypoglycemia. Other gastric factors, such as secretin, enteroglucagon, and gastric inhibitory peptide, may also influence insulin secretion, perhaps even earlier than hyperglycemia.[24] Adrenergic symptoms usually predominate and may be severe, occurring 1½ to 3 hours postprandially.

DIAGNOSTIC STUDIES

Islet cell tumor
  Blood sugar
    Low fasting level

Insulin
  Elevated fasting insulin level

Plasma proinsulin and C-peptide
  Elevated levels

Angiography
  Localization of islet cell tumor

72-Hour fast

Nesidioblastosis
  Blood sugar
    Low fasting level

  Insulin
    Elevated fasting level

  Plasma proinsulin and C-peptide
    Elevated levels

Leucine-induced hypoglycemia
  Blood sugar
    Low fasting and postprandial levels

  Insulin
    Elevated fasting and postprandial levels

  Leucine tolerance test
    Positive for hypoglycemia

Reactive hypoglycemia
  Blood sugar
    Low level 1½ to 5 hours after glucose tolerance test load

Alimentary hypoglycemia
  Upper gastrointestinal series
    Rapid gastric emptying

  Blood sugar
    Low postprandial values

Glucose intolerance
  Tolbutamide test
    Blood sugar values of more than 78% fasting value at 20 minutes

  Insulin tolerance test
    Blood sugar drop of less than 50%

  Plasma proinsulin and C-peptide
    Normal to elevated levels

  Oral glucose tolerance test
    Elevated blood sugar 1½ to 5 hours after glucose load

Exogenous insulin use
  Plasma proinsulin and C-peptide
    Low levels

  Plasma insulin antibodies
    Present

Sulfonylurea use

Plasma proinsulin and C-peptide

Normal to high levels

Plasma or urine screen for sulfonylureas

Positive

Extrapancreatic neoplasm

Blood sugar

Normal to low fasting levels

Insulin

Normal to high fasting levels

Plasma level high

TREATMENT PLAN

Surgical

Subtotal pancreatectomy

Beta-cell pancreatectomy

Nesidioblastosis

Chemotherapeutic

Diazoxide (Hyperstat) for insulinoma and nesidioblastosis: 200 mg tid first day, then 100 mg tid adult
maintenance dose; maintenance dose in children, 12
mg/kg

Antineoplastic agents: streptozocin (Zanosar) for malignant islet cell tumor (see Chapter 14)

Supportive

Diet

ASSESSMENT: AREAS OF CONCERN

Area of Concern	Adult	Child
Circulation	Tachycardia Elevated blood pressure	Cyanosis

Food and fluid	Relief of symp-
	  toms with food
	  intake
	Hunger
	Weight loss
	Weight gain	

Neurosensory concerns	Tremor
	Headache
	Mental dullness
	Confusion
	Amnesia
	Seizures
	Unconsciousness
	Paralysis
	Paresthesias
	Dizziness
	Irritability
	Visual disturbance
		Sluggishness
		Hypotonia
		Intermittent
		  twitching
		Episodic staring
		Frequent yawning
		Remoteness
		Paresthesias
		Visual disturbance
		Loss of concentra-
		  tion

Psychosocial	Change in role
	  performance
	Resents enforced
	  dependency
	Unable to stay
	  alone; related to
	  episodes of loss
	  of conscious-
	  ness
	Past history of
	  destructive be-
	  havior	

NURSING DIAGNOSES and NURSING INTERVENTIONS

Nursing Diagnosis	Nursing Intervention
Nutrition, alteration in: less/more than body requirements	Check blood pressure, pulse, and respiration with occurrence of symptoms. Assess patient for symptoms of low blood sugar and check blood glucose by finger stick using strip or meter determination: fasting, before and 2 hours after meals, at bedtime, and at 3 to 5 AM. Provide patient with 3 AM snack if needed. Arrange a dietary consultation. Assess symptomatology that patient normally experiences with hypoglycemia and whether or not patient is awakened by symptoms at night.
Coping, ineffective individual	Remove potentially dangerous articles from patient's room (factitious use). Encourage maximal independence. Assist individual to communicate with others. Discuss need for restrictions and precautions related to potential loss of consciousness. Give information about disease to enhance feeling of control. See also p. 1897.
Sleep pattern disturbance	Discuss importance of feeding during night if indicated to prevent early morning hypoglycemia. Suggest naps or early bedtime to allow for increased quantity of sleep. Minimize other disturbances during sleeping time.

Patient Education

1. Teach signs and symptoms for early recognition and treatment of hypoglycemia.
2. Teach 24-hour diet plan and importance of adherence.

EVALUATION

Patient Outcome	Data Indicating That Outcome is Reached
Hypoglycemia can be recognized and promptly managed.	There is no loss of consciousness or seizures. The patient verbalizes understanding of diet and signs, symptoms, and treatment of hypoglycemia.
Nutrition is adequate.	The patient complies with dietary prescription including restrictions and snacks. Blood sugar is within normal limits. Weight is in proportion to body height and stature.
The patient copes effectively.	Anxiety is decreased. The family verbalizes adapting to changes imposed by hypoglycemia. The patient accepts support from health professionals. The patient establishes and follows plan to minimize symptoms and maximize functioning. Maximal independence is maintained. There is no self-destructive behavior. The patient complies with precautions and restrictions imposed.
Sleep patterns improve.	The patient verbalizes feeling rested. Total quantity of sleep is increased. Interruptions during sleep are minimized.

HYPERPARATHYROIDISM

Hyperparathyroidism is the hyperactivity of one or more of the parathyroid glands as a result of one of a number of primary or secondary causes.

Hyperparathyroidism is manifested by hypercalcemia. The disease occurs in adults between the ages of 30 and 70. Women present with the disease more frequently than do men (2:1 ratio). Patients with hypercalcemia have chronic elevations in serum calcium levels (above 5.3 mEq/L).

Technical advances and research have created a greater awareness of parathyroid disorders. Symptoms are recognized earlier, and the means for making diagnoses have become more sophisticated in the past decade. New treatments for parathyroid disorders are being used with greater success rates, and diagnostic workups are being made with accuracy as a result of these advancements. Continued research and a strong focus on education of the health care team will ensure early detection and treatment as well as prevention of complications manifested by these disorders.

PATHOPHYSIOLOGY

More than 80% of the patients with primary hyperparathyroidism have a single parathyroid adenoma (a neoplasm of the gland, which may be 2 to 200 times the size of a normal gland). The adenoma is an encapsulated tumor made of chief cells. Primary clear cell hyperplasia is a rare disorder in which all four glands become enlarged 30 to 100 times their normal size. Primary chief cell hyperplasia is more common than clear cell hyperplasia, but it is difficult to differentiate from an adenoma. Chief cell hyperplasia also occurs in patients with multiple endocrine neoplasias, types I and II.[44]

Parathyroid carcinoma occurs rarely. Its progress is more rapid and severe than most hyperparathyroid disorders. Surgical excision and radiation are usually ineffective in its treatment.

The etiology of primary hyperparathyroidism is unclear. It is felt that radiation to the neck might be a possible cause. Secondary hyperplasia may develop as a result of conditions causing a decrease in serum calcium levels, such as chronic renal disease, vitamin D deficiency, pregnancy, rickets, pyelonephritis or glomerulonephritis, hyperphosphatemia, and calcium deprivation.

Clinical manifestations of hyperparathyroidism are based on the effects of increased parathyroid hormone on the target areas: bone, kidney, and gastrointestinal tract. Increased serum calcium levels cause a decrease in parathyroid hormone secretion, resulting in the stimulation of osteoblasts to increase bone resorption. Cysts and fibrous tissue invade bones, causing pain and pathologic fractures. Calcifications form in renal tubules, causing obstructions that inhibit the concentration of urine. Renal colic, dull back pain, and hematuria are symptoms resulting from the formation of calculi.[20]

Other manifestations of increased serum calcium levels include decreased neuromuscular excitability caused by the polarization of cell membranes by high calcium levels and decreased motility of the gastrointestinal tract. Cardiac changes that occur as a result of hypercalcemia include decreased neuronal permeability, defects in conduction, and an increased threshold for stimulation.

DIAGNOSTIC STUDIES

Serum calcium levels
Greater than 5.3 mEq/L in adults; greater than 6.0 mEq/L in children

Serum PO$_4$
Less than 1.8 mEq/L

Urinary calcium levels
Less than 25 mEq/L

Urinary PO$_4$
Greater than 0.6 mEq/L

Creatinine clearance
Decreased

Hydroxyproline
Increased

Urinary cAMP
Increased

TREATMENT PLAN

Surgical
Parathyroidectomy

Chemotherapeutic
Diuretic agents: furosemide (Lasix), 20-80 mg q1-8h, IV or po
Volume expansion up to 3000 ml/d, IV or po
Phosphates, 1-3 g/d, IV or po
Parathyroid hormone agents: calcitonin (Calcimar), 4-8 μg/kg of body weight, IM or subq

ASSESSMENT: AREAS OF CONCERN

Renal concerns
Polyuria
Nephrolithiasis
Nephrosclerosis
Urinary tract infection

Gastrointestinal concerns
Anorexia
Nausea
Vomiting
Weight loss
Constipation

Cardiovascular concerns
Bradycardia
Cardiac irregularities (shortened Q-T interval)

Skeletal concerns
Enlarged skull
Demineralization
Skeletal pain
Pathologic fractures

Central nervous system
Personality disturbances
Disorientation
Paranoia

Disturbed consciousness
Lethargy
Drowsiness
Stupor
Coma

Decreased neuromuscular excitability
Muscle weakness
Hypotonia
Uncoordination

NURSING DIAGNOSES and NURSING INTERVENTIONS

Nursing Diagnosis	Nursing Intervention
Cardiac output, alteration in: decreased	Check vital signs every 4 hours; check pulse for bradycardia. Check ECG strip every 4 hours (flattened or inverted T wave, P wave changes, and Q-T interval changes). Monitor stools, urine, sputum, and emesis for blood. Monitor for petechiae and bruising.
Potential patient problem: alteration in electrolyte balance	Monitor for dehydration. Weigh daily. Record intake and output. Check skin turgor. Encourage fluids to 3000 ml per day. Administer medications to reduce calcium.
Activity intolerance	Observe patient for signs of pain with movement. Observe for steadiness on ambulation. Assist the patient with ambulation when necessary. Splint ribs while the patient turns, coughs, and so on, when fractures are apparent. Handle the patient gently; allow him to move slowly.
Comfort, alteration in: pain	Observe for indications of pain with movement. Avoid extreme temperature changes. Obtain physical therapy consultation. Administer warm packs or soaks to painful areas. Administer pain medications on a schedule rather than as needed. Emphasize good body alignment and posture.
Coping, ineffective individual	Maintain a calm approach if the patient becomes agitated or irritable. Observe for precipitating factors causing stress. See also p. 1897.

Patient Education

1. Teach how to monitor and maintain adequate fluid intake.
2. Teach method for checking urine for stones and hematuria.
3. Stress importance of proper body alignment and mechanics and need for increasing activity to tolerance.
4. Teach how to check pulse and changes to report.
5. Assist patient to develop plan for using alternate pain-relieving methods rather than relying on pain medication.
6. Teach signs and symptoms for early recognition and treatment of hypocalcemia.
7. Ensure that patient understands importance of changing home environment to prevent accidents.

EVALUATION

Patient Outcome	Data Indicating That Outcome is Reached
Cardiac output is adequate.	ECG strip is normal. Vital signs are stable.
Fluid and electrolyte balance is maintained, and calcium levels are normal.	Sodium level is 137 to 145 mEq/L. Potassium level is 3.3 to 4.6 mEq/L. Chloride level is 100 to 110 mEq/L. Calcium level is 4.3 to 5.3 mEq/L. Phosphorus level is 1.8 to 2.6 mEq/L. Intake approximates output. Specific gravity is normal.
Comfort and activity level are increased.	Optimal level of mobility is maintained with little or no pain experienced. The patient follows plan for using alternate pain-relieving methods.

Patient Outcome	Data Indicating That Outcome is Reached
	The patient uses pain medications infrequently.
	The patient verbalizes increased feelings of well-being.
	The patient participates in desired activities.
The patient copes effectively.	The patient expresses feelings and uses effective coping mechanisms for problems surrounding illness.
	The patient is able to identify factors leading to increased stress and possible solutions to prevent these situations.
	Affect is appropriate to the situation.

HYPERPITUITARISM

Hyperpituitarism is the overproduction of one or more anterior pituitary hormones. The most common cause is a pituitary tumor, but other causes, such as hypothalamic lesions or starvation, have been implicated.[20]

Current knowledge regarding hyperpituitarism has been expanded by many recent innovations, including (1) the development of bioassays to measure directly an increasing number of different hormones; (2) the use of sensitive radiologic techniques, especially CT scans, for earlier diagnosis; (3) the use of microsurgical techniques for pituitary surgery; and (4) the ability to synthesize an increasing number of hypothalamic hormones, which is important for diagnosis. Current research includes attempts at exact localization of the tumor (hypothalamic, pituitary, target organ, or ectopic source) and increasing the understanding of the complex rhythmicity of the hypothalamic-pituitary system.

Epidemiologically, pituitary tumors are far more common than is suggested clinically; one study involving autopsies reported an incidence in the general population of 22%,[25] the majority of which were asymptomatic. Among symptomatic patients, men and women are generally equally affected with pituitary tumors.[25] The most common age of the affected person is 35 to 40 years, although this may be decreasing as diagnostic techniques improve.[25] The disease is rare in children under 9 years of age.[20] Pituitary tumors make up 7% of all intracranial tumors.[25] Onset of the disease is often slow and insidious[25] and can be difficult to diagnose, especially in the early phase. A genetic component has been postulated because hyperpituitarism has been seen in more than one member of a single family, but this point remains controversial.

PATHOPHYSIOLOGY

There is no known etiology of pituitary tumors.[20] These tumors are classified by identifying either the staining properties of the tumor or the hormone secreted in excess.

There are four types of tumor according to the former method: (1) basophilic—those that typically secrete adrenocorticotropic hormone (ACTH); (2) eosinophilic—those that usually secrete growth hormone (GH); (3) chromophobic—those formerly thought to be nonfunctioning but now believed to secrete prolactin[25]; and (4) combinations of the other three types. This classification system is subject to controversy because of the variability of staining techniques.[74] It is being replaced by the second classification system, which uses terminology to indicate the hormone that is hypersecreted. With this classification, prolactinomas are most common, followed by GH-secreting tumors, ACTH-secreting tumors, and finally the more rare thyroid-stimulating hormone (TSH) and luteinizing hormone (LH), follicle-stimulating hormone (FSH) secreting adenomas.[72]

Two separate yet related disease entities deserve mention in a discussion of pituitary tumors. The first, Nelson syndrome, is a rare disorder that occurs after bilateral adrenalectomy is used to treat Cushing's disease. It is characterized by hyperpigmentation, caused by excessive production of ACTH and melanocyte-stimulating hormone (MSH) by a pituitary tumor. It is believed that this tumor is the original cause of the Cushing's disease and that it enlarges after adrenalectomy because of the lack of negative feedback. Therefore there is an increase in the production of ACTH and concurrently, MSH. The second disease entity is a type of tumor that occurs in the region of the pituitary but does not secrete hormones.[20] This tumor is called a craniopharyngioma; it is important in the differential diagnosis of any sellar tumor.

The extent of the pathophysiology caused by pituitary tumors is based on two factors: the size of the tumor and the hormone secreted in excess. In terms of the size, the tumors are classified as either microadenomas (diameter less than 10 mm) or macroadenomas (diameter more than 10 mm).[73] The larger tumors cause problems simply by their size; they impinge on the surrounding tissue, including normal pituitary tissue, which can cause varying degrees of hypopituitarism.[73] Other structures that may be affected by a large tumor include the bony sella turcica, which can be enlarged; the optic chiasm, which may be compressed, causing visual field defects; and the hypothalamus, which also may be compressed. The second factor that determines the extent of the pathophysiology is the hormone secreted in excess; the physical manifestations vary greatly (discussed in detail in "Assessment: Areas of Concern").

DIAGNOSTIC STUDIES

Radiologic studies and skull x-ray films, sellar tomograms, head and sellar CT scans
Enlargement of the bony sella
Visualization of the adenoma within the sella or with suprasellar extension

Angiogram
Used to rule out a possible aneurysm

Ophthalmologic examination
Visual field deficits; decreased acuity

Endocrine function testing
Inappropriate baseline hormone levels in blood or urine; inability to suppress or stimulate normal release of pituitary hormones (p. 844)

Neurologic examination
Cranial nerve deficits; unequal pupil size, inappropriate reaction to light

TREATMENT PLAN

Surgical (p. 935)
Removal of the pituitary tumor (intercranial or transsphenoidal approach)
Removal of the target organ (adrenal glands, thyroid; see target organ for discussion)

Chemotherapeutic
Dopamine receptor antagonist: bromocriptine mesylate (Parlodel), used to treat prolactinomas and GH-secreting tumors; usual dosage is 2.5-10 mg/d for prolactinomas; GH-secreting tumors typically require much higher doses, the upper limit being that of patient tolerance

Electromechanical (p. 928)
Radiation therapy

ASSESSMENT: AREAS OF CONCERN[72]

Macroadenomas
Sensory and vision concerns
Bitemporal hemianopsia
Decreased acuity
Blurred vision

Neurologic concerns
Chronic headaches, usually intermittent, of moderate intensity, and variably located; may be associated with nausea and vomiting
Possible neurologic changes, particularly those involving the third cranial nerve (unequal pupil size, inappropriate reaction to light)

Endocrine concerns
Signs and symptoms of hypofunction (in regard to hormones other than those produced by the tumor)

Growth hormone–secreting tumors
Musculoskeletal concerns
Coarse facial features (thick ears, nose)
Prognathism causing chewing difficulties
Thick fingers and toes with concomitant increase in shoe or glove size
Atrophied skeletal muscle
Laryngeal hypertrophy causing voice to deepen
Arthritis, arthralgia, backaches
Osteoporosis
Mobility difficulties related to pain, fatigue

Prepubertal concerns
Rapid increase in height, making patient considerably taller than classmates

Hygiene and skin
Oily skin
Acne
Diaphoresis

Metabolic concerns
Glucose intolerance

Psychosocial concerns
Irritability, hostility, and other psychologic manifestations
Anxiety over "being different" from others
Difficulty with social interactions, including sexual partner and family (acting fearful, hostile, withdrawn)
Incongruity between self-concept and current self-image

Prolactin-secreting tumors
Gynecologic concerns
Galactorrhea involving one or both breasts
Irregular menses
Oligomenorrhea or amenorrhea
Infertility

Androgenic concerns
Decreased libido
Impotence
Gynecomastia

Psychosocial concerns
Anxiety about fertility, sexual performance, and self-image

Melanocyte-stimulating hormone–secreting tumors
Skin
Hyperpigmentation, especially noticeable in skin folds, mucous membranes, and new scars

Past history
Cushing's disease treated with bilateral adrenalectomy

NURSING DIAGNOSES and NURSING INTERVENTIONS

Nursing Diagnosis	Nursing Intervention
Comfort, alteration in: pain	Plan pain control program with patient (following in-depth assessment of type, location, intensity, and frequency of pain and successful or unsuccessful relief measures). Include use and schedule of medications and other physical comfort measures (e.g., heat, cold, light massage).
	Discuss factors that precipitate pain and ways of structuring the environment to decrease or eliminate these factors.
	Instruct patient regarding relaxation techniques (deep breathing, selective focusing).
	Discuss realistic expectations about pain control.
Self-concept, disturbance in: body image	See p. 1820.
Coping, ineffective individual	Discuss with patient and family the relationship of psychologic manifestations to the disease process.
	Encourage family not to "blame" patient for inappropriate behavior.
	See also p. 1897.
Sexual dysfunction	Establish trusting relationship with patient and sexual partner.
	Encourage the patient to verbalize feelings, both with the health care provider and the sexual partner.
	Instruct patient and sexual partner regarding the relationship between the disease process and the sexual dysfunction.
	Provide patient and sexual partner with information about various methods to obtain sexual gratification.
Activity intolerance	Thoroughly evaluate patient's abilities and limitations, both at home and in the community.
	Discuss with patient alternate ways of performing limited activities.
	Help patient structure time to allow for rest periods throughout the day, especially after activities.
	Encourage patient to participate in care to maximal ability.

Patient Education

1. Instruct patient regarding methods for modifying pain control program for use at home (e.g., structuring a supportive physical environment and appropriate self-administration of analgesics).
2. Inform patient about community mental health resources (support groups, individual therapists, etc.).
3. Instruct patient regarding methods for modifying activity program for use at home.
4. Teach and encourage continued performance of range-of-motion exercises at home.

EVALUATION

Patient Outcome	Data Indicating That Outcome is Reached
Comfort is increased.	The patient verbalizes a decreased frequency and amount of pain. The patient verbalizes pain-precipitating factors and means of decreasing or eliminating these factors. The patient demonstrates relaxation techniques. The patient follows a pain control program.
Self-concept improves.	The patient verbalizes acceptance of body changes. The patient maintains relationships with others. Behavior is appropriate during interactions. The patient maintains physical appearance appropriate to age. The patient verbalizes and expresses feelings and concerns about differences between ideal self and realistic self.
The patient copes effectively.	The patient can identify results of ineffective coping mechanisms. The patient uses strengths in planning home care. The patient discusses alternate home care methods and makes positive choices.
Sexual functioning improves.	The patient verbalizes feelings about sexual dysfunction. The patient expresses an understanding of the relationship between prolactinoma and sexual dysfunction or infertility. The patient verbalizes improvement in sexual functioning.
Activity tolerance improves.	The patient identifies increased number of activities performed independently. The patient demonstrates active range-of-motion exercises and performs these three times daily. The patient demonstrates an ability to structure day, including all ADLs and appropriate rest periods.

HYPERTHYROIDISM

Hyperthyroidism is the clinical and biochemical syndrome that results when tissues are exposed to excessive quantities of thyroid hormones.[25]

Hyperthyroidism produces multiple system abnormalities because the thyroid hormones affect all organs and metabolic processes. The clinical signs and symptoms may be mild to severe. The nature of the manifestations depend on the patient's age, the severity of the syndrome, the rate of onset, the presence or absence of concomitant abnormalities in various organ systems, and the additional clinical features presented by the causative agent. Hyperthyroidism is a common disorder and may be transient or permanent. The exact prevalence in the United States is not available, although it is known to be more common in young women regardless of the underlying cause.

PATHOPHYSIOLOGY

Unregulated production of excessive amounts of thyroid hormones may result from (1) intrinsic thyroid disease, (2) unregulated thyroid-stimulating hormone (TSH), or thyroid-releasing hormone (TRH) secretion, (3) production of abnormal thyroid-stimulating hormones, such as thyroid-stimulating immunoglobulins or chorionic gonadotropin, (4) destruction of thyroid tissue with release of hormones, or (5) exogenous thyroid hormone replacement.[25] Varieties of hyperthyroidism are listed in Table 8-10. A brief review of these causes is outlined. Graves' disease is the most common cause of hyperthyroidism.

Graves' disease is defined as a multisystem disease characterized as consisting of one or more of the following: (1) diffuse thyroid enlargement, (2) hyperthyroidism, (3) infiltrative ophthalmopathy, (4) infiltrative dermopathy, and (5) thyroid acropachy. Most patients with Graves' disease have both hyperthyroidism and goiter that develop concurrently. Thyroid disease and infiltrative phenomena may occur singly or concurrently and may run courses largely independent of one another.

There is evidence that hereditary factors predispose to the development of Graves' disease. Thyroid antibodies, abnormalities in thyroid regulation, and thyroid-stimulating immunoglobulins (TSIs) have been found in eu-

Table 8-10
Varieties of Hyperthyroidism

Disorder	Incidence	Cause
Graves' disease (Basedow's disease)	More common in women during third and fourth decades of life; estimated to occur in 0.4% of US population	Believed to be an autoimmune disorder resulting from thyroid-stimulating immunoglobulins
Subacute thyroiditis (granulomatous, giant-cell, or de Quervain's thyroiditis)	Uncommon; more frequent in women; increased incidence during fourth and fifth decades; tendency for seasonal and geographic aggregations; mild hyperthyroidism in about 50% of cases	Probable viral infection of gland results in: Destruction of follicular epithelium; Loss of follicular integrity; Release of large quantities of preformed hormones and abnormal iodinated materials[73]
Painless thyroiditis	Increasing in general population	Subacute thyroiditis or an unusual manifestation of chronic autoimmune thyroiditis[25]
Radiation thyroiditis	Rare: usually occurs 1-2 wk after therapy	[131]I therapy resulting in follicular necrosis and inflammation
Toxic multinodular goiter (Plummer's disease)	Unknown; more frequent in women in the sixth or seventh decade; usually a long history of gradually increasing thyroid enlargement	Hyperfunctioning autonomous thyroid tissue
Toxic uninodular goiter (thyroid adenoma)	Female/male ratio: 3:1 to 6:1; US incidence: 5% of hyperthyroid patients; adults: all ages; especially in younger age group in 30s and 40s; occasionally seen in children	Adenoma functions autonomously; With continued growth, the adenoma assumes a greater share of glandular function and ultimately results in atrophy and complete suppression of the remainder of the gland[73]; Adenoma may infarct, resulting in a change from hyperfunctioning to hypofunctioning nodule with relief from hyperthyroidism[73]
Exogenous hyperthyroidism Iatrogenic		L-Thyroxine in doses of 0.3 mg/d or more; L-Triiodothyronine in doses of 0.1 mg/d or more; Dessicated thyroid in doses of 180 mg/d or more; More likely to develop when T_3 or a combination of T_4 and T_3 is used[56]
Factitious (thyrotoxicosis factitia)	More common in women with background of underlying psychiatric disease, paramedical personnel with access to thyroid hormone, or patients for whom thyroid medications have been prescribed in the past[73]	Chronic ingestion of excessive quantities of thyroid hormone
Iodide-induced hyperthyroidism (jod-basedou)	Iodide-deficient populations (usually in patients with underlying thyroid disorders) or in multinodular goiter	Administration of supplemental iodine to individuals with endemic, iodine-deficiency goiters; hyperthyroidism may be induced in patients with nonendemic goiter when large quantities of iodine are administered in the form of expectorants, x-ray contrast media, medications containing iodine, or any other form[73]
Ectopic hyperthyroidism (struma ovarii)	Very rare	Dermoid tumor or teratoma of ovary that contains a hyperfunctioning thyroid adenoma[25]
Thyroid carcinoma (follicular or mixed papillary follicular)	Uncommon; occurs predominately after 40 yr of age; women are affected 2-3 times more commonly than men	Large, autonomously functioning thyroid tumor
Pituitary thyrotropin (TSH)	Rare	Excessive TSH secretion from a pituitary tumor[25] or inappropriate TSH secretion caused by pituitary resistance to thyroid hormone[62]
Trophoblastic tumor		Tumors of trophoblastic origin: hydatidiform mole, choriocarcinoma or embryonal carcinoma of the testis with very high levels of chorionic gonadotropin
T_3 toxicosis	Unknown; more common in elderly population; occurs in association with Graves' disease, toxic multinodular goiter, toxic adenoma, or carcinoma	Preferential increase in thyroid secretion of T_3

thyroid family members of patients with Graves' disease.[25] Finally, there is an increased evidence of other autoimmune disorders, such as Hashimoto's disease and pernicious anemia, in these patients and their families.[73]

The exact cause of Graves' disease remains unknown. There is general agreement that the thyroid abnormalities result from the action on the gland of immunoglobulins that may be antibodies against components or regions of the thyroid plasma membrane[73] related to the TSH receptor. These autoantibodies, listed below, have been given various names on the basis of the assays used to detect them.

LATS	Long-acting thyroid stimulator
LATS-p	Long-acting thyroid stimulator protector
HTS	Human thyroid stimulator
HTACS	Human thyroid adenylate cyclase stimulator
TSAb	Thyroid-stimulating antibody
TBII	Thyroid-binding inhibiting immunoglobulins
TDII	Thyrotropin displacement activity

These autoantibodies are now usually known as thyroid-stimulating immunoglobulins (TSIs).[25] TSIs bind to the thyroid cell and activate the TSH receptor, which in turn stimulates thyroid function and thyroid growth.[25] Possible mechanisms for TSI production are (1) thyroid injury, (2) an infectious or other agent that stimulates production of the antibodies, (3) suppressed B-lymphocytes, and (4) abnormal T-lymphocyte regulation of B-lymphocytes.[25]

The thyroid gland in Graves' disease is diffusely enlarged (diffuse toxic goiter). The gland has increased vascularity, and there is often infiltration to a varying degree with lymphocytes and plasma cells.[73]

The cause or causes of infiltrative ophthalmopathy, infiltrative dermopathy, and thyroid acropachy remain unknown. Hyperthyroidism may initially develop without these extrathyroidal manifestations, although approximately 20% to 40% of patients have clinical evidence of ophthalmopathy.[25]

Infiltrative dermopathy is an uncommon manifestation seen in approximately 5% to 10% of patients.[73] It usually occurs months or years after treatment for hyperthyroidism and in patients who have significant ophthalmopathy.[25] Thyroid acropachy is seen in patients who have previously treated hyperthyroidism, localized dermopathy, and ophthalmopathy.[25] Generally, no symptoms or deformities occur, but thyroid acropachy may produce contractures.[25]

In general, the actions of the thyroid hormones are stimulatory in nature. The excessive production of thyroid hormones produces a state of hypermetabolism. The manifestations of hyperthyroidism usually reflect (1) increased functions of various organs or tissues and (2) an inability of an organ system to meet the increased demands.[25] Less severe manifestations are seen when the onset is gradual. Hyperthyroidism is tolerated fairly well, especially in younger patients, but it tends to be more debilitating in the elderly.[25]

Excessive heat production, increased neuromuscular activity, and hyperactivity of the sympathetic nervous system account for most of the clinical manifestations.[52] Compensatory mechanisms are called into action in order to meet the demands of the hypermetabolic state. These changes include (1) an increased cardiac output; (2) an increased peripheral blood flow with dilation of superficial skin capillaries; (3) an increased body temperature; (4) an increased oxygen consumption, resulting in an increased respiratory rate; (5) increased absorption of glucose by the gastrointestinal tract; (6) increased cellular use of glucose; (7) hyperinsulinemia; (8) decreased supply of fats and carbohydrates; (9) increased metabolism of vitamins, leading in extreme cases to significant vitamin deficiencies; (10) increased mobilization of bone, leading to a state of hypercalcemia; and (11) increased secretions of ACTH and MSH, leading to skin pigmentation changes.

Apathetic or masked hyperthyroidism may occur in the elderly patient whose hyperthyroidism is manifested primarily by cardiac failure, atrial fibrillation, muscle weakness, or weight loss.[25] These elderly patients do not exhibit the clinical manifestations that are commonly seen in younger patients, such as nervousness, heat intolerance, increased appetite, and general hyperactivity.[25]

Thyroid storm or thyroid crisis is a severe life-threatening form of hyperthyroidism. Thyroid storm is uncommon but is the most severe and dramatic form of hyperthyroidism. It generally occurs in association with Graves' disease but can be seen with toxic multinodular goiter.[73]

DIAGNOSTIC STUDIES

Thyroid suppression test
   No suppression of uptake after T_4 or T_3 administration (no longer a common test)

Thyrotropin-releasing hormone (TRH) stimulation test
   Little or no response of TSH to TRH stimulation (supersedes suppression test)

Laboratory findings
   Serum T_4
      Increased

   Serum T_3
      Increased

Serum free T$_4$ and T$_3$
Increased

Radioactive T$_3$ uptake (RT$_3$U)
High

Radioactive iodine uptake (RAIU)
High in Graves' disease and toxic nodular goiter; low in thyroiditis and thyrotoxicosis factitia

TSH
Suppressed and does not respond to TRH

Thyroid-stimulating immunoglobulins (TSI)
Present in Graves' disease

TREATMENT PLAN

Surgical
Total thyroidectomy
Subtotal thyroidectomy

Chemotherapeutic*
Thioamides
Propylthiouracil (PTU), 50-300 mg po qd for adults; initially 300-600 mg qd; inhibits thyroid hormone synthesis but not release; used to lower thyroid hormone levels; clinical improvement of hyperthyroid is delayed; agranulocytosis may occur in 1.4% of patients during first 2 mo of therapy; skin rashes occur in roughly 3% of patients
Methimazole (Tapazole), 5-20 mg po qd for adults; initially 30-60 mg qd; inhibits thyroid hormone synthesis but not release; similar to PTU
Monovalent cations
Lithium carbonate; dosage not established; 900 mg qd depresses thyroid function in some patients with manic states; inhibits synthesis and release of thyroid hormones by mechanism different from thioamides; when used for treatment of manic states, side effects include nausea and vomiting, twitching muscles, and central nervous system changes; severe intoxication causes convulsions, coma, and death
β-Adrenergic blockers
Propranolol (Inderal), 40-160 mg po qd in divided doses for adults; 5 mg or less IV at 1 mg/min or more slowly for adults; controls symptoms of hyperthyroidism but does not lower T$_3$ and T$_4$ levels; controls palpitations, tremor, sweating, proximal muscle weakness, and cardiac symptoms of hyperthyroidism by competitively blocking β-ad-

renergic receptors; bronchospasm may occur in asthmatics; may precipitate frank heart failure in patient with heart function maintained by sympathetic tone
Iodines
Potassium or sodium iodide (Strong Iodine Solution; Lugol's Solution), 0.1-0.3 ml po tid for adults; 250-500 mg qd for adults in thyrotoxic crisis; produces short-term inhibition of thyroid hormone synthesis by direct action on thyroid; used as presurgical medication to reduce size of thyroid gland after thioamide therapy; used with thioamide and propranolol for hyperthyroid crisis; may produce iodism
Radioactive iodine
^{131}I or ^{125}I as NaI; 4-10 mCi as single dose for Graves' disease; for thyroid carcinoma, single doses of up to 150 mCi; smaller doses used for diagnostic purposes; concentrated in the thyroid and release radiation, which destroys thyroid tissue; used to destroy thyroid tissue without surgery for control of Graves' disease or thyroid carcinoma; hypothyroidism ultimately develops in most patients

Supportive
Treatment of ophthalmopathy (often no cure)
Palliative treatment
Corticosteroids
Surgical decompression
Surgical correction of muscle imbalance
Radiation of orbit
Diet
Control of environment
Psychotherapy

ASSESSMENT: AREAS OF CONCERN

Skin and appendages
Warm and moist; smooth velvety texture; erythema
Increased body temperature (37.8° C or greater may indicate thyroid storm)
Increased sweating
Increased diffuse pigmentation
Localized myxedema

Eyes
Lid retraction and lag
Proptosis
Conjunctival irritation; lacrimation
Characteristic "bright-eyed, frightened, or startled" look

*Data from Clark, J., Queener, S., and Karb, V.: Pharmacological basis of nursing practice, St. Louis, 1982, The C.V. Mosby Co.

Cardiovascular status
  Increased systolic blood pressure; wide pulse pressure
  Tachycardia
  Presence of arrhythmias

Respiratory status
  Changes in rate or depth of respirations
  Increased restlessness

Gastrointestinal status
  Weight loss or modest weight gain (especially if large food intake; seen in younger patients)
  Polyphagia; increased food intake
  Diarrhea

Muscular status
  Generalized muscular wasting and weakness
  Hyperactive deep tendon reflexes
  Noticeable tremor

Nervous system status
  Restlessness; irritability

Decreased ability to concentrate; memory loss; easily distracted
Insomnia

Mental and emotional status
  Emotionally labile; irritable
  Manic behavior
  Family members report changes in performance

Renal status
  Polyuria; urgency and frequency of micturition
  Polydipsia

Reproductive status
  Women
    Hypomenorrhea
    Amenorrhea

  Men
    Reported loss of libido
    Decreased potency

NURSING DIAGNOSES and NURSING INTERVENTIONS

Nursing Diagnosis	Nursing Intervention
Cardiac output, alteration in: potential for increased	Monitor pulse, blood pressure, color, and temperature. Monitor sleeping pulse for more accurate assessment of tachycardia. Measure and record intake and output (I and O).
Breathing pattern, ineffective	Record rate, depth, and character of respirations. Auscultate for breath sounds. Record vital signs every 4 to 6 hours. Provide scheduled uninterrupted rest. Allow minimal exertion during care.
Nutrition, alteration in: less than body requirements	Weigh daily. Monitor daily food intake and serum glucose levels. Stress importance of avoiding coffee, tea, colas, and foods that increase peristalsis. Provide high-calorie, high-protein, high-carbohydrate vitamin B diet with between-meal nourishments. Provide dietary consultation.
Comfort, alteration in	Monitor body temperature and serum electrolytes. Regulate environmental temperature; place patient in cool and quiet room. Have patient wear light clothing; change clothing twice daily. Provide light bed linens (i.e., sheet only). Decrease external stimuli.
Thought processes, alteration in	Monitor level of orientation to person, place, and time. Avoid discrepancies in timing, activities, and methods of performing procedures. Provide physically and emotionally safe environment. Explain procedures slowly and carefully. Repeat instructions. Limit number of instructions. Limit number of care givers.
Skin integrity, impairment of: actual	Inspect skin daily. Monitor for development of localized myxedema. Keep skin and linens clean, dry, and wrinkle free. Lubricate and massage around affected skin. Force fluids (3000-4000 ml/d unless contraindicated by cardiovascular status). Elevate legs.

Patient Education

1. Teach signs and symptoms for early recognition and adjustment of treatment of hyperthyroidism.
2. Teach medication administration: name, dosage, action, frequency of administration, side effects, and importance of taking medicines on schedule.
3. Teach signs and symptoms of hypothyroidism and necessity of reporting to physician.
4. Instruct patient regarding high-calorie, high-protein, high-carbohydrate, vitamin B diet with between-meal nourishment.
5. Stress importance of planned rest and avoidance of stress whenever possible.
6. Prepare patient and family members for emotional outbursts and potential alterations in body image.
7. Stress importance of and necessity for follow-up evaluations.

EVALUATION

Patient Outcome	Data Indicating That Outcome is Reached
Cardiovascular function is normal.	Dysrhythmias are absent or less frequent. Cyanosis is absent or decreased. Skin remains warm and dry. Hourly urine output is 30 ml.
Respiratory function is normal.	The patient demonstrates adequate respiratory depth and effort. There is no cyanosis. Restlessness is absent or decreased. Dyspnea is absent or decreased.
Nutritional intake is adequate.	The patient demonstrates adherence to prescribed diet. The patient maintains stable weight and utilizes measures to increase food intake. The patient verbalizes the importance of a well-balanced diet.
Comfort is increased.	The patient verbalizes a decrease in or relief from heat intolerance. The patient identifies and uses several techniques to control heat intolerance.
Thought processes are normal.	The patient demonstrates orientation to person, place, and time. There is no injury to self, others, or property. The patient validates thought processes with staff. Statements are reality oriented.
Skin is intact.	There are no breaks, cracks, or ulcers. There is no evidence of infection. Skin turgor is normal.

HYPOPARATHYROIDISM

Hypoparathyroidism is a condition in which the parathyroid glands secrete an inadequate amount of parathyroid hormone (PTH) to maintain normal levels of serum calcium.

Hypoparathyroidism is manifested by hypocalcemia. This condition may occur at any age and is usually the result of damage to the parathyroid glands during parathyroid or thyroid surgery.

PATHOPHYSIOLOGY

Although hypoparathyroidism is usually caused by damage to the parathyroid glands during surgical procedures, the disease may also be idiopathic. Idiopathic hypoparathyroidism is a rare autoimmune disorder that usually occurs before 15 years of age. It is sometimes one of a number of endocrine disorders included in a polyendocrine syndrome called HAM (hypoparathyroidism, Addison's disease, and monoliasis). Hypoparathyroidism has been acquired, in a few rare cases, following treatment with ^{131}I therapy. It has also been associated with metastases of malignant tumors to the parathyroid glands.[25]

The signs and symptoms of hypoparathyroidism are associated with hypocalcemia resulting from the decreased level of PTH. Neuromuscular irritability is the most common and recognizable feature of hypocalcemia, causing symptoms which range from mild paresthesias to tetany and hypocalcemic seizures. These symptoms are caused by a decrease in resting ability and increased excitability of nerve and muscle membranes.[11,41]

Bone resorption decreases in hypoparathyroidism, causing a decrease in osteoclastic activity. Bones remain normal or slightly more dense in adults. New growth is suppressed and may cause dwarfism in children. Calcification of the basal ganglion, another clinical manifestation of hypoparathyroidism, results in a Parkinson-like syndrome with bizarre posturing and dystonic choreoathetoid movements.[11] Other characteristics of the disease include dental abnormalities caused by decreased calcium levels, cataracts result from a calcification of the lens, and hypotension caused by decreased cardiac contractility. Pseudohypoparathyroidism is a separate disease entity that is a familial disorder characterized by an atypical phenotype, chemical hypoparathyroidism, and increased circulating PTH levels.[25]

DIAGNOSTIC STUDIES

Serum calcium
Less than 4.3 mEq/L

Urine calcium
Greater than 200 mEq/24 h

Serum PO$_4$
Increased

Urinary PO$_4$
Decreased

TREATMENT PLAN

Chemotherapeutic
Parathyroid hormone, 20-40 USP units q12h, IM, IV, or subq
Vitamins
Dihydrotachysterol, 0.25-1.75 mg every week, po
Vitamin D, 200-400 IU/d, po

Nutritional replenishers
Calcium gluconate, 5 g tid, po (liquid)
Calcium glubionate, 10-60 ml, po or IV
Calcium lactate, 4-10 g bid, po (chewable tablet)

Supportive
Dietary supplement of calcium

ASSESSMENT: AREAS OF CONCERN

Central nervous system
Personality disturbances
Anxiety
Depression
Irritability

Increased neuromuscular excitability
Paresthesias
Tetany
Dysphagia

Headache
Retardation
Bilateral cerebral calcification

Cardiovascular system
Decreased contractility
Decreased output

Gastrointestinal system
Nausea
Vomiting
Diarrhea
Abdominal pain

Soft tissue
Calcification (especially in eyes)

Ectodermis
Exfoliative dermatitis
Coarse, dry, scaly skin
Cutaneous pigmentation
Thin, patchy hair

Skeletal system
Dwarfism
Developmental abnormalities

NURSING DIAGNOSES and NURSING INTERVENTIONS

Nursing Diagnosis	Nursing Intervention
Fluid volume deficit, potential	Monitor intake and output. Force fluid as ordered.
Injury, trauma potential for	Observe the patient for steadiness on ambulation. Assist the patient when necessary.

Nursing Diagnosis	Nursing Intervention
Nutrition, alteration in: less than body requirements	Make high-calcium snacks available to patient at all times. Have the dietitian discuss dietary calcium supplements with the patient. Give calcium replacement medications on time to enhance dietary intake of calcium. Monitor Chvostek's and Trousseau's signs.
Coping, ineffective individual	Maintain a calm approach if the patient is agitated or irritable. Observe for precipitating factors causing stress. See also p. 1897.
Cardiac output, alteration in: decreased	Monitor vital signs. Check rhythm strip for Q-T interval changes and abnormal T wave and P wave changes.

Patient Education

1. Teach how to monitor pulse and importance of reporting irregularities.
2. Teach how to maintain fluid balance especially when nausea, vomiting, and diarrhea are present.
3. Instruct the patient and family in the use of dietary calcium supplements and the reasons for the treatment.
4. Instruct the patient and family in the use and side effects of medications.
5. Teach early recognition and treatment of hypocalcemia.

EVALUATION

Patient Outcome	Data Indicating That Outcome is Reached
Fluid intake is adequate.	Intake and output are within normal limits. Skin turgor is normal.
There is no injury.	There are no bruises or skeletal breaks. The patient states that environment is arranged for safety. Chvostek's and Trousseau's signs are negative.
Nutrition is adequate.	The patient verbalizes adherence to dietary plan. Calcium level is 4.3 to 5.3 mEq/L. Phosphorus level is 1.8 to 2.6 mEq/L. There are no signs or symptoms of hypocalcemia.
Cardiac output is adequate.	Vital signs are stable. Rhythm strip is normal.

HYPOTHYROIDISM

Hypothyroidism is the clinical state resulting from deficient thyroid hormones.

Hypothyroidism is a common disorder affecting both sexes from birth through old age. It occurs more often in women between the ages of 30 to 60 years than in any other group. The incidence of hypothyroidism in infants is estimated to occur in 1 out of every 4000 to 5000 newborns.[73] Population studies have indicated that unrecognized hypothyroidism may be more common in the elderly population than previously thought.[73] Neonatal screening programs have made major contributions toward health care, and it is suggested that screening programs be extended to cover the elderly as well.

The clinical manifestations of hypothyroidism may range from mild, with few signs or symptoms, to severe, culminating in the life-threatening myxedema coma. The clinical manifestations depend on the degree of thyroid hormone deficiency.

Table 8-11
Varieties of Hypothyroidism

Disorder	Incidence	Cause
Idiopathic hypothyroidism	Unknown; occurs more often in women after the fourth decade but may occur at any age	Unknown Antithyroid antibodies may be present Defects in intrathyroidal iodide metabolism resembling chronic autoimmune thyroiditis may be present
Chronic autoimmune thyroiditis (Hashimoto's disease)	Unknown; believed to be very common and increasing in frequency No age is exempt More common in women between 30-50 yr of age Common cause of hypothyroidism in children Often family history of Hashimoto's disease, goiters, hypothyroidism, or Graves' disease Occurs in unexpected frequency in patients with Down's syndrome Patients and their relatives have a higher incidence of other associated autoimmune disorders	Autoimmune disorder
Hypothyroidism after radioiodine therapy and external radiotherapy	Common occurrence; frequency determined by degree of radiation given; incidence increases progressively with time	Radioiodine (^{131}I or ^{125}I) therapy External radiotherapy to neck region
Postoperative hypothyroidism	Following total thyroidectomy: almost immediate occurrence Following subtotal thyroidectomy: less predictable; ranges from 5-30% prevalence rate and then continues to appear indefinitely at a rate of 1-2% per yr[25]	Surgery with loss of or damage to thyroid tissue
Spontaneous hypothyroidism following Graves' disease	Generally occurs following remission of Graves' disease; not associated with antithyroid drugs	May result from concomitant chronic autoimmune thyroiditis that frequently occurs with Graves' disease[25]
Transient hypothyroidism	Exact incidence: unknown	Occurs in patients with subacute or chronic thyroiditis following initial damage to gland
Thyroid dysgenesis	Occurs in 1 out of every 4000-5000 births	Failure of gland to develop Failure of gland to descend properly during embryonic development Causes: largely unknown
Hypothyroidism caused by iodine deficiency	Most common cause of hypothyroidism in many parts of the world	Iodine deficiency resulting in a decreased production of thyroid hormones
Hypothyroidism caused by antithyroid agents	Exact prevalence unknown	Ingestion of compounds with antithyroid potency Drugs: thiocyanates, iodide, lithium, para-aminosalicylic acid Plants: rutabaga, white turnips, soybeans, cabbage, peanuts

Hypothyroidism caused by hereditary defects in thyroid hormone biosynthesis	Rare	Generally autosomal recessive disorders[25]
		Defects may be caused by:
		  Defective iodide transport
		  Defective organification caused by inadequate or defective peroxidase, thyroglobulin, or peroxide
		  Defects in iodotyrosine coupling
		  Defective thyroglobulin biosynthesis and formation of abnormal iodoproteins
		  Defective dehalogenation of iodotyrosines

Table 8-11, cont'd
Varieties of Hypothyroidism

Disorder	Incidence	Cause
Pituitary hypothyroidism (thyroid-stimulating hormone [TSH] deficiency)	Rare; less than 5% of hypothyroidism	Destruction of normal pituitary tissue by tumors, surgery, irradiation, postpartum necrosis, carotid aneurysms, trauma, hemochromatosis, or tuberculosis
Hypothalamic hypothyroidism (thyroid-releasing hormone [TRH] deficiency)	Rare	TRH deficiency resulting from trauma, destruction, or infiltrative diseases of the hypothalamus
Hypothyroidism caused by impaired peripheral sensitivity to thyroid hormones	Rare	Believed to be caused by decreased or abnormal nuclear receptors for T_3

PATHOPHYSIOLOGY

Hypothyroidism results from inadequate peripheral tissue levels of thyroid hormones, usually caused by inadequate thyroid secretion.[25] Hypothyroidism may result from (1) loss or atrophy of thyroid tissue (intrinsic disease), (2) insufficient stimulation of an intrinsically normal gland (resulting from hypothalamic or pituitary disease), or (3) association with compensatory goitrogenesis as a result of defective hormone biosynthesis.[73] Causes of hypothyroidism as well as defining characteristics are listed in Table 8-11.

Clinical manifestations of hypothyroidism are reflections of decreased metabolic processes. Pathophysiologic changes including excessive interstitial glycosaminoglycan deposition occurs throughout all organ systems. Glycosaminoglycan is the highly hydrophilic substance causing the mucinous edema (myxedema) that accounts for the majority of clinical manifestations seen in hypothyroidism.

There are three main forms of hypothyroidism: (1) cretinism, (2) juvenile hypothyroidism, and (3) adult hypothyroidism (myxedema). Cretinism is a state of severe hypothyroidism found in infants. Thyroid hormones are essential for physical and mental growth. They are essential for central nervous system development as well as skeletal maturation. Cretinism is characterized by an interruption in the normal physical and mental development in the infant.[68] It occurs either during fetal life or in the first few months after birth.[68] It is treatable, and permanent retardation may be preventable if treatment begins early.[68] If untreated, however, irreversible cerebral brain damage occurs. If treated during the first 3 months after birth, a better mental prognosis is achieved.[68]

Juvenile hypothyroidism develops during childhood. It is most often caused by chronic autoimmune thyroiditis but may also be caused by medications or defects in thyroid hormone synthesis. Growth and sexual maturation are most often affected. The clinical manifestations usually resemble signs and symptoms similar to those seen in adult myxedema. Myxedema is the term often used to describe adult hypothyroidism.

Myxedema coma is a rare, life-threatening state of hypothyroidism. It is the end stage of neglected or undiagnosed hypothyroidism and has a 50% mortality. Myxedema coma normally requires several years for development, but it has been noted to occur after the administration of sedatives or other psychotropic drugs to patients with undiagnosed hypothyroidism. It is seen more commonly in elderly patients who have been without medical care and has been noted to occur more often during the winter months, suggesting that cold exposure may be a precipitating factor. Myxedema coma is characterized by (1) coma, (2) hypothermia in more than 80% of patients, (3) cardiovascular collapse, (4) hypoventilation, and (5) severe metabolic derangements such as hyponatremia, hypoglycemia, and lactic acidosis. The comatose state is produced by complications such as carbon dioxide retention, reduction in cardiac output, and consequently increasing cerebral hypoxia.[25]

DIAGNOSTIC STUDIES

TRH stimulation tests
Above normal response in patients with primary hypothyroidism; poor or prolonged response in pituitary or hypothalamic disease

TSH stimulation tests
Distinguishes between primary hypothyroidism and secondary hypothyroidism caused by TSH deficiency; normal gland responds by increasing iodine uptake and T_4 release (now used less frequently)

RAIU
Below normal uptake

Serum T₄
Decreased

Serum T₃
Decreased (no value alone)

Serum free T₄ and T₃
Decreased

Serum TSH
Elevated (primary hypothyroidism)

RT₃U
Below normal

TREATMENT PLAN

Chemotherapeutic*
Natural thyroid hormones
  Thyroid U.S.P. (Delcoid; Thyrar; Thyrocrine; Thyro-Teric); 120-180 mg po qd for adults for maintenance; initial doses 15 mg qd; double the dose every 2 wk until appropriate maintenance dose is reached; impure mixture of thyroid components that includes T₃ and T₄; replacement therapy for hypothyroidism; overdose produces symptoms of hyperthyroidism; too large a dose at onset of therapy may cause vascular occlusion, especially in patients with arteriosclerosis
  Thyroglobulin (Proloid), 120-180 mg po qd for adults for maintenance; initial doses are small and are gradually increased to maintenance levels; contains T₃ and T₄, as well as other iodine-containing compounds; replacement therapy for hypothyroidism; overdose produces same symptoms as seen with thyroid U.S.P.
Synthetic thyroid hormones
  Levothyroxine sodium (Cytolen; Levoid; Levothy-

*Data from Clark, J., Queener, S., and Karb, V.: Pharmacological basis of nursing practice, St. Louis, 1982, The C.V. Mosby Co.

roid; Synthroid Sodium), 150-200 μg po qd for adults for maintenance; initial doses are small and are gradually increased to maintenance levels; 3-5 μg/kg/d po for children >1 yr; 0.5 mg with mannitol (Synthroid) or without (Levoid), IV for adults; chemically pure form of T₄; replacement therapy for hypothyroidism; IV form used for myxedemic coma; peak effect 9 d after start of therapy; serum half-life about 11 d
  Liothyronine sodium (Cytomel), 25-75 μg po qd for adults for maintenance; initial doses should be low and gradually increased to maintenance levels; chemically pure form of T₃; replacement therapy for hypothyroidism; peak effect in 2 d; serum half-life 4-6 d
  Liotrix (Euthroid; Thyrolar), 30 μg T₄ with 7.5 μg T₃ or 25 μg T₄ with 6.25 μg T₃ po for adults; doses may be gradually increased as needed; chemically pure T₄ and T₃ combined in a ratio of 4:1; replacement therapy for hypothyroidism
Adenohypophyseal hormone
  Thyroid-stimulating hormone (TSH) (Thytropar), 10 IU IM or subq qd or bid; extract of bovine anterior pituitary contains natural peptide, TSH; diagnostic agent to establish hypothyroidism; may cause release of thyroid hormones that can precipitate adrenal crisis in patient with secondary adrenal insufficiency; may also cause cardiovascular symptoms and rare allergic reactions
  Protirelin (thyrotropin-releasing hormone, TRH) (Relefact TRH; Thypinone) 400-500 μg IV for adults; synthetic preparation of natural hypothalamic tripeptide hormone; diagnostic agent to differentiate pituitary-induced hypothyroidism from other types of hypothyroidism; may transiently produce nausea, facial flushing, hypertension, and urge to micturate

Supportive
Control of environment
Diet: high protein, high fiber, low calorie

ASSESSMENT: AREAS OF CONCERN

	Infant (Cretinism)	Juvenile Hypothyroidism	Adult (Myxedema)
Skin and appendages	Pale, cool to touch, and dry Persistence of physiologic jaundice Hypothermia	Same as adult	Cool, pale, dry, coarse; yellowish tint Rough, scaly skin Puffy, masklike face Periorbital edema Hypothermia Myxedema

	Infant (Cretinism)	Juvenile Hypothyroidism	Adult (Myxedema)
Cardiovascular status	Bradycardia		Bradycardia; decreased blood pressure Decreased exercise tolerance Arrhythmias
Respiratory status	Hoarse or gruntlike cry Signs and symptoms of respiratory distress; peripheral cyanosis		Hypoventilation Hoarseness Sensitivity to narcotics, tranquilizers, sedatives, and anesthetics
Gastrointestinal status	Constipation; abdominal distention with an umbilical hernia Failure to thrive Delay in passage of meconium	Constipation	Anorexia Modest weight gain Constipation; fecal impaction Abdominal distention; myxedema ileus
Muscular status	Poor sucking reflexes Delays in meeting normal developmental milestones	Increase in muscle mass with slow muscle activity Persistent fatigue	Nonspecific fatigue; weakness Slow muscle movement Delayed relaxation of tendon reflexes
Nervous system status	Inactive baby	Dull, apathetic Demonstrates nervousness, aggressiveness, or hyperactivity Short attention span Requires more sleep Fails to complete tasks Poor intellectual functioning	General slowing of all intellectual functions, including speech Decreased hearing Lethargy and somnolence Impaired memory; inattentiveness Loss of initiative
Mental-emotional status	Mental deficiency always present and usually severe	Less severe mental retardation May respond poorly to discipline Experiences frequent temper tantrums Labeled as "problem child"	Paranoia Depression Agitation
Skeletal status	Early sign: large posterior fontanel Dwarfism Head seem disproportionate to large trunk	Short limbs with bone age less than chronologic age	Aches and stiffness of joints
Renal system status			Decreased urine output Slightly impaired ability to concentrate urine
Reproductive status	Sexual immaturity	Delayed or absent sexual maturation If develops before puberty, delayed onset of puberty followed by anovulatory cycle	Women 　Diminished libido 　Failure of ovulation 　Amenorrhea Men 　Diminished libido 　Impotence

NURSING DIAGNOSES and NURSING INTERVENTIONS

Nursing Diagnosis	Nursing Intervention
Cardiac output, alteration in: decreased	Monitor pulse, blood pressure, color, and temperature. Measure and record intake and output; weigh daily. Observe level of consciousness and orientation. Monitor for potentiating effects of drugs (use lower doses of sedatives, narcotics, etc.).

Nursing Diagnosis	Nursing Intervention
Breathing pattern, ineffective	Record rate, depth, and character of respirations. Monitor vital signs. Provide scheduled uninterrupted rest. Allow minimal exertion during care.
Thought processes, alteration in	Monitor level of orientation to person, place, and time. Provide tolerable activity schedule. Provide physically and emotionally safe environment. Explain procedures slowly and carefully. Assist family in accepting dullness and slowness. Time nursing activities to patient's response level to avoid further disorientation.
Skin integrity, impairment of: actual	Inspect skin daily for increased edema, breakdown, signs of infection, and bleeding tendency. Utilize measures to conserve body temperature (i.e., warm blankets, robes, socks, bed jacket). Utilize skin preventive measures.
Bowel elimination, alteration in: constipation	Provide high-protein, high-fiber, low-calorie diet in smaller, frequent meals. Encourage *increased* fluid intake. Monitor the frequency, color, consistency, and amount of stool. Establish daily routine bowel training program. Administer stool softeners and laxatives. Avoid use of enemas.

Patient Education

1. Teach signs and symptoms of hypothyroidism and hyperthyroidism to report.
2. Teach the patient that thyroid hormones are essential for life and that treatment is therefore lifelong.
3. Teach medication administration: name, dosage, frequency of taking, and side effects.
4. Instruct patient regarding maintenance of a well-balanced, high-fiber diet with adequate iodine and fluid intake.
5. Stress importance of adequate rest alternating with increasing periods of exercise.
6. Prepare family members for tolerance of patient's dullness or slowness.
7. Stress importance of avoiding over-the-counter medications without consulting the physician.
8. Emphasize importance of and necessity for follow-up evaluations.

EVALUATION

Patient Outcome	Data Indicating That Outcome is Reached
Cardiovascular function is normal.	The patient demonstrates normal sinus rhythm. Skin remains warm and dry. The patient remains alert and fully oriented. The patient maintains an hourly urine output of 30 ml.
Respiratory function is normal.	Respiratory depth and rate are adequate. Chest expansion is equal. There is no cyanosis.
Thought processes are normal.	The patient is oriented to person, place, and time. The patient validates thought processes with staff. Statements are reality oriented. The patient is interested in work, environment, friends, and family.
Skin integrity is normal.	Skin remains intact. Skin remains free of infection. Edema is absent or decreased. The patient verbalizes or demonstrates skin care measures.

Patient Outcome	Data Indicating That Outcome is Reached
Constipation is absent or decreased.	Bowel movements are regular and of normal consistency, color, and quantity. The patient verbalizes adherence to prescribed diet and fluid intake. The patient identifies high-fiber foods to use in diet plan.

PHENYLKETONURIA

Classic phenylketonuria (PKU) is an inborn error of amino acid metabolism resulting in high levels of serum phenylalanine, which form metabolites that spill into the urine as aromatic phenylketones.[72]

The occurrence of PKU is 1 in every 10,000 live births in northern Europeans. The frequency is highest in those of Irish or Scottish descent and lowest in Ashkenazic Jews and southern Italians.[49]

Phenylketonuria is transmitted as an autosomal recessive trait, meaning there is a one in four chance with each pregnancy of producing an affected infant. Many, but not all, heterozygotes (carriers) can be identified by rapid elution chromatography of a single blood sample.[10] Genetic screening is important in identifying carriers of PKU so that they may be aware of the need for prompt testing and treatment, if indicated, in later progeny.

Diagnosis can now be made in utero as a result of recent success in cloning of the gene for the deficient or absent enzyme in PKU. This has made it possible to test fetal cells from amniotic fluid by using gene-mapping techniques. The fetal genes are then compared to genes of parents and unaffected persons, and an accurate diagnosis can be made. Sibling carriers can also be detected by this new method.

PKU carriers and affected persons can benefit from genetic counseling to learn the risks of future offspring being affected. Informed choices can then be made and preventative measures taken as needed. Discussion with a genetic counselor can also help alleviate guilt feelings common in such families.

The infant with PKU seems normal at birth. Only after feeding has been initiated does the serum phenylalanine level increase. Without early diet therapy there are usually severe neurologic consequences (i.e., mental retardation). Therefore early detection and treatment are imperative.[45]

When diet therapy is started within the first month of life, the chance of the child attaining normal intelligence is statistically significant.[41a] The age of termination of diet therapy remains a controversial issue. The current trend is to decrease restrictions at 8 to 10 years of age but to resume control if there are signs of regression.[72]

The child with phenylketonuria needs frequent medical evaluation to determine phenylalanine blood levels (kept in the range of 2 to 10 mg/dl), growth and development, neurologic status, and dietary adjustments required.[1]

The term *maternal PKU* is applied to a phenylketonuria patient who becomes pregnant. Infants born of PKU mothers no longer on diet therapy are usually severely defective even if they do not have phenylketonuria. PKU mothers who maintain diet therapy before conception and throughout pregnancy have given birth to infants all along a continuum from completely normal infants to those who die from congenital heart disease.[41a] Research in this area is limited.

PATHOPHYSIOLOGY

High serum levels of phenylalanine are the result of a biochemical blockage in the liver enzyme system. The enzyme phenylalanine hydroxylase is either deficient or absent, thereby failing to convert phenylalanine into tyrosine. This causes a buildup of phenylalanine and its metabolites in the bloodstream. When a certain level of phenylalanine is reached, its metabolites are excreted in the urine as phenylketones, giving rise to a musty odor; thus the name phenylketonuria. The etiology of phenylketonuria is unknown.

DIAGNOSTIC STUDIES

Guthrie bacterial inhibition assay
Positive on specimens obtained 48 hours after first feeding and between second and fourth weeks of life

Serum phenylalanine
4 mg/dl or greater

TREATMENT PLAN

Electromechanical
Fluid replacement

Supportive
Diet management (p. 922)

ASSESSMENT: AREAS OF CONCERN

Fluid balance
  Vomiting
  Dry mucous membranes
  Poor skin turgor
  Failure to gain weight

NURSING DIAGNOSES and NURSING INTERVENTIONS

Nursing Diagnosis	Nursing Intervention
Fluid volume deficit, potential	Maintain IV lines as ordered. Record intake and output. Record daily weight. Monitor vital signs. Check for signs and symptoms of dehydration.
Coping, ineffective family	Encourage discussions concerning fears and guilt regarding potential retardation. Make information available about support and counseling groups. Assist with plans for dietary management.

Patient Education

1. Teach parents early recognition and treatment of dehydration.
2. Instruct parents regarding dietary management.
3. Stress importance of genetic counseling for family to enhance decisions regarding reproduction.
4. Stress importance of follow-up medical care and laboratory studies.
5. Instruct parents regarding signs related to slow intellectual and behavioral development to be reported.

EVALUATION

Patient Outcome	Data Indicating That Outcome is Reached
Fluid volume is normal.	Intake equals output. There is no vomiting. There are no signs or symptoms of dehydration. Mucous membranes are moist. Skin turgor is elastic. There is no weight loss. There is a gradual weight gain.
Coping is effective.	Parents express feelings about birth of infant with genetic defect. Parents seek genetic counseling. Parents use support group as necessary. Parents provide care for infant or child appropriate to age. Parents maintain prescribed diet as indicated by laboratory values.

PHEOCHROMOCYTOMA

A pheochromocytoma is a chromaffin cell tumor of the sympathetic nervous system that produces excessive amounts of the catecholamines epinephrine and norepinephrine.

The incidence of pheochromocytoma is rare. Less than 0.5% of all patients with a recent diagnosis of hypertension have pheochromocytoma. The disorder has no predominance for sex or race and occurs more commonly in the third and fourth decades of life. Tumors in children are usually associated with a familial tendency, are frequently bilateral, and are often malignant. Familial tendencies are unusual and inherited as an autosomal dominant trait. Pheochromocytomas are often linked with medullary carcinoma of the thyroid and multiple endocrine neoplasias (MEN II syndromes).[20]

lead to cerebrovascular accidents that can be life threatening. Nephrosclerosis and retinopathy may accompany severe sustained hypertension. Myocarditis, dysrhythmias, and congestive heart failure are seen in patients who develop cardiomyopathies related to the direct effect of high levels of catecholamines on the myocardium.[25]

Elevated levels of circulating epinephrine and norepinephrine create a state of hypermetabolism similar to thyrotoxicosis.[20] The patient may have tachycardia, tacharrhythmias, weight loss, heat intolerance, tremors, and hyperreflexia. Sympathetic overstimulation can give rise to apprehension and emotional instability. Catecholamines suppress insulin secretion and stimulate the conversion of glycogen to glucose in the liver, resulting in hyperglycemia and glycosuria.[25]

PATHOPHYSIOLOGY

Ninety percent of tumors arising from the chromaffin system are found in the adrenal medulla and are called pheochromocytomas. The remainder are extra-adrenal and are classified as paragangliomas; they usually are found in the abdomen. Multiple pheochromocytomas occur in approximately 20% of cases and often in patients possessing the inherited trait. Pheochromocytomas can occur in pregnancy and lead to increased morbidity and mortality for mother and fetus. Malignant pheochromocytomas are a rarity and occur in 5% of patients. Metastatic sites include bone, lung, liver, and lymph nodes.[25]

Pheochromocytomas produce excessive amounts of epinephrine and norepinephrine; however, norepinephrine is more prevalent and is responsible for most of the clinical manifestations. Norepinephrine, an alpha-adrenergic agonist, primarily causes the hypertensive effects of the disorder and is the principal hormone seen in extra-adrenal tumors. Epinephrine, a beta-adrenergic agonist, is responsible for hypertensive as well as hypermetabolic and hyperglycemic effects of the disorder.

Overproduction of norepinephrine causes sustained hypertension, the most outstanding clinical sign in patients. Excess epinephrine production can also bring about hypertension and postural hypotension. Blood pressure measurements can range from 200-300/150-175 mm Hg. Patients may have widely fluctuating blood pressures with or without paroxysmal hypertensive episodes. During a hypertensive crisis the patient may experience severe headaches, palpitations, profuse sweating, pupillary dilation, pallor, or flushing. Hypertensive episodes can be provoked by stimuli such as palpation of the tumor, emotional stress, or increased abdominal pressure (i.e., micturition). Extreme cases of hypertension may

TREATMENT PLAN

Surgical
Vena caval catheterization (p. 930)
Excision of pheochromocytoma (p. 933)

Chemotherapeutic
Alpha-adrenergic blocking agents: used to lower arterial pressure and to increase vascular volume
  Phentolamine (Regitine), 0.5-5.0 mg IV; short acting (carefully monitor blood pressure)
  Phenoxybenzamine (Dibenzyline), 20-40 mg/d, po; long acting
Beta-adrenergic blocking agents*
  Propranolol (Inderal), 40 mg/d, po; used for tumors that secrete epinephrine, which causes tachycardia and dysrhythmias
Tyrosine inhibitors
  Alphamethylparatyrosine (AMPT), 1-2 g/d, po; interferes with catecholamine synthesis and decreases the amount of circulating catecholamines

ASSESSMENT: AREAS OF CONCERN

Respiratory concerns
Increased respiratory rate
Dyspnea

Circulation
Increased heart rate
Palpitations

*Beta-adrenergic blocking agents should be added only *after* alpha blockade has been achieved. Beta-adrenergic blockade alone may exacerbate hypertension.

Postural hypotension
Sustained hypertension
Paroxysmal hypertension

Food and fluid
Weight loss
Nausea
Anorexia
Hyperglycemia

Elimination
Glycosuria
Oliguria
Renal failure
Constipation

Neurosensory concerns
Tremor
Hyperreflexia

Nervousness
Paresthesia

Comfort and pain
Headache

Mobility
Muscle weakness

Sleep and rest
Inability to sleep

Psychosocial concerns
Anxiety

Hygiene and skin
Sweating
Warmth (heat intolerance)

NURSING DIAGNOSES and NURSING INTERVENTIONS

Nursing Diagnosis	Nursing Intervention
Tissue perfusion, alteration in: cardiopulmonary, renal	Monitor blood pressure and pulse (use same arm; routinely take them lying and either sitting or standing). Monitor renal output. In hypertensive crisis: Notify physician. Have emergency cardiac drugs available. Monitor blood pressure and pulse electronically. Perform actions that minimize hypertension: Do not palpate abdomen. Have patient avoid constrictive clothing. Elevate head of bed. Do not allow smoking. Eliminate caffeinated beverages.
Nutrition, alteration in: less than body requirements	Consult dietitian; provide nutritional meals, incorporating patient food preference. Give medications for nausea. Test urine for percent sugar, acetone, and protein.
Activity intolerance	Plan rest and activity schedule with patient daily. Assist with gradual position change from lying or sitting to standing.
Sleep pattern disturbance	Observe quantity of sleep; inquire about quality of sleep. Promote sleep and rest: private, darkened room; quiet, calm environment, and no disturbances while patient is asleep.
Coping, ineffective individual	Collaborate with mental health nurse specialist or psychiatrist as necessary. See also p. 1897.

Patient Education

1. Teach about medication action, schedule, dose, and side effects.
2. Teach importance of regular visits to physician and lifelong follow-up.
3. Instruct patient to carry or wear medical alert information.
4. Teach how to take and record blood pressure measurements.

EVALUATION

Patient Outcome	Data Indicating That Outcome is Reached
Tissue perfusion is normal.	Blood pressure and pulse are within normal range, both lying and standing or sitting. Output is 30 ml/h. There are no paresthesias, tremors, or palpitations.
Nutrition is adequate.	The patient verbalizes a decrease or absence of nausea. The patient maintains body weight in proportion to height and stature. There are no signs of dehydration. Urine chemistry levels are within normal limits.
Activity tolerance and sleep pattern improve.	The patient plans ADL schedule to alternate rest and activity. The patient participates in desired activities without fatigue. The patient verbalizes feeling of well-being after sleep.
The patient copes effectively.	The patient identifies strengths and uses them in ADL. The patient verbalizes ability to manage stressful situations or decrease their frequency. The patient maintains relationships with family and contemporaries. The patient participates in independent self-care.

PRADER-WILLI SYNDROME

The Prader-Labhart-Willi, or Prader-Willi, syndrome is characterized by hypotonia and failure to thrive during infancy, hypogonadism, obesity, short stature, and cognitive and behavioral disabilities. Individuals affected with the syndrome are motivated by the compulsion to eat food and nonfood substances.

The possibility of early death from complications of extreme obesity is a realistic threat. A continuing multidisciplinary approach is essential for diet maintenance and achieving optimal level of cognitive and behavioral abilities.

The cause of Prader-Willi syndrome is unknown. Many patients have abnormalities of chromosome 15. The significance of the chromosome 15 defect is unclear and presently under investigation. The Prader-Willi syndrome is not thought to be of genetic origin since familial incidence is extremely low.[32]

PATHOPHYSIOLOGY

Obesity, hypogonadism, and growth and developmental disorders may be attributed to a central nervous system disorder, possibly originating in the hypothalamus. A prenatal disturbance in the midline structures of the embryo or fetus may cause this hypothalamic dysfunction. Most Prader-Willi patients have delayed puberty and low levels of pituitary gonadotropins and basal luteinizing hormones. Testosterone levels are low in males, yet females may have normal estradiol levels.

Altered pubertal development may be explained as an inappropriate negative-feedback mechanism to the hypothalamic-pituitary axis. Obesity-related abnormalities of carbohydrate intolerance do not appear to have specific etiology related to this syndrome.[32]

The Prader-Willi syndrome may be broken down into two separate phases. The first phase begins in infancy and may last anywhere from a few months to 2 years of age. Characteristics typical of this phase are infantile hypotonia, poor sucking and swallowing abilities, weak or abnormal newborn cry, failure to thrive, and feeding and digestion problems. Physical characteristics such as hypogonadism, acromicria, poorly molded ears, almond-shaped eyes, and triangular mouth are observable in many cases. Treatment and intervention during this first phase are supportive in attempts to maintain nutrition, mobility, hydration, and stimulation needs. Many individuals remain undiagnosed throughout the first phase because signs and symptoms may be associated with a large variety of neonatal and pediatric conditions.[32]

Characteristics, behaviors, and needs associated with the second phase are discussed below.

TREATMENT PLAN

Supportive
Strict dietary management

ASSESSMENT: AREAS OF CONCERN

Musculoskeletal concerns
Short stature
Acromicria
Poor muscle tone

Food and fluids
Food-related behaviors: hoarding, stealing, hiding, and gorging
Frequent ingestion of nonfood stuffs
Continual nonsatiety

Neurosensory concerns
Mental retardation
Decreased pain threshold
Delayed developmental milestones

Sexual development
Hypogonadism
Poorly developed secondary sex characteristics

Safety
Frequent injuries: ingestion of nonfood stuffs
Self-mutilation

Behavioral concerns
Rapid mood swings
Temper tantrums
Poor socialization skills

Body appearance
Extreme obesity
Small forehead
Triangular mouth
Almond-shaped eyes

Family coping
Stresses related to altered physical environment and continual supervision
Unresolved feelings (grief, sorrow, guilt) related to diagnosis, food-related behaviors, and environmental changes

Hygiene and skin
Frequent ecchymosis
Frequent cellulitis
Persistent wounds and infections

NURSING DIAGNOSES and NURSING INTERVENTIONS

Nursing Diagnosis	Nursing Intervention
Self-concept, disturbance in: body image, self-esteem	Provide positive reinforcement for successful behavior. Encourage self-care and responsibility. Encourage appropriate decision making. Encourage appropriate educational and environmental experiences.
Skin integrity, impairment of: actual/potential	Discourage self-mutilating behaviors. Encourage personal hygiene. Provide skin care.
Thought processes, alteration in	Provide safe environment. Structure activities of daily living. Reduce confusing stimuli. Set limits.

Patient Education

1. Instruct parents in methods for maintaining skin integrity and daily hygiene.
2. Stress importance of the following, and assist parents in planning for:
   a. Continual supervision and observation
   b. Educational and environmental stimuli
   c. Environmental changes to increase safety
   d. Setting of behavior expectations and limits
3. Inform parents about and encourage use of support and counseling groups.

EVALUATION

Patient Outcome	Data Indicating That Outcome is Reached
Skin is intact.	Good hygiene is maintained. Patient demonstrates decreased self-mutilation. Wounds heal successfully.
Environment is safe.	Patient remains free of harm to self, others, and property. Behaviors are appropriate for IQ level. Patient demonstrates social behavior and positive coping mechanisms related to intellectual age.
Self-esteem improves.	Verbalizes improved feelings of self-worth. Demonstrates ability to cope with limitations at highest possible level of functioning. Demonstrates pride in self-care. Family participates in socialization experiences. Patient participates in IQ and age-related activities with others.

PRECOCIOUS PUBERTY

Pubertal maturation (Tanner stage II and on) is considered precocious or premature when it occurs earlier than three standard deviations from the norm for chronologic age.

The onset of puberty is influenced by numerous endogenous and exogenous variables, for example, heredity, nutrition, pathologic conditions, and ethnic culture. In the United States, breast development beginning before the age of 7.25 years or menses before 9.25 years is considered early. Testicular maturation before 9.1 years of age or penile development before 10.6 years is considered early for the male.[35] Complete progression of pubertal changes (i.e., growth spurt, rapid bone maturation, presence of sexual hair, genital and breast development) is necessary to conclude true precocious puberty (Fig. 8-20).

The occurrence of premature puberty is estimated at 1 in every 5000 to 10,000 births. The disorder more commonly occurs in girls, in whom it is often idiopathic or caused by a central nervous system (CNS) lesion. Precocious development in boys is generally caused by a hypothalamic hamartoma or other CNS lesion. True precocious puberty is found in a smaller population of children, whose primary diagnosis is congenital adrenal hyperplasia.

The following classifications of the causes of precocious puberty are arranged in descending order of occurrence in the population. These classifications include both true precocious puberty and precocious pseudopuberty.

Causes of Precocious Puberty in Boys

I. Central or peripheral nervous system disorders
   A. Tumors of the hypothalamic (suprasellar) area
      1. Hamartomas (benign)
      2. Astrocytomas
      3. Craniopharyngiomas
      4. Gliomas
      5. Gonadotropin-releasing hormone (GnRH) secreting adenomas
      6. Suprasellar or subarachnoid cysts
   B. Hydrocephalus and other congenital CNS abnormalities
   C. Neurofibromatosis: both central and peripheral lesions may be noted with "coast of California," café au lait skin pigmentation (von Recklinghausen's disease)
   D. Other CNS tumors (i.e., pinealoma, ganglioneuroma, ependymoma, teratomas)
   E. Inflammation or trauma (e.g., encephalitis)
   F. Fibrous dysplasia
II. Adrenal gland disorders
   A. Congenital adrenal hyperplasia (after delayed treatment)
      1. 21-Hydroxylase deficiency
      2. 11-Hydroxylase deficiency
   B. Steroid-producing adenoma or carcinoma (Cushing's syndrome; also from pituitary neoplasms)
III. Testicular disorders
   A. Leydig's cell hyperplasia (unilateral or bilateral)
   B. Familial precocious puberty (high testosterone seemingly independent of low gonadotropins)

Fig. 8-20
Boy and girl with precocious sexual development according to chronologic age (CA). Note discrepancies of height age and bone age (BA). **A,** Boy with familial precocious puberty. CA = 6 $^{10}/_{12}$ years; height = 148.26 cm (height age = 11.5 years); BA = 15 $^{6}/_{12}$ years; Tanner stage: pubic hair = IV; facial hair = light; testes = 23 to 25 cc in volume by orchidometer. Note facial acne, increased muscle bulk, and disproportioned extremities and trunk development. **B,** Girl with idiopathic true precocious puberty. CA = 4 $^{6}/_{12}$ years; height = 124.9 cm (height age = 7.75 years); BA = 11 years; Tanner stage: breasts = Tanner III to IV; pubic hair = Tanner III. Note pubertal pelvic contouring and fat distribution.

Courtesy National Institute of Child Health and Human Development.

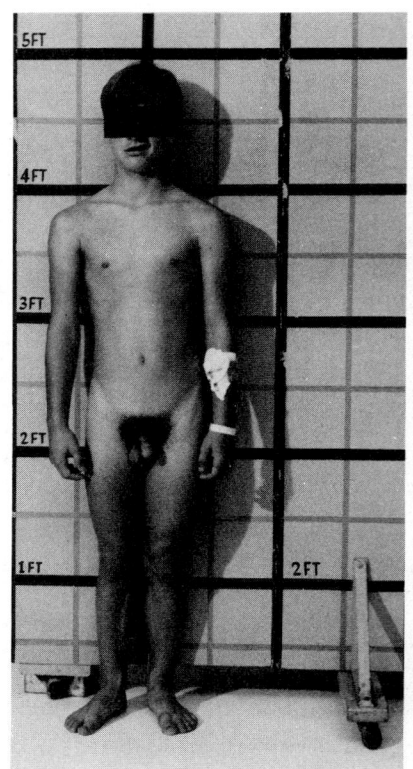
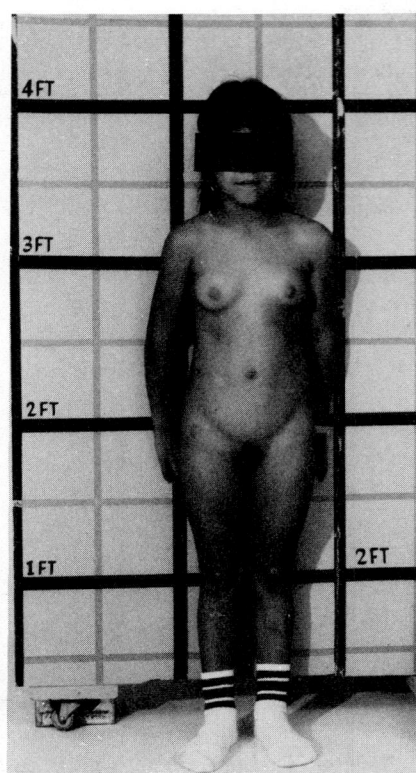

A   B

IV. Gonadotropin-secreting tumors (human chorionic gonadotropin [HCG] secreted)
 A. Hepatoblastomas
 B. Retroperitoneal carcinomas and polyembryomas[35]
V. Exogenous hormones (iatrogenic)
 A. Steroids: androgen creams or tablets
 B. Medications causing hirsutism (e.g., phenytoin [Dilantin])
VI. Hypothyroidism
VII. Idiopathic causes

Causes of Precocious Puberty in Girls

I. Idiopathic isosexual causes (etiology unclear)
 A. Premature breast development alone (thelarche); usually a temporary intermittent occurrence
 B. Premature sexual hair (pubarche)
 C. Complete precocious puberty
II. Central nervous system disorders
 A. Tumors of the hypothalamic (suprasellar) area
  1. Hamartomas (benign)
  2. Astrocytomas
  3. Craniopharyngiomas
  4. Gliomas
  5. GnRH-secreting adenomas
  6. Suprasellar or subarachnoid cysts
 B. Hydrocephalus and other congenital CNS abnormalities
 C. Neurofibromatosis: both central and peripheral lesions may be noted with "coast of California," café au lait skin pigmentation (von Recklinghausen's disease)
 D. Other CNS tumors (i.e., pinealoma, ganglioneuroma, ependymoma, teratomas)
 E. Inflammation or trauma (e.g., encephalitis)
 F. McCune-Albright syndrome: fibrous dysplasia; "coast of Maine," café au lait pigmentation; bilateral or unilateral cystic ovaries; seemingly gonadotropin independent
III. Adrenal gland disorders
 A. Congenital adrenal hyperplasia (after delayed treatment)
  1. 21-Hydroxylase deficiency
  2. 11-Hydroxylase deficiency
  3. Premature adrenarche: elevated urine 17-ketosteroids and plasma dehydroepiandro-

sterone (DHA) and dehydroepiandroste-rone sulfate (DHAS) (possibly from adre-nocorticotropic hormone [ACTH] secreting neoplasms)
  B. Steroid-producing adenoma or carcinoma (Cushing's syndrome; also from pituitary neo-plasms)
IV. Exogenous hormones (iatrogenic)
  A. Steroids: birth control pills and estrogen creams
  B. Medications causing hirsutism (e.g., phenyt-oin [Dilantin])
V. Ovarian disorders
  A. Estrogen-secreting neoplasms
  B. McCune-Albright syndrome (see above)
VI. Hypothyroidism
VII. Gonadotropin-secreting tumors
VIII. Familial true precocious puberty: elevation of go-nadotropins and sex steroids

The most distressing features of precocious puberty are the eventual adult short stature and altered peer re-lationships caused by early development of secondary sexual characteristics. In the presence of elevated sex steroids, namely testosterone and estrogen, these children experience an early adolescent growth spurt with rapid maturation and closure of the epiphyses of the long bones, therefore never reaching their potential height.

Because they appear older than their chronologic age they are often thoughtlessly expected to behave more maturely. Some children possess a high-average to above-average IQ and are comfortably advanced scho-lastically.[51] However, teasing from peers magnifies the emotional turmoil of adolescence, which occurs before its time.

PATHOPHYSIOLOGY

The mechanism controlling the onset of age-appropriate puberty and precocious puberty remains unclear. Puberty occurs when there is an interruption in the inhibitory control of the hypothalamus. This causes a pulsatile re-lease of GnRH to stimulate the pituitary receptors to release luteinizing hormone (LH) and follicle-stimulating hormone (FSH). When pulsations of GnRH reach ap-propriate amplitude and frequency, the gonadotropins are released in pulses to cause gonadal maturation. In turn the gonads secrete sex steroids, which provide negative feedback to the hypothalamus and pituitary.

True precocious puberty is also known as complete or central precocious puberty. It is differentiated from pseu-dopuberty (incomplete) by demonstrable maturation of the hypothalamic-pituitary-gonadal axis. Pubertal levels of serum gonadotropin (LH, FSH) and sex steroids (tes-

tosterone and estrogen) can be measured on assay in true precocious puberty. This evidence suggests that the go-nads are receiving timely hormonal stimulation from the pituitary via LH and FSH and in response secrete sex steroids. The sex steroids in turn provide negative feed-back, as shown in Fig. 8-14. When gonadal hormones decrease, GnRH is secreted from the hypothalamus, causing increased pulsatile secretion of LH and FSH. This sensitive relationship is responsible for maintaining and progressing pubertal development.

In the presence of excessive sex hormones, bone age advances above chronologic age[17] and gonadal tissues mature. Bone age is considered advanced when it falls above two standard deviations for the chronologic age. With rapid longitudinal growth, small muscle and tendon development may not be as quick to mature; although the child has increased muscle bulk, coordination may be delayed, but with time this will improve.

Children with precocious pseudopuberty generally do not possess the mature hypothalamic-pituitary-gonadal axia and elevation of all pubertal hormones. In pseudo-puberty the child may have only breast development or only sexual hair growth. Gonadotropin levels are low, but sex steroid levels are often elevated. The cause may be exogenous sources of sex steroids (e.g., birth control pills), neoplasms, or gonadal disorders. In a young girl with isolated occurrences of vaginal bleeding the cause is often a vaginal foreign body or trauma. Breast devel-opment in pseudopuberty may be of an on-and-off nature. This is a common finding; however, the etiology may not be discernible.

Past treatments for early activation of pubertal hor-mones included synthetic progesterones and antiandro-gens, which were effective in stopping menses. However, they were only somewhat effective in decreasing breast and penile tissue and did little to delay the rapid bone maturation and epiphyseal closure. Current research with GnRH agonists has been more promising.[17] These are administered by subcutaneous injections and nasal sprays. With increased knowledge into the exact patho-physiology of the various forms of true precocious pu-berty and precocious pseudopuberty, more specific and effective treatments are being designed.

DIAGNOSTIC STUDIES

Skull films, cerebral CT scan (sella turcica region), or pneumoencephalogram
  Related to pathologic findings (e.g., dysplasia, neo-plasm, hydrocephalus); otherwise, negative study

Bone age
  Advanced skeletal age compared to chronologic age

Blood and urine baseline levels and stimulated gonadotropins and sex steroids (i.e., GnRH)

Elevated values for age; helpful in differential diagnosis (e.g., male familial precocious puberty shows low gonadotropins in the presence of high testosterone)

Ultrasound

Girls: pelvic ultrasound

Uterus and ovaries large for age and possibly cystic

Boys: testicular ultrasound

Testes large for age and possibly demonstrating hyperplasia or a neoplasm

Maturation index (vaginal smear)

Percent intermediate and superficial cells in pubertal range related to estrogen excess

TREATMENT PLAN

Surgical

Possible excision or biopsy of tumor

Chemotherapeutic

True precocious puberty

Progestational steroids

Medroxyprogesterone acetate (Provera), 50-400 mg/mo, IM, or 5-20 mg/d, po

GnRH agonists (investigational), dose related to agonist and form

Cyproterone acetate (not available for use in United States), approximately 100 mg/m²/d, po

Incomplete pseudopuberty

Congenital adrenal hyperplasia (p. 850)

Sex steroid antagonists and aromatase inhibitors (effectiveness questionable)

The medication of choice is governed by the cause of the precocious puberty and whether it is complete or incomplete. Treatment of complete precocious puberty requires suppression of the pituitary secretion of gonadotropins or use of synthetic progesterones and antiandrogens or both. Investigational LHRH agonists have proven effective in establishing prepubertal gonadotropin levels, presumably by uncoupling of pituitary LHRH receptors. Presently the agonists are administered subcutaneously or intranasally every evening. Synthetic progesterones and antiandrogens are indicated to reduce sex hormone levels. They are also indicated in cases of incomplete precocious puberty in which elevated sex hormones are causing sexual development.

Use of synthetic progesterones is contraindicated in children with adrenal disorders, in whom administration of these progestins may lead to further adrenal suppression. Injections may also cause localized irritation; nasal sprays may cause sinus irritation.

Electromechanical

Radiologic follow-up of precocious puberty

Supportive

Patient and family referrals

Social worker

Dietitian

Pharmacy

ASSESSMENT: AREAS OF CONCERN

Sexual development

Presence of advanced height and sexual development (by Tanner stage) for age; may be isolated (e.g., hirsutism or breast tissue only)

Height and age of onset of puberty in child, parents, and other family members may show familial pattern

Possible consumption of birth control pills or other exogenous form of sex steroids

Neurologic functioning

Age-appropriate milestones met

Child is clumsy, stumbles, has variable muscle strength and tone

Psychosocial concerns

Child is hyperactive or withdrawn, is sexually aggressive, masturbates, and is rebellious, moody, self-conscious, and teased by peers

Incomplete understanding of early development, potential growth, and treatment options by parent and child

Child displays adolescent behavior, prefers older peer group, is easily frustrated with demands of others

NURSING DIAGNOSES and NURSING INTERVENTIONS

Nursing Diagnosis	Nursing Intervention
Knowledge deficit related to diagnosis and treatment	Assess understanding of normal and early puberty and treatment options. Encourage questions and verbalization of concerns. Role play discussing precocious puberty with others and help family identify support systems.

Nursing Diagnosis	Nursing Intervention
	Provide literature and positive feedback.
	Determine acceptable treatment and discuss follow-up care.
	Follow up on identified deficits and assess compliance.
Self-concept, disturbance in: body image	Encourage verbalization of feelings; help to identify frustrations.
	Help patient and family to establish a plan to improve interpersonal relationships.
	Provide teaching regarding early development with parallel to age-appropriate emotional development.
	Provide social work referral as appropriate.
	Assess and help patient to identify problems with interpersonal relationships.
	Encourage contacts with other well-adjusted families of children with precocious puberty.

Patient Education

1. Provide literature outlining treatment, side effects, and follow-up.
2. Inform patient and family of all necessary testing.

EVALUATION

Patient Outcome	Data Indicating That Outcome is Reached
Patient and family display and verbalize acceptance of early development and chosen treatment.	Child is treated age appropriately.
	Child and family comply with treatment regimen.
	Child and family are able to verbalize accurate understanding of early development.
Child and family are comfortable with interpersonal relationships.	Family is able to identify support systems.
	Child is able to establish positive interpersonal peer relationships and displays improved self-concept.

SYNDROME OF INAPPROPRIATE ANTIDIURETIC HORMONE (SIADH)

The syndrome of the inappropriate secretion of antidiuretic hormone is the continuous secretion of antidiuretic hormone when plasma osmolality is low, that is, at a time when ADH secretion should be inhibitied.[73]

Syndrome of inappropriate antidiuretic hormone (SIADH) was first described by Schwartz at the National Institutes of Health in 1957. It is one of the most common causes of hyponatremia. Etiologies include head trauma, central nervous system neoplasms, pulmonary diseases, certain endocrinopathies, and some pharmacologic agents such as morphine and barbiturates. The following outline provides a complete listing of conditions that may predispose a patient to SIADH[71,73]:

1. Central nervous system
   a. Brain tumor
   b. Head trauma
   c. Subarachnoid hemorrhage
   d. Infections
      (1) Meningitis
      (2) Encephalitis
      (3) Abscess
   e. Guillain-Barré syndrome
   f. Acute intermittent porphyria
   g. Cerebellar and cerebral atrophy
   h. Cavernous sinus thrombosis
   i. Neonatal hypoxia
   j. Rocky Mountain spotted fever
   k. Delirium tremens
2. Pulmonary disorders
   a. Pneumonia
   b. Tuberculosis
   c. Cystic fibrosis
   d. Cavitation (aspergillosis)
   e. Abscess
   f. Empyema
   g. Pneumothorax
   h. Asthma
   i. Positive pressure breathing

3. Hypovolemia and hypotension
   a. Sodium-losing renal disease
   b. Adrenal insufficiency
   c. Hemorrhage
4. Endocrinopathies
   a. Addison's disease
   b. Hypopituitarism
   c. Myxedema
5. Tumors producing ectopic ADH
   a. Mesothelioma
   b. Carcinoma of lung, duodenum, pancreas, ureter, bladder
   c. Thymoma
   d. Ewing's sarcoma
   e. Lymphoma
   f. Hodgkin's disease
   g. Prostatic carcinoma
6. Pharmacologic agents
   a. Drugs that increase tubular reabsorption of water
      (1) Vasopressin
      (2) Oxytocin
   b. Drugs that stimulate the release of ADH
      (1) Vincristine
      (2) Nicotine
      (3) Morphine
      (4) Barbiturates
      (5) General anesthesia
   c. Drugs potentiating the action of ADH
      (1) Chlorpropamide
      (2) Carbamazepine
      (3) Thiazide diuretics
      (4) Phenothiazines
7. Acute psychosis
8. Idiopathic causes

Antidiuretic hormone (ADH) can also be secreted by nonpituitary neoplasms such as oat cell carcinoma of the lung. The most common form of treatment is water restriction, but current research in the area is directed primarily at devising improved therapies. For example, lithium salts and demeclocycline have recently been shown to antagonize the effects of ADH and have found a place in the treatment of this syndrome.[42]

PATHOPHYSIOLOGY

The syndrome of inappropriate antidiuretic hormone occurs when there is continuous synthesis and release of ADH in the presence of serum hypo-osmolality. Normally, when plasma osmolality drops, production and release of ADH are reduced, resulting in a diuresis. In SIADH, antidiuretic hormone continues to be released in the face of a subnormal serum osmolality. This also results in a simultaneous urine osmolality that is greater than that of serum. Dilutional hyponatremia occurs in SIADH from an increase in tubular reabsorption of water. The retention of water causes an expansion of plasma volume. This increase in intravascular fluid causes an increase in the glomerular filtration rate, and the reabsorption of sodium and water in the renal tubules is inhibited. The expansion of the plasma volume also inhibits the release of renin and aldosterone. This further increases the loss of sodium in urine and intensifies the dilutional hyponatremia. Because SIADH results in the retention of free water and not salt, edema is not a feature of this disorder.[73]

DIAGNOSTIC STUDIES

Serum osmolality
Below normal

Urine osmolality
Above normal

Serum sodium
Below normal

TREATMENT PLAN

Chemotherapeutic
Diuretics
Furosemide (Lasix), 40-80 mg/d in divided doses, or 20-40 mg/d IV
Hypertonic saline, dosage individually calculated

Supportive
Fluid restriction

ASSESSMENT: AREAS OF CONCERN

Fluids and electrolytes
Decreased volume of urine
Increased specific gravity of urine
Increased weight
Abdominal and muscle cramping

Neurologic changes
Early sign: change in level of consciousness, confusion
Disorientation; uncooperativeness
Hostility
Decreased deep tendon reflexes
Seizure potential
Drowsiness
Lethargy
Headache

Cardiovascular changes
Tachycardia
Orthostatic hypotension

Gastrointestinal changes
Anorexia
Nausea and vomiting
Diarrhea (from water intoxication)
Constiptation (from fluid restriction and hyponatremia motility)

Psychosocial changes
Anxiety
Frustration
Irritability
Uncooperativeness
Hostility

NURSING DIAGNOSES and NURSING INTERVENTIONS

Nursing Diagnosis	Nursing Intervention
Fluid volume, alteration in: excess	Maintain strict fluid limitations; accurate by monitor intake and output. Monitor weight daily. Check specific gravity every 4 hours; assess for symptoms of water intoxication. Monitor environment to control patient's access to fluids; assess compliance.
Thought processes, alteration in	Check orientation to time, place, and person. Set limits as necessary to maintain stable and safe environment. Reduce confusing environmental stimuli. Explain rationale for disturbances in thought processes to family members.
Bowel elimination, alteration in: constipation	Give standard care.

Patient Education

1. Teach patient and family the rationale for fluid restrictions.
2. Teach patient and family the importance of measuring intake and output and how to do it.

EVALUATION

Patient Outcome	Data Indicating That Outcome is Reached
Fluid volume is normal.	Intake is approximately equal to output. Specific gravity is within normal limits. Vital signs are within normal limits. Weight of patient is stable.
Thought processes are normal.	The patient is oriented to time, place, and person. There is no injury to self, others, or property. Statements are reality oriented. The patient performs ADL, within physical limitations, independently.

TURNER'S SYNDROME

Turner's syndrome is a 45,X anomaly resulting in "streaked" gonads, short stature, primary amenorrhea, and sexual infantilism.[38]

This condition affects females and is caused by a genetic error in the formation of one of the sex chromosomes.

The incidence of the 45,X karyotype is estimated at 1 in 10,000 live female births. Approximately 95% of fetuses with this karyotype are spontaneously aborted. The occurrence of Turner's syndrome in a family is usually a sporadic event with no increased risk in later progeny. The prognosis for a normal life span is good, barring complications from cardiovascular defects and gonadal neoplasia.[7]

The affected individual may have some but not necessarily all of the following findings, the first four being the most common[33]:

Sterility
Short stature
Primary amenorrhea
Sexual infantilism
Low nuchal hairline
Hypoplastic, hyperconvex nails
Short or webbed neck
Pigmented nevi
Shield chest
Cubitus valgus
Hearing defects
Short metacarpals or metatarsals
High arched palate
Renal anomalies
Peripheral lymphedema
Micrognathia
Pectus excavatum
Epicanthal folds
Visual defects
Perceptual deficits
Cardiovascular anomalies
Skeletal abnormalities
Ptosis
Keloid formation

Various treatments are available to help improve the condition of the patient with Turner's syndrome. Surgery may be indicated for correction of cardiovascular defects and renal anomalies.[7] Anabolic steroids and growth hormone have been used in the treatment of short stature but do not significantly alter end height.[21] Esthetic surgery is sometimes performed to improve dysmorphic features, although it is not always advisable because of increased risk of keloid formation.[73] Perceptual deficits, such as in space-form recognition and directional sense,[73] can be detected by psychoeducational testing, followed by adjustments in teaching and learning patterns. Sensory defects may be improved by use of corrective lenses and hearing aids. Psychotherapy is beneficial in helping the individual with Turner's syndrome cope with poor self-image often associated with the findings of physical stigmata, short stature, and sterility.[7] Genetic counseling is advisable for the teenager.

The major long-term treatment of Turner's syndrome is the administration of female sex hormones. Secondary sex characteristics and normal menstrual periods can thus be attained. Cyclic hormone therapy should be started at the expected age of puberty or when linear growth has ceased, depending on the psychologic needs of the patient. It is continued until the usual age of menopause.[7]

PATHOPHYSIOLOGY

Complete monosomy for the X chromosome (XO) is most common in Turner's syndrome, yet there are variants and mosaic types with deletion of only part of the short arm of the second X.[22] Clinical findings may be fewer and less severe in these patients.

Karyotyping is the means of obtaining a definitive diagnosis and is of importance in discovering those with a Y-chromosome–bearing line. The Y bearers are at high risk for developing gonadal tumors; hence, early preventative surgery is required.[10]

It is suggested that the chromosomal error in Turner's syndrome results from nondisjunction during meiosis with loss of the sex chromosome from either the sperm or the ovary, or more likely, from an anaphase lag during mitosis (after fertilization), bringing about loss of the X or Y chromosome.[22] These missing genes cause various anomalies and prevent normal female sexual development.

Related disorders in Turner's syndrome include idiopathic hypertension, thyroid antibodies (hypothyroidism), diabetes mellitus, and rheumatoid arthritis.[73]

DIAGNOSTIC STUDIES

Karyotyping
Partial or complete deletion of the short arm of the X chromosome; definition of specific genetic pattern

TREATMENT PLAN

The medical plan depends on clinical findings and associated secondary diseases.

ASSESSMENT: AREAS OF CONCERN

Parent/infant bonding
Negative identification of infant's characteristics
No sensory stimulation given by parents
Difficulty in naming child
Incomplete plans for infant care

NURSING DIAGNOSES and NURSING INTERVENTIONS

Nursing Diagnosis	Nursing Intervention
Parenting, alteration in, actual/potential	Ask parents to tell you what they know about altered development; discuss and encourage questions. Encourage parents to verbalize fears and anxieties. Encourage parent-infant interactions and appropriate sensory stimulation. Discourage parents from discussing altered development as a disease. See also pp. 1919 and 1923.

Patient Education

1. Instruct parents regarding condition, cause, implications, treatments, and options to enhance choice of treatment and life-style.
2. Make information about resource and support groups available.

EVALUATION

Patient Outcome	Data Indicating That Outcome is Reached
Parenting is positive.	Parents verbalize understanding of altered development. Parents verbalize realistic expectations for child. Parents demonstrate positive parent-infant relationship. Parents use appropriate measures in caring for infant.

ZOLLINGER-ELLISON SYNDROME (ZES)

Zollinger-Ellison syndrome (ZES) is gastric acid hypersecretion and recurrent peptic ulcer disease caused by excessive gastrin secretion from pancreatic gamma (G) islet cell tumors or gastrinomas.

Although ZES is uncommon, it is not rare. Multiple endocrine neoplasia, type 1 (MEN I) is present in 25% of patients with ZES. Between 30% and 50% of gastrinomas occur as a single pancreatic tumor, most commonly in the head and tail section of the pancreas.[48] Sixty percent of ZES patients are men, usually between 20 and 50 years of age.[48] Gastrinomas vary in size and location, and up to two thirds are malignant. Usual sites of metastasis are lymph nodes, liver, spleen, bone, skin, and peritoneum.[48]

The mortality from ZES is high, not so much from metastases of the malignant tumor as from the extreme effects of hypergastrinemia and complications of ulcers: perforation, fistula formation, and hemorrhage.[48] Until recently, total gastrectomy was the only relatively successful treatment for ZES. The development of histamine H_2–receptor blocking agents since 1978 has shown promising possibilities for the management of ZES.

PATHOPHYSIOLOGY

The major effect of gastrin is the stimulation of hydrochloric acid secretion from parietal cells, possibly through stimulation of a histamine- or cyclic AMP–mediated process.[27a] The continuous high serum gastrin levels found in ZES produce a state of constant gastric acid hypersecretion, which exceeds the duodenum's capacity to neutralize it. This accounts for the upper gastrointestinal ulcerations found in sites as far distal to the stomach as the jejunum[48] and the presence of large amounts of fluid in both stomach and duodenum even in the fasting state.[27a] Parietal cell mass is increased because of the trophic effect of high serum gastrin levels, ultimately causing the development of prominent rugal folds in the stomach. The increased number of parietal cells in ZES is significant in the development of hyperacidity because a close relationship exists between the number of parietal cells and the amount of gastric acid secreted.[27a]

The diarrhea of ZES is caused by a number of factors:

1. Large amounts of hydrochloric acid irritate the gastrointestinal mucosa and increase peristalsis.

2. Gastrin has a direct influence on increasing intestinal motility.
3. Pancreatic lipase is inactivated in the presence of low intestinal pH and fat breakdown, and absorption is not accomplished.[70]
4. Precipitation of bile salts in the acid environment of the small intestine also prevents fat absorption.
5. The direct effect of gastrin stimulates gastric, pancreatic, liver, and intestinal secretion of water and electrolytes.[27a]
6. The malabsorption of a variety of substances is caused by inactivation of intestinal enzymes in the presence of acidity.

The ultimate results of these factors are diarrhea, steatorrhea, and the severe loss of potassium and magnesium that accompanies diarrhea in the ZES patient.

Gastrin is also known to cause moderate stimulation of pepsin release from gastric chief cells. In the presence of low pH in the proximal and distal duodenum and jejunum, pepsin only contributes to the development of mucosal ulcerations even at points as distal as the jejunum.

The secretion of gastrin by tumor tissue (gastrinomas) is not responsive to the normal inhibitory stimuli (low gastric pH and secretin), as is normal gastrin secretion. In the patient with ZES, secretin paradoxically stimulates gastrin release.

Gastrin also stimulates intrinsic factor secretion. However, in ZES, malabsorption of vitamin B_{12} is thought to result from the low intestinal pH, which may interfere with the action of intrinsic factor in facilitating the absorption of vitamin B_{12}.[48] This condition is not corrected by the administration of the intrinsic factor; only monthly vitamin B_{12} injections can ameliorate it.

DIAGNOSTIC STUDIES

Elevated serum gastrin
Level of 500 to 1000 pg/ml strongly suggestive of ZES; greater than 1000 pg/ml virtually diagnostic of ZES after exclusion of other disorders with hypergastrinemia

Provocative testing
Secretin
Serum gastrin rises by 400 pg/ml over basal value
Calcium infusion
Serum gastrin rises by 50% of basal value or by 500 pg/ml over basal value
Meal test
Positive if meal fails to increase gastrin by more than 50%

Gastric analysis
Basal acid concentration of greater than 15 mEq/hr in previously unoperated patient and greater than 5 mEq/hr in previous operated patients

Radiologic findings
Irregular thick gastric mucosal folds with ulcers at usual and unusual sites; pancreatic G islet cell tumor demonstrated by angiography

TREATMENT PLAN

Surgical
Total gastrectomy
Partial pancreatectomy (tumor excision)

Chemotherapeutic
Histamine H_2–receptor blocking agents
Cimetidine 300-600 mg q6h
Ranitidine 150 mg qid or qid and hs
Streptozoticin, 5-FU, doxorubicin (see cancer section) for treatment of malignant tumors with metastases

ASSESSMENT: AREAS OF CONCERN

Circulation
Decreased blood pressure
Tachycardia
Cold, clammy skin

Food and fluid
Burning, pain in epigastric region between meals
Coffee-ground or frank blood emesis
Thirst
Decreased appetite
Weight loss
Dry mouth

Elimination
Increased frequency of stools
Foul smelling, foamy stools
Abdominal cramping

Neurosensory
Restlessness
Impaired touch and temperature sensation and paresthesias of hands and feet
Unsteady gait
Hyperreflexia

Comfort and pain
Severe upper abdominal pain, may be referred to top of shoulders

Abdomen rigid and tender
Sore mouth

Hygiene and skin
Skin color sallow with lemon-yellow tint
Smooth, red, beefy tongue
Prematurely gray hair

Psychosocial
Feelings of helplessness

Decreased participation in outside-the-home activities because of diarrhea
Embarrassment

Teaching and learning
Lack of exposure to information about or unfamiliarity with Zollinger-Ellison syndrome and associated symptoms

NURSING DIAGNOSES and NURSING INTERVENTIONS

Nursing Diagnosis	Nursing Intervention
Fluid volume deficit: potential	Measure daily fluid loss in stools. Replace fluids with water, tea, carbonated beverages, gelatin, popsicles, and broth. Instruct patient regarding need to include foods high in potassium and magnesium to replace losses in diarrhea.
Nutrition, alteration in: changes in body requirements	Assess patient for symptoms of vitamin B_{12} deficiency. Administer vitamin B_{12} injections as ordered. Stress importance of follow-up and vitamin B_{12} injections as ordered to prevent deficiency.
Bowel elimination, alteration in: diarrhea	Measure fluid losses in diarrhea every day. Check with doctor for medication for perianal irritation from frequent stools. Replace lost fluid and electrolytes. Observe patient for signs and symptoms of dehydration, decreased potassium, and magnesium.
Coping, ineffective individual	Encourage open communication between patient and family members. Assist patient in identifying strengths and positive coping skills. Offer suggestions as to how patient can cope with problem areas and function away from home.

Patient Education

1. Make the patient aware of serious complications or changes that require medical attention (gastric bleeding, vitamin B_{12} deficiency).
2. Teach the patient the importance of fluid and electrolyte replacement for diarrhea to prevent dehydration and changes in electrolyte balance.
3. Teach the patient the need for strict medication compliance to maintain the status of healed ulcers and avoid pain.
4. Teach the patient the dose, schedule, action, and side effects of medication ordered, to ensure safe and effective use of medication.

EVALUATION

Patient Outcome	Data Indicating That Outcome is Reached
Fluid and electrolyte balance is maintained.	There is no hemorrhage. There are no changes in blood pressure or pulse. Patient verbalizes understanding of and complies with fluid and electrolyte (potassium, magnesium) replacement with diarrhea. There is no dehydration.

Patient Outcome	Data Indicating That Outcome is Reached
Patient has normal vitamin B_{12} levels.	Patient verbalizes understanding of and complies with vitamin B_{12} injections as ordered.
Patient has adapted to limitations imposed by disease.	Patient and family demonstrate open communication and problem-solving capabilities. Patient participates in support group. Patient functions at highest level in ADL.
Patient is knowledgeable about disease, symptoms, and treatment.	Patient and family verbalize understanding of disease and the causes of symptoms and their treatment. Patient demonstrates compliance with medication regime.

Medical Interventions

CRISIS INTERVENTION FOR ADRENAL INSUFFICIENCY

Description and Rationale

The patient experiencing adrenal crisis must receive adrenocorticosteroids. The response to IV cortisol can be dramatic. Nelson has reported blood pressure response from an unobtainable diastolic reading to one of over 80 after the initial dose of cortisol was given.[20] Therefore it is vital that the patient be treated with corticosteroids before other interventions, to enable the system to stabilize. The effects of corticosteroids on the electrolyte imbalance, hypovolemia, and blood pressure will become apparent quickly. An IV infusion of 5% dextrose in saline should be part of the therapy, since the patient will likely be hypoglycemic because of the vomiting, diarrhea, and lack of food. Dehydration also compounds the problem. Response to therapy is encouraging, and in fact, within 24 hours most patients are able to resume an oral course of corticosteroids.

Since most glucocorticoids exert some mineralocorticoid effect, additional mineralocorticoid is not always necessary.[20] Also, the sodium present in the IV fluid may be sufficient to restore a normal level.[73] However, if mineralocorticoid replacement is deemed necessary, desoxycorticosterone pivalate can be given intramuscularly.

Antibiotic therapy may also be necessary if the underlying cause of the adrenal crisis is infection.

Volume expanders may or may not be used, depending on how effective the steroid treatment and IV fluid are.

There is controversy in the literature regarding use of vasopressors to treat hypovolemic shock. Response to initial glucocorticoid infusion and IV therapy should be evaluated before employing the use of vasopressors.

Contraindications and Cautions

1. Complications associated with IV therapy
2. Danger of electrolyte imbalance as the potassium level responds to therapy

ASSESSMENT: AREAS OF CONCERN

Circulation
Hypotension
Shock
Hypovolemia

Food and fluid
Vomiting
Hyponatremia
Salt craving

Elimination
Decreased urine output
Diarrhea

Neurosensory concerns
Confusion
Restlessness

Mobility
Weakness

Psychosocial concerns
Anxiety

Teaching and learning
Lack of knowledge about medications and crisis

NURSING DIAGNOSES and NURSING INTERVENTIONS

Nursing Diagnosis	Nursing Intervention
Potential patient problem: susceptibility to infection	Keep patient in environment as free from stress as possible (low lighting, warm temperature, reduced noise level). Encourage frequent rest. Reinforce importance of medications to patient.
Potential patient problem: electrolyte balance, alteration	Encourage patient to choose foods high in sodium and low in potassium. Take apical pulse to detect cardiac arrhythmias. Employ means to combat nausea. Maintain intake and output records.
Tissue perfusion, alteration in: peripheral	Recognize early presyncopal signs (dizziness, lightheadedness, visual changes). Have patient change positions (from lying to sitting to standing) slowly. Take lying and standing blood pressures and pulses. Administer IV fluids as ordered. Monitor intake and output. Monitor vital signs frequently (every 15 to 30 minutes). Explain rationale for IV therapy to patient.
Sleep pattern disturbance	Do not disturb patient when sleeping. Encourage methods of achieving relaxation (back rub, warm milk, dark room). Allow for period of uninterrupted rest during the day. Decrease amount of external stimuli.
Fluid volume deficit, actual	Monitor intake and output. Observe for signs and symptoms of shock. Monitor vital signs frequently. Maintain IV line. Employ means to combat vomiting and diarrhea. Assess skin turgor.

Patient Education

1. Teach the patient the importance of avoiding obvious sources of infection, such as persons with infections.
2. Teach the patient the importance of and how to take medication regularly and in emergency situations.
3. Teach the steps to follow when early symptoms of crises are noted.
4. Teach the importance of regular medical follow-up and wearing medical identification.

EVALUATION

Patient Outcome	Data Indicating That Outcome is Reached
The patient is free of infection.	Temperature is within normal range. The patient has no signs or symptoms of infection. Glucocorticoid and mineralocorticoid levels are within therapeutic range.
Electrolytes are within the normal range.	Sodium and potassium blood levels are within normal limits.
Tissue perfusion is adequate.	The patient makes no statements concerning syncope. Peripheral pulses are adequate. Output equals intake. The patient adheres to activity limitations.
The sleep pattern is undisturbed.	The patient verbalizes and demonstrates methods of achieving relaxation. The patient verbalizes receiving an increased amount of sleep.
Hydration is adequate.	Urine output is greater than 40 ml/h. Blood pressure is maintained within normal limits. Skin is intact, and turgor is normal.

DIETARY MANAGEMENT FOR SELECT DISEASES

Description and Rationale

Diet therapy is the principal medical intervention for patients with Prader-Willi syndrome, glycogen storage diseases, and phenylketonuria (PKU).

In individuals with Prader-Willi syndrome a strict ketogenic diet of less calories than for other types of obesity is required to lose weight and maintain desired weight. Calorie allotment may begin at 6 to 8 kcal/cm of height per day, or it may be 300 kcal/d for children and 600 to 800 kcal/d for adolescents and adults. Weight maintenance may vary from 500 to 700 kcal/d for children and 700 to 1100 kcal/d for adolescents and adults.

The patient with impaired glyconeogenesis is unable to tolerate fasting and has frequent episodes of dehydration and hypoglycemia. Glycogen storage for tissue use is impaired.

Patients with galactosemia must eliminate milk, milk products, and lactose from the diet.

Patients with hereditary fructose intolerance must eliminate fruit, fruit juices, invert sugars, sorbitol, and levulose from the diet.

Patients with glycogen storage diseases must eat small, frequent meals, often requiring nocturnal nasogastric feedings of high glucose content to restore blood glucose levels. They may also require high starch content approximately every 3 hours while awake. The amount of glucose and starch supplements needed varies according to severity of symptomatology and age and weight of the individual.[72,73]

A phenylalanine-controlled diet is required for the child with PKU. This must be balanced with an adequate amount of protein, calories, vitamins, and minerals required for growth and development. Adjustments must be made periodically to allow for growth changes and health status.[1]

Contraindications and Cautions

1. Behavioral modification and exercise are helpful in treatment of Prader-Willi syndrome.
2. Close supervision of food intake is necessary in Prader-Willi syndrome and PKU.
3. Prolonged fasting and limited fluids must be avoided in patients with glycogen storage diseases.
4. Too much phenylalanine causes irreversible neurologic impairment.
5. Too little phenylalanine can cause tissue breakdown, leading to hypoglycemic convulsions and death.
6. Aspartame (Nutra-Sweet) is not allowed for children with PKU.

ASSESSMENT: AREAS OF CONCERN

Food and fluids
Positive vs. negative food-related behaviors
Satiety vs. nonsatiety
Weight loss
Appropriate weight maintenance
Adequate hydration

Psychosocial concerns
Positive vs. negative self-esteem and body image

Growth and development
Normal for age and sex

Family coping
Dietary adherence or noncompliance
Management of diet and child's behavior

Body secretions
Normal or abnormal odor to body secretions

Neurologic status
Normal or abnormal blood values
Normal or abnormal reflexes

Skin
Maintenance or loss of skin turgor

NURSING DIAGNOSES and NURSING INTERVENTIONS

Nursing Diagnosis	Nursing Intervention
Nutrition, alteration in: more than body requirements	For Prader-Willi syndrome: Lock food cabinets and refrigerators. Search for hidden food. Supervise and frequently observe. Weigh daily. For glycogen storage diseases: Give frequent feedings.

Nursing Diagnosis	Nursing Intervention
	Give nocturnal nasogastric feedings every 1 to 3 hours.
	Maintain fluid volume.
	Assess for hypoglycemia.
	For phenylketonuria:
	Use Lofenalac or Phenyl Free.
	Assess for continued signs or symptoms of increased phenylalanine.
	Assess skin condition, and check for eczema.
	Maintain fluid volume.
	Assess growth and development.
Noncompliance	Assess reason for noncompliance.
	Assist with alternate methods for coping with undesired side effects.

Patient Education

1. Teach prescribed diet to patient or care giver.
2. Stress importance of maintaining diet and signs and symptoms of exacerbation of condition to report.
3. Ensure that patient or care giver knows community resources to assist with compliance.
4. Teach integration of exercise into overall care program.
5. Instruct patient or care giver in method of administering nasogastric feedings (for patients with glycogen storage diseases).

EVALUATION

Patient Outcome	Data Indicating That Outcome is Reached
Dietary compliance is achieved.	Weight is toward range of normal for nutritional requirements.
	Environment is safe.
	The patient is fed adequately.
	There is no hypoglycemia.
	Skin integrity is maintained.
	Blood values are normal.
	Growth and development are progressing at optimal level.

FLUID AND ELECTROLYTE REPLACEMENT

Description and Rationale

In diabetic ketoacidosis (DKA) and hyperglycemic hyperosmolar nonketotic coma (HHNC), restoration of circulatory volume is needed to assure delivery of insulin to target tissues and to maintain cardiac output, blood pressure, and pulse and bring osmolarity back to normal.

Electrolytes lost in osmotic diuresis (in HHNC and DKA) must be replaced to prevent serious abnormalities in sodium, potassium, phosphorus, and magnesium.

Contraindications and Cautions

1. Cerebral edema
2. Overhydration
3. Elevated serum electrolytes as measured by laboratory analysis
4. Edema related to sodium excess

TREATMENT PLAN

Chemotherapeutic
Fluid replacement
Diabetic ketoacidosis (DKA)
One to two L of 0.9% normal saline over first 2 to 4 hours (rate: 500 to 1000 ml/h)
Four to five L of 0.45% saline over next 24 hours (rate: 175 to 250 ml/h)
After blood sugar brought to 250 mg/dl range, 5% dextrose in 0.45% saline is given (rate: 175 to 200 ml/h)
Hyperglycemic hyperosmolar nonketotic coma (HHNC)
One to two L of 0.9% normal over first 2 hours (rate: 500 to 1000 ml/h)

Four to six L of 0.45% saline over next 24 hours (rate: 175 to 250 ml/h)

After blood sugar brought to 250 mg/dl range, 5% dextrose in 0.45% saline is given (rate: 175 to 200 ml/h)

Electrolyte replacement

Sodium: replaced as intravenous fluid (normal saline)

Potassium: rate of administration is 20 to 30 mEq of potassium per liter of IV fluid

Phosphorus: replaced as a potassium salt in the intravenous fluid

ASSESSMENT: AREAS OF CONCERN

Circulatory concerns
Tachycardia
Venous distention; edema
Increased blood pressure
Coughing
Shock

Food and fluids
Intestinal cramping
Nausea

Elimination
Diarrhea

NURSING DIAGNOSES and NURSING INTERVENTIONS

Nursing Diagnosis	Nursing Intervention
Tissue perfusion, alteration in	Monitor blood pressure, pulse, and level of consciousness every 30 to 60 minutes.
	Assess for signs of overhydration and notify physician immediately of venous distention, increased blood pressure, coughing, or shortness of breath.
	Assess for signs of cerebral edema and notify physician immediately of headaches, convulsions, decreasing level of consciousness, or varying abnormalities in vital signs.
Potential patient problem: electrolyte imbalance	Assess patient for signs of increased or decreased serum electrolytes.
	Monitor pulse and blood pressure every 30 to 60 minutes.
	Monitor serum electrolyte levels.

EVALUATION

Patient Outcome	Data Indicating That Outcome is Reached
Circulation is normal.	The patient is not dehydrated.
	The patient is not overhydrated.
	Blood pressure and pulse are normal.
	The patient is not short of breath.
	IV fluids are replaced at a rate of 6 to 12 L over 24 hours.
	Intake and output are balanced.
	Level of consciousness is unchanged.
Electrolyte balance is maintained.	Electrolyte balance is maintained.
	Baseline ECG is normal.

GONADOTROPIN REPLACEMENT THERAPY

Description and Rationale

Human chorionic gonadotropin (HCG) is used to treat hypogonadal men interested in fertility. This drug is extracted from the urine of pregnant women; in men it acts like luteinizing hormone (LH) to stimulate androgen secretion by the testes. In partial gonadotropin deficiency only HCG is needed for testicular growth and spermatogenesis.

In complete gonadotropin deficiency, which occurs frequently in hypogonadotropic hypogonadism, the combination of FSH with HCG will allow for complete spermatogenesis. After 18 to 24 months, if the patient remains azoospermic and testicular size has not increased, follicle-stimulating hormone (FSH) is added to HCG. This drug is extracted from the urine of postmenopausal women.

Testosterone enanthate is used to induce virilization in prepubertal boys with hypogonadotropic hypogonadism or adult men who are no longer concerned with procreation.

Contraindications and Cautions

HCG is generally not given in the presence of the following conditions:

1. Precocious puberty
2. Prostatic carcinoma
3. Prior allergic reaction to HCG (rare)

FSH is generally not given in the presence of the following conditions:

1. Normal gonadotropin levels
2. Elevated gonadotropin levels indicating primary testicular failure

Testosterone is generally not given in the presence of the following conditions:

1. Patients with prostatic cancer
2. Patients with cardiac, renal, or hepatic disease

TREATMENT PLAN

Chemotherapeutic

Pituitary hormones

Chorionic gonadotropin (human chorionic gonadotropin; HCG) for injection, 1000-10,000 units; dosages individualized

Menotropins (HMG; human menopausal urinary gonadotropin), 75 units of FSH and 75 units of LH daily for 9-12 d

Androgenic agent: testosterone enanthate (Delatestryl), 200 mg IM q2-4 wk

ASSESSMENT: AREAS OF CONCERN

Testosterone
Genitalia
Initial effects of treatment (4 to 6 months)
Increase in testicular size

Maximum effects of treatment (4 to 5 years)
Increase in phallus size
Increase in libido

Body hair
Increase in Tanner stage in pubic area
Increase in chest, facial, and axillary hair

Muscular concerns
Muscle mass increase
Postinjection induration

Bone
Increase in size and strength

Vocal cords
Voice deepens

Psychosocial concerns
Initial (immediately)
Increase in libido
Increase in self-esteem
Increased confidence with both male and female peers
Improved body image

Human chorionic gonadotropin (HCG)
Testes
Initial (4 months)
Increase in size

Maximum (3 to 4 years)
Increase to 8 ml only if patient has complete hypogonadotropic hypogonadism; if partial hypogonadotropic hypogonadism, testicular size will exceed 8 ml

Leydig's cells
Initial (monthly)
Increased plasma testosterone

Minimum (8 to 12 months)
Sperm production

Maximum (3 to 4 years)

Human chorionic gonadotropin (HCG) and Human menopausal gonadotropin (HMG)
Testes
Initial (3 to 6 months)
Increase in size greater than 8 ml

Leydig's cells
Initial (3 to 6 months)
Sperm production

Maximum (3 to 4 years)

Chest
Gynecomastia possible

NURSING DIAGNOSES and NURSING INTERVENTIONS

Nursing Diagnosis	Nursing Intervention
Anxiety	Help patient identify areas causing anxiety and usual coping mechanisms. Encourage open communications with partner. Explore alternative coping behaviors. Provide patient education covering areas of concern. Ask patient about need for home health nurse visits for continued supervision of injections.

Patient Education

1. Teach name, dosage, action, schedule, side effects, and proper storage of medications.
2. Teach procedure for self intramuscular injection, including preparation and site rotation.
3. Teach method for collection of semen for analysis.
4. Stress importance of follow-up medical care.

EVALUATION

Patient Outcome	Data Indicating That Outcome is Reached
Anxiety decreases.	The patient discusses feelings surrounding need for treatment. The patient continues open communication with partner regarding body changes. The patient complies with medical treatment program.
The patient complies with intramuscular injection of gonadotropins.	The patient is able to prepare medication and do self-injection without hesitancy or difficulty. The spouse demonstrates preparation of medication, injection, site rotation, and disposal of equipment.

PARTIAL PANCREATECTOMY: INSULINOMA AND GASTRINOMA

Description and Rationale

Surgery is the treatment of choice for both insulinoma and gastrinoma. Preoperative localization of the tumor by CT scan or arteriography is preferable and increases the chance of successful surgery, but it is sometimes difficult. In the case of unsuccessful surgery or when the tumor has metastasized, symptoms should be controlled by medical means, diet and medication. In infants with nesidioblastosis, an 80% pancreatectomy usually relieves the hyperinsulinemia. Usually no more than 85% of the pancreas is resected to prevent malabsorption problems.

Contraindications and Cautions

1. With insulinoma, debilitated condition, extrapancreatic neoplasm, reactive hypoglycemia
2. With gastrinoma, active bleeding ulcer

ASSESSMENT: AREAS OF CONCERN

Circulation
Decreased blood pressure
Tachycardia
Pallor
Abdomen rigid and tender
Increasing abdominal girth

Food and fluid
Dry mouth
Nausea
Gas pain

Comfort and pain
Describes incisional pain
Splints, protects, or favors incisional area when moving

Skin

Redness, swelling at incision

Wound disruption

Drainage from incision

NURSING DIAGNOSES and NURSING INTERVENTIONS

Nursing Diagnosis	Nursing Intervention
Cardiac output, alteration in: decreased	Measure blood pressure, pulse, and respiratory rate every 2 to 4 hours. Observe patient for signs or symptoms of bleeding or shock. Check dressing and drainage tube every 1 to 4 hours postoperatively.
Nutrition, alteration in: changes in body requirements (gastrinoma)	Assess bowel sound every shift postoperatively. Stop feeding if pain, vomiting, or nausea occurs.
Comfort, alteration in: pain	Assess type, location, character, and duration of pain. Evaluate effectiveness of pain medication. Report sudden increase in incisional pain or abdominal pain.
Skin integrity, impairment of: actual	Observe incision site every shift for redness, swelling, and drainage. Report signs of wound infection or dehiscence immediately to doctor.

Patient Education

1. Teach the patient the signs and symptoms of wound infection to ensure prompt recognition of infection and increase the chance of early treatment and less spread of infection.
2. Teach the patient proper wound care to decrease the chance of infection.
3. Teach the patient the signs and symptoms and treatment of hypoglycemia (if surgery is unsuccessful) to ensure correct management and no loss of consciousness (insulinoma only).
4. Teach the patient the correct dose, schedule, purpose, and side effects to ensure safe and effective use of medication.

EVALUATION

Patient Outcome	Data Indicating That Outcome is Reached
The patient's normal nutrition requirements are met.	The patient progresses to regular diet postoperatively. There are prompt recognition and correct treatment of hypoglycemia (insulinoma only). The patient's blood sugar is within normal limits (insulinoma only).
The patient has tolerable pain related to incision that allows for activity as needed.	The patient verbalizes a decrease in pain. The patient participates in or initiates coughing, deep breathing activity. The patient requests pain medication as needed.
The incision heals without infection.	The patient has no redness, pain, swelling, or discharge from the incision. The wound edges are well approximated. The wound is afebrile.

RADIATION THERAPY FOR TREATMENT OF PITUITARY TUMORS

Description and Rationale

Radiation therapy is the use of 4500 to 5000 rads[25] of radiation in an attempt to destroy a pituitary adenoma and consequently reduce the elevated hormone levels in the blood to normal range. It is used as an alternative or adjunct to adenomaectomy. Indications include a pituitary tumor with little or no suprasellar extension, incomplete removal of the tumor with hypophysectomy, or regrowth of the tumor. Typically, radiation therapy reduces tumor size, but hormone levels do not always return completely to normal. It may take up to 2 years to see clinical results of radiation therapy.

Contraindications and Cautions

1. Optimally, radiation therapy is not used with tumors large enough to mandate treatment faster than radiation therapy can provide (e.g., those causing pressure on the optic nerve with ensuing partial blindness).
2. Often there is an initial acute inflammatory response[25] with possible hydrocephalus and exacerbation of symptoms.
3. Destruction of normal tissue (pituitary, hypothalamus, or cranial nerves) is possible.[36]
4. Pituitary tumors occasionally turn out to be radioresistant.[25]

ASSESSMENT: AREAS OF CONCERN

Neurologic concerns
Headache

Neurologic status changes: increased blood pressure, pulse, and respirations; unequal pupils; abnormal pupil reaction to light; disorientation to person, place, and time

Skin
Scalp alopecia

Skin changes: scalp and facial dryness, redness, flaking, itching

Psychologic concerns
Level of anxiety initially and as therapy proceeds

Mobility
Decreased energy level

NURSING DIAGNOSES and NURSING INTERVENTIONS

Nursing Diagnosis	Nursing Intervention
Tissue perfusion, alteration in: cerebral (potential)	Monitor neurologic signs every 4 to 8 hours for evidence of increased intracranial pressure (especially important initially). Encourage patient to report headache immediately. Provide analgesics and other supportive measures (quiet environment, cool compresses, etc.) for headaches.
Skin integrity, impairment of: actual/potential	Instruct patient regarding skin care measures, including use of gentle soaps and shampoos and nonirritating creams. Exposure to sun should be minimized. If moist desquamation of the skin occurs, apply treatment (ointments, soaks) as ordered. Encourage use of wigs or scarves for alopecia.
Anxiety	Encourage discussion of concerns and feelings regarding therapy, including the length of time needed to see the results of therapy. Instruct patient and family on the theory of radiation therapy, including safety measures taken to safeguard normal body tissues, length of time needed to see results, and possible side effects. Instruct patient and family on the specifics of therapy, including the use of markings that cannot be washed off and therapy schedule. Instruct patient and family that skin changes, alopecia, and fatigue usually resolve once therapy is completed.
Activity intolerance	Help patient structure day to include frequent rest periods. Encourage patient to limit activities during radiation therapy period.

Patient Education

1. Instruct patient on the importance of returning consistently for follow-up.

EVALUATION

Patient Outcome	Data Indicating That Outcome is Reached
Cerebral tissue perfusion is adequate.	Neurologic signs are within normal limits. The patient will report no headache or no worsening of headache if it is present as baseline.
Skin integrity is unimpaired.	The patient uses appropriate skin care measures. The patient verbalizes decision to use or not use cosmetic devices to disguise alopecia.
Anxiety decreases.	The patient verbalizes concerns regarding radiation therapy. The patient states general and specific facts about radiation therapy. The patient exhibits no observable signs of anxiety.
Activity tolerance improves.	The patient uses stress-reducing methods routinely. The patient structures day to allow for rest periods and desired activities. The patient performs ADL within limitations imposed by underlying disease state. Statements about ''feeling tired'' are reduced.

EXOGENOUS GROWTH HORMONE INJECTIONS

Description and Rationale

Patients with isolated growth hormone deficiency and short stature may be treated successfully with exogenous growth hormone. When this external supply of human growth hormone is maintained in the body, an increased growth rate equal to or greater than 5 cm per year is expected.

Indications for treatment include the following:

1. Height below the first percentile of average growth for chronologic age
2. Delayed bone age of 2 or more years
3. Psychosocial complications related to short stature
4. Euthyroid state

Treatment may continue until significant height is obtained, or bone epiphyses become fused and future bone growth is no longer possible.

Contraindications and Cautions

1. Somatomedin generation disorders
2. Short stature secondary to other physiologic or psychosocial disease
3. Abnormal thyroid function

ASSESSMENT: AREAS OF CONCERN

Mobility
  Increased arm and leg span

Growth
  Increased height
  Attainment of physical and developmental milestones

Psychosocial concerns
  Improved ability to maintain independent ADL
  Improved age-appropriate physical appearance
  Positive self-esteem
  Adult:
  Appropriate onset of puberty
  Appropriate size of genitalia

Other complications related to injections
  Difficulty maintaining injection schedule
  Anxiety related to giving injection

NURSING DIAGNOSES and NURSING INTERVENTIONS

Nursing Diagnosis	Nursing Intervention
Knowledge deficit: (medical treatment)	Teach action, dose, and side effects of medication to be reported. Teach injection technique, time schedule, site rotation, comfort measures after injection, equipment, and medicine storage.

EVALUATION

Patient Outcome	Data Indicating That Outcome is Reached
Exogenous growth hormone is successfully administered.	Two individuals demonstrate proper injection technique. The patient verbalizes no discomfort after injection. Injection site is not infected. Growth continues at expected rate. Physical and developmental milestones are attained.

VENA CAVAL CATHETERIZATION (IN PHEOCHROMOCYTOMA)

Description and Rationale

In vena caval catheterization a radiopaque catheter is introduced into the vena cava through the femoral vein. The catheter is guided into the vena cava with fluoroscopic assistance. The procedure is performed to assist the surgeon to localize the tumor and rule out bilateral and multiple tumors. Venous samples are obtained from different sites along the vena cava for catecholamine determination.

Contraindications and Cautions

Patients with pheochromocytoma should receive alpha blockers before procedure to prevent catecholamine release and hypertensive crisis during the procedure.

Preprocedural Nursing Care

1. Give alpha blockers as prescribed.
2. Have cardiac arrest cart available.
3. Physician or nurse should accompany patient with supply of intravenous phentolamine.

ASSESSMENT: AREAS OF CONCERN

Circulation
Clot formation at catheter insertion site
Interruption in venous return
Blood loss from multiple sampling
Prophylactic IV therapy

Mobility
Flat in bed

Complications
Pulmonary embolus
Hematoma formation at insertion site

NURSING DIAGNOSES and NURSING INTERVENTIONS

Nursing Diagnosis	Nursing Intervention
Tissue perfusion, alteration in: peripheral	Monitor vital signs every 15 minutes for four times, every 30 minutes for two times, and then every hour for two times. Observe affected extremity for color, temperature, edema, and pedal pulses. Observe for hematoma formation, and notify physician. Keep patient flat in bed for 4 hours with no bending at hip.

EVALUATION

Patient Outcome	Data Indicating That Outcome is Reached
Tissue perfusion is normal.	Color and temperature of affected extremity are normal. There is no edema in affected extremity. Pedal pulses are present in affected extremity. There is no hematoma or bleeding at insertion site.

ADRENALECTOMY

Description and Rationale

Adrenalectomy is the removal of the adrenal gland. Unilateral adrenalectomy is the intervention for benign adrenal adenomas involving one gland. Adrenal carcinoma and ectopic adrenocorticotropic hormone (ACTH) producing tumors require bilateral adrenalectomy.

Contraindications and Cautions

1. Bilateral adrenalectomy dictates lifelong glucocorticoid and mineralocorticoid replacement.
2. Patients undergoing unilateral adrenalectomy will be adrenally insufficient immediately postoperative and will require glucocorticoid, but usually not mineralocorticoid, replacement for 6 months to 2 years or until the remaining adrenal recovers.
3. Hyperglycemia should be controlled before surgery.

4. Patients undergoing adrenalectomy may have hypoaldosternism or hyperkalemia after surgery.

Preprocedural Nursing Care

Administration of preoperative steroids

ASSESSMENT: AREAS OF CONCERN

Skin
Poor wound healing
Surgical incision

Complications
Adrenal insufficiency (potential)
Unresolved hypertension from primary aldosteronism may require continued treatment with medication

NURSING DIAGNOSES and NURSING INTERVENTIONS

Nursing Diagnosis	Nursing Intervention
Skin integrity, impairment of: actual	Inspect wound for edema, redness, warmth, induration, and drainage.
Potential patient problem: host defense, ineffective	Follow actions for adrenal insufficiency and for acute adrenal insufficiency when applicable.

Patient Education

1. Teach wound care.
2. Teach early recognition and treatment of adrenal insufficiency.
3. Teach how to use replacement steroids and emergency intramuscular injection of steroids.
4. Instruct patient to wear or carry medical alert information.

EVALUATION

Patient Outcome	Data Indicating That Outcome is Reached
The patient's wound is healed.	The patient's wound closed without redness, edema, warmth, or drainage.
The patient is adrenally sufficient.	The patient displays no symptoms of adrenal insufficiency.

SURGICAL REPAIR OF AMBIGUOUS GENITALIA IN FEMALES

Description and Rationale

Plastic surgery for repair of ambiguous genitalia is recommended before 1 year of age.[20] Because of variation in expression of virilization the repair can range from a minor clitoral recession to a major rebuilding of female genitalia. More complicated cases may require further surgery before puberty so that normal sexual function can be achieved. Early surgical repair helps prevent psychosocial problems for both the parents and child.

Contraindications and Cautions

If a female child is more than 3 years of age and has received wrong gender identification, it is recommended that male role be continued to prevent psychologic disturbances. In such cases external surgical repair to feminize genitalia is inadvisable, but removal of uterus and ovaries is indicated to prevent development of female secondary sex characteristics.[38]

ASSESSMENT: AREA OF CONCERN

Incision site
Redness
Swelling
Abnormal drainage
Fever
Loose or open sutures
Pain

NURSING DIAGNOSES and NURSING INTERVENTIONS

Nursing Diagnosis	Nursing Intervention
Skin integrity, impairment of: actual	Check incision site for signs of infection. Administer wound care as ordered. Do routine urinary catheter care.
Comfort, alteration in: pain	Assess degree of pain. Employ comfort measures. Give pain medications as needed.

Patient Education

1. Teach signs of infection to report: redness, swelling, foul or purulent discharge, and fever.
2. Teach signs and symptoms of urinary tract obstruction to report: pain, burning, urgency, frequency, oliguria, abdominal discomfort or pressure (from full bladder), and anuria.

EVALUATION

Patient Outcome	Data Indicating That Outcome is Reached
Skin is intact.	The surgical site is not infected. The surgical site heals.
Comfort increases.	The patient verbalizes a degree of relief from pain. The patient demonstrates relief from pain and discomfort by functioning at expected level.

EXCISION OF PHEOCHROMOCYTOMA

Description and Rationale

Resection of a pheochromocytoma may involve the removal of one or both adrenal glands.

Contraindications and Cautions

1. Alpha blockers or alpha and beta blockers in combination must be instituted preoperatively to control hypertension before and during the operative procedure.
2. Induction of anesthesia produces a release of catecholamines.
3. Intraoperative hypertension and hypotension occur during manipulation and removal of the tumor.

Preprocedural Nursing Care

Administer alpha and beta blockers

ASSESSMENT: AREAS OF CONCERN

Circulation
Hypotension
Reexpansion of peripheral circulation
Hypovolemia

Elimination
Oliguria

Complications
Postoperative shock

NURSING DIAGNOSES and NURSING INTERVENTIONS

Nursing Diagnosis	Nursing Intervention
Tissue perfusion, alteration in (hypotension, hypovolemia)	Monitor vital signs frequently. Administer adrenergics by IV line to maintain blood pressure in safe range. Note hypotensive effects of narcotics in the continued assessment of the patient. Record intake and output.

Patient Education

1. Teach medication action, schedule, dose, and side effects.
2. Teach signs and symptoms of disorder and need to report change in health status.
3. Ensure that patient understands the importance of regular reevaluations.
4. Stress that hypertension may persist after surgery until peripheral storage of catecholamines is depleted.

EVALUATION

Patient Outcome	Data Indicating That Outcome is Reached
Tissue perfusion is normal.	Vital signs remain stable. Output approximates intake. There are no symptoms of shock.

PARATHYROIDECTOMY

Description and Rationale

Surgical removal of hyperactive parathyroid tissue is the treatment of choice. Surgical techniques vary with different etiologies. When an adenoma is evident, surgical removal of the entire gland is necessary (there may be more than one adenoma present). Hyperplasia usually affects more than one gland; therefore three glands are removed completely, and three fourths of the remaining gland is removed, leaving enough tissue to maintain normal serum calcium levels.

Contraindications and Cautions

1. Contraindications for surgery
   a. Inability to locate the glands
   b. Underlying medical conditions such as renal failure or severe cardiac disorders
   c. Hypercalcemia from nonparathyroid etiology
2. Complications
   a. Hypocalcemia
   b. Edema
   c. Airway obstruction
   d. Paralysis of vocal cords

ASSESSMENT: AREAS OF CONCERN

Renal concerns
Adequate output

Cardiovascular concerns
Blood pressure irregularities
Bleeding

Respiratory concerns
Obstruction of airway
Edema of incisional area

Neuromuscular concerns
Paresthesias
Dysphagia
Laryngeal spasm
Tetany

Pain
Incision
Shoulder
Throat

Gastrointestinal concerns
Dietary tolerance
Calcium intake

Personality disturbances
Anxiety
Depression
Psychoses

NURSING DIAGNOSES and NURSING INTERVENTIONS

Nursing Diagnosis	Nursing Intervention
Potential patient problem: electrolyte imbalance	Monitor for dehydration. Weigh daily. Record intake and output. Check skin turgor. Check urine for pH, glucose, and protein. Monitor electrolytes.
Activity intolerance	Observe the patient for signs of pain with movement. Observe for steadiness on ambulation. Assist the patient with ambulation when necessary. When fractures are apparent, splint ribs while the patient turns or coughs. Handle the patient gently; allow him to move slowly.
Comfort, alteration in: pain	Assess which type of pain is to be treated. Administer pain medications as needed. Provide ice chips for pain from sore throat. Administer throat lozenges. Support neck when patient is turning or in a sitting position.
Nutrition, alteration in: less than body requirements	Monitor Chvostek's and Trousseau's signs for symptoms of hypocalcemia. Make high-calcium snacks available to patient at all times. Keep emergency calcium replacement medications available at bed side. Have dietitian discuss high-calcium diet with the patient.

Patient Education

1. Teach signs and symptoms of hypocalcemia (paresthesias, muscle cramps in extremities, and tingling in fingers and around the mouth) to report.
2. Instruct the patient in incisional care.
3. Teach body mechanics and importance of mobility, especially for patients with irreversible skeletal impairment.
4. Instruct patient about dietary supplements containing calcium and their use in treatment of hypocalcemia.
5. Instruct the patient about calcium replacement medications: actions, uses, side effects, and measures to use in case of emergencies.

EVALUATION

Patient Outcome	Data Indicating That Outcome is Reached
The patient complies with medical plan.	The patient reports decreased incidence of paresthesias and other signs and symptoms of hypocalcemia. Calcium level is 4.3 to 5.3 mEq/L. Phosphorus level is 1.8 to 2.6 mEq/L.
The patient tolerates increased activity.	The patient resumes ADL within limitations of underlying disease parameters.
Comfort increases.	There is no operative pain. The patient does not complain of a sore throat. The patient ambulates without statements of discomfort.

HYPOPHYSECTOMY

Description and Rationale

Surgical resection of the pituitary gland (hypophysectomy) is often necessary to treat tumors of the pituitary gland and craniopharyngiomas and for the palliation of metastatic breast and prostrate cancer.[74] Resection of pituitary microadenomas is often the treatment of choice for Cushing's disease and acromegaly. Emergency hypophysectomy is occasionally required to treat pituitary apoplexy.

The surgical approach to the pituitary gland is by the transsphenoidal or transfrontal approach. The transsphenoidal route is preferred because it provides direct access to the contents of the sella turcica, is relatively safe, and avoids disruption of intracranial structures. It is a well-tolerated procedure that produces no visible scarring. Transsphenoidal hypophysectomy is microscopic surgery performed with the patient in a semisitting position. A gum-line incision is made, a nasal speculum is introduced, and the surgeon has access to the pituitary gland through the sphenoid sinus and floor of the sella turcica.[74] Transfrontal craniotomy may be indicated if the tumor is inaccessible by the transsphenoidal route because of its geometry or because of anomalies of the carotid arteries obstructing access to the pituitary gland.

The indications for hypophysectomy include progressive deterioration of visual fields and increasing hydrocephalus in patients with sellar and parasellar tumors.

Contraindications and Cautions

1. Contraindications
   a. Sphenoidal or nasal infection
   b. Vascular anatomy preventing transsphenoidal approach (threat of damage to carotid arteries)
2. Complications
   a. Diabetes insipidus (40% of patients have transient diabetes insipidus following transsphenoidal hypophysectomy; 10% of patients have persistent diabetes insipidus following transsphenoidal hypophysectomy)[74]
   b. CSF rhinorrhea
   c. Meningitis
   d. Hypothalamic damage (with visual changes)
   e. Uncontrollable hemorrhage (carotid)

Preprocedural Nursing Care

Provide explanations regarding diagnostic testing and procedures (skull x-ray films, tomograms, angiograms, brain scans, urine collection, and blood work). Preoperative teaching specific to transsphenoidal hypophysectomy includes:

Presence of nasal packing postoperatively (2 or 3 days)

Mouth breathing while nasal packing in place

Moustache dressing

Graft site on thigh (muscle plug removed from thigh for packing dura)

Expected decrease in sensation of smell and taste (few months)

No toothbrushing (2 weeks postoperative); mouth care with saline or peroxide solution

Avoidance of coughing, sneezing, nose blowing, and bending over since these may affect muscle graft

Fluid restrictions possibly necessary

Possibly sent to ICU, surgical ICU, or neurosurgical ICU (variable with institution)

ASSESSMENT: AREAS OF CONCERN

Neurologic status

Visual changes

Changes in level of consciousness

Disorientation

Change in extremity strength or coordination

Postnasal drip (CSF rhinorrhea)

Fluid and electrolyte balance

Foley catheter for urine output accuracy

Polydipsia; intake

High fluid intake

Polyuria (200 ml/h)

Urine specific gravity (1.001 to 1.005)

Gum line incision

Redness, swelling, drainage

Thigh (graft site)

Redness, swelling, drainage

Psychosocial concerns

Anxiety

Air exchange

Difficulty breathing due to mouth breathing

Dry mouth

NURSING DIAGNOSES and NURSING INTERVENTIONS

Nursing Diagnosis	Nursing Intervention
Skin integrity, impairment of: actual	Check secretions from nasal drains; assess quality and quantity of drainage.
	Question patient about postnasal drip.
	Perform frequent oral care with normal saline or half strength H_2O_2 solution. Do not allow toothbrushing for 2 weeks, until sutures are healed.
	Apply petroleum jelly to prevent lips from cracking as a result of mouth breathing.
	Instruct patient to avoid sneezing, coughing, nose blowing, straining, and bending over.
Fluid volume deficit, potential	Monitor serum and urine osmolality and electrolytes. Check urine specific gravity.
	Closely measure and record intake and output.

Patient Education

1. Teach patient and family about hormonal replacement that may be indicated postoperatively.

EVALUATION

Patient Outcome	Data Indicating That Outcome is Reached
Healing progresses normally, and there is no infection at the postoperative site.	There are no signs or symptoms of infection at operative sites (gum line, thigh).
	Signs and symptoms of meningitis (i.e., nuchal rigidity, fever, headache) do not develop.
Fluid balance is normal.	Intake approximates output; weight is stable.
	Urine output is less than 200 ml/h.
	Specific gravity is 1.005 to 1.015.

SUBTOTAL THYROIDECTOMY

Description and Rationale

Surgery results in a decrease in excessive quantities of thyroid hormones through permanent removal of thyroid tissue. A subtotal thyroidectomy involves the removal of about five sixths of the gland. The remaining one sixth of the gland is then capable of providing sufficient hormones.[52] Thyroidectomy may be used for (1) patients with hyperthyroidism who do not follow the prescribed medical regimen; (2) patients with large goiters; (3) patients with drug reactions to antithyroid agents; (4) women and men of childbearing age who want to avoid radiation exposure; and (5) pregnant women whose disease cannot be managed with antithyroid drugs.

Contraindications and Cautions

1. Patients must be euthyroid at the time of surgery. They must be prepared before surgery with antithyroid drugs to bring them into a euthyroid state and with iodine preparations to reduce excessive vascularity of the gland.
2. Inadvertent removal or damage to the parathyroid glands may result in hypocalcemia and tetany.
3. Damage to the recurrent laryngeal nerves during surgery may result in aphonia or dysphonia because of vocal cord paralysis.
4. Permanent *hypo*thyroidism occurs in approximately 43% of all the surgical cases. It may develop years after subtotal thyroidectomy and is probably caused by progressive autoimmune thyroiditis of the thyroid remnant.[62]

ASSESSMENT: AREAS OF CONCERN

Respiratory status
 Tachypnea
 Abnormal breath sounds
 Increased restlessness
 Complaints of tightness in throat; inability to swallow; inability to get air; pressure or fullness in neck; dressing too tight
 Change in level of orientation

Circulatory status
 Variations in pulse and blood pressure readings
 Changes in skin condition: cool and clammy
 Increased swelling in tissue surrounding incision
 Decreased peripheral pulses
 Excessive bleeding on surgical dressing
 Hemorrhage

Electrolyte imbalance
 Dysphagia; laryngeal spasms
 Headache
 Positive Chvostek's or Trousseau's sign
 Tetany: muscular twitching
 Personality changes
 Complaints of numbness and tingling of lips, fingers, and toes

Laryngeal nerve damage
 Change in pitch and tone of voice
 Aphonia
 Hoarseness; weakness; "whispery" voice

Incision site
 Redness
 Swelling
 Drainage
 Fever
 Pain
 Guarding behavior
 Distraction behavior (restlessness, moaning)

NURSING DIAGNOSES and NURSING INTERVENTIONS

Nursing Diagnosis	Nursing Intervention
Cardiac output, potential alteration in: decreased (related to hemorrhage)	Monitor serum electrolytes, hemoglobin, and hematocrit values. Monitor pulse, blood pressure, color, and temperature. Monitor level of consciousness and orientation. Check dressing for evidence of excessive bleeding; watch for bleeding at side of neck and at back of head (immediately postoperative: check every hour).
Breathing pattern, potential ineffective	Monitor rate, depth, and character of respirations. Monitor level of consciousness. Monitor for apprehension, restlessness, and cyanosis. Keep suction equipment and tracheostomy set at *bedside*.

Nursing Diagnosis	Nursing Intervention
Sensory-perceptual alteration: electrolyte imbalance related to hypocalcemia	Observe closely for signs and symptoms of hypocalcemia and tetany. Check reflexes every 2 hours; check vital signs every 4 hours. Check Chvostek's and Trousseau's signs every 2 hours. Observe for changes in personality. Have 10% solution of calcium gluconate and equipment for IV administration at bedside or readily available.
Comfort, alteration in: pain	Place in semi-Fowler's position for ease in breathing. Monitor edema surrounding incision; apply ice collar when appropriate. Observe body language for evidence of pain. Log roll head and chest to prevent strain on sutures. Teach patient to support head and neck with folded towel during mobility.
Communication, impaired: verbal	Check pitch and tone of voice every 1 to 2 hours postoperatively. Discourage talking. Monitor for edema of glottis and surgical incision. Establish alternate means of communication (i.e., pad and pencil). Reassure patient that hoarseness (from edema or pressure) will subside in a few days.

Patient Education

1. Teach signs and symptoms of hyperthyroidism, hypothyroidism, and hypocalcemia to report.
2. Teach name, action, dosage, schedule, route of administration, and side effects of thyroid hormone replacement if ordered.
3. Teach care of the surgical incision.

EVALUATION

Patient Outcome	Data Indicating That Outcome is Reached
Cardiovascular function is normal.	Serum electrolytes, hemoglobin, and hematocrit are normal. The patient's skin remains warm and dry. The patient's vital signs remain stable. The patient remains oriented to person, place, and time.
Respiratory function is normal.	The patient demonstrates adequate respiratory depth and rate. The patient does not demonstrate cyanosis, dyspnea, or restlessness. The patient remains oriented to person, place, and time.
Electrolyte balance is normal.	Serum calcium levels are normal. Chvostek's and Trousseau's signs are negative. The patient remains oriented to person, place, and time. There are no signs of tetany.
Comfort increases.	The patient verbalizes decreased pain or relief from pain. Signs of edema at surgical incision are decreased or absent. The patient demonstrates adequate support of head and neck during rest and mobility.
Communication is normal or adequate.	Pitch and voice tone are normal. There are no voice changes (i.e., hoarseness). The patient utilizes alternate means of communication for voice preservation.

RADIOACTIVE IODINE (RAI)

Description and Rationale

The goal of radioactive iodine (RAI) therapy is the reduction in the amount of functioning thyroid tissue. Preparations used for radiation treatment include ^{131}I and ^{125}I. ^{131}I is most often used because it is less expensive and it normally requires only a single dose. Radiation treatment is less traumatic than surgery, causes no cosmetic disfigurement, and has fewer complications. The major disadvantages of this treatment are that a long period of time may be necessary before hyperthyroidism is ameliorated, hypothyroidism may develop, and there may be radiation effects to the body. RAI is the treatment of choice for Graves' disease, patients unable to tolerate antithyroid drugs, and patients whose Graves' disease recurs after thyroid surgery.

^{131}I is given to the patient after determination of the desired therapeutic dose. The dosage is determined by the severity of toxicity, size of the gland, and age of the patient. ^{131}I is available in a capsule form. Small doses may be given on an outpatient basis. Doses greater than 30 mCi (which are unusual) require hospitalization and radiation isolation. ^{131}I is readily taken up and stored in the thyroid gland, where it destroys its ability to synthesize hormones. ^{131}I also exerts a delayed effect on the ability of the thyroid cells to replicate. Full or conventional doses of RAI are recommended for patients over 50 years of age because of their limited life expectancy and their susceptibility to serious complications of hyperthyroidism such as thyrocardiac disease. Smaller doses are recommended for patients between 30 and 50 years of age. RAI is not recommended for use in infants and children because of its carcinogenic potential.

Contraindications and Cautions

1. ^{131}I crosses the placenta and can destroy the fetal thyroid. A pregnancy test should be performed on all women of childbearing age before treatment.
2. Pregnant nursing personnel should be restricted from contact with patients receiving radiation therapy.
3. Hypothyroidism is a consequence of RAI therapy. Rarer complications associated with RAI therapy include hypoparathyroidism, radiation thyroiditis, exacerbations of hyperthyroidism, and thyroid crisis.

4. Antithyroid drugs may be given before radiation therapy. Drug therapy must be discontinued 48 to 72 hours before the ^{131}I uptake is determined.
5. Iodides, iodide-containing drugs, and contrast agents should not be given before therapy.
6. After therapy, saliva, perspiration, urine, feces, vomitus, wound drainage, breast milk, and so on are radioactive.
7. Hyperthyroidism, increased swelling of the gland, pain, tenderness, and sore throat are signs of radiation thyroiditis. These signs may develop 1 to 2 weeks after therapy.

Preprocedural Nursing Care

1. Small doses of RAI are usually given on an outpatient basis. Special instructions are included under Patient Education.
2. Large doses of radioiodine require hospitalization and radiation isolation:
   a. Private room at least 6 feet away from other patients or traffic flow
   b. Special protective measures for caregivers: gowns, gloves, booties, dosimeter, radiation badges and consultation by radiation safety branch of hospital
   c. Special precautions regarding visitors (no children or pregnant women, etc.)

ASSESSMENT: AREAS OF CONCERN

Thyroid gland
Increased swelling
Tenderness and pain with pressure
Difficulty swallowing

Respiratory status
Dyspnea
Difficulty breathing

Psychosocial concerns
Body image alteration
Social isolation
Fear
Anxiety

NURSING DIAGNOSES and NURSING INTERVENTIONS

Nursing Diagnosis	Nursing Intervention
Self-concept, disturbance in: body image	Determine patient's knowledge and understanding of threat. Determine how patient perceives threat. Identify and reinforce patient's coping abilities. Encourage verbalization of fears and anger. Coordinate and mobilize resources to assist patient and family during and after reorganization.
Coping, ineffective individual (related to anxiety, fear, social isolation)	Listen attentively and provide atmosphere of acceptance. Reduce situations that might startle or frighten patient. Avoid discrepancies in timing, activities, and methods of performing procedures. Anticipate and provide for patient's needs. Encourage expression and discussion of feelings. Help patient clarify source(s) of anxiety. Help patient identify strengths and resources. Encourage patient to learn and use diversional activities. Encourage use of telephone to communicate with family and friends. Keep patient informed of daily reductions in radioactivity. Remind patient that isolation is limited.

Knowledge deficit (related to radiation isolation procedures)	Provide private room away from traffic flow. Keep door closed.
	Explain rationale for isolation and visitor limitations.
	Explain purpose of gowns, gloves, booties, dosimeter, and radiation badges.
	Explain all procedures for handling of secretions:
	  1. Saving of urine in special containers or lead pig and flushing of toilet three times after use.
	  2. Use of disposable eating utensils; rinsing sink out after brushing teeth
	  3. Special handling of linens
	  4. Special handling of trash
	  5. Special handling of emesis
	Have patient handle own specimens if able.
	Explain rationale for rotation of nursing personnel.
	Explain rationale for use of Geiger counter.
	Instruct patient concerning signs and symptoms to report.
	Establish and practice procedure for communicating with nursing personnel.
	Check on patient approximately every 2 hours or more often as determined by physical and emotional state.
	Establish patient's plan for diversional activities.

Patient Education

1. For an outpatient, stress:
   a. The importance of urinating frequently during the first 24 hours
   b. The avoidance of contact with others (especially children) (Suggest sleeping alone for at least 2 nights after following dose.)
   c. The avoidance of sharing eating utensils, kissing, and so on
   d. The importance of flushing the toilet three times after use
   e. The avoidance of breastfeeding for 1 week, followed by testing of milk for RAI before resumption
2. For an inpatient or outpatient, explain:
   a. Signs and symptoms of hypothyroidism, hypoparathyroidism, and radiation thyroiditis
   b. Importance of follow-up care

EVALUATION

Patient Outcome	Data Indicating That Outcome is Reached
Patient has adjusted to altered body image.	Patient verbalizes feelings and concerns regarding body image alteration. Patient accepts body image change at highest possible level.

Patient Outcome	Data Indicating That Outcome is Reached
Patient develops strategies for coping with anxiety, fear, or social isolation.	Patient demonstrates ability to cope with restrictions imposed by isolation. Patient verbalizes fears and concerns regarding radiation isolation. Patient identifies source(s) of anxiety and fears. Patient verbalizes decrease in or absence of anxiety and fear. Patient uses strategies to reduce anxiety and fear.
Patient understands radiation isolation procedure.	Patient verbalizes rationale for isolation, visitor restriction, and special radiation precautions. Patient verbalizes procedures for nursing personnel entering and leaving isolation room. Patient verbalizes or demonstrates procedures for handling of secretions. Patient verbalizes signs and symptoms to report. Patient verbalizes or demonstrates method(s) of communicating with nursing staff. Patient verbalizes fears or concerns regarding radiation isolation. Patient verbalizes diversional activities to be used during isolation.

References

1. Acosta, P.B., and Wenz, E.: Diet management of PKU for infants and preschool children, DHEW Pub. No. (HSAO) 78-5209, Rockville, Md., 1978, U.S. Government Printing Office.
2. Allen, M., and Makesh, V., editors: The pituitary: a current review, New York, 1977, Academic Press.
3. Amelar, R., and others: Male infertility, Philadelphia, 1977, W.B. Saunders Co.
4. Anderson, B.J.: Antidiuretic hormone: balance and imbalance, J. Neurosurg. Nurs. 11(2):71, 1978.
5. Arieff, A.I., and Felts, P., editors: Current concepts: hyperosmolar coma, Kalamazoo, Mich., 1974, A Scope Publication, Upjohn Co.
6. Bashan, N., et al.: Glycogenosis due to liver and muscle PK deficiency, Pediatric Research, 15:229, April, 1981.
7. Bergsma, D., editor: Birth defects compendium, ed. 2, New York, 1979, Alan R. Liss, Inc.
8. Biglieri, A., and Baxter, B.: The endocrinology of hypertension. In Felig, P., et al.: Endocrinology and metabolism, New York, 1981, McGraw-Hill Book Co.
9. Bloodworth, J.M.B., Jr.: Endocrine pathology—general and surgical, ed. 2, Baltimore, Md., 1982, The Williams & Wilkins Co.
10. Bondy, P.K., and Rosenberg, L.E.: Metabolic control and disease, ed. 8, Philadelphia, 1980, W.B. Saunders Co.
11. Brickman, A.S.: Diagnosis, classification and treatment of hypoparathyroid disorders, Nutley, N.J., 1982, Hoffman-LaRoche, Inc.
12. Brobeck, J., editor: Best and Taylor's physiological basis of medical practice, ed. 10, Baltimore, Md., 1979, The Williams & Wilkins Co.
13. Brook, C.G.D.: Practical pediatric endocrinology, New York, 1978, Grune & Stratton, Inc.
13a. Brown, J.D., and others: Pituitary pigmentary hormones, JAMA 240(12):1273-1276, 1978.
14. Chiumello, G., and Laron, L., editors: Recent progress in pediatric endocrinology, New York, 1977, Academic Press.
15. Clark, J., et al.: Drugs affecting the parathyroid and thyroid glands, St. Louis, 1982, The C.V. Mosby Co.
16. Cockett, A., and Urry, R., editors: Male infertility, New York, 1977, Grune & Stratton, Inc.
17. Comite, F., et al.: Short term treatment of idiopathic precocious puberty with a long-acting analogue of leuteinizing hormone–releasing hormone, N. Engl. J. Med. 305(26):1546, 1981.
18. Cornblath, M., and Schwartz, R.: Major problems in clinical pediatrics, vol. 3. Disorders of carbohydrate metabolism in infancy, Philadelphia, 1976, W.B. Saunders Co.
19. Daughaday, W.H.: The adenohypophysis. In Williams, R.H., editor: Textbook of endocrinology, ed. 6, Philadelphia, 1981, W.B. Saunders Co.
20. DeGroot, L., editor: Endocrinology, vol. 1-3, New York, 1979, Grune & Stratton, Inc.
21. deGrouchy, J., and Turleau, C.: Clinical atlas of human chromosomes, New York, 1977, John Wiley & Sons, Inc.
22. Dillon, R.S.: Handbook of endocrinology: diagnosis and management of endocrine and metabolic disorders, ed. 2, Philadelphia, 1980, Lea & Febiger.
23. DiMauro, S., and Eastwood, A.B.: Disorders of glycogen and lipid metabolism, Adv. Neurol. 17:123, 1977.
24. Ellenberg, M., and Rifkin, H., editors: Diabetes mellitus: theory and practice, ed. 3, New York, 1983, Medical Examination Publishing Co.
25. Felig, P., et al.: Endocrinology and metabolism, New York, 1981, McGraw-Hill Book Co.
25a. Findling, J.W.: Selective venous sampling for ACTH in Cushing's syndrome, Ann. Intern. Med. 94:647, 1981.
26. Frigley, M.S., and Luttge, W.G.: Human endocrinology: an interactive text, New York, 1982, Elsevier Biomedical.
26a. Galliard, R.C., and others: The antifertility steroid RU486 is an antiglucocorticoid depressing the pituitary-adrenal system in the human, The Ejndocrine Society, 1983 (Abstract).
27. Gotch, P.M.: Teaching patients about adrenal corticosteroids, Am. J. Nurs. 81:78, Jan. 1981.
27a. Greenburgh, N.J.: Gastrointestinal diseases, ed. 2, Chicago, 1981, Year Book Medical Publishers, Inc.
28. Guthrie, D.W., and Guthrie, R.A.: DKA: breaking a vicious cycle, Nurs. '78, p. 54, June 1978.
29. Hazelton Assay Services, Hazelton Laboratories America, Inc.
30. Herbert, P.: Self care after hypophysectomy, J. Neurosurg. Nurs. 11:118, 1979.
31. Hershman, J.M.: Endocrine pathophysiology: a patient oriented approach, ed. 2, Philadelphia, 1982, Lea & Febiger.
32. Holm, V.A., and Laurnen, E.L.: Prader-Willi syndrome and scoliosis, Dev. Med. Child Neurol. 23:192, 1981.
33. Jackson, L.G., and Schmike, R.N., editors: Clinical genetics: a source book for physicians, New York, 1979, John Wiley & Sons, Inc.
34. Joosten, R., et al.: Hyperosmolar nonketotic diabetic coma, Eur. J. Pediatr. 137:233, 1981.

35. Kaplan, S.A.: Clinical pediatric and adolescent endocrinology, Philadelphia, 1982, W.B. Saunders Co.

36. Kelly, P.P., and Tinsley, C.: Planning care for the patient receiving external radiation, Am. J. Nurs. **18:**338, 1981.

37. Kelly, S., editor: Metabolic, endocrine, and genetic disorders of children, vol. 2, New York, 1974, Harper & Row.

38. Kempe, C.H., Silver, H.K., and O'Brien, D.: Current pediatric diagnosis and treatment, ed. 7, Los Altos, Calif., 1982, Lange Medical Publications.

39. Kozak, G., editor: Clinical diabetes mellitus, Philadelphia, 1982, W.B. Saunders Co.

40. Krieger, D.T., and Bardin, C.W.: Current therapy in endocrinology, 1983-1984, Philadelphia and St. Louis, 1983, B.C. Decker, Inc., and The C.V. Mosby Co.

41. Krueger, J., and Ray, J.: Endocrine problems in nursing: a physiologic approach, St. Louis, 1976, The C.V. Mosby Co.

41a. Krupp, M.A., and Chatton, M.J.: Current medical diagnosis and treatment, Los Altos, Calif., 1984, Lange Medical Publications.

42. Loriaux, D.L.: Personal communication, 1983.

43. Loriaux, D.L., and Cutler, G.B.: Diseases of the adrenal gland, Unpublished manuscript, 1983.

43a. Luciano, D.S., Vander, A., and Sherman, J.: Human function and structure, New York, 1978, McGraw-Hill.

44. Lukert, B.P.: Hypercalcemia, Crit. Care Q. **3**(2):11, 1980.

45. Management of newborn infants with phenylketonuria, DHEW Pub. No. (HSA) 79-5211, Washington, D.C., 1979, U.S. Government Printing Office.

46. Marshall, W.A., and Tanner, J.M.: Variations in pattern of pubertal changes in girls, Arch. Dis. Child. **44:**291, 1964.

47. Marshall, W.A., and Tanner, J.M.: Variations in pattern of pubertal changes in boys, Arch. Dis. Child. **45:**13, 1970.

48. McGuigan, J.E.: The Zollinger Ellison syndrome. In Streisenger, M.H., and Fortran, J.S., editors: Gastrointestinal disease, ed. 2, Philadelphia, 1978, W.B. Saunders Co.

49. McKusick, V.: Mendelian inheritance in man: catalogs of autosomal dominant, autosomal recessive, and X-linked phenotypes, ed. 6, Baltimore, Md., 1983, The Johns Hopkins University Press.

50. Miller, P.: Primary aldosterone: a review of assessment, nursing diagnosis, and intervention, Dimensions Crit. Care Nurs., March-April 1984.

51. Money, J., and Walker, P.A.: Psychosexual development, maternalism, nonpromiscuity, and body image in 15 females with precocious puberty, Arch. Sex. Behav. **1**(1):45, 1971.

52. Muthe, N.C.: Endocrinology: a nursing approach, Boston, 1981, Little, Brown & Co.

53. National Diabetes Data Group: Classification and diagnosis of diabetes mellitus and other categories of glucose intolerance, Diabetes **28:**1042, 1979.

54. National Diabetes Data Group, NIADDK, National Institutes of Health: The prevalence and incidence of diabetes in the United States, Bethesda, Md., 1982, National Diabetes Data Group.

55. National Institutes of Health, Clinical Center: Clinical pathology cumulative survey, Bethesda, Md., Dec. 1982, The Institutes.

56. Nelson, D.H.: The adrenal cortex: physiological function and disease, vol. 18, Philadelphia, 1980, W.B. Saunders Co.

57. Nevins, S.K.: Pre and postoperative care of patients undergoing transphenoidal pituitary surgery, J. Neurosurg. Nurs. **8**(1):45, 1976.

58. O'Dorisio, T.M.: Hypercalcemic crisis, Heart Lung **7:**425, 1978.

59. Pang, S., et al.: A pilot newborn screening for congenital adrenal hyperplasia in Alaska, J. Clin. Endocrinol. Metab. **55:**413, 1982.

60. Pediatric laboratory sciences, Tarzana, Calif., 1981, Endocrine Sciences.

61. Reindollar, R.H., and McDonough, P.G.: Delayed sexual development: common causes and basic clinical approach, Pediatr. Ann. **10**(5):30, 1981.

62. Robbins, J.: Personal communication, 1984.

63. Root, A.W., and Reiter, E.O.: Evaluation and management of the child with delayed pubertal development, Fertil. Steril. **27:**745, 1976.

64. Rudolph, A., Hoffman, J., and Axelrod, S., editors: Pediatrics, Norwalk, Conn., 1982, Appleton-Century-Crofts.

65. Russo, L., and Moore, W.V.: A comparison of subcutaneous and intramuscular administration of human growth hormone in the therapy of growth hormone deficiency, J. Clin. Endocrinol. Metab. **55:**1003, 1982.

66. Sanford, S.J.: Dysfunction of the adrenal gland: physiologic considerations and nursing problems, Nurs. Clin. North Am. **15:**481, 1980.

67. Santiago, J.V., and Periera, M.: In Avioli, L.V., editor: Fasting hypoglycemia in adults, Arch. Intern. Med. **142:**465, 1982.

67a. Schulte, H.M., and others: The effect of corticotropin releasing factor on the anterior pituitary function of stalk sectioned cyanomalgus macaques—dose response of cortisol secretion, J. Clin. Endocrinol. Metab. **55**(4):810, 1982.

68. Sharkey, P.L., and Meyer, S.: Hypothyroidism, Crit. Care Update **8**(6):5, 1981.

69. Sharkey, P.L., and Meyer, S.: Hyperthyroidism, Crit. Care Update **8**(5):12, 1981.

70. Silver, H.K., et al.: Handbook of pediatrics, ed. 13, Los Altos, Calif., 1980, Lange Medical Publications.

71. Solomon, B.L.: The hypothalamus and the pituitary gland: an overview, Nurs. Clin. North Am. **15:**435, 1980.

72. Stanbury, J., et al.: The metabolic basis of inherited disease, New York, 1983, McGraw-Hill Book Co.

73. Williams, R., editor: Textbook of endocrinology, Philadelphia, 1981, W.B. Saunders Co.

74. Youmans, J.R., editor: Neurological surgery, vol. 6, ed. 2, Philadelphia, 1982, W.B. Saunders Co.

CHAPTER 9

Female Reproductive System

Overview

The major physiologic function of the reproductive system is the procreation of new life and perpetuation of the human species. This biologic process is primarily under endocrine control but is also influenced by neural and metabolic factors and by human sexuality. Not merely a biologic phenomenon, human sexuality is the sum of physical, functional, and psychologic attributes that are expressed by a person's gender identity and sexual behavior. These factors interact when gynecologic and reproductive processes or conditions threaten, alter, or interfere with female sexual integrity. The focus of this chapter is the female organ system. Selected female organ dysfunctions, interventions based on the nursing diagnosis, and treatment of the patient's responses to actual or potential health problems are discussed, as well as anatomy and physiology.

The comparative incidences of cancers involving the female reproductive organs have changed considerably in recent years. Endometrial cancer has replaced cervical cancer as the most common gynecologic malignancy. Some 39,000 cases of endometrial carcinoma are diagnosed each year, compared with 16,000 cases of invasive cervical cancer.[12,54] Although endometrial cancer can oc-

cur at any age, it is most common in women past the age of 50 years, with the peak incidence occurring at about 55 years. This is in contrast to cervical cancer, which most often occurs between the ages of 40 and 49 for invasive cancer and at an average age of 35 years for preinvasive cancer.[15] Cancer of the endometrium occurs predominantly in middle- and upper-class women, and a major risk factor is long-term unopposed exposure to estrogen. The incidence of cancer of the cervix is higher in sexually active women who began coitus before the age of 20, particularly those who were in their early teens at the age of first coitus. Multiparity increases the occurrence, and a history of multiple sex partners seems to be an important factor.[12,54]

Cancer of the breast is the leading cause of death in women 40 to 55 years of age. In 1982 more than 112,000 new cases were reported and more than 37,000 deaths occurred from the disease. In a small percentage of women breast cancer develops coincident with pregnancy, but most new cases occur in the decade before and the two decades after menopause (40 to 70 years of age).[12,54] Although little is known about the prevention of breast cancer, the chance for survival appears to be good if it is found early and treated promptly. Several factors are associated with an increased risk of breast cancer. The most common are age over 40 years, family history of breast cancer, nulliparity or first parity after age 34, previous cancer of one breast, and precancerous mastopathy type of fibrocystic disease.

There are 3 million pregnancies in the United States each year.[15] The majority result in healthy infants and require relatively little medical attention. However, many pregnancies do have adverse outcomes: at least 1% result in fetal deaths; about 1% of infants die within the first month of life; approximately 7% of infants have low birth weights that threaten survival or lead to complications in development; and nearly 5% of liveborn infants have a significant congenital malformation, birth defect, or genetic disorder.[54] During the past several years a variety of sophisticated techniques have been developed to diagnose fetal disorders and to manage high-risk pregnancies from the time of conception. Some of these techniques have become part of the routine care of all obstetric patients. This increase in the technological management of normal pregnancy has come into conflict with the movement toward natural childbirth and a general increase in concern about the adverse effects of technology, some of which may not be apparent for many years. In addition, techniques for antenatal diagnosis raise serious ethical, legal, and economic issues.

Although most pregnancies end with normal delivery, a sizable number are subject to active obstetric intervention through delivery by cesarean section. The proportion of cesarean deliveries has doubled since the mid-1960s to about 15%. Although the reasons for this are not clear, cesarean delivery is indicated when the intrauterine environment is no longer suitable for fetal development. Balancing the risk of premature delivery against the risk of leaving the fetus in utero is necessary when selecting an optimum time for intervention. Biophysical and biochemical techniques are of utmost importance to the obstetrician in assessing fetal health and maturation before making this decision.

The major risk of premature delivery is respiratory distress syndrome (RDS). The incidence of RDS has been estimated at 40,000 cases per year, and about 30% of these infants die. Prematurity also contributes to mental retardation, cerebral palsy, and other neurologic complications. Although preterm delivery occurs in less than 10% of the obstetric population, it is the cause for approximately 75% of perinatal morbidity and mortality.[11,12,42]

Infant mortality (under 1 year of age per 1000 live births) has steadily decreased from 19.2 in 1971 to 10.7 in 1984. Neonatal mortality (infants under 28 days of age) has declined from 14.3 per 1000 in 1971 to 6.9 in 1984.[39] The incidence of low birth weight infants and infant mortality is twice as high in black women as in white women. As unfavorable social and economic conditions improve, the racial difference in infant mortality and low birth weight infants will doubtless decrease.[42]

Approximately 1.5 million abortions are performed in the United States each year, with a rate of 1.9 abortion-related deaths per 100,000 abortions performed.[21,54] Morbidity associated with first-trimester abortion is less than that associated with all other contraceptive methods combined, causing this procedure to become a method of family planning.

Maternal deaths per 100,000 live births have decreased remarkably in the past half century, from 582.1 per 100,000 live births in 1935 (12,544 maternal deaths) to 8 per 100,000 live births in 1983 (290 maternal deaths).[40] The maternal mortality among black women is three times that among white women, primarily because of economic and social factors such as a relative lack of skilled personnel and appropriate facilities at delivery, lack of antepartum care, lack of family planning services, faulty health education, and dietary deficiencies. It is anticipated that maternal mortality will decrease as economic and social conditions improve.

ANATOMY AND PHYSIOLOGY

The female organ system consists of internal organs in the pelvic cavity and external organs in the perineum. The internal organs are the ovaries, fallopian tubes, uterus, and vagina. The external genitalia are the mons pubis, labia majora, labia minora, and the vestibule of the vagina (Fig. 9-1).

External Structures

The vulva includes all externally visible structures from the pubis to the perineum. These are the mons pubis, labia majora and minora, clitoris, vestibular glands, hymen, urethral opening, and perineum.

Mons pubis. The mons pubis or mons veneris is a cushionlike elevation of adipose tissue over the symphysis pubis. It is covered by pubic hair after puberty.

Labia majora. The labia majora are two rounded folds of adipose tissue with overlying skin that extend from the mons pubis downward and backward, encircle the vestibule, and merge into the perineum. The outer surfaces are covered by hair, and the inner surfaces containing sebaceous follicles are smooth and moist. The labia majora are homologous with the male scrotum.

Labia minora. The labia minora are two flat folds of skin medial to the labia majora. They are devoid of hair and are usually in contact with each other. They come together anteriorly at the frenulum of the clitoris and posteriorly at the frenulum of the labia.

Fig. 9-1

External female genitalia.

From Bobak, I.M., and Jensen, M.D.: Essentials of maternity nursing, St. Louis, 1984, The C.V. Mosby Co.

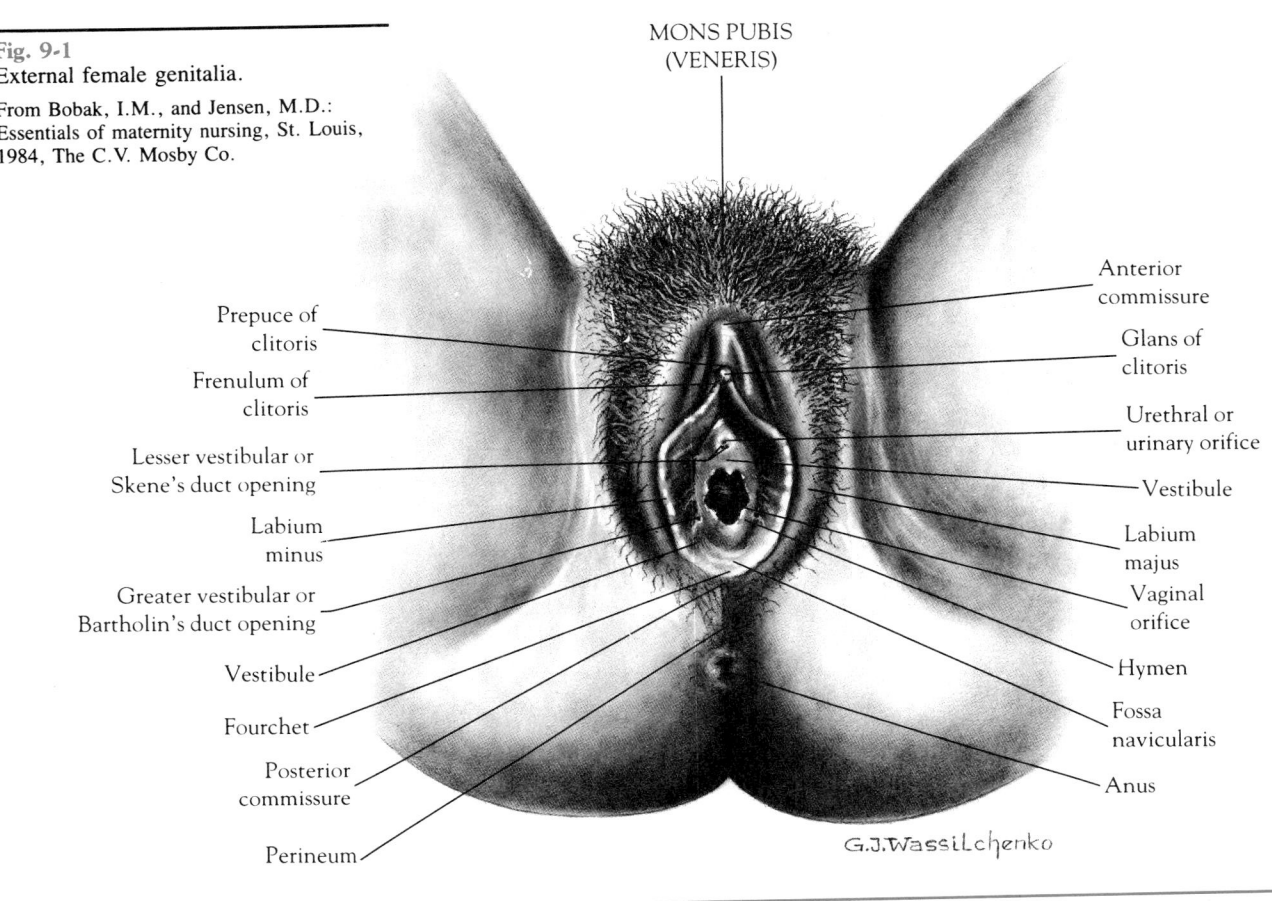

MONS PUBIS (VENERIS)

Prepuce of clitoris
Frenulum of clitoris
Lesser vestibular or Skene's duct opening
Labium minus
Greater vestibular or Bartholin's duct opening
Vestibule
Fourchet
Posterior commissure
Perineum

Anterior commissure
Glans of clitoris
Urethral or urinary orifice
Vestibule
Labium majus
Vaginal orifice
Hymen
Fossa navicularis
Anus

G.J.Wassilchenko

Clitoris. The clitoris, situated at the anterior end of the labia minora, is a small, cylindric, erectile body consisting of a glans, a body (corpus), and two crura. It is partially covered by the anterior ends of the labia minora and is very sensitive to tactile stimulation. It consists of two corpora cavernosa enclosed in a dense fibrous membrane that is made up of smooth muscle and elastic fibers. It is connected to the ischiopubic rami by two crura. The clitoris, which corresponds to the male penis, rarely exceeds 2 cm in length even in a state of erection during sexual arousal. The glans of the clitoris is covered by stratified epithelium that is richly supplied with free nerve endings within the fibers, terminating in small knoblike thickenings in or adjacent to the cells. Genital corpuscles, distributed in the glans and corpora, are considered the main mediators of erotic sensation.

Vestibule. The vestibule is the area between the labia minora. The hymen, vaginal orifice, urethral orifice, ducts of Bartholin's glands, and Skene's ducts are contained within the vestibule. The Bartholin's or greater vestibular glands secrete mucoid material during sexual excitement. They are on either side of the vaginal opening under the constrictor muscle of the vagina.

Urethral opening. The urethral opening or urinary meatus is in the midline of the vestibule posterior to the clitoris and anterior to the vaginal opening. The Skene's or paraurethral ducts open on the vestibule on either side of the urethra. Occasionally these openings are found on the posterior wall of the urethra just inside the meatus.

Hymen. The hymen is a fold of vascularized mucous membrane at the introitus of the vagina. It is not richly supplied with nerve fibers and has no glandular or muscular elements. The hymenal opening is usually very small in virgins who do not use tampons but is rarely imperforate, which would cause a retention of the menstrual discharge. During the first coitus or in certain other situations the hymen generally tears at several points. The edges of the tears soon cicatrize. Bleeding does not always occur when the hymen is ruptured.

Perineum. The perineum is a triangular area that is the inferior end of the trunk. It is situated dorsal to the pubic arch, superior to the tip of the coccyx, and lateral to the pubic and ischial rami. It supports and surrounds the distal portions of the urogenital and gastrointestinal tracts of the body. The central fibrous perineal body between the vagina and the anus divides the perineum into a posterior anal triangle and an anterior urogenital triangle.

Internal Structures

The internal organs include the ovaries, uterine (fallopian) tubes, uterus, and vagina.

Ovaries. The ovaries are two oval structures in the upper part of the pelvic cavity, between the uterus medially and the lateral pelvic wall. They are suspended from the posterosuperior surface of the broad ligaments by the mesovarium. During the childbearing years each ovary is 2.5 to 5 cm in length, 1.5 to 3 cm in breadth, and 0.6 to 1.5 cm in thickness. After menopause the ovaries diminish markedly in size.[12,45] In young women the ovary has a smooth, dull white surface through which glisten several small clear follicles. With advancing age the ovary becomes more corrugated, and in elderly women its exterior may appear convoluted. From the first

stages of development until after menopause the ovary undergoes constant change. From birth to puberty an estimated 200,000 to 400,000 oocytes are present.[24,42] It is evident that a few hundred ova suffice for reproduction, since ordinarily only one ovum is cast off during a menstrual cycle. The glandular elements of the ovaries are described as interstitial, thecal, and luteal cells. The interstitial glandular elements are formed from cells of the theca interna of degenerating follicles. The thecal glandular cells are formed from the theca interna of ripening follicles. Luteal cells are derived from granulosa cells of ovulated follicles and from undifferentiated stroma surrounding them.

The ovarian cycle and its hormones are discussed in greater detail later in the chapter.

Uterine (fallopian) tubes. The uterine (fallopian) tubes are two flexible, trumpet-shaped, muscular tubes that extend from the uterine cornua to the ovaries and provide the ova with access to the uterine cavity. They

Fig. 9-2
Midsagittal view of female pelvic organs with woman lying supine.

From Bobak, I.M., and Jensen, M.D.: Essentials of maternity nursing, St. Louis, 1984, The C.V. Mosby Co.

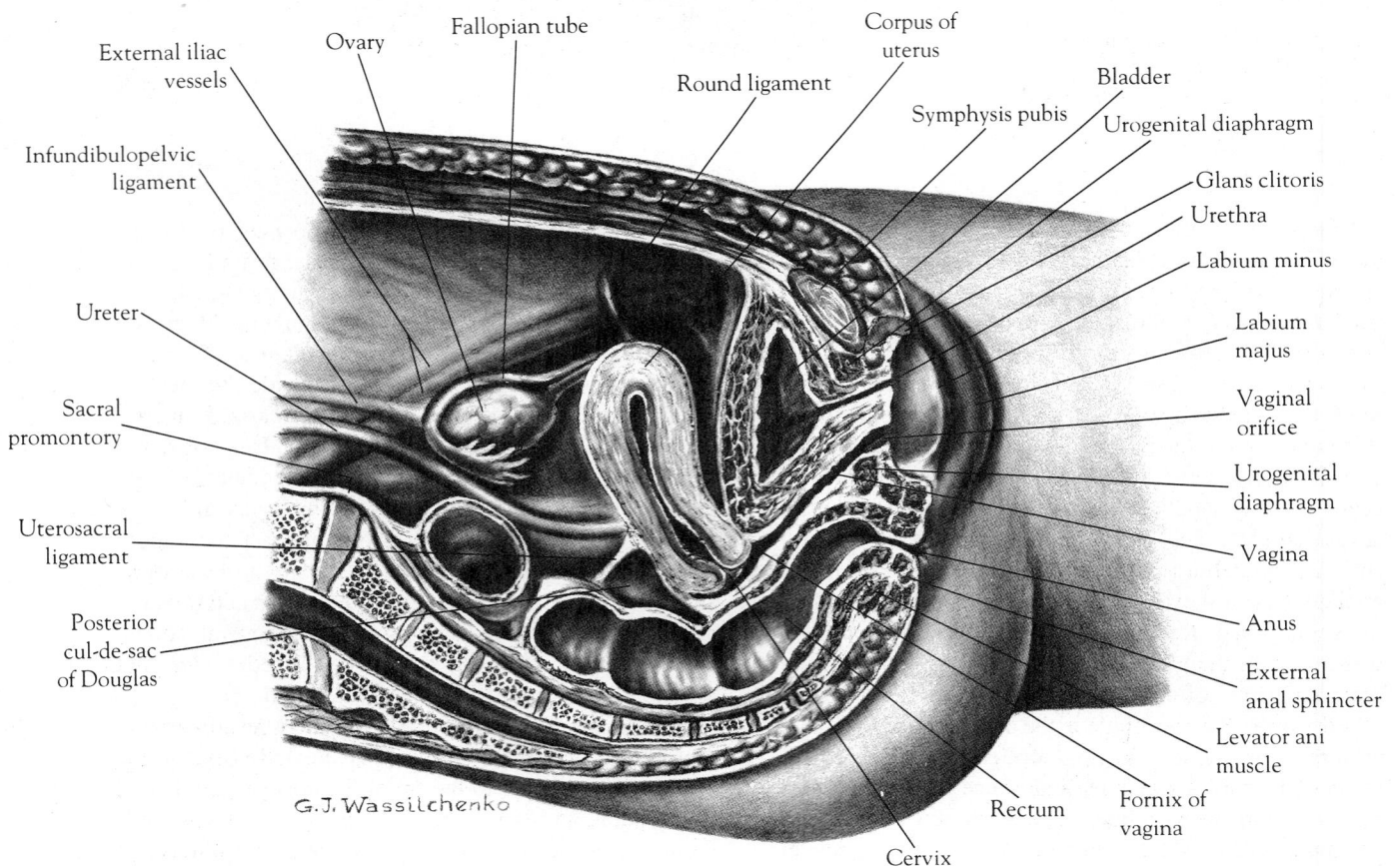

G.J. Wassilchenko

are approximately 10 cm in length in an adult and are suspended by a fold of the broad ligament called the mesosalpinx. The isthmus end of the tube opens into the uterine cavity. The ampulla is the dilated central part of the tube that is continuous with the infundibulum, the fimbriated funnel-shaped opening of the distal end of the tube. This fimbriated portion of the tube, which is adjacent to the ovary, draws the ovum into the tube where fertilization may occur. The tubal musculature undergoes rhythmic contractions that transport the ovum into the uterus.

Uterus (Fig. 9-2). The uterus is a pear-shaped, thick-walled, muscular organ suspended in the anterior part of the pelvic cavity above the bladder and in front of the rectum. It consists of two major but unequal parts: an upper triangular portion, the body or corpus, and a lower cylindric or fusiform portion, the cervix (Fig. 9-3). The isthmus divides these two portions. The uterine (fallopian) tubes emerge from the cornua of the uterus at the junction of the superior and lateral margins. The convex upper segment between the cornua is the fundus uteri. Before puberty the length of the uterus varies from 2.5 to 3.5 cm. In a mature nulliparous woman the uterus is 6 to 8 cm in length, as compared with 9 to 10 cm in a multiparous woman (Fig. 9-4). The uterus is covered with a layer of peritoneum from which arise the broad

ligaments that extend from the lateral margins of the uterus to the pelvic walls and divide the pelvic cavity into anterior and posterior compartments (Fig. 9-5). The base of the broad ligament, which is quite thick, is continuous with the connective tissue of the pelvic floor. The densest portion (cardinal ligament) surrounds the uterine blood vessels. The two round ligaments extend from each side of the uterus below the uterine tubes and hold the organ in the anterior position. During pregnancy the round ligaments undergo considerable hypertrophy and increase in both length and diameter. The uterosacral ligaments extend from the sacrum around the rectum to the cervix of the uterus. They help support the uterus and maintain its position. The uterosacral and cardinal ligaments are the most important ligaments of the uterus; without them the uterus would tend to pass through the vagina or prolapse.

The wall of the uterus is comprised of three layers: serosal, muscular, and mucosal. The serosal layer is formed by the peritoneum covering the uterus. The muscular portion, or myometrium, consists of bundles of smooth muscle that are united by connective tissue containing many elastic fibers. During pregnancy the thickness of the myometrium increases markedly. This occurs because of hypertrophy (actual enlargement of existing fibers) and addition of new fibers derived from transfor-

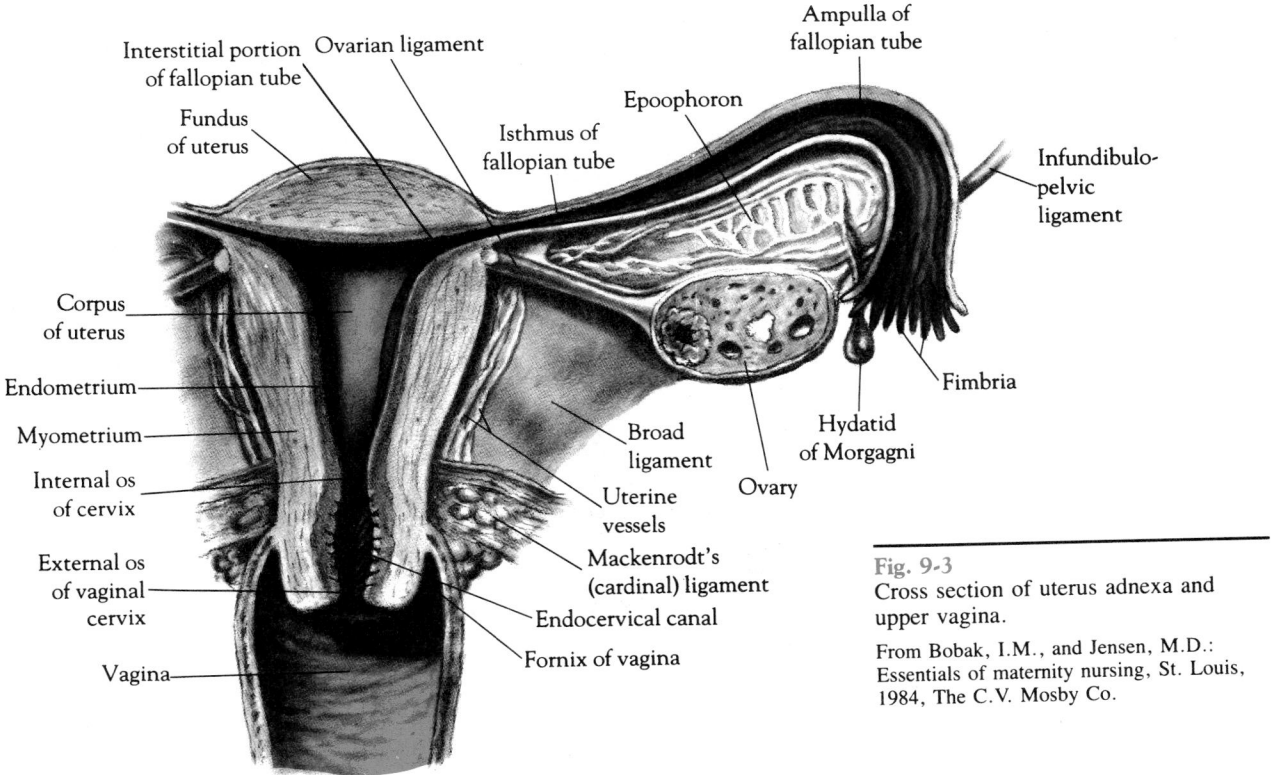

Fig. 9-3

Cross section of uterus adnexa and upper vagina.

From Bobak, I.M., and Jensen, M.D.: Essentials of maternity nursing, St. Louis, 1984, The C.V. Mosby Co.

Fig. 9-4
Comparative sizes of prepubertal, adult nonparous, and multiparous uteruses.

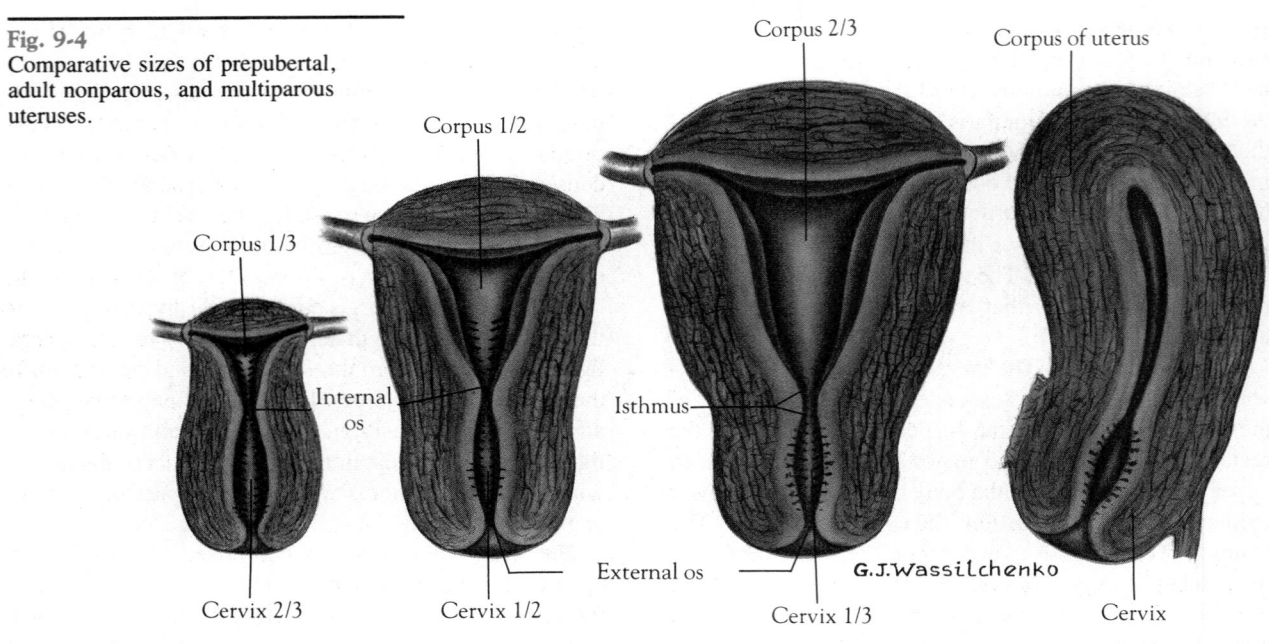

Corpus 1/3

Corpus 1/2

Corpus 2/3

Corpus of uterus

Internal os

Isthmus

External os

G.J.Wassilchenko

Cervix 2/3

Cervix 1/2

Cervix 1/3

Cervix

Fig. 9-5
Female pelvic contents as viewed from above.

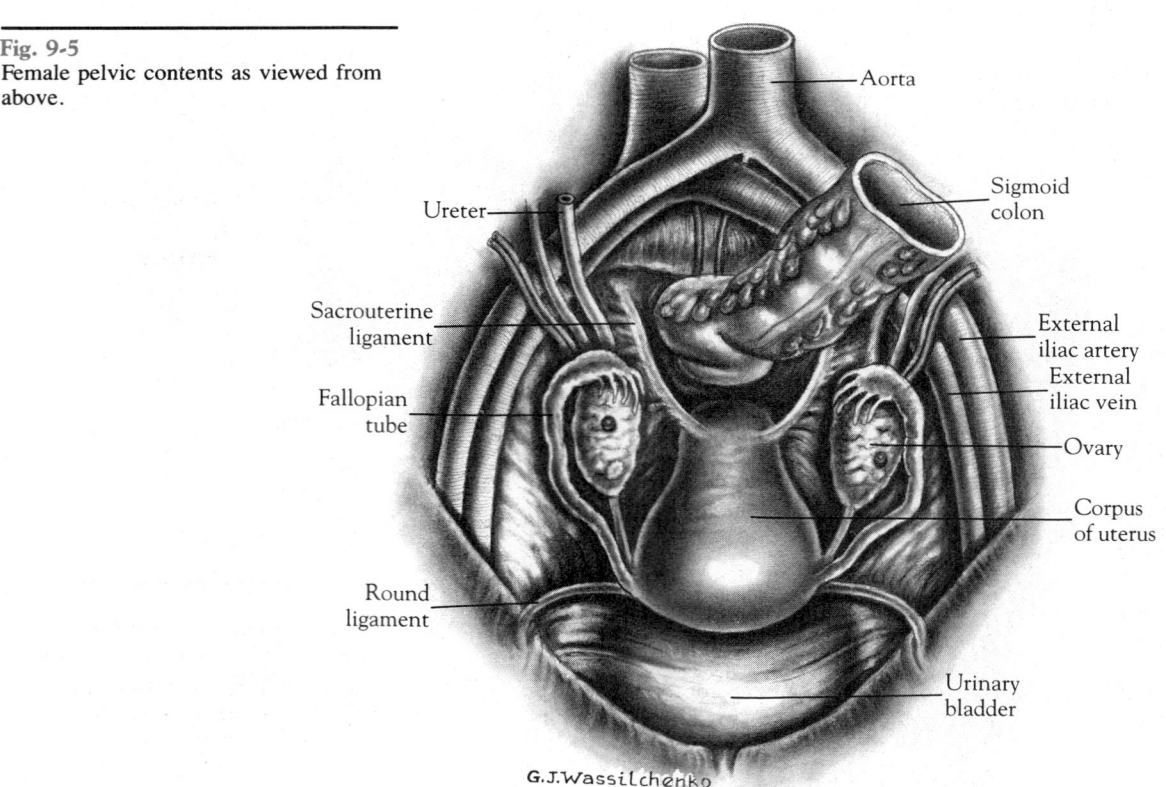

Aorta

Ureter

Sigmoid colon

Sacrouterine ligament

External iliac artery

External iliac vein

Fallopian tube

Ovary

Corpus of uterus

Round ligament

Urinary bladder

G.J.Wassilchenko

mation and division of mesenchymal cells. The innermost or mucosal layer that lines the uterine cavity in the non-pregnant state is the endometrium. It is comprised of surface epithelium, glands, and interglandular tissue. The uterine glands extend through the entire thickness of the endometrium to the myometrium and secrete a thin alkaline fluid that keeps the uterine cavity moist.

Two types of arteries supply blood to the endometrium. The straight basal arteries extend to the basal layer of the endometrium from the radial and arcuate arteries in the myometrium. The coiled or spiral arteries, which are a continuation of the radial and basal arteries, supply the superficial layer of the endometrium. The coiled arteries play an important part in the mechanism of menstruation.

The cervix is the lower part of the uterus. The entrance of the uterus is the cervical os or opening, which changes in size and shape depending on pregnancy or previous deliveries. Hormonal changes influence mucus production by the endocervical glands.

Vagina. The vagina is a tubular canal 10 to 15 cm in length, directed backward and upward and extending from the vestibule to the uterus. It is located between the bladder anteriorly and the rectum posteriorly. It is the female organ of copulation, the birth canal, and the excretory duct of the uterus through which the menstrual flow escapes. In an adult the anterior wall of the vagina is approximately 8 cm long and the posterior wall is 9 to 10 cm long. The difference is due to the projection of the cervix into the anterior aspect of the superior end of the vagina. The anterior, posterior, and two lateral fornices are produced by the cervix projecting into the vagina. The fornices are of clinical importance because the internal pelvic organs can be easily palpated through the thin wall. The mucous membrane lining the vagina forms

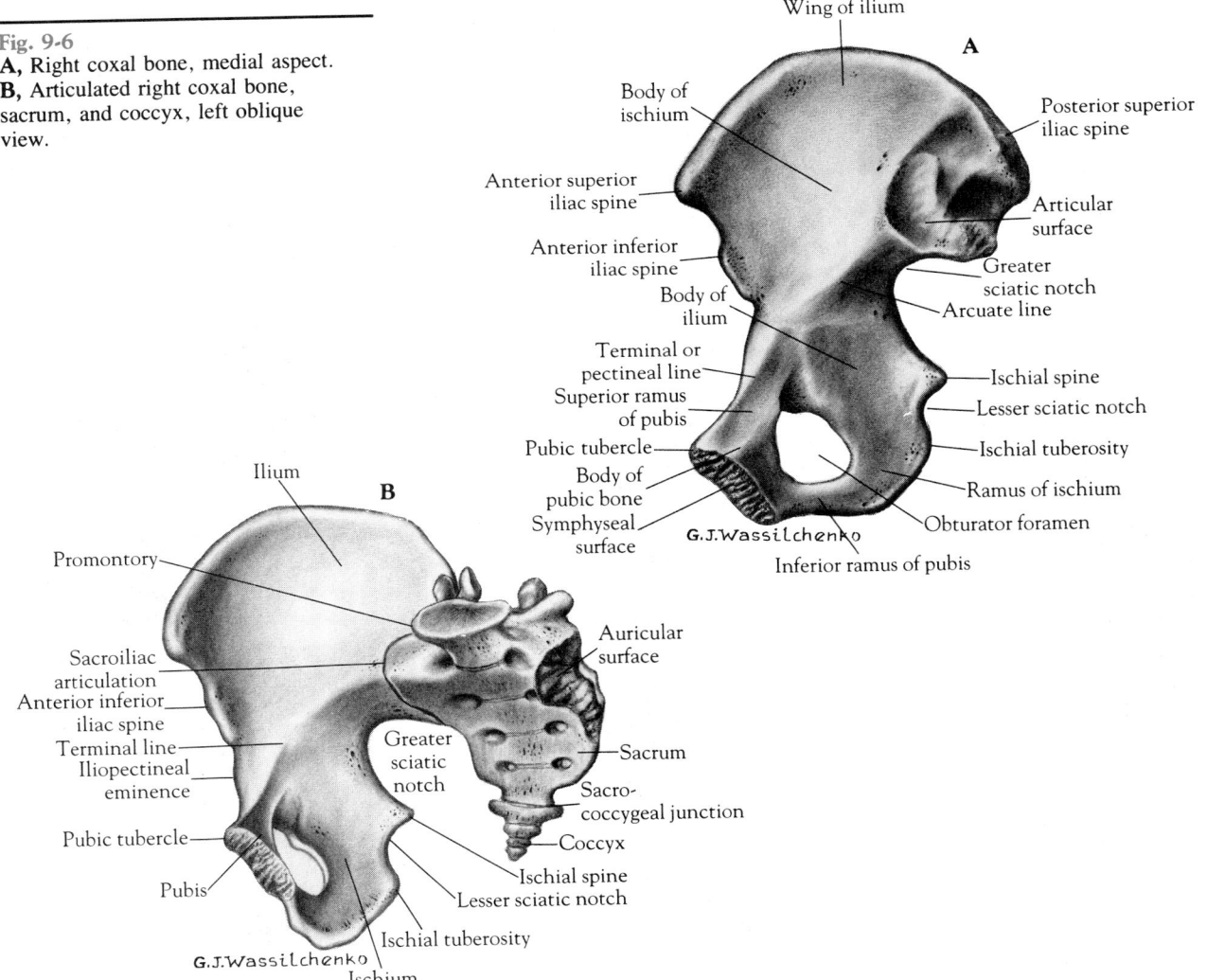

Fig. 9-6
A, Right coxal bone, medial aspect.
B, Articulated right coxal bone, sacrum, and coccyx, left oblique view.

thick folds so that the vaginal walls are in contact with each other and are kept moist by cervical secretions.

Pelvis

The pelvis is composed of the two innominate bones, the sacrum, and the coccyx (Fig. 9-6). The innominate bones are formed by fusion of the ischium, ilium, and pubis and are joined to the sacrum and to each other at the symphysis pubis. The pelvis has two parts: the shallow, upper, or false pelvis and the lower, smaller, or true pelvis. The false pelvis is bounded posteriorly by the lumbar vertebrae, laterally by the iliac fossa, and anteriorly by the abdominal wall. The true pelvis is bounded by the sacrum, the inner surface of the ischial bones, and the pubic bones. The shape and diameter of the true pelvis are important in obstetrics because it must accommodate the fetal head in a vaginal delivery.

Pelvic inlet. The pelvic inlet is bounded posteriorly by the sacral promontory, laterally by the linea terminalis, and anteriorly by the horizontal rami of the pubic bones and symphysis pubis. It has the following anteroposterior diameters (Fig. 9-7):

1. True conjugate (conjugata vera), the distance from the upper margin of the symphysis to the sacral promontory
2. Obstetric conjugate, the distance from the most convex posterior surface of the symphysis to the sacral promontory; this is about 0.5 cm less than the true conjugate and is the shortest anteroposterior diameter through which the fetal head must descend
3. Diagonal conjugate, the distance from the lower border of the symphysis to the sacral promontory; this is the only anteroposterior measurement that can be obtained by clinical examination

The transverse diameter of the pelvic inlet is at a right angle to the obstetric conjugate and represents the greatest distance between the lineae terminales on either side. The oblique diameters extend from each sacroiliac synchondrosis to the opposite iliopectineal eminence.

Midpelvis. The midplane of the pelvis is the roomiest portion of the pelvic cavity. It extends from the middle of the symphysis pubis to the junction of the second and third sacral vertebrae and passes laterally through the ischial bones over the middle of the acetabulum. The interspinous (bispinous) diameter of 10 cm or slightly more in an adult is usually the smallest diameter of the pelvis. The anteroposterior diameter at the level of the ischial spines is normally at least 11.5 cm. The posterior sagittal diameter of the midpelvis is normally approximately 4.5 cm.

Pelvic inclination. In a woman who is standing the upper portion of the pelvis is normally directed downward and backward and the lower portion is directed downward and forward. The tilt of the pelvis, or inclination, is altered with posture. Straightening of the lum-

Fig. 9-7
Planes of pelvic inlet.

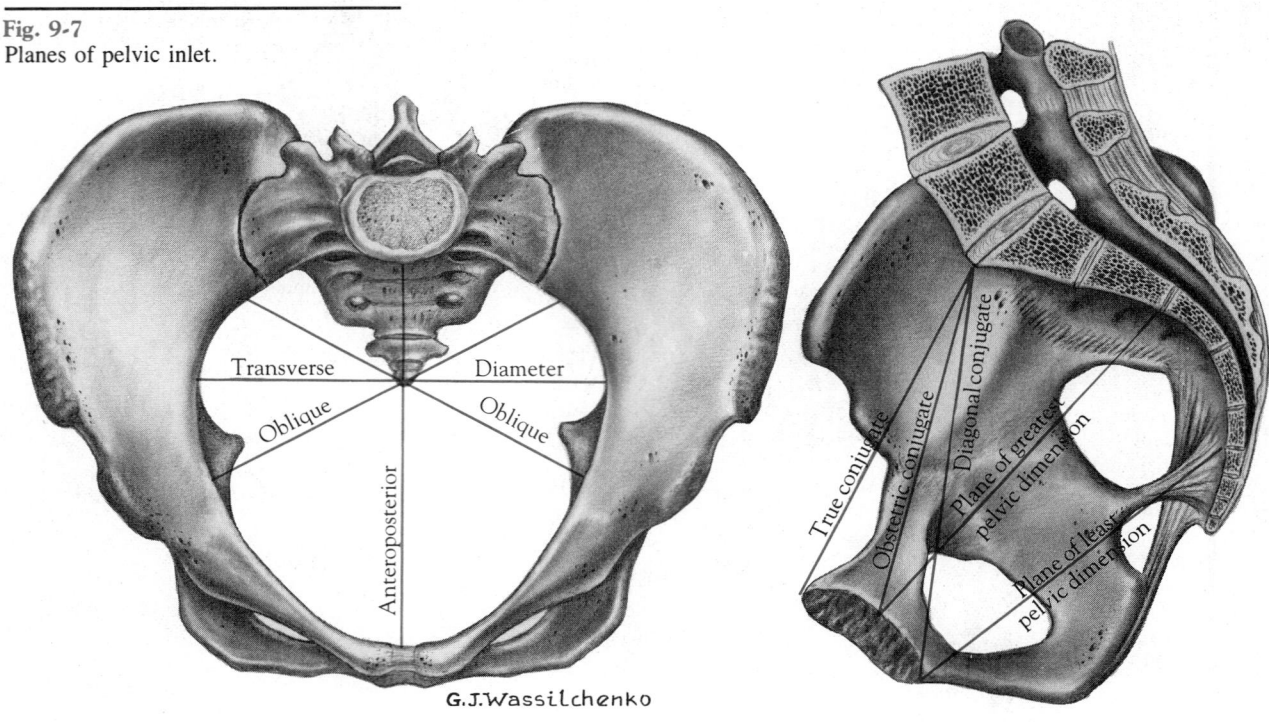

G.J.Wassilchenko

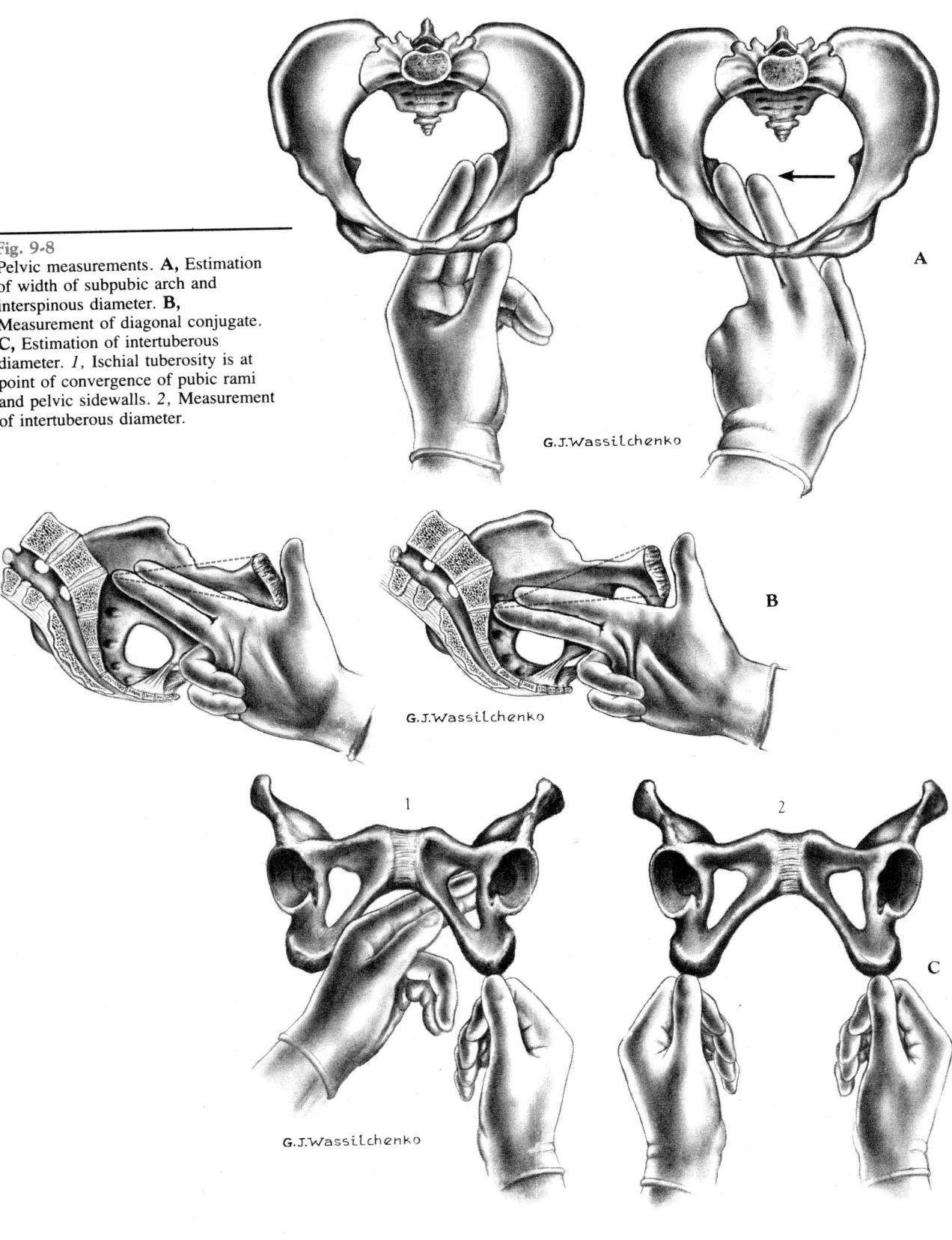

Fig. 9-8
Pelvic measurements. **A,** Estimation of width of subpubic arch and interspinous diameter. **B,** Measurement of diagonal conjugate. **C,** Estimation of intertuberous diameter. *1,* Ischial tuberosity is at point of convergence of pubic rami and pelvic sidewalls. *2,* Measurement of intertuberous diameter.

G.J.Wassilchenko

bar curve reduces the pelvic inclination, and an exaggeration of the lumbar curve increases it. This tilt can influence the progress of labor.

Pelvic outlet. The outlet consists of two triangles having a common base at a line drawn between the two ischial tuberosities. The anteroposterior diameter extends from the lower border of the symphysis pubis to the tip of the sacrum. The transverse diameter is the distance between the ischial tuberosities. This is also called the intertuberous or bi-ischial diameter. The posterior sagittal diameter extends from the tip of the sacrum to a right-angled intersection with a line between the ischial tuberosities (Fig. 9-8).

Pelvic classification. Classification of the pelvis by Caldwell and Moloy in 1933 defined four basic shapes: gynecoid, anthropoid, platypelloid, and android.[42] The classification is based on the configuration of the inlet and the corresponding changes in the midpelvis and lower pelvis. The pelvic inlet is divided into a posterior segment behind a line of the widest transverse diameter and an anterior segment in front of it. The length of the transverse diameter and the anteroposterior length of each segment are assessed to classify the inlet.

The sacrosciatic notch is visualized laterally. A narrow notch indicates a reduced anteroposterior diameter because the sacrum lies forward. A wide notch means that the sacrum is displaced posteriorly. Evaluation of the midpelvis and outlet includes measurement of the bispinous diameter and observation of shape of the spinous processes and the length, width, and curve of the sacrum. The subpubic angle and contour of the arch are noted. The degree of divergence or convergence of the lateral walls is also noted when classifying pelvic shapes.

The four basic types of pelvis are evaluated to assess the adequacy of the pelvic structures for a vaginal delivery. It is uncommon for a pelvis to conform exactly in every dimension to any one type; most pelves are mixed types showing combinations of various characteristics (Fig. 9-9).

Gynecoid pelvis. The gynecoid pelvis is characteristic of the normal female and is associated with the lowest incidence of fetopelvic disproportion. The inlet is nearly round. The sacrum is well curved and has average inclination. The sacrosciatic notch is of average size. The side walls are straight, and the ischial spines are not prominent. The subpubic arch is wide, and the transverse diameter is about 10 cm.

Android pelvis. The android pelvis is characteristic of the normal male. The posterior segment is wide and flat, and the anterior segment is narrow. The sacrum is

Fig. 9-9
Female pelvis—pure types.

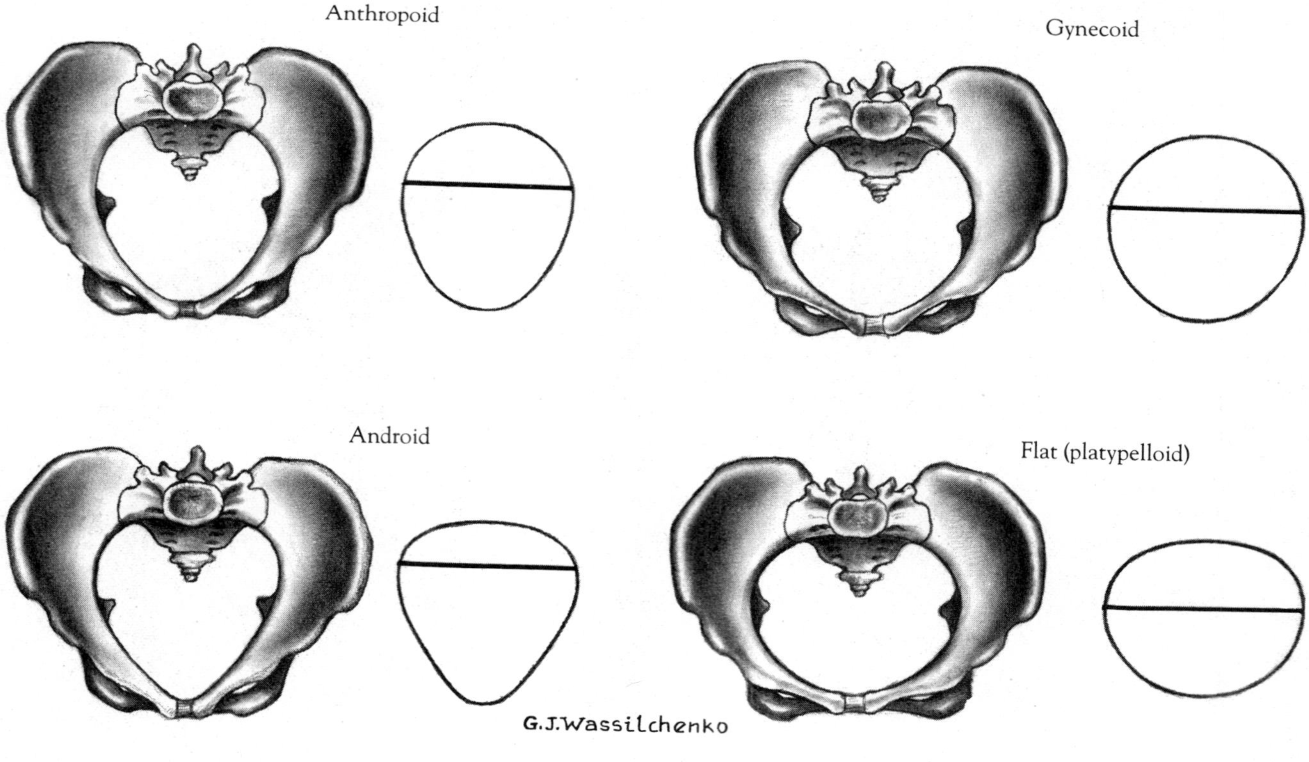

Anthropoid

Gynecoid

Android

Flat (platypelloid)

G.J. Wassilchenko

Fig. 9-10
Perineum. **A,** Superficial components.
B, Deep components.

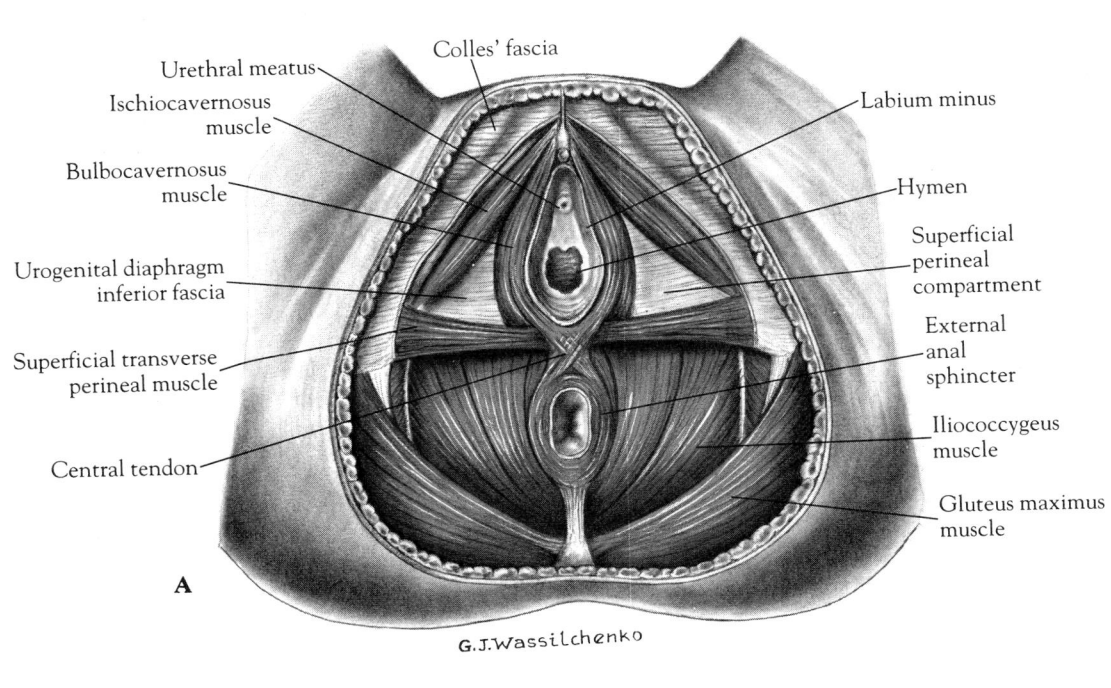

Colles' fascia

Urethral meatus

Ischiocavernosus
muscle

Bulbocavernosus
muscle

Urogenital diaphragm
inferior fascia

Superficial transverse
perineal muscle

Central tendon

Labium minus

Hymen

Superficial
perineal
compartment

External
anal
sphincter

Iliococcygeus
muscle

Gluteus maximus
muscle

A

G.J.Wassilchenko

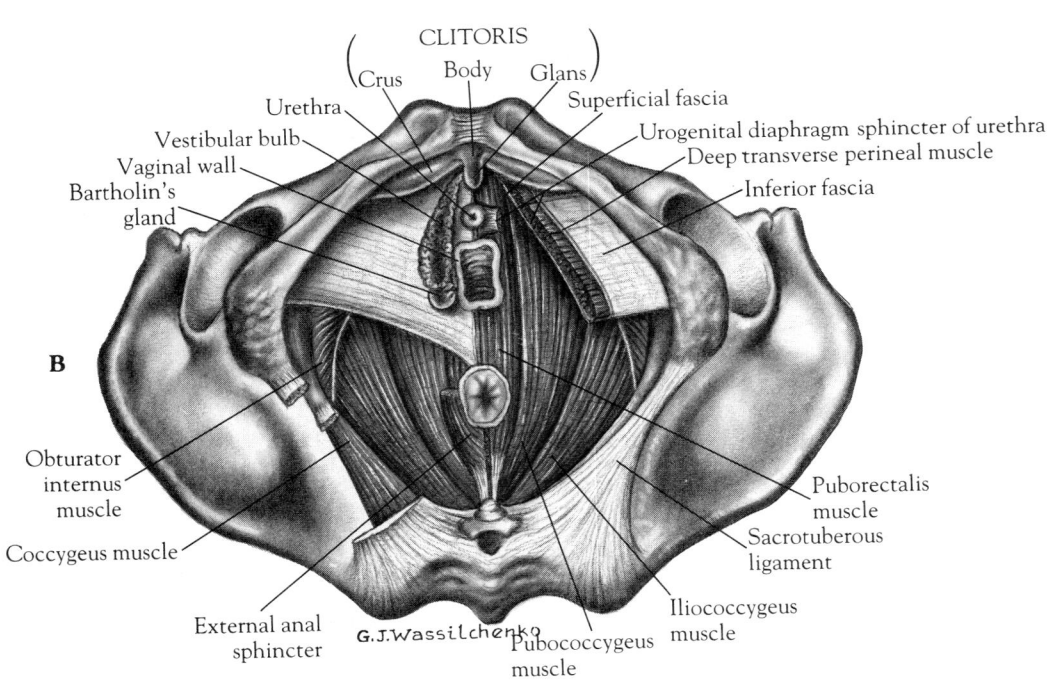

CLITORIS

Crus   Body   Glans

Urethra

Vestibular bulb

Vaginal wall

Bartholin's
gland

Superficial fascia

Urogenital diaphragm sphincter of urethra

Deep transverse perineal muscle

Inferior fascia

Obturator
internus
muscle

Coccygeus muscle

External anal
sphincter

Pubococcygeus
muscle

Iliococcygeus
muscle

Puborectalis
muscle

Sacrotuberous
ligament

B

G.J.Wassilchenko

straight and inclined forward. The sacrosciatic notch is narrow, and the side walls convergent. The ischial spines are prominent, and the subpubic arch is narrow. This is a typical "funnel pelvis."

Anthropoid pelvis. The anthropoid pelvis has a reduced transverse diameter as compared with the gynecoid pelvis, making it a long narrow oval with an elongated anteroposterior segment and a slightly narrowed forepelvis. The sacrum is long and narrow with an average curvature posteriorly. The sacrosciatic notch is wide and shallow, and the side walls are straight. The ischial spines are prominent with a shortened bispinous diameter. The subpubic arch is narrowed.

Platypelloid pelvis. The platypelloid pelvis is similar to the gynecoid pelvis except for narrowing of the anteroposterior diameters at all levels. The inlet appears as a wide transverse oval. The sacrosciatic notch is wide, and the side walls are straight. The ischial spines are prominent, and the subpubic arch is wide.

Pelvic Floor (Fig. 9-10)

A number of tissue layers form the pelvic floor. From the inside outward toward the skin they are the perito-

neum, subperitoneal connective tissue, internal pelvic fascia, levator ani and coccygeus muscles, external pelvic fascia, superficial muscles, and subcutaneous tissue.

The levator ani and the fascia close the lower end of the pelvic cavity and diaphragm and present a concave upper surface. On both sides the levator ani consists of a pubic and iliac portion. The fibers pass backward to encircle the rectum, and a few fibers pass behind the vagina. The posterior and lateral portions of the pelvic floor not covered by the levator ani are covered by the piriformis and coccygeus muscles on either side.

Three layers of fascia fill out the triangular space between the pubic arch and a line joining the ischial tuberosities. This is called the urogenital diaphragm; it forms a compartment in which lie the superficial perineal muscles.

Breasts (Figs. 9-11 and 9-12)

The breasts or mammary glands are accessory organs of reproduction. They consist of a glandular epithelium and a duct system embedded in interstitial tissue and fat. They lie anterior to the pectoralis major muscle and are separated from it by a layer of fat that is continuous with

Fig. 9-11
Lateral view of breast.

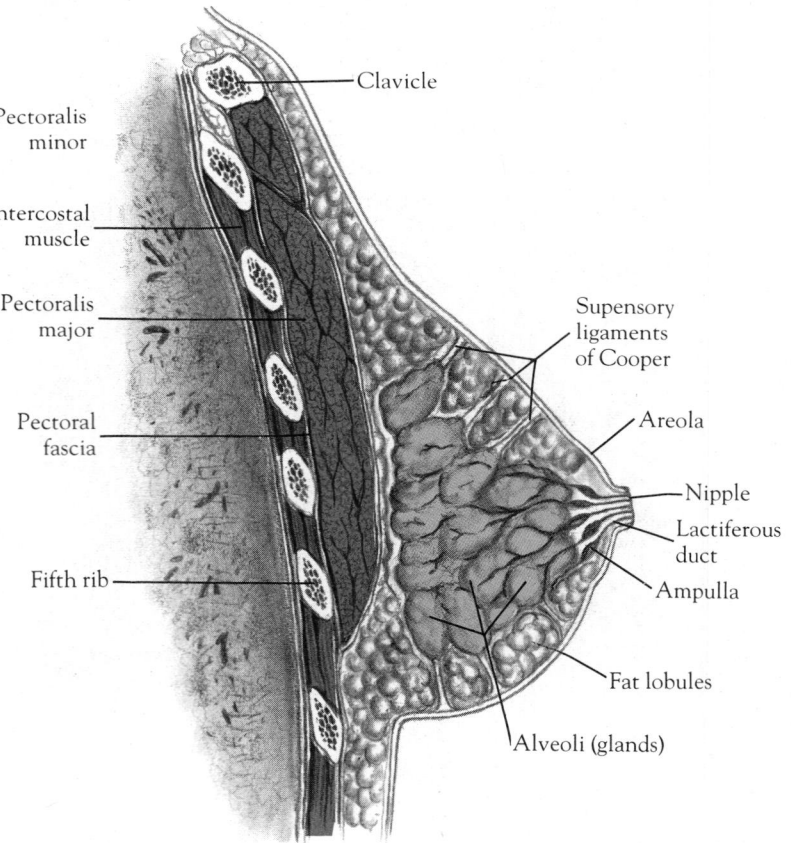

Pectoralis minor

Intercostal muscle

Pectoralis major

Pectoral fascia

Fifth rib

Clavicle

Supensory ligaments of Cooper

Areola

Nipple

Lactiferous duct

Ampulla

Fat lobules

Alveoli (glands)

the fatty stroma of the gland itself. They extend from the anterior border of the axilla to the lateral edge of the sternum. Each gland consists of a comma-shaped mass of fat and collagenous tissue. The tail of Spence extends toward the axilla. The position of the breast is maintained by suspensory (Cooper's) ligaments, which are condensations of connective tissue and are easily stretched, especially if the breasts are large. Lymph drainage is mainly toward the axillary lymph nodes with some drainage directed toward the substernal and diaphragmatic nodes. Some women (as well as some men) have supernumerary nipples or breast tissue that develops along the longitudinal ridges extending from the axilla to the groin, which existed during early embryonic development (Fig. 9-13).

The center of the fully developed breast in an adult woman is the nipple, which is elevated above the breast. Bundles of smooth muscle fibers in the nipple have erectile properties. The areola that surrounds the nipple has a diameter of 1.5 to 2.5 cm. Small sebaceous glands located under the areola give it a rough appearance. Arranged radially under the areola are 15 to 20 lactiferous ducts. In a lactating woman these ducts drain milk from the lobes of glandular tissue embedded in the adipose tissue of the breast. The ducts enlarge slightly before reaching the nipple to form the short lactiferous sinuses in which the milk may be stored. From the sinuses the ducts extend toward the chest wall, uniting various lobules or acinar structures of the breast. Each lobule contains 10 to 100 alveoli or acini, and 20 to 40 lobules compose each of the 15 to 20 lobes that are distributed in each breast. The alveolus is lined by a single layer of milk-secreting epithelial cells, encased in a network of myoepithelial strands; it is surrounded by a dense capillary network.

Secretory alveoli develop in pregnancy as a response to the rising estrogen and progesterone levels. Before puberty the breasts consist mostly of lactiferous ducts. Under the hormonal influence of puberty there are branching and growth of the duct system, as well as extensive distribution of fat. Small masses of cells are formed at the ends of the ducts that are the potential alveoli. During the first trimester of pregnancy a proliferation of the ducts creates a maximum number of epithelial structures for future alveolus formation. In the second trimester the ducts group together to form large lobules, and as the lumens dilate, the alveoli are formed

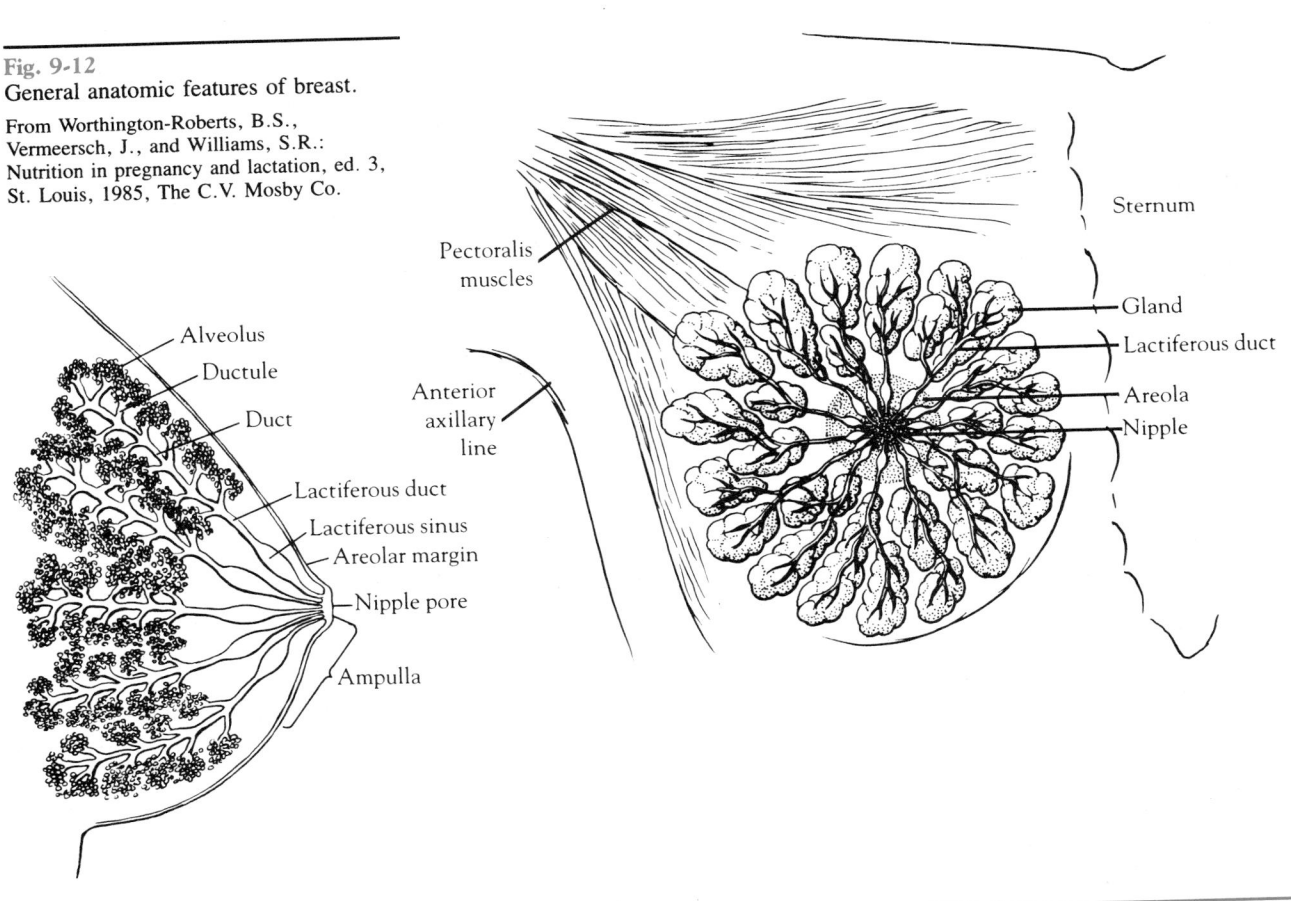

Fig. 9-12
General anatomic features of breast.

From Worthington-Roberts, B.S., Vermeersch, J., and Williams, S.R.: Nutrition in pregnancy and lactation, ed. 3, St. Louis, 1985, The C.V. Mosby Co.

Alveolus
Ductule
Duct
Lactiferous duct
Lactiferous sinus
Areolar margin
Nipple pore
Ampulla

Pectoralis muscles
Anterior axillary line

Sternum
Gland
Lactiferous duct
Areola
Nipple

Table 9-1

Hormonal Contributions to Breast Development and Lactation

Hormone	Origin	Function Before and during Pregnancy	After Delivery
Prolactin	Anterior pituitary	Serum level rises, but estrogen suppresses its effect during pregnancy	Stimulates alveolar cells to produce milk; is probably of primary importance in initiating lactation but of secondary importance in maintaining lactation; may also cause lactation infertility by suppressing release of FSH and LH from pituitary or by causing ovaries to be unresponsive to gonadotropins; levels rise in response to various psychogenic factors, stress, anesthesia, surgery, high serum osmolality, exercise, nipple stimulation, and sexual intercourse
Prolactin-inhibiting factor (PIF)	Hypothalamus	Suppresses release of prolactin into blood; release stimulated by dopaminergic impulses (i.e., catecholamines)	Suppresses release of prolactin from anterior pituitary; agents that increase prolactin by decreasing catecholamines and thus PIF include phenothiazines and reserpine
Oxytocin	Posterior pituitary	Generally no effect on mammary function; sensitivity of myoepithelial cells to oxytocin increases during pregnancy	Causes myoepithelial cells to contract leading to "milk ejection"; release is inhibited by stresses such as fear, anxiety, embarrassment, distraction; also causes uterine contraction and postpartum involution of uterus
Estrogen	Ovary and placenta	Stimulates proliferation of glandular tissue and ducts in breast; probably stimulates pituitary to secrete prolactin but inhibits prolactin effects at mammary cell level	Blood level drops at parturition, which aids in initiating lactation; not important to lactation thereafter
Progesterone	Ovary and placenta	With estrogen, stimulates proliferation of glandular tissue and ducts in breast; inhibits milk secretion	Blood level drops at parturition, which aids in initiating lactation; probably unimportant to lactation thereafter
Growth hormone	Anterior pituitary		May act with prolactin in initiating lactation but appears to be most important in maintaining established lactation
ACTH	Anterior pituitary	Gradually increases in blood during pregnancy; stimulates adrenals to release corticosteroids	High level is believed necessary for maintenance of lactation
Placental lactogen	Placenta	Like growth hormone in structure; stimulates mammary growth; associated with mobilization of free fatty acids and inhibition of peripheral glucose utilization and lactogenic action	
Thyroxine	Thyroid	Normally no direct effect on lactation	Appears to be important in maintaining lactation either through some direct effect on the mammary glands or by control of metabolism
Thyrotropin-releasing hormone	Hypothalamus	Normally no effect on lactation	Stimulates release of prolactin; can be used to maintain established lactation

From Worthington-Roberts, B.S., Vermeersch, J., and Williams, S.R.: Nutrition in pregnancy and lactation, ed. 3, St. Louis, 1985, The C.V. Mosby Co.

Fig. 9-13
Supernumerary nipples.

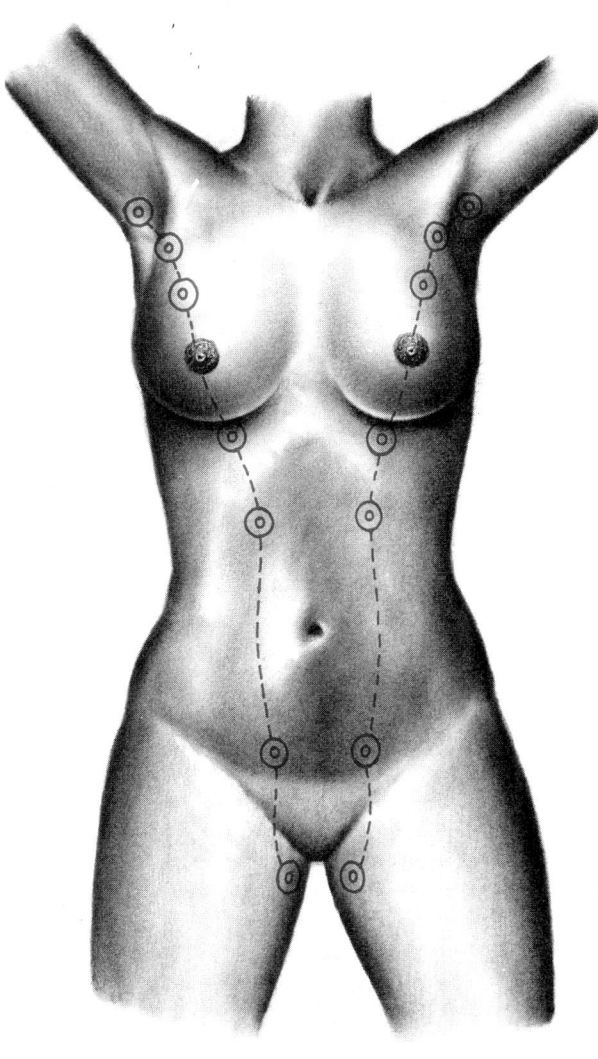

and lined with cuboidal epithelium. In the third trimester the existing alveoli dilate in preparation for lactation. As glandular and duct tissue proliferates during pregnancy, the adipose tissue appears to diminish.[24,55]

Toward the end of pregnancy and until lactation begins 1 to 3 days after childbirth, the mammary glands form colostrum. It is produced at a much lower rate than milk and contains protein and lactose in amounts similar to milk but almost no fat.

Initiation and maintenance of lactation are achieved through a complex neuroendocrine process involving sensory nerves in the nipples and breast tissue, the spinal cord and hypothalamus, and the pituitary gland. See Table 9-1 for hormonal contributions to breast development and lactation.[55]

Table 9-2
Anti-Infectious Factors in Human Milk

Factor	Function
Bifidus factor	Stimulates growth of bifidobacteria, which antagonizes the survival of enterobacteria
Secretory IgA (sIgA), IgM, and IgG	Act against bacterial invasion of the mucosa or colonization of the gut (show bacterial and viral neutralizing capacity; activate alternative complement pathway)
Antistaphylococcus factor	Inhibits systemic *Staphylococcus* infection
Lactoferrin	Binds iron and inhibits bacterial multiplication
Lactoperoxidase	Kills streptococci and enteric bacteria
Complement (C3, C4)	Promotes opsonization (the rendering of bacteria and other cells susceptible to phagocytosis)
Interferon	Inhibits intracellular viral replication
Lysozyme	Lyses bacteria through destruction of the cell wall
B_{12}-binding protein	Renders vitamin B_{12} unavailable for bacterial growth
Lymphocytes	Synthesize secretory IgA; may have other roles
Macrophages	Synthesize complement, lactoferrin, lysozyme, and other factors; carry out phagocytosis and probably other functions

From Worthington-Roberts, B.S., Vermeersch, J., and Williams, S.R.: Nutrition in pregnancy and lactation, ed. 3, St. Louis, 1985, The C.V. Mosby Co.

Removal of the placenta after delivery discontinues a major source of estrogen. The rapid drop in blood concentration stimulates the anterior pituitary to secrete prolactin, the lactogenic hormone. In addition, the suckling movements of the baby on the breast stimulate the release of prolactin from the anterior pituitary gland and oxytocin from the posterior pituitary gland. This stimulates lactation and ejection of milk from the alveoli into the ducts where it is accessible to the infant. Oxytocin then promotes the "milk ejection reflex." An estimated 50% of milk is removed from the breast by the nursing infant within the first 2 minutes of sucking, and some 80% to 90% of breast milk is taken within the first 4 minutes.[55] Stimulation of the lactation process is optimum when the infant is fed on demand.

In the first few days after birth, small amounts of colostrum are secreted from the mammary glands. The yellow appearance of colostrum is attributed to a high carotene content. The caloric content is less than that of mature milk (67 versus 75 kcal/dl). Colostrum contains an abundance of antibodies and facilitates the development of bifidus flora in the neonate's digestive tract.

Table 9-3
Nutrient Content of Human and Cow Milk

Constituent (Per Liter)	Human Breast Milk	Cow Milk	Constituent (Per Liter)	Human Breast Milk	Cow Milk
Energy (kcal)	690	660	Minerals		
Protein (g)	9	35	Calcium (mg)	297	1170
Fat (g)	45	37	Phosphorus (mg)	150	920
Lactose (g)	68	49	Sodium (mg)	150	506
Vitamins			Potassium (mg)	550	1368
Vitamin A (IU)	1898	1025	Chlorine (mg)	385	1028
Vitamin D (IU)	22	14	Magnesium (mg)	23	120
Vitamin E (IU)	2	0.4	Sulfur (mg)	140	300
Vitamin K (μg)	15	60	Iron (mg)*	0.3-0.56	0.5
Thiamine (μg)	160	440	Iodine (mg)	30	47
Riboflavin (μg)	360	1750	Manganese (μg)†	4-5.9	20-40
Niacin (mg)	1.5	0.9	Copper (μg)‡	0.25-0.6	0.3
Pyridoxine (μg)	100	640	Zinc (mg)‡	0.5-4	3-5
Folic acid (μg)	52	55	Selenium (μg)	20	5-50
Cobalamin (μg)	0.3	4	Fluoride (mg)	0.05	0.03-0.1
Ascorbic acid (mg)	43	11			

From Worthington-Roberts, B.S., Vermeersch, J., and Williams, S.R.: Nutrition in pregnancy and lactation, ed. 3, St. Louis, 1985, The C.V. Mosby Co; data from Hambreaus, L.: Pediatr. Clin. North Am. **24:**17, 1977; Siimes, M.A., Vuori, E., and Kuitunen, P.: Acta Paediatr. Scand. **68:**29, 1979; Vuori, E.: Acta Paediatr. Scand. **68:**571, 1979; Vuori, E., and Kuitunen, P.: Acta Paediatr. Scand. **68:**33, 1978; and Nayman, R., et al.: Am. J. Clin. Nutr. **32:**1279, 1979.
*Median iron values at 2 weeks of lactation and 5 months of lactation.
†Median values at 2 weeks and 5 months after which time the manganese content of human milk tends to increase.
‡Median values of copper and zinc after 2 and 37 weeks.

Between the third and the sixth postpartum days, colostrum changes to transitional milk, which has a high protein content. By about the tenth postpartum day the major changes in breast milk have occurred; the protein content has decreased and lactose content is increasing, reaching consistent levels at the end of the first month. Refer to Table 9-2 for a summary of the anti-infective factors in human milk.

Ovarian Cycle and Hormones

The purpose of the ovarian cycle is to provide an ovum for fertilization, whereas the purpose of the endometrial cycle is to furnish a suitable site for the fertilized ovum to implant and develop.

Follicle development. Female primordial germ cells are derived from the germinal epithelium in the embryo. By mitotic division these form primitive ova, or oogonia, until the fifth or sixth month of gestation. Between the second month of gestation and the sixth month of life, some oogonia become primary oocytes through the prophase of meiosis. At birth some 2 million oocytes are in the ovary, decreasing through attrition to about 300,000 by the onset of puberty.

The first stage of follicle development occurs slowly during the childbearing years. The cells of the follicle divide, creating several layers of granulosa cells around the oocyte. Mucopolysaccharides secreted from the gran-

ulosa cells form a protective halo or zona pellucida around the oocyte (Fig. 9-14). The primary oocyte, the surrounding layers of granulosa cells, and the outer basal lamina membrane comprise the primary follicle.

The second stage of development occurs more rapidly, requiring 2 to 4 weeks for completion. During an ovarian cycle approximately six to 12 primary follicles undergo growth and development, but only one reaches maturity and ovulates. All others degenerate and become atretic follicles. The proliferating granulosa cells are separated into two parts. The cavity or antrum is filled with follicular fluid that presses the oocyte to one side. Several cells known as the cumulus oophorus surround the oocyte, forming a stalk that projects into the antrum. The follicle distends with fluid and moves outward to the surface of the ovary. The theca cells surrounding the antrum proliferate, and those nearest the basal lamina are transformed into cuboidal steroid-secreting cells called the theca interna. Spindle cells from the stroma form around this, comprising the theca externa. At this point in development the entire complex is known as the graafian follicle.

The third and last stage of follicular development is completed within 48 hours. Before ovulation a single graafian follicle becomes dominant, and as the follicle ruptures, the oocyte is released into the peritoneal cavity. Since the initial meiotic division is complete at this time, this is called the secondary oocyte. Fertilization of this

Fig. 9-14
Oogenesis. Chromosome content of germ cell is shown at each stage, including sex chromosome shown after comma.

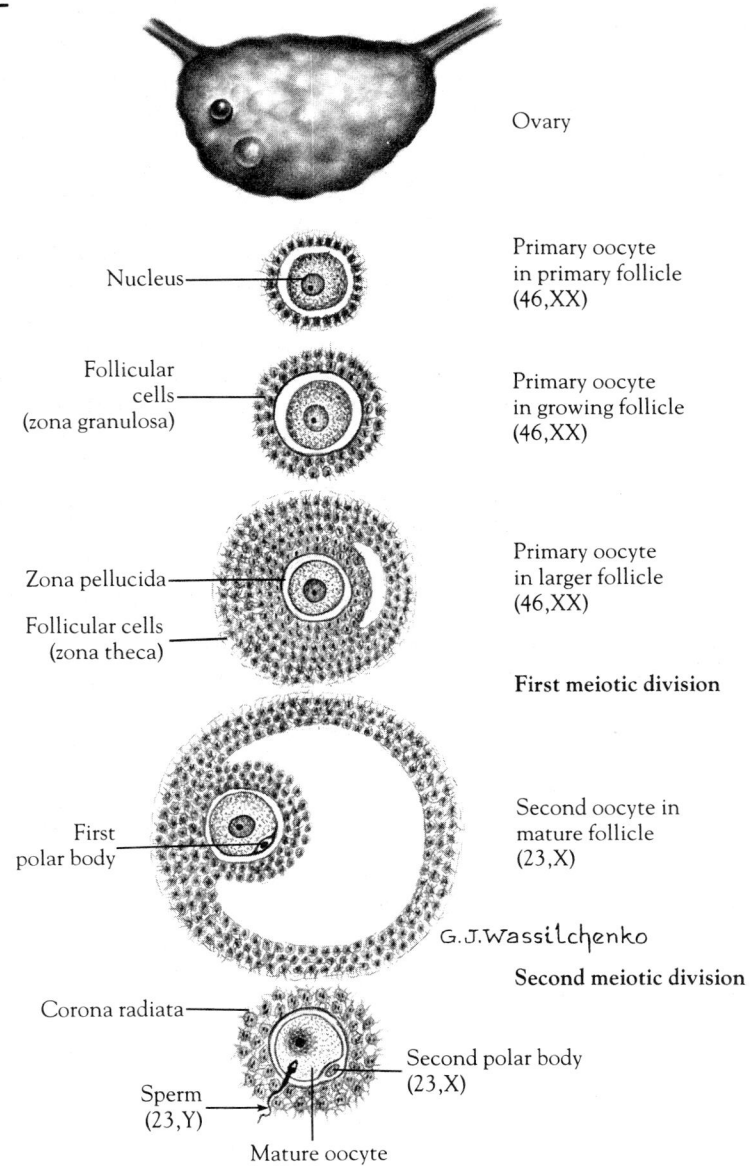

Ovary

Nucleus — Primary oocyte in primary follicle (46,XX)

Follicular cells (zona granulosa) — Primary oocyte in growing follicle (46,XX)

Zona pellucida — Primary oocyte in larger follicle (46,XX)

Follicular cells (zona theca)

First meiotic division

First polar body — Second oocyte in mature follicle (23,X)

G.J.Wassilchenko

Second meiotic division

Corona radiata — Second polar body (23,X)

Sperm (23,Y) — Mature oocyte

oocyte in the fallopian tube causes completion of the second meiotic division, resulting in a haploid ovum.[2]

Ovulation. Ovulation is the actual discharge of the secondary oocyte from the graafian follicle. This usually occurs at the midpoint of both the ovarian and the menstrual cycle. The time from the first day of the menstrual period to ovulation is the follicular phase or preovulatory period. The postovulatory period is the luteal phase.

Some women experience mittelschmerz, a lower abdominal discomfort at the time of ovulation. This is believed to be caused by peritoneal irritation from blood or follicular fluid that has escaped from the ruptured follicle. Another response to ovulation is an increase in basal body temperature caused by the thermogenic action of progesterone. Changes in the cervical mucus near the time of ovulation include decreases in viscosity and opacity, an increase in clarity, and an increase in sodium chloride content, which is demonstrated by arborization or ferning when mucus is allowed to dry on a glass slide. The signs and symptoms of ovulation are important both for women who wish to conceive during a particular cycle and for those who desire to avoid conception.

Corpus luteum. A yellow glandular mass formed at the site of the ruptured follicle is called the corpus luteum. It secretes large amounts of progesterone and lesser amounts of estrogen. If fertilization occurs, the corpus luteum increases in size, remains enlarged for about 3 months until the placenta takes over secreting functions, and then degenerates. If fertilization does not occur, the corpus luteum degenerates and shrinks. The yellow or "luteal" tissue then changes to a white fibrous tissue known as the corpus albicans.

Estrogens. Estrogen is a generic term for substances capable of producing the typical changes of estrus. The common estrogens are estradiol, estrone, and estriol. They are secreted by the developing ovarian follicle and subsequently by the corpus luteum. Estrogens are secreted by the placenta during pregnancy.

Estrogens are responsible for the development of the female secondary sex characteristics, increased growth of the uterus at puberty, and repair of the endometrium after menstruation. They tend to increase uterine sensitivity to oxytocin and uterine motility. In this respect the actions of estrogens are opposite to those of progesterone. Estrogens also increase bone matrix formation and slightly increase sodium and water reabsorption by the renal tubules.

Progesterone. Progesterone is the principal hormone secreted by the corpus luteum. During pregnancy it is secreted by the placenta. Progesterone prepares the uterine endometrium for the reception and development of the fertilized ovum by converting a proliferative endometrium to the secretory stage. It also inhibits the contractility of smooth uterine muscle, which is the opposite action of estrogen. Progesterone is responsible for the development of acini and lobules in the breast during pregnancy and inhibits the action of prolactin. Removal of the placenta, a source of massive progesterone production, removes the inhibitory effect on prolactin, thereby permitting lactation. Progesterone is also called luteo or progestational hormone.

Androgens. Androgens are substances that produce masculine characteristics such as hair growth, lowering of the voice, muscularity, and, in the male, development of the genital system. The major androgen secreted by the female ovary is androstenedione, a biologically weak compound but one that can undergo peripheral conversion to testosterone. The adrenal gland also secretes androgens, androstenedione and dehydroepiandrosterone (dehydroisoandrosterone). Dihydrotestosterone is formed in peripheral tissue by the action of an enzyme on testosterone. In addition, testosterone, which is secreted by

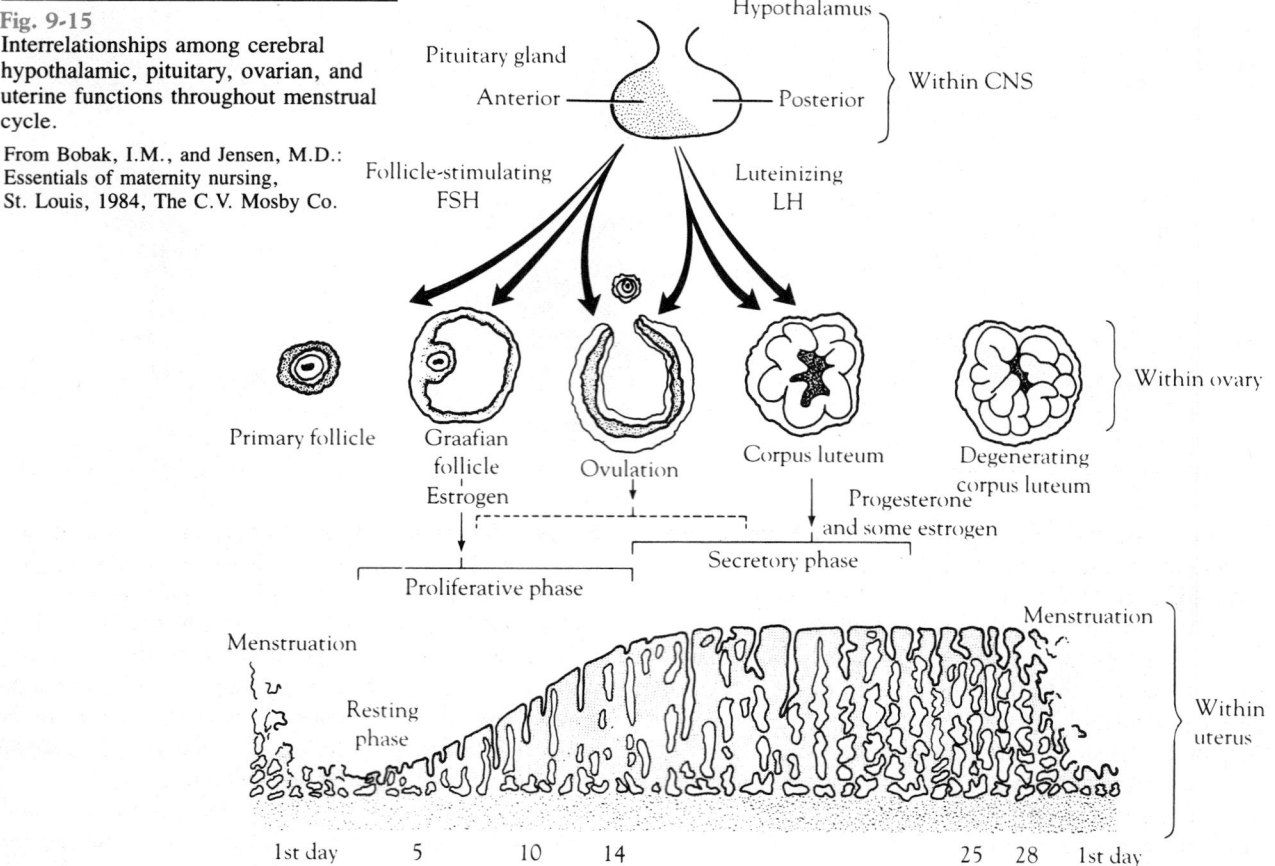

Fig. 9-15
Interrelationships among cerebral hypothalamic, pituitary, ovarian, and uterine functions throughout menstrual cycle.

From Bobak, I.M., and Jensen, M.D.: Essentials of maternity nursing, St. Louis, 1984, The C.V. Mosby Co.

the embryonic testicular cells of Leydig, is required in the male fetus for the differentiation of the genital tubercle, swellings, folds, and urogenital sinus into the penis, scrotum, penile urethra, and prostate. Testosterone stimulates fetal differentiation of the wolffian ducts into the epididymis, vas deferens, and seminal vesicles.

Pituitary gonadotropic hormones. The basophils of the anterior pituitary gland secrete follicle-stimulating hormone (FSH) and luteinizing hormone (LH). The acidophils secrete prolactin, which is also called lactogenic or luteotropic hormone (LTH).

FSH stimulates ovarian follicle growth and maturation. The FSH level rises slightly before both ovulation and menstruation. This hormone is essential to the production of estrogen by the ovary. After menopause the level of FSH in the plasma and the amount excreted in the urine are increased.

LH induces ovulation and stimulates formation of the corpus luteum and progesterone secretion.

Prolactin serves as a luteotropic hormone in helping to maintain the corpus luteum. This hormone stimulates the mammary glands to develop secretory alveoli and secrete milk.

Menstrual Cycle (Fig. 9-15 and Table 9-4)

The menstrual cycle begins at puberty and continues until menopause some 40 years later. The day of onset of menstrual flow is considered to be the first day of the cycle. The cycle ends on the last day before the next onset of menstruation. The cycle can vary from 22 to 35 days but is generally 28 days.

The proliferative or follicular phase begins about the fifth day of the cycle and extends through ovulation. It is also known as the postmenstrual or estrogenic phase. During this phase the uterine endothelium thickens as estrogen secretion rises.

The secreting phase occurs after ovulation. It is also called the postovulatory, luteal, or progestational phase. During this phase the three endometrial zones become well defined. The basal zone is adjacent to the myometrium; the compact zone lies immediately below the endometrial surface; and the spongy zone lies between the compact and basal layers. The endometrium becomes extremely vascular and rich in glycogen, an ideal environment for implantation of the fertilized ovum. The uterine spiral arteries become more coiled and tortuous during this period, growing almost to the surface of the

Table 9-4
Correlation of Ovarian and Endometrial Cycles (Ideal 28-Day Cycle)

	Menstrual (1-3 to 5 days)	Early Follicular (4 to 6-8 days)	Advanced Follicular (9 to 12-16 days)	Ovulation (12-16 days)	Early Luteal (15-19 days)	Advanced Luteal (20-25 days)	Premenstrual (26-32 days)
Ovary	Involution of corpus luteum	Growth and maturation of graafian follicle		Ovulation	Active corpus luteum		Involution of corpus luteum
Estrogen	Diminution	Progressive increase		High concentration Appearing	Secondary rise		Decreasing
Progesterone	Absent			—	Rising		Decreasing Regressive
Endometrium	Menstrual desquamation and involution	Reorganization and proliferation	Further growth and watery secretion		Active secretion and glandular dilation	Accumulation of secretion and edema	
Pituitary secretion Follicle-stimulating hormone (FSH)	Fairly constant until just before ovulation			Moderate increase just before	Rapid decrease to previous levels		
Luteinizing hormone (LH)	Same as above			Marked increase just before	Same as above		

From Pritchard, J.A., and McDonald, P.C.: Williams' obstetrics, ed. 16, New York, 1980, Appleton-Century-Crofts.

endometrium. If implantation of a fertilized ovum does not occur, the corpus luteum loses functional activity and degenerates. If fertilization and implantation occur, the secretion of human chorionic gonadotropin by the placenta maintains the corpus luteum. This promotes the continued secretion of progesterone and estrogen and prevents menstruation.

The premenstrual phase occurs 2 to 3 days before menstruation with infiltration of the stroma by polymorphonuclear or mononuclear leukocytes. The reticular framework of the stroma in the superficial zone disintegrates, resulting in a loss of tissue fluid and thinning of the endometrium. Some 4 to 24 hours before the onset of menstruation a vasoconstriction of the arterioles and coiled arteries causes anoxia and shriveling of the compact and spongy zones. After a period of constriction the coiled arteries relax and bleeding occurs from them or their branches. This marks the onset of menstruation.

The menstrual phase lasts from the first to about the fifth day of the cycle. As the coiled arteries rupture, hematomas form that distend and eventually rupture the superficial endometrium. Fissures develop in adjacent layers and tissues, become fragmented, and detach. The entire functional layer of the endometrium is eventually sloughed, leaving only the deep basal layer intact. Bleeding stops when the coiled arteries return to a state of constriction.

Physiologic Female Sexual Response

Vasocongestion and myotonia are responsible for the phenomena observed during the cycle of sexual response. Vasocongestion is a congestion primarily of venous blood vessels and is the major response to sexual stimulation. Myotonia is a secondary response to stimulation characterized by an increase in muscular tension.

In their classic work published in 1966 Masters and Johnson[30] described the female sexual response cycle as divided into four physiologic phases: excitement, plateau, orgasm, and resolution.

The excitement phase develops as a response to physical or psychic stimuli. The physiologic characteristics include clitoral tumescence, elongation, and widening; vaginal lubrication and expansion; partial uterine elevation; thickening of the labia majora in a multiparous woman; elevation and flattening of the labia majora in a nulliparous woman; erection of the nipples; engorgement of the areolae of the breasts; enlargement of the breasts; spreading of a maculopapular rash or "sex flush" over the epigastric area and breast; and increase in cardiac rate and blood pressure.

The plateau phase occurs if stimulation is maintained. During this period the clitoris retracts and vasocongestion in the labia majora and the outer third of the vagina causes an increase in their size. This is referred to as the or-

gasmic platform. With elevation of the uterus, the cervix produces a tenting effect. The labia minora changes from bright red to wine color, a phenomenon known as "sex skin" that indicates an impending orgasm. A "sex flush" may cover the entire body. There are voluntary and involuntary contractions of the facial, abdominal, and intercostal muscles. Hyperventilation and transient tachycardia and hypertension occur during this phase.

The orgasm phase is characterized by an involuntary release of sexual tension. The primary response occurs in the orgasmic platform with contraction of the perineal, pubococcygeal, and bulbospongiosus muscles. Uterine contractions begin at the fundus and progress to the lower uterine segment. The intensity of the orgasmic experience is paralleled by the sex flush and by excursions of the contracting uterus. Respiratory rate, pulse rate, and blood pressure increase during this phase.

The resolution phase generally parallels the excitement phase in length. The uterus descends, the clitoris descends, and the vagina, labia majora, and labia minora return to their normal sizes. Normal coloring returns to the vaginal wall and the labia minora. The cervical os remains open for 20 to 30 minutes after orgasm. The nipples lose their erection, breast size decreases, and the sex flush disappears. Respiratory and pulse rates and blood pressure return to normal levels. Pelvic vasocongestion and myotonia decrease and eventually disappear.

Parallels between sexual response, birth, and breast feeding were described by Niles Newton in 1973. Labor has been compared with the excitement phase of sexual response and orgasm with birth. In addition, a close resemblance between the emotions experienced during breast feeding and sexual arousal has been described. Birth, breast feeding, and sexual response are all based on neurohormonal reflexes,[2] are sensitive to environmental stimuli,[3] and appear to elicit caretaking behaviors.[41]

Pregnancy and Delivery

Fertilization and implantation (Fig. 9-16). After discharge from the ovary the secondary oocyte is transported through the fallopian tube by the activity of the cilia in the tube and peristaltic contractions of smooth muscles of the tube. The oocyte usually takes 3 to 4 days to reach the uterus. Normally fertilization occurs when the secondary oocyte is one-third the distance down the tube. Once the sperm penetrates the ovum, it releases acrosomal enzymes that disperse the corona radiata and zona pellucida. The tail of the sperm is then shed, and the ovum becomes impenetrable to other spermatozoa. In the presence of the male pronucleus the secondary oocyte proceeds with the second meiotic division, forming a second polar body.

Fig. 9-16
Fertilization and development during first week.

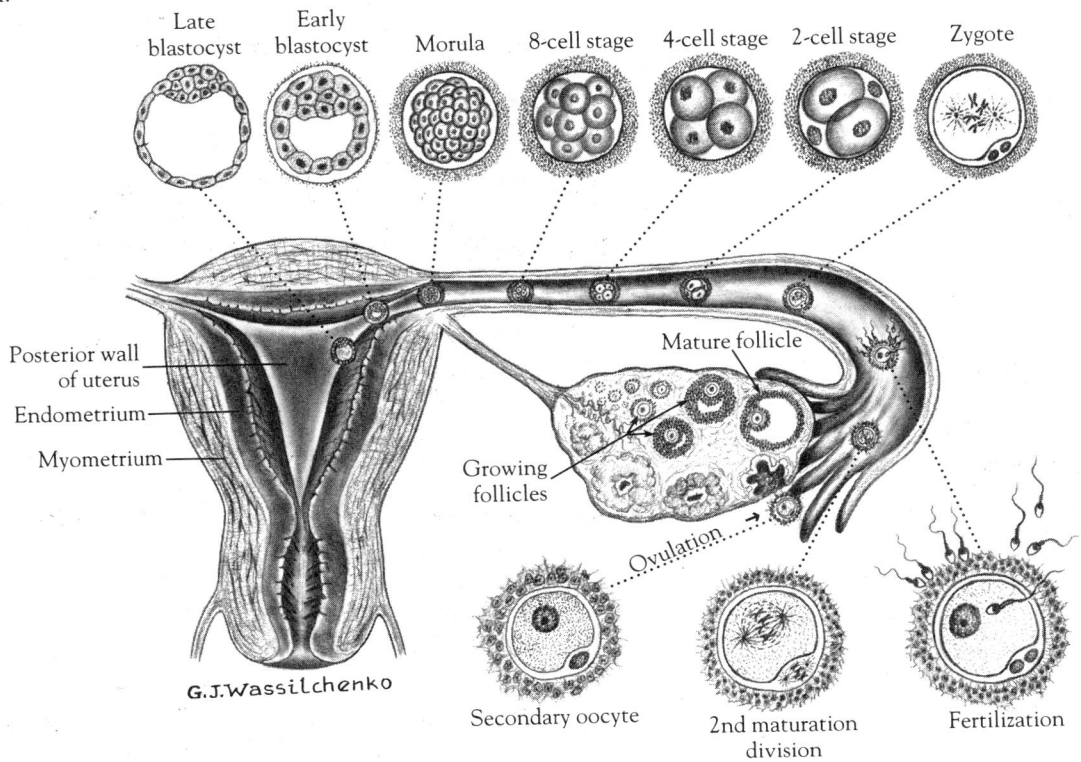

Late blastocyst — Early blastocyst — Morula — 8-cell stage — 4-cell stage — 2-cell stage — Zygote

Posterior wall of uterus
Endometrium
Myometrium

Mature follicle

Growing follicles

G.J.Wassilchenko

Ovulation

Secondary oocyte — 2nd maturation division — Fertilization

Cleavage consists of repetitive mitotic divisions. The first division of the zygote results in two blastomeres. The fertilized ovum undergoes slow cleavage; by the time it reaches the uterus it may contain only 12 blastomeres. The morula is produced after several more divisions of the blastomeres. Gradual accumulation of fluid in the morula results in formation of the blastocyst. The inner cell mass of the blastocyst produces the embryo, and the trophoblast or outer layer of cells provides nourishment to the ovum.

Implantation occurs after the zona pellucida disappears and the blastocyst adheres to the endometrial surface. As the epithelium erodes, the blastocyst sinks into the endometrium with the inner cell mass entering first. The epithelium heals over, and the embryo develops within the tissues of the uterine wall. About 7 to 8 days after fertilization the inner cell mass, now the embryonic disc, differentiates into a thick plate of primitive ectoderm and an underlying layer of endoderm. Cells that will become the amnionic cavity develop between the embryonic disc and the trophoblast. The yolk sac arises from cells that develop below the embryonic disc. Proliferation of cells in the disc causes a thickening of the midline called the primitive streak. The three germ layers become apparent

as cells spread out laterally from the primitive streak. The germ layers give rise to various body organs. They are the ectoderm, from which is derived the nervous system and the skin and its appendages, the mesoderm, which gives rise to the muscles, bones, and connective tissue, and the endoderm, which develops into the lining of the digestive and respiratory tracts and into the derivative organs such as the thyroid, pancreas, and liver.

Placenta and fetal membranes (Fig. 9-17). The placenta develops from the chorion of the embryo and the decidua basalis of the uterus. It is formed when the chorionic villi infiltrate the decidua basalis and is complete by the third month of pregnancy. The villi are tiny vascular branches of the placenta that extend into the intervillous space. Maternal blood is ejected upward from the uterine spiral arterioles and spreads laterally at random into the intervillous space surrounding the villi. The exchange of oxygen and nutrients and the elimination of waste products occur in this space. The mature placenta is a circular disc about 20 cm (8 inches) in diameter and 2.5 cm (1 inch) thick, weighing about 0.5 kg (1 pound). The maternal surface of the placenta is red with about 20 velvety bumps called cotyledons. These are composed of a mainstem villus and its projections. The fetal surface

Fig. 9-17
Advancing pregnancy showing relative
fetal size and proliferation of
chorionic villi into decidua basalis.

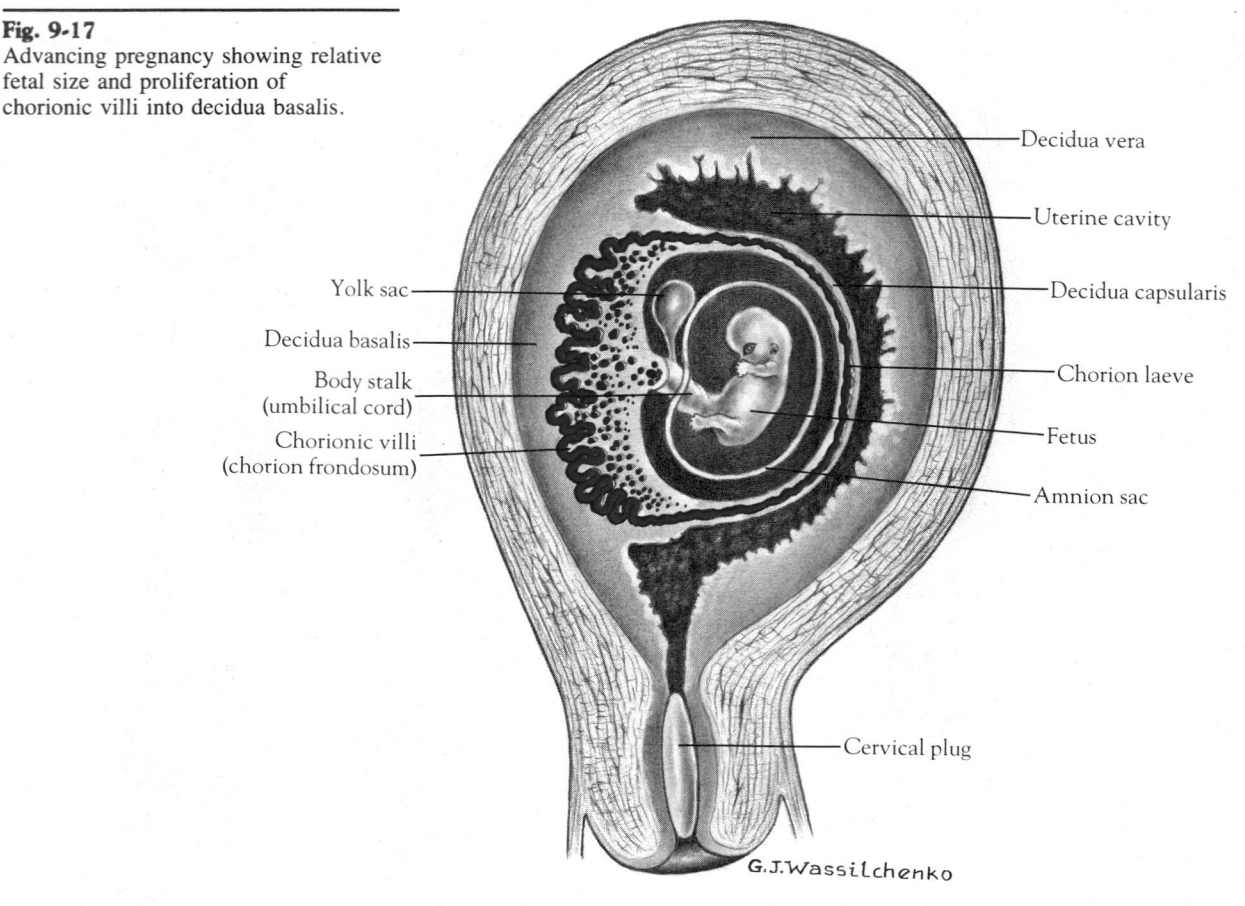

Yolk sac

Decidua basalis

Body stalk
(umbilical cord)

Chorionic villi
(chorion frondosum)

Decidua vera

Uterine cavity

Decidua capsularis

Chorion laeve

Fetus

Amnion sac

Cervical plug

G.J.Wassilchenko

of the placenta is smooth, glistening, and covered with amnion. The umbilical cord usually joins the placenta near the center but may insert at any site (Fig. 9-18).

The amnion is derived from the inner layer of the trophoblast. It enlarges to surround the embryo. As the amnionic sac enlarges, it brings the amnion into apposition with the interior of the chorion. The fluid that fills the amnion is thought to be an extension of the fetal extracellular fluid space during the first half of pregnancy. The control of amnionic fluid volume is modulated during the second trimester as the fetus begins to swallow, urinate, and inspire amnionic fluid. The volume of amnionic fluid increases from an average of 50 ml at 12 weeks' gestation to 400 ml at midpregnancy. It reaches a maximum of about 1 L at 36 to 38 weeks' gestation and decreases as term approaches. Amnionic fluid is a medium in which the fetus can move, be cushioned from external injury, and maintain a constant temperature.

The chorion, the outermost embryonic membrane, is composed of trophoblasts lined with mesoderm. It provides the growing embryo with nourishment and protec-

tion. The chorion forms the fetal part of the placenta as fetal blood vessels develop in the villous portion.

The decidua is the endometrium of the pregnant uterus. It is usually divided into three parts: the decidua basalis, the portion directly under the site of implantation, the decidua capsularis, which lies over the developing ovum and separates it from the rest of the uterine cavity, and the decidua parietalis or decidua vera, which lines the remainder of the uterus. The decidua capsularis and decidua vera fuse at around the fourth month of pregnancy as the growing amnionic sac fills the uterine cavity.

Placental hormones. The placenta functions as a temporary endocrine gland, producing the protein hormones human chorionic gonadotropin and human placental lactogen and the steroid hormones progesterone and estrogen. The trophoblast may also synthesize thyroid-stimulating hormone, and the placenta may form adrenocorticotropic hormone (ACTH or corticotropin).

Human chorionic gonadotropin (HCG) is a glucoprotein with a molecular weight of 39,000. Its primary functions are to maintain the corpus luteum during early preg-

Fig. 9-18
Pregnant uterus showing placenta in situ.

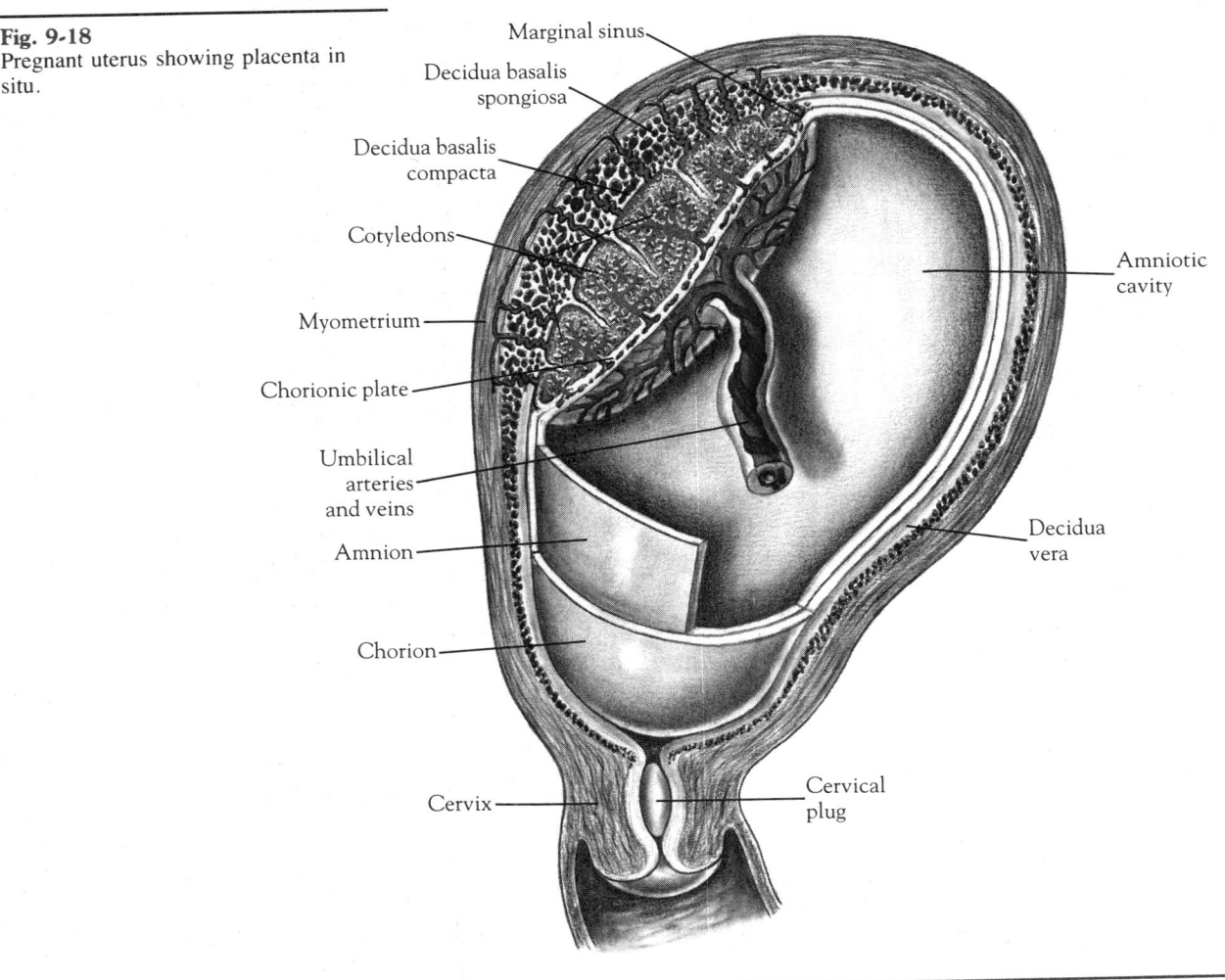

Marginal sinus

Decidua basalis spongiosa

Decidua basalis compacta

Cotyledons

Myometrium

Chorionic plate

Umbilical arteries and veins

Amnion

Chorion

Cervix

Amniotic cavity

Decidua vera

Cervical plug

nancy and to stimulate ovarian secretion of progesterone and estrogens. HCG can be detected in maternal plasma and serum 9 days after conception. It reaches a peak at 9 to 12 weeks and then declines to a plateau for the remainder of the pregnancy.

Human placental lactogen (HPL) or chorionic growth hormone was so named because of its lactogenic activity and resemblance to human growth hormone. It is also called human chorionic somatomammotropin. HPL is synthesized by the placental trophoblasts and can be detected about 4 weeks after fertilization. Maternal blood levels of HPL rise steadily during the first and second trimesters. Each day 1 to 2 g is produced, reaching a level that can be measured by radioimmunoassay of maternal serum in late pregnancy. Negligible amounts are found in the fetal circulation and maternal and neonatal urine. The primary function of HPL, which is mediated through maternal rather than fetal tissues, is to promote a continuous flow of nutrients, primarily glucose, to the fetus. It participates in a number of metabolic activities, including lipolysis and elevation of circulating free fatty acid levels, that provide energy for maternal metabolism and fetal nutrition. It spares glucose and protein by inhibiting glucose uptake and gluconeogenesis. Placental secretion of HPL may be part of a glucose feedback mechanism as suggested by slight elevations of HPL when a person is fasting or has insulin-induced hypoglycemia. The hormone disappears rapidly from maternal serum after delivery and has a half-life of 20 minutes.

During pregnancy the placenta is the site of origin for the secretion of estrogens, which are synthesized from precursor hormones supplied by the maternal and fetal adrenal glands. Estriol is 30% of the unconjugated estrogens circulating in maternal plasma at term and 90% of the total estrogen secreted in the urine. Its measurement provides a valuable clinical index of fetal status.

Rapidly decreasing values suggest placental insufficiency and fetal stress.

Progesterone is synthesized by the placenta beginning at about 6 weeks' gestation, and by 12 weeks the placenta has replaced the corpus luteum as the major producer of this hormone. Progesterone inhibits uterine contractions and stimulates development of the mammary glands. It is produced by the placenta in larger amounts than estrogens, with some 250 mg a day produced at term. This represents a 10-fold increase over the peak rates during the luteal phase of the menstrual cycle.

Stages of labor. The mechanism by which labor begins is unknown. Several theories have been offered, including oxytocin stimulation, progesterone withdrawal, fetal cortisol production, prostaglandin formation by fetal membranes and uterine decidua vera, and uterine stretch. In addition, placental secretion of the hormone relaxin is thought to promote the end of pregnancy by softening the cervical canal and relaxing the pubic ligaments.

Labor has four stages. The first stage lasts from the onset of regular uterine contractions to the complete dilation of the cervix. This is about 12 hours in primigravidas and 6 hours in multigravidas. In the latent or early phase of the first stage there is progress in effacement of the cervix with little descent of the fetal presenting part. During the active phase the cervix dilates rapidly and the presenting part descends.

The second stage of labor lasts from full dilation of the cervix to delivery of the fetus. The mean duration of this stage is 1 hour in primigravidas and 20 minutes in multigravidas.

The third stage of labor lasts from delivery of the fetus to delivery of the placenta. The duration of this stage often depends on the physician or midwife but generally is no more than 10 or 15 minutes.

The fourth stage of labor is a period of about an hour after delivery of the placenta during which the uterus contracts and vessel thrombosis controls bleeding from the placental implantation site.

NORMAL FINDINGS

Area of Concern	Normal Adult Findings	Variations in Child	Variations in Older Adult
External Genitalia			
Surface characteristics	Homogeneous		
Hair distribution	Variable in adults; usually inverse triangle with base over pubis; some hair may extend up midline toward umbilicus	Preadolescent: No hair Average age 10.5 to 11 years: Sparse, lightly pigmented, straight along medial border of labia 11.5 to 12 years: Darker hair, beginning to curl, increased amount 12.5 years average: Coarse, curly, abundant amount but less than adult 13.5 years average: Adult female triangle, spread to medial surface of thighs	Pubic hair thinned, perhaps sparse, often gray
Inguinal and mons pubis skin surface	Smooth; clear		
Labia and vestibule Labia majora, outer surface	Darker pigmentation; shriveled or full; gaping or closed; usually symmetric; skin surface smooth; may appear dry or moist	Pink; smooth surface; symmetric; dry appearance; becomes prominent and covered with hair during puberty	Labial folds flattened or may disappear into surrounding skin; decrease in subcutaneous fat in folds that usually corresponds to degree of loss of subcutaneous fat elsewhere on body; skin appears smooth, often shiny, and paler than in younger adult

Area of Concern	Normal Adult Findings	Variations in Child	Variations in Older Adult
Labia majora, inner surface	Dark pink pigmentation; moist; usually symmetric		Shiny; usually dry; paler than in young adult; fewer folds
Labia minora	Dark pink pigmentation; moist; usually symmetric	Very prominent in infants (may protrude from labia majora); recedes by puberty to adult configuration; light pink, becoming dark by puberty; symmetric	
Vestibule surface	Dark pink pigmentation; moist; usually symmetric		
Palpation of labia and vestibule	Soft, homogeneous consistency; nontender		
Clitoris Size	2 cm length visible; 0.5 cm diameter	3 mm to 1 cm in length depending on age and maturational development	Slightly smaller than in younger adult
Surface	Medial aspect covered by prepuce	Edematous in newborns; prepuce eventually covers clitoris during infancy	Medial aspect covered by prepuce; pink
Urethral meatus and surrounding tissue surface	Irregular opening or slit; may be close to or slightly within vaginal introitus; usually located midline		Relaxed perineal musculature may result in meatus being situated more posteriorly; very near or within vaginal introitus
Milking of urethral duct	Nontender; no discharge		
Vaginal introitus and surrounding tissue Surface	Thin vertical slit or large orifice with irregular edges (hymenal caruncles); moist tissue	Moist tissue; even pink color; hymen may or may not be across or partially across vaginal opening; by menarche, opening should be at least 1 cm wide; vaginal opening present	May be smaller than in younger adult; multiparous client may manifest gaping introitus with vaginal walls rolling toward opening
Palpation of lateral and posterior introitus	Nontender; no discharge	Mucoid or sanguineous discharge in newborn; water discharge as seen in adult present for 2 to 3 years before onset of menstruation and 1 year after	Opening may be very narrow and admit only one finger
Vaginal tone	Nullipara: squeezes tightly around examiner's index and middle fingers; unipara or multipara: squeezes firmly but with less tone than nullipara; no bulging or urinary incontinence when bearing down or pushing		May be relaxed; client has difficulty squeezing examiner's finger with voluntary vaginal constriction; vaginal wall may roll slightly outward; no incontinence
Perineum Surface	Smooth; midline or mediolateral episiotomy scar may be visible	Smooth; pink	Smooth; midline or mediolateral episiotomy scar may be visible
Palpation between index finger and thumb	Nontender; nullipara: thick, smooth; unipara or multipara: thin, rigid, scarring		Thin; rigid

Area of Concern	Normal Adult Findings	Variations in Child	Variations in Older Adult
Anal surface	Increased pigmentation and coarse skin		
Internal Genitalia			
Cervix			
Color	Pink color evenly distributed; bluish in pregnancy; symmetric, circumscribed erythema surrounding os may indicate normal condition of exposed columnar epithelium, but inexperienced examiners should consider any reddened appearance a problem for consultation	Deep pink or red color until puberty	Paler than in younger woman; color evenly distributed
Position	Midline; cervix and os may be pointed in anterior or posterior direction; may project into vaginal tube 1 to 3 cm (resulting in 1 to 3 cm fornices surrounding cervix)		Cervix protrudes less into vaginal tube; may be flush against back of vaginal wall; surrounding fornices diminish or may disappear
Size	Usually 2.5 cm diameter		Cervix decreases in size with age
Surface	Smooth; firm; occasional visible squamo-columnar junction (symmetric reddened circle around os); nabothian cysts (smooth, round, small, yellowish raised areas)		Smooth; may appear paler than in younger woman; occasional visible squamocolumnar junction (symmetric reddened circle around os)
Contour	Evenly rounded or slightly ovoid		Nabothian cysts (smooth, round, yellowish, raised areas) common
Os	Nullipara: small, evenly round; unipara or multipara: slitlike, may be star shaped or irregular		Often very narrow or stenosed; may be obliterated
Cervical discharge	Mucus plug may be present at os; odorless; creamy or clear; thin, thick, or stringy; discharge often heavier at midcycle or immediately before menstruation		Often scanty; if present, should be clear or slightly opaque and odorless
Vagina			
Length			Shortens with aging
Color	Pink		Paler than in younger women
Surface	Transverse rugae (diminish after vaginal deliveries); moist; smooth	Thick and moist mucosa at birth; thin and somewhat atrophic at 2 to 3 months of age	Less moisture; smooth (rugae diminish with aging); shiny
Consistency	Smooth; homogeneous		
Secretions	Minimum to moderate amount; thin; clear or cloudy; odorless		May be absent or sparse; if present, should be clear or slightly opaque
Fornices	Pliable; smooth		Diminish and may disappear with aging; if palpable, should be pliable, smooth, and nontender
Uterus	Mobile; nontender		Diminishes greatly; often not palpable
Position	Fundus anteverted; palpable at level of pubis		If palpated with internal hand, body of uterus should be smooth, firm, freely movable, and nontender

Area of Concern	Normal Adult Findings	Variations in Child	Variations in Older Adult
Contour of fundus	Rounded		
Uterine wall	Firm consistency; smooth surface; pear shaped; 5.5 to 8 cm long		
Ovaries	May not be palpable; slightly tender on palpation; firm; smooth; ovoid; mobile; diameter about 4 cm (size of walnut)		Atrophy with age and rarely palpable in aged women; fallopian tube palpable
Breasts			
Size	Varies	Enlarged for 1 to 2 months in infancy	Increase in adipose tissue
Symmetry	Bilaterally equal; slight asymmetry; breasts hang equally when woman is seated and leaning forward; breasts appear symmetric when woman is seated and pushing hands into hips or pushing palms together	Breasts develop between ages 10 years, 8 months and 13 years, 6 months; each breast may develop at different rate, so size may be unequal during puberty	
Contour	Smooth; convex; even		
Skin color	Even throughout		
Skin texture	Smooth; elastic; movable; striae		
Venous patterns	Bilaterally similar		
Moles, nevi	Long history of presence; nonchanging; nontender		
Areolae			
Size	Bilaterally equal	Small during infancy	
Shape	Round or oval		
Surface characteristics	Smooth; bilaterally similar; Montgomery tubules		
Nipples			
Direction	Bilaterally equal in pointing direction		
Size and shape	Bilaterally equal; long-standing inversion (unilateral or bilateral)	Flat in infancy	
Color	Homogeneous		
Surface characteristics	Smooth or may be slightly wrinkled; skin intact		
Discharge	Absent	Milky appearance during infancy	
Suspensory ligaments	Equal bilateral pull when woman is seated with arms abducted over head		Relaxed; breasts may appear elongated or pendulous
Palpation of breasts			
Tone	Bilaterally firm and equal; sagging of breast tissue may occur with aging or poor bra support		
Tissue qualities	Smooth diffuse tissue bilaterally; nodular, bilateral granular consistency; premenstrual engorgement; elastic; nontender; firm mammary ridge along each breast at approximately 4 to 8 o'clock position		Decrease in glandular tissue
Lymph nodes (including supraclavicular, infraclavicular, central and lateral axillary, pectoral, subscapular, scapular, brachial, intermediate, and internal mammary chains)	Nonpalpable		

PERTINENT BACKGROUND INFORMATION

An additional consideration in assessment of the female organ system is a review of pertinent background information, including the following[15,47,50]:

Concurrent diseases or conditions
  Menstruation
    Age at onset
    Length of cycles (duration)
    Interval between cycles
    Regularity of cycles
    Amount and type of flow
      Number of tampons or napkins used
      Date of most recent douching
      Type of contraceptive used
    Date of last menstrual period (LMP)
    Associated symptoms (such as pain, menorrhagia, or metrorrhagia)
  Pregnancy
    Number of pregnancies and outcome of each
    Complications of pregnancy and delivery or abortion
  Menopause
    When occurred
    Related symptoms
      Hot flashes
      Dry vaginal mucosa
  Gastrointestinal (GI) system
    Constipation
    Hemorrhoids
  Endocrine system
    Hypothyroidism
    Hyperthyroidism
    Stein-Leventhal syndrome

  Blood dyscrasias
  Hypertension
Previous surgery or illness
  Gynecologic surgery
  Other major surgery or illness (for example, of abdomen or endocrine system)
Family history
  Cancer
  Sickle cell disease
  Thyroid disorder
  Diabetes
  Other diseases
  Death from gynecologic-related condition
  Maternal diethylstilbestrol (DES) usage
Social history
  Smoking
  Sexual activity
    Abnormal lesions or discharge in sexual partner
  Contraception
Medication history
  Oral contraceptives
  Estrogen therapy
  Intrauterine contraceptive device (IUD)
  Phenothiazines
  Digitalis
  Diuretics

NORMAL LABORATORY DATA

Laboratory Test	Normal Adult Values
Blood	
Clotting time (Lee-White)	8-15 min
Factor II	83%-117% of normal; term pregnancy 92%
Factor V	50%-150% of normal; term pregnancy 108%
Factor VII	50%-150% of normal; term pregnancy 170%
Factor VIII	50%-150% of normal; term pregnancy 196%
Factor IX	50%-150% of normal; term pregnancy 130%
Factor X	50%-150% of normal; term pregnancy 130%
Factor XI	50%-150% of normal; term pregnancy 69%
Factor XIII	Clot stable in 5M urea for at least 24 hr; if factor XIII deficiency is present, clot usually dissolves in 1-2 hr

Laboratory Test	Normal Adult Values
Fibrinogen	200-400 mg/dl (quantitative); in pregnancy and early puerperium, 300-600 mg/dl
Partial thromboplastin time	25-39 sec (usually stated to be within 10 sec of control); slightly shortened in pregnancy
Prothrombin time	10-13 sec or 60%-100% of control; slightly shortened in pregnancy
Thrombin time	Less than 1½ times control value; term pregnancy 8 sec
Erythrocyte sedimentation rate	Westergren method Females
	Less than 50 yr 0-25 mm/hr
	Over 50 yr 0-30 mm/hr
Zeta sedimentation rate	Less than 50 yr 55%
	50-80 year 40%-60%
Leukocytes	Females 3.9-5.9 10^6/mm³; pregnancy 10,000-15,000/mm³; may increase to as much as 25,000/mm³ in labor and early puerperium

Laboratory Test	Normal Adult Values
Red blood cell (RBC) volume	1355 cells/mm^3 in nonpregnant state; 1790 cells/mm^3 in late pregnancy
α_1-Fetoprotein	Up to approximately 40 ng/ml for serum (interlaboratory differences exist); maternal serum increases to maximum of 500 ng/ml at wk 32, and ranges are stratified by weeks of gestation; normal ranges are available for amniotic fluid by wk
Androstenedione	Less than 250 ng/ml
Bilirubin	Total, 0.3-1 mg/dl; direct, up to 0.4 mg/dl; indirect, 0.1-0.8 mg/dl
Chorionic gonadotropin	3 IU/ml (nonpregnant); 60-70 IU/ml (late pregnancy); 50,000 mIU/ml about 65 days after implantation
Chorionic somatomammotropin	Varies with duration of gestation; may reach 10 µg/ml
Creatine	0.2-0.8 mg/dl; increased in pregnancy
Dihydrotestosterone	None detectable
Estradiol	Menstruating female Early cycle 20-170 pg/ml Midcycle 70-500 pg/ml Late cycle 45-340 pg/ml Patient taking oral contraceptives 12-50 pg/ml Postmenopausal female 1-5 ng/dl Adult male 13-42 pg/ml
Estriol	Nonpregnant female less than 0.5 ng/ml; pregnant female—estriol increases until term and then decreases: 30-32 wk 2-12 ng/ml 33-35 wk 3-19 ng/ml 36-38 wk 5-27 ng/ml 39-40 wk 10-30 ng/ml
Estrogens, total	Menstruating female 15-80 µg/24 hr Postmenopausal female Less than 20 µg/24 hr
Estrone	Menstruating female Early in cycle 50-300 pg/ml Midcycle 100-600 pg/ml Late cycle 80-450 pg/ml Menopausal female 0-30 pg/ml
Follicle-stimulating hormone (normal ranges vary among laboratories)	Menstrual female Before or after ovulation less than 20 IU/L Midcycle less than 40 IU/L Menopausal female 40-160 IU/L
17-Hydroxyprogesterone	Adult female Early cycle 100 ng/dl Late cycle 80-300 ng/dl
Luteinizing hormone	Midcycle 6-30 mIU/ml Follicular phase 2-30 mIU/ml Ovulatory peak 40-200 mIU/ml Luteal phase 0-20 mIU/ml Menopause 35-120 mIU/ml
Magnesium	1.2-1.9 mEq/L

Laboratory Test	Normal Adult Values
Progesterone	Follicular phase 95 ng/dl Luteal phase 1130 ng/dl End of cycle less than 1 ng/ml Wk 20 of pregnancy up to 50 ng/ml
Prolactin	Normal range varies with laboratory
Testosterone	Female 20-100 ng/dl
T_3, triiodothyronine (total circulating)	Approximately 80 to 200-230 ng/dl with some variation among laboratories; increase during pregnancy
T_4, thyroxine (radioimmunoassay)	Cord T_4 and neonatal values much higher, falling over first months and years 10 yr and up approximately 5.8-11 µg/dl, varying somewhat among laboratories
Thyroid-binding globulin	10-26 µg/dl
Transferrin	Approximately 200-360 mg/dl with some variation among laboratories
Urea nitrogen (BUN)	1-40 yr 5-20 mg/dl; gradual slight increase thereafter
Uric acid	Adult female 2.4-6 mg/dl or slightly more
Urine	
Chorionic gonadotropin	Negative; positive in pregnancy
Creatinine	Adult female 0.8-1.8 g/24 hr; creatinine excretion decreases with advanced age as muscle mass diminishes
Estriol	Starting at wk 30, minimum of 9 mg/24 hr
Dehydroepiandosterone	Normal ranges usually provided by laboratories doing such fractionation; ranges often stratified by age and sex
Estrogens	Menstruating female 15-80 µg/24 hr Postmenopausal female less than 20 µg/24 hr
Follicle-stimulating hormone	Follicular phase 5-20 IU/24 hr Luteal phase 5-15 IU/24 hr Midcycle 15-60 IU/24 hr Menopause 50-100 IU/24 hr
Luteinizing hormone	Follicular phase 2-25 IU/24 hr Ovulatory phase 30-95 IU/24 hr Luteal phase 2-20 IU/24 hr Postmenopausal 40-110 IU/24 hr
Pregnanediol	Proliferative phase 0.5-1.5 mg/24 hr Luteal phase 2-7 mg/24 hr Menopause 0.2-1 mg/24 hr 10-12 wk pregnant 5-15 mg/24 hr 12-18 wk pregnant 5-15 mg/24 hr 18-24 wk pregnant 15-33 mg/24 hr 24-28 wk pregnant 20-42 mg/24 hr 28-32 wk pregnant 27-47 mg/24 hr

Laboratory Test	Normal Adult Values
Amniotic fluid	
Osmolality	Decreases about 1 mOsmol/L/wk after 20 wk gestation
Lungs	
Lecithin/sphingo-myelin (L/S) ratio	Mature lung above 2 at term; borderline 1.5-1.9 with risk of respiratory distress syndrome; caution necessary in interpreting results from diabetic patients, in whom misleading evidence for pulmonary maturity has been reported
Disaturated (acetone-precipitated) lecithin	About 70% at term
Phosphatidylinositol (PI)	Decreasing from 25% to 15% at term
Phosphatidylglycerol (PG)	Presence of PG is evidence that fetus is greater than or at least 36-37 wk in development
Creatinine	2 mg/dl at wk 37-38; results higher than 2 mg/dl indicate maturity; concentrations of 1-1.8 mg/dl found at wk 36
Bilirubin (ΔOD 450)	Less than 0.1 mg/dl
Lipid cells	Above 30% indicates fetal age above 36 wk
α-Fetoprotein	Differences exist between laboratories; ranges stratified by wk of gestation, decreasing with increasing maturity
Volume	50 ml at 10 wk gestation 200 ml at 16 wk gestation 1000 ml at 38 wk gestation Decreasing volume postterm

DIAGNOSTIC STUDIES

Papanicolaou (Pap) test

Simple smear method of examining exfoliative cells, particularly malignant and premalignant conditions of cervix; desquamated cells from cervical epithelium obtained during pelvic examination, stained, and examined under microscope; histologic classification includes class I through class V

Class I—normal cells observed

Class II—atypical cells

Class III—mild dysplasia

Class IV—severe dysplasia, suspicious cells

Class V—carcinoma cells observed

Nursing care:

Prepare patient for vaginal examination and validate that patient has not douched or inserted vaginal medications for 24 hours before procedure

Obtain accurate history including following:

Date of last Pap test and results

Date of last menstrual period (LMP)

Frequency and duration of periods

Amount of bleeding with period

Method of contraception

Hormonal drugs

Presence and color of vaginal discharge, pain, or itching

Give patient perineal pad after procedure to absorb any bleeding

Vaginal smears

Vaginal secretions are placed on slide with 1 drop normal saline placed on one side and 1 drop 10% to 20% potassium hydroxide (KOH) on other side; *Trichomonas vaginalis* can be observed at saline end of slide, and *Candida albicans* at KOH side; other organisms can also be identified using this procedure

Endometrial biopsy

Biopsy of endometrial uterine lining; generally performed on first day of menses of premenopausal patients and anytime in postmenopausal patients; tissue specimen may be obtained by (1) Gravlee jet washer (isotonic saline solution is forced through intrauterine cannula, flushing endometrial cells into external collecting reservoir) or (2) Nova curette (curette attached to syringe scrapes endometrium, and cell samples are drawn into syringe)

Nursing care:

Prepare patient for vaginal examination

Explain that she may experience cramping owing to dilation of cervix during procedure

Teach and assist with relaxation and breathing techniques

Give patient perineal pad after procedure

Ensure that menstrual data is noted on laboratory specimen slip for pathologist

Cervical biopsy

Biopsy of cervical epithelium and shallow layer of underlying stroma to diagnose malignant invasion

Nursing care:

Prepare patient for vaginal examination

After procedure give patient perineal pad and inform her that spotting will occur

Cervical conization (cone biopsy)

Surgical removal of cervical tissue in shape of cone for diagnosis or for treatment of cervical infection or carcinoma in situ; done by physician with cold knife scalpel; procedure frequently called cold knife conization (CKC) or cryosurgery

Nursing care:

After procedure assist physician with removal of vaginal packing, usually within 24 hours

Give perineal care with antiseptic solution and change perineal pad every 4 hours and as needed

Instruct patient (1) to avoid coitus, douching, or tampons for 6 weeks or until directed by physician; (2) to report excessive bleeding (more than a period after 7 to 10 days) and symptoms of infection; (3) to avoid constipation; (4) to maintain good perineal hygiene; and (5) to report signs of infection to physician

Colposcopy

Examination of cervix and vagina with colposcope, stereoscopic binocular microscope with various levels of magnification, to evaluate vascular pattern, intercapillary distance, surface pattern, color, tone, opacity, clarity, demarcation, and extent of lesion, to differentiate between inflammatory atypia and neoplasia or between invasive and noninvasive cervical lesions, and to enable follow-up

Nursing care:

Prepare patient for vaginal examination

Show her colposcope and inform her that it will not be inserted into vagina

Inform her beforehand if biopsy is to be performed

Culdoscopy

Visual examination of female pelvic viscera by means of endoscope inserted through posterior vaginal fornix; patient is usually sedated and general anesthesia is not used; procedure is performed with patient in knee-chest position

Nursing care:

Explain to patient that once endoscope is removed she will be requested to exhale as forcefully as possible to force out intraperitoneal air; this maneuver will minimize shoulder pain when patient sits up

Colpotomy (culdotomy)

Excision of posterior vagina with entry into cul-de-sac for visual and manual examination to diagnose obscure pelvic disease; operative procedures that can be performed with this technique include salpingectomy for ectopic pregnancy and tubal ligation

Nursing care:

Provide routine preoperative and postanesthetic recovery care

Explain to patient that she may experience sensations of pelvic fullness and pressure

Instruct patient not to put anything into vagina, including douches and tampons, and not to have intercourse until permitted by physician

Hysteroscopy

Direct visual examination of cervical canal and uterine cavity through hysteroscope to examine endometri-

um, secure specimen for biopsy, remove intrauterine device, or excise cervical polyps; procedure most often performed with patient under spinal anesthesia

Nursing care:

Patient should be maintained in flat position for 8 hours after procedure

Laparoscopy

Visualization and examination of abdominal and pelvic organs with laparascope inserted through small incision in abdominal wall; therapeutic procedures may also be performed, including removal of peritubular adhesions and sterilization through fulguration of oviducts

Nursing care:

Provide routine presurgical and postanesthetic care

Inform patient that she may experience sore throat from intubation and sore chest from insufflation of abdomen; these sensations usually disappear within 48 hours

Tubal insufflation (Rubin test)

Assessment of patency of fallopian tubes by insufflation with carbon dioxide, which is introduced through tight-fitting cannula inserted through cervical os at pressures up to 200 mm Hg; if tubes are open, gas enters abdominal cavity and recorded pressure falls below 180 mm Hg; high-pitched bubbling can be heard through abdominal wall with stethoscope as gas escapes from tubes; shoulder pain from diaphragmatic irritation also indicates that gas has escaped into abdominal cavity; kymographic tracing shows pressure changes and may indicate tubal obstruction, spasm, or leak in system

Nursing care:

Be prepared to assist patient with cramping pain, dizziness, nausea, and vomiting that may occur after procedure

Explain that shoulder pain if present is due to insufflation of gas and will subside

Hysterosalpingography

Injection of radiopaque contrast material, such as iodized oil or water-soluble material, through cervix so it fills cervical canal and body of uterus, flows through fallopian tubes, and spills into peritoneal cavity; procedure most commonly done to determine whether infertility is caused by anatomic defect; can also be used to confirm tubal occlusion and investigate cause of dysmenorrhea, postmenopausal bleeding, or repeated abortion; procedure should be performed no sooner than 6 weeks after delivery, abortion, or dilation and curettage

Nursing care:

Patient should be screened for contraindications to

procedure including active pelvic inflammatory disease, vaginitis, cervicitis, or severe systemic illness

Patient may experience pelvic pain resulting from spillage of contrast material; manage as indicated

If indicated by physician, assist patient to walk for 30 minutes after procedure until another film is taken

Pelvic endoscopy

Visualization and examination of pelvic and abdominal viscera with high-intensity fiberoptic light source; procedure done when hysterosalpingography suggests tubal abnormality and patient does not become pregnant; also done before certain surgical procedures such as tuboplasty and may reveal presence of unsuspected tubal or ovarian disease such as peritubal adhesions and endometriosis

Amniocentesis

Penetration of amniotic cavity through abdominal and uterine walls to withdraw fluid for examination; used to assess fetal health and maturity and to determine genetic karyotype and sex

Nursing care:

Before procedure, ensure that patient has voided

Auscultate fetal heart rate (FHR) to obtain baseline for comparison with FHR after procedure

Explain that procedure is virtually painless and harmless

After procedure apply adhesive bandage to injection site

Auscultate or monitor FHR for 10 to 15 minutes

Explain to patient that she should report any untoward effects including vaginal drainage or discharge and fetal hyperactivity or hypoactivity

Pelvimetry

Measurement of dimensions and capacity of pelvis by radiography

Nursing care:

Accompany patient in labor to radiology department for procedure

Amniography

Injection of radiopaque agents into amniotic sac to identify hydramnios, placenta previa, soft tissue silhouette of fetus, and, after a few hours of swallowing, fetal gastrointestinal tract

Nursing care:

Same as for amniocentesis

Amnioscopy

Direct visualization of amniotic fluid through fetal membranes with cone-shaped hollow tube when cervix is sufficiently dilated; can be used to identify meconium staining of amniotic fluid

Nursing care:

Prepare patient as for vaginal examination

Fetoscopy

Direct observation of fetus in utero using fetoscope introduced through small incision in abdomen with patient under local anesthesia; fetus may be photographed, and amniotic fluid, fetal cells, or blood may be sampled for prenatal diagnosis of congenital anomalies or genetic defects

Nursing care:

Same as for amniocentesis

Ultrasonography

Visualization of deep body structures or fetus by recording reflections of high-frequency sound waves that pass from transducer through abdominal wall, deflect off interfaces, and return to transducer

Doppler ultrasound—measures and displays ultrasound reflected from moving rather than stationary interfaces; used to determine blood flow velocity and movement of fetal heart valves

Real time imaging—shows motion as it occurs; used to observe cardiac, respiratory, and limb movements

A mode display—in amplitude (A) mode echoes are plotted as series of dots along baseline; height of peak correlates with strength of echo; can be used to assess fetal biparietal diameter

B mode—brightness (B) mode gives rough two-dimensional image by amplifying echoes of various tissue densities and displaying them in different shades of gray; transducer is moved over horizontal or vertical plane to obtain slice of anatomic outline of area

M mode—motion (M) mode is used to study moving structures; the ultrasonogram is recorded on continuously moving strip of paper according to time, with distances from transducer shown vertically (for example, echocardiography)

Nursing care:

Ensure that pregnant patient has full bladder before procedure

Thermography

Photography of infrared radiation (heat) coming from any part of body; for breast thermography patient is placed in draft-free room at temperature of about 20° C (68° F); clothing above waist is removed, and patient waits for about 15 minutes until skin cools before infrared photographs are taken

Nursing care:

Explain to patient that room will be cool

Table 9-5
External and Internal Modes of Fetal Monitoring

	External Mode	Internal Mode
Fetal heart rate	Ultrasound transducer: High-frequency sound waves reflect mechanical action of the fetal heart (easiest and most reliable external method to use during the antepartum and intrapartum periods) Phonotransducer: Microphone amplifies sound and reflects excessive noise when woman is in labor; it is used infrequently for antepartum monitoring Abdominal electrodes: Fetal ECG is obtained when electrodes are properly positioned; it is used infrequently for antepartum monitoring because of ease and reliability of ultrasound transducer	Spiral electrode: Electrode converts fetal ECG as obtained from the presenting part to FHR via a cardiotachometer; this method can only be used when membranes are ruptured and cervix is sufficiently dilated during the intrapartum period; electrode penetrates fetal presenting part 1.5 mm and must be attached securely to ensure a good signal
Uterine activity	Tocotransducer: This instrument monitors frequency and duration of contractions by means of a pressure-sensing device applied to the maternal abdomen; it can be used during both the antepartum and intrapartum periods	Intrauterine catheter: This instrument monitors frequency, duration, and intensity of contractions; catheter is filled with sterile water, which is compressed during contractions, placing pressure on a strain gauge that converts the pressure into mm Hg on the uterine activity panel of the strip chart; it can be used when membranes are ruptured and cervix is sufficiently dilated during the intrapartum period

From Bobak, I.M., and Jensen, M.D.: Essentials of maternity nursing, St. Louis, 1984, The C.V. Mosby Co.

Mammography
Soft tissue radiograph of breast with low-energy x-ray and high-contrast film

Nursing care:
Ensure that patient does not have powder, lotion, or ointment on her breasts

Xeromammography
Recording of radiographic image on electrostatically charged plate; image is transferred to plastic-coated paper by pressing plate and paper together and exposing them to heat; all performed automatically in commercial processor

Radionuclide imaging
Evaluation of breast image after intravenous injection of radioactive substance

Galactography
Radiographic breast examination after contrast agent is instilled into mammary duct

Fetal heart rate monitoring
Internal or external monitoring of fetal heart rate and uterine activity for comparison; brief description of internal and external modes of monitoring is supplied in Table 9-5; Table 9-6 contains descriptions of fetal heart rate patterns, their clinical significance, and nursing interventions; Table 9-7 describes fetal distress

Table 9-6
Fetal Heart Rate (FHR) Patterns

	Description	Clinical Significance	Nursing Intervention
Tachycardia	FHR above 160 beats/minute lasting longer than 10 minutes	Persistent tachycardia in absence of periodic changes; does not appear serious in terms of neonatal outcome (especially true if tachycardia is associated with maternal fever); ominous sign when associated with late decelerations, severe variable decelerations, or absence of variability	Dependent on cause; reduce maternal fever with antipyretics as ordered and cooling measures; oxygen* at 10 to 12 L/minute may be of some value; carry out physician's orders based on alleviating cause

Continued.

Table 9-6, cont'd
Fetal Heart Rate (FHR) Patterns

	Description	Clinical Significance	Nursing Intervention
Bradycardia	FHR below 120 beats/minute lasting longer than 10 minutes	Bradycardia with good variability and absence of periodic changes; not a sign of fetal distress if FHR remains above 80 beats/minute; bradycardia caused by hypoxia is ominous sign when associated with loss of variability and late decelerations	Dependent on cause; intervention not warranted in fetus with heart block diagnosed by ECG; oxygen at 10 to 12 L/minute may be of some value; carry out physician's orders for alleviating cause
Increased variability	An increase in irregularity of cardiac rhythm with variance of more than 20 beats/minute from one heartbeat to the next	Significance of marked variability unknown; increase in variability from a previous average variability is earliest FHR sign of mild hypoxia	Observe FHR carefully for any sign of fetal distress including decreasing variability and late decelerations; if using external mode of monitoring, consider using internal mode (spiral electrode)
Decreased variability	Decrease in irregularity of cardiac rhythm from one beat to the next of less than 5 beats/minute	Benign when associated with periodic fetal sleep states, which last 20 to 30 minutes; if caused by drugs, variability usually increases as drugs are excreted; decreased variability considered ominous if caused by hypoxia or asphyxia; when occurring with late decelerations, decreased variability is associated with fetal acidosis and low Apgar scores	Dependent on cause; intervention not warranted if associated with fetal sleep states or temporarily associated with central nervous system depressants; consider application of internal mode (spiral electrode) with physician; assist physician with fetal blood sampling for pH if ordered; prepare for delivery if ordered by physician
Acceleration	Transitory increase of FHR above baseline	Acceleration with fetal movement signifies fetal well-being representing fetal alertness or arousal states	None required
Early deceleration	Transitory decrease of FHR below baseline concurrent with uterine contractions	Reassuring pattern not associated with fetal hypoxia, acidosis, or low Apgar scores	None required
Late deceleration	Transitory decrease in FHR below baseline rate in contracting phase	Nonreassuring, worrisome pattern associated with fetal hypoxia, acidosis, and low Apgar scores; considered ominous if persistent and uncorrected, especially when associated with fetal tachycardia and loss of variability	Change maternal position; correct maternal hypotension; elevate legs; increase rate of maintenance IV; discontinue oxytocin if infusing; administer oxygen at 10 to 12 L/minute with tight face mask; assist physician with fetal blood sampling if ordered; assist physician with termination of labor if pattern cannot be corrected
Variable deceleration	Abrupt transitory decrease in FHR that is variable in duration, intensity, and timing relative to contractions	Occurs in about 50% of all labors and is usually transient, correctable phenomenon not associated with low Apgar scores; mild variable deceleration reassuring; deceleration progressing from moderate to severe associated with fetal acidosis, hypoxia, and low Apgar scores; severe variable deceleration with good baseline variability just before delivery usually well tolerated	Change maternal position; if decelerations do not yet meet criteria for mild variable deceleration, proceed with following measures: discontinue oxytocin if infusing; administer oxygen at 10 to 12 L/minute with tight face mask; assist with vaginal or speculum examination; if cord is prolapsed, examiner will elevate (push up on) fetal presenting part with cord between gloved fingers until cesarean delivery is accomplished; assist with fetal blood sampling if ordered; assist with delivery

Table 9-7
Ominous Fetal Heart Rate (FHR) Patterns and Nursing Interventions

Ominous FHR Pattern	Nursing Intervention
Severe variable deceleration FHR below 70 beats/minute lasting longer than 30 to 60 seconds with any of following: Rising baseline FHR Decreasing variability Slow return to baseline; may be with "overshoot"	With severe variable deceleration: Change maternal position Perform vaginal or speculum examination or both Discontinue oxytocin if infusing Administer oxygen at 10 to 12 L/minute by tight face mask Termination of labor considered by physician if pattern cannot be corrected to meet criteria of mild variable deceleration
Late decelerations of any magnitude—more serious if associated with decreasing variability or rising baseline	Intervene in step-by-step approach proceeding to next step *only* if pattern is uncorrected: Place woman on side Correct maternal hypotension; elevate legs, increase rate of maintenance IV infusion Discontinue oxytocin if infusing Administer oxygen at 10-12 L/minute by tight face mask Assist physician with fetal pH if done; pH >7.20: repeat pH in 10 to 15 minute; pH <7.20: prepare for immediate delivery Expeditious delivery considered by physician if pattern cannot be corrected
Absence of variability	Correct identifiable cause; if uncorrectable, assist physician with termination of labor
Prolonged deceleration	As above
Severe bradycardia	As above

From Bobak, I.M., and Jensen, M.D.: Essentials of maternity nursing, St. Louis, 1984, The C.V. Mosby Co.

Conditions, Diseases, and Disorders

FIBROCYSTIC DISEASE OF THE BREAST

Fibrocystic disease of the breast is the presence of singular or multiple cysts in the breasts. The condition is also called mammary dysplasia or cystic hyperplasia.

Fibrocystic disease is the single most common disease of the breast, accounting for over half of all surgical procedures on the female breast. It affects 10% to 25% of all women, but it is not always clinically apparent and frequently is undiscovered until postmortem examination. Fibrocystic disease occurs primarily in the menopause years and is a rare occurrence before adolescence and after menopause.[45]

PATHOPHYSIOLOGY

Fibrocystic disease is thought to be due to hormonal imbalance in the reproductive years, principally because of estrogen excess and progesterone deficiency during the luteal phase of the menstrual cycle. It is characterized by pain and tenderness of one or both breasts immediately before menses. The cysts may be unilateral or bilateral, firm, regular in shape, and mobile and are most common in the upper outer quadrant of the breasts. Their size may fluctuate during the cycle.[15]

A wide variety of morphologic changes can be found, ranging from an overgrowth of fibrous stroma to a proliferation of epithelium. Four patterns of morphologic change are distinguishable: fibrosis, cyst formation, sclerosing adenosis, and duct epithelial hyperplasia.

Fibrosis is characterized by an overgrowth of stromal fibrous tissue. This type is usually unilateral and occurs most often in women from 30 to 35 years of age. The breast becomes larger before menses and then regresses with a recurrence of pain and tenderness in the next cycle.

Cystic disease is also known as Bloodgood's disease, Schimnelbusch's disease, and blue dome cyst. It is characterized by the formation of cysts, usually over 3 mm in diameter. It is thought to be due to dilation of ducts and hyperplasia of ductal epithelium concurrent with the menstrual cycle. This type of disease is more common in women between 45 and 55 years of age. Multiple bilateral cysts are readily palpable and usually distinguishable from the characteristic solitary focus of carcinoma.[24,45]

The histologic characteristics of sclerosing adenosis are proliferation of small acini and intralobular fibrosis. It is most commonly unilateral and more common in women between 35 and 45 years of age.

Epithelial hyperplasia of the ducts is ill-defined masses found most commonly in women between 35 and 45 years of age. The more atypical the hyperplasia, the greater the risk of carcinoma.[24,45]

Fibrocystic disease must be differentiated from carcinoma and may predispose the woman to carcinoma. Biopsy and examination of the tissue is the only method of specifically differentiating fibrocystic disease from carcinoma.

DIAGNOSTIC STUDIES

Biopsy
Fibrosis: Collagenous stroma engulfing epithelial structures and obliterating periductal and myxomatous stroma
Cysts: Overgrowth of stroma with cystic dilation of ducts filled with serous opaque fluid
Fibroadenosis: Proliferation and compression of small ducts and gland buds

Epithelial hyperplasia: Proliferation of epithelium lining duct, sometimes with solid masses of hyperplastic cells encroaching into lumen of duct

Needle aspiration of cyst
Varying histologic descriptions

TREATMENT PLAN

Surgical
Subcutaneous mastectomy in lieu of multiple diagnostic biopsies and associated discomfort

Chemotherapeutic
Progestins or progestogens
Progesterone (Proluton, others), 5-50 mg IM during second half of cycle

Supportive
Local heat
Support bra
Avoidance of foods with methylxanthines, including tea, coffee, cola, and chocolate, which tend to stimulate cyclic adenosine monophosphate (AMP) and increase metabolic activity in breast[36]

ASSESSMENT: AREAS OF CONCERN

Breast
Palpation of discrete or diffuse nodules; asymmetry; nipple discharge; irregular firmness; cyclic pain of cystic area during premenstrual period

NURSING DIAGNOSES and NURSING INTERVENTIONS

Nursing Diagnosis	Nursing Intervention
Anxiety	Explain rationale for tests and procedures. Encourage verbalization of concerns. Answer patient's questions and explain disease process. See also p. 1839.

Patient Education

1. Ensure that the patient understands the method for breast self-examination (BSE) and can demonstrate this procedure.
2. Explain that only 10% to 15% of masses are malignant and that 90% of cancers confined to the breast are curable.
3. Outline a diet that avoids foods with methylxanthines.

EVALUATION

Patient Outcome	Data Indicating That Outcome is Reached
Anxiety is diminished.	Patient demonstrates adaptive responses to knowledge about and prognosis related to fibrocystic disease.
Patient understands and monitors condition.	Patient demonstrates BSE and lists progression of signs and symptoms to report to health care provider, including increase in dimension of cyst, change in texture, lack of clearly defined margins, nipple discharge, severe pain, immobility of cysts, skin dimpling or retraction, and increasing asymmetry. Patient avoids foods with methylxanthines.

VULVOVAGINITIS

Vulvovaginitis is an inflammation of the vulva and vagina.

Vulvovaginitis is the most common gynecologic complaint among women of all ages. It is most commonly due to infectious processes such as *Trichomonas vaginalis, Candida albicans,* gonorrhea, and *Haemophilus vaginalis;* parasites such as *Chlamydia trachomatis,* pinworms, and *Phthirus pubis;* mechanical irritants; and contact allergens. The infectious causes and the parasitic causes are discussed in detail in Chapter 15. The other common causes of vulvovaginitis are discussed in Table 9-8.

NURSING DIAGNOSES and NURSING INTERVENTIONS

Nursing Diagnosis	Nursing Intervention
Comfort, alteration in	Place cool compresses on perineal area. Provide sitz baths several times a day.
Skin integrity, impairment of	Administer medications as ordered. Advise against scratching. Avoid use of thermal, chemical, or physical sources of inflammation. Reinforce good personal hygiene to remove smegma and perspiration. Pat skin area after washing rather than rubbing with towel.

Patient Education

1. Teach the patient to wipe from front to back.
2. Instruct the patient not to douche routinely to avoid removal of normal vaginal flora.
3. Instruct the patient to avoid using sprays, soaps, powders, and deodorants.
4. Instruct the patient to wear cotton undergarments to permit free airflow to the perineum and to avoid trapping moisture.
5. Instruct the patient to wash undergarments in mild detergent and to rinse them twice.
6. Instruct the patient to avoid sharing towels and washcloths with others.
7. Instruct the patient to use water-soluble lubricants if necessary before intercourse.
8. Instruct the patient to ensure cleanliness of her sexual partner.

EVALUATION

Patient Outcome	Data Indicating That Outcome is Reached
Comfort is achieved.	There is no soreness or itching.
Color and integrity of skin and mucous membrane are good.	There is no vaginal drainage or pruritus or inflammation of vulva and perineum.
Infection and inflammation are controlled.	Patient verbalizes intent to adhere to hygienic practices as described in "Patient Education."

Table 9-8

Common Causes of Vulvovaginitis

Etiology	Epidemiology	Signs and Symptoms	Diagnostic Studies	Medical Plan
Postmenopausal vaginitis (atrophic vaginitis)	Occurs because of decreased estrogen levels	Thin watery discharge; burning and itching	Direct visual examination	Atrophic changes cannot be reversed but can usually be prevented with hormone therapy
Allergic or irritative vaginitis owing to thermal, chemical, and physical causes	Thermal sources: douching with excessively hot water, wearing of nylon undergarments	Redness, burning, and itching of excoriated skin	Direct visual examination; wet smear; detailed history; bimanual examination	Avoidance of source; secondary infection should be treated according to etiology; oral antihistamines for allergic vaginitis; local cortisone ointment; wearing cotton undergarments
	Chemical sources: douche solutions, hygiene sprays, soaps, detergents on undergarments, poor personal hygiene	Increase in type and amount of secretions; rash; burning and itching		
	Physical sources: retained tampon, diaphragm, toilet paper, condom, or pessary	Foul-smelling, serosanguineous, or purulent discharge		

PELVIC INFLAMMATORY DISEASE

Pelvic inflammatory disease (PID) is an infectious process that may involve the fallopian tubes, ovaries, pelvic peritoneum, veins, or pelvic connective tissue.

The incidence of PID is difficult to estimate, since it is not a reportable disease and is not identified in a consistent manner. It is not always treated, especially when symptoms are mild. It most often occurs in sexually active women under 25 years of age and is the result of infection transmitted through sexual intercourse or less commonly through childbirth or abortion. It has been directly or indirectly linked to approximately one fifth of all gynecologic problems.

PID may be confined to one structure or involve the entire pelvis. Infections may be acute, subacute, recurrent, or chronic. PID in the fallopian tubes (the most common site) is referred to as salpingitis.

PATHOPHYSIOLOGY

PID begins in the vulva or accessory glands and spreads upward through the entire genital tract. The principal pathogen is *Neisseria gonorrhoeae*, but gram-negative bacilli, gram-positive cocci, *Mycoplasma*, and viruses are also implicated as causative agents. Salpingitis re-

sulting from tuberculosis has become rare. If PID follows childbirth or an abortion, anaerobic streptococci, staphylococci, coliform bacteria, or *Clostridium perfringens* is usually involved. Infections can also be caused by *Chlamydia trachomatis*, actinomycosis, schistosomiasis, leprosy, oxyurias, sarcoidosis, and foreign bodies (such as radiographic contrast media).

Gonococcal disease is characterized by an acute suppurative reaction with subsequent copious discharge of yellow pus. Hyperemia, edema, and tenseness occur in the involved structures, which are often bilaterally involved. The organisms spread over the mucosal surfaces, eventually involving the tubes and tubo-ovarian region. In an adult the vagina is resistant to the inflammation, but vulvovaginitis may develop in a child because of the more delicate mucosa. The nongonococcal infections spread upward through the lymphatics or venous channels rather than on the surface of the mucosa. As the lumen of the fallopian tube fills with purulent exudate, some leaks out of the fimbriae. Over the course of days or weeks the fimbriae may seal or become adherent to the ovary, causing salpingo-oophoritis. The collection of pus in the sealed tube causes distention of the tube and is referred to as pyosalpinx. In this form the infection may persist for months. The demise of the organisms and sterilization of the infection occur eventually owing to progressive anaerobiasis and increasing acidity. The pus then undergoes a slow proteolysis, and the exudate is transformed to a thin serous fluid in a condition known as hydrosalpinx.

Tubo-ovarian abscesses can occur when exudate collects where the tube is sealed against the ovary. This inflammatory process affects the most superficial layers of the ovary but spares the underlying ovarian tissue. Peritonitis resulting from spread of the exudate to the pelvic peritoneum is common. Infertility caused by mucosal destruction and tubal occlusion is a common sequel of salpingitis.[5,27,29]

DIAGNOSTIC STUDIES

Culture of purulent secretions
Identification of organism and sensitivity to antibiotics

White blood cell count
Elevated

Erythrocyte sedimentation rate
Elevated

Laparoscopic examination
Visualization of pelvic inflammation

Gram stain of secretions
Identification of gram-positive or gram-negative organisms

Ultrasonography
Visualization of abscess or inflammation

Needle culdocentesis
White blood cells or nonclotting blood

TREATMENT PLAN

Surgical
Hysterectomy with bilateral salpingo-oophorectomy—may be required for patients with abscesses, hydrosalpinx, and tubal obstruction if antibiotic therapy is unsuccessful
Laparatomy with incision and drainage of abscesses and lysis of adhesions

Chemotherapeutic
Anti-infective agents
For *Neisseria gonorrhoeae*
Aqueous procaine penicillin, 2.4 million units IM in two separate sites, and probenecid (Benemid) 1 g po
or

cefoxitin (Mefoxin), 1-2 g IM followed by doxycycline (Vibramycin) 100 mg po bid for 10-14 d
Tetracycline (Achromycin, others), 1.5-2 g qd po for 7-10 d; for severely ill patients with acute pain who are hypersensitive to penicillin, 500 mg IV qid for first 24-48 h, then 500 mg po qid to complete 10 d of therapy; should not be given to pregnant patients and those with renal failure
Crystalline penicillin (for severely ill patients with acute pain), 10-40 million units IV over first 24 h; continue treatment for 36-72 h as indicated, follow IV therapy with ampicillin (Amcill), 500 mg po qid for at least 10 d
For gram-negative organisms
Kanamycin (Kantrex), 7.5 mg/kg/12 h IM, *or* streptomycin, 1 g qd IM; kanamycin or streptomycin should be added to initial penicillin therapy and continued until sensitivity of identified pathogens is determined[5,27,32]
For gram-positive organisms and *Bacteroides*
Clindamycin (Cleocin), 300 mg po qid until organisms are identified and sensitivity is determined

Supportive
Bed rest in semi-Fowler's position
Heat applied to abdomen
Warm douches
Parenteral fluids
Nasogastric suctioning if ileus is present
Removal of intrauterine device (IUD)

ASSESSMENT: AREAS OF CONCERN

Subjective data
Abdominal and pelvic pain; low back pain; dyspareunia; menstrual irregularity; urinary discomfort; constipation; malaise; nausea and vomiting; diarrhea; vaginal drainage

Abdomen
Rebound tenderness; normal bowel sounds progressing to ileus in untreated persons

Cervix
Pain with movement; copious purulent discharge

Vulva
Pruritus; maceration

Temperature
Elevated

NURSING DIAGNOSES and NURSING INTERVENTIONS

Nursing Diagnosis	Nursing Intervention
Comfort, alteration in: pain	Maintain complete bed rest; semi-Fowler's position may be most comfortable. Increase activity as tolerated. Explain cause of pain. Instruct patient to request analgesic before pain becomes severe.
Fluid volume deficit, potential	Explain need to increase fluid intake during infectious processes. Encourage fluid intake of 3000 ml daily unless contraindicated. Monitor intake and output.
Skin integrity, impairment of	Explain cause of vaginal discharge and pruritus if present. Assist and teach patient to perform perineal care every 3 to 4 hours or as needed. Blot skin dry; do not rub. Prevent excessive warmth in room; light covers over bed cradle may be indicated.
Knowledge deficit	Explain importance of handwashing before and after contact with perineal area. Explain importance of wiping from front to back after elimination. Explain need to use perineal pads, which should be changed frequently according to amount of vaginal drainage. Instruct patient to avoid use of tampons. Explain that a shower is preferable to a tub bath.
Sexual dysfunction	Encourage patient to share concerns regarding sexual partner as probable source of infection. Explain rationale for removal of intrauterine device (IUD) if this is ordered by physician.

Patient Education

1. Explain the need to avoid using tampons, having intercourse, or douching for at least 1 week after antibiotic therapy.
2. Explain methods to prevent venereal disease if the condition is caused by gonorrhea or *Chlamydia*.
3. Explain the importance of encouraging the patient's sexual partner to be examined and treated.
4. Explain alternative methods of conception control if the condition is related to an IUD.
5. Describe symptoms of recurrence that the patient should report to a physician.

EVALUATION

Patient Outcome	Data Indicating That Outcome is Reached
Comfort is achieved. Pain is gone.	Patient reports that lower abdominal, low back, pelvic, or perineal pain is gone.
Skin and mucous membrane color is good.	There is no vaginal drainage or pruritus, inflammation, or maceration of vulva.
Body temperature is normal.	There is no fever. Temperature is within normal limits. Intake and output are within normal limits.
Infection and inflammation are controlled.	Patient showers rather than taking tub baths. Patient verbalizes intent to prevent venereal disease if condition is caused by gonorrhea or *Chlamydia*. Patient verbalizes intent to avoid douching, intercourse, or use of tampons for at least 1 week after completion of drug therapy. Patient wipes front to back after elimination. Patient verbalizes intent to have sexual partner examined. Patient takes medications at time and dosage prescribed by physician. Patient describes symptoms of PID and expresses intent to notify health care provider in timely manner if they recur.

TOXIC SHOCK SYNDROME

Toxic shock syndrome is an acute bacterial infection generally caused by Staphylococcus aureus *and most frequently associated with the use of tampons during menses.*

National attention was not directed to toxic shock syndrome until the fall of 1980 when some 300 cases were reported to the Centers for Disease Control. These cases occurred from January to September in 285 women among whom 25 deaths were reported. The overall incidence appears to be about 1 in 20,000 menstruating women. Toxic shock syndrome is most common in women who use high-absorbency tampons but has occurred in newborns, children, and men. The incidence in women dropped precipitously in 1981 after widespread publicity and withdrawal of some vaginal tampons from the market.[56]

PATHOPHYSIOLOGY

Almost all cases of toxic shock syndrome have been due to pyrogenic exotoxin-producing strains of phage group I *Staphylococcus aureus*. The organism has been found in the nasopharynx, vagina, and trachea, as well as sequestered in empyema and abscess sites. It is thought that mechanical factors associated with use of high absorbency tampons by a woman with a preexisting *S. aureus* colonization of the vagina increase the risk. As the outflow of menses is obstructed by the tampon, bacterial exotoxins are able to enter the bloodstream through a mucosal break or enter the peritoneal cavity via the uterus. Adult respiratory distress syndrome, which is manifested as pulmonary and peripheral edema despite low central venous pressure, may be a cardiopulmonary complication of toxic shock syndrome.[56]

DIAGNOSTIC STUDIES

White blood cell count
Increased

Blood urea nitrogen
Increased

Creatinine
Increased

Bilirubin
Increased

Serum glutamic oxaloacetic transaminase (SGOT)
Increased

Serum glutamic pyruvic transaminase (SGPT)
Increased

Creatinine phosphokinase (CPK)
Increased

Platelets
Decreased

TREATMENT PLAN

Chemotherapeutic
Anti-infective agents
β-Lactamase-resistant agents
Cefoxitin sodium (Mefoxin), 1-2 g IV or IM q6-8h
Cefazolin sodium (Ancef), 250 mg-1 g q6-8h IM or IV
Cephalothin sodium (Keflin), 500 mg-1 g q4-6h IV or deep IM
Penicillinase-resistant agents
Methicillin sodium (Staphcillin), 1-1.5 g IM q4-6h
Oxacillin sodium (Bactocill), 500 mg q4-6h for at least 5 d
Cloxacillin sodium (Cloxapen), 500-1000 mg q4-6h
Antistaphylococcal agents
Penicillin G (Bicillin), 600,000 units IM at various intervals
Dicloxacillin sodium (Dycill, others), 125 mg po q6h
Methicillin sodium (Staphcillin), 1-1.5 g IM 6h
Corticosteroids
Hydrocortisone sodium succinate (Solu-Cortef), 50-300 mg qd IV or IM

Supportive
Septic shock treatment if indicated
Fluid intake of 3000 ml daily unless contraindicated

ASSESSMENT

Subjective data
Sudden onset of high fever (39° to 40.5° C [102° to 105° F]); myalgia; vomiting; profuse watery diarrhea; sore throat; headache; profound tiredness

Extremeties
Edema; impaired perfusion

Palms and soles
Erythematous rash (sunburnlike); desquamation and sloughing within 1 to 2 weeks

Level of consciousness
Disorientation; intermittent confusion

Blood pressure
Rapid hypotension (within 48 hours); orthostatic syncope

Renal system
Diminished urine output

Conjunctiva
Nonpurulent inflammation

Oropharynx
Hyperemia; edema

Vagina
Hyperemia

NURSING DIAGNOSES and NURSING INTERVENTIONS

Nursing Diagnosis	Nursing Intervention
Tissue perfusion, alteration in	For complete list of nursing diagnosis and interventions, see care of patient in septic shock in Chapter 1 and adult respiratory distress syndrome in Chapter 2 if applicable.
Injury, potential for	Instruct patient to use sanitary napkins rather than tampons during menses.

Patient Education

1. Instruct the patient to avoid using tampons until vaginal culture findings are negative and clearance from a physician is obtained.
2. Instruct the patient to wash hands thoroughly before inserting a tampon.
3. Instruct the patient to avoid the use of high-absorbency, noncotton tampons.
4. Instruct the patient to change tampons frequently during the day, to wear sanitary napkins at night, and to avoid prolonged use of a single tampon.
5. Instruct the patient to avoid using tampons if she has a concurrent skin infection, since there is a possibility of reinfection with *S. aureus*.
6. Instruct the patient to report signs of recurrence to a physician immediately.

EVALUATION

Patient Outcome	Data Indicating That Outcome is Reached
Tissue perfusion is adequate.	There are no symptoms of shock.
Infection is gone.	Vaginal culture findings are negative for causative organism. Patient does not have fever; hyperemia of oropharynx, conjunctiva, or vagina; myalgia; vomiting; diarrhea; sore throat; headache; or malaise.
Patient education is effective.	Patient demonstrates understanding of reasons for health education and expresses intent to maintain behaviors and health practices that will prevent reinfection.

UTERINE BLEEDING

Irregular or excessive bleeding from the uterus is one of the most common gynecologic symptoms.

Abnormalities and variation in uterine bleeding are the most frequently encountered women's health care problems. Patients often view uterine bleeding as life threatening or indicative of a major problem in reproductive or sexual functioning. Abnormal bleeding varying from spotting to the passage of clots may occur at any age and for a variety of reasons.

Dysfunctional uterine bleeding (DUB), which is almost always anovulatory and painless (whereas dysmenorrhea is associated with ovulatory cycles), can occur at any age from puberty through menopause. It generally occurs at the extremes of menstrual life, when disturbances in ovarian function are common. About 50% of dysfunctional bleeding occurs in premenopausal women (age 40 to 50), about 20% during the adolescent years, and about 30% during the reproductive period.[32,35]

The following terms are often used to describe variations in uterine bleeding:

dysfunctional uterine bleeding (DUB) abdominal uterine bleeding not associated with tumor, inflammation, pregnancy, trauma, or hormonal effects.

hypomenorrhea deficient amount of menstrual flow.

menorrhagia (hypermenorrhea) increased amount or duration of menstrual bleeding.

metrorrhagia intermenstrual bleeding.

metrorrhea any pathologic uterine discharge.

oligomenorrhea infrequent menstruation.

polymenorrhea increased frequency of menstruation (not consistently associated with ovulation).

postmenopausal bleeding bleeding from the reproductive tract occurring 1 year or more after menopause.

spotting small amounts of bloody vaginal discharge ranging from pink to dark brown.

PATHOPHYSIOLOGY

The preceding terms used to describe abnormal bleeding do not indicate the cause of the abnormality or reason for bleeding. The following are the most common types of bleeding and their causes:

1. Midcycle spotting—midcycle estradiol fluctuation associated with ovulation
2. Delayed menstruation with excessive bleeding—anovulation or threatened abortion
3. Frequent bleeding—chronic pelvic inflammatory disease, endometriosis, DUB, or anovulation
4. Profuse menstrual bleeding—endometrial polyps, adenomyosis, DUB, submucous leiomyomas, or presence of intrauterine contraceptive device
5. Intermenstrual or irregular bleeding—endometrial polyps, DUB, uterine or cervical cancer, or oral contraceptive use
6. Postmenopausal bleeding—endometrial hyperplasia, estrogen therapy, or endometrial cancer

Other causes of bleeding include foreign bodies, lacerations, and systemic diseases such as leukemia, hypothyroidism, and blood dyscrasias. In addition, precocious puberty may warrant consideration as a cause, as may vaginal adenosis in young women with prenatal exposure to the synthetic estrogen diethylstilbestrol (DES).

DUB is most common before and after the reproductive years and occurs as painless, irregular, heavy bleeding (menometrorrhagia), midcycle spotting, oligomenorrhea, or periods of amenorrhea. In most cases the cause is anovulation, but bleeding may reflect defects in the follicular or luteal phase of the ovulatory cycle.

With anovulation, the persistent unopposed estrogen stimulation may be endogenous from an ovarian tumor such as a granulosa cell tumor, polycystic ovaries (Stein-Leventhal syndrome), or abnormal metabolism of estrogen as in liver disease. Exogenous estrogen taken by the patient can also result in anovulation. Unopposed estrogen stimulation causes endometrial hyperplasia; when the estrogen can no longer maintain the endometrium, sloughing and vaginal bleeding occur.

Follicular phase defects result from premature maturation of the ovarian follicle owing to pituitary hyperstimulation. The cycle is less than 22 days. Increased levels of follicle-stimulating hormone (FSH) and slightly elevated estradiol levels result in a progressively shortened proliferative phase that can cause spotting in perimenopausal women. Oligomenorrhea most commonly occurs in young women and may result from a prolonged proliferative phase.

Luteal phase defects may result in profuse and prolonged bleeding caused by delayed involution of the corpus luteum. A corpus luteum cyst or persistent corpus luteum can cause a delay in menses with premenstrual spotting.[12,54]

DIAGNOSTIC STUDIES

Complete blood count
    To determine the degree of anemia and to detect abnormal leukocyte production

Thyroid function tests
    To assess thyroid function

Dilation and curettage with cervical or endometrial biopsy
    To assess endometrium and identify carcinoma or polyps

Hysterography
    To identify presence of endometrial polyps, submucous myomas, adenomyosis, endometrial carcinoma, and adnexal lesions

Hysteroscopy
    To identify intrauterine abnormalities such as submucous fibroids, endometrial polyps, and foreign bodies

Endocrine profile
    To assess functioning of the adrenal glands, ovaries, and pituitary glands

Tests confirming ovulation
    Endometrial biopsy
        To demonstrate secretory or menstrual endometrium

Basal body temperatures
  Biphasic pattern is indicative of ovulation
Cytologic examination of consecutive vaginal smears
  To show shift from estrogen- to progesterone-dominated smears
Examination of cervical mucus
  To determine presence of ferning
Serum or urine progesterone levels
  To assess progesterone metabolites consistent with progestational phase of menstrual cycle

TREATMENT PLAN

The plan of medical care selected is contingent on the cause of the bleeding.

Surgical
Total abdominal hysterectomy with partial or complete bilateral salpingo-oophorectomy (TAH/BSO) (see p. 1025)
Dilation and curettage (see p. 1028)
Excision of polyps

Chemotherapeutic
Progesterone or progestin
  Medroxyprogesterone (Provera, others), 2.5-10 mg po qd or 100-400 mg IM qd (may be given if patient is anovulatory and infertility is not a concern)

Estrogens
  Conjugated estrogens (Premarin), 0.625-3.75 mg qd followed by high doses of estrogen-progestin combinations (given for excessive anovulatory bleeding)
  Clomiphene citrate can be used when excessive bleeding is due to inadequate luteal phase or to anovulation

ASSESSMENT: AREAS OF CONCERN

Variations depend on the cause of the bleeding.

Bleeding
Heavy menstrual flow; bleeding between periods; infrequent menstruation; increased frequency of menstruation; spotting

Pain
Menstrual cramps or pain with menses; low abdominal pain at midcycle*; uterine cramps at midcycle*

Vaginal secretions
Wet mucoid vaginal secretion at midcycle*

Other complications
Altered sexual function; psychosocial concerns; anemia

*Signs and symptoms suggestive of ovulation.

NURSING DIAGNOSES and NURSING INTERVENTIONS

Nursing Diagnosis	Nursing Intervention
Self-concept, disturbance in	Assess meaning of dysfunction for patient. Encourage patient to ventilate her feelings. Consider nursing interventions associated with loss and grief if results of diagnostic studies confirm anovulatory cycles and infertility.
Comfort, alteration in: pain	Assist in and teach patient pain-relieving techniques.
Sexual dysfunction (related to change)	Explain importance of sharing concerns with sexual partner.

Patient Education

1. Explain the importance of recording dates, type of flow, and number of pads or tampons used.
2. Explain the importance of ongoing care.

EVALUATION

Patient Outcome	Data Indicating That Outcome is Reached
Patient demonstrates adaptive responses related to self-concept.	Patient asks appropriate questions. Patient keeps record of bleeding, including type and date. Patient shows signs of grief if she learns of undesired infertility.

Patient Outcome	Data Indicating That Outcome is Reached
Comfort is achieved; there is no pain.	Patient uses pain-relieving techniques or medication as ordered.
Sexual adjustment is made.	Patient indicates that she has discussed concerns with partner.

PREMENSTRUAL SYNDROME

Premenstrual syndrome is a condition characterized by nervousness, irritability, weight gain, edema, headache, mastalgia, dysphoria, and lack of coordination before the onset of menstruation.

Premenstrual syndrome generally occurs in women in their late twenties and older and increases in incidence and severity as women near menopause. The various behaviors and symptoms described in epidemiologic studies can be placed in the three major categories of edema, emotionality, and headache. The symptoms generally appear 5 to 7 days before menses and sharply decrease with the onset of menses.

PATHOPHYSIOLOGY

The exact cause of premenstrual tension is unknown, but it is believed to be related to decreasing concentrations of estrogen and progesterone and related changes in electrolyte balance. Progesterone stimulates the production of aldosterone, which increases sodium retention and edema formation. Interestingly, no distinct differences in aldosterone levels have been shown between women with and those without premenstrual syndrome. The decrease in brain levels of monoamine oxidase that occurs as estrogen production falls before menses probably accounts for the feeling of depression. Fluctuation of monoamine oxidase and catecholamine levels in the brain may result in the frequently observed symptom of irritability. Studies have shown that carbohydrate metabolism and the adrenal production of corticosteroids change before menses. Premenstrual tension may well be caused by a variety of factors.[14,15,53]

DIAGNOSTIC STUDIES

There are no specific tests for diagnosis of premenstrual syndrome.

TREATMENT PLAN

Chemotherapeutic
Diuretics
    Hydrochlorothiazide, 50-100 mg po qd during 7-10 d before cycle or 24-36 h before onset of expected symptoms

    Diazepam, 5-10 mg po bid
    Medroxyprogesterone (Provera), 10-20 mg po qd during last half of cycle
Vitamins
    Vitamin B_6, 200-800 mg qd
    Vitamin E, 600 units qd

Supportive
Limitation of intake of salt, refined sugars, and animal fats
Emotional and psychologic support

ASSESSMENT: AREAS OF CONCERN

Hydration
Edema; weight gain; backache; breast tenderness; oliguria; palpitations; mastalgia

Gastrointestinal
Abdominal bloating; diarrhea or constipation; nausea; vomiting; food craving; compulsive eating

Affect and behavior
Irritability; anxiety; fatigue; depression; lethargy; agitation; insomnia

Neurologic
Headache; vertigo; fainting; migraine; paresthesias of head and feet

Respiratory
Increase in colds, asthma, or allergic rhinitis

Urologic
Cystitis; enuresis; urethritis

Ophthalmologic
Conjunctivitis; styes

Breasts
Tenderness; enlargement

Dermatologic
Recurrence of herpes; acne; urticaria; boils; easy bruising

NURSING DIAGNOSES and NURSING INTERVENTIONS

Nursing Diagnosis	Nursing Intervention
Anxiety	Reassure patient that her symptoms are temporary and not related to significant disease.
Comfort, alteration in	See ''Patient Education.''

Patient Education

1. Explain that fatigue exaggerates symptoms and that adequate rest and sleep are needed during the premenstrual period.
2. Encourage the patient to avoid stressful activity during the premenstrual period.
3. Instruct the patient to avoid glucose fluctuation by taking small frequent feedings of a high-protein, complex carbohydrate diet and by decreasing sugar intake to less than 5 tablespoons daily.
4. Instruct the patient to reduce salt intake and to avoid foods with ''hidden salt'' such as soy sauce, salted crackers and bread, luncheon meats, dried meats, hot dogs, tomato juice, and cheeses.
5. Instruct the patient to avoid dairy products and animal fats.
6. Instruct the patient to restrict caffeine by decreasing intake of coffee, tea, cola, and chocolate.
7. Instruct the patient to restrict alcohol.
8. Instruct the patient to increase intake of leafy green vegetables and whole grain cereals.
9. Instruct the patient to take medications as prescribed and explain the reasons for taking specific medications. (For example, vitamin B_6 is taken to increase blood progesterone and promote diuresis, and vitamin E is taken to reduce breast tenderness.)

EVALUATION

Patient Outcome	Data Indicating That Outcome is Reached
Comfort is achieved. There is little or no anxiety.	Patient describes feeling of well-being and absence of bloating, weight gain, edema, mastalgia, irritability, anxiety, and other symptoms of premenstrual syndrome.

DYSMENORRHEA

Dysmenorrhea is menstruation that is painful enough to limit normal activity or to cause a woman to seek medical treatment.

Dysmenorrhea is a common gynecologic complaint. It occurs in approximately 10% of high school–age girls, keeping them home from school for 1 or 2 days, and also affects many college students and young women in the work force. Dysmenorrhea is classified as primary or secondary. Primary dysmenorrhea is pain associated with menstruation during ovulatory cycles in the absence of organic disease. Secondary dysmenorrhea is due to a demonstrated disorder.

endometrium under the influence of progesterone in the luteal phase of the cycle. Very little prostaglandin is produced during anovulatory cycles, which are almost never painful. Increased sensitivity of the myometrium and endometrium to prostaglandin F_2 can produce uterine contractions and ischemia, causing the cramping pain of dysmenorrhea.[12,35,54]

Secondary dysmenorrhea is associated with pelvic disorders such as endometriosis, adenomyosis, or chronic pelvic inflammatory disease. It may appear after years of normal menstruation and is characterized by cramping as large clots pass through the cervix.

PATHOPHYSIOLOGY

Primary dysmenorrhea usually develops 1 or 2 years after menarche when ovulatory cycles are established. Increased amounts of prostaglandin are released from the

DIAGNOSTIC STUDIES

Pelvic examination
To rule out or confirm underlying disorders in secondary dysmenorrhea

Laparoscopy
To rule out or confirm underlying disorders in secondary dysmenorrhea

Dilation and curettage
To rule out or confirm underlying disorders in secondary dysmenorrhea

Hysterosalpingography
To rule out or confirm underlying disorders in secondary dysmenorrhea

TREATMENT PLAN

Surgical
Total abdominal hysterectomy and bilateral salpingo-oophorectomy (TAH/BSO)—may be indicated for disorder associated with secondary dysmenorrhea

Presacral neurectomy (severance of nerve trunks in hypogastric plexus)—performed in rare cases when no underlying disorder can be found and there is lack of response to chemotherapeutic agents

Chemotherapeutic
Nonsteroidal anti-inflammatory agents
Ibuprofen (Motrin), 400-600 mg po q4-6h as prostaglandin synthetase inhibitor
Analgesic/antipyretic agents
Aspirin, 650 mg po q3-5h beginning 1-2 d before menses to control mild discomfort

Narcotic analgesics
Meperidine (Demerol), 50-100 mg
Codeine phosphate and sulfate (Methylmorphine), 30-60 mg (not for prolonged use)
Oral contraceptives—may be ordered for hormonal effect to relieve pain by suppressing ovulation

Supportive
Adequate exercise
Balanced diet with increased consumption of fruits and vegetables
Adequate rest and sleep
Attention to personal hygiene

ASSESSMENT: AREAS OF CONCERN

Comfort
Colicky and cyclic pain, infrequently nagging and dull in low pelvis and often with radiation toward vulva, perineum, rectum, and down back of thighs; may be experienced 24 to 48 hours before menses or with start of menstruation; may be associated with symptoms of premenstrual tension including nausea, vomiting, diarrhea, urinary frequency, chills, abdominal bloating, breast tenderness, irritability, or depression

NURSING DIAGNOSES and NURSING INTERVENTIONS

Nursing Diagnosis	Nursing Intervention
Comfort, alteration in: pain	Identify and assist patient to use pain reduction methods including relaxation techniques, heating pad, effleurage (abdominal massage), and orgasm (relieves cramps in some women).

Patient Education

1. Instruct the patient regarding the prescribed dosage and frequency of doses of prostaglandin antagonists or other medications.

EVALUATION

Patient Outcome	Data Indicating That Outcome is Reached
Comfort is achieved. Pain is gone.	Patient uses pain-relieving techniques or medications as ordered.

MENOPAUSE AND CLIMACTERIC

Menopause is the physiologic cessation of menses. The climacteric is the transitional period during which reproductive function diminishes and eventually ceases.

As the average life span has increased in the United States, so has the number of postmenopausal women. In 1970 there were 27.2 million women over 50 years of age, in 1979 there were 32 million, and in 2000 there will be an estimated 49 million. Postmenopausal women constitute one eighth to one sixth of the population. The average life span of women is 76 years, whereas that of men is only 68 years. As the ratio of men to women decreases with age, many women in the climacteric phase of life must cope with societal as well as physical changes.[12,54]

The normal decrease in ovarian function begins during the fourth decade, and the majority of women cease to menstruate between the ages of 45 and 55. The average age at which menses disappears is 51 years, although some women cease to menstruate as early as 35 years and others continue until 55 years or older.

Artificial or premature menopause is the cessation of ovarian function as a result of radiation, surgery, immunologic disease, or bacteriologic or viral agents. Although the signs and symptoms of natural and premature or artificial menopause are similar, the medical management may vary based on the patient's age.

PHYSIOLOGY

A notable event of the climacteric phase of life is menopause, the complete cessation of menses. Before the actual menopause there are usually gradual changes such as a decrease in the amount of menses, lengthening of the interval between menses, periodic amenorrhea, and finally slight spotting. These events are due to a progressive decline in the ovarian secretion of estrogen. When too little estrogen is secreted to cause endometrial growth, bleeding stops permanently. Irregular menses followed by amenorrhea for more than 1 year is indicative of menopause.

With menopause the estrogen fractions change and estrone becomes more available than estradiol. Peripheral conversion of androstenedione, a product of the adrenal glands, to estrone occurs principally in the fat. Some women produce enough estrone to cause endometrial growth and shedding or bleeding. Since obesity is a common factor in women with endometrial cancer, it has been hypothesized that production of estrone in the adipose tissue may contribute to the genesis of a tumor.

Changes in reproductive structures are related directly to decreased estrogen. Labial fat is reabsorbed; the labia majora become flattened and the labia minora disappear.

The vaginal mucosa becomes thinner, the vagina smaller, and the fornices shallower. The myometrium thins, causing the uterus to decrease in size until it resembles that of a prepubertal girl.

Hot flushes, the most characteristic symptom of menopause, coincide with a pulsatile release of luteinizing hormone. A slight increase in core body temperature and a higher increase in skin temperature occur. The sensation of heat is often accompanied by tachycardia, vertigo, palpitation, and a feeling of faintness.

The atrophic changes that result from estrogen deprivation may lead to dyspareunia owing to decreased precoital lubrication or constriction of the introitus or vagina.

Menopausal arthralgia, pain and stiffness in the joints in climacteric women, may be caused by changes in the soft tissues surrounding the joints or by lack of exercise of the muscles and tendons.

Nervousness and other psychologic symptoms are not a direct result of estrogen deficiency. The patient's personality and response to aging are the keys to promoting adaptation to the climacteric.

DIAGNOSTIC STUDIES

Papanicolaou smear
Decrease in estrogen effect noted in vaginal mucosa

Blood chemistry
Estradiol 1-5 ng/dl
Estrogen 0-14 ng/dl
Estrone 25-50 pg/dl
Luteinizing hormone 35-120 mIU/ml
Follicle-stimulating hormone 40-200 mIU/ml

Urine chemistry
Estrogens 1.4-19.6 µg/24 hours
Pregnanediol 0.2-1 mg/24 hours
Luteinizing hormone 40-110 mIU/24 hours
Follicle-stimulating hormone 2-25 mIU/24 hours

TREATMENT PLAN

Chemotherapeutic
Estrogens
Sodium estrone sulfate, 0.3-25 mg po qd, or ethinyl estradiol (Estinyl, others), 0.05-0.2 mg po qd; initial doses should be lowest amount that will control symptoms; drug is taken for first 25 d of month; withdrawal should be gradual over several months to prevent recurrence of hot flushes

Indications: Treatment of hot flushes and senile atrophic vaginitis; prevention of osteoporosis

Contraindications: Presence or history of breast or genital cancer (except cervical cancer in some cases); history of thromboembolism; fluid retention owing to cardiac, renal, or hepatic disease; abnormal liver function

Cautions: Administration is closely monitored in women with uterine fibroids, endometriosis, hypertension, or insulin-dependent diabetes mellitus; annual endometrial biopsy needed for patient receiving long-term estrogen therapy to prevent osteoporosis

Estrogen creams applied to vagina are more effective than oral estrogen in treatment of atrophic vaginitis

Progestins or progestogens

Medroxyprogesterone acetate (Provera), 2.5-10 mg po qd in last 10 d of estrogen cycle

Indications: To prevent endometrial cancer, which may develop with unopposed estrogen stimulation

Cautions: May stimulate withdrawal bleeding; patients receiving long-term estrogen replacement therapy should have annual endometrial biopsies

ASSESSMENT: AREAS OF CONCERN

Subjective complaints

Hot flushes; night sweats; diaphoresis; insomnia; headache; vertigo; syncope; numbness, tingling, or pain in joints; chilly sensation; lack of appetite or weight gain; constipation or diarrhea; nausea or vomiting; flatulence; fatigability; irritability; nervousness; depression or crying spells; fits of anger; forgetfulness; difficulty in concentrating; dyspareunia (resulting from vaginal atrophy)

Vulva

Decreasing labial fat; atrophy of muscle

Vagina

Decreased size with shallow fornices

Abdomen

Abdominal fat deposition

Cardiac rate and rhythm

Tachycardia; palpitations

Breasts

Reduction in size

Body hair

Loss of pubic and axillary hair

NURSING DIAGNOSES and NURSING INTERVENTIONS

Nursing Diagnosis	Nursing Intervention
Knowledge deficit	Explain physiologic process of climacteric and menopause. Explain importance of keeping fit and eating well-balanced diet, getting adequate rest and sleep, avoiding stress and fatigue, and continuing contraception until health care provider indicates it is safe to stop. Inform patient about side effects of estrogen replacement therapy, need to report any vaginal bleeding occurring 6 months or more after last menstrual period, and availability of water-soluble lubricants if needed before coitus.
Self-concept, disturbance in	Encourage patient to verbalize concerns about femininity, sexuality, and aging.

EVALUATION

Patient Outcome	Data Indicating That Outcome is Reached
Patient has acquired knowledge about climacteric.	Patient verbalizes understanding of physiology and desired health behaviors. Patient relates understanding of prescribed medications including dosage, route of administration, frequency, and side effects.
Patient demonstrates progress toward acceptance of altered body image and self-concept.	Patient's verbalization indicates adaptive responses to changes in self-concept and movement toward acceptance of both physiologic and psychologic processes associated with climacteric.

ENDOMETRIOSIS

Endometriosis is an abnormal growth of endometrial tissue outside the uterine cavity.

Endometriosis is a benign disease but has certain characteristics of a malignancy, including the ability to grow, infiltrate, and spread. The ectopic tissue is responsive to hormonal variations of the menstrual cycle and is subject to menstrual-like bleeding.

The incidence of endometriosis is unknown because it exists in many women without causing significant symptoms. Characteristic lesions are found in at least 20% of patients undergoing gynecologic surgery. Endometriosis is a significant finding in only about one third of these patients. Symptoms severe enough to require treatment generally occur between the ages of 25 and 35 years. Endometriosis is very rare in women over 50 years of age. The greatest incidence of the disease seems to be in white women of higher socioeconomic levels, who tend to marry later and have fewer children. However, there is some question about the reliability of these impressions, since the greater demand for medical attention in this higher socioeconomic group may account for earlier and more frequent diagnosis of the condition. The fertility rate of patients with endometriosis is about 66%, compared with 88% for the general population. Endometriosis occurs in young women with congenital obstructions of the vagina or cervix that are associated with reflux menstruation.

PATHOPHYSIOLOGY

Endometriosis has been identified in unusual sites in the body, but the majority of lesions are limited to the pelvis. The most common pelvic sites, in order of frequency, are the ovary, peritoneum of the cul-de-sac or pouch of Douglas, uterosacral ligaments, round ligament, oviduct, and peritoneal surface of the uterus. Isolated lesions in the appendix, bladder, ileum, cecum, cervix, or vagina are far less common. Endometriosis has been identified infrequently in laparotomy or episiotomy scars and in the umbilicus, arms, legs, lungs, kidneys, and nose.

Three major theories exist regarding the pathogenesis of endometriosis:

1. *Transportation.* Endometrium is regurgitated through the fallopian tubes during a normal menses. Following this retrograde flow endometrial fragments implant on the ovary, peritoneal surfaces, and other areas.
2. *Metaplasia or formation in situ.* Celomic epithelium differentiates to endometrial epithelium by inflammatory or hormonal influence and alteration.
3. *Induction.* This is a combination of transportation and metaplasia in which regurgitated endometrium liberates chemical-inducing substances that activate undifferentiated mesenchyme to form endometrial epithelium. This is thought to be the most likely pathogenesis of endometriosis.

The appearance of the lesions varies depending on the stage of the disease and its duration. The foci of endometrial tissue are under hormonal influence and bleed periodically. The foci appear as bluish red to yellow-brown nodules implanted on or lying beneath serosal surfaces. They may be microscopic or 1 to 2 cm in diameter. As individual lesions enlarge and coalesce, they can immobilize the affected structures and form adhesions. Endometriosis of the ovaries is characterized by endometriomas, cystic spaces 8 to 10 cm in size. Since they are filled with brown blood debris, they are also referred to as chocolate cysts.

DIAGNOSTIC STUDIES

Laparoscopy
   To visualize foci and perform a biopsy of lesions

Biopsy of lesions
   To confirm histologic diagnosis by presence of glands, stroma, or hemosiderin pigment (an insoluble form of storage iron that indicates bleeding)

TREATMENT PLAN

The treatment plan is directed toward producing maximum relief of symptoms and minimum interference with childbearing function in patients who desire children in the future.

Surgical
   Total abdominal hysterectomy and bilateral salpingo-oophorectomy
   Resection or cautery destruction of visible lesions

Chemotherapeutic
   Progestational steroids
      Cyclic
         Norgestrel (Lo/Ovral), 0.3-0.5 mg po qd
      Continuous
         Norethynodrel (Enovid), 5-15 mg po qd
      Long-acting
         Medroxyprogesterone acetate (Provera), 2.5-10 mg po for 5 d q 2 mo
         Hydroxyprogesterone (Delalutin), 125-250 mg IM q4 wk
   Antigonadotropic agents
      Danazol (Danocrine), 100-800 mg qd in divided

doses for 6-9 mo; produces hypoestrogenic state similar to menopause with eventual atrophy of endometrial lesions[18]

Bimanual pelvic examination
Tender nodules along uterosacral ligaments; uterus may be immobile

Bleeding
Menses excessive or long or both

ASSESSMENT: AREAS OF CONCERN

Comfort
Pelvic pain with menstruation; vague aching, cramping, or bearing-down sensation in pelvis or lower back; dyspareunia; pain with defecation

NURSING DIAGNOSES and NURSING INTERVENTIONS

Nursing Diagnosis	Nursing Intervention
Comfort, alteration in	Assist with and teach pain-relieving techniques. Instruct patient to take analgesics as ordered.
Self-concept, disturbance in	Explore meaning of condition with patient. Encourage patient to ventilate feelings.
	Refer to nursing interventions for specific surgical procedure if done.

Patient Education

1. Instruct the patient about the importance of ongoing outpatient care.

EVALUATION

Patient Outcome	Data Indicating That Outcome is Reached
Comfort is achieved.	Intervention has relieved pain, ended abnormal bleeding, and preserved fertility if desired.

LEIOMYOMAS

Uterine leiomyomas are well-circumscribed, nonencapsulated, benign tumors also called myomas, fibromyomas, fibromas, or fibroids.

Leiomyomas can be found in at least one fifth of women past 30 years of age and are more common in black women.[54] The incidence of myomas in African blacks is reported to be very low, which implies causative factors other than heredity. An estimated 60% of pelvic laparotomies are performed for leiomyomas, although almost all leiomyomas are asymptomatic.[12]

PATHOPHYSIOLOGY

Leiomyomas are classified according to their location in the uterus as follows:

1. Intramural—central portion of the uterine wall
2. Submucous—beneath the endometrium protruding into the intrauterine cavity; may become pedunculated with growth protruding into the cervix or vagina
3. Subserous—beneath the peritoneal covering and projecting into the abdominal cavity; may become pedunculated with growth
4. Cervical—within the musculature of the cervix
5. Intraligamentous—lateral tumor growth between the leaves of the broad ligament
6. Wandering or parasitic—a subserous growth that has lost its connection to the uterus and receives blood from adjacent viscera, peritoneum, or omentum

Leiomyomas arise from smooth muscle within the myometrium, most commonly during the reproductive years. They increase in size during pregnancy, when estrogen production is high, and with the use of oral contraceptives. They generally regress after menopause.

As the tumor enlarges, it reduces the blood supply, resulting in degenerative changes. The most common type of degeneration is hyalinization in which fibrous and muscle tissue is replaced by hyaline tissue that is smooth and soft and lacks the whorled fascicular pattern. Less commonly, cystic degeneration occurs, with the hyaline material breaking down further and undergoing liquefaction owing to a further decrease in blood supply. Calcification of the leiomyoma may occur after menopause because of calcium deposits. In a large tumor, areas of yellow-brown or red softening, referred to as red or carneous degeneration, may develop because of aseptic necrosis associated with hemorrhage into the tumor. Necrosis may also occur because of twisting or torsion of a pedunculated leiomyoma. Fertility may be impaired when leiomyomas occlude the endocervical canal.

DIAGNOSTIC STUDIES

Pregnancy test
To confirm or rule out pregnancy as a cause of symptoms

Dilation and curettage
To detect submucous leiomyomas

Laparoscopy
To visualize subserous myomas

Ultrasonography
To distinguish between adnexal inflammatory masses and endometriosis from pedunculated or subserous leiomyomas

Laboratory studies
Leukocytosis with degenerating tumor

TREATMENT PLAN

Surgical
Myomectomy to preserve uterus for potential future childbearing in young women
Total hysterectomy

Supportive
Pelvic examinations at regular intervals to monitor status of leiomyoma

ASSESSMENT: AREAS OF CONCERN

Pain
Dull ache, soreness, or colicky pain; acute pain if torsion or twisting of pedunculated leiomyoma has occurred; bilateral pelvic discomfort if large tumor causes pressure on adjacent viscera; cramping pain if uterus attempts to expel submucous tumor; dysmenorrhea from intramural tumors; pelvic heaviness; feeling of bearing down

Elimination
Constipation from pressure on rectum; urinary frequency and urgency if leiomyoma causes pressure on bladder

Abdomen
Firm, irregular nodules palpated in lower abdomen; irregular abdominal contour

Bleeding
Menses excessive or long or both

Temperature
Elevated with degenerating tumor

NURSING DIAGNOSES and NURSING INTERVENTIONS

Nursing Diagnosis	Nursing Intervention
Self-concept, disturbance in	Assess meaning of condition for patient. Encourage patient to ventilate her feelings.
Comfort, alteration in	Assist and teach patient to use pain-relieving methods including relaxation techniques and analgesics as ordered.

Patient Education

1. Instruct the patient about the importance of obtaining follow-up care and regular examinations to check for unusual growths or complications.

EVALUATION

Patient Outcome	Data Indicating That Outcome is Reached
Comfort is achieved.	There is no pain. Menses is normal if myomectomy was performed. There are no subjective or objective signs or symptoms of leiomyomas if hysterectomy was performed.

POLYPS

Polyps are benign neoplasms or protruding growths in the cervix or endometrium.

Cervical polyps are soft, red, pedunculated lesions protruding from the cervical os. Endometrial polyps are small, mostly sessile masses that project into the endometrium and may be pedunculated.

Polyps are usually asymptomatic and are often an incidental discovery during visual examination of the cervix, curettage, or hysterectomy. Because endometrial polyps frequently occur in association with leiomyomas and endometrial hyperplasia, specific symptoms are difficult to identify. The symptoms of cervical polyps are similar to those of chronic cervicitis with irregular bleeding. Polyps are the most common lesions of the cervix and occur most often during the reproductive years. Endometrial polyps can also occur at any age but are more common around the time of menopause. Polyps associated with the use of oral contraceptives tend to regress after the drug is discontinued.[45]

PATHOPHYSIOLOGY

Cervical polyps most commonly arise from the lower end of the endocervix and vary from a few millimeters to 2 cm in diameter. The base of the pedicle is usually small. Polyps develop as a result of inflammatory hyperplasia of endocervical mucosa owing to hyperestrinism, chronic inflammation, or vascular congestion. Microscopic examination shows a surface covered by columnar epithelium with areas of metaplasia and ulcer-ation. The stroma is often congested with blood and infiltrated by inflammatory cells. The polyps may bleed following trauma from coitus or douching.

Endometrial polyps develop as single or multiple soft tumors composed of hyperplastic endometrium. The majority arise from the fundus or cornua, and some may protrude through the cervix. They are usually paler and firmer than cervical polyps. Most frequently the polyp is made up of endometrium similar to that of the basalis and therefore does not show secretory changes. Polyps protruding into the cervix may become necrotic or inflamed, particularly if they are long.[38,45]

DIAGNOSTIC STUDIES

Endometrial polyps are usually an incidental finding with curettage or hysterectomy, but it is possible to diagnose an endometrial polyp from a hysterosalpingogram. Cervical polyps are diagnosed by inspection of the cervix.

TREATMENT PLAN

Surgical
Curettage to remove endometrial polyps
Removal and cauterization of base of cervical polyps; can be performed in outpatient setting
Cryosurgery for cervical polyps (see discussion of cervical conization on p. 972)

FERTILITY CONTROL

Fertility can be controlled by natural, mechanical, chemical, hormonal, and surgical means.

Nearly 80 million infants are born worldwide each year, as compared with 10 million a year in the early 1900s. United Nations researchers project that the world population will grow from the current 4.2 billion to 6.35 billion in 2000. Continued population growth at current rates could have a negative impact on natural resources, food supply, and political stability, especially in Third World countries. The number of people the earth can sustain is unknown. It is known that poverty leads to high fertility, which in turn further increases poverty.[15,42]

Population growth in the United States is currently at a level just over replacement, with a rate of 0.8% or 1 million people per year.[42] Fertility rates are higher among the poor and less educated. The goal of every pregnancy occurring as a result of an informed decision and resulting in a wanted child is far from being achieved.

Many factors affect the selection of a fertility control method, including the person's perception of the risk of pregnancy, knowledge of fertility control methods, and willingness and ability to use them; social pressures; the attitude of health care providers; desires of the partner; and the cost and effectiveness of various methods. The methods most widely used in the United States in order of popularity are oral steroids, condoms, intrauterine devices (IUDs), rhythm, foam, diaphragm, and coitus interruptus.[15] The method of fertility control varies according to the duration of the relationship or marriage. Young couples often use oral contraceptives until their first child is born, change to the use of an IUD until their family is complete, and then select sterilization.

There has been a general decline in the use of oral contraceptives and a fourfold increase in those selecting sterilization in the last decade. Approximately equal numbers of men and women have undergone sterilization. More than 12 million Americans have already undergone voluntary sterilization, and approximately 1 million are sterilized annually.[42]

Abortion, although not a contraceptive technique, is a method of preventing unwanted children. In January 1973 the U.S. Supreme Court declared all restrictive abortion laws by individual states unconstitutional. As a consequence, abortion in both the first and second trimesters is legal in all states, with the decision made by the woman and her physician. States may develop regulations regarding who can perform second-trimester abortions and where they may be done. In some states third-trimester abortions are prohibited except to preserve the life or health of the woman.

Since the Supreme Court decision the numbers of illegal abortions and abortion-related deaths have fallen precipitously. A national trend toward increased abortions appears to have leveled off in 1981, the latest year for which figures are available. In that year 1,300,760 legal abortions were reported in the United States, an increase of 3154 or less than 1% over the number reported in 1980. There were 11 abortion-related deaths, the lowest number since the Centers for Disease Control in Atlanta began keeping records in 1972.[8]

The health care provider has a responsibility to provide information to women or couples choosing a method of contraception. The decision is a voluntary one based on explanation of the methods available, including their action, safety and effectiveness, expected effects, risks, and contraindications. The methods of fertility control can be divided into five major groups: natural or physiologic, mechanical, chemical, hormonal, and surgical.

Natural or Physiologic Methods

Rhythm. In the rhythm method, coitus is confined to phases in the menstrual cycle when conception is unlikely to occur. This can be determined by the calendar method, temperature method, or ovulation method. With the *calendar* method the fertile period is determined by recording the number of days of each menstrual cycle for a year, subtracting 18 days from the length of the shortest cycle to determine the beginning of the fertile period, and subtracting 11 days from the length of the longest cycle to determine the postovulatory safe period. The *temperature* method is based on abstinence from the end of the menses until 4 days after the rise in basal body temperature. The woman must take her temperature the first thing in the morning, since the basal body temperature is the lowest temperature reached by the body during the waking hours. The *ovulation* method is based on the recognition of characteristic changes in cervical mucus. Initially after menstruation there is little mucus and the introitus is dry. The mucus becomes sticky and cloudy as estrogen stimulation increases, and as ovulation occurs it becomes abundant, clear, and slippery and stretches without breaking, the spinnbarkheit phenomenon. Following ovulation and an increase in progesterone the mucus becomes opaque and sticky again with the woman experiencing a sensation of dryness. Coitus should be avoided from first recognition of the sticky mucus until after the watery discharge disappears.

Coitus interruptus. Withdrawal of the penis from the vagina before ejaculation is probably the oldest and most frequently used fertility control method throughout the world. It is associated with a fairly high failure rate, since live sperm may be present in the seminal fluid that leaks from the urethra during coitus.

Mechanical Methods

Condom. The condom or penile sheath must be applied over the erect penis, leaving space at the tip to contain the ejaculate. It must be removed before penile detumescence, with the rim held tightly to prevent leakage.

Diaphragm. The diaphragm is a latex dome-shaped cup that must be fitted to the patient to ensure that the cervix is covered. The woman must be instructed in its use and be able to demonstrate its application.

Cervical cap. The cervical cap is smaller than the diaphragm and made of thick rubber or plastic. It may be applied some time before intercourse and left in place for at least 8 hours after intercourse. It is more difficult to apply than the diaphragm, and some women object to the odor when it is left in place for a long time. Its use, except in a few research centers, is not approved by the Food and Drug Administration.

Intrauterine device (IUD). The IUD is a small plastic device connected to a string that protrudes into the vagina. IUDs are available in various sizes and shapes. A health care provider inserts the device into the uterus, usually during menses when the cervix is partially open.

Chemical Methods

Spermicidal jellies, creams, suppositories, or aerosol foams are placed in the vagina immediately before intercourse and act as a chemical barrier to the sperm. They are often used in conjunction with another method such as a natural or a mechanical method.

Hormonal Methods

The most popular form of hormonal contraception is the oral contraceptive ("the pill"). This is most commonly a combination of estrogen and progestin that inhibits ovulation and changes in the endometrium, cervical mucus, and probably tubal function. Oral contraceptives are extremely effective in preventing pregnancy but are known to affect every body system and may produce significant dangers with long-term use. Generally the benefits and effectiveness outweigh the risk in healthy women below 30 years of age. See Table 9-9 for a summary of current agents.

Diethylstilbestrol (the "morning-after pill") is the postcoital agent most commonly used in the United States. It is not for routine use but should be considered an emergency measure to be taken as soon as possible but no later than 72 hours after unprotected midcycle intercourse. The possibility of an established pregnancy must be ruled out before this drug is administered, since ingestion by the mother is known to cause vaginal adenosis and clear cell carcinoma in daughters.[10]

Surgical Methods

Abortion. First-trimester abortion is done by dilation and curettage, aspiration of intrauterine contents through a suction device, or menstrual extraction. Second-trimester abortion is achieved by dilation and evacuation, intrauterine drug instillation, or hysterotomy.

Dilation and curettage is a painful procedure requiring general anesthesia; a sharp metal curette is inserted into the uterus to remove products of conception.

Vacuum aspiration can be done following a cervical block. The cervix is prepared by instillation of laminaria, an absorbent dried seaweed, into the cervix to expand the cervical canal. After the laminaria is removed, the aspiration curette is inserted and the products of conception are removed.

Menstrual extraction is the aspiration of endometrium and intrauterine contents through a polyethylene catheter that has been inserted into the uterus through the cervix. The procedure seldom requires cervical dilation and is performed no later than 8 weeks after the last menstrual period. Uterine injury and bleeding and continuation of pregnancy are the major risks associated with this procedure, which should not be considered a substitute for contraception.

The cervix must be more dilated for dilation and evacuation than for curettage. Dilation is usually effected with laminaria. The intrauterine contents are evacuated through a crushing instrument, followed by aspiration. The procedure is most frequently done in women who are 13 to 16 weeks pregnant.

Hypertonic saline solution is injected into the amniotic cavity to induce a second-trimester abortion. Complications are inadvertent infusion into the maternal bloodstream, producing salt intoxication; disseminated intravascular coagulation; and infection, especially if there is a long interval between instillation of the drug and uterine evacuation. Prostaglandin can be given by intra-amniotic or intravenous infusion or as a vaginal suppository. This method has virtually replaced use of hypertonic saline solution for abortion. Prostaglandins stimulate contractions of smooth uterine muscle and generally result in abortion within 24 hours. Side effects include nausea, vomiting, diarrhea, and abdominal cramping, which can be controlled with analgesics and antiemetics.[33,42]

Hysterotomy is a surgical incision into the uterus for the removal of products of conception. It is associated with morbidity and is used only rarely for midtrimester abortions.

Sterilization. Sterilization is the ultimate method of fertility control, rendering a person unable to reproduce. This is accomplished by vasectomy in men and tubal ligation or hysterectomy in women.

Vasectomy is a procedure for male sterilization involving the bilateral surgical removal of a portion of the vas deferens. It is most commonly performed on an outpatient basis with the patient under local anesthesia.

Tubal sterilization is the disruption of tubal patency to prevent the union of the ova and spermatozoa. It can be achieved through the vagina or by an abdominal approach through an incision or with laparoscopic visualization. A variety of techniques can be used:

1. *Irving procedure.* The oviduct is severed, and the uterine end is buried in the myometrium posteriorly and the distal or ovarian end is placed in the mesosalpinx.
2. *Pomeroy procedure.* A loop of oviduct is ligated and excised.
3. *Parkland procedure.* A segment of the fallopian tube is separated from the mesosalpinx and ligated proximally and distally, and then the midportion is excised.[42]
4. *Fimbriectomy.* The distal portion of the ampulla, including all of the fimbriae, is resected.

Tubal sterilization can be done at any time but is most convenient during the postpartum period because the uterine fundus is near the umbilicus and the fallopian tubes are readily accessible. Laparoscope sterilization is often referred to as "band aid" surgery, since it can be performed in an ambulatory surgical center with general

Table 9-9
Summary of Methods of Conception Control

Method	Action	Safety-Effectiveness	Effects	Contraindications
Oral Contraceptive ("the pill")				
Combination pill: each pill contains progestin and estrogen; schedule: one pill daily for 21 days, then discontinue for 7 days; placebo may be advised for last 7 days; pill cycle started and repeated on fifth day after onset of menstrual flow	Inhibits ovulation by suppression of pituitary gonadotropin Produces cervical mucus that is hostile to sperm Modifies tubal transport of ovum May have effect on endometrium to make implantation unlikely	100% effective if taken accurately Failure results from failure to take pill regularly If woman forgets to take pill one day, she can "make up" by taking two pills next day Chances of pregnancy increased if pill is missed for even 1 day Highly acceptable to users; easy to take Linked with mortality caused by thromboembolus phenomena Does not alter fertility	Useful Relief of dysmenorrhea in 60% to 90% of cases Relief of premenstrual tension Regulation of menstrual cycles Relief of acne in 80% to 90% of cases Improved feeling of well-being Minor side effects (usually decrease after third cycle) Weight gain Breast tenderness Headaches Corneal edema Nausea Breakthrough bleeding Hypertension Major side effects Thromboembolus disorders May decrease lactation in breast-feeding women	Undiagnosed vaginal bleeding Breast or pelvic cancer Liver disease Cardiovascular disease Renal disease Thyroid disease Diabetes Uterine fibroid tumors Use with caution if history of: Epilepsy Multiple sclerosis Porphyria Otosclerosis Asthma
Intrauterine Contraceptive Device (IUD or IUCD)				
Small objects of various shapes made of plastic, nylon, or steel inserted into uterus; most have nylon string attached that protrudes from cervix into vagina; inserted using aseptic technique; follow-up visits in 1 month, then individualized EXAMPLES Lippes loop Saf-T-Coil Birnberg bow Margulies coil Hall-Stone ring Copper T Copper seven	Unknown Probably modifies endometrium or myometrium to prevent inflammation Probably hastens tubal transport of ovum	Easily inserted, highly effective: 97% to 99% Can be inserted any time during cycle; presence of menstrual flow rules out early pregnancy Can be inserted immediately postpartum, but expulsion rate is higher Can be left in place indefinitely Effectiveness highly dependent on knowing IUD remains in place; women need to be taught to feel for string after each period Spontaneous expulsion occurs most often during menstrua-	Uterine cramping Heavy menstrual flow Irregular menses NOTE: Usually disappear in 2 to 3 months Problems Infection: usually minor and occurs soon after insertion Perforation of uterus: varies with types of device; highest rates in first 6 weeks postpartum; usually occurs at time of insertion	Current infection of reproductive tract Uterine fibroids Undiagnosed vaginal bleeding

Method	Description	Effectiveness	Complications
(continued)		tion (expulsion rates: 10% to 20%) Failure rate (pregnancy) 1.5% to 3% during first year of use; rate declines thereafter Does not alter fertility	Severe uterine prolapse
Diaphragm (with spermicidal foam, cream, jelly)	Rubber dome attached to flexible metal ring; inserted into vagina to cover cervix; available in various sizes (require careful fitting); self-inserted by user; inner surface of diaphragm coated with spermicide before insertion; inserted at least 2 hours before intercourse and left in place at least 6 hours after intercourse. Provides mechanical barrier to sperm. Spermicidal preparation destroys large number of sperm	97% to 98% effective if fitted properly and used correctly. Requires sustained motivation for repeated insertion and removal. Refitting necessary after childbirth, abortion, surgery of cervix and vagina, or weight change of 10 pounds or more	None
Condom ("rubber," "safe," "prophylactic")	Thin, flexible plastic worn over penis; available without prescription; does not require medical supervision. Provides mechanical barrier to prevent sperm from entering vagina. Prevents spread of venereal diseases	Effectiveness increased with use of diaphragm by woman. Effectiveness decreased by tearing or slipping of condom during intercourse. Failure rate 10% to 15%	None
Natural Family Planning (ovulation, symptothermal)	Periodic abstinence from intercourse during fertile periods of menstrual cycle; days 12 to 16 before expected date of menstruation are possible ovulating days; because sperm can survive up to 48 hours, days 11, 17, and 18 added to fertile period. Sexual abstinence around time of ovulation	Safe. 65% to 85% effective. Fertile period varies; precise time of ovulation not known. Effectiveness increased with calculation of fertile period, high motivation to prevent pregnancy, determination of basal body temperature	Frustration. Lack of sexual gratification during period of abstinence. Irregular menstrual cycles. Medical contraindications to pregnancy
Chemical Contraceptive (jellies, creams, foams, suppositories)	Applied inside vagina by means of plunger-type applicator or aerosol spray. Contains spermicidal ingredients. Partial barrier to entrance of sperm into cervix	Effectiveness increased when used with diaphragm or condom. Easily available without prescription. Effectiveness depends on dispersion of substance within vagina	None

From Phipps, W.J., Long, B.C., and Woods, N.F.: Shafer's medical-surgical nursing, ed. 7, St. Louis, 1980, The C.V. Mosby Co.

or occasionally local anesthesia. A pneumoperitoneum is produced with carbon dioxide, and the oviduct is ligated and most commonly electrocoagulated. In a vaginal tubal sterilization the peritoneal cavity is entered through the posterior vaginal fornix (culdotomy, colpotomy) and

a Pomeroy procedure or fimbriectomy is performed. The care of women undergoing tubal ligation is discussed on p. 1029.

A summary of the common methods of conception control is provided in Table 9-9.

INFERTILITY

Infertility is the inability to conceive during a period of 1 year of unprotected intercourse. Primary infertility exists when there has been no prior conception. Secondary infertility follows at least one normal pregnancy.

Infertility affects 10% to 15% of couples in the United States. About 25% of women who do not use contraception and who have coitus regularly conceive within 4 months, more than 60% do so within 6 months, and about 80% within 1 year. The incidence of infertility shows a progression with advancing age of the woman. Fertility peaks between 20 and 25 years of age and decreases after 30 years of age in women and 40 years of age in men.[54]

It is estimated that male factors are responsible for about 40% of infertility problems. The cause of infertility is not identifiable in 10% to 20% of cases. Female factors are responsible for the remaining cases. Of these around 20% to 30% are the result of disorders of the fallopian tubes, 10% to 15% lack of ovulation, and 50% cervical factors.

About 40% of those who seek medical attention for infertility eventually conceive. The identified cause of infertility cannot be corrected in 40% of the couples, and the cause of infertility in the remaining couples is never identified.

PATHOPHYSIOLOGY

Normal fertility is dependent on many factors, including normal ovarian function, endocrine preparation of the uterus for implantation of the fertilized ovum, cervical mucus favorable for transport of sperm, normal anatomic structures, lack of obstruction to sperm and ovum, and normally functioning fallopian tubes. The male partner must have a sufficient number of motile and mature sperm that can be ejaculated without any anatomic or physiologic obstruction and that are capable of penetrating the egg.

The causes of infertility are as follows[15,31]:

Female factors
    Vaginal abnormalities
        Rigid hymen or small hymenal orifice; psychogenic vaginismus; hyperacidity of vaginal secretions

Cervical abnormalities
    Obstructive lesions such as polyps, pedunculated fibroids, or congenital atresia; alterations in cervical mucus owing to bacteria or chemical agents; surgical destruction of endocervical glands
Uterine factors
    Submucous myomas; structural malformations such as bicornuate or septate uterus; hypoplasia owing to endocrine disturbances; synechiae owing to endometritis; pelvic inflammatory disease
Tubal and peritoneal abnormalities
    Peritubal and periovarian adhesions following peritonitis; inflammatory damage owing to intrauterine devices, severe puerperal infections, and pelvic inflammatory disease; endometriosis
Ovarian abnormalities
    Oligo-ovulation or anovulation owing to hypothalamic, pituitary, or ovarian deficits; hyperprolactinemia and galactorrhea associated with anovulation or luteal phase defects; faulty nutrition; metabolic dysfunction; luteal phase defects, which may be due to abnormal stimulation of the graafian follicle, hyperandrogen states, or increased prolactin levels; ovarian tumors (such as Stein-Leventhal syndrome)
Male factors
    Sperm-related factors
        Testicular hypoplasia; endocrine disorders such as hypopituitarism and hypothalamic disorders; cryptorchidism; varicocele; gonadal damage from trauma, surgery, or radiation; exposure of testicles to heat including wearing of tight shorts; systemic infections including mumps, tuberculosis, and syphilis; late descent of testicles; high viscosity of semen; autoimmunity as result of trauma, vasectomy, or infection; low volume
    Ductal obstructions
        Resulting from epididymitis or infection of ejaculatory ducts; congenital absence of ducts
    Transport-related factors
        Hypospadias; ejaculatory problems; impotence

Factors affecting either male or female
  Stress
    Physical or psychic; long-term psychiatric problems
  Nutritional deficiencies
    Malnutrition such as anorexia nervosa and starvation; vitamin, mineral, or fat deficiencies
  Substances
    Exposure to toxins including alcohol, nicotine, metals such as lead, dyes such as aniline dyes, drugs such as narcotics, quinine, hormonal agents, and antineoplastic drugs, radiation
  Congenital anomalies
    Chromosomal abnormalities (such as Turner's and Klinefelter's syndromes)
  Disease processes
    Dysfunctions or disturbances of thyroid, adrenal, or pituitary gland; diabetes mellitus; anemia; chronic nephritis; severe cardiac disturbances; infections; immune responses
Causes of infertility in the couple
  Sexual problems
    Unconsummated relationships; infrequent intercourse; sexual dysfunction; vaginismus; suboptimum technique
  Other problems
    Discordant relationships; immunologic reaction

DIAGNOSTIC STUDIES

Semen analysis
  Standards for fertility are volume of 2 to 6 ml semen per ejaculation; 20 to 300 million sperm/ml; 60% to 80% of sperm actively motile; 60% or more of sperm normally shaped[54]

Tubal patency determination
  Hysterosalpingography
    May indicate obstruction of tube if radiopaque dye fails to spill into peritoneum
  Uterotubal insufflation (Rubin's test)
    May indicate tubal obstruction if pressurized carbon dioxide cannot pass through tubes
  Cervical examination in midcycle
    Cervix not opened; lack of copious mucus; lack of spinnbarkheit and arborization
  Laparoscopy or culdoscopy
    Absence of direct observation of dye passing through fimbriated ends of fallopian tube; peritubal adhesions may be observed

Basal body temperature graph
  Absence of normal biphasic pattern with sustained rise of at least 1° F during last 2 weeks of cycle

Serum progesterone
  Level less than 10 ng/ml indicative of abnormal luteal function; concentration of less than 3 ng/ml suggestive of anovulation

Postcoital test (Sims-Huhner)
  Fewer than five highly motile sperm in mucus from upper cervix; inadequate spinnbarkheit and arborization suggestive of estrogen deficiency and secretory defect of cervical epithelium

Endometrial biopsy
  Findings inconsistent with cycle

Immunologic compatibility tests
  Evaluation of sperm agglutination and immobilization

TREATMENT PLAN

Surgical
  Removal of myomas
  Polypectomy
  Dilation and curettage
  Unilateral or bilateral tuboplasty
  Salpingostomy
  Ovarian wedge resection (for patients with polycystic ovaries)

Chemotherapeutic
  Anti-infective agents
    Therapy based on culture findings
  Ovulatory stimulants
    Clomiphene citrate (Clomid), 50-100 mg for 5-7 d
    Human menopausal gonadotropin (HMG; Pergonal), 1 ampule IM for 9-12 d followed by 10,000 IU human chorionic gonadotropin 1 d after last dose of HMG
  Estrogens
    Estrone (Hormonin, others), 0.7-1.4 mg po qd cyclically
    Conjugated estrogens (Premarin), 0.625-3.75 mg qd po cyclically
  Pituitary-related agents
    Bromocriptine (Parlodel), individually adjusted

Supportive
  In vitro fertilization
  Artificial insemination
  Psychotherapy
  Improvement of coital technique
  Use of condoms and avoidance of orogenital sex for 6 to 12 months to treat immunologic fertility

ASSESSMENT: AREAS OF CONCERN

Couple

Name; age; occupation; religion; ethnocultural influences; years of marriage; previous marriages; duration of involuntary infertility; habits; diet; health status; exposure to alcohol, nicotine, narcotics, quinine, hormones, antineoplastic agents, metals, dyes, and radiation; physical or psychic stress

Female

Health history

Tuberculosis; venereal disease; endometriosis; tumors

Gynecologic history

Menarche; frequency, duration, and amount of menstrual flow; menstrual irregularities; evidence of dysmenorrhea; mittelschmerz; increased midcycle discharge; pelvic inflammatory disease; previous surgical procedure including pelvic operation and appendectomy

Obstetric history

Full-term deliveries; complications; abortions (reason, if elective) or premature deliveries

Conception control history

Type of contraceptives used and duration of use

Sexual history

Frequency of coitus; postcoital practices; libido; orgasm capacity; position during and after intercourse; use of lubricants; sexual involvement with other partners

Male

Health history

Tuberculosis; venereal infection; mumps; orchitis; varicocele; previous surgical procedure including orchiopexy and herniorrhaphy; hydrocele; injury to genitals

Sexual history

Frequency of coitus; technique and position; premature ejaculation; adequacy of erection; timing of coitus; sexual involvement with other partners

Male and female psychosocial factors

Motivation for pregnancy; perception of and feelings related to inability to achieve conception; effect of sociocultural and familial factors related to desired pregnancy

NURSING DIAGNOSES and NURSING INTERVENTIONS

Nursing Diagnosis	Nursing Intervention
Knowledge deficit (regarding optimum sexual technique); sexual dysfunction (related to lack of knowledge)	Ensure that both partners are aware of practices that promote conception, including: 1. Intercourse every 2 days during fertile period 2. Woman in supine position with man astride 3. Woman's hips elevated on pillow with thighs flexed 4. Avoidance of commercial lubricants 5. Penis maintained in vagina without thrusting for short time after ejaculation 6. Woman remaining in bed with hips elevated for approximately 30 minutes after coitus 7. Woman not urinating or douching for at least 1 hour after coitus
Grieving (related to actual or perceived loss)	Support couple's grief through listening and offering explanations about their reactions. Promote cohesiveness; avoid laying ''blame'' on one person. Help couple verbalize their feelings when they find it difficult to do so. Assist couple to explore their feelings and eventually accept the normal ambivalence toward expectations of being a parent. Promote grief work with responses to grieving process of denial, isolation, depression, anger, guilt, fear, and rejection.
Coping, ineffective individual	Assess both partners' coping mechanisms. Explain consequences of prolonged stress. Assist couple to problem solve in constructive manner. Discuss alternatives to treatment. See also p. 1897.
Self-concept, disturbance in	Encourage patient to express feelings about the way that patient views self. Clarify misconceptions. Promote sharing of feelings with partner. Explore patient's personal strengths and resources. Promote discussion regarding resolution of altered body image.

EVALUATION

Patient Outcome	Data Indicating That Outcome is Reached
Realistic self-concept is achieved.	Patient exhibits adaptive responses to altered body image through verbal statements.
Grief is resolved.	Patient has expressed grief, shared concerns with partner, and planned constructively for future.
Knowledge of sexual functions is increased.	Patient indicates practice of optimum sexual technique. Patient relates valid information about sexual function.
Patient uses adaptive coping behavior.	Patient verbalizes feelings about infertility and can identify personal strengths. Patient follows through with decisions and appropriate actions.

ECTOPIC PREGNANCY

Ectopic or extrauterine pregnancy is the implantation of a fertilized ovum outside the corpus of the uterus.

The most common site for ectopic pregnancy is the fallopian tube. Rare forms of ectopic pregnancy include abdominal implantation following tubal rupture, cornual pregnancy at the uterine end of the interstitial portion of the tube, rudimentary uterine horn pregnancy, and implantation in the cervix and ovary.

The incidence of ectopic pregnancy varies with the population and has been reported to range from 1 in 80 to 1 in 200 live births each year. It is more common in the lower socioeconomic strata than in affluent women. The increase in incidence during recent years is related to the greater incidence of pelvic inflammatory disease and the increased use of intrauterine devices and progestin-only oral contraceptives. Ectopic pregnancy is more common in older women who have had previous pregnancies than in teenagers.[12]

PATHOPHYSIOLOGY

The most common cause of tubal pregnancy is thought to be pelvic inflammatory disease, which is reaching epidemic proportions in the United States.[12,54] Between 30% and 50% of women undergoing surgery for tubal pregnancy are known to have had salpingitis, and histologic evidence of chronic salpingitis is found in approximately half of the tubes excised for tubal pregnancy. Other causes of tubal pregnancy include the following:

1. *Peritubal adhesions.* These may result from a postpartum or postabortion infection, appendicitis, or a peritoneal reaction to endometriosis.
2. *Anatomic abnormalities.* Congenital diverticula or atresia of the tube can retard or prevent the passage of a fertilized ovum. Uterine or tubal myomas may cause pressure against or kinking and displacement of the tube.
3. *Zygote abnormalities.* Ectopic pregnancy is more likely if the male has a large percentage of abnormal spermatozoa and an abnormal (high or low) sperm count.
4. *Endocrine disorders.* A decrease in motility of tubal cilia with eventual entrapment of the fertilized ovum in the tube can be caused by an inadequate corpus luteum, delayed ovulation, prostaglandins, catecholamines, or induction of ovulation with pituitary and chorionic gonadotropic hormones.
5. *Previous surgery.* Surgery to restore tubal patency after salpingitis or because of adhesions from previous pelvic or abdominal surgery may result in tubal occlusion.
6. *Prior tubal pregnancy.* Recurrence of tubal pregnancy is between 10% and 20%.
7. *Delayed implantation.* External migration of the fertilized ovum from the producing ovary to the opposite fallopian tube delays implantation of the trophoblast, which can then be too large to pass through the tube.
8. *Endometriosis.* Implants of endometrium within the fallopian tube can prevent passage of the fertilized ovum.
9. *Intrauterine device (IUD).* The exact cause of the 12-fold increase in ectopic pregnancy in women with IUDs is unknown, but tubal infection or decreased tubal motility may be relevant factors. Progesterone-releasing IUDs are associated with more ectopic pregnancies than other types.
10. *Progestin oral contraceptives.* A fivefold increase in ectopic pregnancy is associated with this type of oral contraceptive as compared with combination oral contraceptives.
11. *Tubal ligation.* Formation of fistulas and recanalization may result in pregnancy after tubal ligation. Some 15% of these occur in the tube.

12. *"Morning-after pill."* When on rare occasions the postcoital administration of high doses of estrogen fails, there is a 10-fold increase in ectopic pregnancy.

The trophoblast usually implants between mucosal folds. As the cells proliferate, they invade the muscularis mucosae, destroying tissue and eroding blood vessels. The resulting hemorrhage increases the size of the tube and may rupture it, causing diaphragmatic irritation evidenced by referred supraclavicular pain. The expelled trophoblast may then reinvade the tube from the outside.

The myometrial response to tubal pregnancy is the same as that of an intrauterine pregnancy; the uterus becomes soft and then enlarges because of hypertrophy and hyperplasia of endometrial cells. The endometrial response is also similar, with the development of decidua in response to placental estrogen and progesterone. When the placenta separates from the tubal wall or degenerates, the hormones supporting the endometrium are withdrawn, resulting in shedding of the decidua. Intermittent and sometimes heavy vaginal bleeding accompanied by a soft or enlarged uterus expelling a decidual cast is indicative of an ectopic pregnancy.

A leukocytosis of 15,000 cells/mm^3 and a rapid decrease in hemoglobin and hematocrit may occur in cases of tubal rupture. A positive finding of a human chorionic gonadotropin test confirms the presence of pregnancy but does not reveal its location.

DIAGNOSTIC STUDIES

Physical examination
Deep unilateral lower quadrant tenderness; Cullen's sign (bluish skin discoloration around umbilicus, indicating intra-abdominal hemorrhage); tender boggy mass in cul-de-sac may indicate pelvic hematocele

Ultrasonography
May show extrauterine gestational sac

Culdocentesis
Confirms presence of intraperitoneal bleeding owing to ruptured tubal pregnancy if dark or bright red blood flows freely through needle

Laparoscopy
Confirms unruptured tubal pregnancy through visualization of distended tube or site of implantation

Dilation and curettage
May confirm ectopic pregnancy through pelvic examination under anesthesia or rule it out if placental tissue is obtained from endometrium

Other conditions with similar clinical symptoms must be ruled out. These include threatened or incomplete abortion, corpus luteum cyst, salpingitis, acute appendicitis, degenerating leiomyoma, ruptured graafian follicle, and IUD complications.

TREATMENT PLAN

Surgical
Salpingectomy

ASSESSMENT: AREAS OF CONCERN

Unruptured tube
Low abdominal pain and tenderness that may be generalized or unilateral; signs of pregnancy (such as amenorrhea, nausea, vomiting, and urinary frequency); vaginal bleeding (scanty and dark brown); breast tenderness; pelvic mass may be palpable

Ruptured tube
Severe lower abdominal pain that is sudden and stabbing; dizziness; fainting; referred supraclavicular pain; vaginal bleeding (not always present); pallor; cervical pain during vaginal examination; progressive supine hypotension; tachycardia and tachypnea; decreased hematocrit value; shock

NURSING DIAGNOSES and NURSING INTERVENTIONS

Nursing Diagnosis	Nursing Intervention
Tissue perfusion: alteration in (resulting from hypotension)	See p. 2024.
Fluid volume deficit	See p. 2052.
Comfort, alteration in: pain	Administer analgesics as ordered.
Grieving (related to loss of pregnancy)	Support patient's grief response. Promote cohesiveness between patient and significant others. See p. 1908.

EVALUATION

Patient Outcome	Data Indicating That Outcome is Reached
Shock is resolved.	Vital signs are within normal limits.
Body hydration is normal.	Skin turgor is good, and intake and output are balanced.
Pain is relieved.	Patient denies discomfort.
Patient makes adaptive response to grief.	Patient demonstrates appropriate progression through grieving process, eventually accepts loss, and verbalizes plan for realistic future.

SPONTANEOUS ABORTION

Spontaneous abortion is the termination of pregnancy before the period of fetal viability. This is usually defined as before the end of the twentieth week after the last menstrual period, a fetal weight less than 500 g, and a crown-rump length less than 16.5 cm.

The incidence of spontaneous abortion is about 10% to 15%. The precise incidence is unknown but is hypothesized to be almost half of all pregnancies when human chorionic gonadotropin (HCG) is used as a determinant of pregnancy without other clinical evidence. Some 85% of abortions occur in the first trimester, with early abortions related to fetal causes and later abortions (twelfth to twentieth week of pregnancy) related to maternal factors.[42,54]

When spontaneous abortion is discussed with laypersons, the term ''miscarriage'' may be preferable to ''abortion'' to avoid the connotation of induced, elective, or criminal abortion.

PATHOPHYSIOLOGY

A definite cause of abortion cannot always be established because many closely related fetal, placental, and maternal factors may be involved.

Abnormal development accounts for a large percentage of aborted pregnancies. For example, of 1000 spontaneous abortions 48.9% had degenerated or absent embryos, 3.2% had anomalous embryos, and 9.6% exhibited placental abnormalities.[12,42] Some 61% of abortions occurring in the first trimester demonstrate chromosomal abnormalities as compared with 55% of all abortions. Monosomy and trisomy are the most frequent abnormalities in number of chromosomes. In addition, abnormal development may result from faulty implantation of the fertilized ovum or from a suboptimum intrauterine environment.

Maternal factors responsible for abortion include both systemic and localized conditions. Infectious processes, most notably cytomegalovirus, herpesvirus, and rubella virus, chronic debilitating or wasting diseases, endocrine defects such as deficient corpus luteum, abnormalities of the reproductive organs such as leiomyomas and incompetent cervix, and physical or psychic trauma are all factors that can lead to spontaneous abortion. Other contributing factors include intra-abdominal surgical procedures and exposure to ionizing radiation, drugs, or chemicals. Operating room nurses and anesthetists have a higher incidence of spontaneous abortion and earlier spontaneous abortions than other groups.[12,54]

Morphologic changes depend on the time interval between fetal death and expulsion of products of conception. They are generally focal areas of necrosis resulting from hemorrhage in the decidua basalis. Changes in the ovum or fetus are highly variable; fetal products are absent in many instances.

Hydropic degeneration of the villi is a common finding in abortion owing to retention of tissue fluid after fetal death. These changes are referred to as a blighted ovum.

Hemorrhage around the ovum when expulsion of a dead embryo is delayed is called a carneous or blood mole. Occasionally the loss of placental circulation results in the drying of the fetus, giving it the appearance of parchment. This is called fetus papyraceous.

The types of spontaneous abortion are threatened abortion, inevitable and incomplete abortion, complete abortion, missed abortion, and habitual abortion.

A threatened abortion is bleeding or cramping of the uterus in the first 20 weeks of pregnancy. It is characterized by recurring episodes of scanty bleeding varying from bright red to a dark color, sometimes with pelvic pressure, low back pain, or a dull lower abdominal aching. Tissue is not passed, and the cervix is not found to be open. The prognosis may be determined by real-time ultrasonography to assess any movement, serum levels of the β subunit of HCG in three successive tests done 3 days apart, and assessment of serum estradiol.[12]

An inevitable abortion is characterized by rupture of membranes, cervical dilation, uterine contractions, and an increase in bleeding.

An incomplete abortion is one in which all or part of the placenta remains within the uterus, either attached to the wall or lying free within the uterine cavity. Severe pain may be associated with uterine contractions, and bleeding can lead to profound anemia and shock. The bleeding continues until the products of conception are entirely removed. Once empty, the uterus contracts, compressing the vessels and controlling hemorrhage. This type of abortion generally occurs between the sixth and fourteenth weeks of pregnancy.

A complete abortion is one in which all products of conception are passed with minimum bleeding. This generally occurs before the sixth week of pregnancy or after the fourteenth week.

A missed abortion is the prolonged retention of a dead fetus, generally beyond 8 weeks. There is persistent amenorrhea, often with scanty intermittent brown vaginal discharge, a decrease in breast size, and a cessation of uterine growth progressing to shrinkage as a result of reabsorption of amniotic fluid and maceration of the fetus. Coagulation defects related to a decrease in fibrinogen and platelets and an increase in fibrin degradation products occur in about 25% of women with missed abortion. This is a potentially dangerous situation when the fibrinogen level decreases to 100 mg/dl or less. When the dead conceptus is removed, the coagulation defects are corrected spontaneously.

Habitual spontaneous abortion is the loss of three or more consecutive pregnancies. The causes include structural defects of the cervix and uterus (congenital or acquired), chromosomal abnormalities, hormonal aberrations, psychogenic factors, and possibly some immunologic deficiencies. Cerclage of the cervix may be done if the cause of habitual abortion is an incompetent cervix.

A septic abortion occurs when the uterine contents become infected. The patient may be severely ill with signs and symptoms of an acute infection, including a leukocytosis of 16,000 to 22,000 cells/mm³. Septic or endotoxin shock may develop with profound hypotension, hypothermia, oliguria progressing to anuria, respiratory distress, and vasomotor collapse. The most frequently encountered causative organisms are *Escherichia coli, Enterobacter aerogenes, Proteus vulgaris,* hemo-lytic streptococci, staphylococci, and anaerobic organisms such as *Clostridium perfringens*. Before the 1973 Supreme Court decision on abortion, septic abortions were common in the United States and were almost always associated with illegal abortions.

DIAGNOSTIC STUDIES

The diagnosis is based on the physical examination, clinical evidence of abortion, and laboratory tests.

Human chorionic gonadotropin (HCG)
Presence of this hormone in blood or urine confirms pregnancy

Ultrasonography
May confirm presence of gestational sac or ring

Tissue cytology
Confirms presence of products of conception

TREATMENT PLAN

Surgical
Dilation and curettage—to ensure removal of remaining products of conception from uterus
Cervical cerclage—to close and reinforce incompetent cervix, preferably after first trimester, suture is removed before delivery
Hysterotomy—to remove products of conception not expelled after administration of oxytocin

Chemotherapeutic
Pituitary hormones
Oxytocin (Pitocin), 5-10 units IM or 0.5-20 mU/min IV, to produce uterine contractions and expulsion of products of conception
Rh_o (D) immune globulin (human) (RhoGAM), dosage individually calculated, to prevent Rh isoimmunization in Rh-negative mothers when findings of indirect Coombs' test are negative
Anti-infective agents (indicated for septic abortion; may be indicated for missed abortion)

ASSESSMENT: AREAS OF CONCERN

Type	Area of Concern	Assessment
Threatened abortion	Vaginal drainage	Bleeding varying from bright red spotting to dark brown discharge
	Pain	Abdominal cramps, pelvic pressure, low back pain
	Cervix	Closed

Type	Area of Concern	Assessment
Inevitable abortion	Vaginal drainage Cervix Pain	Heavy vaginal bleeding Dilated Cramping
Incomplete abortion	Vaginal drainage Cervix	Profuse bleeding; evidence of passage of part of products of conception Dilated
Complete abortion	Expelled uterine contents Vaginal drainage	Evidence of passage of entire products of conception Minimum bleeding
Missed abortion	Uterus Ultrasonography Vaginal drainage Breasts Placental hormones	Smaller than expected for presumed duration of pregnancy; absence of fetal heart sounds Absence of fetal activity Scanty intermittent brown discharge Decreased in size Subnormal or decreased concentrations
Septic abortion	Tissue perfusion	Hypotension, tachychardia, fever, cool clammy skin, hemorrhage (see also discussion of septic shock on p. 51)

NURSING DIAGNOSES and NURSING INTERVENTIONS

Nursing Diagnosis	Nursing Intervention
Fluid volume deficit; tissue perfusion: alteration in	Maintain bed rest. Administer blood and blood components as ordered by physician. Increase volume of circulating fluids by oral or intravenous route per protocol. Continually assess for signs of shock. Monitor intake and output. Assist with medical procedures such as dilation and curettage and oxytocin administration. See discussion of hypovolemic shock on p. 50.
Comfort, alteration in: pain	Administer analgesics as ordered. Assist with and teach pain-relieving techniques to use during uterine cramping or contractions, such as massage or effleurage, breathing techniques, cold applications, or distraction.
Patient problem: susceptibility to infection	Administer perineal care with antiseptic solution. Administer antibiotics as ordered. Explain importance of avoiding intercourse or douching if abortion is incomplete.
Grieving (related to loss of pregnancy)	Support patient's reaction. Promote grief work of patient and significant other. If patient desires, refer her to social worker, geneticist, clergyman, or parent support group for counseling. Avoid focusing on possible future pregnancies and favorable outcomes.

Patient Education

1. Instruct the patient to remain in bed until the bleeding becomes minimal.
2. Tell the patient that she may resume normal activities when she feels able.
3. Instruct the patient to avoid pregnancy for two or three normal menstrual cycles.
4. Tell the patient to report vaginal bleeding that persists beyond 10 days or any expulsion of frank red blood.
5. Discuss signs and symptoms of infection, including fever, increased pulse rate, and foul-smelling vaginal drainage.
6. Instruct the patient not to use tampons or douche for at least 2 weeks to avoid infection.
7. Encourage the patient to share her feelings about loss of pregnancy with her partner.

EVALUATION

Patient Outcome	Data Indicating That Outcome is Reached
Body hydration and tissue perfusion are normal.	Skin turgor is good. Vaginal bleeding is diminished or absent. Hemoglobin and hematocrit values are within normal limits. Skin is warm and dry.
Comfort is achieved.	Patient uses pain-relieving techniques or medication when needed. Patient describes feeling of well-being.
Patient demonstrates adaptive response to grief.	Patient expresses grief. Patient describes meaning of loss. Patient shares grief with significant others.

HYPEREMESIS GRAVIDARUM

Pernicious vomiting of pregnancy may lead to fluid and electrolyte imbalance, weight loss, dehydration, and starvation.

Transient nausea and vomiting occur in about half of women during the first trimester of pregnancy but rarely persist beyond the fourteenth week. In a few women nausea continues throughout the pregnancy. Hyperemesis gravidarum, intractable vomiting of pregnancy, occurs in about 1 in 1000 pregnancies. The woman generally requires hospitalization and treatment.[11,42]

PATHOPHYSIOLOGY

The exact cause of hyperemesis gravidarum is unknown, but it is probably related to trophoblastic activity and gonadotropin production that are stimulated or exaggerated by psychologic factors. The incidence and timing of nausea and vomiting parallel gonadotropin levels. Nausea and vomiting are more pronounced in women with hydatidiform mole, who have higher gonadotropin levels; the symptoms disappear when the women abort. Since nausea and vomiting that begin after the tenth to twelfth weeks of pregnancy are probably caused by a medical or surgical condition, health care providers must take steps to diagnose such conditions. Some conditions that cause nausea and vomiting are gastroenteritis, cholecystitis, hepatitis, peptic ulcer, pyelonephritis, vitamin deficiency, and drug toxicity.

Abnormal laboratory data may include the presence of proteins in urine and increased levels of uric acid, urea, and nonprotein nitrogen in the blood. An increase in the hematocrit value and decreases in serum protein, sodium, potassium, and chloride levels can be expected.

Forceful vomiting may cause retinal hemorrhages that impair vision and gastroesophageal tears that bleed and result in hematemesis or melena.

Untreated hyperemesis gravidarum leads to profound dehydration, severe electrolyte imbalance, multiple vitamin deficiencies, hepatic and renal damage, degenerative neuritis of peripheral nerves, scurvylike hemorrhages, encephalopathy, and death. Therapeutic abortion is rarely required to save the life of the mother because the metabolic and nutritional abnormalities can usually be corrected with therapy.

TREATMENT PLAN

Chemotherapeutic

10% dextrose in saline or Ringer's solution with added vitamin B complex, ascorbic acid, and potassium chloride, 3000 ml over first 24 h, followed by sufficient parenteral fluids to maintain urine output of at least 1 L qd; type and volume of fluid based on patient's state of hydration, electrolyte balance, and vitamin requirements

Total parenteral nutrition (TPN) rarely necessary

Antiemetic agents

Prochlorperazine dimaleate (Compazine), 5-10 mg per dose as suppository or IM

Sedative hypnotic agents

Amobarbital sodium (Amytal Sodium), 0.4-0.6 g q6-8h for 2-3 d

Supportive

Complete bed rest

Nothing by mouth for first 2 or 3 days

Progressive diet of dry foods high in carbohydrates, such as crackers, dry toast, and cereal, every 2 hours (five or six times a day); fluids such as 30 ml of hot tea, crushed ice, or carbonated beverages about 1 hour after each dry feeding; meat and vegetables given only when there is no recurrence of nausea

Monitoring of vital signs every 4 hours

Psychiatric consultation and therapy if indicated

ASSESSMENT: AREAS OF CONCERN

Subjective

Nausea, may be severe and often worse in morning; epigastric pain; hiccoughs; thirst; disorientation; heartburn; headache; tiredness; depression; apprehension; confusion

Emesis

Undigested food, mucus, and bile

Body weight

Decreased by as much as 10 to 22 pounds

Skin

Dry; flushed; warm; decreased turgor

Mucous membrane

Dry; coated tongue

Urine

Scanty; may be less than 1000 ml/day; high specific gravity; color amber or darker

Temperature

Elevated

Heart rate

Increased

Electrocardiogram

With severe potassium deficit, prolonged PR and QT intervals and inverted T waves

NURSING DIAGNOSES and NURSING INTERVENTIONS

Nursing Diagnosis	Nursing Intervention
Fluid volume deficit	Administer parenteral fluids at times ordered. Monitor intake and output. Use cooling measures including keeping room cool and eliminating excessive clothing and bed covers. Increase fluid intake as ordered; avoiding fluids high in fat content. Weigh patient daily at same time, on same scale, and with same clothing.
Nutrition, alteration in: less than body requirements	Administer total parenteral nutrition (TPN) as ordered through Hickman or Broviac central catheter or as dilute solution through peripheral line. Give oral hygiene every 2 hours and after meals during waking hours. Serve foods as ordered, preferably those patient desires; present foods attractively and serve at proper temperature. Reduce noxious stimuli including room deodorizers, cleaning solutions, colognes, perfumes, mouthwash solutions, and certain foods. Maintain well-ventilated room. Do not have emesis basin visible during meals. Increase solid foods and fluids as tolerated. Remove meal tray from room as soon as patient has finished eating.
Social isolation	Encourage visitors. If possible, have same nurse care for patient on each night shift to provide continuity and consistency of care. Encourage verbalization of feelings. Identify and assist with diversional activities.

Patient Education

1. Ensure that the patient understands the importance of a well-balanced diet with adequate fluid intake.
2. Explain symptoms of recurrence or any other complications to report to a health care provider.
3. Explain that nausea nearly always disappears by the fourth month of pregnancy.
4. Discuss prescribed medications, including dosage, frequency, purpose, and side effects.
5. Explain that elective termination of pregnancy can be discussed with a health care provider if the patient desires.
6. Reinforce the health care provider's explanation of the effect of the condition on the fetus and emphasize that the prognosis is excellent for both mother and baby.

EVALUATION

Patient Outcome	Data Indicating That Outcome is Reached
Symptoms are resolved.	There is no nausea or vomiting. Patient says she has no subjective symptoms. Patient takes prescribed medications as ordered.
Fluid and electrolytes are within normal range.	Skin turgor is normal. Urine output is more than 1000 ml/day. Fluid intake is between 2000 and 3000 ml/day.
Dietary intake is adequate.	Patient consumes well-balanced meals. Patient has regained lost body weight.
Patient takes part in adaptive social interactions.	Patient verbalizes concerns to significant others and receives emotional support from them.

PREGNANCY-INDUCED HYPERTENSION

Pregnancy-induced hypertension (PIH) is a progressive disease characterized by edema, hypertension, and proteinuria and seen in the last half of pregnancy. If untreated, it can result in eclampsia with generalized convulsions and death.

PIH is also known by other names such as acute hypertension of pregnancy, toxemia, preeclampsia-eclampsia, and EPH (edema, proteinuria, and hypertension).

Hypertension complicates 0.5% to 10% of pregnancies in the United States. It most commonly occurs in primiparas, especially teenagers and women in their late thirties and early forties. Conditions that predispose women to PIH include hydatidiform mole, hydramnios, multiple fetuses, hypertension, cardiovascular disease, chronic renal disease, and diabetes mellitus. About one third of women who have PIH during a pregnancy will have hypertension in subsequent pregnancies. The disease has a familial tendency; daughters of women who had PIH in their first pregnancies have twice the risk of PIH in their own first pregnancies. The incidence of PIH is also higher in women of lower socioeconomic status.

The maternal mortality from PIH in the United States is less than 5%, although in some countries it is as high as 17%. The principal causes of maternal death are heart failure, cerebral hemorrhage, and liver necrosis. Less frequent causes are sepsis, adrenocortical necrosis, and vascular collapse. Perinatal mortality (stillbirths and neonatal deaths) is between 20% and 25% and results from uteroplacental insufficiency, intrauterine anoxia, prematurity, and infection. The objective of care is early identification of high-risk patients to prevent disease progression and the complications of advanced disease.[42,44]

Definitions of terms used to describe PIH include the following[42]:

chronic hypertensive disease presence of persistent hypertension, of whatever cause, before pregnancy or before the twentieth week of gestation, or persistent hypertension beyond the forty-second postpartum day.

eclampsia occurrence of one or more convulsions, not attributable to other cerebral conditions such as epilepsy or cerebral hemorrhage, in a patient with preeclampsia.

edema general and excessive accumulation of fluids in the tissues, commonly demonstrated by swelling of the extremities and face.

gestational edema general and excessive accumulation of fluid in the tissues of greater than 1+ pitting edema after 12 hours' rest in bed, or weight gain of 5 pounds or more in 1 week owing to the influence of pregnancy.

gestational hypertension development of hypertension during pregnancy, or within the first 24 hours postpartum, in a previously normotensive woman. No other evidence of preeclampsia or hypertensive vascular disease is present. The blood pressure returns to normotensive levels within 10 days after parturition. Some patients with gestational hypertension may in fact have preeclampsia or hypertensive vascular disease but do not satisfy the criteria for either of these diagnoses.

gestational proteinuria presence of proteinuria, during or under the influence of pregnancy, in the absence of hypertension, edema, renal infection, or known intrinsic renovascular disease.

hypertension systolic pressure of at least 140 mm Hg (or a rise of at least 30 mm Hg) or diastolic pressure of at least 90 mm Hg (or a rise of at least 15 mm Hg). Hypertension may also be determined by a mean arterial pressure of at least 105 mm Hg (or a rise of at least 20 mm Hg). The levels cited must be measured on at least two occasions 6 or more hours apart, and increases should be based on previously known blood pressure levels.

preeclampsia development of hypertension with proteinuria, edema, or both, during pregnancy or owing to a recent pregnancy. It usually occurs after the twentieth week of gestation but may develop before this time in the presence of trophoblastic disease. Preeclampsia is predominantly a disorder of primigravidas.

proteinuria presence of urinary protein in concentrations greater than 0.3 g/L in a 24-hour urine collection, or in concentrations greater than 1 g/L (1+ to 2+ by standard turbidometric methods) in a random urine collection on two or more occasions at least 6 hours apart. The specimens must be clean, voided midstream, or obtained by catheterization.

superimposed preeclampsia or eclampsia development of preeclampsia or eclampsia in a patient with chronic hypertensive vascular or renal disease. When the hypertension antedates the pregnancy, as established by previous blood pressure recordings, the diagnosis is based on a systolic pressure rise of 30 mm Hg, a diastolic pressure rise of 15 mm Hg, and the development of proteinuria or edema or both.

unclassified hypertensive disorders hypertension about which information is insufficient for classification. Unclassified disorders should be a minority of the hypertensive disorders in pregnancy.

PATHOPHYSIOLOGY

The cause of PIH has not been clearly established despite a century of study by hundreds of investigators. One important factor appears to be the greater amount of trophoblastic tissue as is found in pregnancies with multiple fetuses or hydatidiform mole. Another suggestion is that dietary deficiencies may cause PIH, since it is more common in women of lower socioeconomic status who have a lower protein intake and chronic malnutrition.[54] The hypothesis that immunologic mechanisms are responsible for PIH has been offered; effective immunization by a previous pregnancy is lacking in first pregnancies, whereas previous exposure to the trophoblast may provide protection in subsequent pregnancies.[42] The possibility that PIH is dependent on a single recessive gene has been proposed to account for the increased incidence of PIH in first pregnancies of daughters whose mothers had PIH in their first pregnancies.[42,54] A more recent theory is that a decrease in uterine blood flow alters placental function, permitting the trophoblast to produce thromboplastin, which initiates the vascular changes characteristic of PIH. Uterine ischemia is also a characteristic of women with hypertensive cardiac disease, chronic renal disease, and diabetes, disorders associated with an increased incidence of PIH. A mechanism by which an abnormal placenta initiates or aggravates PIH is disseminated intravascular coagulation (DIC), which occurs subsequent to a release of thromboplastin by the ischemic placenta. Another hypothesis is that inhibition of prostaglandin E synthesis decreases uterine blood flow and increases blood pressure owing to the unopposed vasopressor effects of angiotensin II. This potent vasopressor normally increases uterine prostaglandin E production and uterine blood flow. Further studies may establish whether this is a cause of PIH. The pathophysiologic changes that occur in PIH appear more complex as more is learned about the normal regulation of blood pressure, both in pregnant women and non-pregnant persons. Possibly several factors contribute to the pathophysiology of PIH.

Pathophysiologic changes occurring in PIH affect multiple body systems and functions.

Renal changes. Marked edema of the endothelial cells narrows the glomerular capillary lumen. This is caused by the deposition of amorphous material, a degradation product of fibrinogen, beneath the normal basement membrane of the capillaries and by an increase in the size and number of intercapillary cells. Proteinuria is commonly encountered with this glomerular endotheliosis but may also occur without it. Renal function is reduced as demonstrated by inulin, creatinine, and uric acid clearances that are below normal for pregnancy.

Brain changes. Edema, hyperemia, focal anemia, thrombosis, hemorrhage from rupture of cerebral vessels, and infarction have occurred in 60% of eclamptic patients who died within 2 days of the onset of convulsions. Nonspecific electroencephalographic abnormalities can usually be demonstrated after a seizure.

Liver changes. Fibrin thrombi are found in the blood vessels, and hemorrhagic necrosis occurs in the periphery of the liver lobule. Subcapsular hemorrhage may be caused by a coagulation defect and has the potential to rupture, resulting in massive hemorrhage into the peritoneal cavity.

Retinal changes. Retinal edema and constriction of arterioles occur. Hemorrhage and complete retinal detachment are uncommon, and visual function returns when the patient recovers.

Lung changes. Pulmonary edema is a prominent finding, especially in fatal cases. Caution must be exercised when administering parenteral fluids.

Cardiac changes. Cardiac decompensation can occur because of hypovolemia, decreased cardiac return, and tachycardia. Iatrogenic circulatory overload may lead to cardiac failure.

Adrenal changes. Hemorrhage necrosis may occur, especially in patients who die of vascular collapse.

Placental changes. Uteroplacental blood flow is markedly reduced. Infarction of the placenta is the most common finding after delivery and at autopsy.

Hormonal changes. Levels of renin activity, aldosterone, and angiotensinase may be below those in normal pregnancy. Urinary levels of epinephrine and norepinephrine are increased. The angiotensin II level is normally increased during pregnancy but does not cause an elevation in blood pressure because vascular reactivity is decreased. In PIH, however, the increased angiotensin II results in hypertension because the resistance to decreased vascular reactivity is lost.

Blood volume. Hemoconcentration accompanies severe PIH with an abnormal flow of fluid from intravascular spaces into the tissue spaces. Urine excretion decreases as blood volume decreases, and diuresis is not possible until fluid flows back into the bloodstream from the tissue spaces. The retention of fluid and sodium in the tissue spaces leads to peripheral edema, cerebral edema characterized by convulsions, pulmonary edema, and eventual renal or cardiac failure.[54]

Clinical Course

The onset of PIH is usually gradual with a weight gain of more than 1 kg (2.2 pounds) a week. Edema is an early sign that may go unnoticed because it is common in normal pregnancies. A slow rise in blood pressure frequently precedes the development of proteinuria. Generalized vascular constriction causes resistance to blood flow, resulting in hypertension. The classic signs and symptoms of edema, proteinuria, and hypertension progress at an uneven rate if the condition goes untreated. Late in the disease process the patient notes blurring of vision, scotomas (areas of depressed vision within the visual field surrounded by areas of normal vision), or photophobia. Severe headache and epigastric pain caused by swelling of the liver indicate acceleration of the disease process. Eventually eclampsia develops with seizure activity characterized by clonic and tonic convulsions. Cases of eclampsia occur about equally in the antepartum, intrapartum, and postpartum periods. Anxiety and hyperreflexia usually precede the convulsion, which is first manifested as facial twitching. The body then becomes rigid in a muscular contraction with distortion of the face, protrusion of the eyes, flexion of the arms, clenching of the hands, and inversion of the legs. This tonic contraction phase lasts 15 to 20 seconds. The jaws begin to open and close violently, and similar movements of the eyes occur. In rapid succession the muscles of the body alternately contract and relax for about 1 minute. Unless protected the patient may throw herself out of bed and bite her tongue. Blood-tinged foam may drain from the mouth, and respirations cease during the convulsion because of the fixed diaphragm. The patient may appear to have expired, but after a time she takes a long deep inhalation and breathing resumes. The patient then goes into a coma and eventually awakens in a combative state. Some patients have more than one convulsion and arouse to a semiconscious state between them. In rare instances a patient has many repetitive convulsions, lapses into a coma from which she never emerges, and eventually dies.[12]

After a convulsion the respiratory rate may rise to 50 breaths per minute because of hypercarbia. Lactic acidemia and cyanosis may be present. A temperature above 39.5° C (103° F) is associated with a grave prognosis. Urine output decreases or ceases, and proteinuria is present. There is generally massive edema.

When eclampsia occurs during the antepartum or intrapartum period and the patient delivers, a noticeable sign of improvement is increased urinary output. Within 7 days edema and proteinuria disappear, and within 2 weeks the blood pressure usually returns to normal. Antepartum eclampsia often leads to rapid labor, and intrapartum eclampsia causes uterine contractions to increase in frequency and duration, resulting in shortened labor.[42]

Pulmonary edema, cardiac failure, progressive tachycardia, and hypotension are considered to be terminal events. Death may also occur after a convulsion as a result of massive cerebral hemorrhage.

Rarely after a convulsion visual disturbances including temporary blindness occur because of edema of the retina. The problem may persist for a few hours and or even as long as a week, but in most cases vision returns to normal.

Because of prompt medical management, the full clinical course of PIH seldom occurs. The objectives of care are to terminate the pregnancy in an expeditious manner without trauma to the mother or fetus, to deliver an infant with a high Apgar score who subsequently thrives, and to return the mother to a state of health.

DIAGNOSTIC STUDIES

The diagnosis of mild or severe PIH or preeclampsia is based on the presenting signs and symptoms and diagnostic studies. PIH can be differentiated from a chronic hypertensive state predating the pregnancy through various criteria for a differential diagnosis (Table 9-10).

Laboratory studies
  Urine chemistry
    Amount
      Less than 400 ml/24 hours in severe preeclampsia
    Protein
      More than 0.3 g/L/24 hours or more than 1 g/L in two or more random urine samples collected at least 6 hours apart; in severe preeclampsia protein level more than 5 g/24 hours; albumin (measured by dipstick) may be 1+ or 2+ in mild preeclampsia and 3+ or 4+ in severe preeclampsia
    Uric acid
      Less than minimum normal clearance of 10 mg/minute
    Specific gravity
      Above normal of 1.016 to 1.022
    Creatinine
      Above normal of 0.4 to 1.2 mg/dl
  Blood chemistry
    Plasma uric acid
      More than maximum normal concentration of 6 mg/dl

Table 9-10

Comparison of Pregnancy-Induced Hypertension and Essential Hypertension

Factor	Pregnancy-Induced Hypertension	Essential Hypertension
Onset of hypertension	After 20 weeks' gestation with exception of hydatidiform moles	Antedates pregnancy or is discovered before 20 weeks' gestation
Duration of hypertension	Blood pressure returns to normal in most cases within 2 weeks after delivery	Blood pressure may decrease to normal range during second trimester because of reduced peripheral vascular resistance but rise later in pregnancy to prepregnancy levels and remain at that level after delivery
Family history	Usually negative with exception of primigravida daughters of mothers who had preeclampsia with their first pregnancies	Frequently positive
Age	Most common in teenagers and women in their late thirties and early forties	Generally in older women
Parity	Common in primigravidas	Common in multigravidas
Retina	Vasospasm and edema; infrequent retinal detachment; retinal sheen	Constriction and stenosis of retinal arterioles; hemorrhages; exudates; papilledema
Proteinuria	Usually present with progressive decrease and cessation 2 to 6 weeks after delivery	Usually none except with presence of underlying primary renal disease

Hematocrit

Hemoconcentration owing to lack of hypervolemia that occurs in normal pregnancies; hematocrit value may be as high as 45% or 50%

Blood urea nitrogen (BUN)

Above normal of 10 to 20 mg/dl in severe preeclampsia

Platelets

Below 150,000/mm³

Creatinine

Below normal of 0.08 to 2 g/24 hours

Gant "rollover" test[16]

If blood pressure of woman 28 to 32 weeks pregnant increases more than 20 mm Hg when changing from lateral recumbent to supine position, woman may eventually become hypertensive

Auscultation of blood pressure

In mild preeclampsia blood pressure above 140/90 mm Hg or systolic pressure 30 mm Hg and diastolic pressure 15 mm Hg above normal on two occasions at least 6 hours apart; in severe preeclampsia blood pressure above 160/110 mm Hg or systolic pressure 50 mm Hg and diastolic pressure 35 mm Hg above normal

Quantification of edema

1+: Minimal edema of pedal and pretibial areas

2+: Marked edema of lower extremities

3+: Edema of face, hands, fingers, lower abdominal walls, and sacrum

4+: Generalized massive edema with ascites

Ophthalmoscopic examination

Vasospasm; retinal edema; retinal sheen

TREATMENT PLAN

Termination of pregnancy is the only specific treatment for preeclampsia. This may be done by oxytocin induction of labor or by cesarean delivery when the patient is stable. In cases of mild preeclampsia the preference is to control the symptoms through chemotherapeutic agents, if possible until the fetus reaches term. In cases of severe preeclampsia an expeditious delivery by either the vaginal or cesarean method is preferred.

Chemotherapeutic

Mild preeclampsia

Sedative-hypnotic agents

Sodium phenobarbital (Luminal), 30-60 mg po qid or q6h during waking hours for sedation

Severe preeclampsia

Electrolytes

Magnesium sulfate, 20 ml of 50% solution divided equally into two syringes with 5 g in each, as well as 1 ml 2% lidocaine in each syringe, injected deep into upper outer quadrant of both buttocks through 3-inch-long 20-gauge needle; followed by 10 ml of 50% solution (5 g) divided equally into two syringes with 2.5 g in each and 0.5-1 ml of 2% lidocaine in each injected qid deep into upper outer quadrant of both buttocks through 3-inch-long 20-

gauge needle; continuation of this regimen for 24 h after delivery, predicated on presence of patellar reflex ("knee jerk"), urine flow of at least 100 ml in previous 4 h, and respiratory rate of more than 12 breaths/min and preferably not less than 16 breaths/min

Eclampsia
  Anticonvulsants
    Magnesium sulfate, 20 ml of 20% solution (4 g) IV over 3 min or more, immediately followed by regimen described above for severe preeclampsia or by maintenance dose of about 1 g/h through constant infusion pump; monitor serum magnesium levels; 6-8 mg/dl is therapeutic level; patellar reflexes disappear above 10 mg/dl; respirations are depressed above 16 mg/dl; heart stops in diastole above 30 mg/dl[12,42,54]; calcium gluconate, 10 ml of 10% solution over 3 min only if respiratory depression occurs in response to magnesium sulfate
  Sedative-hypnotic agents
    Amobarbital sodium (Amytal), up to 0.25 g IV over 3 min or more for persistent convulsions
  Antihypertensive agents
    Hydralazine (Apresoline), 5 mg IV for diastolic blood pressure above 100 mm Hg; monitor blood pressure q 5 min after each dose, which may be given q 20 min until diastolic blood pressure of 90-100 mm Hg is achieved; then withhold drug until diastolic pressure is 110 mm Hg

Supportive
  Mild preeclampsia
    Bed rest in lateral recumbent position with bathroom privileges
    Balanced diet with salt content less than 6 g/day
    Daily weighing
    Evaluation of fetal maturity, pelvic measurements, and favorability of cervix
    Daily intake and output measurement
  Severe preeclampsia
    Absolute bed rest in quiet environment
    Intake and output measurement every 8 hours
    Continuous electronic fetal monitoring in some cases
  Eclampsia
    Constant observation
    Absolute quiet in darkened room
    Intake and output measurement every hour
    Fetal heart rate and rhythm every hour
    Seizure precautions
    Nothing by mouth
    Parenteral fluids—usually D5W at rate of 100 ml/

hour or 5% dextrose in lactated Ringer's solution at rate of 60 to 120 ml/hour

ASSESSMENT: AREAS OF CONCERN

Mild preeclampsia
  Blood pressure
    Above 140/90 mm Hg, or systolic pressure 30 mm Hg and diastolic pressure 15 mm Hg above normal on two occasions at least 6 hours apart
  Pedal and pretibial areas
    Edematous
  Urine
    Albumin 1+ or 2+
  Weight
    Gain of more than 1 kg a week

Severe preeclampsia
  Blood pressure
    Above 160/110 mm Hg, or systolic pressure 50 mm Hg and diastolic pressure 35 mm Hg above normal
  Face, hands, fingers, abdominal wall, and sacrum
    Edematous; massive generalized edema
  Urine
    Albumin 3+ or 4+
  Cerebral changes
    Headache; dizziness; tinnitus; drowsiness; change in respiratory rate; tachycardia; fever; anxiety
  Visual changes
    Diplopia; scotomas; blurring; photophobia; temporary blindness
  Gastrointestinal changes
    Nausea; vomiting; epigastric pain; hematemesis
  Renal changes
    Oliguria (less than 30 ml/hour or 400 ml/24 hours); anuria; hematuria
  Reflex response
    Hyperactive

Eclampsia
  Convulsions
    Stage of invasion
      Facial twitching; eyes fixed; pupils dilated for less than 5 seconds
    Stage of contraction
      Distortion of face; protrusion of bloodshot eyes; flexion of arms; clenching of hands; inversion of eyes lasting 15 to 20 seconds
    Stage of convulsion
      Alternate contraction and relaxation of muscles; blood-tinged foaming at mouth; opening and closing of jaws; purple facies; cessation of res-

pirations; lasts about 1 minute until resumption of breathing with deep inhalation and stertor

Coma

Muscular twitching while unconscious with stertorous respirations and nystagmus

Return to consciousness

Disorientation; amnesia; may be combative; respiratory rate may rise to 50 breaths/minute

Fetal heart rate

Temporary bradycardia below 120 beats/minute

Terminal events

Pulmonary edema; cardiac failure; progressive tachycardia; fever above 39.5° C (103.1° F); oliguria progressing to anuria; hypotension

Progressive signs of magnesium sulfate toxicity

Flushing; thirst; diaphoresis; anxiety; drowsiness; lethargy; slurred speech; ataxia; flaccidity; hypotension; hyporeflexia with disappearance of patellar reflex

NURSING DIAGNOSES and NURSING INTERVENTIONS

Nursing Diagnosis	Nursing Intervention	
	Preeclampsia	Eclampsia
Injury: potential for	Maintain seizure precautions including oral airway or padded tongue blade. Position bed height at lowest height. Pad side rails. Have suction and oxygen ready to use. Have available PIH tray of medications: magnesium sulfate, hydralazine, calcium gluconate, and sodium bicarbonate. Keep call light within reach. Keep patient in quiet room with subdued lighting. Have emergency delivery pack ready.	Remove surrounding furniture if patient is on floor. Support and protect head, turning it to side. Gently restrain limbs. Loosen constrictive clothing. Avoid taking temperature other than axillary. Permit nothing by mouth. Maintain darkened room. Protect patient from extraneous stimuli such as sudden noises, jarring of bed, and bright lights. Avoid moving patient unnecessarily.
Gas exchange, impaired	Withhold magnesium sulfate if patellar reflex is absent and notify physician. Have ventilation available if respirations are depressed. Monitor respiratory rate every 30 minutes for 2 hours after each dose of magnesium sulfate.	Insert oral airway or padded tongue blade. Suction mouth and nose as needed. Give oxygen at 10 to 12 L/minute immediately after convulsion to correct fetal hypoxemia and bradycardia.
Fluid volume deficit	Monitor intake and output every 8 hours. Monitor urine albumin as ordered. Administer 2000 to 3000 ml of fluid per day through oral or intravenous route as ordered. Weigh daily at same time and with same scale and clothing.	Monitor intake and output hourly with indwelling bladder catheter. Report output less than 30 ml/hour. Administer parenteral fluids as ordered. Monitor central venous pressure if ordered.
Tissue perfusion, alteration in	Assess edema; observe sacrum for dependent edema if patient is on bed rest. Monitor fetal heart rate every 8 hours. Assist with biochemical and biophysical fetal assessment procedures. Monitor blood pressure every 15 minutes to 4 hours depending on severity of condition; use same arm in same position and same cuff. Maintain complete bed rest or bed rest with bathroom privileges as ordered, with patient lying in left lateral recumbent position to increase renal function and excretion of excess fluid. Ensure availability of cross-matched blood as ordered for undelivered patient.	Monitor fetal heart rate immediately after convulsion when mother is stable. Assess ankle, knee, and biceps reflex response. Prepare for neonatal resuscitation if delivery is imminent. Request that neonatologist be present for delivery, and notify nursery that infant's mother has received magnesium sulfate.

	Nursing Intervention	
Nursing Diagnosis	Preeclampsia	Eclampsia
Diversional activity, deficit	Encourage patient to work on sedentary hobbies, such as needlework, painting, reading, or handicrafts. Limit visitors as indicated by condition; permit visits by patient's other children to reduce patient's anxiety about their welfare.	
Oral mucous membrane, alteration in		After convulsion observe oral cavity for damage. Administer mouth care as needed.
Fear	Encourage patient to discuss fears regarding self and fetus. Assist to auscultate fetal heart rate to reassure self about fetal viability if this is appropriate. Inform patient about procedure for oxytocin induction or cesarean delivery as indicated by physician.	Reorient patient to environment after convulsion.
Self-concept, disturbance in: body image	Encourage expression of feelings and concerns. Clarify misconceptions regarding cause of PIH.	
Health maintenance, alteration in	Continue with same nursing care until at least 48 hours after delivery or as indicated by physician.	Continue with same nursing care for each convulsion and convert to preeclampsia care when danger of convulsions has passed.

Patient Education

Before delivery

1. Instruct the patient to relate any symptoms of disease progression or signs of labor.
2. Instruct the patient to obtain urine specimens as ordered and to notify the nurse after voiding so urine can be measured.
3. Inform the patient about the need to monitor fluid intake.
4. Emphasize the importance of lying in the lateral recumbent position, especially on the left side.

5. Reinforce the physician's explanation about fetal status and prognosis.

After delivery

1. Instruct the patient about the need to monitor vital signs for at least 48 hours after delivery.
2. Instruct the patient to report any symptoms of disease progression.
3. Teach routine postpartum care for vaginal or cesarean delivery as appropriate.

EVALUATION

Patient Outcome	Data Indicating That Outcome is Reached
Body functioning is normal.	Patient is normotensive. There is no edema or retinal vasospasm. Fluids and electrolytes are in balance.
Laboratory findings are within normal limits.	There is no proteinuria. Uric acid and creatinine in urine and specific gravity of urine are within normal limits. Plasma uric acid, hematocrit, BUN, platelets, and creatinine are within normal limits.
Infant is healthy with no or minimum impairment.	Infant is delivered at or near term. Infant's size is appropriate for gestational age. Five-minute Apgar score is 8 or above. There is no hypoglycemia.

DIABETES MELLITUS IN PREGNANCY

Diabetes mellitus is a metabolic disorder in which the ability to oxidize carbohydrates is diminished or absent because of disturbances in insulin production in the islets of Langerhans in the pancreas.

Fluctuation in insulin requirements is one of the primary problems in the management of pregnant diabetic women. In addition, a diabetogenic effect occurs in normal pregnancies because the increased demands on carbohydrate metabolism cause an increase in insulin requirements. Perinatal morbidity and mortality are higher with diabetes than with uncomplicated gestations.

Before the discovery of insulin, diabetes was rarely encountered as a complication of pregnancy because the majority of women with diabetes mellitus were sterile. Mortality of those who became pregnant was 25%, and fetal loss was about 50%. Since that time both maternal and fetal mortality have markedly decreased with earlier identification of the disease and modern management techniques.

Overt diabetes occurs in about 1 in 300 deliveries, and gestational diabetes occurs in 1% to 2% of pregnant women. Some 28% to 29% of those with gestational diabetes develop frank diabetes within 5 to 6 years.[54]

Priscilla White introduced a classification of diabetes in pregnant women in 1965 and updated it in 1978[52]:

A. Chemical diabetes
B. Maturity onset (age over 20 years), duration under 10 years, no vascular lesions
C_1. Age 10 to 19 years at onset
C_2. 10 to 19 years' duration
D_1. Under age 10 years at onset
D_2. Over 20 years' duration
D_3. Benign retinopathy
D_4. Calcified vessels of legs
D_5. Hypertension
E. No longer sought (1965 classification was "Vascular disease is present as evidenced by calcification of pelvic vessels")
F. Nephropathy
G. Many failures
H. Cardiopathy
R. Proliferating retinopathy
T. Renal transplant

Fetal health is closely correlated with the duration of diabetes and the degree of vascular damage it causes. The perinatal mortality is currently about 1.9% in infants of class A diabetic patients and about 4.9% in infants of insulin-dependent diabetic patients.[26,42]

PATHOPHYSIOLOGY

Diabetes mellitus as a metabolic disorder is presented in detail in Chapter 8. The focus of this section is to describe the effect of diabetes on pregnancy and the effect of pregnancy on diabetes.

A diabetogenic effect occurs in normal pregnancy to meet the carbohydrate needs of the fetus. A pregnant patient's fasting blood glucose level is generally 15 to 20 mg/dl lower than that of a nonpregnant woman. Maternal hypoglycemia can become significant if a pregnant patient fasts for a long time, and for this reason a pregnant patient should not engage in a weight reduction program. In addition, plasma insulin levels fall rapidly in response to a decrease in blood glucose, predisposing a fasting patient to ketosis and undesirable transport of ketone bodies to the developing fetus. Another factor predisposing pregnant patients to hypoglycemia is the increase in glomerular filtration rate and lowering of the renal threshold for glucose, which result in a slight glycosuria. Beginning about the twenty-fourth week of gestation the insulin requirement increases. This is caused by the placental hormones, especially human chorionic somato-mammotropin (HCS), which exerts an anti-insulin effect. The β cells of the islets of Langerhans are usually able to meet the demand except in patients who have gestational diabetes. The requirement for insulin declines precipitously in the immediate postpartum period. These changes in glucose production and utilization are known as the diabetogenic effects of pregnancy.

The major effect of pregnancy on diabetes is the fluctuation in insulin requirements. Glucose tolerance varies with the stage of gestation and in response to infections, vomiting, or other complications. The changes are not entirely predictable during labor, since glucose and insulin requirements are altered by depletion of glycogen reserves. Wide variations in glucose tolerance are noted in the puerperium. Hypoglycemia is the most common because of the process of involution and conversion of blood glucose to lactose in lactation. The propensity toward ketosis is evidenced by a decreased carbon dioxide combining power, and the lowered resistance to acidosis is the result of the elevated basal metabolic rate in pregnancy. Oxygen consumption, which normally rises during pregnancy until term, begins to decrease around the thirty-fourth to thirty-fifth weeks of gestation, giving rise to the hypothesis that the fetus of a diabetic woman matures earlier.

Diabetes has several effects on pregnancy, and their control determines the outcome for both mother and baby. Pregnancy-induced hypertension occurs in at least 25% of diabetic pregnancies, as compared with 7% of all pregnancies. Hydramnios affects some 10% of diabetic pregnancies, an incidence 20 times that observed in nondiabetic mothers. The fetus is vulnerable to maternal acidosis and uteroplacental insufficiency in classes D through T of diabetes, resulting in intrauterine growth retardation and small for gestational age infants. The incidence of still births and neonatal deaths is higher in infants of mothers with severe uteroplacental insufficiency; a rise in intrauterine deaths after 36 weeks' gestation has been noted.

Macrosomia, or excessive size of the infant, is a common finding in class A through C diabetic gestations, with infants frequently weighing more than 4000 g. Infants often show evidence of acidosis at birth, with a high PCO_2 and low pH of arterial cord blood and a profound hypoglycemia at 2 to 4 hours of age. Hyperbilirubinemia and hypocalcemia are common in these infants, as is birth trauma for those who are macrosomic or large for gestational age. The incidence of congenital anomalies, particularly of the skeletal, cardiac, and central nervous systems, is increased. Anomalies are three times as common in infants of insulin-dependent diabetics with vascular disease as in infants of diabetic mothers without vascular complications.

DIAGNOSTIC STUDIES

Screening blood glucose level 1 hour after 50 g glucose load[7]

Plasma glucose less than 135 mg/dl indicates less than 1% probability of diabetes; plasma glucose more than 182 mg/dl indicates more than 95% probability of diabetes; plasma glucose between 135 and 185 mg/dl indicates need for further testing such as glucose tolerance test

Glucose tolerance test (GTT)[44,54]

Criteria for abnormal test are met if any two of the following values are equaled or exceeded:
Fasting blood glucose of 90 mg/dl
At 1 hour 165 mg/dl
At 2 hours 145 mg/dl
At 3 hours 125 mg/dl
After 100 g glucose load these values should be increased by 15% if plasma or serum is used rather than whole blood

Urine acetone and protein

Trace to 1+ glucose acceptable by midpregnancy; physician should be notified if value is 3+ or 4+

Urine cultures

Midstream clean-catch specimen should be obtained at first antenatal visit, at 32 to 34 weeks' gestation, and whenever there are symptoms of urinary tract infection

Hemoglobin A_{1c}

May indicate degree of control as fraction of adult hemoglobin combines with glucose; assessment made no later than 13 weeks' gestation; 20% chance of anomalies if values are above 8.5[34]

Fetal surveillance

Ultrasonography
Should be done at about 20 weeks' gestation and again at 26 to 28 weeks as indicated to assess biparietal diameter, number of fetuses, placental location, gross malformations, and fetal size
Nonstress testing (NST)
Done weekly beginning at about 30 to 36 weeks' gestation as indicated by maternal condition; perform contraction stress test if NST is not reactive
Daily fetal movement count
Periodic sampling by patient beginning about 36 weeks' gestation for 1 hour daily after a meal; physician to be notified of substantial decrease
Fetal lung profile
Determination from amniotic fluid initiated after 36 weeks' gestation to assess maturity

TREATMENT PLAN

Chemotherapeutic

Oral hypoglycemic agents not used in pregnancy because they cross the placenta
Insulin
Dosage increased for insulin-dependent diabetic beginning in second trimester and reaching peak at delivery; NPH and lente insulins usually given until patient becomes more labile, at which time preference is to use short-acting insulin; during intrapartum period insulin can be added to D5W, usually in ratio of 1 unit of insulin to 3 g of glucose, titrated according to blood glucose levels; in postpartum period, dosage regulated based on frequent glucose monitoring until long-acting insulin can be safely prescribed

Supportive

Diet—35 cal/kg ideal body weight/day, with daily distribution of 250 g as carbohydrate, 1.3 g/kg as protein, and remainder as fat, half of which is unsaturated, distributed in three meals and three snacks at midmorning, midafternoon, and bedtime[43,44]
Maternal blood glucose control—Chemstrip or dextrose testing performed in hospital or at home; fasting blood glucose level below 90 mg/dl blood; 1 hour after meals blood glucose should be less than 165 mg/dl blood; testing used in conjunction with adjustment of insulin dosage to maintain euglycemia, which will lower incidence of fetal macrosomia and neonatal hypoglycemia
Bed rest—preferably in lateral recumbent position; helps control edema and incipient preeclampsia in patients with signs of pregnancy-induced hypertension; favorably influences uteroplacental circulation and diminishes myometrial tone

ASSESSMENT: AREAS OF CONCERN

Diabetic ketoacidosis

Thirst; abdominal pain; increased urination; constipation; nausea; anorexia; vomiting; hot, dry, flushed skin; drowsiness; weakness; lethargy; air hunger; headache; fruity breath odor; confusion; glucose and acetone in urine; blood glucose greater than 200 to 250 mg/dl

Hypoglycemia

Nausea; hunger; sweating; dizziness; yawning; blurred or double vision; shallow respirations; nervousness

NURSING DIAGNOSES and NURSING INTERVENTIONS

Nursing Diagnosis	Nursing Intervention
Tissue perfusion, alteration in	Give 10 g quick-acting carbohydrate such as 120 ml orange juice or apple juice, 90 ml nondietetic cola, or 2 teaspoons honey for hypoglycemia or insulin reaction.
	For symptoms of ketoacidosis administer insulin as ordered and parenteral fluids as indicated.
	Monitor blood glucose.
	Monitor maternal cardiac rate and rhythm and fetal heart rate.
	Assess level of consciousness and report alterations to physician.
	Measure intake and output.
	Maintain head of bed at 30-degree elevation.
	Administer oral hygiene as indicated.
	Monitor total parenteral nutrition and blood pressure every 1 to 4 hours as indicated by condition.
Noncompliance	Be aware that noncompliance may be related to anxiety or lack of understanding about condition, fetal outcome, or negative side effects of prescribed treatment. Encourage patient to relate concerns about diagnosis and effects on fetus.
	Correct any misconceptions and give appropriate information.
	Involve patient in glucose monitoring and in administration of insulin if appropriate.

For other aspects of care see discussion of diabetes mellitus in Chapter 8.

Patient Education

1. Explain the signs and symptoms of acidosis and hypoglycemia.
2. Have the patient and family demonstrate blood glucose monitoring and administration of insulin as prescribed.
3. Explain the importance of avoiding urinary tract and other infections.
4. Explain the importance of avoiding stress and scheduling rest periods.
5. Explain any fetal evaluation studies that will be done, as well as outcome as appropriate.
6. Emphasize the importance of reporting any untoward signs to a physician.

EVALUATION

Patient Outcome	Data Indicating That Outcome is Reached
Body functioning is normal.	Patient is euglycemic. Laboratory values are within normal limits.
Body hydration is normal.	Intake and output are balanced and insensible water loss takes place through respirations, perspiration, and stools. Skin turgor is good.
Neonatal status is normal.	Size of term infant is appropriate for gestational age with little or no macrosomia. Infant does not have hypoglycemia, respiratory distress, evidence of birth trauma such as fractured

Patient Outcome	Data Indicating That Outcome is Reached
	clavicle or brachial palsy, hyperbilirubinemia, or polycythemia.
Patient complies with prescribed regimen.	Patient correctly describes condition and prescribed treatment. Patient adheres to medication administration schedule. Patient monitors blood glucose regularly. Patient keeps outpatient appointments. Patient follows prescribed diet.

PLACENTA PREVIA AND ABRUPTIO PLACENTAE

Placenta previa is a condition in which the placenta is implanted abnormally over the internal cervical os. Abruptio placentae is the premature separation of the placenta before delivery of the fetus.

Bleeding that occurs in the third trimester of pregnancy may be due to cervical polyps or lesions, invasive carcinoma of the cervix, or rupture of the uterus, but the most common source of significant bleeding in late pregnancy is the placental site, as in placenta previa and abruptio placentae.

Placenta previa occurs in approximately 1 in 200 deliveries and is more common in multiparas. The four degrees of placenta previa are total, partial, marginal, and low lying. In total placenta previa the internal os is covered completely by the placenta. In partial placenta previa the internal os is partially covered by the placenta. In marginal placenta previa the edge of the placenta is at the margin of the internal os. In low-lying placenta previa the placenta can be palpated by the examiner's finger through the cervix. The degree of placenta previa is based somewhat on cervical dilation; a low-lying placenta at 2 cm dilation may become a partial placenta previa at 8 cm.

Abruptio placentae or premature separation of the placenta occurs after 20 weeks' gestation in about 1% of deliveries. The detachment may be partial or complete and may cause overt or concealed hemorrhage.

PATHOPHYSIOLOGY

The cause of placenta previa is unknown. It is seen more frequently in multiparas, in women who have had a previous low cesarean section, and in women carrying multiple fetuses as the large placenta spreads over a large area of the uterus. It is characterized by painless bleeding, a soft and relaxed uterus, and bright red blood. Some 25% of those with placenta previa experience an initial bleeding episode before the thirtieth week of gestation, and more than 50% have initial bleeding between the thirty-fourth and fortieth weeks of gestation.[12]

Abruptio placentae can be caused by trauma, a short

umbilical cord, occlusion of the inferior vena cava, pregnancy-induced or chronic hypertension, a uterine anomaly or tumor, or sudden decompression of the uterus as occurs following delivery of the first twin. It is characterized by extreme uterine tenderness, general or localized pain, progressive uterine rigidity, and signs of shock. The blood flows beneath the placenta and may separate the membranes from the uterine wall, resulting in vaginal bleeding. If the blood cannot escape readily, it may rupture into the amniotic sac or extravasate through the muscle fibers of the myometrium. Severe extravasation of blood gives the uterus a blue or purple appearance and reduces its contractility, eventually rendering it rigid and boardlike (Couvelaire uterus). Retroplacental bleeding can damage the myometrium, releasing large quantities of thromboplastin into the circulation, which results in disseminated intravascular coagulation (DIC).

During a bleeding episode the fetus is initially hyperactive and then demonstrates late deceleration owing to uteroplacental insufficiency and subsequent bradycardia.

DIAGNOSTIC STUDIES

Ultrasonography
Visualization of placenta over internal cervical os; may show sonolucent retroplacental area in occult abruption

Speculum examination
Visualization of placenta or bleeding through examination of cervix

TREATMENT PLAN

Surgical
Cesarean section for fetal distress or to control hemorrhage

Chemotherapeutic
Ritodrine or other tocolytic agents may be given for

placenta previa in normotensive patient when vaginal bleeding is minimal and there is evidence of preterm labor; see p. 1022 for chemotherapeutic treatment plan of preterm labor

Supportive

Infusion of 5% dextrose in lactated Ringer's solution
Typing and cross match for 2 to 4 units of fresh whole blood

Complete blood count and coagulation profile including platelets, fibrinogen, prothrombin time (PT), partial thromboplastin time (PTT), and fibrin split products; repeat every 2 hours and as needed
Continuous monitoring of fetal heart rate and uterine activity
For suspected abruption, periodic measurement of height of uterus fundus

ASSESSMENT: AREAS OF CONCERN

Area of Concern	Placenta Previa	Abruptio Placentae
Comfort	Absence of pain	Extreme uterine tenderness with general or localized pain that progressively becomes more severe; low back pain
Bleeding	Frank red blood	Vaginal bleeding may be present; absent if hemorrhage is concealed
Uterus	Soft and relaxed	Sudden enlargement; may be asymmetric; progressive decrease in relaxation between contractions progressing to boardlike rigidity; fundus may rise in abdomen
Vital signs	Hypotension and tachycardia progressing to signs of hemorrhagic shock	Hypotension and tachycardia progressing to signs of hemorrhagic shock
Fetus	Initial hyperactivity; late deceleration; bradycardia	Initial hyperactivity; late deceleration; bradycardia

NURSING DIAGNOSES and NURSING INTERVENTIONS

Nursing Diagnosis	Nursing Intervention
Tissue perfusion, alteration in	Maintain bed rest. Do not perform vaginal or rectal examinations or stimulate with enemas. Monitor uterine activity. Check blood pressure, pulse, and fetal heart rate every 5 to 15 minutes as indicated by condition. Perform tilt test as necessary.
Fluid volume deficit	Initiate and maintain parenteral fluids as ordered. Maintain intravenous site to ensure its patency at all times. Monitor intake and output. Administer transfusions or volume expanders as ordered. Report saturation of more than one perineal pad every 30 minutes or less. Weigh pads and linen to estimate blood loss as indicated.
Gas exchange, impaired	Monitor fetal heart rate. Administer oxygen to mother at 8 to 12 L/minute. Report signs of fetal distress to physician.

Patient Education

Since patients at term with placenta previa or abruptio placentae are delivered, only a patient who is in the early third trimester and whose bleeding from a placenta previa has stopped may go home.

1. Ensure that the patient lives or can stay within 20 minutes of a hospital in case bleeding recurs.
2. Ensure that the patient has a telephone in working order at home.
3. Ensure that someone will be at home with the pa-

tient at all times and that reliable transportation is immediately available.

4. Instruct the patient to come to the hospital immediately if bleeding recurs.

5. Explain the importance of adequate nutrition and cessation of smoking to avoid placing the fetus at risk for intrauterine growth retardation.

6. Explain the importance of avoiding intercourse, douching, and straining at stool (stool softeners may be prescribed).

7. Explain that the patient must avoid heavy lifting (including lifting children), housework, strenuous activities, or preparation of breasts for breast feeding, since these activities could stimulate contractions and precipitate bleeding.[23]

EVALUATION

Patient Outcome	Data Indicating That Outcome is Reached
There is no maternal hemorrhagic shock.	Vital signs are within normal limits. Bleeding has ceased in patient with placenta previa. Patient with abruptio placentae is delivered of viable fetus and shows no signs of disseminated intravascular coagulation.
Newborn is healthy.	Infant is appropriate for gestational age with 5-minute Apgar score of 8 or above.

PRETERM LABOR

Preterm labor is the onset of labor after the beginning of fetal viability at 20 weeks' gestation and before the end of the thirty-seventh week of pregnancy.

Preterm labor is the most common complication of third-trimester pregnancy and is the major clinical problem in perinatal care. Some 7% of all pregnancies end in preterm labor and delivery, which accounts for 75% of perinatal deaths and 50% of neurologically handicapped infants.[13] The prognosis for fetal survival decreases and morbidity increases with remoteness from term.[9]

Several agents, including sedatives, tranquilizers, hormones, analgesics, and vasodilators, have been used in attempts to arrest preterm labor. Ethanol, in use since the mid-1960s, was for a time one of the most popular drugs. However, it caused side effects ranging from maternal inebriation, nausea, vomiting, headache, and restlessness to severe acidosis, respiratory depression, and aspiration. Infants born within 12 hours after administration of ethanol to the mother had a higher incidence of respiratory distress syndrome and low 1-minute Apgar scores. Its use has been virtually discontinued because other tocolytic agents with fewer side effects have been developed.

PATHOPHYSIOLOGY

Although the exact cause of preterm labor is unknown, the following conditions have been theorized to predispose to the onset of labor before term:

1. Spontaneous rupture of membranes (SROM); the cause of this is usually unknown, but bacterial contamination may play an important role

2. Incompetent cervix, an intrinsic weakness in the cervix that causes premature dilation

3. Uterine anomalies, including bicornuate or diminutive uterus

4. Overdistended uterus, which may occur with multiple gestation or hydramnios

5. Fetal abnormalities, including adrenal hyperplasia, Potter's syndrome (renal agenesis), pulmonary hypoplasia, characteristic facies (such as low-set ears, small chin, and downward turning of tip of nose), and fetal infection (such as rubella or toxoplasmosis)

6. Placental abnormalities, including stasis and edema of the placenta, infarction, hematoma, fibrosis, abruptio placentae, and placenta previa

7. Retained intrauterine device

8. Fetal death

9. Previous preterm delivery or late abortion

10. Systemic maternal disease, including hypertensive cardiovascular disease, anemia, hyperthyroidism, and diabetes mellitus

11. Iatrogenic causes, including elective induction of labor and repeat early elective cesarean delivery

Other clinical and social factors are known to be related to the incidence of premature birth. A scoring system to determine the risk of preterm delivery was developed by Dr. Robert Creasy and others at the University of California, San Francisco Medical Center.[11,22] A high score correlates with an increased risk of preterm labor. The scoring system considers both clinical and social factors, including lack of education, single parent, short stature (below 152 cm), prepregnancy weight less than 45.5 kg, previous birth within 1 year, history of pyelonephritis or cone biopsy, uterine anomaly, diethylstilbestrol (DES) exposure, previous preterm delivery, heavy work, long and tiring commute, more than 11 cigarettes per day, bacteriuria, fibroids, engaged presenting part at 32 weeks' gestation, bleeding after the twelfth week, cervical length less than 1 cm, cervical dilation, uterine irritability, placenta previa, hydramnios or oligohydramnios, multiple pregnancy, febrile illness, weight gain less than 3.3 kg at 22 weeks, weight loss in excess of 2.3 kg before 34 weeks, and hypertension. The scoring system is initiated at the first prenatal visit, and the patient is rescreened at 22 to 26 weeks. Patients who develop additional risk factors after that time are rescreened. All patients are informed of early signs and symptoms to report, and high-risk women are scheduled for frequent regular visits to the health care provider.

A program of prevention of preterm labor for patients at risk includes the following[19,22]:

1. One or two rest periods daily in the lateral recumbent position to increase uterine blood flow
2. Avoidance of strenuous activity, including lifting, heavy cleaning, and physical sports
3. Curtailment of employment if it involves strenuous activity
4. Limitation or discontinuation of sexual activity, especially if uterine contractions persist after orgasm
5. Delay in preparing breasts for nursing until after 37 weeks' gestation to avoid stimulating contractions
6. Avoidance of stressful situations

DIAGNOSIS

The diagnosis of preterm labor must be made rapidly so it can be arrested by appropriate management. Characteristically, preterm labor is the onset of uterine contractions after 20 weeks' gestation and before the end of the thirty-seventh week of gestation, with contractions occurring less than 10 minutes apart, progressive cervical changes or cervical dilation of 2 cm, or effacement of 75%. Preterm labor is usually accompanied by subtle symptoms including menstrual-type cramping, low back pain, pelvic pressure, and vaginal discharge. These symptoms should be given attention, but unfortunately they are often ignored by patients and health care providers until labor is so advanced that it cannot be arrested. No special diagnostic studies are done.[11,22]

TREATMENT PLAN

Surgical

Surgical excision of leiomyomas when absolutely necessary

Cerclage of incompetent cervix during early second trimester

Elective and repeat cesarean section for inevitable delivery and to prevent effects of increased intracranial pressure that would occur with vaginal delivery

Chemotherapeutic

Tocolytic agents

Ritodrine (Yutopar), initial dose 50 μg/min, increasing by 50 μg/min q 10 min up to 350 μg/min; if labor persists more than 30 min at maximum dose, infusion is stopped or concurrent administration of magnesium sulfate may be ordered[20]; if labor is arrested, infusion is maintained at lowest possible dose to maintain tocolysis; ritodrine po initiated 30 min before ending infusion and continued at 10 mg q2h for next 24 h (maximum dose 120 mg/d); 10-20 mg po q4-6h continued until term

Magnesium sulfate, 4 g IV of 10% solution over 15-30 min as loading dose, followed by 1-2 g/h IV for 24 h until uterine contractions stop or drug is discontinued

Terbutaline sulfate (Bricanyl, Brethine), isoxsuprine (Vasodilan), and ethyl alcohol (ethanol)

Refer to institutional protocol

Supportive

Bed rest in lateral recumbent position

Monitoring of uterine activity

Cervical examinations at prescribed intervals

ASSESSMENT: AREAS OF CONCERN

Uterine activity

Regular contractions for longer than 1 hour while at rest; low backache; pelvic pressure (may be rhythmic)

Vaginal examination

Vaginal discharge, especially if watery or blood tinged; leakage of amniotic fluid as assessed by fern test and pH; cervical effacement and dilation; fetal position; station of presenting part

NURSING DIAGNOSES and NURSING INTERVENTIONS

Nursing Diagnosis	Nursing Intervention
Tissue perfusion, alteration in	Maintain bed rest, lateral recumbent position. Monitor uterine activity continuously with tocodynamometer, or note frequency, duration, and strength of contractions every 15 minutes or as needed until uterine activity is arrested and then decrease frequency of monitoring from every hour to every 4 hours based on patient's condition. Monitor fetal heart rate concurrently with uterine activity. Administer tocolytic agent via infusion pump or controller as ordered; use "piggyback" method to attach to main intravenous line. Measure intake and output if patient is receiving ritodrine. Monitor maternal side effects of ritodrine including tachycardia, hypotension, arrhythmias, hypokalemia, palpitations, agitation, elevated blood glucose level, dyspnea, nervousness, tremor, nausea, and vomiting. Be aware that persistent maternal tachycardia over 140 beats/minute may be a sign of impending pulmonary edema, especially after delivery in patients treated concomitantly with corticosteroids. Monitor fetus for tachycardia (or bradycardia if mother is hypotensive), and inform nursery staff of delivery so they can monitor infant for hypotension, hypoglycemia, and hypocalcemia. Reexamine cervix after 1 to 2 hours of parenteral administration of tocolytic agent. If there is no cervical dilation and uterine activity is arrested, reexamine cervix every 12 hours. After oral tocolytic therapy is started, reexamine cervix 12 hours after initial dose. Maintain patient on modified bed rest and monitor uterine activity and fetal heart rate on less frequent but regular basis, such as every 4 hours or as needed during waking hours.
Sleep pattern disturbance	Encourage patient to sleep when possible despite frequent monitoring of uterine activity and vital signs.
Self-concept, disturbance in	Encourage patient to discuss what she thinks or how she feels. Answer patient's questions and be alert to nonverbal indication of patient's concern about her condition, progress, and prognosis. Correct misconceptions about cause of preterm labor. Encourage communication with significant other. Provide anticipatory guidance, especially if delivery is inevitable. Assure patient that feelings of ambivalence toward pregnancy are natural.
Diversional activity, deficit	Encourage participation in nontaxing activities such as reading, watching television, and handicrafts. Encourage visitors as permitted by condition; allow visits by patient's children to reduce her anxiety about their welfare.
Powerlessness	Be aware that a very independent patient, such as a career-oriented woman, may have great difficulty in accepting limitations imposed by others. Provide opportunities for patient to make decisions, express feelings, and participate in care.

Patient Education

1. Discuss prescribed medications, including their dosage, purpose, frequency, route, and side effects.
2. Explain the importance of reporting any signs or symptoms of recurrence of preterm labor.
3. Explain the importance of keeping appointments with a health care provider.
4. Explain the need to avoid activities that decrease uterine blood flow, such as heavy lifting and cleaning, strenuous physical sports, and sitting for long periods, as at work or when traveling.
5. Explain the need to avoid activities that stimulate uterine contractions, including orgasm and nipple preparation for breast feeding.
6. Encourage activities that increase uterine blood flow, such as resting in the lateral recumbent position several times a day.
7. Instruct the patient to avoid stressful situations and, if needed, to use the services of other health care professionals such as a public health nurse, social worker, or psychiatrist.

EVALUATION

Patient Outcome	Data Indicating That Outcome is Reached
Preterm labor is arrested.	Uterine contractions stop, and cervical dilation ceases as assessed by vaginal examination.
Patient demonstrates knowledge about preterm labor.	Patient verbalizes understanding of activities that increase uterine blood flow and lists activities to avoid because they stimulate uterine contractions.

Medical Interventions

TOTAL ABDOMINAL HYSTERECTOMY AND BILATERAL SALPINGO-OOPHORECTOMY

Description and Rationale

Surgical removal of the uterus, both fallopian tubes, and the ovaries is most commonly done to treat malignant neoplastic disease of the reproductive tract and chronic endometriosis. Other indications for hysterectomy are an enlarged myoma, adenomyosis, and hydrosalpinx. If possible, a portion of one ovary is left to prevent symptoms of sudden menopause. The patient is under general anesthesia during the procedure.

Contraindication and Cautions

Abdominal hysterectomy is preferred to vaginal hysterectomy when the diagnosis is in question and exploration is needed, when the uterus is excessively large, when an incidental appendectomy is to be done, and when there is a history of severe pelvic inflammatory disease.

Preprocedural Nursing Care

A douche with an antiseptic solution is usually ordered the evening before or the morning of surgery, or both.

ASSESSMENT: AREAS OF CONCERN

Perineum
Vaginal hemorrhage; vaginal discharge other than serosanguineous; vaginal discharge with foul odor

Temperature
Fever

Abdomen
Redness, pain, swelling, or drainage at site of incision

Pelvic area
Congestion as evidenced by fullness, pain, or thrombophlebitis of legs

Urinary output
Retention of urine, with or without overflow; burning, urgency, and frequency of urination; vaginal leakage of urine

Other complications
Paralytic ileus; pneumonia

Mental status
Emotional investment in value of uterus; signs of depression; misconceptions about procedure

NURSING DIAGNOSES and NURSING INTERVENTIONS

Nursing Diagnosis	Nursing Intervention
Tissue perfusion, alteration in	Provide routine measures for postanesthesia recovery.
	Monitor blood pressure, temperature, pulse, and respiration every 4 hours for 24 hours, then four times a day for 2 days or as ordered.
	Avoid placing patient in high Fowler's position and placing pressure under knees.
	Apply antiembolic stockings as ordered.
	Auscultate abdomen for bowel sounds every 6 to 8 hours. Permit nothing by mouth until bowel sounds are active.
	Assist with initial ambulation as needed.
Fluid volume deficit, potential	Administer parenteral fluids as ordered, progressing to 3000 ml of fluid orally daily.
	Monitor intake and output.
Breathing pattern, ineffective	Assist with turning, coughing, and deep breathing every 2 hours or as needed, decreasing frequency as patient increases general activity.
	Auscultate chest for breath sounds four times a day for 2 days and as needed thereafter.
Skin integrity, impairment of: actual	Observe incision for drainage or hemorrhage every 2 to 4 hours, decreasing frequency as indicated.
	Change or reinforce dressing as indicated.
Bowel elimination, alteration in	Progress to high-protein or high-residue diet as ordered.
	Give Harris flush or insert rectal tube for gas as indicated.
	Give stool softeners or mild laxatives as ordered.
Urinary elimination: alteration in patterns	Connect indwelling catheter to drainage bag.
	Promote micturition when catheter is removed.
Self-care deficit	Assist with bed bath, allowing patient to bathe or shower alone when indicated.
	Administer catheter care twice a day or as needed until removed.
Self-concept, disturbance in	Encourage patient's comments and questions about surgery, progress, and prognosis.
	Reinforce correct information and provide factual information to correct any misconceptions.
	Encourage verbalization with significant others.

Patient Education

1. Instruct the patient to avoid coitus or douching for 6 weeks or as indicated by physician.
2. Instruct the patient to ambulate at regular intervals and to avoid sitting for prolonged periods at home or when traveling.
3. Explain incision care and signs of infection to report to the physician, including redness, swelling, pain, or discharge at the incision site, increase in vaginal drainage, or presence of foul odor.
4. Emphasize the need to avoid heavy lifting and vigorous activities for 6 to 8 weeks after surgery.
5. Instruct the patient to maintain regular outpatient gynecologic examinations.
6. If both ovaries have been removed, explain that surgical menopause will occur and that replacement estrogen may be ordered.
7. If both ovaries have been removed, explain that menstruation will no longer occur and that pregnancy is no longer possible.

EVALUATION

Patient Outcome	Data Indicating That Outcome is Reached
Body functioning is normal.	Wound healing is normal. Vaginal drainage is absent. Bowel and bladder elimination is adequate.
Patient resumes activities of daily living.	Patient walks with erect posture. Patient avoids prolonged sitting and heavy work until physician permits them.
There is no infection.	There is no evidence of inflammation, swelling, pain, or discharge at abdominal site, no fever, and no purulent or odoriferous vaginal discharge.
Comfort is achieved.	Patient says she has no lower abdominal, pelvic, or vaginal pain.
Patient demonstrates adaptive responses related to self-concept.	Patient asks appropriate questions. Patient gives correct information related to procedure and prognosis.
Patient makes sexual adjustment.	Patient indicates that she has discussed concerns with partner.

SALPINGECTOMY

Description and Rationale

Salpingectomy is the removal of one or both fallopian tubes. It is performed for ectopic or tubal pregnancy, chronic salpingitis, and hydrosalpinx.

Nursing Care

The care of a patient undergoing salpingectomy is similar to that of a patient with total hysterectomy, with a few exceptions:

1. Anti-Rh globulin should be administered to an Rh-negative woman following a unilateral salpingectomy for tubal pregnancy.
2. The patient should understand the importance of preventing pregnancy for at least 2 months or as indicated by the physician and that reproductive ability is usually diminished, especially if a tubal pregnancy occurred as a result of acute or chronic salpingitis.
3. Her partner should be included in the discussion of feelings of loss and grief, especially if pregnancy was desired.

DILATION AND CURETTAGE

Description and Rationale

Dilation and curettage is the expansion of the cervix and scraping of the uterine endometrium. It is performed for diagnostic or therapeutic purposes, such as the removal of retained products of conception after an incomplete abortion.

ASSESSMENT: AREAS OF CONCERN

Bleeding
Vaginal hemorrhage

Pain
Pelvic and low back pain

Signs of infection
Foul odor of vaginal drainage; fever; hematuria

NURSING DIAGNOSES and NURSING INTERVENTIONS

Nursing Diagnosis	Nursing Intervention
Tissue perfusion, alteration in	Monitor blood pressure, temperature, pulse, and respirations as indicated by condition until patient is stable.
Potential patient problem: susceptibility to infection	Monitor color and amount of urine. Administer perineal care after elimination. Observe amount and type of vaginal drainage.
Comfort, alteration in: pain	Administer analgesics as ordered.

Patient Education

1. Explain that spotting and bleeding may last a week and may be accompanied by cramping.
2. Explain signs and symptoms of infection that should be reported to the physician.
3. Inform the patient that coitus and douching should be avoided for 2 to 3 weeks.

EVALUATION

Patient Outcome	Data Indicating That Outcome is Reached
Vital signs are within normal limits.	Temperature, pulse, respirations, and blood pressure are within normal limits.
There are no signs of infection.	Color and amount of urine are normal. Vaginal drainage decreases in amount and is not purulent.

TUBAL LIGATION

Description and Rationale

Tubal ligation is tying of the fallopian tubes. Usually the procedure includes excision of a portion of the tubes to ensure that their continuity is disrupted. The procedure is done to provide permanent sterilization.

ASSESSMENT: AREAS OF CONCERN

Pain
Abdominal pain

Signs of infection
Inflammation at site of incision; fever

Other complications
Abdominal distention; absence of bowel sounds; body image disturbances

NURSING DIAGNOSES and NURSING INTERVENTIONS

Nursing Diagnosis	Nursing Intervention
Tissue perfusion, alteration in	Monitor blood pressure, temperature, pulse, and respirations as indicated until patient is stable.
Skin integrity, impairment of	Observe site of incision for inflammation. Keep dressing dry; patient should not shower for at least 24 hours.
Bowel elimination, alteration in	Auscultate bowel sounds to confirm peristalsis before giving food or fluids by mouth. Administer stool softeners as indicated. Give Harris flush or insert rectal tube to relieve abdominal distention.
Comfort, alteration in: pain	Administer analgesics as ordered.
Self-concept, disturbance in: body image	Encourage verbalization of feelings and concerns.

Patient Education

1. Explain that sterility is considered permanent and is rarely reversible.
2. Explain that libido will not be diminished and is often increased by removal of fear of pregnancy.
3. Inform the patient that ovarian function will continue because the ovaries are not removed in this procedure.
4. Explain signs and symptoms of wound infection that should be reported to the physician.

EVALUATION

Patient Outcome	Data Indicating That Outcome is Reached
Incision heals normally.	Site of incision shows no signs of inflammation.
Patient has normal body functioning.	Vital signs are within normal limits. Bowel function is normal.
Patient has no disturbance in self-concept.	Patient does not report adverse changes in body image.

References

1. Babson, S., et al.: Diagnosis and management of the fetus and neonate at risk, St. Louis, 1980, The C.V. Mosby Co.
2. Berne, R.M., and Levy, M.N.: Physiology, St. Louis, 1983, The C.V. Mosby Co.
3. Billings, D.M., and Stokes, L.G.: Medical surgical nursing, St. Louis, 1982, The C.V. Mosby Co.
4. Bobak, I.M., and Jensen, M.D.: Essentials of maternity care, St. Louis, 1984, The C.V. Mosby Co.
5. Brunham, R.C.: Therapy for acute pelvic inflammatory disease: a critique of recent treatment trials, Am. J. Obstet. Gynecol. **148**:235, 1984.
6. Carpenito, L.J.: Nursing diagnosis: application to clinical practice, Philadelphia, 1983, J.B. Lippincott Co.
7. Carpenter, M., and Coustan, D.R.: Criteria for screening tests for gestational diabetics, Am. J. Obstet. Gynecol. **144**:768, 1982.
8. Centers for Disease Control: Statistics on abortion; 1981 end of year figures, Los Angeles Times, July 7, 1984.
9. Check, W.A.: FDA considers a first: approval of drug for inhibiting preterm labor, JAMA **243**:1313, 1980.
10. Chez, R.A., and Yuzpe, A.A.: Postcoital contraception for unprotected intercourse, Contemp. Ob/Gyn. **20**:79, 1982.
11. Creasy, R.K., and Resnick, R., editors: Maternal-fetal medicine, Philadelphia, 1984, W.B. Saunders Co.
12. Danforth, D., editor: Obstetrics and gynecology, Philadelphia, 1983, Harper & Row Publishers, Inc.
13. Fanaroff, A.A., and Martin, R.J.: Behrman's neonatal-perinatal medicine, St. Louis, 1983, The C.V. Mosby Co.
14. Faratian, B., et al.: Premenstrual syndrome: weight, abdominal swelling, perceived body image, Am. J. Obstet. Gynecol. **150**:200, 1984.
15. Fogel, C., Fogel, I., and Woods, N.F.: Health care of women, St. Louis, 1981, The C.V. Mosby Co.
16. Gant, N.F., et al.: A clinical test useful for predicting the development of acute hypertension in pregnancy, Am. J. Obstet. Gynecol. **120**:1, 1974.
17. Gordon, M.: Manual of nursing diagnosis, New York, 1982, McGraw-Hill Book Co.
18. Guzick, D.S., and Rock, J.A.: A comparison of danazol and conservative surgery for the treatment of infertility due to mild or moderate endometriosis, Fertil. Steril. **40**:580, 1983.
19. Harger, J.H., and Caritis, S.N.: What to do if the cervix dilates preterm, Contemp. Ob/Gyn. **20**:201, 1982.
20. Hatjis, C.G., et al.: Addition of magnesium sulfate improves effectiveness of ritodrine in preventing premature delivery, Am. J. Obstet. Gynecol. **150**:142, 1984.
21. Health United States 1979, DHEW Pub. No. 80-1232, Washington, D.C., 1980, U.S. Dept. of Health, Education and Welfare, Public Health Service.
22. Herron, M.A., and Dulock, H.L.: Preterm labor, March of Dimes Staff Development Program Ser. 2, Prog. 5, White Plains, N.Y., 1982.
23. Huff, R.W.: How to handle third trimester bleeding, Contemp. Ob/Gyn. **20**:39, 1982.
24. Jacobs, S.W., and Francone, C.A.: Structure and function in man, Philadelphia, 1982, W.B. Saunders Co.
25. Kim, M.J., McFarland, G.K., and McLane, A.M.: Pocket guide to nursing diagnosis, St. Louis, 1984, The C.V. Mosby Co.
26. Lavin, J.P., et al.: Clinical experience with 107 diabetic pregnancies, Am. J. Obstet. Gynecol. **147**:742, 1983.
27. Loucks, A.: Pelvic inflammatory disease, Nurse Pract. **8**:13, 1983.
28. Malasanos, L., et al.: Health assessment, St. Louis, 1981, The C.V. Mosby Co.
29. Martin, L.: Health care of women, Philadelphia, 1978, J.B. Lippincott Co.
30. Masters, W., and Johnson, V.: Human sexual response, Boston, 1966, Little Brown & Co.
31. McKenzie, C.A., and Edlund, B., editors: Nurs. Clin. North Am. **17**(1), 1982.
32. Merck manual, Rahway, N.J., 1982, Merck Sharp & Dohme Research Laboratories.
33. Methods of midtrimester abortion, Technical Bulletin of the American College of Obstetricians and Gynecologists, No. 56, Washington, D.C., 1979.
34. Miller, E., et al.: Elevated maternal hemoglobin AIC in early pregnancy and major congenital anomalies in infants of diabetic mothers, N. Engl. J. Med. **304**:1331, 1981.
35. Minton, J.P., et al.: Caffeine, nucleotides and breast disease, Surgery **86**:105, 1979.
36. Mishell, D.R., and Brenner, P.F.: Management of common problems in obstetrics and gynecology, Oradell, N.J., 1983, Medical Economics Books.
37. Mosby's medical and nursing dictionary, St. Louis, 1983, The C.V. Mosby Co.
38. Mountcastle, V.B.: Medical physiology, St. Louis, 1980, The C.V. Mosby Co.
39. National Center for Health Statistics: Monthly vital statistics report, Vol. 33, No. 6, Sept. 20, 1984.
40. National Center for Health Statistics: Monthly vital statistics report, Vol. 32, No. 13, Sept. 21, 1984.
41. Newton, N.: Interrelationships between sexual responsiveness, birth and breast feeding. In Zubin, J., and Money, J., editors: Contemporary sexual behavior: critical issues in the 1970's, Baltimore, 1973, Johns Hopkins Press.
42. Pritchard, J.A., and MacDonald, P.C.: Williams' obstetrics, New York, 1980, Appleton-Century-Crofts.
43. Queenan, J.T., editor: Management of high risk pregnancy, Oradell, N.J., 1980, Medical Economics Co.
44. Queenan, J.T.: Protocols for high risk pregnancies, Oradell, N.J., 1982, Medical Economics Books.
45. Robbins, S., and Cotran, R.: Pathologic basis of disease, Philadelphia, 1979, W.B. Saunders Co.
46. Smith, E.D.: Women's health care: a guide for patient education, New York, 1981, Appleton-Century-Crofts.
47. Thompson, J.M., and Bowers, A.C.: Clinical manual of health assessment, St. Louis, 1980, The C.V. Mosby Co.
48. Tilkian, S.M., Conover, M.B., and Tilkian, A.G.: Clinical implications of laboratory tests, St. Louis, 1983, The C.V. Mosby Co.
49. Tucker, S.M.: Fetal monitoring and fetal assessment in high risk pregnancy, St. Louis, 1978, The C.V. Mosby Co.
50. Tucker, S.M., et al.: Patient care standards, St. Louis, 1984, The C.V. Mosby Co.
51. U.S. National Center for Health Statistics: Vital statistics of the United States, Washington, D.C., 1982, U.S. Government Printing Office.
52. White, P.: Classification of obstetric diabetes, Am. J. Obstet. Gynecol. **130**:228, 1978.
53. Willson, J.R., and Carrington, E.R.: Obstetrics and gynecology, St. Louis, 1983, The C.V. Mosby Co.
54. Wilson, M.A.: Menstrual disorders: premenstrual syndrome, dysmenorrhea, amenorrhea, J.O.G.N. **13**(suppl. 2):11s, 1984.
55. Worthington-Roberts, B.S., Vermeersch, J., and Williams, S.R.: Nutrition in pregnancy and lactation, St. Louis, 1981, The C.V. Mosby Co.
56. Wroblewski, S.S.: Toxic shock syndrome, Am. J. Nurs. **81**:82, 1981.

CHAPTER 10

Renal System

Overview

The kidneys are a major part of the urinary system, which also includes the ureters, urinary bladder, and urethra. These latter three components transport and store the urine formed by the kidneys and eventually expel it from the body.

Renal function depends on the normal and interrelated functioning of the cardiovascular, nervous, endocrine, and urinary collecting systems. The cardiovascular system (1) delivers the blood to be filtered, (2) sustains the hydrostatic pressure needed for filtration, and (3) provides specialized capillaries that do the filtering. The nervous system helps regulate blood pressure, thus contributing to the first two functions. The nervous system also controls the process of urination (see Chapter 12) and interacts with the activity of the endocrine system to affect renal function directly through aldosterone and antidiuretic hormone (ADH). The calyces, pelvis, ureters, urinary bladder, and urethra form the urinary collecting system. The urethra provides the exit for urine from the body.

Urine volume varies with food and fluid intake and extrarenal fluid losses through feces, perspiration, and respiration. A diurnal variation in volume that is associated with light-dark periods or sleep-wake patterns occurs.

The kidneys have excretory and nonexcretory functions vital to the regulation of substances essential to the human body.

Excretory functions are (1) excretion of end products of metabolism (urea, creatinine, uric acid, phosphates, sulfates, nitrates, and phenols); (2) excretion of excess normal fluid and electrolyte components (H_2O, Na^+, K^+, HCO_3^-, Cl^-, H^+), thus maintaining the volume and osmolality of the extracellular and intracellular fluids; and (3) excretion of certain drugs and other substances (penicillin and metabolites of hormones).

Nonexcretory functions are (1) secretion of renin, erythropoietin, kallikrein, and prostaglandins; (2) metabolism of carbohydrates, lipids, plasma proteins, and peptide hormones such as insulin and glucagon; and (3) regulation of vitamin D metabolism.

ANATOMY AND PHYSIOLOGY

The kidneys are located in the posterior abdominal cavity in the retroperitoneal area to the right and left of the lumbar spinal column. Each kidney is covered by a tough capsule, surrounded by a cushion of fat, and supported by fascia. Each kidney is partially protected by the ribs. The lower end of each kidney extends below the ribs; the right one is lower than the left (Fig. 10-1). The kidneys move downward during respiration as the diaphragm contracts.

Each kidney has an outer cortex, an inner medulla, and a pelvis, the area in which urine is collected (Fig. 10-2). The fluid filtered from the blood travels through the nephron to reach the large collecting ducts (ducts of Bellini) that form the renal pyramids in the medulla. The ducts empty into a calyx at the papilla. Interspersed be-

Fig. 10-1
Components of the urinary system.

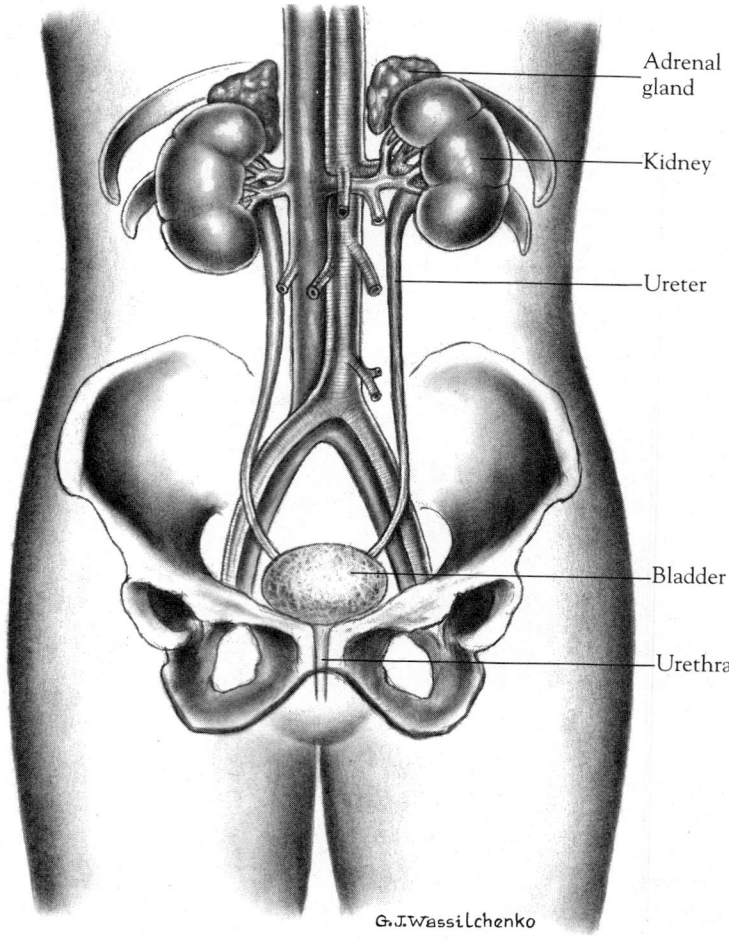

Adrenal
gland

Kidney

Ureter

Bladder

Urethra

G.J.Wassilchenko

Fig. 10-2
Cross section of kidney.

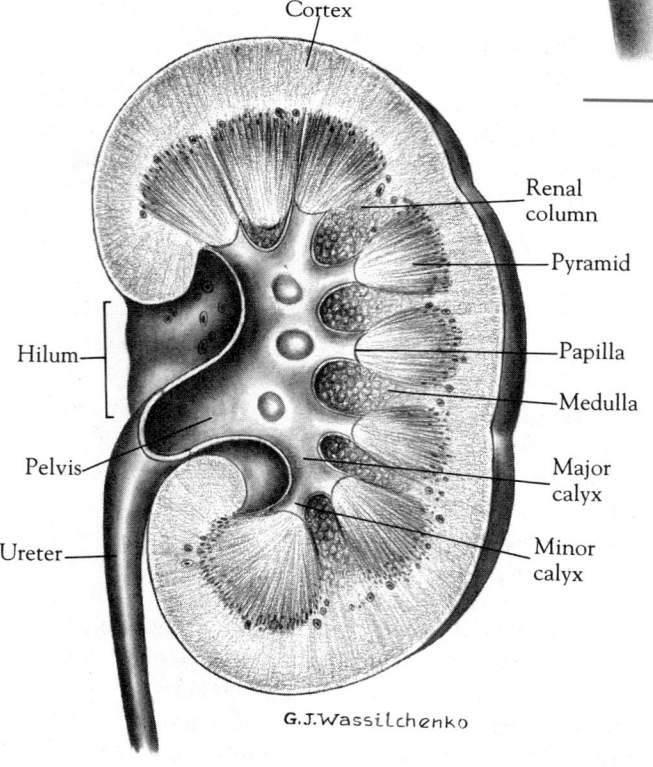

Cortex

Renal
column

Pyramid

Papilla

Medulla

Major
calyx

Minor
calyx

Hilum

Pelvis

Ureter

G.J.Wassilchenko

tween the pyramids is cortical tissue known as the "renal columns" (columns of Bertin). The glomerulus, proximal and distal tubules, and most of the loop of Henle are in the cortex. The deepest part of the loop of Henle and the collecting ducts are in the medulla.

Blood Supply

The renal artery and nerves enter and the renal vein and ureter leave the kidney at the hilum. The blood pumped to the kidneys with each heartbeat equals about one fourth to one fifth of cardiac output. Almost 90% of the blood flows rapidly through the cortex; the rest moves slowly through the medulla. The renal artery branches into interlobar, arcuate, and interlobular arteries (Fig. 10-3). Veins draining the kidneys follow the same pattern as the arteries.

Nephrons are divided into superficial cortical and juxtamedullary nephrons. The efferent arteriole of the su-

Fig. 10-3
Blood supply of nephron.

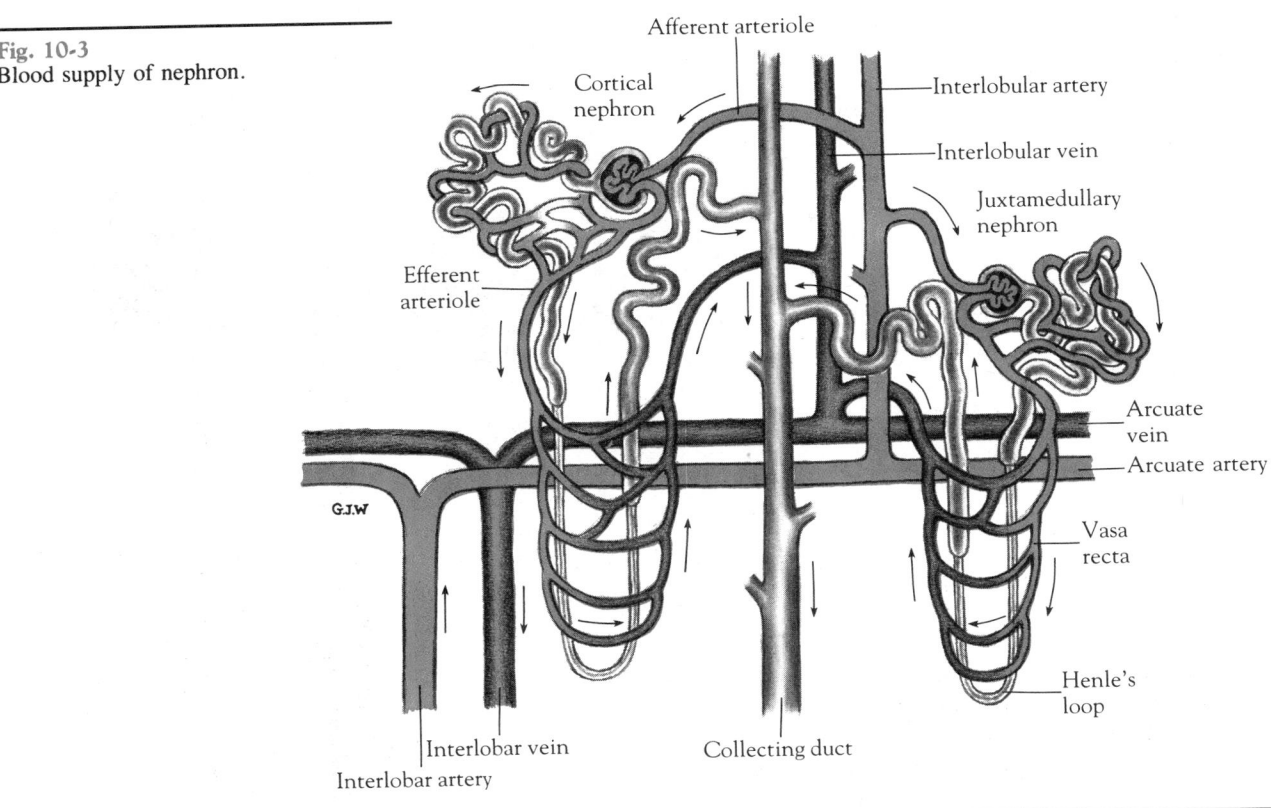

perficial cortical nephron divides to form a peritubular capillary network. The efferent arteriole of the juxtamedullary nephron branches to form a peritubular network and a series of vascular loops, the vasa recta, that form a capillary network around the collecting ducts and ascending limbs of the loop of Henle. Each nephron is perfused by peritubular capillaries arising from the efferent arterioles of many different glomeruli.

Each nephron can control the amount of blood that enters and leaves the glomerulus by means of the afferent and efferent arterioles. Such autoregulation permits the kidney to respond to variations in blood flow and pressure.

Autonomic nerve fibers are found in the kidneys. They are thought to mediate renal vasoconstriction.

The Nephron

The nephron is the functional unit of the kidney (Fig. 10-4). Each nephron is composed of a glomerulus with afferent and efferent arterioles, Bowman's capsule, proximal tubule, loop of Henle, distal tubule, and a collecting duct.

The major functions of the nephron components are as follows: (1) glomerulus: filtration; (2) proximal tubule: reabsorption of Na^+, H^+, H_2O (antidiuretic hormone [ADH] not required), glucose, K^+, amino acids, Cl^-, HCO_3^-, $PO_4^=$, urea secretion of H^+ and foreign substances; (3) Henle's loop: countercurrent flow, concentration of urine; Na^+ is passively and Cl^- is actively reabsorbed; Ca^{++} is reabsorbed; (4) distal tubule: Na^+ reabsorbed (aldosterone increases Na^+ reabsorption); H_2O reabsorbed (ADH required); reabsorption of Cl^-, HCO_3^-, K^+, and urea; secretion of H^+ and K^+; and (5) collecting duct: Na^+, K^+, H^+, and NH_3 may be secreted or reabsorbed; H_2O reabsorbed (ADH required); aldosterone increases Na^+ reabsorption and K^+ secretion.

Each nephron part has a distinctive location, histologic structure, and pattern of vascular network. The glomerulus is discussed in some detail because of its major role in renal disease.

Glomerulus. The glomerulus, a tuft of capillaries invaginated in Bowman's capsule, serves as the filter. The urinary space in Bowman's capsule is continuous with the lumen of the proximal tubule. A parietal (outer) layer of cells and their basement membrane are continuous

Fig. 10-4
Components of nephron.

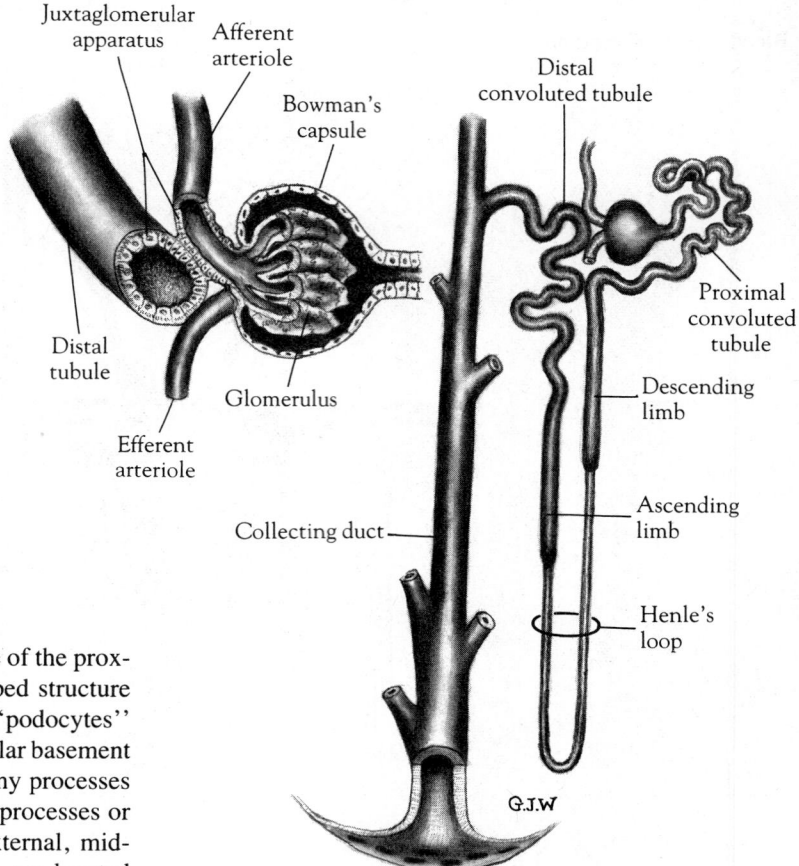

with the epithelium and basement membrane of the proximal tubule. The inner wall of the cup-shaped structure is lined with special epithelial cells called "podocytes" that cover the external surface of the glomerular basement membrane (GBM). The podocytes have many processes that extend from their surfaces to form foot processes or pedicles. The GBM has three layers: the external, middle, and inner. Fenestrated endothelial cells are located on the inner side of the GBM (toward the capillary lumen). Also located on this side of the GBM are the mesangial cells, which are irregularly shaped cells embedded in an amorphous matrix that form a slender branching stalk of specialized connective tissue that supports the capillaries.

Thus the filtration barrier has numerous complex layers. Solutes and water move through the (1) pores in the capillary endothelium, (2) loose matrix of the GBM, and (3) filtration slit membranes of the pedicle layer of the podocytes. Molecules are filtered by size and electrical charge. There are fixed anionic charges in various elements of the capillary barrier. Cationic particles have greater clearance than neutral or anionic particles.[42]

All of these glomerular cells (epithelial, endothelial, and mesangial) can undergo the following pathologic changes: (1) Proliferation of epithelial cells may fuse the foot processes (nephrotic syndrome) or obliterate the space in Bowman's capsule that forms the crescents of cellular-fibrous material found on microscopic examination associated with rapidly progressive glomerulonephritis. (2) Proliferation of endothelial cells may occlude the capillary lumen such as in hemolytic uremic syndrome. (3) Mesangial cell proliferation occurs as part of diabetic nephropathy and membranoproliferative glo-

merulonephritis, causing collapse of the glomerular vessels and damage to the GBM.

The GBM may be damaged by deposits of immune complexes in the mesangial, subendothelial, and subepithelial spaces, as well as by damage to the glomerular cells previously described.

Tubules and collecting ducts.[3] Since the filtering mechanism is nonspecific, provision is made for reabsorption of essential substances and the secretion of excess substances. The tubules and collecting ducts carry out these functions.

The proximal tubule is lined with cells that have interdigitations to increase their area and surfaces covered by microvilli. This segment has high transport capacity and low transepithelial resistance to the movement of molecules being reabsorbed.

The cells of the loop of Henle appear to be simpler, with cells in the thick limb having highly developed active transport properties. This limb can reabsorb sodium against a concentration gradient and is relatively water impermeable. The thin limb appears to lack the transport systems of the thick limb.

The distal tubule passes between the afferent and efferent arterioles of its glomerulus. In the region where the distal tubule lies near the arteriole, specialized cells, the macula densa, are found (see "Juxtaglomerular Apparatus," p.1037). After this segment, the tubular cells become more complex. Cells here can reabsorb sodium ions without an equivalent amount of negatively charged particles. This segment develops both ionic and electrical gradients.

The collecting tubule has two well-defined cell types, light cells and dark cells. The light cells have sparse microvilli. The dark cells have conspicuous microvilli. As the duct descends to the papilla, the number of dark cells decreases until there are none in the papillary region. The significance of this histologic structure is not clear.

Renal interstitium. Cells that form the interstitium lie between the nephrons and their blood supply. More interstitial cells are found in the medulla than in the cortex. The function of these cells is at present unknown.[5]

Urine Formation

Glomerular filtration. Total renal blood flow to both kidneys is approximately 1200 ml/min. Approximately 650 ml of this volume is plasma; of this amount about 125 ml filters through the glomerulus to Bowman's capsule. The renal arteries branch directly off the aorta. Therefore blood perfuses the glomerulus at a high pressure. The filtration force is the result of the pressure gradient between the glomerular capillary and Bowman's space. The rate of glomerular filtration is proportional to filtration pressure. The glomerular filtrate is an isotonic ultrafiltrate of plasma. Large molecules of protein and the cellular elements of the blood are not filtered. The pH of the glomerular filtrate is about 7.4, or equal to that of plasma. The volume of the filtrate decreases with systemic hypotension, localized renal ischemia, urine outflow obstruction, and changes in the filtering surface. Moderate reductions in glomerular filtration also occur with exercise, pain, and dehydration. Extreme reductions in glomerular filtration occur with severe hypotension. Glomerular filtration remains fairly constant even with a marked increase in arterial blood pressure owing to the kidney's autoregulatory mechanisms.

Solute reabsorption and secretion. Solutes and water move by active and passive membrane transport mechanisms.[25] They include (1) simple diffusion—electrochemical potential gradient; (2) convection—hydrostatic or osmotic pressure gradient; and (3) mediated transport—facilitated diffusion, electromechanical potential gradient, and active transport, which requires free energy from metabolism.

"Transport maximum" refers to the amount of a substance that can be reabsorbed per minute. It is a constant value, and when the amount of a substance filtered exceeds this value, the excess is excreted in the urine.

The solutes in the glomerular filtrate are threshold and nonthreshold substances. Urea, sodium, potassium, and others are nonthreshold substances, since the urine always contains at least some of each. Glucose and phosphates are threshold substances, since a certain serum level must be reached before the glomerular filtrate will contain enough that the transport maximum of the substance will be exceeded and the excess will be excreted in the urine.

As the glomerular filtrate moves through the tubules, selective reabsorption of water and solutes and selective secretion of solutes occur. A large volume of isosmotic glomerular filtrate is converted into a small volume of hyperosmotic urine. The composition of the glomerular filtrate triggers appropriate activities in the tubular cells. In the tubules about 87% of the water and electrolytes, all of the glucose, and almost all of the amino acids are reabsorbed in the proximal tubules. The proximal tubule preserves metabolically important components and resists the reabsorption of nitrogenous wastes. It secretes foreign substances. The remaining 13% of the glomerular filtrate passes through the loops of Henle and the distal tubules where variable amounts of the water and electrolytes remaining are absorbed. The exact amounts depend on the needs of the body. The final quantity of urine is about 1 ml/min. The pH of the urine may vary from 4.5 to 8.0, and the osmolality may range from one fourth to four times that of plasma (50 to 1200 mOsm/kg). Urine specific gravity may range from 1.001 to 1.030. The usual range is 1.003 to 1.029 with a normal fluid intake.

Urine concentration and dilution. Obligatory water reabsorption occurs in the proximal tubule since active reabsorption of sodium is accompanied by passive reabsorption of water and anions. Facultative water reabsorption occurs in the distal tubule. Water and solutes are reabsorbed independently, depending on the body's needs. The urine becomes either concentrated, as water without solutes is reabsorbed, or dilute, as solutes without water are reabsorbed. Antidiuretic hormone controls the volume and concentration of the urine by regulating the reabsorption of water.

The medulla increases in hypertonicity with increasing distance from the cortex. The collecting ducts, the long capillary loops (vasa recta), the slower circulation in the medulla, and the impermeability to sodium of the ascending limb of the loop of Henle contribute to the countercurrent mechanism that permits the concentration of urine (Fig. 10-5).

In the juxtamedullary nephrons, the loop of Henle serves as a countercurrent multiplier; that is, it returns

Fig. 10-5

Countercurrent mechanism for concentrating urine. Numbers represent osmotic concentration (in Osm/kg).

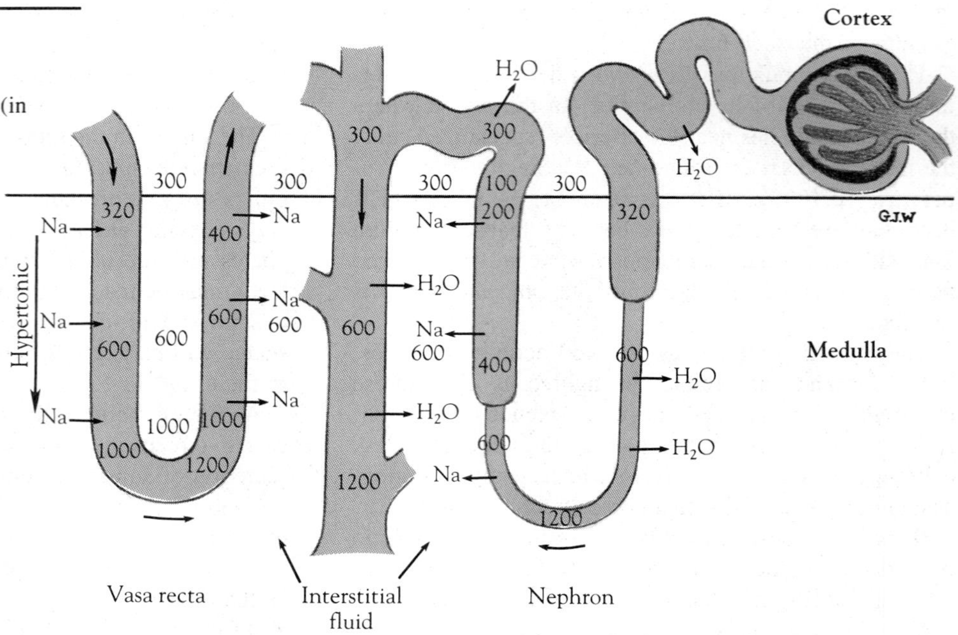

sodium ions to the peritubular fluid of the medulla, creating hypertonic interstitial fluid. The back diffusion of urea (possibly a legacy of an evolutionary stage) adds to the osmolality. The degree of hypertonicity depends on antidiuretic hormone, urine flow rate, and the amount and types of solutes in the tubular fluid in the loops of Henle. The osmotic concentration may become four times that of normal extracellular fluid. The vasa recta loops receive increasing amounts of sodium chloride as the blood flows downward and reaches 1200 mOsm/kg at the bottom of the loop. As the blood flows upward, sodium chloride diffuses into the interstitial fluid, thereby remaining in the medulla. The hypertonic interstitial fluid causes water to be absorbed by osmosis from tubular fluid in the presence of antidiuretic hormone by creating a concentration gradient. Osmoreceptors in the anterior hypothalamus regulate the secretion of antidiuretic hormone, which controls the permeability to water of the distal tubules and collecting ducts. Five hundred milliliters of concentrated urine normally removes the day's solutes. More than 2 L of water would be needed to excrete the same solute load in isotonic urine. Failure of the concentrating mechanism causes polyuria and especially nocturia.

Acid or alkaline urine. The kidneys excrete strong nonvolatile acids and excess alkali. They provide the third line of defense against changes in hydrogen ion concentration. Acid-base buffer systems in all body fluids and the respiratory system respond rapidly, while the

kidneys require several hours to a day or more to readjust the balance. The kidneys excrete excess hydrogen ions and conserve bicarbonate ions. Chloride ions are excreted when bicarbonate ions are needed by the body. Almost all of the bicarbonate in the glomerular filtrate is reabsorbed. Excess bicarbonate ions are excreted when present, causing the urine to become alkaline.

Urine pH may range from 4.6 to 8.3. While the lungs remove the volatile acid, as in the following reaction

$$H^+ + HCO_3^- \rightleftharpoons H_2CO_3 \rightleftharpoons H_2O + CO_2 \uparrow$$

the kidneys excrete strong nonvolatile acids (sulfuric and phosphoric) and strong organic acids (ketone bodies). Hydrogen ions are buffered by bicarbonate ions. The anion base of the acid is balanced electrochemically by sodium ions (Na_2SO_4 and Na_2HPO_4). The tubular cells form bicarbonate ions that combine with the sodium ions of these salts and are reabsorbed. The tubular cell manufactures ammonia, which accepts a hydrogen ion and combines with the sulfate to form $(NH_4)_2SO_4$, which enters the urine. This mechanism permits excretion of hydrogen ions without lowering the urine pH. The Na_2HPO_4 accepts a hydrogen ion to become the acid salt, NaH_2PO_4, which is excreted. The other sodium ion is reabsorbed. Potassium and hydrogen ions compete for excretion in exchange for the reabsorbed sodium ions. The concentration of each ion is important. Acidosis and potassium depletion enhance hydrogen ion secretion. In chronic renal failure, the acid residues of nitrogen metabolism accumulate, and the tubules cannot meet the demand for hydrogen ion secretion. Potassium cannot be excreted since the tubular transport system is overwhelmed and hyperkalemia results.

Juxtaglomerular Apparatus

The juxtaglomerular apparatus is composed of special epithelial cells (the macula densa cells) in the early distal tubule and special myoepithelial cells in the renal afferent arteriole near the glomerulus. These juxtaglomerular cells respond to renal ischemia, low sodium concentration, and activity of the renal sympathetic nerves by secreting renin, which initiates the process that results in the formation of the vasopressor substance, angiotensin II.

Renin is an enzyme that acts on angiotensinogen, a glycoprotein made in the liver, to form angiotensin I. A converting enzyme changes it to angiotensin II. With the loss of an amino acid, angiotensin III is formed. These forms of angiotensin cause (1) peripheral vasoconstriction and (2) increased secretion of aldosterone. The first action elevates blood pressure by increasing peipheral resistance; the second action decreases salt and water loss and therefore increases extracellular fluid volume. Both actions cause an increase in arterial pressure, which relieves renal ischemia. The schema of the renin-angiotensin mechanism is outlined in Fig. 10-6.[22]

The juxtaglomerular apparatus appears to play a role in the autoregulation of renal blood flow and the glomerular filtration rate (GFR) either by responding to the concentration of sodium ions or to the osmolality of the urine in the distal tubule. The conditions of the distal tubule appear to control blood flow in the afferent arteriole.

Other Renal Functions

The kidneys produce erythropoietin, which promotes differentiation, proliferation, and maturation of precursors of red blood cells in the bone marrow. Erythropoietin is produced in response to decreases in oxygen tension and renal perfusion that may arise from anemia, hypoxia, or renal ischemia.

Renal prostaglandins are synthesized in the renal cortex and medulla. They appear to be produced in response to both renal ischemia and vasoconstriction. Observations suggest that they participate in the maintenance of renal vascular resistance and glomerular filtration rate especially when renal hemodynamics are altered.[22] The complex relationships of renal prostaglandins are not yet clearly understood.

The kidneys have a role in the metabolism of vitamin D. Vitamin D_3 is formed in the skin, metabolized in the

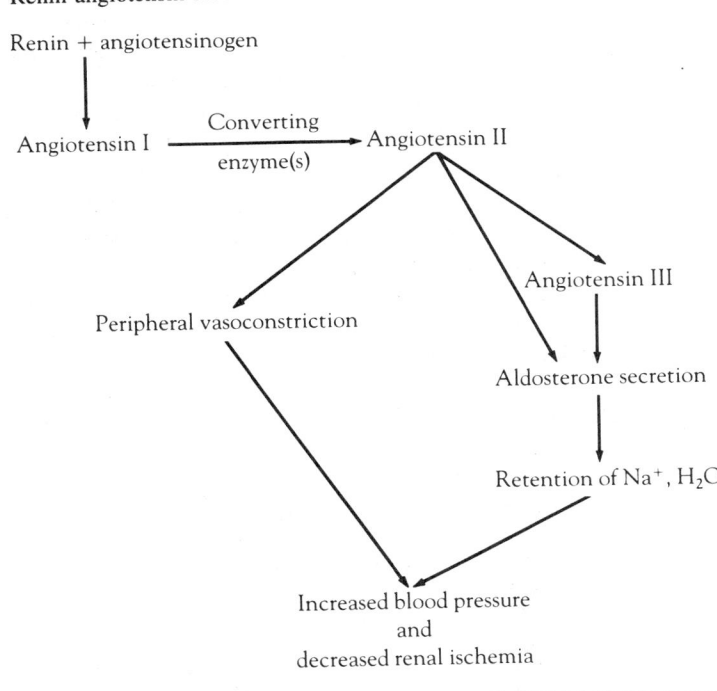

Fig. 10-6
Renin-angiotensin mechanism.

liver to 1,hydroxy D_3, and then metabolized by the kidney to an active form (1,25-dihydroxy D_3 and others). The 1,25-dihydroxy D_3 is produced in response to hypocalcemia or hypophosphatemia. It acts in conjunction with the parathyroid hormone to (1) increase intestinal absorption of calcium and phosphate, (2) mobilize calcium from bones, and (3) increase renal tubular reabsorption of calcium and phosphate. The production of 1,25-dihydroxy D_3 is suppressed by hypercalcemia and hyperphosphatemia. Decreased production of 1,25-dihydroxy D_3 occurs in chronic renal failure and is considered significant in the development of renal osteodystrophy.

Concept of Clearance[22]

Since the kidneys' functions include clearing the plasma of unwanted materials, the concept of renal clearance of a substance is helpful in evaluating renal function. The rate at which a substance is excreted in terms of its plasma concentration is the clearance of that substance.

Clearance of creatinine is used to monitor renal function since it is an endogenous product from muscle creatine phosphate, and its production is relatively independent of protein anabolism and catabolism. The amount of creatinine produced depends on the lean body mass, and this variation is responsible for the differences in serum creatinine levels and creatinine clearances found in men and women. While a small part of the creatinine that appears in the urine is secreted by the tubules, the major portion is filtered by the glomerulus and is not reabsorbed. Creatinine clearance is a practical, clinically useful measure of glomerular filtration rate. Clearances show wide variations between subjects, but are reproducible in the same subject. Serial clearance studies permit the following of a patient's clinical course. Creatinine clearance may be affected by the presence of high glucose concentration, acetone, acetoacetic acid, ascorbic acid, methyldopa, and levodopa in the urine.

Because the total urine for a specified period is required for accurate determinations, patients and staff must understand the procedure: (1) empty the bladder and mark the time; (2) save all urine; (3) void exactly 24 hours later (or the period specified) and save the specimen; (4) measure total volume; and (5) collect serum creatinine once during the 24-hour period.

$$\text{Creatinine clearance (ml/min)} = \frac{\text{Urine creatinine (mg/dl)} \times \text{Urine flow (ml/min)}}{\text{Serum creatinine (mg/dl)}}$$

Inulin clearance is clinically useful as a measure of glomerular filtration rate (GFR). Inulin is freely filtered by the glomerulus and is not reabsorbed or secreted by the tubules so that the amount filtered is the amount excreted. Inulin clearance is used when an exact measure of GFR is required.

$$\text{Inulin clearance (ml/min)} = \frac{\text{Urine inulin (mg/dl)} \times \text{Urine volume (ml/min)}}{\text{Plasma inulin (mg/dl)}} = \text{GFR}$$

Age and Renal Function

Differences in age are associated with differences in renal function that become clinically significant when a young or aged individual has an illness that places excessive demands on the kidneys.

The kidney is immature at birth. Renal blood flow and the glomerular filtration rate of infants are low compared with those of adults. The ability to excrete sodium, potassium, water, and acid loads is limited. The kidneys continue to develop until 1 year of age. Their combined weight continues to increase beyond adolescence (24 g at birth, 140 g at age 6 years, 183 g at age 12 years, and 300 g for adults).[20]

Renal blood flow decreases with age, which is related to a decrease in cardiac output.[11] The loss of renal mass and functioning nephrons also decreases the effective filtering surface and glomerular filtration rate. Creatinine clearance is stable until the fourth decade, when it begins to decrease.[30] Serum creatinine decreases with the decrease in muscle mass associated with aging. Therefore serum creatinine levels may overestimate glomerular filtration rate. To avoid overdoses of drugs in the elderly, creatinine clearance rate is used when dosage of such drugs as digoxin is determined. Also of note is the slower rate of response in elderly patients to acute changes in fluid and electrolyte balances associated with illness. The renin-aldosterone system becomes less responsive with lowered renin levels and an associated reduction in plasma levels of aldosterone. The ability to conserve Na^+ and excrete K^+ is decreased. The decrease in renal response to antidiuretic hormone and in glomerular filtration rate contribute to the inability to conserve water and concentrate the urine.[30] The maintenance of Na^+, K^+, and water balance becomes exceedingly important in elderly patients.

NORMAL FINDINGS

Area of Concern	Normal Adult Findings
General	
Temperature	Normal range
Blood pressure	Normal range
Weight	No marked increase (>2 kg)
Skin	Warm, dry, and normal turgor; no pallor, yellowish color, excoriations, uremic snow, edema, petechiae, ecchymoses, or purpura
Eyes	No periorbital edema, redness, retinal hemorrhages, exudates, or papilledema
Ears	Hearing normal; no tophi in ear cartilages
Mouth	No odor of ammonia; no stomatitis: ulcers, exudate, or bleeding
Neck	Parathyroid glands not palpable
Chest	Normal breath sounds, rate, and rhythm; normal heart sounds, rate, and rhythm

Area of Concern	Normal Adult Findings
Abdomen	Normal bowel sounds; no masses; no tenderness in flank, groin, or costovertebral angle on palpation or percussion; no bruit on auscultation
Neurologic examination	No change in cognitive function, level of consciousness, or behavior; no change in superficial or deep tendon reflexes; no change in muscle action or sensation
Extremities	No edema

NORMAL LABORATORY DATA

Laboratory Test	Normal Adult Values	Variations in Child
Bicarbonate	21-28 mEq/L	
Calcium		
Ionized	4.75-5.2 mg/dl	
Ionized (calculated, blood)	3.9-4.8 mg/dl	
Total	1-30 yr; 8.2-10.5 mg/dl; decreases very slightly with age	Infants, 1 mo: 7-11.5 mg/dl; 1 mo-1 yr: 8.6-11.2 mg/dl; normal range slowly descends
CO_2, total		
Arterial	22-29 mEq/L	
Venous	23-30 mEq/L	Infants, 2 yr: 18-27 mEq/L
Chloride	Children and adults: 97-107 mEq/L	Premature infant: 95-110 mEq/L; full-term infant: 96-106 mEq/L
Cholesterol, total	20 yr and up: 100-210 mg/dl*	Cord blood: <100 mg/dl; 0-1 mo: 45-100 mg/dl
Creatinine	Men: up to 1.2 mg/dl; women: up to 1.1 mg/dl; there are slight differences between the sexes with males higher, since the range relates to the amount of muscle mass present	1-5 yr: 0.3-0.5; mg/dl; 5-10 yr: 0.5-0.8 mg/dl
Glucose, fasting	2 yr-adult: 60-115 mg/dl; normal range increases with age over 50	Premature infants: 40-65 mg/dl; 0-2 yr: 60-110 mg/dl
Glucose tolerance test	Fasting: 60-115 mg/dl; 60 min: <184 mg/dl; 90 min: 100-140 mg/dl; 120 min: <138 mg/dl	
Osmolality	280-300 mosm/kg H_2O	
pH	Venous (children and adults): 7.32-7.43; arterial (children and adults): 7.35-7.45	Newborns with arterialized capillary blood (heel, finger, or big toe) or arterial blood: 7.32-7.49; 2 mo-2 yr (arterialized capillary or arterial blood): 7.34-7.46
Protein (total serum)	6-8 g/dl	6.2-8 g/dl
Albumin	1-31 yr: 3.5-5 g/dl; after age 40, normal range gradually decreases	0-1 yr: 2.9-5.5 g/dl with A/G ratio >1
Phosphorus	2.5-4.5 mg/dl	At birth: 5.6-8 mg/dl; 6-10 days: about 6-10 mg/dl; childhood: approximately 4-7 mg/dl; both low and high ends of the normal range are higher in children than in adults
Potassium (plasma)	3.5-5 mEq/L; add approximately 0.2 to normal ranges if serum is sampled	3.4-4.7 mmol/L

*Sharp inconsistencies are obvious when one studies published normal ranges of serum cholesterol in the United States.

Laboratory Test	Normal Adult Values	Variations in Child
Sodium	135-145 mEq/L	138-145 mmol/L; premature and full-term infants may have levels 5-10 mEq/L lower, but this is controversial
Blood urea nitrogen	1-40 yr: 5-20 mg/dl; gradual, slight increase subsequently occurs	Birth-1 yr: 4-19 mg/dl
Uric acid	Men: 3.4-7 mg/dl or slightly more; women: 2.4-6 mg/dl or slightly more	2-5.5 mg/dl
Hematology		
Hematocrit (%)	Men: 46 ± 3.1; women: 40.9 ± 3	Birth (cord blood): 52 ± 5 1 yr: 39 ± 2 5 yr: 37 ± 3 10 yr: 39 ± 3
Hemoglobin (g/dl)	Men: 15.5 ± 1.1; women: 13.7 ± 1	Birth (cord blood): 17.1 ± 1.8; 1 yr: 11.8 ± 0.5; 5 yr: 12.7 ± 1; 10 yr: 13.2 ± 1.2
Platelet count	150,000-400,000/mm^3	Newborns: 84,000-478,000/mm^3; infants: 200,000-473,000/mm^3
Red blood cell count	Men: 4.6-6.2 million/mm^3; women: 3.9-5.9 million/mm^3	3.8-5.5 million/mm^3
White blood cell count	4500-11,000/mm^3	6200-17,000/mm^3
Coagulation		
Bleeding time	Duke: 1-5 min; Ivy: 2-7 min	
Clotting time (Lee-White)	8-15 min	
Serology		
Antistreptolysin titer	<125 Todd units	<2 yr: <50 Todd units; 2-5 yr: <100 Todd units; 5-19 yr: <166 Todd units
Hepatitis associated antigen (HB$_s$Ag)	Not detected	
Urinalysis		
Calcium (24 hr)	100-250 mg/day (diet dependent; based on average calcium intake of 600-800 mg/24 hr)	
Chloride	110-250 mEq/day	15-40 mmol/day
Creatinine	Men: 1-2 g/24 hr; women: 0.8-1.8 g/24 hr	2-3 yr: 6-22 mg/kg/24 hr; >3 yr: 12-30 mg/kg/24 hr
Glucose	Up to 100 mg/24 hr	
Osmolality	250-900 mOsm/kg	
Protein	30-150 mg/24 hr (method dependent)	Up to 140 mg/m^2 of body surface area is appropriate for small children
pH	4.5-8	5-7
Phosphorus	0.9-1.3 g/day (diet dependent)	
Potassium	26-123 mEq/24 hr (markedly intake dependent)	
Sodium	27-287 mEq/24 hr (diet dependent; output is lower at night)	
Specific gravity	1.003-1.029 (range in SI units)	
Urea nitrogen	6-17 g/day	

Laboratory Test	Normal Adult Values	Variations in Child
Uric acid	250-750 mg/day	
Volume	Men: 800-2000 ml/day; women: 800-1600 ml/day	500-1000 ml/day
Color	Pale to darker yellow	
Clarity	Clear	
Ketones	None	
Red blood count	0-5/high-power field	
White blood count	0-5/high-power field	
Bacteria	None/occasional in voided specimen	
Casts	0-4 hyaline casts/low-power field	
Crystals	Interpreted by physician	
Culture	Negative	
Other		
Creatinine clearance	Men: 85-125 ml/min/1.73 m²; women: 75-115 ml/min/1.73 m²; geriatric: 96.9 ± 2.9 ml/min/1.73 m²	70-140 ml/min/1.73 m²
Renal blood flow	600 ml/min/1.73 m²; geriatric: 300 ml/min/1.73 m²	600 ml/min/1.73 m²
Glomerular rate	120 ml/min/1.73 m²; geriatric: 65.3 ml/min/1.73 m²	120 ml/min/1.73 m²

DIAGNOSTIC STUDIES

Kidney, ureter, bladder examination (KUB)

Plain roentgenogram focused on the KUB area to determine size and location of kidneys and radiopaque stones

Intravenous urogram

Intravenous infusion of contrast medium with serial roentgenograms as the medium is excreted to visualize the kidneys and lower tract

Nursing care:

Avoid dehydration in the elderly, diabetic patient, or person with preexisting renal disease or multiple myeloma; allergic reactions to contrast medium can occur (pruritus, wheezing, dyspnea, and flushed skin)

Renogram and renal scan

Use of radioisotope-labeled chemicals to measure individual kidney function and to trace kidney outlines; useful in identifying vascular problems or space-occupying lesions

Renal arteriogram

Visualization of the renal arteries on a roentgenogram by introducing a radiopaque contrast medium

Nursing care:

Pressure is applied to the injection site; vital signs are monitored and site is observed; serious bleeding may occur; pulses in lower extremities are monitored; bed rest is usually prescribed

Renal ultrasonography

Sound waves travel and return through tissues of varying acoustic impedance; the returning images are turned into an interpretable renal image; noninvasive way to identify dilated collecting system, calculi, cysts, and perirenal collections of blood, pus, lymph, or urine

Conditions, Diseases, and Disorders

ABSCESSES: RENAL AND PERINEPHRIC

A renal abscess is a localized infection found within the cortex of the kidney; a perinephric abscess extends into the fatty tissue around the kidney.

Multiple renal abscesses can occur in a normal or diseased kidney. They can be a complication of subacute bacterial endocarditis and systemic infections.

PATHOPHYSIOLOGY

Renal abscesses may arise from diffuse pyelonephritis or hematogenous transport of bacteria that occur in a systemic infection. Staphylococcal bacteremia, for example, may cause multiple cortical abscesses. Such abscesses may extend into the tissues surrounding the kidney. When infection from the kidney spreads to the fatty and fascial tissues surrounding the kidney, it is known as a "perinephric abscess." Such abscesses are frequently associated with renal calculi or urinary tract obstructions.

DIAGNOSTIC STUDIES

Intravenous urogram
Renal mass and calyceal distortion or renal displacement are shown when radiopaque dye is injected, filtered by the kidneys, and excreted through the urinary tract

TREATMENT PLAN

Surgical
Incision and drainage may be required if the renal abscess is localized; incision and drainage are usually required for perinephric abscesses

Chemotherapeutic
Anti-infective agents
Sulfisoxazole (Gantrisin), po, adults: 1-2 g initially followed by 1 g bid or tid; children: 60-100 mg/kg q8h
Ampicillin (Omnipen), po, patients ≥20 kg: 250-500 mg q6h; patients <20 kg: 50-100 mg/kg/d in equally divided doses q6-8h
Carbenicillin disodium (Geopen), IM, IV, adults: 1-2 g q6h; children: 50-200 mg/kg/d in equally divided doses q4-6h
Gentamicin (Garamycin), IM, IV, adults: 3-5 mg/kg/d q8h; children: 6-7.5 mg/kg/d q8h

Supportive
Bed rest, adequate fluids (2500 to 3000 ml/day), and normal nutrition are important; a normal diet ensures protein, calories, and other nutrients sufficient to meet the needs of the individual's current stage of the life cycle; sterile dressing changes are needed after incision and drainage of abscesses

ASSESSMENT: AREAS OF CONCERN

Signs of infection
Renal abscess
None with solitary abscess; chills and fever; increased white blood count; flank tenderness
Perinephric abscess
Chills and fever; increased white blood count; dull ache in flank; costovertebral angle tenderness on palpation; mass in flank; abdominal pain with guarding

NURSING DIAGNOSES and NURSING INTERVENTIONS

Nursing Diagnosis	Nursing Intervention
Skin integrity, impairment of	Administer antimicrobial agents as ordered by the physician. Monitor temperature and report any changes. Change wound dressing using sterile technique. Observe kind and amount of drainage. Follow isolation precautions if necessary. Explain medications and their purposes.

Nursing Diagnosis	Nursing Intervention
Comfort, alteration in: pain	Administer analgesic drugs as ordered by physician and observe and document response.
Self-care deficit (potential)	Assist as necessary with food and fluid intake, personal hygiene, and rest.

Patient Education

1. Explain the side effects and adverse reactions of chemotherapeutic agents used.
2. Explain care of the incision.
3. Explain the relationship between perinephric abscesses and pyelonephritis, renal calculi, and urinary tract obstruction.

EVALUATION

Patient Outcome	Data Indicating That Outcome is Reached
Infection clears.	Temperature is in the normal range. Patient reports no pain. White blood cell count is normal.
Incision heals.	There is no infection; wound is closed.
Patient demonstrates knowledge of renal or perinephric abscesses.	Patient can describe the nature of renal or perinephric abscess.

RENAL TUBERCULOSIS

Infection caused by Mycobacterium tuberculosis *can occur in the kidneys.*

Renal tuberculosis is much less frequent today than in the past; however, 4135 new cases of extrapulmonary tuberculosis were reported in the United States in 1979. Of these cases 664 were located in the genitourinary system.[37] Prevention is important. About 4% to 9% of persons with active pulmonary tuberculosis develop genitourinary involvement.[10] Contact with persons with active pulmonary tuberculosis should be avoided. Early diagnosis is important. Prophylactic care with isoniazid is ordered for susceptible persons (household members of patients with tuberculosis and persons with positive reactions to the tuberculin skin test).

PATHOPHYSIOLOGY

The tuberculosis organism spreads by the bloodstream from the lungs or gastrointestinal tract. Renal tuberculosis is associated with primary pulmonary infection or occurs during reactivation many years later from infection previously seeded in the kidney. It occurs more frequently in men; the bladder, prostate, epididymis, and testicle may also be involved. An abscess in the cortex may erode into a calyx and spread to the pelvis and downward to the bladder. Early treatment of pulmonary tuberculosis may be reducing the number of patients who develop renal lesions.

DIAGNOSTIC STUDIES

Intravenous urogram

Kidney appears "moth-eaten" when radiopaque dye is filtered through the kidney.

TREATMENT PLAN

Treatment, as for tuberculosis, takes more than 6 months to 2 years (see p. 1518).

Chemotherapeutic
Anti-infective agents

Isoniazid (INH), po or IM, adults: 5 mg/kg/body weight up to 300 mg/d; children: 10-20 mg/kg body weight up to 300-500 mg/d

Rifampin, po, adults: 600 mg/d; children: 10-20 mg/kg/d up to 600 mg/d

Streptomycin, IM, adults: 1 g/d, reduce to 1 g 2-3 times/wk when sputum cultures become negative; children: 20-40 mg/kg/d in divided doses

Supportive

Bed rest is usually prescribed at first; ensure adequate nutrition; observe isolation precautions if sputum or urine is positive for tuberculosis bacilli; proper disposal of urine (flushed down toilet and not bedpan flusher) and other infected material (double-bagged and incinerated) is part of plan of care

ASSESSMENT: AREAS OF CONCERN

General

Fever; weight loss; flank pain; sweating

Urine

Asymptomatic pyuria; tuberculosis organism cultured; hematuria

NURSING DIAGNOSES and NURSING INTERVENTIONS

Nursing Diagnosis	Nursing Intervention
Tissue perfusion, alteration in: renal	Give antimicrobial agents as ordered and observe response. Explain drugs and their purposes. Measure and record intake, output, weight, temperature, pulse, respirations, and blood pressure.
Mobility, impaired physical, and self-care deficit (potential)	Maintain bed rest during acute phase. Implement nursing measures to prevent adverse effects of bed rest. Assist with personal hygiene as needed.

Patient Education

1. Explain the nature of tuberculosis, its cause, spread, and treatment (see p. 1516).

EVALUATION

Patient Outcome	Data Indicating That Outcome is Reached
Infection clears.	Urine culture is negative within 2 months. Temperature is in the normal range.
Renal lesions heal.	Follow-up roentgenograms reveal healing.
Patient complies with long-term drug therapy regimen.	Drugs are taken as directed.
Patient demonstrates knowledge of tuberculosis.	Patient can describe measures to prevent the spread of tuberculosis.

CONGENITAL ANOMALIES

A wide variety of anomalies related to the kidneys can occur. The abnormalities may be in number, volume, form, location, rotation, blood vessels, pelvis, or ureter. These errors in renal development result from failure to develop, abnormal division of the elements, fusion of the elements, or abnormal movement from the pelvis to the lumbar area. These anatomic deviations may range from minor to severe and from easily correctable to incompatible with life. Renal abnormalities are frequently associated with additional anomalies such as low-set ears, imperforate anus, genital anomalies, and abnormalities of the spinal cord and extremities.

Kidney Displacement and Supernumerary Kidneys

Kidney displacement occurs occasionally when the kidneys do not ascend to their normal positions, or one may cross over and cause both kidneys to be on one side. A supernumerary, or extra, kidney, rarely occurs, although duplication of the renal pelvis is common.

PATHOPHYSIOLOGY

The displaced kidneys may be normal except for their abnormal location or rotation. They have increased susceptibility to trauma because they are not protected as well as a kidney in its normal location. Obstruction may occur, as may infection or infarction if the normal blood supply and urinary channel are interrupted. The extra kidney may be small, dysplastic, and infected.

DIAGNOSTIC STUDIES

Intravenous urogram
  Abnormally located or rotated kidney; extra kidney(s) visualized when radiopaque dye filters through the kidney

TREATMENT PLAN

Surgical
  Correction of obstruction to blood supply or urine elimination in displaced kidney and removal of extra kidney(s) may be indicated; function of remaining kidney tissue must be adequate

ASSESSMENT: AREAS OF CONCERN

Renal function
  Asymptomatic; signs of infection or obstruction

NURSING DIAGNOSES and NURSING INTERVENTIONS

Nursing Diagnosis	Nursing Intervention
Potential patient problem: susceptibility to infection	Observe for signs and symptoms of urinary tract infection. Monitor temperature, pulse, and respirations and report any abnormalities.
Skin integrity, impairment of (by surgery)	Prepare for surgery. Explain procedure, diagnostic studies, and postoperative care to be given to patient and family. Prepare the area of skin for incision. Bowel preparation may include enema and nothing by mouth after midnight. *Postoperative care:* Monitor site of incision for drainage and signs of infection. Keep any drainage tubes patent, unkinked, and anchored to avoid inadvertent displacement. Monitor intake (intravenous and oral) and output. Care for urethral catheter. Be alert for and report foul-smelling urine.
Comfort, alteration in: pain	Relieve pain at incision site with analgesics as ordered.
Self-care deficit (potential)	Assist with personal hygiene as needed immediately after surgery.

Patient Education

1. Explain the location of the displaced or extra kidney(s).
2. Explain the signs and symptoms of possible problems (trauma to abdomen, urinary tract infections, or urinary tract obstruction).
3. Explain measures to prevent urinary tract infection: adequate fluid intake (to avoid dehydration), regular emptying of the bladder to avoid overdistention, and good perineal hygiene to prevent the entrance of microorganisms into the urinary tract.
4. Explain postoperative care including care of the incision and self-monitoring skills as needed (intake and output, weight, temperature, and so on).

EVALUATION

Patient Outcome	Data Indicating That Outcome is Reached
Family knows kidney's location.	Family can describe the location of the displaced or extra kidney and its implications.
Incision heals.	No infection is present; wound is closed.
Family knows how to prevent urinary tract infections.	Family can describe measures to prevent urinary tract infections.

Hypoplasia

The hypoplastic kidney is an anomaly that results in a miniature kidney with some functional renal tissue.

PATHOPHYSIOLOGY

The kidneys are small but are normal in structure. They may be dysplastic with malformation of renal tissue. If both kidneys are severely malformed, death occurs during the neonatal period. One kidney usually has poorer function than the other.

DIAGNOSTIC STUDIES

Intravenous urogram
  Small, malformed kidney(s) are seen when radiopaque dye is filtered through the kidneys

TREATMENT PLAN

Surgical
  Elective surgical removal of the dysplastic kidney is usually performed. Careful assessment of the contralateral kidney is essential. If chronic renal failure occurs, renal dialysis or transplantation may be undertaken if technically feasible (see pp. 1085 and 1095).

Chemotherapeutic
  Anti-infective agents (given for infection)
    Parenteral agents (IM or IV)
      Gentamicin (Garamycin), adults: 3-5 mg/kg/d q8h; children: 6-7.5 mg/kg/d q8h
      Cephalosporins: Cefazolin sodium (Ancef), 250-1000 mg q6-8h
      Penicillins
        Sodium ampicillin (Omnipen-N), patients ≥40 kg: 250-500 mg q6h; <40 kg: 25-50 mg/kg/d in equally divided doses q6-8h
      Carbenicillin disodium (Geopen), adults: 1-2 g IM q6h; children: 50-200 mg/kg/d in equally divided doses q4-6h
      Penicillin G potassium (Aqueous penicillin G) Penicillin G sodium, adults: 1-20 million units/d; children: 50,000-250,000 units/kg/d in 4-6 divided doses
    Oral agents
      Sulfonamides: Sulfisoxazole (Gantrisin), 2-4 g initially followed by 1-2 g q4-6h
      Tetracycline (Achromycin), 250-500 mg q6h
      Penicillins
        Amoxicillin (Amoxil), adults and children ≥20 kg: 250-500 mg q8h; <20 kg: 20-40 mg/kg/d in divided doses q8h
        Ampicillin (Omnipen), patients ≥20 kg: 250-500 mg q6h; <20 kg: 50-100 mg/kg/d in equally divided doses
        Penicillin G, adults: 200,000-500,000 units q6-8h; children: 25,000-90,000 units/kg/d in 3-6 divided doses
      Erythromycin (Erythrocin), adults: 25 mg q6h; children: 30-50 mg/kg/d in 4 equally divided doses
      Sulfamethoxazole and trimethoprim (Septra and Bactrim), adults: 2 tab q12h; children: 8 mg/kg trimethoprim and 40 mg/kg sulfamethoxazole/d in 2 divided doses q12h

Electromechanical
  See "Renal Dialysis," p. 1085

ASSESSMENT: AREAS OF CONCERN

Renal function
  May be asymptomatic; bilateral: uremia; unilateral: infection, hypertension, or renal failure

NURSING DIAGNOSES and NURSING INTERVENTIONS

Nursing Diagnosis	Nursing Intervention
Potential patient problem: infection	Observe for signs and symptoms of urinary tract infection. Monitor temperature, pulse, and respirations; report any abnormalities.
Skin integrity, impairment of (if surgery)	Prepare for surgery. Explain procedure, diagnostic studies, and postoperative care to be given to patient and family. Prepare area of skin for incision. Bowel preparation may include enema and nothing by mouth after midnight. *Postoperative care:* Monitor site of incision for drainage and signs of infection. Monitor temperature, pulse, respirations, and blood pressure. Be alert for shock or respiratory complications. Keep any drainage tubes patent, unkinked, and anchored to avoid inadvertent displacement. Monitor intake (intravenous and oral) and output. Care for urethral catheter. Watch for and report foul-smelling urine. Monitor bowel sounds. Patient may take nothing by mouth for 1 to 2 days. Start food and fluid by mouth as ordered and as patient tolerates. Relieve pain at incision site with analgesics as ordered. Implement nursing measures to prevent complications of bed rest.

Patient Education

1. Explain the kidney abnormality.
2. Explain possible problems: urinary tract infection, renal failure, and their signs and symptoms.
3. Explain postoperative care if needed.
4. Explain renal dialysis and transplantation as likely future options.

EVALUATION

Patient Outcome	Data Indicating That Outcome is Reached
Patient and family understand renal abnormality.	Patient and family can describe the renal abnormality and its implications.
Patient and family know how to prevent urinary tract infections.	Family can describe measures to prevent urinary tract infections.

Polycystic Kidney Disease

In polycystic kidney disease the kidney tissue is replaced by grapelike clusters of cysts.

Polycystic kidney disease (PKD) is a genetically transmitted disorder, autosomal dominant in adults. An infant form (autosomal, recessive) occurs; such children rarely live more than a year. The adult form has a similar onset, clinical course, and manifestations within a family.

sion. Cysts may occur anywhere along the nephron. Fluid within the cysts may be yellow, brown, thick, and cloudy. It may contain urine components. Progressive fibrosis of the interstitial tissue occurs. Infection and renal stones often occur because of urinary stasis and compression. Hypertension and renal failure follow the onset of symptoms within 5 to 15 years.[13]

PATHOPHYSIOLOGY

The normal kidney tissue is replaced by grapelike clusters of cysts that destroy the surrounding tissue by compres-

DIAGNOSTIC STUDIES

Flat plate of abdomen

Kidney size is seen on roentgenogram

Intravenous urogram

Renal function and presence of cysts are evaluated when radiopaque dye filters through the kidney and urinary tract

obtained twice a year. Genetic counseling may be suggested for families with polycystic kidney disease. Renal dialysis and transplantation may be indicated when chronic renal failure ensues.

TREATMENT PLAN

No specific treatment is available. Medical goals concentrate on preventing hypertension and infection to preserve renal function. Instrumentation of the urinary tract, which is occasionally followed by a urinary tract infection, should be avoided. If patients do not have symptoms, creatinine clearance and urine cultures should be

ASSESSMENT: AREAS OF CONCERN

Renal function

Intermittent hematuria; infection; hypertension; flank pain (dull or acute) or lateral abdominal pain; palpable kidneys; decrease in renal function tests

NURSING DIAGNOSES and NURSING INTERVENTIONS

Nursing Diagnosis	Nursing Intervention
Tissue perfusion, alteration in: renal	Monitor intake, output, and weight if needed. Monitor blood pressure. Give antihypertensives, if needed as ordered by the physician. Monitor laboratory tests reflective of renal function.
Potential patient problem: susceptibility to infection	Be alert to signs and symptoms of active urinary tract infections. See "Pyelonephritis," p. 1061.
Comfort, alteration in: pain	Analgesics as ordered by physician, rest, and external heat to lumbar area may help.
Family process, alteration in (potential)	Be alert to how the diagnosis of the family member affects others in the family. Help them seek genetic counseling if appropriate.

Patient Education

1. Explain the nature of the kidney abnormality.
2. Explain the need to monitor renal function and blood pressure.
3. Explain measures to prevent urinary tract infection: adequate fluid intake to avoid dehydration, regular emptying of the bladder to avoid overdistention, observation of urine, and good perineal care to prevent entrance of microorganisms into the urinary tract
4. Explain signs and symptoms of urinary tract infections (see "Pyelonephritis," p. 1061).
5. Explain renal dialysis and transplantation as options for the future.

EVALUATION

Patient Outcome	Data Indicating That Outcome is Reached
Early decreases in renal function are recognized.	Urinalysis and blood chemistries are done every 6 months and any change is noted.
Patient and family know how to prevent urinary tract infection.	Patient can describe measures to prevent urinary tract infections.
Infections will be treated promptly.	Patient seeks medical help when signs and symptoms of urinary tract infection occur.
Plans are made for long-term treatment.	Patient describes the anticipated course of the disease and the possible relationship of dialysis and transplantation for the future.
Treatment for hypertension, if present, is followed.	Blood pressure is controlled.

GLOMERULONEPHRITIS

A discussion of glomerulonephritis (GN) is difficult because of the confusion among the older definitions used before renal biopsy was introduced and the newer terms used since. Urizor and Gilboa suggest classifying GN using clinical course (acute, rapidly progressive, and chronic), histopathology (membranoproliferative, for example), and pathogenetic mechanisms (immune complexes and antibodies against kidney antigens).[40]

The kinds of GN include: (1) acute poststreptococcal GN (APSGN) (immune complexes), (2) Goodpasture's syndrome and rapidly progressive GN (antiglomerular basement membrane or anti-GBM antibodies), and (3) membranoproliferative GN. A renal biopsy is necessary to differentiate among the various kinds of GN (see p. 1101). Only APSGN is discussed in this section.

Acute Poststreptococcal Glomerulonephritis (APSGN)

Acute poststreptococcal glomerulonephritis is an infection of the glomeruli that occurs after a streptococcal infection elsewhere in the body.

Glomerulonephritis can follow a respiratory or skin infection. Several strains of group A β-hemolytic streptococci that cause GN have been isolated. In temperate zones the most common nephritogenic strain causing pharyngitis is M-type 12. Only about 5% of such infections are followed by APSGN. Children and young adults are affected most frequently. The incidence of APSGN decreases with age because many children (especially in the urban areas) develop immunities to type 12 β-hemolytic streptococci before reaching adulthood. Renal problems occur abruptly 1 to 3 weeks after the infection. Most patients (95%) recover normal renal function within 2 months.[8,10] The others have irreversible damage that causes long-term problems. Whether prompt treatment of streptococcal infections prevents renal complications of APSGN is unclear.

PATHOPHYSIOLOGY

Antibodies of the host react with circulating antigens that appear to arise from the toxic products of the infecting organism to form immune complexes that then become lodged in the glomeruli. Both kidneys are affected by an acute, diffuse, nonsuppurative inflammation that damages the glomerular basement membrane.

DIAGNOSTIC STUDIES

Kidney, ureter, bladder examination
Normal to slight bilateral kidney enlargement seen on plain roentgenogram

TREATMENT PLAN

The medical plan includes treating the symptoms, attempting to prevent cerebral and cardiac complications, and supporting the patient through a period of decreased renal functioning.

Chemotherapeutic
Antihypertensive agents
Clonidine (Catapres), po, 0.1 mg bid or tid initially, then increase by 0.2-0.8 mg/d (maximum effective dose 2.4 mg/d)
Diazoxide (Hyperstat IV), IV, adults only: 300 mg by bolus in 30 sec or 1-2 mg/kg up to 150 mg at 5-15 min intervals
Hydralazine (Apresoline), po, adults: 10 mg qid for 2-4 d; increase to 25 mg qid, then 50 mg qid; maintenance dose is lowest effective level; children: 0.75 mg/kg initially; increase if needed to 7.5 mg/kg; IM, IV, adults: 10-40 mg repeated as needed (q4-6h); children: 1.7-3.5 mg/kg initially/ d in 4-6 divided doses
Methyldopa (Aldomet), po, adults: 250 mg bid or tid for 48 h; then increase or decrease q2d if needed; maintenance of 500 mg-2 g in 2-4 divided doses (maximum of 3 g); children: 10 up to 65 mg/kg/24 h in 2-4 divided doses
Propranolol (Inderal), po, 40 mg bid at 6-8 h intervals; increase if needed to 160-480 mg/d in divided doses; 640 mg/d may be needed
Diuretics
Furosemide (Lasix), po, adults: 20-80 mg followed by second dose in 6-8 h up to 600 mg; children: 2 mg/kg body weight as single dose; may increase by 1-2 mg/kg and repeat in 6-8 h; IM, IV, adults: 20-40 mg given slowly over 1-2 min; high dose by IV not more than 4 mg/min; children: 1 mg/ kg body weight; may be increased by 1 mg/kg not sooner than 2 h later

Hydrochlorothiazide (Hydrodiuril), po, adults: 25-100 mg/d or bid initially; then maintenance of 25-100 mg/d according to patient's response; children: 2.2 mg/kg/d in 2 divided doses

Spironolactone (Aldactone), po, adults: 25-200 mg/d in divided doses initially for 5 d, then adjust to maintenance level; children: 1.5-3.3 mg/kg body weight in 4 divided doses

Agents for treatment of hyperkalemia[19]

Sodium polystyrene sulfonate (Kayexalate), po or enema, 15 g qd-qid; give po dose in 45-60 ml of water, syrup, fruit juice, or soft drink

Calcium gluconate, IV, 1 g (90 mg Ca^{++}) in 10 ml

Sodium bicarbonate, IV, 2-5 mEq/kg infusion over 4-8 h

Glucose 50% IV, 25-50 g and regular insulin, IV, 10-15 units

Antacids

Aluminum carbonate (Basaljel), po, 30-40 ml 1 h pc and at hs of regular strength (400 mg Al [OH]$_3$/5 ml); 15-20 ml 1 h pc and at hs of extra strength (1000 mg Al[OH]$_3$/5 ml)

Aluminum hydroxide, gel (Amphojel), aluminum hydroxide gel, dried (Amphojel tab), po, 40 ml 1 h pc and at hs; 8 tab 1 h pc and at hs

Anticonvulsive agents

Phenytoin (Dilantin), po, adults: 100 mg tid up to 600 mg/d; children: 4-8 mg/kg/d in 2-3 divided doses

Diazepam (Valium), po, adults: 2-10 mg bid-qid; children: (over 6 mo): 1-25 mg tid-qid

Phenobarbital (Luminal), po, adults: 50-100 mg/d; children: 16-50 mg bid or tid

Anti-infective agents (if infection is still present)

Infection is frequently a complication of acute renal failure

Agents specific to microorganism cultured should be used

Agents whose route of excretion is primarily renal need to be used in smaller doses or at lengthened intervals depending on glomerular filtration rate[10]; agents excreted by only the liver require no change; partial excretion occurs via the kidneys, some adjustment is needed at low glomerular filtration rates

Cardiac glycosides (for congestive heart failure):

Digoxin, po, 1-1.5 mg/d in divided doses; IV, 0.75-1.25 mg initially, maintenance of 0.125-0.5 mg/d

Electromechanical

Hemodialysis or peritoneal dialysis (see pp. 1085 and 1091)

Supportive

Limit sodium intake to 0.5 to 1 g/day

Limit fluids to 500 ml plus amount equal to volume of urine for previous 24 hours

Limit potassium intake (if hyperkalemia) to 60 mEq/day

Limit protein intake (if uremic) to 60 g/day

Provide 2500-3500 calories/day

Prescribe bed rest during acute phase of illness

ASSESSMENT: AREAS OF CONCERN

Infection

Antistreptolysin O (ASO) titer: 200 to 2500 Todd units; fever and chills

Urine

Hematuria (dark brown or rust colored); red blood cell casts; proteinuria; oliguria

Cardiovascular

Hypertension; edema

Blood chemistries

Increased blood urea nitrogen level; increased serum creatinine level

Hematology

Normal or decreased complement (C3); mild anemia

General

Headache; low back pain; malaise

NURSING DIAGNOSES and NURSING INTERVENTIONS

Nursing Diagnosis	Nursing Intervention
Tissue perfusion, alteration in: renal	Monitor renal functions: serum creatinine and blood urea nitrogen. Limit protein and potassium intake. Observe urine for color, presence of blood and protein.
Fluid volume, alteration in: excess (potential)	Monitor intake, output, weight, blood pressure, pulse, and respirations. If volume excess is severe, monitor pulmonary capillary wedge pressure, central venous pressure, and neck veins. Limit sodium and fluid intake.

Nursing Diagnosis	Nursing Intervention
Potential patient problem: susceptibility to infection	Monitor temperature. Observe for signs and symptoms of infection. Avoid exposure to persons with infection.
Nutrition, alteration in: less than body requirements	Ensure adequate calorie intake from carbohydrates and fats to prevent the use of tissue proteins for energy. Be alert to anorexia, nausea, and vomiting. Offer small, frequent feedings.
Mobility, impaired physical	Help patient stay on bed rest. Implement nursing measures to prevent complications of bed rest.
Self-care deficit	Assist with personal hygiene as needed because of malaise, fatigue, or weakness.

Patient Education

1. Explain the diagnosis of APSGN; its signs, symptoms, and the course of the disease.
2. Explain the medical regimen, if any, for discharge.
3. Explain follow-up care: monitoring of blood pressure and urinalysis (hematuria and proteinuria).

EVALUATION

Patient Outcome	Data Indicating That Outcome is Reached
Patient has normal renal function.	Urine output balances with intake. Urine is clear. Edema is gone. Blood pressure is in normal range. Weight is stable. Blood urea nitrogen, serum creatinine, and complement levels return to normal range.
Patient feels well.	Malaise is gone.
Patient is knowledgeable about APSGN.	Patient can describe signs, symptoms, and course of the disease. Patient can describe his level of renal function and possible problems. Patient can outline the medical regimen prescribed.

HEMOLYTIC UREMIC SYNDROME

The group of symptoms that comprise hemolytic uremic syndrome (HUS) are acute hemolysis, thrombocytopenia, and acute renal failure.

HUS primarily affects infants and young children and results in significant morbidity and mortality.

PATHOPHYSIOLOGY

The basic lesion is microangiopathy, which causes focal and diffuse glomerular necrosis. The endothelium is altered, platelets are locally damaged, and coagulation occurs. There appear to be environmental and genetic influences. HUS may be idiopathic or associated with genetic problems, infections, drugs, malignant hypertension of pregnancy, or immunodeficiency. The kidney lesions heal or progress to end-stage renal disease.

DIAGNOSTIC STUDIES

Renal biopsy

Major findings are in glomeruli and arterioles; if dysfunction is mild, swelling of glomerular endothelial cells is seen; oliguria is prolonged, lesions are seen involving the media of the renal arterioles; cortical infarction may be seen with irreversible renal failure

TREATMENT PLAN

Therapy is focused on relief of symptoms and support of bodily systems.

Chemotherapeutic

Anticoagulants

Heparin sodium, IV infusions: 15,000 units initially, 20,000-30,000 units/d; intermittent: 5000 units initially; 5000-10,000 units q4h; sc, 5000 units initially; 10,000-12,000 units q8h or 14,000-20,000 units q12h; depends on clotting time

Warfarin sodium (Coumadin), po, 10-15 mg/d for 2-3 d; IV, IM, initially, 2-10 mg/d maintenance, depending on prothrombin time

Corticosteroids

Prednisone, po, adults: 5-60 mg/d; children: 2 mg/kg/d

Antianginal agents (used as platelet inhibitors)

Dipyridamole (Persantine), po, adults: 50 mg tid used experimentally with aspirin and oral anticoagulants to decrease platelet aggregation[15]; children: 5 mg/kg/d

Fibrinolytic agents[14,21,40]

Fibrinolysin, IV, adults: 250,000-500,000 IU divided into 5 doses/day

Streptokinase (Streptase), IV, adults: 40,000-100,000 IU divided into 4 doses/d followed by 10,000 IU divided into 2 doses/d; children: 250,000 IU/1.73 M^2 body surface area (BSA) initially; then 200,000 IU/1.73 M^2/BSA in 4 h; maintenance: 100,000 IU/1.73 M^2 BSA/h continuously for 36-72 h

Electromechanical

Hemodialysis (see p. 1085)

Supportive

Fluid intake equals the amount needed to replace measurable losses in urine, nasogastric drainage, wound drainage, and the like; avoid fluid overload; daily weights reflect fluid gain or loss

Nutritional support includes maintenance of body weight and positive nitrogen balance[10,29]

Calorie intake should include 100 g of glucose a day

Protein intake may be maintained through hyperalimentation of essential amino acids (50 to 85 g/L solution); oral intake is started as soon as possible (protein 30 to 40 g/day with 75% high biologic value)

Vitamin supplements are needed, since 40 g protein diet is deficient in calcium and folic acid and low in phosphorus and the B vitamins

Sodium intake is 60 to 90 mEq/day if edema or hypertension is present; potassium in diet is restricted to 60 mEq/day if serum levels are more than 5 mEq/L

Blood transfusions may be needed

ASSESSMENT: AREAS OF CONCERN

Renal

Oliguria; hematuria; proteinuria

Vascular

Hemolytic anemia; thrombocytopenia; thrombi in renal arterioles; purpura

Gastrointestinal

Vomiting; diarrhea

Neurologic

Convulsions

Blood chemistries

Elevated blood urea nitrogen and serum creatinine levels

Other

Abdominal pain; hypertension

NURSING DIAGNOSES and NURSING INTERVENTIONS

Nursing Diagnosis	Nursing Intervention
Tissue perfusion, alteration in: renal	Give medications as ordered. Monitor response. Watch K^+ and Ca^{++} levels if diuretics, digitalis, or banked blood is given. Report K^+ levels greater than 5 mEq/L. Watch for electrocardiographic changes: peaked T waves, prolonged PR interval, widened QRS complex, and cardiac standstill. Watch for signs of hypocalcemia (tetany) and Chvostek and Trousseau signs.
Fluid volume excess or deficit (potential)	Monitor weight, intake and output, blood pressure, pulse, respirations, and breath sounds. Observe neck veins and skin turgor. Be alert to electrolyte losses in body fluid losses. Vomitus contains Na^+, K^+, H^+, Cl^-, and water. Diarrhea losses include K^+ and HCO_3^-. Fever and hyperpnea increase water losses. Transudates contain protein-rich fluid.

Nursing Diagnosis	Nursing Intervention
Potential patient problem: susceptibility to infection	Observe for signs and symptoms of infection and temperature. Give meticulous care to any wounds and incisions. Avoid exposure to persons with infections. Establish a routine for deep breathing, coughing, and turning. Give mouth care at regular intervals.
Sensory-perceptual alterations (potential)	Provide safe environment. Assess orientation to time, place, and person. Observe for behavioral changes. Observe level of consciousness. Be alert to possible convulsions.
Thought processes, alteration in (potential)	Provide safe environment. Assess orientation to time, place, and person. Observe for behavioral changes. Observe level of consciousness. Be alert to possible convulsions.
Nutrition, alteration in, less than body requirements	Monitor caloric intake: kinds and amount. Watch for nausea, vomiting, and anorexia. Monitor weight.
Self-care deficit	Give assistance as necessary in feeding, bathing and hygiene, and toileting.
Mobility, impaired physical	Maintain bed rest. Give assistance as needed in feeding, bathing and hygiene, and toileting. Establish routine for changing position.
Knowledge deficit	Help prepare patient understand what is happening: diagnosis, treatment, bodily responses, and expected outcomes.
Family processes, alteration in (potential)	Help family understand what is happening to patient. Help family as needed in meeting the situation.

Patient Education

1. Explain the cause of the episode.
2. Explain the level of renal function after the acute phase is over.
3. Explain diet and fluid restrictions, which may continue, be lessened, or be discontinued.
4. Teach self-observational skills such as measuring temperature, pulse, respirations, blood pressure, intake and output, daily weight, and record keeping.
5. Explain good personal hygiene.
6. Explain how to avoid infections.
7. Explain exercise and rest in the amounts advised.
8. Describe medications, if any, with name, purpose, dosage, time interval, and adverse reactions (discussion and in writing).
9. Explain the schedule for medical follow-up.
10. Explain renal dialysis and transplantation if they are likely options for the future.

EVALUATION

Patient Outcome	Data Indicating That Outcome is Reached
Renal function returns.	Normal urine output balances intake. Urine is free from blood or protein. Serum creatinine and blood urea nitrogen are normal.
Hemolytic lesions are clear.	Hemoglobin level is normal. Platelet count is normal. Bruises disappear.
Gastrointestinal symptoms are clear.	There is no vomiting, diarrhea, or abdominal pain.

HYDRONEPHROSIS

Hydronephrosis is the dilation of the renal pelvis by the pressure of urine that cannot flow past an obstruction of the ureter.

Obstruction can be proximal to the bladder or can occur below the level of the bladder. It is known that hydronephrosis, which is usually on the right side, always occurs during pregnancy and for a time after delivery because of obstruction caused by the enlarged uterus.

PATHOPHYSIOLOGY

Obstruction of the ureter that results in hydronephrosis may be caused by renal calculi, tumors, inflammation associated with infection, fibrous bands that obstruct the ureteropelvic junction, or prostatic urethral valves. The renal pelvis and ureters dilate and hypertrophy. The pressure of the urine, if prolonged, causes fibrosis and loss of function in affected nephrons. The duration and severity of the obstruction are significant. Compression causes ischemia and then atrophy of renal tissue. The kidney may be destroyed without pain.

DIAGNOSTIC STUDIES

Ultrasonography
Dilation of collecting system

Intravenous urogram
Calyceal clubbing is shown after injection of radiopaque dye

TREATMENT PLAN

Management is usually conservative if the condition is not severe.

Surgical
Surgical intervention is used to relieve the obstruction and preserve renal function; pyeloplasty may be indicated; repair of the ureteropelvic junction may be indicated; a nephrectomy may be indicated if the kidney is severely damaged; antimicrobials are used to treat infection if present

Chemotherapeutic
Antiinfectives if infection is present

Parenteral agents (IM or IV)
  Gentamicin, (Garamycin), adults: 3-5 mg/kg/d q8h; children: 6-7.5 mg/kg/d q8h
  Cephalosporins
    Cefazolin sodium (Ancef), 250-1000 mg q6-8h
  Penicillins
    Ampicillin sodium (Omnipen-N), patients ≥40 kg: 250-500 mg q6h; <40 kg: 25-50 mg/kg/d in equally divided doses q6-8h
    Carbenicillin disodium (Geopen), adults: 1-2 g q6h; children: 50-200 mg/kg/d in equally divided doses q4-6h
    Penicillin G potassium (aqueous penicillin G), Penicillin G sodium, adults: 1-20 million units/d; children: 50,000-250,000 units/kg/d in 4-6 divided doses
Oral agents
  Sulfonamides
    Sulfisoxazole (Gantrisin), 2-4 g initially, followed by 1-2 g q4-6h
  Tetracycline (Achromycin), 250-500 mg q6h
  Penicillins
    Amoxicillin (Amoxil), adults and children ≥20 kg: 250-500 mg q8h; <20 kg: 20-40 mg/kg/d in divided doses q8h
    Ampicillin (Omnipen), patients ≥20 kg: 250-500 mg q6h; <20 kg: 50-100 mg/kg/d in equally divided doses
  Erythromycin (Erythrocin, E-Mycin), adults: 25 mg q6h; children: 30-50 mg/kg/d in 4 equally divided doses
  Sulfamethoxazole and trimethoprim (Septra, Bactrim), adults: 2 tab q12h; children: 8 mg/kg of trimethoprim and 40 mg/kg of sulfamethoxazole/d in 2 divided doses q12h

ASSESSMENT: AREAS OF CONCERN

Renal
Hematuria; pyuria

Abdominal
Mass (in child)

General
Fever (with infection)

NURSING DIAGNOSES and NURSING INTERVENTIONS

Nursing Diagnosis	Nursing Intervention
Tissue perfusion, alteration in: renal (potential)	Give antimicrobial drugs, if ordered, and observe for response and side effects. Monitor intake and output. Monitor urine for bleeding that may be present during the first hours after surgery.
Potential patient problem: susceptibility to infection	Observe for signs and symptoms of infection. Monitor temperature, pulse, and respirations.
Skin integrity, impairment of (by surgery)	Prepare for surgery. Explain procedure, diagnostic studies, and postoperative care to be given to patient and family. Prepare area of skin for incision. Bowel preparation may include enema and nothing by mouth after midnight. *Postoperative care:* Monitor site of incision for drainage and signs of infection. Keep any drainage tubes patent, unkinked, and anchored to avoid inadvertent displacement. Monitor intake (intravenous and oral) and output. Care for urethral catheter. Watch for and report foul-smelling urine. Tubes may include a stent (a catheter inserted in the ureter), a nephrostomy tube, and an incisional drain. Observe for flank pain and urine output in relation to intake after nephrostomy tube is removed. Pain, fever, and decreased urine may indicate obstruction or urine leaking into the retroperitoneal space. Observe dressing. Drainage of urine may continue for some time. Keep area clean and dry to avoid skin breakdown.

Patient Education

1. Explain the kidney-ureter abnormality.
2. Explain possible problems: recurrent infection and obstruction.
3. Explain signs and symptoms of urinary tract infection and obstruction.
4. Explain measures to prevent urinary tract infection: adequate fluid intake to avoid dehydration, regular emptying of bladder to avoid overdistention, and good perineal hygiene to prevent entrance of microorganisms into the urinary tract.
5. Explain postoperative care, including care of the incision and self-monitoring skills as needed.
6. Explain plans for medical follow-up of renal function.

EVALUATION

Patient Outcome	Data Indicating That Outcome is Reached
Obstruction is relieved.	Roentgenograms show that hydronephrosis is lessened or does not increase.
Surgical incision heals.	Incision is closed; no signs of infection are present.
Renal function is not impaired.	Renal function tests are normal.
Patient knows how to prevent urinary tract infections.	Patient can describe the measures used to prevent urinary tract infection.
Patient seeks medical follow-up.	Continuing medical supervision is sought.

INTERSTITIAL NEPHRITIS

Interstitial nephritis (IN) is renal disease that involves inflammatory interstitial tissue damage.

Damage to the cortical interstitial tissue is the second most common cause (after glomerular disease) of chronic renal failure. Causes of IN include infections (for example, streptococcal) and drug use (antibiotics such as methicillin and ampicillin, sulfonamides, phenindione, and phenytoin). The cause may be idiopathic. Early detection of drug reactions, infections, and urinary tract obstruction is useful. It is important to be alert to the possibility that selected patients may abuse the use of over-the-counter analgesics, especially those containing phenacetin and acetaminophen (the major metabolite of phenacetin).

PATHOPHYSIOLOGY

Acute inflammation of the interstitium may cause scarring and a rapid decline in renal function. As many as 10% to 15% of the cases of acute renal failure may be associated with acute interstitial nephritis.[27] The inflammatory process is usually diffuse and accompanied by interstitial edema. An immune response appears to cause acute IN that may involve both immune complex and anti–tubular basement membrane antibody deposition.

Chronic IN results in a shrunken kidney with an irregular outline because of scarring and tissue destruction. It follows a slowly progressive course with few clinical manifestations. Changes in renal hormone activity may occur. Renin, erythropoietin, and vitamin D production may decline. Ability to concentrate urine also decreases. Common causes of chronic IN are anatomic abnormalities, such as obstruction in the urinary tract, analgesic use, hyperuricemia, and nephrosclerosis.

DIAGNOSTIC STUDIES

Intravenous urography
Decreased kidney size, irregular cortical outlines, calyceal cupping are seen after injection of radiopaque dye

TREATMENT PLAN

The cause of IN can be removed by treating infection, discontinuing the drugs associated with acute IN, and relieving obstruction. Renal function may gradually im-

prove. Chronic IN requires monitoring as renal function decreases. Changes in the function of the glomeruli and tubules occur as the interstitial inflammation and scarring progress (see ''Chronic Renal Failure,'' p. 1069).

Surgical
Relieve any obstruction

Chemotherapeutic
Anti-infective agents
Parenteral agents (IM or IV)
Gentamicin (Garamycin), adults: 3-5 mg/kg/d q8h; children: 6-7.5 mg/kg/d q8h
Cephalosporins
Cefazolin sodium (Ancef), 250-1000 mg q6-8h
Penicillins
Ampicillin sodium (Omnipen-N), patients ≥40 kg: 250-500 mg q6h; <40 kg: 25-50 mg/kg/d in equally divided doses, q6-8h
Carbenicillin disodium (Geopen), adults: 1-2 g IM q6h; children: 50-200 mg/kg/d in equally divided doses q4-6h
Penicillin G potassium (aqueous penicillin G), penicillin G sodium, adults: 1-20 million units/d; children: 50,000-250,000 units/kg/d in 4-6 divided doses
Oral agents
Sulfonamides
Sulfisoxazole (Gantrisin), 2-4 g initially, followed by 1-2 g q4-6h
Tetracycline (Achromycin), 250-500 mg q6h
Penicillins
Amoxicillin (Amoxil), adults and children ≥20 kg: 250-500 mg q8h; <20 kg: 20-40 mg/kg/d in divided doses q8h
Ampicillin (Omnipen), patients ≥20 kg: 250-500 mg q6h; <20 kg: 50-100 mg/kg/d in equally divided doses
Penicillin G, adults: 200,000-500,000 units q6-8h; children: 25,000-90,000 units/kg/d in 3-6 divided doses
Erythromycin (Erythrocin), adults: 25 mg q6h; children: 30-50 mg/kg/d in 4 equally divided doses
Trimethoprim and sulfamethoxazole (Septra), adults: 2 tab q12h; children: 8 mg/kg trimethoprim and 40 mg/kg sulfamethoxazole/d in 2 divided doses q12h

Electromechanical
Dialysis, if needed

Supportive

Fluid intake to equal amount needed to replace measurable losses in urine, nasogastric drainage, wound drainage, and the like; avoid fluid overload; daily weights reflect fluid gain or loss

Nutritional support includes maintenance of body weight and positive nitrogen balance[10,29]

Calorie intake should include 100 g of glucose/day

Protein intake may be maintained through hyperalimentation of essential amino acids (50 to 85 gm/L solution); oral intake is started as soon as possible (protein of 30 to 40 g/day with 75% having high biologic value)

Vitamin supplements needed, since 40 g protein diet is deficient in calcium and folic acid and is low in phosphorus and the B vitamins

Sodium intake of 60 to 90 mEq/day if edema or hypertension is present; potassium in the diet is restricted to 60 mEq/day if serum levels are more than 5 mEq/L

ASSESSMENT: AREAS OF CONCERN

Renal

Polyuria; nocturia; pyuria; white blood cells and tubular casts; microscopic hematuria; mild proteinuria

Blood chemistries

Elevated blood urea nitrogen and serum creatinine levels

NURSING DIAGNOSES and NURSING INTERVENTIONS

Nursing Diagnosis	Nursing Intervention
Tissue perfusion, alteration in: renal	Give medications as ordered and monitor response. Watch K^+, and Ca^{++} levels if diuretics, digitalis, or banked blood is given. Report K^+ levels greater than 5 mEq/L. Watch for electrocardiographic changes: peaked T waves, prolonged PR interval, widened QRS complex, and cardiac standstill. Watch for signs of hypocalcemia: (tetany) and Chvostek and Trousseau signs.
Fluid volume excess or deficit (potential)	Monitor weight, intake and output, blood pressure, pulse, respirations, and breath sounds. Observe neck veins and skin turgor. Be alert to electrolyte losses in body fluid losses. Vomitus contains Na^+, K^+, H^+, Cl^-, and water. Diarrhea losses include K^+ and HCO_3. Fever and hyperpnea increase water losses. Transudates contain protein-rich fluid.
Potential patient problem: susceptibility to infection	Observe for signs and symptoms of infection and temperature. Give meticulous care to any wounds and incisions. Avoid exposure to persons with infections. Establish a routine for deep breathing, coughing, and turning. Give mouth care at regular intervals.
Sensory-perceptual alteration (potential)	Provide safe environment. Assess orientation to time, place, and person. Observe for behavioral changes. Observe level of consciousness. Be alert to possible convulsions.
Thought processes, alteration in (potential)	Provide safe environment. Assess orientation to time, place, and person. Observe for behavioral changes. Observe level of consciousness. Be alert to possible convulsions.
Nutrition, alteration in, less than body requirements	Monitor caloric intake: kinds and amount. Watch for nausea, vomiting, and anorexia. Monitor weight.
Self-care deficit	Give assistance as necessary in feeding, bathing and hygiene, and toileting.
Mobility, impaired physical	If patient is on bed rest, give assistance as necessary in feeding, bathing and hygiene, and toileting. Establish routine for changing position.

Nursing Diagnosis	Nursing Intervention
Knowledge deficit	Help prepare patient to understand what is happening: diagnosis, treatment, bodily responses, and expected outcomes.
Family process, alteration in (potential)	Help family understand what is happening to patient. Help family as needed in meeting the situation.

Patient Education

1. Explain the nature of interstitial nephritis and the cause in the individual patient.
2. Explain the patient's level of renal function.
3. Explain the need for periodic medical evaluation with tests of renal function.
4. Explain the likelihood of dialysis or transplantation in the future.

EVALUATION

Patient Outcome	Data Indicating That Outcome is Reached
Patient is knowledgeable about interstitial nephritis.	Patient and family describe the nature and extent of interstitial nephritis, the need for follow-up, and implications for the future.

NEPHROTIC SYNDROME

Nephrotic syndrome (NS) encompasses a group of symptoms: proteinuria (primarily albuminuria), hypoalbuminemia, generalized edema, hyperlipidemia, and lipiduria. NS occurs in both adults and children.

NS may occur in various conditions: glomerulonephritis, glomerular lesions associated with such systemic diseases and conditions as diabetes mellitus, infections, circulatory diseases, reactions to allergens and drugs, pregnancy, and renal transplantation. NS is frequently idiopathic in children. Long-term studies are under way to determine the usefulness of corticosteroids and cyclophosphamide in such children.[7]

show minimal changes or marked changes. Most patients with NS who have minimal changes respond well to corticosteroid therapy. Those patients with marked changes are usually unresponsive and progress to end-stage renal disease.

The decrease in plasma proteins may result in less binding proteins for drugs. The usual effect of a drug may occur with half the usual dose. The protein loss may also cause a decrease in vitamin D precursor, transferrin, T_3, and thyroid-binding globulin. Calcium may be required, but thyroid hormone usually is not. Iron may be needed if iron deficiency anemia occurs.

PATHOPHYSIOLOGY

NS results from increased glomerular permeability. The albuminuria causes hypoalbuminemia because the liver cannot replace the losses rapidly enough. The resulting drop in oncotic pressure permits water to escape from the vascular compartment. Adaptive responses to the contraction of fluid volume include increased secretion of antidiuretic hormone and aldosterone, which contribute to the problem of fluid retention. The liver is stimulated to increase the synthesis of many proteins. It also increases production of lipoproteins, thereby causing the hyperlipidemia characteristic of NS.

The results of a renal biopsy in patients with NS may

DIAGNOSTIC STUDIES

Renal biopsy

To identify histologic features of lesion classified as:

Minimal change—podocytes of epithelial cells appear to be fused together on electron microscopy

Membranous change—predominantly thickening of the basement membrane is visible by light and electron microscopy

Proliferative change—glomerular cells appear hypercellular

Membranoproliferative change—there is both hypercellularity and basement membrane thickening

TREATMENT PLAN

Surgical
Renal biopsy may be needed to determine the underlying cause and the appropriate treatment (p. 1101)
Thoracentesis
Paracentesis

Chemotherapeutic
Corticosteroids
Prednisone, po, adults: 5-60 mg/d; children: 1-2 mg/kg/d
Antineoplastic agents (used for immunosuppressive effect)
Cyclophosphamide (Cytoxan), po, adults: 1-5 mg/kg/d; children: 2-8 mg/kg initially; 2-5 mg/kg twice weekly maintenance; IV, adults: 40-50 mg/kg/day initially; 10-15 mg/kg q7-10d, 3-5 mg/kg twice weekly, or 1.5-3 mg/kg/d maintenance; children: 2-8 mg/kg/d initially; 10-15 mg/kg q7-10d or 30 mg q3-4wk maintenance
Azathioprine (Imuran), po (highly individualized): 3-5 mg/kg/d initially; 1-2 mg/kg/d maintenance
Chlorambucil, po, adults: 0.1-0.2 mg/kg/d for 3-6 wk initially; 0.03-0.1 mg/kg/d maintenance; children: 0.1-0.2 mg/kg/d
Plasma expanders and blood components
Albumin human (Albuminate, others) (5 g/100 ml or 25 g/100 ml), IV, adults: 25 g initially; repeated in 15-30 min; children: 25%-50% of adult dose
Diuretics
Furosemide (Lasix), po, adults: 20-80 mg followed by second dose in 6-8 h up to 600 mg; children: 2 mg/kg body weight as single dose; may increase by 1 or 2 mg/kg and repeat in 6-8 h; IM, IV, adults: 20-40 mg given slowly over 1-2 min; high dose by IV not more than 4 mg/min; children: 1 mg/kg body weight; may be increased by 1 mg/kg not sooner than 2 h later
Hydrochlorothiazide (Hydrodiuril), po, adults: 25-100 mg/d or bid initially; then maintenance of 25-100 mg/d according to patient's response; children: 2.2 mg/kg/d in 2 divided doses
Spironolactone (Aldactone), po, adults: 25-200 mg/d in divided doses initially for 5 d; then adjust to maintenance level; children: 1.5-3.3 mg/kg/ body weight in 4 divided doses
Protein diet supplements
Meritene, 8-10 oz bid or tid
Citrotein, 8 oz bid or tid

Immunosuppressive agents are used because they have been shown empirically to decrease or stop the proteinuria. Prednisone, the treatment of choice, is initially given as a single dose at breakfast and may be later given on alternate days. The other immunosuppressive agents are used if corticosteroids cannot be used. Diuretics are often used in conjunction with salt-poor albumin infusions to relieve massive edema. Thoracentesis or paracentesis may be needed if excess fluid accumulates in the chest or abdominal cavities. In minimal disease nephrotic syndrome in children, corticosteroids are started and the responses noted. Often proteinuria clears rapidly. Repeat treatment with corticosteroids is indicated for those children who have a relapse after therapy is discontinued.

Supportive
Protein intake is increased to replace urinary protein losses.[29] If the glomerular filtration rate is normal, adults may have 1.5 to 2 g/kg body weight. For children protein is increased to 2 to 3 g/kg body weight to allow for positive nitrogen balance and growth. If the glomerular filtration rate is decreased, protein intake is lowered. Sodium intake is limited (60 to 90 mEq/day) to control edema. Caloric intake must be sufficient to prevent muscle catabolism and provide energy. The amount varies with height, weight, age, sex, and daily activity. Adults need 35 to 45 kcal/kg ideal body weight/day. Children should have 60 to 80 kcal/kg/ideal body weight/day. The help of a dietitian and the use of exchange lists make implementing these complex diets easier.

Changes in vascular volume are monitored carefully to prevent hypovolemic shock, as well as the hypokalemia and ototoxicity that can accompany diuretic use. Hospitalization is avoided unless the patient has severe generalized edema with ascites, significant hypertension, severe infection, hypovolemic shock, or a persistently low glomerular filtration rate. Bed rest is advised if complications are present. The level of proteinuria is monitored.

ASSESSMENT: AREAS OF CONCERN

Renal
Proteinuria (albuminuria) greater than 3 g/day; urine: foamy, deeper yellow color, oval fat bodies; oliguria

Blood chemistries
Hypoalbuminemia less than 2.5 gm/dl; hyperlipidemia

Cardiovascular
Edema: periorbital, external genitalia, peritoneal and pleural spaces, and extremities

Gastrointestinal
Anorexia; vomiting; diarrhea

General
Weight gain

NURSING DIAGNOSES and NURSING INTERVENTIONS

Nursing Diagnosis	Nursing Intervention
Tissue perfusion, alteration in: renal	Monitor losses of protein in urine. Give medications as ordered and monitor response and side effects. Monitor serum protein, blood urea nitrogen, and serum creatinine levels.
Fluid volume, alteration in: excess	Monitor weight, intake, output, blood pressure, pulse, and respirations. Observe for edema. If edema is severe, monitor neck veins, central venous pressure, and pulmonary capillary wedge pressure. Be alert for side effects of diuretics used. Monitor potassium levels.
Mobility, impaired physical	Maintain bed rest during acute phase and if edema is excessive; otherwise encourage moderate activity. Implement measures to prevent the complications of bed rest, when needed.
Potential patient problem: susceptibility to infection	Be alert to signs and symptoms of infection. Monitor white blood cell count altered by immunosuppressive drugs. Avoid exposure to persons with infections. Encourage good general health habits.
Skin integrity, impairment of	Meticulous skin care of edematous body areas is needed.
Nutrition, alteration in: less than body requirements	Encourage intake as ordered. Provide palatable meals and consider patient's likes and dislikes. Protein diet supplements may be needed.
Self-concept, disturbance in: body image	See p. 1820. Warn patient to expect alopecia as side effect of cyclophosphamide, and recurrence of edema and change in body appearance as side effects of corticosteroids.

Patient Education

1. Explain the nature of nephrotic syndrome, its cause, and the possibility of relapse.
2. Explain the psychologic responses to nephrotic syndrome and its treatment: massive edema, side effects of corticosteroids, and long-term effects of other immunosuppressive agents, which may include aspermia, ovarian fibrosis, and the increased likelihood of malignant tumors.
3. Explain follow-up medical care for monitoring changes in renal function.
4. Explain renal dialysis and transplantation as possible future options.

EVALUATION

Patient Outcome	Data Indicating That Outcome is Reached
Symptoms of nephrotic syndrome are clear.	Patient has normal serum albumin and lipid levels, stable weight, and no edema or gastrointestinal problems.
Renal function is normal.	Patient has normal urine without protein or lipids. Urine volume is normal and balances intake.
Patient is knowledgeable about nephrotic syndrome.	Patient and family describe nephrotic syndrome and its implications for long-term care in their particular situation.

PYELONEPHRITIS

Pyelonephritis (PLN) is an infection of the kidney and pelvis. It is a major problem of the renal system.

Although urinary tract infections, including PLN, cause considerable morbidity, they do not progress to end-stage renal disease unless there is an underlying urinary tract problem such as obstruction. During pregnancy women should be screened for bacteriuria and treated to avoid the development of PLN.[33] Personal health habits should include adequate fluid intake (2500 to 3000 ml/ day) and prompt emptying of the bladder.

PATHOPHYSIOLOGY

The infection is caused by bacteria that spread by hematogenous or lymphatic routes or most commonly by ascending from the lower urinary tract. Obstructive uropathy, glomerulonephritis, polycystic kidney disease, diabetes mellitus, renal calculi, and analgesic abuse appear to lower the kidney's resistance to infection. Without treatment a significant number of pregnant women with asymptomatic bacteriuria will develop PLN.[33]

Damage to the kidneys is caused by inflammation, fibrosis, and scarring that occur because of the infection. Chronic PLN causes tissue destruction and contracted, small kidneys. The medulla is suceptible to the ascending spread of bacteria because of the hypertonic environment and slow blood flow there. Infection spreads through the collecting ducts to the interstitium. Papillary necrosis may be a complication of PLN, and detached pieces of tissue may block the ureters. Infection spreads to the cortex and eventually involves the nephron and blood vessels. The organism most frequently involved is *Escherichia coli*. Other organisms include *Proteus, Enterobacter, Pseudomonas, Klebsiella, Staphylococcus,* and *Streptococcus*.

Most infections are acute. A long-term, smoldering, chronic infection may occasionally occur. One or more of the factors previously mentioned contribute most often to a chronic infection of the kidney.

DIAGNOSTIC STUDIES

Intravenous urography

Small kidneys with an irregular outline and focal clubbing of the calyceal system are seen after injection of radiopaque dye

TREATMENT PLAN

Chemotherapeutic

Anti-infective agents

Parenteral agents (IM or IV)

Gentamicin (Garamycin), adults: 3-5 mg/kg/d q8h; children: 6-7.5 mg/kg/d q8h

Cephalosporins

Cefazolin sodium (Ancef), 250-1000 mg q6-8h

Penicillins

Ampicillin sodium (Omnipen-N): patients ≥40 kg: 250-500 mg q6h; <40 kg: 25-50 mg/kg/ d in equally divided doses q6-8 h

Carbenicillin disodium (Geopen), adults: 1-2 g q6h; children: 50-200 mg/kg/d in equally divided doses q4-6h

Penicillin G potassium (aqueous penicillin G), penicillin G sodium, adults: 1-20 million units/d; children: 50,000-250,000 units/kg/ d in 4-6 divided doses

Oral agents

Sulfonamides

Sulfisoxazole (Gantrisin), 2-4 g initially, followed by 1-2 g q4-6h

Tetracycline (Achromycin), 250-500 mg q6h

Penicillins

Amoxicillin (Amoxil), adults and children ≥20 kg: 250-500 mg q8h; <20 kg: 20-40 mg/kg/ d in divided doses q8h

Ampicillin (Omnipen), patients ≥20 kg: 250-500 mg q6h; <20 kg: 50-100 mg/kg/d in equally divided doses

Penicillin G, adults: 200,000-500,000 units q6-8h; children: 25,000-90,000 units/kg/d in 3-6 divided doses

Nalidixic acid (NegGram), adults: 500-1000 mg q6h for 2 wk; children: 55 mg/kg/d in 4 equally divided doses

Erythromycin (Erythrocin), adults: 25 mg q6h; children: 30-50 mg/kg/d in 4 equally divided doses

Sulfamethoxazole and trimethoprim (Septra), adults: 2 tab q12h; children: 8 mg/kg of trimethoprim and 40 mg/kg of sulfamethoxazole/ d in 2 divided doses q12h

Supportive

High normal (3500 to 4000 ml/day) fluid intake to dilute urine and decrease burning on urination, flush out urinary tract, and prevent dehydration

Bed rest is usual during acute phase

ASSESSMENT: AREAS OF CONCERN

General

Fever and chills; severe flank pain; weakness; anorexia

Renal

Hematuria; bacteriuria; pyuria; urine culture: significant growth; dysuria; nocturia; frequency

In child, in addition, squirming, irritability, foul-smelling urine

NURSING DIAGNOSES and NURSING INTERVENTIONS

Nursing Diagnosis	Nursing Intervention
Tissue perfusion, alteration in: renal	Give antimicrobial agents as ordered and observe response for side effects. Explain drugs and their purpose. Encourage high normal fluid intake; explain why. Measure intake, output, weight, temperature, pulse, respirations, and blood pressure.
Comfort, alteration in: pain	Give analgesics if ordered. External applications of heat may help.
Mobility, impaired physical	Encourage bed rest during acute phase. Implement measures to prevent complications of bed rest when needed.
Self-care deficit (potential)	Assist with personal hygiene as needed; fatigue is common.

Patient Education

1. Explain pyelonephritis; its causes, signs, and symptoms.
2. Explain antimicrobial therapy: drugs, dosage, interval, side effects, and the need to complete course of treatment.
3. Explain the possibility of relapse or reinfection.
4. Explain measures to prevent urinary tract infection, including adequate intake (2000 to 2500 ml/day for adults) to avoid dehydration, regular emptying of bladder to avoid overdistention, and good perineal hygiene for women to prevent the entrance of microorganisms into the urinary tract.

EVALUATION

Patient Outcome	Data Indicating That Outcome is Reached
Signs and symptoms of pyelonephritis are clear.	Temperature, pulse, and respirations are normal, pain is gone, urine is clear of bacteria or pus cells, and problems in urination are gone.
Evaluation of urinary tract is completed.	Intravenous urogram is done to rule out any structural defect.
Patient is knowledgeable about pyelonephritis.	Patient can describe signs, symptoms, and any further treatment needed.

RENAL CALCULI

Renal calculi are stones formed in the kidney, primarily in the pelvis. Stones may be gravel like or formed in the shape of the pelvis, the so-called stag-horn calculus.

Renal stones are often associated with obstructions and infections of the urinary tract. They occur more frequently in men than in women. Geographic areas such as the southeastern United States have a particularly high incidence of renal calculi. Renal tubular acidosis (RTA), the distal form, is frequently associated with the formation of calcium phosphate stones. The alkaline urine and hypercalciuria associated with RTA worsen calcium-phosphate oversaturation and contribute to stone formation (see p. 1074).

PATHOPHYSIOLOGY

The formation of a stone is a physicochemical process involving a nidus of crystals or organic material around which the stone components form. The pH, temperature, ionic strength, and concentration of the urine affect the solubility of the stone-forming substances. The supersaturation of poorly soluble substances, the absence of crystalline inhibitors, and sources of seed crystals contribute to calculus formation.

The primary components of renal calculi include calcium salts, uric acid, cystine, and struvite (magnesium ammonium phosphate). The stones most frequently contain calcium or uric acid.

Hypercalciuria with or without hypercalcemia may be caused by hyperparathyroidism or osteoporosis or may be idiopathic. Calcium and phosphate are more soluble when pH is low. Bacterial infection by urea-splitting organisms causes the urine to become alkaline. Stones composed of struvite are called "infection stones."

Hyperuricemia occurs with idiopathic gout, renal failure, blood dyscrasias, and the use of thiazide diuretics and alkylating agents. Uric acid is less soluble in high concentrations, low urine volume, and with low urine pH.

DIAGNOSTIC STUDIES

Kidney, ureter, bladder examination
   Radiopaque stone visualized on roentgenographic examination

Ultrasonography
   Stones identified

TREATMENT PLAN

The goals of medical care are to (1) remove calculi, (2) relieve effects of the calculi (pain and infection), (3) resolve any causative factors (obstruction, infection and metabolic abnormalities), and (4) prevent future calculous growth.[6] The achievement of these goals should prevent permanent damage to the kidney and recurrence of calculi.

Surgical
   Procedures used may include: pyelolithotomy, nephrolithotomy, ureterolithotomy, cystoscopy-basket extraction of calculi, and percutaneous fragmentation and extraction through a nephroscope; surgical intervention is a last resort with struvite stones because recurrence is so frequent

Chemotherapeutic
   Anti-infective agents
      Parenteral agents (IM or IV)
         Gentamicin (Garamycin), adults: 3-5 mg/kg/d q8h; children: 6-7.5 mg/kg/d q8h
         Cephalosporins
            Cefazolin sodium (Ancef), 250-1000 mg q6-8h
         Penicillins
            Ampicillin sodium (Omnipen-N), patients ≥40 kg: 250-500 mg q6h; <40 kg: 25-50 mg/kg/d in equally divided doses q6-8h
            Carbenicillin disodium (Geopen), adults: 1-2 g q6h; children: 50-200 mg/kg/d in equally divided doses q4-6h
            Penicillin G potassium (Aqueous penicillin G), Penicillin G sodium, adults: 1-20 million units/d; children: 50,000-250,000 units/kg/d in 4-6 divided doses
      Oral agents
         Sulfonamides
            Sulfisoxazole (Gantrisin), 2-4 g initially followed by 1-2 g q4-6h
         Tetracycline (Achromycin), 250-500 mg q6h
         Penicillins
            Amoxicillin (Amoxil), adults and children: ≥20 kg: 250-500 mg q8h; <20 kg: 20-40 mg/kg/d in divided doses q8h
            Ampicillin (Omnipen), patients ≥20 kg: 250-500 mg q6h; <20 kg 50-100 mg/kg/d in equally divided doses
            Penicillin G, adults: 200,000-500,000 units q6-8h; children: 25,000-90,000 units/kg/d in 3-6 divided doses
         Erythromycin (Erythrocin), adults: 25 mg q6h; children: 30-50 mg/kg/d in 4 equally divided doses
         Sulfamethoxazole and trimethoprim (Septra, Bactrim), adults: 2 tab q12h; children: 8 mg/kg of trimethoprim and 40 mg/kg of sulfamethoxazole/d in 2 divided doses q12h
   Diuretics
      Hydrochlorothiazide (Hydrodiuril) (to reduce idiopathic urinary calcium excretion), po, adults: 25-50 mg bid
   Analgesics
      Meperidine (Demerol), po, sc, IM, IV, adults: 50-150 mg q3-4h; children: 1 mg/kg q4h up to 100 mg q4h
      Codeine sulfate, oral, sc, IM, adults: 15-60 mg qid; children: 3 mg/kg/d divided into 6 doses
      Morphine sulfate, po, sc, IM, adults: 5-15 mg q4h prn; children: 0.1-0.2 mg/kg/dose not to exceed 15 mg

Electrolytes (used to ensure alkaline urine)

Sodium bicarbonate, po, adults: 300 mg-1.8 g qd-qid not to exceed 16 g/day

Antirheumatic and anti-inflammatory agents

Allopurinol (Zyloprim), decreases uric acid production, po, adults: 200-800 mg in divided doses if more than 300 mg; children: 100 mg tid; depends on serum uric acid levels

Penicillamine (Cuprimine) (combines with cystine to form a soluble compound), po, adults: 250 mg qid; children: 30 mg/kg/d divided into 4 doses; individualized according to cystine excretion

Supportive

Low-calcium diets (less than 400 mg/day) and extra-high fluid intake (3500 to 4000 ml/day) are helpful but difficult to maintain; patients should avoid dehydration by drinking water rather than fluids that may be high in unwanted substances (such as tea with its high oxylate content); increased fluid intake should be spread out evenly over the 24-hour period including once during the night; low purine diets may help decrease uric acid output; foods extremely high in purines (greater than 150 mg/100 g) are limited; oxalate intake is usually limited to less than 50 mg/day on low oxylate diets

ASSESSMENT: AREAS OF CONCERN

Renal

Hematuria; crystalluria; passage of stone (strain urine); elevated 24-hour urine excretion of Ca^{++}, uric acid, or oxylate; urine pH increases or decreases; cystinuria; nocturia; urinary tract infection

Blood chemistries

Variable levels of serum Ca^{++}, Cl^-, $PO_4^=$, pH, CO_2, uric acid, and creatinine

General

Fever; pain in flank that may extend to groin, labia, or testicle

NURSING DIAGNOSES and NURSING INTERVENTIONS

Nursing Diagnosis	Nursing Intervention
Comfort, alteration in: pain	Note pattern of pain. Give analgesic agents and note responses. Apply external heat to area to relieve discomfort. Ambulation may help.
Potential patient problem: susceptibility to infection	Observe for signs and symptoms of urinary tract infection. Monitor temperature. Give antimicrobial drugs if ordered.
Fluid volume deficit, potential	Monitor blood pressure, pulse, respirations, intake, output, and weight. Force fluids over the 24 hours to high normal level; avoid fluids that contain unwanted substances (such as tea with its high oxylate content).
Nutrition, alteration in; more than body requirements	Lower calcium intake with calcium stones (reduce intake of dairy products). Lower purine intake with uric acid stones (reduce intake of organ meats, meat extracts, shrimp, and dried beans). Lower intake of oxylate-containing foods (such as tea, chocolate, nuts, and spinach) to prevent formation of oxylate stones. Avoid dehydration.
Skin integrity, impairment of (by surgery; potential)	Prepare for surgery by explaining procedure and postoperative care and by preparing the skin and bowels. *Postoperative care:* Monitor site of incision for drainage and signs of infection. Monitor temperature, pulse, respirations, and blood pressure. Keep any drainage tubes patent, unkinked, and anchored to avoid inadvertent displacement. Monitor intake (intravenous and oral) and output. Care for ureteral, urethral, and nephrostomy catheters, record output from each, and be alert for foul-smelling urine.
Self-care deficit (potential)	Assist with personal hygiene as needed after surgery.

Patient Education

1. Explain the nature of renal calculi, their causes, and manifestations.
2. Explain medical management including medications (purpose, dosage, interval, and side effects), diet (low calcium, purine, or oxylate), and fluid intake (amount, schedule, and kinds).
3. Explain medical follow-up to monitor the outcome of treatment.

EVALUATION

Patient Outcome	Data Indicating That Outcome is Reached
Signs and symptoms of renal calculi are clear.	Urine is clear, no infection is present, and pain is gone.
Patient recovers from surgery.	Incision is closed. No infection is present.
Patient is aware of need for life-style changes.	Patient describes any medications, diet, or other instructions given to prevent recurrence of renal calculi.

RENAL FAILURE

Changes in renal function may be considered on a continuum from impairment to failure. Renal impairment may be revealed only by specific urine concentration or dilution tests. Renal insufficiency is revealed when the kidneys cannot meet the extra demands of dietary or metabolic stress. Renal failure occurs when the normal demands of the body cannot be met.

Health professionals can assist in the early detection of renal problems and the prevention of renal failure. Control of environmental factors such as nephrotoxic substances (drugs, organic solvents, insecticides, and cleaning agents) is important. Safe use and disposal of such agents in industry, agriculture, and the home must be encouraged. Avoidance of unnecessary urinary tract instrumentation could prevent infection. Elimination of predisease factors such as (1) excessive or inadequate urination and fluid intake patterns, (2) urinary tract problems, (3) bacteriuria in pregnant women, and (4) streptococcal infections should be supported. Renal function should be monitored in patients with hypertension or diabetes mellitus. Being alert to prerenal problems in patients with surgery, burns, or trauma helps prevent complications. Genetic counseling may be indicated for some families.

Acute Renal Failure

Acute renal failure (ARF) is a sudden, severe impairment of renal function causing an acute uremic episode.

Major causes of ARF include acute tubular necrosis, acute glomerulonephritis, acute urinary tract obstruction, nephrotoxic agents, occlusion of the renal artery or vein, acute pyelonephritis, and bilateral cortical necrosis. A wide variety of substances may be nephrotoxic: antibiotics (aminoglycosides), anesthetics, iodinated radiographic contrast medium, organic solvents, heavy metals, endogenous toxins, and abnormal concentrations of physiologic substances. It is helpful to categorize the causes as prerenal, renal, or postrenal:

Prerenal: dehydration; hemorrhage; shock; burns; trauma

Renal: glomerulonephritis; acute pyelonephritis; occlusion of renal artery or vein; bilateral cortical necrosis; nephrotoxic substances; blood transfusion reactions

Postrenal: acute urinary tract obstruction

Prerenal causes result from a decrease in renal blood flow. Renal causes are those resulting from primary damage to the kidneys. Postrenal causes are those involving obstruction of the urinary tract distal to the kidneys. The mortality from ARF is more than 50%.[4] The prognosis depends on the cause and extent of renal failure. The very young and very old are particularly at risk.

ARF is frequently found in older patients in whom the common inciting events are more common. Dehydration is more frequently a cause of ARF in the elderly or in young persons than in middle-aged adults. Elderly patients with multiple system problems or preexisting renal insufficiency are particularly at risk.

The five stages of ARF according to Muehrcke[26] are as follows: (1) onset: usually a short time from precipitating event to onset of oliguria or anuria; (2) oliguric-anuric: time during which output is less than 400 ml/24 hours

(8 to 15 days, if longer prognosis is poor); (3) diuretic, early: from the time when daily output is greater than 400 ml/day to the time that blood urea nitrogen (BUN) stops rising; (4) late or recovery: from the first day BUN falls to the day it stabilizes or is in the normal range; and (5) convalescent: from the day BUN is stable to the day the patient returns to normal activity; urine volume and BUN are normal; may take several months; some patients develop chronic renal failure.

PATHOPHYSIOLOGY

The current explanations for the pathogenesis of ARF include: (1) leakage of tubular fluid from damaged tubules into the interstitial areas, (2) tubular obstructions owing to an accumulation of intratubular debris or casts, (3) glomerular abnormalities, and (4) renal hemodynamic alterations, primarily excessive vasoconstriction.[4]

Damage caused by nephrotoxins appears to affect the proximal tubular epithelium and leave the tubular basement membrane intact. Damage caused by renal ischemia is more widespread and involves patchy areas of epithelial necrosis. Whatever the damage, the glomerular filtration rate decreases and urine formation is impaired.

In prerenal azotemia, urinary osmolality is high (greater than 900 mOsm/kg) and urinary sodium concentrations are low (less than 20 mEq/L), which is consistent with renal hypoperfusion and well-preserved tubular function. These findings reflect the physiologic response to hypovolemia or ineffective circulating blood volume. Urinary findings with parenchymal disorders reflect glomerular damage and inability to conserve Na^+ (urinary Na^+ greater than 27 mEq/L) or concentrate the urine (urine osmolality less than 250 mOsm/kg). In postrenal problems urinary osmolality and Na^+ levels may be normal.

The management of fluid volume before, during, and after surgery helps protect renal function. The use of crystalloid and colloid volume replacement products and blood products helps prevent volume depletion and renal ischemia. When renal function is at risk, nephrotoxic agents such as the anesthetic methoxyflurane and antibiotics such as the aminoglycosides (gentamicin or kanamycin) should be avoided.

DIAGNOSTIC STUDIES

Kidney, ureter, bladder x-ray film and ultrasonography

Kidney size (normal or enlarged); presence or absence of obstruction

TREATMENT PLAN

Attempts are made to prevent decreased renal perfusion from progressing to ARF. Fluids and osmotic agents may be used. In any case, the cause of the ARF is determined if possible. The major complications of ARF in the oliguric phase include acidosis, hyperkalemia, infection, hyperphosphatemia, hypertension, and anemia. Hypovolemia and hypokalemia may be problems in the diuretic phase. Prompt and adequate management is essential to survival.

Chemotherapeutic
Electrolytes
  Alkalinizing agents (for acidosis)
    Sodium bicarbonate, po, IV, 1-4 g/d; 2-5 mEq/ kg infused over 4-8h
    Sodium citrate and citric acid (Shohl's solution,[14] po, 10-20 ml tid (1 mEq Na^+/ml)
  Treatment for hyperkalemia[19]
    Sodium polystyrene sulfonate (Kayexalate) po or enema, 15 g qd-qid; give oral dose in 45-60 ml of water, syrup, fruit juice, or soft drink
    Calcium gluconate, IV, 1 g (90 mg Ca^{++}) in 10 ml
    Sodium bicarbonate, IV, 2-5 mEq/kg infusion over 4-8h
    Glucose 50%, IV, 25-50 g, and insulin-regular, IV, 10-15 units
Anti-infective agents
  Infection is frequently a complication of ARF
  Agents specific to the microorganism cultured should be used
  Agents whose route of excretion is primarily renal should be omitted or used in smaller doses or at lengthened intervals depending on glomerular filtration rate[10]
  Agents excreted by only the liver require no change; when partial excretion occurs via the kidneys, some adjustment is needed at low glomerular filtration rates
Antacids (used as phosphate-binding agents)
  Aluminum carbonate (Basaljel), po, 30-40 ml 1 h pc and at hs of regular strength (400 mg Al (OH)$_3$/ 5 ml); 15-20 ml 1 h pc and at hs of extra strength (1000 mg Al [OH]$_3$/5 ml)
  Aluminum hydroxide gel, dried (Amphojel tab), 8 tab 1 h pc and at hs
Antihypertensive agents
  Clonidine (Catapres), po, 0.1 mg bid or tid initially, then increase by 0.2-0.8 mg/d (maximum effective dose, 2.4 mg/d)
  Diazoxide (Hyperstat IV), IV, adults only: 300 mg by bolus in 30 sec or 1-2 mg/kg up to 150 mg at 5- to 15-min intervals

Hydralazine hydrochloride (Apresoline), po, adults: 10 mg qid for 2-4 d, increase to 25 mg qid, then 50 mg qid; maintenance dose is lowest effective level; children: 0.75 mg/kg initially; increase if needed to 7.5 mg/kg; IM, IV, adults: 10-40 mg repeated as needed (q4-6h); children: initially 1.7-3.5 mg/kg/d in 4-6 divided doses

Methyldopa (Aldomet), po, adults: 250 mg bid or tid for 48 hr, then increase or decrease q2d if needed; maintenance 500 mg-2 g in 2-4 divided doses (maximum 3 g); children: 10 mg, up to 65 mg/kg/24 hr in 2-4 divided doses

Prazosin (Minipress), po, 1 mg bid-tid initially; maintenance may be increased slowly to a maximum of 20 mg/d in divided doses; up to 40 mg/d may be required

Propranolol (Inderal) po, 40 mg bid at 6-8 h intervals; increase if needed to 160-480 mg/d in divided doses; 640 mg/d may be needed

Diuretics

Furosemide (Lasix), po, adults: 20-80 mg followed by second dose in 6-8 h up to 600 mg; children: 2 mg/kg body weight as single dose; may increase by 1 or 2 mg/kg and repeat in 6-8 h; IM, IV, adults: 20-40 mg given slowly over 1-2 min; high dose by IV not more than 4 mg/min; children: 1 mg/kg body weight; may be increased by 1 mg/kg not sooner than 2 h later

Hydrochlorothiazide (Hydrodiuril), po, adults: 25-100 mg/d or bid initially, then maintenance 25-100 mg/d according to patient's response; children: 2.2 mg/kg/d in 2 divided doses

Spironolactone (Aldactone), po, adults: 25-200 mg/d in divided doses initially for 5 d, then adjust to maintenance level; children: 1.5-3.3 mg/kg body weight in 4 divided doses

Packed red blood cells may be needed if there are symptoms associated with anemia

Particular care is needed in all drug administration: dosage, interval between doses, and recognition of increased sensitivity because of altered renal function

Electromechanical

Dialysis, either hemodialysis or peritoneal dialysis, is used to manage fluid volume and electrolyte imbalances (pp. 1085 and 1091); dialysis is particularly needed in pulmonary edema, hyperkalemia, uremic pericarditis, and convulsions, some nephrotoxic agents are dialyzable

Supportive

Fluid intake to equal amount needed to replace measurable losses in urine, nasogastric drainage, wound drainage, and the like; avoid fluid overload; daily weights reflect fluid gain or loss

Nutritional support including maintenance of body weight and positive nitrogen balance[10,29]

Calorie intake should include 100 gm of glucose/day

Protein intake may be maintained through hyperalimentation of essential amino acids (50 to 85 gm/L solutions); oral intake is started as soon as possible; protein intake is 30 to 40 gm/day with 75% of high biologic value; high biologic value proteins are those that contain the essential amino acids in the proportions needed to promote growth such as milk, eggs, and meat

Vitamin supplements are needed since a 40 gm protein diet is deficient in calcium and folic acid and low in phosphorus and the B vitamins

Sodium intake is 60 to 90 mEq/day if edema or hypertension is present; potassium in the diet is restricted to 60 mEq/day if serum levels are over 5 mEq/L

ASSESSMENT: AREAS OF CONCERN

Cardiovascular

Prerenal: hypotension, flat neck veins, low central venous pressure, pulmonary capillary wedge pressure, dry mucous membranes, and decreased skin turgor

Renal: hypertension, edema, enlarged neck veins, elevated central venous pressure, pulmonary capillary wedge pressure, and tachycardia

Cardiac arrhythmias

Respiratory

Shortness of breath; altered breath sounds; hyperventilation; infection

Gastrointestinal

Vomiting, anorexia, and nausea; hematemesis; melena; stomatitis

Renal

Urine volume in relation to intake: normal, oliguria, or anuria; infection; urinary sediment: normal or hematuria, proteinuria, bacteriuria, pyuria, casts (granular, pigment-stained hyaline, red blood cell; white blood cell), epithelial cells, and crystals; osmolality: hyperosmotic, isosmotic, or hyposmotic in relation to serum osmolality; urine pH lowered

Hematologic

Anemia; platelet deficiency

Blood chemistries

Lowered pH, Na^+, Ca^{++}, and HCO_3^-; and elevated

K^+, Cl^-, $PO_4^=$, and Mg^{++}; elevated blood urea nitrogen and serum creatinine; blood urea nitrogen: serum creatinine ratio greater than 10:1; in prerenal azotemia greater than 20:1; and in parenchymal disease less than 20:1; abnormal glucose tolerance curve

Neurologic

Changes in level of consciousness (somnolence or coma); changes in cognitive function or behavior; asterixis; convulsions

General

Septicemia; bruises; pruritus; dry skin; short-term weight changes

NURSING DIAGNOSES and NURSING INTERVENTIONS

Nursing Diagnosis	Nursing Intervention
Tissue perfusion, alteration in: renal	Give medications as ordered. Dosages of all medications may be less than usual and the intervals between doses may be lengthened. Nephrotoxic drugs are usually avoided. Monitor for responses and side effects. Watch K^+ and Ca^{++}, levels if diuretics, digitalis, or banked blood is given. Watch for rapid changes in K^+ levels. Report changes in K^+ levels less than 3.8 mEq/L or greater than 5 mEq/L. Watch for electrocardiographic changes typical of hyperkalemia: peaked T waves, prolonged PR interval, widened QRS complex, and cardiac standstill Watch for acidosis: HCO_3^- less than 22 mEq/L or Kussmaul breathing. Watch for signs of hypocalcemia (tetany): Chvostek or Trousseau signs.
Fluid volume, alteration in: excess or deficit (potential)	Monitor weight, intake and output, blood pressure (sitting and lying), central venous pressure, pulmonary capillary wedge pressure, pulse, respirations, and breath sounds. Hypervolemia occurs in the anuric phase of acute renal failure. Observe neck veins, skin turgor. Be alert to electrolyte losses in body fluid losses. Vomitus contains Na^+, K^+, Cl^-, and water. Diarrhea losses include K^+ and HCO_3^-. Fever and hyperpnea increase water losses. Transudates contain protein-rich fluid.
Potential patient problem: susceptibility to infection	Observe for signs and symptoms of infection and fever. Give meticulous care to any wounds or incisions. Avoid exposure to persons with infections. Establish a routine for deep breathing, coughing, and turning. Give mouth care at regular intervals.
Sensory-perceptual alteration (potential)	Provide safe environment. Assess patient's orientation to time, place, and person. Observe for behavioral changes. Observe level of consciousness. Be alert to possible convulsions.
Thought processes, alteration in (potential)	Provide safe environment. Assess patient's orientation to time, place, and person. Observe for behavioral changes. Observe level of consciousness. Be alert to possible convulsions.
Nutrition, alteration in: less than body requirements	Monitor caloric intake: kinds and amount. Watch for nausea, vomiting, and anorexia. Monitor weight.
Self-care deficit (potential)	Give assistance as necessary in feeding, bathing and hygiene, and toileting.
Mobility, impaired physical	If patient is on bed rest, give assistance with self-care. Implement measures to prevent adverse side effects of bed rest.
Knowledge deficit	Help prepare patient to understand what is happening: diagnosis, treatment, bodily responses, and expected outcomes.

Nursing Diagnosis	Nursing Intervention
Family process, alteration in (potential)	Help family understand what is happening to patient. Help family as needed in meeting the situation.
Coping, ineffective individual (maladaptive; potential)	Support patient's positive coping mechanisms. Help patient develop new coping mechanisms. See p. 1897.

Patient Education

1. Explain the cause of the episode of acute renal failure.
2. Explain the level of renal function after the acute phase is over.
3. Explain diet and fluid restrictions, which may continue, be lessened, or discontinued.
4. Teach self-observational skills such as the measurement of temperature, pulse, respirations, blood pressure, intake and output, daily weight, and record keeping.
5. Explain good personal hygiene.
6. Explain how to avoid infections.
7. Explain exercise and rest in the amounts advised.
8. Describe medications, if any, with name, purpose, dosage, time interval, and adverse reactions (by discussion and in writing).
9. Explain the schedule of medical follow-up.
10. Explain renal dialysis and transplantation if they are likely options for the future.

EVALUATION

Patient Outcome	Data Indicating That Outcome is Reached
Renal functions returns to normal.	There is stable blood urea nitrogen, no edema, normal blood pressure, normal urine volume, and normal activities.
Patient is knowledgeable about acute renal failure.	Patient and family can describe what has occurred and the implications for long-term follow-up of renal function.

Chronic Renal Failure

Chronic renal failure (CRF) is a slow, insidious, and irreversible impairment of renal function. Uremia usually develops slowly.

Major causes of CRF include polycystic kidney disease, chronic glomerulonephritis, chronic pyelonephritis, chronic urinary obstruction, hypertensive nephropathy, diabetic nephropathy, and gouty nephropathy. Causes can be either primary renal disease or another systemic diseases:

Primary renal disease
  Glomerulonephritis; pyelonephritis; polycystic kidneys; hypernephroma
Secondary to systemic disease
  Hypertensive nephropathy; diabetic nephropathy; gouty nephropathy; lupus nephritis; renal amyloidosis; myeloma kidney; nephrocalcinosis; hereditary nephropathy

Levels of chronic renal failure are identified by changes in the glomerular filtration rate.[10] In early renal failure the rate is 30 to 10 ml/minute; in late renal failure it is 10 to 5 ml/minute; in the terminal stage it is 5 ml/minute. Symptoms are prominent in later renal failure and life threatening in terminal renal failure or end-stage renal disease (ESRD). Because patients vary greatly in their clinical picture, renal function, and performance capabilities, the Renal Section of the Council on Circulation of the American Heart Association developed criteria for the Evaluation of the Severity of Established Renal Disease.[10] These criteria take into account (1) the severity of the signs and symptoms, (2) the level of impairment of renal function (glomerular filtration rate and serum creatinine level), and (3) the performance level (what the patient says he is able to do).

PATHOPHYSIOLOGY

Nephrons are permanently destroyed by various processes that occur in the course of renal disease: ischemia, inflammation, necrosis, fibrosis, sclerosis, and scarring.

The normal nephrons remaining may respond with hypertrophy and hyperplasia. A point is reached, however, when renal deficits become manifest. As many as 50% of the nephrons may be lost before renal deficits are discovered.[16] Such deficits include (1) the inability to respond to excessive salt intake or decreased water or salt intake, (2) decreased synthesis of substances such as erythropoietin by the kidney, and (3) the inability to excrete the end products of metabolism. All the organ systems are eventually affected by renal dysfunction.[18]

DIAGNOSTIC STUDIES

Kidney, ureter, bladder roentgenogram and ultrasonography
Small, contracted kidneys

TREATMENT PLAN

The goal of therapy is to delay end-stage renal disease by conservative management and to begin dialysis or perform a renal transplant at the appropriate point in the course of the disease trajectory. Drug dosages and intervals must be modified when the kidney is involved in the drug's excretion. Rates of excretion, metabolism, and sensitivity to drugs may be altered.

Surgical
Renal transplantation (p. 1095); creation of an internal arteriovenous fistula for hemodialysis or insertion of a Tenckhoff catheter for peritoneal dialysis

Chemotherapeutic
Electrolytes for acidosis
Sodium bicarbonate, po, 1-4 g/d; IV, 2-5 mEq/kg infused over 4-8h
Sodium citrate and citric acid (Shohl's solution),[14] po, 10-20 ml tid (1 mEq Na^+/ml)
Treatment for hyperkalemia[19]
Sodium polystyrene sulfonate (Kayexalate) po or enema, 15 g qd-qid; give oral dose in 45-60 ml of water, syrup, fruit juice, or soft drink
Calcium gluconate, IV, 1 g (90 mg Ca^{++}) in 10 ml
Sodium bicarbonate, IV, 2-5 mEq/kg infusion over 8 h
Glucose 50% IV, 25-50 g, and regular insulin, IV, 10-15 units
Anticonvulsant agents
Phenytoin (Dilantin), po, adults: 100 mg tid up to 600 mg/d; children: 4-8 mg/kg/d in 2-3 divided doses
Diazepam (Valium), po, adults: 2-10 mg bid-qid; children: (over 6 mo): 1-25 mg tid-qid

For status epilepticus, IM, IV, adults: 5-10 mg initially; repeat if necessary at 10-15 min intervals, if necessary up to 30 mg; repeat in 2-4 h if necessary; children (under 5 yr old): 0.2-0.5 mg slowly q2-5min up to 5 mg; children (over 5 yr old): 1 mg q2-5min up to 10 mg; repeat in 2-4 h if necessary
Phenobarbital (Luminal), po, adults: 50-100 mg/d; children: 16-50 mg bid or tid
Phenobarbital sodium, IV, adults: 100-320 mg/d
Antihypertensive agents
Clonidine (Catapres) (functions as a adrenergic blocker), po, 0.1 mg bid or tid initially; then increase by 0.2-0.8 mg/d (maximum effective dose 2.4 mg/d)
Diazoxide (Hyperstat IV) (functions as a thiazide), IV, adults only: 300 mg by bolus in 30 sec or 1-2 mg/kg up to 150 mg at 5-15 min intervals
Hydralazine (Apresoline) (functions as a vasodilator), po, adults: 10 mg qid for 2-4 d; increase to 25 mg qid, and then 50 mg qid; maintenance dose is lowest effective level; children: 0.75 mg/kg initially; increase if needed to 7.5 mg/kg; IM, IV, adults: 10-40 mg repeated as needed (q4-6h); children: initially, 1.7-3.5 mg/kg/d in 4-6 divided doses
Methyldopa (Aldomet) (functions as adrenergic blocker), po, adults: 250 mg bid or tid for 48 h, then increase or decrease q2d if needed; maintenance 500 mg-2 g in 2-4 divided doses/d (maximum of 3 g); children (over 10 yr old): up to 65 mg/kg/24 h in 2-4 divided doses
Prazosin (Minipress) (functions as an α-adrenergic blocker), po, 1 mg bid-tid initially; maintenance may be increased slowly to maximum of 20 mg/d in divided doses; up to 40 mg/d may be required
Propranolol (Inderal) (functions as a β-adrenergic blocker), po, 40 mg bid to 6-8 h intervals; increase if needed to 160-480 mg/d in divided doses; 640 mg/d may be needed
Captopril (Capoten) (functions as an angiotensin converting enzyme inhibitor), po, 25 mg tid initially; increase to 50 mg tid in 2-3 wk if necessary; may be increased to 100 mg tid then 150 mg tid
Diuretics
Furosemide (Lasix), po, adults: 20-80 mg followed by second dose in 6-8 h up to 600 mg; children: 2 mg/kg body weight as single dose; may increase by 1 or 2 mg/kg; IM, IV, adults: 20-40 mg given slowly over 1-2 min; high dose by IV not more than 4 mg/min and repeat in 6-8 h; children: 1 mg/kg body weight; may be increased by 1 mg/kg not sooner than 2 h later

Anti-infective agents

Infection is frequently a complication of chronic renal failure

Agents specific to the microorganism cultured should be used

Agents whose route of excretion is primarily renal should be omitted or used in smaller doses or at lengthened intervals depending on glomerular filtration rate[10]; agents excreted by only the liver require no change; if partial excretion occurs via the kidneys, some adjustment is needed at lower glomerular filtration rates

Antacids (used as phosphate-binding agents)

Aluminum carbonate gel (Basaljel), po, 30-40 ml of regular strength (400 mg Al[OH]$_3$/5 ml) or 15-20 ml of extra strength (1000 mg Al[OH]$_3$/5 ml 1 h pc and at hs

Aluminum hydroxide gel (Amphojel), po, 40 ml 1 h pc and at hs

Aluminum hydroxide gel, dried (Amphojel tab), po, 8 tab 1 h pc and at hs

Androgenic agents

Fluoxymesterone (Halotestin), po, adults: 10-30 mg/d

Methandrostenolone (Dianabol), po, adults: 5-20 mg/d

Nandrolone (Deca-Durabolin), IM, adults: up to 300 mg/wk

Antiemetic agents

Prochlorperazine (Compazine), po, adults: 5-10 mg tid-qid; po and rectal, children: 2.5 mg qd-tid or 5 mg bid; maximum of 15 mg/d

Trimethobenzamide (Tigan), po, adults: 250 mg tid or qid; children (15-45 kg): 100-200 mg tid or qid; (<15 kg): 100 mg tid or qid; IM, adults only: 200 mg tid or qid

Antihistamines (for antiemetic effect)

Cyproheptadine (Periactin), po, adults: 4 mg tid or qid not more than 0.5 mg/kg/d; children: 0.25 mg/kg/d in 3 or 4 doses; (2-6 yr): not over 12 mg/d; (7-14 yr): not over 16 mg/d

Phenothiazine (for antiemetic effect)

Trimeprazine tartrate (Temaril), po, adults: 2.5 mg qid; child (>3 yr): 2.5 mg hs or tid; (6 mo-3 yr): 1.25 mg hs or tid

Laxatives/stool softeners

Methylcellulose (Methulose), po, adults: 5-20 ml tid; children: 5-10 ml/d or bid

Docusate sodium (Colace), po, adults and children over 12 yr: 50-200 mg/d; children: (6-12 yr): 40-120 mg/d; (3-6 yr): 20-60 mg/d; (<3 yr): 10-40 mg/d

Electrolytes, minerals, and nutritional replacements

Calcium supplements

Calcium carbonate (Titralac), po, adults: 0.5-2 g 4-6 times daily; children: 1-2 g or 50-100 mEq if GFR is 20-25 ml/min

Calcium gluconate (Kalcinate), po, adults: 1-5 g tid; children: 500 mg/kg/d in divided doses

Hematinic agents

Ferrous sulfate (Feosol), po, adults: 300 mg-1.2 g/d in divided doses; children: (6-12 yr) 120-600 mg/d in divided doses; (<6 yr): 75-225 mg/d in divided doses

Iron-dextran injection (Imferon), IM, IV, adults and children: varies with weight and hemoglobin level

Vitamins

Multivitamin supplements (water-soluble vitamins), daily requirements: thiamine, 1.5 mg/d; riboflavin, 1.8 mg/d; niacin, 20 mg/d; pantothenic acid, 5 mg/d; pyridoxine, 5 mg/d; vitamin B$_{12}$, 3 mg/d; vitamin C, 100 mg/d

Folic acid (Folvite, Folate sodium), po, sc, IM, IV, adults: up to 1 mg/d; children: up to 1 mg/d

Vitamin D

Calcitriol (1,25 dihydroxycholecalciferol) (Rocaltrol), po, 0.25 μg/d; maintenance is 0.5-1 μg/d

Dihydrotachysterol, 0.2-0.4 mg/d

Electromechanical

Dialysis: peritoneal or hemodialysis (see p. 1085)

Supportive

Fluid intake should balance output: about 400 to 600 ml (about the amount of insensible losses) plus an amount equal to 24-hour urine volume; avoid dehydration and volume excess

Nutritional modifications are made to achieve or maintain adequate nutritional status and to reduce work of diseased kidney[1]

Protein: adults: 0.6 g/kg body weight/d; glomerular filtration rate (GFR) 20 to 25 ml/min-90 g/d; GFR 10 to 15 ml/min—50 g/d; GFR 4 to 10 ml/min—40 g/d; children: not less than 1 to 2 g/kg body weight/d

Sodium: adults: 1 to 2 g/d (45 to 90 mEq/d); children: 1 to 3 g/d (45 to 130 mEq/d); the specific amounts depend on weight, blood pressure, serum creatinine, and 24-hour urine sodium excretion

Potassium: 1560 to 2340 mg/d (40 to 60 mEq/d); no restriction is needed with normal urine output (at least 800 ml/d)

Calories: adults: 35 to 55 kcal/kg body weight; children: 60 to 80 kcal/kg body weight; calories from fat and carbohydrates are used; adequate calories must accompany protein intake to prevent the use of protein for energy and weight loss and to support growth in children
Vitamins

ASSESSMENT: AREAS OF CONCERN

Renal
Oliguria; anuria; infection; urine sediment may contain white blood cells, red blood cells, granular, hyaline, and broad and waxy casts

Cardiovascular
Edema; hypertension; tachycardia; anemia; congestive heart failure; pericarditis; arrhythmias; cardiomegaly; atherosclerosis

Dermatologic
Pruritus; excoriations; yellow-tan or grayish color; uremic frost; pallor; bruises; dry skin; thin, bittle nails

Electrolytes
Increased K^+, H^+, Na^+, PO_4^-, and Mg^{++} and decreased HCO_3^- and Ca^{++}

Gastrointestinal
Urinous odor on breath; metallic taste; stomatitis and gingivitis; loss of sense of smell; anorexia; nausea; vomiting and hematemesis; esophagitis; gastritis; hiccoughs; melena; diarrhea or constipation; thirst

Metabolic
Increased blood urea nitrogen and serum creatinine levels; increased uric acid level; anion gap greater than 9 to 13 mEq/L; carbohydrate intolerance and altered glucose tolerance curve (delayed rate of decrease); altered insulin degradation (decreased renal extraction); hypertriglyceridemia (impaired removal of triglycerides by lipoprotein lipase activity); acidosis; tetany

Neurologic
Changes in cognitive function and behavior; altered levels of consciousness (drowsiness to coma and convulsions); changes in motor function and proprioception; peripheral neuropathy; nocturnal leg cramping; formication and other paresthesias of lower extremities; apathy, lethargy, and fatigue; headaches

Ocular
Retinal changes (hypertension); ''red eyes'' (calcification of conjunctiva); blurred vision

Reproductive
Infertility; impotence; amenorrhea; decreased libido; gynecomastia; failure of children to mature sexually

Respiratory
Pulmonary edema; pneumonia; pleural effusions; hyperventilation; Kussmaul breathing; apnea

Skeletal
Renal osteodystrophy; soft tissue calcification; fractures; bone pain; increased alkaline phosphatase

General
Weight loss; retarded growth rate in children

NURSING DIAGNOSES and NURSING INTERVENTIONS

Nursing Diagnosis	Nursing Intervention
Tissue perfusion, alteration in: renal	Give medications as ordered by physician. Be alert to altered dosages and schedules. Monitor response and side effects. Watch K^+ and Ca^{++} levels. Watch for electrocardiographic changes typical of hyperkalemia: peaked T waves, prolonged PR intervals, widened QRS complex, and cardiac standstill. Watch for signs of acidosis: HCO_3^- less than 22 mEq/L and Kussmaul breathing. Watch for signs of tetany: Chvostek and Trousseau signs.
Fluid volume, alteration in: excess, actual or potential	Monitor weight, intake, output, blood pressure (standing and sitting to detect postural hypotension), pulse, and respiration. Observe for thirst, tachycardia, dry mouth, venous jugular distention, and decreased skin turgor. Observe for dyspnea and edema, and listen for rales. Spread limited fluid intake over 24 hours. Cool liquids help quench thirst. Be alert for electrolyte losses in body fluid losses: Vomitus contains Na^+, K^+,

Nursing Diagnosis	Nursing Intervention
	H$^+$, Cl$^-$, and water. Diarrhea losses include K$^+$ and HCO$_3^-$. Fever and hyperpnea increase water losses.
Potential patient problem: susceptibility to infection	Observe for signs and symptoms of infection and temperature elevation. Note that a hypercatabolic state such as infection can cause life-threatening hyperkalemia. Give meticulous care to any wound or incision. Avoid persons with infections. Establish a routine for deep breathing, coughing, and turning. Give mouth care at regular intervals.
Sensory-perceptual alteration (potential)	Provide safe environment. Assess orientation to time, place, and person. Observe for behavioral changes. Observe level of consciousness. Implement seizure precautions. See p. 1967.
Skin integrity, impairment of	Excoriations of the skin may be related to pruritus. Relieve pruritus: oral drugs may help, as may vinegar or starch baths. Keep fingernails trimmed. Watch for infections. Elevate edematous extremities. Avoid trauma. Use bland soap.
Thought processes, alteration in (potential)	Provide safe environment. Assess orientation to time, place, and person. Observe for behavioral changes. Observe level of consciousness. Use frequent, simple explanations. Do not argue. See p. 1961.
Nutrition, alteration in: less than body requirements	Monitor intake of food to maintain limited protein, sodium, potassium, fluid, and high-calorie diet. Dietary supplements may be ordered. If nausea and vomiting interfere with meals, give antiemetics. Postpone meals. Attractively served foods the patient likes increase intake. Prevent dehydration. Mouth care helps the bad taste in the mouth. Sour candy balls and gum also help. Monitor weight.
Self-care deficit (potential)	Give assistance as necessary in feeding, bathing and hygiene, and toileting. Encourage independence.
Mobility, impaired physical (potential)	See interventions for self-care deficit. If bed rest is needed, implement measures to prevent complications of bed rest. If patient is ambulatory, encourage physical activity to patient's tolerance.
Sleep pattern disturbance	Provide time for rest and sleep. Be aware that uremia can reverse normal sleep-wake patterns.
Knowledge deficit	Help prepare patient to understand what is happening: diagnosis, treatment, bodily response, and expected outcomes. Teach diet, fluid restrictions, self-observational skills (temperature, pulse, respirations, blood pressure, and input and output), record keeping, avoidance of infection, personal hygiene, exercise-rest balance, and medications (dosage, purpose, interval, and adverse reactions).
Self-concept, disturbance in: body image	Observe patient's response to having a chronic illness, altered renal function, alteration in other body systems, or possibility of dialysis or transplantation in the future. Recognize denial, guilt, aggression, fear, displacement, regression, resentment, disbelief, and anxiety in patient. Recognize changes in psychosocial aspects of patient's life: change in social interaction, irritability, hostility, extreme dependence, fear of rejection, inability

Nursing Diagnosis	Nursing Intervention
	to work, loss of job, decreased financial stability, and altered hopes for the future.
	Identify significant aspects of patient's cultural background and religion that may affect responses to chronic renal failure.
	Help patient move through denial and discouragement, to acceptance of the condition, and to rehabilitation by sharing information needed, listening, and offering continuing emotional support. Refer patient to other professional resources as needed.
	See p. 1820.
Sexual dysfunction	Help patient and spouse understand physiologic basis of dysfunction.
	Suggest positive aspects of closeness and touching without intercourse.
	See p. 2004.
Family process, alteration in (potential)	Involve family from the beginning in all items under knowledge deficit and help them understand patient's responses.
	Work with health team as they help family meet illness situation.

Patient Education

1. Explain the nature of chronic renal failure.
2. Explain the medical regimen and its rationale, including diet (restricted protein, sodium, and potassium intake), restricted fluid intake, and medications (purpose, dosage, interval, and adverse reactions).
3. Teach self-observational skills (temperature, pulse, respirations, blood pressure, intake and output, and weight) and record keeping.
4. Explain avoidance of infection.
5. Explain personal hygiene, rest, and exercise.
6. Explain when to call the physician.
7. Explain the plan for medical follow-up.
8. Explain renal dialysis and transplantation.

EVALUATION

Patient Outcome	Data Indicating That Outcome is Reached
Patient is knowledgeable about CRF and its treatment.	Patient and family describe CRF, medical plan of care, and future options for renal dialysis or transplantation.
Conservative management of CRF is effective.	There is no uremia, glomerular filtration rate is greater than 15 ml/minute, and serum creatinine level is less than 10 mg/dl.
If CRF progresses, dialysis or transplantation is instituted when needed.	There are persistent signs and symptoms of uremia, serum creatinine level is greater than 10 mg/dl, and glomerular filtration rate is less than 10 to 15 ml/minute.[31]

RENAL TUBULAR ACIDOSIS

Renal tubular acidosis (RTA) occurs when the kidney is unable to excrete an acid urine because of a defect in the tubules. Hyperchloremic acidosis ensues.

Both infants and adults may have tubular defects in acid handling. Causes of RTA may be hereditary or associated with cystinosis and hyperparathyroidism.

ions. If the defect is in the distal tubule, acidification of the urine is impaired and hypokalemia occurs. Renal function is otherwise normal. A third type of RTA has defects in both parts of the tubule and has a normal or elevated serum K^+ level. Renal calculi occur frequently in patients with distal RTA (see p. 1062).

PATHOPHYSIOLOGY

The tubular defect may be in the proximal tubule, which causes a failure in the usual reabsorption of bicarbonate

TREATMENT PLAN

Chemotherapeutic

Electrolytes (alkalinizing agents)

Sodium bicarbonate, Shohl's solution, or Polycitra; for distal RTA: po, adults: 1-3 mEq/kg/d; children: 0.5-2 mEq/kg/d; for proximal RTA: po, adults: 5-10 mEq/kg/d; children: 3-5 mEq/kg/d

The acidosis must be corrected slowly to avoid further lowering the potassium level

Diuretics (for proximal RTA)

Hydrochlorothiazide (Hydrodiuril) (to decrease Ca^{++} excretion), 1.5-2 mg/kg/d

Potassium supplement (for proximal RTA if serum K^+ <3 mEq/L) KCl (4 mEq K^+/5 ml), po, adults: 20 mEq/kg/d in divided doses; children: 1-3 mEq/kg/d in divided doses

ASSESSMENT: AREAS OF CONCERN

Renal

Distal: urine pH greater than 6.0; hypercalciuria greater than 4 mg/kg/day; nephrocalcinosis

Proximal: urine pH 4.5 to 8.0

Blood chemistries

Hyperchloremic acidosis; hypokalemia less than 3 mEq/L

General

Weakness and lethargy; anorexia; bone pain; impaired growth in children and failure to thrive

NURSING DIAGNOSES and NURSING INTERVENTIONS

Nursing Diagnosis	Nursing Intervention
Potential patient problem: altered acid-base balance	Monitor serum levels of H^+, HCO_3^-, Ca^{++}, K^+, and blood pH. Monitor urinary calcium levels (Sulkowitch test), which become normal (2 to 3 mg/kg/day) when adequate alkali is given for distal renal tubular acidosis. Sulkowitch test: Add a special reagent to a urine sample taken after a meal. Results give a qualitative measure of urine calcium: fine white cloud—normal Ca^{++}; clear solution—decreased Ca^{++}; heavy precipitation—excess Ca^{++}. Watch for tetany caused by hypocalcemia: Trousseau or Chvostek's signs.

Patient Education

1. Explain the nature of the RTA.
2. Explain the treatment regimen: alkalinizing agent with dosage, interval, and side effects.
3. Teach the patient to check urine for pH and calcium.
4. Explain medical follow-up.

EVALUATION

Patient Outcome	Data Indicating That Outcome is Reached
Patient is knowledgeable about RTA.	Patient and family describe RTA and medical management being instituted.
Acid-base imbalance is corrected.	Urine pH is 4.5 to 8.0. Urine calcium is 2 to 3 mg/kg/day. Serum HCO_3^- is 24 to 28 mEq/L. Serum chloride is 97 to 107 mmol/L. Serum potassium is 3.5 to 5.0 mEq/L. Serum pH is 7.32 to 7.43.
Nephrocalcinosis and renal calculi are prevented.	Roentgenograms reveal neither calcifications nor obstruction of urinary tract.

RENAL VASCULAR ABNORMALITIES
Renal Artery Occlusion or Stenosis

Renal artery occlusion is a sudden complete blockage of the renal artery or a branch of it. Stenosis is a narrowing of the artery.

PATHOPHYSIOLOGY

The complete cessation of arterial blood flow causes an infarct with coagulation necrosis in the kidney. If the person has a single kidney, acute oliguric renal failure ensues. Occlusion is most frequently the result of an embolism caused by mitral valve stenosis, subacute bacterial endocarditis, and mural thrombi after a myocardial infarction.

Severe stenosis caused by atherosclerosis leads to ischemic atrophy and fibrosis. Decreased pressure in the arterioles stimulates the juxtaglomerular apparatus to produce an increase in renin secretion and can lead to renovascular hypertension.

DIAGNOSTIC STUDIES

Intravenous urogram or renal arteriogram
   Absence of function in all or part of the kidney is seen as radiopaque dye is filtered by the kidney

TREATMENT PLAN

A conservative approach is used. Patients usually have serious cardiac disease.

Surgical
   Embolectomies not usually performed for renal artery occlusion; renal damage usually has occurred by time diagnosis is made
   Selected patients with renal artery stenosis may have surgical correction; percutaneous transluminal angioplasty may be used[10]

Chemotherapeutic
   Anticoagulants (used for renal artery occlusion)
      Heparin sodium, IV, sc, adults: 10,000-20,000 units initially, (68 kg man); maintenance 8,000-10,000 units q8h or 15,000-20,000 units q12h; IV, children: 50 units/kg initially; 50-100 units/kg q4h maintenance

   Analgesics
      Meperidine (Demerol), po, sc, IM, IV, adults: 50-150 mg q3-4h; children: 1 mg/kg q4h up to 100 mg q4h
      Codeine sulfate, po, sc, IM, adults: 15-60 mg qid; children: 3 mg/kg/day divided into 6 doses
      Morphine sulfate, po, sc, IM, adults: 5-15 mg q4h prn; children: 0.1-0.2 mg/kg/dose not to exceed 15 mg
   Antihypertensive agents (used for renal artery stenosis)
      β-Blockers
         Propranolol (Inderal), po, 40 mg q6 or q8h initially; increased to 160-480 mg/d in divided doses; up to 640 mg/d
      Angiotensin antagonists
         Captopril (Capoten), po, 25 mg tid initially; may be increased to 50 mg tid after 1-2 wk then to 100-150 mg tid as needed

Electromechanical
   Dialysis may be needed (see p. 1085)

Supportive
   Relief of pain of renal artery occlusion
   Monitoring of contralateral kidney function
   Stabilization of cardiac function
   Sodium and fluid restrictions for renal artery stenosis (see discussion of hypertension in Chapter 1)

ASSESSMENT: AREAS OF CONCERN

Renal artery occlusion
   Renal
      Microscopic hematuria; few signs if infarct is small
   General
      Pain in flank or upper abdomen; elevated white blood cell count; elevated lactic dehydrogenase (LDH) level

Renal artery stenosis
   Cardiovascular
      Hypertension
   Renal
      Increased plasma renin activity in renal vein; renal artery bruit

NURSING DIAGNOSES and NURSING INTERVENTIONS

Nursing Diagnosis	Nursing Intervention
Tissue perfusion, alteration in: renal and fluid volume, alteration in: excess (potential)	Monitor intake and output, weight, blood pressures (standing and lying), and urine changes. Monitor heart rate. Monitor Na^+ and fluid intake if necessary. Monitor neck veins, central venous pressure, and pulmonary capillary wedge pressure if necessary. Give medications as ordered. Observe responses for side effects. Watch for side effects of anticoagulants: signs of hemorrhaging, injury, change in stools, localized bleeding, epistaxis, and bruises. Give preoperative and postoperative care, if indicated.
Comfort, alteration in: pain	Give analgesics as needed if ordered and monitor response.

Patient Education

1. Explain the nature of renal artery occlusion or stenosis.
2. Explain the treatment regimen and rationale.
3. Explain follow-up medical care.

EVALUATION

Patient Outcome	Data Indicating That Outcome is Reached
Some function returns after renal artery occlusion.	Patient has improved renal function findings.
Medical therapy or surgery helps renal artery stenosis.	Hypertension is relieved or controlled.

Renal Vein Thrombosis

The renal vein or a branch of it can be blocked by an embolus or thrombus.

Renal vein thrombosis is most frequently associated with nephrotic syndrome (NS). It may also accompany a neoplasm that compresses the renal vein.

PATHOPHYSIOLOGY

A sudden and complete occlusion of the renal vein causes an infarct. The kidney swells, pressing against the capsule. Slow development of an occlusion may permit the development of collateral venous circulation and cause less impairment of renal function.

DIAGNOSTIC STUDIES

Intravenous urogram
  Unilateral change in kidney function when radiopaque dye injected

Venogram
  Demonstrable clot

TREATMENT PLAN

The prevention of pulmonary emboli is vital. The underlying cause of the NS should be treated if possible (see "Nephrotic Syndrome").

Chemotherapeutic
  Anticoagulants
    Heparin sodium, IV, sc, adults: 10,000-20,000 units initially (68 kg man); maintenance of 8000-10,000 units q8h or 15,000-20,000 units q12h; IV, children: 50 units/kg initially; 50-100 units/kg q4h maintenance
    Warfarin (Coumadin), po, IM, IV, 10-15 mg/d for 2-3 days; then maintenance dose of 2-10 mg/d

ASSESSMENT: AREAS OF CONCERN

Renal
  Gross hematuria; signs of nephrotic syndrome: proteinuria (albuminuria) >3 gm/day, foamy, deep yellow urine, oliguria

Other
  Pain in flank

NURSING DIAGNOSES and NURSING INTERVENTIONS

Nursing Diagnosis	Nursing Intervention
Tissue perfusion, alteration in: renal	Monitor urine losses of protein. Monitor serum protein, blood urea nitrogen, and creatinine. Give anticoagulants and watch for side effects: signs of hemorrhaging; bleeding due to injury; change in urine, stools, and other body fluids; and bruises and ecchymoses.
Comfort, alteration in: pain	Give ordered analgesics as needed and observe patient's response.

Patient Education

1. Explain the nature of renal vein thrombosis.
2. Explain the medical regimen and rationale.
3. Explain the plan for medical follow-up.

EVALUATION

Patient Outcome	Data Indicating That Outcome is Reached
Renal function returns.	Renal function tests are normal.
Renal function is impaired.	Renal function findings are abnormal.

Diabetic Nephropathy

Diabetic nephropathy refers to glomerulosclerosis caused by lesions of the arterioles and glomeruli and associated with pyelonephritis and necrosis of the renal papillae.

Diabetic nephropathy (DN) or diabetic glomerulosclerosis is a very important complication of adult onset diabetes mellitus and the most important complication leading to death in juvenile onset diabetes.[35] The changes are related to the duration of the diabetic state. All insulin-dependent diabetic patients can expect the development of DN. Once proteinuria occurs, the renal changes invariably progress. Patients with diabetic nephropathy have increased morbidity and mortality. Although the survival of diabetic patients treated with dialysis or transplantation has improved somewhat in recent years, the outcomes are not nearly as good as in nondiabetic patients.[12] Diabetic patients have particular problems with atherosclerosis, coronary artery disease, peripheral vascular disease, retinopathy, and neurologic deficits. The likelihood of their successful rehabilitation is limited.

PATHOPHYSIOLOGY

The glomeruli are affected by diffuse sclerosis and thickening of the basement membrane and mesangial areas.

Nodular glomerulosclerosis may also occur. Both afferent and efferent arterioles are affected by thickened walls and hyaline deposits. The glomerular filtration rate decreases and azotemia occurs. The diabetic patient may appear clinically uremic at levels lower than the nondiabetic patient. This may be related to their systemic vascular changes.[35]

TREATMENT PLAN

Some authorities believe that control of blood pressure and fluctuations in blood sugar levels slows the deterioration of renal function. Others believe that diabetic nephropathy follows an inexorable downhill course.[35]

Surgical

See "Renal Transplantation" (p. 1095). Diabetic patients who have a renal transplant have more complications, poorer rehabilitation, and a lower survival rate than nondiabetic patients with a renal transplant[35]; the underlying disease process cannot be corrected by transplantation

Chemotherapeutic

Insulin requirements may decrease as renal degradation of the hormone decreases or may increase as resistance to insulin's effects increases; antihypertensive drugs and diuretics may be needed

Electrolytes, minerals

Alkalinizing agents (for acidosis)

Sodium bicarbonate, po, 1-4 g/d; IV, 2-5 mEq/kg infused over 4-8 h

Treatment for hyperkalemia[19]

Sodium polystyrene sulfonate (Kayexalate), po or enema, 15 g qd-qid; give po dose in 45-60 ml of water, syrup, fruit juice, or soft drink

Calcium gluconate, IV, 1 g (90 mg Ca^{++}) in 10 ml

Sodium bicarbonate, IV, 2-5 mEq/kg infusion over 8 h

Glucose 50%, IV, 25-50 g, and regular insulin, IV, 10-15 units

Anticonvulsive agents

Phenytoin (Dilantin), po, adults: 100 mg tid up to 600 mg/d; children: 4-8 mg/kg/d in 2-3 divided doses

Diazepam (Valium), po, adults: 2-10 mg bid-qid; children (over 6 mo): 1-25 mg tid-qid

Phenobarbital (Luminal), po, adults: 50-100 mg/d; children: 16-50 mg bid-tid

Antihypertensive agents

Clonidine (Catapres) (adrenergic blocker), po, 0.1 mg bid or tid initially; then increase by 0.2-0.8 mg/d (maximum effective dose, 2.4 mg/d)

Diazoxide (Hyperstat IV) (thiazide), IV, adults only: 300 mg by bolus in 30 sec or 1-2 mg/kg up to 150 mg at 5-15 min intervals

Hydralazine (Apresoline) (vasodilator), po, adults: 10 mg qid for 2-4 d; increase to 25 mg qid then 50 mg qid; maintenance dose is lowest effective level; children: 0.75 mg/kg initially; increase if needed to 7.5 mg/kg; IM, IV, adults: 10-40 mg repeated as needed (q4-6h); children: initially 1.7-3.5 mg/kg/d in 4-6 divided doses

Methyldopa (Aldomet) (adrenergic blocker), po, adults: 250 mg bid or tid for 48 h; then increase or decrease q2d if needed; maintenance 500 mg to 2 g in 2-4 divided doses/d (maximum 3 g); children: 10 up to 65 mg/kg/24 h in 2-4 divided doses

Prazosin (Minipress) (α-adrenergic blocker), po, 1 mg bid-tid initially; maintenance may be increased slowly to maximum of 20 mg/d in divided doses; up to 40 mg/d may be required

Propranolol (Inderal) (β-adrenergic blocker), po, 40 mg bid at 6-8 h intervals; increase if needed to 160-480 mg/d in divided doses; 640 mg/d may be needed

Captopril (Capoten) (angiotensin converting enzyme inhibitor), po, 25 mg tid initially; increase to 50 mg tid in 2-3 wk if necessary; may be increased to 100 mg tid then to 150 mg tid

Diuretics

Furosemide (Lasix), po, adults: 20-80 mg followed by second dose in 6-8 h up to 600 mg; children: 2 mg/kg body weight as single dose; may increase by 1 or 2 mg/kg; IM, IV, adults: 20-40 mg given slowly over 1-2 min; high dose by IV not more than 4 mg/min and repeat in 6-8 h; children: 1 mg/kg body weight; may be increased by 1 mg/kg not sooner than 2 h later

Anti-infective agents

Infection is frequently a complication of nephropathy/chronic renal failure

Agents specific to the microorganism cultured should be used

Agents whose route of excretion is primarily renal need to be used in smaller doses or at lengthened intervals depending on glomerular filtration rate[10]; agents excreted by only the liver require no change; if partial excretion occurs via the kidneys, some adjustment is needed at lower glomerular filtration rates

Antacids (used as a phosphate-binding agent)

Aluminum carbonate gel (Basaljel), po, 30-40 ml of regular strength (400 mg Al $(OH)_3$/5 ml), 15-20 ml 1 h pc and at hs or extra strength (1000 mg $Al(OH)_3$/5 ml) at same dosage

Aluminum hydroxide gel (Amphojel), po, 40 ml 1 h pc and at hs

Aluminum hydroxide gel, dried (Amphojel tab), po, 8 tab 1 h pc and at hs

Androgenic agents

Fluoxymesterone (Halotestin), po, adults: 10-30 mg/d

Methandrostenolone (Dianabol), po, adults: 5-20 mg/d

Nandrolone decanoate (Deca-Durabolin), IM, adults: up to 200 mg/wk

Antiemetic agents

Prochlorperazine (Compazine), po, adults: 5-10 mg tid-qid; po and rectal, children: 2.5 mg qd-tid or 5 mg bid; maximum 15/kg/d

Antipruritic agents

Cyproheptadine (Periactin) (antihistamine), po, adults: 4 mg tid or qid not more than 0.5 mg/kg/d; children: 0.25 mg/kg/d in 3 or 4 doses; (2-6 yr): not over 12 mg/d; (7-14 yr): not over 16 mg/d

Trimeprazine tartrate (Temaril) (phenothiazine), po, adults: 2.5 mg qid; children: (>3 yr): 2.5 mg hs or tid; (6 mo-3 yr): 1.25 mg hs or tid

Laxatives/stool softeners

Methylcellulose (Methulose), po, adults: 5-20 ml tid; children: 5-10 ml/d or bid

Docusate sodium (Colace), po, adults and children over 12 yr: 50-200 mg/d; children (6-12 yr): 40-120 mg/d; (3-6 yr): 20-60 mg/d; (<3 yr): 10-40 mg/d

Electrolytes, minerals

Calcium (supplement): Calcium carbonate (Titra-lac), po, adults: 0.5-2 g 4-6 times daily; children: 1-2 g or 50-100 mEq if GFR 20-25 ml/min

Calcium gluconate (Kalcinate), po, adults: 1-5 g tid; children: 500 mg/kg/d in divided doses

Hematinic agents

Ferrous sulfate (Feosol), po, adults: 300 mg-1.2 g/d in divided doses; children: (6-12 yr): 120-600 mg/d in divided doses; (<6 yr): 75-225 mg/d in divided doses

Iron-dextran injection (Imferon), IV, IM, adults and children: varies with weight and hemoglobin level

Vitamins

Multivitamin supplements (water-soluble vitamins)
Thiamine, 1.5 mg/d
Riboflavin, 1.8 mg/d
Niacin, 20.0 mg/d
Pyridoxine, 5.0 mg/d
Vitamin B_{12}, 3.0 mg/d
Vitamin C, 100 mg/d

Folic acid (Folvite), folate sodium, po, sc, IM, IV, adults: up to 1 mg/d; children: up to 1 mg/d; adults, maintenance: up to 0.3 mg/d; children (4 yr): up to 0.1 mg/d; infants: up to 0.1 mg/d

Vitamin D

Calcitriol (1,25-dihydroxycholecalciferol) (Ro-caltrol), po, 0.25 μg/d; maintenance: 0.5-1 μg/d

Dihydrotachysterol, 0.2-0.4 mg/d

Electromechanical

See "Hemodialysis" and "Peritoneal Dialysis" (pp. 1085 and 1091); the underlying disease process cannot be corrected by dialysis; vascular complications of diabetes cause major problems in access to vascular system for hemodialysis

Supportive

Fluid intake should balance output: about 400 to 600 ml (about amount of insensible losses) plus amount equal to 24-hour urine volume; avoid dehydration and volume excess; specific amount determined by patient's dry weight (weight at which, after dialysis, patient has normal volume relationships)[24]

Nutritional modifications are made to achieve or maintain adequate nutritional status and to reduce work of diseased kidney[1]

Protein, adults: 0.6 g/kg body weight/day; glomerular filtration rate (GFR), 20 to 25 ml/minute to 90 g/day; GFR, 10 to 15 ml/minute to 50 g/day; GFR, 4 to 10 ml/minute to 40 g/day; children: not less than 1 to 2 g/kg body weight/day

Sodium, adults: 1 to 2 g/day (45 to 90 mEq/day); children: 1 to 3 g/day (45 to 130 mEq/day); specific amounts depend on weight, blood pressure, serum creatinine, and 24-hour sodium excretion

Potassium, 1560 to 2340 mg/day (40 to 60 mEq/day); with normal urine output (at least 800 ml/day), no restriction is needed

Calories, adults: 35 to 55 kcal/kg body weight/day; children: 60 to 80 kcal/kg ideal body weight/day; calories from fat and carbohydrate are used; adequate calories must accompany protein intake to prevent use of protein for energy and weight loss and to support growth in children; control of protein intake takes priority in nutritional management; calories from fat and carbohydrates are increased

ASSESSMENT: AREAS OF CONCERN

Renal

Proteinuria; oliguria; anuria; infection; urine sediment may contain white and red blood cells, granular, hyaline, broad, and waxy casts

Cardiovascular

Hypertension; edema

NURSING DIAGNOSES and NURSING INTERVENTIONS

Nursing Diagnosis	Nursing Intervention
Tissue perfusion, alteration in: renal	Give medications as ordered and monitor response. Be alert to altered dosage and schedules. Watch K^+, and Ca^{++}, levels. Watch for electrocardiographic changes: peaked T waves, prolonged PR intervals, widened QRS complex, and cardiac standstill. Watch for signs of hypocalcemia (tetany) and Chvostek and Trousseau signs.

Nursing Diagnosis	Nursing Intervention
	Radiocontrast medium in diagnostic tests should be avoided. Diabetic patients with renal insufficiency are at risk for severe allergic reactions to the contrast medium. Avoiding dehydration and decreasing the dosage do not appear to prevent renal damage.[12] Avoid nephrotoxic agents.
Fluid volume, alteration in: excess (actual or potential)	Monitor weight, intake, output, blood pressure (standing and sitting to detect postural hypotension), pulse, and respirations. Observe for thirst, tachycardia, dry mouth, venous jugular distention, and decreased skin turgor. Observe for dyspnea and edema and listen for rales. Spread limited fluid intake over 24 hours. Cool liquids help quench thirst. Be alert for electrolyte losses in body fluid losses. Vomitus contains Na^+, K^+, H^+, Cl^-, and water. Diarrhea losses include K^+ and HCO_3^-. Fever and hyperpnea increase water losses.
Potential patient problem: susceptibility to infection	Observe for signs and symptoms of infection and temperature. Note that a hypercatabolic state such as infection can cause life-threatening hyperkalemia. Give meticulous care to any wound or incision. Avoid exposure to persons with infections. Establish a routine for deep breathing, coughing, and turning. Give mouth care at regular intervals.
Sensory-perceptual alteration (potential)	Provide safe environment. Assess orientation to time, place, and person. Observe for behavioral changes. Observe level of consciousness. Implement seizure precautions.
Skin integrity, impairment of	Excoriations of the skin may be related to pruritus. Relieve pruritus; oral drugs may help, as may vinegar or starch baths. Seek order in collaboration with physician. Keep fingernails trimmed. Watch for infections. Elevate edematous extremities. Avoid trauma. Use bland soap.
Thought processes, alteration in (potential)	Provide safe environment. Assess orientation to time, place, and person. Observe for behavioral changes. Observe level of consciousness. Use frequent, simple explanations. Do not argue. See p. 1961.
Nutrition, alteration in: less than body requirements	Monitor intake of food to maintain limited protein, sodium, potassium, fluid, and high-calorie diet. Dietary supplements may be ordered. If nausea and vomiting interfere with meals, give antiemetics as ordered by physician. Postpone meals. Attractively served foods the patient likes increase intake. Prevent dehydration. Mouth care helps the bad taste in the mouth. Sour candy balls and gum also help. Monitor weight.
Self-care deficit (potential)	Give assistance as necessary in feeding, bathing and hygiene, and toileting. Encourage independence.
Mobility, impaired physical	Give assistance as necessary in feeding, bathing and hygiene, and toileting. Encourage independence. Establish routine for changing positions. If patient is ambulatory, encourage physical activity to patient's tolerance.
Sleep pattern disturbance	Provide time for rest and sleep. Be aware that uremia can reverse normal sleep-wake patterns.
Knowledge deficit	Help prepare patient to understand what is happening: diagnosis, treatment, bodily response, and expected outcomes.

Nursing Diagnosis	Nursing Intervention
	Teach diet, fluid restrictions, self-observational skills (temperature, pulse, respirations, blood pressure, and intake and output), record keeping, avoidance of infection, personal hygiene, exercise-rest balance, and medications (dosage, purpose, interval, and adverse reactions).
Self-concept, disturbance in: body image	Observe patient's response to having a chronic illness, altered renal function, alteration in other body systems, and the possibility of renal dialysis or transplantation in the future.
	Recognize denial, guilt, aggression, fear, displacement, regression, resentment, disbelief, and anxiety in patient.
	Recognize changes in psychosocial aspects of patient's life: change in social interaction, irritability, hostility, extreme dependence, fear of rejection, inability to work, loss of job, decreased financial stability, and altered hopes for the future.
	Identify significant aspects of patient's cultural background and religion that may affect response to chronic renal failure.
	Help patient move through stages of denial, discouragement, acceptance of the condition, and rehabilitation. Share information needed, listen, and offer continuing emotional support. Refer patient to other professional resources as needed.
	See p. 1820.
Sexual dysfunction	Help patient understand physiologic basis for dysfunction.
	Help spouse understand.
	Suggest positive aspects of closeness and touching even without intercourse.
	See p. 2004.
Family process, alteration in (potential)	Involve the family from the beginning and help them understand patient's responses.
	Work with health team as they help family meet illness situation.

Patient Education

1. Explain the nature of diabetic nephropathy and chronic renal failure.
2. Explain the medical regimen and its rationale, including diet (restricted protein, sodium, and potassium), restricted fluid intake, and medications (purpose, dosage, interval, and adverse reactions).
3. Teach the patient self-observational skills (temperature, pulse, respirations, blood pressure, intake and output, and weight) and record keeping.
4. Explain avoidance of infection.
5. Explain personal hygiene, rest, and exercise.
6. Explain when to call the physician.
7. Explain the plan for medical follow-up.
8. Explain renal dialysis and transplantation.

EVALUATION

Patient Outcome	Data Indicating That Outcome is Reached
Patient is knowledgeable about diabetic nephropathy and its treatment.	Patient and family describe diabetic nephropathy, medical plan of care, and future options for renal dialysis or transplantation.
Conservative management of nephropathy is effective.	There is no uremia, glomerular filtration rate is 15 ml/min, and serum creatinine level is less than 10 mg/dl.
If nephropathy progresses, dialysis or transplantation is instituted when needed.	Signs and symptoms of uremia persist, serum creatinine level is greater than 10 mg/dl, and glomerular filtration rate is less than 10 to 15 ml/minute.[31]

NEPHROSCLEROSIS

Severe hypertension can cause deterioration in renal function. Nephrosclerosis is the damage to the renal arteries, arterioles, and glomeruli caused by prolonged elevated blood pressure.

PATHOPHYSIOLOGY

A slow, variable progression of vascular changes can occur over the years. The process includes spasm, thickening, hypertrophy, and hyaline degeneration of the renal arterial system. In malignant hypertension renal changes are rapid and include fibrinoid necrosis.

TREATMENT PLAN

Goals of therapy include aggressive control of blood pressure to slow renal deterioration, delay of end-stage renal disease by conservative management, and initiation of dialysis or performance of a renal transplant at the appropriate point in the course of the disease. Drug dosages and intervals must be modified when the kidney is involved in the drug's excretion. Rates of excretion and metabolism and sensitivity to drugs may be altered.

Surgical

Transplantation of donor kidney as described on p. 1095 may be needed; patient may be prepared with adequate dialysis for surgery (see ''Hemodialysis,'' p. 1085); uremic problems are controlled before surgery

Chemotherapeutic

Antihypertensive agents

Clonidine (Catapres) (adrenergic blocker), po, 0.1 mg bid or tid initially; then increase by 0.2-0.8 mg/d (maximum effective dose; 2.4 mg/d)

Diazoxide (Hyperstat IV) (thiazide), IV, adults only: 300 mg by bolus in 30 sec or 1-2 mg/kg up to 150 mg at 5- to 15-min intervals

Hydralazine (Apresoline) (vasodilator), po, adults: 10 mg qid for 2-4 d; increase to 25 mg qid, then 50 mg qid; maintenance dose is lowest effective level; children: 0.75 mg/kg initially; increase if needed to 7.5 mg/kg; IM, IV, adults: 10-40 mg repeated as needed (q4-6h); children: initially 1.7-3.5 mg/kg/d in 4-6 divided doses

Methyldopa (Aldomet) (adrenergic blocker), po, adults: 250 mg bid or tid for 48 h; then increase or decrease q2d if needed; maintenance, 500 mg-2 g in 2-4 divided doses/d (maximum 3 g); chil-

dren: 10 up to 65 mg/kg/24 h in 2-4 divided doses

Prazosin (Minipress) (α-adrenergic blocker), po, 1 mg bid-tid initially; maintenance may be increased slowly to maximum of 20 mg/d in divided doses; up to 40 mg/d may be required

Diuretics

Ethacrynic acid (Edecrin), po, adults: 50-100 mg initially; maintenance 50-100 mg/d or bid pc (up to 400 mg) on continuous or intermittent schedule; children: 25 mg initially, increased by 25 mg increments to maintenance dose

Furosemide (Lasix), po, adults: 20-80 mg followed by second dose in 6-8 h up to 600 mg; children: 2 mg/kg body weight as single dose; may increase by 1 or 2 mg/kg; IM, IV, adults: 20-40 mg given slowly over 1-2 min; high dose by IV not more than 4 mg/min and repeat in 6-8 h; children: 1 mg/kg body weight; may be increased by 1 mg/kg not sooner than 2 h later

Electromechanical

Dialysis by home or in-center hemodialysis, home or in-center intermittent peritoneal dialysis, or continuous ambulatory peritoneal dialysis (CAPD) may be needed; see p. 1091

Supportive

Fluid intake to balance output: about 400 to 600 ml (about the amount of insensible losses) plus amount equal to 24-hour urine volume; patient should avoid dehydration and volume excess

Nutritional modifications to achieve or maintain adequate nutritional status and to reduce work of diseased kidney[1]

Protein: adults: 0.6 gm/kg body weight/day; glomerular filtration rate (GFR) 20 to 25 ml/min-90 g/day; GFR 10 to 15 ml/min-50 g/day; GFR 4 to 10 ml/min-40 g/day; children: not less than 1 to 2 g/kg body weight/day

Sodium: adults: 1 to 2 g/day (45 to 90 mEq/day); children: 1 to 3 g/day (45 to 130 mEq/day); specific amounts depend on weight, blood pressure, serum creatinine, and 24-hour sodium excretion

Potassium: 1560 to 2340 mg/day (40 to 60 mEq/day); with normal urine output (at least 800 ml/day), no restriction needed

Calories: adults: 35 to 55 kcal/kg body weight/day; children: 60 to 80 kcal/kg ideal body weight/day; calories from fat and carbohydrate used; adequate calories must accompany protein intake to prevent use of protein for energy and weight loss and to support growth in children

ASSESSMENT: AREAS OF CONCERN

Renal

Urinary sediment: few white and red blood cells, few casts, and small amount of albumin; nocturia (urinating at night due to loss of ability to concentrate urine); oliguria; anuria; infection

Cardiovascular

Hypertension; see Chapter 1

NURSING DIAGNOSES and NURSING INTERVENTIONS

Nursing Diagnosis	Nursing Intervention
Tissue perfusion, alteration in: renal	Give medications as ordered by physician. Be alert to altered dosages and schedules. Monitor response and side effects. Watch K^+ and Ca^{++} levels. Watch for electrocardiographic changes typical of hyperkalemia: peaked T waves, prolonged PR intervals, widened QRS complex, and cardiac standstill. Watch for signs of acidosis: HCO_3^- less than 22 mEq/L and Kussmaul breathing. Watch for signs of tetany: Chvostek and Trousseau signs.

Patient Education

1. Explain the nature of chronic renal failure.
2. Explain hypertension and its care (see Chapter 1).
3. Explain the medical regimen and its rationale, including diet (restricted protein, sodium, and potassium), restricted fluid intake, and medications (purpose, dosage, interval, and adverse reactions).
4. Teach self-observational skills (temperature, pulse, respirations, blood pressure, intake and output, and weight) and record keeping.
5. Explain avoidance of infection.
6. Explain personal hygiene, rest, and exercise.
7. Explain when to call the physician.
8. Explain the plan for medical follow-up.
9. Explain renal dialysis and transplantation as future options.

EVALUATION

Patient Outcome	Data Indicating That Outcome is Reached
Progression of renal failure is delayed (refer to ''Hypertension'' in Chapter 1).	Renal function findings do not worsen.
Patient is knowledgeable about nephrosclerosis and its treatment.	Patient and family describe nephrosclerosis, medical plan of care, and future options for renal dialysis or transplantation.
Conservative management of nephrosclerosis is effective.	Uremia is not present, glomerular filtration rate is greater than 15 ml/minute, and serum creatinine level is less than 10 mg/dl.
If nephrosclerosis progresses, dialysis or transplantation is instituted when needed.	Signs and symptoms of uremia persist, serum creatinine level is greater than 10 mg/dl, and glomerular filtration rate is less than 10 to 15 ml/minute.[31]

Medical Interventions

RENAL DIALYSIS

Dialysis is the differential diffusion of permeable substances through a semipermeable membrane separating two solutions. Hemodialysis and peritoneal dialysis are two forms of dialysis used clinically to treat patients with acute or chronic renal failure. The dialysate fluid contains electrolytes similar to those in normal blood plasma to permit diffusion of electrolytes into or out of the patient's blood. Glucose is added to the dialysate fluid to raise the osmolality and remove water from the blood channel.

Dialysis replaces some, but not all, of the kidney's functions. Fluid volume, electrolyte balance, acid-base balance, and nitrogenous wastes are controlled.

Dialysis options include home or in-center hemodialysis, home or in-center intermittent peritoneal dialysis, continuous cycling peritoneal dialysis (CCPD), and continuous ambulatory peritoneal dialysis (CAPD). Dialysis plays an important role in renal transplant programs by providing a backup for failed transplants and a pool of potential transplant recipients.

Hemodialysis
Description and Rationale

Hemodialysis involves circulating the patient's blood through semipermeable tubing that is surrounded by a dialysate solution in the artificial kidney (Fig. 10-7).

The blood circuit includes: (1) an access device (cannula or internal arteriovenous fistula); (2) arterial blood lines (with blood pressure monitor); (3) a blood pump; (4) a dialyzer where diffusion, osmosis, and ultrafiltration occur; and (5) venous lines with filter and monitors (for clots or air emboli and pressure), which return blood to the patient.

Fig. 10-7
Components of hemodialysis system.

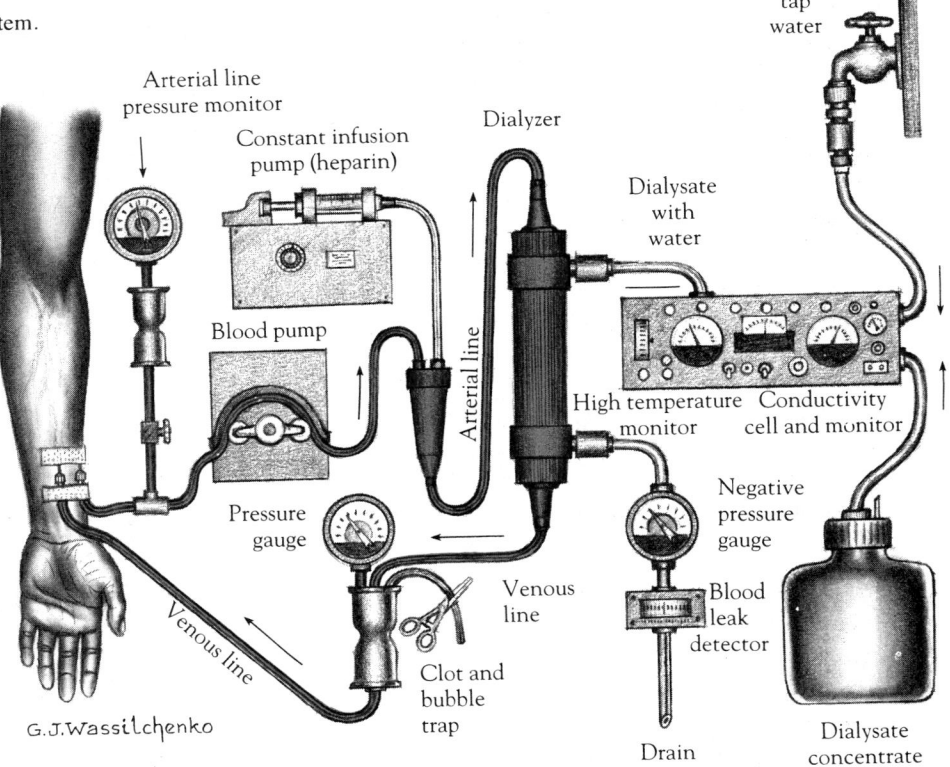

The dialysate circuit includes: (1) a proportioning pump (not shown in Fig. 10-7) that mixes dialysate concentrate with heated water and propels the dialysate through the dialyzer after monitoring it for conductivity, temperature, and pressure; (2) a dialyzer where the dialysate accepts wastes, excess electrolytes, and water; (3) dialysate exit lines, which may have a leak detector (blood-in-effluent lines) or are monitored using Hemastix to detect the presence of blood; (4) a negative pressure gauge on the dialysate lines that controls ultrafiltration; and (5) a bypass circuit (not shown in Fig. 10-7) for diversion of dialysate that is not within the preset temperature, conductivity, or pressure limits.

The composition of the diluted dialysate solution is sodium, 130 to 145 mEq/L; potassium, up to 3 mEq/L; calcium, 2.5 to 4 mEq/L; chloride, 96 to 107 mEq/L; and acetate, 33 to 41 mEq/L.[32]

Blood access is achieved by means of (1) an internal arteriovenous fistula created surgically with the patient's artery and vein, endogenous vein grafts, exogenous vein (bovine) grafts, or grafts made of artificial material such as expanded polytetrafluorethylene or (2) an external arteriovenous fistula or cannula (Fig. 10-8).

Hemodialysis treatment schedules vary with the kind of machine used and the patient's condition. Treatments are usually scheduled three times a week for 3 to 6 hours each.

Major types of artificial kidneys are hollow fiber, flat plate, and coil. The hollow fiber kidney is increasingly used because it can be adapted to the size of the patient. In the hollow fiber kidney the blood flows through narrow filaments that are surrounded by dialysate (Fig. 10-9). The coil kidney is surrounded by dialysate that is pumped through the mesh holding the flattened semipermeable membrane tube containing the blood from the patient. In the flat plate kidney the blood and dialysate flow in opposite directions in alternate layers.

Indications for hemodialysis include (1) rapid efficient treatment if needed; (2) acute poisoning (aspirin, methanol, or phenobarbital); (3) acute renal failure; (4) chronic renal failure; (5) severe edema states; (6) hepatic coma; (7) metabolic acidosis; (8) extensive burns with prerenal azotemia; (9) transfusion reactions; (10) postpartum renal insufficiency; and (11) crush syndrome.

Contraindications and Cautions

1. Other major chronic illness
2. No vascular access
3. Hemorrhagic diathesis
4. Extremes of age
5. Inability to cooperate with treatment regimen

TREATMENT PLAN

Anemia, hypertension, infection, peripheral neuropathy, pericarditis, renal osteodystrophy, reproductive dysfunction, and psychosocial difficulties associated with uremia continue to require treatment (see "Chronic Renal Failure," p.1069). The goal of therapy is to delay end-stage renal disease by conservative management and to begin dialysis or perform renal transplant at the appropriate

Fig. 10-8
Circulatory access. **A,** Internal arteriovenous fistula. Needles are inserted into arterialized vein. **B,** External arteriovenous cannula, with circuit closed *(left)* and attached to tubing from artificial kidney *(right).*

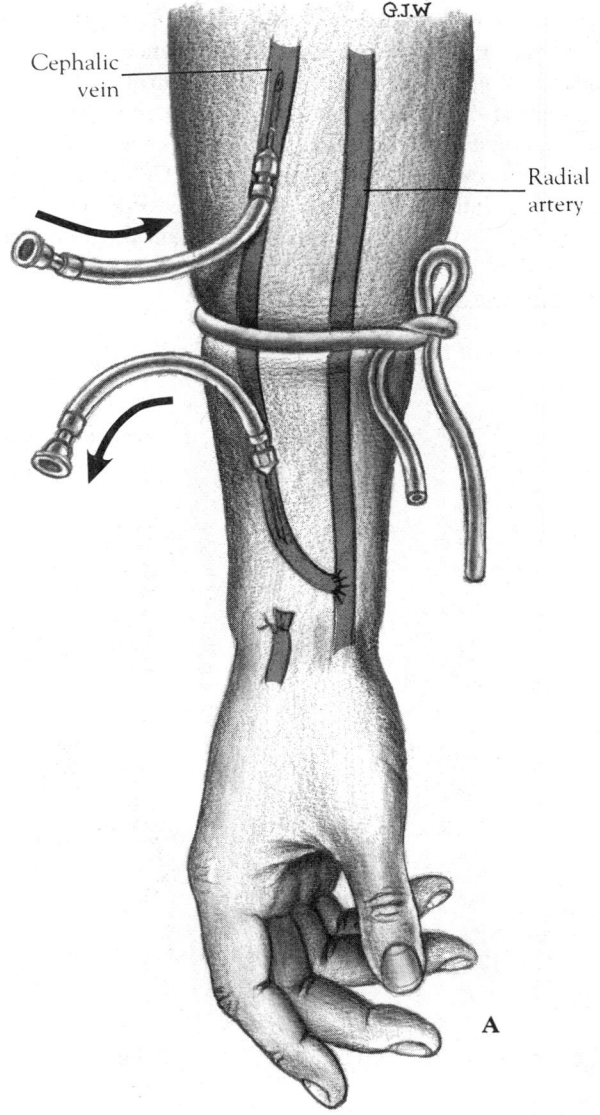

point in the course of the disease. Drug dosages and intervals must be modified when the kidney is involved in the drug's excretion. Rates of excretion and metabolism and sensitivity to drugs may be altered.

Surgical

Internal arteriovenous fistula created or cannula inserted to provide access to arterial and venous circulation

Chemotherapeutic

Anticoagulation agents

Heparin sodium, systemic: (1) intermittent IV injection, priming dose 100 mg/kg body weight with smaller doses repeated as determined by the clotting time, which should be 30-60 min; (2) continuous infusion by pump, 1000-2000 units/

hr determined by the clotting time; regional: inject heparin into blood line to the dialyzer, add protamine to the exit blood line before blood is returned to patient

Antidotes (used as an antiheparin agent)

Protamine sulfate: Amount and kind of heparin determine how much protamine is needed; each 1 mg of protamine sulfate neutralizes activity of about 90-115 units of heparin; keep patient's clotting time normal; monitor clotting time in machine and patient, watch for heparin rebound; this is return of anticoagulation up to 10 h later; more protamine sulfate may be needed

Antihypertensive agents: Omit dosage on day of dialysis to prevent excessive hypotension during treatment

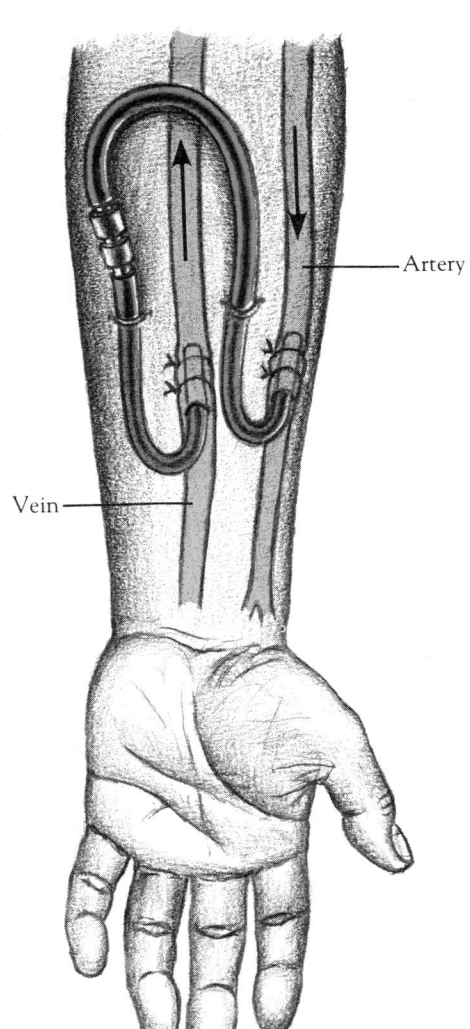

Artery

Vein

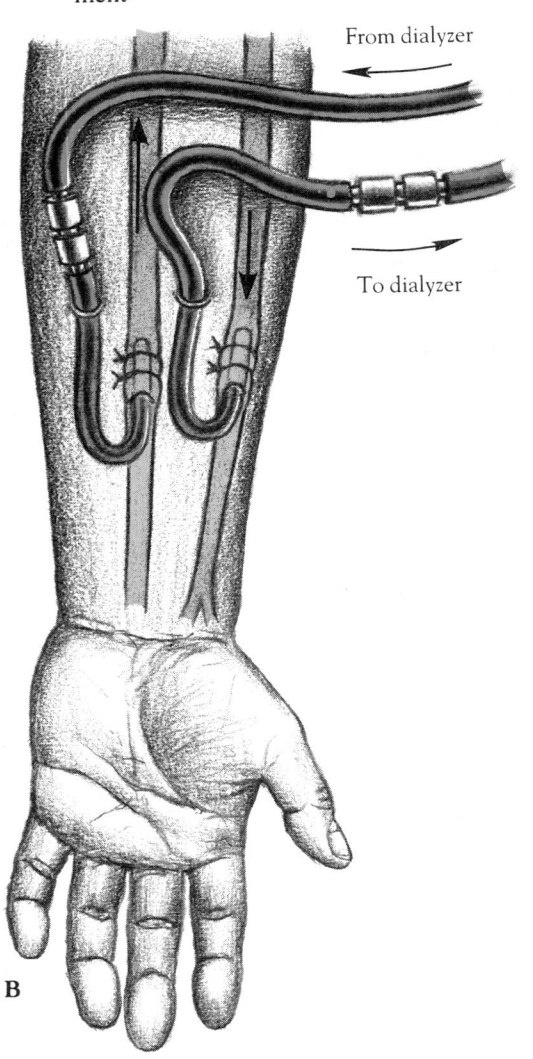

From dialyzer

To dialyzer

B

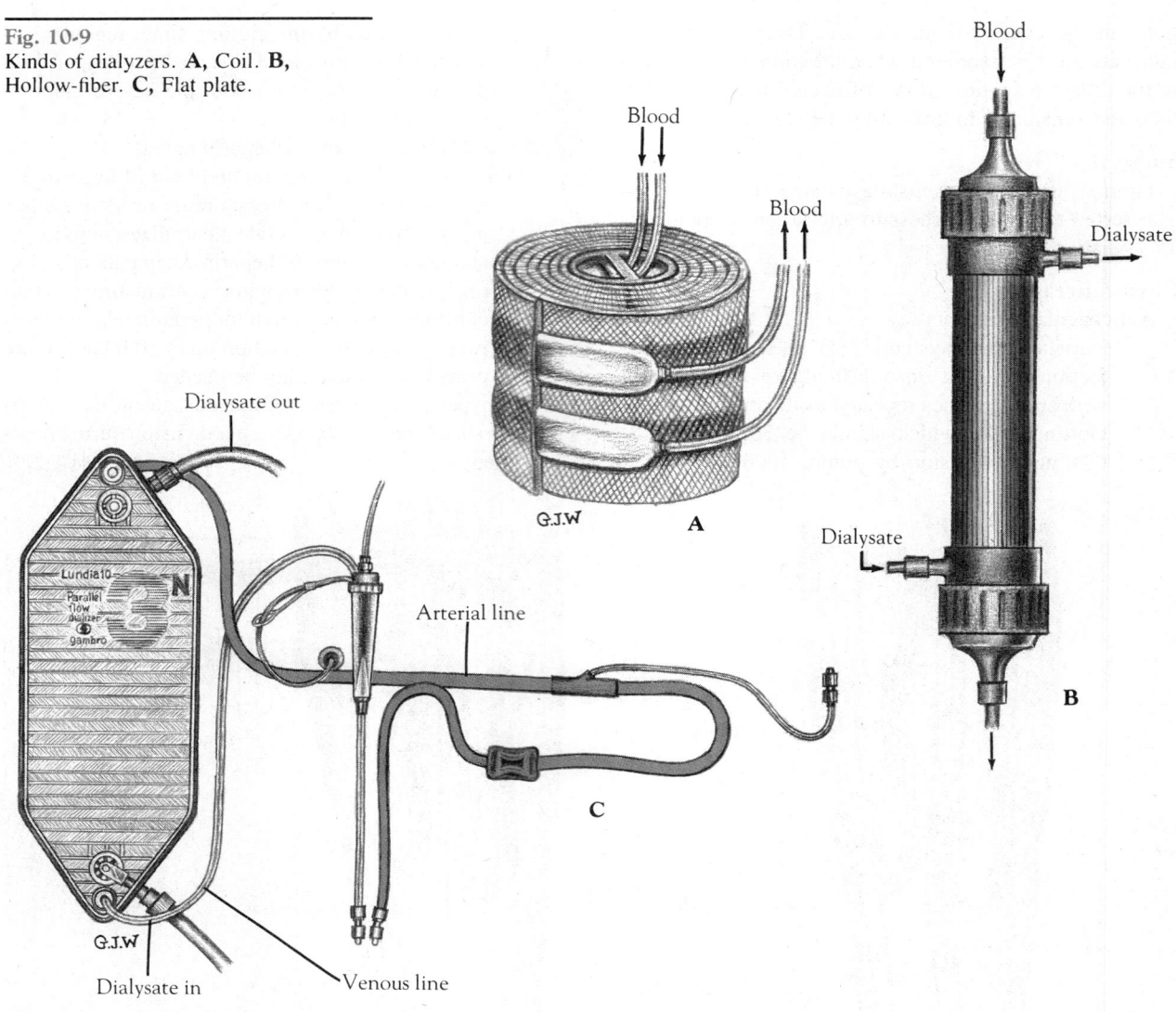

Fig. 10-9
Kinds of dialyzers. **A,** Coil. **B,** Hollow-fiber. **C,** Flat plate.

Vitamins (water-soluble) (lost in dialysate)
   Daily requirements: thiamine, 1.5 mg/d; riboflavin, 1.8 mg/d; niacin, 20 mg/d; pantothenic acid, 5 mg/d; pyridoxine, 5 mg/d; vitamin B_{12}, 3 mg/d; vitamin C, 100 mg/d; folic acid, 1 mg/day

Supportive
   Medical management between dialyses includes: diet: low protein (1.0 g/kg/day, 50% high biologic value); low sodium (1500 to 2000 mg or 65 to 85 mEq/day); low potassium (1560 to 2760 mg or 40 to 70 mEq/day); calories (35 kcal/kg ideal body weight/day); fluids restricted (0.5 to 1 L/day); a specific amount is determined by patient dry weight (weight at which, after dialysis, patient has normal volume relationships)[24]

ASSESSMENT: AREAS OF CONCERN

Cardiovascular
   Vascular access problems: bleeding, infection, and clotting; hypertension; hypotension; hypovolemia; hypervolemia; angina; arrhythmias; hemolysis; pyrogenic reaction

Neurologic
   Headache; dialysis disequilibrium; dialysis dementia; subdural hematoma

Psychological
   Uncooperative; denial, depression, and anger

Other
   Muscle cramps; pruritus; hepatitis B antigen and antibody

Mechanical problems

Electrical outage; hypertonic dialysate; hypotonic dialysate; overheated dialysate; air infusion

Dialysis disequilibrium syndrome may occur near the end of dialysis or after it. The condition is related to the osmotic gradient produced across the blood-brain barrier by the efficient removal of urea from the blood, but not from the brain tissue. The urea draws in water from the plasma and extracellular fluid and causes cerebral edema. Other factors that may be involved are changes in serum pH, rapid ion shifts, and cardiovascular changes. The signs and symptoms of disequilibrium syndrome are headache, nausea, vomiting, agitation, twitching, confusion, and seizures.[16] This syndrome can be prevented by slowing the rate of solute removal by (1) dialyzing at a slower blood flow rate (100 ml/minute) and for a shorter time, (2) using a less efficient dialyzer, or (3) using peritoneal dialysis.

Dialysis dementia, or progressive dialysis encephalopathy, is a syndrome that has emerged as experience with hemodialysis has increased. The clinical picture includes disturbed speech that occurs first during dialysis, myoclonus, dementia, or behavioral changes. It is a progressive condition that ends in death. A number of studies have implicated aluminum accumulation from the water supply or from aluminum hydroxide taken as a phosphate binder.[16]

Dialysis-associated hepatitis B is a major concern for patients (often active carriers of the hepatitis B virus), staff (at risk because of frequent exposure to patient's blood), and families (at risk because of close contact, especially sexual, and from environmental surfaces). It should be noted that special precautions with blood and other bodily fluids are needed to prevent spread of hepatitis B virus (HBV). Health care professionals and patients in dialysis units are particularly at risk because a patient with chronic renal failure receives frequent transfusions and may have a subclinical case of hepatitis B infection owing to impairment of the immune system.

The hepatitis B surface antigen (HB_sAg) is a useful marker for active HBV infections.[9] Transmission occurs by way of some environmental surfaces (toothbrushes, razors, and needles) and by blood, blood products, and other bodily excretions or secretions. The primary sources are infected serum, saliva, and semen. Other sources of HBV can be feces, bile, sweat, tears, breast milk, vaginal secretions, cerebrospinal fluid, synovial fluid, and cord blood.

Programs to prevent the spread of HBV infections focus on identifying persons who are HB_sAg positive. Screening of all dialysis unit personnel and patients is done regularly. Such programs also include hygienic measures: (1) safe, reliable procedures for handling laboratory specimens; (2) procedures for hepatitis B precautions for hospitalized patients including safe care of disposable materials, food handling, and laundry service; (3) segregation of equipment used for patients who are HB_sAg positive; (4) vigilant handwashing practices; (5) sterilization measures appropriate to the material involved; (6) no eating, smoking, or other hand-to-mouth activity in the dialysis unit or laboratory; (7) use of protective clothing, such as masks, goggles, gloves, aprons, shoe covers, gowns, and caps; and (8) policy of reporting and recording any unusual exposure to HBV.

Hepatitis B vaccine is used for active immunization for preexposure prevention in high-risk populations, such as dialysis unit personnel. Hepatitis B immune globulin is used for passive immunization after exposure to HBV.

NURSING DIAGNOSES and NURSING INTERVENTIONS

Nursing Diagnosis	Nursing Intervention
Knowledge deficit	Explain hemodialysis procedure and its purpose. Demonstrate safe aseptic cannula care.
Fluid volume, alteration in: excess (potential)	*Prehemodialysis care:* Measure weight, temperature, pulse, respirations, and blood pressure (lying and standing). Record these prehemodialysis figures. A patient should not gain more than 1.5 kg between treatments. Review blood chemistries (blood urea nitrogen, creatinine, Na^+, K^+, and hematocrit).
Potential patient problem: susceptibility to infection	Wear mask over nose and mouth and place mask over patient's nose and mouth while making connections with dialyzer tubing Use sterile technique to initiate hemodialysis, needle insertions, or cannula connections. Anchor connections securely. Use disposable gloves and plastic apron over clothes to prevent direct contact with blood. Identify HB_sAg status of patient.

Nursing Diagnosis	Nursing Intervention
Fluid volume deficit, potential	Minimize blood loss, since patient with chronic renal failure is anemic. Measure intake and output. Check bleeding and clotting times. Observe hemodialysis system monitors to ensure patient safety (flow rate, pressure, temperature, osmolality, clots, air emboli, negative pressure for ultrafiltration, and blood leaks). Watch for equipment or electrical failures. Monitor vital signs throughout procedure. Check patient's response to the procedure. Infuse normal saline intravenously if patient is hypotensive (nausea and muscle cramps). Check blood pressure, temperature, pulse, respirations, and weight. Patient should weigh less, have lower blood pressure, and higher temperature than before dialysis treatment. Check blood chemistries: blood urea nitrogen, creatinine, and Na^+, and K^+ levels should be decreased.
Skin integrity, impairment of	*After hemodialysis:* Permit no one to take blood pressure or to do intravenous punctures in arm with fistula or cannula (to prevent infection or clotting). Perform regular cannula care. Wear mask. Inspect exit sites for infection. Cleanse gently with hydrogen peroxide and applicator sticks using aseptic technique. Clean cannula with alcohol sponges starting at exit site. Cover with dry sterile dressing and hold in place with paper tape and woven gauze bandage. Avoid trauma to cannula. Check circulation (palpate thrill) on venous side and check for clots. Instruct patient to wear loose sleeves, avoid temperature extremes or lifting heavy objects, avoid prolonged immersion of arm in water (arm may be covered with plastic), and carry clamps to stop bleeding if the cannula separates. Provide fistula care. Apply direct pressure to needle sites for 5 minutes or until bleeding stops. Cover with Band-Aid. Pressure dressing may be used. Watch for signs of bleeding, infection, ischemia of hand, or aneurysm formation. Watch for clotting and formation of scar tissue from repeated venipunctures.
Thought processes, alteration in (potential)	Watch for dialysis disequilibrium and dialysis dementia.
Self-concept, disturbance in: body image	Observe patient's response to having a chronic illness, altered renal function, alteration in other body systems, and the possibility of renal transplantation in the future. Recognize patient's response to dependence on a machine. Patient may feel helpless and hopeless, deny reality, and personalize machine or may accept it as necessary. Be aware of changes in social involvement: fewer social-recreational activities, life-style changes, and withdrawal because of being different. Support patient's strengths: self-confidence, determination, and motivation to live. Help patient develop or continue interests beyond dialysis and return to as normal a life as possible. Be alert to excessive concern with losses, depression, self-neglect, and noncompliance with medical regimen and to possibility of suicide. Be aware of effect loss of libido, impotence, and decreased orgasm has on the marital and sexual life of patient. Try to help patient develop realistic expectations of dialysis. Try to keep lines of communication open. See p. 1820.
Family process, alteration in	Recognize that chronic renal failure and hemodialysis can cause disruption, expense, and considerable alteration in time commitments in family. Try to support family's willing cooperation in patient's care and help them look at ways to decrease domestic tension and unhappiness. Help patient and spouse recognize demands of illness situation on spouse and patient's need for emotional support. Recognize spouse's fears. See p. 1931.

Nursing Diagnosis	Nursing Intervention
Home maintenance management, impaired	Observe the home to see that it is large enough, clean, and adequately supplied with electricity, water, and heat and has a phone to be suitable for home hemodialysis. Recognize patient's inability to continue family role of homemaker or breadwinner, and help patient accept this through discussion of alternatives. In home dialysis recognize stresses that spouse faces and support spouse in learning about dialysis and carrying out hemodialysis in the home.

Patient Education

1. Explain function of normal and artificial kidney.
2. Explain principles of hemodialysis.
3. Explain aseptic technique for needle insertions or cannula care.
4. Teach self-observational skills.
5. Explain components of system with preparation, operation, cleaning, storage (repair and maintenance if home hemodialysis).
6. Explain initiating dialysis, monitoring during dialysis, and discontinuing dialysis.
7. Explain emergencies related to machine and to patient's medical condition.
8. Explain care while off machine: diet, fluid restrictions, medical complications, care of blood access route, medications, and prevention of infection.
9. Explain medical supervision, including help available from medical center, and schedule of return visits, and assistance from the local physician.

EVALUATION

Patient Outcome	Data Indicating That Outcome is Reached
Patient and family have adjusted to life on hemodialysis.	Patient and family have returned to work and social activities as are possible. Children continue to grow and mature sexually and socially. Family and child continue to use support of health team.
Patient and family understand chronic renal failure and hemodialysis.	Patient and family describe chronic renal failure and medical plan of care.
Dialysis is adequate.[17]	Patient and family describe principles of hemodialysis, plan of care, and correct use of hemodialysis machine: good general and nutritional status, normal blood pressure, clinically tolerated anemia, no osteodystrophy and calcifications on roentgenogram; no uremic polyneuropathy and encephalopathy; predialysis plasma concentrations of urea, creatinine, K^+ and Na^+ in desirable range; and good quality of life and rehabilitation.

Peritoneal Dialysis

Description and Rationale

Peritoneal dialysis (PD) involves the introduction of dialysate fluid into the abdominal cavity where the peritoneum acts as a semipermeable membrane between the dialysate and the blood in the abdominal vessels. A machine may be used, or the fluid may be instilled and drained manually from the peritoneal cavity (see Fig. 10-10).

Components of peritoneal dialysis solutions include glucose, 1.5 gm/dl (1.5% solution); sodium, 141 mEq/L; calcium, 3.5 mEq/L; magnesium, 1.5 mEq/L; chloride, 101 mEq/L; lactate, 45 mEq/L; pH, 5.5; and osmolality, 366 mOsm/kg.[33]

Additions may include potassium, 0 to 3 mEq/L; heparin, 150 units/L; and glucose to make 4.5% or 7% solutions.

Continuous ambulatory peritoneal dialysis (CAPD) is under study as an alternative to intermittent peritoneal dialysis for chronic renal failure. CAPD involves four exchanges of 2 L each in 24 hours and dwell times of 4 to 8 hours.[40,41] Dialysate in plastic bags is used. When the solution is infused, the plastic bag is folded up and

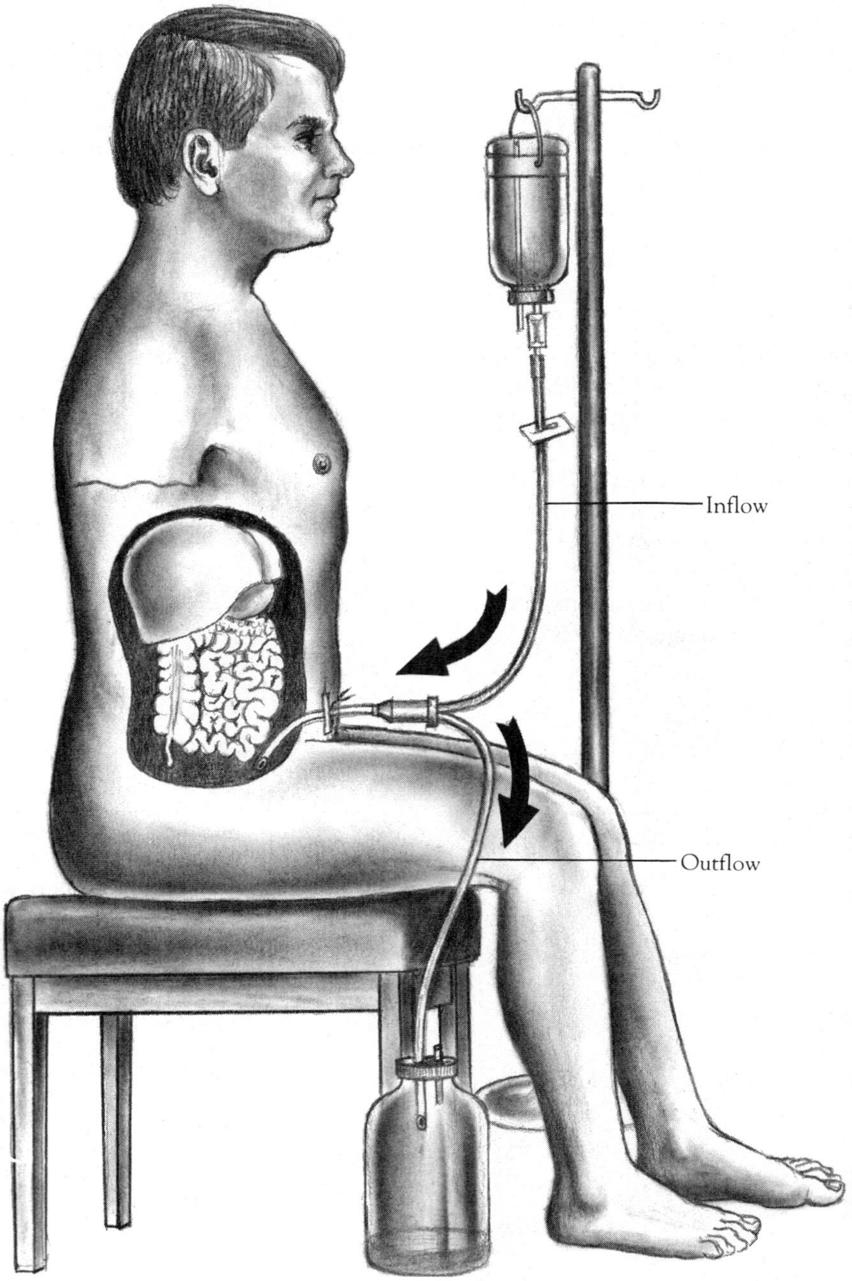

Fig. 10-10
Peritoneal dialysis.

Inflow

Outflow

concealed under the person's clothes. When the fluid is drained, that bag is discarded and a new bag is attached, and its fluid is instilled for the next cycle. CAPD is self-administered and machine free.

Continuous cycling peritoneal dialysis involves connecting the peritoneal catheter to an automated peritoneal dialysis machine that performs 3 to 4 cycles during the night while the patient sleeps. During the day one cycle of fluid is left in the abdomen. The person is free of

dialysis activities during the day and connections are less frequent than in CAPD.

Peritoneal dialysis is indicated when less rapid treatment is needed; equipment and staff for hemodialysis are not available; there is inadequate blood access; the patient is an infant or child; the patient is in shock or has had cardiovascular surgery; severe cardiovascular disease is present; and the patient refuses blood transfusions.

Contraindications and Cautions

1. Peritonitis
2. Abdominal adhesions
3. Recent abdominal surgery

TREATMENT PLAN

Surgical

The peritoneal catheter is inserted into the peritoneal cavity, generally under local anesthetic in the operating room; if the catheter is permanent, it has an internal Dacron cuff that lies between the peritoneum and the abdominal muscles; it has an external cuff that is 1 to 1.5 cm below the skin at the other end of a 3 to 4 cm subcutaneous tunnel[36]

Chemotherapeutic

Anticoagulants

Heparin may be added to dialysate to prevent fibrin formation and obstruction to the fluid flow; antimicrobial agents are used when peritonitis is diagnosed; they usually are given by the intraperitoneal route; vitamins (water-soluble) are lost and must be replaced (see hemodialysis, p. 1085)

Supportive

Medical management of the continuing uremic problems is discussed in the section on chronic renal failure (p. 1069); the use of peritoneal dialysis causes an increased loss of blood proteins and amino acids with the fluid in the outflow; a more generous protein intake is indicated to replace these losses (suggested intake: 1.2 to 5 g/kg/day, 50% of high biologic value; restrictions continue in sodium (1.4 to 2 g/day) and potassium (2.9 to 3.5 g/day); caloric intake may be partly supplied by the glucose in the peritoneal dialysis fluid; patients need 35 kcal/kg ideal body weight/day; fluid restriction ranges from 0.5 to 1 L/day

ASSESSMENT: AREAS OF CONCERN

Abdominal cavity

Peritonitis; infectious or chemical (rebound abdominal tenderness, increase in white blood cells in effluent, and fever); peritoneal access problems (infection and obstruction); leakage of fluid into tissues, thoracic cavity, or scrotum; adhesions

Cardiovascular

Hypovolemia; hypervolemia

Neurologic

Hyperosmolar coma and convulsions

Respiratory

Tachypnea; pulmonary edema and effusions

NURSING DIAGNOSES and NURSING INTERVENTIONS

Nursing Diagnosis	Nursing Intervention
Knowledge deficit	Explain peritoneal dialysis, its purpose, and procedure.
Fluid volume, alteration in excess, actual	*Before peritoneal dialysis:* Have patient empty bladder. Measure weight, temperature, pulse, respirations, and blood pressure (lying and standing). Measure abdominal girth. Record baseline data. Review blood chemistries (blood urea nitrogen, serum creatinine, serum Na^+ and K^+).
Skin integrity, impairment of and susceptibility to infection (potential patient problem)	*During peritoneal dialysis*[23]: Identify HB_sAg status of patient. Wear masks (patient, physician, and nurse). Use sterile technique as acute peritoneal catheter is placed in abdominal cavity. Permanent catheters are inserted in operating room. Use sterile technique during subsequent connections of dialysis fluid to peritoneal catheter and for changing catheter dressings. Anchor connections and tubing securely. Avoid kinks in tubing. Dry off warmed bottle of fluid before hanging it up or use plastic bags of solution warmed in folded heating pad on a low setting. Observe for perforation of bowel (dialysate outflow stained with feces, blood, or watery diarrhea) or bladder (urine pink or bloody). First several exchanges will be pink tinged, but gross blood is not normal. Observe for peritonitis. Collect samples of dialysate outflow for culture and sensitivity whenever it is turbid or bloody or has an odor.

Nursing Diagnosis	Nursing Intervention
Fluid volume, alteration in: excess (potential)	Measure intake, output (inflow, dwell, and outflow times), and weight, as well as temperature, pulse, respirations, and blood pressure regularly and record results. Keep accurate records of dialysis cycles. Record strength of solution used, additions made, and fluid balance (retained or lost). Outflow of dialysate may be obstructed by fibrin or omentum, constipation, or catheter malposition. Observe for respiratory embarrassment (manifested by dyspnea and rales) resulting from abdomen being too full of fluid or leakage of dialysate into the thoracic cavity through defect in diaphragm.
Fluid volume deficit, potential	Do not prolong dwell times, especially with solutions of 4.5% glucose, because water depletion can result. Watch for weight loss during the procedure.
Self-concept, disturbance in: body image	Observe patient's response to having chronic illness, altered renal function, alteration in other body systems, the necessity of renal dialysis, and transplantation as a probability in the future. Recognize denial, guilt, aggression, fear, displacement, regression, resentment, disbelief, and anxiety in patient. Recognize changes in psychosocial aspects of patient's life: change in social interaction, irritability, hostility, extreme dependence, fear of rejection, inability to work, loss of job, decreased financial stability, and altered hopes for future. Identify significant aspects of patient's cultural background and religion that may affect response to chronic renal failure and dialysis. Help patient move through stages of denial, discouragement, acceptance of the condition, and rehabilitation. Share information needed, listen, and offer continuing emotional support. Refer patient to other professional resources as needed. Recognize patient's response to dependence on machine. Patient may feel helpless or hopeless, deny reality, personalize the machine, or accept it as necessity. Support patient's strengths: self-confidence, determination, and motivation to live. Help patient develop or continue interests beyond dialysis and return to as normal a life as possible. Be alert to excessive concern with losses, depression, self-neglect, noncompliance with medical regimen, and possibility of suicide. Be aware of effect loss of libido, impotence, and decreased orgasm has on marital and sexual life of patient. Try to help patient develop realistic expectations of dialysis. Try to keep lines of communication open. See p. 1820.
Family process, alteration in	Recognize that chronic renal failure and dialysis can cause disruption, expense, and considerable alteration in time commitments in the family. Try to support family's willing cooperation in patient's care, and help them look at ways to decrease domestic tension and unhappiness. Help patient and spouse recognize demands of illness situation on spouse and patient's need for emotional support. Recognize spouse's fears. Involve family from the beginning in all aspects and help them understand patient's responses. Work with health team as they help family meet illness situation.

Patient Education

1. Explain the nature of chronic renal failure.
2. Explain the medical regimen and its rationale, including diet; (restricted protein, sodium, and potassium), restricted fluid intake, and medications (purpose, dosage, interval, and adverse reactions).
3. Explain the function of normal and artificial kidneys and the principles of peritoneal dialysis.
4. Teach aseptic technique.
5. Explain components of the system, preparation, operation, cleaning, and storage (repair and maintenance if home dialysis).
6. Explain initiating dialysis, monitoring during dialysis, and discontinuing dialysis.
7. Explain emergencies related to the machine and to the patient's medical condition.
8. Explain care while off the machine: diet, fluid restrictions, medical complications, care of peritoneal access route, medications, and prevention of infection.
9. Teach self-observational skills (temperature, pulse, respirations, blood pressure, intake and output, and weight) and record keeping.
10. Explain ways to avoid infection.
11. Explain personal hygiene, rest, and exercise.
12. Explain when to call the physician.
13. Explain the plan for medical follow-up.

EVALUATION

Patient Outcome	Data Indicating That Outcome is Reached
Patient and family understand chronic renal failure and peritoneal dialysis.	Patient and family describe chronic renal failure and medical plan of care. Patient and family describe principles of peritoneal dialysis, plan of care, and correct use of peritoneal dialysis equipment.
Patient and family have adjusted to peritoneal dialysis.	Patient and family have returned to work and social activities as are possible. Children continue to grow and mature sexually and socially. Family and patient continue to use support of health team.
Dialysis is adequate.[17]	Patient has good general and nutritional status, normal blood pressure, clinically tolerated anemia, no osteodystrophy or calcifications on roentgenograms, no uremic polyneuropathy or encephalopathy, predialysis plasma concentrations of urea, creatinine, K^+, and Na^+ in desirable range, and good quality of life and rehabilitation.

RENAL TRANSPLANTATION

Description and Rationale

Renal transplantation (RT) is the surgical insertion of a human kidney from a living or cadaveric source into a patient with end-stage renal disease, thus replacing the lost renal function. A donor is sought when the patient's serum creatinine is around 5 mg/dl, serum blood urea nitrogen is greater than 70 mg/dl, and creatinine clearance is 15 ml/min.[34] When successful, a transplant restores the recipient to a healthy, useful life. If a transplant is unsuccessful, the patient can return to dialysis or have a second transplant.

The donated kidney is placed in the retroperitoneal area in the iliac fossa on the contralateral side. Thus a donated left kidney is placed in the recipient's right iliac fossa (see Fig. 10-11). The donor's artery is anastomosed end to end to the recipient's hypogastric artery.

The donor's vein is anastomosed to the recipient's internal iliac vein. The donor's ureter is implanted in the recipient's bladder.

The kidney from a living related donor is flushed with a cold solution and then placed in the recipient. A cadaveric kidney may be preserved by flushing followed by cold storage or by constant perfusion with a special solution.

Transplantation is usually the treatment of choice in children. Aging patients may have problems with transplantation because of atherosclerosis or other serious systemic disorders. Patients with diabetes are increasingly considered for transplantation, but the problems with the continuing diabetic condition increase complications such as infection. The use of corticosteroids exacerbates problems in glucose level control.

Fig. 10-11
Renal transplant.

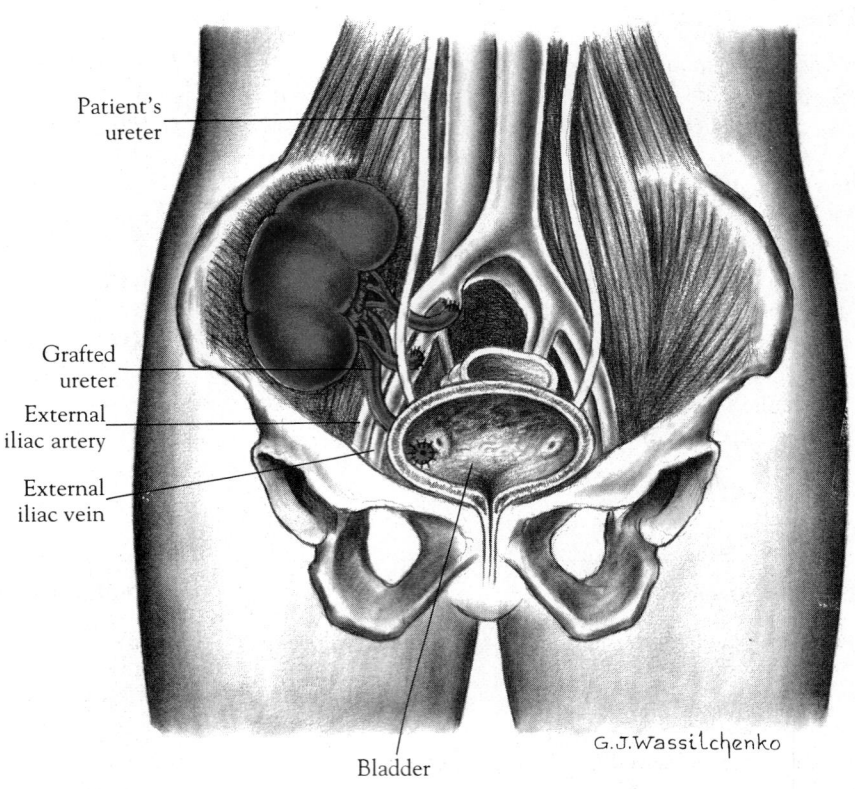

Patient's ureter

Grafted ureter

External iliac artery

External iliac vein

Bladder

G.J.Wassilchenko

Indications for a renal transplant include end-stage renal disease, loss of a solitary kidney through trauma, and the inability to adjust to dialysis.

Contraindications and Cautions

1. Age younger than 5 years or older than 50 years
2. Malignancy
3. Acute uncontrollable infection
4. Hepatic disease
5. Presence of antikidney antibodies
6. Severe psychosis
7. Tuberculosis or peptic ulcer disease
8. Chronic respiratory insufficiency
9. Severe atherosclerosis
10. Severe myocardial dysfunction

Preprocedural Care: Preoperative Assessment

Recipient
Medical examination
History and physical, including blood pressure and weight

Renal-urologic: flat plate abdomen, urinalysis three times, urine culture three times, creatinine clearance two times, 24-hour urine protein and electrolyte excretion, and voiding cystoureterogram

Hematologic: red and white blood cells with differential, platelets, hemoglobin, hematocrit, bleeding-clotting time, prothrombin time, partial thromboplastin time, and thrombin time

Cardiovascular: chest roentgenogram (heart size), electrocardiogram, serum electrolytes, glucose, protein, blood pressure, and eye examination

Respiratory: chest roentgenogram and pulmonary function tests

Gastrointestinal: upper gastrointestinal series and liver function tests

Skeletal: signs of hyperparathyroidism (serum Ca^{++}, $PO_4^{=}$, Mg^{++}, and alkaline phosphatase) and metabolic bone survey

Neuromuscular: nerve conduction time

Infectious: fungal skin tests; urine, blood, skin, nose, throat, and feces cultures

Immunologic: serum electrophoresis, LE cell test, rheumatoid factor (RF) test, anti-streptolysin O (ASO) titer, complement, antinuclear factor, anti–glomerular basement membrane antibodies, blood type (ABO, Rh), tissue type (HLA), serial cytotoxic antibody determinations, and HB$_s$Ag

Psychiatric examination
  Psychologic testing
  Evaluation for psychopathology
  Evaluation of metabolic encephalopathy
Socioeconomic evaluation
  Resources
  Family status
  Potential for return to preillness activities

Donor—living related
Medical examination
  History and physical, including blood pressure and weight
  Immunologic: blood type (ABO, Rh), tissue type, leukocyte cross-matching, antidonor antibody, VDRL, HB$_s$Ag, and mixed lymphocytic culture (MLC) tests
  Renal-urologic: urinalysis, urine culture two times, creatinine clearance, renogram, intravenous urography, and renal arteriogram
  Hematologic: hematocrit, platelet count, white blood cells with differential, prothrombin time, partial thromboplastin time, and thrombin time
  Cardiovascular-respiratory: chest roentgenogram, electrocardiogram, blood chemistries, and electrolytes
  Endocrine: fasting blood sugar and glucose tolerance test
Psychiatric examination
  Emotional maturity and stability
  Motivation
Socioeconomic evaluation
  Resources
  Responsibilities

Donor—cadaveric
No systemic disease such as infection, cancer, or advanced vascular disease including hypertension
No renal-urologic disorders
No prolonged hypoxia or hypotension before death
Relatively young (4 to 55 years old)
Renal function tests normal

TREATMENT PLAN

Surgical
The donor kidney is transplanted as described on p. 1095; the patient is prepared with adequate dialysis for surgery (see "Hemodialysis," p. 1085); the uremic problems are controlled before surgery

Chemotherapeutic
Antiemetics
  Prochlorperazine (Compazine), po, adults: 5-10 mg tid or qid; po and rectal, children: 2.5 mg qd-tid or 5 mg bid; maximum 15 mg/d
  Trimethobenzamide (Tigan), po, adults: 250 mg tid or qid; children (15-45 kg): 100-200 mg tid or qid; (<15 kg): 100 mg tid or qid; IM, adults only: 200 mg tid or qid
Narcotic analgesics
  Meperidine (Demerol), po, sc, IM, IV, adults: 50-150 mg q3-4h; children: 1 mg/kg q4h up to 100 mg q4h
  Codeine sulfate, po, sc, IM, adults: 15-60 mg qid; children: 3 mg/kg/d divided into 6 doses
  Morphine sulfate, po, sc, IM, adults: 5-15 mg q4h prn; children: 0.1-0.2 mg/kg per dose not to exceed 15 mg
Anti-infective agents
  Parenteral agents (IM or IV)
    Gentamicin (Garamycin), adults: 3-5 mg/kg/d q8h; children: 6-7.5 mg/kg/d q8h
    Cephalosporins
      Cefazolin sodium (Ancef), 250-1000 mg q6-8h
    Penicillins
      Ampicillin sodium (Omnipen-N), patients ≥40 kg: 250-500 mg q6h; <40 kg: 25-50 mg/kg/d in equally divided doses q6-8h
      Carbenicillin disodium (Geopen), adults: 1-2 g q6h; children: 50-200 mg/kg/d in equally divided doses q4-6h
      Penicillin G potassium (Aqueous penicillin G), Penicillin G sodium, adults: 1-20 million units/d; children: 50,000-250,000 units/kg/d in 4-6 divided doses
  Oral agents
    Tetracycline (Achromycin), 250-500 mg q6h
    Penicillins
      Amoxicillin (Amoxil), adults and children ≥20 kg: 250-500 mg q8h; <20 kg: 20-40 mg/kg/d in divided doses q8h
      Ampicillin (Omnipen), patients ≥20 kg: 250-500 mg q6h; <20 kg: 50-100 mg/kg/d in equally divided doses
      Penicillin G, adults: 200,000-500,000 units q6-8h; children: 25,000-90,000 units/kg/d in 3-6 divided doses
      Erythromycin (Erythrocin), adults: 25 mg q6h; children: 30-50 mg/kg/d in 4 equally divided doses
      Sulfamethoxazole and trimethoprim (Septra), adults: 2 tab q12h; children: 8 mg/kg trimethoprim and 40 mg/kg sulfamethoxazole/d in 2 divided doses q12h
Antihypertensive agents
  Clonidine (Catapres) (adrenergic blocker), po, 0.1

mg bid or tid initially; then increase by 0.2-0.8 mg/d (maximum effective dose, 2.4 mg/d)

Diazoxide (Hyperstat IV) (thiazide), IV, adults only: 300 mg by bolus in 30 sec or 1-2 mg/kg up to 150 mg at 5-15 min intervals

Hydralazine (Apresoline) (vasodilator), po, adults: 10 mg qid for 2-4 d, increase to 25 mg qid then 50 mg qid; maintenance dose is lowest effective level; children: 0.75 mg/kg initially; increase if needed to 7.5 mg/kg; IM, IV, adults: 10-40 mg repeated as needed (q4-6h); children initially 1.7-3.5 mg/kg/d in 4-6 divided doses

Methyldopa (Aldomet) (adrenergic blocker), po, adults: 250 mg bid or tid for 48 h, then increase or decrease q2d if needed; maintenance, 500 mg to 2 g in 2-4 divided doses/d (maximum, 3 g); children: 10 up to 65 mg/kg/24 h in 2-4 divided doses

Prazosin HCL (Minipress) (α-adrenergic blocker), po, 1 mg bid-tid initially; maintenance may be increased slowly to maximum of 20 mg/d in divided doses; to 40 mg/d may be required

Propranolol HCL (Inderal) (β-adrenergic blocker), po, 40 mg bid at 6-8 h intervals; increase if needed to 160-480 mg/d in divided doses; 640 mg/d may be needed

Captopril (Capoten) (angiotensin converting enzyme inhibitor), po, 25 mg tid initially; increase to 50 mg tid in 2-3 wk if necessary; may be increased to 100 mg tid then 150 mg tid

Antineoplastic agents (used as immunosuppressive agents[2,14,28])

Azathioprine (Imuran), po, 100-150 mg/d; 1.7-2.5 mg/kg/d determined by white blood cell level

Antilymphocyte globulin, IM, IV, 5-10 mg/kg depending on potency of preparation, qd for 5-21 d after surgery with intermittent doses for 4 mo

Cyclophosphamide (Cytoxan), po, 2 mg/kg/d as substitute for azathioprine in patients with liver dysfunction

Cyclosporin A, po, IV, 10-25 mg/kg/d

Corticosteroids (used as immunosuppressive agents[2,14,28])

Prednisone (Deltasone), po, 20-150 mg/d, 0.3-2.5 mg/kg decreasing to 10-15 mg/d by 4 mo; increase to 100-300 mg/d (up to 3 g) to treat rejection

Methylprednisolone (Solu-Medrol), IV, 250-1000 mg qd or alternate days for maximum dose of 3-5 g

Antacids (peptic ulcer disease may be a problem)

Aluminum carbonate gel, basic (Basaljel), po, 300 ml divided into 6 doses

Aluminum phosphate (Phosphajel), po, 180-360 ml divided into 4-12 doses

Insulin preparations (for hyperglycemia resulting from corticosteroid therapy): highly individualized according to blood and urine glucose determinations (see "Diabetes Mellitus," Chapter 8)

Electromechanical

Dialysis may be needed (see p. 1085)

Supportive

No dietary restrictions after gastrointestinal function returns unless renal function is decreased or hypertension continues; if this is the case:

Fluid intake should balance output: about 400 to 600 ml (about the amount of insensible losses) plus amount equal to 24-hour urine volume; patient should avoid dehydration and volume excess

Nutritional modifications to achieve or maintain adequate nutritional status and to reduce work of diseased kidney[1]

Protein: adults: 0.6 g/kg body weight per day; glomerular filtration rate (GFR) 20 to 25 ml/min to 90 g/day; GFR, 10 to 15 ml/min to 50 g/day; GFR, 4 to 10 ml/min to 40 g/day; children: not less than 1 to 2 g/kg body weight/day

Sodium: adults: 1 to 2 g/day (45 to 90 mEq/day); children: 1 to 3 g/day (45 to 130 mEq/day); the specific amounts depend on weight, blood pressure, serum creatinine, and 24-hour sodium excretion

Potassium: 1560 to 2340 mg/day (40 to 60 mEq/day); with normal urine output (at least 800 ml/day), no restriction needed

Calories: adults: 35 to 55 kcal/kg body weight/day; children: 60 to 80 kcal/kg ideal body weight/day; calories from fat and carbohydrate are used; adequate calories must accompany protein intake to prevent use of protein for energy and weight loss and to support growth in children

Vitamins

Routine cultures of likely places for infection (urinary tract, wound, throat, and blood) may be done, since the immunosuppressive agents mask the signs and symptoms of infection. All immunosuppressive agents currently in use affect phagocytosis, cellular immunity, and humoral immunity. Liver function is monitored because azathioprine can cause cholestatic hepatitis. The signs and symptoms of rejection are monitored. These include decreased urine production, hypertension, fever, weight gain, decreased creatinine clearance, increased serum creatinine level, increased blood urea nitrogen level, proteinuria, decreased urine sodium, decreased renal blood flow on renogram, increase in renal size, anxiety, apathy, lethargy, anorexia, and tenderness over the graft site.

ASSESSMENT: AREAS OF CONCERN

Renal

Ischemic damage (acute renal failure, p. 1065); rejection:chyperacute, acute, and chronic (increase in serum creatinine greater than 0.3 mg/dl from previous level; increase in blood urea nitrogen level; proteinuria; hematuria; decrease in creatinine clearance; decrease in urinary sodium, urea, and creatinine; oliguria or anuria; fever and weight gain; edema; enlargement of the graft and decreased renal blood flow; tenderness of graft site; increase in blood pressure and pulse; and anxiety, apathy, and lethargy); spontaneous rupture of the graft (intense pain and shock); reappearance of primary renal disease

Urinary tract

Bacteriuria; ureteral fistula or obstruction or hydronephrosis; perirenal hematoma or lymphocele; perinephric abscess; renal calculi

Cardiovascular

Arrhythmias; cardiac arrest; hypotension; hypertension; congestive heart failure; vascular calcification; renal artery stenosis; renal vein thrombosis

Respiratory

Pulmonary edema; pneumonia and other infections (fever, chills, productive cough, and pleuritic pain); pulmonary emboli; reactivated tuberculosis; "transplant" lung (alveolar-capillary block: fall in arterial Po_2 and O_2 saturation with normal Pco_2 and splotchy pneumonia by roentgenographic and minimal physical findings)

Hematopoietic

Leukopenia (related to azathioprine); neoplasms

Gastrointestinal

Hepatitis (related to azathioprine and HB_sAg positive); pancreatitis; peptic ulcer disease; infections: oral and esophageal (fungal)

Neurologic

Infection

Skin and mucous membrane

Infection; purpura; striae; hirsutism; acne; alopecia; neoplasms; wound infection and delayed healing

Musculoskeletal

Hyperparathyroidism; osteoporosis; avascular necrosis of femur (pain in hip and limp); myopathy (muscular weakness)

Eyes

Infection; increased intraocular pressure; cataracts

Psychologic

Euphoria; excitability; psychosis; appearance changes

Other

Impaired growth in children

Most frequent complications are related to technical problems, effects of preexisting uremia, graft rejection, and side effects of immunosuppression.

NURSING DIAGNOSES and NURSING INTERVENTIONS

Nursing Diagnosis	Nursing Intervention
Tissue perfusion, alteration in: renal (potential)	Measure urine hourly and save to determine urinary creatinine, urea, sodium, potassium, pH, specific gravity, and presence of blood and protein. Report anuria or volumes less than 100 ml/hour. Urine flow starts in 2 to 10 minutes after revascularization at 5 to 10 ml/minute and returns to normal volume in 48 to 72 hours.
	Review daily blood chemistries that reflect renal function: creatinine clearance, serum creatinine, and blood urea nitrogen levels, as well as hemoglobin, hematocrit, and white blood cell count.
	Do not clamp urethral or ureteral catheters. Connect catheters to closed drainage system. Avoid kinks in tubing and anchor them securely.
	Observe urine; it may be blood tinged or quite bloody at first. Sudden cessation of urine may be caused by clot. Urethral catheter irrigation by means of sterile technique may be necessary to dislodge it. Ureteral catheter irrigation is done with particular care when ordered.
	When urethral catheter is removed, patient should void frequently to avoid overdistention of bladder.
	Patients may have bladder spasms as unused bladder is distended.
Fluid volume, alteration in: excess, or fluid volume deficit, potential	Measure intake (intravenous and oral fluids when started) and output. Measure weight every day.

Nursing Diagnosis	Nursing Intervention
	Temperature, pulse, respirations, and blood pressure should be measured every 15 minutes for 4 hours, then every half hour until stable, and then every 2 hours for 24 hours. Measure central venous pressure. Patients are sensitive to fluid volume changes. Try to maintain patency of blood access device by avoiding hypovolemia and blood pressure measurements or intravenous punctures in that arm (dialysis may be needed).
Skin integrity, impairment of and susceptibility to infection (potential patient problem)	Provide aseptic wound care. Little drainage is expected. Provide aseptic care to intravenous lines (peripheral and central venous pressure) and urinary catheters. Watch for signs and symptoms of infection that are masked by immunosuppressive drugs. Temperature may not be elevated. Provide a clean environment. Have patient breathe deeply, cough, and turn (only to operative side) to prevent respiratory complications (Infections of lungs by opportunistic organisms are serious complication and frequent cause of death). Help patient with oral and personal hygiene to prevent infection.
Mobility, impaired physical and self-care deficit (potential)	Maintain bed rest for first 24 hours with patient lying flat (head at 30-degree angle) or on operative side with knees straight to prevent tension on the anastomoses. Ambulate in 24 hours. No sitting is permitted. Sodium excretion is increased in prone position. Thromboembolic disorders may occur. Assist with personal hygiene as needed.
Comfort, alteration in: pain	Give analgesics as ordered and record response.
Nutrition, alteration in: potential for less than or more than body requirements	Nothing by mouth or a nasogastric tube is ordered at first. When bowel sounds return, liquids and food by mouth are begun: normal diet with or without restrictions (see "Chronic Renal Failure," p. 1069).
Self-concept, disturbance in: body image	A major concern is incorporation of new part into body. Acceptance by nurse of the patient's feelings of guilt and concern for donor is helpful. Side effects of azathioprine (alopecia) and prednisone (for example, moonface, acne, body fat redistribution) require marked adjustment. See p. 1820.
Family process, alteration in	Keep lines of communication open with family and assist in family-patient communication. Deal sensitively with feelings of family members concerning transplantation. Family have become used to chronically ill person. Return to real health will modify family-patient expectations. Living related donor, a hero or heroine before transplantation, may feel forgotten afterward. Source of cadaver kidney may be a concern. Recipient may be perceived as too independent or not independent enough. Death of patient after transplant fails is very difficult. Be sure family understands that side effects of corticosteroids can interfere with interpersonal relationships. If family and patient do not already know others who have gone through this situation, offer to introduce them to a patient and family. Refer family to other professional colleagues (social workers or psychologists) when they can better meet family's needs (financial concerns, occupational problems, and need for family counseling beyond nurse's expertise). Assist family when child is transplant recipient to reintegrate "healthy" child into family system. See p. 1931.

Patient Education

1. Preparation for discharge includes teaching the following:
   a. Self-observational skills (temperature, pulse, respiration, weight, intake and output, urine collection, and record keeping)
   b. Medications: name, dosage, strength, schedule, purpose, and side effects
   c. Diet: restriction, if any (patient should avoid becoming overweight)
   d. Fluids: restriction, if any
   e. Signs and symptoms of rejection and infection
   f. Important laboratory values (serum creatinine, blood urea nitrogen level, white blood cell count, calcium, and phosphate); With an arteriovenous fistula, do not have blood pressure taken or blood drawn in that arm

2. Long-term follow-up includes teaching the following:
   a. Medical appointment schedule for routine follow-up; plans for telephone communication between appointments
   b. Personal hygiene, prevention of infection, care of minor trauma, contraceptive device, and need for regular dental and eye examinations
   c. Body changes resulting from uremia and long-term corticosteroid therapy, including increased possibility of malignancies
   d. Physical activity levels (daily exercise, avoidance of contact sports, and avoidance of seat belts across the hips) and return to work and other activities
   e. Resources for rehabilitation (including vocational)

EVALUATION

Patient Outcome	Data Indicating That Outcome is Reached
Renal function returns.	Renal function findings are normal. Red blood count, hematocrit, and clotting time are normal. There is no further bone resorption or progressive neuropathy. Libido improves; menses, ovulation, and potency return.
Patient is aware of susceptibility to drug side effects.	Patient understands risk of hepatitis from azathioprine, and risk of osteoporosis and peptic ulceration from steroids. Patient is aware of increased susceptibility to infection.
Patient and family understand renal transplantation.	Patient and family describe medical plan of care, plan for follow-up, precautions, and any restrictions. Patient and family demonstrate self-care skills.
Patient and family adjust to life after transplantation.	Patient and family return to work and social activities. Child recipient enjoys an active independent life within constraints of medical regimen.

RENAL BIOPSY

Description and Rationale

In a renal biopsy a small piece of tissue is obtained via a special needle inserted through the skin into the kidney (percutaneous) or through a surgical incision (open). The following diagnostic studies may be used to locate the kidney for biopsy: kidney, ureter, bladder roentgenogram, intravenous urogram, and ultrasonography. The examination of the specimen by light and electron microscopy and immunofluorescence techniques helps to determine the specific diagnosis and appropriate treatment, severity of disease, likelihood of return of renal function, feasibility of transplantation or dialysis, and level of function in a transplanted kidney.[39] A renal biopsy is indicated when the results might influence the management of the patient. Indications include persistent proteinuria, nephrotic syndrome, unexplained hematuria, and controlled therapeutic trials of new drugs.

Contraindications and Cautions

Absolute contraindications
   Solitary kidney
   Irreversible hemorrhagic tendencies
Relative contraindications
   Uncooperative patient
   Suspected renal tumor or cysts
   Gross sepsis
   Very small kidneys
   Horseshoe kidney
   Ectopic kidney
   Severe hypertension
   Massive obesity

Severe spinal deformity
Pregnancy

Preprocedural Nursing Care

Prepare the patient for the possibility of pain during the procedure. Instructions include the need for the patient to cooperate by holding the breath on command. Explain the need for 24 hours of bed rest after the biopsy and that some hematuria is normal in the first 24 hours.

Record baseline vital signs. Review the chart for hemoglobin and hematocrit levels, platelet count, prothrombin time, and bleeding and clotting times. Review type and cross-match report for 2 units of blood. Review outcome of any test for pregnancy.

ASSESSMENT: AREAS OF CONCERN

Renal

Microscopic hematuria; gross hematuria; local infection; passage of clots; perirenal hematoma; retroperitoneal hematoma; arteriovenous fistula in kidney; massive hemorrhage from biopsy site (rare); ureteral colic from a clot

Cardiovascular

Hypotension; anemia

Other

Pain: mild, local perforation of other structures; fever

NURSING DIAGNOSES and NURSING INTERVENTIONS

Nursing Diagnosis	Nursing Intervention
Tissue perfusion, alteration in: renal	Measure output carefully and collect voidings individually. Watch for hematuria. Check for microscopic hematuria, which is invariable present in the first few specimens. Urine may appear pink. Report profuse or persistent hematuria.
Skin integrity, impairment of	Tight dressing is applied to biopsy site. Check dressing for bleeding. Apply external pressure for 30 minutes by having patient lie prone with a sandbag placed directly under biopsy site.
Fluid volume deficit, potential	Measure blood pressure, pulse, and respirations every 15 minutes for 4 hours and then every 4 hours for 24 hours. Ensure adequate hydration of 1000 to 2000 ml to ensure good urine flow. Monitor hematocrit 3 to 6 hours after biopsy. Decrease from prebiopsy level suggests perirenal bleeding.
Mobility, impaired physical	Prescribe bed rest for 24 hours. If no hematuria occurs in first 24 hours, bathroom privileges can be instituted for next 24 hours. Permit patient to resume activity as desired after 48 hours.
Comfort, alteration in: pain	Give nonaspirin analgesic agent for mild pain after anesthesia wears off, as ordered by the physician. Report severe loin pain.

Patient Education

1. Explain the reason for the biopsy.
2. Explain the need for observation after biopsy.
3. Explain that the patient should avoid contact sports; lifting or heavy exercise; wrestling; riding bicycles, horses, and snowmobiles; and swimming for several days. Normal activities can be resumed gradually after 48 to 72 hours.
4. Explain the need to call the physician to report any hematuria, drainage from the biopsy site, persistent fever, or pain.

EVALUATION

Patient Outcome	**Data Indicating That Outcome is Reached**
Adequate sample of renal tissue is obtained.	Sample contains four to six glomeruli.
Complications of biopsy do not occur.	No severe bleeding or infection occurs.

References

1. American Dietetic Association: Handbook of clinical dietetics, New Haven, Conn., 1981, Yale University Press.
2. Asscher, A.W., Moffat, D.B., and Sanders, E.: Nephrology illustrated: an integrated text and color atlas, Philadelphia, 1982, W.B. Saunders Co.
3. Beeuwkes, R., III, and Rosen, S.: The structure of the human kidney. In Flamenbaum, W., and Hamburger, R.J., editors: Nephrology: an approach to the patient with renal disease, Philadelphia, 1982, J.B. Lippincott Co.
4. Brenner, B.M., and Lazarus, J.M.: Acute renal failure, Philadelphia, 1983, W.B. Saunders Co.
5. Chapman, W.H., et al.: The urinary system: an integrated approach, Philadelphia, 1973, W.B. Saunders Co.
6. Coe, F.L.: Renal calculi and nephrocalcinosis. In Flamenbaum, W., and Hamburger, R.J., editors: Nephrology: an approach to the patient with renal disease, Philadelphia, 1982, J.B. Lippincott Co.
7. Coggins, C.H.: Nephrotic syndrome. In Flamenbaum, W., and Hamburger, R.J., editors: Nephrology: an approach to the patient with renal disease, Philadelphia, 1982, J.B. Lippincott Co.
8. Couser, W.G., Salant, D.J., and Stilmant, M.M.: Glomerulonephritis. In Flamenbaum, W., and Hamburger, R.J., editors: Nephrology: an approach to the patient with renal disease, Philadelphia, 1982, J.B. Lippincott Co.
9. Deinhardt, F., and Deinhardt, J., editors: Viral hepatitis: laboratory and clinical science, New York, 1983, Marcel Dekker, Inc.
10. Earle, D.A., editor, and Levin, M.L., and Quintanilla, A.P., associate editors: Manual of clinical nephrology, Philadelphia, 1982, W.B. Saunders Co.
11. Feinstein, E.I., and Friedman, E.A.: Renal disease in the elderly. In Rossman, I., editor: Clinical geriatrics, ed. 2, Philadelphia, 1979, J.B. Lippincott Co.
12. Friedman, E.A., and L'Esperance, F.A., Jr., editors: Diabetic renal-retinal syndrome. Vol. 2. Prevention and management, New York, 1982, Grune & Stratton, Inc.
13. Gardner, K.D., Jr.: Cystic disorders of the kidney. In Flamenbaum, W., and Hamburger, R.J., editors: Nephrology: an approach to the patient with renal disease, Philadelphia, 1982, J.B. Lippincott Co.
14. Goodman, A.G., Goodman, L.S., and Gilman, A., editors: Goodman and Gilman's the pharmacological basis of therapeutics, ed. 6, New York, 1980, Macmillan Publishing Co., Inc.
15. Govoni, L.E., and Hayes, J.E.: Drugs and nursing implications, Norwalk, Conn., 1982, Appleton-Century-Crofts.
16. Gutch, C.F., and Stoner, M.H.: Review of hemodialysis for nurses and dialysis personnel, ed. 3, St. Louis, 1979, The C.V. Mosby Co.
17. Hamburger, J., Crosnier, J., and Grünfeld, J.P., editors: Nephrology, New York, 1979, John Wiley & Sons.
18. Hoffsten, P., and Klahr, S.: Pathophysiology of chronic renal failure. In Klahr, S., editor: The kidney and body fluids, New York, 1983, Plenum Medical Book Co.
19. Hummel, R.P., editor: Clinical burn therapy, Boston, 1982, John Wright • PSG, Inc.
20. James, J.A.: Renal disease in childhood, ed. 2, St. Louis, 1972, The C.V. Mosby Co.
21. Johns, M.P.: Pharmacodynamics and patient care, St. Louis, 1974, The C.V. Mosby Company.
22. Klahr, S., editor: The kidney and body fluids in health and disease, New York, 1983, Plenum Medical Book Co.
23. Larson, E., Lindbloom, L., and Davis, K.B., editors: Development of the clinical nephrology practitioner: a focus on independent learning, St. Louis, 1982, The C.V. Mosby Co.
24. Levine, D.Z.: Care of the renal patient, Philadelphia, 1983, W.B. Saunders Co.
25. Massry, S.G., and Glasscock, R.J., editors: Textbook of nephrology, vol. 1, Baltimore, 1983, Williams & Wilkins.
26. Muehrcke, R.C.: Acute renal failure, St. Louis, 1969, The C.V. Mosby Co.
27. Murray, T.G., and Goldberg, M.: Interstitial renal disease. In Flamenbaum, W., and Hamburger, R.J., editors: Nephrology: an approach to the patient with renal disease, Philadelphia, 1982, J.B. Lippincott Co.
28. Papper, S., and Williams, G.R., editors: Manual of medical care of the surgical patient, ed. 2, Boston, 1981, Little, Brown & Co.
29. Pemberton, C.M., and Gastineau, C.F., editors: Mayo clinic diet manual: a handbook of dietary practices, ed. 5, Philadelphia, 1981, W.B. Saunders Co.
30. Rowe, J.W.: Renal system. In Rowe, J.W., and Besdine, R.W., editors: Health and disease, Boston, 1982, Little, Brown & Co.
31. Schmitt, G.W.: Chronic renal failure. In Flamenbaum, W., and Hamburger, R.J., editors: Nephrology: an approach to the patient with renal disease, Philadelphia, 1982, J.B. Lippincott Co.
32. Schmitt, G.W., and Bach, C.: Peritoneal dialysis and hemodialysis: an overview. In Flamenbaum, W., and Hamburger, R.J., editors: Nephrology: an approach to the patient with renal disease, Philadelphia, 1982, J.B. Lippincott Co.
33. Sever, J.L., and Edmonds, J.H.: Urinary tract infection during pregnancy: maternal and pediatric findings. In Kass, E.H., and Brumfitt, W., editors: Infections of the urinary tract, Chicago, 1978, University of Chicago Press.
34. Starzl, T.E., and others: Renal homotransplantation. I., Curr. Prob. Surg., p. 3, April 1974.
35. Takacs, F.J., and Finkel, R.M.: Diabetic nephropathy. In Flamenbaum, W., and Hamburger, R.J., editors: Nephrology: an approach to the patient with renal disease, Philadelphia, 1982, J.B. Lippincott Co.
36. Tenckhoff, H.: Chronic peritoneal dialysis, Seattle, 1974, University of Washington School of Medicine, Department of Medicine, Division of Kidney Diseases.
37. Tuberculosis statistics: states and cities, 1979, Atlanta, 1980, U.S. Centers for Disease Control.
38. Urizar, R.E.: Kidney biopsy and its complications. In Urizar, R.E., Largent, J.A., and Gilboa, N.: Pediatric nephrology: new directions in therapy, New York, 1983, Medical Examination Publishing Co.
39. Urizar, R.E., and Gilboa, N.: The nephritic syndrome. In Urizar, R.E., Largent, J.A., and Gilboa, N.: Pediatric nephrology: new directions in therapy, New York, 1983, Medical Examination Publishing Co.

40. Urizar, R.E., and Largent, J.A.: The uremic syndrome. In Urizar, R.E., Largent, J.A., and Gilboa, N.: Pediatric nephrology: new directions in therapy, New York, 1983, Medical Examination Publishing Co.
41. Van der Hem, G.K., editor: Nephrology, Amsterdam, 1982, Excerpta Medica.

Suggested Readings

Avram, M.W., editor: Prevention of kidney disease and long-term survival, New York, 1982, Plenum Medical Book Co.

Brundage, D.J.: Nursing management of renal problems, ed. 2, St. Louis, 1980, The C.V. Mosby Co.

Levy, N.B., editor: Psychonephrology I: psychological factors in hemodialysis and transplantation, New York, 1981, Plenum Medical Book Co.

Morris, P.J., editor: Tissue transplantation, Edinburgh, 1982, Churchill Livingstone.

Toledo-Pereya, L.H., editor: Basic concepts in organ procurement, perfusion, and preservation, New York, 1982, Academic Press, Inc.

Wright, L.F.: Maintenance hemodialysis, Boston, 1981, G.K. Hall & Co.

CHAPTER 11

Gastrointestinal System

Overview

Diseases of the gastrointestinal system are commonly referred to as digestive diseases. The digestive system is composed of the mouth, esophagus, stomach, small and large intestines, and the accessory organs of digestion: liver, gallbladder, and pancreas. Digestive diseases are disorders or inflammations of any of these organs. Examples of digestive diseases are reflex esophagitis, peptic ulcer disease, ulcerative colitis, pancreatitis, and cancer. The diagnosis, treatment, and management vary with each digestive disease.

More Americans are hospitalized with disorders of the digestive system than any other group of disorders. The National Digestive Disease Advisory Board (NDDAB) reports that 20 million persons are chronically ill with digestive diseases and are absent from work as a result of digestive problems.[48] The NDDAB also reports a $52 billion annual economic cost incurred through lost wages, disability payments, health care expenditures, and lost tax revenues associated with digestive diseases. Approximately 200,000 people die each year from digestive diseases, including malignancies. Thus this group of diseases may have devastating long-term personal, social, and economic effects. The NDDAB is only one national group concerned with digestive diseases. There are 13 lay organizations and 17 professional associations involved in digestive disease programs and education, reflecting the national concern with the management of digestive diseases.

The importance of digestive diseases and their implications for health care have often been minimized. The group of diseases involving the gastrointestinal tract vary from mild to severe. The chronicity of the diseases and the symptoms can affect the person's ability to maintain a desired life-style. Psychosocial stressors often intensify the symptoms.

ANATOMY AND PHYSIOLOGY

The gastrointestinal tract consists of a series of connected organs and accessory organs whose overall purpose is the breakdown of food products that can be used by the body as a source of energy. There are three key processes associated with the gastrointestinal tract: digestion, absorption, and metabolism. Digestion is the mechanical and chemical breakdown of food into amino acids, glucose, and fatty acids that can be used by the body for cellular functions. Absorption is the passage of the digested food products (essential nutrients) from the lumen of the gastrointestinal tract into the blood and lymphatic system. Metabolism is the utilization of the basic food product by the cell. Digestion and absorption can be affected by infections, inflammatory diseases, surgery, or other alterations of the gastrointestinal tract. To adequately assess the effects of digestive diseases, the nurse must first have a basic understanding of the alimentary, or gastrointestinal, system.

Fig. 11-1
Anatomy of the gastrointestinal system.

From Broadwell, D.C., and Jackson, B.S., editors: Principles of ostomy care, St. Louis, 1982, The C.V. Mosby Co.

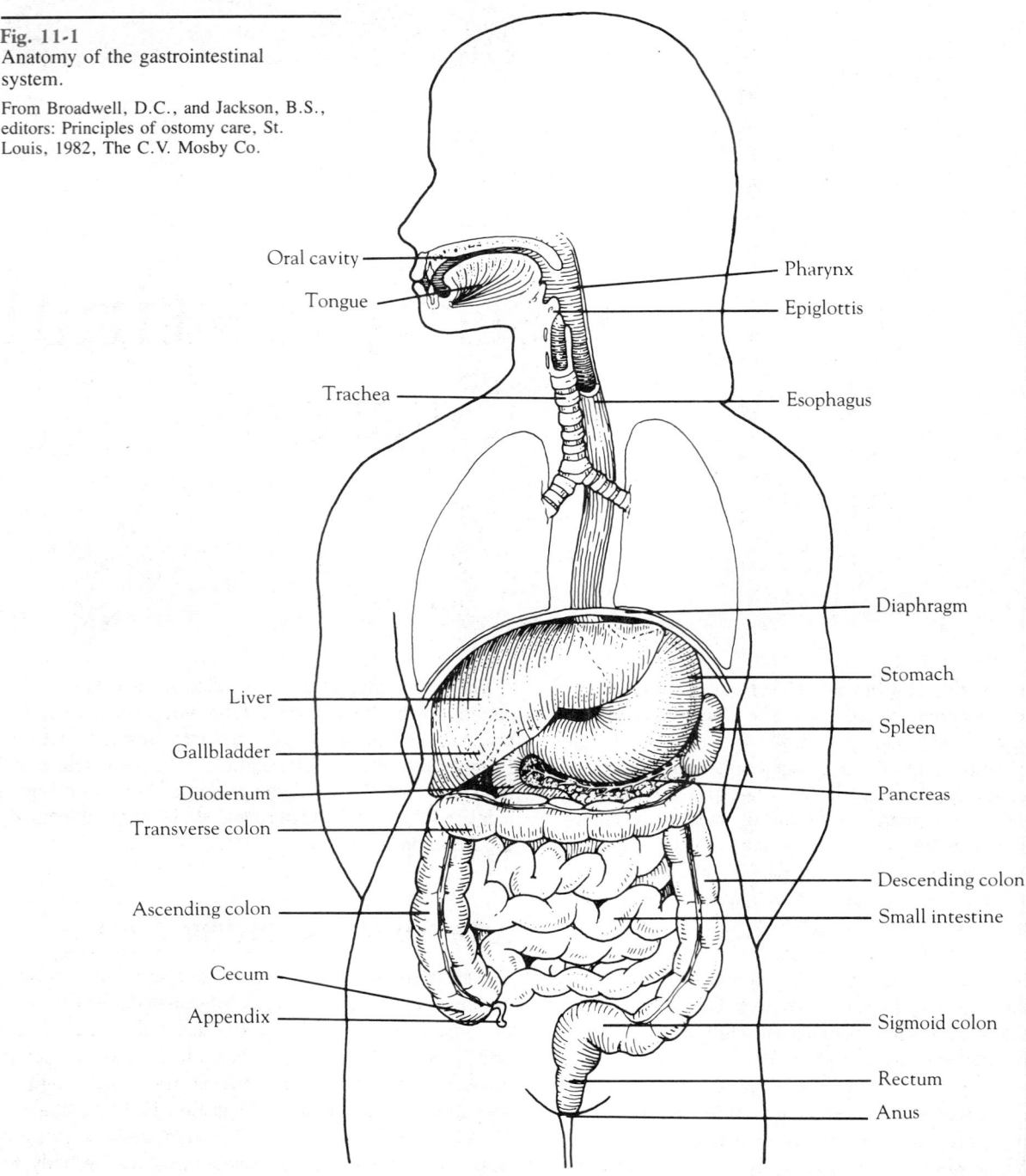

The gastrointestinal system consists of the mouth, pharynx, esophagus, stomach, and small and large intestines. Accessory organs include liver, gallbladder, and pancreas. The accessory organs found in the mouth are the teeth and salivary glands (Fig. 11-1).

The gastrointestinal system produces both exocrine and endocrine secretions. Exocrine secretions prepare food for absorption by diluting it to the osmolality of plasma (isotonic), altering the pH for hydrolysis, and hydrolyzing complex foods. The exocrine secretions also protect the mucosa from physical and chemical irritants. Endocrine secretions play a major role in the control and coordination of secretory and motor activities involved in the digestion and absorption of food. The types and functions of the secretions will be discussed as they appear in the gastrointestinal tract.

Mouth

The mouth, also referred to as the buccal cavity or the oral cavity, is commonly considered the beginning of the gastrointestinal tract. Mechanical and chemical digestion begins in the mouth. The teeth and tongue aid in mechanical breakdown, whereas the secretions of the salivary glands begin basic starch digestion and lubricate food to aid in swallowing.

The vestibule is the region between the lips, cheeks, teeth, and gums. The region posterior to the teeth and gums is the mouth cavity proper. Saliva from the salivary glands is received by the mouth cavity proper and aids in digestion.

The lips keep food and saliva in the mouth during mastication. The lips are sharply demarcated from the surrounding facial skin by the vermilion-cutaneous line. The lips are covered externally by integument and internally by mucous membrane. The bulk of the lips is composed of orbicularis oris, a sphincterlike muscle. The lips play a part in the fine nuances of articulation.

The internal cheeks are composed of muscle, fat, areolar tissue, nerves, vessels, and buccal glands covered by an inner mucous membrane. The gums, or gingivae, are dense fibrous tissue covered by a smooth mucous membrane.

The roof of the mouth is formed by the hard and soft palates. The hard palate is formed by two palatine bones and parts of the superior maxillary bone. The midline of the hard palate is called the linear raphe. The mucous membrane of the hard palate is thick, pale, and corrugated anterior to and to either side of the linear raphe. The posterior mucous membrane is thin, smooth, and a deeper pink. Attached to the posterior portion of the hard palate is the soft palate. The soft palate forms the partition between the mouth and nasopharynx. In a relaxed position the anterior surface of the soft palate is concave and continuous with the roof of the mouth while the posterior surface is convex and continuous with the nasal cavities. The uvula is the conical fingerlike projection of the posterior border of the soft palate. During swallowing the soft palate moves upward, closing off the nasopharynx and preventing foods and fluids from entering the pharynx.

The tongue is a muscular organ anchored to the hyoid bone and the mandible and covered with a mucous membrane. The frenum, or frenulum, is a fold of mucous membrane under the tongue that attaches the tongue to the floor of the mouth. Mucous membrane also attaches the tongue to the epiglottis, soft palate, and pharynx. The tip of the tongue is the apex.

The tongue contains mucous and serous glands. The mucous glands are located behind the apex and secrete mucin. The serous glands are also referred to as Ebner's glands and are found in the back of the tongue. Ebner's glands assist in the distribution of substances to be tasted over the tongue.

The muscles of the tongue are divided into lateral halves by a median fibrous septum. There are two groups of muscles that can be identified by their role in the tongue's functions. The muscles that assist the tongue in protrusion, retraction, elevation, and depression during mastication are the genioglossus, hyoglossus, chondroglossus, styloglossus, and palatoglossus. The muscles that are responsible for altering the shape of the tongue (shortened, curved, narrowed) include the longitudinalis superior, longitudinalis inferior, transversus, and verticalis. These movements are important in the enunciation of different letters and words.

The four types of papillae that contain taste buds are located on the anterior two thirds of the dorsum of the tongue. They are papillae circumvallate, papillae fungiformes, papillae filiformes, and papillae simplices. Papillae circumvallate form an inverted V on the posterior dorsal surface of the tongue. These are the largest papillae and are round and flattened. The taste buds are found on their lateral surfaces.

Papillae filiformes are numerous and are arranged in tight parallel rows. They contain thick, dense epithelium and appear white on the tongue's surface. The filiformes also contain elastic fibers.

The papillae fungiformes are found mainly at the apex and sides of the tongue. They are large and deep red in color.

The papillae simplices are similar to papillae of the skin and cover the entire mucous membrane of the tongue. The papillae simplices play a minor role in taste sensation.

Taste buds are concentrated in the circumvallate and fungiform papillae. Adults have approximately 10,000 taste buds, and children have a few more.[30] As a person ages, the taste buds begin to degenerate and perception of taste becomes less acute.

The four primary sensations of taste are sweet, sour, salty, and bitter. There is a tendency for taste buds detecting a primary taste to be localized to certain areas of the tongue. Sweet taste is primarily on the anterior surface and the tip of the tongue; sour taste on the two lateral sides; bitter taste on the circumvallate papillae; and salty taste over the entire tongue. It is known that taste buds do respond with varying degrees to all four taste sensations. A taste bud may have a greater degree of sensitivity to one or two tastes but will respond moderately to the other taste sensations.

Since taste buds will respond to taste sensations with

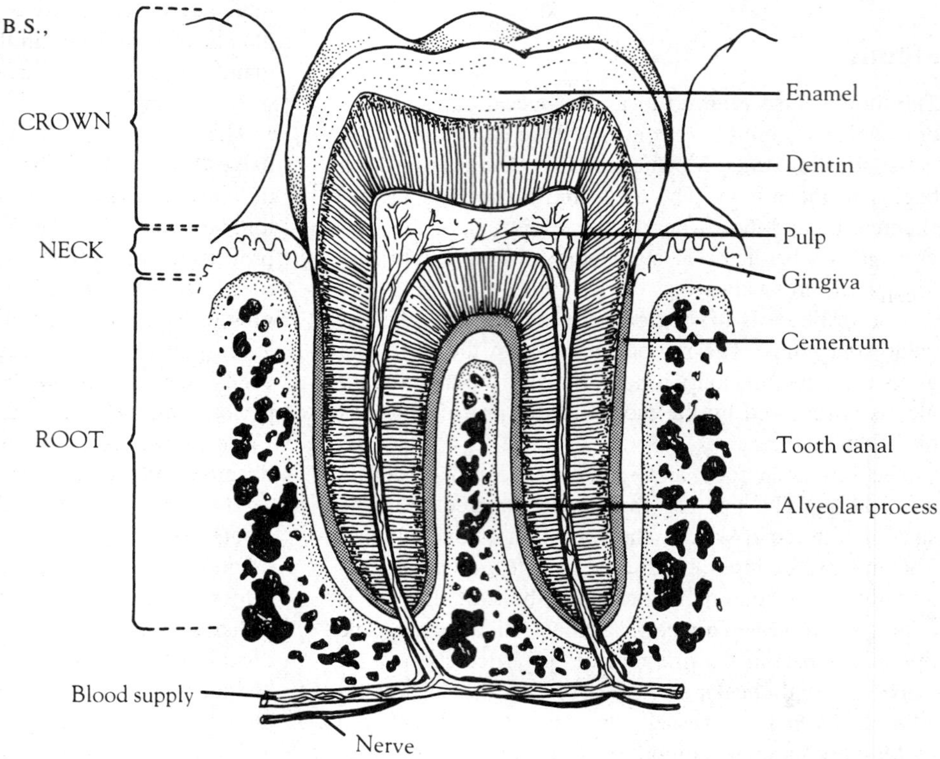

Fig. 11-2
Adult molar.

From Broadwell, D.C., and Jackson, B.S.,
editors: Principles of ostomy care, St.
Louis, 1982, The C.V. Mosby Co.

CROWN

NECK

ROOT

Enamel

Dentin

Pulp

Gingiva

Cementum

Tooth canal

Alveolar process

Blood supply

Nerve

a different degree of sensitivity, the brain determines the taste based on the degree of stimulation of various taste buds. The sense of smell also affects the sense of taste. Odors from food stimulate the olfactory system. When the sense of smell is decreased, the degree of taste is often reported as diminished. Taste preference is used by animals and humans to regulate diet.

Adults have 32 teeth, and children have 20. Teeth cut and mix food, serving as an accessory to digestion. Mechanical breakdown of food occurs when the teeth cut and grind. Mixing the food with saliva begins some chemical digestion and lubricates the food for swallowing.

A tooth consists of three parts: crown, neck, and root (Fig. 11-2). The crown is the visible part of the tooth above the jaw. The root is buried in the alveolus cavity, and the narrow portion between the crown and the root is referred to as the neck. Examination of a cross section of a tooth reveals the following structures: enamel, dentin, cementum, pulp, and periodontal membrane. The enamel is made of small crystals of calcium phosphate and calcium carbonate embedded in keratin fibers. It is the hardest substance in the body and forms a protective covering over the crown.

The dentin, directly below the enamel, forms the bulk of the tooth. It is made up principally of calcium salts of phosphate and carbonate embedded in collagen fibers. Dentin is highly resistant to tensional and compressional forces. Cementum covers the dentin of the root from the enamel junction to the apex. This is a layer of coarse fibrous bone. The pulp is in the center of each crown and root. The soft tissue of pulp is supplied by capillaries, lymph vessels, and nerve fibers. The pulp serves as a cushion to allow slight changes in the circulation of blood into teeth without adding pressure on the nerve fibers. The periodontal membrane covers the root and separates the tooth from the dense bone (lamina dura) that forms the wall of the alveolus.

The primary, or deciduous, teeth begin to erupt during the sixth to ninth month of life. The teeth begin to erupt when calcification of different tissues of the tooth is sufficient to enable it to withstand the pressures of mastication (chewing). The tooth breaks through the gum and becomes firmly implanted in the jaw by the alveoli until eruption of the permanent teeth.

The central and lateral incisors shear and cut food. The canine teeth tear food, and the premolars and molars grind and chew. Fig. 11-3 shows the location of the

Fig. 11-3
Permanent teeth.

From Broadwell, D.C., and Jackson, B.S.,
editors: Principles of ostomy care, St.
Louis, 1982, The C.V. Mosby Co.

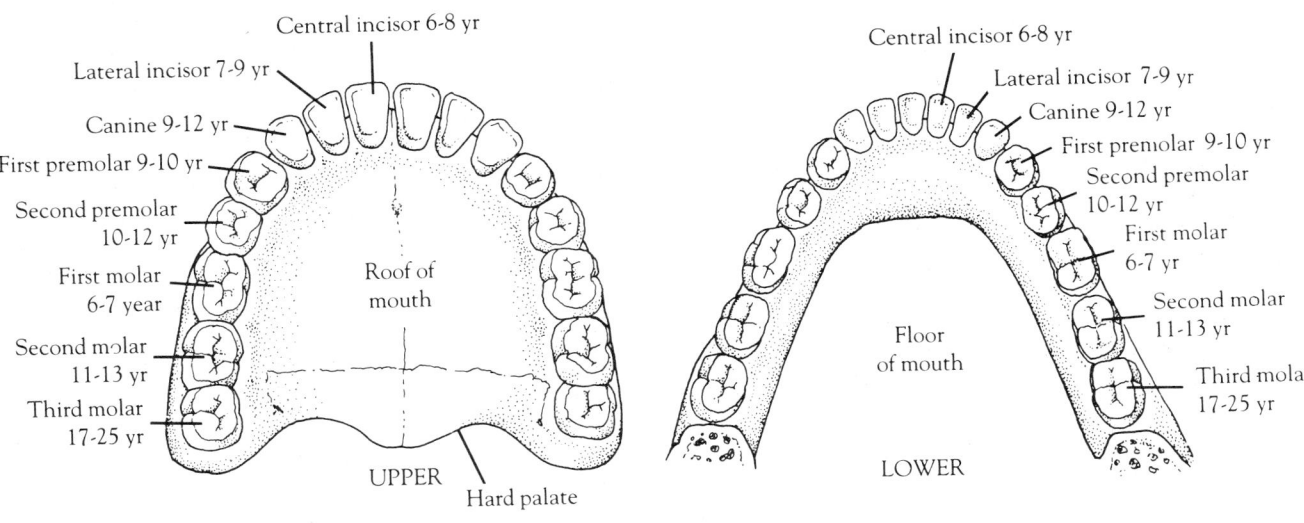

permanent teeth and the age at which they are most likely to appear.

Mastication (chewing) involves the stimulation of jaw muscles. Much of the chewing process is innervated by the motor branch of the fifth cranial nerve. There is also a chewing reflex. The presence of food in the mouth causes a reflex inhibition of the muscles of mastication, which allows the lower jaw to drop. This drop initiates a stretch reflex in the jaw muscles, leading to a rebound contraction: raising the jaw and closing the teeth. The closure of the teeth on the bolus of food inhibits the jaw muscles, allowing the jaw to drop and rebound. This is then repeated.

Since digestive enzymes only work on the surface of food particles, chewing will increase the surface area exposed to the enzymes. Chewing food will also increase the ease with which food is swallowed and affect the ease of emptying of food from the stomach into the small intestine.

Salivary Glands

The salivary glands consist of the parotid, submaxillary, and sublingual glands. There are some small salivary glands found in the lips, buccal mucosa, and palate. These are exocrine glands that secrete a mixture of serous and mucous fluid into the oral cavity.

The parotid gland is located anteriorly to the external ear and wraps around the mandible. The parotids are the largest of the salivary glands; each weighs approximately

14 to 30 g. The parotid (Stensen's) duct enters the mouth at its papillae opposite the second maxillary molar tooth. The parotid gland produces ptyalin (salivary amylase), which begins the chemical breakdown of starches. The ptyalin is released from serous acini. The secretory motor fibers innervate the gland from the otic ganglion via the auriculotemporal nerve, which originates in a branch of the glossopharyngeal nerve.

The action of ptyalin in the mouth will only break down 5% to 10% of the starches. The action of the enzyme continues in the stomach for 30 minutes to several hours, until the pH falls, rendering the enzyme inactive.

The submaxillary gland is smaller, weighing 7 to 10 g, and is located inferiorly to the mylohyoid muscle. It lies adjacent to the body of the mandible. The submaxillary (Wharton's) duct opens on the floor of the mouth adjacent to the base of the frenulum of the tongue. The secretory motor fibers originate in the chorda tympani nerve. The submaxillary gland produces a mixture of mucous and serous secretions.

The sublingual glands are located beneath the floor of the mouth and weigh approximately 3 g. The sublingual glands consist of predominantly mucous acini with a few serous acini. The primary purpose of the sublingual gland secretions is lubrication.

Approximately 1000 to 1500 ml of saliva is produced by the salivary glands in a 24-hour period. The pH of the saliva is between 6.0 and 7.0. The superior and inferior salivatory nuclei are located in the brainstem and

stimulation may be affected by taste and tactile stimuli from the tongue and mouth. Pleasant taste stimuli result in more salivation than unpleasant tastes. Also, smooth-textured foods stimulate more saliva production than rough-textured foods. Less salivation may result in less lubrication of food and more difficulty in swallowing. More saliva is produced when a person is eating a food he likes than when eating a disliked food. Thus some sources have divided salivation into three phases: psychic, gustatory, and gastrointestinal. The psychic phase occurs when the mouth is preparing itself to receive food. It is stimulated by thoughts or smells of pleasant foods. The gustatory phase occurs while one is chewing or swallowing food. The saliva is stimulated to aid in mastication and lubricate the foodstuff for swallowing. The gastrointestinal phase occurs when one has eaten irritating foods. The salivation is a response to reflexes originating in the stomach or upper intestines. The swallowed saliva dilutes or neutralizes the irritant.

Oropharynx

The oropharynx is the midpoint of the upper respiratory tract and digestive tract. The superior boundary is at a horizontal line that would connect the soft palate with the second cervical vertebra. The inferior line would connect horizontally the tip of the epiglottis and the base of the tongue. The nasopharynx lies between the oropharynx and the hypopharynx.

The oropharynx is lined by a mucous membrane of stratified squamous epithelium that is continuous with the lining of the mouth, nasal cavities, and larynx. The contents of the oropharynx include the soft palate, the uvula, the tonsils and their pillars, and the base of the tongue.

Esophagus

The esophagus is a hollow muscular tube approximately 25 cm (10 inches) in length. It begins in the neck at the lower border of the fifth cervical vertebra and connects the hypopharynx to the cardia of the stomach. On each side of the esophagus are the thyroid lobes and parathyroids. The recurrent laryngeal nerves run directly in front of the esophagus. In the thorax the esophagus is found to the left of the midline with the pericardium and left atrium in front. The arch of the aorta crosses the lateral aspect of the esophagus at the level of the fourth thoracic vertebra. The descending aorta runs laterally and slightly posterior to the esophagus. At the level of the tenth thoracic vertebra the esophagus passes through the diaphragm into the abdominal cavity.

The esophagus narrows slightly at three points: near its origin in the region of the cricoid cartilage, at the arch of the aorta, and as it passes through the diaphragm. The esophagus is more vulnerable to perforation and trauma in these areas.

The arterial blood supply of the esophagus comes from the inferior thyroid artery in the neck, from branches of the descending aorta, and from the left gastric artery. The esophageal veins join the vena azygos, which joins the superior vena cava and the systemic circulation. The veins at the lower end of the esophagus communicate freely with the tributaries of the left gastric vein that join the portal vein. The upper part of the esophagus drains into the superior vena cava; the middle part drains into the azygos system; and the bottom third drains into the portal system via the gastric veins. There is no connection here of the portal and systemic venous systems. The hepatic vein drains the liver and empties into the superior vena cava, which is the connection between the two systems. When there is increased pressure in the portal system, there is increased pressure in the esophageal veins, leading to the development of esophageal varices.

The wall of the esophagus has all the characteristics of the gastrointestinal tract except for the serosa. This lack of serosa becomes important when esophageal surgery (i.e., anastomosis) has been performed since there may be an increased chance for leakage postoperatively. The innermost, or mucous, membrane is composed of a stratified squamous epithelium that is continuous with the oral cavity and pharynx. At the lower end of the esophagus the mucous membrane changes to a simple columnar (transitional) epithelium that merges with the gastric mucosa in the cardiac portion of the stomach.

The submucosa layer underlying the squamous epithelium contains the blood vessels, nerves, mucous cells, and connective tissues. The mucous cells secrete mucus to further lubricate the foodstuff and protect the wall of the esophagus. The secretions are amphoteric, neutralizing both acid and base.

The muscle layer is composed of an internal circular and outer longitudinal layer. It differs from the remainder of the alimentary tract in several ways. First, the longitudinal layer is thicker than the inner circular layer. Second, the upper third of the esophagus is striated muscle. This portion of the esophagus receives its innervation from lower motor neurons and is dependent on cholinergic mechanisms. If these nerves are cut, flaccid paralysis of the upper esophagus will occur.[72] The middle third of the esophagus is mixed muscle tissue, and the lower third is primarily smooth muscle. The innervation of the smooth muscle found in the lower two thirds of the esophagus is preganglionic fibers of the autonomic nervous system. No flaccid paralysis will develop if these nerves are cut.

Swallowing

Deglutition (swallowing) can be divided into several phases. The first is voluntary, in which the tongue moves upward and backward, forcing a bolus of food into the pharynx. The following phases are involuntary and involve transfer and transport. Transfer results in changes in the pharyngeal and upper esophagus, while transport involves the middle and lower esophagus.

During the voluntary stage of swallowing, the bolus of food stimulates swallowing receptors around the pharynx and the impulses pass to the brainstem, resulting in a series of autonomic pharyngeal muscular contractions. First, the soft palate is elevated into contact with the posterior pharyngeal wall, closing the nasopharynx. Second, contraction of the suprahyoid muscles elevates the larynx and trachea, increasing the diameter of the pharynx. Third, the epiglottis bends backward and the vocal cords come together, further blocking the respiratory tract.

As the bolus enters the pharynx, the circopharyngeal muscle relaxes, permitting the bolus to enter the esophagus. This stimulates rapid peristaltic waves. These actions increase the size of the pharynx, pull the pharynx up to receive the food, and close the larynx to prevent aspiration. The nerve impulses of the pharynx, which are stimulated by the bolus of food, travel the trigeminal nerve to the medulla oblongata, where the swallowing center is located. Nerve impulses then travel back along the glossopharyngeal and vagus nerves to move the bolus into the esophagus.

The esophageal phase of swallowing moves the bolus from the pharynx to the stomach by peristalsis. There are three types of esophageal peristalsis: primary, secondary, and tertiary. Primary peristalsis is a continuation of the movement begun in the pharynx. If a person is upright, downward gravity will also affect the travel time through the esophagus. If primary peristalsis fails to move all the food that has entered the esophagus into the stomach, secondary peristalsis will be stimulated from the distention of the esophagus by the retained bolus. The only difference is that primary peristalsis is initiated in the pharynx and secondary peristalsis is initiated in the esophagus at the level of the aortic arch.

Tertiary contractions may occur in some individuals, particularly after middle age. These are nonperistaltic contractions and do not assist in transport of food through the esophagus.

Approximately 1 to 3 cm above the junction of the esophagus and stomach is a segment, called the lower esophageal sphincter, that has a higher resting pressure than that in the body of the esophagus and that in the stomach. Under normal circumstances this area relaxes with primary or secondary peristalsis. The purpose of this high-pressure area is to prevent reflux of acid gastric contents into the esophagus. Certain factors* will increase or decrease this high-pressure zone:

1. Increase high-pressure zone
   a. Gastrin
   b. Cholinergic agents
      (1) Methacholine (Mecholyl)
      (2) Bethanechol (Urecholine)
   c. Metoclopramide
   d. Prostaglandin F_2
   e. Gastric alkalinization (antacids)
   f. Alpha-adrenergic agonists
   g. Protein meal
   h. Nonfat milk
   i. Ethanol (low dose)
   j. Bombesin
2. Decrease high-pressure zone
   a. Secretin
   b. Cholecystokinin
   c. Glucagon
   d. Anticholinergics
   e. Gastric inhibitory polypeptide
   f. Vasoactive intestine peptide
   g. Verapamil
   h. Prostaglandins E, E2, A2
   i. Gastric acidification
   j. Alpha-adrenergic antagonists
   k. Fat meal
   l. Whole milk
   m. Ethanol (high dose)

Peritoneal Cavity

The abdomen is the largest cavity in the human body. It contains the stomach, small intestines, kidneys, adrenal glands, and the uterus in women. Also contained here are the liver, colon, gallbladder, pancreas, and major vessels. The abdomen is bordered anteriorly by the abdominal muscles and iliacus, posteriorly by vertebral column and lumbar muscles, inferiorly by the plane of the superior aperture of the lesser pelvis, and superiorly by the diaphragm.

The structures in the cavity are protected and covered by peritoneum, which is made up of serous membrane composed of mesothelium and a thin layer of irregular connective tissue. The parietal peritoneum is the tissue that lines the abdominal wall. The mesentery is a double fold of parietal peritoneum that is fan shaped and encircles the jejunum and ileum (segments of the small intestines) attaching them to the posterior abdominal wall. The blood vessels and nerves of the small intestine pass

*Adapted from Bolt, R.J., et al.: The digestive system, New York, 1983, John Wiley & Sons.

through the mesentery. The organs in the abdominal cavity are covered by a protective lining, the visceral peritoneum. The greater omentum is an apron-shaped double fold of peritoneum that hangs loosely over the intestines. The greater omentum is attached to the upper border of the duodenum, the lower edge of the stomach, and the transverse colon.

A small amount of serous fluid separates the space between the parietal and visceral peritoneum. The fluid provides lubrication between the organs and the abdominal wall.

Stomach

The function of the stomach is to alter the consistency and the composition of ingested foods. The ingested foodstuffs are liquefied into chyme as the stomach mixes the material with gastric secretions. The chyme is then released in a regulated manner into the duodenum for further digestion and absorption.

The stomach connects to the esophagus 3 cm below the diaphragm. The stomach lies obliquely beneath the cardiac sphincter of the esophagus, above the pyloric sphincter next to the small intestine, and under the left lobe of the liver and diaphragm. The size, shape, and portion of the stomach vary depending on body size, posture, degree of gastric retention, degree of gastric muscle development, and effects of pressures from adjacent organs. Its normal capacity is 1 to 2 L. The stomach functions as a reservoir where mechanical and chemical breakdown of foodstuffs continues.

The stomach is divided into the cardia, the fundus, the body, the antrum, and the pylorus (Fig. 11-4). The cardia is the proximal portion of the stomach. The lesser curvature of the stomach extends from the cardiac orifice to the pyloric opening in a downward curve. Attached to this border is the lesser omentum, or gastrohepatic ligament. The greater curvature is almost four times longer than the lesser curvature, and the greater omentum is attached to it.

The fundus is the uppermost portion of the stomach. Although the fundus is distal to the cardia, it is superior to the cardia anatomically. The body of the stomach extends distally from the fundus to the level at which the gastric lumen assumes a transverse direction. The antrum is the peristaltic portion of the stomach and is distal to the body. Not only is the motor activity different in the antrum, the mucosal surface is different. The pylorus is the portion just before the duodenum.

The wall of the stomach is composed of four layers from the innermost lining layer out: the mucosa, the submucosa, the muscle layer, and the serosa. The mucosa layer is separated from the submucosa by the muscularis mucosa and is composed of gastric epithelium. The mucosa is arranged in longitudinal folds called rugae found most predominantly in the fundus and body regions of the stomach. The rugae are low and flat in the lesser curvature and are sometimes absent in the antrum.

Fig. 11-4
Gross anatomy of the stomach.

From Broadwell, D.C., and Jackson, B.S., editors: Principles of ostomy care, St. Louis, 1982, The C.V. Mosby Co.

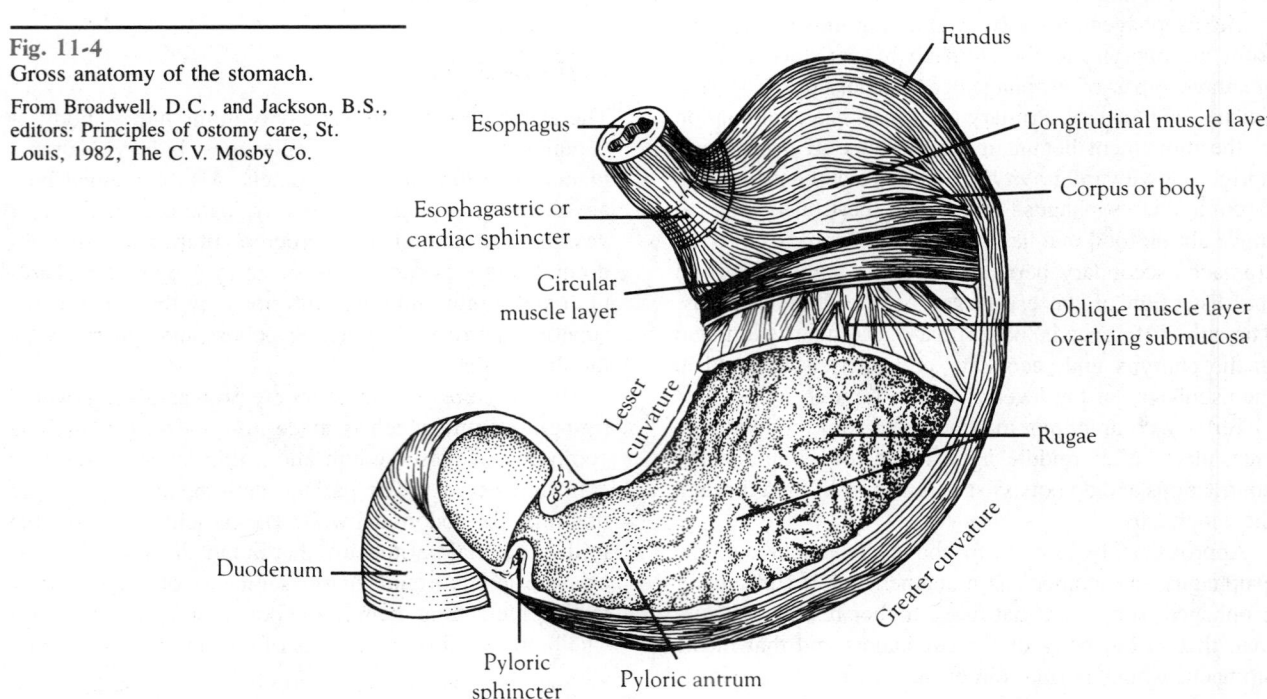

The cells of the mucosa are tall and columnar and contain mucus. The gastric epithelial layer invaginates to form gastric pits or foveolae, which communicate with deeper gastric glands (Fig. 11-5). The gastric glands secrete into the gastric lumen via the gastric pit.

Microscopically, there are three distinct areas of cells within the stomach: the cardia, the oxyntic, and the antral, or pyloric. The mucosa of the cardia is columnar epithelium that secretes mucus. This zone or area has also been referred to as the transitional or junctional mucosa.

The glands of the fundus and body are straight, closely packed, and tubular. These glands contain four cell types: neck cells, parietal (oxyntic) cells, chief (zymogen) cells, and argentaffin cells. Mucous neck cells are most numerous and play a role in mucosal cell renewal. Parietal cells are located at the upper portion of the gland. Parietal cells produce hydrochloric acid (HCl) and intrinsic factor. Chief cells are most abundant in the deeper portion of the gland and secrete pepsinogen (type I). Argentaffin cells are in the deeper portion of the gland and produce serotonin.

The fundus and body are often referred to as the acid-pepsin secreting area. The pepsinogen is activated in a pH below 5. The optimal level of pH is 1.8 to 3.5. The hydrochloric acid provides the acidity necessary for the pepsinogen to convert to its active form, pepsin.

The antrum mucosa is thinner than the oxyntic and the foveolae are deeper. The glands are tubular and coiled. Gastrin-producing G cells are located in the mucosa adjacent to the tubular glands. The tubular glands secrete mucus and pepsinogen II.

The submucosa is composed of loose areolar and elastic tissue. It contains vascular and lymphatic channels and an intrinsic nerve plexus, Meissner's plexus. The muscle layer is thick and is composed of three separate strata of smooth muscle. The outer, longitudinal layer extends downward from the esophagus along the greater and lesser curvatures to the pyloric sphincter. The middle circular muscle forms a uniform layer over the entire stomach. There is a second nerve plexus found between the two muscle layers, Auerbach's plexus. The inner oblique muscle layer is continuous with the circular muscle of the esophagus and is thickest in the fundus region. It extends to the pyloric sphincter. The outermost layer is the serosa and is an extension of the peritoneum.

The blood supply to the stomach is from large branches of the celiac artery. There may be variation in the branching pattern of the celiac axis. In approximately one fourth of all persons, the left hepatic artery may arise in part

Fig. 11-5
Human gastric mucosa. Diagram of tubular gland from fundic area of stomach.

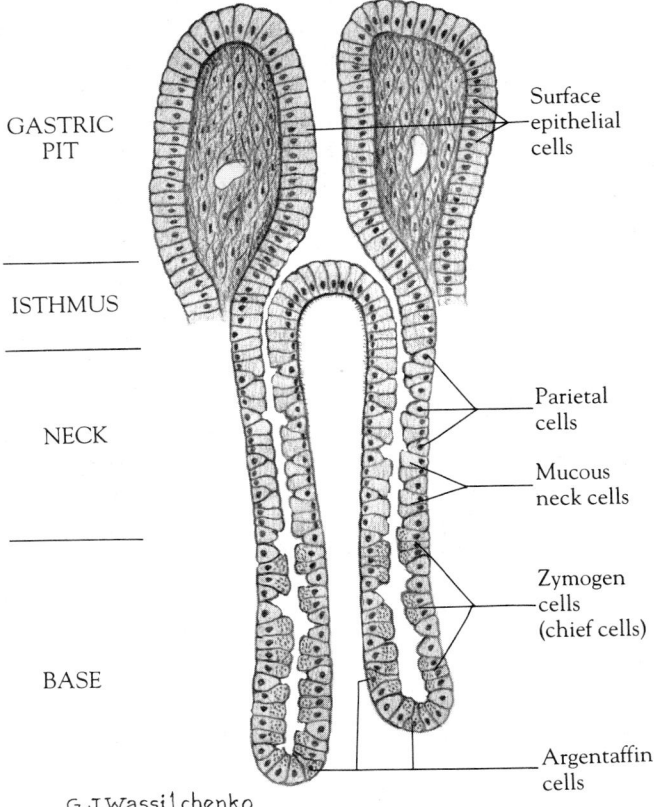

GASTRIC PIT

ISTHMUS

NECK

BASE

Surface epithelial cells

Parietal cells

Mucous neck cells

Zymogen cells (chief cells)

Argentaffin cells

G.J.Wassilchenko

or totally from the left gastric artery. Gastrectomy in this group may lead to necrosis of the left lobe of the liver unless the surgeon first assesses the pattern of arterial blood flow.[4] Arterial branches passing through the muscle layer form an extensive plexus of blood vessels in the submucosa. These vessels then enter the mucosa and subdivide to form a capillary network in the lamina propria surrounding the gastric glands and pits. Blood can be shunted from one area of the stomach to another or from one layer of the stomach to another by submucosa anastomoses and numerous submucosa arteriovenous communications. Mucosal ischemia can be caused by a redistribution of blood flow from vasoconstrictor activity of the sympathetic nervous system and by vasoconstrictor drugs. Bolt and co-workers[4] state that it is not clearly understood if the vagus nerve is capable of directly mediating vasodilation of the gastric vascular supply. Venous blood from the stomach, the right and left gastric veins, empties directly into the portal vein.

Nerve innervation to the stomach arises from the vagus and splanchnic nerves. Branches of the left and right vagus nerves join to form the anterior esophageal plexus, and branches of the right vagus form the posterior esophageal plexus. At the distal esophagus they join to form the anterior and posterior vagal trunk. The anterior trunk provides the anterior gastric and hepatic divisions. The anterior gastric division goes along the lesser curvature to the pyloric sphincter with branches to the anterosuperior wall of the stomach. The hepatic division supplies the gallbladder, biliary tree, and proximal duodenum.

The posterior trunk of the vagus nerve divides into the posterior gastric and celiac divisions. The posterior gastric division goes along the lesser curvature with branches to the posteroinferior wall of the stomach. The celiac division descends with the left gastric artery through the celiac plexus to the superior mesenteric plexus, supplying the small intestine and ascending and transverse colon to the splenic flexure.

The splanchnic nerves contain sensory fibers and postganglionic sympathetic fibers (whose transmitters are catecholamines). The vagi contain sensory fibers, preganglionic parasympathetic fibers (cholinergic), and purinergic fibers (adenosine triphosphetic).[4] These fibers synapse with the ganglion cells of the myenteric (Auerbach's) plexus and the submucosal (Meissner's) plexus. The postganglionic fibers end in the gastric glands and muscle fibers stimulating gastric secretion and muscle contraction.

The reservoir function of the stomach is the capacity of the stomach to accommodate a meal. A vagalmediated reflex relaxes the body of the stomach so that it accepts the ingested meal with minimal increase in intragastric pressure. Once swallowing is completed, the gastric wall tension will increase and intragastric pressure will be proportional to the volume ingested. This also helps to determine gastric emptying. If the normal vagal reflex activity is inhibited or if the capacity of the stomach is reduced, the reservoir function will be altered. People with significantly compromised reservoir functions will need to eat frequent, smaller meals to avoid or minimize symptoms such as early satiety, postprandial epigastric pain, and nausea and vomiting.

Gastric secretions include mucus, pepsinogen, hydrochloric acid, intrinsic factor, and the hormone gastrin. Gastric mucus is composed of proteins, glycoproteins, mucopolysaccharides, and blood group substances. The principal component is glycoprotein. Gastric mucus is a thin layer of mucus adherent to the cell surface. The role of gastric mucus in the mucosal barrier is not well defined. The gastric mucosal barrier helps separate acid in the lumen from bicarbonate on the epithelial cell surface. The mucosal barrier prevents diffusion of hydrogen ions from lumen to mucosa and diffusion of sodium ions from mucosa to lumen.

The surface mucous cells are stimulated by vagus nerve and acetylcholine in response to chemicals (i.e., ethanol) and physical contact and friction from roughage in the diet. They protect the mucosa with an alkaline layer of lubricant.

Pepsinogen is secreted by the chief cells of glands in the body and fundus with a small amount secreted by neck cells and by Brunner's glands in the duodenum (the first portion of the small intestine). Pepsinogen is converted to active pepsin at a pH less than 6. The optimal pH of pepsin is 1.8 to 3.5 with no activity above pH of 5. Pepsinogen is stimulated by both vagal stimulation and a local reflex activity. Pepsinogen secretion is increased by the presence of gastrin, calcium, histamine, and secretin.

Hydrochloric acid is secreted by the parietal cells. Endogenous stimuli for hydrochloric acid production is acetylcholine, gastrin, and histamine. The basal secretion of hydrochloric acid has a biologic cycle with the lowest concentration between 5 and 11 AM and the highest between 2 PM and 1 AM.[34]

The production of intrinsic factor by the parietal cells is an essential function of the stomach. Intrinsic factor, a mucoprotein, binds with vitamin B_{12} and is absorbed at specific receptor cells. This complex attaches to special cells in the terminal ileum. The production of intrinsic factor correlates with the production of acid. Stimuli increasing secretion of intrinsic factor are the same as those stimulating hydrochloric acid production. The failure to secrete intrinsic factor is associated with achlorhydria and the absence of parietal cells. The condition results in vitamin B_{12} deficiency and subsequent pernicious anemia.

Fig. 11-6
Mechanisms for stimulation of acid secretion.

From Johnson, L.R.: Gastrointestinal physiology, ed. 3, St. Louis, 1986, The C.V. Mosby Co.

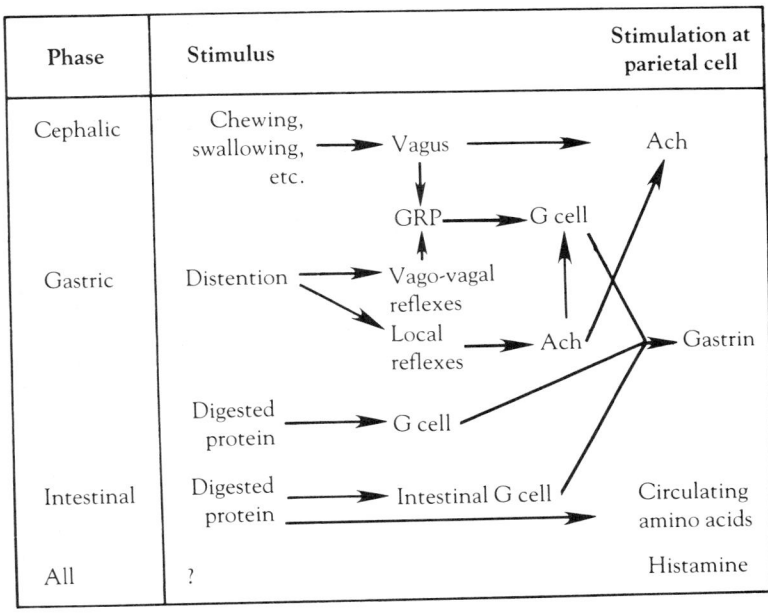

Phase	Stimulus	Stimulation at parietal cell
Cephalic	Chewing, swallowing, etc.	Ach
Gastric	Distention	Gastrin
Intestinal	Digested protein	Circulating amino acids
All	?	Histamine

The hormone gastrin is secreted by the antral G cells and is the primary mediator of gastric acid secretion. Gastrin is also secreted by cells in the duodenum, pancreatic islets, and jejunum. Vagal stimulation, gastric distention, and the presence of amino acids and peptides stimulate the secretion of antral gastrin, which circulates in the blood system with the parietal cells as the target organ. Calcium ions will also stimulate antral gastrin. When the gastric pH is below 1.5, gastrin release is inhibited. Duodenal gastrin is secreted in response to distention and protein.

Gastric secretion has been divided into three phases (cephalic, gastric, and intestinal) that occur almost simultaneously. The cephalic phase includes the sight, smell, taste, thought, and chewing of food as well as conditional reflexes and intracellular hypoglycemia. The vagus nerve releases acetylcholine by postganglionic fibers in the gastric mucosa, causing the secretion of hydrochloric acid, intrinsic factor, and pepsinogen. The gastric phase constitutes the major physiologic stimulus for gastric secretion and is activated by the presence of food in the stomach. The intestinal phase serves mainly to inhibit gastric secretions. The release of gastrin from the duodenum in response to protein digestion products and distention functions in the same way as antral gastrin (Fig. 11-6).

Inhibition of gastric secretions in the intestinal phase is related to the actions of the following: cholecystokinin (CCK), secretin, gastric inhibitory polypeptide (GIP), vasoactive intestinal peptide (VIP), glucagon, and prostaglandins (Fig. 11-7). CCK is stimulated by the presence of L-amino acids and fatty acids in the duodenum. When CCK and gastrin are both present, a competitive inhibition of gastrin occurs since both have the same active terminal tetrapeptide. Thus the secretory function of gastrin is inhibited. Hydrogen ions in the duodenum stimulate the release of secretin. Secretin inhibits acid output and blocks the secretory effects of gastrin and histamine. Secretin stimulates pepsinogen output. Both CCK and secretin stimulate pancreatic secretion of bicarbonate.

Gastric inhibitory polypeptide (GIP) is composed of 43 amino acids and is found throughout the intestinal tract, although it is concentrated in the duodenum. GIP has a wide range of functions, including inhibition of food-stimulated release of gastrin, gastric acid secretion, and pepsinogen secretions. VIP and glucagon inhibit gastric secretion and stimulate intestinal electrolyte secretion.

Prostaglandins are a group of cyclic fatty acid compounds with 20 carbon acids. Approximately 20 subtypes have been identified of which several inhibit gastric secretagogues, including gastrin, histamine, food, acetylcholine, hypoglycemia, and reserpine.

Enterogastrone is a general term often used to designate hormones released from duodenal mucosa in response to acid, fatty acids, and hyperosmotic solutions that inhibit gastric acid secretions.[72] There are still questions regarding gastric inhibition that remain unanswered. Future research should answer many of the uncertainties in the understanding of hormonal inhibition of gastric secretion.

Fig. 11-7
Mechanisms for the inhibition of acid
secretion.

From Johnson, L.R.: Gastrointestinal
physiology, ed. 3, St. Louis, 1986, The
C.V. Mosby Co.

Region	Stimulus	Mediator	Inhibit gastrin release	Inhibit acid secretion
Antrum	Acid (pH < 3.0)	Somatostatin	+	
Duodenum	Acid	Secretin	+	+
		Nervous reflex		+
	Hyperosmotic solutions	Unidentified enterogastrone		+
Duodenum and jejunum	Fatty acids	GIP	+	+
		Unidentified enterogasrone		+

Gastric motility can be divided into tonic, mixing, and peristaltic contractions. Gastric tone controls luminal volume and maintains a relatively constant pressure despite changes in volume. The fundus and body serve as a receptacle and the antrum as a pump. The antrum portion mixes gastric content and empties the contents into the duodenum in a regulated or controlled fashion. Circular muscle contractions in the body of the stomach mix the food with the gastric secretions. Contractions in the antrum are stronger and produce considerable mixing motions as well as propulsion.

Antral peristaltic contractions force the chyme (liquefied food) into the pyloric canal and then into the duodenum. The pyloric sphincter is a high-pressure zone that relaxes with antral peristalsis and contracts in response to acids, fats, amino acids, and nonisotonic solutions in the duodenum. Gastric distention stimulates stretch receptors, which results in increased gastric peristalsis and increased gastric emptying. The stimulus for rapid gastric emptying is gastric distention.

There are three receptors in the duodenum that release substances inhibiting gastric emptying: osmoreceptors, acid-sensitive receptors, and fat-sensitive receptors. Hormones released in the duodenum (gastrin, CCK, secretin, pancreatic polypeptide, gut glucagon, GIP, VIP, calcitonin, prostaglandins, and bulbogastrone) can be shown to inhibit gastric emptying. The complete physiologic role of the hormones is not understood.[4,34]

Gastric emptying can be impaired by drugs, diseases, and surgery. Incomplete emptying may result in early satiety, postprandial epigastric pain, and vomiting. Rapid gastric emptying may occur with duodenal ulcers and following surgery for peptic ulcers.

In summary, the primary function of the stomach is mixing and liquefaction of food to a suitable consistency for the duodenum. The intrinsic factor is an essential substance secreted by the stomach necessary for vitamin B_{12} absorption in the terminal ileum.

Small Intestine

In the small intestine, ingested food is mixed, digested, and absorbed. Anatomically the small intestine is divided into three segments: duodenum, jejunum, and ileum. The small intestine is 6.5 to 7 m (21 to 23 ft) in length and approximately 2 cm (1 inch) in diameter. The first portion is the duodenum, which is the shortest segment (20 to 30 cm). The ligament of Treitz is the dividing point between the duodenum and jejunum, although histologic changes cannot be demonstrated. The jejunum is 2.5 m, and the ileum is 3.5 m. The jejunum and ileum have no specific anatomic division (Fig. 11-8).

The small intestine is divided into four layers: mucosa (innermost layer), submucosa, muscularis externa, and serosa (outer layer). As in outer segments of the gastrointestinal tract, the mucosa is separated from the submucosa by the muscularis mucosae. The submucosa contains the connective tissue, lymphatics, blood vessels, and nerves. Meissner's plexus is in the submucosa. The muscularis externa consists of an inner circular layer and an outer longitudinal layer. Auerbach's (myenteric) plexus lies between the two muscle layers.

Fig. 11-8
Clinical anatomy of the small intestine.

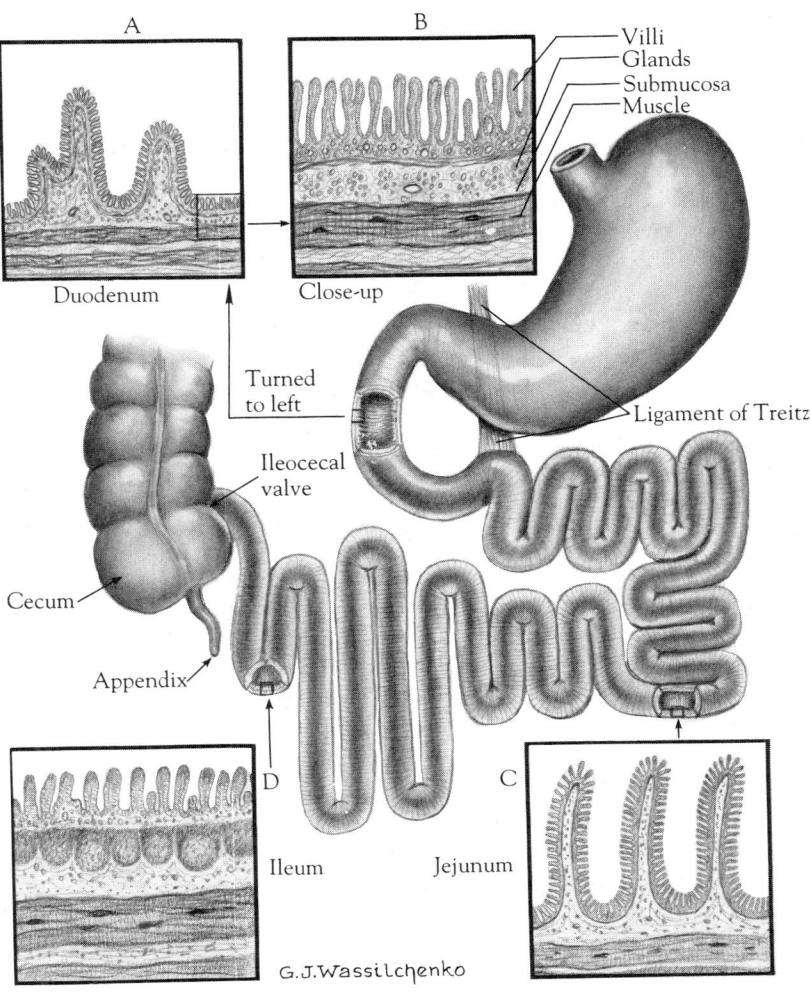

A

Duodenum

B

Close-up

Villi
Glands
Submucosa
Muscle

Turned
to left

Ileocecal
valve

Ligament of Treitz

Cecum

Appendix

D

Ileum

C

Jejunum

G.J.Wassilchenko

The duodenum is shaped like the letter C. The first portion of the duodenum lies behind and below the right and caudate lobes of the liver and gallbladder and in front of the common bile duct and portal vein. This portion is suspended from the lesser omentum and lies within the peritoneal cavity. The remaining duodenum is located retroperitoneally. The second portion of the duodenum descends vertically to the level of the fourth lumbar vertebra and lies in front of the vena cava, right ureter, and psoas muscle. Ventrally, the second portion is related to the right lobe of the liver, transverse colon, and small intestine. The common bile duct and main pancreatic duct empty into the duodenum at the ampulla of Vater, 7 to 10 cm distal to the pyloric sphincter.

The third portion, or horizontal segment, crosses the third and fourth lumbar vertebrae, vena cava, and aorta. The superior mesenteric vessel crosses this segment anteriorly. The fourth segment ascends along the left side of the aorta, turns sharply anteriorly, and then descends

caudally as the jejunum. The ligament of Treitz, a suspensory ligament of the duodenum, is a band of fibers and muscle tissue originating in the right crus of the diaphragm. The portion of the duodenum proximal to the ampulla of Vater receives its blood supply from the celiac axis. The remainder is supplied by the superior mesenteric artery.

The duodenum contains Brunner's glands in the submucosa, which secrete an alkaline fluid containing pepsinogen. The hormones secreted in the duodenum include gastrin, CCK, secretin, GIP, VIP, and enterogastrone. The functions of these secretions in inhibiting gastric secretion and gastric emptying have been previously discussed.

The jejunum and ileum have a greatly increased mucosa and submucosa surface area for absorption. Three characteristic features of this portion of the small intestine are (1) large series of circular folds of mucosa and submucosa; (2) minute, fingerlike projections of the mucosa

...alled villi; and (3) microvilli, or brush border. There are mucosal crypts at the base of the villi extending into the wall of the small intestine to the muscularis mucosae. Epithelial cells migrate from the crypt to extrude from the tip of the villi. As the epithelial cell migrates to the tip of the villus, its absorptive capacity increases. The brush border (microvilli) is covered with a glycocalyx (mucopolysaccharide) cover that contains many of the digestive enzymes of the small intestine. Also found in the microvillus-calyceal area are receptors for vitamin B_{12}.[72] The surface epithelial cells and the microvillus brush border constitute the digestion-absorption unit. Several enzymes are found in this unit including alkaline phosphatase, folic acid, folic acid conjugase, and a number of disaccharides and peptidases, as well as adenyl-cyclase and the "active pump" for sodium.[4,72] In addition to surface epithelial cells, goblet cells (mucin secreting), crypt cells (fluid and electrolyte secreting), and enteroendocrine cells (hormonal) are found in the small intestine.

The mesentery of the small intestine is fixed to the left of the second lumbar vertebra and goes downward and to the right to approximately the level of the right sacroiliac joint. The vascular supply of the entire jejunum and ileum (except for the terminal portion of the ileum) arises from the left border of the superior mesenteric artery. The vessels are contained within the mesentery. The terminal ileum is supplied by the ileocolic artery from the right side of the superior mesenteric artery. Venous drainage is through the superior mesenteric vein to the portal vein.

The small intestine has both sympathetic and parasympathetic stimulation. In addition to the autonomic nervous system, the enteric nervous system also regulates small bowel activities. The enteric nervous system involves purinergic, peptidergic, and serotonergic neurotransmitters. The complexity and interrelatedness of the two systems' regulation of intestinal motility are being studied. The autonomic nervous system stimulation can be interrupted with vagotomy and sympathectomy without significant alteration in intestinal motility. The intactness of the enteric nervous system may be more important for peristalsis than autonomic innervation.

The primary function of the motility of the small intestine is to facilitate the digestive-absorptive process. There are two motions found in the small intestine: mixing, or segmental, and propulsive, or peristaltic. The mixing movements bring the chyme in contact with pancreatic and biliary secretions. The musculature constricts at the rate of 11 to 12 contractions per minute, resulting in segmentation so that it resembles links. Not only does segmentation provide continued mixing with digestive enzymes, it also increases the contact of the chyme with the intestinal villi and microvilli, enhancing absorption. Peristalsis propels chyme forward at a rate of 2 to 20 cm/min. This appears as a progressive moving ring. The myenteric plexus supplies the sympathetic and parasympathetic stimulation for segmentation and peristalsis.

The terms *digestion* and *absorption* emphasize two phases of a single continuing process. The digestion of dietary lipids, carbohydrates, and proteins is initiated in the lumen of the duodenum and proximal jejunum and is completed at the glycocalyx and microvilli plasma membrane of enterocytes (jejunal absorptive cells). Most absorption occurs in the jejunum. Vitamin B_{12} is absorbed in the terminal ileum, and bile salts are reabsorbed by active transport in the terminal ileum. Otherwise, minimal absorption occurs in the ileum unless the jejunum is nonfunctioning or diseased. The processes of absorption in the small intestine are passive absorption and active transport. Passive absorption resembles diffusion of a substance through a membrane, and the rate of movement depends on a higher concentration in the lumen than in the bloodstream. Active transport is more rapid, more complex, and more efficient and requires energy.

Carbohydrate absorption requires conversion of starches to monosaccharides. Starch digestion by pancreatic amylase yields oligosaccharides and disaccharides. Active absorption of sugars occurs primarily in the brush border and at the apex of the epithelial cell. Brush border enzymes include lactose, sucrose, maltose, isomaltose, and trehalase. Lactose is hydrolyzed to glucose and galactose, sucrose to fructose, and dextrins, maltotriose, and maltose to glucose. Disaccharides are further hydrolyzed by brush border enzymes. Disaccharides, sucrose, and lactose are not dependent on pancreatic amylase but are hydrolyzed by the brush border enzymes. Glucose and galactose are transported through a sodium-dependent ATPase process into the epithelial cells. Fructose appears to be absorbed by a nonactive facilitated diffusion transport process.[4] Carbohydrate absorption is in the duodenum and jejunum.

Dietary fat consists of long-chain triglycerides that are insoluble in water. In the stomach, fat is shaken into a very fine emulsion. Gastric pepsin strips fat of its protein wrapper. Lipase secreted in an active state from mouth and tongue remains active in digesting fats in the stomach. In the duodenum and jejunum, pancreatic lipase breaks down triglycerides to diglycerides, then to monoglycerides, and finally to glycerol and fatty acids. Glycerol is absorbed into the epithelial cell and capillaries directly. Monoglycerides, fatty acids, and conjugated bile salts form the micelle. At the brush border the micelle "breaks up," allowing the monoglyceride and free fatty acid to enter the cells. The bile salts return to the intestinal lumen, where they are reabsorbed in the terminal ileum. Bicarbonate from the pancreas is also important because efficient lipolysis occurs in an alkaline pH. At the surface epithelial cell, the conjugated bile salt separates, permitting fatty acids and beta monoglycerides to be absorbed. The bile salts remain in the lumen and are reabsorbed in the terminal ileum. (Reabsorbed bile salts are cycled through the liver and reexcreted in the bile.)

The absorbed fatty acids and beta monoglycerides are resynthesized to triglycerides, are enclosed in a protein covering, forming chylomicrons, are transported through the lymphatics and thoracic duct, and finally reach the blood. Some medium-chain triglycerides are not dependent on micelle formation and after hydrolysis can be asborbed by the epithelial cell as fatty acids and transported directly into the portal venous system.

Although gastric pepsin initiates protein digestion, it is not essential for protein digestion. Pancreatic proteases include the following: trypsinogen, chymotrypsinogen, procarboxypeptidases A and B, leucine aminopeptidase, and nucleases. The hormone cholecystokinin (CCK) is the primary stimulator of the pancreatic acinar cells. CCK is released in the duodenum and jejunum in the presence of amino acids and fatty acids. The presence of hydrogen ions, or a low pH, will stimulate the release of the hormone secretin. Secretin stimulates the bicarbonate and fluid responses of the pancreas. The activation of the pancreatic enzyme trypsinogen depends on the intestinal secretion of the enzyme enterokinase. Thus pancreatic functioning depends on the presence and functioning of a normal proximal small bowel.

The intraluminal protein digestion by-products are peptides of two to six amino acids. The brush border and intracellular enzymes further break down these products to free amino acids, dipeptides, and some tripeptides that can enter the epithelial cell. The enterocyte has at least three carrier-mediated transport systems, including one for neutral amino acids, one for basic amino acids, and one for peptide-linked amino acids. In the cell the small peptides are hydrolyzed into free amino acids, which are absorbed into the capillary, where further protein breakdown occurs.

Vitamin B_{12} binds with intrinsic factor (gastric secretion) to protect it from gastric digestion and bacterial digestion in the small bowel. The intrinsic factor also is essential for attachment of vitamin B_{12} to receptors of the glycocalyx membrane of the ileal absorptive cell. Calcium, magnesium, and pH greater than 5.6 are also necessary for the attachment of vitamin B_{12} and the transport through the cell. The vitamin B_{12} is then transported in the portal blood bound to a carrier (transcobalamin). Pancreatic insufficiency is also associated with a vitamin B_{12} deficiency. This is because R binders found in saliva, gastric secretions, bile, and intestinal secretions can bind with vitamin B_{12} rather than the intrinsic factor. Pancreatic proteases degrade the R binders, making it possible for vitamin B_{12} to bind with the intrinsic factor. Intestinal microflora is capable of synthesizing vitamin

B_{12}. When oral vitamin B_{12} is reduced, the use of antibiotics may alter intraluminal flora, resulting in vitamin B_{12} deficiency. It is important to note that the body stores of vitamin B_{12} may be adequate for years. Thus clinical signs of vitamin B_{12} deficiency are unusual.

Calcium absorption is highest in the upper small intestine where the pH is lowest. Its absorption and transport are enhanced by vitamin D. Calcium is transported against a concentration gradient. Passive absorption occurs when intraluminal concentrations are greater than 6 mM/L. Calcium absorption will be decreased by phosphate ingestion, anticonvulsant drugs, alcohol, and steroids.

Dietary folate is composed of multiple glutamyl units, and the linkage is broken by the mucosal epithelium to monoglutamate. Absorption occurs primarily in the proximal small bowel. The transport mechanism is unclear. It enters the portal circulation and functions as a cofactor in many enzyme systems.

Iron absorption depends on the physiologic demands of the body. When iron stores are low or when red blood cells are being rapidly formed, iron absorption is increased. Iron absorption occurs primarily in the duodenum and proximal jejunum against a concentration gradient. It is absorbed in the ferrous form, bound to globulin (transferrin). It is then released into the portal circulation or stored within cells as apoferritin.

One of the major functions of the small intestine is fluid and electrolyte shifts from gastrointestinal lumen to blood and from blood to lumen. In a 24-hour period, approximately 9 L of fluid enters the lumen of the small intestine. Approximately 7.5 to 8.2 L is endogenous secretions (saliva, gastric, intestinal, pancreatic, and bile). Another 1.0 to 1.5 L is exogenous. The vast majority of the fluid is reabsorbed, and only 500 to 1000 ml will pass through the ileocecal valve into the colon. The duodenum and jejunum are primarily responsible for the large amounts of absorption of fluids, electrolytes, and nutrients because of large pores that allow rapid flow of solutes and water in both directions. Isomolarity in the lumen is rapidly attained and maintained throughout the small intestine. There are several factors that help prevent osmotic disequilibrium, including the relative impermeability of gastric mucosa, the regulation of gastric emptying, the fact that nutrients are largely macromolecules with low osmotic activity, and rapid absorption of products of macromolecule digestion or breakdown. Fat is high in most diets, but since its osmotic potential is low, it does not impede osmotic equilibrium. Maintaining osmolarity requires rapid flow of salt and water through the intestinal membrane. The direction of the flow is determined by hydrostatic and osmotic forces.

Sodium absorption is a major function of the small intestine, with approximately 1145 mEq being reab-

every 24 hours. Sodium absorption plays a part regulating cellular absorption of electrolytes and water. The brush border contain a carrier that binds sodium and glucose. When intraluminal glucose is present, sodium is actively reabsorbed by the shared carrier. Sodium is also absorbed from the lumen by a sodium-hydrogen exchange mechanism. A sodium pump is present at the basolateral border of epithelial absorbing cells transporting sodium from intracellular to intercellular spaces by means of a sodium-potassium ATPase activity. The decrease of intracellular sodium concentration enhances the sodium-glucose carrier mechanism.

In the ileum a chloride-bicarbonate exchange mechanism is present. The bicarbonate concentration in the ileum is much higher than in the jejunum. Potassium is absorbed based on sodium-potassium ATPase and hydrostatic and osmotic forces.

Water transport is passive and depends on osmotic and hydrostatic pressures. Increased solute concentration in the intercellular space (e.g., from sodium pump activity) provides osmotic forces for water absorption. As water flows through the pores it brings small solutes with it. This is referred to as solvent drag. Hydrostatic forces from the serosa layer will restrict passive water and solute absorption. Water from the interstitial fluid will enter the lumen when solutes accumulate in the lumen. The flow continues until osmotic equilibrium exists.

The secretory function of the intestinal epithelium appears to be the result of electrogenic activity. If the secretory function is greater than the absorption function, significant fluid and electrolyte loss can occur. This is frequently seen in diseases or abnormal states (malabsorption syndromes).

Immunologic function of the small bowel through Peyer's patches and lymphoid cells is not clearly documented. Peyer's patches are found in the submucosa and contain small lymphocytes from the mesenteric nodes. Lymphoid cells differing from Peyer's patches are found in the lamina propria. IgA is the prominent immunoglobulin found in the small bowel, but IgM, IgG, IgD, and IgE are also present. The IgA found in the small bowel does differ from serum IgA. An infant is born without secretory or serum IgA. The secretory IgA appears first and reaches adult levels sooner. The secretory IgA has antiviral and antibacterial activities. The immune system of the small bowel appears to be complex, and further investigation may reveal its precise role.

Enzyme activity in the small intestine is located in the brush border of the villi and within the absorbing epithelial cell cytoplasm. The only enzyme secreted by the small intestine with luminal activity is enterokinase. The old concept of succus entericus, luminal intestinal enzymes, is no longer accepted.

Hormonal function of the small intestine is of great interest. The small intestine may be the body's largest and most diffuse endocrine organ. Bolt and associates[4] provide the following criteria for a gut hormone:

- Production of a biologic response in another organ
- Production of a response with no innervation between the gut and another organ
- Similar response in the organ when an extract of the gut tissue is given
- Occurrence of biologic response when pure or synthetic exogenous hormone is given

Four hormones meet this criteria: secretin, gastrin, cholecystokinin (CCK), and gastric inhibitory polypeptide (GIP). Hormone candidates include substances that do not necessarily meet all four criteria. Some of the hor-

Table 11-1
Gastrointestinal Hormones and Their Actions

Hormone	Location	Primary Action	Secondary Action
Gastrin	Antrum, duodenum, proximal jejunum	Stimulates gastric acid secretion	Trophic effect on gastrointestinal mucosa
Cholecystokinin	Throughout small intestine, but primarily found in jejunum	Stimulates contraction of gallbladder Stimulates secretion of pancreatic enzymes	Motility of stomach and small intestine
Secretin	Throughout gastrointestinal tract, except colon; primary sites are duodenum and jejunum	Stimulates pancreatic bicarbonate secretions	Numerous interactions with other gastrointestinal hormones
Gastric inhibitory peptide	Small intestine, primarily jejunum	Increases release of insulin from pancreas	Decreases gastric acid secretion Increases intestinal secretion
Enteroglucagon	Primarily lower ileum and colon	Inhibits motility	May be trophic for mucosa
Vasoactive intestinal peptide	Esophagus to rectum	Increases intestinal and pancreatic secretions	Decreases gastric acid secretion Increases insulin secretion Causes peripheral vasodilation

mone candidates have known structures, while the structures of others have yet to be identified:

1. Known structure
   a. Vasoactive intestinal peptide
   b. Motilin
   c. Pancreatic polypeptide
   d. Somatostatin
   e. Neurotensin
   f. Substance P
   g. Urogastrone
   h. Enkephalins
2. Unknown structure
   a. Chymodenin
   b. Bombesin-like peptides
   c. Gut glucagon–like immunoreactants
   d. Gastrozymin
   e. Anticholecystokinin peptide
   f. Incretin
   g. Villikinin
   h. Entero-oxyntin
   i. Bulbogastrone
   j. Pancreatone

The actions of the hormones are complex, with many having more than one action. The activity may be as a paracrine agent, a neuroendocrine or neurotransmitter substance, or an exocrine agent. Based on amino acid sequence and pharmacologic and physiologic action, two categories of hormones in the small intestine can be identified. Family 1 includes gastrin and CCK. The terminal amino acids in the last four positions are the same in gastrin and CCK. Family 2 includes secretin, enteroglucagon, vasoactive intestinal peptide (VIP), and GIP. Numerous amino acids in similar positions can be found in each of the family 2 hormones.

Table 11-1 summarizes small intestinal hormones and their activities.

Large Intestine (Colon) and Rectum

The colon is approximately 150 cm (4½ to 5 ft) in length. The terminal ileum joins the colon at the ileocecal valve. The appendix arises from the cecum medially, about 2 cm (1 inch) below the junction of the ileum and cecum. The cecum is continuous with the ascending colon, which goes from the cecum to the undersurface of the right lobe of the liver. The colon bends to the left, forming the hepatic flexure. The colon then extends to the left, becoming the transverse colon. The transverse colon has a mesentery and therefore a wide range of movement. The cecum, ascending colon, and proximal half of the transverse colon are derived from the midgut. The innervation and vascular supply are shared with the small intestine.

The transverse colon continues to the left and slightly upward, forming the splenic flexure. The splenic flexure is slightly higher than the hepatic flexure and is in front of and above the left kidney. As the colon turns downward, it becomes the descending colon. The sigmoid colon begins at the point where the descending colon crosses the iliac artery at the rim of the pelvis. The mesentery of the sigmoid colon attaches it to the posterior (retroperitoneal) wall of the pelvis. Near the midsacrum, the sigmoid colon becomes the rectum. The rectum descends in front of the sacrum and coccyx. The rectum becomes the anal canal approximately 2 cm anterior to the tip of the coccyx. The upper portion of the rectum is in the peritoneal cavity, but the distal 12 to 15 cm has no peritoneal covering. This area lies behind the bladder in the male with the seminal vesicles on either side. In the female the distal 12 to 15 cm is found posterior to the uterus. The rectal ampulla is the lowest part of the rectum and is found anterior to the posterior aspect of the prostate in the male. In the female the rectal ampulla is attached to the posterior wall of the vagina.

The distal half of the transverse colon, splenic flexure, descending sigmoid, and rectum are derived from the hindgut. The inferior mesenteric artery supplies this portion of the large intestine and rectum. The nervous innervation is from the sacral parasympathetic fibers.

The wall of the colon is divided into the same four layers as the small intestine: mucosa, submucosa, muscularis externa, and serosa. There are no villi found in the large intestine. The simple columnar epithelial surface is flat and is broken into polygonal units by clefts. Goblet cell openings are found on the epithelial surface. In the center of polygonal units are crypts of Lieberkühn. The crypts of Lieberkühn are lined with goblet cells and extend into the muscularis mucosae. At the bottom of the crypts are proliferating undifferentiated epithelial cells and occasionally argentaffin cells. Cell renewal begins in the crypts. The cells then migrate upward to the surface and extrude into the lumen. The renewal time is approximately 3½ to 4 days.

The mucosa, submucosa, and circular muscle layer form semilunar folds (plicae semilunares) dividing the haustra (sacculations). The semilunar folds are crescent shaped and extend one third of the way around the wall of the intestine. The longitudinal muscle layer is incomplete in the large colon. It is called teniae coli and is the noticeable band in the colon wall. Fatty tags (appendices epiploicae) project from the serosa coat of the colon; this marks another difference between the large and small intestines.

The musculature of the rectum is a continuation of the colonic muscular layers. The outer longitudinal layer spreads from the teniae of the sigmoid colon to form a continuous even coat. The superficial fibers insert into the perianal body and merge with the levator ani muscles of the pelvic floor. The deep fibers insert into the perianal

Fig. 11-9
Arterial and venous blood supply to
primary and accessory organs of the
alimentary canal.

From Broadwell, D.C., and Jackson, B.S.,
editors: Principles of ostomy care, St.
Louis, 1982, The C.V. Mosby Co.

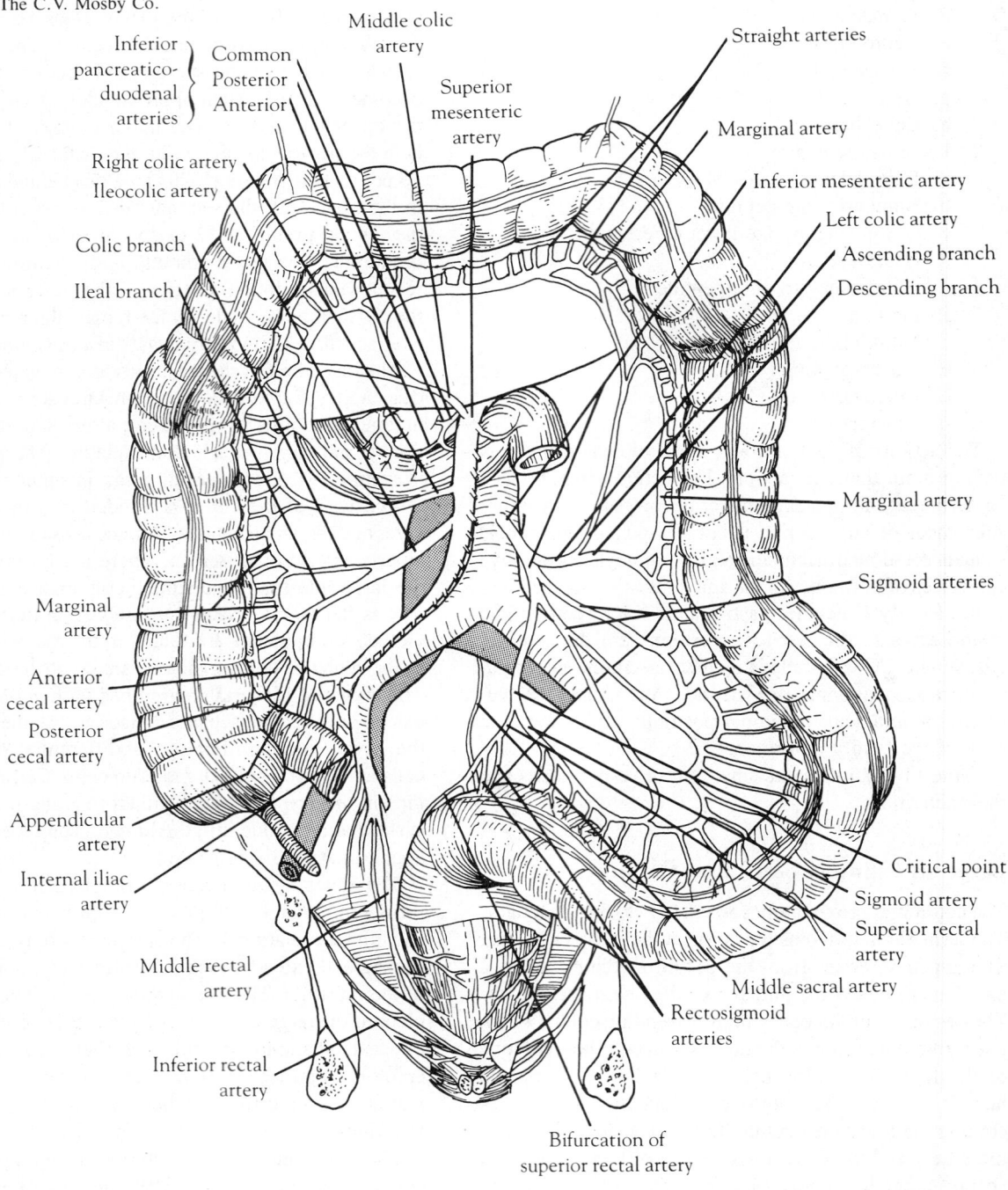

skin. The circular muscle forms the internal sphincter surrounding the anal canal. The pectinate line marks the boundary between the anal canal and rectum. At this anorectal junction, the lining layer changes from columnar to squamous epithelial cells. The external sphincter is striated muscle and lies outside the internal sphincter. The external sphincter encircles the terminal portion of the anal canal.

The mesenteric attachments of the colon permit a considerable amount of mobility of the ileocecal junction and sigmoid colon. A potential problem is a volvulus or twisting of the bowel upon itself. Intussusception can also occur. The hepatic and splenic flexures, descending colon, and rectum are relatively fixed.

The major blood vessels of the large colon and rectum are the superior and inferior mesenteric arteries as previously stated. The superior rectal artery is a branch of the inferior mesenteric and branches as low as the proximal anal canal. The middle and inferior rectal arteries are a branch of the internal iliac and supply the anal canal and subcutaneous perianal area. The superior hemorrhoidal vein empties into the inferior mesenteric vein, which empties into the portal system. The inferior hemorrhoidal veins drain into pudendal veins and the systemic venous system. Because of the venous relationship with the portal system, portal hypertension can lead to congestion and increased size of the hemorrhoidal system and hemorrhoids may occur.

The lymph nodes of the colon include epicolic nodes, found on the surface; paracolic nodes, found on the mesenteric border; and intermediate nodes, associated with superior and inferior mesenteric arteries. The lymphatics from the intermediate nodes join the lymph nodes adjacent to the abdominal aorta (Fig. 11-9).

Nervous innervation includes external sympathetic and parasympathetic fibers and submucosal and myenteric nerve plexuses. Sympathetic innervation is from segments T2 to L2. These form the mesenteric hypogastric nerves. The parasympathetic fibers to the right colon are through the vagus nerve. The left colon parasympathetic fibers are from the second to fourth sacral segments by way of the pelvic nerves.

The integrated functions of the colon, rectum, and internal and external sphincters require both sensory and motor innervation. The sensory pathways for the anal canal and perianal skin go through the somatic nerves to S2, S3, and S4. Proprioceptive spindles are found in the striated muscle of the external sphincter. Autonomic sensory innervation for the rectum passes through the same segments (S2, S3, and S4), but through parasympathetic pathways. The pudendal nerve and coccygeal plexus originating in S2 to S5 form the motor fibers for the external sphincter. The hypogastric nerve provides excitatory motor stimuli of the parasympathetic fibers. The

rectum sympathetic fibers are from L2 through L4 and the parasympathetic fibers are from S2 through S4.

The normal function of the colon includes controlling transit of waste, absorption, and limited secretion. Defecation is the mechanism for eliminating metabolic waste and dietary residue. Colonic motor activity includes segmentation (mixing) and peristaltic movement. Segmentation occurs by alternate formation and relaxation of haustra folds. Peristalsis is a forward movement over longer segments of bowel. Colonic activities increase after a meal. There is an increase in ileal activity resulting in a slow filling of the cecum and ascending colon. The fluid contents of the right colon are moved back and forth (segmentation) over the absorptive epithelium. The proximal colon retains the contents for a longer period of time than the distal colon.

Gradually the sigmoid colon fills and the stool periodically passes into the rectum. Distention of the rectum causes an urge to defecate. Defecation can be a simple emptying of the rectal area, or it may stimulate mass propulsion and empty the distal half of the colon. Defecation in a continent person includes voluntary relaxation of external sphincters, relaxation of internal sphincters, increase in intra-abdominal pressure, tensing of pelvic floor, and colon contraction.

Most absorption of fluid and electrolytes occurs in the right colon. The mechanism for water absorption is passive flow in response to an osmotic gradient. The osmotic gradient is produced by active absorption of sodium. The colon is sensitive to aldosterone and other mineralocorticoids, and the response of the colon is to increase sodium absorption and potassium secretion. Potassium is secreted into the colon lumen. The mucus secreted by the goblet cells can contain high quantities of potassium. If the luminal potassium concentration goes above 15 mEq/L, a shift occurs and potassium is absorbed. Chloride ion is absorbed as a pair with sodium bicarbonate secreted by the colon. The chloride and bicarbonate are related. As chloride is absorbed, bicarbonate is secreted.

The colon has a minimal digestive or synthetic function. Ingested cellulose is not digested and passes into the colon largely unaltered. In constipated people, when feces remain in the lumen for prolonged periods, the colon can digest and absorb the cellulose. The bacteria in the colon can synthesize folic acid, riboflavin, biotin, vitamin K, and nicotinic acid. The importance of this ability is not known.

Enterohepatic circulation involving the colon has been identified. The urea-ammonia enterohepatic circulation is related to the hydrolysis of circulating blood urea in the colonic epithelial wall by bacterial ureases. This produces ammonia, which is absorbed into the blood. Any remaining ammonium ion that enters the lumen is converted to free ammonium as a result of the alkaline pH of the lumen. Free ammonium readily penetrates the mucosa and returns to the liver.

A wide variety of drugs can be administered by enema or suppository. The rectum has a poor absorptive capacity, so that absorption will depend on the level to which the preparation is in the colon and retention time in the colon.

The average amount of gas in the gastrointestinal tract is 100 ml. Gas in the gastrointestinal tract is made up of swallowed air, gas diffusing across the mucosa, and gas produced by bacteria. The major components of flatus are oxygen, nitrogen, carbon dioxide, methane, and hydrogen. Hydrogen and methane are produced by bacteria. The bacteria utilize substrate found within the lumen, related to diet. Carbon dioxide may be formed as a result of neutralization of acid by bicarbonate, or it may be swallowed. Bacterial utilization of oxygen may result in low concentrations of oxygen. Passage of flatus through the colon is more rapid than liquid or semisolid feces since resistance to flatus flow by haustration is less effective.

Liver

The liver is the largest organ in the body, weighing 1.4 to 1.8 kg (3 to 4 lb). It is a complex organ with many functions, including the production of bile, protein metabolism, carbohydrate metabolism, fat metabolism, co-agulation, and detoxification and storage of certain minerals and vitamins. Before examining the functions of the liver, it is necessary to examine its anatomic structure, blood supply, and ductal system.

The liver is located under the diaphragm in the upper right portion of the abdominal cavity (Fig. 11-10). The superior surface of the liver is under the right and left halves of the diaphragm. The inferior surface is above (from right to left) the hepatic flexure of the colon, the upper pole of the right kidney, the first portion of the duodenum, the inferior vena cava, and the stomach. The liver normally extends from the fifth intercostal space to just below the right costal margin. The right lobe is normally palpable on inspiration 1 to 2 cm below the right costal margin. The left lobe is rarely palpable in the epigastric region of a healthy subject.

The liver is divided into two lobes with the right six times larger than the left in an adult, and three times larger in infants. The falciform ligament separates the lobes. The right lobe is further subdivided into quadrate and caudate lobes. Riedel's lobe is a common accessory lobe on the right that is lateral to the gallbladder. This is a functional as well as anatomic division of the liver created by the falciform ligament. The division is determined largely by the liver's vascular supply.

The liver has a dual blood supply: the portal vein and the hepatic artery. The portal vein brings nutrients from the gastrointestinal system, and the hepatic artery pro-

Fig. 11-10
Liver, gallbladder, and pancreas.

From Broadwell, D.C., and Jackson, B.S., editors: Principles of ostomy care, St. Louis, 1982, The C.V. Mosby Co.

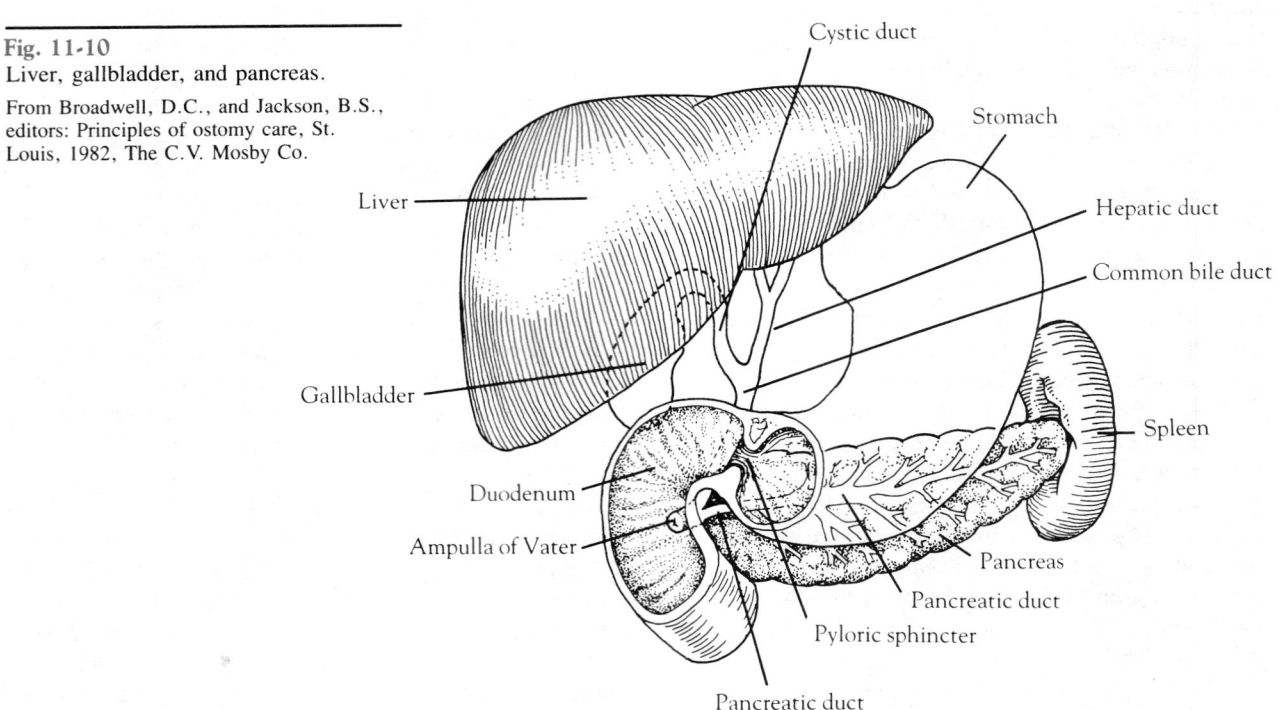

vides the arterial circulation. The origin of the hepatic artery will vary. In approximately 55% of individuals the hepatic artery originates from the celiac artery. The remainder will have hepatic arteries arising from the left gastric or splenic artery. Off the hepatic artery is the gastroduodenal artery; then the hepatic artery enters the porta hepatis, divides into the right and left hepatic arteries, and enters the corresponding lobes of the liver. A middle hepatic artery originates from one branch and supplies the quadrate lobe. In 25% of individuals the left hepatic artery originates from the left gastric artery and this may be the only left hepatic artery present. Occasionally the right hepatic artery arises from the superior mesenteric artery. Another deviation is for the entire hepatic artery to arise from the superior mesenteric artery. The possible variations in blood flow play an important role in surgical interventions in the gastrointestinal tract. Blood flow to the liver can be disturbed if the origin of the hepatic artery is not carefully noted. In reading arteriograms, it is helpful to know of possible alternative patterns of blood flow. Arteriography can be useful before surgery. Also, for effective intra-arterial chemotherapy, a knowledge of possible anomalies of the hepatic arteries is necessary. The right, middle, and left hepatic arteries supply different areas and do not anastomose with each other to any significant degree.

Within the liver, branches of the hepatic artery, the portal vein, and bile ducts in the portal tract, described as the portal triad, accompany each other and empty into sinusoids. The portal vein is formed by the superior mesenteric vein at its junction with the splenic vein. The inferior mesenteric vein also empties into this system. The portal vein has several tributaries, of which the left gastric or coronary vein is the most important. The left gastric vein anastomoses with the esophageal veins, which empty into the vena cava.

The branches of the hepatic artery and portal vein are next to each other within the substance of the liver, with the portal vein emptying into the sinusoids. Approximately 1500 ml of blood passes through the liver every minute. Seventy percent of the blood flow is from the portal vein, which is derived primarily from the inferior and superior mesenteric veins, with one third or less coming from the splenic vein. The remaining 30% of the blood flow is from the hepatic artery.

Sinusoidal outflow is into central veins that flow into the hepatic veins. The three hepatic veins (right, middle, and left) enter the inferior vena cava separately. Normal portal pressure is 8 to 10 mm Hg. Arteriolar resistance, pressure in the aorta, and pressure in the inferior vena cava are important determinants of hepatic blood flow. Exercise reduces hepatic blood flow. Standing or assuming an erect position will also reduce blood flow.

In the liver there is a superficial subcapsular lymphatic network communicating with the gallbladder and a deep lymphatic network that runs in portal triads with branches of the portal vein, hepatic artery, and bile ducts. The lymphatic drainage is primarily to the nodes at the hilum of the liver and eventually into the thoracic ducts.

The innervation of the liver is sympathetic (paravertebral ganglia, T7 to T10) and parasympathetic (vagus). The sympathetic fibers are distributed to the hepatic arterial branches and bile ducts. The parasympathetic fibers innervate the biliary tree. Although neuronal stimulation affects hepatic blood flow and biliary tree pressures, there are no known direct effects on parenchymal cell function.

The stroma is the connective tissue of the liver. It includes Glisson's capsule, which covers the liver and the connective tissue around the vascular and biliary branches. A reticular framework extends into the lobules and lies between the liver plates and sinusoidal lining cells.

The liver is composed of a complex circulatory system involving the hepatic artery, portal vein, sinusoids, central vein, and hepatic vein. The biliary system includes the bile canaliculi, ductules (or cholangioles), hepatic duct, and common duct.

There are several cell types present in the liver. The parenchymal cell, or hepatocyte, is the most important. The chemical actions that occur in the liver take place in the parenchymal cells. Kupffer (reticuloendothelial) cells are those cells that line the sinusoids.

The flow of bile is in the opposite direction of the flow of blood through the liver. The bile canaliculi carry the bile from the central vein area to the portal triads. The bile canaliculi are small intercellular channels between parenchymal cells. The canaliculi join the bile ductules, which are lined by columnar epithelium. The ductules join together to form the bile ducts, which form part of the portal triad with the hepatic artery and portal vein. The bile ducts go toward the hilum of the liver and join, forming the right and left hepatic ducts. The common hepatic duct joins the cystic duct from the gallbladder to form the common bile duct.

The common bile duct is joined by the pancreatic duct, and the two combined ducts form the ampulla of Vater on the duodenal mucosa. Oddi's sphincter at the opening regulates the one-way flow of bile and pancreatic secretions into the duodenum.

Heme, a source of bile pigments, is an end-product of the breakdown of hemoglobin and accounts for 80% to 90% of the bilirubin produced daily in adults.[4] Hemoglobin is broken down into globin, iron, and protoporphyrin heme. The metabolic process for the conversion of protoporphyrin heme to bilirubin is poorly understood. It has been suggested that heme is converted to bilirubin by microsomal heme oxygenase that is found in reticuloendothelial cells of the spleen and liver. This is a multistep process that begins with the oxidation of heme to carbon monoxide and verdoheme. Verdoheme loses its iron to yield biliverdin, which is then reduced to bilirubin. The bilirubin is then taken up by the parenchymal cells (hepatocytes) by active transport. This is unconjugated bilirubin, a lipid-soluble pigment that cannot be excreted by the liver unless it is conjugated, increasing its water solubility. Within the parenchymal cell the bilirubin is conjugated. The enzyme located on the endoplasmic reticulum, glucuronyl transferase, stimulates this process.

Conjugated bilirubin is not absorbed from the intestine or gallbladder. In the colon, bacteria hydrolyze conjugated bilirubin to urobilinogen. Urobilinogen is found in feces, bile, and urine. It is partially absorbed and reexcreted by the liver and kidneys. The majority of urobilinogen is found in the feces.

In the kidneys, urobilinogen is secreted by the proximal tubules and partially reabsorbed. The amount of reabsorption is increased in acid urine. Urine urobilinogen is influenced by the amount of hemolysis of red cells: an increase in hemolysis increases urine urobilinogen. In the presence of decreased bowel motility and stagnation of the small bowel contents, there is an increase in small bowel bacterial colonization and hence bacterial activity. This increases the formation of urobilinogen from bilirubin. Absorption in the small bowel is more efficient, and the absorbed urobilinogen is excreted by the kidney, increasing urine urobilinogen. Hepatocellular disease or transhepatic shunting of portal blood increases the amount of urobilinogen in the systemic circulation, increasing excretion by the renal system. In the presence of biliary tract obstruction, there is less bilirubin entering the intestines, decreasing both fecal and urine urobilinogen.

The formation of bile by the liver is a major function. Hepatic bile has a specific gravity of 1.009 and an alkaline pH. It contains approximately 97% water, cholesterol, bile salts, phospholipids, mucin, conjugated bilirubin, and electrolytes (sodium, potassium, chloride, and bicarbonate). Bile also contains calcium, many enzymes, and drug metabolites. The liver secretes approximately 700 ml of bile per day. Although bile is secreted continuously, a meal will augment the rate of secretion. The volume of bile produced by the liver is determined by the amount of bile salts synthesized. Conjugated bile salts are secreted by the hepatocytes, and this provides an osmotic pressure for the movement of water into bile. The volume of bile increases as it flows through the biliary tree because of active secretion of an electrolyte solution high in bicarbonate by the biliary epithelium.

Secretion of bile is increased by vagal stimulation and by the action of secretin, cholecystokinin-pancreozymin, vasoactive intestinal peptide, gastrin, and glucagon. Vagal stimulation and cholecystokinin-pancreozymin cause relaxation of the sphincter of Oddi. Exogenous agents that increase hepatic bile secretion and contraction of the gallbladder include bile salts, acetylsalicylic acid, pilocarpine, acetylcholine, choline, histamine, and insulin.

Bile is composed of bile acid, phospholipids, cholesterol, and bile pigments. Bile salts are necessary for micellular solubilization of dietary lipids and to maintain biliary cholesterol in solution. Two primary bile salts are cholic (trihydroxy) and chenodeoxycholic (dihydroxy). They are synthesized in the liver from cholesterol, conjugated with glycine and taurine, and then form salts with sodium and potassium. Most bile salts are reabsorbed in the terminal ileum by an active transport process. Bile salts entering the colon are deconjugated and dehydroxylated by bacterial enzymes to form secondary bile acids. Cholic acid is broken down to deoxycholic (dihydroxy) acid, which is absorbed, conjugated in the liver, and secreted into bile. Chenodeoxycholic acid will give rise to lithocholic (monohydroxy) acid, which is poorly absorbed. Bile salts are formed when potassium and sodium combine with conjugated bile acids of which 80% are cholic and chenodeoxycholic acids with the largest percentage of the remaining bile salts being deoxycholic.

There is approximately 5 g of bile salts with a half-life of 3 to 5 days; these salts are recirculated six to ten times a day. New bile acids account for 10% of the total amount each day, replacing the amount lost in the feces.

The formation of bile is only one function of the liver. Protein, carbohydrate, and lipid metabolism are additional functions. The liver is the source of albumin, which is 50% to 60% of the total plasma protein. For protein synthesis the liver uses dietary amino acids, amino acids formed by endogenous protein catabolism, and amino acids formed during carbohydrate and fat metabolism. Deamination of amino acids in the liver releases nitrogen, which is converted to urea. The liver also converts ammonia formed in other parts of the body to urea. Other functions related to protein metabolism include uric acid formation from nucleoprotein, creatine formation from glycine, and synthesis of methionine and arginine. Other proteins of importance to coagulation include haptoglobin, C-reactive protein, several glycoproteins, transferrin, serum enzymes, and ceruloplasmin.

Albumin has two major functions. First, it helps maintain the plasma colloid osmotic pressure because of its small molecular size and high charge. About one third of the body's albumin (4.5 to 5.0 g/kg) is intravascular, and the remaining albumin is extravascular. Second, albumin plays a role in active transport.

Carbohydrate metabolism involves the liver's ability to store glycogen within the hepatocyte. The liver converts glucose, fructose, and galactose to glycogen. If a diet is low in carbohydrates or in the presence of prolonged fasting, the liver can convert protein and fat to glycogen. This is referred to as gluconeogenesis. Glucose that is not stored as glycogen or aminated to amino acid is converted to fatty acids, carbon dioxide, and water.

A normal blood glucose level depends on the ability of the liver to remove glucose from the blood, store glucose as glycogen, break glycogen into glucose, and release glucose into the blood. Glycogenolysis (breaking glycogen to glucose) is increased by a decreased blood glucose, exercise, glucagon, and epinephrine. In a fasting state, glycogen stores can be significantly depleted in approximately 12 hours. In hepatocellular disease, glycogen stores may be reduced, resulting in hypoglycemia. This may also occur during stress and exercise.

Dietary lipid enters the liver in the form of chylomicrons. Triglycerides are hydrolyzed to glycerol and fatty acids. The liver also takes up fatty acids mobilized from fat depots and synthesizes fatty acids from carbohydrates and amino acids. The fatty acids are used in oxidation for energy production, resynthesis of triglycerides, formation of cholesterol esters, and conversion to phospholipids. Hepatic triglyceride accumulation, or fatty liver, may be the result of an excess supply of fatty acids, reduced lipid oxidation, or decreased lipoprotein formation.

Cholesterol is synthesized in the liver from acetate. Other sources of cholesterol are kidneys, adrenals, and small bowel mucosa. The liver will remove cholesterol from the blood and excrete cholesterol into bile, forming a bile acid. Cholesterol may also combine with fatty acids to form cholesterol esters. Serum cholesterol is kept in solution by phospholipids.

The liver plays a major role in coagulation in that it is the site of production of coagulation factors I, II, VI, VII, VIII, IX, and X. Vitamin K is required for the synthesis of factors II, VII, IX, and X. Natural vitamin K is lipid soluble. There are synthetic forms of vitamin K that are water soluble. Vitamin K is stored in the liver. Oral anticoagulants such as coumarin interfere with the action of vitamin K within the parenchymal cell. The liver also removes active clotting factors from the circulation, contributing to coagulation homeostasis.

Plasminogen (profibrinolysin), the inactive form of plasmin (fibrinolysin), is believed to be synthesized by the liver. Plasminogen levels may be decreased in hepatocellular disease. A proteinase inhibitor, antiplasmin, found in plasma and serum is also formed in the liver.

Clotting abnormalities may accompany almost any type of liver disease. The severity of acquired clotting problems associated with hepatic disease depends on the extent of hepatocellular damage. Deficiency of vitamin K is not common since vitamin K is found in food and is synthesized by colonic bacteria. Vitamin K deficiency may be seen in chronically ill persons with limited oral intake who are taking broad-spectrum antibiotics. Chronic alcohol abusers may be vitamin K depleted because of their diets and liver disease. Also, patients on long-term total parenteral nutrition will develop clotting abnormalities if their diet is not supplemented with vitamin K. Malabsorption of vitamin K may result from problems that cause a decrease in lipid absorption, for example, biliary obstruction. Coagulation problems seen in hepatocellular damage are usually caused by one or more of the following: increased utilization of clotting factors, decreased production of clotting factors, production of abnormal clotting factors, or platelet abnormalities.

The liver also plays a role in detoxification of many materials, particularly drugs. Basically, the liver process involves making the substance water soluble for excretion in bile or urine. Enzymes from the smooth endoplasmic reticulum oxidize, reduce, hydrolyze, and conjugate foreign compounds. The enzymes have a low substrate specificity and readily detoxify substances. The processes that determine whether or not a compound is excreted in the urine or the bile are multiple and are not always understood. Substances that are highly polar and those with molecular weights over 200 are excreted in the bile. Substances with smaller molecular weights are excreted via urine.

The effectiveness of lipid-soluble drugs may be altered by the conversion in the liver to a water-soluble state. Some drugs, such as phenylbutazone, become more potent after conversion in the liver to oxyphenylbutazone. However, oxidation of barbiturates results in a loss of effect. A by-product produced may be toxic. Some drugs require metabolic transformation in the liver for a therapeutic action to be produced. In a patient with liver disease it is important to know the effects of a drug. Certain medications should be avoided, and others should be given in reduced dosages.

Gallbladder

The gallbladder (Fig. 11-10) is a pear-shaped sac, 6 to 8 cm (3 to 4 inches) long, and attached to the inferior surface of the liver. It is joined to the biliary tree by the cystic duct at the point where the hepatic duct becomes the common bile duct.

The mucosa of the gallbladder is columnar epithelium overlying a lamina propria. The mucosa is in multiple, irregular folds that increase its absorptive area. The fibromuscular layer forms the framework of the sac. It is a mixture of longitudinal smooth muscle fibers and dense fibrous tissue. The fibromuscular layer is covered by a subserous adventitia. The serous layer is continuous with the serosa of the liver.

The gallbladder is supplied by the superior and inferior cystic artery, which branches off the hepatic artery. The venous system consists of capillary plexuses that drain into superficial veins on the surface of the gallbladder. These superficial veins empty directly into the liver. The gallbladder also has an extensive lymphatic system that connects with the lymphatic channels draining the liver. This system then combines with the lymphatics of the cystic duct and proximal sections of the extrahepatic ductal system and drains into the nodes at the porta hepatis.

Innervation of the gallbladder and biliary tree is from the sympathetic and parasympathetic system. Parasympathetic stimulation causes contraction of the gallbladder. Sympathetic stimulation is inhibitory. Preganglionic sympathetic fibers are from the seventh or tenth thoracic segment and postganglionic fibers from the celiac ganglia.

The hepatic division of the vagal nerve supplies parasympathetic preganglionic fibers that synapse with postganglionic fibers in the wall of the gallbladder. Afferent fibers travel with the splanchnic nerves and the right phrenic nerve. Right referred shoulder pain in gallbladder disease is related to this shared course with the right phrenic nerve.

The function of the gallbladder is to concentrate and store bile. The organ will store 30 to 50 ml of bile. In the presence of cholecystokinin-pancreozymin the gallbladder contracts, forcing bile through the cystic duct into the common bile duct and hence the duodenum (see discussion of bile under ''Liver'').

Pancreas

The pancreas (Fig. 11-10), an important accessory organ of digestion, is located transversely across the posterior wall of the abdomen. It is about 20 cm (10 inches) long and weighs 60 to 160 g. The head of the pancreas is situated in the concavity of the duodenal loop on the right side of the vertebral column at the level of the first lumbar vertebra. The body of the pancreas extends leftward and superiorly to the hilum of the spleen. The terminal portion of the pancreas is the tail.

The pancreas resembles the salivary glands histologically. The difference between the two is the presence of islets of Langerhans within the pancreas. The pancreas has both exocrine and endocrine functions. Acinar cells secrete the exocrine products, bicarbonate and pancreatic enzymes, and the endocrine secretions of insulin, glucagon, and gastrin are from the alpha, beta, and delta cells of islets of Langerhans.

The blood supply of the pancreas is from the superior and inferior pancreaticoduodenal arteries and from branches of the splenic artery. The venous flow from the body and tail of the pancreas is through the splenic vein,

and the head empties directly into the portal vein. The lymphatic system drains through the pancreaticoduodenal nodes to the celiac nodes.

The innervation of the pancreas is sympathetic and parasympathetic. The sympathetic fibers follow the arterial blood vessels and play a part in regulating blood flow to the pancreas. The parasympathetic fibers terminate at the acinar cells, the islet cells, and the smooth muscle cells and regulate pancreatic secretion.

The pancreas is divided into lobules, and each lobule empties into a branch of the main pancreatic duct. The individual lobule is a group of acini formed from acinar cells, drained by a ductule that forms intralobular ducts that empty into the pancreatic duct. In the acinar cells are dark zymogen granules that are the precursors of pancreatic enzymes. The acini are continuous with the excretory ducts and are composed of an epithelial lining layer on a basal membrane.

The exocrine secretion of the pancreas is approximately 2000 ml per day. The secretions are aqueous fluid, rich in bicarbonate, enzymes, and electrolytes. The enzymes formed in the acinar cells are secreted into the ducts. Water and electrolytes are secreted by the ductular epithelium. The major function of the pancreatic exocrine function is digestion and absorption in the small intestines. The bicarbonate, calcium, and magnesium in the pancreatic secretions are necessary for creating an optimal environment for enzyme activity. Interference with the exocrine function may lead to severe malabsorption of the dietary fats, fat-soluble vitamins, protein, and carbohydrates in starch form.

The hormones involved in the regulation of pancreatic exocrine secretions are gastrin, secretin, and cholecystokinin-pancreozymin. Gastrin is released by the antral mucosa in response to the presence of food in the stomach, distention, a decrease in hydrogen ion concentration, and vagal stimulation. In the duodenum, gastrin release is stimulated by distention and the presence of protein. Cholecystokinin-pancreozymin is secreted by the duodenal and proximal jejunal mucosa by the presence of L-amino acids, long-chain fatty acids, and hydrogen ions. The response of the pancreas to gastrin and cholecystokinin-pancreozymin is the secretion of enzyme-rich fluid. There is minimal increase in volume in bicarbonate output, and chloride concentration will decrease slightly. Calcium and magnesium secretions parallel enzyme output. Secretin is released from duodenal and proximal jejunal mucosa in response to hydrogen ion. Secretin stimulates large volumes of pancreatic secretions, which are high in bicarbonate, with little increase in enzyme output. The concentration of cations, sodium and potassium, remains relatively constant. Anion concentration will vary with the flow rate. As bicarbonate concentration increases, chloride concentration decreases. Secretin does interact with gastrin and cholecystokinin-pancreozymin to augment the secretory response.

Vagal stimulation will augment the hormonal stimulation of the exocrine secretions. The sight, smell, and taste of food stimulate the vagus. Also, gastric distention stimulates the vagus nerve. Vagal stimulation of the pancreas results in the secretion of pancreatic enzymes with minimal increase in bicarbonate concentration or volume.

Any disease process that obstructs the duct system or destroys the acinar cells will reduce the secretion of enzymes and bicarbonate and will progress to malabsorption and damage of the duodenal mucosa from unneutralized hydrochloric acid. In the presence of pancreatic disease, secretory functions can be decreased by limiting or eliminating food ingestion, minimizing vagal stimulation with anticholinergics, and reducing acids by nasogastric suctioning and use of cimetidine or antacids. A pancreas that is not secreting properly may be partially compensated for by an increase in fat and protein in the diet, use of medium-chain triglycerides, or administration of pancreatic enzyme extracts.

The islets are spheric cells that are outgrowths from the walls of the pancreatic duct during embryonic life. The hormones released from the islets enter directly into the circulation.

The endocrine functions are the secretion of glucagon (alpha cells), insulin (beta cells), and gastrin (delta cells). Glucagon causes glycogenolysis in the liver. A blood glucose level below 60 to 80 mg per deciliter of blood stimulates the alpha cells to release glucagon, causing the breakdown of glycogen to glucose in the liver. A normal blood glucose level will "turn off" the alpha cells.

The beta cells of the islets of Langerhans secrete insulin, which increases glucose utilization. It carries glucose by active transport through the cellular membrane. An increased blood glucose level, usually following a meal, stimulates the beta cells to release insulin. The insulin carries the glucose across the cell membrane, reducing the blood level to normal.

NORMAL FINDINGS

Area of Concern	Normal Adult Findings	Variations in Child	Variations in Older Adult
Mouth Temporomandibular joint	Mobility: smooth jaw excursion; 3.5-4.5 cm Tenderness: absent on palpation Crepitus: absent Referred pain: absent on closing jaw		
Occlusion	Top back teeth rest directly on lower teeth; upper incisors slightly override lowers	Same as adult when secondary teeth have erupted	May change due to missing teeth Marked overclosure may be associated with edentulous patient Individuals who stoop and thrust head forward tend to habitually protrude lower jaw
Lips	Color: pink Symmetry: vertical and lateral symmetry at rest and on movement Moisture: smooth and moist Surface characteristics: slight vertical linear markings	Breast- or bottle-fed babies may develop a sucking tubercle in middle of upper lip	Decreased saliva production may contribute to drier lips and difficulty swallowing foods Vertical markings increased "Purse-string" appearance associated with edentulism or overclosure of jaws

Adapted from Thompson, J.M., and Bowers, A.C.: Clinical manual of health assessment, St. Louis, 1980, The C.V. Mosby Co.

Area of Concern	Normal Adult Findings	Variations in Child	Variations in Older Adult
Inner lips and buccal membrane	Color: pale coral, pink; increased pigmentation, general or localized, in dark-skinned individuals Landmarks: parotid duct; pinpoint red marking; may be slightly elevated Surface characteristics: where teeth meet, occlusion line may appear on adjacent mucosa; clear saliva over surface	Surface characteristics: smooth; fine grayish ridge; occlusion line may appear where teeth meet; increased salivation in children between 3 mo and 2 yr may be normal If child appears ill, salivation should be considered abnormal until proved otherwise	Surface characteristics: mucosa becomes thinner and less vascular; may appear shinier than in younger adults Fordyce's granules common
Gums	Color: pink, coral Surface characteristics: slightly stippled, clearly defined, tight margin at tooth; patchy brown pigmentation in dark-skinned individuals Hypertrophy may appear during puberty or pregnancy If inflammation (gingivitis) appears, refer to dentist	Surface characteristics: may see downward extension of alveolar frenulum as child's central incisors separate; should self-correct Small pearly white cysts (Epstein's pearls) may be seen along gums of infants; disappear by 2-3 mo of age; called Bohn's nodules when on midpalate	Color: may be slightly paler Surface characteristics: stippling may be decreased

Teeth	Number: 32 (adult); upper and lower third molars may be absent
	Color: white, yellowish, or grayish hues
	Form: smooth edges
	Surface characteristics: smooth; dental restorations
	Movement: none or slight movement
		Baby Teeth
		Central incisors
		  Eruption
		    Upper: 6-8 mo
		    Lower: 5-7 mo
		  Shedding
		    Upper: 6-7 yr
		    Lower: 5-6 yr
		Lateral incisors
		  Eruption
		    Upper: 8-12 mo
		    Lower: 7-10 mo
		  Shedding
		    Upper: 8-9 yr
		    Lower: 7-8 yr
		Canines
		  Eruption
		    Upper: 16-20 mo
		    Lower: 16-20 mo
		  Shedding
		    Upper: 11-12 yr
		    Lower: 9-11 yr
		First molars
		  Eruption
		    Upper: 10-16 mo
		    Lower: 10-16 mo
		  Shedding
		    Upper: 10-11 yr
		    Lower: 10-12 yr
		Second molars
		  Eruption
		    Upper: 20-30 mo
		    Lower: 20-30 mo
		  Shedding
		    Upper: 10-12 yr
		    Lower: 11-13 yr
		
		Eruption of Permanent Teeth
		Central incisors
		  Upper: 7-8 yr
		  Lower: 6-7 yr
			Color: may appear more yellowish or slightly darker
			Form and surface characteristics: teeth may appear elongated as more root surface or neck of tooth is exposed with resorption of supporting bone

Area of Concern	Normal Adult Findings	Variations in Child	Variations in Older Adult
		Lateral incisors 　Upper: 8-9 yr 　Lower: 7-8 yr Canines 　Upper: 11-12 yr 　Lower: 9-11 yr First premolars 　Upper: 10-11 yr 　Lower: 10-12 yr Second premolars 　Upper: 10-12 yr 　Lower: 11-13 yr First molars 　Upper: 6-7 yr 　Lower: 6-7 yr Second molars 　Upper: 12-13 yr 　Lower: 12-13 yr	
Tongue	Symmetry and movement: forward thrust smooth and symmetric; tongue appears symmetric Color: pink Surface characteristics: dorsal and lateral is moist and glistening, with papillae; elongated vallate papillae; fissures; smooth, even tissue Ventral surface: pink and smooth with large veins		Papillae may appear slightly smoother and shinier Epithelium is thin and loosely attached Veins may be varicosed
Floor of mouth	Frenulum is centered Submaxillary duct opening can be found Color: pale, coral pink		
Hard and soft palate	Color: hard palate: pale; soft palate: pink Surface characteristics 　Hard palate: immovable, irregular transverse rugae; midline exostosis (torus palatinus) may be present 　Soft palate: movable, symmetric elevation; smooth	Bohn's nodules in newborn; disappear by 2-3 mo Very high or narrow arch requires further evaluation; may be linked to several syndromes	
Mouth odor	Absent or sweet	Absent	
Oropharynx	Landmarks: anterior and posterior pillars symmetric; uvula midline; tonsils Color: posterior wall pink Surface characteristics: smooth; tonsils may be cryptic; slight vascularity on posterior wall	Tonsils may vary in size from barely visible to very large	
Abdomen Inspection	On inspection the following are normal findings Skin color: may be pale in comparison to body parts that are more exposed Surface characteristics: smooth, soft, silver-white striae Scars: configuration, location, and length Venous network: very faint, fine network Umbilicus: centrally located; usually	Newborn: umbilicus should dry within 5 d; should drop off in 2 wk with dry base remaining; cord should contain two arteries and one vein Umbilical hernia common and is considered normal in white children until 2 yr of age and in black children until 7 yr; hernia	Contour: geriatric patients may have an increase in fat deposits over abdominal area even though subcutaneous fat over extremities is decreased

Area of Concern	Normal Adult Findings	Variations in Child	Variations in Older Adult
	shrunken, but may protrude slightly; should be smooth and noninflamed Contour: flat, rounded, or concave (scaphoid) Symmetry: evenly rounded with maximal height of convexity at umbilicus Surface motion: peristalsis usually not visible but may be visible in thin people; pulsations in upper midline may be visible in thin people Movement with respirations: smooth and even; female primarily exhibits costal movements while males evidence primarily abdominal movements Contour remains smooth and symmetric when patient takes a deep breath and holds it Rectus abdominis muscles are prominent; on tightening muscle, midline bulge may appear	should obtain maximal size by 1 mo of age; size varies from a few millimeters to 3 cm; note if hernia is present during crying or with movements Contour: infant and toddler have round potbelly both standing and lying; school-aged child may show potbelly stance (lordotic) until 13 yr when standing, but on lying, abdomen is scaphoid (concave) Respiration movement: until approximately 7 yr, children are abdominal breathers; after this, boys are chiefly abdominal breathers while girls primarily use costal movements Diastasis recti abdominis is a condition in which the two rectus muscles do not approximate each other; is common in black children and should disappear during preschool years; distance may be 1-5 cm	
Auscultation	Bowel sounds: usually 5-34/min; irregular; gurgles, clicks, and quality vary greatly; all four quadrants Absence of vascular sounds Absence of friction rub		
Percussion Four abdominal quadrants	Tone: general distribution of tympany depending on amount of air and solid material in bowel; suprapubic dullness over distended bladder	Tone: children's abdomens frequently sound louder in tympany tones because children swallow more air	

Liver percussion	Lower border: usually at costal margin or slightly below
	Upper border: begins in fifth to seventh intercostal space
	Midclavicular liver span: 6-12 cm (2½-4½ inches); liver span usually greater in men than women; liver span greater in taller individuals
	Right midaxillary liver: liver dullness; may be heard in fifth to seventh intercostal space
	Midsternal liver span: 4-8 cm (1½-3 inches)
	Liver descent with deep inspiration: lower border should move inferiorly by 2-3 cm (¾-1 inch)
		Lower border: costal margin or 2-3 cm lower (¾-1 inch)
		Upper border: at approximately sixth rib or interspace anteriorly and at ninth rib posteriorly
		Liver span
		  5 yr of age: 7 cm (2¾ inches)
		  12 yr of age: 9 cm (3½ inches)
			Lower border: in elderly patient with distended lungs, liver border is 1-2 cm (½-¾ inches) into abdominal cavity
			Upper border: with distended lung may descend 1-2 cm (½-¾ inch)
			Deep inspiration may be difficult for elderly individual

Spleen percussion*	Left posterior midaxillary line: small area of splenic dullness at sixth to tenth rib, or tone may be tympanic (colonic) Left intercostal space in anterior axillary line: tympanic Left lower rib cage: gastric "bubble"; tympanic; varies in size	Left midaxillary line: small area of dullness above ninth interspace In young infants and children: may extend 1-2 cm (½-¾ inch) below costal margin	

*If an enlarged spleen is suspected, it may be advisable to perform palpation before percussion.

Area of Concern	Normal Adult Findings	Variations in Child	Variations in Older Adult
Palpation Four abdominal quadrants			
Light and moderate palpation	Tenderness: none Muscle tone: abdomen relaxed; muscular resistance may be seen in anxious patients Surface characteristics: smooth, consistent tension opposed to localized area of rigidity (increased tension) Masses: none	In umbilicus area, note size of hernia if present	Muscle tone: often more lax
Deep palpation	Tenderness: often present in midline near xiphoid process over cecum, over sigmoid colon Masses: aorta often palpable at epigastrium and pulsates in forward direction; can palpate borders of rectus abdominis muscles; feces may be palpated in ascending or descending colon; sacral promontory may be palpable Umbilicus: check for bulges, nodes, and umbilicus ring; normal findings include umbilicus ring with no irregularities or bulges; umbilicus may be inverted or slightly everted	In umbilicus area, note size of hernia if present	Muscle tone: often more lax
Liver	Liver border and contour: liver often not palpable; liver may "bump" against fingers on inspiration, especially in thin people Liver border surface: smooth Tenderness: none	Liver border 0-6 mo: palpable 0-3 cm (1 inch) below costal margin 6 mo to 4 yr: palpable 1-2 cm (½-¾ inch) below costal margin Over 6 yr: palpable 1-2 cm (½-¾ inch) or not palpable below right costal margin	Liver commonly palpated 1-2 cm (½-¾ inch) below costal margin in patients with distended lungs, emphysema, and lowered diaphragm
Spleen	Spleen not normally palpable	May feel at costal margin or slightly under ribs in small children Only tip should be palpable	
Kidney	Occasionally lower pole of kidney may be palpable in thin individuals; right kidney most often palpable Contour: smooth, firm Tenderness: none	Palpable periodically; lies adjacent to vertebral column; descends slightly with inspiration	
Inguinal nodes	Note presence of nodes: small, mobile; none tender; nodes often present Contour: smooth or nonpalpable Consistency: soft or nonpalpable		
Assessment for abdominal fluid	None should be found Techniques for assessment include flank bulging and fluid shift		
Rectal-anal region	Skin and surface characteristics: smooth, clear No tenderness in coccygeal area Anus: surface characteristics include increased pigmentation, coarse skin Sphincter muscle: tightens evenly around finger with minimal discomfort for patient Anal muscular ring: smooth, even pressure on finger Rectal wall: continuous, smooth surface (examination should cause minimal discomfort for patient) Stool: brown, soft	Internal rectal examination not routinely done in children unless specific problem exists	

NORMAL LABORATORY DATA

Laboratory Test	Normal Adult Values	Variations in Child
Albumin Whole blood, serum, or plasma	Serum quantitative (1-31 yr): 3.5-5.0 g/dl with A/G ratio greater than 1.0; after age 40, normal range gradually decreases 4.0-5.50 g/dl (electrophoresis)	Serum (0-1 yr): 2.9-5.5 g/dl
Urine	Qualitative: random sample negative Quantitative: less than 20 mg/dl	
Ammonia Whole blood, serum, or plasma	Varies somewhat between laboratories; 11-35 μmol/L	29-59 μmol/L
Urine	Ammonia nitrogen: 20-50 mEq/24 h (500-1200 mg/24 h)	
Amylase	Method dependent	Serum (newborn): little if any
Ascorbic acid (vitamin C) Serum or plasma Urine	0.2-2.0 mg/dl Random sample: 1-7 mg/dl 24 h: >50 mg/24 h	
Bicarbonate	Arterial: 21-28 mEq/L Venous: 22-29 mEq/L	Newborn and infant: 16-24 mEq/L
Bile acids Whole blood, serum, or plasma	Positive: >10 cholesterol monohydrate or calcium bilirubinate crystals per slide Suspicious: 1-9 cholesterol monohydrate or calcium bilirubinate crystals per slide	
Urine	Negative	

Bilirubin
Serum
	Direct (conjugated): up to 0.4 mg/dl
	Indirect (unconjugated): 0.1-1.0 mg/dl
	Total: 0.3-1.0 mg/dl
		For newborns, direct bilirubin varies with age in days and prematurity vs. maturity
		Newborn bilirubin (total serum): up to 2-10 mg/dl depending on age
		Full term
		   24 h: 20-60 mg/L
		   48 h: 60-70 mg/L
		   3-5 d: 40-120 mg/L

Urine	Qualitative: random sample negative	
Calcium Serum	Ionized: 3.9-4.8 mg/dl for one formula available Total (up to 30 yr): 8.2-10.5 mg/dl; decreases very slightly in older years	Infants up to 1 mo: 7-11.5 mg/dl 1 mo to 1 yr: 8.6-11.2 mg/dl Normal range slowly descends
Urine	Qualitative (Sulkowitch; random): 1+ turbidity Quantitative: varies with diet; based on average calcium intake of 600-800 mg/24 h: 100-250 mg/24 h (average diet); <150 mg/24 h (low calcium diet); 250-300 mg/24 h (high calcium diet)	

Laboratory Test	Normal Adult Values	Variations in Child
Chloride Serum	97-107 mEq/L	Premature: 95-110 mEq/L Full term: 96-106 mEq/L

Urine	24-h collection: 110-250 mEq/
	  24 h in adults; lower values
	  in infancy and childhood; re-
	  sults depend on ingestion of
	  chloride	

Cholesterol Serum	See footnote*	0-1 mo: 45-100 mg/dl
Coagulation Bleeding time (Ivy)	2-7 min	
Bleeding time (Duke)	5 min	
Clot reaction	Half in the original mass in 2 h	
Dilute blood clot lysis time	Clot still intact after 2 h is "normal"	
Euglobin clot lysis time	Lysis time >90 min	

Partial thromboplastin time	25-39 s, usually stated to be
	  within 10 s of control; kaolin
	  activated: 35-50 s	

Prothrombin time	10-13 s	
Venous clotting time	8-15 min	
Whole blood clot lysis time	None in 24 h	

Creatine as creatinine
  Serum or plasma
	Male: 0.1-0.4 mg/dl
	Female: 0.2-0.7 mg/dl
		Serum creatine kinase
		  Newborn: 3 times adult values
		  3 wk to 3 mo: 1.5 times adult values
		  >1 yr: at adult values

Urine	Creatine excretion decreases
	  with advanced age as muscle
	  mass diminishes
	Male: 0-40 mg/24 h
	Female: 0-100 mg/24 h (higher
	  in pregnancy)	

Creatinine
  Serum
	Men: up to 1.2 mg/dl
	Women: up to 1.1 mg/dl
	There are slight differences be-
	  tween the sexes with males
	  higher since range relates to
	  amount of muscle mass pres-
	  ent
		1-5 yr: 0.30-0.50 mg/dl
		5-10 yr: 0.50-0.80 mg/dl

Urine	Male: 1.0-2.0 g/24 h Female: 0.8-1.8 g/24 h	2-3 yr: 6-22 mg/kg/24 h >3 yr: 12-30 mg/kg/24 h
Creatinine clearance (endogenous)	Male: 85-125 ml/min/1.73 sq m Female: 75-115 ml/min/1.73 sq m	70-140 ml/min/1.73 sq m

Fatty acids
  Serum
	Total (free and esterified): 9.5
	  mM	

Plasma	Free (nonesterified): 300-480 μEq/L	Newborn: 0-1845 mmol/L 4 mo to 10 yr: 300-1100 mmol/L
Urine	Fat (qualitative): random sample negative	

*Sharp inconsistencies are obvious when one studies published normal ranges of serum cholesterol in the United States. Although 100-210 mg/dl would be regarded as a low normal range for American adults, an increase between ages 25 and 45 of about 25 mg/dl is recognized. Levels above 180 are not desirable but are commonplace in the United States, and adult normal ranges over 300 mg/dl are offered.

Laboratory Test	Normal Adult Values	Variations in Child
Fibrinogen Plasma	200-400 mg/dl	
Folate Whole blood, serum, or plasma	>2.0 ng/ml	
Fructose Urine	24-h collection: 30-65 mg/24 h	

Galactose
    Whole blood
    Urine
	None
	<10 mg/dl
		<20 mg/dl

Gamma globulin Serum	0.5-1.6 g/dl	

Globulins (total)
    Serum
    Urine
	2.3-3.5 g/dl
	No monoclonal gammopathy
	    detected	

Glucose
    Fasting
        Serum or plasma
	60-115 mg/dl (normal range in-
	    creases with age over 50)
		Premature infants: 40-65 mg/dl
		0-2 yr: 60-110 mg/dl
		Serum glucose
		    Preterm: 200-656 mg/L
		    Full term: 200-1100 mg/L
		    Child: 600-1060 mg/L

Whole blood
    Oral glucose tolerance (serum or
    plasma)
	60-100 mg/dl
	Fasting: 60-115 mg/dl (normal
	    range increases with age over
	    50)
	30 min: 30-60 mg/dl above
	    fasting
	60 min: 20-50 mg/dl above
	    fasting
	120 min: 5-15 mg/dl above
	    fasting
	180 min: fasting level or below	

2-h postprandial	0-50 yr: 70-140 mg/dl 50-60 yr: 70-150 mg/dl 60 yr and up: 70-160 mg/dl	
Intravenous glucose tolerance (serum or plasma)	Fasting: 70-110 mg/dl 5 min: maximum of 250 mg/dl 60 min: significant decrease 120 min: <120 mg/dl 180 min: fasting level	
Random glucose	Dependent on time and content of last meal	

Urine	Qualitative: random sample
	    negative
	Quantitative (24 h): copper re-
	    ducing substances: 0.5-1.5 g/
	    24 h
	Glucose: up to 100 mg/24 h	

Glucose-6-phosphate dehydroge- nase (G6PD)	140-280 units/billion cells	
Gamma glutamyl transferase Serum	5-40 IU/L	Premature newborn: 56-233 U/L Newborn to 3 wk: 10-103 U/L 3 wk to 3 mo: 4-111 U/L 1-5 yr: 2-23 U/L 6-15 yr: 2-23 U/L 16 yr to adult: 2-35 U/L

Laboratory Test	Normal Adult Values	Variations in Child
Haptoglobin Serum	40-180 mg/dl but values are method dependent	Newborn: detectable haptoglobin in only 10-20%; newborns reach adult levels at approximately 4 mo
Hematocrit	Male: 40-47 ml/dl Female: 37-42 ml/dl	
Hemoglobin Whole blood, serum, or plasma	Male: 15.5 ± 1.1 g/dl Female: 13.7 ± 1.0 g/dl	1 d: 19.4 ± 2.1 g/dl 1½-3 yr: 11.8 ± 0.5 g/dl 5 yr: 12.7 ± 1.0 g/dl 10 yr: 13.2 ± 1.2 g/dl
Urine	Random sample, negative	

Immunoglobulins
  Serum
	IgG: 564-1765 mg/dl
	IgA: 85-385 mg/dl
	IgM: 53-375 mg/dl
	IgD: 0-40 mg/dl
	IgE: 0.01-0.04 mg/dl
		IgG
		  12-24 mo: 135-1106 mg/dl
		  24-36 mo: 517-1346 mg/dl
		  3-5 yr: 570-1592 mg/dl
		  5-8 yr: 757-1686 mg/dl
		  8-12 yr: 851-1805 mg/dl
		  12-16 yr: 767-1752 mg/dl
		IgA
		  12-24 mo: 18-111 mg/dl
		  24-36 mo: 21-98 mg/dl
		  3-5 yr: 30-178 mg/dl
		  5-8 yr: 74-265 mg/dl
		  8-12 yr: 68-333 mg/dl
		  12-16 yr: 68-250 mg/dl
		IgM
		  12-24 mo: 19-148 mg/dl
		  24-36 mo: 40-151 mg/dl
		  3-5 yr: 28-142 mg/dl
		  5-8 yr: 30-162 mg/dl
		  8-12 yr: 24-161 mg/dl
		  12-16 yr: 26-221 mg/dl

Iron Serum	Total: 42-135 μg/dl Binding capacity: 218-385 μg/dl Saturation: 20-50%	

Ketone bodies
  Serum
  Urine
	Negative
	Random sample negative	

17-Ketosteroids
  Plasma
  Urine
	25-125 μg/dl
	Male: 6-22 mg/24 h
	Female: 4-17 mg/24 h (with decrease in advancing years)
		0-3 d: 0.05 mg/d
		1-3 yr: <2.0 mg/d
		3-6 yr: 0.5-3.0 mg/d
		6-9 yr: 0.8-4.0 mg/d
		10-12 yr male: 0.7-6.0 mg/d
		10-12 yr female: 0.7-5.0 mg/d
		Adolescent
		  Male: 3-15 mg/d
		  Female: 3-12 mg/d

Lactose
  Lactic acid (lactate)
 	
  Lactose intolerance
	Venous: 5-20 mg/dl
	Arterial: 3-7 mg/dl
	Increase of blood glucose <20 mg/dl over fasting level, with symptoms, is considered ab-	

Laboratory Test	Normal Adult Values	Variations in Child
	normal; evidence for lactase deficiency; >30 mg/dl is normal	
Urine	14-40 mg/24 h	
Lipase	Method dependent	
Lipids		
Serum	Total: 400-800 mg/dl Cholesterol* Triglycerides† Phospholipids: 150-380 mg/dl Fatty acids (free): 9.0-15.0 mM/L (300-480 µEq/L) Phospholipid phosphorus: 8.0-11.0 mg/dl	0-1 mo: 45-100 mg/dl
Feces		Fecal fats Full-term newborn: up to 20% extreted 3 mo to 1 yr: up to 15% excreted 1 yr: up to 8.5% excreted
Macroglobulins, total‡		
Whole blood, serum, or plasma	53-375 mg/dl	12-24 mo: 19-148 mg/dl 24-36 mo: 40-151 mg/dl 3-5 yr: 28-142 mg/dl 5-8 yr: 30-162 mg/dl 8-12 yr: 24-161 mg/dl 12-16 yr: 26-221 mg/dl
Magnesium		
Serum	1.2-1.9 mEq/L (may be expressed in mg/dl)	
Urine	5.0-16.0 mEq/24 h	
Mean corpuscular volume	Male: 80-100 μ^3 Female: 79-98 μ^3	
Mucoprotein		
Serum	80-200 mg/dl	
Mucin		
Urine	100-150 mg/24 h	
Osmolality		
Serum	280-300 mOsm/kg H_2O	
Urine	Random sample: 250-900 mOsm/kg H_2O	
pH		
Whole blood	Arterial: 7.35-7.45 Venous: 7.32-7.43	
Serum or plasma	Venous: 7.35-7.45	
Urine	Random sample: 4.8-7.8	
Phenylalanine		
Serum	>3.0 mg/dl	Newborn: 2 mg/dl or less by Guthrie bacterial-inhibition assay; <4 mg/dl by fluorometry in some laboratories

*Sharp inconsistencies are obvious when one studies published normal ranges of serum cholesterol in the United States. Although 100-210 mg/dl would be regarded as a low normal range for American adults, an increase between ages 25 and 45 of about 25 mg/dl is recognized. Levels above 180 are not desirable but are commonplace in the United States, and adult normal ranges over 300 mg/dl are offered.
†Different ranges are in use. Moderate increases from childhood occur. At the 95th percentile: white males, 25-29 yr: up to 250 mg/dl; 35-54 yr: up to 320 mg/dl; 55-64 yr: up to 290 mg/dl; 65 yr and over: up to 260 mg/dl; white females, 35-39 yr: up to 195 mg/dl; 55-64 yr: up to 250 mg/dl.
‡Immunoglobulin M now replaces this; values are for immunoglobulin M.

Laboratory Test	Normal Adult Values	Variations in Child
Phospholipid phosphorus Serum	8-11 mg/dl	
Phospholipids Serum	150-380 mg/dl	
Phosphorus, inorganic Serum	2.5-4.5 mg/dl	At birth: 5.6-8.0 mg/dl 6-10 d: approximately 6-10 mg/dl Childhood: approximately 4-7 mg/dl (Both low and high ends of normal range are higher in children than in adults.)
Urine	Random sample: 0.9-1.3 g/24 h (dependent on dietary intake)	
Potassium Plasma	3.5-5.0 mEq/L; add approximately 0.2 to normal ranges if serum is sampled rather than plasma	Pediatric ranges are sometimes reported as slightly higher than adult levels
Urine	40-80 mEq/24 h	
Platelet count Whole blood, serum, or plasma	150,000-400,000/cmm	

Protein
Serum
	Total: 6.0-8.0 g/dl
	Albumin: 3.5-5.0 g/dl with A/G ratio >1.0
	Globulin: 2.3-3.5 g/dl
	Electrophoresis
	  Albumin: 58.0-74.0%* 4.00-5.50 g/dl†
	  Alpha-1: 2.0-3.5%; 0.15-0.25 g/dl
	  Alpha-2: 5.4-10.6%; 0.43-0.75 g/dl
	  Beta: 7.0-14.0%; 0.50-1.00 g/dl
	  Gamma: 8.0-18.0%; 0.60-1.30 g/dl	

Urine	Qualitative random sample negative 24 h: 30-150 mg/24 h (method dependent)	
Prothrombin time	10-13 sec	
Sodium Serum or plasma	135-145 mEq/L	Premature and full-term infants may have levels 5-10 mEq/L lower than adult values but this is controversial
Urine	27-287 mEq/24 h (varies markedly with dietary intake of sodium); there is also diurnal variation (output lower at night)	

Transferases
Serum
	Asparate amino transferase (AST or SGOT): levels in infancy are two to three times those found in adults; ranges	Gamma glutamyl transferase
		  Premature newborn: 56-233 U/L
		  Newborn to 3 wk: 10-103 U/L
		  1-5 yr: 2-23 U/L

*Percentage of total protein.
†Concentration.

Laboratory Test	Normal Adult Values	Variations in Child
	decrease during childhood years; SMA method: 16 yr and up: 8-42 U/L	6-15 yr: 2-23 U/L 16 yr to adult: 2-35 U/L
	Alanine amino transferase: slightly increased ranges in infancy compared to adult normal range; adult: 3-30 IU/L depending on method	
	Gamma glutamyl transferase (GGT): 5-40 IU/L at 37° C	
Triglycerides Whole blood, serum, or plasma	Different ranges are in use; moderate increases from childhood occur; at 95th percentile: white males: 25-29 yr: up to 250 mg/dl; 35-54 yr: up to 320 mg/dl; 55-64 yr: up to 290 mg/dl; 65 and over: up to 260 mg/dl; white females: 35-39 yr: up to 195 mg/dl; 55-64 yr: up to 250 mg/dl	
Urea nitrogen Blood	1-40 yr: 5-20 mg/dl; gradual slight increase subsequently occurs	Birth to 1 yr: 4-19 mg/dl
Urine	6-17 g/24 h	
Urea clearance Serum and urine	Maximum: 64-99 ml/min Standard: 41-65 ml/min or more than 75% of normal clearance	
Uric acid Serum	Male: 3.4-7.0 mg/dl or slightly higher Female: 2.4-6.0 mg/dl or slightly higher	Increase occurs during childhood
Urine	Approximately 250-750 mg/24 h	

Urobilinogen
    Urine
	2-h collection
	    Male: 0.3-2.1 mg/2 h
	    Female: 0.1-1.1 mg/2 h
	    Results sometimes expressed in Ehrlich units (1 mg urobilinogen = 1 EU)
	    24-h collection: 0.05-2.5 mg/24 h or 0.5-4.0 Ehrlich units/24 h	

Vitamin A Serum	15-60 μg/dl Vitamin A tolerance: fasting 3 h or 6 h after 5000 units: 15-60 μ/dl A/kg/24: 200-600 μg/dl; fasting values are higher	

Laboratory Test	Normal Adult Values	Variations in Child
Vitamin B$_{12}$ Serum	160-950 pg/ml Unsaturated vitamin B$_{12}$ binding capacity: 1000-2000 pg/ml	
Vitamin C Serum or plasma Urine	0.2-2.0 mg/dl Random sample: 1-7 mg/dl 24 h: >50 mg/24 h (as ascorbic acid)	
Zinc Whole blood, serum, or plasma Urine	0.66-1.1 μg/ml 0.15-1.2 mg/24 h	

DIAGNOSTIC STUDIES

Evaluation of contents of gastrointestinal system

Evaluation of pressure systems in gastrointestinal lumen

Involves collection of contents, often through intubation

Nursing care:

Following precautions or concerns are for any test in which nasogastric intubation is necessary:

1. Check location of catheter for placement.
2. Paroxysms of coughing or cyanosis may indicate a catheter in the trachea.
3. Arrhythmias may develop during intubation.
4. Clamp catheter during removal to prevent aspiration from fluids in lumen.
5. Sore throats following intubation may be treated with soothing lozenges, viscous xylocaine, or cetacaine spray.

Esophageal acidity test (pH monitoring)

Evaluates competency of lower esophageal sphincter by measuring intraesophageal pH with an electrode attached to a manometric catheter

Will indicate gastric reflux; normal value: pH of esophagus is 6.0 or higher; 24-hour monitoring involves patient writing down all activities done during that period

Nursing care:

Antacids, anticholinergics, cholinergics, adrenergic blockers, cimetidine, ranitidine, and reserpine should be withheld for 24 hours before test; if medications are not withheld, note this on the laboratory request sheet

Acid perfusion test (Bernstein test)

Test designed to evaluate esophageal mucosa

Patients with gastric reflux often have symptoms of epigastric or retrosternal pain that radiates to the back or arms

Test used to distinguish between chest pain of esophagitis and chest pain of cardiac disorders

Two solutions (saline and acidic) are dripped through a nasogastric tube; presence of pain with acidic solution indicates esophagitis

Nursing care:

Contraindicated in patients with esophageal varices, congestive heart failure, acute myocardial infarction, and other known cardiac disorders

If patient continues to complain of pain or burning after test, antacids may help to relieve discomfort

Esophageal manometry

Measures upper and lower esophageal sphincter pressure

Manometric catheter containing a small pressure transducer along its length is swallowed; baseline measurements are taken and then pressures are recorded before, after, and during swallowing; peristaltic contractions are recorded and used to evaluate patient for achalasia, diffuse spasm of esophagus, and esophageal scleroderma

Normal values: baseline pressure—20 mm Hg; relaxation pressure—18 mm Hg; peristaltic pressure appears as a series of high-pressure peaks

Nursing care:

Provide ice water for swallowing during procedure

Basal gastric secretion test (gastric analysis)

Measures basal secretion under fasting conditions by aspirating stomach contents through a nasogastric tube

Indicated for patients with anorexia, weight loss, and epigastric pain

Normal values: 0.2 to 3.8 mEq/h for females; 1 to 5 mEq/h for males

High values may indicate a duodenaul or jejunal ulcer; depressed values may indicate gastric carcinoma or benign gastric ulcer; absence of gastric secretion indicates pernicious anemia; markedly high levels indicate Zollinger-Ellison syndrome

Nursing care:
   Patient must be relaxed and isolated from sensory stimulations of foods; gastric acid secretions are increased by external factors including sight and smell of food and psychologic stress
   Patient should have nothing to eat for 12 hours; no smoking for 8 hours; and withhold the following drugs for 24 hours: antacids, anticholinergics, cholinergics, alcohol, cimetidine, ranitidine, reserpine, adrenergic blockers, and adrenocorticosteroids
   Stomach contents are aspirated through a nasogastric tube with the patient in supine, left lateral decubitus, and right lateral decubitus positions
   To prevent contamination of gastric contents with saliva, patient should be instructed to expectorate excess saliva rather than swallowing it

Gastric acid stimulation test
   Normally follows basal gastric secretion test
   A drug, usually pentagastrin, is given to stimulate gastric acid output; specimens are collected every 15 minutes for 1 hour
   Normal values: 11 to 21 mEq/h for females and 18 to 28 mEq/h for males
   Clinical diagnosis of the following is indicated by certain results of gastric acid secretion:
      Duodenal ulcers: high values
      Zollinger-Ellison syndrome: markedly high
      Gastric carcinoma: low values
      Pernicious anemia: achlorhydria (Low acid levels are considered normal in patients over 60 years of age.)

Nursing care:
   Prepare patient as for basal gastric secretion test
   Side effects of pentagastrin include abdominal pain, nausea, vomiting, flushing, transitory dizziness, faintness, and numbness of extremities; check history for hypersensitivity to pentagastrin

Peritoneal fluid analysis
   Examines a sample of peritoneal fluid obtained by paracentesis
   Purpose of test: to determine composition of the ascitic fluid, which assists in diagnosis, or to detect abdominal trauma
   Normally, peritoneal fluid is sterile, odorless, clear to pale yellow, and less than 50 ml, with no red blood cells, bacteria, or fungi

Normal values: white blood count—$<300/\mu l$; protein—0.3 to 4.1 g/dl; glucose—70 to 100 mg/dl; amylase—138 to 404 amylase units/L; ammonia—<50 μg/dl; alkaline phosphatase: Male over 18 years—90 to 239 units/L; female under 45 years—76 to 196 units/L; female over 45 years—87 to 250 units/L

Nursing care:
   Record baseline vital signs, weights, and abdominal girth measurements for comparisons with posttest results
   Consent forms generally required
   Patient should void immediately before procedure to avoid injury to bladder
   Patient is usually sitting with feet flat on floor and back supported; if patient cannot tolerate this, use a high Fowler's position
   Check vital signs every 15 minutes during procedure and compare with baseline values; note signs of dizziness, pallor, perspiration, increased anxiety
   Rapid aspiration may induce hypovolemia and shock; slow the rate of aspiration
   After test has been completed, monitor vital signs frequently (every 30 minutes for 2 hours; every hour for next 4 hours; every 4 hours for 24 hours); weight and abdominal girth should be done and compared with baseline
   Cover site with sterile dressing; if site continues to drain requiring frequent dressing changes, consider application of skin barrier and pouch for collection of drainage and accurate measurement of output
   Monitor urinary output for 24 hours and observe for hematuria
   Observe patient closely for signs of hypovolemic shock if large amounts were aspirated
   Complication of procedure is perforation of an abdominal organ or vessels; signs include those for hemorrhage and shock, increasing pain, and abdominal tenderness
   Patients with severe hepatic disease should be observed for signs of hepatic coma, which may be from loss of sodium and potassium with accompanying hypovolemia; observe patient for mental changes, drowsiness, and stupor

Fecal occult blood test
Used to detect gastrointestinal bleeding and as screening test for colorectal cancer
Color usually indicates site of bleeding (e.g., melena is common with esophageal or gastric bleeding; dark maroon color may indicate a lesion below the ligament of Treitz; and bright red may be from a low rectal carcinoma or hemorrhoids)

Procedure consists of patient collecting three separate stool specimens

Nursing care:

Avoid red meats, poultry, fish, turnips, and horseradish for 48 to 72 hours before test begins and throughout collection period

Withhold iron preparations, bromides, iodides, rauwolfia derivatives, indomethacin, colchicine, salicylates, and phenylbutazone for 48 hours before collection begins and throughout the test; if patient is taking steroids, accuracy of test may be affected; do not collect during menses since false positive results may be obtained

Ascorbic acid can interfere with accuracy of test and should be withheld 48 hours before collection period begins

Fecal fat

Steatorrhea, excessive secretions of fecal lipids, may be observed in some malabsorption syndromes

Qualitative (random sample) and quantitative (72-hour collection) tests used

Qualitative tests will identify undigested muscle fibers and various fats, and quantitative tests can confirm steatorrhea

Fecal lipids normally are less than 20% of excreted solids or less than 7 g/24 h

Sudan stain can be done on a sample to test for presence of fat

Nursing care:

Avoid alcohol ingestion for 72 hours before and during stool collection

Maintain high-fat diet, 100 g/d, for 72 hours before and during collection

Avoid use of waxed collection containers since wax can become incorporated into stool and distort results

Specimen container must be refrigerated

Avoid azathioprine, kanamycin, bisacodyl, cholestyramine, neomycin, colchicine, aluminum hydroxide, calcium carbonate, potassium chloride, and mineral oil since they inhibit absorption of fats or affect chemical digestion, producing inaccurate results

Fecal urobilinogen

May be used as an indicator of hepatobiliary and hemolytic disorders

Random stool specimen required

Normal values: 50 to 300 mg/24 h

Low levels may indicate hepatocellular jaundice from cirrhosis or hepatitis or extrahepatic disorders such as tumors obstructing bile flow; low levels are also seen in aplastic anemia with depressed erythropoiesis

Elevated levels are found in hemolytic jaundice, thalassemia, and hemolytic pernicious anemia

Nursing care:

If possible avoid the following for 2 weeks before stool collection:

1. Broad-spectrum antibiotics, which inhibit bacterial growth in the colon and may inhibit fecal urobilinogen levels
2. Sulfonamides, which react with the reagents used in the test
3. Salicylates, which in large doses can raise fecal urobilinogen levels

Stool container must be light resistant since urobilinogen breaks down to urobilin on exposure to light

Keep in mind that serum bilirubin and urine urobilinogen can be measured easily

Endoscopy

Direct visualization of lining of a hollow viscus using an endoscope (a long, flexible tube with a cablelike cluster of glass fibers that transmits light and returns an image to the scope's optical head; used to diagnose a variety of gastrointestinal disorders and allows for biopsy of lesions through the scope)

Esophagogastroduodenoscopy

Permits visual examination of the esophagus, stomach, and upper duodenum

Useful in diagnosing inflammatory disease, ulcers, tumors, structural abnormality, and Mallory-Weiss tears

Nursing care:

Give nothing by mouth for 6 to 12 hours before the procedure is done; during an emergency procedure, a nasogastric tube is used to aspirate gastric contents

Endoscope is passed through the mouth and swallowed

Dentures are removed

Local anesthetic is sprayed into mouth and throat

Saliva may need to be suctioned if patient is unable to adequately allow it to flow out side of mouth

Mouth guard should be used to protect teeth

Anxiety and fear of procedure are expected, and patient should be given emotional support throughout procedures; sedatives and analgesics used to help patient relax

Patient's head is repositioned throughout procedure to facilitate movement of endoscope

Procedure contraindicated in patients with recent ulcer perforations, large aortic aneurysms, cardiac disease or a recent myocardial infarction, and Zenker's diverticulum

Complications include perforations:
1. Cervical esophagus perforation: pain on swallowing and neck movements
2. Thoracic esophagus perforation: substernal or epigastric pain that increases with respirations and trunk movements
3. Diaphragmatic esophageal perforation: shoulder pain and dyspnea
4. Gastric perforation: abdominal or back pain, cyanosis, fever, or pleural effusion

Other signs of complications include difficulty in swallowing, persistent pain, fever, black stools, or hematemesis

Fluids and foods withheld until gag reflex returns

Colonoscopy

Used to examine the colon and rectum to diagnose inflammatory bowel disease including ulcerative colitis and granulomatous colitis

Polyps can be removed through colonoscope

Also helpful in diagnosing or locating source of lower gastrointestinal bleeding

Biopsy of lesions suspected to be malignant may also be performed; also biopsies in patients with ulcerative colitis or Crohn's disease

Nursing care:

Cleansing of bowel with laxatives and enemas; be careful in patients with ulcerative colitis and granulomatous colitis since laxatives can cause exacerbation of disease (special protocols required for this patient group)

Avoid soap suds enemas in all patients since this irritates mucosa

Patient is placed in left lateral decubitus position, and a well-lubricated colonoscope is inserted through anus; air is inserted to help the physician visualize the mucosa and to facilitate advancement of colonoscope; occasionally position changes are required to assist advancement of scope at descending-sigmoid junction and splenic flexure

Specimens for cytology and histology may be obtained as well as for biopsy

Contraindications of the procedure include pregnancy, ischemic bowel disease, acute diverticulitis, peritonitis, toxic megacolon of ulcerative colitis, fulminant granulomatous colitis, and irradiation colitis

Complications include perforation of the bowel; signs and symptoms include abdominal pain and distention, rectal bleeding, fever, and mucopurulent drainage

Barium studies should be done after colonoscopy, or thorough bowel preparation is required for good visualization of mucosa

If bowel is fixed, secondary to irradiation, surgical adhesions, or inflammatory disease, physician may have difficulty during procedure

Procedure is uncomfortable and embarrassing; be supportive; let the patient know that flatus is from air inserted during procedure and cannot be controlled; sedative is given to help patient relax

Proctosigmoidoscopy

Examination of the sigmoid colon, rectum, and anal canal

Sigmoidoscope and proctoscope may be rigid metal instruments or flexible scopes inserted for visualization of the mucosa; biopsy may be performed

Examination usually includes a digital examination of anus and anal canal

Nursing care:

Patients often dread the proctosigmoidoscopy examination because of the embarrassing position and uncomfortable positioning and discomfort caused by the rigid instrument; patients are placed in a knee-chest position on a tilting table; while procedure can be done in a left lateral position, it is important to elevate the right buttocks; most physicians prefer to use a tilting table and the knee-chest position for best visualization

While a proctoscope may be used to examine the rectum and anus, when a sigmoidoscope is removed slowly, rectum and anal canal can be viewed with the sigmoidoscope, eliminating insertion of the proctoscope

Preparation varies with the expected diagnosis; clear liquid diets for 48 hours and a small sodium biphosphate enema may be used

Complications include possible bowel perforation (see discussion of colonoscopy); depressed blood pressure, pallor, diaphoresis, and bradycardia are signs of vasovagal stimulation and require immediate notification of physician

Contrast radiography

Examination of an area of the body using a contrast medium during a radiographic study; barium sulfate is one form of a contrast medium; meglumine iodiopamide is another form of a contrast medium that can be injected or given intravenously or through a tube or catheter; other commercial agents are available

Single-contrast studies use barium alone, whereas double-contrast studies use barium and air

Other than radiography (passage of radiation through the patient to create a radiograph), cineradiography, fluoroscopy, and video are used in many of these procedures; cineradiography is a rapid-sequence x-ray procedure that films motion; fluoroscopy is projection of x-ray films into a screen, or fluoroscope, permitting continuous observation of motion

Nursing care:
Barium as a contrast material precludes effective use of fiberoptic endoscopy for several hours and of arteriography for 24 to 48 hours

Barium retained in intestine may harden and cause an obstruction or fecal impaction; patient with a colostomy should be instructed to irrigate after barium procedure is concluded and should repeat the irrigation the next morning; if it is an upper gastrointestinal series or small bowel follow-through, patient should irrigate after last delayed spot film (approximately 6 hours after ingestion); patient with an ileostomy should never receive a laxative or an enema before or after a barium study; clear liquids for 48 hours before the procedure and forced fluids afterward are sufficient; healthy patients may want to take a mild laxative

Before giving meglumine iodipamide, check for hypersensitivity to iodine, seafood, and contrast media; symptoms of an allergic reaction include nausea, vomiting, flushing, urticaria, sweating, and rarely anaphylaxis; intraductal injection may be accompanied by tachycardia and fever

Barium swallow
Used to diagnose or detect hiatal hernia, achalasia, diverticulum, varices, strictures, ulcers, tumors, motility disorders, and polyps

Examination of the pharynx and esophagus on fluoroscope after ingestion of barium sulfate

Nursing care:
Required fasting after midnight

Once mixture is ingested, patient is placed in various positions; esophagus is also examined fluoroscopically during swallowing of solution

Contraindicated in patient with an intestinal obstruction

Laxative may be given to facilitate expulsion of barium (unless otherwise noted); also, have patient increase fluid intake

Upper gastrointestinal and small bowel series
Fluoroscopic examination of esophagus, stomach, and small intestine after ingestion of barium sulfate; as barium passes through system, fluoroscopy outlines mucosal contours

Spot films used to record significant findings; follow-up spot films after 6 hours can provide some evaluation of gastrointestinal motility

Useful in detecting or diagnosing hiatal hernias, diverticulum, varices, ulcers, strictures, tumors, regional enteritis (also called granulomatous ileitis or Crohn's ileitis), and motility disorders

Nursing care:
Patient is given nothing by mouth past midnight, and a mild laxative may be ordered; patient should also increase fluid intake and maintain low-residue diet for 2 or 3 days before test

Procedure contraindicated in patients with intestinal perforations and intestinal obstructions

Smoking should be avoided from midnight before test and throughout procedure

Anticholinergics and narcotics are withheld for 24 hours before the study if intestinal motility is of concern

Laxatives are used following the procedure to assist in expulsion of barium

Barium enema
Instillation of barium sulfate or barium sulfate and air through anus into large intestine

Used as one method of diagnosing colorectal cancer and inflammatory bowel disease

Will also detect polyps, diverticula, and other changes in colon and rectum

Once the most effective means of identifying colon carcinomas above the level of sigmoidoscope; colonoscopy examination now effectively used for visualization of entire large intestine

Nursing care:
Barium enema should precede barium swallow upper gastrointestinal series with small bowel follow-through

Careful bowel preparation necessary to cleanse bowel of fecal material; ileostomy patient has no large intestine and requires only clear liquids for 24 to 48 hours as a "bowel" preparation; site of colostomy will determine preparation

Patients with suspected inflammatory bowel disease (ulcerative colitis and granulomatous colitis) should not be given a routine preparatory kit for barium enemas; condition can be greatly exacerbated by irritants and may require surgical intervention; double check with physician

Barium enema contraindicated in patients with fulminant inflammatory bowel disease, toxic megacolon, suspected perforations, and suspected obstructions; caution is used with patients with acute inflammatory bowel disease, ischemic bowel disease, acute fulminant bloody diarrhea, and pneumatosis cystoides intestinalis

Laxatives will be required (unless otherwise stated) to facilitate removal of barium

Hypotonic duodenography
Barium sulfate and air instilled through an intestinal catheter for fluoroscopic examination of duodenum

Intravenous infusion of glucagon or intramuscular

ingestion of propantheline bromide used to induce duodenal atony

Examination will demonstrate small duodenal lesions and tumors at head of pancreas

Nursing care:

Catheter inserted through nose and into stomach while patient is sitting; in supine position under fluoroscopy, catheter is advanced into duodenum

Contraindication: administration of anticholinergics in presence of severe cardiac disorders or glaucoma

Oral cholecystography

Radiographic examination of gallbladder

Contrast medium given the evening before the test; iopanoic acid is usually used, but other commercial contrast media are available

Abdomen is examined fluoroscopically to evaluate gallbladder opacification; spot films are taken of significant findings; fat stimulus may also be used during the radiographic procedure

Fluoroscopy is then used to observe emptying of gallbladder; spot films are taken as indicated

Nursing care:

Diet before the test includes a lunch meal containing fats and fat-free evening meal

Check patient for allergies to iodine, seafood, or contrast media before giving tablets; possible side effects include diarrhea, which commonly occurs; nausea, vomiting, abdominal cramps, and dysuria may occur in rare cases

Iopanoic acid, 3 g, given as one tablet with a total of 240 ml (8 oz) of water

Check any emesis or diarrheal stools for undigested tablets

Large intestine generally cleansed by an enema the morning of the test

Procedure not done in presence of severe renal or hepatic disease or jaundice

Intravenous cholangiography

Provides better visualization of biliary ducts than oral cholangiography, which is useful in gallbladder disease

Involves radiography and tomography studies after intravenous infusion of a contrast medium

Generally indicated in patients with right upper quadrant or epigastric pain after cholecystectomy; pain suggests biliary tract disease

Also used with children to evaluate or diagnose congenital abnormalities of biliary system

Nursing care:

Should precede any barium studies since retained barium will cloud x-ray films

Diet should be low residue the day before the test with an evening meal high in simple fats (milk, cream, eggs, butter); patient is given nothing to eat after midnight

Check patient for a history of hypersensitivities to iodine, seafood, and contrast media

Bowel preparations used to cleanse colon

Contraindicated in patients with hyperthyroidism, severe renal or hepatic disease, tuberculosis, or hypersensitivity to iodine

Involves fluoroscopy spot films every 10 minutes until visualization of bile ducts is satisfactory; may take 25 to 40 minutes; tomograms are then done

Films and tomograms are repeated 2 to 2½ hours later, when maximal opacification of gallbladder has occurred (This would be unnecessary in patients with cholecystectomies.)

Delayed films of gallbladder may be taken at 4 and 24 hours

A fatty meal may be given so that with fluoroscopy, emptying may be viewed

Percutaneous transhepatic cholangiography

Fluoroscopic examination of biliary ducts after injection of iodinated contrast medium directly into biliary tree

Liver is punctured by a thin, flexible needle, and contrast medium is injected as needle is slowly withdrawn; contrast medium slowly flows through biliary ducts, outlining biliary tree

Helps to distinguish between obstructive and nonobstructive jaundice; in mechanical obstruction of biliary tree, procedure helps to determine location, extent, and often cause

Catheter used to inject dye is sometimes left in place to drain biliary tree

Nursing care:

Check patient for history of hypersensitivity to iodine, seafood, or contrast media

Check patient for normal bleeding, clotting, and prothrombin times and platelet count

Contraindicated in patients with cholangitis, severe ascites, uncorrectable coagulopathy, and hypersensitivity to iodine

Patient should remain on bedrest for 6 hours after procedure: check vital signs frequently (every 15 minutes for 1 hour, every 30 minutes for 2 hours, every hour for 4 hours, and then every 4 hours); check injection site for bleeding, swelling, and tenderness; check for signs of peritonitis: chills, temperature of 38° to 39° C (102° to 103° F), abdominal pain, tenderness, and distention

Postoperative cholangiography or T-tube cholangiography

Performed 7 to 10 days following cholecystectomy or common bile duct exploration in which a T-tube has been left in the common bile duct to facilitate drainage

Contrast medium injected through T-tube and with fluoroscopy, flow of medium outlining biliary tree can be visualized

Purpose of test: to evaluate patency and size of ducts and to identify calculi, strictures, neoplasms, or fistulae in ductal system

Nursing care:

Some physicians will have the T-tube clamped for 24 hours before procedure to eliminate air bubbles in tube

Cleansing enema to evacuate large intestine may be ordered

Check patient for allergies to iodine, seafood, and contrast media

T-tube may be removed following procedure; sterile dressing is applied; note amount and characteristics of any drainage; if frequent dressing changes are required, consider application of a sterile skin barrier and drainable pouch

Monitor patient for signs and symptoms of sepsis

Endoscopic retrograde cholangiopancreatography (ERCP)

Radiographic examination of pancreatic duct and hepatobiliary ductal system by injection of a contrast medium into duodenal papilla

Endoscopy is done and the duodenal papilla located; cannula filled with contrast medium is passed through endoscope, into duodenal papilla, and into ampulla of Vater; pancreas is visualized first with injection of dye and then fluoroscopy, and then cannula is repositioned for injection of additional contrast medium allowing for visualization of hepatobiliary tree

Purpose: to diagnose cancer of duodenal papilla, pancreas, or biliary ducts; to detect calculi or stenosis of ducts; and to evaluate obstructive jaundice

Tissue biopsy or fluid for histology may be obtained before endoscope is removed

Some centers are able to perform sphincterotomy and snare and remove stones

Nursing care:

See nursing concerns for endoscopic procedures (pp. 1143 and 1144)

Contraindicated in patients with acute pancreatitis, pancreatic pseudocysts, strictures of esophagus or duodenum, obstruction of esophagus or duodenum, cholangitis, infectious disease, or cardiorespiratory disease

Assess patient for a history of hypersensitivity to iodine, seafood, or contrast media

Cholangitis and pancreatitis may develop following ERCP; signs of cholangitis include fever, chills, and hyperbilirubinemia; late symptoms may include hypotension and gram-negative septicemia; pancreatitis may be indicated by upper left quadrant pain, tenderness, elevated serum amylase, and transient hyperbilirubinemia

Frequent vital sign checks are indicated when patient returns to floor (every 15 minutes for 4 hours; every hour for 4 hours; and every 4 hours for 48 hours); check for voiding since urinary retention may be a side effect of anticholinergics

Monitor patient for bleeding after procedure

Splenoportography (transsplenic portography)

Cineradiographic study of the splenic veins and portal system

Contrast medium is injected directly into the splenic pulp

Used to diagnose or assess portal hypertension and to stage cirrhosis

Generally provides a clearer definition of the venous system than superior mesenteric arteriography; superior mesenteric arteriography offers the advantage of outlining the splenic and portal veins during reverse blood flow and has fewer complications; splenoportography may result in excessive bleeding requiring transfusions and occasionally splenectomy

Splenic pulp pressure is measured before dye is injected by attaching a spinal manometer filled with normal saline to a sheath inserted in spleen

Normal splenic pulp pressure is 50 to 180 mm H_2O (or 3.5 to 13.5 mm Hg)

Nursing care:

Assess patient for a history of allergies to iodine, seafood, or contrast media

Contraindicated in patients with ascites, uncorrectable coagulopathy, splenomegaly secondary to infection, hypersensitivity to iodine, or markedly impaired liver or kidney function

Requires frequent assessment of vital signs after procedure (every 15 minutes for 1 hour, every 30 minutes for 2 hours, and every hour for 4 hours); check for bleeding, swelling, and tenderness at site of injection

Patient should remain on left side for 24 hours to minimize risk of bleeding; an additional 24 hours of bed rest is recommended

Hematocrit levels may be obtained every 8 to 12 hours until values have stabilized

Celiac and mesenteric arteriography

In arteriography, contrast medium is injected into celiac, superior mesenteric, or inferior mesenteric artery for visualization of vasculature; superselective angiography permits a detailed visualization of a particular area; as contrast medium is injected, serial radiographs outline abdominal vessels in arterial, capillary, and venous phases of perfusion

Radiologist inserts a needle into the femoral artery; a guide wire is passed through needle into aorta; needle is then removed; angiographic catheter is inserted over guide wire, and placement is checked radiographically and fluoroscopically before guide wire is removed; the catheter, under fluoroscopy, is advanced into one of the three arteries, placement is checked, and an automatic injection of contrast medium is attached; a rapid sequence of serial films is taken as medium is injected; repositioning of catheter is done for superselective visualization

Can be used for locating gastrointestinal bleeding and treating bleeding by infusion of vasopressin at the site or by injection of embolic material to form a clot; embolic material includes aminocaproic acid (Amicar) clot or gelatin sponge (Gelfoam)

Also used to evaluate cirrhosis and portal hypertension, vascular damage after abdominal trauma, intestinal ischemia, or vascular abnormalities; may be used in evaluating tumors (distinguishing between benign and malignant) when other tests are inconclusive

Nursing care:
Assess patient for sensitivities to iodine, seafood, and contrast media

Blood work should include hemoglobin, hematocrit, clotting time, prothrombin time, activated partial thromboplastin time, and platelet count

Patient should remain flat and in bed for at least 12 hours

Check puncture site frequently for bleeding and hematoma; sandbag is often used for 2 to 4 hours to prevent bleeding

Monitor vital signs as ordered: usually every 15 minutes for 1 hour, every 30 minutes for 2 hours, and then every hour for 4 hours or until patient is stable; depending on patient's reactions to test and potential problems of bleeding, this pattern may change

Monitor peripheral pulses with vital signs; compare pulses in each foot; also observe the leg (of the puncture site) for color and temperature; compare to alternate leg if unsure of changes

Notify physician of continued or excessive bleeding, changes in peripheral pulse and temperature, and color changes; also notify physician if vital signs change significantly

Radionuclide imaging

Uses a gamma camera or a rectilinear scanner to record distribution of a decaying radiopharmaceutical (colloid) after intravenous injection

Scanning demonstrates a cold spot or a defect that fails to take up the colloid; focal lesions smaller than 2 cm (1 inch) may not be detected

Tagging RBCs may also be done to detect gastrointestinal bleeding

Liver or spleen scanning

Injection of a radioactive colloid (e.g., technetium sulfide 99m), which concentrates in the reticuloendothelial cells through phagocytosis

Kupffer cells in liver take up to 80% to 90%, spleen takes 5% to 10%, and bone marrow takes 3% to 5%

Used to screen patients for hepatic metastases, cirrhosis, and hepatitis

Will also assist in identifying focal lesions such as tumors, cysts, and abscesses

May demonstrate splenic infarct, hepatomegaly, and splenomegaly

Also used to evaluate liver and spleen following abdominal trauma

Nursing care:
Patient will need to know he will be asked to lie very still; he will be placed in several positions; he also needs to know the procedure will not be painful, with the exception of the intravenous injection

Some patients will have a reaction to a stabilizer added to the colloid; observe for anaphylaxis or for pyogenic response

Do not schedule the patient for more than one radionuclide scan on one day; radionuclides administered in other studies may interfere with liver-spleen imaging

Computed tomography (CT scan)

Uses multiple x-ray beams that pass through patient

Detectors record tissue alteration, and a computer reconstructs information into a three-dimensional image on an oscilloscope screen

CT scan of biliary tract and liver

Can be used to identify focal points found on nuclear scans as solid, cystic, inflammatory, or vascular

Biopsy may be necessary to distinguish between metastatic or primary tumors or to rule out malignancy

Can also identify hematomas after abdominal trauma

Used to determine if etiology of jaundice is obstructive or nonobstructive

CT scan and ultrasound are both effective in biliary tract and liver diagnosis; CT scan proves to be better in obese patients or patients whose liver is located high under rib cage, since bone and excessive fat will hinder ultrasound transmission

Contrast medium is also used during CT scan to intensify vascular structures and liver parenchyma, aiding in visualization of biliary tract

General CT scan of the abdomen is valuable in defining relationship of organs and identifying presence of tumors

Nursing care:

If contrast medium is to be used, assess patient for allergies to iodine, seafood, or contrast media

Barium studies should be done at least 4 days before CT scan or barium will obscure the film

Contrast media excreted in bile used in earlier diagnostic studies may interfere with biliary tree detection

Contraindicated during pregnancy

Patient is given nothing to eat past midnight before the test

CT scan of pancreas

Used to diagnose pancreatic carcinoma and pancreatitis and to distinguish between pancreatic disorders and disorders of the retroperitoneum

Contrast media often used to accentuate differences in tissue density

Preferred over ultrasound as a diagnostic test; although the CT scan is more expensive, results are more accurate

Nursing care:

If contrast medium is to be used, assess patient for allergies to iodine, seafood, or contrast media

Contraindicated during pregnancy

Patient should be instructed to eat nothing past midnight the evening before the CT scan

Recent barium studies can interfere with test results; wait 4 days after barium studies before doing a CT scan

Ultrasonography

Uses focused beams of high-frequency sound waves

Sound waves pass through patient and create echoes that vary with tissue density

Echoes are converted into electrical energy, amplified by a transducer, and appear on an oscilloscope screen

Nursing care:

Overlying bowel gas or retention of barium from a previous study will interfere with ultrasound transmission

In patients who are dehydrated, ultrasound can fail to define boundaries between organs and tissue structures because of a deficiency of body fluids

Ultrasonography of gallbladder and biliary system

Can be used if cholecystography is inconclusive or does not adequately visualize gallbladder

Useful in confirming cholelithiasis, diagnosing acute cholecystitis, and distinguishing between obstructive and nonobstructive jaundice

Sincalide, a hormonal analogue, may be given to cause gallbladder to contract and expel bile; allows an evaluation of gallbladder function

Nursing care:

Give nothing to eat for 8 to 12 hours before procedure; should have a fat-free meal evening before test (allows accumulation of bile in gallbladder)

Side effects of sincalide include abdominal cramping, tenesmus, nausea, dizziness, sweating, and flushing; sincalide should not be given during pregnancy or to children

Ultrasonography of liver

Indicated in patients with jaundice of unknown etiology since it helps to distinguish between obstructive and nonobstructive jaundice

Used as a screening or diagnostic test in hepatocellular disease and in hepatic metastases

Also used after abdominal trauma to detect hematoma

Can be used to define cold spots found on liver scans

Nursing care:

Patient is given nothing to eat for 8 to 12 hours before the test to reduce bowel gas

Ultrasonography of spleen

Used to demonstrate splenomegaly, to evaluate changes in splenic size, to evaluate spleen following abdominal trauma, and to clarify cold spots found on scans of spleen

CT scans often provide more information on splenomegaly than ultrasonography

Nursing care:

Patient is given nothing to eat for 8 to 12 hours before procedure to reduce bowel gas

Ultrasonography of pancreas

Used to detect anatomic abnormalities such as pseudocysts, or pancreatic carcinoma

Detects alterations in size, contour, and parenchymal texture of pancreas

Nursing care:

Patient is given nothing to eat for 8 to 12 hours before procedure to reduce bowel gas

Conditions, Diseases, and Disorders

GLOSSITIS

Glossitis is a chronic or acute inflammation of the tongue.

Glossitis is manifested by a reddened, inflamed, smooth, and sore tongue, which is usually due to one of several causes:

1. Ulcerations, either from stomatitis or lichen planus, can cause glossitis. Carcinomas of the tongue can also produce ulcerations.

2. Anemia (usually iron deficiency or pernicious anemia) is one of the most common causes of glossitis. Other vitamin B–group deficiencies can also produce glossitis, as can the presence of candidiasis.

3. Some patients have a tongue that may appear normal, but the patient complains of soreness. In these cases, anemia must be ruled out, but depression and other psychogenic causes or factors have been known to cause a painful tongue.

4. Geographic tongue, the cause of which is not known, is manifested by irregular, smooth, red areas with sharply defined borders that heal and then reappear in a few days. Examination reveals thinning of the epithelium in the middle of the lesion with mild hyperplasia and hyperkeratosis around the edges. Some chronic inflammatory cells can be found in the underlying tissue. Most patients are asymptomatic, but some complain of soreness and hypersensitivity to certain foods.

A variation of geographic tongue is hairy tongue, in which the filiform papillae become elongated and resemble hair. The papillae can vary in length and color; the cause is unknown but usually only adults are affected. Some drugs, for example, clindamycin, can also cause these papillae.

Treatment for glossitis consists of correcting the underlying cause if known, pain relief, meticulous mouth care, and a bland diet if necessary for patient comfort.

LEUKOPLAKIA

Leukoplakia is commonly described as white patches in the oral mucosa that are persistent and cannot be removed by the patient.

Increased keratin production is known to cause the whitish appearance, but its development can be the result of many factors. A small percentage (about 5%) undergo malignant change and become squamous cell carcinomas. Biopsies should be done on all leukoplakias to determine the probable cause.

PATHOPHYSIOLOGY

The causes of leukoplakia are varied. Friction from cheek biting or prolonged denture wearing can cause lesions that are initially pale and translucent and later become white and thick with a rough surface. Smoking, usually pipe smoking, causes a lesion that is probably formed both from chemical components of the smoke and irritation from the heat.

Syphilis in the tertiary stage produces a characteristic leukoplakia on the dorsum of the tongue that is rarely seen today.

Another uncommon cause is white sponge nevus, which is a familial disorder characterized by large, soft thickening of the superficial epithelial layers. The entire inner surface of the mouth can be affected by the thick, white plaque. Although untreatable, this is a benign condition.

Patients who experience chronic candidal infections in their mouths have plaque formed from epithelial overgrowth. This is another uncommon cause and is treated with local or systemic antifungal agents.

Probably the most common leukoplakias are those of unknown etiology. These patients have a leukoplakia for which the causative factor is undetermined; the degree of hyperkeratinosis ranges from simple to severe. Treatment of choice in these cases may be local excision of the leukoplakia; however, in many cases there is recurrence, so many physicians simply choose to see the patient frequently to observe for any changes in the appearance of the leukoplakia and perform a biopsy periodically if any changes do occur, to assess for malignancy.

Leukoplakia is divided into three types (simplex, verrucous, and erosive), depending on its degree and its likelihood of malignant transformation. Leukoplakia simplex, which is the smooth and nonindurated type, very rarely results in malignant change, while erosive leukoplakia more commonly becomes malignant.

PERIODONTAL DISEASE

The term periodontal disease *refers to diseases of the supporting tissues of the teeth that are usually inflammatory in nature.*

The characteristic feature of chronic periodontitis is the destruction of these supporting tissues; almost every case begins with chronic gingivitis, which, if not treated properly, progresses to the irreversible chronic periodontitis, loosening, and loss of teeth.

Acute Gingivitis

Acute ulceromembranous gingivitis, also called trench mouth, is usually seen in young adults who have neglected oral hygiene but is also frequently seen in parts of Africa where malnutrition, anemia, and malaria are rampant.

Although the exact cause is unclear, two particular organisms, *Bacteroides vincenti* and *Fusobacterium fusiforme,* are thought to be implicated in this infection that may also require lowered host resistance. The inflammation starts at the tips of the interdental papillae and progresses quickly to involve the gingival membranes and periodontal tissues. Crater-shaped ulcers with erythematous, edematous edges are characteristic, with a thick yellowish or grayish material over the surface of the ulcer. Bleeding occurs if this material is removed.

The infection remains localized, although the mouth is very sore and the gums bleed; the patient experiences no fever, malaise, or lymphadenopathy.

Treatment is with antibiotics for the specific organism and oral hygiene measures to reduce the acute oral infection. The patient and family must also be given explicit instructions in the performance of meticulous oral hygiene.

Chronic Gingivitis

Almost everyone has a degree of chronic gingivitis. It is probably caused by the accumulation of plaque around the neck of the tooth, which if not removed adequately by toothbrushing, involves the epithelium and progresses to the periodontal membrane and alveolar bone, causing osteoporotic loss of bone and finally loss of the teeth. Gingivitis can develop in 2 days if plaque is allowed to accumulate, and there is a correlation between the amount of plaque and the severity of the gingivitis.

Although the exact relationship between gingivitis and the destruction of the supporting tissues is not clearly understood, it is probable that the bacteria present in the plaque initiate an inflammatory response that is furthered by interactions between antibodies, complement, neutrophils, lymphocytes, and macrophages. Immunologic responses have also been implicated.

As plaque begins to collect at the neck of the teeth, inflammatory changes occur in the gingiva. The epithelium becomes hyperplastic, blood vessels dilate, and some extend almost to the surface, causing the gums to appear darker than normal, even purplish, as a result of congestion. These inflammatory cells spread so that the gingiva appears edematous, soft, and slightly glazed. The gums bleed easily, and there is usually a collection of calculus, or calcified plaque, above the gingival margins.

Chronic gingivitis, if it has not progressed further than the gingiva, will subside if meticulous oral hygiene is begun and followed strictly. Part of the treatment must be aimed at teaching the patient and family about oral hygiene, diet principles, and the progression of the disease if these instructions are not followed.

Periodontitis

Acute periodontitis is quite uncommon and usually does not last long; it can be caused by trauma, most often from biting on a hard object, which may cause some minor damage and heals quickly; a periodontal abscess, which is a complication of periodontal disease; or progression from ulceromembranous gingivitis if untreated.

Chronic periodontitis is very common, on the other hand, and is also important since it is the main reason for loss of teeth in adults. As discussed in the section on chronic gingivitis, periodontitis is usually a continuation of that process, since untreated infection of the gingiva leads to progressive inflammation and destruction of the supporting structures of the teeth.

The four main features of chronic periodontitis are as follows:

1. Destruction of periodontal membrane fibers
2. Resorption of alveolar bone
3. Migration of the epithelial attachment along the root toward the apex
4. Formation of pockets around the teeth[13]

The pocket formation is characteristic of periodontitis; these pockets form a closed space where bacteria grow and may in fact allow for anaerobic bacterial growth. The infected material cannot drain, and these bacteria cause irritation to the tissues.

Clinical symptoms include bleeding from the gums, a bad taste in the mouth, and foul-smelling breath; later there is gum recession and loosening of the teeth. The gingiva appears purplish and swollen, and plaque and calculus are very evident.

The best treatment is prevention; regular and thorough toothbrushing and removal of plaque would negate the need for any further treatment or surgical intervention. However, surgery is necessary when the disease has been neglected, pockets have formed, and the gingiva cannot be restored to normal without surgical intervention.

Patients who are considered for surgery are those who realize that they will have to expend some effort to maintain their teeth during and after performance of the surgery. The rationale for surgery includes débridement and removal of the pockets and removal of plaque and calculus and restoring soft tissue and bone to its normal contour and state of health.

There are a number of surgical procedures that may be carried out, depending on the severity of the periodontal disease. A local anesthetic is usually used, and patients rarely require hospitalization. Patient education remains a vital part of the overall treatment because patients who are unaware of or fail to comply with meticulous oral hygiene measures will undoubtedly have recurrences or progression of the disease. When the disease has progressed to the point where surgery would not be useful, the teeth must be extracted and the patient will have to wear dentures.

SALIVARY GLAND DISORDERS

Disorders or inflammation can occur in the parotid, sublingual, or submaxillary glands.

Salivary gland disorders can be classified into several categories: inflammation, as in mumps and acute and chronic sialadenitis; obstruction, as in calculi; and degenerative diseases and neoplasms, which will not be discussed here. Dry mouth (xerostomia), which may be caused by damaged salivary glands, is an unpleasant problem and can be the result of local or systemic causes as well as chronic anxiety states.

PATHOPHYSIOLOGY

Inflammation of the salivary glands is most commonly caused by mumps. This is a nonsuppurative type of viral inflammation that is manifested by painful swelling of the parotids and occasionally other glands. One of the commonest of childhood diseases, it is very contagious and frequently occurs in epidemics. It will be discussed further in Chapter 15.

Less common infections are acute ascending parotitis and chronic sialadenitis. Acute ascending parotitis is the result of dehydration and inattention to oral hygiene, sometimes during or immediately following surgery when an endotracheal tube has been used and placed pressure on the salivary ducts. This has also been seen in patients who have nasogastric tubes and causes swelling and severe throat irritation. This produces painful swelling of the glands with fever and malaise. Purulent material can be expressed from the duct. This disorder can be prevented by proper hydration, good oral hygiene, and care taken during surgery to avoid trauma to the duct orifices.

Chronic sialadenitis is usually caused by chronic duct obstruction, which may be due to mucous plugs or other causes. It is usually unilateral, and the patient experiences painful swelling of the gland accompanied by an inflamed duct and purulent discharge from the orifice. Treatment is removal of the obstruction or excision of the gland.

Obstructions of the salivary glands are usually caused by calculi although mucoceles and cysts may also form, and these must be excised. Calculi formation is quite common, and most (80%) of them form in the submandibular gland and Wharton's duct. About 10% to 12% form in the parotid gland or Stensen's duct, and the rest are in the sublingual and minor salivary glands. Children infrequently get salivary calculi, although they do occur at any age, and men are affected twice as often as women.

These stones are composed mainly of calcium and phosphate and may tend to form more frequently in the submandibular gland because its saliva has a high pH and is viscous because of a high mucin content. This gland also receives irritation from the teeth during chewing and is larger in diameter and longer than the parotid duct.

The patient usually experiences pain and swelling that come on suddenly during eating and usually subside within a short period of time. Symptoms may not occur with every meal, and sometimes the patient is asymptomatic until the stone enlarges, moves along the duct, and can be felt in the mouth. Usually there is no inflammation, but occasionally a gland or duct can become infected, indicated by increased swelling and tenderness over the gland and purulent discharge from the orifice. Pain and fever accompany this infection.

Dry mouth can result from a variety of causes, some transient and some chronic. Fear and acute anxiety are the most common causes of transient dry mouth. Chronic conditions can be caused by mouth breathing, heavy smoking, some drugs such as antihistamines and sympathomimetics, chronic anxiety states, and treatment with radiation to the head and neck, which causes damage to the salivary glands. Salivary calculi do not cause xerostomia.

DIAGNOSTIC STUDIES

X-ray films of lateral and oblique views of jaw and upper neck
May demonstrate large stones

X-ray films using dental film to project through floor of mouth from below
Demonstrate small stones

TREATMENT PLAN

Surgical
Surgical removal if stone cannot be removed by manual manipulation

Chemotherapeutic
Narcotic analgesics
Meperidine (Demerol), 50-75 mg IM q4-6h as needed for pain relief
Tylenol with codeine, 30-60 mg q4-6h as needed for pain relief

Electromechanical
Many stones can be removed by manipulation of duct

ASSESSMENT: AREAS OF CONCERN

Inflammation
Localized swelling
Fever; malaise
Purulent discharge from orifice of duct
Dehydration

Obstruction
Pain and swelling related to chewing; may be transient or infrequent
Palpation of stone in gland or duct

NURSING DIAGNOSES and NURSING INTERVENTIONS

Nursing Diagnosis	Nursing Intervention
Comfort, alteration in: pain	Provide analgesia for pain relief and assess and document effectiveness. Provide hard sour candies for patient to suck.
Oral mucous membrane, alteration in	Instruct patient in meticulous mouth care and ways to prevent or minimize dry mouth (i.e., mouthwash, toothettes, or hard sour candies). Observe for signs of infection in opened or excised duct, if stone has been surgically removed.

Patient Education

1. Instruct patient in oral hygiene measures.
2. Inform patient of the symptoms of inflammation and calculi, and encourage patient to seek medical treatment when these occur.
3. Inform patient that calculi tend to recur in some patients.

EVALUATION

Patient Outcome	Data Indicating That Outcome is Reached
Inflammation is resolved.	There is no localized pain, swelling, or fever. Patient verbalizes understanding of symptoms of inflammation and calculi and when to seek medical treatment. Patient verbalizes understanding of oral hygiene measures.

STOMATITIS

Stomatitis is ulceration in the mouth that may be on the gums or the oral mucosa.

Stomatitis may be a single lesion, as from a local injury, or widespread, caused by systemic factors. Stomatitis is mainly inflammatory, and there are several types: viral, bacterial, noninfective, and those caused by drugs. It may result from excessive smoking, spicy foods, poor nutrition, poor oral hygiene, or allergic responses. All types of stomatitis are usually quite painful and may inhibit food ingestion as a consequence; this can be a major problem in an already debilitated patient.

PATHOPHYSIOLOGY

Herpetic stomatitis is the most common form of viral stomatitis; after an initial infection, usually in infancy or childhood, it begins with vesicle formation. After the rupture of the vesicles and the shedding of the cells, an ulcer is visible. These ulcers are usually scattered over the mucous membranes and are circular and about 3 to 4 mm in diameter. The gingivae are swollen and inflamed, and the local lymph nodes are usually swollen. The patient may be febrile and have increased salivation as well as severe mouth pain. These lesions usually clear in 7 to 10 days.

After the primary infection, many people are subject to recurrent infections. These are usually not within the mouth but affect the skin around the lips at the mucocutaneous junctions. These infections are known as herpes labialis, caused by the herpes simplex virus and will be discussed further in Chapter 15.

Angular stomatitis, which is the result of iron deficiency anemia, causes inflammatory changes at the angles of the mouth that vary from reddening to ulcerated, crusting fissures. More common in elderly patients with full dentures, it can cause deep folds at the corners of the mouth, where infection can spread if not treated, making the condition much more extensive. Lack of vitamins such as niacin and riboflavin can cause cellular weakening, since cell growth, oxidation, and metabolism are impaired.

Denture stomatitis is caused by occlusion of the mucous membranes by a tight-fitting denture for a long period of time. This creates a closed environment where organisms can grow. While the patient may be asymptomatic, there is normally a reddened, erythematous area corresponding to the area covered by the denture. These patients should leave their dentures out, at least at night, to allow the mucous membranes to heal.

Aphthous stomatitis is one of the more common diseases affecting the mucous membranes. The underlying cause of these small, yellowish, very painful ulcers is unclear, although several factors have been implicated (virus, allergy, gastrointestinal disease, psychosomatic causes). Women are usually affected slightly more than men, the disease is most troublesome in adolescence or early adult life, and interestingly, it often clears up by early middle age. The first sign of aphthous stomatitis is usually a pricking feeling in the mucous membrane, followed soon after by eruption of painful ulcers that may appear alone or in groups. They appear somewhat craterlike since they have red, raised margins, and they usually heal in a week or so without scarring.

Thrush, or oral candidiasis, is one of the most common types of stomatitis seen in acute care. This type is a mycotic stomatitis characterized by white plaques on the oral mucous membrane, gums, and tongue. It is frequently seen in patients who are malnourished, diabetic, or taking antibiotics (since they destroy the normal oral flora) and in oncology patients.

Although *Candida* is part of the normal mouth flora, some weakening of the body's resistance can permit an increase in its growth (usually *C. albicans* or *C. tropicalis*). Fungal spores lodge between the epithelial cells and cause a gradual separation of the layers, thus spreading the infection to the surface of the mucous membrane and the rest of the mouth. White patchy growths appear in several areas of the mucous membrane and spread so that a continuous membrane forms.

One of the more distressing types of stomatitis is that which appears as a result of drug treatment. It is frequently seen in patients who are taking systemic antibiotics for long periods and who suffer bacterial overgrowth in the mucous membranes or in patients receiving chemotherapy for cancer treatment, and it may be quite debilitating since the patient may already have a lowered resistance to infection. In a severely leukopenic patient, necrotizing ulceration of the mucous membranes, gums, and throat may occur, which can in turn cause septicemia. Usually, these ulcers appear on the mucous membranes in any number, are very painful, may cause increased salivation, and prevent the patient from eating normally.

TREATMENT PLAN

Chemotherapeutic

Anesthetic agents
  Topical anesthetic (viscous lidocaine [Xylocaine] as needed)

Vitamins
  Vitamin replacement if caused by underlying deficiency

Anti-infective agents
  Nystatin (Mycostatin) oral suspension or lozenges for *Candida* every 6 hours

Supportive

Well-balanced diet; bland if necessary; high in protein, calories, and needed vitamins

Mild mouthwashes for comfort

ASSESSMENT: AREAS OF CONCERN

Oral mucous membrane

Painful, ulcerated areas on oral mucous membranes that may appear yellowish with reddened, raised edges

Increased salivation

Halitosis

General well-being

Fever and lymphadenopathy with primary herpetic stomatitis

Malaise

Nutritional status

Sensitivity to spicy foods and discomfort when eating

History of dietary habits; recent or current chemotherapeutic or antibiotic regimen; debilitated physical appearance

Presence of dentures in angular and denture stomatitis

NURSING DIAGNOSES and NURSING INTERVENTIONS

Nursing Diagnosis	Nursing Intervention
Comfort, alteration in: pain	Provide analgesia as prescribed, especially before meals. (Local anesthetic agents [topical] such as viscous lidocaine [Xylocaine] may be helpful.)
Oral mucous membrane, alteration in	Provide mouthwashes (avoid those with alcohol since they are irritating), and assist with thorough but gentle mouth care. Keep lips lubricated. Administer nystatin (Mycostatin) if ordered. (Freezing it may be more tolerable to the patient.) Offer ice or ice chips to suck for a numbing effect.
Nutrition, alteration in: less than body requirements	Provide dietary consultation to produce palatable, nourishing diet that is high in protein, calories, and vitamins. Instruct patient to avoid hot, spicy foods. (A bland or full liquid diet may be more tolerable.) Maintain needed level of hydration, intravenously, as prescribed.

Patient Education

1. Teach the patient the importance of continued meticulous mouth care.
2. Instruct patient and family in maintenance of a proper diet.
3. If stomatitis is herpetic, inform patient of its infective nature and instruct in isolation and hand-washing techniques.

EVALUATION

Patient Outcome	Data Indicating That Outcome is Reached
Stomatitis is resolved.	Oral mucous membranes do not have painful lesions. Patient's weight and hydration are maintained at normal levels. Patient understands infective nature of herpetic lesions and necessity of hand-washing and isolation techniques.

ACHALASIA

Achalasia is a neuromuscular disorder of the esophageal motility that is characterized by failure of the lower esophageal sphincter to relax, esophageal dilation, and hypertrophy.

Achalasia is normally found in adults but may be seen in children and even in infants. In the geriatric patient, achalasia may be related to cancer of the lower end of the esophagus. In the very young individual, achalasia has been associated with familial glucocorticoid deficiency. Trauma of the tissues during vagotomy may result in a transient condition simulating achalasia.

The etiology of achalasia is unknown. Although there are reports of several cases in one family, it has not been classified as hereditary. Emotional factors may exaggerate or trigger a latent defect. Achalasia appears to be of neurogenic origin, but how, where, and why are unknown.

PATHOPHYSIOLOGY

There are three pathophysiologic changes in achalasia:
1. Elevated lower esophageal sphincter pressure
2. Residual pressure after swallowing because of poor relaxation of the lower esophageal sphincter
3. Aperistalsis of the body of the esophagus

The esophageal sphincter pressure is elevated to approximately 50 mm Hg (twice normal level). The normal resting pressure is approximately 20 mm Hg. This high pressure does not relax with swallowing. In a normal situation, the lower esophageal sphincter pressure drops to the level of the stomach pressure. In achalasia the pressure drops but not enough to permit unrestricted passage of food into the stomach.

The lower esophageal sphincter is sensitive to the stimulatory effects of gastrin and cholinergic drugs. Gastrin is responsible for the normal tone of the sphincter. There is some suggestion that oversensitivity to endogenous gastrin results in achalasia. When endogenous gastrin activity is inhibited by infusion of acid into the stomach, lower esophageal sphincter pressure drops in the achalasia patient. Exogenous gastrin in achalasia leads to a significant increase in pressure. This reaction is considered to be the result of denervation of the sphincter. The denervation is the key abnormality, and the sensitivity to gastrin is the reason for the high pressure.

Motility disturbances in the body of the esophagus mean that the peristalsis is weak and ineffectual in pushing a bolus of food through the closed sphincter. Aperistalsis may be located throughout the length of the esophagus. The esophagus may empty only when the hydrostatic pressure of its contents is great enough to overcome the pressure resistance in the lower esophageal sphincter. Since esophageal emptying depends on gravity in this case, emptying is improved if the person is sitting rather than lying down.

In the early stages the body of the esophagus is dilated symmetrically. In later stages the esophagus dilates considerably, lengthens, and curves. The body of the esophagus may bend and rest on the diaphragm. A dilated esophagus in achalasia may hold 1 to 2 L of fluid.

DIAGNOSTIC STUDIES

Splash-down time
Length of time between swallowing and reaching the stomach, normally 8 to 10 seconds, is lengthened or not heard at all

Radiography studies: chest film, barium swallow
Possible aspiration pneumonia
Presence of food in esophagus

Manometry: pressure readings
Elevated lower esophageal sphincter pressure (50 mm Hg or above) and residual pressure after swallowing

Radionuclide scans for esophageal emptying
Decreased or delayed esophageal emptying

Endoscopy
Particularly in geriatric patient, to rule out cancer
Aperistalsis of body of esophagus
Possible presence of tumor

Video or line esophagram
Barium is swallowed and followed on tape

TREATMENT PLAN

Surgical
May be required when dilation cannot be done or is unsuccessful
Surgical procedure utilized is an esophagomyotomy, which divides muscle fibers enclosing esophagus, allowing mucosa to pouch out through divisions in muscle layers; when this surgery includes the cardiac end of the stomach, it is referred to as a cardiomyotomy

Chemotherapeutic*
Sublingual isosorbide dinitrate (Isordil), 5 mg

*Used with varying benefits.

Oral isosorbide dinitrate (Isordil), 10 mg
Slow channel blocking drugs (calcium ion antagonist): verapamil (Isoptin) or nifedipine (Procardia capsules); dosage varies in clinical studies and overall benefits are still uncertain

Electromechanical

Forceful dilation of esophagus is primary treatment and is done to decrease ability of sphincter to react to stretch

Bougienage: simple passage of a mercury-filled bougie; normally the swallowed bougie reaches lower esophageal sphincter and after a pause drops into stomach to prove absence of a tight sphincter

Supportive

Carcinoma following treatment remains a possibility and diagnosis may be more difficult because of lack of early symptoms; a tumor in the dilated esophagus may be large before obstructive symptoms develop; pain and dysphagia associated with carcinomas may be assumed to be part of the primary diagnosis of achalasia

Pulmonary problems may still develop after dilation from overflow at night, and patient instruction should include refraining from oral intake 1 to 2 hours before bedtime

ASSESSMENT: AREAS OF CONCERN

Digestion

Dysphagia, without pain; apparent abrupt onset

Gradual symptoms and adaptation techniques of patients include fullness after meals; swallowing water or bicarbonate of soda after a meal; and using a modified Valsalva maneuver after a meal

Regurgitation of retained material can be recognized as food eaten hours earlier; nocturnal regurgitation may be severe

Dysphagia becomes continuous and annoying with difficulty first with liquids and later with solids

Little belching because of tonic condition of lower esophageal sphincter

Chest pain may be associated with esophageal spasm or esophageal irritation from retained food

Nocturnal regurgitation may be associated with overflow of food and fluids into bronchi, with development of pulmonary disease or aspiration pneumonia

Carcinoma of esophagus more frequent in patients with achalasia

Nutritional status

Gradual weight loss

Vomiting (overflow from esophagus): does not have "sour" characteristics of emesis from stomach (usually undigested or stale food)

NURSING DIAGNOSES and NURSING INTERVENTIONS

If an esophagomyotomy is performed, nursing care will be as for any patient with a chest incision.

Nursing Diagnosis	Nursing Intervention
Nutrition, alteration in: less than body requirements	Determine which foods patient can and cannot swallow. Instruct patient to eat slowly, chew food thoroughly, and arch the back while swallowing. Provide diet that avoids alcohol, spicy foods, or foods at temperature extremes. Request nutritional consultation. Administer medications as ordered to relieve discomfort, thus promoting appetite.
Airway clearance, ineffective	Elevate head of bed while patient sleeps to avoid regurgitation or aspiration.
Anxiety	Allow patient to verbalize concerns and frustration regarding disruption of mealtimes and inability to participate in social functions involving food. See p. 1839.

Patient Education

1. Patient should be instructed to withhold food and fluids at least 2 hours before bedtime. Using more than one pillow, with head and shoulders slightly elevated, may also be indicated.
2. Instruct patient how to perform the Valsalva maneuver to increase hydrostatic pressure in the esophagus and relax the lower esophageal sphincter.

3. Instruct patient in preparation of liquid foods to maintain nutritional status if solid foods cause dysphagia.
4. Inform patient of signs and symptoms of pneumonia or other pulmonary problems.
5. Patient needs to know the relationship of achalasia to a slightly higher incidence of esophageal cancer and the difficulty of distinguishing between the symptoms.

EVALUATION

Patient Outcome	Data Indicating That Outcome is Reached
Nutritional status is adequate.	Patient maintains healthy status.
There are no pulmonary problems.	Patient verbalizes an understanding of the relationship between eating, lying down, and pulmonary problems and verbalizes strategies to prevent aspiration.
	Patient continues to have medical follow-up for managing achalasia and for regular assessments for esophageal cancer.

ESOPHAGEAL CANCER

Malignancy of the esophagus usually arises from squamous epithelium and is epidermoid in type.

Esophageal cancer usually occurs in persons 50 years of age or older and predominantly in men. It is also more common in the black population. There are indications that esophageal cancers are related to tobacco and alcohol use, nutritional deficiencies, and environmental carcinogens. The highest frequency of esophageal cancers is found in the Caspian Sea area, Transkei in southern Africa, and northern China.

Some of the suggested environmental or nutritional factors in the development of esophageal cancer include *nitrosamines* or fungi contaminating pickled vegetables or in grains; chronic addiction to morphine, particularly in areas where opium is eaten; tobacco residue; silica fragments associated with millet bran (northern China); and abuse of alcohol. In associating the above suggested carcinogens with esophageal cancer, alcoholism is the one that has a clear relationship with epidermoid carcinoma of the esophagus. Chronic inflammation of the esophagus is also associated with a higher incidence of carcinomas. There is also an association between cancer of the esophagus and squamous cell carcinoma of the oropharynx or larynx, which is probably a result of exposure of the oral cavity, respiratory tract, and esophagus to the same carcinogenic factors.

PATHOPHYSIOLOGY

Approximately 50% of esophageal cancers are at the esophagogastric junction (these cancers are generally adenocarcinoma and arise from the stomach rather than the esophagus); 25% are in the upper thoracic esophagus; 17% are in the lower esophagus; and 8% are in the cervical esophagus. The preceding three carcinomas are primarily epidermoid, and a small percentage are adenocarcinomas. Lesions above the piriform sinus are transitional cell lesions, or lymphoepitheliomas.

The epidermoid carcinoma begins as a small mucosal patch that eventually grows, ulcerates, and protrudes into the lumen. Local extension to the recurrent laryngeal nerve or tracheobronchial tree is common. Unfortunately, local extension of the cancer is often present at the time of diagnosis. Metastasis to the local lymph nodes includes those around the hilum of the lung and in the neck. Metastases to the abdominal lymph nodes of the celiac axis occur. Metastases to the liver, lungs, kidney, and bone occur with decreasing frequency. Submucosal spread of the carcinoma does occur. Satellite lesions will occur several inches away from the primary lesion.

The esophageal cancer may be clinically staged as follows[72]:
- Stage I: localized tumor involving 5 cm or less of the esophagus; no spreading; no obstruction
- Stage II: involves regional lymph nodes or tumor is greater than 5 cm
- Stage III: distant metastases

Carcinoma of the bronchus or of the stomach will often metastasize to the esophagus. Mediastinal lymph node metastasis from other organ carcinomas may lead to esophageal involvement and symptoms of obstruction. Breast carcinomas may metastasize to the esophagus. Primary adenocarcinoma of the esophagus is rare and should be considered the result of Barrett's esophagus or of spread from an adenocarcinoma of the cardia of the stomach.

DIAGNOSTIC STUDIES

Radiography: barium studies
Source of upper gastrointestinal bleeding
Tumor outline

Chest x-ray film
Pulmonary complications (e.g., fibrosis or fistula)

Endoscopy with biopsy or cytology studies
Tumor invasion
Source of upper gastrointestinal bleeding

Bronchoscopy
Detects bronchial involvement and provides examination of vocal cords

Liver function studies
Detect hepatic involvement

Liver scan; CT scans of liver and chest
Determine tumor size and location and mediastinal involvement

TREATMENT PLAN

The major goal may not be to remove the tumor if it is widely metastasized but rather to provide the patient with a way to eat.

Surgical
Adenocarcinoma of gastroesophageal junction treated by surgical resection of esophagus and cardia, a procedure called gastric pull-up
Epidermoid carcinoma may be resected with colon interposition or esophagogastrectomy

Gastrostomy may be done to provide a route for nutrition

Chemotherapeutic
Chemotherapy in conjunction with irradiation or surgery; no one protocol proven effective; see Chapter 14

Electromechanical
Irradiation, primary form of treatment
Plastic tubes inserted to maintain lumen (Celestin tube)

Supportive
Relief of obstruction
Prevention of aspiration
Nutritional support

ASSESSMENT: AREAS OF CONCERN

Nutritional status
Dysphagia initially with liquids, progressing to solids and odynophagia; swallowing may be difficult or painful; sensation of food taking longer to go through segments of the chest (i.e., reach the stomach) may be described by the patient
Chest pain, which may indicate local extension of the disease
Weakness
Anorexia
Anemia
Profound weight loss

Pulmonary status
Bronchopulmonary symptoms include pneumonia, aspiration, or fistula
Hoarseness from involvement of recurrent laryngeal nerve
Upper gastrointestinal bleeding from tumor or from irritation by stagnant food in esophagus

NURSING DIAGNOSES and NURSING INTERVENTIONS

Nursing Diagnosis	Nursing Intervention
Airway clearance, ineffective	Observe patient's ability to swallow liquids and solid foods. Keep head of bed elevated to prevent regurgitation and aspiration. Encourage patient to refrain from drinking fluids 1 to 2 hours before bedtime. Provide suction if patient is unable to manage saliva.
Nutrition, alteration in: less than body requirements	Request nutritional consultation. Provide patient with meals and fluids that can be tolerated. Weigh patient daily. Maintain accurate intake and output records.

Nursing Diagnosis	Nursing Intervention
	Work closely with other health professionals to provide nutrition. Some possibilities that may be prescribed include the following: Nasogastric tube Liquid supplements before surgery Celestin tube Small feeding tubes placed during endoscopy Gastrostomy tube Total parenteral nutrition in preparation for surgery Provide nasogastric or gastrostomy care per protocols.
Comfort, alteration in: pain	Provide prescribed analgesia as needed and document effectiveness.
Coping, ineffective family: compromised	Assist patient and family in dealing with emotional reactions to the disease, treatment, and possible poor prognosis. Provide opportunities for expression of feelings and concerns. Recommend that home care be provided after discharge for assistance with activities of daily living (ADL). Encourage patient to discuss feelings about possibly not being able to join family members in eating at mealtimes.
Communication, impaired: verbal	Encourage patient to use notepad and pencil or Magic Slate if hoarseness from recurrent laryngeal nerve involvement is severe.

Patient Education

1. When a Celestin or plastic tube is used, the patient must sleep with the head of the bed elevated since the gastroesophageal junction is open and reflux can occur. Also, with the plastic tube, the patient should be instructed to swallow small amounts and not to lie down after eating. Semisolid foods can be eaten. The diet may be pureed. If obstruction occurs, sips of commercial meat tenderizer or dilute hydrogen peroxide may be used to break down the food and unblock the tube.
2. Patients and families should be given information on available support groups in their areas (I Can Cope, American Cancer Society, etc.).
3. Patients should be taught to check placement of gastrostomy, residual gastric contents, and type of feeding before providing gastrostomy feeding. They should also be taught to care for the skin and tube (see p. 1269).

EVALUATION

Patient Outcome	Data Indicating That Outcome is Reached
Nutritional status is maintained.	Patient is comfortable, able to handle secretions, and has sufficient enteral nutrition with a gastrostomy or a plastic (Celestin) tube.
Home care is provided adequately.	Patient and family have available resources mobilized to assist them (home health agency, self-help group, etc.).

ESOPHAGEAL DIVERTICULUM

An esophageal diverticulum is a hollow outpouching of the esophageal wall.

A true diverticulum contains all layers of the esophageal wall, while a false diverticulum lacks a muscular coat. Diverticula in the esophagus are also defined as pulsion or traction. A pulsion diverticulum is pushed out of the esophagus into adjacent structures, tubercupressure.[72] A traction diverticulum is pulled out of the esophagus by adjacent inflammatory tissue. A diverticulum in the posterior pharynx is known as Zenker's diverticulum, and although not esophageal, it is considered in discussions on esophageal diverticulum. Zenker's diverticulum is three times more common than esophageal diverticula and is more common in men than in women. Esophageal diverticula are rare.

PATHOPHYSIOLOGY

The only diverticula of consequence are those that retain food or fluid. Zenker's diverticulum is related to a developmental weakness of the muscular coat of the posterior portion of the pharynx. A small hernia of the esophageal wall is pushed out with swallowing and forms a diverticulum. Zenker's diverticulum can enlarge and obstruct the esophagus.

Most diverticula are found in the middle section of the esophagus. Tuberculosis has been associated with inflammation, which results in traction diverticula. Epiphrenic diverticula are located just above the cardioesophageal junction, are rare, and are associated with motility disorders such as esophageal spasm.

Diverticula may obstruct and perforate.

DIAGNOSTIC STUDIES

Barium swallow
   Herniation of esophageal wall

Endoscopy
   Herniation of esophageal wall (not always recommended since there is an increased incidence of perforation of the diverticulum)

TREATMENT PLAN

Surgical
   Epiphrenic diverticulum: removed with esophagomyotomy; advised if motility problems are also present
   Zenker's diverticulum: one-stage procedure, along the left sternocleidomastoid muscle
   Surgery indicated when other management does not prevent nocturnal regurgitation

Electromechanical
   Patient taught to empty diverticulum before going to bed at night to prevent aspiration

Supportive
   Careful assessment of patient so that other esophageal diseases are not overlooked in managing esophageal diverticulum

ASSESSMENT: AREAS OF CONCERN

Zenker's diverticulum
   Regurgitation of food eaten hours earlier
   Aspiration at night may lead to chronic pulmonary disease
   Dysphagia, late symptom, indicates obstruction of esophagus
   Bad taste in mouth
   Foul odor to breath
   Sloshing of fluid in diverticulum heard as gurgling noises

Esophageal diverticulum
   Regurgitation of food eaten hours earlier
   May have other esophageal disease
   Tracheoesophageal fistula
   Pulmonary symptoms
   Bleeding (rare)
   Abscess formation (rare)

NURSING DIAGNOSES and NURSING INTERVENTIONS

Nursing Diagnosis	Nursing Intervention
Airway clearance, ineffective	Observe patient closely for signs of pulmonary problems (i.e., choking or aspirating). Keep head of bed elevated. Encourage patient to sleep with head and shoulders elevated on at least two pillows. Ensure that patient has emptied diverticulum before lying down, if ordered by physician.
Nutrition, alteration in: less than body requirements	Provide nutritional consultation. Weigh patient daily. Monitor and record intake and output accurately. Ensure that patient's knowledge of food preparation is adequate to facilitate swallowing and emptying of diverticulum.

Patient Education

1. Teach patient to empty diverticulum (if ordered by physician) by postural drainage. Patient should lie on the bed with head on the floor and hips flat on the bed and remain this way for 5 to 10 minutes. Make sure the patient's bed is on a frame and off the floor but not too far off the floor. This procedure drains the diverticulum and prevents regurgitation.

EVALUATION

Patient Outcome	Data Indicating That Outcome is Reached
Nutritional status is maintained.	Patient's weight remains stable.
There are no pulmonary complications.	Airway is clear. There is no evidence of aspiration or other pulmonary complications.

HIATAL HERNIA

Hiatal hernia refers to the presence in the chest, above the diaphragm, of a part of the stomach that has passed through the normal esophageal hiatus.

Hiatal hernia is very common, occurring in an average of 29.6% of persons.[72] It is more common in women, and frequency is much higher in elderly individuals. A hiatal hernia is clinically significant when it is accompanied by a reflux of acid.

PATHOPHYSIOLOGY

Muscle weakness is a primary factor in developing a hiatal hernia. Loss of muscle tone in middle age or after a long illness weakens the muscles around the diaphragmatic opening, predisposing one to hiatal hernia. Increased abdominal pressure helps to push the upper portion of the stomach through the large opening of the diaphragm.

Intra-abdominal pressure may be increased by the effort needed to evacuate firm stools associated with low-residue diets or constipation. Hiatal hernia is uncommon in countries where the diet is high in fibers. Obesity, pregnancy, and ascites are associated with hiatal hernia, as are the use of girdles and tight-fitting belts and clothes. Esophagitis may lead to secondary shortening of the esophagus and spasm, which may pull part of the stomach upward, creating a small hiatal hernia. Esophageal carcinomas may also pull upward on the stomach. This may cause problems in diagnosing the primary etiology. Hiatal hernia is also seen with kyphoscoliosis.

Hiatal hernia may develop after surgical treatment for achalasia. After partial gastrectomy, hiatal hernia may be found because of the straightening and opening of the gastroesophageal junction angle and the elimination of the sphincter.

There are several forms of hiatal hernia, which are difficult to distinguish clinically. Paraesophageal hernia involves the rolling of the cardia of the stomach up into the chest with the gastroesophageal junction remaining below the diaphragm. There is no acid reflux in this type. The complication in paraesophageal hernias is incarceration.

Congenital short esophagus is also referred to as a congenital hiatal hernia. The etiology is probably a spasm rather than an actual short esophagus. The true congenital short esophagus is probably Barrett's esophagus. (Barrett's esophagus refers to an esophagus in which the lower portion is lined with columnar rather than squamous epithelium.)

Sliding hiatal hernia is the most common type. The lower edge of the esophagus and the cardia slide up into the chest through a loose esophageal hiatus. The result is reflux of acid and esophagitis.

Hiatal hernias interfere wtih normal protective mechanisms of the cardia or lower esophageal sphincter, allowing reflux of acid into the esophagus. Also, if the hiatal hernia is fixed above the diaphragm, congestion of the gastric mucosa may lead to gastritis and ulcerations in the herniated portion of the stomach. The size of the hiatal hernia does not matter in the development of esophagitis and the severity of the symptoms.

DIAGNOSTIC STUDIES

Laboratory studies
Stool for diagnosing occult blood
Serum for diagnosing anemia

Chest film

Air shallow behind the heart: presence of pneumonia

Barium swallow

Outpouching, depending on patient's position when test performed

Endoscopy and biopsy

Assessment of degree of esophagitis

Motility studies

Demonstration of reflux and low pressure in lower esophageal sphincter (not routinely done)

pH monitoring of lower esophagus

Increase in acidity

Bernstein test (acid perfusion test)

Differentiation between cardiac chest pain and pain resulting from esophageal origin (Patient has esophageal pain or heartburn if test is positive.)

Radioisotope scintiscan

Diagnosis of nocturnal aspiration

TREATMENT PLAN

Surgical

Conservative medical management usually successful; surgery is indicated in the following situations:

Persistent symptoms not responding to medical treatment

Reflux stenosis not responding to moderately frequent dilation

Strangulation or incarceration

Types of procedures

Nissen's fundoplication: surrounds entire esophagus with a pouch of the stomach

Allison: reconstruction of angle of the stomach and esophagus, narrowing the hiatus posteriorly, and suturing phrenoesophageal ligament to underside of diaphragm

Belsey's Mark IV: holds esophagus in place by plicating fundus around lower end of esophagus for about two thirds of its circumference

Hill: narrows esophagus orifice, pulls gastroesophageal junction below diaphragm, and anchors stomach to median arcuate ligament (posterior gastropexy)

Chemotherapeutic

Antacids used hourly in acute phases with a bland diet

Histamine receptor antagonists

H_2 blockers (cimetidine [Tagamet], 300 mg qid, or ranitidine [Zantac], 100 mg qid, with meals and at bedtime) to relieve the heartburn of reflux esophagitis

Antiemetic agents (used to enhance gastric emptying)

Metoclopramide (Reglan), dopamine depletor, to relieve symptoms of reflux by stimulating gastric emptying and increasing lower esophageal sphincter pressure; neurologic side effects occur

Autonomic agent

Bethanechol (Urecholine), 25 mg four times a day, to increase lower esophageal sphincter pressure

Electromechanical

Instruct patient to use 4-inch bed blocks so that he lies on an inclined plane

Pillows may double the patient in the middle, impeding gastric drainage

Supportive

Bland diet, avoiding foods that are irritating for the individual

Avoid eating 1 to 2 hours before bedtime

Walk around after a meal

Chocolate associated with relaxation of the esophageal sphincter and so is contraindicated, as is smoking

Sip half glass of water after a meal to cleanse the esophagus

ASSESSMENT: AREAS OF CONCERN

Digestion

Reflux esophagitis: symptoms include heartburn or pain made worse by lying down or stooping over; pain relieved by sitting up or by antacids; water brash (mouth filling with fluid from esohpagus); and dysphagia

Epigastric pain

Contortions of neck and arms to reduce discomfort

Hematology status

Upper gastrointestinal bleeding

Anemia from chronic ulcerations

Pulmonary status

Chronic lung disease after nocturnal regurgitation and aspiration; may include hoarseness, chronic laryngitis, inflammation of the arytenoids, bronchitis, and pulmonary fibrosis

Incarceration: symptoms include sudden onset of vomiting, pain, and complete dysphagia

Pediatric

Sucrosuria and mental retardation have been associated with hiatal hernia

Torsion spasms of head and shoulders and recurrent vomiting (Sandifer's syndrome)

NURSING DIAGNOSES and NURSING INTERVENTIONS

Nursing Diagnosis	Nursing Intervention
Comfort, alteration in: pain	Provide 4-inch blocks for head of bed and help patient to identify where they can be purchased for home care. Keep antacids by the bed for frequent use. Administer antacids to patient with poor memory or confusion. Explain relationship between food and pain that patient is experiencing.

Patient Education

1. Instruct patient on relationship between hiatal hernia, reflux esophagitis, and the treatment plan.
2. Provide instructions on use of antacids. If patient has other medical problems and is taking other medications, check with the pharmacist before choosing the antacid to be used.
3. Provide information on the use of 4-inch blocks under the head of the bed; patient may also need help to prevent sliding out of the bed, as will partner, since it is difficult to sleep this way.
4. Other substances that reduce pressure in lower esophageal sphincter include chocolate, peppermint, smoking, and anticholinergics and should be avoided.

EVALUATION

Patient Outcome	Data Indicating That Outcome is Reached
Symptoms of esophagitis are absent.	Heartburn or pain from esophagitis is reduced. There is no perforation or bleeding.

ESOPHAGEAL STRICTURE

An esophageal stricture is a fibrotic process usually at the lower end of the esophagus.

An esophageal stricture is associated with reflux esophagitis. The interesting point is the lack of predictability in determining when an esophageal stricture will occur. Some patients develop strictures after a short history of heartburn, while others have persistent reflux esophagitis for years before developing a stricture.

PATHOPHYSIOLOGY

Esophageal stricture may also be caused by postoperative changes following gastroesophageal surgery, in-lying nasogastric tube, prolonged vomiting, and ingestion of corrosive agents. Esophageal stricture is also associated with mucocutaneous candidiasis and epidermolysis bullosa. The true esophageal stricture involves fibrosis through all layers of the esophagus. Narrowing of the esophageal lumen may also occur with edema and inflammation that stiffen the esophagus or with spasms secondary to inflammation.

DIAGNOSTIC STUDIES

Barium studies
Show tapering

Endoscopy and biopsy
Remove food plugs and help rule out a tumor

TREATMENT PLAN

Surgical
Simple antireflux procedures, with or without dilation of the strictured segment; procedures similar to those for reflux esophagitis (p. 1163)

Chemotherapeutic
Acute dysphagia related to bolus of meat in the esophagus
Solution of commercial meat tenderizer, 2 teaspoons in 8 ounces of water; instruct patient to swallow several spoonfuls, wait 30 minutes, swallow several

sips of soda water, and bear down in modified Valsalva maneuver; use only when food impaction has been present less than 6 hours

Vasodilating agents

Sublingual nitroglycerin or nifedipine (Procardia) may be used to relax spasm around food, *or*

Hypoglycemic agent

Glucagon, 0.25 to 1.0 mg IV

Electromechanical

Esophagoscopy to remove food obstruction

Esophageal dilation can be done with mercury bougies, is usually successful, and prevents need for surgical intervention; if not successful, a guided bougienage (Eder-Puestow technique) may be used

Esophageal dilation can also be done through endoscope

ASSESSMENT: AREAS OF CONCERN

Digestion

History of heartburn

Difficulty in swallowing (solids, steaks, and apples are good tests of esophageal patency)

History of ingestion of caustic agents (lye, ammonia)

History of esophageal surgery

Pediatric

The above assessments plus excessive drooling and abdominal distention the first few days of life

NURSING DIAGNOSES and NURSING INTERVENTIONS

Nursing Diagnosis	Nursing Intervention
Comfort, alteration in: pain	Prepare and administer solution of meat tenderizer as prescribed, and explain its use during acute dysphagia.
Nutrition, alteration in: less than body requirements	Assess patient for weight loss. Provide enteral nutrition high in calories as ordered until esophageal dilation has relieved the underlying problem. Weigh patient daily.

Patient Education

1. Explain the problems related to meat, painful swallowing, and use of meat tenderizer solution. Prevention may involve less meat in diet, particularly steaks, or eating small pieces, chewing well, and waiting between bites.
2. Prepare patient for various medical procedures.

EVALUATION

Patient Outcome	Data Indicating That Outcome is Reached
There are no symptoms of esophageal stricture.	There are no dietary limitations. There is no dysphagia.

ESOPHAGEAL VARICES

Esophageal varices are dilated blood vessels in the esophagus caused by portal hypertension.

Portal hypertension results in the enlargement of collateral blood vessels and the predisposition to ascites. Normally blood flows from the higher pressures of the portal system through the liver sinusoids and then through the hepatic vein to the lower pressure of the vena cava and the systemic venous system. As long as this normal flow is uninterrupted, the potential collateral circulation between the portal and systemic circulations remains closed. Potential collateral circulation exists at the cardioesophageal junction, in the lower rectum, and around the umbilicus. When the normal hemodynamics are disturbed by portal hypertension, the flow of blood that normally goes from the coronary veins into the splenic vein is reversed.[72] This forces open the collaterals between the esophagus and the gastric veins, leading to esophageal varices. Internal hemorrhoids and dilated veins around the umbilicus also occur.

Portal hypertension is the result of blockage or increased resistance to the inflow of blood into the liver or decreased outflow of blood from the portal system into the vena cava. Causes of portal hypertension include the following:

1. Congenital obstruction of portal vein
2. Thrombosis of splenic vein from acute pancreatitis
3. Liver parenchymal disease
4. Occlusion of the hepatic vein
5. Cirrhosis

PATHOPHYSIOLOGY

The veins from the small segment of the abdominal esophagus and the fundus and cardia of the stomach drain into the left coronary vein. These two venous systems are connected by small veins that lie in the esophageal submucosal plexus and normally remain closed. When these veins become dilated, they quickly become tortuous and variceal because of poor support in the esophageal submucosa. In portal hypertension the pressure of the portal system is transmitted through these collateral vessels, which dilate and then produce large esophageal varices. The focus of care is on the management of massive gastrointestinal hemorrhages that occur in these patients.

DIAGNOSTIC STUDIES

Endoscopy
Tortuous protrusions into lower end of esophagus
May show large amount of blood and possibly source of bleeding

Mesenteric angiography
Demonstrates collateral circulation
May demonstrate bleeding site

TREATMENT PLAN

Surgical
Portacaval shunt: portal vein or one of its tributaries is connected to the inferior vena cava, and portal vein blood flow bypasses diseased liver; complication: hepatic encephalopathy

Splenorenal shunt: diverts portion of blood flow away from liver to reduce pressure; lower incidence of hepatic encephalopathy
Mesocaval shunt: unites high-pressure superior mesenteric vein of patient with portal hypertension to low-pressure inferior vena cava, directly or with a synthetic graft
Distal splenorenal shunt: uses spleen to conduct blood from high pressure of esophageal and gastric varices to low-pressure renal vein
Surgery recommended if patient has bled once, since 60% to 90% run a risk of further bleeding
May need to ligate the bleeders

Chemotherapeutic
Focus is on management of the massive gastrointestinal hemorrhages that occur
Correction of electrolyte imbalances; prevention of encephalopathy (e.g., lactulose)
Pituitary hormone
Vasopressin (Pitressin), to reduce portal and mesenteric blood flow, given intravenously or during endoscopy or angiography; side effects include abdominal cramps, diarrhea, hyponatremia, peripheral vasoconstriction, hypertension, decreased cardiac output, angina, arrhythmias, and infarction of bowel; used as adjunctive treatment
Histamine receptor antagonist
Cimetidine (Tagamet), 300 mg qid, or ranitidine (Zantac), 100 mg qid, at meals and bedtime
Antacids
Maalox
Vitamins
Vitamin K, IM
Antibacterial agents
Neomycin (Mycifradin) or lactulose (Cephulac)

Electromechanical
Sclerotherapy of varices may be done by a transhepatic approach or through an endoscope; involves injecting varices with agents that irritate them, causing thrombosis; complications include perforation of esophagus, aspiration pneumonia, pleural effusions, increased ascites, and ulceration of esophagus
Esophageal tamponade to control bleeding
Sengstaken-Blakemore tube: gastric aspiration with two balloons (esophageal and gastric); need additional nasogastric tube to empty esophagus if patient is not alert
Linton tube: two aspiration lumens (esophageal and gastric) and one balloon (gastric)
Boyce's modified Sengstaken-Blakemore tube
Complications of esophageal tamponade include rupture or erosion of esophagus, occlusion of airway by balloon, and aspiration of secretions

Supportive
Blood transfusions
Removal of ascitic fluid (paracentesis)

ASSESSMENT: AREAS OF CONCERN

Gastrointestinal bleeding
Massive hematemesis
Melena
Amount of blood loss

NURSING DIAGNOSES and NURSING INTERVENTIONS

Nursing Diagnosis	Nursing Intervention

Tissue perfusion, alteration in: cerebral, cardiopulmonary, renal, gastrointestinal, peripheral	Assess patient for signs and symptoms of shock:
	  Postural changes in pulse and blood pressure
	  Cool, clammy skin
	  Increase in respiratory rate
	  Change in mental status
	  Decreased urine output
	  Hemoglobin and hematocrit unchanged immediately but decreased within 24 hours
	Start IV line with large-bore catheter and administer IV fluids as ordered by physician.
	Assist with insertion of Swan-Ganz or CVP catheter and perform ongoing hemodynamic monitoring.
	Administer blood transfusions as ordered.
	Monitor patient for possible transfusion reaction per protocol.
	Perform gastric lavage with iced saline or water as ordered by physician.

Bowel elimination, alteration in: diarrhea	Monitor amount, color, and consistency of stools. Administer neomycin, lactulose, or neomycin enemas as ordered. (These agents assist in eliminating blood from patient's gut; if untreated, hepatic encephalopathy could occur from breakdown products of protein metabolism produced by bacterial action in gut.)[67,70] Keep patient clean and dry. Assess skin frequently for potential breakdown. Consider use of rectal pouch or rectal tube if diarrhea is uncontrollable. Monitor intake and output accurately. Assess patient for signs and symptoms of dehydration: skin turgor, elevated temperature.

Thought processes, alteration in	Monitor patient closely for symptoms of hepatic encephalopathy:
	  Apathy
	  Euphoria
	  Asterixis (flapping)
	  Personality changes
	  Confusion
	  Disorientation
	  Stupor progressing to coma
	  Document and report to physician immediately if any of these occur.
	If confusion or disorientation occurs, frequently reorient patient to time, date, and place.
	If patient is disoriented or combative, ensure patient's safety by placing side rails up or restraining patient if necessary.
	Stay with patient or enlist assistance from family members to keep patient from harming self.
	Continue to administer lactulose or neomycin as ordered by physician.
	Provide usual care necessary for comatose patient if hepatic coma should occur.

Skin integrity, impairment of: actual	Assess skin around patient's perirectal area and sacrum frequently since constant diarrhea can be very erosive. Cleanse skin thoroughly with warm water and a mild soap. Rinse well and spray with a skin sealant; then coat the skin with a water-repellant ointment.

Nursing Diagnosis	Nursing Intervention
	If skin breakdown has occurred, cleanse stool from skin gently with a cottonball soaked in glycerin. Apply a mixture of skin cream and ointment over the perirectal area.

Patient Education

1. Prepare the patient for all diagnostic procedures, treatments, or surgery so that he will understand what will be happening and what can be expected.
2. Patient must be instructed on the effects of high-protein diets and alcohol consumption in preventing future complications.
3. Patient needs to know the relationship of the esophageal varices to the primary diagnosis that resulted in portal hypertension.

EVALUATION

Patient Outcome	Data Indicating That Outcome is Reached
There is no gastrointestinal bleeding.	Hematocrit and hemoglobin are normal for patient. Vomiting and diarrhea are not present. Vital signs are stable. Skin turgor is normal for patient.
Mental status is normal for patient.	Patient is alert and oriented to time, date, and place.
Skin integrity is maintained.	There is no skin breakdown in perirectal area or pressure points.

GASTRITIS

Gastritis refers to any diffuse lesion in the gastric mucosa that can be identified histologically as inflamed.

Gastritis may occur as an acute or a chronic disorder and is more common in the elderly population. The reported incidence of chronic gastritis associated with gastrointestinal bleeding has fluctuated over the last few years from 40% to 10%.[72] This shift is probably related to successful utilization of endoscopic diagnostic procedures. The incidence of acute gastritis is undetermined except when associated with gastrointestinal bleeding. Acute gastritis is responsible for 10% to 30% of upper gastrointestinal bleeding.[22,72]

PATHOPHYSIOLOGY

Acute gastritis is a short-lived inflammatory process affecting the mucosa of the stomach. It involves erosion of the mucosa. The mucosa is spotted with submucosal hemorrhages that resemble ecchymoses and may be round or linear. There may also be shallow erosions that appear as brown spots or red petechiae or small breaks in the mucosa. The hemorrhagic erosions usually involve only the glandular layer, are extremely shallow, and are found anywhere in the stomach. Acute gastritis is more common in gastric ulcer than duodenal ulcer. The difference between gastritis erosion and gastric ulcer is that in erosion the muscularis mucosa is uninvolved and healing leaves no scar.

The mechanism that results in erosion and hemorrhage is a back diffusion of hydrogen ions and mucosal ischemia. The disruption of the gastric mucosal barrier allows the back diffusion of the hydrogen ion, which stimulates the release of vasoactive substances, increased capillary permeability, and inflammation.

There are a number of drugs, stimuli, and circumstances associated with acute gastritis, including aspirin, anti-inflammatory agents, alcohol, corticosteroids, major physiologic stress, and intense emotional reactions. The most common cause of acute superficial gastritis is alcohol.[69,72] Stress ulcers are a form of acute gastritis. The term *stress ulcer* is actually a misnomer since the lesions are not ulcers.

Steroids appear to potentiate the action of other factors in acute gastritis. Nonsteroidal anti-inflammatory agents used for the treatment of rheumatoid arthritis probably affect gastric mucosa because they work by inhibiting prostaglandin synthesis. Prostaglandins have a cytoprotective function on the gastric mucosa. It appears that patients taking both nonsteroidal anti-inflammatory agents and aspirin are at a greater risk for bleeding from acute erosive gastritis. The treatment protocol for the patient with rheumatoid arthritis is not stopped, but the patient will need to be observed and treated for erosion as indicated.

Chronic gastritis is often referred to as a nonerosive, nonspecific gastritis that is further differentiated by the histologic appearance of the gastric mucosa into superficial gastritis, atrophic gastritis, or gastric atrophy.

Superficial gastritis is characterized by an inflammatory infiltration of the lamina propria. Lymphocytes, plasma cells, and eosinophils are found in the outer one third of the mucosa. The gastric glands are not involved.

In atrophic gastritis there is loss of fundic glands, parietal cells, and chief cells. The muscularis mucosa is split and thickened, and marked inflammation is present.

Gastric atrophy refers to marked or total gland loss with minimal inflammation. The mucosa is thinned.

Two additional features may be seen in the three types of chronic gastritis: intestinal metaplasia and pseudopyloric metaplasia. Intestinal metaplasia is the replacement of normal gastric cells by cells identical to those of the normal small intestine. Intestinal metaplasia is greater in more severe degrees of gastric atophy. The surface of the normal stomach is columnar, whereas the small intestine has a prominent brush border and may contain goblet and Paneth's cells. When intestinal metaplasia occurs, the stomach acquires the appearance and the absorptive capacity seen in the small intestine. Cancer is much more likely to develop in intestinalized gastric mucosa in comparison to the rare instances of carcinoma of the intestinal epithelium in the small intestine.

In pseudopyloric metaplasia the normal fundic glands are replaced by clear-staining mucous glands that cannot be distinguished from mucous glands in the antral gland or cardial gland mucosa. The replacement may be partial or total. Diagnosis of pseudopyloric metaplasia is made by biopsy. It is imperative that the location of the biopsy be carefully stated on pathology slips so that the pathologist does not mistake normal antral gland mucosa for pseudopyloric metaplasia or vice versa.

Chronic gastritis has also been divided into type A and type B. Type A gastritis involves the fundus. There are circulating parietal cell antibodies and high serum gastrin levels. Pernicious anemia evolves almost exclusively from type A gastritis.[5,72] The relationship of the parietal cell antibodies and intrinsic factor lends support for the hypothesis that type A gastritis has an autoimmune background. Type B gastritis involves the fundus and the antrum. There is a lack of parietal cell antibodies, and approximately 10% of patients with type B gastritis will have gastrin cell antibodies.[72]

In type A gastritis, there is a marked reduction in acid secretion, hypergastrinemia, and eventually impaired vitamin B_{12} absorption. Type B has less reduction of acid secretions, normal gastrin levels, and only rare impairment of vitamin B_{12} absorption. As the mucosa of the stomach changes with atrophy, the acid secretion is reduced, resulting in achlorhydria or hypochlorhydria.

Atrophic gastritis and gastric atrophy are associated with an increase in gastric malignancies. There is a high rate of cell death and increased cell turnover in atrophic gastritis. Evidence is available to document the increased mucosal nuclear activity supporting the premalignant state.[5] The highest mitotic rates are found in areas of intestinal metaplasia.

Although pernicious anemia is discussed at length in Chapter 13, the relationship between the intrinsic factor and vitamin B_{12} absorption should be briefly discussed here. Vitamin B_{12} refers to cyanocobalamin (CN-Cbl). Humans depend on dietary sources of vitamin B_{12} provided by foods of animal origin. The minimal daily requirement is 0.6 to 1.2 μg/d. The vitamin is stored in the liver. The liver stores of vitamin B_{12} are sufficient to last 3 to 5 years.

Under normal conditions of gastric acidity, dietary vitamin B_{12} enters the jejunum bound to proteins. Pancreatic proteases remove the protein, and the vitamin B_{12} binds with the intrinsic factor, secreted in the stomach by parietal cells. Intrinsic factor is crucial to protect vitamin B_{12} from bacterial destruction. In the distal ileum the intrinsic factor–vitamin B_{12} complex attaches to specific brush border receptors. A pH equal to or greater than 5.7 and the presence of divalent cations, particularly calcium, are required for binding (attachment). Once vitamin B_{12} enters the cell, it binds with transcobalamin (II), a transport protein, and is carried to the liver.

Vitamin B_{12} deficiency is difficult to detect early because of the liver stores that continue to supply it. Conditions associated with vitamin B_{12} deficiency include chronic gastritis, ileitis, surgical removal of the ileum, gastrectomy, or loss or deficiency of pancreatic enzymes. Prophylactic intramuscular injections of vitamin B_{12} may be used to prevent the sequelae associated with a vitamin B_{12} deficiency.

DIAGNOSTIC STUDIES

Acute Gastritis

Nasogastric aspiration
Frank blood or heme-positive aspirate

Endoscopy
Erosions, superficial ulcerations, and diffuse oozing

of blood when procedure is done during acute phase; after 3 days, lesions will begin to heal

Angiographic visualization

To detect and treat lesions with infusion of vasopressin

Double-contrast barium study

Superficial gastric erosions
Cannot be used to detect bleeding lesions

Chronic Gastritis

Serum gastrin

Elevated: in a few patients with type B, the level will be normal or low

Serum parietal cell antibodies

Presence suggests gastritis

Pentagastrin stimulation

Normal gastric secretion for person's age and sex would indicate minimal likelihood of gastritis
Diminished gastric secretions increase likelihood of gastritis

Serum pepsinogen I levels

Elevated in superficial gastritis
Low level in atrophic gastritis reflects absence of chief cells

Schilling test

Assessment of vitamin B_{12} absorption by measuring urinary excretion of an oral dose of radiolabeled vitamin B_{12}

Barium swallow with double contrast

Appearance of a "bald fundus" and thinning of gastric rugae

Endoscopy with biopsy and cytology

Biopsy necessary to obtain a definitive diagnosis
Cytology of multiple biopsy sites through the stomach is used to rule out gastric carcinomas

Differential diagnosis

Rule out Zollinger-Ellison syndrome vs. chronic gastritis
High serum gastrin and high serum pepsinogen levels are indicative of Zollinger-Ellison syndrome; may also indicate multiple poorly healed ulcers

TREATMENT PLAN

Acute Gastritis

Surgical

Partial gastrectomy, pyloroplasty, vagotomy, or total gastrectomy may be indicated for managing patients with major bleeding from erosive gastritis

Chemotherapeutic

Histamine receptor antagonists
Ranitidine (Zantac), 100 mg po qid
Parenteral cimetidine (Tagamet), 300 mg q6h in 100 ml of D_5W over 20 min; dosage should maintain gastric pH at 7[72]
Antacids
Antacids recommended to help maintain alkaline pH
Antacids (30 ml q2h) have been shown to be 80% to 90% effective in keeping pH above 4.0
Fluid volume replacement
Intravenous fluid replacement during a bleeding episode to maintain volume
Blood replacement may be required when gastrointestinal hemorrhage is associated with acute gastritis
Pituitary hormone
Vasopressin (Pitressin) per angiography or IV, 20 units in 100 units D_5W over 10 min, may be used in severe cases and may be repeated q3-4h if rebleeding occurs; may lose efficacy after repeated doses

Electromechanical

Ice water or saline lavage used in patient with gastrointestinal bleeding
Laser therapy with direct coagulation of bleeding spots through an endoscopic approach may be utilized

Supportive

Removal of causative agents (alcohol, aspirin, nonsteroidal anti-inflammatory agents)
Withholding of food and fluids until vomiting and inflammation subside; then bland diet of medium temperature in acute gastritis without bleeding will assist healing process

Chronic Gastritis

Chemotherapeutic

Antacids to reduce or alleviate symptoms
Vitamins
Vitamin C (ascorbic acid) to facilitate iron absorption in the patient with achlorhydria[70]
Vitamin B_{12} injections (cyanocobalamin, 1 mg/ml (1000 μg)

Electromechanical

Routine endoscopy to assess formation of gastric polyps and gastric carcinomas in patients diagnosed with atrophic gastritis and gastric atrophy
Routine Schilling tests or serum vitamin B_{12} levels to evaluate intrinsic factor deficiency

ASSESSMENT: AREAS OF CONCERN

Acute Gastritis

Stomach
Asymptomatic; or vague complaints of postprandial distress after a large meal; or vague ulcerlike distress, particularly relieved by food
Massive gastrointestinal hemorrhage
History of aspirin or alcohol intake
History of hematemesis or melena
Nasogastric aspirate or stool heme positive for blood (in hospitalized patient)

Chronic Gastritis

Stomach
Often asymptomatic
Diffuse, epigastric burning or pain that increases after eating large amounts; relieved by a small amount of antacid
Vomiting

Pernicious anemia
May be first clinical sign of chronic gastritis
Weakness; numbness and tingling in extremities; fever; pallor; anorexia; weight loss
Smooth or beefy red tongue

NURSING DIAGNOSES and NURSING INTERVENTIONS

Nursing Diagnosis	Nursing Intervention
Tissue perfusion, alteration in: cerebral, cardiopulmonary, renal, gastrointestinal, peripheral	Give patient nothing by mouth, and keep patient quiet if hemorrhage is considered a possibility. Maintain intravenous fluids and blood as ordered. Monitor vital signs, CVP or Swan-Ganz catheter, blood work, and urinary output. Observe patient for early signs of hypovolemic shock and initiate replacement of fluid volume. Insert a large-bore nasogastric tube. Institute ice water or saline lavage as ordered for gastrointestinal bleeding. Prepare patient for diagnostic procedures.
Nutrition, alteration in: less than body requirements	Provide frequent (approximately six) small feedings of bland food per day. Monitor intake and output. Record nausea and vomiting. Administer antiemetics as ordered.
Oral mucous membrane, alteration in	Notify physician of smooth or beefy red tongue, since this may be an indication of intrinsic factor deficiency.

Patient Education

1. Identify agents that are irritating to the gastric mucosa, including aspirin, aspirin-containing compounds, over-the-counter agents, alcohol, prescription drugs such as indomethacin, phenylbutazone, reserpine, nicotine, ibuprofen, sulindac, and naproxen.
2. Provide patient with information related to the cause-and-effect relationship of above agents and gastritis.
3. Identify need for asymptomatic patient with chronic gastritis to continue to see physician regularly.
4. Discuss bland diets, amounts of food ingested, use of antacids, and their relationship to pain management.

EVALUATION

Patient Outcome	Data Indicating That Outcome is Reached
Gastrointestinal hemorrhage ceases.	Blood pressure, pulse, and respirations are within normal limits. Hematemesis and melena are absent.
Laboratory studies are within normal limits.	Serum vitamin B_{12} level is within normal limits.

Patient Outcome	Data Indicating That Outcome is Reached
	Normal Schilling test (8% to 40% of original oral dose of radioactive vitamin B_{12} appears in a 24-hour urine specimen).
	Endoscopy demonstrates normal mucosa (acute episode) or absence of polyps and carcinoma (chronic gastritis).
There is no pain.	Patient reports a history of frequent, small feedings of bland foods (chronic gastritis).
	Patient identifies causative agents involved in acute gastritis and omits these from his intake.

DYSPEPSIA

Dyspepsia is a vague gastric discomfort that occurs after eating. The person may complain of fullness, pain, heartburn, bloating, and nausea.

The majority of patients (30% to 55%) with dyspepsia do not have obvious pathologic findings in the gastrointestinal system.[69] Dyspepsia has also been divided into two classifications: ulcer-negative dyspepsia and functional dyspepsia.

Ulcer-negative dyspepsia involves classic symptoms of duodenal ulcers. The patient complains of epigastric pain 1 to 3 hours after eating and can obtain relief with antacids. This has also been referred to as Moynihan's disease.[69,72] Spiro reports that 40% of patients with ulcerlike dyspepsia will have a gastric or duodenal ulcer, 40% will have duodenitis, and the remaining group will have a normal endoscopic examination or a gastric cancer. In addition, Spiro reports that patients with ulcer-negative dyspepsia have an increased likelihood of developing duodenal ulcers in the future.

Functional dyspepsia involves epigastric pain shortly after a meal, belching, bloating, and nausea. Antacids offer little if any relief.

PATHOPHYSIOLOGY

The patient with ulcer-negative dyspepsia may be part of a continuum of diseases involving duodenitis and peptic ulcer disease. The functional dyspepsia may be related to poor gastric emptying with gastric distention causing pain or discomfort.

Psychologic factors may play a role in both types of dyspepsia. Gomez and Dally[29] found that 80% of the patients with persistent or recurrent abdominal pain were diagnosed as chronically depressed, suffering from chronic tension, or having hysterical mechanisms. This may indicate a need for early psychologic evaluation of patients with vague recurrent abdominal pain. Although the origin may be psychosomatic, the symptoms are real.

Drugs, prescription and nonprescription, may also produce dyspepsia. The patient may have epigastric pain with or without nausea and vomiting. Anti-inflammatory agents, theophylline, and digitalis are known to produce dyspepsia. Other agents play a role in gastritis and ulcer formation.

DIAGNOSTIC STUDIES

Double-air contrast barium swallow
Negative for ulceration or early carcinoma

Endoscopy
Negative for duodenitis or ulceration

TREATMENT PLAN

Chemotherapeutic
Ulcer-negative dyspepsia
Histamine receptor antagonists
Ranitidine (Zantac), 100 mg po bid
Cimetidine (Tagamet), 400 mg/d po
Antacids
Antacids 1 and 3 h after meals and at bedtime
Antiulcer agents
Sucralfate (Carafate), 1 g po qid, on empty stomach (1 h before meals and at bedtime)
Pirenzepine in clinical trials is effective in relieving symptoms in ulcer-negative dyspepsia
Functional dyspepsia
Antiemetics (used to enhance gastric emptying)
Metoclopramide (Reglan), 10 mg po, 30 min before each meal and at bedtime

Supportive
Low-fat diet

ASSESSMENT: AREAS OF CONCERN

Gastric

Symptoms of fullness, pain, heartburn, bloating, and nausea

Relationship of symptoms to eating

Use of and effectiveness of antacids

History of prescribed medications and over-the-counter drugs that are ulcerogenic

History of ulcer disease

Assessment of emotional status, tension, and stress

NURSING DIAGNOSES and NURSING INTERVENTIONS

Nursing Diagnosis	Nursing Intervention
Comfort, alteration in: pain	Provide symptomatic relief as ordered.
Coping, ineffective individual	Assess life-style with patient, exploring relationship of stress and emotion to symptoms.
	Recommend counseling to physician if appropriate.

Patient Education

1. Patient should be able to identify prescribed medications, dosage regimen, and interactive effects. (For example, antacids cannot be taken 30 minutes before or after sucralfate or they will inactivate sucralfate.)

EVALUATION

Patient Outcome	Data Indicating That Outcome is Reached
There is no dyspepsia, pain, or discomfort.	Patient has no complaints of fullness, pain, heartburn, bloating, or nausea following a meal.
Patient verbalizes sources of psychosocial stress and tension.	Patient is able to verbalize sources of stress and tension and is able to identify coping or adaptation skills.

GASTRIC ULCERS

A gastric ulcer is a well-defined break in the gastric mucosa that extends into the muscularis mucosae.

A gastric ulcer must be differentiated from a duodenal ulcer and from gastric erosion. Often gastric ulcers are included with duodenal ulcers and discussed under the classification of peptic ulcer disease. However, the etiology, incidence, and pathophysiology of gastric and duodenal ulcers are not the same. Duodenal ulcers are three to four times more common than gastric ulcers.[72] In gastric erosions, commonly seen in gastritis, healing occurs without the formation of the scar tissue formed when gastric ulcers heal.

The incidence of gastric ulcers is high in middle-aged and elderly persons, with a predominance of men. Gastric ulcers are strongly correlated with aspirin and alcohol abuse. Causative agents in addition to alcohol and aspirin include other drugs or agents that damage the gastric mucosal barrier. Aspirin abuse is considered to be the ingestion of 15 or more aspirins per week.[72]

Also of interest is that gastric ulcers are more common in people with type A blood (type O is more common in persons with duodenal ulcers). Gastric ulcers also occur within family groups. Patients with gastric ulcers also have an increased chance of developing a gastric malignancy. The relationship of gastritis to gastric ulceration has also been examined (p. 1168).

PATHOPHYSIOLOGY

Gastric ulcers are generally found at the junction of the fundic with the pyloric mucosa. Ulcers in the antrum are usually smaller than ulcers found in the proximal part of the stomach. Gastritis is more common in patients with gastric ulcers and will often be seen around the ulceration. The relationship of gastritis and gastric ulcer can be stated as follows: it appears that a gastric ulcer is more than a localized lesion and that gastritis contributes to the hyposecretion of gastric ulcers and to the susceptibility of the mucosa to ulcerate.

Patients with gastric ulcers have normal to below normal gastric acid secretion. If gastritis is also present, this will contribute to the hyposecretion of acid. An exception to the decreased acid production occurs when the gastric ulcer is close to the pylorus or is associated with a duodenal ulcer, in which case hypersecretion of acid occurs.

There are two proposed processes involved in the formation of gastric ulcers: back diffusion of acid and pyloric dysfunction. The normal gastric mucosa maintains a barrier against back diffusion by the tight junctions of epithelial cells that mechanically prevent reflux. The plasma membrane of the surface epithelial cells is made up of layers of lipids and contributes to the mucosa barrier.

Agents that are barrier breakers (aspirin, alcohol, indomethacin, etc.) disrupt the right junctions and acid flows back into the mucosa. Detergents and toxic agents can destroy the lipid plasma membrane. An example of a detergent is bile salts. When the mucosal barrier is damaged, acid diffuses back from the stomach into the mucosa. Histamine is released, stimulating more acid production, vasodilation, and increased capillary permeability. Bleeding may develop. Protein loss may occur, and an increased sodium content may be found in the stomach.

Bile is generally prevented from contact with the gastric mucosa by a competent pyloric sphincter. In gastric ulcer disease the pylorus does not respond normally to secretin or cholecystokinin and increase the pressure preventing reflux. Bile is allowed to reflux into the stomach.

Antral motility is also decreased in a patient with a gastric ulcer. The delay in gastric emptying may be observed during barium studies. The effect on antral motility appears to be more common in patients with gastric ulcers near the pylorus. The motility returns to normal when healing occurs.

The four layers of a peptic ulcer include the superficial layer, which lines the ulcer with a white fibrinous coat composed of leukocytes and erythrocytes; a second layer of fibrinoid necrosis; the next layer, inflammatory granulation tissue containing blood vessels; and the fourth layer, a dense scar of fibrous tissue lacking elastic tissue. The dense scar forms the base of the ulcer and extends beyond the margins of the mucosal defect. In a rapidly developing ulceration, massive bleeding may develop in asymptomatic patients when the vessel wall erodes. When the ulceration develops at a slower rate, inflammatory responses, thrombosis, and endarteritis occur and inhibit massive bleeding, and the patient experiences symptoms of peptic ulcer disease.

Ulcers heal slowly because of the scarred avascular tissue. The scarred mucosa over a healed ulcer contains patches of atrophic epithelium and scattered glands. The more scar tissue present, the thinner the mucosal layer. Endarteritis is frequent and the muscularis mucosae is interrupted and may be partially obliterated. The mucosa and glands that develop are often a simple pyloric type with areas of intestinalization, rather than gastric glands of the fundic type.

DIAGNOSTIC STUDIES

Double-contrast barium study
Detection of a gastric ulcer; when present, radiologist must determine if lesion is a gastric ulcer or a gastric carcinoma

Gastric analysis
Normal to decreased presence of acid

Gastric cytology
Abnormal findings would indicate gastric carcinoma

Endoscopy and biopsy
May identify gastric ulcer too shallow to detect with barium studies
Biopsy to rule out gastric cancer
Endoscopy repeated in 2 weeks for evaluation purposes

Serum gastrin levels
Normal or slightly elevated

Stool for guaiac
Often positive

TREATMENT PLAN

Surgical
Partial gastrectomy and vagotomy (used to treat complications of gastric ulcers: persistent bleeding; perforations)

Chemotherapeutic
Histamine receptor antagonists
Cimetidine (Tagamet), 300 mg po qid
Ranitidine (Zantac), 100 mg po bid
Antiulcer agents
Sucralfate (Carafate), 1 g po qid on an empty stomach (primary agent in duodenal ulcer, but may be ordered for gastric ulcer)
Antacids
Antacids, prn

Electromechanical
Ice water or saline lavage if bleeding
Arteriography with intra-arterial vasopressin

Supportive
Bland diet of six meals per day
Elimination of barrier breakers (aspirin, steroids, alcohol)
Elimination of smoking
Bed rest

ASSESSMENT: AREAS OF CONCERN

Gastric pain
Complaints of heartburn and dyspepsia
Note absence of duodenal pattern of pain; pain occurs closer to intake of food

Note relief of pain with a few ounces of antacids
Location of pain in left midepigastric area or pain radiating to the back (ulcer on posterior wall)
Vomiting, fullness, and distention may indicate delayed gastric emptying
Weight loss

Upper gastrointestinal bleeding
Hematemesis; melena
Change in vital signs; weakness; dizziness

Perforation
Sudden onset of severe, diffuse abdominal pain

NURSING DIAGNOSES and NURSING INTERVENTIONS

Nursing Diagnosis	Nursing Intervention
Tissue perfusion, alteration in: cerebral, cardiopulmonary, renal, gastrointestinal, peripheral	Give patient nothing to eat, and keep patient quiet if hemorrhage is a possibility. Maintain intravenous fluids and blood replacements as ordered. Monitor vital signs, central venous pressure, Swan-Ganz catheter, laboratory values, and urinary output. Observe patient for early signs of hypovolemic shock and initiate replacement of fluid volume. Institute ice water lavage as ordered. Prepare patient for diagnostic procedures.
Nutrition, alteration in: less than body requirements	Assess nutritional history, note any weight loss (associated with abdominal pain, distention after eating, and patient's limitation of intake) or gain (some patients may eat more in an attempt to decrease the pain). Provide six small meals per day. Monitor intake and output. Record nausea and vomiting. Administer antiemetics as ordered.

Patient Education

1. Teach patient about the relationship of causative agents to the development of gastric ulcers, recurrence rate (approximately 40%), and repeat of endoscopy.
2. Provide written information on medication regimen, and ensure that patient can identify the drugs and when each is to be taken, which require empty stomach vs. after a meal, and so forth.

EVALUATION

Patient Outcome	Data Indicating That Outcome is Reached
Gastric ulcer heals.	Findings on endoscopy are normal. There is no pain.
Patient adheres to plan of care.	Patient resumes a normal diet, avoids causative agents, and continues medical regimen as ordered for prophylaxis against recurrence.

GASTRIC CANCER

Gastric carcinoma refers to malignant neoplasms and tumors found in the stomach. Adenocarcinomas that arise from normal or metaplastic mucosa cells are the most common. Benign neoplasms of the stomach are rare and include leiomyomas and polyps.[69]

The incidence of gastric cancers has significantly decreased in western Europe and the United States. The American Cancer Society[10] estimates approximately 24,700 new cases in 1985. The ACS statistics of gastric cancer deaths decreased in males 59% (22.1 to 9.1 per 100,000) and in females 65% (11.7 to 4.1 per 100,000) from 1952 to 1979.[10] In the 1940s gastric cancer was the most common malignant disease in the United States.[11] No apparent change in the incidence of gastric cancer has occurred in Japan, where it accounts for 60% of all cancers in men and 40% of all cancers in women.[72]

Many questions exist about the decline in gastric cancer. The answers to those questions would provide valuable clues in the early diagnosis, treatment, and ultimately prevention of gastric carcinomas. In addition, interesting geographic variations exist. Gastric cancer is higher in the north central and northeast regions of the United States. It is more common in urban than rural areas in England, but this is not true in the United States. Although it is very common in Japan, gastric cancer is less common in Japanese persons in Hawaii and the incidence decreases with each generation. In 1980 Hawaiian Japanese individuals appeared to have the same low incidence rates as native Hawaiians.[69]

Genetic factors may play a role in the development of gastric cancer. Gastric cancers are more frequent in certain families and in persons with type A blood. In the United States, gastric cancer is more common in blacks than whites and in men than women. In Israel the incidence of gastric cancer is two and a half times higher in Jews of northern European backgrounds than Jews of Mediterranean or Asian descent.

The role of dietary factors has been studied to identify foods or soil contaminants that may lead to gastric cancers. Starches, pickled vegetables, and salted fish and meats have been associated with gastric cancers. However, whole milk, fresh vegetables, vitamin C, and refrigeration are inversely associated with gastric cancers.[35] Increased salt consumption is also seen in patients with gastric cancers. Nitrates, which are converted into nitrites, are commonly found in our diet. Compounds formed with nitrites (nitrosamines and nitrosamides) have been carcinogenic in animals. Although not confirmed as a carcinogen in humans, nitrite-forming bacteria are increased in the upper gastrointestinal tract in persons with hypochlorhydria and achlorhydria and following gastric surgery. Hypochlorhydria and achlorhydria are often found in patients with pernicious anemia and atrophic gastritis. The reduced acid appears to support or allow colonization of the stomach by the bacteria.

Cold temperatures inhibit the conversion of nitrates to nitrites. Better refrigeration and decreased use of nitrates as food additives might explain the decreased incidence of gastric cancers.[67]

Gastric cancer appears to be higher in individuals with late-onset immunoglobulin deficiency. Patients with celiac sprue with reduced IgA are at greater risk for gastric cancer.[72] Other factors associated with gastric cancer are gastric ulcers, atrophic gastritis, gastric polyps, pernicious anemia, and after gastrectomy.

PATHOPHYSIOLOGY

The carcinoma found in the stomach is epithelial growth arising from the mucosa membrane. Microscopically, the cells resemble intestinal metaplasia and contain goblet cells characteristic of the intestines. The parietal and chief glands of the stomach are seldom seen in gastric tumors. Adenocarcinomas in the stomach have been classified in several ways.

First, according to cellular or extracellular characteristics, carcinomas are referred to as papillary, colloid or mucinous, medullary, and signet ring.[69] Papillary refers to cells forming glandular structures in a papillary form. When excessive mucin secretion and extracellular aggregates are present, the adenocarcinoma is referred to as colloid or mucinous. Medullary is a solid band or a mass of undifferentiated cells. The signet ring adenocarcinoma refers to a well-differentiated adenocarcinoma with large amounts of intracellular mucinous material that compresses the nucleus to an unusual location.

Second, an adenocarcinoma of the stomach may be classified histologically according to the degree of cell differentiation from well differentiated to poorly differentiated.

Unfortunately, the preceding two classifications and their parts are not mutually exclusive. Various cellular characteristics and degrees of differentiation may occur within tumor. The third classification system reflects the biologic behavior of the tumor and defines gastric carcinomas as intestinal or diffuse.[41] The intestinal type is a glandular tumor, and the diffuse type is composed of single cells or small groups of cells.

The fourth system is an expansion of the intestinal and diffuse definitions and classifies cancers in the stomach as expanding or infiltrating.[45] The expanding (intestinal) type is characterized by a group of cells that are similar, maintain a coherent relationship, and push aside other cells as they grow. The infiltrative (diffuse) class is characterized by deep, wide infiltration by individual tumor cells.

The intestinal type of gastric cancer is associated with intestinal metaplasia and gastritis. The carcinoma tends to be circumscribed, and spread of the disease is through the bloodstream. The liver is a common site of metastasis. The diffuse type of carcinoma is less circumscribed, spreads by way of the lymphatics, and may take the form of linitis plastica, which is a diffuse fibrosis and thickening of the gastric wall.

The most common site of carcinomas is the lower half of the stomach. An exception occurs when gastric atrophy is a precursor to the cancer, and then the lesion tends to be in the upper portion of the stomach.

In early gastric cancers the disease is confined to the mucosa and submucosa. The symptoms with early gastric cancers may be vague and nonspecific. Early gastric cancers have been divided into three types:

Type I: polypoid or protruded
Type II: superficial
    IIa: elevated
    IIb: flat
    IIc: depressed
Type III: excavated

Advanced gastric cancer denotes involvement of the muscular layer of the stomach. Metastases, local and distant, are common. Advanced gastric carcinomas may be a polypoid or fungating mass, diffuse and infiltrating, or ulcerating.

Gastric ulcers have been associated with gastric cancers. This may be a diagnostic issue.[72] Previously radiologically diagnosed gastric ulcers have later been found to be carcinomas. Occasionally a benign gastric ulcer will have a focal carcinoma at a margin. Also malignant cells may be found at the base of the ulcer as well as at the margin. Most physicians will routinely do a biopsy of gastric ulcers during endoscopy to rule out the presence of gastric carcinoma.

Gastric atrophy and pernicious anemia are associated with achlorhydria. Achlorhydria is a precursor of gastric cancer. Gastric polyps are often found in atrophic mucosa. A polyp may be benign or malignant, and the recommended treatment is removal through an endoscope and histologic examination. Approximately 10% of gastric polyps will be malignant.[72]

DIAGNOSTIC STUDIES

Hematocrit
    Slightly below normal
    Patient may have macrocytic or microcytic anemia

secondary to decreased iron or vitamin B_{12} absorption

Stool for occult blood
    Positive for blood

Serum albumin
    Hypoalbuminemia

Plain chest film
    Distance between base of lung and stomach bubble greater than a few millimeters (gastric infiltration)
    Mass projecting into gas shadow of stomach
    Separation of gas shadow from diaphragm
    Absence of gas bubble

Upper gastrointestinal series (barium swallow)
    Polypoid mass
    Ulceration surrounded by mass
    Thickened, fibrosed gastric wall

Computed tomography
    Thickness of gastric wall
    Presence of metastasis (may assist in differentiating between benign and carcinogenic lesion)

Endoscopy and cytology
    Biopsy and cytology specimens examined for cancer cells
    Can visualize lesion
        Benign: sharply delineated with a white base and regular margins
        Malignant: gray with irregular margins and "heaped-up" edges[72]

Dye-spraying techniques
    During endoscopy, spray gastric mucosa with methylene blue; stains intestinalized mucosa; normal or cancerous mucosa uncolored

Liver function studies
    Abnormal findings may indicate metastasis

TREATMENT PLAN

Surgical
    Subtotal or total gastrectomy

Chemotherapeutic
    Antineoplastic agents
        Combination chemotherapy postoperatively
            5-Fluoruracil (5-FU) IV for 5 d q5wk; dosage: 12 mg/kg
            Methyl-CCNU, po q10wk
            Doxorubicin (Adriamycin), 60-75 mg/sq m IV at 21-d intervals

Electromechanical

Radiation therapy in combination with chemotherapy postoperatively

Immunotherapy: an investigational treatment at this time

Regular follow-up endoscopy procedures (1% to 2% may develop a second primary gastric carcinoma[52])

Supportive

Symptom management

ASSESSMENT: AREAS OF CONCERN

Stomach

Loss of appetite; anorexia

Feeling of fullness with minimal intake

Distaste for meats

Weight loss

Persistent midepigastric pain

Dysphagia

Physical examination

Tenderness in midepigastrium

Mass in epigastrium (late stage)

Enlarged liver

Positive supraclavicular nodes

Ascites (loss of albumin into gastric lumen)

Acanthosis nigricans (rare)

Signs of metastasis: myeloid metaplasia or primary CNS disease

NURSING DIAGNOSES and NURSING INTERVENTIONS

Nursing Diagnosis	Nursing Intervention
Coping, ineffective individual	Provide opportunities for patient to express feelings about diagnosis and prognosis. Assist patient in making adaptations or changes in activities and relationships.
Comfort, alteration in: pain	Provide analgesia for pain as ordered.
Nutrition, alteration in: less than body requirements	Weigh patient daily. Maintain intake and output records. Record symptoms associated with food intake before and after any surgical procedure. Ensure adequate caloric intake after surgery if dietary alterations must be made (i.e., tube feedings; use of high-calorie liquid supplements).
Coping, ineffective family: compromised	Provide opportunities for expression of feelings (gastric cancers may be diagnosed after metastasis has occurred and prognosis is poor). Provide information to assist patients and their families in working through their emotional reactions to disease, the treatment, and the prognosis.
Grieving, anticipatory	Support the patient and family during the dying phase. Identify appropriate resource people for the patient and family; these may include clergy, friends, and lawyers. Provide list of support groups (I CAN COPE; American Cancer Society). See also p. 1908.

Patient Education

1. Instruct the patient on the rationale for combination therapies of surgery, chemotherapy, and radiation therapy in the treatment of gastric cancers. Provide written information in the form of dos and don'ts during chemotherapy and radiotherapy, sequence of treatment, and potential side effects.
2. Instruct patient regarding the necessity for regular follow-up endoscopies.

EVALUATION

Patient Outcome	Data Indicating That Outcome is Reached
Patient can manage pain.	Patient is comfortable and able to relieve pain and symptoms effectively.
Patient adapts to or accepts disease and prognosis.	Patient has mobilized available resources to assist him and his family in handling the emotional, social, and financial stressors of having cancer. Patient attends ''I Can Cope'' groups.
Patient complies with medical regimen.	Patient has regular appointments with physician, maintains treatment sequence of drugs and radiotherapy, and reports signs of side effects. Patient uses home care (visiting) nurse to evaluate progress, reinforce teaching, and provide physical care as needed.
Laboratory findings are normal.	Hematocrit and albumin levels are within normal limits. Stools are negative for occult blood. There is no cancer on repeat endoscopy.
Nutritional status is adequate.	Caloric intake is maintained at level patient can tolerate. Weight loss is minimized.

DUODENAL ULCERS

A duodenal ulcer is a chronic circumscribed break in mucosa extending through the muscularis mucosae that leaves a residual scar with healing. The duodenal ulcer is the most common form of peptic ulcer disease.

The incidence of duodenal ulcers has been decreasing since the 1950s. At this writing, approximately 300,000 to 500,000 new cases of duodenal ulcer will develop each year.[69,72] Approximately 4 to 8 million Americans have active or recurrent ulcers.[69] The ratio of men to women is approximately 2:1. The decrease in duodenal ulcers has been attributed to changing environmental factors such as dietary habits and changing stress levels related to various historical occurrences. For example, urbanization at the beginning of the twentieth century was new and may have been a source of stress that has less effect in the 1980s. A profile of the person who develops duodenal ulcers has also changed. The incidence has declined in young women and increased in older women.

More efficient diagnostic techniques and treatment may also have a role in the decline of duodenal ulcers. The duodenal ulcer can be differentiated from dyspepsia, duodenitis, and gastric ulcer. Medical treatment with H_2 receptor antagonists has been successfully used, and patients often undergo diagnostic techniques and treatment as outpatients. Surgery is used only to manage complications of duodenal ulcers such as perforation.

Regional differences in duodenal ulcers have been recorded. For example, prevalence is higher in Scotland and northern England than southern England. In India, duodenal ulcers are more common in the south. Occupational factors have also been associated with duodenal ulcers. The common myth that duodenal ulcers occur in high-pressured professionals and executives is not true.[48,69] The duodenal ulcer is more common in the unskilled laborer and assembly-line workers. Duodenal ulcers have been found to be inversely related to family income and more frequent in persons with a low level of education.[56]

PATHOPHYSIOLOGY

The duodenal ulcer usually is less than 1 cm in diameter and is located 0.5 to 2.0 cm from the pylorus. Duodenal ulcers occur on both the anterior and posterior walls. The ulcers on the anterior wall appear to have a greater incidence of perforation. Posterior wall ulcers tend to be larger. The four layers of a peptic ulcer are as follows[70]:

1. Superficial layer lining the ulcer with a white fibrinous coat composed of leukocytes and erythrocytes
2. Zone of fibrinoid necrosis
3. Inflammatory granulation tissue
4. Layer of dense fibrosis tissue without elastic tissue (scar), forming the base of the ulcer and extending beyond the margins

Patients with duodenal ulcers secrete more gastric acid than normal in basal states and in response to stimuli. The increased acid production may be the result of an increased capacity to secrete hydrochloric acid because of increased parietal cell mass, or heightened vagal activity increasing the response to stimuli to overproduce acid, or a decreased ability to stop or "turn off" gastric secretions.

The nervous system phase of gastric secretions includes impulses from the cortex (limbic system and hypothalamus) to the vagal nerve. Vagal stimulation acts directly on the parietal cells and indirectly on the antral G cells to release gastrin. Pepsin and hydrochloric acid secretions are stimulated. The stimuli to the nervous system may include food in the mouth (tactile), thoughts and anticipation of food, or the sight of food.

Gastric activity also affects the regulation of secretions. Gastrin is stimulated by peptides and amino acids from digested proteins. Also distention of the antrum may cause a release of gastrin. Gastrin is released by G cells in the antrum and is also produced in the duodenum. A pH of 2.5 to 3.0 directly inhibits the secretion of gastrin and limits the overproduction of acid. Gastrin and acetylcholine directly affect the parietal cells. Histamine increases the parietal cells' response to other stimuli.

Acid chyme in the duodenum inhibits gastric secretions. Cholecystokinin plays a role in inhibiting the effects of gastrin by competing for similar receptors. Fat in the duodenum will also inhibit gastric acid secretions. Secretin and gastric inhibitory peptides inhibit gastric activity. Secretin also stimulates the pancreas, which secretes large amounts of bicarbonate to neutralize acids in the duodenum (see p. 1116 for additional information).

The person with a duodenal ulcer secretes a larger amount of gastric juices and may be unable to stop the release of gastrin in response to normal hormonal stimuli. The concentration of acid in the duodenum is higher than normal. Hypersecretion of acid, in and of itself, does not result in a duodenal ulcer. There appears to be a genetic predisposition to duodenal ulcers. If one or more members of one's immediate family have an ulcer, a person has an increased possibility of developing an ulcer. This relationship appears to be both genetically and environmentally related. People with blood type O are more likely to develop a duodenal ulcer, whereas individuals with blood type A are more likely to develop a gastric ulcer. The emotional aspects of the duodenal ulcer patient must also be considered. Ulcer patients (as a group) tend to repress external expressions of emotions and feelings. It may be that psychosocial stressors and increased susceptibility to stressful life events plus familial or environmental factors may be related to duodenal ulcers.

The more rapid the development of the ulcer, the more likely that blood vessels in the ulcer will show inflammatory changes, medial hypertrophy, or endarteritis. Blood vessels adjacent to the ulcer will have arteriosclerotic changes. The blood vessels 5 cm away from the ulcer will appear normal. In rapidly developing ulcers, bleeding is more common and may be massive because the blood vessel wall may erode in an asymptomic pa-

tient. In instances where the duodenal ulcer develops slowly, thrombosis, endarteritis, and inflammatory changes result in an avascular, scarred area that heals slowly.

In addition to upper gastrointestinal bleeding, other complications of duodenal ulcer disease include gastric outlet obstruction, perforation, and intractable pain. Obstruction of the gastric outlet may be caused by spasms, edema, or scarring. Protracted vomiting may indicate outlet obstruction.

Perforation is a very serious, life-threatening event. Perforation is seen in 2% to 5% of all duodenal ulcers. The overall incidence has been decreasing.

Intractability may develop from other complications of duodenal ulcers, stresses in patients' lives, and other disorders. Primarily, the patient no longer responds to medical management, or recurrences interfere with activities of daily living. Posterior penetration of the ulcer through the duodenal wall and into the pancreas will alter the pain. An increase in pain, loss of antacid relief, and radiation of pain to the back are the primary symptoms. Acute pancreatitis is rare but may occur.

DIAGNOSTIC STUDIES

Double-contrast barium studies
Presence of a crater or scar in duodenum
Delayed gastric emptying of barium (gastric outlet obstruction)
No evidence of marked scarring and minimal deformity of duodenal bulb (posterior penetration)

Abdominal films
Free air under diaphragm (perforation)

Endoscopy
Presence of an ulcer; degree of healing

Gastric analysis
Hypersecretion of gastric acid (also used to evaluate effectiveness of vagotomy in reducing acidity)
Nocturnal acid
Presence of blood in gastric analysis (may indicate bleeding)

Hematocrit and hemoglobin
Decreased (bleeding; microcytic anemia)

Stool for occult blood
Melena (may indicate bleeding)

Pepsinogen levels in blood
High levels associated with duodenal ulcers

Serum amylase
Increased with posterior penetration

TREATMENT PLAN

Surgical

Removal of a portion of gastrin-producing portion of stomach (antrectomy or partial gastrectomy) with attachment of duodenum to stomach (Billroth I) or attachment of stomach to jejunum (Billroth II) and vagotomy

Rarely indicated except for management of complications; there are many postsurgery problems: diarrhea, dumping syndrome, and recurrent ulcers

Chemotherapeutic

Antacids

Antacids (aluminum-magnesium regimen), po: provide 144 mEq buffering capacity 1 and 3 h after a meal and at bedtime (amount required varies based on commercial antacid used; Table 11-2)

Histamine receptor antagonists

Cimetidine (Tagamet), 300 mg qid po for 4-8 wk; with meals and at bedtime; prophylactic treatment: 400 mg at bedtime

Ranitidine (Zantac), 150 mg bid po

Antiulcer agents

Sucralfate (Carafate), 1 g qid on an empty stomach for 4-8 wk; avoid antacids 30 min before and after dose

Supportive

Stop smoking

Delete use of aspirin-containing compounds

Delete coffee (caffeinated and decaffeinated [stimulates gastric acid production])

Small, frequent meals recommended, with no bedtime snacks

Milk is not used as therapy (calcium and protein content stimulates gastric acid)

Avoid calcium carbonate antacids (rebound effect because of calcium content, hypercalcemia, renal stones) and sodium bicarbonate antacids (alkalosis, fluid retention)

ASSESSMENT: AREAS OF CONCERN

Pain

Well-localized epigastric pain occurring when stomach is empty (11 AM, 4 PM, 11 PM, 2 AM), relieved by food or antacids

Bowel habits

Constipation (may be related to diet and drugs)

Diarrhea (may be present from antacid therapy)

Abdominal tenderness

Physical examination; palpation denotes tenderness (anterior duodenal ulcers)

Upper gastrointestinal bleeding

Hematemesis

Melena

Dizziness or syncope

Decreased blood pressure and increased pulse

Decreased hematocrit

Perforation of duodenum

Sudden, severe, diffuse upper abdominal pain

Referred pain to shoulder

Rigid, boardlike abdomen

Rebound tenderness

Rapid, shallow respirations

Pyloric outlet obstruction

Protracted vomiting

Posterior penetration

Increased pain

Pain radiating to back

Loss of antacid relief

Table 11-2
Relative Potency of Liquid Antacids

Antacid	Potency*
Concentrated aluminum and magnesium hydroxides	
Delcid	100
Maalox Therapeutic Concentrates	75
Mylanta II	75
Gelusil II	60
Regular aluminum and magnesium hydroxides	
Maalox	45
Mylanta	40
Gelusil	40
Riopan	40
Aluminum hydroxide	
Alternagel	40
Amphojel	20

Adapted from Sleisenger, M.H., and Fortran, J.S.: Gastrointestinal disease, ed. 3, Philadelphia, 1983, W.B. Saunders Co.
*Millimoles of neutralizing capacity per 15 ml.

NURSING DIAGNOSES and NURSING INTERVENTIONS

Nursing Diagnosis	Nursing Intervention
Comfort, alteration in: pain	Provide frequent small meals and antacids at bedside.
	Observe for changes in nature, location, and relief of pain that would denote impending complications.
Noncompliance (medical therapy)	Evaluate patient's compliance with medical (drug) regimen and treatment plan; look for reasons for noncompliance (i.e., cost of antacids).
	Provide patient information and education to facilitate compliance.
Tissue perfusion, alteration in: cerebral, cardiopulmonary, gastrointestinal, peripheral	Give patient nothing to eat, and keep patient quiet if hemorrhage is actual or anticipated.
	Maintain IV therapy as ordered.
	Monitor vital signs, central venous pressure, Swan-Ganz catheter, laboratory values, and urinary output.
	Observe patients for early signs of hypovolemic shock, and initiate replacement of fluid volume as prescribed.
	Prepare patient for diagnostic procedures.
	Initiate ice water or saline lavages if ordered.

Patient Education

1. Provide instructions (verbal and written) on medication regimen; ensure that patient can identify drugs and when each is to be taken, which requires an empty stomach vs. after a meal, and so forth.
2. Provide information on relationship of duodenal ulcers and smoking, alcohol, coffee, aspirin-containing compounds, milk, and various antacids.

EVALUATION

Patient Outcome	Data Indicating That Outcome is Reached
Duodenal ulcer heals.	Endoscopic examination reveals normal findings and scar. There is no pain.
Patient adheres to plan of care.	Patient resumes a normal diet; avoids coffee, alcohol, aspirin, and smoking; and continues prophylactic medicines as ordered.

APPENDICITIS

Appendicitis is the inflammation of the vermiform appendix and may be classified as simple, gangrenous, or perforated. Simple appendicitis involves an inflamed and intact appendix, whereas in gangrenous appendicitis the appendix may have focal or extensive necrosis with microscopic perforations. Gross disruption of the appendix wall occurs in perforated appendicitis.

Acute appendicitis is one of the most common indications for emergency abdominal surgery. The rate of appendicitis is 1 to 2 per 1000 and is more common in adolescents and young adults. The diagnosis is difficult to determine in very young and elderly individuals. The very young child is often unable to describe the symptoms that are key clues to the diagnosis. In elderly persons the symptoms are vague and may cause a person to delay in seeking medical assistance, and then the physician may not consider appendicitis as a possibility. The abdominal tenderness in the elderly may be mild, making diagnosis more difficult. Acute appendicitis is more common in some families than others. Statistics show acute appendicitis slightly more common in males than females. The incidence for males is from 1.3 to 1.6 per 1000 persons as compared to 1 per 1000 persons for females.[72]

PATHOPHYSIOLOGY

Appendicitis can be compared to a closed loop obstruction in which obstruction occurs first and inflammation and infection second. In acute appendicitis the long narrow tube of the appendix is obstructed, hypoxia develops, the mucosa ulcerates, and bacteria invade the wall. The lumen of the appendix may be obstructed by a kinking of the appendix, edema of the lymphoid tissue, or a fecalith. Kinking of the appendix is uncommon. The lymphoid hyperplasia or edema may develop in response to a viral or bacterial infection. A fecalith is a formed, hard mass of feces. Fecaliths are associated with diets deficient in fiber. After the lumen obstructs, the mucosa continues to secrete fluid until the intraluminal pressure exceeds the venous pressure. Hypoxia develops because blood flow is impeded. The mucosal wall ulcerates and bacterial invasion occurs. The infection results in more edema, which further impedes blood flow. Gangrene and perforation occur in 24 to 36 hours. Perforation of the appendix creates serious complications, including periappendiceal abscess, pelvic abscess, or peritoneal inflammation.

Atypical appendicitis refers to situations in which the symptoms do not follow the classic presentation of appendicitis. The position of the appendix (retrocecal, pelvic, retroileal, preileal, subcecal), the age of the patient, and pregnancy may affect the symptoms of appendicitis, making diagnosis more difficult.

DIAGNOSTIC STUDIES

White blood cells
Elevated, with shift to the left; 10,000 to 16,000/cmm; 75% neutrophils

Abdominal films
Appearance of fecalith in right lower quadrant or localized ileus

Barium enema (under low pressure)
Nonfilling of the appendix and a mass (useful in atypical cases and infants); not commonly used in routine cases

Intravenous pyelogram (IVP)
To differentiate appendicitis from suspected urinary tract disease

Urinalysis
Small number of erythrocytes and leukocytes

TREATMENT PLAN

Surgical
Appendectomy

Chemotherapeutic
Anti-infective agents
Metronidazole (Flagyl) or cefamandole (Mandol) as a single prophylactic dose before surgery or for a period postoperatively (to prevent wound infection or pelvic abscess)

ASSESSMENT: AREAS OF CONCERN

Abdominal pain
Pain in epigastrium or periumbilical area that is colicky, peaks in 4 hours, and subsides
Pain reappears in right lower quadrant, is progressively severe, and is exacerbated by movement

Gastrointestinal functioning
May vomit once or twice; anorexia present
Constipation and failure to pass flatus

Physical examination
  Temperature
    Low-grade fever, does not usually exceed 39° C (102° F)

  Abdomen
    Patient can point to localized pain at McBurney's point (midway between iliac crest and umbilicus)
    Coughing or moving abdominal wall up and out will reproduce or exacerbate pain
    Rebound tenderness; muscle rigidity (palpate abdomen with *one* finger)
    Pain on palpation or percussion can be localized to a spot

  Rectum
    May be normal; if tenderness present, may be sign of obscure or atypical appendicitis

  Respirations
    Shallow, rapid

  Positioning
    Knees bent to reduce tension on abdominal muscles

Atypical appendicitis
  Retrocecal or retroileal
    Pain less intense (no discomfort with walking or coughing) and poorly localized
    Urinary frequency (irritation of ureter)

Pelvic
Very severe, constant pain
Localized pain on left
Urge to urinate and defecate
Tenderness on rectal examination
Absence of muscle rigidity and abdominal tenderness

In infants
Lethargy, irritability; anorexia

Localized tenderness by abdominal and rectal examinations (done under sedation)
May be complication of necrotizing enterocolitis

In elderly persons
Symptoms vague; pain minimal
Pain

In pregnancy
Late in gestation, diagnosis more difficult because of displacement of cecum by uterus

NURSING DIAGNOSES and NURSING INTERVENTIONS

Nursing Diagnosis	Nursing Intervention
Comfort, alteration in: pain	Record patient's description of the type of, duration of, changes in, and location of pain (key to diagnosis).
Tissue perfusion, alteration in: cerebral, cardiopulmonary, renal, gastrointestinal, peripheral	Observe patient carefully for signs of perforation and peritonitis: Fever Sudden relief of pain, followed by increased diffuse pain Increasing abdominal distention Tachycardia Rapid, shallow breathing Abdominal guarding Prepare patient for surgery as ordered. Provide preoperative teaching, keeping in mind that patient will be unable to practice turn, cough, and deep breathing exercises because of acute abdominal pain.
Fear	Provide emotional support for patient and family (pain is acute and frightening). Reassure patient during physical examination of the abdomen. Provide sedation as ordered for infants and young children before abdominal examinations.
Coping, ineffective individual	Assess patient developmentally (occurs most often in adolescents and young adults).

Patient Education

1. Wound or incisional care instructions should be provided.
2. A pattern of increasing activities (i.e., walking, driving) should be provided as recommended by the physician.

EVALUATION

Patient Outcome	Data Indicating That Outcome is Reached
Abdominal incision heals.	There is no abdominal pain. Incision heals with scar and absence of wound exudate, inflammation, and opened edges.
Activity level is normal.	Patient returns to presurgical activities, diet, and interests.

DIVERTICULAR DISEASE

Diverticulosis is an out-pocketing or herniation of the mucosa of the large colon through the muscle layers. At first, the diverticulum is reducible, but it will become fixed as the thin covering of longitudinal muscle fibers is lost. In prediverticular disease the pathologic, physiologic, and clinical features are similar to diverticulosis without the presence of diverticula.

Diverticulitis is the result of an inflammatory process and localized peritonitis following the perforation of a single diverticulum.

It is often difficult to distinguish between diverticulosis and diverticulitis based on symptoms and diagnostic findings. Spiro[72] recommends the use of a generic descriptive term: diverticular disease of the colon.

The incidence of diverticular disease has increased, and the disorder is more common in Western countries. Australia, the United States, the United Kingdom, and France have high rates of diverticular disease, while African, Asian, and Third World countries have low rates. The epidemiology reports based on clinical observations of colon pressures (manometric) related diverticular disease to low-residue diets. When a Western diet is adopted by blacks in Africa, diverticular disease develops.[67,72]

Diverticular disease is seldom seen in persons under 30 years and increases in frequency with age. Approximately one third of individuals over 60 years have diverticular disease and less than 5% of people with diverticular disease are under age 40.[67] Diverticula are most often found in the sigmoid colon.[69] While women are reported to have more diverticular disease than men, autopsy studies demonstrate that the disease is about equal in both sexes.[72] Bleeding from diverticular disease is one of the most common causes of lower gastrointestinal hemorrhage.[69]

PATHOPHYSIOLOGY

The development of diverticula is related to muscle activities and intraluminal pressures. Normal intraluminal pressure is less than 10 mm Hg in the sigmoid colon. The normal pressure can be increased significantly when the bowel is divided into segments by the muscular contraction rings. The muscular activities in the localized segments can exert enough pressure to increase intracolonic pressure to 90 mm Hg, and this high pressure may push out diverticula.

The outer longitudinal muscle layer in the colon forms a continuous sheath around the colon and is concentrated into three narrow bands, or teniae. The diverticula are usually found between the mesenteric teniae and the antimesenteric teniae. When the circular muscle layer is prominent, the neck of the diverticulum will be narrow.

The muscular weakness that develops with age may result in simple asymptomatic diverticulosis in which the mucosa slips through a weakened musculature. The hernias, or out-pockets, are not fixed and may move back and forth, disappearing on occasion. Muscular hypertrophy in the sigmoid colon may cause thick and prominent longitudinal muscles as well as a thick and corrugated circular muscle layer in the colon. The bowel lumen is constricted by the muscular thickening and the redundant folds. No diverticula are present, but clinical symptoms and radiologic studies often lead to a diagnosis of diverticulosis. This disorder is commonly referred to as prediverticulitis.

Constipation has also been associated with diverticular disease. More pressure is required to move hard, dry fecal material through the lumen. High-fiber diets are associated with moist, soft stools. Multiple bowel movements each day are also associated with high-residue diets. The decrease in segmentation and intracolonic pressure with high-residue diets may lessen diverticular disease.

Normal vs. abnormal colonic motility is a key issue in examining diverticular disease. Normal colonic motility has been defined as an absence of abdominal pain, whereas pain is present with abnormal colonic motility.[72] The person with abdominal pain with other symptoms of diverticulosis and without radiologic indications of diverticula may still be classified as having diverticular disease based on colonic motility assessments.

The blood flow to the large colon runs from the mesentery around the bowel and divides into branches that go subserosally. These vessels enter the circular muscle obliquely from the mesenteric side of the bowel between the mesenteric and lateral teniae. There is a rich submucosa plexus around the circumference of the colon. The diverticulum that pushes out under the muscular coat has a prominent vasculature over the dome of the diverticulum and at the antimesenteric border of the orifice of the diverticulum. Major bleeding associated with diverticular disease is associated with the large vessel over the dome. Localized inflammation at the base of the diverticulum with vascular granulation tissue may be the source of minor bleeding from diverticula.

Previously, diverticulitis was believed to be inflammation or abscess formation with a diverticulum that progressed to ulceration and perforation. It is now thought that diverticulitis is the result of a single perforating diverticulum leading to free perforation or a localized pericolic abscess. The etiology leading to the perforation of the diverticulum may include increased intracolonic pressures and abrasions by fecal material.

During episodes of increased intracolonic pressure, fecal abrasions may progress to small diverticular perforations. Fecal material may irritate the mucosa, causing inflammation at the apex or neck of the diverticulum and leading to perforation. Localized peritonitis is more common when the perforation has occurred gradually.

DIAGNOSTIC STUDIES

Barium enema
Demonstrates diverticulum and shortening, narrowing, and haustral deformity

Ultrasonography
May demonstrate mass or abscess

Sigmoidoscopy or colonoscopy
Orifices of the diverticula may be visible (high risk of perforation if instrument enters a diverticulum)

Intravenous pyelogram
To rule out a mass on the left ureter or a colonic vesical fistula

White blood cells
Elevated with a shift to the left in diverticulitis

Urinalysis
A few red cells may be found in urine if left ureter is affected

TREATMENT PLAN

Surgical*
Sigmoid myotomy (allows colon to resume its width and length)
Bowel resection with or without temporary diverting colostomy
Intestinal obstruction: diverting colostomy in transverse colon
Bladder fistula: resection of fistula, portion of bladder and colon removed, reanastomosis of bladder wall, reanastomosis of colon with or without temporary diverting colostomy
Surgical resection if bleeding uncontrolled by medical management

*Most cases are treated medically; surgery is used only in acute diverticulitis with perforation.

Chemotherapeutic
Diverticulosis
Bran, 10 to 25 g/d in divided doses (must slowly increase to develop tolerance; will help relieve abdominal pain; lowers intraluminal pressure)
Laxatives
Hydrophilic colloid laxatives (rather than bran in acute phases may be better tolerated; slowly decrease amount as bran and fiber in diet increase)

Diverticulitis
Intravenous fluid therapy
Narcotic analgesic
Meperidine (Demerol) for analgesia (dose calculated for patient)
Anti-infective agents
Ampicillin (Amcill), 2.0 g, *or*
Cephalexin (Keflex), 1-4 g/d parenterally in divided doses (mild diverticulitis)
Anti-infective agents
Gentamicin (Garamycin) or tobramycin (Nebcin), 5.0 mg/kg/d, and clindamycin (Cleocin), 1.6 to 2.4 g/d parentally in divided doses (severe diverticulitis or perforation)
Chloramphenicol (Chloromycetin), 4 g/d tapering to 2 g/d (severe diverticulitis)
Cefoxitin (Mefoxin), 4 to 6 g/d parenterally in divided doses
All anti-infective agents continued for 7-10 d; not all listed would be used

Electromechanical
Nasogastric tube inserted if nausea, vomiting, and abdominal distention are severe
Radiographic studies and ultrasonography used to evaluate the response to therapy (i.e., resolution of abscess)
Carcinoma: difficult to detect in bowel with narrowed areas and partial obstruction; use colonoscopy procedures to distinguish between acute diverticular disease and carcinoma following an acute episode
Bleeding; angiographic injection of vasopressin, 0.5 to 1.0 ml/min

Supportive
High-fiber diet for managing diverticulosis
Give nothing to eat initially in acute diverticulitis; slowly resume diet; when inflammation has resolved and bowel functioning returns to normal, resume high-fiber diet
For acute diverticulitis, bed rest

ASSESSMENT: AREAS OF CONCERN

Pain

Aching pain in left lower quadrant, tenderness; suprapubic pain may be reported; referred pain from lower colon is to the back

Pain more intense with acute diverticulitis

Urinary system

Dysuria; frequency

Passage of gas or stool through urethra (colovesical fistula)

Abdominal examination

Diverticulosis: tenderness in left lower colon; palpable colon

Diverticulitis: palpable colon, tenderness in left lower quadrant, distended and tympanic abdomen, decreased bowel sounds

Obstructed lumen: increased bowel sounds (if partial) may become an ileus (if total), abdominal distention (p. 1193)

Blood counts

Elevated white count in acute diverticulitis

Bowel habits

Constipation

Dark red (maroon) or bright red blood with bowel movements; blood clots may pass via rectum in massive bleeds

Temperature

Elevated in diverticulitis

Upper gastrointestinal system

Nausea; vomiting; anorexia

Rectal examination

Tenderness, induration, and a mass in cul-de-sac (acute diverticulitis)

NURSING DIAGNOSES and NURSING INTERVENTIONS

Nursing Diagnosis	Nursing Intervention
Tissue perfusion, alteration in: cerebral, cardiopulmonary, renal, gastrointestinal, peripheral	Observe patient for lower gastrointestinal bleeding. Monitor patient for any symptoms of sepsis. Monitor vital signs, intake, and output. Maintain intravenous fluids as ordered to maintain intravascular fluid balance.
Comfort, alteration in: pain	Provide analgesic as ordered. In acute phase, provide low-residue diet (patients with acute and chronic disease should avoid nuts and popcorn). Provide bran or high fiber in diverticulosis. Discuss with patient efficacy of increased fiber, how to increase fluids, and activities to prevent constipation.
Bowel elimination, alteration in: constipation	Provide bran or hydrophilic colloid laxatives as ordered. Increase oral fluid intake. Initiate dietary consultation or provide information on high-residue diets. Assist patient to increase activity. See p. 2062 for management of temporary colostomy and interventions related to care and adaptation.

Patient Education

1. Dietary instructions on high-residue diet should be provided. Teach patient ways to make bran more palatable (e.g., muffins, use on cereals).
2. Discharge instructions should include relationships of diet to diverticular disease, assessment of bowel movements to evaluate dietary intake of bran and fluids, and signs of complications of acute diverticular disease.
3. Instruct patient in bowel training, that is, to set aside a time daily without anxiety or interruption to have a bowel movement.
4. See p. 1273 for colostomy care instructions.

EVALUATION

Patient Outcome	Data Indicating That Outcome is Reached
Body functioning is normal.	Bowel movements are soft and at least once per day. There is no abdominal pain, nausea, vomiting, and anorexia. Temperature is normal. Temporary colostomy, if performed, is closed. Patient is able to describe high-fiber diet, plan meals, and describe medications and relationship of foods and drugs to disease.
Diagnostic findings are normal.	White blood cell count is within normal range. There is no evidence of acute disease or carcinoma on radiologic study or colonoscopy.
Abdominal incision (if surgical intervention required) heals.	There is no abdominal pain; incision heals with scar and absence of wound exudate, inflammation, and open edges.

HERNIATION

A hernia is a protrusion of an organ (usually bowel) through an abnormal opening in the muscle wall. Hernias may be congenital (failure of certain structures to close after birth) or acquired when muscle weakens (associated with obesity, surgery, or illness or from increased abdominal pressure secondary to straining or ascites).

Hernias may be found in any age group. There is a common association between heavy lifting and hernia formation. Regardless of whether the hernia is congenital or acquired, the primary concern is the possibility of obstruction of the bowel lumen, ischemia to the segment or decrease in blood flow, and loss of blood leading to necrosis and perforation. Congenital internal hernias may be diagnosed because of the complication of intestinal obstruction.

PATHOPHYSIOLOGY

Internal congenital hernias are associated with a failure of the intestine to rotate in the usual sequence in the fetus. There are three stages of rotation. Initially the intestine is an unattached, mobile tube; during gestation, as the loop of bowel forming the midgut elongates, it migrates into the umbilicus cord and rotates 180 degrees counterclockwise with the mesenteric vessels as an axis. As the intestines return to the peritoneal cavity, rotation 90 degrees counterclockwise occurs. The cecum will pan from the left side of the abdomen over the superior mesenteric vessels toward the right lower quadrant. The duodenum, descending colon, and the mesentery of the small intestines are fixed to the posterior abdominal wall. The mesentery of the bowel follows an oblique path

across the abdomen from the ligament of Treitz (upper left) to the lower right quadrant. When this series of events does not occur, complications develop. The infant may be born with an omphalocele, nonrotation, reversed rotation, or malrotation. The results are abnormal adhesions, fixations and bands that lead to obstructions, volvulus, and internal hernias.

Internal hernias are associated with malrotation. Paraduodenal hernias develop when the mesentery is not fixed. Left-sided paraduodenal hernias are more common than right-sided paraduodenal hernias. The left paraduodenal hernia forms when the rotation of the midgut was reversed. The duodenum lies posterior to the descending colon and separated from the rest of the peritoneum. Paracecal hernias are also associated with malrotation.[72]

External hernias include inguinal, femoral, umbilical, and incisional hernias. The inguinal hernia is the most common. It is a weakness in the abdominal wall where the spermatic cord (men) or the round ligament (women) emerges. In an indirect inguinal hernia the herniation protrudes through the inguinal ring and follows the round ligament or spermatic cord. A direct inguinal hernia goes through the posterior inguinal wall. Inguinal hernias are more common in men.

A femoral hernia, or protrusion through the femoral ring into the femoral canal, is seen as a bulge below the inguinal ligament. It occurs more frequently in women. Femoral hernias strangulate easily.

The umbilical hernia is more common in children and occurs when the umbilical opening fails to close after birth.

Ventral and incisional hernias are associated with muscle weakness from abdominal incisions. Hernias after surgery are more common in obese persons, those with ascites, and those who have had wound infections or wounds healed by secondary intention.

TREATMENT PLAN

Surgical

Herniorrhaphy (surgical repair of hernia) or hernioplasty (reinforcement of weakened area with wire, fascia, or mesh)

Temporary colostomy (for complications of intestinal obstruction or strangulation of hernia)

Electromechanical

Binder or truss (to reduce hernia and to prevent protrusion; danger: strangulation if not reduced properly)

ASSESSMENT: AREAS OF CONCERN

Physical examination of abdomen

Examine patient supine and sitting

Can often see hernia "bulge" or protrude as person changes position, coughs, or when children cry or laugh (many patients have a history of being able to reduce their own hernias before seeking repair)

Palpate weakened muscle area

Abdominal distention, nausea, and vomiting may be early signs of intestinal obstruction

Pain of increasing severity, fever, tachycardia, and abdominal rigidity are signs of strangulations

NURSING DIAGNOSES and NURSING INTERVENTIONS

Nursing Diagnosis	Nursing Intervention
Tissue perfusion, alteration in: cerebral, cardiopulmonary, renal, gastrointestinal, peripheral	Observe patient for signs of impending intestinal obstruction or strangulation and ischemia of the herniation (pp. 1195 and 1200). Provide preoperative teaching. Assess postoperatively for complications related to anesthesia and surgery: hemorrhage, shock, and respiratory distress. Ambulate patient per physician's order. Apply scrotal support for inguinal hernia repairs. Use ice packs for scrotal edema following surgery.
Urinary elimination, alteration in patterns	Assess urination pattern (may have difficulty voiding postoperatively). Assess bladder for distention. Assist patient in standing to void.
Gas exchange, impaired	Have patient turn and deep breathe following surgery. Avoid coughing since it will increase pressure or strain on muscles. Teach patient to splint incision with hands or pillows if necessary to cough or sneeze.
Skin integrity, impairment of: potential	Assess patient's skin for irritation from binders or from a truss. Evaluate the binder for size, pressure points, and effectiveness in maintaining a reduced hernia.

Patient Education

1. Inform the patient of the necessity for weight reduction if the patient is obese.
2. Patient should avoid heavy lifting for 6 to 8 weeks unless otherwise specified by physician.
3. If patient is discharged using a binder, provide correct instructions for application. Teach patient to observe the skin for irritation and to evaluate the effectiveness of the system.

EVALUATION

Patient Outcome	Data Indicating That Outcome is Reached
Patient recovers from surgical procedures.	Hernia, or bulge is absent. Incision heals with scar and absence of wound infection, open edges, and exudate. Patient returns to presurgical activity with delayed return to lifting objects.

HIRSCHSPRUNG'S DISEASE

Hirschsprung's disease is a congenital disorder in which the autonomic nerve ganglia in the smooth muscle of the colon are absent. The aganglionic segment may be limited or occasionally involve the entire colon. There is absence of peristalsis in the involved narrowed segment progressing to stasis of stool and dilation of the proximal colon, commonly referred to as congenital megacolon.

Hirschsprung's disease is a familial disease, occurring in approximately 1 out of 5000 live births and is more common in males than females with a ratio of 3.8 to 1.[6,72] The incidence of long-segment disease is more common in females and has a greater risk of being found in siblings. Approximately 75% of patients with Hirschsprung's disease have aganglionosis in the rectum and lower sigmoid colon extending proximally above the anorectal junction. In short-segment Hirschsprung's disease, aganglionosis is to and below the anorectal junction. Ultrashort-segment Hirschsprung's disease is limited to the anal canal. The entire colon may be aganglionic in 5% to 8% of the cases.[69,72]

Hirschsprung's disease is associated with Down's syndrome. Although congenital megacolon and Down's syndrome occur in approximately 2% of the cases, Hirschsprung's disease is also associated with other anomalies such as megacystis and megaureter, hydrocephalus, ventricular septal defect, cystic deformities of the kidney, imperforate anus, Meckel's diverticulum and familial polyposis.

Although Hirschsprung's disease is more commonly diagnosed and treated in children, occasionally adults will have previously undiagnosed disease. The older individual generally has a history of chronic constipation and regular use of enemas. Fecal masses may be palpable in the colon.

PATHOPHYSIOLOGY

The primary problem in Hirschsprung's disease is the absence of ganglion cells in the submucosa (Meissner's plexus) and intramuscular (Auerbach's plexus) layers of the bowel wall. The aganglionosis develops when the caudal migration of cells from the neural crest fails. Although the cause is unknown, congenital susceptibility and an ischemic episode (before or after birth) may be responsible for Hirschsprung's disease. Anoxia of the bowel for 4 hours has been found to destroy intramural ganglion cells in the colon of mice and is postulated as a part of the etiology of Hirschsprung's disease.[33]

The aganglionic segment is narrowed and strictured. This segment is permanently contracted. The bowel proximal to the aganglionic segments hypertrophies and dilates, hence the term *megacolon*. The bowel contents fail to enter the aganglionic segment, and a functional obstruction occurs.

The relaxation of the internal anal sphincter is a normal response to rectal distention. This response is absent in Hirschsprung's disease. Rather than relaxing, the internal sphincter contracts. The internal sphincter represents the distal end of the circular smooth muscle, and the aganglionic portion of the colon adjacent to the internal anal sphincter also contracts rather than relaxing. Resting pressure in the internal sphincter is normal or slightly elevated in Hirschsprung's disease, with the inappropriate contraction as a response to rectal distention.

The rectal wall in Hirschsprung's disease has an increased resistance to stretch that has been related to the prognosis of clinical symptoms. The more resistance present, the more severe the clinical symptoms.[2] Acetylcholinesterase has been found in excessive amounts in aganglionic segments. The enzyme is used in nerve impulse transmissions. The presence of acetylcholinesterase in serum and red blood cells and in superficial biopsy specimens may be used as a diagnostic test for Hirschsprung's disease. In Hirschsprung's disease the enzyme cannot be used by the aganglionic segments, resulting in higher levels.

DIAGNOSTIC STUDIES

Full-thickness biopsy of bowel wall
Biopsy should be obtained at least 3 cm proximal to pectinate line
Absence of ganglion cells indicates Hirschsprung's disease

Mucosal suction biopsy
Presence of ganglia in Meissner's plexus excludes Hirschsprung's disease
Absence of ganglia cells does not establish diagnosis and is followed by full-thickness biopsy

Barium enema
Narrowed distal rectal or rectosigmoid segment with dilated proximal colon is indicative of Hirschsprung's disease (exception: infants in which narrowed segment will not have had time to develop significantly)
Retention of barium enema at 24 hours is suggestive of Hirschsprung's disease

Proctosigmoidoscopy
Normal empty rectum with no evidence of organic obstruction indicative of Hirschsprung's disease

Manometry
Loss of normal relaxation response of internal anal sphincter (test is recommended in older children and is supportive but not diagnostic by itself; false negative or false positive in 10% of cases)

Staining biopsy specimens for acetylcholinesterase
Elevated levels in Hirschsprung's disease

Differential diagnosis of acquired megacolon or habitual constipation
Stool present in rectum and fecal soiling more common in acquired megacolon
History of constipation for several weeks

TREATMENT PLAN

Surgical
Diverting temporary colostomy for proximal decompression
Definitive surgery involves removal of the aganglionic segment and a pull-through procedure of the ganglionic bowel to the anus (commonly used pull-through procedures: Swenson, Duhamel, and Soave)

Supportive
Enemas may be used for decompression before surgery but are not recommended for long-term treatment protocols

ASSESSMENT: AREAS OF CONCERN

Infant
Abdomen
Abdominal distention
Functional bowel obstruction
Vomiting
Gas and fluid-filled loops of small intestine on x-ray examination

Rectum
Initial passage of meconium delayed
Absence of stool in rectum (following rectal examination there may be a gush of meconium and a temporary decompression of bowel)

Enterocolitis
Bloody diarrhea
Fever
Explosive, watery diarrhea
Rapid onset of dehydration
Perforation
Pericolic abscess
Septicemia

Young child: abdominal examination and history
Persistent abdominal distention; recurrent fecal impaction and constipation
Fecal mass may be palpable in left colon
Growth and mental retardation
History of congenital anomalies

Adult: abdominal examination and history
Chronic intermittent constipation requiring enemas
Abdominal distention

NURSING DIAGNOSES and NURSING INTERVENTIONS

Nursing Diagnosis	Nursing Intervention
Bowel elimination, alteration in: constipation	Examine the abdomen of neonate who has not passed meconium in the first 48 to 72 hours for signs of intestinal obstruction. Report presence of abdominal distention, repeated vomiting, and constipation or diarrhea (diarrhea may be early sign of associated enterocolitis). Monitor intake and output. Replace fluid losses as ordered. Give enemas as ordered; observe patient carefully for complications of procedure. Amount is determined according to body size: 1. Tap water enemas (greater than 2 L): readily absorbed in dilated, hypertrophied colon; assess for water intoxication 2. Soapsuds enemas: carry risk of causing soapsuds colitis 3. Mineral oil enemas: may be valuable in lubricating very dry stool in colon 4. Saline enemas: shock has been reported from absorption of water from excessive quantities of isotonic saline enemas 5. Hypertonic phosphate enemas: in infants and young children may be a problem; large quantities of water move into colon while sodium or phosphate or both are absorbed; central nervous system changes related to sodium concentrations; tetany related to hyperphosphatemia and hypocalcemia Observe colostomy stoma for mucocutaneous junction, stoma color, and bowel functioning. Apply skin barrier and pouch to protect the skin and contain the stool (see p. 1273 for colostomy care).
Parenting, alteration in: potential	Provide parents with an opportunity to nurture and care for the child during initial and subsequent hospitalizations. Provide ongoing support for families during hospital and outpatient experiences. Coordinate an interdisciplinary approach including the patient, family, primary physician, surgeon, ET nurse, primary nurse, and social worker.
Skin integrity, impairment of: potential	Provide skin protection from colostomy effluent with solid-form skin barriers and open-ended drainable pouches. Provide skin protection for the perineal area following the pull-through procedures (diarrhea is a common postoperative problem and can progress to extremely denuded or severely irritated perineal skin). Use a combination of perineal skin cream and a perineal ointment if diarrhea or incontinence occurs postoperatively.

Patient Education

1. Prepare the parents to care for the colostomy (p. 1273).
2. Teach young child to empty his pouch and progress to self-care as appropriate to age level of child.

EVALUATION

Patient Outcome	Data Indicating That Outcome is Reached
Body functioning is normal.	Patient is continent for bowel elimination. There is no diarrhea, constipation, or skin irritations. Sexual potency (the nerve innervation for erection, ejaculation, and orgasm in males) can be affected by surgery in the rectal area.

INTESTINAL OBSTRUCTIONS

An intestinal obstruction occurs when the contents of the intestines fail to propel forward through the lumen. Intestinal obstructions may be mechanical or functional.

Mechanical obstructions are caused by a blockage of the bowel lumen by adhesion, hernia, volvulus, tumor, inflammation (as in Crohn's disease), impacted feces, or intussusception. Functional obstructions are also referred to as ileus and occur when there is a loss of propulsive peristalsis associated with abdominal surgery, hypokalemia, intestinal distention, peritonitis, severe traumas, spinal fractures, ureteral distention, or the effects of some narcotic drugs and diphenoxylate (Lomotil).

Intestinal obstructions are more common in persons who have undergone abdominal surgery or who have had congenital abnormalities of the bowel. An intestinal obstruction can progress, if untreated, to a serious life-threatening disorder. The severity and types of symptoms will vary according to the etiology and the location of the intestinal obstruction. Ninety percent of intestinal obstructions are the result of adhesions or incarcerated hernias. Intussusceptions are the most common cause of intestinal obstructions in children between the ages of 2 months and 5 years.[70]

Mechanical obstructions can be caused by factors that block the lumen of the bowel wall, in which case they are referred to as obturation obstructions. This category includes intussusception, large gallstones, feces, meconium, or bezoars. Intrinsic factors that may progress to mechanical obstructions include congenital atresia or stenosis; strictures associated with chronic inflammation or neoplasms; iatrogenic strictures following intestinal surgery or radiation therapy; and mesenteric vascular occlusion. Extrinsic factors that may lead to mechanical obstructions of the intestine are the most common cause of intestinal obstructions and include adhesions, hernias, neoplasms, abscesses, and volvulus.

Mechanical obstructions may be simple obstructions in the small bowel or colon or may present as strangulation obstructions. The location of a mechanical obstruction is important in determining the sequelae. Simple mechanical obstructions may resolve medically, whereas strangulation obstructions require surgical intervention.

The paralytic ileus or functional obstruction commonly occurs in patients undergoing abdominal surgery. Prolonged intestinal distention, hypokalemia, peritonitis, narcotic use, and intestinal ischemia are associated with the development of an ileus.

PATHOPHYSIOLOGY

An accumulation of fluid and gas proximal to an obstruction occurs in a simple mechanical obstruction of the small bowel. Initially, the pooled fluids include ingested foods and digestive enzymes. Intestinal gas, in obstruction, is primarily made up of swallowed air that has high concentrations of nitrogens and is not absorbed by the intestinal mucosa. The distention of the bowel by the trapped fluids and gases causes the small bowel to secrete water and electrolytes into the obstructed lumen.

The distention impedes venous return, and the absorptive ability of the mucosa is inhibited. The bowel wall becomes edematous. The bowel continues to secrete water, sodium, and potassium into the obstructed segment. As the obstruction continues, the intestinal distention is self-perpetuating. Distention increases the intestinal secretions of water and electrolytes into the lumen. As fluid and gas pour into the intestine, motility is further compromised and the distention propagates proximally. Successive loops of proximal bowel will distend, fill with fluid, and stop absorbing. Transudation of water through the wall of the obstructed segment may develop, leading to the development of peritoneal fluid. It should also be noted that distention may lead to pressure necrosis of the bowel wall.

Bacteria are not usually found in the small intestine. During intestinal obstructions, an abnormal bacteria flora that rapidly proliferates is found in the intestinal lumen. The bacteria produce some hydrogen or methane gas that contributes to the gaseous distention. Also, the small bowel contents become feculent during obstructions as a result of the bacterial proliferation.

The site and duration of intestinal obstruction will affect the symptoms and potential metabolic effects. Obstructions in the upper jejunal area usually result in vomiting and little abdominal distention. Dehydration and electrolyte depletion occur.

In distal small bowel obstruction or ileal obstructions, constipation is an early symptom. Vomiting, not a prominent symptom, is less effective in reducing intestinal decompression. Reflex vomiting may result from intestinal distention. In distal small bowel obstruction, large quantities of fluid and electrolytes may become trapped in the intestinal lumen, resulting in passage of gas and nausea. As much as 8 L of fluids may be found in the lumen with untreated, prolonged obstructions.[72] The patient has classic signs and symptoms of circulatory shock (severe hypovolemia). Before the development of shock, dehydration and metabolic acidosis accompanied by oliguria, azotemia, and hemoconcentration occur. Early circulatory changes may be detected by tachycardia, low central venous pressure, and hypotension. Hypovolemic shock develops if the obstruction is not treated.

The intestinal distention can impair pulmonary ventilation because abdominal distention causes elevation of the diaphragm. The increased intra-abdominal pressure caused by the intestinal distention may impede venous return from the legs.

Death of the bowel wall, or bowel necrosis, complicates intestinal obstructions. Shock can quickly develop when long loops of bowel are affected. Short-segment involvement progresses quickly to perforation and peritonitis.

Impaired circulation to the bowel wall during obstructions is referred to as a strangulation obstruction. The circulation may be impeded by a closed-loop obstruction that causes occlusion of the lumen at two points along the length of the bowel segment. Volvulus is an example of a closed-loop obstruction. The closed loop obstruction will progress to strangulation more rapidly than a simple mechanical blockage of the lumen. The circulation to the bowel may also be impaired by a sustained increase in intraluminal pressure, as with intestinal distention.

When the circulation is impaired, the venous outflow is impaired and the mural veins become engorged. The bowel wall becomes ischemic. An arterial spasm follows, and the bowel responds to anoxia with increased peristalsis. Within 15 minutes, blood escapes from the engorged veins and infiltrates the submucosa and mucosa, resulting in a hemorrhagic infarction of the tissues. Venous thrombosis occurs, further compromising circulation. The necrosis develops from the mucosa outward. Small intravascular thrombi extend the area of necrosis. The lymph channels dilate and may carry bacteria from the lumen into the serosa. Initially, the fluid accumulating resembles plasma, and it gradually becomes bloody and contains bacteria and toxins.

Strangulation results in loss of blood and plasma from the affected segment. Shock occurs quickly if the patient had been dehydrated before strangulation developed. Gangrene may develop and progress to peritonitis. Perforation of the strangulated segment may occur. The toxic substance released during a strangulation obstruction into the peritoneum and the circulation is lethal when given to normal animals. The toxic material may be absorbed from the peritoneal cavity, producing systemic effects. Bacterial infection and toxemia are generally felt to be responsible for the shock that can quickly develop in strangulation obstructions.

In colonic obstructions the colon may become massively distended by gas. Fluid and electrolyte losses are not as significant as in small bowel obstructions and occur when the obstruction is prolonged. When the ileocecal valve is competent, there will be little if any small bowel

distention present. However, a competent ileocecal valve may resist backward decompression enough to produce a closed-loop obstruction. If this develops, cecal distention may be significant and may progress to perforation of the cecum.

The most common cause of colon obstruction is cancer, and perforation during obstructive episodes is adjacent to the tumor. As in small bowel obstructions, the patient must be carefully observed for signs and symptoms of strangulation obstruction.

DIAGNOSTIC STUDIES

History and physical examination
Crampy abdominal pain, the onset of which is clearly recalled
Vomiting
Obstipation
Abdominal distention and tenderness
Peristaltic rushes

Serial abdominal x-ray films
Abnormally large amounts of gas in the bowel
Films taken with patients standing or sitting; supine; and on left side

Barium enema*
Barium will clear entire colon or stop at site of obstruction

Serum electrolytes
Demonstrates electrolyte losses

White blood cell count
Sudden rise greater than 10,000 indicates strangulation

Serum amylase
Normal value rules out acute pancreatitis

Hemoglobin or hematocrit
Raised values indicate hemoconcentration secondary to fluid losses

TREATMENT PLAN

Surgical
Used when cause of obstruction is thought to be adhesions, necrosis, tumor, or unresolved inflammatory lesions (i.e., strictures found in Crohn's disease)
Surgical resection of mechanical obstruction after pa-

---

*Meglucamine diatrizoate (Gastrografin) used if perforation is suspected.

tient's fluid and electrolytes are stabilized; strangulation obstructions are a surgical emergency

In colonic obstructions, a decompression colostomy to allow relief of the obstruction is the first stage; a cecostomy tube may be rarely used in patients with cecal distention

The second surgical procedure is resection and anastomosis

The third surgical stage is closure of colostomy

Supportive

Nasogastric (for upper or jejunal obstruction) or intestinal suctioning (for distal obstructions); Cantor, or long, tubes used when obstruction is caused by infection or inflammation and can resolve with medical therapy (intravenous fluids and electrolytes; administration of blood or plasma)

ASSESSMENT: AREAS OF CONCERN

History
Abdominal pain

Crampy pain with sudden onset in periumbilicus area, intermittent with pains associated with peristaltic waves (attempting to move the obstruction)

Localized tenderness and continuous severe pain existing between colic attacks and indicative of strangulation

Vomiting

Proximal jejunal obstructions: profuse vomiting unassociated with abdominal distention

Distal small bowel obstruction: less vomiting, feculent odor (secondary to bacterial proliferation in obstructions)

Colonic obstructions: vomiting after prolonged obstructions; usually secondary to pain; may contain fecal material

Constipation

Obstipation and failure to pass gas are signs of a complete obstruction *after* the bowel distal to the obstruction has been evacuated

Previous surgeries

Adhesions, malrotations, and hernias are common causes of mechanical obstructions

History of inflammatory bowel disease

Crohn's disease, ulcerative colitis, diverticulitis, or symptoms of malignancy

Physical examination
Abdomen

Observe for presence of hernias

Note amount of abdominal distention; girth measurements may be beneficial in observing the progress of an obstruction

Mechanical obstruction: peristalsis is high-pitched, tingling sound with rushes

Visible peristalsis: seen moving toward obstruction and reversing

Paralytic ileus: absence of bowel sounds or low infrequent sounds

Auscultate abdomen for full 5 minutes before palpating

Localized tenderness, constant pain, guarding, and rebound tenderness are signs of strangulation obstructions

Additional physical findings

Tachycardia and hypotension may indicate dehydration or peritonitis

Fever and leukocytosis may indicate strangulation

Loss of skin turgor and dry mucous membranes indicate dehydration

Blood in stool may indicate cancer, intussusception, or infarction as obstructing lesions

NURSING DIAGNOSES and NURSING INTERVENTIONS

Nursing Diagnosis	Nursing Intervention
Tissue perfusion, alteration in: cerebral, cardiopulmonary, renal, gastrointestinal, peripheral	Monitor patient carefully for signs and symptoms of severe fluid and electrolyte loss, metabolic acidosis, and hypovolemic shock.
Fluid volume deficit, actual	Replace intravenous fluids and electrolytes, blood, and plasma as ordered. Monitor vital signs, central venous pressure, blood pressure, urinary output, and nasogastric aspirations every hour. Check abdominal girth every 4 to 8 hours. Notify physician of changes in patient's status as they generally indicate a decline in patient's stabilization for surgical intervention.

Nursing Diagnosis	Nursing Intervention
Gas exchange, impaired*	Monitor and document patient's pulmonary status. Elevate head of bed. Provide oxygen therapy as ordered.
Comfort, alteration in: pain	Provide analgesics as prescribed. Assist patient in obtaining a comfortable position.

*Abdominal distention and abdominal guarding may impair pulmonary ventilation, as can metabolic imbalances.

Patient Education

1. Do primary postoperative progression if resection and anastomosis of small bowel obstruction were performed. This would include showering, activity progressions, driving, and returning to work.
2. Colonic obstructions are often treated with a temporary diverting colostomy, and patient requires patient teaching about colostomy care, plans for continued surgical interventions, and education about the primary cause of the obstruction (see p. 1273).

EVALUATION

Patient Outcome	Data Indicating That Outcome is Reached
Body functioning is normal.	Bowel elimination pattern is normal. Colostomy is closed, and patient returns to normal elimination functions.
Fluid balance is maintained.	Patient returns to normal hydration levels as assessed by skin turgor, skin color and mucous membrane, and blood pressure and pulse.
Laboratory studies are normal.	Serum electrolytes, hematocrit, and hemoglobin are within normal limits.
Sepsis is not present.	Patient is not febrile; white blood cell count is within normal limits.

INTESTINAL ISCHEMIA

Intestinal ischemia may develop when the mesenteric vascular supply is insufficient. Acute and chronic occlusion of blood flow to the splanchnic bed, thrombosis or embolus of the superior mesenteric artery, strangulation obstructions, chronic vascular insufficiency, anoxia, or hypotension may lead to intestinal ischemia.

Intestinal ischemia has in the past been difficult to diagnose. The symptoms initially do not correspond with physical examination and laboratory findings. As the ischemia progresses, the severity of the patient's condition becomes apparent and perforation and peritonitis may have already occurred. Advances in angiography have assisted the physician in diagnosing intestinal ischemias. Awareness of intestinal ischemias is increasing, and angiography is being used to rule out acute occlusion of vessels when patients are seen with sudden onset of severe abdominal pain. Poor perfusion of the intestine is known to result in ischemia, and the syndromes of poor perfusion are gaining more attention. The frequency of thrombosis or embolus as the cause of mesenteric ischemia was reported as high as 75%. Diagnosis of poor perfusion syndromes as the pathologic cause of the ischemic episode has decreased the incidence of occlusions of the large vessels to 25%.[72]

Advances in vascular surgery and advances in nutritional and fluid replacement following intestinal resections have allowed a more aggressive approach in the treatment of intestinal ischemias. Although vascular disorders of the intestines are more common in older persons with arteriosclerosis, cases have been reported in children and in pregnant women.

PATHOPHYSIOLOGY

The blood flow to the intestines may be affected by a variety of factors.[7]

The following factors increase splanchnic blood flow:
1. Presence of food
2. Digestive hormones: gastrin, secretin, and cholecystokinin
3. Metabolite-produced muscle activity
4. Beta-stimulating sympathomimetic amines

The following factors decrease splanchnic blood flow:
1. Physical activities
2. Abdominal distention (marked intraluminal pressure)
3. Alpha-stimulating sympathomimetic amines
4. Cardiac glycosides (digitalis)

The response to the alteration in blood flow will depend on the degree of obstruction of blood flow, the rapidity of onset, the duration of the process, and the efficiency of the collateral circulation. Disease processes may affect both large and small vessels. This section will review the normal pattern of blood flow to the intestines, etiology of alteration of blood flow, including a variety of diseases that affect blood distribution to the bowel, and the pathophysiology of events.

The intestine receives its blood supply from the celiac, the superior mesenteric, and the inferior mesenteric arteries. These three major vessels arise from the abdominal aorta. The major three arteries subdivide into a complex collateral circulation. The celiac artery divides into the splenic, left gastric, and hepatic arteries. All three of the above divisions supply the stomach. The splenic artery supplies the greater curvature, and the left gastric supplies the lesser curvature. The hepatic artery divides into the gastroduodenal, which divides to form the superior pancreaticoduodenal. The celiac axis is interconnected with the superior mesenteric through pancreaticoduodenal arcades.

The celiac artery originates from the aorta at the level of the first lumbar and twelfth thoracic vertebrae. It passes next to the median arcuate ligament of the diaphragm. In celiac compression syndrome, one abnormal positioning of the artery and the ligament affects blood flow.

The superior mesenteric artery divides into the ileocolic, middle colic, and right colic arteries. The terminal ileum, cecum, and proximal ascending colon are supplied by the ileocolic artery. The ascending colon and hepatic flexure are supplied by the right colic artery. The middle colic vessel supplies the proximal portion of the transverse colon.

In addition to the above branches, the superior mesenteric artery divides into smaller arteries that supply the jejunum and ileum. The superior mesenteric artery connects with the celiac axis through the pancreaticoduodenal artery. In this way the small intestine receives its blood flow.

The vessels originating from the superior mesenteric artery ultimately enter the wall of the intestine as arteriae rectae, which are end arteries. Few anastomotic connections are found in the bowel wall. Vasculitis may result in the selective occlusion of the distal vessels and may lead to segmental infarction and small bowel ischemia and necrosis.

The superior mesenteric artery is susceptible to atherosclerotic charges and is a common site for thrombosis and embolus. The inverted Y shape of the superior mesenteric artery as it leaves the aorta provides a channel for emboli. Thromboses and emboli tend to occlude the superior mesenteric within 2 cm of its origin off the aorta.

The inferior mesenteric artery supplies blood to the distal transverse colon, the descending and sigmoid colon, and proximal portions of the rectum. The distal transverse colon and the splenic flexure appear to be more vulnerable to ischemia. A "watershed" area refers to branches of the inferior mesenteric artery anastomosing with the superior artery branches in the rectosigmoid area. The branches involved are the inferior mesenteric and the hypogastric.

Vascular occlusion may be the result of thrombosis or embolus to the superior mesenteric artery. The development of emboli is associated with atrial fibrillation in patients with subacute bacterial endocarditis and cardiac valve disease, mural thrombosis of myocardial infarct, and postintracardiac surgery. Thrombosis of mesenteric vessels is associated with polycythemia, sickle cell trait, intra-abdominal sepsis, pancreatic disorders, and blood dyscrasias. It may also occur after bowel surgery, other major surgery, or abdominal trauma, when there may be a decrease in blood flow to the mesentery. Infarction of the bowel results in a sudden onset of severe abdominal pain, distention, fluid loss, and shock.

Intestinal angina is an obstructive vascular disease in which atherosclerotic changes in two of the three major vessels are found. An increase in mesenteric blood flow is required to supply oxygen for the metabolic processes of digestion, absorption, and increased peristalsis. Abdominal pain occurs when the superior mesenteric artery supply is less than the demand of the smooth muscle activity in the intestine. Between meals, the patient is free of pain. Intestinal angina is a chronic problem. The patient may develop a fear of eating and begin losing weight. Diagnosis may be delayed because many physicians first test the patient for cancer since weight loss and pain in older persons are associated with malignancies. Intestinal ischemia may progress to frank infarction of the intestine.

Nonocclusive intestinal ischemia has been reported with increasing frequency. The patient tends to be younger than those with obstructive ischemia. Patients with recent myocardial infarctions, severe congestive cardiac failure, shock, anoxia, or hypotension may develop a nonocclusive intestinal ischemia. An episode of inadequate cardiac output and poor tissue perfusion results in shunting of blood away from the gut to vital organs. The use of alpha-adrenergic vasoconstrictors in patients in shock adds to the effect of the increased secretions of endogenous catecholamines, further reducing mesenteric blood flow. The mucosa layer is the most sensitive to oxygen deprivation since it has the highest energy requirement because of its high metabolic activity and rapid cell turnover. The mucosa will undergo hemorrhagic necrosis. As the anoxia continues, the necrosis becomes transmural (involving all layers of the bowel wall).

The patient who develops nonocclusive intestinal ischemia may have evidence of some degree of occlusive or atherosclerotic changes in smaller splanchnic vessels.

Digitalis has been associated with the development of poor perfusion syndromes. Digoxin constricts splanchnic vessels. In patients with early intestinal infarction, considerations should be made regarding discontinuation of digoxin therapy.[66]

Necrotizing enterocolitis of infancy is a variant of intestinal ischemia. In premature infants, anoxia and hypotension lead to poor perfusion of the intestines. Ischemic enterocolitis develops with its progressing sequelae.

Celiac axis compression by the median arcuate ligament of the diaphragm or by neurofibrous tissue of the celiac ganglion is associated with recurrent epigastric pain and an epigastric bruit (which does not radiate to the lower abdomen). The celiac axis compression is more common in young women and is relieved by surgical division of the ligament or bands. The medical profession has challenged the validity of celiac axis compression as a disorder or a syndrome.[69,72] The etiology of the pain and the absence of symptoms in many patients with stenosis of the celiac axis have raised unanswered questions.

Table 11-3
Systemic Disorders Affecting Splanchnic Perfusion

Disorder	Definition	Gastrointestinal Implications
Periarteritis nodosa	A progressive, polymorphic disease of connective tissue characterized by numerous large, palpable or visible nodules in clusters along segments of medium-sized arteries	Segmental ischemia with ulceration, hemorrhage, or perforation to massive infarction of bowel; may also have hepatic artery thrombosis; nodules obstruct lumen of vessels
Lupus erythematosus	A chronic inflammatory collagen disease affecting many systems; includes severe vasculitis, renal involvement, and lesions of skin and nervous system	Segmental lesions of ischemia progressing to necrosis and perforation; involvement of submucosa and muscularis leads to protein-losing enteropathy; abdominal pain may be caused by serositis or acute pancreatitis; ulcerative colitis and Crohn's disease have been associated with lupus erythematosus; diagnosis of gastrointestinal involvement difficult to evaluate
Dermatomyositis	A disease of the connective tissue characterized by pruritic or eczematous inflammation of skin and tenderness and weakness of muscles	Vasculitis associated with ischemia of bowel; increased incidence of gastrointestinal cancers with this disorder
Rheumatoid arthritis	A collagen disease that affects the connective tissue by inflammation and fibrinoid degeneration	Vasculitis associated with intestinal ischemia; presents with abdominal pain
Scleroderma	A relatively rare autoimmune disease affecting blood vessels and connective tissue; most common in middle-aged women	Bowel symptoms arise from fibrosis of the intestinal wall and loss of muscle; focal areas of vasculitis may lead to ischemia
Anaphylactoid purpura (Henoch-Schönlein syndrome)	A self-limited hypersensitive vasculitis that occurs primarily in young children; palpable purpuric skin lesions appear on lower abdomen, buttocks, and legs; arthritis and abdominal pain are also seen; occasionally seen in adults, whose prognosis is not as favorable as children	Colicky abdominal pain; surgery demonstrates submucosal and subserosal hemorrhages; may have upper or lower gastrointestinal bleeding; segmental ischemic bowel episodes may occur but do not generally progress to gross infarction or perforation
Degos' disease (malignant atrophic papulosis)	A rare syndrome of progressive occlusive vascular disease affecting small and medium-sized arteries; primarily involves the skin (malignant atrophic papulosis) and intestine; skin lesions usually precede gastrointestinal symptoms; primarily affects young men	Lesions (identical to skin lesion) are found in mucosa and serosa of bowel; weight loss and diarrhea develop; progresses to intestinal infarction and perforation

Vasculitis has been associated with mesenteric infarction in approximately 3% of reported cases. However, the vasculitis associated with systemic disorders may be seen as intestinal angina or frank infarction. The systemic disorders include periarteritis nodosa, lupus erythematosus, dermatomyositis, rheumatoid vasculitis, scleroderma, anaphylactoid purpura, and Degos' disease. Table 11-3 examines the bowel involvement that occurs as a result of systemic vasculitis.

Certain surgical procedures such as coarctation of the aorta, excision of abdominal aneurysms, and iliac or femoral grafts are associated with mesenteric vascular insufficiency.

The oxygenation of the bowel depends on patency of the major arterial vessels, arteriolar resistance, adequacy of perfusion pressure, arterial oxygen saturation, and oxygen need. Acute or chronic changes of any or all of the above will affect the blood flow to the bowel.

The events of intestinal ischemia include structural changes in the cells within 5 minutes of the occlusion of the superior mesenteric artery. The epithelium becomes detached from the basement membrane at the villus tips, and subepithelial blebs form. Within 30 to 60 minutes, the villi are denuded of epithelium. The mucosa undergoes necrosis and ulceration with an inflammatory cell infiltration. A secondary bacterial invasion occurs. In acute ischemic necrosis, massive submucosa edema and bleeding into the mucous membrane develop because of an increase in capillary permeability followed by loss of capillary integrity.

The submucosal edema and hemorrhage are seen as the "thumbprint" pattern in radiographic studies. The exudation of protein-rich fluid, and later blood, found in the intestinal lumen is the result of the loss of epithelial and vascular integrity. Fluid loss and hypovolemia further compromise blood flow to the intestine.

The development of peritonitis indicates the involvement of the muscle and serosa layer and that the perforation is imminent or has occurred. If the ischemic episode is self-limited and does not progress to perforation and resection, the acute inflammatory response resolves with granulation tissue, fibrosis, and scarring with potential for development of strictures.

In chronic or gradual reduction of blood flow, the anoxia damages the mucosa initially. The necrosis may be limited to the mucosa, in which event the mucosa will slough with regeneration occurring in 4 to 5 days. The villi may recover, but their shape and functioning abilities are affected and a temporary malabsorption develops that is seen clinically as enterocolitis. As the anoxia continues, the necrosis progresses. A microscopic examination of the bowel may describe a coagulative necrosis of the inner two thirds of the wall with muscle and serosa uninvolved. A scar may form.

The bowel totally deprived of its blood supply will ultimately become black and necrotic. The bowel perforates with leakage of intestinal contents. Bacterial invasion of the necrotic bowel will produce gas cysts, massive sepsis, and shock. Repair cannot take place when this degree of injury has occurred and bowel death usually results. If surgery is done, it is usually a massive bowel resection.

DIAGNOSTIC STUDIES

Abdominal films
Tonic contraction of bowel

Plain films
Complete absence of small bowel air
Generalized distention (later sign)
Thickening of bowel wall with edema and fluid (ischemic colitis)
String or ring of gas outside lumen of bowel (marked necrosis)
Gas in portal vein (evidence of leak of bacteria from infarcted bowel)

Angiography
Abnormal vascular tree (intestinal angina)
Demonstrates site of arterial blockage or spasm (angiographic studies generally indicated only in patients with disorders predisposing to embolization but may be used when other tests are negative and patient is symptomatic; also used preoperatively to map vessels that are narrowed or occluded)

Barium studies
Early stages find appearance of spasm and irritability with narrowing of bowel lumen and thumbprinting

Colonoscopy
Swollen folds and mucosa, dusty color, presence of ulcerations similar to those found in Crohn's disease

Hematocrit
In presence of necrosis, hemocentration (decreased fluid volume)

White blood cell count
Leukocytosis (20,000 and higher)

Amylase and lipase
Elevated (from leakage into peritoneum or from back pressure secondary to development of intestinal obstruction)

TREATMENT PLAN

Surgical

Balloon angioplasty (intestinal angina) to improve blood flow

Bypass graft, embolectomy, endarterectomy, and reimplantation procedures have been used effectively

Resection of necrotic bowel segments with a second-look operation to observe bowel viability 12 to 36 hours after initial exploration

Resection, temporary colostomy or ileostomy, and subsequent reanastomosis (colonic ischemia)

Chemotherapeutic

Anti-infective agents

Agent-specific antibiotics given to reduce bacterial flora of bowel and treat sepsis

Adrenergic agents

Dopamine in low dosages may be used as a vasopressor if fluid replacement does not correct shock (alpha-stimulating sympathomimetic amines [i.e., norepinephrine] should be avoided)

Vasodilators

Intra-arterial infusion of vasodilators (glucagon, isoproterenol, papaverine, histamine, and others) has been used, but effectiveness of this treatment has not been clearly documented[69,72]

Anticoagulation with heparin followed by bishydroxycoumarin (dicumarol) (used in patients with mesenteric venous occlusion that tends to recur); dosages adjusted based on patient's coagulation time

Electromechanical

Electromyography

Doppler ultrasonography

Injection of radioactive microspheres

Intraoperative fluorescein angiography (may be used during surgery to determine viability of bowel and evaluate mesenteric vessels)

Supportive

Intravenous fluid replacements (low molecular dextran, albumin, fresh frozen plasma, blood)

Nasogastric or intestinal suctioning preoperatively

Hyperalimentation postoperatively

Elemental diets (intestinal angina)

ASSESSMENT: AREAS OF CONCERN

This section has been primarily divided into assessments of chronic ischemia of the bowel (i.e., intestinal angina) and acute episodes of ischemia. The acute episodes are similar in progression of symptoms, and therefore not all etiologies will be outlined. Acute occlusive ischemia will be used as the example. Exceptions will be noted. The assessment of abdominal pain is an example of an area where differences do exist in the acute episodes.

Abdominal pain

Intestinal angina: severe crampy or colicky pain around umbilicus; radiates to back; lasts 2 to 4 hours; pain free between meals

Acute occlusive ischemia: severe colicky pain in the periumbilical area; as ischemia progresses, pain becomes more severe and poorly localized

Ischemic colitis: lower abdominal pain of abrupt onset

Mesenteric venous thrombosis: gradual progression of abdominal pain until it resembles acute occlusive ischemia

Gastrointestinal response to ischemia or necrosis

Intestinal angina: nausea and vomiting; abdominal bloating; malabsorption with steatorrhea and diarrhea

Acute occlusive ischemia: copious vomiting and hematemesis indicate necrosis adjacent to ligament of Treitz; gross rectal bleeding

Enterocolitis symptoms: malabsorption; diarrhea, may be hemorrhagic (seen regardless of etiology of ischemia, secondary to sloughing of mucosa and to bacteremia)

Abdominal findings

Absence of significant abdominal findings initially; hyperperistalsis, with no tenderness or resistance

After necrosis occurs: classic signs of peritonitis with rebound tenderness, rigidity, abdominal distention, and ileus

Signs of necrosis

Tachycardia

Fever

Hypotension (may have significant amounts of fluids in bowel lumen)

Changes in laboratory values

Nutritional assessment

Intestinal angina: weight loss; fear of eating because of chronic malabsorption syndrome; malnutrition

Evidence of poor perfusion episodes

Shock; hypotension; anoxia; severe congestive heart failure; recent myocardial infarction or some etiology that results in shunting of blood away from the gut to "vital" organs

NURSING DIAGNOSES and NURSING INTERVENTIONS

Nursing Diagnosis	Nursing Intervention
Tissue perfusion, alteration in: cerebral, cardiopulmonary, renal, gastrointestinal, peripheral	Monitor patient carefully for signs and symptoms of severe fluid and electrolyte loss, metabolic acidosis, and hypovolemic shock.
Fluid volume deficit, actual	Replace intravenous fluids and electrolytes, blood, and plasma as ordered. Provide oxygen therapy as ordered. Monitor vital signs, central venous pressure, blood pressure, urinary output, nasogastric aspirations, and diarrhea every hour. Measure abdominal girth every 8 hours; weigh patient daily. Notify physician of changes in patient's status since they generally indicate a decline in patient's stabilization for surgery.
Comfort, alteration in: pain	Provide analgesics as ordered. Assist patient in obtaining a comfortable position.
Nutrition, alteration in: less than body requirements	Assess through careful history a "fear of eating" vs. other causes of weight loss. Provide enteral nutrition as tolerated. Initiate and monitor hyperalimentation as ordered after operation for significant small bowel resections.

Patient Education

1. Assist patient in understanding relationship of eating and pain in intestinal angina.
2. Following surgery for venous thrombosis, patient may need instructions regarding anticoagulant therapy.
3. In colonic ischemia, a temporary colostomy may be done. If so, the patient will require colostomy teaching and plans for surgical closure at a later date.
4. If the patient has had a massive bowel resection, he may be on home total parenteral nutrition. In these cases, patient and family require extensive discharge preparation (i.e., line care; management of total parenteral nutrition).
5. Assist patient to deal with an increase in diarrhea, especially for the first 6 months postoperatively, caused by rapid transit time or varying degrees of malabsorption.

EVALUATION

Patient Outcome	Data Indicating That Outcome is Reached
Body functioning is normal.	There is no pain or diarrhea; bowel function is normal. Colostomy is closed.
Fluid balance is maintained.	Patient returns to normal hydration levels as assessed by skin turgor, color, mucous membranes, blood pressure, and pulse.
Laboratory studies are normal.	Serum electrolytes, hematocrit, and WBC are within normal limits.
Nutritional status is normal.	Patient returns to "normal" body weight. Nutritional status is maintained through home hyperalimentation (major resection of small bowel).

IRRITABLE BOWEL SYNDROME

Irritable bowel syndrome (IBS), or functional bowel syndrome, is a motor disorder of the large bowel that results in altered bowel habits, abdominal pain, and absence of detectable organic pathologic manifestations.

The patient may have diarrhea or constipation or both. Abnormal motor activity of the large bowel can be measured (see opposite page). It is believed that the small bowel may also be involved, but measurement of motor activity in the small bowel is not as accessible.[69]

It is also important to recognize the mislabeling of IBS in the past. Nervous colon, spastic colon, and mucous colitis are incorrect terms. Nervous colon only recognizes one aspect of the possible etiology of IBS. Spasticity is one sign or response of the colon to the altered motor activity. Inflammation is not present, making "colitis" a misnomer. IBS does not progress or predispose individuals to inflammatory bowel disease or cancer.

The incidence of IBS is considered high, but accurate data on the prevalence are not available. IBS does not lead to death and therefore does not appear on death certificates. Rarely does IBS require hospitalization. Cohen[15] states that it may be the most common disorder for which medical care is sought. IBS is a leading cause of absenteeism from work. Approximately 20% to 50% of referrals to gastroenterologists are for irritable bowel syndrome.[69,72] Not all people with IBS seek medical attention since many have mild symptoms, making it more difficult to estimate the prevalence.

The incidence of IBS is higher in females than males with a 2.3:1 ratio. There is a higher incidence in whites than nonwhites and in Jews than non-Jews. Symptoms generally begin before the age of 35, and in many patients isolated instances of IBS during adolescence can be identified by the patients. A third of the patients can trace IBS to childhood.[23]

In children with IBS, a high familial incidence has been reported. One or both parents and siblings will have reported IBS. The ratio of boys to girls is higher during childhood. As with adults, the incidence of IBS is higher in Jewish than non-Jewish children and in whites than nonwhites.

PATHOPHYSIOLOGY

IBS is a functional disorder of gastrointestinal motility. The abdominal pain and altered bowel pattern are caused by the altered motility. Motility may be affected by emotions, food, neurohumoral agents, gastrointestinal hormones, toxins, prostaglandins, and colon distention.

Two patterns of IBS are identified: painful IBS with diarrhea, constipation, or both and IBS with painless diarrhea. The two types of IBS can be separated based on observations of motility recordings. Patients with painful IBS have a characteristic response to rectal distention that is not found in painless IBS.

Segmental contractions are the predominant form of normal motor activity in the colon, consisting of 90% of recorded motor activity. Segmental contractions slow the forward progress of stool, promoting mixing, absorption, and dehydration. Segmental contractions appear as haustral markings on barium studies. Increasing segmental contractions produces constipation, whereas decreasing segmentation results in diarrhea.

A pattern of hypermotility with high-amplitude pressure waves is common in patients with painful IBS. Studies have also demonstrated that contractions over long segments of colon may be accompanied by abdominal pain.[16] Hypermotility in the small bowel is also associated with abdominal pain. Motility in the pain-free diarrheal-predominant IBS is normal or lower than normal.

Motility of the bowel may be affected by a variety of factors. For example, sleep lowers the motor activity in the colon. This may account for the infrequency of nocturnal symptoms. The presence of nocturnal symptoms usually indicates an organic etiology rather than the functional etiology of IBS.

Emotional factors do affect gastrointestinal motility. Anxiety, depression, fear, and hostility have been identified in IBS as well as other gastrointestinal disorders. Stress and emotions alone do not cause IBS but are related to the clinical course. Stress can be related to the onset of symptoms. Diarrhea can readily be associated with stressful situations such as test taking or job interviews. Constipation is not apparent for several days, and it may be more difficult to pinpoint the source of anxiety or generalized depression.

Meals, or the ingestion of food and caffeine, will stimulate colonic hypermotility in irritable bowel syndrome. The postprandial symptoms are related to this effect. Normally, a meal will lengthen segmental contractions, allowing for additional mixing and absorption and the effect of the meal slows after approximately 50 minutes. In IBS the meal stimulation of segmental contractions is blunted and the effect continues postprandially, gradually becoming stronger.

The gastroileocolic response to food ingestion moves intestinal contents forward, emptying material in the distal colon and creating distention. Colon distention induces exaggerated spastic contractions in IBS. Patients with alternating diarrhea and constipation or diarrhea-predominant IBS often have a bowel movement after every meal. For some this may be the only symptom of IBS. Based on myoelectric studies, the gastrocolic reflex has been divided into two phases: early neurogenic myoelectric and motor reflex and a delayed hormonally mediated phase.

Smooth muscle cells of the bowel act as small electrical oscillators that produce myoelectrical activity. Two types of electrical activity have been recorded: a slow wave (or basic electrical rhythm) and spike action potentials (on electrical response activity). The slow wave results from depolarization and repolarization. The slow wave is sodium dependent, and its predominant rhythmic frequency in the normal distal colon is six cycles per minute. The spike action is superimposed on the slow waves. Short bursts of spike action potentials are commonly associated with phasic motor activity. Longer bursts of spike action are associated with tonic contractions. The spike action potentials are calcium dependent.

The myoelectric activity in IBS is different from the myoelectric activity in normal colons. In IBS the myoelectric frequency is three cycles per minute. The three cycle per minute activity remains constant during symptomatic and asymptomatic periods, regardless of whether the predominant symptom is diarrhea or constipation. The three cycle per minute activity is unaltered by successful treatment. Although researchers are continuing to debate the significance of the three cycles per minute in IBS, it may become a marker for IBS. It should also be noted that three cycles per minute is also seen in neurotic personality disorders (with or without IBS), suggesting that the pattern of three cycles per minute is more characteristic of neurotic disorders than motor disorders.

Myoelectric responses can be tested. In response to a 1000-cal fatty meal, the spike action potentials increase and muscle contractions increase. The activity peaks in 30 minutes and returns to fasting level within 50 minutes. In IBS the response is attenuated the first 30 minutes; then the spike activity continues to rise and peaks at 70 to 90 minutes.[70]

Neurohumoral agents include cholinergic, anticholinergic, adrenergic, and adrenergic-blocking substances. The neurohumoral agents produce hyperactivity of the colon in both normal bowels and in irritable bowel syndromes. In IBS, response to neurohumoral agents is more pronounced and occurs during both symptomatic and asymptomatic periods.

Anticholinergics affect colonic activity induced by meals. Anticholinergics suppress an early neurogenic myoelectric and motor reflex component of the gastrocolic reflex in normal subjects. In IBS the myoelectric and motor reflex is not suppressed, but anticholinergics inhibit the second, delayed component of gastrocolic reflex, which is hormonally mediated.

The gastrointestinal hormones that affect motility include cholecystokinin, gastrin glucagon, and vasoactive intestinal peptide. Cholecystokinin is associated with abdominal pain and colonic hypermotility when given through infusion. Since cholecystokinin is released following a meal, this may account for the postprandial pain in IBS. Also, the delayed hormonally mediated phase of the gastrocolic reflex is dependent on the fatty content of the meal. This indicates a relationship with cholecystokinin that produces colonic contractions.

DIAGNOSTIC STUDIES

Sigmoidoscopy
Spastic contractions that prevent passage of the instrument beyond 10 to 12 cm
Reproduction of symptoms with air insufflation
Mucosa free of ulcers, bleeding, friability, and masses
Do not use enemas or cathartics before sigmoidoscopy (may produce edema, obscuring the normal colon appearance)

Rectal balloon distention
Induces spastic contractions and pain

Manometric studies
May be used to evaluate electric response to colon
Balloons are placed in rectosigmoidal colon (cephalad balloon) and rectum (caudad balloon), and 20 mm of air is instilled into the cephalad balloon every 20 minutes; balloon mimics presence of stool in the area; a graph recording is made of the bowel response to the stimulus
Response in a normal bowel is a brief contraction in rectosigmoid and rectum, with a rapid return to the prestimulus state; in patient with IBS, the distention produces a diffuse spastic contraction in rectosigmoid and rectum
Classically, patients with IBS and diarrhea do not experience significant weight loss as do patients with an inflammatory or viral origin to their diarrhea

Biopsy
To rule out other disorders; not helpful in diagnosing IBS

Stool test for guaiac
To rule out inflammatory bowel diseases and malignancy

Stool stains
To rule out motile amebic trophozoites, leukocytes, and mucus

Stool cultures
To rule out ova and parasites, specifically *Giardia*

Complete blood count
To rule out anemia and inflammation

Differential blood cell count (eosinophilia)
To rule out parasitosis, cytosis (suggests tuberculosis), and vacuolated cells (suggest inflammation)

Three-day trial on lactose-free diet, lactose tolerance test, or breath hydrogen test
To rule out lactose insufficiency in patients with distention and bloating or diarrhea

Double-contrast barium enema
Exaggerated haustral contractions or absence of haustrations; narrow lumen with pellet stones; lumen easily dilated

Cholecystogram or ultrasonography of gallbladder
To rule out gallbladder disease in presence of dyspepsia

Small bowel series
To rule out obstruction of bowel, if diarrhea and symptoms suggest obstruction

Colonoscopy
To rule out inflammatory bowel disease when clinically justified as in change in symptoms in patient with long-standing IBS; uncontrollable exacerbation of IBS

Thyroid function
To rule out hyperthyroidism or hypothyroidism if constipation predominates

Carotene (serum)
To rule out celiac sprue

TREATMENT PLAN

Surgical
Rarely colostomy may be done

Chemotherapeutic
Bulk-forming laxatives
Psyllium preparations (Metamucil, Konsyl, L.A. Formula, Mitrolan) taken at meal times; in obese patients before meals and in thin patients after meals (hydrophilic properties bind water, preventing excessive dehydration of stool and excess liquidity)
Antidiarrheal agents
Diphenoxylate (Lomotil), 2.5 to 5 mg q4-6h
Loperamide (Imodium), 2 mg q6-8h
Paregoric or opium tincture (Parelixir) has been prescribed
Dependency on antidiarrheals can develop; slow withdrawal of medicines as coping abilities are developed is recommended

Cholinergic blocking agents
Antispasmodics (for temporary relief of crampy pain related to intestinal spasm)
For postprandial pain give one of following 30 to 45 minutes before meals:
Dicyclomine (Bentyl), 20 mg
Propantheline (Pro-Banthine), 15 mg
Tincture of belladonna, 10 to 20 drops

Supportive
Patient should be placed on high-fiber (12 to 16 g/d as 2 tablespoons of bran qid; gradually reduced), low-lactose, no-caffeine diet before trying drug therapy
Low-fat diet (to reduce stimulation of cholecystokinin)
Avoid irritating foods (idiosyncratic)
Psychotherapy or counseling
Relaxation techniques

ASSESSMENT: AREAS OF CONCERN

History and physical examination
Presence of lower abdominal pain; small stools, alternating diarrhea and constipation, diarrhea, or constipation
Correlation of onset of symptoms with periods of stress and heightened emotional tension
Symptoms initially appeared during an intercurrent illness and persisted
Tense, anxious patient who may be unaware of features of tenseness
Autonomic lability: rapid, labile pulse; elevated blood pressure; sweaty palms; abdominal tympany
No evidence of weight loss
Palpable, tender sigmoid colon

Constipation
Episodic initially, becomes continuous, increasingly intractable to laxatives and later to enemas
Stools: hard, narrow
Objectively defined as passage of less than three stools per week; sometimes patient will have diarrhea following a week of constipation
Subjectively defined as difficult or painful evacuation

Diarrhea
Defined as loose, mushy, or watery stools
Urgency and tenseness in morning or after meals, followed by evacuation
Initial movement may be of normal consistency and is rapidly followed by a softer, unformed stool and then by increasingly loose stools
Abdominal pain relieved by bowel movement
Postprandial diarrhea correlating with quantity rather than type of food

Patients with diarrheal only–type IBS more likely to have explosive, watery stools; classically these patients experience no weight loss

Pain

Often patient locates pain by using the palm describing a circular motion (rather than finger pointing to one discrete spot)

Pain often precipitated by meals

Pain often relieved by defecation

Abdominal distention

Quantitative measures indicate that patients with IBS who complain about increased gas, bloating, and flatus produce a normal amount but have a decreased tolerance

Mucus

Amount produced varies

Etiology of increased mucus production is unknown, although in the past, it was associated incorrectly with inflammation

NURSING DIAGNOSES and NURSING INTERVENTIONS

Nursing Diagnosis	Nursing Intervention
Bowel elimination, alteration in: constipation and diarrhea	Support patient in recognizing role of emotions, stress, and diet in symptomatology of IBS. Assist patient in identifying sources of stress and relaxation techniques. Assist patient in identifying any secondary gains of illness. Assist patient in identifying irritating or troublesome foods (diet therapy is very important). Support patient and family in understanding that the symptoms are based on functional motility problems and that psychosocial stress accentuates rather than causes the symptoms.

Patient Education

1. Provide information on irritable bowel syndrome. Patient education material is available through the National Digestive Disease Education Information Clearinghouse, NIH, 1555 Wilson Blvd., Suite 600, Rosslyn, VA 22209-2461.
2. Provide patient teaching about necessary diet alterations. Inform patient that often it is possible to manage with diet and stress reduction without using any medications.
3. Provide written instructions for medications prescribed for the management of IBS by the physician. Ensure that patient knows the names, amount, and rationale for the treatment plan.

EVALUATION

Patient Outcome	Data Indicating That Outcome is Reached
Psychosocial stress is reduced.	Patient can identify sources of stress and uses effective coping mechanisms.
Symptoms are managed so that life-style does not center around bowel elimination.	Combination of counseling, relaxation techniques, modification of diet (avoiding irritating foods), and medications is effective in relieving symptoms.
Bowel functioning is normal.	Diarrhea and constipation are relieved, and recurrences are managed through medical regimen and stress reduction.

MALABSORPTION SYNDROMES

Malabsorption syndromes are a complex group of symptoms characterized by anorexia, weight loss, bloating of the abdomen, muscle cramps, bone pain, and steatorrhea. Carbohydrates, proteins, fats, vitamins, and electrolytes may be ineffectively absorbed from the bowel lumen. Temporary malabsorption syndromes are associated with enterocolitis. Lactose intolerance, celiac sprue, tropical sprue, and small bowel resections are disorders that are associated with malabsorption. In Crohn's disease, scleroderma, lymphoma, and acquired immune deficiency syndrome, malabsorption is seen associated with opportunistic infections and Kaposi's sarcoma.

Lactose Intolerance

Lactose intolerance is a disorder that results from a deficiency of the enzyme lactase. Lactase is necessary for the digestion or breakdown of the disaccharide lactose found in the brush border of the intestinal villi. Lactose is found in milk and milk products. Lactose intolerance is a common cause of diarrhea, nonspecific lower gastrointestinal symptoms, and abdominal pain.

Lactose intolerance in the United States is more frequent in Afro-Americans, American Indians, Mexican-Americans, Orientals, and some Jews and Arabs.[49,68] Spiro[72] states that 10% to 20% of the white population of northern European ancestry has a lactase insufficiency and that three fourths of the blacks in Africa, Chinese, Indians, and Mediterranean inhabitants have lactase insufficiency.

Age also plays a part in lactose intolerance. Primary disaccharidase deficiency refers to a congenital, hereditary absence of the lactase enzyme. The symptoms may be present from birth or may become apparent in middle life. By the age of 10 to 20 years, most persons with genetic tendencies for lactase deficiency have the same low level of lactase as adults. Primary lactase insufficiency is associated with a normal bowel mucosa and epithelial cells.

Secondary disaccharidase deficiency occurs when injury or disease damages the brush border of the intestinal mucosa. The secondary lactase deficiency may be temporary or permanent. Diseases or disorders associated with secondary lactase insufficiency include gastroenteritis, ulcerative colitis, Crohn's disease, operative procedures (partial gastrectomy, small bowel resection), and cholera.

PATHOPHYSIOLOGY

The basis of the symptoms found in lactose intolerance is the presence of an excessive amount of sugar in the bowel lumen. Disaccharides form a large part of the dietary carbohydrate, and the three predominant forms are maltose (glucose and glucose), lactose (glucose and galactose), and sucrose (glucose and fructose). The disaccharides are not digested by enzymes in the lumen of the bowel but are taken into the brush border of the intestinal mucosal cell. The disaccharide is split by enzymes in the brush border into the simple sugars (glucose, galactose, and fructose), which can be further absorbed and metabolized. The enzymes of the brush border are lactase, sucrase, and a series of four enzymes that are called maltase.

The lactose absorption begins in the duodenum, and lactase activity is highest in the jejunum and nearly absent in the ileum. The process of lactose digestion is slower, normally, than sucrose and maltose. The blood sugar level after a meal of lactose will show little increase.

Lactase is present in the microvillus membrane of the columnar epithelial cells. In addition, many intestinal bacteria contain lactases. The difference in the two forms of lactase is in their actions. Gut lactase splits the disaccharide, lactose, into glucose and galactose. Bacterial lactase results in the formation of hydrogen gas, carbon dioxide, and short-chain organic acids.

The diarrhea associated with lactose intolerance is caused by the osmotic effect of the lactose in the small bowel. The osmotic load of the lactose increases fluid secretion into the small bowel. The organic acids and fermentation products of the bacteria lactase in the colon impede colonic absorption. The pH of the stools in children may drop to 5.5 in response to the presence of organic acids.

The bloating and gaseous symptoms are the end products of bacterial lactase breaking down lactose.

DIAGNOSTIC STUDIES

Dietary trial: 3 weeks on a lactose-free diet
Absence of gastrointestinal symptoms

Lactose tolerance test
Positive for lactose intolerance: blood sugar rise less than or equal to 20 mg/dl after lactose load of 50 g/sq m in children or 50 g in adults; accompanied by characteristic symptoms

Hydrogen breath test

A rise of more than 20 parts per million is consistent with lactose intolerance (NOTE: oral antibiotics can suppress bacteria that produce hydrogen; smoking increases breath hydrogen concentrations; small percentage of individuals do not normally produce hydrogen gas.)

Stool pH

Drop from the normal pH of 7 or 8 to 5.5 (more common in children)

Small bowel biopsy

Used to determine primary vs. secondary lactose insufficiency; epithelial abnormalities indicate secondary disorder

TREATMENT PLAN

Chemotherapeutic

Commercial lactase preparation can be used in milk for patients with limited tolerance to milk
Lactose-free diet

Supportive

Low-lactose diet (is tolerated well by most individuals; lactose added until symptoms appear and then decreased until asymptomatic)
Calcium supplements (particularly in postmenopausal women)

ASSESSMENT: AREAS OF CONCERN

Infant (congenital)
Nutritional status
Malnourished; failure to thrive

Clinical symptoms
Diarrhea
Irritability
Bloating

Child (acquired)
After the age of 3
Less diarrhea; more abdominal cramping

Child (transient)
Secondary to viral or bacterial infection
Diarrhea; postprandial abdominal pain
Anorexia; weight loss

Adult
Clinical symptoms
Excessive gas and flatus
Abdominal gurgling and pain
Persistent to profuse diarrhea
May vary from mild to extreme

Bone disease
Osteoporosis from low intake of calcium

NURSING DIAGNOSES and NURSING INTERVENTIONS

Nursing Diagnosis	Nursing Intervention
Bowel elimination, alteration in: diarrhea	Record amount, frequency, and consistency of bowel movements. Observe for relationship of foods to onset of abdominal symptoms. Assess past history of milk tolerance or intolerance. Assess for familial tendency for lactose intolerance.
Nutrition, alteration in: less than body requirements	Refer mothers of infants with diarrhea and failure to thrive to physician for evaluation of lactase deficiency vs. other malabsorption syndromes. Provide calcium supplements. Assess patient for bone disease involvement.

Patient Education

1. Provide oral and written instructions on lactose-free or low-lactose diets. Patients should be taught to read all labels to avoid package foods containing milk: milk products, milk solids, whey, lactose, milk sugar, curd, casein, galactose, and skim milk powder. Restricted foods include milk, yogurt, ice cream (also sherbets), cheese, desserts (made from milk and milk chocolate), sauces or stuffings (made with milk, cream, or cheese), and cream soups.

EVALUATION

Patient Outcome	Data Indicating That Outcome is Reached
Bowel elimination is normal.	There are no symptoms with low-lactose or lactose-free diet.
Nutritional status is good.	Calcium level is normal; there are no signs of bone disease.

Celiac Sprue

Celiac sprue is a disease that can result in severe malabsorption. The mucosa of the small intestine is damaged by gluten-containing grains (wheat, barley, rye, and probably oats). The disease has the same clinical features, etiology, pathology, and response to treatment in adults and children.

The most suitable name for this disease is celiac sprue or as an alternative, gluten-sensitive enteropathy. The seriousness of celiac sprue is the potential for severe malabsorption from the small bowel, resulting in marked malnutrition, debilitation, dehydration, and complications of nutrient and vitamin deficiencies.

Celiac sprue was first described in the literature in 1932. In 1950 a landmark study recognized the relationship of certain dietary grains to celiac sprue.[69] The prevalence of celiac sprue is estimated at 0.03% of the general population. It appears that the estimate may be low since asymptomatic celiac sprue patients have been identified during studies of familial and genetic tendencies of the disease.[43] The highest incidence of celiac sprue is in western Ireland, but there are cases of celiac sprue worldwide.[69] Celiac sprue is rare among blacks, Jews, and persons of Mediterranean descent. Women are affected more often than men. Celiac sprue is also higher in people with blood type O and lower in blood type A.

The onset of celiac sprue symptoms occurs at two peak periods. The first peak occurs when the infant's diet is changed to include cereals. There is a period during late childhood where the disease becomes quiescent; however, in the fourth and fifth decades, the second onset of symptoms will occur. Unequivocal evidence of celiac sprue in childhood indicates a need to remain on a gluten-free diet indefinitely to avoid recurrent disease during adult life.

PATHOPHYSIOLOGY

In celiac sprue the interaction of the water-soluble protein moiety (gluten) with the mucosa of the small bowel produces bloating, malaise, abdominal cramps, and diarrhea within a few hours. The fecal fat excretion increases. The mucosal changes of the intestinal segment exposed to gluten develop within 8 to 12 hours.[59] The intestinal absorptive cells are damaged. The dying absorptive cells are sloughed from the mucosal surface more rapidly than normal. The number of proliferating cells increases, and the crypts become hyperplastic to compensate for the excessive loss of absorptive cells. The mucosal layer of the small bowel appears flat, the villi are absent, and the intestinal crypts are markedly elongated and open onto a flat, absorptive surface. These structural changes decrease the amount of epithelial surface available for digestion and absorption. Many of the mucosal enzymes necessary for digestion and absorption are altered in the damaged mucosal cells. Thus the absorptive cells are reduced in number and are functionally compromised. The crypt cells are increased in number, accounting for the elongation of the crypts.

Structural abnormalities of the tight junctions between absorptive cells also occur. The tight junction normally is a barricade separating luminal content from paracellular space and the underlying mucosal vasculature. When damaged in celiac sprue, the barricade is focally disrupted and more permeable.

The cellularity of the lamina propria is regularly increased in the small intestine affected by celiac sprue. The cellular infiltrate consists largely of immunoglobulin-producing plasma cells and lymphocytes.

Celiac sprue may involve varying lengths of small intestines. The amount of involved bowel does correlate with the severity of the clinical symptoms. The proximal bowel is always involved and is usually more severely involved than the distal bowel. In mild cases of celiac sprue, some villous structure will remain even in the proximal bowel.

Treatment with a gluten-free diet results in significant improvements in the intestinal mucosa. The absorptive cells improve in days. The mucosa of the distal small intestine improves more rapidly than the proximal bowel, which was more severely involved. It may take months or years to reach its full recovery. Complete reversion to normal is uncommon. This may be in part related to inadvertent gluten ingestion.

The etiology of how gluten damages the intestinal mucosa is not known. Three possible mechanisms have been postulated, including an immune response to dietary gluten, a genetic disorder, and a metabolic disorder. Circulating antibodies to gluten fractions have been found in patients with celiac sprue. However, there does not appear to be a correlation between the presence of the circulating antibodies and the severity of the disease. Researchers have also found that immunoglobulins synthesized by celiac sprue mucosa have antigluten specificity. Although evidence implicates the immune response etiology, it is inconclusive at this time.

Genetic factors do play a role in celiac sprue. The incidence of disease in relatives is higher than in control populations. Approximately 80% of celiac sprue patients carry the histocompatibility antigen HLA-B8. HLA-DW3 antigen, which is associated with HLA-B8 through linkage disequilibrium, is also found in over 80% of patients with celiac sprue. Not all patients with HLA-B8 or HLA-DW3 have celiac sprue, nor do all patients with celiac sprue have these two antigens.[69]

In addition, antigens have been detected on the surface of B lymphocytes that are identified from antisera of celiac sprue patients. These antigens are present in most patients with celiac sprue and in all the parents of celiac sprue patients. This suggests a recessive inheritance.[54] It may be that the etiology is a combined genetic and immune response.

Some specific peptidases have been found to be reduced in the mucosa of untreated celiac sprue. These peptidases are important in the digestion of gliadin (a complex mixture of proteins obtained by alcohol extraction of wheat gluten). In the treatment of celiac sprue, the peptidase levels return to normal. If the lack of the peptidases caused celiac sprue, the deficiency would be apparent in treated as well as untreated celiac sprue. This does not support the theory of a metabolic disorder as a causative etiology of celiac sprue.

Several factors contribute to the diarrhea in celiac sprue. The stool volume and osmotic load entering the colon are increased by the malabsorption in the small bowel. Water and electrolytes are secreted into the upper small bowel lumen rather than being absorbed. Cholecystokinin and secretin release is impaired in celiac sprue, decreasing pancreatic and biliary secretions and compromising digestion. Thus the digestion and absorption of nutrients and fluids and electrolytes is impaired in the small bowel, resulting in higher stool volume and the osmotic load. The diarrhea is aggravated by the presence of dietary fats and bile salts. The excessive dietary fat content is broken down by the colon bacteria into hydroxy fatty acids, which are potent, irritating cathartics. If the terminal ileum is involved, conjugated bile salts are not absorbed and enter the colon. Bile salts have a direct cathartic action in the colon.

Esophageal cancer and intestinal lymphomas have been associated with celiac sprue. The incidence of carcinomas in celiac sprue patients is approximately 10%.[69]

Patients who have been responding well to a gluten-free diet and who suddenly develop gastrointestinal systems (weight loss, malabsorption, abdominal pain, bleeding) should undergo diagnostic studies to rule out carcinoma. Before the diagnostic work-up, it is necessary to ascertain information from the patient about adherence to the gluten-free diet. Any amount of gluten can damage the mucosa and create symptoms.

Refractory sprue is another complication. In refractory sprue, patients initially respond to a strict gluten-free diet and then relapse despite maintaining the diet. Some of these patients will respond to corticosteroids. If patients do not respond, malabsorption becomes progressive and may lead to death. Since the advent of home total parenteral nutrition, however, death is not as common.

Mucosal ulceration and intestinal strictures can develop in celiac sprue. The ulcers may perforate with ensuing peritonitis. Intestinal strictures may lead to intestinal obstructions.

DIAGNOSTIC STUDIES

Quantitative stool for fat, 72 to 96 hour collection
Normal results: 2 to 7 g of fat per 24 hours while ingesting 100 g/d

Hemoglobin, hematocrit, folic acid, and vitamin B_{12} levels
Anemia common in celiac sprue
Anemia may be related to folic acid or vitamin B_{12} deficiencies

Prothrombin time
Prolonged if vitamin K deficiency present

Xylose tolerance test
Excretion in urine is decreased in severe, untreated celiac disease

Hydrogen breath test for lactose intolerance
Secondary lactase deficiency

Serum electrolytes
Decreased
Metabolic acidosis present

Serum calcium, magnesium, phosphorus, zinc, albumin, globulins, cholesterol, and carotene
Decreased

Alkaline phosphatase
Increased in patients with osteomalacia

Barium contrast studies: barium swallow
Dilation of small intestine

Marked coarsening of mucosal pattern or complete obliteration of mucosal folds
Fragmentation of barium
Delayed transit time of barium

Small bowel biopsy (serial sections)
Most valuable diagnostic procedure
Flat mucosal surface
Absence of villi
Elongated intestinal crypts

Gluten challenge
Following response to gluten-free diet, rechallenge bowel to establish diagnosis unequivocally

TREATMENT PLAN

The major treatment is a gluten-free diet.

Chemotherapeutic
Use to manage effects of malnutrition and malabsorption:
Hematinic agent
Anemia: iron
Vitamins
Anemia: folic acid, vitamin B_{12}
Multivitamins daily to replace vitamins A, C, and E; thiamin; riboflavin; niacin; and pyridoxine
Electrolyte and nutritional replacements
Dehydration: intravenous fluid with potassium chloride added
Calcium: tetany, 1 to 2 g IV calcium gluconate
Magnesium: tetany, 0.5 g magnesium sulfate in dilute solution IV, *or*
100 mEq magnesium chloride po
Osteomalacia: calcium gluconate or calcium lactate, 6 to 8 g/d and oral vitamin D

ASSESSMENT: AREAS OF CONCERN

Malabsorption
Diarrhea: watery, bulky, semiformed, light tan or grayish, greasy-appearing, rancid odor
Constipation: large quantities of "puttylike" stool
Weight loss (some patients lose little weight because of a tremendous intake of calories and enormous appetite until disease becomes severe)
Failure to gain weight and growth retardation in children
Weakness; lassitude; fatigue

Abdomen
Excessive amounts of malodorous flatus
Protuberant and tympanic
"Doughy" consistency
Ascites (hypoproteinemia)

Severe anemia
Weakness; fatigue

Impaired coagulability (vitamin K deficiency)
Purpura
Gastrointestinal, nasal, vaginal, or renal bleeding

Osteomalacia and osteoporosis
Bone pain (low back, rib cage, pelvis)
Pathologic fractures (uncommon but may occur)

Calcium and magnesium depletion
Paresthesias, muscle cramps, tetany; positive Chvostek's or Trousseau's sign

Vitamin A deficiency
Night blindness

Hypokalemia
Severe muscle weakness
Ileus

Secondary hyperparathyroidism
Osteomalacia, bone pain, pathologic fractures

Adrenocortical insufficiency
Sodium depletion: weakness, lassitude, dizziness
Increased skin and mucous membrane pigmentation

Hypotension
Decreased blood pressure, increased pulse (from fluid and electrolyte loss or adrenocortical insufficiency)

Integument
Clubbing of nails
Dry skin
Poor skin turgor
Edema (hypoproteinemia)
Skin pigmentation
Ecchymoses (hypoprothrobinemia)
Hyperkeratosis follicularis (vitamin A deficiency)
Pallor
Dermatitis herpetiformis

Mouth
Cheilosis and glossitis
Decreased papillation of tongue

Extremities
Loss of light touch, vibration, and position (peripheral neuropathy)

NURSING DIAGNOSES and NURSING INTERVENTIONS

Nursing Diagnosis	Nursing Intervention
Nutrition, alteration in: less than body requirements	Do thorough nutritional assessment with a physical assessment. Consult with nutritionist. Weigh patient daily. Provide dietary supplements as ordered; in severe malabsorption, hyperalimentation may be used during initial stabilization period. Observe dietary trays for foods containing gluten. Support patient and family as they learn the implications of a gluten-free diet. Evaluate patient's comprehension of dietary patient education. Evaluate, in outpatient setting, patient's dietary intake and nutritional status (weight gain and stabilization); a diary may be helpful.
Fluid volume deficit, potential	Evaluate weight loss. Monitor vital signs, intake and output (include stools), and daily weights. Replace intravenous fluids and electrolytes, vitamins, and minerals as ordered. Observe patient for signs and symptoms of specific deficiencies: anemia, calcium, and magnesium.
Bowel elimination, alteration in: diarrhea	Assess frequency, volume, and consistency of bowel movements. Assess history or pattern of diarrhea (i.e., onset and duration, symptoms as an infant or child, severity).

Patient Education

1. Provide written and verbal instructions on a gluten-free diet.
2. Encourage patient to purchase a cookbook on gluten-free cooking.
3. Instruct patient to carefully read all labels. Wheat flour is often used as an extender in processed foods and is in many brands of ice cream, salad dressings, canned foods, instant coffee, catsup, mustard, and candy bars.
4. Provide consultation with a nutritionist to teach patient about the presence of gluten in many foods.

EVALUATION

Patient Outcome	Data Indicating That Outcome is Reached
Body functioning is normal.	Bowel elimination is normal with no steatorrhea; quantitative stool specimens for fat are within normal range of 2 to 7 g of fats per 24 hours on 100 g of fat per day diet. Patient gains weight. Blood pressure is within normal limits. Skin turgor is good. There is no edema or ascites. Intestinal biopsy shows recovery of mucosa.
Laboratory values are within normal limits.	Serum, whole blood, or plasma levels of calcium, magnesium, sodium, potassium, folate, zinc, cholesterol, and carotene are within normal limits. Prothrombin time is within normal limits. Hemoglobin level is within normal limits.

Short Bowel Syndrome

Short bowel syndrome refers to the severe diarrhea and significant malabsorption symptoms that develop following small bowel resections. The severity of short bowel syndrome is influenced by the amount of bowel resected and the portion of small bowel resected. Symptoms are related to the diarrhea (fluid and electrolyte losses) and malnutrition (mineral, vitamin, fat, carbohydrate, and protein deficiencies).

Catastrophic malabsorption may develop from massive resections of the small bowel. The total length of resected bowel and the bowel lost must be considered in establishing the prognosis and treatment. Forty percent of the small bowel may be resected and tolerated well, *if* the duodenum, proximal jejunum, distal half of ileum, and ileocecal sphincter are spared. In contrast, resection of 25% of the small bowel can result in severe diarrhea and malabsorption if the distal two thirds of the ileum and ileocecal valve are removed.[69] The advent of hyperalimentation has improved the survival rate of people who have lost significant amounts of small bowel.

PATHOPHYSIOLOGY

The loss of small bowel affects the body's ability to absorb nutrients and vitamins. Intestinal ischemias that compromise the blood flow to the small bowel are the most common clinical conditions that require massive bowel resections. In children, volvulus of the small bowel, aganglionosis of the small bowel, meconium ileus, or necrotizing enterocolitis may lead to resections of large amounts of small bowel. Crohn's disease may also require repeated resections of small bowel. Neoplasms and traumas have also been associated with small bowel resections. Jejunal bypass procedures for obesity are no longer recommended because of the severe malabsorption associated with the surgery.

The pathophysiologic response to resections of small bowel varies depending on length and segments involved. The ileocecal valve plays an important role in reducing contamination of residual small bowel by colonic flora. The valve also increases transit time of the contents. When short bowel syndrome occurs, absorption of water, electrolytes, fat, protein, carbohydrates, vitamins, and trace elements is reduced. Fluid loss is greatest in the initial postoperative days. Fluid loss is also higher when all or part of the colon has also been resected.

The small bowel absorbs nutrients and vitamins in different segments. Resections of small portions of the midintestine do not generally create clinical problems. However, smaller resections involving proximal or distal segments result in more significant clinical symptoms. The duodenum is responsible for iron, folate, and calcium absorption. Resection or bypass of the duodenum may result in anemia. The distal or terminal ileum is responsible for bile salt and vitamin B_{12} absorption. Reduction or absence of the active absorptive sites for bile salts will disrupt the enterohepatic circulation of bile salts. Two forms of diarrhea may develop: cholerrheic or steatorrheic. Cholerrheic diarrhea is a watery diarrhea that is common if less than 100 cm of distal ileum is resected.[69] In cholerrheic diarrhea the hepatic synthesis of bile salts compensates for the bile salts not being absorbed in the ileum. Fat digestion remains normal. The bile salts in the colon impair fluid and electrolyte absorption and stimulate further secretions of fluid into the colon. If more than 100 cm of distal ileum is removed, bile salt loss cannot be compensated by hepatic synthesis and fat digestion is impaired (this can be resolved by using an agent such as cholestyramine). Undigested fat in the colon also impairs fluid and electrolyte absorption and stimulates colonic secretions. Steatorrheic diarrhea contains water, electrolytes, bile salts, and undigested fats. Following ileal resections, gallstones have been reported to be 25% to 32% higher than in the general population. This has been related to the depletion of the bile salt pool.[69]

Interestingly, the small bowel undergoes an adaptative process following bowel resections. The remaining villi enlarge and lengthen, increasing the absorptive surface area. The epithelial hyperplasia is associated with accelerated cell renewal and migration. It appears that exposure to nutrients (oral feedings), exposure to bile and pancreatic enzymes, and response to trophic gut peptides influence the adaptative process. Cholecystokinin and secretin support the adaptative process. The presence of oral feedings is necessary for adaptation to occur, but the oral intake should be gradually started and advanced. Clinically, the patient tends to improve in absorptive ability with time.

Gastric hypersecretion will be found in approximately half of the patients who have massive small bowel resections. This can impair intestinal absorption by damaging the mucosa. This is often a temporary effect and decreases to normal levels.

DIAGNOSTIC STUDIES

Double-contrast barium films
   Estimation of amount of small bowel remaining
   Increase in caliber of remaining segment several weeks
      following surgery (adaptation)

Laboratory studies: folate, iron, vitamin B_{12}, vitamin A, calcium, magnesium, potassium, MCV, MCHC, MCH, sodium, carotene, cholesterol, zinc
   Reduced

Prothrombin time
   Lengthened

Quantitative stool test for fat
   Steatorrhea

Normal: 2 to 7 g of fat per day on diet of 100 g of fat per day

Lactose intolerance
Lactase deficiency (jejunal loss)

Xylose tolerance
Excretion in urine decreased

Culture of intestinal fluid
Bacterial overgrowth

D-Lactate levels (serum)
Elevated

TREATMENT PLAN

Chemotherapeutic
Parenteral replacement of fluid loss
Antidiarrheal agents
    Diphenoxylate (Lomotil), 2.5 to 5.0 mg q4h po
    Loperamide (Imodium), 2 mg q6h po
    Paregoric may be used; dosage varies with degree of resection and diarrhea
Cholinergic blocking agents
    Propantheline bromide (Pro-Banthine), 15 to 30 mg
Anti-infective agents
    Tetracycline (Achromycin) or ampicillin (Amcill) for bacterial overgrowth, 1 g/d for 2 wk
Histamine receptor antagonist
    Cimetidine (Tagamet), 300 mg qid with meals and at bedtime (for gastric hypersection)
Antilipemic agent
    Ileal resections with cholerrheic diarrhea: cholestyramine, 8 to 12 mg/d
Antacid
    Aluminum hydroxide, 15-30 ml qid
Vitamins
    Cyanocobalamin (vitamin B_{12}), 1000 μg IM monthly
    Folate, 1 mg po daily

Supportive
Hyperalimentation for nutrition, especially immediately postoperatively

Gradual oral feedings: elemental diets initially; followed by polymeric supplements; add milk carefully (a low-lactose diet may be preferred)
High caloric intake; six meals per day
Home hyperalimentation

ASSESSMENT: AREAS OF CONCERN

Malabsorption: caloric deprivation
Severe weight loss
Fatigue
Lassitude
Weakness

Calcium and magnesium levels
Tetany; positive Chvostek's or Trousseau's signs
Osteomalacia; osteoporosis; bone pain; spontaneous fractures

Vitamin K
Purpura; generalized bleeding

Protein
Mild or moderate hypoalbuminemia

Iron, folate, vitamin B_{12}
Anemia

Bile salts
Cholerrheic or steatorrheic diarrhea
Gallstones

Dehydration
Poor skin turgor
Hypokalemia
Hyponatremia

Excessive colonic absorption of oxalate
Calcium oxalate kidney stones

Lactic acidosis (D-lactate levels)
Altered personality; confusion; stupor; ataxia (elevated D-lactate is the result of anaerobic colonic bacteria and unabsorbed carbohydrates)

NURSING DIAGNOSES and NURSING INTERVENTIONS

Nursing Diagnosis	Nursing Intervention
Nutrition, alteration in: less than body requirements	Provide nutritional replacements as ordered. Assist patient to design nutrition plan to meet life-style and caloric needs. Observe hyperalimentation catheter site (Broviac, Hickman, central line). Change hyperalimentation dressing three times per week or per protocol. Observe for signs of infection (fever or redness) and if present notify physician immediately.

Nursing Diagnosis	Nursing Intervention
	Monitor vital signs, intake and output, urine for sugar and acetone, and daily weights.
	Record description of stools including frequency, characteristics, and odor.
Fluid volume deficit, actual	Assess patient carefully for signs of fluid loss and shock.
	Assess skin turgor, daily weights, intake and output, and blood pressure (sitting and lying).
	Provide fluid replacement as ordered.
Bowel elimination, alteration in: diarrhea	Assess stools for signs of cholerrheic vs. steatorrheic diarrhea.
	Provide antidiarrheal agents as ordered.
	Record accurate description of stools and frequency.
	Provide fluid replacements as ordered.

Patient Education

1. Provide information, oral and written, on dietary restrictions, dietary supplements, and medications regarding nutritional effects of malabsorption.
2. Teach patient home hyperalimentation if necessary. Provide a home care referral to evaluate and assist patient and family.
3. Teach patient signs and symptoms of key electrolyte, fluid, and nutritional losses and complications from increased acidity and oxalate stones.
4. Instruct patient to notify physician immediately if he gets gastroenteritis as he can become seriously dehydrated quickly.

EVALUATION

Patient Outcome	Data Indicating That Outcome is Reached
Nutritional status is normal.	Dietary plans provide adequate nutrition for absorptive capacity of bowel.
	Degree of diarrhea is minimized.
	Patient gains weight.
Laboratory values are within normal limits.	Hemoglobin level, prothrombin times, MCV, MCHC, and MCH are within normal limits.
	Levels of calcium, magnesium, sodium, potassium, folate, zinc, cholesterol, and carotene are within normal limits.
Home hyperalimentation is performed.	Infusion at night is without incident.
	Line is free of infection.

PERITONITIS

Peritonitis is the inflammation of the peritoneum. The inflammatory response may be localized or generalized.

The etiology of peritonitis is contamination of the peritoneal cavity by bacteria or chemicals. Peritonitis is also classified by primary and secondary etiologies. Primary peritonitis is an acute or subacute bacterial infection of the peritoneum not associated with any underlying bowel disorder. Primary peritonitis is often seen in children with underlying nephrotic syndromes and urinary tract infections. Cirrhosis with ascites has also been associated with primary peritonitis. Secondary peritonitis is the result of contamination of peritoneum from perforation of the gas-

trointestinal tract (peptic ulcer, diverticulum, or appendix), gangrene of the bowel, salpingitis, traumatic injuries, and surgical contaminants. Peritonitis is a common complication of many disease processes that can progress to perforation or rupture of the organs of digestion. In secondary peritonitis the inflammation is a result of bacterial and chemical irritation.

Secondary (generalized) peritonitis is a serious complication of an acutely ill patient. The mortality of generalized peritonitis is 50% even with the use of antibiotics and intensive support systems.[69] Three factors that negatively affect the prognosis are age, type of contamination, and tissue perfusion. The older patient is at a higher risk for a poor prognosis or poor response to treatment. Fecal contamination is the most serious. Poor tissue perfusion indicates a poor prognosis. Poor tissue perfusion is associated with hypotension, acidosis, hypokalemia, or respiratory difficulties. Perforated peptic ulcer, ruptured appendix, trauma, ischemic bowel disease, intestinal obstruction, pancreatitis, and perforated colon are common causes of a generalized peritonitis.

Primary peritonitis accounts for approximately 1% of the incidence of infectious peritonitis.[7] Primary peritonitis may be divided into idiopathic (or spontaneous) and tuberculous peritonitis. Spontaneous bacterial peritonitis is associated with 2% of all pediatric abdominal emergencies and 13% of pediatric diffuse peritoneal sepsis in children.[69]

Tuberculous peritonitis is caused by a reactivation of latent tuberculosis in the peritoneum. The patient may not have active pulmonary, intestinal, or genital tuberculosis. Peritonitis from fungi and parasites is uncommon. *Candida albicans* may cause severe peritonitis, but it requires a contamination of the peritoneum, usually from an occult gastrointestinal perforation. *Coccidioides immitis* may result in granulomatous peritonitis in 1% to 2% of patients with coccidioidomycosis. Parasitic infections rarely lead to clinical symptoms of peritonitis but may closely resemble peritoneal carcinomatosis or tuberculosis during laparotomy.

PATHOPHYSIOLOGY

The peritoneum is a semipermeable membrane enclosing the abdominal viscera and mesentery. The peritoneum forms a closed, saclike structure that is opened in the female at the fallopian tubes. The peritoneum is divided into visceral and parietal peritoneum. The visceral peritoneum covers the intraperitoneal organs and forms the mesenteries of these organs. The parietal peritoneum lines the abdominal wall, the undersurface of the diaphragm, the pelvic floor, and the retroperitoneal viscera (duodenum, ascending and descending colon, portions of the pancreas, kidney, and adrenals). The omentum is formed by a double layer of fused peritoneum and enclosed lymphatic vessels and blood vessels. The omentum plays a primary role in the peritoneal defense mechanism against impending perforations and small perforations.

The nervous innervation of the parietal peritoneum is from the same nerves that supply the abdominal wall. The irritation of the parietal peritoneum stimulates afferent nerves, which are transmitted through the intercostal nerves. The pain is perceived as somatic pain. No pain receptors are identified in the visceral peritoneum,

and afferent stimulation is conducted through the visceral sympathetic nervous system. The different responses or symptoms of irritation are related to the nerve pathways. The symptoms of parietal peritonitis include a sharp, localized pain, whereas the pain in visceral peritonitis is poorly characterized and poorly localized.

The diaphragmatic peritoneum is innervated in the central portion from phrenic nerves and in the peripheral portion by branches of the intercostal nerves. Symptoms will vary depending on the location of the pathologic process. The phrenic nerve stimulation would result in referred pain to either shoulder. Intercostal nerve stimulation may cause pain in the thoracic or the abdominal wall, as occurs in cholecystitis.

The peritoneal defense mechanism is the body's attempt to localize or wall off any contamination of the peritoneal cavity and prevent diffuse peritonitis. The first response is vascular dilation and increased capillary permeability. Large numbers of polymorphonuclear leukocytes pour into the area and through phagocytosis remove bacteria and foreign matter. Fibroplastic exudate is deposited and plasters the adjacent bowel, mesentery, and omentum to the inflamed area, forming a watertight seal. Thus the inflammation is enclosed as an abscess. Peritoneal injuries will heal without fibrous adhesions unless infection, ischemia, or foreign bodies are associated with the peritonitis.

The body's response to secondary (acute bacterial) peritonitis includes removal of the bacteria through diaphragmatic lymphatics; phagocytosis and destruction of bacteria by opsonins, polymorphonuclear leukocytes, and macrophages; and localization by the omentum and fibroplastic exudate. Vascular dilation, hyperemia, and a fluid shift occur. The vascular dilation and hyperemia lead to an increase in polymorphonuclear leukocytes and macrophages. The absorption capacity of the peritoneum is increased, facilitating the absorption of bacteria and toxins. A fluid shift occurs from the extracellular fluid compartment into the free peritoneal space, into the loose connective tissue (as edema), and into the lumen of the atonic gastrointestinal tract. The translocation of water, electrolytes, and protein into this third-space compartment depletes the circulating fluid volume. The rate of fluid shift is proportional to the degree of peritoneal involvement and the success of the body's peritoneal defense mechanism.

Early diagnosis and treatment are necessary to prevent severe shock from the loss of fluid into the peritoneal space. The principal complications of untreated peritonitis include septicemia, shock, ileus, and major organ failure including respiratory, renal, hepatic, and cardiac systems. The patient has symptoms of an acute condition in the abdomen, and it is necessary to rule out other causes of the presenting symptoms.

DIAGNOSTIC STUDIES

Laboratory studies
WBC: increased leukocytes
RBC: hemoconcentration
Metabolic acidosis
Respiratory alkalosis
Electrolytes: vary

Plain abdominal x-ray films
Intestinal distention (small and large)
Air-fluid levels
Free air (perforations)

Peritoneal aspiration
Identification of organisms (primary peritonitis)
Appearance of aspirate (cloudy, blood-tinged, etc.)

TREATMENT PLAN

Surgical
Operative procedure determined by primary etiology
Objectives of surgery are to close perforation, to prevent septicemia, and to prevent abscess formation (or to drain abscess)

Chemotherapeutic
Adequate volumes of electrolytes and colloid solutions to correct hypovolemia
Analgesics to control pain
Antibiotic therapy to cover multiple bacterial flora contaminating the peritoneal cavity; usually includes aminoglycoside (aerobic gram-negative), clindamycin or metronidazole (anaerobes), ampicillin (enterococci), and cephalosporins (broad-spectrum)

Electromechanical
Nasogastric suctioning
Monitoring: CBC, electrolytes, creatinine, arterial pH, Po_2, Pco_2
CVP or Swan-Ganz catheter

Oxygen (increased metabolic demand and respirations decreased because of pain and abdominal distention)
Continuous peritoneal lavage with antibiotics or antiseptic agents (in diffuse, poorly localized peritonitis to remove residual necrotic debris)
Respiratory assist devices or endotracheal intubation

Supportive
Nutritional supplements: total parenteral nutrition (TPN), providing 3000 to 4000 calories per day (to avoid major catabolic losses)

ASSESSMENT: AREAS OF CONCERN

Abdomen
Abdominal pain; diffuse tenderness and rigidity
Diminished or absent bowel sounds
Abdominal distention
Nausea
Vomiting

Respirations
Shallow and rapid
Pain associated with deep respirations

Cardiovascular concerns
Rapid, weak, thready pulse
Decreased blood pressure
Shock

Temperature
Fever
Septicemia

Kidney
Decreased urinary output

General appearance
Lying quietly in bed with knees flexed
Guards abdomen against sudden movements or physical examination
Appears "ill"

NURSING DIAGNOSES and NURSING INTERVENTIONS

Nursing Diagnosis	Nursing Intervention
Tissue perfusion, alteration in: cerebral, cardiopulmonary, renal, gastrointestinal, peripheral	Monitor and record patient's vital signs, central venous pressure, and urinary output every hour until stable. Replace fluids as ordered. Monitor patient's laboratory results as well as signs and symptoms for shock, metabolic acidosis, and respiratory alkalosis.
Breathing pattern, ineffective	Observe patient for breathing difficulties: shallow, rapid respirations secondary to pain; assist with respiratory devices (e.g., incentive spirometer) as appropriate. Monitor oxygen therapy if ordered.

Nursing Diagnosis	Nursing Intervention
Comfort, alteration in: pain	Limit unnecessary physical examinations. Assist patient in maintaining position with minimal stress on abdominal muscles. Provide analgesics as ordered. (Some surgeons will not order analgesia since it may mask signs and symptoms.)
Nutrition, alteration in: potential for more than body requirements	Monitor TPN infusions. Change TPN tubing and dressing per hospital procedures.

Patient Education

1. The patient manages any wounds, abscesses, or incisions that have not closed or continue to drain before and following discharge from the hospital.
2. The patient identifies purpose of discharge medications and appropriate method of administration, including times, route, and length of course of medications.

EVALUATION

Patient Outcome	Data Indicating That Outcome is Reached
Body functions normally.	Pain, fever, and abdominal signs are absent. Urinary output is adequate, and normal bowel pattern is restored. Incision heals without any drains and stab wounds. Blood pressure and pulse are normal.
Laboratory studies are within normal limits.	WBC, hemoglobin, hematocrit, P_{O_2}, P_{CO_2}, and pH are within normal limits.

POLYPS

The term polyp refers to a discrete tissue mass that is elevated above the mucosal surface. A polyp may be described according to histology, presence or absence of a stalk, and whether or not it is one of multiple similar protrusions in the gastrointestinal tract.

The histology of a polyp determines the tissue from which the polyp developed and determines the descriptive name. For example, adenoma develops from epithelium, myoma from smooth muscle, and hemangioma from blood vessels. The most common type of colonic polyp is an adenoma. Pedunculated polyps are attached to the mucosa by a stalk, while sessile polyps rest on a broad base of mucosa. Although polyps may occur throughout the gastrointestinal tract, the predominant site is in the distal 25 cm of the colon. Colonic polyps may be classified as neoplastic or nonneoplastic. Neoplastic polyps include adenomas and carcinomas. Categories of nonneoplastic polyps include mucosal polyps, hyperplastic polyps, pseudopolyps of inflammatory bowel disease, and juvenile polyps. Syndromes that involve multiple gastrointestinal polyps include familial polyposis, Gardner's syndrome, Turcot syndrome, Peutz-Jeghers syndrome, and juvenile polyps.

The frequency of colonic adenomas, although varying widely among populations, tends to be highest in North America and Europe. Autopsy surveys in the United States indicate that 50% of the population have at least one adenomatous colonic polyp. When age is considered as a variable, it is noted that two thirds of those over 65 years of age have colonic adenomas. Adenomas in the colon and rectum are more likely to become malignant. The diagnosis and removal of polyps play an important role in preventing colon and rectal cancers.

Familial polyposis, an inherited autosomal dominant trait, is characterized by progressive development of hundreds of polyps (adenomas) throughout the colon. Familial polyposis is a precancerous condition. The development of colon cancer in familial polyposis is inevitable without surgical intervention. The polyps begin to develop after puberty, and the patient may remain asymptomatic for several years. The presence of multiple cancers at the time of diagnosis is high. Family assessments and genetic counseling are important in reducing the rates of early deaths from colon cancer by identifying family members who have the gene for familial polyposis.

Gardner's syndrome is a variant of familial polyposis

and consists of gastrointestinal polyposis, osteomas of the skull, mandible, and long bones, and soft-tissue tumors. Gardner's syndrome is inherited as an autosomal dominant trait. The gastrointestinal polyps appear in the small and large intestine and are precancerous.

Turcot's syndrome describes the combination of familial polyposis and malignant central nervous system (CNS) tumors. The CNS tumors include glioblastomas and medulloblastomas.

Peutz-Jeghers syndrome involves mucocutaneous pigmentation of the mouth, lips, hands, and feet and multiple polyps in the small and large intestines. The polyps are hamartomas; that is, they develop from glandular epithelium supported by smooth muscle. The pigmentation generally fades following puberty with the exception of those found in the mouth.

Juvenile polyps are distinctive hamartomas found in the rectum of children. The polyps do not tend to be precancerous lesions but are removed because of the associated problems of bleeding, obstructions, and intussusception.

PATHOPHYSIOLOGY

Colonic polyps or adenomas are composed of immature epithelial cells that continue to proliferate. Normally, the lower third of the colonic crypt is the site of cell division. As the cells move upward toward the lumen of the colon, they differentiate into colonic epithelium that secretes mucus. When the normal processes of cell proliferation and differentiation are altered, cells migrate to the surface, where they continue to synthesize DNA and divide. The surface epithelium of undifferentiated cells accumulates and leads to the formation of a polyp. The same steps are found in familial polyposis, where normal-appearing mucosa will be found to be mature, differentiated epithelium and polyps will be composed of proliferative cells.

Adenomatous polyps may develop as tubular adenomas, villous adenomas, or tubulovillous adenomas. Tubular adenoma is used to describe polyps that consist of densely packed colonic cells with some loss of goblet cell mucin, branching of glands, and varying degrees of nuclear atypia. Tubular adenomas are more common and are usually smaller. Villous adenomas contain a proliferation of villi. Villous adenomas are larger than tubular adenomas. The polyps that contain villi and tubular epithelium are referred to as tubulovillous adenomas. The involvement of the villi structures is associated with a higher incidence of cancer.

The relationship between polyps and cancer has been developed through longitudinal observations. Dysplasia, in varying degrees, is found during histologic examination of polyps following biopsy. Evidence supporting the relationship between polyps and colon carcinomas is based on three major findings: location of clusters of cancers within adenomatous polyps, findings in patients with multiple polyposis, and epidemiologic studies. Although small, isolated colon carcinomas are rare, small groups of cancers are found within adenomatous polyps. The development of carcinomas in patients with colonic polyps is usually 10 to 15 years after the appearance of benign adenomas. Data supporting the time span are based on patients with familial polyposis. However, residual adenomatous tissue may be found surrounding malignant tissue in patients with early colon cancer lesions at diagnosis and surgery. The same population groups tend to have high rates of colon cancer and colonic adenomas further supporting the relationship.

When a polyp is removed, cytology and histology studies are performed to carefully assess the patient for further medical or surgical intervention. Polyps may be associated with mild to severe degrees of dysplasia. When the polyp contains foci in which the nuclei are large and irregular, cells are crowded, polarity lost, and cribiform glands are present, the cytologic appearance is malignant. The interpretation of the finding is then made by examining the entire polyp. If the foci do not extend into the muscularis mucosae, the polyp contains carcinoma in situ. If there is extension into the muscularis mucosae and submucosa (and thus lymphatic and blood supply), the polyp is considered invasive carcinoma.

The development of polyps in familial polyposis is through the alteration of the normal cell proliferation and differentiation as previously described. In familial polyposis, young people develop hundreds to thousands of colonic polyps. Cancer, in one or more polyps, will generally develop before 40 years of age.

Studies of skin fibroblasts of patients with familial polyposis and Gardner's syndrome have demonstrated abnormal growth characteristics in culture. The cells have lost normal contact inhibition; they grow in multilayered, crisscrossed patterns and have decreased serum requirements for growth. The study of skin fibroblasts in patients to detect the familial polyposis trait may be a diagnostic tool for the future.[69]

In Gardner's syndrome, polyps may be found throughout the gastrointestinal tract. Duodenal polyps are more common than jejunal or ileal and are precancerous. Multiple polyps may also be found in the stomach. Interestingly, in Japan, gastric polyps are reported as associated with gastric carcinomas, but this is not true in the Western world.[78] Extracolonic manifestations include osteomas of the mandible, skull, and long bones (e.g., epidermoid cysts, fibromas, lipomas, and desmoid tumors), dental abnormalities (e.g., impacted teeth, mandibular cysts), and soft-tissue tumors (e.g., carcinoma of the thyroid and adrenal glands).

DIAGNOSTIC STUDIES

Stool for occult blood
Positive for blood

Proctosigmoidoscopy
Visualization of bowel lumen (flexible fiberoptic sigmoidoscopy is better tolerated, but only 30 cm in length)

Colonoscopy
Visualization and polypectomy; biopsy (total excision of polyp is the accepted method of providing an accurate histologic diagnosis)

Radiography studies
Osteomas found in Gardner's syndrome

Air-contrast barium enema
Used to identify polyps above the rectosigmoid area

TREATMENT PLAN

Surgical
Colonic adenomas: colonic polypectomy for benign polyp or carcinoma in situ; pedunculated polyp treated with polypectomy when confined to head of polyp; invasive carcinoma, sessile polyps, cancer in stalk, cancer at margin of resection, and undifferentiated cancer in any polyp require colon resection with wide margins
Familial polyposis and Gardner's syndrome: total colectomy with ileoanal reservoir (Parks, J-pouch), continent ileostomy (Kock pouch), or conventional ileostomy (Cure is obtained by removing all mucosa in colon and rectum. Rectal mucosal stripping procedures with anal sphincter–saving surgeries are being developed.)
Peutz-Jeghers syndrome: may be required for management of complications (bleeding, intussusception, obstruction)

Electromechanical
Juvenile polyps: colonoscopy (polypectomy)

Supportive
Routine or periodic proctosigmoidoscopy or colonoscopy in patients at risk for developing familial polyposis or Gardner's syndrome
Genetic counseling

ASSESSMENT: AREAS OF CONCERN

Colonic polyp
Intestinal symptoms
Occult or overt rectal bleeding
Constipation or change in caliber of stool (polyps decreasing lumen size)
Diarrhea with hypokalemia and dehydration (villous adenoma)
Crampy, lower abdominal pain (caused by intermittent intussusception)
In presence of above symptoms, must rule out possibility of colon carcinoma

Familial polyposis
History
Family history used to identify asymptomatic individuals at risk
Intestinal symptoms
Hematochezia (rectal bleeding)
Diarrhea
Abdominal pain

Gardner's syndrome
History
Family history to identify asymptomatic individuals at risk
Intestinal symptoms
Bleeding
Diarrhea
Abdominal pain
Extracolonic manifestations (osteomas, soft-tissue tumors)
Careful examination for presence of sebaceous cysts, fibromas of the skin, and bony tumors

Juvenile polyps
Intestinal symptoms
Bleeding
Crampy abdominal pain
Constipation

Peutz-Jeghers syndrome
Intestinal symptoms
Observation for symptoms of intestinal obstruction, intussusception, and gastrointestinal bleeding
Extracolonic manifestations
Macular lesions, brown to greenish black, around mouth, nose, lips, buccal mucosa, hands, feet, and occasionally in perianal and genital regions

NURSING DIAGNOSES and NURSING INTERVENTIONS

Nursing Diagnosis	Nursing Intervention
Potential patient problem: bowel elimination, alteration in	Assess carefully patient's history regarding bowel patterns, changes in pattern, rectal bleeding, and abdominal pain. Prepare patient through preprocedural teaching for colonoscopy examination, barium enemas, and proctosigmoidostomy.
Self-concept, disturbance in: personal identity	Assess patient's level of understanding of genetic factor in familial polyposis and Gardner's syndrome. Assist patient in acquisition of knowledge regarding disease, treatment, and implications for future. Provide genetic counseling. Identify additional family members for workup for familial polyposis and Gardner's disease.
Self-concept, disturbance in: body image	Assist patient by providing information on (1) rationale of total colectomy for familial polyposis and (2) available surgical procedures including conventional ileostomy, continent (Kock) ileostomy, and anal sphincter–saving surgeries. Request a visit from a cured patient who has undergone the same surgical procedure selected by the patient. Refer patient to ET nurse and ostomy organization for support.
Sexual dysfunction (potential)	Evaluate patient's sexual history in relation to the presence of perianal or perirectal disease, which may make sexual activity extremely painful. (Patients may avoid sexual activity because of painful experiences.) Provide patient and partner opportunities to discuss their feelings regarding any actual or feared changes in sexual activities. (The fear of colectomy surgery may be an underlying theme related to changes in self and body image.)

Patient Education

Close follow-up should be planned because of recurrence rates. Evaluation will require barium enema, proctosigmoidoscopy, or colonoscopy. The pattern should be as follows:
1. Benign colonic adenoma: every 2 to 3 years
2. Carcinoma confined to polyp: in 6 months, then yearly
3. Multiple polyps and family history of cancer: yearly
4. Asymptomatic familial polyposis: every 6 months
5. Familial polyposis, following surgery when rectal segment is left: every 6 months

See p. 1273 for instructions on ostomy care.

EVALUATION

Patient Outcome	Data Indicating That Outcome is Reached
Body functions normally.	There is no diarrhea, constipation, rectal bleeding, or abdominal pain.
Patient can care for ileostomy or continent ileostomy (familial polyposis).	For conventional ileostomy, patient is able to manage external pouch, skin is in excellent condition, and diet is normal. For continent ileostomy, patient is able to intubate pouch, and diet is normal.

PSEUDOMEMBRANOUS ENTEROCOLITIS

Pseudomembranous enterocolitis is an inflammation and necrosis of the bowel which primarily affects the mucosa and occasionally the submucosa. Pseudomembranous exudative plaques are found attached to the mucosal surface of the small bowel (enteritis), colon (colitis) or both (enterocolitis).

In 1893, original reports on pseudomembranous colitis indicated intestinal ischemia as the basic etiology. The advent of antibiotics resulted in a series of studies which implicated antibiotic use and *Staphylococcus aureus*. The widespread use of colonoscopy as a diagnostic procedure has improved the detection of pseudomembranous enterocolitis. Stool cultures have ruled out *S. aureus* as the causative agent. At this time, *Clostridium difficile* has been identified as the enteric pathogen responsible for pseudomembranous colitis following antibiotic therapy. Although many antimicrobial agents have been implicated in pseudomembranous colitis, the most common agents include clindamycin, lincomycin, cephalosporins, and ampicillin.

Risk factors for developing pseudomembranous enterocolitis, excluding antimicrobials, include surgery of the colon, stomach, or pelvis region complicated by shock during or following the surgery; spinal fractures; intestinal obstructions; Crohn's disease; neonatal necrotizing enterocolitis; and Hirschsprung's disease. Age also appears to be a risk factor in antibiotic-associated pseudomembranous enterocolitis with older patients at higher risk.

PATHOPHYSIOLOGY

Antibiotic-induced pseudomembranous colitis develops when the normal bowel flora is altered by antibiotic therapy. The *C. difficile* organisms multiply producing two toxins. The toxins damage the membranes of the epithelial cells, leading to cell necrosis. Poor vascular perfusion to the mucosa may also progress to necrosis of the mucosal layer of the gut. Antibiotic-induced pseudomembranous enterocolitis tends to be primarily a disease of the colon, whereas studies of pseudomembranous enterocolitis not associated with antibiotics demonstrated lesions in the small bowel as well.

The pseudomembrane is composed of fibrin, mucin, sloughed epithelial cells, and inflammatory cells. The mildest form of pseudomembranous enterocolitis consists of focal necrosis. A characteristic "summit" lesion develops from a collection of fibrin and polymorphonuclear cells. As the disease progresses, the appearance changes to a "volcanic" lesion that includes glandular cell disruption and the typical pseudomembrane of elevated yellow-white plaques. As the necrosis worsens, there is an extensive involvement of the lamina propria and a thick overlaying of the pseudomembrane. If the pseudomembranes slough, the bowel is left with large denuded areas.

Pseudomembranous colitis can progress to a life-threatening illness. The symptoms may not develop for 4 to 7 weeks after the antibiotic therapy has been discontinued. Patients generally have severe diarrhea, abdominal tenderness, fever, and leukocytosis. As the bowel wall necrosis continues, the patient begins to lose fluids, electrolytes, and albumin. Toxic megacolon may develop. The colon may perforate, leading to the sequelae of peritonitis and sepsis.

Early diagnosis is important in initiating oral treatment and preventing the disorder from becoming fulminant or intractable to medical management. The medical management consists of antimicrobials that are effective against *C. difficile*. In patients with a less severe disease, an anion exchange resin (cholestyramine) has been used to bind the toxins produced by *C. difficile*. Cholestyramine should not be used in combination with antimicrobials since the resin will bind the antimicrobial and reduce the drug levels in the colon.

DIAGNOSTIC STUDIES

Plain films of abdomen
  Markedly edematous colon
  Distorted haustral markings
  Colon distention
  Air fluid levels in toxic megacolon

Barium air-contrast studies
  Rounded filling defects outlining plaques

Colonoscopy
  Yellowish white plaques
  Erythema
  Edema
  Friable mucosa
  Ulcerations
  Hemorrhage

Stool analysis
  C. difficile toxin assay

TREATMENT PLAN

Surgical
  Severely ill patients with fulminant or intractable symptoms may require colectomy or diverting ileostomy (rare)

Chemotherapeutic
Vancomycin, 500 mg to 2 g daily q7-14 d.
Cholestyramine, 12 g/d q5d.
Bacitracin, 2 g/d q7-10d.
Metronidazole, 1.2 to 1.5 g/d q7-15 d.

Supportive
Intravenous fluids; hyperalimentation
Bowel rest

ASSESSMENT: AREAS OF CONCERN

Bowel habits
Diarrhea consisting of watery stools containing mucus; severity varies up to 30 loose stools per day; may begin during antibiotic therapy or after drug is discontinued

Physical examination
Abdominal pain and tenderness on palpation
Signs of severe dehydration and electrolyte imbalance
Abdominal distention and decreased peristalsis (signs of toxic megacolon)

Blood work
Peripheral leukocyte count of 10,000 to 20,000/cu ml or higher

NURSING DIAGNOSES and NURSING INTERVENTIONS

Nursing Diagnosis	Nursing Intervention
Bowel elimination, alteration in: diarrhea	Assess all patients receiving antibiotics for diarrhea, particularly those on clindamycin, ampicillin, and cephalosporins. Report to physician patients experiencing loose, watery, frequent diarrheal stools. Observe patient for signs and symptoms of fluid loss, electrolyte imbalance, abdominal pain or tenderness, and fever. Document number, description, amount, and frequency of bowel movements.
Tissue perfusion, alteration in: gastrointestinal	Assess patient for signs of toxic megacolon, colonic perforation, and intestinal ischemia. Assess patient's blood pressure, pulse, temperature, and respirations, reporting any signs of shock. Assess for presence of maroon stools and abdominal distention. Maintain patient's intravenous fluids as ordered.

Patient Education

1. Patients will be given oral medications, and it is important that the patient understand the rationale for the agent and the importance of compliance with the prescribed protocol.
2. If surgery is required for fulminating disease, the patient and family will require instructions in management of the diverting or permanent ileostomy. The surgery is rarely necessary.

EVALUATION

Patient Outcome	Data Indicating That Outcome is Reached
Body functions normally.	Patient does not experience diarrhea, nor does diarrhea recur after discontinuation of treatment.
Fluid balance is maintained.	Patient returns to normal hydration levels as assessed by skin turgor, mucous membranes, color, blood pressure and pulse.
Laboratory studies	Serum electrolytes, hematocrit, and WBC within normal limits.

CROHN'S DISEASE

Crohn's disease, a chronic inflammatory disorder of the gastrointestinal tract, may occur in any part of the gastrointestinal tract from the mouth to the anus, but the most common sites are the terminal ileum and colon.

Crohn's disease, granulomatous colitis, regional enteritis, transmural colitis, and transmural ileitis all refer to the same disease process. Crohn's disease is segmental in nature, and normal mucosa will be found between diseased segments (skip lesions). Crohn's disease and ulcerative colitis are often called inflammatory bowel diseases (IBD), and differential diagnosis between the two diseases is important in planning treatment. A chronic disorder, Crohn's disease frequently recurs after surgical resection of diseased segments.

The overall incidence of Crohn's disease has increased by a factor of 1.4 to 4 over the past 20 years with a prevalence range of 10 to 70 cases per 100,000 population.[69] The disease has also been increasing in the young.[72] It is hard to determine if the increase is in actual numbers of cases or whether it is related to an increased awareness of Crohn's disease and improved diagnostic techniques. Crohn's disease is more common among Jews than non-Jews and among whites than nonwhites. The age at onset of the disease is the early teens and early twenties with a range of 15 to 30 years of age.[6,69] A positive family history for inflammatory bowel disease may be found in 20% to 30% of the patients.[69] The frequency among siblings is higher than with more distant relatives.

Description of Crohn's disease is by the anatomic location of the disease. Crohn's disease may be limited to the small bowel, involve both small bowel and colon (ileocolitis), be limited to the colon, or be present in the stomach or duodenum. A small group of patients may have Crohn's disease that is limited to the anorectal region. The majority of patients have Crohn's disease involving both the small bowel and colon.

The etiology of Crohn's disease is unknown. Research funded through the National Foundation of Ileitis and Colitis (NFIC) and other digestive disease groups is directed toward discovery of the cause and ultimately the cure for this chronic illness.

PATHOPHYSIOLOGY

Although the etiology of Crohn's disease is unknown, it has been hypothesized that an exogenous agent penetrates the intestinal epithelium, creating a cytopathic immune response in a susceptible individual. Factors that have been examined as possible causes include infectious agents (bacteria and viruses), altered host susceptibility, immune-mediated intestinal damage, psychologic factors, and dietary and environmental factors.

Psychologic factors that have been implicated in the etiology of inflammatory bowel disease have not been documented in patients with Crohn's disease.[6,69,72] This is probably one of the continuing myths about Crohn's disease that is perpetuated in nursing literature. The effect of the chronic illness, its recurrence, and the potential of debilitating symptoms may result in psychologic or social problems. Stress has been associated with clinical exacerbations of the disease.

The role of infectious agents has been studied in order to identify a specific myobacteria or virus responsible for Crohn's disease. Recent studies have explored the possibility of cell wall–defective variants of enteric bacteria, while other research suggests a viruslike agent. Granulomatous lesions have been produced on the footpads of mice by injecting extracts from Crohn's lesions. The same results were discovered when injections were made from intestinal extracts from normal specimens. So far, studies have failed to document a specific etiologic agent in Crohn's disease.

Altered host susceptibility has been considered in the etiology of Crohn's disease. Although a specific infectious agent has not been identified, some researchers suggest that an impaired immune or inflammatory response to an infectious agent might progress to Crohn's disease. Impairment of various manifestations of cell-mediated immunity has been found in a substantial portion of patients with Crohn's disease.[60] Genetic transmission of specific histocompatibility antigens has also been explored without conclusive findings.

Immune mechanisms have been implicated in the etiology of Crohn's disease because of the recurrent inflammatory process, presence of granulomatous lesions, systemic manifestations, and the positive response to corticosteroids. Studies have examined the following as possible immune etiologies: (1) hypersensitivity reaction in the intestines, (2) "autoimmune" antibody–mediated damage to intestinal epithelium, (3) tissue deposition of antigen-antibody complexes, (4) lymphocyte-mediated cytotoxicity, and (5) impairment of cellular immune mechanisms.[6]

Sleisenger and Fordtran[69] identify three weaknesses in the immunity basis for inflammatory bowel disease. First, the cytotoxicity of lymphocytes disappears after surgical removal of the diseased bowel. Second, the antibody-dependent, cell-mediated damage to intestinal mucosa has not been demonstrated in the intact host. Third, it is not confirmed that the K cell–mediated cytotoxicity induced by lymphocytes is specific to inflammatory bowel disease.

Dietary and environmental factors have also been questioned in the etiology of Crohn's disease. Chemical food additives, such as carrageenin, reduced dietary fibers, and increased refined sugars have been studied. No evidence firmly links dietary or environmental factors to Crohn's disease at this time.

In Crohn's disease the inflammatory process extends through the layers of the bowel wall, hence the term *transmural*. Microscopically the following are found in the intestines: transmural inflammation, submucosal infiltration, submucosal thickening and fibrosis, ulceration through the mucosa, fissures, and focal granulomas. As the disease progresses, the bowel wall thickens and the lumen narrows. Stenosis is common. The mucosa shows skip lesions with normal bowel between diseased segments. The mesentery thickens and may extend over the serosal surface toward the antimesenteric border of the bowel. The intestinal segment may become fixed as the mesentery becomes fibrotic and contracts. The mesenteric nodes are enlarged and firm and may come together to form an irregular mass. The lymphatic vessels dilate and may be visible in the involved mesentery and serosal layer of the bowel.

The mucosal layer in advanced Crohn's disease consists of deep mucosal ulcerations and nodular submucosal thickening producing a cobblestone appearance to the surface layer. The ulcers usually extend into the submucosa, and two or more ulcers may coalesce to form deep longitudinal ulcers traversing long segments. These ulcers are often referred to as *rake* ulcers. As the disease progresses, the mucosa becomes denuded.

The inflammation of the serosa and mesentery leads to a characteristic tendency in Crohn's disease for involved loops of bowel to adhere to one another. Fissures extend through the entire wall of the bowel and erode into adjacent loops of bowel or bladder, forming a fistula. It is not unusual for a fistula tract to develop to the skin (enterocutaneous), the umbilicus, or the perineum. When the rectum is diseased, ulcers arising in the rectal crypts may end in the perirectal fat and form abscesses. Rectal abscesses may erode into the anal sphincter and the supporting muscles. Abscesses can occur anywhere in the peritoneum, retroperitoneal area, or pelvis.

The severity of the malabsorption depends on the severity of the Crohn's disease, the amount of gut involved, and the treatment regimen. Crohn's disease in the jejunum and ileum decreases the capacity of the small bowel mucosa to absorb multiple nutrients, including carbohydrates, amino acids, folate, water-soluble vitamins, fats, and fat-soluble vitamins. Disease in the terminal ileum may lead to vitamin B_{12} (cobalamin) malabsorption and bile salt reabsorption, leading to increased diarrhea due to increased osmolality of bile salt in the colon and decreased fat absorption. Lactase deficiency may develop

with small bowel disease. The presence of ulcerations in extensive disease may result in protein loss. Iron deficiency anemia may develop from a chronic, slow blood loss and decrease in iron absorption. Bleeding in Crohn's disease is often mild, and the stool color may not change. The characteristic changes of the lymphatic system in Crohn's disease contribute to an impaired fat absorption.

The strictures and internal fistulas that are common in Crohn's disease may lead to stasis of intestinal contents in the bypassed segment, which results in bacterial overgrowth in the lumen; bacterial overgrowth impairs absorption of carbohydrates, fats, and vitamin B_{12} and alters bile salt metabolism, affecting fat absorption.

Therapy may also affect nutrition. Some patients will self-impose dietary restrictions or limit their oral food intake. Patients should be tested for lactose intolerance before a lactose-free diet is imposed. Surgical resection of disease segments of small bowel and colon may also affect nutrition. Resection or bypass of an intestinal segment may decrease the absorptive surface area. Resection of the terminal ileum may lead to vitamin B_{12} and bile salt malabsorption. The distal ileum is the site for reabsorption of conjugated bile salts, and the loss of ileum results in loss of bile salts through the colon, thereby decreasing the total bile salt pool and thus decreasing biliary secretion of bile salts, resulting in fat malabsorption. Unabsorbed bile salts stimulate the colon mucosal secretion and reduce the net absorption of water and electrolytes in the colon, and the patient experiences increased diarrhea.

Surgeries that result in enteroenterostomies (bowel anastomosis to bowel), surgical blind loops, and loss of ileocecal valve create conditions in which bacterial overgrowth frequently occurs. The effect of overgrowth of enteric microorganisms was discussed previously.

Folate deficiency is common in patients with Crohn's disease. Decreased dietary intake and decreased absorption affect folate levels. In addition, sulfasalazine (which is frequently used in treating Crohn's disease) impairs the absorption of folate. Patients with Crohn's disease may also have an increased requirement for folate because of increased catabolism and chronic blood loss.

Patients with Crohn's disease frequently have increased caloric and protein requirements because of the catabolic effects of the chronic inflammation and superimposed infections. This further depletes the patient's nutritional status. The consequences of the impaired absorption and nutritional deficiencies are more serious in children than adults. Growth retardation and delayed sexual maturation occur in 20% to 30% of young patients. The use of corticosteroids over a prolonged period also contributes to growth retardation.

Complications of Crohn's disease are either intestinal (i.e., small bowel obstructions, abscesses, cancer, perforation, or fistula formation) or systemic. Obstructions are usually the result of inflammation and edema in a strictured or narrowed segment of bowel. The typical obstruction tends to progress slowly to a complete obstruction. Sudden complete obstruction may occur if the bowel becomes kinked by adhesions.

Fistula formation is very common in Crohn's disease and is a characteristic that often distinguishes Crohn's disease from ulcerative colitis. Perianal and perirectal fistulas and fissures can be extremely severe and may cause more problems for the patient than other clinical symptoms. Enterocutaneous fistulas can also cause severe management problems for the patient. A fistula between the bowel and bladder is infrequent, but when it occurs, it leads to chronic urinary infections and if untreated may progress to irreversible renal damage. Free perforation is rare in Crohn's disease because of the more frequent fistula formation and walled-off abscesses.

Systemic manifestations include arthritis, iritis, erythema nodosum, ankylosing spondylitis, pyoderma gangrenosum, aphthous mouth ulcers, and occasionally liver disease. Arthritis is the most common systemic manifestation. Arthritic symptoms may be present several years before bowel symptoms appear. Children with arthritic symptoms should have tests done to rule out inflammatory bowel disease. The arthritis may be migratory arthritis involving large joints, sacroiliitis, or ankylosing spondylitis. In Crohn's disease the arthritis does not seem to reflect the degree of intestinal disease. (However, in ulcerative colitis, arthritis tends to be more severe, and the patient experiences exacerbations or remissions depending on the intestinal state.)

Erythema nodosum and pyoderma gangrenosum are inflammatory disorders of the skin that may occur with Crohn's disease. Pyoderma gangrenosum is the more severe disorder and may be found during a recurrence of active Crohn's disease in a patient following a surgical resection. The lesion may develop before the bowel symptoms.

Although liver disease is unusual in patients with Crohn's disease, mild abnormalities of liver function may be observed in hospitalized patients. Sclerosing cholangitis occurs more frequently in patients with Crohn's disease than in the general population. Renal disorders may also be a complication of Crohn's disease. The infections related to enterovesical fistulas may lead to urinary tract infections. The ureters may also be affected by the bowel and mesenteric inflammation, leading to obstruction and hydronephrosis. Oxalate stones and hyperoxaluria have been associated with steatorrhea in patients with Crohn's disease.

Cancer of the colon occurs three times more often in patients with Crohn's disease than in the general population. This frequency is less than is found in patients with ulcerative colitis. Crohn's disease may vary from a mild to a severely debilitating disease. An individual may experience one acute episode and be asymptomatic for years. Medical management is the primary form of therapy; however, the vast majority of patients will require surgery at some time to manage intestinal complications of the long-term effects of the disease. The recurrence of Crohn's disease following a surgical resection ranges from 75% to 90% in 15 years.[69]

DIAGNOSTIC STUDIES

Differential diagnosis
  Crohn's disease often diagnosed by ruling out other
     disorders with similar symptoms and clinical signs
  Early, acute phase: small or large intestinal involvement
     Viral gastroenteritis
     Appendicitis
     Yersinia enterocolitis
     Salmonella infection
  Chronic, recurrent phase: small or large intestinal involvement
     Giardiasis
     Amebiasis
     Intestinal tuberculosis
     Intestinal lymphoma
     Fungal infection
     Pseudomembranous enterocolitis
     Duodenal ulcer disease
  Involvement limited to colon and rectum
     Ulcerative colitis
     Ischemic colitis
     Cancer of colon
     Diverticulitis

Stool cultures
  Negative (used to rule out infections)

Stool for guaiac
  Positive (slow blood loss)

Blood work
  Serum albumin
     Low (protein loss through lesions and increase in
        protein catabolism)

  Liver function
     Abnormal (pericholangitis or fatty liver)

  Serum cobalamin
     Low (ileal disease)

  Serum folic acid
     Low (malabsorption)

Hemoglobin, hematocrit
Anemia

Lactose tolerance test
To rule out lactase deficiency

Sigmoidoscopy
Rectum: rectal mucosa may be free of disease; perianal or perirectal fissures, fistulas, or abscesses may be found
Distal colon: aphthous ulcers or erosions; deep longitudinal fissures with intervening edematous mucosa

Colonoscopy
Skip lesions; cobblestone mucosa

Biopsy
Presence of granulomas
Also aids in differentiation of pseudopolyposis, ulcerative colitis, adenomatous polyp, and cancer

Barium studies
Upper small bowel, barium enemas
Asymmetric disease, skip lesions, pseudodiverticula, linear ulcerations, transverse fissures, cobblestone mucosa, strictures, fistulas (NOTE: Routine preparation of colon should be omitted since it may initiate an exacerbation of the disease. Prepare patient with a clear liquid diet for 2 to 3 days.)

TREATMENT PLAN

Surgical
Surgical resection of diseased segments of bowel (operative therapy reserved for complications of Crohn's disease or unequivocal failure to respond to medical management)
Total colectomy with ileostomy (when disease is limited to the colon and is not responsive to medical management or cancer is found)
Subtotal colectomy with temporary ileostomy or with ileorectal anastomosis (when the rectum is not involved)

Chemotherapeutic
Sulfasalazine (Azulfidine): acute phase: 3 to 4 g/d in divided doses tid; maintenance: 1 to 2.5 g/d tid
Prednisone: acute phase: 50 to 80 mg/d (intravenously in severely ill patient); maintenance: 5 to 15 mg/d po
6-Mercaptopurine (6-MP): acute phase: 1.5 mg/kg/d po; maintenance: 1.5 mg/kg/d po (has a steroid-sparing effect)
Metronidazole (Flagyl): 20 mg/kg/d in divided doses
Other antibiotics may be indicated in the acute phase

Supportive
Acute phase: intravenous fluids, nothing by mouth, bed rest or limited activity
Complication of small bowel obstruction: nasogastric suctioning
Stenosis or narrowing of lumen: avoid foods containing cellulose or those foods that are not readily digested
Diarrhea: loperamide, Lomotil, codeine; if diarrhea related to bile salt malabsorption: cholestyramine, aluminum hydroxide; metamucil may be used for watery stools in the chronic phase
Nutritional support: vitamin replacement, folic acid, iron, total parenteral nutrition (TPN), enteral alimentation; lactose restrictions (if indicated); some institutions use peripheral amino acids, fat for 1 to 5 days, with bowel rest and then start food or TPN

ASSESSMENT: AREAS OF CONCERN

Gastrointestinal concerns
Initially, diarrhea, abdominal cramping, and fever; as disease progresses, must observe patient for signs of complications
Diarrhea: when disease confined to ileum, five or six loose bowel movements per day; when colon involved, urgency and incontinence frequent
Abdominal cramping: mild to severe, lower quadrant, intermittent periumbilical colic experienced during bowel movements
Fever: low grade
Gastrointestinal complications
Fistulas
Stool in urine
Passing gas via vagina
Fecal drainage through skin (enterocutaneous)
Small bowel obstructions
Toxic megacolon
Cancer
Free perforations (rare)
Hemorrhage (infrequent)

Perianal concerns
Presence of fissures, fistulas, or abscesses

Extracolonic manifestations
Arthritis
Inflammation of eye, skin, or mucous membrane in form of iritis, pyoderma gangrenosum, erythema nodosum, or aphthous ulcers of mouth and tongue

NURSING DIAGNOSES and NURSING INTERVENTIONS

Nursing Diagnosis	Nursing Intervention
Bowel elimination, alteration in: diarrhea	Assess the frequency of bowel movements and the appearance of stools. Note signs of steatorrhea or bleeding. Check stools for occult blood. Provide antidiarrheal medications as ordered.
Fluid volume deficit, potential	Monitor patient's vital signs. Record intake, output, and daily weights. Provide intravenous fluids as ordered.
Nutrition, alteration in: less than body requirements	Evaluate nutritional status. Assist patient in identifying irritating foods. Provide nutritional supplements as ordered. Review blood work for indications of anemia and compare serum levels of folate, vitamin B_{12}, and iron. Observe patient for signs of magnesium deficit (associated with long-standing diarrhea). Observe children for signs of growth retardation.
Skin integrity, impairment of: potential	Assess perianal region for signs of fissures, fistulas, or abscesses. Assess perianal region for irritation from chronic diarrhea. Provide interventions or treatment for perianal fissures as ordered (e.g., sitz baths; keep area clean following bowel movements). Protect perianal skin in patients with frequent bowel movements; use gentle cleansing solutions (Periwash, Uniwash, Tucks, witch hazel pads); if area denuded, cleanse with cotton balls soaked in mineral oil, or use Nupercainal ointment or Anusol suppositories with or without hydrocortisone to decrease perianal pain. Evaluate enterocutaneous fistula for amount and type of drainage. See p. 1268 for specific management suggestions. Protect skin from erosion from fistula drainage.
Comfort, alteration in: pain	Provide analgesic as ordered.
Coping, family: potential for growth	Assist patient and family in supporting each other as they learn to manage the effects of a chronic illness in their lives. Evaluate patient and family needs regarding knowledge of Crohn's disease, compliance with medical treatment, and myths or misconceptions. Provide opportunities for patient and family to express their feelings regarding the illness and to identify their perceptions for a successful outcome. Assess the family background for inflammatory bowel disease. Assist parents and siblings in coping with Crohn's disease and guilt implications if family history is positive. Provide patients with information about support groups: National Foundation for Ileitis and Colitis and United Ostomy Association.
Sexual dysfunction	Evaluate patient's sexual history in relation to the presence of perianal or perirectal disease that may make sexual activity extremely painful (patient may avoid sexual activity because of painful experiences). Provide patient and partner opportunities to discuss their feelings regarding any actual or feared changes in sexual activities. (The fear of colectomy surgery may be an underlying theme related to changes in self and body image.)

Patient Education

1. Provide written schedule for medications and for "tapering" schedule for drugs as dosages are decreased.
2. Provide information on Crohn's disease and the relationship of stress and exacerbations.
3. Provide information on drug toxicities. For example, the patient taking metronidazole (Flagyl) may have an antiabuse reaction with alcohol; metronidazole is also related to peripheral neuropathy. Sulfasalazine is associated with rashes; the patient may be desensitized with small doses.
4. Provide specific instructions for procedures and allow return demonstrations: perianal care, fistula management, dietary instructions, TPN, central line care.

EVALUATION

Patient Outcome	Data Indicating That Outcome is Reached
Disease is in remission.	There is no pain, diarrhea, fever, fistulas, or perianal disease. The patient participates in routine activities of daily living and working.
Nutrition is adequate.	The patient gains weight; there are no signs of malnutrition or vitamin deficiency. Nutrition is maintained by supplements: TPN, vitamins, and minerals.
Fluid balance is maintained.	The patient returns to normal hydration levels as assessed by skin turgor, color, mucous membranes, blood pressure, and pulse.

ULCERATIVE COLITIS

Ulcerative colitis is a chronic mucosal inflammatory disease limited to the colon and rectum.

The disease generally starts in the rectum and progresses uninterrupted through the colon. The mucosa and submucosa layers of the colon and rectum are affected by ulcerative colitis. It is often difficult to differentiate the symptoms of ulcerative colitis from Crohn's disease of the large colon. The distinction between the two diseases is important in planning treatment and long-term prognosis. Ulcerative colitis is cured by total proctocolectomy. Cancer, associated with long-standing ulcerative colitis, is four times greater than in Crohn's disease. Ulcerative colitis is characterized by bloody, frequent, watery diarrhea. Patients report as many as 20 to 30 diarrheal stools per day. Remissions and exacerbations of the disease are common.

The annual incidence of ulcerative colitis in the United States has been relatively stable with six to eight cases per 100,000 persons per year.[6,69] The incidence of ulcerative colitis is more common among Jewish than non-Jewish populations and among whites than nonwhites. Interestingly, the incidence of ulcerative colitis is more common among European and American Jews than Jews living in Tel-Aviv.[26] Diagnosis of ulcerative colitis peaks in the third and fifth decades of life.

There is a higher frequency of additional cases of ulcerative colitis in families than in control populations. It is not uncommon to have family members with ulcerative colitis and Crohn's disease. A small percentage of patients may demonstrate features of both ulcerative colitis and Crohn's disease.

As with Crohn's disease, research continues to focus on discovery of the etiology of ulcerative colitis. Surgery is no longer considered a "last resort," and newer surgical techniques have improved the outlook of patients. Continent ileostomies (Kock pouch) and ileoanal reservoir procedures (Parks pouch) have eliminated the need for conventional ileostomies in selected patient populations.

PATHOPHYSIOLOGY

The etiology of ulcerative colitis is unknown. Proposed etiologies include infectious agents, genetic factors, immunologic mechanisms, and psychosomatic determinants. No specific bacterium or virus has been found to be the exogenous agent producing the inflammatory reaction seen in ulcerative colitis. The genetic hypothesis is suggested because of the familial tendency for the disease, the higher incidence in Jews, and the low incidence among nonwhites.

The immunologic mechanisms have been suggested to be the cause of ulcerative colitis or to contribute to the mucosal inflammation and extracolonic manifestations of the disease. Patients with ulcerative colitis have been found to have alterations of T and B cell lymphocytes, suggesting an immune-deficient state. In addition, the cell-free filtrates of disrupted lymphocytes from patients with ulcerative colitis are cytotoxic to normal colonic epithelium.

Some patients with ulcerative colitis have circulating antibodies to normal colon epithelium that cross react with specific enterobacterial antigens (e.g., *E. coli*).[6] Thus the components of bacteria could change the protein structure, altering the antigenic configuration to create an autoimmune reaction, and the inflammatory bowel disease results from the hypersensitivity to antigens of bacteria.

The association of ulcerative colitis with other autoimmune diseases, such as lupus erythematosus, hemolytic anemia, and vasculitis, strengthens the view that ulcerative colitis is an immunologic reaction.

Research has documented that psychosomatic factors

are not the cause of ulcerative colitis. Controlled studies have shown that patients with ulcerative colitis have no higher incidence of psychiatric problems than a control group.[46] Less than 20% of the sample could document a traumatic emotional experience before the onset of the disease.[46] Social and occupational backgrounds of patients with inflammatory bowel disease do not differ from the general population.

Patients with ulcerative colitis have been labeled in the past with a "colitis personality." It is time to eliminate any reference to personality or psychosomatic mechanisms as the etiology. The effects of chronic illness on a person's life should be explored. Twenty to thirty bowel movements per day with urgency and occasional incontinence may interfere with work, social, and sexual activities. A patient may need help in learning how to cope with his illness and the symptoms. Stress and tension may influence the symptoms of ulcerative colitis and have been known to cause exacerbations.

Ulcerative colitis is an inflammatory disease confined primarily to the mucosa and to a lesser degree to the adjacent submucosa. The primary lesion appears to be crypt abscess formation in the crypts of Lieberkühn. Polymorphonuclear cells accumulate near the tip of the crypt, and degenerative changes occur in the crypt epithelial cells. As the crypt abscess progresses, frank necrosis of the crypt epithelium occurs and the polymorphonuclear infiltrate extends through the colonic epithelium. A more chronic inflammatory infiltrate composed of mast cells, lymphocytes, plasma cells, and eosinophils develops. Vascular engorgement appears in the submucosa. The microabscesses in the crypts are not visible to an unaided eye. However, as the microabscesses coalesce by lateral enlargement, they produce shallow ulcerations of the mucosa extending down to the lamina propria. In some areas the extensions of the abscesses undermine the mucosa on three sides, producing an area of ulceration adjacent to a hanging fragment of mucosa, which is referred to as a pseudopolyp during radiographic or endoscopic procedures.

The body attempts to heal itself even as the destruction of the mucosa is occurring. Highly vascular granulation tissue may develop in ulcerated, denuded areas. Collagen is deposited in the lamina propria. Fibrosis is minimal. In long-standing disease the muscularis mucosae may hypertrophy. The hypertrophy and spasms of the muscularis mucosae may result in shortening and narrowing of the colon, loss of haustral markings, and apparent stricture formation. All of these are reversible in ulcerative colitis since they are not caused by fibrosis.

The two most prominent symptoms of ulcerative colitis are hematochezia and diarrhea. The bleeding is the result of the mucosal changes: ulceration, vascular engorgement, and highly vascular, friable granulation tissue. As

the mucosa is destroyed or damaged, it loses its ability to absorb sodium and water, resulting in watery diarrhea. The absence of involvement of the muscularis and serosa layers accounts for the lack of localized abdominal pain, fistula formation, and well-defined peritoneal signs observed frequently in Crohn's disease.

Complications of ulcerative colitis include perforation, toxic megacolon, adenocarcinoma of the colon, massive hemorrhage, and extracolonic manifestations. Perforation of the colon may develop if the disease process extends through the muscle and serosa layers of the colon. Toxic megacolon is a severe and serious complication of ulcerative colitis. Toxic megacolon is associated with fulminant disease, in which the circular and longitudinal muscles have been destroyed. Damage to the myenteric ganglia in the wall of the colon produces a loss of contractibility, and peristalsis ceases with marked dilatation of the colon developing. The transmural inflammation may lead to necrosis and perforation. Narcotics, anticholinergics, and hypokalemia may precipitate toxic megacolon since they produce atony of the smooth muscles of the colon.

Cancer of the colon and rectum occurs at a much higher rate in patients with ulcerative colitis than in the general population. Two factors appear to be related to the incidence of adenocarcinoma of the colon and rectum. First, the duration of the disease process has been related to the cancers. Ulcerative colitis of 10 years' duration increases the risk, and the risk continues to increase thereafter. Second, the extent of colonic involvement influences the risk of colorectal cancers. The more universal (affecting the entire colon and rectum) ulcerative colitis is, the higher the incidence of cancer. Patients with the disease limited to the rectum have no greater risk of colon cancer than persons of the same age and sex without ulcerative colitis. The cancerous lesions tend to be flat and infiltrative in nature and are multicentric. Early diagnosis is important. In patients with ulcerative colitis of 10 years or longer, double-contrast barium enemas alternating with pancolonoscopy yearly and proctoscopy or flexible sigmoidoscopy with rectal biopsies twice yearly are recommended. Even with close follow-up, colon cancer may be detected too late for curative therapy.

The question often arises of prophylactic colectomy after a duration of 10 years. Colectomy does cure ulcerative colitis and also prevents colon cancer. Of course, the person will have some type of diversional procedure (conventional ileostomy, continent [Kock] ileostomy, ileorectal pouch). One question of length of duration is the actual beginning of the disease. Patients may have ulcerative colitis for a year or two before diagnosis. The decision to have surgery is a serious one with which patients are faced. By the time a patient with long-standing disease is admitted for surgery, he has dealt with a variety of emotions and may be "ready" for surgery. Other patients prefer to wait until it is essential that surgery be done. While it is impossible to generalize and recommend surgical interventions for all patients, the nurse does play an important role in educating patients to the risk of cancer, the long-term effects of a disease, its treatments, and the need for consistent follow-up, even when the patient is asymptomatic.

A medical emergency for a person with ulcerative colitis is a massive hemorrhage, which occurs in approximately 4% of patients.[69] Patients with ulcerative colitis are often severely ill, with high temperatures, tachycardia, and fluid depletion. Massive fluid replacements are required to replace the circulating volume and maintain blood pressure. The hemorrhage usually subsides spontaneously. Surgical intervention (total proctocolectomy) is rarely necessary.

The mortality of an acute initial episode of ulcerative colitis is approximately 5%.[61] The prognosis is negatively affected by total colonic involvement, age at onset over 60 years, and presence of toxic megacolon.

Extracolonic manifestations can also be serious complications of ulcerative colitis. Arthritis, uveitis, and skin disorders reflect the disease process and will have remissions and exacerbations with the disease. The arthritis of ulcerative colitis involves the larger joints and is migratory. The joint is frequently swollen, erythematous, and tender.

Uveitis (iritis) is the most common eye lesion seen accompanying ulcerative colitis. The patient may experience blurred vision, eye pain, and photophobia. An acute attack of iritis may be followed by atrophy of the iris, anterior and posterior synechiae, and old pigment deposits on the lens.

The extracolonic skin disorders consist of erythema nodosum and pyoderma gangrenosum. Erythema nodosum consists of raised, tender, erythematous swellings of 2 to 3 cm on the arms and legs. The condition often develops during an exacerbation of the colitis and is frequently found when arthritis is associated with the exacerbation of the primary disease. Occasionally arthritis and erythema nodosum appear just before the first overt bowel symptoms of ulcerative colitis. Pyoderma gangrenosum is less frequent than erythema nodosum and is usually associated with severe ulcerative colitis. Pyoderma gangrenosum first appears as a pinpoint lesion, a boil, or an infected hair follicle. The lesion collects purulent drainage that contains few polymorphonuclear cells and no bacteria. The lesion may drain spontaneously. There is a characteristic purple border around the lesion. As the lesion becomes gangrenous, progressive necrosis of the dermis occurs and the area is deeply ulcerated. Healing of the lesions required control of the ulcerative colitis through corticosteroids or surgical removal of the colon and rectum.

Liver diseases have also been associated with ulcerative colitis. The pathogenesis is not understood, and the incidence of liver disease is approximately 7%. Liver disease may range from minor abnormalities in one or more liver function tests to more serious changes in liver structure and function. Diseases of the liver associated with ulcerative colitis include fatty infiltrations, pericholangitis, chronic active hepatitis, postnecrotic cirrhosis, amyloidosis, and sclerosing cholangitis. The question remains as to the degree of improvement in liver diseases following colectomy.

Renal stone formation is associated with ulcerative colitis and is probably related to dehydration, inactivity of the patient, and changes in the composition of the urine.

Ulcerative colitis may range from mild to severe. The degree of involvement of the colon influences the severity. For many patients, ulcerative colitis will remain in remission for years after an acute phase of the illness. The treatment and the nursing interventions will be influenced by the degree of involvement and the severity of the colitis.

DIAGNOSTIC STUDIES

Differential diagnosis*

Mild ulcerative colitis with rectal bleeding
Hemorrhoids
Anal fissures
Rectal polyp
Carcinoma of rectum
Factitious proctitis
Crohn's colitis

Mild ulcerative colitis without bleeding
Irritable bowel syndrome

Moderate ulcerative colitis
Irritable bowel syndrome
Diverticular disease
Chronic small bowel diarrhea
Crohn's disease

Severe ulcerative colitis
Acute infectious colitis (salmonellosis, shigellosis, or amebiasis)
Pseudomembranous colitis
Necrotizing colitis

*The diagnosis of ulcerative colitis is often made by the combination of clinical symptoms and an inflamed, abnormal colonic mucosa. The clinical symptoms of ulcerative colitis (chronic, watery diarrhea with intermittent blood and mucus, weight loss, fatigue, and general debility) are associated with other diseases. The disorders listed should be considered in the differential diagnosis.

Stool cultures
Negative

Laboratory studies
Hemoglobin, hematocrit
Anemia

Liver function
Abnormal

Serum albumin
Low

Sigmoidoscopy
Submucosal inflammation and edema
Subepithelium infiltration and edema
Microscopic mucosal erosions
Crypt abscesses
Granular appearance
Friable (bleeds easily)

Rectal biopsy
Inflammatory changes in the mucosa
Helps to differentiate between ulcerative colitis and Crohn's colitis

Colonoscopy
Superficial mucosal changes in early disease: hyperemia, mucosal friability, fine granular pattern, shallow ulcerations
Late disease: coarse, granular appearance; deep mucosal ulcerations; pseudopolyps; shortening of colon; loss of haustrations
NOTE: colonoscopy should be avoided in acute situations because of danger of perforation

Radiography
Plain film of abdomen
Shortening of colon, loss of haustrations
Irregular mucosa caused by pseudopolyps, ulcerations, and mucosa tags
Midtransverse colon dilated with air in toxic megacolon

Double-contrast barium enemas
Evaluates disease above the sigmoidoscopy level (preferred over colonoscopy)
Early disease: study may appear normal, or there may be a reticulated pattern denoting the denudation of the mucosa
Late disease: ulceration of mucosa, shortening of the bowel, pseudopolyps
NOTE: "Under no circumstances should a patient with ulcerative colitis be prepared with irritant cathartics; such treatment may worsen the disease"[51]; barium enemas should be avoided in acute situations because of danger of perforation

TREATMENT PLAN

Surgical
Ulcerative colitis intractable to medical management: proctocolectomy with ileostomy or with continent ileostomy, or colectomy with rectal mucosal stripping and ileoanal reservoir
Surgery will vary depending on complications
Perforation
First stage: subtotal colectomy and ileostomy
Second stage: abdominoperineal resection
Toxic megacolon
First stage: diverting ileostomy (loop stoma or ileostomy and mucous fistula) and a decompression, cutaneous colostomy
Second stage: total colectomy and proctocolectomy
Cancer: proctocolectomy and ileostomy or continent ileostomy

Chemotherapeutic
Corticosteroids
In mild disease (ulcerative proctitis), acute phase: hydrocortisone retention enemas (Contenema), 100 mg in 60 ml daily, should retain for 20 min
In mild disease, remission: hydrocortisone retention enemas several times per week slowly tapering down and discontinuing
In moderate disease, acute phase: prednisone, 40 to 60 mg/d po
In moderate disease, remission: taper off prednisone slowly
In severe disease, acute phase: prednisolone, 100 mg IV over 24 h (need intravenous potassium to prevent steroid-induced hypokalemia) q10-14d followed by Prednisolone, 60 to 100 mg/d po (If patient does not respond, surgery may be indicated.)
Sulfasalazine (Azulfidine): acute phase, 3 to 4 g tid po; maintenance, 2 g po qid
Diarrhea
Loperamide (Imodium), 4 mg/d po and 2 mg after each unformed stool up to a maximum of 16 mg
Diphenoxylate hydrochloride (Lomotil), 5 mg qid (codeine and Lomotil used with caution since opiates and atropine in Lomotil can precipitate toxic megacolon)
Metamucil, 1 tsp qid (used to add bulk to watery stools; avoid in the very ill patient

Supportive
Acute phase: intravenous fluids, limited activity or bed rest, total parenteral nutrition (TPN) (for severe dehydration and cachexia); blood replacement usually required

Nutrition: no general restrictions; patients should avoid foods that they identify as irritating; usually a low-residue diet advanced as tolerated with one food added at a time; milk can be a problem for some patients; need extra calories and protein

ASSESSMENT: AREAS OF CONCERN

Mild disease
  Gastrointestinal symptoms
    Short episodes of anorexia
    Mild lower abdominal cramping
    Small amounts of rectal bleeding
    Frequent stools, small in volume, without gross bleeding
  Extracolonic manifestations
    In absence of diarrhea and colonic bleeding

Moderate disease
  Gastrointestinal symptoms
    Diarrhea: stools are frequent and loose, and contain blood
    Abdominal cramping
  General symptoms
    Intermittent low-grade fever
    Fatigue
    Anorexia and weight loss

Extracolonic manifestations
  Arthritis
  Uveitis
  Erythema nodosum
  Pyoderma gangrenosum

Severe disease
  Gastrointestinal symptoms
    Profuse diarrhea, rectal bleeding, tenesmus, anorexia, weight loss
    Distended, tender, tympanitic abdomen without evidence of localized or generalized peritonitis
    Bowel sounds decreased or absent
  Systemic findings
    High fever, unless on steroids, which may mask fever
    Weakness
    Pallor
    Anemia
    Hypoalbuminemia
    Dehydration
  Extracolonic manifestations
    One or more extracolonic conditions may be present
  Toxic megacolon
    Severe abdominal distention
    Increasing abdominal pain
    Fever
    Tachycardia
    Sharp decrease in number of stools and in gas
    Rectal bleeding
    Hypoactive or absent bowel sounds

NURSING DIAGNOSES and NURSING INTERVENTIONS

Nursing Diagnosis	Nursing Intervention
Bowel elimination, alteration in: diarrhea	Assess the frequency and appearance of bowel movements. Record amounts and presence of blood in chart. Provide antidiarrheal medications as ordered.
Fluid volume deficit, potential	Monitor patient's vital signs. Record intake, output, and daily weights. Provide intravenous fluids as ordered.
Nutrition, alteration in: less than body requirements	Evaluate nutritional status. Identify irritating foods for the individual patient. Provide nutritional supplements as ordered. Review blood work for indications of anemia. Observe patient for signs of magnesium deficit (associated with long-standing diarrhea). Observe children for signs of growth retardation.
Skin integrity, impairment of: potential	Assess perianal region for signs of fissures, fistulas, or abscesses. Assess perianal region for irritation from the chronic diarrhea. Provide interventions or treatment for perianal fissures as ordered; sitz baths; keep area cleansed following bowel movements. Protect perianal skin in patients with frequent bowel movements; use gentle cleansing solutions (Periwash, Uniwash, Tucks, witch hazel pads); if area is denuded, cleanse with cotton balls soaked in mineral oil; use Anusol suppositories or Nupercainal Ointment.

Nursing Diagnosis	Nursing Intervention
Comfort, alteration in: pain	Provide analgesics as ordered. Observe patient with severe disease receiving narcotics, opiates, and anticholinergics for early signs of toxic megacolon.
Coping, family: potential for growth	Assist patient and family in supporting each other as they learn to manage the effects of a chronic illness in their lives. Evaluate patient and family needs regarding knowledge of ulcerative colitis, compliance with medical treatment, or myths regarding disease. Provide opportunities for patient and family to express their feelings regarding the illness and to identify their perceptions for a successful outcome. Assess the family background for inflammatory bowel disease. Assist parents and siblings in coping with ulcerative colitis and guilt implications if family history is positive.
Sexual dysfunction	Evaluate patient's sexual history in relation to the presence of perianal or perirectal disease that may make sexual activity extremely painful. (Patients may avoid sexual activity because of painful experiences.) Provide patient and partner opportunities to discuss their feelings regarding any actual or feared changes in sexual activities. (The fear of ileostomy surgery may be an underlying theme related to changes in self and body image.)

Patient Education

1. Provide written schedule for medications and tapering schedule for drugs as dosages are decreased.
2. Provide information on ulcerative colitis and the relationship of stress and exacerbations.
3. Provide information on drug toxicities. For example, sulfasalazine is associated with rashes and patients may be desensitized with small doses.
4. Provide information on relationship between ulcerative colitis and colorectal cancers.
5. Provide information on various surgical options to patients with ulcerative colitis.
6. Provide specific instructions for procedures and allow return demonstrations: perianal care, ileostomy care, dietary instructions, TPN, central line care.

EVALUATION

Patient Outcome	Data Indicating That Outcome is Reached
There is no active disease.	There is no diarrhea, rectal bleeding, or abdominal cramping. The patient returns to all activities of daily living. There are no signs of cancer of the colon or rectum.
Nutrition is adequate.	The patient gains weight and does not experience anorexia. Protein and calorie intake is adequate (serum albumin level is within normal range by electrophoresis).
Fluid balance is maintained.	Normal hydration levels return as assessed by skin turgor, color, mucous membrane, blood pressure, and pulse.

TUMORS

The term tumor is used to refer to neoplasm, a new growth of tissue characterized by uncontrolled proliferation of cells. A tumor may be malignant or benign.

The benign tumors of the small and large intestines include colonic adenomas (polyps), villous or papillary adenomas, lipomas, leiomyomas, and lymphoid hyperplasia. Polyps have been discussed on p. 1217. A villous adenoma is a rare tumor found most often in the rectosigmoid area; it may be benign or contain foci of carcinoma. Lipomas are smooth, round tumors found in the submucosal layer of the colon. Leiomyomas are found in the small intestine and are submucosal or subserosal growths that protrude intraluminally, extraluminally, or in both directions. Malignant tumors of the colorectal area are covered in Chapter 14.

Benign tumors in the intestines occur equally in men and women. The benign tumors are most often discovered between the ages of 50 and 80. Symptomatic benign tumors are commonly diagnosed between the ages of 30 and 60. The majority of benign tumors in the small and large intestines are asymptomatic and may be discovered during routine examinations or surgery. Symptoms, when present, are generally related to the size of the tumor. A benign tumor may block the lumen, resulting in obstruction or intussusception. If the mucosa covering a tumor is irritated and becomes ulcerated, the patient may have signs of intestinal bleeding.

The etiology of isolated benign tumors of the small intestine is unknown. Benign tumors in the small bowel include adenomas, leiomyomas, lipomas, hamartomas (associated with Peutz-Jeghers syndrome), and neurogenic tumors. Pseudotumors may also be found in the small intestine, and surgical excision is required for histologic studies and differential diagnosis.

The most common benign tumor of the colon is the polyp (or colonic adenoma). Neurofibromas, leiomyomas, and lipomas are found, but the incidence is low. Histologic examination of the tissue is required to determine the type of tumor. Villous adenomas are polyps found in the rectosigmoid area and are associated with more symptoms than other tumors. Both colonic polyps and villous adenomas are associated with malignancies.

PATHOPHYSIOLOGY

Adenomas in the intestines may be tubular, villous, or tubulovillous. Adenomas in the small intestine are generally found near the ileum. Villous adenomas are rare in the small intestine and when they occur are found in the duodenum. The villous adenoma is most often found in the rectosigmoid areas. The rectosigmoid villous adenoma appears as a "frondlike, velvety surface."[72] It tends to recur, to secrete large amounts of mucus, and to be a site for development of cancer.

The primary symptoms of villous adenomas in the rectosigmoid area include increased colonic motility, diarrhea, and electrolyte loss. A villous adenoma higher in the gastrointestinal tract does not seem to have the electrolyte loss, probably because of the reabsorption capacity of the colon distal to the adenoma. Villous adenomas consist of branching papillary fronds lined with goblet cells. The villous adenoma secretes large amounts of mucus. If the villous adenoma is large, the amount of fluid lost through mucous secretions can be significant. Sodium and potassium are lost in the mucous diarrhea. The fluid and electrolyte imbalance may divert attention away from the presence of a villous adenoma as other conditions and etiologies are considered during diagnosis.

Lipomas may occur anywhere in the small and large intestines and are more common in the colon. Lipomas tend to be single lesions averaging 4 cm in diameter. Most lipomas are found incidentally during surgery. Symptoms are associated with intussusception, obstruction, or bleeding. Lipomas in the colon may be detected during water enemas when the returns contain fat. An enlargement of the ileocecal valve may be caused by lipomatosis or by a tumor in the cecum. Lipomatosis is more common, and differential diagnosis can be made by colonoscopy.

Leiomyomas in the small intestine are found in the jejunum and tend to produce more symptoms than other benign tumors of the small intestine. Ulceration of the mucosa is common, and patients' initial complaint is bleeding. Obstruction and intussusception are rare.

Lymphoid hyperplasia of the colon is found more often in children than adults. An enlarged lymphoid follicle may occur in the rectum. No intervention is required. When lymphoid hyperplasia appears in multiple numbers throughout the rectum and colon, it can be confused with familial polyposis. Differential diagnosis is important since treatment is not indicated in lymphoid hyperplasia and total colectomy is used to treat familial polyposis.

DIAGNOSTIC STUDIES

Small bowel
Barium studies
Prograde enteroclysis or retrograde infusion through ileocecal valve
Small isolated tumors
Multiple small tumors

Exploratory laparotomy
Biopsy and removal of tumor for histologic studies

Colon
Sigmoidoscopy, colonoscopy
Visualization, biopsy, and removal of tumor

Double-contrast barium enema
Villous adenoma: reticulated appearance
Presence of tumors in colon and rectum

TREATMENT PLAN

Surgical
Laparotomy may be used for diagnosis and removal of tumors in small bowel when patient is symptomatic
Villous adenoma
Above peritoneal reflection: resection of bowel containing villous adenoma
Below peritoneal reflection: local excision
With evidence of frank invasive carcinoma: abdominoperineal resection

ASSESSMENT: AREAS OF CONCERN

Abdomen
Signs of intestinal obstruction: abdominal pain, distention, nausea and vomiting, absence of peristalsis, absence of bowel movements
Large bowel or distal small bowel obstructions: fecal odor to emesis

Rectum
Occult, blood-tinged, or black tarry stools

NURSING DIAGNOSES and NURSING INTERVENTIONS

Nursing Diagnosis	Nursing Intervention
Bowel elimination, alteration in: constipation	Assess patient for signs and symptoms of intestinal obstructions: abdominal pain, abdominal distention, decreased peristalsis, nausea, vomiting. Determine if patient has regular bowel habits and if his bowel pattern has changed. Observe stool for shape, consistency, color, quantity, and odor. Note and report any signs of blood-tinged stools. Check stool for occult blood.

Patient Education

1. Provide patient with information about the type of tumor and any impact regarding long-term care (e.g., following removal of villous adenoma, regular follow-up required if a foci of carcinoma is present).
2. Provide routine postoperative information on activity, diet, driving, and returning to work associated with any abdominal surgery.

EVALUATION

Patient Outcome	Data Indicating That Outcome is Reached
Body functions normally.	Bowel elimination is adequate. Surgical wound heals.

VOLVULUS

A volvulus is a twisting of the bowel on itself. The two most common sites for the development of a volvulus are the cecum and the sigmoid colon.

The twisting or rotation of the bowel kinks the gut, producing a mechanical obstruction. When the blood supply is also involved, the strangulation leads to acute, early gangrene. The clinical symptoms, diagnosis, and management are similar to those related to any mechanical obstruction of the colon.

A cecal volvulus may occur any time from adolescence but is most common in the fifth decade. Sigmoid volvulus is more common in elderly persons and has been associated with chronic constipation.

PATHOPHYSIOLOGY

A volvulus usually develops in an area where an underlying abnormality exists. A midgut volvulus may develop from a congenital malrotation of the mesentery. If the cecum and ascending colon are poorly fixed on mesentery rather than being retroperitoneal, the cecum may be mobile and able to twist, creating a volvulus. The twisting or torsion is commonly in a clockwise direction and points obliquely toward the left upper quadrant. A sigmoid volvulus develops when the sigmoid colon is long or redundant. It is easy for a long loop to twist about its leash, creating a closed-loop obstruction. A volvulus may also develop when adhesions produce an axis about which the sigmoid colon can twist.

When there is a sudden tight twisting of the mesentery impeding the blood flow to the bowel, gangrene, necrosis, and perforation may develop, resulting in an acute abdominal emergency. A closed-loop obstruction results in marked distention, aperistalsis, and pain. Intermittent, recurrent volvulus produces repeated episodes of abdominal pain, tenderness, and distention.

The reader is referred to the section on intestinal obstruction for the pathophysiology of intestinal obstructions.

DIAGNOSTIC STUDIES

Abdominal radiographic films
Cecal volvulus: marked distention of the cecum
Sigmoid volvulus: large dilated loop, from right to left side of abdomen; two fluid levels can be visualized

Barium enema
Cecal volvulus: conical narrowing at the twist
Sigmoid volvulus: narrowing at the twist

TREATMENT PLAN

Surgical
Cecal volvulus: untwisting bowel; if viable, the cecum and ascending colon are anchored in place; if gangrene is present, bowel resection of involved parts
Sigmoid volvulus: resection of twisted segment if viability is questioned; resection of redundant mesentery or fixation to prevent recurrence

Electromechanical
Reduction of volvulus; if reduction does not occur, colonoscopy will assist by releasing trapped gas and fluids (surgery may be advised following a reduction if the viability of mucosa is in doubt).

ASSESSMENT: AREAS OF CONCERN

Abdomen
Acute abdominal pain, guarding, distention, nausea and vomiting
Sigmoid loop volvulus may be palpable

General physical findings
Auscultation of abdomen for full 3 to 5 minutes before palpating
Signs of strangulation obstructions: localized tenderness, constant pain, guarding, vomiting, rebound tenderness, and absence of gas or bowel movement

Additional physical findings
Tachycardia and hypotension: may indicate dehydration or peritonitis
Fever and leukocytosis: may indicate peritonitis
Loss of skin turgor and dry mucous membranes: dehydration
Blood in the stool: may indicate cancer, intussusception, or infarction of obstructing lesions

NURSING DIAGNOSES and NURSING INTERVENTIONS

Nursing Diagnosis	Nursing Intervention
Tissue perfusion, alteration in: cerebral, cardiopulmonary, renal, gastrointestinal, peripheral	Monitor patient carefully for signs and symptoms of severe fluid and electrolyte loss, metabolic acidosis, hypovolemic shock, and septic shock.
Fluid volume deficit, actual	Replace intravenous fluids and electrolytes, blood, and plasma as ordered. Monitor vital signs, central venous pressure, blood pressure, urinary output, and nasogastric aspirations every hour. Assess abdominal girth every 4 to 8 hours. Do daily weights. Notify physician of changes in patient's status as they generally indicate a decline in patient's stabilization for surgical intervention.
Gas exchange, impaired	Abdominal distention and abdominal guarding may impair pulmonary ventilation as well as creating metabolic imbalances. Monitor patient's pulmonary status. Elevate head of bed.
Comfort, alteration in: pain	Provide analgesics as prescribed. Assist patient in obtaining a comfortable position.

Patient Education

1. Patient should undertake primary postoperative progression if resection and anastomosis of the small bowel were performed. This would include showering, activity progressions, driving, and returning to work.
2. Colonic obstructions are often treated with a temporary diverting colostomy, and patient requires patient teaching about colostomy care, plans for surgical closure, and education about the primary cause of the obstruction.

EVALUATION

Patient Outcome	Data Indicating That Outcome is Reached
Body functions normally.	Pattern of bowel elimination is normal. Colostomy is closed, and normal elimination functions return.
Fluid balance is maintained.	The patient returns to normal hydration levels as assessed by skin turgor, skin color and mucous membranes, blood pressure, and pulse.
Laboratory studies are normal.	Serum electrolytes, hematocrit, and hemoglobin are within normal limits.
Sepsis is not present.	There is no fever; white blood cell counts are within normal limits.

ANORECTAL ABSCESS

An anorectal abscess is a localized infection with pus found in the tissue spaces adjacent to and in the anorectal area.

The classification of anorectal abscesses is according to location:

1. Perianal: beneath perianal skin
2. Ischiorectal: ischiorectal fossa
3. Submucosal: beneath the mucosa of the upper anal canal
4. High intramuscular: below the circular muscle layer
5. Intersphincteric: between internal and external sphincters
6. Pelvirectal or supralevator: above the levators ani and below the pelvic peritoneum

Anorectal abscesses are more common in men. Certain diseases and conditions increase the likelihood of developing anorectal abscesses. Anorectal abscesses are common in patients with Crohn's disease and in homosexual men who engage in traumatic anal intercourse. Hematologic and immune-deficient conditions have also been associated with anorectal abscesses.

PATHOPHYSIOLOGY

Anorectal abscesses develop from infections beginning in an anal crypt and moving along anal ducts through the internal sphincter before spreading in different directions. An infection may also develop in anal fissures, prolapsed internal hemorrhoids, traumatic injuries, and superficial skin lesions that progress to form anorectal abscesses. Extension of the abscess formation is the most common complication. An abscess may eventually progress to an anorectal fistula.

DIAGNOSTIC STUDIES

Differential diagnosis
Rule out pilonidal sinus, carcinoma, Bartholin's gland abscess, and inflammatory bowel disease (Crohn's disease, ulcerative colitis)
Studies used: sigmoidoscopy, barium enema, and small bowel series

Visual inspection of perianal region
Tender, erythematous area that displaces the anus (superficial abscess)
Tender mass in an anatomic space may indicate a deep abscess

Anoscopy (proctoscopy)
Visualization of lesions below the pectinate line

TREATMENT PLAN

Surgical
Surgical drainage of abscess, with or without excision of fistula tracts associated with anorectal abscesses

Chemotherapeutic
Antibiotic therapy based on causative organisms
Stool softeners
Docusate (Colace), 50 to 200 mg/d; dose based on individual's response

Supportive
Sitz baths

ASSESSMENT: AREAS OF CONCERN

Anorectal concerns
Throbbing, constant pain increased by walking or sitting (pain diminishes if abscess drains spontaneously)
Foul-smelling drainage

Systemic concerns
Fever, malaise

Abdomen
Low abdominal pain may occur with a deep anorectal abscess

NURSING DIAGNOSES and NURSING INTERVENTIONS

Nursing Diagnosis	Nursing Intervention
Bowel elimination, alteration in (potential; related to presence of infection)	Assess perianal region for signs of tender mass, purulent drainage, or erythema. Determine patient's bowel habits and any recent change in the pattern (i.e., pain with defecation, purulent discharge, increased odor); also determine patient's last bowel movement and use of laxatives or stool softeners. Keep the perianal area clean. Provide sitz baths for comfort and for cleansing purposes. Monitor patient during sitz bath for hypotension secondary to dilation of the pelvic blood vessels. Apply the dressing over the wound; change frequently, noting color and amount of drainage; dressing may be held in place with mesh "panties" available for use in incontinence management. Keep the surgical wound clean; care is needed following urination and defecation; packing may be used to ensure that the wound heals from the inside out; following bowel and bladder elimination, it is necessary to check the dressing and replace if soiled.

Nursing Diagnosis	Nursing Intervention
	Shave the perianal area weekly to keep hair from the wound (hair will delay wound healing and is often the cause of infection or irritation).
	Irrigate the wound before packing with normal saline or irrigation solution as ordered.
Comfort, alteration in: pain	Provide analgesics as ordered.
	Provide a thick pillow, cushion, or flotation pad for sitting (avoid air rings and rubber donuts since they tend to spread the buttocks apart).
Urinary elimination, alteration in patterns	Keep accurate intake and output records for 24 hours since urinary retention may develop following surgery.
	Have patient stand or sit to void.
	Pour warm water over pubic area or use sitz bath to assist patient in voiding by relaxing the bladder.

Patient Education

1. Teach the patient to irrigate the wound (Water Pik or shower massager may be used) and to reinsert dressing. Family member may need to assist the patient. The patient should comprehend the necessity of keeping the wound clean and free of fecal soiling.

EVALUATION

Patient Outcome	Data Indicating That Outcome is Reached
Body functions normally.	Elimination is adequate; there is no constipation or hard, formed stools.
	Wound heals.
	Temperature is normal.

ANORECTAL FISTULA

An anorectal fistula is a hollow, fibrous tunnel or tract with two openings.

The internal opening of an anorectal fistula is inside the anal canal or rectum and leads to the secondary, or external, opening. The external opening is in the perianal skin. Fistulas from the colon, small bowel, or urethra may exit through the perineum and be mistaken for anorectal fistulas.

Although an anorectal fistula may occur without predisposing conditions, it is more common to find anorectal fistulas associated with Crohn's disease in the large or the small bowel (regional enteritis). Anorectal fistulas are associated with the presence of an anorectal abscess. An anorectal abscess that is drained may reduce the discomfort and pain, but a fistulous tract may remain through which the abscess continues to drain.

preserved as the abscess heals. Anorectal fistulas are associated with traumatic injury, fissures, Crohn's disease, cancer, and radiation therapy. Once the tract is fibrosed, it will not close on its own and surgical intervention is indicated. The terminal opening of the tract is in the perianal skin. Stool, pus, mucus, blood, and flatus may drain through the fistula. Patients may have single or multiple anorectal fistulas. The skin opening may seal over temporarily, but it will reopen spontaneously and drain.

Following treatment, recurrent fistulas in the anorectal area are associated with inadequate exposure of the tract, with primary openings not being identified, and with failure of the tract to heal from the inside out. When a patient has Crohn's disease, recurrent anorectal fistulas are associated with exacerbation of the inflammatory bowel disease.

PATHOPHYSIOLOGY

The primary, or internal, opening of an anorectal fistula is usually at a crypt near the pectinate line. Infection in the crypt progresses to form an abscess that drains (spontaneously or with surgical drainage), and the tract is

DIAGNOSTIC STUDIES

Digital rectal examination
Palpate tract direction internally

Anoscopy (proctoscopy)
May reveal the primary opening in a crypt

Sigmoidoscopy
Used to rule out other sources of fistula formation

Fistulography
Used if the tract is of questionable origin; rules out colonic, small bowel, and urethral fistulas

TREATMENT PLAN

Surgical
Fistulotomy or fistulectomy may be indicated depending on location and depth of the fistula tract

Chemotherapeutic
Antibiotics per sensitive organism
Stool softener
Docusate (Colace), 50 to 200 mg/d; based on individual's response

Metronidazole (Flagyl), 20 mg/kg/d in divided doses (for perianal disease associated with inflammatory bowel disease)

Supportive
Sitz baths as needed and after defecation

ASSESSMENT: AREAS OF CONCERN

Anorectum
Raised, red, papules
Drainage of pus, blood, mucus, or stool through the open skin lesions
Complaints of pain and discomfort; greater when lesions are sealed and not draining
Pruritus
Inundated, "cordlike" pattern may be palpated from cutaneous opening toward anus

History
Anorectal abscesses or inflammatory bowel disease

NURSING DIAGNOSES and NURSING INTERVENTIONS

Nursing Diagnosis	Nursing Intervention
Bowel elimination, alteration in (potential; related to presence of infection, presence of surgical incision)	Assess perianal skin for signs of fistula tracts and drainage. Estimate amount of drainage; note color, odor, and consistency of drainage. Determine patient's bowel habits and record date of last bowel movement, noting consistency of stool; record any changes in bowel habits, such as blood, pus, or odor. Assess patient's use of laxatives, stool softeners, anal intercourse, or anal dilators (e.g., vibrators or other instruments). Keep the perianal area clean following bowel movements with sitz baths and irrigations of the site. Monitor patient for hypotension secondary to vasodilation of the pelvic blood vessels during sitz bath. Replace dressings as soiled and record appearance of wound, signs of healings, and early signs of postoperative infection. Irrigate the wound before packing or dressing. Shave the perianal area regularly to prevent hair from irritating or infecting the wound as granulation tissue develops following surgery.
Comfort, alteration in: pain	Provide pain medication as needed. Provide a thick foam cushion or pillow for patient to use in sitting. (Air rings and rubber donuts should be avoided since they tend to spread the buttocks apart.)

Patient Education

1. Teach the patient to irrigate the wound with a Water Pik or shower massager, to shave the perianal area, and to redress the wound.
2. Teach the patient to use a mirror to inspect the area and look for redness or firm reddened areas of increased itching and tenderness.
3. Mesh panties can be used to hold dressings in place, or sanitary pads or belts may be used in the underwear. Jockey shorts will be more effective than boxer shorts for managing dressings.

4. A family member's help may be needed.
5. Sitz baths can be used for cleansing and for comfort. (The sitz bath does not replace the irrigation procedure.)

EVALUATION

Patient Outcome	Data Indicating That Outcome is Reached
Body functions normally.	Elimination is adequate; there is no constipation or hard, formed stools. Wound heals. Temperature is normal, and there is no purulent, odorous drainage.

ANAL FISSURE

An anal fissure is a small tear in the lining of the anus. The tear resembles a slitlike crack and may extend from the anal verge to the pectinate line.

Fissures are most common in young and middle-aged adults. The posterior midline is the most common site, but occasional anal fissures will be found in the anterior wall. Fissures in other positions on the anal wall are usually associated with Crohn's disease or ulcerative colitis.

PATHOPHYSIOLOGY

Anal fissures are usually caused by trauma from passing large, hard stools. Acute fissures are tears that may become chronic when the patient has an elevated resting anal pressure and contraction of the internal anal sphincter after rectal distention. Defecation stimulates spasms of the internal anal sphincter, which causes the edges of the sphincter to adhere, trapping any drainage. Edema and fibrosis of adjacent tissue develop and progress to hypertrophied anal papillae and a tag of skin at the anal verge.

Loss of elasticity of the anal canal may predispose a person to anorectal fissures. Laxative abuse, scarring from anal surgery, and chronic diarrheal diseases may lead to a loss of elasticity, as will frequent anal intercourse.

DIAGNOSTIC STUDIES

Differential diagnosis
If fissure is not found in midline, rule out inflammatory bowel disease, carcinoma, tuberculosis, syphilis, herpes, and other venereal diseases

Digital rectal examination
Use topical anesthesia before digital examination to decrease pain from the procedure
Induration
Tenderness
Sphincter spasm
Hypertrophied anal papillae

Anoscopy (proctoscopy)
Visualization of the anorectal fissure: a superficial tear that bleeds easily and has a reddish base

TREATMENT PLAN

Surgical
Lateral subcutaneous sphincterotomy (internal sphincter is divided up to the pectinate line, hypertrophied papillae and anal tag are excised, and fissure is left to heal)

Chemotherapeutic
Bulk agents
Psyllium (Metamucil or Effersyllium), 1 tsp. (7 g) one to three times per day
Emollient suppositories
Analgesic ointments
Dibucaine (Nupercaine) prn
Tucks or witch hazel pads to cleanse

Electromechanical
Topical application of silver nitrate solution or cautery with silver nitrate sticks

Supportive
Sitz bath
Warm compresses

ASSESSMENT: AREAS OF CONCERN

Anorectum

Pain during evacuation; may be described as tearing or burning

Evacuation stimulates spasms, which result in prolonged, gnawing discomfort for extended periods

Presence of bright red blood following bowel movements

Rectal tag of skin

Rectal discharge

Pruritus

History

Patient may be able to identify the onset with the presence of constipation and pain with defecation

Bowel movements may be painful and associated with slight bleeding

Delayed onset of pain following a bowel movement

History of anal intercourse, use of laxatives, enema abuse, or diseases such as Crohn's disease or ulcerative colitis

NURSING DIAGNOSES and NURSING INTERVENTIONS

Nursing Diagnosis	Nursing Intervention
Bowel elimination, alteration in: constipation	Obtain a history of patient's bowel habits (i.e., constipation, use of laxatives, dietary history); following surgery, record consistency of stool and effectiveness of stool softeners.
	Record date of last bowel movement. (Patients often postpone or delay having bowel movements because of the pain.)
	Keep the postoperative site clean and free of stool by the use of sitz baths and careful cleansing following surgery.
	Monitor patient for hypotension secondary to vasodilation of pelvic blood vessels during sitz bath.
Comfort, alteration in: pain	Provide warm compresses, sitz baths, and analgesic ointments for pain and discomfort.

Patient Education

1. Provide patient with information on natural methods of relieving or preventing constipation (i.e., diet high in bulk and fiber, increased fluid intake, avoidance of harsh laxatives and constipating medications such as codeine).

EVALUATION

Patient Outcome	Data Indicating That Outcome is Reached
Body functions normally.	Elimination is adequate, and there is no constipation. Wound heals. There is no pain with evacuation or delayed pain.

HEMORRHOIDS

Hemorrhoids are masses of vascular tissue found in the anal canal.[69]

Internal hemorrhoids are found above the pectinate line, arise from the superior hemorrhoidal venous plexus, and are covered with mucosa. External hemorrhoids are found below the pectinate line, arise from the inferior hemorrhoidal venous plexus, and are covered by anoderm and perianal skin. Patients may have a combination of internal and external hemorrhoids.

Internal hemorrhoids may also be classified according to the degree of involvement:

1. First-degree: project slightly into the anal canal
2. Second-degree: prolapse with defecation and reduce spontaneously

3. Third-degree: prolapse with defecation and reduce manually
4. Fourth-degree: irreducible

The usual location of internal hemorrhoids is around the anal circumference, including right anterior, right posterior, and left lateral areas.[69]

The commonly accepted etiology is that hemorrhoids are varicose veins. This etiology has been recently questioned because of weaknesses in the original theory. The basis of the varicose vein theory of hemorrhoids is that increased pressure in the veins results in congestion. Certain occupations, the erect positions of humans, structural absence of valves in the veins, and increased abdominal pressure from straining at defecation, constipation, and pregnancy have been associated with the development of hemorrhoids. The varicose vein and increased pressure etiology has been questioned because internal hemorrhoids may appear in early pregnancy before the uterus is large enough to create increased abdominal pressure and because the blood associated with hemorrhoidal bleeding is bright red, not dark as expected with the venous system.

A hypothesis is that the hemorrhoidal plexus is a rich vascular network with direct arteriovenous shunts. The vascular tissue slides easily and may be displaced downward with the evacuation of stool.[27,69,76] High resting anal pressures and failure of the internal sphincter to relax may contribute to the development of hemorrhoids in some people. In older patients, low resting anal pressures and sliding of tissues during bowel movements have been associated with hemorrhoids.

PATHOPHYSIOLOGY

Based on Thompson's description[76] of the hemorrhoidal plexus as a vascular mound on a cushion, an internal hemorrhoid is a prolapse of normal vascular mounds or a prolapse of normal anal canal lining. The prolapse may be caused by spasms of the internal sphincter that require straining or increased pressure to push the stool through the internal sphincter and at the same time push out the hemorrhoid.

The complications associated with internal hemorrhoids include bleeding, prolapse, and thrombosis. Since the hemorrhoid is composed of spongy vascular tissue, bleeding tends to be an oozing of bright red blood. The blood may appear as a bright spot on toilet paper or on the surface of the stool. Blood may drip from the anus for a few minutes after the stool has been expelled. Iron deficiency anemia may develop if blood loss continues over a period of time.

Prolapse of hemorrhoids is first perceived as a mass of tissue that protrudes from the anus following a bowel movement. Initially, it slips back into the anal canal spontaneously. As the condition continues, the hemorrhoid will later need to be manually replaced and may become irreducible. A mucous discharge is associated with irreducible hemorrhoids because of the mucosal covering of the internal hemorrhoid. Protection of undergarments will be required. Pain is associated with prolapsed and inflamed hemorrhoids but is not a general symptom of internal hemorrhoids. Patients whose initial complaint is pain should be assessed for other anorectal conditions (fissure, abscess) and colorectal diseases.

Thrombosis of prolapsed hemorrhoids can create severe pain. This is also referred to as strangulated hemorrhoids. Ulceration and secondary infections can develop. One or all hemorrhoids may be affected.

A thrombosis of an external hemorrhoid is a blood clot within a hemorrhoidal vein. The pectinate line is visible and separate from the mass or lump that forms. Thrombosis of external hemorrhoids has been associated with heavy lifting, straining at defecation, and childbirth. The patient has a painful lump that appeared suddenly at the anus. Pain may be constant and is increased with sitting and defecation. It usually disappears in a week. The thrombosed external hemorrhoid should not be confused with prolapsed, thrombosed internal hemorrhoids. If the skin covering the clot becomes ulcerated, bleeding may be noted.

DIAGNOSTIC STUDIES

Complete blood count (CBC) and iron studies
  To determine presence of anemia and if it is caused by iron deficiency

Digital rectal examination
  Tone of internal sphincter; usually increased in young men with hemorrhoids; may be low in older patients and women with hemorrhoids
  Palpation of third-degree internal hemorrhoids

Anoscopy
  Visualization of hemorrhoids as instrument is removed

Sigmoidoscopy and barium enema
  To rule out carcinoma and inflammatory disease
  Particularly important in patients over 40 years

TREATMENT PLAN

Surgical
  Injection of sclerosing solutions (5% phenol in vegetable oil) submucosally around hemorrhoid; com-

plications: sloughing of overlying mucosa, infection, reaction to injected material

Rubber band ligation (placement of rubber band over base of hemorrhoid causes necrosis and sloughing of hemorrhoid in 7 days)

Cryosurgery (application of metal probe cooled by liquid nitrogen or carbon dioxide freezes hemorrhoid)

Lateral internal sphincterotomy (partial division of internal sphincter lowers anal pressure); seldom used unless an anorectal fissure is also present

Hemorrhoidectomy (surgical excision of the hemorrhoidal masses); complication: anal stenosis

Excision under local anesthesia of thrombosed external hemorrhoid if seen in a day or two of onset

Chemotherapeutic

Anesthetic ointments and suppositories
Nupercaine (Dibucaine) prn
Stool softeners

Electromechanical

Manual dilation of anus (anus is dilated 4 cm regularly by patient with a special dilator); complication: incontinence

Supportive

High-residue diet, adequate hydration, and exercise to minimize constipation and straining
Warm sitz baths; compresses

ASSESSMENT: AREAS OF CONCERN

Inspection of perianal skin

External hemorrhoids visible in subcutaneous skin at anus; if hemorrhoids are thrombosed, tender, bluish spheric mass at anal verge

Prolapsed internal hemorrhoids: moist, red mucosa covering upper portion; presence of mucoid discharge or staining of undergarments

NURSING DIAGNOSES and NURSING INTERVENTIONS

Nursing Diagnosis	Nursing Intervention
Comfort, alteration in: pain	Assess amount, character, and threshold of pain or discomfort; relate to bowel pattern.
	Use thick foam pillows or pads under buttock; avoid air or rubber donuts since they spread the buttocks apart.
	Promote the use of sitz baths for comfort and for cleansing after bowel movements.
	Monitor patient during sitz bath for hypotension secondary to vasodilation of pelvic blood vessels.
	Provide analgesics as ordered.
	Use ice packs as ordered to reduce congestion and edema.
	Use warm compresses to promote circulation (also soothing).
Bowel elimination, alteration in: constipation	Instruct patient to defecate promptly with the urge, to avoid sitting on the toilet for prolonged periods, and to avoid straining.
	Provide adequate fluids to maintain hydration.
	Encourage patient to exercise (mild at first).
	Give patient medication before first bowel movement.
	Encourage patient to have a bowel movement after surgery even though he may be afraid of increased pain (prevents formation of strictures and preserves lumen size of the anus).
	Monitor patient during first bowel movement for signs of weakness or dizziness.
Urinary elimination, alteration in patterns	Keep accurate intake and output records for 24 hours since urinary retention may develop following surgery.
	Have patient stand or sit to void.
	Pour warm water over pubic area to relax bladder and aid voiding, or use sitz bath.
Injury, potential for: hemorrhage	Monitor vital signs for signs of blood loss (if surgical ligatures slip, blood may collect unnoticed in the rectum).
	Observe perianal area for signs of bleeding.
	Check stools for blood.
	Note frequent unrelieved sensation to defecate (sequestered blood may result in edema, which creates pressure and the urge to defecate).

Patient Education

1. Management and prevention of constipation with diet, fluids, and physical activities should be discussed with the patient.
2. The patient needs to respond to urge to defecate, to avoid straining, and to keep the stool soft and moist.

EVALUATION

Patient Outcome	Data Indicating That Outcome is Reached
Body functions normally.	Elimination is adequate, there is no constipation, and stools are soft.
	The patient does not experience pain, bleeding, or prolapsed hemorrhoids.
Nutrition is adequate.	The patient eats a high-residue diet with good hydration.

IMPERFORATE ANUS

Imperforate anus refers to a group of congenital abnormalities involving the patency of the anorectum and includes stenosis of the anus, imperforate anus membrane, anal agenesis and rectal agenesis, and rectal atresia.

Fistulas are commonly associated with lesions that are translevator and supralevator (low and high lesions as related to the levator ani). Fistulas may occur between the rectum and the urethra, bladder, vagina, or perineum. In the female the perineum and vagina are common sites of fistula formation, while in the male the urinary tract fistula is more common. Anorectal abnormalities that are translevator include anal stenosis and imperforate anus membrane in which the anal opening is at the normal site. In anocutaneous fistula and anterior perineal anus the lesions are translevator and the opening is at a perineal site. Supralevator lesions include anorectal agenesis and rectal atresia. Intermediate lesions include anal agenesis and anorectal stenosis. Fistula formation is more common with anal agenesis and anorectal agenesis.[62]

Imperforate anus occurs in approximately 1 out of 5000 live births.[6] Genitourinary abnormalities, congenital heart disease, tracheoesophageal fistulas, and skeletal abnormalities exist in over half of the infants seen with anorectal abnormalities. The infant with translevator lesions tends to have fewer associated anomalies and a better prognosis.

PATHOPHYSIOLOGY

Anorectal congenital abnormalities result from interruption of the fetal caudal development between the fourth and sixteenth weeks of gestation. The cloaca is the common channel for urinary, rectal, and genital areas at the fifth week of gestation. By the seventh week the urorectal septum descends in a cephalocaudal direction and unites with the cloacal membrane, forming an anterior urogenital sinus and a posterior rectum. The cloacal membrane ruptures during the eighth week, forming urogenital and anal orifices. The levator ani and external sphincter are developed by the ninth week. By the sixteenth week the differentiation between male and female has been completed. Although the etiology is unknown, researchers have associated rectal atresia with vascular ischemia during gestation.[69]

DIAGNOSTIC STUDIES

Rice-Wangensteen invertogram

Allows for a measurement between gas-filled pouch and the radiopaque skin marker: distance greater than 1.5 cm, the defect is high or supralevator; distance less than 1.5 cm, the defect is low or intermediate

Is not always accurate and should be followed by additional diagnostic studies

Radiographic contrast studies

Transcutaneous injection of pouch, vaginograms, cystourethrograms, IVPs

To evaluate anorectal abnormalities and to identify fistulas

TREATMENT PLAN

Surgical

Anorectal membrane: excised or incised followed by digital dilatations

Low lesions with cutaneous fistula: orifice enlarged by perineal anoplasty

Supralevator lesions: divided sigmoid colostomy with sacroabdominal perineal pull-through procedure at 1 year of age and subsequent closure of colostomy

Electromechanical

Anal stenosis: daily dilatations using bougies or fingers for 3 to 6 months

ASSESSMENT: AREAS OF CONCERN

Perineum

Absence or displacement of the anus visualized when thermometer cannot be inserted during newborn assessment

Pigmented depression or anal dimple; elevation of thickened skin; bluish color; usually found on perineal raphe

Stool or gas expelled from urethra or vagina

Unusual numbers or configurations of orifices in the female

Neurologic assessment of pelvic muscles (sacral anomalies may result in neurogenic bladder)

Digital examination of anorectum

Used to detect anorectal stenosis and anal membranes

NURSING DIAGNOSES and NURSING INTERVENTIONS

Nursing Diagnosis	Nursing Intervention
Bowel elimination, alteration in	Carefully inspect perineal area in newborn. Report absence of passage of meconium in newborns. Observe for postoperative complications: mucosal prolapse, anal and rectal stricture, and recurrent fistulas.
Bowel elimination, alteration in: incontinence	Assess patient for continence following pull-through procedure (incontinence occurs in 25% of children with supralevator anomalies). Plan bowel rehabilitation program if incontinence occurs.
Skin integrity, impairment of: potential	Apply colostomy pouch and solid skin barrier in neonate and infant to protect skin from bowel contents. Provide skin protection for the perineal area following pull-through procedure (diarrhea is a common postoperative problem). Use a combination of perineal skin care cream and ointment if diarrhea or incontinence develops to protect the skin.
Grieving, anticipatory	Support parents during the time of initial diagnosis and subsequent treatment phase. A variety of emotional responses occurs when a child is born with congenital anomalies.
Parenting, alteration in: potential	Assist parents in bonding with their infant. Provide parents with an opportunity to nurture and care for the child during initial and subsequent hospitalizations. Provide ongoing support for families during hospitalization and outpatient experiences. Establish support groups for families. Coordinate an interdisciplinary approach to care including patient, parents, primary physician, surgeon, primary nurse, ET nurse, and social worker.

Patient Education

1. Instruct parents in performing digital dilation of the anus daily (if indicated).
2. Instruct parents on colostomy care for infants and toddlers (if indicated).
3. Instruct parents on a bowel regimen to regulate bowel habits if incontinence occurs.

EVALUATION

Patient Outcome	Data Indicating That Outcome is Reached
Body functions normally.	Bowel elimination is continent. Fistulas do not form. There is no diarrhea, constipation, or skin irritation.

PILONIDAL DISEASE

Pilonidal disease occurs in the midline of the upper portion of the gluteal fold. A sinus channel develops that is lined with epithelium and hair.

The sinus channel may appear as a hairy dimple that is asymptomatic unless it becomes infected or inflamed. A cyst or abscess may develop, or the tract may open at the skin, creating a draining fistula. Differential diagnosis between pilonidal disease and anorectal fistula is important. In pilonidal disease the sinus tract does not connect with the anus or rectum.

PATHOPHYSIOLOGY

Pilonidal disease occurs during embryonic development when a small amount of endothelial tissue is included beneath the skin. The penetration of hair beneath the skin and the enlargement of hair follicles irritate the skin, which becomes infected.

DIFFERENTIAL DIAGNOSIS

Rule out anorectal fistula. Refer to diagnostic studies on anorectal fistulas.

TREATMENT PLAN

Surgical
Incision and removal of hair and granulation tissue; wound may be closed or left opened and packed

Chemotherapeutic
Antibiotic therapy to treat the infection per organism

Supportive
Sitz baths

ASSESSMENT: AREAS OF CONCERN

Perineal area
Hairy dimple in gluteal fold
Open, draining lesion in sacral region with hair protruding from sinus opening

NURSING DIAGNOSES and NURSING INTERVENTIONS

Nursing Diagnosis	Nursing Intervention
Comfort, alteration in: pain	Apply hot moist compresses when an abscess is present. Assist patient with sitz bath. Monitor patient during sitz bath for hypotension (related to vasodilation). Position patient on abdomen or side.
Injury, potential for: infection (postoperatively)	Protect surgical wound during urination and defecation. Change dressing as needed if contaminated during elimination. Assess wound for signs of wound healing or wound infection.

Patient Education

1. Prepare patient or family member to change dressing as needed, to keep wound free of fecal and urinary contamination, and to cleanse wound as needed.

EVALUATION

Patient Outcome	Data Indicating That Outcome is Reached
Body functions normally.	There is no infection or drainage. Wound heals. There is no pain and discomfort.

AMYLOIDOSIS

Amyloidosis, a disorder of protein metabolism, is a systemic disease in which an amorphous, protein-polysaccharide complex is deposited in the tissues and organs.

Amyloidosis has been categorized as primary and secondary. Primary amyloidosis may be hereditary or occur sporadically and is also associated with plasma cell dyscrasias such as multiple myeloma; the protein fragments are immunoglobulin. Secondary amyloidosis is associated with other chronic infectious or inflammatory disorders such as Crohn's disease, rheumatoid arthritis, and tuberculosis. The proteins in secondary amyloidosis are called amyloid protein A. Amyloidosis has also been classified according to organ involvement. Pattern I involves heart, tongue, and gastrointestinal tract and has an identified paraprotein M component. The liver, spleen, kidney, and adrenals are involved in pattern II, with only half of the patients having paraproteins.[81]

The incidence of amyloidosis in the overall population is unknown. A higher incidence of amyloidosis is found in groups with chronic inflammatory disease including patients with known leprosy, chronic tuberculosis, and rheumatoid arthritis. Amyloidosis has been associated with familial Mediterranean fever. Hepatic amyloidosis has not been considered significant. Although amyloidosis may be associated with mild jaundice, the most common clinical sign of liver involvement is hepatomegaly.

PATHOPHYSIOLOGY

Amyloid is an amorphous, eosinophilic, glassy, hyaline substance that is extracellular. Small amounts of amyloid cannot be demonstrated in an organ. Large amounts of amyloid cause an organ to become enlarged, rubbery, and firm. The organ may be a waxy pink or gray color. Changes occur in the heart, kidney, and gastrointestinal tract. The most common causes of death in systemic amyloidosis are congestive heart disease, progressive renal failure, and the underlying myeloma.

The etiology of amyloidosis is unknown; several hypotheses have been proposed, including abnormalities of serum proteins with hyperglobulinemia, protein metabolism, or the reticuloendothelial system; excessive antibody production; delayed hypersensitivity; and a combination of the suggested disorders.[63]

The deposits of amyloid are generally extracellular in the connective tissue. The heart may have focal or diffuse deposits in the myocardium, endocardium, or pericardium. The glomerulus is primarily affected in the kidney. Initially, small nodular or diffuse deposits develop near the base membrane. As amyloidosis in the glomerulus

continues, occlusion of the capillary bed may occur. In the gastrointestinal tract, primary and secondary amyloidosis may involve the rich vascular supply of the submucosa of the small bowel. Malabsorption and decreased bowel motility may develop.[69] In the liver, deposits of amyloid are found in the blood vessels or in the parenchyma between the cords of the hepatic cells and sinusoids.[72]

Patients with amyloidosis may be asymptomatic for years. Hepatic amyloidosis will rarely produce clinical or functional changes. Gastrointestinal symptoms may be the most common and include abdominal pain, diarrhea, protein loss, obstruction, and ischemia. Amyloidosis may develop in a variety of organ systems, and symptoms will depend on the site and amount of amyloid deposited.

DIAGNOSTIC STUDIES

Bromsulfophthalein (BSP) retention
Increased in presence of hepatic amyloidosis

Serum alkaline phosphate
Elevated in hepatic amyloidosis

Liver biopsy (Congo red stain)
Characteristic green birefringence (Controversy exists regarding the use of liver biopsy if diagnosis can be confirmed by rectal biopsy because of bleeding complication.)

Rectal biopsy (Congo red stain)
Characteristic green birefringence

Liver scan
Enlarged liver

TREATMENT PLAN

There is no specific medical therapy for systemic amyloidosis. Treatment and eradication of the chronic inflammatory process will slow down the progression of amyloidosis. Refer to the primary reference for the underlying disease (multiple myeloma, rheumatoid arthritis, Crohn's disease, etc.) for treatment plans.

Chemotherapeutic
Hepatic amyloidosis: specific therapy not necessary; significant hepatic dysfunction uncommon

Supportive
Hepatic amyloidosis: replacement of fat-soluble vitamins; pruritus may be treated with cholestyramine

ASSESSMENT: AREAS OF CONCERN

General concerns
Fatigue, weakness, weight loss, dyspnea with exertion, edema

Skin
Brawny, waxy skin lesions

Mouth
Macroglossia (enlarged tongue)

Liver
Hepatomegaly, mild jaundice

NURSING DIAGNOSES and NURSING INTERVENTIONS

Nursing diagnoses and interventions are determined by the underlying condition. Refer to specific diseases (congestive heart failure, renal failure, Crohn's disease, etc.). The following information applies to hepatic amyloidosis.

Nursing Diagnosis	Nursing Intervention
Fluid volume deficit, potential	Assess patient for ascites. Measure abdominal girth daily if ascites is present. Monitor intake, output, and vital signs, and evaluate based on other involved organs and systems (i.e., heart, kidney, gastrointestinal tract).

Patient Education

1. Instruct patient on amyloidosis and its relationship to a primary disease or disorder, the need for regular health checkups, and the treatment plans for the primary disease.

EVALUATION

Patient Outcome	Data Indicating That Outcome is Reached
Body functions normally.	Liver size is normal. There are no signs of mild jaundice. Digestion and absorption are normal. Patient gains weight and does not have signs of malabsorption or diarrhea. Cardiac and renal function are within normal range. Patient does not experience weakness, fatigue, or edema.

CIRRHOSIS

Cirrhosis is a chronic degenerative disease of the liver in which diffuse destruction and regeneration of hepatic parenchymal cells have occurred.

In cirrhosis the lobes are covered with fibrotic tissue, and the lobules are infiltrated with fat. The diffuse increase in connective tissue results in disorganization of the lobular and vascular structure of the liver, affecting the many functions of the liver and its blood flow. Cirrhosis is characterized by nodular regeneration, which is an attempt by the liver to heal itself by fibrosis or scar tissue. Cirrhosis is the end result of pathologic changes associated with liver disease.

A variety of conditions may progress or lead to cirrhosis of the liver and range from genetic disorders to alcohol abuse. The genetic disorders include galactosemia, alpha$_1$-antitrypsin deficiency, and Wilson's disease. Biliary atresia, a congenital malformation of bile ducts, may progress to cirrhosis. Chemical agents that are toxic to the liver include thorazine, ether, amitriptyline (Elavil), and various household cleansers (carbon tetrachloride). Infectious causes, such as viral hepatitis, syphilis, and schistosomiasis, may progress to cirrhosis. Alcoholic cirrhosis is the most common and accounts for approximately 80% of the liver disease in urban areas.

Cirrhosis develops in approximately 10% to 20% of alcoholics. Of interest to clinicians and researchers is why all individuals who abuse alcohol do not develop cirrhosis. One theory is that certain individuals have an increased ability to oxidize alcohol that may be familial or hereditary based.[72] Thus alcohol ingestion in a susceptible host in the presence of an unknown factor may lead to cirrhosis of the liver.

PATHOPHYSIOLOGY

The pathophysiology of cirrhosis will vary according to the initial etiology (viral hepatitis, biliary obstruction, alcohol abuse). The symptoms and the results of cirrhosis are the same. For this reason and because of the high incidence of alcohol abuse–related cirrhosis, the pathophysiology of the alcohol-induced cirrhotic changes will be described. Alcoholic cirrhosis is also referred to as portal cirrhosis, Laënnec's cirrhosis, and micronodular cirrhosis.

Several steps occur before the liver becomes cirrhotic. Initially, subcellular changes develop and may progress to a fatty liver. (Fatty livers are not limited to alcoholic cirrhosis.) The fatty liver is a reversible stage if alcohol intake is eliminated. The fatty liver can be recognized by its increased size and by the marked degree of fatty infiltration seen microscopically. The fatty liver in the presence of continued alcohol ingestion may progress to alcoholic hepatitis. It is the continuing use of alcohol that causes the development of cirrhosis vs. the progression from fatty liver to hepatitis to cirrhosis. These may not be related at all. The patient could have cirrhosis and develop acute hepatitis due to a drinking bout if the patient has cirrhotic changes. In alcoholic hepatitis the fatty infiltration is combined with liver cell necrosis, leukocytic inflammation, and fibrosis. As the disease progresses, the inflammatory changes decrease and fibrotic changes increase. Continued alcohol ingestion leads to chronic changes (i.e., alcoholic cirrhosis).

The microscopic changes in cirrhosis consist of degeneration and death of hepatocytes, proliferation of connective tissue, and regeneration of hepatocytes. The connective tissue spreads from the portal tracts and from the central veins throughout the liver, changing the normal lobular architecture. The extension of fibrous cords throughout the liver alters the relationship between the hepatic veins and the portal veins. Scar tissue and nodular regeneration of hepatocytes may compress small branches of the portal vein. The compression of the vessels leads to an increased alteration in the vascular system. The veins become engorged and dilated, and portal hypertension develops. The nodular regeneration of the hepatic cells produces postsinusoidal obstruction, which causes the portal system to become congested and contributes to portal hypertension.

The overall effects of the structural and vascular changes are seen in the resulting dysfunction of the liver and the changes in the portal circulation. The liver is a very complex organ and plays a major role in metabolism, detoxification, blood-forming functions, storage of iron, copper, and various vitamins, and formation of bile. As the liver functions are altered, various clinical manifestations develop, including bleeding disorders (decreased clotting factors), muscle wasting (decreased protein metabolism), hepatic coma (detoxification of ammonia), jaundice (inability to conjugate bilirubin), and peripheral edema (low serum albumin and an increase in hydrostatic pressure). The changes in the portal circulation result in portal hypertension, one of whose clinical manifestations is esophageal varices. Ascites and mesenteric congestion are other clinical manifestations.

Ascites in chronic liver disease has been associated with portal hypertension, low serum albumin, and abnormalities in the lymphatic system. The transudation of fluid between capillaries and tissue spaces is determined by the equilibrium of hydrostatic and osmotic forces in the two compartments. In the normal situation the hydrostatic pressure is higher at the arterial end of the capillary and promotes the passage of protein-free fluid into the pericapillary space. The hydrostatic pressure is lower than the osmotic pressure and the extravascular tissue pressure at the venous end of the capillary, and reabsorption of the fluid occurs.[63] The patient with advanced cirrhosis and portal hypertension has an increased intravascular hydrostatic pressure (portal hypertension) and decreased vascular osmotic pressure (low serum albumin). The combination of the changes in hydrostatic pressure and osmotic pressure leads to the loss of fluid into the peritoneal cavity, an extravascular space.[63] Abnormalities in the lymphatic system are contributory to ascites formation. In cirrhosis with portal hypertension, the thoracic duct is enlarged and lymph flow is significantly increased. The high lymph flow may decompress the hepatic or splanchnic vessels. Lymph from the liver is generally high in protein. When the lymph flow is greater than the thoracic duct can manage, a hepatic venous outflow obstruction develops with resultant ascites. The ascitic fluid in a venous outflow obstruction is high in protein. When the obstruction is an extrahepatic venous obstruction, the protein concentration is low in the fluid.[72]

The communication between the thoracic duct and the subclavian vein helps to determine the occurrence and the severity of ascites. Thoracic duct drainage can decrease ascitic volume and portal pressure. Fluid exudes from the surface of the liver into the peritoneal cavity when the lymph system is unable to manage it.

The formation of ascites is not a simple reaction to increased hepatic venous outflow obstruction. Interrelated factors include aldosterone, antidiuretic hormone

(ADH), and prostaglandins. The development of ascites results in a decreased blood volume, which stimulates aldosterone secretion. Reexpansion of blood volume stimulates ascites formation, reducing blood volume, re-stimulating aldosterone, and creating a cycle. This traditional hypothesis of the relationship between ascites and aldosterone has been challenged. It has been proposed that sodium retention occurs first followed by fluid retention and then ascites.

ADH has been found to be elevated in the serum and urine of patients with ascites from cirrhosis. The increase in ADH may be the result of a decrease in effective plasma volume. Effective plasma volume has been defined as the portion of the total plasma volume that effectively stimulates volume receptors.[63] ADH in patients with ascites may contribute to the retention of water, resulting in hyponatremia.

Prostaglandins have also been suggested in the complexity of the ascites formation in cirrhosis because of sodium retention. Prostaglandins may play a role in determining renal plasma flow and sodium retention in decompensated cirrhosis. Indomethacin, a potent inhibitor of prostaglandins, decreases renal flow and creatinine clearance in cirrhotic patients with sodium retention. Indomethacin also decreases plasma renin activity and aldosterone levels.[63]

There are three types of jaundice: obstructive jaundice, hemolytic jaundice, and hepatocellular jaundice. Obstructive jaundice develops in association with obstruction of the biliary ductal system. There is marked elevation of alkaline phosphatase, mild elevation of serum glutamic-oxaloacetic transaminase (SGOT) and lactate dehydrogenase (LDH), and significant bile in the urine. Hemolytic jaundice is associated with an increased load of bilirubin from hemolysis that a diseased liver is unable to manage. Large amounts of urobilinogen may be found in the urine. Anemia is generally associated with hemolytic jaundice. Hepatocellular jaundice develops because of a failure of the liver cells to metabolize bilirubin. In acute hepatocellular failure the LDH and SGOT are markedly increased and urine contains both bile and urobilinogen. In chronic cirrhosis or hepatocellular failure there may be no elevation of enzymes and the jaundice may not correlate with the severity of the liver disease. Its presence usually indicates acute disease, and in the patient with chronic cirrhosis the presence of jaundice indicates a poor prognosis. Severe hepatic parenchymal necrosis may develop in the absence of jaundice.[63] Hemolysis is common in cirrhosis and may contribute to jaundice. Biliary obstruction may also occur in cirrhosis.

Hepatic encephalopathy encompasses several stages of mental deterioration culminating in coma. The pathophysiology and treatment are presented on p. 1255 to 1256. Bleeding esophageal varices are a major compli-cation associated with portal hypertension and are discussed on p. 1165.

The healthy liver plays a role in the metabolism of estrogens. In cirrhosis, hyperestrogenism develops, which includes an increase in sex hormone–binding globulin and other hormone-binding proteins and an increase in the secretion of prolactin.[63] Clinically, the patient presents with signs of feminization, including gynecomastia, spider angiomata, palmar erythema, and testicular atrophy. The distribution of body hair changes with less chest hair and axillary hair being noted. In women testosterone may accumulate with some masculinization.

Hematologic disorders associated with cirrhosis include impaired coagulation and anemia. The liver is responsible for the synthesis of proteins needed for coagulation: fibrinogen, prothrombin, and various other clotting factors. The liver uses vitamin K to produce prothrombin. Vitamin K absorption is dependent on bile. Treatment of cirrhosis by wiping out intestinal bacteria will decrease the production of vitamin K.

Anemia in cirrhosis may be microcytic, hypochromic anemia secondary to gastrointestinal blood loss and iron deficiency; macrocytic anemia from folic acid deficiency, leukopenia, or thrombocytopenia; or hemolytic anemia. Hemolysis may be indicated by reticulocytosis, hyperbilirubinemia, or increased levels of serum LDH. Splenomegaly may be associated with leukopenia, thrombocytopenia, and hemolytic anemia.

A major complication of cirrhosis is hepatorenal syndrome. Hepatorenal syndrome occurs when a patient with decompensated cirrhosis develops an acquired, functional renal failure. The usual causes of renal insufficiency are present in hepatorenal syndrome, but the kidneys are normal. The patient has oliguria, azotemia, and a urine of high osmolality and low sodium content. Oliguria and azotemia will persist in hepatorenal syndrome even if blood volume and cardiac output are normal. Hepatorenal syndrome carries a very high mortality and does not respond well to medical management.

Hypotension in liver failure is common and may lead to oliguria, azotemia, hyponatremia, and changes in potassium levels. Clinically, the patient may have a high cardiac output and a low total peripheral resistance. Changes in the liver circulatory system may be responsible for this development, and treatment focuses on improving liver function. In addition, oliguria may be associated with a depletion of circulatory blood volume (decreased cardiac output) and decreased renal perfusion. Treatment requires volume expanders.

The patient with cirrhosis has a complex, interrelated group of clinical manifestations. The symptoms observed in cirrhosis can be correlated with a particular dysfunction in the liver or its vascular system. The nurse must be able to identify potential life-threatening complications of advanced liver failure.

DIAGNOSTIC STUDIES

Laboratory studies
Serum bilirubin
Elevated in jaundice

SGOT, SGPT, LDH
Elevated (SGOT may be higher if alcoholic cirrhosis)

Serum albumin
Decreased (tissue edema)

Prothrombin time
Prolonged

Complete blood count
Anemia, leukopenia, thrombocytopenia

Blood glucose
Hypoglycemia (from impaired gluconeogenesis)

Serum ammonia
Elevated (sign of impending hepatic coma)

Urinalysis
Sodium and potassium levels; urine dark, bile colored; presence of urobilinogen

Bromsulfophthalein (BSP) excretion test
Elevated levels found in cirrhosis (test rarely done; has been replaced by liver enzyme studies and liver scan)

Endoscopic retrograde cholangiopancreatography (ERCP)
May show common bile duct obstruction

Esophagoscopy
Presence of esophageal varices

Percutaneous liver biopsy
Histologic changes found in cirrhosis of liver: fatty infiltration; degeneration and regeneration of hepatocytes (increase in connective tissue)

Ultrasonography
Differentiates biliary obstruction from nonobstructive, parenchymal jaundice

Liver scans
Decreased uptake in liver (caused by intrahepatic shunts that bypass liver cells)
Cold spots of cirrhosis can be differentiated from hepatocellular carcinoma by gallium scans

Barium contrast esophagography
Documents esophageal varices

Angiography
Detects sites of upper gastrointestinal bleeding

Percutaneous transhepatic portography (angiographic study)
Visualization of portal venous system

Paracentesis
Clear, straw-colored fluid; decreased total protein

TREATMENT PLAN

Surgical
Refer to discussions of esophageal varices and hepatic coma
Ascites: peritoneovenous shunt (LeVeen valve, ascites drainage system implanted in abdominal wall and connected to peritoneal cavity and to venous system)

Chemotherapeutic
Diuretics (used to promote fluid loss; recommended weight loss slightly less than 2 pounds/d[63])
  Spironolactone (Aldactone, potassium-sparing diuretic), 100 mg/d (higher dosage may be used initially or given in combination with other diuretics)
  Hydrochlorothiazide (Esidrix) or furosemide (Lasix); dosage varies; given with spironolactone
Digestants
  Pancreatin (Panteric), one or two tablets po with meals; each tablet contains 2400 mg; use in presence of steatorrhea; promotes fat digestion
Vitamins
  Menadiol sodium diphosphate (Synkayvite; vitamin K), 5 to 15 mg IM, subq, or IV; repeat dosage in 12 hours if no improvement or give 10 mg for 3 days
  Vitamin C (decreased vitamin C associated with gastrointestinal bleeding)
  Folic acid, 1.0 mg/d/po (for anemia)
Cathartics and laxatives
  Stool softeners (to reduce straining and thereby reduce chance of bleeding from hemorrhoids); dioctyl (Colace), 50 to 200 mg/day
Antibiotics (as required for infections)

Electromechanical
Paracentesis: indicated for diagnostic purposes, relief of abdominal pain, relief of dyspnea or orthopnea, reduction of intra-abdominal pressure; complications: perforation of abdominal viscera, hemorrhage, infection, shock, hyponatremia syndromes
Ascites reinfusion (as an albumin substitute for expanding plasma volume)
Oxygen and incentive spirometer if respiratory complications develop

Supportive

Intravenous fluids
Fresh whole blood during acute bleeding episodes
Albumin replacement
Vitamin supplements including thiamin, iron, and vitamins K and C
Sodium restrictions
Salt substitutes
Fresh frozen plasma or platelets
Diet: high in protein (70 to 90 g), high in carbohydrates, approximately 3000 calories
Diet: with impending liver failure, restrict protein and fluids

ASSESSMENT: AREAS OF CONCERN

History

Dietary pattern; signs of malnutrition
Drug use, toxic substance ingestion, alcohol use
History of hepatitis or previous liver disease

Physical signs of liver disease

Recent change in weight (loss or gain)
Fatigability
Jaundice
Ascites
Edema of lower extremities
Spider angiomas; spider telangiectasis
Palmar erythema
Nail changes (transverse pale bands)
Anorexia, nausea, vomiting
Fever (more common in alcoholic cirrhosis)
Signs of tissue wasting or loss of muscle mass (often seen in legs)

Estrogen-androgen imbalance

Loss of chest hair
Gynecomastia

Portal hypertension

Splenomegaly
Edema of lower extremities
Distention of collateral circulation (esophageal varices, hemorrhoids)
Caput medusae (dilated veins around umbilicus; also develops around ileostomy, colostomy, and ileal conduit stomas when patient develops portal hypertension)

Urinary output

Changes in volume of output; oliguria
Alteration in sodium and potassium levels; osmolality of urine
Color of urine: dark yellow, amber, mahogany

Psychosocial concerns

Ability to give up alcohol ingestion (if alcoholic cirrhosis)

Gastrointestinal symptoms

Esophageal varices
Change in bowel habits
Gastrointestinal bleeding

Mental status

Changes in thinking and mental function secondary to increased serum ammonia levels; may progress to hepatic coma (Serum ammonia levels do not always correlate with mental functions; that is, some patients with very high levels will have minimal mental function alteration whereas others with low levels may progress to coma.)

NURSING DIAGNOSES and NURSING INTERVENTIONS

Nursing Diagnosis	Nursing Intervention
Injury, potential for: hemorrhage	Observe patient for signs of bleeding: hematemesis, melena, signs of shock. Monitor vital signs and laboratory studies. Provide intravenous fluids as ordered. Prepare patient for endoscopy. Maintain patency of nasogastric tube. If ordered, perform cool saline or water lavage. Record intake and output and color and characteristics of aspirate. Provide medications as ordered: vitamin K, vasopressin, neomycin. Monitor use of Sengstaken-Blakemore tube.
Injury, potential for: altered clotting factors	Assist patient to minimize trauma (i.e., forceful nose blowing, harsh toothbrush, safety razors). Observe for signs of bleeding. Provide stool softener and remind patient not to strain during bowel movements. Use small-gauge needles for injections, and apply pressure following injections. Record any indications of small bleeding sites. Monitor platelet count and prothrombin time.

Nursing Diagnosis	Nursing Intervention
Tissue perfusion, alteration in	Assess patient for alterations in cardiac output and decreased renal perfusion. Monitor and record urinary output. Weigh daily. Monitor urine osmolality and sodium and potassium levels.
Fluid volume deficit, actual	Maintain accurate intake and output records, reporting abnormalities. Record daily weights. Measure abdominal girth daily. Monitor serum and urine electrolytes. Provide diuretics as ordered. Observe for clinical signs of electrolyte imbalance, particularly sodium, potassium, and magnesium. Restrict fluid intake if ordered. Perform frequent mouth care.
Nutrition, alteration in: less than body requirements	Provide small frequent feedings high in calories, carbohydrates, and protein, low in fats, and low in sodium. Provide salt substitutes if ordered.
Skin integrity, impairment of: potential	Assess patient for risk of developing pressure sores. Monitor patient for risk factors: edema, decreased movement or turning. Provide pressure relief device appropriate for patient based on size of patient, bony prominences, and areas of continued stress. Change linens regularly if patient is perspiring or tissues are weepy from edema (moisture contributes to skin breakdown). Manage symptoms of pruritus with calamine lotion and baths. Use preventive protocol for perianal area when patient is to be treated with neomycin or other agents such as lactulose that promote diarrhea. Use vanishing cream and skin sealant (Bard Protective Barrier Film) *before* skin breaks down. Repeat applications with each cleansing of perianal area. The skin may be cleansed with mineral oil and cotton balls to reduce harshness of washcloths and toilet paper. Cleansers are available that soften stool, reduce odors, and are gentle to the skin (Bara Cleanser, Uniwash).
Breathing pattern, ineffective	Place patient in semi-Fowler's or high Fowler's position to increase lung expansion compromised by ascites. Monitor perianal area for signs of pressure sores associated with shearing forces. Turn frequently from side to side. Use pressure relief devices. Monitor blood gases. Monitor vital signs. Assess lung fields for signs of congestion or infection.
Thought processes, alteration in	Observe for early signs of mental changes: lethargy, confusion, drowsiness, and irritability. Avoid use of sedatives or tranquilizers. Refer to section on hepatic coma.

Patient Education

1. Stress the importance of avoiding alcohol and provide information on alcoholic cirrhosis.
2. Assist patient in identifying community resources available for alcohol rehabilitation.
3. Provide patient with information on altered drug effects with cirrhosis and caution to use only physician-prescribed or -approved medications.
4. Provide written dietary instructions. Stress the role of nutrition in recovery. Include any restrictions required, specifically sodium.
5. Instructions should include the need for rest and diversional activities to prevent boredom.
6. Provide written instructions of signs and symptoms that warrant seeing a physician: increased abdominal girth, rapid weight gain or loss, edema, fever, blood in urine or stool, bleeding that does not cease with pressure in a short time (nosebleeds, cuts, gums), gross upper gastrointestinal bleeding, or tarry stools.
7. Instruct the family in all of the above plus signs of mental changes: confusion, untidiness, night wandering, personality changes, irritability, and sleeplessness.

EVALUATION

Patient Outcome	Data Indicating That Outcome is Reached
Blood clotting factors are normal.	Hemorrhage is controlled and recurrence prevented. Platelet count is normal. Prothrombin time is normal.
Tissue perfusion is adequate.	Satisfactory urinary output is maintained.
Fluid volume is maintained.	Serum electrolytes (sodium, potassium, and magnesium) are normal. Fluid weight loss is slightly less than 2 pounds per day. Abdominal girth decreases. Peripheral edema is reduced.
Nutrition is adequate.	Patient does not experience anorexia, nausea and vomiting, indigestion, or muscle wasting. Calorie and protein intake is sufficient for healing. Patient does not drink alcohol.
Breathing pattern is normal.	Patient does not experience atelectasis or pneumonia. Ascites decreases or disappears, therefore lung expansion improves.
Skin integrity is maintained.	There are no signs of irritation, pressure, or broken areas.
Thought processes are normal.	Thought processes are not altered. Serum ammonia levels are controlled.

HEPATIC COMA

In acute and chronic liver diseases, a series of neuropsychiatric manifestations may develop that range from hepatic encephalopathy to precoma to hepatic coma. Hepatic coma is the end stage of the neuropsychiatric manifestations.

The pathophysiology of hepatic coma has become better understood and has been related to the presence of two factors: the shunting of blood around the liver so that substances toxic to the brain are no longer completely metabolized or cleared by the liver, and hepatic insufficiency. The syndrome is currently referred to as portal-systemic encephalopathy (PSE). PSE is characterized by recurrent changes in consciousness, impaired intellectual function, neuromuscular abnormalities, metabolic slowing of electroencephalogram, and elevated serum ammonia levels.[63]

The majority of patients who develop hepatic coma or PSE have cirrhosis. However, PSE may develop in fulminant liver failure, deficiency of urea cycle enzyme, and Reye's syndrome. PSE occurs in patients with cirrhosis who have portal hypertension or portal-systemic shunting. Hepatic coma also develops in half of those patients having portacaval shunts.

Several clinical situations have been associated with the initiation of PSE and include azotemia; medications such as sedatives, tranquilizers, and analgesics; gastrointestinal bleeding; high dietary protein; and hypokalemic alkalosis. An iatrogenic etiology occurs in approximately half of the cases of hepatic coma.

PATHOPHYSIOLOGY

The vast majority of episodes of PSE are caused by ammonia intoxication. Ammonia is a by-product of nitrogen metabolism. Nitrogen is a by-product of amino acid digestion. The bacteria in the colon break down nitrogen to ammonia. The ammonia is absorbed and carried through the portal veins to the liver, where it is converted to glutamine, a nontoxic form. Glutamine is later synthesized by the liver into urea, which is excreted.

The colon, when in a fasting state, is a continuous source of ammonia. The colon bacteria responsible for ammonia formation may also be found in the small bowel of patients with cirrhosis.[72] When the portal vein flow bypasses the liver, such as with a portal-systemic anastomosis, the systemic blood ammonia levels increase to toxic levels.

The following equation refers to the ammonia and ammonia hydroxide balance:

$$NH_4OH \rightleftarrows NH_4^+ + OH^-$$

Only ammonia hydroxide can cross the cell membrane and thus create toxic effects. The pH of the extracellular and intracellular compartments affects this equation. Abnormalities of acid-base balance, primarily alkalosis associated with hypokalemia, result in an increase in ammonia hydroxide and passage of the substance into the cells. Hypokalemia in alcoholic cirrhosis may be related to vomiting, diarrhea, diuretics, and secondary aldosteronism.

Ammonia is also released during muscle activities from the muscles of the extremities. And under normal resting conditions, a small quantity of ammonia uptake occurs. This uptake may increase when arterial levels of ammonia are increased.[63]

PSE may be initiated by conditions that increase nitrogen levels. Endogenous factors include azotemia, blood in the gastrointestinal tract, and constipation. Azotemia affects the kidney's ability to excrete nitrogen. Blood is a source of more ammonia than dietary protein, and the ammonia is liberated from the blood in the colon. Constipation may exaggerate other factors. In constipation the waste products remain in the colon for longer periods, providing more opportunity for colonic bacteria to convert nitrogenous products to ammonia.

Exogenous factors that contribute to the nitrogenous etiology of PSE include dietary protein, ammonia salts, urea, cation exchange resins, amino acids, and diuretics. In addition, potassium depletion is associated with nitrogenous PSE.

Several noncirrhotic clinical conditions in which ammonia levels are associated with PSE include hereditary deficiencies of urea cycle enzymes and Reye's syndrome.

The blood ammonia levels do not correlate well with the clinical manifestations of PSE. Schiff and Schiff[63] have identified several reasons. Venous blood levels do not reflect what is delivered to the tissues. Arterial ammonia blood levels are recommended, and since individuals respond differently to various levels of ammonia, serial studies of ammonia levels would provide a better indication of the relationship of increasing symptoms to blood levels. Blood ammonia levels are also affected by potassium levels and food ingestion. Hypokalemia results in more tissue uptake of ammonia with a resultant low serum ammonia level. Serum levels of ammonia increase after meals and vary according to the amount of protein consumed. Fasting and serial arterial ammonia levels are more likely to correlate with the clinical symptoms of PSE.

Nonnitrogenous factors have also been associated with PSE and include sedatives, tranquilizers, analgesics, hypoxemia, hypoglycemia, fulminant viral hepatitis, and hypokalemia. Although these are not as common as other factors in the etiology of PSE, it is important to identify the cause of PSE in order to appropriately treat the patient.

DIAGNOSTIC STUDIES

Arterial ammonia blood levels (fasting)
Elevated

Serum electrolytes
Hypokalemia
Alkalosis

Blood glucose
Hyperglycemia: iatrogenic hyperglycemia may cause coma; in cirrhosis there is little glycogen stored, so patients are usually hypoglycemic

Electroencephalogram (EEG)
Paroxysms of bilateral, synchronous, symmetric slow waves at a rate of 1½ to 3/sec
Four grades of EEG
Grade 0: normal
Grade 1: mild impairment
Grade 2: moderate impairment
Grade 3: severe impairment
Grade 4: coma
Rule out other causes of coma such as subdural hematomas and nonnitrogenous causes of PSE

TREATMENT PLAN

Surgical
Colectomy (rare)
Ileosigmoidostomy (rare)

Chemotherapeutic
Anti-infective agents (nonabsorbable)
To decrease bacterial action in colon:
Neomycin (Mycifradin) or paromomycin (Humatin), 2 to 6 g/d
Broad-spectrum antibiotics
Ampicillin (Cephulac)
Ammonia detoxicants
Lactulose (synthetic disaccharide), 300 ml syrup diluted with 700 ml water by enema (retain 20 to 30 min), or 30 to 45 ml tid or qid po (acidifies contents of colon)

Electromechanical
Removal of blood from gastrointestinal tract: cathartics
Gastric lavage with cool saline or water
Cleansing enemas with dilute acetic acid or neomycin

Supportive
Discontinuation of any precipitating substance: dietary proteins, sedatives, diuretic therapy, analgesics
Intravenous glucose (minimizes protein breakdown)
Oxygen (respiratory or metabolic alkalosis)
Correction of any electrolyte imbalances

ASSESSMENT: AREAS OF CONCERN

Fetor hepaticus
Sweetish odor detected on breath and in urine

State of consciousness
Hypersomnia, insomnia, or inversion of sleep pattern
Slow responses
Lethargy
Minimal disorientation
Somnolence
Confusion
Semistupor
Stupor
Unconsciousness (coma)

Neuromuscular abnormalities
Metabolic tremor
Muscular incoordination
Impaired handwriting
Asterixis (liver flap)
Slurred speech
Hypoactive reflexes
Ataxia
Hyperactive reflexes
Nystagmus
Babinski's sign (clonus)
Rigidity
Dilated pupils
Opisthotonus (coma)

Intellectual function
Subtly impaired computations (use number connection test (NCT) for assessment [permits serial assessment of minimal changes])
Shortened attention span
Loss of time
Grossly impaired computations
Amnesia for past events
Loss of orientation to place
Inability to compute
Loss of orientation to self
No intellect (coma)

Personality behavioral changes
Exaggeration of normal behavior
Euphoria or depression
Garrulousness
Irritability
Decreased inhibitions
Overt changes in personality
Anxiety or apathy
Inappropriate behavior
Bizarre behavior
Paranoia or anger
Rage
None (coma)

NURSING DIAGNOSES and NURSING INTERVENTIONS

Nursing Diagnosis	Nursing Intervention
Thought processes, alteration in	Observe for early signs of changes in consciousness, intellect, personality behaviors, and neuromuscular activities. Record indications of changes. Have patient do simple arithmetic computations or use NCT. Have patient do serial handwriting in order to compare differences. Monitor arterial ammonia and potassium levels. Observe for clinical signs of hypokalemia and alkalosis. Provide sedatives, tranquilizers, and analgesics as ordered, note any delayed or prolonged reactions, and report immediately; avoid use of above is possible. Protect the patient from injury as personality behaviors become more overt and inappropriate and as neuromuscular activities alter. Identify personality and behavior changes and relate them to the progression of the disease and assist family and staff in their understanding and knowledge of the disease progression. Document treatment ordered by physician as implemented (i.e., retention or cleansing enemas, gastric lavage, medications).
Skin integrity, impairment of: potential	Begin protective perianal skin care before beginning lactulose or neomycin orally or rectally. Diarrheal stools will be more acidic. Cleanse the skin with Periwash (Sween), Uni-Wash (United), or another gentle, nondetergent solution. Cotton balls can be used rather than rough cloth or gauze. Pat the skin dry or use a hair dryer on cool or warm; avoid hot settings. Apply a vanishing cream.

Nursing Diagnosis	Nursing Intervention
	Cover the area with a skin sealant (Bard Protective Barrier Film); spray forms are easiest to use. Allow to dry. Use ointment on top of protective film. Repeat with each bowel movement.
Skin integrity, impairment of: actual	Keep in mind that skin impairment is harder to treat than to prevent.
	Cleanse perianal skin with Domeboro (aluminum acetate) solution and cotton balls; dry with hair dryer.
	Apply vanishing cream and cover with thick ointment-based product. If skin is severely eroded, Karaya and glycerin can be combined to form a paste (commercial paste contains alcohol and will be painful), which should be thick, almost like cookie dough. The paste should be applied rather than the creams and ointments and should be a thin coat. A pectin-based wafer may be used. Be careful that stool does not become trapped underneath the wafer. Pouching the rectum or a rectal tube may help.
	Repeat the procedure with each bowel movement.

Patient Education

1. Provide family with written signs of changes in mental functions that are related to early PSE: confusion, untidiness, night wandering, and personality changes. They should notify the physician if symptoms occur.
2. Provide written dietary instructions for reduced protein intake.

EVALUATION

Patient Outcome	Data Indicating That Outcome is Reached
Thought processes are not impaired.	Thought processes, personality, behavior, consciousness, and neuromuscular activities are not altered. Arterial ammonia levels are normal.
Skin integrity is maintained.	There are no signs of irritation or erosion.

CHOLECYSTITIS WITH CHOLELITHIASIS

Cholecystitis refers to the acute or chronic inflammation of the gallbladder.

Acute cholecystitis is associated with gallstones (cholelithiasis) in 90% of cases. Less than 10% of cases of acute cholecystitis are acalculous or not related to stone formation. Chronic cholecystitis refers to repeated attacks of acute cholecystitis and an abnormal looking gallbladder. Pain often follows a meal in chronic cholecystitis.

Acute cholecystitis is common and accounts for one fourth of all gallbladder surgeries. Although it may occur in all ages, it is more common in middle age. The number of surgeries for acute cholecystitis may increase in the future. The current trend is toward early surgical intervention for cholecystitis.

PATHOPHYSIOLOGY

Acute cholecystitis consists of acute inflammation of the wall of the gallbladder. In calculous cholecystitis an obstruction of the cystic duct by a stone or from edema secondary to the passage of a stone is the underlying problem. The cystic duct is obstructed. The gallbladder distends, and the wall becomes edematous, compressing the capillaries and lymphatics and resulting in ischemia and inflammation. The inflamed mucosa allows bile salt to be reabsorbed, further damaging the mucosa. If the inflammation continues, the wall will become friable and necrosis may develop. Perforation of the gallbladder may occur. The perforation may be small and localized, forming an abscess. In severe acute cholecystitis, inflammation spreads to the serosal layer of the gallbladder and may progress to form inflammatory adhesions to adjacent structures. Bacteria may be found in the bile and is associated with secondary infections.

The gallbladder heals after the acute attack with scarring and decreased absorptive capacity. The mucosa of the gallbladder in a patient with chronic cholecystitis is also ulcerated and scarred. Chronic cholecystitis may develop from repeated intermittent episodes of cystic duct obstruction resulting in chronic inflammation. The gallbladder is contracted, white in color, and thick walled. The bile is turbid and filled with debris.

Acute cholecystitis in the absence of stones has been associated with sudden starvation and immobility. These are changes that affect the regular filling and emptying of the gallbladder. A patient hospitalized for cardiovascular disease, burns, traumas, or biliary surgery may develop acalculous acute cholecystitis. The patient on TPN may also develop cholecystitis secondary to gallbladder distention and biliary stasis.

The primary symptom associated with acute cholecystitis is pain. The pain of acute cholecystitis has been described as colicky. However, this is not a true colic pain that waxes and wanes. The pain of acute cholecystitis is abrupt in onset, reaches a peak intensity quickly, and remains at that level for 2 to 4 hours. Initially, the pain may be poorly localized, but as it becomes more severe it localizes in the right upper quadrant epigastric region. The pain radiates around the midtorso to the right scapular area. Guarding and rigidity represent peritoneal involvement. Tenderness may be elicited at the tip of the ninth costal margin during inspiration (i.e., Murphy's sign). Jaundice may be found in acute cholecystitis. The jaundice may be related to edema of the ducts or to direct involvement of the liver by inflammation since stones are not always found in patients with jaundice.

In acute cholecystitis it is important to rule out concomitant acute pancreatitis, peptic ulcer disease, pneumonitis, hepatitis, and acute appendicitis. In chronic cholecystitis the following must be ruled out: peptic ulcer disease, chronic pancreatitis, and hiatus hernia.

DIAGNOSTIC STUDIES

Acute cholecystitis
Plain films of abdomen
Gallstones visualized

Ultrasound
Gallstones
Thickening of wall

Biliary scintigraphy
Scans 15 to 30 minutes after IV injection of radionuclide show the ducts but not the obstructed gallbladder; recommend repeat scan 4 hours after injection to rule out late filling of gallbladder

Serum amylase
Elevated may indicate concomitant acute pancreatitis; usually indicates common duct stone

White blood count
Leukocyte count of 12,000 to 15,000/cmm

Chronic cholecystitis
Double-dose oral cholecystogram
Nonfunctioning gallbladder

Ultrasound
Presence of gallstones

Upper gastrointestinal series
Excludes peptic ulcer disease and hiatus hernia

TREATMENT PLAN
Acute Cholecystitis with Cholelithiasis

Surgical
Cholecystectomy with exploration of common bile duct
Cholecystostomy (in critically ill patient only a drain is inserted into the gallbladder to drain the abscess, to be removed later when the patient is stable)

Chemotherapeutic
Narcotic analgesics
For acute pain, meperidine hydrochloride (Demerol), 100 mg, and atropine, 0.6 mg, IM
Anti-infective agents
Agent-specific antibiotics for existing or impending secondary infections as indicated by a worsening of clinical condition or acute attack for 4 to 5 days without clinical improvement

Supportive
Intravenous fluids to correct dehydration
Nasogastric tube; give nothing by mouth

Chronic Cholecystitis

Surgical
Cholecystectomy with exploration of common bile duct

ASSESSMENT: AREAS OF CONCERN
Acute Cholecystitis with Cholelithiasis

Jaundice
Mild jaundice of skin noted
Pruritus not commonly a problem

Pain

Severe right upper quadrant pain with referral to right
  scapula
Rebound tenderness; rigidity
Positive Murphy's sign
Gallbladder may be palpable

Gastrointestinal symptoms

Anorexia
Vomiting

Temperature

Fever of 37° to 39° C (99° to 102° F)

Chronic Cholecystitis

Gastrointestinal symptoms

Fat intolerance
Flatulence
Nausea
Anorexia

Pain

Nonspecific abdominal pain and tenderness in right
  hypochondrium

NURSING DIAGNOSES and NURSING INTERVENTIONS

Nursing Diagnosis	Nursing Intervention
Comfort, alteration in: pain	Provide pain medication as ordered and record response of patient. Observe and document characteristics, location, and severity of pain. Allow patient to assume position that is least painful. Provide patient with an opportunity to express feelings and fears.
Fluid volume deficit, potential	Maintain careful intake and output records including emesis and nasogastric aspiration. Observe patient for signs of dehydration: dry mouth and mucous membranes, dry skin. Monitor serum electrolytes. Provide intravenous fluids as ordered. Maintain frequent oral hygiene.
Nutrition, alteration in: less than body requirements	Provide diet that is low fat, high carbohydrate, and high protein when acute phase is ended.
Skin integrity, impairment of: potential	Assess patient carefully for risk factors for developing pressure points. Provide mechanical relief of pressure points: Turn patient following pain medication and assess for changes in skin. NOTE: Elderly patients are at high risk during episodes of acute pain when movement intensifies the pain. Protect the skin from drainage around the T-tube insertion site using pectin-based wafers. If the insertion site leaks for prolonged periods following removal of the T tube, consider a sterile pouching system.

Patient Education

1. During acute phase, patient will need explanation of all procedures and may require pain medication before moving. Patient should be aware that the nurse recognizes the severity of the pain during acute cholecystitis.
2. Following or during the resolution of the acute phase, patient will require data regarding cholecystectomy in order to make an informed decision regarding surgery.
3. Patients electing medical management will need information on (a) chronic cholecystitis, (b) signs and symptoms of recurrence, (c) signs of potential complications (recurrent attacks, jaundice, obstruction of common bile duct, cholangitis, pancreatitis, internal biliary fistula, carcinoma) and (d) low-fat diets.

EVALUATION

Patient Outcome	Data Indicating That Outcome is Reached
Body functions normally.	Patient does not experience jaundice, anorexia, vomiting, pain, or fever. Fluid and electrolyte balance is normal.
There is no infection.	There are no signs or symptoms of secondary infection; white blood count is normal, and there is no fever.

PANCREATITIS

Pancreatitis is an inflammation of the pancreas that may be acute or chronic.

Acute pancreatitis involves a diffuse inflammation caused by premature activation of pancreatic enzymes into active, potent proteolytic enzymes. The acute pancreatitis is a process of autodigestion. The two types of acute pancreatitis are interstitial, or edematous, pancreatitis and hemorrhagic, or necrotizing, pancreatitis. It may be that the two forms are actually a continuum of the same process. Interstitial pancreatitis is milder and is characterized by interstitial edema with exudation. As the disease progresses, frank necrosis develops with disruption and thrombotic occlusion of blood vessels. Bleeding, ischemic necrosis, and fat necrosis are found throughout the pancreas.

Complications of acute pancreatitis include hemorrhage, pseudocysts, pancreatic ascites, and abscesses. A pseudocyst occurs when an accumulation of tissue debris, blood, fat droplets, and pancreatic juice develops within confluent areas of necrosis. A pseudocyst may arise within or adjacent to the pancreas. Pancreatic ascites develops when the accumulation of active pancreatic enzymes and leukocytes imitates the peritoneal surfaces and fluid accumulates in the peritoneal cavity. The same process of irritation through the diaphragmatic lymphatics leads to pleural effusion. Abscesses result from secondary infection of necrotic tissue and fluid collection.

Chronic pancreatitis is progressive functional damage to the pancreas. Removal of the causative factor does not improve the pancreatic function. The primary clinical features are pain, malabsorption, diabetes mellitus, and intraductal calcifications. The primary causative factor is chronic excessive alcohol ingestion. Complications consist of loss of exocrine and endocrine function, pancreatic necrosis, hemorrhage, abscess, and pseudocysts.

Chronic excessive alcohol ingestion and gallbladder disease are associated with acute pancreatitis. The age and sex of the patient will vary according to the primary disease associated with the acute pancreatitis. Gallbladder disease is more common in middle-aged women. Alcohol as an associated agent is seen more often in men. Alcohol ingestion plays a major role in the devel-

opment of chronic pancreatitis. The disease occurs more often in men than women, and the average age is 49. These patients tend to be overweight and have other signs of alcoholic disease such as hepatitis, cirrhosis, or fatty liver. If the patient has signs of malabsorption and diabetes mellitus, he usually is malnourished and has weight loss.

PATHOPHYSIOLOGY

Acute Pancreatitis

Acute pancreatitis is a process of autodigestion, but the causative agent that triggers prematurely the activation of the enzymes is unknown. Several theories have been proposed, including obstruction of the pancreatic ducts, reflux of bile, reflux of duodenal contents, and the toxic effect of alcohol. Unfortunately, none of the proposed theories has proven to be the etiology.

The process of enzyme activation regardless of the etiology is the basis of the disease process. Trypsinogen may undergo spontaneous activation to trypsin in the presence of an alkaline pH. Trypsin is inactivated by a specific trypsin inhibitor found in the pancreatic secretions and in the pancreatic tissue. However, the small amount of trypsin may activate other proteolytic enzymes. Phospholipase A and elastase have been proposed as the primary enzymes responsible for autodigestion. Phospholipase A, in the presence of bile, results in severe pancreatic parenchymal and adipose tissue necrosis. Elastase dissolves the elastic fibers of blood vessels and is implicated in the hemorrhage associated with necrotizing pancreatitis.

Many substances released from the injured pancreas will have systemic effects. Two low–molecular weight vasoactive peptides (kinins) are released and result in vasodilation and increase in vascular permeability, resulting in circulatory shock. Severe pulmonary edema and pain are also associated with the vasoactive peptides.

Hypocalcemia develops when a decreased binding of calcium to serum protein occurs secondary to a drop in albumin levels. In addition, a decrease in ionized serum calcium occurs in acute pancreatitis. Damage to the islet cells results in mild, transient hyperglycemia from release of glucagon and decreased release of insulin. The glucose levels are too high for the insulin production to control.

Patients with acute pancreatitis are at risk for developing adult respiratory distress syndrome (ARDS). Arterial hypoxia occurs when intrapulmonary right-to-left shunting develops. Pulmonary edema from disruption of the alveolar-capillary membrane is a serious complication. In addition, renal function may be altered during acute pancreatitis. Hypovolemia and shock are not always the causative factors in altered renal function. The blood flow may be reduced and the vascular resistance increased in the kidney in the absence of hypovolemia.

Another major potential complication of acute pancreatitis is disseminated intravascular coagulation (DIC), which involves the development of microthrombi and consumption of clotting factors. Mild DIC may play a role in the development of early hypoxia and renal impairment.

Chronic Pancreatitis

Chronic pancreatitis generally develops from an insidious sclerosing process in the pancreas; however, it may develop from repeated bouts of acute inflammation and necrosis. The histologic changes in the pancreas include irregularly distributed fibrosis, reduced number and size of acini and islet cells, and obstruction of the pancreatic ductal system.

The clinical signs of chronic pancreatitis include pain and functional impairment of the pancreas. The pain may be intermittent or chronic and affects the productivity of the patient and his activities of daily living. Nausea and vomiting often accompany the pain. The pain is described as steady, boring, dull, or sharp and radiates from the epigastrium to the back. The pain may be lessened by leaning forward from a sitting position. Eating or lying down may increase the pain.

Malabsorption and weight loss develop during the course of the chronic illness. Patients may limit food intake because of the pain. Secretions of pancreatic enzymes decrease in chronic pancreatitis, and fat and protein are poorly digested. Steatorrhea and azotorrhea are observed. Carbohydrate malabsorption is clinically not seen since salivary amylase is unimpaired. Pancreatic amylase is highly efficient and in fact would have to be reduced by 97% before carbohydrate malabsorption would develop.[69]

Insulin response to glucose is impaired in chronic pancreatitis. Overt diabetes mellitus will occur in the vast majority of these patients. The ability of the pancreas to release glucagon is also affected.

DIAGNOSTIC STUDIES

Acute pancreatitis
Rule out
    Perforated peptic ulcer
    Acute cholangitis
    Mesenteric infarction

WBC
    Greater than 15,000/cmm

Serum glucose
    Greater than 180 mg/dl with no prior history of hyperglycemia

BUN
    Greater than 45 mg/dl after fluid volume replacement

Arterial PO_2
    Less than 60 mm Hg

Serum calcium
    Less than 8.0 mg/dl (in patients with hyperparathyroidism and acute pancreatitis level may be within normal range)

Serum albumin
    Less than 3.2 g/dl

Serum LDH
    Greater than 600 U/L

SGOT or SGPT
    Greater than 200 U/L

Amylase
    Serum: greater than 500 U/dl; highest levels 2 to 12 hours after onset, drop to normal (60 to 180 U/dl) within 48 to 72 hours
    Urine: levels remain elevated for 3 to 5 days; amylase–creatinine clearance ratio (ACR) above 5% indicates acute pancreatitis
    Lipase: elevated; may remain elevated for 5 to 10 days

Chronic pancreatitis
Urinalysis
    Glycosuria (diabetes mellitus)

Serum glucose
    Elevated

Amylase–creatinine clearance ratio
    Normal

Serum amylase and lipase
    Normal
    Increased in presence of pseudocysts and pancreatic ascites

Alkaline phosphate
Increased five times normal for 4 weeks indicates common bile duct stenosis

Lactoferrin levels
Increased (specimens obtained by endoscopic retrograde cannulation)

Exogenous stimulation: secretin-CCK
Decreased stimulation of pancreatic enzymes

Endogenous stimulation: perfusion and feedings
Diminished function

Lundh test meal
Mean trypsin concentration decreased

Para-aminobenzoic acid (PABA) test
Urinary recovery of PABA low in pancreatic insufficiency

Procedures for both acute and chronic pancreatitis
Plain films of abdomen
Peripancreatic, extraluminal gas bubbles indicating pancreatic abscess
Diffuse pancreatitis; calcification of chronic pancreatitis

Ultrasonography
Demonstrates presence of gallstones, pancreatic pseudocyst, pancreatitis abscess, calcification of pancreatic ducts

Computed tomography
Delineates spread of peripancreatic inflammation, pseudocyst, abscess, and localized hematoma formation; presence of calcification

Intravenous cholangiography
Differentiates acute cholecystitis from acute pancreatitis

Upper gastrointestinal series
Used to rule out perforated duodenal ulcer
Demonstrates pancreatic enlargement and inflammation, widening of duodenal C-loop, and enlargement of papilla of Vater
Stomach can be displaced by pseudocyst

Endoscopic retrograde cholangiopancreatography (ERCP)
Not indicated in acute pancreatitis or pseudocyst
Identifies ductal changes in chronic pancreatitis and presence of calculi

TREATMENT PLAN

Acute Pancreatitis

Surgical
Surgical drainage of pancreatic pseudocyst may be indicated if does not resolve spontaneously
Surgical drainage of pancreatic abscesses may be indicated
Laparotomy for common duct obstruction

Chemotherapeutic
Narcotic analgesics
Meperidine hydrochloride (Demerol), 75 to 125 mg IM q4h or prn (Hold analgesics until initial laboratory samples are drawn since many will cause elevations in serum amylase and lipase.)
Antacids
Aluminum-magnesium preparation, 30 to 40 ml (clamp nasogastric tube for 15 min after dosage)
Histamine H_2 receptor antagonists
Cimetidine or ranitidine, 300 mg IV qid if any evidence of upper gastrointestinal bleeding
Anti-infective agents
Cephalothin (Keflin), 2 g q6h IV or with peritoneal lavage
For abscess, chloramphenicol (chloromycetin), 0.5 g q6h IV, and penicillin G, 5 to 10 million units qd IV, or cefoxitin, 1 g q6h IV (used before cultures are known)
Adrenergic agents
For hypotension, dopamine (Intropin), 2-5 µg/kg/min, diluted in solution and titrated as needed or isoproterenol hydrochloride (Isuprel) may be used

Electromechanical
Continuous hemodynamic and arterial blood gas monitoring; Swan-Ganz or CVP catheter
Nasogastric suctioning
Peritoneal lavage for persistent hypotension (removes pancreatic exudate, which contains large amounts of vasoactive kinins)
ARDS: endotracheal intubation and controlled ventilation with positive end-expiratory pressure (PEEP)

Supportive
Restoration and maintenance of intravascular volume including human serum albumin, low–molecular weight dextran 40
Correction of electrolyte imbalances: hypocalcemia, hypomagnesium, hyperglycemia, hyperkalemia, and metabolic acidosis
Nutritional support with TPN or feeding jejunostomy

Chronic Pancreatitis

Surgical

Not primary treatment but may be used to treat intractable pain complications (i.e., pseudocysts or abscesses)

Drainage procedures

Longitudinal pancreaticojejunostomy (modified Puestow procedure)

Caudal pancreaticojejunostomy (Du Val procedure)

Resection

Subtotal or total pancreatectomy

Pancreaticoduodenostomy (Whipple procedure)

To preserve islet cell function

Islet cell autotransplantation by infusion of islet cell preparations into portal system

Segments of pancreas autotransplanted

Insertion of closed-loop insulin infusion system

Chemotherapeutic

Analgesics

Acetaminophen or narcotics prn for pain

Digestants

Pancreatic enzyme supplements (use one of the following)

Pancreatin (Viokase), six tablets with each meal

Pancrelipase (Cotazym), five capsules with each meal

Pancrelipase (Pancrease), enteric-coated, two to three capsules with each meal

Antacids and adsorbents

Sodium bicarbonate or aluminum hydroxide antacids may be used with pancreatic enzyme supplements to improve results

Histamine H_2 receptor antagonists

Cimetidine, 300 mg po 30 min before meals (may be used rather than above to improve effects of pancreatic enzyme supplements)

Medium-chain triglycerides (MCT; Portagen) supplements

Insulin therapy: does vary with individual (remember glucagon deficiency is present and patient may have hypoglycemic reactions easily)

Supportive

Enteral nutritional support or TPN as indicated by nutritional status and weight loss

ASSESSMENT: AREAS OF CONCERN

Acute Pancreatitis

Abdomen

Steady, dull, boring pain in epigastrium or left upper quadrant: poorly localized; reaches peak intensity within 15 minutes to 1 hour; radiates to lower thoracic vertebral area; worsens in supine position

Palpation: localized epigastric tenderness to deep palpation is intense

Soft abdomen (retroperitoneal location of pancreas means that signs of peritoneal irritation, rigidity, and rebound tenderness will not be present initially)

Mild abdominal distention and mild ascites

Gastrointestinal symptoms

Nausea and vomiting hematemesis

Intestinal ileus

General concerns

Fever of 38° C (100° to 101° F)

Circulatory system

Tachycardia, hypovolemia, and hypotension: may progress to circulatory shock and coma

Grey Turner's sign

Bluish brown discoloration of flanks

Cullen's sign

Bluish brown discoloration in periumbilicus area

Jaundice

Seen in some patients; hyperbilirubinemia of 3 mg/dl

Pulmonary concerns

Pleuritic pain; pleural effusion; pulmonary infiltrates

Impaired ventilation

Adult respiratory distress syndrome (ARDS) may develop

Diaphragm

Irritation results in hiccups and referred shoulder pain

Urine

Decreased output (oliguria): less than 400 ml/24 hr; associated with acute tubular necrosis

Pancreatic pseudocyst

Fluid collection in pancreas: may be detected on ultrasound or CT scan

Palpable mass

Fever of 38° C (100° to 101° F)

Pancreatic abscess

Fever above 38° C (101° F)

Increasing pain: palpable mass

Leukocytosis (above 10,000/cmm)

Tachycardia

Chills

Hypotension

Pancreatic cutaneous fistula

Spontaneous drainage of pancreatic abscess through an abnormal tract to skin or following surgical drainage of an abscess

Chronic Pancreatitis

Malabsorption

Weight loss, steatorrhea, voluminous diarrhea, nausea and vomiting (associated with pain and with complications)

Pancreatic endocrine function

Signs and symptoms of diabetes mellitus
Reactive hypoglycemia to insulin therapy

Chronic pain

Intermittent or chronic pain
Boring, dull, or sharp pain that is steady
Epigastric, right or left subcostal region, periumbilical region, or lower abdomen
Radiates to back
Patient observed sitting up and leaning forward to relieve pain

NURSING DIAGNOSES and NURSING INTERVENTIONS

Nursing Diagnosis	Nursing Intervention
Fluid volume deficit, potential	Monitor and record intake and output, central venous pressure, Swan-Ganz catheter, and daily weights. Monitor laboratory values, particularly hematocrit and hemoglobin, which will decrease after volume is restored. Assess vital signs and blood pressure regularly. Monitor for signs of impending cardiac failure. Observe for signs and symptoms of electrolyte imbalance. Provide fluid volume replacement as ordered: intravenous fluids, dextran, fluid expanders.
Comfort, alteration in: pain	Allow patient to assume a comfortable position. Provide analgesics as ordered (pain may be severe and steady). Provide analgesics before procedures to alleviate or minimize discomfort.
Nutrition, alteration in: less than body requirements	Give patient nothing by mouth during acute pancreatitis episodes. Measure and record nasogastric output. Provide frequent mouth care. Monitor blood and urine glucose levels. Provide pancreatic enzyme supplements for patients with chronic pancreatitis. Monitor stools for diarrhea and steatorrhea. Provide insulin as ordered for endocrine dysfunction in chronic pancreatitis. Weigh daily.
Injury, potential for: complications	Observe patient carefully for signs of respiratory distress: breath sounds, cough, sputum, fluid accumulation, elevated diaphragm, shallow breathing. Monitor arterial blood gases. Assess bowel for indications of paralytic ileus: adynamic, fluid accumulation, vomiting. Observe for signs of pseudocyst: upper abdominal pain, mass, tenderness, fever, a general deterioration or no improvement in patient's condition. Monitor output of any fistula. Provide skin protection for a pancreatic fistula with a clean or sterile skin barrier and pouch.

Patient Education

1. Assist patient in understanding the etiology or causal relationships of pancreatitis with alcohol use or gallstones.
2. Plan an appropriate rehabilitation program if alcohol abuse is related to disease process.
3. Provide written dietary instructions.
4. Provide written medication instructions.
5. Teach patient about diabetes mellitus: signs, symptoms, and insulin therapy.

EVALUATION

Patient Outcome	Data Indicating That Outcome is Reached
Pain is absent.	Patient experiences no pain.
Fluid volume is normal.	Hydration and electrolyte balance are adequate.
Nutrition is adequate.	Weight is stable. Patient does not experience steatorrhea or diarrhea. Serum glucose is stabilized. Patient does not experience anorexia, nausea, or vomiting.
Respiratory function is normal.	There are no signs of respiratory distress. Arterial blood gases are within normal range.
Liver function studies are normal.	Laboratory values for SGPT, SGOT, alkaline phosphate, gamma glutamyltransferase (GGT), isocitrate dehydrogenase (ICD), leukocyte alkaline phosphatase, 5′-nucleotidase (5′NT), ornithine carbamoyltransferase (OCT), lactate dehydrogenase (LDH$_5$; accounts for 2% to 11% of total LDH), bilirubin (total), albumin, and urobilinogen are within normal limits.

Medical Interventions

ABDOMINAL SURGERIES FOR SELECTED DISEASES OF GASTROINTESTINAL TRACT

Description and Rationale

Abdominal surgeries involve an incision into the abdomen with the patient under general anesthesia. A variety of different abdominal surgeries may be required under the broad scope of gastrointestinal diseases. Commonalities exist in the preoperative and postoperative patient care assessment and interventions that will be covered in this section. Examples of abdominal surgeries in which a portion of the gastrointestinal tract is surgically removed include appendectomy (appendix), cholecystectomy (gallbladder), colectomy (colon), and gastrectomy (stomach). An intestinal resection may be referred to as an ileotransverse colostomy (ileum is reanastomosed to transverse colon with removal or bypass of the ascending colon: in this particular case there is no externalization of the bowel even though the term colostomy is used).

Surgery is indicated in many gastrointestinal diseases when medical management is not effective or when complications develop. In cholecystitis with cholelithiasis, surgery is the primary choice of treatment. Surgery may be palliative, as in the case of Crohn's disease, or curative, as with ulcerative colitis and familial polyposis.

Contraindications and Cautions

1. Patients with signs and symptoms of an acute condition in the abdomen or an emergency situation will need to be quickly stabilized with fluid and electrolyte replacements.
2. The surgical intervention in an emergency may be considered a first stage, diverting the problem, with a required second operation for definitive treatment.
3. For patients with permanent colostomies, ileostomies, continent ileostomies, and ileoanal reservoirs recommend medical alert card stating: "No rectal temperatures, no rectal enemas, no rectal suppositories: the rectum has been removed." Provide definition of above procedures.

Preprocedural Nursing Care

1. Thorough bowel preparation is required for many abdominal surgeries including oral antibiotics and enemas. Caution must be used with enemas not to deplete weakened or elderly patients with multiple tap water enemas.

2. Drains and tubes are often used and patients should be prepared for their presence after surgery, including nasogastric tubes, T tubes, gastrostomy tubes, and so on.

TREATMENT PLAN

Chemotherapeutic

Bowel preparation (for intestinal surgery); nonabsorbable anti-infective agents

Neomycin (Mycifradin), 500 mg qid

Erythromycin (E-Mycin), 500 mg qid

Postoperatively, broad-spectrum antibiotic prophylaxis

Cefazolin (Ancef), 500 to 1000 mg q6-8h for 24 to 36 h IV

Cephapirin (Cefadyl), 500 to 1000 mg q4-6h for 24 to 36 h IV

Narcotic analgesics

Meperidine (Demerol), 75 to 100 mg IM q3-4h for pain; then po q3-4h for pain

Acetaminophen with codeine phosphate (Tylenol with codeine), one to two tablets po q4h prn for pain

Electromechanical

Incentive spirometry

Postural drainage

Nasogastric drainage

Gastrostomy tubes; T tubes

Transcutaneous electrical nerve stimulation (TENS)

Supportive

Intravenous fluids with electrolytes (particularly potassium)

Total parenteral nutrition

ASSESSMENT: AREAS OF CONCERN

Abdomen

Abdominal pain

Abdominal distention

Absence of bowel sounds, rigidity, rebound tenderness: paralytic ileus, intestinal obstruction, peritonitis; intestinal ischemia

Adhesions

Abdominal incision, surgical site

Hemorrhage

Drainage other than serosanguineous during first 24 hours

Signs of wound infection: redness, pain, edema, drainage

Wound dehiscence or evisceration

Fistula formation

Bowel function

Routine of bowel activity, gas pains, bowel movement

Constipation, diarrhea

Circulatory system

Shock and circulatory failure associated with hemorrhage and fluid and electrolyte imbalance

Thrombophlebitis and pulmonary emboli associated with extensive pelvic surgery (i.e., abdominoperineal resection) and in elderly persons

Fluids and electrolytes

Intestinal obstruction and paralytic ileus and fistulas associated with fluid and electrolyte loss

Nausea, vomiting, diarrhea, and nasogastric and intestinal suctioning may affect fluid and electrolyte balance

Mental status

Evaluation of effects of narcotics: fluid and electrolyte imbalance, insomnia, fatigue

Emotional consideration varies with type of abdominal surgery and changes that result from that surgery (i.e., colostomy or ileostomy vs. appendectomy)

Respiratory system

Hypoxia from respiratory depressants such as narcotics

Shallow breathing and inadequate coughing secondary to abdominal pain

Abdominal distention compromising lung expansion

Temperature

Low grade first 24 to 48 hours common

Fever of 38° C (100° F) or fever that does not subside may indicate pulmonary complications, wound infection, urinary infection, or thrombophlebitis

Fever of 38.3° C (101° F) occurring suddenly and accompanied by chills, weakness, fatigue, rapid respirations, tachycardia, and sudden drop in blood pressure indicates septic shock

Urinary tract signs

Decrease or cessation of urinary output reflects renal dysfunction

Voiding problems following indwelling catheter removal

NURSING DIAGNOSES and NURSING INTERVENTIONS

Nursing Diagnosis	Nursing Intervention
Injury, potential for: infection and hemorrhage	Observe wound dressing frequently for signs of bleeding. Monitor vital signs every 2 hours until patient is stable and then every 4 hours. Assess wound during postoperative period for redness, pain, edema, unusual drainage, odor, and separation of the suture line.
Tissue perfusion, alteration in: cardiopulmonary, renal, gastrointestinal, peripheral (potential)	Monitor patient's vital signs and central venous pressure or Swan-Ganz catheter for changes in cardiac output and tissue perfusion. Assess patient for signs and symptoms of alterations in tissue perfusion associated with major abdominal surgeries for complications of pancreatitis, cholecystitis, ulcerative colitis, and other diseases, including shock, circulatory failure, intestinal ischemia, and renal failure. Encourage patient to do leg exercises, and measure and apply elastic hose to facilitate venous circulation.
Breathing pattern, ineffective	Observe patient for shallow breathing, splinting with respirations, decreased breath sounds, and respiratory distress. Auscultate lungs every 2 hours. Encourage patient to turn, deep breathe, and cough every 2 hours. Encourage use of incentive spirometer to promote maximal inspiratory maneuvers. Provide pain medication and splint abdomen with pillow to decrease abdominal pain associated with deep breathing and coughing.
Fluid volume deficit, potential	Monitor intake and output including all drainage from nasogastric, gastric, intestinal, and T tubes as well as wound drainage or fistula output. Weigh patient daily.

CONTAINMENT OF WOUND DRAINAGE AND FISTULA OUTPUT

1. Determine if a sterile or a clean system is required.
2. Make a pattern of the wound or fistula. The pattern opening should be back ¼ inch from the wound edge. Label the pattern carefully with the following: patient's name, date, patient's left, right, head, and feet, pouch side (the side of the pattern facing the nurse if the pattern is against the skin), and skin side (the side of the pattern that lies against the skin).
3. Select a pectin-based wafer (skin barrier) and an ostomy or wound pouch that will accommodate the pattern. The pouch should have a spout if the drainage is liquid or be able to be attached to a bedside bag.
4. Trace the pattern opening onto the wafer. Take care to place the pattern appropriately or you will cut the pattern inversely. One suggestion is to place the pattern against the patient's abdomen. Lay the wafer down on the pattern as it would be applied to the abdomen (i.e., paper-backing side to abdomen). Lift the two off the patient and turn them over together and trace the pattern.
5. Cut the opening in the pectin-based wafer.
6. Trace the pattern onto the pouch adhesive backing. The same method can be used to avoid inverting the pattern.
7. Cut the opening in the pouch adhesive ¼ inch larger than the line you traced.
8. Remove the paper backing from the pouch and apply the pouch to the "shiny" or top side of the wafer. Press firmly, sealing the two together.
9. Cleanse the patient's skin with warm water and pat dry.
10. Apply a thin coat of paste around the wound edges if the pouch has a spout and no access cap.
11. Remove packing from the skin barrier.
12. Center the pouching system and apply to the skin. Press and seal to the skin.
13. Apply paste to any exposed skin through the access cap or by going up through the bottom of the pouch.
14. Close the spout, and connect to bedside bag or clamp the bottom.
15. Check the system each shift for signs of leakage and change when necessary.
16. Empty according to amount of drainage. Pouch should not fill and pull down against the seal.

Nursing Diagnosis	Nursing Intervention
	Assess patient's hydration status by mucous membrane, skin turgor, and blood pressure.
	Monitor color, consistency, amount, and odor of any drainage; test drainage (i.e., nasogastric aspirate, stool, fistula) for blood or pH if indicated.
	Provide fluid replacement as ordered.
Comfort, alteration in: pain	Assess the location, type, and duration of pain, pattern of pain occurrence, effectiveness of medications, and positioning and alternative methods of pain relief.
	Provide analgesics as ordered as needed for pain.
	Encourage the patient to take the medication postoperatively; reassure the patient that narcotic addiction will not occur.
	Monitor changes in pain associated with signs of abdominal distention, rigidity, and rebound tenderness and with temperature.
Skin integrity, impairment of: potential	Protect the nares when nasogastric tube is to be left in place several days.
	Change wound dressings frequently if output is high to protect skin from moisture maceration.
	Apply a pectin-based (Stomahesive, Hollihesive) wafer to the skin and tape to the wafer rather than applying tape on the skin. Montgomery straps can be applied on top of the pectin-based wafer. Keep in mind that drainage from the gastrointestinal tract continues to contain very irritating digestive enzymes (bile, gastric, pancreatic, intestinal).
	Evaluate patient with wound drainage for a wound pouching system to contain the drainage, protect the skin, allow for accurate measurement, and decrease cost of dressing changes (see box opposite).
	Protect tubes from pulling by adequately taping and provide skin protection if there is leakage around a tube (see box below).
Oral mucous membrane, alteration in (potential)	Provide regular mouth care to prevent problems associated with nasogastric tubes, limited oral intake for several days, and mouth breathing.
	Assist patient in brushing his teeth and rinsing his mouth with nonastringent solutions every 4 hours or more often for patient comfort.
	Provide anesthetic lozenges or hard candy if not contraindicated (use will result in saliva production and stimulate gastric secretions).
Bowel elimination, alteration in: constipation or diarrhea	Monitor patient for first bowel movement after surgery.
	Assess dietary and fluid intake as it relates to normal stool consistency.
	Observe color, consistency, frequency, and amount of stools.
	Evaluate pattern change following gastrointestinal surgery (e.g., diarrhea related to bile in colon following cholecystectomy or small bowel resection).
Self-care deficit: bathing/hygiene	Assist patient with activities of daily living following surgery.
	Allow patient to participate in self-care as tolerated.

GASTROSTOMY TUBE CARE

1. Use a pectin-based wafer (skin barrier) around the tube. Cut a small opening in the wafer ⅛ inch larger than the skin exit site.
2. Cleanse the skin with warm water and pat dry.
3. Apply the wafer, and seal to the skin.
4. Apply a paste (Karaya, Stomahesive) to any exposed skin around the tube. Use a thin coat of paste.
5. Anchor the tube to the wafer with the use of a baby bottle nipple. The end of the nipple is cut open large enough to accommodate the tube. Cut up through the side of the nipple (base to top), open the nipple, and wrap around the tube. The base of the nipple is then taped to the pectin-based wafer.
6. Tape the tube to the top of the nipple.
7. Remove the nipple daily and assess the exit site. If needed, gently cleanse around the tube exit site and dry, reapply paste, and replace nipple. If the skin barrier has drainage leaking under the seal, remove and replace. The wafer should be changed weekly otherwise.

Nursing Diagnosis	Nursing Intervention
	Encourage patient to assume primary responsibility for care as tolerated as nasogastric tube and IVs are removed.
Nutrition, alteration in: less than body requirements	Observe patient for signs of malabsorption: steatorrhea, diarrhea, weight loss.
	Evaluate potential nutritional deficiency based on the gastrointestinal organs involved in the disease process and treatment or interventions.
	Monitor TPN or enteral supplements as ordered.
Urinary elimination, alteration in patterns	Observe for signs of urinary retention associated with anesthesia, pain, anxiety, and removal of indwelling catheter.
	Observe and record intake and output.
	Provide privacy and promote relaxation when patient needs to void.
	Palpate bladder for distention if patient has not voided for 6 to 8 hours or if patient is voiding small amounts frequently (overflow voiding).
	Catheterize patient if ordered.

Patient Education

1. Instruct the patient on routine care following major abdominal surgery: ambulate at regular times, rest frequently, and slowly increase activities as tolerated; keep incision dry, and report any signs of redness, pain, or drainage of incision; avoid heavy lifting for 6 to 8 weeks, and splint abdomen when coughing or sneezing.
2. Provide written instructions on medications and medication schedule.
3. Identify with patient the importance of regular follow-up care.
4. Provide information related to primary diagnosis, type of surgery, and expected outcomes.
5. Provide written instructions for any at-home care: wound, T tube, gastrostomy tube, and so on.

EVALUATION

Patient Outcome	Data Indicating That Outcome is Reached
Body functions normally.	Abdominal incision heals with no drainage; bowel and bladder function normally.
Patient returns to activities of daily living.	Patient resumes activities at home and at work (e.g., driving, exercising).
Patient does not experience pain.	Abdominal pain is resolved; patient no longer requires mild pain medication.
Nutrition is adequate.	Patient tolerates a regular diet or special diet for type of disorder or surgery; patient gains weight.
Skin integrity is maintained.	There are no signs of skin irritation.

DIVERSIONS: COLOSTOMY AND ILEOSTOMY

Description and Rationale

A colostomy is a diversion involving the colon in which a segment of diseased or injured colon is bypassed or removed and an end or loop of colon is brought through a small opening in the abdominal wall and matured, forming a stoma. The anatomic location in the colon is an important description and influences the care. Ascending, transverse, and sigmoid colostomies may be performed. Transverse colostomies are most often loop ostomy stomas and are temporary. A loop means that the intact bowel has been brought through the abdominal wall, a rod placed under the bowel, the incision closed, and a cautery used to open the top wall of the bowel (the lower wall remains intact). The proximal opening will drain the stool while the distal opening may drain mucus and leads to the rectum. The patient may have bowel movements from the rectum that consist of stool in the bowel before surgery or mucus. The stool is semiformed, extremely odorous, and unpredictable.

The sigmoid colostomy is the most common permanent stoma and is indicated for cancer of the colon. The stool from the sigmoid colostomy is similar to normal bowel movements. Generally, stool is evacuated once or twice a day. A regular pattern before surgery is used to predict the possibility of regulation of the sigmoid colostomy with diet or with colostomy irrigations.

The removal of the entire colon and rectum (total proctocolectomy) results in the ileum being brought through the abdominal wall, forming an ileostomy stoma. The stool from the ileostomy is liquid to semiformed and contains residual digestive enzymes. The drainage from the ascending colostomy is similar, and the nursing interventions are the same for both. Fluid and electrolyte imbalance is a potential problem with an ileostomy and may result in significant problems.

Contraindications and Cautions

1. Only a sigmoid colostomy should be irrigated to obtain regular bowel eliminations.
2. An ileostomy lavage for a food blockage refers to the insertion of 30 to 50 ml of normal saline through a small catheter using an Asepto syringe. *This is not a colostomy irrigation.*
3. Laxatives should *never* be given to a patient with an ileostomy. The results can be severe fluid and electrolyte imbalance.
4. Bowel preparation for a person with an ileostomy consists of clear liquids for 2 to 3 days.

Preprocedural Nursing Care

1. Consultation with an enterostomal therapy (ET) nurse is arranged.
2. A preoperative visit by a United Ostomy Association (UOA) trained visitor (rehabilitated person with an ostomy) is recommended.
3. Stoma site selection is marked by ET nurse for the surgeon. This is an important phase to ensure a good pouch seal after surgery.

ASSESSMENT: AREAS OF CONCERN

Perineum
Removal of rectum (abdominoperineal resection) results in large wound
Perineal infection: redness, tenderness, drainage

Intestine
Intestinal obstruction
Food blockage (ileostomy)
Perforation (colostomy irrigation)

Anemia
Vitamin B_{12} deficiency (ileostomy)

Stoma
Peristomal skin irritation or erosion
Parastomal hernias
Stomal stenosis
Stomal prolapse
Stomal retraction
Necrosis of stoma

Colostomy
Constipation
Diarrhea

Ileostomy
Diarrhea
Dehydration
Food blockage

Sexual functioning
Wide resections in perineal area for cancer of rectum may damage nerves responsible for erection, ejaculation, and orgasm in male; no impairment or one or a combination of all functions may be affected
Physiologic effects on women have been poorly studied

Self-concept and body image
Adjustment and integration of ostomy require time and support from family and health care providers
Complications: prolonged use of defense behaviors, noninvolvement in physical care, social isolation

NURSING DIAGNOSES and NURSING INTERVENTIONS

Nursing Diagnosis	Nursing Intervention
Self-concept, disturbance in: body image, self-esteem	Provide patient and family an opportunity to express their feelings regarding the ostomy. Remind patient that an ostomy is an alternative pattern of elimination and will take time to adjust to both physically and emotionally. Provide consistent management of the ostomy, control odor, and prevent leaking, giving patient a sense of control over the stoma.

Nursing Diagnosis	Nursing Intervention

Select a system that is invisible under clothing, is odor proof, and fits the body size.

Encourage the patient to return to all presurgical activities as soon as possible.

Recommend a trained ostomy visitor of same age and sex as patient and preferably one who has had same type of ostomy procedure.

Allow patient to grieve for the loss of a body part and the loss of control of elimination.

Be realistic and positive: negative reactions will be picked up by patient and will make adjustment harder; most people adapt successfully to ostomy surgery.

Sexual dysfunction (potential)

Allow patient to discuss concerns and fears regarding sexual activities. Many patients fear rejection by spouse or significant other.

Discuss positions with patient:
1. Back to belly: pouch is against bed and not as noticeable
2. Missionary: pouch should be empty to prevent leakage
3. Female on top: pouch fully exposed

Suggest material pouch covers; other patients have recommended crotchless panties for women and binders for men to hold pouch in place.

Remind patient that he must first be comfortable with himself. Spouse or significant other is most often kind, gentle, and caring. Communication between partners is extremely important.

Refer men who have had nerve damage and are unable to obtain an erection to a urologist for information on penile prosthesis.

Refer to family and sexual counselors as indicated by poor coping or maladaptation.

Skin integrity, impairment of: potential

Protect the peristomal skin with skin barriers: pectin-based wafers, paste, Karaya washers (Karaya protects skin but does not hold a pouch on and requires tape or belt).

Change pouching system whenever the pouch first begins to leak (an early sign is odor); *do not* tape a leaking pouch seal and plan on changing it later. Skin is damaged within minutes by trapped ileostomy effluent. Prevention is easier than treatment.

Skin integrity, impairment of: actual

Consult an ET nurse at first indication of skin irritation.

Treat skin reactions that are secondary to ileostomy drainage, stool, urine, glue, solvents, and soaps as follows:

Remove the source of the irritation.

Cleanse the skin with warm water and pat dry. A hair dryer on cool may be used.

Expose the skin to air, light, and heat for 15 to 20 minutes. A hair dryer on cool and a 60-watt light 12 to 16 inches away may be used.

Cover the irritated skin with a pectin-based wafer to which the patient is not sensitive.

Apply a pouch.

Repeat every 48 hours.

Treat skin that is eroded or ulcerated as follows:

Cleanse skin with warm water and pat dry.

Apply aluminum acetate (Burow's solution) compresses for 20 to 30 minutes.

Expose skin to light, air, and heat for 15 to 20 minutes. Use hair dryer on cool and 60-watt bulb 12 to 16 inches away.

Cover with a pectin-based wafer and apply a pouch.

Change every 24 to 48 hours.

Avoid mechanical injury to the skin by gentle removal of tape and skin barriers.

Empty pouches rather than changing and discarding pouches that are full.

Observe for monilial *(Candida albicans)* reactions associated with antibiotics and changes in normal bowel flora. Skin appears bright red with weepy papulae, satellite lesions, and secondary crusting.

Assess other sites for monilial infection: under arms, under breasts, and in groin.

Consult physician for order of nystatin (Mycostatin) powder. Powder used in peristomal area must be sealed in with a sealant or water (Bard Protective Barrier, Skin Prep). Ointments will keep pouch from sealing.

Nursing Diagnosis	Nursing Intervention
	Prevent radiation dermatitis by not having any portion of the pouch or pouch adhesive in the field of radiation. If pouch must be removed daily for treatments use a Karaya-only backed pouch that is belted in place. Avoid use of light when treating irradiated skin.
Bowel elimination, alteration in	Observe output for color, consistency, frequency, and amount. Select a pouching system that contains the stool, is easy to empty, is odorproof, and is invisible under the patient's clothing. Clean the spout after each emptying to eliminate odor from a dirty spout. Avoid pin holes in pouches that lead to constant odor release; either empty pouch of gas or use commercial gas release valves added or made into the pouching system.
Fluid volume deficit, potential	Assess patient for dehydration that may develop with high-volume ileostomy output. Observe patient with ileostomy for diarrhea: high volume, watery, hot drainage; pouch emptied every 20 to 30 minutes. Monitor intake and output, vital signs, and daily weights.
Nutrition, alteration in	Instruct patient to chew food carefully and eat slowly. Observe patient for sign of food blockage (ileostomy): history of high roughage in diet and not chewing well; no output and abdominal distention; nausea and vomiting. Perform an ileostomy lavage: 　Remove pouch; stoma will become edematous. 　Apply irrigation sleeve. 　Have patient assume knee-chest position and massage abdomen under stoma; if blockage is removed, stop here and reapply pouching system; if not, continue. 　Insert catheter gently into stoma to level of blockage (usually at fascia level). 　Irrigate with 30 to 50 ml normal saline using Asepto syringe; allow to return. 　Repeat instillation of 30 to 50 ml of saline. 　Procedure may take 1 to 2 hours; may try knee-chest position between irrigations if patient is stable. 　Assess for dehydration; fluid becomes trapped behind food blockage, which acts as an intestinal obstruction. 　Provide intravenous fluids as ordered. NOTE: This procedure is *not* taught to patients. However, patient should be taught to recognize early signs and symptoms and seek medical assistance. Assist patient in returning to regular diet, avoiding only foods that give that person problems.

Patient Education*

1. Colostomy and ileostomy care involves the following:
   a. Stomal and skin assessment: stoma should be red and moist; skin should be free of irritation.
   b. Management of frequently encountered skin problems*:
      (1) Rash can be located under the tape, under the faceplate, and on any part of the skin where the pouch comes in contact with the skin. A generalized reddish appearance that covers an entire area, similar to a diaper rash, will be seen. Cause may be leaking appliance, perspiration, allergies to tape, or hair follicle irritation. Advise patient to use heat lamp or hair dryer to dry the skin. Patient should sprinkle a small amount of powder (Karaya, Stomahesive) on the skin, wipe off the excess, then blot with a skin sealant to seal the powder to the skin. Powder the skin on which the pouch lies after the pouch is applied. Patient should make or buy a pouch cover. Wearing a pouch belt too tight may break the seal.
      (2) Cement or solvent burns can be located anywhere under the faceplate but usually are found at the outside edges. Their cause is chemicals in the cement or solvent that were not allowed to evaporate off the skin surface before applying pouch or cement that was too thick and was unable to dry completely. Pa-

*Portions reprinted with permission from Broadwell, D.C., and Sorrells, S.L.: Summary of your ileostomy care and Summary of your colostomy care, Atlanta, 1978 (revised 1983), Patient Education Booklets.

tient should apply heat lamp or hair dryer to the weeping skin, cover the burn with a pectin-based skin barrier and apply pouch in usual way (advise patient to try to leave the pouch on 24 to 48 hours), and omit using cement on skin or pouch.

(3) Ulcerated area on stoma may be caused by a stomal opening of the pouch that is too small or activities that caused the faceplate to rub or cut into stoma. Patient should enlarge the size of the pouch opening, evaluate his activities (a different size or shaped faceplate may be needed), and loosen belt. The skin should be protected by a skin barrier or paste.

(4) Infected or irritated hair follicles may be located under the faceplate. They are raised red areas (similar to acne) at the shaft of the hair follicle from not keeping the area under the faceplate shaved. Advise patient to let the irritation improve before removing any more hair by shaving or cutting, use hair dryer or heat lamp to dry the skin if oozing is present, and use a skin barrier between skin and faceplate until irritation improves.

(5) Remind patient that weeping skin may prevent a pouch or a skin barrier from adhering to the skin for long periods. If skin is severely irritated and weeping, it may be necessary to change pouch more frequently to prevent leakage and further damage.

(6) Remind patient that the hair under faceplate should be removed by an electric razor or a safety razor.

c. Principles of changing a pouching system should be accompanied by several opportunities for practicing the procedure.

(1) Instruct patient to assemble all equipment: cotton balls, tissues, toilet paper, wash cloths, towels, premoistened towelettes (to cleanse the skin); pouch; skin barriers; pouch closure; tape or belt; and equipment for cleansing or disposing of used pouches.

(2) A paper towel may be used to trace a pattern, which should hug the stoma but not ride up on it and top should be labeled. Outer dimensions of the pattern (avoiding hip bones, pubic area, ribs and folds at waist and navel) should be considered.

(3) For skin barrier (if applicable) wafer size will depend on size of stoma and abdomen. Instruct patient to round the corners or conform the wafer to the shape of the adhesive on the pouch, trace the stomal pattern on the paper

side, cut hole on pattern line, and smooth sides of the opening.

(4) Pouch opening should be slightly larger than opening of skin barrier. Instruct patient to trace pattern on the paper side of the pouch, cut the hole larger than the line of the pattern, remove paper backing from the pouch, center the openings, and apply the shiny side of the skin barrier to the pouch.

(5) Next, empty and remove the pouch being worn. Cleanse and dry the skin.

(6) Patient should note any changes in skin or stoma (color, size, ulcerations, irritations), center and apply skin barrier and pouch, close end, and tape edges.

(7) Instruct patient to check supplies and reorder as necessary.

d. Dietary considerations should be discussed with the patient.

(1) Foods associated with odor are fish, eggs, asparagus, onions, garlic, and some spices.

(2) Foods associated with diarrhea are green beans, broccoli, spinach, raw fruits, highly seasoned foods, and beer.

(3) Foods used to manage diarrhea (low-residue diet) are strained bananas, peanut butter (without nuts), and applesauce.

(4) Foods used to manage constipation are high-fiber foods (bran, celery), increased raw fruits and vegetables, and increased fluid intake (water, fruit juices).

(5) Foods associated with gas are brussels sprouts, cabbage, beans, peas, mushrooms, carbonated drinks, onions, cucumbers, and beer.

(6) Patients are encouraged to eat all above foods in moderation, chewing well, and adding one new food at a time to evaluate tolerance.

e. Provide patient with written instructions for follow-up, and initiate home care referral if indicated.

2. Sigmoid colostomy patient teaching should also include a section on colostomy irrigation that includes adequate opportunity for return demonstrations. Colostomy irrigations are started after the patient has active bowel sounds and has progressed to a low-residue diet.

a. Define colostomy irrigation: an enema through the colostomy stoma that stimulates peristalsis and a bowel movement with the intent of emptying the colon so that no further bowel movements occur until the next irrigation.

b. Remind patient that spillage is common for several weeks. Chemotherapy and radiation therapy will result in spillage and are indications for withholding the colostomy irrigation.

c. Below are general guidelines and tips for colostomy irrigation directed to the patient.

(1) Assemble all equipment: water container and water, irrigating sleeve and belt, items to clean skin and stoma, way to dispose of old pouch, clean, cut pouch, and closure, and skin care items.

(2) Remove old pouch and dispose of it.

(3) Clean skin and stoma with water, and let dry. Observe condition and color of skin and stoma.

(4) Apply irrigating sleeve and belt securely (but not too tight). If you use Karaya washer, dampen and apply this first.

(5) Fill irrigating container with about 1 quart tepid water when you are ready to start.

(6) Suspend the irrigating container so that the bottom of the container is even with the top of shoulder.

(7) Remove air from the tubing (helps prevent the air from increasing gas pains). Do not use a large amount of irrigating water for this, or it will be necessary to refill irrigation container.

(8) Gently insert irrigating cone into stoma, holding it parallel to floor, and start the water slowly. If water does not flow easily, try or check the following:

(a) Slightly change the position or the angle of the cone; cone opening may be blocked by a loop of your bowel.

(b) Check for kinks in tubing from irrigating container.

(c) Check height of irrigating container.

(d) Relax and take some *deep* breaths to relax abdominal muscles.

(e) Stool immediately under skin level may be slightly hard and blocking water flow. Instill *small* amounts of water to loosen it up.

(9) The following are variations in water for irrigations:

(a) People vary in the amount of water they can hold at one time.

(b) The amount of water used can vary daily.

(c) Do not get discouraged. Remember that you want to cleanse as much of the fecal matter out as possible: learn to pay attention to the full feeling and the feeling that you need to expel stool so you do not continue to force water into your bowel.

(d) Do *not* force water into your bowel; if you are cramping, the flow of water stops, or water is forcefully returning around the irrigating cone or catheter.

(e) If you feel bloated or constipated, you may irrigate with about ½ quart more water in the same day or take a mild laxative after consulting physician.

(10) The majority of the stool will return in about 15 minutes. When you feel that you have expelled most of the stool, rinse the sleeve with water, dry the bottom edge, roll it up, close the end, and go about your activities for about 30 to 45 minutes to allow the bowel adequate time to finish emptying.

(11) When you feel that you have obtained complete results, assemble and apply clean pouch and any skin barriers.

(12) Rinse the irrigation sleeve with cold water, hang it up to dry, and put away other equipment.

(13) Check supplies and reorder as necessary.

(14) Try to irrigate within the same 2- or 3-hour period each day so that bowels become regulated; if possible, try to irrigate close to time bowels moved before surgery.

3. Ileostomy patient teaching should include the following:

a. Instruct patient about symptoms of food blockage and what to do if it occurs.*

(1) Discharge changes from semisolid to a thin liquid; food is blocked, but water passes around it.

(2) Total volume of output increases and functions almost constantly; water is drawn from bloodstream in attempt to rid itself of blockage and intestines become hyperactive.

(3) There is an objectionable odor; bacterial overgrowth occurs at the blockage and causes fermentation of foodstuff.

(4) Cramping occurs, usually followed by increase in watery output; this is caused by increased bowel activity to rid itself of blockage.

(5) Abdomen is distended; the blockage traps gas and liquids in the bowel lumen.

(6) Vomiting occurs; this is a further attempt of body to rid itself of blockage by traveling in direction of least resistance.

(7) There is no ileostomy output because of complete blockage.

(8) Instruct patient to get into a knee-chest position for a few minutes or take a hot shower to relax and then try the knee-chest position.

(9) Many blockages will relieve themselves; however, if the blockage persists more than 3 to 4 hours, contact physician.

b. Foods associated with blockage include celery, Chinese foods, corn, nuts, coleslaw, dried fruits, coconut, wild rice, popcorn, whole vegetable skins, and fibrous vegetables. Do not eliminate from diet. Eat in moderate amounts and chew well.

EVALUATION

Patient Outcome	Data Indicating That Outcome is Reached
Patient returns to activities of daily living.	Patient returns to work and to social activities including sex. Patient wears "normal" clothes.
Body functions normally.	Wound (abdominal and perineal) heals with no drainage.
Patient performs self-care.	Patient can care for colostomy or ileostomy. Patient can identify information related to stoma and skin, fluid and electrolytes, diet, and need for regular follow-up.
Personal adjustment is achieved.	Patient verbalizes feelings related to ostomy and external pouching system.

DIVERSION: CONTINENT ILEOSTOMY (KOCK POUCH)

Description and Rationale

The continent ileostomy or Kock pouch was first described by Nils Kock in 1969.[40] The procedure involves the creation of an internal pouch constructed of ileum and of a nipple valve that maintains continency of stool and flatus. The patient has a stoma flush with the skin located in the lower right quadrant, which is intubated with a large-bore tube several times a day to evacuate the stool and flatus. The key to success of the continent ileostomy is the nipple valve.

The continent ileostomy may be recommended for people with emotional problems associated with a conventional ileostomy. Conversion from a conventional to a continent ileostomy may be important for patients who have been unable to cope. Patients do report positive reactions to the continent ileostomy. The lack of an external appliance is the major factor. Also, a flush rather than a protruding stoma is cited as an advantage by patients. Patients do not find the intubation or catheterization procedure bothersome once the pouch capacity increases.

The advantages of the continent ileostomy include the following[25]:
1. No appliance required
2. No noise or odor from stoma except during emptying
3. No skin irritation
4. Improved psychosocial adjustment

The continent ileostomy has a higher risk of complications than conventional ileostomies. Long-term problems are more common and may be associated with loss of continency.

The disadvantages of the procedure are associated with the high percentage of nipple valve dysfunction and the reoperative rate. Even with the high rate of reoperation, patients who have converted to a continent ileostomy state that it is a more satisfactory procedure.

The continent ileostomy is constructed from 45 cm of terminal ileum after the colectomy has been performed. The 45 cm section of ileum is brought through the abdominal incision, maintaining the blood supply to the loop of small bowel. The end 15 cm is left free and will ultimately be used to form the nipple valve. First, the surgeon loops the proximal 30 cm segment back on itself; each side is 15 cm. Then the loop is sutured along its antimesenteric border where the two segments touch. A long U-shaped incision is made around the 30 cm loop close to the the suture line. The ileum then can be opened up into a cuplike shape. The small flaps of tissue on either side of the suture line are sutured together, forming a double suture line. The double suture line produces a smooth internal surface of the reservoir and provides a safeguard against intestinal leakage from the pouch. The nipple valve is then constructed by intussuscepting several centimeters of terminal ileum into the reservoir. The two layers of the valve are anchored by numerous sutures or staples. The pouch is then sutured closed and assessed for adequacy of the valve and the suture line by filling it with a saline solution and air. If no signs of leakage are noted from the valve or from the sutures, the pouch is inserted into the abdominal cavity and anchored. The end portion of the distal ileum is brought through the abdominal wall, and a flush stoma is constructed. A catheter is placed in the reservoir during surgery and remains in the pouch for 3 to 4 weeks.

It should be noted that a similar pouch is being constructed for urinary diversions.

Contraindications and Cautions

1. The diagnosis must be familial polyposis or ulcerative colitis.
2. The patient needs medical alert cards since the continent ileostomy is an uncommon procedure.
3. Obesity is considered a contraindication.

Preprocedural Nursing Care

1. There should be a preoperative consultation with an ET nurse regarding the possible surgical options: conventional ileostomy, continent ileostomy, and ileoanal reservoir.
2. A rehabilitated patient with a continent ileostomy should visit preoperatively.

ASSESSMENT: AREAS OF CONCERN

Continent ileostomy pouch
"Pouchitis": local crampy pain, diarrhea that may be bloody, fever, valve leakage, intubation difficulty
Difficulty intubating pouch
Leakage of nipple valve
Valve prolapse
Skin stricture
Pouch perforation

Intestine
Intestinal obstruction; adhesions
Perforation

Abdominal incision
Wound infection

Perineum
Infection of perineal wound
Poor wound healing; drainage

Sexual functioning
Potential dysfunction in males when rectum resected; rare when performed for inflammatory bowel disease

Body image
Presence of stoma and no external pouch more positive; if valve leaks, requires external pouch (p. 1272)

NURSING DIAGNOSES and NURSING INTERVENTIONS

Nursing Diagnosis	Nursing Intervention
Self-concept, disturbance in: body image	Observe patient's response to presence of flush stoma and intubation. Allow patient opportunity to explore feelings regarding surgery and loss of rectum. Provide trained visitor for patient.
Skin integrity, impairment of: potential	Protect peristomal skin with skin sealant (Bard Protective Barrier, Hollister Gel) from moisture in mucus. Cover stoma with small pad. Protect skin from ileostomy drainage if nipple valve leaks (p. 1272).
Fluid volume deficit, potential	Assess patient for dehydration that may develop with high-volume output. Monitor intake and output, vital signs, and daily weights.
Nutrition, alteration in	Instruct patient to chew foods well and eat slowly. There are no dietary restrictions (see p. 1274 for foods associated with odor, gas, and diarrhea).

Patient Education

1. Intubation and irrigation of continent ileostomy involve the following:
   a. First 3 weeks (catheter in place)
      (1) Irrigate the internal continent ileostomy pouch; insert 30 ml water and allow to drain out by gravity; repeat three or four times; irrigate every 2 hours during day and once at night.
      (2) Attach bedside bag, leg bag, and flushing tubing.
      (3) Clean bedside and leg bags with soapy water; allow to dry; have two and alternate.
      (4) Eat a low-residue diet.
   b. Week 4
      (1) Catheter is removed in outpatient clinic, and patient is taught to intubate the continent ileostomy.
      (2) Intubate and irrigate every 2 hours during day.
      (3) Intubate with catheter to straight drainage at night; irrigate once at night.
   c. Week 5
      (1) Intubate every 3 hours, and irrigate twice a day.
      (2) Connect to gravity drainage at night; irrigate once at night.
   d. Week 6
      (1) Intubate every 4 hours and irrigate twice during day.
      (2) Intubate at night only if sign of fullness or uncomfortable.
   e. Week 7 and thereafter
      (1) Intubate pouch four times each day.
      (2) Irrigate pouch once each day until return is clear.
2. The following procedure is employed for emptying and intubating the continent ileostomy:
   a. The patient sitting on the commode inserts a well-lubricated catheter into the stoma and through the nipple valve. Stool and flatus will drain through the catheter directly into the toilet. If the stool is thick, water can be inserted through the catheter to loosen the stool. The catheter may need to be removed and flushed if the lumen becomes blocked with undigested residue. Grape juice and prune juice are often used by patients to keep their stool "thin."
   b. Several types of catheters are available (Marlen, Atlantic). The patient should have at least two catheters and should know how to order additional ones. It is important that catheters are discarded when they become old. Hard, brittle catheters are more likely to damage the valve or the pouch.
3. The patient should be provided with written instructions on the signs and symptoms of "pouchitis" and procedures if he experiences difficulty intubating pouch or leakage of nipple valve develops.
4. The patient should be given instructions on low-residue diet and advancing to a regular diet.

EVALUATION

Patient Outcome	Data Indicating That Outcome is Reached
Body functions normally.	Wound heals. Pouch functions, and nipple valve is continent; patient empties pouch four times a day; patient eats regular diet.
Patient returns to activities of daily living.	Patient returns to work, to social activities, and to sexual functioning.
Patient performs self-care.	Patient manages continent ileostomy with no or minimal assistance.
Personal adjustment is achieved.	Patient verbalizes positive feelings related to adjustment to continent ileostomy.

DIVERSION: ILEOANAL RESERVOIR

Description and Rationale

The ileoanal reservoir is the procedure that provides the most normal mechanism for maintaining continency and the most natural method of evacuation. The ileoanal reservoir may be the first choice for patients with familial polyposis or ulcerative colitis. However, the patient must be an appropriate candidate for the ileoanal reservoir. Factors that should be assessed when evaluating a patient for this procedure include normal anorectal sphincter mechanism, minimal disease of the rectal mucosa, no evidence of cancer of the colon or Crohn's disease, absence of perianal disease, good physical condition, motivation, maturity, and age. It is important that the patient understand that it is a two- or three-stage procedure and that close follow-up is important throughout. A temporary ileostomy requires that the patient learn stomal care. The patient must also be aware that diarrhea may be a problem for 6 months to 1 year following the closure of the ileostomy. During this time, incontinence may occur but is usually minimal and is more common at night.[58]

Four types of procedures may be done to preserve normal bowel elimination. Each involves removal of the rectal mucosa. The first step in constructing the ileoanal reservoir is the mucosal stripping of the rectal segment to form a muscular cuff through which to bring the ileum. The rectal mucosectomy removes the mucosa and submucosa of the rectum for 4 to 6 cm above the dentate line. The rectal muscle layers and the anal sphincters are left intact while the primary disease is removed. During the abdominal colectomy, the rectosigmoid is removed with care to preserve the autonomic nerves on the posterior and lateral pelvic walls.

When no reservoir is constructed, diarrhea and incontinence are major problems. In 1978, Parks and Nicholls[52] added an ileoanal reservoir to the previously described rectal mucosectomy and ileorectal pull-through. The reservoir provided an important addition, a means by which the liquid effluent could be held until evacuation was appropriate. Thus the patient undergoing total colectomy also will have rectal mucosectomy, construction of an ileal reservoir, ileoanal anastomosis, and a temporary ileostomy during the first stage of the procedure. During the second stage, the ileostomy is closed. The ileoanal reservoir may be constructed in three configurations. It is constructed from 30 to 50 cm of terminal ileum. In the S reservoir, three loops of ileum, approximately 12 to 15 cm in length, are aligned side by side. The reservoir is constructed by suturing the limbs and opening the segments, creating a pouch. A remaining 5 cm of ileum forms a spout that is sutured to the dentate line, completing the ileoanal portion of the procedure. The J reservoir consists of two loops of ileum. The ileum is brought down to the rectal cuff and one limb is looped upward, creating a J shape. The loops are anastomosed in a side-to-side fashion by use of a stapler. The portion where the ileum curves upward is sutured to the anus and opened.

In the isoperistaltic reservoir, a single lumen of 25 to 30 cm of ileum is brought down and through the rectal cuff. The distal end is sutured to the anus, and the proximal end is closed. An ileostomy is performed. In the second stage the ileostomy is taken down and a lateral side-to-side ileal anastomosis is performed to create the reservoir.

The advantages of the ileoanal reservoir include the following:
1. Avoidance of a permanent cutaneous stoma
2. Avoidance of repeated stomal catheterizations
3. Avoidance of body image alterations
4. Decreased incidence of sexual dysfunction
5. Provision of a near-normal pattern of defecation

The disadvantages of the procedure are as follows:
1. Possible residual rectal mucosa
2. Regeneration of rectal mucosa
3. Problems with differentiation of gas, fluids, and solids
4. Tenesmus or fecal urgency
5. Nocturnal incontinence
6. Diarrhea
7. Perianal skin denudation

Contraindications and Cautions

1. Crohn's disease or cancer of the rectum
2. Obesity
3. Short mesentery
4. Decreased sphincter control

Preprocedural Nursing Care

1. Manometric studies of sphincter muscles are done before first and second stages of the procedure.
2. Before second stage, Gastrografin studies of reservoir are performed.

ASSESSMENT: AREAS OF CONCERN

Perineum
Skin erosion from mucus, frequent bowel movements, incontinence, pruritus, and perianal pain

Ileoanal reservoir
Anal stenosis

Ischemia of reservoir
Rectal cuff abscess
Nocturnal leakage
Fecal incontinence
"Pouchitis" (sudden onset of high-volume diarrhea, cramping, and bleeding)

Abdominal surgery
Adhesions; intestinal obstructions
Wound infection
Pain

TREATMENT PLAN

Chemotherapeutic
Bulk-forming agents
  Psyllium (Metamucil), 1 tsp prn for diarrhea
Antidiarrheal agents
  Loperamide hydrochloride (Imodium), one to three capsules po per day for diarrhea
Dermatologic agents
  Balneol cleansing agent (Rowell Co.)
Antifungal agents
  Clotrimazole (Mycelex cream) 1%, prn for pruritus

Supportive
Sitz bath

NURSING DIAGNOSES and NURSING INTERVENTIONS

Nursing Diagnosis	Nursing Intervention
Stage 1: Ileostomy; Ileoanal Reservoir Constructed	
Fluid volume deficit, actual	Monitor fecal output from ileostomy; 800 to 1200 cc is not uncommon. Replace fluid and electrolytes as ordered. Monitor daily weights. Assess patient for signs and symptoms of dehydration: dry mucous membranes, poor skin turgor, dry skin.
Skin integrity, impairment of: actual	Provide perianal skin care since mucus contains residual enzymes, is copious, and is odorous. Use skin sealants and vanishing creams before skin breaks down. Instruct patient in wearing absorbent pads at night. Irrigate the reservoir daily to remove mucous drainage. Protect peristomal skin and maintain pouch seal.
Stage 2: Ileostomy Closure; Ileoanal Reservoir Functioning	
Skin integrity, impairment of: actual	Avoid irritants such as nylon underwear, harsh or deodorant soaps, and fragrant toilet papers. Cleanse skin with water or Domeboro (aluminum acetate) solution and cotton balls; dry with hair dryer. Apply vanishing cream and cover with skin sealant. Protect skin because of frequency of bowel movements and the residual enzymes present in the stool. Provide sitz baths, Balneol cleansing agents, or Tucks pads to help with perianal cleansing and to reduce pruritus.
Bowel elimination, alteration in: diarrhea; incontinence	Monitor frequency of bowel movements and consistency of stools. Expect 10 to 20 bowel movements per day in early postoperative period; frequency slows to 6 to 12 per day as diet increases and averages 3 to 4 per day after 1 year. Provide a regular diet to help manage diarrhea. Provide psyllium (Metamucil) or loperamide (Imodium) as ordered as needed for diarrhea.

Patient Education

The following list applies to stage 1.
1. Teach patient ileostomy management (p. 1273).
2. Teach patient Kegel exercises. Patient is instructed to practice these exercises to increase sphincter tone

before the second stage of the procedure. The patient can be instructed to (a) hold a coin between the buttocks and tighten the sphincter, (b) tape the buttocks together and tighten the sphincter, or (c) practice walking with (a) or (b). The exercises of squeezing and relaxing the perianal muscles can also be done when the patient irrigates the reservoirs, which helps to assess continency.

3. Intubation and irrigation are done daily to remove mucus, which is a source of irritation and odor.
4. Perianal skin care is essential. Mucous drainage through the anus is expected and may be irritating. The skin can be protected by the use of skin sealants and vanishing creams. Minipads may be worn at night to absorb the drainage. Bloody mucous drainage may occur approximately 10 to 14 days after surgery when the sutures are dissolving.
5. Approximately 6 to 8 weeks after surgery, a Gastrografin x-ray film is taken to assess the reservoir, ruling out anastomotic leaks and checking the anatomic position of the reservoir. Gastrografin is water soluble and easier to evacuate from the reservoir than barium would be. Following the gastrograffin study, the reservoir should be irrigated with 100 to 200 ml of tap water.

6. Manometric studies of the sphincter muscle are repeated postoperatively.

The following list applies to stage 2.

1. For perianal skin care:
   a. Avoid nylon underwear, harsh or deodorant soaps, and fragrant toilet papers.
   b. Cleanse the perianal skin with water or Domeboro solution and cotton balls and dry with hair dryer.
   c. Protect the skin with vanishing creams, skin sealants, or ointments.
   d. Manage pruritus with sitz baths, Balneol cleansing agents, or Mycelex cream.
2. Frequency of bowel movements will drop to 6 to 12 per day for first year and then decreases to 3 or 4 per day. Diarrhea associated with flu or viral infection will increase number and amount of bowel movements.
3. Irrigation of reservoir daily may be necessary to reduce incidence of "pouchitis."

EVALUATION

Patient Outcome	Data Indicating That Outcome is Reached
Body functions normally.	Abdominal incision heals. There are no signs of infection. Patient has three or four bowel movements per day.
Perianal skin is normal.	Perianal skin is intact with no signs of irritation or pruritus.

References

1. Appelbaum, P.C., et al.: Intestinal bacteria in patients with tropical sprue, S. Afr. Med. J. **57**:1081, 1980.
2. Arhan, P., et al.: Viscoelastic properties of the rectal wall in Hirschsprung's disease, J. Clin. Invest. **62**:82, 1978.
3. Beahrs, O.H., et al.: Indwelling ileostomy valve device, Am. J. Surg. **141**:111, 1981.
4. Bolt, R.J., et al.: The digestive system, New York, 1983, John Wiley & Sons.
5. Brandt, L.: Gastrointestinal disorders of the elderly, New York, 1984, Raven Press.
6. Broadwell, D.C., and Jackson, B.S.: Principles of ostomy care, St. Louis, 1982, The C.V. Mosby Co.
7. Broadwell, D.C., and McGarity, W.C.: Gastrointestinal disorders. In Kinney, M.D., et al.: AACN's clinical reference for critical care nursing, New York, 1981, McGraw-Hill Book Co.
8. Buls, J.G., and Goldberg, S.M.: Surgical options in ulcerative colitis, Postgrad. Med. **74**:175, 1983.
9. Bussey, H.J.R.: Familial polyposis coli, Baltimore, 1975, Johns Hopkins University Press.
10. Cancer facts and figures, New York, 1985, American Cancer Society.
11. Cancer statistics, Cancer **31**:13, 1981.
12. Canty, T.G., Self, T., and Bonaldi, L.: The lateral reservoir technique of ileal endorectal pull-through for ulcerative colitis and familial polyposis in children, J. Pediatr. Surg. **18**:862, 1983.
13. Cawson, R.A.: Essentials of dental surgery and pathology, ed. 3, London, 1978, Churchill Livingstone.
14. Cohen, S.: Clinical gastroenterology: a problem-oriented approach, New York, 1983, John Wiley & Sons.
15. Cohen, S.: The facts about IBS. DDEIC publication, Bethesda, Md., 1984, National Institute of Health.
16. Connell, A.M., Jones, F.A., and Rowlands, E.N.: Motility of the pelvic colon: abdominal pain associated with colonic motility after meals, Gut **6**:105, 1965.
17. Davenport, H.W.: Physiology of the digestive tract, ed. 5, Chicago, 1982, Year Book Medical Publishers.
18. Delpre, G., et al.: HLA antigens in ulcerative colitis and Crohn's disease in Israel, Gastroenterology **78**:1452, 1980.
19. Donald, P.J.: The oral cavity. In Bolt, J.R., et al.: The digestive system, New York, 1983, John Wiley & Sons.
20. Dworken, H.F.: Gastroenterology: pathophysiology and clinical applications, Boston, 1982, Butterworth.
21. Eastwood, G.L., editor: Core textbook of gastroenterology, Philadelphia, 1984, J.B. Lippincott Co.
22. Farmer, R.G., Achkar, E., and Fleshler, B.: Clinical gastroenterology, New York, 1983, Raven Press.
23. Fielding, J.F.: A year in outpatients with irritable bowel syndrome, Lancet **2**:753, 1969.

24. Fonkalsrud, E.W.: Endorectal ileoanal anastomosis with isoperistaltic after colectomy and mucosal proctectomy, Ann. Surg. **199:**158, 1984.

25. Gerber, A.: The Kock continent ileal reservoir: an alternative to conventional urostomy, J. Enterostomal Ther. **12:**15, 1985.

26. Gilat, T., et al.: Ulcerative colitis in the Jewish population of Tel-Aviv Jafo. I. Epidemiology, Gastroenterology **66:**757, 1974.

27. Goldberg, S.M., Gordon, P.H., and Nivatvongs, S.: Essentials of anorectal surgery, Philadelphia, 1980, J.B. Lippincott Co.

28. Goldman, S.L., and Rombeau, J.L.: The continent ileostomy: a collective review, Dis. Col. Rect. **21:**594, 1978.

29. Gomez, J., and Dally, P.: Psychologically mediated abdominal pain in surgical and medical outpatient clinics, Br. Med. J. **1:**1451, 1977.

30. Guyton, A.C.: Textbook of medical physiology, ed. 6, Philadelphia, 1981, W.B. Saunders Co.

31. Guyton, A.C.: Human physiology and mechanisms of disease, ed. 3, Philadelphia, 1982, W.B. Saunders Co.

32. Hodgson, H.J.F., and Bloom, S.R.: Gastrointestinal and hepatobiliary cancer, Boston, 1983, Butterworths.

33. Hukuhara, T., Kotani, S., and Sato, G.: Effects of destruction of intramural ganglion cells on colon motility: possible genesis of congenital megacolon, Jpn. J. Physiol. **11:**635, 1961.

34. Johnson, L.R., editor: Gastrointestinal physiology, ed. 3, St. Louis, 1986, The C.V. Mosby Co.

35. Joossens, J.V., and Geboers, J.: Nutrition and gastric cancer, Proc. Nutr. Soc. **40:**37, 1981.

36. King, S.A.: Quality of life: the continent ileostomy, Ann. Surg. 1982:29, 1975.

37. Kirsner, J.B.: Observations of the medical treatment of inflammatory bowel disease, J.A.M.A. **243**(6):557, 1980.

38. Klein, K., Stenzel, P., and Katon, R.M.: Pouch ileitis: report of a case with severe systemic manifestations, J. Clin. Gastroenterol. **5:**149, 1983.

39. Klipstein, F.A.: Sprue and subclinical malabsorption in the tropics, Lancet **1:**277, 1979.

40. Kock, N.G., Myrvold, H.E., and Nilsson, L.O.: Progress report on the continent ileostomy, World J. Surg. **4:**143, 1980.

41. Lauren, P.: The two histologic main types of gastric carcinoma: diffuse and so-called intestinal type carcinoma. An attempt at a histo-clinical classification, Acta Pathol. Microbiol. Scand. **64:**31, 1965.

42. Lindeman, R.J., et al.: Ulcerative colitis and intestinal salmonellosis, Am. J. Med. Sci. **254:**855, 1967.

43. MacDonald, W.C., Dobbins, W.O., and Rubin, C.E.: Studies of the familial nature of celiac sprue using biopsy of the small intestine, N. Engl. J. Med. **272:**448, 1965.

44. Mendeloff, A.I., et al.: Illness experiences and life stresses in patients with irritable colon and with ulcerative colitis, N. Engl. J. Med. **282:**14, 1970.

45. Ming, S.C.: Gastric carcinoma: a pathobiological classification, Cancer **39:**2475, 1977.

46. Monk, M.: An epidemiological study of ulcerative colitis and regional enteritis among adults in Baltimore. III. Psychological and possible stress-precipitating factors, J. Chron. Dis. **22:**565, 1970.

47. Morowitz, D.A., and Kisner, J.B.: Ileostomy in ulcerative colitis: a questionnaire study of 1803 patients, Am. J. Surg. **141:**370, 1981.

48. National Institute of Arthritis, Diabetes, and Digestive and Kidney Diseases (NIADDK): Second annual report, DHHS, PHS, NIH Pub. No. 83-2493, Washington, D.C., 1983, U.S. Government Printing Office.

49. Neurcomer, A.D., et al.: Tolerance to lactose deficiency in American Indians, Gastroenterology **74:**44, 1975.

50. Nord, H.J., and Brady, P.G.: Critical care gastroenterology, New York, 1982, Churchill Livingstone.

51. Oster, J.: Recurrent abdominal pains, headache, and limb pain in children, Pediatrics **50:**429, 1972.

52. Parks, A.G., and Nicholls, R.J.: Proctocolectomy without ileostomy for ulcerative colitis, Br. Med. J. **2:**85, 1978.

53. Pemberton, J.H., et al.: A continent ileostomy device, Ann. Surg. **197:**618, 1983.

54. Pena, A.S., et al.: Genetic bases of gluten-sensitive enteropathy, Gastroenterology **75:**230, 1978.

55. Postier, R.G., O'Malley, V., and Pruitt, L.: Continent-preserving operations for ulcerative colitis and multiple polyposis, J. Enterostomal Ther. **11:**237, 1984.

56. Prevalence of selected chronic digestive conditions, U.S., 1975. Vital health and statistics. National health survey. DHHS pub. no. PHS 79-1558, Washington, D.C., 1979, National Center for Health Statistics.

57. Ravitch, M.M., and Sabiston, D.C.: Anal ileostomy with preservation of the sphincter: a proposed operation in patients requiring colectomy for benign lesions, Surg. Gynecol. Obstet. **84:**1095, 1947.

58. Rolstad, B.S.: Ileoanal reservoir: functional results and management, South. Med. J. **77:**1535, 1984.

59. Rubin, C.E., et al.: Biopsy studies on the pathogenesis of celiac sprue. In Wolstenholme, G.E.W., and Cameron, M.P., editors: Intestinal biopsy, Boston, 1962, Little, Brown & Co.

60. Sachar, D.B., Auslander, M.O., and Walfish, J.S.: Aetiological theories of inflammatory bowel disease, Clin. Gastroenterol. **9:**231, 1980.

61. Sales, D.M., and Kirsner, J.B.: The prognosis of inflammatory bowel disease, Arch. Intern. Med. **143:**294, 1983.

62. Santulli, T.V., Kiesewetter, W.B., and Bill, A.H.: Anorectal anomalies: a suggested international classification, J. Peidatr. Surg. **5:**281, 1970.

63. Schiff, L., and Schiff, E.R.: Diseases of the liver, Philadelphia, 1982, J.B. Lippincott Co.

64. Schrock, T.R.: Complications of continent ileostomy, Am. J. Surg. **138:**162, 1979.

65. Sernka, T.J., and Jacobson, E.D.: Gastrointestinal physiology: the essentials, ed. 2, Baltimore, 1983, Williams & Wilkins Co.

66. Shanbour, L.L., and Jacobson, E.D.: Digitalis and the mesenteric circulation, Am. J. Digestive Dis. **17:**826, 1972.

67. Shearman, D.J.C., and Finlayson, N.D.C.: Diseases of the gastrointestinal tract and liver, New York, 1982, Churchill Livingstone.

68. Simons, F.J.: New light on ethnic differences in adult lactose intolerances, Am. J. Digestive Dis. **18:**595, 1973.

69. Sleisenger, M.H., and Fordtran, J.S.: Gastrointestinal disease, ed. 3, Philadelphia, 1983, W.B. Saunders Co.

70. Smith, L., Friend, W.G., and Medwel, S.J.: The superior mesenteric artery: the critical factor in pouch pull-through procedure, Dis. Col. Rect. **27:**741, 1984.

71. Soave, F.: A new surgical technique for the treatment of Hirschsprung's disease, Surgery **56:**1007, 1964.

72. Spiro, H.M.: Clinical gastroenterology, New York, 1983, Macmillan Publishing Co., Inc.

73. Stroehlein, J.R., and Romsdahl, M.M.: Gastrointestinal cancer, New York, 1981, Raven Press.

74. Swenson, O., et al.: Diagnosis of congenital megacolon, J. Pediatr. Surg. **8:**587, 1973.

75. Texter, E.C.: The aging gut, New York, 1983, Masson Publishing Co.

76. Thompson, W.H.F.: The nature of hemorrhoids, Br. J. Surg. **62:**542, 1975.

77. Utsunomiya, J., et al.: Total colectomy, mucosal proctectomy, and ileoanal anastomosis, Dis. Col. Rect. **23:**459, 1980.

78. Watanabee, H., et al.: Gastric lesions in familial adenomatosis coli, Hum. Pathol. **9:**269, 1978.

79. Watt, R.: The J-pouch, unpublished patient education material, Stanford, Calif., 1985, Stanford University Medical Center.

80. Weill, F.S.: Ultrasonography of digestive diseases, St. Louis, 1980, The C.V. Mosby Co.

81. Zakim, D., and Boyer, T.D.: Hepatology: a textbook of liver disease, Philadelphia, 1982, W.B. Saunders Co.

CHAPTER 12

Genitourinary System

Overview

Genitourinary diseases affect the kidneys, ureters, bladder, urethra, or male genitalia. Urologic disorders may result from specific disease states such as infection, hyperplasia, or neoplasia. Other disorders, such as urinary incontinence or male sexual function, are symptoms rather than specific disease states, but they also cause significant health problems related to the genitourinary system.

ANATOMY AND PHYSIOLOGY

Urinary Tract Structures

Kidneys. The kidneys are a pair of reddish brown, symmetrically shaped organs located in the retroperitoneal space, adjacent to the vertebral column at spinal levels T_{12}, and L_1 to L_3 (Fig. 12-1). The lateral aspects of the kidneys are smooth and rounded; the medial aspects are marked by a concave surface known as the renal hilus. The renal veins, arteries, nerve plexus, and renal lymphatics are located at this hilus. The renal pelvis attaches to the kidney at the hilus before tapering into the ureters.[17,61]

The weight of the adult kidney varies from 115 to 175 g. Adult women have slightly smaller kidneys than do adult men. The kidney in the infant or young child is smaller than in the adult. However, a child's kidneys occupy a larger proportion of the child's body weight. The normal adult kidney is approximately 11 cm long, 5 to 7 cm wide, and 2 to 3.5 cm thick. The kidneys are remarkably symmetric in size and shape.[61]

A cross section of the kidneys (Fig. 12-2) reveals two distinct sections: the renal pelvis and renal parenchyma. Within the renal parenchyma, a cortex and medulla are distinguished using the unaided eye. The renal medulla is characterized by pale, striated conical structures called pyramids. The bases of these pyramids are directed toward the periphery of the kidney; the apices face the renal hilus. The renal pyramids end in papillae that project into a minor calix. The kidneys normally contain from eight to eighteen renal pyramids that drain into four to thirteen minor calices. These minor calices drain into two or three major calices, which open into the renal pelvis.[17,116]

The renal medulla is bounded by the renal cortex, which appears darker and has a granular rather than striated appearance. Cortical lobules arch over the pyramids within the medulla. Cortical columns dip between the pyramids. The renal cortex is bounded by the true renal capsule, a layer of dense connective tissue loosely adherent to the parenchyma. The kidneys are supported by the perirenal fascia and perinephric fat. The kidneys, along with the superiorly placed adrenals, are enclosed within Gerota's fascia.[17,116]

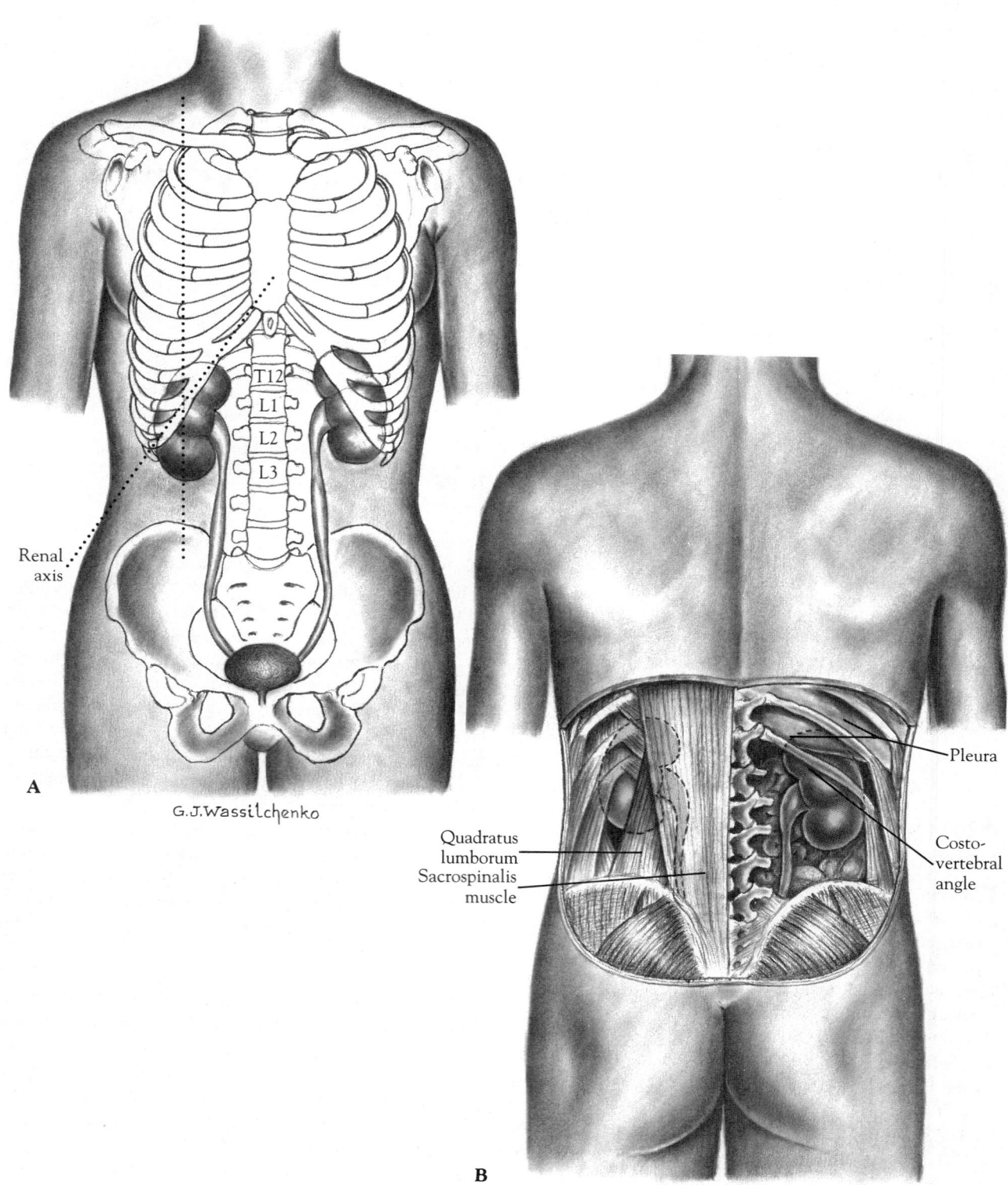

Fig. 12-1
Anatomic relation of kidneys to spinal
column. **A,** Anterior view.
B, Posterior view.

Fig. 12-2
Cross section of kidney.

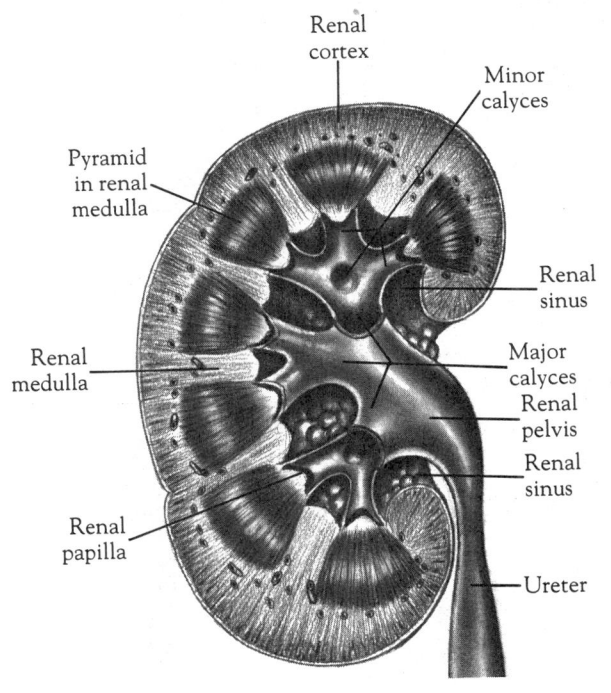

Fig. 12-3
Renal pelvic and calices.

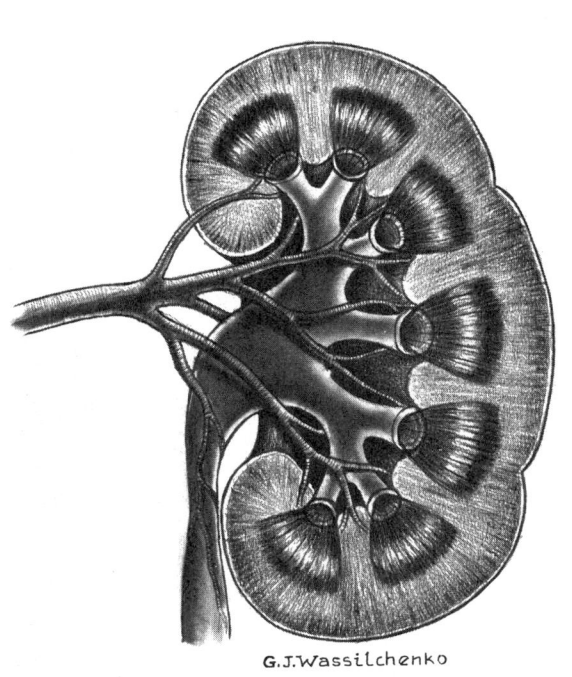

G.J.Wassilchenko

The renal fossa is bounded superiorly by the diaphragm, laterally by the abdominal musculature, and posteriorly by the quadratus lumborum muscle. Because of the presence of the liver, the right kidney lies lower than the left.[61]

The blood supply of the kidneys arises directly from the abdominal aorta. Typically a single renal artery enters the kidney at the renal hilus. However, duplicate renal arteries may be found and are not considered pathologic. After entering the kidney, the renal artery bifurcates into superior and inferior branches, which further divide into the interlobular arteries. These vessels and their branches provide the substantial blood supply necessary for renal function.[61]

The veins that drain the kidneys are paired with arterial vessels. The renal veins exiting the kidney empty directly into the inferior vena cava, and their number corresponds to the number of renal arteries present.[88]

Lymphatics adjacent to the renal cortex and medulla drain into para-aortic and para–vena caval lymph nodes. The sensory and motor neurons that innervate the kidneys arise from the dorsal roots of T_{11} and T_{12}. Autonomic neural control of the kidneys is mediated by fibers from the vagus nerve, splanchnics, semilunar ganglia, and the celiac axis.[61]

The kidneys perform a number of essential functions related to the maintenance of internal homeostasis. These include maintenance of fluid and electrolyte balance, serum pH levels, and excretion of the by-products of metabolism. A detailed discussion of renal physiology is provided in Chapter 10.

Renal pelvis and ureters. The renal pelvis and ureters are a continuous, thick-walled tube that originates at the renal hilus and implants into the bladder wall, connecting the kidneys to the bladder. The renal pelvis is a funnel-shaped structure into which the major calices empty urine for transport to the urinary bladder. After exiting the renal hilus the renal pelvis narrows inferomedially into the ureter (Fig. 12-3).[88]

The ureters are approximately 24 to 30 cm long. The left ureter is slightly longer than the right. The course of the ureters forms an inverted S. After leaving the renal pelvis, the ureters pass medially over the psoas muscle. The ureters then progress medially to the sacroiliac joints before turning laterally to an area near the ischial spines of the pelvis. Finally, the ureters will curve back laterally to insert into the bladder base at the trigone muscle.[18,88]

The internal diameter of the ureters varies from 2 to 10 mm. Three areas of anatomic narrowing have clinical implications: the ureteropelvic junction, the area where

Fig. 12-4
Course of ureter with its varying
internal luminal sizes.

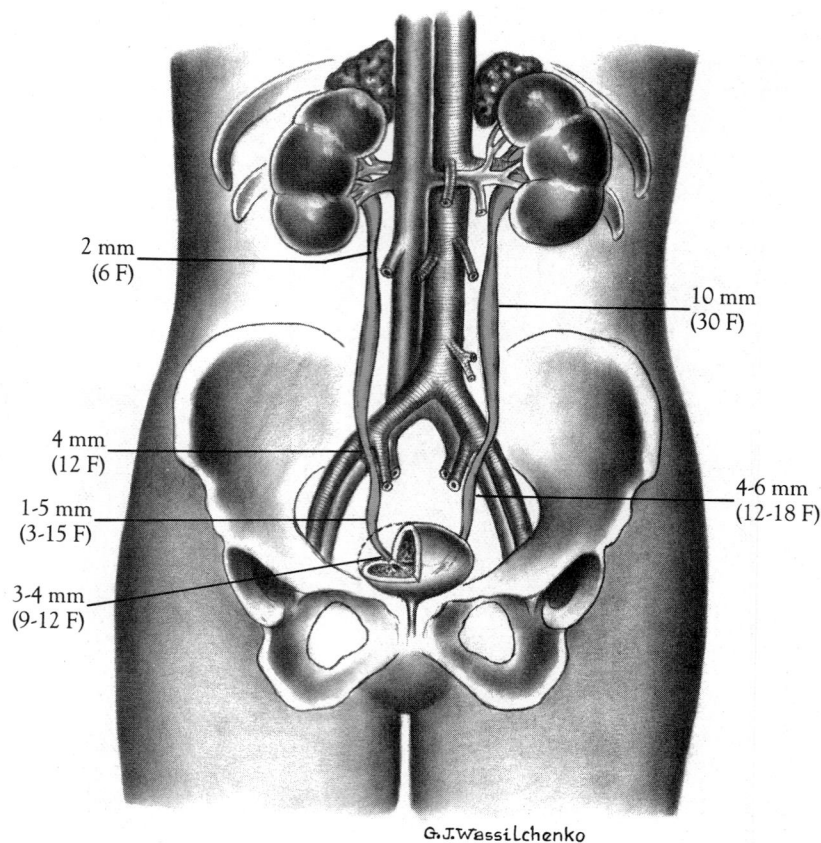

2 mm
(6 F)

10 mm
(30 F)

4 mm
(12 F)

1-5 mm
(3-15 F)

4-6 mm
(12-18 F)

3-4 mm
(9-12 F)

G.J.Wassilchenko

the ureters cross the iliac arteries, and the ureterovesical junction (Fig. 12-4).[49,88]

The ureters and renal pelvis share a common embryologic origin and histologic makeup. The ureter and renal pelvis first appear during the fourth week of life. They arise from the mesonephric duct and grow cranially to meet the metanephric cap.[94]

The ureter and renal pelvis are composed of three histologically defined layers: the external adventitia, a smooth muscle coat, and an inner mucous membrane. The adventitia is a connective tissue sheath that encircles the renal pelvis and ureters to the level of the ureterovesical junction. The adventitial layer blends into the surrounding retroperitoneal tissue, providing support for the ureters. The exact arrangement of these fibers is not known. Two layers of muscle fibers, an inner longitudinal layer and an outer circular layer, have been described.[116] However, histologic studies of ureteral smooth muscle have disputed this theory.[75] Tanagho[94] and Allen[2] describe the muscle fibers as arranged in bundles that are oriented in a helical or spiral fashion. The muscular tissue layer provides peristaltic activity needed to transport urine from the kidneys to the bladder. The mucous membrane

lining the internal ureter is composed of transitional cell epithelium with a supportive lamina propria.[75]

The blood supply of the ureters is variable. The upper portion of the ureter and renal pelvis may receive arterial blood from branches of the renal, gonadal, or adrenal arteries. The pelvic ureters may receive arterial blood from the common iliacs, external iliacs, deferential arteries in the male, uterine arteries in the female, or the obturator artery. Blood enters the ureters via an arterial plexus located within the outer adventitial layer.[18]

Venous blood from the ureters drains into a venous plexus in the ureteral submucosa. This plexus drains into an adventitial venous plexus, which empties into veins closely paired with the arterial supply described previously.

Lymphatic drainage from the ureters is also variable. The upper ureteral and renal pelvic lymphatic channels empty into paraaortic or renal nodes. The mid and lower ureteral lymphatic channels drain into the common or external iliac nodes.[18]

The nerve supply of the ureters arises from the celiacs, mesenteric ganglia, and hypogastrics. Although the exact role of the autonomic nervous system in ureteral function remains unclear, the ureter is known to contain a rich supply of sympathetic and parasympathetic nerve receptors.[18]

The primary function of the renal pelvis and ureters is to transport urine from the kidney to the bladder. In order to accomplish this goal, the ureters must create a peristaltic muscular wave sufficient to drive a bolus of urine from the renal pelvis through the ureters, past the ureterovesical junction.[75]

Although the precise mechanisms of ureteral peristalsis remain unclear, it is influenced by mechanical, chemical, and neural stimuli. Generation of a peristaltic wave does not depend on specific neural firing. Like the smooth muscle of the heart, ureteral smooth muscle will continue to rhythmically contract outside the body. In contrast to the heart, no specialized pacemaker has been clearly defined, although the existence of an intrinsic ureteral pacemaker is well established.[11] Multiple pacemaker cells regulating ureteral activity are thought to exist within the renal calices. The prolonged refractory period of the smooth muscle of the renal pelvis and ureters prevents all caliceal contractions from resulting in ureteral peristaltic waves. The renal pelvis and ureters average two to six peristaltic waves each minute.[49,111a]

Ureteral peristaltic waves typically arise within the renal pelvis. They travel in an antegrade direction from the renal pelvis to the ureterovesical junction. During the resting phase, the renal pelvis assumes a conical shape with an area of narrowing at the pelvic-ureteral junction. At this time both the renal pelvis and ureters maintain a low intraluminal pressure of 2 to 5 cm H_2O. Urine enters the ureter from the renal pelvis passively during the resting phase. During a peristaltic wave, the pressure rises to 20 to 60 cm H_2O, sufficient to force urine past the ureterovesical junction into the bladder. Only 5% of the total renal pelvic contents is evacuated from the renal pelvis during a peristaltic wave. Once the peristaltic wave is propagated into the ureters, urine is pushed ahead of the wave through the length of the ureter and past the ureterovesical junction into the bladder.[49,111a]

An increase in renal output will cause greater pelvic distention, which will increase both the number of peristaltic waves generated per minute and the proportion of renal pelvic contents transported to the bladder with each contraction.[49]

The ureters are also affected by neural influences. Although it has been demonstrated that the normal ureter will continue to contract when removed from the body, the autonomic nervous system does influence ureteral function. The ureters are extensively innervated with alpha- and beta-adrenergic receptors. Stimulation of alpha-adrenergic receptors causes increased ureteral peristalsis. Stimulation of beta-adrenergic receptors results in an inhibition of ureteral peristalsis. The role of the parasym-

pathetic nervous system in ureteral and renal pelvic function is not clearly understood. The parasympathetic nervous system is thought to potentiate ureteral peristalsis directly through cholinergic receptors in the ureteral wall or indirectly through the release of catecholamines.[111a]

Ureteral peristalsis is also influenced by various chemical and pharmacologic agents. For example, the administration of epinephrine or catecholamines will, predictably, increase ureteral peristalsis. Increased histamine levels also stimulate ureteral peristalsis. However, the administration of serotonin, which enhances intestinal peristalsis, does not affect ureteral peristalsis. Upper ureteral dilation, which is commonly seen in pregnant women, was once attributed to fluctuations in the serum levels of the sex hormones. Recent investigation has demonstrated that this dilation was caused by mechanical factors rather than hormonal influences. This hypothesis is further supported by the observation that upper ureteral dilation is not seen in women taking oral contraceptives.[49]

Ureterovesical junction and trigone. The ureterovesical junction is of particular interest in any discussion of genitourinary disease because of its importance in preventing vesicoureteral reflux and associated complications. The ureterovesical junction is located near the base of the bladder in the lateral aspects of the trigone muscle. The ureterovesical junction has three components important to its function: the intravesical ureter, the trigone, and the adjacent bladder wall (Fig. 12-5).[16,95]

Embryologically, the ureterovesical junction is formed in the seventh week of gestation when the caudal end of the ureter opens into the urogenital sinus. The trigone muscle is formed from the same mesonephric tissue that forms the ureter. The intravesical ureter is further connected to the bladder by a continuous connective tissue sheath. Thus, although the intravesical ureter and trigone muscle have different embryologic origins than the bladder, the ureterovesical junction in the fully developed human functions as a single unit to allow for the passage of urine into the bladder while preventing reflux of urine into the upper tracts.[95]

The intravesical ureter enters the bladder at a hiatus in the posterior, lateral aspect of the bladder base and is approximately 1.5 cm long. It is divided into an intramural section surrounded by the detrusor muscle and a submucosal segment that travels under the bladder mucosa. The intravesical ureter terminates at an orifice that opens into the bladder vesicle.[16,95]

The histologic features of the intravesical ureter differ from upper ureteral segments in several ways. The adventitia of the intravesical ureter contains two dense sheaths. The superficial sheath is continuous with the bladder wall. The deep sheath is derived from ureteral adventitia. Between these dense sheaths is a loose connective tissue plane called Waldeyer's sheath. This sheath

Fig. 12-5
Normal ureterotrigonal complex.

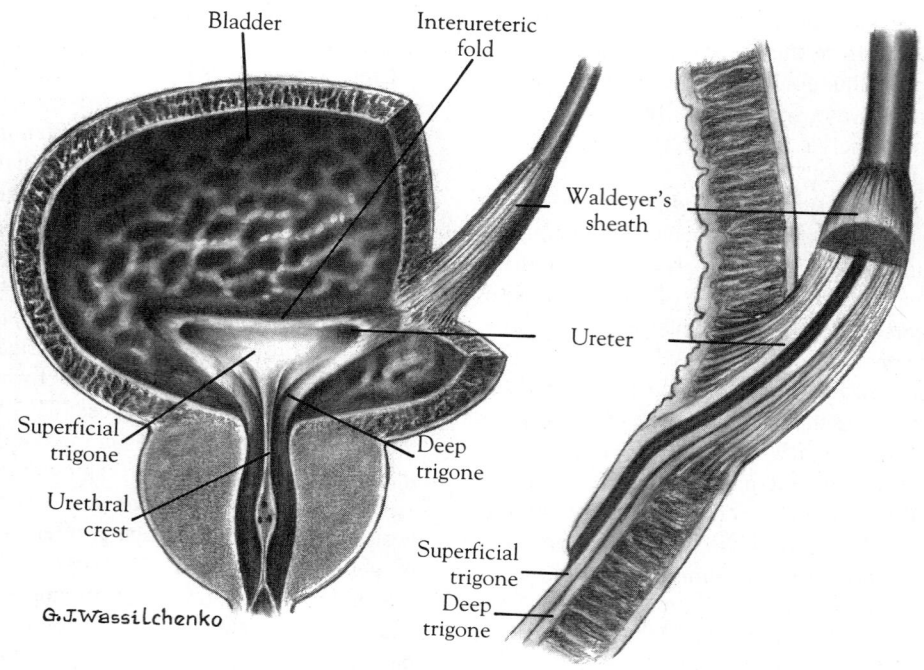

allows for mobility of the intravesical ureter within the adjacent bladder wall and is of surgical significance when performing ureteroneocystostomy.[16]

The arrangement of smooth muscle fibers also differs in the intravesical ureter. Unlike the upper ureters, the intravesical ureter contains longitudinally arranged fibers and is easily collapsible. The ability of the intravesical ureter to seal itself by collapsing is an important mechanism in the prevention of reflux. Muscle fibers from the intravesical ureter decussate inferiorly to fuse with the superficial trigone and medially to form Mercier's bar.[16,38]

The trigone muscle is another essential component of the ureterovesical junction. The muscle is divided into two parts, the superficial trigone and the deep trigone. The superficial trigone is continuous with muscular fibers from the intravesical ureter. It continues along the bladder base and into the proximal urethra. In the male the trigone terminates at the verumantanum. In the female the superficial trigone terminates at the bladder neck.[95]

The deep trigone is characterized by flat, tightly bound, smooth fiber groups. It is continuous with Waldeyer's sheath along the path of the intravesical ureter. The deep trigone is rolled into a tube that is incomplete on its anterior surface. The deep trigone terminates at the bladder neck and continues into the urethra as a layer of circular smooth muscle.[95,108]

The portion of the bladder wall adjacent to the ureterovesical junction is characterized by circular and longitudinal smooth muscle fibers that secure the ureters within the vesical wall. The outer, longitudinal smooth muscle layer is the strongest, most resilient segment of the bladder wall. This strength is vital to the maintenance of continuity between the upper and lower urinary tracts.[95]

The primary functions of the ureterovesical junction are to allow efflux of urine into the bladder and to prevent reflux of urine into the ureters. During bladder filling the ureterovesical junction maintains a relatively low closure pressure between 8 and 15 cm H_2O. This closure pressure is adequate to prevent reflux of urine from the bladder, which also fills at low pressures. However, the closure pressure is easily overcome by a ureteral peristaltic wave, which generates pressure between 20 and 60 cm H_2O. As the bladder fills and intravesical pressure rises, the intravesical ureter becomes progressively compressed against the adjacent bladder wall. The effect of this compression is to carry the ureteral hiatus outward, thus increasing pressure of the intravesical ureter. This compensatory mechanism prevents reflux of urine even when the bladder is filled with urine. At very high volumes the compression of the intravesical ureter becomes functionally obstructed and interferes with normal ureteral peristalsis.[49,95]

Fig. 12-6
Common anatomy of urinary bladder.

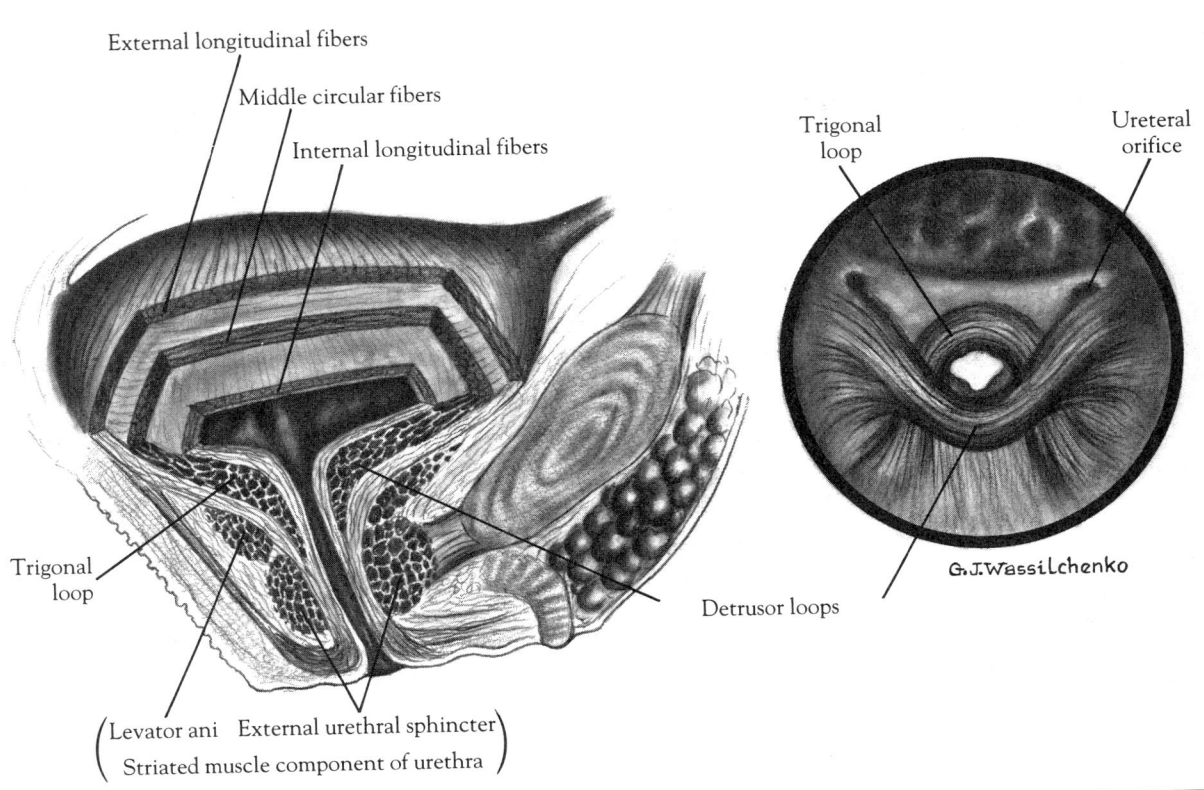

External longitudinal fibers

Middle circular fibers

Internal longitudinal fibers

Trigonal loop

Ureteral orifice

Trigonal loop

Detrusor loops

Levator ani   External urethral sphincter
Striated muscle component of urethra

G.J.Wassilchenko

During the voiding phase the ureterovesical junction must generate even greater resistance to prevent reflux into the upper urinary tract. A few seconds before intravesical pressure rises in response to a detrusor contraction, there is a sharp pressure rise within the intravesical ureter. This high closure pressure at the ureterovesical junction is maintained throughout micturition and persists for a brief period after voiding is completed. The sharp increase in pressure was once attributed primarily to the contractile activity of the adjacent bladder wall. However, recent studies have demonstrated that the trigone is primarily responsible for the prevention of reflux during micturition. The marked pressure rise seen immediately before a detrusor contraction is caused by an increase in the tone of the trigone, which pulls the intravesical ureter tightly closed. The trigonal contraction is maintained for approximately 20 seconds after voiding is completed. As expected, no efflux of urine into the bladder occurs during voiding.[95]

Urinary bladder. The urinary bladder is a hollow muscular organ designed to store and expel urine produced by the kidneys. The size and shape of the bladder vary with its state of fullness and with age. When empty, the bladder assumes the shape of a tetrahedron and lies entirely within the lesser pelvis. As the bladder fills, it becomes more spheric in shape and moves upward and anteriorly toward the abdominal cavity.[85,116]

During infancy the bladder is located in the abdomen; even the bladder neck lies above the symphysis pubis. As the child matures, the bladder will assume its place in the pelvis shortly before puberty. The change in position is not caused by migration of the organ; rather, changes in the size and shape of the vesicle and maturation of the pelvic bone result in the change in relative location of the bladder.[61]

In all individuals the bladder is characterized by two inlets and a single outlet located on the inferior aspect of the organ. Six anatomic areas are seen on gross inspection of the organ: the neck, the base, or fundus, the apex, and the superior, right inferolateral, and left inferolateral surfaces (Fig. 12-6).[85]

The bladder neck is the lowest part of the organ and is located several centimeters from the lower aspect of the symphysis pubis. The bladder neck is a relatively fixed structure regardless of the volume of urine present in the vesicle or the state of the adjacent rectum. The bladder neck is pierced by the internal urethral orifice. In the male it sits directly superior to the prostate gland. In the female it sits posteriorly to the vaginal wall.[85]

The base of the bladder is triangular in shape and oriented posteriorly and downward from the bladder apex. Its borders are rounded and characterized by the junction of the intravesical ureters. In the adult male the bladder is superior to the seminal vesicles and adjacent to the rectum. Denonvilliers's fascia forms an anatomic barrier between the bladder base, rectum, and the vasa deferentia. In adult women the bladder base lies in close proximity to the anterior vaginal wall. Although the female lacks any fascial borders between the bladder and adjacent vagina, the two structures are separate at this point. In contrast, the lower urethra is anatomically continuous with the anterior vaginal wall.[85]

The apex of the bladder is the uppermost surface of the organ and is oriented anteriorly toward the abdominal wall. In the empty bladder of the adult, the apex lies within the pelvis. When the bladder is filled with urine, the apex is pushed upward and anteriorly so that it enters the abdominal cavity. The apex is connected to the abdominal wall via the urachus.[85,88]

The superior surface of the empty bladder is bounded laterally by a line extending from the apex to the exterior borders of the intravesical ureters. The posterior border is formed by a line extending between the external borders of the intravesical ureters. In the adult male a reflection of the peritoneum covers the superior surface. When filled, a prevesical pouch is formed that may contain a segment of the small bowel. In the adult female the superior surface of the bladder is separated from the ureters by the ureterovesical pouch.

The inferolateral surfaces of the urinary bladder are primarily distinguished when the vesicle is empty. They lack any pelvic fascial covering and significantly change shape to accommodate bladder filling. When the bladder reaches capacity, the right and left inferolateral surfaces become a single, convex area lying adjacent to the abdominal wall.

The primary supportive structure of the urinary bladder is the pelvic floor. In addition, the ligaments found adjacent to the bladder are presumed to provide additional support. The true ligaments are thought to play a primary role in maintaining the bladder's position, and the false ligaments are presumed to play a lesser, supplemental role. The arrangement of these ligaments varies between women and men.[85,116]

The true bladder ligaments are dense bands of fascia that arise from the tendinous arch of the peritoneum and connect it with the lateral aspects of the bladder wall. The tendinous arch is a thickening of the peritoneal fascia that lies over the pelvic diaphragm and extends to the symphysis pubis and ischial spines. In the adult male the anterior aspect of this tissue forms the puboprostatic ligaments. The lateral puboprostatic ligaments extend from the anterior end of the tendinous arch to the upper aspect of the prostatic sheath. The medial puboprostatic ligaments extend from the tendinous arch to the back of the pubic bone, near the middle of the symphysis and the back part of the prostatic sheath, forming the retropubic space. In women the analogous structures are the pubovesical ligaments whose attachments are identical to those described in males except that the lower aspects of the ligaments attach to the bladder neck and proximal urethra in contrast to the prostatic sheath. From a neurourologic perspective the bladder neck may be divided from other bladder surfaces, which are collectively referred to as the bladder body.[85,116]

At the apex of the bladder, the allantois forms the median umbilical ligament or urachus, which is a fibrous cord extending to the umbilicus. Normally, the lower portion of the urachus is patent but does not communicate with the bladder vesicle. Occasionally, the inferior urachal remnant will communicate with the vesicle of the bladder; this is not considered pathologic unless infection is present.[85,116]

In addition to the true ligaments, a number of false ligaments are found around the bladder. They are, in reality, reflections of peritoneum that partially envelop the bladder. The three anterior false ligaments are the median umbilical fold, the medial umbilical fold, and the lateral false ligaments. The median fold extends over the urachal remnant near the bladder apex. The medial umbilical fold covers the remaining umbilical arterial remnants, and the lateral false ligaments extend from the bladder to the side walls of the pelvis. Reflections of sacrogenital peritoneum form the posterior false ligaments.[116]

The bladder wall is divided into four distinct histologic layers: the urothelium, lamina propria, tunica muscularis, and outer adventitia. The urothelium of the bladder lines the vesicle and is formed of transitional cell epithelium six to eight layers deep in the empty bladder. As the bladder fills to capacity, the urothelium will become only two to three layers deep. The urothelium has an associated membrane that is impermeable to water, thus preventing the reabsorption of urine stored in the bladder.[12,59]

Under the urothelium is the submucosal layer, or the lamina propria. The lamina propria is only loosely attached to the urothelium and rich with areolar tissues and elastic fibers. The lamina propria is found throughout the distensible portions of the bladder but is absent in the area of the deep trigone. Here, the mucosal lining of the vesicle is attached directly to the tunica muscularis in this nondistensible portion of the bladder.[61]

Unlike its loose connection with the urothelium, the lamina propria is firmly attached to the tunica muscularis of the bladder, which contains only smooth muscle fibers and is called the detrusor. Detrusor muscle fibers are arranged in bundles, interspersed within a collagenous framework. The detrusor muscle is variable in thickness; three muscle layers (inner longitudinal, middle circular, and outer longitudinal) are distinguishable. The middle circular and outer longitudinal detrusor fibers consist of relatively thick smooth muscle fibers. They are most prominent in the body of the bladder and terminate at the internal urethral orifice. The inner longitudinal layer of the detrusor muscle is prominent in the area of the bladder neck. Controversy exists whether detrusor muscle fibers extend into the proximal urethra. Some investigators argue that the inner longitudinal detrusor fibers continue into the proximal urethra as an outer longitudinal smooth fiber layer.[62,108] However, others note that continuity between detrusor fibers and urethral smooth fibers is not seen in fetal tissue specimens. Thus they conclude that vesical smooth muscle and urethral smooth muscle are entirely separate.[19]

The outermost histologic layer of the bladder is the adventitia. The adventitia is composed of fibroelastic tissue and is loosely connected to the various peritoneal coverings of the bladder described previously.[59]

The blood supply of the urinary bladder arises from several sources. Arterial blood reaches the bladder from the superior, medial, and inferior vesical arteries, which are branches of the internal iliac, or hypogastric, artery. Small branches from the obturator and inferior gluteal muscles also supply arterial blood to the bladder. Branches from the uterine and vaginal artery supply vascular nourishment to the bladder in the female. Unlike the kidneys, the veins of the bladder do not follow arterial routes. Venous drainage from the bladder exits anteriorly into the plexus of Santorini and laterally into a neurovascular sheath surrounded by the lateral vesical ligaments. From here venous blood from the bladder is routed into the inferior hypogastric vein.[61,95]

The lymphatic drainage of the bladder originates in the urothelium and drains into the vesical, external iliac, hypogastric, and common iliac nodes. The lymphatic channels in the urinary bladder are not clearly elucidated. Three areas of lymphatic drainage are postulated: the trigone, posterior wall, and anterior wall.[61,95]

The innervation of the bladder represents a deceptively complex discussion; the precise mechanisms of neural control of the urinary bladder are not fully understood. The sensory innervation of the urinary bladder is poorly understood. Sensory impulses from the urinary bladder are both proprioceptive and exteroceptive. Exteroceptive impulses from the bladder include pain, temperature, and touch. Proprioceptive impulses give the person an awareness of various states of vesical fullness. Morphologic studies in animals have demonstrated the presence of free nerve endings throughout the detrusor muscle with the greatest abundance in the trigone. Tension receptors and stretch receptors have also been noted in the detrusor muscle that presumably play an important role in the awareness of bladder filling. The impulses generated by the sensory receptors are thought to travel in the sensory portion of the pelvic nerve.[12,111]

To understand the motor innervation of the urinary bladder, it is necessary to understand that the bladder is a specialized smooth muscular organ. Thus the motor innervation of the bladder is similar to the other smooth muscle structures in the body. Two types of smooth muscle have been described: multiunit and visceral. Multiunit smooth muscle is characterized by extensive innervation and may have a 1:1 ratio of nerve endings to muscle fibers. Examples of multiunit smooth muscles are the ciliary smooth muscles of the body. Spontaneous contractions do not occur in this type of smooth muscle. Visceral smooth muscle is characterized by less extensive innervation of muscle fibers than multiunit smooth muscle. Visceral smooth muscle is also distinguished by its rhythmicity. Examples of visceral smooth muscle are uterine and ureteral musculature. Visceral smooth muscle will contract without discrete neural stimulation; such a contraction is propagated spontaneously throughout the muscle.[111]

The urinary bladder exhibits characteristics of both of these types of smooth muscle. For example, detrusor fibers within the bladder body have considerably less than a 1:1 ratio of nerve endings to smooth muscle fibers. Contraction of the detrusor may occur in response to local irritability such as vesical calculi as well as in response to neurohormonal excitation much like the visceral smooth muscle described above. However, the detrusor fibers at the bladder neck receive much more extensive innervation and exhibit many properties of multiunit smooth muscle.[111]

The motor innervation of the bladder, like all smooth muscle, is provided by the autonomic nervous system. Parasympathetic neural receptors are found throughout the detrusor muscle within the body of the bladder. These receptors are stimulated by acetylcholine and are thus termed cholinergic nerves. Two types of cholinergic receptors are seen in the human body: muscarinic and nicotinic. The bladder contains muscarinic cholinergic receptors. Sympathetic receptors are also found throughout the body of the bladder and are particularly abundant in the bladder neck. The sympathetic nerve endings in the bladder respond to norepinephrine and are called adrenergic nerves. Adrenergic receptors are labeled alpha or beta based on their responses to the various catecholamines found in the body. Beta-adrenergic responses are subdivided into $beta_1$ and $beta_2$ types. In the urinary bladder, both alpha- and $beta_2$-adrenergic receptors are found.

Fig. 12-7
Male urethra.

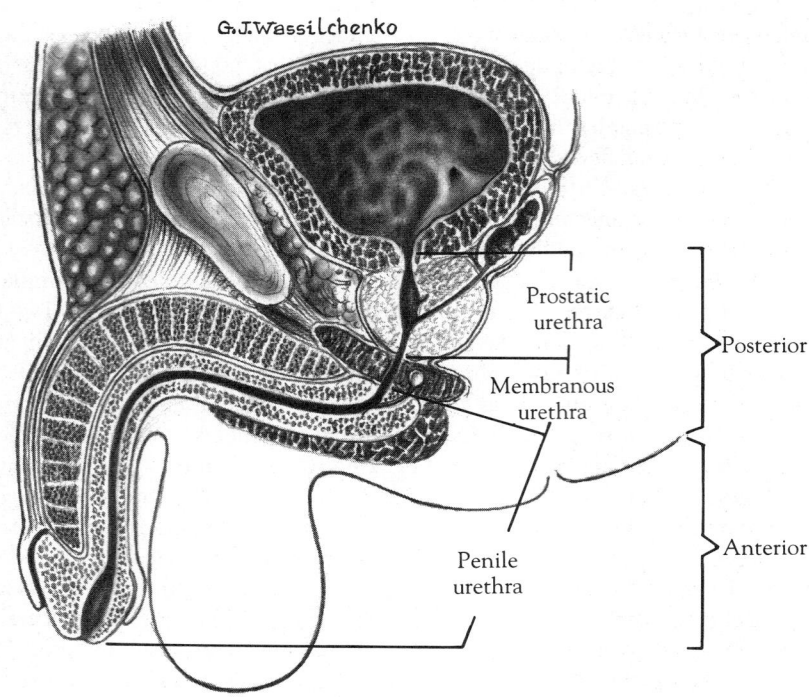

G.J.Wassilchenko

Prostatic
urethra

Posterior

Membranous
urethra

Penile
urethra

Anterior

The alpha-adrenergic receptors are most numerous in the bladder neck and trigone; beta$_2$-adrenergic receptors are most abundant in the body of the bladder.[111]

Sympathetic neural signals are routed to the bladder via branches of the inferior hypogastric nerve. The spinal roots of the sympathetic component of the inferior hypogastric are at T$_{12}$, L$_1$, and L$_2$. Parasympathetic neural signals are routed to the bladder via branches of the pelvic nerve. The spinal roots of the parasympathetic component of the pelvic nerve are located in the interomedial gray matter between the dorsal and ventral horns of spinal levels S$_2$, S$_3$, and S$_4$.

Urethra. The urethra extends from the bladder to an external meatus, serves as a conduit for urine expulsion during micturition, and serves as an aid to the maintenance of continence during bladder filling. In the male the urethra also serves as a conduit for semen expelled at ejaculation.[61,116]

The male urethra is approximately 23 cm long and is divided into two parts: anterior and posterior (Fig. 12-7). The posterior urethra is subdivided into the prostatic and membranous urethra. The prostatic urethra is approximately 3 cm in length and extends from the bladder neck to the origin of the membranous urethral segment at the apex of the prostate gland. It runs through the prostate vertically, lying nearer the anterior surface of the gland. The posterior floor of the prostatic urethra is

elevated at the verumantanum, which tapers inferiorly and superiorly to form the cristae, which are mucous membrane folds that form a depression on the posterior floor known as the prostatic fossa. Secretory ducts from the middle lobe of the prostate enter the urethra at this point (Fig. 12-8).[61]

The membranous urethra is 1.5 to 2.5 cm in length and extends from the apex of the prostate gland to the bulb of the penis. It pierces the area referred to as the urogenital diaphragm, which contains the external urinary sphincter. The external sphincter is a skeletal muscle that completely surrounds the urethra, although its bulk is considerably less posteriorly than on in its anterior surface. During contraction, it occludes the lumen of the urethra, stopping a urinary stream initiated by voiding. Although it is not necessary for the maintenance of continence, it does help prevent urinary leakage during sudden rises in intra-abdominal pressure produced by coughing, laughing, and other activities. The membranous urethra is the least distensible segment of the male urethra since it is securely anchored by the triangular ligament; it is the most susceptible to inflammatory urethral structure.[61,116]

The anterior urethra tunnels the corpus spongiosum of the penis and is divided into the bulbous, pendulous, and glandular urethra. The bulbous and pendulous parts of the urethra together measure 15 cm in length and extend

Fig. 12-8
Prostatic (posterior) urethra.

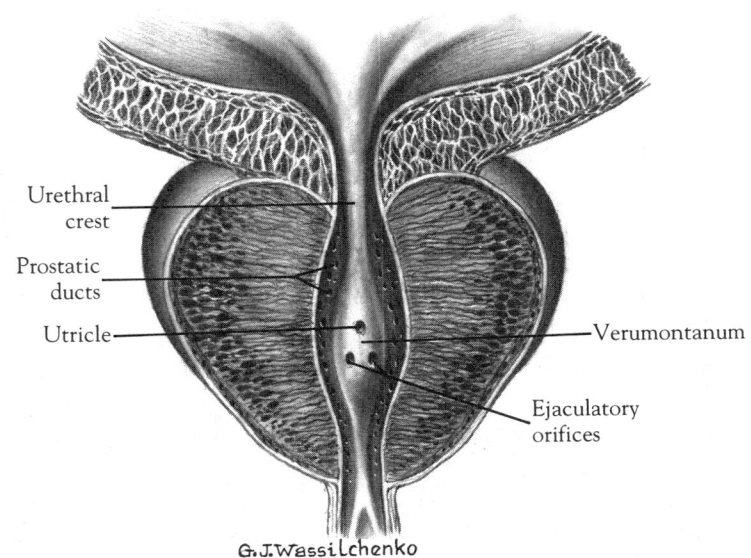

Urethral crest

Prostatic ducts

Utricle

Verumontanum

Ejaculatory orifices

G.J.Wassilchenko

from the distal border of the membranous urethra to the base of the glans penis. The suspensory ligament marks the border between these urethral segments. The bulbous urethra is distinguished by the orifices of the bulbourethral, or Cowper's, glands.[61]

The glandular urethra is the most distal segment in the male that terminates at the external meatus. Immediately before the external meatus, the glandular urethra is marked by a fusiform dilation called the fossa navicularis. It originates at the corona of the glans and is 2.5 cm in length. The external meatus itself is a vertical slit approximately 8 mm in diameter that lies at the summit of the glans.[61,116]

The microscopic anatomy of the male urethra is characterized by an inner mucous membrane composed of columnar cell epithelium persisting throughout the posterior and anterior urethral segments to the level of the fossa navicularis. Here the urethral mucosa changes to a squamous cell epithelium near the external meatus. A submucosal layer composed of connective tissue and elastic fibers lies under the mucosa. The muscular layer of the urethra is composed primarily of smooth muscle fibers. In the prostatic urethra the smooth muscle fibers are indistinguishable from the adjacent musculature to the level of the verumantanum. Below the verumantanum, the urethral smooth fibers are arranged in an outer circular layer and an inner longitudinal layer. Striated muscle fibers have also been noted in the ventral wall of the prostatic urethra.[19,116]

The arterial blood supply of the male urethra arises from the urethral artery, which is a branch of the internal

pudendal artery. Venous blood from the urethra drains into the deep vein of the penis and the pudendal plexus. The sensory innvervation of the urethra is provided by branches of the pudendal nerve. Lymphatic drainage from the male urethra accompanies channels of the glans penis in the anterior segment and empties into the deep subinguinal nodes from the posterior segment.[116]

The female urethra follows a relatively short, straight path when compared to the male urethra (Fig. 12-9). In nulliparous adult women the urethra measures 3.5 to 5.5 cm. The female urethra originates at the internal orifice of the bladder neck and travels at a 16-degree angle to its external meatus at the vestibule. It perforates the urogenital diaphragm and travels through the external striated sphincter near the meatus. In the female the external urethra is not as great in bulk as in the male and does not completely surround the urethra. Like the male urethra it is capable of interrupting a urinary stream and assists in preventing the leakage of urine during sudden increases in intra-abdominal pressure although it is not the primary guardian of continence during bladder filling. The lining of the urethra is marked by longitudinal folds; one such fold that lies along the urethral floor is named the urethral crest.[49,116]

Three histologic elements of the female urethra characterize its microscopic anatomy. The mucous lining of the urethral lumen is lined by columnar cell epithelium that changes to squamous cell epithelium near the external meatus. Unlike the male urethra, the mucous lining is marked by numerous mucus-secreting glands. The muscular lining of the upper urethra is divided into an

Fig. 12-9
Anatomic relations of female urethra.

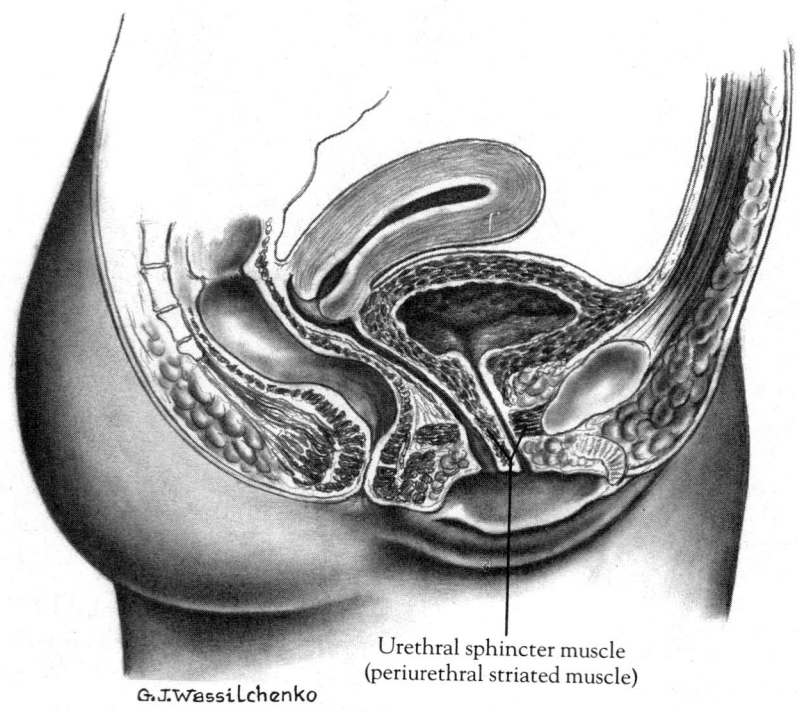

Urethral sphincter muscle
(periurethral striated muscle)

G.J.Wassilchenko

outer longitudinal and an inner circular layer of smooth muscle fibers. However, the lower two thirds of the female urethra is fused with the anterior vaginal wall so that the two muscular layers are not distinguishable. A spongy erectile tissue composed of an extensive venous plexus interspersed with smooth muscle fibers lies between the mucous lining and the muscular layer.[50a,116]

The upper third of the female urethra receives arterial blood from anastomoses of the vesical arteries; the lower two thirds receives arterial blood from the inferior vesical artery as it courses along the posterior vaginal wall. Venous drainage from the urethra empties into the inferior middle and superior vesical veins and the clitoral venous plexus. Branches of the hypogastric neural plexus follow arterial blood supply routes to innervate the urethra. Lymphatic drainage travels to the inguinal, hypogastric, and obturator nodes.[50a]

Lower Urinary Tract Function

The bladder and urethra function as a coordinated unit along with multiple levels of the central and peripheral nervous systems in order to regulate urinary continence and the efficient expulsion of urine during micturition. Although the precise mechanisms governing continence

and micturition are not completely understood, intensive investigation in this area has greatly enhanced our understanding of the physiology of the urinary bladder and urethra.

The innervation of the lower urinary tract can be divided into a central nervous system and a peripheral nervous system component.[8] For the purposes of discussing urinary continence, the urinary bladder, urethra, and pelvic floor musculature are conceptualized as a functional unit.

Central nervous system control

Brain and brainstem. Central nervous system influence on the mechanisms of continence begins in the cerebral cortex. The superomedial portion of the frontal lobes, the cingulate gyrus, and the genu of the corpus callosum interact to modulate detrusor function. The precise mechanisms through which these cerebral areas modulate detrusor function are unknown.[8,111] Kuru[51] extrapolated data gathered from cats and postulated that the net effect of the cerebral detrusor motor area is the inhibition of spontaneous voiding needed to maintain social continence. His theory coincides with the detrusor overactivity seen in patients with neurogenic bladder caused by supraspinal lesions such as cerebrovascular accident.

The external, striated sphincter and adjacent pelvic

floor musculature function is also influenced by the cerebral cortex. The motor area for the external sphincter is geographically separate from the detrusor motor area and located within the sensorimotor cortex at the central sulcus of the frontal lobe. Unlike the detrusor muscle, the external sphincter muscle is a skeletal muscle directly controlled by conscious volition.[8,12]

Communication between the detrusor and periurethral striated muscle areas and lower nuclei in the brain occurs via several pathways. Corticoreticular cells in the detrusor motor area travel through the basal ganglia to synapse at the pontine–mesencephalic–reticular formation center of the brainstem. Axons from the periurethral muscle cortical center travel through the internal capsule and brainstem to synapse with pudendal motor neurons in the ventral gray matter of the spinal cord. In addition to these efferent neural routes, afferent axons from sensory receptors in the bladder wall and periurethral muscles travel to appropriate cerebral areas, providing input from the end organ.[8,12]

Various subcortical brain areas also provide modulatory input for bladder function. The thalamus is the principal relay center between the cerebral cortex and lower areas of the central nervous system. The precise routing of the detrusor and pudendal neural pathways has not been discovered. However, dysfunction of the thalamus has been associated with clinical voiding dysfunction. The basal ganglia are associated with efferent corticoreticular pathways from the detrusor motor area in the cerebral cortex and are presumed to exert an inhibitory effect on detrusor activity. Dysfunction of the basal ganglia (parkinsonism) is associated with detrusor overactivity. Any influence that the basal ganglia may exert on the periurethral striated musculature is not known.[8,111]

The limbic system influences the function of the autonomic nervous system as well as the brainstem reticular formation area and the hypothalamus. In animal experiments, stimulation of the limbic system has resulted in alteration of the detrusor reflex. In humans, however, ablation of the limbic system has not been associated with clinically evident voiding dysfunction. However, urodynamic studies were not performed on these research subjects so subtle voiding dysfunction cannot be excluded.[12]

The hypothalamus is known to affect certain behavior patterns, including those associated with voiding and sexual function. However, the exact mechanisms through which the hypothalamus affects the function of the bladder remain unclear.[12]

The cerebellum's primary function is the modulation of motor activity initiated in other areas of the central nervous system. It influences the urinary bladder and associated structures by the maintenance of tone in the periurethral striated musculature, control of the rate and force of detrusor and pelvic floor muscles, modulatory input to brainstem areas associated with detrusor muscle contractions, and the smooth coordination between contractions of the detrusor and external sphincter muscle.[8] Dysfunction of the cerebellum as seen in cerebellar ataxia is associated with detrusor hyperreflexia or detrusor hyporeflexia. However, none of these patients had detrusor-sphincter dyssynergia (incoordination of detrusor contractions and external sphincter contractions) in the absence of spinal cord lesions.[58]

The pontine-mesencephalic gray matter of the brainstem is the final common pathway to detrusor motor neurons in the intermediolateral cell column of the gray matter of the spinal cord. Clinically, the brainstem is important as a landmark separating those patients at high risk for detrusor-sphincter dyssynergia from those who are not likely to exhibit this symptom from a neurologic lesion. The pontine–mesencephalic–reticular formation center is often referred to as the brainstem micturition center and is given credit for coordinating the detrusor and external striated sphincter. Supraspinal lesions are associated with detrusor hyperreflexia but not detrusor-sphincter dyssynergia. Neurologic lesions caudal to the brainstem micturition center and above the micturition center in the spinal cord (S2 to S4) are associated with detrusor hyperreflexia and a high incidence of detrusor-sphincter dyssynergia.[8,10]

Spinal cord. The spinal tracts important to the physiology of micturition have been partially described in the human and involve the sensory and motor innervation of the detrusor muscle; the other spinal tracts important to micturition are concerned with the sensory and motor innervation of the periurethral striated musculature. Motor axons that make up the spinal pathways for the periurethral musculature travel via corticospinal tracts within the lateral columns to terminate at the pudendal motor nuclei at spinal levels S1 to S3. Sensory impulses enter the spinal cord via pudendal sensory axons located in the pelvic floor musculature. A portion of these sensory axons will synapse at pudendal motor neurons in ventral gray matter of the conus medullaris; others will continue without synapsing and travel in the dorsal columns to synapse with neurons in the cerebellum and sensorimotor center of the cerebrum.[33]

Descending motor axons concerned with detrusor function travel via reticulospinal tracts in the lateral columns located near the corticospinal tracts for periurethral striated muscle innervation described previously. These axons terminate in the conus medullaris. Proprioceptive sensory axons within the detrusor muscle travel to the spinal cord and ascend to the pontine–mesencephalic–reticular formation center of the brainstem without synapsing with other autonomic neurons to any significant degree.[33]

Thus the micturition center for the spinal cord is located in the conus medullaris, which is the terminal tapering of the scleral spinal cord. The detrusor nuclei are located within the intermediolateral portion at spinal levels S2 to S4. Additional detrusor motor neurons are located in the lumbar spine at levels T10 to L1. The pudendal motor nuclei are located more posteriorly than the detrusor motor and are found in the ventromedial portion of spinal levels S1 and S2. Both the autonomic and periurethral muscle spinal pathways are represented bilaterally so that hemisection of the spinal cord does not produce clinically evident voiding dysfunction in experimental animals.[8]

Lapides' "loops of innervation." Many urologists conceptualize central nervous control of the bladder in terms of four "loops of innervation" first outlined by Lapides.[52,55] Integration of the mechanisms involved in normal lower urinary tract function depends on equal contributions from every loop of innervation. Thus significant voiding dysfunction is produced if one or more loops are injured.[8]

Loop I extends from the detrusor motor area in the cerebral cortex to the pontine–mesencephalic–reticular formation center in the brain (Fig. 12-10). The cerebellum and basal ganglia provide input. The primary function to this loop is to regulate volitional control of the

Fig. 12-10
Loops I and II extend from frontal cortex to pelvic nuclei in conus medullaris.

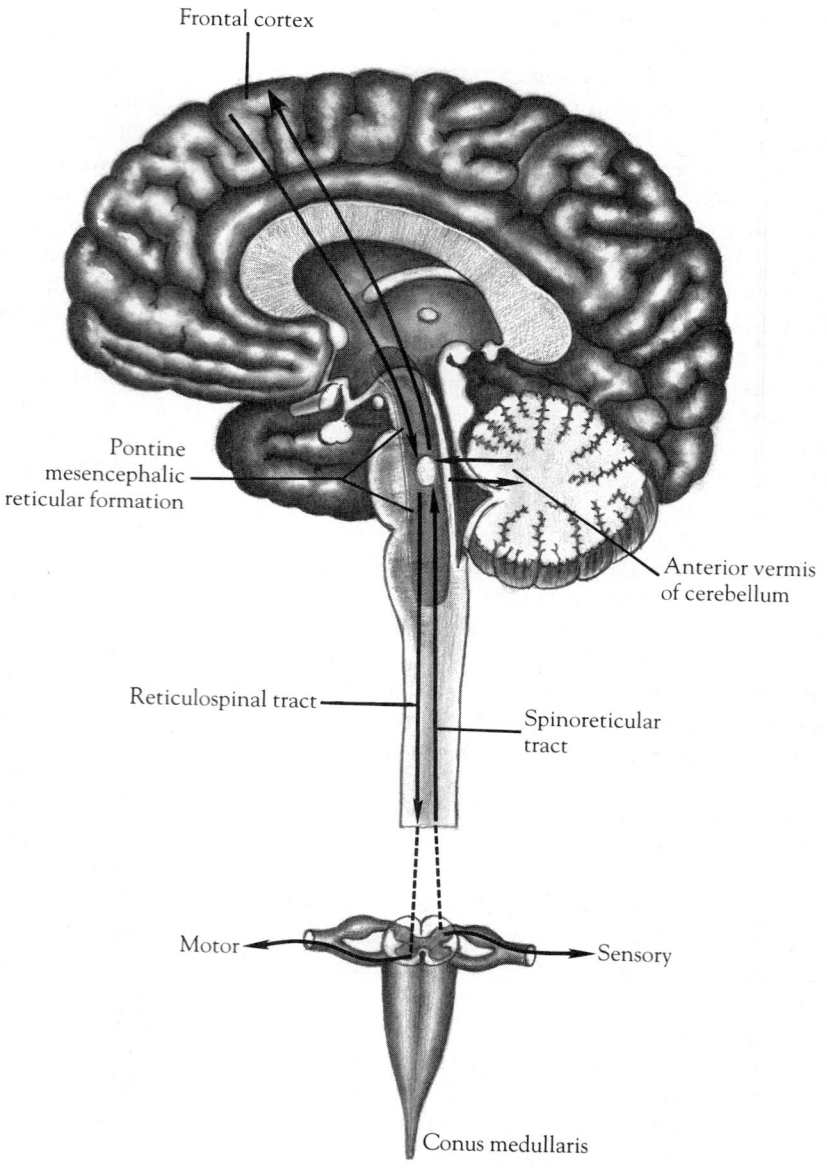

Frontal cortex

Pontine mesencephalic reticular formation

Anterior vermis of cerebellum

Reticulospinal tract

Spinoreticular tract

Motor

Sensory

Conus medullaris

detrusor reflex. Interruption of loop I will result in the loss of the ability to voluntarily suppress detrusor contraction during bladder filling.[33]

Loop II originates in the brainstem micturition center and terminates in the detrusor motor neurons in the conus medullaris (Fig. 12-10). The primary function of loop II is to provide a detrusor reflex of sufficient duration to completely empty the bladder of urine during micturition. Interruption of loop II as seen in spinal cord injury will produce an initial period of detrusor areflexia during spinal shock followed by detrusor hyperreflexia.[33]

Loop III has been described as the pudendal and pelvic nuclei and their interneurons (Fig. 12-11). This loop is responsible for the coordination of the external striated

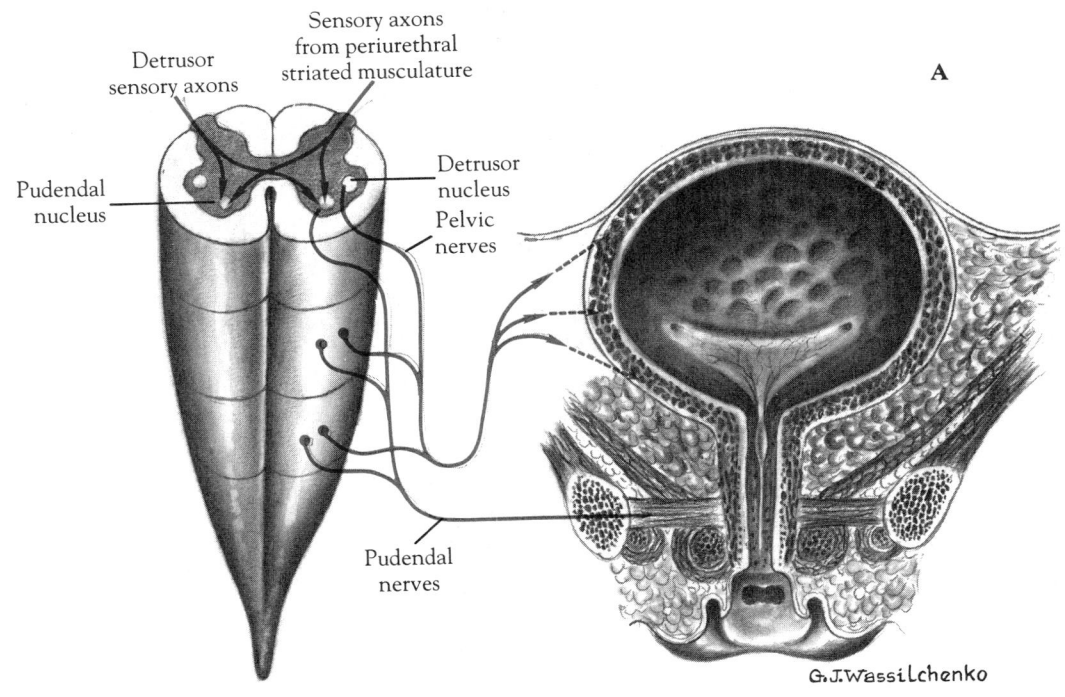

Detrusor sensory axons

Sensory axons from periurethral striated musculature

Pudendal nucleus

Detrusor nucleus

Pelvic nerves

Pudendal nerves

A

G.J.Wassilchenko

Fig. 12-11
A, Sacral micturition center and peripheral bladder innervations. B, Loop III contains pelvic and pudendal nuclei and their interneurons.

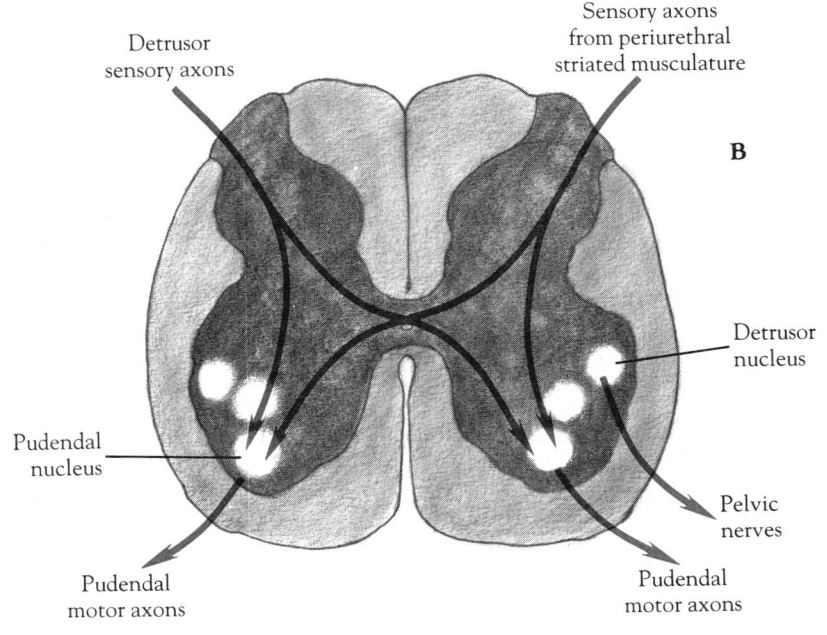

Detrusor sensory axons

Sensory axons from periurethral striated musculature

B

Detrusor nucleus

Pudendal nucleus

Pelvic nerves

Pudendal motor axons

Pudendal motor axons

Fig. 12-12
Lapides' loop IV.

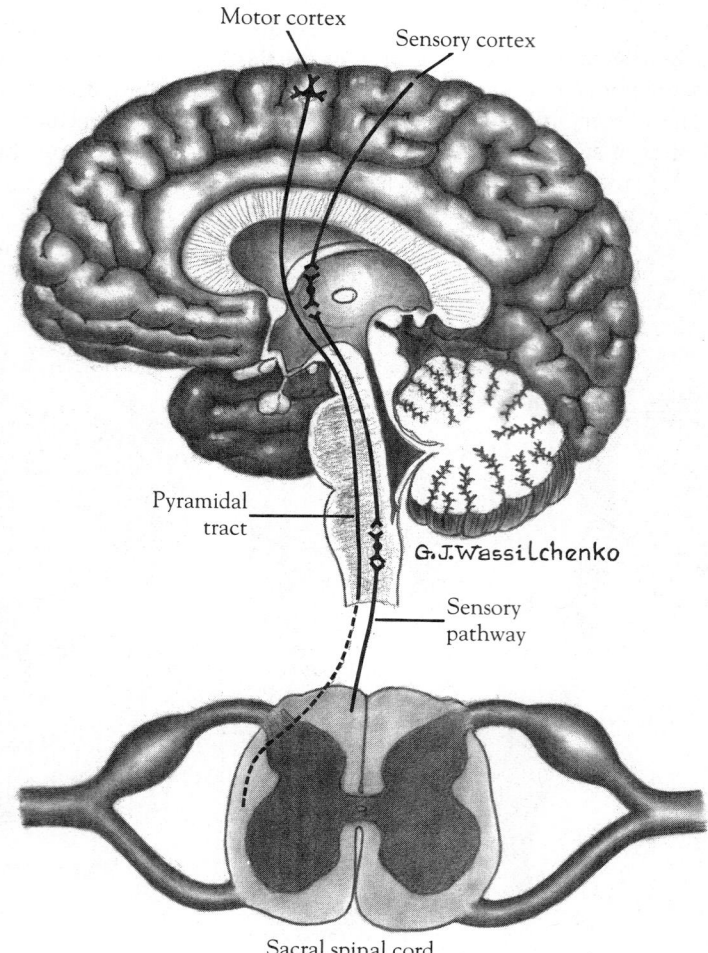

Motor cortex

Sensory cortex

Pyramidal tract

G.J.Wassilchenko

Sensory pathway

Sacral spinal cord

urinary sphincter and the detrusor. Afferent neurons from the detrusor communicate with pudendal nuclei during voiding, which results in inhibition of pudendal firing during detrusor contraction. Therefore, when the pelvic floor fires, the external striated sphincter relaxes, significantly decreasing urethral resistance to urinary outflow. Conversely, during bladder filling the external sphincter is active, causing tone within the external sphincter and adjacent musculature while the motor portion of the pelvic nerve is inhibited. Interruption of loop III will result in incoordination of the detrusor and external sphincter (detrusor-sphincter dyssynergia).[109]

Loop IV extends from the sensorimotor cortex to the periurethral striated musculature (Fig. 12-12). The motor neurons follow the pyramidal tracts in the lateral columns of the spinal cord and synapse on the pudendal nuclei in the conus medullaris. The fourth loop provides for volitional control of the external sphincter during bladder filling and micturition so that the reflexive relaxation of

the third loop can be overcome in the normal adult by a conscious desire to contract the external sphincter.[109]

Peripheral nervous system control. Three major peripheral nerves carry the afferent and efferent neural messages that allow the central nervous system to regulate the function of the lower urinary tract. During bladder filling, the pudendal and hypogastric nerves are active and the motor portion of the pelvic nerve is quiet. Firing of the hypogastric nerve results in a predominance of beta-adrenergic firing in the bladder wall, which relaxes the detrusor muscle to allow urine to fill the vesicle under low intravesical pressures; and it results in a predominance of alpha-adrenergic firing in the bladder neck, preventing leakage of urine into the urethra. In addition, firing of the pudendal nerve causes increased tone at the external sphincter, which plays an important complementary role in continence when intra-abdominal pressure rises sharply.[8]

During bladder filling, sensory receptors that respond

to stretch send signals to the brain via spinal pathways, producing an urgency to void. However, the supraspinal centers will respond to this stimuli by causing further sympathetic predominance in the bladder, resulting in the continuation of bladder filling and the suppression of sphincter and detrusor activity. In the normal adult this process continues until a volitional decision is reached to empty the bladder of urine by voiding.

The first act of micturition is the volitional relaxing of the external striated sphincter and adjacent pelvic floor musculature. The pelvic nerve will fire, causing an inhibition of sympathetic predominance of the detrusor and bladder neck. The bladder relaxes and the detrusor muscle contracts, forcing urine through the urethra and outside the body. If the external urinary sphincter is volitionally contracted, stopping the urinary stream, the detrusor contraction is not immediately stopped: intravesical pressure will initially rise and then fall as the contraction is suppressed by prolonged contraction of the external sphincter. Unless volitionally stopped, a detrusor contraction will continue until virtually all of the urine stored in the bladder is emptied. Once empty, the bladder will begin to refill with urine and the mechanisms to maintain continence are again stimulated.

Other modulators of lower urinary tract function. In addition to the neural regulation of the detrusor muscle, other biochemical substances in the body exert an influence on detrusor function. Specific peptides that affect detrusor activity, such as substance P, have been identified in the bladder walls of experimental animals. Prostaglandins E_1, E_2, and $F_{2\alpha}$ have been identified in the detrusor and urethra in humans and are known to influence both the duration of detrusor contractions and the tone at the bladder neck.[4,102]

Male Genitalia

Scrotum. The scrotum is a cutaneous, fibromuscular sac that is dependent below the pubis bone and houses the testes and lower portion of the spermatic cord. The skin of the scrotum is thin and deeply pigmented and contains abundant sebaceous glands, sweat glands, and hair follicles. The cutaneous layer of the scrotum is bisected by the median ridge or raphe, which extends from the base of the penis to the anus. The skin of the scrotum is further distinguished by rugae. The rugae are formed by parallel dermal muscle fibers and are more clearly seen on younger men, particularly when the testes have retracted because of a certain stimulus. Immediately under the skin is the dartos muscle, which is composed of smooth muscle fibers and elastic tissue. The dartos is a continuation of the suspensory ligament of the penis and superficial fascia of the abdominal, inguinal, and perineal fascia. It sends a sagittal reflection inward, creating an incomplete septum between the median ridge and the radix of the penis, which form the cavities in which the testes lie.[61,116]

The primary functions of the scrotum are to house the testes and provide an adequate environment for the production of sperm. The structure of the dartos allows for considerable variation of scrotal size in response to a variety of stimuli, such as external temperature, physical activity level, and emotions.[61]

Testes. The testes are a pair of ovoid organs that lie in the scrotum. They receive vascular, neural, and lymphatic support from the spermatic cord; the scrotal ligament forms the single scrotal attachment for the testes. Each testis is approximately 4 to 5 cm in length and 2.5 cm in width and weighs from 10.5 to 20 g. The left testis typically lies 1 cm lower than the right.[61,116]

The testes lie under three coverings: the tunica vaginalis, the tunica albuginea, and the tunica vasculosa. The tunica vaginalis arises from the peritoneum and forms a closed sac in which the testis is invaginated. The tunica albuginea is a white, fibrous covering for the testis that helps define the interior architecture of the organ. The posterior border of the tunica albuginea projects into the testis, forming an incomplete vertical septum called the mediastinum testis. From its front and lateral aspects, numerous fibrous projections extend toward the external border of the testis, dividing it into 200 to 300 lobules that contain several seminiferous tubules. The tunica vasculosa is the third testicular covering. It consists of a plexus of blood vessels within a framework of areolar tissue extending over the internal aspect of the tunica albuginea and covering its many septa, providing a vascular supply to each lobule.[61,116]

The functional unit of the testicular cortex is the seminiferous tubule. Each lobule of the testis contains one to three (or sometimes more) seminiferous tubules that are 30 to 60 cm of tortuous length with both ends terminating into a relatively short, straight segment called the canaliculus rectus. The seminiferous tubules occupy 75% of testicular mass; their combined length is almost 1 mile.

A seminiferous tubule is formed of stratified epithelium four to eight cells thick with an identifiable internal lumen. The tubules contain Sertoli cells, spermatogenic cells, and an outer basement membrane with a fibrous tunica propria. The Sertoli cells are columnar in shape and extend radially from just within the outer basement membrane toward the tubular lumen. These interesting cells have indefinite cytoplasmic borders; spermatids and spermatocytes may be completely embedded within the cytoplasm of the Sertoli cells. The Sertoli cells are linked in tight junctions that divide the wall of the seminiferous tubule into two parts: a basal compartment containing spermatogonia and spermatocytes and a luminal compartment containing more advanced stages of testicular germ cells. The exact function of the Sertoli cells remains unclear. They are presumed to provide nourishment and succor for the germinal epithelium, help maintain the blood-testis barrier, secrete the testicular fluid seen in the lumen of the seminiferous tubules, and secrete an androgen-binding protein that promotes the accumulation of androgens in the immediate area of the germinal cell epithelium.[104]

The germinal cell epithelium of the seminiferous tubule is characterized by an ever-changing population of maturing stages of spermatic forms. The more primitive forms are found at the outer borders, and more mature forms are found nearer the inner lumen. Spermatogonia are the most immature cell form seen in the spermatic cycle. Other stages of germ cell epithelium seen in the wall of the seminiferous tubules are primary and secondary spermatocytes as well as spermatids.[104]

The interstitial tissue within the testicular lobules is composed of Leydig's cells, blood vessels, extensive lymphatic channels, and numerous macrophages. Leydig's cells are found in small groups of five to twenty and compose 12% of testicular volume. These are particularly significant because they secrete testosterone, which enters the bloodstream via interstitial capillary beds or goes directly into the seminiferous tubule without going through vascular routes.[104]

The structure and function of the testes in the adult male are significantly different than those seen during infancy and childhood. The germinal elements of the testes have a distinct embryologic origin from the other elements of the gonads. The nongerminal cell components of the testes arise as part of the mesodermic mass that will develop into the urogenital ridge; the germ cells of the testes arise from the entoderm lining the posterior aspect of the yolk sac. Development of both the germinal cell and somatic elements of the testes begins during the fourth week of life.[37]

From their retroperitoneal position, the testes must descend caudally to the scrotal sac in order to mature into viable structures away from the high temperature of the internal abdomen. During the third trimester they begin moving down the posterior aspect of the abdomen, bringing its neurovascular sheath with them. By the seventh month of gestation, the testes enter the internal ring of the inguinal canal and move into their extra-abdominal position at or shortly after birth. The complex factors that regulate this migration are still not fully understood.[37]

At birth the testes are composed of small tubules with poorly differentiated components and few identifiable spermatogonia. Interstitial cells are present at birth but regress over the first several weeks of life to a baseline level that persists throughout the pubescent period. During the period between 4 and 10 years of life, the seminiferous tubules slowly increase in tortuosity. Beginning around age 10 a significant increase in the size, number, and mitotic activity of the germ cell epithelium occurs. This process continues until the onset of puberty around age 12 when the interstitial Leydig's cells mature and begin to produce testosterone levels comparable with adult values and active spermatogenesis begins.[104]

The blood supply of the testes is unique since the temperature of arterial and venous blood must be cooled approximately 2° C from abdominal levels in order to support spermatogenesis. Cooling arises from interactions between arterial and venous vessels in which a countercurrent heat loss mechanism occurs. In addition, the slow, nonpulsating flow of the spermatic artery aids in cooling the vascular beds of the testes.[104]

The arterial blood supply of the testes arises from the internal spermatic artery, the cremasteric artery, and the deferential, or vasal, artery. The latter are important clinically as collateral circulation of the testes. Venous blood from the testes drains into the pampiniform plexus of the spermatic cord, which empties into the internal spermatic veins.[104]

Because of the unique embryologic origins of the testes, the lymphatic drainage is not into local inguinal or pelvic lymph nodes. Rather, the extensive lymphatic channels of the testes drain into the preaortic lymph nodes.[61]

Three adnexa of the testes are of clinical significance; all are composed of vestiges of the embryonic structures relevant to the formation and migration of the testes and spermatic cord. The appendix testes arise in the groove between the head of the epididymis and the testicular remnant of the müllerian duct. It is subject to torsion and must be differentiated from true testicular torsion, which constitutes a urologic emergency. The appendix epididymis is a pear-shaped body attached to the epididymal head, which is a remnant of epigenitalis tubules. The organs of Giraldes are a paragenitalis remnant sometimes noted in the lower spermatic cord anterior to the head of the epididymis.[61]

Epididymis and vas deferens. The epididymis and vas deferens are the efferent routes for sperm leaving the testes after completing the spermatogenic cycle. Along with the prostate and seminal vesicles, the epididymis and vas deferens provide transport, storage, and support for maturing sperm as they migrate toward the male urethra.[116]

The epididymis is a sausage-shaped structure approximately 5 cm long that is attached to the posterolateral aspect of the testis. Three anatomic regions of the epididymis are described: the head, or globus major; the body, or corpus; and the tail, or globus minor. The epididymis contains a single compartment so that injury is likely to entirely ablate the function of the organ. The epididymis is covered by the tunica vaginalis on all except the posterior border, where a fascial reflection forms the epididymal sinus.[61,116]

Inside the compartment of the epididymis is a long, tortuous canal with little muscular tone but abundant cilia lining the tubular lumen folded over on itself and tightly packed so that its total length is 4 to 5 m. The head of the epididymis is directly connected to the efferent ductules, allowing sperm leaving the testis to enter the epididymal tubules via ciliary action. At the tail the tubules have more smooth muscle in their walls as the epididymis opens into the vas deferens.[116]

The vas deferens is a firm, elastic, cylindric tube extending from the termination of the epididymal tail to the ejaculatory duct located near the base of the prostate. The initial segment of the vas deferens is tortuous, although the part of the organ more distal to the testis is straight. From its origin at the epididymal tail, the vas deferens ascends along the posterior wall of the testis adjacent to the medial aspect of the epididymis. The vas then moves upward to the posterior part of the spermatic cord, traversing the inguinal canal to the level of the deep inguinal ring. At this point, the vas deferens leaves the spermatic cord, curves around the lateral aspect of the epigastric artery, and ascends several centimeters to the external iliac artery. The vas then crosses the external iliac obliquely and enters the false pelvis where it becomes a relatively fixed structure attached to the posterior abdominal wall. From this point the vas will cross the ureter and curve at an acute angle to traverse the prostatic base and terminate at the ejaculatory duct (Fig. 12-13). The final segment of the vas deferens is characterized by a spindle-shaped dilation of the tube called the ampulla. It is approximately 10 cm long and contains several false pouches or diverticula that may or may not be clinically significant.[116]

The wall of the vas deferens is composed of an innermost mucosal layer, a middle muscular layer, and an outer layer of areolar tissue. The mucosa of the vas is composed of columnar epithelial cells, which, unlike the tubules of the epididymis, are not ciliated. The muscular tunic consists of an inner longitudinal layer, a middle circular layer, and an outer longitudinal layer of smooth muscle fibers typical of such structures in the body. The outer layer of areolar tissue contains the neural, vascular, and lymphatic supply for the vas.[61,116]

The blood supplies of the vas deferens and the epi-

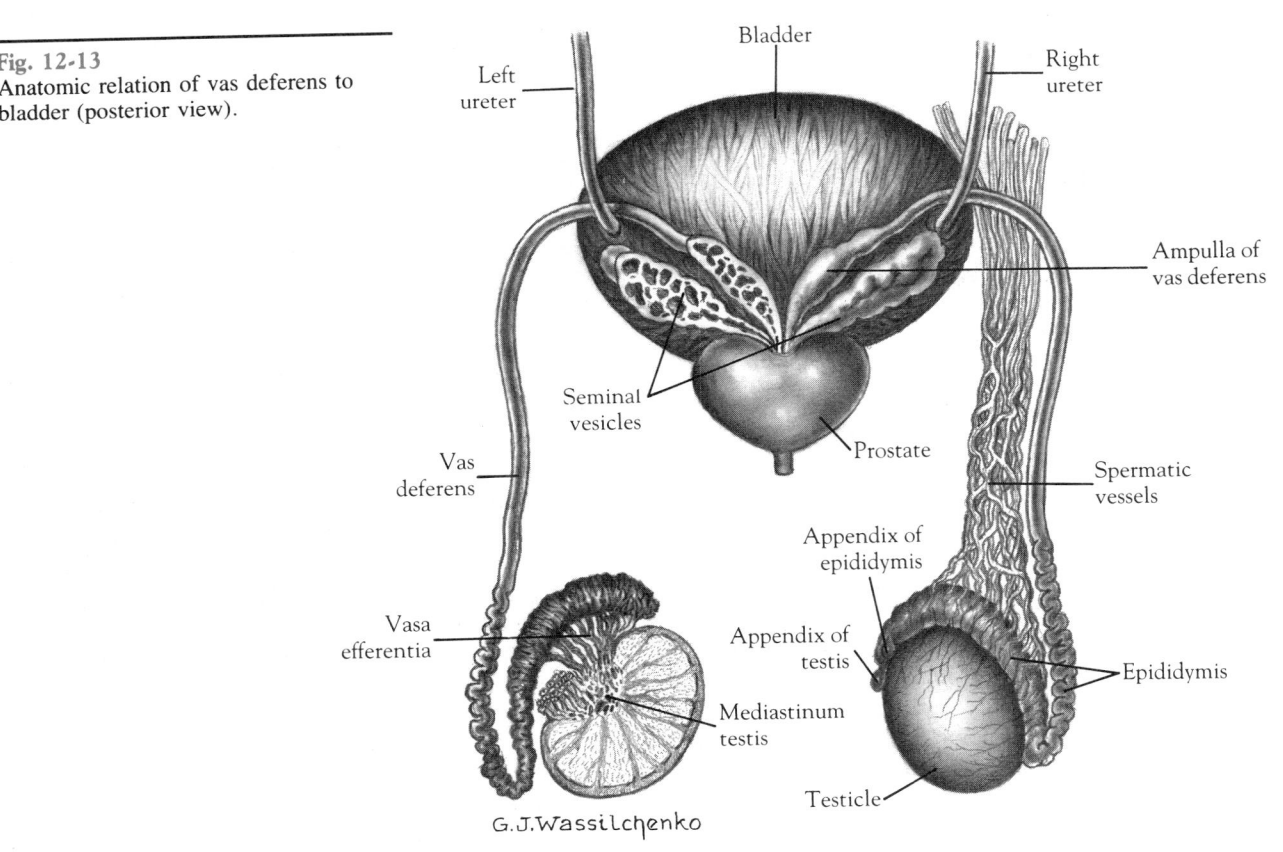

Fig. 12-13
Anatomic relation of vas deferens to bladder (posterior view).

Bladder

Left ureter

Right ureter

Ampulla of vas deferens

Seminal vesicles

Vas deferens

Prostate

Spermatic vessels

Vasa efferentia

Appendix of epididymis

Appendix of testis

Mediastinum testis

Epididymis

Testicle

G.J.Wassilchenko

didymis are closely related. The epididymis receives arterial blood from the internal spermatic artery or the deferential artery; the vas deferens receives arterial blood from the deferential artery. Venous blood from the epididymis and lower segments of the vas drains into the pampiniform plexus of the spermatic cord, which will become the spermatic vein.[61,95]

The motor innervation of the vas deferens arises from the autonomic nervous system. Sympathetic fibers from the hypogastric and parasympathetic fibers from the pelvic nerve provide the powerful contractile pulses seen in the organ associated with ejaculation. Nerve fibers for pain are also found in the sheaths covering the vas and in the coverings of the epididymis.[61,104]

Lymphatic channels from the epididymis drain into the external iliac and hypogastric nodes. Lymphatic channels from the vas deferens drain into the external and internal nodes.[116]

Seminal vesicles and ejaculatory ducts. The seminal vesicles are a pair of saclike structures that lie between the posterior bladder and the rectum. Each vesicle is 4 cm long; they have a pyramidal shape with the superior end oriented laterally and backward from the base. The structure of the seminal vesicles is formed by a single coiled tube that gives rise to irregularly placed diverticula connected by dense fibrous tissue. The diameter of the tube of the seminal vesicle is 3 to 4 mm, and its length is 10 to 15 cm when uncoiled. The seminal vesicles are directed to the posterior bladder surface near the implantation of the ureters and lie in close proximity to the rectum.[65,116]

The walls of the seminal vesicles are composed of an outer areolar layer of connective tissue, a middle layer of muscular tissue, and a luminal layer of mucosal epithelium characteristic of the organs for sperm transport and maturation. The muscular tunic is formed by inner circular smooth muscle fibers and an outer layer of longitudinal smooth muscle. The mucosal layer consists of columnar epithelium with an abundance of goblet cells in the diverticula of the organ and small stellate cells of unknown significance.[116]

The ejaculatory ducts are located along the median plane of the seminal vesicles and are formed by the terminal segment of the vas deferens and the terminal duct of the seminal vesicles. The ejaculatory ducts originate at the prostatic base, run anteroinferiorly between the right and left median prostatic lobes, pass alongside the prostatic utricle, and end in the posterior urethra. The walls of the ejaculatory ducts are thin and characterized by an outer fibrous layer that terminates beyond the prostatic portion of the ducts, a middle layer of nonstriated muscle, and an inner layer of columnar epithelial cells.[116]

The blood supply of the seminal vesicles is similar to

that of the prostate gland. The primary motor innervation arises from sympathetic fibers. The lymphatic channels from the seminal vesicles drain into the hypogastric, sacral, vesical, and external iliacs (Fig. 12-13).[95]

Prostate. The prostate is a partly glandular, partly fibromuscular organ that lies at the base of the bladder and surrounds the initial 2 to 3 cm of posterior urethra. The prostate is conical in shape with an anterior and posterior flattening; its average dimensions are 3.4 cm in length, 4.4 cm in width, and 2.6 cm at its greatest thickness. The organ is securely anchored in its position with only a small degree at its base. The moorings of the prostate are the puboprostatic ligaments, Denonvillier's fascia, and the adjacent pelvic floor musculature. In addition, the resilient, strong prostatic capsule provides support.[61]

The structure of the prostate has been conceptualized in terms of lobes and zones. Anatomists report that there are no anatomic distinctions between the lobes of the prostate; however, the lobes conceptualized by urologists do have clinical significance. Williams and Warwick[116] conceptualize the prostate in terms of four anatomically distinguishable areas: the base, apex, posterior surface, and superior surface. The base of the prostate is contiguous with the bladder neck area. The urethra pierces the prostate at the base near its anterior border. The apex of the prostate is oriented inferiorly to the base; its surface is contiguous with fascia covering the superior aspect of the external urinary sphincter and transversus perinei muscles. The posterior surface is transversely flat and vertically convex. It is separated from the rectum by the prostatic sheath and loose connective tissue external to this sheath. The superior surface is analogous to the median lobe of the prostate; its inferior border is characterized by a sulcus that is used to mark the border between the right and left lateral lobes.[116]

Clinicians conceptualize the prostate in terms of intraurethral and extraurethral lobes: the intraurethral lobes are the anterior, right and left lateral, and subcervical lobes; the extraurethral lobes are the posterior and median lobes. The anterior lobe undergoes atrophy before pubescence and never becomes hyperplastic. The right and left lateral lobes of the prostate form the lateral walls of the prostatic urethra; they have clinical significance since hyperplasia of the glandular tissue of these lobes produces anatomic outlet urinary obstruction and the classic symptoms of benign prostatic hyperplasia. Hyperplasia of the glandular components of the subcervical lobe encroaches the lumen of the prostatic urethra in an upward fashion. The extraurethral lobes of the prostate gland are not as likely to undergo hyperplasia as are the intraurethral lobes. The posterior lobe lies along the posterolateral wall of the prostate between the apex and ejaculatory ducts. The posterior lobe is of great clinical significance because of its affinity for neoplastic degeneration later in life. The median lobe lies between the seminal vesicles and vesical neck; unfortunately, it is inseparable from the posterior lobe anatomically and is only appreciated in a portion of prostates in the adult male.[38]

The microscopic anatomy of the prostate is characterized by glandular components and fibromuscular components. The fibromuscular capsule sends extensions into the interior of the organ, whose apices converge in the posterior urethral surface. The fibromuscular tissue is primarily nonstriated muscle with a relatively small area of skeletal muscle located ventral to and contiguous with the external urinary sphincter. The bulk of muscular tissue is located in the fibromuscular septa found throughout the gland.[116]

The glandular tissue is composed of numerous follicles with frequent papillary elevations that open into long canals seen throughout the organ. These follicles join to form 12 to 20 excretory ducts. The glandular tissue of the prostate is supported by extensions of muscular tissue and delicate areolar stroma that encapsulate a capillary plexus. Three zones of glandular tissue are distinguishable. The peripheral zone contains long branched glands that curve posteriorly to open into prostatic sinuses or directly into the posterior urethra.[116]

The motor and sensory innervation of the prostate gland arises from the lower segments of the inferior hypogastric plexus. The arterial blood supply of the prostate is derived from branches of the internal pudendal, middle rectal, and inferior vesical arteries. Venous blood from the prostate drains into the periprostatic space and into the internal iliacs or deep penile veins. Lymphatic channels from within the prostate drain into the external iliac nodes or the sacral lymph nodes.[116]

Penis. The penis is a cylindrically shaped organ in its flaccid state that contains two portions: a root that attaches to the perineum and a pendulous portion called the corpus, or body. The root of the penis is attached to the pelvic floor via a continuation of Buck's fascia, the pubic rami (crura of the corpora cavernosa), and the suspensory ligament.[61]

The body of the penis contains three elongated bodies of erectile tissue that are capable of considerable enlargement when they become engorged with blood during tumescence (Fig. 12-14). The left and right corpora cavernosa form the majority of the substance of the penile body and lie in close approximation of one another. They are surrounded by an extension of the tunica albuginea containing superficial and deep layers. The superficial layer is composed of longitudinally arranged fibers that surround the two corpora cavernosa as a unit; the deep layer is composed of circularly arranged fibers that encase each corpora separately via a fibrous septum that forms two median grooves of anatomic significance. The larger median groove houses the corpus spongiosum and pendulous urethra; the smaller median groove houses the deep dorsal veins. The corpora cavernosa do not reach the distal end of the penis; instead, they terminate in the proximal portion of the glans.[116]

The corpus spongiosum lies inferiorly to the corpora cavernosa and is pierced throughout its length by the urethra. It is smaller than the paired corpora cavernosa

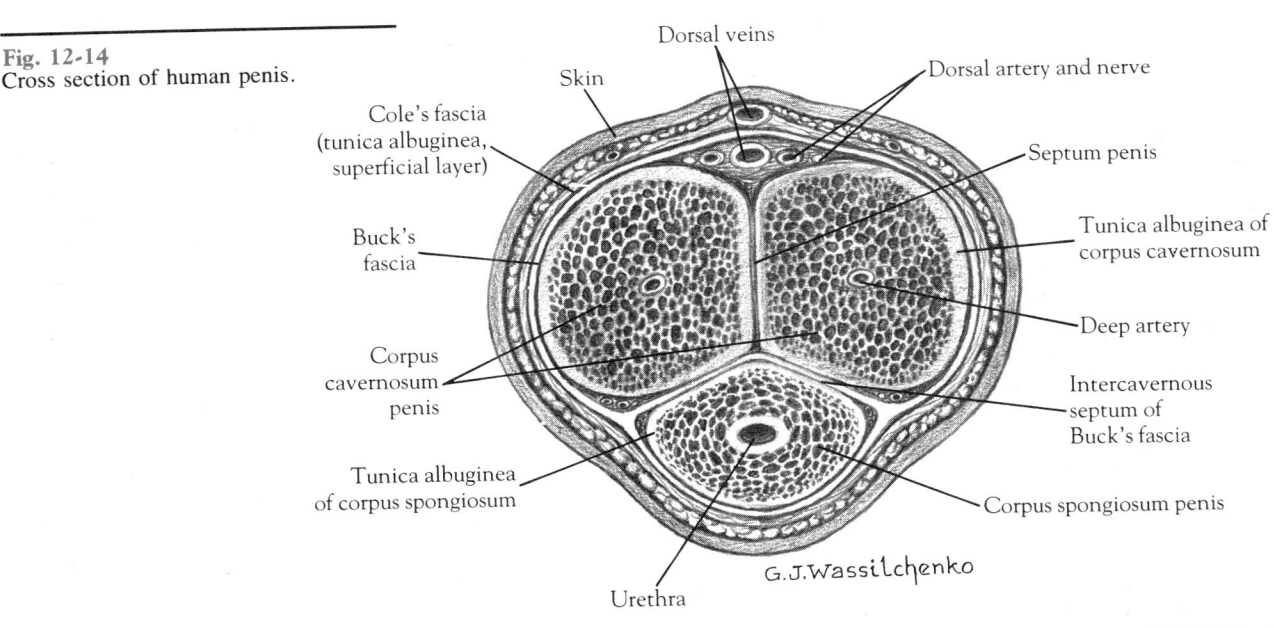

Fig. 12-14
Cross section of human penis.

Dorsal veins

Skin

Cole's fascia (tunica albuginea, superficial layer)

Buck's fascia

Corpus cavernosum penis

Tunica albuginea of corpus spongiosum

Dorsal artery and nerve

Septum penis

Tunica albuginea of corpus cavernosum

Deep artery

Intercavernous septum of Buck's fascia

Corpus spongiosum penis

Urethra

G.J.Wassilchenko

and is also surrounded by a reflection of the tunica albuginea.[116]

The skin of the penis is characterized by its thinness, relatively dark color, and loose connection with the underlying fascia. At the distal portion of the penis, the skin is folded over on itself to form the foreskin covering the glans penis. The internal layer of the foreskin is anatomically to the neck of the penis and the glans and is continuous with the mucous membranes of the external urethral orifice. On its urethral aspect the foreskin contains a small median fold extending from its deep surface to the point of the glans immediately proximal of the urethral meatus, called the frenulum. The glans penis covers the distal portion of the corpora cavernosa and forms their terminal connection. It is pierced by the navicularis fossa of the urethra, which ends at a dorsal slit found on its inferior surface.[116]

The superficial fascia of the penis is characterized by loose areolar tissue and is devoid of any fat. A few fibers of dartos muscle from the scrotum are present as are fibers from the fundiform ligament and the suspensory ligament.[116]

The arterial blood supply of the penis arises primarily from the internal pudendal artery, which branches into the dorsal arteries of the penis to supply the deep structures of the organ. The penile skin also receives arterial blood from the external pudendal and femoral arteries.[61]

The venous drainage of the penis can be divided into deep and superficial groups. The deep veins of the penis drain the erectile bodies via the deep dorsal veins, which empty into the plexus of Santorini and ultimately into the hypogastric vein. The superficial veins of the penis drain venous blood from the skin via the superficial dorsal penile veins that empty into the spahenous vein.[61]

The lymphatic drainage of the penis is also divided into deep and superficial groups. Deep lymphatic channels of the penis are drained by the subinguinal nodes and the external iliac nodes. Superficial lymphatic channels drain into the superficial inguinal nodes.[61]

The nerve supply of the penis has a somatic and an autonomic component. Sensory innervation of the penile skin arises from the pudendal nerve, which has its roots in spinal segments S2 to S4. Motor innervation to the corpora spongiosa and corpora cavernosa arises from the pelvic nerves, which also have their spinal roots at S2 to S4. Sympathetic fibers from the thoracolumbar spinal cord supply the penile vessels and are particularly evident in the vascular component of the corpus spongiosum.[86]

Male Reproductive Function

Spermatogenesis and hormonal regulation. The testes, epididymis, vas deferens, seminal vesicles, and prostate gland function as a coordinated unit to assure the production, maturation, and transport of sperm from the male urethra to the female vaginal tract necessary for propagation of the species. Male reproductive functions are regulated by a hormonal axis that consists of certain extrahypothalamic central nervous system centers, the hypothalamus, pituitary, testes, and gonadal-sensitive end organs.[43, 93]

Extrahypothalamic central nervous system centers are assumed to play an inhibitory and augmentative role in reproduction. The precise interactions by which brain centers influence the male reproductive hormonal axis are unclear, but a correlation between reproductive function and testicular function is postulated.[93]

The more clearly elucidated hormonal axis governing male reproductive function originates in the hypothalamus, where a luteinizing hormone–releasing hormone (LHRH) is produced and travels to the median eminence of the adenohypophysis via a venous portal system. The presence of this releasing factor in the pituitary results in the direct stimulation of luteinizing hormone (LH) and is thought to stimulate the release of follicle-stimulating hormone (FSH).[93]

Both FSH and LH act at receptor sites in the testes to stimulate the gonadal androgens (primarily testosterone and dihydrotestosterone). LH directly stimulates the Sertoli cells to produce testosterone and stimulate spermatogenesis. FSH is not necessary for the production of testosterone although it does play a role in spermatogenic testicular function. FSH and LH are released in a sporadic fashion in response to feedback from the hypothalamic–pituitary–gonadal hormonal axis. When blood levels of the gonadal androgens increase, the production of LHRH in the hypothalamus is inhibited, which suppresses the production of LH by the pituitary. Conversely, decreased serum levels of gonadal androgens will stimulate the hypothalamus to produce LHRH so that more LH is produced and excreted into the systemic circulation. The feedback loop for FSH production is not entirely understood; increased levels of testosterone and estradiol exert negative feedback on the production of FSH. In addition, a substance called inhibin, which is produced in the germinal epithelium of the testes, is postulated to inhibit FSH although its physiologic significance requires further investigation.[43,91]

The gonadal androgens are essential to the genesis, support, and maturation of spermatozoa. In addition to this direct role in male reproductive function, certain androgens, primarily testosterone and dihydrotestosterone, cause the development and maintenance of the secondary male sex characteristics that characterize pubescence.[91]

The process of spermatogenesis occurs within the seminiferous tubule in the testis and is conceptualized in three phases. During the first phase the more primitive spermatogonia will enlarge and undergo mitotic divisions into primary spermatocytes that contain 92 chromosomes. The second phase is characterized by two consecutive meiotic divisions accompanied by only one duplication of chromosomes so that the final product of this phase is four spermatids that contain a haploid number of chromosomes suitable for union with the ovum. The third phase of spermatogenesis is titled spermiogenesis and marks the transformation of spermatid to spermatozoon.[63]

The process of spermiogenesis is relatively slow; it requires 74 days to complete and is divided into four phases. The first phase is the Golgi phase when small granules of hyaluronidase, proteases, and other substances form into a single large acrosomal granule enclosed within a vesicle that attaches to the nuclear membrane at the site of the future sperm head. During the second phase a cap appears around the acrosomal vesicle. The two centrioles of the spermatid now begin to move; the proximal centriole assumes a position at the posterior pole of the nucleus opposite the acrosomal sac while the distal centriole sprouts a flagellum consisting of two central microtubules and nine surrounding pairs of microtubules. The distal centriole will become the tail of the future spermatozoon. The third stage of spermiogenesis is the acrosomal phase, in which the developing sperm cell undergoes extensive metamorphosis so that the acrosome, nucleus, flagellum, and cytoplasm assume the characteristic appearance of the mature spermatozoon. During the acrosomal phase, a mitochondrial sheath is formed to supply energy for the tail of the mature sperm when it becomes motile after ejaculation. The final stage of spermiogenesis is the maturation phase, which is characterized by the completion of the tail of the spermatozoon and the shedding of excess cytoplasm with the assistance of the Sertoli cells (Fig. 12-15).[32,63]

Transport of the sperm from the seminiferous tubule

occurs via the muscular activity of the tubules and fluid movement. Although the sperm that enter the epididymis are mature in appearance, they are not yet capable of motility and not yet able to fertilize an ovum. Thus the epididymis also plays a necessary role in the maturation of sperm. The transit time of sperm through the relatively short epididymis is 12 days. The structure of the epididymis allows relatively slow transit resulting from the slow peristaltic-like activity of the smooth muscle of the organ and the ciliary action of the efferent ductules. Within the time spent within the epididymis, sperm will gain the potential for motility although a substance in the tubular fluid prevents sperm from becoming motile before ejaculation. Although the process by which this maturation occurs is not known, the epididymis is thought to play an active role under the influence of the gonadal androgens (primarily testosterone). The probable maturational functions provided by the epididymis are manipulation of the sodium ion, potassium ion, and chloride ion concentrations in the fluid in the epididymal tubule and the secretion of a variety of compounds such as glycerylphosphorylchlorine and glycoproteins, which are thought to enhance maturation of the spermatozoa.[22,32]

The epididymis also serves as a storage compartment for sperm. The cauda epididymidis may store sperm for a period of several weeks although the storage time in a man who is extremely sexually active is a matter of hours.[22]

After exiting the epididymis the sperm enters the vas deferens in response to smooth muscle contraction associated with ejaculation. Sperm is carried into the ejaculatory ducts, where it is mixed with the nutritive secretions of the seminal vesicles. The seminal vesicles do not, as their name implies, serve as storage compartments for sperm; rather, they secrete a mucoid fluid rich with fructose and other nutritive substances into the ejaculatory duct after the vas deferens empties itself of sperm. In addition to their nutritive support, the seminal vesicles add prostaglandins to the ejaculate that are thought to aid in fertilization of the ovum.[32]

The prostate also supports the male reproductive act by adding its secretions to the ejaculate. During ejaculation the prostatic capsule contracts in synchrony with the vas deferens and secretes a thin, milky fluid that contains a variety of substances including citric acid, calcium, acid phosphate, a clotting enzyme, and profibrinolysin. The pH of this secreted fluid is relatively high (ranging from 6.0 to 6.5), which favors the extended survival of sperm in the harsh, acidic environment created by the vaginal mucosa.[32]

The ejaculated semen thus contains fluid from the vas deferens, the seminal vesicles, and the prostate gland, as well as mucus from the posterior urethral glands, par-

Fig. 12-15
Mature spermatozoon cell.

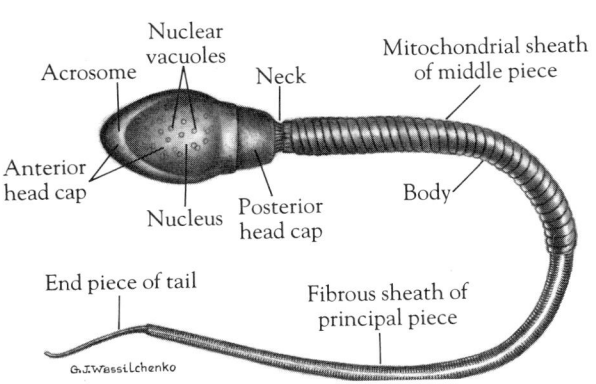

Acrosome
Nuclear vacuoles
Neck
Mitochondrial sheath of middle piece
Anterior head cap
Nucleus
Posterior head cap
Body
End piece of tail
Fibrous sheath of principal piece
G.J.Wassilchenko

ticularly the bulbourethral gland. The pH of the semen is approximately 7.5; the prostatic secretions give the semen a milky appearance, and the seminal vesicle fluid contributes the characteristic mucoid appearance. The normal ejaculate contains 75,000,000 to 400,000,000 sperm cells. After ejaculation a clotting enzyme in the semen will interact with profibrinolysin contributed by the prostate to form a weak coagulum. When this dissolves the sperm will gain their maximal motility as each seeks to fertilize an ovum. Although the sperm cell can survive several months in the male genital ducts, it can survive only 12 to 24 hours in the female genital tract after ejaculation. The relatively short life of sperm in the female genital tract is primarily the result of the acidic nature of the vaginal and fallopian mucosa.[32]

Physiology of erectile activity. The other reproductive function of the male necessary for procreation is the generation and maintenance of an erection in order to introduce semen into the female genital tract. The penis is primarily an organ of copulation with a secondary function as a conduit for the expulsion of urine during micturition. The erectile activity of the penis depends on complex interactions of neural and vascular events within the context of the psychosocial aspects of male sexuality.[61,116]

An erection of the penis is attained when the cavernous bodies become engorged with blood so that the organ assumes a straight line between its root and pendulous portion. Although the corpus spongiosum is involved indirectly with erectile activity, it is the corpora cavernosa that attain the needed volume and rigidity for complete penile erection.[72]

The vascular events that initiate and maintain erections in the male remain unclear. Tumescence depends on the trapping of blood in the corpora cavernosa; whether this is primarily an arterial event or the result of venous constriction is not known. During the flaccid state, blood flow to the corporal bodies is provided by branches of the pudendal arteries and drained via the deep dorsal veins of the penis. Some investigators have postulated that constriction of the deep dorsal veins of the penis is needed for erection. However, others have shown that compression of the dorsal penile vein in dogs does not mimic normal tumescence and opening the dorsal vein to atmospheric pressure does not ablate an erection. More current investigations into the hemodynamics of penile erections have implicated arterial shunting of blood via arteriovenous shunts in the penile vasculature as the cause of tumescence. Three types of arteriovenous anastomoses have been described; the most abundant and functionally significant are the helicine arteries, whose terminal branches open directly into the corpora cavernosa and act as the afferent venous component for the shunting mechanism.[72]

In 1952, Conti[15a] argued that von Ebner's polsters are the physiologic regulators of the arteriovenous shunting that occurs during erection. Polsters, or cushions, are formed of longitudinally arranged smooth fibers and areolar tissue that are found in the walls of the penile vasculature. Great variability in the location, extent, and relative proximity of von Ebner's polsters exists. Polsters are also found in the pudendal vessels outside the penis and in other muscular blood vessels such as the carotid, hepatic, renal, and gastric arteries. Therefore the physiologic importance of polsters in erections is questioned. Several alternate theories concerning the nature of polsters exist; the most prominent theory states that these structures are responses to stress and aging that are not seen in neonates but may be observed in varying degrees in the adult male's penis.[50,72]

The generation and maintenance of an erection cannot be explained as a solely vascular event. Rather, penile tumescence requires the coordination of the central nervous system, peripheral nervous system, and neuroendocrine mechanisms. The motor activity of the corpora cavernosa is modulated by the autonomic nervous system, and stimulation of the pelvic nerve will produce an erection. The pelvic nerve is only the preganglionic portion of the neural tract; thus infusion of atropine will not ablate an erection. The neurotransmitter substance at the postganglionic nerve in the corpora is not known. Sympathetic fibers are present in the penile vasculature and are particularly prominent in the corpus spongiosum. Stimulation of sympathetic fibers produces vascular constriction but not erection. The significance of adrenergic fibers in the corpora cavernosa has not been fully appreciated although they are thought to assume an active role in erectile activity.[86]

The spinal cord is important to male sexual function since it is the origin of the autonomic outflow for the penis. Since both the sympathetic and parasympathetic nervous systems play a role in erections, injury to the spinal cord will produce variations of erectile dysfunction. Injury to the sacral spinal cord is not always connected with impotence. Approximately one third of such patients are able to generate erections using psychogenic stimuli. If the spinal cord is injured, volitional erections are abolished but reflex erections are noted in response to local stimuli.[86]

The brain directly affects penile erections as well as controlling male sexual behavior. A number of brain centers have been found to influence erectile activity, including the temporal lobes, the gyrus rectus of the cerebral cortex, the cingulate gyrus, the hypothalamus, the mammillary bodies, and the hippocampus. The hippocampus and cingulate gyrus influence emotional responses and communicate with the hypothalamus. The mammillary bodies and cingulate gyrus process visual stimuli; the gyrus rectus processes olfactory stimuli. The precise mechanisms through which the brain affects penile erections and human sexuality are complex and poorly understood.[86]

The neuroendocrine mechanisms that influence erectile activity are also poorly understood. Male sexual activity is decreased by serotonin activity and increased by dopamine activity. Male sexual activity is also affected by the presence of testosterone. Castration is connected with decreased sexual function although it does not preclude the ability to produce an erection.[86,97]

Wagner[97] has described four phases of erection that combine existing knowledge of erectile physiology. The first is the resting phase, in which the corporal bodies are maintained at a constant volume, and intracavernous pressure and blood flow rate are significantly less than during an erection. The second phase is called tumescence and is characterized by an increase in the volume in the cavernous spaces of the penis and a subtle increase in intracavernous pressure. On inspection a small increase in penile length precedes a slight increase in circumference. During the third phase the penis becomes fully erect so that intracavernous pressures will exceed 80 mm Hg. The fourth phase is divided into two segments: a slow and a rapid detumescence stage. During the rapid detumescence phase, rigidity of the penis quickly disappears and is followed by a more gradual loss of blood volume in the corpora cavernosa and a return to the values of the first phase.

NORMAL FINDINGS

Area of Concern	Normal Adult Findings	Variations in Child	Variations in Older Adult
Kidney	Overlying skin: edema, bulges, and masses in abdomen absent Palpable only with deep inspiration; may be nonpalpable in obese or muscularly developed persons; smooth, nontender Costovertebral angle tenderness: absent Bruit over costovertebral area or upper abdominal quadrants: absent Transillumination with darkened room and fiberoptic light source: absent	Readily palpable before 6 wk of age; lobulation of organ produces lumpy feeling on palpation	
Bladder	Noted as bulge in abdomen when vesicle contains 500 ml or more urine Noted as dull area under suprapubic skin when vesicle is filled with 150 ml or more urine Inspection of voiding act: steady, straight stream, no spraying, no abdominal straining; postvoid dribble absent; postvoid residual: less than 20% of total bladder volume	Spontaneous act: absent straining; split stream or spraying before age of social continence	Decreased force of stream compared to younger adult years; absent split stream, spraying, and postvoid dribble
Male Genitalia Penis	Skin: may be darker than surrounding integument Ulcers, warts, indurated nodules: absent Foreskin: retractable over glans penis; absent in circumcised males Glans penis: hairless, sagittal slit near apex Penile shaft: absent nontender plaques beneath surface in flaccid state Erect state: even firmness and rigidity over both corpora cavernosa; straight line described between root of penis and glans penis	Foreskin: difficult to retract in infancy or early childhood	Decreased rigidity to corpora cavernosa compared to younger adult years; lateral curvature: absent

Area of Concern	Normal Adult Findings	Variations in Child	Variations in Older Adult
Scrotum	Skin: rugae; hair bearing and loosely mobile Sebaceous cysts: absent Testes: firm, nontender to gentle palpation; masses: absent	Testes: palpable in scrotum; may retract into abdomen when exposed to cool air or examiner's hands	Testes: softer to palpation than in younger adult years
	Epididymis: palpable as comma-shaped structure on posterior aspect of testes; no tenderness, masses, or nodules Spermatic cord: rolled between thumb and forefinger; vas deferens palpable but nontender Varicocele: absent Transillumination: no edema or solid masses that will transilluminate		
Prostate	Posterior aspect of organ accessible beneath anterior rectal wall; two firm, nontender, symmetric, rounded lobes separated by median sulcus (heart shaped and 2.5 cm in length): projects into rectal lumen 1 cm or less Hard, irregular nodes: absent	Difficult to evaluate before 15 yr of age	Increased bogginess noted on digital examination; seen with benign hypertrophy of organ Asymmetric changes in lobe size or discrete nodules: absent

NORMAL LABORATORY VALUES

Laboratory Test	Normal Adult Values	Variations in Child
Acid phosphatase (blood)	Up to 0.8 IU/L; method dependent	
Alkaline phosphatase (blood)	Approximately 35-100 IU/L by SMA 12-60; higher in pregnancy	Higher than adult values
Calcium		
Blood	Up to 30 yr: 8.2-10.5 mg/dl; decreases very slightly in older years	Infants up to 1 mo: 7-11.5 mg/dl 1 mo to 1 yr: 8.6-11.2 mg/dl; normal range slowly descends
Ionized serum	4.75-5.2 mg/dl	
Calculated ionized	3.9-4.8 mg/dl	
Urine	Varies with diet; based on average calcium intake of 600-800 mg/24 h, excretion may be 100-250 mg/24	
Creatinine		
Blood	Male: up to 1.2 mg/dl Female: up to 1.1 mg/dl	1-5 yr: 0.3-0.5 mg/dl 5-10 yr: 0.5-0.8 mg/dl
Urine	Male: 1-2 g/24 h Female: 0.8-1.8 g/24 h	2-3 yr: 6-22 mg/kg/24 h >3 yr: 12-30 mg/kg/24 h
Creatinine clearance test	Male: 85-125 ml/min/1.73 m^2 Female: 75-115 ml/min/1.73 m^2	70-140 ml/min/1.73 m^2
Cystine (urine)	Random sample negative	
Oxalate (urine)	Up to 40 mg/24 h	
Parathormone (blood)	Dependent on individual laboratory and calcium result	
Inorganic phosphorus		
Blood	2.5-4.5 mg/dl	At birth: 5.6-8.0 mg/dl Childhood: approximately 4-7 mg/dl
Urine	0.9-1.3 g/24 h	

Laboratory Test	Normal Adult Values	Variations in Child
Sodium		
Blood	135-145 mEq/L	
Urine	27-287 mEq/24 h (varies significantly with dietary intake)	
Uric acid		
Blood	Male: 3.4-7.0 mg/dl	Increased in childhood
	Female: 2.4-6.0 mg/dl	
Urine	250-750 mg/24 h	
Urea nitrogen		
Blood (BUN)	1-40 yr: 5-20 mg/dl; gradual slight increase subsequently occurs	Birth to 1 yr: 4-19 mg/dl
Urine	6-17 g/24 h	
Urinalysis		
Albumin	<20 mg/dl	
Bilirubin	Negative	
Color	Clear, golden yellow	
Glucose	Negative	
Hemoglobin	Negative	
Ketones	Negative	
Microscopic urinalysis		
Bacteria	Negative	
Casts	0-4 hyaline casts per low-power field	
Crystals	Interpreted by physician	
Mucous threads	Negative	
Red blood cells	0-5 per high-power field	
Squamous epithelial cells	Seen on voided specimen in females; negative on voided specimen in males; negative for catheterized specimens	
White blood cells	0-5 per high-power field	

DIAGNOSTIC STUDIES

Urodynamic studies

A set of clinical/research procedures designed to describe ureteral, urethral, and bladder function; results displayed in graph form

Uroflowmetry

Determines rate, time, and volume of urinary flow

Study requires no catheterization: patient voids into a device that measures characteristics of bladder elimination

Nursing care:

Patient should force fluids and refrain from voiding for 2 hours before testing in order to have at least 300 ml in bladder

Cystometry

Evaluates the two phases of bladder function: filling/storage and expulsion/micturition

One or more catheters is placed in the bladder urethrally or suprapubically; bladder is then filled with a liquid contrast (water or a radiographic material) or carbon dioxide; patient is asked to report sensations of urgency to void and bladder fullness; study is completed by asking patient to void voluntarily

Nursing care:

Instruct patient to watch for signs of cystitis (frequency, dysuria), which should completely disappear within the first 24 hours after testing

Electromyography

Measures electrical activity of external, striated urinary sphincter in response to bladder filling/storage and micturition

EMG needles or hooked wire electrodes are placed directly into external urinary sphincter; or ECG patches are placed over perianal sphincter, measuring activity of pelvic floor musculature

Urethral pressure studies

Measure urethral resistance to urinary outflow

Catheter is pulled through urethra at a given rate while water or carbon dioxide is infused through several side ports; a specialized catheter may be placed at external urinary sphincter to measure urethral response to bladder filling/storage and micturition

Nursing care:

Instruct patient to watch for signs of cystitis (frequency and mild dysuria), which should disappear within the first 24 hours after testing

Pharmacologic testing

A series of two comparative cystometrograms performed before and 30 minutes after administration of a certain drug; most commonly used drugs are bethanechol chloride (Urecholine) and propantheline bromide (Pro-Banthine)

Bethanechol chloride used to assess "denervation" (neuropathic changes in bladder function) vs. functional voiding abnormalities

Propantheline bromide used to assess clinical response of detrusor overactivity to an anticholinergic agent

Nursing care:

Vital signs should be monitored every 15 to 30 minutes for a 2-hour period after testing

Bethanechol chloride may cause nausea and vomiting, hypotension, and shock; atropine given subcutaneously as an antidote if needed

Propantheline bromide may cause hypotension, hypertension, tachycardia, angina, and atrial or ventricular fibrillation; physostigmine salicylate given parenterally as an antidote if needed

Whitaker or Pfister test

Performed to assess ureteral obstruction when other methodologies (IVP, Lasix-enhanced renogram) fail to clearly diagnose or rule out any obstruction

Whitaker test performed by placing a nephrostomy tube percutaneously into renal pelvis of affected kidney; a urethral catheter is also placed to measure bladder pressure; sterile water, saline, or radiographic contrast material is perfused through the nephrostomy tube via a pump at a specific rate; continuous pressure monitoring used to assess presence of ureteral obstruction with bladder empty and full[114]

Pfister test similar to Whitaker test except that a 20-gauge spinal needle is used in place of nephrostomy tube and intermittent rather than continuous pressure monitoring is utilized to assess ureteral obstruction[79]

Nursing care:

Postprocedure complications include bleeding and infection; vital signs should be monitored regularly for the first 24 hours after testing; temperature is an important parameter in assessment of febrile urinary tract infection

Radiographic studies
Kidneys/ureters/bladder (KUB; plain film)

Radiographic film of kidneys, ureters, and bladder without contrast material; important as a scout film when performing an intravenous pyelogram and as a diagnostic study to determine presence of radiopaque calculi

Nursing care:

Preparation not standardized; an "IVP prep" is used when KUB is performed as part of this extensive radiographic study; in other situations, no preparation is indicated

Intravenous pyelogram (IVP; intravenous urogram; excretory urogram)

Contrast-enhanced radiographic study that provides detailed anatomic information about urinary tract; clues to function of kidney are provided by assessment of the organ's ability to concentrate and excrete contrast material; information concerning transport of urine through ureters is provided by use of sequential films after a contrast medium is injected; compression over ureters may be used to provide additional detail; assessment of bladder function is made by obtaining films of the vesicle filled with contrast material and after asking patient to void

Performed after adequate preparation and after a KUB is done

Patient is placed in slight Trendelenburg's position or supine and contrast material is injected intravenously; serial films of kidneys, ureters, and bladder are obtained over a period of time; entire examination requires approximately 30 minutes

Nursing care:

Because of risk of hypersensitivity reactions and potential renal failure secondary to IVP, a number of relative contraindications should be considered before completing the study:

History of allergic reaction when given intravenous iodine-bound contrast material

Patients at higher risk for dehydration, including elderly persons, patients with severe diabetes mellitus, patients with multiple myeloma, or patients with renal insufficiency[60]

Diagnostic value of IVP in first days of life is not clearly established

Postprocedure complications include hypersensitive reactions and acute renal failure; observe for allergic reactions such as urticaria, rhonchi, and shortness of breath; acute renal failure is a rare but serious complication of IVP; observe urinary output (at least 30 ml/h) while ensuring adequate fluid intake[60]

Radiation doses for IVP vary widely, ranging from approximately 1047 mR (milliroentgens) to 1465 mR[64]

Nephrotomogram

Most commonly done as part of IVP

Provides a more detailed reproduction of anatomic detail by focusing on a specific plane of the kidney rather than a nonspecific picture of the entirety of the kidneys

Nursing care:

See IVP

Cystogram, voiding cystourethrogram (VCUG)

Provides a detailed picture of bladder anatomy; vesicoureteral reflux assessed by visualizing area over ureters and right and left renal pelves

Voiding cystourethrogram provides information given by a cystogram along with images of the urethra during voiding phase of bladder function

Cystogram performed by infusing an x-ray medium intravesically under fluoroscopic monitoring

Voiding cystourethrogram performed in same manner; urethral images during voiding are obtained by removing catheter and asking patient to void while under fluoroscope

Nursing care:

Because cystogram and VCUG require placement of an indwelling catheter, cystitis is a potential complication; patient should be encouraged to force fluids for 24 hours following testing; frequency or mild dysuria should disappear completely within 24 hours; may be contraindicated in the presence of urosepsis in infant or child if vesicoureteral reflux is suspected

Retrograde pyelogram (RPG)

Provides a detailed anatomic description of ureter and renal pelvis

Performed in conjunction with cystoscopy because it requires placement of a 4-5 French ureteral catheter within ureter to be studied; radiographic contrast material is then injected into collecting system via gravity infusion or by syringe, and radiographic images are obtained

Nursing care:

Pyelonephritis is a potential side effect of retrograde pyelography; patient should be closely observed for signs of infection (flank pain, fever, chills) for a 24 to 48 hour period after testing

Overdistention of renal collecting system may result in extravasation of contrast medium leading to pain and fever; reaction typically transient; effects should disappear within 48 hours

Retrograde urethrogram (RUG)

Provides a detailed description of urethral anatomy when trauma or stricture is suspected

Performed by injecting contrast material in a retrograde manner into urethra via a catheter-tipped syringe or a Brodney clamp; patient is typically placed in a supine position and oblique films are taken

Nursing care:

Urethritis and cystitis are potential complications; patient should be encouraged to force fluids for a 24-hour period after testing; mild dysuria should cease within 24 hours of testing

Nuclear imaging of the urinary tract (radionuclides)

Set of diagnostic studies that measure certain parameters of renal, ureteral, and bladder function and determine presence of bony metastases in bladder, renal, and prostatic cancer

Renal scans (DTPA scan; DMSA scan)

Provide a functional assessment of glomerular filtration rate (GFR) and effective renal plasma flow (ERPF); DTPA scan also provides an assessment of ureters and bladder; renal scans expose patients to less radiation than does IVP; DMSA scan provides an assessment of individual kidney function

DTPA scan used primarily to assess upper urinary tract obstruction; radionuclide is injected in an intravenous bolus and sequential images are obtained; 30-second film taken to assess cortical blood flow; a 1-minute image and two images are obtained at 5, 10, 15, and 20 minutes; bladder and ureters are included in DTPA scan; DTPA scan assesses GFR and ERPF and provides differential renal function; primary indication is assessment of urinary tract obstruction because radionuclide used is affected by diuretics; furosemide is typically utilized and the change in renal excretion rate is quantified; delays in excretion indicate obstruction

DMSA scan useful in assessing functional renal cortical mass; radionuclide used in DMSA scanning is taken up by renal tubule so that functional cortical mass can be quantified; like DTPA scan, an intravenous bolus of radioisotope is administered and delayed images are obtained; indicated in cases of suspected renal scarring, assessment of segmental renal ischemia, and suspected intrarenal mass

Other radionuclides such as hippurate and radioxenon have been used for renal scans[62a] but are no longer widely used

Nursing care:

Require no preparation

Patients exposed to significantly less radiation than required by IVP; however, since a radioisotope is injected and excreted by the kidneys, patient may continue to excrete radionuclide after study is completed; pregnant women advised not to care for these patients during the initial 24 hours after testing

Bone scan

Methylene diphophosonate radioisotope injected in an intravenous bolus for a bone scan; images are obtained 2 hours after injection

Indicated when bony metastases are suspected in cases of renal, bladder, and prostatic cancer as well as neuroblastoma; bony metastases will demonstrate increased uptake of radionuclide

Nursing care:

Relatively noninvasive test that should produce no side effects other than possible local irritation from dye when injected

Nuclear cystogram (radionuclide cystogram)

Performed in a similar manner to radiographic cystography except that normal saline with a dose of a pertechnetate radionuclide is used rather than an iodine-bound contrast solution; like radiographic cystography, study requires no preparation

An indwelling catheter is passed into bladder via urethra; normal saline is infused into bladder, and radionuclide is injected into solution during bladder filling

May be performed rather than radiographic cystogram because patient is exposed to less radiation; however, nuclear cystogram does not provide anatomic detail seen in standard cystography

Nursing care:

Because catheterization is required for nuclear cystography, cystitis is a potential complication of the study; patient is encouraged to force fluids for a 24-hour period following test and advised that mild dysuria and urinary frequency should disappear completely within this time period

May be deferred in presence of urosepsis in infant or child if vesicoureteral reflux is suspected

Endoscopic studies

Set of diagnostic procedures that allow visualization of urethra, bladder, ureters, and calyces

Cystoscopy and panendoscopy

Cystoscope and panendoscope are instruments that allow direct visualization of bladder and urethra

Cystoscopy and panendoscopy may be performed while patient is under general or spinal anesthesia; in other cases, a local anesthetic, consisting of a lubricant jelly impregnated with lidocaine, is used

To perform cystoscopy, patient is placed in lithotomy position; sterile equipment is used; surgical gowns, gloves, and masks are typically used; a single sheath through which both cystoscope and panendoscope will be passed is inserted into bladder via urethra with adequate lubrication; a telescope is then passed through sheath while bladder is being filled with fluid; using fiberoptic system within the cystoscope, urologist visualizes internal architecture of bladder including bladder neck, urothelial lining, and ureteral orifices; bladder tumors, trabeculation, and inflammatory changes within the internal mucosa are assessed via cystoscopy; panendoscope is utilized to view bladder neck, prostatic urethra (in male), external urinary sphincters, and anterior urethra

Fluid is infused into bladder throughout procedure; infusion is stopped and bladder drained when it becomes filled with 300 to 500 ml of fluid

Cystoscopic and panendoscopic examination may be combined with radiographic diagnostic studies such as retrograde pyelogram or with therapeutic procedures such as transurethral resection of bladder tumor or prostate

Done gently with adequate lubrication so that patient should experience minimal discomfort following procedure

Nursing care:

Mild dysuria and transient hematuria should disappear within first 48 hours after procedure; patient should be able to void normally after routine cystoscopic examination

If general or spinal anesthesia is utilized, patient will be sent to recovery room after procedure and should be closely monitored for potential postanesthesia complications such as low-grade fever ($\leq 38°$ C [101° F]) for 24 to 48 hours

Biopsy of bladder, prostate, and urethra

Biopsy specimens from bladder, urethra, or prostate may be obtained utilizing a cystoscopic/panendoscopic system

A resectoscope, which uses an electrically activated wire loop or a tubular cold knife, is positioned over the lesion and a specimen is obtained

Important to ensure that the bladder is relatively full when a specimen is obtained in order to prevent inadvertent damage to normal mucosal folds

Nursing care:

Postprocedure care is similar to that of routine cystoscopic examination; mild dysuria may be seen with hematuria during the first 48 hours following the procedure; if general anesthesia is used, low-grade fever may occur over the first 24 to 48 hours after procedure; hematuria may recur 5 to 7 days after procedure; patient is assured that lesion is healing and that such hematuria is normal; patient should not experience significant frequency or dysuria at this time

Brush biopsy of renal pelvis and calices

Allows urologist to obtain a tissue biopsy from renal pelvis or calices without an open surgical incision

Ureteral catheter with a steel guide wire is placed using cystoscope as a guide; catheter is then removed and a steel or nylon brush is inserted to level of lesion so that a biopsy is obtained; specimen is then smeared on slides and prepared with a 95% ethanol solution; after specimen is obtained, renal pelvis is irrigated with normal saline[58a]

Nursing care:

Postprocedure care is similar to that of routine cystoscopic examination; low-grade fever may be noted; flank pain secondary to ureteral manipulation is not uncommon and should disappear within 48 hours; fevers greater than 38° C (101° F) and severe flank pain should be reported to physician

Needle biopsy of prostate

Done when prostatic cancer is suspected; transrectal or transperineal needle biopsy is often done in conjunction with cystoscopic examination; in other cases, biopsies may be done in the clinic with only local anesthesia

Transperineal biopsy performed by injecting a local anesthetic into skin of perineum over area where needle will enter; a finger in the rectum is used to guide the needle toward the suspicious area; procedure may be repeated several times to ensure an adequate biopsy

Transrectal biopsy requires no anesthesia; preparation includes cleansing enemas in order to decrease likelihood of introducing intestinal bacteria into bloodstream or prostatic tissue; prophylactic antibiotics are also indicated; when obtaining specimen, tip of needle is placed on examining finger and advanced gently to area over which biopsy is to be obtained; needle is then pushed and a biopsy is taken; procedure may be repeated several times[58a]

Nursing care:

Primary complication of transrectal biopsy (more commonly performed of the two techniques described) is sepsis from perforation of the bowel; fever and chills must be reported to physician at once; prophylactic antibiotic regimens must be strictly adhered to

Ultrasonography of urinary tract

A noninvasive, nonradiographic technique of examining anatomic architecture of urinary tract; utilizes sound waves inaudible to the human ear

Ultrasonography of kidneys

Patient placed in prone position; outline of kidneys obtained and marked on skin; serial scans are then made 1 to 2 cm apart perpendicular to longitudinal axis; additional views may be obtained with patient in supine position, which helps elucidate kidneys' relative position to other abdominal organs

Nursing care:

Noninvasive procedure; patient should experience no side effects

Ultrasound-guided biopsy of kidney

Ultrasonic examination may be combined with placement of a biopsy needle to define makeup of a renal or juxtarenal mass

Routine ultrasonic examination of affected kidney is completed first; mass is located and marked on skin; using sterile drapes, gloves, and local anesthetic, biopsy needle is placed into mass and a tissue sample withdrawn

Aspiration of a renal cyst may be performed in a similar manner

Ultrasonography of bladder and ureters

Ultrasonography of distended bladder provides some detail of vesical outline and may be used to evaluate diverticulum; abdominal ultrasound will detect presence of ureteral dilation although normal ureters may not be completely visualized

Typically combined with examination of kidneys

Nursing care:

Noninvasive and should cause no postprocedure complications

Because of necessity of distending the bladder to evaluate it, patient will wish to void immediately after examination

Ultrasonography of testes

Used to differentiate solid and cystic masses; in addition, torsion of testes is assessed by Doppler ultrasonic techniques, which assess both testicular morphology and blood flow

Nursing care:

> As with other ultrasonic techniques, examination of testes is not invasive and should cause no adverse effects for the patient

Computerized tomography of urinary system (CT scan; reconstructive tomography)

A specialized radiographic technique that presents multiple transverse plane views of organs of urinary system and adjacent structures

Computerized tomography of abdomen

Particularly valuable in defining abnormalities of renal parenchyma

Provides an estimate of density of masses and has the potential to differentiate solid tissue masses from cystic or hemorrhagic structures; varying densities are displayed as Hounsfield units; normal renal parenchyma measures 80 to 100 Hounsfield units; density of a cyst is lower while solid tumors have a similar density to renal parenchyma

Also utilized in evaluation of adrenal masses

An iodine-bound contrast material may be injected before testing in a similar manner to an IVP

To perform abdominal CT, patient is placed in a supine position and asked to lie still while a belt mechanism moves the body in order to obtain the needed images; images are generated and summarized into a series of transverse views of abdominal structures

Nursing care:

> If intravenous contrast material is used, nursing care for patient undergoing intravenous pyelogram is indicated
>
> Because of necessity of remaining still during testing, a general anesthetic may be used when testing infants and children; in these cases, patients should be monitored for side effects of the general anesthetic such as low-grade fever and nausea and vomiting

Computerized tomography of pelvis

Useful technique for evaluating masses (tumors) of pelvic contents and for evaluation of lymphatic enlargement that may be the result of metastatic invasion; pelvic abscesses may be elucidated by CT of the area; may elucidate any mass effect that causes distortion of bladder

Renal arteriography and venography

Provide a detailed description of arterial or venous structures within kidney

Renal arteriography

Provides information concerning arterial and venous blood supply to kidneys

Indications for arteriography include palpable renal masses, potential renovascular hypertension, renal trauma, and acute renal trauma; also used to determine suitability of renal donors

Preprocedure antianxiety/narcotic injection given before procedure; patient is taken to radiologic suite and an additional local anesthetic is given in area over femoral artery; patient is placed in a supine position and a femoral puncture is performed; an opaque catheter is then passed from the femoral artery to the aorta and into the desired renal artery under fluoroscopy; a radiopaque contrast material is then injected into renal artery (If passage into the aorta via the femoral artery is not feasible, the axillary artery may be used as an alternate.)

Rapid radiographic images used to assess the three phases of the arteriogram: arterial phase lasts 2 to 4 seconds and provides a detailed outline of the principal renal arteries; nephrogenic phase is seen as a marked opacification of the renal parenchyma, lasting 15 to 20 seconds; venous phase is of limited value because of kidneys' ability to extract and excrete contrast material (principally useful in assessment of arteriovenous shunting)

Digital subtraction angiography (DSA) is a new method of imaging that allows visualization of kidney's arteries utilizing a significantly smaller dose of contrast material than standard technique; has advantage of being rapid and relatively noninvasive compared to standard techniques so it can be performed on an outpatient basis with an IVP; limitations include poorer visualization of peripheral renal arterial branches[75a]

Nursing care:

> Postprocedure care aimed at preventing complications of procedure; the two major complications are bleeding at site of arterial puncture and allergic reactions to contrast material
>
> Assessment of pedal pulses and capillary filling of nail beds of foot should be done before procedure; after renal arteriogram is completed, femoral puncture site should be assessed regularly (every 1 to 2 hours) for hematoma or external bleeding; assessment of pedal pulses, capillary refill, and general appearance of affected foot is indicated; vital signs and assessment for signs of allergic reaction to contrast material are done frequently (every 1 to 2 hours); signs of allergic reaction include pruritus, wheezing, dyspnea, and flushed skin

Renal venography

Provides a detailed radiographic assessment of kidney's venous system in select instances; indications include renal vein thrombosis, renovascular hypertension, elucidation of renal cell carcinoma, and various congenital abnormalities of renal veins

To perform procedure, a percutaneous catheter is placed into right femoral vein and advanced to opening of renal vein; contrast material is injected, and catheter is then directed upward to enter contralateral (right) renal vein and procedure repeated; imaging may be enhanced by injecting 6 to 10 μg of epinephrine into renal artery followed by renal venography 10 seconds later

Nursing care:

Complications include postpuncture bleeding and allergic reaction to contrast material; assessment of puncture site for signs of hematoma is done routinely for a 24-hour period after testing; assessment for allergic reaction: pruritus, wheezing, dyspnea, and flushed skin

Conditions, Diseases, and Disorders

BENIGN PROSTATIC HYPERTROPHY

Benign prostatic hypertrophy is the progressive enlargement of the prostate gland associated with the aging process. The disease associated with benign prostatic hypertrophy is a result of the obstructive uropathies associated with glandular enlargement rather than a result of the hyperplastic process per se.

Benign prostatic hypertrophy (BPH) is the most common neoplastic growth among men past the fifth decade of life. Autopsy studies have shown that virtually all men over 50 years experience an increase in prostatic weight sometimes defined as BPH. However, when histologic changes are scrutinized, only slightly greater than half of men are diagnosed with a significant degree of BPH.[9,106]

Because of the increasing longevity among individuals in industrialized nations, the incidence of BPH is rising.[9,84] A retrospective study of the male population in the New Haven, Connecticut area between 1953 and 1961 demonstrated that a man aged 50 had a 10% chance of undergoing corrective surgery for obstructive symptoms from BPH within his lifetime. More current data reveal that a 50-year-old man has a 20% to 25% chance of undergoing surgery for prostatism.[84]

Improvements in the surgical treatment of BPH over the past century have significantly decreased the mortality associated with this condition. In Europe the death rate from prostatic surgery is 0.3% to 1.8%, and the overall death rate from conditions occurring as a result of BPH is 23 per 100,000.[9,84]

As the number of males in the United States continues to grow, so will the incidence of BPH and the incidence of corrective surgery. Transurethral resection of the prostate (TURP) is the most commonly performed surgical procedure among men over 50 years. In 1983, approximately 290,000 TURP procedures were performed, generating a total medical cost exceeding 1 billion dollars.[106]

PATHOPHYSIOLOGY

The etiology and natural history of BPH are not clearly understood. The prostate grows relatively slowly during the period between birth and puberty. During pubescence, rapid growth and maturation continue to a steady state attained at age 20.[40] This steady state lasts to age 45 to 50 when another gradual increase in prostatic size and weight occurs.[106]

Contrary to popular beliefs, no persuasive evidence exists concerning risk factors for BPH. Sexual activity (or celibacy), tobacco or alcohol use, diabetes, or social factors are not connected with an increased incidence of BPH. Obstructive symptoms of BPH tend to be seen earlier in black men than among white men, and Japanese men have a lower incidence than white men, but the reason for these racial variances is not known. The two factors necessary for the development of BPH are aging and the presence of functioning testes.[106,117]

The critical role of testicular androgens in BPH is demonstrated by the absence of the condition in males who have undergone castration before puberty and the marked reduction in incidence of BPH among men castrated before 40 years of age. However, the results of castration among men with existing BPH have not produced significant relief of obstructive symptoms in many studies.[106]

Testosterone is the principal hormonal product of the testes. Within the prostate it serves as a precursor for dihydrotestosterone, which is the prominent interstitial androgen that influences prostatic growth. Dihydrotestosterone is known to play a crucial role in normal prostatic growth throughout maturation; however, its role in the development of BPH remains unclear.[106] Wilson and his associates demonstrated that BPH was not produced in a group of male dogs given parenteral dihydrotestosterone. Ironically, spontaneous BPH did develop among some of the control dogs. In human males a gradual decrease in plasma levels of testosterone will logically correspond with a lower level of dihydrotestosterone within prostatic tissue, suggesting that other influences are important in the development of BPH.[106]

Endogenous estrogens have also been implicated in the development of BPH. Walsh and Wilson[105] used a combination of estrogens and dihydrotestosterone to produce BPH in dogs. They found that a combination of androstenediol and dihydrotestosterone produced mild prostatism while administration of estradiol and dihydrotestosterone produced marked hypertrophy. In human males it is important to note that while plasma testosterone levels are falling off, estradiol and androstenediol levels remain relatively unchanged. Thus, argues Walsh,[106] alteration of the synergy between testosterone and its derivatives and the endogenous estrogens in the male is responsible for the proliferation of BPH even though their role in the generation of prostatism is not established.

Although the development of BPH itself is not harmful, the sequelae produced by this condition cause significant morbidity and may prove fatal. The signs and symptoms of BPH are a result of bladder outlet obstruction resulting from gradual encroachment of the prostatic capsule into the proximal urethra. Early changes include hesitancy initiating micturition, decreased force in urinary stream, diurnal frequency, and nocturia. Compensatory hypertrophy of the detrusor muscle will result in trabeculation, diverticula, and hypertrophy of the trigone. Paradoxically, this may produce a reduction in symptoms but does not indicate any objective improvement in bladder outlet obstruction.[87,106]

Later changes produced by bladder outlet obstruction caused by BPH include myogenic decompensation when compensatory hypertrophy is no longer effective. The bladder wall will then become increasingly noncompliant and hypotonic, resulting in increasing postvoid residuals and greater chance of infection. Increased resistance at the ureterovesical junction results in ureteral dilation and progressive hydronephrosis. Unless infection is present in the upper urinary tract, few symptoms are perceived by the individual although renal function is impaired. In certain cases incompetence of the ureterovesical junction combined with increased voiding pressure may result in vesicoureteral reflux that compromises the hydrodynamic function of the renal pelvis and ureters and promotes the likelihood of pyelonephritis.[87]

The two primary complications of BPH are urinary tract infection and acute urinary retention. Urinary tract infection results from the presence of postvoid residuals that cause hypoxemia of the bladder wall and decreased resistance to bacterial invasion.[53] Acute urinary retention is a surprisingly common complication of BPH. Epidemiologic studies in Britain revealed that 44% of all men treated for BPH had acute urinary retention and 54% of those studied experienced at least one episode of acute urinary retention requiring catheterization. Acute urinary retention often results from some other aggravating factor of BPH such as prostatic infarct, or it may be a late result of detrusor decompensation.[9,87]

DIAGNOSTIC STUDIES

Uroflow with postvoid residual
　Decreased peak and mean flow and postvoid residual indicate bladder outlet obstruction

Film of kidneys, ureters, and bladder (KUB)
　Absence of complicating urinary calculi

Intravenous pyelogram (IVP)
　Hydroureteronephrosis, trabeculation, or diverticula of bladder
　Elevation of bladder base due to prostatic enlargement
　Postvoid residual

Urinalysis and urine culture
　Will rule out urinary tract infection, a complication of BPH

Cystoscopy
　Accurate assessment of degree of prostatic invasion into proximal urethral lumen and compensatory changes in bladder wall

Cystometrogram/electromyogram/flow
　Urodynamic studies will accurately assess degree of functional obstruction and severity of detrusor decompensation

TREATMENT PLAN

Surgical
　Transurethral resection of prostate (TURP) remains most widely used surgical intervention for BPH: a cystoscope is passed down urethra through which

a resectoscope is used to remove a portion of the intracapsular tissue

Suprapubic or retropubic prostatectomy (open removal of prostate gland) may be used in selected cases

Cryosurgical technique may be used for patients who are poor risk for anesthesia: an instrument is passed urethrally and the freezing unit placed in the prostatic urethra; liquid nitrogen is passed through the instrument until the prostatic capsule reaches 0° to 10° C, causing slough of prostatic tissue; not as effective as TURP and reserved for select patients

Chemotherapeutic

Antimicrobial therapy indicated if urinary tract infection is present

Exogenous estrogen may be used to reduce prostatic size but is typically contraindicated because of its side effects, which include loss of libido and impotence[88]

Supportive

Intermittent self-catheterization may be used in selected individuals to ensure complete bladder evacuation

Urethral catheterization indicated when acute urinary retention occurs

Suprapubic cystostomy may be necessary if a urethral catheter cannot be passed

Avoid all over-the-counter or prescription cold preparations containing alpha sympathomimetics (will cause increased tone at bladder neck exacerbating outlet obstruction)

Long-term use of antidepressant drugs will exacerbate urinary retention because of their anticholinergic effects

ASSESSMENT: AREAS OF CONCERN

Prostate

Digital examination of rectum will reveal enlargement of all palpable lobes and absence of discrete, hardened nodules

Voiding behavior

Decreased force of urinary stream

Straining or use of Credé's maneuver to void

Postvoid dribble

Diurnal frequency and nocturia with feelings of incomplete emptying

NURSING DIAGNOSES and NURSING INTERVENTIONS

Nursing Diagnosis	Nursing Intervention
Urinary elimination, alteration in patterns	Encourage adequate fluid intake during the 12 hours associated with meal times and restriction or elimination of fluids before sleep to minimize nocturia while providing adequate fluid intake for daily needs.
Noncompliance with medical therapy	Encourage men over 50 years to be aware of signs and symptoms of prostatism. Ironically, after initial obstructive signs appear, an improvement in symptoms is noted that is associated with compensatory detrusor hypertrophy. No improvement in the obstruction has occurred. Earlier treatment for BPH prevents the deleterious complications associated with long-term urinary obstruction (urinary tract infection, bladder trabeculation, upper tract damage).

Patient Education

1. Provide information and assistance in planning a schedule for fluid intake adequate for daily needs, necessity of prompt medical intervention for bladder outlet obstruction, and special instructions for any related drugs taken (e.g., antibiotics).
2. Provide information concerning the true lack of causal relationship between benign prostatic hypertrophy and sexual patterns.

EVALUATION

Patient Outcome	Data Indicating That Outcome is Reached
BPH is surgically repaired.	Peak and mean flow on uroflowmetry improve. Postvoid residual is less than 20% of total bladder volume. Urodynamic results demonstrate negative resistance factors. Cystoscopic examination reveals no urethral obstruction. Subjective improvement in voiding symptoms occurs.

CYSTITIS

Cystitis is defined as any inflammation of the bladder wall. The term is often used synonymously with urinary tract infection even though they are not identical. Many causative agents, including bacteria, viruses, fungi, chemical agents, and radiation exposure, may result in cystitis.

The occurrence of infection in the urinary tract is second only to respiratory tract infections.[15] Infection of the urinary bladder is the most common focus of inflammation in the urinary tract. Women are particularly prone to symptomatic and asymptomatic bacteriuria resulting in cystitis. A study of Jamaican women revealed that 2% of all females between 15 and 24 years of age had bacteriuria on culture. Stamey and associates[90] found that the prevalence of bacterial cystitis in women increased approximately 1% to 2% during each subsequent decade of life until reaching 10% among 54- to 64-year-old women. Gaymons and his associates[27] corroborated these findings in a prospective study of 1758 Dutch women that revealed a 2.7% prevalence of bacteriuria among those 15 to 24 years of age and 9.3% among those 65 years of age and older. Among the general population, a woman can expect a 10% to 20% chance of having at least one episode of cystitis during her lifetime.[90]

Pregnant women and hospitalized women have an increased incidence of urinary tract infection. Among pregnant women the rate of cystitis is approximately 4% to 6%; studies have demonstrated an incidence of urinary tract infection as high as 30% among hospitalized women.[90]

In addition to a significant susceptibility to bacterial cystitis, women are also particularly likely to suffer from interstitial cystitis when compared to their male counterparts. A study in Finland found that the prevalence of interstitial cystitis was 10.6:100,000 with a 10:1 preference of the disease for women.[103] Leach and Raz[58] also report an incidence of 20:100,000 cases of interstitial cystitis among women with a ratio of 10 cases in females for every case reported among men.

The incidence of cystitis among men has not been extensively studied but is generally thought to occur in only 10% as many men as women. Unlike in women, most cases of bacteriuria in men occur as a result of some known infectious focus such as bacterial prostatitis or urinary calculi.[66]

Clearly, the most significant rate of cystitis, resulting in an alarming incidence of associated morbidity and mortality, is that associated with nosocomial urinary tract infection in the presence of an indwelling catheter. In a prospective study of 1458 patients in the United States, 131 patients acquired 136 urinary tract infections during 1474 indwelling bladder catheterizations. Among those studied, 12 deaths may have been caused by acquired urinary tract infections, and another 10 patients died with a retrospective clinical picture compatible with serious infection although no conclusive culture data were available. Thus the authors concluded that acquisition of a nosocomial urinary tract infection was associated with a threefold increase in death rate.[80]

PATHOPHYSIOLOGY

The pathogenesis of cystitis depends on the causative agent. Within this discussion cystitis will be divided into three categories:

1. Infectious cystitis
   a. Bacterial
   b. Viral
   c. Fungal
   d. Tubercular
   e. Parasitic
2. Chemotherapy- and radiation-induced cystitis
3. Inflammatory lesions of the bladder
   a. Cystitis cystica
   b. Cystitis glandularis
   c. Eosinophilic cystitis
   d. Cystitis emphysematosa
   e. Interstitial cystitis

Bacterial cystitis is the most common form of infectious cystitis. The most common causative pathogen in both women and men is *Escherichia coli*. Other common pathogens include strains of *Klebsiella, Enterobacter, Proteus, Pseudomonas,* and *Serratia;* gram-positive organisms such as staphylococci and streptococci are occasionally seen.[66,89]

The three routes of bacterial invasion into the bladder are (1) ascending through the urethra, (2) the hematogenous route, and (3) via lymphatic channels; the most common is the ascending urethral pathway. Bacteria are commonly forced into the bladder without necessarily resulting in infection. The determinants of bacterial cystitis depend on the virulence and inoculum size of invasive bacteria and the adequacy of the host's defense mechanisms. Data concerning the number of bacteria needed to produce a bladder infection are based solely on animal studies which show that an extremely large inoculum (over 1 million) is needed to produce cystitis if host defense mechanisms are not compromised. Fortunately, normal numbers of bacteria that enter the bladder through the urethra are considerably smaller (less than 100).[47]

The human body has two primary defense mechanisms that oppose the establishment of infection when bacteria enter the bladder. The first is the urine itself, which is bacteriostatic or bacteriocidal to the most common pathogens associated with cystitis, such as *E. coli* and a number of other anaerobic bacteria commonly found in urethral flora. The efficiency of this antibacterial activity depends on the size of the bacterial inoculum, the osmolality of the urine, and the concentration of urea nitrogen and ammonium in the urine. A urinary pH of 6.0 or greater will adversely affect antibacterial activity, but the presence of specific antibodies in the urine such as IgA and IgG has not been shown to cause significant effects.[47]

The bladder wall is the second line of defense for bacterial invasion from the urethra, bloodstream, or lymphatic route. Inflammatory changes within the bladder wall are apparent within 30 minutes of invasion when polymorphonucleocytes (PMNs) begin to migrate to the bladder mucosa. Within 2 hours the entire mucosal lining is injected by PMNs, and significant antibacterial activity is measurable by the fourth hour. Inspection at 24 hours will reveal clumps of PMNs throughout the mucosal lining and urine culture will be negative.[47]

Yet the most important defense against bacterial cystitis is the unobstructed flow of urine throughout the urinary tract and regular, complete evacuation of the bladder. This important concept is the basis of the rationale for clean intermittent catheterization. By regularly emptying the bladder, bacteria are flushed from the system that will ultimately colonize the urine if allowed to remain within the bladder.[47]

Abnormalities that interfere with natural host defenses against urinary tract infection include the presence of residual urine, which provides an opportunity for bacteria to reproduce and overwhelm other inherent antibacterial mechanisms. Vesicoureteral reflux also compromises the body's defense mechanisms by allowing the spread of bacteria from the urine into the upper tracts and possibly into the renal parenchyma. Urinary calculi are often obstructive to urinary outflow and serve as a nidus for infection during antibiotic therapy. In addition, any disease or circumstance that interferes with the body's immune system will decrease the efficiency of the bladder wall's reaction to bacteriuria.[47]

Women are particularly susceptible to bacterial cystitis for a number of reasons. Stamey[89,90] studied the problem of bacterial cystitis in women and concluded that much of the nomenclature used to describe the condition does not adequately define this condition. He described four bacteriurial states in women: first infection, unresolved bacteriuria during therapy, bacterial persistence, and reinfection (recurrence).

The etiology of first infection is unclear but is presumed to be similar to reinfections. Unlike recurrent episodes of cystitis, bacteria from the first infection are typically sensitive to any antibiotic and are unlikely to recur within a 2- to 3-year period unless other predisposing factors are present.[89]

Unresolved bacteriuria during therapy may arise from several causes. The bacteria may be resistant to the antibiotic chosen for therapy, or selection of a secondary strain may become predominant as the primary form of bacteria is eliminated. In approximately 6% of patients treated, resistant, mutant bacteria will develop and proliferate. Renal insufficiency may cause inadequate concentrations of antibiotic in the urinary tract even though the correct agent has been chosen. A staghorn calculus may be large enough to support a critical mass of bacteria too great for antibiotics to resolve.[89]

True bacterial persistence may arise after 5 to 10 days of therapy, resulting in culture-proven nonsterile urine from one of two causes. Men with chronic bacterial prostatitis have a persistent focus for ascending urethral infection from the prostatic ductal system. Women or men with struvite stones in the urinary tract have a site of persistent bacteria even after antibiotic therapy.[89]

Reinfection of the bladder accounts for the majority of all occurrences of bacterial cystitis among women. The most common route for bacteria to gain access to the bladder is from the urethra. The colonization of the urethra arises from the vaginal introitus and vestibule rather than from the rectum, as is commonly assumed. Longitudinal studies show that cultures of the vaginal vestibule and distal urethral mucosa are more predictive of recurrent bacterial cystitis than analysis of rectal flora. Ascending infection in the female is particularly problematic because of the relatively short, straight course of the urethra and plentiful flora in the genital area. The relationship between vaginal flora and urethral bacteria is further supported by examining the close anatomic relationship of these two structures, which are confined by the distal labia minora.[90]

The role of sexual intercourse in recurrent urinary infections has been repeatedly studied. Sexual intercourse is associated with an increased incidence of recurrent urinary tract infections and some women will specifically correlate intercourse and recurrence. It is interesting to note that nuns have a 0.4% to 1.6% incidence of urinary tract infection, which is lower than the general population, and that married women have a higher incidence than do their single counterparts. Although sexual intercourse does not cause bacterial cystitis, it does promote the milking of bacteria into the bladder and can cause minor urethral injury that may result in infection among women predisposed to the condition.[90]

Changes in the urinary tract unique to pregnancy also increase a woman's likelihood for having recurring urinary tract infections or experiencing a first infection of the bladder. The primary urologic change noted with pregnancy is the "physiologic hydroureter of pregnancy,'' which is the reversible dilation of the ureters and renal pelvis. This dilation often begins as early as the seventh week of gestation and progresses until delivery. The right ureter is more extensively affected than the left, and ureteral peristalsis is significantly slowed after the second month of gestation so that intraureteral volume may be as great as 25 times normal.[5]

Bacteriuria is more common among pregnant women than in nonpregnant women in the same age group. The presence of ureteral dilation may play a role in this increased incidence. It is known that pregnant women with bacteriuria are at a significantly increased risk (20% to 40%)[40] for developing pyelonephritis and that this risk is dramatically reduced by treating the bladder infection. In addition, catheterization during pregnancy is associated with increased risk of subsequent bacterial cystitis so that the procedure is contraindicated for these women. Although the association between premature delivery and pyelonephritis is well documented, no correlation between bacteriuria and premature delivery exists.[5]

Bacterial cystitis is likely to result in urinary frequency, urgency, and dysuria. Women in particular may complain of suprapubic discomfort and a feeling of pressure in the perineal area. Nocturia and low back pain are also caused by bladder infection. Urge incontinence may take the form of detrusor instability with subsequent painful bladder ''spasms'' and associated leakage; or it may take the form of urethral instability allowing urine passage into the posterior urethra and causing a perception of intense urgency and urinary leakage. Gross hematuria, chills, fever, and flank pain occur only occasionally in the presence of cystitis unless it is also associated with pyelonephritis.[66,89] Approximately one half of patients with significant bacteriuria are asymptomatic.[40] Women with dysuria and frequency who have no bacteriuria or a colony count less than 10,000/ml are typically diagnosed as having an ''acute urethral syndrome.''[83]

Cystitis due to fungal infection is much less prevalent than bacterial cystitis, but its incidence and recognition have greatly increased within the past 25 years. The most common fungal infection of the bladder is candidiasis. *Candida* is endemic to the human body and can often be found in the pharynx, stomach, intestinal tract, and vaginal vault (particularly in pregnant women). The increasing incidence of candidal overgrowth is related to the use of antibiotics. Administration of antibiotics is thought to stimulate the production of *Candida albicans* by altering the pH of gastrointestinal mucosa, suppressing normal bacterial flora that competes with the fungus for food, and inhibiting polymorphonuclear phagocytosis, which helps the body guard against overgrowth.[68]

The body's defenses against candidal infection of the urinary tract include the presence of normal bacterial flora that inhibit fungal growth and the presence of PMNs in the mucosa of the urethra and bladder, which have marked anticandidal effects. In addition, prostatic fluid in the male is fungicidal, which helps explains the relatively low incidence of candidal cystitis in males compared to females. Cell-mediated immunity and other white blood cells also help the body prevent candidiasis.[68]

Candidal cystitis often occurs in the presence of predisposing factors such as diabetes mellitus, obstructive prostatic enlargement, and pregnancy and is often noted after the patient has undergone antibiotic therapy for bacterial infection. Symptoms are similar to bacterial cystitis and include urgency, marked frequency, dysuria, suprapubic pain, and nocturia. Pneumaturia (the expression of gas or air through the urethra during or following micturition) may be seen. The mucosal lining of the bladder is marked by grayish white spots that will result in mucosal bleeding if removed. The ureteral orifices may be affected so that cystoscopic findings may resemble tubercular infection of the bladder. In certain cases asymptomatic candidal colonization of the urine without inflammation of the bladder may be seen.[68]

Tuberculosis of the bladder results from the implantation of the tubercle bacilli into the wall, causing an uneven mix of inflamed areas interspersed with normal mucosal segments. The cystoscopic picture of the bladder may resemble interstitial cystitis or candidal infection with patches of inflamed tissue and reddened ureteral orifices. The anterior urethra is not affected by the infection, but the posterior urethra and prostate are heavily involved in men, representing progression from prostate to bladder. The trigone is relatively spared from inflammatory changes, but the dome of the bladder is extensively affected, resulting in a marked loss in capacity.[56]

The primary symptom of tubercular cystitis is marked frequency and urgency. Bladder volume rapidly decreases and may result in irreversible changes in advanced stages of the infection.[56] Urodynamic assessment in advanced cases may reveal poor compliance of the bladder wall and a functional capacity of 60 ml of urine or less.

Although schistosomiasis is relatively rare in the United States, it is relatively common elsewhere in the world. The ova of this parasite enter the bloodstream via penetration of the skin. The veins of the bladder are a popular breeding site for the parasites. The eggs are then extruded into the vesicle for further spread of the parasitic organisms. The healing of the affected areas of the bladder causes thickening and contraction of the bladder wall. Damage of the ureterovesical junction often occurs, resulting in vesicoureteral reflux. Contracted bands mar the bladder and may extend into the lower ureter. Urinary calculi may be present because of urinary stasis and presence of ova in the urine.[82]

Chemotherapy- or radiation-induced cystitis is characterized by inflammatory changes in the bladder wall in the absence of infection. The symptoms are similar to infectious cystitis and include urgency, frequency, and suprapubic pain. Detrusor instability and urge incontinence may occur.[36,107]

Although the bladder is relatively resistant to radiation, therapeutic doses greater than 6000 to 7000 rads over a 6- to 7-week period may result in cystitis. The bladder's tolerance to radiation will be significantly compromised if schistosomiasis is present. Chemotherapy-induced cystitis may arise from systemic cyclophosphamide (Cytoxan) or intravesical antineoplastic drugs such as mitomycin. Diagnosis is made when symptoms of cystitis are reported in the presence of a normal culture and positive history of exposure to radiation or a chemotherapeutic agent.[36,107]

Cystitis cystica occurs as a result of chronic infection of the bladder or recurrent episodes of cystitis. It is characterized by small, rounded cysts that are seen mostly near the base of the bladder and trigone. These cysts are approximately 1 cm in diameter, have a rounded shape, and may extend into the upper urinary tract. The lesions are benign, and the etiology of the condition is unknown. Because of the gross similarities between these lesions and malignancies of the bladder, biopsy is indicated to rule out cancer.[15]

Cystitis glandularis is a relatively rare, potentially premalignant lesion associated with adenocarcinoma of the bladder. This form of cystitis is particularly common among patients with a history of bladder exstrophy and pelvic lipomatosis. Biopsy is done to rule out malignancy, and follow-up examination for potential cancer of the bladder is recommended.[15]

Eosinophilic cystitis is a severe inflammatory lesion of the bladder that is thought to have an allergic etiology. The bladder mucosa is extensively invaded by eosinophils and exhibits multiple polypoid lesions. The associated signs and symptoms of cystitis are particularly severe.[15]

Cystitis emphysematosa is a rare form of bladder inflammation resulting from infection by gas-forming urinary bacteria or (more commonly) vesicoenteric fistula. The condition may also be observed after urologic instrumentation or urodynamic testing using carbon dioxide. Pneumaturia is associated with this form of cystitis.[15]

Interstitial cystitis is a particularly tenacious form of bladder inflammation characterized primarily by the pain it produces. This pain is centered in the suprapubic area and is typically described as burning and constant. Unlike bacterial cystitis, micturition does not typically relieve the pain, which results in marked urgency, frequency, nocturia, and the despair and frustration seen in patients who must cope with chronic, intractable pain.[103]

Interstitial cystitis occurs in both sexes and all age groups; the most commonly affected are adult women.

The etiology of interstitial cystitis remains unclear. Causative agents may be viral, fungal, or bacterial. Neurosis has been implicated as the cause of the disease although it seems likely that any maladaptive coping patterns are a response to chronic pain rather than the origin of the condition. Recent investigation of possible autoimmune dysfunction may help elucidate the etiology of this difficult clinical syndrome.[103]

The cystoscopic findings are consistent with a "pancystitis" involving all four layers of the bladder wall, which is typically thickened, injected, and friable. The submucosal layer is swollen and marked by enlarged capillaries and hemorrhagic areas. The venous structures of the bladder are engorged and dilated. White blood cell invasion of the bladder wall is common and consists mostly of lymphocytes. Filling of the bladder causes pallor of the mucosa and small tears in the lining. The bladder may be lined with small linear scars because of repeated tears in the mucosa related to normal bladder filling.[103]

DIAGNOSTIC STUDIES

Urine culture and sensitivity
Greater than 100,000/ml bacterial colonies on an agar culture plate or tube indicates clinically significant bacteriuria and associated cystitis

Sensitivity discs indicate bacterial sensitivity, intermediate sensitivity, or resistance to a given antibiotic agent

Urine culture negative in other forms of infectious cystitis and cystitis caused by chemotherapy and radiotherapy

Urinalysis
Color: dark yellow or pinkish red, cloudy with or without sediment

Nitrate/nitrite: positive in bacterial cystitis

Glucose oxidase: positive in bacterial infection

Catalase: positive in bacterial cystitis

Microscopic examination: positive for bacteria, fungus, and parasites in the various forms of infectious cystitis; positive for eosinophils in eosinophilic cystitis; greater than 7 WBCs per high-power field in infectious cystitis; red blood cells with or without gross hematuria

Cystoscopy
Red, inflamed bladder wall

Reddened, swollen trigone

Ureteral orifices may be inflamed

Hemorrhagic patches in urothelial lining

Findings for specific inflammatory lesions of the bladder described under "Pathophysiology"

Biopsy

Cystitis cystica: negative

Cystitis glandularis: negative or positive for adeno-carcinoma of bladder

Eosinophilic cystitis: extensive infiltration of eosino-phils into bladder tissues

Interstitial cystitis: chronic inflammation with extensive invasion of lymphocytes and other white blood cells into submucosa of bladder wall

Urodynamics

Infectious cystitis: urodynamic testing typically contraindicated

Tubercular cystitis: decreased functional capacity with poor compliance of bladder wall; detrusor unstable or areflexic; sensory urgency present

Chemotherapy- or radiation-induced cystitis: sensory urgency with decreased functional capacity; detrusor instability may be present; compliance of bladder wall may be normal or impaired

Interstitial cystitis: marked sensory urgency with decreased functional capacity; detrusor generally stable up to tolerated bladder volume; associated pain may render patient unable to void in testing situation; compliance is typically normal; postvoid residual may be noted

Voiding cystourethrogram (VCUG)

Cystitis emphysematosa: lucent filling defect consistent with gas in vesicle of bladder with or without extravasation of contrast material into vesicoenteric fistula

TREATMENT PLAN

Surgical

Tubercular cystitis: in cases of advanced tubercular cystitis when bladder contraction is irreversible, augmentation cystoplasty may be employed after infection is controlled; colocystoplasty (placing an isolated segment of colon onto the bladder dome in order to enlarge storage capacity) or ileocystoplasty (placing an isolated segment of small bowel on the bladder dome) may be utilized to restore reasonable bladder storage capacity

Cystitis glandularis: transurethral resection of lesion done because of its premalignant potential[15]

Interstitial cystitis: transurethral resection and fulguration of bladder lesions may give temporary symptomatic relief but remain a controversial form of treatment; denervation procedures (bilateral chordotomy, selective sacral neurectomy, or supratrigonal denervation) may be used to manage chronic pain; irreversibility of these procedures (and their

Table 12-1

Common Bacterial Pathogens Encountered in the Urinary Tract and Treatment Options

Pathogen	Commonly Effective Antibiotic Agents*
E. coli	Trimethoprim/sulfamethoxazole, ampicillin
Pseudomonas	Carbenicillin (Geocillin), gentamicin†
Klebsiella	Cephalexin, tetracycline, trimethoprim/sulfamethoxazole
Proteus	Ampicillin, tetracycline, trimethoprim/sulfamethoxazole
Morganelli morganii	Trimethoprim/sulfamethosoxazole
Serratia	Carbenicillin, trimethoprim/sulfamethoxazole
Group D Streptococcus	Ampicillin, nitrofurantoin
Staphylococcus	Cephalexin, tetracycline, trimethoprim/sulfamethoxazole
Staphylococcus saprophyticus	Cephalexin, trimethoprim/sulfamethoxazole, tetracycline

*Antibiotic therapy is guided by individual culture and sensitivity reports.

†Requires parenteral administration.

potential side effects) a significant consideration; bladder substitution such as enterocystoplasty or supratrigonal cystoplasty requires extensive resection of detrusor muscle and replacement with an isolated segment of bowel; urinary diversion has been utilized but is considered a final option when all other treatments have failed[58,103]

Chemotherapeutic

Bacterial cystitis

Treatment of choice is oral antibiotic therapy guided by culture and sensitivity data (Table 12-1)

For first-time infections or recurrent infections, short-term therapy with oral antibiotics favored although single-dose therapy may be utilized

In more severe cases or when resistant bacteria are identified, parenteral therapy is indicated

For recurrent infections, suppressive antibiotic therapy may be used for 6 months up to 24 months (Table 12-2); first choice for long-term antibiotic suppression among women with recurrent bacterial cystitis is nitrofurantoin or trimethoprim/sulfamethoxazole

Nitrofurantoin absorbed in upper intestinal tract so that it does not promote mutation of resistant strains of bacteria in intestinal tract; exerts its antibacterial effects on bacteria that have reached bladder

Trimethoprim/sulfamethoxazole will kill pathogens in vaginal vestibule, preventing bacterial

Table 12-2
Antibiotic Therapy for Bacterial Cystitis

Type of Therapy	Antibiotic Agents*
Single-dose therapy	Amoxicillin (Amoxil), 3.0 g Trimethoprim/sulfamethoxazole (Bactrim DS, Septra DS), one or two double-strength tablets Sulfisoxazole (Gantrisin), 1-2 g
Short-term therapy (5-14 d)	Ampicillin (Amcil), 2 g in four divided doses Amoxicillin (Amoxil), 2 g in four divided doses Trimethoprim/sulfamethoxazole (Bactrim DS, Septra DS), one double-strength tablet bid Nitrofurantoin (Macrodantin), 50-100 mg qid
Suppressive therapy for recurrences (6-24 mo)	Trimethoprim/sulfamethoxazole (Bactrim DS, Septra DS), one regular-strength tablet daily Nitrofurantoin (Macrodantin), 50-100 mg/d

Adapted from Farrar, W.E.: Infections of the urinary tract, Med. Clin. North Am. **67**:193, 1983.
*Antibiotic therapy is guided by individual culture and sensitivity reports.

invasion of bladder but does alter intestinal flora, which can lead to selection of bacteria resistant to drug

Fungal infections
    Two drugs, amphotericin B and 5-fluorocystine, are indicated in cases of nonmucocutaneous infection
    Amphotericin B has disadvantages of requiring parenteral administration and significant side effects such as fever, chills, nausea and vomiting, headache, vertigo, and potential nephrotoxicity with prolonged use
    5-Fluorocystine may be administered orally and is effective against *Candida;* side effects include bone marrow depression, potential nephrotoxicity, and eosinophilia
    Production of resistant strains of fungi is problematic[68]
Tubercular cystitis
    Drug therapy must be long term (2 yr recommended), and multiple agents are often more effective than any single medication
    Combination of isoniazid (INH), ethambutol, rifampin, streptomycin, para-aminosalicylic acid (PAS), cycloserine, or kanamycin is indicated[56]
Parasitic cystitis
    Drugs utilized for schistosomiasis have potentially

dangerous side effects and are not approved by the U.S. Food and Drug Administration
    Current drug of choice is nitrofurantoin given over a period of 5 to 7 d
    Early treatment essential for prevention of irreversible urinary changes from drug
Other chemotherapeutic agents may be utilized to provide symptomatic relief from cystitis due to infection, chemotherapy, or radiotherapy; anticholinergic agents or antispasmodics such as oxybutynin and propantheline may ameliorate sensory urgency and provide greater functional capacity
Eosinophilic cystitis
    Antihistamines and oral steroid agents are indicated
    Antibiotic therapy will control related bacteriuria[15]
Interstitial cystitis
    A variety of pharmacologic agents utilized; currently antibiotics, oral anti-inflammatory agents, antihistamines, analgesics, and vitamins are used with varying success[58]
    Three intravesical agents (silver nitrate, oxychloresene sodium, and dimethyl sulfoxide) may be used; agents are instilled into vesicle per urethral catheter and retained for approximately 30 min before catheter drainage

Electromechanical
Interstitial cystitis: mechanical bladder distention sometimes used in an attempt to increase functional capacity; performed by an intravesical balloon inflated to patient's systolic blood pressure for 1 to 3 hours; therapeutic mechanism of this procedure is the creation of bladder wall ischemia with subsequent lessening of sensory enervation; complications include rupture of bladder[58]

Supportive
Caffeine intake should be restricted because its mild diuretic effect exacerbates frequency
Citrus juices not effective in lowering urinary pH
Cranberry juice only effective in lowering urinary pH if taken in extremely large quantities
Plentiful fluid intake indicated in order to encourage movement of pathogens out of urinary tract

ASSESSMENT: AREAS OF CONCERN

Suprapubic area
Tender on palpation

Costovertebral angle
No tenderness

Voiding behavior
Frequency, urgency, dysuria, nocturia

NURSING DIAGNOSES and NURSING INTERVENTIONS

Nursing Diagnosis	Nursing Intervention
Urinary elimination, alteration in patterns	Encourage copious fluid intake while reassuring patient that urinary frequency is a temporary condition and a positive response to inflammation of the bladder. Inform patient that frequency and dysuria will dissipate after adequate treatment of causative organisms.
Comfort, alteration in: pain	Encourage patient to take a warm bath or a warm sitz bath, which will relieve suprapubic pain associated with cystitis. Teach patient that voiding will relieve pressure associated with bladder filling; retaining urine in the presence of intense urgency is not recommended in infectious cystitis although it is encouraged in interstitial cystitis in order to increase functional capacity.
Noncompliance (medical therapy)	Encourage patient to continue medications for the entire period recommended by the prescriber. Inform patient that 10 days of antibiotic therapy provides a greater chance of complete eradication of bacteriuria than shorter courses. Provide counseling concerning potential adverse effects (e.g., diarrhea and nausea) associated with specific antibiotic agents and preventive strategies such as taking medications with meals.
Coping, ineffective individual	Note that women and men with interstitial cystitis suffer from the adverse effects of a chronic, painful condition associated with discomfort, frustration, disturbances in rest patterns, and social isolation. Sleep patterns are significantly disturbed because of nocturnal voidings that may exceed 12 times in a single night. Attempts at rest during the day are also interrupted by the desire to void and constant feelings of suprapubic pressure and discomfort. Social isolation results from fear of incontinent episodes or painful interludes between opportunities to void and from lack of empathy on the part of family and friends. Social ostracism may result from false perceptions that the person is simply "unwilling" to postpone micturition or that he has "overindulged" the bladder by "giving in" to even mild sensations of urgency. Feelings of frustration and inadequacy may be encouraged by uneducated health caregivers who incorrectly perceive the condition as a form of maladaptive behavior. Encourage the patient to express feelings of fear, frustration, anger, and desperation concerning the condition. Reassurance that others are there to help in coping is indicated. Educate the entire family to the implications of interstitial cystitis and in ways to help the affected member in coping with associated discomfort and alteration in urinary habits.
Knowledge deficit, family (implications of interstitial cystitis)	Educate family members about the implications of interstitial cystitis including physiologic basis of disease, voiding dysfunction, and nature and typical human responses to chronic pain. Include family members in all discussions of surgical, chemotherapeutic, and nursing aspects of care. Reinforce the need of the affected member for family acceptance.

EVALUATION

Patient Outcome	Data Indicating That Outcome is Reached
Bacterial cystitis is resolved.	Urine culture is negative 24 hours after completing antibiotic therapy.
Fungal cystitis is resolved.	Fungal culture is negative after completion of antifungal therapy.
Parasitic cystitis is resolved.	There are no ova or parasites in urine. There are no complications, or they have been surgically repaired.

Patient Outcome	Data Indicating That Outcome is Reached
Chemotherapy- or radiotherapy-induced cystitis is symptomatically improved.	Urgency and frequency are decreased. Functional capacity as measured by urodynamic assessment is increased. Nocturia is decreased or absent. The patient subjectively reports decreased symptoms of suprapubic discomfort. Cystoscopic findings are normal.
Inflammatory lesion of the bladder is resolved.	Cystoscopic findings are normal.
Interstitial cystitis is symptomatically improved.	Functional capacity on urodynamic testing is increased. The patient subjectively reports decreased diurnal frequency (every 3 to 4 hours) and decreased nocturia (less than three episodes per night).

ENURESIS

Enuresis is any involuntary micturition past the age when continence should be present. Nocturnal enuresis is defined as bed-wetting past the age of 4 years, and diurnal enuresis may be defined as involuntary voiding while awake.[77,78] *Current terminology describes enuresis as inappropriate micturition while asleep; this discussion will utilize this definition.*

Enuresis is classified as either primary or secondary. Patients with primary enuresis have never been dry at night, while those with secondary enuresis have been dry for a period of weeks or months before a pattern of bed-wetting begins. The onset of enuresis may be correlated with an identifiable stressor or crisis such as the birth of a sibling or parental divorce.[76,77]

The incidence of enuresis is highest among preschool and school-aged children. At 5 years of age, 15% of all children will be enuretic; the incidence will decrease at a rate of 14% to 16% until reaching a rate of 1% to 2% by the age of 15 years. This relatively low incidence will persist throughout adulthood.[77]

Enuresis occurs in all cultures and social classes but is more commonly found among children of lower socioeconomic status. Children with enuresis are more likely to be middle children, to have a familial history of bed-wetting, and to come from broken homes. The majority of patients with enuresis (85%) have no clinically significant diurnal voiding problems while the remainder will have daytime urinary frequency, urgency, and possibly urge incontinence. Encopresis (involuntary fecal soiling) is found in 10% to 25% of patients with enuresis.[77]

PATHOPHYSIOLOGY

Enuresis is a symptom, not a disease. Therefore multiple factors may contribute to its existence, making a single, straightforward explanation of the condition unrealistic. In addition, the condition is difficult to study because of the lack of suitable animal models. Thus the etiology of enuresis remains poorly understood although a variety of causative associated abnormalities have been advocated.

Perhaps the most popular theory for enuresis supports the existence of a "maturational lag" of neurologic bladder control resulting in enuresis. Incomplete development of the cortical or subcortical tracts concerned with bladder function is implicated, with resulting alteration in sensations of bladder filling and abnormal sleep patterns leading to abnormal arousal in response to the desire to void or a failure of normal detrusor inhibition. This pattern may or may not be noted during daytime hours. The evidence for this explanation of enuresis is largely circumstantial but nonetheless attractive.[77,78]

Subtle urodynamic abnormalities are noted among patients with enuresis; these include a decreased functional capacity, diurnal urgency, and daytime frequency. A subtle form of detrusor instability may be noted among patients who are incontinent only at night, while marked instability is found among those with daytime wetting.[78] These findings are purported to implicate an infantile bladder in the absence of neurologic disease. However, such urodynamic findings must be viewed with caution for several reasons. First, the inclusion of children with abnormal daytime voiding patterns with children who have nocturnal voiding problems may be misleading. The presence of urge incontinence during waking hours is clearly connected with detrusor instability and has been named the unstable bladder of childhood, or the non-neurogenic neurogenic bladder. This condition is significantly different from nocturnal enuresis and is associated with recurrent urinary tract infection, uncoordinated external sphincter activity, and upper tract damage in certain cases.[2,6]

Conclusions of maturational lag in enuretic children based on urodynamic data must also be interpreted with caution because of the technique of testing. Standard urodynamic testing utilizes rapid, provocative filling with carbon dioxide or water in a child who is awake or only moderately sedated. Thus the circumstances unique to nocturnal enuresis are not reproduced. This disparity is demonstrated by Whiteside and Arnold,[115] who found that provocative urodynamic testing was clinically useful among enuretic children with diurnal incontinence but it was not helpful among patients with nocturnal wetting only. Nielsen and his associates[74] examined the relationship between bladder contractions and enuretic episodes. They found that large numbers of contractions were present among children with vesicoureteral reflux (mean of 6.5 to 7.5), which were not all associated with an enuretic episode. Thus the presence of an unstable detrusor alone is not sufficient for enuresis.

Sleep patterns have also been studied among patients with enuresis and have been found to be abnormal. Enuretic children are known to be particularly heavy sleepers. Incontinent episodes typically occur during the transition from deeper to lighter stages of sleep. Enuretic children spend more time in these deeper stages of sleep (stages 3 and 4) when rapid eye movements are absent than do their nonenuretic peers, are more difficult to arouse, and may have greater difficulty suppressing spontaneous bladder contractions.[77,78]

Some studies have found electroencephalographic abnormalities among enuretic children and subtle developmental delays implying a lag in the functional maturity. However, other studies have disputed these findings.[77,78]

Psychosocial factors have also been implicated in the etiology of enuresis and particularly of secondary enuresis. Proponents of this theory point to the association of enuresis with broken homes and identifiable crises connected with the onset of enuresis in certain cases, such as the birth of a sibling. Significant neuroses are not associated with enuresis although enuresis may be a component of the symptoms produced by a deeply rooted psychologic or personality disorder. In these cases treatment is directed toward the underlying psychologic disorder rather than the symptom of enuresis.[78]

Familial patterns of enuresis are well documented. Although the incidence of enuresis is 15% among children with no family history of the condition, children whose parents were enuretic have a 44% chance of bed-wetting. The incidence of enuresis among monozygotic twins is also significantly increased when one sibling develops the condition.[77]

Allergic causes of enuresis have been reported although few children ultimately respond to dietary manipulations. Proponents of this theory believe that certain foods irritate the bladder, resulting in decreased functional capacity and an increased likelihood of enuresis.[77,78]

Only a relatively small percentage of enuretic children have significant associated urologic abnormalities in the absence of diurnal incontinence. Detrusor instability is usually subtle, and a detailed urologic workup is rarely beneficial. The most common associated urologic finding among these children is bacteriuria or symptomatic urinary tract infection. Enuretic girls are two to six times as likely to develop cystitis as their nonenuretic peers although enuretic boys do not have a significantly increased infection rate.[76,77]

Adult enuresis is defined as enuresis that developed in childhood and persists beyond the age of 15 years, or it may develop spontaneously. Unlike bed-wetting in childhood, adults with enuresis are likely to have overt urodynamic abnormalities and often have other underlying urologic or neurologic abnormalities.[34,35]

DIAGNOSTIC STUDIES

Urodynamic testing
Children: not recommended unless other voiding abnormalities exist; studies may be normal or reveal decreased functional capacity with sensory urgency and mild or absent detrusor instability; child is often unable to suppress a volitionally induced contraction
Adults: detrusor instability with or without functional outlet obstruction; other abnormalities may be noted

Urinalysis
Normal
Occasional bacteria or white blood cells may be noted

Urine culture
Normal or asymptomatic bacteriuria among females

TREATMENT PLAN

Surgical
No longer considered prudent

Chemotherapeutic
Tricyclic antidepressants, typically imipramine (Tofranil; 25-50 mg at hs); have several beneficial actions including anticholinergic activity, alpha-sympathomimetic activity that increases tone at the bladder neck, and alteration of sleep patterns decreasing amount of time spent in non-REM sleep

Supportive
If an allergic component of enuresis is suspected, serial deletions of suspected foods are done; dairy products, egg products, chocolate, carbonated beverages, and cola beverages are common causative agents

ASSESSMENT: AREAS OF CONCERN

Abdomen
Normal

External genitalia
Normal

Voiding behavior
Normal

NURSING DIAGNOSES and NURSING INTERVENTIONS

Nursing Diagnosis	Nursing Intervention
Urinary elimination, alteration in patterns	Utilize responsibility/reinforcement therapy if both the child and parents are motivated. Instruct the child to keep a log or calendar of wet and dry nights, and contract goals between the nurse, parents, and child for improvement. After a level of improvement is obtained, provide a previously designated reward to the child. Encourage the patient to develop and record any feelings or emotions that predispose him to enuretic episodes.
	Use bladder training for enuretic children and adults. Employ motivation while using this strategy. Ask the patient to keep a log of diurnal voiding habits. Use this record as a baseline for attempting to increase bladder capacity by delaying voiding for increasing periods of time. Encourage the patient to avoid micturition even if urgency incontinence results.
	Use conditioning therapy, which involves an alarm system that senses the presence of urine and triggers a buzzer that awakens the child. Make certain the alarm device is used and functions properly. Instruct the child to sleep nude or in relatively lightweight pajamas. Provide a thorough explanation of the use and care of the alarm device and caution that old batteries and device malfunction are associated with ulceration of the skin. Counsel parents that this form of therapy requires approximately 16 weeks before enuresis ceases.
	Note that patient noncompliance is a common problem with every approach to enuresis outlined above.
	Be aware that responsibility/reinforcement therapy is undermined if parental support is lacking or if contracted rewards for improvement are not fulfilled. Counsel parents that strict adherence to the terms of the contract is essential to the program. Assess the child's level of maturity to ensure that he is capable of fulfilling his part of the contract. Do not perceive failure to remain dry as worthy of punishment.
	Provide repeated encouragement and reassurance during attempts to increase functional bladder capacity, since bladder training therapy requires considerable motivation and active participation by the patient, family, and nurse. Explain the goals and purposes for the therapy, since the parents and patient may view diurnal incontinence as a striking failure. Assess patients and families carefully for their motivation to undertake this therapeutic program, and provide them with realistic expectations of the time required to control enuresis by this method.
	If the patient is undergoing conditioning therapy, reassure the family of the relatively high success rate of this therapy.
	Forewarn parents of the possibility that the use of an alarm system may initially frighten a child aroused from a deep stage of sleep. Parents should be available to provide emotional comfort as needed during the first several nights the device is used.
	Provide a thorough explanation of the device and a demonstration on its function.
	Provide reassurance of the physiologic root of the problem and offer frequent opportunities to vent feelings and deal with anxiety produced by the condition.
	Inform parents that feelings of shame will be needlessly intensified by parental attempts to humiliate the child into ceasing bedwetting.
	Convince the parents that enuresis does have a physiologic basis and is only complicated by humiliation or punishment.

EVALUATION

Patient Outcome	Data Indicating That Outcome is Reached
Enuresis is absent.	Patient will remain dry every night for a 30-day period.
Recurrences are absent.	Patient will not experience recurrence by the age of 15 years.

EPIDIDYMITIS

Epididymitis is defined as any inflammation of the epididymis; it may be caused by bacteria, viruses, parasites, chemicals, or trauma. Epididymitis is divided into three categories: nonspecific, specific, and traumatic. Complications from this condition include orchitis, testicular infarction, and sterility.[73,113]

Epididymitis is the most common of all intrascrotal lesions. It is almost always unilateral and must be differentiated from testicular torsion, tumor, or trauma.[40] An estimated 600,000 cases occur in the United States each year. In men under 35 years of age, epididymitis is most often associated with sexually transmitted disease and accounts for 20% of all inpatient admissions among military urologic practices. In men over 35 years of age, gram-negative rods associated with some abnormality of the urinary tract or performance of some urologic procedure constitute the most common presentation of the condition. Epididymitis is rarely seen in prepubertal children.[39]

PATHOPHYSIOLOGY

Epididymitis occurs most frequently as a result of reflux of urine or some pathogenic agent through the posterior urethra, prostatic ducts, or seminal vesicles. In rare instances the causative pathogen may reach the epididymis via retrograde lymphatic pathways from the wall of the vas deferens or via hematogenous or metastatic routes. In its earlier stage, epididymitis occurs as a type of cellulitis associated with local pain and edema. In the acute stage the entire hemiscrotum becomes a single erythematous, exquisitely painful mass often associated with an inflammatory hydrocele produced by the tunica vaginalis. Later changes include peritubular fibrosis and occlusion of the epididymis that may result in sterility.[74a,95]

Nonspecific epididymitis refers to a group of common pathogens that typically gain access to the organ via urethral-vasal reflux in the presence of infected urine. Bladder outlet obstruction requiring the individual to strain in order to void is a predisposing factor to this condition. Nonspecific epididymitis is a common complication of prostatitis, urethral stricture disease, and seminal vesiculitis. Occasionally a nonspecific epididymitis may arise from a septic foci such as a pharyngitis. Reflux of sterile urine into the epididymis has been reported to result in inflammation,[73,113] although others dispute this possibility.[39] Strenuous exercise has also been connected with nonpyrogenic epididymitis.[73]

Nonspecific epididymitis also occurs as a complication of certain urologic procedures, particularly transurethral resection of the prostate and urethral catheterization. Postprocedure epididymitis may occur as late as several months following instrumentation because of the persistence of subclinical amounts of bacteria in the urine. It is significant to note that the rate of epididymitis following transurethral resection of the prostate has dropped from 20% to 4% following the institution of routine prophylactic antibiotics after the procedure. Vasectomy has been advocated as a prophylactic measure for men undergoing prostatectomy, but the efficacy of this intervention remains unproven.[113]

Traumatic epididymitis (also referred to as epididymido-orchitis) arises from straining, with reflux of urine into the organ. The etiology of this form of epididymitis remains unclear. Some argue that the trauma only inflames an already present subclinical inflammation of the epididymis, while others propose that the trauma lessens resistance to some more distant foci of infection, allowing invasion of pathogens into the area.[73]

Specific epididymitis refers to a group of known pathogens that invade the epididymis from a urinary focus or via the hematogenous route. The most common causative organisms associated with sexually transmitted epididymitis are *Neisseria gonorrhoeae* and *Chlamydia trachomatis* among heterosexual males and *Escherichia coli* among homosexual males. Prompt, aggressive treatment of these sexually transmitted diseases will help curtail the incidence of subsequent epididymitis as demonstrated by the decreasing incidence of gonococcal epididymitis.[39]

Syphilitic epididymitis may occur more often than has been suspected. This form of epididymal inflammation is typically asymptomatic and connected with the second stage of the disease. Diagnosis of syphilitic epididymitis is presumptive and established when other evidence of syphilis is present while urinary tract infection, prostatitis, and urethritis are absent.[78]

Many forms of specific epididymitis have been reported that have spread to the organ via the hematogenous route. In cases of brucellosis, epididymitis may be the initial symptom of the condition. Meningococcal septicemia, pneumococcal pneumonia, *Haemophilus influenzae,* and other bacterial diseases have been associated with epididymal invasion. Various parasites such as amebae, schistosoma, and various fungi are known to invade the epididymis.[78]

Tubercular epididymitis arises from involvement of the prostate and is one of the few forms of the disease that is painless. Tuberculosis of the epididymis produces a thickened, beaded organ on palpation and leads to occlusion of the epididymal lumen.[23a]

The most common complication of epididymitis is orchitis so that the term *epididymo-orchitis* is used. Infertility is a serious long-term complication of epididymitis. Sterility among men with chronic or recurrent bilateral epididymitis is 40%, while men who suffer from unilateral epididymitis have a 25% chance of sterility. Recurrences of epididymitis are particularly likely when the underlying disease process (e.g., prostatitis) remains unresolved.[113]

DIAGNOSTIC STUDIES

White blood cell count
Generally between 20,000 and 30,000 in an acute episode[95]

Urinalysis
Signs of infection may be present

Urine culture
Will reveal associated bacterial cystitis if present

Urethral discharge culture
Will reveal associated gonococcal or chlamydial urethritis

Prostatic secretion culture
Will reveal associated prostatitis

Doppler stethoscope
Good blood flow will rule out torsion of testis

Testicular radionuclide scan
Good blood flow will rule out torsion of testis

TREATMENT PLAN

Surgical
Epididymectomy rarely indicated as a therapeutic measure in chronic or tubercular epididymitis[95]

Chemotherapeutic
Mild to moderate cases: oral anti-infective agents, which may be guided by culture and sensitivity data

when appropriate; analgesics (ASA gr X q4-6h) used to manage pain and control fever
Severe cases: hospitalization and broad-spectrum antibiotics; combination of ampicillin and aminoglycoside given pending results of blood culture
Very severe cases: spermatic cord block with lidocaine or procaine hydrochloride; use of steroids has been advocated but any beneficial anti-inflammatory activity is outweighed by potential side effects[112]
Antiemetic agent may be required to control associated nausea and vomiting during acute epididymitis; antipyretics may be indicated for associated fever
Administration of antiemetics justified in order to prevent progression of nausea to a severe state that threatens fluid and electrolyte balance

Supportive
Urethral discharge may be copious and is managed by regular cleansing of meatus with hydrogen peroxide[60]

ASSESSMENT: AREAS OF CONCERN

Epididymis
Palpable by rolling contents of spermatic cord between thumb and finger
Early in infection, organ is felt as tender and enlarged; later, becomes indistinguishable because of local inflammation
In chronic epididymitis, organ is firm, nodular, moderately tender

Scrotum
Initial stages of epididymitis: scrotal skin is reddened or normal in appearance; as infection progresses, scrotal skin will become red and hot to touch
Varicocele a common finding
Moderate to severe cases: significant edema of epididymis and adjacent structures (including testis) will cause a large mass in affected hemiscrotum so that epididymitis cannot be distinguished; overlying skin dry, flaky, and without its normal rugated appearance; spontaneous rupture may occur; mass is exquisitely tender
Elevation of scrotum may result in relief from pain (Prehn's sign)[113]

Testis
Testis on affected side may be painful and enlarged
Masses or induration possible

Abdomen
Lower quadrant pain perceived on affected side

Nausea and vomiting
Vomiting may be severe during acute period

NURSING DIAGNOSES and NURSING INTERVENTIONS

Nursing Diagnosis	Nursing Intervention
Comfort, alteration in: pain	Support the scrotum via an athletic support, a towel placed under the scrotum, or a Bellevue bridge.[60,95] Provide analgesics as ordered. Utilize a sitz bath, local heat, or ice pack as prescribed. Provide bed rest during the acute period. Inform patient that sexual activity or any strenuous physical activity is contraindicated in even mild cases.
Fluid volume deficit, potential	Curtail all oral intake to reduce potential for vomiting. Maintain records of intake and output including frequency and amount of vomitus. Administer antiemetics as ordered.
Fear	Reassure patient that epididymitis is not a malignant process and that the mass effect is due to inflammation.

Patient Education

1. Provide instructions on the risk factors associated with epididymitis: prostatitis, urethritis (particularly gonococcal and chlamydial), cystitis, and unusually strenuous physical activity.
2. Emphasize the need for follow-up care aimed at identifying the underlying causes of epididymitis in certain cases.
3. Provide information on the signs and symptoms as well as the natural history of epididymitis and the importance of seeking care promptly.

EVALUATION

Patient Outcome	Data Indicating That Outcome is Reached
Epididymitis is resolved.	There is no pain in affected epididymis. Hemiscrotum is not enlarged. Urethral, prostate, and blood cultures are negative.
There are no recurrences.	Underlying prostatitis, urethritis, cystitis, tuberculosis or the urinary tract, or septic hematogenous focus is resolved.
There are no complications.	Sperm count and motility are normal.

IMPOTENCE

The sexual dysfunction known as impotence is the loss of ability to produce an erection of sufficient duration and rigidity to engage in intercourse.

Both psychogenic and organic factors may contribute to sexual dysfunction. Treatment is aimed at restoring normal erectile and orgasmic function or mimicking the erect penis via a surgically implanted prosthetic device. Other forms of male sexual dysfunction manifested as a loss of libido, premature ejaculation, or inability to achieve orgasm are discussed in Part 2, Pattern 10.

Sexual dysfunction in the male may be noted anytime after the onset of pubescence. The incidence of impo-

tence rises with increasing age. The incidence of men who seek treatment for impotence during the fourth decade of life is 1.5% of the general population; by the seventh decade of life the incidence has risen to 25% of all males. While the aging process is not a direct cause of impotence, sexual activity does generally decrease with increasing age because of a variety of social, cultural, and possibly physical factors. A survey of men revealed that 88% of sexually active males under 20 years of age engaged in intercourse at least once each week. During the fourth decade the proportion of men reporting intercourse at least once per week declined to 80%. During the sixth decade of life only 50% of the men surveyed reported intercourse on a weekly basis; by the seventh decade only one quarter had intercourse each week.[98]

The relative incidence of impotence from psychogenic vs. organic causes has received great attention. Some investigators have reported that 90% to 95% of all cases of impotence are the result of psychogenic causes.[87,92] However, recent data utilizing more sophisticated diagnostic techniques reveal a greater percentage of men whose erectile dysfunction has organic as well as psychogenic components.[92]

PATHOPHYSIOLOGY

A wide variety of organic conditions may cause or be associated with impotence.[87] Within this discussion only a number of the more commonly encountered organic causes of impotence are considered. An in-depth discussion of the psychosocial influences and ramifications of this condition is presented in Pattern 10.

A number of disease processes are associated with erectile dysfunction. These medical disorders may affect the physiologic processes of erection directly, or they may suppress sexual drive without causing true impotence. The psychosocial implications of illness, particularly a chronic condition, may alter a man's self-image and profoundly affect his sexual identity and sexual behaviors. In order to adequately understand and treat this complex problem, the nurse or physician must have an understanding of the underlying influences affecting erectile function in each individual.[99]

Endocrine problems may affect male sexual function by altering normal function of the hypothalamic–pituitary–gonadal hormonal axis. The typical result of this problem is hypogonadism, which is potentially reversible. The range of hypogonadism is significant and includes cases of mildly impaired libido as well as incidences of overt eunuchoidism requiring long-term hormonal replacement.[92]

The severity of impotence related to endocrine disorders is based on the age of onset and related symptoms that influence any medical decision to attempt to establish or restore potency in an affected male. Complete prepubertal gonadotropic failure may be expressed as hypogonadotropic eunuchoidism, Kallmann's syndrome, or a specific luteinizing hormone–follicle-stimulating hormone disorder. In all of the above conditions a failure of the production and propagation of gonadotropins is noted prepubertally and persists throughout the patient's lifetime. Abnormal growth patterns, a high-pitched voice, and a lack of secondary sex characteristics are associated with hypogonadism leading to impaired sexual function and infertility. Kallmann's syndrome is asso-

ciated with significant mental retardation, which may affect the medical approach to treatment of impotence.[92]

Partial prepubertal gonadotropic failure will produce symptoms similar to delayed puberty that actually do stem from an identifiable hormonal deficit rather than normal developmental processes. These males will have significantly decreased testosterone levels arising from a deficiency in the production of FSH and LH or LH only.[92]

Selective postpubertal hypogonadism is associated with a loss of testosterone production and a gradual loss of beard and body hair, declining libido, and resultant impotence and infertility. The eunuchoid aspects of this condition are not as prominent as those associated with prepubertal hypogonadism.[92]

Panhypopituitarism causes erectile dysfunction as well as a number of other hormonal imbalances. The condition is caused by a lesion that renders the pituitary or hypothalamus functionless or by surgical or traumatic ablation.[92]

Several congenital syndromes cause erectile dysfunction along with other medical problems. Prader-Willi syndrome causes neonatal hypotonia, mental retardation, and obesity as well as hypogonadism. Laurence-Moon-Biedl syndrome is an autosomal recessive syndrome that results in retinitis pigmentosa, polydactyly, renal anomalies, cryptorchidism, and erectile dysfunction. Familial cerebellar ataxia is also associated with hypogonadism along with ataxic movements and neural deafness. Other syndromes associated with hypogonadism and impotence include Klinefelter's syndrome, Noonan's syndrome, and Ullrich's syndrome.[92]

Any disease or drug that produces hyperprolactinemia will also interfere with the hypothalamic-pituitary-gonadotropic axis and cause erectile dysfunction. Medical conditions associated with hyperprolactinemia include certain hormone-producing tumors, endocrine disorders, and a number of drugs such as estrogen compounds and certain psychotropic drugs.[92]

Other endocrine-based disorders involving the thyroid or adrenal glands may affect erectile function. Castration has been used since antiquity to decrease libido and ultimately ablate normal male sexual function.[92]

Chronic heart disease has been associated with impotence, which may be attributed to the disease processes involved and to the use of certain antihypertensive drugs or digitalis preparations. Men with heart disease that is reasonably well controlled should consider sexual activity reasonably safe. Erectile dysfunction is best avoided in many of these men by prudent counseling. Sexual dysfunction may be complicated by the use of antihypertensive or antidepressant medications. Digoxin may also adversely affect sexual function by reducing LH and testosterone levels in the body while raising estradiol. Among those men who undergo heart transplant, erectile dysfunction is a potential complication that may be associated with postoperative immunosuppression.[99]

Erectile dysfunction is relatively common among men who suffer from chronic renal insufficiency and renal failure. Multiple factors contribute to the problem, related both to the disease process itself and the use of dialysis as a treatment modality. Impotence is a result of Leydig's cell abnormalities with concomitant decreases in the production of testosterone. Hyperprolactinemia and hyperparathyroidism may further complicate the situation. Erectile dysfunction may worsen after the start of dialysis. Many problems in erectile dysfunction are resolved by renal transplant although transient impotence may be noted in patients who have ligation of the internal artery to provide a blood supply for the transplanted kidney.[99]

Kass and his associates[46] studied a group of men with chronic obstructive pulmonary disease and found that 19% had problems with sexual function. The incidence of impotence in these men was largely attributed to psychosocial aspects of the disease rather than primary organic sexual dysfunction.

Several neurologic conditions are associated with erectile dysfunction. The presence of erectile dysfunction in spinal cord injury is influenced by the level of the lesion, the presence of spinal shock, and the "completeness" of the injury. Following a traumatic injury to the spinal cord, all erectile activity of the penis is inhibited. The generation of posttraumatic erections is typically associated with cessation of spinal shock. The period of time that erectile activity reappears after spinal cord injury is highly variable, ranging from 24 hours to 18 months.[119]

Two types of erections are observed in men with spinal cord injury; reflexogenic erections are mediated by spinal cord centers while psychogenic erections are mediated by supraspinal sexual centers. The incidence of erections among spinal cord–injured men is 63.5% to 94%, but the incidence of consistently successful erections is 23% to 33%.[119] The relatively low rate of successful potency among males with spinal cord injury is largely the result of the characteristics of reflexogenic erections, which are relatively brief and respond to a variety of tactile sensations, rendering penile response significantly altered from previous brain-centered control of sexual response.

Ejaculation is relatively rare among men with spinal cord injury. Ejaculation requires smooth coordination between autonomic and somatic impulses. The likelihood of orgasm among patients with complete spinal cord injuries is between 3% and 19.7%. Lower spinal cord injury is correlated with an increased likelihood of ejaculation but a relatively low incidence of erections (24.2%).[119]

Multiple sclerosis is another neurologic condition associated with male sexual dysfunction. Demyelination of the lateral horns of the lumbar spinal cord is theorized to be the critical underlying organic explanation for impotence among these men. Approximately 91% of all men with multiple sclerosis have significant sexual dysfunction.[119] The relationship between psychogenic factors, organic factors, and sexual dysfunction deserves further investigation.

Epilepsy involving the parietal lobes of the brain is associated with a higher incidence of impotence than other forms of the disease. In most cases the relative contribution of antiseizure medications to sexual dysfunction is negligible. Many men will experience continuing desire for sex with inability to sustain or maintain erections while fewer will experience a loss of libido.[99]

Diabetes mellitus is a causative factor in the development of erectile dysfunction because of a complex interplay of psychologic and organic factors. Erectile dysfunction may be noted near the time a diagnosis of diabetes is established; the diagnosis contributes to psychosocial factors (alterations in self-image and anxiety related to chronic disease) and physiologic factors resulting from insulin deficiency. Sexual dysfunction is generally resolved after the condition is regulated with exogenous insulin.[100]

Later problems related to sexual function have an insidious onset and are generally progressive. Hormonal factors have been theorized but are not supported by objective evidence. Diabetic neuropathies are often implicated in the genesis of impotence among diabetic men based on indirect evidence linking autonomic nervous abnormalities. Vascular compromise associated with diabetic angiopathy may influence potency by affecting the arterial blood supply of the cavernous bodies of the penis.[98,100]

Various vascular disorders may also lead to male sexual dysfunction by adversely affecting the vascular component of erections. Aortoiliac occlusion leads to erectile impairment in approximately 70% of all affected men. Arteriosclerosis is connected with an increased incidence of erectile dysfunction although a causal link is not always apparent. Peripheral arterial insufficiency is most commonly seen in men over 40 years of age so that other factors of aging may exert an influence. However, it is known that arteriosclerosis is the most common cause of occlusion of the penile artery, which may lead to erectile insufficiency, and that as many as 40% to 50% of all men with diagnosed peripheral arterial disease will report sexual dysfunction if questioned closely.[48,101]

Many drugs have been associated with erectile dysfunction. Duration, frequency, and dosage of the drug will affect the likelihood of impotence or loss of libido and secondary erectile dysfunction. It is essential to assess the use of all drugs including prescribed, over-the-counter, and recreational agents a man may be using.[41]

Endocrine drugs are used in a variety of hormonal abnormalities and may be used to treat cancer. Any exogenous estrogens or progestins will ultimately result in impotence if given in sufficient dosages. Anabolic steroids may suppress endogenous steroid levels and cause impotence when the drug is discontinued.[41]

Antihypertensive drugs, particularly the alpha- and beta-adrenergic blocking agents, are associated with impotence although the exact mechanism of sexual dysfunction may be more closely related to a loss of libido rather than a direct side effect of lowering systemic arterial blood pressure.[41] The following antihypertensive drugs are associated with male sexual dysfunction: clonidine (Catapres), guanethidine (Ismelin), hydralazine (Apresoline), monoamine oxidase inhibitors, methyldopa (Aldomet), phentolamine (Regitine), propranolol (Inderal), and reserpine (Serpasil).[41]

Two cardiac agents, digoxin and disopyramide, are commonly linked to male sexual dysfunction. The role of digoxin in erectile function was discussed in Chapter 1; disopyramide is an antiarrhythmic agent with parasympathetic properties that may contribute to erectile difficulties.[41]

The diuretic agents chlorthalidone and spironalactone may cause loss of libido and erectile dysfunction in a few instances. Hydrochlorothiazide is also linked to sexual dysfunction.[41]

Psychoactive drugs affect the central nervous system in many ways that are poorly understood. A significant number of these drugs, including sedatives, amphetamines, antidepressants, and antipsychotic agents, may cause impotence, presumably because of their effects on the central nervous system. The precise mechanisms by which this side effect occurs are not completely understood.[41] These drugs include weight reduction drugs (diethylpropion and phentermine hydrochloride), antidepressant agents (amitriptyline and monoamine oxidase inhibitors), antianxiety/sedative agents (benzodiazapines and glutethimide), and lithium carbonate.[41]

Anticholinergic agents such as propantheline are known to cause impotence as a side effect. Antiparkinson drugs are linked to erectile dysfunction and delayed ejaculation. The immunosuppressives are associated with impotence, but the underlying mechanism may be related to chemically induced psychogenic factors as well as general alterations in metabolism. Indomethacin is related to impotence arising from its antiprostaglandin effects. Metronidazole suppresses libido via some unknown process.[41]

A number of recreational drugs also affect male sexual function. Alcohol has been known to heighten desire while adversely affecting performance. Alcoholism is particularly associated with an increased incidence of impotence. Tobacco use has been linked to erectile dys-

functions in several recent studies. Nicotine may cause impotence by causing vasoconstriction of the penile arteries although the phenomenon requires further study to establish a causal link. Other drugs connected with male sexual dysfunction include amphetamines, barbiturates, opiates, cannabis (the active component of marijuana), and cocaine.[41,97]

A comprehensive discussion of the drugs that affect male sexual function is beyond the scope of this chapter. Inserts of individual drugs are an excellent source for assessing sexual dysfunction as a causative agent when impotence is a problem. However, nurses must be aware that overzealous cautions regarding potential sexual dysfunction are not indicated since such counseling may itself increase performance anxiety and exacerbate impotence.

Certain surgical procedures of the abdomen, thorax, and genital area may result in temporary failure of erectile function; prostatectomy and ileostomy or colostomy are particularly likely to result in alterations in male sexual function. Of all the forms of prostatectomy, open surgery using a perineal approach is the most likely to produce impotence. Transurethral resection of the prostate, the most common approach to prostatectomy, should not result in impotence but is associated with retrograde ejaculation. An open, communicative relationship with the patient including anticipatory guidance of expected postoperative potency is associated with a dramatically reduced likelihood of complaints of erectile dysfunction following the procedure.[99]

Any extensive surgical procedure involving the lower abdomen may lead to the inadvertent destruction of nerves or blood vessels that supply the cavernous bodies in the penis. The incidence of erectile dysfunction is particularly high in men who undergo ileostomy or colostomy with the attendant alteration in body image. Thus sexual dysfunction in these men may have psychogenic and organic components.[99]

Erectile dysfunction in the man may also arise from local disorders of the penis such as priapism, Peyronie's disease, and abnormal leakage of blood from the corpora cavernosa. Priapism is a prolonged, painful tumescent episode caused by the blockage of blood flow from the corpora cavernosa. Underlying causes may be primarily traumatic, neurogenic, vascular, or neoplastic. Some men experience idiopathic episodes of priapism although the condition has been tentatively linked to alcohol and drug use often noted among these men. Peyronie's disease is an abnormal lateral curvature of the penis that is most likely to occur during the fifth and sixth decades of life. The etiology is unclear; curvature is caused by fibroelastic plaques that form in the penis. The plaques may spontaneously regress, or they may persist in spite of various treatment methodologies. Impotence often accompanies Peyronie's disease and may be related to abnormal blood flow through the corpora cavernosa. Mechanical defects of the corpora cavernosa may result in low intracavernous pressure, which causes insufficient rigidity for vaginal penetration. Potency is restored by surgical repair of the defect.[97,98]

DIAGNOSTIC STUDIES

Serum testosterone
Low in impotence because of abnormality of hypothalamic-pituitary-gonadal axis

Serum prolactin
High when testosterone is abnormally low

Serum FSH
Abnormal when impotence is result of abnormality of hormonal axis

Serum LH
Abnormal when impotence is result of abnormality of hormonal axis

Glucose tolerance test
Abnormal in cases of suspected diabetes mellitus[69]

Sacral evoked responses
Increased bulbocavernous latency in diabetic males with autonomic neuropathy

Urodynamic testing
Abnormal sensations of bladder filling on cystometrogram and abnormal urecholine supersensitivity test in males with autonomic neuropathy

Penile systolic blood pressure
Low in cases of vascular impotence

Penile pulse volume recording
Abnormal in cases of vascular impotence

Internal pudendal arteriography
Decreased flow in cases of vascular impotence

NPT
Absent nocturnal erections when underlying cause of impotence is primarily organic rather than psychogenic

Snap-gauge testing
Breakage of three pressure-sensitive plastic bands indicates sufficient pressure for vaginal penetration
Inability to break bands during sleep study indicates erectile dysfunction

Reproduction of erection
19-Gauge scalp vein needle placed into distal portion of one corpus cavernosum and sterile saline is injected via syringe until a complete erection is obtained
Lateral curvature noted in Peyronie's disease

TREATMENT PLAN

Surgical
Corrective surgery of arterial occlusion may correct impotence
Revascularization of penis may be attempted by isolating epigastric artery and reanastomosing it directly to a corporal body[48]
Penile prostheses may be implanted surgically into penis to reproduce penile rigidity sufficient for normal vaginal penetration
Semirigid devices and inflatable penile prosthesis available[26,71]

Chemotherapeutic
Testosterone replacement therapy indicated in cases of hypogonadism
Luteinizing hormone–releasing hormone (LHRH), LH, or FSH may be used in males with identifiable abnormalities of hypothalamic-pituitary-gonadal axis; all other effects of hormonal therapy in males with erectile dysfunction are result of placebo effect[31]
Bromocriptine, zinc, and glyceryl trinitrate have been used to treat erectile dysfunction in selected cases with variable results[41]

Supportive
Discontinue use of any recreational drugs associated with impotence including illicit drugs, tobacco, and excessive alcohol intake (Alcoholism must be controlled to reestablish potency.)

ASSESSMENT: AREAS OF CONCERN

External genitalia
Normal appearance of penis, scrotum, and perineal area
Normal hair distribution, normal phallic size, bilaterally descended testes except in males with endocrine disorders resulting in hypogonadism, in which cases penis will be small, testes small and abnormally soft or cryptorchid, and hair distribution abnormal or absent
Palpation of penis will reveal hard plaques in Peyronie's disease

Polaroid pictures of penile erection obtained by patient will show penile curvature[69]

Rectal examination
Loss of anal sphincter tone with absent bulbocavernous reflex in local neuropathy
Absent saddle sensation with certain partial or complete spinal cord injuries[69]

Peripheral pulses
Decreased or absent in vascular impotence

Neurologic examination
Abnormal in men with underlying neurologic disease

NURSING DIAGNOSES and NURSING INTERVENTIONS

Nursing Diagnosis	Nursing Intervention
Sexual dysfunction	Encourage counseling and assistance in seeking appropriate health care to deal with sexual dysfunction or a surgical procedure likely to alter sexual function because of organic or psychogenic reasons. Open discussion with physician colleagues and clearly stated policies concerning the nurse's roles and responsibilities in cases of existing or potential sexual dysfunction are needed.
Self-concept, disturbance in: role performance	Male sexuality is deeply rooted in ideals of social, athletic/physical, and sexual performance. Any circumstance that significantly alters self-concepts and threatens self-esteem may adversely affect sexual function. Chronic disease, creation of a surgical stoma, and physical changes due to neurologic disease or spinal cord trauma significantly challenge any man's self-image. Empathy and opportunities to express feelings are indicated as the patient reintegrates self-concepts following a change in body image. Psychologic or psychiatric counseling is often a useful adjunct and may be suggested to a patient after a sufficiently trusting relationship has been established.

Patient Education

1. Provide instruction about various implantable prosthetic devices in suitable candidates after consultation with the physician.
2. Instruction of expectations of sexual abilities following specific surgical procedures will help prevent needless loss of sexual function due to anxiety.

EVALUATION

Patient Outcome	Data Indicating That Outcome is Reached
Impotence is resolved.	The patient reports increased satisfaction in sexual life and adequate onset, duration, and rigidity of erections.
Penile prosthesis is successfully implanted.	The patient has an operational semirigid or inflatable penile prosthesis. There is no local infection, pain, or erosion.

PROSTATITIS

Prostatitis is the inflammation of prostatic acini and surrounding tissue that is particularly pronounced in the periurethral portion of the gland.

Inflammation of the prostate is commonly divided into four types: acute bacterial, chronic bacterial, "nonbac-terial," and prostatodynia. Each form of prostatitis has a distinctive clinical presentation and is managed differently.[90]

Prostatitis is most commonly observed in males after the onset of pubescence, but rare cases of the disease have been reported among children and infants.[94] Nonbacterial prostatitis (also named prostatosis) is the most common form of the disease. Acute and chronic bacterial prostatitis are less commonly seen. Rarer forms include viral, fungal, parasitic, and allergic prostatitis.[67,94]

PATHOPHYSIOLOGY

Acute bacterial prostatitis is caused by the ascent of bacteria via the urethra or via the hematogenous route. Acute infection may be precipitated by urethral instrumentation or prostatic massage in the presence of chronic bacterial prostatitis. Common causative pathogens include *E. coli*, *Proteus*, *Klebsiella*, *Pseudomonas*, and *Enterobacter*. An acute episode of prostatic infection is characterized by a sudden onset of fever, chills, myalgia, arthralgia, and general malaise. These symptoms will rapidly progress to localized discomfort in the perineal area or low back associated with irritative voiding symptoms including urgency, frequency, nocturia, dysuria, and a persistent burning sensation in the urethra after micturition. Pain in the prostate will result in varying degrees of functional bladder outlet obstruction that may cause significant urinary hesitancy or even acute urinary obstruction.[3,66]

Histologic examination of prostatic tissue will reveal diffuse glandular inflammation with edema and hyperemia of the stroma. Abscesses are common and may hemorrhage in severe cases. Polymorphonucleocytes, bacteria, and cellular debris are present within the acini of the gland. Rectal palpation of the prostate reveals an exquisitely tender organ. Vigorous massage is contraindicated because of the associated pain and the danger of bacteremia. Acute bacterial cystitis is typically associated so that urine culture provides an excellent clue to the causative prostatic pathogen. An objective diagnosis of acute bacterial prostatitis is made in the presence of evidence of inflammation on expressed prostatic secretions (over 10 leukocytes per high-power field), positive bacterial culture of this expressed prostatic secretion, positive bacterial cystitis, and an abnormal rectal examination.[3,90]

Chronic bacterial prostatitis commonly occurs as a result of ascending infection from the urethra. The condition may arise following an inadequately treated episode of acute bacterial prostatitis, or it may occur via hematogenous bacterial invasion. However, the precise etiology of chronic bacterial prostatitis remains unclear.[94]

The clinical symptoms of chronic bacterial prostatitis vary widely. Some men will have no symptoms of prostatitis other than recurrent urinary tract infections or asymptomatic bacteriuria. More commonly, patients with prostatitis will note recurring irritative voiding symptoms such as urgency, frequency, dysuria, nocturia, and urethral irritation. Perineal pain, postejaculatory pain, hematospermia, and a mucoid urethral discharge may also be noted.[3]

Rectal palpation of the prostate may reveal the presence of prostatic calculi or may be unremarkable. Histologic examination of the prostate shows moderate inflammatory changes that are less localized than in acute infections. Objective diagnosis of chronic bacterial prostatitis requires the presence of inflammatory cells on microscopic examination of expressed secretion, a positive culture of these secretions, and a nontender gland on rectal examination.[3,90]

Unlike acute bacterial prostatitis, the chronically infected prostate is relatively resistant to antibiotic treatment because of the poor absorption of non–lipid soluble substances into the prostatic fluid. The chronically infected prostate has deficient levels of prostatic antibacterial substance. Prostatic calculi may also lower antibiotic susceptibility by serving as a nidus for persistent infection. Thus even extended periods of oral antibiotics may not cure chronic bacterial prostatitis.[66,90]

Nonbacterial prostatitis is the most common form of symptomatic prostatic inflammation. Although the causative agent of nonbacterial prostatitis has not been identified, chlamydia has been implicated as a possible pathogen. Unfortunately cultures are difficult to obtain so that verification of this suspicion will require further investigation.[95]

The symptoms of nonbacterial prostatitis are similar to chronic bacterial prostatitis and include pelvic area pain and irritative voiding symptoms. Objective diagnosis is made by demonstrating the presence of inflammatory cells in expressed prostatic secretions in the presence of negative prostatic secretion and bladder urine cultures. Rectal examination will be normal.[66,90]

Prostatodynia is the presence of symptoms of prostatitis in the absence of any physical findings. The etiology of this form of prostatitis is unknown. Objective diagnosis is made by demonstrating negative inflammatory cells in expressed prostatic secretions, negative bacterial culture of these secretions, and negative urine cultures in the presence of recurrent perineal pain, and irritative voiding symptoms.[90]

Other forms of prostatitis occur rarely and include viral prostatic inflammation following an upper respiratory infection, tubercular prostatitis, or mycotic prostatitis from blastomycosis, coccidioidomycosis, histoplasmosis, and candidiasis. Symptoms are similar to bacterial prostatitis with the presence of perineal area pain and inflammation of the prostate associated with irritative voiding symptoms.[66]

Complications of prostatitis include acute urinary retention, bladder neck contracture, and obstruction in the presence of chronic inflammation. Cystitis is typically associated with the condition, and epididymitis is not uncommon. Pyelonephritis and bacteremia may be associated with acute infection.[94]

DIAGNOSTIC STUDIES

Intravenous pyelogram (IVP)
Normal or evidence of bladder neck obstruction with elevation of bladder base (due to prostatic edema and large postvoid residual)

White blood cell (WBC) count
Acute bacterial prostatitis: 20,000/L

Urinalysis
Bacterial infection: bacteria and WBCs on microscopic examination

Culture: divided specimen
Patient is asked to void his first 10 to 15 ml in a sterile cup and switch to another cup without interrupting the urinary stream, where he will collect the next 50 to 100 ml; voiding completed is cautioned not to squeeze out the last several drops; prostate is then milked for an ''expressed prostatic secretion,'' or all residual urine is expressed by straining if no secretions are obtained

Three portions are obtained from first container of urine (these represent ''urethral discharge''): one portion examined microscopically, one portion used for culture, and remaining portion used for dry mounting on a slide using alcohol

Second container constitutes a midstream urine specimen and is used for routine urine culture and urinalysis

Final specimen is expressed prostatic fluid and is examined microscopically for inflammatory cells and submitted for culture

Bacterial prostatitis diagnosed by presence of over 5000 bacteria/ml with less than 3000 bacteria/ml obtained from bladder and urethral specimens[20]

Urine culture and sensitivity
Acute bacterial cystitis: positive
Chronic bacterial prostatitis: positive
Nonbacterial prostatitis: negative
Prostatodynia: negative

TREATMENT PLAN

Surgical
Open prostatectomy a possible curative measure but generally contraindicated because of associated side effects, including urinary incontinence and impotence[66,67]

Transurethral resection of prostate effective if all of the affected prostatic tissue is removed; clinical results indicate that approximately one third of patients treated in this manner will experience complete resolution of symptoms; remaining two thirds will experience improvement of symptoms or remain the same[20,66]

Chemotherapeutic
Anti-infective agents guided by routine urine culture and sensitivity reports indicated in cases of acute bacterial prostatitis; 30-day course of trimethoprim (Trimpex) or trimethoprim/sulfamethosoxazole (Bactrim DS; 1 tablet po bid) given to prevent occurrence of chronic infection

Mild cases of acute infection may be treated with oral antibiotics

Severe cases will require parenteral antibiotic therapy with gentamicin (Garamycin) or tobramycin (Nebcin) and ampicillin (Amcil) until culture sensitivity reports are available or patient is afebrile[3]

Chronic bacterial prostatitis treated by 30 days of double-strength tablets of trimethoprim/sulfamethoxazole (Bactrim DS) given twice daily; tetracyclines may be substituted if patient is allergic to sulfonamides; combination of erythromycin and sodium bicarbonate may be used although results are not uniformly successful[3]

Antipyretics (ASA) often indicated in presence of acute bacterial prostatitis

Stool softeners may lessen discomfort associated with straining with a bowel movement[66]

Supportive
Alcohol intake often causes exacerbation of symptoms in prostatitis; should be limited to 2 or 3 ounces per day or deleted from diet totally

Foods that contain chili powder or other ''hot'' spices possibly associated with exacerbation of symptoms and are serially deleted from diet to assess their role in relief of symptoms

Dietary manipulation particularly important in management of prostatodynia

Electromechanical
Placement of suprapubic catheter or suprapubic needle aspiration of urine indicated in cases of acute urinary retention from acute bacterial prostatitis[60,66]

ASSESSMENT: AREAS OF CONCERN

Prostate

Acute bacterial prostatitis: firm gland with asymmetry or focal area of enlargement; exquisitely tender to touch

Chronic forms of prostatitis: relatively nontender; may note presence of calculi[90]

Voiding behavior

Frequency, urgency, dysuria, bladder irritability, difficulty initiating stream

NURSING DIAGNOSES and NURSING INTERVENTIONS

Nursing Diagnosis	Nursing Intervention
Comfort, alteration in: pain	Force intake of fluid to decrease irritative voiding symptoms. Provide local heat such as sitz bath as prescribed for symptomatic relief of perineal pain and to encourage urination in patients experiencing discomfort from a distended bladder. Note that gentle prostatic massage is contraindicated during acute infection but may offer relief for chronic prostatitis; massage should be performed no more than once each week. Sexual activity may also afford relief in cases of chronic prostatitis.[60]
Urinary elimination, alteration in patterns (resulting from bladder outlet obstruction)	For acute bacterial prostatitis, monitor intake and output and percuss bladder for signs of overdistention. Provide a warm bath to encourage urination by helping relieve discomfort and relax the pelvic floor musculature. If a suprapubic catheter is placed, monitor intake and output to assess patency of tube and securely tape tube to abdomen to prevent kinking.
Noncompliance with medical therapy	Advise patient to continue antibiotic therapy for the full 30 days in order to achieve optimal therapeutic results.

Patient Education

1. Provide information concerning the prostate's relative resistance to antibiotic therapy.
2. Assure the patient that prostatitis is not associated with an increased incidence of adenocarcinoma of the prostate and that prostatitis is not a form of venereal disease.
3. Provide anticipatory guidance on how to manage acute urinary retention.

EVALUATION

Patient Outcome	Data Indicating That Outcome is Reached
Acute bacterial prostatitis is resolved.	There are no bacteria in expressed prostatic secretion. Bacteriuria is not present. The patient is afebrile. Irritative voiding symptoms are absent.
Chronic bacterial prostatitis is resolved.	There are no bacteria in expressed prostatic secretion. Bacteriuria is not present. Irritative voiding symptoms are absent. There are no complications; urinary flow is unobstructed.
Nonbacterial prostatitis or prostatodynia is resolved.	There are no inflammatory cells in expressed prostatic secretions. Irritative voiding symptoms are absent. Perineal pain is absent.

URINARY CALCULI

Calculi are stones that are formed in the urinary tract.

Calculi that pass spontaneously without discomfort present no serious threat to health. However, many urinary calculi are extremely painful, obstructive, and a focus of infection. The problem of urinary calculi must be addressed by both urologists and nephrologists, since stones have both medical and surgical implications. A detailed discussion of medical aspects of urinary calculi is presented in Chapter 10. This discussion focuses on the two primary urologic complications associated with urinary calculi, infection and obstruction, as well as the surgical and electromechanical therapeutic options available to patients.

The incidence of urinary calculi varies significantly with a number of intrinsic factors such as age, sex, and race, as well as extrinsic factors such as geographic location and climate.

The peak incidence of calculus formation is the third, fourth, and fifth decades of life. Many patients report an onset of symptoms associated with urolithiasis beginning in their twenties; surgical or medical interventions for urinary calculi are most commonly performed in the fifth decade of life. Men are three times more likely to have calculus formation in the upper urinary tract and bladder than are women.[21] The disease is relatively rare among American and African blacks, North American Indians, and native-born Israelis but relatively common among whites and Eurasians.[21]

Throughout the world those persons at greatest risk for urinary calculi live in mountainous areas. The United States, a number of European countries, and Australia have a high incidence of urinary lithiasis, whereas the African and South American countries have a relatively low incidence. The southeastern and arid southwestern United States generally have a higher incidence of calculi than other regions.[21]

Sedentary occupations are associated with an increased incidence of urinary lithiasis. Intake of certain foods can also contribute to stone formation. The patient should be questioned concerning intake of foods containing calcium (dairy products), oxalate (green, leafy vegetables and certain fruits), and purines that are metabolized to uric acid (meat, fish, and poultry).[83] In rare instances medications are responsible for stone disease. Long-term ingestion of calcium carbonate, vitamin D, antacids, megadoses of vitamin C, acetazolamide, probenecid, or triamterene can lead to various types of stone formation.[83]

PATHOPHYSIOLOGY

The five major types of urinary stones occurring in the United States are calcium oxalate, magnesium-ammonium-phosphate (struvite), uric acid, cystine, and mixed calculi. The etiology of calculus formation is complex and not completely understood. The *supersaturation* theory partially explains the etiology of three of the major types of calculi. Uric acid and cystine calculi form in urine that is acidic and oversaturated with the causative substance. Struvite stones form in urine that is alkaline and oversaturated with magnesium, phosphate, and ammonium. The supersaturation theory fails to explain why not all persons whose urine contains high amounts of uric acid, cystine, magnesium, ammonium, and phosphorus form calculi. The *inhibitor lack* theory supposes that individuals who form calculi lack certain innate inhibitor substances. The *matrix initiation* theory places blame on the presence of matrices in the urine that serve as focus for calculus formation. In most urinary calculi the matrix is formed of a mucoprotein derivative that may directly inhibit crystal formation in favor of calculus growth. *Epitaxy of urinary crystals* depends on the resemblance and proximity of structure crystals that will promote oriented overgrowth of one crystal upon another rather than the formation of a calculus. Therapeutic modification of epitaxy may prove beneficial in the prevention of urolithiasis, although no such agents are currently available. The final theory of calculus formation is a combination of the above concepts.[21]

The presence of a urinary calculus is typically discovered when the stone becomes entrapped, resulting in the abrupt onset of acute renal or bladder colic. The most common sites of entrapment are a calyx or calyceal diverticulum, the ureteropelvic junction, the segment of ureter at or near the pelvic brim adjacent to the point where the ureter crosses the iliac vessels, the posterior pelvic portion of the ureter in women, and the ureterovesical junction. Of all the areas of anatomic narrowing, the ureterovesical junction is the most difficult for a calculus to pass.[21]

The renal colic typically occurs at night or during the early morning hours when the patient is sedentary. The pain begins in the flank and radiates to the groin and testes in men or the labia majora and broad ligament in women. As the stone moves to the midureter, the pain radiates to the lateral portion of the flank and lower abdomen. As the calculus moves toward the ureterovesical junction, the pain associated with the initial renal colic may recur, associated with irritable voiding symptoms of urinary urgency or urge incontinence. Colic is perceived most intensely as the calculus moves or if it implants at a certain site. Movement of the stone also causes localized pain resulting from obstruction.[21]

Bladder colic is characterized by bladder pain that crescendoes immediately after micturition. A stabbing pain may be felt when changing position, and urinary urgency and urge incontinence are commonly associated.[21]

Because visceral pain such as renal colic is mediated by the autonomic nervous system via the celiac ganglia, nausea and vomiting, intestinal stasis, and ileus may occur. Patients are typically restless as they change position to reduce discomfort. Grunting respirations signaling distress may be present. The pulse and blood pressure may be elevated in response to pain. Fever is rare unless a urinary tract infection is present.[21]

Many urinary calculi pass spontaneously and do not require urologic intervention, but others need prompt attention. The decision to intervene surgically, endoscopically, or via extracorporeal shock wave lithotripsy is based on prevention of the two significant complications of calculi: obstruction and infection.

Obstruction of the urinary tract in the presence of calculi results in adverse changes in renal and ureteral function associated with hydronephrosis. The adverse effects of acute hydronephrosis have been studied in laboratory animals and divided into the following stages. During the first 90 minutes after the onset of obstruction, ipsilateral renal blood flow is dramatically increased and intramural pressure in both ureters rises. In the second stage, lasting from 90 minutes to the end of the fifth hour, renal blood flow to both kidneys decreases while pressure in the ureters remains high in an attempt to compensate for and overcome the obstruction. From the fifth through the eighteenth hour following acute obstruction, renal blood flow in the affected side and intraureteral pressure decrease as compensatory mechanisms are overwhelmed. Intrarenal changes on the affected side include an early rapid redistribution of blood from the medullary to cortical nephrons during the initial period after obstruction. Later, the renal plasma flow, glomerular filtration rate, and tubular function are all slowed as kidney function is impaired.[21]

Ureteral peristalsis is also adversely affected by obstruction. The creation of acute obstruction in animal models resulted in an initial rise in ureteral pressure and the frequency of peristaltic waves. However, these compensatory mechanisms were soon overcome, resulting in dilation of the ureters and loss of smooth muscle tone and fibrotic replacement in the ureteral wall.[21]

In humans progressive changes from hydronephrosis include renal pelvic dilation and an initial rise in kidney weight because of renal edema. Parenchymal mass decreases as a result of atrophy and adverse changes in the structure and function of the nephron. If hydronephrosis persists for 8 weeks or more, the parenchymal mass may be dramatically compromised with only a thin shell of tissue remaining around a hydronephrotic, distorted collecting system.[21]

Obstruction may be complicated by infection leading to pyelonephritis. In such cases the infection may become the dominant aspect of the disease, requiring immediate intervention before stone manipulation or surgical removal is attempted. Pyelonephritis is characterized by fever, chills, flank pain, and irritative voiding symptoms. Destruction of parenchymal mass by inflammatory changes and sepsis is a serious complication of the condition. Children with pyelonephritis are especially susceptible to renal scarring with subsequent loss of nephric function.[66,90]

Examination of a patient with calculous pyohydronephrosis may reveal a giant or intermediate-size hydronephrotic kidney or an atrophic kidney. The giant hydronephrotic kidney has a massively dilated collecting system with a thin shell of functioning parenchyma. The surface of the kidney is nodular and densely adherent to adjacent perirenal fat. An atrophic kidney is small because of extensive damage. Only a small mass of parenchymal tissue remains in this kidney, and progressive failure of function is likely. The intermediate-size hydronephrotic kidney is not as large as the giant kidney or as severely compromised in its function as the atrophic kidney. Microscopic examination of this type of kidney reveals more nearly normal nephrons than the other types of infected kidney, although inflammatory damage is present.[21]

Multiple factors influence the decision to attempt endoscopic manipulation or surgical removal of a urinary calculus. The patient's occupation and economic status must be considered when contemplating urologic intervention for a calculus. Persons in certain occupations (for example, a pilot) may subject themselves and others to danger if renal colic occurs during the performance of their jobs.[21]

A stone more than 4 mm in diameter is unlikely to pass through the ureter. Even smaller stones that are securely implanted into the wall of a calyx or ureter are less likely to pass and more likely to be obstructive or cause of infection.

Aggressive removal of urinary calculi is considered for any patient who has a single kidney or significant renal insufficiency. Because of age and general health status, however, a patient may be a poor candidate for the anesthesia necessary for calculus manipulation.[21]

DIAGNOSTIC STUDIES

Kidneys, ureters, and bladder (KUB)

Calcifications in urinary tract; calcium phosphate calculi are most densely radiopaque; uric acid stones are radiolucent

Intravenous pyelogram (IVP)

Filling defects in conjunction with calculus; ureteral dilation on affected side if calculus is obstructive;

hydronephrosis may be present with dilation of calyces and renal pelvis; clubbing of calyces in advanced cases of hydronephrosis; signs of pyelonephritis (parenchymal enlargement with impairment of excretion) if calculous pyohydronephrosis is present

Voiding cystourethrogram (VCUG)
Of limited value in diagnosing bladder calculi, which are appreciated as intravesical filling defect

Retrograde pyelography
Useful in cases of radiolucent calculi that cannot be localized by routine radiographic studies[21]

Ultrasonography
Presence of calculi

Analysis of stones
Prominent constituents such as cystine, calcium, oxalate, and uric acid; provides guidance for medical therapy to prevent recurrence

Urine calcium
Elevated in patients with calcium stones or renal tubular acidosis

Urine oxalate
Elevated in patients with calcium oxalate stones

Urine uric acid
Elevated in patients with uric acid stones

Urinary pH
Acidic in patients with uric acid or cystine stones; alkaline in patients who form calcium phosphate, calcium oxalate, and struvite stones

Urine culture
Bacteriuria if infection is due to presence of calculi

Antibody-coated bacteria
Positive in pyelonephritis

Serum calcium
Elevated in hyperparathyroidism

Serum parathormone
Elevated in hyperparathyroidism

TREATMENT PLAN

Surgical
Has been mainstay of urologic interventions throughout twentieth century; surgical procedures for removing calculi are nephrolithotomy, pelvolithotomy, and ureterolithotomy; relative incidence of indications for surgical intervention has been greatly limited owing to refinement of percutaneous, ureteroscopic, and extracorporeal therapy

Chemotherapeutic
Anti-infective agents
Antibiotics guided by urine and blood cultures; pending culture findings: gentamicin, 3-5 mg/kg body weight/d, and ampicillin, 2 g IV q6h
Central nervous system drugs
Narcotic agents for renal colic
For uric acid stones: allopurinol 200-600 mg/d
For cystine stones: penicillamine
For acidic urine: sodium bicarbonate or potassium citrate or sodium citrate
For calcium stones: potassium acid phosphate or neutral sodium and potassium phosphate
For alkaline urine: ascorbic acid, 1 g/d, or ammonium chloride, 0.3-1 g q4h

Electromechanical
Percutaneous removal of renal and ureteral stones using stone baskets or by crushing stones via ultrasonic shock waves, electrical stimulation, or laser techniques

Supportive
Dietary restrictions for preventive therapy
To prevent calcium stones: reduce intake of dairy products and green leafy vegetables
To prevent oxalate stones: reduce intake of foods high in oxalates, including asparagus, beets, plums, raspberries, rhubarb, spinach, almonds, cashew nuts, cranberries, cocoa, cranberry juice, grape juice, grapefruit juice, Worcestershire sauce
To prevent uric acid stones: reduce intake of foods high in purines such as organ meats, lean meats, and whole grains

ASSESSMENT: AREAS OF CONCERN

Pain
Renal colic or bladder colic; may be severe; flank pain noted with pyelonephritis

Voiding behaviors
Irritative voiding symptoms

Fever
Elevated if infection is present

Nausea and vomiting
Associated with renal colic

NURSING DIAGNOSES and NURSING INTERVENTIONS

Nursing Diagnosis	Nursing Intervention
Comfort, alteration in: pain	Provide pain medications as ordered. Minimize environmental noise and activity to promote rest. Observe for intensification of pain, which may indicate impaction of stone or increase in obstructive property of stone. Marked pain relief may indicate passage of stone from relatively narrow ureteral segment to wider segment or passage of calculus through ureterovesical junction.
Noncompliance: potential, associated with medical regimen	Instruct the patient in the need for increased fluid intake (at least 2.5 L/day) to aid the urinary concentration of stone-forming substances. Instruct the patient of the need to strain all urine with proper straining device to secure stone(s) if passed. Reinforce the importance of any dietary measures that are needed in relation to the type of stone suspected. (See "Treatment Plan.")
Tissue perfusion, alteration in: obstruction with renal function compromise	Observe for signs of acute urinary obstruction (marked renal colic) or pyelonephritis (flank pain, fever, and chills). Closely monitor urinary output. Provide fluid hydration.

Patient Education

1. Provide explanation of analysis of stone, adjunct medical therapy aimed at prevention of recurrence, and associated dietary restrictions.
2. Provide instruction concerning options of treatment should manipulation of stones be indicated.

EVALUATION

Patient Outcome	Data Indicating That Outcome is Reached
Spontaneous passage of calculus takes place.	Findings of kidney, bladder, and urine (KUB) are normal. There is no renal colic. Stone is passed in urine and retrieved for analysis.
Calculi do not recur.	Findings of follow-up KUB, 3 to 6 months later, are normal.

URINARY INCONTINENCE

Urinary incontinence is the involuntary leakage of urine after the age of toilet training.

Incontinence is not a disease; it is a symptom that represents a significant health problem and may underlie a serious disease process. Urinary incontinence is a particularly appropriate area of intensive investigation and intervention for nurses who manage patients with genitourinary disease.

The problem of urinary incontinence occurs throughout the life span and is a particularly prevalent and underrated condition among the elderly. The prevalence of urinary incontinence among adults over 65 years of age is approximately 17%.[96] Among nursing home residents the prevalence approaches 50%.[24]

A Welsh study of 1060 women 18 years of age and over revealed that 45% of these women suffered from some degree of incontinence. Symptoms consistent with stress incontinence were reported by 22% of the women, and those of urge incontinence were reported by 10%. A combination of stress and urge incontinence was reported by 14% of those surveyed. In the majority of the women, urinary incontinence was assessed as mild, but 5% related severe enough symptoms to necessitate changing clothing daily. Over 3% of the women reported that urinary incontinence significantly interfered with their daily lives, yet less than half of these had sought medical treatment for the problem.

The prevalence of urinary incontinence in men is less

well documented. In the Danish population, 2% of all adults have urinary incontinence severe enough to prompt them to seek medical help. Among men over 65 years of age, 5% suffer from incontinence; among men under 50 years approximately 20% to 25% will develop symptoms of obstruction and dribble after voiding because of benign prostatic hypertrophy.[33,84]

Urinary continence in childhood is typically accomplished by 5 years of age. Incontinence most often takes the form of enuresis, which is seen in 15% of all 5-year-olds.[76]

PATHOPHYSIOLOGY

Many classification schemes for urinary incontinence have been proposed. Within this discussion, Wheatley's four types of incontinence[112] are used because they offer a simple yet comprehensive conceptual framework for this complex health problem. The four types of incontinence are stress urinary incontinence, instability incontinence, overflow or paradoxical incontinence, and constant incontinence.

Stress urinary incontinence occurs when intravesical pressure exceeds urethral closure pressure and urine is forced through the urethral sphincters in the absence of an inappropriate detrusor contraction. Stress incontinence is more commonly observed in women, although men may also be affected by the condition. The two primary causes of stress incontinence are pelvic relaxation and internal sphincter (bladder neck) incompetence.[54,112]

Pelvic relaxation occurs in a woman's bladder and is influenced by multiple causes. Multiparity, aging, hormonal changes resulting from menopause and the aging process, and impaired innervation of the pelvic floor musculature are associated with anterior pelvic relaxation.[112] Obesity may be an aggravating factor in this condition but may be overemphasized as a primary cause of pelvic relaxation unless there is adequate objective evidence.

Internal sphincter incompetence will also result in stress urinary incontinence, which affects both men and women. Pelvic fracture and radical prostatectomy are associated with increased risk of damage to the internal sphincter. Transurethral prostatectomy may also cause stress urinary incontinence if the entire internal sphincter mechanism is ablated. Bladder neck surgery in women and multiple anti-incontinence procedures are also associated with stress incontinence resulting from internal sphincter incompetence.[112]

The symptom of stress incontinence is leakage of urine noted with coughing, sneezing, or any maneuver that causes a precipitous rise in intra-abdominal pressure. Urinary urgency and nocturia are typically present. Urinary

tract infection may be a problem if pelvic relaxation interferes with efficient bladder emptying owing to the presence of cystocele, rectocele, enterocele, or poor detrusor contraction because of myogenic decompensation. Stress incontinence resulting from internal sphincter incompetence is often severe and may result in failure of bladder storage when the person assumes an upright position.

Instability incontinence refers to urinary leakage resulting from inappropriate detrusor contractions. Detrusor instability is a urodynamic term defined as a spontaneous rise in detrusor pressure during the filling-storage phase of bladder function. Detrusor hyperactivity refers to untimely detrusor contractions. Detrusor hyperreflexia is defined as overactivity of the detrusor muscle in the presence of neuropathic dysfunction.

The primary causes of instability incontinence are neuropathic bladder dysfunction and irritative disorders. The attainment and maintenance of social continence in an adult rely on integration of multiple neural centers in the brain and spinal cord, which influence bladder function. Abnormality of these centers will result in a loss of normal detrusor reflex and subsequent incontinence.[112]

Diseases of the brain may affect its inhibitory function over detrusor reflexes. Cerebrovascular accident, brain tumors, multiple sclerosis, parkinsonism, and Alzheimer's disease may result in loss of normal loop I function.[70] The voiding pattern resembles that of a child who has not been toilet trained; spontaneous micturition with normal sphincter responses occurs at a particular bladder volume, which is unresponsive to the brain's inhibitory signals.

The person who experiences instability incontinence caused by interruption of loop I function has the uninhibited neurogenic bladder described by Lapides.[50,52] The symptoms of uninhibited neurogenic bladder are frequency and urgency with a rapid onset of incontinence. Since the uninhibited bladder typically empties well, urinary tract infection does not occur unless other predisposing factors are present. Nocturia is common, but nocturnal enuresis is rare.

Complete spinal cord injury above the sacral micturition center causes instability incontinence and may result in detrusor–external sphincter dyssynergia. The micturition process shifts from a brainstem-mediated response to a spinal cord–mediated response.[109] A reflex neurogenic bladder is characterized by an unstable detrusor without sensations of urgency. Detrusor–external sphincter dyssynergia is the pathologic contraction of the pelvic floor musculature during voiding resulting from an abnormality in loop III. The reflex neurogenic bladder does not empty completely, and the chronic obstruction may result in cystitis, trabeculation of the bladder wall, diverticulae, and upper urinary tract damage.

Cystitis is also known to cause instability incontinence. These persons have active irritation of the bladder mucosa resulting in overactive afferent signals that may disrupt normal detrusor suppression by the central nervous system.[112] An uninhibited detrusor contraction may follow; the person may become incontinent owing to urethral instability. Urethral instability is the inappropriate relaxation of the urethra resulting in incontinence and an intense perception of urgency.

Causes of irritative instability incontinence include bacterial, tubercular, parasitic, and radiation- or chemotherapy-induced cystitis, as well as specific inflammatory lesions of the bladder. Vaginitis or the female urethral syndrome may also be associated with irritative instability incontinence. Carcinoma of the bladder wall causes instability incontinence in certain individuals.[112] The maintenance of continence depends on the person's general state of alertness and opportunity to move to a toilet rapidly as needed.

Overflow or paradoxical incontinence is the leakage of urine in the presence of a large residual. The two causes of overflow incontinence are deficient detrusor function and bladder outlet obstruction.[112] Deficient detrusor function may result from a variety of causes. Neurologic lesions of the sacral micturition cord such as that noted in myelomeningocele cause an autonomous neurogenic bladder with detrusor areflexia, lack of sensations of urgency, and overflow incontinence. Other central nervous system disorders associated with overflow incontinence are cauda equina syndrome, multiple sclerosis, tabes dorsalis, and poliomyelitis. Peripheral nervous system trauma or abnormalities that compromise parasympathetic innervation of the detrusor muscle also result in overflow incontinence. Examples are herpes zoster, extensive pelvic surgery, pelvic trauma, and diabetes mellitus.[112]

Other factors that result in overflow incontinence and detrusor areflexia are the result of chronic overdistention. The "nurse's bladder," "teacher's bladder," or "librarian's bladder" arises from overdistention of the bladder because of perceived inability to interrupt work for micturition. Acute illness and immobility may also result in deficient detrusor function. Severe constipation or fecal impaction is associated with temporary detrusor failure and overflow incontinence. Certain patients may suffer from urinary retention because of hysterical conversions.

Patients with overflow incontinence may not be aware of their inability to empty the bladder. Symptoms of deficient detrusor function are urgency, frequency, nocturia, and a dribbling, intermittent stream. Urinary tract infection is commonly an associated condition. Low back pain and vague abdominal discomfort may be the result of bladder enlargement.

Bladder outlet obstruction is also a cause of overflow incontinence. Types of bladder outlet obstruction include prostatic enlargement owing to inflammation, benign hypertrophy, or adenocarcinoma. Internal sphincter dyssynergia, bladder neck hypertrophy, and bladder neck contracture are particularly prevalent in men with highly stressful life-styles and may lead to overflow incontinence. Urethral stricture in a man or urethral distortion in a woman may obstruct normal bladder emptying and lead to incontinence.[112]

Patients with bladder outlet obstruction are acutely aware of their problem because of high pressures generated by the detrusor during micturition. Symptoms of bladder outlet obstruction include frequency, nocturia, and poor urinary stream. A dribble after voiding is often noted.

Constant incontinence occurs when a fistulous tract or ectopic bladder, ureter, or urethra bypasses the normal sphincter mechanisms, resulting in relatively continuous leakage. Congenital ectopia of the bladder or urethra is relatively rare but may be associated with severe incontinence. Ectopic ureters associated with ureteral duplication are more common and will result in a constant dribbling discharge superimposed on a normal voiding pattern if the orifice opens outside the bladder vesicle.[112]

Urinary fistula is caused by trauma, cancer, or obstetric complications. Vesicovaginal fistula in women may occur as a persistent watery vaginal discharge or as severe leakage of urine with failure of bladder storage in the upright position. Cystitis is a common finding.[112]

DIAGNOSTIC STUDIES

Marshall test
Performed by placing woman with full bladder in lithotomy position and applying suprapubic pressure; positive findings indicate stress urinary incontinence

Voiding cystourethrogram (VCUG)
Stress incontinence: pelvic descent below pubis; positive urethral excursion with coughing

Incompetent internal sphincter: bladder neck funneling with filling in supine and upright positions

Instability incontinence and uninhibited bladder: normal or trabeculated

Instability incontinence and reflex bladder: narrowing of membranous urethra during micturition, trabeculation, diverticulae, vesicoureteral reflux with ureteral dilation

Overflow/paradoxical incontinence: large capacity; poor filling of proximal urethra with prostatic enlargement; failure of bladder neck funneling with internal sphincter abnormality; urethral narrowing with stricture

Constant incontinence: extravasation of contrast material with urinary fistula

Urodynamic testing

Stress incontinence: normal capacity, sensations, and compliance; stable detrusor; explosive flow with low-pressure detrusor contraction during micturition; normal electromyographic (EMG) findings; residual after voiding in some cases

Instability incontinence: decreased functional capacity; early sensations; normal compliance; unstable detrusor and/or urethra; EMG findings normal or indicative of detrusor–external sphincter dyssynergia

Overflow incontinence with deficient detrusor function: large capacity, delayed sensations, abnormally compliant; with detrusor hyporeflexic or areflexic: urinary stream poor or absent, large residual present after voiding

Bladder outlet obstruction: normal or enlarged capacity; sensations may be delayed; compliance normal or impaired owing to detrusor hypertrophy; detrusor contraction is high pressure with poor urinary flow and positive resistance factor

Constant incontinence: normal or impaired urine storage with large fistulous tract

Intravenous pyelogram (IVP)

Constant incontinence: ureteral duplication with ectopic opening below bladder neck or outside urinary tract; extravasation of contrast material in fistula

Retrograde urethrogram (RVG)

Presence of urethral stricture

Cystoscopy-urethroscopy

Stress incontinence: normal findings in pelvic relaxation or open bladder neck with internal sphincter damage

Urge incontinence: normal findings or signs of vesical irritation

Overflow incontinence: large capacity in deficient detrusor function; localization of obstruction in some cases

Constant incontinence: ectopia or fistulous tract

Urinalysis and urine culture

Instability incontinence: normal findings or presence of bacterial infection

Bladder biopsy

Instability incontinence: normal findings or presence of transitional cell carcinoma or carcinoma in situ

TREATMENT PLAN

Surgical

For stress incontinence

Vesicourethral suspension and repair of cystocele and urethrocele; commonly performed types are the Marshall/Marchetti/Krantz, Lapides' vesicopexy, and Burch's culposuspension

Artificial urinary sphincter for stress incontinence caused by internal sphincter damage; cuff of device is placed at bladder neck, abdominal reservoir is positioned, and pump mechanism is put in scrotum or fascia of labia minora

For overflow incontinence

Radical prostatectomy in certain cases of adenocarcinoma

Correction of female urethral distortion by open surgical reconstruction

For continuous incontinence

Removal or reimplantation of ectopic ureter may preserve significant percentage of renal function in certain cases; otherwise, ectopic ureter is removed

Urinary fistula typically repaired by open surgical procedure

Chemotherapeutic

To affect detrusor contractility

Autonomic drugs

Propantheline, up to 150 mg/d in three divided doses

Oxybutinin, 5 mg bid-tid

Central nervous system drugs

Imipramine, 1.5-2 mg/kg in single dose at bedtime

Spasmolytic agents

Flavoxate, 100-200 mg tid-qid

Dicyclomine, 10-20 mg tid-qid

Drugs that increase detrusor activity and tone

Autonomic drugs

Bethanechol, 15-30 mg tid-qid

Drugs used to increase bladder neck tone

Autonomic drugs

Norephedrine or ephedrine (Sudafed S.A.), 1 tablet bid

Drugs used to decrease bladder neck tone

Autonomic drugs

Phenoxybenzamine, 10-30 mg/d in single dose

Drugs used to decrease external muscle tone

Central nervous system drugs

Diazepam, 5-10 mg qid

Dantrolene, 25-50 mg/d

Baclofen, 5-20 mg tid

ASSESSMENT: AREAS OF CONCERN

Bladder

Suprapubic tenderness associated with cystitis; suprapubic and lower abdominal distention in overflow incontinence

Vaginal vault

Bulge in anterior wall in cystocele associated with anterior pelvic relaxation; inflammation in vaginitis; discharge in vesicovaginal or ureterovaginal fistula or ureteral ectopia in the vagina or uterus

NURSING DIAGNOSES and NURSING INTERVENTIONS

Nursing Diagnosis	Nursing Intervention
Urinary elimination, alteration in patterns: urinary incontinence	For stress incontinence, encourage pelvic floor exercises and weight loss as appropriate in cases of mild to moderate urinary incontinence. Provide options of incontinent pads, briefs, or disposable "diaper" type devices for adults.
	For instability incontinence with uninhibited neurogenic bladder, regulate patient on timed voiding schedule with bulk of oral intake concentrated during daytime hours and curtailment of fluids before hour of sleep. Administer anticholinergic/smooth muscle–relaxing agents as directed.
	For reflex neurogenic bladder, teach patient clean intermittent catheterization technique as directed and regulate acceptable schedule in conjunction with patient.
	Administer anticholinergics as directed. Observe patient for signs of bacterial cystitis.
	For overflow incontinence, provide catheter care or intermittent catheterization as directed. Administer cholinergic agents and bladder neck relaxants as directed. Encourage patient to double void as appropriate.
	For constant incontinence, counsel patient on anti-incontinence collection devices pending definitive repair of fistula or ectopia. Observe patient for signs and symptoms of urinary tract infection.
	For intractable incontinence (that is, not managed adequately by surgery, drugs, or self intermittent catheterization), provide counseling for options of anti-incontinence collection devices.
Self-concept, disturbance in: body image and self-esteem (related to episodes of incontinence)	Offer support and encouragement for maintenance of suggested treatment regimen.
	Encourage feedback to medical personnel as to success of regimen; may need to institute alternative therapy if unsuccessful.

Patient Education

1. Provide instruction on technique of medication regimens and need for continuous therapy in neuropathic bladder cases.
2. Provide a list of signs and symptoms of urinary tract infection and other conditions requiring medical attention.
3. Provide instructions for intermittent catheterization technique or care of long-indwelling Foley catheter.
4. Provide instruction about the relationship of incontinence to fluid intake, various medications, and compliance with medical and nursing strategies for prevention.

EVALUATION

Patient Outcome	Data Indicating That Outcome is Reached
Stress incontinence resulting from pelvic relaxation has been surgically corrected.	Continence is maintained. Residual after voiding is less than 20% of total bladder volume. There is no urinary tract infection.
Stress incontinence has been surgically corrected with placement of artificial urinary sphincter.	Continence is maintained. Sphincter device is functioning. There is no urinary tract infection.

Patient Outcome	Data Indicating That Outcome is Reached
Uninhibited neurogenic bladder is adequately managed.	Continence is maintained.
Reflex neurogenic bladder is adequately managed.	Continence is maintained or patient is using condom device to collect urine.
Instability incontinence caused by irritative disorder is resolved.	Continence is maintained. Underlying irritative disorder is resolved.
Overflow incontinence in bladder with deficient detrusor function is adequately managed.	Continence is maintained. Residual after voiding is less than 20% of total bladder volume.
Overflow incontinence caused by bladder outlet obstruction is resolved.	Continence is maintained. Obstruction is resolved.
Constant incontinence is resolved.	Continence is maintained. Fistula is closed or ectopia is repaired.

Medical Interventions

OPEN UROLOGIC SURGERY

Description and Rationale

Open urologic surgeries include nephrectomy, partial nephrectomy, nephrolithotomy, pyelolithotomy, ureterolithotomy, and cystectomy. The care of the patient during these procedures is similar, and all involve an open surgical incision. Surgery of the kidney is accomplished through a flank incision, while the operative approach for bladder surgeries is an anterior incision.

Indications for nephrectomy include calculus, hemorrhage, hydronephrosis, hypertension, neoplasms, renal donation, trauma, and vascular disease.[28a] Partial nephrectomy is performed to preserve as much renal function as possible in the same conditions that may require nephrectomy. A partial nephrectomy is important when contralateral renal function is impaired. The presence of stones in the kidney, pelvis, or ureter may be removed by an open urologic incision if newer techniques of extracorporeal shock wave lithotripsy (ESWL) and percutaneous ureteroscopic stone removal are ineffective.

Contraindications and Cautions

1. If the condition is bilateral, it is important to preserve total renal function.
2. Nephrostomy drainage may be required following open urologic surgeries through stents or tubes to allow for adequate healing when the tissues are poor, scar tissue is significant, or reconstructive procedures require splinting.

Preprocedural Nursing Care

1. Preoperative teaching concerns the procedure, presence of catheter, and stents for surgery, and turning, coughing, and leg exercises following surgery.
2. Give nothing by mouth past midnight.

ASSESSMENT: AREAS OF CONCERN

Incision
Redness; pain; edema; drainage

Temperature
Fever

Urinary output
Amount of urinary output through nephrostomy tube or catheter
Presence of bright red blood
Absence of urinary output through catheter

Pain
Incisional; postoperative

Hemorrhage
Incisional; through drains, tubes, or catheter

NURSING DIAGNOSES and NURSING INTERVENTIONS

Nursing Diagnosis	Nursing Intervention
Potential patient problem: hemorrhage and infection	Assess patient for signs and symptoms of bleeding. Evaluate amount of drainage through drains and tubes. Observe for signs and symptoms of wound infection.
Fluid volume deficit, potential	Monitor intake and output, daily weights, BUN, and creatinine. Report any indications of decreased renal function.
Comfort, alteration in: pain	Provide analgesics as ordered.
Urinary elimination, alteration in patterns	Monitor urinary output through urethral catheter, nephrostomy tube, or suprapubic catheter.
Skin integrity, impairment of: potential	Protect skin from drainage around Penrose drain or stab wound. Maintain sterile dressing changes. Consider using a sterile wound collection (pouch) system if drainage is copious.

Patient Education

1. Patient education varies with primary etiology; refer to specific discussions of urologic diseases.
2. Patient should be informed about incision care and management of any drains or tubes.

EVALUATION

Patient Outcome	Data Indicating That Outcome is Reached
There is no infection.	There are no signs of redness, edema, or inflammation of incision.
Urinary output is adequate.	Urinary output is sufficient; BUN and creatinine are normal.
The patient returns to activities of daily living.	The patient is able to manage all presurgical activities, including work and recreational activities.

TRANSURETHRAL RESECTION

Description and Rationale

Transurethral resection (TUR) of bladder tumors, prostatic hyperplasia, and bladder neck fibrosis is a common urologic procedure. A resectoscope is inserted through the urethra, and the tissue is removed (resected). The instruments allow for excision and coagulation of tissue with continuous flow of an irrigation solution. The ano-urethral resection of bladder tumors may be indicated for tumors that do not extend through the muscle layer of the bladder and includes radon-seed implantation. Transurethral resection of the prostate (TURP) is indicated for benign prostatic hyperplasia when the urethra is being obstructed by tissue. Transurethral resection of the fibrotic bladder neck is utilized to alleviate obstruction.

Contraindications and Cautions

1. TURP is contraindicated if the prostate gland is more than 40 to 50 g.
2. TURP is contraindicated in the presence of a urinary tract infection.
3. A small-caliber urethra or a urethral stricture may make TUR difficult and an open procedure more appropriate.
4. Physical conditions such as ankylosis of the hip or irreversible scrotal hernia that may interfere with positioning for TUR would be a contraindication.

Preprocedural Nursing Care

1. Preoperative teaching should include the fact that sexual potency is unaffected by retrograde ejaculation but infertility does occur.

TREATMENT PLAN

Chemotherapeutic
Analgesics as ordered
Antibiotics
Gentamicin (Garamycin), 3 mg/kg in three divided
doses per 24 h

Electromechanical
Foley catheter with or without continuous irrigation

ASSESSMENT: AREAS OF CONCERN

Bladder and prostate
Urinary output; presence of clots; adequate drainage
of catheter

Hemorrhage; drop in blood pressure; increase in pulse
rate
Perforation of bladder; drainage of urine into peritoneal
space; fever; pain; peritoneal inflammation
Perforation of prostate; change in blood pressure and
respirations; pain; failure of irrigating fluid to return;
palpable suprapubic mass

Temperature
Fever

Mental status
Acute confusion
Restlessness
Changes in behavior

NURSING DIAGNOSES and NURSING INTERVENTIONS

Nursing Diagnosis	Nursing Intervention
Urinary elimination, alteration in patterns	Evaluate drainage through the Foley catheter frequently; maintain accurate intake and output. Maintain continuous irrigation if ordered. Irrigate blood clots from bladder and tubing as necessary to prevent bladder distention. Provide patient with containers to collect voided urine (string of bottles) after catheter is removed. Evaluate patient for urinary continence after removal of catheter (TURP). Keep catheter anchored to prevent dislodging.
Potential patient problem: hemorrhage	Assess urinary output for bleeding immediately following surgery and after catheter is removed by observation of voided urine specimens. Differentiate between bright red, thick clots, which indicate active bleeding, and dark burgundy clots. Note bleeding with an absence of clots, which may indicate a blood dyscrasia. Monitor vital signs as indicated. Maintain traction on catheter if established by serologist for bleeding.
Comfort, alteration in: pain	Provide analgesics as ordered. Encourage patient to drink large amounts of fluids.
Fluid volume deficit: potential	Monitor intake and output and daily weights. Observe for signs of cerebral edema from absorption of irrigation fluid through venous sinuses in the prostate, including restlessness, confusion, and changes in behavior.
Self-concept, disturbance in: body image, personal identity	Provide male patients opportunity to discuss fears and anxieties related to genitourinary surgery. Provide factual information regarding sexual functioning and infertility; sexual activity can be resumed in 6 to 8 weeks.

Patient Education

1. Encourage patient to maintain adequate fluid intake and report any signs of incontinence, urinary tract infection (burning, urgency), or inability to void to urologist.
2. Follow-up for bladder tumor resections includes radiation and chemotherapy. Refer to sections on cancer management and interventions.

EVALUATION

Patient Outcome	Data Indicating That Outcome is Reached
Vital signs are within normal limits.	There are no signs of infection or hemorrhage.
Urinary elimination is normal.	Urine is clear and amber. The patient does not experience discomfort or difficulty on voiding.
Sexual function in male is unimpaired.	The patient returns to presurgical sexual pattern.

PERCUTANEOUS NEPHROSCOPIC STONE REMOVAL

Description and Rationale

Percutaneous nephroscopic stone removal is a nonsurgical technique to treat urolithiasis. A nephrostomy tube is placed percutaneously into the proper calix under fluoroscopic monitoring, and a dilator system is utilized to allow insertion of a nephroscope with one or more working channels. Several methods may be used to remove calculi percutaneously. A stone basket may be used to retrieve relatively small calculi. Larger stones may be first broken via ultrasonic lithotripter, laser, or electrolysis. Remaining fragments are then removed via a stone basket or flushed from the collecting system mechanically or physiologically.

Contraindications and Cautions

1. Septicemia should be adequately controlled before percutaneous nephroscopic stone removal is attempted.
2. If obstruction is significant, a nephrostomy tube may be placed with the patient under local anesthesia to facilitate adequate pelvic drainage.

Preprocedural Nursing Care

1. Monitor for signs and symptoms of gram-negative septicemia and septic shock including increased fever, pulse, respirations, and blood pressure followed by hypotension and potential cardiovascular compromise.

ASSESSMENT: AREAS OF CONCERN

Pain
   Renal colic
   Acute flank pain

Temperature
   Fever

Urinary output
   Oliguria or anuria in cases of bilateral obstruction

Other complications
   Nausea, vomiting, and ileus secondary to renal colic

Nephrostomy tube
   Hematuria
   Frank bleeding

NURSING DIAGNOSES and NURSING INTERVENTIONS

Nursing Diagnosis	Nursing Intervention
Tissue perfusion, alteration in: renal	Monitor blood pressure, pulse, and respirations. Observe flank for mass, blood, urine, or frank bleeding from nephrostomy tube.
Comfort, alteration in: pain	Administer analgesics as ordered.
Urinary elimination, alteration in patterns	Observe urinary output from nephrostomy tube. Monitor patent nephrostomy drainage system; check tubing for kinks and sediment.

Patient Education

1. Teach techniques for preventing recurrent stone formation including drugs, diet, and fluid intake.

EVALUATION

Patient Outcome	Data Indicating That Outcome is Reached
Hemorrhage is absent.	Urine drainage from nephrostomy tube is clear. Vital signs are within normal limits.
There is no obstruction.	The patient does not experience renal colic. Creatinine and BUN are within normal limits.
Infection is absent.	The patient is afebrile. Urine and blood cultures are negative.

EXTRACORPOREAL SHOCK WAVE LITHOTRIPSY

Description and Rationale

Extracorporeal shock wave lithotripsy (ESWL) is an exciting new technology in urology that crushes renal and ureteral calculi without invasion of the body. The patient is given epidural anesthesia and placed in a lithotripter tub with degassed water. The calculi are located via fluoroscopic techniques, and ultrasonic shock waves are used to crush the stone into powder. The fragments are passed in the urine. The entire procedure requires approximately 1 hour.

Contraindications and Cautions

1. Patients unsuitable for epidural or spinal anesthesia may require general anesthesia.
2. Patients unable to cooperate with requirements of positioning may be managed by other approaches.
3. Children may be too small for equipment.

Preprocedural Nursing Care

1. Preoperative teaching is essential to clarify misconceptions concerning this relatively new intervention.

ASSESSMENT: AREAS OF CONCERN

Urinary output/voiding behavior
Passage of stone particles
Dysuria; bladder colic

Pain
Renal colic

Temperature
Fever

NURSING DIAGNOSES and NURSING INTERVENTIONS

Nursing Diagnosis	Nursing Intervention
Urinary elimination, alteration in patterns	Monitor daily intake and output. Force fluids and strain urine for stone particles. Assess patient for signs of renal colic from ureteral obstruction. Monitor BUN and creatinine.
Potential patient problem: infection	Monitor temperature, pulse, blood pressure, and respirations. Obtain urine culture as ordered.
Comfort, alteration in: pain	Administer narcotics and analgesics as ordered.

Patient Education

1. Teach techniques for preventing recurrent stone formation including drugs, diet, and fluid intake.

EVALUATION

Patient Outcome	Data Indicating That Outcome is Reached
Stones are not present.	Film of kidneys, ureters, and bladder (KUB) and intravenous pyelogram (IVP) are normal.
There is no obstruction.	The patient does not experience pain. IVP is normal.

OPEN PROSTATECTOMY

Description and Rationale

Open prostatectomy refers to the removal of the prostate with or without the prostatic capsule. Several surgical approaches may be used including suprapubic, transvesical, retropubic, perineal, and transcoccygeal. In the suprapubic or transvesical procedures the prostate is removed through the cavity of the bladder. Retropubic prostatectomy is performed through a low abdominal incision without opening the bladder. The most radical of the open procedures for prostatectomy is the perineal approach in which the incision is made between the scrotum and rectum. The transcoccygeal approach allows better surgical access to the posterior lobes of the prostate. The perineal approach is usually associated with loss of erection, orgasm, and ejaculatory function. It is not uncommon for sexual dysfunction to occur when the prostatic capsule is removed.

The suprapubic and retropubic approaches may be used as open surgical approaches when the gland is too large for transurethral resection; they are not generally used for cancer. In these incidences the capsule is left intact.

Perineal prostatectomy is most often performed for cancer of the prostate when it is confined to the capsule. Some controversy exists regarding the use of radical prostatectomy when the tumor extends through the capsule.

Contraindications and Cautions

1. Small fibrous prostate
2. Presence of cancer (suprapubic, retropubic)

Preprocedural Nursing Care

1. Patient teaching is done, including potential sexual impairment if appropriate.
2. Perineum, external genitalia, abdomen, and upper halves of thighs are shaved the night before surgery.
3. Cleansing enemas are given until clear.

ASSESSMENT: AREAS OF CONCERN

Incision
Redness; pain; edema; drainage

Temperature
Fever

Pain
Postoperative pain

Urinary output
Amount of urinary output through urethral catheter or suprapubic catheter
Presence of bright red blood
Incontinence (may last for a few days to 6 months)
Urethral stricture

Other complications
Epididymitis

Sexual dysfunction
Impotence
Retrograde ejaculation

TREATMENT PLAN

Chemotherapeutic
Laxatives (stool softeners)
Docusate (Colace), 100 mg/d po
Analgesics prn

Electromechanical
Urethral catheter, suprapubic catheter, and Penrose drain

Supportive
Intravenous fluids
Clear diet progressing to regular diet
Heat lamp; sitz bath (perineal incision)

NURSING DIAGNOSES and NURSING INTERVENTIONS

Nursing Diagnosis	Nursing Intervention
Potential patient problems: hemorrhage, infection	Observe urinary output for excessive bleeding. Maintain patency of all tubes and catheters. Monitor vital signs. Maintain sterile urinary drainage systems.
Urinary elimination, alteration in patterns	Assess patient's urinary output. Prevent kinking and obstruction of all catheters. Measure urinary output noting color and consistency of blood and clots and amount. Remove urethral catheter as ordered. Provide catheter care; maintain any catheter traction ordered.
Comfort, alteration in: pain	Provide analgesics as ordered. Provide stool softeners to prevent straining with defecation.
Self-concept, disturbance in: body image, personal identity	Discuss the implications of radical or prostatic capsule removal on sexual functioning. Assist patient in exploring his feelings and fears. Provide an opportunity for spouse to be involved in the discussions of sexual concerns. Assess level of sexual functioning. Discuss alternatives available to the patient in the form of penile prosthetic devices.
Skin integrity, impairment of: potential	Change dressing frequently to prevent skin irritation from damp dressing. Cleanse skin gently and pat dry or use a hair dryer to dry. Apply moisture barrier ointments and skin sealants (Bard Protective Barrier Film; Skin Prep) to protect the skin.

Patient Education

1. Incisional care should be discussed with the patient.
2. Skin protection techniques should be discussed with the patient if drainage is still continuing at time of discharge.
3. Urine color will not clear up for 4 to 8 weeks, but the patient should notify physician if it changes and becomes bright red with clots.
4. Provide teaching and counseling regarding sexual concerns.

EVALUATION

Patient Outcome	Data Indicating That Outcome is Reached
Urinary elimination is normal.	Output is adequate. Color is clear. The patient does not experience pain, burning, or bladder spasms.
Sexual functioning resumes.	The patient is able to obtain an erection. Retrograde ejaculation may occur. The patient is scheduled for or has had a penile prosthesis if indicated.

BLADDER NECK SUSPENSION

Description and Rationale

Bladder neck suspension is utilized in women to correct stress urinary incontinence secondary to pelvic relaxation. A number of procedures have been described, including the Marshall-Marchetti-Krantz (MMK) operation, Stamey's vesicopexy, Burch retropubic colposuspension, and the Peyrera needle suspension. The restoration of continence is attained via increasing urethral resistance. Other procedures such as repair of urethrocele, cystocele, or enterocele may be performed to promote bladder emptying and optimal detrusor function.

Contraindications and Cautions

1. Bladder neck suspension is contraindicated in cases of severe stress urinary incontinence as a result of internal sphincter damage.

Preprocedural Nursing Care

1. Preoperative teaching should include information concerning recompensation of detrusor tone and potential for increased difficulty emptying bladder during postoperative period.

ASSESSMENT: AREAS OF CONCERN

Abdomen
Redness, edema, and drainage at wound site if abdominal approach utilized

Perineum
Vaginal discharge
Pain if wound infection present

Voiding behaviors
Decreased force of urinary stream
Perceptions of incomplete bladder emptying or acute urinary retention

Pain
Dysuria
Pelvic pain
Incisional or abdominal pain

NURSING DIAGNOSES and NURSING INTERVENTIONS

Nursing Diagnosis	Nursing Intervention
Urinary elimination: alteration in patterns	Monitor intake and output. Check urine residuals as directed. Teach intermittent self-catheterization as directed. Teach double void technique as directed.
Fear	Reassure patient that retention is probably caused by myogenic decompensation of detrusor and that return of normal voiding patterns is expected unless preoperative urodynamics reveal neuropathic bladder.
Comfort, alteration in: pain	Administer analgesics as directed. Encourage regular bladder emptying during postoperative recuperation.

Patient Education

1. Explain that return of normal voiding patterns may require time.

EVALUATION

Patient Outcome	Data Indicating That Outcome is Reached
Stress urinary incontinence is not present.	Urodynamics are normal. Marshall test is negative.
Bladder emptying is adequate.	Postvoid residual is 20% of total bladder volume or less.

INTRAPENILE PROSTHETIC DEVICES

Description and Rationale

Intrapenile prosthetic devices (IPPs) are utilized when medical, surgical, or psychologic methods are inadequate to restore erectile function. Placement of a device is completed after thorough investigation of organic and psychogenic stigmata of underlying erectile failure and careful psychologic assessment for suitability of the procedure are completed.

A number of devices are available. Semirigid devices include Small-Carrion, Finney Flexirod, and the Jonas Implant. These devices are generally less expensive than the Scott inflatable penile prosthesis but more difficult to conceal. The Scott inflatable penile prosthesis allows the penis to remain in a "flaccid" stage until the device is pumped to produce an erection. This device is more prone to mechanical difficulties than the semirigid devices.

Contraindications and Cautions

1. IPPs are contraindicated in patients with deep-rooted psychologic abnormalities underlying erectile dysfunction.

Preprocedural Nursing Care

1. Sexual counseling of male patient and partner is essential during both preoperative and postoperative periods.

ASSESSMENT: AREAS OF CONCERN

Penis
Redness
Edema
Signs of erosion of prosthetic device

Scrotum/perineum
Hematoma for 2 to 3 weeks; edema for 24 hours postoperatively
Discharge and hemorrhage from incision

Temperature
Fever

Urinary output
Normal voiding patterns after 24-hour catheter drainage

NURSING DIAGNOSES and NURSING INTERVENTIONS

Nursing Diagnosis	Nursing Intervention
Comfort, alteration in: pain	Administer analgesics as ordered.
Potential patient problem: infection	Observe penis and scrotum for signs of infection. Monitor temperature.
Skin integrity, impairment of: potential	Observe operative site for signs of erosion: pallid, stretched skin; appearance of device outline at skin surface; pain.
Self-concept, disturbance in: role performance (potential)	Offer support and encouragement regarding use of implant. Reinforce need for patient and partner to have knowledge and understanding of the use of the device.

Patient Education

1. Instruct patient to abstain from sex for 21 days after surgery to allow for adequate healing if semirigid device is used.
2. Instruct patient to inflate Scott inflatable penile prosthesis repeatedly before use to encourage formation of fibrous sheath around device.
3. Instruct patient on techniques of concealing semirigid device in clothing.
4. Instruct patient about signs of erosion or infection.
5. Instruct patient *and partner* in inflation and deflation of Scott inflatable penile prosthesis.
6. Instruct patient to avoid contact sports or lifting heavy objects for 21 days after IPP is placed.

EVALUATION

Patient Outcome	Data Indicating That Outcome is Reached
There is no infection.	The patient is afebrile. Wound healing is normal.
There is no erosion.	Size, color, and contour of penis are normal.
The patient makes an adequate adjustment to the IPP.	Patient *and* partner give subjective report of satisfaction with device. The patient resumes sexual relations with partner. The patient can demonstrate correct technique for inflating and deflating Scott inflatable prosthesis.

URINARY DIVERSION

Description and Rationale

A urinary diversion refers to the rerouting of the urinary tract when it is necessary to remove or bypass the bladder. The bladder may be removed for cancer. A bypass procedure may be indicated in neurogenic bladder when reflux and hydronephrosis indicate the need to provide a low-pressure system. The most common type of urinary diversion in adults is the ileal conduit. An ileal conduit is not a new bladder but a tube or conduit constructed of small bowel that allows for urine to drain to the outside of the body. The ileal conduit is constructed by taking an isolated segment of ileum with its mesentery intact, reanastomosing the remaining ileum. One end of the isolated segment is sutured closed, and the other end is brought through the abdominal wall to form the stoma. The ureters are anastomosed in an end-to-side fashion into the ileal segment. Urine drains continuously through the stoma and requires an external pouch.

A continent urinary diversion has been described using a procedure similar to the continent ileostomy or Kock pouch (see Chapter 11). This procedure is not common, and the long-term effects of urine in the ileal pouch are unknown.

A ureterostomy may occasionally be seen in adult patients when the ileal conduit cannot be constructed. The ureter is brought to the abdominal wall to form a stoma. The ureterostomy has a higher rate of stenosis, infection, and pouching difficulties.

Contraindications and Cautions

1. Obesity makes it more difficult to construct a good stoma. Obesity is also associated with more tension on the mesentery, leading to stomal necrosis.
2. Radiated bowel should not be used for the conduit and may indicate the use of a higher segment of ileum or jejunum for the conduit.

Preprocedural Nursing Care

1. Intensive bowel preparation is done before surgery.
2. Preoperative stoma site selection is done by ET nurse or surgeon.
3. Preoperative teaching and consultation with ET nurse is important.
4. The patient talks to an ostomy visitor if appropriate.

TREATMENT PLAN

Chemotherapeutic

Anti-infective agents
  Neomycin (Mycifradin), 1 g po q4h for four doses; then 1 g q6h until NPO for surgery (begins 3 d before surgery)
  Erythromycin (Erythrocin), 1 g po q4h for three doses
Laxative agents
  Castor oil, 0.5 mg/kg po 3 d before surgery
Analgesic/antipyretic agents
  Analgesics for pain prn postoperatively
Vitamins
  Vitamin C (ascorbic acid) to maintain acidic pH of urine.

Electromechanical

Bowel preparation: saline enemas for 2 days before surgery

Supportive

Low-residue diet used as part of bowel preparation; liquid diet the day before surgery
Intravenous fluids provided during bowel preparation and following surgery until patient is able to tolerate foods

ASSESSMENT: AREAS OF CONCERN

Incision
Redness, pain, edema, drainage

Temperature
Fever

Pain
Incisional postoperative pain

Hemorrhage
Incisional
Drains
Sumps
Urethral catheter (promotes drainage of operative site)
External pouch

Urinary output
Amount and color
Mucus normal in ileal conduit

Sexual dysfunction (male)
Impotence
Infertility

Stoma
Stoma incision line
Color

Skin
Intact
Early signs of irritation or monilial infections

Intestine
Paralytic ileus; intestinal obstruction; abdominal distention; no bowel movement
Nasogastric suctioning prolonged because of bowel anastomosis

Other complications
Body image alterations
Sexual dysfunction (male)
Pulmonary complications

NURSING DIAGNOSES and NURSING INTERVENTIONS

Nursing Diagnosis	Nursing Intervention
Tissue perfusion, alteration in	Monitor blood pressure and tissue perfusion rate every 4 hours for 5 to 6 days or until removal of nasogastric suctioning and intravenous fluids.
	Apply antiembolic stockings; remove and reapply daily.
	Auscultate abdomen for bowel sounds; note any signs of abdominal distention.
	Assess stoma for color (i.e., blood supply); ileal conduit stoma should be bright red and moist; ureterostomy stoma is pale to dark pink.
	Assist patient with progressive ambulation.
	Encourage patient to turn every 2 hours and to perform leg exercises.
	Observe all drains, sumps, and catheters for amount, color, and consistency of drainage.
	Monitor intake and output; weigh daily.
Potential patient problem: infection	Provide antibiotics as ordered.
	Observe incision for signs of infection: redness, edema, pain, and drainage.
	Assess patient's skin (under the arms and breasts, groin, perineum) for monilial infections associated with prolonged antibiotics, intense bowel preparation, and moisture.
Potential patient problem: hemorrhage	Observe incisional dressing for color and amount of drainage.
	Monitor color, consistency, and amount of drainage from nasogastric tube, sumps, urethral catheter, and stomal output.
	Monitor vital signs for shock.
Breathing pattern, ineffective	Assist patient with turning, coughing, and deep breathing.
	Auscultate chest for breath sounds four times each day.
	Provide analgesics and splinting of abdomen when encouraging patient to deep breathe and cough.
Urinary elimination, alteration in patterns	Evaluate stoma color and suture line.
	Provide an appropriate pouching system with an antireflux valve and a spout; connect to bedside drainage; check frequently to prevent the tubing from kinking.
	Monitor amount and color of urine; if no urine is present in pouch, check all drainage sites (sumps, urethral drain [catheter], Penrose drain) for urine in order to determine if there has been an ileal-ureteral leakage or decreased renal function.

Nursing Diagnosis	Nursing Intervention
	Arrange for enterostomal therapy (ET) nurse to assess stoma and drainage system. Check urine pH every 3 to 5 days, using a fresh urine specimen; do not touch test tape to stoma, an alkaline surface. Obtain all urine specimens for urinalysis or culture and sensitivity by catheterizing the ileal conduit (exception: monitoring urine pH).
Bowel elimination, alteration in: constipation	Monitor patient for first bowel movement. Auscultate abdomen for bowel sounds each shift. Observe for signs of paralytic ileus or intestinal obstruction. Monitor patient for signs and symptoms of peritonitis, which would indicate a leakage or failure of the intestinal reanastomosis: fever, abdominal pain, rebound tenderness, drop in blood pressure, or shallow respirations.
Comfort, alteration in: pain	Provide analgesics as ordered. Assist patient in finding comfortable positions.
Self-concept, disturbance in: body image, personal identity	Provide an opportunity for patient and partner to discuss the implications of the surgery, stoma, and external pouch. Explore the patient's and partner's feelings regarding the presence of the stoma and pouch. Discuss the sexual implications, such as feelings of attractiveness, desirability, and worth. Discuss the presence of the pouch and the inability of detecting it under clothing and how to manage embarrassing leakages and odor. Discuss the potential for sexual dysfunction in the male undergoing radical cystectomy and prostatectomy for cancer, including alternatives for sexual counseling and a penile prosthesis.
Skin integrity, impairment of: potential	Observe peristomal skin with each pouch change. Protect the peristomal skin by gently cleansing with warm water, patting dry, and applying a liquid skin sealant to coat the skin. Change the pouch whenever it appears to be leaking under the faceplate or when there is an overt leakage. Observe solid wafer skin barriers for the degree of melting and absorption of urine with a pouch change, switching barriers if leakage or melting is frequent. Remove the hair in the peristomal area with an electric or safety razor.
Skin integrity, impairment of: actual	Rash can occur under the tape, under the faceplate, and on any part of the skin where the pouch comes in contact with the skin. Cause may be leaking appliance, perspiration, allergies to tape, or hair follicle irritation. Use heat lamp with a 60-watt bulb 1 foot away from skin or hair dryer set on cool to dry the skin. Sprinkle a small amount of powder on the skin, wipe of the excess, and then blot with a skin sealant. Powder the skin on which the pouch lies. Advise patient to make or buy a pouch cover. Advise patient that wearing a pouch belt too tight may break the seal. Cement or solvent burns can occur anywhere under the faceplate but usually are found at the outside edges because chemicals in the cement or solvent were not allowed to evaporate off the skin surface before applying pouch or cement was too thick and was unable to dry completely. Apply heat with heat lamp or hair dryer to the weeping skin. Cover the burn with a skin barrier and apply the pouch in the usual way. Ulcerated area on stoma may occur if stomal opening of the pouch was too small or activities were causing the faceplate to rub or cut into stoma. Enlarge the size of the pouch opening. Evaluate patient's activities; a different-size or -shaped faceplate may be needed. Advise patient to loosen belt; if too tight, the belt may cause the faceplate to ride into stoma. Infected or irritated hair follicles can occur under the faceplate if the area is not kept shaved.

Nursing Diagnosis	**Nursing Intervention**

Let the irritation improve before removing any more hair by shaving or cutting.

Use hair dryer or heat lamp to dry the skin if oozing is present.

Use a skin barrier between the skin and faceplate until irritation improves.

Water-logged skin between opening of the faceplate and the stoma can occur if too much skin is exposed between the stoma and the faceplate and the urine pools on the skin.

Apply heat lamp or hair dryer to area.

Cover area with a pectin-based skin barrier, hugging the stoma.

Decrease the size of stomal opening in faceplate.

Urinary yeast infection on skin surrounding the stoma may extend beyond the faceplate.

Apply heat with heat lamp or hair dryer to the area.

Apply nystatin (Mycostatin) powder to the area, blow off the excess powder, and seal this in with a thin coat of a skin sealant. Apply pouch in the usual manner.

Advise patient to drink sufficient fluids and add buttermilk or yogurt to the diet.

Urine crystals may form on the stoma or around the stoma base if the patient has alkaline urine and a predisposition for stone formation.

Swab vinegar on the stoma when changing the pouch.

Insert vinegar into the pouch while patient is wearing it. For a minor formation, insert twice a day; for an excessive formation, insert four times a day.

Advise patient to use vinyl or plastic pouches until the condition clears, or new rubber pouches.

Remove antireflux valves or vinegar will not come into contact with the stoma.

Monitor urine pH and provide instructions for maintaining an acid urine, including increased fluid intake and ascorbic acid (vitamin C).

Avoid using heat lamps on irradiated skin.

Patient Education

1. Teach pouch-changing procedure (see box on p. 1360). Providing a dry surface is essential to keeping a pouch seal.
2. Review principles in cleaning urinary pouches with patient (see upper box on p. 1361).
3. Instruct patient regarding monitoring urine pH (see lower box on p. 1361).
4. Instruct patient about use of a nighttime drainage system (see box on p. 1362).
5. Instruct patient to inform physician and pharmacist if maintaining acid pH, since it will affect action of certain drugs (such as methotrexate).

EVALUATION

Patient Outcome	Data Indicating That Outcome is Reached
There is no infection.	Temperature is within normal range. There are no signs or symptoms of infection. Incision is healed.
Tissue perfusion is normal.	Stoma is red, healthy, and moist. Blood pressure and pulse are within normal limits.
Bowel elimination is normal.	The patient experiences a return to presurgical bowel habits.
Skin integrity is maintained.	Peristomal skin is intact. There are no signs of irritation.
Sexual functioning is adequate.	Women return to presurgical sexual pattern. Men experiencing sexual dysfunction receive counseling regarding penile prosthesis.

PROCEDURE WHEN PATIENT CHANGES POUCH

1. Assemble all equipment.
   a. The following materials may be used to cleanse the skin: cotton balls, Kleenex, toilet paper, washcloths, towels, premoistened towelettes.
   b. Pouch.
   c. Skin barriers.
   d. Tape and/or belt.
   e. Equipment for cleansing or disposing of used pouches.
2. Pattern
   a. A paper towel may be used to trace a pattern.
   b. The pattern should hug the stoma but not ride up on it.
   c. Always label the pattern for "top" or "skin side."
   d. Not only is the stomal opening important in making a pattern, but the outer dimensions of the pattern should be considered. The pattern should avoid hip bones, pubic area, ribs, and folds at waist or navel.
3. Skin barrier (if applicable)
   a. You may use ½, ¼, or full wafer (4 × 4) depending on the size of the stoma and abdomen.
   b. Round the corners or conform the wafer to the shape of the adhesive on the pouch.
   c. Trace the stomal pattern on the paper side.
   d. Cut hole on pattern line; your line will not be visible when it is cut.
   e. Smooth sides of the opening with your finger.
4. Pouch
   a. Pouch opening should be *slightly* larger (⅛ to ¼ inch) than the opening of the skin barrier (paper can cut the stoma).
   b. Trace pattern on the paper side of the pouch (use the opening from the skin barrier that has already been cut).
   c. Cut the hole larger than the line of the pattern (cut outside the line).
   d. The edges around the opening should be smooth.
   e. Remove paper backing from the pouch, center the openings, and apply the shiny side of the skin barrier to the pouch (when applicable).
5. Remove pouch you are wearing. (If it is disposable, place in Baggie; if reusable, set aside to clean after you have finished.)
6. Cleanse your skin with warm water.
   a. Soaps are not necessary and they leave film residue on the skin.
   b. It is not necessary to remove all the cement or barrier left on your skin—if you cause abrasions by rough cleansing, other barriers will tend to "burn" after applying. This will cease after a few minutes.
7. Dry well.
8. Note any changes of your skin or the stoma (color, size, ulcerations).
9. Use a wick (or tampon) or absorb the urine while you cleanse the skin and apply your skin barriers.
10. Apply skin barrier (if not attached to the pouch in step 4).
11. Center and apply clean pouching system.
12. Close end.
13. Tape and/or belt.
14. Cleanse, dry, and powder your reusable pouch.
15. Check your supplies and reorder as necessary . . . never wait till you have used your last supplies before ordering.

PROCEDURE WHEN PATIENT CLEANS POUCH

I. Commercial products

Commercial products are available from several ostomy specialty companies. The general rule of thumb is to follow the directions on the package.

II. Vinegar solution

A weak vinegar solution of one part white vinegar to three parts water or full-strength white vinegar may be used to cleanse reusable pouches. The vinegar will dissipate the urine odor. The procedure is:

1. Empty the pouch.
2. Rinse the pouch with cool water.
3. Instill the vinegar solution into pouch.
4. Allow to soak for 20 minutes.
5. Rinse with cold water. (The cold water will destroy the vinegar odor.)
6. Allow to air dry.
7. Powder pouch inside and out to prevent sticking.

Note: This entire procedure may be used for the reusable pouch, leg bag, bedside drainage bag, and tubing.

PROCEDURE WHEN PATIENT MONITORS pH

Urine pH (acid or alkaline state) should be checked every week. You can check the pH by touching the tape into urine as it flows from the stoma, but do not let the test tape contact the stoma, which produces alkaline mucus. Alternatively, after changing your pouch, take a specimen of the urine that drains into the pouch within the first 2 to 5 minutes and, using a pH test tape, check the urine. Do not let the urine sit in the pouch before checking the pH, because the urine will become alkaline with time.

Try to maintain a pH of 6 or less. If the urine pH is above 6 (alkaline), increase your fluid intake and (if your doctor agrees) take 500 to 1000 mg of vitamin C (tablets) each day.

Cranberry juice is often used to treat alkaline urine, but it does not work effectively. However, it will help with odor problems.

Disadvantages of prolonged alkaline urine concentration are the destruction of rubber pouches and skin barriers; crystal formation on or around the stoma; greater predisposition to kidney stone formation; formation of an excellent medium for bacteria growth; and odor. An adequate fluid intake (6 to 8 glasses per day) will help prevent concentrated urine.

If there is a tendency toward alkaline urine or crystal formation, it is appropriate to cleanse the pouch while it is worn to decrease odors, decrease bacterial content of the pouch, and/or prevent urine crystals from forming on the stoma or in the pouch. The procedure is as follows:

1. Empty the pouch.
2. Instill ½ ounce of vinegar solution into the pouch (1 part vinegar to 1 part water).
3. Lie down so the solution will bathe the inside of the pouch and stoma for approximately 20 minutes.
4. Empty the pouch and rinse with cool water.

Note: The vinegar solution may discolor the stoma, making it appear "blanched" or "white." It will return to its normal color in a few minutes. Dark vinegar can be used, but it will stain the pouches.

If the pouch has an antiflux valve, the vinegar solution will not come in contact with the stoma, but will help in decreasing odor and bacteria in the pouch. When using the vinegar to treat stomal crystals (with alkaline urine), you must change to a pouch without an antireflux valve or cut a hole in the valve. Your ET nurse will show you how to do this so you do not cut a hole in the pouch itself. Do not substitute commercial cleansers in place of the vinegar. Some commercial cleansers will imitate the stoma. It is best to use commercial products on pouches which you are not wearing.

USE OF NIGHTTIME DRAINAGE SYSTEM

In recent years, several definite advantages of using a nighttime drainage collection system have been found. Urine allowed to remain in the pouch becomes an excellent medium for bacterial growth. During sleep, urine can flow, even around a pouch reflux valve, into the conduit. This may lead to an infection of the kidneys. Also, if the pouch is allowed to fill with urine at night, the pouch seal could be broken by the weight of the urine or the pouch could burst if the patient rolls over on it. With nighttime drainage, the patient is more free to sleep in any position, even on his stomach. The tubing can be run down the pajama leg and off the end of the bed rather than the side, giving more freedom of movement.

Patient Outcome	Data Indicating That Outcome is Reached
Body image is not impaired.	The patient adapts to the presence of the stoma and external pouch. The patient recognizes that adaptation is a continuous process.
The patient resumes activities of daily living.	The patient returns to presurgical activities including work and recreational interests. The patient does not change his style of dress.

References

1. Abrams, H.L., and Adams, D.F.: Renal and adrenal angiography. In Harrison, J.H., et al.: Campbell's urology, Philadelphia, 1978, W.B. Saunders Co.
2. Allen, T.D.: The non-neurogenic neurogenic bladder, J. Urol. **116**:638, 1977.
3. Ambrose, S.S.: Prostatitis. In Hurst, J.W.: Medicine for the practicing physician, Boston, 1983, Butterworth Publishers.
4. Anderssen, K.-E., and Forman, A.: Effects of prostaglandins on the smooth muscle of the urinary tract, Acta Pharmacol. Toxicol. **43**(11):90, 1978.
5. Andriole, V.T.: Urinary tract infections in pregnancy, Urol. Clin. North Am. **2**:485, 1975.
6. Bauer, S.B., et al.: The unstable bladder of childhood, Urol. Clin. North Am. **7**:321, 1980.
7. Bennett, A.H.: Management of male impotence. In Libertino, J.A.: International perspectives in urology, vol. 5, Baltimore, 1982, Williams & Wilkins Co.
8. Bhaita, N.N., and Bradley, W.E.: Neuro-anatomy and physiology: innervation of the lower urinary tract. In Raz, S.: Female urology, Philadelphia, 1983, W.B. Saunders Co.
9. Birkhoff, J.D.: Natural history of benign prostatic hypertrophy. In Hinman, J.F.: Benign prostatic hypertrophy, New York, 1983, Springer-Verlag.
10. Blaivas, J.G.: The neurophysiology of micturition: a clinical study of 550 patients, J. Urol. **127**:958, 1982.
11. Bouarsky, S., and Labay, P.: Principles of ureteral physiology. In Bergman, H.: The ureter, New York, 1981, Springer-Verlag.
12. Bradley, W.E., and Scott, F.B.: Physiology of the urinary bladder. In Harrison, J.H., et al.: Campbell's urology, Philadelphia, 1978, W.B. Saunders Co.
13. Broadwell, D.C., and Sorrells, S.L.: Summary of your urinary diversion, 1976 and 1983.
14. Carlton, C.E.: Initial evaluation including history, physical examination and urinalysis. In Harrison, H.J., et al.: Campbell's urology, Philadephia, 1978, W.B. Saunders Co.
15. Carson, C.C.: Urinary tract infections. In Resnick, M.I., and Older, R.A.: Diagnosis of genitourinary disease, New York, 1982, Thieme-Stratton, Inc.
15a. Conti, G.: L'erection du pénis human et bases morphologio vascularis, Acta Anat. **14**:17, 1952.
16. Cook, W.A., and King, L.R.: Vesicoureteral reflux. In Harrison, J.H., et al.: Campbell's urology, Philadelphia, 1978, W.B. Saunders Co.
17. Crouch, J.E.: Functional human anatomy, Philadelphia, 1982, Lea & Febiger.
18. Davis, J.E., Hagedoorn, J.P., and Bergmann, L.L.: Anatomy and ultrastructure of the ureter. In Bergman, H.: The ureter, New York, 1982, Springer-Verlag.
19. Donker, P.J., Droes, Th.P.M., and van Ulden, B.M.: Innervation of the bladder and urethra. In Chisholm, G.D., and Williams, I.D.: Scientific foundations in urology, Chicago, 1978, Yearbook Medical Publishers, Inc.
20. Drach, G.W.: Prostatitis: man's hidden infection, Urol. Clin. North Am. **2**:499, 1975.
21. Drach, G.W.: Urinary lithiasis. In Harrison, J.H., et al.: Campbell's urology, Philadelphia, 1978, W.B. Saunders Co.
22. Ewing, L.: Physiology of male reproduction. In Harrison, J.H., et al.: Campbell's urology, Philadelphia, 1978, W.B. Saunders Co.
23. Ewing, L.: Testis, epididymis. In Harrison, J.H., et al.: Campbell's urology, Philadelphia, 1978, W.B. Saunders Co.
23a. Farnell, B., and Thomas, P.: Tuberculosis at the epididymis, Can. Med. Assoc. J. **128**:1296, 1983.
24. Farrar, D.J.: Urodynamics in the elderly. In Mundy, A.R., Stephenson, T.P., and Wein, A.J.: Urodynamics: principles, practice, and application, Edinburgh, 1984, Churchill-Livingstone.
25. Farrar, W.E.: Infections of the urinary tract, Med. Clin. North Am. **67**:187, 1983.
26. Furlow, W.L.: Use of the inflatable penile prosthesis in erectile dysfunction, Urol. Clin. North Am. **8**:181, 1981.

27. Gaymans, R., et al.: A prospective study of urinary tract infections in a Dutch general practice, Lancet **2:**674, 1976.

28. Gillenwater, J.Y.: The pathophysiology of urinary obstruction. In Harrison, J.H., et al.: Campbell's urology, Philadelphia, 1978, W.B. Saunders Co.

28a. Glenn, J.F.: Urologic surgery, New York, 1983, Harper & Row Publishers, Inc.

29. Gordon, I.: Renal diagnostic imaging. In Williams, I.D., and Johnston, J.H.: Paediatric urology, London, 1982, Butterworth & Co.

30. Govoni, L.E., and Hayes, J.E.: Drugs and nursing implications, Norwalk, Conn., 1982, Appleton-Century-Crofts.

31. Green, R.: Endocrine therapy of erectile failure. In Wagner, G., and Green, R.: Impotence, New York, 1981, Plenum Press.

32. Guyton, A.C.: Medical physiology, Philadelphia, 1978, W.B. Saunders Co.

33. Hald, T., and Bradley, W.E.: The urinary bladder: neurology and dynamics, Baltimore, 1982, Williams & Wilkins Co.

34. Hindmarsh, J.R., and Byrne, P.O.: Adult enuresis—a symptomatic and urodynamic assessment, Br. J. Urol. **52:**88, 1980.

35. Hindmarsh, J.R., and Byrne, P.O.: Is the enuretic female bladder without instability normal? Urol. Res. **9:**133, 1981.

36. Hope-Stone, H.F.: Radiotherapy in the management of invasive bladder cancer. In Smith, P.H., and Prout, G.R., Jr.: Bladder cancer, London, 1984, Butterworth's International Medical Reviews.

37. Huckins, C.P.: Development of the testes and establishment of spermatogenesis. In Lipschultz, L.I., and Howards, S.S.: Infertility in the male, New York, 1983, Churchill-Livingstone.

38. Hutch, J.A., and Rambo, O.N.: A study of the anatomy of the prostate, prostatic urethra, and the urinary sphincter system, J. Urol. **104:**443, 1970.

39. Ireton, R.C., and Berger, R.E.: Prostatitis and epididymitis, Urol. Clin. North Am. **11:**83, 1984.

40. Isselbacher, K.J., et al.: Harrison's principles of internal medicine, New York, 1980, McGraw-Hill, Inc.

41. Jarowenko, M.V., and Bennett, A.H.: Pharmacology of impotence—sexual dysfunction. In Libertino, J.A.: International perspectives in urology, vol. 5, Baltimore, 1982, Williams & Wilkins Co.

42. Jarvis, J.G.: Bladder drill treatment of enuresis in adults, Br. J. Urol. **54:**118, 1982.

43. Jenkins, A.D., Turner, T.T., and Howards, S.S.: Physiology of the male reproductive system, Urol. Clin. North Am. **5:**437, 1978.

44. Juhan, C.M., Paduta, G., and Huguet, J.H.: Angiography in male impotence. In Libertino, J.A.: International perspectives in urology, vol. 5, Baltimore, 1982, Williams & Wilkins Co.

45. Karacan, I., and Moore, C.A.: Psychodynamics of erectile failure. In Libertino, J.A.: International perspectives in urology, vol. 5, Baltimore, 1982, Williams & Wilkins Co.

46. Kass, I., Updegraff, K., and Muffly, R.B.: Sex in chronic obstructive pulmonary disease, Med. Aspects Hum. Sex. **6:**33, 1972.

47. Kaye, D.: Host defense mechanisms in the urinary tract, Urol. Clin. North Am. **2:**407, 1975.

48. Kedia, K.R.: Vascular disorders and male erectile dysfunction, Urol. Clin. North Am. **8:**153, 1981.

49. Kiil, F.: Physiology of the renal pelvis and ureter. In Harrison, J.H., et al.: Campbell's urology, Philadelphia, 1978, W.B. Saunders Co.

50. Krane, R.J., and Siroky, M.B.: Classification of neuro-urologic disorders. In Krane, R.J., and Siroky, M.B.: Clinical neuro-urology, Boston, 1979, Little, Brown & Co.

51. Kuru, M.: Nervous control of micturition, Physiol. Rev. **45:**425, 1965.

52. Lapides, J.: Structure and function of internal vesical sphincter, J. Urol. **50:**341, 1958.

53. Lapides, J.: Tips on self catheterization, Urol. Dig. p. 11, July 1977.

54. Lapides, J., and Diokno, A.C.: Stress urinary incontinence. In Raz, S.: Female urology, Philadelphia, 1983, W.B. Saunders Co.

55. Lapides, J., Sweet, R.B., and Lewis, L.W.: Role of striated muscle in urination, J. Urol. **77:**247, 1957.

56. Lattimer, J.K., and Wechsler, M.: Genitourinary tuberculosis. In Harrison, J.H., et al.: Campbell's urology, Philadelphia, 1978, W.B. Saunders Co.

57. Leach, G.E., et al.: Urodynamic manifestations of cerebellar ataxia, J. Urol. **128:**348, 1982.

58. Leach, G.E., and Raz, S.: Interstitial cystitis. In Raz, S.: Female urology, Philadelphia, 1983, W.B. Saunders Co.

58a. Leadbetter, G.W.: Diagnostic urologic instrumentation. In Harrison, J.H., et al.: Campbell's urology, Philadelphia, 1978, W.B. Saunders Co.

59. Leeson, C.R., and Leeson, T.S.: Histology, Philadelphia, 1976, W.B. Saunders Co.

60. Lerner, J., and Khan, Z.: Manual of urologic nursing, St. Louis, 1982, The C.V. Mosby Co.

61. Lich, R., Howerton, L.W., and Amin, M.: Anatomy and surgical approach to the urogenital tract in the male. In Harrison, J.H., et al.: Campbell's urology, Phildelphia, 1978, W.B. Saunders Co.

62. Maggio, A.J., and Raz, S.: Why vesicourethral suspension works or fails. In Raz, S.: Female urology, Philadelphia, 1983, W.B. Saunders Co.

62a. Majd, M.: Nuclear medicine. In Kelalis, P.P., King, L.R., and Belman, A.B.: Clinical pediatric urology, Philadelphia, 1985, W.B. Saunders Co.

63. Mann, T., and Lutwak-Mann, C.: Male reproductive function and semen, Berlin, 1981, Springer-Verlag.

64. Marshall, V.F.: Methods in urologic diagnosis. In Emmett, J.L., and Witten, D.M.: Clinical urography, Philadelphia, 1971, W.B. Saunders Co.

65. Mawhinney, M.G.: Male accessory sex organs and androgen action. In Lipschulz, L.I., and Howards, S.S.: Infertility in the male, New York, 1983, Churchill-Livingstone.

66. Meares, E.M.: Urinary tract infections in man. In Harrison, J.H., et al.: Campbell's urology, Philadelphia, 1978, W.B. Saunders Co.

67. Meares, E.M.: Prostatitis, Ann. Rev. Med. **30:**279, 1979.

68. Michigan, S.: Genitourinary fungal infections, J. Urol. **116:**390, 1976.

69. Montague, D.K.: The evaluation of the impotent male. In Libertino, A.J.: International perspectives in urology, vol. 5, Baltimore, 1982, Williams & Wilkins Co.

70. Mundy, A.R., and Blaivas, J.G.: Nontraumatic neurological disorders. In Mundy, A.R., Stephenson, T.A., and Wein, A.J.: Urodynamics: principles, practice, and application, Edinburgh, 1984, Churchill-Livingstone.

71. Narayan, P., and Lange, P.: Semirigid penile prosthesis in the management of erectile impotence, Urol. Clin. North Am. **8:**169, 1981.

72. Newman, H.F.: Physiology of erection. In Krane, R.J., Siroky, M.B., and Goldstein, I.: Male sexual dysfunction, Boston, 1983, Little, Brown & Co.

73. Nickel, W.P., and Plumb, R.T.: Other infections and inflammations of the external genitalia. In Harrison, J.H., et al.: Campbell's urology, Philadelphia, 1978, W.B. Saunders Co.

74. Nielsen, J.B., et al.: Neurourol. Urodynam. **3**(1):7, 1984.

74a. Nistal, M., and Paniagua, R.: Testicular and epididymal pathology, New York, 1984, Thieme-Stratton, Inc.

75. Notley, R.G.: The anatomy of the ureter and pathology of congenital obstructions. In Chisholm, G.D., and Williams, I.D.: Scientific foundations in urology, Chicago, 1982, Yearbook Medical Publishers.

75a. Novick, A.: Renovascular hypertension. In Kendall, A.R., and Karafin, R.: Urology: Goldsmith's practice of surgery, Philadelphia, 1983, Harper & Row, Publishers.

76. O'Brien, D.P.: Enuresis. In Hurst, J.W.: Medicine for the practicing physician, Boston, 1983, Butterworth Publishers.

77. Perlmutter, A.D.: Enuresis. In Harrison, J.H., et al.: Campbell's urology, Philadelphia, 1978, W.B. Saunders Co.

78. Perlmutter, A.D.: Enuresis. In Kelalis, P.P., King, L.R., and Belman, A.B.: Clinical pediatric urology, Philadelphia, 1985, W.B. Saunders Co.

79. Pfister, R.C., Newhouse, J.H., and Hendren, W.H.: Percutaneous pyeloureteral urodynamics, Urol. Clin. North Am. 9(1):41, 1982.

80. Platt, R., et al.: Mortality associated with nosocomial urinary-tract infection, N. Engl. J. Med. 307:637, 1982.

81. Riff, L.J.: Bacteremia arising from the urinary tract, Urol. Clin. North Am. 2:521, 1975.

82. Riley, T.W., et al.: Use of radioisotopic scan in evaluation of intrascrotal lesions, J. Urol. 116:472, 1976.

83. Rose, B.D.: Pathophysiology of renal disease, New York, 1981, McGraw-Hill Book Co.

84. Rotkin, I.D.: Origins, distributions, and risks of benign prostatic hypertrophy. In Hinman, J.F.: Benign prostatic hypertrophy, New York, 1983, Springer-Verlag.

83. Rose, B.D.: Pathophysiology of renal disease, New York, 1981, McGraw-Hill Book Co.

85. Sarma, K.P.: Tumors of the urinary bladder, New York, 1969, Appleton-Century-Crofts.

86. Siroky, M.B., and Krane, R.J.: Neurophysiology of erection. In Krane, R.J., Siroky, M.B., and Goldstein, I.: Male sexual dysfunction, Boston, 1983, Little, Brown & Co.

87. Smith, A.D.: Causes and classifications of incontinence, Urol. Clin. North Am. 8:79, 1981.

88. Smith, D.R.: Tumors of the genitourinary tract. In Smith, D.R.: General urology, Los Altos, Calif., 1981, Lange Medical Publishers.

89. Stamey, T.A.: Urinary tract infections in women. In Harrison, J.H., et al.: Campbell's urology, Philadelphia, 1978, W.B. Saunders Co.

90. Stamey, T.A.: Pathogenesis and treatment of urinary tract infections, Baltimore, 1980, Williams & Wilkins Co.

91. Steinberger, E.: Male reproductive physiology. In Crockett, A.T., and Urry, D.L.: Male infertility: workup, treatment, and research, New York, 1977, Grune & Stratton.

92. Streem, S.B.: The endocrinology of impotence. In Libertino, A.J.: International perspectives in urology, vol. 5, Baltimore, 1982, Williams & Wilkins Co.

93. Swerdloff, R.S.: Physiology of male reproduction. In Harrison, J.H., et al.: Campbell's urology, Philadelphia, 1978, W.B. Saunders Co.

94. Tanagho, E.A.: Anatomy of the genitourinary tract. In Smith, D.R.: General urology, Los Altos, Calif., 1981, Lange Medical Publishers.

95. Tanagho, E.A.: Vesicoureteral reflux. In Smith, D.R.: General urology, Los Altos, Calif., 1981, Lange Medical Publishers.

96. Thomas, T.M., et al.: Prevalence of urinary incontinence, Br. Med. J. 281:1243, 1980.

97. Wagner, G.: Penile dysfunction due to local disorders. In Wagner, G., and Green, R.: Impotence, New York, 1981, Plenum Press.

98. Wagner, G.: Organic causes of impotence. In Libertino, A.J.: International perspectives in urology, vol. 5, Baltimore, 1982, Williams & Wilkins Co.

99. Wagner, G., and Green, R.: General medical disorders and erectile failure. In Wagner, G., and Green, R.: Impotence, New York, 1981, Plenum Press.

100. Wagner, G., Hilsted, J., and Jensen, S.B.: Diabetes mellitus and erectile failure. In Wagner, G., and Green, R.: Impotence, New York, 1981, Plenum Press.

101. Wagner, G., and Metz, P.: Arteriosclerosis and erectile failure. In Wagner, G., and Green, R.: Impotence, New York, 1981, Plenum Press.

102. Walker, D.B.: How important are prostaglandins in the urology of man? Urol. Int. 37:160, 1982.

103. Walsh, A.: Interstitial cystitis. In Harrison, J.H., et al.: Campbell's urology, Philadelphia, 1978, W.B. Saunders Co.

104. Walsh, P.C., and Amelar, R.D.: Embryology, anatomy and physiology of the male reproductive system. In Amelar, R.D., and Dubin, L.E.: Male infertility, Philadelphia, 1977, W.B. Saunders Co.

105. Walsh, P.C., and Wilson, J.D.: The induction of prostatic hypertrophy in the dog with androstanediol, J. Clin. Invest. 54:1093, 1976.

106. Walsh, P.C., et al.: Tissue content of dihydrotestosterone in human prostatic hyperplasia is not abnormal, J. Clin. Invest. 72:1772, 1983.

107. Walton, K.N.: Urinary tract infection. In Hurst, J.W.: Medicine for the Practicing Physician, Boston, 1983, Butterworth Publishers.

108. Waterhouse, K.: Urethral valves. In Glenn, J.F.: Urologic Surgery, Hagerstown, Md., 1975, Harper & Row.

109. Webster, G.D.: Neurogenic bladder disease. In Resnick, M.I., and Older, R.A.: Diagnosis of genitourinary disease, New York, 1982, Thieme-Stratton.

110. Weidman, C.L., and Northcutt, R.C.: Endocrine aspects of impotence, Urol. Clin. North Am. 8:143, 1981.

111. Wein, A.J., and Raezer, D.M.: Physiology of micturition. In Krane, R.J., and Siroky, M.B.: Clinical neuro-urology, Boston, 1979, Little, Brown & Co.

111a. Weiss, R.M.: Effects of drugs on the ureter. In Bergmann, H.: The ureter, New York, 1981, Springer-Verlag.

112. Wheatley, J.K.: Causes and treatment of bladder incontinence, Comprehensive Therapy, 9(8):27, 1983.

113. Wheatley, J.K.: Epididymitis. In Hurst, J.W.: Medicine for the practicing physician, Boston, 1983, Butterworth Publishers.

114. Whitaker, R.: Clinical application of upper tract urodynamics, Urol. Clin. North Am. 6:137, 1979.

115. Whiteside, C.G., and Arnold, E.P.: Persistent primary enuresis: urodynamic assessment, Br. Med. J. 1(5954):364, 1975.

116. Williams, P., and Warwick, R.: Gray's anatomy, Philadelphia, 1980, W.B. Saunders Co.

117. Wilson, J.D.: The pathogenesis of benign prostatic hypertrophy, Am. J. Med. 68:745, 1980.

118. Wilson, J.D., Gloyna, R.E., and Siiteri, P.K.: Androgen metabolism in the hypertrophic prostate, J. Steroid Biochem. 6:443, 1975.

119. Yalla, S.V.: Sexual dysfunction in the paraplegic and quadriplegic. In Libertino, A.J.: International perspectives in urology, vol. 5, Baltimore, 1982, Williams & Wilkins Co.

120. Yarnell, J.W.G., et al.: The prevalence and severity of urinary incontinence in women, J. Epidemiol. Community Health 35:71, 1981.

CHAPTER 13

Hematolymphatic System

Overview

The hematolymphatic system is composed of blood and blood-forming organs, the bone marrow, spleen, liver, and the lymphatics.

Blood, which circulates continuously through the heart and vascular system, performs numerous vital functions: (1) transport of oxygen and absorbed nutrients to cells and waste products, including carbon dioxide, to the kidneys, skin, and lungs; (2) transport of hormones from their origin in the endocrine glands to other tissues; (3) protection of the body from life-threatening micro-organisms; and (4) regulation of body temperature by heat transfer.

Major characteristics of blood include color (arterial blood is bright red, whereas venous blood is dark red); viscosity (blood is three to four times thicker than water); reaction (the pH is 7.35 to 7.40); and volume (adults have approximately 70 to 75 ml/kg of body weight, or 5 to 6 L).

The four physiologic disturbances likely to occur in the hematologic system are decreased number of cells, overproduction of normal or abnormal cells, defects in the clotting mechanism, and disorders of the spleen. Causative factors may be idiopathic (unknown) or one of the following: dietary deficiencies, malabsorption, drug toxicity, metabolic disorders, hemorrhaging, infection, malignancy, genetic predisposition, or immunologic defects.

The lymphatic system has numerous functions that include the transport of lymph, production of lympho-cytes and antibodies, phagocytosis, and absorption of fats and fat-soluble matter from the intestine.

The major characteristics of the lymphatic system are (1) that the formation of lymph is regulated by exchange of fluid between capillaries and tissue spaces; (2) that the muscle pump is responsible for the movement of lymph; and (3) that the amount of lymphoid tissue and the distribution of lymph nodes are related to age. The lymphatic system includes peripheral lymphatics, regional nodes, main lymphatic ducts, and the thoracic duct.

The basic physiologic disturbances that can occur in the lymphatic system, enlargement and swelling of soft tissues, are usually from infection, inflammation, neo-plasm, or obstruction.

ANATOMY AND PHYSIOLOGY

Blood, a suspension of particulate matter in an aqueous solution of colloid and electrolytes, serves as a medium of exchange for body cells between themselves and the exterior. It also has protective properties that are bene-ficial to the body and to the blood itself. The liquid portion, plasma, is a suspension of colloid, electrolytes, proteins, and numerous other substances. The particulate matter includes red blood cells (erythrocytes), white blood cells of several types (leukocytes), and platelets (thrombocytes). All of these cells are believed to be derived from a single stem cell, which divides and matures to produce three distinct types of cells with different functions, properties, and characteristics.

Erythrocytes, of which there are approximately 5 million/mm³ of blood, have as their principal functions the transport of oxygen (which attaches to hemoglobin, the iron-containing substance of the cell) to the tissues; the transport of carbon dioxide to the lungs; and the maintenance of normal blood pH through a series of intracellular buffers. Normal hemoglobin is 15 gm/100 ml of blood. Erythrocytes are produced in the red bone marrow and are found in the ribs, sternum, skull, vertebrae, and bones of the hands, feet, and pelvis. Numerous nutrients are needed for normal cell formation, including iron, vitamin B_{12}, folic acid, and pyridoxine. The young reticulocytes released from the bone marrow circulate for 4 days while maturing into adult erythrocytes. The average life-span of an erythrocyte is 115 to 130 days; dead cells are eliminated by phagocytosis in the reticuloendothelial system, particularly in the spleen and liver.

Hemoglobin is composed of a simple protein called "globin" and a red-colored compound called "heme," which contains iron and porphyrin. Each erythrocyte contains 200 to 300 million molecules of hemoglobin, which combine chemically with oxygen to form oxyhemoglobin. Hemoglobin also combines with carbon dioxide. These two capacities enable the blood to carry oxygen to the tissues and carbon dioxide to the alveoli and thus to the atmosphere.

Total iron in the body ranges from 2 to 6 gm, two thirds of which is contained in hemoglobin; the rest is stored in the bone marrow, spleen, and liver. Iron is obtained from such rich dietary sources as liver, oysters, lean meats, kidney beans, green leafy vegetables, apricots, and raisins.

When hemoglobin is phagocytized in the liver or spleen, it breaks down into its heme and globin factors. The heme's iron is reused by the liver to make fresh hemoglobin, while the porphyrin is converted into bilirubin that is excreted by the body in feces and urine.

Leukocytes, of which there are approximately 5000 to 10,000/mm³ of blood, are divided into three major categories: granulocytes, lymphocytes, and monocytes. Granulocytes, which make up 70% of all white blood cells, are produced by the bone marrow and function based on the type of granule: (1) polymorphonuclear leukocytes (PMNs or neutrophils), whose main function is to fight bacterial infections through a process of phagocytosis (foreign particulate matter, that is, breakdown products from cells, is also digested); these cells are present during the early, acute phase of an inflammatory reaction; (2) eosinophils, which have a similar phagocytic function and are particularly important in digesting bacteria; they appear to play a role in combating allergic reactions; and (3) basophils, which contain many enzymes believed to play a role in combating acute systemic allergic reactions.

Lymphocytes, which are mainly produced in the lymph nodes, compose about 25% of the leukocytes and are primarily concerned with the production of antibodies and maintenance of tissue immunity. Monocytes, which are derived from components of the reticuloendothelial system, are responsible for the phagocytosis of dead erythrocytes and leukocytes in the blood. They are also important in the processing of antigenic information.

There are approximately 250,000 to 500,000 thrombocytes/mm³ of blood. Formed in the bone marrow, their functions are to maintain capillary integrity, initiate coagulation, and retract clots.

The lymphoid system includes lymph nodes, spleen, thymus, lymphoid tissue associated with mucosal surfaces, and bone marrow. Lymph nodes, the most numerous component, are present in virtually every area of the body, the most familiar of which are those palpable in the neck and groin. They serve as filters along the course of lymphatic channels and have a rich blood supply, which is important in the transport of lymphocytes. The spleen is a mass of lymphoid and reticuloendothelial cells found under the ribs in the upper left quadrant of the abdomen. Its structure allows close interaction among lymphocytes, macrophages, and materials carried in the blood stream. The thymus is located in the thorax anterior to the upper part of the heart and great vessels and contains lymphatic follicles and lymphocytes. The bone marrow is considered an important part of the lymphoid system because millions of lymphocytes are scattered throughout it.

The various lymphatic channels in the body drain fluid from organs and tissues, conduct it centrally, and introduce it to the bloodstream via a large vein in the thorax. Many lymphocytes are found in the lymph and are recycled for variable periods of time.

NORMAL FINDINGS[6]

Area of Concern	Normal Adult Findings
Blood	
Erythrocyte	Biconcave disc when viewed laterally, it appears to have lighter center and to be thicker on outer perimeter.
Reticulocyte	Young, nonnucleated cells are formed in bone marrow; stain gray-blue.
Granulocyte	Neutrophil (PMN) has faint, pink, acidophilic granules.
	Eosinophil has refractive, eosinophilic granules.
	Basophil has large blue granules.
Lymphocyte	Single, round nucleus, cytoplasm has faintly basophilic, heavily clumped nuclear chromatin pattern.
Monocyte	Nucleus is folded or indented; often looks lobulated; has clumped nuclear chromatin pattern; cytoplasm is bluish gray or light sky blue.
Thrombocyte	Nucleate, disc-shaped fragments of megakaryocytes of the lymphoid system.
Lymph nodes	They are not normally palpable.
Spleen	It is located in the left upper outer quadrant; not normally palpable.
Thymus	Reticular framework is densely infiltrated with lymphocytes that are arranged in pattern of cortex and medulla.
Lymphoid tissue associated with mucosal surfaces, that is, gastrointestinal and respiratory tracts	It may be distributed diffusely or in nodular aggregates.
Bone marrow	Myeloid tissue is located only in the ribs, sternum, and at the ends of long bones.

NORMAL LABORATORY DATA

Laboratory Test	Normal Adult Values	Variations in Child
Red cell count (10^6/μL)	Men: 5.11 ± 0.38 Women: 4.51 ± 0.36	1 day: 5.30 ± 0.5 11 to 13½ mo: 4.44 ± 0.4 1½ to 3 yr: 4.45 ± 0.4 5 yr: 4.65 ± 0.5 10 yr: 4.80 ± 0.5
Hemoglobin (g/dl)	Men: 15.5 ± 1.1 Women: 13.7 ± 1.0	1 day: 19.4 ± 2.1 11 to 13½ mo: 11.9 ± 0.6 1½ to 3 yr: 11.8 ± 0.5 5 yr: 12.7 ± 1.0 10 yr: 13.2 ± 1.2
Hematocrit (%)	Men: 46.0 ± 3.1 Women: 40.9 ± 3	1 day: 58.0 ± 7 11 to 13½ mo: 39.0 ± 2 1½ to 3 yr: 39.0 ± 2 5 yr: 37.0 ± 3 10 yr: 39.0 ± 3
Mean corpuscular volume (MCV)	Men: 90 (80-100) μm³ Women: 88 (79-98) μm³	
Mean corpuscular hemoglobin (MCH)	Men: 30 (25.4-34.6) pg Women: 30 (25.4-34.6) pg	
Mean corpuscular hemoglobin concentration (MCHC)	Men: 34% (31%-37%) Women: 33% (30%-36%)	
Reticulocyte count (expressed as % of 1000 RBCs)	0.5%-1.5%	Newborns: 7% or less Normal values at birth: 2.5%-6.5%, falling to normal adult level by end of week 2

Laboratory Test	Normal Adult Values	Variations in Child
Erythrocyte fragility test	Hemolysis starts at 0.45%-0.39% saline solution Hemolysis complete at 0.33%-0.30% saline solution	
Erythrocyte life-span determination	Approximately 120 days; half-life, 27-86 days	

Serum
  Serum iron level
  Bilirubin
    Direct
    Indirect
    Total
	
	42-135 μg/dl
	
	Up to 0.4 mg/dl
	0.8 mg
	0.3-1.0 mg/dl	

Fecal and urinary urobilinogen	2 hr urinary urobilinogen Men: 0.3-2.1 mg/2 hr Women: 0.1-1.1 mg/2 hr Results are sometimes expressed in Ehrlich units; 1 mg urobilinogen = 1 EU Fecal: 50-300 mg/24 hr	
Erythrocyte peroxide hemolysis test	<20% hemolysis	
Total white cell count	4500-11,000 cells/mm^3	

Granulocytes
  Neutrophils (%)
  Eosinophils
  Basophils (%)
	
	38-70/mm^3
	50-350/mm^3
	0-2	

Monocytes (%)	1-8	
Lymphocytes (%)	15-45	
Platelets	150,000-400,000/mm^3	
Bleeding time	5 min (Duke) 2-7 min (Ivy)	
Coagulation time	8-15 min	
Capillary fragility	Presence of less than 5 petechiae in men and less than 10 in women in an area with a 2.5 cm radius	Presence of less than 10 petechiae in an area with a 2.5 cm radius

DIAGNOSTIC STUDIES

Peripheral blood smear
  Red cell count
    Number of red blood cells (RBCs) in 1 mm^3 of blood
  White cell count
    Number of white blood cells (WBCs) in 1 mm^3 of blood
  Differential count
    Percentage of various types of WBCs
  Platelet count
    Number of platelets in 1 mm^3 of blood
  Hemoglobin concentration
    Amount of hemoglobin in a given volume of blood
  Hematocrit
    Percentage of blood composed of RBCs
  Mean corpuscular volume (MCV)
    Size/volume of each RBC
  Mean corpuscular hemoglobin (MCH)
    Hemoglobin content in RBC of average size
  Mean corpuscular concentration (MCHC)
    Amount of hemoglobin in packed RBCs (hemoglobin of 100 ml RBCs)
  Reticulocyte count
    Determines effectiveness and speed of RBC production and responsiveness of bone marrow to decreased circulating RBCs.

Erythrocyte fragility test
  Measures rate at which RBCs burst in hypotonic solutions of varied concentrations.

Erythrocyte life-span determination
  Estimates rate at which RBCs tagged with chromium-51 disappear from circulation.
  Patient and normal subject with comparable blood type are injected with tagged cells.

Direct Coombs' test

Used to examine RBCs for the presence of antibodies (agglutinins) that damage RBCs, but will not cause clumping or hemolysis.

Indirect Coombs' test

Used to identify antibodies to RBC antigens.

Fecal and urinary urobilinogen

Determines amount of urobilinogen; result of breakdown of bilirubin by intestinal flora; excreted in urine and feces.

Urine is collected for a 2-hour period in afternoon or for a 24-hour period.

Serum iron level

Amount of iron found in a sample of blood

Bone marrow biopsy

Aspiration of a piece of bone marrow is done by withdrawal through a biopsy needle.

Nursing care:

Preprocedural care: proper positioning, shaving, and cleansing; postprocedural care: application of small sterile dressing

Bilirubin

Venous sample is collected for measurement of total amount of bilirubin; differentiation of conjugate and unconjugate levels can also be done.

Schilling test

Measures absorption of radioactive vitamin B_{12} before and after parenteral administration of intrinsic factor (may be a three-stage procedure).

Gastric analysis

Presence of free hydrochloric acid; histamine may be injected to stimulate flow.

Therapeutic trial with parenteral vitamin B_{12}

Patient is given intramuscular injections of vitamin B_{12} for 10 days; blood work and patient's subjective feeling of well-being are evaluated.

Bleeding time

Small stab wound in earlobe or forearm; time to stop bleeding is noted and measurement is made of rate at which a clot is formed.

Nursing care:

Patient must not take aspirin for at least 5 days before test; patient is also advised not to drink alcoholic beverages before the test.

Coagulation time

Time required for blood to form solid clot in foreign surface such as glass test tube is measured.

Capillary fragility (tourniquet test)

Positive or negative pressure is applied to various areas of the body; relative number of petechiae is noted.

Conditions, Diseases, and Disorders

ERYTHROCYTIC DISORDERS[9]

Two basic pathophysiologic processes can be used to classify all disorders of red blood cells: inadequate numbers of circulating cells (anemia) and increased numbers of circulating cells (polycythemia). Anemias result from insufficient production or defective synthesis, increased destruction, or loss of erythrocytes. Polycythemia results from idiopathic causes or as a compensatory mechanism in response to tissue hypoxia.

While not a disease per se anemia is the primary manifestation of many abnormal states such as dietary deficiencies of iron, vitamin B_{12}, and folic acid; hereditary disorders; damaged bone marrow or an overactive spleen; and bleeding from any tract or organ. The incidence of anemia is quite high; perhaps 50% of the world's population suffers from it at some time.

The major physiologic effect of anemia is to reduce the oxygen carrying capacity of the blood; thus the symptoms of anemia are the result of tissue hypoxia.

Posthemorrhagic Anemia

Posthemorrhagic anemia is a disorder of decreased hemoglobin in the blood as a result of traumatically induced hemorrhage.

Acute posthemorrhagic anemia develops as the result of the rapid loss of large quantities of erythrocytes during a hemorrhage, that is, traumatic severance of blood vessels, rupture of an aneurysm, or arterial erosion by a cancerous or ulcerative lesion. The severity of symptoms and the prognosis depend on the rate of bleeding, site of bleeding, and volume of blood loss. The rapid loss of less blood is more dangerous than is the slower loss of more blood.

PATHOPHYSIOLOGY

During the first 24 to 48 hours after hemorrhage, vasoconstriction and loss of plasma volume distort the erythrocyte count, hemoglobin, and hematocrit, which appear high when they are actually quite low. These laboratory tests more accurately reflect the patient's status after intravenous fluids are infused and extracellular fluid moves into the blood vessels. The red blood cell count and hemoglobin usually return to normal in 4 to 6 weeks, with many reticulocytes observed in the blood.

Chronic blood loss anemia, which is due to bleeding peptic ulcers, menstrual disorders, bleeding hemorrhoids, or gastrointestinal neoplasms, results in continuous losses of erythrocytes and iron. Symptoms and laboratory findings are identical to those of iron-deficiency anemia.

DIAGNOSTIC STUDIES

Erythrocytes
6.1/mm^3 (initial); 4.7/mm^3 (after fluid volume increase)

Hemoglobin
16.5 gm/dl (initial); 14.5 gm/dl (after fluid volume increase)

Hematocrit
50% (initial); 40% (after fluid volume increase)

TREATMENT PLAN

Surgical
If indicated to control source of bleeding

Chemotherapeutic
Hematinic agents
Iron supplements when diet therapy is insufficient, i.e., oral administration of ferrous sulfate (Feosol), 200 mg tid pc (adults); 200 mg tid pc (children, 6 to 12 yr)

Supportive
Intravenous plasma initially; whole blood after typing and cross-matching done
Sedation and rest
Oral fluids as tolerated
Diet high in protein, iron

ASSESSMENT: AREAS OF CONCERN

Sensory function
Restlessness, dizziness, syncope, and severe headache

Mental status
Disorientation

Appearance of skin
Pallor, diaphoresis, and warmth

Level of comfort
Pain in area of bleeding due to tissue distention

Fluid and electrolyte balance
Thirst

Cardiovascular function
Rapid thready pulse
Hypotension

Respiratory function
Rapid deep respirations; later become shallow

NURSING DIAGNOSES and NURSING INTERVENTIONS

Nursing Diagnosis	Nursing Intervention
Cardiac output, alteration in: decreased	Provide rest and anticipate needs. Monitor apical pulse, heart sounds, blood pressure, respirations. Monitor laboratory tests. Avoid stress, that is, high emotions, overexertion, fatigue, coughing, and straining at stool.
Fluid volume deficit, actual	Apply ice bag and manual pressure/dressing over site of blood loss. Elevate and immobilize affected body part. Estimate blood loss. Administer intravenous fluids, including blood, as ordered. Measure intake and output. Increase oral fluid intake as tolerated. Observe for recurrent bleeding.
Tissue perfusion, alteration in: peripheral	Place patient on bed rest in a semi-Fowler position. Maintain warm environment. Inspect for adequate circulation.

Nursing Diagnosis	Nursing Intervention
	Palpate for arterial pulses.
	Protect patient from injury, that is, side rails up.
	Assess level of consciousness and orientation.
	Discourage smoking.
	Encourage exercise, including range of motion exercises.
Nutrition, alteration in: less than body requirements (related to blood loss)	Encourage increased iron and protein food intake.
	Administer iron medication as prescribed.

Patient Education

1. Teach the patient to avoid overexertion, fatigue, and emotional states because they place a strain on the cardiovascular system that may result in respiratory distress, cardiac damage, or impaired peripheral arterial circulation.
2. Instruct the patient to report to the physician serious symptoms such as pain, dyspnea, extreme fatigue, and blood in urine or feces.
3. Instruct the patient in maintenance of normal bowel elimination to avoid strain on the cardiovascular system.
4. Teach the importance of regular exercise to maintain adequate peripheral circulation as well as cardiac and respiratory tone.
5. Teach the maintenance of a diet high in iron and protein, with adequate fluid intake.

EVALUATION

Patient Outcome	Data Indicating That Outcome is Reached
Vital signs are within normal limits.	Respiratory rate and pulse rate are within normal limits.
Laboratory studies are within normal limits.	The hemoglobin level and hematocrit are within normal limits.
The patient's vitality is maintained.	The patient is mentally alert with good concentration and attentiveness. The patient experiences no malaise, fatigue, or weakness.
Color of the skin and mucous membranes is good.	The skin, nails, lips, and ear lobes are warm and moist with a natural color.
Bowel elimination is normal for the individual.	Stools are soft; the abdomen is soft and nondistended. There is no abdominal pressure or cramping.
Body hydration is normal.	There is no edema or thirst.
Daily intake includes the essential food groups.	The diet includes foods high in protein and iron.
The patient participates in daily physical exercise.	The patient participates in activities such as bicycling, tennis, and jogging.

Iron-Deficiency Anemia

Iron-deficiency anemia is caused by an inadequate supply of iron needed to synthesize hemoglobin.

Iron-deficiency anemia, which is high in incidence worldwide and the most prevalent anemia, is caused by inadequate absorption or excessive loss of iron. The disease occurs most frequently among women and young children in underdeveloped countries.

The principal cause of iron-deficiency anemia in adults is acute or chronic bleeding secondary to trauma, excessive menses, gastrointestinal tract bleeding (usually chronic and occult), or blood donation. Another cause is inadequate dietary intake of foods high in iron. A third cause is defective absorption due to malabsorption syndromes, clay-eating (pica), chronic diarrhea, high intake of cereal products with low intake of animal protein, and partial or complete gastrectomy.

PATHOPHYSIOLOGY

Iron-deficiency anemia is a chronic, microcytic, hypochromic anemia; in other words, the erythrocytes are small and pale because of a low hemoglobin level. While the total erythrocyte count is only moderately reduced, the serum iron level may drop dramatically.

DIAGNOSTIC STUDIES[6]

Hemoglobin level
   As low as 3.6 g/100 ml

Total erythrocyte count
   Rarely below 3 million cells/100 ml

Mean corpuscular hemoglobin (MCH)
   <27 pg

Mean corpuscular hemoglobin concentration (MCHC)
   20 to 30 g/100 ml

Serum iron level
   As low as 10 g

TREATMENT PLAN

Chemotherapeutic
   Hematinic agents
      Adults and children 6-12 yr: Ferrous sulfate (Feosol), 0.2 g tid pc.
      Ferrous gluconate (Fergon):
         Adults: 0.3 g bid.
         Children 6-12 yr: 0.3 g qd.
      Iron-dextran (Imferon):
         Adults: 100-250 mg IM qd.
         Children 10-20 pounds: 50 mg IM qd.

Supportive
   Diet high in iron-rich foods

ASSESSMENT: AREAS OF CONCERN

In a mild case the patient generally has no symptoms.

Sensory and motor function
   Dizziness
   Dysphagia

Condition of skin, hair, and nails
   Sensitivity to cold
   Brittle hair and nails

Appearance of oral cavity
   Atrophic glossitis (tongue inflamed and smooth)
   Stomatitis

NURSING DIAGNOSES and NURSING INTERVENTIONS

Nursing Diagnosis	Nursing Intervention
Sensory-perceptual alteration: kinesthetic	Provide safe environment. Assist patient with ambulation and change in position.
Oral mucous membrane, alteration in	Remove dentures if present. Provide soft food and nonirritating fluids. Provide frequent mouth care. Initiate dental consultation.
Nutrition, alteration in: less than body requirements	Administer iron medication as ordered. Monitor laboratory reports. Encourage diet high in iron. Observe for difficulty in swallowing.
Skin integrity, impairment of	Maintain warm and clean environment. Wash hair with care. Provide nail care.

Patient Education

1. Explain the need for correct oral hygiene, including regular dental care.
2. Instruct the patient in the maintenance of a diet high in iron.

3. Explain factors in self-medication with iron supplements, including proper timing, dilution, and awareness of change in the stool color.
4. Explain general hygienic measures, that is, hair and nail care.
5. Explain general safety precautions to prevent injury from dizziness.

EVALUATION

Patient Outcome	Data Indicating That Outcome is Reached
Laboratory studies are within normal limits.	Red blood cells are normocytic and normochromic. The hemoglobin level, MCV, MCH, MCHC, and serum iron level are within normal limits.
Daily intake includes the essential food groups.	Patient's diet includes foods high in iron.
Body temperature is normal.	Patient feels neither hot nor cold.
Patient can easily ambulate.	Patient avoids contact with stable and moving objects. There is no reported dizziness.
General body cleanliness is maintained.	Hair and nails are clean and not brittle. Mouth is clean, with no ulceration or other oral irritation.

Pernicious Anemia

Pernicious anemia is a progressive anemia caused by a lack of intrinsic factor essential for the absorption of vitamin B_{12}.

Pernicious anemia is the most prevalent type of vitamin B_{12} deficiency anemia in the United States. Caused by a deficiency of the intrinsic factor, it is a chronic progressive macrocytic anemia that affects adults, mainly men and women over the age of 50, and blue-eyed persons of Scandinavian origin.

PATHOPHYSIOLOGY

Atrophy of the glanular mucosa of the gastric fundus results in a lack of intrinsic factor. Why this occurs is unknown, but there are several popular explanations: heredity: the disease tends to "run in families"; prolonged iron deficiency, which can cause gastric atrophy; an autoimmune disorder: 90% of patients are diagnosed as having autoantibodies that react against gastric cells, while 40% of patients react against the intrinsic factor.

Other anemias in this category result from a lack of vitamin B_{12}, which is either due to inadequate dietary intake and is corrected by daily oral administration and a more balanced diet, or caused by poor absorption, which is treated with vitamin B_{12} and corrects the malabsorption.

Anemias caused by a deficiency in folic acid are quite common and are usually the result of a poor diet, that is, a lack of green leafy vegetables, liver, citrus fruits, and yeast; malabsorption syndromes; or the increased need during the third trimester of pregnancy. Parenteral and/or oral therapy with folic acid is required. Vitamin C may be used supplementally. The symptoms of this anemia resemble those of pernicious anemia except for the absence of neurologic signs and symptoms.

DIAGNOSTIC STUDIES[6]

Erythrocyte count
Below 3 million/100 ml

Blood film
Red blood cells are oval, macrocytic, and hyperchromic

Bone marrow biopsy
Increased number of megaloblasts

Bilirubin
Unconjugated forms; usually elevated

Schilling test
Abnormal urinary excretion of vitamin B

Gastric analysis
Scanty secretions, elevated pH, and no free hydrochloric acid

Therapeutic trial with parenteral vitamin B_{12}
Large numbers of reticulocytes in blood 4 to 5 days after injection

TREATMENT PLAN[6]

Chemotherapeutic
Lifelong maintenance therapy
Vitamin derivatives
    Cyanocobalamin (Berubigen, Hemocyte, Vitamin B_{12}, and others), 100 mg IM 2 to 3 times/week until 10 doses are given and remission is obtained.
    Cyanocobalamin, 200 mg IM monthly or 100 mg IM every 2 weeks (maintenance therapy).
    Folic acid (Folvite), up to 0.5-1.0 mg po qd in both adults and children.
Hematinic agents
    Ferrous sulfate (Feosol) or ferrous gluconate (Fergon), 0.3 g tid pc po as needed.
Digestants
    Hydrochloric acid (HCL), po in well-diluted water tid pc during first weeks of vitamin B_{12} therapy.

Supportive
Blood transfusions
Nutritious diet, that is, fish, meat, milk, and eggs
Bed rest
Physical therapy

ASSESSMENT: AREAS OF CONCERN

Mental status
Irritability, depression, and psychotic behavior

Appearance of skin
Pallor and jaundice

Oral cavity
Sore mouth
Smooth, beefy red tongue

Respiratory function
Dyspnea or palpitations

Gastrointestinal function
Weight loss, indigestion, constipation, or diarrhea

Sensory and motor function
Tingling, numbness of hands and feet, paralysis, weakness, and fatigue

NURSING DIAGNOSES and NURSING INTERVENTIONS

Nursing Diagnosis	Nursing Intervention
Gas exchange, impaired	Provide bed rest with side rails up. Monitor pulse, blood pressure, and rate and quality of respirations. Observe mood, appropriateness of behavior, and orientation. Restrain as necessary. Assist with increased activity. Ask patient to report dyspnea and palpitations. Monitor laboratory reports.
Mobility, impaired physical	Provide bed rest with gradual ambulation. Provide range of motion exercises progressing to systemic exercise. Use bed cradle or footboard. Massage hands and feet; observe for signs of trauma.
Skin integrity, impairment of: actual	Observe skin color, warmth, texture, moisture, and intactness. Apply heat with extreme caution. Maintain skin with proper hygiene.
Nutrition, alteration in: less than body requirements	Administer vitamin B_{12} and other medications as prescribed. Encourage diet high in vitamins, iron, and protein.
Bowel elimination, alteration in	Offer small, frequent feedings. Observe for diarrhea or constipation and treat as prescribed.

Patient Education

1. Teach precautions in the use of heat therapy, that is, heating pad or hot compress (patient may have impaired sensitivity to heat and pain).
2. Emphasize general hygiene, that is, skin and oral care.
3. Explain physical therapy activities and general exercise (patient may have possible neurologic damage as a result of the disease).
4. Teach the importance of a diet high in vitamin B_{12} and the use of maintenance therapy with vitamin B_{12}.

EVALUATION

Patient Outcome	Data Indicating That Outcome is Reached
Color of the skin and mucous membranes is good.	The skin, nails, lips, and ear lobes are warm and moist with a natural color.
Vital signs are within normal limits.	Respiratory rate, pulse rate, and blood pressure are within normal limits.
Laboratory studies are within normal limits.	Erythrocyte count and serum bilirubin level are within normal limits, red blood cells are normocytic and normochromic.
The patient's vitality is maintained.	Patient is mentally alert, has good concentration, and is attentive. Malaise, fatigue, weakness, or disturbances in the gastrointestinal tract are absent.
Daily intake includes the essential food groups.	Patient's diet is high in iron, protein, and vitamins.
Patient participates in daily physical and therapeutic exercise.	Patient participates in activities such as bicycling, tennis, running, and therapeutic and range of motion exercises.
There is no evidence of physical injury.	There is no evidence of skin damage or physical sign of an accident.
Patient has a positive disposition.	Patient smiles appropriately and uses cheerful conversation.

Aplastic Anemia

Aplastic anemia is the term most frequently used to describe a decrease in the number of circulating erythrocytes caused by a failure of the bone marrow. It is usually accompanied by agranulocytosis and thrombocytopenia, in which case the condition is referred to as "pancytopenia."

PATHOPHYSIOLOGY

In half of all diagnosed cases of aplastic anemia, the cause is unknown; in the other half, it results from exposure to a specific toxin. The myelotoxins are: (1) agents that always cause damage when given in large doses: radiation (x-rays, radium, radioactive isotopes, etc.), benzene and its derivatives, alkylating agents, and antimetabolites; (2) agents that sometimes cause failure: chloramphenicol (Chloromycetin), sulfonamides, diphenylhydantoin, and others; and (3) suspicious agents such as streptomycin, chlorophenothane (DDT), and carbon tetrachloride.

DIAGNOSTIC STUDIES[6]

Erythrocyte count
Usually less than 1 million/mm^3; reticulocyte count also low

Leukocyte count
May be less than 2000/mm^3

Platelet count
<30,000/mm^3

Bone marrow biopsy
Marrow fatty and has few developing blood cells

TREATMENT PLAN

Supportive
Immediate removal of the causative agent
Blood transfusions
Prevention and treatment of complications, that is, infections and bleeding

ASSESSMENT: AREAS OF CONCERN

Energy level
Progressive fatigue, lassitude, and dyspnea

Possibility of infection
Fever, "sniffles," sore throat, severe anorexia, ulcerations on mucous membranes, pain and burning with urination, etc.

Vascular status
Petechiae or ecchymosis
Bleeding from gums, hematuria, occult or frank blood in feces, etc.

NURSING DIAGNOSES and NURSING INTERVENTIONS

Nursing Diagnosis	Nursing Intervention
Gas exchange, impaired	For hypoxia: place the patient in a sitting position; observe respiration rate and dyspnea; observe skin color and temperature; assist with care; plan rest periods; and monitor laboratory values.
Fluid volume deficit, potential	Handle the patient gently since the patient is predisposed to bleeding. Give injections only if necessary and apply pressure afterward. Observe for changes in vital signs and bleeding, that is, urine, stool, gums, or nose wounds. Avoid constipation.
Nutrition, alteration in	Provide food selection and seasonings. Offer small, frequent feedings. Encourage foods that are high in vitamins and protein. Record food intake. Arrange pleasant environment on tray. Provide oral hygiene. Monitor body weight and blood studies.
Skin integrity, impairment of (related to intradermal bleeding)	Apply ice bag or manual pressure. Handle gently. Monitor blood studies. Avoid use of injections. Observe for petechiae and ecchymosis.
Potential patient problem: susceptibility to infection	Maintain reverse isolation. Observe for increases in temperature, pulse, and respirations. Observe the patient for "sniffles," sore throat, anorexia, pain on urination, etc. Administer antibiotics as needed.

Patient Education

1. Patient maintains balance between rest and activity.
2. Patient avoids trauma, that is, use of soft toothbrush and electric razor.
3. Patient maintains adequate nutrition.
4. Patient avoids infection, that is, respiratory or urinary tracts.

EVALUATION

Patient Outcome	Data Indicating That Outcome is Reached
Color of the skin and mucous membranes is good.	The skin, nails, lips, and ear lobes are warm, moist, and a natural color.
Vital signs are within normal limits.	Respiratory rate, pulse rate, and blood pressure are within normal limits.
Patient has normal body functioning.	Elimination is adequate. Healing is prompt. Patient's daily weight is stabilized at a normal level for body build. Digestion is good.
Laboratory studies are within normal limits.	Hemoglobin level and hematocrit are within normal limits. Blood leukocyte count is 5000 to 10,000. No erythrocytes, leukocytes, hemoglobin, etc. are present in the patient's urine. The findings of bacterial culture are negative.
The patient's vitality is maintained.	Patient is mentally alert. Malaise, fatigue, and weakness are absent.
Daily intake includes essential food groups.	Foods high in vitamins and protein are emphasized.
The physical appearance of the patient indicates sufficient rest.	Patient has good concentration and coordination.

Patient Outcome	Data Indicating That Outcome is Reached
Patient participates in daily exercise.	Patient walks, bicycles, etc.
Patient's surroundings are safe.	Patient uses safety precautions.
There is no evidence of physical injury.	Patient does not have cuts, abrasions, etc.
Patient does not have an infection.	Oral temperature reading is 98.6° F (37° C). There is no evidence of inflammation, purulent drainage, pain or aching.

Hemolytic Anemia

Hemolytic anemia is a disorder in which the rate of erythrocyte destruction is greatly accelerated.

PATHOPHYSIOLOGY

Hemolytic anemia is the result of either an intracorpuscular defect or an extracorpuscular factor. This causes a shortened life-span for the erythrocytes, abnormally large numbers of erythrocytes being destroyed by reticuloendothelial cells, and inadequate replacement of lost cells by the bone marrow.

Intracorpuscular defects include a deficiency in glucose 6-phosphate dehydrogenase (G6-PD) and hereditary spherocytosis. Extracorpuscular factors include trauma, that is, burns or surgery; chemical agents or drugs, such as lead poisoning; immune response; infectious organisms, that is, infectious hepatitis, mononucleosis, miliary tuberculosis; systemic diseases such as Hodgkin's disease, leukemia, systemic lupus erythematosus; isoimmune reactions, such as fetalis erythroblastosis; autoimmune disorders; and paroxysmal hemoglobinurias.

Hemolytic anemia may be acute or chronic; hemolytic crises can occur in either form, both of which have the particular danger of acute renal failure.[6,9]

DIAGNOSTIC STUDIES[6]

Red blood cell count
Normocytic anemia

Reticulocyte count
Increased

Red blood cell fragility
Increased

Erythrocyte life-span
Shortened

Bilirubin level
Increased

Fecal and urinary urobilinogen
Increased

Bone marrow biopsy
Hyperplasia

TREATMENT PLAN

Surgical
Splenectomy if steroids fail

Chemotherapeutic
Corticosteroids
Prednisolone (Delta-Cortef, Meti-Derm, and others), 10-20 mg qid (used if autoimmune disease is present).

Supportive
Eliminate causative factors
Maintain fluid and electrolyte balance
Maintain renal function, that is, sodium bicarbonate or lactate to alkalize the blood
Combat anemia and shock with careful administration of blood transfusions

ASSESSMENT: AREAS OF CONCERN

Appearance of skin
Jaundice

Level of comfort
Fever and chills
Back or abdominal pain

Energy level
Weakness and fatigue

Gastrointestinal function
Abdominal pain
Enlargement of liver or spleen
Cholelithiasis

NURSING DIAGNOSES and NURSING INTERVENTIONS

Nursing Diagnosis	Nursing Intervention
Fluid volume deficit, actual	Increase oral fluid intake. Give small but frequent drinks. Monitor intake and output. Observe for adequate renal function: color, specific gravity, volume, and pH of urine. Administer intravenous fluids as ordered. Administer urine alkalizers as ordered. Administer blood transfusions as ordered.
Mobility, impaired: physical	Assist with mobility. Provide walker, wheelchair, or cane as needed. Observe for weakness and fatigue. Medicate for back pain as ordered. Encourage exercise as tolerated.
Nutrition, alteration in: less than body requirements	Provide balanced diet rich in iron and protein. Give small, frequent feedings. Avoid fatty foods. Measure body weight. Observe and record food intake. Palpate liver and spleen. Observe urine color. Monitor laboratory values, that is, bilirubin.
Skin integrity, impairment of	Provide skin care, such as cool water and lubrication. Maintain cool room temperature with adequate humidity. Expose skin to sunlight. Advise patient not to scratch skin.

Patient Education

1. Instruct in the need for adequate balance between rest and exercise.
2. Instruct in the need for well-balanced diet.
3. Teach the patient how to maintain skin cleanliness and integrity.

EVALUATION

Patient Outcome	Data Indicating That Outcome is Reached
Skin and mucous membranes have good color.	The skin, nails, lips, and ear lobes are warm and moist with a natural color.
Vital signs are within normal limits.	Respiratory rate, pulse rate, and blood pressure are within normal limits.
Laboratory studies are within normal limits.	The red blood cell count, reticulocyte count, red blood cell fragility, erythrocyte life-span, and serum bilirubin level are within normal limits. The fecal and urinary urobilinogen levels are within normal limits. Results of bone marrow biopsy are normal. Urine specific gravity and pH are within normal limits.
Body hydration is normal.	Skin turgor and color are good. Patient has thin secretions. Balance between intake and output is maintained.
Daily intake includes essential food groups.	Patient's diet is especially high in iron and protein.
Patient's surroundings are safe and comfortable.	Patient uses safety precautions, especially when ambulating. Room temperature and humidity are appropriate.
Patient maintains general body cleanliness.	Patient's skin is clean. Patient does not complain of itching.

Sickle Cell Anemia

Sickle cell anemia is a severe incurable anemia that occurs in people who are homozygous for hemoglobin S (Hb S).

PATHOPHYSIOLOGY

Sickle cell anemia is the result of a genetic mutation that is transmitted from parent to child. Between 45,000 and 75,000 black persons in this country have the disease, and 2.5 million carry the trait. The incidence of the trait is less than 1% in nonblacks and the disease nonexistent.

The erythrocytes of patients with sickle cell anemia contain more Hb S than Hb A, which causes them to assume a sickle or crescent shape when exposed to decreased oxygen tension. These "sickled" cells are then easily destroyed as they enter smaller blood vessels in the body. The sickle cell trait is usually a mild condition found in heterozygous carriers, who have few or no symptoms.

The exact cause of sickling crises is unknown, but two factors have been identified: hypoxia due to low oxygen tensions (such as climbing to high altitudes, exercising strenuously, or inadequate oxygenation during anesthesia) and elevated blood viscosity due to a concentration of cells and dehydration caused by such factors as vomiting, diarrhea, diaphoresis, or diuretics. Occlusion of the microcirculation then occurs with resultant hypoxia, which causes more sickling. Tissues and organs will develop infarction and thrombosis in the presence of anoxia, such as the brain, kidneys, bone marrow, and spleen.[6,9]

DIAGNOSTIC STUDIES[6]

Stained blood smear
Sickle cells is observed.

Sickle cell slide preparation of blood
Sickling is noted after deoxygenation.

Sickle-turbidity tube test
When patient's blood is mixed with Sickledex, turbid solution indicates the presence of Hg S.

Hemoglobin electrophoresis
Hb S and Hb A indicate the presence of the sickle cell trait; only the presence of Hb S indicates sickle cell anemia.

TREATMENT PLAN

The medical plan of care is generally supportive: rest, oxygen, intravenous fluids and electrolytes, sedatives, and analgesics; urea therapy via a central venous catheter into the superior vena cava is still somewhat controversial.

ASSESSMENT: AREAS OF CONCERN

General
  Integrity of skin
    Jaundice or pallor

  Skeletal integrity
    Joint swelling
    Disproportionately long arms and legs

  Development status
    Delayed sexual maturity
    Retarded growth

  Gastrointestinal function
    Enlargement of liver and spleen

Crisis complications
  Cardiac function
    Systolic murmurs
    Arrhythmias
    Enlargement

  Respiratory function
    Dyspnea
    Acute respiratory distress, that is, shortness of breath, chest pain, and cyanosis

  Sensory and motor function
    Signs and symptoms of increased intracranial pressure due to cerebral hemorrhaging

  Renal function
  Signs and symptoms of uremia, such as decreased urinary output and edema

NURSING DIAGNOSES and NURSING INTERVENTIONS

Nursing Diagnosis	Nursing Intervention
Tissue perfusion, alteration in: cerebral, potential (related to increased intracranial pressure)	Place the patient on complete bed rest with the head elevated. Decrease environmental stimuli. Change the patient's position slowly. Discourage oral stimulants. Monitor neurologic signs, such as level of consciousness, pupillary response, and reflexes. Observe for changes in pulse, blood pressure (BP), and behavior.
Tissue perfusion, alteration in (related to dysrhythmias)	Encourage the patient to rest and avoid strenuous activity. Advise the patient to avoid oral stimulants, such as smoking. Auscultate apical pulse. Monitor BP. Monitor blood studies: enzymes and electrolytes.
Tissue perfusion, alteration in: cardiopulmonary (related to cell sickling)	Auscultate for breath sounds, rate, rhythm, etc. Monitor BP and pulse. Monitor blood studies for gas exchange. Observe for headache, nausea, confusion, dyspnea, cyanosis, etc.
Tissue perfusion, alteration in: renal	Inspect for bleeding and edema. Measure body weight and intake and output. Monitor blood studies for abnormal electrolytes, hematology, and renal function. Monitor urine studies. Monitor temperature and BP. Observe urine for abnormal color, content, and odor. Test urine for protein.
Tissue perfusion, alteration in: peripheral	Place the patient on complete bed rest in a slight sitting position. Remove constrictive clothing. Maintain room and body warmth. Initiate range of motion exercises. Inspect extremities for adequate circulation. Palpate for arterial pulses. Monitor blood studies for gas exchange and hematology.
Skin integrity, impairment of	Place on bed rest. Elevate affected part. Implement cleaning procedure, such as with hydrogen peroxide or saline solution. Apply sterile dressing or expose to air. Apply heat with lamp or cradle. Observe response to therapy. Prepare the patient for skin grafting if necessary.
Comfort, alteration in: pain (related to increased intra-abdominal pressure and discomfort)	Place the patient in a sitting position. Remove constrictive clothing. Change the patient's position frequently. Give small, frequent feedings. Auscultate for abdominal bowel sounds.
Injury: potential for (fracture)	Change the patient's position frequently. Initiate range of motion exercises and physical activity. Encourage the patient to eat foods high in calcium, protein, and vitamins. Observe for pain, swelling, or abnormal alignment.

Patient Education

1. Alert the patient to the need for family testing to determine the presence of Hb S; genetic counseling is available for carriers.

2. Instruct the patient how to avoid sickle cell crises, that is, avoid altitudes, flying in unpressurized planes, and dehydration.

3. Explain to the patient that young pregnant women have a high risk of developing pulmonary and/or renal complications.
4. Teach range of motion exercises and encourage regular physical activity to prevent bone demineralization. Explain the need for balance between rest (physical and mental) and activity, that is, range of motion and isometric exercises.
5. Teach principles of good nutrition, such as the importance of protein, calcium, vitamins, and adequate fluids; the patient should not have oral stimulants.

6. Alert the patient to the signs and symptoms of increased intracranial pressure, to the need to blow the nose gently, to avoid coughing, and to avoid straining on elimination.
7. Monitor the patient's oral intake and urinary output.
8. Advise the patient to avoid trauma and extremes in temperature; patient should not smoke and should protect extremities from injury because of impaired circulation.
9. Monitor urine protein with Combistix or Urostix.

EVALUATION

Patient Outcome	Data Indicating That Outcome is Reached
Tissue perfusion is adequate.	The skin, nails, lips, and ear lobes are warm and moist with a natural color. Vital signs are within normal limits. Hemoglobin level and hematocrit are within normal limits. Levels of serum glutamic-oxaloacetic transaminase, lactic Blood gas values are within normal limits. Levels of serum glutamic-oxaloacetic transaminase, lactic dehydrogenase, and creatine phosphokinase are within normal limits. Electrocardiogram shows a normal tracing.
Fluid-electrolyte balance is adequate.	Skin turgor is good. Edema and ascites are not present. Blood levels of sodium, potassium, chloride, and calcium are within normal limits. Urine specific gravity is within normal limits.
Nutrition is adequate.	Bone development is good. Posture is good. Skin turgor is good. Elimination is adequate. Healing is prompt. Diet includes foods high in calcium, protein, and vitamins.
Acid-base balance is maintained.	Blood and urine pH are within normal limits.
Waste elimination is adequate.	Daily fluid output is equal to fluid intake. Blood urea nitrogen and serum creatinine levels are within normal limits. Results of urine protein test are negative. Results of urine specific gravity, creatinine level, and creatinine clearance are within normal limits.
The patient's energy and vitality levels are good.	Patient is mentally alert. Patient has good concentration and attentiveness. Malaise, fatigue, and weakness are absent.
Patient has adequate performance in work and play.	Patient is able to maintain self-care. Patient can perform household or work activities. Patient can participate in recreation and sports.
Activity and exercise are adequate.	Patient changes position and body movement frequently (walking, sitting, and standing). Patient participates in daily physical exercise (bicycling, tennis, jogging, etc.). Patient participates in range of motion and isometric exercises.

Patient Outcome	Data Indicating That Outcome is Reached
The patient's surroundings are safe and comfortable.	Patient uses safety precautions. Temperature and humidity level are appropriate. There is no evidence that accidents have occurred. There is no evidence of physical injury.
Patient has physical appearance of comfort.	Posture is normal. Patient has freedom of body movement. Patient expresses comfort.

Thalassemias

Thalassemias, which is another group of chronic hemolytic anemias, are caused by an insufficient number of hemoglobin polypeptide chains.

Hemoglobin A (Hb A)
Elevated, may be as high as 6%
(Normal, 1.5% to 3.0%)[6,9]

PATHOPHYSIOLOGY

The thalassemias are inherited disorders most frequently affecting persons of Mediterranean or Southern Chinese ancestry, as well as American blacks and individuals from Southern Asia and Central Africa. Thalassemia major and intermedia, the more serious anemias, appear in homozygotes; thalassemia minor is milder and appears in heterozygotes. The deficiency in hemoglobin polypeptide chains results in extremely thin, fragile erythrocytes called "target cells."

DIAGNOSTIC STUDIES

Blood smear
Target cells and other strangely shaped erythrocytes observed

Serum bilirubin
Greatly elevated

Fecal and urinary urobilinogen
Greatly elevated

Fetal hemoglobin (Hb F)
Elevated; may be as high as 90%

TREATMENT PLAN

The medical plan of care is supportive, such as transfusions of packed red cells on a monthly, bimonthly, and/or "as needed" basis. Splenectomy is necessary if transfused cells are rapidly destroyed by the spleen.

Chelating agents such as diethylenetriamine penta-acetic acid (DTPA) may be used if iron overload results from multiple transfusions.

ASSESSMENT: AREAS OF CONCERN

Integrity of skin
Jaundice
Leg ulcers

Gastrointestinal function
Enlarged spleen
Intolerance of fatty foods and abdominal discomfort

Skeletal integrity
Cranial bone hyperplasia
Mongoloid appearance

NURSING DIAGNOSES and NURSING INTERVENTIONS

Nursing Diagnosis	Nursing Intervention
Tissue perfusion, alteration in: cardiopulmonary (related to dysrhythmia)	Encourage rest and the avoidance of strenuous activity. Avoid oral stimulants, such as smoking. Auscultate apical pulse. Monitor blood pressure, respirations. Monitor blood studies, that is, enzymes, electrolytes, and gas exchange; electrocardiogram.

Nursing Diagnosis	Nursing Intervention
Skin integrity, impairment of: potential	Place the patient on bed rest. Elevate the affected part. Implement cleaning procedure, such as with hydrogen peroxide or saline solution. Apply sterile dressing or expose to air. Apply heat with lamp or cradle. Observe the patient's response to therapy. Prepare the patient for skin grafting if necessary.
Comfort, alteration in: pain (related to an increase in discomfort from intra-abdominal pressure)	Place the patient in a sitting position. Remove constrictive clothing. Change the patient's position frequently. Give small, frequent feedings. Auscultate for abnormal bowel sounds.
Skin integrity, impairment of: actual	Provide skin care using cool water and lubrication. Maintain cool room temperature with adequate humidity. Expose the skin to sunlight. Advise the patient not to scratch the skin.

Patient Education

1. Maintain skin cleanliness and integrity and minimize potential damage from jaundice or stasis ulcer.
2. Monitor the balance between rest and activity.
3. Explain to the patient the need to avoid trauma, extremes in temperature, and smoking to protect the extremities from injury due to impaired circulation.

EVALUATION

Patient Outcome	Data Indicating That Outcome is Reached
Color of the skin and mucous membranes are good.	The skin, nails, lips, and ear lobes are warm and moist with a natural color.
The patient has normal body functioning.	Vital signs are within normal limits. Elimination is adequate. Healing is prompt.
Laboratory studies are within normal limits.	Blood levels of hemoglobin, serum glutamic-oxaloacetic transaminase, lactic dehydrogenase, creatine phosphokinase, bilirubin, sodium, potassium, and carbon dioxide are within normal limits. Oxygen saturation is within normal limits. Urobilinogen levels of feces and urine are within normal limits. Electrocardiogram shows normal tracings.
Patient has adequate performance in work and play.	Patient is able to maintain self-care. Patient can perform household or work activities. Patient can participate in recreation and sports.
Patient has physical appearance of comfort.	The patient's posture is normal. Patient has freedom of body movement. Patient expresses comfort.
Patient has general body cleanliness.	Patient's skin is clean. Patient has no ulceration. Patient does not complain of itching.

Polycythemias

Polycythemia is a term used to describe an increase in the number of circulating erythrocytes and the concentration of hemoglobin in the blood.

PATHOPHYSIOLOGY

The three forms of polycythemia are:
1. Polycythemia vera, a myeloproliferative disorder ("overgrowth of bone marrow"), which usually develops in middle age, particularly among Jewish men; the etiology is unknown, but the overproduction of erythrocytes, myelocytes, and thrombocytes results in increased blood viscosity, blood volume, and congestion of tissues and organs with blood.
2. Secondary polycythemia, a compensatory response to tissue hypoxia in the presence of chronic obstructive lung disease, congenital heart disease, and prolonged exposure to high altitudes (10,000 feet or more).
3. Relative polycythemia, which is a relative increase in erythrocyte concentration in the presence of plasma loss that is due to fluid loss and dehydration; specific causes include insufficient fluid intake, diarrhea, vomiting, burns, excessive diuretics, etc.

DIAGNOSTIC STUDIES[6]

Erythrocyte count
As high as 8 to 12 million/mm^3

Hemoglobin concentration
8 to 25 gm/100 ml

Myelocytes
Increase in polycythemia vera

Thrombocytes
Increase in polycythemia vera

TREATMENT PLAN

Chemotherapeutic
Antineoplastic agents
  Busulfan (Myleran), 4-8 mg po qd.
  Chlorambucil (Leukeran), 4-10 mg po qd.
  Radioactive phosphorus P32 (Phosphotope), 6 μCi po; 3-5 μg IV.
  Mechlorethamine (Nitrogen mustard), 200-600 μ/kg IV in a single or divided dose.

Supportive
Venesection (phlebotomy) with emergency removal of 500 to 2000 ml until hematocrit reaches 45%, then 500 ml every 2 to 3 months
Activity-ambulation used to prevent circulatory stasis; fluid balance

ASSESSMENT: AREAS OF CONCERN

Appearance of skin
Ruddy complexion
Dusky redness of mucosa

Cardiovascular function
Hypertension with dizziness, headache, and sense of fullness in head
Congestive heart failure (shortness of breath, orthopnea, etc.)
Thrombus formation leading to cerebral vascular accident, myocardial infarction, or gangrene of the feet
Bleeding and hemorrhage in gastrointestinal tract, oropharynx, or brain

Gastrointestinal function
Enlargement of liver and spleen
Signs and symptoms of peptic ulcer

Skeletal integrity
Signs and symptoms of secondary gout

NURSING DIAGNOSES and NURSING INTERVENTIONS

Nursing Diagnosis	Nursing Intervention
Tissue perfusion, alteration in: cardiac (related to increased arterial pressure)	Encourage rest and quiet. Massage gently. Discourage oral stimulants, such as smoking. Avoid emotional situations. Administer medication as ordered. Monitor BP. Avoid sodium-rich foods.

Nursing Diagnosis	**Nursing Intervention**
Tissue perfusion, alteration in: pulmonary (related to inadequate pulmonary ventilation)	Change the patient's position frequently; sitting is considered best. Encourage coughing and deep breathing. Ambulate as soon as possible. Observe respiratory rate, breath sounds, etc. Monitor for cyanosis.
Tissue perfusion, alteration in: peripheral	Place on complete bed rest in a slight sitting position. Maintain warm environment, room temperature, and clothing. Initiate range of motion exercises. Avoid applying heat or cold, tight clothing, and pressure under the knee. Inspect extremities for adequate circulation. Monitor blood studies for hematology and gas exchange.
Mobility, impaired physical (related to inflammation of the joints)	Prescribe bed rest and joint rest for the patient. Encourage the patient to drink fluids. Administer medications as ordered, such as analgesics and antigout drugs. Provide soft diet. Provide compresses according to the patient's tolerance.
Comfort, alteration in: pain	Place the patient in a sitting position. Remove constrictive clothing. Change the patient's position frequently. Give small, frequent feedings. Auscultate for abnormal bowel sounds. Observe for evidence of favorable response to therapy. Discourage smoking. Decrease acid-food and gas-forming food intake. Give bland foods, carbonated beverage, and antacids.
Breathing pattern, ineffective (related to thrombus formation)	Encourage patient to perform range of motion and isometric exercises. Administer anticoagulants as ordered. Observe for chest pain, dyspnea, coughing, hemoptysis, changes in pulse, respirations, BP, pupillary response, reflexes, and level of consciousness.
Potential patient problem: hemorrhage	Change the patient's position slowly; handle gently. Place the patient on complete bed rest. Brush teeth with soft toothbrush. Use small gauge needle for injections; apply pressure. Avoid hot liquids, oral stimulants, and straining at elimination. Inspect for bleeding in stool, mouth, and nose. Observe for signs of increased intracranial pressure. Monitor blood studies.

Patient Education

1. Instruct the patient to protect extremities from injury, that is, heat or cold or pressure.
2. Monitor the patient's ability to do range of motion and isometric exercises.
3. Advise the patient to avoid trauma and protect body parts, that is, to use safety precautions, a soft toothbrush, and pressure after injections.
4. Instruct the patient to balance rest with exercise.
5. Teach patient to handle stress in a healthy way.
6. Advise the patient of the need to stop smoking and to avoid oral stimulants.
7. Advise the patient of the need for dietary modification, that is, low sodium, low acid, and low gas-forming foods, foods high in alkaline, and foods low in purines.

EVALUATION

Patient Outcome	Data Indicating That Outcome is Reached
Color of the skin and mucous membranes is good.	The skin, nails, lips, and ear lobes are warm and moist with a natural color.
Vital signs within normal limits.	Respiratory rate, blood pressure, and temperature are within normal limits.
Laboratory studies are within normal limits.	Red blood cell count and thrombocyte count are within normal limits.
Daily intake includes essential food groups.	Patient's diet includes milk, meat, fruits, vegetables, breads, and cereals as required to control gastric irritation, hypertension, and gout.
Patient has physical appearance of comfort.	Patient is calm, contented, and relaxed. Posture is normal. Patient has freedom of body movement.
Patient frequently changes position and body movement.	Patient walks, sits, and stands.
Patient participates in daily physical and therapeutic exercises.	Patient participates in bicycling, tennis, jogging, etc. Patient performs range of motion and isometric exercises.
Patient's surroundings are safe and comfortable.	Patient uses safety precautions. Temperature and humidity are at an appropriate level.
There is no evidence that accidents have occurred.	There is no evidence of physical injury.

LEUKOCYTIC DISORDERS
Agranulocytosis

Agranulocytosis, also referred to as granulocytopenia or malignant neutropenia, is an acute, potentially fatal blood disorder that is characterized by (1) agranulocytic angina, a severe, painful, ulcerative infection of the oral mucosa and throat, whose symptoms are high fever and severe weakness and (2) severe neutropenia.

Agranulocytosis is a worldwide disorder that affects women more often than men. The onset is rapid and prompt treatment is required.

PATHOPHYSIOLOGY

Agranulocytosis is most frequently caused by drug toxicity or hypersensitivity, that is, large dose, long duration drugs such as Nitrogen mustard, radiation, and benzenes and drugs that produce individual sensitivity such as certain tranquilizers (chlorpromazine HCl [Thorazine]), antithyroid agents (propylthiouracil), anticonvulsants (diphenylhydantoin), and antibiotics (chloramphenicol). It may also develop during the course of diseases such as tuberculosis, uremia, and overwhelming infection.

DIAGNOSTIC STUDIES

Leukocyte count
Leukopenia (500 to 3000 white blood cells/mm^3 with extremely low polymorphonuclear (PMN) cell count of 0% to 2%

Bone marrow biopsy
Absence of PMN leukocytes; maturational arrest of young developing cells

Cultures of urine and blood; ulcerative lesions in throat and mouth
Positive for bacteria

History
Exposure to offending drug

TREATMENT PLAN

Chemotherapeutic
Agent-specific anti-infective agent

Supportive
Monitor patient's blood cell count
Observe for infection
Reverse isolation
Bed rest and high-protein, high-vitamin, high-caloric diet

ASSESSMENT: AREAS OF CONCERN

Energy level
Severe fatigue and weakness
High fever, severe chills, and prostration

Gastrointestinal function
Sore throat, ulcerative lesions of pharyngeal and buccal mucosa and dysphagia

Cardiac function
Weak, rapid pulse

NURSING DIAGNOSES and NURSING INTERVENTIONS

Nursing Diagnosis	Nursing Intervention
Oral mucous membrane, alterations in	Give frequent mouth care; irrigate every 1 to 2 hours. Apply ice collar. Offer anesthetic lozenges, analgesics, and sedatives as ordered. Offer soft, bland foods and protein concentrates.
Activity intolerance	Anticipate the patient's needs. Encourage rest and adequate activity. Place objects within reach while the patient is on bed rest. Observe for increasing weakness and dyspnea. Assess pulse and respirations.
Potential patient problem: susceptibility to infection	Place the patient on bed rest. Enforce reverse isolation. Provide high-protein, high-vitamin, high-calorie diet. Encourage the patient to take fluids. Monitor heart rate, respirations, blood pressure, and temperature. Observe for restlessness and irritability. Observe the patient for extreme fatigue, sore throat or mouth, and fever. Observe white blood cell count. Use cooling measures (alcohol rub and tepid baths). Administer antibiotics as ordered. Use enemas and stool softeners as needed.

Patient Education

1. Teach the patient the use of frequent, thorough oral hygiene to treat or prevent mouth and pharyngeal infection.
2. Explain the need for a diet high in protein, vitamins, and calories with soft, bland foods.
3. Teach the importance of normal bowel elimination.
4. Explain the need to avoid self-medication because of the danger of hypersensitivity.
5. Encourage a balance between rest and activity to prevent fatigue and generalized weakness.

EVALUATION

Patient Outcome	Data Indicating That Outcome is Reached
Patient has normal body functioning.	Vital signs are within normal limits. Elimination is adequate. Healing is prompt.
Laboratory studies are within normal limits.	Leukocyte count is 5000 to 10,000 cells/mm^3. The results of a bone marrow biopsy are normal. Cultures of urine and blood are negative.

Patient Outcome	Data Indicating That Outcome is Reached
The patient's vitality is maintained.	Malaise, fatigue, and weakness are absent.
Patient consumes daily intake of essential food groups.	Patient consumes diet high in protein, vitamins, and calories; eats soft, bland foods as needed. Patient drinks adequate fluids.
Bowel elimination is normal for the individual.	Patient's stools are soft.
Patient has frequent changes in position and body movement.	Patient is walking, sitting, and standing.
Patient participates in daily physical exercise.	Patient bicycles, plays tennis, and jogs, etc.
Patient's surroundings are comfortable.	Temperature and humidity are appropriate. Patient has a well-ventilated room.
There is no evidence of physical injury.	There is no evidence of complications arising from drugs or treatment.
Infection is gone.	There is no evidence of inflammation, purulent secretions or drainage, or pain or aching.

Leukemia

Leukemia ("white blood") is usually a fatal cancer that involves the blood-forming tissues of the bone marrow, spleen, and lymph nodes, and is characterized by the neoplastic proliferation of leukocytes and their precursors.

Leukemia represents about 3% of cancers detected each year and causes about 4% of cancer deaths, or about 16,000 persons annually. Although survival rates have improved since the 1950s, mortality rates are still high, especially for those with acute leukemias, that is, acute lymphocytic leukemia (ALL), which is responsible for half of all cancer deaths among children.

Although leukemia is considered a disease that strikes children, most cases occur in adults over 55 years of age, except in blacks, whose median age for leukemia ranges from 35 to 54 years. Men develop leukemia slightly more often than do women.

For reasons as yet unknown, the incidence of leukemia is rising. However, several factors have been implicated: (1) chronic, repeated exposure to relatively small doses of radiation; (2) chloramphenicol; (3) exposure to certain chemicals such as benzene: (4) presence of primary immune deficiency diseases; (5) possible viral etiologies; and (6) a genetic predisposition, such as among siblings or in children with Down's syndrome.

PATHOPHYSIOLOGY

The major effects of leukemia on the body are proliferation of large numbers of abnormal, immature leukocytes, the accumulation of these cells within the lymph nodes, and the eventual infiltration of these cells into tissues all over the body. All organs are eventually involved in the leukemic process.

Leukemias are classified according to the following criteria:

1. Type of cell and tissue involved: the major type of cells are lymphocytes (lymphocytic leukemia: acute and chronic) and granulocytes (myelocytic: acute and chronic; monocytic: acute and chronic). The acute leukemias are sometimes classified as lymphoblastic, myeloblastic, or monoblastic because of the prevalence of immature cell forms. Lymphocytic leukemia causes hyperplasia of the lymphoid tissue, while myelocytic leukemia causes hyperplasia of the bone marrow and spleen. Ninety percent of all leukemias are lymphocytic.
2. Course and duration of disease: acute forms have a rapid onset with progression to death within days or months. The large numbers of leukocytes produced are immature and rapidly cause organ malfunction. Chronic forms have a gradual onset and a slower course. The cells are more mature and function more effectively. Acute leukemia occurs more frequently in children, while chronic leukemia is more prevalent in persons 25 to 60 years of age.
3. Number of leukocytes in blood and bone marrow: if the patient has a normal or lower than normal leukocyte count, the disease is called aleukemic or subleukemic leukemia.

Acute leukemia has its peak incidence in children who are 1 to 5 years of age. There is usually a prodromal period when the child experiences fatigue, headache, sore throat, night sweats, and shortness of breath. These symptoms are followed by severe tonsillitis, ulcerations in the mouth, bleeding from the gums and rectum, bleeding into the skin, and joint and bone pain. The lymph nodes, liver, and spleen enlarge and severe anemia develops. The patient dies from overwhelming infection or severe hemorrhaging. With treatment, the patient may survive 5 years or longer.

Chronic myelocytic leukemia, which is usually found in persons 25 to 40 years of age, is characterized by a massive spleen, enlarged liver, and severe pain in the long bones. The onset is usually insidious, with the patient complaining for months or years of weight loss and weakness. Initial signs of disease may be a heavy sensation in the abdomen, a sense of extreme abdominal distention after meals, sternal tenderness, and mild enlargement of the lymph nodes.

Chronic lymphocytic leukemia is found most often in persons 50 to 70 years of age, many of whom do not have symptoms for years. Early signs and symptoms are chronic exhaustion, anorexia and swollen lymph nodes, and a slightly enlarged liver and spleen. Anemia, fever, increased susceptibility to infections, and mild bleeding tendencies occur as the disease progresses. Visual disturbances, skin lesions, deafness, otitis media, or Meniere's syndrome may develop. Pain and paralysis result from lymph node pressure on the nerves. Respiratory symptoms result from enlargement of the mediastinal lymph nodes. Late complications include hemolytic anemia and hypogammaglobulinemia.[3,6,10]

DIAGNOSTIC STUDIES[6]

During its early stages, leukemia may be accidentally found during a routine physical examination that includes blood work.

Leukocyte count
   Elevated (15,000 to 500,000/mm^3 or higher)
   "Shift to the left" (presence of large numbers of immature neutrophils); one type of white cell predominates

Bone marrow biopsy
   Massive number of white blood cells

Blood smear
   Numerous blast cells

Red blood cells
   Decreased

Platelets
   Decreased

TREATMENT PLAN[1,6]

The goal of treatment is to stop the proliferation and infiltration of abnormal and immature leukocytes and to obtain as long a remission as possible.

Chemotherapeutic
   Dosages are based on body surface area; the following are examples of standard and experimental drugs in use.
Acute lymphoblastic leukemia
   Antineoplastic agents
      Methotrexate (Amethopterin, Mexate), 2.5-5.0 mg/kg/day po or parenterally.
      Mercaptopurine (Purinethol, 6-MP), 2.5 mg/kg/day po.
      Cyclophosphamide (Cytoxan), 40-50 mg/kg IV in divided doses over period of several days then adjusted to lower maintenance dosage; oral dosage 1-5 mg/kg/qd.
      Vincristine sulfate (Oncovin, VCR), 2 mg/m^2 for children; 1.4 mg/m^2 for adults.
      Cytarabine (Cytosar-U), 2 mg/kg IV for 10 days; raised to 4 mg/kg for maintenance.
      Thioguanine (6-TG), 2 mg/kg/day po.
      Asparaginase (Elspar, L-asparagine), 1000 IU/kg/day IV for 10 days, or 6000 IU/m^2 IM intermittently.
      Carmustine (BCNU), 200 mg/m^2 IV every 6 weeks.
      Hydroxyurea (Hydrea), 20-30 mg/kg po qd or 80 mg/kg every third day.
      Dactinomycin (Actinomycin D, Cosmegen), 0.015-0.05 mg/kg IV divided dosages over 1 week; repeat for 3-5 weeks.
   Corticosteroids
      Prednisone (Deltasone), 5-80 mg qd.
Acute myeloblastic leukemia
   Antineoplastic agents
      Methotrexate (Amethopterin), 2.5-5.0 mg/kg/day po or parenterally.
      Mercaptopurine (Purinethol, 6-MP), 2.5 mg/kg/day po.
      Cytarabine (Cytosar), 2 mg/kg IV for 10 days; raised to 4 mg/kg for maintenance.
      Thioguanine (6-TG), 2 mg/kg/day po.
      Daunorubicin (Cerubidine), 30-60 mg/m^2 IV daily for 3 days or weekly.
      Carmustine (BCNU), 200 mg/m^2 IV every 6 weeks.
Chronic lymphocytic leukemia
   Corticosteroids
      Prednisone (Deltasone, Meticorten), 10-100 mg/day po.

Antineoplastic agents
  Chlorambucil (Leukeran), 4-10 mg/day po.
  Cyclophosphamide (Cytoxan), 40-50 mg/kg IV individual doses over period of several days then adjusted to lower maintenance dosage; oral dosage 1-5 mg/kg qd.
  Triethylenemelamine (TEM), 2.5 mg po for 2 or 3 days; then 0.5-5 mg weekly for several weeks.

Chronic myelocytic leukemia
Antineoplastic agents
  Busulfan (Myleran), 4-8 mg/day po.
  Chlorambucil (Leukeran), 4-10 mg/day po.
  Mercaptopurine (Purinethol, 6-MP), 2.5 mg/kg/day po.
  Triethylenemelamine (TEM), 2.5 mg po for 2-3 days; then 0.5-5 mg weekly for several weeks.
  Hydroxyurea (Hydrea), 20-30 mg/kg po each day or 80 mg/kg every third day.
  Dibrommannitol (Mitrobronitol), 250 mg/m^2 for 3 days then 150 mg/m^2 until remission.

Electromechanical
X-ray therapy for the entire body or focused on liver and spleen

Supportive
Bone marrow transplants
Transfusions (whole blood, platelets); reverse isolation techniques; antibiotics

ASSESSMENT: AREAS OF CONCERN

Susceptibility to infection
Ulcerations of mouth and throat
Signs and symptoms of pneumonia
Signs and symptoms of septicemia

Energy level
Fatigue, lethargy, and weakness

Susceptibility to bleeding
Gum bleeding, ecchymoses, petechiae, and retinal hemorrhages

Organ size
Enlargement of liver, spleen, and lymph nodes

Appearance of the skin
Pallor

Renal function
Renal pain
Renal insufficiency, that is, decreased urinary output

Sensory and motor function
Headache and disorientation
Convulsions (late)
Hemiplegia, aphasia, and other deficits due to cerebral vascular accident

Gastrointestinal function
Anorexia, nausea, and vomiting
Weight loss

NURSING DIAGNOSES and NURSING INTERVENTIONS

Nursing Diagnosis	Nursing Intervention
Tissue perfusion, alteration in: cerebral	Place the patient on bed rest with quiet, dim environment. Provide safety, that is, side rails. Provide emergency equipment, such as padded tongue blade. Observe for increased intracranial pressure: vital signs, pupillary response, level of consciousness, reflexes, and orientation. Observe the characteristics of the convulsion if it occurs.
Tissue perfusion, alteration in: cardiopulmonary	Encourage alternate rest and activity as tolerated. Observe pulse, respirations, and blood pressure. Monitor blood studies. Observe for signs of fatigue, lethargy, restlessness, dyspnea, etc.
Urinary elimination, alteration in patterns: potential (related to renal calculi)	Ambulate the patient as tolerated. Change the patient's position frequently. Encourage the patient to take fluids such as carbonated beverages and urine-alkalizing juices. Inspect for bleeding and flank pain. Test pH of urine. Administer allopurinol as ordered. Observe urine studies. Observe blood studies.
Comfort, alteration in	Position comfortably in semi-Fowler position. Remove constrictive clothing.

Nursing Diagnosis	Nursing Intervention
	Handle gently. Discuss possible pain and ways to relieve it with the patient. Administer per the patient's request analgesics as prescribed. Provide oral hygiene and local anesthetic. Observe effectiveness of pain relief measures.
Nutrition, alteration in: less than body requirements (related to increased metabolic rate and anorexia)	Provide balanced diet with emphasis on protein, vitamins, and calories. Monitor caloric intake. Give small, frequent feedings; snacks should be soft, bland, and cold. Encourage the patient to make specific requests. Balance rest with exercise. Discourage smoking and oral stimulants. Measure body weight. Use oral anesthetic and/or antiemetic before eating. Encourage the patient to take fluids.
Fear	Approach the patient calmly and unhurriedly. Express empathy, warmth, and friendliness. Touch the patient as appropriate. Provide frequent contact. Encourage expression of feelings. Listen attentively and offer feedback. Encourage questions. Provide reliable information. Encourage problem solving. Explore with the patient his strengths, resources, and normal coping mechanisms. Encourage interaction with significant others (if the patient views them as a support system). Encourage diversional activities.
Potential patient problem: susceptibility to infection	Place the patient in reverse isolation (may use life island or laminar air flow environment). Encourage rest and limited activity. Maintain warm, clean environment. Encourage increased intake of foods high in protein and fluids. Teach the patient and family proper handwashing and screen visitors with infections. Monitor vital signs: temperature, pulse, respirations, and blood pressure. Observe the patient for restlessness, temperature elevation, sore throat, "sniffles," chills, skin lesions, etc. Check blood studies. Administer antibiotics as ordered. Use cool sponge baths, alcohol rubs, and antipyretic drugs as needed. Administer granulocyte transfusions as ordered. Administer γ-globulin as ordered (for chronic lymphocytic leukemia).
Potential patient problem: hemorrhaging	Protect the patient from falls and other injuries. Apply pressure over the injection site. Prevent constipation; use stool softener, fiber in diet, and fluids. Assess pulse, respirations, blood pressure, level of consciousness, skin color, etc. Observe the skin for petechiae and ecchymosis. Observe for signs of bleeding from mouth, nose, and rectum. Monitor blood studies. Administer transfusions as ordered; whole blood and platelets.

Patient Education

1. Advise the patient to avoid situations in which he/she is likely to contract infection, such as inclement weather or crowds.
2. Teach the patient to maintain a clean body and environment.
3. Teach the patient to maintain a well-balanced diet, especially high in protein, fiber, and fluids.
4. Instruct the patient to observe for and report signs and symptoms of infection.

5. Instruct the patient to take antibiotics as prescribed.
6. Teach the patient how to maintain a safe environment.
7. Instruct the patient to observe for and report signs and symptoms of bleeding.
8. Teach the patient to avoid tissue damage, that is, use soft toothbrush, blow nose gently, and avoid constipation.
9. Instruct the patient to maintain a schedule of alternate rest and activity and to avoid overexertion.
10. Instruct the patient to observe for and report signs and symptoms of anemia.
11. Tell the patient to drink large volumes of fluid, especially carbonated beverages and urine-alkalizing juices.

12. Teach the patient to observe urine for change in color and amount.
13. Teach the patient to use nonaddictive, pain-relief measures as long as possible; pain will increase with progression of the disease and is likely to increase in amount, intensity, types and locations.
14. Teach the patient to avoid smoking and oral stimulants and instruct in the need to stimulate appetite and maintain tissue perfusion.
15. Teach the patient to deal with stress and fear in constructive, healthful ways.
16. Be sure that the patient is aware of support resources available: financial, treatment-related, and psychosocial.

EVALUATION

Patient Outcome	Data Indicating That Outcome is Reached
Color of skin and mucous membranes is normal.	The skin, nails, lips, and ear lobes are warm and moist with a natural color.
Patient has normal body functioning.	Vital signs are within normal limits. Elimination is adequate. Healing is prompt. Daily weight is stabilized at normal level for body build.
Laboratory studies are within normal limits.	Hemoglobin, hematocrit, blood urea nitrogen, and serum creatinine levels are within normal limits. Blood and urine pH are within normal limits. Urine specific gravity and creatinine level are within normal limits. The results of a urine protein test are negative.
Patient's vitality is maintained.	Patient is mentally alert. Patient has good concentration and attentiveness. Patient experiences no malaise, fatigue, or weakness.
Daily intake includes essential food groups.	Protein, vitamins, and calories are emphasized.
Bowel elimination is normal for the individual.	Stools are soft and the abdomen is soft and nondistended; there is no evidence of bleeding. There is no abdominal pressure.
Daily fluid output is equivalent to fluid intake.	Urine output is 1500 to 3000 ml daily or equivalent to intake.
Patient has adequate performance in work and play.	Patient is able to maintain self-care. Patient can perform household or work activities. Patient can participate in recreation and sports.
Patient has the physical appearance of comfort.	Patient is calm and contented and has relaxed facial expression. Posture is normal. Patient has freedom of body movement. Patient expresses comfort.
Patient has frequent changes in position and body movement.	Patient is walking, sitting, and standing.
Patient participates in daily physical exercise and/or therapeutic exercise.	Patient bicycles, plays tennis, jogs, etc. Patient performs range of motion and isometric exercises.
Patient's surrounding are clean, safe, and comfortable.	Patient's environment is free from dust, dirt, etc. Patient uses safety precautions. Room temperature and humidity are appropriate.

Patient Outcome	Data Indicating That Outcome is Reached
Patient has a positive attitude toward utilizing available resources.	Patient accepts suggestion of referral.
Patient follows through on referral.	Patient actively seeks assistance. Patient expresses satisfaction.
Patient prevents accidents, physical injury, deformity, infection, and hypersensitivity response.	There is no evidence that accidents have occurred. There is no evidence of physical injury. There is no evidence of deformity resulting from treatment.
Infection is absent.	There is no evidence of inflammation, purulent drainage or secretions, or pain or aching. Oral temperature is 98.6° F (37° C). Blood leukocyte count is 5,000 to 10,000. There are no urine, red blood cells, white blood cells, or hemoglobin casts. Results of the bacterial culture of γ-globulin are negative: 20% or 0.7 to 1.6 g/dl.
Patient uses healthy coping mechanisms.	Patient reaches out to appropriate support systems. Patient expresses feelings of safety.

MULTIPLE MYELOMA

Multiple myeloma, a neoplastic condition, is a disease that usually strikes adult men over the age of 40 years twice as often as it does women.

PATHOPHYSIOLOGY

Although it used to be a relatively rare disorder, the incidence of multiple myeloma is increasing. The characteristics of the disease are: (1) an abnormal malignant growth of plasma cells; (2) development of single or multiple abnormal plasma cell tumors within the bone marrow; (3) destruction of bone throughout the body; and (4) later dissemination of the disease into the lymph nodes, liver, spleen, and kidneys.

The onset of the disease is usually gradual and often insidious. Many patients experience a presymptomatic period for 5 to 20 years, during which time some persons experience recurrent bacterial infections, especially pneumonia. It is believed that this increased susceptibility to infection is related to disturbed antibody formation due to plasma cell abnormalities.

As symptoms occur, they usually involve the skeletal system, especially the pelvis, spine, and ribs, and produce backache or bone pain that is worse with movement. Some patients may sustain a pathologic fracture that causes severe pain. As skeletal destruction increases, the patient may develop deformities in the sternum and rib cage, with some persons losing stature (5 or more inches). Diffuse osteoporosis with a negative calcium balance is also present. As the diseased bones become

demineralized, the patient develops renal stones, especially if on bed rest.

In addition, impaired production of erythrocytes, leukocytes, and thrombocytes occurs, with resultant anemia, bleeding tendencies, and increased danger of infection.

Complications may be neurologic such as spinal cord compression and/or renal dysfunction due to convoluted tubules' blockage by coagulated protein particles.[1,6]

DIAGNOSTIC STUDIES

X-ray studies
Diffuse bone lesions, demineralization, and osteoporosis

Bone marrow biopsy
Large numbers of immature plasma cells (30% to 95% of cell population)

Blood studies
High concentration of serum globulin, particularly m-type globulin called "Bence Jones protein"

TREATMENT PLAN

Chemotherapeutic
Antineoplastic agents
Melphalan (Alkeran; L-PAM), 6 mg po for 2-3 weeks; maintenance 2 mg qd.

Cyclophosphamide (Cytoxan), 40-50 mg/kg IV in divided doses over a period of several days; then adjust to a lower maintenance dose.

Electromechanical

Reduction of tumor mass by radiation

Supportive

Control of pain
Promotion of adequate ambulation
Treatment of complications: anemia, infection, hypercalcemia, and spinal cord compression

Renal function

Signs and symptoms of calculi

Energy level

Weakness, fatigue, dyspnea, bleeding, and infection

Sensory and motor function

Spinal cord compression as evidenced by loss of sensory and motor function

Fluid and electrolytes

Hypercalcemia as evidenced by lethargy, polyuria, polydipsia, etc.

ASSESSMENT: AREAS OF CONCERN

Skeletal integrity

Backache or bone pain that is worse with movement
Loss of stature
Signs and symptoms of pathologic fractures

NURSING DIAGNOSES and NURSING INTERVENTIONS

Nursing Diagnosis	Nursing Intervention
Comfort, alteration in: pain	Position the patient for comfort. Change the patient's position slowly. Maintain the patient's body alignment. Apply heat. Massage gently. Use firm mattress. Encourage rest. Work with the patient on ways to reduce pain, including analgesics.
Mobility, impaired physical (related to musculoskeletal impairment)	Assist with ambulation. Mobilize as necessary using a walker, cane, or wheelchair. Decrease environmental barriers, that is, chairs, tables, or rugs. Limit the distance that the patient ambulates. Observe gait, coordination, and stability. Utilize good body mechanics. Encourage increased protein and vitamin intake.
Injury: potential for (falling)	Handle the patient gently. Change the patient's position slowly. Avoid jarring the bed. Assess body alignment and complaints of pain.
Urinary elimination, alteration in pattern: potential (related to renal calculi)	Provide adequate hydration of 3000 to 4000 ml of fluid/day. Maintain urinary output of 1500 ml/24 hr. Ambulate the patient as much as possible. Change the patient's position frequently. Encourage a diet with decreased calcium and phosphorus. Give urine-acidifying juices. Avoid bicarbonates and carbonated beverages. Observe intake and output, frequency, and urgency; report findings to the physician.
Activity intolerance	Place the patient in a sitting position. Observe respiration rate and dyspnea. Observe skin color and temperature. Assist with care.

Nursing Diagnosis	Nursing Intervention
	Plan rest periods. Monitor laboratory values.
Mobility, impaired physical, potential (related to spinal cord compression)	Maintain body alignment. Support the spine with brace or traction. Place the patient on bed rest as needed. Log roll the patient. Observe respiratory rate and rhythm. Assess motor function, sensation, and reflexes; report findings to the physician if abnormalities occur.
Nutrition, alteration in, potential (related to hypercalcemia)	Encourage a decrease in intake of foods with calcium and encourage an increase in fluid intake. Monitor blood studies. Observe for complaints of constipation, headache, nausea, thirst, weakness, bone pain, and fatigue; report findings to the physician.
Potential patient problem: bleeding	Handle the patient gently. Give injections only if necessary; apply pressure afterward. Observe for change in VS or bleeding, such as urine, stool, gums, or nose wounds. Avoid constipation.
Potential patient problem: infection	Maintain reverse isolation. Observe for increases in temperature, pulse, and respirations. Observe the patient for "sniffles," sore throat, anorexia, pain on urination, etc. Administer antibiotics as needed.

Patient Education

1. Explain the need for good body balance, good body mechanics, and mechanical support, such as a cane, or brace.
2. Teach methods of pain control: pain-reducing measures and medications.
3. Teach the importance of drinking adequate fluids and controlling intake of high-calcium foods.
4. Explain the need for a diet high in protein and vitamins.

EVALUATION

Patient Outcome	Data Indicating That Outcome is Reached
Color of the skin and mucous membranes is good.	The skin, nails, lips, and ear lobes are warm and moist, with a natural color.
Vital signs are within normal limits.	Respiratory rate, pulse rate, and blood pressure are within normal limits.
Laboratory studies are within normal limits.	Hemoglobin level and hematocrit are within normal limits. Thrombocyte and leukocyte counts are within normal limits. Total protein, albumin, α-globulin, β-globulin, γ-globulin, and calcium levels are within normal limits. Urine pH is within normal limits.
Body hydration is normal.	Skin turgor is good. Mucous membranes are moist. Patient is not thirsty.
Daily fluid output is equal to fluid intake.	Urine output is 1500 to 3000 ml. Patient's diet includes foods high in protein and vitamins.
Patient has physical appearance of comfort.	Patient is calm and contented and has relaxed facial expression. Posture is normal. Patient has freedom of body movement. Patient relaxes muscles when resting and motionless.

Patient Outcome	Data Indicating That Outcome is Reached
Patient verbally expresses comfort.	Patient expresses comfort. Patient stops complaining.
Patient has frequent changes in position and body movement.	Patient walks, sits, and stands.
Patient participates in therapeutic exercise.	Patient participates in range of motion and isometric exercises.
Patient's surroundings are safe.	Patient uses safety precautions, such as side rails, low bed, etc. Patient's movement is not hampered by environmental barriers.
There is no evidence of physical injury.	There is no evidence of pathologic fractures.
Infection is gone.	There is no evidence of inflammation, pain, or aching.

THROMBOCYTIC DISORDERS

Thrombocytopenia is used to describe a platelet count that is below 200,000/mm³, which causes (1) spontaneous bleeding into the skin, mucous membranes, internal cavities, and organs, and (2) oozing for long periods of time from lacerations and punctures.

PATHOPHYSIOLOGY

The major types of thrombocytopenia are: (1) idiopathic thrombocytopenic purpura (ITP), in which platelets are prematurely destroyed (survival decreases from 8 to 20 days to 1 to 3 days); it is believed to be caused by an autoimmune process; the acute form is found mostly in children, whereas the chronic form is found among all ages; it is more common among women; and (2) secondary thrombocytopenic purpura, which results from diseases such as viral infections, bone marrow failure, infectious mononucleosis, and drug hypersensitivity.

DIAGNOSTIC STUDIES[6]

Platelet count
<100,000/mm³

Bleeding time
Prolonged

Coagulation time
Normal

Capillary fragility
Increased

TREATMENT PLAN

Surgical
Splenectomy

Chemotherapeutic
Corticosteroids
Prednisone (Deltasone, Meticorten), 10-20 mg qid.

Supportive
Platelet transfusions

ASSESSMENT: AREAS OF CONCERN

Vascular integrity
Petechiae, ecchymosis, and easy bruising
Epistaxis
Bleeding from gums

Female reproductive function
Heavy menses and bleeding between periods

Sensory and motor function
Cerebral hemorrhage as evidenced by signs and symptoms of increased intracranial pressure
Severe hemorrhaging from nose, gastrointestinal tract, and urinary tract
Bleeding into diaphragm
Nerve pain and anesthesia of extremities and/or paralysis

NURSING DIAGNOSES and NURSING INTERVENTIONS

Nursing Diagnosis	Nursing Intervention
Tissue perfusion, alteration in: cardiopulmonary	Place the patient on bed rest in a slight sitting position. Maintain warm room temperature. Remove constrictive clothing. Apply ice bag and/or manual pressure. Dress patient warmly. Discourage smoking and oral stimulants. Monitor vital signs. Monitor laboratory studies. Observe pulse rate and rhythm, respiration rate and depth and blood pressure.
Tissue perfusion alteration in: cerebral	Observe for signs of increased intracranial pressure: level of consciousness, pupillary response, and reflexes.
Tissue perfusion alteration in: renal	Observe color, amount, and presence of red blood cells in urine.
Mucous membrane, alteration in: oral	Remove dentures. Provide mouth care with soft toothbrush. Give soft foods and iced liquids.
Mucous membrane, alteration in: vaginal	Provide perineal hygiene. Count pads used. Observe amount, color, consistency, and frequency of discharge.
Mucous membrane, alteration in: nasal	Observe amount, color, and consistency of discharge. Position the patient with the head forward and elevated.
Skin integrity, impairment of (related to intradermal bleeding)	Apply ice bag and/or manual pressure over site. Handle gently.
Comfort, alteration in: pain	Position the patient comfortably. Handle the patient gently (massage). Apply bed cradle, lightweight clothing, and blanket. Apply heat lamp, cradle pad, bottle, compress, or apply cold compress bag; do what the patient thinks will make him/her comfortable. Give analgesics as ordered.

Patient Education

1. Explain the need to stop smoking to avoid impairment of arterial circulation.
2. Teach the patient to avoid mechanical trauma:
   a. General safety precautions.
   b. Soft toothbrush.
   c. Gentle nose blowing.
   d. Stool softeners and maintenance of diet high in roughage and fluids.
3. Teach the patient to detect and report signs and symptoms of bleeding.

EVALUATION

Patient Outcome	Data Indicating That Outcome is Reached
Vital signs are within normal limits.	Respiratory rate, pulse rate, blood pressure, and temperature are within normal limits.
Laboratory studies are within normal limits.	Platelet count and bleeding time are within normal limits. Capillary fragility test shows occasional petechiae or none.
Daily intake includes essential food groups.	Diet includes milk, meat, fruits, vegetables, bread, and cereals.
Bowel and bladder elimination are normal.	Stools are soft. There is no evidence of bleeding.
Patient is mentally alert.	Patient has good concentration.

Patient Outcome	Data Indicating That Outcome is Reached
Patient has physical appearance of comfort.	Posture is normal. Patient has freedom of body movement. Patient has changes position and body movement frequently. Patient walks, sits, and stands.
Patient's surroundings are safe.	Patient uses safety precautions. Room temperature and humidity are appropriate.
There is no evidence that an accident or physical injury has occurred.	There are no signs of infection.

MALIGNANT LYMPHOMA

Malignant lymphoma is a neoplasm of the lymphoid tissue.

Malignant lymphomas include lymphosarcoma, reticulum cell sarcoma, and Hodgkin's disease. While the cause of these cancers is unknown, a viral etiology is believed responsible for several types, particularly Burkitt's lymphoma (a childhood disease) and Hodgkin's disease. A genetic factor may also be a factor in Hodgkin's disease.

PATHOPHYSIOLOGY

Lymphosarcoma and reticulum cell sarcomas account for about 40% of malignant lymphomas; the incidence increases with age, primarily striking middle-aged people. Early widespread dissemination is common, with oropharyngeal lymphoid tissue, the gastrointestinal tract, and bones frequently affected. The earliest sign is painless lymphadenopathy, usually unilateral and in the neck. The disease spreads via lymphatic channels to other nodes and in the case of lymphosarcoma invades the bone marrow. Other organs that may be involved are the skin and nervous system. Pressure and organ obstruction produce symptoms such as abdominal pain, nerve pain, and paralysis. Other patient problems include anemia, fever, sweating, pruritus, weight loss, and malaise. Diagnosis and treatment of these lymphatic malignancies are similar to those of Hodgkin's disease.

Hodgkin's Disease

A chronic and progressive cancer, Hodgkin's disease primarily affects young adults aged 20 to 40 years. Men are affected twice as often as women and boys five times more than girls.

The disease is characterized by the abnormal proliferation of histiocytes called "Reed-Sternberg cells," which eventually replace the normal cellular structure of the lymph nodes and cause areas of necrosis and fibrosis to develop. Malignant reticulum cells are also present.

While Hodgkin's disease initially affects one lymph node and then travels by lymphatic channels to nodes throughout the body, it may also appear in the liver and spleen, vertebrae, ureters, and bronchi. Staging of the disease is based on microscopic appearance of the lymph nodes, extent and severity of the disease, and prognosis. Table 13-1 shows one method of staging.

Prognosis for untreated patients is about 5 years; those diagnosed in stage I or II have a 95% cure rate while those with stages III or IV have a poor prognosis.[1,3,6]

DIAGNOSTIC STUDIES[6]

Lymph node biopsy
Presence of Reed-Sternberg cells

X-ray film of chest
Mediastinal or hilar lymphadenopathy

Blood studies
Normocytic normochromic anemia

Table 13-1
Staging of Hodgkin's Disease[6]

Stage*	Definition
I	Single lymph node region
II	Two or more node regions limited to one side of the diaphragm
III	Disease on both sides of the diaphragm, but limited to the lymph nodes and spleen
IV	Involvement of the bones, bone marrow, lung parenchyma, pleura, liver, skin, gastrointestinal tract, central nervous system, renal, etc.

*All stages are subclassified as A or B to describe the absence (A) or presence (B) of systemic symptoms.

Skin tests for tuberculosis
Abnormal reaction

TREATMENT PLAN[1,6]

Surgical
The tumor that is causing pressure on an organ or nerve is excised.

Chemotherapeutic
Antineoplastic agents in combination therapy (See Chapter 14):
MOPP
Mechlorethamine (Nitrogen mustard).
Vincristine (Oncovin).
Prednisone (Deltasone).
Procarbazine (Matulane).
MVPP
Mechlorethamine (Nitrogen mustard).
Vinblastine (Velban).

Procarbazine (Matulane).
Prednisone (Deltasone).
COPP
Cyclophosphamide (Cytoxan).
Vincristine (Oncovin).
Prednisone (Deltasone).
Procarbazine (Matulane).

No specific drug dosages are given for the chemotherapy combinations for the following reasons: (1) Doses may change when used in combination; (2) doses differ depending on the patient's physical status, that is, white blood cell and platelet counts and Karnofsky scale rating (Table 13-2); and (3) individual drug protocols differ from one institution to another.

Electromechanical
Wide-field megavoltage radiation (3500 to 4000 roentgens over 4- to 6-week period can be curative for stages I or II)
Combined radiotherapy and chemotherapy for stages III and IV

ASSESSMENT: AREAS OF CONCERN

Skin integrity
Severe pruritus
Jaundice
Edema and cyanosis of face and neck
Irregular fever

Sensory and motor function
Bone pain, vertebral compression, fracture, paraplegia, and nerve pain

Respiratory function
Cough, stridor, dyspnea, chest pain, and pleural effusion
Laryngeal paralysis

Energy level
Anemia with fatigue, malaise, anorexia, etc.
Increased susceptibility to infection

Gastrointestinal function
Splenomegaly and hepatomegaly with resultant abdominal distention and discomfort

Table 13-2
Karnofsky Performance Scale

Activity Status	Point	Description
Normal activity	10	Normal, with no complaints or evidence of disease
	9	Able to carry on normal activity but with minor signs or symptoms of disease present
	8	Normal activity but requiring effort; signs and symptoms of disease more prominent
Self-care	7	Able to care for self, but unable to work or carry on other normal activities
	6	Able to care for most needs but requires occasional assistance
	5	Considerable assistance required, along with frequent medical care; some self-care still possible
Incapacitated	4	Disabled and requiring special care and assistance
	3	Severely disabled; hospitalization required but death from disease not imminent
	2	Extremely ill; supportive treatment, hospitalized care required
	1	Imminent death
	0	Dead

NURSING DIAGNOSES and NURSING INTERVENTIONS[2]

Nursing Diagnosis	Nursing Intervention
Skin integrity, impairment of	Bathe in cool water or apply cool, moist compresses. Apply calamine lotion, cornstarch, soda-bicarbonate, and medicated powder. Use a bed cradle and lightweight blankets and clothing. Lubricate skin with baby oil, bath oil, body lotion, or petrolatum. Maintain adequate humidity and cool room. Encourage adequate rest and fluids. Avoid adhesive, alkaline soap, and local heat.
Fluid volume, alteration in	Elevate head of bed. Remove constrictive clothing. Apply heat using a hot water bottle and warm moist compresses. Handle and massage the patient gently. Lubricate the skin with cocoa butter, glycerine, lanolin, or mineral or olive oil. Report increase in edema or cyanosis; indicate increasing pressure on superior vena cava.
Mobility, impaired physical: potential	Maintain body alignment. Move body as a single unit. Provide mechanical support during ambulation. Observe respiratory rate and rhythm and motor function in extremities; monitor complaints of numbness and tingling; report findings to the physician.
Comfort, alteration in: pain[7]	Handle the patient gently and in an unhurried manner. Position the patient comfortably and change position gradually. Support affected body part. Encourage adequate rest. Provide pain relief measures based on the patient's choice. Give medications as ordered. Avoid ingestion of alcohol. For intraabdominal pressure: place in a sitting position; remove constrictive clothing; change the patient's position; and give small, frequent feedings.
Breathing pattern, ineffective (related to airway edema)[8]	Place the patient in a sitting position. Remove constrictive clothing. Encourage deep breathing. Administer oxygen as needed. Provide standby emergency equipment. Inspect chest for respiratory rate and rhythm and symmetrical expansion. Auscultate for abnormal breath sounds, lung aeration, rales, and rhonchi. Observe for hoarseness, cough, stridor, and pain. Observe skin color. Monitor blood studies for abnormal gas exchange. Plan rest periods. Monitor laboratory values.
Potential patient problem: susceptibility to infection	Maintain reverse isolation. Observe increases in temperature, pulse, and respirations. Observe the patient for "sniffles," sore throat, anorexia, pain on urination, etc. Administer antibiotics as needed.
Potential patient problem: body temperature, alteration in	Apply cool, damp cloth to face. Bathe in cool water and apply ice bag or alcohol. Cover with lightweight blankets and clothing. Maintain cool room temperature. Encourage rest. Increase fluid intake, especially iced liquids. Monitor oral temperature level and pattern.

Patient Education

1. Explain the need to avoid scratching and correctly care for skin in order to reduce susceptibility to infection and mechanical skin damage.
2. Teach correct maintenance of body alignment, use of body mechanics and the danger of vertebral compression and paralysis.
3. Teach ways to relieve pain without the use of medications as often as possible; bone, nerve, and abdominal pain is chronic in nature and increases with pressure of disseminated disease.
4. Emphasize the importance of respiratory exercises to prevent or decrease severity of mediastinal lymph node enlargement, involvement of lung parenchyma, and invasion of pleura.
5. Teach the need for adequate rest and exercise and a balanced diet.

EVALUATION[2]

Patient Outcome	Data Indicating That Outcome is Reached
Color of skin and mucous membranes is color.	The skin, nails, lips, and ear lobes are warm and moist with a natural color.
Vital signs are within normal limits.	Respiratory rate, pulse rate, blood pressure, and temperature are within normal limits.
Laboratory studies are within normal limits.	The hemoglobin level, hematocrit, oxygen saturation, and leukocyte count are within normal limits.
Body hydration is normal.	Skin turgor is good. Mucous membranes are moist.
Patient has physical appearance of comfort.	Patient is calm and relaxed. Posture is normal. Patient has freedom of body movement. Patient verbally expresses comfort. Patient ceases previous complaining.
Patient's surroundings are comfortable.	Room temperature is appropriate. Humidity level is appropriate. Room is well ventilated.
There is no evidence of physical injury.	There is no evidence of complications arising from drugs, treatment, disease process, or nursing care.
There is no infection.	There is no evidence of inflammation, pain or aching, or purulent secretions.

Medical Interventions

BLOOD TRANSFUSIONS

Infusion of blood may be lifesaving for the patient with anemia due to acute blood loss whose hemoglobin is less than 10 gm because of the immediate increase in the body's ability to receive oxygen and avoid severe tissue damage. Transfusions are used less frequently for patients with severe chronic anemia (hemoglobin <6 gm) because of potential complications.

Contraindications and Cautions

1. Reaction to hemolytic transfusions is caused by the administration of mismatched blood.
2. Bacterial reactions are usually due to contaminated blood.
3. Allergic reactions can occur. Their exact cause is unknown, although in some cases donor may have ingested drugs or foods to which the recipient is allergic.

4. Circulatory overload results from too rapid an infusion or too great a quantity.
5. Transmission of infectious agents such as hepatitis virus can occur.

TREATMENT PLAN

Supportive

Medications and other interventions are administered as needed in response to reactions to transfusions.

ASSESSMENT: AREAS OF CONCERN[6]

Hemolytic reaction

Chills and fever

Hematuria or oliguria
Jaundice
Headache
Backache
Dyspnea
Cyanosis
Chest pain

Bacterial (febrile) reaction

Fever, chills, lumbar pain, headache, malaise, bloody vomitus, diarrhea, or red shock (skin warm, dry, and pink)

Allergic reaction

Mild edema, hives, bronchial wheezing, or anaphylaxis

Circulatory overload

Cough, dyspnea, edema, tachycardia, hemoptysis, and frothy pink-tinged sputum

NURSING DIAGNOSES and NURSING INTERVENTIONS

Nursing Diagnosis	Nursing Intervention
Injury: potential for (related to hemolytic reaction)	Discontinue blood transfusions immediately. Notify the physician and laboratory. Send remaining blood and sample of the patient's blood to the laboratory for repeat type and cross-matching. Administer intravenous fluids (to maintain patency of line), oxygen, and drugs, that is, vasopressor agents, epinephrine, sedatives, and mannitol. Monitor vital signs. Insert Foley catheter. Measure intake and output. Provide reassurance to patient.
Injury: potential for (related to bacterial reaction)	Discontinue blood; notify the physician. Send remaining blood and sample of the patient's blood to the laboratory for repeat type and cross-matching. Monitor vital signs; use cooling measures as needed. Start intravenous fluids. Insert Foley catheter. Measure intake and output. Administer medications as ordered, such as vasopressors, corticosteroids, and broad-spectrum antibiotics.
Injury: potential for (related to allergic reaction)	Slow blood flow if mild (mild edema, hives, or bronchial wheezing). Stop blood if severe (bronchospasm or severe dyspnea). Start intravenous fluids. Give medications as ordered. Provide reassurance to the patient.
Fluid volume, alteration in: excess	Stop transfusions and notify the physician. Give digitalis as ordered. Prepare for venesection or rotating tourniquets as ordered.

EVALUATION[2]

Patient Outcome	Data Indicating That Outcome is Reached
Color of the skin and mucous membranes is good.	The skin, nails, lips, and ear lobes are warm and moist with a natural color.
Vital signs are within normal limits.	Respiratory rate, pulse rate, and blood pressure are within normal limits. Breathing pattern is regular.
Laboratory studies are within normal limits.	The hemoglobin level, hematocrit, and leukocyte count are within normal limits.
Patient has normal body hydration.	Secretions are thin. Mucous membranes are moist. There is no edema.
Daily fluid output is equal to fluid intake.	Urine output is 1500 to 3000 ml daily, or equivalent to intake. Patient feels neither hot nor cold.
There is no evidence of physical injury.	There is no evidence of complications arising from drugs, treatments, or nursing care.
There are no signs of infection.	There is no evidence of inflammation, purulent drainage or secretions, pain or aching.

BONE MARROW TRANSPLANTATION

For a discussion of bone marrow transplantation, see pp. 1722 to 1730.

SPLENECTOMY

Although it serves various important functions, the spleen can be surgically removed from adults without harm. If the procedure must be performed on a child, prophylactic antibiotics are given after surgery. Hypersplenism, the destruction of excessive numbers of blood cells by the spleen, is a major reason for its surgical removal. Another frequent indication is splenic rupture with severe hemorrhage, often caused by trauma. The procedure is relatively simple unless the spleen is greatly enlarged or is surrounded by adhesions.[6]

TREATMENT PLAN

Surgical
   Removal of the spleen

ASSESSMENT: AREAS OF CONCERN

Vascular function
   Signs and symptoms of hemorrhaging and shock

Gastrointestinal
   Abdominal distention and discomfort

Metabolic activity
   Elevated temperature

NURSING DIAGNOSES and NURSING INTERVENTIONS

Nursing Diagnosis	Nursing Intervention
Fluid volume deficit, actual (related to hemorrhaging)	Apply ice bag and manual pressure/dressing over site of blood loss. Estimate blood loss. Administer intravenous fluids, including blood as ordered. Measure intake and output. Increase oral fluid intake as tolerated.
Fluid volume deficit, actual (related to fever)	Monitor oral temperature. Apply cool, damp cloth to the face. Bathe in cool water, apply ice bag or alcohol, and cover with lightweight blankets and clothing. Maintain cool room temperature. Encourage rest. Increase fluid intake, especially iced liquids.
Comfort, alteration in	Give bland foods and/or warm full liquids and carbonated beverages. Identify the patient's preferred pain relief measures; implement when feasible. Apply abdominal binder. Apply warmth, such as heating pad. Administer medication as ordered, such as neostigmine (Prostigmin) and mild analgesics. Observe for increased complaints of pain, nausea, vomiting, diarrhea, and abdominal distention. Evaluate effectiveness of pain-relief measures.

EVALUATION[2]

Patient Outcome	Data Indicating That Outcome is Reached
Color of the skin and mucous membranes is good.	The skin, nails, lips, and ear lobes are warm and moist with a natural color.
Vital signs are within normal limits.	Respiratory rate, pulse rate, blood pressure, and temperature are within normal limits.
Laboratory studies are within normal limits.	The hemoglobin level and hematocrit are within normal limits.
Without verbalizing, patient has the physical appearance of comfort.	Patient has calm, relaxed facial expression. Posture is normal. Patient expresses comfort.

References

1. American Cancer Society: A cancer source book for nurses, New York, 1981, American Cancer Society.
2. Campbell, C.: Nursing diagnosis and intervention in nursing practice, New York, 1978, John Wiley & Sons.
3. Cancer Facts and Figures, New York, 1984, American Cancer Society.
4. Donovan, C.F.: Protective isolation, Oncology Nurs. Forum 9(3):50, 1982.
5. Kim, M.J., McFarland, G.K., and McLane, A.M.: Pocket guide to nursing diagnoses, St. Louis, 1984, The C.V. Mosby Co.
6. Luckmann, J., and Sorensen, K.C.: Medical-surgical nursing. A psychophysiologic approach, Philadelphia, 1981, W.B. Saunders Co.
7. Oncology Nursing Society, Clinical Practice Committee: Guidelines for the nursing care of patients with altered comfort, Oncology Nurs. Forum 10(4):93, 1983.
8. Oncology Nursing Society, Clinical Practice Committee: Guidelines for nursing care of patients with altered ventilation, Oncology Nurs. Forum 10(2):113.
9. Quick guide to common anemias, Nursing '83 83:24, 1983.
10. Wiley, F.M., and De-Cuir-Walley, S.: Allogenic bone marrow transplantation for children with acute leukemia, Oncology Nurs. Forum 10(3):49.

CHAPTER 14

Neoplasia

Overview

Cancer, the second most common cause of death in the United States, kills about 450,000 persons annually. Cancer is the leading cause of death in children 3 to 14 years of age, and it is estimated that 870,000 new cases of cancer are diagnosed in Americans every year. Earlier diagnosis and treatment of certain cancers and better health practices have improved the outlook for persons with cancer: three out of eight persons whose cancer is diagnosed in 1984 will be alive 5 years later.[2]

Cancer is a universal disease that affects people without regard to race, sex, socioeconomic status, or culture; however, different forms of cancer strike specific age, racial, and sexual groups. For example, cancer mortality increases rapidly with aging; some researchers believe that anyone who lives long enough will eventually develop cancer. Social and environmental factors are thought to explain racial differences in cancer. Both incidence and mortality are higher in blacks than in whites. Although women are more likely than men to develop cancer, more men die of the disease. The sites in men that are associated with the greatest mortality are the lung, colon and rectum, and prostate. In women the leading sites are the breast, lung, colon, and rectum.[2] Another interesting variable is heredity. Certain cancers, such as those of the stomach, breast, colon and rectum, uterus, and lung, occur in a familial pattern. Whether this is indicative of "an inherited susceptibility or common exposure to an etiologic factor"[1] is unknown. In addition, certain diseases that are cancer precursors, such as multiple familial polyposis and Gardner's syndrome, seem to be hereditary.

Cancer is probably caused by many interacting factors (initiators and promoters) rather than a single one, and its development appears to be a multistep process. Some causative agents have been found and others are suspected. One predisposing factor is chronic irritation such as frequent, prolonged exposure to sunlight or sustained alcohol consumption. Some benign lesions, such as leukoplakia of the oral cavity, colon and rectal polyps, and pigmented moles, may undergo malignant transformation. Persons whose cancer is already diagnosed are at risk for later development of the disease at the same or another site. Environmental carcinogens that have been identified include cigarette smoke, asbestos, uranium, asphalt, and aniline dye. Iatrogenic factors that have been implicated are radiation and drugs, for example, diethylstilbestrol (DES), certain cancer chemotherapeutic agents, radioisotopes such as phosphorus (^{32}P) and radium, and immunosuppressive drugs.

Among the factors theorized to cause cancer are (1) oncogenes that are normally dormant but may be activated by external agents and (2) viruses such as the Epstein-Barr virus (EBV) and hepatitis B virus, which are associated with neoplasms and with impaired immune surveillance.

ANATOMY AND PHYSIOLOGY

In describing the nature and possible causes of cancer, it is important to understand that cancer cells, unlike normal cells, proliferate without organization and often without differentiation. Certain stimuli are believed to initiate this process, which subsequently overpowers the normal control mechanism. The results are uninhibited growth (autonomy), uncontrolled function (anaplasia), and uncontrolled motility, permitting spread to other parts of the body (metastasis) via blood or the lymphatic system. Cancer metastasis is a complex series of events involving interactions among malignant cells from the primary tumor and between those cells and the normal cells. The steps that lead to tumor colonization in a distant site are as follows[7]:

1. Extension into surrounding tissues
2. Penetration of body cavities and vessels
3. Release of tumor cells for transport to other sites
4. Reinvasion of tissue at the site of arrest
5. Manipulation of the new environment to promote tumor cell survival, vascularization, and tumor growth

Only a small fraction of the cells that extend from a primary tumor overcome the body's numerous defense mechanisms and survive to complete the metastatic process. However, one cannot easily predict whether host immunity, as well as chemotherapy and immunotherapy, will inhibit or enhance tumor spread in a patient.

Neoplasms are described as benign or malignant. Benign tumors have little or no invasive activity, are generally encapsulated, usually grow more slowly, and are rarely fatal. Malignant tumors not only invade surrounding tissues but also produce metastases. If untreated these tumors usually result in death.

There are four types of cancer: carcinomas, usually solid tumors that arise from epithelial cells; sarcomas, derived from muscle, bone, and fat and other connective tissues; lymphomas, originating in lymphoid tissue; and leukemias, cancers of the hematologic system.

NORMAL FINDINGS

For assessment of a specific body system, see that chapter.

Area of Concern	Normal Adult Findings		Variations in Child	Variations in Older Adult
Respiratory rate	16-20 breaths/min		Child 20-30 breaths/min Adolescent 15-24 breaths/min	
Pulse rate	70-82 beats/min		Child 70-140 beats/min Adolescent 50-110 beats/min	
Blood pressure	18-44 yr 45-64 yr 65 yr and older	140/90 mm Hg 150/95 mm Hg 160/95 mm Hg	7-10 yr 110/70 mm Hg 11-17 yr 130/80 mm Hg	
Temperature	36°-37.5° C (96.8°-99.5° F)			
Normal Laboratory Data				
Blood				
Glycosylated hemoglobin	5.7%-8.8%			
Plasma hemoglobin	1-5 mg/dl			
Hemoglobin	Men 15.5 ± 1.1 g/dl Women 13.7 ± 1 g/dl		11-13.5 mo 11.9 ± 0.6 g/dl 1.5-3 yr 11.8 ± 0.5 g/dl 5 yr 12.7 ± 1 g/dl 10 yr 13.2 ± 2.1 g/dl	
Hematocrit	Men 42%-52% Women 35%-47%		Male (2 yr) 35%-44% Male (6 yr) 31%-43% Female (2 yr) 35%-44% Female (6 yr) 31%-43%	
pH	Arterial 7.35-7.45 Venous 7.32-7.43		2 mo-2 yr (arterialized capillary or arterial blood) 7.34-7.46	
Blood urea nitrogen (BUN)	Under 40 yr 5-20 mg/dl		Birth-1 yr 4-19 mg/dl	Gradual slight increase after 40 yr
O_2 saturation	95%-99%		Infant-2 yr 18-27 mEq/L	
CO_2	Arterial 22-29 mEq/L Venous 23-30 mEq/L			
Po_2	80-95 mm Hg			

Area of Concern	Normal Adult Findings	Variations in Child	Variations in Older Adult
P_{CO_2}	Arterial 35-45 mm Hg Venous 38-50 mm Hg		
Calcium	Under 30 yr 8.2-10.5 mg/dl		Decreases very slightly in older years
Potassium	3.5-5 mEq/L		
Serum creatinine	Men <1.2 mg/dl Women <1.1 mg/dl	1-5 yr 0.3-0.5 mg/dl 5-10 yr 0.5-0.8 mg/dl	

Urine
  Specific gravity
  pH
  Protein
  Creatinine
	1.001-1.035
	4.8-7.8
	Negative
	Men 1-2 g/24 hr
	Female 0.8-1.8 g/24 hr
		2-3 yr 6-22 mg/kg/24 hr
		>3 yr 12-30 mg/kg/24 hr
			Decreases with advancing age as muscle mass diminishes

Creatinine clearance	Male 85-125 ml/min/1.73 m² Female 75-115 ml/min/1.73 m²		

DIAGNOSTIC STUDIES[8]

Enzyme studies
  Serum acid phosphatase
    Elevation indicates possibility of prostate cancer
  Serum alkaline phosphatase
    Elevation indicates possibility of bone or liver metastases
  Hemoccult slide test
    Can give indication of gastrointestinal cancer
  Free acid in stomach
    Absence indicates likelihood of cancer of stomach

Oncofetal antigens such as carcinoembryonic antigen (CEA)
  Serum levels elevated in many malignancies, such as cancers of colon, pancreas, stomach, lung, and breast

Protein or hormonal products such as human chorionic gonadotropin (HCG) and adrenocorticotropic hormone (ACTH)

Cytologic techniques
  Body secretions collected and examined for sloughed cancer cells, which are stained and evaluated; examples are Papanicolaou smear and examinations of cervical discharge, sputum, gastric washings, pleural fluid, and urinary washings

Conventional x-ray film with or without contrast medium
  Chest film; upper gastrointestinal film; barium enema may show tumors

Scanning x-ray film
  Radioactive substance administered orally or intravenously; machine records concentration of radionuclide in targeted tissues, such as thyroid, spleen, lymph nodes, kidneys, central nervous system, liver, pancreas, lungs, and bones

Computed tomography (CT)

Dye contrast studies
  Injection of contrast medium into appropriate artery (arteriography of brain, kidney, liver, adrenal gland), femoral vein (venography), or lymph node of toe (lymphangiography)

Mammography
  Low-dose x-ray study of soft tissues of breast

Xerography
  Use of dry photoelectric process to make radiographs

Ultrasound
  Use of high-frequency sound waves to detect deep tumors

Thermography
  Measures and plots areas of localized elevation of skin temperature over inflammatory or malignant lesions

Histologic examination of tissue obtained by biopsy
  Biopsy can be incisional (surgical excision of tumor section), excisional (removal of entire growth), aspiration (removal of small tumor plug or fluid); frozen section involves freezing questionable tissue removed during surgery for microscopic study

Cystoscopy, bronchoscopy, sigmoidoscopy, proctoscopy
  Direct visualization of internal organs

Conditions, Diseases, and Disorders

PRIMARY CARCINOMA OF THE LUNG

Carcinoma of the lung is an uncontrolled growth of ana-plastic cells in the lung. Types are epidermoid (squamous cell), adenocarcinoma, small cell undifferentiated (oat cell), and large cell undifferentiated.

Carcinoma of the lung is the leading cause of death from cancer in men in the United States.[2] The incidence among women is steadily increasing, and more blacks than whites develop the disease. More than 90% of persons with lung cancer will die of it.

Approximately 80% of lung tumors are linked to cigarette smoking. The persons at highest risk began smoking in their teens, inhale deeply, and smoke at least half a pack a day. Persons who quit smoking have a gradual decline in risk, eventually reaching levels similar to those of nonsmokers.

Another etiologic factor in the development of carcinoma of the lung is occupational exposure to such substances as asbestos, uranium, nickel, and chromate. Air pollutants have not yet been proved a cancer risk factor, but the incidence of the disease is higher in urban populations.[2]

PATHOPHYSIOLOGY

The major histologic types of lung cancer are[8]:
1. Epidermoid (squamous cell)—the most common, comprising 40% to 50% of all lung tumors; 90% occur in men; tend to be centrally located; often produce bronchial obstruction
2. Adenocarcinoma—25% of lung cancers; often peripherally located; a common scar carcinoma that arises in area of fibrosis resulting from previous pulmonary damage; less association with smoking than other types
3. Small cell undifferentiated (oat cell)—20% to 25% of lung cancers; usually centrally located; most aggressive with lymphatic and distant metastases at time of diagnosis; most responsive to chemotherapy
4. Large cell undifferentiated—10% of malignant lung tumors; may appear in any part of lung

All types have lymphatic metastasis early in the course of the disease, beginning in the bronchial and mediastinal nodes and extending upward to supraclavicular nodes and downward to nodes below the diaphragm and to the liver and adrenal glands. Distant metastasis via the blood-stream to brain, bones, and contralateral lung may occur.

A chronic cough and wheezing are the most common early symptoms; other symptoms are fatigue, chest tightness, and aching joints. Late but clinically significant signs include hemoptysis, clubbing of the fingers, weight loss, and pleural effusion. Invasion of the superior vena cava causes edema of the neck and face. Phrenic nerve involvement results in paralysis of the diaphragm. A superior sulcus tumor involving the brachial plexus may be manifest as shoulder and arm pain and paresthesias.

The chest lesion may be relatively asymptomatic, with the chief complaint caused by metastatic disease. Metastasis to the brain may result in headache, unsteady gait, and other neurologic signs. Weight loss, jaundice, or anorexia may occur with liver involvement. Localized bony pain or pathologic fractures may accompany skeletal involvement.

Paraneoplastic syndromes may be associated with lung cancer. For example, inappropriate antidiuretic hormone (low serum sodium) or Cushing's syndrome from ectopic adrenocorticotropic hormone production occurs in some patients with small cell cancer. Other syndromes include hypercalcemia resulting from production of ectopic parathormone-like substance (epidermoid lung cancer); carcinomatous neuropathy and myopathy; dermatomyositis; and hypertrophic pulmonary osteoarthropathy.[8]

DIAGNOSTIC STUDIES[3]

Chest roentgenogram (lateral and posteroanterior views), chest tomography, and computed tomographic scanning
Outline shape, size, and position of lesion

Sputum collection for cytology, bronchoscopy with biopsy, brushings, or washings, and percutaneous biopsy under fluoroscopy
Cells gathered for histologic examination show evidence of malignancy

Scalene node biopsy
Evidence of spread to scalene nodes

Mediastinoscopy
Evidence of spread to ipsilateral and contralateral mediastinal lymph nodes

Radioisotope scanning
Reveals size, shape, and position of lesion

Liver function studies and scans, brain and bone scans
Evidence of metastases

Skin tests, absolute lymphocyte counts
Evidence of immunocompetence

TREATMENT PLAN[8]

Surgical
Lobectomy (see Chapter 2 for details)
Pneumonectomy for centrally located lesions (see Chapter 2)
Segmental and wedge resection based on patient tolerance and absence of spread (see Chapter 2)

Chemotherapeutic
For small cell lung cancer
Antineoplastic agents
Cyclophosphamide (Cytoxan), 40-50 mg/kg IV in individually determined doses over several days and then adjusted to lower maintenance dosage; po 1-5 mg/kg/d
Methotrexate (Mexate), 2.5-5 mg/kg/d po or parenterally
Doxorubicin (Adriamycin), 60-75 mg/m² at intervals of 21 d, or 30 mg/m²/d for 3 d repeated every 4 wk
Vincristine sulfate (Oncovin; VCR), 2 mg/m² for children, 1.4 mg/m² for adults
Carmustine (BCNU), 200 mg/m² IV q6 wk
Procarbazine (Mastulane), 2-4 mg/kg/d po initially and then 4-6 mg/kg/d until maximum response occurs; maintain at 1-2 mg/kg/d
Hexamethylmelamine (HXM), in combination therapy; dose individually determined
These agents only slightly useful in non–small cell cancer; partial regression with cisplatin-based regimens

Electromechanical
Radiation therapy—sole modality for patient who has clinically resectable lesion but is medically nonoperable and for patient with locally advanced, nonresectable tumor without demonstrable distant metastases but with such symptoms as cough, wheezing, obstructive infection, hemoptysis, pain, dysphagia, or superior vena cava syndrome; may be used preoperatively or postoperatively[3]

The prognosis for persons with lung cancer is correlated with tumor cell type. Those with well-differentiated squamous cell cancer have the best chance of survival; those with undifferentiated small cell cancer have the poorest. Peripheral tumors are more curable than central lesions. The presence of lymph node and distant metastases reduces the chance of cure. The stage of disease, patient's performance status, and immunologic state of the patient are important prognostic signs. Patients with gross supraclavicular adenopathy, a malignant pleural effusion, massive local extension, or distant metastases usually survive less than 1 year.

ASSESSMENT: AREAS OF CONCERN[6]

Respiratory function
Chronic cough, nonproductive or productive; wheezing; chest tightness; hemoptysis; dyspnea; hoarseness

Comfort level
Aching joints; clubbed fingers; bony pain

Sensory and motor function
Shoulder and arm pain; paresthesias; headache; unsteady gait

Systemic function
Fatigue; weight loss; edema of neck and face; anorexia

NURSING DIAGNOSES and NURSING INTERVENTIONS

Nursing Diagnosis	Nursing Intervention
Tissue perfusion, alteration in: pulmonary	Place patient in sitting position and change position frequently. Encourage coughing and deep breathing with splinting of chest. Ambulate patient as soon as possible. Encourage fluids. Administer oxygen therapy as prescribed. Anticipate patient's needs. Inspect chest for respiratory rate and rhythm and symmetric expansion.

Nursing Diagnosis	Nursing Intervention
	Auscultate for abnormal breath sounds, lung aeration, rales, and rhonchi. Percuss chest for abnormal resonance or decreased diaphragmatic descent. Monitor blood studies for abnormal gas exchange. Observe for cyanosis and change in amount or character of sputum. Discourage smoking.
Mobility, impaired: physical	Assist with ambulation; encourage efforts to move about. Move patient as necessary with walker, wheelchair, or cane. Minimize environmental barriers. Observe for complaints of weakness, fatigue, abnormal gait, and impaired coordination. Encourage range of motion and isotonic exercises that can be done in bed.

Comfort, alteration in: pain	For headache:
	    Position patient comfortably; change position slowly.
	    Elevate patient's head.
	    Apply cold, moist compress or ice bag.
	    Massage patient's neck and shoulders.
	    Subdue room lighting.
	    Provide quiet and encourage patient to rest.
	For chest pain:
	    Remove constrictive clothing.
	    Administer respiratory therapy as prescribed.
	For joint or bone pain:
	    Maintain body alignment.
	    Apply heating pad, hot water bottle, warm, moist compress, or mentholated ointment.
	    Exercise gently in range of motion.
	    Massage gently.
	    Be alert for complaints of pain and assess its duration and radiation.
	    Provide pain relief measure of patient's choice, such as relaxation therapy, diversion, or distraction.
	    Administer pain medications as ordered.
	    Evaluate pain for intensity and quality.
	    Evaluate effectiveness of pain relief measures.

Nutrition, alteration in: less than body requirements	Provide pleasant surroundings. Provide attractive meal tray. Postpone feeding when patient is fatigued. Give small, frequent, nutritious feedings. Provide selection of foods. Provide foods at appropriate temperature. Encourage family and friends to bring food. Season food to patient's taste.

Patient Education

1. Discourage smoking.
2. Teach the patient to cough productively and to perform breathing exercises and other respiratory therapy as prescribed.
3. Assist the patient to ambulate and instruct the patient in the use of assistive devices such as canes and walkers.
4. Teach the patient to self-administer medication for pain.
5. Inform the patient of the need for adequate nutrition (high-calorie, high-protein diet).
6. Inform the patient of the signs and symptoms of complications or adverse reactions to therapy.
7. Discuss with the patient the availability of resources and support systems.

EVALUATION

Patient Outcome	Data Indicating That Outcome is Reached
Skin and mucous membrane color is normal.	Skin, nails, lips, and earlobes are warm and moist and have natural color.
Vital signs are within normal limits.	Respiratory rate; pulse rate; and blood pressure are within normal limits.
Laboratory findings are within normal limits.	Blood oxygen saturation, carbon dioxide, P_{O_2}, and P_{CO_2} are within normal limits.
Body hydration is normal.	Skin turgor is normal, secretions are thin, and there is no edema.
Body functioning is normal.	Weight is stabilized.
Vitality is good.	There is no malaise, fatigue, or weakness.
Patient has daily intake of essential food groups.	Milk, meat, fruits, vegetables, breads, and cereals are included in daily diet.
Patient is comfortable.	Facial expression is calm, contented, and relaxed. Posture is normal. Patient has freedom of body movement and expresses comfort.

CANCERS OF THE COLON AND RECTUM

Cancer of the colon and rectum is an uncontrolled growth of anaplastic cells in the colon or rectum. Types are adenocarcinoma, carcinoid tumor, leiomyosarcoma, and lymphoma.

Each year approximately 114,000 new cases of colon or rectal cancer are diagnosed in the United States. These tumors occur almost equally in men and women, usually after 40 years of age.[2]

No definite external etiologic factors have been identified, although dietary habits such as frequent ingestion of refined carbohydrates are suspected. Conditions that increase the risk of colorectal cancers include familial polyposis of the colon or rectum, chronic ulcerative colitis, diverticulosis, and villous adenomas of the colon. Exposure to asbestos has also been identified as a possible cause of these diseases.[8]

PATHOPHYSIOLOGY[3]

The most common symptom of colorectal cancer is rectal bleeding, followed by changes in bowel pattern (constipation or diarrhea), excessive flatus, distention, cramps, obstruction, and unexplained anemia. The presence of symptoms depends on the location of the tumor. Right-sided colonic lesions may be manifest as unexplained iron-deficiency anemia and gastrointestinal tract bleeding. Tumors of the sigmoid are characterized by obstruction from napkin ring growth. Rectal tumors are evidenced by rectal pain, gross rectal blood, and tenesmus with a feeling of incomplete evacuation.

The majority of colorectal cancers are adenocarcinomas; others are carcinoid tumors, leiomyosarcomas, and lymphomas. Regional lymph nodes are involved in at least half of the patients. Most colon cancers spread to periaortic nodes. Anal carcinomas spread into perineal nodes. Distant metastasis is most often to the liver and lungs.

The 5-year survival rate for patients with localized disease is 75% for colon tumors and 70% for rectal lesions. These rates are reduced by half with regional or distant involvement. The earlier the diagnosis and treatment, the more curable the cancer. Even with a large tumor and invasion of adjacent structures, the prognosis is favorable if appropriate treatment is provided. Only the presence of distant metastases precludes the possibility of cure. For early detection the American Cancer Society recommends annual digital rectal examination for all persons 40 years and older, an annual stool guaiac test at 50 years and older, and sigmoidoscopy every 3 to 5 years after two initial negative ones 1 year apart.

DIAGNOSTIC STUDIES[3]

Digital rectal examination
Palpation of suspect lesion

Proctosigmoidoscopy with fiberoptic scope
Visualization and biopsy of suspect lesion

Barium enema
Visualization of suspect lesion

Testing of stool for occult blood
Presence of blood may be indicative of ulcerating malignancy

TREATMENT PLAN[8]

Surgical
Depends on cancer's location and invasive characteristics

End-to-end anastomosis with or without temporary colostomy

Abdominoperineal resection with permanent colostomy

Transverse colostomy to relieve distal bowel obstruction with later resection

Oophorectomy in women because of possible ovarian involvement

Resection en bloc of other organs attached to primary tumor, such as small bowel loops, urinary bladder, uterus, and adnexa

Electrocoagulation of tumor transanally (experimental approach)

Chemotherapeutic
No proven effective adjuvant therapy; palliation for liver or lung metastases with 5-fluorouracil produces 20% response rate

Electromechanical
Radiation therapy for prevention of local recurrence after surgery, preoperative reduction of tumor, intraoperative sterilization of operative field, and relief of symptoms such as bleeding, discharge, tenesmus, and pain

ASSESSMENT: AREAS OF CONCERN[6]

Gastrointestinal function
Rectal bleeding; constipation or diarrhea; excessive flatus; distention; cramps; rectal pain; tenesmus

NURSING DIAGNOSES and NURSING INTERVENTIONS*

Nursing Diagnosis	Nursing Intervention
Bowel elimination, alteration in: constipation	Ambulate patient frequently, and encourage physical exercise. Encourage increased intake of high-bulk foods and fluids. Give fresh fruits, prune juice, hot coffee, and warm and iced liquids. Place patient in sitting position. Give stool softeners and laxatives. Administer enemas. Measure intake and output.
Bowel elimination, alteration in: diarrhea	Provide fluids so intake equals output. Cover patient with warm blankets. Encourage adequate rest. Discourage oral stimulants. Discourage intake of high-bulk foods. Give tea, carbonated beverages, clear-liquid or full-liquid diet, and dry crackers. Administer antidiarrheal drugs as ordered. Refrain from giving hot or iced liquids, enemas, or laxatives. Refrain from inserting rectal tube or taking rectal temperature. Check for impaction. Employ caution with pancytopenic patients. Ausculate abdomen with abnormal bowel sounds. Measure body weight and intake and output. Monitor blood studies for acid-base and electrolyte abnormalities. Be alert for complaints of pain.
Comfort, alteration in: pain (related to abdominal distention)	Change patient's position frequently; increase movement if tolerated. Discourage smoking. Give small, frequent feedings. Encourage decreased intake of gas-forming foods. Restrict liquids at mealtime; give warm liquids after meals. Refrain from giving iced liquids and carbonated beverages. Avoid use of straws. Give nonprescription drugs such as simethicone.

*Refer to Chapter 11 for postoperative nursing interventions.

Nursing Diagnosis	**Nursing Intervention**
	Insert rectal tube.
	Encourage moderate physical activity.
	Remove restrictive clothing.
	Inspect abdomen for distention.
	Auscultate abdomen for abnormal bowel sounds.
Comfort, alteration in: pain (related to cramping)	Encourage decreased intake of fatty foods.
	Give bland foods.
	Apply heat to abdomen.
	Involve patient in selection of other pain relief measures.
	Evaluate effectiveness of pain relief measures.
Comfort, alteration in: pain (rectal)	Position patient comfortably.
	Apply warm, moist compress to rectal area or provide sitz bath.
	Increase fluid intake to 2000 ml daily.
	Encourage decreased intake of high-bulk food.
	Involve patient in selection of pain relief measures.
	Evaluate pain for duration, intensity, and quality.
	Evaluate effectiveness of pain relief measures.
Potential patient problem: bleeding	Apply ice bag to rectal area.
	Change patient's position slowly.
	Cover patient with warm blankets.
	Maintain complete bed rest if bleeding is severe.
	Elevate foot of bed.
	Refrain from giving enemas or laxatives, inserting rectal tube, or taking rectal temperature.
	Estimate blood volume loss.
	Monitor blood pressure and blood studies.

Patient Education

1. Inform the patient of the need to maintain adequate gastrointestinal function.
2. Instruct the patient in pain relief measures.
3. Explain bowel changes (such as bleeding) the patient should report.
4. Instruct the patient in the care of an ostomy if present.

EVALUATION

Patient Outcome	Data Indicating That Outcome is Reached
Vital signs are within normal limits.	Respiratory rate, pulse rate, and blood pressure are within normal limits.
Laboratory findings are within normal limits.	Blood values for hemoglobin, hematocrit, and potassium are within normal limits.
Body hydration is normal.	Skin turgor is normal. There is no edema. Body functioning is normal. Elimination is adequate. Weight is stabilized at normal level for body build.
Vitality is good.	Patient is not fatigued or weak.
Patient has daily intake of essential food groups.	Diet includes milk, meat, fruits, vegetables, breads, and cereals (as tolerated).
Bowel elimination is normal for patient.	Stools are soft. Abdomen is soft and not distended.
Patient is comfortable.	Facial expression is calm, contented, and relaxed. Posture is normal. Patient expresses comfort and satisfaction. Patient no longer complains. Patient frequently changes position and walks, sits, and stands with normal body movement.
Patient participates in daily physical exercise.	Patient bicycles, jogs, or exercises in some other way.

CARCINOMA OF THE BREAST

Carcinoma of the breast is an uncontrolled growth of anaplastic cells in the breast. Types include ductal, lobular, and nipple adenocarcinomas.

Although lung cancer is increasing in prevalence, the breast is the most common site of cancer in women between 25 and 75 years of age. Each year breast cancer is diagnosed in approximately 115,000 women in the United States, and it is the leading cause of death in women 40 to 44 years of age. Breast cancer also develops infrequently in men. Symptoms and treatment are the same for men and women.

Most breast lesions are first detected by a woman during breast self-examination or by her sexual partner. The possibility for cure is 85% for women with localized disease at the time of diagnosis. Half of breast cancers are in the upper outer quadrant, 20% in the central portion, 20% in the medial quadrants, and 10% in the lower outer quadrant.

Risk factors that have been cited in the incidence of breast cancer include previous breast cancer, a family history of breast cancer, nulliparity, or a first pregnancy after 30 years of age. Irradiation, particularly as therapy for postpartum mastitis or as multiple chest fluoroscopies, is believed to contribute to breast cancer development. Obesity and total fat content in the diet, especially animal fat, may be factors. Total lifetime exposure to endogenous estrogen is a major risk factor. This disease is more common among white women, but the incidence among blacks is rising.[2,8]

PATHOPHYSIOLOGY[3]

The most common initial sign of carcinoma of the breast is a mass, usually painless. Bloody discharge is more indicative of cancer than is spontaneous unilateral serous nipple discharge in a nonlactating breast. Signs of advanced breast cancer include dimpling of the skin, nipple retraction, change in breast contour, fixation to the pectoral fascia or chest wall, edema and erythema of the breast skin, and axillary adenopathy. Dermatitis of the nipple or areola may be indicative of Paget's disease. Important associated findings are described in "Assessment: Areas of Concern."

DIAGNOSTIC STUDIES[8]

Monthly breast self-examination and annual examination by a physician are important for early diagnosis. Mammography offers the potential for the identification of occult breast cancer. The following are current recommendations of the American Cancer Society and the National Cancer Institute:

1. Annual or other periodic mammography for asymptomatic women 50 years of age and older
2. Annual or periodic mammography for women between 40 and 49 years of age if they are at high risk, that is, have a history of breast cancer, have had prior breast biopsy results of lobular carcinoma in situ or an atypical proliferative process, or have been successfully treated for carcinoma of the ovary or endometrium
3. Annual or other periodic mammography in women less than 40 years of age if they have a history of breast cancer or a premenopausal mother or sister with breast cancer, especially if bilateral
4. Baseline mammogram for women 35 to 50 years of age

A person of any age with a suspect breast mass should undergo mammography and biopsy.

Other procedures being used or studied as adjuncts in the diagnosis of breast cancer include thermography, ultrasonography, and identification of tumor markers. Biopsy for histologic diagnosis is by needle aspiration, core or cutting needle, or open excision. The histologic type of breast cancer is adenocarcinoma, usually of the duct (in situ, invasive, inflammatory, medullary, mucinous, papillary, scirrhous, or tubular), lobule, or nipple (Paget's disease). In addition to the procedures already cited, the following tests may be used to diagnose this disease:

1. Level of estrogen receptor protein, which predicts response to hormonal manipulation of metastatic disease, as well as prognosis for primary cancer
2. Level of carcinoembryonic antigen (CEA), which is elevated 6 months to 1 year before other evidence of hepatic involvement is noted
3. Gross cystic disease protein (investigational)
4. Metastatic evaluation, including bone scanning, liver function studies, brain or computed tomography (CT) scan, and chest roentgenograms

TREATMENT PLAN[3,8]

Surgical

Controversial, with various options

Radical mastectomy (rarely used now)

Modified radical mastectomy (total mastectomy with partial axillary dissection) for stages I and II

Lumpectomy, segmental mastectomy, or quadrantectomy with axillary node dissection; primary irradiation of remaining breast tissue

Resection of local recurrences or metastases to opposite breast; stabilization of fractures by orthopedic devices; decompression laminectomy

Chemotherapeutic

As initial treatment before radiation or surgery; as adjuvant for premenopausal patients with axillary node metastases

Hormone therapy with antiestrogens; hormone ablation by oophorectomy

Chemotherapy with cyclophosphamide, methotrexate, 5-FU with or without prednisone, and vincristine; doxorubicin as single agent

Antineoplastic agents

Hormones

Tamoxifen citrate (Nolvadex), 10-20 mg bid (indicated for women who are estrogen receptor protein positive)

Phenylalanine mustard or other alkylating agent

Other antineoplastic agents

Cyclophosphamide (Cytoxan), 40-50 mg/kg IV in divided doses over period of several days, then adjusted to lower maintenance dosage; po 1-5 mg/kg/d

Fluorouracil (5-FU, Adrucil, others), 12 mg/kg IV for 4 d followed by 6 mg/kg on alternate days for approximately 12 d

Methotrexate (Amethopterin; Mexate), 2.5-5 mg/kg/d po or parenterally

Doxorubicin (Adriamycin), 60-75 mg/m^2 at intervals of 21 d; or 30 mg/m^2 on each of 3 successive d repeated q4h

Vincristine sulfate (Oncovin), 2 mg/m^2 for children, 1.4 mg/m^2 for adults

Vinblastine (Velban), 0.1 mg/kg increased weekly by 0.05 mg/kg up to 0.5 mg/kg

Electromechanical

For recurrent disease

Radiation therapy for pain control, prevention of pathologic fractures, and control of local soft tissue disease preoperatively or postoperatively (adjuvant), cerebral metastases, and localized symptoms

Supportive

Ablative surgery such as bilateral oophorectomy, adrenalectomy, or hypophysectomy

Additive therapy with large doses of estrogen, androgen, or progestin (in women more than 10 years past menopause)

Patients with stage I tumors and no involvement of axillary nodes have a 10-year survival greater than 80%; those with stage II tumors have greater than 60% 10-year survival. If the lymph nodes are involved, the 10-year survival is 30% to 40% in the absence of adjuvant chemotherapy. Recent studies have shown that patients whose cancers are estrogen receptor protein negative have a much poorer prognosis. Patients with stage IV disease have a 10-year survival of less than 10%.

Follow-up care includes early detection of second primary breast cancers and recurrent disease. Breast self-examination, yearly mammography, and physician's examination of the intact breast and nodes are important. Rehabilitation is an essential intervention after primary treatment.

ASSESSMENT: AREAS OF CONCERN[3]

Breast tissue

Presence of mass; bloody discharge; dimpling of skin; nipple retraction; change in breast contour; fixation; edema and erythema; enlarged axillary or supraclavicular nodes

Comfort

Bone pain (indicative of bony metastases); headache (indicative of brain metastases)

Gastrointestinal function

Anorexia; nausea; hepatomegaly; jaundice; clay-colored stools; mahogany-colored urine; ascites; edema (indicative of liver metastases)

Respiratory function

Dyspnea; increased respirations; tachycardia

NURSING DIAGNOSES and NURSING INTERVENTIONS

Nursing Diagnosis	Nursing Intervention
Skin integrity, impairment of: potential	Cleanse skin. Apply warm, moist compress. Apply antibiotic ointment and sterile dressing if indicated. Expose draining area to air (depends on patient's immunocompetence). Elevate arm. Observe for increased discharge, skin changes (color, dimpling), swelling, enlarged nodes, and dermatitis.

Nursing Diagnosis	Nursing Intervention

	For jaundice related to liver metastasis:
	  Apply cornstarch or sodium bicarbonate.
	  Bathe patient in cool water.
	  Lubricate patient's skin.
	  Minimize patient's clothing.
	  Increase daily fluid intake to 2000 ml.
	  Maintain adequate atmospheric humidity and cool room temperature.
	  Observe patient's skin for change in color.
	  Note patient's complaints of itching.

Comfort, alteration in: pain	For bone pain related to bony metastasis:
	  Handle patient gently.
	  Position patient comfortably and change position slowly.
	  Support affected body part(s).
	  Apply warm, moist compress or place in whirlpool bath.
	  Encourage adequate rest.
	  Provide pain relief measure of patient's choice.
	  Be alert for complaints of pain and assess pain for duration and radiation.
	  Evaluate effectiveness of pain relief measures.
	For headache related to brain metastasis:
	  Elevate head.
	  Apply cold, moist compress or ice bag.
	  Massage gently.
	  Subdue room lighting.
	  Provide quiet.
	  Encourage adequate rest.
	  Provide pain relief measure of patient's choice.
	  Be alert for complaints of pain and assess pain for duration and radiation.
	  Evaluate effectiveness of pain relief measures.
	For abdominal discomfort:
	  Change patient's position frequently.
	  Give small, frequent feedings.
	  Handle gently.
	  Place patient in sitting position.
	  Remove constrictive clothing.

Nutrition, alteration in: less than body requirements (related to anorexia)	Arrange pleasant surroundings and provide attractive meal tray. Postpone feeding when patient is fatigued. Balance nutritional intake. Give small, frequent feedings. Provide selection of foods. Provide foods at appropriate temperature. Encourage family and friends to bring in food. Measure body weight daily. Observe and record food intake.
Nutrition, alteration in: less than body requirements (related to nausea)	Elevate patient's head. Encourage deep breathing. Feed slowly. Give bland food or carbonated beverages or hot tea. Give nonprescription antiemetics or drugs as prescribed. Observe effectiveness of interventions.
Tissue perfusion, alteration in (related to respiratory metastasis)	Position patient comfortably with head elevated. Suction airway as needed. Administer vaporized air. Encourage adequate rest. Remove constrictive clothing. Maintain adequate humidity and ventilation. Discourage smoking. Inspect chest for respiratory rate and rhythm and symmetric expansion. Auscultate for abnormal breath sounds, voice sounds, rales, and rhonchi. Monitor blood studies. Be alert for complaints of pain, cyanosis, dyspnea, and fatigue.

Patient Education

1. Emphasize the need for safety precautions.
2. Teach the patient how to perform pain relief measures.
3. Stress the need for adequate nutrition.
4. Explain how to assess the body for further breast disease or evidence of spread by performing breast self-examination.
5. Provide information about resources and support systems such as the Reach to Recovery program of the American Cancer Society.

EVALUATION

Patient Outcome	Data Indicating That Outcome is Reached
Vital signs are within normal limits.	Respiratory rate and pulse rate are within normal limits. There is no respiratory distress.
Laboratory findings are within normal limits.	Blood values for hemoglobin and hematocrit are within normal limits.
Body hydration is normal.	There is no edema or ascites.
Body functioning is normal.	Weight is stabilized at normal level for body build. Incision is healed.
Patient has daily intake of essential food groups.	Milk, meats, fruits, vegetables, breads, and cereals are included in daily diet.
Vitality is good.	There is no malaise, fatigue, or weakness.
Patient is comfortable.	Facial expression is calm, contented, and relaxed. Posture is normal. Patient has freedom of body movement. Patient expresses comfort and satisfaction and demonstrates acceptance of loss of breast. Patient frequently changes position and walks, sits, and stands with normal movement.
Patient's surroundings are safe.	Patient uses safety precautions.
Patient shows no evidence of physical injury.	There is no evidence of complications arising from drugs, treatments, or nursing care.

CANCERS OF THE URINARY TRACT
Wilms' Tumor

Wilms' tumor is a malignant embryonal neoplasm of the kidneys that affects primarily children under 5 years of age.

Sixty-five percent of children with Wilms' tumor are less than 3 years of age. In most cases the child has an abdominal swelling or mass initially detected by a parent. These tumors grow quickly and metastasize most frequently to the lungs and regional lymph nodes and occasionally to the brain and liver.

The 5-year survival rate is 70% with localized tumors but falls to 39% with regional involvement. The sexes are equally affected, as are the left and right kidneys.

Lung metastases can be successfully treated, with a cure rate of more than 50%.[2]

PATHOPHYSIOLOGY

This nephroblastoma, usually a single expanding mass, is thought to arise from the metanephric blastema. Infiltration through the renal capsule into adjacent structures is common, and frequently there is direct extension into the pelvis and ureter or renal vein and vena cava. Metastasis to hilar lymph nodes is common.

About 40% of these tumors are believed to be hereditary, transmitted as an autosomal dominant disorder. All bilateral tumors are heritable.[8]

DIAGNOSTIC STUDIES

Abdominal ultrasonography and intravenous urography

To determine patency of inferior vena cava, renal status, and presence of bilateral involvement

Chest radiography and computed tomography evaluation

To detect pulmonary disease

Blood pressure determination

Hypertension may be present

24-hour quantitative vanillylmandelic acid (VMA) test

To exclude neuroblastoma

Serum hepatic studies

To detect liver metastases

TREATMENT PLAN[8]

Surgical

Exploratory laparotomy and transperitoneal nephrectomy with node sampling from renal hilar and para-aortic areas, hepatic evaluation, and examination of opposite kidney

Chemotherapeutic

Adjuvant therapy

Antineoplastic agents

Vincristine sulfate (Oncovin), 2 mg/m[2] for children, 1.4 mg/m[2] for adults

Dactinomycin (Cosmegen), 0.015-0.05 mg/kg IV in divided dosages over 1 wk; repeat for 3-5 wk

Doxorubicin (Adriamycin), 60-75 mg/m[2] at intervals of 21 d; or 30 mg/m[2] on each of 3 successive days repeated q4wk

Cyclophosphamide (Cytoxan), 40-50 mg/kg IV in divided doses over several days and then adjusted to lower maintenance dosage; po 1-5 mg/kg/d

Electromechanical

Radiation therapy for large primary lesions, capsular involvement, lymph node disease, or residual disease at primary site or in lung or opposite kidney

ASSESSMENT: AREAS OF CONCERN[3]

Gastrointestinal function

Abdominal mass; pain; nausea and vomiting; anorexia

Energy level

Fever; malaise

Urinary function

Hematuria

Respiratory function

Dyspnea

Cardiovascular function

Hypertension

NURSING DIAGNOSES and NURSING INTERVENTIONS

Nursing Diagnosis	Nursing Intervention
Comfort, alteration in: pain (abdominal)	Approach patient with reassurance and calmness. Give bland or full-liquid foods, warm liquids, and carbonated beverages. Offer patient pain relief measures of choice. Give medications as ordered. Evaluate effectiveness of pain relief measures. Measure abdomen at least once a day. Check for bowel sounds. Record bowel movements. Be alert for complaints of increased pain, nausea, vomiting, diarrhea, and fever.
Urinary elimination, alteration in patterns	Inspect urine for bleeding; test with Hemastix. Encourage adequate rest and moderate exercise. Increase fluid intake. Monitor intake and output.

Nursing Diagnosis	Nursing Intervention
Tissue perfusion, alteration in: cardiopulmonary	Change patient's position frequently; place in sitting position. Encourage coughing and deep breathing. Observe respiratory rate and rhythm. Auscultate chest. Monitor blood studies. Administer oxygen and respiratory therapy as ordered. Elevate head. Change patient's position frequently as needed (children are often naturally active). Provide quiet, restful environment. Discourage oral stimulants and smoking; avoid emotional situations. Monitor blood pressure.
Potential patient problem: body temperature alteration (fever)	Apply cool, damp cloth to face. Bathe in cool water or apply ice bag or alcohol to skin. Cover with lightweight clothing. Maintain cool room temperature. Encourage rest. Give antipyretics as indicated. Increase fluid intake. Measure temperature and intake and output. Obtain bacterial cultures as indicated.

Patient Education

1. Emphasize need for balanced diet as tolerated, such as bland foods, full-liquid diet, and foods high in calories and protein.
2. Emphasize need for adequate fluid intake.
3. Explain pain-relieving measures such as position change, warmth, and analgesics.
4. Explain changes to report to physician: respiratory problems, headache, fever, blood in urine, or increased pain.

EVALUATION[4]

Patient Outcome	Data Indicating That Outcome is Reached
Vital signs are within normal limits	Respiratory rate, pulse rate, blood pressure, and temperature are within normal limits.
Laboratory findings are within normal limits.	Blood values for hemoglobin, hematocrit, oxygen saturation, and carbon dioxide are within normal limits.
Body hydration is normal.	Skin turgor is normal. Secretions are thin. Mucous membranes are moist. Patient is not thirsty.
Patient has daily intake of essential foods.	Diet includes milk, meat, fruits, vegetables, breads, and cereals.
Daily fluid output is equal to fluid intake.	Urine output is 1500 to 3000 ml daily or equivalent to intake.
Vitality is good.	There is no malaise.
Performance at work and play is adequate.	Patient is able to maintain self-care. Patient is satisfied with work and play performance.
Patient is comfortable.	Facial expression is calm and relaxed. Patient has freedom of body movement. Patient expresses comfort. Patient ceases to complain.

Adult Renal Tumors

Renal cancer is an uncontrolled growth of anaplastic cells of the kidney. Types include hypernephroma, parenchymal tumors, papillary tumors, and nephrotic carcinomas.

Renal cancer usually occurs in persons over 40 years of age, is twice as common in men as in women, and has a lower incidence in blacks. Signs and symptoms develop late in the course of the disease; the most common sign is painless, intermittent hematuria.

PATHOPHYSIOLOGY

Hypernephroma, or adenocarcinoma of the renal parenchyma, is the most common renal neoplasm in adults. It grows slowly but may metastasize at any stage. Metastasis via the bloodstream results in spread to the lungs, bone, regional lymph nodes, liver, and other visceral organs. Parenchymal tumors infiltrate more rapidly than hypernephroma and have a poor prognosis. Papillary tumors of the renal pelvis (transitional cell, squamous cell, adenocarcinoma) are usually multiple, involving the ureter and often the bladder, as well as lymphatics.

Nephrotic carcinomas are usually large and encapsulated; as many as 50% may perforate the apparently intact capsule. Hematogenous metastasis results from early invasion of renal venules. The neoplasm often extends into the renal vein and vena cava. Distant metastases occur in the lung, lymph nodes, liver, bone, adrenal gland, opposite kidney, brain, and heart (in decreasing frequency).

The kidney is the site of more metastatic than primary tumors. The most frequent sites of origin are the lung and breast.[3,8]

DIAGNOSTIC STUDIES[8]

Retrograde pyelogram, ultrasonography, and computed tomography
Visualization of lesion

Cyst aspiration
Determination of whether process is benign or malignant

Selective renal angiography
Clear visualization of renal vascular anatomy

Cystoscopy with surface biopsy, washings for cell block, and Papanicolaou smear
Evidence of malignant cells or tissue

Blood studies
Normochromic, normocytic anemia; polycythemia in some patients; leukocytosis; hypercalcemia; elevated erythrocyte sedimentation rate

Alkaline phosphatase, bilirubin, and transaminase levels
Elevated

Prothrombin time
Prolonged

Urine LDH
Elevated

TREATMENT PLAN[3]

Surgical
Radical nephrectomy
Nephroureterectomy
Palliative nephrectomy for bleeding and pain control
Resection of solitary metastatic site such as in brain or liver

Chemotherapeutic
Progestins
Medroxyprogesterone acetate (Provera, Depo-Provera), 2.5-10 mg po or 100-400 mg IM
Antineoplastic agents
Cyclophosphamide (Cytoxan), 40-50 mg/kg IV in divided doses over several days, then adjusted to lower maintenance dosage; po 1-5 mg/kg/d
Vinblastine (Velban), 0.1 mg/kg, increased weekly by 0.05 mg/kg up to 0.5 mg/kg
Hydroxyurea (Hydrea), 20-30 mg/kg/d po or 80 mg/kg every third day

Electromechanical
Preoperative radiation therapy
Palliative radiation therapy
Postoperative radiation therapy for patients with high risk of local recurrence

Improved survival rates (5-year survival of 65% for early hypernephroma) have been attributed to thoracoabdominal nephrectomy with node dissection, as well as earlier diagnosis of "incidental" carcinomas. Spontaneous regression has prompted investigational therapy with biologic response modifiers such as the histamine H_2 antagonist cimetidine.

ASSESSMENT: AREAS OF CONCERN

Urinary function
Painless hematuria; bladder retention

Comfort
Chronic aching pain; renal colic; nerve or bone pain

Systemic function
Unexplained weight loss; reflex gastrointestinal disturbances such as nausea and vomiting; fever; hypertension; seizures

Cardiovascular status
Abdominal bruit; ascites; edema of lower extremities and scrotum; dilated abdominal veins; high-output heart failure

NURSING DIAGNOSES and NURSING INTERVENTIONS

Nursing Diagnosis	Nursing Intervention
Urinary elimination, alteration in patterns	Measure intake and output. Inspect urine for bleeding; check with Hemastix. Inspect abdomen for distention; palpate bladder. Encourage adequate rest and exercise. Ambulate patient often. Apply heating pad or hot water bottle. Catheterize only if necessary.
Comfort, alteration in: pain	Be alert for complaints of pain; assess duration, radiation, intensity, and precipitating and relieving factors. Approach patient unhurriedly; provide reassurance. Position patient comfortably and handle gently. Encourage adequate rest. Discuss possible pain-reducing measures such as guided imagery, relaxation, distraction, and hypnosis. Administer medications as ordered, such as nonsteroidal anti-inflammatory agents and narcotics. For chronic, aching pain, apply heating pad, hot water bottle, or warm moist compress. For renal colic, increase fluid intake, remove constrictive clothing, and provide sitz bath. For nerve pain, apply heat or cold, apply bed cradle, decrease drafts, and massage gently. For bone pain, change patient's position slowly, support affected body part, and place in whirlpool bath.
Nutrition, alteration in: less than body requirements	Estimate required daily calories. Give small, frequent feedings. Grant special food requests. Encourage adequate rest. Encourage increased fluid intake. Supplement protein and caloric intake. Provide mouth care. Monitor intake and output and temperature. Measure body weight. Administer medications as ordered, such as antiemetics and antipyretics.
Injury, potential for (related to chemical agent or seizure)	Maintain bed rest. Provide quiet environment with subdued lighting. Remove constrictive clothing. Minimize environmental danger. Provide emergency equipment such as padded tongue blade. Inspect patient for abnormal body movements. Observe for confusion and reduced level of consciousness. Monitor neurologic vital signs.
Tissue perfusion, alteration in: cardiopulmonary	Remove constrictive clothing. Raise head of bed.

Nursing Diagnosis	Nursing Intervention
	Elevate extremities without elevating bed at knee gatch or placing pillow under knees.
	Apply elastic stockings.
	Change position frequently.
	Perform range of motion exercises.
	Ambulate patient as much as possible.
	Inspect extremities for adequate circulation.
	Palpate for pulses.
	Measure abdominal growth, circumference of extremities, and scrotal size.
	Auscultate abdominal sounds.
Potential patient problem: alteration in arterial blood pressure	Elevate patient's head.
	Change patient's position frequently.
	Provide restful, quiet environment.
	Tell patient to avoid oral stimulants, emotional situations, and smoking.
	Monitor blood pressure.

Patient Education

1. Emphasize need for balanced diet, adequate fluid intake, and high-calorie, high-protein diet.
2. Explain pain-relieving measures such as exercise, warmth, and analgesics.
3. Discuss changes that should be reported to physician: headache, seizures, fever, blood in urine, increasing pain, increasing edema, and respiratory distress.

EVALUATION

Patient Outcome	Data Indicating That Outcome is Reached
Skin and mucous membrane color is normal.	Skin, nails, lips, and earlobes are warm and moist and of natural color.
Vital signs are within normal limits.	Respiratory rate, pulse rate, blood pressure, and temperature are within normal limits.
Body hydration is normal.	Skin turgor is normal. Secretions are thin. Mucous membranes are moist. There is no edema, ascites, or venous distention.
Patient has daily intake of essential foods.	Diet includes milk, meat, fruits, vegetables, breads, and cereals.
Daily fluid output equals fluid intake.	Urine output is 1500 to 3000 ml daily or equivalent to intake.
Vitality is good.	There is no malaise, fatigue, or weakness.
Patient has physical appearance of comfort.	Patient expresses comfort and satisfaction. Patient ceases to complain.
Patient frequently changes position.	Patient walks, sits, and stands with normal body movement.
Patient participates in therapeutic exercise.	Patient performs range of motion exercises.
Patient's surroundings are safe and comfortable.	Patient uses safety precautions. Temperature, humidity, and ventilation of patient's room are appropriate.
There is no evidence of physical injury.	Patient shows no evidence of complications arising from drugs or treatments.

Carcinoma of the Bladder

The bladder is the most common site of urinary tract malignancy.

Cancer of the bladder occurs most often in men between 50 and 70 years of age. In the past 25 years the incidence in men has increased while the incidence in women has decreased; now the prevalence is nearly twice as great in men. The most frequent sign of bladder cancer is hematuria, although some patients are asymptomatic until uretheral obstruction occurs.

The second most common symptom complex is marked urgency, dysuria, and frequency with small volumes of urine in an older patient. Low back pain may be indicative of sacral or lumbar metastases.[8]

PATHOPHYSIOLOGY[3]

Ninety percent of bladder tumors are transitional cell carcinoma, 6% to 7% are true squamous cell carcinoma, and only 1% to 2% are glandular cancer. Some of these tumors are undifferentiated. Depth of invasion (stage) is more important than grading in predicting prognosis.

Lymph node involvement is present in half of the patients with deep muscle infiltration and has a poor prognosis. The disappointing long-term survival rate of patients with deeply invasive tumors has led to an integrated form of therapy in which irradiation is followed by cystectomy.

The best way to reduce the incidence is elimination of known carcinogens, especially cigarette smoke.

DIAGNOSTIC STUDIES[8]

Urine culture
  Sterile urine in patient with symptoms of cystitis

Urinary tract cytology
  Examination of midmorning specimen or bladder washings to detect abnormal cells

Intravenous urography
  Dilated ureter or nonfunctioning kidney

Intravenous pyelography
  Filling defects, halo or dye around base of bladder, flattening or rigidity of bladder wall

Cytoscopy with multiple biopsies
  Evidence of malignant tissue

Bimanual examination
  Revelation of firm or hard nodularity

Chest and skeletal roentgenograms, bone scans, and liver function studies
  Evidence of metastatic disease

TREATMENT PLAN[3]

Surgical
  Endoscopic resection and fulguration; cystectomy, prostatectomy and urethrectomy
  Cystectomy with urinary diversion

Chemotherapeutic
  Antineoplastic agents
    Thiotepa (Triethylenethiophosphoramide), IV 60 mg initially, usually at 1- to 4-wk intervals
    Cyclophosphamide (Cytoxan), 40-50 mg/kg IV in divided doses over several days, then adjusted to lower maintenance dosage; po 1-5 mg/kg/d
    Doxorubicin (Adriamycin), 60-75 mg/m² at intervals of 21 d, or 30 mg/m²/d for 3 d and repeated q4wk
    Cisplatin (Platinol), 50-80 mg/m² IV q3wk or individually determined dosage

Electromechanical
  Hydrostatic pressure from intravesical balloon
  Hyperthermia (investigational)
  Open diathermy
  External radiation—preoperative, radical alone, or palliative for local recurrence and bone pain

ASSESSMENT: AREAS OF CONCERN[3]

Urinary function
  Hematuria; urgency; dysuria; frequency; azotemia; pelvic mass

Comfort
  Low back pain

NURSING DIAGNOSES and NURSING INTERVENTIONS

Nursing Diagnosis	Nursing Intervention
Urinary elimination, alteration in patterns	Measure intake and output. Inspect urine for blood; check with Hemastix. Inspect abdomen for swelling and distention. Encourage adequate rest and exercise. Increase patient's fluid intake. Apply heating pad or hot water bottle to abdomen as ordered. Catheterize patient only if necessary. Monitor blood studies: acid-base balance, hemoglobin level, hematocrit value, blood urea nitrogen, and creatinine level. Monitor urine studies: acid-base balance, creatinine level, specific gravity, and protein level.
Comfort, alteration in: pain	Change patient's position slowly. Place patient in whirlpool bath or apply heat. Provide safety measures. Administer bladder antispasmodics as ordered. Discuss possible pain-relieving measures with patient; use those possible. Evaluate effectiveness of pain relief measures.

Patient Education

1. Emphasize the need for adequate fluid intake, exercise, and rest.
2. Discuss pain-relieving measures such as exercise, warmth, safety, and medication.
3. Instruct the patient in self-care.

EVALUATION

Patient Outcome	Data Indicating That Outcome is Reached
Daily fluid output is equal to fluid intake.	Urine output is 1500 to 3000 ml daily or equivalent to intake.
Laboratory findings are within normal limits.	Blood urea nitrogen, serum creatinine, hematocrit, hemoglobin, and blood pH values are within normal limits. Creatinine clearance and urine creatinine level, pH, and specific gravity are within normal limits; no protein is found in urine.
Patient is comfortable.	Facial expression is calm and relaxed. Patient has freedom of body movement. Patient expresses comfort and ceases to complain.

CANCERS OF THE MALE REPRODUCTIVE SYSTEM
Cancer of the Prostate

Cancer of the prostate is a malignant tumor arising from the parenchyma of the prostate gland.

The prostate is the third most common site of cancer in men, accounting for 17% of all male cancers. The incidence and mortality of this cancer are increasing, especially in blacks.[2]

Most prostatic cancers are adenocarcinomas discovered by a physician during rectal examination, which should be done yearly on all men over 50 years of age.

These slow-growing tumors arise in the posterior portion of the prostate and eventually involve the entire gland. They spread via the lymphatics throughout the pelvic region and into the pelvic bones.

Early symptoms resemble those of benign prostatic hypertrophy and include weak urinary stream, urinary frequency, dysuria, and difficulty in starting and stopping urination. Some patients initially report pain in the lower back, pelvis, or upper thighs. Bilateral ureteral obstruction with renal insufficiency is not uncommon at the time of diagnosis.[8]

PATHOPHYSIOLOGY[3]

The cellular appearance of these adenocarcinomas is a definite glandular pattern with small gland size or lack of papillae in a disorderly connective tissue framework. By the time of diagnosis, most prostatic cancers have already invaded the base of the bladder, seminal vesicles, or perivesicular fascia or moved laterally into the levator ani muscles.

Grading of these tumors—well, moderately, or poorly differentiated—correlates with the prognosis.

DIAGNOSTIC STUDIES[8]

Digital rectal examination
Fifty percent of palpable prostatic nodules are cancer

Closed needle biopsy via perineal or transrectal route or open biopsy
Evidence of malignant cells

Prostatic acid phosphatase (PAP)
Elevated in localized disease

Serum total acid phosphatase
Elevated in two thirds of cases of metastatic spread; bone marrow acid phosphatase more accurate indicator

Alkaline phosphatase
Elevated with bony metastases

Bone survey, bone scan
Detection of bony metastases

Excretory urogram
Bladder outlet involvement; ureteral obstruction or displacement

Pelvic computed tomography scans
Local extensions; nodal involvement

Lymphangiography
Para-aortic and pelvic node involvement

TREATMENT PLAN[3]

Treatment is based on clinical assessment, stage of disease, anticipated tolerance to therapy, morbidity, and expected longevity.

Surgical
Radical prostatectomy by perineal, retropubic, or transpubic route
Orchiectomy

Chemotherapeutic
Estrogens
Diethylstilbestrol (DES, Stilbestrol), 1.5-15 mg po
Corticosteroids
Prednisone (Deltasone, others), 10-100 mg po

Electromechanical
Supervoltage radiotherapy for palliation

ASSESSMENT: AREAS OF CONCERN[5]

Urinary function
Weak urinary stream; urinary frequency; dysuria; difficulty starting and stopping urination; renal insufficiency (azotemia, decreased output)

Comfort level
Pain in lower back, pelvis, or upper thighs

NURSING DIAGNOSES and NURSING INTERVENTIONS

Nursing Diagnosis	Nursing Intervention
Urinary elimination, alteration in patterns	Measure intake and output. Be alert for patient's complaints of frequency, pain, and urination difficulties. Encourage adequate rest and activity. Increase patient's fluid intake. Catheterize patient only if necessary.
Urinary elimination, alteration in patterns (related to renal insufficiency)	Monitor blood studies: blood urea nitrogen, creatinine, acid-base balance, hemoglobin, and hematocrit. Monitor urine studies: acid-base balance, creatinine, and specific gravity. Inspect for edema. Weigh daily and measure intake and output. Monitor blood pressure and oral temperature. Test urine for protein.

Nursing Diagnosis	Nursing Intervention
Comfort, alteration in: pain (bone)	Change patient's position slowly. Support affected body parts. Place patient in whirlpool bath or use heat applications. Provide safety measures. Discuss possible pain-relieving measures with patient; use those possible or ordered. Evaluate effectiveness of pain relief measures.

Patient Education

1. Inform the patient of the need for adequate fluid intake, exercise, and rest.
2. Instruct the patient in pain-relieving measures such as exercise, warmth, and medication.
3. Tell the patient to notify the physician if signs and symptoms of renal insufficiency appear. Discuss these with the patient.

EVALUATION

Patient Outcome	Data Indicating That Outcome is Reached
Laboratory findings are within normal limits.	Blood urea nitrogen, hemoglobin, hematocrit, blood pH, and serum creatinine are within normal limits. Creatinine clearance and urine specific gravity, pH, and creatinine are within normal limits; urine test for protein is negative.
Body hydration is normal.	There is no edema.
Fluid output equals fluid intake.	Urine output is 1500 to 3000 ml daily or equivalent to intake.

Testicular Carcinoma

Testicular cancer is a malignant neoplastic disease of the testis occurring most frequently in men between 20 and 35 years of age.

The incidence of testicular carcinoma is higher in men with undescended testes (cryptorchidism). The first sign of the disease is usually a small, hard, painless lump in the testicle; symptoms are a sensation of heaviness in the testicle, sudden fluid accumulation in the scrotum, and perineal pain or discomfort.[2]

PATHOPHYSIOLOGY[8]

Most testicular tumors are of germ cell origin and are malignant. The basic categories are the seminoma and heterogeneous, nonseminomatous germ cell tumor. Para-aortic lymph node involvement, ureteral obstruction, and pulmonary metastases may be present.[3]

DIAGNOSTIC STUDIES[8]

Palpation of testes
Presence of mass

Examination of breasts
Presence of gynecomastia

Transillumination
Detection of intrascrotal lesions

Abdominal examination
Palpable mass

Excretory urogram
Ureteral deviation from para-aortic or paracaval nodal involvement

Radioimmunoassay (RIA)
Elevated serum α-fetoprotein (AFP) and human chorionic gonadotropin (HCG)

Abdominal computed tomography scan
For staging

Chest roentgenogram and computed tomography scan
To detect metastatic disease

TREATMENT PLAN[3]

Surgical
Inguinal exploration and orchiectomy
Bilateral retroperitoneal lymph node dissection

Chemotherapeutic
Antineoplastic agents
For seminomas
Cyclophosphamide (Cytoxan), 40-50 mg/kg IV in divided doses over several days; then adjust to lower maintenance dose
Chlorambucil (Leukeran), 4-10 mg po qd
For nonseminomas
Cisplatin (Platinol), 50-80 mg/m^2 IV q3wk, or dosage individually determined
Vinblastine sulfate (Velban), 0.1 mg/kg increased weekly by 0.05 mg/kg up to 0.5 mg/kg
Bleomycin sulfate (Blenoxane), 0.25-0.5 units/kg, or 10-20 units/m^2 IV, IM, or subcutaneously 1 or 2 times/wk
Dactinomycin (Cosmegen), 0.015-0.05 mg/kg IV divided doses over 1 wk; repeat for 3-5 wk

Electromechanical
Radiation
For seminomas—irradiation of retroperitoneal and homolateral iliac nodes to level of diaphragm; may also include mediastinum and supraclavicular node area
For nonseminomas—occasionally used for localized metastases that cannot be excised and do not respond to chemotherapy

Dramatic responses to single agent and combination drug chemotherapy have made even advanced cases of testicular cancer curable. Radiation therapy is still used for seminomas but has been replaced by chemotherapy for nonseminomatous tumors. Tumor markers (AFP and HCG) are useful not only in early diagnosis but also in follow-up monitoring for recurrent disease.

ASSESSMENT: AREAS OF CONCERN[3]

Scrotum
Small, hard, painless lump; sensation of heaviness; fluid accumulation; pain or discomfort

Urinary function
Renal insufficiency (azotemia); decreased output

Cardiovascular function
Dyspnea; tachycardia; confusion

NURSING DIAGNOSES and NURSING INTERVENTIONS

Nursing Diagnosis	Nursing Intervention
Comfort, alteration in: pain (scrotal)	Approach patient unhurriedly and provide reassurance. Handle patient gently. Position patient comfortably. Apply heat as ordered with heating pad, hot water bottle, warm moist compress, or warm water bath. Discuss pain-relieving measures such as scrotal support and analgesics; implement them as feasible. Evaluate effectiveness of pain-relieving measures. Be alert for complaints of pain and assess duration and radiation.
Urinary elimination, alteration in patterns (related to renal insufficiency)	Monitor blood studies: blood urea nitrogen, creatinine, acid-base balance, hemoglobin, and hematocrit. Monitor urine studies: acid-base balance, creatinine, and specific gravity. Inspect for hematuria and edema. Measure blood pressure and oral temperature. Test urine for protein.
Tissue perfusion, alteration in: pulmonary	Elevate patient's head. Place patient in sitting position. Monitor rest and activity. Encourage coughing and deep breathing.

Nursing Diagnosis	Nursing Intervention
	Inspect chest for respiratory rate and rhythm.
	Auscultate for abnormal breath sounds, lung aeration, rales, and rhonchi.
	Monitor blood pressure and pulse.
	Monitor blood studies and gas exchange.
	Observe for confusion and dyspnea.

Patient Education

1. Inform the patient of the need for adequate fluid intake, exercise, and rest.
2. Instruct the patient in the use of pain relief measures such as exercise and warmth.
3. Tell the patient to notify the physician if signs of respiratory distress or renal insufficiency appear.
4. Emphasize the need for follow-up evaluation.

EVALUATION[4]

Patient Outcome	Data Indicating That Outcome is Reached
Vital signs are within normal limits.	Respiratory rate, rhythm, and depth are normal; pulse rate and blood pressure are within normal limits.
Laboratory findings are within normal limits.	Blood urea nitrogen, hemoglobin, hematocrit, blood pH, oxygen saturation, and serum creatinine are within normal limits. Creatinine clearance and urine specific gravity, pH, and creatinine are within normal limits; findings of urine test for protein are negative.
Body hydration is normal	There is no edema.
Body functioning is normal.	Elimination is adequate.
Daily fluid output is equal to fluid intake.	Urine output is 1500 to 3000 ml daily or equivalent to intake.
Patient is comfortable.	Facial expression is calm and relaxed. Posture is normal. Patient has freedom of body movement. Patient expresses comfort and ceases to complain.
Patient frequently changes position and has normal body movement.	Patient walks, sits, and stands with normal body movement.

GYNECOLOGIC CANCERS

Cancer of the uterus, both endometrial and cervical (including in situ), accounts for 14% of all female cancers. Cancers of the female genital organs—uterus, ovaries, vulva, and vagina—are second only to breast cancer in causing morbidity and mortality in women.

Cancer of the Cervix

Cancer of the uterine cervix is a neoplasm of the uterine cervix that can be detected in the early, curable stage by the Papanicolaou (Pap) test.

Cancer of the uterine cervix has its highest incidence in women who are 35 years of age or older, began sexual activity in puberty, and have had multiple partners. Other risk factors include low socioeconomic status, poor prenatal and postnatal care, and in utero exposure to diethylstilbestrol (DES). Women in urban, industrialized areas and white or Jewish women have a lower incidence of the disease than do those in rural, underdeveloped areas and nonwhites. Celibate women and those in religious groups that encourage male circumcision and monogamy also have a lower incidence. Women with multiple genital infections such as herpes, *Trichomonas* infection, and gonorrhea are at greater risk.

Improved general and genital hygiene and cytologic screening with the Papanicolaou (Pap) smear have contributed to decreased mortality of cervical cancer. The

American Cancer Society now recommends that, after two negative Pap tests 1 year apart, women over 20 years who are not at high risk should be tested at least every 3 years. Sexually active women under 20 years should also follow this schedule. Women at risk are encouraged to have a yearly Pap test.

Changes in cells of the cervical epithelium may be present for 10 years before invasive cancer develops. However, a Pap smear can detect even the earliest changes, so regular Pap tests, as well as manual pelvic examinations, are the most important means of reducing mortality from cervical cancer.[2,3]

PATHOPHYSIOLOGY[3]

The first sign of uterine cancer is unusual bleeding or vaginal discharge between menstrual periods, after intercourse, or after menopause. When symptoms appear, the cancer has usually progressed beyond its early stages. Squamous cell carcinoma accounts for 95% of all invasive tumors diagnosed, and adenocarcinomas account for most of the rest. Clear cell carcinoma develops in the cervix and vagina of women exposed in utero to DES. Invasive carcinoma of the cervix spreads by direct extension to the vaginal wall, laterally into the parametrium toward the pelvic wall, and anteroposteriorly into the bladder and rectum. Metastases to the pelvic lymph nodes are more common than those to distant nodes.

DIAGNOSTIC STUDIES[8]

Pathologic examination of multiple cervical biopsy specimens by Schiller test with endocervical curettage or colposcopy; conization when colposcopic examination unsatisfactory
  Evidence of malignant cells by Pap test

Cystoscopy
  Establishes normal bladder anatomy

Intravenous pyelogram
  Ascertains that ureters are unobstructed and that kidney and upper collecting system are normal

Lymphangiography
  Screening for lymph node metastases

TREATMENT PLAN[3]

The clinical stage of the tumor at the time of diagnosis is used to determine therapy and prognosis.

Surgical
  For mild to moderate dysplasia
    Cryocautery
    Thermocauterization
    Laser surgery
  For carcinoma in situ
    Simple hysterectomy if patient is beyond childbearing age or does not want more children
    Excision of mucocutaneous junctional tissue and regular examinations for women who wish to have children
  For invasive carcinoma
    Total hysterectomy
  For central recurrent or persistent pelvic cancer
    Pelvic exenteration

Chemotherapeutic
  Poor results when patient has far advanced disease
  Antineoplastic agents
    Drugs used in combination; dosages of combination drugs individually determined (see Chapter 13 for criteria)
      Methotrexate (Amethopterin, Mexate, MTX)
      Bleomycin (Blenoxane)
      Mitomycin (Mutamycin)
      Cisplatin (Platinol), 50-80 mg/m^2 IV q3wk or by individually determined dosage

Electromechanical
  Radiation therapy—combination of external and intracavity (radium) therapy; doses determined by tolerance of surrounding organs (rectum, bladder, and small intestine)

The prognosis for stage I (vaginal wall) invasive cancer is similar for pregnant and nonpregnant women, but pregnancy seems to have an unfavorable effect on the prognosis of more advanced disease. Caesarean section is the indicated delivery method for these patients.

There is no proof that postoperative pelvic or para-aortic radiation is effective in improving the prognosis for patients with lymphatic metastases, although further studies are in progress.

More than 55% of treated patients live 5 years. Radical surgery can now be performed safely with limited morbidity. The overall cure rate is 29%.

ASSESSMENT: AREAS OF CONCERN[5]

Perineal hygiene
  Unusual bleeding or vaginal discharge; profuse, malodorous discharge

Circulatory function
  Lymphedema

Level of comfort
 Back and leg pain; inability to lie with leg straightened; feeling of pressure; heavy, aching abdominal pain

Gastrointestinal
 Rectal discharge; feeling of pressure

NURSING DIAGNOSES and NURSING INTERVENTIONS

Nursing Diagnosis	Nursing Intervention

Comfort, alteration in: pain	For abdominal pressure:
	    Change patient's position frequently.
	    Give small, frequent feedings.
	    Place patient in sitting position.
	    Remove constrictive clothing.
	    Insert rectal tube per policy.
	    Auscultate abdomen for abnormal bowel sounds.
	For back pain, leg pain, or lymphedema:
	    Position comfortably, and change position slowly.
	    Maintain body alignment.
	    Apply heating pad, hot water bottle, or warm, moist compress.
	    Bathe in warm water.
	    Massage gently.
	    Encourage adequate rest.
	    Provide pain relief measure of patient's choice.
	    Be alert for complaints of pain and assess duration and radiation.
	    Evaluate effectiveness of interventions.

Skin integrity, impairment of: potential (related to vaginal or rectal infection)	Anticipate needs. Bathe locally. Change dressings or pads frequently. Maintain dry, clean linen and dry skin. Provide clean clothing. Position patient comfortably. Observe skin for irritation. Observe quality and quantity of drainage. Administer antibiotics as ordered. Monitor vital signs.

Patient Education

1. Teach the patient to carry out comfort measures.
2. Teach the patient ways to avoid unnecessary pain to abdomen, back, legs, and other areas.
3. Emphasize the need to maintain skin hygiene.

EVALUATION

Patient Outcome	Data Indicating That Outcome is Reached
Vital signs are within normal limits.	Respiratory rate, pulse rate, blood pressure, and temperature are within normal limits.
Body is clean.	Skin is clean. There is no unpleasant body odor. Patient feels clean and refreshed.
Patient is comfortable.	Facial expression is calm, contented, and relaxed. Posture is normal. Patient has freedom of body movement. Patient expresses comfort and satisfaction.
Patient does not have infection.	There is no evidence of inflammation, purulent drainage or secretions, pain, or aching. Blood leukocyte count is 4500 to 11,000 cells/mm^3.

Other Gynecologic Cancers

Malignant diseases occur in all parts of the female reproductive system. They include cancers of the uterine endometrium, the vagina, the vulva, the ovaries, and the fallopian tubes, as well as gestational trophoblastic neoplasms.

Endometrial cancer. Endometrial cancer is less common than cervical cancer in young women, but the diseases occur with equal frequency in postmenopausal women. Etiologic factors include infertility, late menopause (after 55 years of age), obesity, diabetes, and hypertension. Long-term diethylstilbestrol (DES) therapy may also be a factor. Cancer of the endometrium occurs with higher frequency in urban, white, and Jewish women. The benefits of maintaining an ideal weight and careful management of estrogen therapy for menopause should be emphasized.[2]

The most common initial symptom is intermenstrual or postmenopausal bleeding. The diagnosis of endometrial cancer is based on histologic tissue examination.

The usual treatment for cancer limited to the fundal portion of the uterus is preoperative intracavity radiation therapy followed by total hysterectomy and bilateral salpingo-oophorectomy. External radiation is added to the treatment plan when the cancer extends beyond the fundus.

The 5-year survival rate for patients with early endometrial cancer is greater than 85%. The cure rate drops to 50% when the cancer has metastasized.

Vaginal cancer. Vaginal carcinoma is rarely a primary lesion, although it does occur in both menopausal and postmenopausal women. It is related to in utero DES exposure in younger women. Vaginal cancer is rare in black and Jewish women. The primary signs and symptoms are vaginal spotting and discharge, pain, groin masses, and changes in urinary pattern.

Radiation therapy consists of intracavity irradiation combined with total pelvic external irradiation. Radical surgery includes complete vaginectomy, pelvic node dissection, and anterior exenteration as indicated. Grafting may be used to avoid vaginal stenosis, especially in younger patients.

Vulvar cancer. Fewer than 1% of female genital cancers are found in the vulva. Vulvar cancer occurs most commonly in women who are between 50 and 70 years and in lower socioeconomic strata. Symptoms include vaginal discharge, pruritus, and bleeding.

The leukoplakic changes (whitish, plaquelike or ulcerated lesions) that precede carcinoma can be eliminated by simple vulvectomy. Once carcinoma develops, invasion of the inguinal nodes and the lower vagina is common.

Surgery for this form of cancer may be preventive to remove precancerous lesions (hemivulvectomy or local excision with a wide margin of normal tissue), curative (radical vulvectomy), or palliative (extent depends on the patient's symptoms).

The 5-year survival rate is greater than 80% for women with early, localized lesions but is much lower when nodal or distant metastasis is present.

Ovarian cancer. Ovarian cancer has replaced cervical cancer as the leading cause of death from genital cancer. Its development is closely linked to breast cancer, which suggests abnormal endocrine activity. The peak incidence is between 60 and 80 years of age.

These tumors do not usually produce symptoms until intra-abdominal metastasis has occurred, with outward signs such as ascites. Therefore the mortality is high; only 34% of patients survive the disease. When symptoms do occur, they include increasing abdominal girth, weight loss, abdominal pain, dysuria or urinary frequency, and constipation.

Treatment of ovarian cancer consists of hysterectomy and bilateral salpingo-oophorectomy. Radiation therapy and chemotherapy may be used in conjunction with surgery or when the cancer is inoperable.

Cancer of the fallopian tube. Fallopian tube cancer is the rarest of the gynecologic malignancies. It is difficult to diagnose, and diagnosis is usually at time of surgery. Most are adenocarcinomas. Patients are usually in their midfifties when fallopian tube cancer is detected. The most common symptoms are pelvic pain, abnormal vaginal bleeding, and a heavy, watery vaginal discharge. Colicky pain may be associated with bleeding.

Removal of the uterus, fallopian tubes, ovaries, and omentum is the usual treatment. Radiation and chemotherapy have been used postoperatively with some success. Survival rates are as high as 90% with early disease, although the overall 5-year survival rate is 38%.

Gestational trophoblastic neoplasms. The gestational trophoblastic neoplasms include hydatidiform mole, invasive mole (chorioadenoma destruens), and choriocarcinoma. Molar pregnancy, the most common of these tumors, occurs in approximately 1 in 1500 live births in the United States; locally invasive disease develops in 16% of these patients and metastatic disease in 31%. These neoplasms can also develop after abortal, ectopic, and term gestations.

The measurement of human chorionic gonadotropin (HCG) by the β subunit radioimmunoassay test is essential for diagnosis, monitoring of therapy, and follow-up. Early diagnosis is facilitated by amniography and ultrasonography.

Hydatidiform mole is treated with suction curettage when preserving fertility is desirable. Actinomycin D, given prophylactically, reduces the incidence of sequelae when the uterus is larger than the fruit dates, the serum HCG titer is over 100,000 mU/dl, and the ovaries are cystic. Postevacuation monitoring of HCG levels is done weekly for 3 consecutive weeks and then monthly for 6 months or until HCG is undetectable. During this time pregnancy should be avoided. If fertility is not desired, total abdominal hysterectomy is the treatment of choice when the mole is in situ.

Locally invasive mole or choriocarcinoma is diagnosed by elevated HCG level, pelvic angiography, ultrasonography, and curettage. If fertility is desired, intermittent courses of single agent chemotherapy, such as methotrexate with citrovorum rescue or actinomycin D, yield a cure rate of 100%. When fertility is not desired, hysterectomy is the treatment of choice.

Metastasis is most common with choriocarcinoma; the most frequent sites are the lung, vagina, oral cavity, gastrointestinal tract, central nervous system, and liver. The treatment of choice is chemotherapy with a single agent or a combination of drugs. Surgery or adjunctive radiation therapy may be required. The overall survival with metastasis is still good, although the prognosis is poor with metastases to the liver or brain.[3,8]

CANCERS OF THE HEAD AND NECK

Cancers of the head and neck are neoplasms characterized by the uncontrolled growth of anaplastic cells in the larynx, oral cavity, pharynx, or salivary glands.

Although less than 5% of all cancers are neoplasms of the head and neck, they are important because surgical treatment may result in extensive cosmetic deformities and may impair such vital functions as eating and speaking. Patients with head and neck cancers represent 15% of cancer admissions to large medical centers.[2]

The most common site is the larynx, followed by the oral cavity, pharynx, and salivary glands. Etiologic factors for oral and laryngeal cancers include wood dust (nasal cavity cancer), chronic irritation, poor oral hygiene, prolonged heavy use of alcohol, snuff, or tobacco, and Epstein-Barr virus (associated with nasopharyngeal cancer).

PATHOPHYSIOLOGY

Most head and neck cancers grow as malignant ulcerations on surface mucosa. The infiltrative, endophytic lesions are more aggressive and difficult to control than the less common elevated, fungating, exophytic growths. The signs and symptoms depend on the location and are as follows:
1. Oral cavity—swelling or ulcer that fails to heal and bleeds easily
2. Oropharynx—"silent" area; dysphagia, local pain, pain on swallowing, referred pain to ear, enlarging cervical mass
3. Hypopharynx—another "silent" area; dysphagia, painful swallowing of food, referred ear pain, or neck mass
4. Nasopharynx—bloody nasal discharge, obstructed nostril, neurologic problems such as facial pain, diplopia, or hoarseness, conductive deafness
5. Nose and sinuses—bloody nasal discharge, nasal obstruction, diplopia, facial pain or swelling
6. Parotic and submandibular glands—painless local swelling, hemifacial paralysis
7. Larynx—persistent hoarseness, pain, referred ear pain, dyspnea, stridor[3,8]

DIAGNOSTIC STUDIES[8]

Inspection, directly and via mirror, of oral cavity, nasopharynx, oropharynx, larynx, and hypopharynx
Visualization of suspect lesion

Fiberoptic aerodigestive endoscopy
Visualization and biopsy of suspect lesion

Palpation of cervical lymphatics
Metastatic nodes hard, oval, or round

Biopsy of suspect lesions
Histologic evidence of malignancy

Radiographic studies for staging workup; plain films of skull and its base, sinuses, and lateral neck soft tissue; computed tomography for staging
Visualization of suspect lesion and metastatic process

Chest roentgenograms
Presence of metastasis or second primary tumor

Bone scan
Evidence of metastasis

Anti-Epstein-Barr virus (EBV) antibody titers
Elevation of immunoglobulin G (IgG) and immunoglobulin A (IgA) fairly specific indicators for nasopharyngeal carcinoma

TREATMENT PLAN[3]

The goals of treatment for head and neck cancers are (1) eradication of both clinically demonstrated disease and microscopic subclinical disease; (2) maintenance of adequate physiologic function by reversal of present dysfunction and posttreatment dysfunction in the special senses, chewing and swallowing, respiration, and speech; and (3) socially acceptable cosmesis including sufficient surgical, radiation, plastic surgical, and prosthesis rehabilitation.

Treatment decisions involve a multidisciplinary approach with emphasis on such factors as age, general physical condition, other morbidity (such as extensive dental disease, premalignant mucosa, leukoplakia, erythroplasia, or second primary lesion), habits and lifestyle, occupation, and the patient's desires.

Surgery and radiation therapy are the major curative modalities. Chemotherapy is employed as adjuvant therapy or sequentially before radiation or surgery.

More than 75% of head and neck cancer patients whose treatment fails have the first recurrence in areas above the clavicles. The most common failure pattern is recurrent primary tumor with neck metastasis and subsequent carotid erosion or rupture. Distant metastasis to the lung, bone, and elsewhere occurs in long-term survivors of local or regional disease. Intercurrent disease such as alcoholism or chronic lung disease, accidents, and suicide account for 10% to 30% of deaths.

Cancers of the Oral Cavity

Cancers of the oral cavity are neoplasms that may invade the tongue, buccal mucosa, and hard palate.

Small, localized lesions of the oral cavity may be treated with radiation therapy or surgery or both. Larger lesions may be irradiated before surgical excision. Tumors that spread to cervical lymph nodes require radical neck dissection. Overall survival for carcinoma of the oral cavity is 40% to 65%, depending on site. Early primary lesions have the best prognosis.

ASSESSMENT: AREAS OF CONCERN[3]

Oral cavity appearance and function
Leukoplakia (white patch); erythroplasia (red patch); chronic, nonhealing ulcer; localized pain; dysphagia

Lymphatic function
Enlarged nodes

NURSING DIAGNOSES and NURSING INTERVENTIONS

Nursing Diagnosis	Nursing Intervention
Oral mucous membrane, alteration in	Provide frequent oral hygiene; use soft brush. Offer nonirritating (nonacidic) foods. Refrain from giving hot or iced liquids. Apply local analgesics as needed.
Nutrition, alteration in: less than body requirements	Place patient in sitting position. Feed slowly with small, frequent feedings; provide high-calorie, high-protein diet. Give clear liquid, full-liquid, pureed, or soft foods as tolerated. Have suction equipment available.

Patient Education

1. Emphasize the need for adequate oral hygiene and dietary management.
2. Discuss signs and symptoms of progressive disease or side effects of treatment that should be reported to the physician.

EVALUATION

Patient Outcome	Data Indicating That Outcome is Reached
Mucous membrane color is normal.	Mucous membrane is warm, moist, and of natural color.
Body hydration is normal.	Mucous membranes are moist. Patient is not thirsty.
Body functioning is normal.	Digestion is adequate.
Patient is comfortable.	Facial expression is calm and relaxed. Patient expresses comfort.

Cancer of the Larynx

Cancers of the larynx arise from the epithelial lining of the laryngeal mucous membrane.

Carcinoma of the supraglottic larynx (epiglottis, aryepiglottic folds, arytenoids, and false cords) has a lower incidence than glottic carcinoma; 60% to 65% of laryngeal carcinomas occur in the glottic larynx (true vocal cord). Ninety percent occur in men, with highest incidence in those between 60 and 70 years of age. The early warning sign of progressive hoarseness, caused by a change in the phonating edge of the vocal cord, has led to 5-year survival rates of nearly 80% for localized lesions.[2,8]

Early cancer can be treated by radiation therapy or surgery. Extensive lesions, which cause necrosis of cartilage or glottic extension, require total laryngectomy.[3]

ASSESSMENT: AREAS OF CONCERN[3]

Respiratory function
Hoarseness; dyspnea; stridor; hemoptysis

Gastrointestinal function
Dysphagia

Level of comfort
Pain referred to ear (otalgia)

NURSING DIAGNOSES and NURSING INTERVENTIONS

Nursing Diagnosis	Nursing Intervention
Breathing pattern, ineffective	Place patient in sitting position. Encourage deep breathing. Inspect chest for respiratory rate, rhythm, and expansion. Auscultate for abnormal breath sounds and lung aeration. Palpate and percuss chest. Monitor blood studies. Suction airway as necessary. Provide standby emergency equipment (oxygen and tracheostomy tray). Provide tracheostomy or laryngectomy care as indicated.
Nutrition, alteration in: less than body requirements	Place patient in sitting position. Feed slowly with small, frequent feedings. Give clear-liquid, full-liquid, pureed, or soft foods as tolerated. Have suction equipment available.
Comfort, alteration in: pain	Apply heating pad, hot water bottle, or warm, moist compress to ear. Maintain warm room temperature. Provide pain relief measure of patient's choice. Evaluate effectiveness of pain relief measures. Encourage adequate rest. Be alert for complaints of pain and assess duration and radiation.

Patient Education

1. Explain methods of maintaining respiratory function, such as deep breathing and use of oxygen; provide a list of emergency resources.
2. Emphasize the need for adequate dietary management.
3. Discuss the value of speech therapy and put the patient in touch with support groups such as the Lost Cord Club.
4. Teach the patient methods of managing pain.
5. Discuss signs and symptoms of progressive disease and side effects of treatment that should be reported to the physician.

EVALUATION

Patient Outcome	Data Indicating That Outcome is Reached
Skin and mucous membrane color is normal.	Skin, nails, lips, and earlobes are warm and moist and have natural color.
Vital signs are within normal limits.	Respiratory rate, rhythm, and depth are normal. Breathing pattern is regular. Patient does not have respiratory distress.
Laboratory findings are within normal limits.	Blood oxygen saturation and carbon dioxide are within normal limits.
Body hydration is normal.	Mucous membranes are moist. Patient is not thirsty.
Body functioning is normal.	Digestion is adequate.
Patient is comfortable.	Facial expression is calm and relaxed. Patient expresses comfort.

CARCINOMAS OF THE DIGESTIVE AND ENDOCRINE GLANDS

Approximately 6% of cancers detected in the United States affect the digestive and endocrine glands. Some are easily detected because of their location and secretory patterns, whereas others are more difficult to diagnose. The 5-year survival rate varies from 1% for pancreatic carcinoma to 95% for localized thyroid cancer.[2]

Digestive Tumors

Carcinomas of the digestive glands are neoplasms that may involve the pancreas, liver, or gallbladder.

Carcinoma of the gallbladder, with its insidious onset, may be diagnosed only during surgery for presumed acute cholecystitis. The only possibility of cure is with complete removal of the gallbladder; often a partial hepatectomy is also required because of early liver invasion. Mortality is as high as 75%; four times as many women as men are dead 1 year after diagnosis.

Carcinoma of the liver is usually metastatic; primary tumors constitute only 1% of hepatic cancer. One primary tumor, hemangiosarcoma of the liver, is a rare disease believed to be caused by vinyl chloride exposure. The risk of hepatocellular carcinoma is about 40 times greater in patients with cirrhosis. Early signs and symptoms of hepatic cancer are often absent or insidious and slow to localize. The most common complaints are vague upper abdominal pain and generalized weakness. Other indications of liver involvement are anemia, anorexia, jaundice, weight loss, pain, and respiratory distress. Obstruction of the portal vein, sometimes occurring suddenly, may cause splenomegaly, esophageal varices, and ascites. Patients may also have fever of unknown origin and dependent edema. Diagnosis is based on laboratory data obtained from a liver profile, scanning, angiography, and biopsy.

The only possibility for cure is lobectomy to remove the diseased tissue. In some major medical centers, liver transplantation is being used as an alternative procedure for eligible patients. If surgery is contraindicated by the extent of the disease or the patient's condition, radiation therapy and chemotherapy via implantable infusion pump may be used. The prognosis is poor, and few patients are alive 5 years after the initial diagnosis.

Carcinoma of the pancreas has increased more than 20% in recent years. The reason for this is unknown, although cigarette smoking and coffee may be causative factors. As in liver and gallbladder disease, the onset is insidious and the diagnosis is made late in the course. Clinical signs indicating the tumor's location include the following:

1. Head of the pancreas—obstructive jaundice resulting from blockage of the common bile duct
2. Body and tail of the pancreas—vague abdominal or back pain, progressive weight loss, anorexia, and a variety of gastrointestinal symptoms
3. Islet cells—hypoglycemia and insulin-shock syndrome resulting from production of large quantities of insulin

As many as half of these patients have occult blood in the stools. The pain is steady, dull, and aching and unrelated to digestive activity. Because of the vagueness of the signs and symptoms, few pancreatic tumors are diagnosed at a curable stage. The diagnosis is usually based on tomographic scanning, ultrasonography, and biopsy.

Pancreatoduodenectomy (Whipple's procedure) is rarely used because of its high morbidity and mortality, although it has been helpful in cancer of the head of the pancreas. Palliation may be effected with radiation therapy or chemotherapy. The prognosis is extremely poor; only 10% of patients are still alive 1 year after diagnosis.

Salivary gland tumors grow slowly and are often diagnosed late. Complete excision, although difficult to accomplish without producing facial nerve damage, is important to prevent recurrence. If the tumor cannot be removed surgically, radiation therapy may be used to shrink it.

Endocrine Gland Tumors

Endocrine gland tumors may occur in the parathyroid, thyroid, or adrenal glands.

Parathyroid tumors are rare. When they do occur, they produce excessive amounts of parathyroid hormone, which causes bony deformities and renal calculi. These tumors are treated by surgical excision.

Carcinoma of the thyroid has its highest incidence (37% of endocrine cancers) in persons 25 to 44 years of age. It occurs most frequently in women and in whites.

High-risk persons are those who as children received radiation therapy to the neck for such conditions as hypertrophy of the tonsils, adenoids, or lymphatic tissue, enlarged thymus gland, or skin disorders such as acne.

The initial sign of a thyroid tumor is a lump in the gland, which may first be palpated during a routine physical examination. More extensive local involvement causes hoarseness, dysphagia, or dyspnea. Thyroid scanning, ultrasonography, and biopsy are used to diagnose the lesion, which is most commonly papillary carcinoma of the thyroid, a slow-growing, easily removed tumor. Even without total surgical eradication, many patients live 10 to 15 years with few symptoms. The 5-year survival rate is 97% for patients with localized disease and 86% if the disease has spread. Spread is usually to adjacent cervical lymph nodes.

Undifferentiated thyroid cancers are more likely to cause tracheal compression and metastasis to cervical lymph nodes. For these patients treatment is lobectomy or total thyroidectomy and en bloc dissection of lymph nodes. Radioactive iodine (^{131}I) and radiation therapy may also be used.

Neoplasms of the adrenal glands cause changes in body functioning depending on the affected component. Cortical neoplasms may alter the body's sex characteristics and cause complex steroidal changes such as Cushing's syndrome. Medullary neoplasms may precipitate attacks of hypertension.

The median age for occurrence is 40 years, although persons of any age may be affected. The tumors may be benign or malignant and may be linked with a specific pituitary tumor.

Signs and symptoms, such as pain, distention, and hemorrhage, are usually noted at a late stage when local extension obstructs or destroys the kidneys. Pheochromocytoma, a tumor of the adrenal medulla, secretes an adrenalin-like substance that causes paroxysmal or sustained hypertension. The diagnosis is based on intravenous pyelography, tomography, ultrasonography, and urinalysis of hormones such as 17-ketosteroid.

Surgical excision, the treatment of choice, necessitates temporary or permanent cortisone replacement therapy. Radiation and chemotherapy may also be used, but since the diagnosis is rarely made before extension of the tumor has occurred, the prognosis is poor.[3,8]

Ovarian and testicular tumors are discussed elsewhere in this chapter.

CANCERS OF THE ESOPHAGUS AND STOMACH

Cancers of the esophagus and stomach account for 4% of all cancers. Unfortunately, many of the early symptoms of these diseases (dysphagia, epigastric discomfort, anorexia, and weight loss) are nonspecific, and therefore affected persons often delay seeking treatment. Cancers of the esophagus and stomach are discussed in detail in Chapter 11.

CANCERS OF BONE AND CONNECTIVE TISSUES

Sarcomas of bone and soft tissue, although relatively uncommon, are of particular interest because of their tendency to occur in young persons, their generally poor prognosis, and the major surgery usually required. The prognosis has been improved in recent years by the combination of local surgery and chemotherapy. In addition, in many patients the primary lesion can be successfully treated by more conservative surgical procedures combined with high-dose radiation therapy. However, 60% to 65% of bone cancers are metastatic from other primary lesions and thus are more difficult to treat successfully. In 1984 there were approximately 7000 new cases of these cancers and 4200 deaths.[2]

Bone Sarcomas

Bone cancer is a skeletal malignancy occurring as a primary sarcomatous tumor in an area of rapid growth.

Persons at high risk for development of bone sarcomas are those with Paget's disease of bone, Ollier's disease, multiple exostoses, retinoblastoma, or previous high-dose radiation therapy to bone. Osteosarcoma and Ewing's sarcoma occur most commonly in persons under the age of 20 years. This is in contrast to reticulum cell sarcoma, fibrosarcoma, and chondrosarcoma, which occur later in life but with a much wider age distribution.

PATHOPHYSIOLOGY[3]

The patient's complaints are initially subtle and intermittent with gradually increasing severity. An initially painless mass is the most common symptom; others include pain, functional deficit, or pathologic fracture. The pain is usually described as mild and brief and is often associated with a minor injury. It may increase in severity but is often reported as being a localized dull ache. It usually does not increase with activity or decrease with rest but may be greater at night. This pain rarely responds to simple analgesic medication but requires narcotics for relief.

There may not be any symptoms; if they are present, they are dependent on the size, site, and patterns of local infiltration. The site and extent of pathologic fractures dictate the severity of symptoms. Metastases to regional lymph nodes are uncommon, but systemic illness may be related to pulmonary, visceral, and subcutaneous tissue involvement.[3,8]

DIAGNOSTIC STUDIES[8]

Roentgenograms of involved bones and soft tissues
Visualization of suspect lesion

Chest roentgenogram
Evidence of metastasis

Bone scan
Evidence of primary lesion or metastasis

Computed tomography
Evidence of cortical bone destruction

Blood studies
Increased alkaline and acid phosphatase; increased calcium

Urine study
High calcium excretion

TREATMENT PLAN[3]

Surgical
Amputation with limb salvage to degree possible
  Foot and ankle—below-knee amputation or knee disarticulation
  Proximal tibia—thigh amputation
  Distal femur—hip disarticulation
  Proximal end of femur—modified hemipelvectomy
En bloc resection for low-grade malignant lesions; reconstruction with bone autografts, cadaver hemografts, or metal or plastic devices

Chemotherapeutic

Antineoplastic agents

Preoperative and postoperative systemic chemotherapy for osteogenic sarcoma; high-dose methotrexate (Amethopterin; Mexate) with leucovorin rescue; doxorubicin (Adriamycin) by intra-arterial perfusion; dosages individually determined

Systemic chemotherapy for metastatic disease

Electromechanical

Radiation therapy for treatment of Ewing's sarcoma before surgery

Supportive

Immunotherapy with interferon (investigational)

Disease-free survival rates for patients whose osteogenic sarcoma is treated with surgery and chemotherapy appear to be greater than 50% at 5 years. Among patients with localized Ewing's sarcoma the disease-free survival at 5 years is 50% following chemotherapy and radiation therapy.

ASSESSMENT: AREAS OF CONCERN[3]

Musculoskeletal function

Presence of mass; functional deficit; pathologic fracture

Pain

Mild and fleeting; dull and aching; increased at night; not affected by activity or rest; need for narcotics to obtain relief

Systemic function

Fever; malaise, easy fatigability; anorexia; weight loss

Respiratory function

Dyspnea; cough

NURSING DIAGNOSES and NURSING INTERVENTIONS

Nursing Diagnosis	Nursing Intervention
Mobility, impaired physical	Assist patient with ambulation; control distance. Have patient use walker, cane, or wheelchair as needed. Minimize environmental barriers. Encourage use of involved limb. Observe for deficits, weakness, or abnormal gait.
Comfort, alteration in: pain	Change patient's position slowly. Provide whirlpool or use heat applications. Provide patient safety. Discuss possible pain-relieving measures with patient; use those possible. Observe for increasing pain and dysfunction.
Nutrition, alteration in: less than body requirements	Balance nutritional intake. Supplement protein intake. Give small, frequent feedings and snacks. Grant patient requests. Provide selection of foods. Weigh patient daily. Observe and record food intake and diet tolerance.
Tissue perfusion, alteration in	Change patient's position frequently; place in sitting position. Encourage coughing and deep breathing. Monitor respiratory rate and rhythm and pulse. Auscultate chest. Monitor blood studies. Administer oxygen and respiratory therapy as ordered.
Activity intolerance	Ambulate patient or seat patient in armchair. Encourage moderate physical exercise, adequate rest, and performance of range of motion exercises. Balance nutritional intake; supplement protein. Observe for increased nutritional requirements and weakness.
Potential patient problem: body temperature elevation	Apply cool, damp cloth to face. Bathe in cool water or apply ice bag or alcohol to skin.

Nursing Diagnosis	Nursing Intervention
	Dress patient in lightweight clothing.
	Maintain cool room temperature.
	Encourage rest.
	Give antipyretics.
	Increase daily fluid intake to about 2000 ml.
	Measure temperature and intake and output.

Patient Education

1. Discuss the principles of safe ambulation: wide supportive stance, well-fitting low-heeled shoes, good body mechanics, and weight bearing on unaffected side.
2. Discuss the principles of good nutrition, especially protein supplementation.
3. Instruct the patient to report changes in respiratory status.

EVALUATION

Patient Outcome	Data Indicating That Outcome is Reached
Skin and mucous membrane color is normal.	Skin, nails, lips, and earlobes are warm and moist and have natural color.
Vital signs are within normal limits.	Respiratory rate, pulse rate, and temperature are within normal limits.
Laboratory findings are within normal limits.	Blood calcium, hemoglobin, hematocrit, oxygen saturation, carbon dioxide, and calcium are within normal limits.
Body functioning is normal.	Weight is stabilized. Digestion is adequate.
Vitality is good.	Patient is mentally alert and without malaise, fatigue, or weakness.
Patient has daily intake of essential food groups.	Milk, meat, fruits, vegetables, breads, and cereals are included in daily diet.
Patient is comfortable.	Facial expression is calm and relaxed. Posture is normal. Patient has freedom of body movement. Patient expresses comfort and ceases to complain.
Patient frequently changes position and has normal body movement.	Patient walks, sits, and stands with normal body movement.
Patient participates in therapeutic exercises.	Patient performs range of motion and isometric exercises.
Patient is receiving sufficient rest.	Coordination is good. Patient is not fatigued.
Patient's surroundings are safe.	Patient uses assistive devices such as walker or cane. There is no physical sign of accident having occurred. There is no evidence of complications arising from drugs or treatments.
No deformity has resulted from health treatment.	Hands, feet, limbs, and spine are in good alignment and functional. Patient has little or no pain.

Soft Tissue Sarcomas

Soft tissue sarcomas are neoplasms that arise in soft tissue, parenchymatous organs, or hollow viscera and include fibrosarcoma, malignant fibrous histiocytoma, liposarcoma, rhabdomyosarcoma, leiomyosarcoma, angiosarcoma, synovial sarcoma, mixed mesenchymal sarcoma, and unclassified or spindle cell sarcoma.

Only among children are soft tissue tumors, especially rhabdomyosarcoma, relatively frequent.[8]

PATHOPHYSIOLOGY[3]

A painless mass is the most common initial symptom. Masses in the thigh area are suspect because of the high number of sarcomas occurring there. Advanced local disease is rare except for large tumors arising in the retroperitoneal or pelvic areas. Lymph node metastases are uncommon except in patients with rhabdomyosarcoma, high-grade synovial sarcoma, and epithelioid sarcoma.

Rhabdomyosarcoma arises from the embryonic mesenchymal cells that form striated muscle. It may develop in almost any body site; the most common primary sites are the head and neck, extremities, genitourinary tract, trunk, and orbit. The prognosis depends on the primary site and the stage of the disease (histologic grade), which is in turn based on extent of disease and resectability. Genitourinary lesions generally have the most favorable prognosis, and extremity tumors have one of the worst prognoses.

DIAGNOSTIC STUDIES[8]

Radiographic study of affected part (computed tomography, xerography, arteriography)
Visualization of suspect lesion and vasculature

Chest tomography or chest computed tomography
Evidence of metastasis

Excisional, incisional, or needle biopsy
Histologic evidence of malignancy

TREATMENT PLAN[3]

Surgical
Radical surgical excision—amputation, muscle group resection, radical local excision

Chemotherapeutic
Antineoplastic agents
Vincristine sulfate (Oncovin), 2 mg/m² for children, 1.4 mg/m² for adults
Doxorubicin (Adriamycin), 60-75 mg/m² at intervals of 21 d or 30 mg/m² on each of 3 successive d repeated q4wk
Cyclophosphamide (Cytoxan), 40-50 mg/kg IV or individual doses over several days, then adjusted to lower maintenance dosage; po 1-5 mg/kg qd
Cisplatin (Platinol), 50-80 mg/m² IV q3wk or by individually determined dosage

Electromechanical
Radiation therapy—used with more conservative surgery, preoperatively and postoperatively

ASSESSMENT: AREAS OF CONCERN[3]

Body contours
Painless mass

Sensory and motor function
Peripheral neuralgia; paralysis

Vascular status
Ischemia

Gastrointestinal function
Bowel obstruction

Urinary function
Ureteral obstruction

Respiratory function
Dyspnea

NURSING DIAGNOSES and NURSING INTERVENTIONS

Nursing Diagnosis	Nursing Intervention
Mobility, impaired physical	Assist patient with ambulation; control distance. Use walker, cane, or wheelchair as needed. Minimize environmental barriers. Encourage use of involved limb. Observe for deficits, complaints of weakness, and abnormal gait. Test for impaired coordination.

Nursing Diagnosis	Nursing Intervention
Comfort, alteration in: pain	Change patient's position slowly. Support affected part(s). Place patient in whirlpool or use heat applications. Provide safety measures. Discuss possible pain-relieving measures with patient; use those possible. Monitor effectiveness of pain relief methods. Administer analgesics as ordered. Observe for increases in pain and dysfunction.
Urinary elimination, alteration in patterns	Inspect urine for bleeding. Encourage adequate rest and activity. Increase fluid intake to about 2000 ml daily. Monitor intake and output. Inspect abdomen for distention. Palpate bladder. Catheterize only if necessary.
Bowel elimination, alteration in	Place patient in sitting position. Change patient's position frequently. Handle patient gently. Remove constrictive clothing. Give small, frequent feedings. Insert a rectal tube if necessary. Auscultate abdomen for abnormal bowel sounds. Inspect abdomen for distention and absence of bowel sounds. Record bowel movements.
Tissue perfusion, alteration in: cardiopulmonary (related to potential for pulmonary ventilation)	Change patient's position frequently; place in sitting position. Encourage coughing and deep breathing. Observe respiratory rate and rhythm and pulse. Auscultate chest. Monitor blood studies. Administer oxygen and respiratory therapy as needed.

Patient Education

1. Explain the principles of safe ambulation.
2. Discuss the management of disease-related pain.
3. Instruct the patient to report any change in respiratory status and urinary and bowel function.

EVALUATION[4]

Patient Outcome	Data Indicating That Outcome is Reached
Vital signs are within normal limits.	Respiratory rate and pulse rate are within normal limits.
Laboratory findings are within normal limits.	Blood hemoglobin, hematocrit, oxygen saturation, and carbon dioxide are within normal limits.
Body hydration is normal.	There is no edema, ascites, or venous distention.
Body functioning is normal.	Elimination is adequate. Weight is stabilized. Digestion is adequate.
Vitality is good.	There is no malaise or fatigue.
Bowel elimination is normal for patient.	Stools are soft. Abdomen is soft and not distended. There is no abdominal pressure or cramping.
Daily fluid output is equal to fluid intake.	Urine output is 1500 to 3000 ml daily or equivalent to intake.
Patient is comfortable.	Facial expression is calm and relaxed. Posture is normal. Patient has freedom of body movement. Patient expresses comfort.
Patient frequently changes position with normal body movement.	Patient walks, sits, and stands with normal body movement.

Patient Outcome	Data Indicating That Outcome is Reached
Patient participates in therapeutic exercise.	Patient performs range of motion and isometric exercises.
Patient's surroundings are safe.	Patient uses safety precautions.
Patient shows no evidence of accident or physical injury.	There is no physical sign of accident or evidence of complications arising from drugs or treatment.
Patient shows no evidence of deformity resulting from treatment.	Patient's hands, feet, limbs, and spine are in good alignment and functional.

CANCERS OF THE CENTRAL NERVOUS SYSTEM

Tumors of the central nervous system are neoplasms of the brain or spinal cord.

Tumors of the central nervous system (CNS) account for more than 2% of annual cancer deaths. Eighty percent of CNS tumors involve the brain, with as many as half of these metastatic from primary cancers of the lung, breast, kidney, melanoma, and gastrointestinal tract; the other 20% involve the spinal cord.

Many CNS tumors occur in children and young adults. In children, brain tumors are second only to leukemia as a cause of death. In contrast to brain tumors in adults, those in children are largely infratentorial and involve the cerebellum, midbrain, pons, and medulla.[8]

PATHOPHYSIOLOGY[3]

The majority of CNS tumors are gliomas, which are peculiar because they rarely spread beyond the CNS. There are no known etiologic factors, although childhood tumors are believed to be developmental in origin.

Spinal cord tumors are gliomas (23%), meningiomas or schwannomas (56%), or miscellaneous other forms such as epidermoid and dermoid cysts, hemangioblastomas, and chordomas. These tumors produce symptoms in the body below the level of tumor location in the cord: difficulty in walking, postural disturbances, back pain, and changes in sensation and muscle power. The pain of a spinal cord tumor is worse at night.

Brain tumors in adults are divided as follows:
1. Gliomas (50%), of which 50% are glioblastomas; occur most often in the cerebrum of persons between 40 and 60 years of age
2. Meningiomas, the most common of nongliomatous tumors; average host age is 50 years; common sites are parasagittal area and anterior part of base of skull
3. Pituitary adenomas (12% to 18%), which are almost never malignant
4. Neurilemomas (schwannomas), which are usually benign

Brain tumors in children are divided as follows:
1. Medulloblastomas (30%)
2. Astrocytomas (30%) such as optic pathway gliomas
3. Ependymomas (12%), the most common fourth ventricular tumors
4. Posterior fossa tumors
5. Craniopharyngiomas
6. Pineal tumors

Brain tumors cause nonlocalized signs and symptoms by increasing intracranial pressure. Localized signs and symptoms are caused by direct compression, invasion, or irritation of regions of the brain (see "Assessment: Areas of Concern").

DIAGNOSTIC STUDIES[8]

Physical and neurologic examinations
Identification of specific neurologic deficits

Visual field examination
Alterations caused by optic nerve lesion

Funduscopic examination
Alterations caused by optic nerve lesion

Computed tomography; skull roentgenograms
Visualization of suspect lesion

Electroencephalography
Altered tracings in presence of central nervous system lesion

Technetium pertechnetate brain scanning
Visualization of suspect lesion

Cerebral angiography
Visualization of suspect lesion

Air study, pneumoencephalography, and ventriculography
Cytologic evidence of malignant lesion

Spinal fluid examination
Visualization of suspect lesion

Nuclear magnetic resonance (NMR)
Visualization of suspect lesion

TREATMENT PLAN[3]

Surgical
Excision—initial treatment for all intracranial tumors, with removal limited by location of lesion and its invasiveness

Chemotherapeutic
Of limited value because of blood-brain barrier
Antineoplastic agents
Procarbazine (Matulane), 2-4 mg/kg/d po initially, then maintained at 4-6 mg/kg/d until maximum response occurs; maintain at 1-2 mg/kg/d
Carmustine (BiCNU), 200 mg/m² IV q6wk
Vincristine sulfate (Oncovin), 2 mg/m² for children, 1.4 mg/m² for adults
Corticosteroids
Prednisone (Deltasone, others), 10-100 mg po for metastatic brain tumors

Electromechanical
Radiation therapy—external irradiation for malignant brain tumors; usually postoperative; used when tumor is centrally located and surgery is likely to aggravate it or when vital structures are involved, for example, brainstem tumor, metastatic deposit, uncomplicated pituitary adenoma, or medulloblastoma

Combination therapy
May include surgery, chemotherapy, and radiation therapy

Despite therapeutic advances, CNS tumors have high morbidity and mortality. About 40% of persons with brain tumors can return to a useful life, and another 30% gain good palliation. The neoplasms vary in their aggressiveness and consequently their prognosis. The earlier the diagnosis, the better the patient's chances for maximum restoration of function.

ASSESSMENT: AREAS OF CONCERN[3]

Increased intracranial pressure
Early headache; nausea and vomiting; decreased level of consciousness; failing vision; changing pupillary response

Localized signs
Contralateral homonymous hemianopsia; jacksonian seizures or weakness; convulsions; headache; suboccipital tenderness; personality change such as irritability or bizarre behavior; dizziness; disturbances in gait and balance

NURSING DIAGNOSES and NURSING INTERVENTIONS

Nursing Diagnosis	Nursing Intervention
Sensory-perceptual alteration: visual	Anticipate patient's needs. Reassure patient. Arrange environment to minimize barriers. Illuminate room adequately. Place objects within sight and reach. Provide frequent patient contact. Express empathy and acceptance. Demonstrate calmness. Encourage expression of feelings, listen attentively, and offer feedback. Reduce demands placed on patient. Observe for irritability or unusual behavior.
Injury: potential for (related to increased intracranial pressure)	Maintain complete bed rest. Provide quiet. Lower bed height. Subdue room lighting. Elevate patient's head, and change position slowly. Discourage oral stimulants. Refrain from jarring bed and performing nonessential procedures. Place padded side rails up; place airway or padded tongue blade on bed for use in case of seizure. Inspect eyes for pupillary response and observe for papilledema. Monitor blood pressure.

Nursing Diagnosis	Nursing Intervention
	Observe for confusion, lethargy, restlessness, vomiting, and complaints of headache and nausea. Palpate pulse rate and rhythm and monitor volume.
Injury: potential for (related to falling)	Minimize environmental barriers. Assist patient with mobility. Safeguard patient with side rails. Place safety helmet on patient's head. Cover bed with netting as needed.
Comfort, alteration in: pain (related to headache or suboccipital tenderness)	Position patient comfortably. Massage gently. Provide pain relief measures of patient's choice. Evaluate the effectiveness of pain relief measures. Encourage adequate rest. Apply cold, moist compress or ice bag. Monitor blood pressure. Assess pain duration, intensity, and quality.

Patient Education

1. Emphasize the need to avoid injury.
2. Explain ways of adjusting to potential visual changes.
3. Teach the patient to carry out various pain relief measures.
4. Tell the patient and family to report difficulty with mobility or changes in behavior.

EVALUATION[4]

Patient Outcome	Data Indicating That Outcome is Reached
Vital signs are within normal limits.	Respiratory rate, pulse rate, and blood pressure are within normal limits.
Vision is adequate.	Pupillary response and size are normal.
Vitality is good.	Patient is mentally alert and shows good concentration and attentiveness.
Performance of work and play is adequate.	Patient is able to maintain self-care.
Patient ambulates safely.	Patient avoids contact with stable and moving objects when walking.
Patient is comfortable.	Facial expression is calm, contented, and relaxed. Posture is normal. Patient has freedom of body movement. Patient expresses comfort and satisfaction and ceases to complain.
Patient has positive disposition.	Patient smiles appropriately.
Patient's ability to communicate is adequate.	There is no evidence of frustration in communication.
Patient's surroundings are safe.	Safety precautions such as side rails and low bed are used. There is no physical sign or subjective evidence of accident.

Neuroblastoma

Neuroblastoma is a highly malignant tumor composed of primitive ectodermal cells derived from the neural plate during embryonic life.

Neuroblastoma, the most common malignancy in the first year of life, commonly occurs as an abdominal mass.

In nearly 70% of those affected, metastasis occurs to lymph nodes, bone marrow, bone, and liver. Originating in neural crest tissue, the tumor may arise either in the adrenal gland or in the sympathetic ganglia at any anatomic site along the craniospinal axis.

Common symptoms of neuroblastoma include fever, malaise, irritability, and weight loss. Severe bone pain, anemia, and pallor may also occur. Invasion of the tissues behind the eye causes periorbital swelling, ecchymosis, and sometimes proptosis of the eyes.

Diagnostic evaluation includes intravenous pyelography, bone scanning, 24-hour quantitative vanillylmandelic acid (VMA) assessment, and computed tomography.

Patients with limited diseases should have surgical resection of the tumor. If there is no evidence of lymph node or other residual regional disease, additional therapy is usually not indicated. Older children with limited residual disease or with regional residual tumor (mediastinal or intraspinal) may benefit from radiation. The use of either radiation therapy or chemotherapy in a child less than 13 months of age with residual disease is controversial.

Children less than 13 months of age who have limited primary lesions but involvement of the liver, skin, or subcutaneous tissues have a good prognosis, with the focus on prevention of locally distressing or functionally destructive tumor growth and without specific therapy. Unfortunately, most children with neuroblastoma are older and have widespread subdiaphragmatic lesions. Chemotherapy combined with surgery or radiation or both increases survival, but over the past decade the number of cured patients has not increased significantly.

Retinoblastoma

Retinoblastoma is a relatively rare congenital malignant tumor of the retina.

Retinoblastoma occurs once in every 25,000 live births but is expected to double in frequency within the next century because of increased exposure to mutagenic agents and prolonged survival of affected children with subsequent genetic transmission to their children.

Retinoblastoma is characterized by leukokoria (white or cat's eye reflex), strabismus, red painful eye, or "squint." Evaluation consists of bilateral indirect ophthalmoscopy with the patient under anesthesia, bone marrow biopsy, and lumbar puncture for spinal fluid examination. The treatment of choice for any eye that is blind or in which restoration of vision is impossible is surgical enucleation with removal of the longest possible segment of optic nerve. Radiation therapy may be used to preserve remaining vision. Patients with bilateral disease usually receive radiation therapy alone or in combination with surgical enucleation of a blind eye. Chemotherapy is most frequently used for children with locally advanced or metastatic disease. As many as 90% of children with retinoblastoma are cured.[3,8]

CANCERS OF THE SKIN
Basal Cell and Squamous Cell Carcinoma

Basal cell carcinoma is a malignant, epithelial cell tumor that begins as a papule and enlarges peripherally. Squamous cell carcinoma is a slow-growing malignant tumor of squamous epithelium.

Skin cancer is the most common human malignancy. An estimated 400,000 cases are discovered each year. The vast majority are the highly curable basal cell and squamous cell carcinomas. These lesions are more common among persons with lightly pigmented skin and those at latitudes near the equator. Additional risk factors are excessive exposure to the sun and occupational exposure to coal tar, pitch, creosote, arsenic compounds, and radium.[2]

Basal cell carcinoma is usually a pearly gray nodule on the face, neck, or back of the hand.[2] Invasion is usually local, although metastatic disease occurs rarely. The histologic appearance is that of small undifferentiated basal cells with minimal nuclear atypia. Recurrence indicates initial incomplete tumor destruction; however, 90% to 95% of patients are considered cured.[8]

Squamous cell carcinoma is a scaly, slightly elevated lesion with or without a cutaneous horn. The prognosis with complete tumor destruction is excellent. Tumors more difficult to treat are those arising in a scar, a chronically ulcerated area, or a site of radiation damage or in an immunosuppressed patient. Squamous cell carcinoma can metastasize, with 2% to 3% spreading to regional lymph nodes. The cure rate for this cancer is 75% to 80%.[8]

DIAGNOSTIC STUDIES[8]

Physical examination

Careful inspection, particularly of lesions showing biologic activity such as change in size, shape, or color; bleeding and ulceration seen in more advanced lesions

Simple shave or dermal punch biopsy
For histologic confirmation of malignancy

TREATMENT PLAN[3]

Surgical
Scalpel excision with wide margin of skin and subcutaneous tissue; may be supplemented with split-
thickness graft, adjacent flaps, distant pedicles, or
free graft
Chemosurgery (Moh's procedure)

Chemotherapeutic
Antineoplastic agents
Fluorouracil (5-FU), topical application to skin bid
for several weeks

Electromechanical
Radiotherapy by beam electron and superficial x rays,
especially for cancers around face

Cryotherapy—tumor tissue with margin of normal skin
frozen to 20° to 40° C by liquid nitrogen; excellent
cosmetic results
Electroexcision—use of diathermy for repetitive coagulation and curettage

Lesions greater than 20 cm in diameter, those in such
critical areas as the central third of the face, recurrent
lesions, and lesions with histologic signs of sclerosis are
associated with a poor prognosis. Treatment for cure at
the time of initial therapy and frequent examination for
at least 2 years are essential.

ASSESSMENT: AREAS OF CONCERN[3]

Skin integrity
Raised, hard, red or red-gray, pearly lesion on forehead, eyelid, cheek, nose, preauricular fold, or lip;
scaly, slightly elevated lesion with irregular border;
ulceration

NURSING DIAGNOSES and NURSING INTERVENTIONS

Nursing Diagnosis	Nursing Intervention
Skin integrity, impairment of: actual	Bathe patient in warm water or apply warm, moist compress. Clean skin with agents appropriate to therapy. Maintain dry skin. Use paper or transparent tape over dressing. Observe lesions for change in shape, size, and color and bleeding.

Patient Education

1. Inform the patient of the need for regular physical examinations and self-examination.
2. Inform the patient of the need for careful protection of the skin with use of sunscreens, avoidance of excessive exposure to sun, and limited exposure to ionizing radiation.

EVALUATION[4]

Patient Outcome	Data Indicating That Outcome is Reached
Skin is healed.	Skin integrity is maintained without infection or ulceration.
Patient has physical appearance of comfort.	Facial expression is calm and relaxed.
Patient shows no evidence of physical injury.	There is no evidence of complications arising from drugs or treatments.

Malignant Melanoma

Malignant melanoma is a skin cancer that is composed of melanocytes.

Seventy-five percent of deaths from skin cancer, an average of 5500 deaths a year, are due to malignant melanoma. This cancer develops from melanocytes that migrate into the skin, eye, central nervous system, and mucous membranes during fetal development. Only 40% of melanomas develop from nevi; the majority arise de novo from melanocytes.

The exact cause of malignant melanoma is unknown. A hereditary factor is involved in 10% of patients. Other theories suggest possible hormonal factors, ultraviolet light exposure, or an autoimmunologic effect.

Malignant melanoma is easily recognized in its early stages and should be suspected in any patient with a history of change in a preexisting nevus or with a new pigmented lesion that has irregularities such as the following:

1. Various shades of brown and black plus red, white, or blue and the half tones of pink or gray
2. Notching or indentation of the border and pigment streaming from the lesion's edge
3. Loss of skin markings or development of a nodule, especially with erosion or ulceration
4. Bleeding of mole or change in color, size, or thickness[2,8]

PATHOPHYSIOLOGY[3]

The four distinct forms of malignant melanoma, in order of decreasing incidence, follow:

1. Superficial spreading melanoma (70%) occurs anywhere on the body surface. The average patient age is 50 years. The lesion has a haphazard combination of colors and irregular shapes.
2. Nodular melanoma (15%) also occurs anywhere on the body surface and has a wide age distribution. It may be small and usually is darkly pigmented. Invasion is usually into the dermis with resultant lymph node metastasis.
3. Acral (extremity) lentiginous melanoma (10%) occurs on palms, soles, nail beds, and mucous membranes. It is usually flat to slightly raised with an irregular pigment pattern and border.
4. Lentigo malignant melanoma (5%) is a slowly evolving lesion occurring on exposed surfaces (especially face and hands) of elderly persons. It usually undergoes many color changes.

DIAGNOSTIC STUDIES[8]

Total excisional biopsy
Deep margin to include subcutaneous fat preferred; performed to determine presence, type, and stage of malignancy

Punch or incisional biopsy
Followed by wide excision if findings are positive; incisional biopsy performed for large lesions and those in areas of cosmetic concern; done to determine presence, type, and stage of malignancy

Measurement of tumor thickness and depth of invasion

Physical examination and symptom- or organ-oriented diagnostic tests
Ordered as needed to detect metastases in lung, liver, bone, or brain (or anywhere in body); examples are chest roentgenogram, liver function test, and baseline liver and spleen scan

The prognosis is poorer with increased depth of invasion, lymphatic and vascular invasion, high number of mitotic figures per high-power microscopic field, little or no lymphocytic infiltration at the tumor base, and ulceration. The overall prognosis is better in women.

TREATMENT PLAN[3]

Surgical
Wide, deep excision of primary lesion
Regional lymph node dissection

Chemotherapeutic
Antineoplastic agents
Dacarbazine (DTIC), 2-4.5 mg/kg/d IV for 10 d or 250 mg/m^2/d IV for 5 d
Tamoxifen citrate (Nolvadex), 10-20 mg bid (morning and evening)
Anti-infective agents
BCG vaccine, active specific forms used as investigational drug

Electromechanical
Radiotherapy for palliation of metastases
Hyperthermic isolation perfusion

ASSESSMENT: AREAS OF CONCERN[3]

Skin integrity
Dark brown or black pigmentation; ulceration and bleeding; enlarged regional lymph nodes

Respiratory function
Dyspnea; cough and wheezing

Abdominal girth
Hepatomegaly

Skeletal structure
Pathologic fractures; pain

Sensory and motor function
Confusion; lethargy

NURSING DIAGNOSES and NURSING INTERVENTIONS

Nursing Diagnosis	Nursing Intervention
Skin integrity, impairment of: actual	Bathe patient in warm water or apply warm, moist compresses. Clean skin with agents appropriate to therapy. Maintain dry skin. Observe lesions for change in shape, size and color and bleeding.
Tissue perfusion, alteration in: pulmonary (potential)	Change patient's position frequently; place patient in sitting position. Encourage coughing and deep breathing. Monitor respiratory rate and rhythm and pulse. Auscultate chest. Monitor blood studies. Administer oxygen and respiratory therapy as ordered.
Tissue perfusion, alteration in: cerebral (potential)	Maintain bed rest as needed. Provide quiet environment with subdued lighting. Remove constrictive clothing. Ensure patient's safety, for example, by using padded tongue blades. Inspect for abnormal body movements. Observe for confusion, lethargy, and headache. Monitor vital signs, pupillary response, and reflexes.

Comfort, alteration in: pain	For adominal discomfort:
	  Discuss possible pain-relieving measures with patient; use those possible and monitor their effectiveness.
	  Give bland foods, full-liquid foods, warm liquids, and carbonated beverages.
	  Observe for distention, nausea, vomiting, and diarrhea.
	For bone pain:
	  Change patient's position slowly.
	  Support affected body part(s).
	  Place patient in whirlpool bath or use heat applications.
	  Ensure patient's safety.
	  Be alert for pain.

Patient Education

1. Emphasize the need for regular physical examinations.
2. Inform the patient of the need for meticulous skin care and assessment and the importance of avoiding ultraviolet light.
3. Instruct the patient to report changes such as those in respiratory status, abdominal girth or comfort, mobility, and level of consciousness.

EVALUATION

Patient Outcome	Data Indicating That Outcome is Reached
Vital signs are within normal limits.	Respiratory rate, rhythm, and depth and pulse are within normal limits.

Patient Outcome	Data Indicating That Outcome is Reached
	Breathing pattern is regular.
Patient is comfortable.	Facial expression is calm and relaxed. Posture is normal. Patient expresses comfort and no longer complains.
Patient's surroundings are safe.	Safety precautions such as side rails are used.
Patient shows no physical sign of injury.	There is no evidence of accident, physical injury, or complications arising from drugs or treatments.

ONCOLOGIC EMERGENCIES

Oncologic emergencies are the result of advanced cancer's impact on body functioning. Among the most serious but most treatable acute conditions that can occur are hypercalcemia, obstruction of the superior vena cava, spinal cord compression, and cardiac distress.

Hypercalcemia. Hypercalcemia occurs when the bones release more calcium into the extracellular fluid than can be excreted in the urine. This occurs most frequently in patients with multiple myeloma or cancer of the breast, lung, or prostate. In addition, some tumors produce parathyroid hormone or a substance with the same physiologic effects, which include increased resorption of calcium from bone, increased intestinal absorption of calcium, and reduced renal excretion.

The most common cause of hypercalcemia is thought to be bone destruction by invasive metastases. Other causes are tumor production of vitamin D–like substances and osteoclast-activating factors, dehydration, and immobilization.

Excessive calcium can cause bradycardia, increased cardiac contractility, depression of the central and peripheral nervous system (mild lethargy that may progress to coma), fatigue, muscle weakness, anorexia, nausea and vomiting, confusion, or irritability. Interference with reabsorption of water from the distal tubules leads to nocturia, polyuria, and dehydration.

Acute hypercalcemia is treated initially with intravenous saline. Furosemide may also be given intravenously to encourage diuresis. Careful recording of intake and output, monitoring of electrolyte levels, and frequent cardiopulmonary assessment are necessary. Mithramycin inhibits bone resorption of calcium; given as a rapid intravenous infusion at 25 μg/kg body weight, it can lower serum calcium levels in 48 hours.

Steroid administration and restriction of dietary calcium are thought to be of little therapeutic value. Orally administered phosphates and calcitonin injections may be used. Use of vitamin D, thiazides, absorbable antacids, and estrogens should be avoided.

External compression of the superior vena cava. Compression of the superior vena cava can occur slowly or quickly owing to pressure from an adjacent tumor mass or enlarging lymph node. The majority of patients with superior vena cava syndrome have bronchogenic cancer; other causes of this syndrome are lymphoma, breast cancer, and gastrointestinal tract metastases.

Prompt diagnosis and treatment are needed to relieve the distressing symptoms, which are progressive shortness of breath, cough, distention of neck veins, and edema of the face and hands. Dilated veins may appear on the upper chest wall. The patient may complain of headache and visual disturbances.

The patient must be kept in Fowler's position. Diuretics may be of some help. However, the obstruction must be relieved to prevent cerebral anoxia, hemorrhage, or strangulation. Radiation therapy is the treatment of choice for this. If the obstruction is not accessible, chemotherapeutic agents such as cyclophosphamide (Cytoxan) can produce good results.

Spinal cord compression. Compression of the spinal cord is extremely dangerous because of the possibility of a permanent neurologic deficit. The usual cause of compression is a tumor, such as lymphoma or cancer of the breast, lung, or prostate, that metastasizes to the bony vertebral body and grows into the epidural space.

Pain, localized in the spinal region or radicular, is almost always an early symptom. The pain may be constant and aggravated by movement or coughing. Relief is usually obtained with morphine, meperidine (Demerol), or an analgesic agent. Bed rest is recommended, and transfer and position change should be done by multiple personnel.

A careful neurologic examination should be performed to check motor and sensory function and the autonomic nerve tracts. Roentgenograms or myelograms should be done immediately to localize the destruction and determine its extent. The prognosis appears to be related to the patient's ability to walk at the time of diagnosis; if he is unable to do so, motor function is not recoverable, even with emergency radiotherapy or laminectomy.

Severe or prolonged cord compression can lead to extremity paralysis and loss of sphincter control, which is manifest as difficulty starting urination or as bowel incontinence.

Treatment must be prompt. Corticosteroids such as dexamethasone in high doses reduce swelling and inflammation around the cord. Surgical decompression or radiotherapy may be required. Early diagnosis is important for recovery.

Cardiac tamponade. Cardiac tamponade results from excessive amount and pressure of fluid in the pericardial sac, which is a response to metastasis or direct invasion by tumor. The normal diastolic filling is impaired, and stroke volume is reduced. If tamponade is untreated, circulatory collapse occurs.

Signs and symptoms depend on how quickly the fluid accumulates. Frequent signs of tamponade include rapid and weak pulse, distended neck veins during inspiration (Kussmaul's sign), pulsus paradoxus (inspiratory decrease in arterial blood pressure of greater than 10 mm Hg from baseline), ankle or sacral edema, pleural effusion, lethargy, and altered consciousness.

The diagnosis is confirmed with echocardiography and pericardiocentesis; the latter also provides immediate symptomatic relief. Palliative measures such as surgical construction of a pericardial window must also be taken; total pericardectomy is usually not practical. Newer techniques include catheter drainage of fluid and instillation of a sclerosing agent such as tetracycline.

PSYCHOSOCIAL ASPECTS OF CANCER

Cancer evokes deep fears of pain, suffering, dependence, disfigurement, and death. Indeed, the fear of the disease is often so strong that a person may delay examination and diagnosis in hopes that the signs or symptoms will go away. This lag time between awareness of a problem and seeking medical attention can affect the impact of therapy and the prognosis. Thus awareness of attitudes toward cancer and efforts to influence them in a more hopeful direction through education are an important part of the nurse's role.

Variables that have been identified as shaping attitudes toward cancer are life experiences, especially those related to this disease; parental and cultural values and attitudes toward illness; society's emphasis on youth, health, and beauty; social pressures for early sexual experience, smoking, and other harmful behaviors; and portrayals of people with cancer in the mass media. Positive experiences and hopeful presentations of cancer and its treatment will give the individual, group, or community a clear perspective on the value of prevention, early diagnosis, and treatment.

The following are some of the myths regarding cancer that should be dispelled or at least clarified:

1. "Cancer is contagious." There is no clear evidence that this is true, although a human leukemic virus has been identified and some cancers do seem to occur with greater frequency in family members.
2. "All cancer patients have pain." Pain is highly variable and is related to the type, size, and location of the malignancy as well as the patient's pain tolerance.
3. "The treatment is worse than the disease because of disfiguring surgery and side effects of chemotherapy." This may be true in patients who are asymptomatic or relatively free of symptoms at the time of diagnosis.
4. "Sexual activity and other aspects of normal life must be forfeited." This is certainly not true if the patient and significant others are willing to consider modifications in life-style.
5. "Cancer is a death sentence." There are hundreds of thousands of cured cancer patients (almost 50% of persons with cancer) in the United States today. With early diagnosis and treatment, most persons with cancer could live a long and productive life.

The most common concerns of cancer patients are fear of alienation from family, friends, or health care providers; mutilation, particularly if surgery is the treatment of choice; vulnerability, dependence, or lack of control; and mortality. The emotional responses of a patient to these and other concerns related to the disease may be feelings of hopelessness, helplessness, and guilt, denial, apathy, hostility, self-blame, withdrawal, and a sense of unreality. The nature and severity of these behaviors depend on the patient's usual behavior, attitudes toward illness in general and cancer in particular, the site of the disease, therapeutic options, and the expected outcome. All of these factors must be recognized as influencing the response of the patient and family.

All persons with cancer have certain basic needs that transcend their individual responses to cancer. These are:

1. To know what is happening and talk about its reality with someone who will listen
2. To participate in decisions affecting how the patient will live and die
3. To experience the pain of "feeling bad" rather than having to hide feelings from others

Not to be ignored are the effects of employability and insurability, potential loss of support systems, and the unfamiliarity of terms, procedures, drugs, and other aspects of therapy.

The ways in which patients cope with cancer are as

varied as their reactions to the diagnosis. Some of the more positive coping strategies that have been identified and described by researchers include the following:

1. Seeking more information about the disease and its treatment
2. Using humor to lighten the situation
3. Using various distraction techniques
4. Sharing concerns with others, for example, in self-help groups
5. Negotiating feasible alternatives such as treatment options

Coping strategies that are generally considered to be less positive include:

1. Reducing tension and anxiety with excessive drinking, drugs, or dangerous activities
2. Withdrawing into isolation
3. Blaming others, the situation, or the Supreme Being
4. Becoming fatalistic
5. Blaming self and expressing guilt feelings

The nurse and other health care providers should assess the patient's coping style, evaluate its effectiveness, and intervene when there is increasing distress or a continuing problem.

General nursing interventions that have been identified as helpful to cancer patients during the various stages of the illness include maintaining hope while avoiding false optimism, using a gentle, unhurried manner, expressing caring and concern, and focusing on the patient's strengths rather weaknesses.

Many patients find self-help groups useful in dealing with the effects of cancer and its treatment. The value of receiving help from another person who has undergone a similar experience is well documented. The functions of such groups are to provide special information and successful coping techniques to persons with similar problems, encouragement to maintain prescribed regimens, normalization of a behavior, and education of health care professionals and the public about cancer patients' special needs. The most useful aspects of this approach to coping are believed to be the modeling aspects ("You can do it—I did!") and the observation that helping someone else benefits the helper.

The family of the cancer patient may also need the assistance of health care team members. Factors to be assessed when determining the impact of cancer on the family include the age of the patient and other family members, family dynamics, communication style, family background, and practical matters of concern to the patient and family. Specific nursing interventions that are of value to the family are:

1. Giving the patient quality care
2. Communicating frequently with the family
3. Listening to the family
4. Making the family comfortable, as by orientation to the institutional setting and policies
5. Referring the family to other members of the health care team as appropriate
6. Using touch to comfort family members as appropriate
7. Preparing the family for home care of the patient
8. Doing small things that are important to the family, such as rearranging mealtime to permit a special dinner from home

Additional coping strategies that patients and their families may wish to learn about and use include relaxation exercises, meditation, imagery, self-hypnosis, music therapy, and humor. The nurse may serve as teacher or provide referral to resources for instruction in these techniques.

As previously mentioned, disfigurement is a particular concern of cancer patients. A change in body image may be actual (as with mastectomy) or perceived (as with hysterectomy). The visibility of the alteration may not affect the patient's reaction to it; perhaps of more significance is the function of the part or system and the patient's emotional attachment to it.

Patients may react to a change in body image in a variety of ways:

1. Denying the existence of the change, minimizing its presence, or deemphasizing its importance
2. Increased perception of phantom sensations
3. Use of unrealistic goal-setting
4. Use of inappropriate defenses, such as denial, inappropriate dress, self-imposed isolation, aggression, or dissociation

The nurse should assist the patient in developing more realistic responses to the change in body image. Some suggestions that may be beneficial to the patient include:

1. Resumption of prealteration life-style
2. Confinement of the effect of the disability to the area of loss
3. Emphasis on assets rather than liabilities
4. Solicitation of support from others
5. Reevaluation of personal and professional goals

Another area of concern to patients and their families that may be less readily discussed is sexuality and feelings regarding gender and gender role identity. Many beliefs (cultural, religious, personal, and societal) affect a person's ability to deal with alteration in sexuality. Some that have been identified as especially influential are:

1. The duty of a man to satisfy a woman and vice versa
2. The man as the aggressor and the woman as the passive recipient
3. The obsession of both sexes with performance
4. The use of sexual intercourse for procreation

These beliefs, as well as the other attitudes regarding masculine and feminine behaviors, may confuse and depress both the patient and partner. In addition, the symptoms of cancer, such as fatigue, malaise, fever, discharge, and odor, may adversely affect libido and the patient's general view of his or her sexuality. This is further complicated by hospitalization with the resultant lack of privacy.

The nurse's role in this sensitive area is to assess the patient's readiness to discuss sexual concerns, identify appropriate resources, provide oral and written information that will assist the patient in understanding sexual concerns and possible solutions, and respect the patient and partner's need for privacy.

This section has included a few of the psychosocial issues confronting the cancer patient. Not discussed here but of equal concern is the experience of dying, which is faced by many cancer patients and their families. The nurse's support during this phase of the illness is invaluable. The hospice movement has been particularly useful to patients and their families who desire terminal care at home.

Meeting the psychosocial needs of the cancer patient and family is one of the greatest challenges facing the nurse. The roles of counselor, teacher, consultant, and resource person are used to their maximum to enhance the patient's and family's coping with this complex of diseases and therapies.

Medical Interventions

SURGERY

Surgery has historically been the treatment of choice for most cancers. A decision to use this therapy is based on analysis of a variety of data, including a thorough history and physical examination; laboratory, radiologic, and other specialized procedures; and biopsy proof of cancer.

A radical surgical approach to operable tumors is no longer routinely used because of an increased variety of surgical procedures and more sophisticated disease staging. The current treatment of choice is excision of the primary tumor and enough surrounding tissue and lymph nodes to offer maximum protection against local recurrence. These are termed curative resections. Palliative resections may be done when there is spread to distant, previously (preoperatively) undetected sites.

A tumor is considered inoperable if it is large or in a difficult-to-reach place or if there is evidence of extensive local growth or metastasis.

Staging operations such as laparotomy may be performed to determine appropriate therapy. Secondary operations may be done for local recurrence. "Second look" operations may be performed in the absence of clinical evidence of recurrent disease, but the effectiveness of this procedure for finding recurrent disease is questionable.

Distant metastasis (for example, pulmonary or hepatic) may respond to direct surgical resection. Indirect ablative procedures such as adrenalectomy and hypophysectomy may be useful in the palliation of hormonally sensitive cancers of the breast or prostate. Other indirect palliative procedures include cordotomy for relief of intractable pain and ostomy to relieve gastrointestinal obstruction.[3]

CHEMOTHERAPY

Chemotherapy is a relatively new cancer treatment modality, the first patient having been treated with nitrogen mustard in 1942. The use of chemical agents is especially important in the treatment of systemic disease. Researchers continue to discover drugs that kill cancer cells without causing extensive damage to normal tissues. In addition, combinations of chemotherapeutic agents, as well as the combination of chemotherapy with other treatment modalities, have increased the cancer cure rate.

Chemotherapy is used to cure patients, prolong life, increase the disease-free interval, and palliate symptoms, thus improving the quality of life.

Chemotherapeutic agents are highly toxic, attacking all rapidly dividing cells, both normal and malignant. Thus the contraindications and cautions are a reflection of the patient's pretreatment condition, stage of disease, response to therapy, and allergies or sensitivities. The nurse involved in drug administration and monitoring of

Table 14-1
Cancer Chemotherapeutic Agents

Classification	Agents	Mechanism of Action
Alkylating agents	Mechlorethamine (nitrogen mustard); cyclophosphamide (Cytoxan); phenylalanine mustard (Alkeran, L-PAM, Melphalan); chlorambucil (Leukeran); bulsulfan (Myleran); dacarbazine (DTIC); thiophosphoramide (Thiotepa)	Produce breaks in DNA module and cross-linking of strands and thus interfere with DNA replication
Antimetabolites Folic acid analog	Methotrexate (MTX)	Competitively inhibit enzymes necessary for cell function and replication
Pyrimidine analogs	5-Fluorouracil (5-FU); cytosine arabinoside (Cytosar)	
Purine analogs	6-Mercaptopurine (6-MP); 6-thioguanine (Thioguanine)	
Vinca alkaloids	Vinblastine (Velban); vincristine (Oncovin)	Bind to substances needed for formation of mitotic spindle and thus prevent cell division
Antibiotics	Doxorubicin (Adriamycin); daunorubicin (Daunomycin); bleomycin (Blenoxane); dactinomycin (actinomycin D); mithramycin (Mithracin); mitomycin C (Mutamycin)	Bind with DNA to inhibit DNA and RNA synthesis
Nitrosureas	Bis-chloroethyl nitrosourea (BCNU); lomustine (CCNU)	Action similar to that of alkylating agents
Hormonal agents		Alter cellular environment
Corticosteroids	Prednisone; prednisolone; methylprednisolone (Solu-Medrol); hydrocortisone (Solu-Cortef); dexamethasone (Decadron)	
Estrogens	Ethinyl estradiol (Estinyl); fosfestrol (Stilbestrol); diethylstilbestrol (DES); diethylstilbestrol diphosphate (Stilphostrol); conjugated estrogens (Premarin)	
Antiestrogens	Clomiphene; nafoxidine; tamoxifen	
Androgens	Testosterone; calusterone; fluoxymesterone (Halotestin); nandrolone	
Progestins	17-Hydroxyprogesterone (Delalutin); medroxyprogesterone acetate (Provera); megestrol acetate (Megace)	
Miscellaneous agents	Cisplatin diamine dichloride (Platinol); hydroxyurea; L-asparaginase; procarbazine (Matulane)	

the patient's responses must have a comprehensive baseline assessment to use in evaluating the patient's condition and ability to tolerate the treatment.

The most commonly used chemotherapeutic agents are listed in Table 14-1. Many others are being developed and tested for possible therapeutic value.[1,3,8]

ASSESSMENT: AREAS OF CONCERN[3,8]

Gastrointestinal

Nausea and vomiting; diarrhea; constipation; stomatitis; esophagitis; anorexia

Dermatologic

Alopecia; dermatitis; changes in skin color; extravasation; hyperpigmentation of nail beds

Hematologic

Anemia owing to decreased RBCs; bleeding owing to thrombocytopenia (petechiae); infection owing to leukopenia

Reproductive

Sterility; amenorrhea; decreased libido

Urinary

Hemorrhagic cystitis as evidenced by hematuria, burning during urination, and backache; nephrotoxicity as evidenced by renal failure

Neurologic

Ototoxicity (vertigo, tinnitus, loss of hearing); peripheral neuropathies as evidenced by muscle weakness; numbness and tingling; jaw pain; absence of deep tendon reflexes

Respiratory

Pulmonary fibrosis as evidenced by dyspnea, chest pain, or cyanosis

Musculoskeletal

Myalgia; muscle weakness; osteoporosis; gout

Cardiac

Congestive heart failure as evidenced by exertional dyspnea, cough, and rales; ECG changes

Hepatic

Jaundice

Emotional and mood changes

Depression; anger; withdrawal; preoccupation with self

NURSING DIAGNOSES and NURSING INTERVENTIONS

Nursing Diagnosis	Nursing Intervention
Fluid volume deficit (related to nausea and vomiting)	Administer antiemetic (prochlorperazine, thiethylperazine, trimethobenzamide, mitoclopramide, intravenous dexamethasone, or δ-9 tetrahydrocannabinol [THC]) prophylactically before chemotherapy and on regular schedule after therapy per physician order. Withhold food and fluids for 4 to 6 hours before treatment. Provide small feedings and increased fluids. Provide frequent mouth care. Provide clean environment with fresh air and no odors. Monitor intake and output, weight, and electrolytes. Administer intravenous therapy as ordered.
Bowel elimination, alteration in: constipation	Use relaxation techniques, guided imagery, self-hypnosis, and distraction as indicated. Offer fluids and foods high in fiber and bulk. Offer stool softener or laxatives. Avoid enemas.
Bowel elimination, alteration in: diarrhea	Offer clear liquids. Offer antidiarrheal agent such as Kaopectate or diphenoxylate (Lomotil) per physician order. Maintain good perineal care. Test stools for occult blood. Record number and consistency of stools. Observe for dehydration and electrolyte imbalance.
Oral mucous membrane, alteration in (related to stomatitis)	Encourage good oral hygiene. Discourage spicy or hot foods. Offer topical agents for relief of pain (lidocaine or dyclonine) per physician's order. Apply K-Y Jelly to lips. Offer popsicles.
Oral mucous membrane, alteration in (related to infection)	Administer nystatin oral suspension or suppository or clotrimazole (Mycelex) troche per physician's order. Have patient postpone dental work if possible, brush teeth gently, and use toothettes.
Nutrition, alteration in: less than body requirements (related to esophagitis)	Offer bland or pureed foods. Have patient avoid spicy foods, alcohol, and tobacco. Offer antacids.
Nutrition, alteration in: less than body requirements (related to increased body requirements)	Identify food preferences. Encourage patient to eat. Offer small frequent feedings. Do not rush meals. Keep room free of odors and clutter. Provide meticulous mouth care. Use enteral feeding tube or total parenteral nutrition if necessary. Weigh daily.
Skin integrity, impairment of	For alopecia: Help patient plan for wig, scarf, or hat before hair loss. Offer tourniquet or ice cap preventive therapy based on policy and diagnosis. Have patient wash and comb remaining hair gently. Reassure patient that hair will grow back after therapy.

Nursing Diagnosis	Nursing Intervention

	For dermatitis:
	   Use cornstarch, Alpha Keri, calamine lotion, or other agent to relieve itching.
	   Warn against overexposure to sun.
	   Keep skin clean and dry.
	 For changes in color of skin or nail beds:
	   Assure patient that discoloration will fade with time.
	   Use nail polish according to patient's wishes.
	 For jaundice:
	   Monitor hepatic enzymes.
	   Assess skin and sclera daily.

Gas exchange, impaired (related to anemia)	Have patient change position slowly. Encourage adequate rest. Observe patient for dyspnea and increased weakness. Administer oxygen therapy as needed. Monitor hemoglobin and hematocrit. Administer transfusions as ordered.
Gas exchange, impaired (related to fibrosis)	Monitor respiratory function with pulmonary function tests. Note limitation of lifetime dosage of bleomycin. Assist with pulmonary function studies. Observe for dyspnea and shortness of breath; report to physician as ordered.
Tissue perfusion, alteration in: cardiac	Limit cumulative dosage of doxorubicin. Monitor cardiac function with gated blood pool scan and ejection fraction.
Potential patient problem: susceptibility to infection	Warn patient to avoid crowds and persons with cold, flu, or cold sore. Use sterile technique whenever needed. Initiate reverse isolation as indicated. Monitor temperature and leukocyte count. Encourage careful hygiene. Discourage fresh-cut flowers. Avoid using indwelling catheters or performing rectal procedures or examination. Administer antibiotics as prescribed.
Potential patient problem: bleeding	Protect patient from injury; for example, use precautions when shaving with razor blade, do not permit cluttered environment, and do not administer rectal suppositories. Have patient avoid using aspirin and aspirin products. Avoid giving injections; if they are necessary, apply pressure at site for 3 to 5 minutes afterward. Use toothettes for oral care. Monitor petechiae, ecchymoses, and stools. Evaluate neurologic status. Have nasal packing available. Administer platelet transfusions as necessary. Observe for redness, tenderness, drainage, or discharge.
Sexual dysfunction	Help patient explore alternatives for sterility, such as sperm banking, hormonal therapy during treatment, and postponement of conception and childbearing. Refer to sexual counselor as needed and explore partner's feelings.
Urinary elimination, alterations in patterns	Force fluids. Monitor blood urea nitrogen, serum creatinine, creatinine clearance, and electrolytes. Monitor intake and output and edema. Administer diuretics as ordered. Encourage foods high in potassium. Administer normal saline and mannitol before cisplatin therapy per physician's order. Observe for signs of inflammation and infection. Administer allopurinol as prescribed with high fluid intake. Encourage patient to empty bladder frequently, especially at night.
Sensory-perceptual alteration: auditory	Provide adequate hydration. Monitor hearing with baseline and periodic audiograms.

Nursing Diagnosis	**Nursing Intervention**
Sensory-perceptual alteration: tactile	Assess patient for numbness and tingling in extremities.
	Encourage patient safety, for example, by prohibiting smoking.
Mobility, impaired physical	Monitor calcium level.
	Plan frequent rest periods.
	Provide safety measures.
	Be alert for complaint of pain over bony area; if patient has such a complaint, maintain bed rest until roentgenograms are taken for fracture.
	Use assistive devices for ambulation.
	Encourage range of motion exercise.
	Position patient in proper anatomic alignment.
Coping, ineffective individual	Assess coping behavior.
	Reassure patient that mood changes are temporary.
	Allow independence in self-care.
	Maintain supportive, nonjudgmental attitude.
	Encourage use of resources such as support group.

Patient Education

1. Encourage maintenance of adequate nutrition and hydration.
2. Emphasize the need for self-regulation of medication to control nausea, vomiting, constipation, diarrhea, or itching.
3. Discuss the warning signs of bleeding and infection that the patient should report to a physician.
4. Emphasize the need for thorough personal hygiene and oral care.

EVALUATION

Patient Outcome	Data Indicating That Outcome is Reached
Skin and mucous membrane color is normal.	Skin, nails, lips, and earlobes are warm and moist and have natural color.
Vital signs are within normal limits.	Respiratory rate, pulse rate, blood pressure, and temperature are within normal limits.
Laboratory findings are within normal limits.	Blood urea nitrogen, hemoglobin, hematocrit, blood pH, sodium, potassium, and serum creatinine are within normal limits.
	Urine creatinine clearance specific gravity, pH, and creatinine are within normal limits. Blood leukocyte count is 5000 to 10,000 cells/mm^3.
Body hydration is normal.	Skin turgor is normal. Mucous membranes are moist. There is no edema or ascites.
Body functioning is normal.	Elimination is adequate. Healing is prompt. Weight is stabilized.
Vitality is good.	Patient is mentally alert and without malaise, fatigue, or weakness.
Patient has daily intake of essential food groups.	Diet includes milk, meat, fruits, vegetables, breads, and cereals. High-calorie, high-protein foods are included.
Bowel elimination is adequate.	Stools are soft and normal for individual.
Daily fluid output is equal to fluid intake.	Urine output is 1500 to 3000 ml daily.
Hearing is adequate.	Patient performs appropriate actions or gives appropriate verbal response. Audiometry findings are within normal limits.
Touch is adequate.	Patient feels pinprick, heat, cold, and touch.

Patient Outcome	Data Indicating That Outcome is Reached
General body cleanliness is good.	Patient has clean hair, eyes, ears, nose, mouth, skin, nails, teeth, and clothes. Patient has no unpleasant body odor.
Patient's disposition is good.	Patient's conversation is cheerful. Patient smiles appropriately.
Patient's surroundings are clean, safe, and comfortable.	Room is free from dust, dirt, and clutter. Safety precautions such as side rails and low bed are in effect. Temperature and humidity are appropriate. Room is well ventilated. No unpleasant odors are noticeable.
Patient has not suffered accidents or physical injury.	There is no physical sign or subjective evidence of accident or injury.
Patient does not have infection.	There is no evidence of inflammation, purulent drainage or secretions, pain, or aching.

RADIATION THERAPY

The goal of radiation in the treatment of cancer is the local destruction of malignant cells or their reproductive capability with minimal damage to normal tissue. This treatment modality is used in the prevention, treatment, and palliation of cancer, either alone or with chemotherapy or surgery. Radiation therapy can be administered either externally or internally.

The substances used most often for radiation therapy include:

1. X rays—the higher the voltage, the deeper the penetration; for example, high voltage is used for bladder cancer and low voltage is used for superficial tumors such as skin cancers
2. Radioactive elements such as radium and cobalt, which occur in nature
3. Radioactive isotopes such as iodine, gold, and phosphorus, which are produced in atomic reactors

External radiation, the treatment of choice for such cancers as early laryngeal cancer, early retinoblastoma, and some brain tumors, is delivered by x ray or radioisotope via sophisticated equipment with refined delivery, such as the linear accelerator. External radiation is also used as adjuvant therapy and for palliation through reduction of tumor mass.

Internal radiation may include temporary or permanent implants, intracavitary or interstitial instillation, or parenteral or oral administration. Specific uses for these forms of therapy are:

1. Implants (such as radon, iodine, and gold seeds) sutured into the tumor via tubes or needles for cancers of the tongue, lip, breast, and vagina and small bladder tumors
2. Intracavitary or interstitial instillation via "seeding" with radioactive gamma ray–emitting beads such as radium or cesium for localized but inoperable lung cancers and invasive tumors of the uterus; "afterloading" with an applicator that provides channels through which to place the radioisotope may be used to reduce exposure
3. Radioactive isotopes administered orally or parenterally for thyroid cancer, chronic leukemia, or myeloma

The nurse involved in the care of patients receiving internal irradiation should avoid radiation damage by adhering to the principles of time (by being efficient but brief), distance (by standing as far as possible from the source), and shielding (by wearing a lead apron or using other precautions as determined by the radiation safety officer).

Radiosensitive cells—those most likely to be adversely affected by radiation—include relatively undifferentiated and rapidly dividing cells such as those of genes, the mucosa of the gastrointestinal tract, and lymphoid tissue. The most radioresistant cells are those originating from the connective tissue. At the cellular level the degree of sensitivity is related to the degree of cell differentiation, rate of mitosis, and mitotic potential. The degree of vascularity and oxygenation are also important in determining tissue responsiveness.

The side or toxic effects of radiation therapy depend on the site of irradiation, the volume of tissue irradiated, the total dosage delivered, and the time frame within which it is administered. Although newer technology has increased the therapist's ability to treat the cancer more precisely, surrounding or underlying healthy tissue may still be damaged.

The dose of radiation that can be delivered to any tumor is limited by the radiation tolerance of the adjacent normal tissues. One method of improving the therapeutic ratio is fractionation of treatment, or dividing the total dosage of radiation into multiple doses. This allows four processes to occur: repair of sublethal tissue damage, repopulation of clonogenic cells, reassortment of cells in the cell cycle, and reoxygenation of hypoxic cells. The best results are achieved with predetermined doses given five times a week for 4 to 6 weeks.

Before initiating therapy the therapist may localize the treatment portals with a simulator, such as an x-ray machine that produces the geometric factors of actual therapy or computed tomography scanning that defines both the tumor-bearing volume and critical normal structures. The information obtained is used to produce, with computer assistance, an individualized treatment plan.

In combining surgery with radiation, the relative merits of preoperative or postoperative radiation for many cancers are still a matter of controversy. The use of chemotherapy with radiation requires careful monitoring of peripheral blood counts and observation for exacerbation of drug-induced disorders such as severe dysuria (cyclophosphamide), enhanced mucositis (methotrexate), or carcinogenesis such as leukemia. Actinomycin D and doxorubicin produce a recall phenomenon in which reactions appear in previously irradiated tissues when the drug is given as late as 1 year after the patient's radiation exposure.

ASSESSMENT: AREAS OF CONCERN[3]

Gastrointestinal tract
Nausea and vomiting; anorexia; taste changes; esophagitis; diarrhea; xerostomia; mucositis; radiation tooth decay

Genitourinary
Urinary frequency; vaginal discharge; amenorrhea; impotence

Skin
Hair loss; dry reaction-reddened area; dry, itchy feeling; moist desquamation—blistering and sloughing of skin surface

Central nervous system
Headache

Neuromuscular
Transient paresthesia; paresis or paralysis

Cardiovascular
Pneumonitis—dry, hacking cough; dyspnea; pericarditis; chest pain, ECG changes; myocarditis; friction rub

Hemopoietic
Anemia; infection; bleeding

NURSING DIAGNOSES and NURSING INTERVENTIONS

Nursing Diagnosis	Nursing Intervention
Fluid volume deficit (related to nausea and vomiting)	Administer antiemetic as needed. Plan rest periods before and after meals. Provide small bland feedings and increased fluids. Offer frequent mouth care. Provide clean environment with fresh air and no odors. Administer intravenous therapy as ordered. Monitor intake and output, daily weight, and electrolytes.
Nutrition, alteration in: less than body requirements (related to anorexia and taste changes)	Encourage patient to eat high-calorie, high-protein diet. Offer small frequent feedings. Do not rush meals. Keep room free of odors and clutter. Provide meticulous mouth care. Use enteral feeding tube or total parenteral nutrition if necessary. Monitor weight daily.
Nutrition, alteration in: less than body requirements (related to esophagitis or rectal mucositis)	Encourage clear liquids and low-residue diet. Offer antidiarrheal agents per physician's order. Maintain good perineal care. Test stools for occult blood. Record number and consistency of stools. Observe for dehydration and electrolyte imbalances.
Oral mucous membrane, alteration in (related to mucositis, xerostomia, or radiation tooth decay)	Encourage good oral hygiene with use of dental floss or Water Pik. Discourage spicy or hot foods and dry, thick foods. Offer topical relief of pain with lidocaine ointment, Aspergum, or ice chips. Apply K-Y Jelly to lips. Offer popsicles.

Nursing Diagnosis	Nursing Intervention
	Offer artificial saliva.
	Encourage increased fluid intake with meals.
	Use mouth irrigations or sprays such as half-strength hydrogen peroxide and saline.
	Encourage use of sugarless lemon drops or mints.
	Discourage smoking, alcohol, or ginger ale.
	Assess mouth for dryness, lesions, bleeding, discharge, and tooth decay.
	Consult with dentist as needed for dental care, including fluoride therapy.
Urinary elimination, alteration in patterns	Force fluids.
	Encourage patient to empty bladder completely.
	Catheterize for residual urine as indicated.
	Administer urinary antiseptics as prescribed.
	Observe for signs of infection such as burning, cloudy urine, hematuria, and fever.
Skin integrity, impairment of	For alopecia:
	Help patient plan for wig, scarf, or hat before hair loss.
	Have patient gently wash and comb remaining hair.
	Reassure patient that hair will grow back after therapy.
	For dermatitis:
	Observe irradiated area daily.
	Apply baby oil or ointment as prescribed: lanolin or Aquaphor.
	Keep reddened area dry and aerated.
	Use cornstarch, A & D Ointment, or hydrocortisone ointment to relieve dryness and itching.
	For moist desquamation:
	Provide saline soaks, exposure to air, topical vitamins, steroids, or antibiotic ointments.
	Avoid use of adhesive tape.
	Assist patient with bathing to maintain markings.
	Have patient avoid excessive heat, sunlight, tight restrictive clothing, and soap.
	Provide special skin care to tissue folds such as buttocks, perineum, groin, and axilla.
	Avoid application of deodorant or after-shave lotion to treated area.
Comfort, alteration in: pain (headache)	Assess presence and characteristics of headache.
	Administer medications such as steroids and analgesics as prescribed.
	Offer patient other pain relief measures if desired.
Mobility, impaired physical (related to fatigue and impaired motor function)	Plan frequent rest periods.
	Avoid injury.
	Use assistive devices for ambulation.
	Assess reflexes, tactile sensation, and movement in extremities and report abnormal findings.
	Observe for Lhermitte's sign (sensation of electric shock running down back and over extremities), which is indicative of cervical cord compression.
Tissue perfusion, alteration in: cardiopulmonary (related to pneumonitis)	Auscultate lungs and report signs of pleural rub.
	Observe for cough, dyspnea, and pain on inspiration.
	Treat with antibiotics and steroids as prescribed.
Tissue perfusion, alteration in: cardiopulmonary (related to pericarditis or myocarditis)	Auscultate heart and report signs of friction rub, arrhythmias, or hypertension.
	Observe for chest pain and weakness.
	Monitor ECG reports.
	Administer drugs as prescribed.
Gas exchange, impaired (related to anemia)	Encourage adequate rest; alternate rest and activity periods.
	Observe patient for dyspnea and increased weakness.
	Administer oxygen therapy as needed.
	Monitor hemoglobin and hematocrit.
	Administer transfusions as ordered.
Potential patient problem: susceptibility to infection	Warn patient to avoid crowds and persons with cold, flu, or cold sore.

Nursing Diagnosis	Nursing Intervention
	Use sterile technique whenever needed. Initiate reverse isolation as indicated. Monitor temperature and leukocyte count. Encourage careful hygiene.

Sexual dysfunction	For sterility:
	    Help patient explore alternatives such as sperm banking and hormonal therapy.
	    Refer patient to sexual counselor as necessary.
	For vaginal discharge:
	    Encourage patient to douche as needed and to perform thorough perineal care.
	    Observe for redness, tenderness, discharge, or drainage.

Potential patient problem: hemorrhage	Protect patient from injury when shaving or ambulating. Have patient avoid aspirin and aspirin products.

Patient Education

1. Discuss the need for skin care such as maintenance of dye markings, avoidance of soap and other ointments, and avoidance of sunbathing or heat applications.
2. Emphasize the need to avoid injury to the skin.
3. Explain the maintenance of adequate nutrition.
4. Explain the patient's "radioactive state," if present, and precautions to be taken.
5. Discuss the management of fatigue and the maintenance of mobility.

EVALUATION

Patient Outcome	Data Indicating That Outcome is Reached
Skin and mucous membrane color is normal.	Skin, nails, lips, and earlobes are warm and moist and have natural color.
Vital signs are within normal limits.	Respiratory rate, pulse rate, blood pressure, and temperature are within normal limits. There is no respiratory distress.
Laboratory findings are within normal limits.	Blood hemoglobin, hematocrit, sodium, potassium, chloride, and pH are within normal limits. Leukocyte count is 5000 to 10,000 cells/mm^3. Urine output is 1500 to 3000 ml daily or equivalent to intake. There are no erythrocytes or leukocytes in urine, and findings of bacterial culture are negative.
Body hydration is normal.	Skin turgor is normal. Secretions are thin. Mucous membranes are moist. Patient is not thirsty.
Body functioning is normal.	Elimination is adequate. Healing is prompt. Weight is stabilized. Digestion is good.
Vitality is good.	Patient has no malaise, fatigue, or weakness.
Patient has daily intake of essential food groups.	Diet includes milk, meat, fruits, vegetables, breads, and cereals (as tolerated). High-calorie, high-protein foods are included.
Patient has positive attitude toward food.	Use of salt and spices is not excessive. Patient indicates that foods taste good.
Patient gives physical appearance and verbal expression of comfort.	Facial expression is calm, contented, and relaxed. Patient expresses comfort.
Patient frequently changes position with normal body movement.	Patient walks, sits, and stands with normal body movement.
Surroundings are clean and safe.	Room is free from dust, dirt, and clutter. Safety precautions are in effect. There is no evidence that accident has occurred.
Patient has not suffered physical injury.	There is no evidence of complications arising from treatment.
Patient does not have infection.	There is no evidence of inflammation, purulent drainage or secretions, pain, or aching.

BLOOD COMPONENT THERAPY

The goal of blood component therapy is to administer only the component needed by the patient. This minimizes transfusion reactions and increases the number of patients who can benefit from a single unit.

Granulocytes are used to treat granulocytopenic patients with severe infection, particularly those in whom severe bone marrow depression develops during chemotherapy. Granulocytes are collected from a single donor by means of a machine that withdraws donor blood, removes the granulocytes, and returns the rest of the blood to the donor. This procedure, called leukopheresis, requires several hours. Administration of steroids before donation can increase the cell yield.

Although granulocytes can be stored up to 24 hours, immediate transfusion is recommended. Because of the short posttransfusion cell life, frequent transfusions are usually needed, for example, daily for at least 4 days, administered slowly over 2 to 4 hours period.

The most common untoward reactions are shaking chills and temperature elevation, which are treated symptomatically with acetaminophen 30 minutes before subsequent transfusions and with reduction of the flow rate.

Hives are another minor reaction and are usually treated with an antihistamine. Life-threatening reactions include hypotensive response, anaphylactic response, and respiratory reaction. Emergency intervention is necessary.

Platelets are usually given to patients with thrombocytopenia and bone marrow depression resulting from chemotherapy or radiation therapy. Platelet concentrates are obtained through platelet pheresis of a single donor or prepared from units of platelets collected from as many as four to 10 donors. Blood is removed from the donor into a machine with a centrifuge bowl, where platelets are separated, and red cells and plasma are then returned to the donor. The procedure takes 1½ to 2 hours. Pheresis donors may give as many as 12 units of platelets at a time. The platelets should be administered within 24 hours.[3,8]

The nurse is an essential member of the team involved in this therapy; it is often the nurse who identifies the patient's need for blood components, recruits donors, obtains the blood components from the donors, and administers the therapy to the patient.

IMMUNOTHERAPY

Immunotherapy is still considered an investigational treatment for cancer. Its usefulness in treating a wide variety of tumors is being studied, but its value in improving long-term survival will require many years of evaluation.

The rationale for the use of immunotherapy in cancer care is based on animal studies, as well as clinical observations such as the following:

1. Postoperative patients are often found to have malignant cells in circulating blood and in operative wound washings but may never receive a diagnosis of cancer.
2. Among transplant patients who receive immunosuppressant therapy, cancer occurs at a rate at least 80 times that of the general population.
3. Rapidly progressive recurrent cancer sometimes appears 10 to 20 years after cure.
4. Patients with congenital or acquired immunologic deficiencies have a greater incidence of cancer than that of the general population.
5. Persons with faulty immune systems cannot be sensitized to certain chemicals such as 2,4-dinitrochlorobenzene (DNCB) and are thus classified as anergic. An anergic cancer patient usually has a rapidly growing tumor and a poor prognosis.

The three types of immunotherapy are active, passive, and adoptive. Active therapy involves administration of an antigen to stimulate the patient's immune system, with subsequent development of immunity (antibody).

Specific active immunotherapy stimulates an immune response to a tumor-associated antigen:

1. Autologous vaccine produced from the patient's own tumor and injected intradermally at various sites
2. Allogeneic vaccine—a mixture of tumor cells that are of the same type as the patient's but that may be more immunogenetic because they are new to the patient's immune system
3. Modified tumor cells—cells treated artificially to increase their antigenicity; cells may be irradiated or treated with neuramidinase, a chemical found to stimulate the immune system by removing a coating on tumor cells

Nonspecific immunotherapy stimulates the immune response to a wide variety of antigens, including tumor-associated antigens. Most frequently used is BCG (bacillus of Calmette and Guérin), which has some benefit as local treatment for superficial or subcutaneous melanoma metastases on the extremities. BCG immunotherapy is accomplished by scarification, intradermal injection into the tumor nodule, or a multiple puncture tine technique (which is quicker and causes less discomfort).

Corynebacterium parvulum is a gram-positive anaerobic bacillus also used for nonspecific immunotherapy. Other agents are 2,4-dinitrochlorobenzene (DNCB), pertussis vaccine, MER (methanol-extracted residue of BCG), and bacterial endotoxins.

Passive immunotherapy involves the direct transfer of transient immunity from person to person. Substances used include the antisera of patients with similar tumors, close family members, or associates and lymphocytes from cured cancer patients; cross-immunization and cross-transfusion are also performed.

Adoptive immunotherapy is based on the transfer of passive immunity and subsequent development of active immunity by the host. Transfer factor and immune RNA are the substances used.

Recent developments in immunotherapy include the synthesis of interferon, a substance discovered as natural body protein that has anticancer growth activity. Having already been proved active against viral diseases such as herpes zoster and hepatitis, interferon is believed to activate the immune system. It has been used with some success in the treatment of lymphomas and other cancers.

Monoclonal antibodies are the result of the genetic fusing of cancer cells with leukocytes to produce specific antibodies, which provide passive immunity and serve as carriers of cytotoxic agents to cancer cells.

Tumor cell vaccines (active immunotherapy) are administered in small intradermal injections and may produce reddened or pruritic injection sites and painful ulcerations. The sites should be washed at least twice a day with soap and water. If excoriation occurs, they may be cleansed with hydrogen peroxide and covered with a dressing. Fever, chills, and general malaise can usually be effectively treated with an analgesic such as acetaminophen.

When BCG is used for nonspecific immunotherapy, an inflammatory reaction occurs at the injection site after the patient becomes sensitized. Intradermal injection may cause fever, chills, and general malaise, as well as localized abscesses and drainage. Pretreatment with antihistamines and acetaminophen is helpful. If symptoms persist, isoniazid (INH) is effective. These same side effects may occur, although with less severity, after tine technique treatment. The lymph nodes that drain BCG may become enlarged and painful; SGOT or alkaline phosphatase levels may rise, and jaundice may appear. These reactions are usually temporary.[3,8]

References

1. American Cancer Society: A cancer source book for nurses, New York, 1981, The Society.
2. American Cancer Society: Cancer facts and figures, Boston, 1985, The Society.
3. American Cancer Society, Massachusetts Division: Cancer: a manual for practitioners, Boston, 1982, The Society.
4. Campbell, C.: Nursing diagnosis and intervention in nursing practice, New York, 1978, John Wiley & Sons, Inc.
5. Kim, M.J., McFarland, G.K., and McLane, A.M.: Pocket guide to nursing diagnoses, St. Louis, 1984, The C.V. Mosby Co.
6. Luckmann, J., and Sorensen, K.C.: Medical-surgical nursing: a psychophysiologic approach, Philadelphia, 1984, W.B. Saunders Co.
7. Nicholson, G.: Cancer metastasis, Sci. Am. **240**:66, 1979.
8. Rubin, P., editor: Clinical oncology for medical students and physicians: a multidisciplinary approach, New York, 1983, American Cancer Society.

Suggested Readings

CANCER OF THE LUNG

Boyer, Marjorie W.: Treating invasive lung cancer, Am. J. Nurs. **77**:1916, 1977.
Mier, J.W.: Management of metastatic carcinoma of the lung, Hosp. Formul. **18**:856, 1983.

CANCERS OF THE COLON AND RECTUM

Cullen, P.P.: Patients with colorectal cancer: how to assess and meet their needs, Nursing 76 **6**:42, 1976.
Dericks, V.C., and Donovan, C.J.: The ostomy patient really needs you, Nursing 76 **6**:30, 1976.
Lamanske, J.: Helping the ileostomy patient to help himself, Nursing 77 **7**:34, 1977.

CARCINOMA OF THE BREAST

Burger, D.: Breast self-examination, Am. J. Nurs. **79**:1088, 1979.
Thomas, S.G., and Yates, M.M.: Confronting one's changed image: breast reconstruction after mastectomy, Am. J. Nurs. **77**:1438, 1977.
Toal, D.R.: Tumor cell kinetics and cancer chemotherapy, Am. J. Nurs. **80**:1802, 1980.
Tully, J.P., and Wagner, B.: Breast cancer: helping the mastectomy patient live life fully, Nursing 78 **8**:18, 1978.
Warren, B.: Adjuvant chemotherapy for breast cancer: the nurse's role, Cancer Nurs. **2**:32, 1979.

CANCERS OF THE SKIN

Jepsen, L.: Malignant melanoma: rare cancer, unique problems, Nursing 77, **7**:38-43, 1977.
Sullivan, B.P.: BCG in cancer therapy: patient responses to BCG therapy for malignant melanoma, Am. J. Nurs. **79**:320, 1979.

CANCERS OF THE URINARY TRACT

Barrett, N.: Cancer of the bladder: a case history, Am. J. Nurs. **81**:2192, 1981.
Gault, P.L.: Six patients with bladder cancer . . . and how they fared after surgery, Nursing 77 **7**:48, 1977.

CANCERS OF THE MALE REPRODUCTIVE SYSTEM

Hoeft, R.T., and Jones, A.G.: Cancer of the prostate: treating metastasis with estramustine phosphate, Am. J. Nurs. **82**:829, 1982.
Jones, A.G., and Hoeft, R.T.: Cancer of the prostate, Am. J. Nurs. **82**:826, 1982.

GYNECOLOGIC CANCERS

Hamilton, M.S., and Schlapper, N.B.: Pelvic exenteration, Am. J. Nurs. **76**:266, 1976.
Kalbarcyk, J.A.: Cancer of the uvula, Nursing 75 **5**:28, 1975.
Winer, W.K.: Laser treatment of cervical neoplasia, Am. J. Nurs. **82**:1384, 1982.

CANCERS OF THE DIGESTIVE AND ENDOCRINE GLANDS

Gotch, P.M.: Are you ready for a total pancreatectomy patient? RN **44**:54, 1981.

CANCER OF THE HEAD AND NECK

Larsen, G.L.: Rehabilitation for the patient with head and neck cancer, Am. J. Nurs. **82**:119, 1982.

McConnell, E.A.: How to truly help the patient with a radical neck dissection, Nursing 76 **6**:58, 1976.

ORAL CANCER

Daly, K.M.: Oral cancer: everyday concerns, Am. J. Nurs. **79**:1415, 1979.

Oser, J.: Oral cancer: coping with the changes, Am. J. Nurs. **79**:1418, 1979.

CANCER OF THE BONE

Levitt, D.Z.: Multiple myeloma, Am. J. Nurs. **81**:1345, 1981.

McNally, J.: Bone metastasis, Oncol. Nurs. Forum **8**:50, 1981.

Megliola, B.: Multiple myeloma, CA Nurs. **3**:209, 1980.

Rickel, L.: Emotional support for the multiple myeloma patient, Nursing 76 **6**:76, 1976.

Rose-Williamson, K., and Rathburn, S.: Planning discharge for a patient with osteogenic sarcoma, Oncol. Nurs. Forum **8**:38, 1981.

CANCERS OF THE CENTRAL NERVOUS SYSTEM AND CHILDHOOD CANCERS

Cleveland, M.J.: Nursing care in childhood cancer: brain tumor, Am. J. Nurs. **82**:422, 1982.

Craft, M., et al.: Nursing care in childhood cancer: coping, Am. J. Nurs. **82**:440, 1982.

Gaddy, D.S.: Nursing care in childhood cancer: update, Am. J. Nurs. **82**:418, 1982.

Greene, P., and Fergusson, J.: Nursing care of childhood cancer: late effects of therapy, Am. J. Nurs. **82**:443, 1982.

Wong, D., and Dornan, L.R.: Nursing care in childhood cancer: retinoblastoma, Am. J. Nurs. **82**:425, 1982.

ONCOLOGIC EMERGENCIES

Doogan, R.A.: Hypercalcemia of malignancy, CA Nurs. **4**:299, 1981.

Spross, J., and Stern, R.: Nursing management of oncology patients with superior vena cava obstruction syndrome, Oncol. Nurs. Forum **6**:3, 1979.

Valentine, A.S., and Stewart, J.A.: Oncologic emergencies, Am. J. Nurs. **83**:1281, 1983.

Yarbro, J.W., and Borstein, R.S.: Oncologic emergencies, New York, 1981, Grune & Stratton, Inc.

PSYCHOSOCIAL ASPECTS OF CANCER

Accola, K.M., and Sommerfield, D.P.: Helping people with cancer consider parenthood, Am. J. Nurs. **79**:1580, 1979.

Adams, J.: Mutual help groups—enhancing the coping ability of oncology clients, CA Nurs. **2**:95, 1979.

Aiken, S.: Family structure and utilization of cancer support groups, Oncol. Nurs. Forum **9**:22, 1982.

Coping with cancer: a resource for the health professional, Bethesda, Md., 1980, U.S. Department of Health and Human Services, Public Health Service, National Institutes of Health.

Freidenbergs, I., et al.: Assessment and treatment of psychosocial problems of the cancer patient: a case study, CA Nurs. **3**:111, 1980.

Friedman, B.D.: Coping with cancer: a guide for health care professionals, CA Nurs. **3**:105, 1980.

Herzoff, N.E.: A therapeutic group for cancer patients and their families, Cancer Nurs. 469, 1979.

Kelley, P.P., and Ashby, G.C.: Group approaches for cancer patients: establishing a group, Am. J. Nurs. **79**:914, 1979.

Miller, M.W., and Nygren, C.: Living with cancer-coping behaviors, Nurs. **1**:297, 1978.

Ostchega, Y., and Jacob, J.G.: Providing "safe conduct": helping your patients cope with cancer, Nursing 84 **14**:42, 1984.

Osterlund, H.: Humor: a serious approach to patient care, Nursing 83 **13**:46, 1983.

Shubin, S.: Cancer widows, Nursing 78 **8**:56, 1978.

Watts, R.J.: Dimensions of sexual health, Am. J. Nurs. **79**:1568, 1979.

Weisman, A.: Coping with cancer, New York, 1979, McGraw-Hill Book Co.

Welch-McCaffrey, D.: When it comes to cancer, think family, Nursing 83 **13**:32, 1983.

Whitman, H.H., Gustafson, J.P., and Coleman, F.W.: Group approaches for cancer patients: leaders and members, Am. J. Nurs. **79**:910, 1979.

CANCER CHEMOTHERAPY

Barlock, A., et al.: Nursing management of adriamycin extravasation, Am. J. Nurs. **79**:94, 1979.

Bersani, G., and Carl, W.: Oral care for cancer patients, Am. J. Nurs. **83**:533, 1983.

Brager, B.L., and Yasko, J.: Care of the client receiving chemotherapy, Reston, Va., 1984, Reston Publishing Co., Inc.

Burns, N.: Cancer chemotherapy: a systemic approach, Nursing 78 **8**:56, 1978.

Fredette, S.L., and Gloriant, F.S.: Nursing diagnoses in cancer chemotherapy: in theory, Am. J. Nurs. **81**:2013, 1981.

Fredette, S.L.: Nursing diagnoses in cancer chemotherapy: in practice, Am. J. Nurs. **81**:2021, 1981.

Maxwell, M.B.: Scalp tourniquets for chemotherapy-induced alopecia, Am. J. Nurs. **80**:900, 1980.

Oncology Nursing Society: Cancer chemotherapy: guidelines and recommendations for nursing education and practice, Pittsburgh, Pa., 1984, The Society.

Petton, S.: Easing the complications of chemotherapy: a matter of little victories, Nursing 84 58, 1984.

Rose-Williamson, C.: Cisplatin: delivering a safe infusion, Am. J. Nurs. **81**:320, 1981.

Scogna, D.M., and Smalley, R.V.: Chemotherapy-induced nausea and vomiting, Am. J. Nurs. **79**:1562, 1979.

Wroblewski, S.S., and Wroblewski, S.H.: Caring for the patient with chemotherapy-induced thrombocytopenia, Am. J. Nurs. **81**:746, 1981.

RADIATION THERAPY

Breeding, M.A., and Wollin, M.: Working safely around implanted radiation sources, Nursing 76 **6**:58, 1976.

Elliott, C.S.J.: Radiation therapy: how you can help, Nursing 76 **6**:34, 1976.

Kelley, P.P., and Tinsley, C.: Planning care for the patient receiving external radiation, Am. J. Nurs. **81**:338, 1981.

Varricchio, C.G.: The patient on radiation therapy, Am. J. Nurs. **81**:334, 1981.

IMMUNOTHERAPY

Bochow, A.J.: Cancer immunotherapy: what promise does it hold? Nursing 76 **6**:50, 1976.

Croft, C.L.: BCG administration and nursing implications, Am. J. Nurs. **79**:315, 1979.

Dodd, M.J.: BCG in cancer therapy: theoretical bases of immunotherapy, Am. J. Nurs. **79**:310, 1979.

BLOOD COMPONENT THERAPY

Kazak, A.: Blood therapy: processing blood for transfusion, Am. J. Nurs. **79**:931, 1979.

Thoms, S.F.: Blood therapy: transfusing granulocytes, Am. J. Nurs. **79**:942, 1979.

CHAPTER 15

Infectious Diseases

At the beginning of the nineteenth century no infectious disease was controlled in America. Major efforts in environmental sanitation, advances in immunization and antibiotic therapy, and application of antimicrobial technology to disease agents have resulted in control of many of the dreaded infectious diseases of the past. Today, most health professionals in the United States never see cases of the major killers such as yellow fever, cholera, typhus, smallpox, malaria, typhoid fever, or plague. That is not meant to suggest that infectious disease has been eradicated or even controlled. Some infectious diseases, such as hepatitis and the sexually transmitted diseases, are increasing in the United States. Others, such as measles and mumps, persist despite the availability of preventive measures. Antibiotic-resistant organisms flourish, and new infectious disease agents continue to be identified. While many of the major killers have been controlled in the United States, these diseases continue to cause death and destruction in other parts of the world, necessitating a vigilant attitude toward these diseases.

Because all infectious disease have characteristics in common, this overview will discuss the following aspects:

1. Nature of infectious disease
2. Pathogenic agents
3. Agent, host, and environmental interaction for disease transmission

Nature of Infectious Disease

Definitions. Contamination, infection, infectious disease, communicable disease, and contagious disease are not synonymous terms. Contamination is merely the presence of a microorganism on an inanimate object, whereas infection is the implantation and successful reproduction of a microorganism on or in the tissue of a human host. If no physiologic response occurs, the organisms have merely colonized the host. The colonized host who also sheds the organisms is a carrier. If physiologic response occurs without overt symptoms, the process is termed a subclinical or inapparent infection. If tissue injury or body responses result in symptoms of illness, an infectious disease is present. Communicable disease is an infectious disease that results from transmission of an infectious microorganism or its products to a susceptible human host either directly or indirectly, through an intermediate animal host, a vector, or the inanimate environment. Contagious diseases are communicable diseases transmitted by direct contact.

Stages of infection. The progression from infection to infectious disease in human beings follows definable stages. The duration of the stages and the potential outcomes vary with infectious disease agents and disease processes. A latent stage follows invasion of the cells by a microorganism and lasts until infection is patent and the organism can be shed (i.e., the beginning of com-

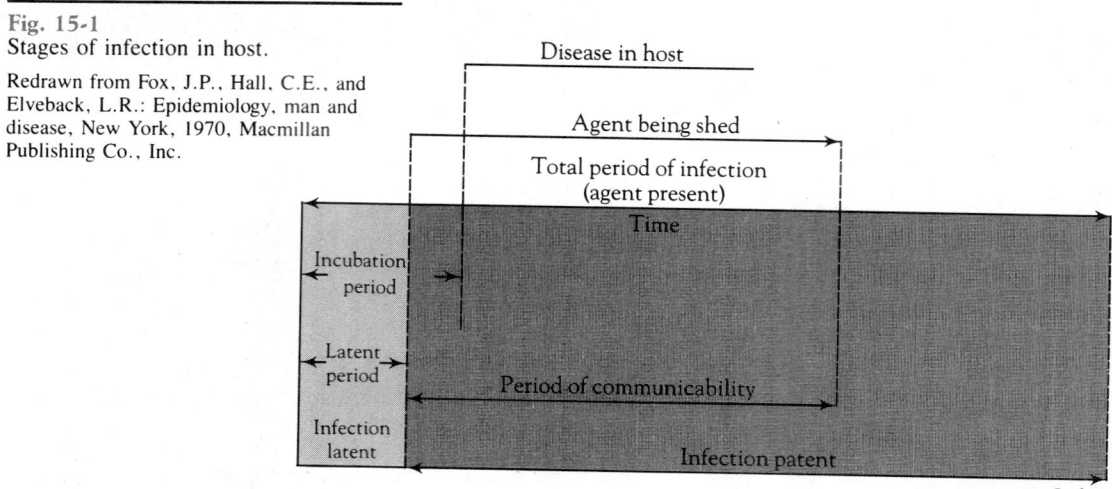

Fig. 15-1
Stages of infection in host.

Redrawn from Fox, J.P., Hall, C.E., and
Elveback, L.R.: Epidemiology, man and
disease, New York, 1970, Macmillan
Publishing Co., Inc.

municability). The incubation stage, during which the organism is multiplying, also starts with microorganism invasion and persists until the disease process is present. The disease stage may be asymptomatic (subclinical) or may present overt symptoms. The length of the disease stage is extremely variable, sometimes extending beyond the period of communicability. Resolution of the infectious disease may precede or coincide with termination of the infection. The infectious process may terminate completely or revert to the latent stage. In the latter case intermittent infectious disease may result or the host may become a carrier, continuing to harbor and shed the incubating infectious agent.[37] Fig. 15-1 depicts the stages of infection in the host.

Spectrum of occurrence of cases. The frequency of occurrence of cases of infectious disease can be characterized as sporadic, endemic, or epidemic. Sporadic refers to occasional and irregular occurrence of cases in a population over a specified period of time. Endemic means that the disease occurs with a constant frequency in a specified population over a definite time period. Epidemic refers to a definite increase in disease incidence over its expected endemic occurrence.

Pathogenic Agents

Infectious diseases have one characteristic in common: a pathogenic agent is a necessary factor to the development of the disease. Although the agent must be present, it is not a sufficient cause for disease; disease development also depends on host susceptibility and pathogen characteristics to be discussed here.

Symbiotic relationships with humans. Pathogenic agents are living parasites, maintaining themselves at the expense of their human host. Parasitic relationships can be differentiated from other types of relationships between living organisms and humans. The human has a constant symbiotic relationship with a normal flora of organisms, some of which are harmless and others of which are pathogenic only under certain conditions. If the relationship benefits both the organism and the human host, as is the case with *Escherichia coli* in the intestinal tract, the relationship is one of mutualism. If the relationship only benefits the organism but causes no harm to the host, it is termed commensalism. Some organisms may have a commensal relationship on one part of the body but become pathogenic elsewhere, as is the case with alpha streptococci in the nasopharynx becoming pathogenic to heart valves. Some pathogens that normally have a commensal relationship with the host may produce disease only under conditions of host susceptibility. These pathogens are opportunists, producing opportunistic infections. In addition to establishing one of the symbiotic relationships, many organisms are transient residents on or in the human. These organisms, some of which are pathogenic, are picked up and shed regularly, possibly producing disease in a more susceptible host.

Intrinsic characteristics of agents. One characteristic common to all pathogenic agents is their ability to establish a parasitic relationship in humans. Generally, the greater the dose of the pathogen, the greater the risk for disease. Pathogenic agents vary according to observable intrinsic characteristics such as their morphology and chemical composition, their growth requirements, and their viability.

Morphology (size, shape, and structure) of the organism and the chemical composition (nucleic acids, enzyme system, and antigenic proteins) of living agents provide

Table 15-1
Characteristics of Categories of Pathogens with Representative Diseases[20,41]

Category	Characteristics	Pathogen	Diseases
Protozoa	Animal-like, single cell organism; breaks down and absorbs nutrients from host; can grow outside living cells	*Plasmodium* *Entamoeba histolytica* *Giardia* *Trichomonas vaginalis*	Malaria Amebic dysentery Enteritis Vulvovaginitis
Fungi	Plantlike organism; lives on decaying matter	Dermatophytes *Histoplasma*	Athlete's foot Ringworm Histoplasmosis
Yeast	Plantlike organism; a type of fungus	*Candida albicans*	Moniliasis Candidiasis
Bacteria	Plant and animal like; can grow outside living cell; 19 different categories; differentiated according to morphology, staining characteristics, motility, colony formation, nutritional requirements, biochemical activity, and antigenic makeup	*Bacillus anthracis* *Bordetella pertussis* *Clostridium botulinum* *Clostridium tetani* *Corynebacterium diphtheriae* *Haemophilus influenzae* *Klebsiella pneumoniae* *Staphylococcus aureus* *Streptococcus pyogenes* *Mycobacterium tuberculosis* *Neisseria gonorrhoeae* *Salmonella typhi* *Shigella* *Treponema pallidum* *Vibrio cholerae*	Anthrax Pertussis Botulism Tetanus Diphtheria Meningitis Pneumonia Septicemia Strep throat Tuberculosis Gonorrhea Typhoid fever Shigellosis Syphilis Cholera
Rickettsiae	Sometimes classified with bacteria but smaller than bacteria; must live inside a cell, like viruses; carried by vectors	*Rickettsiae rickettsii* *Rickettsia typhi*	Rocky Mountain spotted fever Typhus
Chlamydiae	Like viruses, can only obtain energy from living cell; sometimes classified with bacteria; spread by person-to-person contact	*Chlamydia trachomatis*	Trachoma Lymphogranuloma venereum
Mycoplasmata	Smallest cellular microbes; sometimes classified with bacteria; can grow outside living cell as can bacteria	*Mycoplasma pneumoniae*	Atypical pneumonia Sinusitis Conjunctivitis
Viruses	Small particles (not classified as living cells); lack ability to produce energy; depend on ribosomes of infected cells for energy production; possess DNA or RNA (not both); replication directed by nucleic acids (RNA or DNA); action: injects RNA or DNA into cell, altering metabolism of host cells; if cells die, all viruses are released at once; if cells do not die, viruses are released one at a time; local reaction: cells undergo hyperplasia or hyperplasia and necrosis; differentiated according to nucleic acid core, according to biologic, chemical, or physical properties, and according to the way they enter the body	Pox virus Herpes simplex 1 Herpes simplex 2 Adenovirus Rhinovirus Polio virus Hepatitis A; B; non-A, non-B Coxsackievirus *Enterovirus* Myxovirus parotids Paramyxovirus Rhabdovirus Orthomyxovirus, types A and B	Smallpox Cold sores Venereal herpes Pneumonia, conjunctivitis Colds Poliomyelitis Hepatitis Meningitis Intestinal infection Mumps Rubeola Rabies Influenza
Helminths	Multicellular; large enough to be seen without microscope; migrate within host; induce eosinophilia; unable to multiply in the host; transmitted by ingestion, skin penetration, injection by insects	Nematodes (roundworms, hookworms, and pinworms) *Trichinella* worms Filarial worms Cestodes (flatworms and tapeworms) Trematodes (flukes)	Anemia Anal pruritus Trichinosis Filiariasis Anemia Biliary obstruction Hepatomegaly

the basis for classification and laboratory identification of specific categories of agents and for differentiation within categories. Morphology alone permits identification of the larger parasitic worms. Identification of the microorganisms depends on knowledge of morphology, colony formation, staining characteristics, nutritional requirements, and the antigenic proteins of specific organisms.

Pathogens can also be differentiated according to their growth requirements. Because they cannot synthesize their own amino acids, they rely on their host to supply their nutritional requirements. Some pathogens, such as bacteria, have a metabolic structure enabling them to sustain themselves outside the human cell for varying lengths of time depending on the organism. Viruses have no metabolic activity and must receive all sustenance for survival from the host cell.

Viability is the ability of the pathogenic agent to survive in an adverse environment by resisting physical, chemical, or thermal agents. Viability is determined by the morphology and chemical composition of various pathogens. The ability of some organisms, such as the tetanus bacilli, to produce spores or to undergo genetic change, as with the antibiotic-resistant strains of bacteria, increases their viability. Antigenic changes in some pathogens, such as the influenza viruses, permits parasitism in previously immune hosts, thus extending the viability of the pathogen.

The microorganisms pathogenic to humans are classified as protozoa, fungi and yeasts, bacteria, rickettsiae, chlamydiae, mycoplasmata, and viruses, in order of decreasing size. A larger group of organisms, also parasitic to humans, are the helminths, or worms. Table 15-1 describes basic characteristics of each of the categories of pathogens with examples of the organisms and diseases they produce.

Agent characteristics interacting with humans. Pathogenic agents also vary according to the manner in which they interact with the human host as to their mode of action, infectivity, pathogenicity, virulence, toxigenicity, and antigenicity.

The mode of action may be direct damage to cells by causing hyperplasia, necrosis, and death to the cells; or the action may be through the production of poisonous toxins that cause local or systemic reactions in the host.

Infectivity of the agent is its ability to invade and multiply in the host. It is affected by host defenses and enzymes produced by the organism to facilitate invasiveness. Coagulase, an extracellular enzyme, enables organisms such as staphylococci to clot plasma and form a sticky fibrin layer around themselves to protect against the host's defenses. Another enzyme, streptokinase, lyses or dissolves fibrin clots, allowing streptococci to spread through host tissue. Hyaluronidase causes breakdown of connective tissue and increases tissue perme-

ability of organisms such as streptococci, pneumococci, and clostridia. Collagenase breaks down collagen, allowing deep invasion of organisms such as *Clostridium perfringens* into tendons, cartilage, and bones. Agents have been graded according to their infectivity potential.[37] Poliomyelitis virus is a highly infective agent; rubella virus is an intermediate infective agent; and *M. tuberculosis* is an agent of low infectivity.

Pathogenicity, the ability of an agent to produce disease, depends on the speed with which the agent multiplies, the extent of tissue damage, and the production of a toxin. Agents can be graded according to this characteristic also.[37] Agents causing smallpox and rabies are highly pathogenic, and infection with them generally results in disease. The rubella virus has intermediate pathogenicity, and the poliomyelitis virus has low pathogenicity.

Virulence, or potency, of the pathogenic agent determines the severity of the disease process. It is measured in terms of the number of microorganisms or micrograms of toxin necessary to kill a given host.[61] Gradation of agents according to virulence is possible.[37] The rabies virus is a highly virulent agent; the poliomyelitis virus is intermediate; measles virus is low; and the virus causing the common cold has very low virulence.

The toxigenicity of agents is an important factor in determining virulence. Agent products associated with toxigenicity are hemolysin, leucocidin, and toxins. Hemolysin causes destruction of the host's erythrocytes; and leucocidin destroys leukocytes. Both are factors in the virulence of some streptococci and staphylococci. Agents vary in the amount and destructive potential of the toxins they produce. Some bacteria secrete water-soluble antigenic exotoxins that are quickly distributed by the blood, causing potentially severe systemic and neurologic manifestations. Diseases associated with exotoxins are tetanus, botulism, and diphtheria. Endotoxins make up the cell wall of some bacteria and cause local inflammation and destruction of host tissue. They are weakly toxic, are relatively stable, and are not antigenic. Diseases associated with endotoxins include staphylococcal food poisoning and cholera.[61]

Antigenicity is the ability of a pathogen to induce an immune response in the host. Pathogens vary according to this characteristic. Some have intrinsic antigens (proteins, polypeptides, or polysaccharides) that causes the host to produce antibodies against the antigen. This host response will be discussed under immunity.

Agent, Host, and Environment Interaction for Disease Transmission

The ability of a pathogenic agent to produce infectious disease in humans depends on the agent characteristics discussed in the previous section plus an intact chain of transmission. The chain includes a host reservoir, mode of escape from the reservoir, environment conducive to transmission of the pathogen, entry into a new host, and susceptibility of the new host to the infectious disease.

Reservoir. A reservoir is a person, animal, arthropod, plant, soil, or organic substance, alone or in combination, in which an infectious agent lives and multiplies. The agent depends on the reservoir for its reproduction and consequent survival.[7] Humans are the only reservoir for some pathogens, whereas other pathogens require an intermediate animal or chain of animal or inanimate reservoirs. The human reservoir may have a frank or a subclinical infection, or the person may be a carrier.

Escape. The organism escapes from the reservoir at the site of the multiplication of the organism. Portals of exit may be the genitourinary tract, the gastrointestinal tract, the oral cavity, the respiratory tract, open lesions, or mechanical escape of blood. There may be more than one portal of exit for any one disease process. The duration of escape coincides with the period of communicability and varies with each disease. Generally, there is an inverse relationship between the length of the communicable period and the infectivity of the organism. Highly infectious organisms such as the influenza virus have a short duration of escape, whereas the less infective *M. tuberculosis* has a long duration of escape.

The portal of exit determines the mode of transmission and is therefore an important consideration for health workers in contact with infectious agents. An outline* of the types of pathogens usually associated with each portal of exit is included here:

I. Oral and respiratory tracts
   A. Bacteria
      1. Gram-positive cocci (pneumonia, *Streptococcus pneumoniae;* scarlet fever, *S. pyogenes*)
      2. Gram-negative cocci (epidemic meningitis, *Neisseria meningitidis*)
      3. Gram-positive rods
         a. Diphtheria *(Corynebacterium diphtheriae)*
         b. Tuberculosis *(M. tuberculosis)*
      4. Gram-negative rods (laryngitis, *H. influenzae;* whooping cough, *B. pertussis*)
      5. Spirochetes (Vincent's angina, syphilis)
      6. Psittacosis organisms
   B. Viruses
      1. Smallpox
      2. Mumps
      3. Measles
      4. Chickenpox
      5. Rabies

      6. Myxoviruses
      7. Adenoviruses, rhinoviruses
      8. Poliovirus
   C. Fungi (see V)
II. Intestinal and/or urinary tract
   A. Bacteria
      1. Enterobacteriaceae (typhoid, dysentery)
      2. *Brucella* (undulant fever)
      3. *Leptospira* (leptospirosis)
      4. *Clostridium* (gas gangrene and tetanus; see V)
   B. Viruses
      1. Poliomyelitis
      2. Coxsackie
      3. ECHO
      4. Hepatitis A
   C. Protozoa
      1. *E. histolytica* (dysentery)
      2. *Trichomonas hominis* (enteritis)
      3. *Giardia lamblia* (enteritis)
   D. Helminths
      1. Hookworm
      2. *Ascaris*
      3. Pinworms
      4. Whipworm
      5. Flukes
      6. Tapeworms
III. Genital tract
   A. Bacteria
      1. *T. pallidum* (syphilis)
      2. *N. gonorrhoeae* (gonorrheal infection)
      3. *Haemophilus ducreii* (chancroid)
      4. *Calymmatobacterium granulomatis* (granuloma inguinale)
      5. *Chlamydiaceae* (lymphogranuloma venereum organisms)
   B. Protozoa
      1. *T. vaginalis* (vulvovaginitis)
IV. Pathogens of humans usually transmitted in blood
   A. Mainly by sanguiferous arthopods
      1. Bacteria
         a. *Yersinia pestis* (bubonic plague)
         b. *Pasteurella tularensis* (tularemia)
         c. *Borrelia* (relapsing fever)
      2. Rickettsiae (Rocky Mountain spotted fever, typhus)
      3. Viruses
         a. Yellow and dengue fevers
         b. Other arboviruses
      4. Protozoa
         a. *Plasmodium* (malaria)
         b. *Trypanosoma* (trypanosomiasis)
         c. *Leishmania* (leishmaniasis)
      5. Helminths
         a. Filarias (filariasis)

*Adapted from Frobisher, M., and Fuerst, R.: Microbiology and disease, ed. 13, Philadelphia, 1973, W.B. Saunders Co.

B. Mainly by artificial vectors (e.g., hypodermic needles, syringes, autopsy instruments, surgical instruments, and some blood derivatives [plasma, serum whole blood])
   1. Viruses (notably those of epidemic hepatitis and of homologous serum hepatitis [i.e., hepatitis viruses A and B]), which may be circulating in the blood at the time the blood is drawn or the instruments used
   2. Bacteria that frequently cause bacteremia: *Brucella*, *Salmonella*, *Streptococcus*, *Staphylococcus*, *Neisseria*, *Pasteurella*, *Diplococcus*, *Leptospira*, *Treponema*

V. Pathogens commonly found in the soil
   A. Bacteria
      1. Genus *Clostridium* (anaerobes)
         a. Gas gangrene group
         b. *Cl. tetani* (tetanus)
         c. *Cl. botulinum* (food poisoning)
      2. Genus *Bacillus* (aerobes)
         a. *B. anthracis* (anthrax)
   B. Fungi
      1. *Coccidioides immitis* (coccidiodomycosis)
      2. *H. capsulatum* (histoplasmosis)
      3. *Sporotrichum* (sporotrichosis)
      4. *Blastomyces*
   C. Helminths (see II)

Transmission. The organism may have a single or multiple routes of transmission. In general, the organism may be transmitted directly through person-to-person contact or indirectly through an animate or inanimate vehicle of transmission. Direct contact occurs when there is actual physical contact between the source and the victim as is the case with sexual, fecal-oral, or mucous droplet transmission. Indirect transmission requires that the organism survive outside the human on or in animate or inanimate vehicles. Animate vehicles include animals and vectors. Inanimate vehicles are air, food, water, milk, soil, fomites, or biologic materials. If an inanimate vehicle has the potential of infecting many persons, it is called a common vehicle.[7]

Entry. Portal of entry into a new host corresponds frequently with the portal of exit from the reservoir. Entry may be by ingestion, by inhalation, by percutaneous injection, through the mucous membranes, or across the placenta. The duration of the exposure and the numbers of organisms necessary to start the infectious process in the new host vary with each disease.

Host susceptibility. Susceptibility refers to those host conditions that increase the probability that disease may develop in the host. Susceptibility is affected by specific resistance factors such as the immunologic responses and nonspecific body defenses against disease agents, both of which will be discussed in the next section. Host

Table 15-2
Chain of Transmission of Infectious Disease

Transmission Chain	Factors
Agent (living parasite)	Bacteria, rickettsiae, fungi, chlamydiae, mycoplasmata, viruses, helminths
Reservoir (where agent lives and multiplies)	Humans (frank cases, subclinical cases, carriers) Inanimate organic matter Animals
Portal of exit	Genitourinary tract, gastrointestinal tract, respiratory tract, oral cavity, open lesions, blood
Transmission	Direct: person to person (fecal-oral, sexual, droplet) Indirect: through a vehicle (animate: animal or vector; inanimate: food, water, soil, milk, air, intravenous therapy or catheters)
Modes of entry	Ingestion, inhalation, percutaneous injection, transplacental entry, mucous membranes
Susceptible host	Specific immune reactions Nonspecific body defenses Host characteristics: age, sex, ethnic group, heredity, behaviors Environmental and general health status

susceptibility is also affected by general human characteristics such as age, sex, ethnic group, and heredity; behaviors regarding eating and personal hygiene; geographic and environmental living conditions; and general health status, including nutritional status, hormonal balance, and the presence of concurrent disease. All of these factors either determine the type of pathogenic agent to which the person is exposed or determine the extent of the host response and resistance to the pathogens.[7] The chain of transmission is summarized in Table 15-2.

Control. Control of infectious disease relies on procedures aimed at breaking the chain of transmission at one or more of its links. The point of the chain most amenable to control varies with the organism and its reservoirs, the disease process, and available technology. Control measures may be directed to killing or altering the virulence of the agent, destroying nonhuman reservoirs and vectors, isolating the infected persons, using precautions with infected body fluids and contaminated inanimate objects, and altering host resistance, defenses, and immunity.

Effective control is also based on monitoring of disease occurrence to facilitate early intervention. Certain diseases must be reported to the local health authority. These are identified in the section on conditions, diseases, and disorders.

ANATOMY AND PHYSIOLOGY

Certain anatomic and physiologic characteristics of the human operate to increase resistance to infectious diseases and to fight the infectious process once it occurs. These characteristics can be considered as lines of defense against pathogenic agents. The first two lines are nonspecific to any agent; they result from the body's attempt to prevent the invasion of and to destroy foreign substances. The third line of defense, the immune response, is specific to specific pathogens. In addition to these defenses the human characteristically responds to an infectious process with a change in body temperature.

First Line of Defense: Nonspecific Body Defenses Against Infectious Agents

Mechanical barriers. Certain anatomic characteristics prevent the invasion of microorganisms. These include the intact skin and mucous membranes and oil and perspiration on the skin. Ciliary action in the respiratory tract, reflexes such as coughing and sneezing, and peristalsis in the gastrointestinal tract act to remove an organism before its penetration into tissue. The flushing action of body secretions such as tears, saliva, and mucus further protects against invasion. Compromise in any of these barriers increases susceptibility to invasion of infectious agents.

Chemical barriers. In addition to the mechanical barriers, the chemical composition of body secretions is protective. The pH of saliva, vaginal secretions, urine, and digestive secretions prevents or inhibits growth of some microbes. Bile acts to decrease the surface tension causing changes in the cell wall of some bacteria. This renders the organisms more digestible by other digestive enzymes. Oil and sweat secretions contain chemicals that are bactericidal to some microbes. The normal flora of microorganisms on the skin and in the intestinal and vaginal tracts is a further means of protection against invasion of pathogenic agents.

Second Line of Defense: Cellular Response

If a microorganism penetrates the first line of body defenses and invades cells, a response is initiated at the cellular level to protect the human cell from death and to prevent further invasion of the microorganism. The cellular response leads to the inflammatory process (the second line of defense).

Mechanisms of cell injury. The cell responds to an invading microorganism in a manner similar to its reaction to nonlethal physical, chemical, or thermal trauma. A biochemical lesion forms within the cell, reflecting a change in one or more cellular metabolic reactions. This may or may not be accompanied by a detectable morphologic change in the cell or impairment of function. The injured cell swells because of its inability to pump out sodium ions. If cellular metabolic activity is severely compromised, intracellular enzymes may digest portions of the cell. The resulting cellular atrophy reduces metabolic demands on the cell. Cell death results if metabolism can no longer be maintained. Enzymes are then released from the dead cell to further dissolve the cellular contents. These enzymes seep into the circulation and are the basis for laboratory tests to detect tissue necrosis in the body. The enzymes also act to stimulate the inflammatory process in surrounding tissue.

Inflammation. Inflammation, an active and aggressive response of tissue to cellular injury, serves to wall off, destroy, or neutralize infectious agents and to prepare the tissue for repair. It involves blood vessels, the fluid and cellular components of the blood, the lymphatic system, and the surrounding connective tissue.

The arterioles, venules, and capillaries dilate, resulting in hyperemia to the injured area. This increases the filtration pressure of the blood and increases permeability of the capillaries, causing a leakage of proteins and of fluid exudate into the interstitial spaces. The leakage of proteins increases the tissue colloid osmotic pressure, further attracting fluid into the interstitial spaces and resulting in visible edema and walling off of the inflamed area from other tissues.

With the leakage of fluid from the blood there is a concomitant slowing of the blood flow resulting in a "pavementing" or margination of leukocytes along the vascular endothelium. Leukocytes emigrate through the endothelium (diapedesis) to the injured tissue, attracted to the tissue by chemicals released by the injured cells or by the enzymes of necrotic cells. These chemicals include histamine, prostaglandins, and plasma kinins. The process of attracting the leukocytes is called chemotaxis.

Leukocytes are the cellular components of the blood associated with the inflammatory response to the infectious process. Leukocytes originate in the bone marrow, where most remain in an immature state until needed during infection. The number of mature leukocytes circulating in the blood is closely controlled to between 4500 and 11,000/cu mm of blood during noninfection states. Leukocytosis, an abnormal increase in circulating white blood cells, is symptomatic of many bacterial infections. Leukopenia, an abnormal decrease in circulating white blood cells, severely hampers the body's de-

Table 15-3

Differentiation of Leukocytes According to their Characteristics and Functions[41]

Leukocytes	Characteristics	Functions
Polymorphonuclear or granulocytes	Segmented lobular nucleus and granules in cytoplasm that contain enzymes and antimicrobial particles	
Neutrophils	First at scene of injury; ameboid motion to engulf agents; contain opsonins: substances that coat agent to be ingested; also contain antibacterial chemicals and enzymes; increase markedly during bacterial infections	Phagocytosis: engulf, digest living agents
Eosinophils	Same as above plus contain enzymes that counteract inflammatory process in allergic reactions	Weak phagocytosis
Basophils	Granules contain heparin and histamine	Respond to immunologic reactions
Mononuclear or agranular leukocytes	No granules in cytoplasm	
Lymphocytes	Large, round nuclei with scanty cytoplasm	Antibody production
Monocytes	Abundant cytoplasm and kidney-shaped nuclei; emigrate to site slowly but remain three or four times longer than granulocytes; not a mature cell when released from bone marrow; therefore they divide within injured tissue and increase their metabolic activities there	Phagocytosis

fenses against infectious agents. Leukopenia is characteristic of some adverse drug reactions and of conditions that depress bone marrow production of leukocytes. This latter condition is called agranulocytosis.

Blood leukocytes are differentiated according to their cellular characteristics and according to their various functions. The most numerous are the granulocytes or polymorphonuclear leukocytes with horseshoe-shaped nuclei that become multilobed as the cells age. Most of these cells contain neutrophilic granules in their cytoplasm (neutrophils), but some contain granules that stain with acid dyes (eosinophils), and some have basophilic granules (basophils). The other two cell types, lymphocytes and monocytes, have no granules in their cytoplasm. Table 15-3 outlines types of leukocytes with their characteristics and functions.

The various types of blood leukocytes can be identified and differentiated by hematologic tests, which report each type as a proportion of 100%. An increase in the percentage of one type will result in a decrease in the percentage of the other types even though the actual number of the other types does not change. As the total count of leukocytes increases during an acute bacterial infection, the percentage of polymorphonuclear neutrophils increases with a corresponding decrease in the percentage of mononuclear lymphocytes.

In addition to the circulating blood leukocytes there are mature monocytes called macrophages that are ordinarily fixed in tissue. The tissue macrophage system is referred to as the reticuloendothelial system. Macrophages adhere to tissue in the blood vessels, lymph nodes, spleen, and liver sinuses, destroying infectious agents that enter those systems. Macrophages can become mobile as needed or can produce phagocytosis directly in the involved tissue.[49]

Phagocytosis is the process of engulfing, digesting, and destroying infectious agents, primarily accomplished by circulating neutrophils and monocytes and tissue macrophages. This process occurs at the site of invasion of an infectious agent into tissue and continues into the lymph and blood circulation if organisms permeate those systems. Intracellular digestion of microorganisms by the phagocytic cells eventually results in further release of enzymes that induce lysis to some of the leukocytes. These dead leukocytes together with dead organisms and fluid from the blood make up the inflammatory exudate.

Four types of inflammatory exudates may be present in or on tissue during inflammation. The serous exudate contains only blood fluid and proteins and is characteristic of edema during early inflammation. Mucinous or catarrhal exudates represent an increase in secretions from inflamed mucous membranes. They may contain live or dead microorganisms. Fibrinous exudates are formed on tissue, particularly mucous membranes, when large amounts of fibrinogen are extravasated into the tissue. Purulent exudates consist of living and dead leukocytes, living and dead microorganisms, fluid exudate from the blood, and the liquefied digestive products of the dead, necrotic tissue. Pus is an example of a purulent exudate. Some inflammatory conditions produce combinations of exudates. A fibrinopurulent exudate, resulting from necrosis of the mucous membrane of the throat, is characteristic of diphtheria.

Inflammation and inflammatory exudates may remain

localized, may permeate the tissue, or may spread through the blood or lymph. An abscess is an example of an infection and inflammatory process with purulent exudate in a localized stage. Leukocytes form a wall around the infectious agent in the tissue. The area of abscess deepens into the tissue as more leukocytes are drawn to the area, more organisms are killed, and more necrotic tissue is dissolved. The exudate may eventually be autolyzed and reabsorbed by the body, leading to resolution of the inflammation and abscess. Resolution may leave a cavity or ulcer at the site of the inflammation, may prepare the way for regeneration of cells, or may leave scar tissue. In some cases calcification occurs around the exudate, serving to wall off living infectious agents in the tissue. Such is frequently the case with tuberculosis.

The abscess may rupture or be mechanically ruptured and drained. Rupture of an abscess into a pleural cavity is called empyema; rupture into the peritoneal cavity leads to peritonitis. An abscess may also drain through a sinus or tract to another organ or tissue causing inflammation there. The spread of a purulent inflammatory process diffusely through tissue may result in cellulitis. If the infectious agent enters the bloodstream, bacteremia is present. Septicemia results if a pathogenic agent multiplies or releases toxin in the blood. If the infectious agent enters lymph vessels and initiates inflammation, lymphangitis is present. Lymphadenitis describes inflammation of lymph nodes.

Factors affecting the outcome of the inflammatory defense process include host and agent factors. Age, nutritional status, and general health status of the human host greatly affect the person's ability to successfully initiate and resolve an inflammatory process. Agent factors, such as the ability to produce enzymes and fibrin, promote spread of the organism in spite of an aggressive inflammatory defense.

There may be both local and systemic symptoms of inflammation present in the infected human. Local symptoms include erythema, heat, edema, and pain from pressure on nerve endings. A purulent exudate may or may not be visible. Systemic symptoms may include fever and chills, diaphoresis, malaise, and nausea and vomiting. Alterations can be seen in blood leukocyte levels, blood proteins, and the erythrocyte sedimentation rate.

At the cellular level of defense two additional systems of blood and tissue products are important in preventing the spread of invading organisms: the properdin system and cellular interferon. The properdin system is made up of a group of serum components (properidine, magnesium ions, and a complement of 11 interacting proteins) that act as enzymes to inactivate viruses and to directly destroy bacteria. Interferon is a cellular protein produced by cells when viral DNA or RNA is introduced into the cell. Interferon is released by the infected cells and transferred to noninfected cells, thus preventing the spread of the virus to other cells.[41]

Third Line of Defense: Specific Resistance or Acquired Immunity

Whereas the first two lines of defense are nonspecific for any one type of infectious agent, the third line of defense, acquired immunity, is a host response to a specific agent. Those agents that have antigenic characteristics are capable of eliciting an immune response in the human host. Not all agents are antigenic or immunogenic. Some agents, although not antigenic by themselves, combine chemically with substances produced by the host to form an antigen that elicits an immune response.

Nature of the immune response. The human immune response has certain general properties. First, antibodies or specific lymphocytes are produced in response to specific antigens. Antigens are the chemical compounds of agents or their toxins that are different from all other chemical compounds. In general, these compounds are proteins, large polysaccharides, or large lipoprotein complexes. Second, the immune system generally recognizes host cells as nonantigenic and thus responds only to foreign proteins or polysaccharides as antigens (autoimmune diseases are an exception to this rule). Third, the immune system remembers the antigens that have invaded in the past. Host cells have a memory for the antigen and respond more rapidly with successive invasions.

Differentiating types of immunity. This section deals with immunity acquired directly as a response to a specific pathogenic and antigenic agent. This can be

Table 15-4

Types of Acquired Immunity

	Natural	**Artificial**
Active	Resistance resulting from natural contact with the pathogenic agent and infection with the agent; may be temporary or permanent	Resistance resulting from injection of dead or attenuated pathogens or toxoids; may be temporary or permanent
Passive	Temporary resistance resulting from transfer of antibodies from mother to infant congenitally, transplacentally, or through colostrum	Temporary resistance resulting from injection of antiserum, antitoxin, or gamma globulins produced in another host

Fig. 15-2

Cellular and humoral immunity.
Formation of antibodies and sensitized
lymphocytes by a lymph node in
response to antigens. This figure also
shows the origin of thymic (T) and
bursal (B) lymphocytes, which are
responsible for the cellular and
humoral immune processes of the
lymph nodes.

From Guyton, A.C.: Human physiology
and mechanism of disease, ed. 3,
Philadelphia, 1982, W.B. Saunders Co.

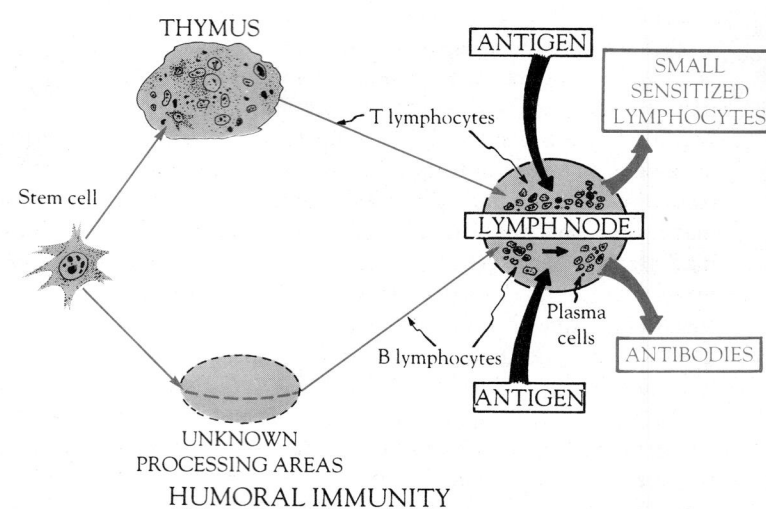

CELLULAR IMMUNITY

THYMUS

T lymphocytes

ANTIGEN

SMALL SENSITIZED LYMPHOCYTES

Stem cell

LYMPH NODE

Plasma cells

B lymphocytes

ANTIBODIES

ANTIGEN

UNKNOWN
PROCESSING AREAS

HUMORAL IMMUNITY

contrasted with innate immunity that may result from heredity. Acquired immunity can be subdivided into natural immunity (active and passive) and artificial immunity (active and passive). Table 15-4 defines and illustrates these categories of acquired immunity.

Components of the immunologic system. Active acquired immunity results from activity of the body's lymphoid tissue in the lymph nodes, spleen, submucosal areas of the gastrointestinal tract, and bone marrow. Two types of lymphocytes, found in lymphoid tissue and in circulating lymph and blood, are responsible for the immune response. The T lymphocytes, which originate from cells in the thymus gland, are responsible for forming the sensitized lymphocytes important to cellular immunity. The B lymphocytes, originating elsewhere, produce the antibodies important to humoral or antibody-mediated immunity. Both types of immunity may be operative during an infectious process. Fig. 15-2 illustrates these two types of immunity.

Stages in the development of immunity. Phagocytosis of an antigenic agent by leukocytes is the first stage in the development of the active immune response. Lymphocytes in the circulating blood, lymph, or tissue exudate recognize the structure of the antigen as different from the body and set up a chain of responses to destroy or neutralize the antigen. The type of response depends on whether T lymphocytes or B lymphocytes or both are operative.

Cell-mediated immunity. The cellular immune response results from the activity of T lymphocytes, which proliferate and are disseminated widely during inflammation. There is a different type of T lymphocyte for

each type of antigenic compound. T lymphocytes may attack a specific antigen directly or may secrete chemotactic substances to attract other leukocytes to the area to destroy the antigen. The T lymphocytes differ from other leukocytes in that they are sensitized to a specific type of antigen. This characteristic enables the T lymphocytes to respond more quickly to successive invasions by the specific antigenic agent. Cellular immunity provided by sensitized T lymphocytes persists indefinitely in the host. The cellular response is the basis for skin testing for tuberculosis, which will be discussed later in this chapter. Cellular immunity cannot be transferred passively to another host.

Humoral or antibody-mediated immunity. Antibodies are protein molecules produced by the B lymphocytes in response to a specific antigen. First, an antigen stimulates B lymphocytes dormant in lymph tissue. Then lymphocytes specific to the antigen enlarge and divide into plasma cells that produce gamma globulin antibodies. These antibodies circulate from the lymph to the blood and tissue exudate and attach themselves to the specific antigen that stimulated their production. The amount and types of antibodies produced depend on the nature and amount of the antigen, the site of the antigen stimulus, and the number of times a person has been exposed to the specific antigen.

Antibodies have three major activities. The first, although not the major function, is direct attack of the antigen. Through direct attack, antibodies destroy or neutralize antigens through processes of agglutination or clumping of the antigens, precipitation of toxins out of solution, neutralization of antigenic substances, and lysis of the cell wall of the organism. The second major action of antibodies is to activate the complement system of the host. The complement system is composed of nine different enzyme precursors that are normally inactive in the blood. The activated enzymes then attack the antigen directly by lysis, opsonization (attaching to the surface of the antigen to enhance phagocytosis), agglutination, and neutralization. Activated enzymes also promote chemotaxis (by attracting other leukocytes to the area) and inflammation in surrounding tissue. Many diagnostic tests for antibody activity are based on the action of the complement system. The third action of antibodies is to activate the anaphylactic system by releasing histamine in tissue and blood. The resultant inflammation of the area acts to localize the antigenic agent to prevent spread through the body.[49]

There are five classes of antibodies, all with different actions. They are listed here with their major actions and the areas where they are likely to be found[61]:

IgG: slower to develop during infection but persists for years; activates complement system; attacks antigens; most abundant in blood; crosses placenta

IgM: first to form during infection; same actions as IgG; found in blood

IgA: secretory antibody; found in blood and secretions (tears, colostrum, saliva)

IgE: sensitizing; releases histamine; tissue bound

IgD: function not clear; found in serum

Not all of the available B lymphocytes form plasma cells to produce antibodies at the time of invasion by an antigen. Some become sensitized and remain dormant so as to be activated quickly with subsequent exposure. These B lymphocytes are called memory cells.

Humoral immunity is faster acting than cellular immunity and is more frequently a factor in resistance to acute bacterial infections. In contrast to cellular immunity, the antibodies in humoral immunity can be transmitted to another human passively, either by artificial injection or by transfer through the placenta or breast milk.

Some few individuals are born without the ability to produce antibodies, a condition called agammaglobulinemia. The condition of producing insufficient antibodies is referred to as hypogammaglobulinemia.

Artificial immunity. Artificial immunity, as discussed earlier, is immunity intentionally induced in a person. In active artificial immunity dead organisms, attenuated organisms, or toxoids are injected in the form of vaccines to induce an active immune response in the human. Such immunity may be temporary or permanent, depending on the disease and vaccine. In passive artificial immunity, antibodies or antitoxins produced by an animal or another human are infused into a person. Passive ar-

tificial immunity is temporary, lasting approximately 2 to 3 weeks. Vaccines, antitoxins, and antibody injections available for specific infectious diseases will be discussed later in this chapter.

Body Temperature Response

A change in body temperature is a characteristic systemic symptom of infectious diseases. The regulation of body temperature and the etiology of fever in infectious diseases are discussed here. Fever patterns associated with specific infectious diseases will be described later.

Body temperature regulation. The temperature of the body is regulated primarily by nervous system feedback mechanisms, most of which operate through a temperature-regulating center located in the hypothalamus. The feedback mechanisms consist of heat-sensitive neurons in the preoptic area of the hypothalamus, on the skin, in the spinal cord, and in the abdomen. Signals from the peripheral receptors are transmitted to the posterior hypothalamus, where they are integrated with the receptor signals from the preoptic area. Efferent signals are transmitted from the hypothalamus throughout the body to control heat loss, heat conservation, and heat production.

Heat loss is promoted (1) by stimulation of the sweat glands to cause evaporative heat loss through the skin and (2) by inhibiting sympathetic centers in the posterior hypothalamus, resulting in peripheral vasodilation. Heat conservation is promoted by stimulation of the hypothalamus to send efferent signals for vasoconstriction and abolition of sweating. Heat production is increased in three ways. First, a primary motor center for shivering in the hypothalamus becomes activated as a response to cold. Impulses are transmitted to the anterior motor neurons, which stimulate tone and shivering in skeletal muscle, thus increasing heat production. Heat production can also be increased by stimulation of cellular metabolism by circulating epinephrine and norepinephrine. This means of heat production is more common in infants than adults. A third method of increasing heat production results in a slower response than the first two. Cooling of the preoptic area stimulates release of the thyrotropin-releasing hormone of the hypothalamus. This neurosecretory hormone stimulates release of thyrotropin, which in turn stimulates the production of thyroxine. Thyroxine, from the thyroid gland, acts to increase cellular metabolism, thus increasing heat production.[49]

Etiology of fever in infectious diseases. Fever, a sustained temperature above normal, can be caused by abnormalities of the hypothalamus, brain tumors, dehydration, or toxic substances affecting the temperature-regulating center of the hypothalamus. Certain protein substances and toxins can cause the ''set point'' of the hypothalamic thermostat to rise. This results in activation of the hypothalamus to conserve heat and to increase heat production. Substances that cause these effects are called pyrogens. In infectious diseases the endotoxins of some bacteria and the extracts of normal leukocytes are pyrogenic. They act to raise the "thermostat" in the hypothalamus, thus raising the body temperature.[61]

Distinct patterns of fever onset and resolution and characteristic temperature curves are associated with different infectious diseases. Fever onset may be abrupt or gradual. A persistent elevation may be maintained throughout the disease, or there may be remissions at specific times of the day or certain days in the illness. Fever associated with some diseases follows a "saddle back" curve with a high fever initially, followed by a few days of remission and then another high elevation. A habitual fever is a low-level fever present in some diseases for years. Intermittent fevers have predictable cycles of paroxysms and remissions. Relapsing fevers are those that recur after apparent recovery. Fevers may resolve suddenly by crisis or gradually by lysis.

For each degree Fahrenheit of temperature elevation there is a 7% increase in body metabolism, necessitating fluid and calorie supplements to meet metabolic needs.

NORMAL FINDINGS

Please refer to specific chapters in this book to obtain normal findings pertinent to each body system.

Area of Concern	Normal Adult Values	Variations in Child	Variations in Older Adult
Body temperature: varies with time of day, exercise, room temperature, method of measurement, and accuracy of thermometer	36.3-37.1° C (97.3-98.8° F): AM oral 36.8-37.6° C (98.3-99.9° F): rectal	0.5° C (1.0° F) higher than adults	More sensitive to changes in environmental temperature
Respiratory rate	12-20/min	Newborn: 30-50/min 1 yr: 20-40/min 6 yr: 16-22/min 17 yr: 14-20/min	
Pulse rate	60-90/min	Newborn: 120-170/min 1 yr: 80-160/min 2 yr: 80-130/min 3 yr: 80-120/min 4 yr: 80-120/min 6 yr: 75-115/min >6 yr: 70-110/min	

NORMAL LABORATORY DATA[20,28,43,103]

Laboratory Test	Normal Adult Values	Variations in Child	Variations in Older Adult
Complete white blood count (WBC)	4500-11,000/cmm	Newborn: 9000-35,000/cmm 2 mo to 2 yr: 6000-18,000/cmm Gradually decreases to adult levels	Undocumented decrease with age
Differential WBC	Expressed as a percent of total WBC		

Laboratory Test	Normal Adult Values	Variations in Child	Variations in Older Adult
Granulocytes Neutrophils	62.0% (range of 60-70%)	40-50% by day 4 after birth, gradually shifting with increasing age	
Eosinophils Basophils	50-350/cmm 0.4%		

Nongranular leukocytes
  Monocytes
  Lymphocytes
	
	5.3%
	30.0%
		
		45% by day 4 after birth, gradually shifting to adult values by age 19	

Erythrocyte sedimentation rate (Westergren method)	Men (<50 yr):
	  0-15 mm/h
	Women (<50 yr):
	  0-25 mm/h
		0-20 mm/h	Men (>50 yr):
			  0-20 mm/h
			Women (>50 yr):
			  0-30 mm/h

Erythrocyte sedimentation rate (microsedimentation method)		<2 yr: 1-6 mm/h >2 yr: 1-9 mm/h	
Zeta sedimentation ratio	<50 yr: <55%		>50 yr: 40-60%
Lactic acid dehydrogenase (LDH)	18-44 yr: 115-200 IU/L 44 yr and up: 115-225 IU/L	0-2 yr: up to 450 IU/L 2-5 yr: up to 320 IU/L 5-8 yr: up to 270 IU/L 8-14 yr: up to 260 IU/L 14-15 yr: up to 235 IU/L 15-18 yr: up to 225 IU/L	
Serum albumin	1-31 yr: 3.5-5.0 g/dl with A/G ratio >1.0; after 40 yr, normal range gradually decreases	0-1 yr: 2.9-5.5 g/dl	
Partial thromboplastin time	25-39 sec (usually stated to be within 10 sec of control)		
Fibrinogen	Quantitative: 200-400 mg/dl		
RBC	Men: 4,600,000-6,200,000/cmm Women: 3,900,000-5,900,000/cmm		
Sodium (serum or plasma)	135-145 mEq/L		
Potassium (plasma)	3.5-5.0 mEq/L		
Chloride (serum)	97-107 mEq/L	Premature infant: 95-110 mEq/L Full-term infant: 96-106 mEq/L	
Magnesium (serum)	1.2-1.9 mEq/L		

Laboratory Test	Normal Adult Values	Variations in Child	Variations in Older Adult
Calcium (serum)	1-30 yr: 8.2-10.5 mg/dl	Infant to 1 mo: 7-11.5 mg/dl 1 mo to 1 yr: 8.6-11.2 mg/dl Normal range slowly descends	Decreases very slightly
Blood urea nitrogen (BUN)	1-40 yr: 5-20 mg/dl Gradual slight increase subsequently occurs	Birth to 1 yr: 4-19 mg/dl	
Fibrin split products	<10 μg/ml		
Serum complement C₃	900-2000 μg/ml		
Reticulocytes (expressed as a percentage of 1000 RBCs)	0.5-1.5%	Newborn: 7% or less	
Direct bilirubin	Up to 0.4 mg/dl	Newborn: varies with age in days and prematurity vs. maturity	
Total bilirubin	0.3-1.0 mg/dl	Newborn: up to 2-10 mg/dl, depending on age	
Serum creatinine	Men: up to 1.2 mg/dl Women: up to 1.1 mg/dl	1-5 yr: 0.30-0.50 mg/dl 5-10 yr: 0.50-0.80 mg/dl	
Coagulation factors V VII VIII IX X	60-140% 70-130% 50-200% 60-140% 70-130%		
Glycosylated hemoglobin	5.7-8.8%		
Plasma hemoglobin	1-5 mg/dl		
Hemoglobin	Men: 15.5 ± 1.1 g/dl Women: 13.7 ± 1.0 g/dl	Birth (cord blood): 17.1 ± 1.8 g/dl 1½-3 yr: 11.8 ± 0.5 g/dl 5 yr: 12.7 ± 1.0 g/dl 10 yr: 13.2 ± 1.2 g/dl	
Hematocrit	Men: 42-52% Women: 35-47%	Birth to 2 d: 54-68% Male (2 yr): 35-44% Male (6 yr): 31-43% Female (2 yr): 35-44% Female (6 yr): 31-43%	
Blood pH	7.35-7.45		

Laboratory Test	Normal Adult Values	Variations in Child	Variations in Older Adult
Serum iron	42-135 µg/dl		
Serum enzymes SGOT SGPT CPK	 8-42 U/L 3-30 U/L Men: 55-70 U/L Women: 15-57 U/L		
Serum aldolase	1.3-8.2 mU/ml		
Serum alkaline phosphatase	35-100 IU/L		
Blood platelets	150,000-400,000/cmm		
Prothrombin time	10-13 sec		
Prothrombin levels	60-140%		
O_2 saturation	95-99%		
Bleeding time	Ivy: 2-7 min Duke: 5 min		
CO_2	Arterial: 22-29 mEq/L Venous: 23-30 mEq/L	Infant to 2 yr: 18-27 mEq/L	
Po_2	80-95 mm Hg		
Pco_2	35-45 mm Hg		
Urine output	1500-3000 ml/24 h		
Urine specific gravity	1.001-1.035		
Urine protein (electrophoresis)	No monoclonal gammopathy detected		
Cerebrospinal fluid Glucose Protein IgG Pressure	 50-80 mg/dl in fasting patients 6 mo and up: approximately 15-50 mg/dl 0-11% of total protein 80-180 mm H_2O	 0-1 mo: 30-170 mg/dl	
Serum proteins Immunoglobulins IgG	 1140 mg/dl (75% of total; range of 564-1765 mg/dl†)	Levels gradually increase until teens 1-3 mo: 161-713 mg/dl 12-24 mo: 135-1106 mg/dl 24-36 mo: 517-1346 mg/dl 3-5 yr: 570-1592 mg/dl 5-8 yr: 757-1686 mg/dl 8-12 yr: 851-1805 mg/dl 12-16 yr: 767-1752 mg/dl	

Laboratory Test	Normal Adult Values	Variations in Child	Variations in Older Adult
IgA	214 mg/dl (10-15% of total; range of 85-385 mg/dl†)	1-3 mo: 0-30 mg/dl 12-24 mo: 18-111 mg/dl 24-36 mo: 21-98 mg/dl 3-5 yr: 30-178 mg/dl 5-8 yr: 74-265 mg/dl 8-12 yr: 68-333 mg/dl 12-16 yr: 68-250 mg/dl	
IgM	168 mg/dl (7-10% of total; range of 40-120 mg/dl)		
IgD	0.5-3 mg/dl (<1% of total)		
IgE	0.01-0.04 mg/dl (<1% of total)		

DIAGNOSTIC STUDIES

Culture or microscopic examination of slides containing smears of body secretions or exudates[20,43,61]

Body secretions are cultured and examined to detect presence of pathogenic agents and to determine the organism's sensitivity to specific antibiotic agents. Some specimens are placed into a culture medium at the bedside. Others are cultured in the laboratory.

Time for laboratory culture varies from 36 hours to 10 days.

Some antibiotic sensitivity tests are available in 24 hours.

Different laboratory procedures are used to detect specific organisms. Among these are (1) the Gram stain and (2) the acid-fast bacilli stain.

Nursing care:

General considerations for collection, handling, and processing of specimens:

1. Collect in a manner to prevent contamination by normal flora and airborne organisms.
2. Place in sterile or clean container as indicated.
3. Obtain specimen before antibiotic therapy has begun.
4. Obtain during acute stage of disease if possible.
5. Prevent embarrassment of patient.
6. Give complete instructions to the patient who is expected to collect his own specimen.
7. Collect as much of the specimen as necessary for the tests.
8. Protect specimen from heat and cold and deliver to the laboratory as soon as possible to prevent death of organism.
9. Protect oneself and others from contamination.
10. Label to identify patient and body source of the specimen, date and time collected, and test to be performed.

Blood culture[20,43,61]

Culture for bacteria in blood; may do an aerobic and an anaerobic culture; three to five cultures during a 24 to 48 hour period; blood is normally sterile.

Nursing care:

Use sterile technique: prepare patient's skin with an effective antiseptic in widening circles. Apply tourniquet. Do not palpate vein after disinfecting the arm. Withdraw 10 ml venous blood with a 21-gauge needle into a sterile syringe. Using sterile technique replace needle on syringe with a new sterile needle. Inject 3 to 5 ml blood into each bottle containing 50 ml of culture medium (one bottle for anaerobic and one bottle for aerobic culture). Transport immediately to the laboratory. Keep at room temperature.

Urine culture[20,43,61]

Microscopic examination for bacteria or culture for specific bacteria: urine is normally sterile, but microorganisms may be present due to method of collection. Bacteria less than 10,000/ml urine indicates no infection; 10,000 to 100,000/ml is inconclusive; greater than 100,000/ml indicates infection.

Nursing care:

Collect a midstream, clean-catch specimen (5 ml) after thorough cleansing of area around urethra. Place in a sterile container. If a sterile specimen is desired, catheterize patient using sterile technique and place urine in a sterile container. Catheterization should be avoided, if possible. Process within an hour or refrigerate at 4° C (39.2° F) up to 5 hours.

Cerebrospinal fluid culture[20,43,61]

Microscopic examination and culture for bacteria, particularly meningococci. Cerebrospinal fluid is normally sterile. Specimens are obtained through a lumbar puncture performed by a physician under surgically aseptic conditions. Lumbar puncture procedure is described in Chapter 3.

Nursing care:

Send specimen to laboratory immediately. Do not refrigerate specimens for bacterial culture. Specimens for viral culture must be kept frozen at $-20°$ C $(-4°$ F) until cultured.

Sputum culture[20,43,61]

Culture for specific bacteria, particularly *Mycobacterium tuberculosis;* must distinguish from normal flora; physician may aspirate a specimen through bronchoscope.

Nursing care:

Have patient cleanse mouth and deeply cough up at least 1 tsp. of mucus into a sterile wide-mouthed bottle with a lid. Place container in a sealed plastic bag to avoid contamination of health care workers. Specimens may be refrigerated for several hours.

Mucous membrane swab culture[20,43,61]

Secretions of throat, nose, ear, eye, urogenital openings, genital lesions, rectum, wounds, operative sites, and ulcerations are cultured. Must distinguish from normal flora.

Nursing care:

Use sterile polyester (not cotton) disposable swabs to collect specimen. Secretion specimens must be good representatives of secretions being produced.

Throat: take from tonsillar area as well as posterior pharyngeal wall.

Ear: specimens must be of drainage from middle ear.

Nasal pharyngeal: specimen must be immersed in a broth medium to preserve viruses.

Place swab directly in a sterile tube containing a transport medium with swab suspended above the medium. Most may be refrigerated up to 2 to 3 hours. Secretions may be highly infectious.

Fecal culture[20,43,61]

Many different types of culturing procedures used, dependent on the infectious agent that is suspected. Must distinguish pathogens from normal flora.

Nursing care:

Use a tongue depressor to place a small amount of feces in a special container with a tight-fitting lid. Avoid contaminating the outside of the container. Transport immediately to the laboratory. The laboratory should be informed which disease is suspected.

Culture of fluid from peritoneal or pleural cavities

Normally sterile. Physician removes fluid using sterile technique for paracentesis or thoracentesis.

Nursing care:

Paracentesis: usually performed in the patient's room. Explain the procedure and obtain signed consent. Instruct patient to void. Obtain necessary supplies. Assist patient into a sitting position with back supported at the side of the bed or in a chair. Prepare the puncture site on the midline of the abdomen below the umbilicus by shaving and application of an antiseptic solution. Reassure the patient during the procedure. Monitor for hypotension and syncope during and following the procedure. Maintain a dry dressing on the puncture wound. Record characteristics of the peritoneal fluid and patient reactions to the procedure. Send specimen immediately to laboratory.

Thoracentesis: usually performed in the patient's room. Explain the procedure and obtain signed consent. Instruct the patient to avoid coughing and to remain immobile during the procedure. Explain that patient will experience feeling of deep pressure. Obtain appropriate supplies, such as thoracentesis tray, sterile gloves, local anesthetic, antiseptic solution, extra culture tubes and tape to identify tubes, and drainage bottle if a large amount of fluid is expected. Position patient sitting on the side of the bed with feet supported and arms and head resting on an overbed table. Alternate position: sitting straddling a chair with the patient's arms stretched over the back of the chair. Open gown to expose patient's back. Obtain baseline vital signs and breath sounds. Prepare puncture site with antiseptic wash.

During procedure: instruct patient to hold breath during needle insertion. Provide reassurance.

During and following procedure: monitor for dyspnea, tachypnea, tachycardia, hypotension, vertigo, cyanosis, chest pain, hemoptysis, uncontrollable cough, and absent or diminished breath sounds. Record characteristics of fluid removed. Send specimen immediately to the laboratory. Maintain a dry dressing on the puncture wound. Observe for signs of bleeding. Have patient lie on nonaffected side for 1 hour; then position for comfort. Monitor vital signs and breath sounds and compare with baseline every 30 minutes for three times or until stable.[13,30]

Serology: antigen-antibody reaction tests[43,103]

Detect antibodies and/or antigens in serum, depending on technique used.

Laboratory test of serum to detect antibodies or antitoxins to specific antigens. The presence of specific antibodies indicates that the person has the disease, is immune to the disease, or has an allergy to the antigen. Antibody response may take up to 2 weeks in a primary infection with a specific agent. The antibody response is generally more rapid in a second infection with the same agent. Many of these tests are performed twice (during acute stage and during convalescence) to detect a rise in antibody titer. Generally, a fourfold increase indicates concurrent infection. Antigen-antibody reactions can be used to detect organisms in serum also. Antibodies measured by different techniques do not necessarily give parallel results. Techniques of analysis make use of the following antibody-antigen reactions.

Hemagglutination inhibition (HI): Coombs', Widal, VDRL (Venereal Disease Research Laboratories), RPR (rapid plasma reagin), Weil-Felix tests

Agglutination of antigen in test tube or on slide by serum antibodies. Results are reported as a certain titer, which is the last dilution where a reaction occurred. The higher the dilution, the greater the antibody titer. A rise in titer between tests at two time periods is more significant than one high titer.

Precipitin tests

For exotoxins of diphtheria, tetanus, scarlet fever.
Precipitation of antibodies and antigen in test tube.

Complement fixation (CF) tests: Wasserman

Complement found in normal serum produces lysis when combined with antibody-antigen complexes. Serum is incubated with antigen and a specific amount of complement. Complement fixes to antigen-antibody complexes if antibodies are present. Erythrocytes coated with antibodies are added to the serum. If no lysis of erythrocytes occurs, this indicates that complement was used up during the first phase of the test in the presence of antibodies. The titer is defined as the highest dilution of serum giving a 2+ or greater fixation. (If a 2+ occurs at a dilution of 1:80, the titer is 1:80.)

Immunofluorescent antibody tests (IFA): IFA for toxoplasmosis, FTA-ABS test for syphilis

Antibody attachment to antigens observed on a slide under the fluorescent microscope through use of a fluorescent dye; quantifies antibodies.

Opsonization tests

For confirming presence of bacteria.
Opsonization and phagocytosis of bacteria if antibodies are in serum.

Quellung reaction

For *Haemophilus influenzae* and *Streptococcus pneumoniae*.
Capsular swelling of organism in presence of serum.

Microscopic examination for immobilization

Immobilization of pathogens in presence of serum.

Neutralization tests for viruses

Incubated known virus and test serum are inoculated into tissue culture. If antibody is present against the virus, there is no tissue destruction by the virus.

Radioimmunoassay (RIA)

For hepatitis B surface antigen or its antibody.
These tests are based on competition for antibody between a radioactive labeled indicator (the antigen) and its unlabeled counterpart in the sample serum. The higher the level of unlabeled antigen in the specimen, the less radioactive labeled antigen will be bound.

Enzyme-linked immunoabsorbent assay (ELISA)

These tests have the sensitivity of RIA with the advantages of low cost, rapidness of testing, and the absence of health risks associated with the use of radioactive isotopes.

Immunodiffusion

Visualization of multiple antigen-antibody systems precipitating in agar gel.

Counterimmunoelectrophoresis (CIE)

Variation of the agar gel diffusion test. Can be used to detect certain antigens before antibody is produced in detectable amounts.

Skin tests for toxin neutralization by specific antibodies or for antibody reaction to the antigen[43,103]

Antigens are injected into the skin, and the site is observed for a localized reaction indicating the presence of circulating antibodies or antitoxins. Conversion from negative to positive test indicates recent infection.

Nursing care:

Proper technique for subcutaneous administration: entire test volume (usually 0.1 ml) must be injected.

Reading the test: usually the size of the induration is more important than the presence of erythema. The optimal time for reading the test varies with the test. See section on conditions, diseases, and disorders for specific skin tests.

Antibiotic sensitivity tests: tube dilution methods and agar diffusion methods[43,103]

Sensitivity depends on the growth characteristics of the organisms and diffusion characteristics of the antibiotic. Test results determine whether organism is sensitive, intermediate, or resistant to an antibiotic.

Please refer to chapters on body systems for additional diagnostic procedures appropriate to those systems.

Conditions, Diseases, and Disorders

There are many schemes in common practice for categorizing infectious diseases. They include categorizing as to the type of pathogenic agent, as to the mode of transmission, according to the body system affected, and according to alphabetical order. The infectious diseases presented here are ordered as to body system, whenever possible, to allow the reader to refer to other body system chapters for additional information on pathophysiology, assessment, diagnostic studies, and nursing diagnoses and interventions pertinent to the system. The exceptions to this scheme are (1) all childhood or communicable diseases for which there is a routine immunization schedule are grouped together even though they have neurologic, skin, or respiratory symptoms; (2) the nosocomial (hospital-acquired) infections are grouped together although they cross all systems; and (3) enteric infections are subdivided to include food poisonings, gastroenteritis, and parasitic infections where eggs are ingested or found in the stool even though the diseases may affect other body systems.

CHILDHOOD COMMUNICABLE AND IMMUNIZABLE INFECTIOUS DISEASES

The infectious diseases presented in this section, with the exception of chickenpox, are all preventable with routine immunization. All except tetanus affect primarily children. For these two reasons these diseases have been grouped together (Table 15-5).

Chickenpox

Chickenpox (varicella) is an acute, highly communicable viral disease common in childhood. It is characterized by a sudden-onset fever, mild malaise, and a skin eruption that is maculopapular for a few hours and vesicular for 3 to 4 days, leaving a granular scab. Lesions generally occur in successive crops with several stages of maturity present at one time. They are generally more abundant on covered areas of the body, but they may appear everywhere including the scalp, conjunctivae, and upper respiratory tract.

PATHOPHYSIOLOGY

The varicella-zoster (V-Z) virus, a herpesvirus, enters the body by way of the respiratory mucous membranes and produces systemic disease. As is characteristic of herpesvirus lesions, the skin lesions of chickenpox consist of eosinophilic intranuclear inclusions and contain giant multinucleated cells. The lesions are generally superficial unilocular vesicles, with the fluid containing more polymorphonuclear cells than mononuclear cells. Lesions have been found in the lungs, liver, spleen, adrenal glands, and pancreas. Complications include secondary bacterial infections, viral pneumonia, encephalitis, aseptic meningitis, myelitis, Guillain-Barré syndrome, and Reye's syndrome. Disease is severest in neonates and those with deficiencies in cell-mediated immunity. After recovery the virus is believed to remain in the body in an asymptomatic latent stage, possibly localized in the dorsal root ganglia.[18]

Table 15-5
Childhood Communicable and Immunizable Infectious Diseases[7]

	Chickenpox	Tetanus	Diphtheria	Pertussis (Whooping Cough)
Occurrence	Worldwide; in metropolitan areas 75% of the population has had chickenpox by age 15 yr, and 90% by young adulthood	Worldwide; occurs sporadically and affects all ages; rare in United States with immunization; common among agricultural workers and parenteral drug abusers	Formerly a prevalent disease; rare in United States with immunization; affects unimmunized children under 15 yr	Common in children; worldwide; decline in incidence in areas with active immunization programs
Etiologic agent	Varicella-zoster (V-Z) virus, a member of the *Herpesvirus* group	*Clostridium tetani*, the tetanus bacillus (an anaerobic pathogen)	*Corynebacterium diphtheriae*, with many toxigenic strains	*Bordetella pertussis*, the pertussis bacillus
Reservoir	Humans	Intestines of humans and animals	Humans	Humans
Transmission	Direct and indirect contact with droplets from respiratory passages; an extremely contagious disease	Tetanus spores enter body through a wound contaminated with soil and feces; necrotic tissue favors the growth of the bacillus	Direct or indirect contact with exudate from mucous membranes of infected person or carrier; raw milk may also be a vehicle	Direct contact with droplets from respiratory passages
Incubation period	2-3 wk; commonly 13-17 d	4-21 d; commonly 10 d	2-5 d	7-21 d; commonly 7 d
Period of communicability	1-2 d before onset of rash and until lesions have crusted over	Not directly transmitted	Variable; until bacilli have disappeared from discharges and lesions (usually in 2 wk); a carrier may shed bacilli for 6 mo	7 d after exposure to 3 wk after onset; highly communicable in early catarrhal stage before cough; not communicable after 3 wk even though cough may persist
Susceptibility and resistance	General; one attack confers long immunity; second attacks are rare; neonates whose mothers are not immune suffer severe disease	General; recovery from tetanus does not confer permanent immunity; temporary active immunity provided by tetanus toxoid	Unimmunized children most susceptible; infants born of immune mothers have passive immunity for 6 mo; recovery from clinical disease confers temporary immunity	General; children under 7 yr most susceptible; no passive immunity from mother; attack confers prolonged, but not lifetime, immunity
Report to local health authority	In some areas	Case report required	Case report required	Case report required

DIAGNOSTIC STUDIES[18]

Electron microscopy or tissue culture of vesicular fluid from lesions

Visualization of V-Z virus during first 3 days after eruption

Giemsa-stained scrapings from lesions

Multinucleated giant cells

Immunofluorescence

Increase in long-lasting antibodies 2 weeks after rash

Complement fixation

Increase in antibodies up to 2 months after infection, with subsequent decrease of antibodies

Poliomyelitis	Mumps (Infectious Parotitis)	Rubella (German Measles)	Rubeola (Hard Measles)
Worldwide; commonly in summer and early autumn; highest in children and adolescents but does affect nonimmune adults; United States incidence decreasing with immunization	Occurs less than other childhood communicable diseases; greatest in winter and spring; one third of those exposed have subclinical infections	Worldwide and endemic; most common in winter and spring; primarily a disease of children but does occur in unimmunized adolescents and adults	Worldwide and common in children before immunization; endemic and epidemic occurrences; seen more in adolescents and adults since routine immunization of children
Polio virus, types 1, 2, and 3; all are paralytogenic	A type of paramyxovirus; antigenically related to parainfluenza viruses	Rubella virus	Measles virus, a type of paramyxovirus
Humans, particularly children with subclinical infections	Humans	Humans	Humans
Direct and indirect contact with respiratory discharges and feces; fecal-oral route more common than respiratory transmission	Direct contact with saliva droplets from infected person	Direct or indirect contact with nasopharyngeal secretions of infected persons; transplacental transmission leads to congenital rubella syndrome	Direct or indirect contact with nasal secretions from infected persons; highly communicable
3-35 d; commonly 7-14 d	2-3 wk; commonly 18 d	14-21 d; commonly 16-18 d	Commonly 10 d; 8-13 d until fever; 14 d until rash
Highly communicable during first days after onset of symptoms; virus is in throat secretions in 36 h and in feces in 72 h after infection and remains 1 wk in throat and 6 wk in feces	6 d before parotid symptoms to 9 d after; most communicable 48 h before parotid swelling	From 1 wk before and 4 d after appearance of rash; highly communicable; infants with congenital rubella syndrome may shed virus for months after birth	A few days before fever to 4 d after appearance of rash
General; paralytic infections are rare and risk increase with age; infection confers long-term immunity; second attacks are result of another virus type	General; immunity is lifelong and develops after clinical and subclinical disease; placental transfer of antibodies occurs	General; infants born with passive immunity from mother; one attack confers lifetime immunity	General; acquired immunity from infection is permanent; artificial active immunity may not be permanent
Case report required	Case report required in some areas	Case report required	Case report required

TREATMENT PLAN[18]

Chemotherapeutic

Immunologic agents
Zoster immune globulin (ZIG), 2 ml within 3 d of exposure to varicella

Supportive

Relief of pruritus

Prevention of superinfection through proper hygiene
Treatment of complications: encephalitis (p. 1566), Reye's syndrome (Chapter 3), Guillain-Barré syndrome (Chapter 3), viral pneumonia (Chapter 2)
Strict isolation of hospitalized patients until all lesions have crusted (p. 1620)

ASSESSMENT: AREAS OF CONCERN

Skin and mucous membranes

Lesions in various stages of development; erythematous macules forming over a 4- or 5-day period progress rapidly to vesicles and crusts; start on scalp and trunk and spread in a centrifugal fashion to the extremities; may have lesions on buccal mucosa, palate, or conjunctivae

Body temperature

Fever: 38° to 39° C (101° to 103° F)

Subjective symptoms

Headache, anorexia, malaise

NURSING DIAGNOSES and NURSING INTERVENTIONS

Nursing Diagnosis	Nursing Intervention
Skin integrity, impairment of: actual and potential	Bathe or encourage patient to bathe regularly. Caution patient against scratching lesions. Ensure smoothness of bed linen and clothing.
Comfort, alteration in: pain	Apply calamine lotion or cornstarch. Use minimal clothing and bed linen. Maintain cool room temperature with adequate humidity.[18]
Potential patient problem: transmission of infection	Observe strict isolation until all lesions have crusted (p. 1620).

Patient Education

1. Teach parent to care for child at home as described above.
2. Explain that fever can be lowered with tepid sponge baths.
3. Explain that antipyretics should be given only under the direction of a physician.

EVALUATION

Patient Outcome	Data Indicating That Outcome is Reached
Skin and mucous membrane functions are good, with minimal scarring.	Crusts are shed, and warm, moist natural color returns to skin and mucous membranes.
Complications and infection are absent.	There are no respiratory or neurologic pathologic findings. Body temperature is normal.

Tetanus

Tetanus (lockjaw) is an acute neurointoxication induced by the tetanus bacillus growing anaerobically at the site of an injury. It is manifested by tonic rigidity and painful, intermittent tonic spasms of the masseter and cervical muscles and muscles of the trunk and extremities. Abdominal rigidity, a position of opisthotonus, generalized spasms induced by sensory stimuli, and a facial expression known as risus sardonicus *are characteristic. Fatality is high.*

PATHOPHYSIOLOGY

Tetanus spores enter through a trivial or extensive injury to the skin. The anaerobic organism multiplies in the wound, even after the injury has healed, producing a lethal toxin. The toxin (tetanospasmin) reaches the central nervous system by the bloodstream or by centripetal passages along peripheral motor nerves. The toxin binds with central nervous system tissue and spinal motor ganglia. There it interferes with the release of an inhibitory transmitter and induces a hyperexcitability of motor neurons, resulting in tonic rigidity and spasms of facial, cervical, masseter, respiratory, abdominal, and extremity muscles. The bound toxin cannot be neutralized by an antitoxin.[98]

The permanency of pathologic changes in the central and peripheral nervous system in patients who recover has not been determined. Neonatal tetanus generally leaves no permanent neurologic sequelae. Central nervous system findings in fatal cases range from mild congestion to definite hemorrhage, perinuclear chromatolysis, and perivascular areas of demyelination and gliosis with confluent areas of tissues necrosis in the cerebral hemispheres.[98]

Pathologic changes in other parts of the body result from anoxia caused by respiratory impairment, asphyxial convulsions, toxic degeneration, and inanition. Pulmonary complications are frequent in tracheotomized patients. Changes in striated muscles such as hemorrhage and rupture also occur throughout the body. The risk for further pathologic change increases with duration of the disease. Cardiac, pulmonary, and musculoskeletal complications are common.[98]

DIAGNOSTIC STUDIES

There are no definitive diagnostic studies. The organism is rarely recovered from the site of the lesion, and there is no detectable antibody response. Clinical findings are important for differential diagnosis.

Tetanus must be differentiated from meningitis, poliomyelitis, encephalitis, rabies, strychnine poisoning, reactions to phenothiazides, tetany, peritonsillar abscess, and peritonitis.[64] Abnormal laboratory and physiologic data[98] include the following:

Increased spinal pressure
Moderately elevated WBC count
Slight decrease in blood platelets and prothrombin time
Low prothrombin levels, impaired thrombin generation, and increased fibrinolytic activity
Increased serum enzymes: SGOT (serum glutamic oxaloacetic transaminase), SGPT (serum glutamic pyruvate transaminase), CPK (creatinine phosphokinase), serum aldolase, alkaline phosphatase
Decreased serum iron and iron-binding capacity
Metabolic acidoses
Hypoxemia
Sinus tachycardia and transient electrocardiographic (ECG) changes
Electroencephalographic (EEG) changes

TREATMENT PLAN

Surgical[98]

Tracheostomy or laryngotracheal intubation as needed to aid respiration
Surgical care of local lesion by removal of foreign bodies only (débridement or amputation of locus of infection is not indicated)

Chemotherapeutic[98]

Antitoxin serum therapy (two types)
Hyperimmune human tetanus immune globulin, 1500-6000 units IM (one dose), or hyperimmune equine or bovine serum, 10,000-20,000 IU (neonates: 1500-10,000 IU) IV or IM (one dose)
Sensitivity test dose of 0.01-0.05 ml undiluted antitoxin should be administered IM and patient observed for 15-30 min for anaphylactic-type reaction before administering full dose
Sedative-relaxant therapy
  Sedatives
    Thiopental sodium (Pentothal sodium), 0.4% IV drip
    Phenobarbital (Luminal), 3-5 mg/kg of body weight, IM, IV, or po q3-6h
    Paraldehyde (Panal), 0.15 mg/kg IM q4-6h
  Psychotherapeutic agents
    Chlorpromazine (Thorazine), 0.5 mg/kg IM or IV q4-8h; 100 mg IV (up to 300 mg/24 h) used for relaxant effect and emergency control of seizures in adults; 25-50 mg po q6h for mild cases
  Antianxiety agents
    Meprobamate (Miltown Injectable), 200-400 mg for patients over 5 yr; 100-200 mg for patients 2-5 yr; 50-100 mg for children under 2 yr; IM q3h
    Diazepam (Valium), 0.2 mg/kg/q3-4h IM or IV; dosage may be increased with severity of seizures up to 9.5 mg/kg/24 h for adults
  Muscle relaxants
    Methocarbamol (Robaxin), IM or IV; initial dose of 15 mg/kg; maximal dose of 50 mg/kg/24 h divided into four to six doses to be infused at rate of 3 mg/min
    Neuromuscular block is only indicated in severe cases when above agents are ineffective; these agents include tubocurarine chloride, demethyl tubocurarine chloride, gallamine triethiodide, and succinylcholine chloride; assistive or controlled respiration must be available
Beta-adrenergic blockers
  Propranolol (Inderal), 0.2 mg aliquots, to a total of 2 mg IV for adults or 10 mg q8h intragastric; used for treatment of cardiovascular sympathetic overactivity syndrome
Active or passive immunization (p. 1617)

Electromechanical

Intermittent positive pressure breathing (IPPB)
Suction of respiratory secretions

Supportive[98]

Control of environment to reduce stimulation

Hyperalimentation, nasogastric feedings, or IV fluids; plus liquid feedings as patient's condition warrants

Indwelling catheter to control urinary retention

Physical therapy to prevent contractures and to facilitate return of muscle function and ambulation during convalescence

Care of vertebral compression fractures

Control of delayed allergic anaphylactic reactions to antitoxin

Treatment of local lesions and tetanus prophylaxis in wound management to prevent tetanus

Aseptic care of umbilical stump and circumcision wound to prevent tetanus

ASSESSMENT: AREAS OF CONCERN[41]

Skin
Pain, tingling at site of injury
Profuse perspiration

Musculoskeletal concerns
Early: stiff neck, tight jaw, incipient stiffness of arms and legs
Later: locked jaw (trismus); spasms of facial muscles with raising of eyebrows, wrinkling of forehead, and drawing out of mouth corners (risus sardonicus)
Difficulty in swallowing, rigid muscles

Neurologic concerns
Early: restlessness, irritability
Later: convulsions; paralysis of one or more cranial nerves in cephalic tetanus

Respiratory concerns
Dyspnea; asphyxia and cyanosis result from viselike constriction of chest muscles

Urinary elimination
Urinary retention

Body temperature
Early: 38° to 40° C (101° to 104° F) or afebrile
Terminal: 43° to 44° C (110° to 112° F)

Bowel elimination
Constipation

Hematopoietic concerns
Increased risk for hemorrhage

Cardiovascular concerns
Arrhythmias
Tachycardia
Hypertension

NURSING DIAGNOSES and NURSING INTERVENTIONS[98]

Nursing Diagnosis	Nursing Intervention
Airway clearance, ineffective	Maintain patent airway by frequent aspiration of secretions and care of tracheostomy or endotracheal tube.
Breathing pattern, ineffective	Observe for signs of respiratory failure in sedated patients; provide respiratory assistance as needed. Administer oxygen as prescribed.

Injury, potential for	Protect from injury from convulsions with padded side rails and headboard on bed and padded tongue blade and by removing dentures.
	Provide continuous supervision.
	Monitor for signs of internal trauma and hemorrhage.
	Minimize convulsions precipitated by environmental stimuli:
	    Maintain quiet, nonstimulating environment to reduce seizures.
	    Minimize physical handling of patient during acute stage.
	Take vital signs and perform any procedures while patient is in a sedated state.
	Monitor patient closely for anaphylactic reaction to antitoxin therapy.
	Provide standby emergency equipment and be prepared to resuscitate and provide life support.

Fluid volume deficit, potential	Administer IV therapy as prescribed. Monitor intake and output.
Nutrition, alteration in: less that body requirements	Administer alimentation therapy as prescribed.
Urinary elimination, alteration in patterns	Monitor urinary output, or maintain indwelling catheter to relieve urinary retention.
Bowel elimination, alteration in: constipation	Administer enemas as prescribed to avoid patient straining to defecate.

Nursing Diagnosis	Nursing Intervention
Skin integrity, impairment of: potential	Turn frequently during convalescence. Place on air mattress or lamb's wool.
Mobility, impaired physical	Position sedated patients to maintain proper body alignment. Administer range of motion exercises, and supervise gradually increasing movement during convalescence.
Cardiac output, alteration in: decreased	Monitor vital signs for tachycardia and hypertension. Monitor for symptoms of arrhythmias. Administer prescribed therapy (Chapter 1).
Potential patient problem: fever	Sponge patient while sedated to lower body temperature.
Potential patient problem: susceptibility to infection	Use aseptic technique to prevent secondary infection. Monitor temperature and respiratory function for signs of secondary infection.

EVALUATION

Patient Outcome	Data Indicating That Outcome is Reached
Respiratory function is normal.	Patient is breathing on own without mechanical assistance. There are no periods of cyanosis or labored breathing or signs of pulmonary complications such as pneumonia. Respiratory rate is normal.
Neurologic function is normal.	There are no convulsions. Reflexes, including cough and gag reflexes, are normal.
Neuromuscular function is normal.	Spasms, muscular rigidity, posturing, or spasmodic facial expressions are not present.
Musculoskeletal function is normal.	Fractures, contractures, or prolonged muscle weakness is not present. Mobility returns.
Cardiovascular function is normal.	Heart rate is normal, without tachycardias or arrhythmias. Blood pressure is normal.
Body temperature is normal.	Temperature is normal.
Essential nutrients are part of daily intake.	Patient is able to eat a regular diet during convalescence.
Bowel elimination is normal for individual.	Stools are soft; abdomen is soft and not distended.
Urinary elimination is normal.	Patient is able to empty bladder completely without assistance; urine output equals fluid intake.
Integrity of skin and mucous membranes is maintained.	Injuries that may have been sustained during convulsions are healed. There are no decubiti. Skin is warm and moist with good color.
Laboratory studies are within normal limits.	WBC count is normal. Spinal pressure decreases to normal. There is no acidosis. Serum iron and serum enzyme levels are normal. Blood platelet count is normal. Prothrombin time is normal. Prothrombin levels are normal.

Diphtheria

Diphtheria is an acute communicable disease in which a bacterial toxin affects the mucous membranes of the respiratory tract. The disease is manifested by fibropurulent exudative membranes, commonly on the tonsils and pharynx but also on the larynx, nasal passages, skin, conjunctivae, and genitalia; and by systemic symptoms resulting from toxin dissemination.

PATHOPHYSIOLOGY

The *Cornynebacterium diphtheriae*, widely available in the nasopharynx of carriers and persons with inapparent infection, invades and multiplies in the nasopharynx of susceptible persons. The pathogen produces a toxin that is disseminated by the blood and lymph throughout the body. The toxin first causes necrosis of the local tissue, resulting in a fibrinopurulent exudative membrane characteristic of this disease. The membrane appears as grayish membrane patches surrounded by a red zone of inflammation on the tonsils, pharynx, larynx, nasal mucosa, or skin. Edema is present in adjacent and underlying tissue and in the cervical lymph nodes. Laryngeal edema and the extension of the membrane into the trachea, bronchial tree, and alveoli may result in suffocation. Nasopharyngeal diphtheria and laryngeal diphtheria are the most severe types. Nasal diphtheria is mild and marked by one-sided nasal excoriations and discharge. Cutaneous diphtheria lesions are variable and may resemble impetigo.

Disseminated toxin inhibits protein synthesis primarily in heart, peripheral nerves, and muscle tissue. Effects of toxin absorption appear early and include fatty degeneration, edema, and interstitial fibrosis in the myocardium and in the myelin sheath of peripheral nerves. Damage to peripheral nerves results in peripheral motor and sensory palsies. The spleen and kidneys also may be affected. Otitis media, peritonsillar abscess, and albuminuria are less serious complications. Severe toxemia may result in a life-threatening myocarditis, motor or sensory paralysis, pharyngeal and respiratory paralysis, and pneumonia. ECG changes and an increase in SGOT levels may be present.[7,106]

DIAGNOSTIC STUDIES[12,64,106]

Bacteriologic examination of lesions using Loeffler's methylene blue stain
Positive for *C. diphtheriae*

Test for toxigenicity by inoculation of an animal with serum from patient
Necrosis at site of inoculation; animal will become ill if toxin is present in patient's serum

Hemagglutination and radioimmunoassay
Positive for agglutinating antibodies

Schick skin test
0.1 ml of active diphtheria toxin and 0.1 ml of an inactive toxin (for a control) are injected at two different sites on person

Read at 24 and 48 hours; increased redness, edema, and flaking of skin at test site between two readings indicates no circulating antitoxin

A test for susceptibility

Differential diagnosis
Rule out acute tonsillitis, septic sore throat, infectious mononucleosis, and scarlet fever

TREATMENT PLAN

Surgical
Tracheostomy

Chemotherapeutic[106]
Immunologic agents
Diphtheria antitoxin administered IM in mild infections and IM and IV (diluted) in severe infections; dosages vary with severity of infection and number of days since disease onset:
Tonsillar: 20,000 units
Pharyngeal: 20,000-40,000 units
Tonsillar and uvular: 40,000 units
Nasopharyngeal: 60,000-100,000 units
Laryngeal: 20,000 units
Laryngeal with other: 20,000-100,000 units
Corticosteroids
May be used to prevent or ameliorate myocarditis
Anti-infective agents
Local application of pencillin solution plus IM antitoxin for cutaneous diphtheria
Erythromycin (Robimycin), 50 mg/kg body weight/d for 1 wk for carrier state
Active or passive immunization for prevention (p. 1617)

Electromechanical
Laryngeal and tracheal suction
Intubation
Nasogastric feedings if pharyngeal paralysis occurs
Positive pressure ventilation if respiratory paralysis occurs

Supportive

Bed rest with minimal exertion for 4 to 6 weeks

IV administration of glucose and amino acids if oral feeding is impossible; otherwise, soft diet[106]

Strict isolation until two nasopharyngeal cultures 24 hours apart are negative; for cutaneous diphtheria, contact isolation (p. 1620)

ASSESSMENT: AREAS OF CONCERN[106]

Body temperature

Moderately elevated: 38° to 39° C (100 to 102° F)

Head and neck

Edema of neck and lymph nodes

Nasopharynx

Presence of edema and gray membranous patches on tonsils, pharynx, larynx, or nasal passages

Difficulty in swallowing

Breathing pattern

Noisy, labored; may be sudden obstruction; neck muscle retraction; suprasternal and substernal retraction

Activity patterns

Restlessness as a sign of impaired oxygenation

Cardiovascular concerns

Sudden slowing of pulse and beginning irregularity; pallor

Neurologic: peripheral nerves

Palatal paralysis: nasal tone to voice (tenth day)

Oculomotor paralysis: strabismus (third week)

Ciliary paralysis: dilation of pupils and blurring of vision (third week)

Facial paralysis: loss of tone of cheek muscles; flattening of one side of face; inability to blow out cheeks equally (third week)

Pharyngeal paralysis: difficulty in swallowing; regurgitation of food through nose (third or fourth week)

Laryngeal paralysis: hoarseness or aphonia (third to fifth week)

Paralysis or paresis in extremities: weakness, numbness, and tingling in extremities

Paralysis of diaphragm: difficulty in breathing; cyanosis (fifth or sixth week)

NURSING DIAGNOSES and NURSING INTERVENTIONS

Nursing Diagnosis	Nursing Intervention
Airway clearance, ineffective	Monitor for symptoms of obstruction, particularly neck muscle retraction, suprasternal and substernal retraction, dyspnea, and signs of restlessness. Have tracheostomy tray available; administer tracheostomy care. Increase humidity of inspired air; administer oxygen as prescribed.
Cardiac output, alteration in: decreased	Monitor for changes in pulse (rate, rhythm, and quality) and changes in blood pressure. Look for sudden decrease in pulse rate and onset of irregularity and pallor. Employ complete bed rest. Minimize anxiety. Perform care for cardiac complications as prescribed (Chapter 1).
Nutrition, alteration in: less than body requirements	Provide frequent, small feedings of soft foods and liquids as can be swallowed. Nasogastric feedings may be necessary if patient cannot swallow.
Sensory-perceptual alteration	Monitor for onset of peripheral nerve paralysis as listed under assessment.
Fluid volume deficit, potential	Monitor intake and output. Administer IV fluids, as prescribed, for patient who cannot swallow.
Activity intolerance	Employ complete bed rest for up to 6 weeks. Provide total hygiene and feeding.
Oral mucous membrane, alteration in	Provide frequent use of mouth rinses; avoid swabbing or any oral hygiene procedure that induces gagging. Lubricate nostrils in nasal diphtheria with zinc oxide ointment.[106]
Communication, impaired: verbal	Anticipate needs of patient who is unable to communicate because of labored breathing and swallowing.
Potential patient problem: fever	Sponge bathe patient, or administer antipyretics as prescribed.
Potential patient problem: transmission to others	Employ strict isolation precautions until two nasopharyngeal cultures 24 hours apart are negative (p. 1620). Collect specimen for culture (p. 1481).

EVALUATION

Patient Outcome	Data Indicating That Outcome is Reached
Body hydration and oxygenation are normal.	Skin, nails, lips, earlobes, and mucous membranes are warm and moist, with natural color. Skin turgor is good. Secretions are thin. The patient is not restless.
Vital signs are within normal limits.	Pulse rate, respiratory rate, blood pressure, and temperature are normal.
Airway clearance and breathing patterns are effective.	The patient can swallow secretions. Breathing is unlabored, with normal rhythm.
Sensory function is normal. Visual tests are positive.	The patient correctly identifies letters on Snellen eye chart from distance of 20 feet. Pupils are normal and reactive.
Touch test is positive.	The patient responds to touch of extremities. There are no feelings of tingling or numbness. The patient feels pinprick, heat, and cold.
Motor function is normal.	The patient moves extremities and changes body position in bed. There are no signs of facial paralysis: the patient is able to blow out cheeks equally. The patient can swallow without difficulty. The patient is able to speak coherently, without nasal tone to voice.
Rest and sleep are adequate.	The patient gets adequate sleep: 18 to 20 hours for infant, 10 to 14 hours for children, and 7 to 9 hours for adult. Bed rest is maintained.
Patient is in a relaxed state while resting.	Facial expression is calm and serene; breathing is regular; there are periods of motionlessness. There is no startle response to stimuli.
Mucous membranes return to prepathogenic state.	There is no secondary infection in nasopharynx. There is no edema, erythema, or membranous patches. Two nasopharyngeal cultures are negative.

Pertussis (Whooping Cough)

Pertussis (whooping cough) is an acute communicable bacterial infection of the mucous membranes of the tracheobronchial tree, characterized by paroxysms of repeated and violent coughing. Paroxysms are terminated by a prolonged, high-pitched inspiratory whoop and the expulsion of clear, tenacious mucus. This disease is severest in children under 1 year of age and in persons living in poverty.

PATHOPHYSIOLOGY[64,113]

The toxigenic *Bordetella pertussis* bacillus enters the respiratory passages by airborne droplets of respiratory secretions from persons with asymptomatic infections or with clinical disease. The organism reproduces in the mucous membranes of the trachea, bronchi, and bronchioles, producing a toxin that causes necrosis to the ciliated mucosa. There are three stages of the disease: catarrhal, paroxysmal, and convalescent. A serous exudate is produced initially in the catarrhal stage, lasting 1 to 2 weeks. This is followed by a viscid mucopurulent exudate that is irritating to the mucosa. This exudate, which is difficult to expel, initiates severe spasmodic coughing (paroxysms) that may persist for 1 to 2 months. Coughing may also be initiated by toxin stimulation to the central nervous system.

Local necrosis of the tracheal and bronchial epithelium is extensive—with an associated peribronchial and interstitial inflammatory infiltrate. Unexpelled mucous plugs may produce areas of atelectasis and emphysema. Paratracheal and bronchial lymphadenopathy may be present. Edema, congestion, and hemorrhage may be present in lung tissue; and edema and petechial hemorrhages are commonly found in brain tissue. These pathologic findings result from anoxia during the prolonged paroxysms of coughing. Paroxysms may also result in epistaxis, scleral hemorrhage, periorbital edema, vomiting, exhaustion, aspiration, and aspiration pneumonia. Also, umbilical and inguinal hernias and rectal prolapse may result from increased intra-abdominal pressure during paroxysms.

Additional complications include secondary bacterial infections such as otitis media or pneumonia. Convulsions occur in small children as a result of high temperature and anoxia caused by prolonged paroxysms.

A marked hyperleukocytosis and lymphocytosis are characteristic. WBC count may range as high as 175,000 to 200,000; and lymphocytes increase to 90% in the differential count.[113]

The convalescent stage is characterized by a cessation of whooping and vomiting with a gradual decrease in the number of paroxysms over a 2- to 3-week period. Some patients will develop exacerbations of paroxysms of cough, whooping, and vomiting during subsequent respiratory tract infections.[64]

DIAGNOSTIC STUDIES[7,113]

Direct fluorescent antibody staining of nasopharyngeal secretions during catarrhal stage
Positive for *B. pertussis*

WBC count
Leukocytes: 15,000 to 40,000/cmm; may be as high as 175,000 to 200,000/cmm

Differential WBC count
90% lymphocytes

Agglutination tests
Variable results; of questionable value

TREATMENT PLAN

Chemotherapeutic[113]
Immunologic agents
  Human hyperimmune pertussis globulin, 1.25 ml/24 h IM q3-5d (for small infants with severe disease); authorities disagree as to the efficacy of this treatment
Anti-infective agents
  Erythromycin (Erythrocin), 35-50 mg/kg/24 h po in four divided doses for 14 d
Betnesol, 0.075 mg/kg/24 h, po
Corticosteroids
  Hydrocortisone sodium succinate (Solu-Cortef), 30

mg/kg/24 h for 2 d, IM; to be reduced gradually and discontinued by eighth day
Active immunization for prevention (p. 1617)

Electromechanical
Suction of respiratory secretions
Ventilatory assistance, if needed

Supportive
Oxygen administration
Parenteral fluid and electrolyte therapy
Small, frequent feedings
Postural drainage following paroxysms[113]
Respiratory isolation for 3 weeks after onset of paroxysms or 7 days after antimicrobial therapy (p. 1620)

ASSESSMENT: AREAS OF CONCERN[113]

Respiratory concerns
Catarrhal stage: normal respirations; dry, hacking cough
Paroxysmal stage (after 1 or 2 weeks): paroxysms of cough (40 to 50/24 h in severe cases) followed by high-pitched inspiratory whoop; vomiting frequently follows paroxysm
Convalescent stage: paroxysms and vomiting become gradually less frequent and prolonged

Mucous membranes
Catarrhal stage: serous rhinorrhea, sneezing, lacrimation, conjunctivitis
Paroxysmal stage: tenacious mucus; epistaxis

Skin
Color may be cyanotic following paroxysms
Loss of turgor because of dehydration

Body temperature
Normal or low-grade fever; elevated in secondary infection

Head and neck
Venous engorgement of face and neck during paroxysms
Scleral hemorrhages and periorbital edema may be present

Neurologic concerns
Anoxic convulsions

Activity patterns
Exhaustion following paroxysms

Abdomen
Umbilical or inguinal hernia complications

NURSING DIAGNOSES and NURSING INTERVENTIONS

Nursing Diagnosis	Nursing Intervention
Airway clearance, ineffective	Place infant on stomach, head down, on lap during paroxysms to reduce risk of aspiration. Suction pooled secretions if necessary. Maintain patent airway.
Breathing pattern, ineffective	Restore breathing after paroxysms with oxygen by mask. Assist respiration if necessary. Monitor breathing for signs of atelectasis or pneumonia. Monitor temperature for secondary infection.
Fluid volume deficit, potential	Give frequent, small liquid feedings or parenteral fluids if vomiting is excessive.
Gas exchange, impaired	Monitor for symptoms of anoxia. Administer oxygen as prescribed following paroxysms.
Activity intolerance	Provide for rest in a nonstimulating environment to compensate for exhaustion from paroxysms.
Injury, potential for	Provide convulsion precautions: padded bed, side rails, and tongue blade.[113]
Potential patient problem: transmission of infection	Employ respiratory isolation (p. 1620) for 3 weeks after onset of paroxysms or 7 days after onset of antimicrobial therapy. Collect nasopharyngeal specimen for culture (p. 1481).

EVALUATION

Patient Outcome	Data Indicating That Outcome is Reached
All cells receive oxygen.	Skin, nails, lips, and earlobes are warm and moist, with natural color.
Respirations are normal.	Breathing pattern, rhythm, rate, and depth are regular.
Laboratory studies are within normal limits.	Oxygen saturation, carbon dioxide, P_{O_2}, and P_{CO_2} are normal.
Body hydration is normal.	Skin turgor is good; secretions are thin. Urine output equals intake. Urine specific gravity is normal.
There is no evidence of infection.	Blood leukocyte count is normal. Bacterial culture is negative. Breathing patterns are normal. Body temperature is normal.
Energy level is adequate.	Patient moves and cares for self at level of development. There is no weakness or malaise. Breathing during activity is regular.

Poliomyelitis

Poliomyelitis is an acute communicable systemic viral disease affecting the central nervous system with variable severity ranging from subclinical infection, to a nonfebrile illness, to an aseptic meningitis, to paralytic disease, and possibly to death.

PATHOPHYSIOLOGY[64,105]

Three immunologically distinct polioviruses produce poliomyelitis, an infection that occurs 100 times more frequently in a subclinical form than in clinical disease. The polioviruses are all enteroviruses; that is, they multiply in the intestinal tract and can be recovered from the feces of cases and subclinical cases. Transmission of the virus is primarily by the fecal-oral route and sometimes by direct contact with respiratory secretions.

Once in a susceptible host, the virus multiplies in the lymphoid tissue of the throat and ileum, producing a lymphocytic hyperplasia and follicular necrosis there. A transient viremia follows with subsequent viral invasion of the central nervous system producing cell damage primarily in the anterior horn cells of the spinal cord, in the medulla and pons, in the midbrain, and in the motor area of the precentral gyrus. Damage to the motor neurons results from destruction within the body of the cells. Diffuse chromatolysis of the Nissl substance of the cytoplasm occurs first, followed by nuclear changes and pericellular infiltration of polymorphonuclear leukocytes and monocytes. Damage may be reversible at this point, with complete recovery, or it may progress to necrosis and phagocytosis of the neurons resulting in clinical disease concomitant with the extent and concentration of neuron destruction.

Clinical paralysis results when there is extensive damage to motor neurons associated with any one functional motor group. Skeletal muscle fiber groups atrophy rapidly from absence of innervation from associated destroyed motor neurons. Paralysis is characteristically asymmetric, involving the lower extremities and muscles of respiration and swallowing.

Clinical poliomyelitis may be seen in three phases: a systemic stage, a phase of central nervous system involvement, and the paralytic stage. The onset of the systemic phase is acute, with low-grade fever, headache, nausea, abdominal tenderness, occasional vomiting, and the presence of a mild tonsillitis or pharyngitis. These symptoms subside within 24 to 36 hours, and the infectious process is terminated for about 80% of patients.

A small percentage of patients manifest signs of the second phase within 1 to 4 days, with a higher fever, frontal headache, vomiting, strained anxious expression on the face, dermal hypersensitivity, and a hyperhidrosis, particularly around the head and neck. The symptoms may end here or progress to the paralytic stage, with nuchal and spinal stiffness from spasm of back and hamstring muscles, positive spinal fluid findings (protein levels of 80 to 200 mg/dl), hypertension, and paralysis.

Paralysis may affect different parts of the body depending on the area of central nervous system damage, giving rise to the differentiation of types of paralysis as spinal, spinobulbar, bulbar, ataxic, encephalitic, or meningitic. Complications are associated with the areas of muscle paralysis or weakness and the effect on body functioning. They include intercostal and respiratory paralysis, pharyngeal, facial, and palatal paralysis, and paralysis of eye muscles and of the urinary bladder.

DIAGNOSTIC STUDIES[64,105]

Culture of feces
Positive for poliovirus 5 days after exposure to 1 to 4 months after exposure

Culture of nasopharyngeal secretions
Positive for poliovirus 5 days after exposure to 14 days after disease onset

Neutralization and complement fixation tests
Increase in IgA antibody titer 7 days to 4 months after exposure
Antibodies persist for a few years

Differential diagnosis
Rule out aseptic meningitis, suppurative meningitis, toxic neuronitis, brain trauma, encephalitis, diphtheria

TREATMENT PLAN[105]

Chemotherapeutic
Active immunization for prevention (p. 1620)

Electromechanical
Respiratory assistance
Tracheostomy
Suction
Indwelling catheter for urinary bladder paralysis
Oxygen

Supportive
IV fluids; nasogastric feeding
Complete bed rest
Hot, moist packs to muscles in spasm
Passive range of motion exercises for paralytic disease
Muscle reeducation during convalescence
Stabilizing prosthesis may be used later in convalescence
Enteric precautions for 7 days after disease onset (p. 1481)

ASSESSMENT: AREAS OF CONCERN[105]

Systemic stage
Body temperature
37° to 38° C (99° to 101° F)

Abdomen
Abdominal tenderness; nausea

Head and pharynx
Erythema of throat and tonsils
Headache

CNS involvement
Body temperature
38° to 39° C (100° to 102° F)

Abdomen
Vomiting

Head and neck
Strained, anxious expression
Frontal headache

Skin
Hypersensitive to touch
Profuse perspiration, particularly around head and neck

Neuromuscular system
Pain and stiffness in neck, back, and legs

Paralytic stage
All of above plus:

Level of consciousness
Drowsiness, stupor, or restlessness

Neuromuscular concerns
Pain and spasm (neck, back, and legs)
Hyperactive deep tendon reflexes followed by absence of reflexes
Asymmetric paralysis (variable parts of body): legs, arms, abdomen, back, face, urinary bladder, pharyngeal, and respiratory

Blood pressure
May be elevated

Breathing patterns
Dyspnea, respiratory stridor

Rib cage fixed in inspiration because of spasm of sternocleidomastoid, platysma, and trapezius muscles
Movement of diaphragm and intercostal muscles may be absent

Head and neck
Paralysis of face may be observed by an inability to pull up the corner of the mouth when smiling, flattening of one side, or an inability to close one eye

Oral pharynx
Patient may be unable to stick out tongue; or tongue may deviate to one side
Palate and uvula may deviate to one side; voice may have nasal tone
Liquid may be regurgitated through nose
Difficulty in swallowing

Speech
Aphonia may be present

Urinary elimination
Distended bladder
No urinary output

NURSING DIAGNOSES and NURSING INTERVENTIONS

Nursing Diagnosis	Nursing Intervention
Breathing pattern, ineffective	Monitor for dyspnea, avoidance of speech, abnormal chest movement, respiratory stridor, or cyanosis. Initiate ventilatory assistance with respirator or positive pressure breathing and oxygen as prescribed. Gradually wean from respirator, as prescribed, during convalescence.
Airway clearance, ineffective	Monitor for inability to swallow. Provide suctioning or tracheotomy care as prescribed. Feed, using nasogastric tube if swallowing is impaired.
Mobility, impaired physical	Position (on a firm mattress with a footboard) in a dorsal or prone position with extremities extended, with no pillow, in perfect alignment.
Activity intolerance	Employ complete bed rest in a quiet, nonstimulating environment.
Comfort, alteration in: pain	Handle and move as little as possible. Support body parts completely when moving patient. Apply hot, moist packs to muscles in spasm.
Self-care deficit	Feed patient, starting with fluids and increasing toward normal diet as tolerated. Provided frequent oral hygiene. Bathe daily during convalescence; omit during acute stage. Refer for home nursing care if needed at time of hospital discharge.
Communication, impaired: verbal	Anticipate the patient's needs. Observe and encourage nonverbal communication.
Urinary elimination, alteration in patterns	Monitor output. Maintain indwelling catheter. Provide bladder retraining during convalescence.
Potential patient problem: transmission of infection	Employ enteric precautions for duration of hospitalization (p. 1620). Collect fecal and nasopharyngeal specimens.

Patient Education

Patient teaching will depend on the amount of physical function the patient has at discharge. Refer for home nursing and physical and occupational therapy, if necessary.

EVALUATION

Patient Outcome	Data Indicating That Outcome is Reached
There is no infection.	Fecal and nasopharyngeal cultures are negative. Body temperature is normal.
Blood pressure is normal.	Blood pressure is within normal range.
Breathing pattern is effective.	Breathing pattern, rhythm, and depth are regular. Respiratory rate is normal.
Urinary elimination is normal.	Urine output is normal. The patient empties bladder completely on own during convalescence.
Laboratory studies are within normal limits.	O_2 saturation and carbon dioxide levels are normal.
The patient appears to be physically comfortable.	Facial expression is calm and relaxed; posture is normal; muscles are relaxed when patient is resting and motionless.
The patient participates in therapeutic exercise.	The patient participates in muscle-building physical therapy. Mobility is adequate. The patient ambulates independently with mechanical devices if needed.
There is no evidence of deformity resulting from treatment.	Arms, legs, feet, and spine are in good alignment. There are no contractures.
The patient is able to function independently or with assistance when discharged from hospital.	Patient can carry out all activities of daily living. Arrangements have been made for home help if needed.

Mumps (Parotitis)

Mumps (parotitis) is an acute, communicable systemic viral disease characterized by localized unilateral or bilateral edema of one or more of the salivary glands, with occasional involvement of other glands.

PATHOPHYSIOLOGY

The paramyxovirus invades and multiplies in the parotid gland or the superficial epithelium of the upper respiratory passages, invades the blood, and subsequently localizes in glandular or nervous tissue. Interstitial tissue edema and infiltration with lymphocytes occur in the affected gland. Cells of the glandular ducts degenerate, producing an accumulation of necrotic debris and polymorphonuclear leukocytes in the lumina, resulting in plugging of the ducts or tubules. The parotid and testes are the glands most frequently involved; but mumps may also affect the pancreas, other salivary glands, ovaries, breast, and thyroid. Meningoencephalitis is a common complication; pericarditis and permanent deafness are less common complications. Testicular atrophy follows mumps orchitis, but sterility is rare. The intensity of symptoms in mumps is extremely variable, with at least 30% of infections asymptomatic. Elevated cerebrospinal fluid protein concentrations are common even in the absence of clinical symptoms of meningoencephalitis. Depressed glucose levels may also be present.[19]

DIAGNOSTIC STUDIES[19,64]

Cell cultures from saliva, urine, cerebrospinal fluid specimens (not ordinary procedures)
Positive for virus up to 7 days after onset of infection; in urine up to 2 weeks after infection onset

Serum amylase determination
Elevated early in acute illness

Serology: complement fixation; hemagglutination; neutralization*

Fourfold increase in antibody titer between acute and convalescent stages

TREATMENT PLAN

Chemotherapeutic

Steroids for treatment of orchitis
Analgesics for pain
Active immunization for prevention (p. 1617)

Supportive

Relief of pain with heat or cold applications
Fluid diet until patient tolerates solid food
Support of scrotum (small pillow or Alexander bandage)[19]
Respiratory isolation of hospitalized patients for 9 days after onset of swelling (p. 1620)

ASSESSMENT: AREAS OF CONCERN[19]

Body temperature

38° to 39° C (100° to 103° F) for 3 or 4 days; higher if orchitis is present

Head and neck

Variable parotid swelling lasting up to 1 week; severe parotid pain aggravated by eating, particularly sour substances

*More time consuming and expensive.

Parotid gland (or other glands) tender to the touch; hooked lobe of the parotid (extending under ear lobe) can be palpated

Abdomen

Pain from pancreatitis or oophoritis

Breasts

Inflammation and pain associated with mastitis

Sensory concerns

Photophobia and headache associated with meningo-encephalitis
Unilateral mild transient hearing loss to permanent deafness possible

Testes

Swollen and tender to touch; patient has severe pain

Neuromuscular concerns

Stiff neck
Convulsion in severe cases
Ataxia
Symptoms of transverse myelitis (rare complication)

Cardiovascular concerns

Dyspnea, tachycardia, and bradycardia (symptoms of myocarditis; a rare complication)

Urinary concerns

Symptoms of nephritis (a rare complication)

Skeletal concerns

Symptoms of arthritis (a rare complication)

NURSING DIAGNOSES and NURSING INTERVENTIONS

Nursing Diagnosis	Nursing Intervention
Comfort, alteration in: pain	Administer analgesics as prescribed. Give liquid or soft diet as prescribed. Apply warm or cold compresses, whichever is most comfortable to patient. Support scrotum with small pillow, nest of cotton (for a child), or an adhesive tape bridge between the thighs.
Anxiety	Allay anxiety and concern regarding effects of orchitis: inform patient that testicular atrophy does not result in impotence; and sterility is extremely rare.[19, 64]
Nutrition, alteration in: less than body requirements	Encourage liquid or soft bland diet as prescribed. Allow patient to drink from a straw.
Potential patient problem: transmission of illness	If patient is hospitalized, employ respiratory isolation for 9 days after onset of swelling (p. 1620).

Patient Education

1. Teach parent or patient to perform nursing care as listed above for the patient who remains at home.

EVALUATION

Patient Outcome	Data Indicating That Outcome is Reached
The patient appears physically comfortable.	Facial expression is calm and relaxed; posture is normal; muscles are relaxed when patient is resting and motionless. There is no pain in any glandular area.
The patient is not anxious regarding sexual function after orchitis.	The patient has not developed distress mannerisms. The patient discusses any concerns about future sexual functions.
Body hydration and nutrition are normal.	Skin turgor is good; elimination is adequate; intake is adequate for needs.
Glandular inflammation is absent.	There are no signs of glandular edema or pain. Body temperature is normal.

Rubella (German Measles)

Rubella (German measles) is a mild, febrile, highly communicable viral disease characterized by a diffuse punctate macular rash. Symptoms in the prodromal period include low-grade fever, coryza, malaise, headache, lymphadenopathy, and conjunctivitis. Infection during the first trimester of pregnancy may lead to infection in the fetus and may produce a variety of congenital anomalies: the congenital rubella syndrome.

PATHOPHYSIOLOGY[44,64,104]

Rubella is usually a mild disease caused by a specific virus that invades and is present in nasopharyngeal secretions, blood, urine, and feces. The virus is transmitted primarily through contact with nasopharyngeal secretions of clinical and subclinical infectious persons 7 days before to 5 days after the appearance of the rash. The virus may also be transmitted transplacentally, producing active infection in the fetus. This may result in death to the fetus or congenital damage (the congenital rubella syndrome). Infants born with congenital rubella syndrome generally have the virus in their nasopharyngeal secretions, stools, and urine for up to 1 year after birth, indicating the presence of a chronic infection.

In postnatal rubella the virus invades the lymph glands from the nasopharynx, producing a lymphadenopathy. It subsequently enters the blood, stimulating an immune response that is responsible for the development of the rash. Once the rash appears, the virus can no longer be found in the blood, and prodromal symptoms of a viremia subside. There may be a temporary leukopenia during acute infection. Complications are rare. They include a transitory arthritis, an extremely rare encephalitis, and hemorrhagic manifestations that subside in 2 weeks. In the latter case there is a decrease in blood platelets and an increase in clotting time.

Congenital rubella syndrome is a much more serious manifestation, affecting about 25% of infants born to mothers who were infected with rubella virus during their first trimester. Infection later in the pregnancy carries a lesser risk for congenital damage. The syndrome is characterized by a variety of permanent or transitory defects including cataracts, microphthalmia, microcephaly, mental retardation, deafness, patent ductus arteriosus, arterial or ventral septal defects, congenital glaucoma, retinopathy, purpura, hepatosplenomegaly, neonatal jaundice, and bone defects. There is a high risk for death during the first 6 months, generally from congenital heart disease and sepsis.

The pathologic mechanisms producing the syndrome are not clear, but they appear to be the direct result of viral invasion and infection of developing tissue of the placenta and embryo. One hypothesis is that persistent infection with the virus may lead to mitotic arrest of cells, causing retardation in organ growth. Maternal infection may also result in placental and fetal vasculitis resulting in retarded growth of the fetus. Also, chromosomal breakage has been found in cultured cells from children with congenital rubella syndrome.

DIAGNOSTIC STUDIES[64]

Culture of pharyngeal secretions (also blood, urine, or stool)

Positive for rubella virus in pharyngeal secretions 7 days before rash in postnatal rubella
Virus present up to 1 year following birth in congenital rubella syndrome; decreasing with age

Postnatal infections

Hemagglutination inhibition (HI)

Fourfold increase in antibody titer between acute and convalescent stages; hemagglutination antibodies develop quickly and are long lasting; used to determine immunity

Complement fixation (CF)

Complement fixation antibodies develop slowly; can be detected within 2 weeks of onset

Titers of 1:8 to 1:64 indicate recent infection

Solid-phase radioimmunoassay (SPRIA)

Increase in IgG and IgM antibodies; increase in short-lasting IgM indicates recent infection

Congenital rubella: hemagglutination

Increase in IgM antibodies from birth to 5 months is diagnostic

Passively acquired maternal IgG antibodies will decrease after 1 month in infant's serum

Increase in IgG within 6 months to 1 year indicates active immune response in infant

TREATMENT PLAN

Acquired Rubella

Chemotherapeutic

Antipyretics for temperature control

Antibiotic treatment of otitis media, an infrequent complication

Active immunization for prevention (p. 1617)

Congenital Rubella Syndrome

Surgical

Correction of various anomalies

Chemotherapeutic

Treatment of sepsis

Treatment of congestive heart failure

Supportive

Rehabilitation of children who survive infancy

Strict isolation of neonates with rubella until throat culture is free of virus (p. 1620)

ASSESSMENT: AREAS OF CONCERN[44,64,104]

Acquired rubella

Body temperature

37° to 38° C (99° to 101° F) during 1- to 5-day prodrome in adult and adolescent; subsiding after rash appears

Elevated temperature with rash in children

Upper respiratory concerns

Coryza, sore throat, cough during prodrome

Head and neck

Postauricular, postcervical, and occipital lymphadenopathy (small, shotty, and occasionally tender nodes can be palpated during prodrome and a few days after rash fades)

Mild conjunctivitis and headache possible later complication

Skin

Light pink to red, discrete macular rash, rapidly becoming papular; appearing on the first day of the rash on face and trunk and by the second day on the upper and lower extremities; rash fades within 3 days

Purpura is a rare complication, appearing several days to several weeks after the rash

Oral cavity

Reddish spots, pinpoint or larger, on soft palate during prodrome or on first day of rash (Forchheimer spots)

Musculoskeletal concerns

Self-limiting polyarthritis possible complication

Inflammation and pain in proximal interphalangeal and metacarpophalangeal joints of hand and knee and ankle joints (begins within 5 days of rash and persists for less than 2 weeks)

Neurologic concerns

Symptoms of complicating encephalitis very rare; occur usually during first few days after rash

Congenital rubella syndrome

A variety of defects may be present and some are listed here; please refer to chapters on specific systems for assessment

Central nervous system

Encephalitis

Psychomotor retardation

Head and neck

Microencephaly

Large anterior fontanelle

Ears
Deafness

Eyes
Cataracts
Retinopathy
Corneal clouding
Glaucoma

Lungs
Interstitial pneumonitis

Cardiovascular concerns
Patent ductus arteriosus
Septal and aortic arch defects
Pulmonary artery and valvular stenosis
Myocardial necrosis

Hematopoietic concerns
Anemia
Hepatitis
Thrombocytopenia

Skin
Purpura
Jaundice

Abdomen
Inguinal hernia
Hepatomegaly
Splenomegaly

Lymphatic concerns
Generalized lymphadenopathy

Skeletal concerns
Metaphyseal rarefaction
Growth retardation

NURSING DIAGNOSES and NURSING INTERVENTIONS

Nursing Diagnosis	Nursing Intervention
Comfort, alteration in: pain	Administer antipyretics and analgesics as prescribed.
Anxiety	Reassure parents and patient of the benign nature of this condition.
Potential patient problem: transmission of infection	Isolate child from pregnant women. If patient is hospitalized, employ contact isolation for 5 days after rash (p. 1620).
Congenital Rubella Syndrome* Parenting, alteration in: potential	Explain and interpret infant's disease to parents. Allow parents to express feelings of anxiety and guilt. Allow parents to have adequate contact with isolated infant and to participate in infant's care as much as possible. Support bonding. (Refer to support group if needed. Reassure parents that defects are not hereditary.)
Potential patient problem: transmission of infection	Employ contact isolation until three throat cultures after 3 months are free of virus. Select nursing personnel who are not at risk for rubella infection to care for infant.

*Remainder of diagnoses depend on needs of infants and on the type of anomaly present. These will not be dealt with here.

Patient Education

1. For patient with postnatal rubella, teach parent to care for child at home as described above.

EVALUATION (postnatal acquired rubella)

Patient Outcome	Data Indicating That Outcome is Reached
There is no infection.	Temperature is 37° C (98.6° F). Joints are not inflamed or tender. There are no signs of encephalitis or purpura. Lymph nodes are not palpable. Skin is free of rash.
Laboratory values are within normal limits.	Leukocyte and platelet counts and bleeding time are normal.

Rubeola (Measles)

Rubeola (hard measles or red measles) is an acute, highly communicable viral disease manifested by a prodromal fever, conjunctivitis, coryza, bronchitis, Koplik's spots on the buccal mucosa, and a characteristic red blotchy rash. The rash appears on the third to seventh day on the face, becomes generalized, lasts 4 to 7 days, and sometimes ends in a branny desquamation.[7]

PATHOPHYSIOLOGY[45,64]

The virus of rubeola (measles) is a paramyxovirus that can be found in the blood, urine, and pharyngeal secretions of infected persons. It is transmitted directly and indirectly through contact with respiratory secretions of infected persons during the catarrhal phase of the illness (from 4 days before to 5 days after the onset of the rash). The virus invades the respiratory epithelium and multiplies there. It spreads by way of the lymph system, producing hyperplasia of lymphoid tissue. A primary viremia results and spreads the virus in leukocytes to the reticuloendothelial system. The infected reticuloendothelial cells necrose; an increased amount of virus is released; and a reinvasion of leukocytes with a secondary viremia results. With the secondary viremia the entire respiratory mucosa becomes infected, producing upper respiratory symptoms. Edema of the mucosa may predispose to secondary bacterial invasion and complications such as otitis media and pneumonia.

Within a few days after the occurrence of generalized involvement of the respiratory tract, Koplik's spots appear on the buccal mucosa and a dermal rash develops. The virus appears to invade the cells of the epidermis and oral epithelium, producing histologic changes there and stimulating a cell-mediated immune response manifested by the rash. The onset of the rash, following respiratory prodrome, coincides with the production of serum antibodies. Uncomplicated disease lasts 7 to 10 days. There is frequently a leukopenia and lymphocytosis. A leukocytosis later in the disease occurs if there is a secondary bacterial infection.

Complications of measles involve the respiratory tract and central nervous system. Pneumonia may result from direct invasion of the virus or by secondary bacterial infection. Encephalitis resulting from direct viral invasion of the brain affects many persons subclinically. Pathologic specimens of brain tissue show demyelination, vascular cuffing, gliosis, and infiltration of fat-laden macrophages near blood vessel walls. Gross evidence of edema, congestion, and petechial hemorrhages can be seen in the brain and spinal cord. Symptoms range from mild to severe. A large number of patients who recover are left with neurologic sequelae.

DIAGNOSTIC STUDIES[45]

Tissue culture of secretions from nasopharynx, conjunctiva, and culture of blood or urine
   Positive for measles virus

Hemagglutination inhibition
   Detects long-lasting antibodies; therefore useful for determining immune status
   Fourfold increase in antibodies between acute and convalescent stages is diagnostic

Complement fixation tests
   Detect short-lasting antibodies during and shortly after rash
   Titer as high as 1:512

Neutralization tests
   Lack of antibodies indicates susceptibility

TREATMENT PLAN

Chemotherapeutic
   Anti-infective therapy for secondary infections only
   Antipyretics for temperature control
   Active immunization for prevention (p. 1617)

Supportive
   Bed rest during febrile period

ASSESSMENT: AREAS OF CONCERN[45,64]

Body temperature
Up to 40° C (104° F) during prodrome; decrease in 3 to 5 days (when rash appears)

Upper respiratory concerns
Hacking cough; coryza within 24 hours of fever, increasing in intensity until rash appears, gradually subsiding within 5 to 10 days

Eyes
Periorbital edema
Conjunctivitis, subsiding with appearance of rash
Photophobia

Head and neck
Lymphadenopathy possible

Oral cavity
Koplik's spots on buccal mucosa, most often opposite the second molars; appear 2 to 4 days after onset of prodrome; resemble tiny grains of bluish-white sand surrounded by an inflammatory areola

Skin
Irregular macules appear on face and neck and in front of and behind the ears 3 to 4 days after onset of prodrome

Rash rapidly becomes maculopapular, spreading to trunk and extremities within 24 to 48 hours; at this time it begins to fade from the face
Rash is brownish pink in color and irregularly confluent
Petechiae or ecchymoses may be present in severe cases
Rash fades in 4 to 7 days, leaving a brownish desquamation
An acute thrombocytopenic purpura with hemorrhage may be a complication

Neurologic concerns
Symptoms of an encephalitis, a rare complication, occurring within 2 days to 1 week after onset of rash
Secondary elevation of temperature
Headaches, seizures, altered state of consciousness

Ears
Otitis media may result as a secondary infection

Abdomen
Symptoms of secondary acute appendicitis

Activity level
Severe lethargy or prostration after onset of rash may indicate a secondary bacterial infection

Breathing patterns
Dyspnea may indicate secondary bacterial infection

NURSING DIAGNOSES and NURSING INTERVENTIONS

Nursing Diagnosis	Nursing Intervention
Skin integrity, impairment of: potential	Provide tepid baths as necessary to keep skin clean.
Activity intolerance	Provide bed rest during febrile period.
Fluid volume deficit, potential	Provide adequate oral fluids of a variety that appeals to age of patient.
Sensory-perceptual alteration: visual	Dim lights if photophobia is present. Cleanse eyelids with warm water to remove crusts or secretions.
Potential patient problem: fever	Administer antipyretics as prescribed. Give cool sponge baths to lower body temperature.
Potential patient problem: transmission of infection	If patient is hospitalized, employ respiratory isolation for 4 days after onset of rash (p. 1620).
Potential patient problem: susceptibility to infection	Protect from exposure to bacteria, particularly streptococcus. Monitor for secondary increase in temperature, ear pain, dyspnea, chest pain, lethargy, and increased coughing.

Patient Education

1. Teach parent to do all nursing care listed above for the child who remains at home.

EVALUATION

Patient Outcome	Data Indicating That Outcome is Reached
There is no infection.	Body temperature is normal.
Laboratory studies are within normal limits.	Leukocyte and lymphocyte counts are normal.
There is no secondary otitis media.	There is no pain in ear: tympanic membrane is normal.
There is no secondary pneumonia.	Respiratory rate, rhythm, and depth are normal. Breath sounds are clear.
Skin and mucous membranes are normal.	Skin and mucous membranes are warm and moist, with natural color.

Table 15-6
Overview of Respiratory Infectious Diseases[7]

	Streptococcal Throat	Scarlet Fever	Rheumatic Fever
Occurrence	More common in temperate zones; may be endemic, epidemic, or sporadic in occurrence; highest in late winter or spring; ages 3-15 most often affected; no sex or racial difference		Females at greater risk for certain characteristics
Etiologic agent	Streptococcus pyogenes (group A streptococcus of approximately 70 serologically distinct types)	Erythrogenic toxin	
Reservoir	Humans	Humans	Humans
Transmission	Direct or intimate contact with patient or carrier; may follow ingestion of contaminated food		
Incubation period	1-3 d	2-4 d (range: 1-7 d)	3-35 d after clinical strep throat (average: 19 d)
Period of communicability	Untreated, uncomplicated cases: 10-21 d; complicated: weeks to months; antibiotic treated: 24-48 h		
Susceptibility and resistance	General; many develop antitoxic or antibacterial immunity to one of the types of streptococci through inapparent infection	Permanent acquired immunity from active disease	Persons who have suffered one attack are predisposed to a recurrent episode following group A streptococcal upper respiratory infections
Report to local health authority	Epidemics only		

RESPIRATORY INFECTIOUS DISEASES

The respiratory infectious diseases discussed in this section are those acute and chronic respiratory pathologic conditions that are caused by a specific pathogenic agent that is transmitted by inhalation or by direct contact with infectious respiratory secretions. Although diphtheria, pertussis, and measles fit this definition, they are discussed in this chapter under childhood and immunizable infectious diseases. Rheumatic fever and scarlet fever are discussed here, because of their etiologic agent, the group A streptococcus, causing streptococcal throat (Table 15-6). Nonspecific lower respiratory infections such as pneumonia are discussed in Chapter 2. Nonspecific upper respiratory infections such as pharyngitis and tonsillitis are discussed in Chapter 7.

Streptococcal Throat, Scarlet Fever, Rheumatic Fever

Streptococcal throat is an acute exudative tonsillitis or pharyngitis caused by group A beta-hemolytic streptococci. Coincident or subsequent otitis media or peritonsillar abscess may be present. Rheumatic fever, chorea, and acute glomerulonephritis are possible sequelae.

Scarlet fever is a group A beta-hemolytic streptococcal disease characterized by a skin rash. It occurs when the infecting strain of streptococcus produces a toxin causing a sensitivity reaction in the infected host. Clinical characteristics may include those of streptococcal sore throat plus enanthem, strawberry tongue, and exanthema.

Histoplasmosis	Influenza	Legionellosis (Legionnaires' Disease)	Tuberculosis
Worldwide; higher in eastern and central United States; increases with age to 30 yr; no differences by sex; outbreaks in groups with common exposure	Worldwide in pandemics, epidemics, localized outbreaks, and sporadic cases; highest in winter in temperate zones	Europe, United States, and Canada; first recognized in 1977; sporadic cases and outbreaks in summer and autumn; increases with age	Worldwide; mortality and prevalence decreasing in many places; highest in males and poor; most active disease arises from a latent infection
Histoplasma capsulatum (a fungus)	Three types of viruses (A, B, and C), each with many strains	*Legionella pneumophila* (a bacteria with subgroups)	*Mycobacterium tuberculosis* and *M. bovis*
Soil around chicken houses, caves harboring bats, and around starling roosts and decaying trees	Humans; some mammals suspected as sources of new strains of viruses	Unknown, but probably environmental; organism survives in hot and cold tap water and distilled water for months	Humans; *M. bovis* in diseased cattle
Inhalation of airborne spores	Direct transmission by inhalation of virus in airborne mucous discharge	Common source, airborne transmission suspected	Inhalation of bacilli in airborne mucous droplets from sputum of persons with active disease; less frequent: ingestion or skin penetration
5-18 d after exposure	24-72 h	2-10 d	4-12 wk after exposure or anytime when disease is in latent stage
Not transmitted from person to person	3 d from onset of symptoms	No documented person-to-person transmission	As long as bacilli are in sputum; some are intermittently communicable for years
General; inapparent infections common, and result in increasing resistance	Universal; infection produces immunity to a specific strain of virus	General; rare in those less than 20 yr; greatest in males, smokers, and immunosuppressed persons	General; highest in children less than 3 yr, those greater than 65 yr, chronically ill, silicone and asbestos workers, and malnourished and immunosuppressed individuals
In some states	Mandatory case report	In some states	Mandatory case report

Rheumatic fever is a sequela of group A streptococcal infection of the upper respiratory tract, occurring in about 2.8% of those having a streptococcal throat infection. The condition is thought to result from an altered immune reaction to the streptococcus. Rheumatic heart disease is a potential complication.

PATHOPHYSIOLOGY

Infection with group A streptococci results in a number of related clinical disease entities such as streptococcal throat, scarlet fever, erysipelas, and nonsuppurative complications such as nephritis and rheumatic fever. The type of disease resulting from group A streptococci depends on the site of tissue invasion, the antigenic characteristics of the infecting strain of streptococcus, and the immune status of the host. There are 60 to 70 serologically distinct strains of group A streptococci, producing a variety of different enzymes and at least three different erythrogenic toxins. These antigenic characteristics determine the type of enzyme-specific and toxin-specific antibodies produced by the host. A host with adequate antibodies against a particular serotype with or without antitoxic immunity may develop no clinical disease if reinfected with the same serotype. A person with antitoxic immunity resulting from previous group A infections but with no antibodies against a particular invading serotype may develop a clinical streptococcal throat. A person with no antitoxic immunity and no antibodies against an invading toxigenic group A streptococcus may develop clinical scarlet fever. In all clinical streptococcal disease a leukocytosis is present.[64]

Streptococcal throat (septic sore throat) results when the streptococcus invades and remains in the lymphoid tissue of the oropharynx, rapidly producing inflammation with edema, erythema, and infiltration with polymorphonuclear leukocytes. The mucosal surfaces, particularly over the tonsils, become ulcerated, releasing a mucopurulent exudate. Cervical lymphadenopathy is present. Severity of symptoms increases with age.[64] Untreated, uncomplicated disease lasts a few days to a week. The streptococcus may invade surrounding tissue producing suppurative complications such as peritonsillar cellulitis and abscess, retropharyngeal abscess, sinus empyema, otitis media, mastoiditis, meningitis, cervical lymphadenitis, pneumonia, and periorbital abscess. Toxin dissemination may result in rheumatic fever or nephritis.[110]

Scarlet fever results if the invading streptococcus releases an erythrogenic toxin stimulating a sensitivity reaction in the host. Dilation of small capillaries and toxic injury of the vascular epithelium may be widespread in the body, particularly in the liver, myocardium, and kidneys. The pathologic changes are most visible on the skin, with an erythematous rash and desquamation, and in the oral cavity, with the strawberry tongue and an enanthem. Hepatocellular damage and destruction of red cells may result in jaundice, increase in bilirubin, mild anemia, and an increase in reticulocytes. In rare situations, toxins may be disseminated in the bloodstream, producing a severe toxic illness. Streptococcus may invade adjacent tissue and the bloodstream, producing a severe septic scarlet fever.[110]

Rheumatic fever is a delayed complication of upper respiratory infection with group A streptococci producing nonsuppurative inflammatory lesions in connective tissue of the heart, joints, subcutaneous tissues, and central nervous system. Symptoms may be present in all or some of those systems. The exact causal mechanism is not known. The following have been hypothesized: (1) there is direct tissue invasion by group A streptococci or by cell wall antigens of the microorganism; (2) streptococcal enzymes, particularly streptolysins S or O, induce tissue injury; (3) antigen-humoral antibody reactions localize in affected tissue; and (4) an autoimmune reaction is operative. The autoimmune theory is supported by the detection of heart-reactive antibodies (HRA) in the sera of patients with rheumatic heart disease. A genetic predisposition to this disease is suggested by the fact that rheumatic fever consistently affects only 2.8% of those with a clinical upper respiratory streptococcal infection.[14]

Cardiac connective tissue lesions show early fragmentation of collagen fibers, cellular lymphocytic infiltration, and fibrin deposits. These changes are followed by the development of the Aschoff nodule, a perivascular locus of inflammation with an area of central necrosis surrounded by large mononuclear and polymorphonuclear leukocytes. Cardiac findings include pericarditis, myocarditis, and left-sided endocarditis. Valvular lesions begin with edema and cellular infiltration of the leaflets and chordae with small verrucae forming along the closure lines. With healing the valves become thickened and deformed, the valve commissures become fused, and the chordae become shortened. These changes result in valvular stenosis and insufficiency, varying in extensiveness and severity. Carditis may result in long-term disability or death.[14]

Joint lesions are characterized by a fibrinous exudate over the synovial membrane and a serous effusion without joint destruction. Subcutaneous nodules form that resemble the Aschoff nodules described above.

Laboratory tests demonstrate the presence of C-reactive proteins in the blood and an increased erythrocyte sedimentation rate. Electrocardiogram readings may exhibit an elongation of the P-R interval before the development of symptoms.[110]

A later neurologic sequela of rheumatic fever is Sydenham's chorea. The latent period for this condition may be so long as to occur in the absence of laboratory changes associated with rheumatic fever.[14]

DIAGNOSTIC STUDIES[14, 110]

Streptococcal throat
Culture of throat exudate
Positive for group A hemolytic streptococci (10 or more colonies)

Scarlet fever
Schultz-Charlton reaction skin test
Rash blanches at site of intradermal injection of antitoxin

Dick skin test for susceptibility
Erythema and induration greater than 3 mm within 24 hours of intradermal injection of 0.1 ml exotoxin; reaction is compared with a control site where 0.1 ml of a control substance is injected intradermally

Rheumatic fever
Antistreptolysin O (ASO)
Increase in ASO suggests recent infection with streptococcus; ASO peaks 2 to 5 weeks after strep infection and decreases thereafter; 80% to 85% of patients with rheumatic fever develop high ASO titers; ASO titers exceeding the following may be diagnostic:
Preschool: 1:85
5-18 years: 1:170
Adults: 1:85

Deoxyribonuclease B (ADN-B) test
ADN-B develops later and persists longer than ASO; titers greater than the following are diagnostic:
Preschool: 1:60
5-18 years: 1:170
Adults: 1:85

Streptozyme test
Measures five different streptococcal enzymes
Titers of 100 to 200 are equivocal; titers greater than 300 indicate recent streptococcal infection

C-reactive protein (CRP)
Normally not present in serum
Presence of CRP in serum is diagnostic

Sedimentation rate
Elevated:
Greater than 120 mm/h in Westergen method
Greater than 50 mm/h in Wintrobe test

TREATMENT PLAN

Chemotherapeutic[14]
Anti-infective agents
Benzathine penicillin G (Bicillin), 1,200,000 units IM one time for adults (children: 600,000-900,000 units), *or*
Oral penicillin, 250,000 units tid q10d, *or*
Procaine penicillin (Wycillin), 600,000 units IM q10d for severe scarlet fever
Erythromycin (Erythrocin, others), 40 mg/kg/24 h in young children; 250 mg po qid q10d for patients allergic to penicillin[110]
Antipyretic agents
Aspirin, 90-100 mg/kg/d q2wk; 60-70 mg/kg/d for subsequent 6 wk for treatment of polyarthritis of rheumatic fever
Antipyretics for management of fever
Corticosteroids
Prednisone (Deltasone, others), 40-60 mg/d q2-3wk for treatment of carditis, *or*
Methyl prednisone sodium succinate (Solu-Medrol), IV, in severe cases; decrease to complete withdrawal in 3 wk[14]
To prevent recurrent streptococcal infections in post–rheumatic fever patients:
Anti-infective agents
Benzathine penicillin G (Bicillin), 1,200,000 units IM q4wk during and following convalescence for life (recommended duration is controversial), *or*
Erythromycin (Erythrocin, others), 250 mg bid po for those allergic to penicillin

Supportive[14]
Bed rest during febrile stage of all streptococcal diseases; bed rest for 3 weeks for patients without carditis; for an additional month after carditis is detected
Nonstimulating environment and sedation for patients with chorea
Fluid therapy as indicated
To prevent transmission to others: secretion precautions of hospitalized patients with an upper respiratory streptococcal infection for 24 hours following initiation of antibiotic therapy

ASSESSMENT: AREAS OF CONCERN[14,110]

Body temperature
38° to 39° C (100° to 103° F)

Pulse
Rapid

Head and neck

Enlarged, tender cervical lymph nodes

Symptoms of suppurative complications: mastoiditis, otitis media, periorbital abscess, sinus empyema

Oropharynx

Edema, erythema (fiery red to dull red), and petechiae of uvula, tonsils, and posterior oropharynx

Confluent, easily removable mucopurulent exudate

May be suppurative complications

Subjective symptoms

Pain on swallowing

Headache

Anorexia

Malaise

Chills[110]

Respiratory concerns

Complications: symptoms of pneumonia (Chapter 2)

Neurologic concerns

Complications: symptoms of meningitis (p. 1561)

Scarlet fever

All of the above plus the following:

Skin

Erythematous and punctate rash appearing within 2 days of streptococcal throat, becoming generalized rapidly; appearing first on upper chest and back and then on the lower back, upper extremities, abdomen, and lower extremities

Extensiveness of rash is variable; it may be better felt (like sandpaper) than seen

Petechiae may precede the rash on the lower extremities; more common in skin folds

Desquamation may develop between 5 days to 4 weeks after appearance of the rash, starting on the neck, upper chest, back, fingertips, or toes; skin peels in large sections, particularly on the palms and soles

Flushing of cheeks with circumoral pallor

Oral cavity

Tongue is inflamed and heavily coated at first; after the rash appears, the papillae become swollen and appear as red bumps on a gray background (strawberry tongue); within a few days the tongue peels, first at the tip and margins; by day 6 the tongue is completely denuded, beefy red, moist, and glistening (raspberry tongue); tongue returns to normal by the end of the second week

Enanthem: for a few days around the time of rash appearance on the skin there may be a hemorrhagic rash on the soft palate and anterior pillars of the fossae

Abdomen

Liver may be slightly enlarged and tender

Musculoskeletal concerns

Tender, slightly inflamed, and edematous joints possible

Septic scarlet fever

Body temperature

40° to 42° C (104° to 108° F)

Pulse

Rapid and weak

Oropharynx

Throat manifestations more severe but same as those for streptococcal throat and scarlet fever

Ulceration and perforation on uvula, soft palate, and tonsils

Seropurulent or mucopurulent nasal discharge

Excoriations on lips, mouth, and nares

Skin

Rash may be slight to severe

Head and neck

Cervical lymphadenopathy

Mastoid and middle ear pain

Breathing patterns

Labored, due to swelling and occlusion

Toxic scarlet fever (fulminating scarlet fever)[110]

Body temperature

41° to 42° C (105° to 108° F)

Pulse

Very rapid

Skin

Heavy punctate or erythematous hemorrhagic rash: bright to purple-red

Vascular concerns

Capillary fragility as seen by hematuria, epistaxis, and hematemesis

Oropharynx

Edema without exudate

Systemic concerns

Intense headache

Vomiting

Cardiovascular concerns

Symptoms of toxic myocarditis

Mental status

Delirium

Irrationality

Coma

Rheumatic fever[14]

Body temperature

Low-grade fever: 38° C (100° F)

Musculoskeletal concerns

Acute onset of mild to severe symptoms of polyarthritis: heat, swelling, redness, and severe tenderness affecting mainly the knees, ankles, elbows, and wrists; migratory, with multiple joint involvement at one time; inflammation subsides in each joint in 1 to 2 weeks; entire episode subsides in 4 weeks

Cardiovascular concerns

Insidious onset of symptoms of carditis within 3 weeks: cardiac enlargement, pericardial friction rubs, congestive heart failure, signs of effusion, tachycardia, gallop rhythm, and diastolic and possibly systolic murmurs

Three types of murmurs associated with acute carditis: (1) high-pitched blowing holosystolic apical murmur of mitral regurgitation, (2) low-pitched apical middiastolic flow murmur, (3) high-pitched decrescendo diastolic murmur of aortic regurgitation heard at the secondary and primary aortic areas

Mitral and aortic stenotic murmurs associated with chronic rheumatic valvular disease

Skin

One to two dozen firm, painless, variable in size (3 mm to 2 cm), subcutaneous nodules; usually over bony prominences and tendons; lasting 1 to 2 weeks

Nonpruritic, erythematous macular eruption on the trunk or proximal extremities (erythema marginatum); lesions appear to be a vasomotor phenomenon, moving over the skin with a tendency to advance at the margins and clear at the center; individual lesions clear within hours, but the process persists intermittently for weeks or months

Neurologic concerns

Symptoms of chorea: involuntary, purposeless, rapid motions; irritability; emotional lability; weakness; restlessness; fretfulness; gradually increasing in intensity over a 2-week period, reaching a plateau, and gradually subsiding

Subjective symptoms

Malaise

Abdominal pain

NURSING DIAGNOSES and NURSING INTERVENTIONS

Nursing Diagnosis	Nursing Intervention
Oral mucous membrane, alteration in	Provide frequent oral fluids and oral hygiene. Provide high humidity in room. Lubricate lips and nares.
Activity intolerance	Maintain complete bed rest of scarlet fever and rheumatic fever patients to prevent complications. Provide all care including hygiene and feeding.
Fluid volume deficit, potential	Encourage frequent oral fluids that patient is able to swallow. Administer IV fluids as prescribed.
Skin integrity, impairment of: actual	Give sponge baths with a solution of sodium bicarbonate or calamine lotion to relieve pruritus associated with desquamation in scarlet fever.
Cardiac output, alteration in: decreased	Monitor for symptoms of carditis and congestive heart failure in rheumatic fever patients. Administer therapy as prescribed (Chapter 1).
Mobility, impaired physical	Monitor for symptoms of polyarthritis. Maintain rest of involved joints. Administer salicylates, as prescribed.
Potential patient problem: fever	Give tepid sponge baths. Administer antipyretics as ordered to decrease elevated temperature.
Potential patient problem: transmission of infection	Maintain respiratory secretion precautions of hospitalized patients for 24 hours after antibiotic therapy is initiated.

Patient Education

1. Oral antibiotics must be taken for prescribed length of time. Follow-up throat cultures may be necessary.
2. Compliance with prescribed long-term antibiotic therapy is necessary to minimize risk for recurrence of rheumatic fever with subsequent streptococcal infections.
3. Upper respiratory infections should be diagnosed and treated promptly in post–rheumatic fever patients.
4. Continued rest during convalescence is necessary for post–rheumatic fever patients.
5. Medical monitoring for cardiac complications is necessary after rheumatic fever.

EVALUATION

Patient Outcome	Data Indicating That Outcome is Reached
Laboratory values are within normal limits.	Leukocyte count and sedimentation rate are normal. There is no C-reactive protein in serum.
There is no infection.	Cervical lymph nodes are not palpable. There are no subjective symptoms of malaise, abdominal pain, or pain on swallowing. Body temperature is normal.
Skin and mucous membranes are normal.	Skin and mucous membranes are warm and moist, with natural color. There is no edema, inflammation, or exudate in oropharynx. Exanthema and enanthem of scarlet fever are not present. Exanthema and subcutaneous nodules of rheumatic fever are not present.
Physical activity patterns are normal.	There is no limitation of joint movement. The patient can move all joints without pain. The patient exhibits purposeful movement, indicating no signs of chorea.
Cardiac function is normal.	Pulse rate is normal. There is no fatigue on exertion. Electrocardiogram is normal. No murmurs are auscultated.

Histoplasmosis

Histoplasmosis is a pulmonary and systemic infection, similar to tuberculosis, resulting from inhalation of the spores of Histoplasma capsulatum, *which are frequently found in the soil. Infection is common, but overt clinical disease is rare. Five clinical forms of the disease have been recognized.*

PATHOPHYSIOLOGY[7,10]

Spores of *H. capsulatum*, a fungus, are inhaled when soil containing them is disturbed. A lesion is formed within the lung parenchyma where the spores convert to a yeast phase and are phagocytized by macrophages. Lesions may also be formed in the hilar or mediastinal lymph nodes as a result of migration of yeast-laden mac-rophages to those areas. Dissemination and lesion formation may also occur in the spleen and liver. These primary lesions become necrotic at the center, build up a fibrotic capsule, and frequently calcify. In most cases where calcification occurs there is no reactivation of the infection and the host manifests no symptoms except an immune response to histoplasmin.

Four other clinical forms of the disease are possible: (1) acute benign respiratory disease, (2) acute disseminated disease, (3) chronic disseminated disease, and (4) chronic pulmonary disease. In acute benign respiratory disease the primary pulmonary lesion remains active, resulting in a spreading infiltration pneumonia. In acute disseminated disease, inflammatory and necrotic lesions may result in septic-type fever, hepatosplenomegaly, severe prostration, and death. Chronic disseminated histoplasmosis results when there is extensive invasion of yeast-laden macrophages by way of the reticuloendothelial system to bone marrow, spleen, liver, and lungs. The inflammatory and necrotic reaction in those tissues is subacute but progressive and may eventually result in death. Chronic pulmonary histoplasmosis is manifested by a progressive emphysema. Fluid-filled cysts surrounded by chronic inflammation progress through stages of caseation necrosis and cavitation, continuing to disseminate the yeast through pulmonary tissue.

The clinical symptoms are quite varied but are generally more severe in infants, immunosuppressed persons, and chronically debilitated persons.[7,10]

DIAGNOSTIC STUDIES[25]

Sabouraud's agar culture; Giesma- or Wright-stained smears of respiratory exudate, blood, or exudate from ulcerated lesions
Positive for *H. capsulatum*
Results are frequently erratic, necessitating the culture of many specimens

Precipitation and complement fixation tests; agglutination test
Increase in antibodies within 3 to 4 weeks; fourfold increase suggests disease progression
Agglutinins greater than 1:8

Skin test
Induration greater than 5 mm in 24 hours indicates past or present infection

Chest x-ray film
Acute: transient parenchymal pulmonary infiltrates resembling lobar pneumonia
Chronic: progressively enlarging areas of necrosis with or without cavitation

TREATMENT PLAN

Chemotherapeutic[25,101]
Anti-infective agents
Amphotericin B (Fungizone), 0.5-0.6 mg/kg/d for 11 wk or 1-1.2 mg/kg every other day for 10 wk given IV in 500 ml 5% dextrose and water; may be gradually increased, starting with 10 mg/d, increasing to 50 mg/d, and further increasing to 2.5 g three times a week
Corticosteroids
Corticosteroids, 10-20 mg may be mixed with the infusion to minimize the side effects of amphotericin B

Antihistamines
Diphenhydramine hydrochloride (Benadryl), 25-50 mg added to IV to control side effects

ASSESSMENT: AREAS OF CONCERN[25,101]

Pulmonary, acute
Mild to severe; duration: days to weeks

Respiratory concerns
Pleural and substernal chest pain
Dry or productive cough with a metallic tone, suggesting tracheobronchial obstruction

Subjective symptoms
Malaise
Weakness
Anorexia

Body temperature
Low-grade fever

Skin
Erythema multiforme
Erythema nodosum

Cardiovascular concerns
May have complicating symptoms of a pericarditis

Pulmonary, chronic
May have above symptoms plus:

Respiratory concerns
Purulent sputum; hemoptysis
Increasing signs of pulmonary insufficiency

Disseminated, acute
Abdomen
Enlarged liver and spleen

Body temperature
High fever

Disseminated, chronic
Symptoms vary depending on site of dissemination

Abdomen
Symptoms of gastrointestinal ulcers, hepatitis, and peritonitis

Oropharynx
Ulcerated lesions in larynx, mouth, nose, or pharynx, resembling epidermoid cancer

Skin
Purpura

Neurologic concerns
Symptoms of meningitis (p. 1561)

Respiratory concerns
Symptoms of pneumonia (Chapter 2)

Cardiac concerns
Symptoms of endocarditis (Chapter 1)

NURSING DIAGNOSES and NURSING INTERVENTIONS

Nursing Diagnosis	Nursing Intervention
Potential patient problem: adverse chemo-therapeutic response	Monitor for cyanosis, changes in pulse and respiratory rate, and signs of renal dysfunction; resulting from amphotericin toxicity. Administer antihistamines and corticosteroids as prescribed. Encourage fluids high in potassium if nausea and vomiting persist. Prevent phlebitis by using small-gauge needle for IV line. Agitate IV fluid bag every 15 to 20 minutes while chemotherapeutic agent is being administered to ensure even distribution of drug and fluid in bag and in intravenous line. Give infusion over a 5- to 6-hour period.
Comfort, alteration in: pain	Frequently reposition the patient for comfort during prolonged painful IV infusions. Provide diversional activities. Administer analgesics before IV administration, as prescribed.

Other diagnoses will depend on extent of dissemination and of pulmonary dysfunction (see Chapters 1 and 2).

Patient Education[7]

1. Medical follow-up for 1 year after treatment to prevent relapses is necessary.
2. Patients can protect themselves from reinfection by avoiding infected sites, by wearing a protective mask, or by sterilizing the site with 3% formalin.

EVALUATION

Patient Outcome	Data Indicating That Outcome is Reached
Patient is free of complications from treatment.	There are no signs of phlebitis, renal dysfunction, electrolyte imbalance, pain, or neuritis.
Patient is aware of need for protection from reinfection.	Patient states methods to use to avoid reexposure.
Patient is aware of need for medical surveillance.	Patient states intent to see physician on a regular basis for 1 year after hospitalization.
Breathing patterns are normal.	There is no cough, dyspnea, sputum, or hemoptysis.
Oropharynx is normal.	There are no lesions in mouth, larynx, pharynx, or nose.
Skin is normal.	There is no purpura, erythema multiforme, or erythema nodosum.
Energy levels are adequate.	Patient has energy to carry out all daily activities.
Gastrointestinal function is normal.	Patient does not have abdominal pain; patient is able to eat all desired foods. Patient is not jaundiced.
There is no infection.	Sputum cultures are negative. Body temperature is normal.

Influenza

Influenza is a generalized, acute, febrile disease associated with upper and lower respiratory infection; it is characterized by a severe and protracted cough, fever, headache, myalgia, prostration, coryza, and mild sore throat. The disease may be unrecognizable clinically from the common cold. Complications include bacterial pneumonia, particularly in elderly and debilitated persons.

PATHOPHYSIOLOGY

Influenza viruses A, B, or C, each with many mutagenic strains, are inhaled in aerosolized mucous droplets shed from infected persons. The viruses are deposited on and penetrate the surface of upper respiratory tract mucosal cells, producing cell lysis and destruction of the ciliated epithelium. Viral neuraminidase decreases the viscosity of the mucosa, thus facilitating the spread of virus-containing exudate to the lower respiratory tract. An interstitial inflammation and necrosis of the bronchiolar and alveolar epithelium result, filling the alveoli with an exudate containing leukocytes, erythrocytes, and hyaline membrane.[64]

Regeneration of epithelium, following necrosis and desquamation, slowly begins after the fifth day of illness. Regeneration reaches a maximum within 9 to 15 days, at which time mucous production and cilia begin to appear. Before complete regeneration the compromised epithelium is prone to secondary bacterial invasion resulting in bacterial pneumonia usually caused by *S. aureus.*[71]

The initial invasion of the virus can be aborted at the portal of entry if virus-specific secretory antibodies (IgA) are present in mucous secretions and if virus-specific serum antibodies are adequate.[64]

The disease is usually self-limiting. Acute symptoms last 2 to 7 days and are followed by a convalescent period of about a week. The disease is important because of its cyclic epidemic and pandemic nature and because of the high mortality associated with pulmonary complications resulting from secondary bacterial pneumonia. This risk is highest in elderly and chronically diseased persons.

Laboratory findings show an elevated sedimentation rate, leukopenia or a slight leukocytosis, and a febrile albuminuria.

DIAGNOSTIC STUDIES[71]

Tissue culture of nasal or pharyngeal secretions
Positive for influenza virus

Sputum culture
Positive for bacteria in secondary infections

Fluorescent antibody staining of secretions
Positive for influenza virus

Hemagglutination inhibition or complement fixation tests
Fourfold increase in antibody titer between acute and convalescent stages

TREATMENT PLAN

Chemotherapeutic
Agent-specific anti-infective agents for bacterial complications or for patients with chronic pulmonary disease
Antipyretics
ASA, 600 mg orally q4h for adults
Adrenergic agents
Phenylephrine (Neo-Synephrine), 0.25%, 2 drops in each nostril for nasal congestion
Antitussive agents
Terpin hydrate with codeine, 5-10 ml orally q3-4h for adults for cough

Supportive
Oxygen and IV fluid and electrolytes for complications
Steam inhalation for congestion
Amantadine, 100 mg po bid for duration of epidemic (3-6 wk) for high-risk persons over the age of 9 yr for prevention; 2-4 mg/lb/d (not exceeding 150 mg/d in two or three doses for young children)
Vaccine, 0.5-1 ml IM for adults; 0.25 ml IM for infants 6-35 mo; 0.5 ml IM for children 3-12 yr; for infants and children give two doses at 4-wk intervals; must be repeated yearly in the fall for viral strain expected in the winter; recommended for elderly individuals, chronically ill adults, children with chronic heart or pulmonary disease, residents of nursing homes and chronic care facilities, and health care providers with contact with high-risk patients[6,7]

ASSESSMENT: AREAS OF CONCERN

Body temperature
Sudden-onset fever (38° to 39° C [102° to 103° F]) that gradually falls and rises again on the third day

Subjective symptoms
Prostration

Myalgia, particularly in back and legs
Anorexia and malaise
Headache, photophobia, and retrobulbar aching

Respiratory concerns

Mild at first: sore throat; substernal burning; nonproductive cough; coryza
Later: severe and productive cough; erythema of soft palate, posterior hard palate, tonsillar pillars, and posterior pharynx; increased respiratory rate

Head and neck

Conjunctivitis may be present
Flushed face
Anterior cervical lymphadenopathy may be present

Complicating viral pneumonia

Dyspnea
Cyanosis
Hemoptysis
Crepitant and subcrepitant rales
See Chapter 2

Complicating bacterial pneumonia
Respiratory concerns

Same as for viral pneumonia plus purulent or bloody sputum
See Chapter 2

Body temperature

Secondary rise in fever

NURSING DIAGNOSES and NURSING INTERVENTIONS

Nursing Diagnosis	Nursing Intervention
Airway clearance, ineffective	Administer decongestants as prescribed. Provide cool, humidified air. Suction if necessary. Monitor for signs of viral or bacterial pneumonia. Provide oxygen as prescribed.
Fluid volume deficit, potential	Encourage fluids as much as patient can tolerate (3000 ml for adult). Administer IV fluids as prescribed.
Activity intolerance	Maintain bed rest for 2 or 3 days after temperature returns to normal. Provide for diversional activity to maintain quiet during convalescence.
Comfort, alteration in: pain	Administer analgesics and antipyretics as prescribed. Give tepid sponge baths to reduce fever. Provide cool, humidified air.
Potential patient problem: susceptibility to infection	Protect from exposure to bacteria. Monitor for a subsequent increase in temperature accompanied by chest pain, dyspnea, hemoptysis, purulent sputum, or ear pain. See discussion of pneumonia in Chapter 2.
Potential patient problem: transmission of infection	Employ contact isolation for duration of the illness for hospitalized infants and children (p. 1620).

Patient Education

1. Maintain bed rest for 2 or 3 days after temperature returns to normal.
2. Force fluids.
3. Continue to take antibiotics for duration as prescribed for bacterial complications.
4. Report symptoms of secondary infection (ear pain, purulent or bloody sputum, chest pain, increase in temperature) to physician.

EVALUATION

Patient Outcome	Data Indicating That Outcome is Reached
There is no secondary bacterial infection.	Energy returns. There is no otitis media, cyanosis, dyspnea, chest pain, hemoptysis, or mucopurulent sputum.

Patient Outcome	Data Indicating That Outcome is Reached
	Sputum cultures are negative.
	Body temperature is normal.
Laboratory values are within normal limits.	Leukocyte count and sedimentation rate are normal.
Airway clearance is effective.	Secretions are clear and thin. There is no cough.
Respirations are normal.	Rate, depth, and rhythm of respirations are normal.

Legionellosis (Legionnaires' Disease)

Legionellosis (Legionnaires' disease) is an acute bacterial infection so named because it caused an outbreak of pneumonia at a convention of American Legionnaires at a Philadelphia hotel. The acute disease is a patchy pulmonary infiltrate and consolidation, with a high fever, malaise, myalgia and headache, nonproductive cough, and a high risk for respiratory failure and death.

PATHOPHYSIOLOGY

Inhalation of the *Legionella pneumophila* causes two distinct clinical syndromes: (1) Pontiac fever, which resembles influenza, and (2) Legionnaires' disease, with pathologic changes characteristic of lobar pneumonia. In the latter there is a cellular exudate consisting of polymorphonuclear leukocytes and macrophages with extensive necrosis of the exudate and alveolar septa. Bronchi are clear of the necrotic process. Rarely is a purulent sputum produced. The disease progresses rapidly during the first 4 to 6 days of clinical illness. Complications include renal failure, bacteremic shock, and respiratory failure resulting in death to 15% of patients.[38]

Chest radiographs show a patchy pattern of pneumonia and small pleural effusions. There may be a normal or slight leukocytosis, markedly elevated sedimentation rate, hematuria, proteinuria, and laboratory evidence of liver dysfunction.[39]

DIAGNOSTIC STUDIES[39]

Culture of blood, sputum, pleural fluid, lung tissue
Positive for *L. pneumophila*

Direct immunofluorescent stain of respiratory secretions
Positive for *L. pneumophila*

Enzyme-linked immunosorbent assay (ELISA) on urine
Positive for *L. pneumophila* antigen

Indirect immunofluorescence
Fourfold or greater rise in antibody titer to 1:128 within 21 days of onset of illness

TREATMENT PLAN[39]

Chemotherapeutic
Anti-infective agents
Erythromycin (Robimycin), 0.5-1.0 g/6 h for adults; 15 mg/kg/6 h for children, IV or oral, for 14 d
Rifampin (Rifomycin, others; as adjunct therapy)

Electromechanical
Assisted ventilation
Oxygen therapy
Temporary renal dialysis

Supportive
IV fluids and electrolytes

ASSESSMENT: AREAS OF CONCERN[39]

Body temperature
38° to 41° C (102° to 105° F) within a day

Subjective symptoms
Anorexia
Malaise
Myalgia
Chills
Abdominal pain

Respiratory concerns
Nonproductive cough
Dyspnea
Tachypnea
Pluritic chest pain
Rales or rhonchi

Cardiovascular concerns
Tachycardia
Symptoms of shock

Digestive concerns
  Diarrhea
  Sometimes vomiting

Neurologic concerns
  Confusion, slurring of speech, and falling: infrequent
    symptoms

Elimination
  Renal insufficiency
  Hematuria

NURSING DIAGNOSES and NURSING INTERVENTIONS

Nursing Diagnosis	Nursing Intervention
Breathing pattern, ineffective	Monitor for signs of respiratory failure; assist ventilation and administer oxygen as prescribed (Chapter 2).
Tissue perfusion, alteration in	Monitor for symptoms of shock. Administer vasoactive drugs as prescribed.
Urinary elimination, alteration in patterns	Monitor for edema and decreased urine output. Record intake and output. Assist with dialysis as prescribed.
Fluid volume deficit, potential	Administer IV therapy as prescribed. Monitor intake and output.
Injury, potential for: falling	Protect the confused, ataxic patient from falls: use side rails; monitor closely.

EVALUATION

Patient Outcome	Data Indicating That Outcome is Reached
Body temperature is normal.	Oral adult temperature is 37° C (98.6° F).
Breathing patterns are normal.	Respiratory rate is normal. There is no dyspnea, cough, rales, or rhonchi.
All cells receive oxygen.	Skin color is normal and warm.
Laboratory values are within normal limits.	Leukocyte count, sedimentation rate, urine specific gravity, carbon dioxide, Po_2, and Pco_2 are normal.
Urine elimination is normal.	Urine output is adequate.

Tuberculosis

Tuberculosis is a chronic pulmonary and extrapulmonary infectious disease acquired by inhalation of a dried-droplet nucleus containing a tubercle bacillus into the alveolar structure of the lung; it is characterized by stages of early infection (frequently asymptomatic), latency, and a potential for recurrent postprimary disease.[7]

PATHOPHYSIOLOGY

Tuberculosis infection can be differentiated from tuberculosis disease. Tuberculosis infection is characterized by the presence of mycobacteria in the tissue of a host who is free of clinical symptoms and who demonstrates the presence of antibodies against the mycobacteria. Tuberculosis is manifested by pathologic and functional symptoms indicating destructive activity of mycobacteria in host tissue. Both infection and disease result from tissue invasion by either the *Mycobacterium tuberculosis*, *M. bovis*, or a variety of atypical mycobacteria. All are spore formers capable of remaining viable and virulent for long periods of time inside or outside host tissue. *M. tuberculosis*, the tubercle bacilli, is the most frequent etiologic agent in human tuberculosis. Transmission is primarily by inhalation of minute dried-droplet nuclei (each containing a single tubercle bacillus), coughed or sneezed into the air by a person whose sputum contains virulent tubercle bacilli.[67] Less commonly, transmission may occur by ingestion or by invasion of the skin or mucous membranes.[64]

The pathologic condition of the infection and disease occurs in three stages: (1) initial or primary infection, (2) latency, and (3) postprimary disease. In the initial infection the bacilli invade the tissue at the portal of entry, usually the mid or lower zones of the lungs; multiply there over a 3-week period; and create a small inflammatory lesion. Bacilli immediately enter the lymphatic system and are carried to the nearest group of lymph nodes, where they also produce inflammatory lesions. In addition, hematogenous dissemination of bacilli results in a subclinical bacteremia and the production of inflammatory lesions throughout the body. The sites and the extensiveness of the systemic lesions depend on the numbers of disseminated bacilli and the speed with which the host produces an immune response. These early lesions at the portal of entry, in the lymph nodes, and disseminated are referred to as the *primary complex*.[64]

The extent of inflammatory response at the sites of tissue invasion increases with the number of invading bacilli. Nonspecific cellular resistance permits some phagocytosis of tubercle bacilli producing suppuration and necrosis in the central portion of the lesion. Bacilli continue to replicate at the periphery of the lesion. This initial or primary infection stage is generally symptom free.

Within 3 to 12 weeks a cellular and humoral immune response can be detected. *Mycobacterium*-specific lymphocytes and antibodies stimulate a fibroblastic response at the periphery of the lesion, resulting in a dense connective tissue enclosure and the formation of a noncaseating granuloma. The focal lesions continue to harbor viable tubercle bacilli, with the potential for reactivation under conditions of decreased host resistance.[67]

The specific immune response results in successful encapsulation of all lesions in 85% to 95% of those persons infected. These people enter the latent stage of the disease, remaining disease free for variable periods of time, dependent on their ability to maintain specific and nonspecific resistance. The specific immune response does not preclude reinfection with subsequent exposure.[35]

For 5% to 15% of infected persons, host responses are not adequate to contain the infection, and active disease progresses in the portal of entry lesion or in all lesions in the body. Necrosis and cavitation continue in the lesions, forming caseation. The lesions may rupture, spreading necrotic residue and bacilli throughout the tissue and throughout the body. Disseminated bacilli establish new focal lesions that progress through stages of inflammation, noncaseating granulomas, and caseating necrosis.[67]

The disease symptoms vary with the body tissue affected. Extrapulmonary tuberculosis in the meninges, blood vessels, kidneys, bones, joints, larynx, skin, intestines, lymph nodes, peritoneum, or eyes is much less common than pulmonary tuberculosis.[7]

Reactivated disease following latency accounts for most of the active tuberculosis diagnosed today. It occurs most frequently in aged persons and persons with chronic and debilitating disease. Although reactivation may occur in any of the focal lesions, it most commonly occurs in those in the upper lobes or at the apex of the lower lobes of the lungs, forming abscesses and tuberculous cavities at those sites. Untreated reactivated disease has a variable course with many exacerbations and remissions. Complications caused by excessive cavitation are common.

DIAGNOSTIC STUDIES[7,67]

Sputum culture
Positive for *M. tuberculosis* within 2 to 3 weeks of active disease; will not be positive during latency

Acid-fast with Ziehl-Neelsen stain smear of sputum (cerebrospinal fluid or blood in extrapulmonary disease)
Positive for acid-fast bacilli

Histologic examination or culture of tissue in extrapulmonary disease
Positive for *M. tuberculosis*

Skin tests: intradermal injection of antigen
PPD: five tuberculin units of purified protein derivative (PPD)
Heaf test: old tuberculin (OT) injected with pressure gun
Mantoux test: PPD or OT injected intradermally
Tine test: OT pressed into skin with tine unit
Volmer patch test: OT on gauze strip applied to skin
Tuberculin reaction begins 3 to 6 weeks after infection; an area of induration greater than 10 mm in 48 to 72 hours indicates past infection and presence of antibodies; does not indicate active disease; nonspecific reactions during first 48 hours can be overlooked

Pleural needle biopsy
Positive for granulomas of tuberculosis; giant cells indicating caseation necrosis

Chest x-ray film
Findings may show calcification at the original site, enlargement of hilar lymph nodes, parenchymal infiltrate representing extension of the original site of infection, or the appearance of pleural effusion or cavitation
Not diagnostically definitive of tuberculosis

TREATMENT PLAN[7,35,67]

Surgical

Intervention for complications

Resectional procedures for persisting cavitary lesions (less common since antimicrobial therapy)

Surgical intervention for massive hemoptysis, spontaneous pneumothorax, abscess drainage, intestinal obstruction, or ureteral stricture

Chemotherapeutic

A combination of anti-infective agents is recommended: a primary plus a secondary drug. Initial dosages are higher, followed by prolonged therapy at reduced dosages. The combination of drugs used, the dosage, and duration of administration depend on the stage of the infection or disease, the presence of extrapulmonary disease, and the sensitivity of the patient to certain chemotherapeutic agents.

Anti-infective agents

Primary drugs

Isoniazid (INH), 10-20 mg/kg/d po for 1-2 yr

Ethambutol (Myambutol), 15 mg/kg/d po for 1-2 yr

Rifampin (Rifomycin, others), 20 mg/kg/d po for 6 mo to 2 yr

Streptomycin, 30 mg/kg/d IM q2-3mo

Secondary drugs

Pyrazinamide (Aldinamide), 20-30 mg/kg/d

Ethionamide (Trecator), 10-30 mg/kg/d

Para-amino salicylic acid (PAS), 0.2 mg/kg/d po for 1-2 yr

Cycloserine (Seromycin), 0.5-1.0 g/d in divided doses po

Capreomycin (Capastat), 0.75-1.0 g/d IM for 30 d; twice weekly thereafter

Kanamycin (Kantrex), 1 g IM qd

Viomycin (Viocin), 1 g IM qd

An example of recommended treatment plans

Preventive therapy for contacts: isoniazid, 10 mg/kg/d q3mo for 1 yr

Primary pulmonary tuberculosis infection: isoniazid, 10 mg/kg/d for 1 yr

Chronic pulmonary tuberculosis

Isoniazid, 10-20 mg/kg/d for 18 mo or more, plus

Rifampin, 20 mg/kg/d for 18 mo or more, or

PAS, 0.2 mg/kg/d for 18 mo or more, or

Ethambutol, 15 mg/kg/d for 18 mo or more

Corticosteroids

May be used in conjunction with the anti-infective agents for overwhelming and life-threatening disease

Supportive

After stabilization most patients can be effectively managed on an outpatient basis with monitoring for compliance with drug taking, drug side effects, and patient response to the drug therapy.

AFB isolation until antimicrobial therapy is successfully initiated for sputum-positive patients to prevent spread to others (p. 1621).

Secretion precautions until wounds stop draining for patients with external tuberculosis lesions (p. 1622).

Skin testing: identify recent converters to tuberculosis skin tests; trace their contacts to identify persons with active disease; isoniazid therapy for 1 year for recent converters and for close household contacts of persons with active disease (not routine for those over 35 years); tuberculosis skin testing is recommended for children at school entry and again at age 14 years

BCG vaccine for those persons who are at high risk for contact with active cases, who are skin test negative, and who are not immunosuppressed (benefits of BCG vaccine are controversial)[7,35]

ASSESSMENT: AREAS OF CONCERN[67]

Body temperature

Slight continued elevation with chills and night sweats

Respiratory concerns

Initially a nonproductive cough

Later mucopurulent secretions

Advanced: hemoptysis; dyspnea on exertion and at rest; rales over apex of lung; chest pain with respiratory movement if pleura is involved; hoarseness with involvement of larynx; dysphagia with pharyngeal involvement; sibilant and sonorous rhonchi

Cardiovascular concerns

Tachycardia

Subjective symptoms

History of weight loss

Anorexia

Generalized weakness and fatigue

Assessment of extrapulmonary tuberculosis depends on the system involved. The onset of symptoms is generally insidious, as is the onset of pulmonary tuberculosis.

Tuberculosis pericarditis

Precordial chest pain, fever, and pericardial friction rubs

Jugular venous distention, hepatic congestion, ascites, and peripheral edema

Tuberculosis peritonitis
  Abdominal pain simulating that of appendicitis
  Abdominal distention
  Anorexia, vomiting, and weight loss
  Night sweats
  Abdominal tenderness when palpated
  Ascites

Miliary tuberculosis
  More severe symptoms of respiratory involvement: dyspnea, hyperventilation, and cough
  Hypoxemia
  Spontaneous unilateral or bilateral pneumothorax (manifested by sudden chest pain and breathlessness) and fever
  Painful, nodular cutaneous lesions, which may ulcerate, may be present

Tuberculosis meningitis
  Headache, vomiting, fever, and anorexia
  Alterations in intellectual function, diminishing levels of consciousness, and neurologic deficits
  Cerebrospinal fluid leukocytes of 100 to 400 cells/cmm, and increase in protein

Tuberculosis lymphadenitis
  Palpable enlargement of supraclavicular and cervical lymph nodes

Osteoarticular tuberculosis
  Pain aggravated by movement, in joints
  Swelling, minimal erythema, and tenderness to palpation
  Limitation of motion and gross deformities (most common in vertebral column, hip, and knee joints)

Tuberculosis of gastrointestinal tract
  Symptoms depend on the area involved
  May have gastrointestinal bleeding, pain, constipation, or diarrhea
  Partial or complete obstruction
  Perforation with peritonitis

Tuberculosis of genitourinary organs
  Urgency, frequency, dysuria, hematuria, and pyuria
  Salpingitis with lower abdominal pain and infertility
  Amenorrhea
  Abnormal vaginal discharge or bleeding

NURSING DIAGNOSES and NURSING INTERVENTIONS

Nursing Diagnosis	Nursing Intervention
Airway clearance, ineffective	Assist patient to turn, cough, and deep breathe every 2 to 4 hours.
Breathing pattern, ineffective	Monitor breathing for dyspnea and signs of pneumothorax. Initiate respiratory assistance as needed. Observe sputum for hemoptysis.
Fluid volume deficit, potential	Force fluids to 2000 to 3000 ml daily unless contradicted.
Anxiety	Explain that tuberculosis is a completely curable condition with proper long-term antimicrobial therapy.
Nutrition, alteration in: less than body requirements	Maintain high-protein, high-carbohydrate diet with frequent, small feedings.
Potential patient problem: transmission of infection	Employ AFB isolation until antimicrobial therapy is successfully initiated for sputum-positive patients (p. 1621). Employ secretion precautions until wounds stop draining for patients with external tuberculosis lesions (p. 1622). Teach hospitalized patient to cough and sneeze into paper tissues and to properly dispose of tissues. Collect sputum specimens according to procedures on p. 1481.

There may be other nursing diagnoses if the patient has extrapulmonary tuberculosis complicated with other chronic disease.

Patient Education

1. Teach care of sputum if discharged patient still has positive sputum cultures.
2. Teach hand washing and good hygiene.
3. Drug therapy must be continued uninterrupted for the designated time period. Explain dosage, frequency of administration, and purpose for prolonged treatment.

4. Explain medication toxic and side effects:
   a. INH: infrequent toxic effects; peripheral neuropathy, convulsions, ataxia, dizziness, optic neuritis. Older patients may experience a drug-related hepatitis with fatigue, malaise, and anorexia.
   b. Ethambutol: reduced visual acuity with inability to perceive the color green.

c. Streptomycin: skin rash, fever, malaise, vertigo, and deafness; gastrointestinal disturbances and central nervous system symptoms.
d. PAS: toxic reactions more common with this drug and include symptoms of hypersensitivity, hepatic damage, gastrointestinal disturbances, and renal failure.
e. Rifampin: red-orange colored urine common, jaundice, nausea, anorexia, vomiting, diarrhea, cramps, occasional central nervous system disturbances, and hypersensitivity reactions. May interfere with actions of oral contraceptives.
f. Ethionamide: gastrointestinal irritation and symptoms of hepatotoxicity.

g. Pyrazinamide: hepatotoxicity.
h. Cycloserine: central nervous system effects including seizures, somnolence, and muscle twitching.
5. Report side effects to physician immediately.
6. Emphasize need for periodic reculturing of sputum during period of therapy: monthly until cultures are negative; then every 3 months for duration of therapy.
7. Report to physician: hemoptysis, chest pain, difficulty in breathing, hearing loss, or vertigo.
8. Maintain adequate fluid and caloric intake.

EVALUATION

Patient Outcome	Data Indicating That Outcome is Reached
There is no active infection.	Sputum cultures are consistently negative. X-ray findings show a reduction in the size of cavities and decrease in the thickness of cavity walls. Body temperature is normal. The patient does not experience chills or night sweats.
Laboratory values are within normal limits.	Serum alkaline phosphatase levels, hematocrit, hemoglobin, and leukocyte count are normal. Urine does not contain erythrocytes.
Patient contacts are free of infection.	Contacts do not convert to a positive skin test.
Breathing patterns are normal.	The patient does not experience dyspnea, cough, or pain on breathing.
There is no extrapulmonary disease.	See p. 129.

ENTERIC INFECTIOUS DISEASES

A wide range of enteric infectious diseases are caused by bacteria found in contaminated food or water. Food poisoning can be caused by infectious agents that have already multiplied in food (food intoxications such as staphylococcal food poisoning and botulism and enteric infections) or by bacteria that multiply in the body after ingestion (bacterial and viral gastroenteritis and parasitic enteritis). Food and water can also be sources of *Salmonella* infection, which can produce a variety of clinical entities. Intestinal infections caused by parasitic worms (helminths) are also discussed in this section.

Food poisoning is the generic term applied to illnesses acquired through consumption of food or water contaminated with chemicals, bacteria and bacterial toxins, or organic poisons naturally present in some edible substances. The food poisonings caused by bacteria and bacterial toxins will be discussed here. In all cases disease

is produced in the host shortly after ingestion of food containing bacteria that have already multiplied in the food. These diseases are not directly communicable. If the bacteria have produced a toxin in the food, the resulting disease in the host is intoxication; as in staphylococcal food poisoning and botulism. If the bacterial cells are antigenic, they produce an infection in the host, as in *Clostridium perfringens* and *Vibrio parahaemolyticus*[7] (Table 15-7).

Staphylococcal Food Poisoning

Staphylococcal food poisoning is an enteric intoxication of acute onset, presenting with severe nausea, intestinal cramps, vomiting, diarrhea, prostration, and, occasionally subnormal temperature and hypotension. The inten-

Table 15-7
Overview of Food Poisoning: Intoxications and Enteric Infections[7]

	Intoxications		Enteric Infections	
	Staphylococcal Food Poisoning	**Botulism**	**Clostridium perfringens**	**Vibrio para- haemolyticus**
Occurrence	Widespread and frequent; one of the principal acute food poisonings in United States	Sporadic; family-grouped cases occur	Widespread and frequent in countries with cooking practices that favor growth of organism	Sporadic cases and outbreaks occur in warm months of the year
Etiologic agent	Several enterotoxins of staphylococci; stable at boiling temperature	Toxins produced by Clostridium botulinum in anaerobic conditions; destroyed by boiling	Type A strains of C. perfringens (C. welchii)	V. parahaemolyticus (many types)
Reservoir	Humans; cows with infected udders	Soil, water, and intestinal tract of animals and fish	Soil and gastrointestinal tract of humans and animals	Marine silt, coastal waters, fish, and shellfish
Transmission	Ingestion of food containing staphylococcal toxin	Ingestion of food in which toxin has formed; generally home-canned vegetables, fruits, and meats	Ingestion of food, especially meat, contaminated by soil or feces; spores survive normal cooking temperatures, germinate, and multiply during cooling and reheating	Ingestion of raw or undercooked contaminated seafood
Incubation period	1-6 h	12-36 h	6-24 h; usually 10-12 h	4-96 h; usually 12-14 h
Period of communicability	Not applicable	Not applicable	Noncommunicable	Noncommunicable
Susceptibility and resistance	General; no immune response	General; no immune response	General; no resistance develops from exposure	General
Report to local health authority	Prompt report of outbreaks	Report of cases and outbreaks	Prompt report of outbreaks	Report outbreaks

sity of the disease depends on the quantity of the ingested toxin and host susceptibility. The duration of the illness is 1 to 2 days; and recovery is generally complete.

PATHOPHYSIOLOGY

The ingested enterotoxin acts on the abdominal viscera, creating a sensory stimulus that reaches the vomiting center of the brain by way of the vagus and sympathetic nerves. The action of the enterotoxin on the gastric mucosa produces a patchy hyperemia, erosions, petechiae, and a purulent gastric exudate. Diarrhea results from inhibition of water absorption from the intestinal lumen and from increased transport of fluid into the lumen.[97]

DIAGNOSTIC STUDIES[97]

Culture of stomach contents, feces, or suspected food

10^6 enterotoxin-producing staphylococci per gram of specimen

Enterotoxin tests
Not routinely available

TREATMENT PLAN

Supportive
Oral or IV fluids and electrolytes

ASSESSMENT: AREAS OF CONCERN

Digestive system
Acute-onset nausea, vomiting, intestinal cramps, and diarrhea

Vital signs
Subnormal temperature
Hypotension

Energy level
Weakness
Prostration

NURSING DIAGNOSES and NURSING INTERVENTIONS

Nursing Diagnosis	Nursing Intervention
Fluid volume deficit, potential	Encourage oral fluids as tolerated. Administer IV fluids and electrolytes as prescribed. Monitor for signs of dehydration.

EVALUATION

Patient Outcome	Data Indicating That Outcome is Reached
Body hydration is normal.	Skin turgor is good. Urine output is adequate.
Digestive function is normal.	Stools are soft, formed, and normal colored. Patient tolerates regular diet.
Laboratory studies are within normal limits.	Urine specific gravity is normal. Measurements of sodium, potassium, chloride, magnesium, and calcium in blood are normal.

Botulism

Botulism is a severe neurointoxication with a wide range of neurologic symptoms and severity of symptoms. In the United States 10% of cases under treatment result in death, primarily from respiratory failure. Three types of botulism have been recognized: (1) food borne, (2) wound, and (3) infant botulism.

PATHOPHYSIOLOGY[9]

Clostridium botulinum, a spore-forming anaerobe capable of withstanding boiling, produces a potent toxin in anaerobic conditions. A common source of botulinal toxin is improperly processed canned foods. Less commonly, *C. botulinum* enters the body through a wound and produces toxin in traumatized, necrotic tissue. Ingestion of *C. botulinum* spores does not result in toxin production in adults and children but does result in toxin production in the bowel lumen of some infants, producing infant botulism.

The botulinal toxin is hematogenously disseminated to peripheral cholinergic synapses, where it becomes irreversibly bound. This action blocks the release of acetylcholine, producing impaired autonomic and voluntary neuromuscular transmission and muscular paralysis. Gradual recovery occurs over a period of weeks from the regeneration of terminal motor neurons to reinnervate noncontracting muscle fibers.

Intestinal stasis predisposes to the colonization of any ingested viable spores of *C. botulinum*. Additional toxin is produced in vivo, prolonging the course of the disease.[9]

Complications in hospitalized patients with botulism are similar to those affecting other critically ill paralyzed persons who are dependent on mechanical support to sustain life.

DIAGNOSTIC STUDIES[9]

Culture of feces
Positive for *C. botulinum*

Serum
Positive for toxins; circulating toxins found in about one third hospitalized patients with botulism

Differential diagnosis
Electromyography (EMG)
Demonstrates a defect in transmission at neuromuscular junction
Cerebrospinal fluid cultures and chemistries
Normal
Serology
Normal

TREATMENT PLAN[7,9]

Chemotherapeutic
Immunologic agents
Trivalent (ABE) botulinal antitoxin (not used for infants)

Anti-infective agents
   Penicillin for wound botulism
   Agent-specific anti-infective agents for secondary
      bacterial infection

Electromechanical
Gastric lavage initially
Mechanical ventilation in the event of respiratory paralysis
Suction of secretions
Intubation or tracheostomy

Supportive
Nasogastric feedings
IV fluid and electrolytes
Must be reported to local health authority immediately
All patient contacts known to have eaten the same food
   should have gastric lavage, high enemas, and cathartics and should be kept under close medical supervision
Public education
   Proper home canning methods
   Boiling all home canned food before eating
   Not feeding honey to infants under 1 year old

ASSESSMENT: AREAS OF CONCERN[9]

Neurologic concerns
Head and neck
   Abrupt onset, bilateral, and symmetric: ptosis, blurred vision, diplopia, dry mouth, dysphagia, dysphonia, dysarthria, nasal regurgitation

Gastrointestinal concerns
Vomiting
Diarrhea
Constipation

Respiratory concerns
Paralysis of muscles of respiration

Large muscles
Symmetric flaccid paralysis
No sensory disturbances, only motor

Temperature and pulse
Normal

Wound botulism
Same as above except there are no gastrointestinal symptoms

NURSING DIAGNOSES and NURSING INTERVENTIONS

Nursing Diagnosis	Nursing Intervention
Airway clearance, ineffective	Provide patent airway. Suction secretions. Provide tracheostomy care. Offer nasogastric tube feedings per protocol.
Breathing pattern, ineffective	Monitor for signs of respiratory paralysis and oxygen insufficiency. Initiate mechanical ventilation and oxygen as prescribed. Monitor patient on respirator for signs of hyperventilation or hypoventilation.
Mobility, impaired physical	Position to prevent contractures. Assist with range of motion exercises.
Nutrition, alteration in: less than body requirements	Administer nasogastric tube feeding or alimentation as prescribed. Offer frequent small oral feedings as patient tolerates.
Fluid volume deficit, actual	Administer IV fluids as prescribed. Offer frequent, small oral liquids as patient can tolerate.
Self-care deficit	Provide total hygiene care as needed.
Potential patient problem: susceptibility to infection	Protect patient from a complicating bacterial infection: Suction to prevent aspiration of secretions. Monitor for signs of pneumonia and urinary tract infection. Turn every 2 hours. Provide skin care and catheter care. Ensure adequate fluid intake.

Patient Education[7]

1. Destroy all canned food and containers from same batch that contained the *C. botulinum* by burying deep in soil or boiling 3 minutes before discarding. Commercial canned foods should be submitted for laboratory examination.
2. Contaminated cooking utensils should be sterilized by boiling for 3 minutes before reuse.
3. No questionable canned food should ever be tasted. Foods containing *C. botulinum* do not necessarily have off odors or a spoiled taste.
4. Recommended processing times and temperatures for home canning must be followed to ensure killing of all *C. botulinum* spores. This information is available through state agricultural extension services.
5. Home-canned vegetables and meats should be boiled for 3 minutes to destroy botulinal toxin.

EVALUATION

Patient Outcome	Data Indicating That Outcome is Reached
Breathing patterns are normal.	Respiratory rate is normal. Respirations are of normal depth; there is no dyspnea. Skin and mucous membranes are warm and moist, with normal color.
Airway clearance is effective.	Airway is open; secretions are thin and easily coughed up by patient. Patient swallows without difficulty.
There is no secondary infection:	Body temperature is normal.
Respiratory	Secretions are thin; there is no cough, rales, or rhonchi; breathing patterns are normal.
Urinary	Urinary output is normal.
Skin	Skin is warm and moist; there are no lesions or decubiti.
Neuromuscular function is normal.	Neuromuscular innervation and muscle control are regained. The patient can see, speak, swallow, breath, cough, and move around at will. Gastrointestinal tract peristalsis is normal.
Laboratory studies are within normal limits.	Blood leukocytes, O_2 saturation, CO_2, PO_2, and PCO_2 are normal. Urine is negative for protein, blood, or bacteria.

Food Poisoning: Enteric Infections

Clostridium perfringens *generally causes a mild intestinal infection characterized by sudden onset of abdominal colic, nausea, and diarrhea. Fever and vomiting are rare.*[7]

Vibrio parahaemolyticus *is a moderately severe intestinal infection characterized by sudden-onset abdominal cramps and watery diarrhea lasting 1 to 7 days. Nausea, vomiting, fever, and headache may be present.*[7]

The two enteric infections discussed here are both caused by ingestion of food contaminated with specific bacteria that have already multiplied in the food. Disease is produced in the host shortly after ingestion of the food and is manifested by symptoms of enteritis.

PATHOPHYSIOLOGY

C. perfringens, a spore former widely distributed in feces, soil, and water, multiplies rapidly in foods that have been cooled and reheated. The organism produces an enterotoxin in the intestinal tract within 6 to 24 hours after ingestion. The enterotoxin acts on the epithelial layer of the ileum, increasing the secretion of sodium, chloride, and fluid and inhibiting the absorption of glucose.

V. parahaemolyticus multiplies in uncooked, contaminated seafood. When ingested, the pathogen directly invades intestinal tissue to produce necrosis, ulceration, possible hemorrhage, and granulocytic infiltration of the mucosa. Disease intensity ranges from asymptomatic to severe; duration ranges from 2 hours to 10 days.[97]

DIAGNOSTIC STUDIES[97]

These conditions are most commonly diagnosed by identification of the pathogen in a food or fecal culture.

Quantitative culture of food or fecal specimen to estimate the number of organisms
Greater than 10^5 spores of *C. perfringens* per gram of specimen, or positive for *V. parahaemolyticus*

TREATMENT PLAN[97]

Supportive
Oral fluids if tolerated
IV fluids and electrolytes if needed

ASSESSMENT: AREAS OF CONCERN[97]

Digestive concerns
Acute-onset abdominal cramping and diarrhea
Diarrhea may be watery and bloody and persist up to 7 days in *V. parahaemolyticus*
Nausea and vomiting are less common symptoms but may occur

Body temperature
Usually normal

NURSING DIAGNOSES and NURSING INTERVENTIONS

Nursing Diagnosis	Nursing Intervention
Bowel elimination, alteration in: diarrhea	Obtain stool specimen. Provide privacy for patient. Eliminate odors. Protect skin around anal opening from irritation: wash and lubricate frequently.
Fluid volume deficit, potential	Monitor for symptoms of dehydration and electrolyte imbalance. Administer frequent liquids as tolerated. Administer IV electrolytes as prescribed.

Patient Education[7]

1. Cooked foods should not be held at room temperature; they should be kept hot or should be refrigerated. Reheating should be done rapidly.
2. All seafood should be cooked at a temperature above 60° C (140° F) for 15 minutes.

EVALUATION

Patient Outcome	Data Indicating That Outcome is Reached
Digestive wastes are eliminated normally.	Stools are soft and formed. Abdomen is not distended. There is no cramping.
Fluid and electrolyte balance is normal.	Skin turgor is good. Mucous membranes are moist. Urine output is normal. Secretions are thin.
Laboratory studies are within normal limits.	Blood levels of sodium, potassium, chloride, magnesium, and calcium are normal. Urine specific gravity is normal.

Acute Bacterial and Viral Gastroenteritis[7]

Campylobacter *enteritis is an acute bacterial enteric infection lasting from 1 to 10 days and is considered to be an important cause of "traveler's diarrhea."*

Diarrhea caused by E. coli *is another cause of "traveler's diarrhea." Three types of pathogenic* E. coli *are capable of producing a self-limiting enteritis of varying intensity.*

Shigellosis (bacillary dysentery) is an acute bacterial infection of the large intestine with severity ranging from asymptomatic infection to fulminating diarrheal disease and death.

Epidemic viral gastroenteritis is usually a self-limited mild gastric and intestinal infection lasting from 24 to 48 hours. Disease often occurs in outbreaks.

Table 15-8
Overview of Acute Bacterial and Viral Gastroenteritis[7.114]

	Campylobacter Enteritis (Traveler's Diarrhea)	Diarrhea Caused by E. coli (Traveler's Diarrhea)	Shigellosis (Bacillary Dysentery)	Epidemic Viral Gastroenteritis	Rotavirus Gastroenteritis
Occurrence	Worldwide; common-source outbreaks occur; highest in warmer months	Worldwide; common-source outbreaks occur; high in areas of poor sanitation and during warm months	Worldwide; highest in children under 10 yr old; outbreaks common in crowded living conditions	Worldwide and common; epidemics and outbreaks occur	Worldwide; sporadic and in outbreaks; highest in infants and young children
Etiologic agent	*Campylobacter jejuni*	Enterotoxigenic, invasive, or enteropathogenic strains of *E. coli*	From different groups of *Shigella* bacteria, with many strains	Many serotypes of parovirus-like agents	Many types of rotaviruses
Reservoir	Domestic and wild animals and birds	Infected humans, who are often asymptomatic	Humans	Humans	Humans; pathogenicity of animal viruses undetermined
Transmission	Ingestion of water or food contaminated with organism from feces; contact with infected animals or infants; fecal-oral	Fecal contamination of food, water, or fomites; transmitted to infant during delivery; fecal-oral, by hand	Direct or indirect fecal-oral transmission from infected person or carrier	Fecal-oral route; food-borne and water-borne transmission	Fecal-oral; possibly fecal-respiratory
Incubation period	3-5 d; range: 1-10 d	12-72 h	1-7 d; usually 1-3 d	Usually 24-48 h; range: 10-51 h	48 h
Period of communicability	Several days to weeks throughout course of infection; usually 2-7 wk; carriers are rare	Duration of fecal excretion of organism, possibly weeks	During acute infection to 4 wk after illness; carrier state may persist for months	During acute stage and shortly thereafter	During acute stage and shortly thereafter
Susceptibility and resistance	General	Infants very susceptible; duration of acquired immunity unknown	General; more severe in children and elderly and debilitated individuals; strain-specific antibodies develop	General; short-term (14 wk) immunity may follow infection with specific serotypes	By age 2 yr most individuals have acquired antibodies against most serotypes
Report to local health authority	In some endemic areas	Report epidemic only	Mandatory case reporting	Report epidemics; no individual case reports	Report epidemics; no individual case reports

Rotavirus gastroenteritis is a sporadically occurring gastric and intestinal infection of infants and young children ranging in severity from asymptomatic to severe disease and occasionally to death.

Many forms of acute gastroenteritis are caused by ingestion of food and water contaminated with pathogenic agents or by fecal-oral transmission directly or indirectly from an infected person. These infections differ from the food poisonings previously discussed in the following ways:

1. The pathogenic agents causing these diseases invade, colonize, and multiply in the human intestinal tract.
2. The incubation periods are slightly longer, ranging from 1 day to several weeks.
3. Direct and indirect fecal-oral transmission is possible.
4. Acquired immunity of varying duration results from many of these infections.

In addition, the predominant manifestation of these diseases is acute-onset diarrhea of varying intensity and duration. The bacterial- and viral-caused gastroenteritises are usually self-limiting diseases (Table 15-8).

PATHOPHYSIOLOGY[7,64,66,114]

Bacterial and viral agents that produce gastroenteritis produce pathologic conditions in one of three ways:

1. Toxigenic agents, such as some *Shigella* strains and enterotoxigenic *E. coli*, release an enterotoxin that acts on the small intestine to produce a local inflammation and a secretory diarrhea with rapid loss of electrolytes.
2. Invasive pathogens, such as *Shigella, Campylobacter,* and invasive strains of *E. coli,* penetrate the small or large intestine, producing cellular destruction, necrosis, and potential ulceration. The diarrheal stools in these conditions frequently contain leukocytes and erythrocytes.
3. Some pathogens such as the rotaviruses attach to the mucosal epithelium without invasion. They destroy cells of the intestinal villi, resulting in malabsorption of electrolytes and the potential for electrolyte imbalance.

The general effect of all of the above pathologic conditions is to increase gastrointestinal motility and to increase the secretory rate of fluids and electrolytes into the intestines. The result may be rapid dehydration, electrolyte imbalance, circulatory failure, and death. Fluid and electrolyte loss in other forms of gastroenteritis may develop more gradually or may not occur at all. Infants, small children, and debilitated individuals are at greater risk for severe dehydration.

The attachment of the pathogens to the mucosa may be altered by nonspecific resistance factors in the host:

1. The normal bacterial flora of the intestinal tract acts to prevent attachment by competing for attachment sites or by production of volatile organic acids. If the normal flora is diminished as a result of antibiotic therapy or malnutrition, this host defense is ineffective.
2. The pH of the gastrointestinal tract acts to impede the growth of some microbes. Altering the pH through the ingestion of antacids reduces the effectiveness of this defense.
3. Normal gastrointestinal motility purges the intestinal tract of many pathogens; and interference with this function increases the risk for invasion of pathogens.

Specific immune responses of varying duration occur in the host following infection with *Shigella*, parovirus-like agents, rotavirus, and *E. coli.*[7, 66]

DIAGNOSTIC STUDIES[7, 114]

The diagnosis of these conditions relies on identification of the pathogen in a specimen of feces and by a fourfold or greater rise in serum antibody titer between acute disease and convalescence.

Campylobacter
Direct examination of stool with phase-contrast microscopy
  Positive for leukocytes and erythrocytes and *C. jejuni*

Serology: immunofluorescence or agglutination tests
  Fourfold increase in antibody titer

E. coli diarrhea
Stool culture
  Positive for enterotoxigenic or invasive strains of *E. coli*

Serology
  Fourfold increase in antitoxic antibodies

Shigellosis
Examination of stool specimen
  Pus cells in specimen

Fecal culture
  Positive for *Shigella*

Epidemic viral gastroenteritis
Immune electron microscopy or radioimmunoassay of feces specimen
  Positive for virus

Serologic tests using immune electron microscopy, immune adherence hemagglutination assay, or radioimmunoassay
Fourfold or greater increase in antibody titer

Rotavirus gastroenteritis
Electron microscopy or immunologic examination of feces or rectal swabs
Positive for rotavirus (10^6 per gram of feces)

Serology: complement fixation, ELISA, or immunofluorescent techniques
Fourfold increase in antibody titer; 80% to 90% of children have detectable antibodies by age 3 years

TREATMENT PLAN

Chemotherapeutic
Agents that suppress intestinal motility are not given for bacterial gastroenteritis
For shigellosis
Anti-infective agents
Trimethoprim-sulfamethoxazole (Septra, Bactrim), adults, one tablet (80 mg trimethoprim and 400 mg sulfamethoxazole) q12h for 5 d; children: trimethoprim, 10 mg/kg/24 h, and sulfamethoxazole, 50 mg/kg/24h, in two divided doses for 5 d[66]

Supportive[7,66]
IV fluids and electrolyte replacement
For shock: rapid infusion of 20 to 30 ml/kg of Ringer's lactate, isotonic saline, or similar isotonic solution given within an hour
For complete rehydration after circulation is restored: glucose electrolyte solution (oral or IV hypotonic electrolyte solutions in amounts equal to estimated fluid loss)[7, 66]
No immunization available for *Campylobacter, E. coli,* shigellosis, or viral gastroenteritis
Avoidance of contaminated food and water is best protection against all water- and food-borne gastroenteritis[7]

ASSESSMENT: AREAS OF CONCERN[7, 64, 114]

Campylobacter
Gastrointestinal concerns
Days 1 and 2: nausea, vomiting, abdominal pain
Days 2 to 4 (sometimes lasts 10 days): foul-smelling, or liquid diarrhea; sometimes 20 or 30 stools per day; blood in stools after day 4

Day 7: ulcerative colitis may occur
Body temperature
38° to 41° C (100° to 105° F)

Neurologic concerns
Later in course of disease: febrile convulsions

E. coli diarrhea
Gastrointestinal concerns
Day 1: vomiting
Day 2 (lasting 7-10 days:) mucoid and bloody diarrhea or profuse watery diarrhea without blood or mucus

Fluids and electrolytes
Anytime during disease: poor skin turgor, dry mucous membranes, faint pulse, hypotension

Body temperature
Days 1 and 2: fever possible

Shigellosis
Gastrointestinal concerns
Day 1: nausea, abdominal pain, colic, vomiting, painful diarrhea
Days 2 to 5: stools contain blood and mucus; rectal irritation and tenesmus

Fluids and electrolytes
Days 2 to 5: loss of turgor, oliguria, hypotension, weak pulse, shock

Body temperature
Days 1 to 5: 38° to 41° C (101° to 105° F); may have febrile convulsions in children

Epidemic viral gastroenteritis
Gastrointestinal concerns
Day 1 (lasts 24 to 48 hours): nausea, vomiting, diarrhea, abdominal pain

Body temperature
Day 1: low-grade fever

Subjective symptoms
Myalgia
Headache
Malaise

Rotavirus gastroenteritis
Gastrointestinal concerns
Day 1: vomiting for 48 hours
Days 2 to 8: watery diarrhea, rectal bleeding may occur

Fluids and electrolytes
Days 2 to 8: severe dehydration possible, particularly in infants

Body temperature
   Day 1: usually low-grade fever (up to 39° C [102° F]); may go higher

Upper respiratory concerns
   Anytime during course of disease: pharyngeal exudate, cough, and rhinitis may be present

NURSING DIAGNOSES and NURSING INTERVENTIONS

Nursing Diagnosis	Nursing Intervention
Fluid volume deficit, actual	Monitor blood pressure, temperature, pulse, and respirations for symptoms of circulatory collapse. Administer IV fluids and electrolytes as prescribed. (Once circulation is stabilized, the initial rate of IV infusion and type of IV electrolytes may be altered to provide for rehydration.) Continue monitoring for symptoms of dehydration (oliguria, loss of skin turgor). Measure all fluid output (emesis, urine, diarrhea). Measure all intake. Ensure that intake compensates for output. Provide oral liquids as tolerated.
Bowel elimination, alteration in: diarrhea	Obtain stool specimens for culture. Measure watery diarrhea output to estimate rapidity of fluid loss. Cleanse perianal area and lubricate after each diarrheal stool. Provide adequate air circulation and room deodorization.
Nutrition, alteration in: less than body requirements	Provide patient with oral glucose electrolyte solution as soon as patient can take oral fluids. Oral fluids can usually be tolerated once electrolyte imbalance is corrected. Gradually add clear fluids and soft foods (milk and cream products are to be avoided at first; apple juice and 7-up are usually well tolerated).
Potential patient problem: fever	Monitor temperature. Sponge with tepid water. Employ convulsion precautions for febrile children and infants.
Potential patient problem: transmission of infection	Use enteric precautions until three consecutive fecal cultures are negative for infecting organism for *Shigella*. Use enteric precautions for duration of illness for others (p. 1622).

Patient Education

For children being cared for at home, teach parents:
1. Signs of dehydration and the importance of prompt medical attention should dehydration occur
2. Measurement of intake and measurement or estimation of output
3. Maintenance of oral fluid intake equal to output
4. Types of clear, high-glucose oral fluids that may be tolerated by the child (apple juice; defizzed carbonated beverages such as 7-Up)
5. Scrupulous hand washing; avoidance of contamination of food

EVALUATION

Patient Outcome	Data Indicating That Outcome is Reached
Fluid and electrolyte balance is achieved: Circulating fluid is adequate.	Blood pressure and pulse are normal.
Body hydration is normal.	Skin turgor is good. Mucous membranes are moist. Urine output is equal to intake.
Laboratory values are normal.	Blood levels of sodium, potassium, chloride, magnesium, and calcium are normal. Urine specific gravity is normal.
Bowel elimination is normal.	Stools are soft, formed, and brown colored.
There are no signs of infection.	Body temperature is normal.

Acute and Chronic Parasitic Enteritis

Amebiasis (amebic dysentery) is an infection with an amoeba. This parasite may form a commensal relationship with the host or invade the intestinal mucosa, producing an enteritis ranging from asymptomatic to fulminating diarrheal and systemic disease. The parasite may persist in the host for years (Table 15-9).

Giardiasis is a protozoan infection of the upper intestinal tract ranging in severity from asymptomatic infection to chronic damage to the duodenal and jejunal mucosa resulting in a malabsorption syndrome[7] (Table 15-9).

Parasitic enteritis is similar in several ways to the bacterial and viral forms of gastroenteritis described on p. 1526, but it may become chronic under some conditions.

PATHOPHYSIOLOGY

Amebiasis

Ingested cysts of the *Entamoeba* develop into trophozoites that penetrate by mechanical and proteolytic activity into the mucosa and submucosa of the large intestine. Edema, fibrin formation, and necrosis occur, creating necrotic lesions that may extend laterally in the submucosa, giving a flasklike appearance. These discrete lesions appear primarily in the cecal area, sigmoid colon, and rectum. Hematogenous dissemination may occur to the liver, peritoneum, pleura, lung, pericardium, vagina, cervix, skin, and brain, with microabscesses produced in those tissues. Symptomatic onset may be acute or ill defined, or the infection may be asymptomatic. Untreated patients develop symptoms similar to a chronic persistent colitis. Complications include perforated bowel, hemorrhage, systemic deterioration, anemia, or extraintestinal disease resulting from abscesses in other organs and tissue. Antibody titers increase and persist following infection but do not confer protection against reinfection.[50]

Giardiasis

Ingested cysts of the *Giardia lamblia* protozoan develop into trophozoites that attach by a powerful ventral sucker to the mucosa of the jejunum and ileum without producing an inflammatory response. Diarrhea and malabsorption are thought to occur as a result of mechanical obstruction in the intestinal mucosa. Trophozoites and cysts are both excreted in the stool of ill individuals. Cysts may continue to be excreted for months in untreated persons. The disease is characterized by acute-onset diarrhea that may progress to a chronic intermittent diarrhea with malabsorption of fats and the fat-soluble vitamins. There is no invasion beyond the bowel lumen.[7,114]

DIAGNOSTIC STUDIES

Amebiasis[50]
Microscopic examination of feces, rectal secretions, aspirates of abscesses, or tissue sections
　　Positive for trophozoites of protozoan

Serology: agglutination tests
　　Increased titer may persist for some time after infection

Table 15-9
Overview of Acute and Chronic Parasitic Enteritis[7]

	Amebiasis	Giardiasis
Occurrence	Widespread; higher in areas with poor sanitation, in homosexual communities, and in institutions	Worldwide; more common in children, institutions, and where sanitation is poor
Etiologic agent	*Entamoeba histolytica* (a parasitic amoeba)	*Giardia lamblia* (a protozoan)
Reservoir	Humans, usually an asymptomatic carrier	Humans; possibly beaver and other animals
Transmission	Water contaminated with human feces of infected persons; fecal-oral by hand or contaminated food; oral-rectal sexual contact	Ingestion of contaminated water; fecal-oral by hand contamination or by homosexual activity
Incubation period	Variable: 3 d to months; usually 2-4 wk	1-4 wk; average: 2 wk
Period of communicability	As long as cysts are in feces, probably years	Entire period of infection; could persist for months
Susceptibility and resistance	General, although most people harboring the organism do not develop disease	General; asymptomatic carrier rate is high
Report to local health authority	In some endemic areas	Case report in endemic areas

Liver scan
Detection of abscesses

Giardiasis[114]

Examination of feces or duodenal contents
Positive for cysts or trophozoites of the *Giardia lamblia* protozoan

TREATMENT PLAN

Chemotherapeutic

Amebiasis[50]: treatment regimens will depend on the severity of the illness and the location and dissemination of the parasite. Some combination of the following amebicides and antibiotics is used. The number of drugs and potency of the drug used will increase with the severity of the symptoms.

Anti-infective agents
Emetine hydrochloride, 1 mg/kg IM (not to exceed 65 mg/24 h) for 7-10 d; not to be repeated for 8 wk

Dehydroemetine, 1.5 mg/kg (not to exceed 80 mg/24 h)

Chloroquine (Aralen) (to be used concurrently with one of the above), 0.25 g qid for first day; 0.5 g/24 h for next 14 d (adults)

Metronidazole (Flagyl), 750 mg po tid for 10 d (adults)

Diiodohydroxyquin (Diodoquin), 650 mg po tid for 20 d (adults)

Diloxanide furoate (Furamide), 0.5 g po tid for 10 d (adults)

Tetracycline, 250 mg po q6-8h for 10 d (adults)

Giardiasis
Anti-infective agents[70]
Quinacrine hydrochloride (Atabrine), 100 mg po tid for 7 d (adults)

Furazolidone (Furoxone) liquid (children)

Metronidazole (Flagyl), 250 mg tid for 7 d (is not currently licensed for giardiasis use)

Household and sexual contacts should be examined and treated. Pregnant women should only be treated if they show significant symptoms.

ASSESSMENT: AREAS OF CONCERN

Amebiasis[50]
Gastrointestinal concerns
Nondysenteric colitis: recurring episodes of loose stools; vague abdominal pain; tenesmus; hemorrhoids with occasional rectal bleeding; constipation alternating with diarrhea
Dysenteric colitis: intense intermittent bloody, mucoid diarrhea
Rigid abdomen symptomatic of appendicitis

Systemic manifestations
Signs of dehydration, anemia, or hemorrhage

Body temperature
May have fever

Skin
May have ulceration of perianal area

Abdomen
Enlarged, tender liver (with hepatic abscess)

Respiratory concerns
Expectoration of reddish brown odorless pus suggesting rupture of hepatic abscess to lung

Giardiasis[114]
Gastrointestinal concerns
Acute: explosive, foul-smelling diarrheal stool (frothy appearance with steatorrhea); abdominal cramping and flatulence; nausea (no vomiting)
Chronic: intermittent loose stools; increased flatulence and distention; vague abdominal discomfort

NURSING DIAGNOSES and NURSING INTERVENTIONS

Nursing Diagnosis	Nursing Intervention
Bowel elimination, alteration in: diarrhea	Obtain stool specimen for examination. (Specimen obtained within 3 days of a barium enema or of a soapsuds, oil, hypertonic, or water enema cannot be examined.) Administer amebicide therapy as prescribed. Observe stool for signs of bleeding. Monitor patient for symptoms of perforation, obstruction, or liver disease.
Fluid volume deficit, potential	Monitor for signs of dehydration. Encourage oral fluids as tolerated.

Nursing Diagnosis	**Nursing Intervention**
	Administer IV line as prescribed.
	Measure intake and output and patient's weight.
Injury, potential for: poisoning (etiology related to chemotherapeutic agent)	Amebicides are toxic. Monitor for symptoms of toxicity to gastrointestinal, cardiovascular, muscular, and neurologic systems.
Activity intolerance	Enforce restricted activities during amebicide therapy.
Potential patient problem: transmission of infection	Employ enteric precautions for duration of the infection (p. 1622).

Patient Education

1. Cyst passers must wash hands thoroughly after defecating to prevent recontamination or transmission to others.
2. Travelers to areas where the water supply is not chemically treated or protected from sewage contamination should boil all water used in cooking, drinking, or making ice.
3. Relapses after treatment for amebiasis are common. Patient should be monitored by a physician at 6 weeks and 6 months.
4. Household and sexual contacts should seek medical examination and treatment.
5. Patients on amebicides should be taught side effects of drug and the importance of restricting their activities during treatment and to abstain from alcohol if on metronidazole (Flagyl).

EVALUATION

Patient Outcome	Data Indicating That Outcome is Reached
There is no infection.	Stool culture is negative for protozoan cysts.
	There are no signs of hepatic abscesses.
	There are no skin, vaginal, or lung abscesses or drainage.
	Body temperature is normal.
Bowel elimination is normal.	Stools are soft, formed, and normal colored.
	Abdomen is soft and nontender; liver is normal sized.
	Bowel sounds are normal.
Body hydration is normal.	Skin turgor is good; mucous membranes are moist.

Water-Borne and Food-Borne Salmonella Infections

Salmonellosis is manifested by an acute gastroenteritis and sometimes a septicemia. It is frequently classified as a food poisoning because of the short incubation period following ingestion of food contaminated with Salmonella. The greater the number of organisms present in the food, the shorter the incubation period.

Paratyphoid fever is an acute systemic infection manifested by an enteric fever generally of less severity than typhoid fever. Mild and asymptomatic infections occur.

Typhoid fever is an acute enteric fever manifested by a sustained bacteremia, reticuloendothelial involvement, and microabscess formation and ulceration of the distal ileum. Gastrointestinal symptoms generally follow the systemic manifestations. Mild and asymptomatic infec- *tions occur. Acute typhoid is less common than other* Salmonella *infection.*[7]

Salmonella bacteria multiply in food and water contaminated with feces from an infected person, carrier, or, in the case of salmonellosis, an animal. Person-to-person transmission is least common. Once ingested, the organisms invade and multiply in the gastrointestinal mucosa, producing systemic as well as enteric pathologic findings and symptoms. Four overlapping clinical entities are possible, dependent on the type of *Salmonella* ingested and on host defenses. They are (1) acute gastroenteritis, (2) enteric fever, (3) septicemia, with or without localized infection, and (4) asymptomatic carrier state[64] (Table 15-10).

Table 15-10
Overview of Water-Borne and Food-Borne Salmonella Infections[7]

	Salmonellosis	Paratyphoid Fever	Typhoid Fever
Occurrence	Worldwide; frequently classified as a food poisoning; small outbreaks in institutions; 2 million cases per year in United States	Worldwide; sporadic cases and small outbreaks	Worldwide; rare; sporadic cases occur in United States; usually associated with unsanitary conditions
Etiologic agent	2000 serotypes of *Salmonella*	*Salmonella paratyphi* with many serotypes	96 types of *Salmonella typhi* (the typhoid bacillus)
Reservoir	Humans and domestic and wild animals	Humans	Humans; carriers are common
Transmission	Ingestion of food contaminated with feces from an infected person or animal; ingestion of meat and animal products; fecal-oral	Ingestion of food, particularly milk contaminated with feces from an infected person or carrier; direct or indirect contact with urine or feces	Ingestion of food or water contaminated with feces or urine from infected person or carrier; sewage-contaminated shellfish
Incubation period	6-72 h; usually 12-36 h	1-3 wk	1-3 wk
Period of communicability	Throughout infection; days to weeks; temporary carrier state may continue up to 1 yr	As long as bacilli are in excreta; weeks to months; commonly 1-2 wk after recovery	As long as bacilli are in excreta; first week to 3 months; 2-5% of cases become permanent carriers
Susceptibility and resistance	General; increased risk for those with achlorhydria, antacid therapy, gastrointestinal surgery, and immunosuppression	General; some immunity follows infection	General; increased risk with gastric achlorhydria; susceptibility usually declines with age; lifelong immunity sometimes follows infection as long as antibiotic therapy was not used
Report to local health authority	Mandatory case report	Mandatory case report	Mandatory case report

PATHOPHYSIOLOGY

Salmonella organisms ingested in contaminated food or water invade and multiply in deep mucosal layers of the stomach and small intestine, lodging in the lamina propria. An inflammatory response in the tissue with many polymorphonuclear leukocytes produces a gastroenteritis if the *Salmonella* is not *S. typhi* or *S. paratyphi*. The mesenteric lymph nodes become edematous, and the Peyer's patches show edema and superficial ulceration. The disease may be contained here, or the organism may invade beyond the lymph system and be disseminated into the vascular circulation, producing a septicemia or lesions in other organs.[64]

S. typhi and *S. paratyphi* stimulate a mononuclear leukocyte reaction in the lamina propria, facilitating early hematogenous dissemination of the organisms. Disease is manifested as an enteric fever. Invasion of other organs results in lesion formation with disease manifestations dependent on the organ involved. Endocarditis, meningitis, pneumonia, pyelonephritis, osteomyelitis, cholecystitis, and hepatitis may result from the invasion of any type of *Salmonella*.[64]

Complications of gastroenteritis may include intestinal perforation and hemorrhage. Secondary infections such as otitis media, pneumonia, skin infections, and septicemia sometimes occur with all types of *Salmonella*.

A leukocytosis (10,000 to 15,000 WBC/cmm) is generally present in the gastroenteritis form of *Salmonella* infections. Leukopenia is present in enteric fevers, although children with typhoid fever sometimes show a leukocytosis.[64]

Thrombocytopenia (50,000 platelets/cmm) and anemia frequently occur in typhoid fever.[79]

Several nonspecific host defenses affect the type and severity of clinical disease produced by *Salmonella*. Gastric acidity impedes *Salmonella* growth, and persons with hypochlorhydria or achlorhydria or who have had gastric surgery are more susceptible to infection. Normal intestinal peristalsis, intact mucous membranes, and the normal intestinal flora all act to prevent invasion. Anything interfering with these defenses increases the risk for more severe infection.

Cellular and humoral immunity appears also to interfere with invasion of *Salmonella;* and persons with an impaired immune system are more susceptible to systemic disease with *Salmonella*. In addition, systemic focal lesions most commonly appear in those tissues that are damaged or devitalized or in those persons with altered immune systems.[91]

About 2% of acute cases of typhoid fever result in the chronic carrier state (excreting *S. typhi* for 12 months or longer following infection). Subclinical infections or other *Salmonella* disease may also result in the chronic carrier state.[79]

DIAGNOSTIC STUDIES[79]

Culture of feces
Positive for *Salmonella* during first week

Culture of feces and/or urine
Positive for *S. typhi* or *S. paratyphi* during second week

Culture of blood
Positive for *S. typhi* or *S. paratyphi* during first week

Serology: Widal agglutination test
Not specific for *Salmonella* organisms
Increase in antibody titer to 0 antigen after 10 days to 2 weeks
Titer greater than or equal to 1:160 or fourfold increase to 1:640 by 4 weeks is presumptive
Initial high antibodies to H antigen suggests past infection
Gradual increase during acute disease suggests concurrent infection

WBC count
Leukocytosis in salmonellosis
Leukopenia in typhoid and paratyphoid fever

TREATMENT PLAN[7,40,64,79,91]

Chemotherapeutic*
Anti-infective agents
Chloramphenicol (Chloromycetin), 100 mg/kg/d in four divided doses IV or po until defervescence; then 50 mg/kg/24 h until a total 14-d course has been completed
Ampicillin, 1-2 g IV qid for 2 wk (adults)
Ampicillin, 8 g/d po in divided doses for 6 wk for carrier state
Trimethroprim-sulfamethoxazole (for organisms resistant to above drugs)
Corticosteroids
Prednisone, 40-50 mg/d for 3 d (adults)
Large prolonged doses of ampicillin and surgical removal of gallbladder, if it is the site for focal infection, for treatment of carriers

*For typhoid fever and paratyphoid fever (anti-infective agents are not used with salmonellosis unless there is systemic disease).

Supportive
IV fluids and electrolytes
Bed rest
Hyperalimentation
Treatment of complications such as perforation and hemorrhage
Avoidance of antispasmodics, laxatives, and salicylates
Prevention of carriers from handling food for general consumption
Typhoid vaccine given in a primary series of two injections, 4 to 6 weeks apart, with boosters in 3 to 5 years; recommended only for those living in or traveling to areas of high endemicity; confers only partial immunity

ASSESSMENT: AREAS OF CONCERN[7,64]

Salmonellosis
Gastrointestinal concerns
Acute-onset abdominal pain, diarrhea, nausea, and vomiting persisting for several days
Stool is green-brown, slimy, watery, and foul; may contain mucus, pus, or blood
Bloody diarrhea more common in children

Fluids and electrolytes
Dehydration may be severe in infants: loss of skin turgor, dry mucous membranes, prostration, circulatory collapse, and death are possible

Body temperature
Low grade to 41° C (105° F); chills; lasting 2 to 7 days

Neurologic concerns
Vertigo

Skin
May have rose spots on trunk

Typhoid fever
Gradual onset of symptoms

Body temperature
Stair-step rise in temperature during first week to 40° C (104° F; (slightly lower in morning)
Sustained at 40° C (104° F) for 3 to 4 weeks

Subjective symptoms
Early: headache, malaise, anorexia

Pulse
Slower than expected with fever

Abdomen
Enlarged spleen

Abdominal pain
Distention

Skin

Discrete rose spots that blanch on pressure, on trunk after first week
Secondary skin infections frequently occur

Respiratory concerns

Nonproductive cough

Gastrointestinal concerns

Constipation more common than diarrhea
Acute cholecystitis is a complication

Sensory concerns

May have slight deafness or otitis media

Musculoskeletal concerns

Pain in joints

Urinary tract

Urinary retention

Cardiovascular concerns

Tachycardia, hypotension, and shock if hemorrhage, secondary infection, or septicemia develops

Central nervous system

Delirium to stupor
Personality change
Catatonia
Aphasia

Paratyphoid fever

Some symptoms of salmonellosis and some of typhoid fever

Body temperature

Acute-onset fever 39° to 40° C (102° to 104° F), spiking to 41° C (105.8° F)

Gastrointestinal concerns

Similar to salmonellosis
Early: nausea and vomiting in children; abdominal pain and diarrhea in adults; abdominal distention; enlarged spleen

Central nervous system

Meningeal symptoms similar to typhoid

Septicemia with localized infection

Symptoms depend on site of systemic lesions caused by any of the *Salmonella* organisms
Symptoms of appendicitis, cholecystitis, peritonitis, otitis media, meningitis, pneumonia, osteomyelitis, pyelonephritis, cystitis, and endocarditis (refer to specific chapters for assessment of those conditions)

Septicemia without localized infection

Intermittent fever
Chills
Anorexia
Weight loss

NURSING DIAGNOSES and NURSING INTERVENTIONS

Nursing Diagnosis	Nursing Intervention
Potential patient problem: transmission of infection	Employ enteric precautions for duration of diarrhea with salmonellosis. Employ enteric precautions until three consecutive fecal cultures, after cessation of antibiotic therapy, are negative for *S. typhi* and *S. paratyphi* (p. 1622).
Salmonellosis Bowel elimination, alteration in: diarrhea	Obtain stool specimen. Measure output so that fluids can be replaced equal to output. Apply heating pad to abdomen to help cramping (antispasmodics are to be avoided). Use room deodorizers and adequate ventilation.
Fluid volume deficit, actual	Administer IV fluids and electrolytes as prescribed or clear liquids as tolerated.

Further diagnosis will depend on whether bacteremia, septicemia, or systemic focal abscesses are present and where they are located.

Typhoid Fever and Paratyphoid Fever Bowel elimination, alteration in: constipation	Obtain stool specimen. Administer small low enema or glycerin suppositories as ordered (do not give laxatives). Observe stool for blood. Check for and prevent abdominal distention. Monitor for signs of perforation and hemorrhage.

Nursing Diagnosis	Nursing Intervention
Urinary elimination, alteration in patterns	Monitor for bladder distention. Measure output. Catheterize if necessary.
Injury, potential for: trauma	Protect delirious patient from injury with padded headboard and side rails. Supervise closely.
Oral mucous membrane, alteration in	Provide frequent oral fluids and mouth care. Lubricate lips to prevent cracking.
Skin integrity, impairment of: potential	Provide skin care and frequent position changes to prevent skin pressure and breakdown.
Fluid volume deficit, potential	Give oral fluids as tolerated. Administer IV fluids, if prescribed, very cautiously.
Activity intolerance	Maintain bed rest.
Potential patient problem: fever	Sponge bathe to reduce temperature (do not give salicylates).

Additional diagnoses will depend on the presence of complications and the area of localized lesions.

Patient Education

1. Scrupulous hand washing following defecation and before preparing food is necessary.
2. Carriers must not handle food for consumption by others until six consecutive fecal and urine cultures taken 1 month apart are negative for *S. typhi* and *S. paratyphi*.
3. Family and close contacts should be examined and treated if specimens from them are positive for any *Salmonella* bacilli.
4. All foods of animal origin, including eggs, must be thoroughly cooked; cross contamination of cooked and uncooked foods must be avoided; and foods must be refrigerated below 8° C (46° F) to avoid infection with *Salmonella*.
5. Protect food and water supply from contamination with sewage containing *S. typhi*. Screen food against flies or other mechanical vectors.

EVALUATION

Patient Outcome	Data Indicating That Outcome is Reached
There is no infection.	Blood, stool, or urine cultures are negative for *Salmonella*. The patient is mentally alert and oriented and has good concentration. There are no symptoms of complications or secondary infection. There is no pain anywhere. Temperature and pulse are normal.
Laboratory data are normal.	Leukocyte count, hemoglobin, hematocrit, platelets, and blood measurements of sodium, potassium, chloride, magnesium, and calcium are normal.
Bowel elimination is normal for individual.	Stools are soft, formed, and brown colored. Abdomen is soft and nondistended. There is no abdominal cramping or pain.
Body hydration is normal.	Skin turgor is good; mucous membranes are moist.
Urinary elimination is normal.	There is no bladder distention; urine output equals intake.
Digestive function is normal.	Patient eats regular diet and fluids without nausea, vomiting, or abdominal distention.

Intestinal Parasitic Worm Infections[7,111]

Ancylostomiasis is a chronic debilitating disease manifested by an iron deficiency anemia and hypoproteinemia that result from intestinal blood loss to the hookworm.

Ascariasis, the most common roundworm infection of the small intestine, is a chronic infection producing vague gastrointestinal symptoms and sometimes acute and severe manifestations of infection in other organs, commonly the lung. Bowel obstruction is a potential complication.

Enterobiasis (pinworm) is a mild infection of the cecum and colon producing mild symptoms of anal pruritus.

Strongyloidiasis is a chronic, frequently asymptomatic infection of the duodenum and upper jejunum manifested by (1) a dermatitis in which larvae penetrate the skin, (2) respiratory symptoms caused by migration through the lungs, and (3) gastrointestinal symptoms.

Taeniasis is a mild infection of the small intestine with the adult stage of the large tapeworm. It is manifested by variable gastrointestinal symptoms and loss of weight.

Toxocariasis is a chronic and usually mild infection of young children with systemic and local symptom manifestation dependent on the organs and tissues where the nematode has migrated.

Trichinosis is a chronic disease, ranging from asymptomatic to acute, caused by migration of the Trichinella *larvae to striated muscles where they become encapsulated. Severity of symptoms depends on the number of larvae and the organ system involved.*

Trichuriasis is an infection of the cecum and colon resulting in enteritis and potential rectal prolapse.

Helminths, or worms, differ from other agents pathogenic to humans in the following ways: (1) they are large enough to be seen directly; (2) they migrate within the host; (3) their life cycles are more complex; (4) they replicate by means of egg production, the eggs being shed through the feces; and (5) they are capable of producing an eosinophilia. There are three groups of helminths: the nematodes (roundworms), trematodes (flukes), and cestodes (tapeworms). The portal of entry into the host is by ingestion, skin penetration, or injection into the blood by an insect. The portal of entry is not related to group membership.

Trematode (fluke) infections are not commonly found in the United States and therefore will not be discussed here. The most common roundworm and tapeworm parasitic enteric infections will be discussed (Table 15-11).

PATHOPHYSIOLOGY

The helminths discussed here produce pathologic conditions in the human by one or more of the following ways: (1) feeding on the host's blood, resulting in anemia; (2) feeding on nutrients in the intestinal tract, thus depriving the host of those nutrients; (3) growing in numbers or size, causing blockage in the intestinal tract or ducts in other organs where they have migrated; (4) causing inflammation and necrosis in tissue; or (5) causing an allergic response in tissue with a resulting eosinophilia. The site of their damage depends on their life cycle migratory patterns within the host, which in turn is specific for each type of helminth. The extent of pathologic findings is greatly affected by the numbers of helminths present in the host. Unless treated, helminths remain for long periods. Reinfection or autoinfection greatly adds to the worm burden in the host, particularly in a host whose defenses are compromised by the presence of the worms, malnutrition, and debilitation.[111]

In both *ancylostomiasis* and *strongyloidiasis* the larvae of the respective hookworm and threadworm, present in the soil, penetrate the skin of the host. An erythema and papular vesicular rash appear at the site of the penetration, possibly resulting in a generalized urticaria. The larvae migrate through the blood to the lungs, producing an eosinophilia and transitory respiratory inflammation. From the lungs the larvae migrate to the pharynx and are swallowed to the small intestine. There the hookworms attach and the threadworms burrow in the intestinal mucosa. Localized irritation is manifested with symptoms of burning or colicky abdominal pain and diarrhea. The adult hookworm may remain attached to the intestinal mucosa for as long as 5 years. It ingests 15 ml of the host's blood per worm per day, resulting in weight loss, anemia, and hypoalbuminemia. Eggs from the hookworm pass through the feces as long as the hookworm is attached. The threadworm produces the same pathologic findings as the hookworm, with the additional ability to lay eggs that hatch within the mucosa of the duodenum and upper jejunum. The larvae may be excreted in the feces or may invade the bloodstream directly from the mucosa, reinitiating the life cycle to produce an autoinfection. Septicemia and death may be complications of threadworm infections in immunosuppressed individuals.[7,68]

In *ascariasis* the eggs of the roundworm are ingested, hatch in the small intestine, penetrate the mucosa, and migrate by way of the blood to the lungs. There they produce inflammation, transitory respiratory symptoms, and an eosinophilia similar to that produced by the hookworm and threadworm. The larvae then penetrate the alveoli and migrate to the pharynx, where they are swallowed to the small intestine. They attach to the mucosa, where they impair digestion and protein absorption. They may also travel to the biliary duct and attach there. The irritating presence of the worms may produce vomiting,

Table 15-11

Overview of Intestinal Parasitic Worm Infections[7]

	Strongyloidiasis (Threadworm)	Taeniasis (Tapeworm)	Toxocariasis
Occurrence	Common in warm wet climates; endemic or epidemic where hygiene is poor, particularly in institutions	Particularly high where beef and pork are eaten raw or undercooked; pork tapeworm rare in United States	Worldwide; highest in children 14-40 mo; some infection in adults
Etiologic agent	*Strongyloides stercoralis*, a roundworm (nematode)	*Taenia saginata* (beef tapeworm); *Taenia solium* (pork tapeworm); cestodes	
Reservoir	Humans and dogs	Humans, swine, and cattle	Dogs and cats; almost 100% of newborn puppies are infected
Transmission	Infective larvae in soil penetrate skin, usually the foot, migrate through blood to lungs, migrate up to pharynx, and are swallowed to intestines	Ingestion of inadequately cooked, infected meat; anal-oral transfer from person to person; contaminated food or water with eggs from feces	Direct or indirect transmission of eggs in soil (from animal feces) to mouth
Incubation period	2-3 wk	8-14 wk	Weeks or months
Period of communicability	As long as living worms remain in intestine; up to 35 yr	As long as worm is in intestine; up to 30 yr	Not directly communicable
Susceptibility and resistance	General; no acquired immunity has been demonstrated	General; no resistance follows infection	Adults have lower exposure or decreased susceptibility
Report to local health authority	No	Reportable in some areas	No

abdominal distention, and cramps. Blockage of the biliary duct results in colicky epigastric pain, nausea, and vomiting. Because of the size of these roundworms a large mass may obstruct the bowel lumen.[68]

The roundworms causing *enterobiasis* (pinworm) and *trichuriasis* (whipworm) have simpler life cycles in the human host. Ingested eggs hatch in the small intestine, and larvae migrate directly to the cecum. The tiny gravid female pinworm migrates at night to the perianal area to deposit eggs, which embryonate within 6 hours. Perianal and perineal irritation and pruritus are the only symptoms. Occasionally appendicitis, salpingitis, or ulcerative lesions result from migrating pinworms. Embryo-

nated eggs remain infective on the skin, clothing, and bedclothes for 29 days and may be reingested by the host.[68]

Once in the cecum, the whipworm larvae embed their heads in the mucosa and consume 0.005 ml of blood per worm per day, producing a mild anemia. The adult female worms discharge eggs in 1 to 3 months, which are eliminated in the feces.[68]

The roundworms causing *toxocariasis* and *trichinosis* produce more severe systemic pathologic findings because of the ability of the larva to invade and encyst in organs beyond the intestinal tract. In *toxocariasis* eggs from animal feces (particularly puppies) are ingested and

Ancylostomiasis (Hookworm)	Ascariasis (Roundworm)	Enterobiasis (Pinworm)	Trichinosis	Trichuriasis
Endemic in tropic and subtropic areas where disposal of human feces is inadequate	Worldwide and common; in United States, most common in the south; greatest in moist, tropical areas; greatest in children	Worldwide and very high in some areas; most common helminth infection in United States; highest in school-aged and preschool-aged children and in mothers of infected children	Worldwide in areas where pork is eaten	Common in warm, moist regions
Necator americanus and *Ancylostoma duodenale*, roundworms (nematodes)	*Ascaris lumbricoides*, a common roundworm (nematode)	*Enterobius vermicularis*, roundworm (nematode)	Larvae of *Trichinella spiralis*, an intestinal roundworm (nematode)	*Trichuris trichiura* (human whipworm), a roundworm (nematode)
Humans	Humans	Humans; pinworms of animals not transmitted to humans	Swine, rats, dogs, cats, and many wild animals	Humans
Infective larvae in soil penetrate skin, usually foot, and migrate through blood to intestine; may be ingested directly	Ingestion of infective eggs from soil contaminated with feces	Direct transmission of infective eggs from anus to mouth; indirect transmission through contaminated food, clothing, or dust	Ingestion of inadequately cooked flesh of infected animals	Ingestion of eggs from soil contaminated with human feces
Weeks to months, depending on health status of host	Worms reach maturity 2 mo after ingestion	Life cycle of worms requires 4-6 wk	1-45 d; usually 10-14 d	Indefinite; eggs appear in feces 90 d after ingestion; symptoms may be earlier
Infected persons can excrete larvae for years; larvae remain infective in soil for weeks	As long as mature, fertilized female lives in intestine (10-18 mo); embryonated eggs viable in soil for years	As long as gravid females are depositing eggs on perianal skin; continuous reinfection occurs	Not directly communicable; animal hosts are infective for months	As long as eggs reach the soil, probably years
General; immunity unknown	General	General	General; infection probably results in immunity	General
No	No	No	Mandatory case report	No

hatch in the intestinal tract. The larvae penetrate the intestinal mucosa and migrate through the blood to the eye, skin, liver, lung, kidney, brain, or muscles. The larvae invade those tissues, producing a localized inflammatory reaction and granulomatous nodules. The larvae remain viable in the nodules for years. Systemic manifestations include an eosinophilia (3000/cmm), a leukocytosis (100,000/cmm), an increase in IgG, IgM, and IgE antibodies, and an increase in isoagglutinin titers to A and B blood group antibodies. Specific pathologic findings depend on the organ sites of invasion but may include hepatomegaly, an elevated SGOT, respiratory symptoms, blindness and central nervous system manifestations.[78]

In *trichinosis* the ingested larvae from improperly cooked infected meat attach to the intestinal mucosa within 2 to 3 weeks after infection. The body responds by producing an inflammatory exudate containing polymorphs, eosinophils, lymphocytes, and macrophages. Intestinal symptoms may be present. Each female *Trichinella* releases about 500 larvae over a 2-week period. The adult females are then discharged in the feces. The larvae penetrate into the bloodstream, migrate, and invade striated muscle. There they increase in length tenfold during a 3-week period. Muscle fibers become edematous, lose their cross striations, and undergo basophilic degeneration and nuclear proliferation. An acute toxemia results from inflammatory destruction of larvae in the blood. The toxemia subsides when the larvae become encysted in the muscles during the fourth to sixth week. Although most infections are subclinical, disease manifestations may be severe, dependent on the numbers and sites of invading larvae. Muscles and organs most frequently affected are the intercostals, diaphragm, eye, masseter, neck, pectoral, and limb flexors. Laboratory findings show an eosinophilia and an increase in serum creatinine phosphokinase and lactic dehydrogenase, indicating muscle destruction. Death may result from respiratory failure or pneumonia, myocarditis, or encephalitis caused by the toxemia.[48]

Taeniasis (tapeworm) infections may be local or systemic. If eggs of the pork tapeworm are ingested, they hatch in the intestine, and the larvae penetrate the intestinal mucosa and migrate and form cysts in subcutaneous tissue, striated muscles, or other vital organs. Disease may be severe if larvae localize in the eye, central nervous system, or heart. When larvae from the beef or pork tapeworm are ingested directly, the larvae attached to the intestinal mucosa where they feed and grow. The adult may remain attached for more than 30 years, discharging segments (proglottids) containing eggs into the feces. This form of the disease is less severe than the systemic form.[62]

DIAGNOSTIC STUDIES

The diagnosis of the parasitic infections where the worm localizes in the intestinal tract is confirmed when eggs or larvae are detected in a fecal specimen or at the anal opening. Toxocariasis and trichinosis are confirmed by biopsy of affected tissue together with the demonstration of elevated serum antibodies.

Ancylostomiasis[68]
  Fecal specimen
    1200 hookworm eggs/ml

  Microscopic examination of cultured specimen
    Positive for larva

Ascariasis[68]
  Fecal specimen
    Eggs of *Ascaris lumbricoides*

Enterobiasis[68]
  Fecal specimen
    Adult pinworms

  Transparent adhesive tape to perianal region
    Eggs can be visualized
    Five examinations will detect 99% of infections

Strongyloidiasis[68]
  Fecal specimen
    Visualizes motile threadworm larvae; after 24 hours adults may be visualized

Trichuriasis[68]
  Fecal specimen
    Eggs of whipworm

  Sigmoidoscopy
    Visualizes adult worms attached to colon wall

Taeniasis[62]
  Fecal specimen
    Visualizes worm segments (proglottids)

Toxocariasis[78]
  Liver biopsy
    Toxocara larvae

  Serology: ELISA
    Increase in IgG, IgM, and IgE antibodies

Trichinosis[48]
  Skeletal muscle biopsy
    Trichinella larvae 10 days after exposure

  Serology: complement fixation, precipitin, fluorescent antibody
    Fourfold increase in antibody titer 2 weeks after infection

  Bentonite flocculation
    Antibody titer greater than 1:5

  Differential WBC count
    Increase in eosinophils

TREATMENT PLAN

Chemotherapeutic[7,68,108,111]
  Anti-infective agents
    Antihelminthic agents are toxic substances and should not be used for small worm burdens.
    Ancylostomiasis (hookworm)
      Mebendazole (Vermox), 100 mg bid for 3 d
      Pyrantel pamoate (Antiminth), single oral dose of 11 mg/kg up to total of 1 g/d
    Ascariasis (roundworm)
      Mebendazole (Vermox), 100 mg bid for 3 d
      Piperazine citrate (Antepar), 150 mg/kg initially followed by six doses of 65 mg/kg for 12 h through nasogastric tube for intestinal or biliary obstruction
    Enterobiasis (pinworm)
      Mebendazole (Vermox), 100 mg po one time, *or*

Pyrantel pamoate (Antiminth), *or*

Pyrvinium pamoate (Povan), *or*

Piperazine citrate (Antepar)

Treatment should be repeated after 2 wk

Strongyloidiasis (threadworm)

Thiabendazole (Mintezol), 25 mg/kg bid for 2 d, *or*

Mebendazole (Vermox), 100 mg bid for 3 d

Repeated treatment may be required

Taeniasis (tapeworm)

Niclosamide (Yomesan), 2 g in one dose (adults)

Paromycin (Humatin), 1 g q15min for four doses (adults); 75 mg/kg in one dose (children)

Quinacrine (Atabrine), 800 mg in one dose or 400 mg in two doses; 30 min apart for adults

Toxocariasis

Diethylcarbamazine (Banocide), 2 mg/kg tid q1-3wk

Thiabendazole (Mintezol), 50 mg/kg/d for 7-10 d (questionable effectiveness; infections recur after treatment)

Trichinosis

Thiabendazole (Mintezol), (within 24 h of eating infected meat), 25 mg/kg/d for 1 wk

No treatment available once larvae are in bloodstream and muscle

Trichuriasis

Mebendazole (Vermox), 100 mg bid for 3 d po

Supportive

Correct anemias with iron therapy

Nutritional supplements

Follow-up examination of stool

Examination and treatment of contacts

ASSESSMENT[48,62,68,78]

Area of Concern	Worm Infection	Assessment
Skin	Ancylostomiasis, strongyloidiasis	Erythematous papular or vesicular eruption at site of invasion (generally soles of feet); may become generalized
	Trichinosis	Petechial rash; periorbital edema
	Toxocariasis	Pallor; nodular skin eruptions
Respiratory concerns	Ancylostomiasis, strongyloidiasis, ascariasis	Transitory cough and irregular respirations (Loeffler's syndrome) during migration of larvae
	Trichinosis	During third to sixth week: painful breathing; dysphagia; cough, shortness of breath
	Toxocariasis	Continual cough; rales; rhonchi
Gastrointestinal concerns	Ancylostomiasis, strongyloidiasis	Colicky abdominal pain; diarrhea
	Trichuriasis	Bloody diarrhea; rectal prolapse
	Ascariasis	Vomiting; abdominal distention; cramps; acute abdominal symptoms
	Taeniasis	Mild abdominal discomfort
	Trichinosis	Abdominal discomfort and diarrhea (first week only)
	Toxocariasis	Abdominal pain; hepatomegaly
Musculoskeletal concerns	Trichinosis	Edema and pain in affected muscles, including eye, diaphragm, intercostal, pectoral, masseter, neck, limb flexors, and lumbar muscles
Sensory concerns	Toxocariasis	Strabismus; loss of vision
	Trichinosis	Periorbital edema; subconjunctival and subungual and retinal hemorrhage; photophobia
Perianal area	Enterobiasis	Pruritus at night; may be localized erythema
Central nervous system	Toxocariasis	Seizures
	Trichinosis	During third to sixth week: symptoms of encephalitis
	Taeniasis (systemic)	Seizures; psychiatric symptoms
Cardiovascular concerns	Trichinosis	Symptoms of myocarditis during fourth to eighth week
Body temperature	Toxocariasis	Fever throughout infection
	Ancylostomiasis, strongyloidiasis, ascariasis	Fever during migration of larvae through lungs
	Trichinosis	Fever during second week (40° C [104° F]); profuse sweating
Systemic manifestations	Ancylostomiasis, trichuriasis, ascariasis, taeniasis	Anemia; weight loss; impaired growth
	Trichinosis	Weakness and headache persisting for varying periods of time beyond migratory phase of larvae; prostration during acute phase

NURSING DIAGNOSES and NURSING INTERVENTIONS

Nursing Diagnosis	Nursing Intervention
Nutrition, alteration in: less than body requirements (related to ancylostomiasis, trichuriasis, ascariasis, taeniasis)	Administer iron and nutritional supplements as prescribed. Encourage frequent high-protein feedings. (Blood transfusions may be necessary in ancylostomiasis.)
Injury, potential for: trauma (related to toxocariasis, trichinosis, taeniasis)	Monitor for signs of central nervous system involvement. Closely supervise these patients. Protect from injury during seizures with padded tongue blade, padded headboard, and side rails.
Breathing pattern, ineffective (related to toxocariasis, trichinosis)	Monitor for signs of pneumonia. Administer oxygen and respiratory assistance if required. Aid patients to deep breath.
Bowel elimination, alteration in: diarrhea (related to ancylostomiasis, strongyloidiasis, trichuriasis, trichinosis, taeniasis)	Monitor diarrhea output for fluid replacement. Collect stool specimen for laboratory analysis.
Comfort, alteration in: pain (related to ascariasis, trichinosis)	Report to physician symptoms of acute abdominal pain and distention that may suggest obstruction. Encourage rest to relieve muscle pain. Administer analgesics as prescribed.
Sensory-perceptual alteration: visual (related to toxocariasis, trichinosis)	Reassure patient that visual symptoms will disappear in 3 months. Assist patient as needed with mobility. Protect from injury.
Potential patient problem: fever (related to toxocariasis, trichinosis)	Provide tepid sponge baths. Administer antipyretics as prescribed. Encourage fluids.

Patient Education[7]

1. Follow-up examination of stools 2 weeks after therapy is necessary in ascariasis, ancylostomiasis, strongyloidiasis, and taeniasis. Monthly examinations for 3 months are necessary for taeniasis.
2. Toxocariasis and strongyloidiasis tend to recur following treatment. Patients should be monitored by a physician.
3. Anemias and protein deficiencies from ancylostomiasis, trichuriasis, ascariasis, and taeniasis may take time to correct. Patients should receive nutrition counseling and be encouraged to take iron and vitamin supplements until deficiencies are corrected.
4. Treatment for enterobiasis should be repeated in 2 weeks following first treatment. Daily machine washing with hot water of underwear and bedclothes during that time is necessary. Thorough hand washing following defecation is necessary.
5. Family members and close contacts of patients with any of these intestinal parasitic infections should be examined and treated for parasites.
6. Thorough hand washing following defecation is necessary.
7. Treatment of puppies for worms may prevent toxocariasis in humans.
8. Prevent children from eating dirt.
9. Proper cooking of pork to 65.6° C (150° F) is necessary.
10. Home freezing of meat for 3 weeks at −25° C (−13° F) destroys larvae.
11. Employ sewage disposal of contaminated feces. No human feces should be used as fertilizer.
12. Wear shoes in areas where human or animal feces may be on soil.
13. Bury animal feces deep in an area where children do not play.

EVALUATION[28]

Patient Outcome	Data Indicating That Outcome is Reached
There is no infection.	Stool specimen is negative for larvae of pinworms or threadworm; negative for eggs of hookworm, ascariasis, and whipworm; negative for tapeworm segments. There is no perianal pruritus. Respiratory patterns are normal without cough, rales, or rhonchi. There is no muscle or abdominal pain. Spleen and liver are not palpable. There are no signs of myocarditis, encephalitis, meningitis, or visual loss. Body temperature is normal.
Bowel elimination is normal.	Abdomen is soft; stools are soft, formed, and normal colored.
All cells receive nutrition.	Energy is at preinfection level. The patient is mentally alert. Growth, development, and weight are normal for age of person. Skin and mucous membranes are warm and moist, with natural color. Skin turgor is good.
Laboratory values are within normal limits.	Leukocyte and eosinophil counts are normal. For toxocariasis and trichinosis, SGOT, CPK, and lactic dehydrogenase levels are normal. For ancylostomiasis, trichuriasis, ascariasis, and taeniasis, hemoglobin, hematocrit, and erythrocyte levels are normal.

VIRAL HEPATITIS

Viral hepatitis is an inflammatory primary infection of the liver with three distinct clinical forms, each caused by a different hepatitis virus.

Depending on the etiologic agent, the diseases differ in their transmission and in their immunologic, pathologic, and clinical characteristics. Treatment is similar for each disease, but prevention and control vary greatly. Hepatitis may also occur as a secondary infection during the course of viral diseases caused by the cytomegalovirus, Epstein-Barr virus, herpes simplex virus, varicellazoster virus, coxsackie B virus, and rubella virus[7,64] (Table 15-12).

PATHOPHYSIOLOGY

Although the etiologic agents, mode of transmission, and course of the disease vary with each type of hepatitis, the pathologic condition produced in the liver is the same with all types. The similarities in disease pathologic findings will be presented first, followed by the variations.

The hepatitis virus, regardless of its mode of transmission, invades, replicates, and produces damage only in the liver. Inflammation and mononuclear cell infiltration in the parenchyma and portal ducts, hepatic cell necrosis, proliferation of Kupffer cells, cellular collapse, and accumulation of necrotic debris in the lobules and portal ducts all act to produce architectural changes in the lobules and portal ducts. The result is disturbance in bilirubin excretion.[60,64,69]

Cellular regeneration and mitosis are usually concurrent with hepatocyte necrosis; complete regeneration usually occurs within 2 to 3 months. Failure of the liver cells to regenerate while the necrotic process progresses results in a severe, fulminant, frequently fatal hepatitis. This occurs more often in hepatitis B. Continuation of the inflammatory response and necrosis, also more common in type B and in non A, non B, results in chronic active or chronic persistent hepatitis. In chronic active hepatitis the necrotic process, fibrosis, and architectural destruction continue throughout the hepatic lobes and portal ducts. In chronic persistent hepatitis the inflammatory process is limited to the portal tracts with little or no evidence of hepatocellular necrosis. There is a great deal of variability in clinical manifestations of hepatitis. All types of hepatitis may present with or without icterus; and all types may have a clinical severity ranging from subclinical infection to acute fulminating disease. Only hepatitis A does not lead to chronic disease or the chronic carrier state. All types stimulate an antibody response specific to the type of virus causing the disease.[64]

Hepatitis A virus (HAV) is acquired by ingestion of the HAV in food, water, or uncooked shellfish contam-

Table 15-12
Overview of Viral Hepatitis[7]

	Hepatitis A	Hepatitis B	Non-A, Non-B Hepatitis
Occurrence	Worldwide; sporadic and epidemic, with a tendency toward cyclic recurrence; outbreaks in institutions	Worldwide; endemic; highest in young adults, narcotic users, and health care workers	Worldwide; most common form of posttransfusion hepatitis; sporadic outbreaks occur
Etiologic agent	Hepatitis A virus (HAV)	Hepatitis B virus (HBV)	One or several viral agents distinct from type A and type B (NANB)
Reservoir	Humans and captive primates	Humans and possibly captive primates	Suspected to be the same as type B
Transmission	Person to person by fecal-oral route; contaminated food, water, shellfish	Direct and indirect contact with blood, saliva, and semen; sexual contact; perinatal	Percutaneous; transmission similar to HBV is suspected but not documented
Incubation period	15-50 d; average: 28-30 d	45-160 d; average: 60-90 d	15-180 d; average: 60 d
Period of communicability	Latter half of incubation period to 1 wk after onset of jaundice	During incubation period and throughout clinical course of disease; carrier state may persist for years	Suspected to be the same as for type B but is not known definitely
Susceptibility and resistance	Usually affects children and young adults; immunity after infection probably lasts for life; 45% of population has hepatitis A antibodies	All age groups; disease is mild in children; lifetime immunity follows infection	All age groups; degree of immunity following infection is not determined
Report to local health authority	Mandatory case report	Mandatory case report	Mandatory case report

inated with feces containing the virus or by direct fecal-oral transmission. The virus localizes in the liver, replicates there, enters the bile, and is carried to the intestinal tract where it is shed in the feces. Fecal shedding occurs late in the incubation period, usually before onset of clinical symptoms. Antibodies develop during acute disease and later during convalescence.[69]

Hepatitis B virus (HBV) is viable in blood and secretions containing serum (oozing cutaneous lesions) or derived from serum (saliva, semen, vaginal secretions). Transmission may be by one of the following routes: (1) direct percutaneous inoculation of infective serum or plasma by needle or transfusion of infective blood or blood products; (2) indirect percutaneous introduction of infective serum or plasma, such as through minute skin cuts or abrasions; (3) absorption of infective serum or plasma through mucosal surfaces, such as those of the mouth or eye; (4) absorption of other potentially infective secretions such as saliva or semen through mucosal surfaces, as might occur following sexual (heterosexual or homosexual) contact; and (5) transfer of infective serum or plasma via inanimate environmental surfaces or possibly vectors. Fecal transmission of HBV does not occur. HBV may be transmitted transplacentally, or the infant may become contaminated with the mother's infective blood at birth.[3,69]

Several complex antigen-antibody systems have been identified with the HBV. These will be described subsequently in this section. HBV antigens infect the blood within 30 to 60 days of exposure to HBV and are at their peak before disease onset. They persist for varying lengths of time; and their presence is useful for determining the course of the disease and the carrier state. Antibodies, specific for the antigens, develop at different times during convalescence. Detection of serum antibodies is useful for predicting the course of the disease and for determining immune status.[3]

Non-A, non-B hepatitis is a clinical disease similar to hepatitis B, for which an antigenically distinct agent (or agents) is suspected but has not yet been identified. Percutaneous transmission has been documented. Other modes of transmission similar to hepatitis B are suspected but not proven. The disease is generally milder than hepatitis B but has a greater risk for chronicity. It is the most common form of posttransfusion hepatitis, possibly because serologic screening for hepatitis B in potential donors has decreased this mode of transmission for hepatitis B.

The identification of serologic markers for virus type–specific antigens and antibodies has been important in the diagnosis, prevention, and control of viral hepatitis. The standard nomenclature and abbreviation with char-

Table 15-13
Standard Nomenclature, Abbreviations, and Characteristics of Hepatitis[3,5,83]

Abbreviation	Term	Characteristics and Implications
HAV	Hepatitis A virus	Etiologic agent with one serotype
Anti-HAV	Antibody to HAV	Detectable at onset of symptoms and persists for lifetime, probably confers life-time immunity
IgM	Immunoglobulin M	The anti-HAV present early in the infection; it represents current infection and is used to establish the diagnosis; serum levels drop during convalescence and disappear in 4-6 mo.
IgG	Immunoglobulin G	The anti-HAV that develops late in the infection and persists for years; its presence in serum indicates past infection and present immunity
HBV	Hepatitis B virus	Etiologic agent of hepatitis B; also called Dane particle
HBsAg	Hepatitis B surface antigen	Previously known as Australian antigen; detectable in large quantities in serum 2-7 wk before and during acute clinical disease, during chronic disease, and in carriers; its presence indicates blood is infectious
HBeAg	Hepatitis Be antigen	Soluble antigen that correlates with HBV replication; indicates a high titer of HBV in serum and consequent infectivity of serum; it rises 2-7 wk before clinical disease onset and usually drops before acute disease; its persistence is associated with progression to chronic hepatitis; found only in HBsAg-positive serum
HBcAg	Hepatitis B core antigen	Found in liver cells; cannot be detected in sera with present technology
Anti-HBs	Antibody to HBsAG	Rises in serum during convalescence; its presence indicates immunity to HBV either from past infection, passive antibody from HBIG, or active immune response from HBV vacccine
Anti-HBe	Antibody to HBeAg	Its presence in serum of person with continuing levels of HBeAg suggests chronic presence of HBV and infectivity of blood
Anti-HBc	Antibody to HBcAg	Increases during clinical disease, peaks during convalescence, and persists for years; presence indicates past infection with HBV
NANB	Non A, non B hepatitis	Disease similar to hepatitis B with etiologic agents that are neither HAV or HBV
IG	Immunoglobulin	Formerly called immune serum globulin (ISG) or gamma globulin; given before and within 2 wk after exposure to HAV and NANB; given in large doses after exposure to HBV
HBIG	Hepatitis B immune globulin	Contains a higher titer of HB immune globulins than does IG; preferred for use after exposure to HBV
HB vaccine	Hepatitis B vaccine	Inactivated vaccine prepared from carriers of HBsAg; stimulates production of anti-HBs; series of three injections recommended for those at risk for hepatitis B

acteristics and implications are presented here for easy reference (Table 15-13).

DIAGNOSTIC STUDIES[5,60,64,69]

Serum enzymes
Asparate aminotransferase (AST, SGOT) and alanine aminotransferase (ALT, SGPT)
At least eight times normal during clinical disease
Indicators of liver damage
Peak at onset of jaundice and fall during recovery
May be 20 to 50 times normal for hepatitis B and 10 to 20 times normal for non-A, non-B hepatitis, persisting at two to five times normal for months

Alkaline phosphatase
One to three times normal

Lactic dehydrogenase (LDH)
One to three times normal

Creatine phosphokinase (CPK)
Normal

Serum bilirubin
Elevated: measures extent of liver dysfunction
Ratio of direct to indirect fraction—1:1

Prothrombin time
Normal
Elevated only in severe fulminating hepatitis

VDRL
False positive

Hepatitis A
Stool specimen: immune electron microscopy, radioimmunoassay, or enzyme immunoassay
Positive for HAV 2 to 4 weeks after exposure, remains until onset of clinical disease, then is negative
HAV may be absent from stool by time patient is hospitalized

Serology: radioimmunoassay or ELISA test

Fourfold rise in anti-HAV antibodies between early disease and convalescence

Identification of IgM antibodies during early disease indicates present infection

IgG peaks after clinical disease and persists for life; high levels indicate past infection and present immunity

Hepatitis B

Serum antigen tests: radioimmunoassay, enzyme immunoassay

HBeAg and HBsAg in serum 1 to 2 weeks after exposure and 2 to 7 weeks before onset of clinical disease; peak and begin to drop during clinical disease

HBsAg will remain in serum of chronic carriers for life; positive tests indicate present infection or carrier state

Positive test in carrier with disease symptoms may misdiagnose infection with HAV or NANB

Serum antibody tests: radioimmunoassay

Anti-HBc increases during clinical disease and peaks during convalesence; anti-HBs begins rising during convalescence; both persist and gradually decrease over time

Carriers are always HBeAg positive and/or HBsAg positive and anti-HBs negative

For screening purposes: anti-HBs greater than 10 RIA sample ratio units indicates immunity

Non-A, non-B hepatitis

If above tests are negative in patient with clinical symptoms of viral hepatitis, non A, non B is suspected

TREATMENT PLAN[3,5,60,69,83]

Chemotherapeutic

There is no direct chemotherapeutic treatment for viral hepatitis. (There is no evidence that corticosteroids are helpful.)

Supportive chemotherapeutics may be used for fulminating hepatitis:

Anti-infective agents

Neomycin (Mycifadrin) 1.0-1.5 g po q6h until loose stools are achieved

Histamine-receptor antagonist

Cimetidine (Tagamet) 300-500 mg IV q6h or vigorous antacid therapy for gastrointestinal bleeding

Preventive chemotherapeutics may be used for preexposure prophylaxis against hepatitis A (HAV) for those traveling to high risk areas outside tourist routes for up to 2-3 months:

Immunologic agent

Immune globulin (gamma globulin), 0.02 ml/kg in a single dose IM

For prolonged travel

Immunologic agent

Immune globulin (gamma globulin), 0.06 ml/kg IM for 5 mo

Postexposure prophylaxis within 2 wk of close personal contact with hepatitis A–infected person in the home, day-care center, institution for custodial care, or hospital

Immunologic agent

Immune globulin (gamma globulin), 0.02 ml/kg in a single dose IM

Preexposure prophylaxis against hepatitis B (HBV) for high-risk groups (health care workers in contact with blood or blood products, clients and staff of institutions for the mentally retarded, hemodialysis patients, homosexual males, illicit injectable drug users, patients with clotting disorders who receive factor VII or IX concentrates, household and sexual contacts of HBV carriers, classroom contacts of deinstitutionalized mentally retarded carriers, and inmates of long-term correctional facilities)

Prevaccination serologic screening to identify HBV carriers and those already immune; one anti-HBc test will identify both; anti-HBs test will identify those immune

Hepatitis B vaccine (Heptavax-B)

Vaccinate those with negative Anti-HBc or negative anti-HBs tests

Adults: three doses of 1.0 ml vaccine (20 µg/ml) IM at 0, 1, and 6 mo

Hemodialysis patients: three doses of 2.0 ml vaccine (40 µg) IM at 0, 1, and 6 mo

Children under 10 yr: three doses of 0.5 ml vaccine (10 µg) IM at 0, 1, and 6 mo[5]

Do not accept blood from HBsAg-positive donors

Post-exposure prophylaxis

Infants born to mothers who are HBsAg positive: HBIG 0.5 ml IM within 12 h of birth; HB vaccine given IM in three doses of 0.5 ml (10 µg): first dose at birth (or within 7 d), then at 1 mo and 6 mo after first dose

Household contacts of acute hepatitis B cases and health workers who receive needle sticks from HBsAg-positive cases

Hepatitis B immune globulin (HBIG), 0.06 ml/kg IM or 5.0 ml for adults within 24 hr of exposure (repeat in 1 mo if hepatitis B vaccine is not given at time of exposure) *plus*

Hepatitis B vaccine (Heptavax B), 1.0 ml (20 µg)

IM at same time as HBIG in another site (or within 7 d); repeat 1 mo and 6 mo after initial dose

Immune globulin in same dose and schedule if HBIG B unavailable[3,5]

Sexual contacts should receive HBIG, 0.06 ml/kg IM or 5.0 ml for adults within 14 d of sexual contact

Supportive

For nonfulminating hepatitis:

Hospitalization for those with bilirubin concentrations greater than 10 mg/dl or greater than 10 times normal and for those with a prolonged prothrombin time

Bed rest until symptoms subside.

Diet as tolerated: small frequent low-fat, high-carbohydrate feedings may be better tolerated.

Symptomatic treatment for nausea (avoid chlorpromazine)

Symptomatic treatment for pain (acetaminophen preferred over aspirin)

All unnecessary medications, particularly sedatives, to be avoided.

For fulminating hepatitis:

Hospitalization and bed rest

Low protein diet: 20-30 mg protein/day

Enemas

Discontinue any sedatives

IV fluids and electrolytes

Central venous pressure line

Nasogastric tube feedings

Urinary catheter

Fresh frozen plasma to correct coagulation defects

ASSESSMENT: AREAS OF CONCERN[60,64]

Preicteric phase (3 to 10 days)

Onset

Acute for hepatitis A

Insidious for hepatitis B and non-A, non-B

Subjective symptoms

Malaise, weakness, dull headache, anorexia, intermittent nausea and vomiting, myalgias, chills

Right upper quadrant abdominal pain

Body temperature

38° to 40° C (100° to 104° F) for hepatitis A

Low grade or absent for hepatitis B and non-A, non-B

Skin

For hepatitis B and non-A, non-B

Urticarial pruritic hives or maculopapular lesions or fleeting, irregular patches of erythema in some patients

Multiple forearm needle pricks in drug users

Exacerbation of acne

Excoriations with severe pruritus

Musculoskeletal concerns

For hepatitis B and non-A, non-B: mild to moderate, nondeforming polyarticular arthritis: migratory, affecting elbows, wrists, knees, small joints of hands

Abdomen

Bowel sounds normal

Slightly enlarged, tender liver (9 to 13 cm)

Edges smooth, regular, and firm

Icteric phase (bilirubin greater than 2.5 mg/dl; lasts 1 to 3 weeks)

Skin

Jaundice with or without pruritus may be present or absent; can be observed under the tongue

Eyes

Scleral icterus

Urine

Dark

Stools

May be clay colored

Vital signs

Normal, although there may be a bradycardia with severe hyperbilirubinemia

Subjective symptoms

Nausea and vomiting frequently abate and appetite returns, or they may worsen

Malaise continues

Temperature

Normal or low grade

Complications: fulminant hepatitis with encephalopathy

Level of consciousness

Patient becomes lethargic and somnolent with personality changes; may show mild confusion, sexual or aggressive activity, loss of usual inhibitions

Lethargy may alternate with excitability, euphoria, or unruly behavior

Worsening of the condition leads to stupor and eventual coma

An early sign is asterixis (the irregular flapping of forcibly dorsiflexed outstretched hands)

Circulatory system

Prothrombin time is prolonged: abdominal bleeding; epistaxis; prolonged bleeding from puncture sites; blood in vomitus, stool, or urine; easy bruising

NURSING DIAGNOSES and NURSING INTERVENTIONS

Nursing Diagnosis	Nursing Intervention
Fluid volume deficit, potential	Provide frequent high-carbohydrate fluids as tolerated during acute symptoms. Administer IV fluids for patients with persistent vomiting or for those with hepatic encephalopathy, as ordered.
Nutrition, alteration in: less than body requirements	Encourage frequent small feedings as patient tolerates. Administer nasogastric tube feedings for patients with hepatic encephalopathy and coma.
Activity intolerance	Maintain bed rest during acute symptoms. (Patients need not be limited in their activity during convalescence.)
Knowledge deficit	Educate patient about disease and disease transmission. Emphasize the self-limiting nature of most hepatitis but the need for follow-up of liver function tests and serum HBsAg. Explain precautions.
Potential patient problem: hemorrhage	Monitor and report signs of gastrointestinal bleeding. Provide care as warranted by bleeding (Chapter 11).
Potential patient problem: encephalopathy	Monitor for signs of encephalopathy. Monitor and report as described under assessment. Monitor, also, progress of icterus. Provide care as warranted by level of consciousness of patient.
Potential patient problem: transmission of infection	Employ enteric precautions for 7 days after onset of jaundice for hepatitis A. Employ blood and body fluid precautions until patient is HBsAg serum negative for hepatitis B and for the duration of illness for non-A, non-B (see p. 1620 and next section).

Patient Education[60,83]

1. Follow-up serology in 1 or 2 months is necessary for all hepatitis B patients to determine the presence or absence of HBsAg.
2. Patients should follow precautions with blood and secretions until they are determined to be free of HBsAg. Close personal contacts should be examined and receive HBIG or HB vaccine.
3. HBV carriers should be aware that their blood and secretions are infectious. Close contacts of HBV carriers should receive HB vaccine. Carriers should not share razors or toothbrushes and must be cautious in handling cuts and lacerations. HBV carriers and patients with a history of NANB should not donate blood.
4. Patients caring for themselves at home during the acute stage of the disease should avoid alcohol and any nonprescribed medications, particularly sedatives and aspirin.
5. Severity of symptoms can determine patterns for bed rest and diet. Frequent small feedings of low-fat, high-carbohydrate foods may be better tolerated; but it is not necessary to limit the diet in any way.
6. Liver function tests should be monitored until normal.
7. Hepatitis A patients must wash hands thoroughly following toileting, must disinfect articles soiled with feces (boil 1 minute), and must not prepare foods for others during symptomatic disease. They should avoid sharing eating utensils, toothbrushes, toys, and so on.
8. Sexual activity should be avoided during acute stage of hepatitis B and non-A, non-B. Ideally, hepatitis B patients should not resume sexual activity until tests for HBsAg are negative or until partner has received HB vaccine or HBIG, if HB vaccine is unavailable.

EVALUATION

Patient Outcome	Data Indicating That Outcome is Reached
There is no infection.	Serum HBsAg and HBeAg tests are negative. Close personal contacts of hepatitis B patients have received HBIG or HB vaccine.

Patient Outcome	Data Indicating That Outcome is Reached
Liver function is normal.	There is no icterus. Patient has full appetite, energy, and no right upper quadrant abdominal pain. Urine and stool are normal colored. There are no changes in personality or level of consciousness.
Liver function tests are normal.	SGPT (ALT), SGOT (AST), alkaline phosphatase, LDH, serum bilirubin, and prothrombin time are all within normal limits.
Patient is knowledgeable about need for follow-up, means of preventing transmission to others, and convalescent self-care.	Items listed in "Patient Education" are met.

INFECTIOUS DISEASES OF THE HEMATOLYMPHATIC SYSTEM

The infectious diseases grouped here produce either primary pathologic findings in the lymphatic system or disseminated infection with lymphadenopathy as part of the clinical picture. Two of the diseases can be transmitted transplacentally with serious consequences to the fetus (Table 15-14).

Mononucleosis

Mononucleosis is an acute viral infectious disease producing a generalized lymph node hyperplasia and characterized by fever, exudative pharyngitis, lymphadenopathy, and splenomegaly.

PATHOPHYSIOLOGY[90]

The Epstein-Barr virus (EBV) is transmitted in saliva by prolonged direct contact, probably through kissing with salivary exchange. The pathogen invades B lymphocytes in lymphatic tissue, stimulating the development of a surface membrane antigen on the infected lymphocytes. T lymphocytes actively proliferate in response to the antigen, producing a generalized lymph node hyperplasia. Atypical T lymphocytes infiltrate into the spleen, tonsils, lungs, heart, liver, kidneys, adrenal glands, central nervous system, and skin. The circulating T cells are not infective and do not therefore produce necrosis in these systems. Their infiltration does cause enlargement, particularily of the spleen, and disturbance in function of those organs.

There is great variability in the severity of the disease, from asymptomatic disease (usually in children) to severe systemic and localized organ involvement. Lymphadenopathy, splenomegaly, and exudative pharyngitis are characteristic. More serious manifestations of the disease include hepatitis, pneumonitis, and central nervous system involvement. Rare but serious complications include splenic rupture, hematologic complications (hemolytic anemia, agranulocytosis, thrombcytopenic purpura), pericarditis, and orchitis.

Saliva remains infective for 18 months in spite of the development of EBV-specific antibodies early in the disease. The virus has been cultured from the throats of 10% to 20% of normal, healthy adults, suggesting that the disease may be contacted from asymptomatic viral shedders.[90]

DIAGNOSTIC STUDIES[34,64,90]

Differential white blood count
  Lymphocytes and monocytes greater than 50% with over 10% being atypical lymphocytes

Leukocyte count
  Normal early in disease; rises to 10,000 to 20,000/ cmm in second week

Serology: heterophil agglutination antibody tests
  Rapid forms of this test are Monospot, Monoscreen, and Monotest, all commercially prepared kits
  Heterophil antibody titer greater than 1:40 to 1:128 (depending on the laboratory), usually by the end of the first week; usually disappears by the fourth week, although disappearance may be delayed
  May be false negative reactions to this test
  If the heterophil antibody test is negative but there is strong clinical evidence for mononucleosis, the following EBV-specific antibody tests may be performed. Both IgM antibodies and IgG antibodies are present early in the disease.

Table 15-14
Overview of Infectious Diseases of the Hematolymphatic System[7]

	Mononucleosis	Cytomegalovirus Infections	Toxoplasmosis	Brucellosis
Occurrence	Worldwide; highest in adolescents and young adults in developed countries; asymptomatic infection in children	Worldwide; many asymptomatic infections; congenital infection may be severe	Worldwide; common in humans, mammals, and birds; many asymptomatic infections; congenital infection may be severe	Worldwide; an occupational disease of those working with infected animals; about 170 cases per year in United States
Etiologic agent	Epstein-Barr virus, one of the herpesviruses	Cytomegalovirus, one of the herpesviruses	*Toxoplasma gondii*, a protozoan	*Brucella abortus, B. canis, B. melitensis, B. suis*
Reservoir	Humans and possibly primates	Humans	Cats; other mammals and birds are intermediate hosts	Cattle, swine, sheep, horses, dogs
Transmission	Direct contact with saliva; through blood transfusions	Direct contact with secretions and excretions; blood transfusions and transplacentally	Transplacental if mother has active infection; eating infective meat; water contaminated with cat feces	Contact with blood, tissues, urine or vaginal discharges of infected animals; ingestion of raw milk from infected animals
Incubation period	4-6 wk	Unknown; 3-8 wk following transfusion; in neonate, 3-12 wk following delivery produced infection	Unknown; probably between 5-23 d	Variable: 5-30 d
Period of communicability	Prolonged; pharyngeal excretion may persist for years; 15-20% of adults are carriers	Virus excreted in saliva and urine for months to years	Not directly transmitted except transplacentally; cysts in infected meat remain infective as long as meat is edible and uncooked	Not communicable person to person
Susceptibility and resistance	General; infection confers a high degree of resistance	General; fetuses, immunosuppressed individuals, and those with debilitating disease have more severe disease	General, but risk for infection increases with age; immunity after infection persists indefinitely	Children have less severe symptoms; duration of immunity unknown
Report to local health authority	No	No	In some states	Mandatory case report

EBV-specific antibody tests: immunofluorescence

Elevated EBV–IgM antibody titers of 1:80 to 1:160; may be false positive reactions; titers drop rapidly after clinical disease

Elevated EBV–IgG antibody: 1:80 is suggestive; persists for life; titer greater than 1:5 suggests immunity

Liver function tests

Serum transaminases (AST [SGOT], ALT [SGPT])

All elevated in hepatic involvement, two to three times upper normal limits

Bilirubin

Elevated if there is hepatic involvement

Throat culture

Positive for group A hemolytic streptococci in 10% of patients

Platelet count (in complications)

Below 140,000/cmm occurs frequently
Below 1000/cmm in severe complications

TREATMENT PLAN[34,64]

Surgical
For splenic rupture: surgical removal of the spleen

Chemotherapeutic
Corticosteroids
    Prednisone (Deltasone, others), 30 mg/24 h in divided doses, decreasing for 5 d, for severe neurologic complications, airway obstruction, thrombocytopenic purpura, or hemolytic anemia

Supportive
Bed rest during acute stage
Saline throat gargle
Aspirin or acetaminophen for sore throat and fever

ASSESSMENT: AREAS OF CONCERN[34]

Prodromal symptoms
Fatigue
Anorexia
Chilliness
Retro-orbital headache

Body temperature
Marked elevation, sometimes persisting for 1 to 2 weeks
38° to 41° C (101° to 105° F)
Peaks in afternoon

Head
Photophobia with headache
Periorbital edema

Throat
Painful, exudative tonsillitis
Exudate either white, pasty, and discrete or greenish gray membrane with a bad odor
Inflammation and tonsillar edema may be extreme
Dysphagia

Oral cavity
Bleeding gums
Palatine petechiae

Lymph nodes
Cervical adenopathy of posterior cervical chain, anterior cervical, submandibular, and axillary nodes
Nodes are discrete and slightly tender

Abdomen
Splenomegaly
Tenderness of liver

Skin
Jaundice in 5% of patients
Measleslike rash in 5% of patients
Purpura in complicated disease

Respiratory complications
Symptoms of pneumonia

Neurologic complications
Symptoms of meningitis or encephalitis

NURSING DIAGNOSES and NURSING INTERVENTIONS

Nursing Diagnosis	Nursing Intervention
Activity intolerance	Encourage bed rest during acute symptomatic disease.
Comfort, alteration in: pain	Administer analgesics per order or saline gargle for sore throat.
Anxiety	Assist patient in developing a realistic plan for returning to work or school during convalescence. (The prolonged malaise accompanying this disease may produce anxiety in the patient, particularly college students.)
Potential patient problem: ruptured spleen	Monitor for signs of neurologic or purpuric complications or splenic rupture. Protect patient from activity that may risk splenic rupture.
Potential patient problem: fever	Administer antipyretics. Bathe with tepid water or alcohol to reduce high fever. Encourage adequate fluid intake.

Patient Education

1. Although complete bed rest is not usually necessary during acute disease or convalescence, the patient caring for himself at home should be encouraged to rest as symptoms dictate. Convalescence may be long, lasting 3 to 4 weeks.
2. The patient with splenomegaly should avoid heavy lifting, contact sports, or any activity

that may increase the risk of injury to the spleen. Children must be protected in their play from injury.

3. Report to physician any jaundice, excess bruising or bleeding, or central nervous system symptoms.

EVALUATION

Patient Outcome	Data Indicating That Outcome is Reached
There is no infection.	Cervical lymph nodes are nonpalpable and nontender. Throat and tonsils are normal colored and not swollen. There is no exudate on tonsils. Patient swallows without pain. Body temperature is normal.
Laboratory findings are within normal limits.	Leukocyte, lymphocytes, and platelet counts, bilirubin level, and serum transaminase (SGOT; SGPT) levels are normal.

Cytomegalovirus Infections

Cytomegalovirus infections are extremely common viral infections that are ordinarily asymptomatic. Clinical disease in the adult resembles mononucleosis. Congenital and perinatal acquired infections are serious in the neonate, leading to irreversible central nervous system damage.

PATHOPHYSIOLOGY[51,56,64]

The cytomegalovirus (CMV), with several antigenically related strains, is a member of the herpesvirus group and has characteristics common to other herpesviruses. Like the Epstein-Barr herpesvirus, CMV produces a frequently asymptomatic mononucleosis-type infection in children and adults. CMV remains latent in body tissue, similar to herpes types I and II, with the potential for producing recurrent infection. CMV, like herpes I and II, also crosses the placental barrier and is shed in cervical secretions. Therefore it has the potential for producing congenital infection with severe congenital anomalies and perinatal infection acquired during vaginal delivery. Like herpes II, the CMV is suspected of having oncogenic properties.

CMV can be found in all body secretions including saliva, blood, urine, semen, cervical secretions, and breast milk, even in the presence of CMV-specific antibodies. Transmission requires prolonged direct contact with secretions. Although the exact mechanism for postnatal transmission is not known, sexual, oral, and blood transfusion transmission is suspected in postnatal acquired infections.

Irrespective of the mode of transmission, CMV may invade the cells of most tissues in the body. An inflammatory response with focal tissue destruction, areas of calcification, and hyperplasia of the reticuloendothelial system develops. Typical cellular lesions are characterized by enlarged cells containing intranuclear and cytoplasmic inclusion bodies. These lesions are disseminated widely, particularly in the brain, liver, lungs, kidney, and spleen.

A humoral and cell-mediated anti-CMV antibody response occurs, which does not appear to alter the course of the spread of the virus from the cell to cell or alter the presence of the virus in body secretions. Circulating maternal antibodies in the fetus also do not appear to impede the infectious process or the development of congenital anomalies.

Dependent on the mode of transmission, three different forms of the infection have been identified: congenital, perinatal, and postnatal acquired. All three forms can be asymptomatic or occur as either mild or severe clinical disease.

Congenital CMV infection is acquired by transplacental transmission, usually resulting from a primary infection of the mother acquired during pregnancy. Ninety-five percent of infants with congenital infections are asymptomatic at birth. The virus can be detected in the infant's urine for up to 15 months; and maternal antibodies are present in cord blood at birth. In utero viral invasion is most destructive to the developing fetal central nervous system, particularly the cerebellum and cerebral cortex. Neurologic defects such as microcephaly, psychomotor retardation, and severe mental retardation result. The infant born with symptomatic CMV infection will also have evidence of a severe generalized infection plus symptoms of organ involvement of the liver, lung, kidney, or eye. This extraneural organ involvement is usually self-limiting. If the child lives, there will invariably be neurologic sequelae. Congenital CMV infections need to be differentiated diagnostically from toxoplasmosis, rubella, herpes, hemolytic anemias, and bacterial sepsis.

Perinatal infection is acquired at the time of delivery from a serologic-positive mother who had either a primary infection during pregnancy or a reactivation of a latent infection. Cervical secretions of CMV are high during the last trimester, having increased as the pregnancy progressed. Perinatally infected infants develop signs of infection (virus in urine and an antibody response with or without clinical evidence of organ involvement) 4 to 8 weeks following birth. The long-term effects on neurologic development are not known.

Postnatal acquired infection requires close contact with body secretions containing the virus, usually from an asymptomatic person. Blood transfusions and renal and bone marrow transplants (possibly because of immunosuppression) have been linked with CMV transmission. Sexual transmission and kissing are also suspected as modes of transmission. The disease may be asymptomatic, or there may be symptoms of liver and lung involvement or a mononucleosis-like syndrome. There is no evidence of chronic organ impairment in acquired CMV infection. Primary or reactivation infection can be severe and life threatening in the immunosuppressed individual. Such patients may develop a progressive pneumonitis, hemolytic anemia, purpura, gastrointestinal ulceration, hepatitis, or pericarditis.

DIAGNOSTIC STUDIES[51,56,64]

Cell culture of specimen of urine, oral secretions, cervical secretions, or biopsied tissue
Positive for specific cytopathic effect of CMV
Presence of CMV in urine of infant at birth suggests congenital infection

Biopsy of liver tissue
Histologic evidence of typical inclusion bodies

Complement fixation
Presence of IgG antibody in infant blood during first 6 months represents maternal antibodies; levels persisting after 6 months suggest congenital CMV infection
Fourfold rise in titer in adult or child suggests current infection

Indirect fluorescent antibody, immunofluorescence, anticomplement immunofluorescent test
Presence of IgM in cord blood at birth suggests congenital CMV infection
Elevated titer in adult or child suggests current infection

Serum transaminase (AST)
Elevated in CMV hepatitis but rarely higher than 800 units

Platelets
May be as low as 5000/cmm

Differential WBC count
Increase in lymphocytes, many atypical

Differential diagnosis: heterophil agglutination
Negative in CMV (positive in mononucleosis)

TREATMENT PLAN[7,51,56,64]

Chemotherapeutic
Results of clinical trials using antiviral drugs, corticosteroids, or immune globulins in treating CMV infections are equivocal at this time. Antiviral drugs do suppress viruria in neonates but do not alter the course of the infection.

Supportive
Transfusion of sedimented RBCs for anemia
Transfusion of platelet-rich plasma for thrombocytopenia
Antipyretics for fever in CMV mononucleosis–like syndrome
Experimental live CMV vaccines currently being evaluated for prevention
Infants born of antibody-free mothers should not receive breast milk from a woman serologically positive for CMV antibodies since the virus may be in the milk[7]

ASSESSMENT: AREAS OF CONCERN[51,56,64]

Congenital CMV
Skin
Jaundice
Transient petechial rash (subsides if child lives)

Abdomen
Hepatosplenomegaly (persists for months)

Activity
Lethargy

Breathing patterns
Respiratory distress

Head
Microcephaly possible

Neurologic concerns
Seizures in severe cases, usually followed by death in a few days or weeks

Laboratory findings
Anemia; thrombocytopenia
Increased protein in cerebrospinal fluid

Eye
Progressive chorioretinitis

There is a long list of congenital anomalies associated with congenital CMV infections in addition to those listed above. The majority of CMV-infected infants are asymptomatic at birth but develop varying degrees of neurologic sequelae later in life.

Sequelae to congenital CMV
Neurologic concerns
Spasticity; diplegia
Epileptiform seizures
Blindness; deafness

Mental concerns
Retardation

Postnatal acquired CMV
Body temperature
Fever lasting 2 to 5 weeks

Skin
Rubelliform rash

Musculoskeletal concerns
Migratory polyarthritis in knees, fingers, and toes

Subjective symptoms
Headache
Myalgia; malaise
Nausea (with hepatitis)

Abdomen
Hepatomegaly and splenomegaly

Respiratory concerns
Paroxysmal cough or symptoms of pneumonia

Like congenital CMV, postnatal acquired CMV is usually asymptomatic. When clinical disease is present, the symptoms are variable and similar to mononucleosis without the lymphadenopathy and exudative pharyngitis. Complications include the following:

Respiratory concerns
Progressive pneumonitis

Neurologic complications
Sensory and motor weakness; photophobia
Pyramidal tract signs

Cardiac complications
Symptoms of myocarditis

Eye complications
Retinitis

NURSING DIAGNOSES and NURSING INTERVENTIONS

Nursing Diagnosis	Nursing Intervention
Potential patient problem: transmission of infection	Encourage pregnant nursing staff not to care for neonates with congenital CMV, although CMV is not highly communicable.

Diagnoses and interventions for neonates with congenital CMV are beyond the scope of this chapter. Children and adults with CMV infections are generally not hospitalized and rarely have symptoms requiring medical intervention. The care of those who do is similar to that of mononucleosis (p. 1549) or is dependent on the complications (pneumonitis, myocarditis, hepatitis, meningoencephalitis, or chorioretinitis).

Toxoplasmosis

Toxoplasmosis is a systemic protozoan infection, ranging from subclinical to severe to chronic. Four different clinical syndromes can be identified depending on where the pathogen localizes in the body. Transplacental transmission results in congenital toxoplasmosis, which may be fatal to the fetus or neonate.

PATHOPHYSIOLOGY[8,36,64]

Toxoplasmosis, like the cytomegalovirus (CMV) infections, may be congenital or acquired. Unlike CMV, there is not a risk for perinatal acquired toxoplasmosis. Both forms of toxoplasmosis may present with clinical patterns ranging from subclinical infection to severe generalized infection (with neurologic and sensory sequelae) to death. Both may occur in latent or recurring forms under conditions of reduced host defenses.

The pathogen producing toxoplasmosis, *Toxoplasma gondii*, is a protozoan that is pathogenic to animals and humans. The pathogen can multiply only in living cells. This parasite exists in three forms: trophozoites, tissue cysts, and oocysts. Trophozoites are capable of invading, multiplying, and necrotizing all host cells. Trophozoites can remain viable extracellularly in body secretions such as peritoneal fluid, breast milk, urine, saliva, or tears for a few hours to days. They cannot survive drying, heating, freezing, or contact with digestive juices.

Tissue cysts are formed within host cells. A surrounding membrane produced by the pathogen encapsulates up to 3000 organisms. This enables the parasites to maintain their viability, in spite of circulating host antibodies, for the life of the host. Tissue cysts are responsible for recurrent infection in humans and for transmission of the pathogen from animal reservoirs. Tissue cysts also cannot survive freezing, drying, or heating.

Oocysts are a form in the life cycle of *T. gondii* that occurs only in cats. Oocysts, a noninfectious form, are discharged in the feces of infected cats. Oocysts sporulate in 1 to 21 days in environmental temperatures of 4° to 37° C (39° to 99° F). They remain infectious in the soil for up to 1 year, given favorable environmental conditions.

Transmission of *T. gondii* can occur by one of two modes: (1) ingestion of tissue cysts in uncooked meat or ingestion of sporulated oocysts by hands or food contaminated with cat feces or (2) transplacental transmission of trophozoites in maternal circulation during acute infection acquired by the mother during the pregnancy.

In ingestion-acquired toxoplasmosis the capsule surrounding ingested cysts is digested by gastric juices, permitting viable trophozoites to invade intestinal mucosa and to be disseminated throughout the body by way of blood and the lymphatics. Organ cell invasion produces foci of necrosis surrounded by intense inflammatory reaction with mononuclear cell infiltration. The spleen, liver, brain, lung, myocardium, and eye are most frequently involved. The development of cysts and tissue calcifications may impair organ functioning.

An early antibody response destroys many parasites before they form tissue cysts and supports cyst formation by the remainder. Thus the infection is limited to its mild or subclinical forms for the majority of infected persons. Failure of an immune response, as is the case with immunosuppressed patients or those with debilitating disease, is more likely to result in progressive, life-threatening infection with multiple organ involvement and extensive damage.

Transplacentally transmitted *T. gondii* is disseminated to every organ in the developing fetus, particularly to the brain, heart, lungs, adrenal glands, striated muscle, and eye. Focal necrotic and inflammatory lesions are produced with cyst formation and calcification. Extensive destruction may occur in the central nervous system, affecting the cortex, subcortical white matter, caudate and lenticular nuclei, midbrain, pons, medulla, and spinal cord. Obstruction of the foramina of Monro or the aqueduct of Sylvius may result in an internal hydrocephalus. Microcephalus, hydrocephalus, or varying degrees of central nervous system impairment may occur.

Infection in the eye produces edema and necrosis of the retina, necrosis and disruption of the pigmented layer of the rods and cones, and infiltration of the retina and choroid with inflammatory cells. Granulation tissue and exudate may spread to the vitreous. This chorioretinitis may be manifested within weeks after birth or at some time later in life when the latent infection becomes reactivated.

Maternal infection early in the pregnancy is usually associated with fetal death or severe disease at birth. Infection later in the pregnancy results in less severe or no manifestations at birth. Only 11% of maternal infections result in infants damaged at birth. The majority, 60% of infants, are not affected; 29% have subclinical infections that will be manifested by neurologic or sensory defects as the infant develops.

DIAGNOSTIC STUDIES[8,64]

Inoculation of mice with specimens from blood, spinal fluid, lymph nodes, muscle tissue; morphologic examination of mouse tissue after 4 weeks

Identification of *T. gondii* cysts or trophozoites in mouse tissue is presumptive evidence of present infection.

Electron microscopic examination of tissue sections or smears

Identification of trophozoites present during acute infection.

Identification of cysts does not differentiate between acute or chronic infection.

Indirect fluorescent antibody test or Sabin-Feldman dye test

IgG antibodies (1:4) appear within 1 to 2 weeks after acute infection; reach high titers (over 1:1000) in 6 to 8 weeks; and then gradually decline over months or years to titers of 1:4-1:64.*

False positive results may follow blood transfusions. Fourfold rise in titers or slow decline after the peak is diagnostic. A rapid decline in these antibodies in the neonate suggests the presence of maternal antibodies and the absence of infant infection. A titer of 1:256 at 4 months suggests congenital infection.*

Indirect hemagglutination test

Becomes positive for IgG antibodies (1:16) in 2 to 4 weeks; reaches peak (1:1000) in 8 to 16 weeks and stays positive longer (1:16 to 1:64). There are many false negative results in congenital toxoplasmosis. Fourfold rise in titer is diagnostic.*

IgM fluorescent antibody test

Detects IgM antibodies (1:10) in 5 days, which peak (1:80) in 2 to 4 weeks. These antibodies decrease (1:10 to 1:40) during convalescence and are negative in 3 weeks to 4 months.

Test is useful for diagnosing acute infection.

Persistent IgM antibodies in neonate suggest active infection; a rapid drop suggests maternal antibodies.*

Radioimmunoassay, agglutination tests, and enzyme-linked assay (ELISA)

Detects both IgG and IgM antibodies.*

Cerebrospinal fluid

Congenital: protein: 2000 mg/dl; increase in RBC and WBC counts.

Acquired: glucose and protein normal.

TREATMENT PLAN

Chemotherapeutic[8,36]

Sulfadiazine (or sulfamerazine and sulfamethazine) in combination with pyrimethamine synergistically affects trophozoites but not cysts. Treatment will not prevent recurrence of chorioretinitis. It is indicated

*These tests may show false negative results in immunosuppressed hosts.

for severe, protracted disease, for those with chorioretinitis, for immunosuppressed individuals, and for active infections in the newborn. Pyrimethamine is contraindicated for pregnant women.

Anti-infective agents

Sulfadiazine (Suladyne), or triple sulfonamides po for 4 wk

Adults: initial dose of 50-75 mg/kg followed by 75-100 mg/d in four equal doses

Infants: initial dose of 75-100 mg/kg followed by 100-150 mg/kg/d in four equal doses

Pyrimethamine (Daraprim), for 4 wk

Adults: First day: 100-200 mg in two divided doses, followed by 1 mg/kg/d in two divided doses (maximum: 25-50 mg/d)

Children: first 2-3 days: 2 mg/kg/d in two divided doses, followed by 1 mg/kg/d in two divided doses

Vitamins

Folinic acid (calcium leucovorin), IM or po, 2-10 mg/d to prevent bone marrow suppression; 6-10 mg/d if platelets are less than 100,000/cmm

Baker's yeast, three or four cakes per day

Supportive

To prevent spread, reject leukocyte or organ donors who are antibody positive

ASSESSMENT: AREAS OF CONCERN[64]

Congenital disease

Ranges from mild or asymptomatic generalized infection to symptoms of irreversible central nervous system damage

Head

Hydrocephalus or microcephalus

Neurologic concerns

Convulsions

Respiratory concerns

Pneumonitis: cough, dyspnea, cyanosis

Skin

Jaundice

Purpura

Petechial or maculopapular rash

Abdomen

Splenomegaly

Hepatomegaly

Lymph nodes

Generalized lymphadenopathy

Gastrointestinal concerns

Vomiting, diarrhea

Eye

Bilateral chorioretinitis developing within a few weeks of birth; lesions can be visualized on the macula or periphery of the retina

Acquired disease

Ranges from subclinical to a variety of clinical syndromes, occurring singly or in combination; four syndromes outlined below

Systemic syndrome

Subjective symptoms

Weakness and malaise for 6 to 10 days preceding following symptoms

Body temperature

Fever up to 41° C (106° F)

Skin

Generalized, bright red to pink, maculopapular rash, blanching on pressure; rash not seen on scalp, palms, or soles

Respiratory concerns

Pneumonitis: coarse rales; dullness over both lung bases; cough, dyspnea, cyanosis

Progresses to prostration and death in 2 to 4 weeks

Cardiovascular concerns

Myocarditis

Neurologic syndrome

Encephalitis: headache, vomiting, generalized convulsions, ataxia, transitory confusion

Neurologic sequelae common

Lymph node syndrome

Generalized lymphadenopathy: firm, smooth, discrete, movable, enlarged nodes; tender early, painless later; no involvement of overlying skin; self-limiting

Abdomen

Splenomegaly

Eye syndrome

Chorioretinitis (more frequently associated with congenital infection or recurrence of congenital chorioretinitis): blurred vision, pain, photophobia, loss of central vision, tearing; results in permanent loss of visual acuity

NURSING DIAGNOSES and NURSING INTERVENTIONS

The diagnoses and care of infants born with symptomatic toxoplasmosis depend on the type of anomaly. Care of acutely ill neonates is beyond the scope of this chapter.

Nursing Diagnosis	Nursing Intervention
Grieving, anticipatory	Encourage parents to express feelings of guilt and fears that infant will die or that future pregnancies will be impaired. Assist with grief process (also see ''Patient Education'').
Injury, potential for (etiology: chemotherapeutic agent)	Monitor for signs of bone marrow depression caused by pyrimethamine: purpura, epistaxis, bleeding at injection site (see ''Patient Education'').
Sensory-perceptual alteration: visual	Provide a safe environment for patients with chorioretinitis. Assist patient with interpreting the environment, with personal care, and with ambulation as needed. Refer for rehabilitation for vision loss.

For persons with encephalitis, see p. 1569. For persons with pneumonitis or myocarditis, see Chapters 1 and 2.

Patient Education

1. Patients treated with pyrimethamine (which depresses bone marrow) should have peripheral blood cell and platelet counts twice a week during therapy. Explain medication regimen, particularly the use of folinic acid and/or baker's yeast to counteract effects of pyrimethamine.

2. Infants born with asymptomatic toxoplasmosis should be evaluated periodically for visual problems and developmental delays.

3. Refer families of infants with congenital toxoplasmosis to counseling, support, or rehabilitation resources as needed. Provide information about the resource and its services and how to access the resource.

4. The congenital anomalies do not represent a hereditary defect.
5. There is not a risk for congenital toxoplasmosis in subsequent pregnancies. The risk is only present when toxoplasmosis is acquired during the pregnancy.[64]
6. Immunocompromised persons and pregnant women can avoid exposure by cooking all meat to 60° C (140° F), washing fruits and vegetables, washing hands thoroughly after handling uncooked meat, wearing gloves while working in soil, and avoiding cat feces. Children's sandboxes should be kept free of cat feces.[7]

EVALUATION

Patient Outcome	Data Indicating That Outcome is Reached
There are no toxic effects from therapy.	Leukocyte, reticulocyte, and platelet counts and bilirubin level are normal.
Parents of infected children are aware of needs and able to use resources.	Parents express plans to have child medically evaluated periodically for early detection of ocular or neurologic complications. They are aware of counseling, support, or rehabilitation resources and have phone numbers and names of people to contact at those services.

Brucellosis

Brucellosis is an acute or subacute systemic bacterial infectious disease of the reticuloendothelial system, with a variety of toxic manifestations that mimic other diseases.[7]

PATHOPHYSIOLOGY[7,15,94]

The microorganism causing brucellosis is a bacterium appearing as a coccus, a bacillus, or a coccobacillus, with six species pathogenic to specific animals. Four of the species found in cattle, swine, sheep, buffaloes, goats, horses, and dogs are pathogenic to humans.

Brucella is transmitted to humans by ingestion of infected milk, milk products, or uncooked meat; by skin or conjunctival contact with tissues, blood, urine, vaginal discharges, aborted fetuses, and placentas from infected animals; or by inhalation of airborne *Brucella* organisms in pens or stables.

The transmitted organism invades the lymphatics, bloodstream, and reticuloendothelial system and is disseminated throughout the body. Lesions infiltrated with large mononuclear cells are formed. The lesions may be suppurative or nonsuppurative, depending on the species of infecting *Brucella*. Focal necrotic and granulomatous lesions develop in the endocardium, bones, central nervous system, gallbladder, lungs, spleen, liver, kidneys, and intestinal mucosa. A fatal septicemia is possible. Brucellosis may be asymptomatic or be manifested as an acute systemic disease, a chronic relapsing disease, or an infection localized in one or more organs. *Brucella* contains an endotoxin that is liberated when the organism dies. The endotoxin may be responsible for the systemic symptoms of pain, fever, and mental changes associated with the disease.

An immune response develops early in the disease and is sustained at low levels for years after acute disease. Antibodies do not prevent reinfection, the development of chronic disease, or relapses of acute symptoms during convalescence. It appears that *Brucella* organisms are able to survive within the phagocytes of the reticuloendothelial system, producing relapses of the disease in spite of high antibody titers.

DIAGNOSTIC STUDIES[15,94]

Culture of blood, lesions, or exudate
Positive for *Brucella*

Widal agglutination test
Titer greater than 1:80 (preferably 1:160 to 1:320) is presumptive; a fourfold rise to 1:640 to 1:1280 is diagnostic
May be false negative in localized brucellosis
Agglutination antibodies should begin a gradual decrease during convalescence and have faded after 1 year
Rapid increase suggests a relapse during chronic brucellosis

Erythrocyte sedimentation rate
Elevated

Differential WBC count
Relative or absolute lymphocytosis

Skin test: intradermal injection of 0.1 ml antigen
Induration and erythema at injection site within 48 hours indicate antibodies from present or past infection
Of questionable use for diagnosis

TREATMENT PLAN[7,15,95]

Surgical (depends on complications)
Splenectomy
Drainage of abscesses

Chemotherapeutic
Adults
  Anti-infective agents
    Tetracycline (Achromycin), 2 g/24 h po in four divided doses of 500 mg, plus
    Dihydrostreptomycin or streptomycin, 1-2 g/24 h po, plus
    Triple sulfonamides, 4-6 g/24 h po in four divided doses
Children
  Anti-infective agents
    Tetracycline, 30 mg/24 h, plus
    Streptomycin or dihydrostreptomycin, 25-40 mg/ kg/24 h po, plus
    Triple sulfonamides, 0.15 g/kg/24 h
In uncomplicated, acute cases, the combined therapy is given for 3 weeks followed by 2 weeks of tetracycline (1-2 g/24 h) alone; for chronic cases or cases with complications, combined therapy is given for 4-6 wk
Corticosteroids
  Steroids in severe disease

Supportive
Bed rest in severe and complicated cases
Additional supportive therapy depending on the complications
Diet: 3000 to 3700 cal/d; 2 g protein/kg/d

ASSESSMENT: AREAS OF CONCERN[15,95]

Early: subjective symptoms
Gradual-onset weakness and malaise; worsens as day progresses

Acute stage
  Body temperature
    Gradual rise in temperature (38° to 40° C [101° to 104° F]), showing sharp remissions
    Chills
    Continues for weeks, declines, and may spike again during a relapse

Subjective symptoms
Myalgia, severe in back and legs
Headache
Insomnia
Pain in joints, particularly hip, knee, ankle, and shoulder

Skin
Heavy perspiration with a disagreeable odor

Gastrointestinal concerns
Indigestion
Diarrhea or constipation
Weight loss
Bleeding

Lymph nodes
Lymphadenopathy: anterior and posterior cervical, axillary; small, firm, discrete, nontender

Oral mucous membranes
Gums become spongy and bleed easily when pressed

Respiratory concerns
Dry cough

Abdomen
Painful, enlarged spleen
Hepatomegaly less common

Mental status
Depression
Hysterical episodes

Complications
Symptoms of pneumonia and pleurisy, neurasthenia, meningoencephalitis, orchitis, epistaxis, extremely high fever, spondylitis, endocarditis

NURSING DIAGNOSES and NURSING INTERVENTIONS

Nursing Diagnosis	Nursing Intervention
Comfort, alteration in: pain	Administer analgesics as prescribed. Position for comfort. Apply heat to painful joints.
Oral mucous membrane, alteration in	Provide frequent oral hygiene. Observe gums for bleeding.
Activity intolerance	Maintain bed rest during acute illness; gradually increase activity during convalescence.
Skin integrity, impairment of: potential	Bathe; change position frequently; massage skin over bony prominences. Provide intermittent pressure mattress.
Thought processes, alteration in	Monitor for signs of depression or increasing irritability. Assure patient that these reactions are normal and temporary. Provide for safety, diversional activity, and opportunities for patient to verbalize concerns. Monitor for changes in mentation or consciousness indicating a complicating encephalitis; report to physician (p. 1566).
Nutrition, alteration in: less than body requirements	Offer frequent food and fluids in a variety that will encourage patient to eat. Measure intake and output to ensure adequate intake. Provide vitamin supplements and 3000 to 3700 cal/d diet, which is required because of increased metabolism due to fever.
Sleep pattern disturbance	Control the environment to facilitate sleep. Allow patient opportunities to relieve anxiety, such as by talking or listening to music before bedtime. Provide for relaxation techniques, such as bathing and massage.
Sensory-perceptual alteration: visual and auditory	Monitor for changes indicating an encephalitis and report to physician. Continuously monitor patient's safety. Interpret the environment to the patient.
Anxiety	Encourage patient to verbalize anxiety about prolonged illness and lost work and income. Refer to social service or to other community agencies if financial aid is needed.
Injury, potential for (chemotherapeutic agent)	Monitor for toxic reactions and temporary increase in severity of symptoms, which is sometimes precipitated by antimicrobial therapy. Note changes in temperature, other vital signs, levels of pain, and mood. Reassure patient and report changes to physician. Administer steroids, if ordered. Observe also for drug reactions such as hearing loss caused by streptomycin or severe diarrhea caused by tetracycline.
Potential patient problem: fever	Bathe patient frequently to lower body temperature and to remove perspiration. Administer oral fluids freely. Maintain comfortable environmental temperature with freely circulating air.

Patient Education

1. Premature resumption of activity during convalescence aggravates symptoms and predisposes to relapses. Convalescence may take 6 to 8 weeks in treated patients.
2. Patient must complete the entire medication regimen.
3. Patient should report to the physician any symptoms recurring after completion of the therapy, since another course of therapy will be required.
4. Duration of acquired immunity from the disease is uncertain. Patient should protect himself from exposure and reinfection and others from exposure:

   a. Drink only pasteurized milk and milk products.
   b. Boil milk if pasteurization is not possible.
   c. Animals suspected to be diseased should be tested and slaughtered if infected. Diseased meat should not be eaten.
   d. Placenta, discharges, and fetus from aborted animals should be handled with care (with gloves).
   e. Farmers, slaughterers, and butchers should handle carcasses or products of potentially infected animals with gloves.[7]

EVALUATION

Patient Outcome	Data Indicating That Outcome is Reached
Body temperature is normal.	Oral adult temperature is normal for 2 to 7 days.
Laboratory findings are within normal limits.	Erythrocyte sedimentation rate, differential WBC count, leukocyte count, RBC count, hematocrit, and hemoglobin are normal.
Nutrition and fluids are adequate for body requirements.	Patient has not lost weight, or daily weight is stabilized for body build. Skin color and turgor are good. Mucous membranes are moist. Urinary output equals fluid intake. Stools are soft, formed, and normal colored.
There is no chronic infection.	There is no malaise, weakness, or fatigue. Patient can perform all ADL without tiring and is mentally alert and attentive. There is no adenitis, arthritis, neurosensory alterations, or signs of other complications.
Patient is aware of needs and able to use resources.	Patient verbalizes intent to take entire course of antimicrobial therapy and to report to physician any recurrence of symptoms. Patient has plans for gradual return to normal activities and has realistic expectations for progress during convalescence. Patient has adequate income to support him through work lost during illness.

NEUROLOGIC INFECTIOUS DISEASES
Meningitis

Meningococcal meningitis is an acute communicable inflammation of the meninges caused by Neisseria meningitidis. *It frequently occurs in epidemic form.*

Haemophilus meningitis is an acute communicable inflammation of the meninges caused by Haemophilus influenzae. *It is the most common form of bacterial meningitis in general and is the most common type in neonates and small children.*

Pneumococcal meningitis is an acute inflammation of the meninges caused by Streptococcus pneumoniae. *The meningitis frequently results from an extension of a primary infection in the upper respiratory tract. This form of meningitis has a high risk for fatality.*

Viral (aseptic or serous) meningitis is an acute meningeal inflammation that occurs as a sequela to many viral diseases. The condition is usually self-limiting and benign.[7,64]

Meningitis is an inflammation of the meninges covering the brain and spinal cord. The inflammation may result from an acute infection of the meninges caused by the invasion of bacteria, viruses, fungi, or parasitic worms into the tissues or from the iatrogenic introduction of a substance that is irritating to the meninges. The forms of meningitis discussed in this section are those caused by bacterial and viral invasion.

The invasion may produce a primary or secondary infection. Some bacteria produce a primary focal infection in the meninges. Such is the case with the *N. meningitidis* and *H. influenzae*, which cause meningococcal and *Haemophilus* meningitides, respectively. Other bacterial and viral pathogens are capable of producing a secondary infection in the meninges following hematogenous dissemination from a primary focal infection elsewhere in the body. *H. influenzae, S. pneumoniae* (pneumococcal meningitis), many viruses, and other bacteria have this pathogenic potential.[112]

In addition to the differentiation as to primary and secondary infection, two clinical forms of meningitis, suppurative and nonsuppurative, can be identified. Suppurative (purulent) meningitis results from bacterial invasion and is manifested by a characteristic high leukocytosis in cerebrospinal fluid with the majority of the leukocytes being neutrophils. In nonsuppurative (aseptic or serous) meningitis, cerebrospinal fluid leukocytes are less and are made up primarily of lymphocytes. Viruses from an antecedent infection elsewhere in the body are the predominant causes of nonsuppurative meningitis[112] (Table 15-15).

Although many bacteria are capable of producing a suppurative meningitis, the most common forms are *Haemophilus,* meningococcal, and pneumococcal meningi-

Table 15-15
Overview of Meningitis[7]

	Meningococcal Meningitis	Pneumococcal Meningitis	Haemophilus Meningitis	Viral Meningitis (Aseptic)
Occurrence	Endemic and epidemic; worldwide; greatest during winter and spring; greatest in males, in children less than 5 yr, and in persons in crowded living conditions	Endemic; greatest in infants, elderly persons, and alcoholics; follows pneumococcal pneumonia	Worldwide; most common bacterial meningitis in children 2 mo to 3 yr	Worldwide; epidemics and sporadic cases associated with other infections
Etiologic agent	*Neisseria meningitidis,* with many subgroups	*Streptococcus pneumoniae,* many serotypes	*Haemophilus influenzae,* six serotypes; type B responsible for 90% of *Haemophilus* meningitis	Most viruses produce the syndrome: mumps, herpes, polio, etc.
Reservoir	Humans	Humans; many carriers	Humans	Humans
Transmission	Direct contact with droplets from respiratory passages of infected persons and carriers	Direct and indirect contact with discharges from respiratory passages	Direct contact with droplets from respiratory passages	
Incubation period	2-10 d; usually 3-4 d	1-3 d for pneumonia	2-4 d	
Period of communicability	Until organism is not present in discharges: within 24 h of treatment with sulfonamides	Until organism is not present in respiratory discharges: 24-48 h after antibiotic treatment	Prolonged; until organism is not present in nasal discharge	Depends on virus and associated viral disease
Susceptibility and resistance	Susceptibility to clinical disease is low; many carriers; group-specific immunity of unknown duration follows infection	Infants and elderly most susceptible; immunity for specific type persists for years	Children most susceptible; otitis media may be a precursor; immunity of unknown duration follows infection	
Report to local health authority	Mandatory case report	Only epidemics; no individual case reports	Yes in certain endemic areas	Yes in endemic areas

tides. They will be discussed together since their pathologic manifestations and symptomatology are similar. Viral meningitis will be discussed as a separate disease entity regardless of the viral disease that preceded the meningitis.

PATHOPHYSIOLOGY

Bacteria causing the suppurative meningitis being considered here are inhaled in mucous droplets from infected persons or carriers, invade the respiratory passages, and are disseminated by way of the blood to meninges of the brain and spinal cord. The respiratory phase is generally subclinical in meningococcal meningitis, although organisms present in respiratory secretions can be transmitted to another host. The respiratory phase is usually symptomatic in pneumococcal and *Haemophilus* menin-

gitides. The bacteremia produced during dissemination gives rise to toxic manifestations. In the case of meningococcus the organism penetrates and damages vascular endothelium, resulting in petechial and purpuric lesions of the skin.[112]

Bacteria in the meninges elicit an inflammatory response and the production of an exudate consisting of leukocytes, fibrin, and bacteria in the subarachnoid space. Cerebrospinal fluid may be thin or thick with plaquelike accumulations. In untreated disease the cerebrospinal fluid may become so thick as to interfere with its circulation and reabsorption. An internal or external hydrocephalus may result. Extension of the bacteria into brain tissue may produce a bacterial encephalitis.[112]

Meningococcal infections may be so severe in the systemic stage as to produce an acute meningococcemia, either leading to death or to the initiation of therapy before meningeal involvement. Meningococcemia may become chronic with toxic symptoms persisting intermittently for weeks or months. Recurrent meningitis is usually of the pneumococcal form and is frequently associated with an undetected skull fracture.[112]

Complications of bacterial meningitis include internal hydrocephalus, deficits of cranial nerve function leading to blindness and deafness, arthritis, myocarditis, pericarditis, and neuromotor and intellectual deficits. Symptomatic and asymptomatic infection with bacterial meningitis does result in a protective immune response of unknown duration.[112]

Aseptic (viral, serous, or nonsuppurative) meningitis is a syndrome generally associated with an existing systemic viral disease, the most common one being mumps. Inflammation and lymphocytic infiltration of the meninges occur with a wide gradient in clinical severity depending on the infectious agent. Toxic and meningeal symptoms are usually less severe than in suppurative meningitis. This form may also progress to clinical encephalitis. The disease is usually self-limiting with complete recovery, although patients may experience muscle weakness and malaise during a prolonged convalescence.[112]

DIAGNOSTIC STUDIES[64,112]

Cerebrospinal fluid examination
Gross appearance
Turbid: bacterial
Clear: viral (aseptic)

Leukocytes
500 to 20,000/cmm: bacterial
10 to 500/cmm: viral (aseptic)

Cell types
Neutrophils: bacterial
Lymphocytes: viral (aseptic)

Protein
Increased for both

Glucose
Low to normal: bacterial
Normal: viral (aseptic)

Cerebrospinal fluid culture or Gram's stain or serologic techniques (counterimmunoelectrophoresis, coagulation, latex agglutination, or fluorescent antibody techniques)
Positive for bacteria
Absence of bacteria with cerebrospinal fluid cell changes would suggest viral (aseptic) meningitis

Gram's stain of scrapings from petechial skin lesions
Positive for meningococci

Blood culture
Positive for *H. influenzae* or *N. meningitidis* (meningococci)

Serology
Increase in antibody titer with specific viral infections

TREATMENT PLAN[7,112]

Chemotherapeutic*
Anti-infective agents
  Initial therapy until organism is identified
    Ampicillin, 200 mg/kg/24 h IV plus chloramphenicol if *H. influenzae* is suspected for patients over 2 mo of age
    Ampicillin, 75-150 mg/kg/24 h IV, plus gentamicin (Garamycin), 6 mg/kg/24 h for infants under 2 mo of age
  Definitive therapy: meningococci or pneumococci
    Ampicillin (Amcill), 200 mg/kg/24 h IV, or chloramphenicol (Chloromycetin), 100 mg/kg/24 h IV to a maximum of 4 g
  Definitive therapy: *H. influenzae*
    Ampicillin or chloramphenicol (Chloromycetin), 100 mg/kg/24 h IV to a maximum of 4 g
  All of the above are administered by rapid intravenous infusion. Initial dose should be one third of daily dose, the remainder divided into six equal doses. Therapy should continue for 5 days after temperature is normal and clinical signs have cleared. Barbiturates may be given for seizures.
Analgesics for headache and muscle pain (nonnarcotic)[112]
Immunologic agents for prevention of bacterial meningitides
  Meningococcal polysaccharide vaccine against group A and C serotypes for those over age 2 yr at risk for epidemic disease; given in single dose (0.5 ml subq)
  Meningococcal vaccine against group A serotype can be given to children 3 mo to 2 yr; given in two doses 3 mo apart
    Routine immunization of civilians not recommended
Anti-infective agents for meningococcal contacts
  Rifampin (Rifamycin, others), 600 mg bid (adults) for 2 d; 10 mg/kg bid (children over 1 mo of age);

*For bacterial meningitis.

5 mg/kg (children under 1 mo of age); may be used to treat carriers

Sulfadiazine, 1 g bid for 3 d for mass prophylaxis during meningococcal epidemics or for close patient contacts if strain is proven susceptible

Electromechanical
Intratracheal tubation
Ventilatory assistance

Supportive[7,112]
IV therapy and dopamine if shock is present
Fluid restriction to two thirds of daily needs if excess secretion of ADH
Control of intracranial pressure
Close monitoring for early diagnosis of patient contacts

ASSESSMENT: AREAS OF CONCERN[7,64,112]

Subjective symptoms
Severe throbbing headache
Muscle pains
Stiff neck
Backache
Chills

Body temperature
38° to 41° C (100° to 106° F), starting in systemic phase

Pulse
May be slow as intracranial pressure increases

Cardiovascular concerns
Symptoms of shock with increase in intracranial pressure

Level of consciousness
Alert early in disease but may show delirium progressing to deep coma later

Neurologic concerns
Reflex changes: absence of abdominal reflexes; absence of cremasteric reflexes in male; alteration of tendon reflexes
Resistance to neck flexion

Brudzinski's sign positive: attempted flexion of neck will elicit flexion of knees and hips

Kernig's sign positive: limitation in angle at which a straight leg may be raised from bed with patient in supine position

In addition to the above symptoms of meningitis some symptoms are characteristic of specific forms of the disease:

Pneumococcal
Symptoms of pneumonia or otitis media frequently precede the meningitis

Meningococcal
Petechial and purpuric skin lesions preceded by a rash resembling measles on trunk and extremities
Large ecchymotic lesions on face and extremities in severe disease

Haemophilus
Respiratory concerns
Symptoms of pneumonia or otitis media frequently precede the meningitis

Head
Bulging fontanelle in infants

Chronic meningococcemia
Musculoskeletal concerns
Swelling and pain in large joints, particularly knees and ankles

Skin
Recurrent macular or petechial lesions

Subjective symptoms
Headache
Malaise
Irritability

Body temperature
Intermittent low-grade fever

Aseptic meningitis
Symptoms preceding meningeal signs depend on the disease and its etiologic agent; may have parotid swelling of mumps, respiratory or gastrointestinal symptoms, skin manifestations of measles or chickenpox

NURSING DIAGNOSES and NURSING INTERVENTIONS

Nursing Diagnosis	Nursing Intervention
Tissue perfusion, alteration in: cerebral	Monitor patient carefully, particularly after lumbar puncture.
	Have patient lie flat for 4 to 6 hours or as ordered after lumbar puncture.
	Watch for changes in pulse.

Nursing Diagnosis	Nursing Intervention
	Monitor for signs of intracranial pressure throughout course of the disease: slowing of pulse, increase in blood pressure, decreased level of consciousness, arrhythmic breathing, altered pupillary response, facial weakness (see also Chapter 3 for further neurologic assessment).
	Monitor vital signs and neurologic findings every 5 to 30 minutes for patient with intracranial pressure.
	Report changes to physician immediately.
	Avoid any position or movement of patient that would increase intracranial pressure.
	Provide for bed rest.
	Elevate patient's head slightly.
	Prevent any sudden or unnecessary movements of patient's head and neck and avoid neck flexion.
	Assist patient with all activities and movement to prevent muscle straining.
	Administer stool softeners as prescribed (avoid enemas).
	Instruct patient to exhale while turning or moving in bed.
	Position to avoid knee or hip flexion.
	Time and space nursing procedures to coincide with periods of relaxation or sedation.
	Avoid unnecessary environmental stimuli.
	Administer hypertonic agents as prescribed.
	Evaluate during convalescence for motor, sensory, and intellectual impairment.
Airway clearance, ineffective	Maintain fully patent airway for patient with increased intracranial pressure.
	Suction secretions; perform endotracheal care.
	Continually supervise patient having convulsions.
Gas exchange, impaired	Monitor blood gases.
	Preoxygenate before suctioning, and limit suctioning to 10 to 15 seconds for apneic patients.
	Employ mechanical ventilation if necessary.
	Continually monitor delirious or convulsive patient.
Injury, potential for: trauma	Pad bed and provide restraints for delirious patient.
	Prevent aspiration or injury during convulsions.
Fluid volume deficit, potential	Administer frequent oral or continuous IV fluids.
	Monitor intake and output and signs of fluid retention.
	Restrict IV fluids to two thirds of needs if signs of fluid retention occur.
Nutrition, alteration in: less than body requirements	Provide high-calorie liquids and nasogastric tube feedings if needed.
Comfort, alteration in: pain	Administer analgesics as prescribed. (Do not give narcotics or sedatives that will depress vital functions in patients with increased intracranial pressure.)
	Provide moist heat for muscle aches and pains in absence of high fever.
	Place blanket roll under knees in absence of elevated intracranial pressure.
Mobility, impaired physical	Administer range of motion exercises to patient without signs of elevated intracranial pressure.
	Frequently change position to prevent contractures and decubiti.
Self-care deficit	Provide all feeding and hygiene measures for patient.
Urinary elimination, alteration in patterns	Assess for retention.
	Maintain indwelling catheter if necessary.
Potential patient problem: fever	Take rectal temperature every 2 hours.
	Administer antipyretics as prescribed.
	Sponge with tepid water or alcohol in water.
Potential patient problem: transmission of infection	Employ respiratory isolation for 24 hours after initiation of antimicrobial therapy for bacterial meningitis (p. 1621).
	Employ excretion precautions for duration of hospitalization for viral meningitis (p. 1621).
	Assist in collection of cerebrospinal fluid specimens.
	Record amount and character of cerebrospinal fluid.
	Administer IV antibiotics as prescribed.

EVALUATION

Patient Outcome	Data Indicating That Outcome is Reached
Body temperature is normal.	Oral adult temperature and rectal adult and children's temperatures are normal for 5 days.
Cerebrospinal fluid findings are normal.	There are less than 30 cells/cmm. Glucose, protein, and pressure are normal. There are no organisms in cultures. Color is clear.
Blood pressure, pulse, and respirations are normal.	Blood pressure, pulse, and respirations are normal.
All cells receive oxygen.	Blood levels (O_2 saturation, carbon dioxide, and PO_2) are normal.
There is no systemic infection.	There are no skin petechiae or purpura. Blood cultures are negative for bacteria.
Patient returns to premorbid level of consciousness.	Patient is alert, responds appropriately to questions and environmental stimuli, and is oriented to person and place. Patient has memory for recent and past events.
Patient exhibits appropriate motor responses to stimuli.	Pupils are equal and reactive to light. There is no resistance to neck flexion. Straight legs may be raised from the bed with patient in a prone position. Abdominal, cremasteric, and tendon reflexes are normal. Patient is able to walk and carry out all functions without residual weakness or impairment.
Patient does not experience pain.	Patient does not have headache or pain in neck and back.

Encephalitis

Amebic meningoencephalitis is an acute and severe inflammation of the brain and meninges caused by invasion of the tissues by a free-living ameba usually found in water, soil, and decaying vegetation. The disease is frequently fatal.

Mosquito-borne viral encephalitides are a group of acute inflammatory diseases of the brain, spinal cord, and meninges caused by a variety of viruses transmitted to humans through the bite of infected mosquitoes.

Infectious viral encephalitides are acute inflammations of the central nervous system associated with, and as a sequela to, systemic viral infections; they are caused commonly by the genus Herpesvirus.[7]

Whereas meningitis is an inflammation of the meninges covering the brain and spinal cord, encephalitis is an inflammation of the tissues of the brain and spinal cord, resulting in altered function of various portions of these tissues. Encephalitis is frequently also accompanied by signs of systemic infection. Clinical disease manifestations range from mild to severe to death; and disease may be followed by temporary or permanent neurologic sequelae or complete recovery.[64]

Like meningitis, encephalitis may result from a variety of causes: (1) a toxemia accompanying an infectious disease, (2) an allergic response to microbial antigens, (3) direct invasion of central nervous system tissue by pathogens as a primary focal infection, or (4) direct invasion of central nervous system tissue secondary to hematogenous dissemination from a primary focal infection elsewhere in the body. Direct invasion, either primary or secondary, is usually caused by a virus, a great many of which are capable of producing encephalitis.[26]

The majority of viruses producing encephalitis as a primary focal infection are transmitted by mosquitoes and will be discussed together. Encephalitides occurring secondary to other viral diseases will be discussed as infectious encephalitis. A rarer form of meningoencephalitis caused by direct invasion of an ameba will also be described (Table 15-16).

PATHOPHYSIOLOGY

Amebic meningoencephalitis. Two types of amebae, *Naegleria* and *Acanthamoeba*, are capable of producing meningoencephalitis in humans. *Naegleria* infection is acquired when water containing the pathogen is forced into the nasal passages, usually by diving or swimming in water containing large amounts of organic matter. The organism colonizes and invades the mucosa and travels along olfactory nerves to the meninges and brain, pro-

Table 15-16
Overview of Encephalitis[7]

	Amebic Meningoencephalitis	Mosquito-Borne Viral Encephalitides (Equine and St. Louis Encephalitis)	Infectious Viral Encephalitis
Occurrence	Worldwide, but rare; greatest in young persons, in warm climates, and during summer	Warm, moist climates; summer and early fall when mosquitoes are greatest	Worldwide; epidemic and sporadic; associated with other viral diseases
Etiologic agent	*Naegleria fowleri; Acanthamoeba culbertsoni*	A variety of diseases, each caused by a different virus	A variety of viruses, commonly the *Herpesvirus*
Reservoir	Amebae are free living in water and soil	Birds, rodents, bats, reptiles, amphibians; differing for each virus	Humans
Transmission	Water infected with *N. fowleri* forced into nasal passages while swimming; *Acanthamoeba* enters a skin lesion	Bite of infective mosquitoes	Direct contact with droplets from respiratory passages or other excretions harboring the virus
Incubation period	3-7 d or longer	5-15 d	Depends on viral disease
Period of communicability	Not communicable person to person	Not communicable person to person; mosquitoes are infective for life	Depends on viral disease
Susceptibility and resistance	Unknown; immunosuppressed persons are susceptible to infection with *Acanthamoeba*	Highest susceptibility to clinical disease is infancy and old age; in endemic areas, adults are immune to local strains of virus because of subclinical infections	Depends on viral disease
Report to local health authority	Only for means of surveillance	Mandatory case report	In select endemic areas

ducing a severe and rapidly fatal fulminating pyogenic meningoencephalitis. *Acanthamoeba* colonizes a skin lesion and travels to the central nervous system along peripheral nerves to produce a meningoencephalitis with a more insidious onset and prolonged course. Immunologic investigations have shown many people to have a natural antibody against these organisms, suggesting that more subclinical than clinical infections may occur.[7,50]

Mosquito-borne viral encephalitis. A variety of viruses capable of infecting animals and birds can be carried to humans by vector mosquitoes that feed on the infected animals. The virus, injected into humans from a mosquito bite, rapidly localizes in the central nervous system and produces congestion, edema, and small hemorrhages in the brain. Neuronal lesions with nerve cell necrosis and destruction and foci of cellular infiltration are widespread throughout the brain and spinal cord. Disease severity depends on the virus and on host resistance factors. Generally, older persons are more severely affected and have the highest fatality. Disease onset may be acute or insidious, depending on the virus involved. Infants generally have a more acute-onset encephalitis

than do other age groups. Infants and children are also more likely to develop motor and mental disabilities (seizures, hydrocephalus, and mental retardation) as a sequela to mosquito-borne encephalitis.

An antibody response can be seen within 7 days. Duration of the disease is variable, depending on the virus. Blood leukocytes are generally normal or slightly elevated with some viruses. The virus cannot be recovered from blood, secretions, or discharges and is therefore not communicable from person to person.[7,26]

Infectious encephalitis. A variety of directly transmittable viruses are capable of producing encephalitides either as a concomitant to or as a sequela to clinical viral disease (e.g., measles, mumps, rubella, and chickenpox) or as a result of a subclinical viral infection such as herpes. In both cases the pathologic manifestations of the encephalitis may result from a postinfection autoimmune response to the virus or from direct invasion of the central nervous system by the virus. Timing of the onset of central nervous system manifestations in relationship to the associated disease symptomatology and the ability to isolate the virus from cerebrospinal fluid allow differentiation as to postinfection or direct invasion encephalitis.[64]

Disease onset may be acute or insidious, and disease severity may be mild to severe depending on the virus and on the distribution, location, and concentration of the neuronal lesions. Mumps virus usually produces a more benign disease whereas herpes encephalitis is frequently fatal. Permanent neurologic sequelae are also more common in herpes infections.[64]

DIAGNOSTIC STUDIES

Amebic meningoencephalitis[50]
Phase contrast microscopic examination of fresh spinal fluid mount
Mobile amebae can be visualized

Cerebrospinal fluid examination
Large number of polymorphonuclear leukocytes; may be RBCs

Mosquito-borne viral encephalitis[7,26]
Neutralization, complement fixation, hemagglutination inhibition, fluorescent antibody, or agar gel precipitation
Fourfold increase in antibody titer between early disease and convalescence

Blood count
Leukocytes vary with virus: range from 10,000 to 66,000/cmm

Cerebrospinal fluid examination
Not diagnostic
Leukocytes: 50 to 500/cmm; sometimes as high as 1000/cmm in infants; usually lymphocytes

Infectious viral encephalitis[7,26]
Complement fixation, hemagglutination inhibition, or neutralization
Fourfold decrease in antibody titer between early disease and convalescence

Cerebrospinal fluid examination
Virus isolation
Increase in protein: 50 to 150 mg/dl
RBCs; leukocytes: 50 to 500/cmm, predominantly lymphocytes

TREATMENT PLAN[26,50,64]

Chemotherapeutic
Anti-infective agents
Amebic meningoencephalitis: combination of the following drugs (individual dose calculation)
Amphotericin B (Fungizone), IV

Sulfadiazine, IV
Miconazole (Monistat), IV
Rifampin (Rifamycin; others), po
Mosquito-borne: no specific treatment
Infectious viral encephalitides: no specific treatment except for herpes infections; adenine arabinoside (Vidarabine, ara-A) IV 15 mg/kg/24 h for 10 d

Electromechanical
Tracheostomy
Assisted ventilation
Suction

Supportive
Sedatives for hyperexcitability and seizures
IV fluids and electrolytes
Nasogastric tube feedings

ASSESSMENT: AREAS OF CONCERN[26,50,64]

Body temperature
39° to 41° C (102° to 105° F)
May be acute-onset fever accompanying central nervous system symptoms, or there may be a 1- to 4-day prodromal period with fever and chills before central nervous system symptoms

Central nervous system
Signs of meningeal irritation: severe frontal headache, nausea, vomiting, dizziness, nuchal rigidity

Level of consciousness
Alterations in consciousness: mild listlessness progressing to confusion, stupor, and eventual coma
May have extreme irritability
Bizarre behavior with temporal lobe involvement of herpes encephalitis
Seizures, particularly in infants with postinfectious encephalitis

Neurologic concerns
Focal neurologic signs
Aphasia
Olfactory hallucinations

Motor concerns
Weakness, accentuated deep tendon reflexes, extensor plantar response
Ataxia, spasticity, and tremors
In herpes encephalitis there may be a flaccid paralysis and depression of tendon reflexes with spinal cord involvement and bowel and bladder paralysis
Postinfectious encephalitis may not manifest motor signs

Regulatory mechanisms
Excess or deficient antidiuretic hormone secretion
Increasing hyperthermia

NURSING DIAGNOSES and NURSING INTERVENTIONS

Nursing Diagnosis	Nursing Intervention
Tissue perfusion, alteration in: cerebral	Monitor patient carefully, particularly after lumbar puncture. Have patient lie flat for 4 to 6 hours or as ordered after lumbar puncture. Watch for changes in pulse. Monitor for signs of intracranial pressure throughout course of the disease: slowing of pulse, increase in blood pressure, decreased level of consciousness, arrhythmic breathing, altered pupillary response, and facial weakness (see Chapter 3 for further neurologic assessment). Monitor vital signs and neurologic findings every 5 to 30 minutes for patient with intracranial pressure. Report changes to physician immediately. Avoid any position or movement of patient that would increase intracranial pressure. Provide for bed rest. Elevate patient's head slightly. Prevent any sudden or unnecessary movements of patient's head and neck and avoid neck flexion. Assist patient with all activities and movement to prevent muscle straining. Administer stool softeners as prescribed (avoid enemas). Instruct patient to exhale while turning or moving in bed. Position to avoid knee or hip flexion. Time and space nursing procedures to coincide with periods of relaxation or sedation. Avoid unnecessary environmental stimuli. Administer hypertonic agents as prescribed. Evaluate during convalescence for motor, sensory, and intellectual impairment.
Airway clearance, ineffective	Maintain fully patent airway for patient with increased intracranial pressure. Suction secretions; provide endotracheal care. Continually supervise patient having convulsions.
Gas exchange, impaired	Monitor blood gases. Preoxygenate before suctioning, and limit suctioning to 10 to 15 seconds for apneic patients. Employ mechanical ventilation if necessary. Continually monitor delirious or convulsive patient.
Injury, potential for: trauma	Pad bed and provide restraints for delirious patient. Prevent aspiration or injury during convulsions.
Fluid volume deficit, potential	Administer frequent oral or continuous IV fluids. Monitor intake and output and signs of fluid retention. Restrict IV fluids to two thirds of needs if signs of fluid retention occur.
Nutrition, alteration in: less than body requirements	Provide high-calorie liquids and nasogastric tube feedings if needed.
Comfort, alteration in: pain	Administer analgesics as prescribed. (Do not give narcotics or sedatives that will depress vital functions in patients with increased intracranial pressure.) Provide moist heat for muscle aches and pains in absence of high fever. Place blanket roll under knees in absence of elevated intracranial pressure.
Self-care deficit	Provide all feeding and hygiene measures for patient.
Urinary elimination, alteration in patterns	Assess for retention. Maintain indwelling catheter if necessary.
Potential patient problem: fever	Take rectal temperature every 2 hours. Administer antipyretics as prescribed. Sponge with tepid water or alcohol in water.
Breathing pattern, ineffective	Monitor closely for signs of respiratory paralysis, and initiate ventilatory assistance as needed.
Sensory-perceptual alteration: visual, auditory, olfactory	Minimize environmental stimuli; give clear, concise explanations to patient. Clarify stimuli that patient may be misperceiving. Monitor for reflex and sensory changes.

Nursing Diagnosis	Nursing Intervention
Thought processes, alterations in	Supervise closely; disoriented patients cannot be responsible for their actions. Protect from injury: side rails and so on. Monitor for changes in level of consciousness, orientation, and memory. Reorient the confused patient as appropriate.
Mobility, impaired physical	Use intermittent-pressure mattress, foot board, and frequent turning of comatose patients. Administer range of motion exercises. Give attention to body alignment. Gradually increase physical activity during convalescence. Monitor for impaired motor ability during convalescence. Refer for graded rehabilitation therapy, and reinforce and support patient's relearning efforts on the unit.
Potential patient problem: transmission of infection	The viral disease associated with infectious viral encephalitis can be transmitted, and isolation procedures specific for the disease should be instituted (see specific diseases in this chapter and p. 1620). Only general principles of asepsis are necessary for amebic meningoencephalitis or mosquito-borne encephalitis.

Patient Education

1. Amebic meningoencephalitis can be prevented by swimming in chlorinated pools only.
2. Mosquito-borne encephalitis can be prevented by environmental control of mosquitoes, particularly through elimination of their breeding places in stagnant pools of water and by avoidance of exposure to mosquitoes by wearing protective clothing, screening living quarters, and using repellants.
3. Sequelae of encephalitis include mental deterioration, paralysis, and possible convulsive disorders, particularly in children. Families should be informed of the need for periodic evaluation and long-term physical therapy and of potential resources to help them cope with a handicapped family member.

EVALUATION

Patient Outcome	Data Indicating That Outcome is Reached
Cerebrospinal fluid findings are normal.	There are less than 30 cells/cmm. Glucose, protein, and pressure are normal. There are no organisms in cultures. Color is clear.
Vital signs are normal.	Blood pressure, temperature, pulse, and respirations are normal.
All cells receive oxygen.	Blood levels (O_2 saturation, carbon dioxide, and P_{O_2}) are normal.
Motor responses to stimuli are appropriate.	Pupils are equal and reactive to light. There is no resistance to neck flexion. Straight legs may be raised from the bed with patient in a prone position. Abdominal, cremasteric, and tendon reflexes are normal. Patient is able to walk and carry out all functions without residual weakness or impairment.
There is no pain.	Patient does not have headache or pain in neck and back.
Motor function is normal, or patient is participating in therapeutic exercise.	Patient has full range of motion and is increasing in muscle strength and in purposeful movement and coordination. Patient is able to or is increasing in ability to ambulate and to carry out all activities of daily living.

Patient Outcome	Data Indicating That Outcome is Reached
Sensory perceptions are normal.	Patient responds appropriately to all stimuli. Visual, hearing, smell, and touch tests are positive. There is no hallucinatory behavior.
Mental status is normal.	Patient is oriented to person, place, and time and exhibits recall of recent and past events. Affect is appropriate to environmental stimuli. Patient is awake and responds to environmental stimuli. Adults demonstrate cognitive ability, ability to problem solve, concentration, and attentiveness.
The patient or family is aware of needs and able to use resources.	Patient or family of patient with a residual limitation in physical or mental function has been referred for appropriate therapy during convalescence. Parents of disabled infants and children have been given an opportunity to express their concerns and have been referred for counseling and to support groups if necessary. Parents understand the need for periodic reevaluation of their child's limitations and progress.

INFECTIOUS DISEASES OF THE SKIN

The two diseases discussed in this section are manifested primarily with skin lesions with potential or actual systemic pathologic findings. They are differentiated from skin infections discussed in Chapter 5 because a distinct pathogen causes each of these conditions (Table 15-17).

Leprosy

Leprosy is a chronic systemic infection characterized by lesions of the skin and mucous membranes, involvement and palpable enlargement of peripheral nerves, and trophic changes in skin, muscle, and bone.[7]

PATHOPHYSIOLOGY[17,65]

The exact transmission of the *Mycobacterium leprae* is uncertain. The organism can be found in the skin lesions, nasal passages, blood, and breast milk of infected persons, suggesting that transmission may be possible through routes other than skin contact. The disease is not

Table 15-17
Overview of Infectious Diseases of the Skin[7]

	Leprosy	Erysipelas (Necrotizing Cellulitis)
Occurrence	11 million cases in world; highest in low socioeconomic areas; endemic in some tropic and subtropic areas; increasing in United States	Sporadic; most common in people over 20 yr and in infants
Etiologic agent	*Mycobacterium leprae* (Hansen's bacillus)	*Streptococcus pyogenes,* group A, with 70 serologically distinct types
Reservoir	Humans; infection has been found in armadillos in Louisiana and Texas	Humans
Transmission	Prolonged intimate contact; agent gains entrance through broken skin and respiratory passages	Direct contact with person infected with organism or with a carrier
Incubation period	3-6 yr; shortest known is 7 mo	1-3 d
Period of communicability	As long as bacilli are present; not communicable after 3 mo of treatment	10-21 d; months in untreated cases with purulent discharge
Susceptibility and resistance	Resistance depends on ability to develop a cell-mediated immunity; children may be more susceptible	General; one attack predisposes person to subsequent attacks; women and those with debilitating conditions more susceptible
Report to local health authority	Mandatory case report	Only outbreaks; no individual case reports

highly contagious. Because the incubation period is long, there is speculation that adult-onset disease may actually have been acquired in childhood.

The disease is differentiated into two forms, lepromatous and tuberculoid, with borderline classifications representing the clinical expressions between the two distinct forms. The exact clinical expression of the disease may be determined in part by cell-mediated immune responses in the host; a cellular immune response is lacking in those persons developing lepromatous leprosy.

Both forms produce progressively destructive granulomatous skin and mucous membrane lesions, which can be differentiated histologically, and sensory and autonomic peripheral nerve damage.

The course of the lepromatous type is progressive and malignant with continual activity of the organism in the lesions causing an extensive, gradually developing granulomatous condition in the skin and peripheral nerves and a continuous bacteremia. Nerve destruction leads to atrophy of skin and muscles and eventual absorption of small bones with extensive deformity. Erythema nodosum and eye damage, secondary to corneal insensitivity, are possible complications.

The course of the tuberculoid type is benign and less progressive, with few bacteria in the lesions but with acute-onset asymmetric nerve involvement.

DIAGNOSTIC STUDIES[65]

Microscopic examination of stained tissue from lesion
Positive for acid-fast bacilli

Biopsy from periphery of skin lesion
Foamy lepra cells plus acid-fast bacilli in lepromatous leprosy
Damage to peripheral nerves in tuberculoid leprosy

Lepromin skin test for patients with known leprosy to distinguish the types
Positive test: hard nodule in 3 to 4 weeks after intradermal injection; majority of the population shows a positive test
Positive in patients with tuberculoid leprosy
Negative in patients with lepromatous leprosy

TREATMENT PLAN

Surgical
Plastic surgery to correct deformities

Chemotherapeutic[7]
Anti-infective agents
Dapsone (DDS), 6-10 mg/kg/wk, po, given in daily doses for 10 yr in lepromatous leprosy and for 5 yr in tuberculoid disease
Rifampicin, po, may be given daily for a few months for new cases to supplement DDS

Supportive[7]
Counseling to cope with stigma attached to the disease
Orthopedic aids
Prevention: immunization of close contacts with BCG; prophylactic treatment of contacts with dapsone for 3 years

ASSESSMENT: AREAS OF CONCERN[7,65]

Skin
Initial: flat pigmented or erythematoid skin lesions
Lepromatous: Symmetric lesions consisting of numerous macules, with diffuse infiltrations and margins shading into the surrounding skin; lesions may be nodular and may ulcerate; they are not anesthetic; usually appear on earlobes, nose, eyebrows, forehead, cheeks, lips, elbows, and fingers; loss of hair, particularly eyebrows
Tuberculoid: asymmetric, circumscribed dry macules or plaques; always anesthetic

Neurologic concerns
Peripheral nerves: local or widespread anesthesia; muscle weakness, atrophy, and paralysis; trophic ulcers; disfigurement on extremities resulting from traumatic injury
Eye: photophobia, conjunctivitis, paralysis of eyelids; corneal injury

Upper respiratory tract
Nasal stuffiness or obstruction
Epistaxis
Perforated septum
Collapse of nasal bridge
Ulceration in any mucous membrane
Difficulty in breathing or swallowing
Change in timbre of voice

Systemic concerns
Manifestations of erythema nodosum leprosum: malaise, fever, lymphadenopathy, and arthralgia

NURSING DIAGNOSES and NURSING INTERVENTIONS

Nursing Diagnosis	Nursing Intervention
Noncompliance (potential)	See ''Patient Education.''
Self-concept, disturbance in: body image	Refer for or provide the long-term support and rehabilitative help that is needed for patients with disfigurement. (See p. 1820 for additional intervention.)
Potential patient problem: transmission to others	See ''Patient Education.''

Patient Education[7]

1. Compliance with therapy is necessary. Explain side effects of long-term drug treatment.
2. Patient should report medication reactions to physician immediately.
3. Household contacts of patient should be examined every 6 to 12 months for at least 5 years.
4. Assure patient that continuing with therapy can minimize disfigurement.

EVALUATION

Patient Outcome	Data Indicating That Outcome is Reached
Patient is complying with treatment.	Patient is taking prescribed medication and is returning for periodic evaluation. Close contacts are being evaluated.
Patient is aware of needs and able to use resources.	Patient is using rehabilitative or counseling services as needed.

Erysipelas

Erysipelas is an acute inflammatory reaction of the superficial lymphatics of the skin accompanied by fever and systemic symptoms.

PATHOPHYSIOLOGY

Erysipelas is an acute, rapidly progressive inflammatory reaction of superficial lymph vessels. It is frequently associated with a previous respiratory or systemic infection with group A streptococcus or with preexisting lymph obstruction. Lymph channels become filled with the streptococci, leukocytes, and fibrin. The inflammation spreads peripherally through the lymph channels, creating a lesion characteristic of the condition. The infection may remain localized in the dermis or may extend into subcutaneous tissue, forming a cellulitis, or it may be disseminated into the blood to produce a bacteremia. Leukocytosis is always present. There is a tendency for the condition to recur.[64,102]

DIAGNOSTIC STUDIES

There are no tests to diagnose erysipelas definitively since the group A streptococcus is rarely isolated or cultured from lesion exudate. A history of a streptococcal infection plus the characteristics of the lesion is used for diagnosis.

TREATMENT PLAN

Chemotherapeutic[102]
Anti-infective agents
  Mild cases in adult
    Procaine penicillin (Wycillin), 600,000 units IM once or twice daily, or
    Penicillin V (V-cillin), 250-500 g po q6h, or
    Erythromycin (Erythrocin), 0.25-0.5 mg po q6h
  Extensive cases: penicillin G, 600,000-2,000,000 units IV q6h

ASSESSMENT: AREAS OF CONCERN[7,64,110]

Skin
Abrupt-onset, hot, stinging, itching of skin
Painful, red, indurated thickening, which begins as a small lesion that spreads marginally for 4 to 6 days; margins have a raised, firm, palpable border

Rash on face may have a butterfly distribution; central point of origin may clear as periphery extends; face and legs are common sites; raised portion may contain superficial blebs with clear yellowish fluid

Systemic symptoms
Fever
May have sore throat and cervical adenopathy, headache, vomiting

NURSING DIAGNOSES and NURSING INTERVENTIONS

Nursing Diagnosis	Nursing Intervention
Skin integrity, impairment of: actual	Administer antibiotics as prescribed. Apply cool, sterile saline dressings to decrease pain. Observe for symptoms of systemic spread of infection. Elevate and immobilize extremity if lesion is on an extremity.

Patient Education

1. Patient must take complete course of antibiotic therapy.
2. Report recurrence of pain, erythema, or edema to physician.

EVALUATION

Patient Outcome	Data Indicating That Outcome is Reached
There is no infection.	Temperature is normal. Blood leukocyte count is normal. There is no heat, erythema, pain, or edema of skin.

ARTHROPOD-TRANSMITTED FEVERS

The diseases presented in this section are severe systemic infections of the blood caused by pathogens transmitted to humans by an infected arthropod. The rickettsial fevers, caused by rickettsiae that are transmitted by infected body lice, fleas, mites, or ticks, are presented first. The mosquito-borne fevers, malaria and dengue, caused by protozoa and viruses, are discussed second. Table 15-18 summarizes arthropod-borne fevers.

Rickettsial Fevers: Rocky Mountain Spotted Fever, Epidemic and Endemic Typhus

Rocky Mountain spotted fever is an acute rickettsial infectious disease transmitted to humans by infected ticks and manifested by severe systemic symptoms and a macular or maculopapular rash. The disease is severe, with a 10% to 20% fatality, increasing with age, in the untreated.

Epidemic typhus is an acute rickettsial infectious disease transmitted from person to person by infected body lice during epidemics. It is characterized by acute-onset, severe systemic symptoms and a macular rash. Fatality in untreated individuals is 10% to 40%.

Endemic (murine) typhus is an acute rickettsial infectious disease transmitted to humans by fleas that have fed on infected rats. It is clinically similar to epidemic typhus, but milder, with a fatality rate of 2% in untreated individuals.[64]

Ten immunologically distinct, but clinically similar, infectious diseases are caused by different types of rickettsiae. Five of these diseases have occurred in the United States: epidemic typhus, endemic (murine) typhus, Rocky Mountain spotted fever, rickettsialpox, and Q fever. Rocky Mountain spotted fever and endemic typhus occur with the greatest frequency. Although epidemic typhus is now rare, it will be discussed together with endemic typhus because of the clinical similarities (Table 15-18).

Table 15-18
Overview of Arthropod-Transmitted Fevers[7]

	Rickettsial Fevers			Mosquito-Borne Fevers	
	Rocky Mountain Spotted Fever	**Epidemic Typhus Fever (Louse Borne)**	**Endemic Typhus Fever (Flea Borne; Murine Typhus)**	**Malaria**	**Dengue**
Occurrence	United States: spring and summer; in western United States incidence is highest in adult males; in eastern United States, highest in children; two thirds of cases are from North and South Carolina, Virginia, Maryland, Georgia, Tennessee, and Oklahoma	Endemic in underdeveloped areas; epidemics occur; last outbreak in United States in 1921	Worldwide; found in areas where rats are uncontrolled; increases in late summer and autumn; 80 cases/yr in United States	Endemic in tropics and subtropics; acquired by travelers to those areas; 400-800 cases/yr in United States	Endemic in tropical areas; recent epidemics in Central America, Mexico, the Caribbean, and Rio Grande valley; migrating north; most cases in United States are presently acquired by travelers to endemic areas
Etiologic agent	*Rickettsia rickettsii*	*Rickettsia prowazekii*	*Rickettsia typhi*	*Plasmodium vivax, P. malariae, P. falciparum, P. ovale*	Flavivirus, four immunologically distinct serotypes (types 1, 2, 3, and 4)
Reservoir	Ticks	Humans	Rats	Humans	Mosquitoes and humans as one reservoir
Transmission	Bite of infected tick	Infected body louse	Infected rat fleas carry agent to humans	Bite of infected female *Anopheles* mosquito, blood transfusion, or congenital	Bite of infected mosquito; *Aedes* species
Incubation period	3-14 d	1-2 wk; average of 12 d	1-2 wk; average of 12 d	Dependent on strain of *Plasmodium* agent; average of 12-30 d; may be as long as 8-10 mo	3-15 d; average of 5-6 d
Period of communicability	Not communicable person to person	Not directly communicable; body louse acquires organism from infected person during febrile illness and for 3 d after fever	Not directly communicable; infected fleas remain so for life (up to 1 yr)	Untreated cases may be a source of mosquito infection for 1-3 yr; stored blood is infected for 16 d	Infected persons are a source of infection for mosquitoes 1 d before and 5 d after disease onset; mosquitoes are infective for the remainder of their lives (1-4 mo)
Susceptibility and resistance	General; infection confers lifetime immunity	General; infection confers long-lasting immunity	General; infection confers immunity; cross immunity with epidemic typhus	General; tolerance present in adults in endemic areas; black Africans show a natural resistance	General; children have less severe cases; immunity to one subtype of virus follows infection with that type
Report to local health authority	In some states where disease is endemic	Mandatory case report	Mandatory case report	Mandatory case report	Report during epidemics

PATHOPHYSIOLOGY[64,115,117]

The pathophysiology, although not completely understood, appears to be the same for all of these rickettsial infections. Differences in severity of disease manifestations are the result of differences in degree of the pathologic process and not of differences in the process.

Rickettsiae, like viruses, are intracellular parasites that replicate and metabolize only within host cells. The pathogens are carried in the feces of their respective arthropods and are deposited on the skin while the arthropod feeds on humans. Rickettsiae are subsequently rubbed or scratched into the open skin lesion produced by the arthropod bite.

Initially, a local neutrophilic inflammatory response occurs at the site of skin inoculation. Later, mononuclear cells infiltrate and phagocytize the rickettsiae. This local tissue reaction may result in an eschar. The rickettsiae then replicate and are disseminated within mononuclear cells throughout the vascular system.[115]

Once in the blood, rickettsiae invade the cytoplasm of vascular endothelial cells, replicate there, and cause the cells to burst. A rapidly progressive systemic angiitis with severe systemic manifestations develops, heralding the acute onset of these diseases. Vascular endothelial edema, fibrin and platelet deposition, and microthrombi development lead to obstruction and occlusion of small blood vessels with resultant hemorrhage, tissue infarction, and necrosis.

Other vascular changes include increased permeability with perivascular accumulation of neutrophils, macrophages, and lymphocytes, and plasma loss into tissues. The mechanism for this process is not known. It is hypothesized that the vascular permeability results from an allergic response of the host from the action of toxin produced by the pathogen.

Vascular lesions are widely disseminated, most frequently affecting the skin, myocardium, skeletal muscles, kidneys, and central nervous system. Disease symptoms, following the initial systemic manifestations, are the result of the localization of the vascular lesions and tissue infarctions and the loss of circulating plasma. A petechial skin rash that becomes purpuric, clouded sensorium, edema, hypotension, and peripheral vascular circulatory collapse are characteristic. Myocardial involvement with symptoms of myocarditis results from the focal vascular lesions plus a diffuse mononuclear cell infiltration. A shift in intracellular water and electrolytes in terminal stages of the disease may result in increases in circulating volume and tissue edema.

Complications include shock, disseminated intravascular coagulation, gangrene of distal extremities and genitalia in cases of severe local thrombosis, renal failure, pneumonia, coma, and death. Fatality generally is associated with delay in diagnosis and treatment rather than with treatment failure.

Both antibiotic therapy and the development of circulating antibodies during the second week of acute disease arrest the progression of rickettsiae but do not completely eradicate them. The pathogen remains latent in cells; and relapses, although uncommon, do occur. Recurrence of epidemic typhus in the form of Brill-Zinsser disease is seen in US immigrants who contacted typhus in Europe during World War II.[115,117]

Neurologic or myocardial sequelae are uncommon in survivors of typhus but are common in survivors of Rocky Mountain spotted fever. Potential sequelae include deafness, disturbances in vision and speech, mental confusion, cardiac arrhythmias, and amputations.[64]

Common laboratory findings include decreased platelets, normocytic anemia, hyponatremia, hypochloremia, and hypoalbuminemia. The WBC count is normal; and liver function tests are normal or slightly abnormal. In disseminated intravascular coagulation there is a thrombocytopenia, hypofibrinogenemia, and prolonged prothrombin and partial thromboplastin times.[115,117]

DIAGNOSTIC STUDIES[64,87,117]

Immunofluorescence of biopsied skin tissue
Identification of rickettsiae during third or fourth day of Rocky Mountain spotted fever

Weil-Felix agglutination test
Does not differentiate Rocky Mountain spotted fever from typhus
Increase in antibody titers can be detected after 7 to 10 days of illness in the untreated but may be delayed for 4 weeks if antibiotic therapy is begun early
Titers decrease rapidly during late convalescence
Strong reaction to *Proteus* OX-19 strain is diagnostic of typhus
Weaker reaction to *Proteus* OX-19 and OX-2 strains is suggestive of Rocky Mountain spotted fever

Complement fixation
Fourfold rise in antigen-specific antibodies by end of second week

TREATMENT PLAN[7,64,117]

Chemotherapeutic
Anti-infective agents
Tetracycline (Achromycin; others), 25-50 mg/kg/d po in four divided doses until patient is afebrile for 48 h, or for 5-7 d, *or*
Chloramphenicol (Chloromycetin), 50-100 mg/kg/d po in four divided doses until patient is afebrile for 48 h, or for 5-7 d

Either of above may be given IV in appropriate doses during initial toxic stage

Doxycycline (Vibramycin), 5 mg/kg po in a single dose is curative for epidemic typhus

Delousing epidemic typhus patients with dusting with an insecticide powder (10% DDT or 1% lindane)

Cardiac glycosides

Digitalis for cardiac decompensation

Narcotic analgesics

Codeine or meperidine (Demerol) for severe headache

Supportive*

IV fluids and electrolytes (to be administered cautiously)

Sedation of delerious patients with paraldehyde or chloral hydrate

High-protein, high-calorie diet

Transfusion of serum albumin

Packed red cells for anemia

Oxygen for pulmonary complications

Refrigerated blanket for fever control

Prevention: epidemic typhus patient contacts should be deloused

*Depends on severity of disease and complications.

ASSESSMENT: AREAS OF CONCERN[64,87,115,117]

	Rocky Mountain Spotted Fever	Epidemic Typhus	Endemic Typhus
Onset	Sudden	Sudden	Gradual and less severe
Subjective symptoms	Chills; severe headache; extreme myalgias and arthritic-type pain; prostration	Chills; severe headache; extreme myalgias and arthritic-type pain; prostration	Chills; severe headache; extreme myalgias and arthritis-type pain; prostration
Body temperature	39-40° C (102-104° F); AM remissions; fever lysis in 2-3 wk if untreated	40-41° C (104-106° F); unremitting; fever lysis in 2-3 wk if untreated	39-40° C (102-104° F); fever lysis in 2-3 wk if untreated
Eyes	Injected and suffused conjunctiva; photophobia	Injected and suffused conjunctiva; photophobia	
Skin	Eschar at site of tick bite Macular rash (3-5 mm) on mucous membranes, face, palms, and soles, beginning on third to fifth day; red to purple colored; blanches on pressure; begins on face and extremities; spreads in a centripetal fashion, involving the trunk last; if untreated, rash becomes maculopapular to petechial to purpuric; areas coalesce with possible necrosis and gangrene Jaundice	No eschar Macular rash (3-5 mm) beginning on fourth to seventh day; pink to rose colored; blanches on pressure; begins in axillary folds and upper trunk; spreads to involve the whole body except face, palms, and soles; if untreated, rash becomes maculopapular to petechial to purpuric; areas coalesce with possible necrosis and gangrene	Macular rash (3-5 mm) beginning on fourth to seventh day; pink to rose colored; blanches on pressure; begins on upper thorax and abdomen; remains central in distribution; becomes maculopapular, lasting 4-8 d; rash is more sparse and discrete than in epidemic typhus
Respiratory concerns	Nonproductive cough may be present; rapid respirations	Nonproductive cough may be present	Nonproductive cough may be present
Lymph nodes	Unilateral postauricular adenopathy if bite was on the head		
Abdomen	Hepatosplenomegaly, gastrointestinal distress, anorexia; constipation	Splenomegaly; constipation	
Central nervous system	Early: mental dullness and lethargy, progressing to delirium, stupor, convulsions, coma, and death;	Early: mental dullness and lethargy, progressing to delirium, stupor, convulsions, coma, and death;	Rare to have central nervous system symptoms

	Rocky Mountain Spotted Fever	Epidemic Typhus	Endemic Typhus
	may have focal neuro-logic signs such as deaf-ness, tinnitus, nuchal ri-gidity, tremor, vertigo; hallucinations, paranoid behavior, and extreme ir-ritability	may have focal neuro-logic signs such as deaf-ness, tinnitus, vertigo; hallucinations, paranoid behavior, and extreme ir-ritability	
Cardiovascular concerns	Early: bradycardia Later: tachycardia, gallop rhythm; hypotension and intractable shock may lead to death	Early: bradycardia Later: tachycardia, gallop rhythm; hypotension and intractable shock may lead to death	Rare to have cardiovascular symptoms
Urinary concerns	Oliguria or anuria in the event of circulatory col-lapse; incontinence in se-verely ill	Oliguria or anuria in the event of circulatory col-lapse; incontinence in se-verely ill	
Complications	Pneumonia; hemorrhage; iritis; nephritis; hemiple-gia; deafness; impaired vision; persistent tachy-cardia	Pneumonia; otitis media; parotitis	

NURSING DIAGNOSES and NURSING INTERVENTIONS

Nursing Diagnosis	Nursing Intervention
Tissue perfusion, alteration in	Administer antibiotics *as soon* as ordered to prevent vascular damage. Regularly check vital signs and intake and output. Monitor for signs of shock: hypotension, cyanosis, tachycardia, absent peripheral pulses, urinary output less than 30 ml/h. Administer oxygen. Maintain patient in a supine position, and give nothing by mouth. Prepare for cardiopulmonary resuscitation. Maintain indwelling urinary catheter.
Comfort, alteration in: pain	Administer analgesics regularly as prescribed for severe headache.
Sensory-perceptual alteration: visual and auditory	Minimize unnecessary environmental stimuli if patient is excitable or halluci-nating. Continuously interpret the environment for the patient. Supervise closely. Restrain, if necessary to prevent injury. Administer sedatives as prescribed.
Skin integrity, impairment of: actual	Turn frequently and position to prevent pressure over bony prominences or purpuric or necrotic areas. Monitor distal extremities, nose, and genitalia for signs of gangrene.
Fluid volume deficit, potential	Administer IV fluids slowly in enough quantity to maintain 1500 ml urine output.
Fluid volume, alteration in: excess	Monitor IV infusion rate hourly. Monitor for signs of overhydration: edema. Measure intake and output. Stop IV line if anuria occurs.
Nutrition, alteration in: less than body requirements	Offer frequent small high-protein, high-calorie feedings. Administer nasogastric feedings if necessary.
Oral mucous membrane, alteration in	Administer frequent oral hygiene to prevent parotitis. Monitor for hemorrhage in patients with Rocky Mountain spotted fever.
Urinary elimination, alteration in patterns	Monitor for oliguria and anuria. Monitor intake and output (hourly output should be at least 40 ml).

Nursing Diagnosis	Nursing Intervention
Injury, potential for: trauma	Constantly supervise delirious or convulsing patient. Use padded headboard and side rails. Administer sedatives as prescribed.
Activity intolerance	Provide opportunity for adequate rest until patient's energy returns. Reassure patient that the loss of energy is temporary.
Bowel elimination, alteration in: constipation	Administer small enemas to relieve constipation and rectal tube to relieve flatulence.
Potential patient problem: transmission of infection	Search for ticks in warm dark areas on patients suspected of having Rocky Mountain spotted fever. Wear gloves and do not touch ticks with hand. Attached ticks cannot be removed directly but must be induced to release their hold on skin. Apply a drop of kerosene, lighter fluid, gasoline, or alcohol; or barely touch with a hot match. Remove loosened tick with tweezers or forceps. Disinfect patient's clothing. Thoroughly bathe patient with epidemic typhus and delouse patient weekly until discharged. Wear gown and gloves when handling patient until delousing is complete. Disinfect patient's clothing with heat.
Potential patient problem: fever	Sponge bathe frequently to lower and maintain temperature at 39° C (102° F). Use refrigerated blankets if necessary.

Patient Education

1. Explain that relapses may occur and recurrence of symptoms should be reported to physician immediately so that antibiotic therapy can be resumed rapidly.

EVALUATION

Patient Outcome	Data Indicating That Outcome is Reached
Body temperature is normal.	Oral adult temperature is 37° C (98.6° F).
All cells receive oxygen.	Skin and mucous membranes are warm, moist, and normal colored. There are no purpuric or necrotic skin lesions. Peripheral pulses are palpable. Blood pressure, pulse, and respirations are normal. Patient is awake and oriented and communicates coherently; sensory and visual perceptions are normal.
Urinary elimination is normal.	Urinary output is between 1500 and 3000 ml or equal to intake. There is no edema.
Laboratory findings are within normal limits.	Serum albumin, sodium, and chloride levels are normal. Prothrombin time, partial thromboplastin time, platelets, fibrinogen, and RBC count are normal.
There are no complications.	Pneumonia, renal failure, gangrene, mental or neurosensory sequelae, or cardiac arrhythmias are not present.
Nutrition is adequate for body requirements.	Patient has not lost weight during course of the illness. Energy level is adequate, following convalescence, to enable patient to perform all activities of daily living. There are no signs of anemia or hypoalbuminemia.

Malaria

Malaria is a severe systemic infection caused by one of four protozoan parasites of the Plasmodium *family. The parasite is transmitted from person to person by the bite of a mosquito. Disease severity varies with the type of plasmodium causing the infection, with some plasmodia causing death to over 10% of untreated individuals. The duration of acute malarial disease is long, sometimes lasting months, with recurrent fever in treated individuals. Irregularly occurring relapses persist for years in untreated persons.*

PATHOPHYSIOLOGY[27,118]

Four species of plasmodia produce malaria in humans, with more than one species possibly present in any given malarial infection. The life cycle of the plasmodium is important to the pathophysiology of the disease. The sexual stage of the cycle occurs only in the intestines of the *Anopheles* mosquito, producing sporozoites that are discharged in mosquito saliva. The asexual development of the pathogen takes place in humans. There are two phases to the asexual cycle within humans, the exo-erythrocytic and the erythrocytic. The exoerythrocytic phase begins when plasmodium sporozoites from mosquito saliva are inoculated into human blood and are carried to the liver, where they invade hepatocytes. There they form cystlike structures, which, when mature, rupture and release hundreds of merozoites into the blood. Once in the blood the parasite never reinvades the liver. Two of the species, *P. vivax* and *P. ovale,* may not release all of the merozoites at once but may retain some in the liver in a dormant form. Release of these at a later time causes relapsing malaria. Infection induced by transfusion of blood containing the life cycle form of merozoites does not progress through the exoerythrocytic phase but begins directly with the erythrocytic phase.

The erythrocytic phase of the plasmodium life cycle is responsible for pathologic findings in the human host. Plasmodium merozoites invade select erythrocytes that contain surface receptors that attract the plasmodia. The absence of these RBC receptors in black Africans protects them from symptomatic malaria. Once in erythrocytes the merozoites feed and grow into trophozoites. Trophozoites feed on hemoglobin, metabolizing the globin fraction and depositing the heme fraction as hematin granules into the cytoplasm. Trophozoites sexually segment into numerous merozoites. This causes the erythrocytes to rupture and release merozoites into the circulation, enabling them to reinvade additional erythrocytes within seconds.

The process of erythrocytic invasion, asexual multiplication of the plasmodia, and erythrocytic rupture continues until antibodies develop within the host to control the parasite or until the host is treated with sufficient antimicrobial agents. An antibody response is adequate to limit all malarial plasmodia except *P. falciparum,* which, in the absence of treatment, may overwhelm the host with severe fulminating disease resulting in death.

Symptomatic attacks of chills, fever, and diaphoresis coincide with completion of the erythrocytic life cycle of the plasmodium in humans. The length of time between attacks varies with the *Plasmodium* species: every 42 to 48 hours in *P. vivax,* 48 hours in *P. falciparum,* 50 hours in *P. ovale,* and 72 hours in *P. malariae.*

The erythrocytic activity of the parasite produces the following pathophysiologic changes: (1) fever and its physiologic consequences, (2) hemolytic anemia, (3) tissue hypoxia resulting from anemia and alterations in the microcirculation, and (4) coagulation defects resulting from immunopathologic events.

Fever, with marked vasodilation, leads to a decrease in effective plasma volume with a resultant orthostatic hypotension and an increased secretion of ADH and aldosterone. Diaphoresis and vomiting that accompany the toxic fever result in fluid and electrolyte loss and possible hyponatremia.

Anemia triggers the spleen to store erythrocytes, resulting in splenomegaly. Anemia also results in tissue hypoxia, particularly in the kidneys, lungs, liver, and central nervous system, with resultant dysfunction to those systems. Erythrocyte invasion also causes erythrocytes to adhere to vascular endothelium, slowing the blood flow and accentuating tissue hypoxia, edema, and vascular pathologic findings and hemorrhage.

The immune response is pathologic as well as protective. Excess immunoglobulin production triggers hypersplenism and plays a role in the further development of anemia and in the development of neutropenia and thrombocytopenia. Laboratory evidence of coagulation defects in some patients can be observed. These include decreases in fibrinogen and platelets (platelets less than 50,000/cmm), decreases in factors V, VII, VIII, and X, and prolonged prothrombin and partial thromboplastin times.

Specific organ system complications resulting from the previously described pathologic conditions include renal and hepatic failure, pulmonary edema, and central nervous system disturbances resulting from perivascular edema and hemorrhage in the cerebral cortex. Laboratory evidence of renal failure includes proteinuria and increased serum creatinine. Laboratory findings in hepatic failure include increases in serum transaminase and indirect serum bilirubin.

Laboratory findings present in uncomplicated malaria include leukopenia, relative or absolute monocytosis, a normochromic, normocytic hemolytic anemia, decreased platelets, and a false positive VDRL.[27,118]

DIAGNOSTIC STUDIES[27,118]

Microscopic examination of stained peripheral blood smear taken at least twice daily, within 6 to 12 hours after a chill
    Identification of plasmodia in blood
    Detection of granular brownish pigment within monocytes or neutrophils or identification of parasitized RBC
    If more than 5% of RBCs are affected, *P. falciparum* should be suspected

Indirect fluorescent antibody or ELISA test
    Increase in antibody titer after 1 week of illness
    Useful for screening blood donors but should not be relied on for diagnosis

TREATMENT PLAN

Uncomplicated infections with *P. ovale, P. vivax,* and *P. malariae* can be treated in an outpatient setting. Patients infected with *P. falciparum* should be hospitalized.

Chemotherapeutic
Anti-infective agents[7]
    Uncomplicated infection with all species except chloroquine-resistant *P. falciparum:* chloroquine phosphate (Aralen), po, 25 mg/kg (base) administered over a 3-d period: 15 mg/kg the first day (10 mg initially and 5 mg 6 h later), 5 mg/kg the second day, and 5 mg/kg the third day
    For emergency treatment of severe infections or for persons unable to retain orally administered medications
        Chloroquine hydrochloride (Aralen hydrochloride), IM, 300 mg base repeated in 6 h; no more than 900 mg base/24 h (maximum of 10 mg/kg/24 h), *or*
        Quinine dihydrochloride, 650 mg (10 gr), diluted in 1 L of normal saline, glucose, or plasma, administered slowly IV (Never push and never give IM); repeat in 6 h (no more than three doses per 24 h); pediatric dosage is 25 mg/kg, half given over ½ h and the other half 6-8 h later
    For infection caused by chloroquine-resistant *P. falciparum*
        Quinine sulfate, po, 25-30 mg/kg/24 h in three divided doses for 7-10 d, plus
        Pyrimethamine (Daraprim), po, 0.85 mg/kg/24 h in divided doses for 3 d, plus
        Sulfadoxine, po, 15 mg/kg the first day, followed by 10 mg/kg 24 h later
    Prevention of relapses from *P. vivax* and *P. ovale*
        Primaquine phosphate, po, 0.3 mg base/kg/d for 14 d (26.3 mg/d for average adult) following treatment with chloroquine phosphate[7]
    Chemoprophylaxis for persons traveling to areas where malaria is endemic[22]
        Chloroquine phosphate (Aralen), po, 300 mg (base) once weekly for 2 wk before entering and 6 wk after leaving an endemic area, *plus*
        Fansidar (a fixed combination of pyrimethamine, 24 mg, and sulfadoxine, 500 mg), one tablet po per week together with chloroquine phosphate (The pyrimethamine in Fansidar is contraindicated for pregnant women. Sulfadoxine is contraindicated for those with allergies to sulfonamides.)

Supportive[118]
    IV fluids and electrolytes; restrict fluids in cerebral edema
    Assisted ventilation and intubation in pulmonary edema
    Transfusion of packed RBCs in anemia
    Transfusion of whole blood in shock
    Corticosteroids in cerebral edema
    Heparin, low–molecular weight dextran, or fresh frozen plasma in coagulopathy

ASSESSMENT: AREAS OF CONCERN[27,118]

Prodrome: subjective symptoms
    Myalgia
    Fatigue, malaise
    Slight chills

Chill phase: skin
    Cold, pale skin
    Cyanotic nail beds
    Severe shaking chills lasting 1 to 2 hours

Fever phase
  Body temperature
    Fever of 39° to 41° C (103° to 106° F) lasting 3 to 6 hours, decreasing suddenly by lysis

Vital signs
    Tachycardia
    Tachypnea
    Hypotension

Systemic manifestations
    Severe headache, nausea, and vomiting
    Cough

Diaphoresis phase
  Skin
    Profuse sweating

Systemic concerns
Weakness leading to sleep

Between attacks
Abdomen
Hepatomegaly in *P. vivax* and *P. falciparum*
Splenomegaly in *P. vivax*
Abdominal pain

Lungs
Scattered rales

Systemic concerns
Energy returns to normal between attacks in all but *P. falciparum* infections

Vital signs
Tachycardia persisting between fever episodes

Additional symptoms in P. falciparum infections
Gastrointestinal concerns
Severe prolonged vomiting and diarrhea leading to dehydration and electrolyte imbalance

Skin
Jaundice resulting from hepatic dysfunction

Neurologic concerns
Delerium, convulsions, coma
Altered intellectual function, behavior changes, focal neurologic signs, positive Babinski's sign, tremors, and hemiparesis

Respiratory concerns
Pulmonary congestion and respiratory distress

NURSING DIAGNOSES and NURSING INTERVENTIONS

Nursing Diagnosis	Nursing Intervention
Fluid volume deficit, potential	Encourage oral fluids. Administer IV fluids and electrolytes cautiously per protocol. Monitor body weight, intake and output, and skin for edema.
Injury, potential for: trauma	Protect from splenic rupture; palpate gently. Caution patient against lifting heavy objects.
Injury, potential for (chemotherapeutic agent)	Monitor patient receiving IV drugs for evidence of cardiotoxicity, hypotension, and widening of QRS complex. Monitor for toxic reactions to oral quinine (tinnitus, headache, nausea, altered vision) and for hypersensitivity (bronchospasm, hemolytic anemia, thrombocytopenia).
Tissue perfusion, alteration in: cerebral	Monitor and report changes in level of consciousness, behavior, or neurologic signs. Protect delerious patient from injury.
Tissue perfusion, alteration in: pulmonary	Monitor for signs of pulmonary edema. Limit fluid intake if necessary. Prepare to assist ventilation if needed.
Tissue perfusion, alteration in: renal	Monitor intake and output and body weight; report edema or urinary output less than intake.
Potential patient problem: transmission of infection	Employ blood and body fluid precautions for duration of illness (p. 1623).
Potential patient problem: chills	Provide hot drinks and application of external heat to provide comfort.
Potential patient problem: fever	Administer tepid water or alcohol sponge bath; ice cap to head; and analgesics and antipyretics as ordered. Bathe patient and change clothing following diaphoresis.

Patient Education

1. Patients infected with *P. vivax* or *P. ovale* may still have plasmodia in the liver after treatment; remissions are possible. They should continue with prescribed medication for 14 days following initial treatment and should report recurrence of symptoms immediately.
2. All patients should return for blood examination 4 or 5 days after completion of treatment.

EVALUATION

Patient Outcome	Data Indicating That Outcome is Reached
There is no infection.	No parasites are detected in peripheral blood smears 4 or 5 days after treatment.
Body temperature is normal.	Adult oral body temperature is consistently around 37° C (98.6° F) for 4 to 5 days after treatment. Paroxysms of chills and diaphoresis that accompany fever are absent.
Laboratory findings are within normal limits.	Leukocyte, monocyte, erythrocyte, and platelet counts are normal. Coagulation factors V, VII, VIII, and X are normal. Prothrombin time and, partial thromboplastin time are normal. Serum transaminase, indirect bilirubin, and creatinine levels are normal. Serum sodium level is normal. Urine protein is normal.
Patient is aware of need for follow-up.	Patient expresses intent to return to physician for follow-up blood cultures as advised.
All cells receive oxygen.	Patient is alert and oriented to surroundings, speaks coherently, and has memory for recent and past events; behavior and affect are appropriate to the situation. All neurologic signs are normal.
Respiratory function is normal.	Breath sounds are clear. There is no dyspnea or cyanosis.
Urinary elimination is normal.	Urine output is 1500 to 3000 ml or equal to input. There is no evidence of edema.
Vital signs are normal.	Blood pressure, pulse, and respirations are normal.

Dengue

Dengue (breakbone fever) is an acute viral febrile illness of short duration that is transmitted to humans by the bite of an infected mosquito. The disease has clinical characteristics similar to other arthropod-borne viral fevers such as yellow fever, Colorado tick fever, and Venezuelan equine fever. The risk for dengue is increasing in the southern United States because of movement of infected mosquitoes northward from Mexico. Dengue is presented here as a prototype of the arthropod-borne viral fevers. Two forms of the disease, benign and a hemorrhagic form, occur.

PATHOPHYSIOLOGY

The pathologic agents producing dengue are four immunologically distinct viruses that require both *Aedes* mosquitoes and humans for their viability. The *Aedes* mosquito that feeds on an infected person during the symptomatic viremic stage of dengue becomes infective after an incubation period of 8 to 10 days. Infective mosquitoes transmit the virus to every person they bite. In tropical and subtropical areas where *Aedes* organisms

survive year-around, dengue is an endemic, and sometimes epidemic, disease in the population. Epidemics or disease outbreaks may occur anywhere that *Aedes* mosquitoes are present by the introduction of either infective mosquitoes or persons into the area.[7]

Dengue occurs in two clinical disease forms: classic (benign) dengue and the more severe dengue hemorrhagic fever. Either form may be produced by any of the four viral serotypes. The mechanism for the development of two different dengue diseases is not known. One hypothesis is that the form of the disease varies with differences in virulence within viral strains. A second hypothesis is that a primary infection with one viral serotype may result in the benign form of the disease but predispose one to an immunopathologic response to a subsequent infection with another serotype resulting in dengue hemorrhagic fever.[72,85]

The pathologic process is similar in both disease forms although more extensive and life threatening in dengue hemorrhagic fever. Once injected, the virus replicates at the site of inoculation and in local lymphatic tissue. Viruses invade the blood within days, producing a viremia that lasts 4 to 5 days after symptomatic disease onset.

The viremia results in endothelial swelling, mononuclear cell infiltration, increased vascular permeability, and perivascular edema. Extravasation of blood from dermal vessels produces a maculopapular or petechial rash. Leukopenia and lymphadenopathy are common. Symptom severity varies in the benign form.

In the hemorrhagic form of the disease the increased vascular permeability is more severe, with extensive extravasation of blood and fluid into serous cavities and hemorrhage and congestion within many organs, particularly the spleen, liver, kidneys, pleura, and peritoneum. Blood changes include a thrombocytopenia, increase in platelet agglutinability, mild or moderate disseminated intravascular coagulation, and hemoconcentration. A rising hematocrit concentration on the third day of illness is a sign of impending life-threatening hypovolemic shock, the dengue shock syndrome. Vascular and blood component pathologic findings coincide with the development of an immune response and may result from the action of circulating antigen-antibody complexes, the activation of complement, or the release of vasoactive amines.[72,85]

Laboratory findings in dengue hemorrhagic fever include decreased serum albumin and sodium; decreased platelets, fibrinogen, and coagulation factors V, VII, IX, and X; decreased C3 serum complement; a 20% or greater increase in hematocrit; the presence of fibrin split products in plasma and an increase in prothrombin time; and an increase in BUN and serum transaminase proportional to kidney and liver dysfunction, respectively.[7,72]

Patients may spontaneously recover from dengue hemorrhagic fever or progress to hypovolemic shock. Untreated shock leads to tissue anoxia, coma, metabolic acidosis, hyperkalemia, and death within 12 to 24 hours.

Virus serotype–specific IgM antibodies develop early during the febrile period of both forms of the disease and persist for 8 weeks. This initial antibody response is followed within 1 or 2 days by a rise in IgG antibodies that persists for over 40 years and confers lifetime immunity against the specific dengue serotype. Secondary infections with another dengue serotype initiate an early and extremely high IgG antibody response that cross reacts against the infecting serotype, the initial serotype, and other flaviviruses. This immune response is thought to play a role in the pathogenesis of dengue hemorrhagic fever.[85]

DIAGNOSTIC STUDIES[86]

Animal or cell culture of serum: plaque reduction neutralization method
Isolation of dengue virus subtypes
Takes 1 to 2 weeks for test

Useful for diagnostic confirmation and epidemiologic surveillance

Neutralization, hemagglutination inhibition (HI), radioimmunoassay (RIA), or complement fixation tests
Fourfold rise in titer to one serotype in a series of paired sera or a single HI titer greater than 1:640 or CF titer greater than 1:32 suggests primary infection

Single HI titer greater than 1:1280 or CF titer greater than 1:256 without fourfold change suggests secondary infection

Fourfold change in titer to more than one serotype with HI titer greater than 1:640 or CF titer greater than 1:128 also suggests secondary infection

TREATMENT PLAN[7,72,85]

Chemotherapeutic
Analgesic/antipyretic agents
Acetaminophen (Tylenol) (salicylates should not be used) 325-600 mg q4-6h
Anticoagulants
Heparin for disseminated intravascular coagulation

Supportive
IV fluids and electrolytes
Frequent monitoring of hematocrit
Shock
IV lactated Ringer's solution, 10-20 ml/kg/h, plus plasma or plasma expanders (Discontinue IV line when hematocrit decreases to 40% to prevent hypervolemia and pulmonary edema.)
Central venous pressure line
Whole blood transfusions in severe hemorrhage
Oxygen

ASSESSMENT: AREAS OF CONCERN[72,85]

Benign dengue
Subjective symptoms
Prodrome: 12 hours; malaise, anorexia
Abrupt onset: chills, severe frontal headache, ocular pain, severe and incapacitating myalgia, arthralgia, and backache

Throat
Mild pharyngitis

Gastrointestinal concerns
Nausea and vomiting
Epigastric pain

Body temperature

Fever of 40° C (104° F), unremitting and persisting for 3 to 7 days

Diaphasic course with "saddle back" temperature curve

Heart rate

Tachycardia for first few days of fever

Bradycardia during last days of fever

Eyes

Injected conjunctivae

Lymph nodes

Generalized tender lymphadenopathy

Skin

First 1 or 2 days: transient erythematous flush over face, neck, and upper trunk, disappearing within a day

Third to fifth day: distinct macular or maculopapular rash on trunk, spreading centrifugally to face and extremities; petechiae on palate, in the axilla, and on the lower extremities at the end of the febrile period

Subjective symptoms during convalescence

Prolonged fatigue and depression

Laboratory values

Leukopenia during febrile period

Hemorrhagic dengue

Same symptoms as benign dengue with the following additions:

Skin and mucous membranes

Hemorrhagic symptoms during the febrile period: positive tourniquet test, purpura, epistaxis, gingival bleeding, hematemesis, melena, hematuria

Jaundice

Abdomen

Hepatomegaly

Severe epigastric or generalized abdominal pain

Shock phase
Vital signs

Rapid, weak pulse

Hypotension; narrow pulse pressure

Rapid drop in body temperature

Skin

Cool, clammy edematous skin

Circumoral cyanosis

Laboratory values

Profound thrombocytopenia

Increased hematocrit concentration

NURSING DIAGNOSES and NURSING INTERVENTIONS

Nursing Diagnosis	Nursing Intervention
Tissue perfusion, alteration in	Monitor vital signs and intake and output. Monitor for signs of internal hemorrhage and for signs of shock: hypotension, cyanosis, cold edematous skin, tachycardia, absent peripheral pulses, and urinary output less than 30 ml/h. Administer oxygen. Discontinue IV line in presence of pulmonary edema.
Comfort, alteration in: pain	Regularly administer analgesics, as prescribed, during acute symptomatic phase. Frequently reposition patient for comfort. Provide diversional activities as tolerated.
Fluid volume deficit, potential	Give IV fluids and electrolytes or oral fluids as tolerated during fever. Monitor intake and output for output equal to intake.
Anxiety	Inform that prolonged weakness and depression may extend into convalescence; reassure that this is expected and that it will not affect the eventual prognosis.
Potential patient problem: fever	Administer antipyretics (avoid salicylates), tepid sponge baths, and adequate fluids.
Potential patient problem: transmission of illness	Utilize blood and body fluid precautions for duration of hospitalization.

Patient Education

1. During illness, patient must protect self from mosquito vectors to prevent transmission to others.

2. Patient can prevent future infections by protecting self from mosquito vectors by screening living quarters, wearing protective clothing, and using insect repellants on exposed skin and clothing when in the proximity of mosquitoes. *Aedes* mosquitoes enter homes and usually bite during the day.
3. Mosquitoes can be controlled around living quarters by eliminating potential breeding places, particularly any water-filled containers.
4. Persons living close to the patient may have been exposed to mosquito vectors infected with dengue. They should be monitored for early diagnosis of dengue.
5. Prolonged weakness and depression are characteristic of the convalescent period.

EVALUATION

Patient Outcome	Data Indicating That Outcome is Reached
All cells receive oxygen.	Skin is warm and normal colored; there is no edema, cyanosis, or purpura. Peripheral pulses are strong. Urinary output is 3000 ml or equal to intake.
There is no infection.	There are no signs of internal hemorrhage or dermal bleeding. Vital signs are normal.
The patient appears physically comfortable.	During acute stage, patient is able to rest without signs of pain.
The patient returns to preillness energy level.	During convalescence, patient gradually increases self-care and activities of daily living.
Laboratory findings are within normal limits.	The following measurements are all in the normal range: hematocrit; platelets; leukocytes; serum albumin; serum sodium; coagulation factors V, VII, IX, X; fibrinogen; serum complement C3; prothrombin time; fibrin split products; serum transaminase; BUN; and blood pH.

SEPSIS

Bacteremia refers to the presence of bacteria in the circulating blood as demonstrated by blood culture. It is asymptomatic; it may be transient and abate spontaneously or become sustained, leading to septicemia.

Septicemia is a bacteremia with clinical manifestations of the pathogenic activity of bacteria in the blood. Symptoms vary with the pathogen.

Septic shock is a syndrome of circulatory insufficiency with hypoperfusion of body tissues caused by the effects of pathogenic bacterial toxins on peripheral blood vessels. It frequently results in death.[70]

The infections manifesting a clinical picture consistent with the presence of bacteria or bacterial toxins in circulating blood (and not discussed elsewhere in this section) are grouped under sepsis (Table 15-19).

PATHOPHYSIOLOGY

Bacteria may enter the blood directly through contaminated needles, catheters, monitoring transducers, or perfusion fluid to produce a primary bacteremia. In this situation there is no evidence of infection elsewhere in the body. About one third of diagnosed bacteremias are primary, and most are caused by gram-negative bacteria that are part of the normal flora of the skin or intestinal tract. Immunocompromised patients are at greatest risk for primary bacteremia (p. 1615). Secondary bacteremia results from dissemination of bacteria from a localized infection at another body site. Usually, clinical symptoms of infection precede the bacteremia. Urinary tract infections with gram-negative bacteria (usually catheter induced), surgical wound infections with gram-positive *Staphylococcus aureus,* and pneumonia (particularly with gram-negative *Pseudomonas*) are the infections that most frequently precede secondary bacteremias. Bacteremia may also be polymicrobial.[10,100,119]

Bacteremia may abate spontaneously; or the multiplying bacteria in the blood may overwhelm host defenses and produce a symptomatic septicemia or metastatic bacterial abscesses at other organ sites, particularly in the brain, endocardium, kidneys, bones, and joints. Renal

Table 15-19
Overview of Sepsis[7,11,119]

	Bacteremia and Septicemia	**Septic Shock**
Occurrence	Bacteremia is common and transient; associated with medical procedures on hospitalized patients, colonization and dissemination of normal flora in debilitated persons, or dissemination of bacteria from a locus of infection; sustained bacteremia leads to septicemia	25-30% of septicemias lead to shock; highest in hospitalized neonates and chronically ill persons
Etiologic agent	Gram-positive bacteria, particularly *S. aureus* and group B streptococci; gram-negative bacteria, particularly *Pseudomonas, Klebsiella, Proteus, E. coli, Serratia,* and *Enterobacter*	75% caused by gram-negative bacteria and their endotoxins; most common bacteria in order of frequency: *E. coli, Klebsiella, P. aeruginosa, Serratia, Enterobacter,* and *Proteus;* 25% caused by exotoxins of gram-positive bacteria, particularly *S. aureus*
Reservoir	Humans	Humans
Incubation period	Variable	Variable
Transmission	Bacteria may be introduced directly into blood as a primary bacteremia or may be secondary to an infection elsewhere in the body	Results from a primary or secondary septicemia
Period of communicability	Not directly transmittable; organism in draining lesions or respiratory secretions may be transmitted	Not directly transmittable
Susceptibility and resistance	Primary: invasive medical procedures increase susceptibility Secondary: urinary tract infections and pneumonia; neonates and elderly persons at greatest risk	Susceptibility greatest in neonates and chronically ill and immunocompromised individuals
Report to local health authority	No	No

failure and endocarditis are serious complications of untreated bacteremia-produced metastatic abscesses.

Bacteremia in the newborn is almost always accompanied by metastatic focal lesions of the meninges, lungs, or heart. Infection early in the neonatal period is usually acquired from the mother's vagina and is associated with a difficult delivery, premature rupture of membranes, or prematurity. Infection appearing later is usually acquired from the environment and is frequently associated with invasive procedures in the hospital.[64]

Progression of a bacteremia to septicemia or septic shock depends greatly on host characteristics and defenses. Premature infants, elderly persons, individuals with chronic debilitating diseases (cirrhosis, diabetes, renal disease, collagen diseases), and immunocompromised persons are at greatest risk.[100]

Symptoms of septicemia result from the release of bacterial toxins and enzymes in the blood. In the case of gram-positive *Staphylococcus aureus*, exotoxins and enzymes cause RBC hemolysis, aggregation of platelets, leukocyte destruction, and increase in cell membrane permeability with protein leakage. Gram-negative bacterial endotoxins appear to activate at least four interacting humoral systems responsible for the pathologic findings in septicemia and progression to septic shock:

1. Activation of complement results in release of anaphylotoxins, which enhance the inflammatory reaction and increase vascular permeability.

2. Activation of the coagulation system by stimulation of the conversion of fibrinogen to fibrin with resultant clotting. Consumption of clotting factors II, V, and VII and platelets may produce clinical bleeding. Other complications include thrombosis with tissue ischemia, necrosis, and organ failure and disseminated intravascular coagulation.

3. Activation of the plasmin fibrinolytic mechanisms lyses fibrin into fibrin split products, which have anticoagulant properties. This results in prolonged prothrombin time and partial prothrombin time.

4. Activation of the bradykinin system is thought to be partially responsible for progression to shock. Bradykinin, a vasoactive peptide, stimulates vasodilation and increased vascular permeability.[76,94,119]

Two processes appear to produce skin lesions in septicemia. The lesions may be the result of direct bacterial invasion into dermal vessels with vessel damage and necrosis. They may also be manifestations of the vasoactive effect of toxins.[119]

About 30% of gram-negative and 5% of gram-positive septicemias progress to septic shock. Gram-negative septic shock is the more severe type with a high risk for death.[94,119]

The shock syndrome is precipitated by the complex action of bacterial toxins on peripheral blood vessels and blood components, with an end result of microcirculatory failure and cellular anoxia similar to shock of any cause. The sequence of events is as follows:

1. Vasoactive toxins induce spasm of precapillary sphincters and venules, especially in visceral organs. This results in reduced capillary perfusion and hypoxic damage to capillaries as well as organ tissue.

2. The precapillary sphincters eventually dilate while the venules remain constricted, causing blood to stagnate in the capillaries, the capillary pressure to increase, and fluid to be lost from the vascular system.

3. Blood stasis in the capillary bed plus decreasing blood volume potentiates intravascular clotting and impairment of venous return.

4. Anoxia to the capillaries causes them to lose their integrity and to release whole blood as well as fluid into the tissues. This further decreases venous return.

5. Loss of venous tone with dilation further impairs venous return. The end result is reduced cardiac output, extreme hypotension, further impairment of tissue perfusion with severe tissue anoxia, metabolic acidosis, renal and brainstem dysfunction, heart failure with pulmonary edema, respiratory insufficiency, and potential death.[42,49,70,119]

There is a wide spectrum of cardiovascular and laboratory findings in septic shock depending on the organism and the stage in the progression and on the patient's hemodynamic compensation mechanisms. Initially, the patient may be warm with peripheral vascular dilation and normal or decreased peripheral resistance, normal or increased cardiac output with tachycardia, and respiratory alkalosis and hypotension. Progression of the vascular pathologic conditions leads to higher peripheral resistance, worsening hypotension, acidosis, heart failure, and anuria. Gram-positive septic shock may not progress beyond peripheral vasodilation with no anoxia or acidosis.[100,119]

Laboratory findings in both gram-positive and gram-negative septicemia and septic shock are as follows:
Hematology
  Leukocytes: 15,000 to 30,000/cmm (There may be an early leukopenia in gram-negative infections, increasing in 6 to 12 hours. A persistent leukopenia is a poor sign in gram-positive infections.)
  Differential: increase in neutrophils and decrease in lymphocytes (In elderly persons, the shift may be present without leukocytosis.)
  Hemoglobin: 10 g/dl in *S. aureus* infections
  Hematocrit: less than 30% in *S. aureus* infections
  Decrease in platelets (less than 100,000)
  Prolonged prothrombin time and partial thromboplastin
  Low fibrinogen concentration
  Presence of fibrin split products in the blood
Renal function tests

Increased BUN greater than two times normal
Increased serum creatinine greater than two times normal
Decreased creatinine clearance
Blood electrolytes
  Hyponatremia
  Hypochloremia
  Potassium may be high or low depending on status of kidney function
Arterial blood gases
  Decreased P_{CO_2} and increased serum lactate early in shock
  P_{O_2} less than 70 mm Hg and acidosis later
Urine
  High specific gravity
  Albuminuria and hematuria in *S. aureus* infections

DIAGNOSTIC STUDIES[95]

Blood culture for both anaerobic and aerobic bacteria

Two or three sets of temporally separated blood cultures should be drawn before antibiotics are administered
One or more cultures positive for bacteria are diagnostic of bacteremia
Septicemia diagnosed based on positive cultures with clinical evidence of toxicity

Gram stain

Differentiates gram-positive from gram-negative bacteria

Limulus amebocyte lysate test on blood specimens

Positive for gram-negative endotoxins

Counterimmunoelectrophoresis or Ouchterlony gel diffusion tests

Positive for serum antibody to *S. aureus* cell wall antigen
Tests take only 40 minutes to perform and are useful for rapidly differentiating *S. aureus* from other bacteria

TREATMENT PLAN

Surgical

Incision and drainage of any suppurative lesion containing staphylococci
Removal of intravenous catheter or any foreign body that may be a source of the infection (prosthesis, stitches, etc.)

Chemotherapeutic[70,76,95]

Anti-infective agents

Antibiotic therapy will depend on the type of bacteria that is present in the blood or that is releasing a toxin from a localized infection elsewhere in the body and on the sensitivity of the organism to the antibiotic. A series of blood cultures should be drawn before antibiotic therapy is initiated.

Anti-infective agents should be administered IV every 4 to 6 hours.

Combinations of agents may be used in severe disease before culture and sensitivity results are obtained. An effective regimen for bacteremia of unknown etiology is as follows:

Gentamicin (Garamycin), 3-5 mg/kg/d IM or IV, plus either

Methicillin (Staphcillin), 6-12 g/day IV, or

Cephalothin (Keflin), 6-8 g/d IV, plus

Carbenicillin (Geopen), 30 g/d IV if *Pseudomonas* is suspected

Duration of therapy will be long (2-6 wk dependent on the presence of a primary source of the infection, host defenses, and the response of the pathogen to the antibiotic).

For treatment of shock

Adrenergic agents

Dopamine

Phenoxybenzamine

Isoproterenol (Chapter 1)

Corticosteroids

Methylprednisone (Medrol), 30 mg/kg as a bolus; repeat at 6-12 h intervals q12-48h

Control of hemorrhage

Fresh frozen plasma if there is a clotting factor deficiency

Platelets if thrombocytopenia is present

Diuretics

Mannitol (Osmitrol), 50-100 mg IV in 15-20% solution, or ethacrynic acid (Edecrin), 25-200 mg orally per day

Heart failure: digitalis (Chapter 1)

Intravascular coagulation: heparin (Chapter 1)

Supportive

Monitoring of central venous pressure or pulmonary artery pressure

IV fluids until central venous pressure reaches 10 to 12 cm water or until pulmonary wedge pressure is 12 to 15 mm Hg

Blood volume replaced with blood, plasma, dextran, human serum albumin, or dextrose saline with bicarbonate

Respiratory assistance with nasal oxygen, tracheal intubation, or tracheostomy as required

ASSESSMENT: AREAS OF CONCERN[70,95,119]

Septicemia

Body temperature

Fever: may be intermittent with wide diurnal variations; high in evening

Subjective symptoms

Chills

Prostration

Myalgia and headache

Hypothermia sometimes present in gram-negative septicemia

Respiratory system

Tachypnea

Gastrointestinal concerns

Nausea

Diarrhea

Skin

Petechial, purpuric, papular, pustular, or vesicular skin eruptions depending on type of bacteria present

There will be additional symptoms if septicemia is secondary to a localized infection elsewhere in the body (genitourinary or gastrointestinal tract, skin, or lungs). Symptoms may be insidious in elderly persons and neonates (elderly persons: hypothermia, lethargy, confusion; infants: poor sucking, failure to thrive, respiratory distress, symptoms of central nervous system irritation).

Septic shock

Cardiovascular concerns

Tachycardia

Hypotension (systolic blood pressure less than 90 mm Hg)

Congestive failure

Respiratory concerns

Tachypnea

Skin

Cool, pale, or cyanotic extremities (In gram-positive or early gram-negative septic shock, skin is likely to be warm and flushed.)

Mental status

Confusion and disorientation rapidly leading to coma

Urinary elimination

Oliguria (urinary output less than 20 ml/h)

Abdomen

Hepatosplenomegaly in some patients

NURSING DIAGNOSES and NURSING INTERVENTIONS

Nursing Diagnosis	Nursing Intervention
Tissue perfusion, alteration in	Administer IV antibiotic as soon as ordered because untreated septicemia may rapidly lead to septic shock. Monitor for adverse reaction to drugs. Monitor for signs of impending shock: decreased blood pressure, tachycardia, pale cool skin, alteration in consciousness, and urinary output less than 30 ml/h. (for nursing interventions for patients in shock, refer to Chapter 1).
Potential patient problem: fever	Administer tepid water or alcohol sponge baths. Administer antipyretics as ordered. Maintain room temperature at 17° to 20° C (63° to 68° F) to decrease metabolic needs, particularly during shock.
Potential patient problem: transmission of illness	If the bacteremia or septicemia is secondary to a major skin, wound, or burn infection, maintain contact isolation for duration of the illness. Maintain drainage and secretion precautions for a minor skin wound or burn infection or pulmonary infection for duration of the illness. Collect at least two blood specimens for culture and sensitivity tests before administration of antibiotics.

Patient Education

1. Take antibiotics as directed for prescribed length of treatment.
2. Report recurrence of symptoms or side effects of medication to physician immediately.

EVALUATION

Patient Outcome	Data Indicating That Outcome is Reached
There is no infection.	Blood cultures are negative for bacteria. Cultures of secretions, excretions, or exudates (from a primary source of infection) are negative for bacteria. Body temperature is normal. There are no skin lesions.
Laboratory findings are normal.	Hematologic findings (leukocyte count, hemoglobin, hematocrit, platelet count, fibrinogen, prothrombin time, and partial thromboplastin time) are within normal limits. Findings of renal function tests (blood urea nitrogen and serum creatinine) are normal. Blood electrolytes (sodium, chloride, and potassium) are normal. Arterial blood gases (Pco_2 and Po_2) are normal. Urine specific gravity is normal. There is no albuminuria or hematuria.
Oxygen reaches all body cells.	Patient is alert and oriented and responds appropriately to environmental stimuli. Skin is warm and of normal color, with no petechiae or purpuric skin manifestations.
Vital signs are normal.	Blood pressure, pulse, and respirations are normal.
Urinary output is normal.	Urinary output is equal to intake.
Gastrointestinal function is normal.	Patient is able to eat regular diet without nausea or vomiting. Stools are soft, formed, and of normal color.
Patient is comfortable.	Patient does not have a headache or myalgia. Energy returns to preillness level.

SEXUALLY TRANSMITTED DISEASES

The term *sexually transmitted diseases (STDs)* refers to a large group of disease syndromes that can be transmitted sexually irrespective of whether the disease has genital pathologic manifestations. STD is more encompassing than the previously used "venereal disease" categorization. The STDs, like other infectious diseases, can be classified as to their etiologic agent or according to their disease manifestations. The following pathogens are known or thought to be sexually transmitted[7,58]:

Bacteria: *Neisseria gonorrhoeae; Chlamydia trachomatis; Mycoplasma hominis; Ureaplasma urealyticum; Treponema pallidum; Gardnerella vaginalis; Haemophilus ducreyi; Shigella; Calymmatobacterium granulomatis*

Viruses: Herpes simplex virus; *Papillomavirus;* hepatitis A, B, and non-A, non-B viruses; molluscum contagiosum virus; cytomegalovirus

Protozoa: *Trichomonas vaginalis; Entamoeba histolytica; Giardia lamblia*

Fungi: *Candida albicans*

Ectoparasites: *Pthirus pubis; Sarcoptes scabiei*

The list of disease syndromes produced by the above pathogens is equally extensive. Many pathogens produce multiple disease syndromes, and many of the disease syndromes may be caused by more than one pathogenic agent. The STDs are grouped in this section according to the disease manifestations that the patient is most likely to present to the health care provider. These categories can be seen in Table 15-20. Some of these diseases have been discussed elsewhere in this chapter but are included in the table for completeness. It must be noted that patients with symptoms of a sexually transmitted disease frequently have multiple sexually transmitted diseases and should be evaluated accordingly (Table 15-20).

Table 15-20
STD Categories According to Disease Manifestations[7,32]

Disease Manifestations	STD
Urethritis, cervicitis with an inflammatory pyogenic exudate, salpingitis and related sequelae	Gonorrhea Nongonococcal urethritis Pelvic inflammatory disease
Ulcerative lesions with systemic dissemination of pathogen	Syphilis Lymphogranuloma venereum Herpes
Ulcerative lesions only	Chancroid Granuloma inguinale (donovanosis)
Nonulcerative lesions	Molluscum contagiosum Condylomata acuminata
Vulvovaginitis	Trichomoniasis Candidiasis *Gardnerella vaginalis* vaginitis
Systemic infections without lesions	Cytomegalovirus Hepatitis
Enteric infections	Giardiasis *Campylobacter* enteritis Shigellosis Amebic dysentery
Pubic infestations (Chapter 5)	Scabies Pediculosis

Congenital and perinatal infections and anomalies (see specific infection in this chapter)	TORCH organisms (syndrome):
	  *T*oxoplasmosis
	  *O*ther (e.g., syphilis)
	  *R*ubella
	  *C*ytomegalovirus
	  *H*erpes simplex
	Others
	  Gonorrhea
	  C. trachomatis infections
	  Candidiasis
	  Trichomoniasis

Gonorrhea, Nongonococcal Urethritis, and Pelvic Inflammatory Disease

Gonorrhea (clap, strain, gleet, dose, jack) is an inflammation of the columnar and transitional epithelium caused by the sexually transmitted gonococcus. Symptoms, course of disease, and severity differ between males and females. Chronic and severe complications may result from untreated infections.

Nongonococcal urethritis is a sexually transmitted urethritis in males (cervicitis and salpingitis in females) caused by an agent other than the gonococcus, most commonly Chlamydia trachomatis.

Pelvic inflammatory disease is an acute salpingitis caused by an extension of gonococcal or nongonoccal infection from the vagina and endocervix. Peritonitis, infertility, and ectopic pregnancy are possible sequelae.

The diseases discussed in this section are manifested with urethritis or cervicitis with an inflammatory pyogenic exudate. Salpingitis and other related sequelae may be present (Table 15-21).

PATHOPHYSIOLOGY

In *gonococcal infections*, the gonococcus attaches to and penetrates columnar epithelium, producing a patchy inflammatory response in the submucosa with a polymorphonuclear exudate. Affected areas in the male are the urethra, Littre's and Cowper's glands, the prostate, seminal vesicles, and the epididymis. Affected areas in the female include the glands of Bartholin and Skene, the urethra, the cervix, and the fallopian tubes. The stratified and transitional squamous epithelia are resistant to the gonococcus; therefore the bladder, upper urinary tract, preputial sac, vulva, vagina, and uterus are infrequently involved. The only exception is prepubescent girls who are susceptible to a gonococcal vulvovaginitis before changes in the vaginal epithelium that accompany puberty. In both sexes, primary infections may also affect the pharynx, conjunctivae, and anus. Homosexual males are at risk for primary infections in the anus. Anal infections in females result from an extension of the infection to the anus.[7,63]

Direct extension of the infection occurs by way of lymph vessels. In the female, extension most frequently occurs unilaterally or bilaterally to the fallopian tubes, bypassing the uterus. It appears that the cell surfaces of gonococci are extremely variable, some having greater ability to attach to the fallopian tube mucosa. Thus not all gonococcal cervicitis leads to salpingitis. Direct extension in the male most frequently occurs to the epididymis.[75]

Table 15-21
Overview of STDs Manifested with Urethritis or Cervicitis[7]

	Gonorrhea	Nongonococcal Urethritis (NGU)	Pelvic Inflammatory Disease (PID)
Occurrence	Worldwide; increasing in incidence; highest in 15-30 yr olds and among male homosexuals	Worldwide; increasing more rapidly than is gonorrhea; higher in upper socioeconomic bracket	10-20% of women with gonorrhea develop PID; highest rates in sexually active adolescents
Etiologic agent	*N. gonorhoeae*, the gonococcus	*C. trachomatis, U. urealyticum, T. vaginalis, C. albicans*	*N. gonorrhoeae, C. trachomatis*, or other organisms not sexually transmitted
Reservoir	Humans	Humans	Humans
Transmission	Contact with exudates from mucous membranes of infected persons, usually by direct contact	Direct contact with exudates	Sequela to infection with *N. gonorrhoeae, C. trachomatis*, or other organisms
Incubation period	2-7 d	Range of 2-35 d	Variable
Period of communicability	Months, if untreated	Unknown	Until treated
Susceptibility and resistance	Universal	Universal; no acquired immunity	Women with untreated gonococcal and nongonococcal cervicitis or with an IUD are most susceptible
Report to local health authority	Mandatory case report	No	No

Localized infection in any of the above areas may produce cysts and abscesses. The infection may infrequently resolve without treatment if an adequate cellular immune response develops and if there is adequate drainage of the purulent exudate containing the organism. More commonly, the inflammatory exudate is replaced with fibroblasts; and fibrous tissue fills in the inflamed tissue. Hardening of the fibrous tissue causes strictures of the lumen of the urethra, epididymis, or fallopian tubes. Complete or partial occlusion of the fallopian tubes results in sterility or increased risk for ectopic pregnancy.[63,75]

Infection of the fallopian tubes may also result in an acute pelvic inflammatory disease. Exudate may be released into the pelvic cavity, causing a severe peritonitis; or the pelvic inflammatory disease may become chronic, with recurrent inflammatory flare-ups that predispose to pelvic inflammation with normal flora organisms.

One to three percent of gonococcal infections become disseminated in the blood, producing a septicemia, arthritis, endocarditis, meningitis, or skin lesions. Most disseminated infections are asymptomatic before the dissemination. Occasionally, an extension of a salpingitis in a female will lead to a perihepatitis.[64]

Infection with gonorrhea does result in a short-lived cellular immune response and a longer-lasting humoral immune response, neither of which protects against future infections.[75]

Nongonococcal urethritis and cervicitis are most frequently caused by strains of *Chlamydia trachomatis* that are pathogenic to columnar epithelium in a manner similar to *Neisseria gonorrhoeae*. Symptomatic manifestations are generally less severe than with gonorrhea, with many subclinical infections. Extension of the inflammation into the fallopian tubes with the potential for a pelvic inflammatory disease is a potential complication of infection with *C. trachomatis*. Transmission of the pathogen during birth can result in ophthalmia neonatorum and pneumonia in the neonate. Infection with *C. trachomatis* stimulates a cellular and humoral immune response, neither of which is protective against future infections.[89]

DIAGNOSTIC STUDIES[23]

Culture of exudate from urethra, vagina, or fallopian tubes

Positive for *N. gonorrhoeae* or *C. trachomatis* associated with gonorrhea, nongonococcal urethritis, cervicitis, or pelvic inflammatory disease

Microscopic examination of gram-stained exudate

Positive for gram-negative intracellular diplococci of gonorrhea

In nongonococcal urethritis there will be excess WBCs in urethral smear in absence of gram-negative diplococci

Nongonococcal cervicitis cannot be diagnosed by Gram's stain

Serology for systemic gonococcal infections: complement fixation or immunofluorescent test

Fourfold rise in antibody titer between onset of infection and later disease

Laparotomy

Direct visualization of inflamed fallopian tubes and exudate in pelvic inflammatory disease

Sonogram

Abscess may be visualized in pelvic inflammatory disease

TREATMENT PLAN[23]

Surgical

Hysterectomy possibly indicated in a severe pelvic inflammatory disease to prevent septicemia

Chemotherapeutic

Anti-infective agents

Uncomplicated gonococcal infections in adults

Tetracycline hydrochloride (Achromycin; others), 500 mg po qid for 7 d, or

Doxycycline hyclate (Vibramycin), 100 mg po bid for 7 d, or

Amoxicillin (Amoxil; others), 3.0 g po, single dose with 1.0 g probenecid po, or

Ampicillin (Amcill; others), 3.5 g po, single dose with 1.0 g probenecid po, or

Aqueous procaine penicillin G, 4.8 million units IM at two sites with 1.0 g of probenecid po

For gonococcal infections with chlamydial infection

Amoxicillin or ampicillin (as above), plus tetracycline or doxycycline (as above; tetracycline is effective against *Chlamydia*)

For anorectal gonorrhea

Aqueous procaine penicillin (as above)

For pharyngeal gonorrhea

Tetracycline or aqueous procaine penicillin

For penicillin-allergic patients who cannot tolerate tetracycline or for treatment failures: spectinomycin hydrochloride (Trobicin), 2.0 g IM in one injection

For treatment failures resulting from penicillinase-producing *N. gonorrhoeae*

Spectinomycin (Trobicin), 2.0 g IM in one injection, plus

Tetracycline (Achromycin; others) (for *Chlamydia*), or

Cefoxitin (Mefoxin), 2.0 g IM in one injection plus probenecid, 1.0 g po, or

Cefotaxime (Claforan), 1.0 g IM in one injection without probenecid

For pharyngeal infections with penicillinase-producing *N. gonorrhoeae*

Trimethoprim/sulfamethoxazole (Septra, Bactrim), 80 mg trimethoprim and 400 mg sulfamethoxazole po in a single dose of 9 tablets daily for 5 days

Gonococcal infections during pregnancy

Amoxicillin or ampicillin (as described above), or

Spectinomycin (Trobicin), 2.0 g IM

Disseminated gonococcal infections, excluding meningitis and endocarditis

Aqueous crystalline penicillin G, 10 million units IV/d until improvement, followed by

Amoxicillin (Amoxil), 500 mg, or ampicillin (Amcill; others), 500 mg po qid to complete 7 days of antibiotic treatment, or

Amoxicillin (Amoxil), 3.0 g, or ampicillin (Amcill; others), 3.5 g po; each with probenecid, 1.0 g, single dose followed by amoxicillin or ampicillin, 500 mg po qid for 7 d, or

Tetracycline hydrochloride (Achromycin; others), 500 mg po qid for 7 d, or

Cefoxitin (Mefoxin), 1 g IV, or

Cefotaxime (Claforan), 500 mg IV either given qid for 7 d, or

Erythromycin (Erythrocin), 500 mg po qid for 7 d

Nongonococcal urethritis

Tetracycline hydrochloride (Achromycin; others), 500 mg po qid for 7 d, or

Doxycycline (Vibramycin), 100 mg po bid for 7 d, or

Erythromycin (Erythrocin), 500 mg po qid for 7 d

Pelvic inflammatory disease: combination of antimicrobials is used until the etiologic agent in the infection is established. Effective against *N. gonorrhoeae*, penicillinase-producing *N. gonorrhoeae*, and *C. trachomatis:*

Inpatient treatment

Doxyclycline (Vibramycin), 100 mg IV bid, plus

Cefoxitin (Mefoxin), 2.0 g IV qid; both to be given for 4 d, then

Doxycycline (Vibramycin), 100 mg po bid to complete 10-14 d therapy

Outpatient treatment

Cefoxitin (Mefoxin), 2.0 g IM, or

Amoxicillin (Amoxil), 3.0 g po, or

Ampicillin (Amcill; others), 3.5 g po, or

Aqueous procaine penicillin G, 4.8 million units IM at two sites; each along with

Probenecid, 1.0 g po, followed by

Doxycycline (Vibramycin), 100 mg po bid for 10-14 d[23]

All sexual partners of patients with gonorrhea, nongonococcal urethritis (or cervicitis), or pelvic inflammatory disease should be examined and treated

All persons treated for gonorrhea should be recultured 4-7 d after completion of treatment. Rectal cultures should be obtained from women treated for gonorrhea[23]

ASSESSMENT: AREAS OF CONCERN[7,64]

Gonorrhea: males

2 to 7 days after exposure

Urinary tract

Purulent yellow-white discharge from anterior urethra

Dysuria

Inflammation around urinary meatus

Pain and urinary retention with prostatitis

Severe pain and swelling with epididymitis

Rectum

Pruritus, tenesmus, and discharge (homosexuals)

Gonorrhea: females

2 to 7 days after exposure: may be asymptomatic

Urinary tract

Dysuria sometimes occurs

Vagina

Purulent discharge (may go unnoticed)

Uterus

Abnormal and painful menses

Symptoms of endometritis

Rectum

Tenesmus

Bloody mucoid diarrhea

Burning and discharge

Gonorrhea: males and females

Oropharynx

Pharyngitis possible

Eyes

Conjunctivitis possible

Systemic manifestations (possible)

Septicemia

Endocarditis

Meningitis

Arthritis

Painful vesicular pustular skin lesions on an erythematous base
Petechial skin lesions

Nongonococcal urethritis: males
Opaque discharge from urethra
Dysuria
Urethral pruritus

Nongonococcal cervicitis: females
Asymptomatic usually

Pelvic inflammatory disease
Vagina
Abnormal uterine bleeding

Foul-smelling vaginal discharge
Pain with coitus

Abdomen and pelvis
Pain and tenderness in lower abdomen
Palpation of soft, tender, fluid-filled pelvic abscess
with bimanual examination

Body temperature
Fever and chills

Laboratory values
Elevated WBC count and erythrocyte sedimentation
rate

NURSING DIAGNOSES and NURSING INTERVENTIONS

Nursing Diagnosis	Nursing Intervention
Potential patient problem: transmission of illness	See "Patient Education" below. Collect specimen for culture. Administer antibiotics as prescribed.
Sexual dysfunction	See "Patient Education."

See Chapter 11 for care of patients with pelvic inflammatory disease.

Patient Education[23]

1. Avoid sexual activity until follow-up cultures are negative for *N. gonorrhoeae* organisms or until treatment
   is completed for other organisms.
2. Sexual contacts must be examined and treated to prevent reinfection of the patient.
3. Course of antibiotic therapy must be completed to
   avoid chronic infection and subsequent complications. If tetracycline is prescribed, it should be taken
   1 hour before or 2 hours after meals. Patient should
   avoid dairy products, antacids, iron, or other mineral-
   containing preparations and sunlight.

4. Condoms provide some protection.
5. Individuals who are high risk for reinfection should
   be encouraged to be screened periodically. All treated
   patients should return for evaluation 4 to 7 days after
   completion of therapy.
6. Care should be taken with vaginal or urethral discharges to avoid contamination of eyes.
7. Following treatment for pelvic inflammatory disease,
   patients who use an IUD should consult with physician for reevaluation of IUD as a contraceptive
   method.

EVALUATION

Patient Outcome	Data Indicating That Outcome is Reached
There is no infection.	Cultures are negative for gonococcus. There is no urethral or vaginal discharge, dysuria, tenesmus, urethral pruritus, or abdominal pain. Menses are normal, with no dysmenorrhea.
There are no chronic complications.	Female is able to conceive. Male is free of urinary retention and pain of epididymitis.
Body temperature is normal.	Oral adult temperature is 37° C (98.6° F).
Laboratory values are within normal limits.	Leukocyte count and sedimentation rate are normal.
The patient complies with recommendations.	Sexual partners have been examined and treated.

Syphilis

Syphilis (lues) is a chronic systemic disease characterized by a primary lesion, a secondary eruption involving skin and mucous membranes, long periods of latency, and late seriously disabling lesions of skin, bone, viscera, central nervous system, and cardiovsacular system.

Syphilis is one of several sexually transmitted diseases that have both ulcerative lesions and systemic dissemination. Others are herpesvirus infections and lymphogranuloma venereum (Table 15-22).

PATHOPHYSIOLOGY

Syphilis is a systemic infection of the vascular system characterized by five distinct stages: incubation, primary and secondary stages, latency, and late syphilis. Incubation begins with the penetration of *Treponema pallidum* into intact mucous membranes or abraded skin. Some of the pathogens remain at the site of invasion while others migrate, within hours, to regional lymph nodes, where some remain while others are disseminated throughout the body. *Treponema* can invade and multiply in any organ system, producing lesions wherever the concentration of the microorganism is the greatest. During this incubation period, blood containing the *Treponema* organisms is infectious.[84,107]

Vascular pathologic manifestations are the consequence of treponemal tissue invasion at all stages. The inflammatory response in the endothelial tissue produces perivascular infiltration of lymphocytes and plasma cells, resulting in endothelial swelling and an obliterative endarteritis of terminal arterioles and small arteries. Concentric fibroblastic proliferative thickening occurs in the vessels, resulting in eventual foci of tissue necrosis.[84,107]

Table 15-22
Overview of STDs with Ulcerative Lesions and Systemic Dissemination[7]

	Syphilis	**Genital Herpes**	**Herpes Type 1**	**Lymphogranuloma Venereum**
Occurrence	Worldwide; increasing in incidence; highest in 15-30 yr olds and in males, particularly male homosexuals	Worldwide; increasing rapidly; highest in 15-30 yr olds; most common STD in United States	Worldwide; 70-90% of adults have antibodies against herpes type 1; primary infection probably occurs by age 5 yr	Worldwide; higher in tropical and subtropical climates
Etiologic agent	*Treponema pallidum*, a spirochete	Herpes simplex virus 2; possibly Herpes simplex virus 1	Herpes simplex virus type 1	Several strains of *C. trachomatis*
Reservoir	Humans	Humans	Humans	Humans
Transmission	Direct contact with exudates from lesions on skin and mucous membranes; blood transfusion; congenital	Direct contact with saliva or secretions from mucous membranes and lesions; congenital	Contact with saliva of carriers and active lesions; may be transmitted sexually	Direct contact with open lesions
Incubation period	10 d to 10 wk; usually 3 wk	2-12 d; average of 6 d	2-12 d	4-21 d; usually 7-12 d
Period of communicability	Variable; during primary and secondary stages and in mucocutaneous recurrences; 2-4 yr if untreated	Transient shedding of virus in absence of lesions probably occurs; 7-12 d with lesion	During lesions; virus in saliva found as long as 7 wk after recovery of lesions; transient shedding of virus is common	Variable; weeks to years as long as lesions are present
Susceptibility and resistance	Universal, although only 10% of exposures result in infection; no natural immunity; infection leads to gradually developing resistance to new infections	Universal; immune response does not prevent recurrence	Universal susceptibility	General
Report to local health authority	Mandatory case report	No	No	In some states

The primary stage is characterized by a single lesion containing the *Treponema* at the site of initial invasion, appearing 10 to 90 days after infection. The lesion is firm and hard as a result of intense cellular infiltration accompanied by serum accumulation in connective tissue. The lesion heals spontaneously within 1 to 5 weeks (average of 2 to 3 weeks). A satellite lesion, or bubo, may develop in an inguinal lymph node.[64]

The secondary stage begins as the primary lesion is resolving, lasts 2 to 6 weeks, and is manifested with parenchymal, systemic, and mucocutaneous symptoms that indicate treponemal pathologic manifestations throughout the body. *Treponema* can be recovered from all skin and mucous membrane lesions.[107]

A period of latency, ranging from 1 to 40 plus years, follows the secondary stage. During the first year of latency there may be recurrence of secondary stage manifestations. Subclinical infection with progressive arterial damage continues for some number of infected persons.

About one third of infected, untreated persons manifest symptoms of late syphilis with clinical evidence of degenerative lesions of the cardiovascular and central nervous systems, the skin, and the viscera. These lesions, called gummas, may be the result of a hypersensitive cellular immune response to the *Treponema* in the tissue. Gummas are granulomatous lesions consisting of a necrotic, coagulated center with obliterative endarteritis of small vessels in the tissue. Lesions of late syphilis, including open gummas on the skin, do not contain *Treponema*. They are therefore not infectious.[84,107]

Disease manifestations of late syphilis depend on the area of arterial lesions and the extent of circulatory insufficiency. Central nervous system disease may be asymptomatic, meningovascular, or parenchymatous. Parenchymatous neurosyphilis can be seen clinically as paresis (resulting from progressive cortical neuron degeneration) or tabes dorsalis (resulting from posterior column degeneration).[64]

Cardiovascular symptoms frequently result from aortic necrosis with resultant aortic insufficiency.

The immune response in syphilis is not completely understood. Humoral antibodies develop early and persist in untreated persons, but they do not seem to alter the course of the disease. The cell-mediated immune response increases during latency. This may account for the lack of progression to late syphilis for a large portion of untreated persons. Antibody levels will gradually decrease in persons treated in primary and secondary stages.[84]

Congenital transmission of *Treponema* may occur at any time during pregnancy, but the fetus does not develop an inflammatory response to the pathogen until around the fifteenth week of gestation. Treatment of infected pregnant women before the fifteenth week may prevent damage to the fetus. Evidence of congenital syphilitic damage includes early malformations, observed at birth or during the first 2 years of life, and later evidence of developmental deformities. Infants with congenital syphilis born to untreated or inadequately treated mothers will have active infection and must be treated.[64]

DIAGNOSTIC STUDIES[64,84,107]

Dark-field or phase-contrast microscopic examination of exudate or cells from lesions or regional lymph nodes
  Positive for *T. pallidum* in primary and secondary stages
  Not useful for latent or tertiary stages

Nontreponemal serologic tests: VDRL (most common), Kline, Kahn, Hinton, Mazzini tests; RPR (rapid plasma reagin), ART (automated reagin test), RST (reagin screen test)
  Useful for screening; many false positive results
  Increase in nonspecific antibodies 1 to 3 weeks after appearance of the chancre or 4 to 6 weeks after infection
  Become negative in 6 to 12 months after treatment of primary syphilis; 12 to 18 months after treatment of secondary syphilis
  Serologic tests may not revert to negative if treatment is delayed beyond 2 years

Treponemal serologic tests: FTA-ABS (fluorescent Treponema antibody absorption); TPHA-TP (T. pallidum hemagglutination assay); TPI (T. pallidum immobilization; rarely done), MHA-TP (microhemagglutination assay)
  Useful for confirmation of positive screening tests
  Reported as nonreactive, borderline, or reactive
  These tests become reactive earlier in the primary stage and remain reactive longer in latent and late syphilis
  More sensitive and specific but expensive

TREATMENT PLAN

Chemotherapeutic[23,64]
  Anti-infective agents
    Primary, secondary, or early syphilis of less than 1 yr duration: benzathine penicillin G, 2.4 million units IM
    Of more than 1 yr duration: benzathine penicillin G (Bicillin), 7.2 million units total; 2.4 million units IM weekly for 3 successive weeks
    Patients allergic to penicillin: tetracycline hydrochloride (Achromycin; others), 500 mg po qid for 15 d for infections of less than 1 yr; for 30 d for

infections of longer duration (Pregnant women should not receive tetracycline.)

For penicillin-allergic pregnant women: erythromycin (stearate, ethyl succinate or base), 500 mg po qid for 15 d for infections of less than 1 yr; for 30 d for infections of longer duration (Infants born to women treated with erythromycin should be treated with penicillin.)

Infants suspected of having syphilis with abnormal cerebrospinal fluid findings: aqueous crystalline penicillin G, 50,000 units/kg IM or IV in two divided doses daily for 10 d

Infants with normal cerebrospinal fluid findings: benzathine penicillin G, 50,000 units/kg IM in a single dose

ASSESSMENT: AREAS OF CONCERN[64,84,107]

Primary stage
Within 10 to 90 days after exposure (average of 21 days); lasts 1 to 5 weeks

Genitalia
Single painless papule erodes to become a hard, painless indurated chancre without an exudate; usually located on the glans penis of the male and on the cervix or external genitalia of the female; may be on the scrotum, anus, rectum, lips, tongue, tonsils, nipple, and fingers

Inguinal lymph nodes
Hard, nonfluctuant, painless, enlarged inguinal lymph node

Secondary stage
Within 6 weeks of onset of primary infection; lasts a few days to 1 year

Skin
Local or generalized, papulosquamous, macular, papular, or pustular rash; bilateral and symmetric, beginning on trunk and proximal extremities; frequently on soles of feet and palms of hands

Lesions: 3 to 10 mm; nonpruritic

Condylomata lata: lesions on moist areas coalesce and erode to produce painless, moist, gray-white raised plaques

Alopecia: nonscarring, temporary hair loss in patches on head and eyebrows

Mucous membranes
Mucous patches: silver-gray superficial erosion surrounded by red periphery on mucous membranes

Systemic symptoms
Malaise
Fever
Headache

Gastrointestinal concerns
Epigastric pain or vomiting associated with ulceration

Latent stage
May have relapses of mucocutaneous symptoms of secondary stage early in latency; otherwise, no symptoms

Late stage
Symptoms may be manifested in one or more systems

Neurologic concerns
Asymptomatic
No symptoms except leukocytes and protein in cerebrospinal fluid

Meningovascular symptoms
Focal neurologic signs depending on area of lesions
Seizures

Parenchymatous symptoms
Paresis: personality changes ranging from minor to severe psychosis; alteration in intellect and judgment; hyperactive reflexes
Tabes dorsalis: ataxia, areflexia, paresthesias, bladder disturbance, impotency; sharp, tearing pain
Trophic joint changes
Optic atrophy with small, irregular pupils that are not reactive to light but respond normally to accommodation

Cardiovascular concerns
Signs of aortic insufficiency

Skin and mucous membranes
Gummas: lesions varying from small to large tumorlike masses or ulcers

Early congenital syphilis
Abdomen
Hepatosplenomegaly

Skeletal concerns
Osteochondritis, particularly of the femur and humerus, seen on x-ray examination
Periostitis

Nasopharyngeal concerns
Rhinitis and coryza within first week of life
Frequently bloody mucus

Skin and nails

Dark red, copper-colored maculopapular rash: appears slowly over 3-wk period and is followed by a branny desquamation; coppery pigmentation may persist

Suppuration and exfoliation of nails

Loss of hair and eyebrows

Mucous membranes

Fissures on lips, nares, and anus, which bleed easily

Mucous patches on any mucous membrane

Raised moist lesions (condylomata) on areas of skin where there is moisture or friction

Lymph nodes

Generalized lymphadenitis

Late congenital syphilis

Developmental deformities of bones and teeth

Hutchinson's teeth and mulberry molars

Saddle nose

Interstitial keratitis

Enlarged frontal bossae

Saber shins

Scaphoid scapulae

Short maxilla, high palatine arch, protuberant mandible, and perforation of the hard palate

Neurologic concerns

Deafness

Taboparesis

Mental deficiency

NURSING DIAGNOSES and NURSING INTERVENTIONS

Nursing Diagnosis	Nursing Intervention
Potential patient problem: transmission of infection	Employ drainage and secretion precautions and blood and body fluid precautions for hospitalized patients with primary, secondary, or congenital syphilis (p. 1622).

Patient Education[23,107]

1. All sexual partners should be referred for examination and treatment (sexual contacts up to 3 months preceding primary infection, up to 6 months preceding secondary stage, and up to 1 year preceding latent stage).
2. Sexual activity should be avoided until patient and partners are adequately treated and all lesions are healed.
3. Condoms may prevent future infections.
4. Treated patients should return for follow-up serologic tests 3, 6, 12, and 24 months after therapy.

5. If tetracycline is administered, it must be taken for the full prescribed course. It should be taken 1 hour before or 2 hours after meals. Dairy products, antacids, iron, other mineral-containing preparations, and sunlight should be avoided.[23]
6. A systemic reaction (fever, chills, headache, tachycardia) 1 or 2 hours after onset of antibiotic treatment is due to endotoxin release from dying spirochetes. The condition is benign and self-limiting. Bed rest and aspirin will help.

EVALUATION

Patient Outcome	Data Indicating That Outcome is Reached
There is no infection.	Lesions have cleared; cerebrospinal fluid is normal. Patient and sexual contacts have been adequately treated with antibiotics. Follow-up serologic tests indicate decreasing antibody titers.

Herpesvirus Infections

Herpes simplex is a systemic viral infection characterized by a localized primary lesion, latency, and a tendency to localized recurrence. Two serologically distinct herpes viral agents, 1 and 2, generally produce distinct clinical syndromes. Herpes simplex virus type 2 (HSV-2) is most often implicated in genital herpes.

Both types of herpesvirus infections are summarized with other sexually transmitted diseases with ulcerative lesions and systemic dissemination in Table 15-22.

PATHOPHYSIOLOGY

Two antigenically distinct herpes simplex viruses (HSV), types 1 and 2, are responsible for herpes infections. Both are capable of producing infection in epithelial tissue anywhere in the body, but HSV-1 is most often associated with oral, labial, ocular, or skin herpes above the waist, whereas HSV-2 is implicated in 90% of genital, anal, and perianal herpes or oral herpes associated with genital, oral, or sexual transmission.[74] Infections caused by both types of HSV will be discussed in this section because of the potential for sexual transmission of both agents and because both produce essentially the same pathologic findings.

All HSV infections have two characteristics in common:

1. Once present in tissue, HSV produces a chronic infection initiated with active self-limiting tissue destruction. The lesions heal, but the organism continues to be viable in the body in the presence of circulating antibodies and in the absence of symptomatic disease.

2. There is a latent period during which the genome of the virus is present in tissue in a nondestructive form. Infectious virions cannot be recovered until the virus becomes reactivated and produces recurrent infectious disease. Active infection, either initial or recurrent, need not be symptomatic.[29]

Initial infection refers to the first infection with the HSV type. Initial infection with HSV-1 usually occurs by age 4 years and is manifested by a clinical or subclinical gingivostomatitis. Initial infection with HSV-2 usually occurs during the ages of sexual activity and is usually manifested by clinical or subclinical genital herpes.

The organism is transmitted by close contact with saliva or genital secretions of persons with active clinical or subclinical infections either directly or by hand.

The transmitted virus invades and replicates in the parabasal and intermediate epithelial cells of mucous membranes or traumatized skin. Intracellular and extracellular edema and cell lysis cause the cells to lose their intercellular bridges and to undergo a ballooning degen-

eration. Polymorphonuclear cells infiltrate, forming a thin-walled intradermal vesicle on an erythematous base. Multiple grouped vesicles can be visualized at the sites of tissue inoculation. The superficial epithelium collapses and sloughs, leaving single shallow ulcers; or the vesicles may coalesce into large painful ulcers. Crusting may occur on non-mucous-membrane ulcers. All ulcers spontaneously granulate without scarring in about 12 days in initial infections.[29,55,74]

The virus may enter the lymphatic system, producing localized lesions there. Rarely, the virus is disseminated to visceral organs, particularly the liver, adrenal glands, lungs, or central nervous system, producing discrete focal areas of necrosis in epithelial tissues in those organs. The virus may also be spread to other external body sites by autoinoculation.[74]

Cellular immune response and nonspecific host defenses appear to inhibit dissemination. Circulating humoral antibodies develop but do not appear to be protective against reinfection or recurrent infection.[55,74]

Following the primary infection the HSV travels along sensory nerve pathways to a sensory nerve ganglion where it remains in a latent stage. The viral DNA is stored in ganglion neurons in the absence of other viral products. The virus is not pathogenic in this form. It appears that the transient viral shedding may occur during this stage.[23,55]

The exact mechanism for reactivation of the virus to produce recurrence of lesions is not known; but there are two predominant hypotheses. The *ganglion trigger theory* suggests that a stimulus to latently infected ganglion neurons stimulates the replication of the virus in the neurons. The virus migrates along peripheral nerves to reinvade epithelial cells, producing focal and cellular destruction as in initial infections. The *skin trigger theory* proposes that virus replication in the ganglion neurons is continuous, with viruses regularly reaching the epidermis by way of peripheral nerves. Cellular immune responses block the development of a cellular infectious process unless an external stimulus, such as trauma, overwhelms the defenses.[29]

Recurrence of HSV lesions is generally in the area of initial inoculation. Genital recurrence is usually associated with HSV-2 and is usually less severe, lasting 4 or 5 days. Genital recurrence is common in women with asymptomatic cervical lesions. Oral HSV-1 infections frequently recur on the lips. Recurrence of either type may be triggered by another infectious disease, menstruation, emotional stress, and immunosuppression.[29,55]

Potential complications of herpes infections include neuralgia, meningitis (HSV-1), encephalitis (HSV-2), ascending myelitis, urethral strictures, and lymphatic suppuration. In females there is the possibility of an increased risk for spontaneous abortion and cervical cancer. Neonates may become infected during vaginal delivery. Congenital herpes ranges from subclinical infections to severe infections of the skin, eyes, mucous membranes, visceral organs, or central nervous system. Congenital herpes has a high mortality. Many survivors have ocular or neurologic sequelae.[23]

DIAGNOSTIC STUDIES[23,74]

Virus tissue culture of specimen from base of vesicles using fluorescent antibody or neutralization techniques
Identification of type 1 or type 2 viral cytopathogenic effect in tissue culture

Microscopic examination of stained smear from base of vesicles
Direct identification of multinucleated giant cells with intranuclear inclusions

Complement fixation or neutralization tests
Fourfold increase in antibody titer in convalescent serum; difficult to differentiate type 1 from type 2

Indirect immunofluorescence and radioimmunoassay
IgM antibodies detected in primary and recurrent infections

TREATMENT PLAN[23,74]

Surgical
Caesarean delivery before membranes rupture when primary or recurrent genital herpes occurs in late pregnancy

Chemotherapeutic
Anti-infective agents
For first clinical episode of genital herpes: acyclovir ointment (Zovirax), 5% topically applied to cover all genital lesions q3h, six times a day for 7 d
For ocular herpes: topical vira-A or trifluorothymidine or topical iododeoxyuridine

ASSESSMENT: AREAS OF CONCERN[74]

Gingivostomatitis
Initial HSV-1 infection

Oral cavity
Multiple vesicular and ulcerative lesions on labial and buccal mucosa, tongue, and larynx
Erythema of gums; excessive salivation
Infection heals in 7 to 10 days; recurrent infections rare in mouth

Cervical lymph nodes
Enlarged and palpable

Lips
Recurrent "cold sore" or "fever blister" preceded by 1 or 2 days of paresthesia; lesions crust and heal within 3 to 10 days

Ocular herpes
Eyes
Keratitis and conjunctivitis (unilateral or bilateral)

Lymph nodes
Periauricular lymphadenopathy

Cutaneous
Skin
Clustered vesicular lesions anywhere on body
Deep burning pain; skin edema

Lymph nodes
Regional lymphadenopathy

Genital herpes
Genitourinary: females
Asymptomatic or extensive vesicular lesions with deep ulceration and marked hyperplasia and erythema of cervix, labia, fourchette clitoris (sometimes vagina); may extend to anal area, buttocks, and thighs
Dysuria, leukorrhea, and marked genital tenderness

Genitourinary: male
Scattered vesicles over glans, prepuce, and shaft of the penis
Urinary retention
Urethritis may occur without genital lesions
Anal lesions in homosexual males

Inguinal lymph nodes
Bilateral lymphadenopathy in 50% of initial genital infections

Systemic manifestations
Fever in initial infections

Oral cavity
Genital lesions may be sexually transmitted to oral cavity

NURSING DIAGNOSES and NURSING INTERVENTIONS*

Nursing Diagnosis	Nursing Intervention
Comfort, alteration in: pain	Keep involved area clean and dry.
Potential patient problem: transmission of infection	See "Patient Education" below. Employ drainage and secretion precautions for hospitalized patient. Employ contact isolation for neonates with perinatal exposure (p. 1620). Health care workers must wear gloves when in contact with secretions and lesions.

*For genital herpes only.

Patient Education[23]

1. Abstain from sex while lesions are present during initial and recurrent infections. Condoms may offer protection during latency.
2. Pregnant women should inform physician of history of genital herpes.
3. Annual Papanicolaou smears are recommended.

EVALUATION

Patient Outcome	Data Indicating That Outcome is Reached
Infection does not spread.	Herpes is not spread to health care workers, newborn infants, or sexual partners of the patient.

Lymphogranuloma Venereum

Lymphogranuloma venereum is a systemic and disabling bacterial infection beginning with a small, painless evanescent erosion on the penis or vulva. Regional lymph nodes undergo suppuration, spreading the inflammatory process into adjacent tissue. The disease is disseminated further by way of the lymph system. There are usually systemic symptoms of the lymphadenitis and serious complications in untreated individuals.[7]

For an overview of lymphogranuloma venereum with other sexually transmitted diseases characterized by ulcerative lesions and systemic dissemination, see Table 15-22.

PATHOPHYSIOLOGY

Lymphogranuloma venereum is a systemic infection produced by mucosal invasion of a number of closely related strains of *Chlamydia*. The disease has three stages: a primary lesion, regional and disseminated lymphadenitis, and late complications resulting from progression of the regional lymphadenitis.[54]

A primary transient nodular or vesicular lesion forms at the site of inoculation. Dissemination of the organism to regional lymph nodes (primarily inguinal lymph nodes) results in lymph node lesions that are initially similar to the inoculation lesion. The lesions are composed of small masses of epithelioid cells with multinucleated cells scat-

tered throughout, and a necrotic center filled with polymorphonuclear leukocytes. Satellite lesions are formed in the lymph node, surrounded by a narrow layer of epithelioid cells. The nodes show hyperplasia with an inflammatory cellular infiltration consisting of plasma cells, polymorphonuclear leukocytes, large mononuclear cells, and lymphocytes. Spread of the inflammation throughout the nodes causes the nodes to become matted together and form a large abscess. These abscesses develop in one or more areas along the lymphatic system. Untreated, the abscesses may rupture through the skin or other epithelial surfaces to produce chronic draining sinuses or fistulas. If the condition is not treated, it progresses, producing complications resulting from the impaired lymph and draining sinuses.[54]

Complications include elephantiasis of the genitalia, and perianal abscesses and fistulas resulting in eventual rectal stricture. Advanced stages of rectal stricture may be manifested by symptoms of painful ileus, distention, complete obstruction, perforation, and peritonitis.[54]

DIAGNOSTIC STUDIES[54]

Cell culture of lesion exudate or bubo aspirate (not widely available)
Positive for *C. trachomatis*

Complement fixation

Antibody titer of 1:16 or higher within 1 to 3 weeks of infection; fourfold rise in titer between early infection and convalescence

Nonspecific, since it detects antibodies against all *C. trachomatis* strains

TREATMENT PLAN[23]

Surgical

Aspiration of fluctuant lymph nodes as needed (Incision and drainage or excision is contraindicated.)

Strictures or fistulas may require surgery

Chemotherapeutic

Anti-infective agents

Tetracycline hydrochloride (Achromycin; others), 500 mg po qid for 14 d, or

Doxycycline (Vibramycin), 100 mg po bid for 14 d, or

Erythromycin (Erythrocin; others), 500 mg po qid for 14 d, or

Sulfamethoxazole (Gantanol), 1 g po bid for 14 d (other sulfonamides can be used in equal doses)

ASSESSMENT: AREAS OF CONCERN[23,54]

Primary lesion (genitalia)

2-3 mm painless, discrete, superficial vesicle or non-indurated ulcer at site of inoculation; frequently unnoticed

Usually on glans or shaft of the penis in males and on the labia, vagina, or cervix in females

May be in the rectum or mouth

Rectal inoculation produces bloody discharge and tenesmus at first; mucopurulent discharge, cramps, and diarrhea later

Regional lymph nodes

7 to 30 days after primary lesion

Initially a firm, tender, discrete, movable inguinal lymph node, which later becomes indolent, fixed, and matted; may be unilateral or bilateral; may subside spontaneously or proceed to form an abscess that may rupture to produce a draining sinus or fistula

Female lymph node involvement may be mainly in the pelvic nodes with extension to the rectum and rectovaginal septum

Systemic symptoms

Fever

Chills

Headache

Joint pains

Anorexia

Abdominal pain

Urinary retention

Complications

Genitalia

Elephantiasis of prepuce, penis, scrotum, or vulva

Rectum

Perianal abscess; rectovaginal, rectovesical, and ischiorectal fistulas

Rectal stricture 1 to 10 years after infection

NURSING DIAGNOSES and NURSING INTERVENTIONS

Nursing Diagnosis	Nursing Intervention
Potential patient problem: transmission of infection	Handle exudates with caution. See "Patient Education" below.

Patient Education

1. The sequelae of untreated lymphogranuloma venereum are serious. Patient must complete the prescribed antibiotic regimen and return for evaluation 3 to 5 days after treatment is begun and weekly or biweekly until the infection is entirely healed.
2. Tetracycline should be taken 1 hour before or 2 hours after meals. Dairy products, antacids, iron, other mineral-containing preparations, and sunlight should be avoided.
3. Sexual partners should be examined and treated.

EVALUATION

Patient Outcome	Data Indicating That Outcome is Reached
There is no infection.	Lymph nodes are not swollen, hot, or tender. Mucopurulent exudate no longer drains from sinuses. Body temperature is normal.
There are no complications.	Rectum and anal opening are patent. There is no abdominal distention or cramping. Defecation is normal.

Chancroid and Granuloma Inguinale

Chancroid, also called "soft sore" or "soft chancre," is an acute, localized, autoinoculable bacterial infection of the genitalia. Necrotizing ulceration occurs at the site of inoculation, frequently accompanied by suppuration of regional lymph nodes. Systemic dissemination does not occur.

Granuloma inguinale (donovanosis) is a mildly communicable, chronic and progressive, autoinoculable bacterial infection of the skin and mucous membranes, external genitalia, inguinal and anal regions, face, and oral cavity. Lesions first appear as small, painless papules or vesicles that become ulcerated and slowly develop into bleeding granulomatous masses. The disease may be difficult to differentiate from carcinoma[7] (Table 15-23).

PATHOPHYSIOLOGY

Although both chancroid and granuloma inguinale are manifested by ulcerative lesions, their pathophysiologies differ. In *chancroid* the transmitted pathogenic bacteria initially invade genital skin or mucous membranes at sites traumatized by sexual contact. A preexisting abrasion facilitates invasion. A small papule is formed, surrounded by a zone of erythema. This erupts to form a shallow and painful ulcer. The lesions histologically show three layers. The shallow surface layer contains many polymorphonuclear cells, erythrocytes, and necrotic debris. The middle layer is edematous and shows endothelial proliferation of blood vessels. In the deep layer there is dense infiltration of plasma cells and lymphocytes. A purulent exudate results from the extensive necrotic process. The ulcers may enlarge and continue to erode and destroy tissue or become secondarily infected, producing even more rapid destruction of tissue. Fresh lesions may occur from autoinoculation. Extragenital lesions may occur on fingers, tongue, lips, breasts, and eyelids.[52]

Lymphatic dissemination results in a unilateral or bilateral painful inguinal adenitis within 7 to 10 days of the primary lesion. The enlarged lymph gland (bubo) softens, becomes fluctuant, and may rupture spontaneously. Long-term complications include phimosis and urethral fistulas in males. Females are frequently asymptomatic.

Table 15-23
Overview of STDs With Ulcerative Lesions[7,52,53]

	Chancroid	Granuloma Inguinale (Donovanosis)
Occurrence	Most common in tropical and subtropical climates	Most common in tropical and subtropical climates and in males
Etiologic agent	*Haemophilus ducreyi*, a bacterium	*Calymmatobacterium granulomatis*
Reservoir	Humans	Humans
Transmission	Direct sexual contact with exudate from lesions; indirect transmission is rare	Direct sexual contact with lesions or with organism in rectum of nondiseased carriers
Incubation period	3-14 d	8-80 d
Period of communicability	Until lesions heal (can be weeks)	Duration of open lesions
Susceptibility and resistance	General, but highest in uncircumcised males; no evidence of resistance, although women may have more subclinical infections	No evidence of immunity
Report to local health authority	Mandatory case report	Mandatory case report

The transmission of *granuloma inguinale* is less well understood. The pathogenic bacterium can be found in the rectum of nondiseased patients, suggesting that the organism may be part of the normal gastrointestinal flora of some persons. Lesions may result from autoinfection, possibly following trauma to the genitalia. The pathogen in the lesions is transmitted sexually, but repeated exposure seems to be necessary for transmission. The disease is rare in heterosexual partners of patients. Clinical disease is highest in homosexual males.[53,96]

The organism invades mononuclear endothelial cells, forming a small, painless papule or nodule at the site of dermal invasion. The prickle cell layer becomes thickened, and a dense dermal infiltrate containing plasma cells, histiocytes, and polymorphonuclear cells forms in the lesion. The epithelium overlapping the lesion softens, erodes, and ulcerates, producing a gradually enlarging granulomatous ulcerating lesion that bleeds easily. Pronounced marginal epithelial proliferation may simulate early epitheliomatous changes of cancer. The raised mass of granulation tissue looks more like a tumor than an ulcer. Single or multiple lesions may coalesce, or lesions may spread to contiguous tissue. Lesions have variable clinical appearances depending on the area located, mode of spread, tissue resistance, and texture of the skin (p. 549). Secondary infection and expanding necrosis in untreated lesions may result in complete genital erosion.[53,96]

The lesions heal by fibrosis at the same time that tissue destruction is occurring in expanding lesions. Resultant scarring may produce urethral occlusion.

Hematogenous spread of the pathogen to bones, joints, and liver is rare but has been reported. Lymphatic spread is questionable. The inguinal swelling that is sometimes seen with this disease is not a lymphadenopathy, but rather a subcutaneous granuloma.[53,96]

DIAGNOSTIC STUDIES[23]

Chancroid
Culture or microscopic examination of exudate from bubo or lesions
Positive for *H. ducreyi* bacilli

Ducrey skin test
In 72 hours, induration of at least 8 mm indicates past infection
Antibody reaction may persist for years

Granuloma inguinale
Microscopic examination of scrapings from ulcer margin
Donovan bodies can be visualized

TREATMENT PLAN

Surgical
Chancroid: fluctuant lymph nodes should be aspirated through adjacent normal skin (Incision and drainage or excision of nodes is contraindicated.)[23]

Chemotherapeutic[23]
Anti-infective agents
Chancroid
Erythromycin (Erythrocin), 500 mg po qid, or
Trimethoprim/sulfamethoxazole (Septra; Bactrim), tablet containing 160 mg trimethoprim and 800 mg sulfamethoxazole, po bid for at least 10 d or until ulcers or lymph nodes have healed
Granuloma inguinale
Tetracycline (Achromycin; others), 0.5 g po qid for 21 d or until lesions heal, or
Streptomycin, 0.5 g IM bid for at least 21 d, or
Chloramphenicol (Chloromycetin), 0.5 g po tid for at least 21 d, or
Gentamicin (Garamycin), 40 mg IM bid for at least 21 d

ASSESSMENT: AREAS OF CONCERN[52,53,63,96]

Genitalia
Chancroid
One to ten primary lesions: inflamed macule/papule/pustule; irregularly shaped and of variable size (1 mm to 2 cm); surrounded by a zone of inflammation; erupts to produce a sharply circumscribed, nonindurated ulcer with a granulating base and ragged edges; abundant, purulent exudate; location: frenulum, prepuce, coronal sulcus, glans and shaft of penis, and urinary meatus in males; cervix, vagina, fourchette, labia, and perianal area in females
Variations in clinical appearance of lesions:
1. Follicular pustules rupture forming ulcers.
2. Dwarf chancroid lesions look like herpes lesions.
3. Transient chancroid lesion resolves quickly but is followed by an inguinal bubo.
4. Papular chancroid starts as an ulcer but becomes raised.
5. Giant chancroid frequently follows rupture of inguinal abscess and grows rapidly.
6. Phagedenic chancroid, a small lesion, rapidly extends and becomes necrotic and destructive.

Granuloma inguinale

Single or multiple, indurated, sharply defined but irregular papules/nodules; erode to form a beefy, exuberant granulomatous, heaped, clean ulcer, progressing slowly and coalescing with adjacent lesions; serous exudate; location: glans, prepuce, urethra, shaft of penis, and perianal area in males; labia and fourchette in females; lesions bleed easily; if secondarily infected, may have odorous necrotic exudate

Variations in clinical appearance:

1. Oral lesions are painful and look like malignancies.
2. Vaginal and cervical ulcers produce profuse, purulent discharge and irregular bleeding.
3. Cervical ulcers are soft, friable, irregular, and not well fixed to tissue; resemble cancer.
4. Male genital ulcers may be hypertrophic and verrucose, destructive and necrotic, discoid (buttonlike), or chronic and indolent.
5. Inguinal ulcers and ulcers on female genitalia are generally fleshy and exuberant.
6. Anal ulcers are hypertrophic and verrucose or chronic and indolent.

Inguinal area

Chancroid

Single, unilateral (can be bilateral), tender, and unilocular lymphadenopathy with overlying erythema

Suppuration and rupture of fluctuant nodes in 5 to 10 days may occur, leaving a single large ulcer

Granuloma inguinale

Rarely any inguinal involvement

May have a subcutaneous granuloma that suppurates, mimicking a lymphadenopathy

Subjective symptoms

Chancroid

Pain

Granuloma inguinale

Rarely any pain

NURSING DIAGNOSES and NURSING INTERVENTIONS

Nursing Diagnosis	Nursing Intervention
Potential patient problem: transmission of infection	See "Patient Education" below.

Patient Education[7,23,63,96]

1. Antibiotics must be taken for complete course of treatment.
2. Tetracycline is to be taken 1 hour before or 2 hours after meals. It is not to be taken with dairy products, antacids, iron, or other mineral-containing preparations. Patient should avoid sunlight.
3. Patient should return for evaluation within 3 to 5 days of beginning therapy and weekly or biweekly thereafter until all lesions are healed. Total healing of granuloma inguinale takes 3 to 5 weeks. If treatment is stopped prematurely, lesions may become reactivated.
4. Sexual partners should be examined and treated as soon as possible. Sex contacts 2 weeks before or after onset of chancroid lesions must be treated. Females may be asymptomatic but should be treated.
5. In chancroid the prepuce should remain retracted during therapy and the lesions cleansed three times daily. Retraction is contraindicated if there is preputial edema.
6. Use of condoms may prevent future infections.

EVALUATION

Patient Outcome	Data Indicating That Outcome is Reached
There is no infection.	All lesions are healed without scarring.
The patient complies with recommendations.	Sexual partners have been examined and treated. Patient is returning for follow-up examination.

Molluscum Contagiosum and Condylomata Acuminata

Molluscum contagiosum is a viral disease of the skin resulting in pearly pink to white papules with a central exudative pore. Multiple lesions appear on the genitalia and clear spontaneously in 6 to 9 months. Children develop lesions on skin elsewhere on the body.

Condylomata acuminata constitute one of the four major categories of virus-produced warts; this category occurs primarily on the genitalia or perineum. The warts appear as single or multiple, soft pink to brown, elongated lesions, usually in clusters and sometimes as large cauliflower-like masses. The warts sometimes heal spontaneously. Malignant transformation has been reported[7,46] *(Table 15-24).*

Complications from warts occur. Laryngeal papillomatosis may develop in infants born to mothers with vaginal warts. Also, the enlarged size of some warts may lead to difficulty during a vaginal birth. Secondary infection and bleeding of warts are common. Enlarged or giant condylomata of the penis, although benign, may destroy large areas of the penis. Cancer must be ruled out in this situation. Malignant transformation, both invasive and intraepithelial, has been observed in some warts.[77]

The papules of molluscum contagiosum clear spontaneously in 6 to 9 months as a result of an immune response. Warts sometimes clear spontaneously, suggesting an immune response.[7,46]

PATHOPHYSIOLOGY

The viruses of both these diseases invade superficial layers of the epidermis, infecting single epithelial cells and stimulating the cells to divide. In the case of condylomata there is excessive proliferation of the prickle cells of the stratum spinosum, constituting the bulk of the wart. There is marked papillomatosis but no hyperkeratosis. Microscopic examination of the infected cells shows aggregates of the virus particles plus basophilic inclusions. In the case of molluscum contagiosum, a central pore containing the virus and exudative material develops in the papules.[7,46,77]

Both molluscum papules and genital warts appear as multiple lesions on the external genitalia. Genital warts may also be found in the vagina and cervix of females and anterior urethra of males. Perineal and anal warts in females are generally caused by spread, whereas anal warts in males are associated with anal coitus among homosexuals. Genital warts that resemble skin warts suggest hand-to-genital transmission of another category of skin warts.[77]

DIAGNOSTIC STUDIES

Molluscum contagiosum: microscopic examination of material in core of lesion

Pathognomonic molluscum inclusion bodies can be visualized

Condylomata

Biopsy necessary for definitive diagnosis to rule out malignancy

Rule out condylomata lata of syphilis with serologic test for syphilis

TREATMENT PLAN

Surgical

Alternative therapies for warts may include cryotherapy, electrosurgery, or surgical removal (scissors or curette)

Table 15-24
Overview of STDs with Nonulcerative Lesions[7]

	Molluscum Contagiosum	Condylomata Acuminata (Anogenital Warts)
Occurrence	Worldwide; 90% of adults have antibodies; four times higher in prepubertal males	Worldwide
Etiologic agent	A member of the poxvirus group	*Papillomavirus*
Reservoir	Humans	Humans
Transmission	Direct sexual contact and indirect contact	Direct sexual contact
Incubation period	2-7 wk	1-20 mo (usually 4 mo)
Period of communicability	Unknown; probably as long as lesions persist	Unknown; probably as long as lesions persist
Susceptibility and resistance	Usually occurs in small children	General
Report to local health authority	No	No

Molluscum lesions may resolve spontaneously or be removed by curettage after cryoanesthesia or cryotherapy or by the use of caustic chemicals

Chemotherapeutic
Keratolytic agents
Condylomata acuminata: podophyllum, 10-25% in compound tincture of benzoin to wart only; to be washed off in 1-4 h; four weekly treatments (not to be used during pregnancy or with urethral, oral, cervical, or anorectal warts)[23]

ASSESSMENT: AREAS OF CONCERN

Anogenital area
Molluscum: multiple papules, 1 to 10 mm, pearly pink to white, with a central pore
Condylomata: multiple or single, soft pink to brown, elongated lesions, usually in clusters; may be in large masses

NURSING DIAGNOSES and NURSING INTERVENTIONS

Nursing Diagnosis	Nursing Intervention
Potential patient problem: transmission of illness	See "Patient Education" below.

Patient Education[23]
1. Sexual partners should be examined and treated.
2. During therapy, patient should abstain from sex or should use a condom.
3. Follow-up examination should take place 1 month after treatment for molluscum so that new lesions can be removed.
4. Follow-up examinations should be done weekly until all warts have been resolved.
5. All women with anogenital warts should have a Papanicolaou smear.

EVALUATION

Patient Outcome	Data Indicating That Outcome is Reached
There is no infection.	Lesions have been removed or are resolved.
The patient complies with recommendations.	Sexual partners have been examined and treated, if necessary. Females have negative Papanicolaou smear.

Vulvovaginitis

Vulvovaginitis is an inflammation of the superficial mucous membranes of the vulva and vagina caused by a number of microorganisms that are frequently part of the normal vaginal flora in adult women. The inflammation is accompanied by a purulent exudate with characteristics that differ with causative agents. The etiologic agents most frequently associated with vulvovaginitis are Trichomonas vaginalis *(a protozoan),* Candida albicans *(a yeast form of fungus), and* Gardnerella vaginalis *(Corynebacterium vaginale, Haemophilus vaginalis) (a bacterium). They are responsible for trichomoniasis, candidiasis, and* Gardnerella vaginalis *vaginitis, respectively (Table 15-25).*

PATHOPHYSIOLOGY

The presence of estrogen in women supports a normal flora of microorganisms in the vagina and anterior urethra. Under certain conditions (alterations in hormonal levels during the menstrual cycle, pregnancy, antibiotic therapy, immunosuppression), imbalance occurs in the normal flora. Certain opportunistic organisms become pathogenic or may be sexually transmitted in large enough numbers to become pathogenic. They colonize on the superficial mucosal layers, producing patches of inflammation and exudate containing large numbers of the pathogens. The infection rarely extends beyond the

Table 15-25
Vulvovaginitis[7,32,73]

	Trichomoniasis	Candidiasis	Gardnerella vaginalis Vaginitis
Occurrence	Worldwide; highest in females 16-35 yr; often accompanies other STDs	Worldwide; fungus is part of normal flora in 50% of women 15-45 yr; most common cause of vaginitis	Worldwide; bacteria are part of normal vaginal flora in many asymptomatic women
Etiologic agent	*Trichomonas vaginalis*, a protozoan	*Candida albicans*, a fungus	*Gardnerella vaginalis (Haemophilus vaginalis, Corynebacterium vaginale)*, a gram-negative coccobacillus
Reservoir	Humans	Humans	Humans
Transmission	Direct and indirect contact with vaginal and urethral discharges; transmitted to infant during birth	Direct and indirect contact with excretions from mouth, skin, vagina, and rectum of infected persons and carriers; transmitted to infant during vaginal delivery	Direct contact with vaginal and urethral discharges
Incubation period	4-20 d; average of 7 d	2-5 d in thrush in newborn	5-7 d
Period of communicability	Duration of infection	Duration of lesions	Duration of infection
Susceptibility and resistance	General, but clinical disease is mainly in females; exacerbated during menstruation and pregnancy	Low level of pathogenicity or high level of natural resistance because many persons have organism but few acquire infection	General, but clinical disease is only in females; many women have the organism but not all acquire symptomatic infections
Report to local health authority	No	No	No

endocervix. There is a wide range in severity of infections, with many being asymptomatic. The organism may be transmitted to a male sexual partner, who may or may not develop symptomatic urethritis. Reinfection of the female from untreated males is common.

The organisms may be transmitted to an infant during birth. Infections in newborns are generally temporary, limited to the time period before maternal estrogens are metabolized by the newborn.

Certain physiologic changes in the host support the pathogenic growth of different organisms. Trichomoniasis is exacerbated during and after menstruation, whereas bacterial infections such as *G. vaginalis* vaginitis are not associated with hormonal changes during the menstrual cycle. *G. vaginalis* vaginitis is associated with an altered vaginal pH; the organism usually does not grow in the normal acid secretions. Yeast infections, such as *candidiasis*, are greatly exacerbated preceding menstruation, during pregnancy, and in women taking oral contraceptives. Candidiasis is also exacerbated by the elimination of normal flora bacteria with antibiotic therapy or with any other condition that compromises skin or mucous membrane defenses.[81,82]

Whereas *Trichomonas* and *Gardnerella* rarely extend beyond the vulvovaginal or anterior urethral area, *Candida* has the potential for producing infection anywhere in the body where normal defenses are altered. *Candida* is part of the normal gastrointestinal, oral, and cutaneous flora of many persons; and it may become pathogenic in those areas. Severe infection with invasion and abscess formation, particularly in the gastrointestinal tract, may lead to hematogenous dissemination of the yeast to other organs. The organism may also be introduced iatrogenically to internal organs through surgical procedures, catheters, or implanted devices, producing multiple microabscesses in infected tissue. The areas most commonly infected are the central nervous system (particularly the meninges), lungs, peritoneum, heart (myocardium, pericardium, and endocardium), endometrium, eyes, ears, joints, oral cavity, esophagus, skin, and nails. Deep tissue infection is more common in patients with neoplastic disease. Cutaneous infections are more commonly associated with skin injury or continual wetting of the skin. *Candida* infections may involve multiple organs and tissue simultaneously, a particular risk for immunosuppressed individuals.[33]

Vaginal candidiasis may be transmitted to the infant during delivery. A common manifestation of such an infection in the newborn is thrush, an infection in the oral cavity. Creamy white, curdlike patches consisting of desquamated epithelial cells, leukocytes, bacteria, keratin, necrotic tissue, and food debris are formed on the oral mucosa. Scraping of the patches leaves a raw, bleeding, and painful surface. Thrush may be acquired in the adult also.

DIAGNOSTIC STUDIES[23]

Trichomoniasis
Culture of vaginal secretions
Positive for *T. vaginalis*

Microscopic examination of saline wet mount of vaginal secretions
Visualization of motile protozoa

Candidiasis
Culture of vaginal secretions
Positive for *C. vaginale* in symptomatic women
Because *Candida* is part of normal oral flora, culture is not useful in thrush

Microscopic examination of Gram's stain or KOH wet mount preparation of vaginal secretions
Visualization of yeast cells

Gardnerella
Culture of vaginal secretions
Positive for *G. vaginalis* in symptomatic women

Microscopic examination of Gram's stain or KOH wet mount preparation of vaginal secretions
Identification of "clue" cells

TREATMENT PLAN

Chemotherapeutic
Anti-infective agents
Trichomoniasis: metronidazole (Flagyl), 2.0 g po at one time (contraindicated during first trimester of pregnancy; asymptomatic women should be treated to prevent sexual transmission)[23]
Candidiasis
Nystatin (Mycostatin), one vaginal suppository bid for 7-14 d, or
Miconazole nitrate 2% vaginal cream (Monistat), one applicator intravaginally at bedtime for 7 d (and applied externally for vulvitis), or

Clotrimazole (Lotrimin), one vaginal suppository daily for 7 d[23]
Gardnerella vaginitis
Metronidazole (Flagyl), 500 mg po bid for 7 d, or
Ampicillin (Amcill; others), 500 mg po qid for 7 d[23]
Systemic *Candida* infections: amphotericin B (Fungizone), 5-10 mg IV first day, increasing the dosage 5 mg as tolerated to 0.7 mg/kg every other day for 6-10 wk[33]
Prevention
Sexual partners should be examined and treated. Treatment of candidiasis during third trimester of pregnancy to prevent oral thrush in newborn.[7]

ASSESSMENT: AREAS OF CONCERN[59,81,82]

Vulvovagina
Trichomoniasis
Inflammation of vaginal walls and endocervix; punctate hemorrhagic lesions
Painful coitus
Copious loose discharge with an odor
One third of patients have yellow-green discharge with bubbles

Candidiasis
Pale or erythematous labia; labial excoriations; erythema extending into vagina and toward anus
Tiny papulopustules beyond main area of erythema
Severe perivaginal pruritus
Discharge: thick and adherent, containing curds, or thin and loose; without an odor

Gardnerella vaginalis
Milder symptoms; less erythema
Mild or moderate discharge; thin white or gray white; uniformly adheres to vaginal walls; 25% have gas bubbles in discharge; fishy or aminelike odor to discharge

Urinary concerns
Candidiasis
Dysuria

Trichomoniasis
Dysuria or frequency

Lymph nodes
Trichomoniasis
Inguinal adenopathy possible

NURSING DIAGNOSES and NURSING INTERVENTIONS

Nursing Diagnosis	Nursing Intervention
Potential patient problem: transmission of infection	Collect vaginal specimens for culture. Teach self-medication administration to patients (See "Patient Education" below.)

Patient Education[23]

1. Sexual partners, even though asymptomatic, should be referred for treatment.
2. Recurrent infections are common. Patient should return for treatment if symptoms recur.
3. Condoms are protection against reinfection.
4. Alcohol should be avoided until after 3 days following metronidazole therapy.
5. If tetracycline is given for *Gardnerella* it should be taken 1 hour before or 2 hours after meals. It should not be taken with dairy products, iron, or other mineral-containing preparations. Patient should avoid sunlight.
6. Vaginal suppositories for candidiasis should be stored in a refrigerator. Treatment should continue during menstruation. Sanitary pads can be worn to protect clothing.

EVALUATION

Patient Outcome	Data Indicating That Outcome is Reached
There is no vaginal infection.	There are no symptoms of inflammation, pruritus, or dysuria. Vaginal discharge is thin, clear white, nonfrothy, and nonirritating.
The patient complies with recommendations.	Sexual partners have been treated so as to minimize risk for reinfection.

NOSOCOMIAL INFECTIONS

Nosocomial describes infections that are hospital acquired in contrast to community acquired. An infection classified as nosocomial is not present nor is the microorganism incubating (unless the organism was acquired during a previous hospitalization) at the time of admission to an inpatient health care facility. Symptoms of the nosocomial infection need not be present during the hospitalization but may become evident after discharge.

Any infectious disease, whether transmitted directly or indirectly from person to person, has the potential for becoming a nosocomial infection. Infections that develop from microorganisms carried as part of the patient's normal flora or from normally nonpathogenic microorganisms in the hospital environment and that invade and colonize in a susceptible patient are also considered to be nosocomial.

A community-acquired infection is one that is present or incubating at the time of hospital admission. The known incubation period of a disease is used to determine whether an infection that becomes clinically apparent during or after hospitalization is hospital or community acquired. A disease occurring in the hospital with an unknown incubation period is generally classified as nosocomial. Also classified as nosocomial are infections occurring in newborns that are acquired during birth from an infected mother.[99]

Iatrogenic infections are those arising from treatment or other actions of health care providers. They may be nosocomial or community acquired, depending on where the pathogen was encountered. Many nosocomial infections are iatrogenic. Neither iatrogenic nor nosocomial classifications imply provider negligence or error.[10]

Extent. Reported occurrences of nosocomial infections in the United States range from 3% to 15.5% of hospital discharges, depending on the type of hospital, type of patients, and completeness of the reporting system. On the average, 5% to 7% of people who are admitted to a general hospital acquire a nosocomial infection. The extent of nosocomial infections in hospital personnel has not been quantified. The incidence is thought to be high, especially for tuberculosis and hepatitis.[99]

Nosocomial infections have been studied according to body sites and to the hospital services where they occur most frequently. The results of the National Nosocomial Infections Study by the Center for Disease Control (1975-1978) demonstrated that 41.2% of all nosocomial infections involve the urinary tract, 22.6% involve the lower respiratory tract, and 15.6% involve surgical wounds. The remaining 20% of infections affected the skin, blood, and gynecologic, upper respiratory, gastrointestinal, cardiovascular, and central nervous systems. The hospital service with the highest incidence of infection is the surgical service followed by medicine, gynecology, obstetrics, nursery, and pediatrics.[99]

Etiology. Certain interacting agent, host, and environmental characteristics of the hospital contribute to the risk for nosocomial infections. A large number of individuals (patients, families, and personnel) are brought together in close proximity in one environment. Some portion of these individuals have community-acquired overt or subclinical infections. Patient care necessitating close contact with body fluids and excretions increases the risk of transmission of pathogens from person to person and to the hospital environment. Thus a greater variety of microorganisms of greater virulence are likely to be present in hospitals. The increase in antibiotic-resistant strains of bacteria in hospitals is an example of this phenomenon. Hospitals also contain a wide range of potential reservoirs for microorganism growth such as infusion liquids, foods, biologic materials, and equipment.

Patients, already weakened by existing disease or treatment, are susceptible to invasion and infection by normal flora microorganisms, opportunistic organisms in the environment, and pathogens. Use of invasive diagnostic and treatment technologies further increases opportunities for microorganism invasion. Treatments that result in immunosuppression compromise patient resistance and further increase the risk for infection.

Epidemiology of Transmission

Nosocomial infections are transmitted according to the same chain of transmission as described on p. 1468 of this chapter. Select hospital factors associated with the chain are listed below.

Agents: endogenous (part of patient's flora) or exogenous (part of environment)

Aerobic and anaerobic bacteria, particularly gram-positive *S. aureus*, streptococci, and *Legionella pneumophila*

Gram-negative bacteria, particularly *E. coli*, *Proteus*, *Pseudomonas*, *Klebsiella*, *Enterobacter*, and *Serratia*

Fungi, particularly *Candida* and *Aspergillus*

Viruses, particularly hepatitis B and non-A, non-B, herpes, cytomegalovirus, varicella, rubella, influenza, and respiratory syncytial virus

Reservoir

Patients, visitors, health care personnel, equipment, products, or the environment

Human reservoirs may be frank cases, subclinical cases, or carriers

Portal of exit

Genitourinary tract

Gastrointestinal tract

Respiratory tract

Skin or mucous membranes

Blood

Mode of transmission

Direct contact with secretions, excretions, exudates, or blood in provision of direct patient care or from mother to infant or from patient to patient

Indirect contact through handling of specimens, contaminated equipment, infusion fluids, biologic materials, or food or by the hands of health care workers

Portal of entry

Ingestion

Inhalation

Percutaneous injection or infusion

Surgical incision

Invasive diagnostic procedures

Susceptible host

Characteristics of hospitalized patients that increase their susceptibility: chronic disease, malnutrition, dehydration, stasis of body fluids, traumatized tissue, leukopenia, preexisting infection, and any condition or treatment that interferes with host defenses and immune responses

Control

Control of nosocomial infections, as with community-acquired infections, relies on efforts to break the chain of transmission at one or more of its links. The point of the chain most amenable to control will vary with the microorganism and disease process. General hospital procedures for control are outlined below.

Agent

Sterilization and disinfection of inanimate reservoirs and vehicles of transmission

Reservoir

Antibiotic treatment of patients and employees

Limitation of visitors

Policies that encourage ill employees to stay home

Portal of exit and mode of transmission

Isolation procedures and secretion and excretion precautions

Hand washing by personnel between patients

Proper handling of specimens

Environmental air control, sanitation, proper waste disposal, and proper laundry practices

Portal of entry

Protective isolation of high-risk patients

Sterile techniques

Recommended procedures that minimize organism invasion (see recommendation for each body system discussed in this section)

Susceptible host

Nursing procedures that minimize stasis of body fluids (i.e., coughing, turning, ambulating), that prevent compromise in body defenses (i.e., skin and mucous membrane care, hydration, nutrition), and that improve immunologic status (i.e., active and passive immunization of patients and employees)

Hospital infection control also requires systematic monitoring and complete reporting to the hospital infection control committee of *all* infections occurring in the hospital. In addition, select infections must be reported to the local health authority. These infections are identified in the tables in each disease section in this chapter.

The Joint Commission for Hospital Accreditation requires that hospitals have an effective infection-control program in order to qualify for accreditation. The program must contain the following components[99]:

1. Infection-control committee
2. Systematic surveillance of nosocomial infections
3. Employee health program
4. Isolation policies
5. In-service education on infection control for employees
6. Regular procedures for environmental sanitation
7. Microbiology laboratory
8. Implementation of accepted infection control procedures in patient care

Urinary Tract Infections

The urinary system, except for the distal urethra, is normally sterile. Endogenous or exogenous microorganisms enter the system from devices that enter it or have contact with it. Approximately 75% of nosocomial urinary tract infections have been preceded by urologic implementation, including catheterization. The organisms most frequently associated with urinary tract infections are gram-negative organisms usually found in the colon, including *E. coli*, *Klebsiella*, *Proteus*, and *Enterobacter*. Bacteriuria increases the risk for septicemia and nephritis and should be treated.[99]

Criteria for classification. Urinary tract infections meeting the following Center for Disease Control (CDC) criteria are classified as nosocomial[10]:

1. Asymptomatic bacteriuria with colony counts greater than 100,000 organisms/ml urine where patient had had a previous negative culture at a time when the patient was not receiving antibiotics; or colony counts of a new organism greater than 100,000/ml even if patient had previous positive cultures of a different organism
2. Symptomatic urinary tract infection (fever, dysuria, costovertebral angle tenderness, suprapubic tenderness) with onset after admission and a prior negative urinalysis or present urinalysis with one or both of the following:
   a. Colony counts greater than 10,000 microorganisms/ml of midstream urine specimen
   b. Pyuria greater than 10 WBCs per high-power field in an uncentrifuged specimen

Urinary system alterations that increase risk for infection[10]

1. Obstructions: urethral strictures, calculi, tumors, blood clots
2. Trauma: injury to abdomen, ruptured bladder
3. Congenital anomalies: polycystic kidneys, exstrophy of bladder, horseshoe kidney
4. Disorders of other symptoms: abdominal or gynecologic surgery, rectovesicular fistula, meningomyelocele, spina bifida
5. Acute or chronic renal failure
6. Postpartum state
7. Aging changes, particularly in the female

Procedures that increase risk[10]

1. Urethral catheterization
   a. Indwelling (continuous): risk increases greatly after 7 days. A closed system is superior to an open system in delaying colonization of urine. Disconnecting a closed system increases the risk.
   b. Straight catheterization: less risk than with indwelling catheter. Intermittent urethral catheterization, using clean technique and performed by the patient, has less risk than indwelling catheterization.
2. External (condom) catheter can cause urinary tract infections, but the risk is less than with urethral catheterization.
3. Suprapubic catheterization: risk for infection may be lower than for urethral catheterization.
4. Ureteral catheterization: microorganisms from urethral colonization or contaminated instruments increase the risk for urinary tract infection.
5. Irrigations: irrigation equipment and solutions have great potential for contamination. Frequent

disconnection of system further increases risk for infection.

6. Urethral dilation: the procedure may introduce bacteria and produce tissue trauma.
7. Cystometrography: same risks as those with urethral catheterization.
8. Cystoscopy: septicemia may result if urine is not sterile before the procedure.
9. Transurethral resection of the prostrate: bacteremia may result if urine is not sterile before the procedure.
10. Operative procedures on the bladder and kidneys: microorganisms introduced at the time of the procedure or from a subsequent wound infection increase the risk for a urinary tract infection
11. Urinary diversion procedures: chronic infections are common as a result of colonization of bacteria at the stomal site.

Recommendations for prevention[10,116]

1. Avoid unnecessary catheterization.
2. Use aseptic techniques for insertion of devices and for opening the drainage system.
3. Use closed indwelling catheter system in preference to an open system.
4. Decrease the duration of indwelling catheters.
5. Use external catheter for males who can empty bladder but cannot control micturition.
6. Use clean-catch midstream method of collecting urine specimens in preference to catheterization.
7. Use straight rather than indwelling catheter whenever possible.
8. Use smallest catheter possible to minimize trauma.
9. Avoid leg bags in acute care setting.
10. Obtain specimens by aspirating urine from catheter or sampling port rather than by disconnecting catheter from drainage tubing.
11. Use silicone catheters rather than latex for long-term catheterization.
12. Anchor the catheter to stabilize and reduce irritation of the urethra.
13. Maintain a continual downward flow of urine.
14. Routinely empty drainage bags, but do not change unless entire closed system is changed. The addition of disinfecting agents in the bag is still controversial.
15. Use a separate, clean measuring container for each patient.
16. Gently and regularly clean perineum. Meatal care with antimicrobial agents has not been found to be helpful and in some cases has produced infection.
17. Avoid irrigations unless obstruction is anticipated. Use continuous irrigation in a closed system in preference to intermittent irrigation in an open system.

Surgical Wound Infections

The intact integumentary system provides the first line of defense against the invasion of microorganisms; and any disruption in the integrity of the system increases the risk for infection. The risk is increased with the extensiveness and severity in the disruption of the skin integrity and the length of time until the disruption is repaired. Repair and healing are further influenced by host factors. Postoperative wound infections vary substantially by hospital, suggesting that hospital practices and surgical skill may also greatly affect the occurrence. The incubation period for surgical wound infections is 3 to 8 days after the operation, suggesting that many infections are acquired in the operating suite.[10,99]

Criteria for classification. A surgical wound is classified as the site of a nosocomial infection if it drains purulent material with or without a positive culture for bacteria.[10]

Alterations in the host that increase risk for infection

1. Impaired immune response
2. Age (newborns and elderly individuals)
3. Diabetes mellitus with accompanying degenerative blood vessel changes
4. Corticosteroids, which reduce inflammatory response
5. Chemotherapy, which decreases immune response
6. Neurologic deficits causing loss of sensation and potential tissue pressure and anoxia
7. Infection elsewhere in the host
8. Malnutrition resulting in inadequate nitrogen for tissue repair
9. Obesity
10. Presence of *Staphylococcus aureus* on patient, particularly in the anterior nares

Surgical variables that increase risk for infection[10,99]

1. Class of operation (the risk for infection increases from class I to class IV procedures.)
   a. Class I (clean wound): no break in sterile technique; the gastrointestinal or respiratory tract is not entered; if genitourinary or biliary tract is entered, their contents are sterile
   b. Class II (clean, contaminated wound): gastrointestinal, genitourinary, or respiratory tract is entered with no spillage of contents; minor breaks in technique
   c. Class III (contaminated wound): acute inflammation without pus encountered; spillage from a hollow viscus occurs; trauma from a clean source

d. Class IV (dirty): pus or a perforated viscus is encountered; trauma from a dirty source

2. Duration of preoperative stay: prolonged presurgery hospitalization increases the risk for microbial colonization in or on the patient before the surgery.
3. Location of the surgery: infection increases if surgery is in body areas with impaired circulation or in areas with microorganisms already present.
4. Surgical technique: delayed wound closure, excess tissue trauma, improper suture tension, excess blood loss, and presence of a drain increase the risk.
5. Presence of bacteria at closure: the single most common agent causing postoperative wound infections is *S. aureus*, which is part of the normal flora for some people and has been found in the respiratory passages of 21% of operating suite personnel. Other gram-negative bacteria, accounting for 60% of infections, are transient on the hands of hospital employees and may be transmitted after surgery as well as in the operating suite.

Recommendations for prevention[93]

1. Surveillance and classification: all surgical procedures should be classified and recorded; and surveillance should be maintained on all postsurgical infections by classification. Surgeons should be appraised of their infection rates.
2. Preoperative preparation: the preoperative hospital stay should be as short as possible. Preexisting bacterial infections, excluding those for which the operation is performed, should be treated and controlled. Malnourished patients should receive oral or parenteral hyperalimentation before elective surgery. The patient should be bathed the night before elective surgery with an antiseptic soap. Hair should not be removed unless it will interfere with the procedure. If hair removal is necessary, it should be done immediately before surgery. Skin preparation includes scrubbing with a detergent solution followed by application of an antiseptic solution, preferably tincture of chlorhexidine, iodophors, or tincture of iodine. The patient should be completely covered with sterile drapes.
3. Postoperative wound care: use aseptic technique in dressing changes. A drain for an infected wound should be placed in an adjacent stab wound and attached to a closed suction system. Dressings should be changed if wet or if patient has signs of infection. Exudate should be cultured. Personnel must wash hands before and after caring for a surgical wound.
4. Prophylactic antibiotics: parenteral antibiotic prophylaxis should be started 2 hours before operations that are associated with a high risk of infection. They should be discontinued between 12 and 48 hours after the surgery.

Bacteremia and Septicemia

See description of sepsis in this chapter.

Vascular system alterations that increase risk for infection

1. Thrombophlebitis caused by mechanical or chemical irritation from IV cannula or infusate
2. Decreased blood volume
3. Circulatory stasis caused by immobility or pressure
4. Immunosuppression of host
5. Vascular changes associated with diabetes, collagen diseases, and other chronic diseases

Procedures that increase risk for cannula-related infection[92]

1. Type of cannula used for IV therapy (plastic cannulas generally associated with higher rate infection than steel "scalp vein" cannulas)
2. Method of insertion: cutdown has greater infection risk than percutaneous insertion
3. Duration over 48 to 72 hours
4. Purpose of the cannula: CVP lines are associated with high risk for infection
5. Microbial contamination of infusion fluid: rare and usually caused by gram-negative bacteria

Recommendations for prevention of secondary bacteremia

1. Prevention of original underlying infection
2. Early recognition and treatment of underlying surgical wound, urinary tract, and pulmonary infections

Recommendations for prevention of primary bacteremias induced by intravenous catheters[10,92]

1. Wash hands before insertion.
2. Use sterile gloves and antiseptic hand wash for cutdowns or central lines.
3. Use upper extremity veins; lower extremity veins develop phlebitis more readily.
4. Use an antiseptic preparation before venipuncture (in declining order of preference: tincture of iodine, chlorhexidine, iodophors, 70% alcohol, avoid quaternary ammonium compounds and hexachlorophene).
5. Use plastic catheters for cannulation of central veins and steel needles for IV infusions.
6. Secure catheter and apply sterile dressing.
7. Inspect daily.
8. Insert new cannula every 48 to 72 hours.
9. Change dressing and apply antibiotic ointment every 48 hours.
10. Change IV tubing every 48 hours and after blood products or lipid emulsions.
11. Avoid irrigations or blood drawing.

Lower Respiratory Tract Infections

As many as 1% to 2% of hospitalized patients develop nosocomial bacterial pneumonias, with 30% of those infected persons dying even with adequate antimicrobial therapy. Certain factors contribute to the risk for pneumonia in hospitalized patients[10]:

1. The integrity of normal respiratory defense mechanisms may be disrupted, thus permitting the invasion of oropharyngeal normal flora microorganisms into the lung alveoli.
2. Medical diagnostic and treatment procedures may introduce microorganisms from the oropharynx or from the equipment or solutions into the lower respiratory tract.
3. Ill persons with altered respiratory clearance mechanisms are susceptible to rapid oropharyngeal colonization of pathogens from the hospital environment, equipment, or the patient's normal flora. The pathogens that frequently colonize in hospitalized patients and are most often associated with nosocomial pneumonia are *Klebsiella*, *S. aureus*, *Pseudomonas*, *E. coli*, *Enterobacter*, *S. pneumoniae*, and *H. influenzae*. Opportunistic organisms such as *Candida*, *Aspergillus*, cytomegalovirus, and *Pneumocystis carinii* cause pneumonia in immunocompromised hosts.[88,109]

Microbial invasion of lung alveoli can occur from one of three routes:

1. Aspiration from the oropharynx
2. Inhalation of aerosolized droplets or gas containing suspended organisms
3. Lymphohematogenous spread

Aspiration is probably the most frequent route in nosocomial pneumonia.[88,109]

Criteria for classification. The criteria used by the Hospital Infections Branch of the Centers for Disease Control for classifying nosocomial pneumonia are as follows[88]:

1. Purulent sputum developing 48 hours or more after admission, or increased production of purulent sputum with recrudescence of fever in a patient hospitalized with pulmonary disease; plus one of the following:
2. Cough, fever, and pleuritic chest pain, or
3. Infiltration seen on chest roentgenography or physical findings of infection

An infection present on admission can be classified as nosocomial if it is related to a previous hospitalization.

Host factors that increase the risk for nosocomial pneumonia[10,109]

1. Airway obstruction caused by tumors, foreign bodies, edema, fluid, or chronic obstructive pulmonary disease
2. Impairment of mucociliary defenses as a result of

dehydration, inhalation of chemical irritants, viral infection, or anticholinergic drugs
3. Impaired immunologic function
4. Traumatic injury to respiratory tract or surgery to abdominal or thoracic cavity
5. Altered swallowing, clearing, or coughing caused by central nervous system disorders, alcoholism, depressed levels of consciousness, dysphagia, nasogastric tubes, anesthesia, sedation, or medications that alter the cough reflex; immobilization
6. Oropharyngeal colonization of bacteria (Colonization increases with length of hospital stay, prolonged intubation, and preceding antibiotic therapy.)

Procedures that increase risk for infection[10,88,109]

1. Large-volume nebulizers: the major source of aerosolized bacteria; humidifiers do not have the same risk
2. Any device or airway that may carry bacteria from the oropharynx to the lower respiratory tract including nasogastric tubes and endotracheal tubes
3. Ventilation equipment including intermittent positive pressure machines
4. Administration of oxygen or anesthesia
5. Pulmonary function testing
6. Bronchoscopy
7. Surgical procedures, including lung biopsy and tracheostomy

Recommendations for prevention of nosocomial pneumonia associated with respiratory care equipment[10,109]

1. Use sterile, adequately disinfected, or disposable breathing circuits (mouthpieces, tubing, cannulae) that come in contact with the patient.
2. Replace circuitry for patients on continuous assisted or controlled ventilation and on intermittent therapy every 24 to 48 hours. Remove fluid buildup in the tubing.
3. Use high-efficiency bacterial filters on ventilators and intermittent positive pressure machines between the machine and the patient. Use in-line filters to prevent contamination of internal parts of anesthesia machines and ventilators from patient's exhaled air.
4. Change or sterilize or disinfect aerosol-producing equipment between patients and every 24 hours for the same patient. Do not use spinning disc nebulizers.
5. Use sterile solutions in fluid reservoirs, dispensed under aseptic conditions. Fill water reservoirs at the time needed, not in advance. Unused portions should be discarded every 24 hours at the time the reservoir is sterilized or replaced.

6. Do not add to fluid levels in nebulizers or humidifiers. If additional fluid is needed, empty reservoir and fill with sterile water.

7. Use sterile medications in single-use vials for nebulization.

8. For suctioning, use sterile catheter and sterile glove. Change suction catheter after each use. Use intermittent rather than continuous suctioning.

Medical Interventions

IMMUNIZATIONS

Some infectious diseases are preventable with artificial active immunization. In some cases artificial passive immunization can be used to provide temporary immunity. Clinical considerations for active and passive immunization, general recommendations for administration of vaccines, and a schedule for administration of vaccines for the diseases discussed in the section on childhood communicable and immunizable infectious diseases (p. 1483) will be presented here. (Refer to "Anatomy and Physiology" in this chapter for an overview of the development of specific immune responses.)

Clinical Considerations for Active and Passive Immunization

Active immunization. Vaccines used for active immunization are prepared from bacteria or viruses, or their derivatives, that have been modified to stimulate antibody production without causing disease. Modification is accomplished by two methods: (1) inactivation or killing of the organism and (2) alteration of the organism so that it retains its antigenicity while losing its virulence.

Inactivated vaccines must be given in multiple first doses to stimulate an adequate antibody response; and a periodic booster must be given to maintain serum antibody levels. Attenuated vaccines stimulate lifetime antibody levels with one administration.

Routine immunizations are given according to a schedule that facilitates administration at a time earliest in life when the vaccine will be effective. The health care provider administering the immunization should fully inform the patient or parent of the reason for the immunization, the schedule, side effects that may occur, and actions to take in the event of side effects. Informed consent must be obtained.[31]

Passive immunization. Active immunization is preferred to passive in most situations. Passive immuniza-

tion with serum antitoxins prepared in animals or with human immune globulins is only recommended for those situations where (1) active immunization procedures have not been developed; (2) exposure has already occurred, leaving insufficient time for active immunization; or (3) concurrent active and passive immunization is required for immediate and future protection.

The use of human immune globulins for passive immunization is preferred to use of serum antitoxins from animals. The risk for anaphylaxis-like reactions and serum sickness is greater when animal prepared sera are used. Anaphylaxis-like reactions affect principally the cardiovascular and respiratory systems, producing dyspnea, asthma, respiratory decompensation, and possible death. These reactions occur in minutes to a few hours after administration of the serum, and they range from mild to severe. The much more common serum sickness reactions develop in 7 to 12 days after injection of the serum, producing mild to severe symptoms of fever, urticaria, or arthralgia. The severity of the symptoms depends on the type of serum and the route of administration (IV administration leads to more severe reactions). Individuals previously sensitized to the serum may react within 1 to 3 days of receiving the serum.[31]

General Recommendations[2]

Multiple dose vaccines. Some vaccines must be administered in more than one dose for full protection. If the intervals between doses are longer than recommended, there is usually not a reduction in final antibody levels. It is therefore not necessary to restart an interrupted series or to add extra doses.

Simultaneous administration of certain vaccines. Most of the widely used vaccines can be safely and effectively administered simultaneously. Inactivated vaccines can be administered simultaneously at different

Table 15-26
Immunization Schedule[1,4,21]

	Tetanus	Diphtheria	Pertussis	Polio (Trivalent Oral Polio Vaccine [TOPV])	Measles (Rubeola)	Mumps	Rubella
Vaccine	Toxoid (detoxified toxin)	Toxoid (detoxified toxin)	Killed vaccine	Live attenuated virus	Live attenuated virus	Live attenuated virus	Live attenuated virus
Administration		1. Primary (under 7 yr) One dose diphtheria, pertussis, tetanus toxoid (DPT) IM q4-8wk; give three times Fourth dose 1 yr later Booster: school entry and q10yr (DT only) 2. Primary (7 yr and older) Two doses DT IM separated by a 4-8 wk period Third dose 6-12 mo later Booster q10yr		One dose at 6-8 wk followed by a second dose 6-8 wk later; third dose 8-12 mo later; booster at school entry	Single dose	Single dose Give combined as MMR	Single dose
Recommendations	Ideally begin at 2-3 mo of age		Do not give pertussis after 7 yr	Not recommended over 18 yr	Must be given after age of 15 mo	All persons over 12 mo with no history of mumps	All persons over 12 mo with no evidence of immunity
Major adverse reactions	Rare: neurologic reactions including neuritis and transverse myelitis		Convulsions; loss of consciousness	Rare: paralysis within 2 mo	Rare: central nervous system reactions (encephalitis)	Rare: encephalomyelitis	In older children and adults, transient arthralgias and arthritis 2 wk after immunization
Less severe reactions	Fever within 24-48 h; soreness, swelling, and redness at injection site; lump may persist for weeks but gradually disappears; may also have urticaria and malaise		Thrombocytopenia	None	Anorexia, malaise, rash, and fever within 7-10 d	Brief, mild fever	Mild rash lasting 1 or 2 d after immunization
Passive immunization	Immune globulin following injury for those without active immunization	Antitoxin for unimmunized contacts with an active case	Hyperimmune pertussis globulin for active cases	None	When active immunization is contraindicated in exposed person, give immune globulin	Not recommended	Not recommended

sites unless the person is known to have experienced past side effects to one or more of the vaccines. In that case the vaccines should be administered on separate occasions. An inactivated vaccine and a live attenuated virus vaccine can be administered simultaneously at different sites.

Hypersensitivity to vaccine components. Vaccine antigens produced in systems or with substrates that contain allergenic substances may cause hypersensitivity reactions and possible anaphylaxis. Antigens grown in eggs of chickens or ducks should not be given to anyone with a history (or questionable history) of allergy to eggs. Influenza vaccine antigens, although produced from viruses grown in eggs, are highly purified and are associated with only rare hypersensitivity reactions. Influenza vaccine should not be administered to anyone with a history of an anaphylactic reaction to eggs.

No hypersensitivity reactions have been reported from administration of live attenuated measles, mumps, or rubella (MMR) vaccine prepared from viruses grown in cell cultures.

Some vaccines that are derived from organisms grown in bacteriologic media frequently produce local or systemic reactions that are not allergenic. These vaccines—including cholera; diphtheria, pertussis, and tetanus (DPT); plague; and typhoid—should not be given to persons who have a history of serious side effects from the vaccine.

Those vaccines that contain preservatives or trace amounts of antibiotics, as indicated on the package insert, should not be given to any person with a history of hypersensitivity to those substances.

Contraindications for immunization[2]

1. Altered immunity: immunosuppressed persons should not receive live attenuated virus vaccines because of the risk for multiplication of the virus within those persons. Also, individuals living in the same household with an immunocompromised person should not be given oral polio vaccine (OPV) because vaccine viruses are excreted and may be transmitted to other persons.

2. Severe febrile illnesses: although the presence of mild illnesses does not preclude vaccination, immunization should be deferred for those with severe febrile illnesses.

3. Pregnancy: attenuated virus vaccines, particularly MMR, should not be given to pregnant women or women who may become pregnant within 3 months of the vaccination. OPV and yellow fever vaccines may be given if there is a high risk for acquired infection. There is no contraindication for administration of inactivated viral vaccines, bacterial vaccines, or toxoids to pregnant women.

4. Recent administration of immune globulin: live attenuated virus vaccines should not be administered within 3 months of passive immunization. Similarly, immunoglobulins should not be administered for at least 2 weeks after a vaccine has been given. These precautions reduce the risk that high serum levels of immunoglobulins would prevent the development of active acquired immunity.

5. All adverse reactions to vaccines should be reported to the local or state health authority and to the manufacturer of the vaccine.

Tetanus prophylaxis in wound management is as follows. Medical treatment regarding the administration of active or passive tetanus immunization following a skin injury depends on the severity of the injury and on the patient's history of active tetanus immunization. Complete active immunization provides long-lasting immunity so that booster injections of toxoid are not necessary more often than every 5 years in the event of a wound and every 10 years without injury. Serum antitoxin develops rapidly following a toxoid booster in persons who

Table 15-27

Recommendations for Tetanus Prophylaxis in Wound Management[1]

History of Tetanus Immunization	Clean Minor Wounds		All Other Wounds	
	Toxoid (Detoxified Toxin; Td)	Tetanus Immune Globulin (TIG)	Toxoid; (Detoxified Toxin Td)	Tetanus Immune Globulin (TIG)
Uncertain history	Yes	No	Yes	Yes
No dose or one dose	Yes	No	Yes	Yes
Two doses	Yes	No	Yes	No*
Three or more doses				
Last dose within past 5 yr	No	No	No	No
Last dose 5-10 yr ago	No	No	Yes	No
Last dose over 10 yr ago	Yes	No	Yes	No

*Unless wound is more than 24 hr old.

have received at least two doses of tetanus toxoid out of the four doses recommended for primary immunization. In this situation it is important to administer the toxoid within 24 hours of injury.[1]

For persons without a full series of tetanus toxoid in the past and with a wound over 24 hours old it may be necessary to administer tetanus antitoxic antibodies together with tetanus toxoid. If such passive immunization is to be used, tetanus immune globulin (TIG), 250 units, is recommended rather than antitoxin because TIG provides longer immunity with no undesirable reactions. Toxoid and TIG, given concurrently, should be administered with separate syringes in separate sites. There would be no indication for giving TIG without also giving toxoid. The recommendations for tetanus prophylaxis in wound management are described in Table 15-27.

ISOLATION PROCEDURES

Isolation procedures are designed to prevent the spread of microorganisms among hospitalized patients, personnel, and visitors. Most of the infectious diseases discussed in this chapter have the potential for being transmitted to others. For those infections that can be transmitted, the recommended hospital isolation category precautions were specified in this chapter under "Nursing Diagnoses and Interventions." These recommendations are those published in 1983 by the Center for Disease Control (CDC).[24]

The 1983 CDC guidelines provide for two isolation systems: one based on revised categories of isolation and a new system based on disease-specific isolation precautions. The disease-specific isolation system differs from the category system by specifying only the necessary precautions to interrupt the transmission of each disease. Only a single instruction card is used, on which specific precautions may be checked or written.

The category system specifies seven categories of isolation based on the major modes of transmission of infectious diseases. Each disease has been assigned to one of the categories. Precautionary procedures have been specified for each category. Color-coded category-specific instruction cards are available for use with this system.

Hospitals may choose one of these systems, modify one of these systems, or develop their own system. The CDC recommendations are not meant to restrict hospitals or medical and nursing personnel from requiring more stringent precautions. Nurses are advised to follow isolation procedures that are operative within their institution of employment and to use the material presented here for reference and clarification. The isolation precautions presented here may also require modification for patients who need constant care or require emergency intervention.

Hospital policy usually designates the personnel responsible for placing a patient on isolation precautions and the personnel who have ultimate authority to make decisions regarding isolation precautions when conflicts arise; but all personnel are responsible for complying with isolation precautions to protect themselves, coworkers, patients, and visitors.

The category-specific isolation system* is presented here.

Strict Isolation

Strict Isolation is an isolation category designed to prevent transmission of highly contagious or virulent infections that may be spread by both air and contact.

Specifications for strict isolation
1. Private room is indicated; door should be kept closed. In general, patients infected with the same organism may share a room.
2. Masks are indicated for all persons entering the room.
3. Gowns are indicated for all persons entering the room.
4. Gloves are indicated for all persons entering the room.
5. Hands must be washed after touching the patient or potentially contaminated articles and before taking care of another patient.
6. Articles contaminated with infective material should be discarded or bagged and labeled before being sent for decontamination and reprocessing.

Diseases requiring strict isolation
Diphtheria, pharyngeal
Lassa fever and other viral hemorrhagic fevers, such as Marburg virus disease†
Plague, pneumonic
Smallpox†
Varicella (chickenpox)
Zoster, localized in immunocompromised patient or disseminated

Contact Isolation

Contact Isolation is designed to prevent transmission of highly transmissible or epidemiologically important infections (or colonization) that do not warrant Strict Isolation.

---

*From Centers for Disease Control: CDC guideline for isolation precautions in hospitals. HHS pub. no. (CDC) 83-8314, Atlanta, 1983, The Centers.
†A private room with special ventilation is indicated.

All diseases or conditions included in this category are spread primarily by close or direct contact. Thus, masks, gowns and gloves are recommended for anyone in close or direct contact with any patient who has an infection (or colonization) that is included in this category. For individual diseases or conditions, however, 1 or more of these 3 barriers may not be indicated. For example, masks and gowns are not generally indicated for care of infants and young children with acute viral respiratory infections; gowns are not generally indicated for gonococcal conjunctivitis in newborns; and masks are not generally indicated for patients infected with multiply-resistant microorganisms, except those with pneumonia. Therefore, some degree of "over-isolation" may occur in this category.

Specifications for contact isolation

1. Private room is indicated. In general, patients infected with the same organism may share a room. During outbreaks, infants and young children with the same respiratory clinical syndrome may share a room.
2. Masks are indicated for those who come close to patient.
3. Gowns are indicated if soiling is likely.
4. Gloves are indicated for touching infective material.
5. Hands must be washed after touching the patient or potentially contaminated articles and before taking care of another patient.
6. Articles contaminated with infective material should be discarded or bagged and labeled before being sent for decontamination and reprocessing.

Diseases or conditions requiring contact isolation

Acute respiratory infections in infants and young children including croup, colds, bronchitis, and bronchiolitis caused by respiratory syncytial virus, adenovirus, coronavirus, influenza viruses, parainfluenza viruses, and rhinovirus
Conjunctivitis, gonococcal in newborns
Diphtheria, cutaneous
Endometritis, group A *Streptococcus*
Furunculosis, staphylococcal in newborns
Herpes simplex, disseminated, severe primary or neonatal
Impetigo
Influenza, in infants and young children
Multiply-resistant bacteria, infection, or colonization (any site) with any of the following:
1. Gram-negative bacilli resistant to all aminoglycosides that are tested. (In general, such organisms should be resistant to gentamicin, tobramycin, and amikacin for these special precautions to be indicated.)
2. *Staphylococcus aureus* resistant to methicillin (or nafcillin or oxacillin if they are used instead of methicillin for testing).
3. *Pneumococcus* resistant to penicillin.
4. *Haemophilus influenzae* resistant to ampicillin (beta-lactamase positive) and chloramphenicol.
5. Other resistant bacteria may be included if they are judged by the infection control team to be of special clinical and epidemiologic significance.
Pediculosis
Pharyngitis, infectious, in infants and young children
Pneumonia, viral, in infants and young children
Pneumonia, *Staphylococcus aureus* or Group A *Streptococcus*

Rabies
Rubella, congenital and other
Scabies
Scalded skin syndrome, staphylococcal (Ritter's disease)
Skin wound or burn infection, major (draining and not covered by dressing or dressing does not adequately contain the purulent material) including those infected with *Staphylococcus aureus* or group A *Streptococcus*
Vaccinia (generalized and progressive eczema vaccinatum)

Respiratory Isolation

Respiratory Isolation is designed to prevent transmission of infectious diseases primarily over short distances through the air (droplet transmission). Direct and indirect contact transmission occurs with some infections in this isolation category but is infrequent.

Specifications for respiration isolation

1. Private room is indicated. In general, patients infected with the same organism may share a room.
2. Masks are indicated for those who come close to the patient.
3. Gowns are not indicated.
4. Gloves are not indicated.
5. Hands must be washed after touching the patient or potentially contaminated articles and before taking care of another patient.
6. Articles contaminated with infective material should be discarded or bagged and labeled before being sent for decontamination and reprocessing.

Diseases requiring respiratory isolation

Epiglottitis, *Haemophilus influenzae*
Erythema infectiosum
Measles
Meningitis
  Haemophilus influenzae, known or suspected
  Meningococcal, known or suspected
Meningococcal pneumonia
Meningococcemia
Mumps
Pertussis (whooping cough)
Pneumonia, *Haemophilus influenzae*, in children (any age)

Tuberculosis Isolation (AFB Isolation)

Tuberculosis Isolation (AFB Isolation) is an isolation category for patients with pulmonary TB who have a positive sputum smear or a chest X-ray that strongly suggests current (active) TB. Laryngeal TB is also included in this isolation category. In general, infants and young children with pulmonary TB do not require isolation precautions because they rarely cough, and their bronchial secretions contain few AFB, compared with adults with pulmonary TB. On the instruction card, this category is called AFB (for acid-fast bacilli) Isolation to protect the patient's privacy.

Specifications for tuberculosis isolation (AFB isolation)

1. Private room with special ventilation is indicated; door should be kept closed. In general, patients infected with the same organism may share a room.

2. Masks are indicated only if the patient is coughing and does not reliably cover mouth.
3. Gowns are indicated only if needed to prevent gross contamination of clothing.
4. Gloves are not indicated.
5. Hands must be washed after touching the patient or potentially contaminated articles and before taking care of another patient.
6. Articles are rarely involved in transmission of TB. However, articles should be thoroughly cleaned and disinfected or discarded.

Enteric Precautions

Enteric Precautions are designed to prevent infections that are transmitted by direct or indirect contact with feces. Hepatitis A is included in this category because it is spread through feces, although the disease is much less likely to be transmitted after the onset of jaundice. Most infections in this category primarily cause gastrointestinal symptoms, but some do not. For example, feces from patients infected with "poliovirus" and coxsackieviruses are infective, but those infections do not usually cause prominent gastrointestinal symptoms.

Specifications for enteric precautions

1. Private room is indicated if patient hygiene is poor. A patient with poor hygiene does not wash hands after touching infective material, contaminates the environment with infective material, or shares contaminated articles with other patients. In general, patients infected with the same organism may share a room.
2. Masks are not indicated.
3. Gowns are indicated if soiling is likely.
4. Gloves are indicated if touching infective material.
5. Hands must be washed after touching the patient or potentially contaminated articles and before taking care of another patient.
6. Articles contaminated with infective material should be discarded or bagged and labeled before being sent for decontamination or reprocessing.

Diseases requiring enteric precautions

Amebic dysentery
Cholera
Coxsackievirus disease
Diarrhea, acute illness with suspected infectious etiology
Echovirus disease
Encephalitis (unless known not to be caused by enteroviruses)
Enterocolitis caused by *Clostridium difficile* or *Staphylococcus aureus*
Enteroviral infection
Gastroenteritis caused by
  Campylobacter species
  Cryptosporidium species
  Dientamoeba fragilis
  Escherichia coli (enterotoxic, enteropathogenic, or enteroinvasive)
  Giardia lamblia
  Salmonella species
  Shigella species

  Vibrio parahaemolyticus
  Viruses—including Norwalk agent and rotavirus
  Yersinia enterocolitica
  Unknown etiology but presumed to be an infectious agent
Hand, foot, mouth disease
Hepatitis, viral, type A
Herpangina
Meningitis, viral (unless known not be caused by enteroviruses)
Necrotizing enterocolitis
Pleurodynia
Poliomyelitis
Typhoid fever *(Salmonella typhi)*
Viral pericarditis, myocarditis, or meningitis (unless known not be caused by enteroviruses)

Drainage/Secretion Precautions

Drainage/Secretion Precautions are designed to prevent infections that are transmitted by direct or indirect contact with purulent material or drainage from an infected body site. This newly created isolation category includes many infections formerly included in Wound and Skin Precautions, Discharge (lesion), and Secretion (oral) Precautions, which have been discontinued. Infectious diseases included in this category are those that result in the production of infective purulent material, drainage, or secretions, unless the disease is included in another isolation category that requires more rigorous precautions. For example, minor limited skin, wound, or burn infections are included in this category, but major skin, wound, or burn infections are included in Contact Isolation.

Specifications for drainage/secretion precautions

1. Private room is not indicated.
2. Masks are not indicated.
3. Gowns are indicated if soiling is likely.
4. Gloves are indicated for touching infective material.
5. Hands must be washed after touching the patient or potentially contaminated articles and before taking care of another patient.
6. Articles contaminated with infective material should be discarded or bagged and labeled before being sent for decontamination and reprocessing.

Diseases requiring drainage/secretion precautions

The following infections are examples of those included in this category provided they are not (a) caused by multiply-resistant microorganisms, (b) major draining (and not covered by a dressing or dressing does not adequately contain the drainage) skin, wound, or burn infections, including those caused by *Staphylococcus aureus* or group A *Streptococcus*, or (c) gonococcal eye infections in newborns. See Contact Isolation if the infection is one of these three.

Abscess, minor or limited
Burn infection, minor or limited
Conjunctivitis
Decubitus ulcer, infected, minor or limited
Skin infection, minor or limited
Wound infection, minor or limited

Blood/Body Fluid Precautions

Blood/Body Fluid Precautions are designed to prevent infections that are transmitted by direct or indirect contact with infective blood or body fluids. Infectious diseases included in this category are those that result in the production of infective blood or body fluids, unless the disease is included in another isolation category that requires more rigorous precautions, for example, Strict Isolation. For some diseases included in this category, such as malaria, only blood is infective; for other diseases, such as hepatitis B (including antigen carriers), blood and body fluids (saliva, semen, etc.) are infective.

Specifications for blood/body fluid precautions

1. Private room is indicated if patient hygiene is poor. A patient with poor hygiene does not wash hands after touching infective material, contaminates the environment with infective material, or shares contaminated articles with other patients. In general, patients infected with the same organism may share a room.
2. Masks are not indicated.
3. Gowns are indicated if soiling of clothing with blood or body fluids is likely.
4. Gloves are indicated for touching blood or body fluids.
5. Hands must be washed immediately if they are potentially contaminated with blood or body fluids and before taking care of another patient.
6. Articles contaminated with blood or body fluids should be discarded or bagged and labeled before being sent for decontamination and reprocessing.
7. Care should be taken to avoid needle-stick injuries. Used needles should not be recapped or bent; they should be placed in a prominently labeled, puncture-resistant container designated specifically for such disposal.
8. Blood spills should be cleaned up promptly with a solution of 5.25% sodium hypochlorite diluted 1:10 with water.

Diseases requiring blood/body fluid precautions

Acquired immunodeficiency syndrome (AIDS)
Arthropod-borne viral fevers (for example, dengue, yellow fever, and Colorado tick fever)
Babesiosis
Creutzfeldt-Jakob disease
Hepatitis B (including HBsAg antigen carrier)
Hepatitis, non-A, non-B
Leptospirosis
Malaria
Rat-bite fever
Relapsing fever
Syphilis, primary and secondary with skin and mucous membrane lesions

References

1. Advisory Committee on Immunization Practices: Diphtheria and tetanus toxoids and pertussis vaccine, Morbidity and Mortality Weekly Report **26**:401, Dec. 9, 1977, and **26**:440, Dec. 30, 1977 (reprinted Sept. 1980).
2. Advisory Committee on Immunization Practices: General recommendations on immunizations, Morbidity and Mortality Weekly Report **26**:81, Feb. 22, 1980 (reprinted Sept. 1980).
3. Advisory Committee on Immunization Practices: Immune globulins for protection against viral hepatitis, Morbidity and Mortality Weekly Report **30**:423, Sept. 4, 1981.
4. Advisory Committee on Immunization Practices: Measles prevention, Morbidity and Mortality Weekly Report **31**:218, May 7, 1982.
5. Advisory Committee on Immunization Practices: Inactivated hepatitis B virus vaccine, Morbidity and Mortality Weekly Report **31**:317, June 25, 1982; and Postexposure prophylaxis of hepatitis B, Morbidity and Mortality Weekly Report **33**:285, June 1, 1984.
6. Advisory Committee on Immunization Practices: Influenza vaccines 1982-1983, Morbidity and Mortality Weekly Report **31**:349, July 9, 1982.
7. American Public Health Association: Control of communicable diseases in man, ed. 13, Washington, 1980, The Association.
8. Anderson, S.: Toxoplasma gondii. In Mandell, G.L., Douglas, R.G., Jr., and Bennett, J.E., editors: Principles and practice of infectious diseases, New York, 1979, John Wiley & Sons, Inc.
9. Arnon, S.S., and Chin, J.: Botulism. In Wehrle, P.F., and Top, F.H., Sr., editors: Communicable and infectious diseases, ed. 9, St. Louis, 1981, The C.V. Mosby Co.
10. Association for Practitioners in Infection Control: The APIC curriculum for infection control practice, Iowa, 1981, Kendall/Hunt Publishing Co.
11. Barrett, T.: Cardiovascular system. In Axnick, K., and Yarbrough, M., editors: Infection control: an integrated approach, St. Louis, 1984, The C.V. Mosby Co.
12. Beare, P.G., Rahr, V.A., and Ronshausen, C.A.: Nursing implications of diagnostic tests, Philadelphia, 1983, J.B. Lippincott Co.
13. Beland, I.L., and Passos, J.Y.: Clinical nursing: pathophysiological and psychosocial approaches, ed. 4, New York, 1981, Macmillan Publishing Co., Inc.
14. Bisno, A.L.: Rheumatic fever. In Mandell, G.L., Douglas, R.G., Jr., and Bennett, J.E., editors: Principles and practice of infectious diseases, New York, 1979, John Wiley & Sons, Inc.
15. Borts, I.H., and Hendricks, S.L.: Brucellosis. In Wehrle, P.F., and Top, F.H., Sr., editors: Communicable and infectious diseases, ed. 9, St. Louis, 1981, The C.V. Mosby Co.
16. Boyce, J.M.: Francisella tularensis. In Mandell, G.L., Douglas, R.G., Jr., and Bennett, J.E., editors: Principles and practice of infectious diseases, New York, 1979, John Wiley & Sons, Inc.
17. Bullock, W.E.: Mycobacterium leprae (leprosy). In Mandell, G.L., Douglas, R.G., Jr., and Bennett, J.E., editors: Principles and practice of infectious diseases, New York, 1979, John Wiley & Sons, Inc.
18. Brunell, P.A.: Chickenpox. In Wehrle, P.F., and Top, F.H., Sr., editors: Communicable and infectious diseases, ed. 9, St. Louis, 1981, The C.V. Mosby Co.
19. Brunell, P.A.: Mumps. In Wehrle, P.F., and Top, F.H., Sr., editors: Communicable and infectious diseases, ed. 9, St. Louis, 1981, The C.V. Mosby Co.
20. Burton, G.R.: Microbiology for the health sciences, Philadelphia, 1979, J.B. Lippincott Co.
21. Centers for Disease Control: CDC monograph: immunization against disease 1980, Atlanta, Sept. 1980, The Centers.
22. Centers for Disease Control: Revised recommendations for malaria chemoprophylaxis for travelers to East Africa, Morbidity and Mortality Weekly Report **31**:328, June 25, 1982.
23. Centers for Disease Control: Sexually transmitted diseases treatment guidelines 1982, Morbidity and Mortality Weekly Report **31**:35s, Aug. 20, 1982.
24. Centers for Disease Control: CDC guideline for isolation precautions in hospitals. HHS pub. no. (CDC) 83-8314, Atlanta, 1983, The Centers.
25. Chick, E.W., and Dillon, M.L.: Histoplasmosis. In Wehrle, P.F., and Top, F.H., Sr., editors: Communicable and infectious diseases, ed. 9, St. Louis, 1981, The C.V. Mosby Co.
26. Chin, T.D.: Encephalitis, infectious. In Wehrle, P.F., and Top, F.H., Sr., editors: Communicable and infectious diseases, ed. 9, St. Louis, 1981, The C.V. Mosby Co.
27. Chin, W., and Coatney, G.R.: Malaria. In Wehrle, P.F., and Top, F.H., Sr., editors: Communicable and infectious diseases, ed. 9, St. Louis, 1981, The C.V. Mosby Co.

28. Corbett, J.V.: Laboratory tests in nursing parctice, East Norwalk, Connecticut, 1982, Appleton-Century-Crofts.

29. Corey, L.: Herpes simplex virus. In Holmes, K.K., and Mardh, P.-A., editors: International perspectives on neglected sexually transmitted diseases, New York, 1983, McGraw-Hill Book Co.

30. Duke University Hospital Nursing Services: Quality assurance: guidelines for nursing care, Philadelphia, 1980, J.B. Lippincott Co.

31. Dull, H.B., and Wehrle, P.F.: Prevention of communicable diseases: general considerations. In Wehrle, P.F., and Top, F.H., Sr., editors: Communicable and infectious diseases, ed. 9, St. Louis, 1981, The C.V. Mosby Co.

32. Dunkelberg, W.E.: Gardnerella (haemophilus) vaginalis. In Holmes, K.K., and Mardh, P.-A., editors: International perspectives on neglected sexually transmitted diseases, New York, 1983, McGraw-Hill Book Co.

33. Edwards, J.E., Jr.: *Candida* species. In Mandell, G.L., Douglas, R.G., Jr., and Bennett, J.E., editors: Principles and practice of infectious diseases, New York, 1979, John Wiley & Sons, Inc.

34. Evans, A.S.: Mononucleosis. In Wehrle, P.F., and Top, F.H., Sr., editors: Communicable and infectious diseases, ed. 9, St. Louis, 1981, The C.V. Mosby Co.

35. Farer, L.S.: Mycobacterium tuberculosis: bacteriology, epidemiology and treatment. In Mandell, G.L., Douglas, R.G., Jr., and Bennett, J.E., editors: Principles and practice of infectious diseases, New York, 1979, John Wiley & Sons, Inc.

36. Feldman, H.A.: Toxoplasmosis. In Wehrle, P.F., and Top, F.H., Sr., editors: Communicable and infectious diseases, ed. 9, St. Louis, 1981, The C.V. Mosby Co.

37. Fox, J.P., Hall, C.E., and Elveback, L.R.: Epidemiology, man and disease, New York, 1970, Macmillan Publishing Co., Inc.

38. Fraser, D.W.: Legionella pneumophila (Legionaires' disease). In Mandell, G.L., Douglas, R.G., Jr., and Bennett, J.E., editors: Principles and practice of infectious diseases, New York, 1979, John Wiley & Sons, Inc.

39. Fraser, D.W.: Legionellosis. In Wehrle, P.F., and Top, F.H., Sr.: Communicable and infectious diseases, ed. 9, St. Louis, 1981, The C.V. Mosby Co.

40. Freitag, J.J., and Miller, L.W., editors: Manual of medical therapeutics, ed. 23, Boston, 1980, Little Brown & Co.

41. Frobisher, M., and Fuerst, R.: Microbiology in health and disease, ed. 13, Philadelphia, 1973, W.B. Saunders Co.

42. Ganong, W.F.: Review of medical physiology, ed. 11, Los Altos, Calif., 1983, Lange Medical Publication.

43. Garb, S.: Laboratory tests in common use, ed. 6, New York, 1976, Springer Publishing Co.

44. Gershon, A.A.: Rubella. In Mandell, G.L., Douglas, R.G., Jr., and Bennett, J.E., editors: Principles and practice of infectious diseases, New York, 1979, John Wiley & Sons, Inc.

45. Gershon, A.A.: Rubeola. In Mandell, G.L., Douglas, R.G., Jr., and Bennett, J.E., editors: Principles and practice of infectious diseases, New York, 1979, John Wiley & Sons, Inc.

46. Greer, K.E.: Papillomavirus (warts). In Mandell, G.L., Douglas, R.G., Jr., and Bennett, J.E., editors: Principles and practice of infectious diseases, New York, 1979, John Wiley & Sons, Inc.

47. Griffin, D.G., and Johnson, R.T.: Encephalitis, myelitis and neuritis. In Mandell, G.L., Douglas, R.G., Jr., and Bennett, J.E., editors: Principles and practice of infectious diseases, New York, 1979, John Wiley & Sons, Inc.

48. Grove, D.I.: Tissue nematodes (trichinosis, filariasis). In Mandell, G.L., Douglas, R.G., Jr., and Bennett, J.E., editors: Principles and practice of infectious diseases, New York, 1979, John Wiley & Sons, Inc.

49. Guyton, A.C.: Human physiology and mechanisms of disease, ed. 3, Philadelphia, 1982, W.B. Saunders Co.

50. Hamilton, H.E.: Amebiasis and primary amebic meningoencephalitis. In Wehrle, P.F., and Top, F.H., Sr., editors: Communicable and infectious diseases, ed. 9, St. Louis, 1981, The C.V. Mosby Co.

51. Hanshaw, J.B.: Cytomegalovirus. In Wehrle, P.F., and Top, F.H., Sr., editors: Communicable and infectious diseases, ed. 9, St. Louis, 1981, The C.V. Mosby Co.

52. Hart, G.: Chancroid. In Wehrle, P.F., and Top, F.H., Sr., editors: Communicable and infectious diseases, ed. 9, St. Louis, 1981, The C.V. Mosby Co.

53. Hart, G.: Granuloma inguinale (donovanosis). In Wehrle, P.F., and Top, F.H., Sr., editors: Communicable and infectious diseases, ed. 9, St. Louis, 1981, The C.V. Mosby Co.

54. Hart, G.: Lymphogranuloma venereum (LVG). In Wehrle, P.F., and Top, F.H., Sr., editors: Communicable and infectious diseases, ed. 9, St. Louis, 1981, The C.V. Mosby Co.

55. Hirsch, M.S.: Herpes simplex virus. In Mandell, G.L., Douglas, R.G., Jr., and Bennett, J.E., editors: Principles and practice of infectious diseases, New York, 1979, John Wiley & Sons, Inc.

56. Ho, M.: Cytomegalovirus. In Mandell, G.L., Douglas, R.G., Jr., and Bennett, J.E., editors: Principles and practice of infectious diseases, New York, 1979, John Wiley & Sons, Inc.

57. Holloway, N.M.: Nursing the critically ill adult, Menlo Park, Calif., 1979, Addison-Wesley Publishing Co.

58. Holmes, K.K.: Introduction: classification of sexually transmitted diseases. In Holmes, K.K., and Mardh, P.-A., editors: International perspectives on neglected sexually transmitted diseases, New York, 1983, McGraw-Hill Book Co.

59. Holmes, K.K.: Vaginitis, cervicitis and urethritis. In Holmes, K.K., and Mardh, P.-A., editors: International perspectives on neglected sexually transmitted diseases, New York, 1983, McGraw-Hill Book Co.

60. Hoofnagle, J.H.: Acute hepatitis. In Mandell, G.L., Douglas, R.G., Jr., and Bennett, J.E., editors: Principles and practice of infectious diseases, New York, 1979, John Wiley & Sons, Inc.

61. Jawetz, E., Melnick, J.L., and Adelberg, E.A.: Review of medical microbiology, ed. 13, Los Altos, Calif., 1978, Lange Medical Publications.

62. Jones, T.C.: Cestodes (tapeworms). In Mandell, G.L., Douglas, R.G., Jr., and Bennett, J.E., editors: Principles and practice of infectious diseases, New York, 1979, John Wiley & Sons, Inc.

63. King, A., Nicol, C., and Rodin, P.: Venereal diseases, London, 1980, Bailliere Tindall.

64. Krugman, S., and Katz, S.L.: Infectious diseases of children, ed. 7, St. Louis, 1981, The C.V. Mosby Co.

65. Levan, N.E., and Freedman, R.I.: Leprosy. In Wehrle, P.F., and Top, F.H., Sr., editors: Communicable and infectious diseases, ed. 9, St. Louis, 1981, The C.V. Mosby Co.

66. Levine, M.M.: Shigellosis. In Wehrle, P.F., and Top, F.H., Sr., editors: Communicable and infectious diseases, ed. 9, St. Louis, 1981, The C.V. Mosby Co.

67. Locks, M.O.: Tuberculosis. In Wehrle, P.F., and Top, F.H., Sr., editors: Communicable and infectious diseases, ed. 9, St. Louis, 1981, The C.V. Mosby Co.

68. Mahmoud, A.: Intestinal nematodes (roundworms). In Mandell, G.L., Douglas, R.G., Jr., and Bennett, J.E., editors: Principles and practice of infectious diseases, New York, 1979, John Wiley & Sons, Inc.

69. Maynard, J.E.: Hepatitis. In Wehrle, P.F., and Top, F.H., Sr., editors: Communicable and infectious diseases, ed. 9, St. Louis, 1981, The C.V. Mosby Co.

70. Merck manual of diagnosis and therapy, ed. 14, New Jersey, 1982, Merck & Co., Inc.

71. Mogabgab, W.J.: Influenza. In Wehrle, P.F., and Top, F.H., Sr., editors: Communicable and infectious diseases, ed. 9, St. Louis, 1981, The C.V. Mosby Co.

72. Monath, T.P.: Flavirus (St. Louis encephalitis and dengue). In Mandell, G.L., Douglas, R.G., Jr., and Bennett, J.E., editors: Principles and practice of infectious diseases, New York, 1979, John Wiley & Sons, Inc.

73. Muller, M.: Trichomonas vaginalis and other sexually transmitted protozoan infections. In Holmes, K.K., and Mardh, P.-A., editors: International perspectives on neglected sexually transmitted diseases, New York, 1983, McGraw-Hill Book Co.

74. Nahmias, A.J., and Kohl, S.: Herpes simplex. In Wehrle, P.F., and Top, F.H., Sr., editors: Communicable and infectious diseases, ed. 9, St. Louis, 1981, The C.V. Mosby Co.

75. National Institute of Allergy and Infectious Diseases Study Group: Gonorrhea. In Sexually transmitted diseases 1980: status report, U.S. DHHS, PHS, NIH pub. no. 81-2213.

76. Norden, C.W., and Ruben, F.L.: Staphylococcal infections. In Wehrle, P.F., and Top, F.H., Sr., editors: Communicable and infectious diseases, ed. 9, St. Louis, 1981, The C.V. Mosby Co.

77. Oriel, J.D.: Genital warts. In Holmes, K.K., and Mardh, P.-A., editors: International perspectives on neglected sexually transmitted diseases, New York, 1983, McGraw-Hill Book Co.

78. Ottesen, E.A.: Visceral larva migrans and other migratory helminths. In Mandell, G.L., Douglas, R.G., Jr., and Bennett, J.E., editors: Principles and practice of infectious diseases, New York, 1979, John Wiley & Sons, Inc.

79. Overturf, G.D., and Underman, A.E.: Typhoid and enteric fevers. In Wehrle, P.F., and Top, F.H., Sr., editors: Communicable and infectious diseases, ed. 9, St. Louis, 1981, The C.V. Mosby Co.

80. Poland, J.D.: Tularemia. In Wehrle, P.F., and Top, F.H., Sr., editors: Communicable and infectious diseases, ed. 9, St. Louis, 1981, The C.V. Mosby Co.

81. Rein, M.F.: Trichomonas vaginalis. In Mandell, G.L., Douglas, R.G., Jr., and Bennett, J.E., editors: Principles and practice of infectious diseases, New York, 1979, John Wiley & Sons, Inc.

82. Rein, M.F.: Vulvovaginitis and cervicitis. In Mandell, G.L., Douglas, R.G., Jr., and Bennett, J.E., editors: Principles and practice of infectious diseases, New York, 1979, John Wiley & Sons, Inc.

83. Robinson, W.S.: Hepatitis. In Mandell, G.L., Douglas, R.G., Jr., and Bennett, J.E., editors: Principles and practice of infectious diseases, New York, 1979, John Wiley & Sons, Inc.

84. Rudolph, A.H.: Syphilis. In Wehrle, P.F., and Top, F.H., Sr., editors: Communicable and infectious diseases, ed. 9, St. Louis, 1981, The C.V. Mosby Co.

85. Russell, P.K.: Dengue. In Wehrle, P.F., and Top, F.H., Sr., editors: Communicable and infectious diseases, ed. 9, St. Louis, 1981, The C.V. Mosby Co.

86. Rymzo, W.T., Jr., et al.: Dengue outbreaks in Guanica-Ensenada and Villalba, Puerto Rico, 1972-1973, Am. J. Trop. Med. Hyg. **25**(1):136, 1976.

87. Saah, A.J., and Hornick, R.B.: Rickettsiosis. In Mandell, G.L., Douglas, R.G., Jr., and Bennett, J.E., editors: Principles and practice of infectious diseases, New York, 1979, John Wiley & Sons, Inc.

88. Sanford, J.P., and Pierce, A.K.: Lower respiratory tract infections. In Bennett, J.V., and Brachman, P.S., editors: Hospital infections, Boston, 1979, Little, Brown & Co.

89. Schacter, J.: Chlamydia trachomatis. In Holmes, K.K., and Mardh, P.-A., editors: International perspectives on neglected sexually transmitted diseases, New York, 1983, McGraw-Hill Book Co.

90. Schooley, R.T., and Dolin, R.: Epstein-Barr virus (infectious mononucleosis). In Mandell, G.L., Douglas, R.G., Jr., and Bennett, J.E., editors: Principles and practice of infectious diseases, New York, 1979, John Wiley & Sons, Inc.

91. Seals, J.E.: Nontyphoidal salmonellosis. In Wehrle, P.F., and Top, F.H., Sr., editors: Communicable and infectious diseases, ed. 9, St. Louis, 1981, The C.V. Mosby Co.

92. Simmons, B.P.: Guideline for prevention of intravenous therapy related infections, Oct. 1981 (reprinted Feb. 1982), Center for Infectious Diseases, Centers for Disease Control.

93. Simmons, B.P.: Center for Disease Control guideline for prevention of surgical wound infections, Infect. Control **3**(3):187, 1982.

94. Smith I.M.: Brucella species (brucellosis). In Mandell, G.L., Douglas, R.G., Jr., and Bennett, J.E., editors: Principles and practice of infectious diseases, New York, 1979, John Wiley & Sons, Inc.

95. Smith, I.M.: Staphylococcus aureus. In Mandell, G.L., Douglas, R.G., Jr., and Bennett, J.E., editors: Principles and practice of infectious diseases, New York, 1979, John Wiley & Sons, Inc.

96. Socomini, C.N.: Donovanosis. In Holmes, K.K., and Mardh, P.-A., editors: International perspectives on neglected sexually transmitted diseases, New York, 1983, McGraw-Hill Book Co.

97. Sours, H.E.: Food poisoning, bacterial. In Wehrle, P.F., and Top, F.H., Sr., editors: Communicable and infectious diseases, ed. 9, St. Louis, 1981, The C.V. Mosby Co.

98. Spaeth, R.: Tetanus. In Wehrle, P.F., and Top, F.H., Sr., editors: Communicable and infectious diseases, ed. 9, St. Louis, 1981, The C.V. Mosby Co.

99. Stamm, W.E., and Bennett, J.V.: Nosocomial infections. In Wehrle, P.F., and Top, F.H., Sr., editors: Communicable and infectious diseases, ed. 9, St. Louis, 1981, The C.V. Mosby Co.

100. Steere, A.C., et al.: Gram-negative rod bacteremia. In Bennett, J.V., and Brachman, P.S., editors: Hospital infections, Boston, 1979, Little, Brown & Co.

101. Sutliff, W.D., and Bennett, J.E.: Histoplasma capsulatum. In Mandell, G.L., Douglas, R.G., Jr., and Bennett, J.E., editors: Principles and practice of infectious diseases, New York, 1979, John Wiley & Sons, Inc.

102. Swartz, M.N.: Cellulitis. In Mandell, G.L., Douglas, R.G., Jr., and Bennett, J.E., editors: Principles and practice of infectious diseases, New York, 1979, John Wiley & Sons, Inc.

103. Tilkian, S.M., Conover, M.B., and Tilkian, A.G.: Clinical implications of laboratory tests, ed. 3, St. Louis, 1983, The C.V. Mosby Co.

104. Top, F.H., Jr.: Rubella. In Wehrle, P.F., and Top, F.H., Sr., editors: Communicable and infectious diseases, ed. 9, St. Louis, 1981, The C.V. Mosby Co.

105. Top, F.H., Sr., Johnson, K.M., and Wehrle, P.F.: Enteroviruses: poliomyelitis. In Wehrle, P.F., and Top, F.H., Sr., editors: Communicable and infectious diseases, ed. 9, St. Louis, 1981, The C.V. Mosby Co.

106. Top, F.H., Sr., and Wehrle, P.F.: Diphtheria. In Wehrle, P.F., and Top, F.H., Sr., editors: Communicable and infectious diseases, ed. 9, St. Louis, 1981, The C.V. Mosby Co.

107. Tramont, E.C.: Treponema pallidum. In Mandell, G.L., Douglas, R.G., Jr., and Bennett, J.E., editors: Principles and practice of infectious diseases, New York, 1979, John Wiley & Sons, Inc.

108. Underman, A.E.: Tapeworm disease. In Wehrle, P.F., and Top, F.H., Sr., editors: Communicable and infectious diseases, ed. 9, St. Louis, 1981, The C.V. Mosby Co.

109. Veasey, J.M., Jr., and Wenzel, R.P.: Nosocomial pneumonia. In Mandell, G.L., Douglas, R.G., Jr., and Bennett, J.E., editors: Principles and practice of infectious diseases, New York, 1979, John Wiley & Sons, Inc.

110. Wannamaker, L.W., Rammelkamp, C.H., and Top, F.H., Sr.: Streptococcal infections. In Wehrle, P.F., and Top, F.H., Sr., editors: Communicable and infectious diseases, ed. 9, St. Louis, 1981, The C.V. Mosby Co.

111. Warren, K.S.: Introduction to diseases due to helminths. In Mandell, G.L., Douglas, R.G., Jr., and Bennett, J.E., editors: Principles and practice of infectious diseases, New York, 1979, John Wiley & Sons, Inc.

112. Wehrle, P.F., and Mathies, A.W., Jr.: Meningitis. In Wehrle, P.F., and Top, F.H., Sr., editors: Communicable and infectious diseases, ed. 9, St. Louis, 1981, The C.V. Mosby Co.

113. Wilkins, J., and Bass, J.: Pertussis. In Wehrle, P.F., and Top, F.H., Sr., editors: Communicable and infectious diseases, ed. 9, St. Louis, 1981, The C.V. Mosby Co.

114. Wilson, R.: Enteric infections. In Wehrle, P.F., and Top, F.H., Sr., editors: Communicable and infectious diseases, ed. 9, St. Louis, 1981, The C.V. Mosby Co.

115. Wisseman, C.L., Jr.: Rickettsial diseases. In Wehrle, P.F., and Top, F.H., Sr., editors: Communicable and infectious diseases, ed. 9, St. Louis, 1981, The C.V. Mosby Co.

116. Wong, E.C.: Guideline for prevention of catheter-associated urinary tract infections. In Center for Infectious Diseases: Guidelines for prevention and control of nosocomial infections, Feb. 1981, The Center.

117. Woodward, W.E., and Hornick, R.B.: Rickettsia rickettsii (Rocky Mountain spotted fever). In Mandell, G.L., Douglas, R.G., Jr., and Bennett, J.E., editors: Principles and practice of infectious diseases, New York, 1979, John Wiley & Sons, Inc.

118. Wyler, D.J., and Miller, L.H.: Plasmodium species (malaria). In Mandell, G.L., Douglas, R.G., Jr., and Bennett, J.E., editors: Principles and practice of infectious diseases, New York, 1979, John Wiley & Sons, Inc.

119. Young, L.S.: Gram-negative sepsis. In Mandell, G.L., Douglas, R.G., Jr., and Bennett, J.E., editors: Principles and practice of infectious diseases, New York, 1979, John Wiley & Sons, Inc.

CHAPTER 16

Immunologic System

Overview

The immune system is a highly specialized group of cells and tissues that protects the internal milieu of the host. Immune responses are initiated when cellular components of the system recognize an agent as foreign and attempt to eliminate it. One role of the immune system is defense against invasive microorganisms. A second function is to maintain homeostasis by removing effete or damaged cellular elements from the circulation. Recently it was also appreciated that the immune system serves as a surveillance network to guard against the development, growth, and dissemination of tumor cells.

When the immune system responds appropriately to a foreign stimulus, the host's integrity is maintained. If the immune response is too weak or too vigorous, a derangement in homeostasis results. Certain hypersensitivity reactions and autoimmune diseases can occur when the regulatory cells of the immune system do not adequately control effector cell activities. Similarly, a depression in immune reactivity caused by regulatory or effector cell dysfunction can result in host susceptibility to recurrent infections and malignant disease.

Knowledge of basic immunology is increasing at a rapid rate and has had a profound influence on current medical and surgical practice. Immunomodulatory agents are being widely used to augment immune function in cancer patients and persons with immunodeficiency diseases. Histocompatibility matching and the development of pharmacologic agents that selectively depress immune reactivity have had a major impact on organ transplantation. Since a number of diseases, such as cancer, rheumatoid disorders, and certain hematologic and gastrointestinal problems, have been associated with immunologic changes, therapies involving immunologic manipulation may soon play a pivotal role in all clinical specialty fields.

ANATOMY AND PHYSIOLOGY
Cellular Components and Their Anatomic Organization

The cellular constituents of the immune system include granulocytes, mononuclear phagocytes, and lymphocytes (Fig. 16-1). White cells have been grouped into these three general categories on the basis of cell morphology, functional activities, and stem cell derivation.

Cells of the granulocyte series, that is, basophils or mast cells, eosinophils, and neutrophils, are derived from a common bone marrow progenitor cell, the myeloblast. *Basophils* comprise 0.5% to 1% of the circulating white blood cell (leukocyte) population. *Mast cells*, tissue counterparts of the blood basophil, are found adjacent to smooth muscle in the perivascular and peribronchiolar tissues. Mast cells and basophils play an important role

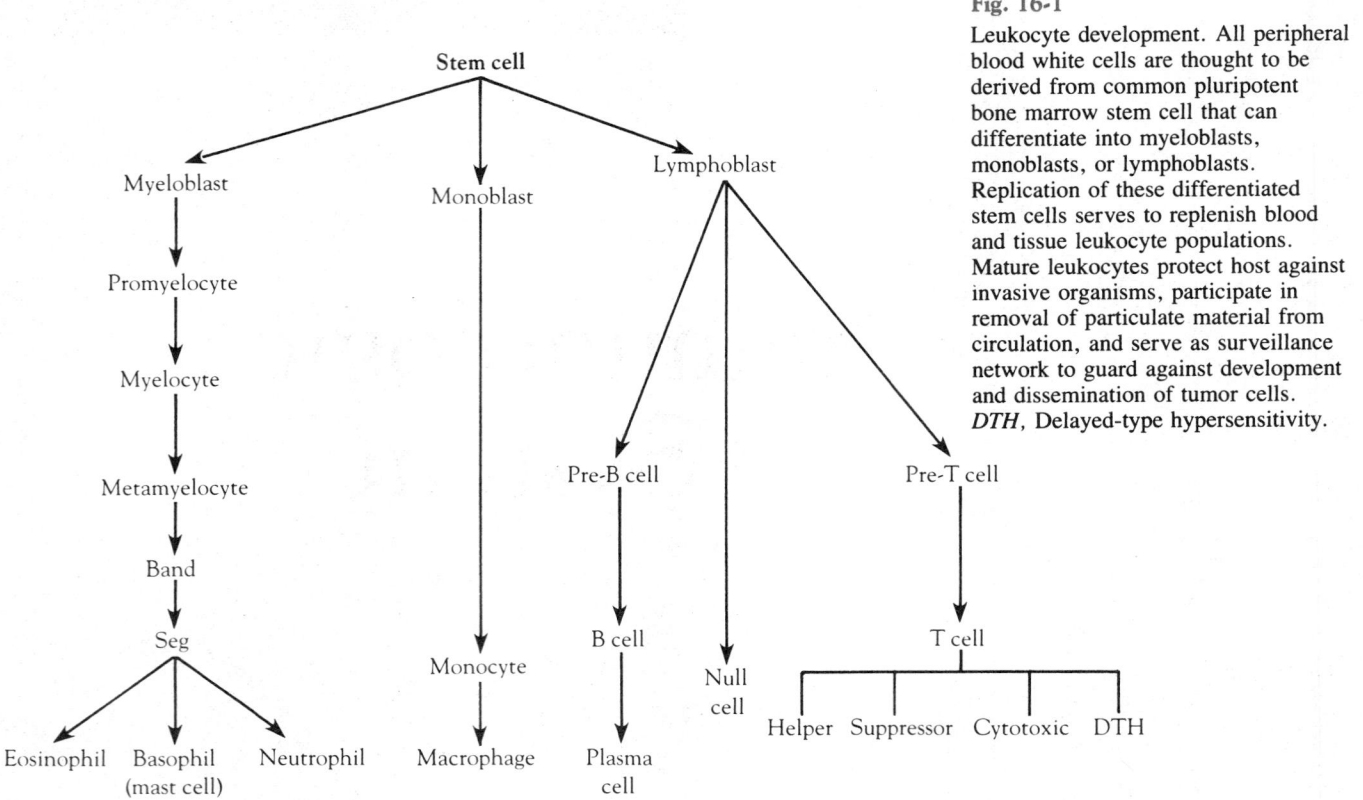

Fig. 16-1

Leukocyte development. All peripheral blood white cells are thought to be derived from common pluripotent bone marrow stem cell that can differentiate into myeloblasts, monoblasts, or lymphoblasts. Replication of these differentiated stem cells serves to replenish blood and tissue leukocyte populations. Mature leukocytes protect host against invasive organisms, participate in removal of particulate material from circulation, and serve as surveillance network to guard against development and dissemination of tumor cells. *DTH*, Delayed-type hypersensitivity.

in allergic reactions. *Eosinophils* make up 1% to 3% of peripheral blood leukocytes. They accumulate at sites of anaphylaxis and in addition may influence the host response to parasitic infections. *Neutrophils* comprise up to 70% of the blood leukocyte population. Neutrophils are actively phagocytic cells that leave the vascular compartment and rapidly accumulate within the tissue spaces at sites of inflammation.

Cells of the mononuclear phagocyte series, all originally derived from the bone marrow monoblast, are distributed throughout the body. *Monocytes* comprise approximately 5% of the circulating leukocyte population. Following a brief interval in the blood, monocytes migrate into the tissues where they mature into *macrophages,* the metabolically and functionally mature cells of this series. Macrophages are present in the brain (microglial cells), spleen, and lymphoid tissues. They also line the lung alveoli, the blood sinusoids of the liver (Kupffer cells), and most extravascular tissue spaces. Mononuclear phagocytes help to protect the host from invasive organisms, clear tissue debris from sites of tissue injury, and may serve as surveillance cells in antitumor host defense.

Cells of the lymphoid series play a key role in the development of acquired immunity. All *lymphocytes* (T, B, and null cells, which do not have surface markers identifying them as either B or T lymphocytes) are derived from a common bone marrow progenitor cell. Certain immature lymphocytes leave the bone marrow and populate the thymus, where under the influence of thymic hormones they proliferate and differentiate into mature *T lymphocytes*. Other immature lymphocytes proliferate and differentiate into mature *B lymphocytes*. In birds this maturation takes place in an organ called the bursa of Fabricius. No mammalian bursal equivalent tissue has been identified. It is thought that B cell maturation in humans may take place in the bone marrow or in the lymphoid tissues lining the gastrointestinal tract.

After maturation, T and B lymphocytes, now capable of interacting specifically with foreign materials and participating in immune responses, are released into the circulation and populate the peripheral lymphoid tissues, including the spleen, lymph nodes, and tonsils. Mature lymphocytes are also localized in lymphoid tissues directly associated with the mucosal surfaces of the body. Such organized tissues comprise the appendix, Peyer's

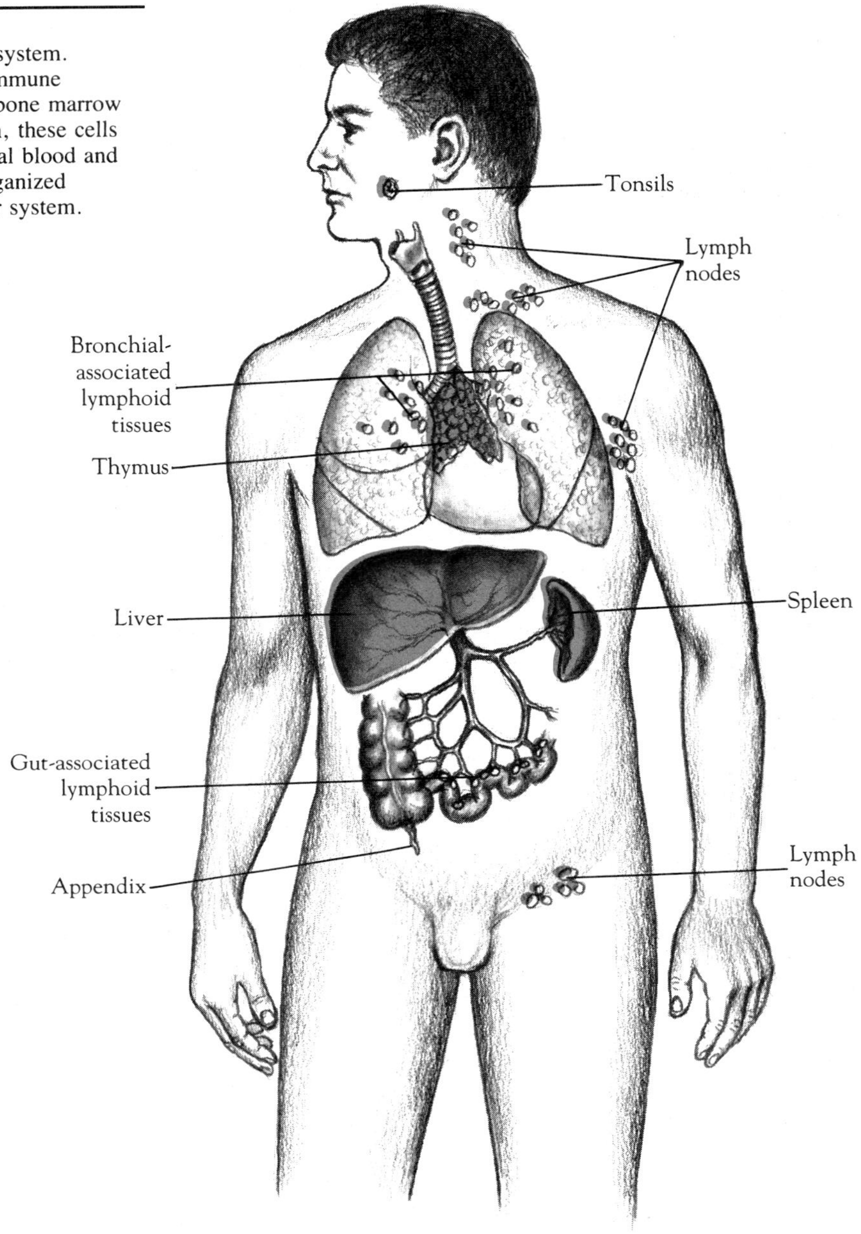

Fig. 16-2

Organization of immune system. Cellular constituents of immune system are derived from bone marrow stem cells. On maturation, these cells are released into peripheral blood and subsequently populate organized tissues of lymphoreticular system.

patches of the ileum, and bronchial-associated lymphoid tissue. The major organs housing the cellular elements of the immune system are illustrated in Fig. 16-2.

Nonspecific Immune Mechanisms

Physical and chemical barriers. The first line of defense against invasive organisms is provided by intact skin and mucous membranes. These structures not only serve as a physical barrier to invasion but also provide a chemically unsuitable milieu to support microbial growth. Certain skin and mucosal secretions, such as lactic acid, gastric acid, and lysozyme, have bactericidal properties. Mechanical factors, such as ciliary action in the respiratory tract, also act to protect the host in a nonspecific manner.

Microbial factors. Resident normal flora of the skin and mucous membranes also provide a defense against colonization with pathogenic bacteria. These resident microorganisms suppress growth of infectious agents by competing for essential nutrients, producing growth-inhibiting substances, and altering pH. When normal flora are reduced by antibiotic treatment, a person is more susceptible to infection with pathogenic microorganisms.

Inflammatory response. When a microorganism transcends the physical, chemical, and microbial barriers afforded by the host, or the body is injured by mechanical or chemical means, an inflammatory response is generated. At the onset of inflammation a rapid vasodilation occurs. Within minutes, blood neutrophils accumulate near the site of injury, migrate to the junctional zones between the vascular endothelial cells, and extravasate into the tissue spaces. Neutrophils within an inflammatory site represent the first line of cellular defense against invasive microorganisms.

If neutrophils do not neutralize the inflammatory focus within a few hours, monocytes and lymphocytes begin to accumulate at the site of tissue injury. These cells attempt to localize the inflammatory response, providing a cellular barrier against the migration of the infectious organism into the lymphatic compartment or blood vessels. When neutrophils, lymphocytes, and monocytes neutralize the inflammatory focus, granulation tissue is laid down and inflammation subsides. If the acute inflammatory response is unsuccessful at eliminating the infectious agent or tissue repair is incomplete, chronic inflammation results.

The persistence of an infectious agent during chronic inflammation results in granuloma formation. *Granulomatous lesions* are characterized by accumulations of lymphocytes and macrophages surrounding a central core of foreign material. Fibrotic tissue laid down on the periphery of the granuloma acts as a physical barrier, separating the lesion from surrounding normal tissues.

Accompanying the cellular responses that occur during inflammation are elevations in serum levels of certain proteins. These *acute phase proteins*, which include C-reactive protein and serum amyloid A protein, are used clinically to detect the presence of an infectious or inflammatory process. *C-reactive protein* may play a protective role by activating the complement pathway and influencing certain leukocyte responses. Large increases in the serum concentrations of globular proteins and fibrinogen may also accompany episodes of infection, inflammation, and tissue necrosis. In vitro, an elevation in the levels of these plasma proteins increases the aggregation and precipitation of erythrocytes suspended in plasma. This phenomenon, manifested in the laboratory as an elevation in *erythrocyte sedimentation rate* (ESR), is indicative of an ongoing inflammatory process.

Other serum proteins that play a major role in inflammation include the kinins, vasoactive amines, prostaglandins, and certain complement components (C3a, C4a, and C5a). These factors increase *vasodilation* and induce a widening of the junction between adjacent vascular endothelial cells, thus facilitating the exudation of fluid and cellular elements into the tissue spaces. *Chemotactic factors,* molecules that attract leukocytes toward an inflammatory focus, also contribute to the generation of inflammatory processes. These mediators include bacterial products, certain fluid phase components of the complement system (C5a), and products of stimulated leukocytes.

Lymphoreticular system. When an infectious agent is able to permeate the barriers afforded by the local cellular response that occurs during acute or chronic inflammation, it enters the vascular compartment or the lymphatic channels. The lymphoreticular system, comprised of organs housing both tissue macrophages and lymphoid cells, functions to remove bacteria, tissue debris, or tumor cells from the lymph and blood.

When foreign materials enter the lymphatics, they are filtered by, and become lodged within, the lymph nodes (Fig. 16-3). Within the nodes they may be engulfed and destroyed by fixed phagocytic cells or, alternatively, may activate a specific immune response. In a corresponding fashion, when a foreign agent enters the blood, it is phagocytosed by macrophages lining the blood sinusoids of the liver and spleen. If these macrophages do not completely destroy or neutralize the foreign material, they present it in a modified form to lymphoid cells, initiating a specific immune response.

Phagocytosis. Granulocytes and mononuclear phagocytes are key cellular participants in the nonspecific immune response. Monocytes and neutrophils that have migrated into an inflammatory site and tissue macrophages that encounter foreign materials within the respiratory, vascular, or lymphatic compartments protect the host largely by their phagocytic capabilities.

Phagocytosis is a multistep process that is initiated by the attachment of a damaged or foreign material to the surface of the phagocytic cell (Fig. 16-4). Particle recognition may occur at nonspecific membrane receptors or may be mediated by *opsonic proteins,* such as immunoglobulins and certain complement components that coat particles and facilitate their attachment to specific receptors on phagocytic cells. After particle attachment the cell membrane on the surface of the phagocyte invaginates, encloses the particle, pinches off, and is internalized. The phagocytic vacuole subsequently fuses with lysosomal granules, vacuoles within the cell containing potent hydrolytic enzymes.

During the process of phagocytosis a number of metabolic changes occur within the cell. These include a stimulation in glucose oxidation via glycolysis and the hexose monophosphate shunt and an elevation in oxygen consumption. These metabolic changes are tightly linked to the activities of certain cellular enzymes, NADPH

Fig. 16-3

Lymph node structure. Lymph enters node via afferent lymph vessels, percolates through cortex and medulla, and leaves via efferent lymphatics. Foreign materials are trapped by macrophages in cortex, digested, and presented to lymphoid cells to initiate specific immune response. Superficial cortex is comprised primarily of B lymphocytes clustered into follicles. Interfollicular regions of superficial cortex and bulk of deep cortex are populated by T lymphocytes.

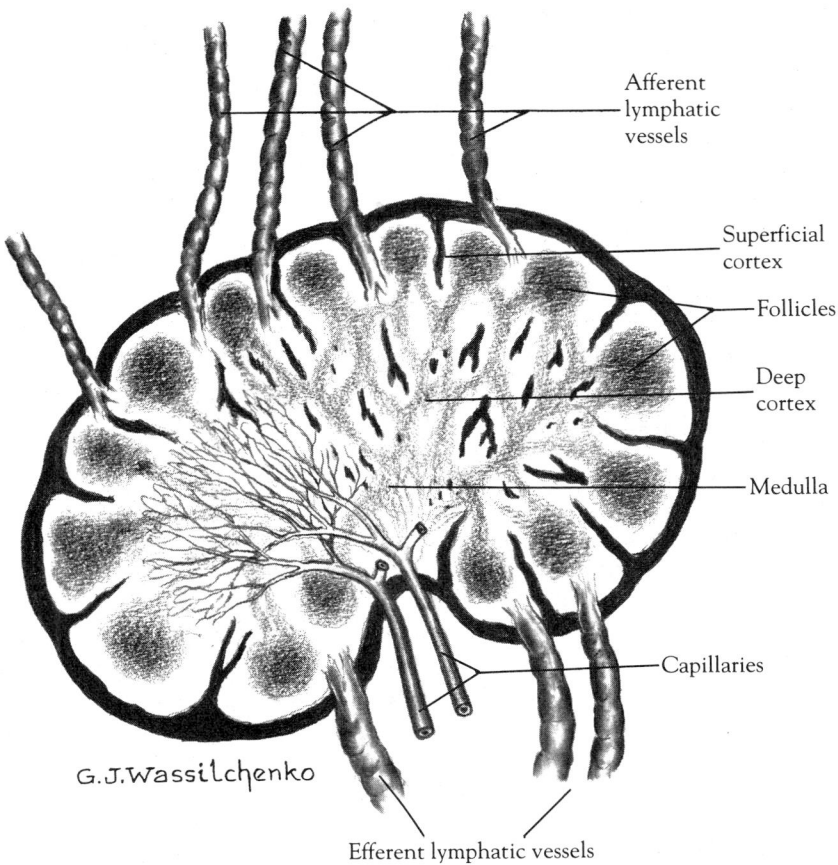

G.J.Wassilchenko

Fig. 16-4

Phagocytosis. This multistep process is used by granulocytes, monocytes, and macrophages to remove foreign materials from body. These materials come in contact with digestive enzymes and destructive oxygen metabolites within phagocytic vacuole. Incompletely digested materials, lysosomal enzymes, and toxic oxygen products may be released from cell.

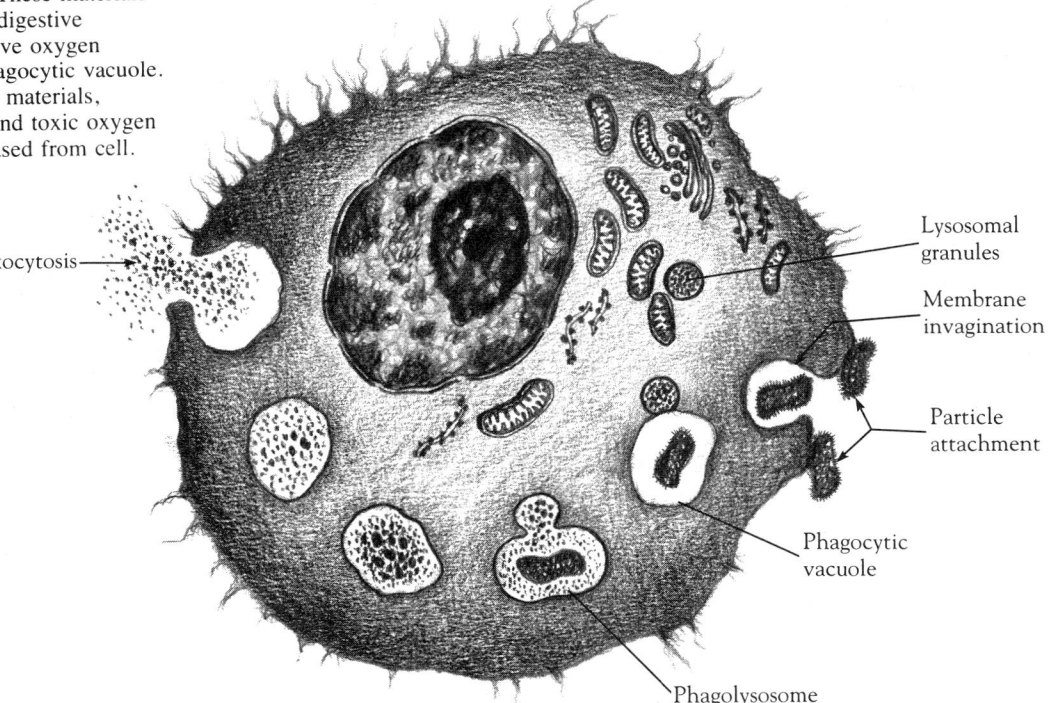

oxidase and glucose 6-phosphate dehydrogenase. Associated with these biochemical events is the increased production of lactic acid, hydrogen peroxide, superoxide anion, hydroxyl radical, and singlet oxygen. These oxidative products of the *respiratory burst,* in concert with lysosomal granule constituents such as myeloperoxidase, lysozyme, lactoferrin, and granular cationic proteins, are important antimicrobial agents employed by phagocytic cells. Under certain conditions, lysosomal enzymes and toxic oxygen products are released from the phagocytic cell. These events are responsible for much of the tissue damage that occurs in an ongoing inflammatory process.

Specific Immune Mechanisms

Antigenicity. An *antigen* (or immunogen) is a substance capable of evoking an immune response. To qualify as an antigen a molecule must be recognized as foreign by the immune system. Antigens present on bacteria, viruses, molds, and pollens can induce a detectable immune response.

Similarly, antigens found on mammalian cells and tissues can be immunogenic. *Autologous antigens* are tissue determinants that under normal conditions do not evoke an immune response. When these "self" antigens are altered by infectious or inflammatory processes, the immune system recognizes its own tissues as "foreign" and produces an autoimmune response. *Alloantigens* are genetically determined antigens that discriminate individuals within a given species. Red cells, for example, have on their surface a number of determinants, including A, B, and Rh antigens, that may precipitate an immunologic reaction following the transfusion of incompatible blood. Similarly, human leukocyte antigens (HLA), present on

the surface of all nucleated cells, have a profound influence on allograft survival. The human *major histocompatibility complex* (MHC) is a genetic region on chromosome 6 that codes for these human alloantigens. Gene products of the HLA-A, HLA-B, and HLA-C loci appear on all nucleated cells, whereas HLA-D region products are found primarily on lymphocytes, macrophages, epidermal cells, and sperm.

Induction of a specific immune response. Antigen-specific responses are designated as either humoral or cellular immunity (Table 16-1). *Humoral immunity* is mediated by B lymphocytes that synthesize and secrete γ-globulins in response to antigenic challenge. *Cell-mediated immune mechanisms* involve the participation of effector T lymphocytes and macrophages. Humoral immunity can be transferred from an immune to a nonimmune host with cell-free globulin-bearing serum, whereas cellular immunity is transferred with sensitized cells. Although the body's response to an antigenic challenge usually involves both cellular and humoral immune mechanisms, one response may predominate.

A specific immune mechanism involves the participation of T and B lymphocytes that have been genetically programmed to recognize and interact with unique antigenic determinants on a foreign material. A specific immune response is triggered after the clearance of foreign materials from an inflammatory site, the lymph, or the vascular compartment by tissue macrophages. These phagocytic cells internalize and degrade the foreign antigens. The processed antigens are reexpressed on the macrophage surface in a highly immunogenic form for presentation to lymphocytes that continuously circulate through the lymphoid organs. Recognition of antigen by specific receptors on lymphocytes results in their stimulation and sequestration within the tissue.

Humoral immunity. When confronted with an antigen, B lymphocytes synthesize and secrete specifically reactive γ-globulins called *antibodies* or *immunoglobulins.* On first exposure to a given antigen, a *primary humoral immune response* is evoked. This response occurs after a lag period of 1 to 7 days during which only trace amounts of specific antibody can be detected. During this induction period, antigen is processed and specific clones of B lymphocytes are stimulated to divide and differentiate ultimately into two different cell types. The first type, *plasma cells,* synthesizes and secretes antibodies. Other B lymphocytes, *memory cells,* remain quiescent until secondary exposure to a given antigen.

The *secondary,* or *anamnestic, response* that occurs after subsequent exposure to a particular antigen has a short lag period, produces high levels of antibody, and is more sustained than the primary response. This memory property of the immune system increases resistance

Table 16-1

Humoral and Cell-Mediated Immune Responses

	Humoral	Cell-Mediated
Effector cells	B lymphocytes	T lymphocytes and macrophages
Regulatory cells	T helper cells and T suppressor cells	T helper cells and T suppressor cells
Effector mechanisms	Elaboration of antibody	Generation of factors that are directly toxic to target cells
Host protection	Against many gram-positive and certain gram-negative bacteria	Against mycobacteria, fungi, protozoa, and tumors

to infection in persons who have been immunized to, or previously infected with, a particular antigen.

The humoral immune response offers protection against many gram-positive and certain gram-negative organisms. Specific antibody generated during a humoral immune response facilitates viral neutralization, enhances bacterial ingestion and destruction by phagocytic cells, and results in activation of the complement system.

When a humoral immune response is generated against soluble antigens, small antigen-antibody complexes form. These *immune complexes* may be rapidly cleared from the circulation by fixed macrophages in the liver and spleen or, alternatively, may be deposited within tissues. Tissue-bound immune complexes can activate the complement system and provoke inflammatory destruction of normal cells.

Regulation of the humoral immune response. Certain antigens are capable of stimulating B cells directly or after presentation on the macrophage surface. These *T-independent antigens* have a primary structure of repeating identical units.

Most antigens, however, require the activation of a subpopulation of lymphocytes, *T helper cells,* in addition to B lymphocytes, to effect an antibody response. The antibody response to a *T-dependent antigen* is initiated by macrophage presentation of antigen to T helper cells and secretion of interleukin 1, a T cell growth–promoting substance. T helper cells, stimulated in this way, interact with B lymphocytes and promote their growth and differentiation. B cell growth factor, derived from T cells, may play a role in B cell activation (Fig. 16-5).

The antibody response to T-dependent antigen is under the control of the major histocompatibility complex (MHC). To interact with antibody-presenting macrophages, helper T cells have to recognize and bind "self" antigens, called Ia antigens, on the macrophage surface. These self antigens are coded for by genes of the HLA region. Similarly, T cell binding to B lymphocytes involves their recognition of a genetically determined marker on the B cell surface.

In addition to T lymphocytes that provide help in the induction of an immune response, certain other T lym-

Fig. 16-5

Humoral immune responses. Antibody response to T-dependent antigens involves interaction between macrophages, T cells, and B cells. Macrophages ingest foreign materials, reexpress processed antigen on their surface, and present it in context of Ia molecule to T helper cells. T helper cells facilitate B lymphocyte proliferation and differentiation. On primary exposure to given T-dependent antigen, memory cell generation occurs, although little antibody is generated. During anamnestic response, plasma cells synthesize large quantities of specific antibody. Humoral response to T-independent antigens may be macrophage-dependent or independent process. This response generally produces only antibody of IgM class and has little or no memory. *IL-1,* Interleukin 1.

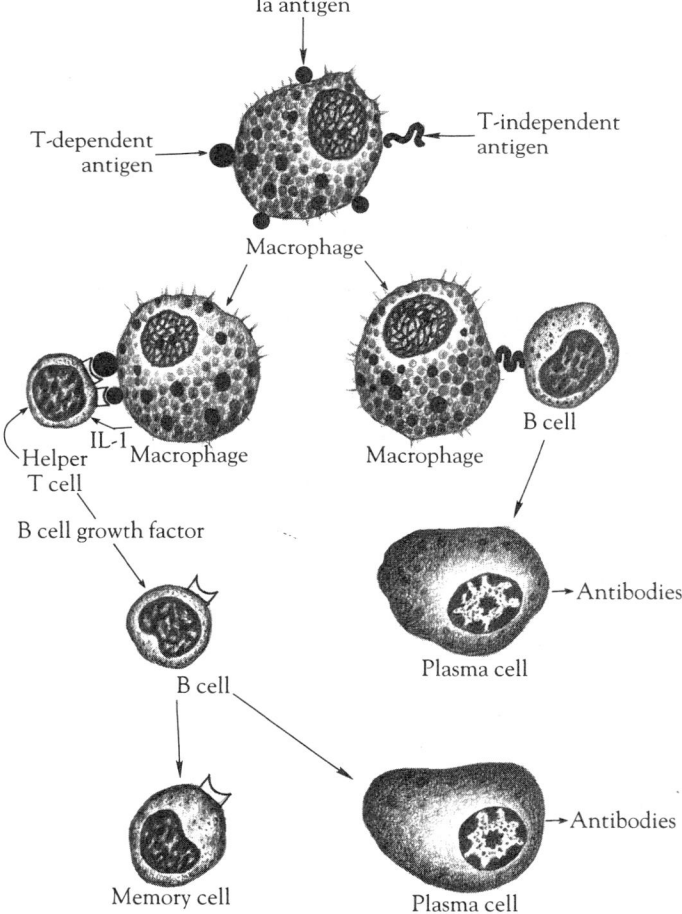

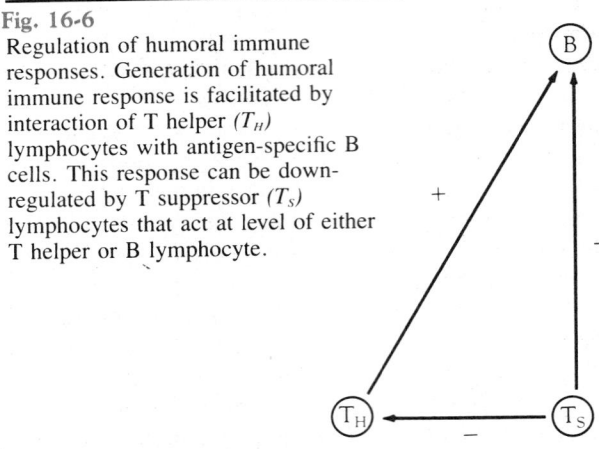

Fig. 16-6

Regulation of humoral immune responses. Generation of humoral immune response is facilitated by interaction of T helper *(T$_H$)* lymphocytes with antigen-specific B cells. This response can be down-regulated by T suppressor *(T$_s$)* lymphocytes that act at level of either T helper or B lymphocyte.

phocytes have distinct surface markers and can be readily discriminated in the laboratory, immune function can be estimated by measuring the T helper/T suppressor cell ratio. Normally a person has roughly twice as many T helper cells as T suppressor cells. In contrast, patients with acquired immunodeficiency syndrome (AIDS) frequently demonstrate a T helper/T suppressor cell ratio of 1:1 or less.

Biologic activities of immunoglobulins. The γ-globulin-bearing or antibody-bearing fractions of serum are referred to as *immunoglobulins*. The immunoglobulins are a highly heterogeneous population of proteins, not a singular molecular species. Currently five physicochemical classes of immunoglobulins are recognized: IgG, IgM, IgA, IgE, and IgD.

Immunoglobulin molecules are made up of a four-chain polypeptide (protein) unit consisting of two identical high–molecular weight (heavy) chains and two identical low–molecular weight (light) chains. The immunoglobulins have been assigned to their respective classes on the basis of their heavy chains, gamma (γ), mu (μ), alpha (α), epsilon (ε), and delta (δ). There are two different light chain types, kappa (κ) and lambda (λ). A schematic representation of the five major immunoglobulin classes is shown in Fig. 16-7.

When a humoral immune response is triggered, one or more classes of antibody may be elaborated. The nature of the antibody response is dependent on the chemical and physical nature of the antigen, route of administration, and immunization history of the host.

IgG is the predominant serum antibody and represents a large proportion of the immunoglobulin found in internal secretions (for example, pleural, synovial, and peritoneal fluids). Specific IgG is produced only in small

phocytes depress immune reactivity. *Suppressor T cells* have an important role in homeostatic control, since they maintain the humoral immune response at a level appropriate for the stimulus. Suppressor T cells are activated during the generation of all immune responses. They limit the immune response by acting at the level of the helper T cell or B lymphocyte (Fig. 16-6). The modulatory activity of suppressor T cells may be mediated by direct cell-to-cell contact or, alternatively, may involve the release of suppressor factors.

The relative numbers and functional reactivities of helper and suppressor cells determine the strength and persistence of an immune response. When the delicate balance between T helper and T suppressor cell populations is disrupted, autoimmune or immunodeficiency disease may result. Since helper and suppressor T lym-

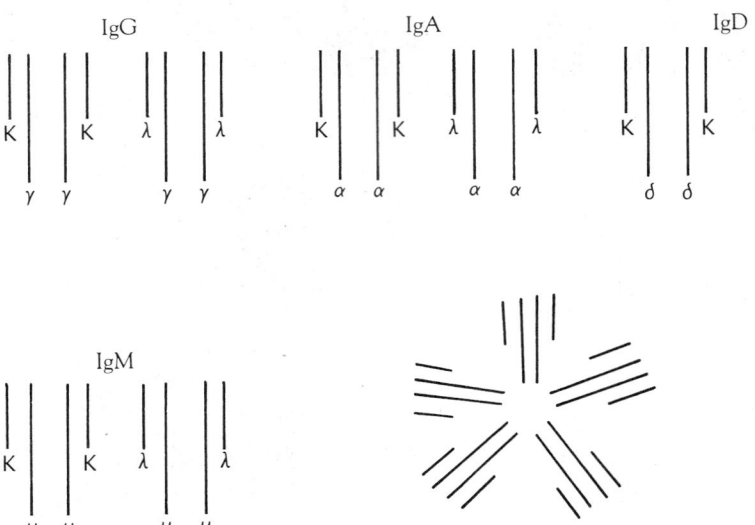

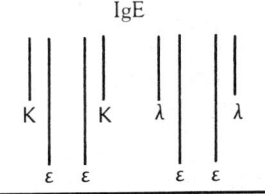

Fig. 16-7

Antibody structure. All immunoglobulins are comprised of four-chain polypeptide unit. Differences among immunoglobulin classes reside in heavy chain structure. IgM, found in serum and external secretions, is pentamer consisting of five identical subunits.

Modified from Unaue, E.R., and Benacerraf, B.: Textbook of immunology, Baltimore, 1984, Williams & Wilkins.

Fig. 16-8

Cell-mediated immune reactions are initiated by macrophage presentation of processed antigen to helper T lymphocytes. Stimulated T helper cells release interleukin 2 *(IL-2)* that activates DTH and cytotoxic T lymphocytes. Targets, such as tumor or virus-infected cells, are lysed directly by cytotoxic T cells. Following infection with intracellular pathogens, activated macrophages are major effector cell population generated. *IL-1*, Interleukin 1.

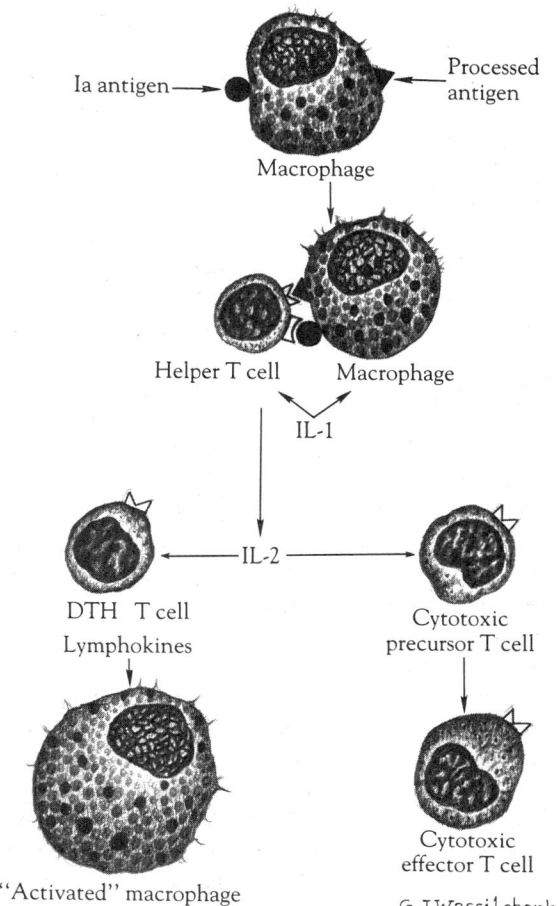

amounts late in the primary immune response, but it is the major antibody generated during a *secondary challenge* with antigen. The generation of IgG protects the host, since this class of immunoglobulin has a number of biologically significant properties. For example, IgG can neutralize toxins produced by various strains of bacteria and induces the agglutination of infectious organisms, facilitating their uptake by phagocytic cells. In addition, IgG has opsonic activity and can activate complement, resulting in the lysis of certain strains of bacteria. IgG is thought to play a crucial role in neonatal host defense, since it is the only immunoglobulin class to be transferred across the placenta.

IgM, comprising approximately 10% of the serum immunoglobulins, is the first antibody to appear during the *primary immune response*. Exposure to antigen via the respiratory or gastrointestinal tract results in the elaboration of IgM into the external secretions. IgM shares many of the biologic properties of IgG: it can neutralize bacterial toxins, can agglutinate certain microorganisms, and is a potent activator of the complement system.

IgA, comprising only a small proportion of the serum antibody pool, is the predominant immunoglobulin in all *serous* and *mucous secretions*. Secretory IgA interferes with bacterial attachment to mucosal surfaces, impedes colonization, and virtually prevents bacterial penetration into the general circulation. In addition, IgA is capable of neutralizing certain bacterial toxins but does not have opsonic or complement-fixing properties. Secretory IgA in maternal milk affords protection to infants before maturation of their secretory immune system.

IgE antibodies, present in the serum in trace amounts, are found attached to mast cells and basophils. These immunoglobulins play a major role in the generation of anaphylactic reactions. When an *allergen*, a substance capable of inducing an allergic reaction, binds to IgE on the surface of basophils or mast cells, mediators such as histamine, serotonin, and leukotrienes are released. These products stimulate bronchial smooth muscle contraction and precipitate systemic vasodilation. Although

IgE is generated in small amounts during conventional humoral immune responses, the physiologic significance of IgE production is not well understood. Evidence suggests that IgE may afford protection against parasitic infections by facilitating eosinophil recognition and destruction of the parasite.

IgD is only a minor component of the serum immunoglobulin pool and is not found in appreciable amounts in external or internal secretions. The biologic function of IgD has not been elucidated.

Cell-mediated immunity. Whereas humoral immune mechanisms afford protection against many gram-positive and certain gram-negative organisms, *cell-mediated immunity is important during host infection with intracellular pathogens such as mycobacteria, fungi, viruses, and protozoa.* Cell-mediated reactions are also elicited as a component of the host response to *tumors* and *tissue transplants*.

Cell-mediated immune responses have been classically characterized as either *delayed-type hypersensitivity* (DTH) or *cytotoxic T lymphocyte* (CTL) reactions (Fig. 16-8). CTL responses play a major role in host defense against tumors, virally infected cells, and allogeneic tissue transplants, whereas DTH reactions are activated by host infection with intracellular pathogens.

Generation of a DTH response involves the participation of macrophages, T helper cells, and DTH-effector T cells. During a primary infection the organisms are ingested by macrophages that process and reexpress antigen on their surface for presentation to helper cells. T helper cells, stimulated by antigen presentation and macrophage release of interleukin 1, induce proliferation of a pool of antigen-specific DTH-precursor T cells. The major portion of these cells remain quiescent until secondary challenge with antigen.

On secondary exposure an anamnestic response develops. Macrophages present processed antigen to antigen-specific T helper cells that rapidly stimulate large numbers of DTH-effector T cells, previously generated by clonal expansion. The activated DTH-effector cells release factors, called lymphokines, that stimulate other cells, particularly macrophages. Most tissue macrophages are incapable of killing intracellular pathogens; however, macrophages activated by exposure to lymphokines are avidly bactericidal.

The duration and magnitude of a DTH response are regulated by T suppressor cells. In general, a secondary DTH reaction can be demonstrated within a few hours of antigen challenge, peaks at 24 to 48 hours, and gradually recedes as the inflammatory focus is eliminated. A person's capacity to generate a secondary DTH response can be measured by intradermal injection with a battery of skin test antigens. If, for example, a person with normal immunity and a history of tuberculosis is tested with purified tuberculoid antigen (PPD), he demonstrates a classic wheal-and-flare reaction. This positive response is evidence of a functionally intact cell-mediated immune system.

CTL reactions are mediated by a subpopulation of T lymphocytes known as *cytotoxic T lymphocytes*. These lymphocytes have surface receptors that recognize genetically different MHC markers on allogeneic tissues and mediate tissue rejection. Similarly, cytotoxic lymphocytes recognize tumor- and virally infected host cells as foreign. On primary exposure to genetically different or altered cells, a population of cytotoxic T precursor cells is expanded with the participation of T helper cells. On secondary exposure an anamnestic response is generated. The cytotoxic T lymphocyte, once activated, attaches to its target and lyses it, employing an unknown mechanism. CTL reactions, like all classic immune responses, can be down-regulated by T suppressor cells.

The recognition and destruction of tumor- and virally infected target cells are not limited to cytotoxic T lymphocytes. Other categories of effector cells include mononuclear phagocytes, killer (K) cells, and natural killer (NK) cells.

Killer cells, often called null cells, are mature lymphoid cells that do not bear the classic markers found on B or T lymphocyte surfaces. They do have receptors that bind antibody-coated target cells. Target cell lysis by K cells requires antibody and is thus described as an antibody-dependent cellular cytotoxic (ADCC) mechanism. Immunization has no effect on the generation of K effector cells but may enhance their reactivity as the result of increased antibody production.

Natural killer cells are large granular lymphocytes that are distinct from CTL and K cells. They bind to and lyse target cells in the absence of antibody. This killing occurs naturally and is not enhanced by immunization. Although NK cells do not have immunologic memory, their functional activities can be modified. Interferons, protein products of stimulated leukocytes, increase NK killing of target cells. In contrast, certain prostaglandins depress NK function.

Cells of the mononuclear phagocyte series can kill target cells directly or by an ADCC mechanism. Peripheral blood *monocytes* and resident tissue *macrophages* exhibit low levels of antitumor activity. Following activation with T lymphocyte–derived products such as γ-interferon, macrophage lysis of tumor- and virally infected target cells increases.

Since immunization is not generally required for the activities of K, NK, and mononuclear phagocytic cells, these populations are thought to play an important host defense role in early stages of infection and tumor growth, before CTL effector cells have been generated. Interferon, shown experimentally to increase both NK cell and macrophage cytotoxic activities, is being used in clinical trials to treat certain malignancies and immunodeficiency disorders.

Complement System

The complement system is comprised of a series of proteins that when activated serve to amplify an immune response. Activation of the complement system leads to the elaboration of potent inflammatory mediators, facilitates particle opsonization and clearance, and may result in the direct lysis of altered mammalian cells and certain bacteria. The complement system may be activated by a number of immunologic and nonimmunologic stimuli. Complement activation proceeds by two mechanisms, the classical and alternative pathways (Fig. 16-9).

The *classical complement pathway* is comprised of 11 distinct proteins. The early-acting components are numbered according to the order of their discovery, and the later-acting components according to their order of reaction. Thus the sequence of action of these components is C1, C4, C2, C3, C5, C6, C7, C8, and C9. C1 is made up of three distinct proteins, C1q, C1r, and C1s.

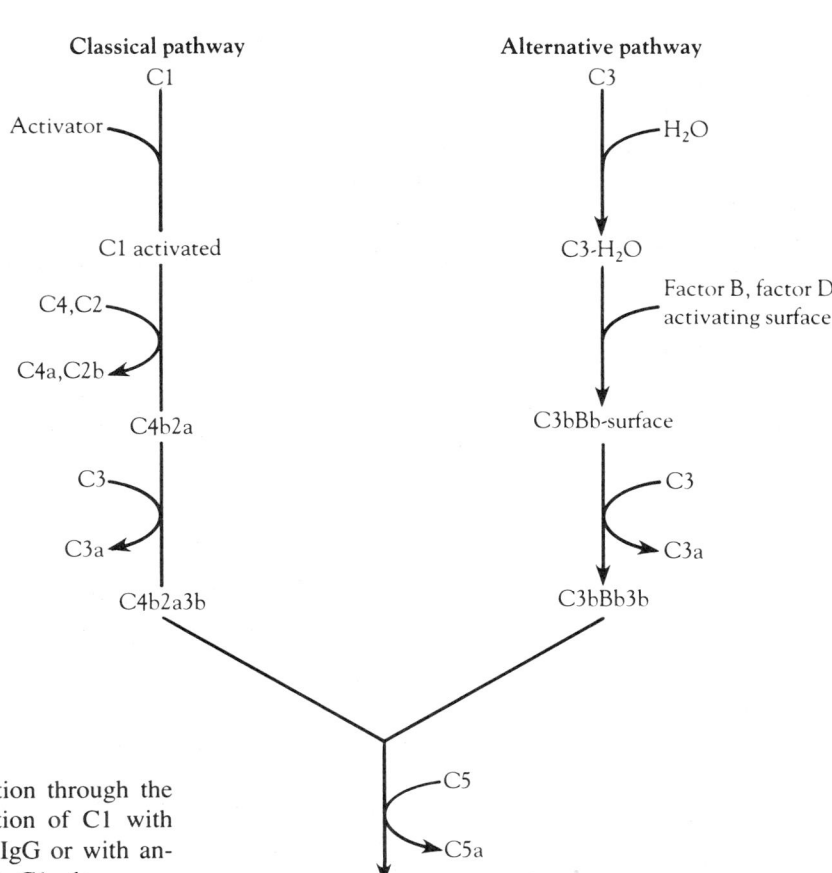

Fig. 16-9

Complement activation. Complement activation can proceed by either classical or alternative pathway. Activation of these pathways results in generation of chemotactic factors (C5a), anaphylatoxins (C3a, C5a), and membrane attack complex (C5b6789).

The first step of complement activation through the classical pathway involves the interaction of C1 with immune complexes containing IgM or IgG or with antibody-coated particles. When activated, C1, the recognition complex of the classical pathway, cleaves C4 and C2. Two protein fragments subsequently combine and form an active enzyme (C4b2a) that cleaves C3 molecules. C3a generated in this way is a potent anaphylatoxin, a substance capable of stimulating basophils and mast cells and thus provoking release of vasoactive amines. A portion of the C3b fragments elaborated during this cleavage is deposited on the activating surface and facilitates particle attachment to phagocytic cells. Certain other C3b molecules combine with C4b2a to form an enzyme (C4b2a3b) that cleaves C5 into two fragments. C5a released into the fluid phase has both anaphylatoxic and chemotactic properties. C5b has an affinity for membranes and, when deposited on a surface, facilitates the binding of C6 and C7. This trimolecular complex (C5b67) provides a binding site for C8, the complement component responsible for initiating target cell lysis. Although some membrane damage occurs following the formation of the C5b-8 complex, lysis is accelerated by the binding of C9. C5b-9, on the surface of a target cell, is called the membrane attack complex.

Before the generation of specific antibody, the complement system can be activated via the *alternative pathway*. Known activators of the alternative pathway include bacterial lipopolysaccharide, virus-infected cells, yeasts, fungi, and certain bacterial cell walls. The constituents of the alternative pathway include all the classical complement components except C1, C4, and C2. Two other proteins, factor B and factor D, contribute to activation of the alternative pathway.

The alternative pathway is activated with the formation of an enzyme that cleaves C3 molecules. This enzyme (C3bBb), distinct from the classical pathway enzyme (C4b2a), is generated following the spontaneous hydrolysis of C3, which in the presence of factor D cleaves factor B. C3bBb generated in this way and bound to an activating surface (such as a bacterium) is capable of cleaving many more C3 molecules, resulting in the generation of C3bBb3b, an enzyme that cleaves C5 into C5a and C5b. The subsequent steps of the alternative pathway are identical to those of the classical pathway and lead to the elaboration of anaphylatoxins, chemotactic factors, and target cell lysis.

Although the complement system protects the host against infectious organisms and may play a role in tumor cell destruction, the uncontrolled activation of this system would result in inflammatory changes and lytic destruction of host tissues. These potentially devastating effects are modulated by a number of control proteins including C1 inhibitor, factors H and I, C4 binding protein, S protein, anaphylatoxin inhibitor, and inhibitors of the membrane attack complex.

NORMAL FINDINGS[4,5,17,32]

Since certain alterations in immune status appear to be genetically determined, a *family history* of recurrent infections, malignancies, allergies, immunodeficiency, and autoimmune diseases should be elicited.

A detailed *patient history* is an essential component of the immune status profile. In addition to documentation of the patient's age, race, sex, and ethnic background, the following information should be obtained:

1. Past history—allergies, childhood and recurrent infections, malignancy, autoimmune disease, primary disorders known to suppress immune function, immunization profile, medications
2. Social, occupational, and nutritional habits
3. Abnormal signs and symptoms—fever, diaphoresis, rashes, joint pain, unusual masses, lymphadenopathy, overt signs of infection, poor wound healing, eczema, hepatosplenomegaly

Since immunologic and inflammatory diseases can involve many organ systems, a complete physical examination is warranted. Particular attention should be paid to signs of infection (abscesses, persistent lesions, and so on), inflammatory tissue changes, wheezing, joint swelling, and skin integrity.

Alterations in vital signs may indicate the presence of an ongoing inflammatory process. (Geriatric patients however, frequently demonstrate a reduced febrile response to infection.)

Area of Concern	Normal Adult Findings	Variations in Child
Liver	Usually located completely under rib cage; may be palpated just below right costal margin with deep inspiration	Easily palpable to 1-2 cm below right costal margin
Spleen	Not generally palpable	Easily palpable in left upper quadrant
Thymus	Can be detected only by radiologic examination; size varies with age (between birth and 20 years, thymic mass increases; after age 20, thymus progressively decreases in size until age 60, when thymic involution is complete)	
Lymph nodes (head and neck, axillary, inguinal, epitrochlear)	Generally not palpable; small, nontender nodes may be found in cervical or inguinal chain of persons with history of local infection	Small, discrete, movable, cool, nontender nodes up to 3 mm in size at all sites normal; cervical and inguinal nodes up to 1 cm in diameter may be observed before 12 years of age

Fig. 16-10

Serum protein electrophoresis. Electrophoresis is clinical laboratory test used to estimate gross levels of certain proteins in serum sample. Specimen is spotted on paper and exposed to electric field, and protein separation is determined using a densitometer. With this technique, normal human serum is separated into five major bands corresponding to albumin, α_1-globulin, α_2-globulin, β-globulin, and γ-globulin. The γ-globulin peak is comprised of the antibody-bearing fraction of serum. Serum protein electrophoresis is used in diagnosis of hypogammaglobulinemic and hypergammaglobulinemic disorders.

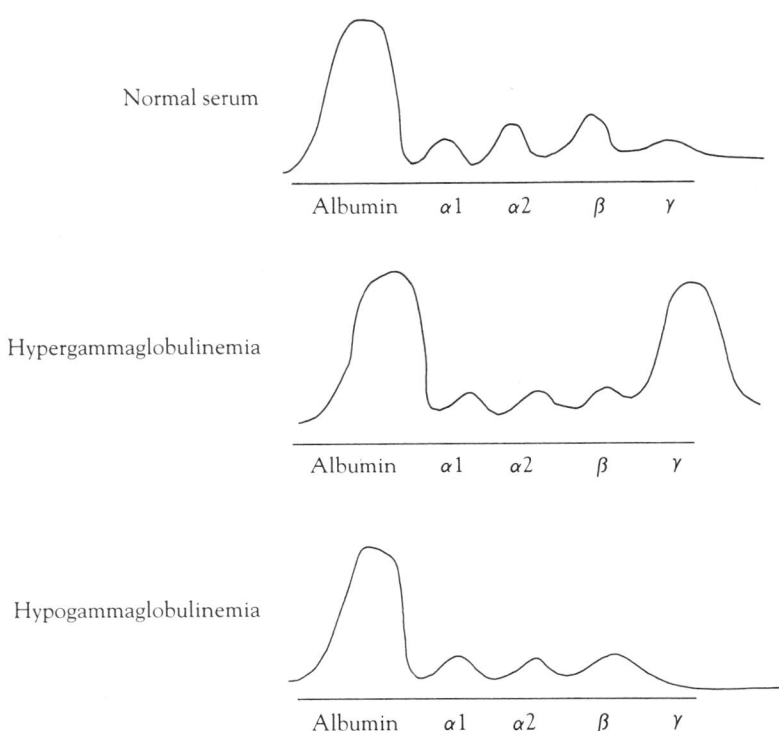

NORMAL LABORATORY DATA[11,19]

Patient history and physical examination will determine which laboratory tests are indicated. For example:

1. If a patient has persistent fungal or viral infections, one may suspect a defect in cell-mediated immunity.
2. A history of gram-positive bacterial infection may indicate a potential humoral immune deficit.
3. Recurrent infections with organisms that do not elicit a strong antibody response, such as *Pseudomonas aeruginosa* or *Staphylococcus aureus,* are frequently observed in persons with phagocytic cell defects.

When interpreting laboratory data, be aware that certain diseases may alter white cell numbers and functional activities. Other processes may be associated with impaired cell function despite normal leukocyte numbers. Alternatively, perturbations in cell numbers may be observed in association with normal cell function.

Laboratory Test*	Normal Adult Values	Variations in Child	
		Newborn	Infant
White blood cell counts			
Total WBC ($\times 10^3$/mm^3)	5-10	9-30	6-17.5
Differential counts (%)			
Segmented (mature) neutrophils	26-60	52	28
Band cells (immature neutrophils)	2-20	9	3
Lymphocytes	35-40	31	61
Monocytes	5-10	5.8	4.8
Eosinophils	0-7	2.2	2-3
Basophils	0-1.5	0.6	0.6
Lymphocyte populations (%)			
Total B cells	5-11		
Total T cells	75-90		
T helper cells (T$_4$ positive)†	40-58		
T suppressor/cytotoxic cells (T$_8$ positive)†	19-30		
Bone marrow differential cell counts (%)			
Erythroblasts	22.5	35.0	20.0
Myeloblasts	1.0	2.5	1.5
Promyelocytes	3.0	3.0	2.5
Myelocytes	15.0	6.0	10.0
Metamyelocytes	15.0	12.5	8.0
Stab cells	15.0	12.5	8.0
Segmented cells	7.0	15.0	7.0
Eosinophils	4.0	1.0	4.0
Basophils	<0.5	0.05	<0.05
Monocytes	2.0	7.5	2.0
Lymphocytes	7.5	—	—
Reticular cells	6.5	5.0	35.0
Plasmacytes	1.0	0.1	<0.5
Megakaryocytes	<0.5	0.1	<0.5
Serum immunoglobulin levels			
IgG (mg/dl)	600-1600	662-1793	296-1004
IgM (mg/dl)	50-250	0-19	21-104
IgA (mg/dl)	80-350	0	10-70
IgE (units/ml)	<125	<10	<100
IgD (mg/dl)	0-30	Not detectable	0
Autoantibody titers‡			
Anti-DNA	Low levels of antibody or none; units and reference range depend on laboratory and method		
Antinuclear antibody (ANA)	Negative at 1:20 dilution		
Rheumatoid factor (RF)	Negative		
Sjögren's antibody	Negative		
Nonspecific indicators of inflammation			
Erythrocyte sedimentation rate (ESR)	<20 mm/hr		
C-reactive protein (CRP)	<6 μg/ml		
C3 complement (serum)	800-1800 μg/ml		
Circulating immune complexes			
C1q binding assay	<25 μg/ml aggregated human γ-globulin (AHGG) equivalents		
Raji cell assay	0-12 μg/ml AHGG equivalents		

*Many of these analyses are not performed in smaller hospitals. Complete diagnostic workups may be obtained from the immunology laboratory of a major medical center.

†In normal persons the T helper/T suppressor cell ratio is approximately 2:1.

‡A profile of tests to identify and discriminate autoimmune diseases is available in many clinical laboratories. In addition to screening for antinuclear antibody and rheumatoid factor, these panels screen for erythrocyte sedimentation rate and C-reactive protein as nonspecific indicators of inflammation, measure functional complement, and quantitate C3 and C4.

DIAGNOSTIC STUDIES

Bone marrow aspiration and biopsy

Needle biopsy of marrow performed after entering marrow cavity of sternum, iliac crest, posterosuperior iliac spine, spinous process, rib, or tibial head; bone marrow cellularity determined

Nursing care:

1. Exert immediate pressure over biopsy site.
2. Apply occlusive dressing.
3. Check biopsy site for bleeding, erythema, or purulent drainage.
4. Maintain bed rest for 1 hour.
5. Administer analgesics as needed.

Lymph node biopsy

Excision of peripheral lymph node performed to assess immunologic function in suspected immunodeficiency diseases and to stage certain malignancies

Nursing care:

1. Provide occlusive dressing.
2. Check surgical site for bleeding, erythema, or purulent drainage.

Lymphangiography

Radiopaque medium introduced into peripheral lymphatics to allow visualization of deep femoral, iliac, and periaortic lymph nodes

Spleen and liver scan

Radiolabeled colloids injected intravenously to allow visualization of liver and spleen; organ size and shape and any potential lesions are identified

Chest roentgenogram

Left anterior oblique view to visualize thymus

HLA typing

Venous blood specimen collected for use in identification of HLA-A, HLA-B, and HLA-C histocompatibility antigens; used for screening patients and potential donors for tissue transplantation

Delayed-type hypersensitivity (anergy) testing (cell-mediated immunity testing)

Measures capacity to generate DTH response; patient is injected intradermally with four common soluble recall antigens (for example, PPD, *Candida, Trichophyton,* and tetanus) and examined for induration and erythema after 48 hours; most young, healthy persons respond positively to at least one antigen; reactivity may decline with age and protein-calorie deficiency states

Nursing care:

1. Check for local erythema and induration at 48 hours.

Allergy skin testing

Antigen introduced by scratching or pricking skin surface or by intradermal injection

Nursing care:

1. Check for erythema at site of antigen introduction after 20 minutes.
2. Observe for potential anaphylactic reactions following antigen introduction.
3. Antihistamines may be administered as comfort measure.

In vitro leukocyte function tests

Used in evaluation of patients with recurrent infections and suspected immunodeficiency diseases; normal values determined in each laboratory

Lymphocyte stimulation

Lymphocytes incubated with particular antigen or mitogen (polyclonal activator), and cell proliferation determined; alterations may be seen in genetic or acquired immunodeficiency states

Cytotoxicity

Lymphocytes incubated with tumor cells or virally infected cells, and target cell lysis measured; in absence of antibody, NK cell function measured; if donor has been sensitized to target cell in vivo, secondary CTL response can be determined; K cell cytotoxicity can be assessed by adding antibody to incubation mixture

Chemotaxis

Phagocytic cells incubated in chamber that permits cells to migrate through filter toward chemoattractant; when samples from patient are incubated with standard chemotactic factors, chemotactic capabilities of phagocytic cells are assessed; alternatively, one can incubate normal phagocytes with patient serum to test ability of that serum to generate chemotactic factors

Phagocytosis

Particle uptake assays to measure phagocytic cell function or opsonizing capacity of patient serum; to assess phagocyte function, patient monocytes or neutrophils incubated with test particle in presence of normal human serum; to examine opsonization, normal phagocytic cells incubated with particles in presence of patient's serum; phagocytosis can be assessed by direct visualization or use of radiolabeled particles

Bactericidal activity

Phagocytic cells incubated with appropriately opsonized bacteria, washed, lysed, and numbers of live intracellular bacteria determined

NBT dye reduction

Phagocytic cells incubated with particles in presence of oxidized nitroblue tetrazolium (NBT); on stimulation of respiratory burst activity, reducing equivalents generated and NBT converted into deep blue insoluble precipitate; NBT dye reduction does not occur in certain patients with genetic phagocytic cell defects

Chemiluminescence

Phagocytes incubated with opsonized particles, and light emission measured in spectrophotometer; during phagocytosis, normal monocytes and neutrophils generate highly unstable oxygen intermediates that emit light during decay to the ground state; chemiluminescence is reduced in patients with certain phagocyte dysfunctions

Conditions, Diseases, and Disorders

IMMUNODEFICIENCY DISEASES
X-Linked Infantile Hypogammaglobulinemia (XLIH) (Panhypogammaglobulinemia, Bruton's Disease, Congenital Agammaglobulinemia)

X-linked infantile hypogammaglobulinemia (XLIH) is a rare congenital disturbance of the humoral immune system that is first noted in 5- to 6-month-old male infants.

The onset and chronic course of XLIH are characterized by marked deficiency or absence of all classes of immunoglobulin, absence of circulating B cells, recurrent pyogenic infections, and a dramatic response to exogenous γ-globulin.

Agammaglobulinemia occurs with a frequency of 1:50,000 live births.[6] Twenty percent of patients have affected male maternal relatives.[27] Recurrent or chronic infection is a classical clinical feature of this disease. The most common types of infection are sinusitis, pneumonia, otitis, meningitis, and septicemia. Patients often have malabsorption, sometimes resulting from giardiasis. In some cases persistent viral or parasitic infections have been reported, although these findings are somewhat controversial.[6,27] With early medical treatment, patients often survive beyond childhood. However, the disease course is frequently complicated by persistent sinopulmonary bacterial infections and chronic lung disease, potentially fatal central nervous system infections with echoviruses, autoimmune disease, and lymphoreticular malignancies. In addition, varying degrees of response to therapy contribute to a questionable prognosis.

PATHOPHYSIOLOGY

In birds the bursa of Fabricius is known as the organ of production and maturation of B lymphocytes. Removal of this organ results in agammaglobulinemia. Researchers have theorized that depletion or congenital absence of bursa-equivalent tissue in humans (gut-associated lymphoid tissue) similarly results in infantile hypogammaglobulinemia. At present the defect associated with XLIH is presumed to be at the level of pre–B cell and B cell differentiation. Consequently, severe depression or absence of plasma cells and peripheral B lymphocytes is a hallmark feature of this disorder. Cell-mediated immunity remains intact.

The bacterial infections associated with XLIH reflect the absence of humoral immunity. For example, the severe depletion or absence of IgA, an important defense at mucosal surfaces, is manifested by recurrent sinopulmonary and gastrointestinal infections.

DIAGNOSTIC STUDIES

Serum protein electrophoresis
Decreased or absent γ-globulin

Total Ig quantitation
Less than 100 mg/dl

Selective Ig quantitation
IgG, IgM, IgA, IgD, and IgE each less than 200 mg/dl or absent

B cell quantitation
Less than 10% to 15%

Peripheral blood lymphocytes
Absence of circulating B cells; normal to increased T cell levels

Anergy profile

Positive response to cutaneous recall antigens; distinguishes XLIH from T cell disease

Lymphoid tissue biopsy

Hypoplasia of adenoids, tonsils, and peripheral lymph nodes; rare or absent plasma cells and immunoglobulin; lymph nodes depleted in B cell–dependent areas

Bone marrow biopsy

Pre–B cells present

Chest roentgenogram

Chronic lung disease

Sinus roentgenogram

Chronic sinusitis

Pulmonary function tests

Abnormal findings

Malabsorption studies

Blunting of gastrointestinal villi on biopsy; abnormal findings on D-xylose absorption test; lack of normal intestinal enzymes

Stool for ova parasites

To rule out giardiasis

Antinuclear antibody, biopsies, and so on

Optional studies to detect presence of autoimmune disease and lymphoreticular malignancies

During evaluation for the presence of XLIH, the following diseases should be considered as differential diagnoses: juvenile-onset arthritis, cystic fibrosis, asthma, alpha-1 antitrypsin deficiency, and, most important, transient hypogammaglobulinemia.

TREATMENT PLAN

Chemotherapeutic

Serum agents

Intramuscular γ-globulin[*][2] (contains primarily IgG); loading dose 200 mg/kg IM; maintenance dose 100 mg/kg IM q4wk; dose titrated to control symptoms rather than Ig levels, since metabolism varies between patients; at higher increments, total dose may be administered weekly in divided amounts; patient should be monitored for anaphylactoid reaction

Intravenous γ-globulin[*] (contains primarily IgG); newly developed therapy; treatment of choice over IM IgG; 100-200 mg/kg body weight/mo produces increase of 200 mg/dl in serum IgG; patient should be monitored for anaphylactoid reactions; other side effects are chills, neuralgias, and flushing, which are often related to rate at which dose is administered; enables large amounts of immunoglobulin to be administered to adults; achieves nearly normal blood levels that are unattainable with IM preparations

Anti-infective agents

Continual administration of low-dose broad-spectrum antibiotics such as Bactrim may prove useful as prophylaxis against recurrent infections

Supportive

For malabsorption, treatment with γ-globulin and dietary regulation to control diarrhea and prevent malnutrition

Chest physical therapy, breathing exercises, postural drainage, and oxygen therapy as prophylaxis or treatment for chronic pulmonary disease

Serial sinus and chest roentgenograms and pulmonary function tests to follow disease course and determine adequacy of treatment

Follow-up for, and treatment of, concomitant autoimmune or neoplastic disease as needed

Only irradiated, cytomegalovirus-negative blood products should be administered

ASSESSMENT: AREAS OF CONCERN

Recurrent infection[*]

Otitis; conjunctivitis; osteomyelitis; pneumonia; meningitis; pharyngitis; septicemia; sinusitis; furunculosis; hepatitis; enterovirus infections

Skin integrity

Eczema

Joint integrity

Polyarthritis

Gastrointestinal status

Malabsorption, often caused by recurrent giardiasis

---

[*]The most common organisms are pneumococci, streptococci, and *Haemophilus*. Infections with meningococci, staphylococci, and *Pseudomonas* occur less frequently. Infections are unremitting, with no recovery between episodes, and response to treatment is slow and incomplete.

---

[*]Treatment schedules may vary; optimal dosage and frequency are unknown.[27] No data are available on the dosage or serum levels to be maintained to prevent later infection recurrences.

NURSING DIAGNOSES and NURSING INTERVENTIONS

Nursing Diagnosis	Nursing Intervention
Gas exchange, impaired (related to recurrent sinopulmonary infections)	Assess respiratory status: monitor rate, rhythm, and quality of respirations, presence of cyanosis, adventitious breath sounds, and restlessness. Monitor results of sputum cultures and pulmonary function studies (arterial blood gases and so on), and chest roentgenograms. In collaboration with physician, administer appropriate antibiotics, oxygen therapy, bronchodilators, and chest physiotherapy. Assess effectiveness and note side effects.
Skin integrity, impairment of (related to eczema)	In collaboration with physician, administer appropriate topical or systemic medications as ordered and assess patient's response (see Chapter 5). Monitor skin lesions for evidence of infection. Assess changes in skin integrity in response to treatment of the underlying humoral deficiency.
Comfort, alteration in: pain (related to polyarthritis and infection)	In collaboration with physician, administer appropriate analgesic or anti-inflammatory medication as ordered; assess patient's response and note side effects. Provide joint support for affected areas throughout the night. Provide thermal therapy to affected joints as needed. Assess patient's response to treatment of underlying cause of pain.
Bowel elimination, alteration in: diarrhea (related to giardiasis and other intestinal infections)	Monitor intake and output to assess for volume depletion. Monitor for electrolyte imbalances. Maintain adequate hydration and oral intake as tolerated. Determine need for tube feeding and parenteral alimentation. In collaboration with physician, administer appropriate antimicrobial therapy. Assess effectiveness and note side effects.
Nutrition, alteration in: less than body requirements (related to malabsorption)	Assess degree of nutritional deficit. Provide high-protein, high-calorie diet as tolerated. Provide small, frequent feedings as tolerated. Encourage family members to provide patient's favorite foods. Provide vitamin supplements. Determine need for parenteral nutrition if oral intake is deficient.
Coping, family: potential for growth	Assess family's anxiety related to limited understanding of diagnostic procedures, disease process and prognosis, and therapies employed. Explain relationship of disease process and rationale for various therapeutic interventions at level appropriate for comprehension and degree of anxiety. Involve family in care as appropriate. Encourage family to verbalize questions, fears, and anxieties.
Potential patient problem: susceptibility to infection	Assess for anorexia, failure to thrive, pain, weakness, and lethargy. Assess for evidence of infection at sites of invasive procedures. Assess for breaks in skin integrity, particularly over pressure areas and oral mucosa. Assess pulmonary status: auscultate lung fields to determine presence of adventitious breath sounds. Maintain optimal nutritional status and fluid intake. Assess ocular integrity for evidence of conjunctivitis: erythematous, pruritic conjunctiva. Assess mentation for evidence of central nervous system infection: decreased level of consciousness, headache, and visual disturbances. Assess for evidence of gastrointestinal infection: abdominal pain, fever, and diarrhea. Monitor temperature and vital signs for evidence of fever and sepsis. Maintain body hygiene. Limit environmental stress. Monitor laboratory data: white blood cell count and differential, erythrocyte sedimentation rate, C-reactive protein, urinalysis, and cultures. In collaboration with physician, administer appropriate antimicrobial, antipyretic, or analgesic medication. Assess patient's response and monitor for side effects.

Nursing Diagnosis	Nursing Intervention
	Promote pulmonary toilet: breathing exercises, postural drainage, and chest physical therapy.
	Maintain normal sleep and rest patterns.
	Protect patient from physical injury.
	Provide clean environment.
	Maintain protective isolation based on hospital policy.
	Restrict contact with family and health care providers who have infectious diseases.
	Maintain good handwashing before and after contact with patient.

Patient Education

1. Teach parents signs and symptoms of infection.
2. Teach techniques to prevent recurrent pulmonary infection: prophylactic antibiotics, breathing exercises, postural drainage, and chest physiotherapy.
3. Discuss with the parents the patient's increased risk for the development of vaccine-associated poliomyelitis. This vaccine should be administered only after consultation with the primary physician.
4. Teach the importance of compliance with regular follow-up examinations for γ-globulin level and clinical evaluation.

5. Teach the parents about the avoidance of risk factors associated with infection.
6. Teach principles of good nutrition.
7. Teach facts about and the importance of prescribed medications.
8. Refer the parents for genetic counseling to explain the inheritance pattern.
9. Stress the importance of wearing medical alert identification.

EVALUATION

Patient Outcome	Data Indicating That Outcome is Reached
Infection is decreased or gone following chemotherapy.	There are no signs or symptoms associated with recurrent pyogenic infections.
Laboratory data return to normal limits.	IgG, IgE, IgD, white blood cell count, erythrocyte sedimentation rate, and C-reactive protein level are within normal limits. (IgA and IgM may not return to normal limits.) Cultures findings are negative. Urinalysis findings are within normal limits.
Unnecessary complications are avoided.	No live vaccines are administered.

COMMON VARIABLE IMMUNODEFICIENCY (ACQUIRED HYPOGAMMAGLOBULINEMIA, AGAMMAGLOBULINEMIA WITH IMMUNOGLOBULIN-BEARING B LYMPHOCYTES)

Common variable immunodeficiency (CVID) is an immune disorder of unknown cause that predominantly affects the B cell system. The clinical features and treatment of this disease are very similar to those of X-linked hypogammaglobulinemia.

The immunologic feature of acquired hypogammaglobulinemia that is shared with the X-linked form is the marked depression or absence of all five classes of immunoglobulin. Consequently, recurrent bacterial infections are also observed in this disorder, although these infections tend to be less severe that with the X-linked form. Other common features include malabsorption syndromes (usually resulting from *Giardia lamblia* infestation) and an increased incidence of autoimmune and lymphoreticular malignancies. A predilection for autoimmune and neoplastic disease in first-degree relatives of these patients suggests a hereditary influence.

CVID is distinguished from X-linked hypogamma-globulinemia by the presence of B lymphocytes. Also in contrast, patients with CVID may manifest hyperplasia of lymphoid tissue, including the tonsils, nodes, and spleen. In addition, acquired hypogammaglobulinemia occurs at any age and in both sexes equally, whereas X-linked hypogammaglobulinemia occurs only in male infants and is rarer than CVID.

PATHOPHYSIOLOGY

The pathogenesis of acquired hypogammaglobulinemia is unknown. The presence of normal numbers of B cells together with markedly depressed amounts of immuno-globulin suggests that decreased synthesis or release of antibody is the problem. Researchers have suggested that faulty differentiation of the B lymphocyte to the plasma cell may be the primary defect. It is also speculated that this defect occurs as the result of increased T suppressor cell activity or failure of T cell cooperation.[27]

DIAGNOSTIC STUDIES

B cell quantitation and function
B cells low, normal, or increased; cells clonally diverse and relatively immature; fail to respond to most antigens and mitogens by differentiating into plasma cells; in some patients B cells synthesize but do not secrete immunoglobulin[27]

Immunoglobulin quantitation
Total greater than 300 mg/dl

T cell studies
Levels may be normal or reflect increased numbers of T suppressor cells with decreased numbers of helper cells; B cells are unable to function without T helper cell feedback; generally, T cell function deteriorates with time[27]

Lymphoid tissue biopsy
Absence of plasma cells in B cell–dependent areas; hyperplasia of lymphoid tissue

Chest roentgenogram
Chronic lung disease

Sinus roentgenogram
Chronic sinusitis

Pulmonary function tests
Findings abnormal

Malabsorption studies
Blunting of villi on biopsy; abnormal findings on D-xylose absorption test; lack of normal intestinal enzymes

Stool examination for ova and parasites
Giardia lamblia detected most frequently

Antinuclear antibody and other optional studies
To detect presence of autoimmune disease or lymphoreticular malignancies; antinuclear antibody present in autoimmune disease

ASSESSMENT: AREAS OF CONCERN

Recurrent infection
Sinusitis; pharyngitis; pneumonia; osteomyelitis; conjunctivitis; abscesses; otitis

Gastrointestinal tract
Chronic diarrhea; malabsorption

Lymphatic system
Lymphadenopathy; splenomegaly

Presence of concomitant autoimmune disease
Signs and symptoms associated with systemic lupus erythematosus, dermatomyositis, and hemolytic anemia

Presence of concomitant neoplastic disease
Signs and symptoms associated with leukemia, lymphoma, and gastric carcinoma

• • •

The treatment plan, nursing diagnoses, nursing interventions, and evaluation are the same as for X-linked hypogammaglobulinemia.

SELECTIVE IgA DEFICIENCY

Selective IgA deficiency is the presence of serum IgA in quantities less than 10 mg/dl while other immunoglobulins are present in normal amounts.

Selective IgA deficiency is the most common immunodeficiency disease. In the United States the incidence is approximately 1 in 700. Although the disease is most commonly detected during the first decade of life, patients often survive until the sixth or seventh decade. It cannot be diagnosed before 1 year of age because infants may not produce IgA until then.

As discussed previously, IgA is the predominant immunoglobulin of external secretions. Therefore bacterial infections of the respiratory, gastrointestinal, and urogenital tracts are the major clinical manifestations associated with this disorder.

Many affected persons are asymptomatic. Autoimmune disease develops in 25%. Recently IgG subclass deficiencies were reported in association with IgA deficiency.[27]

Morbidity is associated with recurrent sinopulmonary infections, autoimmune disease, and, rarely, neoplastic disease. Spruelike disease may also complicate the disease course.

PATHOPHYSIOLOGY

The immunopathogenesis of this disorder is unclear. The presence of normal numbers of IgA B cells suggests that the underlying defect involves decreased synthesis or release of IgA. However, lymphocyte culture studies have demonstrated that IgA B cells synthesize but do not secrete immunoglobulin. Therefore the underlying defect probably occurs in the transformation of the IgA B lymphocyte to the plasma cell. T suppressor mechanisms may influence this process.[2] The presence of antibodies to IgA in up to 44% of cases of IgA deficiency implies that an autoimmune process is involved as well.[6] See p. 1635 for a description of the role of IgA.

A genetic predisposition has also been postulated. Autosomal recessive and autosomal dominant modes of inheritance have been implicated. IgA deficiency appears with greater than normal frequency in families with a variety of immunodeficiency diseases. In addition, the presence of HLA-A1, HLA-B8, and HLA-DW3 is associated with IgA deficiency and autoimmune disease.[2]

Whatever the cause, the lack of secretory IgA antibody promotes the attachment of infectious microbes at the mucosal surfaces and explains the occurrence of gastrointestinal, urogenital, and sinopulmonary infections. In addition, IgA probably acts to prevent absorption of other foreign proteins such as those in the diet. Its absence

may explain the spruelike syndrome associated with selective IgA deficiency.

The deficiency of IgA may not be primary. Instead it may follow the administration of certain drugs such as phenytoin. In this case the decreased serum levels may result from induction of T suppressor cells that interfere with B cell maturation.[27]

DIAGNOSTIC STUDIES

Ig quantitation
IgA level less than 10 mg/dl; IgG, IgM, IgD, and IgE normal or increased

Immunization
Normal antibody response

B cell quantitation
Normal numbers of B cells, including IgA-bearing lymphocytes

T cell studies
Normal findings

Chest roentgenograms
Pneumonia

Sinus roentgenograms
Sinusitis

Pulmonary function tests
Findings abnormal

Gastrointestinal studies
Findings abnormal in celiac disease; abnormal D-xylose absorption in malabsorption

Antinuclear antibody
Positive findings in presence of autoimmune disease

Differential diagnoses that must be excluded include chronic mucocutaneous candidiasis, Nezelof syndrome, and drug-induced IgA deficiency.

TREATMENT PLAN

Since no replacement therapy is yet available, treatment is aimed at management of recurrent infections and serial assessment for the presence of autoimmune and neoplastic disease.

Chemotherapeutic
γ-Globulin for selected patients who also demonstrate IgG subclass deficiency
Antibiotic therapy according to system involved and culture results

Supportive

Gluten-free diet for celiac disease

Chest physical therapy, breathing exercises, postural drainage, and oxygen therapy as prophylaxis or for treatment of chronic pulmonary disease

Serial sinus and chest roentgenograms and pulmonary function tests to follow the disease course and determine adequacy of treatment

Follow-up for, and treatment of, concomitant autoimmune or neoplastic disease as needed

Administration of IgA-deficient blood products to prevent future antigen-antibody reaction

ASSESSMENT: AREAS OF CONCERN

Recurrent infection

Sinusitis; pneumonia; urogenital infections; gastrointestinal infections

Gastrointestinal status

Celiac disease

Presence of concomitant autoimmune disease

Signs and symptoms associated with systemic lupus erythematosus, rheumatoid arthritis, dermatomyositis, hemolytic anemia, Sjögren's syndrome[2]

Presence of concomitant neoplastic disease

Signs and symptoms associated with squamous cell carcinoma of the esophagus and lung[2] or thymoma

NURSING DIAGNOSES and NURSING INTERVENTIONS

The majority of IgA-deficient patients are asymptomatic; the rest may have infections. See Chapter 15 for nursing care related to specific infections.

Patient Education

1. Teach techniques to prevent recurrent pulmonary infection: breathing exercises and postural drainage.
2. Teach methods to prevent recurrent urogenital infection: adequate hydration, intake of fluids (such as cranberry juice) to maintain urine acidity, frequent voiding (every 2 to 3 hours), meticulous perineal care, voiding before and after intercourse, antibiotic prophylaxis, use of condom, and limited exposure to multiple or anonymous sex partners.
3. Teach the patient a gluten-free diet (if celiac disease is present).
4. Teach methods of self-assessment for infection: signs and symptoms associated with sinopulmonary, urogenital, and intestinal infections. Teach the patient to report significant symptoms.
5. Teach the patient the importance of medical alert identification that specifies the need for IgA-deficient blood products.

EVALUATION

Patient Outcome	Data Indicating That Outcome is Reached
Number of recurrent sinopulmonary, intestinal, and urogenital infections is decreased.	Serial follow-up indicates decreased incidence of infections.
Complications of recurrent infections are avoided.	Evidence of chronic, progressive lung, kidney, and intestinal disease is limited or absent.
Complications associated with IgA deficiency (autoimmune disease, malignancies) are detected early or are absent.	Serial monitoring for autoimmune phenomena and malignancies reveals early disease, or results of studies are negative.

CONGENITAL THYMIC APLASIA (DiGEORGE SYNDROME)

The DiGeorge syndrome is a cellular immunodeficiency disorder resulting from aberrant fetal development of the thymus and parathyroid glands.

Congenital thymic aplasia is manifested immediatedly after birth in both sexes. It is characterized by the classic findings of hypoparathyroidism, abnormal facies, congenital heart disease, and minimal or absent T cell function. The thymus gland is commonly absent; however, some neonates possess a gland, although it may be small or in an abnormal location. In these cases spontaneous remission may occur following late thymic hypertrophy. In general, the DiGeorge syndrome should be suspected in infants with severe congenital heart disease and hypocalcemia. Total reconstitution of cellular immunity can be achieved in some cases when the diagnosis is made early and a fetal thymus graft is performed, although patients may die of heart disease.

PATHOPHYSIOLOGY

The cause of interference with normal fetal development of the thymus gland is unknown. The defect probably occurs during the eighth week of gestation when the thymus and parathyroid glands normally develop from a common source of fetal tissue. Facial and cardiac structures are differentiated at this time as well and are probably also affected by the defect, as illustrated by the facial and cardiac abnormalities associated with this disease.

DIAGNOSTIC STUDIES

Chest roentgenograms
  Lateral view of anterior mediastinum shows absence of thymic shadow

Parathyroid studies
  Low serum calcium level; elevated serum phosphorus level; absence of parathyroid hormone

Cardiac studies
  Right-sided aortic arch; persistent truncus arteriosus; tetralogy of Fallot; aberrant subclavian artery

Evaluation of cellular immunity
  Total lymphocyte count decreased; absence of response (anergy) to delayed hypersensitivity skin test (with killed viruses); T cells less than 65% of total lymphocytes; T cell response to mitogens, antigens, and allogeneic lymphocytes decreased

Evaluation of humoral immunity
  B cell numbers normal; B cell function variable

TREATMENT PLAN

Surgical
  Fetal thymus transplant—effective but available only in a few centers; should be performed as soon as possible after diagnosis; provides needed humoral factors and stem cells or thymic epithelial cells for further T cell development; gland tissue should be less than 14 weeks' gestation to prevent graft-versus-host disease; tissue is from abortuses obtained via hysterotomy or prostaglandin-induced abortions; tissue is implanted in the rectus abdominis muscle, or minced tissue is injected intraperitoneally; thymus transplant has largely been replaced by administration of thymosin and other thymic hormones
  Surgical correction of congenital heart defects—irradiated transfusions should be used for blood replacement to prevent graft-versus-host reaction in patients who have not yet received thymus transplantation

Chemotherapeutic
  Hormonal agents
    Thymosin and other thymic hormones have improved immunity in some patients
  Vitamins and minerals
    Calcium po in conjunction with vitamin D or parathyroid hormone for hypocalcemia
    Calcium gluconate IV for hypocalcemia
  No live attenuated vaccines should be administered
  Only irradiated cytomegalovirus-negative blood products should be administered

Supportive
  Low-phosphorus diet if needed for hypocalcemia
  Diagnosis, treatment, and follow-up of congenital abnormalities as needed

ASSESSMENT: AREAS OF CONCERN

Recurrent infection
  Variable, multiple viral, mycobacterial, fungal, and protozoal, or gram-negative infections; diarrhea; thrush; failure to thrive

Parathyroid function
  Hpyocalcemia resistant to conventional therapy, occurring within first 24 hours of life; associated findings including tetany, seizures, congestive heart failure, and hyperphosphatemia

Congenital defects
  Tetralogy of Fallot; right-sided aortic arch; persistent truncus arteriosus; septal defects; aberrant subclavian artery; patent ductus arteriosus

Abnormal facies
  Low-set ears; "fish-shaped" mouth; hypertelorism; notched ear pinnae; micrognathia; antimongoloid slant of eyes

Graft-versus-host reaction (in response to blood transfusions and marrow or thymus transplant)
  Rashes; thrombocytopenia; diarrhea; jaundice; hepatosplenomegaly; alopecia; fingernail ridging; pulmonary infiltrates; secondary infection

NURSING DIAGNOSES and NURSING INTERVENTIONS

Nursing Diagnosis	Nursing Intervention
Cardiac output, alteration in: decreased (potential; related to certain congenital heart defects or hypocalcemia)	Assess for signs and symptoms associated with congestive heart failure: pallor, easy fatigability, difficulty feeding, tachypnea, cyanosis, rales, frothy sputum, cough, hepatomegaly, edema, and diaphoresis. In collaboration with physician, institute appropriate interventions for management of heart failure: digitalization, oxygen, bed rest, fluid restriction, diuretics, and low-sodium diet. Assess effectiveness. Monitor for development of heart murmur(s), mottling of skin, growth retardation, and other symptoms consistent with congenital heart defect. Monitor electrocardiogram, chest roentgenogram, and blood gas results.
Comfort, alteration in: pain (related to anxiety, invasive procedures, sleep deprivation, immobility, sensory overstimulation, infection, or fever)	Assess degree of discomfort and determine cause. Institute appropriate interventions based on assessment (for example, range of motion exercises, analgesics, antipyretics, skin care, and massage). Assess effectiveness. Comfort child during procedures. Encourage family members to visit as often as feasible. Provide child with familiar articles and toys from home. Plan care to allow for periods of rest and sleep. Allow time for holding, cuddling, feeding, and rocking that are unrelated to other treatments or procedures.
Coping, ineffective family (related to prolonged hospitalization and questionable prognosis)	Assess family's anxiety related to limited understanding of diagnostic procedures, disease process and prognosis, and therapies employed. Provide information in areas needed. Explain relationship of disease process and rationale for various therapeutic interventions at level appropriate for comprehension and degree of anxiety. Involve family in care as appropriate. Encourage family to verbalize questions and fears. Encourage parents to leave hospital to attend to family matters. Allow parents to call hospital at any time when they cannot be there.
Patient problem: susceptibility to infection	Assess for anorexia, failure to thrive, pain, weakness, and lethargy. Assess for evidence of infection at sites of invasive procedures. Assess for breaks in skin integrity, particularly over pressure areas and oral mucosa. Assess pulmonary status: auscultate lung fields to determine presence of adventitious breath sounds. Maintain optimal nutritional status and fluid intake. Assess ocular integrity for evidence of conjunctivitis: erythematous, pruritic conjunctiva. Assess mentation for evidence of central nervous system infection: decreased level of consciousness, headache, and visual disturbances. Assess for evidence of gastrointestinal infection: abdominal pain with fever and diarrhea. Monitor temperature and vital signs for evidence of fever and sepsis. Maintain body hygiene. Limit environmental stress. Monitor laboratory data: white blood cell count and differential, erythrocyte sedimentation rate, C-reactive protein, urinalysis, and cultures. In collaboration with physician, administer appropriate anti-infective, antipyretic, or analgesic medication as ordered. Assess patient response and monitor for side effects. Promote pulmonary toilet: breathing exercises, postural drainage, and chest physical therapy. Maintain normal sleep and rest patterns. Protect patient from physical injury. Provide clean environment. Maintain protective isolation based on hospital policy. Restrict contact with family and health care providers who have infectious diseases. Maintain good handwashing before and after patient contact.

Nursing Diagnosis	Nursing Intervention
Potential patient problem: hypocalcemia (related to congenital parathyroid dysfunction)	Monitor for tetany, seizure activity, congestive heart failure, and hyperphosphatemia. In collaboration with physician, administer calcium, vitamin D, and parathyroid hormone orally or calcium gluconate intravenously. Assess effectiveness and monitor for side effects.
Potential patient problem: graft-versus-host reaction (related to blood transfusion or marrow or thymus transplant)	Monitor for rashes, thrombocytopenia, diarrhea, jaundice, hepatosplenomegaly, alopecia, fingernail ridging, and pulmonary infiltrates. See p. 1722.

Patient Education

1. Teach techniques that would enable family members to participate in the child's care as much as possible.
2. Inform the parents that counseling is available to assist them in coping with the child's illness.
3. Encourage the parents to seek genetic counseling to explain inheritance patterns.
4. Teach facts about and importance of medications and other therapies and diagnostic procedures.
5. Teach methods to limit the child's risk for infection: handwashing, skin and oral hygiene, environmental control, and nutrition.
6. Teach the parents about surgical interventions used to correct congenital heart defects.

EVALUATION

Patient Outcome	Data Indicating That Outcome is Reached
Hypocalcemia is corrected.	Calcium level is within normal limits.
Congenital heart defect is corrected.	Patient has no signs or symptoms of heart failure.
Cell-mediated immunity is restored.	T cell numbers increase. Findings of delayed hypersensitivity skin test are positive (anergy is reversed).

DISORDERS OF COMPLEMENT

Primary deficiency or dysfunction of complement components in the classical pathway increases host susceptibility to infection. In acquired complement disorders, particularly immune complex disease, activation of complement and subsequent inflammatory mediator involvement may cause increased tissue damage.

The classical and alternative complement systems (Fig. 16-9) play an integral role in the amplification of nonspecific host defense mechanisms to invading organisms and in clearance of circulating immune complexes from the serum.

Complement proteins are present in the serum in inactive form, and activation leads to biologic activity. Activation occurs in a cascade fashion and is regulated by four complement proteins.

Certain complement components, when activated, generate chemotactic factors, enhancing the accumulation of leukocytes at an inflammatory site. Other components are deposited on the surface of bacteria, enhancing their ingestion by phagocytic cells (opsonization). The terminal components (C5 to C9) have the capacity to mediate direct lysis of certain bacteria. Complement attaches to circulating immune complexes, decreasing their solubility and thus increasing their removal from the serum.

Primary complement disorders account for less than 1% of primary immunodeficiencies. Deficiency or dysfunction has been identified for each of the classical complement components; none have been identified in the alternative pathway. Certain of these disorders, especially those late in the cascade, have a benign clinical course, but up to 5% of these patients have severe *Neisseria* infections.

In contrast, defects involving key complement components that regulate the complement cascade or components early in the cascade may be associated with severe, recurrent infections or autoimmune diseases.

Secondary complement deficiencies arise when a disease process causes decreased synthesis or triggers increased consumption. With increased activation, as occurs in immune complex disease, tissue damage often occurs because of the inflammatory mechanisms modulated by complement.

PATHOPHYSIOLOGY

A brief schema of the sequence of activation is shown in Fig. 16-11.

With deficiency or dysfunction in one of the classical complement components, activation of the normal cascade can occur only up to the deficient component. Activation of the remainder of the pathway theoretically should not occur. However, because the classical and alternative pathways share the same terminal components, activation through a different regulatory point in the cascade can compensate for the deficiency.

Deficiencies in the C1, C4, and C2 proteins are the most commonly reported. C2 deficiency occurs in 1 in 10,000 persons. Persons with these deficiencies may be in good health and usually do not have difficulties with recurrent infections. When infections do develop, bacterial rather than viral organisms are involved. In addition, up to 50% of persons with C2 deficiency have autoimmune disease, particularly systemic lupus erythematosus and juvenile rheumatoid arthritis.

Clinically, C3 is one of the most important complement components because of its place in the complement cascade, and C3 deficiency is the most severe disorder identified. Patients with this abnormality have recurrent, fulminant, pyogenic bacterial infections. C3 deficiency may result from a genetic defect in production. Some persons, including those with nephritic factor, have serum factors that continuously activate and thus deplete C3. Other persons lack C3bI, a regulatory protein that prevents continuous consumption of C3 once the alternative pathway is activated.

Terminal complement component deficiencies (C5 through C9) have also been identified. Many affected persons are asymptomatic. Others may manifest an increased incidence of infection with *Neisseria gonorrhoeae* and *N. meningitidis*. Although persons with C9 deficiency have been identified, this abnormality has not been associated with clinical disease. These persons show normal resistance to infection with bacterial, viral, and fungal organisms.

In C5 dysfunction, all levels of complement components including C5 are normal, but serum chemotactic and opsonic activities are reduced because of a defect in C5 activity. Clinical features of C5 dysfunction resemble those of C5 deficiency. Susceptibility to recurrent infections, particularly of the skin and gastrointestinal tract, is increased.

C1 inhibitor deficiency is also known as hereditary angioedema. C1 inhibitor is a regulatory protein that controls activation of C1. Continuous activation of C1 with resultant depletion of C2 and C4 may be due to a failure of this control protein to "turn off" primary pathway activation once initiated. Possibly deficiency of C1 inhibitor, which also inhibits kinin activation, allows kinin formation with subsequent vascular permeability and tissue edema, leading to angioedema.

Association of primary complement disorders with various autoimmune diseases is common (Table 16-2), although the cause is unknown.

Secondary disorders of complement have multiple pathophysiologic mechanisms. The degree of complement disorder will vary with the severity of the underlying disease process. In extreme protein deficiency states, decreased synthesis results in overall depression of the total complement component quantities resulting in inadequate host defense.

Various disease states may result in increased complement consumption. In fulminant bacterial infections, complement is consumed and production cannot meet demand.

Complement activation is an integral component of the pathophysiology of diseases associated with circulating immune complexes. With involvement of complement, and resultant inflammatory response, tissue damage occurs. Degree of complement activation correlates with activity of disease and is often monitored as an indicator of disease activity or response to therapy.

Fig. 16-11
Sequence of complement activation.

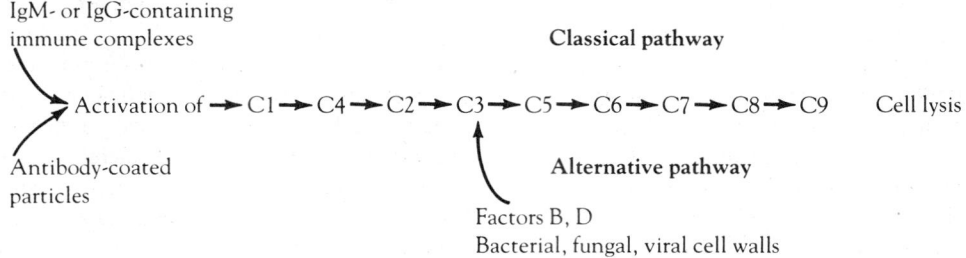

Table 16-2
Complement Component Deficiencies and Associated Diseases

Component	Collagen-Vascular Diseases*	Infections†	Other
C1q	+	+	Glomerulonephritis; immunodeficiencies
C1r	+	−	Glomerulonephritis
C1s	+	−	
C4	+	−	
C2	+	+	Glomerulonephritis
C3	+	+	Nephritis
C5	+	+	
C6	+	+	
C7	+	+	
C8	+	+	
C9	−	+	
I‡	−	+	
H‡	−	−	Hemolytic uremic syndrome
Properdin‡	−	−	
C1INH‡	+	+	Hereditary angioedema

*A variety of autoimmune diseases have been described.
†A variety of infective organisms have been identified.
‡Control proteins.

The following are some of the factors associated with secondary disorders of complement:

Decreased synthesis
  Asplenia
  Sickle cell disease
  Protein-deficient states
    Cirrhosis
    Malnutrition
    Severe burns
    Anorexia nervosa
  Newborns (up to 6 months)
Increased consumption
  Acute nephritis
  Partial lipodystrophy
  Immune complex diseases, especially systemic lupus erythematosus
  Bacteremia, endotoxins
  Dialysis (renal, plasmapheresis, heart-lung)

DIAGNOSTIC STUDIES

History
  Recurrent bacterial infections, especially meningitides; associations with autoimmune disease

Physical examination
  Dependent on disease process
  Serum complement protein levels*
    Classical pathway†
      C1q, 7 mg/dl
      C1r, 3.4 mg/dl
      C1s, 3.1 mg/dl
      C4, 50 mg/dl
      C2, 2.5 mg/dl
      C3, 160 mg/dl
      C5, 8 mg/dl
      C6, 7.5 mg/dl
      C7, 5.5 mg/dl
      C8, 8 mg/dl
      C9, 5.8 mg/dl
    Alternative pathway
      Factor B, 20 mg/dl
      Factor D, 0.2 mg/dl
      Properdin, 1.5 mg/dl
    Control proteins
      C1q inhibitor, 12.5 mg/dl
      C3b inactivator (factor I), 2.5 mg/dl
      Anaphylatoxin inactivator, 5 mg/dl
      C4 binding protein, 25 mg/dl
      S protein, 50 mg/dl
      Factor H, 50 mg/dl
    CH50, 20 to 40 units/ml‡

*C3, C4, and CH50 assays are available in most laboratories. Reference laboratories generally perform other assays. Numbers will be decreased in specific complement deficiency. With control protein abnormalities, succeeding components will be depressed.
†Detects quantity and not functional capacity. Ranges vary among laboratories.

‡Indicative of classical pathway integrity; measures the dilution of serum required to lyse 50% of a standard number of antibody-coated sheep red blood cells; normal values determined within each laboratory.

TREATMENT PLAN

No therapy is available for direct treatment of complement disorders. With primary complement disorders, aggressive management of infections is indicated. Management of hereditary angioedema is discussed elsewhere in this text.

In secondary complement disorders, management of the disease process should restore normal complement levels. The reader is referred elsewhere in this text for management of individual diseases.

SEVERE COMBINED IMMUNODEFICIENCY DISEASE

In severe combined immunodeficiency disease (SCID), the most severe type of immune system aberrancy, there is total congenital absence of both B and T cell immunity.

SCID is inherited in an X-linked recessive form or an autosomal recessive form. Seventy-five percent of patients are male. The diagnosis must be made early so bone marrow transplantation may be attempted. Without successful intervention, chances for survival beyond 1 year of age are poor.

Infants with SCID have frequent episodes of polymicrobial infections in the first few months of life. Bacterial infections are common, as are fungal *(Candida)*, protozoal *(Pneumocystis carinii)*, and viral (cytomegalovirus, measles, herpes) infections. Recurrent otitis, pneumonia, sepsis, intractable diarrhea, cutaneous infections (especially moniliasis), wasting, hepatosplenomegaly, and failure to thrive are classic features of this disease.

PATHOPHYSIOLOGY

The basic defect of this disorder is unknown; probably several defects are involved. One explanation is that stem cells fail to differentiate into B and T lymphocytes. This concept is supported by the successful transplantation of histocompatible bone marrow. Another theory implicates failure of the thymus and bursa equivalent tissue to develop normally, thus interfering with T and B cell maturation.[2] In the autosomal recessive form of severe combined immunodeficiency, approximately half of the cases are thought to be the result of a genetic deficiency of adenosine deaminase, an enzyme found in all mammalian cells that plays a key role in DNA synthesis.[27] Its absence results in inhibition of lymphocyte function.

Whatever the cause of this life-threatening disease, its manifestations result from profound decrease or absence of humoral and cellular immunity. Humoral deficiency is demonstrated by recurrent bacterial infections. Cell-mediated immune deficiency is reflected by recurrent or chronic viral, fungal, and protozoal infections.

DIAGNOSTIC STUDIES

Lymphocyte count
  Markedly depressed (less than 1000/mm³)

T cell studies
  T cells absent or markedly depressed; some patients may have normal numbers of circulating T cells, but these are of immature form[27]; absence of lymphocytic response to mitogens, antigens, and allogeneic cells (mixed lymphocyte culture [MLC]); absent response (anergy) to delayed hypersensitivity skin test

B cell studies
  Peripheral B cells absent or markedly depressed; immunoglobulin titers absent or markedly depressed (during first 3 to 6 months of age, maternal IgG may be detected)

Biopsy of lymph nodes
  Severe depletion of lymphocytes with corticomedullary depression and no follicular formation[2] (lymph nodes may be absent)

Thymus gland biopsy
  Presence of islands and nests of endodermal cells that have not developed into lymphoid tissue[27]

Biopsy of intestinal tract
  Complete absence of plasma cells[27]

Chest roentgenogram
  Absence of thymic shadow; evidence of pneumonia

Cultures and biopsy
  Evidence of polymicrobial infections

TREATMENT PLAN

The goals of the medical plan include prevention and treatment of infection and reconstitution of the immune system.

Surgical

Bone marrow transplantation (see p. 1722)

Chemotherapeutic

Anti-infective agents
  Agent-specific antimicrobial agents for recurrent infections
Serum agents
  γ-Globulin, 100-400 mg/kg IV q1-4wk depending on symptoms

Supportive

Avoidance of complications: vaccines should not be administered; only irradiated cytomegalovirus-negative blood products should be administered
Protective isolation
Family counseling to assist family members in coping with prolonged hospitalization and potentially fatal complications of disease course and treatment
Chest physiotherapy, postural drainage, breathing exercises, or oxygen therapy as prophylaxis or treatment for recurrent pulmonary infections

ASSESSMENT: AREAS OF CONCERN

Recurrent infections

Persistent recurrent infections by viral, protozoal, bacterial, and fungal organisms such as candidiasis, pneumonia (especially *Pneumocystis* and cytomegalovirus), otitis media, sepsis; common viral infections (measles, herpes, chickenpox) often fatal

Graft-versus-host reaction

Occurs in response to administration of foreign tissue (such as blood products); may include rashes, thrombocytopenia, diarrhea, jaundice, hepatosplenomegaly, alopecia, fingernail ridging, pulmonary infiltrates, and renal failure

Nonspecific symptoms

Failure to thrive; alopecia; unusual skin eruptions; excessive seborrhea; cutaneous laxity: redundant skin folds, hyperelastic joints, large umbilical hernias

NURSING DIAGNOSES and NURSING INTERVENTIONS

Nursing Diagnosis	Nursing Intervention
Gas exchange, impaired (related to recurrent pulmonary infections)	Assess respiratory status: monitor rate, rhythm, and quality of respirations, presence of cyanosis, adventitious breath sounds, and restlessness. Monitor results of sputum cultures, pulmonary function studies (such as arterial blood gases), and chest roentgenograms. Be alert for development of *Pneumocystis* or cytomegalovirus infections. In collaboration with physician, administer appropriate antibiotics, oxygen therapy, bronchodilators, and chest physiotherapy. Assess effectiveness and note side effects.
Bowel elimination, alteration in: diarrhea (related to antimicrobial therapy or intestinal infection)	Monitor intake, output, and weight. Monitor for dehydration. Force oral fluids (oral electrolyte solution may be ordered). Determine need for tube feeding and hyperalimentation. Monitor for electrolyte imbalance. In collaboration with physician, administer appropriate anti-infective therapy. Assess effectiveness and note side effects (especially if diarrhea is exacerbated). Avoid use of antidiarrheal agents if intestinal infection is present. Institute enteric isolation precautions. Monitor nutritional status.
Comfort, alteration in: pain (related to restricted mobility, invasive procedures, frequent diarrhea, oral pain, or fever)	Assess degree of discomfort and determine cause. Institute appropriate interventions based on assessment: range of motion exercises, analgesics, antipyretics, frequent diaper changes, skin care and massage, and oral hygiene. Assess effectiveness. Comfort child during procedures. Encourage family members to visit as often as feasible. Provide child with familiar articles and toys from home. Plan care to allow for periods of rest and sleep. Allow time for holding, cuddling, feeding, and rocking that are unrelated to other treatments or procedures.

Nursing Diagnosis	Nursing Intervention
Oral mucous membranes, alteration in (related to moniliasis or graft-versus-host reaction)	Maintain meticulous oral hygiene. Provide liquids and soft foods served at moderate temperatures. Administer antifungal suspension as ordered for treatment of thrush. Inspect oral cavity frequently for evidence of secondary infection.
Anxiety (related to hospitalization, fear of death, or invasive procedures)	Encourage family interaction: allow family members to touch, hold, rock, and cuddle child as frequently as possible, particularly after invasive procedures. Provide pleasant diversional activity such as mobile, reading aloud, and television cartoons. Provide reassurance before, during, and after diagnostic procedures and treatments. Involve family and child in care as much as possible.
Coping, family: potential for growth (related to prolonged hospitalization and poor prognosis)	Assess family's anxiety related to limited understanding of diagnostic procedures, disease process and prognosis, and therapies employed. Provide information in areas needed. Explain relationship of disease process and rationale for various therapeutic interventions at level appropriate for family's comprehension and degree of anxiety. Involve family in care as appropriate. Encourage family to verbalize questions and fears. Encourage parents to leave hospital to attend to family matters. Allow parents to call hospital at any time when they cannot be there.
Parenting, alteration in (related to prolonged hospitalization and inability to normalize parent-child relationship)	Support parents' efforts to maintain nurturing, loving relationship with their child. Allow parents to leave hospital to attend to patient's siblings.

Patient Education

1. Teach the parents assessment skills related to the monitoring of systemic infections.
2. Teach about bone marrow transplantation (see p. 1722).
3. Teach techniques to prevent recurrent pulmonary infections: chest physiotherapy, postural drainage, and breathing exercises.
4. Teach facts about and importance of medications and other therapies and diagnostic procedures.
5. Explain that no live viral vaccines should be administered to the child.
6. Explain that the child should receive only irradiated blood products.
7. Teach methods to limit the child's risk for infection: handwashing, skin and oral hygiene, environmental control, proper nutrition, and supervision during activity to prevent skin trauma.
8. Refer parents for genetic counseling to explain inheritance pattern.

EVALUATION

Patient Outcome	Data Indicating That Outcome is Reached
Immunocompetence is restored following bone marrow transplantation.	B and T cell levels return to normal.
Complications of therapy are avoided.	Graft-versus-host disease is self-limited, reversed, or absent. Side effects of chemotherapy are minimized.
There are fewer or no recurrent infections in response to antimicrobial therapy.	There are no signs or symptoms of recurrent pyogenic and opportunistic infections.

ACQUIRED IMMUNE DEFICIENCY SYNDROME

Acquired immune deficiency syndrome (AIDS) is characterized by dysfunction of cell-mediated immunity. The cell-mediated immune defect is manifested clinically as the development of recurrent, often severe, opportunistic infections (such as Pneumocystis carinii *pneumonia) or unusual malignancies (such as Kaposi's sarcoma).*

Various hypotheses explaining the pathogenesis of AIDS have been proposed since it was first recognized in 1981. Early in the study of this syndrome alleged causative agents included the use of recreational drugs, homosexual activity, cytomegalovirus, and the introduction of sperm into the bloodstream. None of these theories, however, fully explained the incidence of the disease in various populations affected. As the epidemiology of the disease was clearly defined, the theory that AIDS is an infectious disease transmitted via intimate contact with body fluids and blood or blood products was widely accepted as the most plausible explanation.

April 1984 brought news of a breakthrough in AIDS research. Dr. Robert Gallo of the National Institutes of Health announced his discovery of the probable AIDS virus, a strain of the human T cell leukemia/lymphoma virus (HTLV-3). The original virus, discovered by Gallo in 1980, is known to induce hematologic malignancies by infecting T cells and altering their genetic structure. A similar virus was previously isolated by French researchers at the Pasteur Institute.

Gallo believes that HTLV originated in Africa and traveled via slave trade to Europe, Latin America, and the Caribbean. Subsequently, a new strain of HTLV evolved. According to Gallo, "the virus may have been in the bush for some time, but with mass migration into cities, crowding, and prostitution, what was contained at a low level became a problem."[37] Evidence supporting his hypotheses includes the fact that Kaposi's sarcoma, a connective tissue cancer to which AIDS patients are prone, has been prevalent in Central Africa for decades. In addition, AIDS itself is common in that region.

How the AIDS virus entered the United States remains a mystery. One intriguing theory is that the virus, existing in the Caribbean, may have been brought into the country by vacationers returning from Haiti or by Haitian immigrants. This proposed "Haitian connection," however, remains speculative.

The signs and symptoms of AIDS vary greatly. Clinical manifestations depend on the degree of immunosuppression and the particular infection or neoplasm that develops secondarily. Nonspecific constitutional complaints may also occur and are usually exacerbated as the disease progresses.

A syndrome referred to as pre-AIDS, AIDS-related complex (ARC), or chronic lymphadenopathy syndrome has been described. Essentially, it is one way of describing immunosuppression in a person from a high-risk group who has not yet developed the sequelae of recurrent infections and neoplastic disease. Up to 19% of these patients may go on to develop AIDS. Signs and symptoms of ARC may include severe fatigue, malaise, weakness, persistent unexplained weight loss, persistent lymphadenopathy, fevers, arthralgias, and persistent diarrhea. Laboratory and other diagnostic measures are important because such observations are nonspecific.

By far the most common manifestations associated with full-blown AIDS are two life-threatening diseases: Kaposi's sarcoma and *Pneumocystis carinii* pneumonia.

Kaposi's Sarcoma

Named after a turn-of-the-century dermatologist, Kaposi's sarcoma (KS) is a malignant tumor of the endothelium, the layer of epithelial cells that lines the cavity of the heart, blood vessels, lymphoid tissues, and serous cavities. In its most benign form KS is usually limited to the skin, particularly of the lower extremities. Lesions are characteristically soft, vascular, bluish purple, painless areas of discoloration. Lesions may be either macular or papular or may appear as plaques, keloids, or ecchymotic areas. In this classic form the course of the disease is usually indolent with a high rate of survival at 10 years. This form until recently affected only select populations. In the United States these included Jewish and Italian males over 50 years of age and severely immunocompromised persons such as organ transplant recipients and cancer patients receiving immunosuppressive drug therapy. The disease was rare; fewer than 40 cases were reported to the Centers for Disease Control (CDC) between 1976 and 1980.

Late in 1980 physicians in New York City began to notice an alarming increase in the number of KS patients. Approximately 30 cases were reported over a period of months.

Two findings were disturbing to investigators. First, KS was identified in apparently healthy persons, not persons with known histories of or predispositions for immunosuppression. Moreover, these patients were sexually active homosexual males between 25 and 50 years of age.

Second, the KS described by clinicians was not the classic, chronic form limited to the skin. Rather, the syndrome mimicked the invasive form previously detected only in a population inhabiting Central Africa. It was initially characterized by diffuse cutaneous spread of lesions to the upper extremities and trunk. In addition, multicentric lesions were found in the endothelium of the gastrointestinal tract and other organs such as the lungs, liver, viscera, bones, and lymph nodes. More recent data suggest that, although KS in AIDS patients tends to resemble the aggressive African form, patients have varying degrees of systemic and cutaneous involvement. Possibly the invasiveness of the KS reflects the degree of immunodeficiency.

Diagnosis of KS is based on biopsy of suspect tissue or skin lesions. Before therapy is started, a staging work-up is also performed to identify involvement elsewhere and to assist in determining the type and dosage of systemic chemotherapy. Pharmacologic agents used have included vinblastine, bleomycin, VP-16 (Etoposide), doxorubicin, and interferon. All have been used in various protocols with variable results.

Generally AIDS patients with KS have a milder immunodeficiency. However, severe immunosuppression and invasive KS carry a poor prognosis, although survival rates are longer than for patients with recurrent opportunistic infections. Other malignancies that may be associated with AIDS are non-Hodgkin's lymphomas, leukemias, and squamous cell carcinomas of the mouth and rectum.

Pneumocystis carinii Pneumonia

About the same time the CDC began to receive reports of KS, cases of another relatively rare condition, *Pneumocystis carinii* pneumonia (PCP), were reported from San Francisco and Los Angeles. As in the KS cases, patients affected were young homosexual men without known history of immunosuppression.

P. carinii is a one-celled protozoan that is ubiquitous in the environment. Usually a benign flora in the healthy population, it becomes an aggressive pathogen in immunocompromised hosts. Infestation can result in death from respiratory failure. Until the advent of AIDS, PCP was considered a relatively rare complication in cancer patients receiving chemotherapy, transplant patients, and patients with congenital defects of cellular immunity.

Probably spread by person-to-person transmission via the respiratory route, this opportunistic organism assaults pulmonary tissue, resulting in diffuse, bilateral interstitial infiltrates and alveolar infiltration by exudates of many clumped organisms, or cysts. PCP is usually slow to manifest itself, and the duration of symptoms varies from 2 weeks to 8 months.

Early symptoms often include increasing dyspnea on exertion, dry cough, and weight loss. Fever is sometimes present. Chest roentgenograms are unremarkable initially, and lung fields are clear to percussion and ausculta-

tion. Abnormal findings of pulmonary function studies may be the only way to confirm early suspicions that an infection is brewing. Patients have low Po_2 when arterial blood gases are measured. PCP can be definitively diagnosed only by bronchoscopy with transbronchial lung biopsy or by open lung biopsy.

The later course of PCP can be rapid and associated with clinical findings compatible with respiratory failure. The death rate of untreated persons with PCP is approximately 60%.

Two drugs are available to control this disease. The first-line defense is trimethoprim-sulfamethoxazole (Bactrim) given intravenously and later orally. Unfortunately, for as yet unexplained reasons, severe allergic reactions to this sulfa drug occur in many AIDS patients.

Pentamidine isethionate is the second drug of choice. It is administered intramuscularly over 10 to 14 days. Potential complications with this medication include hypotension, severe nausea and vomiting, renal insufficiency, and hepatotoxicity.

Use of the aforementioned drugs usually decreases the mortality associated with PCP to 3% to 5%. However, AIDS patients tend to clear the organism very slowly despite therapy, and relapses are common. Prolonged treatment is required in AIDS patients.

Listed below are a few of an ever-growing number of opportunistic infections associated with AIDS*:

Protozoal
    Pneumocystis carinii pneumonia
    Toxoplasmosis
    Cryptosporidiosis
    Giardiasis
Fungal
    Candidiasis
    Cryptococcosis
    Histoplasmosis
    Coccidioidomycosis
    Aspergillosis
Viral
    Cytomegalovirus (CMV)
    Progressive multifocal leukoencephalopathy
    Herpes (HSV)
Bacterial
    Mycobacterium avium intracellulare
    Miliary mycobacterial tuberculosis
    Salmonellosis

Despite the variety, these organisms have one commonality: all are intracellular pathogens. As discussed previously, this has significance in that cell-mediated immune defenses are responsible for clearing these organ-

---

*Most infections are disseminated, tend to recur, and do not respond well to therapy.

isms. T lymphocytes and macrophages are important cells responsible for this defense. The occurrence of these pathogens in AIDS patients is consistent with findings that the immune deficiency is characterized by dysfunction of T cells.

Antimicrobial drugs are poorly effective against intracellular pathogens because most of these agents are unable to penetrate cell membranes. Thus, if the immune system cells (T cells) responsible for clearing these microbes are not functioning properly, these infections will clear much more slowly, if at all, despite attempts to facilitate a response with currently available pharmacologic agents.

Autoimmune Phenomena

AIDS may also be associated with several disorders characterized by the development of hemolytic anemia and thrombocytopenia. The significance of these findings is unclear. A possible explanation is that, because of abnormal regulation of immunity in AIDS, the large numbers of B cells and immunoglobulins present may react with self-tissues or blood components. In any case the presence of autoantibodies generally reflects the overall immune system dysfunction that characterizes this disease.

Populations at Risk

AIDS has been identified in diverse populations (Table 16-3). Further dissemination of AIDS outside these groups seems possible considering that its transmission is similar to that of hepatitis B. The incidence of AIDS in these populations supports the theory that the disease is transmissible via direct contact with body fluids and blood or blood products of known AIDS patients. In addition, there appears to be a carrier state associated with AIDS transmission. That is, exposure may occur from direct contact with persons who are infected with the virus but remain asymptomatic. Evidence supporting the existence of a carrier state suggests that the incubation period of the AIDS virus may be as long as 5 years.

Most children with AIDS have been offspring of high-risk parents and apparently contract the disease during the birth process or through later close contact with family members. In addition, children have acquired AIDS because of transfusions.

Most heterosexual AIDS patients report exposure to members of the high-risk groups. It is possible that the disease will spread beyond the current risk groups through heterosexual contacts.

Over 95% of AIDS patients are male. All races and major ethnic groups have been affected. Cases have been reported in virtually every state and many foreign countries. Eighty-five percent of patients are less than 45 years of age; the median age is 35.

Prognosis

Although annual mortality stands at approximately 40%, if death rates are broken down according to year of diagnosis, the ultimate mortality associated with AIDS approaches 100%. No one has fully regained immunocompetence. Patients typically die of recurrent infections and malignancies that are poorly responsive to therapy. If HTLV is proved conclusively to be the AIDS virus, a vaccine may be developed to halt the spread of this life-threatening disease. Current management is aimed at control rather than cure.

PATHOPHYSIOLOGY

Viruses are generally successful pathogens because of their ability to invade host cells and utilize the metabolism and genetic material of the host cells to produce copies of themselves. HTLV is no exception. According to Gallo's theory, HTLV-3 infects T helper lymphocytes, which are normally present in a ratio of 2:1 over T suppressor cells. When the virus decreases the number of T helper cells, this ratio is reversed and T suppressor mechanisms dominate. Clinical findings are compatible with profound immunosuppression. Because T cell–mediated immunity is important in tumor surveillance and in defense against intracellular pathogens such as viruses, protozoa, mycobacteria, and fungi, deregulation within this component of the body's defensive network results in the development of characteristics of AIDS, such as the following:

Table 16-3
Populations at Risk for AIDS

Population	Incidence (% of Total Cases)
Homosexual and bisexual men	73
Intravenous drug abusers	17
Hemophiliacs	4
Heterosexuals	4
Transfusion recipients	1
Pediatric (under 13 years)	1
Unknown/other	7

Cutaneous anergy
Leukopenia
Lymphopenia
Decreased T cell function and reactivity
Reduced or absent T helper cells
Increased percentage of T suppressor cells
Depressed natural killer cell activity
Depressed interferon production by peripheral blood
  leukocytes
Normal or increased immunoglobulin levels
Abnormal immunoglobulin function in some cases
Normal phagocytic function

DIAGNOSTIC STUDIES

No test points to a diagnosis of AIDS with 100% accuracy. Laboratory data are nonspecific and merely support a diagnosis of immunosuppression, which can occur for a variety of reasons.

White blood cell count
Depressed

Lymphocyte count
Depressed

T cell studies
T cell numbers and function depressed; delayed hypersensitivity skin test shows decreased or absent response to cutaneous recall antigens (anergy); T helper/T suppressor cell ratio reversed (less than 0.5)

B cell studies
B cell numbers and function normal or increased; immunoglobulin levels normal or increased

Natural killer cell activity
Usually depressed

Cultures
Polymicrobial (fungal, viral, protozoal, and bacterial) infections

Tissue biopsy
Kaposi's sarcoma; *Pneumocystis carinii* pneumonia; lymphoreticular malignancies

Viral titers
Document exposure to herpes simplex, hepatitis, Epstein-Barr virus, cytomegalovirus; elevated titers may explain panhypergammaglobulinemia

Chest roentgenogram
Used in initial evaluation of respiratory complaints; pneumonia, pneumonitis, pulmonary infiltrates detected (causative agents determined via culture, bronchoscopy with brushings, or biopsy)

Gallium scan
Useful in early detection of interstitial pneumonias

Stool for ova and parasites
Variety of parasites, including *Giardia lamblia* and *Cryptosporidium*

Neurologic workup (cerebrospinal fluid analysis, brain CT scan, brain biopsy, electromyography, nerve conduction studies, ophthalmic examination, electroencephalogram)
Indicated for evaluation of changes in mentation and fever of unknown etiology; variety of AIDS-associated disorders may be detected, including progressive multifocal leukoencephalopathy, cryptococcal meningitis, encephalitis, organic brain syndrome, and toxoplasmosis

Staging workup for Kaposi's sarcoma[20]
Skin: Photographs and biopsies of representative lesions
Nodes: Biopsy of accessible nodes, CT scan of abdomen and pelvis
Gastrointestinal tract: Endoscopy, colonoscopy, and gastrointestinal contrast studies
Lung: Bronchoscopy (if chest roentgenogram shows abnormalities)
Liver: CT scan or radioisotope scan
Bone: Bone scan when alkaline phosphatase level is elevated
See Table 16-4

TREATMENT PLAN

The goals of the medical plan include rapid detection and treatment of opportunistic infections and neoplastic disease, management of signs and symptoms, and prevention of complications from treatment. The ultimate objective for treatment of AIDS is reconstitution of the immune system. However, all attempts to correct the underlying immune defect, including bone marrow transplantation, have been unsuccessful.

Treatment for individual AIDS patients varies considerably and depends on the degree of immunosuppression and systemic involvement.

Surgical
Placement of Hickman or Raaf catheter to facilitate frequent blood drawing, hyperalimentation, transfusions, and administration of chemotherapy
Surgical intervention for treatment of malignancies in certain cases

Table 16-4
Staging System of Kaposi's Sarcoma

Stage	Description
Stage I	Cutaneous, locally indolent
Stage II	Cutaneous, locally aggressive with or without regional lymph nodes
Stage III	Generalized mucocutaneous or lymph node involvement
Stage IV	Visceral

Subtypes
A. No systemic signs or symptoms
B. Systemic signs: 10% weight loss or temperature greater than 100° F orally, unrelated to identifiable source of infection, and lasting more than 2 weeks
Generalized: more than upper or lower extremities alone; includes minimal gastrointestinal disease defined as more than five lesions and greater than 2 cm in combined diameters

From Laubenstein, L.J.: Staging and treatment of Kaposi's sarcoma in patient with AIDS. In Friedman-Kien, A.E., and Laubenstein, L.J., editors: AIDS: the epidemic of Kaposi's sarcoma and opportunistic infections, New York, 1984, Masson Publishing USA, Inc.

Chemotherapeutic

Directed at treatment of opportunistic diseases associated with AIDS; no pharmacologic agent has been identified that corrects underlying immunodeficiency

Supportive

Maintenance of adequate hydration, particularly during acute febrile episodes and with administration of nephrotoxic medications

Maintenance of optimal nutritional status with high-calorie, high-protein diet; use of supplemental feedings such as Isocal and Ensure if needed; parenteral feedings if needed

Physical therapy for immobilized patients; regular program of rest and exercise for ambulatory patients

Mechanical ventilation if periods of respiratory failure occur as result of pulmonary infections

In patients with recurrent pulmonary infections, serial chest roentgenograms, arterial blood gases, and pulmonary function studies if needed; chest physiotherapy, postural drainage, and oxygen therapy in conjunction with antimicrobial therapy if needed for pulmonary infections

Neurologic workup if changes in mentation indicate organic disease; may include cerebrospinal fluid analysis, brain scans, brain biopsy, and electroencephalogram; frequent attempts to maintain patient's orientation and safety indicated in event of central nervous system disturbances

Support services as indicated: social worker, clergyman, psychologist, psychiatrist, clinical nurse specialist; involvement of significant others in care

Local support groups as indicated

Reduction of risk factors for infection: malnutrition, exposure to infectious sources such as contaminated equipment, frequent venipuncture, and other invasive procedures such as Foley catheterization

ASSESSMENT: AREAS OF CONCERN

The signs and symptoms of AIDS vary. Clinical manifestations depend on the degree of immunosuppression and the opportunistic infections and neoplasms that develop secondarily. Nonspecific complaints may also occur and are usually exacerbated as the disease progresses. Why such a variety of conditions develops remains a mystery. Genetic predisposition may play a role, and exposure to certain risk factors may also be important.

Recurrent infections

Protozoal infections
  Pneumocystis carinii pneumonia
  Toxoplasmosis
  Cryptosporidiosis
  Giardiasis
Fungal infections
  Candidiasis
  Cryptococcosis
  Histoplasmosis
  Coccidioidomycosis
  Aspergillosis
Viral infections
  Herpes
  Progressive multifocal leukoencephalopathy
  Cytomegalovirus (CMV)
Bacterial infections
  Mycobacterial infection
  Salmonellosis

Malignancies

Kaposi's sarcoma; non-Hodgkin's lymphomas; leukemias; squamous cell carcinomas of mouth and rectum

Nonspecific complaints

Malaise; weakness; persistent weight loss; persistent lymphadenopathy; fever; arthralgias; persistent diarrhea

NURSING DIAGNOSES and NURSING INTERVENTIONS

Nursing Diagnosis	Nursing Intervention
Gas exchange, impaired (related to pulmonary infection)	Assess respiratory status: rate, rhythm, and regularity of respirations, use of accessory muscles, presence of adventitious breath sounds on auscultation, cough, and cyanosis. Encourage patient to report cough and progressive dyspnea on exertion. Monitor results of pulmonary function studies. In collaboration with physician, administer appropriate anti-infective medications. Assess effectiveness and side effects. In collaboration with physician, administer oxygen therapy. Assess effectiveness. Provide chest physiotherapy and postural drainage as indicated. Provide preprocedural teaching before bronchoscopy, lung biopsy, CT scans, pulmonary function tests, and other procedures. Instruct patient in breathing exercises and encourage patient to perform them. Encourage patient to stop smoking. Obtain sputum specimens as needed. Maintain patent airway at all times. In collaboration with physician, determine need for mechanical ventilation if respiratory status worsens.
Nutrition, alteration in: less than body requirements (related to protracted diarrhea, malabsorption, anorexia, or stomatitis)	Assess nutritional status: height and weight, caloric intake, total protein, serum albumin, hematocrit, and hemoglobin level. Determine need for dietary changes, enteral feedings, and parenteral alimentation. Provide vitamin supplements for deficiencies. Provide small, frequent, high-calorie, high-protein feedings. Encourage patient to eat. Provide or encourage patient to perform frequent oral hygiene. Correct stomatitis.
Bowel elimination, alteration in: diarrhea (related to chemotherapy or gastrointestinal infection)	Assess elimination pattern: quality and quantity of stool and presence of gross blood, fat, or undigested food. Monitor intake and output. Monitor stool culture results. Monitor guaiac or Hemoccult tests. Avoid use of antidiarrheal medications. Monitor for signs and symptoms associated with fluid and electrolyte imbalances. Maintain patient's safety should weakness become problem. Monitor vital signs for evidence of hypovolemia.
Skin integrity, impaired (related to malnutrition, Kaposi's sarcoma, frequent venipunctures, or side effects of chemotherapy)	Assess skin integrity: presence of lesions, texture, temperature, moisture, color, vascularity, and evidence of poor wound healing. Monitor lesions for signs of infection, dissemination, and other abnormal changes. Provide or encourage patient to perform meticulous hygiene in involved areas. For stomatitis: perform regular oral care, avoid acidic oral fluids, provide topical viscous anesthetic, and serve bland foods at medium temperatures. If Kaposi's lesions are present, assess response to chemotherapy; note changes in size, color, and configuration. Provide or encourage use of mild, hypoallergenic, nondrying soaps for skin cleansing. Avoid trauma to the skin; do not allow long periods of immobilization. Consider placement of Hickman or Raaf catheter if frequent venipunctures are necessary.
Comfort, alteration in: pain (related to side effects of chemotherapy, infections, frequent venipunctures, or immobility)	Assess pain: location, onset, duration, and precipitating or alleviating factors. Have patient describe intensity on scale of 0 to 10. In collaboration with physician, provide appropriate anti-inflammatory and analgesic agents. Assess effectiveness and note side effects. Provide thermal therapy for affected muscles and joints as needed. Provide diversional activities as tolerated. Consider placement of Hickman or Raaf catheter if frequent venipuncture is necessary.

Nursing Diagnosis	**Nursing Intervention**
Activity intolerance (related to weakness, fatigue, arthralgias, myalgias, side effects of therapy, dyspnea, fever, malnutrition, or fluid and electrolyte imbalances)	Assess degree of activity intolerance. Encourage regular exercise and rest as tolerated; confer with physical or occupational therapist to determine optimal approach. In collaboration with physician, provide appropriate treatment for underlying causes of activity intolerance (such as pain, infections, or malnutrition). Assess effectiveness.
Anxiety (related to diagnosis, fear of death, or hospitalization)	Avoid false reassurances but encourage hope; inform patient of promising research findings. Encourage patient to participate in care as much as possible to promote feelings of self-control. Provide accurate information about AIDS and related treatment; include information about diagnostic procedures. Encourage patient to use available resources. See also p. 1839.
Self-concept, disturbance in: body image (related to diagnosis, Kaposi's lesions, side effects of chemotherapy, depression, or social stigmatization and isolation)	Provide accurate information as indicated; focus on correcting myths and clarifying controversial information the patient might have seen, heard, or read. Direct patient to appropriate resources: clergyman, social worker, psychologist, psychiatrist, or AIDS clinic counselor. Encourage patient to participate in AIDS support groups. See also p. 1820.
Knowledge deficit: AIDS disease process, life-style implications, and therapy (related to anxiety, unavailable resources, poor communication skills, or fear)	Assess patient's understanding of disease process, life-style implications, and therapy. Provide information based on assessment (see ''Patient Education''). Refer patient to available resources. Include significant others in teaching sessions if appropriate.
Potential patient problem: susceptibility to infection	Assess for signs and symptoms associated with opportunistic infections. Institute AIDS isolation precautions. Assess for anorexia, failure to thrive, pain, weakness, and lethargy. Assess for evidence of infection at sites of invasive procedures. Assess for breaks in skin integrity, particularly over pressure areas and oral mucosa. Assess pulmonary status. Auscultate lung fields to determine presence of adventitious breath sounds. Maintain optimal nutritional status and fluid intake. Assess ocular integrity for evidence of conjunctivitis: erythematous, pruritic conjunctiva. Assess mentation for evidence of central nervous system infection: level of consciousness, headache, and visual disturbances. Assess for evidence of gastrointestinal infection: abdominal pain, fever, and diarrhea. Monitor temperature and vital signs for evidence of fever and sepsis. Maintain body hygiene. Limit environmental stress. Monitor laboratory data: white blood cell count and differential, erythrocyte sedimentation rate, C-reactive protein, urinalysis, and cultures. In collaboration with physician, administer appropriate anti-infective, antipyretic, or analgesic medication. Assess patient's response. Monitor for side effects. Promote pulmonary toilet: breathing exercises, postural drainage, and chest physical therapy. Maintain normal sleep and rest patterns. Protect patient from physical injury. Provide clean environment. Maintain protective isolation based on hospital policy. Restrict contact with family and health care providers who have infectious diseases. Maintain good handwashing before and after contact with patient.

AIDS ISOLATION PRECAUTIONS

In Hospital

1. The door to the patient's room need not be closed, since airborne transmission is unlikely.
2. Gloves should be worn only if in *direct* contact with specimens, linen, and items or surfaces exposed to blood or body fluids. Gloves need *not* be worn if one is merely conversing with the patient or walking into the room.
3. A mask is not indicated, since airborne transmission is unlikely. A mask should be worn if secretions may be aerosolized onto the face during suctioning, oral hygiene, and other procedures. A mask may be indicated if a health care worker with a respiratory infection must enter the room of a severely immunosuppressed patient.
4. Protective eyewear may be indicated if aerosolization of secretions or blood may contact the conjunctiva (as during suctioning or blood drawing).
5. A gown should be worn if clothing is likely to become contaminated with blood or body fluids, as during bathing of the patient, linen changes, some specimen collections, or dressing changes.
6. Proper isolation technique should be used. Gown and gloves should be removed in the room.
7. Soiled linen and dry waste should be bagged and discarded.
8. Specimens should be bagged and labeled properly.
9. Special care in handling contaminated needles is essential. Attempts to recap needles should be avoided, since most needle-stick injuries occur this way. Needles should be disposed of in a puncture-resistant container, which should be sealed, bagged, and labeled before being taken from the room.
10. Handwashing should be performed in the room before and after contact with the patient.
11. Contaminated nondisposable items should be cleaned with soap and water and bagged (using paper bags) for autoclaving. Items that cannot be autoclaved should be washed with soap and water (or other solution recommended in the hospital procedure manual).
12. A private room may be indicated for patients unable to maintain scrupulous hygiene (those with intractable diarrhea, incontinence, or central nervous system infections leading to altered sensorium).
13. Ancillary services should be alerted to isolation precautions required for the patient. A duplicate door card attached to the chart with which the patient travels is suggested. Other methods vary depending on hospital protocol.
14. Usually no precautions are needed when handling food trays. However, if the patient has copious oral or respiratory secretions or if diarrhea is a problem, the use of disposable utensils and paper trays should be considered.
15. Disposable resuscitation equipment (Ambu bags, airways, and so on) should be available at all times.
16. Postmortem handling of the body may include the use of gown and gloves. Bodily remains should be double wrapped and clearly labeled. Morgue personnel may need to be notified of the transport of the body (this varies depending on hospital policy).

At Home*

1. Disposable gloves should be worn by family members who come in direct contact with the patient's blood and body fluids.
2. Linen and clothing soiled with secretions or excretions should be washed separately with a 1% bleach solution (1 cup bleach to 9 cups water).
3. Dishes and eating utensils do not require separate handling but should be washed in hot, soapy water.
4. Dry waste contaminated with blood or body fluids should be disposed of in a separate container and bagged securely.
5. Any needles used for the administration of medication should be placed in an impervious container before disposal.
6. Meticulous handwashing before and after contact with the patient is essential.

*Recommendations of New York Red Cross Nursing Service.

Patient Education

1. Teach the principles of a balanced diet. Encourage the use of dietary supplements, such as Ensure, for weight gain. Encourage the patient to take a multivitamin daily.
2. Teach the patient to avoid alcohol in excess and other recreational drug use.
3. Teach the patient to modify sexual habits: decrease number of partners, avoid contact with anonymous partners, use condoms, explore alternative sexual activities that limit direct contact with mucous membranes; avoid analingus.
4. Teach the patient to maintain a balanced program of rest and exercise as tolerated.
5. Teach methods of self-assessment for recurrent infections.
6. Teach the patient that smoking further limits resistance to respiratory infections.
7. Teach the patient to limit contact with persons with known infections.
8. Teach the importance of meticulous hygiene.
9. Teach the patient to avoid accidental injury to skin or mucous membranes and to inspect all wounds for signs of infection.
10. Teach the patient to refrain from donating blood.
11. Teach the importance and side effects of medications.
12. Teach that travel outside the United States may increase the risk for amebic infections and may require antibiotic prophylaxis.
13. Teach that the patient's dentist should be made aware that the patient has AIDS.
14. Teach home care to the family (see box).
15. Teach Hickman catheter care if indicated.
16. Teach home hyperalimentation or tube-feeding administration if indicated.
17. Teach the importance of regular follow-up by a physician.
18. Teach the patient to keep a log of medical history (diary of symptoms and treatment).
19. Teach the importance of obtaining up-to-date factual information about AIDS.
20. Teach the importance of medical alert identification.

EVALUATION

Patient Outcome	Data Indicating That Outcome is Reached
Optimal nutritional status is maintained.	Albumin and total protein are within normal limits.
Complications of therapy are avoided.	There is no evidence of severe myelosuppression, Stevens-Johnson syndrome, neurotoxicity, nephrotoxicity, hepatotoxicity, retinopathy, ototoxicity, gastrointestinal hemorrhage, psychosis, secondary infection, or severe malnutrition.
Patient complies with recommendations for life-style adjustments.	Patient reports making sexual behavior modification, having balanced nutritional intake, and limiting recreational drug use, including alcohol. Patient reports significant symptoms and observations early. Complications of therapy are limited.
Kaposi's sarcoma is responsive to treatment.	Lesions are decreased in size and number; biopsy results are improved.
Opportunistic infections are responsive to treatment.	There is absence of or decrease in clinical findings associated with infections.

INFLAMMATORY DISEASES
Wegener's Granulomatosis

Wegener's granulomatosis is a multisystem disorder of unknown cause characterized by diffuse granuloma formation and vasculitis involving primarily the respiratory tract.

Wegener's granulomatosis occurs in both sexes equally. It may appear at any age, with a peak incidence in the fourth and fifth decades of life.

Signs and symptoms may be widespread but usually occur in the upper or lower respiratory tract. For example, a patient may have headache, sinusitis, rhinorrhea, and otitis media. Other manifestations include hearing loss (resulting from recurrent otitis), renal disease, pericarditis, myocarditis, granulomatous lung disease, ocular inflammatory disease, arthralgias, and some dermatologic manifestations associated with vasculitis.

Once considered a fatal disease, Wegener's granulomatosis now has a good prognosis when detected early and treated with cyclophosphamide, which is capable of inducing prolonged remission in most cases. However, extensive renal disease is indicative of a poor prognosis.

PATHOPHYSIOLOGY

Any organ may become involved, with granuloma formation and vasculitis. Although the immunopathogenesis remains an enigma, these manifestations suggest that delayed-type hypersensitivity or cell-mediated reactions may be involved. Immune complex deposition may also occur.[15]

Histologic features include widespread necrotizing vasculitis of small arteries, venules, arterioles, and some capillaries, together with granuloma formation. Almost all patients have pulmonary involvement. Paranasal sinuses and the nasopharynx demonstrate granuloma formation. Pansinusitis may result in erosion of adjacent bones and septum perforation. Sinuses often become secondarily infected with bacteria. Saddle-nose deformity may be observed as well. Diffuse, bilateral, nodular lesions that tend to cavitate are found in lung tissue. When renal tissue is affected, focal glomerulitis may progress to diffuse proliferative disease.

DIAGNOSTIC STUDIES

Biopsy of affected tissue
Granuloma formation; vasculitic lesions

Complete blood count
Mild anemia (normochromic, normocytic); leukocytosis in presence of superimposed infection

Erythrocyte sedimentation rate
Elevated during active disease

Serum protein electrophoresis
Mild hypergammaglobulinemia (especially IgA)

Differential diagnoses include other vasculitides, connective tissue diseases, infectious and noninfectious granulomatous diseases, pulmonary neoplasia, and lymphomatoid granulomatosis.

TREATMENT PLAN

Chemotherapeutic
Antineoplastic agents (used as immunosuppressant)
Cyclophosphamide (Cytoxan), 1-2 mg/kg po qd; dosage adjusted to maintain total WBC at >3000/mm^3; treatment continued 1 yr after remission is achieved
Corticosteroids
Prednisone; may be added to above regimen if disease course is fulminant; 60 mg recommended as starting dose and should be continued until cyclophosphamide produces therapeutic effect (within 14 d); prednisone should then be tapered and eventually discontinued unless disease course accelerates

ASSESSMENT: AREAS OF CONCERN

Respiratory status
Paranasal sinus pain; purulent or bloody rhinorrhea; nasal mucosa ulceration; septal perforation; saddle-nose deformity; serous otitis media; epistaxis; chronic cough; pleurisy; dyspnea; chest pain; sinusitis; hemoptysis

Ocular integrity
Mild conjunctivitis; episcleritis; granulomatous sclero-uveitis; ciliary vessel vasculitis; proptosis

Skin integrity
Vasculitic dermatitis

Neurologic status
Cranial neuritis; mononeuritis multiplex

Renal status
Hematuria; abnormal urinalysis findings; progressive glomerulonephritis on biopsy

NURSING DIAGNOSES and NURSING INTERVENTIONS

Nursing Diagnosis	Nursing Intervention
Cardiac output, alteration in: decreased (related to pericarditis or myocarditis)	Monitor for signs and symptoms of pericarditis and myocarditis: edema, ascites, rales, angina, friction rub, pulsus paradoxus, electrocardiographic changes. See p. 2038.

Nursing Diagnosis	Nursing Intervention
Gas exchange, impaired: (related to sinusitis, chest pain, saddle-nose deformity, or granulomatous lung disease)	Assess degree of impairment: monitor blood gases, note presence of cyanosis or respiratory distress, auscultate lungs for presence of adventitious sounds, monitor chest roentgenograms, and note presence of hemoptysis, epistaxis, and sinus pain. Report significant abnormal findings to physician. Assess response to cyclophosphamide therapy. In collaboration with physician, institute other interventions (such as oxygen therapy) for related conditions. Assess effectiveness.
Comfort, alteration in: pain (related to sinusitis, ocular inflammation, dermatitis, arthralgias, headache, pleurisy, or angina)	Assess pain: location, onset, duration, and precipitating or alleviating factors. Have patient describe intensity on a scale of 0 to 10. Assess response to cyclophosphamide therapy. In collaboration with physician, administer appropriate analgesic and anti-inflammatory agents. Assess effectiveness and note side effects.
Tissue perfusion, alteration in: renal (related to glomerulonephritis)	Assess renal status: blood urea nitrogen, serum creatinine, blood pressure, urinalysis results, presence of edema, and rapid weight gain. Assess response to cyclophosphamide. In collaboration with physician, institute appropriate interventions related to treatment of glomerulonephritis (diet, fluids, and so on). Assess effectiveness.
Tissue perfusion, alteration in: cranial and peripheral (related to cranial neuritis or mononeuritis multiplex)	Assess degree of neurologic impairment. Monitor for cranial neuropathy: diplopia, ptosis, headache, and so on. Monitor for peripheral neuropathy: changes in sensation and motor ability, paresthesias, and so on.
Sensory-perceptual alteration: visual (related to conjunctivitis, episcleritis, or proptosis)	Assess degree of visual impairment. In collaboration with physician, administer appropriate analgesics and anti-inflammatory medications as ordered. Assess effectiveness. Assess response to cyclophosphamide therapy. Provide for patient safety.
Skin integrity, impairment of: potential (related to vasculitis dermatitis)	Assess skin integrity: texture, lesions, temperature, moisture, color, and vascularity. Monitor lesions for signs of infection, dissemination, and other abnormal changes. Provide or encourage patient to maintain meticulous hygiene in involved areas. Monitor skin for evidence of impaired circulation or necrosis.
Anxiety	See p. 1839.
Self-concept, disturbance in: body image	See p. 1820.

Patient Education

1. Teach the importance of and information about cyclophosphamide and steroid therapy (see p. 1732).
2. Teach the importance of regular follow-up by a physician.
3. Teach the patient to report significant changes: visual impairment, hematuria, oliguria, pyuria, sinusitis, hemoptysis, dyspnea, and pain.
4. Teach the importance of semiannual eye examinations.
5. Teach the importance of medical alert identification.

EVALUATION

Patient Outcome	Data Indicating That Outcome is Reached
Complications and medical crises are avoided.	There are no repeated sinus infections, progressive glomerulonephritis, visual loss, or respiratory insufficiency.
Laboratory findings are within normal limits or improved.	Erythrocyte sedimentation rate and urinalysis findings are within normal limits or improved. Tissue biopsy findings are normal or show decreased evidence of granulomatous and vasculitic changes.

Polyarteritis Nodosa (Periarteritis Nodosa)

Polyarteritis nodosa, a multisystem inflammatory disorder of unknown cause, is characterized by necrotizing inflammation of segments of medium and small arteries.

Polyarteritis nodosa is a disease of adulthood and affects two to three men for every woman. The onset and clinical presentation of this disorder vary greatly depending on the location of the arteries affected and the severity of the involvement. Widespread lesions may involve arteries of the heart, abdominal mesentery, kidneys, muscles, and vasa vasorum. Involvement of the central nervous system and pulmonary tissue is unusual.

Although the cause remains an enigma, some evidence suggests that this type of vasculitis may result from immune complex deposition in tissues following exposure to an infectious antigen. The finding of hepatitis B surface antigen (HbsAg) in the sera of 30% to 40% of these patients further suggests that this may be true.[15,22]

The prognosis of polyarteritis nodosa is guarded. Renal involvement denotes rapid disease progression. Death often occurs from renal failure, myocardial infarction, heart failure, infection, or gastrointestinal bleeding.

PATHOPHYSIOLOGY

The inciting agent that leads to inflammation within the blood vessels is unknown. The inflammatory process is characterized by early infiltration of polymorphonuclear leukocytes. New lesions are often surrounded by older lesions characterized by cells that respond late in the inflammatory reaction—monocytes, lymphocytes, and plasma cells. This suggests that the inflammatory process involved in polyarteritis is chronic, although subjected to repeated insults, perhaps by antigen that is continuously available.[22]

Chronic inflammation within the vessel walls leads to occlusion and necrosis with possible hemorrhage. Blood supply to major organs and other structures diminishes. Tissue ischemia and infarction are the notable outcomes.

DIAGNOSTIC STUDIES

No specific laboratory tests exist for polyarteritis nodosa. The abnormalities observed depend largely on the organ systems affected. Differential diagnoses include systemic lupus erythematosus, trichinosis, heart failure, and infection.

White blood count
Elevated owing to neutrophilia

Erythrocyte sedimentation rate
Elevated during acute phase

Angiography
Detects characteristic aneurysms at bifurcation points of arteries in kidneys, mesentery, liver, pancreas, and so on (acute), or narrowing and thrombosis of involved arteries (late)

Tissue histologic studies
Necrotizing inflammation of segments of medium and small arteries; aneurysms at areas of arterial bifurcation; invasion of tissue by polymorphonuclear leukocytes and monocytes

TREATMENT PLAN

Chemotherapeutic
Corticosteroids
   Prednisone, 40-60 mg to start; tapered gradually
Antineoplastic agents
   Used as immunosuppressants; use controversial and poorly documented but has been successful in some cases, particularly when corticosteroid therapy has failed

ASSESSMENT: AREAS OF CONCERN

Nonspecific manifestations
Fever; weakness; anorexia

Cutaneous
Subcutaneous nodules (5 to 10 mm) along course of arteries in extremities; purpuric, urticarial exanthemata; subcutaneous hemorrhage; ulcerations; livedo reticularis; ischemic changes of distal digits

Muscles
Muscle weakness; myalgias

Joints
Migratory arthralgias

Peripheral nervous system
Mononeuritis multiplex; paresthesias; hemiparesis

Kidneys
Glomerulitis; glomerulosclerosis; progressive renal failure; hypertension

Eyes
Retinopathy

Gastrointestinal tract
"Surgical abdomen"; abdominal pain; anorexia; nausea and vomiting; mucosal ulceration and hemorrhage; appendicitis; cholecystitis; hepatitis

Brain
  Headache; seizures; papillitis

Testes
  Pain; edema

Heart
  Coronary arteritis; myocardial ischemia or infarction; pericarditis; congestive heart failure

NURSING DIAGNOSES and NURSING INTERVENTIONS

Nursing Diagnosis	Nursing Intervention
Tissue perfusion, alteration in: cerebral (related to cerebral arteritis)	Assess for development of headache, changes in sensorium, seizures, and papilledema. Perform mental status examination. Perform ophthalmic examination of fundus and disc. Provide for patient's safety. In collaboration with physician, administer treatment for conditions detected during assessment. Assess effectiveness.
Tissue perfusion, potential alteration in: renal (related to polyarteritis of kidneys)	Assess for development of glomerulonephritis, renal failure, and hypertension. Monitor blood urea nitrogen, creatinine, hemoglobin, hematocrit, blood pressure, urinalysis results, presence of edema and rapid weight gain, and symptoms associated with hypertension: headache and visual disturbances. Report significant findings to physician. In collaboration with physician, institute appropriate treatment as ordered. Assess effectiveness.
Tissue perfusion, potential alteration in: eye (related to retinal arteritis)	Assess presence of retinopathy. Monitor for visual disturbances: changes in acuity, scotomas, and so on. Perform ophthalmic examination; determine presence of retinal exudates. Report significant findings to physician.
Tissue perfusion, alteration: muscles (related to vasculitis of vessels supplying musculature)	Assess for presence of muscle weakness. Assess muscle strength.
Tissue perfusion, potential alteration in: gastrointestinal (related to mesenteric arteritis, intestinal mucosal arteritis, or vasculitis in liver, gallbladder, or appendix)	Assess for presence of abdominal pain, anorexia, nausea, vomiting, and findings compatible with gastrointestinal ulceration or hemorrhage, appendicitis, cholecystitis, or hepatitis. Palpate abdomen to detect areas of tenderness. Perform Hemoccult or guiaic test of stool. Monitor oral intake. Report significant findings to physician. In collaboration with physician, institute appropriate treatment as ordered. Assess effectiveness.
Tissue perfusion, potential alteration in: cardiopulmonary (related to coronary arteritis, pericardial arteritis, or vasculitis of pleural sac)	Assess for myocardial ischemia, infarction, pericarditis, pleuritis: Monitor for presence of pleuritis, chest pain. Monitor serial electrocardiograms and chest roentgenograms. Auscultate chest for presence of pericardial friction rub. Monitor serial cardiac enzymes. Monitor vital signs. Report significant findings to physician. In collaboration with physician, institute appropriate treatment as ordered. Assess effectiveness.
Mobility, impaired physical (related to neuritis, paresthesia, paresis, myalgias, or muscle weakness)	Assess degree of physical limitations: perform neuromusculoskeletal assessment. In collaboration with physician, provide appropriate corticosteroid therapy. Assess effectiveness and note side effects. Provide progressive physical and occupational therapy. Encourage patient's participation. Provide for patient's safety. Assist with activities of daily living as needed.

Nursing Diagnosis	Nursing Intervention
Comfort, alteration in: pain (related to tissue and organ ischemia resulting from vasculitis)	Assess pain: location, onset, duration, and precipitating and alleviating factors. Have patient describe intensity on scale of 0 to 10.
	In collaboration with physician, provide appropriate analgesic agents. Assess effectiveness and note side effects.
	In collaboration with physician, institute appropriate other measures relative to the tissues and organs involved. Assess effectiveness.
Skin integrity, impairment of (related to impaired perfusion of cutaneous tissue resulting from peripheral vasculitis)	Assess skin for presence of ecchymosis, purpura, ulcerations, gangrene, and vasculitic lesions.
	Monitor lesions for signs of infection, dissemination, and other abnormal changes.
	Provide meticulous skin care using mild, nondrying, hypoallergenic soaps for cleansing.
	In collaboration with physician, provide appropriate treatment for lesions as ordered. Assess effectiveness.
	Protect skin from further injury: use paper or cloth tape; apply dressings loosely; avoid venipunctures.
	Gently massage skin to promote circulation to area.
Cardiac output, alteration in: decreased (related to myocardial ischemia)	Assess for signs and symptoms associated with changes in cardiac output: hypotension, dyspnea, edema, jugular venous distention, rales, and pulse irregularities.
	Monitor electrocardiogram for rate, rhythm, and ectopy.
	Report significant irregularities to physician.
	In collaboration with physician, administer appropriate medication as ordered. Assess effectiveness and note side effects.
	Adjust patient's activity to reduce oxygen demands and provide rest periods.
	Assess response to oxygen therapy and other interventions.
Sensory-perceptual alteration: visual (related to retinopathy resulting from retinal arteritis)	Assess degree of visual impairment.
	Provide for patient's safety.
	Perform regular ophthalmic examinations.
Anxiety	See p. 1839.
Self-concept, disturbance in: body image, role performance	See p. 1820.

Patient Education

1. Explain that many specialists will be involved in care, since this disease is multisystemic.
2. Teach the importance of regular physician follow-up.
3. Teach methods of self-assessment, and emphasize the importance of reporting significant changes to the physician.
4. Teach the method of self-assessment to detect early crises: monitoring of blood pressure, pulse, weight, proteinuria, edema, intake, and output. Instruct the patient to report dyspnea, unexplained weight gain, proteinuria, oliguria, hematuria, hypertension, abnormal changes in the eyes, paresis, new pain and melena.
5. Stress the importance of medications and provide information about them.
6. Emphasize the need for regular eye examinations.
7. Teach alternative methods for pain relief: relaxation techniques, biofeedback, guided imagery, and so on.
8. Teach the patient to keep a log of disease course, treatments, and other disease-related information.
9. Teach the patient to carry medical identification (especially if taking steroids).

EVALUATION

Patient Outcome	Data Indicating That Outcome is Reached
Medical crises are prevented.	There is no deterioration of renal function: blood urea nitrogen and creatinine levels and urinalysis results stabilize or improve. Major organ involvement remits.
Signs and symptoms are managed.	Signs and symptoms related to involved organ system(s) diminish or disappear in response to therapeutic maneuvers.
Laboratory values return to within normal limits in response to steroid therapy.	C-reactive protein, erythrocyte sedimentation rate, C3, and C4 are within normal limits.

Giant Cell Arteritis (Temporal Arteritis)

Giant cell arteritis is an inflammatory disorder of unknown etiology that affects large and medium-sized arteries in the elderly population.

Giant cell arteritis affects persons of both sexes over 50 years of age. It is twice as common in women as men. This disease is rarely seen in blacks. Any artery or the aorta may be involved, but the diagnosis is often made through biopsy of the temporal artery. Patients initially show nonspecific systemic signs, including fever. Morning headaches are frequent. Other clinical findings are related to the arteries involved.

Although the etiology is unknown, the disease may have some basis in immunologic dysfunction similar to that of other vasculitides such as polyarteritis nodosa. Cellular and humoral mechanisms reactive against elastic arterial tissue may play a role.[22]

The prognosis for giant cell arteritis is good, particularly when major vessels are uninvolved. The disease tends to be self-limiting in 2 to 5 years, but the threat of blindness makes treatment imperative. Patients respond dramatically to corticosteroid therapy with remission of clinical manifestations and lowering of the erythrocyte sedimentation rate, which can be serially monitored for recurrence of inflammatory episodes.

PATHOPHYSIOLOGY

Giant cell arteritis is distinguishable from other vasculitides because small vessels such as arterioles and capillaries are not involved. Histologic characteristics include the accumulation of histiocytes, epitheloid cells, multinucleated giant cells, lymphocytes, and plasma cells in the interna and media adjacent to the internal elastic lamina of medium-sized arteries. The elastic lamina is fragmented and may be absent in some areas. In large arteries and the aorta the media tends to be inflamed, with fragmentation of the elastic fibers. The intima is thickened more than would be expected from age alone.

The lesions are spotty and do not involve long stretches of arteries. Thrombosis may occur at inflammation sites.[22]

DIAGNOSTIC STUDIES

Giant cell arteritis should be suspected in any elderly person who has a fever of unknown origin and an elevated erythrocyte sedimentation rate. It is often associated with polymyalgia rheumatica.

Erythrocyte sedimentation rate
Greater than 50 mm/hour

Temporal artery biopsy
Positive; demonstrates inflammation of superficial temporal artery

Muscle enzymes
Normal

Electromyography
Normal

Muscle biopsy
Normal

Complete blood count
Anemia

TREATMENT PLAN

Chemotherapeutic
Corticosteroids
Prednisone, 60 mg po tapered over 4 wk until symptoms abate and erythrocyte sedimentation rate returns to normal; maintenance dose 10 mg or less po qd; alternate-day therapy not successful; can be discontinued eventually in most patients; monitor for side effects associated with steroid therapy

ASSESSMENT: AREAS OF CONCERN

Temporal artery
Temporal pain; headache; marked scalp tenderness; intermittent claudication of jaw and tongue

Aorta
Aneurysm; dissection

Internal and external carotid arteries and vertebral arteries
Transient ischemic attacks

Ophthalmic artery and central retinal artery
Visual loss (insidious or sudden onset)

Coronary arteries
Myocardial ischemia and infarction

Iliac and femoral arteries
Claudication of lower extremities

Mesenteric arteries
Abdominal pain; gastrointestinal bleeding; bowel infarction or obstruction

Systemic signs and symptoms
Fever; malaise; anorexia

NURSING DIAGNOSES and NURSING INTERVENTIONS

Nursing Diagnosis	Nursing Intervention
Tissue perfusion, potential alteration in: cerebral (related to carotid arteritis)	Assess for development of headache, transient ischemic attacks, and other changes in sensorium. Perform mental status examination. Maintain patient's safety. In collaboration with physician, administer appropriate treatment for headache and other symptoms detected during assessment. Assess effectiveness. Assess patient response to steroid therapy.
Tissue perfusion, potential alteration in: temporal aspect of head (related to temporal arteritis)	Assess for presence of temporal pain, headache, scalp tenderness, and intermittent claudication of jaw and tongue. Assess patient response to steroid therapy. In collaboration with physician, administer appropriate analgesics as ordered. Assess effectiveness.
Tissue perfusion, potential alteration in: eye (related to ophthalmic or central retinal arteritis)	Assess for presence of retinopathy, visual disturbances, and changes in acuity. Report significant findings to physician.
Tissue perfusion, potential alteration in: gastrointestinal (related to mesentery arteritis)	Assess for presence of abdominal pain, anorexia, nausea and vomiting, gastrointestinal ulceration, and hemorrhage. Palpate abdomen to detect areas of tenderness. Perform Hemoccult or guaiac test of stool. Monitor oral intake. Report significant findings to physician. In collaboration with physician, institute appropriate treatment of above conditions as ordered. Assess effectiveness.
Tissue perfusion, potential alteration in: cardiac (related to coronary arteritis)	Assess for myocardial ischemia and infarction: monitoring for angina, monitoring of serial electrocardiograms, monitoring of chest roentgenograms, auscultation of heart to determine rate, rhythm, and regularity of pulse, monitoring of cardiac enzymes, monitoring of vital signs. Report significant abnormal findings to physician. In collaboration with physician, institute appropriate treatment (oxygen, vasodilators, and so on) as ordered. Assess effectiveness.
Tissue perfusion, potential alteration in: lower extremities (related to iliac and femoral arteritis)	Assess for claudication: presence of pain during ambulation. Report claudication to physician. Assess response to steroid therapy.
Mobility, impaired physical (related to claudication)	Assess degree of impairment. Encourage regular program of walking distances slowly and Beurger-Allen exercises.

Nursing Diagnosis	Nursing Intervention
Comfort, alteration in: pain (related to myocardial ischemia, temporal arteritis, or claudication)	Assess pain: location, onset, duration, and precipitating and alleviating factors. Have patient describe intensity on scale of 0 to 10. In collaboration with physician, provide appropriate analgesic agents as ordered. Assess effectiveness and side effects. Assess response to steroid therapy. In collaboration with physician, institute appropriate other measures relative to tissues and organs involved. Assess effectiveness.
Sensory-perceptual alteration: visual (related to ophthalmic and retinal arteritis)	Assess degree of visual impairment. Provide for patient safety. Encourage patient to receive regular ophthalmic examinations.
Cardiac output, alteration in: decreased (related to aortic aneurysm or aortic dissection)	Assess for findings associated with aortic aneurysm. Assess for findings associated with aortic dissection. Report significant abnormal findings to physician. In collaboration with physician, institute appropriate interventions. Assess effectiveness.
Anxiety	Counsel patient that this disorder is often self-limiting and is highly responsive to chemotherapy (see p. 1671).

Patient Education

1. Emphasize the importance of steroid therapy and provide information about it (see p. 1732).
2. Teach the patient complications and crises for which to monitor: transient ischemic attacks, claudication, visual loss, gastrointestinal bleeding, and myocardial infarction.
3. Teach the importance of medical alert identification.

EVALUATION

Patient Outcome	Data Indicating That Outcome is Reached
Complications and medical crises are avoided in response to steroid therapy.	There is no evidence of progressive pain, visual loss, aortic aneurysm or dissection, gastrointestinal bleeding, cerebral ischemia, or myocardial infarction.
Laboratory values return to normal in response to steroid therapy.	Erythrocyte sedimentation rate is within normal limits.

Polymyalgia Rheumatica

Polymyalgia rheumatica is a well-defined inflammatory disorder of the proximal muscles that usually affects men and women over 50 years of age.

Polymyalgia rheumatica is accompanied by a highly elevated erythrocyte sedimentation rate and is often diagnosed on the basis of a rapid clinical response to corticosteroid therapy. The onset may be acute or insidious and is associated with pain and morning stiffness in the back and neck, as well as in the pelvic and shoulder girdles. Anorexia, weight loss, fever, and mild anemia may be present as well. Temporal arteritis also develops in many patients.

PATHOPHYSIOLOGY

The origin and pathogenesis of polymyalgia rheumatica are unknown. Although elevation of the erythrocyte sedimentation rate is indicative of an inflammatory process, and despite the severe pain associated with the muscle involvement, findings of muscle examinations are normal.

DIAGNOSTIC STUDIES

Erythrocyte sedimentation rate
Elevated (often greater than 100 mm/hour)

Corticosteroid challenge
Rapid, dramatic response

Creatine phosphokinase
Normal; to distinguish from polymyositis

Muscle biopsy
Normal; to distinguish from polymyositis

Serum protein electrophoresis
Normal; to distinguish from myeloma

Rheumatoid factor
Normal; along with absence of synovitis, to distinguish
from arthritis

TREATMENT PLAN

The goal of the treatment plan is to induce a remission
of the disease using low-dose corticosteroid therapy.

Chemotherapeutic
Corticosteroids
Prednisone, 10 mg qd, or equivalent low-dose corticosteroid; larger doses may be employed but are
usually tapered rapidly; although some patients
are able to discontinue drug after several months,
most require prolonged maintenance therapy with
small doses

ASSESSMENT: AREAS OF CONCERN

Musculoskeletal system
Pain in proximal muscles: shoulder girdle, back, neck
and pelvis, unassociated with deformity or synovitis; elevated erythrocyte sedimentation rate; normal creatine phosphokinase level (above findings in
combination in elderly patient are classic diagnostic
features of polymyalgia rheumatica)

NURSING DIAGNOSES and NURSING INTERVENTIONS

Nursing Diagnosis	Nursing Intervention
Comfort, alteration in: pain (related to proximal muscle involvement)	Assess pain: location, onset, duration, and provocative and palliative factors. Have patient rate intensity on scale of 0 to 10. Assess response to corticosteroid therapy. Supplement with aspirin or acetaminophen as prescribed. Administer hot or cold thermal therapy to affected muscles. Perform limited range of motion exercises as tolerated to combat stiffness and prevent atrophy from immobilization.
Activity intolerance (related to proximal muscle weakness and pain)	Assess patient's limitations. Employ interventions listed above to limit pain. Encourage patient to explore alternative methods of performing activities of daily living. Encourage balanced program of rest and exercise as tolerated.
Anxiety	Counsel patients that this disorder responds well to steroid therapy; activity intolerance may be short lived.
Self-concept, disturbance in: role performance	See p. 1820.

Patient Education

1. Teach the importance and side effects of prednisone (see p. 1732).
2. Explain that family members may find it difficult to accept the patient's illness, since patients often do not appear to be sick. Encourage honest, open communication between family members. Include the family when giving information about polymyalgia.
3. Teach that temporal (giant cell) arteritis may be a complication of the disease. Alert the patient to associated symptoms, including headache, scalp tenderness, and intermittent claudication of the jaw or tongue.
4. Teach the importance of medical alert identification.

EVALUATION

Patient Outcome	Data Indicating That Outcome is Reached
Laboratory findings are within normal limits.	Erythrocyte sedimentation rate is within normal limits.
Pain is relieved or minimized.	Subjective distress is decreased. Objective decrease is based on rating scale.

SARCOIDOSIS

Sarcoidosis is a multisystem granulomatous disorder of unknown cause.

In the United States approximately 34 cases of sarcoidosis per 100,000 population are diagnosed each year. Cases are equally distributed between both sexes. Although all races and age groups may be affected, sarcoidosis occurs most commonly in adults, especially blacks younger than 40 years of age.

The prognosis of sarcoidosis varies depending on the degree of systemic involvement and the intensity of steroid therapy. Sarcoidosis may be staged according to international standards, based on chest roentgenograms of patients with pulmonary involvement, the major clinical finding (Table 16-5). The disease is fatal in about 5% of cases. Current research focuses on determining the immunologic pathogenesis of the disease through detailed studies of immune function of cells derived from sarcoid tissue.

PATHOPHYSIOLOGY

No single factor has been convincingly identified as the etiologic agent, although several have been proposed: viruses, organic dust, pine pollen, fungi, and beryllium, to name a few. Immune system abnormalities include lymphopenia with decreased T cell numbers, impaired lymphocyte function, anergy, and panhypergammaglobulinemia. Although the exact role of such mechanisms is unknown, these findings suggest a problem of the T cell population and perhaps, more specifically, with lymphokine production. In other granulomatous diseases,

such as tuberculosis, granuloma formation occurs as a result of inadequate clearance of a pathogen by macrophages. These macrophages require the help of T cells that secrete lymphokines that, in turn, activate poorly effective macrophages to become aggressive phagocytic cells. The lack of lymphokine secretion may help to explain the granuloma formation in sarcoidosis.

DIAGNOSTIC STUDIES

Differential diagnoses include tuberculosis, mediastinal lymphoma, and other granulomatous lung diseases.

Delayed-type hypersensitivity skin test
  Absence of response (anergy)

Chest roentgenogram
  Varies from prominent hilar lymphadenopathy to diffuse pulmonary infiltrates with fibrosis

Serum protein electrophoresis
  Polyclonal hypergammaglobulinemia: usually increased IgG, but IgA and IgM may also be elevated

Kviem test
  Intradermally injected sarcoid tissue suspension; positive in 60% to 80%

Tissue biopsy
  Noncaseating granulomas

C-reactive protein
  Elevated in associated acute arthritis

Erythrocyte sedimentation rate
  Elevated in associated acute arthritis

Table 16-5
Staging, Prognosis, and Treatment of Sarcoidosis

Stage	Chest Roentgenogram	Prognosis	Corticosteroid Therapy
1	Bilateral hilar adenopathy	Resolves in 60% of cases	None
2	Bilateral hilar adenopathy with parenchymal pulmonary infiltration	Resolves in 46% of cases	Yes, to decrease pulmonary fibrosis and relieve symptoms
3	Advanced parenchymal pulmonary infiltration with nodular densities	Resolves in 12% of cases	Same as stage 2

TREATMENT PLAN

Chemotherapeutic
Corticosteroids
   Prednisone in doses adjusted to relieve symptoms and reverse fibrosis of pulmonary tissue
Optic agents
   Methylcellulose eye drops and assorted ophthalmic ointments to treat ocular manifestations
Antiarrhythmic agents
   For ventricular ectopy
Treatment of arthritis manifestations varies depending on their severity; salicylates used first, followed by nonsteroidal anti-inflammatory agents, and finally corticosteroids, including intra-articular injections

Supportive
Chest physiotherapy, breathing exercises, postural drainage, and oxygen therapy as necessary for prophylaxis or as treatment for chronic pulmonary disease
Serial sinus and chest roentgenograms and pulmonary function studies as necessary to follow disease course and determine adequacy of treatment
Thermal therapy and joint supports for arthritis

ASSESSMENT: AREAS OF CONCERN

Constitutional signs and symptoms
Malaise; fever; weight loss; anorexia

Pulmonary status
Parenchymal lesions (in asymptomatic patients or associated with dyspnea and nonproductive cough); pulmonary fibrosis; cough; superinfection; restrictive disease; decreased vital capacity

Skin and mucous membrane integrity
Small skin nodules over face, neck, and extremities; vitiligo; alopecia; erythema nodosum

Ocular integrity
Blurred vision; lacrimation; ocular pain; conjunctival infection; uveitis; Sjögren's syndrome; iritis

Salivary gland status
Nontender enlargement of parotid and other salivary glands

Reticuloendothelial system status
Lymphadenopathy; bilateral hilar adenopathy; mediastinal or peripheral lymphadenopathy; splenomegaly with or without anemia, leukopenia, and thrombocytopenia

Cardiovascular status
Arrhythmias: bundle-branch block or ventricular ectopy; cor pulmonale

Hepatic manifestations
Chronic granulomatous hepatitis: jaundice, hepatomegaly, increased alkaline phosphatase

Musculoskeletal status
Arthritis (symmetric, migratory); arthralgias (diffuse); muscle weakness, soreness, and wasting (symmetric)

NURSING DIAGNOSES and NURSING INTERVENTIONS

Nursing Diagnosis	Nursing Intervention
Gas exchange, impaired (related to pulmonary fibrosis, infection, restrictive disease, or parenchymal lesions)	Assess respiratory status: note respiratory rate, rhythm, and quality, presence of hemoptysis, cough, adventitious breath sounds, or dyspnea. Monitor results of pulmonary function studies. Obtain sputum specimens for culture to determine presence of secondary pulmonary infection. Reinforce teaching related to proper positioning, body mechanics, and breathing exercises. In collaboration with physician, administer appropriate respiratory medications and oxygen therapy for treatment of restrictive lung disease or infection. Assess effectiveness and note side effects.
Cardiac output, alteration in: decreased (related to arrhythmias or cor pulmonale)	Assess for signs and symptoms associated with decreased cardiac output: hypotension, dyspnea, edema, jugular venous distention, rales, and pulse irregularities. Monitor electrocardiograms for rate, rhythm, and ectopy. Report significant electrocardiographic irregularities and other abnormal assessment data to physician. In collaboration with physician, administer appropriate cardiac medications. Assess effectiveness and note side effects.

Nursing Diagnosis	Nursing Intervention
	Adjust patient's activity to reduce oxygen demands and provide rest periods. Assess response to oxygen therapy and other interventions.
Comfort, alteration in: pain (related to ocular discomfort, infection, arthralgias, erythema nodosum, or synovitis)	Assess pain: location, onset, duration, and provocative and palliative factors. Have patient rate pain on scale of 0 to 10. In collaboration with physician, institute appropriate interventions and administer analgesics based on underlying cause of pain. Assess effectiveness, and note side effects.
Sensory-perceptual alteration: visual (related to Sjögren's syndrome, lacrimation, conjunctivitis, iritis, or uveitis)	Assess degree of visual impairment. Provide for patient safety. Encourage patient to have regular ophthalmic examinations. In collaboration with physician, administer appropriate ocular medication as ordered. Assess effectiveness.
Tissue perfusion, alteration in: liver (related to hepatitis granulomatous disease)	Assess for hepatic dysfunction: monitor serum glutamic oxaloacetic transaminase, serum glutamic pyruvic transaminase, lactic dehydrogenase, alkaline phosphatase, and total bilirubin. Monitor for associated jaundice, lethargy, and weakness.
Potential patient problem: susceptibility to infection	Assess for anorexia, failure to thrive, pain, weakness, and lethargy. Assess for evidence of infection at sites of invasive procedures. Assess for breaks in skin integrity, particularly over pressure areas and oral mucosa. Assess pulmonary status: auscultate lung fields to determine presence of adventitious breath sounds. Maintain optimal nutritional status and fluid intake. Assess ocular integrity for evidence of conjunctivitis: erythematous, pruritic conjunctivae. Assess mentation for evidence of central nervous system infection: level of consciousness, headache, and visual disturbances. Assess for evidence of gastrointestinal infection: abdominal pain, fever, and diarrhea. Monitor temperature and vital signs for evidence of fever and sepsis. Maintain body hygiene. Limit environmental stress. Monitor laboratory data: white blood cell count and differential, erythrocyte sedimentation rate, C-reactive protein, urinalysis, and cultures. In collaboration with physician, administer appropriate antimicrobial, antipyretic, or analgesic medication. Assess patient response. Monitor for side effects. Promote pulmonary toilet: breathing exercises, postural drainage, and chest physical therapy. Maintain normal sleep and rest patterns. Protect patient from physical injury. Provide clean environment. Maintain protective isolation based on hospital policy. Restrict contact with family and health care providers who have infectious diseases. Maintain good handwashing before and after contact with patient.
Anxiety	See p. 1839.
Self-concept, disturbances in: body image	See p. 1820.

Patient Education

1. Teach facts about, and the importance of, prescribed medications.
2. Provide information related to system involvement: assessment and reporting of signs and symptoms.
3. Teach the importance of chest physiotherapy, postural drainage, steroid therapy, and other methods of dealing with pulmonary compromise.
4. Teach signs and symptoms of infections.
5. Teach about the avoidance of risk factors associated with infection.
6. Teach the principles of good nutrition.
7. Teach the importance of medical alert identification.

EVALUATION

Patient Outcome	Data Indicating That Outcome is Reached
Pulmonary involvement is reversed.	Chest roentgenogram shows clear or improved lungs fields.
Other symptoms are resolved or prevented.	There are no symptoms associated with individual system involvement.
Laboratory findings are within normal limits.	There is positive response to cutaneous recall antigens (anergy is reversed). Serum protein electrophoresis findings return to normal. Kviem test findings are negative.
Medical complications and crises are prevented.	There is no respiratory failure, secondary infection, vision loss, or hepatic failure.

REITER'S SYNDROME

Reiter's syndrome is a relatively common, chronic, multisystem inflammatory disease characterized by the development of seronegative asymmetric arthropathy that may be associated with urethritis, cervicitis, dysentery, inflammatory eye disease, or mucocutaneous disease involving the penis, oral mucosa, or skin.

Reiter's syndrome has been a subject of worldwide research since the discovery of its link with HLA-B27 in 1973. This finding suggested a genetic predisposition. A search for the environmental factor or factors that act as inciting agents ensued. Although such an agent remains elusive, current data suggest that enteric infection may play a role. Microbes that have been implicated include *Shigella flexneri*, *Shigella dysenteriae*, and *Yersinia enterocolitica*.[7] Venereal infections with *Chlamydia* and *Mycoplasma* have also been associated with Reiter's syndrome.

Based on this evidence it is theorized that patients with a specific genetic background (HLA-B27) may develop Reiter's syndrome following infestation by a variety of microbes. Research continues with the goals of improving its recognition, defining etiologic factors, and ultimately, finding a cure.

The incidence of Reiter's syndrome is difficult to assess for a variety of reasons. Current research indicates that this disease occurs primarily in white males throughout the world. Although it may be detected at any age, it is usually diagnosed in the third decade. Reiter's syndrome may be the most common inflammatory arthropathy detected in young men. The pathogenesis of Reiter's syndrome is unknown.

DIAGNOSTIC STUDIES

Differential diagnoses include infective arthritis, rheumatic fever, and psoriatic arthropathy.

History
Recent history of dysentery or venereal disease combined with inflammatory monarthropathy or oligoarthropathy, urethritis, cervicitis, and ocular and cutaneous inflammatory changes

Roentgenograms of muculoskeletal system
Erosive joint changes; juxta-articular osteoporosis; plantar spurs

Erythrocyte sedimentation rate
Variable from 1 to 130 mm/hour

HLA typing
HLA-B27 (this test is costly and unnecessary and is usually performed only as an academic endeavor)

TREATMENT PLAN

The goals of the treatment plan include management of signs and symptoms and early detection of disabling complications. This disease has no cure, and current treatment is empiric and inadequate.

Chemotherapeutic
Nonsteroidal anti-inflammatory agents
To treat synovitis and arthralgias; any agent may be tried; one clinician reports success with indomethacin (Indocin), 25-50 mg tid, and phenylbutazone (Butazolidin), 100 mg tid or qid[7]
Corticosteroids
Methylprednisone (Medrol), 40-80 mg intralesionally for arthropathy, tendinitis, etc.
Steroid eye drops or subconjunctival ointments for conjunctivitis
Antineoplastic agents[7]
Azathioprine (Imuran), 0.75-2.5 mg/kg body weight qd for immunosuppression until symptomatic improvement, usually 2-12 wk, then tapered dosage

Methotrexate

Anti-infective agents

Use is controversial and varies depending on existing infection

Analgesics and nonsteroidal anti-inflammatory agents

To reduce pain associated with arthritis and ocular inflammation

Optic agents

Methylcellulose eye drops for symptomatic relief of ocular discomfort

Supportive

Physical therapy for arthritis complications

Rest to conserve energy during acute exacerbations

Counseling to allay feelings of guilt or anxiety about sexual misconduct

Use of condom to protect patient from postvenereal exacerbation[7]

Discouragement of use of topical steroidal medications for skin involvement, since atrophy may occur

Meticulous skin care of involved areas

Periodic assessment for symptoms associated wth uveitis, spondylitis, and cardiac or pulmonary involvement

ASSESSMENT: AREAS OF CONCERN

Musculoskeletal involvement

Arthritis, particularly of weight-bearing joints; tendonitis, especially of Achilles tendon; plantar fasciitis; back pain such as sacroiliitis and ankylosing spondylitis; costochondritis, often manifested as pleuritic chest pain; dactylitis

Genitourinary involvement

Urethritis; cervicitis; cystitis; balanitis

Gastrointestinal involvement

Stomatitis; diarrhea: acute passage of bloody, loose stools over 24-hour period, precedes rheumatic syndrome by 1 to 3 weeks

Ocular involvement

Conjunctivitis; uveitis; optic neuritis; intraocular hemorrhage; blindness (late)

Skin integrity

Keratoderma blennorrhagica (hyperkeratotic nodules); balanitis: painless, superficial lesions of coronal margins of prepuce and adjacent glands; nails: subungual corny material that accumulates under and may lift nail plate, which becomes yellow and thickened

Cardiovascular status

Electrocardiogram: increased PR interval, heart block, ST segment changes, abnormal Q waves; palpitations; transient murmurs; pericardial rub; aortic regurgitation

NURSING DIAGNOSES and NURSING INTERVENTIONS

Nursing Diagnosis	Nursing Intervention
Mobility, impaired physical (related to arthritis)	Assess degree of physical immobility resulting from arthritis.
	In collaboration with physician, provide nonsteroidal anti-inflammatory agents. Assess effectiveness.
	Encourage patient to rest joints during periods of acute inflammation. Otherwise, encourage program of regular exercise, including range of motion exercises, as tolerated. Confer with physical or occupational therapist to determine other beneficial interventions.
Comfort, alteration in: pain (related to inflammatory conditions of eye, genitourinary tract, joints, and gastrointestinal tract)	Determine location of pain.
	Assess degree of discomfort using subjective data and objective measurement on 0 to 10 rating scale.
	In collaboration with physician, provide analgesic agents as ordered. Assess effectiveness and note side effects.
	In collaboration with physician, institute other appropriate measures relative to system involved. Assess effectiveness.
Sensory-perceptual alteration: visual (related to conjunctivitis and uveitis)	Assess degree of visual impairment.
	Provide for patient's safety.
	Provide methylcellulose 1% eye drops as needed.
	In collaboration with physician, provide steroidal eye drops and anti-infective agents as ordered. Assess effectiveness.

Nursing Diagnosis	Nursing Intervention
Skin integrity, impairment of (related to multiple skin lesions)	Assess skin for presence of lesions and hyperkeratotic nodules. Monitor lesions for signs of infection, dissemination, and other abnormal changes. Provide or encourage patient to perform meticulous foot care with special attention to nail integrity. Provide mild, nondrying, hypoallergenic soaps for skin cleansing, and encourage their use. Assess effectiveness of treatment of lesions.
Bowel elimination, alteration in: diarrhea (related to gastrointestinal infection)	Assess severity of diarrhea: monitor for passage of bloody stools and quantify output. Assess for signs and symptoms associated with electrolyte imbalance. Provide fluids and encourage adequate fluid intake. Provide for patient's safety if weakness becomes a problem. In collaboration with physician, administer appropriate anti-infective agents. Assess effectiveness and note side effects.
Urinary elimination: alteration in patterns (related to urethritis or cystitis)	Assess for signs and symptoms associated with urethritis or cystitis: dysuria, pyuria, hematuria, and fever. In collaboration with physician, administer appropriate anti-infective agents. Assess effectiveness and note side effects.
Cardiac output, alteration in: decreased (related to Reiter's syndrome)	Assess patient for presence of palpitations, murmurs, and pericardial rub. Assess electrocardiogram for prolonged PR interval, heart block, ST segment changes, and abnormal Q waves. In collaboration with physician, institute appropriate measures based on assessment. Assess effectiveness of specific interventions.
Anxiety	See p. 1839.
Self-concept, disturbance in: body image	See p. 1820.

Patient Education

1. Teach the importance of reporting symptoms associated with significant complications of Reiter's syndrome: spondylitis, uveitis, ocular hemorrhage, and cardiopulmonary disease.
2. Teach that the use of a condom during sexual activity will limit exposure to venereal disease, which could exacerbate Reiter's syndrome.
3. Teach the importance of physician follow-up to monitor the disease course. The physician should also be consulted for management of acute episodes.
4. Teach facts about and the importance of prescribed medications.
5. Teach the importance of keeping a personal log of the disease course, treatments, and other disease-related information.
6. Teach the importance of medical alert identification.

EVALUATION

Patient Outcome	Data Indicating That Outcome is Reached
Symptoms resolve in response to therapeutic measures.	There are no symptoms associated with individual system involvement.
Pain is relieved or minimized.	There is decrease in subjective distress. Objective decrease is based on rating scale.
Medical crises are prevented.	There are no life-threatening side effects of chemotherapeutic interventions. Blindness, crippling spondylitis, and cardiopulmonary compromise do not occur.
Patient complies with treatment.	Patient verbalizes understanding of importance of compliance, adherence to prescribed regimens, and symptom control.

SJÖGREN'S SYNDROME

Sjögren's syndrome is a chronic inflammatory disorder of unknown etiology that affects primarily the lacrimal and salivary glands.

The major symptoms of Sjögren's syndrome are keratoconjunctivitis and xerostomia, which result from decreased lacrimal and salivary gland secretion, respectively. The syndrome is often associated with other connective tissue diseases, especially rheumatoid arthritis, systemic lupus erythematosus, and progressive systemic sclerosis (scleroderma). Twenty percent of patients with Sjögren's syndrome manifest Raynaud's phenomenon. Ninety percent are middle-aged women, with a mean age of 50 years. All races may be affected. There is evidence that sex hormones play an etiologic role in the disease, and research in this area continues.

PATHOPHYSIOLOGY

Biopsy specimens from glandular lesions demonstrate infiltration by lymphocytes, plasma cells, and macrophages, which replace secretory acinar tissue. Anti–salivary duct antibodies have been observed. The factors precipitating such autodestruction of host tissue are unknown. Destruction of tissue results in decreased secretion by involved glands. In addition, dryness of the nose, pharynx, and tracheobronchial tree may occur.

DIAGNOSTIC STUDIES

Differential diagnoses include Felty's syndrome, Raynaud's phenomenon, chronic thyroiditis, hepatomegaly, chronic active hepatitis, gastric achlorhydria, acute pancreatitis, adult celiac disease, polymyositis, drug-induced xerostomia, irradiation xerostomia, diabetes, sarcoidosis, salivary duct stones, and mumps.

Salivary scintigraphy
Decreased uptake, concentration, and excretion of intravenous ^{99m}Tc pertechnetate by major salivary glands; measured by means of sequential scintophotographic technique

Sialography
Dilations and other changes such as atrophy within intrasalivary duct system[1]

Labial salivary gland biopsy
Infiltration of tissue by lymphocytes, plasma cells, and macrophages; replacement of acinar tissue

Schirmer test
Decreased tear production; less than 15 mm of filter strip wetted

Complete blood count
Mild anemia; leukopenia

Erythrocyte sedimentation rate
Elevated

Serum protein electrophoresis
Hypergammaglobulinemia

Rheumatoid factor
Elevated (90%)

Antinuclear antibody
Greater than 1:80 (70%) anti–salivary duct antibodies, thyroid antibodies, gastric-parietal cell autoantibodies

TREATMENT PLAN

The goals of the treatment plan are to provide palliative measures and prevent complications of this chronic disorder.

Chemotherapeutic
Corticosteroids
Prednisone; dose titrated for relief of *severe* symptoms; usually administered only late in course of disease when symptoms are unrelieved by supportive approaches
Antineoplastic agents
Cyclophosphamide; success varies and use is controversial[1]
Optic agents
Artificial tears (0.5% methylcellulose eye drops) as needed

Supportive
Avoidance of sour or sweetened drinks or candies
Mouth rinses of 1% methylcellulose
Oral hygiene with frequent brushing, flossing, and fluoride rinses
Regular dental examinations
Regular conjunctival cultures to detect ocular infections

ASSESSMENT: AREAS OF CONCERN

Oral cavity
Xerostomia: dental caries (multiple), oral candidiasis, dysphagia, difficulty chewing, changes in phonation, adherence of food to buccal mucosa, hoarseness, fissures and ulcerations of tongue, buccal mucosa, and lips, frequent ingestion of liquids with meals

Eyes

Conjunctivitis: foreign body sensation, "grittiness," burning, accumulation of thick ropy strands at inner canthus, decreased tearing, redness, photosensitivity, eye fatigue; pruritus; filmy sensation that interferes with vision; (late) corneal ulceration, vascularization, and opacification

Skin

Dryness

Ears

Recurrent otitis media

Respiratory tract

Nasal mucosal dryness; epistaxis; bronchitis; pneumonia

Parotid gland

Episodic, unilateral parotitis (often associated with fever, tenderness, and erythema)

In addition to the above, a relatively small percentage of patients with Sjögren's syndrome show symptoms associated with pancreatitis, hepatomegaly, renal tubular defects, thyroiditis, glomerulonephritis, myositis, and lymphoreticular malignancies.[1]

NURSING DIAGNOSES and NURSING INTERVENTIONS

Nursing Diagnosis	Nursing Intervention
Sensory-perceptual alteration: visual (related to keratoconjunctivitis)	Assess degree of visual deficit. Administer 0.5% methylcellulose eye drops as needed. Obtain regular cultures of eye. In collaboration with physician, administer antimicrobial ointments for ocular infections as needed. Administer hot or cold therapy to eyes as needed. Encourage use of sunglasses as needed. Encourage patient to have semiannual ophthalmic examinations.
Oral mucous membrane, alteration in (related to xerostomia)	Assess oral skin integrity for presence of ulcerations, fissures, and candidiasis. Provide or encourage patient to perform frequent oral hygiene: brushing, flossing, and fluoride rinses. Force fluids as tolerated; avoid sour or sweetened liquids. Encourage semiannual dental examinations.
Comfort, alteration in: pain (related to parotitis, conjunctivitis, and otitis)	Assess pain: location, onset, duration, and provocative and palliative factors. Have patient rate intensity on scale of 0 to 10. In collaboration with physician, administer appropriate analgesics as ordered. Assess effectiveness, and note side effects.
Gas exchange, impaired (related to nasal mucosal dryness, bronchitis, and pneumonia)	Assess degree of respiratory impairment: monitor rate, rhythm, and quality of respirations, and monitor for epistaxis, hemoptysis, dyspnea, and cough. Obtain sputum specimens for culture. In collaboration with physician, administer appropriate anti-infective therapy and other respiratory-related medications for treatment of bronchitis or pneumonia. Assess effectiveness and note side effects. Administer saline soaks for nasal dryness.
Skin integrity, impairment of: potential (related to skin dryness)	Assess skin integrity: color, moisture, lesions, vascularity, and so on. Provide and encourage use of lotions, creams, or ointments for skin dryness. Provide and encourage use of lubricants such as K-Y Jelly for vaginal dryness.

Patient Education

1. Teach the use of artificial tears.
2. Teach the importance of obtaining regular eye examinations.
3. Teach the importance of meticulous oral hygiene: frequent brushing of teeth and use of dental floss and mouth rinses.
4. Teach the importance of increasing fluid intake to control xerostomia.
5. Teach the patient to avoid sour or sweetened drinks and candies.
6. Teach the importance of regular dental examinations for presence of dental caries and the need for fluoride treatments.
7. Teach self-assessment of the oral cavity for development of lesions, fissures, and ulcerations.
8. Teach the importance and side effects of medications.

9. Teach the importance of regular follow-up to detect presence of underlying autoimmune or neoplastic disease.
10. Teach that the use of unnecessary antibiotics should be avoided (owing to increased incidence of drug allergy, especially to penicillin).
11. Teach that regular application of saline soaks for nasal dryness may be beneficial. Oil-based lubricants should be avoided to limit the risk of lipoid pneumonia.
12. Teach that skin dryness often responds to a variety of lotions, creams, and emollients. Vaginal dryness leading to dyspareunia usually responds to lubricants such as K-Y Jelly.

EVALUATION

Patient Outcome	Data Indicating That Outcome is Reached
Pain is relieved or minimized.	Patient reports subjective decrease. Objective decrease is based on rating scale. Patient has fewer subjective complaints of oral and ocular dryness.
Medical complications and crises are avoided.	There is no evidence of corneal abrasions, oral ulcerations, recurrent otitis, or respiratory infections.

AMYLOIDOSIS

Amyloidosis is a syndrome characterized by deposition of amyloid (proteinaceous material) in tissues.

Amyloidosis occurs as an acquired or hereditary disorder and may be a primary disease or be associated with a variety of other illnesses. Although its etiology is unknown, at least two observations suggest that amyloidosis represents immunologic dysfunction: the presence of immunoglobulin proteins in amyloid deposits and the syndrome's increased incidence in inflammatory, infectious, and neoplastic diseases.

The term ''amyloid,'' which means starchlike, is a misnomer. The syndrome is actually characterized by the diffuse deposition of insoluble proteinaceous material in the extracellular matrix of one or more organs. The accumulation of amyloid encroaches on parenchymal tissues, compromising organ function. Clinical manifestations of amyloidosis vary widely and depend on the organs involved and the severity with which they are affected. Specific immunotherapy to treat the underlying cause of organ failure is lacking, so treatment is restricted to management of signs and symptoms. For this reason amyloidosis is usually fatal. Renal failure and cardiac diseases are the most frequent causes of death.[16,25]

Types of Amyloidosis[16]

Primary generalized amyloidosis (PGA) occurs in the absence of associated diseases, although most patients exhibit some type of plasma cell dyscrasia. PGA accounts for 50% to 60% of all cases of amyloidosis. Deposits of amyloid are found in mesenchymal tissues of the heart, tongue, carpal tunnel, gastrointestinal tract, peripheral nerves, skin, joints, and skeletal muscle. Although this type of amyloidosis may occur as early as the second decade, the mean age at diagnosis is approximately 60 years. Men are affected more often than women, and whites more than nonwhites. Virtually all patients with classic PGA demonstrate a monoclonal immunoglobulin in their serum or urine and bone marrow plasmacytosis.

Multiple myeloma-associated amyloidosis (MMA) accounts for approximately 30% of cases. In roughly 15% of myeloma patients, clinical findings are consistent with a diagnosis of amyloidosis.[13] Serum and urine paraproteins are found. The clinical presentation, age, and sexual predilection are similar to PGA. Amyloidosis contributes to early morbidity in myeloma disease.

Secondary generalized amyloidosis (SGA), detected in 10% of the patients, occurs as a result of a variety of long-term or poorly controlled inflammatory, infectious, or neoplastic diseases. Adult and juvenile rheumatoid arthritis may be the most frequent predisposing factor. SGA has also been reported in other inflammatory conditions, including ankylosing spondylitis, Reiter's syndrome, psoriatic arthritis, chronic rheumatic heart disease, dermatomyositis, scleroderma, Behçet's disease, and systemic lupus erythematosus.

Neoplastic diseases associated with the development of amyloidosis include gastrointestinal, pulmonary, and genitourinary carcinomas, non-Hodgkin's lymphomas, malignant melanomas, and most frequently, hypernephroma and Hodgkin's disease. Chronic, systemic infections are a significant factor associated with worldwide distribution. Such infectious diatheses include tuberculosis, pyelonephritis, osteomyelitis, inflammatory bowel disease, and chronically infected burns.

In addition to the above types, amyloidosis is also described as a hereditary illness detected with increased frequency in various countries and some well-defined areas of the United States. Neuropathic, nephropathic, and cardiopathic syndromes have been described.

PATHOPHYSIOLOGY

Only limited insight has been gained into the pathogenesis of this syndrome. Histologic staining techniques and electron microscopy have provided some clues. Fibers formed from laterally aggregated protein fibrils have been detected in amyloid deposits. Some of these fibrils are apparently derived from free immunoglobulin light chains. In addition, amyloid deposits are further constructed of globular glycoprotein subunits (pentagonal, or ''P'' components) absorbed from the serum into the fibrillar units.

An explanation for the deposition of the proteinaceous substance has not yet been found. Whatever the reason, accumulation of amyloid in extracellular spaces results in pressure atrophy and eventual necrosis and destruction of underlying tissue. Organ dysfunction and failure are responsible for clinical manifestations. Amyloid deposition occurs in the following areas:

Articular
  Glenohumeral junction
  Synovial villi
Neurologic
  Dural blood vessels
  Autonomic ganglia
  Spinal nerve roots
  Peripheral nerves
Renal
  Glomeruli
  Arteriolar walls
  Tubular basement membranes
Cardiac
  All layers of the cardiac walls (predominantly myocardium)
  Conduction tissue
  Intramural coronary arterioles
Pulmonary (any area)
  Upper nasal passages
  Vocal cords
  Tracheobronchial submucosa
  Parenchyma
Gastrointestinal (any area)
  Gingiva
  Tongue
  Oropharyngeal muscles
  Liver
  Voluntary muscles of upper third of esophagus
  Diffuse esophageal infiltrates
  Small bowel
Integumentary
  Face
  Upper trunk

DIAGNOSTIC STUDIES

Tissue biopsy
  Apple-green birefringence of Congo red–stained tissue specimens under polarization microscopy; tissue from organ suspected to be infiltrated with amyloid preferred, but rectal biopsy findings positive in approximately 80% of cases of generalized amyloidosis[16]

Serum and urine electrophoresis
  Paraproteins detected in presense of associated plasma cell dyscrasia

Bone marrow aspiration and biopsy
  Plasmacytosis in presence of associated multiple myeloma

TREATMENT PLAN

The goals of therapy in amyloidosis are to prevent further deposition of amyloid material and to promote or accelerate its resorption.

Surgical
  Serial biopsies to determine regression of amyloid deposition

Chemotherapeutic
  Antineoplastic agents
    May be used to reduce the serum concentration of amyloid precursor light chains if underlying B cell dyscrasia is present
  Colchicine, dimethyl sulfoxide (DMSO), and corticosteroids have met with some success, although their use remains controversial; corticosteroids are used primarily to treat underlying inflammatory or neoplastic disorder

Electromechanical
  Plasmapheresis may interrupt dissemination of amyloid precursor light chains (see p. 1730)

Supportive
  Family and patient counseling to assist in coping with fatal illness
  Supportive approaches for complications
    For congestive heart failure: conservative management; avoid use of digitalis unless closely mon-

itored in hospital setting (usually cardiac amyloid is unresponsive to treatment with digitalis)

For neuropathic hypotension: elastic stockings

For malabsorption syndromes: broad-spectrum antibiotics

For macroglossia: supplemental Keo-Feed gastrostomy feeding; tracheostomy for upper airway obstruction

For respiratory tract amyloidosis: bronchoscopy with curettage of amyloid deposits

For renal failure: dialysis

ASSESSMENT: AREAS OF CONCERN

Neurologic status

Idiopathic, sensorimotor, peripheral neuropathy with autonomic neuropathy; depressed pain and temperature sensation, and motor dysfunction of lower extremities

Cardiovascular status

Restrictive cardiomyopathy with low-voltage electrocardiogram; chest pain; myocardial infarction; conduction disturbances in absence of other recognized causes

Skin integrity

Waxy, indurated papules and purpura; skin thickening; ''orange-peel'' skin; alopecia; periorbital purpura

Joint integrity

Rheumatoid-like arthritis

Renal status

Proteinuria; idiopathic nephrotic syndrome

Pulmonary status

Nasal lesions; vocal cord nodules; bronchiectasis; airway obstruction; wheezing; dyspnea; hilar adenopathy

Gastrointestinal status

Macroglossia: dysphagia, deglutination, and dysphonia; impaired esophageal peristalsis: gastric accumulation, mobility disturbances, hemorrhage, obstruction achlorhydria, and vitamin B_{12} deficiency; small bowel impairment: diarrhea, constipation, malabsorption, hemorrhage, protein-losing enteropathy, perforation, and ischemic necrosis; hepatomegaly without portal insufficiency or hypertension

NURSING DIAGNOSES and NURSING INTERVENTIONS

Nursing Diagnosis	Nursing Intervention
Gas exchange, impaired (related to amyloid deposition in pulmonary tissue)	Assess degree of respiratory distress: note rate, rhythm, and quality of respirations, auscultate lung fields for presence of adventitious breath sounds, and note use of accessory muscles. Maintain open airway at all times. In collaboration with physician, institute appropriate interventions, relative to type and severity of pulmonary compromise. Assess effectiveness.
Cardiac output, alteration in: decreased (related to amyloid deposition in cardiac structures and subsequent myopathy and ischemia)	Assess for signs and symptoms associated with decreased cardiac output: hypotension, dyspnea, edema, jugular venous distention, rales, and pulse irregularities. Monitor electrocardiogram for rate, rhythm, and ectopy. Note in particular presence of ischemia, infarction, and conduction abnormalities. Report significant electrocardiographic changes and other abnormal assessment data to physician. In collaboration with physician, institute appropriate interventions (such as oxygenation) relative to type and severity of cardiac compromise. Assess effectiveness and note side effects of chemotherapy. Adjust patient's activity to reduce oxygen demands and provide rest periods.
Tissue perfusion, alteration in: renal (related to amyloid deposition in kidneys)	Assess for renal insufficiency: Monitor blood urea nitrogen and creatinine, 24-hour urine for creatinine clearance, blood pressure, urinalysis result, presence of edema and rapid weight gain, and intake and output. Report significant abnormal findings to physician. Institute dialysis in event of renal failure.
Nutrition, alteration in: less than body requirements (related to amyloid deposition in gastrointestinal tract)	Assess degree of malnutrition. Note presence of hypoalbuminemia, hypoproteinemia, negative nitrogen balance, protein and calorie deficit, and weight loss. Assist physician in determining underlying cause of malnutrition, such as malabsorption, dysphagia, and impaired esophageal peristalsis.

Nursing Diagnosis	Nursing Intervention
	Provide and encourage patient to maintain nutritionally balanced diet. Determine need for parenteral nutrition. Weigh patient weekly. In collaboration with physician, institute appropriate interventions relative to underlying causes of malnutrition. Assess effectiveness.
Comfort, alteration in: pain (related to arthritis, cardiac ischemia, or gastrointestinal distress)	Assess pain: location, onset, duration, and provocative and alleviating factors. Have patient describe intensity on scale of 0 to 10. In collaboration with physician, administer appropriate analgesics. Assess effectiveness and note side effects. In collaboration with physician, institute other appropriate interventions relative to tissues and organs involved. Assess effectiveness.
Sensory-perceptual alteration: tactile (related to peripheral neuropathy)	Assess degree of sensory impairment: perform sensory neurologic examination. Provide for patient's safety. Discuss loss or alteration with patient and provide appropriate reassurance. In collaboration with physician, institute appropriate interventions relative to severity of neurologic impairment. Assess effectiveness.
Mobility, impaired physical (related to peripheral and autonomic neuropathy)	Assess degree of motor impairment: perform motor neurologic examination. Provide for patient's safety. In collaboration with physician, institute appropriate interventions relative to severity of neurologic impairment. Assess effectiveness.
Skin integrity, impairment of (related to amyloid deposition in dermis)	Assess skin integrity: color, temperature, moisture, and presence of lesions. Protect skin from injury or infection.
Coping, family: potential for growth (related to poor prognosis)	Assess family's anxiety related to limited understanding of diagnostic procedures, disease process, prognosis, and therapy. Provide information in areas needed. Explain relationship of disease process and rationale for various therapies at level appropriate for comprehension and degree of anxiety. Involve family in care as appropriate. Encourage family to verbalize questions and anxieties.
Anxiety	See p. 1839.
Self-concept, disturbance in: body image	See p. 1820.

Patient Education

1. Teach facts about and the importance of managing signs and symptoms and frequent physician follow-up.
2. Teach care and methods of self-assessment relative to the systems involved.
3. Refer the patient and family for counseling to assist in coping with this potentially fatal illness.
4. Teach the importance of medical alert identification.

EVALUATION

Patient Outcome	Data Indicating That Outcome is Reached
Pain is relieved or minimized.	There is decrease in subjective distress. Objective decrease is based on rating scale.
Laboratory findings improve.	Paraprotein level detected in serum and urine electrophoresis is decreased.
Medical crises are avoided.	There is no evidence of renal failure, myocardial infarction, paralysis, airway obstruction, or gastrointestinal obstruction.

SERUM SICKNESS

Serum sickness is a relatively uncommon, acute reaction that was originally noted in persons who had received antisera made from animal sources.

Today serum sickness occurs most commonly following the administration of a variety of drugs, particularly penicillin. However, it may also occur after injection of heterologous antiserum used in the treatment of rabies, venomous snake bites, gas gangrene, botulism, and tetanus.

Serum sickness is characterized by the abrupt onset of a skin rash or urticaria, fever, arthralgias, edema (particularly of the face), and hepatosplenomegaly 7 to 15 days after an inoculation. Its course is self-limited, lasting 1 to 3 weeks. Although complications are rare, vasculitis, glomerulonephritis, and neuropathies may occur secondarily. Serum sickness can develop in anyone. Its severity increases with age. The following agents are known to cause serum sickness[13]:

Animal serums	Penicillins
Barbiturates	Phenylbutazone
Griseofulvin	Probenecid
Hydralazine	Procainamide
Insulin	Quinidine
Iodides	Quinine
Mercurial diuretics	Salicylates
Nitrofurantoin	Streptomycin
Oxyphenbutazone	Sulfonamides
Para-aminosalicylic acid	

PATHOPHYSIOLOGY

The basic mechanism responsible for the development of serum sickness is antibody reaction against foreign protein with subsequent immune complex formation. The antigen-antibody complexes are deposited in the endothelium and basement membranes of vessel walls, and the subsequent inflammatory response results in vascular injury, thrombosis, and hemorrhage. Such widespread inflammation accounts for the clinical findings associated with this disease.

DIAGNOSTIC STUDIES

History
Exposure to inciting agent

White blood cell count
Mild leukocytosis

Erythrocyte sedimentation rate
Mildly elevated or within normal limits

Complement (C3 and C4)
Decreased during acute phase

TREATMENT PLAN

The goals of treatment include symptomatic relief and prevention of medical crises.

Chemotherapeutic
Before chemotherapeutic intervention, serum or drug that allegedly caused reaction should be discontinued

Antihistamines

Contraindicated in acute asthmatic attacks; caution patient to avoid alcohol ingestion, driving, and other hazardous activities; coffee or tea may reduce drowsiness; gum, sour hard candy, or ice chips may relieve dry mouth

Brompheniramine maleate (Dimetane, Spentane, Veltane); adults: 4-8 mg po tid or qid; children over 6 yr: 2-4 mg tid or qid, or 0.5 mg/kg qd IM, IV, or SC divided tid or qid; children under 6 yr: 0.5 mg/kg qd po IV, IM, or SC divided tid or qid

Tripelennamine (Pyribenzamine, Ro-Hist); adults: 25-50 mg po q4-6h; children: 5 mg/kg qd po in 4-6 divided doses

Diphenhydramine (Benadryl); adults: 25-50 mg po tid or qid; 10-50 mg IM or IV to 400 mg maximum qd; children: 5 mg/kg qd po IM or IV qid in divided doses

Antipruritic agents
See p. 1719

Corticosteroids
Prednisone, 10-40 mg qd for 4-5 d; response often remarkable within 24 h

Nonsteroidal anti-inflammatory agents
May be used to treat accompanying myalgias, arthralgias, or synovitis

ASSESSMENT: AREAS OF CONCERN

Skin integrity
Urticarial rash (often the first sign and starts at site of injection); petechial pruritic rash; erythematous pruritic rash; angioedema of face, lips, glottis, and eyelids; lymphadenopathy (begins in area of injection)

Musculoskeletal integrity
Arthralgias; synovitis; stiffness; myalgias

Constitutional signs and symptoms
Fever; malaise; headache; abdominal pain; nausea and vomiting

NURSING DIAGNOSES and NURSING INTERVENTIONS

Nursing Diagnosis	Nursing Intervention
Skin integrity, impairment of (related to urticaria, pruritic rash, or angioedema)	Assess skin integrity: lesions, texture, temperature, moisture, color, and vascularity.
	Monitor lesions for signs of infection, dissemination, and other abnormal changes.
	Provide and encourage meticulous hygiene to involved area.
	Provide and encourage use of mild, nondrying, hypoallergenic soaps for skin cleansing.
	Apply antipruritic medication as needed.
	In collaboration with physician, administer appropriate antihistamines. Assess effectiveness and note side effects.
Comfort, alteration in: pain (related to arthritis and myalgias)	Assess pain: location, onset, duration, and precipitating and alleviating factors. Have patient describe intensity on scale of 0 to 10.
	In collaboration with physician, provide appropriate anti-inflammatory and analgesic agents. Assess effectiveness and note side effects.
	Administer thermal therapy to affected muscles and joints as needed.

Patient Education

1. Teach side effects of medication.
2. Teach the patient to avoid subsequent exposure to the inciting agent.
3. Teach the patient to request skin desensitization before administration of drugs listed on p. 1687.
4. Teach the importance of medical alert identification.

EVALUATION

Patient Outcome	Data Indicating That Outcome is Reached
Laboratory findings are within normal limits.	Erythrocyte sedimentation rate is within normal limits.
Medical crises are prevented.	There is no vasculitis, neuropathy, or glomerulonephritis.
Abnormal clinical findings are resolved in response to therapeutic measures.	Initial signs and symptoms have disappeared.

SYSTEMIC LUPUS ERYTHEMATOSUS

Systemic lupus erythematosus (SLE) is a chronic, multisystem, autoimmune, inflammatory disorder characterized chiefly by antibody formation directed against autologous tissues and serum factors.

SLE has no cure. Although its origin remains elusive, increasing evidence suggests that multiple factors—genetic, hormonal, immunologic, and possibly viral—may play a role in the onset and perpetuation of the disease.

In the United States approximately 500,000 persons have this disease. Although virtually anyone may be affected, SLE has a predilection for women of childbearing age. Nine times more women than men are affected. Three times as many blacks as whites have SLE. Late-onset (sixth decade or later) SLE accounts for 12% of cases.

SLE was once considered a fatal illness of young women, but 85% of patients now survive longer than 15 years after diagnosis. This improved prognosis reflects advances in the diagnosis and treatment of the disease. Patients with central nervous system involvement and renal failure have poorer prognoses. Complications, especially infections, associated with the long-term use of steroids used to control the disease also significantly contribute to early mortality.

Despite the significant improvements in the treatment of SLE, it can be a serious and potentially life-threatening illness. Because of this, as well as the recognition that SLE is a prototype of autoimmune disease, it has been a subject of worldwide research.

The cause of SLE remains unknown, but several etiologies have been proposed. It is unlikely that any single factor is the cause. Most researchers conclude that SLE is probably caused by an unknown inciting agent coupled with a genetic "lupus diathesis."

Drugs

Over the past 30 years many drugs have been implicated in the development of a reversible lupuslike syndrome that includes elevated antinuclear antibody (ANA) titers and well-defined clinical features. Perhaps certain drugs alter tissues to such a degree as to make them act as immunogenic stimuli. Both hydralazine and procainamide can bind to and alter the physical properties of DNA, perhaps enhancing its immunogenicity. There may also be some correlation between an individual's ability to metabolize certain drugs and a predisposition for SLE.[29]

The following outline lists drugs thought to induce lupuslike syndromes.[29] Once these drugs are discontinued, clinical manifestations disappear:

Definite
  Hydralazine
  Procainamide
  Isoniazid
Possible
  Dilantin
  Chlorpromazine
  Methyldopa
  Penicillamine
  Quinidine
  Propylthiouracil
  Practolol
  Acebutolol
  Lithium carbonate

Unlikely
  Griseofulvin
  Phenylbutazone
  Oral contraceptives
  Gold salts
  Sulfonamides
  Penicillin

PATHOPHYSIOLOGY

The pathogenesis of SLE is characterized by the development of antibodies directed against "self" tissues, cells, serum proteins, or all of these. The presence of autoantibodies reflects a loss of tolerance, or autoimmunity, and constitutes a serious defect in the regulatory components of the immune system. As discussed on p. 1628, the T lymphocytes are the primary group of white cells responsible for control of the immune response. In SLE the number of T suppressor cells is decreased. In addition, T suppressor cell activity is inhibited. Polyclonal hypergammaglobulinemia occurs as a result, since B cells proliferate unrestrained by normal suppressor mechanisms.

In most SLE patients, antibodies develop directed against native, double-stranded DNA, as well as other

Table 16-6
Autoantibodies in SLE

Autoantibody	Clinical Manifestations
Antinuclear Anti–double-stranded DNA (ds-DNA) Antineuronal	Nephritis; vasculitis; pleuritis; pericarditis; synovitis; peritonitis Cerebritis; organic brain syndromes; peripheral neuropathies
Anticoagulant	Coagulopathies
Anti-RBC	Anemia
Anti-WBC	Leukopenia; lymphopenia; immunosuppression; infection
Antiplatelet	Thrombocytopenia
Anti–basement membrane	Dermatitis; nephritis

antigens. The combination of autoantibodies and autoantigens, or immune complexes, may circulate or be deposited within capillary plexi, near basement membranes, and in other tissues such as glomeruli, renal interstitia, serosal (pleural, pericardial, or peritoneal) membranes, the choroid plexus, and the vasculature of the lungs. Immune complex formation triggers the inflammatory response, which is the primary mechanism by which tissue destruction and subsequent clinical disease occur. Chronic deposition of immune complexes leads to chronic destruction of host tissue. *The intensity and location of the inflammatory process dictate the severity of the clinical response and organ involvement, respectively.*

A variety of autoantibodies may be detected by serologic assay. Some of these are listed in Table 16-6. Further discussion of the pathogenesis of SLE by systems is summarized here:

Musculoskeletal
  Deposition and accumulation of fibrin along synovial surfaces; arteriolar and venular inflammation; perivascular inflammation; inflammation of tendon sheaths; interstitial inflammation of muscle tissue leading to necrosis, degeneration, and fibrosis (late)
Gastrointestinal
  Ulceration of mucosal membranes associated with collagen degeneration and vasculitis; vasculitis leading to infarction, necrosis of tissue, and organ rupture; arteritis of mesenteric circulation
Renal: "lupus nephritis"
  Immune complex deposition and inflammation of the glomerular basement membrane and mesangium; glomerular sclerosis
Hematologic
  IgG and IgM against erythrocytes (cells destroyed

by macrophages and complement); IgM antibodies against leukocytes; antibodies detected against platelets (cells destroyed by splenic macrophages); periarterial fibrosis and inflammatory infiltration of lymph nodes; circulating anticoagulant proteins

Pulmonary

Inflammation of pleura; infiltration of parenchyma; interstitial vasculitis leading to infarction, necrosis, and fibrosis

Cardiovascular

Diffuse vasculitis; inflammation and scarring of SA and AV nodes; inflammation of pericardial sac

Cutaneous

Immune complex deposition and inflammation of dermal-epidermal junctions; vasculitis

Neurologic

Immune complex deposition and inflammation in choroid plexus; antineuronal antibody action

DIAGNOSTIC STUDIES

Antinuclear antibody (ANA)

Positive in titers greater than 1:80

Anti–double-stranded DNA antibody (ds-DNA)

Positive in titers greater than 1:80

Rapid plasma reagin (RPR) test

Falsely positive

Fluorescent treponemal antibody absorption (FTA-ABS)

Negative

Complement (C3 and C4)

Decreased during flares, indicative of acute inflammation; otherwise within normal limits

Skin or muscle biopsy

Evidence of inflammation with or without tissue necrosis; deposits of immunoglobulin and complement at dermal-epidermal junctions

Kidney biopsy

Focal or diffuse proliferative nephritis; also membranous or interstitial disease

Complete blood count

Pancytopenia or selective deficits; lymphopenia during flare

C-reactive protein

Elevated during flares, indicative of acute inflammatory state

Erythrocyte sedimentation rate

Elevated during flares, indicative of acute inflammatory state

Coombs' test

Positive in presence of hemolytic anemia because of autoantibody production against erythrocytes

Coagulation profile

Prolonged prothrombin time and partial thromboplastin time if circulating anticoagulant antibodies are present

Rheumatoid factor (RF) (anti-IgG antibody)

Usually positive in titer greater than 1:40

Circulating immune complexes

Present during flares

Urinalysis

Abnormal casts and sediment associated with renal damage

Antibodies to single-stranded DNA (ss-DNA)

May be present in ANA-negative lupus and associated with congenital heart block in lupus patients' neonates

The 1982 revised classification of SLE is based on the 11 criteria defined below. For the purpose of identifying patients in clinical studies, a person should be said to have SLE if any four or more of the 11 criteria are present, serially or simultaneously, during any interval of observation.

1. Malar rash: fixed erythema, flat or raised, over malar eminences, tending to spare nasolabial folds
2. Discoid rash: Erythematous raised patches with adherent keratotic scaling and follicular plugging; atrophic scarring may occur in older lesions
3. Photosensitivity: skin rash as result of unusual reaction to sunlight, based on patient history or physician's observation
4. Oral ulcers: oral or nasopharyngeal ulceration, usually painless, observed by physician
5. Arthritis: Nonerosive arthritis involving two or more peripheral joints, characterized by tenderness, swelling, or effusion
6. Serositis: pleuritis—convincing history of pleuritic pain or rub heard by a physician or evidence of pleural effusion—or pericarditis—documented by electrocardiogram, rub, or evidence of pericardial effusion
7. Renal disorder: Persistent proteinuria greater than 0.5 g/day or greater than 3+ if quantitation not performed or cellular casts—may be red cell, hemoglobin, granular, tubular, or mixed
8. Neurologic disorder: seizures in absence of offending drugs or known metabolic derangements

(such as uremia, ketoacidosis, or electrolyte imbalance) *or* psychosis in absence of offending drugs or known metabolic derangements

9. Hematologic disorder: hemolytic anemia with reticulocytosis *or* leukopenia—less than 4000/mm³ total on two or more occasions *or* lymphopenia—less than 1500/mm³ on two or more occasions *or* thrombocytopenia—less 100,000/mm³ in absence of offending drugs

10. Immunologic disorder: Positive LE cell preparation *or* anti-DNA—antibody to native DNA in abnormal titer *or* anti-Sm—presence of antibody to Sm nuclear antigen *or* false positive serologic test for syphilis known to be positive for at least 6 months and confirmed by *Treponema pallidum* immobilization or fluorescent treponemal antibody absorption test

11. Antinuclear antibody: abnormal titer of antinuclear antibody by immunofluorescence or equivalent assay at any point in time and in absence of drugs known to be associated with "drug-induced lupus" syndrome

TREATMENT PLAN

The goals of the treatment plan include management of signs and symptoms, induction of remission, prevention of untoward complications of therapy, and early recognition of flares.

Surgical

Joint replacement may be indicated if chronic synovitis and pain have been problematic.

Chemotherapeutic[29]

Nonsteroidal anti-inflammatory agents. Acetylsalicylic acid (aspirin) may be given in a daily oral dosage of 3 to 6 g for adults. Indomethacin (Indocin) is given orally, 25 to 50 mg three or four times a day for adults. The patient should be monitored for evidence of gastrointestinal bleeding.

Anti-infective agents. Hydroxychloroquine (Plaquenil), 200 to 400 mg orally twice a day for adults, or chloroquine, 250 mg orally daily to twice weekly for adults, is given. The patient should be started on therapy slowly. Gastrointestinal intolerance may occur when full doses are used initially. The beneficial effect of these drugs is usually demonstrated within a month or two. Nonsteroidal anti-inflammatory agents should be continued until this time. Retinal toxicity may occur at higher doses, so patients should receive pretreatment and annual ophthalmic examinations.

Corticosteroids. Prednisone (Orasone, Deltasone, Meticorten) is given orally in low doses (15 mg/day), moderate doses (16 to 40 mg/day), or high doses (41 to 120 mg/day). Alternate-day dosage may be instituted as maintenance therapy (see p. 1732). The amounts listed above may be given in divided doses to provide more sustained anti-inflammatory action.

Any amount of prednisone given as a single oral dose in the morning has *less* adrenal suppressing activity than the same amount given in divided doses throughout the day. However, any given amount of this drug, taken in divided doses, has greater lupus-suppressing activity than does the same amount of drug given as a single morning dose.[31] Fever, cutaneous involvement, arthropathy, and serositis are usually managed with 20 to 30 mg of prednisone orally each day. Major organ involvement (cardiac and vascular systems and kidneys) often requires 15 to 20 mg prednisone orally (or intravenous equivalent) every 6 hours until attenuation of disease activity is achieved.

Methylprednisolone (Solu-Medrol, A-methaPred) is given intravenously in a dosage of up to 1000 mg/day for adults. One gram may be administered in divided doses. The use of intravenous therapy is limited to situations of acute exacerbations of the disease or when the patient is unable to tolerate oral administration. Central nervous system involvement (psychosis, grand mal seizures) requires 35 to 40 mg methylprednisolone intravenously every 6 hours. The dose should be doubled if no response is attained in 48 hours.

In addition, bolus or "pulse" steroid therapy may be administered, though its use remains controversial. The usual course involves the intravenous infusion of 1 to 1.5 g of methylprednisolone daily for three doses. Oral medications, which may include up to 60 mg of prednisone daily, may be continued right through the treatment episode. Pulse therapy has been used with varying success during acute exacerbations of the disease, involving renal failure and central nervous system and hematologic "crises." This treatment is not without inherent hazards. Sudden death has been reported.

Topical steroids include hydrocortisone (Cortaid), fluocinonide (Lidex), betamethasone dipropionate (Diprosone), flurandrenolide (Cordran), betamethasone valerate (Valisone), and fluocinolone acetonide (Synalar).

Once remission is achieved on moderate to high divided dose therapy, the steroids are gradually tapered (decreased 5 mg per week). After reaching 40 mg, the dose should be consolidated to a single morning dose and tapered to 20 mg/day. The dose is then decreased by 2.5 mg a week until a 10 mg/day schedule is reached. The dose may be further decreased by 1 mg per week until the patient is totally weaned from the drug. If the disease flares while the dose is being decreased, the prednisone will be increased back to the last dosage at which the patient was asymptomatic and laboratory findings were within normal limits.

Alternate-day therapy is usually not successful during acute phases of SLE. Once the disease is under control, the physician may place the patient on an alternate-day schedule (which has less adrenal suppressing activity) using the following protocol[31]:

1. The patient initially receives 2x (x = daily dose) on the "on" day and ¾x on the "off" day.
2. One week later, the "off" day dose is switched to ½x.
3. One week later, the "off" day dose is switched to ¼x.
4. One week later, the "off" day dose is discontinued.

Patients receiving long-term steroid therapy should be assessed for the following signs and symptoms: hyperglycemia, central fat distribution, arrhythmias, hypertension, edema, electrolyte imbalances, violaceous striae, alopecia, glaucoma, cataracts, infections, osteoporosis, myopathies, seizures, gastrointestinal ulceration, and pancreatitis.

In addition, patients should be assessed frequently for signs and symptoms associated with adrenal crisis, particularly when tapering of dosages is begun: sudden fatigue and profound weakness, muscle weakness, arthralgias, fevers, anorexia, dizziness, syncope, dyspnea, lethargy, and hypotension.

Antineoplastic agents. Azathioprine (Imuran) is given in an oral dosage of 150 mg/day to 25 mg thrice weekly for adults. The patient should be monitored for pancytopenia, gastrointestinal distress, skin rash, hepatic toxicity, and hyperuricemia. Cyclophosphamide (Cytoxan, Neosar) is given as 150 mg/day to 25 mg thrice weekly for adults. The patient should be monitored for pancytopenia, cardiotoxicity, gastrointestinal distress, hemorrhagic cystitis, and hyperuricemia. Chlorambucil (Leukeran) is given orally as 10 mg/day to 2 mg thrice weekly for adults. The patient should be monitored for pancytopenia, exfoliative dermatitis, and hyperuricemia.

Other medications. A variety of anti-infective agents may be used to treat infections associated with SLE or immunosuppressive therapy. Treatment of renal disease includes the use of antihypertensive agents and aluminum derivatives. Raynaud's phenomenon may respond to biofeedback or sympatholytic drugs such as guanethidine, nifedipine, reserpine, and tolazoline. Intra-articular steroid injections may prove useful in the alleviation of synovitis and joint pain.

Electromechanical

Plasmapheresis (see p. 1730) has been shown to decrease circulating immune complexes and autoantibodies. After the procedure, which may be done two or three times a week, a rebound effect may be noted. This is characterized by elevated antibody or immune complex titers. To circumvent this problem, a brief course of cytotoxic medication, often cyclophosphamide intravenously, may be administered after the plasmapheresis series. Although the use of plasmapheresis as a therapeutic modality remains controversial, it has been suggested for extremely ill patients who do not respond well to conventional treatment.

Peritoneal dialysis or hemodialysis may be indicated in the treatment of renal insufficiency or failure.

Supportive

A balanced diet should be encouraged. A weight reduction diet may be indicated for patients receiving steroids. Salt restriction often prevents fluid retention. Vitamins are useful during pregnancy and dieting.

A balance is needed between rest and exercise. Flares probably warrant temporary rest. Otherwise, a regular exercise program should be implemented to increase and maintain strength, endurance, and muscle tone. Aerobic exercises such as walking, swimming, and bicycling are recommended. Jogging should be avoided because it places stress on joints, but swimming is particularly beneficial because it avoids this problem. For patients unable to engage in the aforementioned activities, a regular program of exercise, including range of motion, should be planned with the aid of a physical therapist.

Many patients with SLE cannot tolerate sun exposure. Flares have been associated with photosensitivity. Patients are especially intolerant of type B ultraviolet light. Therefore they should be encouraged to avoid the sun, wear protective clothing, and liberally apply sunscreens with a sun protection factor of 15 or above.

Patients with SLE should not take birth control pills or use intrauterine devices (IUDs). Use of diaphragm and foam is the preferred contraceptive method.

ASSESSMENT: AREAS OF CONCERN

Skin and mucous membrane

Facial erythema; butterfly dermatitis; alopecia; "lupus hair"—thin unruly hair that fractures easily around frontal hairline; periorbital edema; Raynaud's phenomenon; photosensitivity; oral and nasal ulcers; purpura; petechiae; periungual erythema; leg ulcers; digital gangrene; diffuse, transient rashes; urticarial lesions; livedo reticularis; "discoid" lesions: demarcated, annular, erythematous plaques with atrophy, scaling, and telangiectasia; scale is adherent and "plugs" dilated hair follicles, with classic distribution over sun-exposed areas of skin

Neuropsychiatric status

"Lupus cerebritis"; encephalitis; aseptic meningitis; progressive multifocal leukoencephalopathy; seizures (usually grand mal); cranial neuropathies: ophthalmoplegias, visual disturbances, papilledema, facial weakness, dysarthria, vertigo, nystagmus, trigeminal neuralgia; cytoid bodies; aphasia; hemiparesis; headache; peripheral neuropathies; anxiety; depression; mania; insomnia; confusion; hallucinations; disorientation; emotional lability; psychosis

Musculoskeletal integrity

Arthralgias; arthritis: Polyarticular, often episodic, may or may not result in deformities; tenosynovitis; synovial Baker's cysts; diffuse myalgias; polyfocal myositis; steroid-induced osteoporosis, aseptic bone necrosis, or myopathy; pseudothrombophlebitis

Gastrointestinal status

Dysphagia; gastric and duodenal ulcerations (may also be steroid induced); pancreatitis; hepatomegaly; peritonitis; "acute abdomen"

Hematologic status

Anemia: autoimmune hemolytic anemia, iron deficiency anemia, chronic anemia; granulocytopenia; leukocytosis; lymphocytopenia; thrombocytopenia; lymphadenopathy; splenomegaly; hepatomegaly; coagulopathies; potential infection

Cardiovascular status

Diffuse vasculitis; pericarditis; myocarditis; endocarditis; atherosclerosis (also steroid induced); thrombophlebitis; arrhythmias

Pulmonary status

Pleurisy; pleural effusions; pneumonitis; interstitial fibrosis; decreased pulmonary function; pulmonary hypertension; pulmonary emboli

Renal status

"Lupus nephritis": focal (mild), diffuse proliferative (severe), membranous, interstitial fibrosis, tubular necrosis; edema; retinopathy; hypertension; anemia; electrolyte imbalances

See Table 16-7

Table 16-7
Frequency of Clinical Symptoms in SLE

Symptoms	Percent
Fever	83
Weight loss	62
Arthritis, arthralgia	90
Skin	74
Butterfly rash	42
Photosensitivity	30
Mucous membrane lesions	12
Alopecia	27
Raynaud's phenomenon	17
Purpura	15
Urticaria	8
Renal	53
Nephrosis	18
Gastrointestinal	38
Pulmonary	47
Pleurisy	45
Effusion	24
Pneumonia	29
Cardiac	46
Pericarditis	27
Murmurs	23
Electrocardiographic changes	39
Lymphadenopathy	46
Splenomegaly	15
Hepatomegaly	25
Central nervous system	32
Psychosis	15
Convulsions	15
Cytoid bodies	11

From Schur, P., editor: The clinical management of systemic lupus erythematosus, New York, 1983, Grune & Stratton, Inc.

NURSING DIAGNOSES and NURSING INTERVENTIONS

Because of the multiple systemic effects of SLE, nursing care must be structured to cope with the patient's individual requirements. Therefore nursing care often varies greatly, ranging, for example, from minor application of topical steroids to aggressive pulmonary toilet for an intubated patient. The following is meant to provide a generalized perspective. Refer to other chapters for a detailed approach to systems involved.

Nursing Diagnosis	Nursing Intervention
Breathing pattern, ineffective (related to pulmonary complications of SLE)	Assess respiratory status: monitor respiratory rate and rhythm, auscultate lungs for presence of adventitious breath sounds, and monitor for subjective distress (chest pain and dyspnea). Maintain bed rest during acute phase. In collaboration with physician, administer oxygen, analgesics, inhalants, bronchodilators, and steroids as appropriate. Provide chest physiotherapy and postural drainage. Teach deep breathing exercises and encourage patient to perform exercises as often as needed. Monitor chest roentgenograms and sputum culture results. Monitor results of pulmonary studies: VQ scan, pulmonary function tests, lung biopsy, and so on.
Cardiac output, alteration in: decreased (related to cardiovascular complications of SLE)	Assess cardiac status. Auscultate apical pulse for irregularities, presence of murmurs, tachycardia, and bradycardia. Auscultate for pericardial friction rub. Monitor for subjective distress: syncope, palpitations, and dyspnea. Monitor electrocardiographic results. Monitor for presence of peripheral edema. Auscultate lung for presence of rales or rhonchi. Auscultate arterial pulses for presence of bruits. In collaboration with physician, administer oxygen, steroids, and antiarrhythmic agents if appropriate. Assess patient's response.
Coping, ineffective individual (related to organic brain syndrome associated with SLE or difficulty dealing with diagnosis and its implications)	Assess changes in neurologic status: orientation, judgment, and intellectual function. Assess degree of patient's ability to cope. Assess for suicidal ideation. Work with patient to identify resources for support and coping mechanisms that have proved helpful in past. Provide emotional support and attempt to limit patient's fears through frequent explanations of tests and procedures. Provide patient education (see p. 1696). Encourage visits by family and friends. If orientation is problem in hospital, provide familiar articles from home. Provide clock and calendar to orient patient to time. Maintain patient's safety. Encourage participation in local chapter of Lupus Foundation.
Tissue perfusion, alteration in: renal (related to the renal complications of SLE)	Assess renal status. Monitor for presence of dyspnea, hypertension, edema, weight gain, anorexia, and nausea. Monitor urinalysis results, blood urea nitrogen, serum creatinine, hemoglobin, hematocrit, and urine and serum electrolytes. Modify diet as indicated. In collaboration with physician, administer antihypertensive medications. Assess patient's response. Monitor for symptoms of electrolyte imbalance.
Mobility, impaired physical (related to arthritis and general weakness)	Assess degree of limitation: range of motion, joint integrity, presence of pain (location, duration, quality, severity, and precipitating or alleviating factors), deformity, and muscular atrophy. Perform range of motion exercises as tolerated. In collaboration with physician, administer analgesics according to appropriate and regular time schedules. Assess patient's response. Administer thermal therapy to muscles and joints. Confer with physical or occupational therapist to determine other beneficial interventions.

Nursing Diagnosis	Nursing Intervention
Skin integrity, impairment of (related to integumentary manifestations of SLE)	Assess skin and mucous membranes. Inspect and palpate noting color, vascularity, lesion size, configuration, and distribution, edema, moisture, temperature, texture, thickness, mobility, and turgor. Monitor skin lesions for signs of infection. In collaboration with physician, administer topical steroidal or anti-infective creams and ointments as indicated. Assess response. Provide hypoallergenic, nondrying soaps and mild shampoos. Encourage use of sunscreen products if patient is photosensitive.
Nutrition, alteration in: less than body requirements (related to anorexia, electrolyte imbalance, or chemotherapy side effects)	Assess nutritional status. Monitor serum protein and albumin values. Monitor for evidence of poor wound healing. Determine weight loss and compare to ideal body weight. Encourage balanced diet with supplements if indicated. Encourage weight reduction diet for patients who have gained weight while taking steroids. Low-sodium, high-potassium diet may be indicated for patients receiving steroids. Encourage intake of vitamin supplements for patients who are pregnant or dieting.
Activity intolerance, potential (related to flare, chronic anemia, arthralgias, and other effects of SLE)	Assess degree of activity intolerance. Encourage balance between rest and exercise. Flares warrant temporary rest. During periods when disease is quiescent, encourage program of regular, aerobic exercise that places as little stress on joints as possible.
Self-concept, disturbance in: body image (related to multisystem disturbances, including skin changes)	See p. 1820.
Potential patient problem: susceptibility to infection	Assess for anorexia, pain, weakness, and lethargy. Assess for evidence of infection at sites of invasive procedures. Assess for breaks in skin integrity, particularly over pressure areas and oral mucosa. Assess pulmonary status: auscultate lung fields to determine presence of adventitious breath sounds. Maintain optimal nutritional status and fluid intake. Assess ocular integrity for evidence of conjunctivitis: erythematous, pruritic conjunctiva. Assess mentation for evidence of central nervous system infection: changes in level of consciousness, headache, and visual disturbances. Assess for evidence of gastrointestinal infection: abdominal pain, fever, and diarrhea. Monitor temperature and vital signs for evidence of fever or sepsis. Maintain body hygiene. Limit environmental stress. Monitor laboratory data: white blood cell count and differential, erythrocyte sedimentation rate, C-reactive protein, urinalysis, and cultures. In collaboration with physician, administer appropriate antimicrobial, antipyretic, or analgesic medication. Assess patient's response. Monitor for side effects. Promote pulmonary toilet: breathing exercises, postural drainage, and chest physical therapy. Maintain normal sleep and rest patterns. Protect patient from physical injury. Provide clean environment. Maintain protective isolation based on hospital policy. Restrict contact with family and health care providers who have infectious diseases. Maintain good handwashing before and after contact with patient.

Patient Education

1. Teach side effects of medication(s).
2. Teach the importance of avoiding contact with persons who may expose the patient to infection.
3. Teach the importance of frequent assessment for signs and symptoms associated with infection. While steroids are being given, many of these findings will be masked, so the slightest change in temperature, wound characteristics, or other parameters should be reported immediately.
4. Teach the importance of skin care. Tell the patient to avoid dryness and use of irritant soaps, shampoos, chemical coloring, or permanent waving of hair. Encourage use of hypoallergenic makeup and wearing wig if there is hair loss. Teach photosensitive patients to avoid sun exposure: limit outdoor activities between 10 AM and 4 PM, wear long sleeves, pants, and hats, and use PABA sunscreen products with a sun protection factor of at least 15.
5. Teach methods to cope with arthralgias and myalgias: range of motion exercises, balance between rest and exercise, use of analgesics and nonsteroidal anti-inflammatory agents, joint supports at night, contacting Arthritis Foundation.
6. Teach the importance of regular follow-up by a physician and the need for blood tests.
7. Teach the importance of recognizing factors that lead to a flare: psychologic and physical stress, use of drugs that induce a lupuslike syndrome (see p. 1689), abrupt cessation of medications, and photosensitivity.
8. Teach warning signs of a flare: fever, chills, excessive fatigue and malaise, nausea, muscle weakness, increased joint pain, chest pain, oliguria, and dysuria—essentially, exacerbation of an old symptom or development of a new one.
9. Teach the importance of maintaining a balanced diet; include restrictions associated with medications.
10. Teach family planning. Pregnancy is usually allowed during remissions with close monitoring. Barrier contraceptives such as a condom or diaphragm are recommended.
11. Teach the importance of keeping a log of the disease course, treatments, and other disease-related information.
12. Teach the importance of obtaining up-to-date information about SLE.
13. Teach the patient to carry medical alert identification.
14. Direct the patient to available resources.

EVALUATION

Patient Outcome	Data Indicating That Outcome is Reached
Laboratory findings are within normal limits.	Anti–double-stranded DNA (anti-dsDNA) and antinuclear antibody (ANA) are less than 1:80. Complement (C3 and C4), C1q binding, CH50, complete blood count, white blood cell count, erythrocyte count, hematocrit, hemoglobin level, and platelet count are within normal limits. Prothrombin time and partial thromboplastin time are within normal limits. Urinalysis findings, blood urea nitrogen, and creatinine levels are within normal limits.
Symptoms resolve in response to therapeutic measures.	There are no symptoms associated with individual system involvement.
Patient maintains independence in activities of daily living.	Patient returns to baseline ability to perform activities of daily living.
Pain is relieved or minimized.	There is decrease in subjective distress. Objective decrease is based on rating scale.
Medical crises are prevented.	There are no life-threatening side effects of chemotherapeutic interventions: cardiopulmonary failure, renal failure, sepsis, or psychosis.
Patient complies with treatment.	Patient verbalizes understanding of importance of compliance and adheres to prescribed regimens and methods of symptom control.
No infection occurs.	There are no signs or symptoms associated with infections. Patient says there is no malaise, fatigue, weakness, anorexia, dysuria, or pain. There is no evidence of rhinitis; productive

Patient Outcome	Data Indicating That Outcome is Reached
	cough; pyuria; erythema, heat, edema, or purulent drainage at wound site(s); breaks in skin integrity; rales; rhonchi; or wheezing. Temperature and vital signs are within patient's normal limits. Culture findings are negative. White blood cell count, erythrocyte sedimentation rate, C-reactive protein, and urinalysis findings are within normal limits.

ATOPIC DISEASE

The term "allergy" was initially used to describe "altered reactivity" and has evolved over the years to refer broadly to any immunologic reaction to a foreign substance that produces detrimental consequences to the body. It is often used interchangeably with atopy.

Atopy is an abnormal immune response mediated by IgE antibody produced against substances that normally occur in the environment. Atopic diseases include anaphylaxis, allergic rhinoconjunctivitis, allergic asthma, atopic dermatitis, gastrointestinal allergy, and occasionally urticaria or angioedema. Allergy to a drug or an insect bite or sting can cause anaphylaxis or hives by an immunologic IgE mechanism in persons with or without other allergic symptoms (atopic or nonatopic).

Atopy appears in approximately 20% of the population and is thought to be inherited through genes linked to HLA antigen haplotypes. The expression of atopy has been linked to multiple factors including hormonal changes, antigen exposure, and concurrent illness. Expression of symptoms can occur at any time during life and varies from mild to life threatening in severity.

PATHOPHYSIOLOGY

The genetic defect is thought to be in T suppressor cell modulation, which allows increased or unmodulated production of IgE antibody.

The antigens precipitating the IgE response are restricted to either complete protein antigens with specific carrier and antigenic determinants or low–molecular weight substances that function as haptens by combining with serum or tissue proteins to form a complex. Antigens may be inhaled (tree, grass, or weed pollens, mold spores, dust, animal proteins), ingested (food, drugs), injected (venom, drug), or touched.

On initial exposure the antigen (allergen) is processed by a macrophage and then presented to the appropriately responsive T lymphocyte. Interaction then occurs with B lymphocytes, which, when stimulated, develop into mature plasma cells and secrete the antigen-specific IgE antibody.

Only a very small amount of IgE antibody circulates in the serum. Most IgE is found fixed to the surface of mast cells (fixed in tissue) or basophils (circulating). There may be 5000 to 500,000 IgE molecules on a single mast cell. A mast cell may have a large variety of antigen-specific IgE antibodies on its surface.

Mast cells and basophils contain several potent chemical mediators of inflammation, including histamine, arachidonic acid metabolites such as prostaglandins and leukotrienes (slow-reacting substance of anaphylaxis [SRS-A]), eosinophil chemotactic factors of anaphylaxis (ECF-A), and platelet-activating factor (PAF). Mediators may exert a direct pharmacologic effect or release or activate other mediators potentiating the response. Mediators initiate a sequence of physiologic events in various organ systems, resulting in such responses as vasodilation, enhanced vasopermeability, smooth muscle contraction, and increased mucus production (Fig. 16-12).

On reexposure and entry the antigen binds to IgE antibodies. This causes degranulation of the mast cell and release of the mediators that initiate the pathophysiologic responses. Symptoms of atopic disease are the result of the tissue response to the mediators. Symptoms may be generalized (anaphylaxis) or localized (for example, in bronchi, conjunctiva, nasal membranes, skin, or gut). This mechanism of tissue reaction occurs immediately on exposure to the antigen and is identified as a type I anaphylactic or immediate hypersensitivity reaction by the Gell and Coombs nomenclature.

Anaphylactoid reactions mimic allergic reactions and clinically may be identical to IgE-mediated responses. However, no IgE is involved and symptoms may result from direct action on mast cells causing release of chemical mediators (occurs with dextran and radiocontrast media), prostaglandin activation (occurs with acetylsalicylic acid and some nonsteroidal anti-inflammatory agents), or complement activation (occurs with aggregated IgG). The exact trigger mechanism and pathways of inflammatory responses are not fully understood. However, these reactions are treated in the same manner as anaphylactic reactions. The only clinical difference is that, since IgE is not involved, skin testing is of no value and reactions can occur with the first exposure; prior sensitization is not required.

Fig. 16-12

Mediators of immediate hypersensitivity. Interaction of allergen-antibody reaction, complement system, clotting system, and kinin system (→ indicates stimulation; —/— indicates inhibition).

From Lawlor, G., et al., editors: Manual of allergy and immunology, Boston, 1981, Little, Brown, & Co.

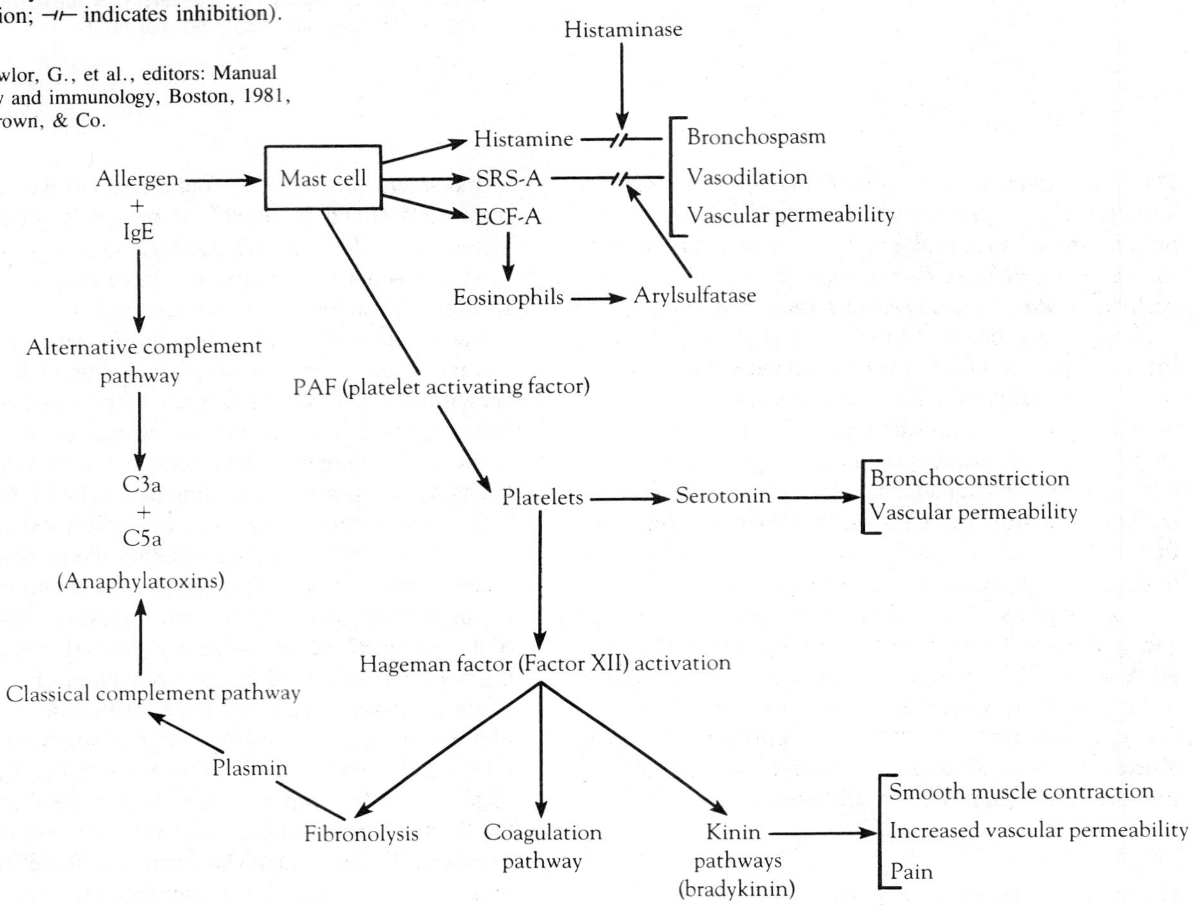

DIAGNOSTIC STUDIES

A thorough history is by far the most important diagnostic tool. The physical examination focuses on all areas of potential atopic manifestations. Laboratory studies may be useful in supporting the diagnosis and in monitoring response to therapy but are not in themselves diagnostic.

History

Onset, nature, and progression of symptoms; aggravating and alleviating factors; frequency, time, and duration of symptoms; complete environmental history including occupational, chemical, smoking, animal, and hobby exposures; household description including heating and cooling systems, pets, and bedding; past medical history; medications; family history including atopic history

Physical examination

Skin; middle ear; conjunctiva; nasal membranes; naso-oropharynx; chest

Laboratory studies

Complete blood count
  Within normal limits
Differential
  May have eosinophil percentage, up to 5%
Eosinophil count
  Within normal limits or increased up to 10% (up to 700 cells/mm), but range of normal is wide and increases may also occur in other diseases that have similar symptoms

Smears for eosinophils
  Generally predominate in secretions (up to 90% of total) during symptomatic periods
Total serum IgE levels
  Within normal limits or increased (up to 700 units/ml), but there is wide range of normal and increases can also occur in other diseases
Skin testing
  Demonstrates presence of specific IgE antibody; most reliable test for allergy; reliable correlation for inhalants, much less reliable for foods; false positive findings may result from irritant response; false negative findings may result from poor skin response or antihistamines; findings must correlate with history; drug may be hapten or metabolite; testing currently limited to penicillin, horse serum, insulin, and egg-based vaccines
Radioallergosorbent test
  Demonstrates presence of specific circulating IgE antibody; less reliable than skin testing (not as sensitive; difficulty in standardization of test and reproducibility of tests among reference laboratories)
Provocative testing
  Specific antigen challenges performed under controlled conditions to demonstrate clinical reactivity
Elimination testing
  Demonstration of clinical sensitivity to antigen by removing and then reintroducing it while monitoring clinical symptoms

TREATMENT PLAN

The goals of the treatment plan include symptom management through medications, environmental control, and immunotherapy. Specific plans are discussed with each disease.

Chemotherapeutic

Medications are used to prevent the tissue response and resultant symptoms. The choice of medication is to some extent organ specific, since the tissue response differs in specific organ systems, and these are discussed with the specific allergic disease.

Antihistamines are competitive antagonists of histamine and compete for cell surface receptors. Thus better symptom control is achieved by using the drug on a regular basis or as needed before allergen exposure. Six classes of older H_1 antihistamines are available; all have central nervous system and anticholinergic side effects.

The side effects, drowsiness and dryness, may limit their use in susceptible patients. Occasionally central nervous system excitation, palpitation, urinary retention, or constipation occurs. A newer H_1 antihistamine that would eliminate these side effects is now available (terfenadine [Seldane], 60 mg). Topical preparations should be avoided because of the potential for sensitization. They may be given orally or intramuscularly depending on preparation and with dose adjustments to patients of any age over 3 months, including pregnant women (who may receive selected antihistamines, including chlorpheneramine).

Cromolyn sodium stabilizes the mast cell membrane, preventing mediator release. It has no known side effects other than occasional sore throat or hoarseness after inhalation. It must be used preventively, either before exposure or on a regular basis. Topical nasal, otic, and bronchial cromolyn preparations are currently available for any age range; oral administration preparations are undergoing clinical trials. Available agents include the following:

  Intal, via Spinhaler every 6 hours or as needed before exposure for adult and child over 6 years
  Nebulizer solution, 1 ampule via nebulizer every 6 hours or as needed before exposure for adult and child over 2 years
  Nasalcrom, 1 spray every 4 to 6 hours or as needed before exposure for adult and child over 6 years
  Opticrom, 1 drop in each eye as above

Environmental Control

Environmental control is the preferred method of treatment because complete avoidance of the offending allergen affords total relief of symptoms. Efforts to decrease the amount of allergen exposure will reduce symptom severity. Removal of the offending antigens, especially those of an inhalant perennial nature, often seems to have an ameliorative effect on the progression of disease. The following is a representative list of allergens and possible measures:

  Tree, grass, and weed pollens—air-conditioning, closing bedroom and car windows during pollen season (times of pollination are dependent on geographic area)
  Mold spores—removal of source (such as plant dirt), application of mold retardant solutions for damp areas (for example, crawl spaces, bathrooms), air filtration by a high-efficiency particulate arresting (HEPA) filter or electrostatic air cleaner
  House dust and mites—plastic mattress casing, removal of carpets, damp dusting and face masks while dusting, air filtration
  Epidermals (feather, animal protein)—removal of source

Foods—avoidance
Drugs—avoidance
Stinging or biting insects—avoidance

Immunotherapy

The response to immunotherapy with inhaled antigens is well known, but the mechanism is not definitely elucidated. Proposed mechanisms include the following[8]:

Development of IgG serum "blocking" antibodies
Induction of tolerance in IgE-producing B cells
Impairment of T helper cell function
Restoration of antigen-specific or isotype-specific T suppressor cells or factors
Decreased IgE synthesis by anti-idiotypic autoantibodies
Decreased sensitivity of mediator-releasing cells

The major risk of immunotherapy is anaphylaxis from antigen overdose. The clinical efficacy of immunotherapy varies with different antigens, depending on the antigen involved, potency and dose of the antigen preparation, and complete match of antigens used with those clinically important to the patient. Currently the minimal length of therapy is 3 years. Immunotherapy is recommended for inhalant antigens (for example, tree, grass, and weed pollens) and venoms but not for foods. Gradual diminution of symptoms occurs during the therapy. When no further clinical improvement is noted, therapy is discontinued but may be reinstituted over the life span as necessary. Current investigations center on specifically identifying the antigenic components of various allergens and preparing immunotherapy extracts that increase the antigen load, require fewer injections, and minimize adverse effects.

Desensitization for insulin and penicillin requires special protocols performed under close supervision and is done only when medically indicated.

Supportive

Although atopy should be considered a chronic illness, adequate patient education and motivation, coupled with a specific medical plan, should enable the patient to manage the disease adequately.

If the inflammatory response is prevented or blocked, sequelae such as fatigue, malaise, and secondary bacterial infections will be minimized.

ASSESSMENT: AREAS OF CONCERN

Allergic responses may involve one or more organ systems, and symptoms may range from mild to severe. Symptoms may be episodic or perennial depending on exposures. Assessment must also discriminate among possible concurrent diseases. Specific assessment is discussed with each allergic disease.

NURSING DIAGNOSES and NURSING INTERVENTIONS

Because of the variable expression of atopic disease, the following is included as part of the comprehensive overview of the disease. Specific interventions are addressed with discussion of each disease.

Nursing Diagnosis	Nursing Intervention
Injury, potential for (related to exposure to antigen)	Obtain complete allergy history and record in appropriate places. Emphasize potential harm of repeat exposure. Identify and teach patient the measures to institute if patient is reexposed to antigen. Emphasize need for medical alert identification.
Activity intolerance, potential	Modify activity prescriptions based on current symptom status. Encourage full activity schedule for growth and developmental age. Make appropriate medication adjustments and apply environmental control measures.
Potential patient problem: susceptibility to infection	Assess for signs and symptoms of infection. Maintain optimal nutritional intake. Maintain appropriate rest patterns. Monitor use of medications to control or eliminate symptoms.
Self-concept, disturbance in: role performance, body image	Assess patient for current restrictions in life-style and work, adjustment to illness, self-management behaviors, and family's adjustment to illness. Coordinate with physician and patient modifications in medical therapeutic prescriptions as indicated.

Patient Education

1. Review the disease process with the patient to assess the accuracy of the patient's understanding.
2. Review with the patient medication use and expected response to therapy.
3. Teach the patient self-responsibility for allergen identification and avoidance measures.
4. Direct the patient to support and educational groups.

EVALUATION

Specific criteria are identified with discussion of each atopic disease. The following are general outcome measures for any atopic disease.

Patient Outcome	Data Indicating That Outcome is Reached
Symptoms are resolved in response to therapeutic measures.	There are no symptoms associated with individual system involvement.
Normal activity and exercise are maintained.	Patient performs activities appropriate for growth and developmental age.

Allergic Rhinitis/Allergic Rhinoconjunctivitis

Allergic rhinitis/allergic rhinoconjunctivitis is a complex of symptoms resulting from an antigen–IgE antibody reaction occurring in the nasal membranes, conjunctiva, or nasopharynx. The antigen is generally inhaled and deposited on the mucous membrane surface. Symptoms may also result from antigen injected or ingested and transported to the site.

Approximately 18.6 million infants, children, and adults in the United States have seasonal or perennial allergic rhinitis. An estimated $224 million is spent annually for physician services and $300 million for medications, and some 28 million days each year are lost because of restricted activity or absence from school or work.

Symptoms may develop as early as infancy but can occur at any time throughout the life span. A positive family history may be obtained in the majority of cases. Without intervention, symptoms may remain constant, increase, or diminish over time.

PATHOPHYSIOLOGY

With antigen-antibody linkage, mast cell degranulation and chemical mediator release occur, resulting in slowing of ciliary action, stimulation of mucosal glands, vasomotor instability, leukocyte infiltration (primarily eosinophilic), and tissue edema because of vasodilation and capillary permeability. Histamine is the major mediator of the inflammatory response, although other mediators such as slow-reacting substance of anaphylaxis (SRS-A), eosinophil chemotactic factor of anaphylaxis (ECF-A), and bradykinin participate.

With prolonged exposure, basement membrane destruction and foamy cell formation occur. More chronic and irreversible changes include hyperplasia and thickening of the mucosal epithelium, mononuclear cellular infiltration, and connective tissue proliferation.

Symptoms generally result from inhalant allergen exposure or occasionally, especially in infants, from food ingestion. The inflammatory response may be confined to the nasal membranes or extend to the conjunctiva or oropharynx.

Acute ocular manifestations may include bilateral conjunctival edema, hyperemia, photophobia, profuse tearing, blurring, and occasional superficial keratitis. With chronic exposure, dryness, itching, and photophobia are more pronounced than hyperemia, and the conjunctivae may appear pale.

Serous otitis occurs because swelling of the eustachian tube meatus prevents normal serous drainage. Although otitis is more prevalent in childhood, any age group may be affected. Decreased hearing and a sensation of fullness or ear popping are common symptoms. In young children otitis is often asymptomatic, and therefore regular ear examinations are mandatory.

Seasonal inhalant exposures may generate intense, acute symptoms including nasal congestion, paroxysmal sneezing, itching, and clear, watery secretions. When these secretions drain into the pharynx, dry cough or hoarseness may occur. Occasionally epistaxis or headache may be present. Seasonal allergic rhinitis may be confused with viral infection, since the symptoms are similar.

Chronic or perennial exposure generally results in attenuated responses manifested by pressure, congestion, mucoid secretions, and chronic postnasal drip with cough, hoarseness, or recurrent throat clearing. Snoring or obligatory mouth breathing may be present. Perennial allergic rhinitis may be misdiagnosed as vasomotor rhinitis, perennial nonallergic rhinitis, or sinusitis.

Particularly with adults, allergic rhinitis may occur with other nasal diseases. A primary vasomotor response or one resulting from the inflammatory reaction may intensify symptoms. Allergic rhinitis may aggravate existing nasal polyps. Increased sensitivity to nonspecific irritants occurs during an allergic episode. Occasionally secondary bacterial infections occur with prolonged nasal congestion, mucus production, and host fatigue. The sense of smell may diminish but usually remains intact during allergic episodes.

DIAGNOSTIC STUDIES

See p. 1698.

Skin tests
Positive responses that correlate with history

Sinus roentgenograms
Within normal limits; may be necessary to rule out other diseases such as cysts, nasal polyps, infective rhinitis, and structural defects

TREATMENT PLAN

The goal of the treatment plan is to block symptoms, maintain optimal function, and prevent sequelae such as fatigue, infections, serous otitis, and restricted activity (see also pp. 1699 to 1700).

Chemotherapeutic
Antihistamines
May be used prn or round the clock; long-acting compounds generally best; tolerance avoided by using different antihistamines; often combined with decongestants; see also p. 1699
Cromolyn sodium, prn before known antigen exposure (cat, dog, dusting) but more effective round the clock; short half-life often requires doses q4-6h or concomitant nocturnal antihistamine; see also p. 1699
Sympathomimetic agents
Topical decongestants; over-the-counter; should not be used for more than 3 consecutive d; useful for severe acute symptoms until other medications take effect
Oral decongestants; agents available (phenylephrine, phenylpropanolamine, pseudoephedrine); may be obtained over-the-counter or by prescription; age-dependent dosage; may be used from 3 mo of age; often used in combination with antihistamines and in long-acting preparations for decreased dosage schedule; must be used with caution in patients with hypertension or glaucoma; blood pressure monitoring needed
Corticosteroids
Topical; excellent for controlling more severe symptoms; must be used on regular basis; prn use ineffective; flunisolide and beclomethasone have no systemic effects, but occasional local effects of stinging dryness or irritation may occur; may be used on long-term basis
Flunisolide (Nasalide), 1 spray q8h for adult or child over 6 yr
Beclomethasone (Vancenase, Beconase), 2 sprays q8h for adult or child over 12 yr
Decadron (Decadron Turbinaire), 2 sprays q8h for adult; 1-2 sprays bid for child over 6 yr
Oral; Rarely used since advent of topical agents; should be considered only when symptoms are severe and other measures have failed
Ocular; because of side effects, even short-term use severely restricted and closely monitored
Anti-infective agents
Used for secondary bacterial infections; synthetic penicillins, sulfa, or erythromycin generally recommended and should be used for 10 d to 2 wk
Analgesic agents
Used to reduce symptoms of pressure headache until appropriate medications achieve symptom control

Environmental control
Allergic rhinitis responds dramatically to removal of allergen; see p. 1699 for control of antigen exposure

Immunotherapy
Allergic rhinitis responds well to appropriately designed immunotherapy program; see p. 1700

Supportive
Increased fluid intake to liquefy secretions and counter loss from obligatory mouth breathing
Steam or topical nasal saltwater solutions to decrease irritability and help loosen secretions

ASSESSMENT

The goal of assessment is to confirm the extent and severity of organ involvement and establish a baseline for later evaluation.

Conjunctival inflammation
Hyperemia; edema (chemosis) involving either palpebral or bulbar membranes; secretions in palpebral

fissures; superficial keratitis; edema; hyperplasia of papillae

Facial changes

Dark discoloration in orbital-palpebral groove beneath lower eyelids ("allergic shiners"); adenoidal facies consisting of elongated maxilla, narrow chin, gaping expression, possible dental malocclusion, and transverse crease across top of nose

Nasal membrane inflammation

Swollen, wet, pale turbinates; mucosal edema; glis-

tering, clear, watery or serous discharge; more variability in chronic disease

Oropharyngeal inflammation

Nasal secretions; erythema; edema; high-arched palate; overbite

Tympanic membrane involvement

Bulging or retracted; prominent bony landmarks or none present; membrane thick, dull, or wrinkled, with gray, pink, amber, slightly yellow, or deep blue color; injected; evidence of fluid levels or bubbles

NURSING DIAGNOSES and NURSING INTERVENTIONS

Nursing Diagnosis	Nursing Intervention
Breathing pattern, ineffective	Assess for obligatory mouth breathing, paroxysmal nocturnal dyspnea, snoring, or sleep apnea that may contribute to "allergic fatigue." Elevate head of bed to 45 degrees to facilitate mucus drainage. Humidify air as needed. Monitor medication schedule to block symptoms adequately. Assess environment for presence of offending allergens and remove if possible. Emphasize importance of nasal breathing.
Health maintenance, alteration in (potential)	Discuss chronicity of disease process and reinforce need to prevent symptoms through medications and environmental control.
Injury: potential for	Emphasize importance of avoiding antigens known to cause severe reactions, and explain potential for severe reactions to people who are likely to have contact with patient. Adhere strictly to immunotherapy protocols, and monitor patient for 20 minutes after injections.
Activity intolerance, potential	Explain that normal activities of work, exercise, and recreation should and can be maintained through medications and environmental control.
Potential patient problem: susceptibility to infection	Assess for signs and symptoms of infective rhinitis, infective otitis, and infective conjunctivitis. Maintain adequate nutritional intake and appropriate rest. Discuss rationale for adequately controlling symptoms and self-monitoring for secondary infections.

Patient Education

1. Assess the patient's current knowledge of the disease process and reinforce the concept of self-care and self-management of the disease.
2. Assess the patient's current knowledge of medications, side effects, and rationale for the use of medications, and reinforce the concepts of prophylaxis and prevention of symptoms.
3. Teach the importance of environmental control measures and the patient's responsibility for implementing recommended measures.
4. Teach the patient the importance of monitoring symptom response to therapies, recording any difficulties, new symptoms, and untoward effects, and communicating this on an ongoing basis to those prescribing the therapies.

EVALUATION

Patient Outcome	Data Indicating That Outcome is Reached
Symptoms are resolved in response to therapeutic measures.	There are no symptoms associated with inflammatory response or infective process.
Health is maintained at optimal level.	Patient can identify all recommended therapies and provide information related to self-management.
Optimal functional levels are maintained.	Patient engages in normal work, school, or recreational activities without restrictions.

Anaphylaxis

Anaphylaxis results from a systemic IgE-mediated antigen-antibody response. It is an immediate and often life-threatening event in which massive release of mediators triggers a sequence of events in target organs throughout the body, resulting in a variety of symptoms that may include respiratory embarrassment or circulatory collapse.

As with other IgE antigen-antibody reactions, prior sensitization to the antigen must have occurred for anaphylaxis to take place. Anaphylactoid reactions and blood transfusion reactions are mediated by a non-IgE mechanism with the same final common pathway as IgE-mediated reactions. Reactions must be differentiated from vasovagal reactions, syncopal attacks, myocardial infarctions, insulin reactions, hysterical reactions, and shock or respiratory obstruction from other causes.

A history of atopic disease is often not elicited from patients with anaphylaxis. Previous exposures to the offending antigen may or may not have caused an untoward reaction.

Anaphylactoid reactions, through direct mast cell destabilization, immune complex aggregation, or prostaglandin-activating mechanisms, may also cause the release of mediators that results in a systemic reaction clinically similar to anaphylaxis. Anaphylactoid reactions appear frequently in hospital settings. The following are some mechanisms that have been proposed for anaphylactoid reactions:

Direct mediator release (agents such as dextran and radiopaque eyes)

Immune complex aggregation (agents such as γ-globulin administered intramuscularly or intravenously)

Cytotoxic antibody transfusion reactions (agents such as whole blood and cryoprecipitate)

Prostaglandin-induced (agents such as aspirin and nonsteroidal anti-inflammatory agents)

Anaphylaxis may result from injection of antigen (subcutaneous, intravenous, or intramuscular drugs or venom stings), although enough antigen may be absorbed from the gut (ingested food or drug) or from the respiratory tract (inhaled antigen) to precipitate the reaction. The antigen is distributed via the bloodstream and fixes to IgE antibody on mast cells and basophils, triggering mediator release.

A systemic reaction is any organ involvement away from the site of antigen deposition. Reactions are classified as mild, moderate, or severe and may involve the respiratory tract, cardiovascular system, gastrointestinal tract, or skin (Table 16-8). Symptoms may progress in minutes from mild to severe, or severe reaction may occur without warning. Reactions may occur up to 2 hours after exposure. Reactions that occur immediately are the most life threatening. Resolution of symptoms may be immediate or take several days. Resolution depends on the severity of the reaction, the promptness of medical intervention, and any complications occurring during the reaction. Early recognition and rapid intervention may prevent progression to severe reactions.

PATHOPHYSIOLOGY

On reexposure to antigen and its subsequent linkage with IgE antibody, mediator release occurs and affects the end organ responses (Table 16-9).

Almost any drug may precipitate an anaphylactic reaction. Subcutaneous, intramuscular, and intravenous routes provide sufficient antigen for overwhelming systemic reactions. Anaphylaxis produced by insect venom may account for over 100 deaths annually. Foods may generate an anaphylactic reaction, particularly in adults, although this is not common. The following are some common antigens of anaphylaxis[34]:

Drugs
    Proteins (presumably complete antigens)
        Foreign serum
        Vaccines
        Allergen extracts
        Enzymes
    Nonprotein drugs (presumably haptens)
        Penicillin and other antibiotics
        Sulfonamides

Table 16-8
Potential Symptom Complex of Anaphylaxis

Target Organ	Mild	Moderate	Severe
General status (prodromal)	Malaise; sense of illness	Greater malaise and sense of illness	Deep malaise and strong sense of illness
Skin	Hives; erythema; tingling; warm sensation; itching	Generalized urticaria; flushing; generalized pruritus; periorbital edema	Cyanosis; pallor
Upper respiratory tract	Nasal congestion; sneezing; rhinorrhea; conjunctivitis	Profuse congestion and rhinorrhea	Periorbital edema; obligatory mouth breathing
Upper airway	Fullness in mouth or throat	Edema of tongue, larynx, and pharynx; hoarseness	Stridor; completely occluded airway
Lower airway	—	Bronchospasm; dyspnea; cough; wheezing; air trapping	Severe dyspnea; hypoxia; respiratory arrest
Gastrointestinal tract	—	Nausea; vomiting; increased peristalsis	Dysphagia; intense abdominal cramping; diarrhea
Cardiovascular system	Tachycardia	Hypotension; syncope	Coronary insufficiency; cardiac arrhythmias; shock; circulatory collapse
Central nervous system	Anxiety	Intense anxiety; confusion	Seizures; coma

    Local anesthetics
    Hormones
  Venoms
    Hymenoptera (honeybees, wasps, hornets, yellow jackets)
    Deerfly
    Fire ant
  Foods
    Legumes (especially peanuts)
    Nuts
    Berries
    Seafood
    Egg albumin

DIAGNOSTIC STUDIES

The diagnosis is based on a history of signs and symptoms of anaphylaxis immediately after exposure to a likely offending agent, as well as supportive laboratory data.

Complete blood count
  Within normal limits or increased hematocrit value resulting from hemoconcentration

Blood chemistries
  Within normal limits unless myocardial or renal damage has occurred owing to circulatory collapse

Chest roentgenogram
  Normal appearance or hyperinflation with or without atelectasis; pulmonary edema

Electrocardiogram
  Normal unless myocardial damage or hypoxemic changes are present

Skin tests
  Must be done at least 4 weeks after anaphylactic episode to ensure adequate repopulation of IgE antibody; requires extreme caution; usefulness limited to egg-based vaccines, venom, foods, horse serum, insulin, and penicillin

Table 16-9
Physiologic Response to Mediators

Mediator	Effect	End Organ Response
Histamine	Vascular permeability	Edema of larynx, gut, and airways; urticaria
Leukotrienes	Vascular smooth muscle relaxation	Decreased peripheral volume; decreased peripheral resistance
Kalikrein	Vasodilation and vascular engorgement	Decreased blood pressure; bronchospasm
Platelet-activating factor	Increased bronchial smooth muscle tone	Rhinorrhea; bronchorrhea
Others	Mucous gland secretion; irritability of peripheral nerve endings; intestinal smooth muscle tone	Pruritus; gut motility; rhinorrhea; bronchorrhea

TREATMENT PLAN

The goal of the treatment plan is swift, aggressive management of symptoms. Establishment of an airway and maintenance of blood pressure are crucial. Therapy is individualized based on organ involvement and severity of reaction.

Chemotherapeutic

Medications used to counteract effects of mediator release, block additional mediator release, and protect organ system involved; continued until all symptoms have completely resolved; given over sufficient time to prevent further symptom development; withdrawn with careful monitoring

Supportive

Maintained until all symptoms of anaphylaxis are resolved

Respiratory status

Airway maintained in position; suctioning as appropriate

Monitoring of laryngeal involvement

Airway patency maintained with endotracheal tube or tracheostomy if indicated

Arterial blood gas monitoring as indicated

Treatment of acidosis, if present; administration of oxygen if hypoxemic

Monitoring for bronchospasm, rales, and bronchorrhea by peak flow assessment and physical assessment

Monitoring of pulmonary edema and treatment if present

Vascular status—blood pressure maintained through volume replacement or vasopressors

Renal status

Monitoring of urine output

Treatment of oliguria if present

Cardiac status

Monitoring of electrocardiograms

Treatment of arrhythmias if present

Mental status

Monitoring for orientation three times

Explanation of therapies

Monitoring for seizure activity and coma

Preventive

Avoidance of known offending agents mandatory

Complete drug allergy history before administration of any new drug

For patient with history of episodes, reemphasis on avoidance of allergens and labels listing allergy in appropriate places

Parenteral therapy avoided if possible

If parenteral therapy must be instituted, close monitoring needed for first 20 minutes

If parenteral therapy must be instituted, all emergency equipment ready to use

Human serum preparations preferred if antiserum indicated

If indicated, skin testing for vaccines, venoms, antivenoms, insulin, and penicillin

Use of pretreatment protocols and close monitoring required in the special circumstances when patients at risk must be exposed (to radiocontrast media, insulin, or penicillin)

Appropriate identification carried by patients at risk and information shared with significant others

Teaching self-administration of epinephrine and subsequent measures to take to patients at risk

Attempts to identify causative agent, and sharing of information with patient

ASSESSMENT: AREAS OF CONCERN

Because of multisystem involvement, anaphylactic or anaphylactoid reactions may initially have a variety of manifestations.

Laryngeal involvement

Hoarseness; stridor; use of accessory muscles; difficulty in speech

Respiratory status

Dyspnea; substernal tightness; use of accessory muscles; cough

Bronchospasm

Mucus production; rales; wheezing; decreased breath sounds; anxiety; inability to lie supine; evidence of air trapping or atelectasis on chest roentgenogram

Pulmonary edema

Wet rales at base; frothy clear or blood-streaked secretions

Respiratory arrest

No air movement

Circulatory status

Hypotension; weak, thready pulse; tachycardia; oliguria; mental confusion

Cardiac status

Arrhythmias; tachycardia; cardiac arrest

Central nervous system status

Anxiety; malaise; sense of illness; mental confusion; obtundation; coma

Dermal status

Pruritus; erythema; flushing; urticaria; angioedema; cyanosis; pallor

Gastrointestinal status
  Nausea; vomiting; diarrhea; gastrointestinal cramping

Upper respiratory status
  Rhinorrhea; congestion; sneezing; conjunctivitis; tearing

NURSING DIAGNOSES and NURSING INTERVENTIONS

Nursing Diagnosis	Nursing Intervention
Breathing pattern, ineffective	In collaboration with physician, maintain airway patency; administer epinephrine, aminophylline, antihistamines, and oxygen; and assess and document patient's response. Maintain endotracheal tube or tracheostomy if instituted. Assess and record ventilation pattern, including rate, rhythm, use of accessory muscles, and length of expiratory phase. Monitor for mouth breathing and rhinorrhea. Maintain 45-degree elevation of patient's head if possible. Assess for laryngeal involvement, including stridor, hoarseness, and difficulty in swallowing or speech.
Gas exchange, impaired	Monitor blood gases in collaboration with physician. Administer oxygen at indicated rate. Assess for presence of breath sounds including rales, rhonchi, cough, and wheezing. Assess for absence shortness of breath, dyspnea, and substernal tightness. Monitor fluid replacement and assess for pulmonary overload.
Airway clearance, ineffective	Suction if necessary.
Tissue perfusion, alteration in: cerebral	Assess for symptoms of anxiety, confusion, obtundation, or coma. In conjunction with physician administer fluid replacement.
Tissue perfusion, alteration in: renal	Monitor and record intake and output. In conjunction with physician, administer epinephrine, vasopressors, or fluid as indicated.
Tissue perfusion, alteration in: gastrointestinal	Monitor for nausea, vomiting, abdominal cramping, and diarrhea. Record findings. In conjunction with physician administer antihistamines as indicated.
Tissue perfusion, alteration in: peripheral	Monitor for cyanosis, pallor, and pulse abnormalities. Record findings. In conjunction with physician, administer epinephrine, fluids, or vasopressors as indicated.
Tissue perfusion, alteration in: cardiac	Monitor electrocardiogram for arrhythmias. In conjunction with physician, administer epinephrine or antiarrhythmic agents as indicated.
Tissue perfusion, alteration in: dermal	In conjunction with physician, administer epinephrine or antihistamines as indicated. Assess for pruritus, erythema, flushing, angioedema, and urticaria. Record findings.
Injury: potential for (anaphylaxis related to exposure to inciting agent)	Obtain complete drug allergy history before administering new drug. Put labels noting allergic drug history in all appropriate places. Closely monitor patient for 30 minutes after administering new drug.

Patient Education

1. Reassure patient during procedures.
2. Explain reason for each procedure.
3. Explain relationship of symptoms to anaphylactic reaction.
4. Explain absolute necessity of avoiding causative agent.
5. Explain patient's responsibility in interactions with care givers.
6. Explain need to carry appropriate identification and to share information with appropriate others.
7. Provide information on medical alert identification.
8. Teach self-administration of epinephrine and subsequent measures, including oral administration of antihistamine and seeking immediate medical care.

EVALUATION

Patient Outcome	Data Indicating That Outcome is Reached
Symptoms resolve in response to therapeutic measures.	Patient is symptom free. Patient expresses feeling of well-being. There is no evidence of urticaria or angioedema or subjective complaint of pruritus or swelling. There is no evidence of rhinoconjunctivitis, asthma, pulmonary edema, or laryngeal edema. Bowel sounds and elimination pattern are normal. Blood pressure and pulse rate are normal. There is no evidence of hypoxia.
Recurrence is prevented.	Patient can identify triggering agent and explain all appropriate avoidance measures.

FOOD ALLERGY

Food allergy is an IgE-mediated hypersensitivity disease. It may be manifest in the respiratory, integumentary, or gastrointestinal system as rhinitis, asthma, atopic dermatitis, urticaria, nausea, vomiting, diarrhea, or cramps or may result in anaphylaxis. An adverse food reaction is any untoward symptom complex resulting from food ingestion.

Adverse reaction to food is a complex diagnostic problem. There are various causes for adverse food reactions. True food allergy is mediated by IgE antibody (type I hypersensitivity reaction) in sensitized individuals on exposure to the offending antigen. Antibody-antigen linkage occurs, resulting in mediator release and symptoms.

Food intolerance is any abnormal physiologic response to an ingested food or food additive that is nonimmunologic in nature. Other immunologic mechanisms have been identified in adverse food reactions, including IgA deficiency, cytotoxic responses (type II), immune complex formation (type III), and cell-mediated reactions (type IV). Adverse reactions to foods may have multiple origins, with a variety of nonimmunologic mechanisms resulting in a clinically abnormal host response. An idiosyncratic response in an individual may result in an anaphylactoid reaction, as with ingestion of monosodium glutamate. A metabolic defect such as lactose enzyme deficiency may cause foods to be improperly digested, or a metabolic problem such as diabetes may result in an abnormal response. Toxic responses to spoiled food are well known. Pharmacologic properties such as those of caffeine may exert a direct untoward effect. All these reactions are well documented and reproducible in controlled settings.

Other clinical syndromes are ascribed to foods or food additives, but this cannot be substantiated by reproducible, objective studies. While anecdotal evidence exists to support a relationship between food ingestion and behavior, other causal relationships have not been adequately ruled out. Tension-fatigue syndrome, hyperactivity syndrome, and psychiatric disorders such as mood swings are among the many disorders identified as being linked to food. Similar reports linking foods to rheumatoid arthritis or vasculitis and other physical syndromes also have not been substantiated. Other causes of vomiting, diarrhea, and stool abnormalities must also be excluded.

The prevalence of food allergy is unknown. Estimates range from 0.1% to 7% of the population, with a male/female ratio of approximately 2:1. If one sibling has a documented food allergy, a 50% probability of food hypersensitivity exists in other siblings. Anaphylactic episodes are most common in adults but may occur at any age. Non-immunologic-mediated adverse food reactions have a much higher prevalence than immunologic reactions.

In exquisitely sensitive persons merely inhaling the antigen in cooking odors can precipitate a massive allergic reaction. Reactions are often dose related and may vary with time in the same individual. The foods most commonly associated with allergic reactions are milk, eggs, wheat, and soybeans in children and fish, shellfish, peanuts, nuts, and seeds in adults, although virtually any food may cause an allergic response. Families of foods may share allergenic features, and thus cross-reactivity among those foods (for example, shellfish) is more common. Because of absorption characteristics, the reaction may be immediate or delayed up to 2 hours after ingestion.

PATHOPHYSIOLOGY

As with other antigen–IgE antibody–mediated responses, prior exposure with sensitization in the atopic individual must occur. On reexposure, antigen-antibody linkage occurs with resultant mediator release. For reasons unknown, one end organ may be affected with a localized response, as in urticaria, or loss of sensitivity may occur over time.

Why different individuals become sensitized to particular foods is also unknown. Allergenicity of the protein correlates with its heat-labile or enzyme-resistant properties. Although cooking or digestion may alter the protein, rendering it less allergenic, the altered protein may still precipitate an allergic response. An alteration in the original protein may contribute to false negative skin test findings if the unaltered food is used as the test antigen.

The gastrointestinal tract plays an important role in food allergy. The gut normally reaches maturity by 2 years of age. Before maturation there is a greater likelihood of absorption of food protein prior to complete digestion. Increase in absorption of potentially antigenic substances may also occur in IgA deficiency, malabsorption disease, and chronic inflammatory bowel diseases and after viral, parasitic, or bacterial diseases when the normal protective barriers have been damaged. These clinical syndromes may also contribute to adverse food reactions by decreasing normal flora, decreasing digestive enzymes, bile salts, and other secretions, reducing peristalsis, and interfering with cell renewal.

When the gut mucosal wall is damaged, protein may be absorbed and may precipitate IgE and IgG involvement or immune complex formation. Increased immunologic reactivity involving IgG and immune complex formation may result in enteropathies. Aspiration of milk in infancy may stimulate an IgE host defense response.

Genetic factors, amount of food ingested, food-drug interactions, contaminants, infections, pharmacologic properties, and nonimmunologic mechanisms have all been identified as contributing to adverse food reactions (Table 16-10).

Because of the multiple pathophysiologic mechanisms involved, clinical manifestations of adverse food reactions are widely variable (Table 16-10). Depending on the mechanism, amount, and duration of exposure, symptoms may vary from episodic to chronic and from mild to severe, and consequences may be reversible or irreversible.

DIAGNOSTIC STUDIES

Diagnostic studies are chosen based on the presentation of the adverse food reaction. The history is by far the most important diagnostic tool. The physical examination focuses on the clinical presentation.

Laboratory tests are chosen based on the suspected mechanism of the adverse food reaction. Cytotoxic testing, sublingual testing, and red blood cell lysis have no proven efficacy in diagnosis and should not be employed.

History
Frequency, duration and seasonality of symptoms; onset, severity, progression, and nature of symptoms; timing between ingestion and symptom onset; amount and nature of provoking food; concomitant illnesses; nutritional history; drug history; atopic history; infectious disease history

Physical examination
Skin; upper and lower respiratory tract; gastrointestinal tract; oropharynx; weight and height; growth and development; general appearance; vital signs; muscle mass and amount of subcutaneous tissue; texture and amount of hair; hepatomegaly

Laboratory tests
Type I hypersensitivity
Skin tests
May have false positives or negatives; not diagnostic; must be used in conjunction with challenge tests
Radioallergosorbent test (RAST)
May be less sensitive and has more limited panel than skin tests; may also have false positives or negatives; not diagnostic; must be used in conjunction with challenge tests
Total serum IgE
Not specific indicator, not helpful
Eosinophil count
Not specific indicator, not helpful
Elimination diets
Aid in diagnosis by symptom response; used in conjunction with rechallenge; strict elimination diets difficult and cannot be used for more than 7 days
Food rechallenge
Confirms diagnosis; not to be used if there is history of anaphylaxis
Types II, III, and IV hypersensitivity
Biopsy of involved tissue
Demonstrates presence of IgG, IgM, complement activation, or T cell involvement
Hemagglutination
May be present in persons without disease or absent in persons who have disease
IgA deficiency
IgA level
Wide range of normal (80 to 350 mg/dl); may be low normal or depressed
Natural pharmacologic agents
Diet diary and elimination diet
Correlates symptoms with suspected agents
Food rechallenge
Confirms diagnosis

Table 16-10

Adverse Reactions to Foods

Type	Mechanism	Food (Examples)	Host Response
Type I Hypersensitivity			
Food allergy	IgE antibody–antigen linkage	Shellfish; nuts	Urticaria; angioedema; rhinitis; bronchospasm; nausea; vomiting; diarrhea, anaphylaxis
Metabolic Reactions			
Enzyme deficiencies	Lactase deficiency	Milk	Bloating; diarrhea; cramps
	Glucose 6-phosphate dehydrogenase (G6-PD) deficiency	Fava beans	Hemolytic anemia
	Phenylketonuria		Central nervous system changes
Severe chronic inflammatory bowel disease	Loss of enzymes through diarrhea and decreased production	Saccharides	Bloating; diarrhea; cramps; malabsorption
Medication interactions	Monoamine oxidase inhibitors	Cheese	Hypertensive crisis
Celiac disease	Probable type IV reaction	Wheat	Bloating; diarrhea; malabsorption
Gallbladder disease	Decreased bile salts	Several	Bloating; indigestion; diarrhea; cramping
Diabetes	Decreased insulin	Sugar	Hyperglycemia
Cystic fibrosis	Inadequate pancreatic function	Fats; proteins	Fatty, foul-smelling stools; malabsorption
Natural Pharmacologic Agents			
Psychoactive agents	Direct sympathetic stimulation	Caffeine; theobromine	Central nervous system stimulation
Vasoactive amines (e.g., tryptamine, tyramine)	Direct action on end organ or autonomic stimulation	Cheese; chocolate	Headaches
Food Contamination by Infectious Agents, Microbes, and Toxins			
Bacteria; viruses; parasites; fungi	Endotoxins; neurotoxins; toxic alkaloids; damage to gut wall	Contaminated foods	Nausea; vomiting; diarrhea; bloating; weight loss; liver dysfunctions; headaches; fever; chills
Natural Toxic Agents			
Licorice	Sodium retention	Licorice	Hypertension
Glycoalkaloids	Probable direct blood vessel effect	Green potatoes; lima beans	Angioedema; urticaria
Anaphylactoid Reactions			
Chemical mediator release	Direct action on mast cell	Strawberries; tomatoes	Urticaria; angioedema; diarrhea
Nonimmunologic	Unknown	Tartrazine (FD & C yellow #5)	Urticaria; angioedema; rhinitis; asthma
	Unknown	Sodium metabisulfite	Urticaria; angioedema; rhinitis; asthma; anaphylaxis
	Unknown	Monosodium glutamate	Headache; flush; asthma
Types II, III, and IV Hypersensitivity			
Immune complexes with food antigen	Complement activation	After acute viral gastroenteritis	Diarrhea; cramping
Weiner's syndrome	IgG-antigen complexes; also type IV reaction	Milk	Respiratory symptoms; failure to thrive
Enteropathies	IgG precipitating antibodies	Milk; soy	Gastrointestinal bleeding; malabsorption; diarrhea; cramping
IgA deficiency	Failure to regulate antigen absorption	Variable	Malnutrition; diarrhea; increased with severity of disease

Food contamination by infectious agents
  Stool cultures
    Document infection agent
Natural toxic agents
  Diet diary and elimination diet
    Correlate symptoms with suspected agent
  Food rechallenge
    Confirms history
Anaphylactoid reactions
  Diet diary and elimination diet
    Correlate symptoms with suspected agent
  Food rechallenge
    Confirms history
Metabolism
  Disease-specific workup (refer to discussion of specific disease elsewhere in text)

TREATMENT PLAN

The goal of the treatment plan is to eliminate the offending food, thus preventing recurrence of symptoms. Types I, II, III, and IV hypersensitivity, reactions to natural pharmacologic agents and natural toxic agents, and anaphylactoid reactions respond completely to elimination of the offending food.

Often symptoms are time limited and resolve without therapy. Choice of medications and supportive therapy are dependent on the nature and severity of symptoms, organ system involved, and mechanism of the reaction.

Chemotherapeutic
  Based on severity and nature of symptoms, organ system involved, and mechanism of reaction (Table 16-11)

Supportive
  Based on nature and severity of symptoms and mechanism of adverse drug reaction; goal of supportive therapy is to facilitate healing process; see elsewhere in text for further organ specific-supportive measures
  For type I hypersensitivity, anaphylactoid reactions, drug contamination (IgE), glycoalkaloids, and types III and IV hypersensitivity
    See specific therapy for rhinitis, angioedema, and anaphylaxis
    Maintenance of appropriate elimination diet
    Monitoring for further symptom involvement
    High-caloric replacement therapy if needed
    Keeping affected skin dry and clear and preventing further injury
    Restriction of activity while symptoms are acute
  For metabolic reactions
    See specific therapy for underlying disease process
    Maintenance of appropriate elimination diet
    Monitoring for further symptom development
    High-caloric replacement therapy as appropriate
    Restricted activity while symptoms are acute
  For reactions to natural pharmacologic agents
    Restful, calm, quiet environment
    Restricted activity while symptoms are acute
  For reactions to infectious agents
    See specific therapy for underlying disease process
    Analgesics if appropriate
    Adequate hydration
    Restricted food intake until gastrointestinal healing has occurred
    Restricted activity while symptoms are acute

Prevention
  Avoidance of known offending foods mandatory; patient should be taught relationship of foods to symptom development
  For patient with history of atopic reaction reemphasis

Table 16-11
Medications Used in Treatment of Adverse Food Reactions

Mechanism	Potential Organ Involvement	Class of Medication
Type I hypersensitivity	Skin	Antihistamines
Anaphylactoid reactions	Upper respiratory tract	Sympathomimetic agents
Penicillin, drug contamination	Lower respiratory tract	Bronchodilators
Glycoalkaloids	Upper airway; gastrointestinal tract; multiorgan	Corticosteroids
Types II, III, and IV hypersensitivity (IgG-mediated, immune complex, and T cell sensitization, respectively)	Gastrointestinal tract Skin; respiratory tract	Topical or oral corticosteroids Nonsteroidal anti-inflammatory agents
Infectious agents (bacterial, fungal, parasitic, viral)	Multisystemic response; gastrointestinal tract	Anti-infective agents
Metabolic reactions (enzyme deficiencies [cystic fibrosis], chronic inflammatory bowel disease)	Gastrointestinal malabsorption; protein-calorie deficiencies	Enzyme replacement; see specific therapy for disease process

on avoidance of agent and labels warning of reaction posted in appropriate places

Emphasis on carrying appropriate identification and sharing information with significant others

For patients at risk, education about self-administration of epinephrine and subsequent measures to take

Patient education about self-monitoring of symptoms using cause-effect approach

Emphasis on patient's responsibility in interactions with care givers

Immunotherapy has no proven efficacy in food allergy

Breast feeding with some maternal dietary restriction and delay in introduction of new foods to prevent or minimize food allergy in infants

ASSESSMENT: AREAS OF CONCERN

Response to therapy is based on the underlying mechanism, degree, and length of exposure. The symptom complex may vary among individuals.

Type I hypersensitivity, anaphylactoid reactions, reactions to glycoalkyloids
Laryngeal involvement
  Hoarseness; stridor; use of accessory muscles; difficulty in speech
Respiratory involvement
  Dyspnea; substernal tightness; use of accessory muscles; cough
Bronchospasm
  Mucus production; rhonchi; wheezing; decreased breath sounds; anxiety; inability to lie down; evidence of air trapping or atelectasis on chest roentgenogram
Dermal involvement
  Pruritus; erythema; flushing; urticaria; angioedema; cyanosis; pallor
Upper respiratory involvement
  Rhinorrhea; congestion; sneezing; tearing; conjunctivitis
Gastrointestinal involvement
  Nausea; vomiting; bloating; distention; diarrhea; cramping
Anaphylaxis
  All the above

Immunogenic (type II [IgG], type III [circulating immune complexes], type IV [T cell sensitization], IgA deficiency)
Gastrointestinal involvement
  Nausea; vomiting; bloating; distention; diarrhea; cramping; gastrointestinal bleeding; malabsorption; failure to thrive; hepatomegaly
Dermal involvement
  Vasculitic lesion; contact dermatitis; hair thinning
Musculoskeletal involvement
  Muscle mass loss; subcutaneous tissue loss
See IgA deficiency assessment

Infective agents
Gastrointestinal involvement
  Nausea; vomiting; bloating; distention; diarrhea; cramping; gastrointestinal bleeding; malabsorption
Systemic
  Fever; arthralgias; malaise

Reactions to natural pharmacologic agents
Psychoactive agents
  Central nervous system stimulation
    Palpitations; anxiety; tachycardia; irritability
Vasoactive amines
  Central nervous system
    Vascular headaches; migraines

Metabolic reactions (cystic fibrosis, diabetes, phenylketonuria, glucose 6-phosphate dehydrogenase deficiency, chronic inflammatory bowel disease, celiac disease, gallbladder disease)
See specific disease process
Gastrointestinal involvement
  Nausea; vomiting; diarrhea; cramps; bloating; flatulence; fatty, foul-smelling stools; presence of occult blood in stool; failure to thrive; malnutrition; hepatomegaly; protuberant abdomen
Dermal involvement
  Sparse hair; lanugo
Musculoskeletal
  Loss of muscle mass; subcutaneous tissue

NURSING DIAGNOSES and NURSING INTERVENTIONS

The nursing diagnosis and interventions are based on the mechanism of the adverse food reaction and the severity of symptoms.

Nursing Diagnosis	Nursing Intervention
Injury: potential for	Obtain complete history of adverse food reactions and put labels specifying allergies in appropriate places.
	Maintain elimination diet.
	Teach patient self-management behaviors.
Nutrition, alteration in: less than body requirements (potential)	Assess current dietary intake for caloric and nutritional requirements.
Bowel elimination, alteration in: diarrhea	Monitor intake, output, and weight.
	Assess for signs and symptoms of dehydration.
	Assess for signs and symptoms of electrolyte imbalance.
	Provide fluid supplementation.
	Monitor stool for occult blood, character, and pathogens.
	Provide adequate hygiene.
	Monitor for further symptom development.
	In conjunction with physician, administer medication as appropriate.
Activity intolerance	Restrict activity during acute and convalescent phases.
Comfort, alteration in: pain	Assess for bloating and other symptoms.
	Provide calm, quiet, restful environment.
	Maintain hygiene and skin care.
	In conjunction with physician, administer analgesics and other medications as needed.

Patient Education

1. Assess the patient's current knowledge of the disease process and reinforce the concept of self-care and self-management of the disease.
2. Explain that the disease is a chronic one, and reinforce the need to prevent symptoms through avoidance of foods that cause them.
3. Teach the patient the importance of monitoring the response of symptoms to therapies, recording any difficulties, new symptoms, and cause-effect relationships noted, and communicating this on an ongoing basis to those prescribing the therapies.
4. Emphasize the importance of carrying appropriate identification and sharing information with significant others.
5. For patients at risk of anaphylaxis, teach self-administration of epinephrine and subsequent measures to take.

EVALUATION

Patient Outcome	Data Indicating That Outcome is Reached
Symptoms resolve in response to therapeutic measures.	Patient is symptom free.
Recurrences are prevented.	Patient can identify causative food and explain appropriate measures to avoid it.

Drug Allergy

An adverse drug reaction is any noxious or unintended effect of a drug. True drug allergy is mediated by IgE antibody–antigen interaction. Adverse reactions may also be mediated by other immunologic or nonimmunologic mechanisms.

Adverse drug reactions have steadily increased with the increase in available pharmacologic preparations. Drug allergy is one of the most common iatrogenic problems.

The incidence of adverse reactions is unknown. Three percent of hospitalizations are attributed to adverse drug reactions, and approximately 15% to 30% of hospitalized patients have an adverse drug reaction. Hospitalized patients not uncommonly receive 10 or more drugs, which obviously increases the risk of adverse drug reaction. The contribution of most additives or contaminants in adverse reactions is unclear, although idiosyncratic responses to tartrazine, sodium metabisulfite, and sodium benzoate have been well described.

Table 16-12
Adverse Drug Reactions

Reaction	Mechanism	Example
Non-Drug-Related (symptoms dissimilar to expected pharmacologic effects)		
Psychogenic	Vasovagal	Syncope; anxiety
Coincidental symptoms	Disease process itself	Viral rash with antibiotics
Drug-Related in Any Patient (symptoms similar to expected pharmacologic effects)		
Overdose	Increased intake, lowered metabolism, overdose, decreased liver excretion, toxic pharmacologic effect	Digoxin toxicity in elderly
Side effects	Undesirable pharmacologic effect of drug, often unavoidable with normal dose	Sleepiness with antihistamine
Secondary effects	Indirectly related to primary pharmacologic action	Vaginal infection after orally administered antibiotics
Drug interactions	Alter normal physiology of host, e.g., changes in absorption, metabolism, excretion; additive effects	Erythromycin changes liver metabolism and thus slows metabolism of theophylline
Disease-associated effects	Decreased absorption, metabolism, excretion; alteration in metabolic pathways	Digoxin toxicity
Drug-Related in Susceptible Patients (symptoms, except for intolerance, dissimilar to expected pharmacologic response)		
Intolerance	Quantitively greater effect at normal dosages	CNS excitation with pharmacologic dose of adrenergic drug
Idiosyncracy	Qualitatively abnormal response that is different from pharmacologic effects (nonimmunologic)	Adverse response to local anesthetics
Genetic	Lack of enzyme or metabolic pathway	Hemolytic anemic in G6-Pd deficiency
Anaphylactoid	Nonimmunologic	Aspirin-induced bronchospasm
Allergy	IgE antigen-antibody	Penicillin allergy
Cytotoxic	Cytoxic antibody-mediated against cell membranes with involvement of complement, IgG, and IgM	Coombs' test–positive hemolytic anemia
Immune complex	Drug-IgG, IgM-drug immune complexes, complement	Serum sickness, drug-induced lupus
Cell-mediated	T lymphocyte sensitization	Fixed drug eruption, photosensitivity eruptions

Symptoms may affect any organ system of the body and may have a short or protracted course. Symptoms may range from mild to severe, and resolution of symptoms depends on the initiating mechanism, amount of drug, and host response.

Drug and host factors can influence the development of an adverse drug reaction:

Drug factors

Nature of drug—class; weight; size; metabolites; ability to bind as hapten to protein (generally low molecular weight [500-1000])

Route of administration—intravenous, topical, oral (in descending order of risk)

Degree of exposure—prolonged course, high doses, and intermittent exposures increase risk; risk increases in first 2 to 3 weeks of therapy

Host factors

Age—adult at greater risk than child, probably because of total exposures and greater need for drugs

Sex—no difference except that women at greater risk with muscle relaxants and chymopapain

Atopic history—no greater incidence but appears to be associated with more severe reactions

Genetic—may contribute by influencing metabolic pathways or increased mediators

Prior drug reactions—increased tendency with new drugs

Underlying disease state—may compromise immunologic mechanisms or alter metabolic pathways

PATHOPHYSIOLOGY

Adverse drug reactions may be classified according to mechanism of reaction (Table 16-12).

Non-drug-related reactions of the psychogenic type generally occur only with fear of pain, as with the intramuscular or subcutaneous route of administration. Coincidental symptoms are more easily distinguished with knowledge of disease symptoms.

Adverse drug reactions that any patient may experience are the most common and most predictable. Overdosage results in toxic pharmacologic effects of the drug and occurs most commonly in pediatric or geriatric populations with dosage miscalculations or with failure to recognize concurrent drug or host factors that delay the metabolism and excretion of the drug.

Side effects vary among patients and with drugs. They are most commonly seen with drugs that directly or indirectly affect the central nervous system or gastrointestinal system.

Drug interactions are complex, and thoughtful analysis is required before administration of more than one drug.

Drug interactions may potentiate, decrease, or negate the desired therapeutic effects and may place the patient at risk of overdose.

Disease-associated effects generally result in toxic overdose as a result of decreased metabolism or excretion. In gastrointestinal diseases, drugs may be poorly absorbed, resulting in lack of therapeutic response.

Intolerance is a common problem. Many patients exhibit increased side effects or gastrointestinal sensitivity to numerous drugs at normal doses.

Idiosyncratic responses of an anaphylactoid nature are nonimmunologic. Direct action on mast cells resulting in release of chemical mediators, prostaglandin activation, or IgG aggregation result in clinical symptoms similar to IgE antibody hypersensitivity. The following are some mechanisms of anaphylactoid reactions:

Mast cell degranulation (for example, codeine, morphine, radiocontrast media)

Prostaglandin-induced reactions (for example, dextran and other plasma expanders, aspirin, nonsteroidal anti-inflammatory agents, tartrazine)

Immune complex aggregation (for example, intramuscular or intravenous γ-globulin)

Cytoxic antibody transfusion reactions (for example, mismatched blood transfusions)

In anaphylactoid reactions, prior exposure is not required, the host response may be variable over time, reactions can be produced with minute quantities, and the reaction resolves after the drug is discontinued.

Allergic, IgE antibody mechanisms account for a large proportion of adverse drug reactions because of the frequency with which drugs that fall in this category are prescribed. Some examples of such drugs are penicillin and synthetic penicillins, sulfonamide antibiotics, sulfonylurea hypoglycemics, thiazide diuretics, carbonic anhydrase inhibitors, insulin and other hormones, egg-based vaccines, enzymes including chymopapain, antitoxins, and allergen extracts. The drug may act directly, it may bind with serum or tissue protein as a hapten, or a metabolite of the drug may be the offending antigen.

The allergic response requires prior exposure, can be reproduced by agents with cross-reacting structures, and can be produced by minute quantities. The reaction resolves after the drug is discontinued.

In cytotoxic or type II hypersensitivity, IgG or IgM antibody activates complement, resulting in damage to cell membranes. A drug may act as a hapten by binding to a cell surface, a drug-antibody complex may be absorbed to the cell surface, or a drug may change or modify a cell membrane leading to cell destruction.

In circulating immune complex or type III hypersensitivity, drug or drug hapten bound to protein may bind with antibody, forming circulating immune complexes.

In cell-mediated reactions or type IV hypersensitivity,

T lymphocytes are sensitized, resulting in skin or organ damage. A drug may elicit symptoms through more than one mechanism, for example, penicillin allergy or serum sickness.

In allergic, cytotoxic, immune complex, and cell-mediated reactions the evolution of symptoms often suggests an immunologic mechanism, although the exact mechanism may be impossible to establish and the diagnosis is commonly made on clinical grounds.

DIAGNOSTIC STUDIES

There are no simple, rapid, and predictable in vitro tests, nor is there safe and reliable in vivo testing for most adverse drug reactions. Demonstration of IgE antibody is limited to selected cases. No test is available for non-drug-related reactions, drug-related intolerance, or anaphylactoid adverse drug reactions. The clinical history is the most important tool in diagnosing adverse drug reactions.

Drug history
All drugs taken by patient within last 2 weeks, including over-the-counter preparations; time between exposure and symptom onset (delay of 7 to 10 days is common); route of administration and duration of treatment; prior drug exposure; onset, progression severity, and nature of symptoms; clinical course after drug is discontinued; concomitant diseases; infectious disease history

Skin testing
Limited because of lack of knowledge of true antigen-inducing response; available only for penicillin, toxoids, antisera, insulin, ACTH, egg-based protein; must be done under strict protocol with close supervision

Patch testing
Useful in diagnosing contact sensitivity to topical preparations only

Radioallergosorbent test (RAST)
Not generally useful for drug allergy

Enzyme assays
See specific enzyme deficiency disease

Eosinophil levels
May be elevated in inflammatory tissue response

Anti-DNA (12%)
May be elevated (single stranded) in certain drug-induced reactions

Antinuclear antibody (ANA) (1:20)
Speckled or homogeneous pattern

Complete blood count with differential
Leukocytosis in serum sickness

Erythrocyte sedimentation rate
May be elevated in inflammatory tissue response

Direct challenge
Can confirm suspected drug but is generally not done because of potential morbidity and mortality

TREATMENT PLAN

The goal of the treatment plan is to eliminate the offending drug and thus prevent further symptoms. Most symptoms respond quickly to removal of the offending drug and resolve without therapy. Choice of medications and supportive therapy is dependent on the nature and severity of symptoms, organ system involved, and mechanism of the reactions.

Chemotherapeutic
See Table 16-13

Supportive
Maintained until resolution of symptoms; see elsewhere in text for organ-specific therapy
Forcing fluids to increase renal clearance of drug

Table 16-13
Medications Used in Treatment of Adverse
Drug Reactions

Mechanism	Potential Organ Involvement	Categories of Medications
Type I hypersensitivity, anaphylactoid reactions	Skin Upper and lower respiratory tract Upper airway Gastrointestinal tract	Antihistamines Sympathomimetic agents Bronchodilators Corticosteroids
Type II, cytotoxic	Gastrointestinal tract, skin	Rarely immunosuppressive agents, e.g., azathioprine, cyclophosphamide, nonsteroidal anti-inflammatory agents
	Renal Hematologic	Corticoteroids Oral corticosteroids
Type III, immune complex	Vascular, skin, kidney, heart, liver	Nonsteroidal anti-inflammatory agents
Type IV, cell mediated	Skin	Antihistamines, topical corticosteroids

Plasmapheresis to remove circulating immune complexes

Hemodialysis or peritoneal dialysis in severe overdose to remove drug rapidly

Emesis or stomach lavage to remove drug in overdose

Prevention

Patient with allergic drug reaction should not receive that drug or cross-reacting one, if possible

If drug must be given, informed consent and administration under strict protocol necessary

ASSESSMENT

Adverse drug reactions have multiple mechanisms. Coincidental symptom assessment varies, since it is based on manifestations of the disease process. Drug-related reactions of overdose toxicity, side effects, intolerance, and secondary effects are related to specific drugs, and knowledge of the drug mechanism makes it possible to identify potential symptoms. In immunologic mechanisms, organ system involvement may also be variable. The reader is referred elsewhere in this text for specific organ assessment.

Type I hypersensitivity, anaphylactoid reactions

See section on anaphylaxis

Type II cytotoxic

Hematologic involvement

See assessment for hemolytic anemia, thrombocytopenia, agranulocytosis

Renal involvement

See assessment for interstitial nephritis

Type III, immune complex

Serum sickness

See serum sickness assessment

Drug fever

Systemic

Low-grade fever, malaise

May be associated with serum sickness

See serum sickness assessment

Vasculitis

See vasculitis assessment

Drug-induced lupus

See lupus assessment

Vasculitis

See vasculitis assessment

Type IV, cell mediated

Contact dermatitis

See assessment for contact dermatitis

Photosensitivity eruptions

See assessment for photosensitivity eruptions

NURSING DIAGNOSES and NURSING INTERVENTIONS

Nursing interventions are based on the mechanism and the organ involved. The reader is referred to the discussion of the specific organ involved for the nursing diagnosis and nursing interventions.

Nursing Diagnosis	Nursing Intervention
Injury: potential for	Obtain complete drug allergy history before administering new drug.
	Put labels concerning allergic drug history in appropriate places.
	Closely monitor patient for 30 minutes after administering new drug intramuscularly, subcutaneously, or intravenously.
	Maintain emergency equipment and drugs.
	Maintain high index of suspicion with patients receiving any medications.
	Monitor patient for development of new symptoms during course of medication therapy and for 2 weeks after drug administration ends.
Activity intolerance	Restrict activity level through acute and convalescent periods.
Anxiety	Provide explanations of disease process and expected course of symptoms. See also p. 1839.

Patient Education

1. Explain the relationship of symptoms to the adverse drug reaction.
2. Explain the absolute necessity of avoiding use of the causative agent.
3. Explain the patient's responsibility in interactions with care givers.
4. Explain the need to carry appropriate identification and to share information with appropriate others.
5. Provide information on medical alert identification.

EVALUATION

Patient Outcome	Data Indicating That Outcome is Reached
Symptoms resolve in response to therapeutic measures.	Patient is symptom free.
Recurrence is prevented.	Patient can identify causative drug and explain appropriate avoidance measures.

URTICARIA/ANGIOEDEMA

Angioedema is soft tissue swelling in submucosal or sub-cutaneous tissues as the result of increased local vascular permeability and serum transudation. Urticarial lesions occur in the upper stratum corneum of the dermis, whereas angioedema lesions occur in the deeper subcutaneous tissues.

Urticaria (discussed in detail in Chapter 5) and angio-edema have the same pathophysiologic features. Urticaria is more common; angioedema may be associated with urticaria or may occur independently. Why some patients have urticaria and others have angioedema is not known.

Angioedema may occur anywhere on the skin, but the periorbital area, lips, throat, tongue, larynx, area around joints, and tips of the extremities are the most common sites. Urticaria and angioedema may occur at any age, and up to 20% of the population may be affected with acute, self-limited episodes. Episodes greater than 6 weeks in duration are defined as chronic. Symptoms may be mild to life threatening, and death may result from laryngeal involvement.

PATHOPHYSIOLOGY

With antigen-antibody linkage, mast cell or basophil de-granulation and chemical mediator release occur. His-tamine and other mediators interact with receptors along the lymphatic, capillary, and venule walls, resulting in dilation, engorgement, and increased capillary perme-ability with a perivascular mononuclear cell infiltrate in which eosinophils may predominate. This inflammatory response usually resolves within 2 to 6 hours after insult, although in soft tissues nonpitting edema may be more diffuse and reabsorption of fluid may take up to several days. Complaints of burning pain or tightness are more commonly associated with angioedema than is pruritus.

Other immunologic mechanisms may precipitate the same pathophysiologic response.

Physical or environmental factors may also trigger or exacerbate urticaria and angioedema (Table 16-14). In addition, urticaria and angioedema may occur in different disease states (Table 16-15). In up to 60% of cases, no causative agent can be identified.

DIAGNOSTIC STUDIES

History

Exceptionally important: onset; distribution; aggra-vating and ameliorating factors; time sequencing; food history; past, current, and infective history; contactant or insect exposures; family and atopic history; occupational, hobby, and environmental history; travel

Drug history

Any medications, including over-the-counter and oral contraceptive preparations, may precipitate urticaria and angioedema

Clinical examination

All areas of potential involvement: periorbit, oro-pharynx, joints, tips of extremities

Tests

See Table 16-16

TREATMENT PLAN

The goal of the treatment plan is to prevent symptoms of angioedema. Obviously, with removal of the causative agent, no further therapy is necessary.

Chemotherapeutic

Unless symptoms are sporadic, regular medication ther-apy is advised. Decongestants may be added to coun-teract the sporific effects of antihistamines. Side effects may prevent optimal dosage schedules. Two different classes of antihistamines may be given in an effort to decrease side effects while maximizing the total amount given. Long-acting preparations require less frequent doses. The physician dictates the specific drug protocol. In hereditary angioedema, in addition to treatment of existing symptoms, certain drugs are used to prevent symptoms or treat acute symptoms.

Table 16-14
Mechanisms of Angioedema

Mediator	Example	Proposed Mechanism
Immunologic		
Circulating immune complexes	Autoimmune phenomena	Activation of complement cascade
Cytotoxic antibodies	Transfusion reactions	Activation of complement cascade
Antigen-antibody complexes	Serum sickness reactions; malignancies	Activation of complement cascade
Drugs—directly or as haptens	Opiates; muscle relaxants; dextran	Direct mast cell degranulation
Foods—directly or as haptens	Tomatoes; strawberries; citrus fruits	Direct mast cell degranulation
Chemicals—directly or as haptens	Radiocontrast media; thiamine; bile salts	Direct mast cell degranulation
Drugs	Aspirin; indomethacin	Alteration of arachidonic acid metabolism
Chemical additives	Tartrazine	Alteration of arachidonic acid metabolism
Nonimmunologic		
Pressure	Tight garments; sitting	Unknown
Vibratory	Electric shavers; steering wheels	Unknown; autosomal dominant; genetically transmitted
Solar (five types)	Exposed areas	Unknown except for type IV, production of erythrocytic protoporphyria
Aquagenic	Water contact, regardless of temperature	Unknown
Heat	Direct contact	Unknown
Cholinergic	Heat exposure; emotional stress; vigorous exercise	Release of acetylcholine from cholinergic sympathetic nerve fibers
Cold	Delayed onset (30 minutes to 4 hours)	Autosomal dominant inheritance
	Exposed areas, immediate response	Unknown
	Associated with underlying disease	Presence of abnormal proteins with cold-dependent properties: cold hemoglobins, cryofibrinogens, cold agglutinins, cryoglobulins

Table 16-15
Diseases Association with Angioedema

Type	Proposed Mechanisms
Systemic mastocytosis	Accumulation of mast cells that spontaneously or easily degranulate in dermis, bone marrow, and gastrointestinal tract
Infections: viral parasitic (infectious mononucleosis, hepatitis), rarely bacterial	Circulating antigen-antibody complexes with activation of complement cascade
Endocrinopathies: hyperthyroidism, pregnancy, menses	Unknown
Hereditary angioedema	Autosomal dominant, genetically inherited deficiency or malfunction of C1 esterase inhibitor with activation of complement cascade
Malignancies	In addition to antigen-antibody complexes, interference with C1 esterase inhibitor and resultant activation of complement cascade
Psychogenic	Rarely primary but may be exacerbating factor through hormonal and neural secretory mediators

Drugs used in hereditary angioedema
Hormones
  Danazol (Danocrine), 200 mg tid; androgen derivative; contraindicated in children and pregnancy
Hemostatic agents
  Aminocaproic acid, 3.5 mg qid for adults; antifibinolytic agent, plasminogen inhibitor
  Tranexamic acid, 1 g tid for adults before dental procedures etc.
Blood products
  Fresh-frozen plasma during acute attacks

Drugs used in urticaria and angioedema
Antihistamines*
  Cyproheptadine (Periactin), 4-8 mg po q6h
  Chlorpheneramine (Chlortrimeton), 2 mg/kg/24 h po in 4 divided doses
  Clemastine (Tavist), 1.34 or 2.68 mg po q8-12h
  Diphenhydramine (Benadryl), 25-100 mg po q6h or 5 mg/kg/d
Histamine receptor antagonists*
  Cimetidine (Tagamet), 300 mg po q6h
Tranquilizers*

*Available in syrup form; dosage calculated by patient's weight.

Table 16-16
Diagnostic Tests for Urticaria and
Angioedema

Condition Suspected	Test*
Atopic: food or drug (inhalant or contactant) sensitivity	Elimination of offending agent; daily symptom diary; challenge with suspected foods; skin tests to food or selected drugs; total serum IgE determination; eosinophil count; skin tests or radioallergosorbent tests of suspected antigens
Cutaneous vasculitis or systemic collagen vascular disease	Immunoglobulin analysis; antinuclear antibody; rheumatoid factor; cryoglobulins; cryofibrinogens; complete complement profile; skin biopsy with immunofluorescence
Hereditary angioedema	C4; C2; C3; total hemolytic complement (CH50); C1-esterase inhibitor (immunochemical and functional assays)
Physical urticaria Dermatographia	Firm stroke on skin with tongue blade
Cold	Ice cube test; cryoglobulins; cryofibrinogens; VDRL test
Cholinergic urticaria	Exercise challenge; methacholine skin test
Solar urticaria	Exposure to various wavelengths of light; protoporphyrin and coproporphyrin determinations
Pressure urticaria and angioedema	Application of pressure with weights for 10 minutes
Vibratory angioedema	Vibratory stimulation of skin for 4 minutes
Aquegenic urticaria	Tap-water challenge at various temperatures
Infections	Appropriate cultures and x-rays; stool for ova and parasites; hepatitis B antigen and antibody
Urticaria pigmentosa	Test for dermatographia; skin biopsy
Malignancy with angioedema	Total hemolytic complement (CH50); C1; C1-esterase inhibitor
Idiopathic urticaria	Skin biopsy with immunofluorescence

From Fineman, S.: Urticaria and angioedema. In Lawlor, G.J., et al.,
editors: Manual of allergy and immunology. Copyright 1981 by Little,
Brown & Co., p. 210. Used with permission of Little, Brown & Co.
*General screening consists of complete blood count, urinalysis, and
erythrocyte sedimentation rate determination.

Hydroxyzine (Atarax), 25 mg po q6h to maximum
total of 400 mg
Adrenergic agents
Appear to be of limited value in long-term therapy
but may be employed for control of acute symptoms
Epinephrine
Aqueous (Adrenalin), 0.2-0.3 ml sc q 30 min or
0.01 mg/kg
Long-acting (Sus-Phrine), 0.1-0.3 ml sc q4-6h or
0.005 mg/kg (maximum dose 0.15 ml)
Ephedrine (Bronkaid), 20-50 mg q4h or 3 mg/kg/
24 h in 4 divided doses
Corticosteroids
May be used if symptoms are unresponsive to above
therapy but should be limited to lowest possible
dose and alternate-day therapy with monitoring
of side effects
Prednisone (Deltasone, Orasone, Liquid Pred), 2
mg/kg/d up to 100 mg in adult; 1 mg/kg/d in
child
Topical agents
Sun blockers with sun protection factor of at least
15 (Total Eclipse [15-18], Super Shade [15], Coppertone [15], Pre Sun [15]); used to block ultraviolet light in solar urticaria
Mild analgesics for pain associated with swelling

Supportive

Cool compresses to reduce periorbital edema
Support for involved joints as necessary
Restricted activity during acute episodes
Monitoring for full response to medication therapy
Monitoring to prevent further progression of symptoms
Avoidance of physical or environmental agents and food
or chemical additives
Endotracheal tube placement or tracheostomy for extensive laryngeal involvement

ASSESSMENT: AREAS OF CONCERN

Because angioedema may have multiorgan involvement,
careful assessment should be made of all potential organ
systems.

Laryngeal involvement
Hoarseness; stridor; use of accessory muscles; difficulty in speech

Dermal status
Concurrent urticaria

Ocular status
Periorbital edema

Gastrointestinal status
Nausea; vomiting; diarrhea; gastrointestinal swelling

Oropharyngeal status
Swelling of lip, tongue, and uvula

Articular status
Swelling at tips of extremities, in soft tissue, and around joints

NURSING DIAGNOSES and NURSING INTERVENTIONS

Nursing Diagnosis	Nursing Intervention
Breathing pattern, ineffective	Maintain endotracheal tube or tracheostomy if instituted. In collaboration with physician, administer appropriate medications and assess and record patient's response. Assess and record ventilation pattern including rate, rhythm, and use of accessory muscles. Assess for presence of laryngeal involvement, including stridor, hoarseness, and difficulty in speech or swallowing. Record if present.
Tissue perfusion, alteration in: gastrointestinal	In collaboration with physician, administer appropriate medications as indicated. Assess for presence of nausea, vomiting, abdominal cramping, and diarrhea. Record if necessary.
Tissue perfusion, alteration in: peripheral vasculature	In collaboration with physician, administer appropriate medications as indicated. Assess and record involvement in periarticular areas and tips of extremities.
Injury: potential for	Obtain complete history of drug allergies before administering new drug. Put labels indicating allergic drug history in all appropriate places. Closely monitor patient for 30 minutes after administering each new drug.

Patient Education

1. Explain to the patient the relationship between symptoms and exposure to the causative agent.
2. Explain the necessity of avoiding use of the causative agent.
3. Explain the patient's responsibility in interactions with health care givers.
4. Explain the need, if appropriate, to carry appropriate identification and to share information with appropriate others.
5. Provide information on medical alert identification.
6. Teach self-administration, if appropriate, of epinephrine and subsequent measures including oral administration of antihistamine and seeking immediate medical care.

EVALUATION

Patient Outcome	Data Indicating That Outcome is Reached
Symptoms resolve in response to therapeutic measures.	Patient is symptom free, with no evidence of soft tissue swelling, joint restriction or subjective feelings of tightness or swelling, hoarseness, or difficulty in swallowing, speech, or air movement. Bowel sounds and elimination pattern are normal.
Recurrence of symptoms is prevented.	Patient can identify triggering agent and explain appropriate avoidance measures. Patient can identify appropriate medications to use, dosage, and length of therapy if symptoms occur. Patient can identify nondrug therapeutic measures to institute if symptoms occur.

Medical Interventions

BONE MARROW TRANSPLANTATION

Description and Rationale

Bone marrow transplantation (BMT) is the treatment of choice for patients with severe aplastic anemia who are under 40 years of age and have a compatible donor. Marrow transplantation is also a treatment modality for severe immunodeficiency disorders, and recently it has been used with increasing success in the treatment of patients with leukemia, lymphoma, and selected solid tumors.

Bone marrow is harvested in the operating room with the donor under general or spinal anesthesia. Multiple aspirations from the posterior iliac crests are performed; if necessary the anterior iliac crests and sternum may be used. A small volume of bone marrow is collected with each aspiration and placed into tissue culture medium containing heparin. This solution is filtered through stainless steel screens to remove bone chips, fat globules, and clots and then is transferred to a blood transfusion bag.

The amount of bone marrow aspirated depends on a number of factors: the donor's weight, the concentration of cells in donated marrow, and the processing procedure employed before the marrow is transfused. If no special processing is done, the volume of marrow obtained is approximately 10 to 15 ml/kg of the recipient's body weight. In the typical adult a volume of 500 to 750 ml of blood and marrow contains 10 to 20 $\times$ 10^9 nucleated marrow cells.[36]

After harvesting, the marrow is either administered intravenously to the recipient through a central venous access device such as a Hickman or Raaf catheter or is cryopreserved and stored for future use. In the latter case, which occurs only with autologous bone marrow transplantation, the harvested marrow may be treated before cryopreservation to eliminate any occult tumor cells that may be present, especially in lymphohemopoietic malignancies. Ex vivo treatment with 4-hydroperoxyclophosphamide (4-HC), an analog of cyclophosphamide, is one method used to treat the marrow. More recently, immunologic approaches using monoclonal antibodies are being tested in clinical trials for diseases such as T cell lymphoma and common acute lymphocytic leukemia (ALL).

Until recently most marrow transplants have involved donors of two types, an identical twin or an HLA-matched, mixed lymphocyte culture (MLC)–compatible sibling. A syngeneic transplant, using marrow from an identical twin, is ideal because donor is matched with the recipient at all genetic loci.

Transplantation using marrow from anyone other than an identical twin or the patient himself is called an allogeneic transplant. In most allogeneic bone marrow transplants a sibling who matches at HLA-A, -B, -C, and -D loci is the donor. The HLA loci are on a small chromosomal region, and these loci are usually inherited as a unit known as a haplotype. Each parent has two haplotypes, and a child inherits one haplotype from each parent. A 25% probability exists that two siblings will be HLA identical.

A partially matched donor (such as a sibling, parent, or uncle) may be selected when no HLA-identical sibling is available, or an HLA-identical unrelated donor may be used. Preliminary reports using partially matched donors are encouraging, but further investigation in this area is needed.

A third form of bone marrow transplantation, the autologous graft, involves use of the patient's own marrow. As with the identical twin situation, in this circumstance no clinically significant graft-versus-host disease will occur. However, with autologous grafts, tumor cells may be present in marrow harvested during remission; therefore attempts to purge marrow of occult tumor cells before cryopreservation are being investigated. Autologous bone marrow transplants are experimental and are indicated only when a genetically identical donor is not available.

The rationale for bone marrow transplantation is to replace defective or missing host hemopoietic stem cells with healthy stem cells. In the treatment of neoplasm the transplant is done after therapy designed to rid the patient of the tumor. The patient's normal bone marrow is destroyed with high-dose therapy, and the transplant is designed to repopulate the patient's hemopoietic system.

Graft-Versus-Host Disease

Graft-versus-host disease (GVHD) presumably results from the attack of host tissue by immunocompetent donor T lymphocytes. In acute cases the peak onset occurs 30 to 50 days after the transplant.[23] In chronic cases the onset occurs 100 days after the transplant.[35] Tables 16-17 and 16-18 give two systems for the clinical staging of GVHD.

Table 16-17
Proposed Clinical Stage of Graft-Versus-Host Disease According to Organ System

Stage	Skin	Liver	Intestinal Tract
+	Maculopapular rash over 25% of body surface	Bilirubin 2-3 mg/dl	Greater than 500 ml diarrhea/day
+ +	Maculopapular rash over 25%-50% of body surface	Bilirubin 3-6 mg/dl	Greater than 1000 ml diarrhea/day
+ + +	Generalized erythroderma	Bilirubin 6-15 mg/dl	Greater than 1500 ml diarrhea/day
+ + + +	Generalized erythroderma with bullous formation and desquamation	Bilirubin greater than 15 mg/dl	Severe abdominal pain with or without ileus

From Thomas, E.D.: N. Engl. J. Med. **292**:896, 1975.

Table 16-18
Overall Clinical Grading of Severity of
Graft-Versus-Host Disease

Grade	Degree of Organ Involvement
I	+ to + + skin rash; no gut involvement; no liver involvement; no decrease in clinical performance
II	+ to + + + skin rash; + gut involvement or + liver involvement (or both); mild decrease in clinical performance
III	+ + to + + + skin rash; + + to + + + gut involvement or + + to + + + + liver involvement (or both); marked decrease in clinical performance
IV	Similar to grade III with + + to + + + + organ involvement and extreme decrease in clinical performance

From Thomas, E.D.: N. Engl. J. Med. **292**:896, 1975.

Conditioning Regimen

Pretransplant conditioning regimens include high-dose chemotherapy with or without radiotherapy. The purposes of conditioning are (1) to eliminate defective stem cells, (2) to provide immunosuppression to minimize the possibility of rejection, and (3) to eliminate any residual malignant cells.

The conditioning regimen used before bone marrow transplantation varies depending on the disease being treated. The use of multiple-day chemotherapy (with cyclophosphamide, busulfan, or other agents) may or may not be preceded or followed by local or total body irradiation (TBI).

In the case of leukemias or lymphomas, intrathecal methotrexate (approximately 10 mg/m^2) is given for central nervous system prophylaxis before transplantation.

With allogeneic transplants, prophylaxis for graft-versus-host disease includes additional treatment with agents such as cyclosporin A (dosage and route of administration vary). Use of cyclosporin A may continue for several months after marrow transplantation.

The following is an example of a schedule using cyclophosphamide and TBI conditioning. Days before transplant are indicated by negative numbers, with day 0 being the day of transplant.

Monday	Day − 8	Admission
Tuesday	Day − 7	Cyclophosphamide
Wednesday	Day − 6	Cyclophosphamide
Thursday	Day − 5	Rest
Friday	Day − 4	TBI
Saturday	Day − 3	TBI
Sunday	Day − 2	TBI
Monday	Day − 1	TBI
Tuesday	0	Bone marrow infusion

Preprocedural Nursing Care

Immediate concerns are related to the conditioning regimen using chemoradiotherapy. The patient, family, donor, and significant others are instructed on the procedure, its course, and complications.

Radiation. Dosage varies, in general from 800 to 1200 rad. For example, 1000 rad may be given in fractioned doses (250 rad per day). Single-dose whole body irradiation may be used. Typical side effects include nausea, vomiting, diarrhea, erythema of the skin, and parotitis. These side effects are usually of short duration when moderate fractioned radiotherapy is used. With the exception of erythema of the skin, they usually resolve within 7 days.

Cyclophosphamide. Nausea and vomiting may occur 6 to 8 hours after administration of cyclophosphamide and may last 8 to 10 hours. The drug may cause hemorrhagic cystitis in the bladder. Uric acid is released as cells are destroyed, resulting in deposition and accumulation of uric acid crystals in the kidney. Cardiotoxicity is a further problem with cyclophosphamide.

TREATMENT PLAN

Infusion of bone marrow is used to restore defective or missing stem cells. For autologous marrow, blood bags containing approximately 50 ml of cryopreserved marrow are thawed quickly, one at a time, in a basin of warm water at approximately 100° F. The contents of the blood bag are removed using a 50 ml syringe with a 16-gauge needle and then administered rapidly through a central line (double-lumen Raaf catheter or Hickman catheter). A solution of 0.9 normal saline is infused during the procedure. Epinephrine, diphenhydramine, and hydrocortisone are kept at the bedside.

For a syngeneic or allogeneic donation, a standard-type blood bag containing fresh bone marrow just obtained from a donor is transported from the operating room. The donated marrow is administered slowly (over a period of 4 hours) through a Raaf catheter without a filter.

ASSESSMENT: AREAS OF CONCERN

Fluid overload
Increased respiratory rate; dyspnea; rales; rhonchi

Micropulmonary emboli
Shortness of breath; chest pain; increased heart rate

Reaction to white cells in marrow
Chills; fever; urticaria; chest pain

Hematuria
Hemastix-positive urine normal for first 24 hours after bone marrow transplant

Bacterial contamination of marrow
Hypotension; fever; shaking chills

Engraftment
No evidence of hematologic recovery 2 to 4 weeks after bone marrow transplant

Infection
Fever; pain; redness; swelling of any site; wound drainage; cough; dyspnea; sore throat; headache; dysuria; frequency; urgency; positive blood culture findings; change in mental status

Anemia
Decreased red blood cell count, hematocrit, and hemoglobin level; excessive fatigue

Stomatitis
Oral soreness; dryness; burning or tingling; taste changes; erythema; ulcerations or patches on oral mucosa

Thrombocytopenia
Petechiae; purpura; bleeding from any body orifice or site of catheter; hemoptysis; hematemesis; hematuria; hematochezia; seizures; change in mental status

Nutritional status
Anorexia; decreased weight; nausea; vomiting; diarrhea

Psychosocial status
Anger; depression; frustration; anxiety

Graft-versus-host disease (GVHD)
Mild maculopopular rash; generalized erythroderma with desquamation; increase in serum bilirubin, serum glutamic oxaloacetic transaminase (SGOT), or alkaline phosphatase; abdominal cramping; diarrhea (green, watery); hematochezia

Veno-occlusive disease (VOD)
Sudden weight gain; right upper quadrant pain; jaundice; hepatomegaly; ascites; encephalopathy

NURSING DIAGNOSES and NURSING INTERVENTIONS

Nursing Diagnosis	Nursing Intervention
Nutrition, alteration in: less than body requirements (related to nausea and vomiting from total body irradiation)	Administer antiemetic drug before treatment and at frequent intervals after treatment as ordered. Choice of drug is largely empiric. Drugs should be administered intravenously. Consider use of behavioral relaxation techniques. Provide frequent oral hygiene. Instruct patient to avoid quick movements while nauseated. Encourage patient to eat or drink when not nauseated regardless of the time. Encourage patient to eat slowly and chew thoroughly. Suggest high-protein, high-calorie diet. Suggest small, frequent, low-fat meals.

Nursing Diagnosis	Nursing Intervention
	Encourage patient to drink liquids (clear, cool beverages or soups) slowly through a straw before, not during, meals.
	Provide patient with beverages or foods that may curb nausea: carbonated beverages such as cola or ginger ale; dry crackers or toast; tart foods such as lemons or sour pickles; ice pops and gelatin desserts.
	Instruct patient to avoid favorite foods during periods of nausea.
	Instruct patient to avoid lying flat for at least 1 hour after eating.
Comfort, alteration in: pain (related to fever)	Maintain adequate hydration.
	Administer antipyretics as ordered.
	Inform patient that fever usually disappears in 4 to 6 days following total body irradiation.
Comfort, alteration in: pain (related to parotitis)	Encourage increased fluid intake.
	Encourage frequent oral hygiene.
	If xerostomia is present, suggest hard candies, sugarless gums, or commercial product such as Xero-Lube.
	Avoid use of irritants such as alcohol or tobacco.
	Use measures for oral pain according to physician's order; narcotic analgesics may be required.
Bowel elimination, alteration in: diarrhea (related to effects of total body irradiation on gastrointestinal mucosa)	Administer antidiarrheal agents as ordered.
	Maintain adequate hydration.
	Suggest bland, low-residue diet that is high in potassium.
	Instruct patient in meticulous perianal skin care.
	Apply soothing lubricant to perianal area after each bowel movement.
Skin integrity, impairment of: potential (related to erythema of skin)	Instruct patient to keep skin clean and dry. Use mild soap such as Dove or Dial for bathing, rinse skin well, and pat dry.
	Avoid use of perfumed powders or lotions.
	Avoid extremes of temperature to skin, that is, hot or cold baths, ice packs, and heating pads.
	Avoid pressure from constricting clothing.
Tissue perfusion, alteration in: bladder (hemorrhagic cystitis related to local effect of cyclophosphamide)	Begin intravenous hydration 4 hours before cyclophosphamide administration and continue for 24 hours after therapy. Intravenous fluids should be administered 1½ to 2 times maintenance rates.
	Perform continuous bladder irrigations using three-way Foley catheter if ordered. If patient can void every hour to eliminate toxic products of cyclophosphamide that irritate bladder lining, catheter is unnecessary.
	Monitor urine for blood every 4 hours.
	Maintain accurate intake and output records.
Tissue perfusion, alteration in: renal	As above, administer hydration fluids.
	Check urine output hourly.
	Administer furosemide as ordered.
	Check urine pH every 4 hours; maintain at or above 7.
	Administer sodium bicarbonate as ordered.
	Administer allopurinol as ordered, if needed. Allopurinol may increase incidence and degree of bone marrow suppression by prolonging half-life of cyclophosphamide.
Cardiac output, alteration in: decreased (potential; related to cardiotoxicity)	Check results of electrocardiogram (ECG) for decreased voltage. (ECG is taken daily while patient is treated with high-dose cyclophosphamide.)
Potential patient problem: infection, potential for (related to leukopenia)	Maintain protective environment. (Reverse isolation protocols vary among centers from simple protective isolation to sterile laminar airflow rooms.)
	Monitor white blood cell count and absolute granulocyte count daily.
	Monitor vital signs every 4 hours.
	Check skin and mucous membranes.
	Inspect all body orifices daily for redness, swelling, and pain.
	Auscultate lungs every 8 hours. Check for increased or decreased breath sounds, rhonchi, and rales.

Nursing Diagnosis	Nursing Intervention
	Inspect site of insertion of venous access device for redness, swelling, and pain.
	Assess patient for complaints of dysuria and frequency.
	Note any change from patient's baseline vital signs, behavior, or appearance.
	Encourage turning, coughing, and deep breathing exercises.
	Maintain integrity of skin and mucous membranes. (Skin care measures vary among centers from use of povidone-iodine to use of antibacterial soap.)
	Maintain meticulous mouth care. (Mouth care varies among centers).
	Use strict aseptic technique when changing dressings.
	Use strict aseptic technique in intravenous preparation and administration.
	Avoid bladder catheterization.
	Avoid administering enemas and suppositories and taking rectal temperatures.
	Encourage patient to use deodorant rather than antiperspirant. (Axillary sweat glands are blocked by antiperspirants, which may promote infection.)
	Obtain surveillance cultures of throat, urine, stool, skin, and other areas as ordered. (Need for surveillance cultures to detect colonization before infection is controversial.)
	Maintain dietary restrictions as ordered. (Efficacy of low-bacteria diets has not been established.)
	Eliminate stagnant water in patient's room.
	Do not allow fresh-cut flowers or plants in patient's room.
	Limit number of visitors, and screen them for infection, recent vaccinations, or exposure to communicable diseases.
	Provide mask, gloves, and gown for patient when patient leaves room.
Potential patient problem: infection (related to leukopenia)	Obtain culture and sensitivity tests and Gram's stain of all potential sites of infection per physician's order.
	Administer antibiotics on schedule per physician's order.
	Monitor vital signs every 4 hours. (Subtle changes may be early sign of septic shock.)
	Control fever with tepid sponge baths and acetaminophen.
	Maintain adequate hydration of patient.
Potential patient problem: hemorrhage, potential for (related to thrombocytopenia)	Monitor platelet count regularly. Risk of bleeding is high when platelet count is under 10,000 cells/mm³.
	Inspect skin and mucous membranes daily. Monitor for increased bruising tendencies, petechiae, bleeding gums, and epistaxis.
	Test stool, urine, and emesis for occult blood.
	Note any changes in patient's vital signs or behavior. Changes may indicate intracranial hemorrhage.
	After invasive procedures such as bone marrow aspiration and biopsy, monitor site frequently for any oozing of blood.
	Avoid giving intramuscular subcutaneous injections.
	Avoid taking rectal temperatures and administering rectal suppositories and enemas.
	Encourage adequate fluid intake and use of stool softener to prevent constipation and straining.
	Avoid invasive procedures.
	Place sign indicating bleeding precautions over patient's bed.
	Administer medroxyprogesterone acetate as ordered to control menses.
	Instruct patient to avoid cutting, bruising, or bumping self. Eliminate sharp objects in environment.
	Instruct patient to use electric razor rather than hand razor.
	Instruct patient to wear shoes or slippers—no bare feet while walking.
	Instruct patient to use soft-bristled toothbrush. If platelet count is below 20,000/mm³, use toothette rather than a toothbrush.
	Flossing may be contraindicated. Instruct patient to discontinue if bleeding occurs.
	Instruct patient to avoid use of toothpicks.
	Discourage patient from having elective dental work.
	Teach patient to avoid use of aspirin and products containing aspirin.
	Teach patient to avoid use of all beverages containing alcohol.
	Instruct patient to avoid blowing the nose forcefully or sneezing forcefully.

Nursing Diagnosis	Nursing Intervention
Potential patient problem: hemorrhage (related to thrombocytopenia)	If epistaxis occurs, keep patient in sitting position. Application of ice helps to constrict small vessels. Local application of pressure may control bleeding. Nasal packing may be indicated if these measures fail. Apply topical agents such as thrombin, aminocaproic acid, cocaine, or Gelfoam to bleeding sites per physician's order. Bleeding in oral cavity may be controlled with iced saline mouth rinses. Administer irradiated platelet transfusions rapidly as ordered. (Families are encouraged to find donors for blood products.) Monitor posttransfusion platelet counts.
Activity intolerance (related to anemia, inadequate nutritional status, disruption of sleep, anxiety, or depression)	Administer irradiated red blood cell transfusions as ordered. Monitor hemoglobin levels and hematocrit values regularly. Maintain optional nutritional status. Arrange nursing care so patient has uninterrupted periods of rest and sleep, especially during the night. Encourage progressive activity program as tolerated. Encourage patient to verbalize feelings and concerns. Explain reasons for fatigue.

Oral mucous membrane, alteration in (related to conditioning regimen or infection)	Implement nursing care for stomatitis based on assessment using grading system developed by Capizzi[9]:
	Grade 1—generalized erythema of oral mucosa
	Grade 2—isolated small ulcerations or white patches
	Grade 3—confluent ulcerations with white patches covering more than 25% of oral mucosa
	Grade 4—hemorrhagic ulcerations
	For grade 1 or 2 stomatitis:
	1. Perform oral hygiene regimen every 2 hours while awake and every 6 hours during night, as follows:
	  a. Use normal saline mouthwash if crusts are absent. (One teaspoon of salt in 1 L of sterile water may be used.) If crusts and debris are present, use *either* one part hydrogen peroxide* diluted† with three parts water‡ *or* sodium bicarbonate solution (1 teaspoon mixed in 8 ounces of water.‡) Perform mouth care every 2 hours while patient is awake. Alternate *either* hydrogen peroxide or bicarbonate solution with normal saline. Rinse with normal saline after the use of either.
	  b. Floss gently with unwaxed dental floss every 24 hours; discontinue if bleeding occurs.
	  c. Brush using soft toothbrush and nonabrasive toothpaste, such as Colgate, after each meal and before sleep.
	  d. Remove dentures or partial plates. Replace only for meals.
	  e. Apply lip lubricant such as Vaseline, Blistex, or K-Y Jelly four times a day and as needed.
	2. Use measures for oral pain per physician's order. Suggestions are:
	  a. Dyclonine (Dyclone) 0.5% or 1% (available in spray or gargle), 5 to 10 ml every hour
	  b. Viscous lidocaine (Xylocaine) 2%, 10 ml every 2 hours
	  c. Hydrocortisone (Orabase) or carbamide peroxide (Gly-Oxide) applied to affected sites
	  d. "Stomatitis cocktail"—equal parts viscous lidocaine (Xylocaine), diphenhydramine (Benadryl) elixir, and magnesium and aluminum hydroxide mixture (Maalox), 30 ml every 2 to 4 hours
	  e. One part diphenhydramine (Benadryl) elixir mixed with one part kaolin and pectin (Kaopectate), every 2 to 4 hours

*Hydrogen peroxide should not be used if the patient has fresh granulation tissue.

†Hydrogen peroxide solutions should be prepared immediately before use, since hydrogen peroxide decomposes rapidly in water.

‡Sterile water or normal saline should be used for mouthwash or dilution of agents when patients are immunosuppressed. Whether using nonsterile solutions for dilution increases the number of infections is unknown.[9]

Nursing Diagnosis	Nursing Intervention

3. Implement dietary measures including the following:
   a. Instruct patient to avoid abrasive foods such as toast, apples, and celery.
   b. Encourage intake of pureed, bland foods.
   c. Instruct patient to avoid tart or acid foods such as hot beverages or iced drinks.
   d. Instruct patient to avoid spices and vinegar.
   e. Instruct patient to avoid alcohol.
   f. Arrange for dietary consultation.
4. Discourage smoking.
5. Recommend use of artificial saliva for xerostomia. No comparative research on various agents is available.

For grade 3 or 4 stomatitis:
1. Obtain samples from suspicious area and culture—one culture for bacteria and one for fungus—per physician's order.
2. Institute oral hygiene regimen:
   a. Alternate antifungal or antibacterial suspension with warm saline mouthwash every 2 hours while patient is awake and every 4 hours during night.
   b. Do not floss.
   c. Brush gently using toothettes or cotton-tipped applicators.
   d. Remove dentures or bridge. Do not replace for meals.
   e. Apply lip lubricant every 2 hours.
3. In addition to local measures as indicated for grade 1 and 2 stomatitis, systemic analgesics may be indicated, especially before eating.
4. Liquid diet may be indicated. If not, use pureed diet. See other measures as indicated in no. 3 for grade 1 and 2 stomatitis.
5. Discourage smoking.

Nutrition, alteration in: less than body requirements (related to inability to ingest or digest food)

Maintain optimal nutritional status.
Check weight daily.
Monitor calorie counts.
Arrange dietary consultation.
Administer total parenteral nutrition (TPN) as ordered.
Monitor serum electrolytes daily.
Check urine for glucose, ketones, and protein.

Potential patient problem: graft-versus-host disease (GVHD)

Assess skin integrity daily.
Assess level of pain and pruritus and administer analgesics and antihistamines as needed.
Provide meticulous skin care, including daily bath with povidone-iodine and normal saline or other antibacterial solution. Oatmeal baths may be indicated for pruritus.
Apply creams or lotions (Aquaphor or A & D Ointment with mineral oil) on intact skin to minimize breakdown.
Apply mixture of silver sulfadiazine and nystatin on open areas of skin. (Other creams and ointment such as fluocinonide, hydrocortisone, and petroleum gauze may be used.)
Explain need to prevent scratching. Use mittens if necessary on infant or child.
Use Clinitron bed for patient who has extensive skin involvement.
Use bed cradle to prevent linens from touching skin if patient has extensive skin involvement.
Assist patient frequently with active and passive range of motion exercises.
Note character and quantity of stool.
Administer antidiarrheal agent as ordered. (Antidiarrheal agents are usually not helpful in controlling diarrhea with GVHD.)
Provide meticulous perianal skin care.
Test all stools for occult blood.
Permit nothing by mouth as ordered to allow bowel to rest.
Reinstitute oral feedings with isosmotic, low-fat, lactose-free beverages as ordered; increase diet as tolerated.
Monitor closely for dehydration, electrolyte imbalance, and weight change.
Auscultate bowel sounds every 8 hours to monitor for development of ileus.

Nursing Diagnosis	**Nursing Intervention**
	Monitor bilirubin and serum glutamic oxaloacetic transaminase (SGOT) levels daily.
	Measure abdominal girth twice a day.
	Position patient on left side to decrease pressure on liver.
	Administer drugs (such as steroids, cyclosporin A, methotrexate, and antithymocyte globulin) as ordered according to protocol.
Potential patient problem: veno-occlusive disease (related to fibrous obliteration of small hepatic venules)	Assess for sudden weight gain, right upper quadrant pain, ascites, jaundice, and disorientation.
	Measure abdominal girth twice a day at level of umbilicus with patient supine.
	Restrict sodium intake as ordered.
	Administer all intravenous medication in minimal volume of fluid.
	Monitor urine sodium levels.
	Monitor blood pressure for orthostatic change daily.
	Monitor patient closely for toxic side effects of medications because of impaired liver function.
	Monitor blood urea nitrogen levels frequently.
Self-concept, disturbance in: body image (related to alopecia, weight loss, sterility, and so on)	Encourage patient and significant others to verbalize feelings and concerns.
	Explore perceived meaning of loss with patient and significant others.
	Help patient and significant others recognize that alopecia and weight loss are temporary.
	Assist patient to identify methods to improve appearance (such as use of clothing, scarves, hats, or hairpieces).
	Assist patient to identify strengths.
	Convey attitude of acceptance and understanding.
	Emphasize that negative reactions to altered body image are normal and expected.
	Consult other health care providers in planning comprehensive approach to patient.
Fear (related to uncertain outcome of treatment, threat of death, isolation, treatment protocols, and so on)	Encourage patient and significant others to express feelings and concerns.
	Encourage patient and significant others to ask questions to dispel misconceptions and reduce fear.
	Assist patient to cope with isolation through use of radio, television, tape recorder, or video cassette recorder.
	Reinforce and restate information given to patient and significant others to promote understanding.
	Encourage patient and significant others to discuss hopes for positive outcome.

Patient Education

1. Teach daily care for the central venous access device to maintain the patency of the catheter and prevent infection and bleeding.
2. Explain diet for optimal nutritional status. (Ideally the patient must be able to tolerate 1000 calories a day to be discharged.)
3. Teach measures to prevent the occurrence of infection. Precautions are more rigid during the first 3 months after bone marrow transplantation and are relaxed as the year progresses.
   Wear face mask when outside home.
   Avoid contact with young children who attend school.
   Avoid contact with anyone who has a cold or illness.
   Avoid crowds; go to grocery stores, theaters, restaurants, and other public places when they are not crowded.
   Avoid restaurant food for the first 3 months.

   Wear a mask. (Walks can be taken without wearing a mask, but one should be carried in case of contact with other pedestrians.)
   Use good handwashing technique before eating, after using the toilet, and after contact with someone who has a cold.
   Avoid contact with any pets in living quarters for the first 3 months. Do *not* clean litter boxes or come in contact with animal feces.
   Avoid contact with plants and flowers.
   Children should not attend school for the first year after a bone marrow transplant.
   Do not swim in private or public pool for the first year after bone marrow transplant.
   Maintain good dental hygiene.
   Do not have immunizations without the physician's approval.

Take prophylactic antibiotics as prescribed.
4. Tell the patient to take temperature daily and notify the physician of an elevation 2° above baseline.
5. Tell the patient to report appearance of rash, change in color or consistency of bowel movements, change in color of urine, nausea or vomiting, appearance of pain, dysphagia, and xerostomia.
6. Tell the patient to report cough and dyspnea immediately.

EVALUATION

Patient Outcome	Data Indicating That Outcome is Reached
Patient demonstrates proficiency in care of catheter.	Line is patent and site is free from infection.
Patient tolerates diet.	Ideal body weight is maintained.
There is no evidence of active infection.	Patient is afebrile, with no local or generalized findings and a clear chest roentgenogram.
There is no evidence of graft-versus-host disease.	There are no skin, gastrointestinal, or liver abnormalities.
Engraftment is successful.	Peripheral blood counts are in normal range.

PLASMAPHERESIS

Apheresis is the separation of whole blood into its various components by passage through automated centrifugation devices or membrane filters. After fractionation, certain blood constituents are discarded, while others are returned to the donor. Apheresis can be performed as a therapeutic protocol or to obtain donor blood products.

Plasmapheresis is the procedure by which plasma is selectively removed from whole blood. This experimental therapeutic manipulation is employed in certain diseases to remove an abnormal constituent from the plasma or replenish a deficient plasma factor. During therapeutic plasma exchange, patient plasma is removed and the cellular elements of the blood are reinfused following reconstitution with normal plasma or a suitable colloidal substitute.

Although not many well-controlled scientific studies concerning the therapeutic efficacy of plasmapheresis have been performed, it is being employed to treat a number of immunologic and nonimmunologic disorders. Conditions commonly treated with plasma exchange are outlined in Table 16-19.

Patients treated with plasmapheresis may expect to experience only temporary clinical improvement. Since therapeutic plasma exchange is designed to relieve the manifestations of a clinical disease process without affecting the underlying disorder, repeated treatments are usually indicated. Patients undergoing therapeutic plasma exchange to remove plasma antibodies or circulating immune complexes are treated concomitantly with immunosuppressive drugs to retard the recovery of immunoglobin levels.

Although plasmapheresis is generally believed to be a benign procedure, a number of complications are associated with this treatment. These untoward effects and suggested patient management* are described in Table 16-20.

*References 14, 18, 21, 30, 33, 38.

Table 16-19
Disorders Treated with Therapeutic Plasma Exchange

Disorder	Rationale
Autoimmune hemolytic anemia	Removal of antiplatelet antibodies
Myasthenia gravis	Removal of antibodies directed at acetylcholine receptor
Goodpasture's syndrome	Removal of anti–basement membrane antibodies
Multiple sclerosis	Removal of putative anti-myelin antibodies
Systemic lupus erythematosus	Removal of circulating immune complexes
Amyloidosis	Removal of immunoglobulin
Thrombotic thrombocytopenia purpura	Replenishment of plasma factor

Table 16-20
Complications of Therapeutic Plasma Exchange

Complication	Nursing Care	Complication	Nursing Care
Trauma or infection at site of vascular access	Keep entry site clean and dry; inspect regularly for signs of infection	Temporary paresthesias, muscle twitching, nausea, and vomiting owing to administration of citrated plasma	Provide comfort measures and reassurance; add calcium gluconate to replacement fluids
Disequilibrium syndrome (nausea, diaphoresis, lightheadedness, tachycardia, and hypotension resulting from hypovolemia)	Monitor fluid balance and vital signs closely; administer fluids as needed; offer patient orange juice or saltines	Anemia owing to hemolysis	Replace erythrocytes in combination with fluids or plasma
Hypokalemia, hypocalcemia (which may predispose to cardiac irregularities)	Monitor electrolyte balance and replace electrolytes as needed	Increased risk of infection owing to depletion of certain plasma proteins	Observe for signs of infection
Bleeding owing to temporary depletion of platelets and clotting factors	Maintain safe environment; observe for signs of bleeding or bruising	Transient peripheral edema owing to fluid shifts	Symptoms are transient and no further treatment is warranted
		Hypothermia owing to infusion of cool fluids	Provide extra blankets; prewarm replacement fluids

γ-GLOBULIN THERAPY

γ-Globulin administration is indicated as replacement therapy for immunodeficiency diseases affecting the humoral or antibody-mediated immune system. Recurrent, severe, sinopulmonary infections are hallmark clinical manifestations of the humoral immunodeficiency diseases. The frequency and severity with which these infections occur assist the clinician in evaluating the effectiveness of γ-globulin therapy. γ-Globulin is also used to provide passive immunity against a variety of infectious agents, such as the hepatitis virus.

For the past 30 years, human immune serum globulin (HISG) has been available for intramuscular administration. Its use has effectively limited both the severity and frequency of infections in antibody immune deficient patients. The usual dose of HSIG ranges from 100 to 200 mg/kg/month. Only IgG is present in significant quantities in HSIG.

Although untoward side effects are uncommon, rare anaphylactic reactions to the intramuscular injections have been reported. Patients who have such reactions should be treated immediately with epinephrine and antihistamines. Later, therapy may resume, but HISG from a different manufacturer should be used following a skin test of HSIG from the new lot.

Long-term monthly injections produce local pain.

HISG is slowly degraded within the injection sites. The risk of entering the intravenous compartment in infants and malnourished patients is high. In addition, large doses of γ-globulins require multiple injections.

Recently, modified preparations of intravenous immune serum globulin (Gamimmune, Intraglobin) have been available for experimental use in the United States. Data indicate that these products are effective as replacement therapy.[2,12,28] Larger doses of γ-globulin may be delivered with greater efficacy. Serum levels of IgG are reached early and maintained longer. In addition, minimal side effects are associated with its administration.

Doses of intravenous γ-globulin preparations range from 100 to 300 mg/kg/month to maintain IgG serum levels at a minimum of 200 mg/dl. The therapy is usually well tolerated,[28] although chills, fever, and transient leukopenia have been reported.[12] Several researchers indicate that intravenous γ-globulin therapy is highly superior, in terms of clinical efficacy, to intramuscularly administered immunoglobulin.[2,12,28] Intravenous γ-globulin therapy appears to be useful for the treatment of patients who require large doses of immunoglobulin, debilitated patients who might not tolerate monthly intramuscular injections, and Wiskott-Aldrich patients who are prone to hemorrhage.

CORTICOSTEROIDS

Synthetic corticosteroids are chemotherapeutic agents that mimic the effects of the major endogenous glucocorticoid, cortisol. They are used in the treatment of many immunologic diseases because of their potent anti-inflammatory and immunosuppressive effects. Corticosteroids exert their widespread effects by initially binding to a specific cytoplasmic receptor protein that is present in most cells. This complex then enters the nucleus where alteration of the rate of synthesis of specific proteins occurs.

Synthetic corticosteroids should be used with caution in persons with hepatic disease or hypoalbuminemia or in patients who are receiving phenytoin, barbiturates, or rifampin. Lower-dose therapy is recommended in these cases. In addition, care should be exercised in prescribing steroid therapy for persons who are predisposed to or have known histories of diabetes, osteoporosis, peptic ulcer disease, infections, hypertension, psychosis, or coronary artery disease.

A major concern with the use of corticosteroid therapy is suppression of the hypothalamic-pituitary-adrenocortical axis (HPAA). Exogenous steroids provide negative feedback to this mechanism, which promotes total body homeostasis via the regulation of cortisol production. Therefore suppression of the HPAA results in widespread systemic manifestations. To limit this untoward effect, steroids are administered in as low a dosage as possible to control the disease for which they are being prescribed. However, to control acute exacerbations of many inflammatory disorders, usually corticosteroids are prescribed initially in relatively high doses (greater than 40 mg daily), so HPAA suppression is unavoidable. Once the disease is under control, the dosage is lowered at a rate of 2.5 to 5 mg per week. *Gradual* tapering of the dosage of corticosteroids is necessary, since the body cannot respond quickly to changes in cortisol levels owing to the initial suppression of the natural HPAA feedback mechanism. It may take as long as 12 months for adaptation to occur when the patient has received high-dose therapy for a month or more.[3] Although useful in controlling many clinical manifestations, steroid therapy is not without inherent dangers. Because these agents exert such widespread systemic effects, their adverse effects are diverse and often complicate the course of the disease for which they are being used.

The type and severity of side effects are dose dependent and related to the duration of therapy. Although alternate-day therapy (single doses every other day) has been associated with fewer side effects, it is not recommended for control of acute disease.

Table 16-21
Comparison of Various Glucocorticoids with Hydrocortisone

Glucocorticoid	Anti-Inflammatory Potency	Equivalent Potency (mg)	Sodium-Retaining Potency	Duration of HPAA Suppression (hours)
Hydrocortisone	1.0	20	2	12
Cortisone	0.8	25	2	12
Prednisolone	4.0	5	1	24-36
Prednisone	3.5	5	1	24-36
Methylprednisolone	5.0	4	0	24-36
Triamcinolone	5.0	4	0	24-36
Paramethasone	10.0	2	0	24-36
Betamethasone	25.0	0.60	0	Greater than 48
Dexamethasone	30.0	0.75	0	Greater than 48

IMMUNOTHERAPY

Immunotherapy has a role in the treatment of allergic and immune deficiency diseases, some autoimmune disorders, and cancer. In allergic diseases immunotherapy is used to hyposensitize the patient. (Desensitization is discussed elsewhere.) In immunodeficiency disease the aim is to restore absent or deficient products; for example, in X-linked hypogammaglobulinemia, treatment involves administration of γ-globulin. Patients with autoimmune disorders such as systemic lupus erythematosus may benefit from therapeutic plasmapheresis (a type of immu-notherapy), with removal of circulating immune complexes. (Immunodeficiency and autoimmune disorders are discussed elsewhere.) Immunotherapy in the treatment of cancer, whether it is the sole form of treatment or used as adjunct therapy, is currently experimental. Cancer immunotherapy is manipulation of the immune system to control or eliminate the growth of neoplastic cells.

Table 16-22 lists several immunotherapeutic agents that are being intensively investigated.

Table 16-22
Experimental Immunotherapeutic Agents

| Agent | Results in Humans | | |
	Disease	Response	Side Effects
Nonspecific			
BCG (several types)	Malignant melanoma	Regression of dermal metastases after intralesional injection; no effect on visceral metastases; effect on survival rates unknown	Chills, fever, malaise; granulomatous hepatitis, immune complex renal disease; anaphylaxis (rarely) due to antibody formation; persistent BCG infection at injection site in immunodepressed patients; side effects vary, depending on route of administration
	Childhood acute lymphoblastic leukemia	Prolongation of disease-free interval after induction of remission by chemotherapy	
	Lung carcinoma (intrapleural injection)	Prevention of relapse (?)	
	Lymphoma (after radiotherapy)	Prolongation of remission, prevention of relapse (requires confirmation)	
	Colorectal cancer	Increase in disease-free interval (in some patients)	
	Metastatic breast cancer	Increase in survival	
Muramyl dipeptide	—	Results not available	—
C. parvum (heat-killed and formaldehyde-treated)	Malignant melanoma (cutaneous metastases)	Regression of lesions after intralesional injection; effects on survival unknown	Fever (up to 40.5° C), headache, nausea, vomiting; mild hypertension, peripheral vasoconstriction
	Lung cancer (intrapleural)	No effect on survival	
	Other solid tumors, acute leukemia (in combination with other agents or with irradiated leukemic cells)	Trials in progress	

Modified from Fudenberg, H.H., and Wybran, J.: Experimental immunotherapy. In Stites, D.P., et al., editors: Basic and clinical immunology, Los Altos, Calif., 1984, Lange Medical Publications.

Continued.

Table 16-22, cont'd
Experimental Immunotherapeutic Agents

Agent	Results in Humans		Side Effects
	Disease	**Response**	**Side Effects**
Thymic hormones (thymosin fraction V, facteur thymique sérique (FTS), thymopoietin, thymosin polypeptides α_1, β_1, α_5, α_7, β_3, β_4, and others)	Hereditary deficiencies of cell-mediated immunity Oat cell carcinoma Other malignancies (e.g., melanoma, in combination with chemotherapy)	Immunologic normalization, clinical improvement Increase in survival Trials in progress	Allergic reactions (rarely severe)
Fetal thymus (13-week) or fetal liver (8-week) transplants	DiGeorge syndrome, severe combined immunodeficiency	Restoration of immune function, reduced infections, increased survival (better success with fetal liver than fetal thymus)	Mild or none
Cultured thymic epithelium; autologous T cells cultured with fetal thymic epithelium	Severe combined immunodeficiency	Restoration of immune function, reduced infections, increased survival	None reported
Immunoglobulins (plasma, immune serum globulins, Cohn fraction V)	Hypogammaglobulinemia, severe combined immunodeficiency, Bruton's disease, complement deficiencies Malignancies (plasma therapy)	Temporary improvement in immune function and clinical course; repeated injections required to maintain humoral immunity Trials in progress	None reported
Levamisole	Rheumatoid arthritis Aphthous stomatitis Bronchogenic carcinoma Malignant melanoma Juvenile periodontitis SLE	Improvement in some Marked improvement Results controversial No significant increase in survival rates Improvement Trials in progress	Neutropenia (occasionally severe) in rheumatoid arthritis
Interferon	Osteosarcoma, lymphomas, myeloma, breast cancer, laryngeal papillomatosis Herpes infections	Induction of remissions Healing of the lesions	Occasional leukopenia, anemia, fever
Inosiplex	Herpes labialis, herpes progenitalis, shingles, rhinovirus infection, influenza A infection, cytomegalovirus infection Viral hepatitis (both type A and type B) Subacute sclerosing panencephalitis Rheumatoid arthritis	Marked reduction in duration of illness and severity of symptoms Possible effect Prevention of further deterioration Rapid response in 60% of patients	None reported
Pyrimethamine (antimalarial)	No trials in humans	—	—
Glucan	Metastatic malignancy (intralesional injection)	Prompt tumor cell necrosis and regression of lesions	None reported
Tilorone	Trials in progress	—	—
L-Fucose	No trials in humans	—	—
Synthetic polynucleotides (e.g., poly A·U/poly I·C)	Poly A·U, trial in breast cancer	Increased survival after conventional therapy	—

Table 16-22, cont'd
Experimental Immunotherapeutic Agents, cont'd

| Agent | Disease | Results in Humans | |
		Response	Side Effects
Specific			
Active specific immunotherapy (tumor antigen in Freund's adjuvant)	Bronchogenic carcinoma (stage I) after chemotherapy	Marked prolongation of survival	Local ulceration at injection site
	Colon carcinoma, breast carcinomas	Trials pending	
Enzyme-treated (neuraminidase) autochthonous tumor cells	Leukemia (in combination with other agents)	Increased survival (in some trials)	None reported
	Stage III breast carcinoma (in combination with BCG)	Trials in progress	
	Malignant melanoma (without concomitant therapy)	Apparent cessation of local tumor growth	
Irradiated tumor cells	Acute leukemia (in combination with BCG or *C. parvum*)	Trials in progress	—
Immune RNA (xenogeneic)	Metastatic renal cell carcinoma	Regression or complete disappearance of metastases in some patients	None reported in phase I studies
Dialyzable leukocyte extracts (transfer factor)	Genetically determined immune deficiency	Dramatic decrease in parasitic, viral, and fungal infections	Remarkably few: severe pain at site of primary or metastatic bone tumors; occasionally hypersensitivity pneumonia if pulmonary metastases are present
	Recurrent infections with a single organism unresponsive to antibiotic therapy: fungal (e.g., *Candida*), viral (e.g., cytomegalovirus, herpes zoster), parasitic (e.g., *Leishmania*), mycobacterial (e.g., lupus vulgaris, *Mycobacterium fortuitum*, progressive BCG infection)	Excellent clinical results, provided proper donors are used and recipients are monitored by appropriate immunologic tests for frequency and amount of administration	
	Malignancies (especially those presumed to be of viral origin): e.g., epidermodysplasia verruciformis with squamous cell carcinoma and osteosarcoma	Clinical improvement, prevention of metastases, prolongation of survival	
	Multiple sclerosis	Decrease in incidence of relapses, especially in mild disease	

References

1. Alspaugh, M.A., and Whaley, K.: Sjogren's syndrome. In Kelley, W.N., et al., editors: Textbook of rheumatology, Philadelphia, 1981, W.B. Saunders Co.
2. Ammann, A.J., and Fudenberg, H.H.: Immunodeficiency diseases. In Fudenburg, H.H., et al., editors: Basic and clinical immunology, ed. 3, Los Altos, Calif., 1980, Lange Medical Publications.
3. Axelrod, L.: Steroids. In Kelley, W.N., et al., editors: Textbook of rheumatology, 1981, W.B. Saunders Co.
4. Bates, B.: A guide to physical examination, Philadelphia, 1983, J.B. Lippincott Co.
5. Brown, M.S., and Hudak, C.M.: Student manual of physical examination, Philadelphia, 1984, J.B. Lippincott Co.
6. Buckley, R.H.: Immunodeficiency, J. Allergy Clin. Immunol. **72:**627, 1983.
7. Calin, A.: Reiter's syndrome. In Kelley, W.N., et al., editors: Textbook of rheumatology, Philadelphia, 1981, W.B. Saunders Co.
8. Cantani, A., et al.: A three year controlled study in children with pollenosis treated with immunotherapy, Ann. Allergy **53:**79, 1984.
9. Capizzi, R.L., et al.: Methotrexate therapy of head and neck cancer: improvement in therapeutic index by the use of leucovorin "rescue," Cancer Res. **30:**1782, 1970.

10. Daeffler, R.: Oral hygiene measures for patients with cancer, Cancer Nurs. **4:**29, 1981.

11. Diem, K., and Lentner, C.: Scientific tables, Ardsley, N.Y., 1970, Geigy Pharmaceuticals.

12. Eibl, M.M., et al.: Safety and efficacy of a monomeric, functionally intact intravenous IgG preparation in patients with primary immunodeficiency syndromes, Clin. Immunol. Immunopathol. **31:**151, 1984.

13. Harvey, A.M., et al.: The principles and practice of medicine, New York, 1976, Appleton-Century-Crofts.

14. Huestis, D.W.: Mortality in therapeutic haemapheresis, Lancet **1:**1043, 1983.

15. Hunder, G.G., and Conn, D.L.: Necrotizing vasculitis. In Kelley, W.N., et al., editors: Textbook of rheumatology, Philadelphia, 1981, W.B. Saunders Co.

16. Ignaczak, T.F.: Amyloidosis. In Kelley, W.N., et al., editors: Textbook of rheumatology, Philadelphia, 1981, W.B. Saunders Co.

17. Judge, R.D., and Zuidema, G.D., editors: Methods of clinical examination: a physiologic approach, Boston, 1974, Little, Brown & Co.

18. Keller, A.J., Chirnside, A., and Urbaniak, S.J.: Coagulation abnormalities produced by plasma exchange on the cell separator with special reference to fibrinogen and platelet levels, Br. J. Haematol. **42:**593, 1979.

19. Lab Comp: clinical laboratory user's guide, Stow, Ohio, 1984, Lexi-Comp, Inc.

20. Laubenstein, L.J.: Staging and treatment of Kaposi's sarcoma in patients with AIDS. In Friedman-Kien, A.E., and Laubenstein, L.J., editors: AIDS: the epidemic of Kaposi's sarcoma and opportunistic infections, New York, 1984, Masson Publishing USA, Inc.

21. Levy, J.: Safety and standards in therapeutic apheresis, Plasma Ther. **3:**195, 1982.

22. Mannick, M., and Gillilund, B.C.: Vasculitis. In Petersdorf, R.G., et al.: Harrison's principles and practice of internal medicine, vol. 1, New York, 1983, McGraw-Hill Book Co.

23. Parker, N., and Cohen, T.: Acute-graft-versus-host-disease in allogeneic marrow transplant, Nurs. Clin. North Am. **18:**570, 1983.

24. Price, D.M., and Scimeca, A.M.: The epidemic of the 80's: AIDS, Cancer Nurs., August 1984, p. 283.

25. Primer on the rheumatic diseases, ed. 7, Atlanta, 1973, Arthritis Foundation.

26. Rocklin, R.E.: Clinical and immunologic aspects of allergic-specific immunotherapy in patients with seasoned allergic rhinitis and/or allergic asthma, J. Allergy Clin. Immunol. **72:**323, 1983.

27. Rosen, F.S., et al.: The primary immunodeficiencies, N. Engl. J. Med. **311:**235, 1984.

28. Schiff, R.J., et al.: Use of new chemically modified intravenous IgG preparation in severe primary humoral immunodeficiency: clinical efficacy and attempts to individualize dosage, Clin. Immunol. Immunopathol. **31:**13, 1984.

29. Schur, P., editor: The clinical management of systemic lupus erythematosus, New York, 1983, Grune & Stratton, Inc.

30. Shumak, K.H., and Rock, G.A.: Therapeutic plasma exchange, N. Engl. J. Med. **310:**762, 1984.

31. Sontheimer, R.D.: Lupus erythematosus. In Rackel, R.E., editor: Conn's current therapy, Philadelphia, 1984, W.B. Saunders Co.

32. Stites, D.P., et al., editors: Basic and clinical immunology, Los Altos, Calif., 1984, Lange Medical Publications.

33. Sutton, D.M.C., et al.: Complications of extensive plasma exchange, Plasma Ther. **2:**19, 1981.

34. Terr, P.: Allergic diseases. In Stites, D.P., et al., editors: Basic and clinical immunology, ed. 5, Los Altos, Calif., 1984, Lange Medical Publications.

35. Thomas, E.D.: Marrow transplantation for malignant diseases, J. Clin. Oncol. **1:**526, 1983.

36. Thomas, E.D.L.: Marrow transplantation for acute leukemia, Cancer **42:**895, 1978.

37. Wallis, C., and Thompson, D.: Knowing the face of the enemy, Time, April 30, 1984, pp. 66-67.

38. Wallace, D.J., and Klinenberg, J.R.: Apheresis, Chicago, 1984, Year Book Medical Publishers, Inc.

Suggested Readings

AIDS: achieving optimal care through interagency cooperation (syllabus), Nursing Education and Research. Nursing Services, University of California, San Francisco.

AIDS: an update (syllabus), Nursing Education and Research. Nursing Services, University of California, San Francisco.

AIDS: fear and loathing, Emergency Med. **15:**157, 1983.

Alexander, J.W., and Good, R.A.: Fundamentals of clinical immunology, Philadelphia, 1977, W.B. Saunders Co.

Becker, T.M.: Cancer chemotherapy, a manual for nurses, Boston, 1981, Little, Brown & Co.

Behrman, R.E., and Vaughn, V.C., editors: Nelson textbook of pediatrics, Philadelphia, 1983, W.B. Saunders Co.

Bellanti, J.A.: Immunology II, Philadelphia, 1978, W.B. Saunders Co.

Benenson, A.S., editor: Control of communicable diseases in man, Washington, D.C., 1980, American Public Health Association.

Blau, S.P., and Schultz, D.: Lupus: the body against itself, New York, 1978, Doubleday & Co., Inc.

Brown, M.H., and Kiss, M.E.: Standards of care for the patient with "graft-versus-host disease" post bone marrow transplant, Cancer Nurs. **4:**191, 1981.

Brundage, D.: Nursing management of renal problems, St. Louis, 1980, The C.V. Mosby Co.

Campbell, C.: Nursing diagnosis and intervention in nursing practice, New York, 1978, Wiley Medical Publications.

Crow, S.: Nursing care of the immunosuppressed patient, Infection Control **4:**465, 1983.

Current, W.L., et al.: Human cryptosporidiosis in immunocompetent and immunodeficient persons, N. Engl. J. Med. **308:**1252, 1983.

Davis, B.D., et al.: Microbiology, Hagerstown, Md., Harper & Row Publishers, Inc.

Delp, M.H., and Manning, R.T.: Major's physical diagnosis: an introduction to the clinical process, Philadelphia, 1981, W.B. Saunders Co.

Diem, K., and Lentner, C.: Scientific tables, Ardsley, N.Y., 1970, Geigy Pharmaceuticals.

Dominick, N.P.: The methanol extract residue (MER) of bacillus Calmette-Guerin in cancer immunotherapy, Nurs. Clin. North Am. **13:**369, 1978.

Douglas, G.N.: Complement system, LaJolla, Calif., Calbiochem-Behring.

Fine, D.P.: Complement and infectious diseases, Boca Raton, Fla., 1981, CRC Press, Inc.

Ford, R., McClain, K., and Cunningham, B.A.: Veno-occlusive disease following marrow transplantation, Nurs. Clin. North Am. **18:**563, 1983.

Friedman-Kien, A.E., and Lauberstein, L.J., editors: AIDS: the epidemic of Kaposi's sarcoma and opportunistic infections, New York, 1984, Masson Publishing USA, Inc.

Fries, J.F.: Arthritis, Reading, Mass., 1980, Addison-Wesley Publishing Co.

Fudenburg, H.H., et al., editors: Basic and clinical immunology, ed. 3, Los Altos, Calif., 1980, Lange Medical Publications.

Grieco, M.H., and Meriney, D.K.: Immunodiagnosis for clinicians: interpretation of immunoassays, Chicago, 1983, Year Book Medical Publishers, Inc.

Guidelines for the nursing care of patients with altered protective mechanisms, Oncol. Nurs. Forum **9:**69, 1982.

Hammond, W.P., et al.: IV: Infections in the compromised host, part I, Hosp. Med. **19:**132, 1983.

Hammond, W.P., IV: Infections in the compromised host, part II, Hosp. Med. **19:**13, 1983.

Harder, L.: Primers assist patients in managing chemotherapy side effects, Oncol. Nurs. Forum **10:**74, 1983.

Hutchison, M.M., and King, A.H.: A nursing perspective on bone marrow transplantation, Nurs. Clin. North Am. **18:**511, 1983.

James, K.: Complement: activation, consequences, and control, Am. J. Med. Tech. **48:**735, 1982.

James, K.: The laboratory evaluation of the complement system, Chaska, Minn., Kallestad Laboratories, Inc.

Jawetz, E., Melnick, J.L., and Adelberg, E.A.: Review of medical microbiology, Los Altos, Calif., 1976, Lange Medical Publications.

Kadota, R.P., and Smithson, W.A.: Bone marrow transplantation for diseases of childhood, Mayo Clin. Proc. **59:**171, 1984.

Kaposi's sarcoma and pneumocystic pneumonia: new phenomenon among gay men (syllabus), Nursing Education and Research, Nursing Services, University of California, San Francisco.

Kim, M.J., McFarland, G., and McLane, A.M.: Pocket guide to nursing diagnosis, St. Louis, 1984, The C.V. Mosby Co.

Knobf, M.D., et al.: Cancer chemotherapy, treatment and care, Boston, 1981, G.K. Hall Medical Publishers.

Koren, M.E., and Hermann, C.S.: Cancer immunotherapy, what, when, how, Nursing 81 **11:**34, 1981.

Lawler, G.J., and Fisher, T.J., editors: Manual of allergy and immunology: diagnosis and therapy, Boston, 1981, Little, Brown & Co.

Lint, T.F.: Laboratory detection of complement activation and complement deficiencies, Am. J. Med. Tech. **48:**743, 1982.

Loebl, S., et al.: The nurses' drug handbook, ed. 3, New York, 1983, John Wiley & Sons, Inc.

Lorig, K., and Fries, J.F.: The arthritis helpbook, Reading, Mass., 1980, Addison-Wesley Publishing Co.

Luskin, A.T., and Tobin, M.C.: Alterations of complement components in disease, Am. Soc. Med. Tech. **48:**749, 1982.

Ma, P., and Armstrong, D., editors: The acquired immune deficiency syndrome and infections of homosexual men, New York, 1984, Yorke Medical Books.

Mayer, K., and Pizer, M.: The AIDS factbook, New York, 1983, Bantam Books.

Muller-Eberhard, H.J.: Complement abnormalities in human disease, Hosp. Pract. **12:**65, 1978.

Myers, M.C.: Hematopoietic system. In Judge, R.D., and Zuidema, G.D., editors: methods of clinical examination: a physiologic approach, Boston, 1974, Little, Brown & Co.

Myrvik, Q.N., and Weiser, R.S.: Fundamentals of immunology, Philadelphia, 1984, Lea & Febiger.

Myskowiski, P.L., et al.: Treatment of Kaposi's sarcoma: a review. In Ma, P., and Armstrong, D., editors: The acquired immune deficiency syndrome and infections of homosexual men, New York, 1984, Yorke Medical Books.

Porter, S.F.: Arthritis care: a guide for patient education, Norwalk, Conn., 1984, Appleton-Century-Crofts.

Potter, D.O., et al.: Nurse's reference library: assessment, Springhouse, Pa., 1982, Intermed Communications, Inc.

Rackel, R.E., editor: Conn's current therapy, Philadelphia, 1984, W.B. Saunders Co.

Richter, M.A.: Clinical immunology: a physician's guide, Baltimore, Md., Williams & Wilkins Co.

Roberts, R.B.: Treatment of opportunistic infections in patients with AIDS. In Ma, P., and Armstrong, D., editors: The acquired immune deficiency syndrome and infections of homosexual men, New York, 1984, Yorke Medical Books.

Rose, N.R., and Friedman, H.: Manual of clinical immunology, Washington, D.C., 1980, American Society for Microbiology.

Schur, P.H., editor: The clinical management of systemic lupus erythematosus, New York, 1983, Grune & Stratton, Inc.

Scipien, G.M., et al., editors: Comprehensive pediatric nursing, ed. 2, New York, 1979, McGraw-Hill Book Co.

Shahinpour, N.: The patient with systemic lupus erythematosus: prototype of autoimmunity, Heart Lung **9:**682, 1980.

Siegal, F.P., and Siegal, M.: AIDS: the medical mystery, New York, 1983, Grove Press, Inc.

Steele, R.W.: Immunology for the practicing physician, Norwalk, Conn., 1983, Appleton-Century-Crofts.

Steinberg, A.D.: Immunoregulatory agents. In Kelley, W.N., et al., editors: Textbook of rheumatology, Philadelphia, 1981, W.B. Saunders Co.

Thomas, E.D.: Marrow transplantation for malignant diseases, J. Clin. Oncol. **1:**517, 1983.

Trester, A.K.: Nursing management of patients receiving cancer chemotherapy, Cancer Nurs. **5:**201, 1982.

Unanue, E.R., and Benacerraf, S.: Textbook of immunology, Baltimore, Md., 1984, Williams & Wilkins.

Update: treatment of cryptosporidiosis in patients with acquired immune deficiency syndrome, MMWR **33:**117, 1984.

Whaley, L.F., and Wong, D.L.: Nursing care of infants and children, St. Louis, 1979, The C.V. Mosby Co.

Wiley, F.W., and Decuir-Whalley, S.: Allogeneic bone marrow transplantation for children with acute leukemia, Oncol. Nurs. Forum **10:**49, 1983.

Wintrobe, M.M., et al.: Clinical hematology, Philadelphia, Pa., 1974, Lea & Febiger.

Yasko, J.M., and Lauffer, B.E.: Infection in the cancer patient. In Donovan, M.I., editor: Cancer care, a guide for patient education, New York, 1981, Appleton-Century-Crofts.

Ziebell, B.: Wellness: an arthritis reality, Dubuque, Ia., 1981, Kendall/Hunt Publishing Co.

CHAPTER 17

Mental Health

Overview

Mental health is an elusive concept with diverse definitions. Not all theorists identify the same personality traits as indicators of healthy functioning, but their definitions are not necessarily contradictory. The diversity is related to the complexity of human beings and the beliefs each theorist has about human nature. Theorists recognize that biologic, social, and psychologic influences all contribute to healthy personality functioning, but each theorist emphasizes one dimension over the others.

Characteristics of healthy personality functioning compiled from psychoanalytic, interpersonal, and cognitive theories are listed below. The list is not exhaustive and is not in order of importance, but all characteristics are indicators of mental health.

1. Positive self-identity
2. Awareness of oneself as a separate individual
3. Responsibility for oneself and own actions
4. Acceptance of emotions and ability to correct faulty ones
5. Constructive use of cognitive processes
6. Achievement of satisfying interpersonal relationships
7. Autonomy, which includes use of self-supports
8. Flexibility to adapt to change

PERSONALITY THEORIES

An overview of normal personality development as seen by psychoanalytic and interpersonal theorists will be presented to provide a basic background for understanding concepts relevant to healthy functioning. Since Beck,[4] the major cognitive theorist discussed, has no theory of personality development, his theory will be described mainly in terms of "here and now" functioning.

Psychoanalytic Theory

Freud defined the personality as developing intrapsychically in relation to instincts and drives. The three major structures of the personality are the id, ego, and super-ego.[11] The id is the source of all psychic energy (libido). It operates on the "pleasure principle" in that it discharges tension and anxiety immediately and thrives on unrealistic, uncompromising, and insatiable narcissism.[53] As the infant interacts with the world of reality, the ego develops as the "reality principle" of the personality. It foregoes immediate pleasure by delaying gratification and reducing anxiety in socially acceptable ways. Logically organized behavior replaces impulsive self-gratification. The superego serves as the self-evaluative dimension of the personality and begins as the child introjects parental standards of behavior. It inhibits id impulses, imposes moralistic standards that are often

1739

unrealistic, strives for perfection, and demands self-punishment or repentance for wrongdoing.[11]

Freud believed that the first 6 years of life are crucial periods of development and that future development is an elaboration of these early periods. The psychosexual phases during the first 6 years are the oral, anal, and phallic. These phases are not discrete but overlap, and fragments of them continue throughout life.

The newborn can be viewed as an instinctual creature who is totally dependent on the mothering one for gratification of all needs. The mother gives unconditional love to ensure the infant's comfort. During the oral phase, the mouth is the source not only of nourishment but also of pleasure. The infant moves from a symbiotic relationship with the mother during the first 6 months to taking an active role in the process of differentiating the self from the nonself. During this time the infant begins to view himself as separate from the mother as he experiences alternating periods of gratification and frustration in having his needs met.

In the anal phase, 18 to 36 months of age, the child surrenders some of his freedom by responding to the demands of parents to control bowel and bladder functions through toilet training. With much ambivalence and conflict, the child accepts the parent's requests as his own. Gaining control over the elimination processes leads the child to achieve mastery over other processes of life.

The genitalia become the erotogenic zone during the phallic phase of development from 3 to 6 years of age. The child develops interest in his own and others' sexual organs. Resolution of the oedipal complex occurs during this phase in which the child represses sexual desires for the parent of the opposite sex and identifies with the parent of the same sex. Sexual activities such as masturbation are diminished or abandoned by the end of this phase; they reappear during adolescence.[11]

Freud had little to say about later periods of development. The latency period, 6 to 12 years of age, is a period when the child has opportunities to consolidate previous achievements and to increase social interactions with peers. The genital phase of development occurs during the adolescent years; sexual impulses are intensified and increase anxiety. The tasks the adolescent faces are to adapt the personality to the biologic changes that disrupt equilibrium and to accept sexuality as part of the personality.

The ego becomes stronger as the person successfully resolves the issues of early development and also as the personality develops in its ability to think, make judgments, experience emotions, and become aware of self. In the ego's mediator role it balances conflicting demands of the superego, the id, and the external world. Defense mechanisms such as repression, identification, and dis-placement are used by healthy persons in the service of the ego to manage overwhelming anxiety and conflicts. The normal adult deals effectively with anxiety and aggressive impulses and can consciously and logically choose a course of action to achieve satisfying relationships with self and others.

The ego-analytic theorists, such as Mahler, Hartmann, Rapaport, and Erikson, as a group view themselves as logically extending and elaborating Freud's theory. They give increased emphasis to ego development and to healthy behavior in their study of normal individuals.

Mahler, Pine, and Bergman[49] focus on the intrapsychic separation-individuation process that evolves between 4 and 36 months of age, at the same time as Freud's psychosexual phases of development. The infant moves from the autistic and symbiotic phases of development to become a psychologically separate and distinct human being. Locomotor abilities and other aspects of ego functions ordinarily develop concurrently with the separation-individuation process, but when they lag behind or spurt ahead, the child encounters additional difficulties and anxieties in resolving the issues. The child needs a stable relationship with an emotionally and physically available parent or significant other to master the psychologic tasks of this period.

In separation the infant begins to disengage himself from the mother and to differentiate himself from other objects. By the end of this process he conceives of himself as a separate individual with ego boundaries. In individuation, which occurs concurrently with the separation process, the child develops abilities to function autonomously, use cognitive processes, and achieve self-identity. The child needs positive experiences to stabilize the goodness in himself and others so he can develop positive self-identities and object relationships. Only toward the end of this process can the child tolerate mixed emotions toward a single person and make qualitative evaluations about the self and others.[49]

The separation-individuation process of adolescence is in response to major biologic and psychologic changes.[9a] The adolescent separates psychologically from the parents as support and value givers and turns to peers and others outside the family. Peers share his experiences and ease the emancipation from early dependencies and loyalties. The adolescent needs intense subjective experiences to differentiate himself from others. Vacillation from apathy to self-certainty and from dependence to independence is common in the adolescent. In preparation for the establishment of his social, personal, and sexual identity, he tries out new roles with no permanent commitment. During this time the adolescent develops close relationships with members of his own sex to develop his own sexual role before he reaches out to become comfortable with the opposite sex.[9a]

Toward the end of this period the adolescent establishes firm ego boundaries, accepts responsibility for what he is and does, develops increased decision-making capacities, establishes the capacity for mature relationships with males and females, and develops an autonomous life-style.

Interpersonal Theory

Interpersonal theory, developed by Harry Stack Sullivan, emphasizes interpersonal interactions and communication as the keys to development. Interpersonal theorists view the environment as influencing the personality throughout the individual's lifetime.[17]

Crucial learning experiences begin in infancy in relation to the mother's caretaking activities. An anxious mother evokes anxiety in the infant. Anxiety in the mother interferes with her ability to comfort the infant and the infant's ability to gain relief. According to Sullivan,[71] the educative influence of anxiety cannot be overestimated in modifying behavior and achieving satisfaction of needs, although severe anxiety causes confusion and no learning takes place.

The self-system is the organization of educative experiences that develops to avoid or minimize the occurrence of anxiety in interpersonal situations. As the self-system becomes increasingly complex in later childhood, it protects the individual's self-esteem and defines the characteristics of the individual. It has the advantage—or the disadvantage if the person evaluates the self negatively—of being relatively resistant to change.

Communication through the use of language is important to the development of the personality. Language provides the means for consensual validation of thought processes, since it arises in interpersonal interactions. In early infancy the infant experiences life in a prototaxic mode; that is, unrefined, undifferentiated momentary states of awareness occur. By the age of 18 months the child begins to acquire language to communicate needs and wishes, and thinking is in the parataxic mode; the child is aware that events occur together, either sequentially or at the same time, but does not recognize that events are not logically related to one another. The ability to think and experience in the syntaxic mode develops after 7 years of age. Older children reflect and compare events through the use of language according to the principles of logic. They gain capacities to deal with abstract concepts rather than be limited to concrete experiences. Consensual validation becomes a tool for clarifying perceptions and conclusions by talking with others. By sharing and comparing information with others the person increases awareness of himself and the world.[71]

A healthy adult is able to think logically and abstractly and examine and verify observations, assumptions, and conclusions. The ability to use anxiety and other emotions as an educative experience enables the person to perceive himself and the environment, experience feelings, anticipate events, recall past experiences, and establish satisfying interpersonal relationships with others.

Cognitive Theory

Cognitive theorists such as Ellis, Meichenbaum, Beck, and Seligman are a diverse group; however, they generally believe that individuals use their cognitive processes to resolve problems throughout the life cycle. Behaviorists who previously ignored cognitive processes such as thinking, recalling, intellectualizing, problem solving, and judging because they are inaccessible to empirical validation now recognize these important processes in the acquisition of knowledge.[49a]

Cognitive appraisals of internal (mental) or external stimuli precede emotional responses, although not necessarily at a conscious level. Arieti,[3] an interpersonal theorist, believes as cognitists do that cognitions and emotions are intertwined: some type of cognitive appraisal intervenes between the stimulus and emotional response. Specific emotions, appropriate or faulty in relation to the stimulus, are experienced because the person assigns a meaning or value to aspects of the experience.

Anxiety and depression are key factors in emotional distress. Beck,[7] a cognitive theorist, posits that people sometimes use "automatic thinking," which may result in faulty conceptions, self-signals, and emotions. An educative approach is used in therapy to restructure cognitions by helping the person become aware of his thoughts and then correct inaccurate judgments and emotional responses. In addition to learning problem-solving approaches, the person learns adaptive coping skills as part of the educative approach. Some of these skills are relaxation techniques, meditation, self-distraction, and preperformance rehearsals, as through role playing.

Ordinarily a person is able to use cognitive abilities to deal with events even under adverse conditions. In complex societies the person is expected to adapt to haphazard changes in the environment and to make rapid decisions, often in threatening situations. When interacting with others, even in aggressive, confrontation-type situations, the person attends to subtle cues in the interaction to differentiate between sincere and insincere and between logical and illogical messages. A wide variety of techniques are used to make observations, resolve conflict, examine alternative courses of actions, and manage rejections, failures, and threats. Restructuring and reinterpreting an event, for example, identifying humor in a situation, is one technique. The person gains increased understanding of himself and others and the world around them as he uses his cognitive abilities. The healthy person holds a positive view of himself and has positive expectations of the environment and future.[7]

. . .

The theories that have been discussed are not necessarily contradictory; they focus on different dimensions of the personality, with some overlapping of conceptualizations. Psychoanalytic and interpersonal theorists believe that early childhood experiences strongly influence later development and functioning. Interpersonal theorists believe more than psychoanalytic theorists that a person is able to make changes in his personality throughout the lifetime as a result of new life experiences. Cognitive theorists believe the person can help himself to adapt to new situations, but they do not address developmental influences explicitly.

MENTAL DISORDERS

When personality growth and development go awry because of psychologic, social, cultural, or biologic influences, the person may become mentally ill. The American Psychiatric Association's *Diagnostic and Statistical Manual of Mental Disorders,* ed. 3 (DSM-III)[1] is the official classification system for diagnosing mental disorders. The manual offers clinicians a common language to communicate with one another about disorders and a basis for planning a treatment program.

The third edition of the manual provides a multiaxial evaluation to assess patients in a comprehensive manner.[72a] Axes I and II of the DSM-III describe the patient's current condition by addressing all of the mental disorder classifications and conditions not associated with a mental disorder. Axis III indicates physical disorders and conditions that may be relevant to the understanding or treatment of the patient. Axis IV, an assessment of the severity of psychosocial stressors that contributed to the current disorder, and Axis V, an assessment of the highest level of adaptive functioning during the past year, complete the evaluation. The DSM-III multiaxial evaluation is outlined as follows.

DSM-III MULTIAXIAL EVALUATION*

AXIS I: Clinical Syndromes
Conditions not Attributable to a Mental Disorder that are a Focus of Attention or Treatment
Additional Codes
AXIS II: Personality Disorders
Specific Developmental Disorders

All official DSM-III codes and terms are included in ICD-9-CM. However, in order to differentiate those DSM-III categories that use the same ICD-9-CM codes, unofficial non-ICD-9-CM codes are provided in parentheses for use when greater

*From American Psychiatric Association: Diagnostic and statistical manual of mental disorders, ed. 3, Washington, D.C., 1980, pp. 15-19, 27, 29-30. Reprinted with permission from the American Psychiatric Association.

specificity is necessary. The long dashes indicate the need for a fifth-digit subtype or other qualifying term.

Disorders Usually First Evident in Infancy, Childhood or Adolescence

Mental retardation
Code in fifth digit: 1 = with other behavioral symptoms [requiring attention or treatment and that are not part of another disorder], 0 = without other behavioral symptoms.

317.0(×) Mild mental retardation, _____
318.0(×) Moderate mental retardation, _____
318.1(×) Severe mental retardation, _____
318.2(×) Profound mental retardation, _____
319.0(×) Unspecified mental retardation, _____

Attention deficit disorder
314.01 with hyperactivity
314.00 without hyperactivity
314.80 residual type

Conduct disorder
312.00 undersocialized, aggressive
312.10 undersocialized, nonaggressive
312.23 socialized, aggressive
312.21 socialized, nonaggressive
312.90 atypical

Anxiety disorders of childhood or adolescence
309.21 Separation anxiety disorder
313.21 Avoidant disorder of childhood or adolescence
313.00 Overanxious disorder

Other disorders of infancy, childhood or adolescence
313.89 Reactive attachment disorder of infancy
313.22 Schizoid disorder of childhood or adolescence
313.23 Elective mutism
313.81 Oppositional disorder
313.82 Identity disorder

Eating disorders
307.10 Anorexia nervosa
307.51 Bulimia
307.52 Pica
307.53 Rumination disorder of infancy
307.50 Atypical eating disorder

Stereotyped movement disorders

307.21 Transient tic disorder
307.22 Chronic motor tic disorder
307.23 Tourette's disorder
307.20 Atypical tic disorder
307.30 Atypical stereotyped movement disorder

Other disorders with physical manifestations

307.00 Stuttering
307.60 Functional enuresis
307.70 Functional encopresis
307.46 Sleepwalking disorder
307.46 Sleep terror disorder (307.49)

Pervasive developmental disorders

Code in fifth digit: 0 = full syndrome present, 1 = residual state.

299.0 × Infantile autism, _____
299.9 × Childhood onset pervasive developmental disorder, _____

299.8 × Atypical, _____

Specific developmental disorders
Note: These are coded on Axis II.

315.00 Developmental reading disorder
315.10 Developmental arithmetic disorder
315.31 Developmental language disorder
315.39 Developmental articulation disorder
315.50 Mixed specific developmental disorder
315.90 Atypical specific developmental disorder

Organic Mental Disorders

Section 1. Organic mental disorders whose etiology or pathophysiological process is listed below (taken from the mental disorders section of ICD-9-CM).

Dementias arising in the senium and presenium

Primary degenerative dementia, senile onset,

290.30 with delirium
290.20 with delusions
290.21 with depression
290.00 uncomplicated

Code in fifth digit:
1 = with delirium, 2 = with delusions, 3 = with depression, 0 = uncomplicated.

290.1 × Primary degenerative dementia, presenile onset, _____

290.4 × Multi-infarct dementia, _____

Substance-induced
Alcohol

303.00 intoxication
291.40 idiosyncratic intoxication
291.80 withdrawal
291.00 withdrawal delirium
291.30 hallucinosis
291.10 amnestic disorder

Code severity of dementia in fifth digit: 1 = mild, 2 = moderate, 3 = severe, 0 = unspecified.

291.2 × Dementia associated with alcoholism, _____

Barbiturate or similarly acting sedative or hypnotic

305.40 intoxication (327.00)
292.00 withdrawal (327.01)
292.00 withdrawal delirium (327.02)
292.83 amnestic disorder (327.04)

Opioid

305.50 intoxication (327.10)
292.00 withdrawal (327.11)

Cocaine

305.60 intoxication (327.20)

Amphetamine or similarly acting sympathomimetic

305.70 intoxication (327.30)
292.81 delirium (327.32)
292.11 delusional disorder (327.35)
292.00 withdrawal (327.31)

Phencyclidine (PCP) or similarly acting arylcyclohexylamine

305.90 intoxication (327.40)
292.81 delirium (327.42)
292.90 mixed organic mental disorder (327.49)

Hallucinogen

305.30 hallucinosis (327.56)
292.11 delusional disorder (327.55)
292.84 affective disorder (327.57)

Cannabis

305.20 intoxication (327.60)
292.11 delusional disorder (327.65)

Tobacco

292.00 withdrawal (327.71)

Caffeine

305.90 intoxication (327.80)

Other or unspecified substance

305.90 intoxication (327.90)
292.00 withdrawal (327.91)
292.81 delirium (327.92)
292.82 dementia (327.93)
292.83 amnestic disorder (327.94)
292.11 delusional disorder (327.95)
292.12 hallucinosis (327.96)
292.84 affective disorder (327.97)
292.89 personality disorder (327.98)
292.90 atypical or mixed organic mental disorder (327.99)

Section 2. Organic brain syndromes whose etiology or pathophysiological process is either noted as an additional diagnosis from outside the mental disorders section of ICD-9-CM or is unknown.

293.00 Delirium
294.10 Dementia
294.00 Amnestic syndrome
293.81 Organic delusional syndrome
293.82 Organic hallucinosis
293.83 Organic affective syndrome

310.10 Organic personality syndrome
294.80 Atypical or mixed organic brain syndrome

Substance Use Disorders

Code in fifth digit: 1 = continuous, 2 = episodic, 3 = in remission, 0 = unspecified.

305.0× Alcohol abuse, _____
303.9× Alcohol dependence (Alcoholism), _____
305.4× Barbiturate or similarly acting sedative or hypnotic abuse,
304.1× Barbiturate or similarly acting sedative or hypnotic dependence, _____
305.5× Opioid abuse, _____
304.0× Opioid dependence, _____
305.6× Cocaine abuse, _____
305.7× Amphetamine or similarly acting sympathomimetic abuse, _____
304.4× Amphetamine or similarly acting sympathomimetic dependence, _____
305.9× Phencyclidine (PCP) or similarly acting arylcyclohexylamine abuse, _____(328.4×)
305.3× Hallucinogen abuse, _____
305.2× Cannabis abuse, _____
304.3× Cannabis dependence, _____
305.1× Tobacco dependence, _____
305.9× Other, mixed or unspecified substance abuse, _____
304.6× Other specified substance dependence, _____
304.9× Unspecified substance dependence, _____
304.7× Dependence on combination of opioid and other non-alcoholic substance, _____
304.8× Dependence on combination of substances, excluding opioids and alcohol, _____

Schizophrenic Disorders

Code in fifth digit: 1 = subchronic, 2 = chronic, 3 = subchronic with acute exacerbation, 4 = chronic with acute exacerbation, 5 = in remission, 0 = unspecified.

Schizophrenia
295.1× disorganized, _____
295.2× catatonic, _____
295.3× paranoid, _____
295.9× undifferentiated, _____
295.6× residual, _____

Paranoid Disorders

297.10 Paranoia
297.30 Shared paranoid disorder
298.30 Acute paranoid disorder
297.90 Atypical paranoid disorder

Psychotic Disorders not Elsewhere Classified

295.40 Schizophreniform disorder
298.80 Brief reactive psychosis
295.70 Schizoaffective disorder
298.90 Atypical psychosis

Neurotic Disorders

These are included in Affective, Anxiety, Somatoform, Dissociative, and Psychosexual Disorders. In order to facilitate the identification of the categories that in DSM-II were grouped together in the class of Neuroses, the DSM-II terms are included separately in parentheses after the corresponding categories. These DSM-II terms are included in ICD-9-CM and therefore are acceptable as alternatives to the recommended DSM-III terms that precede them.

Affective Disorders

Major affective disorders
Code major depressive episode in fifth digit: 6 = in remission, 4 = with psychotic features (the unofficial non-ICD-9-CM fifth digit 7 may be used instead to indicate that the psychotic features are mood-incongruent), 3 = with melancholia, 2 = without melancholia, 0 = unspecified.

Code manic episode in fifth digit: 6 = in remission, 4 = with psychotic features (the unofficial non-ICD-9-CM fifth digit 7 may be used instead to indicate that the psychotic features are mood-incongruent), 2 = without psychotic features, 0 = unspecified.

Bipolar disorder
296.6× mixed, _____
296.4× manic, _____
296.5× depressed, _____

Major depression
296.2× single episode, _____
296.3× recurrent, _____

Other specific affective disorders
301.13 Cyclothymic disorder
300.40 Dysthymic disorder (or Depressive neurosis)

Atypical affective disorders
296.70 Atypical bipolar disorder
296.82 Atypical depression

Anxiety Disorders

Phobic disorders (or Phobic neuroses)
300.21 Agoraphobia with panic attacks
300.22 Agoraphobia without panic attacks
300.23 Social phobia
300.29 Simple phobia

Anxiety states (or Anxiety neuroses)
300.01 Panic disorder
300.02 Generalized anxiety disorder
300.30 Obsessive compulsive disorder (or Obsessive compulsive neurosis)

Post-traumatic stress disorder
308.30 acute
309.81 chronic or delayed
300.00 Atypical anxiety disorder

Somatoform Disorders

300.81 Somatization disorder

300.11 Conversion disorder (or Hysterical neurosis, conversion type)
307.80 Psychogenic pain disorder
300.70 Hypochondriasis (or Hypochondriacal neurosis)
300.70 Atypical somatoform disorder (300.71)

Dissociative Disorders (or Hysterical Neuroses, Dissociative Type)

300.12 Psychogenic amnesia
300.13 Psychogenic fugue
300.14 Multiple personality
300.60 Depersonalization disorder (or Depersonalization neurosis)
300.15 Atypical dissociative disorder

Psychosexual Disorders

Gender identity disorders
Indicate sexual history in the fifth digit of Transsexualism code: 1 = asexual, 2 = homosexual, 3 = heterosexual, 0 = unspecified.

302.5× Transsexualism, _____
302.60 Gender identity disorder of childhood
302.85 Atypical gender identity disorder

Paraphilias
302.81 Fetishism
302.30 Transvestism
302.10 Zoophilia
302.20 Pedophilia
302.40 Exhibitionism
302.82 Voyeurism
302.83 Sexual masochism
302.84 Sexual sadism
302.90 Atypical paraphilia

Psychosexual dysfunctions
302.71 Inhibited sexual desire
302.72 Inhibited sexual excitement
302.73 Inhibited female orgasm
302.74 Inhibited male orgasm
302.75 Premature ejaculation
302.76 Functional dyspareunia
306.51 Functional vaginismus
302.70 Atypical psychosexual dysfunction

Other psychosexual disorders
302.00 Ego-dystonic homosexuality
302.89 Psychosexual disorder not elsewhere classified

Factitious Disorders

300.16 Factitious disorder with psychological symptoms
301.51 Chronic factitious disorder with physical symptoms
300.19 Atypical factitious disorder with physical symptoms

Disorders of Impulse Control not Elsewhere Classified

312.31 Pathological gambling
312.32 Kleptomania
312.33 Pyromania
312.34 Intermittent explosive disorder
312.35 Isolated explosive disorder
312.39 Atypical impulse control disorder

Adjustment Disorder

309.00 with depressed mood
309.24 with anxious mood
309.28 with mixed emotional features
309.30 with disturbance of conduct
309.40 with mixed disturbance of emotions and conduct
309.23 with work (or academic) inhibition
309.83 with withdrawal
309.90 with atypical features

Psychological Factors Affecting Physical Condition

Specify physical condition on Axis III.

316.00 Psychological factors affecting physical condition

PERSONALITY DISORDERS	
Note: These are coded on Axis II.	
301.00 Paranoid	301.82 Avoidant
301.20 Schizoid	301.60 Dependent
301.22 Schizotypal	301.40 Compulsive
301.50 Histrionic	301.84 Passive-Aggressive
301.81 Narcissistic	301.89 Atypical, mixed or other
301.70 Antisocial	personality disorder
301.83 Borderline	

V Codes for Conditions not Attributable to a Mental Disorder That are a Focus of Attention or Treatment

V65.20 Malingering
V62.89 Borderline intellectual functioning (V62.88)
V71.01 Adult antisocial behavior
V71.02 Childhood or adolescent antisocial behavior
V62.30 Academic problem
V62.20 Occupational problem
V62.82 Uncomplicated bereavement
V15.81 Noncompliance with medical treatment
V62.89 Phase of life problem or other life circumstance problem
V61.10 Marital problem
V61.20 Parent-child problem
V61.80 Other specified family circumstances
V62.81 Other interpersonal problem

Additional Codes

300.90 Unspecified mental disorder (nonpsychotic)
V71.09 No diagnosis or condition on Axis I
799.90 Diagnosis or condition deferred on Axis I

V71.09 No diagnosis on Axis II
799.90 Diagnosis deferred on Axis II

AXIS III: Physical Disorders and Conditions

AXIS IV: Severity of Psychosocial Stressors

Code	Term	Adult Examples	Child or Adolescent Examples
1	None	No apparent psychosocial stressor	No apparent psychosocial stressor
2	Minimal	Minor violation of the law, small bank loan	Vacation with family
3	Mild	Argument with neighbor; change in work hours	Change in schoolteacher; new school year
4	Moderate	New career; death of close friend; pregnancy	Chronic parental fighting; change to new school; illness of close relative; birth of sibling
5	Severe	Serious illness in self or family; major financial loss; marital separation; birth of child	Death of peer; divorce of parents; arrest; hospitalization; persistent and harsh parental-discipline
6	Extreme	Death of close relative; divorce	Death of parent or sibling; repeated physical or sexual abuse
7	Catastrophic	Concentration camp experience; devastating natural disaster	Multiple family deaths
0	Unspecified	No information, or not applicable	No information; or not applicable

AXIS V: Highest Level of Adaptive Functioning During the Past Year

Levels	Adult Examples	Child or Adolescent Examples
1 *SUPERIOR*—Unusually effective functioning in social relations, occupational functioning and use of leisure time.	Single parent living in deteriorating neighborhood takes excellent care of children and home, has warm relations with friends, and finds time for pursuit of hobby.	A 12-year-old girl gets superior grades in school, is extremely popular among her peers, and excels in many sports. She does all of this with apparent ease and comfort.
2 *VERY GOOD*—Better than average functioning in social relations, occupational functioning, and use of leisure time.	A 65-year-old retired widower does some volunteer work, often sees old friends, and pursues hobbies.	An adolescent boy gets excellent grades, works part time, has several close friends, and plays banjo in a jazz band. He admits to some distress in "keeping up with everything."
3 *GOOD*—No more than slight impairment in either social or occupational functioning.	A woman with many friends functions extremely well at a difficult job, but says "the strain is too much."	An 8-year-old boy does well in school, has several friends, but bullies younger children.
4 *FAIR*—Moderate impairment in either social relations or occupational functioning, or some impairment in both.	A lawyer has trouble carrying through assignments; has several acquaintances, but hardly any close friends.	A 10-year-old girl does poorly in school, but has adequate peer and family relations.
5 *POOR*—Marked impairment in either social relations or occupational functioning, or moderate impairment in both.	A man with one or two friends has trouble keeping a job for more than a few weeks.	A 14-year-old boy almost fails in school and has trouble getting along with his peers.
6 *VERY POOR*—Marked impairment in both social relations and occupational functioning.	A woman is unable to do any of her housework and has violent outbursts toward family and neighbors.	A 6-year-old girls needs special help in all subjects and has virtually no peer relationships.
7 *GROSSLY IMPAIRED*—Gross impairment in virtually all areas of functioning.	An elderly man needs supervision to maintain minimal personal hygiene and is usually incoherent.	A 4-year-old boy needs constant restraint to avoid hurting himself and is almost totally lacking in skills.
0 *UNSPECIFIED*	No information.	No information.

NORMAL LABORATORY DATA

Laboratory Test	Normal Adult Values	Laboratory Test	Normal Adult Values
Serum tests—sequential multiple analyzer with computer (SMAC)		Alkaline phosphatase	5-13 units/100 ml (King-Armstrong units)
Triglycerides		Acid phosphatase	1-5 units/100 ml (King-Armstrong units)
Ages 1-29 years	10-140 mg/100 ml	Total protein	6-8 g/100 ml
Ages 30-39 years	10-150 mg/100 ml	Albumin	3.3-4.5 g/100 ml
Glucose	80-120 mg/100 ml	Blood urea nitrogen (BUN)	8-20 mg/100 ml
Carbon dioxide (CO_2)	22-34 mEq/L	Creatinine	0.6-1.2 mg/100 ml
Calcium (Ca)	4.5-5.5 mg/100 ml	Uric acid	
Chloride (Cl)	100-108 mEq/L	Males	4.3-8 mg/100 ml
Potassium (K)	3.5-5 mEq/L	Females	2.3-6 mg/100 ml
Sodium (Na)	135-145 mEq/L	Bilirubin	
Phosphorus (P)	3-4.5 mg/100 ml	Direct	0.1-0.4 mg/100 ml
Creatine phosphokinase (CPK)		Total	0.2-0.9 mg/100 ml
Males	23-99 units/L	Iron	
Females	15-57 units/L	Males	80-160 μg/100 ml
Lactic dehydrogenase (LDH)	48-115 IU/L (total)	Females	50-150 μg/100 ml
Serum glutamic oxaloacetic transaminase (SGOT)	5-40 units/ml (Frankel)	Urinalysis	
		Color	Straw
		Appearance	Clear
		Specific gravity	1.005-1.030
Serum glutamic pyruvic transaminase (SGPT)	5-35 units/ml (Frankel)	pH	4.5-8.0
		Cells and protein	None
		Sugars and acetone	Negative

Conditions, Diseases, and Disorders

Mental health problems nurses are likely to encounter in any psychiatric setting in which they interact with patients are presented in this section. The organizing framework for the mental disorders is DSM-III,[1] since it is the standard diagnostic classification that is accepted by mental health professionals. The diagnoses are based on criteria that have been field tested for reliability and validity. Although the classification system is not free of controversy, the definitions and descriptions provide a common frame of reference for communication among professionals. The manual attempts to describe clinical manifestations of mental disorders comprehensively without linking the defining criteria to a theoretic framework. The justification for the atheoretic approach is that clinicians, regardless of theoretic persuasion, can agree on the identification of disorders based on clinical manifestations without agreeing on how and why the disturbances developed.

Since the classification system is atheoretic and useful to clinicians in various mental health professions with diverse theoretic perspectives, it is logical to assume that the system has relevance for nurses.[76] Conceptual frameworks in nursing are applicable to the atheoretic classification system. By sensitizing themselves to the clinical features of each disorder, nurses can use the nursing assessment to identify problems. Since the plan of patient care is derived from both medical and nursing diagnoses, familiarity with the commonly accepted diagnostic system permits knowledgeable participation in devising intervention strategies to achieve individualized goals for patients.

The major diagnostic classes are included in this section with brief descriptions of mental disorders within each class. The decision to present a complete discussion of mental disorders within a class is based on its representing that diagnostic class (for example, schizophrenia), being the more frequently occurring condition, or being a management problem for nurses and other staff. The last two conditions listed under "Adaptive and Maladaptive Behavior" are not diagnostic categories of mental disorders. They do have serious implications for mental health if preventive strategies are not implemented.

DISORDERS USUALLY FIRST EVIDENT IN INFANCY, CHILDHOOD, OR ADOLESCENCE

The disorders in this class usually begin or are evident in infancy, childhood, or adolescence, but they can develop in later adulthood.[1] For example, eating disorders usually develop in older children or adolescents but may develop as an adult disorder. Anorexia nervosa and bulimia, two subclasses of this class, are included because of the frequency of their occurrence in the general population and their apparent increase in incidence. Since they frequently are associated with similar dysfunctional behaviors, they are discussed together.

Anorexia Nervosa and Bulimia

Anorexia nervosa is a formidable disorder affecting mainly young women and characterized by a determination to lose weight despite emaciation. Bulimia is insatiable appetite.

Although anorexia is usually viewed as an eating disorder and a distorted drive to thinness, these are secondary to achieving a sense of control and rejection of a mature feminine body.[32] The anorexic person has a history of being a high achiever, a compliant pleaser of others, and a model child to her parents. When she begins to diet, she is aware of hunger but denies it in her obsession about weight loss.

Major categories of disordered eating exist: strict restriction of food intake, cycles of starvation and overeating with purging, and overeating with purging (bulimia).

Some persons are extremely self-disciplined in restricting their food intake to 600 calories or less per day because of their fear of overeating and losing control. These persons are unrelenting in their avoidance of eating, although they are preoccupied with food.

Other persons alternate between periods of starving and bingeing. Time intervals of restrictive food intake vary from days to weeks, and those of severe overeating from hours to days. Purging is done through induced vomiting, laxatives, and diuretics.

The third type of eating disorder is bulimia. Other terms used for this disorder are bulimia nervosa, bulimia syndrome, and more recently, bulimarexia. The bulimic person has an average intake of 5000 calories per day and may take in as much as 20,000 calories during a binge. She purges her body to avoid gaining weight. Forms of purging include self-induced vomiting several times a day, misusing laxatives (up to 50 per day), and misusing diuretics.[10,32]

Theorists disagree about the differentiation between the patterns of eating disorders. Some regard the various eating disorders as subtypes of anorexia nervosa and others as separate entities.[58] However, overlap of the three major patterns generally exists.

Eating is a source of anxiety for both anorexics and bulimics. Some anorexics never engage in binge eating and purging because of their great self-discipline; bingers are more impulsive and unable to maintain the strict self-control. Anorexics, whether or not they binge, are likely to become emaciated, whereas bulimics are usually nearer their normal weight. A further difference between the two is that purging behaviors are less pervasive in anorexics than in bulimics. Persons with the various eating disorder patterns tend toward chronicity in their ability to hold on to the dysfunctional behaviors. They avoid eating with others around them; purging is also performed out of the view of others.

Bulimic persons are more outgoing and sensitive to others and less likely to reject their mature-appearing bodies and feminine roles than the more ascetic anorexics. As the disorders develop, relationships tend to become more superficial and distant. Social contact is avoided because of the fear of being invited to eat and being discovered. They are preoccupied with food, meal planning (especially for others), their calorie intake throughout the day, and methods to avoid eating food themselves. Eating, whether normally, in tiny quantities, or by gorging, becomes a private endeavor rather than a socially enjoyable activity. The "model child" becomes defiant, aggressive, and irritable when the pattern becomes well ingrained.

Severe physiologic complications result from the nutritional deficits and emotional disturbances. Some of these are bradycardia, arrhythmia, hypotension, renal changes such as elevated blood urea nitrogen and reduced glomerular filtration rate, electrolyte imbalance such as hypokalemia and hypochloremic alkalosis, and neurologic complications such as convulsions. A decrease in gonadotropins leads to amenorrhea in women and reduced testosterone in men. Skeletal maturation is delayed when anorexia nervosa is tenaciously maintained. A mortality of 15% to 20% is associated with this eating disorder.[1,32,46]

Anorexia nervosa should be differentiated from other mental disorders such as depression, schizophrenia, hysteria, and obsessive-compulsive disorders. In these disorders weight loss occurs because of lack of interest in food or delusions, not because of a fundamental drive for thinness. Physiologic diseases also need to be differentiated from anorexia nervosa on the basis of a thorough history and physical examination. Such conditions include chronic wasting owing to tumors and hypothalamic diseases and endocrine disorders such as hyperthyroidism, diabetes mellitus, and Addison's disease. An anorexic person does not consult a physician with complaints of weight loss but for treatment of amenorrhea, gastrointestinal disturbances, and disturbances in sleep and concentration. Occasionally she seeks help for emotional disturbances.

Prevalence

The estimated incidence of anorexia is 1 of every 250 adolescents. Approximately 95% are female. Possibly because of greater medical and public awareness in the last decade, an enormous increase in the incidence of anorexia has been reported. The prevalence figure is probably much higher than the estimated incidence figure of 50,000, since there is little information on the number of chronically ill persons with anorexia. Bulimia is more difficult to identify in the population because the bulimic person seldom loses more than 20% of her ideal body weight and is more able to hide bingeing-purging behaviors than the restrictive anorexic.[1,32,65]

Population at Risk

The onset of anorexia nervosa ranges from prepuberty to middle age. The incidence is greatest between 12 and 22 years of age, and it is uncommon after 30 years of age. The 5% of anorexics who are males has remained stable and is related to gender identity problems or fears of obesity.[40] Until 1976 the disorder was seen almost exclusively in the upper social classes, but it is now observed almost equally in all socioeconomic levels. Recently anorexia has appeared in blacks, mainly from upper-class professional families. A high incidence is observed among models and dancers, especially ballerinas.[32,46]

Persons with anorexia and bulimia are characteristically perfectionists in their appearance, scholastic endeavors, and work situations. They are high achievers who are never satisfied with their accomplishments. Since they appear to be self-sufficient and strong, parents refrain from giving them the needed guidance and emotional support. Anorexics think that they cannot rely on others; therefore they overorganize to gain control of every minute of the day and every aspect of their lives.[32,46]

Hospitalization

Hospitalization is recommended when a person with anorexia nervosa or bulimia evidences severe medical complications such as weight loss of more than 20% of normal body weight and electrolyte and acid-base imbalances resulting from endless cycles of starvation and bingeing-purging. The patient may continue to deny any physical dangers and need for hospitalization even when emaciated. The fear of losing control looms large in her mind. To decrease resistance, the protective nature of and reasons for hospitalization should be emphasized.

The patient's cooperation may be gained by involving her in the treatment plan and criteria for discharge. Weight gain to 80% of ideal body weight, or stabilization of weight for a nonemaciated patient, should be a part of the discharge criteria.

The patient needs to believe that the staff is interested in helping her deal with other areas of her life in addition to her weight. Although steady weight gains are essential before psychotherapy can be initiated, the patient needs to feel supported and nurtured by staff from the beginning. Development of a safe, trusting relationship within a consistently supportive environment provides the patient with a sense of security.

If weight gain does not occur and electrolyte and acid-base values are abnormal, tube feeding may be prescribed. High-protein and high-caloric feedings are instilled by tube every hour. As the patient begins to drink the liquid diet, the tube feeding may be discontinued after 48 hours.[65] Daily weight gains of ¼ to ½ pound are generally expected for the emaciated patient, and weight stabilization without gorging-purging behaviors for the bulimic patient.

A dietitian is involved in the treatment to discuss food preferences, teach nutrition, and plan a well-balanced diet for the patient. Food intake is limited to regular meals and prescribed snacks, and the family is prohibited from bringing food in and visiting or calling during mealtimes. Close supervision of meals is necessary initially, with a nurse in attendance to monitor food intake. Obsessional discussions of food and power struggles about eating should be avoided. The nurse should be cognizant of the patient's anxiety about eating and weight gain; reassurance that weight gain is being controlled to prevent obesity is vital. Assisting the patient to interpret weight gain or stabilization of weight as a sign of being in control can decrease her sense of powerlessness and lack of control.

The nurse should challenge the patient's misconceptions about her illness and herself by questioning her assumptions and irrational conclusions. As the relationship develops, the nurse should help the patient increase her self-awareness and self-acceptance by encouraging her to clarify her own thinking and trust her own thought processes and self-evaluations.

Since parents may convey to their daughter that her growing maturity is a threat to the family system, they should be included in the therapy for an adolescent girl.

Goals of family therapy are to decrease patterns of overinvolvement within the family and to strengthen the marital relationship. The therapist encourages new interactional patterns by having each family member accept responsibility for his or her own perceptions and behaviors, listen and respond to messages, and participate in the resolution of conflict.

PSYCHOPATHOLOGY

Psychoanalytic Theory

Psychoanalytic theorists view anorexia nervosa and bulimia as oral fixations in which eating disturbances and gastrointestinal disturbances can be traced to infancy.[32] Affected persons had anxious, compulsive mothers and continue to have disturbed mother-child relationships.

Oral fixation is the persistent concentration of psychic energy on the objects of the infant developmental phase. The focus is on taking in or spitting out, as evidenced by overeating, rejecting food, smoking excessively, vomiting, and oral conceptions of sexuality and pregnancy. These individuals may hold ascetic views, believing self-indulgence in eating and other behaviors to be sinful and starvation to be superior and saintly.

Interpersonal Theory

Interpersonal theorists believe that anorexia arises because of family relationships. They view the family as an emotionally closed system that "traps" members in intense relationships with one another. Individual ego boundaries and identities of members are blurred. By focusing on the child, parents avoid dealing with their own tensions and conflicts. As the child moves into adolescence and begins to seek independence and autonomy, the parents are unwilling to give up their accustomed pathologic interpersonal patterns of behavior. They become more overcontrolling and demanding, which foils the adolescent's efforts to achieve autonomy.

The parents expect selfless conformity from the child but are emotionally inaccessible; they demand that the child deny and mistrust perceptions that are incongruent with theirs. As the adolescent responds to the parents by offering support and strength, she perceives herself as loved for what she gives rather than for herself. She overorganizes her life to become perfect in her parents' eyes and to assume responsibility for her own physical and emotional safety. These dynamics within the family prohibit maturation of the adolescent to maintain the family's status quo.[64]

Although family characteristics predispose to the development of anorexia, environmental, constitutional, and psychologic factors also enter into the determination of whether a person develops this eating disorder.

Cognitive Theory

Cognitive and behavioral theorists say that the behaviors of the anorexic person are learned. The glorification of thinness in Western society results in attempts to conform to cultural ideals of physical appearance. Thinness is equated with self-control, beauty, and success. Models resembling prepubertal girls in high-fashion magazines are considered elegant beauties. These magazines and other media bombard women with reduction diets, exercises, and recipes.

The preanorexic, who may or may not be slightly overweight, is told by parents, teachers, or friends that she would look much better if she lost a little weight. The positive reinforcement she receives for dieting and losing weight and the pleasure she experiences in her new shape encourage her to lose more. If she happens to eat more than she deems correct, she learns from peers to purge her body by vomiting and misusing laxatives and diuretics. The elation of controlling caloric intake and losing weight leads her to compete with others to be the thinnest in her peer group. She devotes herself to activities related to food, weight, and exercise, with no time or energy left for social relationships and activities. The young woman's perceptions of her body size and self-appraisals are distorted so that low self-worth is related to fatness, and high self-worth to thinness.[32]

DIAGNOSTIC STUDIES

Serum test
Sequential multiple analyzer with computer (SMAC); if electrolyte and acid-base values are abnormal, repeat once a day until stable

Electrocardiography
To rule out cardiopathy

Urinalysis
To screen for urinary and systemic abnormalities

TREATMENT PLAN

Chemotherapeutic
Antidepressants
Doxepin (Sinequan), 25 mg bid and hs; acts as tricyclic antidepressant; reported incidence of side effect is low, and drug appears well tolerated

Supportive

Diet

Consultation with dietitian; high-protein and high-caloric diet; for severely emaciated client, 1200-calorie diet gradually increased to 3000-calorie diet

Occupational therapy

Recreational therapy

ASSESSMENT: AREAS OF CONCERN

Signs and symptoms of anorexia and bulimia vary from individual to individual; no one experiences all of those listed.

Emotional

Anxiety; depression; lability of mood; irritability; anger

Thought processes

Denial of hunger; fear of eating and weight gain; mistrust of self and others; low self-esteem; shame at being discovered bingeing and purging; sense of failure even when successful; perfectionism; rejection of feminine role; fear of psychosexual maturation; lack of interest in sex and opposite sex; impairment in concentration

Power and control

Powerlessness; struggle for control; helplessness; non-assertiveness

Body image

Denial of thinness or emaciated appearance; rejection of feminine body; self-loathing; delusions about body size

Fluid volume

Decreased fluid intake; excessive loss of fluids through (1) induced vomiting (possibly 18 times a day) with finger, toothbrush, or use of emetics such as Ipecac, especially after eating, (2) diarrhea caused by lax-atives (up to 50 a day), or (3) diuretics; altered electrolytes such as hypokalemia or hypochloremic alkalosis; muscle weakness; convulsions or muscle tetany; altered kidney function such as elevated blood urea nitrogen; altered cardiac function such as bradycardia or arrhythmias

Skin integrity

Skeletal prominence; bruised skin; altered circulation with cyanosis of extremities; dry, cracked skin; loss of scalp hair; lanugo on cheeks, neck, forearms, and thighs; peripheral edema; delayed skeletal maturation related to duration of emaciation

Sleep patterns

Disturbances in sleeping such as early morning wakening and restlessness

Nutrition

Fasting; starvation diet; bingeing (up to 20,000 calories a day with average of 5000); aversion to eating; weight loss to 20% of normal body weight and occasionally to 50%; frequent checking of weight, such as 10 times a day; nausea; bloating of abdomen; grossly distended stomach and duodenum because of bingeing; disposing of meals by feeding to dog and placing in garbage or toilet; hiding food for binges; eating secretly; amenorrhea; esophageal abrasions from vomiting; dental caries, loss of teeth, and buccal erosion because of hydrochloric acid from stomach; diarrhea; constipation; abdominal pain

Social activities

Sense of social inadequacy and ineffectiveness; insecurity; withdrawal from social relations to isolation; fear of interpersonal closeness

Family processes

Fear of abandonment and engulfment; overinvolvement of parents; overprotectiveness or lack of protectiveness by parents; denial of family conflict

NURSING DIAGNOSES and NURSING INTERVENTIONS

Nursing care should be implemented selectively based on severity and type of symptoms and behaviors.

Nursing Diagnosis	Nursing Intervention
Anxiety	Begin to develop safe, trusting relationship with patient.
	Continue to develop relationship through working and termination phases. (See also p. 1839.)
	Explain treatment plan explicitly to allay anxiety and decrease resistance. Review plan with patient at regular intervals.
	Assist patient to become aware of feelings such as anxiety. Encourage identification and acceptance of feelings.

Nursing Diagnosis	Nursing Intervention
	Encourage patient to begin to express feelings. Reaffirm her right to feelings including anger.
	Assist patient to feel comfortable expressing feelings and to work through inappropriate feelings.
	As patient begins to gain weight or stabilizes weight, help her deal with anxiety (which sometimes reaches almost panic level). Remain with patient, encouraging slow, deep breathing. Reinforce relaxation breathing when anxiety is severe.
Coping, ineffective individual	Assist patient to identify emotions that precede bingeing and past alternatives to bingeing. Help patient accept that she can deal with uncomfortable feelings.
	Reinforce use of substitutes for binge eating: relaxation techniques, reinterpretation of emotions, and diversionary activities such as watching television or talking to friend.
	Reinforce healthy coping skills as pleasurable alternative to bingeing or starving.
	Administer antidepressant such as doxepin as prescribed. Explain purpose of medication, effects, and side effects. If medication is continued, teach importance of compliance.
	If patient uses denial, encourage her to examine difficulties in other areas of life and eventually relate these to preoccupations with eating.
	Begin to help patient identify fears associated with starvation, bingeing, and purging.
	Correct misconceptions about bingeing-purging behaviors; for example, laxatives will *not* prevent absorption of calories. Teach patient to use problem-solving approach to examine issues, and to assess possible consequences.
	Encourage patient to implement and evaluate new behaviors.
	Assist patient to become aware of her needs and self-expectations and to differentiate these from others' expectations of her.
	Encourage patient's acceptance of and confidence in her thinking abilities.
	Teach patient how to get needs met by herself and others rather than meeting others' needs.
	Begin to explore functions and dysfunctions of starving, bingeing, and purging. Correct distortions and examine alternative ways of attaining satisfying experience. Encourage implementation of alternative satisfying experiences.
	Begin to identify patient's strengths and assist patient to enlarge on these.
	Help patient assess abilities and accomplishments realistically using problem-solving approach. Encourage acceptance of abilities and choices patient makes. Teach patient to evaluate decisions realistically and to trust her thoughts and feelings.
	Teach patient to develop realistic self-expectations including acceptance of limitations and mediocre performance.
	Teach patient to function comfortably in ambiguous situations.
Nutrition, alteration in: less than body requirements	After assessing patient's eating pattern, discuss food preferences.
	Have dietitian discuss nutritional plan and rationale, as well as body's nutritional needs. Teach importance of well-balanced diet that contains wide variety of foods. Encourage patient as able to assume responsibility for planning well-balanced meals.
	If patient has been on starvation diet, be alert for gastric dilation if refeeding is rapid. To prevent this, 1200- to 1500-calorie, well-balanced diet, sometimes divided into more than three feedings, may be prescribed initially.
	Teach patient to eat slowly to taste and enjoy food.
	To allow more supervision, have patient eat alone rather than in unit dining room. When patient develops control over eating, encourage eating in dining room with others.
	To prevent vomiting permit patient's use of bathroom only if accompanied by staff for 1 to 2 hours after eating.
	Explain nasogastric feedings and rationale in matter-of-fact yet sensitive, supportive manner. (Nasogastric feedings may be prescribed if patient does not gain or electrolyte balance is viewed as unsafe.) After each instillation of high-protein, high-caloric fluid (such as Isocal), observe patient for at least 30 minutes to prevent vomiting. As patient is willing, allow drinking of feeding instead of instilling in tube.

Nursing Diagnosis	Nursing Intervention
	Inform patient that abdominal discomfort or bloating will be experienced with increased food intake and that symptoms will disappear.
	Allay patient's fears of becoming obese by informing her that uncontrolled weight gain is not the goal. With assistance of dietitian, teach patient weight maintenance diet.
	Explain that, as caloric intake is increased, the amount will not make patient fat because metabolism is slowed as protective mechanism on starvation diet.
	Avoid getting into obsessional discussion of food and diet with patient. Avoid casual conversation about your eating preferences and habits.
	Avoid power struggles over food to prevent reenactment of food struggles at home.
	Encourage good oral hygiene to prevent oral disease.
	Begin to help patient identify role low weight plays in patient's life (for example, as way of avoiding dealing with frightening adolescent issues). Continue to explore meaning of weight loss, expectation and reality of weight loss, and restrictions in areas of life resulting from preoccupation with food.
	Monitor patient's weight as prescribed, possibly daily, but prevent patient from indiscriminate frequent self-weighing. Remain nonjudgmental about weight gains and losses. (Weight monitoring will continue with less frequency.)
Self-concept, disturbance in: body image	Encourage patient to wear loose clothing to avoid focus on body size and weight gain. Encourage patient to give "skinny" wardrobe away to avoid longing for thinness and relapsing. Suggest new life-style for patient in nonthreatening way.
	Begin to correct patient's distorted perceptions about body size. Assist patient to perceive body size correctly and accept appearance.
	Encourage patient to accept positive self-appraisals and take pride in appearance.
	As patient gains more mature-appearing body, assist in dealing with sexual identity issues including menses. Explore meanings of sexuality and feminine role. Encourage self-acceptance.
Fluid volume deficit, actual	Monitor fluid intake and output.
	Maintain adequate hydration.
	Monitor vital signs as prescribed and as deemed advisable.
	Administer replacement fluids and electrolytes such as potassium if indicated and as prescribed.
	Limit physical activity initially to decrease stress on body, such as stress on cardiac function when arrhythmias and muscle weakness are present.
Skin integrity, impairment of: potential	Teach patient that skin conditions such as bruises, loss of scalp hair, lanugo, and dry skin are related to malnutrition.
	Encourage good skin hygiene. Instruct patient to use body lotion for dry skin.
	Attend to skin lesions and bruises as indicated.
Powerlessness	Convey to patient that treatment plan is way of helping and protecting and not of control.
	Encourage patient to make decisions, when able, about treatment regimen to provide sense of control and to increase self-confidence.
	Help patient reinterpret eating-purging patterns as signs of being out of control rather than in control.
	Begin to teach patient how to become assertive with others and, as able, with parents. Emphasize that patient can assume responsibility for herself and that she is not responsible for others' happiness or discomfort.
	Practice assertiveness skills with awareness of possible outcomes of behaviors. Help patient identify her wants and make choice not to binge or starve.
	Teach patient how to deal with conflict, for example, by negotiating, assessing importance of issue, or clarifying issue with others.
Bowel elimination, alteration in: constipation	If patient is accustomed to laxative abuse, provide high-fiber diet to prevent constipation.
	Recommend adequate fluid intake.
	Teach methods for adequate elimination, such as diet, fluid intake, and proper exercise. (See also p. 2062.)

Nursing Diagnosis	Nursing Intervention
Sleep pattern disturbance	After assessing sleep pattern, explore methods that have been conducive to sleep in past. Reinforce healthy methods. If applicable, explain that malnourishment contributes to sleep disturbances. Teach relaxation routines that promote sleep, including warm bath, quiet activities such as reading and watching television, and breathing techniques.
Social isolation	As medical condition stabilizes, suggest that patient participate in activities with other patients. Encourage occupational therapy to develop skills such as crafts and sewing. Encourage development of enjoyable minor personal activities to replace focus on exceptional ones. Encourage recreational therapy such as group games and participation in graded exercise program. Assist patient to deal with free periods and to learn to enjoy relaxing times. Assist patient to identify and discuss discomfort in social interactions. Encourage patient to assess social interactions and to pursue satisfying ones. Assist patient to differentiate her responsibilities in interactions from others'. Emphasize personal satisfaction in social interactions and activities rather than perfectionism. Encourage patient to initiate contact with friends, as able, and to engage in activities patient enjoys with friends.
Family process, alteration in	Discourage family from discussing patient's dietary intake, bringing in food, and phoning during mealtimes. Assist parents to understand illness without blaming each other. In family sessions, begin to help family members alter their interactional patterns, for example, by speaking for self only and not for others and by responding to one another's messages. In family sessions help parents become aware of overprotectiveness and overinvolvement. Facilitate disengagement and foster relationships that encourage autonomy of family members.

Patient Education

1. Reinforce use of problem-solving technique to correct misconceptions of self and performance.
2. Teach planning of well-balanced weight maintenance diet.
3. Reinforce compliance with medical regimen.
4. Teach assertiveness skills.
5. Reinforce need for continued psychotherapy.

EVALUATION

Patient Outcome	Data Indicating That Outcome is Reached
Patient establishes normal eating habits and achieves increased sense of self-control.	Patient participates actively in making decisions about treatment plans. Patient makes decision not to binge or starve. Patient views weight maintenance diet as evidence of self-control. Patient states that preoccupation with food has diminished. Patient identifies and accepts relationship between preoccupation with eating and problems in other areas of life.
Patient achieves weight gain or weight stabilization near ideal body weight.	Patient perceives body size accurately and states acceptance of more mature-appearing body. Patient makes plans to engage in new life-style without continual concerns about losing weight.
Patient implements problem-solving approach to dealing with issues.	Patient practices problem-solving approach in dealing with issues such as feminine role, sexuality, and control. Patient develops more realistic expectations for self and performance.

Patient Outcome	Data Indicating That Outcome is Reached
Patient demonstrates ease in interpersonal relationships by assertive behaviors and ability to initiate interactions with others.	Patient practices assertiveness when interacting with family and friends. Patient verbalizes increased self-confidence during interactions with family. Patient initiates and engages in relaxing activities with friends and family. Patient verbalizes awareness and increased acceptance of own needs and wants.
Patient makes plans to continue treatment after discharge.	Patient states actions of medicine and plans to self-administer medicine as ordered. Patient schedules appointment to continue counseling after discharge.

SUBSTANCE USE DISORDERS

Substance use disorders are those in which maladaptive behaviors result from regular use of chemical substances that affect the central nervous system and adversely affect health.[1] Such substances include depressants, stimulants, hallucinogens, and analgesics. Some substances, such as alcohol, over-the-counter drugs, and medically prescribed drugs, are obtained legally; others such as cocaine and marijuana are obtained illicitly.

Substance use disorders are divided into two general groups: substance abuse and substance dependence. Substance abuse is the pathologic use of chemical substances that continues for at least 1 month and often impairs work or social functioning. Substance dependence is a more severe form of substance use disorder that involves physiologic dependence on a drug.[1] Dependence is evidenced by tolerance for the drug or withdrawal symptoms when the drug is discontinued.

Types of dependence on chemicals include the following[47]:

1. *Tolerance*. Drug dosage must be increased progressively to reproduce the original physical and psychologic effects.
2. *Physiologic dependence*. Physiologic changes that occur with repeated use result in withdrawal symptoms when the dose is reduced or discontinued abruptly.
3. *Psychologic dependence*. Feelings of pleasure and satisfaction are experienced with drug use. These produce intense cravings for repetitive use of the substance.

Substance abuse and dependence most commonly begin during adolescence and young adulthood. Persons between 18 and 25 years of age are the heaviest users of illegal chemicals.[9] The reasons for becoming involved in the use and abuse of chemical substances are many and include influence of peers, rebellion against parents and society, and attempts to bolster self-esteem. Most of these young adults are able to discontinue use as they take on responsibilities of adulthood, but some become chronic abusers.

Substance abuse and dependence or addiction may be also associated with relief of pain, especially among immature, easily frustrated persons, those with psychic disorders, and those with countercultural life-styles. Viewing substances as a way for coping with life stresses and experiences is one factor in continued abuse.[1,21]

Since chemical substances affect the central nervous system, abuse may cause transient or permanent brain dysfunction and other physical illnesses. Deterioration of physical health is due in part to inadequate diet, poor personal hygiene, and inattention to physical disorders. Infections such as hepatitis and septicemia can occur when substances are administered with contaminated needles. Since the potency and purity of illicitly obtained substances are often unknown, fatal overdoses and toxic reactions occur.[21,47]

The mood-altering effects of substances may cause erratic, impulsive, and irresponsible behavior. Relationships with family and friends become disturbed and are sometimes severed. The alcohol or drug habit may drain the financial resources of the person's family. The person may also engage in criminal behaviors to support the use of substances or violate laws when in an intoxicated alcohol or drug state (for example, causing an automobile accident).

Changes in occupational and scholastic functioning occur with substance abuse. The person loses interest in job or school activities, fails to strive to achieve, and is less able to perform tasks.[1,21]

Table 17-1 lists some commonly used types of chemical substances, their uses, and intoxication and withdrawal effects.[1,47,55]

Between 5% and 10% of the employed population in the United States suffer from alcoholism, and an estimated 3% to 7% use some type of illicit drug. The annual cost for health care, absences from work, and decreased productivity of workers related to alcohol and drugs is approximately $70 billion. Almost half of work fatalities and injuries are due to alcohol abuse.[62] At least half of automobile accidents involve alcohol use by the driver

Table 17-1
Effects of Intoxication and Withdrawal of Substances

Drug	Usual Route of Administration	Use
Opiates		
Opium	Oral; sniffed; smoked	Analgesic, antidiarrheal
Morphine	Oral; injected	Analgesic
Diacetylmorphine (heroin)	Injected; sniffed; smoked	Analgesic (illegal)
Hydromorphone (Dilaudid)	Oral; injected	Analgesic
Meperidine (Demerol)	Oral; injected	Analgesic
Propoxyphene (Darvon)	Oral; injected	Analgesic
Codeine	Oral; injected	Analgesic; antitussive
Methadone	Oral; injected	Detoxification of opiates
Depressants		
Alcoholic beverages (e.g., liquor, beer, wine)	Oral	Tension relief; analgesic
Sedative-hypnotics		
Barbiturates		
Amobarbital (Amytal)	Oral; injected	Anesthetic; anti-convulsant; sleep
Secobarbital (Seconal)	Oral; injected	
Pentobarbital (Nembutal)	Oral; injected	
Other		
Meprobamate (Equinal, Miltown)	Oral	Anti-anxiety; sedation
Diazepam (Valium)	Oral; injected	Anti-anxiety; anticonvulsant
Glutethimide (Doriden)	Oral	Hypnotic
Chloral hydrate (Noctec and others)	Oral	Hypnotic
Stimulants		
Cocaine	Oral; sniffed; injected	Local anesthetic
Amphetamine (Benzedrine, Dexedrine)	Oral; injected	Narcolepsy; attention deficit disorder; weight control
Methylphenidate (Ritalin)	Oral	Attention deficit disorder with hyperactivity
Phenmetrazine (Preludin)	Oral	Weight control
Hallucinogens		
Lysergic acid diethylamide (LSD)	Oral	None
Phencyclidine (PCP)	Oral; smoked; injected	Animal tranquilizer
Mescaline	Oral	None
Psilocybin	Oral	None
Cannabis sativa		
Marijuana, hashish	Oral, smoked	Stimulant and sedative (illegal drug)

or a pedestrian. Aside from the damage the alcohol does to the one who abuses substances, family stresses with marital and family dysfunction occur.

Alcoholism

Alcoholism is dependence on excessive amounts of alcohol, associated with a pattern of deviant behaviors.

This discussion focuses on alcohol because it appears to be abused more than other chemicals. Use of alcohol is accepted at social gatherings and business meetings and as part of cultural and religious celebrations such as marriages and births. About 70% of the adult population consumes at least one drink during a 1-year period, but about 1 in 10 will become a problem drinker.[55,57] Among the many reasons for dependence on alcoholic beverages are stress, family- and work-related problems, economic

Intoxication Effect	Withdrawal Effect
Euphoria with tranquility; emotional lability; drowsiness; clouding of consciousness; psychomotor retardation; slow, shallow respiration; constricted pupils; decreased muscle tone; with circulatory collapse and cyanosis, dilated pupils; coma; possible death	Runny nose; watery eyes; severe anxiety to panic; gooseflesh; hot and cold flashes; yawning; irritability; loss of appetite; muscle cramps; tremors; nausea and vomiting; tachycardia; hypertension; increased respirations and temperature; insomnia; after 24 hours diarrhea and dehydration; symptoms peak 48 to 72 hours after last dose
Slurred speech; lack of coordination; unsteady gait; talkativeness; euphoria or depression; emotional lability; impaired attention	Hyperactivity; tremors; psychomotor agitation; hypertension; tachycardia; irritability or depression; impaired attention and memory; illusions (misinterpretation of stimuli); hallucinations, auditory or visual; disorientation; delusions; delirium; orthostatic hypotension; convulsions
Slurred speech; irritability; impaired attention, memory, and judgment; emotional lability; talkativeness; lack of coordination; confusion; tremors; cold, clammy skin; dilated pupils (with barbiturates, constricted pupils)	Nausea and vomiting; weakness; hypertension; tachycardia; orthostatic hypotension; gross tremors; agitation; disorientation; anxiety; nightmares; visual hallucinations; hyperthermia; delirium; convulsions; coma
Psychomotor agitation; mood lability; hypervigilance; tachycardia; hypertension; dilated pupils; perspiration and chills; impaired judgment; psychotic symptoms; insomnia; tremors; confusion; convulsions; possible death	Fatigue; depression; disturbed sleep; apathy
Tachycardia; hypertension; hyperthermia; dilated pupils; hyperreflexia; nausea; visual hallucinations; extreme emotional lability; poor time perception; feeling of depersonalization; psychic numbness; psychosis; violent outbursts; amnesia; convulsions; possible death	None reported; flashbacks occur for 5 days after use of PCP, with catalepsy, agitation, and unpredictable violent outbursts
Panic; depression; disorientation; hallucinations; delusions; flashbacks; psychotic symptoms; apathy; impaired attention and judgment	Irritability; insomnia; loss of appetite; tremors; perspiration; nausea

difficulties, and feelings of social inadequacy. Genetic factors have been implicated in the development of alcoholism, but their significance is unclear.[1,55] It is uncertain whether personality traits such as dependence and self-doubt predispose a person to chronic alcoholism or are the result of alcoholism.[55]

A careful assessment of the drinking patterns and use of other chemicals by all patients, including those being treated for other conditions, is essential. Attention must be given to abuse of multiple drugs, since a person found to be dependent on one substance is probably also dependent on others that potentiate or inhibit the effects of the first. Although denying use or minimizing the amount consumed is common, a nonjudgmental attitude will help the nurse elicit the necessary information.[45]

A person who drinks moderately experiences minor symptoms during the 24 hours after the last drink. These include irritability, anxiety, slight increase in heart rate and blood pressure, gastric irritation, and restless sleep.[47,55,77] A person who consistently consumes large amounts of alcohol over a long period is likely to develop a more severe withdrawal syndrome characterized by agitation, tachycardia, hypertension, tremors, anorexia, abdominal cramps, insomnia, sweating, and blushing. Memory lapses (blackouts) concerning events that occurred while the person was drinking may occur. A minority of persons have seizures, typically grand mal, within 48 hours after the last drink.[55] Delirium tremens may occur 72 to 96 hours after the person's last drink. Symptoms of delirium tremens include confusion, disorientation, delirium, frightening hallucinations that are usually visual, illusions in which stimuli are misinterpreted, nightmares, diaphoresis, and elevated temperature. The mortality for persons with delirium tremens is approximately 10%; death is often due to hyperthermia or cardiovascular collapse.[55] If adequate preventive treatment is instituted during the early signs and symptoms of alcohol withdrawal, delirium tremens will not develop.

Some physiologic problems of chronic alcoholism are the following[12,19,47]:

Cardiovascular system
    Anemia
    Hypertension
    Tachycardia
    Arrhythmias
    Cardiomegaly
    Edema
Liver
    Hepatomegaly
    Edema
    Ascites
    Cirrhosis
Gastrointestinal system
    Gastritis
    Esophagitis
    Duodenal and gastric ulcers
    Nausea
    Malabsorption syndrome
    Pancreatitis
    Colitis
Neurologic system
    Fatigue
    Depression
    Irritability
    Memory and learning deficits
    Tremors
    Polyneuropathy that typically occurs in feet first
    Wernicke-Korsakoff syndrome

Alcoholic Family

Family members may initially accept drinking alcoholic beverages and occasional drunkenness as normal social behavior. However, as the frequency of use increases, the problem drinking begins to have detrimental effects on the drinker and family members. The drinker's personality changes with severe mood swings, he may be arrested for driving while intoxicated, and his employment behavior changes, with frequent absences and tardiness.[12,28,55] Family relationships deteriorate, and family members feel trapped between the sober and intoxicated phases of the alcoholic. They experience shame, anger, confusion, and guilt. Family conversations are increasingly focused on the alcohol-dependent behavior and issues related to it. Family members unconsciously engage in enabling behaviors to protect the family reputation and keep the family secret. Such behaviors include making excuses to friends and employers, attempting to keep the alcoholic out of trouble, and sometimes buying liquor for the alcoholic. The person with a drinking problem offers alibis for his behavior or is unwilling to discuss it. If the spouse threatens to leave or no longer make excuses, the alcohol-dependent person may promise never to touch another drop. These promises are usually broken. The family may feel locked into dysfunctional behaviors or may sever their relationship with the drinker.

Alcoholism among Professionals

Health professionals have recently become aware of the severity of problems of substance abuse among their colleagues. State nurses' associations have established peer assistance programs to guide nurses into treatment and provide support during the recovery phase. These programs often depend on volunteer nurses to assist their colleagues into rehabilitation programs.[36]

DIAGNOSTIC STUDIES

Serum: SMAC
    To screen for systemic abnormalities (see above for possible pathologic conditions)

Urinalysis
    To screen for urinary and systemic abnormalities

Electrocardiogram
    To screen for cardiopathy

Chest roentgenogram
    To screen for pulmonary infection and cardiac disease

TREATMENT PLAN

Chemotherapeutic
Antianxiety agents

Diazepam (Valium), 10 mg IM stat and q4h if necessary for severe withdrawal symptoms during first 24 h, thereafter 10 mg po qid; for elderly or adolescent, 5 mg IM stat and q4h if necessary for severe withdrawal symptoms during first 24 h, thereafter 2 mg po qid; acts to reduce anxiety and seizures and promotes drowsiness and hypotension

Vitamins

Added Protection III, multivitamin and multimineral supplement, 2 tabs po tid with meals

Supportive
Bland diet; introduction of regular diet as able to tolerate

ASSESSMENT: AREAS OF CONCERN

Emotional
Anxiety; emotional lability; depression

Thoughts
Denial of alcoholism; guilt; shame; sense of inadequacy; impairment of judgment and memory; suicide ideation (correlation exists between alcoholism and suicide)

Physical
Type of drinking pattern established; duration and amount of last alcohol consumed; irritability to psychomotor agitation; demanding behavior; memory lapses (blackouts); tachycardia; hypertension; increased respirations; tremors; fatigue; nausea and vomiting; anorexia; abdominal cramps; insomnia; elevated temperature; illusions; hallucinations (most frequently visual, sometimes auditory); seizure potential

Social and occupational
Argumentativeness with family, friends, and co-workers; aggressiveness with others; tardiness at work; work absences because of "not feeling well"; sensitivity to criticism; mistakes at work

NURSING DIAGNOSES and NURSING INTERVENTIONS

Nursing Diagnosis	Nursing Intervention
Potential patient problem: alcohol withdrawal	Provide quiet environment, since excess stimuli may increase agitation or tremors. In collaboration with physician, administer diazepam if needed for agitation and tremors. Because of patient's tolerance to sedative effects of alcohol, larger doses are needed than for nonalcoholic. Briefly explain effects of medicine. Provide physical protection in bed as needed such as side rails. If suicidal ideation exists, assess seriousness. See also discussion of suicide for nursing interventions. Maintain light in room, especially at night, to decrease possibility of misinterpreting environmental stimuli.
Fluid volume, alteration in: excess	Monitor and record intake and output. Avoid forcing fluids to prevent overhydration, since alcohol initially exerts antidiuretic effect. Monitor blood pressure, pulse, and respirations hourly until stable and then as ordered. Monitor temperature every 4 hours. Observe for infection such as respiratory, since resistance is low.
Mobility, impaired physical	Maintain bed rest until patient regains stability and vital signs are normal. Assist patient to ambulate as needed and when permitted.
Self-care deficit: self-bathing and hygiene	Assist with bathing and personal hygiene as needed until patient is able to care for self. Observe for infections, bruises, and broken skin when providing care and treat as per order.
Nutrition, alteration in: less than body requirements	Help to ensure adequate nutritional diet in collaboration with physician and dietitian. Offer bland foods for gastric distress. Teach patient essentials of nutritionally balanced diet and importance of compliance.

Nursing Diagnosis	Nursing Intervention
Coping, ineffective individual	Establish supportive, nonjudgmental relationship. Assist patient to identify feelings of anxiety and relate them to stress-producing situations. Help patient identify methods for coping with anxiety instead of relying on alcohol. Such methods include problem solving, relaxation techniques such as slow, deep breathing, and diversionary activities such as physical exercise. Assist patient to identify needs and learn how to have them met. Teach assertiveness skills and evaluation of effects of skills. Encourage patient to learn to ask for support and to deal with positive and negative responses. Help patient learn to socialize without use of alcohol and develop skills in refusing alcohol in social situations. Refer patient to Alcoholics Anonymous for support of nondrinking behavior and prevention of relapse. Correct patient's misconceptions about physiologic, psychologic, and social effects of alcohol. Assist patient to identify evidence of own drinking patterns if patient denies problem. Encourage patient to examine consequences of drinking behavior on self, family, and social and work functioning and to identify alternative behaviors.
Family process, alteration in	Assist patient and family members to identify expectations of one another within the family and willingness to meet these expectations. Assist each to hear and respond to the others and to compromise on or negotiate differences. Refer family for counseling if indicated. Suggest attendance at Al-Anon for spouse and Alateen for children for support and information to deal with patient's alcoholism.

Patient Education

1. Reinforce healthy coping behaviors for dealing with anxiety.
2. Teach use of self-support and support from others.
3. Reinforce importance of nutritionally balanced diet.
4. Teach patient to accept responsibility for own behavior and sobriety.

EVALUATION

Patient Outcome	Data Indicating That Outcome is Reached
Recovery from withdrawal symptoms of alcohol is uncomplicated.	Vital signs are stable. Patient performs self-care activities. Patient responds appropriately to people and other stimuli. Patient eats regular, well-balanced meals.
Patient demonstrates knowledge of adverse effects of alcohol.	Patient states physiologic effects of prolonged alcoholism. Patient discusses psychologic effects of alcohol. Patient discusses social effects of alcohol on self and others.
Patient is aware of alternative behaviors for coping with stress-producing situations.	Patient practices relaxation techniques and engages in physical exercise. Patient practices assertiveness skills and evaluates effects on self and others. Patient practices refusal of alcoholic beverages in social situations.
Patient demonstrates ability to obtain support from family and others.	Patient verbalizes awareness of needs and is able to ask for support. Patient listens and responds to family members. Patient contacts Alcoholics Anonymous and begins to attend meetings.

SCHIZOPHRENIC DISORDERS

A diagnosis of schizophrenia is made if the person at some phase of the illness has experienced delusions, hallucinations, or certain thought disturbances with continual signs of the illness for at least 6 months. The following types of schizophrenia are identified in DSM-III[1]:

1. *Disorganized.* Marked incoherence and flat, inappropriate, or silly affect are present. Delusions and hallucinations occur but are not systematized. The person engages in peculiar behaviors such as grimacing and mannerisms. Childlike behavior may also be evident. This type has an early and insidious onset and generally becomes chronic.

2. *Catatonic.* The main feature of this type is stupor in which the person appears almost nonresponsive to the environment and shows little movement or activity. Mutism is common. Negativism is apparent as an inability to respond to instructions. Excitement, the opposite of stupor, is sudden, extreme, apparently purposeless, motor activity. In catatonic posturing the person assumes inappropriate and bizarre postures that at times appear uncomfortable. At present this type is rarely seen in the United States.

3. *Paranoid.* The prominent dysfunctions of the paranoid type are persecutory or grandiose delusions or hallucinations. Additional dysfunctions are anxiety, anger, and argumentativeness.

4. *Undifferentiated.* Psychotic symptoms that are not characteristic of any type of schizophrenia or that meet the criteria of more than one type are assigned to this diagnostic category.

5. *Residual.* This category is used when the person has had at least one schizophrenic episode in the past but has no apparent psychotic symptoms. Signs of the condition are apparent in such behaviors as flat affect, social withdrawal, and eccentricity.

Symptoms frequently change while a schizophrenic person is in long-term therapy, and as symptoms change, the diagnostic type also changes. The symptoms the person develops are the best solution he is capable of in restoring equilibrium. The presentation of schizophrenia is not specific to a diagnostic type but deals with the dysfunctional behaviors that are common to persons with schizophrenia.

Schizophrenia

Schizophrenia is a disorder in which a person exhibits psychotic symptoms including disturbances in perception, thought, affect, and psychomotor behaviors during an acute phase. The person's social and psychologic abilities are impaired.[1,2]

Schizophrenia is characterized by the following:

Thoughts

Associations—irrational, illogical, and bizarre

Delusions—false beliefs that are usually negative, persecutory, and injurious; may be grandiose

Ideas of reference—belief that events or conversations are related to individual or have special significance to him, for example, that others are making negative comments about him

Thought broadcasting—belief that others can hear person's thoughts

Loosening of associations—irrational, illogical, and bizarre thoughts, for example, shifts from one to another unrelated or obliquely related idea

Incoherence—incomprehensibility, inability to think or express thoughts in a clear, orderly manner

Poverty of content—paucity of ideas and thoughts; vague, repetitive, overly concrete ideas

Information processing and attention—limited ability to process incoming information with slow reaction time; impaired ability to select relevant from irrelevant aspects of communication

Projection—disowning of perceived or actual attributes of self while attributing them to someone or something in the environment

Perception

Hallucinations—false sensory perceptions with no external stimulus; auditory is most frequent form of perceptual disturbance; voices may be negative, insulting, or commands; especially in chronicity, voices may be friendly and helpful; visual hallucinations occur occasionally in acute phase and involve seeing nonexistent things such as insects or people; smell (olfactory), taste (gustatory), and touch (tactile) are less common

Illusions—misidentification or distortion of stimulus

Affect

Blunting—reduction of affective, emotional expression

Flatness—impoverishment of emotional reactivity; emotionally dull, cold, colorless; monotonous voice

Apathy—apparent absence of emotions

Inappropriateness—incongruence between emotions and content or ideas, for example, laughing in response to news of death of significant other

Activity level

Psychomotor activity—decreased reaction to environment; stereotypic, purposeless movement such as rocking or pacing

Spontaneity and activity—markedly decreased activity to withdrawal; repetitive, stereotypic activity; apathy; immobility

Posture—rigid, inappropriate, manneristic

Other

Self-identity—impairment or loss of ego boundaries; impairment of self-identity

Volition—impaired ability to will self to act; disturbance in goal-directed activities

Role behaviors—impairment in work and social roles; lack of social skills

Personal appearance—neglect

The onset of schizophrenia may be slow and insidious or sudden. In some persons the onset is preceded by a significant external event such as loss of a friend, marriage, or leaving home; in others the onset is not related to an identifiable external event. External events, if identified, are insufficient to evoke a psychosis if the internal processes such as relatedness to self and environment are not impaired.

Psychotic symptoms are present during the active phase. The person loses contact with reality.[2] Behaviors are unpredictable, in part because the person responds to internal processes such as hallucinations and delusions. He may hear voices that order him to protect himself from the evil and harmful world. Projection, the externalization of rejected, undesirable thoughts, feelings, and behaviors onto others, is a common defense mechanism. The secondary processes of mental integration that is based on logic and the reality principle deteriorate and give way to the primary processes of illogical, disorganized mental activity of the unconscious system that is normal during infancy.

Although a few persons recover completely, a majority have residual effects of the schizophrenic process with acute relapses. Vulnerability to stressors remains and may trigger relapses.[2,48] The person lacks the psychologic and social resources to cope with the stress of overstimulation from the environment. However, too little stimulation may result in withdrawal, underactivity, and impaired motivation. The person is unable to initiate interactions with others and to establish relationships that are neither too intrusive nor too distant. Social skills are lacking, and development of social networks is limited.[8]

Prevalence

In Europe and Asia the prevalence of schizophrenia ranges from 0.2% to 1%. Since criteria used by researchers in the United States generally have been broader than those used in Europe and Asia, the prevalence appears higher in the United States. When narrower diagnostic criteria were used to estimate the rate among psychiatric populations, the U.S. rate was 6%; when researchers used broader criteria, the rate was around 30%.[1,35]

Population at Risk

The onset of schizophrenia is usually during adolescence and young adulthood. The disease is almost equally distributed between males and females. A relationship appears to exist between social class and schizophrenia; the prevalence is greatest in low-status socioeconomic groups and in poor neighborhoods of large cities. Whether schizophrenia-prone persons are products of these environments or drift toward inner cities when they lose economical and social status is unknown. Some socioeconomic groups are more tolerant than others of persons who are different from themselves or who engage in eccentric behaviors.[68]

Responses of Nurses to Schizophrenics

Schizophrenia is a chronic disorder in which the person appears cold, distant, and apathetic. Response to therapy is extremely slow, and obvious signs of success are few. The schizophrenic is emotionally unnourished and is unnourishing to the nurse and others around him. Nurses often find it easier to withdraw from the withdrawn schizophrenic than to experience a sense of helplessness, hopelessness, and inadequacy in dealing with the patient. The nurse needs to establish small goals with the patient such as having the patient speak to her, share an activity, or ask to have a need or want met. If unrealistic goals are established, the nurse is bound to experience frustration and hopelessness. If the goal is attainable, specific, and immediate, the nurse's frustration is reduced.

Maintaining the nurse's own good health is part of good care to the patient. The nurse must keep in mind that the problems are the patient's and that change is very slow. By maintaining her own physical and psychologic comfort, the nurse has energy to devote to the patient. One way of increasing energy is to focus on one's own breathing while taking several slow, deep breaths. A "time-out" between patients renews the nurse's energy. Support from colleagues is essential to have her needs met and to receive recognition for what she has attempted to do or succeeded in doing with a patient. Outside of work the nurse should develop hobbies and engage in social activities that are unrelated to work.

PSYCHOPATHOLOGY

The discussion of the psychopathology of schizophrenia will be preceded by a brief presentation of constitutional and biochemical theories.[68]

Inheritance of a defective gene or genes is thought to be a factor, as evidenced by the greater risk for schizophrenia among children whose parents, siblings, or other relatives have the disease. Another hypothesis is that the person's temperament is related to genetically based neurophysiologic differences. A hypersensitive infant who is very difficult to satisfy is at greater risk for schizophrenia than an easy-going, adaptable infant.

A promising biochemical theory is that an overabundance of dopamine, a neurotransmitter, is present in the brain of a schizophrenic.[68] Dopamine has a disinhibiting effect that causes the person to become conscious of countless associations and therefore results in fragmentation of these associations. It is known that antipsychotic medicines block dopaminergic activity, although the exact pathways of change are unknown. These drugs may act by blocking the dopamine receptors, lowering the store of dopamine, or inhibiting the synthesis of dopamine. Whether the biologic aberrations leading to schizophrenia are primary or secondary is unknown. The changes could be mediated by physiologic or psychologic factors.[68]

Psychoanalytic Theory

The functions of the ego include the ability to differentiate the self from objects in the environment, reality testing, organization of affect, and development of cognitive processes such as perception, thinking, remembering, and learning. The organizing processes operate in integrating the id, ego, and superego and in differentiating the self from objects outside the self.

Since the functions of the ego develop in stages, traumatic experiences do not affect all functions adversely. Those functions affected negatively are subject to regression to an earlier phase of development and reflected in symptoms. Since the secondary processes of cognition that are reflected in abstract, logical thinking develop later in the person's development, these are among the first to be lost. The person regresses to the early primary processes of infancy, including memory traces, lack of differentiation between subjective imagery and reality, and illogical connections between experiences.[59]

The ego, as mediator of the id's instinctual drives, libido and aggression (death instinct), neutralizes the aggressive energy and puts the energy into the service of itself. The ego uses the energy to maintain the various ego functions. If aggression is unneutralized, disorganization occurs when the person entertains angry thoughts or acts on them. When aggression is deneutralized, the person has a low tolerance for his own aggressive feelings and a tendency toward acting out violently.[59] The aggressive energy regresses to an instinctual drive, is no longer available to maintain some of the ego functions, especially the cognitive processes, and conse-

quently plays a role in the initiation of schizophrenic symptoms.

Interpersonal Theory

Interpersonal theory stresses that the personality develops through relationships with others. Sullivan[72] assumed that the mother of the future schizophrenic is more intensely anxious than the average mother. Because she transmits anxiety to the infant, severe anxiety, experienced as dread and terror, is evoked in the infant. To avoid overwhelming panic and with few resources, the infant attempts to get rid of the discomfort by dissociating from it as a "not-me" experience. The infant with excessive "not-me" experiences is vulnerable to future excessive anxiety.[72] Although dissociation serves to protect the person from extremely uncomfortable experiences, it also prevents him from recalling, examining, and correcting perceptions of these experiences and limits his capacity to deal with future ones. To avoid the sense of terror, the person urgently gets rid of situations that may evoke anxiety without determining if the event is frightening and what aspect of it is. No learning can take place when the person is busy defending against anxiety.

Regression occurs when the feelings of self are compromised and weakened. The self-system is actively warding off or decreasing anxiety, and the dissociated experiences are no longer available for learning. Since complex cognitive processes of thinking, learning, and remembering are compromised, the person reverts to earlier modes of experiencing such as the momentary reverie of infancy or the distorted thinking of the young child in which illogical connections are made between experiences. The severity of the schizophrenic processes is related to the strength of the self-system and the degree of regression to more primitive functioning of the infant or young child.[2,72]

Cognitive Theory

Although all human beings are biologically predisposed to think illogically at times, to be self-destructive, and to experience inappropriate feelings, a seriously ill person may have a greater predisposition to disordered thinking. The person underestimates his abilities and emphasizes problems. Because past traumatic events are exaggerated, the person overreacts to even minor problems.[4] Even when new information makes possible a different perspective, the person resists and continues to think about the self and others illogically.

Thinking and emotional disturbances are also related to social learning. The child is taught to please his parents even when the directive appears illogical and begins to accept directives without thinking. When told often enough that he is worthless to himself and to others, he accepts the idea. Self-defeating beliefs are rigidly held and become strongly habituated patterns of thinking, feeling, and acting.[4,25]

TREATMENT PLAN

Chemotherapeutic
Psychotherapeutic agents
Haloperidol (Haldol)
For severely disturbed patient: 5 mg bid by tablet or concentrate
For acute agitation: 2 mg IM prn
For elderly disturbed patient: 2 mg bid by tablet or concentrate
Major initial side effect is orthostatic hypotension

Supportive
Occupational therapy
Recreational therapy

ASSESSMENT: AREAS OF CONCERN

Thoughts
Disturbance in orientation to person, place, and time; retarded thought processes; impaired ability to process incoming information; blocking of thoughts; autistic thinking, that is, inability to distinguish between reality and fantasy; suspiciousness; distorted, illogical thinking; false beliefs, such as of being persecuted or poisoned; projection, that is, disowning aspects of self while ascribing them to something or someone in environment; poor judgment; fear of rejection and of interpersonal and physical closeness; lack of trust; vulnerability to stress

Perception
Appearance of listening to voices observed as movement in vocal cords and lips and head and facial movement

Affect
Anxiety; loneliness; depression; apathy; colorless speech and monotonous voice; incongruity between emotional responses and idea

Activity
Withdrawal from relationships and contact with others; impairment in goal-directed activity; purposeless movement such as pacing and mannerisms; unpredictable behavior that may be related to delusions or hallucinations; impairment or absence of social skills; poor work history

Self-care
Neglectfulness; lack of motivation; impairment in bathing, grooming, and hygiene

Nutrition
Unawareness of hunger or thirst; apathy to food at mealtime; fear of eating, for example, belief that food is poisoned

Sleep
Disturbed sleep patterns; reluctance to go to bed at night or inability to awaken in morning

NURSING DIAGNOSES and NURSING INTERVENTIONS

Nursing Diagnosis	Nursing Intervention
Social isolation	Begin to establish a trusting relationship. Convey trust in patient and in his capacity to improve. Orient patient, as needed, to person, place, and time, for example, "My name is Jean. I am a nurse. You are in City Hospital." Be aware of patient's fears and sense of terror of physical and interpersonal closeness. Maintain appropriate physical distance when with patient and avoid sense of personal rejection by patient. Visit patient frequently for brief time periods. Speak slowly to patient, using brief statements. Emphasize your presence, for example, by saying "I will stay with you for 10 minutes," "I came to see you," or "I want to help you." Tell patient when you are leaving and let him know when you will return. Avoid asking a nonverbal patient questions to push him to talk, since this may result in further withdrawal. Comment on neutral subjects such as patient's immediate environment, for example, color of the room or activities of others in the room. Look at pictures in a magazine with patient and comment on them without asking patient to respond. As patient begins to gain a sense of security, he

Nursing Diagnosis	**Nursing Intervention**

will begin to comment on magazines or tell you you are talking too much. Accept comments or criticism as sign of improvement.

Pace with patient, as appropriate, maintaining adequate distance between patient and yourself.

As you and patient are able to tolerate longer time periods together, increase time gradually.

Observe patient when alone for hallucinatory experiences. Distract patient by sitting with him and commenting at intervals on immediate environment or by engaging patient in activity.

If patient becomes increasingly agitated and distracting techniques do not decrease behavior, medication may be administered as needed in collaboration with physician. Briefly explain reason for medication and major effects and side effects.

Be alert to your sense of helplessness and anxiety with patient and obtain help from social network.

As patient improves, encourage interaction with at least one other patient by sharing activity such as watching television or playing cards or other games.

Assist patient to examine experiences of interactions with others.

Teach social skills, such as how to interact, initiate a conversation, or make requests, since these skills are often impaired or lacking.

Assist patient to deal with rejections or refusals from others. Teach patient that others have responsibilities in interactions and that patient is responsible only for his own behavior.

Encourage patient to identify and accept skills. Assist patient to elaborate on and build on strengths.

Assist patient to attend and participate in occupational therapy as prescribed.

Assist patient to identify and begin using support from significant others.

Teach assertiveness skills and encourage practice. Examine attempts to be assertive and assist patient to become aware of successes, even if attempts were awkward.

As patient is able to tolerate interactions with others, encourage recreational therapy for enjoyment, exercise, and development of skills.

Thought processes, alteration in

Listen attentively and patiently to patient's seemingly incomprehensible speech to increase his willingness to relate to another human being. Do not pretend understanding. Let patient know you are listening and trying to understand.

Listen for themes, feeling tones, or reality-oriented phrases or thoughts. Comment on understandable conversation, for example, "I sense loneliness in what you're saying."

Assist patient, as able, to elaborate on reality-oriented ideas.

Assist patient to correct misconceptions about his environment, self, and experiences through recall of event and use of problem solving.

Avoid reinforcing ideas of reference and delusions by having patient repeat false beliefs, arguing with patient, or agreeing with him. "I find that hard to believe" may be appropriate comment.

Assist patient to examine what he was experiencing before delusional thoughts began or to reexperience delusions. Attempt to identify patient's thoughts and feelings toward himself and determine if patient was feeling threatened. Gradually assist patient to recognize delusional content of thoughts and feelings.

When patient shows signs of anxiety or expresses discomfort, change topic to less anxiety-provoking one. If patient is able to discuss anxiety-provoking topic, help him identify his feelings (awareness of feelings will evolve slowly).

Administer medication as ordered. If you suspect patient is not swallowing tablets, concentrates may be administered in collaboration with physician.

Briefly explain reason for medication, as well as its effects and side effects. Inform patient of possible sleepiness and dizziness, especially when standing up. Caution patient to stand up slowly.

Observe patient closely for effects and side effects of medication and report to physician for dose adjustments as needed. Check vital signs four times a day initially.

As patient is able to comprehend, teach effects and side effects of medication, reasons for medication, and continued compliance with medical regimen.

Nursing Diagnosis	Nursing Intervention
Sensory-perceptual alteration: auditory	When patient is observed moving lips and vocal cords or cocking head as if listening, ask patient, "Do you hear voices?" or "Who is talking to you?" Use distractive techniques such as involving patient in conversation or activity if patient is unable to examine reality of voices. If "voices" are chronic, teach patient to hum or whistle to prevent him from using vocal cords for "voices." Gradually assist patient to examine thoughts and feelings just before hallucinations. Help patient recognize eventually that he expects to hear voices. Accept patient's protests and denials as his understandings now. As patient is able to accept connection between thoughts or feelings and expectation of voices, he will begin to be aware that he has ability to control his experiences and correct thoughts and feelings about himself. Continue examination of hallucinatory experience.
Nutrition, alteration in: less than body requirements	When patient is suspicious of food, emphasize that food is nutritious and has not been tampered with. Have patient participate in choosing foods and liquids. When patient is preoccupied or hallucinating, obtain his attention and suggest eating. If necessary, direct patient to take each mouthful, for example, "Take a spoonful. Now eat it." Offer fluids between meals to maintain hydration. Teach ingredients and importance of good nutrition when patient is able to process information.
Self-care deficit: bathing, hygiene, dressing, grooming	Assist patient with bathing, grooming, and personal hygiene as needed. Wash patient if he is unable to bathe himself or to follow directions such as "Wash your left arm." Offer each article of clothing to put on, and direct patient to complete grooming and hygiene care. Assist patient as needed. Encourage patient to initiate self-care activities as able. Acknowledge patient's self-care activities and encourage patient to identify and eventually accept appearance and positive characteristics.
Sleep pattern disturbance	If patient has fears of going to sleep, assist him to talk about fear and to begin to correct misconceptions. Offer warm milk to assist sleeping. Encourage slow, deep breathing while focusing on number "1." If helpful, turn radio at low volume to soothing music to decrease panic or fears. Discourage naps during day to enhance restful sleep at night.

Patient Education

1. Teach beginning skills in use of problem-solving technique.
2. Reinforce patient's strengths.
3. Teach social skills.
4. Discuss use of social supports and resources in community, such as continuing care program in community or mental health centers.
5. Teach compliance with medication therapy and encourage continuation of counseling.

EVALUATION

Patient Outcome	Data Indicating That Outcome is Reached
Patient no longer has psychotic symptoms.	Patient is oriented to person, place, and time. Patient states that he no longer hears "voices." Patient uses problem-solving method to correct misconceptions. Patient performs self-care.
Patient participates in social activities with staff and other patients.	Patient initiates activities with others. Patient spends less time alone in unit. Patient says that he enjoys participating in some of the planned activities.

Patient Outcome	Data Indicating That Outcome is Reached
Patient complies with medication regimen.	Patient describes effects and side effects of medication and refers to handout on drug information as needed. Patient has developed system to keep track of self-administration of medication. Patient states action he will take when adverse effects of medication are experienced.
Patient plans to continue counseling after discharge.	Patient has made appointment with health professional for counseling after discharge. Patient has visited day care center and plans to attend regularly after discharge.

PARANOID DISORDERS

Paranoid disorders are a general classification of conditions in which the person experiences delusions of persecution and jealousy. Such delusions persist for at least 1 week. The symptoms lack the bizarreness, incoherence, and loose associations of schizophrenia. Excluded from this category are persons who are acutely depressed or manic or have organic disease.

DSM-III[1] presents four types of paranoid disorder:
1. *Paranoia.* The criteria include those described above and a chronic, stable persecutory delusional system for at least 6 months.
2. *Shared paranoid disorder.* The criteria include those described above and a persecutory delusional system that develops as a result of a close relationship with another person with whom the patient shares at least some delusions.
3. *Acute paranoid disorder.* The criteria are those described above that have been present for less than 6 months.
4. *Atypical paranoid disorder.* This is a paranoid disorder that does not fit into the preceding three diagnoses.

Paranoid Disorder

A person with a paranoid disorder exhibits delusions of persecution, suspiciousness of others, intolerance of ambiguity, superior and aloof attitude, and anger that may lead to violence. Beneath this exterior is an insecure, vulnerable, and inferior-feeling person.[53]

Symptoms of paranoid disorder are as follows:

Thoughts
  Delusions of persecution—false belief that others are conspiring to harass or destroy individual
  Delusions of jealousy—false belief concerning the loss of valued possession or loved one
  Delusions of grandiosity—false belief of having power, wealth, and prestige
  Ideas of reference—events or conversations incorrectly interpreted as related to self
  Projection—disowning perceived or actual self-attributes and attributing them to someone else
  Prejudice—incorrect and inflexible generalization directed at an individual or group and influenced by emotions
  Sense of superiority
  Self-righteous resentment of others
  Suspiciousness, secretiveness
  Intolerance of uncertainty and ambiguity
  Vindictiveness
  Facade of self-sufficiency and competence
  Fear of loss of control
  Sense of vulnerability
  Sense of inadequacy
Feelings
  Anxiety
  Anger
  Hostility
  Depression
Behavior
  Social isolation
  Seclusiveness
  Eccentricity
  Litigiousness—initiates legal actions for perceived injustices
  Distance, coldness, aloofness

The person may appear normal on the surface until the paranoid theme is identified. Judgment may be impaired only in relation to the single theme or intricately connected themes involved in the delusional system. The prominent ideas are persecution or expansive grandiosity or both. The paranoid person has a self-righteous attitude and avoids feelings of insecurity and inadequacy by affirming confidently that his ideas are correct.[53] If the person perceives an injury to his self-esteem, he may attempt to retaliate. When seeking revenge, the person experiences no guilt, remorse, or responsibility for the consequences of his behavior. The verbal or physical behaviors arise from the need to defend the self from imaginary or actual threats of humiliation and injustices to the self-esteem.

Prevalence

The occurrence of paranoid disorders is rare, although delusions of jealousy in paranoia may be more common.[1]

Population at Risk

Paranoid disorders generally develop in middle or late adult life; the true paranoias have a poor prognosis.[1] Paranoid persons are seldom hospitalized unless severe disorganization occurs. They generally live within the bounds of society, although they may appear eccentric in their attempts to redress the injustices and wrongs in society.

PSYCHOPATHOLOGY

Psychoanalytic Theory

The paranoid process is influenced by genetic factors and developmental patterning of the personality.[54] The person cannot tolerate hostile, aggressive, and omnipotent impulses that are unintegrated in the ego structure. To stabilize a sense of self, the person externalizes the aggressive, hostile impulses and attributes them to others or forces outside the self. The person becomes the victim of projected aggression in the form of hostile persecutors. The omnipotent components, which arise from the narcissism that reaches its peak between 12 and 18 months of age, are expressed as a sense of superiority, privilege, and even perfection. The projections are organized into a set of coherent and sustaining beliefs so that the delusional system exists along with the person's clear and orderly thinking.[53,54]

Interpersonal Theory

Deviations in development that begin in childhood may have dysfunctional effects in later life. The parent punishes the child either because the child deserves it or because the child does not measure up to the parent's demands.[56] The child often makes complex discriminations of the situation and may decide to deceive the authority figure by concealing his anger, since he has learned that anger aggravates the situation. Instead he develops the covert response of resentment. Because even the resentment must be concealed to avoid punishment and receive love and tenderness, the feeling is excluded from awareness.[71]

The exclusion of anger and other negative attitudes from awareness lays the groundwork for malevolent attitudes toward life and other people, who are viewed as enemies. The behavior inhibits the development of close, reciprocal, interpersonal relationships in which the person can consensually validate and correct feelings and thoughts. The person learns to protect his self-esteem by noting how unworthy everyone else is. By projecting the defects and weaknesses he perceives in himself onto other people, the person can renounce the actual or imaginary negative aspects of his own personality. The paranoid transformation of the personality occurs through this transfer of blame to others.[56]

Cognitive Theory

The cognitive theorists postulate that the person's conceptualization or definition of an event, rather than the event itself, determines the emotional response.[4] Cognitive appraisals precede emotional responses; therefore incorrect conceptions derived from faulty learning are the basis for emotional upsets and problems. The person concerned with rules, standards, and rights is likely to respond angrily to violations of his rights and unjust criticisms. The person's self-esteem is maintained because he views himself as right and others as wrong. He attributes malevolent motives to the perceived attacks or intrusions on his boundaries. This thinking escalates as the paranoid person views his rules as unconditional and absolute and believes that others are deliberately opposing or sabotaging him.[4]

TREATMENT PLAN

Chemotherapeutic
Psychotherapeutic agents
Haloperidol (Haldol), 2 mg po tid; for elderly patients, 1 mg po tid; side effects are drowsiness and hypotension

ASSESSMENT: AREAS OF CONCERN

Feelings
Anxiety; anger; depression

Thoughts
Delusions of persecution; projection; intolerance of uncertainty and ambiguity; suspiciousness; facade of self-confidence; sense of vulnerability; sense of inadequacy; inappropriate expression of anger

Behavior
Aloofness; seclusiveness; isolation from others

NURSING DIAGNOSES and NURSING INTERVENTIONS

Nursing Diagnosis	Nursing Intervention
Coping, ineffective individual	Begin to establish a nonthreatening relationship with patient.
	Be scrupulously truthful with patient.
	Allow patient to ventilate feelings of anger.
	If emotional state escalates, assist patient to engage in diversionary activities, such as table tennis or walking, or change subject.
	Convey acceptance of patient's right to experience anger.
	Avoid criticizing patient. Suggest alternatives without negating a behavior.
	Administer medication as ordered (see "Treatment Plan").
	Explain effects and side effects of medication.
	Assist patient to focus on current realities that can be validated more easily than past events and abstract concepts; for example, avoid discussions about the Communists' secret weapon or that Big Brother is watching.
	Assist patient to identify and describe events or thoughts that evoke tension.
	Begin to assist patient to explore issues.
	Assist patient in using problem solving. It may be necessary to begin with assumption underlying issue if patient uses problem solving to reinforce distorted thinking.
	Be careful not to reinforce distorted thinking. Appropriate comment is "I hear what you are saying, but it does not seem so to me." Intervention may begin at process level, that is, when patient believes his thinking is correct, with comments such as "How did you decide you are right?" "What's it like to always be right?" "What would it be like for you if you were wrong?"
	Avoid becoming defensive when patient criticizes or directs anger at you; these patients often become aware of others' vulnerable areas or weaknesses. Use "I" statement when responding, for example, "I become uncomfortable when I hear you say . . ."
	If patient makes accurate observation about you, acknowledge it and, if appropriate, ask how the behavior affects patient or what patient thinks about your shortcomings or behaviors.
	Slowly begin to help patient become aware of and accept feelings of discomfort.
	Encourage patient to identify and accept imperfections without evaluating himself negatively. For example, encourage patient to say "I don't like my behavior when I . . . but I like myself."
	Encourage patient to accept thoughts and feelings rather than disowning them through projection onto others.
Social isolation	Encourage development of social skills, including satisfying leisure activities, to increase self-confidence.
	Teach assertiveness skills to replace aggressive behavior, and encourage their implementation.
	Encourage patient to examine interactions with others, including his part in the interaction.
	Teach relaxation techniques such as slow, deep breathing when tension is experienced.

Patient Education

1. Teach the patient to accept his strengths.
2. Reinforce the patient's participation in leisure activities for enjoyment.
3. Teach the patient the effects and side effects of medication and the reasons for compliance with the treatment plan.

EVALUATION

Patient Outcome	Data Indicating That Outcome is Reached
Patient demonstrates relief of symptoms.	Patient practices relaxation techniques twice a day. Patient appears comfortable talking with staff, other patients, and significant others. Patient verbalizes strengths in self-confident way.
Patient demonstrates increased satisfaction in social relationships.	Patient initiates interactions with others. Patient engages in social activities and expresses enjoyment.

AFFECTIVE DISORDERS

Affective disorders are those in which a disturbance of mood is sufficiently intense to be dysfunctional.[1] The two major groups are manic and depressive syndromes. Another way of classifying affective disorders is as bipolar or unipolar. A person with a bipolar disorder has experienced at least one manic episode or has alternated irregularly or regularly between manic and depressive episodes. A person with a unipolar disorder experiences only depressive episodes. The manic and depressive phases are compared in Table 17-2.[1,3]

The bipolar disorders are discussed first with a focus on manic behavior. This is followed by a discussion of depression.

Table 17-2

Comparison of Manic and Depressive Phases

Mania	Depression
Elation, expansiveness, irritability	Melancholia, sense of despair
Inappropriate laughing, joking, punning	Tearfulness, crying
Accelerated, sharpened thinking, flight of ideas	Retarded thinking, impaired attention and concentration
Unlimited self-confidence	Lack of self-confidence
Overoptimism	Pessimism, hopelessness
Loquacity	Decreased talkativeness
Exhibitionism	Inhibition
Extroversion to environment	Introversion
Rapid shift to aggression toward environment	Self-destructiveness
Gregariousness	Social withdrawal
Hedonism	Limited or absence of pleasure
Licentiousness	Limited or absence of sexual interest
Reduced need for sleep	Insomnia or hypersomnia
Unlimited energy	Fatigue, psychomotor retardation
Appetite ravenous but "no time" to eat	Appetite decreased or lost
Flight from superego	Submission to superego

Three types of bipolar disorders, as well as another cyclic condition that is milder, are included in the category of bipolar disorders in DSM-III[1]:

1. *Bipolar disorder, mixed.* Both manic and depressive episodes are involved in the current picture, with both occurring at one time or alternating rapidly.
2. *Bipolar disorder, manic.* The current episode fulfills the criteria for mania.
3. *Bipolar disorder, depressed.* The current phase is depression, and at least one manic phase has occurred in the past.
4. *Cyclothymic disorder.* This is milder than bipolar disorder. The depressive and manic phases are cyclic but do not attain the severity and duration to meet the criteria for a bipolar disorder.

Manic Behaviors in Bipolar Disorders

Manic behavior is excessive mental and physical activity.[1]

Thought is accelerated and expansive, mood is labile with rapid sequences of euphoria, irritability, depression, elation, and rage, and physical activity is excessive with boundless energy, little need for sleep, constant motion, and assaultiveness in response to limit setting. Persons in manic states have pressured speech and flight of ideas and are self-indulgent, impatient, humorous, extroverted, friendly, impulsive, and distractible. They appear to have unlimited self-confidence and self-assurance as they propel their energy outward into the environment. The levels of mood disturbance vary from a mild form, hypomania, to a psychotic level of delirious mania.

Prevalence

The prevalence of mania is not clearly known. Inconsistencies in diagnostic criteria and standards used in different countries and cultures and even within one hospital make the true incidence and prevalence difficult to determine. The estimated prevalence of bipolar disorders is 2% in Western countries, with wide variations between these countries. For example, the rate is higher in England than in the United States. American psychiatrists tend to diagnose certain conditions as schizophrenia rather than bipolar disorder as psychiatrists would in England. Whether the differences are due to a diagnostic bias or true differences in the distribution of the bipolar condition is unknown. Carpenter and Stephens[16] believe that, since some symptoms of mania overlap with other psychiatric conditions, attention must be given to multiple features of the condition, including personal and family history, to establish a more accurate diagnosis. Of persons whose disorder is diagnosed as bipolar, approximately 20% do not recover completely and possibly 10% have chronic disease with deterioration.[16,42]

Population at Risk

The findings of researchers as to which sex is at greater risk for bipolar disorder are variable. Some researchers report that the female/male ratio is 2:1, others found parity for the sexes, and still others found males to be at greater risk than females.[21,31] These variations may be related in part to the difficulties of diagnostic bias or to true differences in distribution of the condition, as described in the discussion of prevalence.

Relatives of manics are known to have a high prevalence (10% to 40%) of bipolar or cyclothymic personalities. A relationship between social class and bipolar disorder exists. Manic persons are three times as likely to come from the upper social classes and wealthy families as from the poor and lower strata. Thus manics are more commonly seen in private health facilities. Manic persons are often highly productive and respected in their society.[42]

The onset of manic episodes usually occurs between 20 and 25 years of age, with women having a younger age at onset than men. The first depressive episode usually occurs 10 years later. The onset of each phase can be sudden, especially in mania, in which symptoms escalate within several hours; however, both phases can have slower onsets. The duration of a phase may be as brief as 1 day but is highly variable. The average duration for untreated manics is 6 months and for untreated depressives is 9 months. Modern treatment methods including drugs have obscured the phases and blurred the development of symptoms.[42]

Biologic factors contribute to the development of manic depressive conditions and may even be causative. Since there is a high prevalence of bipolar and cyclothymic personalities among relatives of manic persons, genetic factors such as the dominant X-chromosome may

be a factor. Many theories of biochemical factors as causative or contributory are being studied. These include alterations in catecholamine and norepinephrine metabolism and electrolyte disturbances, including hypocalcemia. That lithium carbonate alters a variety of neurochemical and electrolyte systems supports a pathophysiologic condition. However, the importance of stressful environmental events preceding the onset of manic symptoms cannot be dismissed. Clinical and other systematic studies support a relationship between stressful experiences and the onset of depressive and manic episodes, with stress causing biochemical changes.[23,31]

The cyclothymic disorder is viewed as a mild form of bipolar disorder. To fit this diagnosis, the person must experience hypomanic and depressive mood disturbances for at least 2 years. This disorder may be relatively common among outpatients.[1]

The phases of mania and depression usually occur irregularly but may alternate regularly. They may be separated by symptom-free periods or follow each other with no appreciable interval between them.

Behaviors associated with the manic phase overlap with those of other psychiatric conditions and, when mild, those of nonpathologic deviations of normal behavior. Bipolar disorder should be differentiated from schizophrenia, personality disorders, unipolar depressions, and drug states. Drugs such as steroids, for example, cortisone and amphetamines, can produce elation. Organic disease such as multiple sclerosis must also be ruled out.

Levels of Manic Mood Disturbances

Hypomania is a pathologic state that is less severe than mania. The person has intensified energy, a stable elated mood, self-indulgence, distractibility, pressured speech, poor judgment, and increased motor activity.[3] Hypomanic persons radiate good health, appear tireless, and are humorous and friendly to the point of being unacceptably personal with others. Intolerance to limit setting is observed as irritability or anger.

Mania or acute mania is a more intense and disturbed level in which propriety and discretion are absent. Persons in this state tease and joke, often making others the butt of their jokes. Their good humor can change rapidly to vicious anger. They flit from one activity to another without ever completing anything. Talk may be incessant, since impulses are expressed in words with flight of ideas proceeding to incoherence and clang association (mental association between dissociated ideas made because of similarity in sounds of words used to describe the ideas). These persons have delusions of grandeur concerning their wealth and power and have lost control of their behavior, but do not have severe disturbances of self-identity as in schizophrenia.

Persons with delirious mania or psychosis evidence all of the symptoms of the previous levels plus loss of contact with reality. Speech is incoherent, activity is constant and purposeless, and delusions and hallucinations are present. At times incontinence of urine and feces occurs.[3]

Interactions with manics, and less so with hypomanics, are stressful to others because of their exploitative behaviors, which include the following:

1. Manipulating the self-esteem of others by praise and deflation
2. Striking exploitatively at vulnerable areas
3. Projecting responsibility onto others
4. Testing limits of rules by trying to extend them
5. Alienating others, especially family members

PSYCHOPATHOLOGY

Psychoanalytic Theory

Persons with bipolar disorders have an oral-dependent character and the basic psychopathologic characteristic of unipolar depressives: the introjection of anger and hostility. Depression is repressed hostility, and mania, a defensive behavior, is a massive denial of depression. Manic behavior is a flight from the superego with an abatement of ego restraints, whereas depressed persons submit to the superego.

The apparent warmth and social responsiveness of persons with bipolar disorders may be related to satisfying early relationships with their mothers. However, these persons are unable to master the intrapsychic separation-individuation processes of development to become separate individuals with a sense of self-identity. Psychoanalysts think that biologic factors operate in the alternating moods of manic-depressives, since the condition recurs in successive generations.[27,42]

Interpersonal Theory

The family environment is extremely important in the development of manic depression. The mother enjoys her relationship with the helpless, dependent infant but attempts to control the independent and rebellious strivings of the toddler with threats of abandonment. As the young child develops, the mother or both parents expect compliance and conformity to extremely high standards of behavior and achievements to improve the family's social position and reputation rather than to instill a sense of self-achievement and pride in the child. The child receives favoritism and special attention because of either the child's superior ability to achieve or the child's greater

effort to please and to remain dependent. The child grows into adulthood learning to use others for unlimited help and support, yet fears competitiveness and confrontation because he is afraid to alienate others. Mania is an escape from the burdens of the duty-bound self into superficial liveliness and freedom. Although these persons appear warm and sincere in interpersonal relations, they are shallow and nonempathetic.[3]

Cognitive Theory

According to Beck,[5] manic and hypomanic persons, in contrast to depressives, unrealistically evaluate their efforts as decidedly positive and their accomplishments as impressive. The euphoria they experience because of their inflated evaluations of their superiority and superb performance drives them into uninterrupted motion. When questioned about their inaccurate self-appraisals and fantasies, these persons become inappropriately angry or belligerent.

TREATMENT PLAN

Chemotherapeutic
See also discussion of psychotropic drugs in Appendix C

Psychotherapeutic agents

Haloperidol (Haldol), 5 mg tid po; may order IM injection or po concentrate initially; dosage will be reduced and may be discontinued when patient becomes stable

Lithium carbonate (Lithane),* 300 mg qid po or 600 mg tid po; lithium citrate syrup may be ordered initially instead of tablets

Supportive
Occupational therapy

Recreational therapy as condition permits

Regular diet with normal sodium intake; sometimes high-carbohydrate supplements are ordered

---

*Serum lithium level determination is made before initiating lithium therapy, especially if the patient was formerly receiving medication. Normally no lithium is present without medication. After therapy is initiated, serum levels are examined frequently, for example, every other day until level has stabilized and just before a lithium dose. Therapeutic serum lithium levels are 0.6 to 1.2 mEq/L. Toxic symptoms may occur at slightly more than or even at therapeutic levels. Early signs of lithium intoxication are diarrhea, vomiting, drowsiness, and weakness. The patient should be closely monitored for signs of interaction effects of haloperidol and lithium carbonate, especially tardive dyskinesia and early neurologic toxicity such as weakness, lethargy, fever, confusion, and elevated serum enzyme levels, blood urea nitrogen, and fasting blood sugar.

ASSESSMENT: AREAS OF CONCERN

The mental and physical activities of manic persons vary with the severity of the mood disturbance.

Physical activity

Hyperactivity (moving rapidly from one activity to another, bustling about, restlessness, pacing, fidgeting); limited ability to complete tasks owing to distractibility; eyes bright; face flushed; head erect; animated facial expression; increased metabolism; unrestrained playfulness and mischievousness; uninhibited activity (singing, dancing, and so on); expansive gesturing; dramatic self-expression in movement; colorful appearance (wearing bright colors, jewelry); telephone abuse (calls at all hours); acting out of impulses; sexual acting out without discretion; alcohol abuse; giving money and possessions away; assaultiveness, especially when requests are denied and limits are set; violation of rules; abusiveness; destruction of belongings or bedclothes to be busy; violent motor excitement in severely disturbed

Thought processes

Enhanced sensory acuity (stimulated by other people, objects, and environment); flight of ideas (skipping from one idea to another without completing any); distractibility; expansive, vivid, intense thoughts; impaired judgment; intact memory and orientation to person, place, and time (except when severely disturbed); lack of motivation to change based on "feeling well"; self-confidence, self-centeredness; enthusiasm; self-will; overvaluing of abilities and performance; projection of responsibility onto others; loose associations evidenced in incoherence; paranoid ideation (emerges from anger); arrogance; haughtiness; vengeful ideas; criticism of others; delusions of grandeur (false beliefs of power, wealth, achievements; wish-fulfilling type); clang association of thoughts (words with similar sounds but no relation of meaning, such as ring, ding, and ling); loss of contact with reality; clouded consciousness; visual and auditory hallucinations when severe

Communication

Loquacity to logorrhea; pressured rapid speech; speaking with vigor, excitement, animation, emphasis; flowery, witty, loud, lewd, or pompous speech; superficial content; manipulativeness (pleas and threats, praise and deflation, ingratiating manner, excuses, bargaining, demanding, deception, verbal abuse, trying to extend limits)

Affect

Labile mood (elation, euphoria, exhiliration, irritability, anger, laughter, cheerfulness, tearfulness, tremulousness, depression, sadness)

Social interactions

Appearance of warmth and likability; entertaining, humorous affect; joking, making others the butt of joke; fear of interpersonal intimacy; meddling; interference with and intrusion in others' interaction; attempts to dominate others; exploitation of others' vulnerable areas; destructiveness in group interactions

Self-care

Obliviousness concerning infections and other physical illness as disturbance increases; neglect of personal needs and grooming

Nutrition

Decrease in appetite but no major weight loss; dehydration possible with hyperactivity

Family processes

Promises to spouse made and broken; demeaning of family with anger and blame; family conflicts and instability; spouse perceives patient as spiteful, lacks understanding and knowledge of condition, and has diminished self-esteem

NURSING DIAGNOSES and NURSING INTERVENTIONS

Nursing care should be implemented selectively based on severity of symptoms and presenting behaviors. Nurses need to be alert to their own responses to these patients and their behavior. These patients can evoke frustration and anger in nurses because of their hyperactivity, verbal abuse, and attempts to manipulate staff.

Nursing Diagnosis	Nursing Intervention
Patient problem: activity, alteration in: excess	Identify degree of hyperactivity. Provide quiet, nonstimulating environment. If patient is highly excited, restrict from general patient population areas. Explain restrictions simply and make use of distractibility.

Nursing Diagnosis	Nursing Intervention
	Begin to develop supportive relationship through consistent, frequent opportunities for interpersonal interchange.
	Administer medication as prescribed.
	Be certain patient swallows oral medication.
	Do not allow patient to bargain to take medication later.
	State reason and effects of medication briefly, including signs of hypotension.
	Monitor for effects and possible adverse reactions to medication, including vital signs.
	Teach effects and side effects of medication when condition stabilizes and patient is able to hear instruction.
	Teach importance of maintenance dose of medication and ongoing compliance (be aware that patient is concerned about losing sense of well-being).
	As excitement begins to decrease, involve patient in gross motor activities such as walking and exercise. Be aware that activities often increase excitement rather than produce tranquility and fatigue.
	Set firm, consistent limits on behavior with short explanation as needed. Staff members need to understand and conform to uniform limits. Encourage patient, when able, to set own limits of behavior consistent with treatment goals.
	Allow patient opportunity to express anger about restriction in appropriate way. If anger is inappropriate, use distraction to change focus.
	Gradually help integrate patient into general unit milieu. Be alert for overstimulation.
Violence, potential for	Be alert for possible physical aggression against other patients and staff. If patient is in general unit area, remove from situation giving short, firm, directions for "time out." Use distraction before aggressiveness escalates.
	Protect patient from other patients' aggressiveness.
	If necessary, obtain order for medication as needed (for example, haloperidol).
	Evaluate patient for suicide potential. If patient is suicidal, institute precautions.
	Encourage patient, when able, to identify and accept angry feelings for greater self-understanding.
	Encourage use of problem-solving approach to relate feelings to events that evoked them and develop appropriate ways to resolve issues.
	Assist patient to attend occupational therapy activities and recreational activities when ready and as prescribed.
	Provide opportunities to talk about activities to resolve problem areas.
	Encourage patient to identify enjoyable activities.
	Direct patient to appropriate activities to discharge energies, such as punching bag or exercise.
Thought processes, alteration in	Identify orientation to time, place, and person. (Usually it is intact.)
	Identify seriousness of thought disturbances.
	Acknowledge that you hear patient. If patient's ideas are incoherent, let patient know, as by saying, "I'm having trouble understanding you."
	Listen for themes in flight of ideas and clarify them with patient, for example, "Are you saying you're . . ."
	If patient denies, do not disagree. Remain silent or say "That's the way you see it now."
	Convey acceptance of patient without agreeing with and reinforcing distortion.
	Help patient, as able, to focus on one idea. Allow some digressions and then bring patient back to topic.
	Observe closely for increased excitement.
	Reinforce realistic thoughts.
	Assist patient to identify role and responsibility in situations.
	Since patient often rejects responsibility, use humor to suggest patient's role and responsibility.
	Be aware of resistance to accepting responsibility because of threat to self-esteem.
	Encourage patient to accept responsibility for positive and negative events. Assure patient that it is all right to make mistakes.
	Help patient examine distortions in thinking and correct them without negating patient's self-esteem.
	Teach patient to use problem-solving approach to develop alternative ways for dealing with situations and to evaluate possible consequences.

Nursing Diagnosis	Nursing Intervention
Communication, impaired: verbal	When patient's specch is pressured, rapid, and loud, respond in soft, assertive voice, make short statements, and speak slowly.
	Respond to appropriate humor, but be careful not to escalate excitement and hostility.
	When patient is able, explore inappropriate humor. For example, when humor is inconsistent with content, assist patient to express self directly.
	Let patient know what you will do and will not do in interactions and in treatment plan when patient makes requests.
	Be firm and consistent in maintaining limits even when requests appear reasonable.
	During acute phase, schedule frequent brief sessions with patient, for example, 15 minutes. Increase length of sessions as excitement decreases and patient is able to use the time.
	When patient verbally strikes out at you, help patient identify underlying feelings. If patient continues, communicate your discomfort and let patient know that you will leave if abuse continues. Leave if patient does not stop.
	Teach assertiveness skills to give patient sense of control and influence.
	Convey acceptance of patient without patient's entertaining and pleasing you.
Coping, ineffective individual	As patient is able, identify frequency and duration of mood changes.
	Assist patient, as able, to identify underlying feelings.
	Encourage patient to accept feelings of sadness and euphoria.
	Help patient identify stressful life experiences that preceded excitement and other feelings.
	Assist patient to deal with stressors in healthy ways.
	Assist patient to accept strengths and resources.
	Explore coping mechanisms for dealing with illness.
	Teach patient about illness and treatment.
	Assist patient to develop coping strategies to deal with chronicity and cyclic nature of illness and to increase self-awareness and compliance with treatment regimen.
Self-care deficit: bathing, hygiene, dressing, grooming	Help patient with activities of daily living and hygiene activities (which patient may ignore because "pressed for time").
	During hygiene activities, observe for skin integrity, infections, and other health problems.
	Give clear, concise directions to patient to participate in self-care activities. Use patient's distractibility constructively.
	Allow patient, as able, to make decisions in self-care activities.
	Recognize patient's attempts to initiate and participate in own care.
	Teach patient good hygiene and grooming practices as needed.
Sleep pattern disturbance	Assess patient's inability to sleep and have quiet periods. If needed, obtain order for sedative or neuroleptic agent (haloperidol).
	As patient is able, help identify methods that produce rest and sleep.
	Teach relaxation exercises such as deep breathing to induce sleep.
Nutrition, alteration in: less than body requirements	When patient is highly excited, provide food in small unbreakable containers or finger foods to eat while standing or pacing. If necessary, provide food in liquid form.
	Provide diet with normal sodium level because of lithium administration.
	Ensure that patient's fluid intake is at least 2000 ml daily and preferably 2500 ml to prevent lithium toxicity.
	Teach patient importance of good nutrition with normal sodium intake and fluid intake of at least 2500 ml each day.
	Teach patient need for continued hydration because of lithium therapy. If oral intake of fluids is to be restricted before medical treatments such as surgery or laboratory tests, nurse should inform physician so intravenous fluids can be given to prevent dehydration and lithium toxicity.
	Have dietitian provide additional information on diet as needed.
	Encourage patient to participate in selecting foods for meals.
Social isolation	When patient is highly excited, restrict from other patients in unit to prevent overstimulation.
	Convey your accessibility by your presence and comments.

Nursing Diagnosis	Nursing Intervention
	As patient's excitement decreases, gradually introduce patient to unit for brief periods of time.
	Participate with patient in social activities.
	Observe interactions with other patients. Provide feedback on interactions with other patients and staff.
	Help patient work through difficulties in interactions.
	Assist patient to share information on friends and past activities.
	Encourage patient to begin making contact with friends.
	Teach patient healthier coping strategies and interpersonal skills.
Family process, alteration in	Allow patient's spouse and other family members to talk about experiences, including feelings, with patient. They often think patient is spiteful and willful in hurting them rather than ill.
	Be supportive with spouse and family members as they express their concerns and feelings, but do not participate in blaming patient.
	Teach spouse and other family members about the illness, its cyclic nature, and importance of patient's compliance with medical regimen.
	Begin sessions with family and patient to talk about their experiences generally and responses to illness.
	Help patient and family identify unhealthy interactions such as hostility, blaming, and talking for each other, and help them change these.
	Remain neutral; avoid siding with a family member.
	Encourage members to talk about effects of illness on entire family and how they deal with these.
	Help all family members to recognize need for continued family therapy, if appropriate, after patient leaves hospital.

Patient Education

1. Teach the patient about the chronic and cyclic nature of the illness and the importance of complying with the medical regimen.
2. Teach the patient the signs of increasing mood disturbances in depressive and manic behaviors.
3. Reinforce the patient's awareness of effects and adverse effects of medicine and the need for regular assessments of serum lithium levels (for example, at 1- to 2-month intervals when stabilized).
4. Teach the patient the importance of a normal diet and an adequate daily fluid intake.

EVALUATION

Patient Outcome	Data Indicating That Outcome is Reached
Patient attains persistent mood level nearing healthy state for self.	Patient carries on normal conversation with others. Patient accepts realistic limits and delays. Patient sits quietly for periods of time. Patient is able to engage in an activity for long periods of time. Patient carries out own self-care activities.
Patient demonstrates knowledge of illness.	Patient verbalizes knowledge of illness. Patient identifies patterns of own mood changes. Patient states symptoms that indicate beginning of own manic and depressive phases.
Patient demonstrates knowledge of treatment.	Patient verbalizes knowledge of effects and side effects of prescribed medicine. Patient states knowledge of accurate self-administration of prescribed medicine and importance of compliance. Patient states importance of daily sodium and fluid intake to prevent adverse effects of medication. Patient verbalizes importance of regular serum lithium tests.
Patient demonstrates importance of continued counseling.	Patient makes arrangements to continue counseling to work on personal issues and family relationships. Patient continues to work on listening skills with spouse and other family members.

Depressive Behaviors in Bipolar Disorders

Depression is an abnormal response to psychosocial stressors or loss in which a person characteristically has a sense of worthlessness and despair, morbid thoughts, and psychomotor retardation.

Physiologic and psychologic components operate in all depressions; genetic factors have been implicated as predisposing to some. Suicide is the most serious consequence of depression.

Depression is the polarity of mania and as such occurs as one phase of the bipolar disorder. It frequently occurs as a unipolar disorder in which a person experiences only depressive symptoms. To be diagnosed as a major depressive episode, symptoms must be intense with at least some interference in social and occupational functioning.

The more frequently occurring categories of depression listed in DSM-III[1] are listed below:

1. *Major depression, single episode.* The features are a one-time severe disturbance characterized by depression and loss of interest or pleasure in usual activities for at least 2 weeks. Impairment in thinking and psychomotor agitation or retardation are present.
2. *Major depression, recurrent.* Intense symptoms occur more than one time.
3. *Dysthymic disorder.* This is a milder depressive disturbance than the above and is of at least 2 years' duration in adults.

Depression is the most frequently occurring disturbance in the general population and is viewed as the "common cold" of mental disorders.[67]

Prevalence

Depression is the single most prevalent psychiatric condition and accounts for approximately 75% of all psychiatric hospitalizations. In any 1 year, 15% of the adult population experiences notable depressive symptoms.[7] Reports of the prevalence of pathologic depression in children and adults vary widely. Some researchers state that 25% of their child and adolescent clinic population was depressed, and at an adolescent clinic the figure was 40%. A few have stated that under 5% of their child and adolescent clinic population was given a primary diagnosis of depression.[24] According to the DSM-III,[1] in 30% of cases depression becomes chronic with social or occupational impairment and residual symptoms.

Population at Risk

Some categories of individuals are more susceptible to depression than others. Women are more likely to experience depression than men by a 2:1 ratio. This is related in part to traditional socialization practices of women such as reinforcement of dependent, compliant, and submissive behaviors.[41] The middle years, between 45 and 60 years of age, are a common period for the development of symptoms. The elderly are prone to depression because of shrinking social roles and responsibilities, loneliness, and increasing physical impairment.[18] Although depression is common among adolescents as a result of maturational crises, severe depression is often unnoticed.[24] Depression is also a part of unresolved grief.

Types of Depression

Depression may be primary or secondary to other factors such as a medical or mental disorder or use of medicine and other chemicals. The primary type of depression is an underlying component of the syndrome rather than superimposed on other conditions. It may be a major depressive episode, the depressive phase of manic-depressive episodes, or a cyclothymic disorder. Depression may range in severity from a mild type, such as a dysthymic disorder with a duration of symptoms of 2 years in adults, to a psychotic level.[1]

Precipitating events such as psychosocial stressors or loss are identifiable in 75% of depressive episodes; the onset in these cases is usually sudden and referred to as reactive depression.[67] In some persons a lifelong pattern of many mild depressive episodes is unnoticed until severe symptoms develop in response to an apparent mild stressor. The onset of this latter type, referred to as endogenous depression, is often insidious.

The distinction between reactive and endogenous depression was meant to differentiate depression in response to environmental stressors or events from depression with no discernible precipitant. This distinction may be an artificial one. There is little justification for stating that no precipitant exists just because it has not been identified. During the course of careful interviewing patients are often able to identify stressors. In addition, sometimes stressors or losses are viewed as minor or as nonstressors by the observer but as major by the depressive patient. The patient's self-awareness and definition of an event enter into the identifiability of a precipitant. In both endogenous and reactive depressions with no psychotic features, responses to chemotherapy and psychotherapy are similar. Beck and co-workers[7] state that some kinds of depression, such as bipolar depression, depression with psychotic features, and depression with severe somatic symptoms, appear to require chemotherapy or electroconvulsive therapy rather than psychotherapy alone.

Some depressions are masked by physical symptoms such as psychophysiologic disorders and hypochondriacal symptoms with no reports of feeling sad or depressed. The depressive symptoms are often missed, resulting in unnecessary or harmful medical and surgical treatments.

Depression resulting from severe or chronic physical conditions may be due to an etiologic link or to the discomforts of treatment or chronicity. Depressive symptoms are common with neurologic diseases such as epilepsy and endocrine disorders such as arthritis and cancer. Depression may be evident with other mental disorders such as general anxiety and schizophrenia.[3] Side effects of medicine and chemicals such as antihypertensive drugs, steroids, cardiac drugs (for example, propranolol), antianxiety drugs, and alcoholic beverages can also cause depressive symptoms.

Degrees of Depression

Mild depression is often undiagnosed, and persons who have it may be labeled "prophets of gloom." Those with severe depression are easier to identify. Some symptoms of mild and severe depression, differentiated by Arieti and Bemporad,[3] are listed below:
   Mild
       Unpleasant feelings about self and the environment
       Self-sacrificing, especially in relation to giving to others
       Inhibition of normal pleasurable activities
       Inhibition of spontaneous behavior
       Extra effort needed to concentrate
       Preoccupation with trivial failures and underestimating ability
       Pessimistic outlook toward life
       Self-reproach and irritability for not living up to an ideal standard
       Dependence on others for gratification
       Somatic symptoms
   Severe
       Utter despair and hopelessness
       Sense of emptiness
       Unrelieved sense of guilt and feeling of worthlessness
       Severe immobility or agitated behavior that is purposeless and lacks conscious control
       Catastrophic expectations
       Lack of interest in self and environment
       Retarded thought processes to process and respond to stimuli
       Retardation of bodily processes
       Preoccupation with bodily functions
       Delusional thinking that becomes severe when contact with reality is greatly impaired or lost

PSYCHOPATHOLOGY

Psychoanalytic Theory

Psychoanalysts theorize that persons experience ambivalent feelings of love and hate toward a former love object. Psychic energy (libido) is withdrawn from the lost object; hate or aggression felt for the love object is turned inward toward the self. The person then feels worthless, guilty, and depressed.[27]

Interpersonal Theory

Interpersonal theorists believe that depressive patterns develop within an interpersonal context and may begin in childhood. The child introjects an exaggerated sense of duty and responsibility. The duty and responsibility along with dependence on others are often emphasized by parents so that the child is unaware of self and his own resources. The inability to live up to parents' expectations provokes anxiety in the child; the anxiety becomes guilt, self-criticism, and lowered self-esteem. The child experiences many mild episodes of depression throughout life with no identifiable major stressor.[3]

Cognitive Theory

Cognitive and behavioral theorists are similar in their belief that depression is a consequence of faulty logic. Persons blame themselves for actual or perceived loss of an object and become self-critical and self-rejecting. They generalize their feelings of self-blame to viewing themselves as failures, inferior, and helpless and as having bleak futures. Successes and achievements are disowned. Behaviorists view depression as a consequence of negative reinforcement or no reinforcement of positive, successful behavior.[5]

DIAGNOSTIC STUDIES

Dexamethasone suppression test (DST)
   Dexamethasone, 1 mg administered orally at bedtime; on following day specimens obtained for serum cortisol at 4 PM and 11 PM (if outpatient, 4 PM specimen only); serum cortisol greater than 5 μg/100 ml at either 4 PM or 11 PM is indicative of depression (administration of dexamethasone, a synthetic steroid similar to cortisol, suppresses adrenal cortisol secretion in most normal persons); NOTE: this test is still experimental, and false negatives and positives have been reported[37]

TREATMENT PLAN

Chemotherapeutic

Psychotherapeutic agents

Amitriptyline (Elavil), 50 mg tid po (rarely doses to 300 mg/d); may be given initially as 30 mg qid IM for more rapid effects; for elderly and adolescent patients, 10 mg tid and 20 mg at hs; when depression lifts, single dose at hs

Lithium carbonate, 300 mg tid po, along with antidepressant if depression is part of bipolar disorder; serum lithium levels must be assessed frequently until condition is stabilized, then at 1- to 2-mo intervals, to determine therapeutic serum levels and current toxic levels; blood is drawn for testing just before administration of next lithium dose; therapeutic serum lithium levels are 0.6 to 1.2 mEq/L; if bipolar disorder, observe closely for rapid change to manic phase

Electromechanical

Electroconvulsive therapy, *only* if patient does not respond to antidepressant or if suicidal risk is severe[30]

Supportive

Occupational therapy

Recreational therapy

ASSESSMENT: AREAS OF CONCERN

According to Seligman,[67] no one symptom is experienced by all patients with depression, since the illness is a convenient diagnostic label for a family of symptoms. The severity of symptoms is related to the depth of depression.

Physical

Activities

Low energy; fatigue; lack of ability or motivation to perform tasks; slow movements; eyes downcast and avoidance of eye contact; agitated, purposeless behavior evidenced by pacing and restlessness; substance abuse such as alcohol

Self-care

Lack of interest and ability to perform activities of daily living such as bathing, dressing, and hygiene

Nutrition

Lack of appetite or interest in food (occasionally increased appetite); indigestion; weight loss, usually not critical but may be when condition is very severe or psychotic

Bowel elimination

Constipation

Sleep pattern

Inability to fall asleep, especially with anxiety, or waking early in morning; restless sleep; hypersomnia, occasionally to most of day owing to fatigue or withdrawal

Self-esteem

Low self-esteem; self-rejection; guilt; emptiness; extreme sadness; tearfulness; despair; irritability; low frustration level; sulkiness in adolescents; excessive cheerfulness, especially in adolescents, to hide perceived inadequacies

Power

Sense of lack of power or control; hopelessness, usually greatest when awakening in the morning; helplessness; feeling that nothing patient can do will make a difference

Affect

Agitation; trembling; repeated requests for help ("Will I get better?") or reassurance ("I'm not worth bothering with"); worry; ruminations

Cognitive

Self-harm

Seriousness of suicidal risk: suicidal thoughts and threats, previous self-harming behavior, statements indicating intent and development of a plan (see also discussion of suicidal behavior, p. 1794)

Thought processes

Morbid thoughts; narrow and repetitive range of thoughts; forgetfulness and inability to concentrate; self-rejection and criticism of self and others; somatic complaints; delusions about body and environment, especially bizarre in severe depression; narrow view of self, environment, and the future; failures exaggerated; achievements disowned; paranoid ideation

Communication

Impaired ability to process and respond to verbal stimuli; slow thinking; slow speech; low voice; monotonous tone; limited ability to concentrate

Social interactions

Withdrawal from social interactions and activities because of sense of unworthiness; limited social skills; loneliness; apathy concerning others

NURSING DIAGNOSES and NURSING INTERVENTIONS

Nursing care should be implemented selectively based on severity of symptoms and presenting behaviors.

Nursing Diagnosis	Nursing Intervention
Violence, potential for: self-directed or directed at others	Institute suicide precautions: safe environment, removal of harmful objects, and close observation. Continue close observation as depression lifts, since patient has energy, and as it deepens, since patient may commit suicide before losing energy. Begin to establish trusting, caring relationship. Observe for verbal and nonverbal clues to self-harm. Administer medication as ordered. Briefly state effects and side effects of medication, such as hypotension with lithium. Regardless of serum levels, observe for toxic symptoms such as muscle twitching, ataxia, vomiting, diarrhea, perspiration, dizziness, coma, and seizure. Teach effects and adverse effects of medications and importance of taking as ordered.
Communication, impaired: verbal	Speak slowly, using short sentences. Address patient by name when seeking patient's attention. Give concrete directions. Let patient become aware of your accessibility. Repeat comments if necessary. Schedule frequent, brief (10-minute) therapeutic periods daily so that they are tolerable for both patient and nurse. Schedule longer (50-minute) therapeutic sessions as patient becomes more verbal and tolerates more.
Coping, ineffective individual	Accept patient's feelings as being indicative of what patient is experiencing. When patient is agitated, accept pacing and inability to sit still. Pace with patient as appropriate. Acknowledge patient's discomfort or pain. Let patient know of your presence, as by saying "I am here and want to help you." Teach patient to use relaxation techniques such as slow deep breathing and focus on number "1" with exhalation. Teach diversionary techniques such as an activity, or change subject to decrease emotional discomfort. Assist patient to express feelings. Accept patient's expression of irritability and anger. Teach appropriate expression of feelings rather than, for example, inappropriate cheerfulness. Encourage expression of feeling "hurt" and eventually verbally express anger. Help patient work through feelings of irritability and anger and encourage appropriate expression. Help patient, as able, to identify strengths and positive feelings about self and experiences. Encourage acceptance of self and strengths. Teach assertiveness techniques to give patient sense of control.
Self-care deficit: bathing, hygiene, dressing, grooming	Acknowledge patient's low energy. Assist patient with activities of daily living such as bathing, dressing, and personal hygiene. Give directions one at a time. Recognize efforts to perform activities of daily living. Encourage patient to accept ability to perform task and to make decisions about self-care activities. Acknowledge improvements in appearance, and encourage patient's acceptance of improved appearance.
Nutrition, alteration in: less than body requirements	Monitor food and fluid intake. Do not give patient opportunity to avoid eating or taking fluids. Discourage dieting until condition stabilizes. Ensure adequate fluid intake; with lithium administration, intake should be 2500 ml per day. If patient is nauseated, offer bland diet. Normal sodium intake should be maintained during lithium therapy.

Nursing Diagnosis	**Nursing Intervention**
	Stay with patient during meals, assisting as needed. Remind patient to take another bite of food and chew well. Offer small, frequent meals if necessary. Teach good nutrition and emphasize adequate fluid intake.
Bowel elimination, alteration in: constipation	Monitor bowel elimination. Administer laxatives as ordered and if needed. Teach patient how to prevent constipation by diet with roughage, fluid intake, and exercise. Be alert for diarrhea, especially if patient is receiving lithium.
Urinary elimination: alteration in patterns	Inform patient that medication may cause urinary retention and inhibition of urinary response. Teach patient to begin flow by concentration and pressure on area above pubic bone.
Sleep pattern disturbance	Assist patient, as able, to identify methods of promoting sleep that have been successful in the past. Give warm milk at bedtime. If patient unable to sleep after 30 minutes, suggest that patient get out of bed and assist in diversionary activities. Correct any misconception that insufficient sleep endangers patient's health. Teach patient to develop a relaxation routine before bedtime. Teach patient to breathe slowly and deeply for relaxation. If patient has hypersomnia, encourage patient to get out of bed and participate in simple diversionary activities.
Thought processes, alteration in	Interrupt ruminations by diversion, for example, changing subject or helping patient focus on the topic. Examine one experience at a time using problem-solving approach. Assist patient to learn to monitor his subject changes and to make conscious decisions about changing subject. Acknowledge and question conclusions, especially when based on negative misconceptions or illogical thought. Evaluate whether somatic symptoms have physical basis. Acknowledge hearing patient's complaints. Use diversionary tactics when patient ruminates about somatic symptoms. Explore meaning symptoms have for patient, and correct distortions. Help patient develop healthy coping strategies to replace somatic symptoms. Help patient identify positive thoughts about self and experiences. Encourage patient to think about self and experiences realistically and to accept positive appraisals. Teach problem-solving method, evaluating possible consequences of alternative solutions. Teach assertiveness skills to help patient express self and let others know needs and desires. Acknowledge patient's lack of interest in sexual activities. Convey to patient that interest in sex usually returns when depression lifts. Identify and correct inaccurate thoughts about sexuality. Inform patient that medication may cause impotence. Assist patient to anticipate problems he may encounter after discharge and to examine possible responses to and consequences of each.
Powerlessness	Communicate to patient your hopes for patient's future. Allow patient to be dependent initially. Identify patient's strengths and support system. Identify and reinforce realistic goals for patient's future. Encourage independent and interdependent functioning with family and friends. Teach patient to ask for and accept help from others. Teach assertiveness skills. Teach patient to accept others' refusals to give help without feeling rejected, guilty, or self-critical.
Social isolation	Identify patient's interests and skills as patient is able to participate. Participate with patient in simple social activities such as looking at pictures and commenting about them. Give recognition for patient's efforts to socialize with others.

Nursing Diagnosis	Nursing Intervention
	Structure patient's activities, and give patient copy of plan.
	Encourage patient to make changes in plan or develop own plan (goal).
	Assist patient to develop interests and social skills.
	Participate with patient in activities as needed.
	Encourage patient to attend occupational therapy as scheduled.
	Reinforce attendance at recreational therapy to promote enjoyment of activities and development of social and physical skills.
	Teach patient to initiate interactions and participate with others.
	Help patient to evaluate social skills realistically and to make changes as needed.
	Support patient's decision to engage or not engage in activities when decision is not counter to treatment goals. If it is, discuss with patient.
	Encourage family to be supportive of patient's efforts to interact with them.
	Assist patient to learn adaptive skills for interaction with family and others.
	Help patient and family members listen and respond to one another's messages. Teach them to negotiate and to develop healthier communication patterns.

Patient Education

1. Reinforce problem-solving approach to correct faulty thinking.
2. Teach use of support system for help; for example, write down crisis center name and telephone number or names of significant others who could be called on to help.
3. Reinforce use of self-supports and resources.
4. Review effects and side effects of medication, importance of taking medicine as prescribed, and importance of reporting adverse effects to physician.
5. If patient is receiving lithium, reinforce need to monitor serum lithium levels as prescribed by physician.
6. As termination of nurse-patient relationship nears, review patient's progress and teach patient to deal with loss of relationship.

EVALUATION

Patient Outcome	Data Indicating That Outcome is Reached
Patient demonstrates relief of symptoms.	Patient verbalizes positive feelings about self. Patient expresses enjoyment in participating in activities. Patient initiates interactions with others. Patient sleeps soundly and awakens rested.
Patient demonstrates use of problem solving to correct thinking.	Patient consciously monitors and corrects misconceptions about self and others.
Patient evidences knowledge of depression and importance of continued treatment.	Patient verbalizes awareness of depressive thoughts and feelings and importance of obtaining help early. Patient states effects, side effects, and methods of self-administration of medication. Patient has made plans to continue counseling.

ANXIETY DISORDERS

Anxiety disorders are a group of disturbances in which anxiety is the predominant symptom that is experienced or defended against, as by avoiding the anxiety-provoking object.[1] Anxiety is a subjective experience that can be inferred by observing the person's behavior and physiologic responses and by subjective reports. Apprehension, dread, and intense alertness to an unspecified source of danger are symptoms of anxiety. Unlike fear that is a response to an actual object or event, anxiety is a response to no specific source or actual object. The two categories of anxiety disorders are phobic disorders and anxiety states.

Phobic Disorders

Phobic disorders, the more specific subclass of anxiety disorders, are experienced as morbid, irrational fear when the person confronts the dreaded object or situation onto which the morbid anxiety has been displaced.

The major types of phobic disorders are agoraphobia, social phobia, and simple phobia.[1]

Agoraphobia is a severe, pervasive, morbid fear of being alone, in open spaces, or in public places such as elevators, bridges, tunnels, or public transportation. When exacerbated, the avoidance behavior increases until the person becomes housebound to avoid panic states. Agoraphobia can occur with or without panic attacks.

Social phobia is a persistent irrational fear of being observed or scrutinized by others for fear of acting in a humiliating or embarrassing manner. To avoid the severe anxiety the person avoids speaking, performing, eating, or writing in public.

Simple phobia is a specific morbid fear such as the following:

Claustrophobia: Fear of closed spaces or confinement
Acrophobia: Fear of heights
Nosophobia, pathophobia: Fear of disease
Mysophobia: Fear of filth
Zoophobia: Fear of animals
Scopophobia: Fear of being looked at
Aviophobia: Fear of flying
Demophobia, ochlophobia: Fear of crowds
Nyctophobia, scotophobia: Fear of darkness
Pyrophobia: Fear of fire
Algophobia: Fear of pain
Ophidiophobia: Fear of snakes
Arachnephobia: Fear of spiders
Genophobia: Fear of sex
Coitophobia: Fear of sexual intercourse
Catagelophobia: Fear of being ridiculed
Graphophobia: Fear of writing
Gynephobia: Fear of women

Phobic reactions severe enough to interfere with social or role functioning are relatively uncommon. They are displacement of anxiety arising from an unrecognized source onto a specific idea or object.

Anxiety States

Anxiety states or anxiety neuroses are another subclass of anxiety disorders.[1] Anxiety is the predominant disturbance or is experienced if the person resists giving in to the symptoms. In an obsessive compulsive disorder, anxiety is experienced if the person does not give in to obsession or compulsion.

The major types of anxiety states are panic disorder, generalized anxiety disorder, obsessive compulsive disorder, and posttraumatic stress disorder.[1]

Panic disorder is the experience of recurrent intense anxiety or panic attacks. The sudden, unpredictable attacks are usually experienced as intense apprehension or terror, often with feelings of impending disaster. Common symptoms are palpitations, chest discomfort, dyspnea, choking sensation, dizziness, feelings of unreality, sweating, trembling, hot or cold flashes, and fear of dying or loss of control. Attacks usually last for a few minutes.

Generalized anxiety disorder is the experience of a persistent, free-floating type of anxiety for at least 1 month. To meet the criteria for this diagnosis, the person must have at least three of the following characteristic features of anxiety:

1. Motor tension—jumpiness, trembling, shakiness, jitteriness, tension with muscle aches, eyelid twitch, easy startle
2. Autonomic hyperactivity—dizziness, racing heart, rapid respirations, paresthesias, flushing, pallor, nausea, frequent urination, clammy hands, dry mouth
3. Apprehensive expectation—anxious rumination, worrisome expectation of catastrophe to self or others
4. Vigilance and scanning—hyperattentiveness, darting eyes, impatience, irritability, difficulty concentrating, insomnia, restless sleep with fatigue on awakening

Obsessive compulsive disorder is the presence of recurrent obsessions or compulsions that are distressing to the person or interfere with social or role functioning. Obsessions are recurrent, persistent ideas, thoughts, or impulses that are involuntarily produced, invade the consciousness, and are experienced as senseless. The person attempts to exercise control to suppress the mental activities. Compulsions are repetitive behaviors that are performed according to certain rules or in a stereotyped manner. The seemingly purposeful behaviors are designed to cause or prevent some event and are usually recognized as senseless by the person. If the compulsion is not carried out, tension mounts; if it is, tension decreases. Common compulsions are handwashing, counting, checking, and touching.

Posttraumatic stress disorder (PTSD) is a reaction to a traumatic or catastrophic event. Traumatic stressors include military combat, rape, assault, tornadoes, strong earthquakes, and airplane crashes.[1,39] The subtypes are acute and delayed or chronic. In the acute type, symptoms begin within 6 months after the traumatic event and last no longer than 6 months. The prognosis for this type is good. In the delayed or chronic type, symptoms develop more than 6 months after exposure to trauma or last more than 6 months. Characteristic symptoms are reexperiencing the traumatic event, psychic numbing, and detachment. Additional symptoms are anxiety (especially with flashbacks), anger and even rage, irritability, depression, impaired memory and ability to concentrate, guilt, shame, recurrent nightmares, impaired interpersonal relationships, and aggressive, impulsive behaviors, especially among combat veterans. Some persons may engage in self-destructive and substance abuse behaviors. PTSD is more likely to develop among persons with preexistent psychopathologic disorders.

The discussion and treatment plan focus on severe anxiety or panic attack, since this is one of the most common forms of anxiety.

Prevalence

It is estimated that 2% to 4% of the population has at some time experienced a disturbance sufficient to have been diagnosed as an anxiety disorder.[1]

Population at Risk

Psychologic and interpersonal factors that predispose a person to anxiety disorders include early psychic trauma such as separation anxiety in the infant, pathogenic parent-child relationships, pathogenic family patterns, disturbed interpersonal relationships, and sudden object loss. The panic attacks occur more commonly in women than in men.[1,21]

The person may experience chronic anxiety that is punctuated at intervals by acute anxiety attacks, that is, panic states. These panic attacks are sudden and intense and may subside in a few minutes or last an hour or more. The person may have them several times a day, once a week, or less than once a month. The attacks occur during the day or night. The person may awake from a sound sleep with intense apprehension or terror. During the attack the person has fears of imminent death or physical catastrophe. Other fears include humiliation or appearing foolish and stupid. The fears arise in the absence of any apparent cause such as marked physical exertion or a life-threatening event.

Types of Anxiety

Anxiety is a person's subjective response to actual or perceived threats to the self and lack of confidence in ability to cope with the threats. Persons with *trait* anxiety have a personality structure that shows continual anxiety with no apparent or immediate danger.[52] The foundations for this type of anxiety were laid by experiences in infancy and childhood so that minor threats trigger anxiety. *State* anxiety is episodic and is a response to stressful or threatening stimuli.

Perceptions and interpretations of threatening situations influence how a person responds. Some react disproportionately to the threat by panicking or use nonadaptive defenses such as repression, denial, displacement, and somatization. Some use chemicals such as alcohol. The response is related in part to the person's ego strengths and the types of coping strategies used.[52]

In addition to anxiety disorders, anxiety occurs in other mental disorders such as somatization disorder, schizophrenic disorders, psychophysiologic condition, and various depressive disorders.[1]

Organic disorders must be ruled out, since symptoms of these disorders can be confused with symptoms of anxiety. For example, in cardiopulmonary disorders symptoms may include angina pectoris, palpitations, and breathing difficulties. Endocrine disorders such as hyperthyroidism are characterized by rapid pulse, perspiration, tremors, and restlessness. Some medicines such as epinephrine, antidepressants, thyroid tablets, and dextroamphetamine produce symptoms associated with anxiety.

PSYCHOPATHOLOGY

Psychoanalytic Theory

In psychoanalytic theory, anxiety, an intrapsychic phenomenon, develops as an automatic response to the ego's perception of a traumatic situation, that is, the ego's inability to master or discharge the overwhelming influx of stimuli. It initially develops in infancy when the ego is too weak and immature to deal with the stimuli. As the young child learns to anticipate dangerous stimuli that originate usually from the id (drives) but also from external situations, he reacts to avoid trauma. The maturing ego uses psychic energy (libido) to cope with dangerous events. The dangers and concomitant anxiety are characteristic of situations children face, particularly during the first 6 years of life, and persist throughout life in varying degrees and to an excessive degree in psychoneurotic conditions. Intrapsychic conflicts are present in all psychoneurotic anxiety.[11]

The ego, the reality principle of the personality, attempts to neutralize the energy of the dangerous id by dealing with anxiety rationally and by developing healthy adaptive strategies, including identification and sublimation. When the ego is unsuccessful in dealing with anxiety adaptively, it overuses defense mechanisms. Less healthy defenses and their overuse require continuous expenditure of psychic energy and decrease the ego's strength. Since repression is part of all defense mechanisms, repressed experiences are functionally separate from the ego but continue to operate unconsciously by falsifying or distorting reality.[11]

Interpersonal Theory

In interpersonal theory, anxiety is viewed as developing within an interpersonal context. It is transmitted from the mother in infancy; later it is a response to real or imagined threats to the person's self-system. Anxiety is experienced as apprehension and discomfort, which the person attempts to avoid by developing defensive strategies. The self-system begins to develop to protect the person by excluding painful, threatening experiences from awareness. However, as the organization of the self-system becomes more complex in late childhood, experiences that provoked severe anxiety are out of awareness of or dissociated from the rest of the personality. The person is unable to examine dissociated experiences, correct distortions, and integrate these experiences into the personality. The dissociated material impairs the person's ability to perceive, remember, and think rationally. Persons are able to increase awareness of self and the environment when they integrate dissociated material into their personality.[17]

Cognitive Theory

Cognitive theorists view anxiety as a painful or unpleasant response to actual or imaginary threats of physical harm, economic disaster, social rejection or failure, or humiliation; danger to principle or values; and anticipated loss of friends through separation, illness, or death. (Depression is related to actual or perceived losses, whereas anxiety is related to anticipated losses.) Seligman[67] states that highly anxious persons have a sense of lack of control over events in their lives.

At the core of anxiety is faulty thinking. Anxious persons have impaired ability to examine repetitive dangerous thoughts logically and evaluate them objectively. They may generalize dangers to almost any other stimulus or to perceived changes in their world. Anxiety evoked in response to the initial danger is also evoked in response to the generalizations. They respond automatically to dangerous thoughts and their generalizations without examining their validity. Correction of faulty thinking brings about appropriate emotional responses to dangers that do not negate feelings about the self.[4,7]

TREATMENT PLAN

Chemotherapeutic

Sedative-hypnotics

    Chlordiazepoxide (Librium), 25 mg qid po for severe anxiety; 5 mg bid to qid po for geriatric patients and adolescents; when anxiety level decreases, dosage decreased gradually, e.g., to 10 mg tid po; since half-life of chlordiazepoxide is 24-48 h, 1 dose/d may be advantageous; drowsiness is frequent side effect; convulsions may occur after abrupt discontinuation, especially of high doses

Supportive

Occupational therapy
Recreational therapy

ASSESSMENT: AREAS OF CONCERN

Not all dysfunctional responses are experienced by all anxious persons.

Affect

Apprehension; dread; terror; tearfulness; sobbing; irritability; anger; helplessness; frustration; sometimes laughter; nervousness

Thoughts

Scattering of thoughts or focus on details; preoccupation with self, behavior, and bodily functions; lack of confidence in abilities; low self-esteem; worry; anticipation of adversity; jealousy; envy of others; lack of control to effect or influence outcome; impaired sense of responsibility for self and behavior; sense of worthlessness and rejection by others; distractibility; indecisiveness; vacillation, especially in conflict; forgetfulness; somatization

Communication

Stuttering; blocking; rapid, pressured speech; selective inattention to stimuli observed in limited ability to hear; frequent requests, for example, in hospital for water, medication, information on physician's visit, or laboratory tests; repetitive questioning about treatments, procedures, activities, and so on; petty complaining

Physical

Dizziness; light-headedness; hyperventilation; chest pain; difficulty breathing; palpitation; perspiration; weakness; heartburn; flushing or pallor of face; tachycardia; muscle ache, especially in neck and back; jitteriness; tremulousness; restlessness to agitation; pacing; dry mouth; dilated pupils; blurred vision; darting eyes; headache; accident proneness; impaired sexual functioning

Nutrition

Increased (occasionally decreased) appetite; nausea; belching

Bowel and bladder elimination

Diarrhea or occasionally constipation; urinary urgency and frequency

Sleep pattern

Insomnia; difficulty falling asleep; restless or interrupted sleep

Social interactions

Discomfort interacting with others because of fear of rejection or humiliation; decreased social activities because of fear of failure, especially in competitive activities

NURSING DIAGNOSES and NURSING INTERVENTIONS

Before severely anxious patients can learn, levels of anxiety must be reduced. Anxiety is contagious, affecting others by increasing their anxiety. Nurses need to be aware of their responses to anxiety and how they deal with their own feelings to be able to intervene therapeutically with patients. They can use changes in their anxiety level as indicators of changes in a patient's anxiety.

Nursing Diagnosis	Nursing Intervention
Anxiety	Provide quiet, comfortable environment.
	Begin to establish supportive, safe relationship.
	Allow temporary dependence.
	Remain with patient during panic attack.
	Acknowledge painfulness of patient's feelings.
	Allow patient to pace. If appropriate, pace with patient.
	Listen to patient's complaints of physical problems, and convey hope that these will decrease as anxiety level decreases.
	Encourage patient, as able, to get in touch with body sensations and relate them to level of anxiety.
	Inhibit patient's ventilation of feelings if escalation to nonconstructive level occurs; change focus, for example, to comfort measures such as offering juice or water.
	Instruct patient to breathe slowly and deeply. Breathe with patient as needed to demonstrate. Briefly explain that breathing slowly will help patient become more comfortable.
	Teach patient to monitor own breathing pattern, and reinforce importance of slow, deep breathing to increase oxygen supply, energy, and relaxation.
	When appropriate, teach effects and side effects of medication and precautions such as not operating machinery; potentiating effects with central nervous system depressants such as alcohol; and caution against abrupt discontinuation (convulsion is major danger).
	Teach patient that reframing event can be useful, for example, thinking of boss as "purring kitten" instead of "growling big cat." Teach patient to redefine anxiety as pleasant, exciting sensation.
	Teach patient to monitor own restlessness and engage in diversionary activities to decrease anxiety, such as exercise (for example, walking or table tennis) or problem solving.
	Encourage patient to develop self-supports by identifying and accepting strengths and weaknesses.
	See also p. 1839.
Thought processes, alteration in	When patient is in severe anxiety or panic, minimize environmental stimuli.
	Speak calmly and authoritatively, using patient's name frequently.
	Using short sentences, acknowledge thoughts that patient expresses.
	Give clear, concise directions.
	Teach patient to focus on one topic and to monitor self to stay with one topic or consciously choose to change topic.
	Assist patient to identify thoughts just before anxiety experience and begin to correct misconceptions about experience.
	Teach patient to monitor thoughts realistically about anxiety-evoking experience, using problem-solving approach.
	Teach patient to become aware of automatic thoughts when anticipating negative experiences, to examine evidence for and against distorted thoughts using problem-solving approach, and to anticipate possible consequences of alternative solutions.

Nursing Diagnosis	Nursing Intervention
	Help patient, as able, to decrease fear in decision making by identifying the worst thing that might happen and the best when anticipating adversity. Teach patient to anticipate realistically possible negative and positive outcomes of anxiety-evoking event. Assist patient to identify strengths, support system, and past successes in influencing events. Encourage patient to accept ability to influence events. Teach patient to set realistic goals and not to expect too much of self. Teach patient to ask for help in work and home situations without viewing self as weak or incompetent.
Communication, impaired: verbal	Initially answer repetitive questions simply and concisely. Accept petty complaints without criticism. Try to anticipate areas of concern in treatment, daily schedule, and so on. Inform patient of plans and schedules and write them down so patient can refer to the paper. Teach patient to write down own schedules and so on rather than rely on own memory, especially when anxious. As patient is able, help identify anxiety when patient questions repetitively, has petty complaints, stutters, and blocks. Teach patient to relate anxiety to questioning, complaining, and verbalizing difficulties. Suggest that patient speak more slowly when stuttering. Encourage patient to breathe slowly and deeply to increase energy, decrease stuttering and blocking, and be able to complete sentences. State matter-of-factly that patient will remember blocked material later (this acknowledges strengths). Reinforce speaking slowly and deep breathing. Inform patient that saying ''I stutter when I get excited or uncomfortable'' to others may help decrease stuttering and embarrassment.
Nutrition, alteration in: potential for more or less than body requirements	Monitor food and fluid intake. If needed, obtain order for soft, bland diet to decrease belching and nausea. Small, more frequent meals may be advisable. Encourage patient to eat slowly and chew food well. If patient is unable to sit still, provide food in unbreakable containers that can easily be carried. If needed, remind patient to take another bite or spoonful of food. Administer medication such as antacid as ordered and needed for nausea and belching. Teach good nutrition and ways to increase or decrease caloric intake as needed. Delay weight reduction diet until condition is stable and patient has sense of control of own life.
Urinary elimination, alteration in patterns	Identify and monitor urinary difficulties. Help patient, as able, to relate urinary difficulty to anxiety level. Inform patient that urinary difficulty will diminish as patient becomes more comfortable. Encourage adequate fluid intake.
Bowel elimination, alteration in: diarrhea or constipation	For diarrhea, administer antidiarrheal medication (such as diphenoxylate) as ordered and indicated. For constipation caused by antianxiety drug, encourage adequate diet and fluid intake and exercise. Obtain temporary order for laxative if indicated. Teach patient importance of adequate fluid intake, roughage in diet, and exercise, along with routine for bowel elimination to prevent constipation.
Sleep pattern disturbance	If patient is able, identify previous methods used to promote sleep and assist patient to implement if appropriate. Assist patient to engage in relaxing activities before bedtime. Teach fixed routine in evening that promotes sleep, such as warm bath, watching television, and reading. Assist patient to practice focusing on breathing slowly and deeply to promote relaxation. Encourage patient to listen to tape recordings on relaxation when settled in bed.

Nursing Diagnosis	**Nursing Intervention**
Social isolation	Initially share with patient activities such as walking and table tennis.
	As patient is able, encourage interaction with others.
	Identify patient's social skills and activities enjoyed in past.
	Encourage patient to state and accept social skills and likeable social characteristics.
	Encourage participation in recreational therapy for enjoyment, physical stimulation, and increased confidence in social activities.
	Teach patient that responsibility in social activities is shared and that successes or failures are not entirely patient's.
	Help patient begin to identify social network and apprehension in social interactions.
	Teach assertiveness skills and practice them with patient.
	Teach patient to share feelings with significant others and to ask for help.
	Teach patient to accept positive feelings about interactions with significant others, and help patient examine interactions in which patient expects rejection or disapproval to identify evidence and resolve the issue.
	Assist patient to differentiate between rejection of patient's behavior and rejection of patient as person.
	Encourage patient to accept self, including strengths, abilities, and imperfections.

Patient Education

1. Reinforce knowledge of antianxiety medications, especially affects that impair alertness and dangers of abrupt discontinuation.
2. Reinforce self-management strategies for decreasing anxiety, such as relaxation techniques, physical activities, and diversionary activities.
3. As termination of nurse-patient relationship nears, review patient's progress, strengths and resources, and ability to ask others for help. Assist patient to anticipate and deal with end of this relationship.
4. Teach patient to deal realistically with issues to be faced immediately after discharge.

EVALUATION

Patient Outcome	Data Indicating That Outcome is Reached
Patient evidences relief of severe symptoms.	Patient practices relaxation techniques and engages in diversionary activities to relieve anxiety. Patient is able to relate anxiety to physical sensations and incorrect thinking. Patient uses problem-solving approach to correct misconceptions about events and self. Patient verbalizes sense of increased confidence in ability to perform tasks and interact with others. Patient states ability to fall asleep more easily than in past and awaken feeling rested.
Patient demonstrates knowledge of medication and importance of compliance with treatment plan.	Patient states effects and side effects of medicine, including danger of abrupt discontinuation. Patient develops system to ensure accurate self-administration of medicine as prescribed after discharge. Patient schedules appointment with health professional to continue counseling after discharge.

PERSONALITY DISORDERS

Personality disorders are a category of conditions in which a person evidences enduring personality traits that are inflexible and maladaptive. These traits are stable patterns of perceiving, thinking, feeling, and relating to the person's world and self.[1] The inflexibility of the personality may remain unnoticed until adaptation to environmental changes or pressures is expected.

The personality disorders differ from other classifications of mental disorders in that they are seldom expressed in grossly regressive disturbances or in psychologic defenses such as the affective disorders or anxiety disorders. Significant impairment is experienced in social or occupational functioning or subjective distress. The disorders are recognizable during adolescence or earlier and continue into adulthood.

Since a person frequently exhibits features of more than one type of personality disorder, more than one diagnosis is given. The major types of personality disorders are grouped into the following three clusters based on their main features[1]:

Eccentric features

Paranoid personality disorder is the diagnosis applied to a person who evidences pervasive, unwarranted suspiciousness and mistrust, hypersensitivity, and limited affectivity.

Schizoid personality disorder is evidenced when a person is emotionally cold and aloof, indifferent to praise, criticism, or the feelings of others, and limited in his capacity to form close relationships.

Schizotypal personality disorder is the diagnosis applied when at least four of the following characteristics are present: magical thinking; social isolation; recurrent illusions in which a force or person perceived as present is not; odd speech that is vague, overelaborate, and circumstantial although coherent; inadequate interpersonal relations; paranoid ideation, and hypersensitivity to real or imagined criticism.

Dramatic, emotional, or erratic features

Histrionic personality disorder is characterized by overly dramatic emotional reactions with shallow, demanding, dependent, or egocentric interpersonal relationships.

Narcissistic personality disorder is characterized by a grandiose sense of self-importance; fantasies of unlimited success and brilliance; exhibitionism with a constant need for attention; feelings of rage, humiliation, or emptiness in response to criticism or defeat; and exploitativeness in relationships with a lack of empathy for others.

Antisocial personality disorder is characterized by chronic violations of the rights of others that begin before 15 years of age. During adolescence there are persistent resistance toward authority, delinquency, vandalism, sexual promiscuity, lying, and substance abuse.

Borderline personality disorder is characterized by impulsivity, unstable and intense interpersonal relationships, intense anger, identity disturbance, emotional lability, and chronic feelings of emptiness.

Anxious or fearful features

Avoidant personality disorder is the diagnosis applied when a person avoids desired close relationships because of a fear of rejection or humiliation. The person wants uncritical acceptance and is socially isolated.

Dependent personality disorder is characterized as subordination of a person's needs to those of the individual on whom the person depends. The person allows others to make decisions and assume responsibility for major areas of his life.

Compulsive personality disorder is evidenced by limited expression of warm emotions, perfectionism, being unduly conventional, preoccupation with details and rules, stubborn insistence on own way of performing, and indecisiveness.

Passive-aggressive personality disorder is characterized as passive resistance to demands of others by procrastination, intentional inefficiency, stubbornness, or forgetfulness. Behaviors are nonassertive and ineffective, although more adequate behavior is possible.

The borderline personality disorder is discussed here because its occurrence is increasing and its management creates difficulties for health professionals.

Borderline Personality Disorder

Borderline personality disorder is a condition in which the person exhibits enduring patterns of behavior that do not change with experiences.[1] The person may appear to function adequately until exposed to personal or environmental stressors.

Behaviors associated with borderline personality disorder are intolerance to frustration, impulsivity in which the person acts destructively toward self and others, and instability of affect, with anger the prominent expression rather than anxiety or depression. Anger and hostility are expressed in irritability, sarcasm, demandingness, and projection of feelings onto others. The borderline is vulnerable to brief, mild psychotic episodes that are triggered by stress.

Although the person forms intense relationships, he has difficulty with intimacy and maintaining close relationships; he shifts from idealizing to devaluing others. Being unable to hold an integrated view of self and others with degrees of good and bad, the borderline personality splits objects and thus holds compartmentalized, polarized views of either positiveness or negativeness at any one time.[70] Because of feelings of loneliness and emptiness, the borderline personality avoids being alone and spends most of his time in the presence of others. His relationships are strongly dependent, masochistic, sadistic, and manipulative. Through manipulation he exploits others to gain control and support.[50,70]

Distorted perceptions are related to self-centeredness and inability to empathize with others. Denial is a common ego defense against uncomfortable feelings and relevant past experiences.

When the person is questioned about or confronted with his contradictory actions and feelings, he uses denial to avoid awareness of himself and his behavior.

Hospitalization

The decision to hospitalize a person with a borderline personality disorder may be based on severe anxiety or panic, self-destructive acts including suicidal threats, or transient psychosis. While in the hospital the patient provokes conflict and tension among staff members.[50] Contradictory views of the patient held by staff lead to strong disagreement about the patient and his behavior. The strong emotional reactions evoked in the staff by the patient, countertransference, confirm the patient's projections. Some staff members receive positive projections from the patient and may respond in a nurturing, permissive way; other staff members receive negative projections from the patient and may respond in a punitive, controlling, and hostile manner. The nurse needs to be aware that the flattery and criticism are ego defenses used by the patient in his shifting projections of the self.[34,61]

An understanding of the dynamics of the condition and open communication among staff members with regular staff meetings are essential to implement consistent care.

The hospital structure can provide the patient with a sense of security and protection. However, care must be taken not to overwhelm the borderline personality with too much nurturing and closeness because this evokes feelings of suffocation from which the patient needs to escape. Setting limits consistently and nonpunitively establishes expectations of responsibility and accountability for the patient. Since the borderline personality's tolerance for frustration is low, he responds to limit setting with hostility and rage. The nurse helps the patient examine the factors leading to the hostility, explore alternative responses, and handle feelings. The nurse clearly communicates the patient's behaviors that will and will not be permitted; for example, verbal expressions of anger may be allowed but not physical ones.[22,34,50]

Prevalence

Borderline personality disorder is common, affecting an estimated 30% of the general population and an estimated 17% to 25% of the psychiatric population.[34] Some mental health professionals think the prevalence is increasing, possibly because society is becoming less structured and there is increasing emphasis on individualism and violence.[1,44]

Population at Risk

The borderline personality disorder begins in childhood or adolescence and occurs more commonly in women than men.[1,34] The symptoms frequently overlap with other disorders, especially those within the personality disorder classification. Borderline personality disorder is most difficult to differentiate from the histrionic and antisocial disorders, since they are all characterized by impulsivity, dramatization, and emotionalism.

Motivation for psychotherapy is low, and dropout rates are high. When the patient's stress is decreased, motivation for continuing in therapy frequently declines until the next crisis. Outcomes expected are increased adaptability in interpersonal relationships and to environmental events and increased openness in communications with others.

PSYCHOPATHOLOGY

Conceptualizations of the borderline personality disorder have been developed most clearly and extensively by psychoanalytic theorists. The interpersonal and cognitive theorists have not specifically addressed this disorder. Without an understanding of the dynamics of the borderline personality, it is difficult to intervene therapeutically to interrupt the psychopathologic condition.

Psychoanalytic Theory

The borderline personality has impaired development of object relations that have been conceptualized in the separation-individuation process. In this process, which occurs from 4 to 36 months of age, the child develops a sense of self as a psychologically separate object with clear boundaries differentiating him from other objects in the environment. In the identity of self the child has integrated stable inner images of himself and other objects as having both good and bad qualities. He has the ability to function independently, that is, without his mother's presence.[38,49]

In the borderline personality the separation-individuation process is arrested during the rapprochement phase, which occurs between 16 to 24 months of age. The rapprochement phase occurs concomitantly with the anal phase of development during which aggression and ambivalence are experienced in response to the powerful parent figures. Issues of dependence and independence and control are intertwined with fears of abandonment, loss of love, or engulfment or being "swallowed up" by the mother. The toddler with his growing autonomy experiences conflicts between the desire to be separate and omnipotent and the wish to have needs magically fulfilled. His own feelings and wishes are still poorly differentiated from what he perceives as his mother's; that is, he believes his thoughts and feelings are similar to his mother's as evidenced by her meeting his needs. The mother's empathetic understanding is viewed by the toddler as reading his mind.[38]

The anger and aggression of this period are unstructured and outside of ego control; no cohesive, integrated mental images of self and others have emerged within the personality. The split in mental images of good or bad precludes the development of evocation of memories and past experiences. In the borderline personality the images of self and others are predominantly bad. The arrest in this developmental phase in the borderline personality is generally attributed to the mother who rewards clinging, regressive behaviors and withdraws and is unavailable when the child shows healthy development. Possibly constitutional and other environmental factors also contribute to the arrest of the child's development in this phase.[49]

Interpersonal Theory

According to interpersonal theory, anxiety originates in interpersonal relations initially with the mother and later in interactions with others. It occurs when the person experiences a threat to the self or is unable to cope with an incident. The powerlessness and helplessness experienced in severe anxiety are evidenced in the person's perceptions of his inability to influence or affect others in interpersonal situations, thereby contributing to lowered self-esteem. To eliminate the sense of powerlessness and unbearable tension and achieve a sense of importance, the person learns that anger and aggression are potent forms of behavior.[51,56] Aggression with its impulsivity relieves the child's frustrations. Being intimidated, others respond defensively and allow themselves to be manipulated in the situation, thereby feeding the person's sense of power and control. The feeling of anxiety is no longer recognized as the person automatically responds aggressively and then justifies the aggression to himself. These irrational behaviors prevent the person from examining his response and thereby learning healthier ways of living.

Cognitive Theory

The cognitists believe that conscious thoughts occur in response to an event before the person responds emotionally. Involved is a cognitive appraisal of internal events such as reminiscing and mental images and external events that produce an emotion. The appraisal may become automatic as if by reflex. The expression may be related to how the person expects others to react to him rather than how the others actually respond. The person attempts to conclude what others think by perceiving outward reactions without validating their thoughts. The person acts on the meanings he has attributed to the behaviors.

In some instances the person perceives a nonexistent danger or offense to him as a threat and reacts excessively and inappropriately. The person may also label incidents as either good and accepting or bad and rejecting rather than as a point on a continuum of goodness and badness. The person on the basis of a single incident may unjustifiably generalize to other incidents, reacting automatically to them without validating or making a conscious effort to respond appropriately to the events. This faulty thinking results in habitual faulty emotional responses.[4,7]

These conceptualizations can be applied to the patient with a borderline personality disorder. However, they are limited in explaining borderline behavior. The automatic thinking continues without any reassessment of the original assumptions and responses toward the stimulus. When questioned about his interpretations of the event, the person states his strongly held conclusions. Until the person can be directed to examine perceptions and initial thoughts, he will continue to have inappropriate emotional responses.

TREATMENT PLAN

Chemotherapeutic
Sedative-hypnotics
Oxazepam tablets (Serax), 15 mg bid and hs; for elderly, 10 mg bid and hs; appears to reduce hostility better than other benzodiazepines; causes drowsiness and occasionally dizziness; half-life 5-15 h

ASSESSMENT: AREAS OF CONCERN

Signs and symptoms vary in type and severity among patients.

Emotions

Anger; hostility; depression; anxiety; emptiness; loneliness; emotional shallowness

Thoughts and actions

Denial of contradictory feelings; denial of responsibility for behavior; intolerance of stress and frustration; demandingness; acting out of tensions and feelings; poor judgment; projection of hostile feelings onto others; misinterpretation of stimuli; impaired problem solving; sense of inadequacy and insecurity; ambivalence; polarized views of others as good or bad; sense of specialness; masochistic and sadistic behavior; destructive behavior toward self and others

Communication

Demanding; sarcasm; criticism; verbally striking out at others' vulnerabilities; manipulativeness by evoking rescue fantasies in some individuals or hostility with subsequent counterattacks from others; evoking disagreements and competitive behaviors among others

NURSING DIAGNOSES and NURSING INTERVENTIONS

Nursing care should be implemented selectively based on severity and type of behavior. Since hospitalization is likely to be brief and change is slow, usually interventions only begin to have positive effects on the patient's healthy adaptation.

Nursing Diagnosis	Nursing Intervention
Coping, ineffective individual	Develop trusting relationship with patient without being too nurturing or overinvolved.
	Involve patient in treatment plan by having him identify how he wants you and other staff members to help him. Ask patient to state needs rather than anticipate they will be met "magically."
	Communicate unit routines and expectations to comply in matter-of-fact way.
	Help patient structure his days.
	Encourage patient to describe events that lead to impulsive behaviors, including patient's thoughts and actions.
	Be alert to patient's omissions of own behaviors and his focus on others.
	Gradually assist patient to identify feelings.
	Help patient correct distortions in perceptions, thought processes, and definitions of an event.
	Encourage patient to identify and evaluate consequences of impulsive behavior, for example, how behavior achieved or did not achieve desired outcome.
	Assist patient to examine and evaluate alternative behaviors to achieve satisfying outcome.
	Ask patient what help he wants in controlling or preventing impulsive behaviors.
	If patient is unable to control impulsivity, prevent or interrupt behavior when patient shows signs of losing control, such as changes in activity level, argumentativeness, irritability, or increased muscle tension.
	Use diversionary techniques such as escroting patient to quiet area, going for walk, or changing subject. After patient is away from situation, encourage discussion of details of issue and patient's feelings. Teach problem-solving approach for dealing with situation and examination of possible consequences of alternatives.
	Communicate clearly to patient behaviors that will not be permitted, and emphasize that you will set limits to intervene if needed. After setting limits (for example, that certain verbal behaviors such as disagreeing are permitted but physical ones such as threatening others or striking out are not), protect patient and others from harmful acts.
	Be alert to self-destructive acts. Take suicide threats and even minor suicidal acts seriously. If indicated and in collaboration with physician, institute suicide precautions. (See also p. 1797 for interventions.)
	Administer sedative-hypnotic medication per physician's order. Teach patient effects and possible side effects. Observe for adverse reactions such as increase in impulsive or hostile behaviors.

Nursing Diagnosis	Nursing Intervention

Teach patient to use relaxation techniques, such as slow deep breathing and focus on breathing or the number ''1.'' Listening to quiet music on the radio can have hypnotic effect to decrease panic and promote sleep and relaxation.

Point out that patient avoids talking about his part in an interaction (for example, ''I hear you talk about what John did, but I hear nothing about what you did.'').

Avoid empathetic understanding of patient's thoughts and feelings, since patient may think you can read his mind. Help patient recognize reality of his separateness.

Comment on overt behavior and ask for patient's thoughts or feelings (for example, ''I notice the tightness of the muscles in your face and your clenched hands. Are you upset?''). If patient denies being upset, ask what patient is experiencing now. If patient continues to deny feelings, say nothing or say ''I am available when you want to talk about this with me'' in nonthreatening manner.

Patiently reintroduce issue of whether patient's feelings are appropriate.

As patient identifies feelings, help him to experience and accept them. Eventually help patient to connect feelings with thoughts and acts.

When patient projects his thoughts and feelings onto others, ask patient to share evidence he has. If patient is unable to present evidence, question his opinions or assumptions (for example, ''From what I hear you saying, I don't agree with your conclusions about . . .'').

Matter-of-factly point out inconsistencies or contradictions in patient's actions and expressions of thoughts and feelings to increase patient's awareness of behavior.

Set limits in nonpunitive way when patient makes demands to stretch rules and asks for special favors. Be explicit in responding that you will not comply. If appropriate give reasons. If patient continues to make same demands, remind patient that you have told him no before. Be firm and consistent without getting into discussion or argument. If patient tells you that another nurse gave permission, do not allow yourself to be manipulated. Merely repeat your refusal without being defensive.

Be alert to patient playing one staff member against another. Keep in mind that patient's negative and positive appraisals of others are patient's defenses and are not accurate.

When patient's appraisal is accurate, tell him he is correct to validate reality (for example, ''Yes, I do enforce rules.'').

When patient complains about another staff member, encourage patient to work problems out with that person rather than tell you.

Point out disproportionate anger or other reaction in interaction. Explore what the anger is about (for example, ''I don't understand the anger you're expressing. Tell me about it.'').

Regular staff meetings are essential to clarify or modify treatment plans and to support one another.

Assess whether patient is able to accomplish requested task. Assist patient, as able, to examine request.

Support patient's ability to perform tasks by stating that he has that ability.

Encourage patient's identification and acceptance of strengths. Have patient reinforce strengths by acting on them.

Patient Education

1. Teach the patient to monitor responses to events by thinking before acting out and using diversionary techniques.
2. Teach the patient to focus on his own behavior in situations rather than on others only.
3. Teach the importance of compliance with the medical regimen and long-term psychotherapy.

EVALUATION

Patient Outcome	Data Indicating That Outcome is Reached
Patient demonstrates reduction in symptoms	Patient monitors own behavior to control impulsive behavior. Patient is able to state needs and accept delays. Patient verbalizes decrease in uncomfortable feelings. Patient begins to use problem-solving approach to deal with issues.
Patient evidences acceptance of need for continuing treatment.	Patient verbalizes value of examining own behavior. Patient states effects and side effects of medication and knowledge of accurate self-administration after discharge. Patient makes plans to continue counseling by scheduling appointment after discharge.

ADAPTIVE AND MALADAPTIVE BEHAVIOR

Two conditions, potential for self-harm and crisis, are presented in this section. Although these related conditions are not classifications of mental disorders, they have serious implications for mental health. Crisis intervention services arose from suicide prevention programs of the 1950s and 1960s.[20] Preventive strategies are emphasized in both. In potential for self-harm the immediate goal is prevention of suicide; in crisis intervention a goal is prevention of the maladaptation of mental illness. Alternative effective coping responses are sought when intervening in these conditions.

Stressors play an important part in the development of dysfunctional responses. DSM-III[1] takes into account psychosocial stressors (ranging in influence from "none" to "catastrophic" depending on severity) as contributors to the development or exacerbation of dysfunctional behaviors. Therapeutic interventions are directed toward fostering adaptive rather than maladaptive responses. Adaptation is the ability to mobilize the resources needed to make changes in the self or in the external environment to cope effectively with stress. Maladaptation is the inability to mobilize the necessary resources to manage stress.

Potential for Self-Harm

Suicide is an act to terminate one's life. The term can be broadly categorized as including completed suicide, suicide attempt, and suicide ideas.

Completed suicide is the cessation of life resulting from self-destructive behavior, whereas attempted suicide is an apparently life-threatening act that does not result in death.[75] Persons with suicide ideas are preoccupied with thoughts of ending their lives and may indicate these directly or indirectly by behavior such as making a final will or saying "Others would be better off without me." The term "suicide" does not explain the cause of death but only the mode of death or the presence of life-threatening thoughts and acts.

The seriousness of suicidal acts and thoughts is related to the lethality and intent. Lethality of an act or contemplated act is ranked from zero to high depending on its destructiveness and reversibility. Suicide attempts by firearms and hanging are highly lethal, whereas ingesting 15 aspirin is not. Sometimes ignorance of the consequences of a method enters into the lethality; that is, persons who lack information may incorrectly choose a method that is or is not fatal.[75]

Intent to commit suicide is a determination to end one's life. Extremes of intent range from absolute determination to none. The degree of intent is difficult to assess accurately, since people exaggerate or deny their intent to kill themselves. Some persons may state a strong desire to commit suicide in order to manipulate others, with no intention of committing suicide. Others deny their intentions even though they have well-formulated plans and serious intent to kill themselves.[75] However, all threats and attempts must be taken seriously.

Families are often reluctant to admit that a member intended to commit suicide because of the stigma attached to such behavior. Religious beliefs and societal values in many countries prohibit self-destructive behavior. Contrary to popular belief, however, the Bible does not prohibit or condemn suicide.[29,75]

Accidental suicides occur for a variety of reasons. A "suicidal gesture" used as a manipulative ploy to gain favors and influence others may inadvertently result in death. Conditions that cloud consciousness such as chronic pain, organic disease, dysfunctional states (panic, severe depression, psychosis, and high stress), and drugs may lead to unintentional self-destructive behavior. For example, persons with severe pain may take repeated doses of analgesics until they no longer remember if or how much medicine was ingested. Psychotic suicides in depression or schizophrenia may be in response to delusional ideas or hallucinatory orders to punish the self through self-destructive behaviors.[3]

Some suicidal acts are conscious, logical decisions persons make when they view life as less desirable than death. These persons have no hope that their life circumstances will change, and they carefully plan and carry out their suicides. Altruistic suicides are carried out for the welfare of others and are often viewed as honorable acts.[7,29]

In any suicide ideation and act, health professionals must take the viewpoint of the attemptor and not superimpose their own views and judgments on the individual and the act. This is so regardless of whether the threat and act are manipulative ploys or serious attempts in response to mild or severe stressors. All suicidal thoughts and acts must be taken seriously and responded to accordingly.

Prevalence

The official statistics on attempted and completed suicides are unreliable and thought to be understated by 25% to 50%. Unless the evidence clearly points to suicide, attempted and completed suicides are usually attributed to other causes. The number of deaths by suicide is approximately 25,000 to 30,000 annually in the United States, with an estimated eight to 10 attempts for each successful suicide. Suicide is one of the 10 leading causes of death among adults and the second leading cause of adolescent deaths.[29,75]

Population at Risk

Many people have had at least fleeting thoughts of killing themselves at some point in their lives. Men are more likely to commit suicide than women by a 3:1 ratio, but women are more frequent attemptors than men, with a reverse ratio of 3:1. Male adolescents also outnumber females in completed suicides, but female adolescents are more frequent attemptors. A sharp rise in suicides occurs in 15- to 19-year-old adolescents as compared with the 10- to 14-year-old group.[26,75] Another sharp increase occurs among young adults, with a much higher rate among college students than others in their age group. Medical students and physicians, especially psychiatrists, have a surprisingly high suicide rate when compared with the general population. This group has the medical knowledge and access to lethal methods to complete the act successfully.

Separation from and death of loved ones, divorce, loss of health, loss of jobs and money, and sickness are powerful factors in suicide. The suicide rate increases with advancing age; midlife and old age are particularly difficult periods.

Persons whose significant others have commited suicide or who have attempted suicide themselves in the past are more prone to suicide. The suicide may be related to a significant date such as an anniversary, a birthday, or becoming the same age as the lost person. A history of previous suicide attempts is an important predictor of future suicidal behavior; many of those who successfully complete a suicide have attempted suicide previously.[75]

Family disruptions affect younger family members more than older ones. Conflicts and arguments within the family create suicidal pressures on members. The potentially suicidal member is often isolated within the family and becomes the "bad" one. When working therapeutically with families, it is important to avoid prematurely correcting pathologic family relationships, since this may push the suicide-prone person to follow through with suicide.[26,63]

Sequelae in the Family

Family members, loved ones, and friends of those who commit suicide are survivor-victims of suicide. They are tortured by guilt, shame, hatred, and confusion for years after the episode. Obsessional thoughts about the death and the search for reasons are often attempts to relieve self-blame. Significant others may deny that the cause of death was suicide despite the evidence and may continue to believe that the death was accidental or due to natural causes.

Shneidman,[69] one of the pioneers of suicidology, coined the word "postvention" for techniques to intervene in and alleviate the survivors' emotional distress and prevent suicide among this group. Abnormal grief response is the continuation of symptoms for years after the death. Shneidman believes interventions with the survivor-victim should begin as quickly as possible, preferably within the first 72 hours.

PSYCHOPATHOLOGY

Psychoanalytic Theory

Psychoanalytic theorists view suicide from the psychopathology of depression. Ambivalent feelings of love and hate experienced toward the lost love object are withdrawn from the object, and the hate or aggression are turned inward toward the self. Suicide is the extreme response of self-hatred. The self-destructive act is carried out as self-punishment with the hope of gaining forgiveness from the sadistic component of the developing superego.[27]

Interpersonal Theory

In interpersonal theory, suicide stems from depression in which the person believes that it is better to die than to suffer emotional pain and emptiness. Through self-punishment the person hopes to gain relief from guilt, feelings of helplessness, and failure. Often through self-destructive behavior the person gains relief from negative self-feelings and, if he survives, may begin to improve.[3]

Suicide in children is markedly different from that in adults. Before 9 years of age, children have no concept of the permanence and irreversibility of death. The rarity of suicide in children is due to their cognitive immaturity to plan and implement it. When suicide occurs, it may be related to fears of punishment, especially by parents. Adolescents attempt suicide because of self-hatred and losses, especially of love objects; some do so as a desperate cry for help, often to others beyond their family. In some adolescents coercive manipulation is involved to obtain revenge or peer approval.[3]

Delusions and hallucinations in psychotic persons reinforce and support self-redemption and forgiveness through the self-punishment of suicide.

Cognitive Theory

Petrie and Chamberlain[60] found in their own and others' studies that suicidal behavior and ideation are not significantly related to depression per se but that hopelessness is the important explanatory variable in suicide. These studies support Beck's finding that persons experiencing hopelessness and negative views of their future are at high suicidal risk. Depressed persons with hope are less likely to engage in suicidal behavior.

Hopeless persons see no escape from their unbearable feelings and situation. The sense of no escape gives rise to suicidal ideas and behavior as the only solution and as an end to emotional distress.

Beck and others[7] state that realistic problems related to environmental factors such as work and school performance, loss of job by the head of the family, and unsatisfying interpersonal relationships may contribute to a person's hopelessness and wish to end it all. It is true that the expectation of regaining a lost loved one, wealth, status, or health is unrealistic unless the person is able to accept alternative solutions. Persons who view suicide as the only solution may carry it out in a logical, rational manner or may perform it as a highly illogical response to a situation.

The nurse should be aware that the tranquillity and peacefulness observed in a formerly distressed or agitated person may not be a sign of improvement but rather a sign of having made a decision and plans to commit suicide.

TREATMENT PLAN

Chemotherapeutic
Psychotherapeutic agents
  Amitriptyline (Elavil) for depression or personality disorder; 50 mg bid for adults; 10 mg bid for elderly or adolescents; if there is suspicion that patient is not swallowing pills or is hoarding them, IM medication may be substituted, e.g., 20 mg tid
  Chlorpromazine (Thorazine) for psychotic disorder; 25 mg tid for adults; 25 mg bid for elderly and adolescents; IM or liquid may be substituted to prevent hoarding

Supportive
Suicide precautions
Seclusion if deemed necessary for patient's protection

ASSESSMENT: AREAS OF CONCERN

Signs and symptoms will vary among individuals.

Violence*
Instability or changes in life situation; thoughts that life is not worthwhile; presence, duration, and strength of self-harm thoughts; contemplation of ways of harming or killing self; development of well-formulated plans; strength of motive or serious intent to follow through with plans; availability of chosen suicide method; factors, such as family, religion, and additional stress, that may push person toward or deter suicide; previous thoughts and attempts of suicide along with intent and lethality of attempts or ideas; loss of significant other through suicide

Power and control
Hopelessness; inability to influence or alter interpersonal or life situation

Affect
Sadness or depression; inappropriate feelings such as laughter; anger; distress; tranquillity once decision and plan are finalized

Thoughts
Negative view of the future; humiliation (for example, feeling of being a failure); perceived or actual recent losses, stressors, or changes; ambivalence; fantasies about how others may react (for example, "They'll be sorry"); vengeful thoughts; delusions or auditory hallucinations of sin, self-punishment, and atonement

*These may be used for a graded level of assessment to determine whether suicide is likely.

Communication

Comments such as saying good-bye instead of good night, "I won't be seeing you again," or "Next time you see me I'll be riding in a hearse"; informing family or spouse of whereabouts of important papers, such as insurance papers, bankbooks, and will; threats of suicide as cry for help or to manipulate interactions

Activities

Making or changing will; increasing life insurance; visiting or phoning relatives and friends for intense conversations; giving away prized possessions; demonstrating increased concern or care for others; obtaining tools needed to implement suicide, such as buying a gun, rope, or prescription refills; acting-out behavior; writing farewell note

Social interactions

Perceived or actual lack of support from others; loss of valued relationships through separation, divorce, death, or romantic breakups

Family process

Dysfunctional patterns of interactions such as conflict, arguments, and blaming; others not perceiving and responding to needs or wishes

NURSING DIAGNOSES and NURSING INTERVENTION

Although the environment should be made as safe as possible by removing any materials suicidal patients might use to harm themselves, it is not possible to make the environment completely suicide proof.[14] The importance of developing a concerned, supportive interpersonal relationship with the patient cannot be overemphasized.

When working with suicidal patients, even when they are manipulative, nurses need to be aware of and manage their own feelings while empathizing with the patients' point of view. Nursing care should be implemented selectively based on seriousness of symptoms and presenting behaviors.

Nursing Diagnosis	Nursing Intervention
Violence, potential for: self-directed or directed at others	Identify seriousness of suicidal intent. Begin to establish supportive, trusting relationship with patient. Convey empathy and concern. Institute precautions such as removing all harmful objects from environment (glass containers, drugs, clothing, possessions, and so on) and closely observing patient (initially one-to-one observation day and night if necessary, later, observation every 15 minutes and frequent interactions while awake, and eventually hourly checks). Allow patient to keep more possessions as deemed safe and as precautions become less stringent. Continue close observation with knowledge of patient's whereabouts. While suicide precautions are in effect, engage patient, as able, in simple activities such as exercises or looking at magazine. Evaluate patient's condition frequently at first and at least once a day later. Administer medication with simple explanation including possible side effects, such as orthostatic hypotension and drowsiness. Teach patient effects and side effects of medication.
Powerlessness	As patient is able, explore reasons for suicide attempts or suicidal feelings and sense of hopelessness. During interactions convey sense of hope in patient's ability to control own behavior. Assist patient to begin to identify solutions other than suicide. Convey to patient that you are there to help control behavior and to provide relief and sense of security. Encourage patient to explore current situation, identify aspects that can be changed and ways of changing them, explore positive elements in unchangeable situation and ways of dealing with negative aspects, including obtaining support and help. Evaluate possible consequences of choices. Encourage patient to identify and accept strengths and self-resources. Teach assertiveness techniques to express self and ask for help. Encourage patient to develop healthy coping strategies to deal with uncomfortable feelings in situations.

Nursing Diagnosis	Nursing Intervention
Thought processes, alteration in	Convey acceptance of patient and take suicidal thoughts seriously.
	Help patient identify reasons for and meaning of suicide threats (or suicide attempt) and what patient expected to happen to self and others.
	Acknowledge pain and distress when talking about suicide ideas or attempt.
	Examine losses and stressors that evoked suicidal behavior.
	Help patient recall and identify reasons for living when life was better than currently.
	Avoid reinforcing delusions and hallucinations.
	Assist patient to examine experiences before delusions or hallucinations. Gradually help patient to connect thoughts and feelings with false beliefs or perceptions.
	Question inaccurate comments.
	Encourage patient to use problem solving to correct illogical thoughts.
	Help patient to identify advantages and disadvantages of dying and to assess them objectively.
	Teach patient to anticipate future problems and to develop methods, other than suicide, for handling them.
Communication, impaired: verbal	Help patient recall people with whom patient could share problems and feelings.
	Help patient identify when and why he stopped sharing information and problems with others.
	Encourage patient to correct faulty thinking and negative expectations about sharing.
	Explore with patient what happened when he shared thoughts and feelings and how he handled this.
	Encourage patient to communicate needs and feelings directly, and teach patient to do this.
	If patient denies suicidal intent, ask what *was* going on with patient at time of suicide attempt.
	If patient continues denials, ask patient what others would think of him if he had suicidal thoughts.
	If patient says suicidal behavior was accidental, help him identify way to prevent future "accidents."
Coping, ineffective individual	Allow patient to ventilate feelings.
	Identify patient's feelings about what was happening when patient began having suicidal ideas.
	If you feel patient's tone is inappropriate to situation or verbal content, comment on this, as by saying "I notice you're smiling as you talk about your family's distress."
	Examine appropriateness of patient's feelings to event, using problem-solving approach.
	Teach patient to express feelings directly and that feelings such as sadness and anger are all right.
	Use role playing to help patient learn to express feelings.
	When patient shows signs of increased tension, encourage patient to breathe slowly and deeply to decrease tension.
	Observe for change in patient's mood, such as calmness or tranquillity, as prelude to suicide act.
Social isolation	Assist patient to identify enjoyable interactions with others. Determine what patient enjoyed about interaction.
	Encourage patient to identify and accept social skills.
	Teach patient that others have responsibilities in interactions instead of patient alone.
	Assist patient to deal with discomfort experienced in interactions.
	Encourage patient to decide what and how to tell others about suicidal ideations or attempts. Use role playing to rehearse the telling.
	Assist patient to avoid sharing suicidal behaviors when he does not want to and to realize that he has a right not to share information.
Family process, alteration in	Identify relationships from patient's point of view.
	Allow patient to decide whom he wishes to see.
	Assist family to perceive patient's point of view.

Nursing Diagnosis	Nursing Intervention
	If suicidal behavior was manipulative, assist patient to be more direct in seeking fulfillment of needs. For example, ask patient how he stopped himself from asking for help.
	Meet with patient and family to identify interaction patterns.
	Assist family to identify positive aspects of relationships, such as warmth and caring, as they interact.
	Point out dysfunctional patterns as they occur, for example, ''How is it you speak for Joe? Joe, why do you let them?''

Patient Education

1. Reinforce alternative solutions and methods for handling situations instead of suicide: identification of feelings and thoughts when the patient experiences loss of control and asks for help, reaching out to supports within the family and among friends, problem-solving approach, and self-supports and strengths.
2. Teach the patient to write down names, addresses, and phone numbers of the local suicide prevention center and 24-hour help lines. Encourage the patient to use them day or night to obtain support or to talk with someone when the therapist is not available.
3. Reinforce the need for continued counseling or psychotherapy, and emphasize that this is a sign of strength rather than weakness.
4. Review effects and side effects of medicine.
5. Review possible ways of dealing with situations after discharge. Help the patient learn to share or avoid sharing aspects of suicide and hospitalization with others.

EVALUATION

Patient Outcome	Data Indicating That Outcome is Reached
Patient demonstrates ability to manage stressors without resorting to suicide.	Patient verbalizes coping strategies for dealing with issues. Patient evidences increased self-assurance in behavior. Patient verbalizes desire to live and states plans for resolving similar problems in future.
Patient develops plans to increase satisfaction by changing life situation.	Patient is able to use self-supports. Patient identifies and voices acceptance of supportive social network. Patient sets aside time for leisure activities. Patient identifies more realistic goals for performance in work and play.
Patient plans to continue treatment plan after discharge.	Patient states accurate information about actions and self-administration of medication. Patient verbalizes commitment to continue counseling and makes appointment.

Crisis

Crisis is a turning point in a person's life or an upset in a steady state. It may occur when a person is confronted with a problem that cannot be resolved by the person's usual methods.[15] The generally accepted view is that a crisis is not a pathologic state.

Not all persons react to similar events in the same way, and a person reacts differently to similar events in different life phases. The person's perceptions of an event influence his definition of it. If the person perceives an event as a severe threat, he is likely to respond to it as a crisis. However, another may perceive the same event as a challenge. Ego strengths and resources affect the way people manage crises.[73] For example, a person with a strong ego usually can more easily resolve a crisis than a person with a weak ego. Previous success or failure influences the person's ability to respond favorably to crisis stimuli.

Often when a crisis occurs the person is already in a vulnerable state because of previous stressors.[33] Despite being in a state of moderate anxiety or depression, the person is able to mobilize the resources to cope, although at a reduced level, with the initial stressors. However, when an overpowering experience, the precipitant, occurs, it produces the disorganizing effect of a crisis state. For example, the initial stressor may be a surgical procedure that produces a vulnerable state, and the crisis-precipitating event may be the discovery that the excised tumor is cancerous. Sometimes a person experiences just one stressor of sufficient force to precipitate the crisis.

Persons commonly view the precipitant as their problem without awareness that earlier stressors put them into a vulnerable state and increased the impact of the crisis-precipitating event. Some counselors believe that dealing with the thoughts and feelings resulting from the precipitant alone is sufficient to restore equilibrium and that helping the patient work through the initial stressors is unnecessary.[33]

Acute crisis is a subjective state of psychologic and physical disorganization in which the person experiences temporary loss of control. This is called a panic state. Since emotional reactions to the stimulus are overwhelming and nonintegrated, the cognitive processes such as assessing, thinking, decision making, and judging are inoperative.[43] Thinking is scattered with no ability to attend to anything or to fix on one narrow point; affectional ties to others are severely disrupted or severed so that the person feels isolated.[72] The person is immobilized or moves about aimlessly.

Korner[43] differentiates two types of crisis on the basis of their causes. In exhaustion crisis the person has coped effectively under emergency conditions for some time and suddenly reaches a point of exhaustion when all energy and resources have been spent. In shock crisis the person experiences a sudden change and is overwhelmed by an explosive release of emotions. Too much has happened unexpectedly and rapidly for the person to cope with the flooding of stimuli. Nursing interventions for these two crisis types differ. A person in exhaustion crisis is unable to gain control over emotions and is apathetic and indifferent to interpersonal contact or intervention techniques. This person needs a calm, supportive environment to regain energy slowly before attempting to deal with the crisis. A person in shock or acute crisis is open to change and highly motivated to accept and use help in resolving the crisis.

Although theoretically it is possible to isolate the phases of crisis—hazardous or precipitating event, acute crisis, and reorganization—they usually overlap in the individual. A crisis generally lasts 4 to 6 weeks but may be much longer or shorter depending on the type of precipitating event, the level of stress experienced, and the person's ego strengths and resources.

Incidence

Crisis situations occur episodically throughout a person's lifetime because of normal developmental stages and the demands associated with anticipated life situations. In addition, unanticipated crisis situations occur during the life span. Many crises do not come to the attention of health professionals but are resolved with the help of family, friends, or the clergy. Since crises are time limited, the person may successfully deal with them or may maladaptively resolve them, resulting in a reduction in functioning from the precrisis level.[13,33]

Population at Risk

From birth to death a person is exposed to crisis situations that are anticipated and predictable or unanticipated. Anticipated crises are ones that most people experience during the developmental stages of the life cycle and in other transitional phases of life.

According to Erik Erikson,[33] the eight developmental phases are basic trust versus mistrust; autonomy versus shame and doubt; initiative versus guilt; industry versus inferiority; identity versus role confusion; intimacy versus isolation; generativity versus stagnation; and ego integrity versus despair. The identity crisis of adolescents has been given considerable attention because of their rapid physiologic and cognitive changes and high vulnerability to stress. Parents who have difficulty dealing with their children in this age group may themselves be experiencing midlife crises in the generativity versus stagnation phase of development. The elderly, who are in the ego integrity versus despair phase of development, are particularly susceptible to crisis because of decreases in physical and cognitive functioning, roles, and sense of purpose.

A person who has not resolved the conflicts engendered in previous phases of development may find the expectations of the current phase fraught with stress and may have a greater predisposition to crises.[13,33]

The expected transitional life crises, such as toilet training, beginning and changing schools, entering and later retiring from the work force, marriage, parenthood, the "empty nest" syndrome when children leave home, and loss through death of elderly parents, produce upheavals in roles and status and necessitate adaptation to new conditions.

Unanticipated events may affect individuals, communities, and countries. They include natural catastrophic events, such as tornadoes, floods, and earthquakes, and man-made catastrophes, such as economic depressions with unemployment and bank failures. Loss of a job and money creates a crisis not only for the person experiencing the loss but also for family members, who are suddenly faced with changes in life-style and status.

Loss or threatened loss of a loved one through an untimely death or reduced capacity to function because of an accident or illness creates havoc for all involved. Although death of any loved person is stressful, the loss of a child or young adult is especially shocking to survivors. Unanticipated traumatic stress occurs in "victim crisis," in which physically or emotionally aggressive acts are perpetrated on a person. These include persecution of an individual or group and violent crimes such as assault, rape, and murder. The crisis situation can have a lifelong effect because of the intense emotional trauma and possible irreversible physical disability such as paralysis or loss of an extremity. The person may have flashbacks in which the violence or aggressiveness of the precipitating event is reexperienced. This can happen in persons who have successfully resolved the crisis issues.

In some instances a preexisting psychopathologic condition in the person or family may be a factor in precipitating a crisis or may impair successful resolution. A person with schizophrenia, general anxiety disorder, or a personality disorder has lowered ego strength and is less able than others to resolve crises.[13,73]

Approaches to Crisis Intervention

Generally persons experiencing crises have healthy personalities, and interventions are focused on the current crisis situation. Even when an underlying psychopathologic condition exists, interventions remain issue oriented to alleviate the crisis situation; the patient can be referred later to other resources for further help. If treatment is continued to deal with problems other than those related to the crisis, interventions are no longer viewed as crisis ones.

General goals of crisis intervention are to reinforce strengths, to resolve the crisis, and to assist the patient to integrate the crisis experience into the personality. A minimum expectation of crisis intervention is the person's return to a precrisis level of functioning.

Golan[33] discusses two general approaches to crisis intervention: generic and individual. In the generic approach the intervener assumes that a specific crisis will follow a characteristic course (such as that of grief) and directs interventions toward the identified phases of the crisis situation. Little or no attention is directed toward the patient's personality and dynamics. Treatment is focused on the precipitant of the crisis, using a brief, supportive approach. Nonprofessionals or paraprofessionals such as trained volunteers at a 24-hour hotline or a crisis center are frequently charged with the responsibility for generic intervention. Although this approach is effective for many persons, dangers may exist when individual personality differences are not considered.

The individual approach also focuses on crisis issues but emphasizes in addition the personality of the individual. Stressors before the precipitating event, previous coping behaviors, and reactivated conflicts that are contributing to the current reactions are identified. Resolution includes not only relief of symptoms but also development of effective coping skills to deal with similar situations in the future.

Korner[43] presents three general approaches that can be used in crisis intervention. Emotional responses can be controlled after emotions are freely discharged through crying, yelling, and expressing anger. If anger is the only emotion experienced, it may be nonconstructive when it is used to deny fear and emotional pain but may also be constructive when it counteracts feelings of helplessness. A second approach is to enhance the patient's use of the cognitive processes and thus give the patient a sense of control. The patient is helped to remember details of the situation, including painful ones, to correct distortions, and to provide factual information when appropriate. Thus the patient gains a realistic perspective and is able to regain cognitive functioning and neutralize emotional reactions. A third approach is to allow the patient to experience security and hope through a supportive relationship. When anxiety has been reduced, the patient can begin to cope with the crisis events. The supportive approach may be particularly useful in exhaustion crisis, when the person must regain energy before beginning to deal with the crisis. Although providing support to the patient can be helpful, too much support can prolong the patient's dependence beyond a useful point. In addition, the patient may misinterpret support as sympathy or pity or perceive it as shallow. Korner's three approaches generally overlap to some extent, and depending on the patient, all three can be used during different phases of crisis intervention.

Since crisis has built-in time limits, the nurse takes an active, involved role to discover what kind of help the patient wants and the extent to which cognitive functions and emotions are out of control.[13,33] The nurse assists the patient in acute crisis in the following ways:

1. Allowing the patient to be dependent initially by satisfying basic needs such as directing the patient to a chair and giving water, tissues, damp washcloth, and so on
2. Providing the patient with opportunities to express emotions in his own way as long as it is not destructive, that is, providing a safe, supportive relationship by conveying acceptance of emotional outbursts and possibly encouraging expressions of anger
3. Increasing use of cognitive processes by helping the patient review details of stressful events and,

if appropriate, offering additional facts related to the event to expand the patient's perspective

4. Assisting the patient to examine alternative choices and the possible consequences of each choice
5. Encouraging the patient to identify supportive relationships and assisting the patient to interact with these individuals by inviting them to visit
6. Helping the patient to deal with reactions to the crisis situation such as emotional upsets and to accept and integrate the crisis experience

Support for Nurses Involved in Crisis Intervention

Because of their intense involvement with patients in crisis, nurses experience high levels of pressure and stress. The need for a fast, accurate assessment and rapid intervention requires a great expenditure of energy and can be emotionally and cognitively exhausting. Nurses continually involved in crisis interventions with patients need their own support system to deal with their responses to emotion-laden situations and to receive emotional nourishment.

PSYCHOPATHOLOGY

Psychoanalytic Theory

In psychoanalytic theory crisis is viewed as occurring in persons who have low stress tolerance and inadequate skills to deal with stressors. These persons may have been unsuccessful in resolving conflicts of early development and have not established a clear self-identity. The goals of therapy include working through unresolved conflicts related to the crisis situation and rebuilding and strengthening defenses through an intensive, long-term psychotherapeutic relationship.[73]

Interpersonal Theory

According to interpersonal theory, persons are influenced by others and their environment throughout their lives. Persons who have excluded a significant number of anxiety-provoking experiences from awareness are less able to respond to events, since these dissociated processes are no longer accessible to consciousness. These persons may have decreased ability to assess new situations, especially stressful ones, and respond to them adequately. The goals of therapy are helping the patient to perceive the situation accurately, resolve reactivated conflicts, and develop skills to deal with the situation and future stressful events. Therapy is a growth-producing experience for the patient.[2,73]

Cognitive Theory

In cognitive or learning frameworks crisis is considered to be a result of sensory overload that interrupts the cognitive processes of perceiving, thinking, decision making, and evaluating. The overload may be related to a perceived or actual bombardment with stressful stimuli the person is unable to process logically. The person's definition of the situation determines whether it is interpreted as a crisis or as a challenging, exciting experience. Thus the person's definition also determines the person's response and methods of dealing with the situation. Intervention is directed toward correcting cognitive distortions, learning new skills to resolve the problem, unlearning inappropriate thinking patterns, and reinforcing gratifying patterns of behavior.[7,33]

TREATMENT PLAN

Chemotherapeutic
Psychotherapeutic agents
Trazodone (Desyrel) for depression; 50 mg tid po; has high sedative action and low anticholinergic action
Alprazolam (Xanax) for anxiety; 0.5 mg tid po for adults; 0.25 mg tid po for elderly; belongs to benzodiazepine class of drugs; may be effective in panic attacks and purportedly in depression

Supportive
Occupational and recreational therapy after initial acute phase if patient is hospitalized and there are no contraindicating medical conditions

ASSESSMENT: AREAS OF CONCERN

Persons may seek help 1 to 2 weeks after the precipitating event; however, some do so immediately after the onset of acute crisis. These persons ask for assistance in a variety of health care facilities such as hospital emergency rooms, community agencies, including mental health centers, and private physicians' offices. Acute crisis often affects hospitalized patients and their families as the result of a change in the seriousness of an illness, discovery of a poor prognosis, family responses to the patient's illness or death, or family difficulties unrelated to the ill member.

In crisis, rapid assessment is necessary and intervention often begins before the assessment has been completed. Each person responds to crisis in an individual way.

Affect

Severe anxiety to panic; depression; anger; apathy; tearfulness to convulsive crying; feeling of alienation; emptiness; motionless state; temporary lowered self-esteem

Thoughts

Paralysis of cognitive processes; impaired recall of crisis event; misinterpretation of events; forgetfulness; blocking; confusion; indecisiveness; frustration; conflicting thoughts; denial; guilt; psychophysiologic symptom complaints; suicidal or homicidal thoughts

Power and control

Helplessness; hopelessness; vulnerability; lack of control

Activities

Paralysis or aimless, automatic behavior; agitation; tremors; stiffness of body as if trying to hold self together; clenched fists; contorted facial features; limpness of body, sometimes with impaired balance; impaired performance of tasks; regressive childlike behaviors such as tantrums

Sleep patterns

Impaired sleep; inability to sleep; restless sleep; hypersomnia

Nutrition

Change in eating pattern, such as overeating or inability to eat; picking at food; nausea; vomiting

Social interactions

Withdrawal from social support network; loosening of ties with loved ones

NURSING DIAGNOSES and NURSING INTERVENTIONS

Nursing care should be implemented selectively based on seriousness of symptoms and presenting behaviors. Because of the time limits of crisis, patients may be seen for only one or as many as eight sessions.

Nursing Diagnosis	Nursing Intervention
Anxiety: moderate to panic	Assess emotional state rapidly to determine whether acute crisis and panic state exist.
Provide quiet, nonstimulating environment.
Convey concern and caring through temporary taking charge of activities to reduce panic and loss of control; for example, direct patient to comfortable chair and provide comfort measures such as cool wet cloth, drink, and tissues.
Speak calmly in short sentences using authoritative voice.
Encourage patient to express feelings through words and behavior.
If patient is crying, acknowledge tears and offer tissues. If appropriate and acceptable to patient, reach out to touch patient.
Help identify and clarify feelings about crisis (such as despair, anger, or hopelessness) during or after expression; for example, say "Tell me what you're feeling as you're crying."
If exhaustion crisis is present, be supportive and giving to help patient regain energy.
When appropriate after initial expression of feelings of anxiety or despair, encourage expression of anger.
Identify previous painful emotions and successes in dealing with them.
Help patient develop ways to deal with current feelings, for example, relaxation techniques such as breathing slowly and deeply, diversionary activities, and talking with others about feelings.
Administer medication if ordered and as needed to relieve emotional discomfort. Briefly inform patient of effects and side effects, such as drowsiness and lightheadedness. More fully discuss effects and side effects if medication is to be continued, and emphasize need for medical follow-up.
Allow patient to pace as needed while conveying your presence and desire to help.
Observe patient closely for appearance, dress, general demeanor, and muscle tightness.
Acknowledge signs of discomfort, for example, by saying "I notice you're holding your body tightly. You seem uncomfortable."

Nursing Diagnosis	Nursing Intervention
	Encourage expression of what patient is experiencing, for example, by saying "What are you experiencing now while holding your body tightly?" Assist patient to explore meaning of behaviors such as tightness, pacing, and limpness.
	Encourage patient to become aware of behaviors and to relate behaviors to feelings and thoughts.
	If patient is in hospital, encourage participation in occupational therapy as ordered for diversion and learning new skill. (If there is no physical or emotional contraindication, recreational therapy may also be ordered to reduce anxiety, expend excess energy, and teach new skills.)
	Encourage patient to identify relaxing activities enjoyed before crisis, such as hobbies, exercises, and physical activities.
	Help patient make plans to engage in these activities or to learn new ones.
Coping, ineffective individual	Identify type of crisis (for example, anticipated or unanticipated) and precipitating event.
	In developmental crisis, assist patient to come to terms with and accept phase of life and self.
	If crisis was unanticipated, assist patient to resolve issues related to crisis and underlying conflict reactivated because of crisis events.
	Determine phase of crisis by learning duration since onset and what patient has experienced so far.
	Clarify perceptions of problem and events before crisis.
	Help patient correct distortions in perceptions and interpretation of events.
	In exhaustion crisis, when able, identify various stressors along with their patterns and use problem-solving approach to resolve issues or alleviate impact of events.
	In problem solving, help patient identify possible consequences of various choices.
	Provide factual information, as appropriate, to alter and broaden patient's perspective of issues, for example, helping patient understand crisis phases, tasks involved in patient's developmental stage, and factors related to crisis situation.
	Help patient anticipate similar events in the future and develop ways of resolving them and examining possible consequences of alternative choices.
	Assist patient to deal with long-term impact of crisis events, for example, in cancer, changes in body image such as facial disfigurement, mastectomy, or other losses.
	Assess whether physical basis exists for complaints such as headache and abdominal pain. Medication may be ordered for symptomatic relief such as analgesic for headache or antacid for gastritis.
	Help patient identify relationship between physical symptoms and anxiety or tension.
Powerlessness	Assist patient to identify sense of helplessness and aspects of events that provoked feelings.
	Convey realistic sense of hope in that alternative ways of viewing and dealing with issues exist.
	Assist patient to recall and accept previous successful coping strategies.
	Assist patient to identify strengths and areas in current situation in which patient has control, especially control over self.
	Examine problem areas in similar past events along with current situation to determine similar factors that evoke feelings of vulnerability.
	Teach coping strategies for dealing with vulnerability such as strengthening or developing defenses, avoidance, redefining situations, and relaxation techniques.
	Encourage patient to accept own strengths and resources.
Sleep pattern disturbance	Assist patient to identify sleep disturbances and what patient thinks about or does when unable to sleep.
	If patient is obsessed about problem or restless, suggest that patient get out of bed after 30 minutes and engage in relaxing, diversionary activities such as reading, watching television, and writing letters.

Nursing Diagnosis	Nursing Intervention
	Teach patient to establish relaxation routine before bedtime such as reading, watching television, or taking warm bath. Encourage patient to practice slow, deep breathing and listen to relaxation tape to promote sleep.
Nutrition, alteration in: less than body requirements	Identify changes in fluid and food intake and eating difficulties. Help identify how patient has handled eating difficulties in past. Assist patient to identify possible alternative methods, such as soft bland food, frequent small meals, and adequate fluid intake. Explore relationship between emotional discomfort and changes in eating pattern. Administer medication as ordered and needed for symptom relief, such as antacids for nausea. Inform patient that, as emotional state returns to near normal, usual eating patterns can be reestablished. Teach importance of nutritious diet and adequate fluid intake.
Social isolation	Explore social relationships and learn whom patient views as supportive. Discuss how supportive persons might be helpful now. Suggest that patient call supportive person, or if unable to call, allow you to make phone call to invite person to visit. Assist patient to rehearse sharing problems and asking for help from significant others. Explore patient's ability to ask others for help and deal with others' responses to requests. Assist patient to accept help or refusal to help from others. Evaluate overall social skills and teach as needed. If patient is in emergency room or a community agency and alone, arrange to have someone drive patient home if patient will not be hospitalized. If patient lives alone, encourage staying at someone else's home or having someone stay with patient. Identify community resources, write down names, addresses, and phone numbers, and encourage patient to use them.

Patient Education

1. To relieve any embarrassment the patient may be experiencing, teach the patient to accept emotional expressions during the acute crisis as a normal response to the stressor.
2. Reinforce the use of self-supports and support from significant others.
3. Reinforce the use of a problem-solving approach to deal with stressors.
4. Teach the importance of follow-up care after discharge.

EVALUATION

Patient Outcome	Data Indicating That Outcome is Reached
Patient evidences return to precrisis level of functioning.	Patient verbalizes awareness of events leading to crisis. Patient practices use of problem-solving approach to deal with crisis and related issues. Patient asks for and receives support from significant others. Patient verbalizes ability to cope with changes in life situation. Patient sleeps peacefully at night and awakens rested. Patient no longer experiences physical manifestations of crisis reactions.
Patient demonstrates knowledge of treatment plan.	Patient describes effects and side effects of medicine. Patient accurately states information about self-administration of prescribed medicine after discharge. Patient makes plans to continue treatment after discharge.

Medical Interventions

The major therapeutic interventions for psychiatric disturbances are counseling and drug therapy. Counseling techniques have been discussed in detail throughout this chapter. Specific chemotherapeutic interventions have been presented with each disease. A more detailed discussion of the categories and classes of drugs used is presented in Appendix C. The specific categories and classes of chemotherapeutic agents used for psychiatric disturbances include antidepressants, tranquilizers, and sedative-hypnotics.

ELECTROCONVULSIVE THERAPY

Electroconvulsive therapy (ECT) or electroshock therapy is the production of a generalized motor seizure by the application of electrical stimulation to the temporal region of the brain. The placement of the electrodes that are covered with moistened cotton pads may be bilateral or unilateral. In bilateral ECT the electrodes are applied to both temples, whereas in unilateral ECT one electrode is placed on the scalp on the patient's nondominant hemisphere, that is, the same side as the dominant hand. Unilateral ECT is thought to produce less amnesia and confusion than the bilateral treatment.[30,74] A series of ECT ranges from five to 12 treatments. They are administered every 2 to 4 days until the series prescribed is complete.

Studies have demonstrated that ECT is highly effective in certain psychiatric conditions such as agitated depressions. However, it is viewed as a controversial form of treatment, in part because of concerns about the development of organic brain disease and past misuse.[66] Studies have shown that patients recover most of their memory for events before ECT within 6 to 9 months after completion of the treatment.[30] In hospitalized patients, estimates of ECT use are 5% of depressed patients and 1% of those with schizophrenia.[74]

Mode of Action[30,66]

No consensus exists on the precise action of ECT, although it is thought to be similar to antidepressant drugs. It produces changes in the central nervous system including increase in serotonin and dopamine levels and increase in postsynaptic neurotransmitter receptor sensitivity.

Indications[30]

1. Poor response to medications
2. When containment of symptoms is needed immediately (for example, when there is high suicidal risk, severe mania, severe depression with self-care and food or fluid intake impairment, or extreme agitation and assaultiveness)
3. When medication is contraindicated because of significant medical disorders such as some cardiovascular diseases
4. Some types of schizophrenic disorders such as catatonia
5. Good response to ECT in the past

Contraindications[66]

1. Some severe cardiovascular diseases such as recent myocardial infarction
2. Active pulmonary inflammation
3. Central nervous system tumors
4. Organic brain disease

Preprocedural Care

1. If the patient has previously had ECT, encourage him to talk about experience as able to do so.
2. Explain the procedure as needed.
3. Provide opportunities to discuss fears of and hopes for the expected treatment.
4. Correct misconceptions and provide accurate information.
5. Discuss the treatments with family members, explaining the procedure as needed and correcting misconceptions.
6. On the day before initiating ECT:
   a. Check the patient's record, including physical examination, laboratory findings, and signed informed consent form by patient, family member, or guardian.
   b. Call the physician's attention to laboratory findings that differ from these normal findings:
      (1) Red blood cell count: males 4.5 to 6.2 million/μl, females 4.2 to 5.4 million/μl
      (2) Hemoglobin: males 14 to 18 g/dl, females 12 to 16 g/dl

(3) White blood cell count: 4100 to 10,900 cells/μl

(4) Urine color: straw

(5) Urine appearance: clear

(6) Urine specific gravity: 1.005 to 1.030

(7) Urine pH: 4.5 to 8.0

(8) Urine cells and protein: none

(9) Urine sugars and acetone: negative

7. On the evening before treatment:

   a. Record vital signs.

   b. Permit nothing by mouth after midnight as ordered.

8. On the morning of treatment:

   a. Record vital signs.

   b. Have patient empty bladder.

   c. Ask patient to remove dentures.

   d. Administer anticholinergic medication as ordered ½ hour before scheduled treatment (for example, atropine 0.4 mg IM).

   e. Remain with patient. Offer support in ways acceptable to patient, such as restating purpose of ECT. Allow patient to talk about expectations of treatments and other topics to help patient relax.

Procedure

1. Anesthesiologist starts intravenous therapy and administers

   a. Short-acting sedative-hypnotic, such as amobarbital (Amytal Sodium), intravenously to induce sleep

   b. Muscle relaxant such as succinylcholine (Anectine) intravenously after amobarbital

   c. 100% oxygen to assist ventilation because of muscle paralysis

2. Physician applies electrode(s) bilaterally or unilaterally to temporal region prepared with conduction jelly. Electrical stimulus is administered.

3. Since succinylcholine relaxes muscles, blood pressure cuff inflated above patient's last systolic reading is placed on the arm opposite the one with the intravenous line before administration of drug to monitor seizure activity.

4. When muscle relaxant is insufficient to prevent generalized seizure activity, nurse observes for seizure activity during treatment while protecting joints in upper and lower extremities.

5. Patient begins to awaken minutes after the treatment and is fully awake in about 20 minutes.

TREATMENT PLAN

Chemotherapeutic

Anticholinergic agents

   Scopolamine or atropine, 0.4 mg IM ½ h before ECT treatment

Supportive

Nothing by mouth after midnight before treatment

ASSESSMENT: AREAS OF CONCERN

Cognitive

Confusion; amnesia

Physical

Elevated blood pressure and pulse immediately after treatment; unsteadiness; impaired ability to meet self-care needs

NURSING DIAGNOSES and NURSING INTERVENTIONS

Nursing Diagnosis	Nursing Intervention
Sensory-perceptual alteration	Monitor blood pressure, pulse, and respirations closely until elevated pressure returns to normal and signs stabilize, and then as ordered.
	As patient begins to awaken, call by name, reassure patient by orienting to environment, and let patient know treatment is over, as by saying "Mary, you are all right. Your treatment is over. You are at City Hospital. My name is Amy. I am your nurse."
	Continue reorientation, since some amnesia will be present.
	As able, assist patient to talk about ECT and eventually to integrate negative and positive aspects of experience.
	Help family deal with patient's amnesia and their own reactions.
	Assist patient to participate in daily activities as able.
Self-care deficit: feeding, bathing, hygiene, dressing, grooming, toileting	When patient is awake, assist out of bed.
	Help with breakfast as needed.
	Give directions using short, concrete sentences.
	Assist with self-care activities.

Nursing Diagnosis	**Nursing Intervention**
	Support patient's efforts to perform self-care activities and give reassurance that patient will remember.

Patient Education

1. Reinforce participation in prescribed medical and counseling regimen after discharge.

EVALUATION

Patient Outcome	**Data Indicating That Outcome is Reached**
Patient demonstrates decrease in psychiatric symptoms.	Patient states increase in positive feelings toward self. Patient talks about positive and negative aspects of electroconvulsive therapy. Patient participates in activities with staff, family, and other patients. Patient makes plans to continue with treatment after discharge.

References

1. American Psychiatric Association: Diagnostic and statistical manual of mental disorders, ed. 3, Washington, D.C., 1980, The Association.
2. Arieti, S.: Interpretation of schizophrenia, ed. 2, New York, 1974, Basic Books, Inc., Publishers.
3. Arieti, S., and Bemporad, J.: Severe and mild depression: the psychotherapeutic approach, New York, 1978, Basic Books, Inc., Publishers.
4. Beck, A.T.: Cognitive therapy and the emotional disorders, New York, 1976, The New American Library, Inc.
5. Beck, A.T.: Beck's cognitive therapy. In Millman, H.L., Huber, J.T., and Diggins, D.R., editors: Therapies for adults, San Francisco, 1982, Jossey-Bass, Inc., Publishers.
6. Beck, A.T.: Techniques of cognitive therapy. In Goleman, D., and Speeth, K.R., editors: The essential psychotherapies: theory and practice by the masters, New York, 1982, The New American Library, Inc.
7. Beck, A.T.: et al.: Cognitive therapy of depression, New York, 1979, The Guilford Press.
8. Beels, C.C.: Social supports and schizophrenia, Schizophr. Bull. 7:58, 1981.
9. Bennett, G.: Substance abuse in adulthood. In Bennett, G., Vourakis, C., and Woolf, D.S., editors: Substance abuse: pharmacologic, developmental, and clinical perspectives, New York, 1983, John Wiley & Sons, Inc.
9a. Blos, P.: The second individuation process of adolescence. In Esman, A.H., editor: The psychology of adolescence: essential readings, New York, 1975, International Universities Press, Inc.
10. Boskind-White, M., and White, W.C., Jr.: Bulimarexia: the binge/purge cycle, New York, 1983, W.W. Norton & Co.
11. Brenner, C.: An elementary textbook of psychoanalysis, ed. rev., Garden City, N.Y., 1974, Doubleday & Co., Inc.
12. Brodsley, L.: Avoiding a crisis: the assessment, Am. J. Nurs. 82:1865, 1982.
13. Burgess, A.W., and Baldwin, B.A.: Crisis intervention theory and practice, Englewood Cliffs, N.J., 1981, Prentice-Hall, Inc.
14. Busteed, E.L., and Johnstone, C.: The development of suicide precautions for an inpatient psychiatric unit, J. Psychosoc. Nurs. Ment. Health Serv. 21(5):15, 1983.
15. Caplan, G.: An approach to community mental health, New York, 1961, Grune & Stratton, Inc.
16. Carpenter, W.T., Jr., and Stephens, J.H.: The diagnosis of mania. In Belmaker, R.H., and van Praag, H.M., editors: Mania: an evolving concept, Jamaica, N.Y., 1980, Spectrum Publications, Inc.
17. Chapman, A.H.: The treatment techniques of Harry Stack Sullivan, New York, 1978, Brunner/Mazel, Inc.
18. Chenitz, W.C.: Primary depression in older women: are current theories and treatment of depression relevant to this age group, J. Psychiatr. Nurs. Ment. Health Serv. 17(8):20, 1979.
19. Ciske, S.J.: Assessment and management of physical consequences. In Bennett, G., Vourakis, C., and Woolf, D.S., editors: Substance abuse: pharmacologic, developmental, and clinical perspectives, New York, 1983, John Wiley & Sons, Inc.
20. Cohen, L.H., and Nelson, D.W.: Crisis intervention: an overview of theory and technique. In Cohen, L.H., Claiborn, W.L., and Specter, G.A., editors: Crisis intervention, ed. 2, New York, 1983, Human Sciences Press, Inc.
21. Coleman, J.C., Butcher, J.N., and Carson, R.C.: Abnormal psychology and modern life, ed. 7, Glenview, Ill., 1984, Scott, Foresman & Co.
22. Danzinger, S.: Major treatment issues and techniques in family therapy with the borderline adolescent, J. Psychosoc. Nurs. Ment. Health Serv. 20(1):27, 1982.
23. Dixson, D.L.: Manic depression: an overview, J. Psychiatr. Nurs. Ment. Health Serv. 19(6):28, 1981.
24. Easson, W.H.: Depression in adolescence. In Feinstein, S.C., and Giovacchini, P.L., editors: Adolescent psychiatry, vol. V, New York, 1977, Jason Aronson, Inc.
25. Ellis, A.: How to live with—and without—anger, New York, 1977, Reader's Digest Press.
26. Evans, D.L.: Explaining suicide among the young: an analytical review of the literature, J. Psychosoc. Nurs. Ment. Health Serv. 20(8):9, 1982.
27. Fenichel, O.: The psychoanalytic theory of neurosis, New York, 1945, W.W. Norton & Co., Inc.
28. Finley, B.G.: The family and substance abuse. In Bennett, G., Vourakis, C., and Woolf, D.S., editors: Substance abuse: pharmacologic, developmental, and clinical perspectives, New York, 1983, John Wiley & Sons, Inc.
29. Fitzpatrick, J.J.: Suicidology and suicide prevention: historical perspectives from the nursing literature, J. Psychosoc. Nurs. Ment. Health Serv. 21(5):20, 1983.

30. Frankel, F.H.: The use of electroconvulsive therapy in suicidal patients, Am. J. Psychother. **38**:384, 1984.

31. Gagrat, D.D., and Spiro, H.R.: Social, cultural, and epidemiologic aspects of mania. In Belmaker, R.H., and van Praag, H.M., editors: Mania: an evolving concept, Jamaica, N.Y., 1980, Spectrum Publications, Inc.

32. Garfinkel, P.E., and Garner, D.M.: Anorexia nervosa: a multidimensional perspective, New York, 1982, Brunner/Mazel, Inc.

33. Golan, N.: Treatment in crisis situations, New York, 1978, The Free Press.

34. Gunderson, J.: Borderline personality, Paper presented at Conference in Akron, Ohio, December 2, 1983.

35. Haier, R.J.: The diagnosis of schizophrenia: a review of recent developments. In Special report: schizophrenia 1980, Washington, D.C., 1980, U.S. Government Printing Office.

36. Harakal, B.M.: What the SNA's are doing in Ohio, Am. J. Nurs. **82**:582, 1982.

37. Harris, E.: Dexamethasone suppression test, Am. J. Nurs. **82**:784, 1982.

38. Horner, A.J.: Object relations and the developing ego in therapy, New York, 1979, Jason Aronson, Inc.

39. Huppenbauer, S.L.: PTSD: a portrait of the problem, Am. J. Nurs. **82**:1699, 1982.

40. Kiecolt-Glaser, J., and Dixson, K.: Postadolescent onset male anorexia, J. Psychosoc. Nurs. Ment. Health Serv. **22**(1):10, 1984.

41. Klerman, G.L., and Weissman, M.M.: Depressions among women: their nature and causes. In Guttentag, M., Salasin, S., and Belle, D., editors: The mental health of women, New York, 1980, Academic Press, Inc.

42. Kolb, L.C., and Brodie, H.K.H.: Modern clinical psychiatry, ed. 10, Philadelphia, 1982, W.B. Saunders Co.

43. Korner, I.N.: Crisis reduction and the psychological consultant. In Spector, G.A., and Claiborn, W.L., editors: Crisis intervention, vol. 2, New York, 1973, Behavioral Publications, Inc.

44. Kramer, R., and Weiner, I.: Psychiatry on the borderline, Psychology Today **17**:70, 1983.

45. Kurose, K., et al.: A standard care plan for alcoholism, Am. J. Nurs. **81**:1001, 1981.

46. Levenkron, S.: Treating and overcoming anorexia nervosa, New York, 1982, Charles Scribner's Sons.

47. Luckmann, N.J., and Sorensen, K.C.: Medical-surgical nursing: a psychophysiologic approach, ed. 2, Philadelphia, 1980, W.B. Saunders Co.

48. Lukoff, D., et al.: Life events, familial stress, and coping in the developmental course of schizophrenia, Schizophr. Bull. **10**:258, 1984.

49. Mahler, M.S., Pine, F., and Bergman, A.: The psychological birth of the human infant, New York, 1975, Basic Books, Inc., Publishers.

49a. Mahoney, M.J., and Arnkoff, D.B.: Cognitive and self-control therapies. In Garfield, S.K., and Bergin, A.E., editors: Handbook of psychotherapy and behavioral change: an empirical analysis, ed. 2, New York, 1978, John Wiley & Sons, Inc.

50. Mark, B.: Hospital treatment of borderline patients: toward a better understanding of problematic issues, J. Psychiatr. Nurs. Ment. Health Serv. **18**(8):25, 1980.

51. May, R.: Power and innocence: a search for the sources of violence, New York, 1972, W.W. Norton & Co., Inc.

52. May, R.: The meaning of anxiety, ed. rev., New York, 1977, W.W. Norton & Co., Inc.

53. Meissner, W.W.: The paranoid process, New York, 1978, Jason Aronson, Inc.

54. Meissner, W.W.: The schizophrenic and the paranoid process, Schizophr. Bull. **7**:611, 1981.

55. Mirin, S.M., and Weiss, R.D.: Substance abuse. In Bassuk, E.L., Schoonover, S.C., and Gelenberg, A.J., editors: The practitioner's guide to psychoactive drugs, ed. 2, New York, 1983, Plenum Medical Book Co.

56. Mullahy, P., and Mellinek, M.: Interpersonal psychiatry, New York, 1983, Spectrum Publications, Inc.

57. Naegle, M.A.: The nurse and alcoholic: redefining an historically ambivalent relationship, J. Psychosoc. Nurs. Ment. Health Serv. **21**(6):17, 1983.

58. Neuman, P.A., and Halvorson, P.A.: Anorexia nervosa and bulimia: a handbook for counselors and therapists, New York, 1983, Van Nostrand Reinhold Co., Inc.

59. Pao, P.: Schizophrenic disorders: theory and treatment from a psychodynamic point of view, New York, 1979, International Universities Press, Inc.

60. Petrie, K., and Chamberlain, K.: Hopelessness and social desirability as moderator variables in predicting suicidal behavior, J. Counseling Clin. Psychol. **51**:485, 1983.

61. Platt-Koch, L.M.: Borderline personality disorder: a therapeutic approach, Am. J. Nurs. **83**:1666, 1983.

62. Quayle, D.: American productivity: the devastating effect of alcoholism and drug abuse, Am. Psychol. **38**:454, 1983.

63. Richman, J.: The family therapy of attempted suicide, Fam. Process **18**:131, 1979.

64. Rudolph, E.: Anorexia nervosa: some multigenerational hypotheses, Family **9**:43, 1981.

65. Sanger, E., and Cassino, T.: Eating disorders: avoiding the power struggle, Am. J. Nurs. **84**:31, 1984.

66. Schoonover, S.C.: Depression. In Bassuk, E.L., Schoonover, S.C., and Gelenberg, A.J., editors: The practitioner's guide to psychoactive drugs, ed. 2, New York, 1983, Plenum Medical Book Co.

67. Seligman, M.E.P.: Helplessness: on depression, development, and death, San Francisco, 1975, W.H. Freeman & Co.

68. Shapiro, S.A.: Contemporary theories of schizophrenia: review and synthesis, New York, 1981, McGraw-Hill Book Co.

69. Shneidman, E.S.: Suicide. In Freeman, A.M., Kaplan, H.I., and Sadock, B.J., editors: Comprehensive textbook of psychiatry II, ed. 2, Baltimore, 1975, The Williams & Wilkins Co.

70. Stone, M.H.: The borderline syndromes, New York, 1980, McGraw-Hill Book Co.

71. Sullivan, H.S.: The interpersonal theory of psychiatry, New York, 1953, W.W. Norton & Co., Inc.

72. Sullivan, H.S.: Schizophrenia as a human process, New York, 1962, W.W. Norton & Co., Inc.

72a. Taylor, C.T.: Mereness' essentials of psychiatric nursing, ed. 11, St. Louis, 1982, The C.V. Mosby Co.

73. Umana, R.F., Gross, S.F., and McConville, M.T.: Crisis in the family: three approaches, New York, 1980, Gardner Press, Inc.

74. Weiner, R.D.: Electroconvulsive therapy: contemporary issues, Carrier Foundation Letter, No. 105, March, 1985.

75. Wekstein, L.: Handbook of suicidology: principles, problems and practice, New York, 1979, Brunner/Mazel, Inc.

76. Williams, J.B.W., and Wilson, H.S.: A psychiatric nursing perspective on DSM-III, J. Psychosoc. Nurs. Ment. Health Serv. **20**(4):14, 1982.

77. Woolf, D.S.: CNS depressants: alcohol. In Bennett, G., Vourakis, C., and Woolf, D.S., editors: Substance abuse: pharmacologic, developmental, and clinical perspectives, New York, 1983, John Wiley & Sons, Inc.

PART TWO

Nursing Diagnoses

Self-Perception– Self-Concept

The self-perception–self-concept pattern involves one's consciousness of being, of existence. "Clients have perceptions and concepts of themselves, such as body image, social self, self-competency, and subjective mood states. . . . The objective of assessment in this pattern area is to describe the client's pattern of beliefs and evaluations regarding general self-worth and feeling states."[1]

An initial attempt at grouping nursing diagnoses under functional health pattern areas is described by Gordon.[1] Included under the self-perception–self-concept pattern are fear and disturbance in self-concept. Anxiety was added to this list because it is so closely linked to fear. Powerlessness was added because it concerns one's perception of whether or not one's own actions will affect an outcome. As work on the taxonomy continues, other arrangements for clustering the diagnostic labels will undoubtedly evolve.

Reference

1. Gordon, M.: Nursing diagnosis: process and application, New York, 1982, McGraw-Hill Book Co.

SELF-CONCEPT, DISTURBANCE IN: BODY IMAGE, SELF-ESTEEM, ROLE PERFORMANCE, PERSONAL IDENTITY

THEORY AND ETIOLOGY

Man's self-concept has profound effects upon his thinking processes, emotions, behaviors, desires, values, and goals. To understand man, one must understand his self-concept and the standards by which he judges himself.[5]

Importance of Self-Concept

The assessment and nursing management of patients who demonstrate disturbances in self-concept are extremely important. In clinical practice nurses are frequently confronted with patients who have a disturbed body image, lack of self-esteem, role performance difficulties, and problems with personal identity. Since a person's self-concept is the single most significant key to understanding his behavior, nurses must incorporate strategies into their plans of care to evaluate and enhance patients' self-concept. Combs, Avila, and Purkey[6] stressed the importance of self-concept in the helping professions by stating that to ignore self-concept and its impact upon behavior seriously hinders a practitioner's therapeutic effectiveness, and that "patients judge the value of their experiences with helpers from the frame of reference of the self-concept."

Fitts[13] emphasized the importance of self-concept in relation to the rehabilitation and self-actualization of individuals. He stated:

> . . . Self concept is the frame of reference through which the individual interacts with his world. Thus, the self concept is a powerful influence in human behavior. We can never completely understand another person's actions or perfectly predict his behavior, but knowledge of his self concept can advance such understanding and prediction. The rehabilitation of individuals is dependent upon the understanding and prediction of their behavior. If the self concept is a means toward better understanding and prediction of behavior, then it should be a significant variable in rehabilitation.

Since rehabilitation of patients—returning patients to their maximum level of independent functioning—is one of the main concerns of nursing, aspects relating to patients' self-concept need to be addressed when planning care. Roy's work[32] in the area of a conceptual adaptation model for nursing practice stresses the importance of self-concept. In describing the relevance of self-concept to adaptation and nursing, Roy contended that, if nurses have a framework for assessing patients' self-concept, they will be better able to predict potential problems in temporary or permanent adaptations to stressful situations along the health-illness continuum. In addition, nurses would be better able to help patients use the strengths of their self-concept to cope with these situations. In turn, nurses would be promoting patients' adaptation skills.

In summary, self-concept is (1) the most prominent aspect of an individual's perceptual world; (2) a stable feature in humans that is learned from experience but that can be modified through intervention; (3) a central construct that facilitates one's ability to understand individuals and to predict their behavior; (4) an idea that influences how one confronts and manages the emergencies of daily living; and (5) a primary concern for nurses who care for patients.

Theories of Self-Concept

Several divergent schools of thought have defined and explained the development of self-concept. A controversy still remains as to its definition and formulation. Efforts describing self-concept date back to the late nineteenth century literature of social philosophers and psychologists such as Pierce,[29] James,[16] and Balwin.[2] These individuals, prior to the symbolic interactionism movement, emphasized self as a product and reflection of social life. In the early twentieth century, when the theory of symbolic interactionism evolved, theorists such as Cooley,[8] James,[17] Mead,[26] Lecky,[20] Rogers,[30] Sullivan,[34] Combs and Snygg,[7] and Kinch[19] attempted to define self-

concept within the theoretical framework of symbolic interactionism. Other theorists of the late twentieth century who have attempted to explore the notion of self and self-concept include Sarbin,[33] Allport,[1] Epstein,[11] and Driever.[10] A summary of how each of these theorists views the nature of self-concept is presented.

Cooley[8] is credited with being the first symbolic interactionist, and he introduced the concept of *looking-glass self,* which refers to an individual perceiving himself in the way others perceive him. He posited that self is inseparable from social life and necessarily involves some reference to others. He believed that concepts of self from early childhood developed from seeing how others responded to us. "In the presence of one whom we feel to be of importance there is a tendency to enter into and adopt by sympathy his judgment of one self" (p. 175). He stated that self can be designated by the pronouns *I, me, my, mine,* and *myself,* and that which is labeled by the individual as self produces stronger emotions than what is labeled as nonself. He stressed that it is only through subjective feelings that self can be identified.

James[17] identified two different theoretical approaches to the theory of self: self as a knower and self as an object of knowledge. He saw no value to self as a knower for understanding behavior and felt it should be placed in the realm of philosophy. He valued self as an object of knowledge and felt that it consisted of whatever the individual viewed as belonging to himself. He stated that self as an object of knowledge consists of three empirical selves: material self (an individual's own body, family, and possessions), social self (how others view the individual), and spiritual self (an individual's emotions and desires). He viewed self as having unity as well as being differentiated and saw it as intimately associated with emotions as mediated through self-esteem.

Mead[26] expanded on Cooley's looking-glass self. He highlighted the development of the ability to take the role of the *generalized other,* i.e., one's whole sociocultural environment, and particularly to perceive the attitude of the other toward the perceiver as essential to the genesis of self. He amplified the view of self as a product of social interaction by stating: "The individual experiences himself as such, not directly, but only indirectly, from the particular standpoints of other individuals of the same social group, or from the generalized standpoint of the social group as a whole to which he belongs." He indicated that by incorporating estimates of how the generalized other might respond to certain actions, the individual acquires a source of internal regulation, which serves to guide his behavior in the absence of external pressures.

Lecky[20] identified self-concept as the nucleus of one's

personality. He stressed that it plays a key role in determining which concepts are acceptable for assimilation into one's overall personality organization. The major motive for this selective assimilation is to maintain unity and preservation of personality organization.

Rogers[30] postulated that self-concept includes only those characteristics an individual is aware of and over which he believes he exercises control. He believed that persons have a basic need to maintain and enhance self and that threats to the organization of self-concept produce anxiety. If the threat and subsequent anxiety cannot be defended against, catastrophic disorganization to a person's self-concept will result.

Sarbin[33] noted that behavior is organized around cognitive structures, one of which is the structure of self. He stated that self was hierarchically organized and subject to change, usually from lower to higher order constructs. He indicated that self can be divided into three selves: empirical self, somatic self, and social self. An *I*, or *pure ego*, serves as the cross section of an individual's total cognitive organization, including his different selves, at any moment in time.

Sullivan's beliefs[34] were similar to those of Cooley[8] and Mead[26] in that self arises out of social interaction. However, unlike Cooley and Mead, he emphasized that interactions with significant others (especially the mother figure), rather than interactions with society at large, are the key to formulating a person's self-concept. He identified significant others as those who provide rewards and punishments in a person's life. Based on these reward and punishment interactions, the person forms a *reflected appraisal* of himself. Thus how a person is treated and judged by significant others influences and determines how he perceives himself.

Allport[1] questioned the need for the construct of self-concept and felt that all activities and relationships could be explained without ever referring to it. Instead he coined the word *proprium* and defined it as "all the regions of our life that we regard as peculiarly ours." According to Allport, a person's proprium consists of those aspects which he regards as centrally important and which contribute to his sense of inward unity.

The pivotal point in the Combs and Snygg[7] theory of self-concept is perception. What one thinks and how one behaves are largely determined by the beliefs one holds about oneself and one's abilities. They stressed that each person continuously tries to achieve an adequate concept of self to preserve psychic integrity and that perceptions of self influence behavior. For these two theorists, self-concept is a basic variable that affects and controls our perceptions and eventual behaviors. In turn these perceptions and behaviors affect our concept of self, setting into place a perpetual circular pattern regarding the for-

mation and existence of one's self-concept. They describe the nature of self-concept in three parts: (1) *inner cell of the self-concept*, which includes those perceptions about self which are most vital, fundamental, and significant; (2) *phenomenal self*, which encompasses all of 1 plus those perceptions an individual holds about self that are not significant; and (3) *perceptual field of the self-concept*, which encompasses all of 1 and 2 plus those perceptions which are outside the self (the *not* self). They postulated the following characteristics of the phenomenal self: (1) perceptions of the phenomenal self have the feeling of being very real to the individual, but an individual is never fully able to perceive the total organization of his self-perceptions and only perceives those concepts of self which emerge from time to time as he attempts to satisfy needs; (2) perceptions of self vary in intensity and sharpness for the individuals; and (3) phenomenal self has a high degree of stability and consistency and is very resistive to change.

Kinch[19] summarized and systematized symbolic interaction theory and stated that self involves the interrelationship of four components: our self-concept, our perception of others' attitudes and responses to us, the actual attitudes and responses of others to us, and our behavior.

Epstein[11] defined self-concept as self-theory. He stated: "It is a theory that an individual has unwittingly constructed about himself as an experiencing, functioning individual, and it is part of a broader theory which he holds with respect to his entire range of significant experiences." He stressed that the major purposes for self-theory are to "optimize the pleasure/pain balance of an individual over the course of a life time . . . facilitate the maintenance of self-esteem, and organize the data of experience in a manner that can be coped with effectively."

Driever[10] incorporated many of the essential elements identified by past symbolic interactionist phenomenologists and behaviorists in defining self-concept. She stated that "self-concept is the composite of beliefs and feelings one holds about one self at a given point in time, formed from perceptions, particularly of others' reactions, and directing one's behavior." She believed that self-concept was an ongoing process that directed behavior.

A synthesis of the theories just presented shows that the major characteristics associated with self-concept are as follows:

1. It is inseparable from social life and develops out of experience, particularly out of social interaction with significant others.
2. It is perpetual and circular in its formation and existence. It affects and controls our perceptions and behaviors over time.

3. It contains different empirical selves, namely a material or body self, a social self, and a spiritual self.

4. It is the nucleus of one's personality and plays a key role in determining which perceptions and experiences are acceptable for assimilation into one's overall personality organization.

5. It is essential to the psychic functioning of an individual to maintain the organization of self-concept. When the organization of an individual's self-concept is threatened, the individual experiences anxiety. If the threat and subsequent anxiety cannot be defended against and are prolonged, catastrophic personality disorganizations results.

6. It is a dynamic organization that changes with the assimilation of new experiences. However, once the phenomenal self is established, it serves as the fundamental frame of reference for an individual and therefore has a high degree of stability and consistency.

7. It has two main functions: (1) it organizes the data of daily living experiences, especially those involving social interactions, into predictable sequences of action and reaction; and (2) it attempts to fulfill needs while minimizing disapproval and anxiety.

A conceptual formulation of self-concept is presented in Fig. 1. The circle represents a person's self-concept as an open system with arrows going in both directions to demonstrate that self-concept development is a continuous process. Self-concept is viewed as developing from perceptions of inner, phenomenal, and perceptual-field self as described by Combs and Snygg.[7] The circle is divided into four quadrants to show that self-concept consists of four selves: physical self (body image), psychologic self (personal identity, self-esteem), social self (role performance), and moral self (spiritual beliefs and values). The large circle reflects variables that influence a person's self-concept and that can produce tension and stress, resulting in subsequent anxiety and eventual disorganization of a person's self-concept. These variables are physical and personality characteristics present at birth, family and environmental factors, and emotional-social-cultural interactive experiences.

Etiology

At the Third and Fourth National Conferences on the Classification of Nursing Diagnoses four components of self-concept were identified: body image, self-esteem, role performance, and personal identity. These four com-

Fig. 1

Conceptual formulation of self-concept.

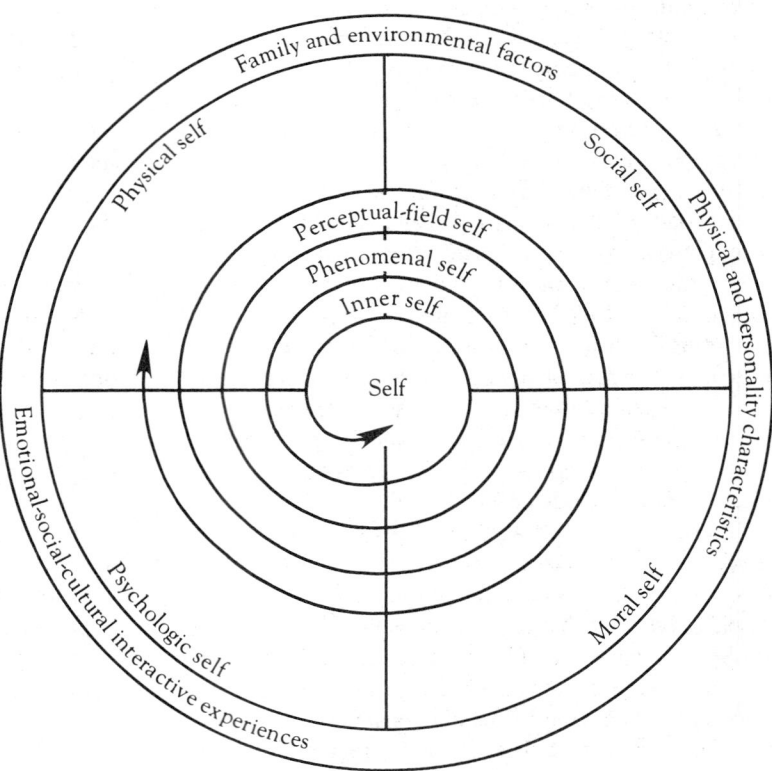

ponents are discussed in relation to their etiological development.

Disturbance in body image. The development of a person's body image is a continuous process that does not end with childhood or adolescence but rather continues to develop and change throughout a person's life cycle. As an individual's physical appearance changes, as in adolescence and aging, the person strives to readjust his body image and integrate these changes into the overall self-concept. If this process is completed without disruption, the person's body image becomes consistent with reality. If a person fails to adjust and integrate the body image in relation to accompanying physiologic changes, disturbances in body image can result.

McCloskey[24] identified two major types of body image (body boundary) disturbances in hospitalized patients. Such a condition exists when, through accident or surgery, "the body wall changes but the patient keeps the old body boundary." Examples of this type of disturbance include phantom limb pain after amputation and colostomy or mastectomy patients who have not adjusted well to the new and changed body wall image. The second type of disturbance occurs when "the patient changes a body boundary even though his body wall remains intact."[24] Examples of this include a stroke patient who is unaware that a portion of his body is paralyzed and remains unaware in spite of efforts to make him conscious of it, and the schizophrenic patient whose ego boundaries (body boundaries) have become distorted, resulting in an inability to discriminate between stimuli coming from inside and that coming from outside the self.

Potential for disturbance in body image is especially heightened in adolescence. Adolescents often go through a stage of narcissism during which they reevaluate themselves in light of new physical changes and sensations. This period is often characterized by feelings of irritability, self-aggrandizement, and overdramatized self-perception. Adolescents continuously compare themselves to peers and become overly concerned with body image because of common problems such as acne, obesity, and dysmenorrhea.

In summary, major etiological factors associated with disturbance in body image include the following:

1. Cognitive-perceptual difficulties
2. Inability to adjust to and integrate body changes

The latter may be the result of accompanying physiologic or psychologic changes or to changes in body wall (structure) or body boundary (function).

Disturbance in self-esteem. The terms *self-concept* and *self-esteem* are often used interchangeably yet are defined differently by various authorities. In defining self-esteem Rogers[31] stated: "Self-esteem is the estimate one places on oneself. It is the single most crucial value judgment for an individual's ultimate psychologic de-

velopment and motivation." Integrated within the concept of self-esteem are the characteristics of self-worth, self-respect, self-approval, and self-confidence.

How a person develops self-esteem is contingent on the number of repetitive positive experiences encountered in interactions with significant others in the environment. Sullivanian theory stressed the importance of the parental relationship and the reflected appraisal the child receives from parents. Rogers related[31]:

. . . The state of a person's self-esteem is not the product of a single issue or happening but is formed gradually over time. Therefore the collapse of self-esteem is not something which is reached in a day or even a month. It is the cumulative result of a long succession of failures. . . . Self-esteem represents the reputation a person has acquired within himself.

In examining the etiology of how a person develops low self-esteem one realizes that it occurs through repeated negative experiences and attacks on self-worth, self-respect, self-confidence, and self-appraisal systems.

Maslow[23] postulated that all people have a need to esteem or value themselves and that positive values of self help persons seek and deal with their environmental experiences constructively. A person with a low value of self tends to perceive environmental stimuli as negative and threatening. In turn, the ability to deal with environmental experiences positively is disrupted in an effort to ward off further threats to an already damaged self-esteem.

To repeat, major etiological factors associated with disturbance in self-esteem include the following:

1. Repeated negative interpersonal experiences with significant others
2. Cognitive-perceptual difficulties

Disturbance in role performance. Meleis developed a conceptual framework relating role theory to the nursing process. She stressed the importance of role and its relevance to nursing by stating[27]:

Role as a sociopsychological construct is particularly useful in assessing nursing problems and in planning nursing intervention modalities. Because professional nurses deal with clients as biopsychosocial beings, the ability to understand the behavior of clients is imperative for making appropriate diagnosis and intervention. Nurses and other health workers can no longer separate psychosocial influences on clients' health and wellbeing. In caring for patients, nurses encounter numerous situations of role change, such as the transition from wellness to illness, birth, or death. Nurses, therefore, are in the most opportune position to assess the client's psychosocial needs during role transitional periods and provide the necessary interventions based upon the individual's needs and deprivations created by role transitions.

Currently three schools of thought exist in the area of role theory. The Lintonian approach views roles as culturally given prescriptions.[21] The second view indicates that roles can be defined in terms of actions and expectations of individual members of society.[28] The third school of thought contends that roles stem from interactions with others in a social system.[3,15]

After examining the importance of role in relation to self-concept, Meleis[27] indicated that through social interaction and role-taking processes with significant others, each person's roles are discovered, created, defined, and modified. In turn these roles become incorporated into a person's self-concept. The roles that one chooses to assume become a reflection of how one perceives oneself. In conceiving the function of roles as stemming from interaction with others in a social system, Meleis reported[27]:

The role that the actor elects to play is a derivative of his voluntary actions that are motivated by the returns expected, and, indeed, received from others. In addition, the role assumed by an interactant in a given situation is validated when others indicated acceptance of that role allocation. Thus, roles chosen by the patient are validated by the acceptance of his significant others such as the nurse. . . .

Problems associated with role functioning include role insufficiency, role distance, interrole conflict, intrarole conflict, and role failure. These role-functioning problems are defined as follows:

1. *Role insufficiency:* Occurs whenever an individual has difficulty in the cognizance and/or performance of a role or of the sentiments and goals associated with the role behavior as perceived by the self or by significant others.[27]
2. *Role distance:* Implies that an individual demonstrates both instrumental and expressive behavior appropriate to his role, but these behaviors differ significantly from prescribed behaviors for the role.[22]
3. *Interrole conflict:* Occurs when the individual demonstrates instrumental and expressive behaviors incompatible with the expected behaviors for his role as a result of occupancy of one or more roles that require incompatible expected behaviors.[22]
4. *Intrarole conflict:* Occurs when the individual demonstrates instrumental and expressive behaviors incompatible with the expected behaviors for his role as a result of incompatible expectations from one or more persons in the environment concerning his expected behavior.[22]
5. *Role failure:* Occurs when there is an absence of feelings or expressive behavior and/or a lack of action or instrumental behaviors.[22]

Each of these role functioning problems can develop in relation to developmental transitions (such as moving from adulthood to old age, accompanied by gerontologic problems relating to identity, retirement, and chronic illness), situational transitions (such as the addition or loss of a member of the family through birth or death or transition from nonparental to parental status), and health-illness transitions (such as going from a well state to an acute or chronic illness state). Each of these role transitions denotes a change in role relationships, expectations, and abilities. To adjust successfully to the role transitions, an individual must be able to incorporate new knowledge, alter expressive and instrumental behaviors, and thus change the concept of self. If a person cannot adjust to these encountered role transitions, several types of role-functioning problems can result.

In sum, major etiological factors associated with disturbance in role performance include the following:
1. Absence of significant role models
2. Cognitive-perceptual difficulties
3. Inability to learn new role-functioning behaviors in response to developmental, situational, and health-illness transitions.

Disturbance in personal identity. This component of self-concept refers to how a person recognizes himself as a unique being, separate from the rest of the world. In psychoanalytic theory it concerns a person's ability to distinguish self from nonself. In Freudian terminology it is a person's ego.

Personal identity formation is greatly influenced by an individual's developmental needs, capabilities, consistent role models, identifications, and successful ego defenses.[36] Its development starts in early infancy when the child begins to differentiate self from the environment. Through this differential process the child begins to experience his own separateness and uniqueness from the rest of the world. It is through personal identity that one recognizes what belongs to self. If this process of differentiation does not occur (for example, if a pathologic symbiotic relationship exists between the child and mother, from which the child never learns or experiences separateness and autonomy from the mother), the person's ego becomes fused, or undifferentiated. The person then loses a sense of coherent self with a resultant inability to actualize abilities. There are accompanying feelings of confusion and indecisiveness.

The concept of personal identity in relation to psychosexual development has been addressed by Freud,[14] Erikson,[12] and Sullivan.[34] Each perceived personal identity as evolving on a developmental continuum with successful resolution resulting in the development of integrated psycho-social-sexual behaviors. If the process of a person's psychosexual development is interfered with, several problems may result, such as unsuccessful resolution of Oedipus or Electra complexes, verbalizations of feelings of uncertainty, dissatisfaction, and confusion about sexual identification and preference.

When examining personal identity from a nonpsychoanalytic framework, one realizes that personal identity concerns can sometimes be associated with developmental life crises. For example, in adolescence the individual experiences personal identity concerns such as "Who am I?" and "What direction is my life taking?" In midlife persons become concerned with what accomplishments they have made in life. Concerns of this nature are normal, but if the person becomes overly anxious, resolution of problems may require professional intervention.

In summary, major etiological factors associated with disturbance in personal identity include the following:
1. Poor ego differentiation
2. Faulty resolution of Oedipus or Electra complexes
3. Biochemical body changes

DEFINING CHARACTERISTICS*

Subjective	Objective
Body Image	
Change in life-style	Missing body part
Fear of rejection by others	Actual change in structure and/or function
Focus on past strength, function, or appearance	Not looking at body part
Negative feelings about body	Not touching body part
Feelings of helplessness, hopelessness, or powerlessness	Hiding or overexposing body part (intentional or unintentional)
Feelings of depersonalization and/or derealization	Trauma to nonfunctioning part
Feelings of grandiosity relating to physical size and strength	Change in social involvement
Preoccupation with change or loss	Change in ability to estimate spatial relationship of body to environment
Emphasis on remaining strengths, heightened achievement	Inability to discriminate stimuli from inside or outside self (loss of ego boundaries)
Extension of body boundary to incorporate environmental objects	Inability to accept a change in body wall (such as a patient with an amputation, mastectomy, colostomy)
Personalization of part or loss by name	Inability to accept a change in body boundaries (such as a stroke patient who is unaware of his paralysis despite efforts to make him conscious of it)
Depersonalization of part or loss by use of impersonal pronouns	
Refusal to verify actual change	
Self-Esteem	
Feelings of hopelessness, helplessness, powerlessness, despair, guilt, inferiority, inadequacy, failure, defeatism, frustration, disappointment, worthlessness, and isolation	Appearance of signs of depression: psychomotor retardation, retarded thought processes, lack of energy, etc.
Expression of suicide intention with accompanying feelings of sadness, loss, depression, anxiety, and anger	Slouched or drooping posture
Frequent expression of body aches and pains and an overconcern with somatic woes	Anorexia or obesity
Perception of minimal strengths and assets with refusal to accept positive feedback	Withdrawal from activities and interpersonal-social relationships
Denial of past and present successes and accomplishments	Decrease in sexual relationships and drive
Frequent ruminations of past problems	Decrease in motivation and spontaneous behavior
Fear of handling change, making decisions, taking risks, expressing anger, and relating to others	Inability to communicate one's needs and concerns, to defend oneself, and to confront and overcome difficulties
Feelings of self-deprecation, inadequacy, and self-dislike; judging self harshly and punitively	Homicidal and/or suicidal behavior
Self accusation	Inability to initiate, follow through, or complete task in a timely fashion
	Inability to assume responsibilites for self-care
	Inability to accept and/or extreme sensitivity to criticism
	Avoiding situations of self-disclosure; tending to assume passive, nonparticipatory roles; tending to be a wallflower in social situations
	Misperception and misinterpretation of real self from self-ideal
	Nonparticipation in therapy
	Lack of eye contact
Role Performance	
Feelings of grief, loss, powerlessness, anger, anxiety, depression, and withdrawal	Denial of role
Lack of knowledge of role	Failure to assume role (role failure)
Change in self-perception or role	Conflict in roles:
	Behaviors that are appropriate for the role but that differ from prescribed behaviors for the role (role distance)

*References 9, 18, 22, 24, 25, 27.

Subjective	Objective
Change in others' perception of role Dislike of role Ambivalence of role	Behaviors that are incompatible with the expected role due to the occupancy of one or more roles that require incompatible expected behaviors (interrole conflict) Behaviors that are incompatible with the expected role due to incompatible expectations from one or more persons in the environment concerning the expected behavior(s) (intrarole conflict) Change in physical capacity to resume role Change in usual patterns or responsibility Lack of knowledge of how to perform role (role insufficiency)
Personal Identity Feelings of confusion, uncertainty; indecisiveness about one's sense of self, purpose, and direction in life Feelings of anxiety, dissatisfaction, depression, and confusion over one's sexual identity and sexual preference	Distorted or blurred ego boundaries Demonstration of dependent behaviors (inability to make decisions, fear of making changes, uncertainty, inability to articulate one's feelings, clinging to others) Sexual behaviors and/or mannerisms that are in conflict with one's sexual preference

NURSING INTERVENTIONS

Patient Goal	Nursing Intervention*
Body Image Maintain a positive, accepting, and realistic body image.	Assess the patient's perception of his body image. What aspects of his body does he find pleasing? Not pleasing? Explore with the patient how he came to perceive his body image as negative (as in past experiences with significant others). Acknowledge and give positive reinforcement whenever the patient attempts to improve personal body image (for example, improved hygiene, wearing make-up, wearing new clothes, wearing cosmetic devices after disfiguring surgery). Help the patient to realistically accept and value his present physical self. Stress that certain physical characteristics of a person cannot be changed but that a person has other, more important, positive strengths unique to that individual. List these strengths with the patient. Teach the patient ways he might go about improving his body image (such as how to dress, apply makeup, perform exercises to improve physical tone, use cosmetic devices).
Accept the body wall or body boundary change and incorporate the change into body image and self-concept.	If a patient has had an amputation, mastectomy, colostomy, or stroke and is experiencing a body boundary disturbance because of a change in body wall or body boundary, the following interventions should be used: 1. Encourage the patient to verbalize his feelings of concern, anger, anxiety, loss, and fear over the change in his body wall or body boundary. 2. Encourage the patient to verbalize and explore his feelings regarding what impact the missing body part or changed body boundary has had on his assuming activities of daily living (family, work, and social relationships). 3. Encourage the patient to look at and touch the changed body wall or body boundary area. Ask the patient to verbalize feelings after performing these behaviors. 4. Encourage the patient to assume normal social activities as soon as possible without hiding or overexposing the changed body wall area. 5. Reinforce to the patient the reality of the changed body wall or body boundary area and that it may or may not be permanent. 6. Encourage the patient to use rehabilitative and physical therapy services to improve functioning of the affected body wall or body boundary area. 7. Encourage the patient to use cosmetic services available for disfiguring surgery and mechanical devices for improved functioning of the affected body boundary area.

*References 4, 22, 24, 25, 27, 31, 35, 36.

Patient Goal	Nursing Intervention
	8. Encourage the patient to use support services or reference groups in the community (such as a visit by a former colostomy, mastectomy, or stroke patient).
Reintegrate ego functions and boundaries so that they are congruent with reality and self-concept.	When ego boundaries become distorted and the patient no longer can discriminate between inside and outside stimuli, the following interventions should be used:
	1. Provide the patient with a structured, quiet, nonstimulating environment. As the person's ego strength improves, increase environmental stimuli.
	2. Help the patient to discriminate between real and unreal environmental and internal stimuli.
	3. Encourage the patient to verbalize his feelings and anxieties over his distorted perceptions of reality.
	4. Reinforce and maintain the patient's contact with reality. Engage him in reality-oriented activities.
	5. Encourage the patient to participate in all treatment modalities (pharmacologic therapy, individual or group therapies, etc.). Discuss the therapeutic benefits of these modalities.
	6. When the patient has regained control of his ego boundaries, encourage him to critically examine and evaluate what caused him to experience a disturbance in his body boundaries.

Self-Esteem

Patient Goal	Nursing Intervention
Improve and maintain a constructive level of self-esteem.	Communicate acceptance of the patient as a worthwhile, trusted human being who has intrinsic value.
	Show genuine interest in and concern for the patient. Spend time with the patient in groups and in one-to-one relationships.
	Avoid judgmental attitudes when working with the patient. Do not criticize or belittle the patient's feelings, actions, or ideas.
	Assist the patient in developing an attitude of not always having to be perfect to feel adequate and good about oneself. Point out that he is as worthy as anyone else despite imperfections.
	Encourage the patient to identify his strengths, assets, and potential and how they are currently being used.
	Help the patient to list his current and past successes.
	Encourage the patient to identify and participate in experiences he finds satisfying and rewarding.
	Encourage the patient to develop new interpersonal and social skills and to initiate activities in which he will be reasonably successful.
	Encourage the patient to participate in various treatment modalities (such as group or family therapy) in which support, acceptance, and the concern of others are the major emphases, and in which the patient learns that he is not alone in experiencing fears and failures.
	Teach the patient assertive techniques and communication skills such as:
	1. Use of "I" statements
	2. Conveying clear expectations of others
	3. Use of negotiation as a viable tactic
	4. Use of body posture, facial expression, and tone of voice consistent with verbal communication
	5. Remaining firm but gentle and unyielding when appropriate
	Encourage the patient to accept responsibility for his own personal opinions and behavior and to evaluate their outcome in relation to the options available.
	Encourage the patient to identify his disappointments and dissatisfactions. In turn, have the patient develop constructive problem-solving steps, with action behaviors and realistic time frames and goals to successfully lessen or correct these problem areas. Encourage the patient to use this same approach when confronted with future problems.
	Offer supportive, positive, and genuine comments and feedback to the patient when appropriate. Focus on specific changes in his behavior and appearance when making these statements. Offer positive reinforcers for actual achievements. Avoid false praise.
	Maintain a therapeutic environment that will foster the patient's level of self-esteem. Emphasis should be on:
	1. Helping the patient recognize that self-respect is first related to one's ability to respect self and then to respect and understand others

Patient Goal	Nursing Intervention
	2. One's feelings of self-worth need to be based on current life experiences and relationships, rather than on those from the distant past. Encourage the patient to develop and maintain good grooming habits and personal hygiene.

Role Performance

| Develop role mastery in newly acquired roles. | Determine which type of role-functioning problem the patient is experiencing: role insufficiency, role disturbance, interrole conflict, or role failure.
Determine the condition(s) predisposing the patient to the problematic role-functioning behavior: developmental, situation, or health-illness transition.
Encourage the patient to verbalize feelings, concerns, fears, and anxieties associated with assuming the new role.
Help the patient to assess what impact this new role will have when assuming present and future roles.
Once the type of role-functioning problem has been identified, use the following role supplementation strategies:
  1. Role clarification: emphasis should be on what the role entails in terms of behavior, sentiments, costs, and rewards, and whether a significant other reinforces the role negatively or positively.
  2. Role taking: emphasis should be on helping the patient imaginatively assume the position or point of view of another person taking on the new role.
  3. Role modeling: emphasis should be on helping the patient enact and play out the new role so that he can understand and emulate the intricacies of behavior associated with the new role.
  4. Role rehearsal: emphasis should be on helping the patient fantasize, imagine, and mentally enact how an encounter might take place and how the new role might evolve and develop.
  5. Reference groups: emphasis should be on exposing the patient to other individuals or groups who have successfully assumed role mastery of the new role.
Provide a therapeutic environment that will allow for opportunities to learn and practice new role behaviors. Emphasis should be on helping the patient practice with feedback the role behaviors they have failed to assume or perform before. |

Personal Identity

| Develop and maintain a positive concept of personal identity. | Encourage the patient to verbalize his concerns and anxieties regarding personal identity.
Help the patient develop problem-solving skills and subsequent strategies that will facilitate his achieving a sense of personal identity.
Encourage the patient to take responsibility for personal behavior and to take risks in exploring new behaviors.
Encourage participation in peer group activities and in the development and maintenance of meaningful interpersonal relationships.
Provide a therapeutic environment that will foster the patient's sense of personal self.
Teach the patient principles of normal growth and development. Emphasize that certain phases of development (such as adolescence) are accompanied by *normal* crises in personal identity. |
| Achieve satisfaction with own sexual identity and sexual preference. | Encourage the patient to verbalize anxieties concerning sexual identity and sexual preference for companionship. In a nonjudgmental manner support the patient in his choice of sex role.
Explore with the patient the meanings of being a man or woman. Stress that sexuality is only one component of a person's identity.
Encourage the patient to explore the positive and negative consequences as perceived in making a decision to assume a particular sexual role. Stress that the decision is a personal choice, but that consequences of the choice must be accepted. |

In formulating appropriate intervention strategies for disturbance in self-concept (body image, self-esteem, role performance, and personal identity), one must first assess and determine which type of disturbance(s) is being manifested by the patient. The patient must be assessed for subjective and objective characteristics. In addressing overall disturbances in self-concept, the nurse should use certain major interventions. These consist of the following:

1. Assessment questions should include:
   a. What is the patient's perception of himself? How does the patient perceive and evaluate his physical, psychologic, social, and moral self?
   b. Is the patient satisfied with his present perception of self? What would he like to change? Does he feel he can change his self-concept? How does he feel he might best go about changing his self-concept?
   c. How does the patient establish standards/goals for himself? What are these standards/goals? Are they realistic?
   d. What are the patient's assets and strengths as he perceives them? Does he use these in daily social-interpersonal interactions and relationships?
   e. What are significant others' perceptions of the patient's strengths and assets?
2. Communication techniques useful in caring for a patient experiencing disturbance in self-concept include:
   a. Talking with the patient in a nonjudgmental, empathetic manner. The patient's feelings and perceptions in relation to his evaluation of his self-concept should not be rejected, belittled, criticized, or demeaned.
   b. Communicating acceptance of the patient as a worthwhile human being.
   c. Listening to the patient and demonstrating genuine interest, concern, and empathy.
   d. Fostering communication that allows for consensual validation of interpersonal experiences and perceptions.
3. Focusing on the patient's assets and strengths. Reinforce these when the opportunity arises.
4. Helping the patient set realistic, achievable goals and standards for himself.
5. Planning activities for and with the patient that will foster and promote the patient's self-concept in relation to his physical, psychologic, social, and moral self.
6. Verbalizing and reinforcing the patient's past and present successes.
7. Encouraging the patient to accept responsibility for his own behavior and to evaluate its outcome in a fair, noncritical, nonjudgmental manner.
8. Providing a therapeutic environment that will foster and improve the patient's self-concept.

EVALUATION

Patient Outcome	Data Indicating That Outcome is Reached*
Body Image	
Positive, accepting, and realistic body image	Decrease in manifestation of subjective and objective defining characteristics as presented previously
	Positive expression of the acceptance of body image
	Understanding of how the negative body image possibly developed in relation to growth and development, social, cultural, and interpersonal experiences
	Problem-solving skills with subsequent strategies that promote and maintain a positive body image
Body wall or body boundary change accepted and incorporated into body image and self-concept	Decrease in manifestation of subjective and objective defining characteristics as presented previously
	Positive expression of the acceptance and reality of the changed body wall or body boundary area
	Ability to look at, touch, and discuss with others the changed body wall or body boundary area
	Describes the impact the changed body wall or body boundary has had on the assumption of activities of daily living and in family work and social relationships
	Use of appropriate cosmetic or mechanical devices as well as reference support groups
	Use of all available treatment modalities to improve functioning of the affected body wall or body boundary area

*References 4, 13, 22, 24, 27, 35.

Patient Outcome	Data Indicating That Outcome is Reached
Reintegration of ego functions and boundaries so that they are congruent with reality and self-concept	Decrease in manifestation of subjective and objective defining characteristics as presented previously Improvement in mental functioning (absence of or decrease in psychosis and regressive behaviors) Discrimination between environmental stimuli and external stimuli

Self-Esteem

Improvement and maintenance of a constructive level of self-esteem	Decrease in manifestation of subjective and defining characteristics as presented previously Acceptance of self-worth, self-respect, self-approval, and self-confidence Improvement in personal appearance (hygiene and grooming) Improvement in psychologic test scores that measure self-concept and self-esteem (for example, Tennessee Self-Concept Scale) Demonstrates problem-solving skills with subsequent strategies that can promote and maintain a positive level of self-esteem Identification and use of existing strengths, assets, and successes Recognition of value and use of various treatment modalities (such as group and family therapy) Appropriate assertive behaviors and communication skills

Role Performance

Development of mastery of newly acquired roles	Decrease in manifestation of subjective and objective defining characteristics as presented previously Positive expression of acceptance of new role Understanding of the appropriate cognitive, instrumental, and expressive behaviors, goals, and sentiments associated with the role Understanding of the impact the new role will have in assuming other role behaviors Use of various role supplementation strategies with the resultant ability to perform the role without difficulty Problem-solving skills with subsequent strategies that can promote and maintain mastery of the newly acquired role and possible future roles

Personal Identity

Development and maintenance of a positive concept of personal identity	Decrease in manifestation of subjective and objective defining characteristics as presented previously Positive acceptance of who he is Problem-solving skills with subsequent strategies that can promote and maintain the development of personal identity Understanding of what are considered to be normal crises in growth and development associated with personal identity issues
Satisfaction with sexual identity and sexual preference	Decrease in manifestation of subjective and objective defining characteristics as presented previously Acceptance of sexual identity and sexual preference Understanding of the consequences in their choice of a particular sexual identity and sexual preference

References

1. Allport, G.W.: Becoming, New Haven, 1955, Yale University Press.
2. Baldwin, J.M.: Social and ethical interpretations in mental development: a study in social psychology, New York, 1897, Macmillan Co.
3. Blau, P.M.: Exchange and power in social life, New York, 1964, John Wiley & Sons, Inc.
4. Bonham, P.A., and Cheney, A.M.: Concept of self: a framework for nursing assessment. In Chinn, P., editor: Advances in nursing theory development, Rockville, Md., 1983, Aspen Systems.
5. Brandon, N.: The psychology of self-esteem, Los Angeles, 1969, Nash.
6. Combs, A.W., Avila, D.L., and Purkey, W.W.: Helping relationships, ed. 2, Boston, 1971, Allyn & Bacon, Inc.
7. Combs, A.W., and Snygg, D.: Individual behavior: a perceptual approach to behavior, New York, 1959, Harper & Brothers.
8. Cooley, C.H.: Human nature and the social order, New York, 1902, Scribner's.
9. Driever, M.: Problem of low self-esteem. In Roy, Sr. C., editor: Introduction to nursing: an adaptation model, Englewood Cliffs, N.J., 1976, Prentice-Hall, Inc.
10. Driever, M.: Theory of self-concept. In Roy, Sr. C., editor: Introduction to nursing: an adaptation model, Englewood Cliffs, N.J., 1976, Prentice Hall, Inc.
11. Epstein, S.: The self-concept revisited, Am. Psychol. 28(5):404-416, 1973.
12. Erikson, E.H.: Childhood and society, ed. 2, New York, 1963, Norton.

13. Fitts, W.H.: The self-concept and self-actualization, Nashville, 1971, Dede Wallace Center.
14. Freud, S.: Three essays on sexuality. In Strachey, J., editor: The standard edition of the complete psychological works of Sigmund Freud, London, 1962, Hogarth Press.
15. Gouldner, A.W.: The norm of reciprocity: a preliminary statement, Am. Sociol. 25:161-178, 1960.
16. James, W.: The principles of psychology, New York, 1890, Holt.
17. James, W.: Psychology: the briefer course, New York, 1910, Holt.
18. Kim, M.J., and Moritz, D.A., editors: Classification of nursing diagnoses, New York, 1982, McGraw-Hill Book Co.
19. Kinch, J.W.: A formalized theory of the self-concept, Am. J. Sociol. 68:481-486, 1963.
20. Lecky, P.: Self-consistency: a theory of personality, New York, 1945, Island Press.
21. Linton, R.: Cultural background of personality, New York, 1945, D. Appleton-Century.
22. Malaznik, N.: Theory of role function. In Roy, Sr. C., editor: Introduction to nursing: an adaptation model, Englewood Cliffs, N.J., 1976, Prentice-Hall, Inc.
23. Maslow, A.H.: Motivation and personality, New York, 1954, Harper & Brothers.
24. McCloskey, J.C.: How to make the most of body image theory in nursing practice, Nursing 76 6(5):68-72, 1976.
25. McFarland, G.K., and Wasli, E.L.: Care of the adult psychiatric patient. In Brunner, L.S., and Suddarth, D.S., editors: The Lippincott manual for nursing practice, ed. 3, Philadelphia, 1982, J.B. Lippincott Co.
26. Mead, G.H.: Mind, self and society, Chicago, 1934, University of Chicago Press.
27. Meleis, A.: Role insufficiency and role supplementation, Nurs. Res. 24(4):264-271, 1975.
28. Parsons, T.: The social system, Glencoe, Ill., 1951, Free Press.
29. Pierce, C.S.: Questions concerning certain faculties claimed for man, J. Speculative Philosophy 2:103-114, 1868.
30. Rogers, C.R.: Client-centered therapy, New York, 1951, Houghton-Mifflin.
31. Rogers, J.A.: The need for acceptance of self and others. In Yura, H., and Walsh, M.B., editors: Human needs and the nursing process, Norwalk, Conn., 1983, Appleton-Century-Crofts.
32. Roy, C.: Introduction to nursing: an adaptation model, Englewood Cliffs, N.J., 1976, Prentice-Hall, Inc.
33. Sarbin, T.R.: A prefect to a psychological analysis of the self, Psychol. Rev. 59:11-22, 1952.
34. Sullivan, H.S.: The interpersonal theory of psychiatry, New York, 1953, Norton.
35. Taylor, M.C. Sr.: The need for self-esteem. In Yura, H., and Walsh, M.B.: Human needs and the nursing process, Norwalk, Conn., 1982, Appleton-Century-Crofts.
36. Wilson, H.S., and Kneisl, C.R.: Psychiatric nursing, Menlo Park, Calif., 1979, Addison-Wesley.

Suggested Readings

Coopersmith, S.: The antecedents of self-esteem, San Francisco, 1967, Freeman.
Guller, I.B.: Stability of self-concept in schizophrenics, J. Abnorm. Psychol. 71(4):275-279, 1966.
Kolb, L.: Disturbances in body image. In Arieti, S., and Reiser, M., editors: American handbook of psychiatry, ed. 2, New York, 1975, Basic Books.
Murray, R., editor: The concept of body image, Nurs. Clin. North Am. 7(4):593-707, 1972.
Offer, D., Ostrov, E., and Howard, K.I.: The adolescent, New York, 1981, Basic Books.
Randell, B.: Development of role function. In Roy, Sr. C., editor: Introduction to nursing: an adaptation model, Englewood Cliffs, N.J., 1976, Prentice Hall, Inc.
Schofield, A.: Problems of role function. In Roy, Sr. C., editor: Introduction to nursing: an adaptation model, Englewood Cliffs, N.J., 1976, Prentice-Hall, Inc.
Schrauger, J., and Schoeneman, T.: Symbolic interactionist view of self-concept, Psychol. Bull. 86(3):549-573, 1979.

POWERLESSNESS
THEORY AND ETIOLOGY

Relevant Theories and Concepts

Rotter's expectancy-value theory. Rotter,[25] an expectancy-value theorist, differentiated between internal and external locus of control. A person high in internal locus of control perceives that his or her own life and circumstances are controlled primarily by self-determined activity, actions, and characteristics. A person high in external locus of control, on the other hand, perceives his or her own life and circumstances to be primarily controlled by external events, such as fate, chance, luck, powerful people, or unpredictability caused by the complexity of situations. Increased external locus of control reflects a sense of helplessness[13,25,33] and a general expectancy of powerlessness.[9] This general expectancy of powerlessness can be measured by Rotter's internal-external locus control scale.[25]

Locus of control is a relatively stable personality characteristic, acquired over time from numerous social experiences, but subject to change with new experiences. Locus of control—a generalized expectancy—influences a person's perception of a given situation. Arakelian has stated[2]:

Individuals have a choice in how they will behave, and before deciding on a particular action they first must consider both their valuation of the outcome (reinforcement value) and their estimation of the likelihood or probability of its occurring (expectancy). In any specific event, people judge their chances for success by assessing immediate situations (situational expectancy), but they also draw upon what they have learned from past experiences that seem similar to present experiences (generalized expectancies).

Seeman's concept of alienation. Seeman[30] perceives powerlessness as a variety of alienation and describes it as a sense of low control rather than a sense of mastery over events. A sense of powerlessness arises from an individual's belief that outside forces such as chance govern what happens in life and that personal resources are not available to influence consequences of one's own actions and control of one's situation. Other types of alienation identified by Seeman are meaninglessness, normlessness, cultural estrangement, and self-estrangement.

Seligman's theory of learned helplessness. Seligman's theory[32] of learned helplessness proposes that feelings of helplessness result from repeated, unremitting hardships in some people. Minor mishaps result in such feelings of helplessness in other people. A sense of helplessness versus mastery and control over circumstances develops over time as one experiences uncontrollable events. The perceived control over the environment leads the child to learn about and experience being an effective person. Experience of successful control of outcomes is essential in human development because it immunizes the person against the effects of later hardships. Early, repeated exposure to uncontrollable events may lead to a lack of trust and hope and eventual depression.

Seligman views helplessness as a learned response to repeated exposure to uncontrollable events, which generalizes across situations but which can be unlearned. Helplessness decreases motivation to respond in a more constructive way that would improve one's comfort. Even if more adaptive responses are tried and produce relief, the person experiencing helplessness has difficulty learning and perceiving that the response actually worked. Depression and anxiety eventually predominate.

The learned helplessness hypothesis is reformulated in an extensive analysis by Abramson and Seligman.[1] Seligman's original hypothesis stated the following[32]:

. . . that learning the outcomes are uncontrollable results in three deficits: motivational, cognitive, and emotional. The hypothesis is "cognitive" in that it postulates that mere exposure to uncontrollability is not sufficient to render an organism helpless; rather, the organism must come to expect that outcomes are uncontrollable in order to exhibit helplessness. In brief, the motivational deficit consists of retarded initiation of voluntary responses and is seen as a consequence of the expectation that outcomes are uncontrollable. If the organism expects that its responses will not affect some outcome, then the likelihood of emitting such responses decreases. Second, the learned helplessness hypothesis argues that learning that an outcome is uncontrollable results in a cognitive deficit, since such learning makes it difficult to later learn that responses produce that outcome. Finally, the learned helplessness hypothesis claims that depressed affect is a consequence of learning that outcomes are uncontrollable.

The reformulated hypothesis of learned helplessness includes the notion that when a person experiences helplessness, he begins to ask *why* this helplessness is occurring, that is, the person attributes helplessness to a cause. "This cause can be stable or unstable, global or specific, and internal or external. The attribution chosen influences whether expectation of future helplessness will be chronic or acute, broad or narrow, and whether helplessness will lower self-esteem or not."[1]

The concept of power. McFarland, Leonard, and Morris[16] define power "as the generalized capacity or potential to get others to do something one wants them to do and which they would not ordinarily do otherwise." Although power can be abused, these authors point out that power has a positive aspect and exists within the context of interpersonal relationships. "Power is based, to an extent, on empowering responses, interpersonal expectations, and interpersonal attitudes."

French and Raven[11] identify five bases for personal social power:

1. *Expert power:* based on skill or knowledge
2. *Reward power:* based on ability to give positive rewards to others
3. *Referent power:* based on personal characteristics with which another person identifies
4. *Legitimate power:* based on the right to be influential over others
5. *Coercive power:* based on the ability to administer punishment

In Emerson's social exchange theory power is viewed as a property of social relationships—group-group, group-person, person-person—which are characterized by ties of mutual dependence between actors. Emerson[10] states:

A *depends* upon B if he aspires to goals or gratifications whose achievement is facilitated by appropriate actions on B's part. . . . These ties of mutual dependence imply that each party is in a position, to some degree, to grant or deny, facilitate or hinder, the other's gratification. . . . The power to control or influence the other resides in control over the things he values. . . . In short, *power resides implicitly in the other's dependency.* . . . [That is] the dependence of actor A upon actor B is (1) directly proportional to A's *motivational investment* in goals mediated by B and (2) inversely proportional to the availability of those goals to A outside of the A-B relation.

Stephenson[35] identifies two types of powerlessness—trait and situational. Trait powerlessness refers to the general affect, attitude, and life-style of person. Situational powerlessness, on the other hand, refers to a lack of control, in an otherwise empowered person, regarding a specific circumstance or series of events. Three sets of factors are identified as affecting situational powerlessness: focal, contextual, and residual stimuli. Focal stimuli refer to the situation leading to feelings of powerlessness. Contextual stimuli refer to related factors such as the environment or interpersonal climate. Residual stimuli refers to demographic variables and other factors such as education, income, and occupation.

Characteristics of the powerless person, according to Stephenson, are manipulation; apathy; withdrawal; resignation; lack of decision-making activity; reviving old feelings of inadequacy; perceiving loss of continuity between past, present, and future; protest; noncompliance; lack of knowledge about illness; perceiving self and/or environment as different from what was expected; insomnia; depression; uneasiness; perceiving interpersonal relationships as less gratifying or severe; perceiving self as less intact or in control; restlessness; aimlessness; unpleasant feelings of distress ascribed to a sense of personal helplessness; resignation; fatalism; and malleability.

Miller[18] defines powerlessness as a

. . . perception that one's own actions will not affect an outcome. . . . Powerlessness is a perceived lack of control over a current situation or immediate happening. The greater the individual's expectation to have control and the greater the importance of the desired outcomes to the individual, the greater the perceived powerlessness experienced when the individual does not, in fact, have control.

A patient's powerlessness can be diminished by power rebuilding, augmenting, or improving power resources—physical strength, psychologic stamina, support networks, self-concept, energy, knowledge, motivation, and a belief system (hope). Effective coping strategies must be preserved, augmented, and developed. (See discussion of ineffective individual coping elsewhere in text.) Effective coping strategies result in a decrease in uncomfortable feelings, generation of hope, enhancement of self-esteem, maintenance of positive interpersonal relationships, and maintenance of or improvement in the state of coping.

Miller views powerlessness as situationally determined and related to locus of control, a long-term tendency to perceive situations in a certain way. Miller formulates theoretical propositions regarding powerlessness and learning: (1) powerlessness can cause difficulty in learning control-relevant information; (2) learning can be enhanced by involving the client in making decisions about content to be included in client teaching programs; (3) locus of control can influence one's ability to use control-relevant information.

Practice guidelines that evolve from this are (1) to assess the degree of powerlessness prior to patient teaching and (2) to provide information that gives patients with an internal locus of control a sense of control, using different strategies of content presentation. For those with an external locus of control provide structured approaches, teach in small increments, and involve them in determining what aspects of health care they are ready to learn.

Studies indicate that persons show less anxiety and physiologic response in aversive situations in which they believe that personal competence and action affect outcome. That is, even in stressful situations the person can remain relatively calm or experience only mild to moderate anxiety if the person feels that what he does will influence consequences for himself.

Theoretical propositions identified by Miller follow:

1. An illusion of control leads to a less harmful evaluation of threats and less physiologic arousal during stressful situations than do situations in which the person perceives himself as not being in control.
2. If freedom of choice is offered, an illusion of control can result.
3. Helplessness can result from repeated exposure to threatening stimuli.
4. If there is a degree of predictability about the consequences of one's actions, the threat of aversive stimuli is decreased.
5. Success experiences can reverse learned helplessness.
6. Helplessness can result from repeated no-control experiences.

Practice guidelines formulated from these propositions include the following:

1. Help patients feel a sense of control.
2. Stimulate an illusion of control by providing the patient with alternatives.
3. Assess factors causing a sense of helplessness.
4. Decrease unpredictability by providing appropriate information.
5. Facilitate patient awareness of personal feelings that accompany threatening experiences.
6. Help patient recognize and control those aspects of experience that are within control.

Relevant Research

Seeman's research[29] supported the proposition that a person's "generalized expectancy for control of his outcomes (i.e., his sense of powerlessness) governs his attention to, and acquisition of, information available in the environment . . . [in other words] those who are high in powerlessness . . . have inferior knowledge in control-relevant areas of their experience." A study cited by Seeman reported that patients high in powerlessness were less knowledgeable about relevant health matters and demonstrated ward behavior indicative of this low level of knowledge. Studies support the finding that persons with low powerlessness are sensitive to helpful cues in the environment and learn relevant information. Poorer learning for control-relevant information takes place, however, in persons experiencing high levels of powerlessness.

Arakelian[2] summarized research studies and showed that initial health information is mastered more readily by persons with an internal locus of control. Learning is enhanced for persons with an internal locus of control when health is a valued aspect of life and "when information is presented in programs consistent with their preference for control and information."

Lowery and DuCette's nursing research[15] among diabetic patients provided support for the notion that those with an internal locus of control are more active as seekers of information than those with an external locus of control. Internals were found to know more about diabetes than did externals.

Chang's nursing research[8] indicated that, on an average, institutionalized residents in nursing homes who

perceived situations to be self-determined had higher morale than those who perceived situations to be other-determined. . . . Those who were external (chance in orientation) scored significantly . . . higher in morale when situations were perceived to be self-determined than other-determined. . . . Perceived self determination, regardless of orientation, resulted in higher morale for respondents than other-determination. Under conditions of other-determination, morale was lower for those with chance orientation than it was for either the powerful-other or internal orientation groups.

Significance of this research to nursing is the tool developed to measure residents' perceived control of daily activities (SCDA) and the suggestion that institutionalized nursing home residents be given increased control over their activities of daily living.

Powerlessness in Selected Age Groups

Children. When faced with threatening situations, children may reduce the threat, set limits to control threat, destroy the threat, or balance the threat with security operations.[21] Baumann[4] adds that "the individual child displays variations in coping methods depending on problems encountered (degree of perceived threat), previous experiences, maternal involvement, and the child's unique coping repertoire."

Using Johnson's Behavioral Systems Model of Nursing, Baumann described nursing intervention strategies designed to help a toddler cope with feelings of powerlessness. Strategies identified in the achievement subsystem included the following:

1. Provide choices for activities such as play.
2. Avoid shaming for regressive behavior.
3. Provide positive feedback when the toddler shows evidence of performing previously mastered tasks.
4. Engage in manipulative play with art and toys.
5. Encourage self-care to the extent possible.

Suggested strategies in the affiliative system included:

1. Interpret the child's behavior to staff members as necessary.
2. Use the peek-a-boo game to resolve separation anxiety.
3. Encourage maintenance of feelings of relatedness

with home by talking with child about family or leaving a family album, article of clothing, or toys with the child.

Pounding bench toys, punching bags, toy drums, drawing, and pull-push toys were used to deal with interruptions in the aggressive subsystem.

Obviously, each child must be assessed for the degree of powerlessness with close attention given to the developmental stage. Baumann provided a summary of general guidelines for working with children with a nursing diagnosis of powerlessness:

1. Permit children a time to prepare for an event to give them a sense of control.
2. Demonstrate confidence while providing nursing care.
3. Encourage the child to work together with nurse, permitting choice of time and order of treatment.
4. Permit crying.
5. Provide constructive outlets for anger, aggression, or withdrawal.
6. Offer interpretation of the child's attempts to communicate.
7. Provide as much consistency in nursing care as possible.

The elderly. The elderly are particularly vulnerable to feelings of powerlessness.[11] A number of contextual factors may contribute to the development of such feelings. False labels, myths, or characteristics may be ascribed to elderly persons. The elderly may, for example, be described as senile, worthless, rigid, or inferior. Such beliefs may be internalized and lead to powerlessness. Elderly persons may be assigned demeaning tasks in certain settings, such as nursing homes, or they may no longer be engaged in reinforcing and valued activities. Such constricted spheres of control, influence, and engagement in valued activities can result in powerlessness.[26] Miller and Oertel[19] cited numerous research studies which demonstrate that lack of control, choice, responsibility, and social interaction can have detrimental results.

Powerlessness is frequently experienced by aging persons in our culture and is a prominent nursing diagnosis of elderly persons admitted to acute care facilities. "The aging person is vulnerable to powerlessness because of physiologic and psychosocial changes inherent in the aging process."[19] Sensory changes can occur in aging. An altered body image occurs because of multiple physiologic changes. Many other physiologic changes, especially if accompanied by lack of knowledge about the aging process or a chronic illness, can make the elderly vulnerable to powerlessness.[19] Losses may be multiple and can include loss of friends, roles, family, income, health, home, and an adequate physiologic reserve and energy level.

Etiology

In addition to the etiological factors identified by the National Conference Group in Kim, McFarland, and McLane,[14] possible causes of powerlessness were identified in particular from Bennett,[5] Neal and others,[22] Stephenson,[35] Miller,[18] Ball and Wyman,[3] Gottesman and Gutstein,[13] Schmidt,[27] Seeman,[30,31] and Mills.[20]

Etiological factors for the nursing diagnostic label—powerlessness—are included in the following list:

Institutional environment and staff behavior
  Stripping of personal possessions
  Excessive surveillance
  Assault on privacy
  Lack of individuation
  Castelike separation from persons in authority
  Misuse of rewards
  Misuse of punishment
  Staff monopoly of scarce or strategic resources
  Misuse of power, authority, or force
  Absolute power of staff to structure conditions of negotiation
  Deployment or blocking of resources by staff
Situational crises
Parental influences and parenting styles
Social conditions
Peer influences
Repeated interpersonal failures and problems
Actual or potential loss of significant other
Lack of available or accessible social and personal resources
  Lack of ability to reward a favor
  Lack of ability to extort a concession or do without
  Belief in lack of control over resources
Altered state of physical wellness
Diagnosis of acute or chronic illness
Threat to physical integrity
Progressive physical deterioration
Loss of control over body
Loss of control over mental ability
Loss of independent role
Hospitalization
Alterations in mental status
Loss of autonomy
Weak ego identity
Spoiled identity/stigma
Life-style
Extremely hostile environment
Delay or distortion in accomplishing developmental tasks
Developmental changes
Perception of authority figures as distant or unapproachable
Alterations in schedule
Lack of knowledge
Lack of participation in decision-making
Excessive threatening experiences
Unsupportive environment
Living in battering relationship

DEFINING CHARACTERISTICS*

Verbal expression of having no control or influence over situation†
Verbal expression of having no control or influence over outcome†
Verbalizes feelings of loss of control and powerlessness†
Low orientation to learning control-relevant information
Lack of knowledge about own illness
Inability to seek information about care
Low orientation to achievement in control-relevant area
Verbal expression of having no control over self-care
Frustration about inability to perform previously mastered activities
Doubtful about role performance
Inability to carry out activities of daily living
Low planned use of health services
Acknowledges failure readily
Expresses feelings of inadequacy
Rationalizes failure
Displays aggression when goal achievement frustrated
Devalues desired goal when achievement frustrated
Apathy
Passivity
Withdrawal
Feelings of despair
Resignation
Fatalism
Aimlessness
Lack of participation in decision-making
Feelings of depression
Anxiety
Restlessness and uneasiness
Sleeplessness
Malleability
Sadness or crying
Inappropriate aggression
Low self-esteem
Resentment
Irritability
Mistrust of others
Anger or hostility toward others or environment
Overly dependent on others
Low self-reliance
Fears alienation from care-givers
Fluctuating or low energy levels
Asks many questions
Asks no questions
Loss of control over environment
Loss of control over self-functioning
Loss of control over personal behavior
Inappropriate or immature coping abilities for developmental stage

*References 2, 14, 20, 22, 24, 26, 27, 31, 35.

†Critical defining characteristic.

Projects blame on others and environment
Negative feedback
Little ability to benefit from assistance of authority figures

Feels little responsibility for behavioral outcomes
Inability to influence others
Seeks immediate rewards in favor of long-term goals

NURSING INTERVENTIONS

Patient Goal	Nursing Intervention*
Control or influence outcomes in current situations	Make change within institutions or residential settings.

Make change within institutions or residential settings.
1. Decrease surveillance of patient unless essential for safety.
2. Minimize rules and regulations; permit patient input in their development.
3. Enhance individuality and autonomy.
4. Increase patient control over rewards.
5. Preserve privacy; increase territorial rights.
6. Allow patient to wear own clothes.
7. Prevent a castelike separation between staff and patients.
8. Vary setting and routine of daily activities based on patient input.
9. Do not block patient's attainment and use of resources (within limits of safety).
10. Do not use coercion.
11. Support patient's efforts to increase resources, such as benefits that can be shared with other patients or allies that can be mobilized.
12. Decrease dependency on staff; encourage independent behavior.
13. Maintain patient's sense of dignity; permit exploration of environment.
14. Be less directive and overprotective.
15. Foster personal powerfulness by putting bedside stand, call light, telephone, etc. within reach.
16. Promote active involvement in appropriate decision making in ADL.
17. Involve patients in other decision-making opportunities.
18. Provide patients with positive and predictable events, such as group experiences.
19. Provide opportunities for engagement in meaningful activities.

Help patient reduce feelings of powerlessness.
1. Help patient recognize and describe powerlessness; identify the behavior with patient.
2. Help patient separate controllable from uncontrollable events.
3. Help patient set realistic goals.
4. Teach patient to problem-solve and try out alternative coping strategies.
5. Help patient identify personal preferences, wants, feelings, values, attitudes.
6. Help patient identify and use strengths and potential; identify improvement in condition.
7. Encourage verbalization of feelings and concerns about feelings of powerlessness.
8. Improve self-esteem.
9. Provide situations in which patient can succeed and experience control.
10. Assess patient's perception and knowledge of treatment program, encouraging expression of views *before* giving information.
11. Assess internal versus external locus of control prior to patient teaching.
12. For those with an internal locus of control, provide information that gives patient a sense of control, using different strategies of content presentation.
13. For those with an external locus of control, provide structured approaches, teach in small increments, and involve in determining readiness for learning.
14. Provide needed information.
15. Encourage patient to ask questions; reinforce the right to ask questions.
16. Help patient seek and master relevant health information.
17. Help patient use health care personnel.
18. Help patient develop long-term valued health goals and take fewer risks.

*References 2, 4, 8, 17-19, 22-24, 27, 28, 31, 34, 35.

Patient Goal	Nursing Intervention
	19. Restore energy imbalance.
	20. Teach assertive communication skills.
	21. Involve in decision-making and planning own care.
	22. Allow patient to assume more complicated decision-making when ready.
	23. Provide positive reinforcement and acknowledgment for active participation in own care.
	24. Help patient develop increased internal locus of control by encouraging participation in sensitivity training, behavior modification, brief psychotherapy, encounter groups, community action programs; altering perception of life situation; using behavioral rehearsal and role playing; rewarding manifestations of internality; challenging external locus of control–oriented verbalizations; examining possible outcomes of alternative approaches.
	25. Facilitate improvement in life circumstances—returning to work, constructive significant other influences, successful therapy experiences.
	26. Involve significant others in care of patient within realm of capability.
	27. Sensitize significant others to the importance of their reactions.
	28. Build trusting relationship; be consistent and dependable.
	29. Use active listening.

A sound data base is needed to determine the defining characteristics present and to analyze and synthesize the data to determine the nursing diagnosis of powerlessness. Additional assessment parameters to consider in assessing a patient for powerlessness include the following questions[19,20]:

1. Does the patient belong to a high-risk group? Women? Elderly? Educationally/economically disadvantaged? The chronically ill or handicapped? Ethnic/racial minorities?
2. Are perceived or actual abilities to influence personal outcome and control the situation present?
3. Are there verbal expressions of:
   a. Having no control/influence over situation?
   b. Having no control or influence over outcomes?
   c. Feelings of loss of control and powerlessness?
4. Does the patient experience characteristics such as lack of decision-making? Lack of knowledge about illness and treatment? Withdrawn? Fatalistic?
5. Are coping strategies currently or previously used?
6. Are environmental factors, staff behaviors, or other etiological factors present? Excessive surveillance? Assault on privacy? Lack of individuation?

Planning involves determination of goals and priorities with the patient and formulating a plan of nursing interventions. The major overall goal for the patient with this nursing diagnosis is for the patient to be able to control or influence outcomes in current situations.

EVALUATION

Patient Outcome	Data Indicating That Outcome is Reached
Control or influence outcomes in current situations	Verbalization of ability to control or influence situation and outcomes
	Verbalization of feelings of powerfulness
	Seeking control-relevant information
	Knowledge about control-relevant situation
	Adequate role-functioning and coping skills
	Feelings of adequacy
	Goal-directed behavior
	Hope
	Involvement in decision-making
	Appropriate mood
	Welcoming assistance from others when needed but not overly dependent
	Working toward long-term goals
	Sense of responsibility over behavioral outcomes
	Holding self responsible when appropriate; no projecting of blame on environment

References

1. Abramson, L., and Seligman, M.: Learned helplessness in humans: critique and reformulation, J. Abnorm. Psychol. **87**(1):49-74, 1978.
2. Arakelian, M.: An assessment and nursing application of the concept of locus of control, Advances Nurs. Sci. **3**(1):25-42, Oct. 1980.
3. Ball, P., and Wyman, E.: Battered wives and powerlessness: what can counselors do? Victimology: An International Journal **2**(3-4):545-552, 1977-1978.
4. Baumann, D.: Coping behavior of children experiencing powerlessness from loss of mobility. In Miller, J., editor: Coping with chronic illness: overcoming powerlessness, Philadelphia, 1983, F.A. Davis Co.
5. Bennett, R.: The meaning of institutional life, Gerontologist **3**(3):117-125, 1963.
6. Blau, P.: Exchange and power in social life, New York, 1964, John Wiley & Sons, Inc.
7. Bloch, D.: Alienation. In Carlson, C., and Blackwell, B., editors: Behavioral concepts and nursing interventions, Philadelphia, 1978, J.B. Lippincott Co.
8. Chang, B.: Generalized expectancy, situational perception, and morale, Nurs. Res. **27**(5):316-324, Sept.-Oct. 1978.
9. Crawford, T., and Naditch, M.: Relative deprivation, powerlessness, and militancy: the psychology of social protest, Psychiatry **33**:208-223, 1970.
10. Emerson, R.: Power-dependence relations, Am. Sociol. Rev. **27**(1):31-41, 1962.
11. French, J., and Raven, B.: The bases of social power. In Cartwright, D., editor: Studies in social power, Ann Arbor, 1959, The University of Michigan Press.
12. Fuller, S.: Inhibiting helplessness in elderly people, J. Gerontol. Nurs. **4**:18, July-Aug. 1978.
13. Gottesman, D., and Gutstein, S.: The course and duration of crisis, J. Consult. Clin. Psychol. **47**(1):128-134, 1979.
14. Kim, M., McFarland, G., and McLane, A.: Pocket guide to nursing diagnoses, St. Louis, 1984, The C.V. Mosby Co.
15. Lowery, B., and DuCette, J.: Disease-related learning and disease control in diabetics as a function of locus of control, Nurs. Res. **25**(5):358-362, Sept.-Oct. 1976.
16. McFarland, G., Leonard, H., and Morris, M.: Nursing leadership and management: contemporary strategies, New York, 1984, John Wiley & Co.
17. Meldman, M., McFarland, G., and Johnson, E.: The problem oriented psychiatric index and treatment plans, St. Louis, 1976, The C.V. Mosby Co.
18. Miller, J.: Coping with chronic illness: overcoming powerlessness, Philadelphia, 1983, F.A. Davis Co.
19. Miller, J., and Oertel, C.: Powerlessness in the elderly: preventing hopelessness. In Miller, J., editor: Coping with chronic illness: overcoming powerlessness, Philadelphia, 1983, F.A. Davis Co.
20. Mills, W.: Alienation: a basic concept underlying social isolation. In Kim, M., McFarland, G., and McLane, A., editors: Classification of nursing diagnoses: proceedings of the Fifth National Conference, St. Louis, 1984, The C.V. Mosby Co.
21. Murphy, L.: Vulnerability, coping and growth: from infancy through adolescence, New Haven, 1976, Yale University Press.
22. Neal, M., and others: Nursing care planning guides for psychiatric and mental health care, Monterey, 1981, Wadsworth Health Sciences.
23. Pfister-Minogue, K.: Enabling strategies. In Miller, J., editor: Coping with chronic illness: overcoming powerlessness, Philadelphia, 1983, F.A. Davis Co.
24. Robinson, G., and Owen, J.: No one told me to, Nurs. Outlook **22**(3):182-183, March 1974.
25. Rotter, J.: Generalized expectancies for internal versus external control of reinforcement, Psychological Monographs: General and Applied **80**(1):1-28, 1966 Whole No. 609.
26. Roy, Sister Callista: Introduction to nursing: an adaptation model, Englewood Cliffs, N.J., 1976, Prentice-Hall Inc.
27. Schmidt, M.: Exchange and power in special settings for the aged, Int. J. Aging Hum. Devel. **14**(3):157-166, 1981-1982.
28. Schultz, R., and Hanusa, B.: Long term effects of control and predictability-enhancing interventions: findings and ethical issues, J. Pers. Soc. Psychol. **36**:1194, 1978.
29. Seeman, M.: Powerlessness and knowledge: a comparative study of alienation and learning, Sociometry **30**:105-123, 1967.
30. Seeman, M.: Alienation and engagement. In Campbell, A., and Converse, P., editors: The human meaning of social change, New York, 1972, Russell Sage.
31. Seeman, M.: Alienation studies, Annu. Rev. Sociol. **1**:91-123, 1975.
32. Seligman, M.: Helplessness: on depression, development and death, San Francisco, 1975, W.H. Freeman Co.
33. Smith, R.: Changes in locus of control as a function of life—crisis resolution, J. Abnorm. Psychol. **75**:328-332, 1970.
34. Stapleton, S.: Decreasing powerlessness in the chronically ill: a prototype. In Miller, J., editor: Coping with chronic illness: overcoming powerlessness, Philadelphia, 1983, F.A. Davis Co.
35. Stephenson, C.: Powerless and chronic illness: implications for nursing, Baylor Nurs. Educ. **1**(1):17-23, 1979.

Suggested Readings

Bandura, A.: Self-efficacy: toward a unifying theory of behavioral change, Psychol. Rev. **84**(2):191-215, 1977.

Gatchel, R., McKinney, M., and Kolbernick, L.: Learned helplessness, depression, and physiological responding, Psychophysiol. **14**(1):25-31, 1977.

Glass, C., and Levy, L.: Perceived psychophysiological control: the effects of power versus powerlessness, Cogn. Ther. Res. **6**(1):91-103, 1982.

Goodstadt, B., and Hjelle, L.: Power to the powerless: locus of control and the use of power, J. Personality Social Psychol. **27**(2):190-196, 1973.

Hanes, C., and Wild, B.: Locus of control and depression among noninstitutionalized elderly persons, Psychol. Rep. **41**:581-582, 1977.

Hiroto, D., and Seligman, M.: Generality of learned helplessness in man, J. Personality Social Psychol. **31**(2):311-327, 1975.

Jenkins, L.: The concept of assertion: from theory to practice, Issues Ment. Health Nurs. **4**:51-63, 1982.

Johnson, D.: Powerlessness: a significant determinant in patient behavior? J. Nurs. Educ. **6**:39-44, April 1967.

Lowery, B.: Misconceptions and limitations of locus of control and the I-E scale, Nurs. Res. **30**(5):294-298, Sept./Oct. 1981.

Lowery, B., Jacobsen, B., and Keane, A.: Relationship of locus of control to preoperative anxiety, Psychol. Rep. **37**:1115-1121, 1975.

Miller, W., and Seligman, M.: Learned helplessness, depression and the perception of reinforcement, Behav. Res. Ther. **14**:7-17, 1976.

Reid, D., Haas, G., and Hawkings, D.: Locus of desired control and positive self-concept of the elderly, J. Gerontol. **32**(4):441-450, 1977.

Rodin, J., and Langer, E.: Long-term effects of a control-relevant intervention with the institutionalized aged, J. Personality Social Psychol. **35**(12):897-902, 1977.

Rotter, J.: Some problems and misconceptions related to the construct of internal versus external control of reinforcement, J. Consult. Clin. Psychol. **43**(1):56-67, 1975.

Ryden, M.: Energy: a crucial consideration in the nursing process, Nurs. Forum **16**(1):71-82, 1977.

Schulz, R.: Effects of control and predictability on the physical and psychological well-being of the institutionalized aged, J. Personality Social Psychol. **33**(5):563-573, 1976.

Schulz, R., and Hanusa, B.: Long-term effects of control and predictability-enhancing interventions: findings and ethical issues, J. Personality Social Psychol. **36**(11):1194-1201, 1978.

Taylor, S.: Hospital patient behavior: reactance, helplessness, or control? J. Social Issues **35**(1):156-184, 1979.

Wallston, B., and others: Development and validation of the health locus of control (HLC) scale, J. Consult. Clin. Psychol. **44**(4):580-585, 1976.

Ziegler, M., and Reid, D.: Correlates of locus of desired control in two samples of elderly persons: community residents and hospitalized patients, J. Consult. Clin. Psychol. **47**(5):977-979, 1979.

FEAR AND ANXIETY: MILD, MODERATE, SEVERE, EXTREME (PANIC)

THEORY AND ETIOLOGY

Sigmund Freud

Freud[2,3] viewed anxiety as an automatic affective response occurring under certain situations of danger. When the ego senses impending or real danger, anxiety can result. According to Freud, real, or objective, anxiety is a reaction to a danger from outside the individual, such as death. Neurotic anxiety, on the other hand, stems from an unknown source of danger that is not necessarily external and that is frequently out of proportion to the danger.

Anxiety arises from two anxiety-provoking situations, according to Freud.[12] In a type 1 situation the person's ego is unable to handle excessive instinctual stimulations. The person feels helpless, and panic or traumatic states may result. Although more common in infancy and childhood, this type of anxiety can occur in adulthood. In type 2 situations anxiety arises in anticipation of danger from external or internal sources.

"Each stage of the child's development is accompanied by characteristic danger situations that are phase specific or appropriate to the issues pertinent to that particular developmental phase."[12] Freud discusses the anxiety related to birth trauma, to the separation anxiety felt by the young child on loss of the mother, and to the anxiety felt by the child on the loss of the love of a significant other. Later, in the phallic phase, anxiety can result from a threatened loss of a body part, for example, the penis. During the latency period the source of anxiety can stem from a perceived loss of approval or punishment from parental internalizations in the superego. In adulthood anxiety can stem from a threat to life or anticipated death.

The emotional response experienced in anxiety is painful. "Excitations in the internal organs of the body . . . result from internal or external stimulation and are governed by the automatic nervous system."[4] In anxious states the heart begins to beat faster, respirations increase, the mouth often becomes dry, and the palms perspire. The anxiety signals the ego to mobilize defensive mechanisms such as avoidance mechanisms or psychologic defenses.

Karen Horney

Horney[6-9] viewed normal anxiety as follows[19]:

. . . implicit in the human situation of contingency in the face of death, powers of Nature, and so forth. . . . [Normal anxiety] does not connote hostility on the part of Nature or the conditions which make for human contingency; it does not provide inner conflict or lead to neurotic defense measures.

Basic anxiety, on the other hand, is a reaction to a threat to the core or essence of personality patterns, upon which feelings of safety depend. Basic anxiety is characterized by feelings of isolation, diffuseness, helplessness, and a surrounding hostility that increase insidiously and pervade all.[7] In contrast, Horney describes fear as "a reaction to a specific danger, to which the individual can make a specific adjustment."[19]

Basic anxiety is fundamental in Horney's theory. It has its roots in early childhood in adverse influences and the resultant hostility, but it can be experienced throughout life during adverse conditions and stress. These adverse influences include the absence of respect and love along with severe criticism and rejection on the part of significant others.

In an attempt to cope with and protect against basic anxiety, the person can use three basic behavioral patterns—moving toward people, moving against people, and moving away from people. *Moving toward people* is characterized by the behavioral pattern of being compliant, agreeable, and self-effacing; searching for acceptance by developing those qualities that are acceptable; being dependent and leaning on others for advice; and demonstrating sensitivity and unselfishness toward others. True feelings are repressed to such an extent that inner turmoil exists. The person views the self negatively and is often used by others for their own gains. *Moving against people* is characterized by behaviors such as use of power and achievement of control and mastery over the environment and self; aggression; toughness and endurance; rebellion; and defiance. *Moving away from people* is characterized by withdrawal from people, a search for privacy and freedom, self-sufficiency, and lack of competitiveness or requests for assistance.

If more than one of these patterns become intense, internal conflict can result. Auxiliary approaches to tension and conflict reduction are then employed. Ford and Urban[1] summarize these as follows:

1. Selecting one pattern predominantly while repressing its opposite
2. Detached character structure—extreme emotional withdrawal from others
3. The idealized self-image—building up a good image of oneself
4. Externalization (blaming others)

Harry Stack Sullivan

H.S. Sullivan,[30-33] the founder of the interpersonal theory of psychiatry, believed that "personality is the relatively enduring pattern of recurrent interpersonal situations which characterize a human life.''[31] The personality evolves out of the interpersonal relationships of the infant and developing human being with significant others in the environment.

Tension arises mainly from two sources. First are the basic organic needs such as food, air, and water. The goal of such activities as eating and breathing is to reduce tension and to gain satisfaction. Second is the need to reduce tensions arising out of one's social behavior and interpersonal interactions. Man has the potential for the expansion of abilities and for activities used in the pursuit of security and the reduction of anxiety. These anxiety-reduction activities affect an individual's self-respect and self-esteem, as well as overall personality development.

Anxiety is an innate response that is a part of each human being's repertoire of responses. During infancy anxiety is elicited by the behavior (that is, disapproval) of significant others. Sullivan states: ''The first of all learning is . . . beyond doubt in immediate connection with *anxiety*.''[31] That is, learning begins to occur on the basis of the anxiety gradient. The infant and developing human being learn to modify social behavior in a manner that reduces anxiety. Thus the developing human being begins to increasingly engage in activities that bring approval from significant others and attempts to avoid those which bring disapproval and concomitant anxiety. As Sullivan states: ''Anxiety, as a phenomenon of relatively adult life, can often be explained plausibly as anticipated unfavorable appraisal of one's current activity by someone whose opinion is significant.''[31] The self develops out of the interpersonal experiences resulting in approval and disapproval. Those experiences which are rewarded are incorporated into the self. In summary, mild to moderate anxiety results in learning and modification of learning.

Sullivan equates severe anxiety, however, to a blow on the head. Severe anxiety prohibits any clear comprehension of the immediate situation. From experiences of intense anxiety the personification of the *not-me* evolves.

The not-me is literally the organization of experience with significant people that has been subjected to such intense anxiety, and anxiety so suddenly precipitated, that it was impossible for the then relatively rudimentary person to make any sense of, to develop any true grasp on, the particular circumstances which dictated the experience of this intense anxiety.[31]

The self tends to limit awareness of, and engagement in, anxiety-provoking experiences. Mental disorders can result from severe anxiety and the reliance on dissociations and ineffective security operations to deal with it. Clarification of anxiety, awareness of self, expansion of one's abilities, and effective anxiety- and tension-reduction strategies contribute, on the other hand, to mental health.

Each stage of human development is characterized by commonly occurring interpersonal responses and experiences. At any given level of development, anxiety can arise out of disturbed interpersonal relationships. Ford and Urban[1] describe the characteristics of Sullivan's stages of development as follows:

1. *Infancy:* articulate, but uncommunicative speech
2. *Childhood:* interpersonal patterns of interactions with playmates begin to develop
3. *Juvenile:* interpersonal patterns of intimacy with persons of the same sex begin to develop
4. *Preadolescence:* the beginning of interest in persons of the opposite sex and genital sexuality
5. *Early adolescence:* the development of semistable patterns of sexual interaction
6. *Late adolescence:* the development of a love relationship with another person
7. *Adulthood*

Sullivan[31] differentiates between anxiety and fear, especially in relation to childhood. He describes the ''felt component'' of both of them to be identical. The difference lies in the fact that ''anxiety is something which . . . is acquired by an empathic linkage with the significant older persons, whereas fear is that which appears when the satisfaction of general needs is deferred to the point where these needs become very powerful.''

O. Mowrer

Anxiety is a conditioned part of fear according to learning theorists such as Mowrer.[23] The theory maintains that an unconditioned stimulus causes an unconditioned response such as fear. Fear stimulates escape behavior, which, if successful, reduces fear and reinforces the use of escape behaviors. Klein[14] further explained:

Stimuli that often precede the unconditioned stimuli become conditioned stimuli by simple, classical, Pavlovian contiguity conditioning. Conditioned stimuli serve as signals of the oncoming, unconditioned stimuli and release a conditioned response, anxiety, which then serves as a secondary drive. The secondary drive incites avoidant behavior. Successful avoidance of the unconditioned stimulus reduces the secondary drive of anxiety and thereby reinforces the avoidant behavior. Phobic avoidance behavior, then, is a learned avoidance maintained by a decrease in anxiety.

Carl Rogers

The major propositions of Rogers' theory of personality follow[28]:

1. Every individual exists in a continually changing world of experience of which he is the center.
2. The organism reacts to the field as it is experienced and perceived. This perceptual field is, for the individual, ''reality.''

3. The organism has one basic tendency and striving—to actualize, maintain, and enhance the experiencing organism.

4. Behavior is basically the goal-directed attempt of the organism to satisfy its needs as experienced, in the field as perceived.

5. Emotion accompanies and in general facilitates such goal-directed behavior, the kind of emotion being related to the seeking versus the consummatory aspects of the behavior, and the intensity of the emotion being related to the perceived significance of the behavior for the maintenance and enhancement of the organism.

6. As a result of interaction with the environment, and particularly as a result of evaluational interaction with others, the structure of the self is formed.

7. As experiences occur in the life of the individual, they are either (a) symbolized, perceived, and organized into some relationship to the self, (b) ignored because there is no perceived relationship to the self-structure, (c) denied symbolization or given a distorted symbolization because the experience is inconsistent with the structure of the self.

Mild to moderate fear is described as an emotion that facilitates goal-directed behavior, as, for example, mobilizing the organization of the person to escape a danger. Anxiety is defined by Rogers as a state of tension or uneasiness that is an innate response pattern. Anxiety occurs when a person experiences a threat to the self, as, for example, from an experience that is perceived in the self as bad when, in fact, it is innately satisfying. Ford and Urban,[1] in a comparative analysis and comparison of major psychotherapists, note that when responses elicit both negative and positive evaluative thoughts of self, anxiety results.

Two types of defenses are used to avoid this anxiety: denial of awareness and distortion of awareness. In denial the person's responses are ignored or repressed. In distortion the responses are distorted so they are more in line with the self-concept. Maladaptive behaviors and emotional ill health can result from such a pattern of avoiding anxiety.

Rollo May

May[18] defines anxiety as "the apprehension cued off by a threat to some value that the individual holds essential to his existence as a personality." Anxiety is a vague, diffuse, objectless, nonspecific apprehension that grips at the essence or inner aspect of our personality. Characteristics include a sense of helplessness, uncertainty, powerlessness, worthlessness, and lowered self-esteem. In anxiety the security pattern—the foundation on which the person distinguishes himself from the environment—is threatened. These threats can be directed toward anything the person holds essential to that central core or security pattern, whether it be a threat to physical safety, to the ability to meet physiologic needs, or to the ability to meet higher level needs such as self-esteem, belonging, meaning, freedom, patriotism, or goal achievement.

Anxiety originates in the fact that human organisms are born with the capacity to respond to threats. "This capacity is innate and has its inherited neurophysiological system."[18] What stimuli will be perceived as threats, as well as in what form and to what extent anxiety occurs, depends on the individual's experience and consequent learning.

May makes a clear distinction between anxiety and fear. Fear is a specific protective response to a definable, specific danger. If the person adequately copes with these specific dangers, his inner core or being remains intact and is not threatened. "If, however, one cannot cope with dangers in their specific forms, one will be threatened on the deeper level which we call the "core" or "essence" of personality."[18] The response to this threat to one's essence is anxiety.

As the human being matures, the capacities for exhibiting more differentiated types of responses to danger are developed. May contends that "after the first reflexive protective reactions, there emerge the diffuse, undifferentiated emotional responses to threat–namely, anxiety; and last to emerge in maturation are the differentiated emotional responses to specific, localized dangers—namely, fears."[18]

Normal anxiety differs from neurotic anxiety. Normal anxiety is proportionate to the actual threat, can be confronted consciously and constructively, can be relieved by altering or removing the threat, and does not require defense mechanisms, such as repression, for its management. Neurotic anxiety, on the other hand, is disproportionate to the actual threat, involves repression, involves intrapsychic conflict, and is managed by retrenchment of awareness and activity (symptoms, inhibitions, repression).

Fear and Anxiety in Nursing Literature

A number of nurse-authors address the topic of anxiety and fear. A classic work on anxiety was done by Peplau.[25] The sources of anxiety are threats to the security of the person, such as threats to one's biologic integrity or to one's values, patterns of behavior, and views of self.

Peplau describes the effects of anxiety, differentiating between mild and moderate anxiety, which increase one's capabilities, and severe or extreme anxiety, in which capabilities and structures are paralyzed or overworked. Physiologic changes, such as the release of epinephrine, can cause manifestations such as anorexia, urinary urgency, shifts in blood pressure, temperature, and menstrual flow, increased heart rate, and increased respiration. Observational capacity is increased in mild anxiety, whereas in moderate anxiety the perceptual field is somewhat narrowed but attention is directed to the situation of concern. In severe anxiety attention is focused on scattered detail, whereas in extreme anxiety the detailed focus is blown out of proportion or the speed of focusing on scattered details is increased. In mild anxiety the person is aware, alert, and perceives connections between elements of a situation. In moderate anxiety the person does not notice peripheral details. In severe and extreme anxiety the person displays dissociating tendencies, failing to notice what goes on in a situation. In mild and moderate anxiety the person can learn; "i.e., is able to observe, describe, analyze, formulate meanings and relations, validate with another person, test, integrate, use the learning product."[25] In severe and extreme anxiety learning is diminished and the person seeks means of reducing the discomfort of anxiety. Four major behavior patterns can occur in coping with anxiety: acting out, somatizing, withdrawal or depression, or learning from the anxiety.

From Canada comes a current and extensive research project on nursing diagnoses, including anxiety and fear. Jones and Jakob define anxiety as[10]:

. . . a vague, uneasy sense of worry, nervousness, anguish, or marked ambivalence. The client appears not to have yet expressed the underlying feelings involved, such as fear, grief, conflict, insecurity. The client may or may not be aware of the particular display pattern of the anxiety or the factors contributing to it.

Fear, on the other hand, is defined as a "client-expressed or client-confirmed response of apprehension or dread of the presence of a recognized, usually external, threat or danger to one's limb, autonomy, self-image, or community with others."[10] The findings revealed the following, in terms of frequency of occurrence among nursing diagnoses[10]:

. . . *Anxiety* ranked third (148 incidents, 5.3% of the total) and *fear* ranked fourth (140 incidents, 5.0% of the total). . . . In terms of clients affected, *anxiety* was reported for 35% and *fear* for 33% of the total of the 427 clients. *Anxiety* and *fear* were diagnosed in persons of all ages with health status at all levels and were associated with all categories of medical diagnoses. Furthermore, these client/patients were reported from a wide range of health care settings.

Mereness and Taylor[22] point out that anxiety can occur in situations that threaten a person's self-esteem or personal identity and result in insecurity, helplessness, and isolation, along with such vague, uneasy feelings as dread, apprehension, and nervousness. In anxiety the person is prepared for fight or flight by the autonomic nervous system in varying degrees. In mild anxiety, for example, the person's alertness increases and performance may be actually enhanced. In extremely high anx-

iety, on the other hand, the person's behavior can become dysfunctional. Normal anxiety, linked to realistic situations, is differentiated from neurotic anxiety, arising out of the person's own unacceptable thoughts. Attempts to cope with intolerable neurotic anxiety include several dysfunctional behavioral patterns. The basic origin of the disorders, according to Mereness and Taylor, is an unconscious conflict (with its origin most likely in childhood) that has been repressed. At some point later in life the person's ego is not able to compromise between elements in the unconscious conflict. Certain behavioral patterns are sometimes engaged in to cope with the resultant anxiety. Of particular interest are the etiological factors and characteristics manifested by persons experiencing anxiety reactions. Etiological factors include loss of love, threat to personal security, and loss of prestige. Characteristics can include perpetual exhaustion, tightness in throat and/or stomach, lack of appetite, diarrhea, tachycardia, palpitations, shortness of breath, tight feelings in the head, and an abdominal feeling of heaviness.

Kalkmann and Davis[11] describe acute anxiety as characterized by an inability to pinpoint any reason for its existence. The characteristics of acute anxiety can include restlessness, tenseness, sense of impending doom, uneasiness, panic, agitation, tachycardia, palpitations, diarrhea, urinary frequency, dyspnea, tremors, and excessive perspiration. The authors point out that anxiety is experienced by the elderly particularly, since there may be more times when they feel helpless and dependent on others. If the anxiety remains unresolved, sometimes dysfunctional defense mechanisms are manifested, such as somatic complaints.

Topalis and Aguilera[34] note that anxiety can be aroused by internal or external dangers, either imagined or unreal. Fear, on the other hand, "is a response to a real or threatened danger." Mild anxiety can serve as a stimulus for action and as a motivator. Extreme or severe anxiety can be destructive and overwhelming. Physical symptoms associated with anxiety include dry mouth, constipation or diarrhea, vomiting, loss of appetite, gastric hyperactivity, tachycardia, palpitations, alterations in blood pressure, diaphoresis, and urinary frequency. Psychologic symptoms can include self-absorption, alertness, feelings of impending danger, exhaustion, powerlessness, and overactive/agitated or frozen/immobile motor tension.

Wilson and Kneisl[35] differentiate between fear and anxiety. "*Fear is* the feeling aroused by the accurate perception of a genuine external danger. The intensity of the fear is proportionate to the degree of that danger." Anxiety is an unexplained discomfort that is generally not objectively realistic and can, for example, stem from a threat to one's biologic integrity or self-concept. Physiologic reactions to fear and anxiety include increased heart rate, blood pressure, and respirations, urinary frequency and urgency, dilated pupils, and dry mouth. The authors cite four levels of anxiety: mild, moderate, severe, and extreme (panic). Perception is altered with changing levels of anxiety. The person experiencing mild anxiety is unusually alert and makes detailed observations. Attention is focused on immediate details and connections between detail are more readily perceived. The person experiencing moderate anxiety concentrates even more on sensory data relevant to the immediate situation, demonstrates selective inattention, and is motivated to do something about the anxiety and the current situation. The person with severe anxiety, however, becomes preoccupied with the discomfort felt, experiences greatly reduced perceptions, focuses on scattered details, dissociates anxious feelings from oneself, and engages in dysfunctional behavior. In panic the person cannot concentrate, experiences feelings of personal disintegration, distorts the situation, and perceives the experience unrealistically.

Manfreda and Krampitz[15] differentiate between fear and anxiety. Fear is defined as a response to an objective, recognized external threat. Anxiety, on the other hand, is defined as a subjective, unpleasant, vague, diffuse, unexplainable apprehensive feeling, arising from a threat, and resulting in defensive behaviors. Behavioral manifestations of anxiety include tremor, diarrhea, vomiting, exhaustion/fatigue, restlessness, increased heart rate, increased respiration, preoccupation with and increased talk about the situation, change in voice tone and rate of speech, blocking, perspiration, and insomnia. In severe anxiety helplessness and immobility may be experienced.

Stuart and Sundeen,[29] in their model of anxiety, identify predisposing factors—genetic endowment, present needs, thoughts, feelings, and resources, and past experiences—which affect the actual internal or external stimuli that the person then cognitively evaluates as a threat. The central nervous system is aroused and anxiety is felt. The sympathetic reaction appears to prepare the body for a flight or fight reaction in most persons. Upon perception of the threat in the cortex, the sympathetic branch of the autonomic nervous system is stimulated and the adrenal glands are activated. Epinephrine is released. Blood flows to the central nervous system, muscle, and heart from the stomach and intestines. The heart beats faster, blood pressure rises, breathing becomes more rapid, and blood glucose levels increase. Other physiologic manifestations include anorexia, constipation, dry mouth, perspiration, facial pallor, weakness, dilated pupils, exhaustion, hyperventilation, breathing difficulties, and muscular tension. The parasympathetic reaction, coexisting or predominating in some individuals, causes urinary frequency, diarrhea, decreased blood pressure, and decreased heart rate. Other physiologic and psychomotor reactions can include headaches, blurring of vision, nausea and/or vomiting, sleep disturbances, interference with sexual functioning, abdominal discomfort, restlessness (which may progress to agitation), physical tension, tremors (varying from fine, digital tremors to gross shaking of the entire body), startle reaction, rapid speech, lack of coordination of actions and movements, and accident proneness.

Etiology

A number of variables contribute to the development of fear and can be identified as a major cause. Other variables contribute toward the development of anxiety. By drawing from the previous theoretical discussion, especially contributions by Kim, McFarland, and McLane[13] and McFarland and Wasli,[20] possible causes of fear and anxiety can be listed. Both the diagnostic label and the identified etiology form the total nursing diagnosis, for example, fear related to knowledge deficit.

Fear
- Definable, specific danger
- Powerful unmet needs
- Natural dangers, such as sudden noise, loss of physical support, height, pain
- Sensory impairment
- Language barrier
- Knowledge deficit
- Lack of social support in threatening situation
- Learned response, as by conditioning or identification

Anxiety: mild, moderate, severe, extreme (panic)
- Perceived or actual threat to personal security pattern
- Perceived or actual threat to core/essence of personality
- Perceived or actual threat to self-concept
- Perceived or actual threat to value system, beliefs, ideals
- Perceived or actual threat to meaningful interpersonal relationships/patterns and belonging
- Adverse interpersonal relationships
- Perceived or actual threat to biologic integrity
- Perceived or actual failure to adaptive coping skills
- Perceived or actual threat to physical safety
- Unmet needs
- Perceived or actual threat to the ability to meet physiologic needs
- Interpersonal transmission/contagion
- Perceived or actual threat to goal achievement
- Situational or maturational crises
- Perceived or actual threat to stable environment

Perceived or actual change in role functioning

Perceived or actual change in socioeconomic status

Unconscious conflict

Arousal of both positive and negative evaluative thoughts

Perceived, actual, or anticipated disapproval by significant others

Empathic linkage with significant other

Terminal illness or potential death

Adverse influences (especially in childhood)

    Absence of love from significant other(s)

    Absence of respect from significant other(s)

    Criticism by significant other(s)

    Rejection by significant other(s)

    Disapproval by other person(s)

DEFINING CHARACTERISTICS[13,20]

Fear

Differentiated emotional response to definable specific danger*

Increased tension, jittery

Apprehension

Scared, frightened

Terrified, panic

Increased alertness

Concentration on danger

Fight behavior (aggression)

Flight behavior (withdrawal)

Pupil dilation

Increased respiratory and heart rates

Goal-directed behavior facilitated (during mild or moderate fear)

Organization of person enhanced to flee or fight danger

Increased muscle tension

Diaphoresis

Mild Anxiety

Mild, vague, diffuse, objectless, apprehensive response to threat*

Mild, vague, diffuse, objectless, apprehensive response to threat to personality core*

Slight discomfort or tension

Slight uneasiness

Irritability

Restlessness

Repetitive questioning

Attention seeking

Belittling

Misunderstandings

Increased alertness

Enhanced problem-solving ability

Increased awareness and perception

Increased learning

Increased involvement in activities approved by others (especially during childhood)

Tension-relieving behaviors

    Lip chewing

    Finger tapping

    Foot shuffling

    Nail biting

Moderate Anxiety

Moderate, vague, diffuse, objectless, apprehensive response to threat*

Moderate, vague, diffuse, objectless, apprehensive response to threat to personality core*

Moderate discomfort or tension

Moderate uneasiness

Moderate feeling of diffuseness

Shakiness

Rattled

Pacing

Increased verbalizations

Increased alertness

Moderate sense of isolation

Slightly lowered self-esteem

Slight sense of worthlessness

Narrowing of perceptual field

Selective inattention

Increasing concentration on problem situation

Increased concentration on sensory data relevant to problem

Increased learning

Increasingly engaging in activities that elicit approval from significant others (especially during childhood)

Voice tremors

Change in voice pitch

Increased heart rate

Increased respiratory rate

Increased muscle tension

    Trembling

    Hand tremors

    Facial tension

Diaphoresis

Frequency

Urgency

Somatic complaints

Sleeplessness

Severe Anxiety

Severe vague, diffuse, objectless, apprehensive response to threat*

Severe vague, diffuse, objectless, apprehensive response to threat to personality core*

Sense of impending doom

Severe uneasiness

Severe discomfort, distress, tension

Dissociation of anxious feelings from self

Denial of existence of uncomfortable feelings

Painful sense of helplessness and inadequacy

Severe feeling of being in hostile environment

Moderately low self-esteem

Moderate sense of worthlessness

Moderate feeling of powerlessness

Uncertainty

Severe sense of isolation

Severe feeling of diffuseness

Inability to learn

Purposeless activity

Ineffective functioning

Difficult and/or inappropriate verbalizations

Reduced range of perception

    Inability to concentrate

    Focus on scattered or small details

---

*Critical defining characteristic.

Selective inattention
Inability to see connections between events or details
Lack of clear comprehension of immediate situation
Hyperventilation
Tachycardia
Urinary frequency
Urinary urgency
Nausea
Headache
Dizziness
Insomnia

Extreme Anxiety (Panic)

Extremely severe vague, diffuse, objectless, apprehensive response to threat*
Extremely severe vague, diffuse, objectless, apprehensive response to personality core*
Extremely severe discomfort, tension
Extremely severe uneasiness
Severe shakiness
Severe hyperactivity
Immobility
Extreme sense of helplessness and inadequacy
Extreme feeling of isolation
Extreme feeling of diffuseness
Extreme sense of being in hostile environment
Severely lowered self-esteem
Severe worthlessness
Severe powerlessness
Extreme uncertainty
Inability to communicate
Unintelligible communication
Inability to learn
Disruption of perceptual field
    Distortion or unrealistic perception of situation
    Enlargement of detail
Feeling of personality disintegration
Mental disorders
Dilated pupils
Pallor
Vomiting
Sleeplessness

The nursing diagnosis of fear or anxiety is formulated from a synthesis of data, which are collected by means of clinical assessment. Assessment parameters for consideration for fear follow:

1. Identify and observe for definable specific dangers.

2. What behavioral and physiologic changes indicating fear are present?
3. How does the patient perceive the danger and describe the discomfort?
4. Identify maladaptive or adaptive coping responses to fear.
5. What strategies has the patient used to cope with past fear?
6. What resources are available to deal with the fear?

Assessment parameters to consider in relation to anxiety follow:

1. Observe for perceived or actual threats to:
   a. Personal security pattern
   b. Core or essence of personality
   c. Self-concept
   d. Value system, beliefs, ideals
2. What behavioral and physiologic changes indicating anxiety are present?
3. What degree of anxiety is manifested? Physiologic and psychologic signs and symptoms present?
4. What does the patient say about this state of discomfort?
5. Identify maladaptive and adaptive current responses to anxiety.
6. What strategies has the patient used to cope with anxiety in the past?
7. What strengths and resources are available to cope with the anxiety: problem-solving skills, decision-making skills, significant others, religion, professional assistance, recreational activities, hobbies?

Determination of the diagnosis of fear or anxiety is based on the presentation of a set or cluster of defining characteristics.[13,20] The defining characteristics manifested by a client are useful in determining the nursing diagnosis. Not all characteristics need be present at a given time, but the patient must experience at least those characteristics defined as critical. To complete the nursing diagnosis, the nurse then adds the identified etiology to the diagnostic label, for example, fear or moderate anxiety, when possible. An example is ''moderate anxiety related to perceived threat to goal achievement.''

NURSING INTERVENTIONS[10,20,21,24]

Patient Goal	Nursing Intervention
Reduce or prevent fear.	Help patient in identify danger that is causing fear; use indirect and open-ended questions.
	Assist patient in identifying major response pattern to danger—fight or flight.
	Encourage verbalization, when timing is appropriate, about:
	1. Feelings experienced.
	2. Perception of danger.
	3. Perception of ability to cope with danger.
	4. Questions about progress and/or outcome of diagnoses or treatment.

Patient Goal	Nursing Intervention

Help patient use most appropriate approach to cope with present fear:
1. Clearly identify danger.
2. Use strategies to avoid danger.
3. Use strategies to work around danger.
4. Develop alternative goals, resources, etc.
5. Engage in problem-solving activities to cope with danger.
6. Facilitate realistic or alternative perception of danger.

Help patient identify strengths and adaptive skills to cope with fear(s):
1. Scrutinize types of learning involved.
2. Gain more constructive facts about the feared situation.
3. Engage in stimulus exposure or systematic desensitization to reduce and eliminate fear.

Avoid situations that could aggravate the fear and related feelings:
1. Give careful explanations of what is to happen to patient in health care setting.
2. If fear cannot be reduced, make appropriate referrals, for example, a surgeon who may postpone surgery.
3. Involve and provide information to patient's family and/or friends.

Reduce anxiety.

For patient with severe or extreme anxiety:
1. Employ comfort measures such as warm bath, restful environment.
2. Keep in calm, nonstimulating milieu: remove any stress or threat; limit contact with other anxious patients.
3. Use short, simple sentences.
4. Use calm, firm tone of voice.
5. Administer tranquilizers or sedatives as prescribed.
6. Observe for and institute needed protective measures.
7. Use nonverbal behavior, such as quiet physical presence or touch, to offer reassurance.
8. Avoid asking patient to make decisions.
9. Avoid probing for cause of anxiety.
10. Avoid interpreting behavior or confrontation.

Develop constructive, positive interpersonal relationship with patient:
1. Be empathetic.
2. Convey unconditional positive regard.
3. Be congruent.

Intervene early to prevent escalation of anxiety to severe or extreme levels.

Use active listening skills.

Facilitate patient's participation in recreational and diversional activities aimed at decreasing anxiety:
1. Group singing or instrumental groups
2. Simple games
3. Housekeeping chores
4. Grooming
5. Routine tasks
6. Walking or jogging
7. Simple concrete tasks
8. Swimming

Remain calm:
1. Avoid reciprocal anxiety.
2. Recognize own anxiety.
3. Develop control over own responses.

Encourage ventilation of feelings when ready; permit crying.

Offer brief and clear information about experiences during hospitalization.

Offer, clarify, and validate information as needed.

Offer reassurance.

Convey attitude that there is hope and that a constructive resolution can be found.

Prevent further escalation of anxiety by *avoiding* threats, indifference, rejection, judgmental attitude, impatience, unrealistic demands, insincerity, focusing on weakness.

Mutually develop daily schedule of activities, incorporating patient's strengths, abilities, preferences, and goals.

During short-term hospitalization offer additional support and assistance in dealing with anxiety on admission, on about the fifth day, and on notification of discharge.

Patient Goal	Nursing Intervention
Recognize anxiety, develop insight, and use adaptive coping strategies.	If anxiety is at mild or moderate levels, help patient to: 1. Recognize presence of anxiety by providing feedback on characteristics indicating anxiety and asking questions such as, "Are you uncomfortable right now?" 2. Explore similarity between present and past experiences. Ask questions such as, "Have you felt like this before? What was happening to you then? What did you do to reduce your discomfort?" 3. Identify thoughts or expectations prior to becoming anxious. 4. Identify relationship between anxiety and consequent adaptive or maladaptive responses. 5. Clarify nature of threat to self. 6. Develop adaptive strategies to reduce anxiety. 7. Problem-solve. 8. Evaluate results of strategies used. 9. Seek and implement alternatives for unsuccessful results. Reduce any secondary gains from maladaptive strategies used in coping with anxiety. Permit patient to set pace in solving problems. Reduce negative expectations. Facilitate development of constructive and optimistic view of existence, especially if view is distorted, closed, or deadened. Facilitate choice of effective, objective environmental interventions to cope with anxiety, especially if patient is already optimistic, open to new experiences, and flexible. Encourage participation in new interests and hobbies. After establishing relationship with patient and extreme or severe anxiety has been reduced: 1. Encourage social activities despite reluctance and fears. 2. Attend activities with patient initially. Permit patient to leave if anxiety is greatly increased. Gradually encourage attendance independent of staff support. Use role playing to deal with anxiety-provoking situations. With children, try role-play strategies using puppets, dolls, or other playthings, art, or play requiring large motor activities. Teach patient: 1. About the constructive aspects of mild or moderate anxiety in learning, growth, and movement toward self-actualization. 2. To recognize personal characteristics indicating presence of anxiety. 3. To describe present state of anxiety. 4. To analyze current expectations, goals, beliefs, and values versus what is perceived as actually happening. 5. Assertive communication skills. 6. Problem-solving and decision-making skills. 7. Progressive muscle relaxation. 8. To increase repertoire of strategies to reduce severe anxiety; talking or being in presence of someone; simple, concrete tasks; walking; noncompetitive sports; professional assistance.

EVALUATION

Patient Outcome	Data Indicating That Outcome is Reached
Reduction or absence of fear	Absence or reduction of defining characteristics indicating presence of fear
Reduction of anxiety	Absence or reduction of defining characteristics indicating presence of anxiety
Anxiety recognized, insight developed, and adaptive coping strategies used	Recognition of anxiety in self Demonstration of insight about cause of anxiety Use of adaptive coping strategies to reduce anxiety Use of mild or moderate anxiety for personal change or growth

References

1. Ford, D., and Urban, H.: Systems of psychotherapy: a comparative study, New York, 1965, John Wiley & Sons, Inc.
2. Freud, S.: Inhibitions, symptoms, and anxiety, 1925. In Strachey, J., editor: Standard edition, vol. 20, London, 1959, Hogarth Press.
3. Freud, S.: The problem of anxiety, H. Bunker (translator), New York, 1963, W.W. Norton Co.
4. Hall, C.: A primer of Freudian psychology, New York, 1979, New American Library.
5. Harp, D.: Teaching a concept of anxiety to patients, Nurs. Res. **10:**108-113, Spring 1961.
6. Horney, K.: New ways in psychoanalysis, New York, 1939, W.W. Norton Co.
7. Horney, K.: Neurotic personality of our times, New York, 1937, W.W. Norton Co.
8. Horney, K.: Our inner conflicts, New York, 1945, W.W. Norton Co.
9. Horney, K.: Neurosis and human growth: the struggle toward self-realization, New York, 1950, W.W. Norton Co.
10. Jones, P., and Jacob, D.: Anxiety revisited—from a practice perspective. In Kim, M., McFarland, G., and McLane, A., editors: Classification of nursing diagnoses: proceedings of the Fifth National Conference, St. Louis, 1984, The C.V. Mosby Co.
11. Kalkman, M., and Davis, A.: New dimensions in mental health–psychiatric nursing, ed. 5, New York, 1980, McGraw-Hill Book Co.
12. Kaplan, H., Freedman, A., and Sadock, B.: Comprehensive textbook of psychiatry, Baltimore, 1980, Williams & Wilkins.
13. Kim, M., McFarland, G., and McLane, A., editors: Pocket guide to nursing diagnoses, St. Louis, 1984, The C.V. Mosby Co.
14. Klein, D.: Anxiety reconceptualized. In Klein, D., and Rabkin, J., editors: Anxiety: new research and changing concepts, New York, 1981, Raven Press.
15. Manfreda, M., and Krampitz, S.: Psychiatric nursing, Philadelphia, 1977, F.A. Davis Co.
16. May, R.: The meaning of anxiety, New York, 1950, The Ronald Press.
17. May, R.: Historical roots of modern anxiety theories. In Hoch, P., and Zubin, J., editors: Anxiety, New York, 1964, Hafner Publishing Co.
18. May, R.: The meaning of anxiety, New York, 1977, W.W. Norton Co.
19. May, R.: The meaning of anxiety, New York, 1979, Pocket Books.
20. McFarland, G., and Wasli, E.: Mild anxiety, moderate anxiety, severe anxiety, extreme anxiety (panic). In Kim, M., McFarland, G., and McLane, A., editors: Pocket guide to nursing diagnoses, St. Louis, 1984, The C.V. Mosby Co.
21. Meldman, M., McFarland, G., and Johnson, E.: The problem-oriented psychiatric index and treatment plans, St. Louis, 1976, The C.V. Mosby Co.
22. Mereness, D., and Taylor, C.: Essentials of psychiatric nursing, ed. 10, St. Louis, 1978, The C.V. Mosby Co.
23. Mowrer, O.: Learning theory and behavior, New York, 1960, John Wiley & Sons, Inc.
24. Neal, M., and others: Nursing care planning guides for psychiatric and mental health care, Monterey, Calif., 1981, Wadsworth Health Sciences.
25. Peplau, H.: A working definition of anxiety. In Burd, S., and Marshall, M., editors: Some clinical approaches to psychiatric nursing, New York, 1966, The Macmillan Co.
26. Rogers, C.: Counseling and psychotherapy, Boston, 1942, Houghton Mifflin Co.
27. Rogers, C.: On becoming a person: a therapist's view of psychotherapy, Boston, 1961, Houghton Mifflin Co.
28. Rogers, C.: Client-centered therapy: its current practice, implications, and theory, Boston, 1965, Houghton Mifflin Co.
29. Stuart, G., and Sundeen, S.: Principles and practice of psychiatric nursing, St. Louis, 1979, The C.V. Mosby Co.
30. Sullivan, H.: Conceptions of modern psychiatry, New York, 1953, W.W. Norton Co.
31. Sullivan, H.: The interpersonal theory of psychiatry, New York, 1953, W.W. Norton Co.
32. Sullivan, H.: The psychiatric interview, New York, 1954, W.W. Norton Co.
33. Sullivan, H.: Clinical studies in psychiatry, New York, 1956, W.W. Norton Co.
34. Topalis, M., and Aguilera, D.: Psychiatric nursing, ed. 7, St. Louis, 1978, The C.V. Mosby Co.
35. Wilson, H., and Kneisl, C.: Psychiatric nursing, Menlo Park, Calif., 1979, Addison-Wesley Publishing Co.

Suggested Readings

Archer, R., and Kutash, K.: Anxiety response to psychological feedback among psychiatric inpatients, Psychol. Rep. **50:**547-551, 1982.
Burrows, G., and Davies, B., editors: Handbook of studies on anxiety, Amsterdam, 1980, Elsevier/North-Holland Biomedical Press.
Hartfield, M., Cason, C., and Cason, G.: Effects of information about a threatening procedure on patients' expectations and emotional distress, Nurs. Res. **31**(4):202-206, July/Aug. 1982.
Highland, A.: Anxiety: a summary of past and present research and theory, Child Welfare **60**(8):519-528, Sept.-Oct. 1981.
Johnston, M.: Recognition of patients' worries by nurses and by other patients, Br. J. Clin. Psychol. **21:**255-261, 1982.
Johnston, M., and Carpenter, L.: Relationship between preoperative anxiety and post-operative state, Psychol. Med. **10:**361-367, 1980.
Kelly, D.: Anxiety and emotions, Springfield, Ill., 1980, Charles C Thomas, Publishers.
Kerr, N.: Anxiety: theoretical considerations, Perspect. Psychiatr. Care **16**(1):36-39, 40, 46, Jan.-Feb. 1978.
Kim, M., McFarland, G., and McLane, A., editors: Classification of nursing diagnoses: proceedings of the Fifth National Conference, St. Louis, 1984, The C.V. Mosby Co.
Kirschenbaum, H.: On becoming Carl Rogers, New York, 1979, Delacorte Press.
Lintel, A.: Physiological anxiety responses in transcendental meditators and nonmeditators, Percept. Motor Skills **50:**295-300, 1980.
Marks, I.: Living with fear: understanding and coping with anxiety, New York, 1978, McGraw-Hill Book Co.
McCaul, K.: Sensory information, fear level, and reactions to pain, J. Personality **48**(4):494-504, Dec. 1980.
McHenry, L.: Situational anxiety levels and the intensive care unit staff nurse, Issues Ment. Health Nurs. **3:**341-351, 1981.
Mishel, M.: The measurement of uncertainty in illness, Nurs. Res. **30**(5):258-263, Sept./Oct. 1981.
Mullins, L., and Lopez, M.: Death anxiety among nursing home residents: a comparison of the young-old and the old-old, Death Educ. **6:**75-86, 1982.
Pease, V.: Anxiety into energy, New York, 1981, Hawthorn.
Ricci, M.: An experiment with personal-space invasion in the nurse-patient relationship and its effect on anxiety, Issues Ment. Health Nurs. **3:**203-218, 1981.
Sarason, I., and Spielberger, C., editors: Stress and anxiety, vol. 7, New York, 1980, Hemisphere Publishing Corp.
Shimko, C.: The effect of preoperative instruction on state anxiety, J. Neurosurg. Nurs. **13:**318-322, Dec. 1981.
Shipley-Miller, L.: Covert anxiety in the acute MI patient, Crit. Care Update **8:**21-23, Nov. 1981.
Solomon, S., Holmes, D., and McCaul, K.: Behavioral control over aversive events: does control that requires effort reduce anxiety and physiological arousal? J. Personality Social Psychol. **39**(4):729-736, 1980.
Spielberger, C., Sarason, I., and Milgram, N., editors: Stress and anxiety, vol. 8, New York, 1982, Hemisphere Publishing Corp.
Suess, W., and others: The effects of psychological stress on respiration: a preliminary study of anxiety and hyperventilation, Psychophysiology **17**(6):535-540, Feb. 1980.
Toth, J.: Effect of structured preparation for transfer on patient anxiety on leaving the coronary care unit, Nurs. Res. **29**(1):28-34, Jan.-Feb. 1980.
Yocom, C.: The differentiation of fear and anxiety. In Kim, M., McFarland, G., and McLane, A., editors: Classification of nursing diagnoses: proceedings of the Fifth National Conference, St. Louis, 1984, The C.V. Mosby Co.

Value Belief

SPIRITUAL DISTRESS

THEORY AND ETIOLOGY

Recognition of some of the assumptions underlying the concept of spiritual distress is a prerequisite to understanding its potential usefulness as a nursing diagnosis. Many of the assumptions are embedded in the numerous definitions of related concepts, such as spiritual health, spiritual integrity, spiritual need, spiritual growth, spiritual vulnerability, spiritual crisis, spiritual healing, spiritual help, and spiritual well-being, which are found in the literature on spiritual nursing care and pastoral care. Two major assumptions are that individuals experience spiritual health and that nurses are able to recognize spiritual health and its deviations, that is, a person's need for spiritual help. Nurses can be prepared to offer spiritual help and may be willing to focus care on the spiritual dimension of nursing.

According to Colliton,[5] Friedlander defines spirituality as the "life principle that pervades a person's entire being, including volitional, emotional, moral-ethical, intellectual and physical dimensions, and generates a capacity for transcendent values. The spiritual dimension of a person integrates and transcends biological and psychosocial nature. . . ." The premise that people have a need for transcendence provided the stimulus for Ellison and Paloutzian to develop an instrument to measure spiritual well-being. "The need for transcendence refers to reaching beyond oneself, with the outcome being a sense of well-being that we experience when we find purposes to commit ourselves to."[50] According to these two authors, spiritual well-being is not the same as spiritual health. Rather, it refers to a psychological-experiential

dimension, whereas spiritual health pertains to the creeds and codes of a religious group. Spiritual well-being is viewed as arising "from an underlying state of spiritual health and is an expression of it. . . ."[9] Spiritual well-being is conceptualized as a continuous rather than dichotomous variable with multiple factors influencing "how much" spiritual well-being.

In a compelling discussion of three general modes of knowing (body, mind, and spirit), Wilber[68] differentiates two ways of knowing about the spiritual dimension: first, the mind attempting to reason about the spirit and, second, the "eye of contemplation," that is, spirit's knowledge of spirit. He states that the latter "is the most direct, clearcut, impactful knowledge imaginable—it simply transcends conceptualization and therefore resists neat hypothetical categorizations and mental mappings."[68] If one accepts Wilber's analysis, then it becomes clear that it is mind's apprehension of spirit that is pertinent to a discussion of spirituality and spiritual distress, not spirit's direct knowledge of spirit.

Tubesing[65] believes that all stress-related illness is fundamentally a spiritual disorder, "often growing from a conflict of values, beliefs and goals" and that differences in stress levels may be determined by the answers persons give to a series of spiritual questions. He proposes that beliefs serve to organize individuals' lives and help them make decisions about how to use their time and focus their energies. "The bottom line of the spiritual dimension of stress is how we 'spend' ourselves."[65] In a similar manner, Linn and Linn[33,34] view emotional responses to stress as triggers that precipitate illness. Their success in treating physical and emotional illness by means of a five-stage process for the healing of memories is well documented.

The National Interfaith Coalition of Aging proposed the following definition of spiritual well-being: "Spiritual well-being is the affirmation of life in a relationship with God, self, community and environment that nurtures and celebrates wholeness."[45] The two-dimensional definition, a religious component and a social-psychologic component, is consistent with the theoretical notions of Moberg,[42] who conceptualized spiritual well-being as having both vertical and horizontal dimensions. The vertical dimension refers to a person's relationship to God, whereas the horizontal dimension refers to a sense of purpose in life and life satisfaction. The instrument developed by Ellison[9] and Paloutzian[50] was based on Moberg's two-dimensional conceptualization of spiritual well-being.

Highfield and Cason[19] constructed a two-dimensional framework, religious-existential, to assess nurses' awareness of the spiritual needs of patients: need for meaning and purpose in life, need to give love, need to receive love, and need for hope and creativity. Although no validity and reliability were reported for the instrument, the finding that less than one third of patients' spiritual problems were identified by the sample suggests that nurses often may fail to recognize problems of a spiritual nature.

Some of the earlier contributors to nursing's literature on the spiritual dimension of care view spiritual needs or spirituality as a single dimension. Fish and Shelly[12] defined spiritual need as the "lack of any factor(s) necessary to establish and/or maintain a dynamic personal relationship with a God." A unidimensional approach was also taken by Stallwood and Stoll[61] when they defined spiritual needs as "any factors necessary to establish and maintain a person's dynamic personal relationship with God (as defined by that individual)." The writings of O'Brien clearly reflect a unidimensional concept of the spiritual, one limited to a person's relationship with God. She defines spiritual health in the following way[47]:

. . . a state of well-being and equilibrium in that part of a person's essence and existence which transcends the realm of the natural and relates to the ultimate good. Spiritual health is recognized by the presence of an interior state of peace and joy; freedom from abnormal anxiety, guilt, or a feeling of sinfulness; and a sense of security and direction in the pursuit of one's life goals and activities.

Instead of spiritual distress, O'Brien proposed an overall diagnostic category—alterations in spiritual integrity—with seven subcategories of diagnostic labels: spiritual pain, spiritual alienation, spiritual anxiety, spiritual guilt, spiritual anger, spiritual loss, and spiritual despair. The definitions in each subcategory are consistent with O'Brien's one-dimensional approach to spiritual concerns. That is, each label represents an alteration in spiritual integrity that is a consequence of a person's failure in his relationship with God. Each of the subcategories could be viewed as a cause of the overall category label (alterations in spiritual integrity) rather than as a separate diagnosis. A decision about whether to call the seven subcategories labels or etiologies should be based on clinical research on the relationships among labels, etiologies, interventions, and evaluation.

The etiologies or spiritual sources of stress that Tubesing described reflect a more existential notion of the spiritual: unclear values, beliefs, and goals, conflicting values, sloppy time management habits, incongruence of life-style and values, incongruence of image of self and others, unwillingness to surrender, belief conflicts with others, and burn-out syndrome. The sources are consistent with his notion that stress-related illness is fundamentally a spiritual disorder growing from a conflict in values, beliefs, or goals. The etiologies defined by participants at the Fifth National Conference,[27] that is, separation from religious and cultural ties and a challenged belief and value system resulting from moral and ethical implications of therapy or resulting from intense suffering, are the result of illness rather than the factors producing the illness.

Using Stallwood and Stoll's five major areas in which humans could experience distress of the spirit as a framework, Flesner[13] developed an instrument to assess spiritual distress in the responsive adult. Although the instrument needs additional validation and testing, the proposed indicators of different etiologies of spiritual distress, developed from an extensive review of the literature, provide more conceptual clarity to a rather abstract and ambiguous area of nursing practice. Indicators of spiritual distress were proposed for five etiologies and their subcategories: forgiveness, love, hope, trust, and meaning and purpose in life. Indicators for the following subcategories of etiologies in the area of forgiveness were proposed: inability to feel God's forgiveness, inability to forgive self, and inability to forgive others. In the area of love, indicators for subcategories of etiologies reflected an absence of a desired state: lack of loving relationships, lack of healthy self-love, and lack of an ability to give and receive love with others. There were no subcategories identified in the areas of hope, trust, and meaning and purpose in life, but indicators were specified for each overall category. It is interesting to note that the cluster of indicators in each of the given areas (hope, trust, and meaning and purpose in life) reflects absence of a desired state, which contributes to spiritual distress.

The possibility and issues of a viable theology of spiritual growth were explored by Neuman,[45] who identified spiritual growth as one of four constitutive elements that are always operative within a given spirituality. He called for caution in the accurate following of theories of growth and development and suggested that the most they can do for an individual is to provide awareness points along the way:

In the making of a human life, the setting of attitudes, actions and hopes is as much the result of the particular and unique events which happen to an individual as it is of the unfolding of any chronologically structured growth scheme.

Neuman sees the absence of any methodologic statement of spiritual growth in the Bible as an indication that there is not supposed to be one. The writings are open-ended; they provide no absolute goal; they are examples of men and women who are "on the spiritual way." Being on the way requires beginnings, and Neuman[45] makes a powerful argument for the formulation of a theory of religious initiative and provides an outline of three major tasks that a developed theory of religious initiative would include: forming a religious personality; sharpening one's awareness of shaping a personal faith; and the reorganization of life's activities toward a concrete religious belief.

Although the theoretical speculations about aspects of spirituality related to health and wellness are many and varied, shifting from a focus on the purely faith and religious aspects of spirituality on one end of the continuum to the existential on the other, it was Moberg's idea of spiritual well-being as having both vertical (religious) and horizontal (existential) dimensions that sparked the imagination of Ellison[9] and Paloutzian.[50] They developed measures of both aspects in the Spiritual Well-Being (SWB) Index.

The SWB Index is currently being used in a cluster of studies by faculty and graduate students at Marquette University College of Nursing. Three of the studies have been completed,[10,11,41] and manuscripts have been submitted for publication. Other studies are at various stages in the research process, among them a qualitative study of indicators of spiritual well-being in older adults[22] and a comparison study of 180 older adults living in three different environments (home, high rise, and nursing home) in two geographic areas.[39]

In the first study[11] 435 randomly selected undergraduate students responded to a depression and life change inventory and the SWB Index. The researchers found a modest but significant positive relationship between life changes and depression, and a positive relationship between depression and spiritual well-being, with religious well-being contributing the most to the predicted relationship.

Two correlation studies[10] of 95 freshman nursing students and 75 randomly selected college students were reported. The researchers found a strong inverse relationship between indicators of spirituality (spiritual well-being, existential well-being, and spiritual outlook) and negative psychologic states. Miller[41] studied a group of chronically ill adults and compared them with healthy adults to determine the relationship between loneliness and spiritual well-being. She found no statistical difference between the groups in terms of loneliness but did find a negative relationship between loneliness and spiritual well-being in both groups. Leasor[31] studied 50 patients with chronic obstructive pulmonary disease and found a significant inverse relationship between spiritual well-being and negative mood states. Although the studies are limited to correlations, they are the beginning of a research program that might establish a more solid base of knowledge on which nursing practice can be based.

In several other health-related studies O'Brien, Swaim, and Comstock and Partridge found that aspects of spirituality influenced positive health states. O'Brien[47] studied dialysis patients and reported that subjects with a positive attitude toward their religion showed a decreased degree of alienation, a positive degree of interactional behavior, and a positive assumption of sick role behavior. Swaim[63] studied individual patients with rheumatoid arthritis and found that subjects who improved their spiritual well-being also improved their remission status. In the Comstock and Partridge[6] study, church attendance was found to exert a positive influence on health.

In summary, there is no solid base of research to guide the recognition and treatment of the phenomenon of spiritual distress. The theoretical speculations and practice wisdom of nurses and other professionals committed to providing spiritual care to persons seeking health were used in the following sections as the base for assessment, planning, intervention, and evaluation.

Etiological factors for the diagnostic label—spiritual distress—are included in the following list:

Separation from religious and cultural ties
Challenged belief and value systems
Sense of meaninglessness or purposelessness
Remoteness from God
Disrupted spiritual trust
Moral or ethical nature of therapy
Sense of guilt and shame
Intense suffering
Unresolved feelings about death
Anger toward God

DEFINING CHARACTERISTICS

Expresses concern with meaning of life or death or any belief system*

Anger toward God

Questions meaning of suffering

Verbalizes inner conflict about beliefs

Verbalizes concern about relationship with deity

Questions meaning for own existence

Unable to participate in usual religious practices

Seeks spiritual assistance

Questions moral or ethical implications of therapeutic regimen

Gallows humor

Displacement of anger toward religious representatives

Nightmares or sleep disturbance

Alteration of behavior or mood evidenced by anger, crying, withdrawal, preoccupation, anxiety, hostility, apathy, etc.

Loss of or separation from God and/or institutionalized religion†

The experience of evil or disillusionment†

A sense of failing God; the recognition of one's own sinfulness†

Lack of reconciliation with God†

A perceived loneliness of spirit†

Experiences a disturbance in belief system‡

    Questions credibility of belief system

    Is discouraged

    Is unable to practice usual religious rituals

    Has ambivalent feelings (doubts) about beliefs

    Feels a sense of spiritual emptiness

*Critical defining characteristic.
†O'Brien.[47]
‡Waterhouse.[66]

Expresses concern (anger, resentment, fear) over meaning of life, suffering, death‡

Requests spiritual assistance for a disturbance in belief system‡

Thirteen of the preceding defining characteristics were approved by participants of the Fourth National Conference on Classification of Nursing Diagnosis held in 1980.[28] The historical development of the label is of interest, particularly since nursing's concern for the spiritual nature of human beings was expressed in two different categories at the First National Conference, which was held in 1973. The overall categories identified at the first conference were faith, alteration in, with three subcategories: Faith in self, Faith in others, and Faith in God; and spiritual comfort, alteration in, a subcategory of the category, Comfort, alteration in. In 1978, at the Third National Conference, new labels were added: spiritual concern, spiritual distress, and spiritual despair. At the Fourth National Conference in 1980 the old labels in both categories were deleted by participants and only one label, spiritual distress (distress of the human spirit) was recommended for use and testing. Recommendations for refinement of the category were made at the Fifth National Conference and were reported in the proceedings.[27] Distress of the human spirit is a disruption in the life principle that pervades a person's entire being and integrates and transcends one's biologic and psychosocial nature.[28]

NURSING INTERVENTIONS

The following nursing interventions flow from the plan addressed in the following section. Each plan is specific to the proposed etiologies for the diagnosis of spiritual distress. The following interventions, however, are speculative and need validation through practice, research, and evaluation.

Patient Goal	Nursing Intervention
Alleviate the sense of powerlessness and loneliness related to separation from religious ties.	Take time to listen and be open to patient's expressions of loneliness and powerlessness.
	Be an available advocate to patient's needs.
	Refer to spiritual advisor of patient's choice.
	Prepare patient for religious rituals of choice.
	Provide patient with an atmosphere conducive to prayer, for example, provide religious articles and prayer pamphlets.
	Help patient pray.
	Share appropriate religious readings that convey a message of hope in dealing with loneliness and doubt, if patient is open and ready.
Clarify beliefs and values.	Value clarification[38]
	1. Have patient get in touch with self through use of prayer, meditation, and relaxation (centering prayer).

Patient Goal	Nursing Intervention
	2. Have patient make lists of what is important and how much time is spent on things that are important and not important. 3. Delineate long- and short-term goals. 4. Plan short-term tasks to meet short-term goals. 5. Suggest that patient imagine self asking God or an inner advisor to help clarify doubts and to ask what the person should do and be. 6. Have patient act on advice from inner advisor. Provide opportunity for patient to meet with spiritual advisor.
Find meaning and purpose in illness and diversity.	Be available to listen to and be empathetic to patient's feelings. Suggest and teach the use of meditation and centering prayer. Use religious or other readings (such as Frankl's *Man's Search for Meaning*[14]) that describe others who have found meaning in life in difficult situations. Help patient put problems into a wider perspective. Have patient select and write down positive labels for each stressor of life. Aid patient in replacing negative thoughts and labels with positive ones. Help patient take risks and make commitment to something or someone.
Increase relationship with God and satisfaction in prayer.	Be present and available to patient. Offer to obtain for patient religious articles that could aid in praying. Teach simple quieting and relaxation skills so patient can relax and experience the presence of God. Offer to pray with patient. Suggest the need to find God's presence in self and others. Remind patient that many people have experienced remoteness from God (give appropriate examples of people in religious stories and writings). Refer to clergy if patient is open to spiritual experts.
Decrease sense of alienation with God, self, and others.	Develop trust with patient by listening and by being present and responsive to patient's needs. Be empathetic and understanding of patient's feelings. Provide quiet times for patient to do meditation and centering. Help patient find in illness a means to grow and develop depth in understanding life. Express that God accepts and loves people for who they are. Facilitate patient's use of meditation, prayer, and other religious traditions and rituals.
Find understanding and comfort in moral and ethical decisions.	Help patient solve problem openly and to act on decisions. Include patient in decision process about treatments and illness. Teach patient the use of prayer and meditation and to imagine bringing problems to a loving God. Help patient obtain advice from pastoral care and experts in moral and ethical decisions.
Decrease sense of guilt by healing past hurts.	Be open and present when patient is willing to share past hurts and guilt. Suggest the use of reflective prayer and keeping journals to analyze past hurts. Teach patient the use of centering prayer and healing of memory prayers. Have patients imagine themselves sharing with a loving God their painful memories and hurts, ask God to take the hurt away, heal them, and to allow themselves to be filled with love.
Experience feelings that God will help to endure and relieve suffering.	Assure patient that nurse will be available to support patient in times of suffering. Offer to pray with patient in times of suffering. If patient is comfortable with your touch, hold patient's hand or place your hand gently on the patient's arm or other part of the body that is causing pain. If patient desires, form a praying team; while touching, pray for God's healing presence. Other members of the health team and a person close to the patient might be included in the praying team. Ask them to pray in a way that is comfortable in asking for God's healing of the patient's suffering. After about 5 minutes of prayer conclude with a simple closing prayer. While praying, have the patient imagine the presence of a loving God healing part of the body that is painful, injured, or diseased.

Patient Goal	Nursing Intervention
Reduce fear of death.	Be open, present, and empathetic to patient's feelings about death. Support patient's beliefs of an afterlife in the presence of a loving God. Have patient visualize own death while relaxing and meditating; include in the image being in the presence of God and past friends and family that have died before. Refer patient to clergy or other spiritual advisor for religious rites. Refer patient to religious writings that support concept of afterlife.
Decrease anger toward God.	Mention to patient that anger towards God is a normal (or common) part of the process of healing past hurts. Help patient get in touch with feelings of anger. Help patient share feelings of anger with self or trusting friend. Problem solve ways to properly express and relieve anger. Use prayer and imagery to heal past hurts. Encourage patient to adopt attitude of gratitude for getting deeper insights into life.

The following plan, designed for the diagnosis of spiritual distress, contains nursing-ordered interventions directed toward treating etiologies taken from the Fourth and Fifth Conferences on the Classification of Nursing Diagnoses.

Etiology	Goal
Separation from religious and cultural ties	Alleviate the sense of powerlessness and loneliness related to separation from religious/cultural ties.
Challenged belief and value systems	Clarify beliefs and values.
Sense of meaninglessness or purposelessness	Find meaning and purpose in illness and diversity.
Remoteness from God	Increase relationship with God and satisfaction in prayer.
Disrupted spiritual trust	Decrease sense of alienation from God, self, and others.
Moral and ethical nature of therapy	Find understanding and comfort in moral and ethical decisions.
Sense of guilt and shame	Heal past hurts and find a sense of forgiveness from God, self, and others.
Intense suffering	Endure, find meaning in suffering, and experience feeling that God will help them cope with any suffering they will endure.
Unresolved feelings about death	Reduce fears of death and increase acceptance and meaning in death and an afterlife.
Anger toward God	Decrease anger toward God and self.

Developing a plan of care for a person with the nursing diagnosis of spiritual distress is difficult because of its abstract nature. Spiritual distress has never been clinically validated nor have there been reports of clinical or research-based interventions to treat the diagnosis. The diagnosis exists because it was retrospectively identified by nurses interested in spiritual matters who attended national or regional nursing diagnosis conferences. The nursing literature, however, does include articles and books that deal with unvalidated nursing diagnoses and spiritual needs that have some association with the diagnosis of spiritual distress. The articles offer some ideas for plans of care that could be used in treating spiritual distress. For example, O'Brien[47] defined spiritual pain and gave a case example of possible treatment. Fish and Shelly[12] discussed a number of spiritual needs in their book on spiritual care and presented chapters on the use of prayer and scripture to meet the patient's spiritual needs.

Although there is scant literature on the diagnosis of spiritual distress and although the diagnosis has not been clinically validated, it is appropriate to discuss the role of the professional nurse in the area of spiritual care. A plan of care is presented here to stimulate thought, clinical testing, and formal research. Although the provision of spiritual care by nurses has a historical basis, the diagnosis and treatment of spiritual matters are not common practice for nurses and might be more controversial than in other areas of nursing care.

Roles in Spiritual Care

Fish and Shelly[12] addressed the roles of nurses and pastoral ministers in providing spiritual care and compared them in four areas: (1) availability, (2) involvement, (3) education and experience, and (4) context and authority. The main point is that a nurse has an opportunity to be more intimately involved with a patient and is more fa-

---

SPIRITUAL BELIEFS

As nurses, we can help our patients with their spiritual beliefs. By this, we are not referring necessarily to religion, which is an organized group experience. By spiritual, we mean the personal experience of feeling balance and connections. By our very actions and qualities of honesty, caring, and compassion, we can help patients balance their lives and decrease their stress.

There are many ways that people can have spiritual experiences which allow them to connect with that energy often referred to as God, Buddha, creator, supreme being, higher power, or universal life force—whatever the individual preference happens to be. It may be through music, meditation, or prayer. A person may describe such connections as a peak experience, a shift in consciousness, moving out and beyond, or a sense of oneness with the universe. All people have their own interpretation of the meaning of spirituality. As nurses, we can help patients decrease their stress and increase their balance by engaging them in discussions of their feelings and thoughts. During the discussions we can assess body reactions and mannerisms to help them move toward balance and relaxation.

From Guzzetta, C.E., and Dorsey, B.M.: Cardiovascular nursing: bodymind tapestry, St. Louis, 1984, The C.V. Mosby Co.

---

miliar with hospital settings and procedures. The nurse's education, experience, and expertise, however, are usually not in spiritual matters. On the other hand, ministers, rabbis, and other clergy are expert in matters of spirituality and provide and perform religious rituals, but they are not immediately available on a 24-hour basis, are often uncomfortable in hospital settings, and do not usually develop the type of intense intimate contact with a patient characteristic of a nurse. The preceding statements are obviously generalizations. Many clergy and others who provide spiritual guidance develop close relationships with patients and are comfortable with the hospital setting. What is important is that nurses and clergy recognize that their roles do overlap and that they collaborate and communicate with one another in providing the best spiritual care for a patient. Nurses, because of their familiarity with health care settings and close contact with a patient and family, can often facilitate the role of clergy in a hospital or nursing home setting.

Members of the clergy and nurses both share the responsibility of helping patients decide what is best for them in relation to their illness and what they perceive their spiritual response should be. Travelbee[64] believed that the essence of nursing is helping patients find meaning in illness, suffering, and death. The role of the nurse also overlaps with that of the clergy in regard to other important areas of health management, such as grief counseling, preparing patients for death, alleviating suffering, fears, and loneliness, and answering ethical questions.

The types of spiritual interventions that nurses provide might also induce controversy. Most nurses, clergy, and patients probably believe it is proper for nurses to help prepare patients for religious rituals, to be aware of spe-

cial religious needs of patients with different religious backgrounds, to be available to listen to patients' concerns about spiritual matters, to refer patients to spiritual experts, and to pray with them occasionally. Interventions beyond these are open to controversy and speculation. Martin, Burrows, and Pomilio[36] asked 90 patients how they thought nurses might help patients meet spiritual needs. A majority of the respondents said by listening, being present, and referring to clergy. O'Brien[47] stressed that all nurses may not be or feel comfortable in dealing with spiritual matters. She stated that no level of spiritual assessment should be attempted without an initial expression of need by a patient. It has also been suggested that nurses who do not share a patient's religious and spiritual convictions should not attempt to provide spiritual guidance.

Probably the most compelling and common argument for the role of the nurse in providing spiritual care is that nurses profess to treat patients from a wholistic perspective. If nurses purport to treat the total patient, then they must deal with the patient's spiritual side as well as the mind and body. If not, nurses are ignoring an important dimension of their patient's well-being.

The role of the nurse in providing spiritual care is dictated by what the nursing profession defines and uses in practice, research, and education. If the profession follows the American Nurses Association's Social Policy Statement,[30] then it seems that spiritual responses to actual and potential health problems should be a core concern of nursing. The spiritual responses to illness may be more appropriately dealt with by nurses than by religious caregivers because nurses are the best equipped persons to recognize responses to illness and are more available to treat the responses. Spiritual responses to health problems, however, need to be identified and validated by nurses so that they become part of the common language and practice of nursing.

Assessment

Before developing a plan of care, nurses should do a comprehensive assessment to determine the nursing diagnoses. An assessment of a patient's spiritual well-being might be part of an overall general assessment or an indepth secondary assessment after spiritual concerns have been elicited. An assessment will not only help nurses detect spiritual problems but also provide them with baseline data for further analysis and evaluation.

A number of spiritual assessment guides and spiritual measurement tools are available in the literature, but not all of them are specific for the diagnosis of spiritual distress. Colliton,[5] in her chapter in a textbook by Beland and Passos, included a spiritual assessment guide that is essentially a listing of labels and characteristics of spiritual matters from the Fourth National Conference on Classification of Nursing Diagnoses. Being aware of the characteristics of spiritual distress can help a nurse assess whether a patient merits the diagnosis. It must be emphasized that the defining characteristics have not been validated in practice or research. Use of the guide, however, is a step in that direction.

O'Brien[47] developed a spiritual assessment guide to provide a broad overview of spiritual beliefs and behaviors. The guide is used to assess areas of general and personal spiritual beliefs, religious support systems, religious rituals, identification with institutionalized religion, and spiritual deficit or distress. Under spiritual distress there are questions related to spiritual pain, spiritual alienation, spiritual anxiety, spiritual guilt, spiritual anger, spiritual loss, and spiritual despair. Several of the labels coincide with the etiologies of spiritual distress on the National Conference listing—specifically anger, guilt, and alienation from God.

Stoll[62] developed guidelines for spiritual assessment based on four areas: (1) a concept of God, (2) sources of hope and strength, (3) religious practices, and (4) relationship between spiritual beliefs and health. She provided specific questions that a nurse might ask patients to assess each of the four areas. Use of such an assessment guide might indicate etiologies and characteristics of spiritual distress. Fish and Shelly[12] gave tips on detecting spiritual needs by observing cues from patients' affects and attitudes, behaviors, verbalizations, interpersonal relationships, and environments. Flesner[13] developed a 20-item measurement tool for the specific diagnosis of spiritual distress. Each item is based on a five-point Likert scale. The tool was developed for a master's essay and needs further testing and validation.

The Spiritual Well-Being (SWB) tool developed by Paloutzian and Ellison[51] could also be useful in assessing a person's spirituality. Their test, like Flesner's, is a 20-item Likert-type scoring instrument. Besides obtaining a total SWB score, religious well-being (RWB) and existential well-being (EWB) subscores can be obtained. The RWB score is a measure of the strength of a person's relationship with God, and the EWB score a person's satisfaction with self and purpose in life. Although the SWB tool does not assess spiritual distress, a low SWB score might indicate spiritual problems and a need for further assessment.

A final suggestion for spiritual assessment is a set of five questions that Tubesing[65] proposed to assess a person's spiritual outlook. Spiritual outlook concerns a person's goals, faith, value, commitments, and ability to let go and to receive forgiveness from self and others. Tubesing's five questions are: What is the aim of life? What beliefs guide me? What is important to me? What do I choose to spend myself on? What am I willing to let go? The questions and other spiritual assessment tools, however, must be used with caution by a nurse and only with proper training and understanding.

In assessing spiritual matters, a number of authors mention the need to be sensitive to cues from patients that might indicate a desire to talk about spiritual problems.[8,12] The cues might be verbal, nonverbal behaviors, or inanimate objects. The authors encouraged nurses to develop their own spirituality, thereby becoming more sensitive to patients' spiritual problems and better equipped to manage them. Nurses might develop their own spirituality through the practice of religion, or spiritual development might be of a humanistic nature and involve taking time to listen to classical music or to enjoy the beauty of nature. It might also mean the realization by nurses of the importance of the spirit in health and illness. Some authors of books on wholistic health believe that the spirit may suffer when a person does not take care of the body and mind.[32,54] There is also a corollary to this, that is, a person's spiritual self develops as the body suffers from an acute or chronic illness. Many persons use religion and prayer to cope with illness, and there is some indication that patients with chronic illnesses who have high levels of SWB will also have high levels of psychologic well-being.[23,31,41] This evidence suggests that it is important for nurses not to ignore the influence of spirituality and religion in health care. Finally, nurses have been helped to be more sensitive to patients' spiritual needs through hospital-sponsored prayer groups and conferences on spiritual needs.[3] Such groups are most appropriate in hospitals with formal religious affiliations and are best held in conjunction with hospital chaplains and other spiritual care personnel to maintain good relationships with them and to encourage use of their expertise in matters of spirituality.

Treatment Plan

The literature is a source of ideas that could be used to develop a treatment plan for spiritual distress. Campbell[4] devised a common plan for treating spiritual diagnoses related to spiritual distress: disrupted spiritual rites, disrupted spiritual trust, difficulty in achieving desired spiritual dependence, spiritually restricted health maintenance, and difficulty maintaining a religious diet. The common treatment plan included comfort, protection from psychologic threat, warm communicating relationships, and religious-philosophic satisfaction. Fish and Shelly's suggestions[12] are broad in scope and do not provide direction for a specific diagnosis or etiology. They recommended planning to help patients establish and maintain a dynamic relationship with God, establish continuity of care and communication with other health care providers, outline patients' spiritual needs with appropriate interventions, and determine the best person to assume responsibility for meeting a patient's spiritual needs. They also addressed the use of prayer, scripture readings, and clergy referrals. Stallwood and Stoll[61] contributed guidelines for use of prayer and scripture in a general nursing text. Pumphrey[55] proposed giving spiritual support and reinforcement by suggesting that patients talk with clergy and try meditation and prayer. Dickinson[7] viewed spiritual care from a broad perspective and spirituality as the force that activates individuals. She believed that spiritual care was an integral part of a nurse-patient relationship provided through common nursing measures such as support, awareness, empathy, nonjudgmental understanding, and helping persons find meaning in suffering and death.

O'Brien[47] included listening, support, and referral as interventions in spiritual care. Ellis[8] also suggested the use of active listening and gave suggestions for nurses to help patients with religious rituals, prayer, spiritual concerns, and preparing a patient for a chaplain. Assisting patients at religious rituals and practices, arranging visits from key religious persons, and providing encouragement and support of spiritual values were viewed as appropriate nursing interventions by Keining.[26] Finally, Hubert[21] concluded that helping patients recognize meaning in illness, helping them to strengthen their relationships with God, and helping them to appreciate spiritual values were part of the spiritual care that could be provided by nurses. She believed that this was accomplished through frequent contacts with the patient, by appropriate attitudes, with wholesome uplifting readings, and through prayer.

From the nursing and spiritual care literature it is evident that several broad areas are appropriate for nursing intervention: providing spiritual support through active listening, caring, and being available and sensitive to patients' spiritual needs; making referrals to qualified spiritual experts, using meditation, prayer, and religious readings; and preparing patients for religious practices. Nurses concerned with specific religious practices for hospitalized patients should refer to Henderson's chapter[17] on worship or articles by Kelly[25] and Pumphrey.[55]

Most of the literature on nursing and spiritual care suggests the use of listening, being supportive of spiritual values and concerns, being sensitive to spiritual needs, and being available as a means of providing spiritual care. This is probably the minimal amount of spiritual intervention that all nurses should and could provide, since a therapeutic relationship is the essence of nursing practice. Dickinson[7] described nursing practice as a therapeutic spiritual relationship and suggested that nursing could be a spiritual ministry. Being present, available, and an empathetic listener could do much to help a person who is spiritually distressed, especially those patients suffering from loneliness and expressing doubts, fears, and feelings of alienation. As Padovano[49] expressed, an aspect of humanity is the ability to be healed through the presence of another.

In hospitals and other settings with pastoral care departments, referral to pastoral care is another commonly suggested intervention because the department's staff are viewed as experts in spiritual and pastoral care. They, however, are not necessarily the experts on spiritual responses to health problems. It is of benefit to patients that nursing and pastoral care have a close relationship and confer on the spiritual care of a patient. It is often a nurse who first detects a spiritual problem, and a nurse might be the person who has developed the intense trusting relationship that is needed for spiritual intervention or that is needed for the patient to be receptive to spiritual care. In settings without religious affiliations or for patients whose spiritual beliefs differ from those of the hospital staff, spiritual counsel may be provided by the patient's own clergy or spiritual adviser or by clergy from local churches and synagogues. When spiritual counselors are from outside the hospital and are not familiar with the hospital setting or patient, then helping them to be comfortable, informed, and welcome is an important role for the nurse to assume.

There are other settings besides the hospital in which the nurse and pastoral minister work closely for the health and wholistic well-being of patients. Westberg[67] and others[20] have modeled wholistic health clinics in which a member of the clergy, nurse, and physician work as an integral team in providing health care. Westberg has recently advocated that nurses assume the role of health ministers in church-based settings.[1]

The use of prayer, meditation, and scripture and other religious readings can be another powerful source of spir-

OPENING THE ENERGY CENTERS

This is a meditation for healing and purifying your body, and for getting your energy flowing. It is an excellent one to do in the morning when you first wake up, or at the beginning of any meditation period, or anytime you want to be relaxed and refreshed:

Lie down on your back with arms at your sides or with hands clasped on your stomach. Close your eyes, relax and breathe gently, deeply and slowly.

Imagine that there is a glowing sphere of golden light surrounding the top of your head. Breathe deeply and slowly in and out five times while you keep your attention on the sphere of light, feeling it radiate from the top of your head.

Now allow your attention to move down to your throat. Again imagine a golden sphere of light emanating from your throat area. Breathe slowly in and out five times with your attention on this light.

Allow your attention to move down to the center of your chest. Once again imagine the golden light, radiating from the center of your chest. Again take five deep breaths, as you feel the energy expanding more and more.

Next put your attention on your solar plexus; visualize the sphere of golden light all around your midsection. Breathe into it slowly, five times.

Now visualize the light glowing in and around your pelvic area. Again take five deep breaths, feeling the light energy radiating and expanding.

Finally, visualize the flowing sphere of light around your feet, and breathe into it five more times.

Now imagine all six of the spheres of light glowing at once so that your body is like a strand of jewels, radiating energy.

Breathe deeply, and as you exhale, imagine energy flowing down along the outside of the left side of your body from the top of your head to your feet. As you inhale, imagine it flowing up along the right side of your body to the top of your head. Circulate it round your body this way three times.

Then visualize the flow of energy going from the top of your head down along the front of your body to your feet as you slowly exhale. As you inhale, feel it flow up along the back of your body to the top of your head. Circulate the flow in this direction three times.

Now imagine that the energy is gathering at your feet, and let it flow slowly up through the center of your body from your feet to your head, radiating from the top of your head like a fountain of light, then flowing back down the outside of your body to your feet. Repeat this several times, or as long as you wish.

When you finish this meditation you will be deeply relaxed, yet energized and exhilarated.

Excerpted from *Creative Visualization* by Shakti Gawain, copyright © 1978 by Shakti Gawain. Reprinted by permission of Whatever Publishing, Inc., Mill Valley, California.

itual care and comfort and the alleviation of spiritual distress. Some nurses find the use of prayer uncomfortable, and others think it inappropriate as a nursing intervention. However, for many patients it is the most common method used to cope with and face adversity. Learning to feel comfortable with prayer—a simple, safe, and available method to treat spiritual distress—to provide an environment conducive to prayer, and to provide prayer books or other religious objects to aid in prayers are minimum expectations of a professional nurse.

Many forms of prayer and meditation could be used to help a patient develop a feeling of oneness with the universe or a better relationship with God, comfort the patient, and help relieve spiritual distress. The type of prayer, however, should be tailored to a patient's own style, comfort, and needs. Sometimes patients might be too sick to pray for themselves and need the support from others. If the patient's family, close friends, or spiritual advisor is not available, then a nurse who shares the patient's spiritual beliefs might be the person best suited for the task.

Many forms of meditation, both religious and secular, can be used by patients to help them relax, clear their mind, achieve a feeling of oneness with a deity or the universe, promote peaceful acceptance of painful memories or decisions, and gather energy and hope that may enable them to overcome spiritual distress. The meditation technique described in the box above is an example of meditation that can be used by many patients and can be adapted to fit a particular patient's situation and spiritual beliefs.

Centering prayer is similar to a secular meditation or relaxation technique, except that the person focuses on the presence of God. A prayer such as this might provide a sense of relaxation while the patient develops and maintains a relationship with God. While centering and relaxing, patients might try imagining a loving God and then imagine themselves bringing their doubts, painful decisions, past hurts, loneliness, and lack of meaning to Him and then asking Him what He wants them to do and be. This form of prayerful imagination could be helpful for patients trying to find meaning in their suffering or for those who have painful decisions about their health problems. Bringing divine guidance into the decision process might be comforting to a patient, provide the loving authority of God, and bring a transcendence to the decision process. A daily journal of the patient that included feelings, insights, and a dialogue with God and self could augment the prayer process.

Certain types of prayers might be particularly appropriate for the diagnosis of spiritual distress in caring for the Christian client. A prayer form called *healing of memories* has been popularized and developed by two Catholic priests, Dennis and Mathew Linn.[33-35] Healing of memories is a type of prayer that helps give a person a deeper insight into self, a sense of forgiveness, and an inner healing of past hurts. The prayer essentially entails sharing with Christ painful memories, asking Him to take away the hurt, and filling oneself with the love of His spirit. Healing of memories might also entail imagining past stages of development, imagining the specific hurts at those given times, and imagining Christ's healing presence at each stage of life. Schlientz[57] found this type of prayer helped people to understand and decrease their anger. Healing of memories might be particularly helpful for persons suffering from spiritual distress and the accompanying anger, fears, guilt, loneliness, and distrust.

Healing of memories or other types of prayers could be extended to prayer teams in which several people touch and pray over the person seeking healing. A team made up of a nurse, attending physician, clergy, and a person close to the patient might not only be beneficial for a patient but also could benefit the health team by bringing a common spiritual dimension into their work. Barbara Shlemon,[59] a nurse, participated in such prayer teams and prayed for not only a spiritual healing but physical healing as well. Shlemon provided healing workshops for nurses and other health care professionals throughout the country. Use of touch with prayer might also provide the benefits of healing touch, as described by Montague,[43] Krieger,[29] and others.[15]

The use of religious and inspirational readings by the nurse to help a person heal spiritual distress might be particularly beneficial. This form of intervention requires openness by the patient and knowledge of appropriate religious literature by the nurse. Scripture should never be used by a nurse to push ideas or individual interpretations, but rather to support a patient's spiritual values or to alleviate the person's sense of loneliness, powerlessness, suffering, or lack of meaning. Many religious works illustrate characters who have had the same doubts and feelings. Relaying these passages might be of benefit

and comfort to the spiritually distressed patient. Shelly[58] suggested that nurses use scriptural passages that have been most meaningful to them. Travelbee[64] illustrated the use of scripture in helping patients find meaning in their illness and suffering, and Stallwood and Stoll[61] and Fish and Shelly[12] described the use of scripture in spiritual care. Scripture can be useful in reinforcing patients' beliefs and provide a message of hope. Examples of comforting and inspirational works and their relevance to certain forms of forgiveness, hurts, doubts, and values can be found in some of the suggested readings at the end of this pattern.

There are several other types of interventions that might be useful in treating patients with spiritual distress. For example, the use of value clarification by the nurse might be helpful for a patient who is ambivalent about his or others' beliefs. There are self-help workbooks available that patients or nurses could use to help clarify values and beliefs. Use of value clarification in a religious context by referring to readings, meditation, or prayer to reinforce values might also be worthwhile.[38]

The use of music helps to calm or comfort some persons with intense suffering and can help a person feel closer to God or at one with nature or the universe. A wide variety of religious, inspirational, and secular music may have a calming effect and may be spiritually uplifting to a patient. Norbet[46] and the monks of the Weston Priory have recorded music that was specifically composed to heal the spirit. It would be relatively easy for a hospital to have tape recorders and cassette tapes of music available to meet a patient's choice and tastes.

Tubesing[65] offers a number of spiritual treatment plans for people with stress-related illnesses that grow from an inappropriate spiritual outlook. Although the eight spiritual skills that he lists are treatment plans for stress-related illness, the skills seem particularly applicable for persons with the diagnosis of spiritual distress. The eight spiritual skills as proposed by Tubesing are as follows. Some of these skills have been delineated in earlier discussions.

1. *Valuing:* the art of choosing between alternatives
2. *Personal planning skills:* the art of setting goals and making steady progress toward them
3. *Commitment skills:* the art of saying "yes" and investing self
4. *Surrender skills:* the art of saying "goodbye," letting go, and closing doors
5. *Faith skills:* the art of accepting the mysterious and the unknowable
6. *Relabeling skills:* the art of calling a spade a diamond in the rough and seeing the promise in every problem
7. *Imagination skills:* the art of creativity and laughter
8. *Whisper skills:* the art of talking to self and giving self positive messages

EVALUATION

The following are suggested outcome criteria based on treating the previously listed causes of spiritual distress. Some of the outcomes are rather abstract and exist as a matter of degree. Quantifiable outcomes are presented when possible.

Patient Outcome	Data Indicating That Outcome is Reached
Sense of control related to religious cultural ties	Identification of available religious and cultural resources Comfort in religious and cultural rituals and objects Low score on loneliness scale[51]
Clear beliefs and values	Delineation of short- and long-term goals Plans to meet these goals Value clarification complete
Sense of purpose and meaning in illness	Positive thoughts about life and self High score (40-60) on the RWB scale of the SWB index
Closeness with God	Ability to pray or meditate. Satisfaction in prayer and/or meditation High score (40-60) on the RWB scale of the SWB index
Trust in God, self, and others	Feeling that God and others love and accept them for who they are
Understanding of ethical nature of illness and/or therapy	Understanding of ethical choice of treatment Active involvement in decision process of therapy Identification of support systems in making ethical decisions (pastoral care, ethical committees)
Sense of forgiveness	Sharing of past hurts and guilt Acceptance of forgiveness from God and others Sense of God's and others' love
Relief from and/or acceptance of suffering	Feeling that God will help relieve and/or endure suffering Sense of comfort
Decreased fear of and/or acceptance of death	Ability to image and talk about death without undue anxiety
Relief of anger toward God	Understanding of God's will High score (40-60) on the RWB scale

Several approaches can be taken in evaluating the effectiveness of interventions for treating spiritual distress. The three discussed in this chapter are (1) the simple and direct approach, (2) the relief of symptoms approach, and (3) the amelioration of etiologies approach.

The simple and direct approach to evaluation entails a test that directly or indirectly measures spiritual distress. For example, the Spiritual Distress Scale has been designed as a direct measure of the nursing diagnosis of spiritual distress.[13] Although the tool needs further validation and more reliability, total scores can indicate a patient's level of spiritual distress. If a nurse has diagnosed a patient as spiritually distressed through the use of the tool (that is, the patient had a high spiritual distress score), then the tool could be readministered through the course of treatment to determine if the spiritual distress is decreasing or was relieved. A low score on the spiritual distress scale indicates successful treatment.

Another example of a paper and pencil measurement tool is the SWB Index developed by Paloutzian and Ellison.[51] Although it provides a measure of spiritual well-being rather than spiritual distress, a high SWB score would indicate that a person is spiritually well and not spiritually distressed. The two subscales of the SWB scale also help determine the effects of treatment. A person who has been effectively treated for spiritual distress would have a high RWB score and would give an indication of a good relationship with God. A high EWB score, on the other hand, indicates that a person is comfortable with a purpose in life and has a satisfying self-concept. Again, meaning, purpose, and self-concept are related to the etiologies of spiritual distress. Use of measurement tools by the nurse, however, requires understanding them and employing sensitivity in administration.

If a patient is too sick to have a paper-and-pencil test

administered or if it would be inappropriate, a simple spiritual titre might be used. Jourard[24] has indicated that everybody has a spiritual titre on a continuum from 1 to 100, with 100 indicating a high spirit of life and 1 being a person very low in spirit. A nurse who is evaluating the patient's spiritual distress or the effectiveness of treatment could simply explain the spiritual titre scale and have the patient periodically indicate his spiritual level on a scale from 1 to 100.

Another approach to evaluation of treatment of spiritual distress is through the absence of symptoms or characteristics common to spiritual distress, such as anger, guilt, depression, anxiety, and crying. This is a good indication that a patient is no longer spiritually distressed. A more formal evaluation of a given set of symptoms of spiritual distress could be accomplished with reliable measurement tools. For example, a patient's anxiety could be evaluated with the State-Trait Anxiety Inventory (STAI),[60] anger could be evaluated with the Profile of Mood State (POMS)[40] inventory, and depression through Beck's Depression Inventory.[2] Use of the tools, however, requires expertise in administration and interpretation. Some of the tests require professional psychological supervision.

A third approach is through evaluating the given etiologies of the problem. For example, a patient who is spiritually distressed because of an unclear belief or value system might benefit from value clarification. The patient's ability to identify short- and long-term goals consistent with previously expressed values and beliefs would indicate the effectiveness of the intervention. In another example, a nurse who treats spiritual distress related to expressed remoteness from God through prayer, meditation, and spiritual counseling could get an indication of the effectiveness of treatment through the patient's expression of satisfaction with prayer and feelings of closeness to God. In other words, each plan or intervention could be evaluated by assessing the influence of treatments on the presenting cluster of indications for a given etiology.

A more formal approach to evaluation of treatment effectiveness is through research, including single-case experimental designs. This approach might be particularly appropriate because of the abstract nature of the diagnosis. Formal evaluation through the use of single-case designs lends experimental validity to the existence of the diagnosis. Single-case experiments are also very practical because nurses with graduate degrees are able to use the method to evaluate a treatment program for an individual patient.

There are many examples of single-case experimental designs. The simplest and most practical is the *AB* design, where *A* is the baseline phase and *B* represents evaluation of the treatment phase. The design is practical because it follows the normal course of evaluation for a single patient. The *AB* design, however, has some drawbacks in that there could be many explanations for the effectiveness of a treatment other than the treatment itself. To overcome this drawback, reversal designs such as the *ABA* or *ABAB* design are preferred. Another type of single-case design requires the use of several *AB* designs extended across either subjects, settings, or dependent variables.

A simple example of the use of an *AB* single-case evaluation for spiritual distress is for healing prayers. A nurse could measure a patient's symptoms of anger, guilt, depression, and anxiety through the use of the STAI, POMS, and Beck's Depression Inventory. The variables are measured two or three times daily over a baseline period of 2 or 3 days and through an intervention period during which some form of healing prayer is used daily. Analysis of effectiveness is accomplished through graphing the measures and analyzing the graphs or through use of statistical techniques designed for single-cased experiments.[18]

The use of single-case experimental designs requires some knowledge of research design and methodology and may also require formal patient consent and review by the hospital's research committee. Use of the designs, however, could provide an effective means of evaluation. The nurse who does not have the required knowledge of research methodology or who does not have time or energy could use other evaluation approaches mentioned earlier.

References

1. Anderson, D.E.: Health may be next for church ministry, The Milwaukee Journal, June 11, 1983.
2. Beck, A.T., and Beamesderfer, A.: Assessment of depression: the depression inventory, Psychological Measurements in Psychopharmacology **7:**151, 1974.
3. Buys, A.M.: Discussion series sensitizes nurses to patients' spiritual needs, Hosp. Prog. **62:**44, Oct. 1981.
4. Cambell, C.: Nursing diagnosis and intervention in nursing practice, New York, 1978, John Wiley & Sons, Inc.
5. Colliton, M.A.: The spiritual dimension of nursing. In Beland, I.L., and Passos, J.Y., editors: Clinical nursing: pathophysiological and psychosocial approaches, ed. 4, New York, 1981, Macmillan Publishing Co.
6. Comstock, G.W., and Partridge, K.B.: Church attendance and health, J. Chronic Dis. **25:**665, 1972.
7. Dickinson, S.C.: The search for spiritual meaning, Am. J. Nurs. **75**(10):1789, 1975.
8. Ellis, D.: Whatever happened to spiritual dimension? Can. Nurse **76:**42, Sept. 1980.
9. Ellison, C.W.: Spiritual well-being, Paper presented at Duke University, Jan. 1982.
10. Fehring, R., and Brennan, P.: Psychological and spiritual well-being in college students, Unpublished paper, Milwaukee, 1983, Marquette University.
11. Fehring, R., Brennan, P., and Keller, M.: Life change, depression and spiritual well-being in college students, Unpublished paper presented to graduate students in nursing, Milwaukee, 1983, Marquette University.

12. Fish, S., and Shelly, J.A.: Spiritual care: the nurse's role, Downers Grove, Ill., 1978, InterVarsity Press.

13. Flesner, R.S.: Development of a measure to assess spiritual distress in the responsive adult, Master's essay, 1982, Marquette University.

14. Frankl, V.: Man's search for meaning, Boston, 1963, Beacon Press.

15. Heidt, P.: Effect of therapeutic touch on anxiety level of hospitalized patients, Nurs. Res. **30**:32, Jan./Feb. 1981.

16. Helleberg, M.M.: Beyond TM, New York, 1980, Paulist Press, Inc.

17. Henderson, V., and Nite, G.: Principles and practice of nursing, ed. 6, New York, 1978, Macmillan Publishing Co.

18. Hersen, M., and Barlow, D.H.: Single case experimental design: strategies for studying behavior change, Elmsford, N.Y., 1976, Pergamon Press, Inc.

19. Highfield, M.F., and Cason, C.: Spiritual needs of patients: are they recognized? Cancer Nurs. **6**:187, 1983.

20. Holinger, P.C., and Tubesing, D.A.: Models of health and wholeness, J. Religion Health **18**:3, 1979.

21. Hubert, M.: Spiritual care for every patient, J. Nurs. Ed. **2**:9, 1963.

22. Hungelmann, J., and others: Harmonious interconnectedness: indicators of spiritual well being in older adults, Conference on Spirituality: A New Perspective on Health, Marquette University, Milwaukee, Aug. 15-16, 1984.

23. Jalowiec, A., and Powers, M.: Stress and coping in hypertensive and emergency room patients, Nurs. Res. **30**:10, 1981.

24. Jourard, S.M.: The transparent self, New York, 1971, Van Nostrand.

25. Kelly, L.Y.: Dimensions of professional nursing, ed. 3, New York, 1975, Macmillan Publishing Co.

26. Kiening, M.: Spiritual needs of the psychiatric patient. In Dunlap, L., editor: Mental health concepts and nursing practice, New York, 1978, John Wiley & Sons, Inc.

27. Kim, M.J., McFarland, G., and McLane, A.M.: Classification of Nursing Diagnoses: Proceedings of the Fifth National Conference, St. Louis, 1984, The C.V. Mosby Co.

28. Kim, M.J., and Moritz, D.A.: Classification of Nursing Diagnoses: Proceedings of the Third and Fourth National Conferences, New York, 1982, McGraw-Hill Book Co.

29. Krieger, D.: The therapeutic touch, Englewood Cliffs, N.J., 1979, Prentice-Hall, Inc.

30. Lang, N., and others: Nursing: a social policy statement, Kansas City, 1980, American Nurses' Association.

31. Leasor, M.: Spiritual indicators and psychological variables in chronically ill patients, Master's thesis, 1983, Marquette University.

32. Legere, T.E.: Thoughts on the run: glimpses of wholistic spirituality, Minneapolis, 1983, Winston Press, Inc.

33. Linn, D., and Linn, M.: Healing of memories, New York, 1974, Paulist Press.

34. Linn, D., and Linn, M.: Healing life's hurts: healing memories through five stages of forgiveness, New York, 1978, Paulist Press.

35. Linn, M., and others: Prayer course for healing life's hurts, New York, 1983, Paulist Press.

36. Martin, C., and others: Spiritual needs of patients study. In Fish, S., and Shelly, J.A., editors: Spiritual care: the nurse's role, Downers Grove, Ill., 1978, Inter Varsity Press.

37. McGee, N.: Health care ministers, Minneapolis, 1982, Winston Press, Inc.

38. McKay, M., and others: Thoughts and feelings, the art of cognitive stress intervention, Richmond, Calif., 1981, New Harbinger Publications.

39. McLane, A.M., and others: Spiritual well-being, morale and living environments of older adults, research in progress.

40. McNaire, D.M., Lorr, M., and Deoppleman, L.: Profile of mood states, San Diego, 1971, Educational and Industrial Testing Service.

41. Miller, J.F.: Loneliness and spiritual well-being in chronically ill and healthy subjects, manuscript submitted for publication.

42. Moberg, D.O.: The development of social indicators of spiritual well-being for quality of life research. In Moberg, D.O., editor: Spiritual well-being: sociological perspectives, Washington, D.C., 1979, University Press of America.

43. Montagu, A.: Touching! The human significance of the skin, New York, 1971, Columbia University Press.

44. National Interfaith Coalition on Aging, Inc.: Spiritual well-being: a definition, Athens, Ga., 1975, National Interfaith Coalition on Aging.

45. Neuman, M.: Am I growing spiritually? Elements for a theology of growth, Review for Religious, Jan.-Feb., 1983, pp. 38-49.

46. Norbet, G.: Spirit alive! Songs of the healing spirit, Weston, Vt., 1977, Weston Priory Productions.

47. O'Brien, M.E.: The need for spiritual integrity. In Yura, H., and Walsh, M.B., editors: Human needs and the nursing process, Norwalk, Conn., 1982, Appleton-Century-Crofts.

48. O'Brien, M.E.: Religious faith and adjustment to long-term hemodialysis, J. Religion Health **21**:68, Spring 1982.

49. Padavano, A.: Belief in human life, New York, 1971, Paulist Press.

50. Paloutzian, R.E.: Research directions on spiritual well-being, Paper presented at S.S.S.R. Convention, Providence, R.I., Oct. 1982.

51. Paloutzian, R., and Ellison, C.: Loneliness, spiritual well-being, and quality of life. In Peplau, L., and Perlman, D., editors: Loneliness: a sourcebook of current theory, research and therapy, New York, 1983, John Wiley & Sons, Inc.

52. Perlberg, M.: There's more to patient care than medicine, Hospitals **52**(10):62, Aug. 1978.

53. Piepgras, R.: The other dimension: spiritual help, Am. J. Nurs. **68**(12):2610, 1968.

54. Pilch, J.J.: Wellness: your invitation to full life, Minneapolis, 1981, Winston Press, Inc.

55. Pumphrey, J.B.: Recognizing your patient's spiritual needs, Nursing **7**(12):64, 1977.

56. Ryan, T.: Fasting rediscovered: a guide to health and wholeness for your body-spirit, New York, 1981, Paulist Press.

57. Schlientz, M.A.: A study of the decrease of unresolved anger through a teaching protocol and healing prayer as a nursing intervention in spiritual care, Doctoral dissertation, 1981, University of Pittsburgh.

58. Shelly, J.A.: Spiritual care workbook, Downers Grove, Ill., 1978, InterVarsity Press.

59. Shlemon, B.L., and others: To heal as Jesus healed, Notre Dame, Ind., 1978, Ave Maria Press.

60. Spielberger, C.D., and others, STAI manual for the state-trait anxiety inventory, Palo Alto, Calif., 1970, Consulting Psychologists' Press, Inc.

61. Stallwood, J., and Stoll, R.: Spiritual dimension of nursing practice. In Beland, I.L., and Pasos, J.Y., editors: Clinical nursing: pathophysiological and psychosocial approaches, ed. 3, New York, 1975, Macmillan Publishing Co., Inc.

62. Stoll, R.I.: Guidelines for spiritual assessment, Am. J. Nurs. **9**:1574, Sept. 1979.

63. Swaim, L.: Arthritis, medicine and the spiritual laws, Philadelphia, 1962, Clinton Book Co.

64. Travelbee, J.: Interpersonal aspects of nursing, Philadelphia, 1966, F.A. Davis Co.

65. Tubesing, D.A.: Stress, spiritual outlook and health, Specialized Pastoral Care J. **3**:17, 1980.

66. Waterhouse, J.: Spiritual distress. In Nursing diagnosis: application to clinical practice, Philadelphia, 1983, J.B. Lippincott Co.

67. Westberg, G.E.: Dissemination of wholistic health centers. In Allen, D.E., and others, editors: Whole-person medicine, Downers Grove, Ill., 1980, Inter Varsity Press.

68. Wilber, K.: Eye to eye: the quest for a new paradigm, Garden City, N.Y., 1983, Anchor Press/Doubleday.

Suggested Readings

Appel, G.: A philosophy of mizvot: the religious-ethical concepts of Judaism, their roots in biblical law and the oral tradition, New York, 1975, Ktav Publishing House, Inc.

Buscaglia, L.F.: Personhood: the art of being fully human, New York, 1978, Charles B. Slack, Inc.

Donin, H.H.: To be a Jew: a guide to Jewish observance in comtemporary life, New York, 1972, Basic Books, Inc., Publishers.

Donin, H.H.: To pray as a Jew: a guide to the prayer book and the synagogue service, New York, 1980, Basic Books, Inc., Publishers.

Ferrucci, P.: What we may be: techniques for spiritual growth through psychosynthesis, Los Angeles, 1982, J.P. Tarcher, Inc.

Frankl, V.: Man's search for meaning, Boston, 1983, Beacon Press.

Gibran, K.: The prophet, New York, 1972, Alfred A. Knopf, Inc.

Kon, A.: Prayer, London, 1972, Soncino Press.

Linn D., and Linn, M.: Healing life's hurts: healing memories through five stages of forgiveness, New York, 1978, Paulist Press.

Linn, M., and others: Prayer course for healing life's hurts, New York, 1983, Paulist Press.

Maslow, A.: Religions, values and peak experiences, New York, 1970, Viking Press, Inc.

McGee, N.: Health care ministers, Minneapolis, 1982, Winston Press, Inc.

Shelly, J.A.: Spiritual care workbook, Downers Grove, Ill., 1978, InterVarsity Press.

Communication

IMPAIRED COMMUNICATION THEORY

Communication is a dynamic, complex, continuous series of reciprocal events through which messages are exchanged, primarily to produce a response from a person or a group. Communication includes all modes of behavior used by a person, consciously or unconsciously, to affect another person. Hence communication is an integral part of interpersonal relationships. According to Satir, "communication is the largest single factor determining what kinds of relationships [a person] makes with others and what happens to him in the world about him."[34] All persons experiencing emotional disorders encounter problems in interpersonal relationships. Communication and interpersonal relationship difficulties can be etiologic factors, manifestations, or consequences of an emotional disorder.

The nurse-patient relationship provides the vehicle for nursing care and is the major tool of the psychiatric nurse. The effectiveness of this relationship depends on the strength of the communication process.[19] Therefore it is essential for the nurse to become more aware of the complexity of the communication process.[4]

A person's communication pattern is the particular sequence of communication behaviors practiced over time by that person. The nurse ascertains a patient's pattern of communication through analysis of clinical data acquired from history taking, interaction, and observation. The objective in assessing the communication pattern is to obtain data about how, when, where, what, and with whom the patient communicates. Specific details assessed include the components of the communication process, the variables affecting the communication process, and the characteristics manifested.

Components of the Communication Process

To evaluate whether communication is effective or impaired, it is necessary to understand the communication process. Communication has no beginning or end. The events in communication are in dynamic interaction. Here the components are identified and discussed in sequence: sender, message, receiver, and feedback.

Sender. The sender generates and sends a message. The source of the message is an idea, event, or situation reviewed via sensory input from the internal or external environment. The input functions of human communication are mediated by the sensory end organs and the afferent nerve fibers. "Therefore, infectious, toxic, degenerative, traumatic, and neoplastic conditions and congenital malformations can alter or obstruct input."[32]

The sender can consciously focus on only a few of the many signals being received at any one moment in time. The selected input is then analyzed and evaluated before a message can be developed. This phase of *covert rehearsal* involves, according to Wilson and Kneisl,[41] the sender's review of information about self and others and internal rehearsal of possible actions to take and possible reactions of the other. The sender decides what to say, how to say it, and to whom to address the message.

Covert rehearsal is mediated by psychosocial factors such as self-concept, values, anxiety, and social norms. Those parts of the central nervous system which connect input with output, regulate the magnitude of excitation, accelerate or retard responses, store and recall information, process data, and make decisions also affect the covert rehearsal phase of communication.[32] After internal rehearsal of several alternative messages, the sender transmits the one that will, in his or her opinion, have the highest chance for success.[41]

Message. The message is, according to Berlo,[1] the translation of ideas, purpose, and intention into a code that is carried through a channel to the receiver. Ruesch describes two basic systems of codification of a message: "The analogue system rests on some similarities in shape, color, or proportion to the events it purports to represent; the digital system is purely arbitrary in that a number or letter is assigned to a given event and a legend has to indicate what these signs refer to."[32]

Analogue communication. Analogue communication has been present since preverbal humankind. It is a self-explanatory likeness and therefore involves a one-to-one correspondence between the communication and what it represents. The primitive picture-writing by cavedwellers in which concepts were represented by their physical likeness is an example of analogue communication. It is not possible in analogue communication to express negation, qualification, or logical relationships such as "if-then," and "either-or." Analogue communication is nonverbal.

Nonverbal communication is any form of communication that does not use words; it is as effective and important as verbal communication. In fact, in some circumstances "the nonverbal message predominates so strongly that it completely overrides the words another person may be speaking."[24]

Nonverbal communication serves a variety of functions, such as to supplement verbal signals, to substitute for verbal signals, to display affect, to regulate the flow of verbal messages, and to reflect the relationship between sender and receiver.[12] It is expressed through a variety of channels. Wilson and Kneisl[41] describe some nonverbal components: kinesic behavior, paralanguage, proxemics, touch, and the use of cultural artifacts.

Kinesics is the study of body movement. This form of nonverbal communication includes facial expression, eye contact, and gestures.

Facial expression is often used as a general indicator of the emotion a person is experiencing. Lewis[24] cautions, however, against inaccurate interpretation of facial expression. The facial expression for the same emotion can vary with each person according to the degree of the emotion experienced and the extent to which a person demonstrates that emotion.

Eye contact can indicate a willingness to interact with another. Yet aggression and the purposeful inducement of anxiety in another can be the motivation for extended eye contact. Lack of eye contact can communicate dislike, poor self-esteem, competition, embarrassment, or hurt feelings.[24] Culture, in part, determines the meaning of eye contact.

Gestures are defined by Lewis as "any movement of the body or of part of the body which is used to express

or emphasize ideas in conjunction with verbal expression."[24] Clues are provided about how a person may feel toward another by gestures such as positioning of the body and the placement and movements of eyes, hands, and feet. We learn gestures through imitation of others; hence culture dictates the significance of the gesture. Birdwhistell[2] states that there is no one gesture that has the same social meanings in all societies.

Paralanguage or *paralinguistics* includes vocal phenomena such as voice qualifiers (pitch and range), vocal differentiators (crying and laughing), vocal identifiers ("ah" and "un-hun"), and conveyance of emotion through voice quality.[5] Personality characteristics and emotional states are inferred through paralanguage. The ear, as a sound receiver, plays a dual role in communication, according to Lewis[24]: a physiologic role for the reception of sound and a psychologic role for the perception of the attitude(s) associated with the spoken words.

Proxemics, the study of the relationship of space to social interaction, is the third channel of nonverbal communication. Hall,[16] who coined the term, describes four main distances: intimate, personal, social and public.

The *intimate zone* can range from 3 inches to 12 inches. Low tones of voice or whispers are used to communicate intimate or secret messages. In American culture the intimate zone is usually reserved for lovers, spouses, family members, and very close friends. The *personal zone* ranges from 12 to 36 inches. In this zone confidential or personal information is communicated in a soft tone of voice. Americans use this zone for conversations at parties, certain work relationships, and close friendships. In the *social zone* communicators stand 4 to 8 feet apart and talk in full voice. Nonpersonal information is exchanged between business acquaintances or casual friends. The *public zone* can range as far as 100 feet. This space is used for activities such as public speaking, business presentations, and entertainment performances.

Touch has been described as an integral component of nonverbal communication in many studies.[17,28,40] Touch has been credited with establishment of rapport, decrease in confusion, personality development, and decrease in anxiety. Because the use of touch is governed by social norms, it is important to consider the meaning of touch to a given individual within a given culture.

Therapeutic touch has been demonstrated empirically as an effective intervention for the reduction of anxiety.[23,28] The healer enters into a meditative state in which she concentrates on directing energy to the patient through her hands. After receiving therapeutic touch, patients have described sensations such as lessening of pain, tingling, and relaxation. Laboratory indexes such as EEG, electromyograph, galvanic skin response, and temperature, as well as a self-evaluation questionnaire measuring the degree of A-state anxiety, have corroborated the patients' subjective reports of relaxation after therapeutic touch.[17,23]

Cultural artifacts are items or substances that reflect a certain culture or subculture, such as clothing, cosmetics, scents, or jewelry. Cultural mores must be considered when interpreting cultural artifacts.

Digital communication. "Verbal codification rests on the digital principle."[32] Digital communication was launched when humans learned how to represent concepts, ideas, items, and objects by arbitrarily selected signs or symbols, such as *t-r-e-e* for tree. These signs and symbols can be manipulated to create a syntax of language, which in turn allows for versatility and abstract expression. Language is composed of a multitude of signs or symbols that must be known to a number of interpreters and that retain the same meaning in different situations.[31]

Denotation and connotation describe differences in the meaning of words. A denotative meaning is the one that is in most general use, whereas a connotative meaning is an additional meaning for a word that is specific to a person. Derived from personal experience, connotative meaning includes emotions, associations, and referents added to the denotative meaning of a word. People can communicate only to the extent that they share similar meanings, so words must be selected that best describe the intended meaning and that the other person understands.

Highlights of Watzlawick, Beavin, and Jackson's comparison of analogue and digital communication are included in Table 1. These authors summarize with the axiom of communication[39]:

> Human beings communicate both digitally and analogically. Digital language has a highly complex and powerful logical syntax but lacks adequate semantics in the field of relationship, while analogic language possesses the semantics but has no adequate syntax for the unambiguous definition of the nature of relationships.

Translation from the digital to the analogue form of communication, or vice versa, presents dilemmas that can lead to dysfunctional communication. Loss of information occurs with translation from the digital into the analogue mode. The human brain uses both analogue and digital communication in a complementary and highly complex manner.[25] Edwards[11] reported on the split-brain studies conducted by Roger W. Sperry and his associates during the 1950s and 1960s. This research concluded that both hemispheres of the brain are involved in higher

Table 1

Comparison of Digital and Analogue Communication

Digital Communication	Analogue Communication
Words used to name a concept or thing	Concept can only be represented by its physical likeness
Verbal communication	Nonverbal communication
Possesses high degree of complexity, versatility, and abstraction	Lacks ability to express logic, syntax, qualification, negation, and tense
Lacks adequate language for contingencies of relationships	Expresses contingencies of relationships

cognitive functions but employ different methods or modes of processing information. Springer and Deutsch[38] stated that the left hemisphere of the cortex controls language (digital communication) and the right cerebral cortex processes spatial information (analogue communication). Table 2 depicts additional characteristics of left-brain and right-brain communication.

Messages can also be described as having a content level that is usually verbal (the data of communication) and a relationship level that is usually nonverbal (how this communication is to be taken). Watzlawick, Beavin, and Jackson[39] point out that the relationship aspect of a communication is a communication about a communication, or "metacommunication;" thus the axiom: "Every communication has a content and a relationship aspect such that the latter classifies the former and is therefore a metacommunication."

The subtleties of the variations of metacommunication are learned through different social contexts and situations. Therefore understanding metacommunicative statements "requires knowledge of the social matrix or the culture in which the exchange of messages takes place."[30]

When there is lack of agreement between the content and relationship level of a communication, the relationship message takes precedence over the content message. A higher level of importance is attached to the relationship message because, according to McFarland, Leonard, and Morris,[25] it tells a person what to do with the content message.

Receiver. The receiver, the recipient of the message, perceives and interprets the communication. The receiver then responds, based on personal perception and interpretation, thereby providing feedback and becoming the sender.

Stimuli in the receiver's perceptual field include those

Table 2

A Comparison of Left-Mode and Right-Mode Characteristics

L-mode	R-mode
Verbal: Using words to name, describe, define.	*Nonverbal:* Awareness of things, but minimal connection with words.
Analytic: Figuring things out step-by-step and part-by-part.	*Synthetic:* Putting things together to form wholes.
Symbolic: Using a symbol to *stand for* something. For example, a drawing of an eye stands for *eye,* the sign + stands for the process of addition.	*Concrete:* Relating to things as they are, at the present moment.
Abstract: Taking out a small bit of information and using it to represent the whole thing.	*Analogic:* Seeing likenesses between things; understanding metaphoric relationships.
Temporal: Keeping track of time, sequencing one thing after another; doing first things first, second things second, etc.	*Nontemporal:* Without a sense of time.
Rational: Drawing conclusions based on *reason* and *facts.*	*Nonrational:* Not requiring a basis of reason or facts; willingness to suspend judgment.
Digital: Using numbers, as in counting.	*Spatial:* Seeing where things are in relation to other things, and how parts go together to form a whole.
Logical: Drawing conclusions based on logic; one thing following another in logical order, for example, a mathematical theorem or a well-stated argument.	*Intuitive:* Making leaps of insight, often based on incomplete patterns, hunches, feelings, or visual images.
Linear: Thinking in terms of linked ideas, one thought directly following another, often leading to a convergent conclusion.	*Holistic:* Seeing whole things all at once; perceiving the overall patterns and structures, often leading to divergent conclusions.

From Edwards, B.: Drawing on the right side of the brain. Copyright © 1979 by Betty Edwards. Reprinted by permission of J.P. Tarcher, Inc., and Houghton-Mifflin Co., Souvenir Press, Ltd.

present in the verbal and nonverbal communication of the sender and the immediate environment (context). These stimuli are selectively received by receiver organs such as eyes, taste buds, olfactory sensors, skin, ears, and kinesthetic sensors and are sent, via afferent nerve fibers, toward the brain. In the brain perception is further affected by the input of psychologic factors such as the receiver's concept of self, others, and society, as well as the sender's feelings and values. Interpretation of the communication received, then, depends on the receiver's review of this input.

To organize input for interpretation and action, the receiver "punctuates" the interactional sequence by organizing it into a linear sequence, that is, with a beginning and an end. Punctuation is neither good nor bad, but practical in that it simplifies the complex and dynamic series of reciprocal events of a communication sequence. However, disagreement about how to punctuate a sequence of events often results in conflict and impaired communication. Consider the following example of a couple having marital problems (Fig. 2). A husband states that he engages in extramarital affairs because his wife is jealous and accuses him of infidelity. "I may as well do what I am accused of doing," states the husband. The wife views the situation differently. She is jealous and accusatory in response to his behavior. The husband perceives the sequence of events as 2-3-4 and 4-5-6, whereas the wife punctuates the sequence as 1-2-3 and 3-4-5.

The primary problem in a communication pattern such as this is "their inability to metacommunicate about their respective patterning of their interaction. . . . The nature of a relationship is contingent upon the punctuation of the communicational sequences between the communicants."[39]

Feedback. During the phase of covert rehearsal the receiver reviews information about self and others, rehearses possible actions to take, and anticipates possible reactions of the other. The receiver decides the response, or feedback, to the sender's communication. Feedback performs a regulatory function in the communication process. It is that process by which performance is checked and malfunctions are corrected.

Feedback is composed of the information the original sender receives about the receiver's reaction to the message that has been generated by the original sender. Feedback that is helpful is clearly stated with tact and tolerance, relevant to the persons and context, and appropriately timed.

Properly operating feedback processes facilitate understanding and agreement between communicators. Ruesch[30] outlines four possibilities for the correspondence of the information between two persons. The first possibility is *acknowledgment of receipt of statement with understanding.* The receiver communicates that the sender's statements are fully understood and appreciated. If this acknowledgment of the receiver matches the expectancies of the sender and the sender indicates this, acknowledgment of understanding has occurred. The sender feels pleasure and satisfaction.

The second possibility for correspondence of information is *acknowledgment without understanding.* In this

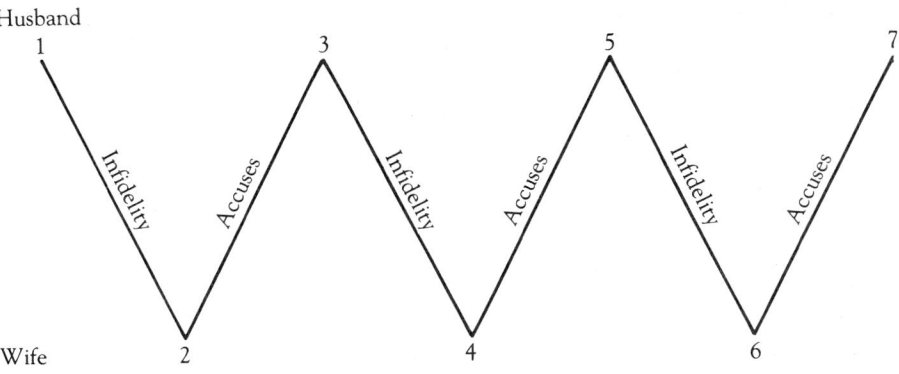

Fig. 2
The nature of a relationship is contingent on the punctuation of the communicational sequences between the communicants.

case, the receiver's feedback implies lack of understanding but a willingness to explore the sender's intentions. To encounter readiness to be understood is gratifying to the sender, whether or not understanding or agreement is reached.

Correspondence of information between communicators can also take the form of *acknowledgment of mutual agreement*. Ruesch states that it is easier to reach a limited agreement than it is to be fully understood, since understanding requires a benevolent attitude in another individual. Pleasure is experienced when an agreement is reached. In mutual agreement both communicators, via feedback, make statements that convey the idea, "I am of the same opinion as you are," or "We made a deal."

The last possibility for correspondence of information is *acknowledgment of mutual disagreement*. This may be carried out in a variety of ways: by the lack of any acknowledgment, by an unexpected hostile response, by factitious mutual claims of agreement, by overt declaration that no agreement can be reached but the door remains open for future negotiation, and by overt declaration that agreement is impossible now and forever. The reactions of an individual to disagreement are variable. In general, the stronger an individual's ego, the better he can tolerate disagreement.

Watzlawick, Beavin, and Jackson[39] state that no matter what the content of the communication, there is some metacommunication contained that is reflective of the communicator's self-definition. For example, Ms. Avery, a nurse, takes her dog to a veterinarian who prescribes ampicillin. Ms. Avery interrupts the veterinarian's explanation of the effects of this medication by angrily saying, "I'm a nurse." She is communicating that she views herself as knowledgeable about medication and is insulted by his explanation.

Possible receiver responses to the sender's self-definition include confirmation, rejection, and disconfirma-

tion.[39] *Confirmation* is a process by which an individual is strengthened or validated through acknowledgment of his worth or existence. A confirming response results in feelings of endorsement, acceptance, and enhanced self-image in the recipient.[19] It is possible to disagree with a person yet confirm his worth.

Rejection is the second possible response of the receiver to the sender's self-definition. Although difficult to accept, rejection assumes at least minimal recognition of that which is being rejected. When communicating, "You are wrong," the communicator also sends the message, "You exist." At times, forms of rejections may be constructive, as in the example of a nurse refusing to accept a patient's negative self-concept.

The message of *disconfirmation,* the third response to self-definition, is, "You do not exist." Disconfirmation leads to loss of self, lack of interpersonal growth, and impaired communication patterns. The disconfirmed person feels misunderstood, alienated, frustrated, and irritated. Over time, disconfirmation results in psychologic damage. The following categories of disconfirmation are identified by Heineken.[19]

Indifferent responses disavow the person's attempt to communicate and thereby convey the idea that the speaker does not matter. Examples of indifferent responses include inappropriate silence, change of topic, foot or finger tapping, and interruption of the speaker.

Tangential responses steer the communication in another direction. The receiver responds to a fortuitous aspect of the sender's communication, thereby disregarding the speaker's original intent. Examples include the sender shifting the focus of the communication, drifting into personal accounts, and moving from the content to the personality of the sender.

Ambiguous responses contain double messages that are often conflicting, for example, "I don't want to get involved." These responses can also take the form of incompatible verbal and nonverbal communication, for example, "I want to hear your views on the subject," followed by the speaker leaving the room.

Impervious responses imply that the receiver can read the sender's mind and therefore can judge the accuracy of the sender's perceptions and feelings. Responses such as, "I know what you're thinking," and "You have no reason to feel that way," are examples of impervious responses.

Responses that derogate, denounce, or put down the speaker are *disparaging responses*. These responses represent an attack. Profanity, sarcasm, and laughing at the sender are examples of such responses.

Included in the category of *inadequate responses* are overqualified statements (perhaps, maybe) and redundant statements. Inadequate responses contain a paucity of meaning in that they are incomplete or contain much trivia.

Feedback from the receiver can lead to changes in the original sender's behavior. These changes or corrections can be viewed as part of the total feedback process. The original receiver thus becomes the sender by communicating feedback or by responding to the corrections in communication made by the original sender. Thereby the process of communication is perpetuated.

Successful Communication

The following characteristics of successful communication are drawn from the foregoing discussion.
1. Both the sender and receiver have the physical ability to receive, analyze, and send messages.
2. The relationship between the sender and receiver is considered in all components of the communication process.
3. Selective attention is given to appropriate input.
4. Both the digital/verbal and the analogic/nonverbal form of communication are employed.
5. The sender selects and organizes words to best describe the intended meaning of the message.
6. The sender and receiver have similar meanings for words.
7. All channels of nonverbal communication are synchronized.
8. Nonverbal behavior is consistent with verbal communication.
9. The message sent is appropriate to the context.
10. The message is complete, that is, not overloaded with or insufficient in information.
11. The timing of the message is appropriate to its content and the context.
12. The receiver listens actively.
13. The sender and receiver agree on the punctuation of a communication sequence.
14. Feedback is requested and accepted.
15. Feedback is relevant to the persons and context, clearly stated, and appropriately timed.
16. The sender is able to correct the information or message.
17. Both the sender and receiver assume responsibility for their communication.
18. Concordant information is established between the sender and receiver.
19. Both the sender and receiver attain confirmation and gratification.

ETIOLOGY

Many variables affect the process of communication. Variables can act alone or together. Although a variable considered alone is neutral, it has a potential valence in that it can act either positively or negatively in a communication sequence. When a variable exerts a negative influence in a given situation, communication is ineffective at that moment. However, when variables *consistently* exert a negative influence on a person's communication, a pattern of impaired communication results. The variables affecting communication to be discussed include growth and development, physical condition, stress, feelings, perception, self-concept, culture, and communication skills.

Growth and Development

Communication is a major human function to be mastered. Mastery occurs through learning a series of progressive tasks over time. Interference at any stage leaves a mark, especially during an individual's formative years. During these years human adaptation is focused on growth of the body systems as well as on the environmental demands. During periods of peak growth—early childhood and adolescence—more energy and focus are directed toward the growth of organ systems. Therefore the individual is less able to respond to the demands of the environment.

Communication with children requires knowledge of the salient features of their specific age level. A child under the age of 3 has a limited ability to communicate verbally, as well as a limited sense of past or future. During this period a child learns responses to sensory input and muscular coordination and locomotion. Children between the ages of 4 and 7 learn much about themselves and how to communicate with one person at a time. A child's vocabulary increases dramatically during this period. During later childhood (ages 7 to 12) communication opportunities increase because a child has peers with whom to interact. A child's interests at this stage of development are primarily on same-sex

Table 3
Developmental Influences on Communication

Age Level	Salient Features of Development	Age-Specific Interference with Communicative Behavior
Intrauterine period (40 weeks)	Organism responds to thermal, mechanical, and chemical stimuli.	Toxic, infectious, vascular, hormonal, and mechanical interference with communication apparatus of fetus.
Neonatal period (12 weeks)	Infant learns to respond to tactile, auditory, and visual stimuli.	Stimulation exceeding the tolerance limits of the baby, including neglect and erroneous timing.
Infancy (3 to 24 months)	Mastery of head, eye, and hand movements (second quarter); trunk and fingers (third quarter); legs and feet (fourth quarter); speech (second year).	Interference with muscular system and locomotion; premature training, insufficient exercise; absence of nonverbal exchange, particularly in terms of action, may prevent the establishment of feedback processes.
Early childhood (2 to 5 years)	Interpersonal communication with one person at a time (mother, father, sibling, or other relative or friend).	Interference with speech and social action: selective and tangential responses; separation from mother; and interference with perception.
Later childhood (6 to 12 years)	Group communication with several persons at a time; learning communication with children of the same age, with emphasis on members of the same sex.	Interference with group behavior; broken families, nonparticipation in school; separation from father; erroneous setting of limitations; lack of transmission of skills at home; lack of responsiveness of parents in verbal terms.
Adolescence (12 to 18 years)	Interpersonal communication with members of opposite sex resumed; growing attempts to communicate with members of out-groups.	Interference with participation in autonomous groups, with premating behavior, with attempts to make decisions and to be independent; inadequate provisions for athletic activities and the acquisition of information.
Young adulthood (19 to late 20s approximately)	Mastery of the complexity and heterogeneity of adult communication and the multiplicity of roles and diversity of rules; communication with age superiors; the young adult is occupationally placed in a position of subservience; observes and follows orders.	Interference with mating behavior, with the acquisition of skills and the learning of multiple roles; changeover from family system of communication to other systems may be interfered with by relatives; nonconformance to group practices may jeopardize support from the group.
Middle adulthood (30 to middle 40s approximately)	Peak of communication with age inferiors and children; switch from role of perceiver and transmitter to position of greater responsibility.	Interference with communication vis-à-vis youngsters; position between two generations is delicate and ill defined when pull from either side is too strong.
Later adulthood (45 to 65 approximately)	Intake of information and learning now displaced in favor of output of information, teaching, governing and ruling; participation in decision-making groups.	Interference with independence and decision-making; realization of failure to implement self-chosen ideals; collapse of wishful thinking; interference with identification with younger generation.
Age of retirement (65 to 80 approximately)	Preparation for relinquishment of power and gradual retirement from decision-making; philosophical considerations after completion of life cycle; symbolic and global treatment of events.	Inactivity; sudden withdrawal from participation on communication networks; lack of stimulation.
Old age (80 +)	Life in retrospect, with emphasis on early memories.	Interference with equilibrium; tolerance limits for over- and understimulation and over- and underactivity quickly reached.

peers. Independence gradually increases as a child moves into adolescence. Communication is affected in this insecure period by the adolescent's self-consciousness. Communication is resumed with the opposite sex.

Adulthood brings with it a demand for mastery of complex communication abilities so that adults can engage in activities such as planning for their life, choosing a career, selecting a mate, and producing children. Early adulthood (ages 19 to 29) often includes an increase in number and complexity of roles. These roles may include spouse, parent, and worker. In addition, the age superiors with whom the young adult interacts increase from primarily family members and close friends to neighbors and fellow workers. An individual in middle adulthood (ages 30 to 44) often assumes more responsibility in the work place and in the rearing of children.

The late adulthood period contains events that also impinge on the individual's communication. The individual often reflects on accomplishment of life goals. Communication networks are narrowed through retirement, illness, and loss of friends or family. Presbyacusis, the hearing loss associated with the aging process, affects 39% to 50% of the U.S. population over the age of 65.[8] This, as well as other results of the aging process, may result in depression and withdrawal from others. Table 3 summarizes salient features of development and the possible interferences with communicative behavior relative to age level.

Physical Condition

Since communication is a process involving the whole person, a physical condition may affect a person's ability to communicate. Physical conditions that directly affect communication are any that interfere with an individual's ability to receive and process sensory input or send a message (output). Examples of such conditions are (1) mental retardation, (2) trauma, (3) infections, (4) neoplasms, (5) toxic reactions, (6) metabolic disturbances, (7) vascular conditions, and (8) chronic brain syndromes. There may be a direct relationship between the physical condition and communication, such as an inability to speak as a result of a left hemisphere cerebral vascular accident, or an indirect relationship, such as withdrawal from communication opportunities related to the stress of a physical illness.

Ruesch[32] discusses communication disturbances associated with diseases of the organs of communication. Reception of sensory input depends on the functioning of the sensory end organs, the afferent nerve fibers, and the peripheral nerves. Impairment of these input functions results in disturbances in the five main sensory channels (sight, hearing, gustation, olfaction, palpation), as well as senses of pain, temperature, and vibration.

The processing of sensory input is carried out by the central nervous system with the brain playing the primary role. The cerebellum affects balance, coordination, muscle tone, and speech. The cortex controls the interpretation of sight, hearing, and touch data, purposive movements, spoken and written language, and gestures. The coordination of auditory and visual input data with speech and certain skeletal movement, the level of consciousness, memory, and the regulation of emotions are also mediated by the cerebellum. Impairment in processing sensory input can result in communication-related disorders such as ataxia, tremors, apraxia, aphasia, loss of consciousness, loss of memory, and unrestrained emotional expression.

Generation of communication output is regulated primarily by the motor system, including the motor cranial nerves (III, IV, VI, VII, IX, X, XI, and XII), efferent neurons, muscles, and glands. Impairment in the output functions affects a person's ability to communicate verbally and nonverbally and is manifested through behavior such as lack of control of movements of the eye, face, tongue, and pharynx, involuntary movements, and the inability to produce voluntary movement.

Stress

Communication is also affected by stress. Stress is a complex phenomenon that is precipitated by internal or external demands that result in neurocognitive, affective, physiologic, and behavioral responses.[25]

The cortical and subcortical areas of the brain are involved in the thinking and reasoning components of the neurocognitive activation process. Included in the thinking and reasoning components are mental structure (such as memory and concept formation) and mental operations (such as level of alertness and problem-solving).[37] The mental structure and operations evaluate the personal impact of the stressor(s). The perceived relevancy of the stressor(s) in turn affects the affective, physiologic, and behavioral responses.

Affective responses to stress are the emotions experienced during a given stressful situation. These emotions may include anxiety, fear, suspicion, or depression and are manifested in behavioral and related physiologic responses.[25]

The outcome behavioral response may include directly observable actions, self-reports, and end-organ responses to glandular secretory changes and autonomic nervous system activation. Behavioral responses may be adaptive or inadequately adaptive. Adaptive behavioral responses enable the person to cope with the stressor(s), whereas inadequate adaptive responses lead to continuation, or possibly augmentation, of the stress. A moderate level of stress can increase a person's motivation, learning, and productivity. However, excessive or uncontrolled stress can contribute to mental or physical dysfunction.[14]

Successful communication with a person experiencing stress requires (1) recognition of the existence of stress, (2) determination of the source of the stress, and (3) reduction of the stress. Stress can be recognized and its source determined by careful attention to verbal and non-verbal communication. Reduction of stress may be accomplished by elimination of the stressor, recognition and development of the person's inherent ability to cope with stress, or direct assistance by another person.

Feelings

A feeling is a state of mind or a condition of being that can facilitate or impede communication. Although feelings such as love, anger, anxiety, and depression are universal experiences, each individual is unique in how each feeling is experienced and in the significance of that feeling for that person.

Expressing feelings can enhance communication and produce growth in interpersonal relationships in that expression of feelings enables another to know more about us as individuals and more about what we are experiencing. Thereby channels of communication are kept open and the other person is allowed a chance to change his behavior.

On the other hand, expression of feelings can impair communication. More often than not, it is the manner in which feelings are expressed that results in negative consequences. It is truly a skill to be able to express anger, for instance, in a socially acceptable manner that the other person can accept.

A person experiences anxiety when faced with a real or imagined threat to self or basic need fulfillment, an unknown or unfamiliar situation, or a loss or crisis. The resulting manifestations of anxiety are many and may include physiologic symptoms such as increased heart rate, blood pressure and respirations, diaphoresis, tremors, and flushing of the skin; interference in the rest-activity level, such as insomnia and increased motor activity; somatic complaints such as vertigo, fatigue, and headache; and other responses such as irritability, inability to concentrate, and exaggerated emotions. Anxiety can be quantified as mild, moderate, and severe. Mild anxiety can motivate a person, enhance problem-solving, and sharpen perception. The person experiencing mild anxiety can identify options and learn from experience. In moderate anxiety perception is narrowed so that all factors or options for action are not considered. Choices are available but will not be made as thoughtfully as in mild anxiety. Severe anxiety lowers intellectual functioning, reduces perception, and renders the individual incapable of making choices.

Depression also has profound influence on a person's ability to communicate effectively. Depression is often accompanied by feelings of sadness, helplessness, hopelessness, worthlessness. Precipitants to the state of depression include a real or imagined loss, dependence on others, and a sense of powerlessness. Because most of the depressed individual's energy is internalized, the behavioral manifestations of depression are characterized by an absence of vitality. The depressed individual withdraws from interaction with others, is mute or speaks in monosyllables or short phrases, may experience anorexia, weight loss, insomnia, and constipation, and may express numerous somatic complaints.

The withdrawal and isolation experienced by the depressed individual may be compounded by the reactions of others. Frequently those attempting to communicate with a depressed person experience sadness, guilt, and frustration. These feelings lead to withdrawal from or avoidance of the depressed person. However, communication with others facilitates the resolution of depression. Through an interpersonal relationship in which effective communication techniques are used the depressed individual can be assisted in verbally expressing his thoughts and feelings, thereby gaining understanding of the dynamics of the depression.

Perception

The behavior of a person is directly related to his perceptual field at a given moment in which the behavior occurs.[6,9] Effective communication depends on understanding the meaning intended by the communicator. The meaning of a communication, in turn, depends on understanding the communicator's perception. Perception is a process that includes reception, selection, organization, and interpretation of sensory data.

At any given time a person may receive numerous sensory impressions. Only input that is evaluated as relevant is perceived. Furthermore, only some of the input perceived will be responded to by the recipient.

The selection of and response to input is influenced by such factors as the functioning of the nervous system, past experience, values, and needs and emotional states. A person's *nervous system* must function adequately to receive, interpret, and respond to sensory stimuli. When the sensory organs, brain, and nerves are dysfunctional, however, perception is limited or altered. Any substance or condition affecting the central nervous system can affect perception. Many drugs alter perception, for example, phencyclidine (PCP) and cocaine. *Past experience* can bias a person to certain "sets" of perception, that is, perceiving certain events in a stereotyped way. These sets of perception can result in a person neglecting differences or changes in a given individual or situation or lead a person to faulty conclusions about another's behavior. Differentiations in perceptual field are also made according to the perceiver's *values*. Values are derived from an individual's culture. An individual's *needs and emotional state* also affect perception. Maslow's theory is based on the concept that hierarchic needs motivate an individual to behave in a certain manner. Clues to a person's need state are found in his perceptions. Emotional states can result in the distortion or blocking of certain sensory input. In experiences producing intense emotional reactions, such as a fire or a physical assault, participants are sometimes unable to attend and respond to stimuli that might save their lives. When one or more of the factors influencing perception produces a distortion, omission, or falsification of sensory input, perception is limited. Limited perception can result in impaired intrapersonal or interpersonal communication.

Self-Concept

Included in an individual's perceptual field is the self. The perceptions an individual has of personal physical, social, and psychologic characteristics comprise that individual's self-concept. Self-esteem is the evaluative component of the self-concept that expresses an attitude of approval or disapproval toward self and reflects the individual's appraisal of his capabilities, significance, and worth.

Self-concept develops in the context of an interpersonal relationship and is enhanced or impaired through that relationship and through communication. It is also developed through internalization of the reflected attitudes and appraisals that result from interaction with significant others and the environment. Early childhood is a critical period in the development of self-concept. A child incorporates into self observations of personal behavior and increasingly attributes to self descriptions made by others, such as pretty, naughty, good, smart.

According to Coopersmith[10] as an individual matures, the self-concept reflects more experiences and the person becomes more selective as to which experiences are assumed to be self-referring. In early writings Mead[27] emphasized the importance of social activity to the development of self-concept. Attitudes, values, and behaviors of social groups in which an individual holds, or wishes to hold, membership contribute to that individual's self-definition. The evaluations and reactions of these groups can be a potent determinant of self-concept.

Another phase crucial to the development of self-concept is the adolescent phase.[24] Adolescence is accompanied by heightened emotions, new experiences, and changes in interpersonal relationships, all of which affect the self-concept of the individual at that time. Reeval-uation of self is a primary task of the adolescent, who is launching an independent life as an adult.

Negative self-concept is a result of numerous negative interactions over time and is reflected in the inability to take criticism, hypercritical and pessimistic attitudes, self-derogatory remarks, ineffective coping behaviors, and impaired communication.

Three patterns of impaired communication related to a negative self-concept are described by Goldberg and Stanitis[13]: *invalidation* is a communication that negates the person's view of himself; *inflexibility* allows only stereotyped behavior in interpersonal relationships; and *incongruence* reflects incongruent verbal and nonverbal behavior.

Conversely, the individual possessing a positive self-concept has feelings of self-confidence and adequacy. The individual is able to select, process, and assimilate information in an adaptive manner. Successes approximate aspirations. A positive self-concept contributes to an individual's ability to interact and communicate effectively with others.

Culture

Each communicator learns to communicate within a certain cultural context. A culture is made up of groups that provide a frame of reference for behavior. Within that frame of reference are the rules, values, mores, and norms that govern what, how, and to whom a person communicates. Cultural influences that affect development of values, perception of others, and communication include economic position, occupation, race, religion, political views, and education.[24]

Verbal as well as nonverbal behaviors take on different meanings within different cultural groups. Culture dictates interpretation of all forms of nonverbal behavior (kinesic behavior, paralanguage, proxemics, touch, and cultural artifacts). The meaning of verbal communication also reflects the culture. Translation from one language to another is often difficult because of a lack of comparable words. Furthermore, within a given culture different meanings may exist among subcultural groups for the same word or phrase.

It is customarily the family unit that passes on the values, mores, norms, and rules of a culture. Communication patterns, functional or impaired, are learned initially within the family unit and vary according to culture.

Rugg[33] identified two factors found within lower socioeconomic families that interfere with the learning of functional communication: impermanence and unpredictability. A sense of *impermanence* develops as a result of transient marital and familial relationships. There is often a lack of private possessions or space for an individual in a lower socioeconomic family. Relationships are frequently competitive and devoid of dialogue. A sense of *unpredictability* evolves from erratic household events and inconsistent rewards and punishments from the parents. It is often difficult to predict arrival of family members, meal and bedtimes, and responses of family members. Material items are frequently given to express love. The amount of attention a child receives may differ greatly from one point of time to another. The feelings that result from such unpredictable circumstances can include confusion, uncertainty, and insecurity.

The impermanence and unpredictability in a lower socioeconomic family may contribute to a pattern of impaired communication, characteristics of which are an inability to keep communication channels open, lack of questioning and clarification, suppression of feelings, and an inability to discriminate and attend to relevant stimuli.[33]

Communication Skills

Successful communication depends on the use of effective communication skills. The effective communicator uses a style and specific skills that enhance the communication process. Several methods of categorizing communication skills and styles have been identified.

According to Satir[34,35] a person's communication style is related to stress. When a behavior occurs in a meaningful relationship that is perceived as unloving or untrusting, stress results. The five styles of communication used when stress is experienced include placating, blaming, super-reasonable, irrelevant, and congruent.

The *placator* agrees and tries to be nice no matter what the circumstances are. The verbal and nonverbal behavior together send a message of peace at any cost. In so doing the placator ignores personal feelings and needs while assuming responsibility for the other and the context.

The *blamer* frequently disagrees, dominates, and attempts to wield power irrespective of the situation. The blamer uses accusatory and hostile words and nonverbal behavior—a pointed finger, clenched teeth, tight muscles, and a lording posture. Self becomes the predominant focus in the blaming style of communication. The feelings and needs of the other and the context are not taken into account.

The *super-reasonable* style of communication promotes rational thought and excludes feelings. This person communicates in an impersonal manner, relies on facts and figures, and focuses on the content of communication. The nonverbal behavior lacks vitality. The super-reasonable person stands straight and rigid, avoids eye contact, and speaks in a monotone. In this style the feeling and needs of both persons are ignored, thereby making the context the focus of communication.

The person choosing the *irrelevant* style of commu-

nication selects words that are unrelated to the circumstances. The subject is changed and feelings are avoided in this style. The nonverbal behavior is that of motion and distraction. The irrelevant style of communicating ignores self, others, and the context.

Placating, blaming, super-reasonable, and irrelevant styles of communication are incongruent styles in that each denies self, other, or context. In the *congruent* style "the words and actions in a communication fit the inner experience of self and are appropriate to the context."[3] The needs and feelings of the other person are considered in a congruent response. The verbal and nonverbal behaviors are in synchrony. Tension is reduced, self-worth is maintained, and communication is effective when a congruent style is employed. Implications of congruent responses cited by Satir, Stachowiak, and Taschman[36] include maintenance of the conviction of the universality of human beings, restoration of full use of the senses, and opportunity for multiple options.

Assertive communication, according to Clark,[7] "is direct, honest, and appropriate; its goal is to convey to others what you expect from others and what can be expected from you." The assertive communicator determines goals, acts on those goals in a clear and consistent manner, and assumes responsibility for the outcomes of those actions.[25] A person who uses assertive communication skills is sensitive to the feelings and rights of others, is able to negotiate, accepts workable outcomes, is firm but gentle, and assumes an unyielding position when it is appropriate.[29] The assertive person is also sensitive to personal feelings and rights. Edwards and Brilhart[12] list the personal rights of the assertive person. A person has the right to:

1. Judge my own behavior, thoughts, and feelings.
2. My own needs and to have these accepted as being just as important as those of any other person with whom I interact.
3. Refuse requests without having to apologize or feel guilty.
4. Feel and express competitiveness and achievement of goals.
5. Make honest mistakes without having to make excuses or feel guilty.
6. Stay out of other people's business.
7. Change my mind.
8. Not know and to say, "I don't know."
9. Not understand.
10. Decide when to communicate assertively.

Persons using aggressive patterns of communication, on the other hand, disregard the rights and feelings of others, attempt to control or manipulate others, and assume little responsibility for the consequences of their behavior. Verbal messages often begin with "You" and contain threats, demands, or hostilities. Nonverbal behavior may include fist-waving, finger-pointing, a loud voice, grimaces, or even physical assault.[7]

In the nonassertive/recessive,[29] or acquiescent/avoiding[7] pattern of communication conflict and confrontation are avoided. Instead, the person attempts to smooth things over through complete agreement with the other person. Behavior is passive and reactive rather than independent and goal directed. The person often feels frustrated, insecure, inadequate, and depressed. These feelings can build and ultimately lead to aggressive behavior.

The following list of etiological factors of impaired communication is derived from the foregoing discussion of theoretical considerations of the communication process:

1. Developmental or age-related stage(s)
2. Mechanical impairment(s)
3. Physical condition(s)
4. Severe physical or psychosocial stress(es)
5. Extreme anger
6. Severe anxiety or panic
7. Moderate to severe depression
8. Significant impairment of perception
9. Unrealistic or inadequate self-concept
10. Cultural differences
11. Faulty communication skills

DEFINING CHARACTERISTICS[20,21]

Disorientation
Too little or too much attention to stimuli
Speech impediments
Physical conditions
Inability to speak dominant language
Inability or reluctance to speak
Disregard for speaker
Reliance on nonverbal communication
Inability to organize words
Inappropriate selection of words
Use of unfamiliar words
Inconsistent nonverbal messages
Inconsistent verbal and nonverbal messages
Message inappropriate to context
Excessive or insufficient verbiage
Ill-timed message
Inadequate listening skills
Disparity of punctuation
Absent or inappropriate feedback
Discordant information
Disconfirmation
Absence of gratification
Inability or reluctance to express feelings
Withdrawal from interaction
Unrestrained or inappropriate emotional expression
Imaginary or false perceptions
Incongruent communication styles
Lack of assertive skills

NURSING INTERVENTIONS

The overall goal for the client with impaired communication is to reduce or resolve impaired communication. Subgoals or short-term goals can include the following:
1. Attend to appropriate input.
2. Transmit clear, concise, understandable messages.
3. Use congruent analogue/nonverbal and digital/verbal communication.
4. Send and receive feedback.
5. Experience gratification from communication.

Patient Goal	Nursing Intervention
Reduce or resolve impaired communication.	Reduce or increase environmental stimuli.
	Encourage patient to seek assistance in correcting, modifying or preventing physical conditions that interfere with communication.
	Teach patient to identify and focus on relevant stimuli.
	Encourage interaction with others.
	Assist patient in increasing or modifying language skills.
	Assist in correction of faulty perception.
	Teach and support patient's use of appropriate communication techniques.
	Teach and support patient's use of assertive communication skills.
	Teach and encourage expression of feelings.
	Increase self-esteem.
	Teach and encourage use of stress-reduction techniques.
	Help patient examine effects of his behavior.
	Increase awareness of strengths and limitations in communicating with others.
	Point out discrepancies in nonverbal behaviors.
	Point out discrepancies in verbal and nonverbal behavior.
	Point out discrepancies in the message sent and the context within which it is sent.
	Help patient develop understanding of dynamics of relationships.

Continued on page 1872.

Table 4
Useful Communication Techniques

Technique	Definition	Purpose	Example
Reflection	Conveying to the patient his expressed thoughts and implied feelings.	Allow patient to develop and evaluate thoughts. Clarify unspoken or incongruent impressions. Explore new information.	Patient (P): "I feel so depressed." Nurse (N): "You feel depressed?" P: "My thoughts are disjointed." N: "Disjointed?"
Focusing	Concentrating on a specific thought or feeling in reference to a particular point.	Sustain goal-directed communication. Draw attention to significant data.	P: "Every morning I feel so bad." N: "Describe how you feel." P: "My husband always puts me down." N: "Give me an example."
Validation	Confirming one's observations and interpretations.	Accurately appraise patient and message. Prevent inaccurate assumptions.	P: "I don't want to do what my mother tells me to do." N: "It must be hard to disagree with your mother."
Silence	Communicating without verbalization.	Communicate concern, interest, or acceptance. Allow time for collection of thoughts. Allow patient to assume initiative. Relieve emotionally charged content.	P: "Diabetes is going to upset my whole life." N: (remains silent)
Summarizing	Highlighting the main ideas.	Review progress. Focus thinking. Facilitate conscious learning. Recall important points.	P: "I must leave soon." N: "Today you and I have discussed. . . ."
Clarification	Attempting to find the meaning of a communication.	Establish mutual understanding. Promote further communication. Assist patient to be more specific.	P: "Life's not fair." N: "I'm not sure what you're telling me." P: "They are always telling me what to do." N: "Who are they?"
Open-ended questions	Questions that allow multiple options for response.	Encourage expression of ideas and feelings. Allow patient freedom to structure conversation.	P: "The nurses don't have much to say to me." N: "What would you like to talk about?"
Stating observations	Verbalizing what is observed.	Explain corrections between verbal and nonverbal behavior. Correct perception.	N: "While you were talking about your daughter's graduation plans, you began to fidget and sweat."
Confrontation	Description and examination of discrepant behaviors.	Promote self-understanding. Evaluate consequences of behavior. Encourage exploration.	N: "Your words say 'yes' but your body language says 'no.'"
Exploring	Obtaining all pertinent data on a specific subject or feeling.	Establish mutual understanding. Allow patient to develop and evaluate thoughts.	P: "My husband and I had a fight." N: "Tell me what happened." P: "I want to move to Dallas with my parents, but I just don't know." N: "You seem unsure. You don't know what?"
Providing feedback	Description of some aspect of an individual's communication and its impact on the receiver.	Become aware of the effects of behavior. Verify, modify, or correct perception.	P: "When you do everything for me I feel helpless. I can feed and bathe myself."

References 15, 18, 22, 26, 41.

Patient Goal	Nursing Intervention
	Describe, demonstrate, and encourage use of active listening skills. Request patient to ask for feedback when communicating with others. Assist and encourage patient efforts to accept positive and negative feedback. Assist patient in mastering tasks appropriate for age or developmental level. Demonstrate and support responsibility for communication. Use facilitative communication techniques in interacting with patient (see Table 4).

EVALUATION

Patient Outcome	Data Indicating That Outcome is Reached
Successful communication	Attendance to appropriate input: 1. Oriented to person, place, and time. 2. Selects and responds to relevant stimuli. 3. Perception is accurate. 4. Absence or control of physical symptoms. Clear, concise understandable messages: 1. Absence of speech impediments. 2. Selects and organizes words appropriate to the receiver and context. 3. Speaks dominant language. 4. Uses effective communication techniques. 5. Uses appropriate amount of verbiage. 6. Expresses feelings appropriately. Congruent nonverbal and verbal communication: 1. Expresses congruent nonverbal behaviors. 2. Expresses congruent verbal and nonverbal behavior. 3. Balances use of verbal and nonverbal behavior. Sends and receives feedback: 1. Listens actively. 2. Examines effects of behavior on others. 3. Asks for and receives feedback. 4. Sends feedback to others. Experiences gratification from communication: 1. Reports satisfaction from communication. 2. Reports a sense of high self-esteem. 3. Reports or shows a willingness to assume responsibility for communication. 4. Sends and receives confirmation when communicating.

References

1. Berlo, D.: The process of communication: an introduction to theory and practice, New York, 1960, Holt, Rinehart, & Winston.
2. Birdwhistell, R.: Kinesics and context, Philadelphia, 1970, University of Pennsylvania Press.
3. Bradley, J., and Edinberg, M.: Communication in the nursing context, New York, 1982, Appleton-Century-Crofts.
4. Bridge, W., and Clark, J., editors: Communication in nursing care, London, 1981, H.M. & M. Publishers.
5. Brooks, W.: Speech communication, ed. 2, Dubuque, Iowa, 1971, William C. Brown Co., Publishers.
6. Bruner, J.: Beyond the information given, New York, 1973, W.W. Norton Co.
7. Clark, C.: Assertive skills for nurses, Wakefield, Mass., 1978, Contemporary Publishing Inc.
8. Clark, C., and Mills, G.: Communicating with hearing impaired adults, J. Gerontol. Nurs. 5(3):40-44, 1979.
9. Combs, A.: The professional education of teachers, Boston, 1965, Allyn & Bacon, Inc.
10. Coopersmith, S.: The antecedents of self-esteem, San Francisco, 1967, W.H. Freeman & Co.
11. Edwards, B.: Drawing on the right side of the brain, Los Angeles, 1979, J.P. Tarcher, Inc.
12. Edwards, B., and Brilhart, J.: Communication in nursing practice, St. Louis, 1981, The C.V. Mosby Co.
13. Goldberg, C., and Stanitis, M.: The enhancement of self-esteem through the communication process in group therapy, J. Psychiatr. Nurs. 15(12):5-8, 1977.
14. Greenwood, J., and Greenwood, J.: Managing executive stress: a systems approach, New York, 1979, John Wiley & Sons, Inc.
15. Haber, J., and others: Comprehensive psychiatric nursing, ed. 2, New York, 1982, McGraw-Hill Book Co.
16. Hall, E.: The hidden dimension, New York, 1966, Doubleday & Co.
17. Heidt, P.: Effect of therapeutic touch on anxiety level of hospitalized patients, Nurs. Res. 30:32-37, 1981.
18. Hein, E.: Communication in nursing practice, ed. 2, Boston, 1980, Little, Brown & Co.
19. Heineken, J.: Treating the disconfirmed psychiatric client, J. Psychiatr. Nurs. Ment. Health Services 21(1):21-25, 1983.
20. Kim, M., McFarland, G., and McLane, A.: Pocket guide to nursing diagnoses, St. Louis, 1984, The C.V. Mosby Co.
21. Kim, M., and Moritz, D.: Classification of nursing diagnoses: proceedings of the third and fourth national conferences, New York, 1982, McGraw-Hill Book Co.

22. Kreigh, H., and Perko, J.: Psychiatric and mental health nursing: commitment to care and concern, Reston, Va., 1979, Reston Publishing Co.
23. Krieger, D., Peper, E., and Ancoli, S.: Therapeutic touch: searching for evidence of physiological change, Am. J. Nurs. **79**:660-662, 1979.
24. Lewis, G.: Nurse-patient communication, ed. 3, Dubuque, Iowa, 1978, William C. Brown Co., Publishers.
25. McFarland, G., Leonard, H., and Morris, M.: Nursing leadership and management: contemporary strategies, New York, 1984, John Wiley & Sons, Inc.
26. McFarland, G., and Wasli, E.: Psychiatric nursing. Part 2. In Brunner, L., and Suddarth, D., editors: The Lippincott manual of nursing practice, Philadelphia, 1982, J.B. Lippincott Co.
27. Mead, G.: Mind, self and society, Chicago, 1934, The University of Chicago Press.
28. Miller, L.: An explanation of therapeutic touch using the science of unitary man, Nurs. Forum **18**:279-287, 1979.
29. Moskowitz, R.: Assertiveness for career and personal success, New York, 1977, AMACOM.
30. Ruesch, J.: Disturbed communication, New York, 1972, W.W. Norton Co.
31. Ruesch, J.: Therapeutic communication, ed. 2, New York, 1973, W.W. Norton Co.
32. Ruesch, J.: Communication and psychiatry. In Kaplan, H., Freedman, A., and Sadock, B., editors: Comprehensive textbook of psychiatry, vol. 1, Baltimore, 1980, Williams & Wilkins.
33. Rugg, J.: Communication patterns of disorganized lower socioeconomic families: nursing assessment and intervention, Military Med. **145**:776-779, 1980.
34. Satir, V.: People making, Palo Alto, Calif., 1972, Science and Behavior Books.
35. Satir, V.: Making contact, Millbrae, Calif., 1976, Celestial Arts.
36. Satir, V., Stachowiak, J., and Taschman, H.: Helping families to change, New York, 1975, Jason Aronson, Inc.
37. Scott, D., Oberst, M., and Dropkin, M.: A stress-coping model, Adv. Nurs. Sci. **95**(2):99-108, 1980.
38. Springer, S., and Deutsch, G.: Left brain, right brain, San Francisco, 1981, W.H. Freeman & Co.
39. Watzlawick, P., Beavin, J., and Jackson, D.: Pragmatics of human communication, New York, 1967, W.W. Norton Co.
40. Weiss, S.: The language of touch, Nurs. Res. **28**(2):76-79, 1979.
41. Wilson, H., and Kneisl, C.: Psychiatric nursing, Menlo Park, Calif., 1979, Addison-Wesley.

Suggested Readings

Bandler, R., and Grinder, J.: Frogs into princes: neurolinguistic programming, Moab, Utah, 1979, Real People Press.
Bashor, P.: A nursing communication assessment guide, Rehab. Nurs. **8**(1):20-21, 30, 1983.
Berne, E.: Games people play, New York, 1964, Grove Press.
Ceccio, J., and Ceccio, C.: Effective communication in nursing: theory and practice, New York, 1982, John Wiley & Sons, Inc.
Doona, M.: Travelbee's intervention in psychiatric nursing, ed. 2, Philadelphia, 1979, F.A. Davis Co.
Duldt, B., Giffin, K., and Patton, B.: Interpersonal communication in nursing, Philadelphia, 1983, F.A. Davis Co.
Gazda, G., Childers, W., and Walters, R.: Interpersonal communication: a handbook for health professionals, Rockville, Md., 1982, Aspen Systems Corp.
Hardin, S., and Halaris, A.: Nonverbal communication of patients and high and low empathy nurses, J. Psychiatr. Nurs. Ment. Health Services, **21**(1):14-19, 1983.
Henrich, A., and Bernheim, K.: Responding to patient's concerns, Nurs. Outlook **29**:428-433, 1981.
Jourard, S.: The transparent self (Rev. ed.), New York, 1971, Van Nostrand Reinhold.
Key, M.: Paralanguage and kinesics (nonverbal communication), Metuchen, N.J., 1975, Scarecrow Press.
MacKay, R.: Hearing and responding: communicating with the critically ill, Dimensions Health Service **58**(8):18-19, 1981.
Macleod, J.: Communication in nursing, Nurs. Times **77**(1):12-18, 1981.
Palmer, M., and Deck, E.: Teaching assertiveness to seniors, Nurs. Outlook **29**:305-310, 1981.
Pluckham, M.: Human communication: the matrix of nursing, New York, 1978, McGraw-Hill Book Co.
Shanks, S., editor: Nursing and the management of adult communication disorders, San Diego, 1983, College-Hill Press.
Shanks, S., editor: Nursing and the management of pediatric communication disorders, San Diego, 1983, College-Hill Press.
Springer, S., and Deutsch, G.: Left brain, right brain, San Francisco, 1981, W.H. Freeman & Co.
Yura, H., and Walsh, M.: The nursing process, ed. 3, New York, 1978, Appleton-Century-Crofts.

Health-Perception Response

NONCOMPLIANCE

THEORY

Noncompliance, or the extent to which a person's behavior deviates from a prescribed regimen, exists in one third to one half of all treated persons.[40] At the turn of the century noncompliance was not a significant problem, since few diagnoses could be made with accuracy and a scientific rationale for treatment was rare. The activities of persons with contagious diseases, such as tuberculosis, were controlled by law. Health care has changed significantly! Now patients are being discharged earlier from acute care facilities and are expected to assume increasingly greater responsibility for the management of their therapeutic regimens. A gap exists between the health care system's expectations of the patient and the patient's adherence to the therapeutic regimen, as evidenced by the high percentage of noncompliance. This discrepancy needs to be reduced. Using the nursing diagnosis of noncompliance allows the practitioner to identify the specific cause of the problem and to choose those strategies which have been identified to positively affect the specific cause of noncompliance.

Initially it was suggested that persons noncompliant with health care regimens could be identified by sociodemographic characteristics.[40,72] The influence of age, sex, socioeconomic status, race, religion, education, marital status, and mental status were examined; results were often contradictory and inconclusive. For each study which demonstrated that a particular variable had a statistically significant effect on compliance, there was at least one other study with conflicting results. Many studies produced inconclusive evidence for all demographic variables except age and mental status, which were generally accepted as having a significant impact on compliance.

Noncompliance has been frequently reported in the young and the aged. Mothers were thought to have difficulty administering medication to their children, especially if their symptoms had abated, and the elderly have problems such as alteration in thought patterns, limited resources, alteration in energy and mobility, and isolation, all of which adversely affect compliance. Another group in which noncompliance has been reported is patients with schizophrenia, paranoid features, and personality disorders.

One of the first models to be studied to predict noncompliance was the medical model.[40,72] Through this model attempts to predict compliance are made on the basis of characteristics of the regimen (type of illness for

1875

Fig. 3

Summary health belief model for predicting and explaining sick role behavior.

From Becker, M.: Health belief model and sick role behavior, Health Education Monograph **2**:416, Winter 1974.

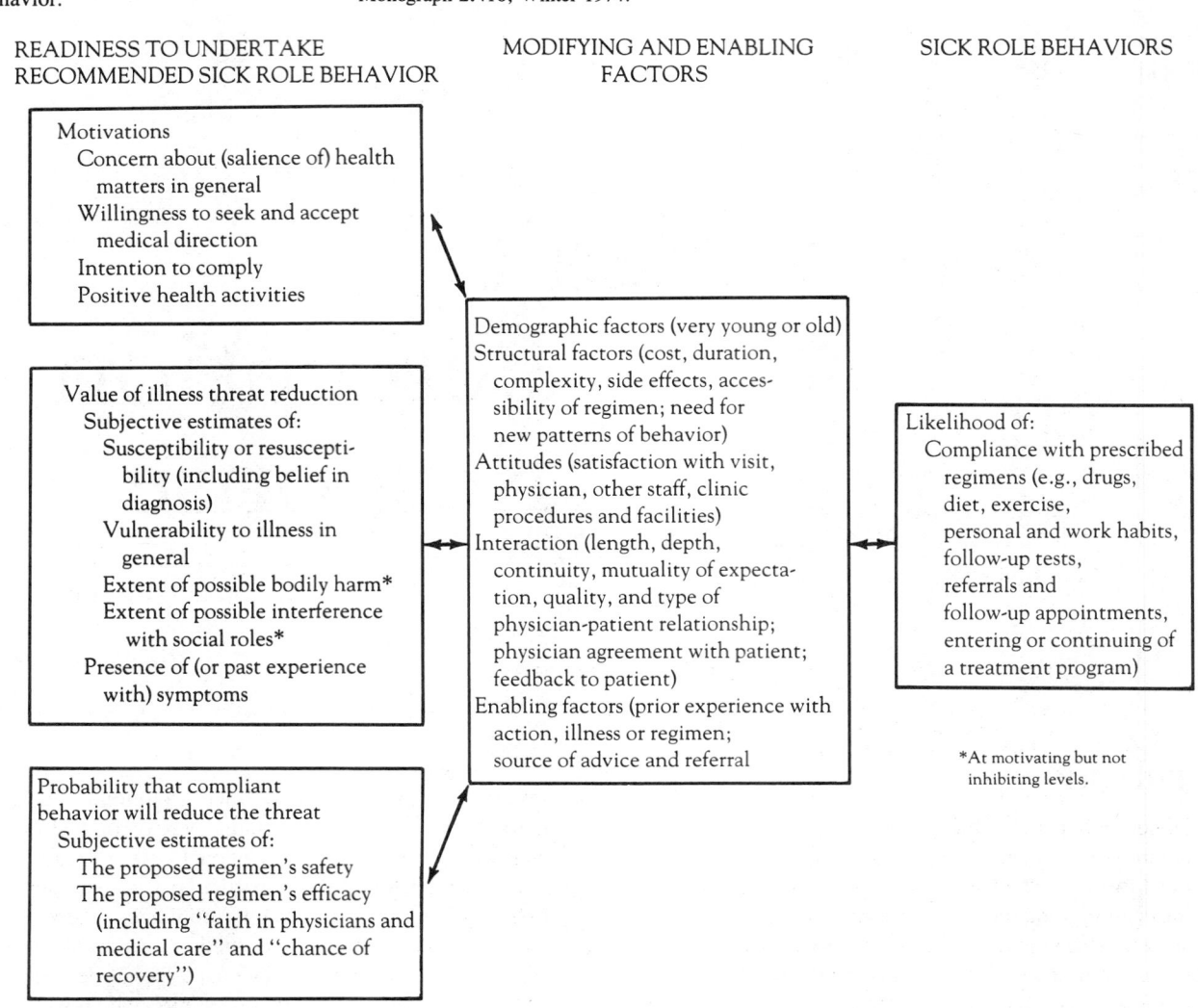

READINESS TO UNDERTAKE RECOMMENDED SICK ROLE BEHAVIOR

Motivations
   Concern about (salience of) health
      matters in general
   Willingness to seek and accept
      medical direction
   Intention to comply
   Positive health activities

Value of illness threat reduction
   Subjective estimates of:
      Susceptibility or resuscepti-
         bility (including belief in
         diagnosis)
      Vulnerability to illness in
         general
      Extent of possible bodily harm*
      Extent of possible interference
         with social roles*
      Presence of (or past experience
         with) symptoms

Probability that compliant
behavior will reduce the threat
   Subjective estimates of:
      The proposed regimen's safety
      The proposed regimen's efficacy
         (including "faith in physicians and
         medical care" and "chance of
         recovery")

MODIFYING AND ENABLING FACTORS

Demographic factors (very young or old)
Structural factors (cost, duration,
   complexity, side effects, accessibility of regimen; need for
   new patterns of behavior)
Attitudes (satisfaction with visit,
   physician, other staff, clinic
   procedures and facilities)
Interaction (length, depth,
   continuity, mutuality of expectation, quality, and type of
   physician-patient relationship;
   physician agreement with patient;
   feedback to patient)
Enabling factors (prior experience with
   action, illness or regimen;
   source of advice and referral

SICK ROLE BEHAVIORS

Likelihood of:
   Compliance with prescribed
      regimens (e.g., drugs,
      diet, exercise,
      personal and work habits,
      follow-up tests,
      referrals and
      follow-up appointments,
      entering or continuing of
      a treatment program)

*At motivating but not
inhibiting levels.

which treatment is prescribed, complexity of the regimen, discomfort associated with the illness, and duration of the therapy) and gravity of the illness (medically defined seriousness, duration, and associated disability). Again, this model does not accurately predict noncompliance. Clinical prediction of noncompliance based on the perception of the health care worker is no more accurate than are random predictions.

The health belief model[6,8,50,85] is based on the perceptions of the client rather than those of the health care professional. This model assumes that an individual will cognitively decide to choose a goal based on (1) the attractiveness of the goal to the individual, (2) the pa-

tient's estimation of his ability to attain the goal, and (3) the occurrence of a cue. Basically, the health belief model states that motivation = reward − (perceived cost + barriers). As seen in Fig. 3, the health belief model has several components: motivation, value of illness threat reduction, probability of threat reduction, and modifying and enabling factors.

This model has been very popular, both clinically and in research. The components of the health belief model have been demonstrated to have a statistically significant relationship with compliance. Persons who feel motivated, value risk reduction, or believe that the health care system is safe and effective will be compliant. However, the health belief model does not appear to be predictive of compliance.[8] That is, the measured beliefs do not always precede the behavior, but rather behavior can be changed prior to a change in beliefs. For example, a reformed smoker may be adamant about the dangers of smoking, but in the first week of abstinence these beliefs are not so strong.

Many promising models in the literature offer hope of prediction and measurement of noncompliance,* but they have not yet been adequately tested. Much, however, has been learned about compliance by observing the effects of different approaches to the treatment of noncompliance. For instance, Sackett and Haynes[39,90] found behavioral approaches to the management of noncompliance

*References 4, 19, 23, 24, 27, 47, 59, 100.

more effective than patient education, increasing convenience, and reducing the expense of treatment. They reported increased compliance with the use of the behavioral methods of self-monitoring, tailoring, and reinforcement. Another behavioral approach rigorously tested is contracting, or a systematic arrangement for granting a reward in return for performance of a specific behavior. Steckel[96,101] has clearly identified the efficacy of contracting in altering the compliance of patients with hypertension, diabetes, and arthritis.

At this point there is no proven theory for compliance. However, extremely valuable contributions have been made by the current models and the specific therapeutic behavioral approaches; and it is through both the inductive and deductive approaches that the clinician receives direction and perspective for clinical practice.

ETIOLOGY AND DEFINING CHARACTERISTICS

General and Specific Etiology	Defining Characteristics
	Behavior indicative of failure to adhere by direct observation or statements by patient or significant others
	Objective tests (physiologic measures, detection of markers)
	Evidence of development of complications
	Evidence of exacerbation of symptoms
	Failure to keep appointments
	Failure to progress
	Inability to set or attain mutual goals[51]
Alteration in cognition Inadequate knowledge	Has never been taught
	Unable to accurately answer questions
	States, "I don't know."
	Does not want information
	Makes inaccurate statements
	Holds myths and fantasies to be true
	Information has not been updated by new knowledge
Alteration in thought process	Disturbance in recent or remote memory
	Inability to solve problems
	Inability to concentrate
	Inability to follow directions
	Presence of psychopathology
Inability to read or write	Illiteracy
	Neuromuscular deficits
Sensory deficits	Hearing deficit
	Visual deficit
Alteration in perception Inadequate motivation	Does not perceive illness or risk to be serious
	Does not feel susceptible to the risk or effects of the illness
	Does not feel vulnerable in terms of the risk
	Does not believe in the efficacy of therapy
	Prefers illness to treatment
	Cultural beliefs are opposed to prescribed regimen
Alteration in affective state	Behavioral denial
	Verbal denial
	Depression
	Anger

General and Specific Etiology	Defining Characteristics
	Fear and anxiety
Conflict to value system	Agrees that behavior is desirable but "not for me" or "not now"
	Identifies desired behavior as being of low priority
Belief in therapy but inability to change behavior	History of making behavior change but returning to undesirable behavior
	Has made repeated attempts to do something but cannot
Inadequacies in social system	
Inadequate social support	Significant other does not:
	1. Possess accurate information
	2. Believe in the efficacy of therapy
	3. Have the necessary time, energy, or resources
	4. Perceive support of the health care regimen as part of his role responsibilities
	Failure of social systems to provide necessary support
Inadequate resources	Financial difficulty
	Lack of personal energy
	Inadequate transportation
	Lack of proper material or equipment
Deficits in health care system	
Complexity of regimen	Patient perceives regimen as too complex
	Therapy effective for one health problem is contraindicated for coexisting health problem
System inadequacy	Complaints of failure to provide specific and comprehensive information
	Failure of individual members of the health care team to endorse behavioral change
	Failure of the system to provide:
	1. Accurate feedback
	2. Adequate follow-up referral
	3. Specifics on how to make a behavioral change
Nontherapeutic relationship with health care professional	Verbalizes dissatisfaction with the professional
	Inconsistent caregivers

The preceding list has been derived from theory, practice, and research. The etiologies were clustered for similarities, and four general etiologies emerged: alteration in cognition, alteration in perception, inadequacies in the social system, and deficits in the health care system. The validity of these etiologies and defining characteristics is currently under investigation.[87]

Alteration in Cognition

The specific etiologies included in the general etiologic category of alteration in cognition are related to the patient's ability to obtain or process information.

Inadequate knowledge is listed as the first etiology for several reasons. Patient education has long been considered the solution of the noncompliance problem. It has now been clearly demonstrated that knowledge alone does not change compliance.* However, inadequate knowledge is a reason at times for noncompliance, and it is easily diagnosed and treated.

*References 4, 32, 33, 36, 67, 83, 93, 103, 106.

Patients with inadequate knowledge make statements such as, "I've never been told that's important," or "No one ever showed me how to do that." Throughout assessment or discussion they are unable to verbalize the key information or cannot answer questions. Included in this etiology are those patients who do not want information: "I don't want to know anything that they are going to do to me."

Patients who are noncompliant because of *inaccurate knowledge* make inaccurate statements (for example, "The government wouldn't subsidize tobacco fields if smoking was truly harmful."), hold myths or fantasies to be true (copper bracelets for arthritis), or have inaccurate information because it has not been updated by new information.

The characteristics of *alteration in thought process*[23,114] include disturbances in memory, recent or remote (the patient can't remember if she took her pill this morning). Another characteristic is the inability to problem solve (the patient can't decide what to do when he misses a medication or runs out of medication).

Another etiology is appropriate for any person who is unable to use written language. Clinically, the *inability to read and/or write* could stem from illiteracy, neuro-muscular difficulties, or neurologic deficits.

Those individuals who have visual and/or hearing difficulties that affect their ability to comply are considered under the *sensory deficits* etiology.

Alteration in Perception

The specific etiologies included in the general etiological category of alteration in perception relate to the patient's beliefs, feelings, and values.

Inadequate motivation[7] can be identified by the patient's belief that the illness is not serious or that he does not feel susceptible to the illness. People have particular illnesses that they feel susceptible to. This feeling of susceptibility increased with (1) actually experiencing the illness or (2) a significant other experiencing the illness.

Another cause of decreased motivation is the patient's belief that the therapy is not effective, or the patient actually prefers the illness to the treatment ("I'd rather have high blood pressure than take a pill for the rest of my life.").

Strong religious or cultural beliefs and traditions can oppose the therapeutic regimen (for example, a Christian Scientist patient who refuses blood despite critical medical indications for a transfusion).

Alterations in one's affective state[4,11,54,105,115] have been clinically noted and reported to influence compliance. Denial is a defense mechanism used to protect an individual against unmanageable anxiety levels. The individual discounts part of the experience or the distress accompanying the experience. Denial can be verbal, behavioral, or both. An individual using verbal denial behaves in accord with the prescribed regimen but verbally discounts the experience. Such a person might discount the need to quit smoking, discuss all the reasons why the need for smoking cessation does not apply to them, but *not* smoke. A person using behavioral denial would verbally agree, but the behavior would be inconsistent with the goals of therapy. Such a person would talk about the importance of not smoking but *continue* to smoke. The patient using a combination of verbal and behavioral denial discounts the significance of the information and continues to behave in a noncompliant fashion.

Obviously, treatment interventions and goals for each of these types of patients differ, and thus the specific cause of noncompliance must be differentiated in the diagnostic phase.

Persons who are clinically depressed, angry, or anxious also experience barriers to compliant behavior (for example, the patient who is anxious because of increasing angina uses medications excessively and inappropriately, and fails to contact medical help).

Another reason for noncompliance is *value conflict*.[14] Persons can agree with the desirability of a behavior; yet when considered with all of life's other demands, the resources (time, money, energy) necessary to enact the behavior just are not available. Or persons simply consider the goal to be of low priority to them.

Some patients believe in the therapy but are unable to change their behavior. The defining characteristics of this etiology include a history of making behavior changes but returning to the undesirable behavior.[48,96,82,107] As Mark Twain said, "It's easy to quit smoking. I've done it a thousand times." Failure to identify specific behavioral plans is also a cause of *inability to make behavioral change*. Habitual behaviors, such as smoking and overeating, are difficult to alter. Success is closely associated with a specific, predetermined method of changing behavior. Repeated failures at altering behavior are also included in this category, and this may occur in even the best motivated and best informed clients.

Inadequacies in the Social System

Inadequate social support concerns the patient as he relates to others and to the environment. Any factor related to a significant other, job, church, community, or material resources belongs in this category.

The magnitude of the role of the significant other in compliance[11,12,23-25,98] is currently unknown, but it is believed to be great. However, the relationship of individuals to the significant people in their lives is very difficult to evaluate and measure clinically. When the significant other is uniformed, has misconceptions, or is doubtful of the efficacy of the therapy, compliance is more difficult to attain and maintain. The significant other who does not have the necessary resources or does not feel a responsibility to support the individual also offers a barrier to compliance.

Also included in this category is the failure of social systems (for example, work, church, clubs) to provide support.

Research clearly demonstrates that adequate financial resources do not lead to compliance.[41,90] In countries where national health insurance is available to all persons, compliance with antihypertensive regimens is not increased when compared with settings in which national health insurance is not available. However, *inadequate resources* can be a barrier to compliance, easily identified in the patient on a fixed income who requires multiple expensive medications. Lack of transportation and equipment also can lead to noncompliance.

Deficits in the Health Care System

The specific etiologies that are concentrated under this general etiologic category are concerned with deficits in the persons, processes, facilities, or resources of the health care system.

A health care regimen that the patient perceives as too complex is associated with noncompliance.[10,13,29,92,102] Compliance is less likely in a patient taking medications four times per day than in someone taking medications three times per day.[45] Therapy effective for one health problem can be contraindicated for a coexisting health problem. For example, a patient with both coronary artery disease and peripheral vascular disease is frequently unable to accomplish the recommended exercise program for the former condition because of claudication.

Failure of the health care system to provide specific and comprehensive information retards compliance.[3,18,23] Also, verbal or nonverbal behavior of a member of the system to endorse a behavioral change can erode the motivation or belief of the patient (for example, the patient who has been told that she must quit smoking by the cardiologist but is given permission to smoke by the nurse). In addition, any system that fails to provide feedback, supervision, or appropriate referral promotes noncompliance.

The *patient/professional relationship* has received considerable attention for its effect on compliance. Like social support, however, the complexity of the patient/professional relationship is difficult to evaluate and measure in a clinical setting.*

*References 10, 20, 21, 23, 34, 38, 45.

NURSING INTERVENTIONS

Patient Goal	Nursing Intervention
Alteration in Cognition	
Demonstrate accurate performance of specific health-related behavior.	Offer patient education accommodating for personality characteristics, coping styles,* and locus of control.†
	Engage in discussion.
	Correct patient misconceptions.
	Provide reminders.
	Encourage self-monitoring.
	Help the person use a structured method of remembering and performing routine aspects of the therapeutic regimen (a fishing tackle box to set up medications).
	Teach problem-solving skills.
	Help the patient use resources appropriately (Meals on Wheels).
	Provide information in multiple forms (written, audiotapes, pictures).
Alteration in Perception	
Engage in behaviors consistent with goals of therapeutic regimen.	Engage in discussion groups.
	Inform about reference groups.‡
	Participate in value clarification techniques.
	Use reminders.
	Provide cues.
	Use prompts.
	Encourage self-monitoring.
	Use applied analysis of behavior.
	Use framing.
	Assist with shaping behavior.
Inadequacies in Social System	
Use alternative sources of social support.	Provide alternative sources of support and resources.
Engage in activities to strengthen and/or maintain coping ability.	Offer assertiveness training.
	Involve appropriate social support.
	Encourage participation in reference group.
	Use problem-solving.
	Assist with goal-setting.
	Imagery.
	Use relaxation therapies.
	Use thought-stopping.

*References 16, 55, 57, 65, 66, 75, 105.
†References 1, 52, 58, 61, 69, 86, 112, 113.
‡References 5, 31, 37, 77, 81, 107.

Patient Goal	Nursing Intervention

Deficits in Health Care System

Report that the health care system recognizes and provides for individual needs and abilities.

Use foot-in-the-door.
Demonstrate graduated regimen.
Use tailoring.
Use self-monitoring.
Provide opportunities for negotiation.
Use reinforcement.
Use contracting.
Simplify the regimen.
Provide referral.

Comprehensive Program

The components of a comprehensive program are listed in the following outline and include strategies directed at the actual change of behavior and the maintenance of this behavior. Components necessary to make a behavioral change are organizational factors, educational methods, behavioral strategies,[25] and cognitive/affectual therapies. The long-term maintenance of compliance is much more challenging, but the results of current theory and research suggest that the problem can be managed by involvement of the significant others in the therapeutic regimen, a regular exercise program, and stress reduction.[11]

A. Organizational components
 1. Consistent care
 2. Appointment times
 3. Waiting time
 4. Reminders
 5. Allied health workers
B. Educational components
 1. Methods
  a. Individual instruction
  b. Lecture
  c. Programmed learning
  d. Skill development
  e. Simulation and games
  f. Inquiry learning
  g. Audiovisual modalities
 2. Process
  a. Repetition
  b. Primacy
  c. Organization
  d. Specificity
  e. Brevity
  f. Readability
C. Behavioral techniques
 1. Cues
 2. Reminders
 3. Self-monitoring
 4. Applied analysis of behavior

D. Cognitive restructuring
 1. Assertiveness training
 2. Problem-solving
 3. Thought-stopping
E. Maintenance
 1. Stress reduction
 2. Regular exercise
 3. Involvement of significant others

Organizational Components

Organizational factors known to be associated with compliance include consistent care, appointment times, waiting time, reminders, and the use of allied health workers.

Educational Components

Patient education is effectively accomplished by a variety of methods. The method chosen should fit the needs of the clients and the resources of the system. Alternative methods include individual instruction, lecture, programmed learning, skill development, simulation and games, inquiry learning, and audiovisual modalities.

Ley[62] identified characteristics of the process of patient education that increase compliance: (1) primacy—information should be given first; (2) brevity—the more information presented to a person, the less is retained, so the message should be brief; (3) organization—material should be organized into subheadings or categories; (4) readability—vocabulary should be consistent with the reading level of the audience; (5) specificity—information must be presented in specific behavioral terms; and (6) repetition—important information should be repeated.

Behavioral Techniques

Specific behavioral techniques are discussed under strategies. The effectiveness of behavioral techniques in altering habitual behavior has been clearly demonstrated.

Examples of behavioral techniques are cuing, reminders, self-monitoring, and applied analysis of behavior.

Cognitive Restructuring

Although the effectiveness of the cognitive strategies has not been tested specifically in relation to compliance, their effectiveness has been demonstrated in other areas. Examples of cognitive restructuring are assertiveness training, problem-solving, and thought-stopping.

Maintenance

Once compliance has been obtained, maintenance of the behavior continues to remain a significant challenge. At this time continual supervision is the most effective strategy known. However, the effect on compliance of stress reduction, exercise, and involvement of the significant other is being investigated.

Not all patients require each component of a comprehensive program. However, being prepared to offer any component increases flexibility and preparedness of the system to meet the needs of the majority of their clients. If a particular health care system is unable to provide the various components, personnel should be prepared to offer appropriate referral.

Sequencing of Strategies

Sequencing of strategies is intended to maximize the impact of the professional in the minimal amount of time necessary to attain compliance. Once the diagnosis of noncompliance has been made, strategies can be sequenced, beginning with the easiest and progressing to the more complex.[88] Easily adjusted factors include attention and supervision (that is, increasing the length of the visit or decreasing the interval between appointments), modification of the regimen (see Tailoring under Strategies), and use of allied health members. If noncompliance continues to be a problem, the behavioral and cognitive strategies should be enforced.

Expected Patient Outcomes and Nursing Strategies

Once the cause(s) of noncompliance has been determined, specific strategies can be selected to treat the cause. However, three preconditions need to be met prior to deliberate use of a strategy to alter behavior: (1) the diagnosis must be correct; (2) therapy must do more good than harm; and (3) the patient must be an informed, willing partner.[89]

There are numerous interventions available to alter noncompliant behavior. The strategies, which are discussed in the following section, have been demonstrated to be effective in altering noncompliance in various medical conditions (such as hypertension and diabetes). Within this chapter, however, the strategies are discussed as they specifically effect the etiologies of the nursing diagnosis of noncompliance.

Value clarification. "Value clarification is the process of examining alternatives and deciding what is important to you."[108] It is a process[9,109] that assists an individual to increase consistency between beliefs and actions. According to Raths[84] the following steps or tasks are necessary to the process of value clarification:

1. Choosing freely
2. Choosing from alternatives
3. Choosing after consideration of the consequences
4. Prizing and cherishing
5. Publicly affirming
6. Acting on one's choice
7. Acting repetitively and with consistency

Numerous tools enable a client to progress through the process as outlined. An example of a value clarification technique is the "pie of life." A patient is asked to cut a pie (circle) into slices that represent his current activity. He is then asked to slice a second pie into slices representing what he would really like to be doing. As differences in the circles become apparent, the patient is able to clearly see the discrepancy between doing and believing. The patient is ready to begin work on decreasing the differences between what is actually occurring and what he wants to occur.

The purpose of value clarification is to provide the patient with an experience that allows him to explore beliefs about a specific aspect of his life. Once the patient has been helped to identify the discrepancies between intellectual beliefs and actual behavior, he will be better able to make a choice about future behavior.

Reminder, prompts, cue. A reminder* is a stimulus that serves as the antecedent for a desired behavior. A variety of reminders have been successfully used to improve compliance. Written reminders, as well as telephone calls, serve equally well as appointment reminders. Medication reminders, calendars, reminder systems, and special packaging have all been shown to be effective.

Reminders are most effective for problems of forgetting. Their effectiveness decreases rapidly over a short period of time, and there is some evidence to suggest that a combination of reminders even further increases the effectiveness of this technique.

Self-monitoring. Self-monitoring is the process of recording one's own behavior to allow specific behavioral

---

*References 23, 25, 30, 43, 63, 68, 74, 76.

patterns to become observable.* Behavioral patterns can effectively be identified by recording the specific behavior (smoking, overeating) in relation to specific variables (time, environment, persons). Generally, the patient is provided with a graph or chart that facilitates both the recording and the recognition of a behavioral pattern. A graph can be as simple as the time and a check mark indicating the occurrence of the behavior, or it can be as complex as identifying surroundings, persons, present position, feelings, and so on. Once the behavior has been observed and recorded, those factors associated with the behavior can be identified (such as nibbling when preparing dinner). Through discussion the professional can guide the client to identify the antecedents and consequences of the behavior (for example, nibbling was at its height when dinner was late, the children were noisy, and the individual was hungry). Behavior can be changed by identifying alternatives to the identified antecedents and consequences. Planning with the patient to change conditions that are associated with the behavior changes the antecedents to the behavior and therefore the behavior. Self-monitoring identifies the when, where, how, and frequency of a behavior.

Various authors have pointed out that behavior changes, once recording or observation starts (even before any deliberate change has been planned), and that the benefits of self-monitoring are self-limiting, that is, they do not continue much beyond the period of recording. Some evidence also exists to suggest that observing one's behavior rather than an outcome is more effective in achieving compliance (for example, eating behaviors rather than weight change).

Applied analysis of behavior. Applied analysis of behavior[82,99,116,117] is the combination of self-recording, functional analysis, and tailoring. Applied analysis of behavior is a five-step process:

1. Identify target behavior.
2. Patient records the behavior.
3. Patient learns patterns identification and explores feelings, perceptions, and barriers.
4. Alternative behaviors are developed as a result of the analysis.
5. Effectiveness of alternatives is evaluated, and they are locked into place.

This behavioral technique has been recommended in particular for increasing medication compliance.

Thought-stopping. "Thought-stopping or covert assertion is a cognitive technique in which the client deliberately and consciously develops a method to reduce or obliterate negative, unproductive thoughts that can lead to unwanted emotions and a perception of helplessness."[20] Thought-stopping is a five-step process:

*References 2, 15, 23, 25, 26, 49, 56, 70, 74, 77, 80, 82, 94, 110.

1. Stressful thoughts are identified in terms of their frequency and effect on the patient.
2. The stressful thought is imagined.
3. Deliberate interruption of the thought occurs.
4. Alternative behaviors are developed as a result of the analysis.
5. Effectiveness of alternatives is evaluated, and they are locked into place.

To demonstrate the impact of this cognitive technique on compliance, consider the following example: "I just can't make it without a cigarette." The thought itself is a cue to the behavior of smoking. Deliberately blocking that thought and replacing it with an alternate thought changes the antecedent or cue to the behavior. "I am really proud of myself. I find deep breathing much more relaxing than a cigarette."

Tailoring. Tailoring[25] is the process of fitting the prescribed regimen and intervention strategies to an individual's life-style, value system, and circumstances (for example, the modification of a standard 2-gram sodium diet to include particular favorites). Modification of this kind decreases the life-style changes being requested of the patient and demonstrates to the patient that his needs are recognized and that compromise is possible.

Graduated regimen implementation. Graduated regimen implementation,[23,25,74,78,110] or shaping, is the process of introducing components of the regimen sequentially as the patient successfully masters prior steps in the sequence. The steps are graded in order of difficulty to the patient. For example, if the patient's goal is to lose 25 pounds, the sequential steps could start with (1) returning for the next appointment, (2) recording food intake for 3 days, (3) increasing fluid consumption, and (4) including vegetables with the dinner meal twice a week. This technique is helpful for a patient who is overwhelmed or has had an experience with a regimen and "just can't do it."

Contracting. "Contract is a systematic arrangement for granting a reward in return for performance of a specific behavior."[96] A contract has three elements:

1. The desired behavior
2. The consequences of a behavior (reward)
3. Identification of roles

The sample contract on p. 1884 has been adapted from the work of Steckel.[96]

According to Mahoney and Thoresen[71] five conditions are necessary for a contract to be successful:

1. It must be fair.
2. Its terms must be clear.
3. It must be generally positive.
4. It must identify procedures clearly, and those procedures must be carried out consistently and systematically.
5. At least one other person should participate.

I, _____, will _____
                (Name of client)

_____

In return I expect _____ to
                              (Nurse's name)

_____

_____

Signed: _____

Signed: _____

Dated: _____

A contract does not challenge an individual to live up to its terms but rather is made knowing that the patient will be successful in meeting its terms. A contract can be written or verbal; however, there is evidence that the written contract has a higher success rate in terms of increasing compliance.*

Nursing care includes the provision of a comprehensive program designed to facilitate compliance, sequentially applying strategies beginning with the easiest and progressing to the most complex, and selecting strategies specific to the cause of noncompliance. Strategies are chosen to provide success; if this goal is not achieved,

*References 11, 23, 25, 42, 53, 60, 73, 74, 95, 96, 101, 107.

alternative strategies should be selected. Finally, patients do not merely participate in a single behavior-oriented program but also learn the rationale and methods so that they can acquire skills to alter their behavior in other circumstances.

Foot-in-the-door is a strategy borrowed from marketing in which the patient is asked to participate in some aspect of the therapy that she "can't" refuse, for example, a request to read a one-page brochure or acceptance of a telephone call by a nurse 1 week following their initial contact. This continual contact keeps the individual in touch with the health care system, and other innocuous changes can gradually be introduced without alienating the patient.

EVALUATION

Patient Outcome	Data Indicating that Outcome is Reached
Accurate performance of specific health-related behavior	Accurate knowledge of specific health-related behavior Verbalization, in concrete terms, of plan to carry out desired health-related behavior Verbalization of errors or misconceptions in prior thoughts and/or behavior Ability to compensate for problems with memory, vision, and/or hearing by using alternative materials or resources
Behaviors consistent with goals of therapeutic regimen	Active participation in therapy Freedom to express feelings and beliefs Goals and priorities consistent with therapeutic regimen
Uses alternative resources and social support	Through discussion, identification of help obtained from alternative sources of support Verbalization of behavioral plan to deal with social situation that opposes therapeutic regimen
Engages in activities to strengthen and/or maintain coping ability	Use of specific cognitive therapy and identification of times when it was effective and times when it was not Requests for more information related to specific therapy

Patient Outcome	Data Indicating That Outcome is Reached
Reports that health care system recognizes and provides for individual needs and abilities	Use of available resources Acceptance of referral Active contribution to establishment of goals, priorities, and methods of evaluation Positive intention Noncompliance reported, with the expectation of further negotiation or assistance

The evaluation of compliance focuses on the methods of evaluation, the process of nursing care, and the outcomes of care. Compliance measurements have been fraught with problems.[17,23,34,72] The specificity and accuracy of different measurements vary. Such variables continue to pose a serious impediment to increasing the accuracy of diagnosis and determining the effectiveness of specific strategies.

Compliance can be measured directly or indirectly. Direct measurements are most frequently used in compliance research. For example, smoking cessation has been measured by thiocyanate, nicotine/cotinine, carbon monoxide, and carboxyhemoglobin levels.[64] Although physiologic measurements offer a high level of reliability and validity, they are not without problems[26,34]: they are expensive; individual variation in metabolism can interfere with the outcomes; and they frequently measure behavior for only a short time prior to the test. Other factors not related to compliance may alter the measurements. Glycosylated hemoglobins provide information on approximately 6 weeks of compliance for diabetics; however, even with this test, factors other than compliance (such as, superimposed infection) may affect this measurement.

Indirect measurements are inexpensive and accessible; but their accuracy is a significant problem. Studies of the accuracy of clinical judgment indicate that clinicians are not able to accurately assess compliance. They generally overestimate it. Failure to achieve treatment goals may or may not be associated with compliance. Failure to achieve a lowered blood pressure might indicate noncompliance, or it might indicate ineffective medication. Conversely, achieving goals may reflect changes in physiology more than compliance.

Absence of pharmacologic effects or side effects is not a reliable indicator of compliance because of individual variability in pharmacokinesis.[104] However, if a patient achieves a therapeutic level of anticoagulation on a stabilized maintenance dosage under close supervision and fails to maintain this as supervision decreases, noncompliance is strongly indicated.

Compliance with a specific therapeutic regimen does not correlate with adherence to all regimens. If, however, a pattern of nonadherence has been previously estab-lished, the accuracy of the diagnosis of noncompliance increases.

Pill counts or measurements of remaining medication have been used to assess compliance with some success.[28,79] This can be accomplished through self-medication programs, counting remaining medication during a clinic visit or home health visit, or in collaboration with a pharmacist. Problems occur if the patient has several sources of medication or if prescription and nonprescription medications are mixed together in the same container.

The original research on self-reporting found that patients and significant others overreport compliance. Later studies have indicated that nonthreatening interviews attain a greater accuracy.[91] Rather than ask if the person took medications as directed, it is better to use a nonthreatening statement, such as, "Most people have difficulty remembering to take their medication. Some people have difficulty when they change their schedule, some when they are busy. When do you notice that you have problems with your medications?"

Another clinically useful method of measurement is self-monitoring records.[26,46] The efficacy of this method has been clearly demonstrated for weight loss[70] and diabetic management,[56,70,80,94] but it is not as effective for monitoring blood pressure.[15,50]

Great care must be exercised in evaluating compliance because the methods available are plagued with problems. Because of this, the practitioner must use multiple measurements. We also need to clearly identify the patient's perceptions, intentions, and specific behaviors.

References

1. Averill, J.: Personal control over aversive stimuli and its relationship to stress, Psychol. Bull. **80**(4):286, 1973.
2. Baile, W., and Engel, B.: A behavioral strategy for promoting treatment compliance following myocardial infarction, Psychosom. Med. **40**:413, Aug. 1978.
3. Baksaas, I., and Helgeland, A.: Patient reaction to information and motivation factors in long term treatment with antihypertensive drugs, Acta Med. Scand. **207**:407, 1980.
4. Bartlett, E.: Behavioral diagnosis: a practical approach to patient education, Patient Counsel. Health Educ. **4**(1):29, 1982.
5. Bebbington, P.E.: The efficacy of Alcholics Anonymous: the elusiveness of hard data, Br. J. Psychiatr. **128**:572, 1976.

6. Becker, M., Drachman, R., and Kirscht, J.P.: A new approach to explaining sick-role behavior in low-income populations, Am. J. Public Health **64:**205, March 1974.

7. Becker, M.: The health belief model and sick role behavior, Nurs. Digest vol. 35, Spring 1978.

8. Becker, M., and others: Patient perceptions and compliance: recent studies of health belief model. In Haynes, R.B., Taylor, D.W., and Sackett, D., editors: Compliance in health care, Baltimore, 1979, Johns Hopkins University Press.

9. Berger, B., Hopp, J., and Raettig, V.: Values clarification and the cardiac patient, Health Education Monographs **3:**191, Summer 1975.

10. Blackwell, B.: Patient compliance, N. Engl. J. Med. **289:**249, Aug. 1973.

11. Blumenthal, J., and others: Continuing medical education: cardiac rehabilitation: a new frontier for behavioral medicine, J. Cardiac Rehab. **3:**637, Sept. 1983.

12. Bowler, M., Morisky, D., and Deeds, S.: Needs assessment strategies in working with compliance issues and blood pressure control, Patient Counsel. Health Educ. vol. 22, First Quarter, 1980.

13. Brand, F., Smith, R., and Brand, P.: Effect of economic barriers to medical care on patients' noncompliance, Public Health Rep. **92:**72, Jan. 1977.

14. Brown, N., and others: The relationship among health beliefs, health values, and health promotion activity, West. J. Nurs. Res. **5**(2):1550, 1982.

15. Carnahan, J., and Nugent, C.: The effects of self-monitoring by patients on the control of hypertension, Am. J. Med. Sci. **269:**69, Jan.-Feb. 1975.

16. Cohen, F., and Lazarus, R.: Active coping process, coping dispositions, and recovery from surgery, Psychosom. Med. **35:**375, Sept.-Oct. 1973.

17. Coronary Drug Project Research Group: Influence of adherence to treatment and response of cholesterol on mortality in the coronary drug project, N. Engl. J. Med. **303:**1038, Oct. 1980.

18. Covington, T., and Porter, M.: Improper prescription instructions: a factor in patient compliance, Patient Counsel. Health Educ. vol. 97, Winter/Spring 1979.

19. Cox, C.: An interaction model of client health behavior: theoretical prescription for nursing, Adv. Nurs. Sci. **41:**41, Oct. 1982.

20. Davis, M.: Variations in patients' compliance with doctors' orders: analysis of congruence between survey responses and results of empirical investigations, J. Med. Educ. **41:**1037, Nov. 1966.

21. Davis, M.: Variations in patients' compliance with doctors' advice: an empirical analysis of patterns of communication, Am. J. Public Health **58:**274, Feb. 1968.

22. Davis, M., Eshelman, E., and McKay, M.: The relaxation and stress reduction workbook, Richmond, Calif., 1980, Harbinger Publications.

23. DiMatteo, M., and DiNicola, D.: Achieving patient compliance: the psychology of the medical practitioner's role, New York, 1982, Pergamon Press.

24. Dracup, K., and Meleis, A.: Compliance: an interactionist approach, Nurs. Res. **31:**31, March 1982.

25. Dunbar, J., Marshall, G., and Hovell, M.: Behavioral strategies for improving compliance. In Haynes, B., Taylor, D., and Sackett, D., editors: Compliance in health care, Baltimore, 1979, Johns Hopkins University Press.

26. Epstein, L., and Masek, B.: Behavioral control of medicine compliance, J. Appl. Behav. Anal. **11:**1, Spring 1978.

27. Fishbein, M.: Attitude and the prediction of behavior. In Fishbein, M., editor: Readings in attitude theory and measurement, New York, 1967, John Wiley & Sons, Inc.

28. Fletcher, S., Papius, E., and Harper, S.: Measurement of medication compliance in a clinical setting, Arch. Intern. Med. **139:**635, June 1979.

29. Francis, V., and Harris, L.: Gaps in doctor-patient communication, N. Engl. J. Med. **280:**535, 1969.

30. Gabriel, M., Gagnon, J.P., and Bryan, C.: Improved patient compliance through use of daily drug reminder chart, Am. J. Public Health **67:**968, Oct. 1977.

31. Garb, J., and Stunkard, A.J.: Effectiveness of a self help group in obesity control: a further assessment, Arch. Intern. Med. **134:**716, 1974.

32. Given, B., Given, C., and Simoni, L.: Relationships of processes of care to patient outcomes, Nurs. Res. **26:**85, March-April 1979.

33. Glanz, K., and Schall, T.: Intervention strategies to improve adherence among hypertensives: review and recommendations, Patient Counsel. Health Educ. **4**(1):14, 1982.

34. Gordis, L.: Conceptual and methodologic problems in measuring patient compliance. In Haynes, R., Taylor, D., and Sackett, D., editors: Compliance in health care, Baltimore, 1979, The Johns Hopkins University Press.

35. Gordis, L., Markowitz, M., and Lilienfeld, A.: The inaccuracy in using interviews to estimate patient reliability in taking medications at home, Medical Care **7:**49, Jan.-Feb. 1969.

36. Green, L.: Educational strategies to improve compliance with therapeutic and preventive regimens: the recent evidence. In Haynes, B., Taylor, D., and Sackett, D., editors: Compliance in health care, Baltimore, 1979, The Johns Hopkins University Press.

37. Gussow, Z., and Tracy, G.S.: The role of self help clubs in adaptation to chronic illness and disability, Nurs. Digest **6:**23, 1978.

38. Hayes-Bautista, D.: Modifying the treatment: patient compliance, patient control and medical care, Social Sci. Med. **10:**233, 1976.

39. Haynes, B., and others: Improvement of medication compliance in uncontrolled hypertension, Lancet **2:**1265, June 1976.

40. Haynes, R.B.: Determinants of compliance: the disease and the mechanics of treatment. In Haynes, R.B., Taylor, D.W., and Sackett, H.D., editors: Compliance in health care, Baltimore, 1979, The Johns Hopkins University Press.

41. Haynes, R.: Strategies to improve compliance with referrals, appointments, and prescribed medical regimens. In Haynes, B., Taylor, D., and Sackett, D., editors: Compliance in health care, Baltimore, 1979, Johns Hopkins University Press.

42. Herje, P.: Hows and whys of patient contracting, Nurse Educ. Jan.-Feb. 1980, p. 30.

43. Hladik, W., and White, S.: Evaluation of written reinforcements used in counseling cardiovascular patients, Am. J. Hosp. Pharm. **33:**1277, Dec. 1976.

44. Hulka, B.: Patient clinician interactions and compliance. In Haynes, B., Taylor, D., and Sackett, D., editors: Compliance in health care, Baltimore, 1979, The Johns Hopkins University Press.

45. Hulka, B., and others: Communication, compliance, and concordance between physicians and patients with prescribed medications, Am. J. Public Health **66:**847, Sept. 1976.

46. Hyman, M., and others: Assessing methods for measuring compliance with a fat-controlled diet, Am. J. Public Health **72:**152, Feb. 1982.

47. Icek, A., and Fishbein, M.: Understanding attitudes and predicting social behavior, Englewood Cliffs, N.J., 1980, Prentice-Hall, Inc.

48. Jaccard, J.A.: Theoretical analysis of selected factors important to health education strategies, Health Education Monographs **3:**152, Summer 1975.

49. Johnson, A., and others: Self-recording of blood pressure in the management of hypertension, CMA J. **119:**1034, Nov. 1978.

50. Kasl, S.: The health belief model and behavior related to chronic illness, Health Education Monographs **2:**433, Winter 1974.

51. Kim, M.J., McFarland, G., and McLane, A.: A pocket guide to nursing diagnosis, St. Louis, 1984, The C.V. Mosby Co.

52. Kirscht, J.: Perceptions of control and health beliefs, Can. J. Behav. Sci. **4**(3):225, 1972.

53. Knapp, T., and Peterson, L.: Review of the literature: behavior analysis for nursing of somatic disorders, Nurs. Res. **26:**281, July-Aug. 1977.

54. Konecni, V.: Some effects of guilt on compliance, J. Personality Social Psychol. **23**(1):30, 1972.

55. Krely, W.F.: Coping with severe illness, Adv. Psychosom. Med. **8:**105, 1972.

56. Krosnick, A.: Self-management, patient compliance and the physician, Diabetes Care **3**:124, Jan.-Feb., 1980.

57. Lazarus, R.: Psychological stress and coping in adaptation and illness, Int. J. Psychiatr. Med. **5**(4):321, 1974.

58. Lefcourt, H.: The function of the illusions of control and freedom, Am. Psychol. **28**:417, May 1973.

59. Leventhal, H., Meyer, D., and Gutman, M.: The role of theory in the study of compliance to high blood pressure regimens (Report), Washington, D.C., 1980, National Institutes of Health.

60. Lewis, C., and Michnich, M.: Contract as a means of improving patient compliance. In Barofsky, I., editor: Medication compliance: a behavioral management approach, Thorofare, N.J., 1977, Charles B. Slack, Inc.

61. Lewis, F., Morisky, D., and Flynn, B.: A test of the construct validity of health locus of control: effects on self-reported compliance for hypertensive patients, Health Education Monographs **6**:138, Spring 1978.

62. Ley, P.: Towards better doctor-patient communication. In Bennett, A., editor: Communications between doctors and patients, London, 1976, Oxford University Press.

63. Liberman, P.: A guide to help patients keep track of their drugs, Am. J. Pharm. **29**:507, June 1972.

64. Lichtenstein, E.: The smoking problem: a behavioral perspective, J. Clin. Psychol. **50**:804, 1982.

65. Lipowski, Z.: Psychosocial aspects of disease, Ann. Intern. Med. **71**:1197, Sept. 1969.

66. Lipowski, Z.: Physical illness, the individual and the coping process, Psychiatr. Med. **291**:91, 1970.

67. Lowe, M.: Effectiveness of teaching as measures by compliance with medical recommendations, Nurs. Res. **19**:59, Jan.-Feb. 1970.

68. Lowther, N.B.: How to increase compliance in hypertensives, Am. J. Nurs. **81**:963, May 1981.

69. MacDonald, A.: Internal-external locus of control: a promising rehabilitation variable, J. Counsel. Psychol. **18**:111, March 1971.

70. Mahoney, M.: Self-reward and self-monitoring techniques for weight control, Behav. Ther. **5**:46, 1978.

71. Mahoney, M.J., and Thoresen, C.E.: Self control: power to the person, Calif., 1974, Brooks-Cole.

72. Marston, M.V.: Compliance with medical regimens: a review of the literature, Nurs. Res. **19**:312, July-Aug. 1970.

73. Masserman, J.: Survey of behavior therapies. In Masserman, J., editor: Current psychiatric therapies, vol. 20, New York, 1981, Grune & Stratton.

74. McKenney, J.: Method of modifying compliance behavior in hypertensive patients, Drug Intell. Clin. Pharm. **15**:8, Jan. 1981.

75. Meichenbaum, D.: Toward a cognitive theory of self-control. In Schwartz, G.E., editor: Consciousness and self regulation: advances in research, New York, 1974, Plenum Press.

76. Moulding, T.: Preliminary study of the pill calendar as a method of improving the self-administration of drugs, Am. Rev. Resp. Dis. **84**:284, 1961.

77. Nessman, D., Carnahan, J., and Nugent, C.: Increasing compliance: patient operated hypertension groups, Arch. Intern. Med. **140**:1427, Nov. 1980.

78. Oldridge, N.: Compliance and exercise in primary and secondary prevention of coronary heart disease: a review, Prev. Med. **11**:56, 1982.

79. Park, L., and Lipman, R.A.: Comparison of patient dosage deviation reports with pill counts, Psychopharmacologia **6**:299, April 1964.

80. Peterson, C.M., Forhan, S.E., and Jones, R.: Self management: an approach to patients with insulin-dependent diabetes mellitus, Diabetes Care **3**:82, Jan.-Feb. 1980.

81. Piper, G., Jones, J., and Matthews, V.: The Saskatoon smoking study: results of the second year, Can. J. Public Health **65**:127, 1974.

82. Pomerleau, O., Bass, F, and Crown, V.: Role of behavior modification in preventive medicine, N. Engl. J. Med. **292**:1277, June 1975.

83. Powers, M., and Wooldridge, P.: Factors influencing knowledge, attitudes, and compliance of hypertensive patients, Res. Nurs. Health **5**:171, 1982.

84. Raths, L., Harmin, M., and Simon, S.: Values and teaching, Columbus Ohio, 1966, Charles E. Merrill Publishing Co.

85. Rosenstock, I.M.: Why people use health services, Milbank Mem. Fund Q. **44**:94, 1966.

86. Rotter, J.B.: Generalized expectancies for internal vs. external control of reinforcement, Psychological Monographs 80 (1 Whole No. 609), 1966.

87. Ryan, P.: A pilot study to determine the validity of the etiologies and defining characteristics of the nursing diagnosis of noncompliance, Nurs. Clin. North Am. (In press.)

88. Sackett, D.: Introduction. In Sackett, D., and Haynes, R., editors: Compliance with therapeutic regimens, Baltimore, 1976, The Johns Hopkins University Press.

89. Sackett, D.: A compliance practicum for the busy practitioner. In Haynes, R., Taylor, D., and Sackett, D., editors: Compliance in health care, Baltimore, 1979, Johns Hopkins University Press.

90. Sackett, D., and others: Randomized clinical trial of strategies for improving medication compliance in primary hypertension, Lancet **79**:18, May 1975.

91. Sackett, D., and others: Patient compliance with antihypertensive regimens, Patient Counsel. Health Educ. First Quarter 1978, p. 18.

92. Schwartz, D.: Medication errors made by elderly chronically ill patients, Am. J. Public Health **52**:2018, Dec. 1963.

93. Sechrist, K.: The effect of repetitive teaching on patients' knowledge about drugs to be taken at home, Int. J. Nurs. Studies **16**:51, 1979.

94. Sonksen, P.H., Judd, S., and Lowy, C.: Home monitoring of blood glucose: new approach to management of insulin-dependent diabetic patients in Great Britain, Diabetes Care **3**:100, Jan.-Feb. 1980.

95. Steckel, S.: Contracting with patient-selected reinforcers, Am. J. Nurs. **80**:1596, Sept. 1980.

96. Steckel, S.: Patient contracting, New York, 1982, Appleton-Century-Crofts.

97. Steckel, S., and Swain, M.A.: Contracting with patients to improve compliance, Hosp. J.A.H.A. **51**:51, Dec. 1977.

98. Steidl, J., and others: Medical condition, adherence to treatment regimens, and family functioning, Arch. Gen. Psychiatry **37**:1025, Sept. 1980.

99. Stunkard, A.: Adherence to medical treatment: overview and lessons from behavioral weight control, J. Psychosom. Res. **25**(3):187, 1981.

100. Suchman, E.: Preventive health behavior: a model for research on community health campaigns, J. Health Soc. Behav. **8**:197, 1967.

101. Swain, M.A., and Steckel, S.: Influencing adherence among hypertensives, Res. Nurs. Health **4**:213, 1981.

102. Taggart, A., Johnston, G., and McDevitt, D.: Does the frequency of daily dosage influence compliance with digoxin therapy? Br. J. Clin. Pharm. **1**:31, 1981.

103. Tagiacozzo, D., and Ima, K.: Knowledge of illness as a predictor of patient behavior, J. Chronic Dis. **22**:765, 1970.

104. Tempero, K.F.: Biological variability and drug response variability as factors influencing patient compliance: implications for drug testing and evaluation. In Barofsky, I., editor: Medication compliance: a behavioral management approach, Thorofare, N.J., 1977, Charles B. Slack, Inc.

105. Thornburg, K.: Coping: implications for health practitioners, Patient Counsel. Health Educ. **4**(1):3, 1982.

106. Tirrell, B., and Hart, L.: The relationship of health beliefs and knowledge to exercise compliance in patients after coronary bypass, Heart Lung **9**:487, May-June 1980.

107. Ureda, J.: The effect of contract witnessing on motivation and weight loss in a weight control program, Health Educ. Q. **7**:163, Fall 1980.

108. Uustal, D.: Searching for values, Image **9**:15, Feb. 1977.

109. Uustal, D.: The use of values clarification in nursing practice, J. Cont. Ed. Nurs. **8**(3):9, 1977.

110. Wenerowicz, W.: Behavior modification technique for the treatment of hemodialysis patient noncompliance, J. ANNNT 7(4):373, 1980.
111. Williams, A., and Duncan, B.: A commercial weight reducing organization: a critical analysis, Med. J. Austr. 1:781, 1976.
112. Winefield, H.: Reliability and validity in health locus of control scale, J. Personality Assess. 46(6):616, 1982.
113. Wise, T., Hall, W., and Wong, O.: The relationship of cognitive styles and affective status to post-operative analgesic utilization, J. Psychosom. Res. 22:513, 1978.
114. Wolanin, M.O., and Phillips, L.F.: Confusion, prevention and care, St. Louis, 1981, The C.V. Mosby Co.

115. Yanagida, E., Streltzer, J., and Siemsen, A.: Denial in dialysis patients: relationship to compliance and other variables, Psychosom. Med. 43:271, June 1981.
116. Zifferblatt, S.: Increasing patient compliance through the applied analysis of behavior, Prev. Med. 4:73, 195.
117. Zifferblatt, S., and Curry, P.: Patient self-management of hypertension medication. In Barofsky, I., editor: Medication compliance: a behavioral management approach, Thorofare, N.J., 1977, Charles B. Slack, Inc.

HEALTH MAINTENANCE, ALTERATION IN

THEORY

Alteration in health maintenance, or the inability of an individual to identify, manage, or seek help to maintain health, can be caused by a variety of physical, psychologic, social, and situational factors.[14] This nursing diagnosis is encountered in persons with mental retardation,[19] chemical addiction, emotional disorders, inadequate finances, inadequate information, and in persons consciously choosing not to engage in primary health prevention.

The 1980 ANA Social Policy Statement[1] clearly identified health maintenance as a responsibility of the nursing profession. This responsibility affects every nurse/patient encounter. As such, the nursing diagnosis alteration in health maintenance transcends disease-related categories and requires development by nurses in all facets of nursing practice. A listing of the multiple etiologies and defining characteristics currently developed for the nursing diagnosis of alteration in health maintenance is presented following a discussion of the etiology and characteristics. The etiologies have been clustered into categories, and defining characteristics are listed for each general etiological category. Since the diagnosis encompasses such an extensive population, the remainder of this chapter focuses on a specific etiology: failure to assume responsibility for primary prevention.

Failure to assume responsibility for primary prevention of health maintenance is a person's failure to identify, manage, or use the information and resources necessary to prevent disease. "Life-styles seem responsible for at least 51% of our health problems."[8] Major risk factors associated with cardiovascular illness, cancer, and hypertension have been identified, and their causal relationships are currently being investigated. Many authorities agree that a decrease in the incidence of specific diseases would occur with a decrease in risk factor behavior. The nursing diagnosis alteration in health maintenance: failure to assume personal responsibility for primary prevention is concerned with those individuals who fail to alter their life-styles to prevent disease.

The three levels of prevention are primary, secondary, and tertiary.[17] Primary prevention occurs prior to any sign of symptom of an illness and serves to prevent or delay the occurrence of a disease. A diet low in saturated fat and cholesterol, regular exercise, no smoking, and managing stress are the primary preventative behaviors to maintain cardiovascular health.

Secondary prevention is concerned with the early detection and treatment of a disease. In this case disease is manifested as signs, but the individual is not experiencing symptoms. Secondary prevention serves to minimize the impact of the illness. A hypertensive person who practices secondary prevention regularly takes medication, controls his weight, limits salt intake, exercises regularly, and uses specific measures to control stress.

Tertiary prevention occurs once an acute illness has stabilized as the individual attempts to return to the maximum level of function. A patient who experiences a cerebral vascular accident participates in tertiary prevention as he assumes self-care and undertakes physical, occupational, and speech therapy programs; secondary prevention as the patient takes diuretics to control blood pressure; and primary prevention as the patient stops smoking to minimize the risk of associated coronary artery disease. Although the demarcation between the levels of prevention is not always clear, this arbitrary distinction is helpful in discussing the individual's responsibility for health maintenance.

The reasons a person chooses to engage in primary health prevention are unclear. Originally, the health belief model[4,5] was developed to explain why people choose to engage in preventative health behavior. This model is presented in its entirety in the section on noncompliance. The health belief model states that an individual will decide to use preventative health behavior based on personal judgment about (1) the attractiveness of the goal to the individual, (2) the person's estimation of his ability to attain the goal, and (3) the occurrence of a cue. Basically, the health belief model states that motivation = reward − (perceived cost + barriers). The

Table 5
Comparison of Sick-Role and At-Risk Role

Sick Role	At-Risk Role
1. Duties—Must want to get well, try to get well, and seek and follow medical advice. Advantages—Exempt from social responsibilities; it is legitimate to expect help from others.	1. Duties—Must continue to fulfill social obligations; must change some existing behavior without help or social recognition.
2. Sick role is legitimatized by society.	2. At-risk role is not formally recognized by society; behavior change depends on the individual.
3. Payoff (return to usual role) will occur in limited time.	3. Payoff (possibility of avoiding or minimizing disease) in distant future and often unrecognized.
4. Positive reinforcement for sick-role behaviors.	4. New behavior not formally reinforced by medical profession or society; rather society is a continual source of stimuli to revert to prior behavior.
5. Symptoms decrease with sick-role behaviors.	5. Symptomless—Relies on abstract beliefs or statistical probability.
6. Person not held responsible for illness.	6. Person held responsible for behavior.

Modified from Baric, L.: Recognition of the ''at-risk'' role: a means to influence health behavior, 1969, International Seminar on Health Education, 1970, Hamburg, Federal Republic of Germany.

components of this model include the individual's motivation, value of illness threat reduction, probability of threat reduction, and modifying and enabling factors. This model is popular with clinicians and researchers; however, it has not been shown to predict preventative health behavior.

In the early 1950s Parsons[18] proposed a model describing the behavior of persons with an acute illness or sick-role behavior. In Parsons' terms

a sick role implies certain rights and obligations that can be briefly summed up:
1. The sick person is exempt from certain social responsibilities.
2. He cannot be expected to take care of himself.
3. He should want and do everything to get well.
4. He should seek medical advice and cooperate with medical experts.

This concept of sick-role behavior provides a description of the role assumed during an acute period of illness and, with minor modification, chronic illness. It does not adequately explain the behavior of persons who are at

risk of developing an illness. Baric[3] compared and contrasted the concept of sick-role behavior to the at-risk role (Table 5).

Persons who are ill have a duty to both want and try to get well. They must seek and follow medical advice. During their illness they are exempt from social responsibilities and may legitimately expect help from others. Persons at risk must continue to fulfill their social obligations and role responsibilities. They are expected to change an existing behavior without help or social recognition. A working parent continues with responsibilities for child care, home, work, and the ''should'' of regularly participating in an exercise program.

The sick role is a legitimate role in our society. Professionals, facilities, and equipment exist solely to care for the ill. Society has not uniformly recognized behavior required by primary prevention. Currently, it is easy to obtain equipment for aerobic exercise but difficult to remain on a diet low in saturated fats, cholesterol, sugar, and salt and still eat in a restaurant.

If the ill person behaves in the appropriate fashion, the payoff, or return to usual role, occurs within a relatively short time. Persons are asked to modify at-risk behavior for benefits that will not materialize for years or to prevent problems that may never occur even without health maintenance behavior.

Persons with an illness receive positive reinforcement for sick-role behaviors. But the individual who modifies ''risk'' behavior does not receive consistent reinforcement by either the medical profession or society. Slowly, some exceptions are appearing, such as in insurance rate reductions. However, there exists a significant amount of social pressure to smoke and to improperly eat and drink.

An acute illness is usually manifested by symptoms that are distressing to the individual. These distressing symptoms abate with enactment of sick-role behavior. Persons at risk do not experience symptoms. In fact, it is often not until they begin to modify their risk behaviors that they begin to experience distressing symptoms, such as the anxiety, cravings, and weight gain that occur with smoking cessation. Additionally, the decision to modify behavior is made because of abstract beliefs and reliance on statistical probability.

A person with an acute illness is generally not held responsible for the illness. However, persons who engage in at-risk behaviors are held responsible for their behavior.

At this time there is no theory to explain the use of primary preventative behaviors for health maintenance. Comparing and contrasting the sick-role theory with at-risk behavior provides a perspective of the multiple factors that make primary prevention difficult. In addition to these factors, a number of variables also have been identified by clinicians and researchers to be associated with the use of primary health behaviors. These variables are accessibility of information and services,[12] conflicting information,[3] health beliefs and motives,* value and norm conflict within social groups,[3,6,12] change in role behavior, conflict with personal autonomy or one's control over one's behavior,[9] and inadequate resources of time and money.

*References 2, 4-6, 12, 21, 23.

ETIOLOGY AND DEFINING CHARACTERISTICS

General Etiology	Specific Etiology	Defining Characteristics
Alteration in cognitive ability (pathologic causes)	Lack of or significant alteration in communication skills Lack of ability to make deliberate and thoughtful judgments Perceptual/cognitive impairment Complete/partial lack of gross and/or fine motor skills Ineffective individual coping Unachieved developmental task Ineffective family coping[14]	Lack of knowledge regarding basic health practices Lack of adaptive behaviors to internal/external environmental changes Inability to take responsibility for meeting basic health practices Lack of health-seeking behavior Lack of expressed patient interest in improving health behaviors Impaired personal support system
Alteration in cognitive ability (addictive behaviors)	Perceptual/cognitive impairment related to alcohol and/or drugs	Need for alcohol or drugs directing behavior
Inadequate resources	Inadequate finances Inadequate or limited insurance Inadequate material resources	Lack of equipment, financial, and/or other resources
Inadequate information	Inadequate knowledge	Unable to correctly answer questions Verbalizes inaccurate information Verbalizes inaccurate information Verbalizes discrepancies in content form different informational sources Illiteracy Does not have access to or use television, radio, or newspaper
Emotional difficulties	Dysfunctional grieving Ineffective coping Depression	See specific nursing diagnoses related to those etiologies for an in-depth discussion of defining characteristics.
Failure to assume responsibility for primary prevention	Conflicting information Inadequate time and energy Health beliefs and motives inconsistent with desired behavior Lack of personal autonomy Inaccessibility of information and services Desired behavior poses conflict with social norms Value conflict	Diet high in saturated fats and cholesterol Diet high in salt Diet low in fiber Lack of regular exercise Obesity Cigarette smoking Failure to manage stress Failure to have periodic medical examination

NURSING INTERVENTIONS

Patient Goal	Nursing Intervention
General Public	
Receive consistent, accurate information.	Use mass media, printed material, closed circuit television, and teaching methods requiring patient interaction. Provide positive reinforcement.

Patient Goal	Nursing Intervention
Assume responsibility for primary health maintenance.	Provide information. Use problem-solving techniques. Use assertiveness training. Help clarify values* and establish personal health goals.
High-Risk Individuals	
Use behavior modification techniques.	Use self-monitoring,* guided practice and reinforcement, contracting,* cuing,* and tailoring.* Help establish patterns of environmental control.
Use cognitive restructuring.	Encourage positive self-control of preferences.* Use relaxation training, biofeedback, meditation, imagery, and thought-stopping.*
Use support systems.	Encourage participation in reference groups.* Provide information on community resources. Use small group discussion and support groups.*

*These nursing interventions have been discussed in the section on noncompliance.

The primary goal for an individual with alteration in health maintenance is to establish behavior patterns that maintain health. Nursing interventions are designed (1) to provide large numbers of individuals with a cue or message identifying the behaviors necessary to maintain health and (2) to provide individuals at high risk with the specific information on how to modify the behavior.

Messages appropriate for the general public need to be kept simple, identifying a global theme while avoiding complex, specific behavior.[10,11] Some evidence supports increased effectiveness of the message with professional reinforcement.

Primary prevention is the responsibility of the "healthy individual" who generally has limited contact with the health care system. A large percentage of health information is acquired from mass media, sources known for persuasive messages, fictionalization, and opinion. Personal encounters with a health care professional may take place, but they are infrequent, irregular, and generally during an acute health crisis. Receptiveness to information not directly related to the acute crisis is limited.

Nursing interventions to assist the general public in health maintenance should communicate clear, concise, and meaningful information. In addition, positive reinforcement of health information by a nurse validates the significance of the health message. Such positive reinforcement could occur during routine activities, such as contact with visitors by nurses in acute care facilities, with families by nurses in home health care agencies,[7] at work and school settings by occupational and school health nurses, and by professionals speaking to lay groups.

In addition to providing information and positive reinforcement, nurses can identify persons at high risk for specific diseases.[23] For example, persons who smoke are at high risk for developing both cancer and heart disease. These high-risk individuals require general information and information related to methods of behavioral alteration. Specifically, they would benefit from learning behavior modification and cognitive restructuring techniques. They need encouragement and assistance to strengthen their social support. Persons with alteration in health maintenance and those with noncompliance require changes in their behavior. Many of the nursing interventions that follow have already been discussed in the section on noncompliance and are so indicated.

Behavior modification techniques are based on the *ABC's* of behavior. *A* is the antecedent or cue to a particular behavior; *B* is the actual behavior; and *C* is the consequence of the behavior. A cup of coffee or drink can be the antecedent to the particular behavior of smoking. The consequences are the pleasurable sensations that the person experiences when smoking. Advocates of behavior modification theory suggest that to alter behavior to quit smoking, the antecedents and consequences of a behavior need to be changed. An individual needs to alter his environment to eliminate or reduce the cues to the targeted behavior. Additionally, the individual needs to identify other sources of pleasure that are congruent with the targeted behavior and replace the old reward with a new one.

The use of cognitive restructuring techniques allows the individual to control thoughts and therefore feelings and behavior related to a specific problem. For example, the newly reformed smoker who continually tells herself that she cannot stand being without a cigarette and fantasizes about the next cigarette can be taught to stop those provocative thoughts, which are inconsistent with the goal of smoking cessation. In addition, this individual can be taught to use one of several alternative methods of relaxation to reduce the stress associated with behavior change.

Since the number of persons with alterations in health maintenance is so great, it is important that health care professionals encourage use of community resources, lay reference groups, and support of family and friends.

Effectiveness of the general messages needs to be de-termined in terms of accuracy, clarity, and the impact on the general public. For individuals at high risk, evaluation needs to include their ability to incorporate the use of behavior modification technique into their lives, their ability to use cognitive restructuring techniques, and their use of social support and resources.

EVALUATION

Patient Outcome	Data Indicating That Outcome is Reached
Responsible for health maintenance	Personal health goals identified Appropriate decisions Problem-solving strategies Desired health goals attained
Controls antecedents and consequences of targeted behavior	Behavior modification techniques used Specific behavior plan to alter targeted behavior Multiple personal reinforcers identified
Controls thoughts related to targeted behavior	Cognitive restructuring technique Personal preference in relaxation techniques identified
Uses social support and alternative resources	Community resources used Sources of long-term support identified

References

1. American Nurses Association: Nursing: a policy statement, Kansas City, 1980, The American Nurses Association.
2. Anderson, S.V.D., and Bauwens, E.E.: Patterns of chronic health problems. In Anderson, S., and Bauwens, E., editors: Chronic health problems: concepts and application, St. Louis, 1981, The C.V. Mosby Co.
3. Baric, L.: Recognition of the "at-risk" role: a means to influence health behavior, 1969, International Seminar on Health Education. In Behavior change through health education: problems of methodology: reports on fundamental research in health education, Hamburg, Federal Republic of Germany, 1970.
4. Becker, M., and Mauman, L.: Sociobehavioral determinants of compliance with health and medical care recommendations, Med. Care 13:10-24, Jan. 1975.
5. Becker, M.H., and others: A new approach to explaining sick role behavior in low-income populations, Am. J. Public Health 84:250-216, March 1974.
6. DiMatteo, M.R., and DiNicola, D.D.: Achieving patient compliance: the psychology of the medical practitioner's role, New York, 1982, Pergamon Press.
7. Flynn, J.B., and Giffin, P.A.: Health promotion in acute care setting, Nurs. Clin. North Am. 19:2:239-250, June 1984.
8. Fritz, W.: Maintaining wellness: yours and theirs, Nurs. Clin. North Am. 19:263-270, June 1984.
9. Goodrick, K.: An alternative approach to risk reduction, Health values: Achieving High Level Wellness 2:297-300, Nov.-Dec. 1978.
10. Goorasser, S.C., and Craft, B.J.G.: The patient's approach to wellness, Nurs. Clin. North Am. 19:195-206, June 1984.
11. Green, L., and others: Health education planning: a diagnostic approach, Palo Alto, Calif., 1980, Mayfield Publishing Co.
12. Kar, S., and others: A psychosocial model of health behavior: implications for nutrition education, research and policy, Health Values: Achieving High Level Wellness 7:2, March-Apr. 1983.
13. Kim, M.J., and Moritz, D.A.: Classification of nursing diagnoses: proceedings of the third and fourth national conferences, St. Louis, 1982, The C.V. Mosby Co.
14. Kim, M.J., and others: Pocket guide to nursing diagnosis, St. Louis, 1984, The C.V. Mosby Co.
15. Lovvorn, J.: Types of preventive health cues given to high-risk individuals, Heart Lung 10:3, May-June 1981.
16. McAlister, A., and others: Behavioral science applied to cardiovascular health: progress and research needs in the modification of risk-taking habits in adult populations, Health Education Monographs 4:45-73, Spring 1976.
17. Moore, P., and Williamson, G.: Health promotion: evolution of a concept, Nurs. Clin. North Am. 19:195-206, June 1984.
18. Parsons, T.: Definitions of health and illness in the light of American values and social structure. In Jaco, E.G.: Patients, physicians and illness, New York, 1958, Free Press.
19. Peret, K., and Stachowiak, B.: Alteration in health maintenance: conceptual base, etiology, and defining characteristics. In Kim, M.J., and others, editors: Classification of nursing diagnoses: proceedings of the fifth national conference, St. Louis, 1984, The C.V. Mosby Co.
20. Raths, L., and others: Values and teaching, Columbus, Ohio, 1966, Charles E. Merrill Publishing Co.
21. Rosenstock, I.M.: What research in motivation suggests for public health, Am. J. Public Health 50:3, March 1960.
22. Shultz, C., and Smith, M.: Lifestyle assessment: a tool for practice, Nurs. Clin. North Am. 19:271-282, June 1984.
23. Warr, W.: Toward a higher level of wellness: prevention of chronic disease. In Anderson, S., and Bauwens, E., editors: Chronic health problems: concepts and application, St. Louis, 1981, The C.V. Mosby Co.

Coping-Stress-Tolerance

The coping-stress-tolerance pattern is described by M. Gordon[23a] as follows. Stress is viewed as a normal part of living. A stressor is an event that challenges or threatens a person's integrity. The stressor "produces a psychophysiological response that can lead to growth and further development or to disorganization manifested as anxiety, fear, depression, and other changes in self-perception or roles and relationships." Gordon cites the loss of a family member as such a stressor. Coping patterns are ways in which people generally respond to stressful situations, and the stress-tolerance pattern "describes the amount of stress the client has handled effectively."

Since a significant loss is a stressor and normal grieving can be viewed as a coping pattern in response to such a stressor, both nursing diagnoses—anticipatory grieving and dysfunctional grieving—are included for discussion under the coping-stress-tolerance pattern in addition to ineffective individual coping. The decision was made to focus the discussion regarding coping on ineffective individual coping. As explained later the word *coping* used in relation to the family as a functioning unit does not seem appropriate.

COPING, INEFFECTIVE INDIVIDUAL

Response to actual and potential health problems is the focus of nursing.[1] Responses to daily life situations or major life events are commonly referred to as coping, an individual's effort to prevent or overcome problems. Coping implies the ability to handle a situation and effect change.

As a person confronts health problems, he may find himself less able to care for himself, unable to sleep, experiencing pain, feeling lonely and rejected, suspicious of his friends, thinking "I am no good now. . . . the only cure is rest and medicine," and being very dependent on others or completely alone. How an individual deals with these problems or focuses on only one of them can be identified as his coping response. The response may be judged by self and others as reflected in the use of the terms effective and noneffective, adaptive and maladaptive, and functional and dysfunctional.

Holroyd and Lazarus[12] identified the ways coping affects health. First, the neuroendocrine stress response is influenced. Problem-focused coping may either help a person prevent the stress event, avoid or resolve the issues, or generate additional concerns. Emotion-focused coping can relieve or intensify one's emotions and physiologic responses. Certain patterns of response are associated with neuroendocrine responses that predispose a person to a particular type of disorder.

Second, the symptoms of illness or illness behaviors relieve the stress and assist in management of the problems. Third, changes in health behavior, as a person responds to the situation, may expose the person to other injurious substances or stresses, for example, a person with an ulcer who drinks more alcohol as stress at work increases. Finally, consider the ways in which an individual copes with the treatment process: he may seek help when the symptoms are life threatening; he may take the medication only when he is fearful; or he may carefully follow the physician's instructions. These behaviors in turn affect the medical care given.

The nursing profession's concern about responses to health problems that involve coping, coping behaviors, and coping strategies is further validated by actions taken at the National Conference on Nursing Diagnoses. The label *coping, ineffective individual* was accepted in 1978. "Ineffective coping is the impairment of adaptive behaviors and problem-solving abilities of a person in meeting life's demands and roles."[18] The literature reviewed to develop the diagnostic label focused on one aspect of coping—seeking and using information. Currently the literature in the area of coping is prolific and complex. It is closely related to concepts of stress and adaptation.

As developed, the nursing diagnosis is broad, perhaps providing a working diagnosis until more data about a patient are collected and processed.

THEORY AND ETIOLOGY

Currently there is no accepted typology of coping responses. However, Moos and Billings[29] have organized appraisal and coping processes into three major groupings. *Appraisal-focused coping* concerns defining the meaning of the situation. *Problem-focused coping* involves dealing with reality by modifying the source of threat, by handling consequences of the problem, and by changing the self and developing new satisfactions. *Emotion-focused coping* attempts to manage the aroused emotions. Moos and Billings[29] present the following outline of components:

1. Appraisal-focused coping
   a. Logical analysis
   b. Cognitive redefinition
   c. Cognitive avoidance

Fig. 4
Model of response to illness and treatment.[23]

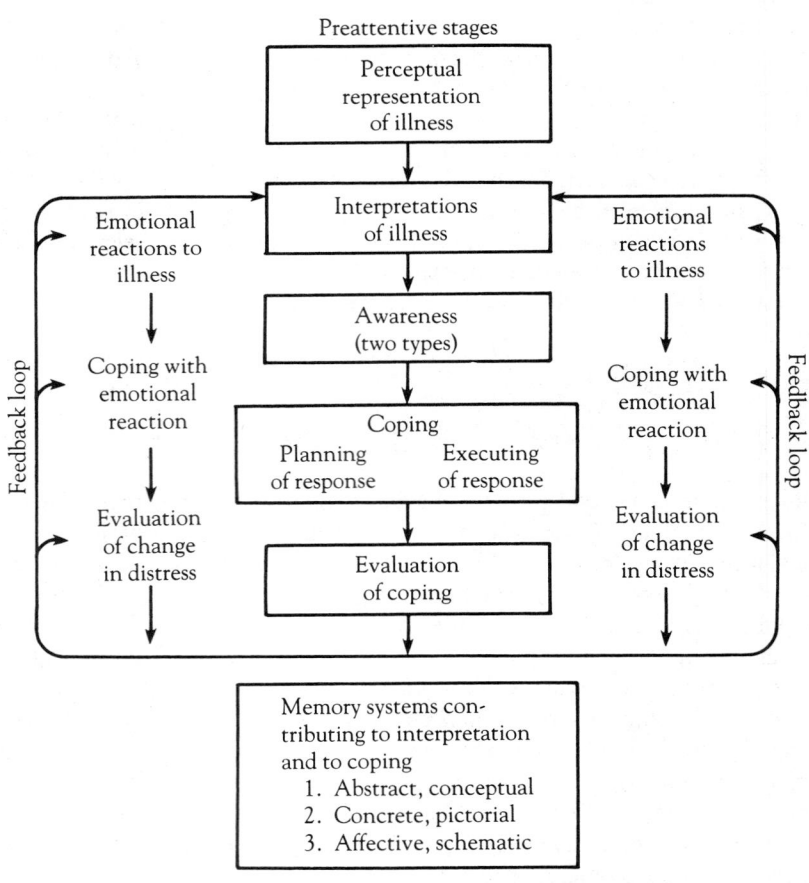

2. Problem-focused coping
   a. Seek information or advice
   b. Take problem-solving action
   c. Develop alternative rewards
3. Emotion-focused coping
   a. Affective regulation
   b. Resigned acceptance
   c. Emotional discharge

Another perspective is reflected in Erikson's eight life stages.[8] Each stage of life brings a new crisis with concomitant opportunity to acquire additional skills. Healthy resolution of preceding stages is prerequisite to the healthy resolution of later stages. The development of basic trust in the first stage is essential to mastering the next stage involving autonomy and so on. Personal coping resources or strengths are developed over the life span. Coping resources are a "complex set of personality, attitudinal, and cognitive factors that provide the psychological context for coping."[29]

The transactional model of stress emphasizing cognitive appraisals and coping responses offers another way to integrate complex concepts.[21,22] Following a primary cognitive appraisal that a response to avoid or reduce physical or psychologic harm is needed and a secondary appraisal that a response which is fully effective is not available, the individual makes the best possible response. The response affects the environment, another reappraisal is made of the situation, and the coping response follows.

Leventhal and Nerenz[23] proposed a model of response to illness and treatment (Fig. 4). The model describes the self-regulative processes that result in adaptation to stress: the preattentive stage or input stage, the response or coping stage, and a monitoring stage; each stage is a feedback loop. Coping refers to the processes of planning and action. The following example illuminates the model:

A physician begins to stumble occasionally. He notes a slight foot drop on the right side. He is worried because he cannot determine a feature of the physical environment that should cause him to stumble. In the past he feared dying of a heart attack, as his father had at the age of 50. Now he wonders about cancer. His mother died after having a colostomy for cancer of the rectum; he was unable to be with her at the time because of travel restrictions during World War II. He also recalls his medical knowledge and experience with helping others in pain. His fears mount. Then he remembers falling downstairs 2 years before and having a compacted fracture of a vertebra. This previous injury offers an explanation, and the questions and concerns decrease.

The occasional falling continues, and a severe headache develops in the left temporal area. The information finally is shared with his wife and then with a friend who is a physician. Medication is suggested as well as further tests. His fear is abated as the pain is controlled.

He continues to believe the stumbling is related to the back injury and begins to visit the physical therapy department occasionally. He tries numerous medications to help ease the severe headaches. There is no lessening of his busy daily activities. His increasing fear is shared with his wife, and he begins to contact his physician more frequently to relate symptoms and to submit to various tests for brain disorders.

The first stage of the model of Leventhal and Nerenz[23] is the preattentive stage/appraisal process in which perceptual representation and interpretation occur. The stimulus first enters the perceptual system through the sense organs, where it is registered and a perceptual representation is generated. The sense organs then relay the input to the central nervous system. Emotions affect the process by intensifying body sensations. By further processing, aspects of the stimulus event stimulate the recall and perception memories, which again may activate other memories. The relationships among memory structure, the input, and one's attending to the information determine when the information reaches conscious awareness. It is recognized that emotional memory structures are more powerful and demand greater attention.

Interpretation of the event is assisted by the schemata of past experiences, in other words, mental images about what was felt, seen, heard, and smelled, what the symptom was called, how long it lasted, its cause, and its prognosis. The interpretation of the stimulus occurs as it is given labels, causal relationships, time structures, and consequences.

Leventhal and Nerenz stress the importance of distinguishing between the types of memory for the effect on the coping process. Perceptual memory—memory of the visual, auditory, and tactile sensations of an event—is associated with automatic responding; therefore interpretation of an event using more of the emotional schemata leads to automatic responding. Abstract and conceptual memory is related to more conscious, volitional responding.

In Leventhal and Nerenz's model the response or coping stage follows the complex appraisal process. The representation of the illness in an individual's conscious awareness directs the plans and actions. It is important that the plan include goals for dealing with emotional reactions as well as goals for managing objective features of the illness or event. The person can make more objective long-range plans if he can identify whether he is responding to the emotional or objective aspects of the situation and if he can postpone or refocus his goals and actions.

Folkman and Lazarus[9] believed that, among life situations, health problems are particularly demanding of emotional coping resources. The threat to the self is great. The dependence on others for assistance of all types is increased. Therefore particular attention needs to be given to planning for the emotional reactions.

What enables a person to generate coping responses? Bandura,[2] as well as Leventhal and Nerenz,[23] identified the importance of self-esteem and "self-effectance." Self-effectance implies the ability to perceive self as able to identify problems, make plans, and act. Experiences increase the person's knowledge and ability to cope. In addition, observing others making successful plans and actions as well as other forms of social support contribute to coping responses.

The last stage of the model of Leventhal and Nerenz is the monitoring stage, which involves the appraisal process again. An evaluation of the change in distress, of the coping responses, and of the objective impact on the illness or event is made.

The appraisal made is related to several factors. First, the setting of reasonable goals is important. When goals are set too high, are unrealistic and very abstract, are extremely concrete and minute, or demand an unreasonable time sequence, the person may conclude that he cannot make a difference and thus effect change. Second, the feedback system is important in the appraisal process. The model has two basic types of feedback: emotional and objective. Leventhal and Nerenz proposed that the key sign of disruption of problem-solving behavior is awareness of affect. As the problem-solving behavior becomes less effective in coping with the stresses, the person focuses less on acquiring and processing information and more on emotional responses. Emotional expressions are pleas for assistance or social support. Reevaluation is signaled by the intense emotions.

A model developed by Cameron and Meichenbaum[3] considers the process of effective coping. It is a linear model based on cognitive functional analysis. Four prerequisites for effective coping are given: (1) accurate appraisal of world and self, (2) adequate response repertoire (such as assertive behavior, communication skills, palliative skills), (3) appropriate deployment of coping resources, and (4) recovery from a stress-coping episode. Failure at any stage represents noneffective coping.

Following are possible etiologies for this nursing diagnosis.[5,17,18,24]

Impaired self-concept
Life cycle stage of development
Impairment of nervous system
Memory loss
Severe pain or overwhelming threat
Sensory impairment
Unresolved memories of past threats or negative experience
Conflict
Perceptual impairment
Multiple repetitive stressors over time
Lack of social support
Impaired thought processes

DEFINING CHARACTERISTICS*

Impairment of adaptive behaviors and problem-solving abilities for meeting life's demands†
Inaccurate appraisal
    Inability to make valid appraisal of situation
    Inability to recognize source of threat
    Inability to redefine or interpret threat correctly
    Inability to find meaning for the event
    Inability to identify the skills, knowledge, and abilities self has to cope with the threat
    Lack of clear realistic goals or outcomes
Inadequate response repertoire
    Difficulty in expressing feeling, especially anger, guilt, fear
    Use of behavior destructive to self or others, such as attempting suicide, aggressive acts toward others, use of alcohol and other drugs
    Inability to seek out or to learn new skills and knowledge needed to resolve stress/event/illness
    Inability to deal with tangible consequences of stress/event/illness
    Increasing emotional responsiveness or lack of objective responsiveness
    Defensive avoidance of dealing with threatening situations
    Lack of assertiveness behaviors
    Impaired communication skills
    Lack of palliative skills
Inappropriate deployment of coping resources
    Inability to develop alternative goals, plans, actions, and rewards
    Lack of ability to transfer knowledge and skills to actual problem resolution
    Giving up hope and spiritual values
    Social withdrawal
    Difficulty in using problem-solving skills and decision-making skills
    Concerns and/or fears about initiating action
    Lack of an appropriate coping response because there is not a cognitive cue to action
    Lack of supportive social network
Inability to recover from stress-coping episode
    Overdependence on significant others, professional help, or institutions
    Nonproductive life-style
    Nonperformance of activities of daily living
    Lack of functioning in usual social roles
    Inertia or apathy
    Hypervigilance

To establish the nursing diagnosis, any number of combinations of the defining characteristics can be manifested by a client. However, the critical defining characteristic—impairment of adaptive behaviors and problem-solving abilities for meeting life's demands—must be present. The list further specifies how the main characteristic can be manifested.

Parameters to consider in assessing a patient and formulating the diagnosis include the following:
1. What is the nature of the stress?
2. What is the patient's interpretation of the stress/event/illness?

---

*References 3, 12, 13, 17, 18, 28, 29.
†Critical defing characteristic.

a. How does he describe the situation?
b. What are the emotional factors in the situation?
c. What concepts does he use to interpret the situation?
d. What are the knowledge gaps?
3. What are the patient's coping responses?
   a. How is he coping with the objective features of the situation?
   b. What specific plans and actions are being made?
c. How is he coping with the emotional reactions?
4. What is the patient's evaluation of his total response?
   a. How is he evaluating his response to the objective features of the situation?
   b. How is he evaluating his coping responses?
   c. How is he evaluating his response to the distress of the situation?

NURSING INTERVENTIONS

Patient Goal	Nursing Intervention*
Develop an objective appraisal of the stress/event/illness.	Explore the perception of the event by encouraging description. Provide factual information about the threatening stimulus. Provide preparatory information to patients undergoing new procedures and experiences, especially describing the physical sensations and causes of the sensations. Raise questions, encourage data gathering, and promote an attitude of openness to new information. Avoid evaluative statements when providing information. Work through unresolved memories of past events; image-based reconstruction. Encourage medical, social work, legal, and other consultation to assist in interpretations. Make referral for spiritual counseling as a way to assist patient in finding meaning for a situation.
Develop an awareness of the emotional reactions to the stress/event/illness.	Give empathetic responses to expressions of feelings to encourage acceptance of these feelings in self. Elicit what the patient fears and what makes him angry. Give feedback about the behavior observed and the feelings expressed. Assist in identifying feelings with names that are acceptable and understandable to the patient. Assist in developing ideas about the relationship of his emotional state and consequent thought patterns and behaviors.
Develop coping responses to the objective features of the stress/event/illness.	Assist in identifying and making changes in health behaviors that are necessary because of the stress. Serve as a role model and/or social support when helping patient perform activities of daily living.
Develop plans and actions in response to the stress/event/illness.	Teach patient problem-solving skills, decision-making skills, assertive communication skills, goal-setting skills, evaluation skills, study skills, palliative coping skills, and relaxation skills. Assist in identifying coping responses he is using and other coping responses that are possible. Engage patient in role rehearsal and mental imagery for active social role participation. Encourage socialization and social support. Teach patient to monitor self for noneffective thoughts about self or maladaptive behaviors. Explore past situations in which effective coping behaviors were demonstrated.
Develop coping responses to the emotional reactions to the stress/event/illness.	Assist patient in reduction of anxiety by use of recreational and diversional activities as well as working through feelings of anxiety. Foster constructive outlets for anger and hostility by teaching warning signs of outbursts, ways to gain self-control, and ways to express anger appropriately. Assist patient in working through denial or other defensive mechanisms, or to understand and accept it as a coping response useful at a point in time. Teach patient to observe for coping responses of defensive avoidance and hypervigilance, which may impede decision-making. Encourage an attitude of realistic hope as a way to deal with feelings of helplessness.

*References 4, 5, 7, 10, 14-16, 19, 23-28, 30-32.

Patient Goal	Nursing Intervention
	Teach effect of negative self-reflections and derogatory ideas on emotional reactions.
	Foster expression of feelings through open communication.
Evaluate the impact of coping response on the objective aspects, on the emotional distress level, and on the plans and actions.	Confront the patient about impaired judgment when appropriate.
	Assist patient in getting reasonable goals.
	Provide feedback to patient and assist him in eliciting feedback from others.
	Assist patient in developing cues for self to indicate whether he is reacting automatically or objectively.
	Give patient a conceptual model for understanding the event or treatment regimen: model of emotion, model of stress.

EVALUATION

Patient Outcome	Data Indicating That Outcome is Reached
Accurate appraisal of stress/threat/illness	Valid appraisal
	Recognition of source of stress
	Use of new facts and/or knowledge to redefine threat/cognitive model of stress-coping
	Finds meaning for the event
	Identification of skills, knowledge, and abilities within self to cope with threat
	Clear, realistic goals
Adequate response repertoire	Appropriate expression of feelings
	No behaviors destructive to self or others
	Seeks new knowledge and skills to resolve stress/event/illness
	Decreased emotional responsiveness
	Increased objectivity and ability to problem solve
	Assertiveness
	Adequate communication skills to convey needs and plans
	Skills to reduce anxiety, aggressive feelings, and so on
Appropriate deployment of coping resources	Development of alternative goals, plans, actions, rewards
	Use of knowledge and skills learned in past or in training sessions to achieve problem resolution
	Use of support system and/or development of a supportive network
	Use of hope and spiritual values
	Use of problem-solving and decision-making skills
	Initiates action
	Cognitive cues to indicate appropriate actions
Recovery from stress-coping episode	Appropriate use of others and professional help
	Productive life-style
	Performance of activities of daily living
	Performance of usual social roles and work roles
	Approaches next problem with sense of accomplishment

References

1. American Nurses' Association: Nursing: a social policy statement, Kansas City, 1980, American Nurses' Association.
2. Bandura, A.: Self-efficacy toward a unifying theory of behavior change, Psychol. Rev. 84(2):191-215, March 1977.
3. Cameron, R., and Meichenbaum, D.: The nature of effective coping and the treatment of stress related problems: a cognitive-behavioral perspective. In Goldberger, L., and Breynitz, S., editors: Handbook of stress: theoretical and clinical aspects, New York, 1982, The Free Press.
4. Craft, M., and others: Nursing care in childhood cancer: coping, Am. J. Nurs. 82(3):440-442, March 1982.
5. Dean, A., and Lin, N.: The stress-buffering role of social support, J. Nervous Ment. Dis. 165(6):403-417, June 1977.
6. Dunn, J.: Distress and comfort, Cambridge, Mass., 1977, Harvard University Press.
7. Elliott, S.: Denial as an effective mechanism to allay anxiety following a stressful event, JPN Ment. Health Services 18(10):11-15, Oct. 1980.
8. Erikson, E.: Childhood and society, ed. 2, New York, 1963, W.W. Norton Co.
9. Folkman, S., and Lazarus, R.S.: An analysis of coping in a middle-aged community sample, J. Health Social Behav. 21(3):219-239, Sept. 1980.

10. Fraser, J., and Spicka, D.: Handling the emotional response to disaster: the case for American Red Cross/community mental health collaboration, Ment. Health J. **17**(4):255-264, Winter 1981.

11. Haan, N.: Coping and defending: processes of self-environment organization, New York, 1977, Academic Press, Inc.

12. Holroyd, K., and Lazarus, R.: Stress, coping, and somatic adaption. In Goldberger, L., and Breynitz, S., editors: Handbook of stress: theoretical and clinical aspects, New York, 1982, The Free Press.

13. Jalowiec, A., and Powers, M.J.: Stress and coping in hypertensive and emergency room patients, Nurs. Res. **30**(1):10-15, Jan.-Feb. 1981.

14. Janis, I.: Decision making under stress. In Goldberger, L., and Breynitz, S., editors: Handbook of stress: threoetical and clinical aspects, New York, 1982, The Free Press.

15. Janis, I.: Stress inoculation in health care. In Meichenbaum, D., and Jaremko, M., editors: Stress reduction and prevention, New York, 1983, Plenum Press.

16. Kendall, P.: Stressful medical procedures. In Meichenbaum, D., and Jaremko, M., editors: Stress reduction and prevention, New York, 1983, Plenum Press.

17. Kim, M., McFarland, G., and McLane, A.: Pocket guide to nursing diagnoses, St. Louis, 1984, The C.V. Mosby Co.

18. Kim, M., and Moritz, D.: Classification of nursing diagnoses: Proceedings of the Third and Fourth National Conferences, New York, 1982, McGraw-Hill Book Co.

19. Korner, I.: Hope as a method of coping, J. Consult. Clin. Psychol. **34**(2):134-139, April 1970.

20. Lazarus, R.: Psychological stress and the coping process, New York, 1966, McGraw-Hill Book Co.

21. Lazarus, R., and Launier, R.: Stress related transactions between persons and environment. In Pervin, L., and Lewis, M., editors: Perspectives in interactional psychology, New York, 1978, Plenum Press.

22. Lazarus, R.S., and others: Psychological stress and adaption: some unresolved issues. In Selye, H., editor: Selye's guide to stress research, vol. 1, New York, 1980, Van Nostrand Reinhold Co.

23. Leventhal, H., and Nerenz, D.: A model for stress research with some implications for the control of stress disorders. In Meichenbaum, D., and Jaremko, M., editors: Stress reduction and prevention, New York, 1983, Plenum Press.

24. Lin, N., and others: Social support, stressful life events, and illness: a model and empirical test, J. Health Social Behav. **20**(2):108-119, June 1979.

25. McFarland, G., and Wasli, E.: Psychiatric nursing. Part 2. In Brunner, L., and Suddarth, D., editors: The Lippincott manual of nursing practice, Philadelphia, 1982, J.B. Lippincott Co.

26. McHugh, N., Christman, N., and Johnson, J.: Preparatory information: what helps and why, Am. J. Nurs. **82**(5):780-782, May 1982.

27. Meichenbaum, D., and Cameron, R.: Stress inoculation training. In Meichenbaum, D., and Jaremko, M., editors: Stress reduction and prevention, New York, 1983, Plenum Press.

28. Miller, J.: Coping with chronic illness: overcoming powerlessness, Philadelphia, 1982, F.A. Davis Co.

29. Moos, R., and Billings, A.: Conceptualizing and measuring coping resources and processes. In Goldberger, L., and Breynitz, S., editors: Handbook of stress: theoretical and clinical aspects, New York, 1982, The Free Press.

30. Murgatroyd, S.: Coping and the crisis counselor, Br. J. Guidance Counsel. **10**(2):151-166, July 1982.

31. Smith, M., and Selye, H.: Reducing the negative effects of stress, Am. J. Nurs. **79**(11):1953-1955, Nov. 1979.

32. Wollert, R., Levy, L., and Knight, B.: Help-giving in behavioral control and stress coping self-help groups, Small Group Behav. **13**(2):204-218, May 1982.

Suggested Readings

Averill, J.R.: A selected review of cognitive and behavioral factors involved in the regulation of stress. In Depue, R.A., editor: The psychobiology of the depressive disorder, New York, 1979, Academic Press, Inc.

Garfield, S.L., and Bersin, A.E., editors: Handbook of psychotherapy and behavior change: an empirical analysis, New York, 1978, John Wiley & Sons, Inc.

Henry, J.P., and Mechan, J.P.: Psychosocial stimuli, physiological specificity and cardiovascular disease. In Weiner, H., Hofer, M.A., and Stunkard, A.J., editors: Brain, behavior and bodily disease, New York, 1981, Raven Press.

LaRocco, J.M., House, J.S., and French, J.R.: Social support, occupational stress, and health, J. Health Social Behav. **21**(9):202-218, Sept. 1980.

Miller, J.F.: Coping with chronic illness: overcoming powerlessness, Philadelphia, 1982, F.A. Davis Co.

Scott, D.W., Oberist, M.T., and Dropkin, M.J.: A stress-coping model, Adv. Nurs. Sci. **3**(1):9-23, 1980.

Strain, J.J.: Psychological reactions to chronic medical illness, Psychiatr. Quart. **51**(3):173-183, 1979.

Turk, D.C., Meichenbaum, D., and Genest, M.: Pain and behavioral medicine: a cognitive behavioral perspective, New York, 1983, Guilford Press.

Weiner, H.: Brain, behavior and bodily disease: a summary. In Weiner, H., Hofer, M.A., and Stunkard, A.J., editors: Brain, Behavior and Bodily Disease, New York, 1981, Raven Press.

Zubin, J.: Discussion. Part IV: an overview. In Barrett, J.E., editor: Stress and mental disorder, New York, 1975, Raven Press.

COPING, INEFFECTIVE FAMILY: COMPROMISED; COPING, INEFFECTIVE FAMILY: DISABLING; COPING, FAMILY: POTENTIAL FOR GROWTH

Use of the concept of coping in understanding the behavior and treatment of families is in question. As presented here coping is a process within the regulatory system in an individual, not a family. In the model of response to illness and treatment[12] the coping process is activated by stress. The person makes an appraisal, followed by plans and actions (coping process), and then an evaluation of the event, goals, actions, and level of distress is made.

Descriptions of responses of persons to specific stressful events, such as spouses of alcoholics, divorce, death, occupational and marital strains, and health crises, are found in the literature, and some examples follow. Fitting into corporate life-style, developing oneself and interpersonal relationships, and establishing independence and self-sufficiency are coping responses of wives responding to routine absences of husbands in the writings of Boss, McCubbin, and Lester.[3] Discussion of denial of obvious differences and labeling as ways to cope with multiple infants was presented by Goshen-Gottstein.[5] Sahu[20] discussed the grief process of parents coping with perinatal death. Escape, preoccupation, religiousness, altruism, role replacement, and child replacement are dimensions of a coping scale to examine parental responses to a child's death.[22] McCubbin[13] identified the basic coping response in family separations as establishing independence and self-sufficiency.

Efforts have been made to relate family concepts to stress or crisis intervention theories. The relationship of the concepts used in the assessment of the family to individual assessments can be noted. Walkup[23] proposed a family assessment model for a crisis in which coping mechanisms are separate from the family constellation comprising perception of event, value orientation, role relations, expectations, and situational support. Oehrtman[17] identified areas of family assessment in a crisis as perception of event, role relations, expectations, value orientation, and situational supports.

Several writers in the field of family therapy were reviewed for discussion of stress-coping response, and these concepts were not included in their conceptual frameworks.[2,6,7] Only one writer in Kaslow's book[10] dealt with stress and coping. Reiss and Oliveri[19] identified nine tasks of family coping of stress: owning up, family identity, reference to past, exploration, organization of response, novelty of response, response to outcome, consensus on decision, and self-evaluation. These tasks appear to be related to individual tasks also.

Laird and Allen[11] presented an approach to categorizing family theories related to most appropriate target of change in the family. First, the communication processes were an area of focus for some theorists. The importance of clarity of communication and of having an open system to permit communication is based on a belief that family rules, roles, interactions, and beliefs are basic to family functioning. Theorists and therapists primarily interested in communication are Watzlawick, Beavin, and Jackson[24] and Satir.[21] Second, the rule-governing processes are another area of focus. Rules function as a way to regulate the family system. The family's transactions are patterned after rules and may be labeled, games that members know and obey. Palazzoli and others[18] helped families to change the rules of the game and thus improve functioning.

Third, family organization and structure are recognized as vital. Having family structure and boundaries clear and the family being able to reorganize during the life stages are both essential to family functioning. Therapists working to enhance these processes are Minuchin,[14] Haley,[8] and Haley.[9] Fourth, the differentiation and growth processes are noted in intergenerational levels, and the current family experiential levels are viewed as another area for change. Concepts of differentiation, multigenerational transmission or projection processes, triangles, unresolved events and losses assist in understanding emotional processes. For an example see Bowen.[4]

Fifth, the transactional processes with the extended environment are targeted. This focuses on the interaction of family with the larger social system or ecologic perspective. Auerswald[1] uses this approach in helping families. Finally behavior and social learning processes are areas all therapists seek to change. Napier and Whitaker[16] assist family members in a growth experience as a primary focus.

Perhaps a more congruent concept than using the term *coping* could be to identify the nursing diagnoses for families. For example the nursing diagnosis coping, ineffective family: compromised might be more conceptually identified as family organization and structure, impaired. The six concepts targeted as areas of change in families by therapists might serve as a beginning and be explored for relevance to nursing as actual and potential health problems.

References

1. Auserwald, E.H.: Interdisciplinary versus ecological approach, Family Process **7**:202-215, 1968.
2. Berger, M.: Beyond the double bind, New York, 1978, Brunner-Mazel.
3. Boss, P., McCubbin, H., and Lester, G.: The corporate executive wife's coping patterns in response to routine husband-father absence, Family Process **18**(1):79-86, March 1979.
4. Bowen, M.: Family therapy in clinical practice, New York, 1978, Jason Aronson.
5. Goshen-Gottstein, E.: The mothering of twins, triplets, and quadruplets, Psychiatry **43**(9):189-204, 1980.
6. Guerin, P.J., editor: Family therapy, theory and practice, New York, 1976, Gardner Press.
7. Gurman, A., and Kniskern, D., editors: Handbook of family therapy, New York, 1981, Brunner-Mazel.
8. Haley, J.: Problem solving therapy, San Francisco, 1977, Jossey-Bass Publishers.
9. Haley, J.: Leaving home, New York, 1980, McGraw-Hill Book Co.
10. Kaslow, F.W., editor: The international book of family therapy, New York, 1982, Brunner-Mazel.
11. Laird, J., and Allen, J.: Family theory and practice. In Rosenblatt, A., and Waldfogel, D., editors: Handbook of clinical social work, San Francisco, 1983, Jossey-Bass Publishers.
12. Leventhal, H., and Nerenz, D.: A model for stress research with some implications for the control of stress disorders. In Meichenbaum, D., and Jaremko, M., editors: Stress reduction and prevention, New York, 1983, Plenum Press.
13. McCubbin, H.: Integrating coping behavior in family stress theory, J. Marriage Family **41**(2):237-244, 1979.
14. Minuchin, S.: Families and family theory, Cambridge, Mass., 1974, Harvard University Press.
15. Moos, R., and Billings, A.: Conceptualizing and measuring coping resources processes. In Goldberger, L., and Breynitz, S., editors: Handbook of stress: theoretical and clinical aspects, New York, 1982, The Free Press.
16. Napier, Y., and Whitaker, C.A.: The family crucible, New York, 1978, Harper & Row.
17. Oehrtman, S.E.: Assessment and crisis intervention: a model for the family. In Hall, J., and Weaver, B., editors: Nursing of families in crisis, Philadelphia, 1974, J.B. Lippincott Co.
18. Palazzoli, M., and others: Paradox and counterparadox, New York, 1978, Jason Aronson.

19. Reiss, O., and Oliveri, M.: Family paradigm and family coping: a proposal for linking the family's intrinsic adaptive capacities to its response to stress. In Kaslow, F.W., editor: The international book of family therapy, New York, 1982, Brunner-Mazel.
20. Sahu, S.: Coping with perinatal death, J. Reproduct. Med. **26**(3):129-132, March 1981.
21. Satir, V.: Conjoint family therapy (revised ed.), Palo Alto, Calif., 1967, Science and Behavior Books.
22. Videka-Sherman, L.: Coping with the death of a child: a study over time, Am. J. Orthopsychiatr. **52**(4):688-698, Oct. 1982.
23. Walkup, L.: A concept of crisis. In Hall, J., and Weaver, B., editors: Nursing of families in crisis, Philadelphia, 1974, J.B. Lippincott Co.
24. Watzlawick, P., Beavin, J., and Jackson, D.: Pragmatics of human communication, New York, 1967, W.W. Norton Co.

GRIEVING, ANTICIPATORY; GRIEVING, DYSFUNCTIONAL

THEORY

Normal Grieving

Normal grieving is a universal human phenomenon accompanied by psychologic and physiologic reactions. Normal grieving is the process by which a person adapts to a significant loss. A significant loss refers to being without something which one possessed and which was personally meaningful and valued. There are several types of losses. One of the major types of loss that can trigger normal grieving is the loss of a significant person, whether through actual death, divorce, geographic separation, or through a perceived or actual negative change in a significant relationship. Death of a significant person is one of the most difficult losses.

Grief can result from the loss of a pet animal through death,[47] loss, or separation. Grieving can also result from the loss of material objects that have been prized by the person, such as loss of heirlooms through fire or theft. In addition, there are intangible material losses such as leaving a familiar environment and moving to a new one.

The loss of a part of the self, for instance, the loss of vision, the loss of a limb, or the loss of a body function, can lead to grieving. The mental image component of self loss can include "ideas and feelings about one's attractiveness, lovability, and worth" or "loss of positive attitudes, such as independence and control, and loss of social role, such as mother, husband, wife, or breadwinner."[26]

Finally, there are losses during the process of human psychosexual development (developmental losses) or during other transitional periods in life. Examples include the loss experienced by some mothers when their last child leaves home, the loss of energy or strength, and the loss of physical well-being in the aging process.

A number of variables affect one's perception of and response to a loss. The very same loss can be of great significance to one person and of little importance to another. Each individual's frame of reference and life situation must be assessed to determine the real significance of the loss. Does the grieving person suffer from the loss of a role, for example, interpersonal roles, responsibilities, functions, and status when a family member dies, in addition to the loss of any particular person or object?

Previous experience with loss may provide strength through already developed coping skills, although negative experiences may have the opposite effect. Problem-solving and coping skills, including the availability of and ability to use social and environmental supports and resources developed over the course of life's experiences, can influence the grief reaction. General physical and mental health, along with health habits, also can be influencing variables. Physical and mental illness are additional burdens during a time when energies are needed to cope with the experience of a significant loss. Poor health habits, such as inadequate rest and sleep, poor nutrition, or misuse of alcohol or drugs, can adversely affect normal grieving. On the other hand, cultural, ethnic, and religious backgrounds are also of significance. Attitudes and family support systems can influence an easier acceptance of death[10]:

The Amish people see death as a part of the natural rhythm of life, within a religious belief system based on the teachings of the New Testament, which sees the person's relationship to death as one of human temporality and divine eternity. This concept of the transcendental nature of life can take much of the fear out of death and dying. The relational systems within their traditional society provide the Amish people with a sense of *Gemeinschaft,* of community.

A number of major theories address the topic of normal grieving. Freud,[19] discussing the normal process of grieving as early as 1917, pointed out that normal grieving is triggered by a significant loss and is a process that can be expected after such a loss. Normal grieving comes to a satisfactory resolution with time, generally in 1 to 3 years. Characteristics describing the person experiencing normal grieving include loss of capacity to love, self-centered, painful dejection, decrease in other-centered activities, and focus on thoughts about the loss. Other theorists that help us understand normal grieving are Lindemann,[35,36] Bowlby,[6] Engel,[18] Glaser and Strauss,[23] and Kübler-Ross.[33,34]

E. Lindemann. The characteristics and stages of normal grieving have been described by Lindemann,[35,36] the first major theorist to devote attention to grieving. Initially, the person may experience shock, disbelief, and an inability to accept loss. Attempts may be made to avoid focusing on the dead. The loss may be denied. Sensations of somatic distress occurring in waves of 20 to 60 minutes, decreased muscular power, feelings of emptiness in the stomach, tightness of the throat, choking sensations, shortness of breath, sighing, perspiration, flushed face, and exhaustion may take place.

As the person begins to accept the loss, the working phase of normal grieving is begun. Internal preoccupation with the memory of the loss and disinterest in daily affairs may follow, along with anger; hostility and irritability toward others; guilt, including self-accusation of negligence; weeping; feelings of loss and loneliness; emotional distance from and a desire not to be bothered by others; a slight sense of unreality; insomnia; loss of appetite; restlessness; speech pressure; aimless moving about; continual drive for activities, but apathy and inability to initiate and engage in organized activities; adhering to and carrying out activities of daily living with difficulty; and reduced abilities to interact socially. The person may begin to look to others for suggestions for meaningful activities to follow.

As the person unties the emotional bonds with the significant object or person, readjustments to the environment are made. In the final stage of normal grieving the person establishes new relationships and interests and gradually reenters an active life-style in which energies are no longer focused on the loss.

J. Bowlby. Bowlby's theory[6,7] encompasses normal grieving resulting from a loss of others, loss of a part of self, or a loss of objects. Three phases are described. The first—protest—is characterized by anger, disbelief, denial, shock, and yearning. The person may focus thoughts toward the loss and direct anger and hostility toward that loss. The person might cry, search consciously or unconsciously to recover the loss, make appeals for help, sigh, and experience changes or disturbances in sleep, digestion, and appetite. The second phase—disorganization—is characterized by despair, depression, withdrawal, regression, social isolation and inhibition, and psychomotor retardation. In reorganization, the third phase, the person begins to break away from attachments to that which was lost, develop new interests and attachments, restructure his life-style, and return to a preloss level of functioning.

G. Engel. The sequence of events of normal grieving as identified by Engel[18] are shock and disbelief, developing awareness, restitution, and resolving the loss. On learning that a significant loss has taken place, the person may refuse to accept or comprehend reality, be stunned, experience a numbness in which thoughts and feelings about the loss are not accepted, become immobile, and be difficult to distract to other interests. The person may attempt to carry out usual activities of daily living without

acknowledging the loss, but periods of despair and anguish may be experienced as the person begins to realize the loss.

Some persons may accept the loss intellectually and engage in meaningful activities while denying its emotional reality. The initial phase of shock and disbelief is an attempt to protect self "against the effects of the overwhelming stress by raising the threshold against its recognition or against the painful feelings evoked thereby."[18] The shock and disbelief phase is influenced by a person's previous reaction to loss, sociocultural factors, and the intensity of the loss. This initial phase is important because eliminating denial before a person is ready can lead to difficulties in the normal grieving.[26]

Within minutes to hours of the loss experience the person begins to perceive its reality and develop awareness. Characteristics of this phase include painful awareness of the loss, painful emptiness, feelings that the environment is empty and frustrating, anger directed toward self or toward those held responsible for the death, crying, and great anguish and despair. Expressed anger is not meant as a personal attack.

The rituals surrounding death initiate the restitution phase. Funeral rites, such as viewing the body, emphasize the reality of the death. The ceremony often helps the mourner identify with the dead person, and the griever may idealize the deceased. The gathering of friends and family permits the sharing of ordinarily guarded feelings. Religious beliefs can offer a great deal of comfort and support during this time. Sustenance, provided by religion and significant others, permits the mourner to continue the work of grieving.

As the process of normal grieving (which can take up to 2 years) continues, the person begins to loosen the emotional ties to the lost person and builds a new life. As Engel states[18]: "The clearest evidence of successful healing is the ability to remember comfortably and realistically both the pleasures and disappointments of the lost relationship."

Glaser and Strauss. Rather than focusing on the process of normal grieving per se, Glaser and Strauss[23] discuss various types of social contexts that may surround a dying patient in a hospital. They also evaluate contexts as to the degree they support anticipatory grieving. In the *closed awareness context:*

The patient does not recognize his impending death even though the hospital personnel have the information. . . . The patient who is dying but who has not yet discovered or been told of his terminality faces a peculiar problem in getting an accurate assessment of his condition from the medical and nursing personnel. . . . To keep the patient unaware of his terminality, the staff members must construct a *fictional* future biography for him, and they must sustain his belief in that biography by getting and keeping his trust.

This context is maintained to reduce expression of emotions and avoid sensitive situations that are perceived as disrupting delivery of care.

Five structural factors contribute to the maintenance of closed awareness, according to Glaser and Strauss:

1. In general, patients do not know enough about medicine to recognize signs and symptoms of gradual, impending death.
2. Physicians often do not freely disclose to their patients that death is inevitable.
3. Family members tend not to deliberately disclose information about the patient's dying status.
4. The organization of hospitals and the hospital staff tend to keep medical information from patients. For example, medical records are generally inaccessible, staff withhold information or discuss only surface aspects of the illness with patients, and medical jargon is often used.
5. The patient generally has nobody to serve as an advocate and help him discover the staff's knowledge about his impending death.

The consequences of closed awareness are frequently negative. As the patient's health deteriorates further, it becomes increasingly difficult for nursing and medical staff to offer plausible explanations. In addition, treatment that now becomes necessary might make little sense to a patient who is unaware of impending death. Unless nurses explain symptoms, the patient might be severely stressed in coping with a severely deteriorating physical status. Furthermore, the closed awareness situation does not foster the patient's ability to talk familiarly to other patients or staff about a fatal condition and give each other support, review their lives and plan realistically for their family's future, or close their lives by finishing important tasks and engaging in meaningful rituals. A patient in a closed awareness situation may initiate plans that make little sense or refuse treatments that are absolutely essential to extending life. The closed awareness situation can be painful to family members who cannot express their grief openly. The considerable burden of dealing with the patient and his family in the closed awareness situation falls primarily on the nurse. Finally, closed awareness can change explosively to another type of awareness context, a process that can be quite disruptive.

In the *suspicion awareness context* "the patient does not know, but only suspects with varying degrees of certainty, that the hospital personnel believe him to be dying."[23] A contest is set up, with the staff on the defensive and the patient on the offensive. The patient attempts to confirm suspicions, either by detecting or eliciting signs that confirm the suspicion. Direct or indirect means may be used. For example, the patient may attempt to look at his chart or directly confront the staff. He may indirectly seek the information by making the statement that he is dying and then observing staff response. Information is also gained accidentally. Unless the information gained is clear beyond doubt, the patient must interpret it and create his own meaning. Staff members use countertactics to deny the patient's claim "to be told about his terminality. They deny his claim by refusing his invitations to talk, to drop hints or even to disclose, and by rejecting his efforts to force them into unwanted interactional stances, as when he demands a straight answer or attempts to trap them into a revealing cue."[23]

The consequences of a suspicion awareness context can be negative. Patients can needlessly spend a great deal of energy trying to deal with the staff's evasiveness and the runaround they are given. Needless to say, a patient can become sad or even depressed and may die without being given the opportunity to take care of important matters. The quantity and quality of nursing care offered a patient who is suspicious may suffer. Considerable strain is on both the patient's family and the nurse, and a mood of tenseness can pervade the ward.

In the context of *mutual pretense awareness* the patient and the staff are fully aware that the patient is dying, but nothing is said about it openly. "At least one interactant must indicate a desire to pretend that the patient is not dying and the other must agree to the pretense, acting accordingly."[23] Interactions in the mutual pretense awareness context tend to be subtle. Props are used to sustain the pretense, with both staff and patient playing according to certain implicit rules:

1. Dangerous topics should not be discussed, but if they are, neither the patient nor the staff must break down.
2. The focus should be deliberately on safe topics.
3. If a slip-up that tends to expose the pretense occurs, then both the patient and staff must pretend that nothing has happened to destroy the mutual pretense awareness.

The mutual pretense awareness context is fragile and can change to the open awareness context, either suddenly or gradually.

In the *open awareness context* the patient and staff both openly display knowledge about the impending death. Other aspects related to the death, for example, the time death is expected or the mode of death, may not be fully known by the patient. Staff and patient may have differing ideas about the mode of dying, but the open awareness context permits the exchange and confrontation of ideas and facilitates open expression of anticipatory grief.

Once a patient has indicated awareness of impending death, he becomes responsible for his actions as a dying human being. First, it is expected by staff that he will not do anything to shorten his own life. Second, he must meet certain obligations. Implicit standards for dying that may be expected of patients by staff are to remain composed, cheerful, and dignified, to continue to interact with family members and other patients, to cooperate with hospital staff, and to avoid embarrassing hospital staff.

E. Kübler-Ross. Kübler-Ross[33,34] posited five stages in the grieving process of dying patients. In stage 1—denial and isolation—the reaction is, "No, not me! It can't be true!" and the patient feels shock and disbelief. "Denial functions as a buffer after unexpected shocking news, allows the patient to collect himself and, with time, mobilize other, less radical defenses."[33] Although it may be reverted to from time to time, denial is generally temporary, especially if the person is in a social environment that permits him to talk about the loss when ready. Other factors that lessen the need for denial are the manner in which the person is told about the terminal illness, how much time remains to acknowledge eventual death, and what coping strategies the person has used throughout life.

In stage 2—anger—the person asks, "Why me?" and may express anger, rage, envy, and resentment. The anger might be displaced and projected to anyone or anything in the environment. Loud complaints may be voiced. The patient is generally difficult to deal with by both family and staff, but it should be understood that the anger is not directed toward staff or family and should not be taken personally. As Kübler-Ross states[33]:

A patient who is respected and understood, who is given attention and a little time, will soon lower his voice and reduce his angry demands. He will know that he is a valuable human being, cared for, allowed to function at the highest possible level as long as he can. He will be listened to without the need for a temper tantrum, he will be visited without ringing the bell every so often because dropping in on him is not a necessary duty but a pleasure.

The third stage is bargaining. The theme is "Yes, me, but . . .!" The patient tries to enter into some type of agreement to postpone death. "The bargaining is really an attempt to postpone; it has to include a prize offered 'for good behavior'; it also sets a self-imposed 'deadline' . . . and it includes an implicit promise that the patient will not ask for more if this one postponement is granted."[33]

In stage four—depression—the theme is, "Yes, me." The inevitable can no longer be denied and the multiple losses become recognized as a reality. After some time the patient may become silent, withdraw socially, and be depressed. The depression could be reactive, responding to the multiple losses already experienced in the course of terminal illness. The patient, however, can also experience "preparatory depression," which is part of the anticipatory grief for his own death.

The final stage is acceptance. With assistance in working through earlier stages the patient will begin to accept fate and contemplate death with a degree of quiet acceptance. This state is almost void of feelings and diminishing interests. "It is as if the pain has gone, the struggle is over, and there comes a time for 'the final rest before the long journey.'"[33]

Anticipatory Grieving

Anticipatory grieving is the initiation and actual process of grieving that takes place when anticipating a significant loss, before the significant loss actually takes place. The significant loss can refer to the potential death of a significant person who is facing terminal illness, the potential loss of a limb in upcoming surgery, the potential loss of a friend who is planning to move away, or anticipation of one's own impending death.[11] David[13] concludes: "There is a general consensus among writers that where there is an impending death, the 'mourning process' or 'grief work' begins well before the actual loss."

The feelings and behaviors exhibited by a person experiencing anticipatory grief are similar to those experienced in normal grieving.[15,16,26,35,44] Fulton and Gottesman,[22] however, cite an author who states that anticipatory grieving differs from grieving following death in both form and duration. Aldrich[2] points to differences between anticipatory grieving, such as that experienced by the terminally ill, and the normal grieving process that follows a significant loss in end point, acceleration, hope, and ambivalence. The anticipatory grief of the terminally ill has a definitive end point—death, whereas postloss grieving can be prolonged. Anticipatory grieving may not accelerate in the terminally ill as death approaches because of defense mechanisms. During anticipatory grieving there can always exist some hope that action can be taken to prevent the significant loss. In normal grieving after a significant loss, action cannot change the extent of the loss. Ambivalence appears to be more pronounced during anticipatory grieving. In addition, for the terminally ill person experiencing anticipatory grieving there is no period of reestablishment, but this may be replaced by a realization or resolution of the impending death. Finally, the intensity of some of the emotions expressed during anticipatory grieving may differ from those in normal grieving. As Fulton and Gottesman[22] point out, anticipatory grieving can be influenced by psychologic, interpersonal, and sociocultural variables.

Hampe's research[25] showed that a spouse experiencing anticipatory grieving has the following needs: to be with and be helpful to the significant other who is terminally ill; to be accepted, supported, and reassured by nursing staff and family members; to assist the dying loved one; to express feelings; to be informed about the loved one's condition and status or nearness of death; and for assurance of the spouse's comfort. Breu and Dracup's research[8] added to this list the need to be relieved of initial anxiety.

Anticipatory grieving can serve as a safeguard or protection against the experience of the actual loss, that is, anticipatory grieving can help a person adjust to the actual loss and lighten the burden of grieving after the loss.*

Anticipatory grieving can also result in negative consequences. Clayton and others[11] found that anticipatory grieving and immediate postmortem depression in the person grieving were positively related; that is, "those with 'anticipatory grief' did worse in the first month of bereavement and no better at one year than those without such a reaction." Anticipatory grieving may be functional or dysfunctional for an individual or family depending on the manner in which it is experienced and responded to by others in the environment.[22]

Fulton and Gottesman also note the complexity of factors that interplay in the outcome of anticipatory grieving. Psychologic variables may intensify some emotions in the anticipatory grieving process and diminish others. Interpersonal variables, such as how other family members and health care professionals react, influence its process. In addition, sociocultural variables such as the lack of norms or appropriate behavior can have an effect.

Dysfunctional Grieving

Dysfunctional grieving represents a distortion of normal grieving. In dysfunctional grieving the normal process of grieving is delayed or prolonged. (The acute phase of normal grieving is 6 to 8 weeks—longer in older adults—but the process of reorganization may take up to 3 years.) Or there is an exaggeration or persistence of one or a combination of symptoms found in normal grieving. Dysfunctional grieving can thus be defined as[27]:

The intensification of grief to the level where the person is overwhelmed, resorts to maladaptive behavior, or remains interminably in the state of grief without progression of the mourning process toward completion. . . . [It] involves the processes that do not move progressively toward assimilation or accommodation but, instead, lead to stereotyped repetitions or extensive interruptions of healing.

Characteristics of dysfunctional grieving are identified by a number of authors.† Included are the following:

1. Excessive grief that is protracted
2. Protracted apathy, hyperactivity, irritability, or withdrawal along with inappropriate affect
3. Protracted symptoms similar to those experienced by the deceased
4. Excessive self-blame, self-reproach, or guilt related to the loss

5. Severely impaired self-esteem
6. Severe feelings of loss of identity or hopelessness
7. Irrational despair
8. Loss of interest in and planning for the future
9. Excessive ambivalence and inability to deal with it
10. Severe or agitated depression
11. Prolonged panic attacks or intense separation anxiety
12. Unabated searching behavior or yearning for the lost object
13. Recurrence of searching behavior, depressive symptoms, or other changes in behavior on specific dates, anniversaries, or holidays
14. Feeling or behaving as if the loss occurred yesterday
15. Inability to remove material possessions of the deceased
16. Inability to discuss a loss wth equanimity if it has happened up to 2 years ago
17. Overactivity of an expansive or adventurous nature without a sense of loss
18. Psychosomatic conditions
19. Furious, persistent hostility against specific persons
20. Social withdrawal or isolation or schizophrenic-like features
21. Lasting loss of patterns of social interaction
22. Engaging in activities that are detrimental to self
23. Suicidal thoughts or fantasies
24. Unusual dependence

Dysfunctional grieving can result from lack of a social network, social involvement, social support, and alternative social options; difficulty or inability in expressing feelings freely; unresolved guilt connected with deceased person; a sudden or untimely, unexpected death or loss; prolonged or stressful anticipated loss; previous unresolved or interlocking grief reactions; unrevealed secrets or unfinished business with the deceased person; occurrence of a loss when the person is confronted with important tasks or a need to emotionally sustain others; an anniversary date or other life circumstance that leads to a recall of the circumstances surrounding the loss; a history of delayed or dysfunctional grief reactions; secondary gain from others to maintain grieving; powerful but silent contracts with the deceased person; and overidentification with the deceased person.*

Grieving in Selected Age Groups

Children. "Grief and loss stimulate painful emotions in the child, for they are aimed at the security system that is rooted in utter dependence on others. Feelings of aban-

*References 13, 15, 16, 20, 26, 35, 41, 43, 45.
†References 13, 15, 24, 27, 35, 36, 39, 44.

*References 21, 26, 35, 36, 39, 44.

donment are related to fears of death, for the young child cannot make it on his own."[28] Death-concept formation progresses with developmental age[28] and can be correlated to Piaget's theories of intellectual development.[29] In Piaget's preoperational thought stage of development (ages 2 to 7) death is viewed in terms of structure (death is real and the person is immobile; separation is experienced), and much magical thinking occurs. In the concrete operational thought stage of development (ages 7 to 11) death is viewed as specific, concrete, and irrevocable. Although both specific internal and external causes are recognized, the focus appears to be on the physical means by which death may occur. In the formal operations stage (ages 11 and above) death is viewed more abstractly, and the various components of death begin to be interrelated. For example, the child can now grasp the notion of the aging process and the gradual decline of body systems.

A number of age-related variables affect the grieving process as it is experienced by children. Developmental age is obviously an important variable. "Because their ego-strengths may not yet be fully established and because their love may not yet be invested in balanced, stabilized relationships, children will need to mourn differently than adults. Children may accomplish the 'work' of grieving through play or art rather than through verbalization of feelings."[46] Other variables include parents' own grieving process and response to the death, prior losses, supportive significant others, the significance of the loss, preparation given in anticipation of a significant loss, and other variables described previously.

Separation anxiety, hostility, ambivalence, and guilt frequently plague children faced with the death of a significant other. Dysfunctional grieving may result if these feelings are not worked through. The parent's own dysfunctional grief reaction may prohibit meeting the needs of their children and thus prohibit the child's normal grieving process. Krell and Rabkin[32] point out that surviving siblings may become the focus of unconscious family maneuvers to alleviate guilt and control fate by a conspiracy of guilt in which communication about the death is evaded, by according special status to the surviving child through overprotection and shielding, or by selecting one of the surviving children to play the role of the deceased child.

The elderly. Early old age is the arbitrary category of the life span from about 65 to 75, and later old age refers to those older than 75. The aging process brings with it major changes and losses. Brown[9] categorized the changes and losses experienced by the elderly into those associated with body image, social role, and personality integration.

The body can be altered, with a resultant disturbance in body image. Body changes include decreasing sensory organ functioning (loss of hearing, presbyopia, reduction of temperature and kinesthetic sensitivity, loss of taste sensation), loss of tissue elasticity (causing wrinkles and musculoskeletal rigidity), reduction in reaction time and memory, diminishing energy levels, and the beginning of a number of common chronic conditions.

Changes and losses surround the older adult's social roles. Retirement can be perceived as a significant loss if adequate preparation for this time in life has not been initiated earlier. Financial losses can have an impact here. As Agee[1] points out: "The shrinking of the elderly person's world is accomplished through the loss of family and friends . . . and the loss of human contact. . . ." The death of a spouse means adjustment to widowhood, and other significant persons may die. A shrinking social network requires adjustment.

The elderly must cope with personality integration and achieve ego integrity. Old age is the final chance to evaluate one's accomplishments and contributions. A negative appraisal can result in despair, but a more positive appraisal can result in ego integrity, a sense of satisfaction with one's life, and a more matter-of-fact acceptance of one's ultimate death.

It is critical to keep in mind, however, that the extent and perception of loss and change vary among the elderly. For example, some elderly people do not experience widowhood. Of course, the grieving process is affected by a number of variables as it is in other age groups. In particular, Dimond[14] argued that the grieving process among the elderly depends on social support networks, congruent losses, and coping skills. Particularly in adjusting to widowhood the presence, quality, and source of social support are important for the elderly. Bankoff[5] identified five types of social support that are essential for the widowed (including younger adults): intimacy, social integration, reassurance of worth, nurturance and assurance of assistance, and guidance. Bankoff found that in the early stages of the grieving process the widowed benefited most from support from married friends in the form of providing social companionship, listening to personal problems, generalized support, and providing emergency support. Later in the grieving process the widowed benefit most from others who are widowed or single in the form of approval for developing a new, active social life, guidance, social companionship and intimacy, but not assurance of dependability in emergencies or stress.

The nature of potential losses faced by many elderly has already been described. The elderly widowed may be particularly vulnerable because alternatives to meeting needs following a major loss may be difficult to find. In general, the elderly may be more at risk for dysfunctional grieving because they may not have time to finish the "grief work" associated with one loss before another loss occurs.[14] This accumulation of losses in the elderly has been referred to by Kastenbaum[30] as "bereavement overload." Thus the grieving process, especially related to the death of a spouse, may be experienced somewhat differently by the elderly than by middle-aged adults. The grieving process may be delayed initially in the elderly and continued beyond the first year after bereavement, even into the third or fourth year.[48]

ETIOLOGY[31,38]

Anticipatory Grieving

Perceived potential loss of significant person
Perceived potential loss of significant animal
Perceived potential loss of prized material possession(s)
Perceived potential loss of body part(s) or function(s)
Perceived potential loss of physiopsychosocial well-being
Perceived potential loss of social role
Perceived potential developmental or role-transition loss(es)
Perceived impending death of self

Dysfunctional Grieving

Perceived or actual loss of significant person
Perceived or actual loss of significant animal
Perceived or actual loss of prized material possession(s)
Perceived or actual loss of body part(s) or function(s)
Perceived or actual loss of physiopsychosocial well-being
Perceived or actual loss of social role(s)
Perceived or actual developmental or role-transition loss(es)
Multiple previous or concurrent losses
Previous unresolved or interlocking grief reactions
Lack of adequate social supports
Difficulty or inability in expressing feelings freely
Unresolved guilt related to deceased person
Sudden, untimely, unexpected death or loss
Prolonged or stressful anticipated loss
Unrevealed secrets or unfinished business with the deceased person
Loss sustained when confronted with important tasks or need to emotionally sustain others
Previous pattern of delayed or dysfunctional grief reactions
Secondary gain from others to maintain grieving
Powerful but silent contracts with the deceased
Overidentification with the deceased
Dysfunctional grieving process of parents
Unconscious family maneuvers to alleviate guilt or control fate

DEFINING CHARACTERISTICS[31,38]

Anticipatory Grieving

Normal grieving initiated on anticipation of a significant loss*
Denial of potential loss
    Shock

Disbelief
Avoiding focusing on loss
Physiologic symptoms
    Decreased muscular power
    Feeling of emptiness in stomach
    Tightness in throat
    Choking sensation
    Shortness of breath
    Sighing
    Perspiration
    Flushed face
    Exhaustion
    Changes in eating habits, such as decreased appetite
Internal preoccupation
Disinterest or difficulty in carrying out activities of daily living
Anger
Hostility or irritability toward others
Guilt
Self-accusation of negligence
Weeping
Feelings of loss and loneliness
Emotional distance from others
Sense of unreality
Alterations in sleep patterns
Social isolation and inhibition
High ambivalence
Altered communication patterns
    Speech pressure
    Reduced communication
Alterations in activity level
    Psychomotor retardation
    Restlessness with inability to engage in organized activities
    Withdrawal
Decreased acceleration of grieving, increased defense mechanisms as death or loss approaches
Hope regarding action(s) to prevent actual loss
Realization or resolution of impending death or loss

Dysfunctional Grieving

Arrested or excessive time in any step of normal grieving*
Excessive distorted, exaggerated, and/or delayed emotional reaction*
Prolonged or excessive denial of loss
Extreme difficulty in concentration and/or pursuit of tasks
Prolonged developmental regression
Maladaptive behavior interfering with life functioning
Continuous reliving of past experiences
Excessive idealization of lost person
Severely impaired self-esteem
Excessive self-blame or self-reproach
Protracted withdrawal
Protracted symptoms similar to those of dead person
Protracted hyperactivity or irritability
Stereotyped, repetitive behaviors
Being overwhelmed by protracted grief
Severe feelings of loss of identity
Loss of interest in and planning for the future
Resurrection-of-the dead syndrome
Unabated searching behavior or yearning for the lost object
Feeling or behaving as if loss occurred yesterday
Inability to remove material possessions of the deceased

---

*Critical defining characteristic.

Psychosomatic conditions
Social withdrawal or isolation
Engaging in self-detrimental activities
Unusual dependency
Expansive, adventurous overactivity without sense of loss
Prolonged depression, agitated depression
Irrational despair, severe hopelessness
Suicidal thoughts and fantasies
Extremely labile affect
Extreme anger or hostility
Furious, persistent hostility toward specific persons
Prolonged guilt
Protracted apathy
Inappropriate affect
Excessive ambivalence along with inability to deal with it
Prolonged panic attacks
Intense separation anxiety
Schizophrenic-like features
Refusal to follow prescribed treatment regimen, especially in clients with chronic mental illness

A nursing diagnosis of anticipatory grieving (normal grieving initiated on anticipation of a significant loss) or dysfunctional grieving (an excessive, distorted, exaggerated, or delayed grief response) is formulated from a synthesis of data collected by means of a thorough clinical assessment of the patient. Assessment parameters for consideration follow:

1. What is the nature of the loss? Significance to client? Time of occurrence?
2. Does the patient display characteristics of normal grieving? Anticipatory grieving? Dysfunctional grieving?

3. Describe the patient's behavior between the time the loss took place and the present.
4. What are the patient's strengths and limitations in coping with the loss?
5. Is the patient at high risk for dysfunctional grieving?
   a. Traumatic relationship with deceased?
   b. Poor social network or supports?
   c. History of dysfunctional grieving?
   d. Multiple losses?
   e. Previous unresolved or interlocking grief reactions?
   f. Difficulty or inability in expressing feelings freely?
   g. Sudden, untimely, unexpected death or loss?
   h. Sustaining loss when confronted with important tasks or need to emotionally sustain others?
   i. Secondary gain from others to maintain grieving?
   j. Overidentification with the deceased?
   k. Existence of dysfunctional grieving process of parents?
   l. Presence of unconscious family maneuvers to alleviate guilt or control fate?

Determination of the diagnosis of anticipatory grieving is based on the timing of grief. Dysfunctional grieving is based on the presentation of a set or cluster of defining characteristics. The patient need not experience all the characteristics at any one time but must experience at least those characteristics defined as critical.

NURSING INTERVENTIONS

Patient Goal	**Nursing Intervention**
Resolve grief reaction to loss through normal grieving process.	Help the patient through the denial phase: 1. Use caring, soft tone of voice. 2. Be empathetic. 3. Be genuine and realistic about loss. 4. Explain that others respond similarly when grieving a loss. 5. Permit visual and tactile contact with body where and when appropriate. 6. Offer support in dealing with bewilderment experienced after loss. 7. Encourage seeking of help from others. 8. Permit reasonable period of denial. 9. Provide news of death in family group setting and in privacy, as much as possible. 10. Respect the cultural, religious, and social customs of the mourner. Help the patient through the anger phase: 1. Be tolerant, patient, and understanding. 2. Realize source of anger and do not take it personally. 3. Facilitate patient's constructive expression of anger. 4. Assist in working through guilt feelings; offer reassurance that guilt feelings are a part of normal grieving. 5. Work through remaining conflicts about the deceased. 6. Assist staff and patient to develop open awareness context (for patient experiencing anticipatory grieving). 7. Offer attention and recognition as needed for patient.

Patient Goal   **Nursing Intervention**

8. Encourage enrollment in grief intervention program.
9. Validate and clarify feelings.
10. Use action-orientation/behavioral counseling techniques.

Help the patient through the bargaining and depression phases:
1. Allow reminiscing about the lost or soon to be lost person, object, etc.
2. Use active listening.
3. Encourage expression of feelings and thoughts.
4. Point out reality in a gentle manner, for example, do not argue with patient.
5. Encourage patient to participate in planning and attending funeral rites and ceremonies.
6. Encourage sharing of feelings with friends and relatives.
7. Observe for suicidal ideation or acts.
8. Increase self-esteem by conveying personalized deference and respect.
9. Use action-oriented/behavioral counseling techniques.

Help patient accept reality of loss:
1. Facilitate contact with nursing staff so as to correct misinformation about cause of loss.
2. Reinforce strengths and coping skills.
3. Permit expression of feelings, such as crying.
4. Observe for depression.
5. Facilitate discussion of both negative and positive aspects regarding lost person or object.
6. Encourage social interaction and companionship.
7. Foster environment in which loss can be experienced within a spiritual context.
8. Use insight-oriented counseling techniques

Help patient accept reality of loss, develop appropriate adaptive changes in lifestyle, and develop a constructive life-style.
1. Provide guidance as needed; refer to appropriate self-help groups.
2. Facilitate exploration of available options.
3. Discuss availability of useful resources and development of additional ones.
4. Encourage role-playing to try out new patterns of behavior.
5. Provide information as sought.
6. Encourage development of new interests.

Encourage and teach patient about good health habits.

Use additional interventions when assisting children and parents to resolve normal grieving.
1. Use art or play therapy with children.
2. When working with children:
   Do not deny death; acknowledge the occurrence of death.
   Do not tell children things that are false or half truths.
   Keep child in normal setting; do not send away to relatives.
   Include child in events surrounding death and funeral; give support and help feel accepted.
   Talk at child's level of understanding; be a good listener; do not cut off questions.
   Do not equate death with punishment, going away, or old age.
   Help child recall good things about dead person's life.
3. Help parents work through their own anticipatory grief response about terminally ill child.
4. Encourage family therapy to work through unconscious family maneuvers to alleviate guilt and control fate.
5. Recognize the effect of the grieving process on parents experiencing the loss of one twin on the slowing down of the ability to become involved with the remaining infant.
6. Avoid comments to parents who lost a child about their fortune in having a living child remaining.
7. Encourage parents of SIDS victim to enroll in grief intervention program.

Use additional interventions when helping the elderly resolve normal grieving:
1. Support verbalizations about body image changes.
2. Provide guidance regarding the availability of community resources.
3. Permit and encourage review of life's achievements and experiences.
4. Support past achievements, current strengths, and coping skills.

Patient Goal	Nursing Intervention
	5. Respect the worthiness of the elderly person. 6. Encourage involvement in socialization groups. 7. Encourage involvement in bereavement crisis intervention groups.
Engage in constructive anticipatory grieving (for patients experiencing anticipatory grieving).	Support anticipatory grieving: 　1. Help the patient through the denial phase. 　2. Offer support in dealing with bewilderment experienced about potential loss. Help the patient through the anger phase. 　1. Work through other feelings and interpersonal difficulties. Help the patient through the bargaining and acceptance phase. 　1. Foster an environment in which potential loss can be experienced within a spiritual context. 　2. Offer *realistic* hope. 　3. Support verbalizations about ambivalence. 　4. Support use of defense mechanisms as needed in patient who is terminally ill. 　5. Assist terminally ill patient to resolve feelings about impending death by permitting an open awareness context to develop. Assist spouses during anticipatory grieving: 　1. Permit spouse or parent (within limits of tolerance) to be with, and to be helpful to, terminally ill person; help spouse accept fact that he or she cannot be perfect. 　2. Be accepting, supportive, and reassuring. 　3. Encourage expression of feelings. 　4. Offer needed information about the loved one's condition and status or nearness of death. 　5. Facilitate patient's comfort. Provide anticipatory guidance.
Experience less or no dysfunctional grieving.	Use interventions listed for normal grieving. Assess current state of grieving. Assist patient in moving through phase in which stuck; use graded flooding approach as follows: 　1. Present patient with increasing significant facts about loss. 　2. Rework feelings generated, such as, through role-playing. 　3. Use principles of behavior modification, such as rewards for more adaptive behavior. 　4. Use mental imagery techniques. Work through exaggerated, excessive, distorted, and delayed emotional reactions: depression, anger, apathy, inappropriate affect, hopelessness, anxiety, or suicidal ideation. Teach patient to: 　1. Identify and develop alternative potential strategies to deal with problems. 　2. Discuss potential consequences of using each strategy. 　3. Develop priority of strategies to plan for future. Encourage patient to seek assistance from friends, relatives, professionals, and self-help groups. Support self-esteem, for example, by pointing out strengths and potentials. Help patient regain identity. Guide patient in developing new patterns of social interaction. Work through interlocking grief reactions. Point out universality and need for normal grieving. Encourage and engage in brief psychodynamic psychotherapy where indicated.

Fundamentally, the overall goal for nurses who work with patients experiencing either anticipatory grieving or dysfunctional grieving is to facilitate normal grieving. The patient experiencing dysfunctional grieving should be assisted in resolving dysfunctional grieving. Patients who have had a significant loss should be assisted in maintaining their own health and preventing dysfunctional grieving.

In planning nursing interventions the nurse must consider the unique needs of each individual patient. The preceding list was developed from clinical expertise and the work of McFarland and Wasli,[38] Armstrong,[4] Earnshaw-Smith,[17] Wilson and others,[49] Constantino,[12] Lowman,[37] Pisarcik,[42] Alexy,[3] and Morrison.[40]

EVALUATION

Patient Outcome	Data Indicating That Outcome is Reached
Grief reaction to loss resolved	Absence or reduction of objective and subjective defining characteristics, indicating: 1. Resolution of denial phase 2. Resolution of anger phase 3. Resolution of bargaining phase 4. Resolution of depression 5. Acceptance of reality of loss 6. Use of adaptive coping skills 7. Constructive life-style 8. Scores indicating resolution of grief on tools measuring presence of grieving
Constructive anticipatory grieving (for patients experiencing anticipatory grieving)	Successful progress of anticipatory grieving process with absence of characteristics of dysfunctional grieving Maintenance of constructive relationship with terminally ill or the recovering significant other (who triggered the anticipatory grieving)
Diminished or no dysfunctional grieving	Absence or reduction of objective or subjective defining characteristics, indicating resolution or reduction of dysfunctional grieving Moving through phases of normal grieving at a normal pace without remaining stuck in one phase Absence of exaggerated, excessive, distorted or delayed emotional reactions

References

1. Agee, J.: Grief and the process of aging. In Werner-Beland, J., editor: Grief responses to long-term illness and disability, Reston, Va., 1980, Reston Publishing Co., Inc.
2. Aldrich, C.: Some dynamics of anticipatory grief. In Schoenberg, B., and others, editors: Psychological aspects of terminal care, New York, 1974, Columbia University Press.
3. Alexy, W.: Dimensions of psychological counseling that facilitate the grieving process of bereaved parents, J. Counsel. Psychol. 29(5):498-507, 1982.
4. Armstrong, S.: Dual focus in brief psychodynamic psychotherapy, Psychotherapy Psychosomatics 33:147-154, 1980.
5. Bankoff, E.: Effects of friendship support on the psychological well-being of widows. In Lopata, H., and Maines, D., editors: Research in the interweave of social roles: friendship, vol. 2, Greenwich, Conn., 1981, JAI Press, Inc.
6. Bowlby, J.: Processes of mourning, Int. J. Psychoanal. 42:317-340, 1961.
7. Bowlby, J.: Loss: sadness and depression-attachment and loss, vol. 3, New York, 1980, Basic Books.
8. Breu, C., and Dracup, K.: Helping the spouse of critical patients, Am. J. Nurs. 78(1):51-53, Jan. 1978.
9. Brown, M.: Maturational losses. In Bower, F., editor: Nursing and the concept of loss, New York, 1980, John Wiley & Sons, Inc.
10. Bryer, K.: The Amish way of death: a study of family support systems, Am. Psychol. 34(3):255-261, March 1979.
11. Clayton, P., and others: Anticipatory grief and widowhood, Br. J. Psychiatry 122:47-51, 1973.
12. Constantino, R.: Bereavement crisis intervention for widows in grief and mourning, Nurs. Res. Nov./Dec. 30(6):351-353, 1981.
13. David, C.: The resurrection-of-the-dead syndrome, Am. J. Psychotherapy 34(1):119-126, Jan. 1980.
14. Dimond, M.: Bereavement and the elderly: a critical review with implications for nursing practice and research, J. Adv. Nurs. 6:461-470, 1981.
15. Doyle, P.: Grief counseling and sudden death, Springfield, Ill., 1980, Charles C Thomas, Publisher.
16. Dracup, K., and Breu, C.: Using nursing research findings to meet the needs of grieving spouses, Nurs. Res. 27(4):212-216, July-Aug. 1978.
17. Earnshaw-Smith, E.: Emotional pain in dying patients and their families, Nurs. Times Nov. 3, 1982, pp. 1865-1867.
18. Engel, G.: Grief and grieving, Am. J. Nurs. 64(9):93-98, Sept. 1964.
19. Freud, S.: Mourning and melancholia (1917). In Strachey, J., and Freud, A., editors: Standard edition of the complete psychological works of Sigmund Freud, London, 1964, Hogarth Press.
20. Friedman, S., and others: Behavioral observations of parents anticipating the death of a child, Pediatrics 32(4):610-625, 1963.
21. Fulton, R., and Gottesman, D.: Anticipatory grief, Br. J. Psychiatry 139:79-80, 1981.
22. Fulton, R., and Gottesman, D.: Anticipatory grief: a psychosocial concept reconsidered, Br. J. Psychiatry 137:45-54, 1980.
23. Glaser, B., and Strauss, A.: Awareness of dying, Chicago, 1968, Aldine Publishing Co.
23a. Gordon, M.: Nursing diagnosis: process and application, New York, McGraw-Hill Book Co.
24. Greenblatt, M.: The grieving spouse, Am. J. Psychiatry 135(1):43-47, Jan. 1978.
25. Hampe, S.: Needs of the grieving spouse in a hospital setting, Nurs. Res. 24:113-120, March-April 1975.
26. Hess, P.: Loss and grief. In Bower, F., editor: Nursing and the concept of loss, New York, 1980, John Wiley & Sons, Inc.
27. Horowitz, M., Wilner, N., and Marmar, C.: Pathological grief and the activation of latent and self-images, Am. J. Psychiatry 137(10):1157-1162, Oct. 1980.
28. Jackson, E.: The pastoral counselor and the child encountering death. In Wass, H., and Corr, C., editors: Helping children cope with death: guidelines and resources, New York, 1982, Hemisphere Publishing Co.
29. Kane, B.: Children's concepts of death, J. Gen. Psychiatry 134:141-153, 1979.
30. Kastenbaum, R.: Death and bereavement in later life. In Kutscher, A., editor: Death and bereavement, Springfield, Ill., 1969, Charles C Thomas, Publisher.
31. Kim, M., McFarland, G., and McLane, A., editors: Pocket guide to nursing diagnoses, St. Louis, 1984, The C.V. Mosby Co.
32. Krell, R., and Rabkin, L.: The effects of sibling death on the surviving child: a family perspective, Family Process 18:471-477, Dec. 1979.
33. Kübler-Ross, E.: On death and dying, New York, 1969, The Macmillan Co.
34. Kübler-Ross, E.: What is it like to be dying? 71(1):54-61, Jan. 1971.
35. Lindemann, E.: Symptomatology and management of acute grief, Am. J. Psychiatry 101(2):141-148, 1944.

36. Lindemann, E.: Beyond grief: studies in crisis intervention, New York, 1979, Jason Aronson.

37. Lowman, J.: Grief intervention and sudden infant death syndrome, Am. J. Commun. Psychol. 7(6):665-677, 1979.

38. McFarland, G., and Wasli, E.: Potential dysfunctional grieving. In Kim, M., McFarland, G., and McLane, A., editors: Pocket guide to nursing diagnoses, St. Louis, 1984, The C.V. Mosby Co.

39. Melges, F., and DeMaso, D.: Grief-resolution therapy: reliving, revising, and revisiting, Am. J. Psychotherapy 34:51-61, Jan. 1980.

40. Morrison, J.: Successful grieving: changing personal constructs through mental imagery, J. Ment. Imagery 2:63-68, 1978.

41. Parkes, C.: Anticipatory grief, Br. J. Psychiatry 138:183, Feb. 1981.

42. Pisarcik, G.: Psychiatric emergencies and crisis intervention, Nurs. Clin. North Am. 16(1):85-94, March 1981.

43. Pollock, G.: Mourning and adaptation, Int. J. Psychoanal. 42:341-361, 1961.

44. Rando, T.: Module III: concepts of death, dying, grief and loss. In Hospice education program for nurses, DHHS Pub. No. HRA 81-27, Washington, D.C., 1981, U.S. Government Printing Office.

45. Richmond, J., and Waisman, H.: Psychological aspects of management of children with malignant diseases, Am. J. Dis. Child. 89:42, 1955.

46. Salladay, S., and Royal, M.: Children and death: guidelines for grief work, Child Psychiatry Hum. Devel. 11(4):203-212, Summer 1981.

47. Thomas, G.: Human grief when a pet dies. Part 1. Cincinnati Horizons 12(4):8-11, April 1983.

48. Weiner, A., and others: Process and phenomenology of bereavement. In Schoenberg, B., editor: Bereavement: its psychological aspects, New York, 1975, Columbia University Press.

49. Wilson, A., and others: The death of a newborn twin: an analysis of parental bereavement, Pediatrics 70(4):587-591, Oct. 1982.

Suggested Readings

Busse, E., and Pfeiffer, E., editors: Behavior and adaptation in late life, Boston, 1977, Little, Brown & Co.

Carruth, G., and Blankenship, J.: Grieving the loss of alcohol: a crisis in recovery, J. Psychiatr. Nurs. Ment. Health Services 20(3):18-21, March 1982.

Demi, A., and Miles, M.: Understanding psychologic reactions to disaster, J. Emergency Nurs. 5(2):11-16, March-April 1983.

Faschingbauer, T., Devaul, A., and Zisook, S.: Development of the Texas Inventory of Grief, Am. J. Psychiatry 134(6):696, 1977.

Freihofer, P., and Felton, G.: Nursing behaviors in bereavement: an exploratory study, Nurs. Res. 25(5):332-337, Sept.-Oct. 1976.

Johnson-Soderberg, S.: Grief themes, Adv. Nurs. Sci. 3(4):15-26, July 1981.

Kavanaugh, R.: Facing death, Baltimore, 1974, Penguin Books.

Kellner, K., and others: Perinatal mortality counseling program for families who experience a stillbirth, Death Educ. 5(1):29-35, Spring 1981.

Lipe, H.: The function of weeping in the adult, Nurs. Forum 19(1):26-44, 1980.

Parkes, C.: Effects of bereavement on physical and mental health: a study of the medical records of widows, Br. Med. J. 2:274, 1964.

Parkes, C.: Bereavement and mental illness. Part 1. A clinical study of the grief of bereaved psychiatric patients, Br. J. Med. Psychol. 38:1, 1965.

Parkes, C.: Bereavement and mental illness. Part II. A classification of bereavement reactions, Br. J. Med. Psychol. 38:13, 1965.

Parkes, C.: The first year of bereavement, Psychiatry 33:444-467, 1970.

Parkes, C.: Bereavement: studies of grief in adult life, New York, 1973, International Universities Press.

Parkes, C.: Determinants of outcome following bereavement, Omega 6(4):303-323, 1975.

Parkes. C., Benjamin, B., and Fitzgerald, R.: Broken heart: a statistical study of increased mortality among widowers, Br. Med. J. 1:740, 1969.

Sease, S.: Grief associated with a prison experience: counseling the client, J. Psychiatr. Nurs. Ment. Health Services 20(7):25-27, July 1982.

Simos, B.: Grief therapy to facilitate healthy restitution, Social Casework 58:337-342, June 1977.

Stoller, E.: Effects of experience on nurses' responses to dying and death in the hospital setting, Nurs. Res. 29(1):35-38, Jan.-Feb. 1980.

Towns, J.: How to understand and communicate with a person in sorrow, Nurs. Forum 19(3):301-309, 1980.

Wylie, N., and Kustaborder, M.: Helping caregivers cope with loss, especially dying, J. Gerontol. Nurs. 7(8):469-473, Aug. 1981.

Role-Relationship

PARENTING, ALTERATION IN: ACTUAL AND POTENTIAL

Parenthood is an experience known to most people. To formulate a workable model for using the nursing diagnosis of alterations in parenting, actual and potential, the disciplines of psychology, sociology, and child development need to be integrated into nursing theory.

Parenting has been most recently defined in nursing diagnosis literature by Kim, McFarland, and McLane[28] as the ability of a nurturing figure(s) to create an environment that promotes the optimum growth and development of another human being. It is important to state as a preface to this diagnosis that adjustment to parenting in general is a normal maturational process that elicits nursing behaviors of prevention of potential problems and health promotion.[28] Parenting behaviors include both physical and emotional aspects, such as love, protection, interaction, giving of self, and enjoyment of the child. The emotional quality in parenting enables the child to grow and develop into a physically and emotionally healthy individual.[33]

This nursing diagnosis was approved by the Third and Fourth National Conferences on the Classification of Nursing Diagnoses. The group recommended at that time that it be developed further and actual parenting alteration be differentiated from potential. Further research is still needed to identify critical data.[28] The etiologies of alteration in actual and potential parenting are discussed together because overlap is obvious. The defining characteristics, nursing care, and evaluation sections are presented separately to further define specific characteristics, interventions, and evaluation for each.

THEORY AND ETIOLOGY

Infancy to Preschool

Many factors affect the ability to effectively parent a child. Initially, labor and delivery may stand out in the parents' minds as a measurement of early success or failure in the parenting role. If the birth process was a positive experience for the mother, the potential is there for increased self-esteem.[34] A negative birth experience may decrease confidence in the parenting role. For example, a painful or difficult delivery might interfere with the mother's immediate visual contact with her infant or with her feelings for him.

The complexity of maternal-infant attachment has been recognized in recent years.[26] Cropley states that, at the same time the mother is getting acquainted with her infant, she is concerned with the infant's acceptance of her.[26] Positive responses from the infant can foster maternal bonding. An in-depth review of maternal attachment and bonding is presented in Johnson[26] and Klaus and Kennell.[29]

The lack of an available or effective role model can also influence an individual's ability to learn acceptable parenting skills. Katz[27] states that individuals are the result of their parents' upbringing. The Bernhardts[3] state that attitudes, moral standards, manners, ways of thinking, and patterns of behavior are absorbed by the child from his or her social environment. Thus the individual integrates a concept about parenting primarily from those behaviors learned from parents. If the parent role model is unavailable or ineffective, the individual may have difficulty being an effective parent himself.

1913

Klaus and Kennell[29] suggest major influences on parental behavior such as the following:

1. Parent's care by his or her own mother
2. Endowment or genetics of parents
3. Practices of the culture
4. Relationships within the family
5. Experiences with previous pregnancies
6. Planning, course, and events during pregnancy

Unrealistic expectations for self, infant, or partner also interfere with the ability to effectively parent. For example, a new parent who desires to be perfect is being unrealistic and may be setting himself up for failure.

Child abuse can be divided into the categories of physical and emotional abuse. Physical abuse has been discussed in depth in recent years.[26,33] Parents who abuse their children are often unaware that children develop slowly over time and thus may have unrealistic expectations of the child's abilities.[26]

The presence of outside stressors, such as a new family location, lack of supportive persons, and a financial or legal crisis, impinge on the individual's ability to effectively parent in high-risk situations.[26,33] The type and degree of problems seem to be related to several common variables. These include the family's coping abilities in crises, health problems, other stress situations, and quality of interaction.

After initial parenting behaviors are learned, the continued success of the individual in the parent role depends on multiple factors. Absence or loss of the other parent or support person affects the emotional stability and responsibilities of the remaining parent. Any new family crisis or health problem may complicate or interfere with the coping mechanisms that were effective prior to the crisis. Self-concept disturbances related to job or financial problems also have an impact.

Individuals become parents on the birth of an infant. Yet few are prepared for the constant, exhausting and time-consuming role. The change of roles or taking on of new roles may produce anxiety and temporarily cause disequilibrium within the family system. The effect of this change varies according to the individual's ability to adapt, communicate, and use coping mechanisms effectively.

Roles in parenting are culturally defined. In the nineteenth to midtwentieth century the father was recognized as more than an economic provider and strict disciplinarian. Fathers began participating in caretaking after simultaneous social forces combined to change their role. Lynn[31] lists these as democratization, industrialization, the feminist movement, and immigration. Sons ceased to follow in the occupation of their father and began considering upward mobility.[31] Fathers began to participate in the intimate life of the family because they had more leisure time.[3]

When father and mother are in partnership, they can mutually help and support each other in the parenting role. In addition, the father can be an understanding friend and guide for his children, an interesting, entertaining member of a group, and an example of adult adjustment. An added benefit is that fathers are finding deep satisfaction in their role.[3]

Several factors stimulate parents to want to care for their infant. Some of the factors are parent initiated, such as seeing their infant as a duplication of themselves. Some of the factors are infant produced and are called care-eliciting behaviors.[26] The infant responds to the care given to him by quieting, feeding or sucking, and smiling. These behaviors encourage the parent to continue to satisfy his needs. If this positive reciprocal interaction does not occur, both infant and parent suffer.

Not only the mother but also the father is affected by the infant's care-eliciting behaviors: "If the infant does not respond to the father's caregiving tasks, or if the father is unaware of the infant's positive responses, the father will begin to experience feelings of inadequacy and failure."[26]

Distinguishing actual from potential parenting alterations presents some difficulties. Johnson states[26]:

Certain risk problems may actually cause other risk situations. For example, premature birth has shown to be associated to later child abuse. Families in which one of the parents is alcoholic are more likely to end in divorce than non-drinking families and therefore more likely to have a single parenthood problem. A high-risk fetal situation frequently leads to a premature birth or an infant with a congenital anomaly. Adolescent pregnancy and single parenthood frequently occur together. The nurse identifies signs of the initial risk situation so that she can help reduce the initial problem, prevent family difficulties and therefore prevent any resulting risk situations.

Except in cases of obvious physical or emotional abuse, the nurse's assessment must show multiple or repeated maladaptive parenting behaviors before the nursing diagnosis of actual alterations in parenting is validated.

Mercer[33] states:

Immature parents have difficulty placing the needs of another person before their own, or in considering options from the viewpoint of another person, or in giving to a demanding infant while postponing their own desires. . . . If parents experience a crisis involving loss, their grief presents the barrier of separation to early acquaintance and attachment. During the initial phase of grief, when parents are experiencing shock, they are unable to respond to their infant except in a mechanical manner.

Johnson[26] points out that "too much or too forceful discipline occurs in some families such as the abusive family. Extremely forceful discipline that harms the child becomes a problem in itself for the abusive family." Chronic fatigue caused by an irritable infant can be a cause of this.

Alcoholic parents demonstrate complex parenting problems. Almost all children from alcoholic homes show ill effects.[44] These children are not only at greater risk of becoming alcoholics themselves but are also at greater risk for both physical and emotional neglect and abuse. Alcoholic parents have difficulty maintaining a relationship with their child because of inconsistencies in their behavior related to alcohol consumption. Often, when the child looks for recognition for a job well done in school or at home, the parent is unable to give it. Thus the child's self-esteem suffers and development can be hindered. The child may actually learn to parent the adult in an effort to cope.

Each of these variables indicates that the nurse has a critical role in helping families recognize and deal constructively with stressful situations and therefore prevent risk situations.

How does one become a successful parent? Katz[27] states that knowledge of the child's emotional development is the parent's greatest asset. The mere fact of becoming a mother or father does not call forth natural instincts that give the parent knowledge of the child's feelings. Katz stresses that one must learn how to become a successful parent.

Gordon[21] describes the amazing transformation from "persons" to "parents" when an infant is born. Parents may forget they are still humans with human faults, personal limitations, and real feelings. Forgetting one's humanness is the first serious mistake one can make on entering parenthood. An effective parent lets himself be a person. Children deeply appreciate this quality of realness and humanness in their parents.

Gordon also discusses the power of the language of acceptance. He says that when a person is able to feel and communicate genuine acceptance of another, he possesses a capacity for being a powerful helping agent for the other. This acceptance for the other—his child—as he is fosters a relationship in which the child can grow, develop, make constructive changes, learn to solve problems, move in the direction of psychologic health, become more productive and creative, and actualize his fullest potential.[21] Unfortunately, Katz[27] points out, most parents rely heavily on the language of unacceptance in rearing children, believing this is the best way to help them.

The Bernhardts[3] state that successful parenting is a real challenge, does not just happen, and requires effort, study, and a number of attitudes and personality traits that can be cultivated. He lists love, patience, clear objectives, intelligence, skill, and knowledge as components of successful parenting.

Honig[25] asks: What particular parenting practices promote the optimal development of children? She refers to hundreds of research studies to suggest that specific kinds and qualities of family functioning, teaching techniques,

and rearing conditions have differential effects. Among those cited are Ainsworth's studies.[1] The "strange situation" technique is used to assess the security of attachment of infants to mothers by coding behaviors after the mother leaves the infant alone with a stranger several times and then rejoins the baby. Ainsworth found that babies whose mothers have been sensitive to their signals of distress, have ministered promptly and capably to their needs, and have given them freedom to explore the home environment scored higher on developmental tests at the end of the first year of life. These babies communicated with the mother using coos, tugs, and smiles instead of crying. The courage to explore was found to be related to nurturant mothering. Babies whose mothers were fairly insensitive to infant needs for care and comfort and delayed meeting these needs promptly cried more in the last quarter of the first year of life and were more irritable. Ainsworth[1] concluded that these babies had not learned to trust that comfort was consistently given or available from their mother.

Secure attachment early in a baby's life has been positively related to child compliance and cooperativeness in the toddler years. Honig includes other studies that reinforce the finding that children who are self-reliant, confident, curious, and exploring were securely attached to tender, responsive mothers. Children who in infancy had avoided or resisted maternal comforting at their reunion with their mother were described as either overcontrolled or undercontrolled.[25]

School Age

Certain parenting styles have been found to characterize those children who are good learners and good friends in school. Baumrind[1b] concluded that there are three main types of parenting styles: authoritative, authoritarian, and permissive. *Authoritative* parents set firm rules, use reason and explanation when directing the child, encourage competence, and exhibit personal warmth, concern for, and interest in the child. Children of authoritative parents were more responsible, active, successful in schoolwork, and popular with peers. In contrast, *authoritarian* parents were more dominating and punitive and had unrealistically high or low standards. *Permissive* parents were lax and exhibited little control. Both authoritarian and permissive parenting practices were found to shield the child from the opportunity to engage in vigorous interaction with people.

Swan and Stavros[43b] studied highly motivated, achieving kindergarten children from black, low-income families. These parents reported a strong positive enjoyment of their children. They frequently read to their children, engaged in animated dinner conversations, and respected the abilities and unique interests of each child. These parents felt comfortable and competent in child rearing.

In contrast, Carew's studies[10b] found that ineffective children tended to come from families with high permissiveness and the use of physical harshness to discipline. These parents had sometimes arbitrary rules and enforcements and often denigrated or ignored their children's needs.

Honig[25] provides a model, based on the previously cited theory and research, which integrates six areas of parenting patterns to help parents develop children to be altruistic, prosocial people.

1. *Infants need dominion over a caregiver's body.* Infants and young children need skin contact from their parents to enhance closeness.[9,29] Kaplan[26a] concluded that physical assurances of love allow toddlers to become more comfortable about separating from adults when inner urges for growth lead to adventures of creeping and toddling and pattering into the world. Then the young child will find it easier to venture into the wider world of neighborhood and school. Body-loving promotes secure attachment that fuels courage to be curious, to explore, and to concentrate.

2. *Families need to be responsive to child signals.* It is difficult for adults unaccustomed to the ways of small creatures and busy with adult occupations and preoccupations to be sensitive to children's needs, unless the adults become fine-tuned noticers. A downcast face, sagging shoulders, tense grinding teeth, fearful eyes, angry fists, restless wanderings are signs for families that all is not well. Honig suggests that adults who are responsive in appropriate ways to child signals of joy and distress teach the child a model of caring concern. Altruism and compassion for those in distress take shape early in the behaviors of toddlers whose families model empathetic caring and courtesies coupled with strong disapproval if the child ever hurts others.

3. *Families need to cultivate authoritative parenting styles.* High expectations for achievement, firm household rules, and clear reasons for those rules coupled with sincere interest and attention to the child as a person nourish competence and altruism in children. Musson and Eisenberg-Berg[35a] found that altruists are likely to be children of nurturant parents who are good models of prosocial behaviors, use reasoning in discipline, maintain high standards, and encourage their children to accept responsibility for others early.

4. *Mastery of language gives a child the power to succeed in learning and communicating in school.* Families who talk with, listen to, sing with, and respond verbally to children are promoting the power of language. Honig and Wittmer[25a] found that posing Socratic, open-ended questions and choice questions allows children to reason and think about their ideas as they respond to adults. Honig further stated that reading to children promotes intellectual competence. Carew[10a] found that rich provision of early language mastery experiences is the single variable most frequently found correlated with later cognitive ability on developmental tests.

5. *Families need to arrange learning experiences that allow children to engage in, struggle with, persist at, and master both socialization tasks and intellectual tasks.* Parents should challenge but not overwhelm the child with demands beyond present capabilities nor shame the child for clumsy tries. Honig found that encouragement which matches family requirements to the ever-developing potential of the child will ensure competent rather than discouraged children. Psychologic space is needed to allow for early tries and failures and bumps that occur while trying to master knowledge and skills.

6. *Families need to feel crazy about their kids!* As children feel loved, delighted in, admired for their being, okay as they are, they feel the courage to use life energies to grow, to explore, to learn, and to cope with their lives.

Ginott[18] identifies parents' goals in relation to children and suggested methods of achieving those goals. He discussed 10 areas in which parent and child interact and can either successfully develop their relationship, foster child development, and effectively solve problems or fail to communicate, become frustrated, and hinder development of the parent-child relationship and the child's self-esteem. His findings are based on 15 years of work with children and parents in individual and group guidance and psychotherapy.

Conversing with children is ''a unique art with rules and meanings of its own. . . . Children are rarely naive in their communications and their messages are often in a code that requires deciphering.''[18] Children often resist dialogues with parents because they resent being preached to, talked at, and criticized. Children feel that parents talk too much. To reach children and reduce parental frustration, a new code of communication, based on respect and skill, is called for. It requires that messages preserve the child's as well as the parents' self-respect and that statements of understanding *precede* statements of advice or instruction. When a child is in the midst of strong emotions, he cannot listen to anyone. The child cannot accept advice or consolation or constructive criticism, and he wants parents to understand him.

Children also love and resent their parents at the same time, just as they do all persons who have authority over them. Parents find it difficult to accept ambivalence as a fact of life. Ginott suggests emotional education to help children to know what they feel. It is more important for a child to know what he feels than why he feels it. The parent should serve as an emotional mirror to reflect feelings as they are without distortion. For example, if the child is screaming at and calling a brother names, the parent can start by saying, ''It looks as though you are very angry.'' Showing the child clearly what the feelings are provides an opportunity for self-initiated grooming and change.

Praises should deal not with the child's personality and attributes but with efforts and achievements. Comments should be "phrased so that the child draws from them positive inferences about his personality."[18] Praise has two parts: our words and the child's inferences. The words should clearly state that the child's effort, work, achievement, help, consideration, or creation is appreciated. From these words the child pictures a positive image of himself, one of the building blocks of mental health.

Criticism, on the other hand, can be destructive because it may cause the child to lose confidence in abilities. Constructive criticism confines itself to pointing out how to do what has to be done, entirely omitting negative remarks about the personality of the child. The problem, however, is that a parent becomes angry and is not always able to deal with the anger appropriately. Ginott suggests three ways to deal with anger: (1) accept the fact that children will make us angry; (2) a parent is entitled to anger without guilt or shame; (3) a parent is entitled to express feelings provided the parent does not attack the child's personality or character. For example, a parent can say, "I feel very, very angry when you hit your brother." This allows a parent to vent anger without causing the child emotional damage.

Self-defeating patterns include threats, bribes, promises, sarcasm, sermons on lying and stealing, and rude teaching about politeness. Threats are invitations to misbehavior because they challenge the child's autonomy. Bribes may spur the child toward an immediate goal but seldom, if ever, inspire him toward continued efforts. Promises should neither be made to, nor demanded of, children. Trust should be the basis of a parent's relationship with a child. Sarcasm simply serves as a barrier to effective communication. Children sometimes lie because they are not allowed to tell the truth about their feelings, be they positive, negative, or ambivalent. Last, a parent often points out to the child in front of other people that he has forgotten to be polite: "You didn't say thank you." This response itself is impolite.

"Responsibility cannot be imposed. It can only grow from within, and be fed and directed by values absorbed at home and in the community."[18] Responsibility in children starts with the attitude and skills of the parent. Attitudes include a willingness to allow children to feel all their feelings, and the skills include an ability to demonstrate to children acceptable ways of coping with feelings. There are three ways for a parent to initiate favorable changes in the child. First, listen with sensitivity. Children experience frustration and resentment when parents seem uninterested in their feelings and thoughts. They feel their ideas are stupid or unworthy. Second, a parent should consciously avoid words and comments that create hate and resentment. Third, state

feelings and thoughts without attacking. A sympathetic atmosphere draws the child nearer to the parents and the attitudes of fairness, consideration, and civility are noticed and emulated. Then the child is willing to be involved in learning how to do jobs that will help shape responsibility at different levels of maturity.

The new approach to *discipline* is the distinction between wishes and acts. Limits are set on acts, but wishes are not restricted. Each part has to be handled differently. Feelings have to be identified and expressed; acts may have to be limited and redirected. Ginott stresses that a limit should be stated so that it tells the child clearly what constitutes unacceptable conduct and what substitute will be accepted, when the parent makes the feelings about a restriction crystal clear and the restriction is phrased in inoffensive language. Ginott finds that the child will usually conform. If a limit is violated, the parent should not become argumentive and verbose. The parent should reinforce the rule and state his feelings about the violation. For more discussion on discipline, refer to Gordon[21] and the Bernhardts.[3]

A parent must say no to many of the small child's greatest pleasures. Ginott reinforces the importance of parents not overplaying the role of "policemen for civilization" or the child may become resentful and hostile. Routines such as getting up in the morning, getting dressed, going to school, eating breakfast, bedtime, and television viewing all need some guidelines, but overmoralizing or overcontrolling behaviors or verbalizations by parents produce resentment by the child.

"In contrast to their parents, children do not question the existence of *jealousy* in the family. They have long known its meaning and impact."[18] Ginott suggests parents resist the temptation to explain the situation or defend their position about the fairness or unfairness of decisions. Rather, spend time with each child individually to give undivided attention and make those moments memorable.

Ginott discusses several *sources of anxiety* in children, including fear of abandonment, guilt, denial of autonomy and status, friction between parents, interference with physical activity, and death.

A child should never be threatened with abandonment. Unnecessary guilt should be prevented by dealing with children's transgressions in a positive manner. Parental support and sympathy lead to greater intimacy between parent and child when new tasks are tried by the child and either success or failure results.

Ginott stresses that when parents fight, children feel anxious and guilty: anxious because their home is threatened, and guilty because of their actual or imagined role in the family friction. The child sides with either mother or father and the consequences are harmful to the child's psychosexual and character development.

Lack of space for muscle activity creates anxiety in the child. Young children need to release their tension in physical activity and materials for play.

Death is a mystery to young children. A child should be given honest, simple answers to questions about death. A child should not be deprived of his right to grieve and mourn.

Sex education starts with the parents' own attitudes toward their sensuality. Whatever the parents' unspoken feelings are, they will be conveyed to the children. From birth on, infants are equipped to feel body pleasures, and sex attitudes are in the process of forming. The organs of sex and eliminating are so close to each other that attitudes acquired in toilet training are likely to have an effect on sexual development. Masturbation also occurs at this age of development. The parents should so involve the child with their love, affection, and interest in the outside world that self-gratification will not remain the child's only means of satisfaction.

Ginott states that *identification* is the crucial process whereby boys become men and girls women. Identification is facilitated when parental relationships with children are based on respect and love.

Adolescence

Ginott[19] describes adolescence as a time of turmoil and turbulence, of stress and storm. Rebellion against authority and against convention is to be expected and tolerated for the sake of learning and growth. Ginott stresses that parents can help by tolerating the restlessness, respecting the loneliness, and accepting the discontent. Silent love and being available for the adolescent to come to are Ginott's recommendations because adolescents are preoccupied with existential questions and the search for identity. It is important to differentiate between acceptance and approval: unpleasant behavior is tolerated, but it is neither encouraged or welcomed.

Gordon[21] states that, as a young person moves into adolescence, he will dismiss his parents, write them off, and sever his relationship with them because many parents try to change their children's cherished beliefs and values. Adolescents dismiss their parents when they feel they are being denied basic rights. A parent is effective if he demonstrates continuous modeling by living his values. Sharing ideas, knowledge, and experience guides the adolescent without preaching and imposing on him. If this approach is not taken by a parent, the adolescent discharges or "fires" the parent.

From the theoretical discussion, support is lent to the following etiologies of potential or actual alterations in parenting by the work of Carpenito[11] and Kim, McFarland, and McLane[28]:

Lack of available role model
Ineffective role model

Physical abuse of nurturing figure
Psychosocial abuse of nurturing figure
Lack of support from significant other(s)
Unmet social maturation needs of parenting figures
Unmet emotional maturation needs of parenting figures
Interruption in bonding process (maternal, paternal, other)
Perceived threat to own survival (physical or emotional)
Mental or physical illness
Presence of stress (such as financial or legal problems)
Family relocation
Change in family unit
Lack of knowledge
Limited cognitive functioning
Lack of role identity
Lack of appropriate response of child to relationship
Multiple pregnancies
Unrealistic expectations for self, infant, partner
Alcoholism
Cultural practices
Absence of infant care behaviors
Chronic fatigue
Congenital anomaly
Prematurity
Inability to show humanness as a parent
Absence of acceptance
Inability to show love
Inability to set clear objectives
Extreme authoritarianism
Extreme permissiveness
Lack of respect for child/adolescent
Lack of responsiveness to infant/child/adolescent
Depression
Inability to facilitate learning for child
Lack of psychologic space
Ineffective communication skills
Negative self-concept
Inappropriate release of anger
Lack of trust
Frequent family conflict

Potential Alteration in Parenting
DEFINING CHARACTERISTICS

Infancy to Preschool
Lack of parental attachment behaviors*:
  Inappropriate visual, tactile, auditory stimulation
  Negative identification of characteristics of infant/child
  Negative attachment of meanings to characteristics of infant/child

*Critical defining characteristic.

Constant verbalization of disappointment in gender or physical characteristics of infant/child.
Verbalization of resentment toward infant/child.
Verbalization of role inadequacy.
Disgust at body functions of infant/child.
Does not ask to hold, talk to, or ask questions about infant.
Affect sad, angry, or without expression.
Does not hold infant to neck or face.
Does not spontaneously rock, stroke, or kiss infant.
Absence of eye-to-eye contact.
Visits or calls hospitalized infant less than every other day.
Noncompliance with health appointments for self and/or infant/child.
Frequent accidents.
Frequent illness.
History of child abuse or abandonment by primary caretaker.
Verbalizes desire to have child call parent by first name despite traditional cultural tendencies.
Care provided by multiple caretakers without consideration for the needs of the child.
Compulsive seeking of role approval from others.

School Age

Demonstrates extreme authoritarian or permissive parenting style.
Demonstrates arbitrary rules and enforcements.
Provides poor model of prosocial behavior.
Demonstrates lack of respect in conversing with child.
Expresses anger inappropriately; attacks child's personality or character.
Self-defeating patterns (bribes, sarcasm).

Adolescence

Refuses to accept adolescence as developmental stage.
Unable to give "silent love."
Hassles, harangues adolescent.
Unable to demonstrate verbalized values.
Dictates adolescent's life.

Parenting behaviors are assessed during different developmental stages—at the time of delivery, at 1 week, at several months or years, or during adolescence. Finely tuned assessment skills are necessary to identify critical factors appropriate for each developmental stage. Valid assessments can be made only after more than one or two parent-infant interactions.[11,28]

NURSING INTERVENTIONS

Patient Goal	Nursing Intervention

Infancy to Preschool

Patient Goal	Nursing Intervention
Maintain satisfactory/adequate parenting role.	Listen attentively.
	Sit down, talk with parent.
	Validate, offer feedback.
	Provide nonthreatening environment.
	Encourage role-playing.
	Assist with identification of strengths, weaknesses, resources.
	Identify disturbing topics.
	Observe nonverbal communication.
	Provide reality orientation.
	Assist with value clarification.
	Provide positive reinforcement for adequate parenting behaviors.
	Foster self-esteem and a positive self-concept.
	Observe contact behaviors.
	Assess affect.
	Demonstrate/assist with chosen feeding method.
	Touch, share concerns.
	Point out root and suck reflexes.
	Answer questions.
	Provide consistent nurse for mother and baby.
	Promote trust relationship.
	Provide father or significant other with opportunities to feed infant.
	Avoid gender-specific behavior.
	Set goals with patient for infant care.
	Assist with feeding.
	Provide information and teaching needs, such as what to expect from the infant, reflexes, feeding, infant care, role change, time management after discharge, rest and nutrition needs for self and infant.
	Encourage individual responsibility for amount of time spent with infant (open visitation).
	Assess family structure and roles and support system.
	Discuss concerns regarding new parenting role.
	Teach stress-reduction techniques.

Patient Goal	Nursing Intervention
	Demonstrate and observe parents' bathing, shampoo, cord care, diapering, handling, positioning infant in crib.
	Teach recognition of infant illness.
	Discuss need for rest.
	Prepare for feeling of disorganization first month at home.
	Refer to appropriate resources, such as the Public Health Nurse or Social Services.
	Assess self-confidence in patients' parenting role.
	Teach to be sensitive to signals of distress.
	Explain importance of skin contact (closeness, touching, cuddling).
	Teach to talk, listen, sing with, and respond verbally to infant/child.
	Provide space for gross motor activity.

School Age

Patient Goal	Nursing Intervention
Maintain satisfactory/adequate parenting role.	Review developmental stage of child.
	Encourage reading and learning about emotional development of children.
	Explain importance of seeing self as a real person with real feelings.
	Encourage positive enjoyment of child.
	Explain importance of reading to and responding to child verbally.
	Explain importance of challenging but not overwhelming child.
	Explain importance of psychologic space for early tries and failures.
	Encourage parent to serve as an emotional mirror to reflect feelings of child.
	Explain importance of conversing with child based on respect and skill at deciphering hidden messages.
	Explain importance of praising efforts and achievements.
	Explain use of constructive rather than destructive criticism.
	Reinforce fact that verbally expressing anger is acceptable as long as it does not attack child's personality or character.
	Explain importance of avoiding self-defeating patterns (threats, bribes, promises, sarcasm, sermons).
	Explain importance of trust as the basis of parent-child relationship.
	Teach to listen with sensitivity to feelings and thoughts.
	Explain importance of avoiding words that create hate and resentment.
	Explain importance of role-modeling, consideration, and civility.
	Explain importance of some flexibility in daily routines.
	Teach importance of not using abandonment as stimulus to get cooperation.
	Explain importance of support and sympathy.
	Encourage parents to respect own and each other's sexual roles.
	Explain authoritative parenting: sets firm rules, uses reason and explanation when directing child versus authoritarian and permissive parenting.
	Discuss discipline techniques: consistency, firm but fair rules, and consequences.
	Encourage attendance at parenting classes and groups.
	Discuss importance of mutual respect between parent and child.
	Assess ability to balance independence and limit-setting for child.
	Encourage need for close contact despite age of child.
	Teach about play and toys that are appropriate for age.
	Discuss necessity and ability to provide food, comfort, closeness appropriate for age of child.

Adolescence

Patient Goal	Nursing Intervention
Maintain satisfactory/adequate parenting role.	Review developmental stage of adolescence.
	Reinforce adolescence as stage of turmoil, turbulence, stress, and storm.
	Teach parent to expect and learn to tolerate rebellion.
	Explain importance of silent love.
	Teach ways to differentiate between acceptance and approval.
	Avoid hassling to change beliefs and values.
	Encourage parents to continuously model by living those values.
	Explain importance of sharing ideas, knowledge, and experience open endedly.

To work with parents, the nurse must first convey a genuine concern for each individual in the new family. The establishment of a trust relationship is necessary before learning can occur. Many new parents are fearful, unsure of what their role and responsibilities are, and have expectations of themselves in that role.

The birth of a normal, healthy baby after a planned pregnancy and successful labor and delivery helps begin the process of parenting. However, frequently the pregnancy is not planned, the labor and delivery do not meet the expectations of the individuals, or the infant has some problem. Even a slight problem may augment fears that the parents had up to this point. The parents are vulnerable and need careful attention. It is important to prevent threat to the parents' self-image. This includes generating anxiety associated with inability to meet one's own or one's spouse's expectations in the parenting role or feelings of failure if the infant does not meet the parents' expectations.

To foster the "taking in role," as described by Rubin,[39] parents must be given responsibility for their infant. This means that within minutes after delivery the parents must have the opportunity to unwrap, touch, hold, and feed their infant. This maternal sensitive and paternal engrossment period, described by Klaus and Kennell,[29] facilitates instinctive cues and begins the attachment process. Mercer[34] acknowledges that "early interaction [with the infant] serves as an immediate reward, providing the woman with relief and joy."

The nurse must make every effort to point out the positive aspects of the infant and answer questions during this time. Johnson[26] points out that "in progressive institutions, both parents and children are being included as essential members of the treatment team, since it is apparent that their involvement in the plan directly influences the outcome." Thus providing closeness at birth, as well as later in the child's life, facilitates nurturing. In the infant the attachment process is stimulated. This is a reciprocal process between parent and infant.

Once the initial contact has been made between parents and infant, identification with and claiming of the infant can begin. Again, it is the responsibility of the nurse to provide consistent care, such as mother-baby care, a system in which one nurse per shift takes care of the mother *and* the baby through the postpartum hospitalization, to promote trust. Likewise it is important to provide accurate information to the parents about the infant, assess parenting problems, or deal with potential problems when teaching the parents what to expect from their infant.

Ideally, this is begun in prenatal classes when the parents' image of the anticipated infant is forming. Pointing out that infants focus on and respond to the human face and voice within the first week of life makes the parents aware of the need for sensory and auditory stimulation. The infant has basic needs: food, air, water, elimination, comfort, closeness, and safety. Positive feeding experiences provide the basis for reciprocal satisfaction of needs for parent and infant. For example, parents need to be told that the infant's cry can be irritating, but it is a communication of need. Ongoing reinforcement of positive parenting behaviors provides the mechanism for support and helps ensure continued mutually satisfying experiences for parent and infant.

The caretaking role is usually thought of as the primary parenting role. Demonstration of bathing, hair washing, cord care, diapering, handling, and positioning the infant in a crib is best accomplished in a nonthreatening environment. New parents feel insecure and often frightened at the thought of providing this care on the first or second postpartum day. Asking the parents to participate in the care, to the extent that they desire, in a supportive manner inspires confidence. Reinforcement on subsequent days provides them with a chance to develop the parenting skills they may have been most frightened of. Fathers and other significant persons in the family system need special encouragement to learn these skills. Validation with the parents and praise prior to discharge from the hospital reinforce their successful achievement of parenting goals. This interaction facilitates a supportive environment for maintaining the health of the infant.

EVALUATION

Patient Outcome	Data Indicating That Outcome is Reached
Positive feelings about own parenting role	Identifies strengths and weaknesses in own parenting; focuses on strengths. Communicates concerns clearly. Shares troublesome memories from own childhood parenting experience. Verbalizes desire to learn more about parenting role. Verbalizes knowledge of developmental stage. *Infancy:* Reviews the birth experience. Ventilates concerns regarding individual performance during labor and delivery. *School age:* Verbalizes feelings of self-worth. Identifies supports.

Patient Outcome	Data Indicating That Outcome is Reached
	Adolescence: Verbalizes any frustration over turmoil/stress in dealing with ups and downs of adolescent. Identifies solutions for and approaches to frustration.
Constructive interpersonal relationship with offspring	*Infancy:* Demonstrates en face position. Fingertip touches infant's face and body. Proceeds to finger and palm touch. Expresses joy or other appropriate emotions. Verbalizes desire to breastfeed. Demonstrates positive attitude toward the child. Brings infant to own neck and face. Talks to infant. Asks questions about infant. Makes positive statements about infant. Verbalizes knowledge of and preferred method of feeding infant. Demonstrates comfortable positions for feeding. Verbalizes knowledge of root and suck reflexes. Verbalizes feelings of adequacy during feeding. Asks questions about frequency and amount of feeding. Verbalizes knowledge of sleep/wake cycles. Exhibits eye-to-eye contact. Verbalizes knowledge that infant's burp, falling asleep, and relaxation in arms after feeding indicates satisfying experience. Demonstrates ability to comfort infant during or after feeding. Verbalizes preparations for infant homecoming and necessary supplies. Identifies roles in family. Discusses taking on of new role(s) in family. Verbalizes feelings of role adequacy. Verbalizes coping mechanisms for stress. Calls physician if infant shows signs of illness. Verbalizes knowledge and demonstrates ability to bathe, shampoo, provide cord care, diaper, handle, and position infant in crib. Verbalizes need to nap when infant sleeps during first month. Expresses satisfaction with infant or acceptance of infant's limitations. Verbalizes ability to assume new or modified roles in family system. Provides food, comfort, closeness for child. Child receives care from one or two primary caretakers. *School age:* Verbalizes knowledge of developmental stage. Verbalizes feelings of self-worth. Identifies supports. Demonstrates authoritative parenting style. Demonstrates humanness. Verbalizes positive enjoyment of child. Responds to child appropriately. Reads to child at least every other day. Challenges but does not overwhelm child. Allows psychologic space. Verbalizes comfort and mutual respect in conversing with child. Praises child's efforts and achievements. Demonstrates constructive criticism. Verbalizes anger and frustration appropriately. Demonstrates trust in parent-child relationship. *Adolescence:* Verbalizes any frustration over turmoil or stress in dealing with ups and downs of adolescent. Identifies solutions for and approaches to frustration. Differentiates between acceptance and approval. Avoids hassling to change beliefs and values. Demonstrates values cited in own life. Shares ideas in "consultant" manner.

Actual Alteration in Parenting
DEFINING CHARACTERISTICS

Infancy to Preschool
Abandonment*
Runaway
Cannot control child*
Evidence of physical trauma*
Evidence of psychologic trauma*
Does not assume en face position despite encouragement
Refuses to hold infant
When infant placed in arms, muscles become tense; does not touch infant; looks away
Repeated negative comments about infant*
Predominant affect sad, angry, expressionless
Conflicting attitudes
Inconsistent behaviors
Insists infant has a defect or problem, when none is present*
Distorted perceptions of childrearing
Absence of reciprocal behaviors between parent and infant
Father and child show signs of frustration and emotional distress
Predominance of own needs
Does not talk to infant
Does not want to feed infant at delivery
Inappropriate caretaking behaviors (toilet training, sleep, rest, feeding)
Inappropriate or inconsistent discipline practices
Growth and development lag

---

*Critical defining characteristics.

Child receives care from multiple caretakers without consideration for his needs
Inattention to infant/child needs*

School Age
Abandonment*
Runaway
Cannot control child*
Evidence of physical trauma*
Evidence of psychologic trauma*
Verbalizes or demonstrates nonacceptance of child
Absence of response to, reading to, or sincere interest in and attention to child
Denies child psychologic space for early tries and failures
Unable to praise efforts and achievements
Uses destructive rather than constructive criticism
Uses words that create hate and resentment

Adolescence
Abandonment*
Runaway
Cannot control child*
Evidence of physical trauma*
Evidence of psychologic trauma*
Ignores adolescent's feelings, thoughts
Refuses to negotiate with adolescent

Defining characteristics are limited for actual parenting alterations. More research is needed to establish thorough defining characteristics for each age group.[11,26,28,33]

NURSING INTERVENTIONS

Patient Goal	Nursing Intervention
Infancy to Preschool	
Promote adequate parenting behaviors.	Listen attentively.
	Foster trust relationship.
	Encourage verbalization of childhood experiences.
	Encourage discussion of self-concept and self-esteem.
	Reduce anxiety.
	Discuss infant's birth as needed.
	Identify any interruption in attachment process.
	Encourage verbalization of feelings when with infant (sadness, fear, repulsion).
	Point out positive characteristics of infant.
	Discuss goals for attainment of parenting skills.
	Reinforce all positive parenting behaviors.
	Provide ongoing follow-up and support system during first month after discharge.
	Stress importance of improving self-esteem and self-concept.
	Refer to clinical nurse specialist, social worker, or psychologist as needed.
	Encourage attendance at parenting classes and groups.
	Assist parents to become effective problem-solvers.
	Sit down and discuss child's developmental stage, any physical abnormalities or delays, and emotional concerns.
	Collaborate and discuss with physician treatment plans, discharge dates, patient goals, appropriate referrals.
	Set goals with parent for attaining beginning or improved parenting skills.
	Demonstrate appropriate behaviors to meet infant or child's physical and emotional needs.
	Reinforce fact that feelings of guilt, anger, and depression over abnormality are normal and may last 4 to 6 months.

Patient Goal	Nursing Intervention
	Discuss coping mechanisms.
	Assess and foster support social systems.
	Include significant other(s) in modeling behavior.
	Observe behaviors over several days.
	Facilitate learning of reciprocal behaviors for mutual satisfaction.
	Reinforce all positive parenting behaviors.
	Encourage touch, holding, relaxation.
	Provide ongoing follow-up during first month after discharge, and minimally at 3, 6, and 12 months.
	Initiate protective services intervention if maladaptive parenting behaviors observed.
	Encourage stress reduction by appropriate venting of anger.
	Use Brazelton Neonatal Scale to demonstrate infant's capabilities.
	Use Carey Temperament Questionnaire to identify annoying infant behaviors.
School Age Promote adequate parenting behaviors.	Discuss feelings about being a parent. Review developmental stage. Identify stressors in parent-child relationship. Identify activities parent and child engage in and frequency of activities. Identify reasons for nonacceptance of child. Evaluate ability to show sincere interest in and give attention to child. Set goals for improving parenting skills together. Explain authoritative discipline style. Explain importance of using constructive rather than destructive criticism. Explain communication techniques and identify blocks to communication. Evaluate if undercontrolling or overcontrolling child and set goals to improve.
Adolescence Promote adequate parenting behaviors.	Listen attentively. Assist parent to identify conflict or problem. Evaluate parents' knowledge of adolescence. Review developmental stage of adolescence. Examine parents' own experience as adolescents (negative feelings, guilt, anger, role model). Identify parents' goal in their relationship with adolescent. Suggest family counseling to facilitate communication and problem-solving abilities. Discuss authoritative discipline techniques. Identify style of discipline and effectiveness.
Alcoholism Identify and resolve parenting problems resulting from alcoholism.	Refer to appropriate health care and voluntary resources to deal with problem of alcoholism (AA, alcohol treatment programs). Provide accepting environment, trust. Encourage verbalization of fears regarding parenting. Provide support system, such as Alcoholics Anonymous. Reinforce fact that recovery process takes time; set realistic goals. Encourage parent to show love verbally and physically to child. Discuss role-modeling; teach how. Discuss acceptable discipline techniques. Encourage giving praise and recognition to child in large quantities. Provide ongoing follow-up at least monthly to discuss parenting concerns.

Parents who display actual parenting alterations need expert help. Careful identification of the cause of the parenting problem may take several interactions or observation periods. Often, when caring for patients in an acute care setting, there is little time to accomplish the necessary change of behavior. Identification and implementation of a plan of action must be made as soon as possible.

The parents and the nurse need to establish mutual goals to effectively change parenting behaviors. These goals primarily focus first on identification of the cause for maladaptive attachment behaviors. Once a trust relationship is formed, the history of the parent, including childhood experiences with parents and role models, must be discussed. Parents who were abused as children are more prone to abuse their children.[26] The nurse's responsibility in child abuse is to carefully assess any maladaptive parenting behaviors that might seem connected to physical injuries and to report these to the appropriate child protective services department.

Emotional abuse or neglect is more difficult to determine. The child's basic needs are physical care and protection, affection and approval, stimulation and teaching, discipline and control that are consistent and appropriate to the child's age, and opportunity and encouragement to acquire gradual autonomy.[45] If the parent is indifferent, ignores the child, or refuses to give emotional warmth, the child does not grow and develop normally, and emotional needs are not met.

If the unmet social or emotional needs stem from a specific risk situation such as prematurity or congenital anomaly, nursing interventions need to be specific to that problem. "High risk parents and their children are particularly susceptible to problems in their reciprocal behaviors."[26]

Many of these infant problems can cause emotional difficulties for parents. Parental behaviors indicative of grief and mourning, extreme guilt, or depression over having produced such a child may become apparent. These feelings interfere with the parent's ability to respond positively to the infant.

Another problem may be unrealistic expectations of self or child. Providing the parent with knowledge of the developmental stage of the child, realistic expectations, comfort, play, and learning needs will promote the ability to parent effectively. Assessment and discussion of appropriate discipline techniques must also be included. If the parents are either very young or relatively old, their developmental level and self-concept needs must be considered when analyzing solutions.

The child who is cared for by multiple caretakers may not form adequate attachments. Withdrawal or poor self-esteem may be seen in the child. Careful family assessment, including thorough knowledge of child development, is essential.

Parents who are alcoholic need help for themselves as well as their children. Careful attention is required to communicate in a nonthreatening manner with alcoholic parents. They view themselves as dual failures, to themselves as well as to their children. Effective nursing care must be provided. A sensitive, caring approach with mutual goal setting is essential.

EVALUATION

Patient Outcome	Data Indicating That Outcome is Reached
Admission of unmet social or emotional needs	Identifies childhood experiences that affect parenting behaviors. Identifies fears about infant/child/adolescent and self. Reality orientation. Verbalizes need to work to improve parenting skills. *School age:* Acceptance of child. Interest in and attention to child. Authoritative parenting style. Constructive criticism. Effective communication techniques. *Adolescence:* Identifies conflict/problem. Attends family counseling if set as goal for improving parenting ability. Authoritative parenting style. Verbalizes feelings of frustration.
Knowledge of developmental stage and realistic expectations of infant/child/adolescent	Knowledge of risk situation. Knowledge of basic needs of infant/child/adolescent appropriate to developmental stage. Appropriate discipline techniques.
Attachment behaviors to infant/child/adolescent	Assumes en face position. Holds infant in relaxed manner. Constructive comments about infant/child/adolescent. Appropriate affect; able to show sadness if discussing abnormality, but when interacting with infant, shows pleasure, smiles. Expresses concerns about mothering/fathering behaviors. Changes diapers; disgust over body excretions absent. Verbalizes a plan for dealing with inconsistencies.

Patient Outcome	Data Indicating That Outcome is Reached
	Comprehension of any physical defect or abnormality.
	Realistic perceptions of childrearing.
	Ability to deal constructively with stress, feelings of guilt, depression.
	Knowledge of resources, supports.
	Reciprocal behaviors with infant/child.
	Infant/child receives care from one or two primary caretakers.
	Ability to interact and accomplish mutual goal with adolescent.
Admission of parenting problems related to alcoholism	Verbalizes fears and feelings of failure in parenting role.
	Willingness to seek professional help for alcoholism.
	Discusses disease with family and children.
	Mutual goals for improving parenting skills with family.
	Attends Alcoholics Anonymous.
	Recognizes child's/adolescent's need for increased self-worth.
	Verbal and physical expressions of love to child/adolescent.
	Role model to child/adolescent.
	Consistent appropriate discipline for developmental age.
	Praises child's/adolescent's successes.

References

1. Ainsworth, M., Bell, S., and Stayton, P.: Infant-mother attachment and social development: socialization as a product of reciprocal responsiveness to signals. In Richard, M., editor: The integration of a child into the social world, London, 1974, Cambridge University Press.

1a. Anthony, E.J., and Benedek, T.: Parenthood, Boston, 1970, Little, Brown & Co.

1b. Baumrind, D.: Some thoughts about childrearing. In Cohen, S., and Cominskey, T.J., editors: Child development: contemporary perspectives, Itasca, Ill., 1977, F.E. Peacock.

2. Belsky, J.: The interrelation of parenting, spousal interaction and infant competence: a suggestive analysis, Syracuse, N.Y., 1979, ERIC Document Reproduction Service, ED. 168719.

3. Bernhardt, K.S., and Bernhardt, D.K.: Being a parent, Toronto, 1970, University of Toronto Press.

4. Bettelheim, B.: Love is not enough, New York, 1950, The Free Press.

5. Bettelheim, B.: Dialogues with mothers, New York, 1962, The Free Press.

6. Bettelheim, B.: The empty fortress, New York, 1967, The Free Press.

7. Bettelheim, B.: The children of the dream, London, 1969, Collier-MacMillan Ltd.

8. Bossard, J.H.: The sociology of child development, New York, 1954, Harper & Brothers, Publishers.

9. Brazelton, T.B.: Toddlers and parents, New York, 1974, Delacorte Press/Seymour Lawrence.

10. Campbell, C.: Nursing diagnosis and intervention in nursing practice, New York, 1984, John Wiley & Sons, Inc.

10a. Carew, J.V.: Experience and the development of intelligence in young children at home and in day care, Monogr. Soc. Res. Child Dev., Sec. No. 187, p. 45, 1980.

10b. Carew, J.V., Chan, I., and Halfar, C.: Observed intellectual competence and tested intelligence: their roots in the young child's transactions with his environment. In Cohen, S., and Cominskey, T.J., editors: Child development: contemporary perspectives, Itasca, Ill., 1977, F.E. Peacock.

11. Carpenito, L.: Nursing diagnosis: application to clinical practice, Philadelphia, 1983, J.B. Lippincott Co.

12. Chinn, P.: The game of parenthood, J. N.Y. State Nurses Assoc. **13**(4):30-45, 1982.

13. Curry, M.A.: Maternal attachment behavior and mother's self-concept: the effect of early skin-to-skin contact, Nurs. Res. **31**(2):73-77, 1982.

14. Erikson, E.H.: Childhood and society, New York, 1963, W.W. Norton Co.

15. Farrell, M.: Familial factors: a critical dimension of early identification, Syracuse, N.Y., 1978, ERIC Document Reproduction Service, ED. 157636.

16. Gesell, A.: The child from five to ten, New York, 1946, Harper & Brothers, Publishers.

17. Gesell, A.: Studies in child development, New York, 1948, Harper & Brothers, Publishers.

18. Ginott, H.G.: Between parent and child. New York, 1965, The Macmillan Co.

19. Ginott, H.G.: Between parent and teenager, New York, 1969, The Macmillan Co.

20. Gordon, M.: Nursing diagnosis: process and application, New York, 1982, McGraw-Hill Book Co.

21. Gordon, T.: P.E.T.: parent effectiveness training, New York, 1975, New American Library.

22. Graybill, D.: Relationship of maternal child-rearing behaviors to children's self-esteem, J. Psychology **100**:45-47, 1978.

23. Greenberg, S.: Right from the start, Boston, 1978, Houghton-Mifflin Co.

24. Hall, J.E., and Weaver, B.R.: Nursing of families in crisis, Philadelphia, 1974, J.B. Lippincott Co.

25. Honig, A.S.: The gifts of families: caring, courage and competence, Syracuse, N.Y., 1981, ERIC Document Reproduction Service, ED. 208972.

25a. Honig, A.S., and Wittmer, D.S.: Teacher questions and toddler responses, Paper presented at biennial meeting of the International Society for the Study of Behavior Development, Toronto, July, 1981.

26. Johnson, S.H.: High-risk parenting: nursing assessment and strategies for the family at risk, Philadelphia, 1979, J.B. Lippincott Co.

26a. Kaplan, L.J.: Oneness and aloneness: from infant to individual, New York, 1978, Simon & Schuster.

27. Katz, B.: How to be a better parent, New York, 1953, The Ronald Press.

28. Kim, M., McFarland, G., and McLane, A., editors: Pocket guide to nursing diagnoses, St. Louis, 1984, The C.V. Mosby Co.

29. Klaus, M.H., and Kennell, J.H.: Parent-infant bonding, St. Louis, 1982, The C.V. Mosby Co.

30. LaRossa, R., and LaRossa, M.M.: Transition to parenthood, Beverly Hills, Calif., 1981, Sage Publications.

31. Lynn, D.B.: The father: his role in child development, Monterey, Calif., 1974, Brooks/Cole Publishing Co.

32. McGillicuddy-DeLisi, A.V.: Parental beliefs about developmental processes, Human Development 25:192-200, 1982.

33. Mercer, R.T.: Nursing care for parents at risk, Thorofare, N.J., 1977, Charles B. Slack, Inc.

34. Mercer, R.T.: A theoretical framework for studying factors that impact on the maternal role, Nurs. Res. 30(2):73-77, 1981.

35. Mercer, R.T.: Relationship of psychosocial and perinatal variables to perception of childbirth, Nurs. Res. 32(4):202-207, 1983.

35a.Musson, P., and Eisenberg-Berg, N.: The roots of caring, sharing, and helping: the development of prosocial development in children, San Francisco, 1977, W.H. Freeman & Co.

36. Nuttall, E.V., and Nuttall, R.L.: Parent-child relationships and academic motivation, Syracuse, N.Y., 1976, ERIC Document Reproduction Service, ED. 127542.

37. Perry, S.E.: Parents' perceptions of their newborn following structured interactions, Nurs. Res. 32(4):208-212, 1983.

38. Roberts, F.B.: Infant behavior and the transition to parenthood, Nurs. Res. 32(4):213-217, 1983.

39. Rubin, R.: Attainment of the maternal role. Part I. Processes, Nurs. Res. 16(3):237-245, 1967.

40. Rubin, R.: Attainment of the maternal role. Part II. Models and referrants, Nurs. Res. 16(4):342-346, 1967.

41. Segal, J.: The mental health of the child: program reports of the national institute of mental health, Rockville, Md., 1971, National Institute of Mental Health.

42. Siefert, K., and others: Perinatal stress: a study of factors linked to the risk of parenting problems, Health Social Work 18(2):107-121, 1983.

43. Solnit, A.J., and Provence, S.A.: Modern perspectives in child development, New York, 1963, International Universities Press, Inc.

43a.Stayton, D.J., Hogan, R., and Ainsworth, M.D.S.: Infant obedience and maternal behavior: the origins of socialization reconsidered, Child Dev. 42:1057-1069, 1971.

43b.Swan, R.W., and Stavros, H.: Childrearing practices associated with the development of cognitive skills of children in low socioeconomic areas, Early Childhood Development and Care 2:23-28, 1973.

44. Triplett, J.L., and Arbeson, S.W.: Working with children of alcoholics, Pediatr. Nurs. Sept./Oct. 1983, pp. 317-320.

45. Trowell, J.: Emotional abuse of children, Health Visitor 56:252-254, 1983.

46. Ventura, J.N.: Parent coping behaviors, parent functioning and infant temperament characteristics, Nurs. Res. 31(5):269-273, 1982.

47. Wong, D.L., and Whaley, L.F.: Clinical handbook of pediatric nursing, St. Louis, 1981, The C.V. Mosby Co.

FAMILY PROCESS, ALTERATION IN

THEORY AND ETIOLOGY

The family has been most recently described as a "human group with significant emotional bonds, usually living together in the same household."[16] Alterations in family process is the state in which a normally supportive family experiences a stressor that challenges its previously effective functioning ability.[2]

The family is a structural unit or system in which the majority of human beings are born, nurtured, and socialized. Although the nuclear family remains typical, the number of single-parent and alternate life-style family units, including members of the same or opposite sex, is significant. Various sociologists have speculated as to the future of the traditional family in modern society. However, others feel that because belongingness and love needs (see section on Social Isolation) are listed third in Maslow's hierarchy of basic human needs, the family will continue to be an active force. Schuster and Ashburn list the following as functions of the family[19]:

1. Reproduction
2. Socialization (education of the young)
3. Protection and safety
4. Economic security (provision of food and shelter)
5. Conferral of roles
6. Social contact
7. Sexual fulfillment
8. Conferral of status
9. Belongingness, love, and affection
10. Physiologic needs
11. Recreation
12. Religious needs

Duval discusses the functions of the family in terms of developmental tasks.[23] Foley[8] describes these tasks in terms of stages or crises that begin with courtship of a couple and proceed to the disintegration of a family system with the death of the couple:

The fantasy of the engagement period yields to the reality of daily life. The birth of a child changes a dyadic system into a triad, and presents the possibility of alliances and splits in the family. The departure of the last child for school brings about a definitive shift into middle age for a couple. The marriage of a child brings still another period of adjustment and initiates the process of a return to the former dyadic state.

All these transitions can be described as normal or developmental. These tasks are a difficult undertaking, and the family that does not succeed may need professional help. What seems to happen in disturbed families is that several factors cluster at the same time. "A combination of events produce symptomatic behavior in one or more members of a given family."[8]

A well-functioning family is flexible and can shift roles, levels of responsibility, and patterns of interaction as it passes through periods of varying stressful life changes.[20] Even if a well-functioning family is under prolonged or acute stress and a family member shows symptoms of the stress, the unit is able to rebalance itself in such a way that the functions of all family members are restored. Fogarty[7] and Minuchin[17] described the characteristics of a functional family.

1. Homeostatic balance is maintained along with flexibility.

Table 6
Family Therapy Models[5,21]

Model	Normal Family Process	Dysfunctional Family Process

Structural
Minuchin
Montalvo
	Boundaries are firm.
	Family hierarchy has strong parental cohesiveness.
	Family system is flexible in allowing for:
	   Autonomy and interdependence of members
	   Individual growth and system maintenance
	   Continuity
	   Adaptive restructuring in response to change or internal (developmental) and external (environmental) stress
		Symptoms are caused by family structural imbalance:
		   Boundaries unclear
		   Hierarchical arrangement diffused
		   Maladaptive reaction to changes internally and/or externally

Strategic
Haley
Bateson
Jackson
	Family is flexible.
	Family has many behaviors to:
	   Resolve problems
	   Pass through developmental stages
	Rules are clear in regard to the family's governing hierarchy.
		The origin of family problems or symptoms is family's inability to:
		   Problem solve
		   Adjust to life cycle transitions
		   Maintain clear hierarchical rules
		Symptoms are result of inadequate communication and interaction patterns.

Family systems
Bowen
Satir
Whitaker
	Differentiation of self.
	Intellectual/emotional balance.
	High self-esteem.
	Clear, specific, honest communication.
	Family rules are flexible and appropriate.
	Family is linked to society in an open way.
		Functioning impaired by relationships with family of origin:
		   Poor differentiation
		   Anxiety
		   Family projection process
		   Triangulation
		Symptoms are seen in nonverbal messages, as reaction to family's communication dysfunction.

2. The family is able to adapt to external (environmental) and internal (developmental) stress or changes.
3. Levels of authority are not blurred; family hierarchy is fair and clear.
4. Emotional contact is maintained between family members and across generations.
5. Emotional problems are viewed as product of the family as a whole, not blamed entirely on one family member.
6. Overcloseness (fusion-enmeshment) is avoided.
7. Distance (disengagement) is avoided or not used to solve problems.
8. Problems between two family members (spouses, spouse and child, children) are resolved by the two people. A third person is not involved to take sides or become triangulated.
9. Individual differences are encouraged to promote growth.
10. Preservation of a positive emotional climate is encouraged.
11. Children have age-appropriate expectations, responsibility within the family; parents negotiate openly with their children for age-appropriate privileges.

12. Each spouse functions within his or her respective role, and spouses maintain a balance of effective expression, rational thought, caretaking, object orientation, and relationship focus.

Family process, alteration in can be viewed as the lack of one or more of the previously described characteristics. A number of stressors can challenge the family's functioning. Some of the stressors come from within the family structure itself or can be attributed to individual family members' inability to cope within the family unit or from extended, sociocultural events impinging on the family unit or on an individual family member.

Much of the theory about normal and altered family process comes from family therapy models (Table 6).

Another way in which these models can be conceptualized is as follows:

Systems	Structural	Communication-strategic
Bowen	Minuchin	Bateson
Jackson		Haley (communication and power)
Haley		Satir (communication and feeling)
Satir		Jackson (communication and cognition)

Often a theorist borrows certain ideas and builds on one theory to develop another. In some ways the models overlap, but there are distinctions. For the purpose of this discussion, the systems, structural, and communication-strategic models are examined.

Systems Model

The systems model was the first to be developed in terms of family therapy by Bowen in the 1950s. A premise of this therapy and the others is that a family is a homeostatic system. Literally speaking, homeostasis means staying the same. The term refers to the ability to restore steady states after an upset to the balance. In systems theory the term is conceived as a more dynamic and open concept. "It does not operate to restore a previous balance or level of functioning, but is the principle which allows for change and growth within a given system."[8] Homeostasis is not a principle for maintaining the status quo, but for allowing a controlled instability or change within the system.[8] A healthy family can withstand stress and change with it, whereas a dysfunctional family cannot.

In Bowen's family systems theory there are seven interlocking concepts. Three of these concepts—differentiation of self, triangles, and the nuclear family emotional system—are core concepts to the overall characteristics of family systems and are discussed in detail. The other four concepts are elaborations of the central or core family characteristics. These four follow:

1. *Multigenerational transmission process.* A symptom in one family member in one generation has its origin several generations before, although the symptom is presented as a nuclear family problem.
2. *Family projection process.* Anxiety about specific issues is transmitted through the generations. These issues are emotionally powerful. Family members polarize around these issues, taking either the family position or the opposite. Neither position allows for freedom or flexibility of thought. This also refers to the process that labels and assigns characteristics to individual members. The labels may be overpositive (genius) or overnegative (dummy). They are always unrealistic and confusing.
3. *Sibling position.* Sibling rank and birth order and sex help to develop personality characteristics in an individual. This can be a source of conflict to a married couple and to the family unit.
4. *Emotional cutoff.* This is a way in which some families deal with intense, unresolved attachment between children and parents. It can be manifested as emotional isolation or physical distance. This cutoff produces an illusion of having achieved separation from one's parents and can be repeated over generations.

All seven of these concepts refer to the family process that may inhibit or promote an individual family member's ability to disengage from the fusion that binds a person to their family. Bowen purports that the higher the level of differentiation in a person, the higher the level of functioning.

Differentiation of self. Differentiation of self is a concept developed by Bowen to measure human functioning on a continuum from the greatest emotional fusion of self boundaries to the highest degree of differentiation or autonomy[8,21]:

Undifferentiated Self	**Differentiated Self**
Intellect and emotions fused	Intellect and emotions separate
Not adaptable	Adaptable
Inflexible	Flexible
Emotionally dependent on family	Emotionally independent of family
Quickly stressed to dysfunction	Not easily stressed to dysfunction
Unable to recoup from stress; fixed	Can recoup from stress rapidly

This continuum model is important when viewing relationships. In all relationships there is a back-and-forth movement of closeness and then distancing. Relationships cycle through these phases based on stress levels. If the person is undifferentiated, often the relationship stops at the distancing phase and the two people become fixed at an angry standoff. This is because one or the other or both of their intellects and emotions are so fused that they are dominated by the automatic emotional system.

Triangles. This is a key concept in understanding the systems approach to emotional function. Bowen calls the triangle the building block of an emotional system. There are triangles in all families and groups. Triangulation is a natural emotional process that takes place in any significant relationship in which there is difficulty.

The triangle can exist between three people, between two people and a group (such as a religious affiliation), between two people and an issue (such as drinking), or between two people and an object (a house, drugs).[6] The balance is tenuous between two people who are attempting to maintain a comfortable distance so that there is emotional closeness without fusion. One illustration of a family triangle follows:

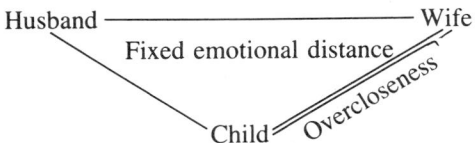

Fogarty states: "All members of a triangle participate equally in perpetuating the triangle and no triangle can persist without the active cooperation of all its members.''[6] Triangles form and reform rapidly and are a daily occurrence. Problems arise when the triangle and a person's position in it become fixed. This is viewed as dysfunctional. Fixed triangles are a way to maintain a homeostatic balance and to avoid stress.[1] However, it causes increased distancing and more stress in the family.

Nuclear family emotional system. This term refers to ''patterns of interaction between individual family members and the degree in which these patterns promote emotional fusion.''[20] Patterns of interaction, or operating principles, are the ways in which an individual behaves in most significant relationships. All marriage relationships reflect a balance of operating principles and reciprocal function.[11] The differences in the operating principles provide an attraction and the balancing stability to the marriage relationship. One spouse becomes the object overfunctioner, and the other the emotional overfunctioner. The difficulty arises when dependence on the attributes of the spouse reduces functional attributes in oneself. Self boundaries become blurred, and this is ego fusion. When the reciprocal functions become fixed positions of overfunction-underfunction, emotional dysfunction and symptoms occur. Emotional fusion is normal. It occurs in all marriages to a greater or lesser extent. If the relationship is unstressed, the reciprocal function works. When stress occurs, each person becomes more like oneself, and to handle personal anxiety he or she may become fixed in personal operating principles, and the relationship can become dysfunctional. Bowen[1] describes three ways in which spouses maintain sufficient emotional distance from each other to handle the anxiety associated with fusion: (1) marital conflict, (2) dysfunction in one spouse, and (3) projection of the problem onto one or more children.

Structural Model

The structural family therapy model has components that are both similar and dissimilar to the systems therapy model. Minuchin[17] was the forerunner in structural family therapy theory. He described three components to this model.

The first component is that the family is a social system in transformation. This means that the family members can grow while the system adapts to internal and external stresses. If the family is unable to adapt to stresses, it becomes dysfunctional.

The second component is that the family undergoes predictable stages of development over time that require adaptive restructuring. As discussed previously, each family has basic developmental tasks it must accomplish to move on and grow. This is similar to Erikson's stages of individual personality development (see section on Social Isolation).

The third component to this model of a viable functioning family relates to the structure of the family. The elements of the structure are power and influence, sets of relationships, and boundaries (individual, sexual, generational). Minuchin states that the structure can become dysfunctional in any or each of the elements. For example, families with extreme boundary problems are described as either enmeshed or disengaged. Enmeshed boundaries are weak; the diffuseness of boundaries inhibits autonomy and competence. Disengaged families have rigid boundaries. Communication is poor between members, and they have a skewed sense of independence. This produces lack of feelings of loyalty and the capacity for interdependence.

Communication-Strategic Model

Communication theory is an offshoot of systems theory. It is the cornerstone to the development of strategic family therapy. Strategic family therapy is a short-term or problem-solving approach to viewing dysfunctional families. ''Communication theorists contend that all behavior, not only verbal productions, is communication, and since there is no such thing as nonbehavior, it is impossible not to communicate.''[22] It is believed that there is a multiplicity of levels of communication between sender and receiver. With the communications model, when a system is dysfunctional in its communication, there is potential for pathology. In families, complex and highly patterned repetitive interactions become established. These interactions can become fixed in an unhealthy way, and then the family becomes dysfunctional.

Within the communications model, as a whole, there are a number of theorists who emphasize specific elements of communication. Jackson's emphasis[14a] is on the cognitive aspects of communication. He believes that what a person thinks influences what he does or says. Haley[12,13] looks at communication in terms of power or control. The family communicates in relation to control issues or the power structure. Satir[18a] is concerned about emotions and feelings in a family system and is considered an experiential theorist. How one individual thinks and who is in control are issues, but she believes that how one feels toward oneself and others in the family system is the main concern.

A family system becomes dysfunctional if the communication within the system is dysfunctional, for example, double messages, behavior incongruent with what is verbalized, inconsistent family roles, continuous skewed negative or positive messages or behaviors, disqualification in communication (self-contradictions, incomplete sentences). The following are etiologies for alteration in family process[2,15]:

Situation transition and/or crises
   Poverty
   Disaster
   Relocation
   Economic crisis
   Change in family roles
   Conflict
   Breech of trust between members
   Social deviance by family member
Development transition and/or crises
   Birth of infant with a defect
   Loss of family member
   Gain of new family member
Pathophysiologic factors
   Illness of family member
      Discomforts related to illness symptoms
      Change in member's ability to function
      Time-consuming treatments
      Disabling treatments
      Expensive treatments
      Psychiatric illness
   Trauma
      Surgery
      Loss of body part or function

DEFINING CHARACTERISTICS

Family system unable to meet physical needs of its members
Family system unable to meet emotional needs of its members
Family system unable to meet spiritual needs of its members
Parents who do not demonstrate respect for each other's view on child-rearing practices
Parents who do not respect children's age-appropriate abilities
Inability to express or accept wide range of feelings
Inability to express or accept feelings of members
Family unable to meet security needs of its members
Inability of family members to relate to each other for mutual growth and maturation
Family uninvolved in community activities
Inability to accept help appropriately
Rigidity in function, rules, and roles
Family that does not demonstrate respect for individuality and autonomy of its members
Family inability to adapt to change and deal with traumatic experience constructively
Family that fails to accomplish current and past developmental tasks
Ineffective family decision-making process
Family enmeshment
Family disengagement
Fixed triangulation
Blurred hierarchical system
Members who use distance to maintain homeostasis
Use of member scapegoating
Spouses who do not maintain a balance in relationship
Failure to send and receive clear messages
Inappropriate boundary maintenance
Inappropriate or poorly communicated family rules, rituals, symbols
Impaired communication
Unexamined family myths
Inappropriate level and direction of energy

NURSING INTERVENTIONS

Patient Goal	Nursing Intervention
Reduce or resolve alterations in family process.	Assess family structure, role relationships.
	Listen attentively and promote trust.
	Encourage verbalization of needs/crisis/fears.
	Assist member to problem-solve.
	Discuss ability to adapt in various situations.
	Ascertain with member strengths and weaknesses of family's ability to adapt.
	Identify stressors.
	Identify overt and covert rules.
	Assess degree of interdependence and bonding among members.
	Teach coping skills and ways to decrease stress.
	Reassure that some family conflict is healthy.
	Encourage members to mutually set goals for providing reciprocal needs.
	Assess ability to give and receive love.
	Discuss sexuality.
	Identify spiritual supports and make referrals if needed.
	Discuss child-rearing practices, beliefs, and discipline techniques.
	Encourage open communication between parents and children.
	If child is acting out
	1. Evaluate if the parenting is ineffective.
	2. Evaluate if one is consistent and stronger and one is inconsistent and lenient.

Patient Goal	Nursing Intervention
	3. Evaluate if parents are locked in triangle with acting-out child.
	4. Explain that the person who sets the rule must be present to enforce it.
	5. If two-parent household, divide areas of responsibility for allowances, bedtime, etc., so it is clear with whom child must negotiate.
	6. Encourage parent to control emotion; maintain calmness and ability to think clearly.
	7. Help parent to calmly determine consequences of child's disobedient behavior.
	8. When acting out occurs, help parent carry out consequences without fail.
	9. After child's behavior is controlled, the nurse may form the third person in the triangle to keep the focus of the problem between the spouses.
	Teach communication techniques.
	Encourage verbalization of each member's feelings and concerns about potential or actual crisis.
	Identify the immediate stressors.
	Discuss possible solutions through use of problem-solving techniques.
	Teach problem-solving techniques and ways to prevent or reduce situation.
	Validate cause of stressors.
	Evaluate effectiveness of problem-solving skills (immediate and over time).
	Give positive reinforcement for constructive family behaviors.
	Provide opportunities for family to give or participate in the care of the hospitalized family member.
Reduce or resolve family crisis.	Identify if crisis is situational or developmental.
	Discuss impact of crisis on all members.
	Discuss role adjustment, ability to adapt, and expectations of other members.
	Encourage family to ventilate feelings regarding effectiveness of their problem-solving skills.
	Provide ongoing support or appropriate referral after crisis.
	Role-play possible situations and ways of dealing constructively with crisis.
	Reinforce the feeling of satisfaction or closeness resulting from working together rather than anger and disruption.

Assessment of the family may be difficult because often not all members are available to interact with the nurse. It is of utmost importance that nurses provide early intervention for families at risk because alterations in family process, such as relationship problems and communication barriers, can be prevented. Leavitt[16] suggests that the nurse become attuned to the family's environment so that she can exchange information with the family system. Three major categories for family assessment are described in the Calgary Family Assessment Model by Wright and Leahey[24]: structural, developmental, and functional.

1. Structural: who is in the family and what is the connection among household members versus those outside the family
   a. Internal structure
      (1) Family composition
      (2) Rank order
      (3) Subsystem (delineated by generation, sex, interest, or function)
      (4) Boundary (defines who participates and how)
   b. External structure
      (1) Culture
      (2) Religion
      (3) Social class status and mobility
      (4) Environment
      (5) Extended family
   c. Effective tool (genogram)
2. Developmental: how this family came to be at this stage in its developmental life cycle
   a. Identify developmental stage family is in
   b. Identify tasks requiring completion during this developmental stage
3. Functional: details of how individuals actually behave in relation to one another
   a. Instrumental functioning (routine, mechanical activities of daily living)
   b. Expressive functioning
      (1) Emotional communication
      (2) Verbal communication
      (3) Nonverbal communication
      (4) Circular communication
      (5) Problem-solving
      (6) Roles
      (7) Control
      (8) Beliefs
      (9) Alliances/coalitions

Wright[24] states that facilitating change within the family system is the primary goal in family work; thus a thorough knowledge of change theory is essential. The role of nursing in the care of families also includes teaching and helping families to develop adaptive skills. For example, careful family assessment is necessary to intervene effectively when the crisis is a chronically ill individual in the family. Family roles must be revised and strengths and weaknesses identified. Dysfunctional coping mechanisms must be replaced with effective ones. Family members can be supportive of each other by communicating needs and adapting roles to meet reciprocal physical, emotional, spiritual, and mutual respect needs.

The nurse can help the family identify and work toward mutual goals by becoming involved with the family from the onset of the health care situation. For instance, if the family is dealing with painful news, the nurse can acknowledge that the news was unfavorable, encourage and listen to angry or distraught family members, recognize the need to discharge feelings, and facilitate the family's awareness of the nurse's ability to assist in identifying coping strategies. Regular patient-nurse interactions, particularly at crisis times, are necessary to reinforce stress-reducing techniques and problem-solving efforts. Giving choices helps the family feel the important need of control over what is happening. The nurse can often assist best by being the liaison between other health care professionals involved in the care of the family. Later, helping the family examine realistic approaches or expectations of the situation provides structure and support in spite of the disequilibrium being experienced.

The process of review of the negative experience can help the family sort out what has happened and help them verbalize fears. Guilt feelings may surface and can be dealt with realistically at this time.

Family participation in the care of an ill family member helps meet the needs of closeness, love, sharing and order in their lives. Separation is extremely threatening and causes pain and anxiety. Even small tasks can be of great comfort to both the hospitalized member and other family members. Family members should be given the opportunity to participate whenever hospitalization occurs.

Preparation for resuming family interactions after a crisis must be made and ongoing follow-up provided. Families lacking nursing support after having received it before flounder and may again become ineffective. Follow-up at 1, 3, and 6 months helps them make the transition to independent role relationships within the family system and provides a time for evaluating the coping mechanisms they are using.

Another important nursing role is to provide family therapy by a qualified family therapist, who has usually had additional education in this area, or intervention that helps clients solve problems now and in future crises. This involves identifying how the family obtains and uses information from the environment.[16] Evaluating the family's ability to seek and use help gives clues to the ability of the family to resolve problems. Dysfunctional families do little or no negotiating when problem-solving. The family's cognitive capacity—their ability to realistically and competently appraise a situation and their own capabilities in relation to it—depends on their openness and their respect for each other's unique capabilities.[16] The nurse must help the family adapt to change, deal with the crisis constructively, accomplish developmental tasks, readjust roles to accommodate situational and developmental crises, and use problem-solving techniques. If difficulty is observed with either the family's or the individual's ability to function in the family system when the problem is an acting out adolescent, an anorexic, a young person with bulimia, or a violent or sexually abusing member, family therapy is indicated and referral to a qualified family therapist necessary. A family unable to effectively negotiate rules or demonstrating continued enmeshment, disengagement, fixed triangulation, use of distance to maintain homeostasis, or scapegoating also needs family therapy.

EVALUATION

Patient Outcome	Data Indicating That Outcome is Reached
Mutual support in family	Effective communication of physical, emotional, spiritual needs Adapt roles to meet reciprocal needs Mutual respect Belongingness, love, affection Sexual fulfillment Provision of protection and safety Coping mechanisms
Ability to negotiate	Effective discussion and agreement about rules Openness to others

Patient Outcome	Data Indicating That Outcome is Reached
	Verbalize values involved in negotiation
	Ability to accept help appropriately
Family cohesiveness	Verbalize/demonstrate emotional bonding
	Verbalize boundaries
	Verbalize/identify mutual interest
	Effective decision-making as a unit
Ability to adapt to change	Deal constructively with crisis
	Accomplish developmental tasks
	Readjust roles to situational or developmental crises
	Problem-solving techniques
	Verbalize need for continued guidance at 1, 3, and 6 months
	Ability to seek help if family ineffective in crisis

References

1. Bowen, M.: Intrafamily dynamics in emotional illness. In D'Agostino, A., editor: Family, church and community, New York, 1961, P.J. Kennedy & Sons.
2. Carpenito, L.: Nursing diagnosis: application to clinical practice, Philadelphia, 1983, J.B. Lippincott Co.
3. Craven, R.F., and Sharp, B.H.: The effects of illness on family functions, Nurs. Forum 11(2):186-193, 1972.
4. Cromwell, R.E., and Peterson, G.W.: Multisystem-multimethod family assessment in clinical contexts, Family Process 22(2):147-163, 1983.
5. Fogarty, T.: Family structure in terms of triangles. In Bradt, J., and Moynihan, C., editors: Systems therapy, Washington, D.C., 1972, The Groome Child Guidance Center.
6. Fogarty, T.: Triangles, The Family 2:165, 1975.
7. Fogarty, T.: Systems concepts and dimensions of self. In Guerin, P., editor: Family therapy theory and practice, New York, 1976, Gardner Press.
8. Foley, V.D.: An introduction to family therapy, New York, 1974, Grune & Stratton, Inc.
9. Ford, F.R.: Rules: the invisible family, Family Process 22(2):135-145, 1983.
10. Green, C.P.: Assessment of family stress, J. Adv. Nurs. 7:11-17, 1982.
11. Guerin, P.: Theoretical aspects and clinical relevance of the multigenerational model of family therapy. In Guerin, P., editor: Family therapy theory and practice, New York, 1976, Gardner Press.
12. Haley, J.: Uncommon therapy: the psychiatric techniques of Milton H. Erickson, M.D., New York, 1973, W.W. Norton Co.
13. Haley, J.: Problem solving therapy, San Francisco, 1976, Jossey-Bass, Inc.
14. Hall, J.A., and Weaver, B.R.: Nursing of families in crisis, Philadelphia, 1974, J.B. Lippincott Co.
14a. Jackson, D.: The question of family homeostasis. In Jackson, D., editor: Communication, family, and marriage. Palo Alto, Calif., 1968, Science & Behavior Books.
15. Kim, M., McFarland, G., and McLane, A., editors: Pocket guide to nursing diagnoses, St. Louis, 1984, The C.V. Mosby Co.
16. Leavitt, M.B.: Families at risk: nursing assessment and strategies for the family at risk, Philadelphia, 1982, J.B. Lippincott Co.
17. Minuchin, S.: Families and family therapy, Cambridge, Mass., 1979, Harvard University Press.
18. Otto, H.A.: Criteria for assessing family strength, Family Process 2(2):329-337, 1963.
18a. Satir, V.: Conjoint family therapy, Palo Alto, Calif., 1964, Science & Behavior Books.
19. Schuster, C.S., and Ashburn, S.S.: The process of human development: a holistic approach, Boston, 1980, Little, Brown & Co.
20. Stuart, G.W., and Sundeen, S.J.: Principles and practice of psychiatric nursing, St. Louis, 1979, The C.V. Mosby Co.
21. Walsh, F.: Normal family processes, New York, 1982, The Guilford Press.
22. Watzlawick, P.: Some basic issues in interaction research. In Framo, J., editor: Family interaction, New York, 1972, Springer Publishing Co.
23. Wilson, H.S., and Kneisel, C.R.: Psychiatric nursing, Palo Alto, Calif., 1983, Addison-Wesley Publishing Co.
24. Wright, L.M., and Leahey, M.: Nurses and families: a guide to family assessment and intervention, Philadelphia, 1984, F.A. Davis Co.

Suggested Readings

Corsini, R.J., and others: Current psychotherapies, Itasca, Ill., 1979, F.E. Peacock Publishers, Inc.

Ferrari, M., Matthews, W.S., and Barabas, G.: The family and the child with epilepsy, Family Process 22(2):53-59, 1983.

Hoffman, L.: Foundations of family therapy, New York, 1981, Basic Books, Inc.

Johnson, S.H.: High-risk parenting: nursing assessment and strategies for the family at risk, Philadelphia, 1979, J.B. Lippincott Co.

Jones, S.L., and Dimond, M.: Family theory and family therapy models: comparative review with implications for nursing practice, J. Psychosoc. Nurs. Ment. Health Services 20(1):12-19, 1982.

Morello, P.A., and Factor, D.C.: Therapy as prevention: an educational model for treating families, Can. Ment. Health Sept. 1981, pp. 10-11.

Olson, D.H., Russell, C.S., and Sprenkle, D.H.: Circumplex model of marital and family systems. VI. Theoretical update, Family Process 22(1):69-83, 1983.

Satir, V.: Conjoint family therapy, Palo Alto, Calif., 1967, Science and Behavior Books, Inc.

Swanson, A.R., and Hurley, P.M.: Family systems: values and value conflicts, J. Psychosoc. Nurs. Ment. Health Services 21(7):24-30, 1983.

SOCIAL ISOLATION
THEORY AND ETIOLOGY

Kim, McFarland, and McLane[12] define social isolation as the condition of aloneness, perceived as being imposed by others and as a negative or threatening state. Carpenito[4] defines it as the state in which the individual has a need or desire for contact with others but is unable to make that contact because of psychologic, biologic, or sociocultural factors. Social isolation is a negative state of aloneness.

Lynch[14] states that human relationships are important to mental and physical well-being. Actually, social isolation, the lack of human companionship, death or absence of parents in early childhood, sudden loss of love, and chronic human loneliness are significant contributors to premature death and to abnormal human functioning.

To realize the consequences of social isolation, it is important to understand relevant personality theory. A number of personality theorists—Adler, Freud, Horney, Sullivan, Erikson, and Fromm—contributed to an understanding of this diagnosis.[9,18] Erikson, Horney, and Sullivan are more recent theorists, whose ideas are based on those of Freud and Adler.

Psychologic

K. Horney. Horney defines basic anxiety as follows[11]:

> . . . the feeling a child has of being isolated and helpless in a potentially hostile world. A wide range of adverse factors in the environment can produce this insecurity in a child: direct or indirect domination, indifference, erratic behavior, lack of respect for the child's individual needs, lack of real guidance, disparaging attitudes, too much admiration or the absence of it, lack of real warmth, having to take sides in parental disagreements, too much or too little responsibility, overprotection, isolation from other children, injustice, discrimination, unkept promises, hostile atmosphere, and so on and so on.

Anything that disrupts the security of a child in relation to his parents produces basic anxiety. A child will attempt to cope, to decrease this anxiety that causes him to feel isolated and helpless. Any way in which a child finds to cope may become a permanent characteristic in the child's adult personality. A child may learn to cope neurotically (by using irrational means) or normally (by using rational means) in a home where there is security, trust, love, respect, tolerance, and warmth.[9] "The person who is likely to become neurotic is one who has experienced the culturally determined difficulties in an accentuated form mostly through the medium of childhood experience."[10]

H. Sullivan. Sullivan developed the interpersonal theory of personality. He believed that an individual cannot exist apart from his relationships with other people.[9] An individual learns to behave in a particular way as a result of interactions with people, and not because he possesses innate imperatives for certain kinds of action. Like Horney, Sullivan based his theory on the premise that each person seeks to avoid anxiety.[16] Coping mechanisms are developed in childhood to reduce anxiety. Some of the coping mechanisms are healthy and help the person to develop intimate relationships and some do not.

Sullivan delineated six states in the development of personality prior to maturation.[9,18] In each of the stages an individual needs to learn coping mechanisms to deal with the particular anxieties of each stage.

Infancy: Major task is maturation of the capacity for language behavior; lasts from birth to 3 or 4 years of age.

Childhood: Major task is maturation of the capacity for getting along with peers; lasts from infancy to 5 or 6 years of age.

Juvenile: Major task is maturation of the capacity for isophilic intimacy; affection for others of the same sex; lasts from childhood to age 9 or 10.

Preadolescence: Major task is maturation of the genital lust dynamisms, chumships, first reciprocal love relationship; lasts from juvenile stage until 10 to 13 years of age.

Early adolescence: Major task is maturation of the patterning of lustful behavior; lasts to 17 years of age.

Late adolescence: Major task is maturation on the whole; lasts until 20 to 23 years of age.

E. Erikson. Erikson also viewed society as having a profound impact on the emerging personality. Development is seen as a gradual process, the ultimate goal being an individual who not only feels comfortable with his own identity, but who is also sensitive to the needs of others in his environment.[16] Erikson, like Sullivan, divided the developmental process into stages. However, Erikson's stages begin with infancy and progress throughout the life cycle. Each stage has a particular task that must be met for a person to move successfully to the next stage. The basic virtues listed in Erikson's stages are the ideal. If a person successfully completes a task, he will have that virtue as part of his personality. For example, if a teenager struggling with identity versus role diffusion passes through that conflict feeling confident in his identity, he will be a person who can also exhibit devotion and fidelity.

Erikson believed that an individual may need to rework certain stages throughout his life. Table 7 lists these stages.[9,18]

Social isolation can be a result of faulty development in the life span. The psychologic ramifications are mul-

Table 7
Erikson's Life Stages

Basic Task		Negative Counterpart	Developmental Level	Basic Virtue
Trust	vs.	Mistrust	Infant	Drive and hope
Autonomy	vs.	Doubt	Toddler	Self-centered and will-power
Initiative	vs.	Guilt	Preschooler	Direction and purpose
Industry	vs.	Inferiority	Schoolager	Method and competence
Identity	vs.	Role diffusion	Adolescent	Devotion and fidelity
Intimacy	vs.	Isolation	Young adult	Affiliation and love
Generativity	vs.	Self-absorption	Middlescent	Protection and care
Integrity	vs.	Despair	Older adult	Renunciation and wisdom

tiple. If an individual does not learn to cope with the stress and anxieties of life in a healthy manner, he may end up with grave psychologic difficulties. These difficulties can be limiting in that they can lead to social isolation and difficulties in interpersonal relationships. Some include depression, dependent personality, autism, sociopathy, antisocial behavior, and schizophrenia.[20]

Considering the social-psychologic personality theories, one can understand that certain disruptions are possible in the development of mature, interdependent, interpersonal relationships. Some individuals might find it difficult to establish or maintain close relationships. Three basic disruptions can occur in the area of relatedness: withdrawal from others, excessive dependency on others, which causes others to move away, and manipulation of others.[20] Individuals who have difficulties in relatedness are likely to have difficulty trusting others.

Loneliness is likely to be a component of the lives of people who experience disruption in relatedness. The loneliness or lack of intimacy with others is very painful. Loneliness is a characteristic of social isolation, a state in which an individual is aware of not relating to other people, but at the same time experiences a need for other people.[15] Lynch[14] points out that every segment of our society seems to be deeply afflicted by one of the major diseases of our age—human loneliness.

The exceedingly unpleasant and driving experience of loneliness results from the frustration of a basic need for personal intimacy.[22] Humans have a definite need for relatedness, and if a particular individual does not have this need met and satisfied, then loneliness becomes a prominent part of his state of being.

It is important to distinguish between loneliness and aloneness. If a person feels loneliness, he has withdrawn involuntarily and feels separated and isolated by forces that are outside of himself.[22] Aloneness is voluntary and can be constructive. Loneliness is usually destructive.

Biologic

Often it is difficult to completely separate biologic etiologies of isolation from psychologic because a biologic cause can lead an individual to exhibit psychologic manifestations of isolation. Conversely, a psychologic cause can lead to a biologic outcome. Both biologic outcomes and etiologies are discussed.

A minimum rate of information inputs to a system must be maintained for it to function normally. Moreover, individuals strive to get such inputs.[6] The effects of social isolation, or a lack of variability in information inputs on people, such as truck drivers who spend long hours driving, prisoners in solitary confinement, and patients on respirators, have been described as an isolation syndrome. Often extreme subjective experiences such as hallucinations have been reported with even relatively mild sensory deprivation, such as is experienced in a long drive alone at night.[21] The states of isolation syndrome can be described as follows[6]:

1. Person able to pass time thinking, but finally becomes sleepy and may fall asleep.
2. As time goes on, individual is unable to direct thoughts or think clearly.
3. Becomes irritable, restless, hostile.
4. May make attempt to use fantasy material as an adjustment process to substitute for needed information inputs.
5. Becomes childlike in emotional variability and behavior.
6. State of vivid musical and auditory or kinesthetic hallucinations.
7. Finally, sensation of otherness (depersonalization).

If an individual does receive some sensory input after he has been deprived for a long time, he will not necessarily recover quickly. There may be residual effects from the deprivation.[6]

Conversely, information or input overload can cause ill effects on humans and animals. Studies with rats in overcrowded conditions have been conducted.[6] The overpopulation caused various disorders. The input overload, according to Spitz,[19] elicited various abnormal internal cognitive and affective processes and behaviors. Especially observed was frenetic activity and pathologic withdrawal. Luby[13] suggested that schizophrenic withdrawal may be an attempt by the patient to use escape as an adjustment process to reduce the rate at which information comes in to him.

Physical deprivation and/or physical ailments can cause social isolation and pathologic disorders in individuals. Physical deprivation can be reviewed as removal of an individual from social supports, such as loss of parents, institutionalization, and loss of physical functionings.

In one study[6] monkey infants living with their mothers and peers were first separated from their mothers at about 180 days of age and then secondarily separated from their peers at 205 days. This procedure produced a double despair syndrome, first elicited by maternal separation and then by playmate separation. It is clear that an anaclitic depression may be induced by the loss of any social object to which the animal is deeply attached, not only by the loss of the mother.

Spitz,[19] Harlew,[6] and Bowlby[3] all found that children who were physically separated from parents had difficulty in forming attachments to others in their adult life. Severe adult depression, dependency, psychosis, varied neuroses, and suicide all have been frequently reported among individuals who suffer early parental loss.[14]

Many physical illnesses, for example, Alzheimer's disease, mental retardation, frequent surgeries, cancer treatments, and paraplegia, have a major isolating influence for both the affected individual and the family. Sometimes the individual may need to be physically removed from the home into an institution. If this is not necessary, the isolation may be caused by the affected person's withdrawal from society because of the psychologic ramifications of the physical ailment.

Sociocultural

Sociocultural etiologies of social isolation overlap the psychologic and biologic causative factors. A number of broad influences can be classified as sociocultural etiologies that can result in social isolation: loss either by death, divorce, or separation (mobile society); the decline of the extended family and society[6]; prejudice[9]; ramifications of urbanization[6]; lessened adult social contact experienced by mothers of young children[7]; social breakdown syndrome in the elderly. The manifestations of the syndrome are either a withdrawal syndrome, anger and hostility, or some combination of the two.[8]

Research[17] has shown that isolation has a negative impact on the aged: it desocializes them, hampers social adjustment, and seems to reduce independence. Isolation is not synonymous with mental disorder in the aged, although it may result in some behavior patterns associated with mental disorders, specifically poor social adjustment and poor cognitive functioning. The effects of isolation may be reversed through resocialization, remotivation, and friendly visiting programs. Rathbone-McCuan and Hashimi[17] identified four broad isolating influences: biophysical, psychoemotional, economic, and social. These particular influences have an impact not only on the elderly but also on all age groups. Within each heading a number of specific isolating influences are listed.

Biophysical: Lessened physical vigor, endurance, sensory losses, limitations on mobility, and organic brain disorders.

Psychoemotional: Shifts in developmental tasks, low self-esteem, internalized social stereotypes, fear of decline and institutionalization, loss of control over life, separateness from others, deprivation of sexual needs.

Economic: Insufficient personal financial resources, which control availability of housing, adequate nutrition, recreation, and transportation.

Social: Loss of work role and family roles, loss of family and/or friends through death, lack of knowledge of social resources, victim of criminal attack.

It is important to separate the different types of isolating influences to focus specifically on social isolation as a nursing diagnosis. The following are etiologies for social isolation[4,12]:

Psychologic
    Emotional illness (extreme anxiety, depression, paranoia, phobias, psychosis)
    Unaccepted social behavior
    Inability to engage in satisfying personal relationships
    Delay in accomplishing developmental tasks
    Immature interests
    Obesity, anorexia, bulimia
    Drug or alcohol addiction
    Alterations in physical appearance
Physiologic
    Altered state of wellness
    Drug or alcohol addiction
    Obesity, anorexia, bulimia
    Cancer
    Hospitalization or terminal illness
    Physical handicaps (paraplegia, amputation, arthritis, hemiplegia)
    Incontinence (embarrassment, odor)
    Sensory loss

Sociocultural
Death of a significant other
Divorce
Extreme poverty
Moving into another culture
Homosexuality
Loss of usual means of transportation
Unaccepted social values
Inadequate personal resources
Single parent

DEFINING CHARACTERISTICS[4,12]

Adults

Absence of supportive significant other(s): family, friends, group
Sad, dull affect
Inappropriate or immature interests and activities for developmental age or stage
Uncommunicative
Withdrawn
No eye contact
Preoccupation with own thoughts, repetitive, meaningless actions
Projects hostility in voice, behavior
Seeks to be alone or exists in subculture
Evidence of physical and/or mental handicap or altered state of wellness
 Obesity
 Anorexia
 Paraplegia
Shows behavior unaccepted by dominant cultural group
Feelings of uselessness
Doubts about ability to survive
Expresses feeling of aloneness imposed by others
Expresses feelings of rejection
Experiences feelings of difference from others

Expresses values acceptable to subculture but unable to accept values of dominant culture
Inadequacy in or absence of significant purpose in life
Altered thought processes
Agoraphobia
Inability to meet expectations of others
Insecurity in public
Excessive sleeping
Expresses interests inappropriate to developmental age or stage
Self-absorbed
Sleep disturbances
Inability to make decisions
Change in nutritional intake (overeating or anorexia)
Paranoia
Mistrust
Hallucinations: auditory, visual, kinetic
Feelings of inferiority
Depersonalization
Feeling of otherness
Lack of attention

Children

Absence of appropriate language capability
Lacks eye contact
Rocking
Absence of play
Unaccomplished developmental tasks
Failure to thrive
Physical growth below minimum for age group
Acting out destructive behavior
Imagining playmates instead of peer relationships
Lack of friendships of same sex

Adolescents

Consistently daydream in school
Inattentive to studies
Poor academic accomplishments
Not being included socially by peers
Frequently pointing out inadequacies of others
Acting out destructive behavior
Lack of friends

NURSING INTERVENTIONS

Patient Goal	Nursing Intervention
Reduce or eliminate social isolation.	Establish trust. Assess social history. Identify limitations and barriers in ability to form meaningful relationships with others. Discuss feelings of loneliness. Explain relationship between loneliness and unmet intimacy needs. Encourage verbalization of loneliness. Discuss potentials for a meaningful relationship to decrease loneliness. Identify with patient possible social outlets. Promote increased self-esteem. Explore ways of reaching out to others. Assess and assist with balancing independence and dependence in family roles. Encourage involvement in peer groups, social activity, or evening out at least weekly. Support individual experiencing a loss.

Patient Goal	Nursing Intervention

Validate normalcy of grieving.

Encourage support group participation for widows and widowers.

Use grandparent programs, day care centers (for children and elderly), retirement communities, house sharing, pets, telephone contacts to decrease isolation.

Recognize and use churches as a valued resource.

Encourage physical closeness (touch).

Help identify and obtain transportation options.

Identify diversional activities that decrease feelings of loneliness.

Assist with development of alternate means of communication, if sensory impairment exists.

Identify and suggest solutions for physical impairments that affect body image (ostomy, cancer odor, incontinence, disfiguring surgery).

Children:
1. Provide daily opportunities for play and play therapy.
2. Encourage play with peers to promote socialization skills.

Adolescents:
1. Develop one-to-one relationship built on openness and trust.
2. Explore ideas about an ideal relationship with peers.
3. Assist in developing skills necessary to strive toward the ideal relationship in a safe environment.
4. Reassure that feelings of isolation are common for young adolescents and are often temporary.
5. Discuss with parents reason for adolescent's behavior and encourage verbalization of their frustrations.
6. Encourage liberal visitation in institutional setting for acutely ill adolescents.

Elderly:
1. Introduce self and call patient by name.
2. Establish trust and mutual respect.
3. Locate and inform about neighborhood social groups and self-help groups specific to the patient's needs.
4. Teach the family and older person about the process of aging.
5. Encourage to select and perform productive activities that promote self-esteem.
6. Teach problem-solving techniques.
7. Encourage selection of activities that broaden the social network and facilitate personal growth.
8. Find ways to maintain a life-style that allows personal freedom.
9. Provide interpreters to assist the elderly Hispanic or other non-English-speaking person to locate appropriate social support resources.
10. Determine the upper and lower levels of the mentally disabled patient's functional capacity.
11. Thoroughly assess the social history of the mentally disabled patient.
12. Evaluate physical health problems.
13. Identify social supports available to the mentally disabled patient.
14. Assess diet and exercise.
15. Teach self-management skills prior to inpatient discharge and weekly follow-up after discharge.
16. Assess onset, frequency, and impact of manifestations of Alzheimer's disease.
17. Teach caregiving relatives ways to deal with difficult or inappropriate behavior.
18. Provide ongoing support to caregiving relatives and encourage social relationships outside the family group.

The formation of effective human relationships affects the health and well-being of all patients nurses come in contact with. Therefore it is essential that the nurse assess carefully the patient's social history when limitations or barriers are found in the ability to form relationships with others. Carpenito[4] states that since social isolation is a subjective state, all inferences made regarding a person's feelings of aloneness must be validated. The nurse must possess skilled interview and communication techniques to effectively help patients identify and overcome social isolation.

It is important for the nurse to discuss any feelings of

loneliness the patient expresses. Loneliness is the result of unmet intimacy needs. After a therapeutic nurse-patient relationship is established, these feelings can be discussed and ways of meeting intimacy needs explored. To do this effectively, the nurse must accept and deal with any of her own feelings of loneliness.

Possible etiologies of social isolation must be explored with the patient in an open, direct, and supportive manner. Problem-solving techniques need to be discussed and taught to the patient with the ultimate decision-making process focusing on the patient to promote behavioral change. Follow-up care is absolutely necessary for the patient's continued support and accomplishment of the outcomes desired.

Children who suffer from social isolation require intense multidisciplinary intervention. The age of the child will affect the success of the treatment and amount of residual effects.

Isolated older persons pose a complex problem for nursing care because the likelihood that they will seek assistance depends on several factors.[17] A painful physical disorder that cannot be ignored is more likely to lead the individual to seek help. Second, the more isolated older persons are, the less likely they are to seek help. Third, the social support resource must be familiar and acceptable to the person. Last, unsuccessful, uncaring, or inappropriate experiences with the social resources will discourage older persons from seeking future contact.

The elderly person often lacks the social skills to find supports and use referral services. It is important to increase the patient's awareness of appropriate resources that best meet his specific needs. The nurse can help develop adequate communication and assertiveness skills to facilitate the use of available social resources to decrease social isolation. Encouraging the elderly person to accept the need for a broader support system can be challenging. The nurse must establish mutual respect and trust to promote continued self-esteem and openness to outside resources. Family members can often assist in this process. The patient, however, must be encouraged to make his own decision to maintain pride and self-respect, unless he is cognitively incapable of making appropriate decisions. Peer groups and other social organizations in close proximity to the patient can also help increase awareness of and openness to social support resources.

Assessment of the older woman should include two parameters,[17] the rhythm of isolation, which refers to an individual's pattern of social involvement and withdrawal, and the relativity of isolation, an individual's pattern of cognitive and comparative assessment of the usual behavior of those considered as peers. Rathbone-McCuan and Hashimi[17] suggest focusing on the following:

. . . (a) the extent to which dyadic and multiple networks may complement or substitute for each other; (b) the extent to which cognitive awareness and perceptions of the various networks change over time; (c) whether an increase in the degree of commitment in one or more networks may compensate for age-linked losses in others; and (d) whether past commitments have symbolic significance, thus compensating at least in part for the lack of current behavioral involvement.

Cultural differences also affect the social isolation of the elderly. Separation from their extended family, low expectations of service providers, language differences from those of the larger population, limited education, language deficits, and noncitizen status are other barriers that contribute to lack of knowledge of social service resources. The nurse must assess for the presence of these barriers and find ways to promote social interaction.

The chronically mentally disabled elderly face long-standing isolators, including broken family relationships and community ties, limited social coping skills, limited education, and limited employability.[17] These patients need complex multidisciplinary intervention guided by the nurse.

EVALUATION

Patient Outcome	Data Indicating That Outcome is Reached
Can identify causes of feelings of isolation	Verbalization of fears, limitations, barriers to interaction with others Verbalization of feelings of loneliness Recognition of need for intimacy Admission of concerns about low self-esteem Verbalization of negative experiences in past that may have ended relationships
Verbalization and demonstration of ways to promote meaningful relationships	Desire to increase meaningful relationships Increased self-esteem Participation in routine activities as inpatient Talking to others Approaching others to socialize Plan to join social peer group or activity at least once a week

Patient Outcome	Data Indicating That Outcome is Reached
	Increased social skills Admission of fears and concerns regarding social interaction Participation in support group Recognition of need for personal freedom and growth Ability to function as a part of a group
Identification of activities that provide diversion and stimulate interest and self-esteem	Listing at least five activities that provide enjoyment and increased self-worth Participation in one or more of these activities at least biweekly Positive feeling elicited from these activities Increased feelings of involvement

References

1. Benson, E.R.: Care for the elderly in Yugoslavia, Int. Nurs. Rev. 23(2):55-56, 1976.
2. Block, B.: Preparing students for physical restraint, J. Psychiatr. Nurs. 14(1):9-10, 1976.
3. Bowlby, J.: Attachment and loss, vol. 1: Attachment, New York, 1969, Basic Books, Inc.
4. Carpenito, L.J.: Nursing diagnosis: application to clinical practice, Philadelphia, 1983, J.B. Lippincott Co.
5. Dunlop, B.D.: Need for and utilization of long-term care among elderly Americans, J. Chronic Dis. 29(2):75-87, 1976.
6. Freedman, A.M., Kaplan, H., and Sadock, B.J., editors: Comprehensive textbook of psychiatry, vols. 1 and 2, Baltimore, 1975, The Williams & Wilkins Co.
7. Griffey, D.: The health visitor and the isolated mother, Health Visitor 48(4):111-112, 1975.
8. Gunter, L.: Do nurses have the power to cause, prevent, and cure "Social Breakdown Syndrome?" (editorial) J. Gerontol. Nurs. 6(11):648-651, 1977.
9. Hall, C.S., and Lindzey, G.: Theories of personality, ed. 2, New York, 1970, John Wiley & Sons, Inc.
10. Horney, K.: Neurotic personality of our times, New York, 1937, W.W. Norton Co.
11. Horney, K.: Our inner conflicts, New York, 1945, W.W. Norton Co.
12. Kim, M., McFarland, G.K., and McLane, A.M., editors: Pocket guide to nursing diagnosis, St. Louis, 1984, The C.V. Mosby Co.
13. Luby, E.D., and others: Model psychoses and schizophrenia, Am. J. Psychiatr. 119:61-67, 1962.
14. Lynch, J.J.: The broken heart, New York, 1977, Basic Books, Inc.
15. Mahon, N.E.: Developmental changes and loneliness during adolescence, Topics Clin. Nurs. 5(1):66-76, 1983.
16. Pasquali, E.A., and others: Mental health nursing: a biocultural approach, St. Louis, 1981, The C.V. Mosby Co.
17. Rathbone-McCuan, E., and Hashimi, J.: Isolated elders, Rockville, Md., 1982, Aspen Systems Corp.
18. Schuster, C.S., and Ashburn, S.S.: The process of human development, Boston, 1980, Little, Brown & Co.
19. Spitz, R.A.: The derailment of dialogue: stimulus overload, action cycles, and the competition gradient, J. Am. Psychoanal. Assoc. 12:752-775, 1964.
20. Stuart, G.W., and Sundeen, S.J.: Principles and practice of psychiatric nursing, St. Louis, 1979, The C.V. Mosby Co.
21. Wheaton, J.L.: Fact and fancy in sensory deprivation studies, Aeromed Rev. 5:59, 1959.
22. Wright, L.M.: A symbolic tree: loneliness is the root, delusions are the leaves, J. Psychiatr. Nurs. 13(3):30-35, 1975.

Suggested Readings

Carser, D.L., and Doona, M.E.: Alienation: a nursing concept, J. Psychiatr. Nurs. 16(9):33-40, 1978.
Ingenito, J.E.: Patterning for a constructive relationship in problem isolation, J. Psychiatr. Nurs. 12(6):29-33, 1974.
Managan, D., and others: Older adults: a community survey of health needs, Nurs. Res. 23(5):426-432, 1974.
Mealey, A.: Provision of a multi-range program for clients in a downtown hotel by baccalaureate nursing students, J. Psychiatr. Nurs. 19(2):11-16, 1981.
Miles, H.S., and Hays, D.R.: Widowhood, Am. J. Nurs. 75(2):280-282, 1975.
Rogers, R.E.: The challenge of gerontological nursing, J. Practical Nurs. 32(9):18-21, 1982.
Svanborg, A.: Seventy-year-old people in Gothenburg—a population study in an industrialized Swedish city. II. General presentation of social and medical conditions, Acta Med. Scand. Suppl. 611:5-37, 1977.
Taggart, M.: When your elderly patient is withdrawing—what can you do? J. Practical Nurs. 26(12):16-19, 1976.

VIOLENCE, POTENTIAL FOR
THEORY AND ETIOLOGY

Potential for violence is a state in which an individual has aggressive feelings that can be directed either at oneself or others and result in physical injury. The causes of human violence are complex and as yet remain unclear. Much of the literature describes the derivation of violent behavior by using the term *aggression*. Aggressive behavior does not necessarily lead to violent behavior, but when an individual behaves violently, he is also being aggressive. It is a matter of degree. By definition the term *violence* means an act of destructiveness. Violence is not an emotion. Violence can be viewed as an end result of a number of psychologic (emotional), biologic, and sociologic influences.[12] No one theory explaining these influences is more valid than the other. Moreover, a combination of theories is often employed to explain the etiology of violent behavior because the potential for violent behavior needs to be assessed on an individual basis.

Fig. 5
Anger continuum.

MILD	MODERATE	SEVERE	EXTREME
Part of everyday life	Interference with an	Interference with	(Perceived or real)
Experienced as small	accomplishment of a	goal or seen as	threat to personal
annoyances	goal or threat to	threat to being	value system or
Feelings simply expressed;	personal value system	Experienced as intense	self
reaction without	Experienced as feelings	frustration/fear	May occur because of
thought	of frustration/disappointment	Alternatives difficult	continuous inter-
Experience forgotten	Alternatives usually	to find	ference to goal
quickly or easily	at hand and goals	or cannot be found	or threat to
handled without much	reestablished	Difficult to	personal value
emotional strain	Feelings remembered,	express feelings	system or self
	but quickly resolved	May need help to	Also called rage,
		find equilibrium	or fury
			Totally consumed
			by feelings
			Unable to control
			expression of feelings
			Potential for violence
			Depleted coping
			mechanisms

Psychologic

One theory[12] hypothesizes that the experience of certain emotions may lead the person to a violent act. Some of these emotions are frustration, anger-aggression (often these terms are used interchangeably in the literature), rage, and fury. Anger is defined as "a strong feeling excited by a real or supposed injury; often accompanied by a desire to take vengeance or to obtain satisfaction from the offending party."[12]

Stuart and Sundeen define anger as a "feeling of resentment that occurs in response to heightened anxiety when the individual perceives a threat."[12] Anger can be described in terms of degrees or as a continuum similar to the way in which anxiety is often described. Stuart and Sundeen's discussion of anger is the basis for the anger continuum in Fig. 5.

Another continuum model (Fig. 6) illustrates a psychologic paradigm for violence.[14] This particular model can further explain Fig. 5 because it illustrates the extreme anger segment of that continuum. It shows what the physiologic and psychologic ramifications might be if a person experienced the internal reaction of rage and anxiety-panic.

Dollard's psychologic approach to the etiology of aggressive behavior is the frustration-aggression theory.[3] According to this author all aggressive behavior results

from the feeling of frustration. Frustration occurs, as seen in the anger continuum, when a goal cannot be achieved. The sense of frustration and the degree of frustration are increased if the goal is highly valued or if the individual has repeatedly attempted and failed to achieve it.

Behaviorists view aggression and possibly violence as a learned response that has been reinforced by facilitating goal achievement.[12] Learning theorists postulate that positive and negative reinforcements learned in childhood determine future behavior in adulthood. An example might be a child who throws a temper tantrum; because his parents cannot tolerate the behavior, they give into his demands to stop the aggressive behavior. If the child continues to throw tantrums when he wants something and his parents continue to give in to him, the child has learned that aggressive behavior, possibly violent behavior, will be rewarded. Another example of how learning theory may explain potential for violence or aggression was documented in a study.[8] It was found that the television programs preferred by an 8-year-old boy were the best predictors of how aggressive he would be when he was 19 years of age, due to the copying of aggressive behaviors viewed on television.

Freud hypothesized that human aggression evolves from instinctual drives. He believed human beings were under the influence of two instinctual drives: *eros,* the

Fig. 6
The continuum of violence.

From Duggan, M.: Violence in the family.
In Getty, C., and Humphreys, W., editors:
Understanding the family: stress and
change in American family life, Norwalk,
Conn., 1981, Appleton-Century Crofts.

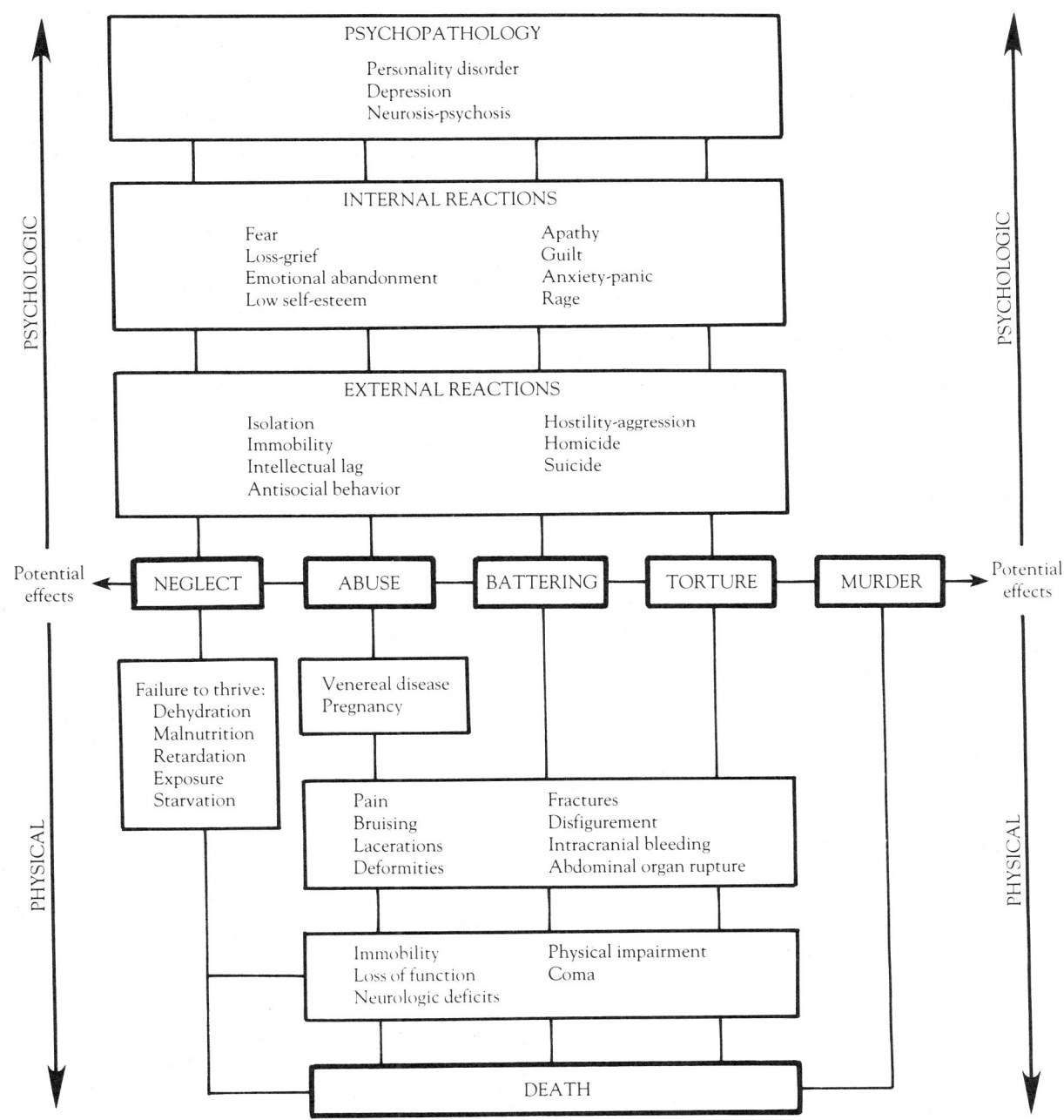

life drive expressed through sexuality; and *thanatos*, the death drive expressed through aggression. The theory maintains that life is the constant struggle between *eros* and *thanatos*. It was Freud's belief that suicide, homicide, and other violent and destructive behaviors occurred when the death drive gained supremacy.

Konrad Lorenz's theory[9] is based on his observations of animals. He believed that there is an instinctual aggressive drive that is common to all animals regardless of species. His theory includes the hypothesis that man "suffers from insufficient discharge of his aggressive drive."[9] If a person is unable to release aggression, then various self-destructive behaviors are exhibited, such as neurosis, accidents, and possibly suicide.

Biologic

Some theorists believe that aggressive or violent behavior is caused by somatic and organic phenomena, such as a neurologic disorder. Specific internal physiologic causes include endocrine imbalance (hyperthyroidism or hypoglycemia), hunger, fatigue, brain tumors, and convulsive disorders.[12] Researchers have found areas in the brain that, when stimulated, cause aggressive outbursts. Fromm[5] links the neural response to the fight-or-flight mechanism in the body and sees it as a method of self-preservation.

Neuropsychologists have made strides in brain research. This has been difficult, however, because the areas in the brain that cause certain responses, such as aggression, are deeply buried and difficult to reach.[12] The following research findings appear to substantiate the organic theory of violence[4]: of 100 people on trial for murder, 18 were epileptics; of 29 people who committed sudden impulse murders, 5 had gross organic disease; studies of convicted murderers showed that when there seems to be normal brain functioning, a higher percentage of those convicted of unmotivated murders have abnormal EEGs than those who killed in self-defense.

The feeling of anger is physically uncomfortable, probably because of the activity of the sympathetic fibers of the autonomic nervous system in response to the secretion of epinephrine.[12] The physiologic response to anger is the same as the body's response to anxiety—the fight-or-flight mechanism. The specific responses are discussed in the Defining Characteristics section.

Sociocultural

Sociocultural factors can also contribute to an individual's potential for violence. Cultural norms aid in defining acceptable and unacceptable means of expressing anger and aggressive feelings. A society's legal system, whatever it may be, applies sanctions to violators of the established norms. The legal system is a mechanism to control violent behavior. Even before civil law, religious law was a way to control unacceptable aggressive acts. If someone harmed a person, the consequences for the behavior were high. The thought was that people would then think twice before becoming violent again. Christian religious ethics taught nonaggression: "Turn the other cheek."

"Urban life tends to foster increased aggressive behavior."[12] In some respects this may be related to the theory of personal space. City dwellings are in close proximity. "When people have little privacy or when they feel that their area of personal space has been invaded, there is frequently an aggressive response."[12] The riots of the 1960s in ghetto areas exemplified this theory.

Similar to the learning behavior theory, it is thought that humans model behaviors that they see or experience repeatedly. Adults who engage in family violence tend to have experienced violence, neglect, or other forms of pathologic parenting in their families of origin.[13] In a study of 84 prisoners, 74% had a history of exposure to brutal and extreme violence, child arson, and cruelty to animals. Children tend to model the behaviors they see in the home or experience in their environment. If an individual is abused as a child, he is also likely to abuse his children.

May[10] discusses violence in relation to the feeling of lack of power. He contends that powerlessness, which leads to apathy, promotes violence and that deeds of violence are performed largely by those trying to establish self-esteem, defend their self-image, and demonstrate that they, as individuals, are significant. One can see this exemplified in adolescent street gangs.

In American culture today the family is recognized as one of the most common environments for violence.[13] Most sources agree that parents are usually the people who abuse children. Younger parents more frequently abuse their children than do older ones. Low income, lower educational level, inadequate housing, unemployment, and social isolation increase the likelihood of child abuse. Abusive parents tend to exhibit mental illness, alcoholism, and a variety of personality defects. Children under age 6 are at greatest risk. Illegitimate children or children with malformations, handicaps, or other imperfections are more likely to be abused.

Four broad patterns were found when child abuse was studied nationwide: (1) psychologic rejection from parental inability to love and accept the child; (2) impulsive uncontrolled discipline style; (3) personal inabilities in meeting stress; and (4) child's stubbornness, willfulness, or other problems.[13]

Spouse abuse is prevalent. Pregnant women are three

times more likely to be battered than are nonpregnant women. Sibling abuse, a violent attack by one child on another, occurs in four out of five families with siblings ages 3 to 17; 53% of these attacks are severe.

Elderly abuse is estimated at 4% of the total elderly population. There appear to be three predominant situational causes.[13] The first occurs in an initially loving home, but with increasing disability the stress and abuse can take place. In the second situation the elderly person is taken in reluctantly and has a marked physical disability. In the third situation family stress creates a potential for violence even before the elderly person moves in. The following are etiologies for potential violence[1,2,6]:

Psychologic
    Antisocial behavior
    Physical abuse in the family
    Rage reactions
    Suicidal behavior
    Homicidal behavior
    Panic states
    Drug or alcohol abuse
    Depression
    Increase in stressors within a short period of time
    Physical immobility
    Real or perceived threat to self
    Fear of the unknown
    Response to a catastrophic event
    Misperceived messages from others
    Response to dysfunctional family through developmental stages
    Dysfunctional communication patterns
Physiologic-biologic
    Organic brain syndrome
    Temporal lobe epilepsy
    Toxic reaction to medication (prescribed and unprescribed)
    Toxic reaction to alcohol
    Hormonal imbalance (such as premenstrual syndrome)
    Alteration in biochemical functioning leading to depression or manic-depressive illness
    Physical trauma (result of accidents or battering)
Sociocultural
    Battered spouse
    Child abuse
    Homicidal behavior
    Environmental controls
    Response to a dysfunctional family
    Dysfunctional communication pattern

DEFINING CHARACTERISTICS[1,2,6]

Loss of control*
    Physical assault
    Forcefully damages inanimate objects
    Forcefully injures others
    Injures self
Body language
    Clenched fists
    Clenched jaw
    Rigid posture
    Tautness indicating intense effort to control
    Agitation
    Increased motor activity
    Pacing
Hostile threatening verbalizations*
Possession of destructive means (gun, knife, other weapon)*
Rage
Self-destructive behavior resulting in minimal injury*
Suspicion of others, paranoid attitude
Delusions, hallucinations
Perception of self as worthless or hopeless
Perception of environment as frightening or hostile
Poor impulse control
Provocative behavior
    Argumentative
    Dissatisfied
    Overactive
    Hypersensitive
    Poor impulse control
Vulnerable self-esteem
Extreme anger
Increasing anxiety levels
Fear of self or others
Inability to verbalize feelings
Repetition of verbalizations such as continued complaints, requests, demands
Minimal tolerance to anxiety or stress
Surface appearance of overcontrol, inhibition
Proneness to action rather than words
Inability to remember all or part of recent or past events
Disconnected thoughts
Disorientation to time, place, and person
Staring eye contact or avoidance of eye contact

To ascertain an individual's potential for violence, any number of defining characteristics can be observed or manifested verbally or physiologically by a patient. However, there are certain critical characteristics that, if present, represent more immediate, imminent danger to the client or others. Once these critical characteristics are seen, intervention should be undertaken immediately.

*Critical defining characteristic.

NURSING INTERVENTIONS

Patient Goal	Nursing Intervention

Reduce or eliminate potential for violent behavior.	Encourage patient to talk rather than act out physically.
	Use positive reinforcers when patient has reduced or not used profanity for 1 day.
	Reward the positive behavior by complimenting or spending extra time with patient.
	Function as role model:
	  1. Be calm.
	  2. Verbalize feeilngs.
	  3. Demonstrate positive interpersonal relationships.
	  4. Discuss importance of caring about self and others.
	Do not threaten patient's self-esteem or sense of control.
	Assist with external controls when needed:
	  1. Remove easily accessible items that could be used as weapons.
	  2. Do not confront patient with issue of control.
	  3. When possible, allow the patient to make decisions about own actions if not currently being harmful to others; explain what will happen if acting out or violence occurs (security will be called, additional personnel will be called, medications may be used).
	Help person maintain control by discussing frustrations, thus decreasing physical and verbal aggression.
	Assure patient that he will be assisted in controlling violent impulses.
	Set limits for each aggressive episode.
	Place patient in seclusion if dangerous to self or others.
	If seclusion is necessary, maintain safety.
	Remove individual from situation if environment is contributing to aggressive behavior; use least amount of control needed (for example, ask others to leave and take individual to a quiet room).
	When using seclusion, institutional policy will provide specific guidelines. The following are general:
	  1. Observe individual every 15 minutes.
	  2. Search patient before secluding to remove harmful objects.
	  3. Check seclusion room to see that safety is maintained.
	  4. Offer fluids and food periodically.
	  5. When going into seclusion room, have sufficient staff present.
	  6. Explain precisely what is happening and why; give individual a chance to cooperate.
	  7. Assist person in toileting and personal hygiene.
	Assist in verbalization of depressed feelings.
	Assist in finding alternatives to deal with depressed feelings.

Eliminate or reduce precipitating factors.	Provide and document accurate information concerning the relationship of the physiologic alteration and the disturbing feelings or thoughts. Provide short, concise, honest statements concerning hospital routines and procedures. Remove excess equipment. Decrease noise volume. Use same personnel. Discuss rationale for fear, if known, if person can verbalize. Identify available support systems. Allow person to verbalize feelings about hospital environment. Allow person to arrange personal belongings to promote sense of security. Reinforce reality during each interaction; orient individual to time, place, person. Provide calendar and clock for person's room. Set realistic day-to-day goals. Give short, consistent statements when explaining case. In collaboration with physician, begin medical regimen to counteract effects of toxic medication. Remove any medications patient may have brought. Present alternative physical ways to deal with family and community frustrations.

Patient Goal	Nursing Intervention
	Demonstrate genuine caring, support, and respect when helping family members integrate the violent experience.
	Listen and provide empathy when patient discusses pain and trauma of family.
	Have person role-play family communication with personnel and practice problem-solving techniques.
	Discuss how communication can be misperceived by others.
	Provide frequent 10-minute interactions rather than one 30-minute interaction.
	Give feedback on positive changes in communication pattern.
	Administer medications as prescribed.
	Provide a trusting relationship with patient to help patient feel more comfortable:
	1. Be honest, clear, concise during interactions.
	2. Recognize that defensive, manipulative behavior has meaning for the person.
	3. Maintain a stable physical environment.
	4. Establish short-term goals; use contracts, such as spending a certain amount of time with patient; follow through.
	Help to decrease agitation in the patient if it occurs:
	1. Allow physical activity to channel aggression in accordance with person's ability.
	2. Administer medications as prescribed by physician.
	3. Interact with patient on one-to-one basis.
	4. Do not touch patient until you explain what the procedure or rationale is for such an intervention.
	5. Allow patient to maintain personal space.
	6. Use calm, nonverbal and verbal behavior.

The nurse must provide controls to prevent violent behavior. Setting limits, seclusion, and restraints (chemical and physical, which are not often used today) are all methods of controlling behavior, if the patient loses control. The nurse must understand that the potentially violent patient often has low self-esteem, may be lonely, and may feel hopeless. Thus it is of utmost importance to establish trust and rapport by approaching calmly and allowing personal space. Helping the patient think and talk about his problems can correct distorted perceptions and ideas. The violent threatening patient fails and believes violence to be the sole exit from his stress-bound box of life. The patient is unable to perceive any alternatives other than violence. Complex, long-term supportive or deterrent measures may be required.

Because fear is a possible source for violent behavior, the nurse must help to eliminate the patient's fears. One way to decrease fear is to discuss it and try to find ways to eliminate or deal with it. The nurse can also help to control the environment by minimizing noise and traffic (by other patients or visitors) and by carefully explaining procedures that require equipment or medication.

A person who commits a violent act frequently has tremendous feelings of guilt and remorse. Those family members or staff who witnessed or were victims of the violent behavior also need time to verbalize their feelings, fears, and anger. How a person sees and interprets the world about him is crucial to the future eruption of violent behavior.[10]

The nurse must encourage and allow verbal expressions of anger. The key to prevention of violent aggression is finding out what precipitates feelings of anger, frustration, or rage. Then, after careful discussion, the nurse and patient can find ways to decrease or eliminate the etiologic factors and develop alternative coping mechanisms. Encouraging physical expenditure of energy by exercise, unit jobs, games, or discussion helps decrease anxiety and increase self-esteem.

Parents who feel aggressive tendencies toward their child must learn to deal constructively with their feelings and retain control. Teaching the parents realistic expectations of their child by discussing growth and development in detail helps them recognize and deal with frustrations in childrearing. Also, finding acceptable alternate coping mechanisms for those frustrating times is essential in preventing aggressive violence. This must be done on an individual basis for each parent. Trust is again essential to effectively work toward changing behavior.

To work with abusive families, the nurse must first work through her own feelings and be nonjudgmental and accepting of the family members as persons. She must be able to use confrontation when necessary. Parents who abuse their children generally have not received the love or "mothering" they needed as children and actually lack a basic trust in people. Their basic needs have not been met. Consequently, the parents place unrealistic expectations on the child; the child cannot meet these expectations and in turn becomes neglected or abused. The parent is looking for gratification of needs from the child instead of the reverse—providing the child with these needs. The role of the nurse is to provide support and education for the parents to understand themselves, motivation for behavioral change, and strategies for interacting effectively with others. Parent modeling is equally important for abusive adults. Lay therapists who go into the home and provide a warm parent model for the abusing parent have been found to help reduce the tendency for future abuse and neglect. Intensive work with the nurse, psychiatric clinical nurse specialist, psychotherapist, caseworker, and lay therapist is required for any hope of changing behavior.

The etiology of spouse abuse is similar to that for child abuse. Each spouse may have a tremendous amount of unmet needs, and violence occurs when spouses fail to meet each other's needs. The victim of this abuse must understand that the behavior might not change until the violent person seeks help. The victim may need to get out of the situation. This is a long process and requires maximal support from the nurse.

The first step in nursing care is the assessment process. The nurse must assess a number of factors to know how to intervene. Assessment may be done by verbal interview, visual observation, or information gathered from significant others. The nurse can assess any of the following factors:

1. History of previous homicides, physical or verbal assaults, or suicides
2. Relationships with significant persons and factors in environment that could trigger violent response

3. Conscious awareness of hostile or violent feelings
4. Life experiences that create resentment and bitterness
5. Family history of severe emotional deprivation
6. History of alcohol or drug use or abuse
7. Inability to control behavior following drug or alcohol ingestion
8. Exposure to violent person
9. History of repeated frustrations
10. History of psychiatric treatment
11. Self-concept in relation to others
12. History of medical problems such as epilepsy, head injuries, brain tumor
13. Family violence
14. The nurse's feelings regarding violent behavior
15. Abnormal diagnostic studies performed in conjunction with physician's orders:
    a. Thyroid function
    b. EEG
    c. CT scan
    d. Electrolyte levels
    e. Blood gases
    f. Blood alcohol levels
    g. Blood glucose
    h. Drug levels (blood, urine, gastric)
    i. Renal function
16. Medical history (may be obtained from physician's medical history):
    a. Epilepsy
    b. Head injury
    c. Brain disease
    d. Hormonal balance
    e. Alcohol abuse
    f. Drug abuse
    g. Insomnia

EVALUATION

Patient Outcome	Data Indicating That Outcome is Reached
Self-control	Body relaxed
	Eye contact when communicating
	Verbalization of precipitating factors to incident
	Verbalization of feelings of hopelessness, loneliness, decreased self-esteem
	Verbalization and demonstration of alternatives to violent, aggressive behavior
	Allows trusted person to approach boundaries of personal space
	Knowledge of rationale for limit setting or seclusion, if required
	Verbalization of fears
	Desire to control self
	Admission of remorse or guilt
Verbalization of specific aggressive behavior, feelings of anger, and hostility	Verbalization of sources of anger, frustration or rage
	Verbalization of stress tolerance capacity
	Recognition of perceptual distortions resulting from anger
	Knowledge of physiologic or chemical causes of alterations in behavior (if appropriate)

Patient Outcome	Data Indicating That Outcome is Reached
	Desire to control aggressive behavior Identification and demonstration of appropriate aids to decrease anger and hostility (physical exercise, visual imagery, relaxation techniques)
No overt or covert dangerous behavior	Verbalizes feelings of anger and hostility rather than acting out physically Participation in therapy Ability to effectively cope in conflict situations or role play Verbalization of supports
Adaptive coping mechanisms in conflict situation	Knowledge of alternative ways to deal with aggressive feelings in role playing Ability to maintain self-control Use of thought processes rather than physical response Has perception of violence; acceptable vs. unacceptable in own value system Verbalization of feelings when self-esteem is threatened Ability to effectively cope with threats to self-esteem Identification of constructive ways to increase power Identification of supportive person(s) or groups in environment

References

1. Campbell, C.: Nursing diagnosis and intervention in nursing practice, New York, 1984, John Wiley & Sons, Inc.
2. Carpenito, J.J.: Nursing diagnosis: application to clinical practice, Philadelphia, 1983, J.B. Lippincott Co.
3. Dollard, J., and others: Frustration and aggression, New Haven, Conn., 1939, Yale University Press.
4. Fawcett, J.: Dynamics of violence, Chicago, 1972, American Medical Association.
5. Fromm, E.: The anatomy of human destructiveness, New York, 1973, Holt, Rinehart & Winston, Inc.
6. Kim, M.J., McFarland, G.K., and McLane, A.M., editors: Pocket guide to nursing diagnosis, St. Louis, 1984, The C.V. Mosby Co.
7. Kolb, L.C.: Modern clinical psychiatry, Philadelphia, 1973, W.B. Saunders Co.
8. Liebert, R.M., Neale, J.M., and Davidson, E.S.: The early window: effects of television on children and youth, New York, 1973, Pergamon Press.
9. Lorenz, K.: On aggression, New York, 1966, Harcourt, Brace & World, Inc.
10. May, R.: Power and innocence: a search for the sources of violence, New York, 1972, W.W. Norton Co.
11. Office for Children, Youth and Families: Annual Report to the Governor and the Legislature on the Wisconsin Child Abuse and Neglect Act, Madison, Wisc., 1983, Division of Community Services, Department of Health and Social Services.
12. Stuart, G.W., and Sundeen, S.J.: Principles and practice of psychiatric nursing, St. Louis, 1979, The C.V. Mosby Co.
13. Warner, C.G., and Braen, G.R.: Management of the physically and emotionally abused: emergency assessment, intervention and counseling, Norwalk, Conn., 1982, Appleton-Century-Crofts.
14. Wilson, H.S., and Kneisl, C.R.: Psychiatric nursing, Menlo Park, Calif., 1983, Addison-Wesley Publishing Co.

Suggested Readings

Agee, V.L.: Treatment of the violent incorrigible adolescent, Lexington, Mass., 1979, D.C. Heath & Co.

Anders, R.L.: When a patient becomes violent, Am. J. Nurs. 77(7):1144-1148, 1977.

Basque, L.O., and Merhige, J.: Nurse's experience with dangerous behavior: implications for training, J. Continuing Ed. Nurs. 11(5):47-51, 1980.

Christensen, M.L., Schommer, B.L., and Velasquez, J.: Child abuse. I. An interdisciplinary approach to preventing child abuse, Am. J. Matern. Child Nurs. 9(2):108-112, 1984.

Christensen, M.L., Schommer, B.L., and Velasquez, J.: Child abuse. II. Intensive services help prevent child abuse. Am. J. Matern. Child Nurs. 9(2):113-117, 1984.

DeFelippo, A.M.: Preventing assaultive behavior on a psychiatric unit, Supervisor Nurse 7(6):62-65, 1976.

Erickson, M.D., and Realmuto, G.: Frequency of seclusion in an adolescent psychiatric unit, J. Clin. Psychiatry 44(7):238-241, 1983.

Holding, T.A.: Suicide and "The Befrienders," Br. Med. J. 3:751-753, 1975.

Johnson, R.N.: Aggression in man and animals, Philadelphia, 1972, W.B. Saunders Co.

Levenseler, S.: Role of victim counseling coordinator, J. Emergency Nurs. 6(5):57-59, 1980.

Levy, P., and Hartocollis, P.: Nursing aides and patient violence, Am. J. Psychiatr. 133(4):429-431, 1976.

Penningroth, P.E.: Control of violence in a mental health setting, Am. J. Nurs. 75(4):606-609, 1975.

Phillips, M.: Aggression control in the psychiatric hospital, Dimensions Health Service 54(3):39-41, 1977.

Pisarcik, G.: Violent patient, Nurs. 81 Sept. 1981, pp. 63-65.

Schwab, P.J., and Lahmeyer, C.B.: The uses of seclusion on a general hospital psychiatric unit, J. Clin. Psychiatry 40(5):228-231, 1979.

Shuman, S.I.: Psychosurgery and the medical control of violence, Detroit, 1977, Wayne State University Press.

Sines, D.: The mentally handicapped: a group at risk, Nursing (Oxford) 14:597-600, 1980.

Weissman, M.M., and Klerman, G.L.: Sex differences and the epidemiology of depression, Arch. Gen. Psychiatry 34:98-111, 1977.

Whitman, R.M., Armao, B.V., and Dent, O.B.: Assault on the therapist, Am. J. Psychiatry 133(4):426-429, 1976.

Cognitive-Perceptual

KNOWLEDGE DEFICIT
THEORY AND ETIOLOGY

Knowledge deficit has been defined as an inability to state or explain information or demonstrate a required skill related to disease management procedures, practices, or self-care health management.[5] Knowledge deficit is very common. The patient may have entered a new health condition, such as pregnancy, be undergoing newly prescribed treatments or diagnostic tests, be taking new medications, or beginning a new developmental phase, such as adolescence, parenthood, or old age. If one has not experienced these states before or learned about them from others in the culture, knowledge deficit is possible. In general, health practitioners have not been inclined to consider teaching a prominent part of their practice. Exacerbating this problem are the facts that health care technology has become increasingly complex and difficult to understand and more patients are using it at home for self-care under medical direction.

Standards and Theories

A major point in the preceding definition is the standard for determination of adequate information or required skill. This standard may be changing rapidly as more self-care is required, not only of those with chronic illness, but also to contain health care costs in general and to maintain patients in their normal social settings.

One must distinguish as clearly as possible between the knowledge needed by health professionals and that needed by patients. Patient knowledge is more oriented toward adaptation to living with a health problem, how to seek assistance, or just healthful living. Knowledge of diagnosis, treatment alternatives, physiology, and pathophysiology is relevant only insofar as it promotes better coping and adaptation but not as a mandatory knowledge base.

Sometimes knowledge deficit is defined by a legal standard. The court decision in *Rogers v. Okin*[23] held that committed mental patients are presumed competent to make decisions regarding their treatment in nonemergency situations. Yet only 8% of patients in a state psychiatric hospital who were asked about medications they were taking knew the name of at least one medication, its dosage schedule, and intended effect, and 47% showed no understanding of their medications.[4] In general, a standard of knowledge is justified if it is necessary for safe self-care, if the patient has agreed to it or if it is legally mandated.

Within the context of educational theory, knowledge is the lowest level of cognitive learning—recalling or remembering information as opposed to applying and synthesizing information in problem-solving.[1] In general, it has been found that recalling or remembering is not sufficient for most significant health behavior changes. Attitudinal change, a higher level of understanding, and practiced behavioral sequences with adequate reinforcement are necessary. Much health teaching is still knowledge oriented, probably because it is much easier to teach information than it is to change behavior.

Important behavioral goals in health in which knowledge deficits are of concern include compliance, coping, and decision-making, both within a professional-patient relationship and outside of it. Every person suffers from knowledge deficit in health situations repeatedly. Much can be resolved by the patient himself or by his family or in the natural course of patient-professional interchange if information and interpretation of its application to a particular health care problem are available to patients. Some patients may not know where to seek information; others may have providers who are not interested in teaching them or whom they cannot understand because of cultural or language differences. Knowledge deficit as a diagnostic category is more likely to be used when a person has a temporary or permanent defect in his ability to learn from cues most people find adequate, when he has these abilities but is not motivated to learn, or when information has been misinterpreted or forgotten, causing a clinical crisis. Learning and educational theory provides direction on how to handle each of these problems.

Deficits in knowledge and ability to learn may be reversible with return of normal physiologic function, as with a high blood urea nitrogen concentration or low oxygenation of the blood. Chemical substances such as alcohol and drugs produce not only alterations in thought processes but also knowledge and skill deficits, only some of which may be reversible.

Other deficits, such as brain damage from trauma or cerebral vascular accident, may reverse for a time and then stabilize. Specialized techniques that compensate for the learning deficit are used to help patients relearn skills they once had.

Patients with various levels of mental retardation have knowledge deficits but frequently can remedy these deficits through teaching techniques of operant conditioning. Use of reinforcement, shaping, and other techniques in sustained, persistent learning have been successful in developing knowledge and skill in these people.

Motivation etiologies are less clearly defined but are common among "normal" patients. Again, the question of standard becomes important. It would be fair to say that there has been an implicit medical standard of patient motivation, which is to comply with the medical regimen, and that in general at least a third of patients have not adhered to that standard. Although only a portion of this nonadherence could be said to be the result of knowledge deficits or lack of motivation to obtain the necessary knowledge, lack of will to reach this standard is no doubt involved.

Anxiety that interferes with perception and ability to learn, depression, and denial are common sources of alteration in motivation to remove knowledge deficits. Excessive anxiety often responds to supportive relationships and attainment of knowledge, which allows one to perceive that one is in control of the anxiety-producing situation.

Misinterpretation of health information seems unfortunately to be common and often attributed to lack of ability or interest on the part of health care providers to use any but their own language and conceptual systems. Even though forgetting is normal, apparently an interference of new material learned, both patients and practitioners can do much to avoid forgetting important material. Much material is forgotten because it was never thoroughly learned to begin with. Also, material is remembered if it is rehearsed regularly in one's mind and used. Health professionals' habit of giving a great deal of complex information at once often invites misinterpretation and forgetting because the information is not understood initially. The solution is obvious.

Two major areas of theory underlie the diagnostic area of knowledge deficit. One is learning theory, which speaks to the basic mechanisms by which deficits can be avoided or removed. Much more complete treatises on this subject can be found elsewhere.[22]

The second area of theory is the value base for definition of a knowledge deficit on the part of the health consumer or patient. The literature of informed consent elucidates the predominant cluster of these values. Autonomy is seen as the goal of informed patients, so they can participate in decision-making about their care in a way that meets the concept of informed consent. Knowledge is presumed to be with the physician. Suffering is an undesirable evil or one to be borne only temporarily. Action and control are valued over passivity. Rationality, forthright communication, and self-determination are highly valued, and the doctrine of informed consent (which is the main societal standard, embodied in the law) manifests, promotes, and protects these interests.[21]

Another cluster of values with which nursing theory is more compatible is embodied in the concept of coping. In many ways this cluster forms a dialectic with those of informed consent. Its goals are to attain a sense of acceptance; the process is one of contending with the problem; and the relationship with the professional is on equal terms. This means that a knowledge deficit is not presumed but is jointly diagnosed by the professional and the patient from the skills and knowledge necessary to meet an adequate coping resolution. Clinicians can see both value clusters used and should realize that they conflict.

Assessment in Determination of Etiology

Assessment must include gathering of data about the patient's perception of his health condition, his theory for why it occurred, and what might be done about it. Objective data include his ability to correctly answer questions and perform tasks, his level of cognitive and psychomotor development, presence of sensory deficits (vision, hearing, touch), and basic physiologic func-

1. **Discovery of learning needs from individual family members themselves.** A questionnaire in which family members are asked to project themselves into a certain situation reveals many needs. For example:

   a. As you were preparing to come to visit the stroke patient today, what worries about the patient, medical-nursing treatment, or rehabilitation came into your mind?

____ Tests (what's going to happen)	____ How can another stroke be prevented?
____ Quality of nursing care today	____ Can I talk with the doctor?
____ Test results	____ Patient's eating
____ Condition of the stroke patient	____ Bowel and bladder problems
____ Therapy (when and how often)	____ My own health
____ Recovery	____ Other (please explain) _____

   b. What do you wish you understood better about stroke?

____ Causes of stroke	____ How to cope
____ Could it have been prevented?	____ The effects on the person
____ How the brain works	____ Behavior
____ What actually happens when you have a stroke	____ Other (please explain) _____
____ What to expect	

   c. Since the stroke, what problems do you feel least adequate to deal with?

____ Patient's behavior, temper	____ My own feelings
____ Patient's emotions	____ Daily activities
____ Patient's depression	____ Money matters at home
____ Physical disabilities	____ Car problems
____ Speech problems	

   d. When you think about life a year from now, what do you feel most insecure about?

____ Handling the patient's needs	____ Having friends
____ Lifting the patient	____ Having a meaningful life
____ The "changes" in the person	____ Our sexual relationship
____ Having enough money	____ Loneliness
____ Taking care of the house	____ Being unable to cope
____ Family-marriage relationship	____ Other (please explain) _____

2. **Discovery of learning needs from people in helping roles with the stroke patient.** Draw from your own experience and from the experiences of those on your advisory committee to whom patients and family members have brought questions. Ask the following questions of yourself and of your committee:
   - What questions do patients and family members most often ask?
   - What kinds of complaints do we receive?
   - What procedures do we perform that families seem most anxious about?

   Answers to these questions in a brainstorming session, along with results from patient-family questionnaires, will help you diagnose learning needs of patients and families and generate main topic areas for your stroke education program. Here are examples of main topic areas that may have resulted from your work in Step 1:

   a. The brain and how it works
   b. Cause and effects of stroke
   c. Risk factors in stroke
   d. Medical and nursing procedures
   e. Occupational and physical therapy
   f. Communication problems
   g. Emotional reactions to stroke
   h. Leisure, recreational, and community programs

From VanMeter, M.J.: Neurologic care: a guide for patient education, New York, 1982, Appleton-Century-Crofts.

tions necessary for cognition, such as circulation, respiration, nutrition, and hydration.

The questionnaire on p. 1953 gathers more subjective than objective information but clearly shows how an assessment can be used to plan educative programs.

Examples of assessment of knowledge deficit portray the kind of thinking involved in obtaining evidence of knowledge and comparing it against a standard, at least an implicit one. This standard forms the base for decisions about whether an intervention is needed and, if so, what its goals should be.

A study[14] in Britain found that in a sample of 50 women aged 40 to 53 years, drawn from a general practice list, 40% had incorrect ideas about menopause. This was used as justification for starting a menopause information group. The implicit standard is that all women should understand menopause at least in experiential terms, if not its scientific basis.

In a second example, a study[8] found that 60% of a group of low-income women reported becoming pregnant at least one time when they did not want to be. Sixty-four percent did not know when it is possible to become pregnant; 60% did not know if women can become pregnant while breastfeeding; and 37% did not know if pregnancy can occur during menopausal years. About 65% reported what was judged by the investigators to be incorrect use of oral contraceptives. The presumption of the study is that these knowledge deficits probably played a role in ineffective contraception, although the study provided no direct evidence of this.

A final example comes from a series of studies in the nursing literature about knowledge deficits among parents about growth and development in infants. In one study[24] about 13% of the mothers expected their babies to be aware from birth; some did not expect to begin teaching their babies until 1 year of age; and some thought talking to the child was not especially important until 2 years of age. Those who expected their children to develop at later ages provided significantly less stimulating environments for them, and these children showed lower indicators of development at 1 and 2 years of age. The question unanswered by this study but strongly implied is whether appropriate instruction would change parents' expectations and thus their stimulation of their babies and the babies' developmental levels. The study found no relationship between the mother's expectations and the number of antepartal classes they attended and surmised that this content was probably not taught in these classes.

Jarrett[7] studied mothers aged 15 to 21 years, largely from low socioeconomic groups. Half these mothers expected their child to sit without support before 6 months; the norm is 7 to 8 months. Most thought their child would take its first step before 12 months; the norm is 12 to 15 months. The concern was that some parents physically

punished their children for not being able to do these developmental tasks long before the child was biologically ready.

A final study[11] done with middle class mother-father pairs found incorrect knowledge of half of the 20 developmental milestones in motor, language, and social development in the first 2 years of life.

The implicit standard used in these studies of knowledge deficit of infant development is a futuristic one based to some extent on new knowledge about infant development. The evidence that must be obtained is what kind of intervention would wipe out the knowledge deficit *and* also yield the outcome desired (that is, adequate stimulation of infants, thus hastening their development; or lack of punishment for inappropriate developmental expectations, thus leading to better mental health and parent-child relationships).

Since the kinds of knowledge deficits demonstrated in these studies are not at all uncommon in multiple areas of health care, a second question would be in which of those many situations one would wish to invest intervention resources. Snyder[25] believes that assessing parents' expectations should be a routine part of prenatal care, that this takes little time, and that administering the Brazleton test of development with parents is highly instructive.

DEFINING CHARACTERISTICS

Verbalization of a problem, which can point out lack of knowledge or perception of inability to cope[9]

Inaccurate or no follow-through of instructions[9]

Inadequate performance of a test or a task[9]

Inappropriate or exaggerated behaviors, such as, hysterical, hostile, agitated, apathetic[9]

Occurrence of a preventable and undesired event

Inability to make a decision about own care

Not seeking needed services

Infant or child not meeting developmental norms because of actions of caregiver

Living with a health problem, below level of potential well-being

Overdependence on others for self-care

Essentially all evidence of knowledge deficit is more or less indirect. What one tries to do with assessment is set up situations in which the quality of the inference obtained from verbalizations or behaviors is as strong and direct as possible: ask the patient directly or set up an unobtrusive test for him. Since most meaningful health behaviors require knowledge, motivation, and skill, it is important in the assessment to seek evidence in each of these areas to obtain as complete a diagnosis as possible. This means data gathered must be both objective, to determine adequacy of present knowledge and behaviors, and subjective, which is the source of crucial information about motivation, the patient's frame of reference, and cognitive schemata.

A diagnosis of knowledge deficit means the evidence gathered does not meet the standard of adequate knowledge, but as indicated in the discussion of theory, one must be quite certain that the standard is justified and that one intends to provide an opportunity for the patient to learn.

NURSING INTERVENTIONS

Patient Goal	Nursing Intervention
Increase knowledge or decrease cognitive deficit.	Communities and institutions provide freely available information through reading materials, hotlines, mass media.
	At every provider-patient interaction, assess for knowledge deficit.
	Talk to the patient's significant other to obtain evidence of knowledge deficit.
	Use the patient's theories about his illness as a starting point for teaching.
	During interactions check frequently to see if the patient understands.
	See if the patient accepts his diagnosis.
	Simplify the information to conform to the patient's terms and thought patterns and daily routines.
	Give explicit directions.
	Be accessible to the patient when he has a question; this may require new structures of care such as a diabetes education center.
	Demonstrate to patient and family how to use the information.
	Reinforce correct use of information, and get others in the patient's natural environment to do so.
	Teach the patient how to set up a system of cues in his environment to remember health actions.
	Teach the patient how to mentally rehearse a health action he should take.
	Teach the patient how to use rewards for positive health behaviors.
	Call the patient to remind him, show support, and see if he has questions.
	Make certain the patient is actively involved in decisions about his care.
	Provide opportunities for him to gain a sense of control over his illness.
	Offer a peer support network and opportunity for patient to watch others successfully mastering health care problems.
	Ask the patient if he is satisfied with his care.
	Use practice of knowledge and skill, perhaps with role-playing, until the patient feels satisfied and has met the standard.
	Use special teaching approaches to deal with neurologic learning deficits.

In general, nursing goals include helping the patient attain the knowledge and skills needed through the teaching and learning process, which includes assessing readiness, planning realistic goals, developing a teaching plan using appropriate multiple verbal, behavioral, and audiovisual instructional strategies, and evaluation of learning and reteaching when necessary.[24]

Active involvement of the patient is essential, as is practice of the thoughts and behaviors to be learned. For many, psychologic support and follow-up are important, as are a feeling of personal reward sometimes developed through a contract with the provider and involvement of the family.

Not all the interventions necessary for knowledge deficit have been seen to be within the purview of nursing. An unclear boundary divides information transfer assumed to be the prerogative and responsibility of the physician from that available to other direct care providers. The old model of total control by the physician of all information flow to the patient has broken down because of increasing assignment of responsibility for patient welfare to institutions, such as hospitals.

What has replaced this old model is not a clear division of responsibility among professions but rather a large variety of institutional policies and programs that usually incompletely allocate responsibility for certain areas of patient knowledge and skill deficit. Perhaps the best that can be said is that under this new scheme, nursing departments often take major responsibility for development and implementation of programs in which patients obtain needed information.

Preventive Care

It is clear that knowledge deficits can be prevented, if sources from which to obtain the knowledge are made available and if the patient is motivated enough to learn. One approach is to invest in general health knowledge development by many individuals in schools, work sites, churches and other social institutions, and community programs of health care institutions. These programs are increasingly available although frequently targeted to that knowledge which can be used to prevent a particular health disorder. An example is hypertension education and screening efforts, in which those who do not have hypertension learn about risk factors and how to control them. Businesses have found that such prevention programs can save them money in time lost from work and in insurance benefits. Since making information available costs money, social institutions with purposes other than education or health are likely to provide such information when it has a fairly direct payoff of employee health and good will. And, within health and education institutions, one has to compete with other subject matter.

A second way in which information can be made available to prevent knowledge deficits is to provide it to individuals as part of their health care. Again, it would seem much more likely that the time would be taken to provide this information if a specific and probable payoff from the information was identified. Although general health education is available through mass media, availability of this information through counseling by health professionals is highly variable. Some examples from the research literature seem pertinent.

One study[13] of patients with coronary artery disease tried to track retrospectively the types of preventive recommendations these patients had received during the 5 years prior to development of symptoms. During this time they had had two or more risk factors. Health practitioners were in many cases identifying individuals at risk for coronary artery disease but often failed to provide for them action structures and reinforcers, two important mechanisms for achieving behavior change.

Another example of preventive care to prevent knowledge deficit is the strongly research-based practice of preparation of patients for diagnostic or therapeutic procedures. The research base has shown that provision of objective and subjective sensory information apparently provides realistic mental schemata that help patients interpret the procedures as they experience them. Johnson's research[8] provides guidelines for giving the sensory information: (1) physical sensations should be described but not evaluated; (2) patients should be told what causes the sensations so they will be less apt to misinterpret them and conclude something has gone wrong; (3) patients should be prepared only for those aspects of the experience which are noticed by the majority of patients.

We suggest that nurses on units develop their message by talking to patients until they have identified those aspects of the messages that are noticed by 50% of the patients, and to note also the words often used by patients to describe the sensations. After the message is developed, its effect can be evaluated by the amount of sedation needed, facial and verbal expressions, degree of cooperation, and length of hospitalization.[16]

Supportive Care

Sometimes efforts to remove a knowledge deficit are primarily supportive but essential to other therapeutic interventions that are ongoing. Indeed, the search for meaning and understanding is an inevitable part of any encounter with a health concern. The usefulness of work on these knowledge deficits sometimes can be documented in relation to an important outcome. An example is a study of 12 families who had at least one teenage child with severe hemophilia on a home treatment program. Especially with mothers and patients less than 15 years of age, the better informed the individual was about the disease, the less psychologic distress he or she reported.[10]

The strong drive people have to assign causality and to search for meaning can be seen in the stages that Horan[6] summarized about parents with a defective baby. The environment of prospective parents is saturated with information they use to form thoughts about their expected baby; very little of the information concerns the possibility of a defective baby. At first parents recall the pregnancy and investigate immediate and extended families, trying to assign blame for the defect. This is an effort to gain a feeling of control, since knowing the cause suggests that the problem can be prevented from happening again. Eventually, parents begin to accept the negative feelings and finally reach out to each other and to social supports for coping with both the present and the future.

Patients who had had myocardial infarctions, and their spouses, engaged in a similar perceptual-interpretive process whereby a succession of causal explanations were explored and evaluated. Interactions with health professionals were evidently extremely influential direction-setting experiences for these people and moved them onto a postattack course.[24]

There is concern that a wider array of resources be available to provide supportive information. Overlook Hospital in Summit, New Jersey, opened its Consumer Health Information Library in 1981, following a survey which found that 38% of respondents were unable to locate medical information they needed.[18] The President's Commission for the Study of Ethical Problems in Medicine, in its study of informed consent, recommended that hospital and public libraries be available to assist individuals with access to whatever medical information they desire.[21]

Education as a Direct Intervention

It is often unclear whether an educational intervention is primarily preventive, supportive, or a major thread of intervention in the care of a patient. For example, the ability of a chronically ill patient to maintain the quality of his life depends on his constant ability to continue to affirm himself, to collaborate in his care through learning, to endure certain pathologic and technical givens, and to actively negotiate and bargain for his needs.[20] This kind of need requires preventive, supportive, and direct work to alleviate knowledge deficits, with the patient often taking the major role within the context of available medical knowledge and skills.

Other educational needs require specialized skills. The 300,000 persons who survive a stroke each year should be tested for (1) ability to deal with all aspects of language (speaking, writing, understanding spoken words, and reading), (2) performance modalities of visual-motor perception and spatial coordination, (3) auditory and visual retention spans, and (4) ideational and problem-solving abilities that require integration of new stimuli with past learning. In general, left brain damage affects language skills, so the patient must learn through nonverbal modalities such as pantomime, demonstration, and imitating steps. Those with right brain damage have visual-motor perception impairment, often with impulsive behavior, lack of organization and ability to initiate planned actions, and without insight into personal difficulties. The patient must be taught through detailed schedules of daily events with verbal instructions to initiate activities. Since none of the predictors is precise enough to predict individual outcome, it is believed that no patient should be excluded from rehabilitation unless he is too ill or has had too much cognitive damage to participate.[2]

Sufficient research has now been done on patient education interventions, particularly with certain health problems or treatments, to allow summarization of studies. Summarizing 34 studies of psychologic intervention effects on recovery from surgery and heart attacks, Mumford[19] found (1) on the average, patients provided information or emotional support did better than patients who received only ordinary care and reduced hospitalization 2 days below control groups; and (2) a combination of approaches to offer emotional support and relieve anxiety *and* educational approaches were clearly superior to either of these approaches alone.

In summarizing studies on the effect of patient education in chronic disease, Mazzuca[15] found it to be significantly effective over control groups in altering compliance, physiologic progress, and health outcome. Didactic emphasis with invariant presentation of medical facts intended for all patients with a single chronic medical problem was rarely successful alone. Patient education with a behavioral emphasis was more successful, especially if the patient's own regimen and daily routine were the content of instruction and if the intervention tried to affect the patient's work or home environment in ways that promoted self-management, such as memory aids, social support, medication monitoring, or phone follow-up.

The recent interest in educational interventions for cognitive deficits represents a turning of theory toward more complex cognitive variables as explanations for complex behavior.

Learning in health care settings as they exist at present has many constraints for adequate knowledge and skill development. This has occurred in part because what was reimbursed and therefore rewarded were medical procedures, not adapted patients. At the same time it is clearly possible to alter delivery of care so that teaching and learning are expected and rewarded components of care and consistent over sufficient periods of time so that complex learning can occur. Diabetes education and detection centers and oncology centers are examples of these new organizations of services in which education and learning are central. These interventions cluster to deal with the etiologies discussed earlier.

EVALUATION

Patient Outcome	Data Indicating That Outcome is Reached
Adequate knowledge and skill to support needed self-care activities, including procedures, medications, when to seek care, use of appropriate community resources	Can explain how and why he will take an action or perform a skill Takes appropriate action when necessary and can explain appropriate reasoning process
Use of knowledge in a health care decision satisfactory to the patient, such as whether to have surgery, what kinds of regimens to which he can agree	Can describe how he assesses the benefits and costs to him of a particular health action Can describe why he made a decision and that he is prepared to follow through with the required treatment activities
Knowledge of how to guide own and others' development in the area of health	Monitors body and mental state for signs and symptoms of illness Acts on the basis of realistic expectations in guiding the development of self and others
Competent to carry out health care activities necessary to his well-being	Can describe how to use verified health knowledge in daily living Moves ahead to take health actions when satisfied they are worthwhile

Patient Outcome	Data Indicating That Outcome is Reached
Knowledge to cope adequately with health stresses	Knows where to get sources of health care information efficiently and does so when needed Can describe the problem-solving process to successfully deal with an injury, a threatening diagnosis, a persistent symptom Describes how his action met his standards of adequate coping

Evaluation means to make a judgment about the quality of the outcomes obtained, in this case from an intervention designed to alleviate a cognitive or skill deficit. In general, evaluation is done informally as part of the interaction of clinical practice, with questioning, patient demonstration of skills, and patient reporting of use of knowledge and skills in everyday living. Although there is concern that these methods are not standardized enough to ensure that patients are adequately taught, there is little movement toward development of strong measurement tools.

Evaluation of instruction commonly finds significant knowledge deficits remaining. For example, patients who had undergone open heart surgery were asked to recall what information they had been given. The results were heart function (55%), surgical procedure (65%), diet (75%), drugs (90%), care of incision (45%), activity (55%), and complications (50%). The question, "Was there anything you were not told you would have found helpful during recovery?" resulted in an outpouring of patient anxieties and uncertainties. About 27% wanted information about pain and 69% about activity, including specifics on how to increase activities, low cholesterol and sodium diets, signs and symptoms of complications, and when to report them.[17]

After sessions for informed consent for cardiac catheterization it was found that the risk of significant arrhythmias, heart damage, length of the catheter, and other items were not well understood by many patients. About 15% did not understand that a heart attack is a form of heart damage.[3]

Parents who had had genetic counseling were questioned regarding their understanding of rate information. Although information was recalled accurately by parents, they overwhelmingly perceived the chance of recurrence in binary form—it either will or will not happen. This appeared to be a simplifying strategy to deal with ambiguous medical information in which there is often no 1:1 correspondence between a diagnosis and level of health functioning it would permit, and to meet the couple's need for normalization. Parents dealt not with chances but with scenarios in which the worst of the acceptable events and consequences happened.[12] So the gap was not in knowledge but in how it was used. Is this an acceptable outcome from the intervention?

The above criteria may seem ambitious. They are meant to incorporate the many knowledge-deficit-removal activities that are part of everyday care. They also are meant to reflect the fact that we have generally been satisfied with a very low level of independent thinking and knowledge in health on the part of the public. The status quo is not likely to be an effective strategy. We know that good health habits and the patient's ability to care for himself and to use health professionals as consultants increase his commitment to doing so and are likely to decrease demand for costly health care services.

References

1. Bloom, B.S., editor: Taxonomy of education objectives: the classification of educational goals. Handbook I. Cognitive domain, New York, 1956, David McKay Co., Inc.
2. Delisa, J.A., and others: Stroke rehabilitation. Part I. Cognitive deficits and prediction of outcomes, Am. Fam. Physician **26:**207-214, 1982.
3. Freeman, W.R., Pichard, A.D., and Smith, H.: Effect of informed consent and educational background on patient knowledge, anxiety, and subjective responses to cardiac catheterization, Catheter. Cardiovasc. Diagnosis **7:**119-134, 1981.
4. Geller, J.L.: State hospital patients and their medication: do they know what they take? Am. J. Psychiatr. **139:**611-615, 1982.
5. Gordon, J.: Manual of nursing diagnosis, New York, 1982, McGraw-Hill Book Co.
6. Horan, M.L.: Parental reaction to the birth of an infant with a defect: an attributional approach, Adv. Nurs. Sci. **5:**57-68, 1982.
7. Jarrett, G.: Childrearing patterns of young mothers: expectations, knowledge and practices, Matern. Child Nurs. **7:**119-121, 1982.
8. Johnson, S.M., and Snow, L.F.: Assessment of reproductive knowledge in an inner-city clinic, Soc. Sci. Med. **16:**1657-1662, 1982.
9. Kim, M.J., and Moritz, D.A.: Classification of nursing diagnoses: proceedings of the Third and Fourth National Conferences, New York, 1982, McGraw-Hill Book Co.
10. Klein, R.H., and Nimorwica, P.: The relationship between psychological distress and knowledge of disease among hemophilia patients and their families: a pilot study, J. Psychosom. Res. **26:**387-391, 1982.
11. Linde, D.B., and Engelhardt, K.F.: What do parents know about infant development? Pediatr. Nurs. **5**(1):32-36, 1979.
12. Lippman-Hand, A., and Fraser, F.C.: Genetic counseling: the post-counseling period. I. Parents' perceptions of uncertainty, Am. J. Med. Genet. **4:**51-71, 1979.
13. Lovvorn, J.: Types of preventive health cues given to high-risk individuals, Heart Lung **10:**520-524, 1981.
14. Martin-Burnham, L.A.: The menopause: how much do women know? Health Visitor **54:**200-201, 1981.
15. Mazzuca, S.A.: Does patient education in chronic disease have therapeutic value? J. Chronic Dis. **35:**521-529, 1982.
16. McHugh, N.G., Christman, N.J., and Johnson, J.E.: Preparatory information: what helps and why? Am. J. Nurs. **82:**780-782, 1982.
17. Meyer, R.M., and Latz, P.A.: What open heart surgery patients want to know, Am. J. Nurs. **79:**1558-1560, 1979.
18. Moeller, K.A., and Deeney, K.E.: Documenting the need for consumer health information: results of a community survey, Bull. Med. Libr. Assoc. **70**(2):236-239, 1982.
19. Mumford, E., Schlesinger, H.J., and Glass, G.V.: The effects of psychological intervention on recovery from surgery and heart attacks: an analysis of the literature, Am. J. Public Health **72:**141-151, 1982.

20. Olbrisch, M.E., and Ziegler, S.W.: Psychological adjustment to inflammatory bowel disease: informational control and private self-consciousness, J. Chronic Dis. **35:**573-580, 1982.
21. President's Commission for the Study of Ethical Problems in Medicine and Biomedical and Behavioral Research: Making health care decisions, Washington, D.C., 1982.
22. Redman, B.K.: The process of patient education, ed. 5, St. Louis, 1983, The C.V. Mosby Co.
23. *Rogers v Okin,* F. Supp. 1342 (D. Mass. 1979).
24. Rudy, E.B.: Patients' and spouses' causal explanations of a myocardial infarction, Nurs. Res. **29:**352-356, 1980.
25. Snyder, C., Hures, S.J., and Barnard, K.: New findings about mothers' antenatal expectations and their relationship to infant development, Matern. Child Nurs. **4:**354-357, 1979.

THOUGHT PROCESSES, ALTERATION IN

THEORY AND ETIOLOGY

The essence of who we are as human beings apart from other animals evolves from the existence of mental faculties that allow us to think, to feel, to remember, to believe, to create, to dream. The hows and whys of this essence have been a focal point of study and exploration for centuries. Yet much of the knowledge about the mind and its functioning remains elusive, controversial, and the focus of multiple theoretical explanations.

Certain characteristics, however, have proven to be common denominators in most theoretical discourse on the mind[6]:

1. The mind is housed in the brain, a complexly functioning physical and chemical entity.
2. The principal functions of the mind are storage, organization, interpretation, and retrieval of internal and external data.
3. These functions are accomplished through processes such as thinking, learning, remembering, feeling, perceiving, creating, imagining, willing, and other, yet to be identified, phenomena.
4. These processes are active in nature and are highly interrelated.
5. These processes are internal and explainable more in a phenomenologic rather than an empirical sense.

Theoretical exploration of the mind and its functions and processes has spawned an entire branch in a discipline. It is known as cognitive psychology and is dedicated to the study of higher mental processes (thinking, perceiving, remembering, learning, language) using the scientific method. Information processing has become a major paradigm used to direct such studies. Neobehaviorism, learning theories, human engineering, communications engineering, and linguistics have all influenced the development of the information processing paradigm.[15] Information processing essentially formulates theories in the format of programs to be run on computers. The aim is to have the computer go through the actions that simulate cognitive actions underlying specific human behavior. Unlike behavioral models of the past, which focused on finer analysis of progressively simpler behavior, the information processing theorists have attempted to synthesize complex behaviors. Thus there is an attempt to observe and measure internal processes.[10,15]

The major body of work on cognitive functioning is that of Piaget. His work spans nearly 60 years and represents a developmental approach to the study of cognition. His focus is on the structure of cognition as opposed to its content or function. However, he addresses all three issues. Cognitive content is viewed as raw, uninterpreted behavioral data. Cognitive function is viewed as an active organized process of adaptation. Adaptation is comprised of accommodation and assimilation (of reacting to and acting on the environment). Content varies with time, but the functions of organization and adaptation are invariant.[9]

Interposed between content and function is Piaget's idea of cognitive structure (schema). These structures are the organizational properties of cognition. They are created through functioning and are inferred from the behavioral contents whose nature they determine. Piaget states that structures are "mediators interposed between the invariant functions on the one hand and the variegated behavioral contents on the other."[9]

Structures form the basis for Piaget's developmental stages, and at any given stage they represent cognitive organization. Through a process of equilibration, in the course of development, old structures are modified and replaced by new structures. In general, the movement is from concrete to abstract, specific to general, static to dynamic, egocentric to universal.

Bruner[2] also contributed greatly to cognitive theory. Like Piaget, Bruner has a developmental focus and his theory of cognitive growth contains three modes of thinking that occur in orderly stages: the enactive mode is cognition through action; the iconic mode is perceptual in nature; and the symbolic mode enables the translation of experience into language, thus allowing transformations similar to those discussed by Piaget. Unlike those of Piaget, Bruner's stages, while appearing in an orderly developmental sequence, do not replace one another. Thus an adult has access to all three cognitive modes. Adult thinking in fact is characterized by the simultaneous interplay and processing of the three modes.[2]

Unlike Piaget, Bruner attaches major importance to language for its role in cognition. For Bruner and others, such as Whorf,[4] language is a basic structure of thought. Bruner viewed the role of language as guiding and amplifying thought. Whorf stated that thought was most mysterious, with the greatest understanding of the thought processes coming through the study of language. He saw the structure of language as influencing the way we think and ultimately behave in relation to our environment. We also represent and symbolize our thoughts through language.

Chomsky,[5] a leading linguist, proposed the transformative generative theory. He attempted to relate sound and meaning by positing an underlying structure that governed language and speech. His model constituted a representation of the process that we go through to translate and communicate our experience. When we wish to speak, we form a linguistic representation of our experience called a deep structure. As we speak we make a series of choices (transformations) about the form in which we will speak. These choices are generally unconscious. Thus the structure of the spoken word (surface structure) can be analyzed for fuller understanding of the deep structure because the transformations or choices are rule governed.

Although interest in the specifics of Chomsky's theory has waned, his views of the relationship between thought and language have changed the paradigms in psychology and linguistics. His theory has also given rise to a new form of psychotherapy known as neurolinguistic programming.[1]

At this point there is little argument that thought and language are closely tied and interrelated. Therefore it is logical to assume that alterations in thought are reflected in the language behavior of the individual. The nursing interventions presented in this chapter are based on this tie between cognitive processes and language.

It is a paradox that the same cognitive processes that allow survival, growth, and change can also block growth, inhibit change, and produce limitations in living. Through the cognitive processes (thought, perception, memory, judgment) we create our own unique representation or model of reality. That model is bounded by physical, social, and psychologic factors that make each of our representations unique.

Three chief mechanisms are used in our model making: (1) generalization, (2) deletion, and (3) distortion.[1] Generalization is the process by which elements from an experience structure themselves to represent a category of which the experience is an example. For example, we generalize from the experience of being cut that knives are sharp and must be used with care. This is a useful and necessary coping skill. If, however, we were to refuse to use knives at all or to even have knives in the house as a result of being cut, then our generalization has become limiting.

Deletion is a process of selective attention to certain parts of an experience, for example, the ability to read while the television is on. Deletion allows us to manage our world and not be overwhelmed. However, we can also use deletion in ways that are limiting, such as not hearing compliments about our accomplishments and hearing only criticism.

Distortion is a process of experience shifting. It allows us to interpret experience under a different set of circumstances or to project an experience into the future, for example, fantasizing. Distortion can also be limiting if experiences are shifted in a limiting fashion: compliments about accomplishments might be heard but shifted to mean that the purveyor of the compliment must want something.

These three mechanisms work together to create our model of reality. An alteration in cognitive processes then disrupts or distorts our model. These alterations can be detected by viewing the individual's model of reality as expressed symbolically in language behavior. Exploration of the individual's use of generalization, deletion, and distortion can clarify his reality model. Limiting uses of generalization, deletion, and distortion can then be challenged. This allows individuals to broaden their models of reality.

An issue that should be addressed when considering the nursing diagnosis alteration in thought process is the subsuming of the diagnosis altered levels of consciousness under it.[13] The prevailing view at the Fifth National Conference was to call consciousness, altered levels of, a diagnosis in its own right, complete with specified defining characteristics. Therefore altered levels of consciousness was listed as a diagnosis to be developed and presented for action at a later conference.[11] Thus the development of the diagnosis alteration in thought processes here is done in light of the action at the Fifth National Conference.

Alterations in thought processes and sensory-perceptual alterations as nursing diagnoses are closely aligned. Many of the defining characteristics and nursing strategies are similar. This is to be expected because perception and thought are both higher order cognitive processes. Because the two processes are internal and highly interrelated, an alteration in either process is likely to produce an alteration in the other. (See section on sensory-perceptual alteration for a full discussion.)

Carpenito[3] makes a distinction between the two diagnoses on the basis of etiology. She states that sensory-perceptual alterations result from environmental, sensory, physical, or motor alterations. Alterations in thought processes are seen as stemming from personality and mental disorders. This may serve as a viable distinction, although it should be noted that both diagnoses share some common etiological ground (for example, chemical alteration). Based on this distinction, Carpenito offers the following definition of alteration in thought processes: "A state in which an individual experiences a disruption in such mental activities as conscious thought, reality orientation, problem-solving, judgment, and comprehension related to coping disorders."

The following are etiologies for alteration in thought processes[3,8,12,16]:

Physiologic changes
Biochemical change
Genetic predispositions
Psychologic conflicts
Ineffective coping
Loss of memory
Sleep deprivation
Substance abuse
Mental disorders and illnesses

DEFINING CHARACTERISTICS

Disruption of thinking process
   Disorientation in time, place, person, circumstances, or
      events
   Disordered sequencing of thought
   Impaired ability to think abstractly
   Impaired ability to solve problems and make decisions
   Impaired reasoning ability
   Impaired ability to grasp ideas
   Impaired ability to calculate
   Concretizing of ideas
Memory disruption
   Memory deficit
   Changes in remote, recent, immediate memory
   Confabulation
Changes in attention span
   Distractibility
   Difficulty concentrating
   Inability to follow flow of conversation
Emotional changes
   Feelings of worthlessness
   Extreme sadness
   Mistrust
   Guilt

Anger
Anxiety
Lability
Exaggerated response
Fear of others, of losing control, of falling apart
Decreased or shallow affect
Apathy
Inaccurate interpretation of stimuli
   Hallucinations
   Delusions
   Ideas of reference
   Obsessions
Changes in routine patterns and habits
   Altered sleep pattern
   Insomnia
   Too much sleep
   Change in grooming habits
   Change in eating habits
   Change in motor activity: repetition, agitation
   Hypervigilance
   Inappropriate social behavior
Bizarre thinking as noted by language use
   Inappropriate use of global pronouns, global adjectives
   Evidence of automatic thinking: universal "you know,"
      assumption that listener knows omitted details
   Circumstantiality: inability to get to the point
   Lack of verbal distinction between thoughts, feelings, ac-
      tions
   Use of indirect statements, extensive use of modifiers and
      qualifiers
   Overgeneralization
   Imputing intentions to others
   Loose connection of ideas
   Use of neologisms

A disruption in thought processes, whether in the area of comprehension, judgment, memory, problem-solving, or other aspects, creates a disruption in the way we perceive reality. Thus our thinking processes become non–reality based, the critical defining characteristic for this nursing diagnosis. (Note the similarity of this critical defining characteristic and that for sensory perceptual alterations.)

Additional defining characteristics assist in the evaluation of severity of non–reality-based thinking and the extent of the thought alteration. Any number or combination of defining characteristics can be manifested by a client. These additional characteristics are grouped and subgrouped by the nature of the characteristic.[3,12,17]

NURSING INTERVENTIONS

Patient Goal	Nursing Intervention
Prevent physical injury to self and others.	Maintain patient safety; prevent suicide and aggression: 1. Assess for suicide potential (history, plans for self-harm, verbalization of desire to die, disposal of possessions, viewing self in the past tense). 2. Institute suicide precautions as indicated. 3. Assess potential for aggressive behavior. 4. Identify early signs of aggressive behavior.

Patient Goal	Nursing Intervention
	5. Remove environmental factors that contribute to aggression.
	6. Promote individual control (set limits on destructive behavior, encourage verbalization and safe acting-out behaviors within limits, allow choice within constraint, use seclusion if indicated).
	7. Help patient set limits on own behavior (substitute verbalizations and physical activity for behavioral acting out, set incremental goals, recall and repeat successful ways of coping).
Reduce anxiety or stress.	Approach in calm, nurturing manner (use calm, level voice, lower tone, familiar terms, avoid sudden movements, compose facial expression).
	Provide physical and emotional structure as needed (physical: environment altered to provide for safety and comfort; emotional: prediction of feelings and occurrences, imaging of situations that evoke safety and comfort).
Enhance realistic and constructive interpretations of reality.	Explore patient's representation of reality by analyzing language behavior:
	1. Listen intently to patient's verbal and nonverbal communication.
	2. Analyze communication for generalizations (use of global pronouns and adjectives), deletions (automatic knowing), distortions (imputing intentions to others, loose connections of ideas).
	Assist patient in clarifying representation of reality by:
	1. Clarifying generalizations ("Nobody pays any attention to what I say." Clarify who specifically. What specifically do you say?)
	2. Eliciting deletions in communication ("I am scared." Scared about what?)
	3. Clarifying nominalizations. Change statements of event into statements of process ("I hate my relationship with my wife." Explore "relating" as a process versus "relationship" as an event.)
	4. Challenging distortions of control ("Steve makes me act up." Repeat statement with emphasis on "Steve makes?" Explore how that is possible.)
	5. Challenging distortions that impute intentions to others ("The doctor hates me." Analyze basis for statement: "What was said or done that makes you feel your doctor hates you?")
	Use reality orientation where indicated:
	1. Orient to person, time, and place.
	2. Use direct terminology, clear sentence structure.
	3. Avoid generalization.
	4. Use terms that help patient maintain individuality (such as "I" instead of "we").
	5. Avoid vagueness, asides, whispered comments.
	6. Have patient focus on real things and people.
Increase ability to relate with others positively.	Provide group process situations that allow patients to experience relating in a controlled setting.
	Encourage validation of thoughts and feelings.
	Encourage patient to ask for wants and to express feelings.
	Help patient examine the effect of behavior on others.
	Help patient recognize use of and need for personal space and distance.
Enhance responsibility for self-care.	Provide opportunity for patient to contribute to own treatment plan.
	Encourage acceptance of responsibility for actions and interactions.
	Encourage acceptance of responsibility for seeking help, following treatment plans, and changing behaviors.

The goal of nursing intervention for persons with alteration in thought processes is to improve the individual's ability to define and communicate reality. This goal is achieved primarily through a patient-nurse dyadic interaction or small group process. Such encounters frequently occur in, but need not be limited to, mental health care settings. Nursing intervention strategies are aimed at reducing or eliminating etiological factors and/or presenting defining characteristics.

EVALUATION

Patient Outcome	Data Indicating That Outcome is Reached
Safety maintained: no injury to self or others	No reported or physical evidence of injury to self or others Absence of or decrease in violent response Absence of or decrease in suicidal behavior Ability to control own behavior
Anxiety and stress reduced	Verbal statement that patient feels less anxious Physical signs of stress and anxiety decreased or absent
Model of reality more realistic and constructive	Verbalizations clearer, more well rounded (decrease in generalizations, deletions, nominalizations, distortions of control, distortions of intent) Oriented to environment, self, time, and space Decrease in or absence of hallucinations and delusions Increased signs of problem-solving, abstraction
Ability to relate with others positively	Functions as group member (expresses thoughts and feelings, makes wants and needs known to the group, uses group response as guide to monitoring behavior) Increased interaction with others Appropriate interaction process observed
Assumes responsibility for self-care	Makes contribution to treatment plan Follows through on assumed responsibility Seeks increasing responsibility for own activity and behavior Increase in self-monitoring

References

1. Bandler, R., and Grindler, J.: The structure of magic, Palo Alto, Calif., 1975, Science and Behavior Books, Inc.
2. Bruner, J., Goodnow, J., and Austin, A.: A study of thinking, New York, 1956, John Wiley & Sons, Inc.
3. Carpenito, L.: Nursing diagnosis: application to clinical practice, Philadelphia, 1983, J.B. Lippincott Co.
4. Carroll, J.: Language, thought and reality: selected writings of Benjamin Lee Whorf, New York, 1956, The Technology Press.
5. Chomsky, N.: Language and mind, New York, 1968, Harcourt-Brace-Jovanovich.
6. Delgado, J.: Physical control of the mind: toward a psychological society, New York, 1969, Harper & Row.
7. Dixson, B.: Intervening when the patient is delusional, J. Psychiatr. Nurs. Mental Health Services 7(1):25, 1969.
8. Dubovsky, S., and Weissberg, M.: Clinical psychiatry in primary care, Baltimore, 1978, Williams & Wilkins.
9. Flavell, J.: The developmental psychology of Jean Piaget, New York, 1963, D. Van Nostrand Co.
10. Hilgard, E., and Bower, G.: Theories of learning, Englewood Cliffs, N.J., 1975, Prentice-Hall, Inc.
11. Kim, M., McFarland, G., and McLane, A., editors: Classification of nursing diagnoses: proceedings of the Fifth National Conference, St. Louis, 1984, The C.V. Mosby Co.
12. Kim, M., McFarland, G., and McLane, A.: Pocket guide to nursing diagnosis, St. Louis, 1984, The C.V. Mosby Co.
13. Kim, M., and Moritz, D.: Classification of nursing diagnoses: proceedings of the Third and Fourth National Conferences, New York, 1982, McGraw-Hill Book Co.
14. Knowles, R.: Disputing irrational thoughts, Am. J. Nurs. 81(4):735, 1981.
15. Lachman, R., Lachman, J., and Butterfield, E.: Cognitive psychology and information processing: an introduction, Hillsdale, N.J., 1979, Lawrence Erlbaum Associates.
16. Pincus, J., and Tucker, G.: Behavioral neurology, New York, 1974, Oxford University Press.
17. Schroder, P.: Nursing intervention with patients with thought disorders, Perspect. Psychiatr. Care 17(1):32, 1979.
18. Schwartzman, S.: The hallucinating patient and nursing intervention, J. Psychiatr. Nurs. Mental Health Services 13(6):23, 1975.
19. Tyler, S.: The said and the unsaid: mind, meaning and culture, New York, 1978, Academic Press, Inc.

SENSORY-PERCEPTUAL ALTERATION: VISUAL, AUDITORY, KINESTHETIC, GUSTATORY, TACTILE, OLFACTORY

THEORY AND ETIOLOGY

Sensory experiences transformed to input form the raw data that human beings use to interpret the world around them. Through the process of perception, we define and represent reality. We give meaning to our experiences, thereby shaping out interactions and influencing our goals, directions, and decisions. Thus an interruption of or alteration in this sensory-perceptual process ultimately affects how we interact and behave.

Before exploring alterations and their effects however, an examination of the concept of sensory perception is necessary. A review of the literature on perception reveals a wealth of information and a mass of contradiction. The following sections are designed to provide an overview of the concept of perception and the theoretical trends that have occurred.

The question of how we come to know reality has ancient philosophic roots. The rise of scientific theories of perception can be traced as far back as the sixteenth century. Between the sixteenth and the early twentieth century three views were predominant. The first was based on an additive learning model whereby complex ideas were formed by a learned association among simple sensory elements. Knowledge of reality was learned and came only from information that had been processed through the sensory apparatus. The second approach was nativistic in nature. Perception was viewed as an innate process "wired in" at birth. This process was simply triggered by sensory stimuli. The final view of this period held that the process of perception was an internal carbon copy of the external stimulus pattern. Here an internal stimulus-response pattern was thought to occur, resulting in recognition.[7,28]

Recent theoretical viewpoints have become increasingly complex. However, influences from the earlier approaches still remain. Two major theoretical thrusts seem to predominate in the current movement in perception: (1) information processing theories and (2) transactional person-centered theories.

Stimulus-response approaches gave rise to information processing and extraction models. The human need to adapt to the environment is a key assumption in this theoretical approach. To adapt effectively, knowledge of the environment is of primary importance. Such knowledge is acquired by the extraction of information from a vast array of sensory stimuli. Information is defined as those stimuli which have the ability to trigger an adaptive reaction. This process is labeled perception and is continuously modified by experience with the environment. Learning and thinking are viewed as processes that aid in extraction of information. This occurs as learning and thinking modify the organism (human), who in turn modifies perceptions of incoming stimuli.[7,8] Thus information processing theories are heavily influenced by behavioral and learning theories.

Transactional theories are influenced by *gestalt* ideas and existential philosophic notions. Ames stated that individuals develop a defined set of percepts to deal with the infinite variety of sensory data being received.[28] This development occurs through transactions with each individual's unique environment. As these transactions occur, assumptions are made about reality. These assumptions in turn determine what the individual perceives. Thus perception becomes a learned act of constructing reality to fit a set of assumptions about it.

Ittleson and Cantril[11] espoused three transactional characteristics of perception: (1) "the facts of perception always present themselves through concrete situations"; (2) perception occurs within each individual from a unique position in time and space in combination with past experience and present needs; (3) each individual creates a personalized psychologic environment independent of experience.

Klein[16] viewed perception as a process influenced by and influencing a person's goals, cognitive processes, and needs. The process is an interactive one whereby an interaction is drawn between internal and external elements. Transactional theories, then, view humans as unique individuals, each possessing a separate view of reality colored by past, present, and future considerations. The whole of the perceptual process is seen as greater than the parts.

Using these theoretical viewpoints as a foundation, it is possible to identify a set of characteristics for the concept of perception.

Perception is a process. As a process, the act of perception is inferred and unobservable except in a phenomenologic sense. The process is psychologic in nature with parallel physiologic events that are isomorphic to the process. The end result of the process is a percept. The process of perception is generally judged as accurate when the percept agrees with other indicators about an object, person, or event's character.[28]

Perception is universal. All human beings engage in the act of perception as a way of surviving in and ordering the physical world around them. Categories of percepts are formed as we test out our perceptions, coming to a common understanding of concrete concepts such as dog, cat, and cow and more abstract concepts such as animal. All human beings possess similar equipment with which to interpret the environment. We all possess the same sense organs, neurologic systems, and electrochemical relay systems.[14]

Perception is individual.[14,15,20] The process of perception is subjective, selective, and influenced by a vast array of factors. These factors can be broadly classified as physiologic, psychologic, and sociocultural.[15] Physiologic influences include chemical imbalances (hunger, thirst, fatigue, drugs, fever, pain), constitutional variations (height, weight), and ranges in sense modalities (coordination). Psychologic factors include psychogenic needs (motivation), adaptive and defense mechanisms, and ordering mechanisms (beliefs, values, attitudes). Sociocultural factors include roles, positions, social strata (class, ethnic, origin), customs, mores, and folkways.[15]

Perception is interactive.[11] The perceptual act involves a reaction to the environment and action on the environment. There is an interplay between external events and stimuli and internal neurologic functions. This interaction occurs within a defined time-space position for each individual and creates a unique psychologic environment for that individual.

Perception is continuous and present oriented.[14] Humans are in a constant state of participation in the perceptual act. Perception occurs in the present and is influenced by past events, current needs, and future goals.

Perception is an interrelated cognitive function.[7,14] The concepts and processes of perception, thinking, and learning are interrelated. All are cognitive processes separable only in a theoretical sense rather than a practical sense. (This becomes increasingly evident when comparing the two nursing diagnoses alteration in sensory perception and alteration in thought processes.)

Perception is maturational and developmental.[28] The ability to perceive becomes more complex with age and experience. The process begins with simple reflexive actions at birth and moves to an increasingly abstract and conceptual level as the individual interacts with the environment.

Using the theory presented thus far it is possible to forge an operational definition of perception. The following definition is stated as a serial order of emergent behaviors. This technique is described by Peplau[22] as a method for defining abstract concepts.

1. An individual with physiologic, psychologic, and sociocultural sets who has certain assumptions, motivations, and expectations encounters a concrete situation.
2. Stimuli bombard one or more of the sense organs. Categories of senses[7,19]:
   a. Exteroceptors (distance senses)
      (1) Vision
      (2) Audition
   b. Proprioceptors (near senses)
      (1) Tactile sense
      (2) Taste (gustatory)
      (3) Smell (olfactory)
   c. Interoceptors (deep senses)
      (1) Kinesthetic (muscle, bone, joint sense)
      (2) Vestibular (sense of balance)
      (3) Visceral (hollow organ sense)
3. Sense organs transduce the stimuli (transduction is the sensory transformation of raw stimulus data into informational messages/nerve impulses).
4. Nerve impulses are relayed to the brain and reticular activating system (RAS),* which creates an aroused state.

---

*For a full explanation of the functioning of the RAS see Lindsley, D.: Common factors in sensory deprivation, sensory distortion and sensory overload. In Solomon, P.: Sensory deprivation, Cambridge, Mass., 1961, Harvard University Press.

5. Impulses are automatically forwarded *or* impulses are selected, reorganized, and modified based on perceptual set, past experience, present needs, and future goals and then forwarded (transformation).
6. Meaningful impulses are integrated and a percept is formed.
7. Resulting percept may have direct or indirect affect on subsequent emotions and/or behavior.

Percepts, the product of the perceptual process, have certain characteristics. These characteristics can be divided into six major classes[2]:

1. Sensory quality and dimensions: hue, color, pressure, temperature, intensity, strength, shading, size, volume, depth
2. Configuration: shape, outline, figure versus ground, form
3. Constancy: things remain the same regardless of angle, distance, lighting
4. Frame of reference: standard for judging abstract nature (lighter versus heavier) of the percept
5. Concrete object character: attaches meaning to the percept
6. Prevailing "set" or "state": attaches current need of percept

Percepts addressed by the first three characteristics are likely to be universal in nature (red is red; a square is a square). Percepts defined by characteristics 4 and 5 are likely to be similar for individuals of common background and experience. The subjective influence of perception is best seen as percepts are influenced by the final characteristic.

An alteration in sensory perception occurs when there is an interruption at or during one or more of the steps set forth in the operational definition. The extent and severity of the alteration depend on the point or points of interruption and the etiological nature of the interruption. The classification of etiological factors also spells out those persons who are at risk for an alteration in sensory perception.

The etiologies for the diagnosis of sensory-perceptual alterations can be categorized in a number of ways. Carpenito[5] divides etiological factors into pathophysiologic, situational, and maturational. The National Conference group[12,13] cites four categories: altered environmental factors, altered sensory reception, transmission, and/or integration, chemical alterations, and psychologic stress. Other classification schemes might include those factors which are external processes versus those which are internal processes or those factors which affect the senses and sensory input versus those factors which affect the internal perceptual process. No one scheme seems clearly superior, nor does the literature give any clear guidance for classification. Thus, in some attempt at consistency the classification scheme devised by the National Conference group is used here[12]:

Altered environments (excessive or insufficient stimuli)

Therapeutically restricted (isolation, intensive care, bed rest, traction, confining illnesses, incubator)

Socially restricted (institutionalization, homebound, aging, chronic illness, dying, infant deprivation)

Stigmatized (mentally ill, retarded, handicapped)

Bereaved

Altered sensory reception, transmission, or integration

Neurologic disease, trauma, deficit

Altered states of sense organs

Inability to communicate, understand, speak, or respond

Sleep deprivation

Pain

Chemical alteration

Endogenous (electrolyte imbalance, elevated BUN, elevated ammonia, hypoxia)

Exogenous (CNS stimulants/depressants, mind-altering drugs)

Extreme anxiety or panic (narrowed perceptual fields caused by anxiety)

DEFINING CHARACTERISTICS

Changes in thought processes
  Disorientation in time, place, or person
  Disordered sequencing in thought, time, or events
  Altered abstraction or conceptualization
  Change in problem-solving abilities
  Bizarre thinking
  Hallucinations
  Hypersuggestibility
Changes in attention span
  Diminished concentration
  Daydreaming
  Restlessness
  Increased distractibility
  Inability to follow the flow of conversation
Emotional lability
  Rapid mood swings
  Exaggerated responses
  Ambivalence
  Apathy
  Flattened affect
  Emotional detachment
  Anger
  Depression
  Fear
  Irritability
  Anxiety
Changes in routine patterns or habits
  Change in behavior pattern
  Change in response to stimuli

Altered communication patterns
Change in sleeping patterns
Altered eating habits
Changes in sensory capabilities
  Vision
    Diminished visual capacity
    Visual distortion
    Photosensitivity
  Audition
    Hypersensitivity or hyposensitivity
    Auditory distortion
    Distortion of verbal messages
  Tactile sense
    Hyperesthesias or hypoesthesias
    Inability to tell nature of object by feel
  Taste
    Increased taste sensitivity
    Diminished sense of taste
    Altered taste sense
    Loss of appetite
  Smell
    Diminished sense of smell
    Hypersensitivity to odor
    Distortion of odor
  Kinesthetic sense
    Motor incoordination
    Inability to tell where body parts are located
    Paralysis
    Muscular weakness, flaccidity, rigidity
    Surgical joint replacement
  Vestibular sense
    Diminished sense of balance
  Visceral sense
    Feelings of emptiness, hollowness
Presence of any of the etiological factors associated with the diagnosis
Changes in percept characteristics
  Distortion of color, hue, intensity, light, size
  Distortion of environment
  Growth of inanimate objects
  Failure to notice stimuli
  Disregard of normally ''important'' percepts

An interruption in the perceptual process results from whatever etiological factor produces an alteration in sensory perception. This alteration, by definition, affects the way we make sense of the world and the way we define reality. Thus the critical defining characteristic for this nursing diagnosis is evidence of reality distortion as judged against some set of normative criteria. These criteria are both objective and subjective just as the perceptual process contains objective and subjective elements.

The extent of reality distortion varies widely in this diagnostic category. A person recovering from surgery in a recovery room atmosphere, groggy from anesthesia and bombarded with meaningless stimuli, may display signs of gross disorientation and confusion. Reality distortion in this case is rated severe. A person with a diminished sense of smell may fail to detect certain odors and confuse the tastes of certain foods. Reality distortion in this instance is mild.

Additional defining characteristics assist in evaluating the severity of reality distortion and the extent of the perceptual alteration. Any number or combination of defining characteristics can be manifested by a patient. These additional defining characteristics are grouped and subgrouped by the nature of the characteristics.[5,12,23,26]

NURSING INTERVENTIONS

Patient Goal	Nursing Intervention
Prevention	
Enhance the ability to identify factors that increase risk for sensory-perceptual alteration.	Assess patient for risks and potential risks for alteration (see Etiologies). Present resulting risk profile to patient when possible.
Identify ways to reduce risks of alteration.	Provide strategies for reduction or elimination of identified risk factors (altering sleep pattern to reduce sleep deprivation; altering drug habits; rearranging environment).
Identify stimuli needed for daily functioning.	Explore the source, type, amount, and patterns of stimuli needed by the individual for optimum functioning.
Identify methods for maintaining adequate stimuli in the environment.	Provide strategies for maintaining adequate amounts of meaningful stimuli in identified therapeutically or socially restricted environments (introducing pattern and structure in environment, orienting features, noise control, presence of familiar objects and/or persons).
Acute Care*	
Prevent injury.	Maintain safety precautions (bed rails up, bed lowered, sharp objects out of reach, call bell in reach).
Decrease or eliminate presence of defining characteristics.	Restore sensory-perceptual function by: 1. Assessing stimuli present in environment: intensity, quantity, quality, repetitiveness, movement, change, novelty, incongruity, clarity, ambiguity. 2. Altering environmental factors to increase meaningful stimuli and decrease extraneous stimuli: a. Use orienting features such as clocks, calendars, windows, name tags, favorite objects. b. Maintain verbal contact, eye contact, touch. c. Reduce unnecessary traffic, personnel, noise. d. Structure routines. e. Structure input by giving clear, concise explanations of surroundings, treatments, procedures. f. Allow frequent short visits by significant others. 3. Orienting to reality: a. Address by name, introduce self frequently, regularly state time and place. b. Explain and allow participation when possible in all tasks and treatments. c. Interpret sights, sounds, smells present in environment. d. Explain routines and policies. 4. Obtaining feedback of perception of events, objects, and clarifying misperceptions. 5. Assisting in clarifying reality (see Alteration in thought processes for more detailed intervention with hallucinations, delusions).
Chronic Care†	
Maintain orientation to surroundings.	Use reality orientation techniques: 1. Address by name, orient to time. 2. Point out surroundings, identify self. 3. Structure input with concrete, concise explanations. 4. Maintain eye contact. 5. Reinforce behavior that is reality oriented, such as responding to meaningful comments.

*References 1, 3-6, 9, 20, 23.
†References 5, 9, 17, 20, 24, 25.

Patient Goal	Nursing Intervention
	Provide meaningful stimuli and reduce extraneous stimuli in environment: 1. Keep clocks and calendars in view. Make use of windows and the out-of-doors. 2. Observe holidays and significant occasions. 3. Provide structured routines. 4. Place familiar objects in plain sight. 5. Structure experiences that make use of all the senses.
Increase appropriate social interaction.	Promote social interaction: 1. Arrange physical environment to encourage interaction (open spaces, circles instead of rows), increase mobility with wheelchairs, walkers, carts, etc. 2. Encourage exploration of surroundings; encourage verbalization of experiences, desires, thoughts. 3. Set up interactions with others in structural settings with defined purpose. 4. Encourage reminiscence. 5. Encourage decision-making. 6. Use small group sessions to widen interaction.

Perceptual adequacy and accuracy are necessary prerequisites to enable nurses and patients to engage in mutual goal setting and exploration of means for goal achievement.[14]

This nursing diagnostic category is an encompassing one. Alterations range from mild to severe; manifestations can be acute or chronic; age of persons affected ranges from infancy to old age. Thus many specific nursing interventions depend on individual patient characteristics, identified etiological factors for a particular patient, and presenting defining characteristics for a particular patient.

Nursing care as described in this chapter is divided into three major modes: prevention, acute care, and chronic care. Prevention requires careful assessment of the client and environment for risk factors. Patient education plays a major role. Once a pattern of defining characteristics appears and a diagnosis of sensory-perceptual alteration is made, the alteration may be classified as acute or chronic.

Acute alterations tend to be abrupt in onset and temporary in nature. The degree of alteration tends to be severe and dramatic in presentation of defining characteristics (for example, sudden confusion and disorientation, rapid large mood swings, bizarre behavior). Etiologies for acute alterations include trauma, drug intoxication, sudden sensory loss (blindness, deafness), acute pain, panic, and placement in intensive care units or recovery rooms.

Chronic alterations are progressive in onset and are subject to recurrence because of the long-term or permanent nature of the etiological factors. The degree of alteration may range from mild to severe, and defining characteristics may be subtle and ambiguous. When chronic alterations are left untreated, defining characteristics become more clear-cut and overt. Etiologies for chronic alterations typically include socially restricted environments such as nursing homes, children's homes, and prisons, declining sensory equipment, neurologic disease, chronic pain, prolonged immobility, social isolation, and chronic illness.

In all cases the ultimate goal is to promote, maintain, and restore optimum contact with reality. Nursing interventions are aimed at preventing, reducing, or eliminating etiological factors and presenting defining characteristics.

EVALUATION

Patient Outcome	Data Indicating That Outcome is Reached
Prevention	
Identifies risk factors.	States risk factors. Recognizes self-risk profile.
Identifies risk reduction methods.	States or demonstrates use of strategies for reduction or elimination of identified risk factors.
Identifies daily stimulus needs.	States source, type, amount, and patterns of usual daily stimulation. Recounts life-style and role patterns.
Identifies stimulus maintenance methods.	Verbalizes or demonstrates use of strategies for maintaining and altering environment. Lists changes planned for or already made.

Patient Outcome	Data Indicating That Outcome is Reached
Acute Care	
No injury sustained.	No physical or reported evidence of injury.
Decrease in or elimination of defining characteristics.	Increased ability to test reality. Orientation to person, place, time. Absence of hallucinations, delusions. Stabilization of emotions. Increased participation in care. Accurate perception of stimulus input as evidenced by verbal feedback and appropriate behavior. Appropriate responses to the environment. Absence of bizarre behavior. Increased decision-making and problem-solving abilities. Lowered anxiety levels.
Chronic Care	
Oriented to surroundings.	Oriented to person, time, place. Can recall past, present events. Can verbalize future plans. No evidence of confusion. Communicates in a meaningful fashion: responds appropriately to questions, cues, initiates interaction.
Social interaction increases and is appropriate.	Interaction time increases. Interaction is meaningful. Verbalizes about time spent with others. Verbalizes plans for future outings, social times. Verbalizes choices for dyad, group plans.

References

1. Aiello, J.: The concept of sensory deprivation, Austral. Nurs. J. 7(10):38, 1978.
2. Allport, F.: Theories of perception and the concept of structure, New York, 1955, John Wiley & Sons, Inc.
3. Ashworth, P.: Sensory deprivation: the acutely ill, Nurs. Times 75(8):330, 1979.
4. Bolin, R.H.: Sensory deprivation: an overview, Nurs. Forum 13:241, 1974.
5. Carpenito, L.: Nursing diagnosis: application to clinical practice, Philadelphia, 1983, J.B. Lippincott Co.
6. Chodil, J., and Williams, B.: The concept of sensory deprivation, Nurs. Clin. North Am. 5:453, 1970.
7. Forgus, R.: Perception, New York, 1966, McGraw-Hill Book Co.
8. Gibson, E.: Principles of perceptual learning and development, New York, 1969, Appleton-Century-Crofts.
9. Hahn, K.: Using 24 hour reality orientation, J. Gerontol. Nurs. 6(3):130, 1980.
10. Hochberg, J.: Perception, Englewood Cliffs, N.J., 1978, Prentice-Hall, Inc.
11. Ittleson, W., and Cantril, H.: Perception: a transactional approach, Garden City, N.Y., 1954, Doubleday & Co.
12. Kim M., McFarland, G., and McLane, A.: Pocket guide to nursing diagnosis, St. Louis, 1984, The C.V. Mosby Co.
13. Kim M., and Moritz, D.: Classification of nursing diagnosis: proceedings of the Third and Fourth National Conferences, New York, 1982, McGraw-Hill Book Co.
14. King, I.: A theory for nursing: systems, concepts, process, New York, 1981, John Wiley & Sons, Inc.
15. King, S.: Perceptions and medicine, New York, 1962, Russell Sage Foundation.
16. Klein, G.: Perception, motivation and personality, New York, 1970, Alfred A. Knopf.
17. Kratz, C.: Sensory deprivation in the elderly, Nurs. Times 75(8):330, 1979.
18. Lipowski, Z.: Sensory and informational inputs overload: behavioral effects, Comprehensive Psychiatr. 16(3):199, 1975.
19. Mitchell, P., and Loustau, A.: Concepts basic to nursing, New York, 1981, McGraw-Hill Book Co.
20. Nordmark, M., and Rohweder, A.: Scientific foundations of nursing, Philadelphia, 1975, J.B. Lippincott Co.
21. Oatley, K.: Perceptions and representations, New York, 1978, Free Press.
22. Peplau, H.: Theory: the professional dimension, Unpublished paper, 1972.
23. Roberts, S.: Behavioral concepts and the critically ill patient, Englewood Cliffs, N.J., 1976, Prentice-Hall, Inc.
24. Smith, M.: Changes in judgment of duration, Nurs. Res. 24:93, 1975.
25. Voelkel, D.: A study of reality orientation and resocialization groups with confused elderly, J. Gerontol. Nurs. 4(3):13, 1978.
26. Watson C., and Wyatt, N.: Altered levels of awareness. In Hart, L., Reese, J., and Fearing, M., editors: Concepts common to acute illness: identification and management, St. Louis, 1981, The C.V. Mosby Co.
27. Woods, N., and Falk, S.: Noise stimuli in the acute care area, Nurs. Res. 23:144, 1974.
28. Zimbardo, P., and Ruch, F.: Psychology and life, Glenview, Ill., 1975, Scott Foresman and Co.
29. Zubek, J.: Sensory deprivation: 15 years of research, New York, 1969, Appleton-Century-Crofts.

Suggested Readings

Ashworth, P.: Sensory deprivation: the acutely ill, Nurs. Times 15(7):290, 1979.
Cohen, S.: Contact deprivation in infants, Psychosomatics 7:85, 1966.
Fleming, J.: Sensory losses in children, Curr. Concepts Clin. Nurs. 1:339, 1967.
Kratz, C.: Sensory deprivation in the elderly, Nurs. Times 75(8):330, 1979.
Saller, C.D., and Salter, C.A.: Effects of individualized activity program on elderly patients, Gerontologist 15(5):404, 1975.
Taulbee, L., and Folsom, J.: Reality orientation for geriatric patients, Hosp. Commun. Psychiatr. 17:133, 1966.

Comfort

COMFORT, ALTERATION IN: PAIN

THEORY AND ETIOLOGY

The diagnostic category comfort, alteration in: pain concerns the phenomenon of pain and the nurse's role as a patient advocate in its management. Pain is an abstract concept. It is an invisible yet complex personal experience. It acts like a warning to the body because it occurs whenever there is tissue damage. Pain is defined by the International Association for the Study of Pain as "an unpleasant sensory and emotional experience associated with actual or potential tissue damage or described in terms of such damage."[3]

Even in like situations the pain experience varies from individual to individual and includes both sensory and affective components. It is described both in terms of the sensation of pain and the distress or degree of suffering that an individual experiences. Feldman[9] describes the total pain response as being "determined by such factors as threshold, tolerance, attention to pain, action of pain relievers, counterirritation measures (such as heat or cold), summation, expectations, and perceptions." These factors help determine an individual's perception of pain, response to the pain, effectiveness of the pain control measures, and tendency to report pain.

An individual may have difficulty describing the pain to others; pain is a personal experience. McCaffery[20] defines pain as "whatever the experiencing person says it is."

Primary Etiologies

This diagnostic category has four primary etiologies: biologic, chemical, physical, and psychologic.[1] The four etiologies of pain can act alone or in combination with each other. Knowing the etiology is helpful but not es-

sential for the treatment of pain. At times the etiology is unknown but the pain is very real.

Biologic etiologies of pain are changes in life processes caused by disease, microorganisms (as in inflammation), or cell injury (as in ischemia). The pain is caused by actual or impending tissue damage. For example, prolonged pressure on a bony prominence can cause a decubitus ulcer because of the diminished blood flow to the skin where it is compressed by the body weight. Individuals with normal sensation shift their weight when they become uncomfortable, which prevents the development of an ulcer. In contrast, people with diminished or absent sensation risk developing decubitus ulcers because they cannot feel pressure and therefore do not change their position. Individuals may experience pain of biologic origin because of alterations in essential life processes such as cell growth, oxygenation, nutrition, transport, metabolism, and regularity of response mechanisms. Pain caused by biologic etiologies includes angina in coronary artery disease, leg pain from claudication in peripheral vascular disease, joint pain in rheumatoid arthritis, and the pleural pain of pneumonia.

Chemical etiologies of pain include cytotoxic agents that damage or destroy tissue and cells. Most agents are man made and include noxious chemicals such as lead, insecticides, tobacco, alcohol, drugs, and poisons.[1] Internal chemical imbalances can cause stomach pain with a peptic ulcer and bone pain because of the progressive deossification in Paget's disease.

The *physical* etiologies of pain include trauma, temperature extremes, electricity, and radioactive rays. Trauma encompasses minor abrasions and contusions, surgical trauma, and major injuries that threaten the function of critical organs and tissues.[5] Burns and frostbite are

1971

examples of temperature extremes. Both electricity and radioactive rays can also cause burns and tissue damage.

The *psychologic* etiologies of pain are best described as emotions or subjective feeling states that cause an individual to feel distressed. It is difficult to identify the psychologic etiologies of pain because, according to Davis, Buchsbaum, and Bunney[8]: ''Perceptual experience has a physiological basis and all physiological stresses have psychological effects.'' Pain is neither purely psychologic nor purely somatogenic. The pain experience includes both the sensation of the pain and the distress, or degree of suffering perceived by the individual. Almost all types of pain have some psychologic overlay and have the potential to evoke an emotional response.

Pain that is purely psychogenic is rare. The diagnosis of psychologic pain may be used in reference to an individual whose apparent discomfort exceeds that which is usually expected with a given noxious stimulation.[10]

Persons diagnosed with conversion reaction, hysteria, and hypochondriasis may experience psychologic pain.[2] These psychiatric diagnoses carry a negative connotation. People with a diagnosis of psychologic pain are often considered ''crocks,'' malingerers, and manipulative. Pain of a psychologic origin is as real as any other pain. Therefore it is the primary responsibility of the nurse to treat the pain and not try to determine whether it is psychologic.

In some psychophysiologic disorders an individual's emotions can affect the degree of pain. These include tension headaches, peptic ulcers, and ulcerative colitis. Tension and stress evoke an emotional response. ''Chronic muscle contraction headaches or tension headaches are considered to be the most common type of headache in our society.''[21] Emotions can also cause an exacerbation of a peptic ulcer or ulcerative colitis. Pain is secondary to the disorder and is not of a psychologic origin.[19] It is best, therefore, to view psychologic etiologies of pain as the power of the emotions to precipitate, aggravate, and prolong pain.

Pain Mechanisms

Pain receptors, or nociceptors, are free nerve endings in the tissues that are sensitive to painful or noxious stimuli. These receptors are stimulated by tissue damage, extremes in temperature, and chemical changes in the body, such as those produced by prostaglandins, histamines, kinins, and serotonin. Therefore pain receptors are mechanosensitive, thermosensitive, and chemosensitive. Most pain receptors are sensitive to more than one stimulus.

Two types of peripheral nerve fibers are responsible for the transmission of pain sensations from the tissues to the central nervous system: the A-delta fibers and the C fibers. The *fast* pain signals are transmitted by the A-delta pain fibers, and the slower pain signals are transmitted by C fibers. When a sudden pain experience occurs, a double pain sensation may be experienced. For example, if an object falls on your foot, you feel a fast pricking pain that alerts you to the injury. This is caused by stimulation of the A delta fibers. After you remove the object from your foot, a slow, burning, dull, aching sensation occurs. The discomfort may also feel more diffuse and cause a more intense suffering. Stimulation of the C fibers causes this type of pain.

Different sensations are felt because the A-delta fibers and the C fibers are associated with different aspects of the pain experience. A-delta fibers send impulses to pathways that deal with the temporal and spatial aspects of the pain experience. C fibers send impulses to pathways that deal with the emotional and autonomic aspects.[7] The pain transmitted by C fibers is of a low intensity, but the summation of impulses makes this pain difficult to tolerate.[21] Although the initial stimuli for pain may occur in the tissues, the pain is not experienced as such until the higher cortical levels of the brain interpret it as pain and identify the location of the pain.

There are numerous pain pathways to the brain. The pain fibers enter the spinal cord through the dorsal roots, then either ascend or descend one or two segments to the dorsal horn of the spinal cord. In the dorsal horn they synapse in the substantia gelatinosa. The pain impulses then pass one or more short-fibered neurons and cross to the other side of the spinal cord by way of long fibers and ascend to the cortex by way of the dorsal column system and the spinothalamic system.[13,21]

The dorsal column system transmits information very rapidly and precisely. It is able to discriminate small changes in the intensity and the precise locations of the sensation. Some of the sensations transmitted by the dorsal system include fine gradations in the intensity of touch and pressure, vibration, position, and movement against the skin.[13]

The spinothalamic tract transmits sensations of pain, temperature, gross information on touch and pressure, sexual sensations, tickle, and itch. It divides into three tracts: the ventral spinothalamic tract, the lateral spinothalamic tract, and the spinoreticular tract.[7,13,21] The ventral spinothalamic tract begins after the spinothalamic and dorsal column fibers cross and ends in the thalamus. General sensations of touch and pressure are transmitted through it. The tract lacks the ability to identify intensity or to localize the involved area. The lateral spinothalamic tract also ends in the thalamus and transmits sensations of aching and burning and thermal sensations. The spinoreticular tract ascends through the reticular formation in the brainstem and then to areas of the midbrain. The fibers eventually enter the thalamus. The reticular activating system is composed of the reticular formation and a portion of the thalamus. This system is important because it activates most of the nervous system. It can create a sense of excitement, urgency, or self-defense associated with pain.

Neurotransmission of Pain

During the 1970s endogenous peptides with opiate-like properties were discovered. These peptides were given the name *endorphins,* meaning ''morphine within'' because of their apparent analgesic properties. Endorphins are activated in stressful and painful experiences. In some situations placebos can also activate the release of endorphins.[21] Endorphin levels are also found to deviate from normal during depression. Endorphins modify neural activity by indirectly influencing the effects of some neurotransmitters.

Endorphins are classified into three groups: beta-lipotrophin, enkephalin, and dynorphin. The beta-lipotrophin group is composed of beta-endorphin, gamma-endorphin, and alpha-endorphin. The beta-endorphins can produce potent analgesia. There is a small amount of beta-endorphin in the brain and a larger concentration in the pituitary. The beta-endorphins are attracted to the opiate receptors in the hypothalamus and the pituitary gland. The gamma-endorphins and alpha-endorphins have less analgesic effects.[21]

Enkephalins are found throughout the central and peripheral nervous systems in nerve fibers and nerve endings. It is interesting to note that high concentrations are found in areas associated with pain perception, including the limbic system.[15] Within the limbic system the affective nature of sensations is differentiated as either pain or pleasure.[13] Enkephalins may affect the modulation or the transmission of pain impulses because they are found in vast quantities within the pain pathways. It is also suggested that they may interfere with or inhibit the release of substance P, which transmits noxious stimuli.[21]

Dynorphin means ''dynamite endorphin.'' As the name describes, it is thought to have strong analgesic properties. It is considered to be 50 times stronger than beta-endorphin in providing analgesia.[21]

Clinical application of much of the information concerning endorphins is still tentative. Researchers are optimistic about future findings concerning these peptides.

Pain Theories

Because the transmission and modulation of pain impulses are complex, there are still many unanswered questions. Several theories of pain have been proposed, each adding contributions to piece together this compli-

cated puzzle. None of the theories has been able to adequately explain the total pain experience.

The specificity theory (Descartes, 1644; VonFrey, 1894; and others) was one of the earliest proposed.[7] This theory viewed pain as being separate and independent of other sensations such as touch. Pain occurs because of the stimulation of fibers along specific pathways from the receptors to the spinal cord. Proponents of this theory believe that there is a direct relationship between the receptor type, fiber size, and the pain experienced. This is a stimulus-response relationship. It has been criticized because it assumes that when certain fibers are stimulated, pain is produced. In reality, pain production and perception vary between individuals and even within the same individual at different times. This theory does not explain the pain that occurs after a nerve is severed, such as phantom limb pain after an amputation.

The pattern theory was originally proposed by Goldschneider in 1894 and arose because of deficiencies in the specificity theory. The theory proposed that the ''sensations of pain experience by an individual are primarily related to the transmission of nerve impulse patterns originating from and coded at the peripheral stimulation site.''[11] Later, other pattern theories developed, including the reverberating circuit theory, the specialized input-controlling system, and the nonspecific receptors.[21] The pattern theories have not been able to account for physiologic evidence of nerve fiber specialization.

More recently, the gate control theory (Fig. 7) was developed by Melzack and Wall.[22-24] This theory incorporated some aspects of both the specificity and pattern theories, such as the specificity of fibers and the patterns created by those fibers. Although some deficiences were found in this theory, its advent brought about a renewed interest in pain research. The research by Melzack and Wall did not support the stimulus-response relationship between the degree of intensity of the stimulus and the pain experienced, but instead proposed that the pain experienced was determined by numerous physiologic and psychologic variables.[4] This theory was summarized by Melzack[23]:

> The theory proposes that: (1) the substantia gelatinosa functions as a gate control system that modulates the amount of input transmitted from the peripheral fibers to the dorsal horn transmission (T) cells; (2) the dorsal column and dorsal lateral systems of the spinal cord act as a central control trigger, which activates selective brain processes that influence the modulating properties of the gate control system; and (3) the T cells activate neuromechanisms that constitute the action system responsible for both response and perception.

Simplistically, this theory implies that when the gate is open, pain impulses flow through and pain is felt; when the gate is closed, the pain impulses are stopped. The

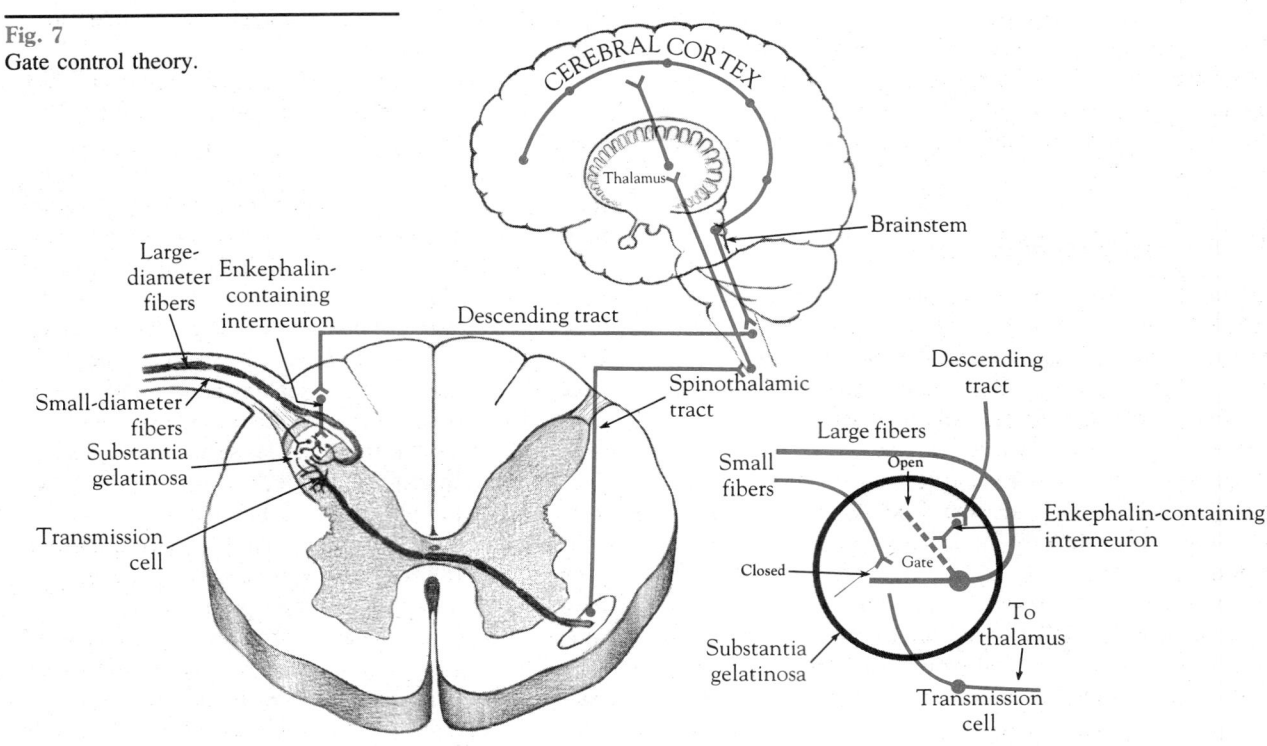

Fig. 7

Gate control theory.

opening and closing of the gate are influenced by the activity of the large A-delta fibers, the small C nerve fibers, the brainstem reticular formation, and the cerebral cortex.

As mentioned earlier, the C fibers transmit potentially painful sensations. When the gate is open, these sensations travel from the periphery to the dorsal column and to the cerebral cortex and thalamus. When the C fibers are excited, the activity of the substantia gelatinosa is inhibited. The substantia gelatinosa is the proposed location of the gating mechanism. When its activity is inhibited, the gate is open and the painful impulses flow through. On the other hand, the large-diameter A-delta fibers, when stimulated, increase the activity of the substantia gelatinosa and close the gate, thus preventing the impulses from reaching the level of awareness in the brain. These A-delta fibers are stimulated by interventions such as massage, heat, cold, and transcutaneous electrical nerve stimulation.[21]

The brainstem reticular formulation serves as the central biasing mechanism, which means that it controls sensory input. If sufficient or excessive sensory input is present, the reticular formation sends signals to the spinal cord to close the gate. Few or no pain sensations are able to reach the level of awareness in the cortex. A reduction of sensory input, such as a monotonous environment or a long sleepless night, may open the gate. Distraction

and imagery are examples of interventions that theoretically close the gate. It may be that these interventions do not close the gate but rather make the pain more tolerable by placing it away from the center of attention.[21]

The cerebral cortex and thalamus store information regarding past experiences, thoughts, and emotions. Impulses sent via the descending fibers of the cerebral cortex and thalamus have the potential to open or close the gate. Because of this, the individual interprets the meaning of the sensations. It is important to evaluate what pain has meant to the individual in the past and how the individual dealt with the pain experience. Past memories of pain can create learned responses that influence future pain experiences.

Psychosocial Factors

For pain to be experienced, the pain impulses must reach the higher cortical levels of the brain. In an unconscious person these areas may not be functioning. As mentioned, gate control theory suggests that past experiences can influence how potentially painful stimuli are perceived. For example, a person who has had uncontrolled pain in the past may have perceptions of uncontrolled pain in any future painful events. An individual who has not encountered severe pain may have less fear concerning the sensation of pain.

Pain might be viewed and expressed differently by children and adults because of the level of cognitive development. Children usually have reached a well-developed level of cognition by age 8.

The part of the body involved also can influence the perceived meaning of pain. Chest pain may be perceived as more threatening than back pain. An individual may be less likely to offer information about hemorrhoid pain than knee pain because knee pain is less embarrassing to discuss.

The individual's sex may be a factor in pain expression. In general, our society permits women to express their pain more freely than men. Men are expected to be less expressive and exhibit more control.

Early studies on elderly white men from four ethnic groups in the United States indicated that people from different cultures react very differently to pain.[26] Pain expression is dictated to some degree by cultural norms. This may also be true of patients with chronic pain who have learned to cover it up. Therefore pain expression is not always a true indicator of pain.

Acute and Chronic Pain

Acute pain is intense and of short duration. The pain lasts less than 6 months. Generally acute pain provides a warning to the individual of actual or potential tissue damage. It creates an autonomic response commonly referred to as the fight or flight response. When healing occurs, the pain also resolves. There is usually anxiety associated with the pain. Since the pain is of short duration, physicians are more likely to prescribe narcotics and analgesics.

Chronic pain is generally characterized by pain lasting longer than 6 months. The pain can be continuous or intermittent and can be as intense as acute pain. Habituation of the autonomic response occurs so that the fight or flight response is no longer present. Chronic pain does not serve as a warning of tissue damage. In rheumatoid arthritis for example, joint pain may still be present when the disease process is no longer active, because of the structural damage that has already occurred in the joint. The reason for some forms of chronic pain may not be known. Chronic pain does not necessarily serve a purpose. Fortin[12] provides a vivid description of the effects of the chronic pain:

Eventually the debilitating effects of the chronic pain experience and loss of coping reserves alters the individual's perceptions, personality and social functioning. As the person changes, the environment to which he responds changes; that is, personal variability in pain sensation and psychophysiologic responses become intrinsically woven into the situational milieu. Problems of altered self-esteem, social identity, changes in roles and social interaction, and the responses that feed back into the problems, depression, anxiety, and irritability become integral to the chronic pain experience.

Fortin suggests a beginning model for viewing chronic pain. Acute pain has traditionally been viewed from a sensory-reactive model, which does not encompass the chronic pain experience. She uses the gate control theory to depict the psychophysiologic aspects of pain and describes the psychosocial aspects using an interactional approach. Viewing these models together, Fortin has reformulated a model for describing chronic pain and defines the model as:

. . . an integrated pattern of sensory, sentiment and interactive components. Sensory refers to the quality and intensity of the pain sensation. Sentience refers to the motivational and affective qualities of the experience. Interactive refers to the simultaneous interaction between the individual and the environment. It is suggested that in the experience of chronic pain, these forces act collectively to repattern the person and the environment in a transactional process.

From reviewing the general differences between acute and chronic pain, it becomes apparent that some aspects of nursing care may differ depending on the acute or chronic nature of the pain.

DEFINING CHARACTERISTICS*

Acute Pain	Chronic Pain
Guarding, protective behavior Hands placed over painful area	Guarding, protective behavior

Autonomic response (may have periods of physiologic adaption/
   potential of shock)
   Diaphoresis
   Pallor
   Changes in BP, pulse rate, stroke volume, respiratory rate,
     muscle tone
	Habituation of autonomic response

*References 4, 7, 13, 14, 16-18, 20, 21.

Acute Pain	Chronic Pain
Dry mouth Pupillary dilatation	
Decreased appetite	Increase or decrease in appetite (usually decreased with depression, increased if activity limited by pain)
Fatigue	Fatigue
Distraction behavior (moaning, crying, pacing, seeking out other people and/or activities, restlessness)	Preoccupation with pain
Self-focusing	Self-focusing
Shortened attention span	Shortened attention span
Altered time perception	Altered time perception
Impaired thought process	Impaired thought process
Facial mask of pain (eyes lack luster), "beaten look," fixed or scattered movement, grimace	Facial mask of pain (eyes lack luster), "beaten look," fixed or scattered movement, grimace
May or may not verbalize: Pain descriptors (may deny them) Fear, anxiety, anger, helplessness Hope that pain will end Frustration at lack of treatment Increased irritability	May or may not verbalize: Pain descriptors (may deny them) Fear, anxiety, anger, helplessness, depression, hopelessness, suicidal thoughts Hope that pain will end or possibility that pain may persist Frustration at lack of treatment Increased irritability, feeling like a burden, feelings of guilt, anger at others Does not verbalize anger at caretakers when dependent
Occasional difficulty sleeping or awakening from sleep because of pain	Disturbed sleep pattern with difficulty falling asleep; awakens from sleep because of pain
Social isolation	Social isolation
Family/marital dissonance	Family/marital dissonance Reduced sexual activity Uses unproven remedies or visits quacks Discontinues or reduces employment Financially dependent on external sources

To establish a diagnosis of comfort, alteration in: pain, any number of defining characteristics can be identified. Defining characteristics are either subjective or objective. Subjective defining characteristics are verbal or nonverbal communications of pain. The defining characteristics are divided into acute and chronic. To determine the defining characteristics, the nurse must assess the individual's comfort status by completing a pain assessment. Whenever possible both subjective and objective data should be assessed. Several factors must be considered when doing a pain assessment:

1. The nurse and the individual have perceptions of pain based on past experiences, cultural influences, and other factors.
2. The individual may assume that the nurse, being a health care provider, is aware of how the individual is experiencing pain so therefore may not readily offer information about it.
3. Individuals will provide honest information if they know that this information will be used to help control their pain. People need reassurance that their complaints of pain are believed and that the nurse will continue to provide control interventions.
4. The individual may not offer information about the pain experience because of a desire to be a "good patient."
5. The meaning of pain for each individual influences that person's response to pain.
6. Pain can cause fatigue; therefore a complete pain assessment is not always practical. Eliciting information on changes since the last pain assessment may help conserve the individual's energy.

Keeping these factors in mind, it becomes apparent that the key component in any pain assessment is good communication. Since the pain experience affects all as-

PAIN ASSESSMENT FLOWSHEET

Date and time

Location/characteristics Where is your pain located? Does it shoot/radiate? (explain) Is it deep/superficial? (explain)							
Onset Where did the pain begin? (explain) (ask on admission)							
Frequency Is your pain constant/intermittent? (explain)							
Intensity Use subjective 0-5 scale: 0 = not present; 5 = very intense How severe is your pain at the present time? (scale) How severe has the pain been, taking the last 3 days into consideration? (scale) Is the intensity of your pain always the same or does it vary? (explain)							
Quality What words best describe your pain at the present time?							
Precipitating factors Is there anything that causes or aggravates this pain? (explain) Is there anything to warn you that the pain will be starting? (explain)							
Pain control measures Effective Is there anything that you have done that helped reduce or control the pain? (explain)							
Ineffective Is there anything you have used to reduce or control the pain that did not help, or that made the pain worse? (explain)							
Desired interventions Is there anything that you have not tried that you feel may be effective? (explain)							
Pain expression style Stoic, verbal, crying, moaning, other							

PHYSIOLOGIC PARAMETERS							
Date and time							
Level of consciousness Alertness, wakefulness, orientation							
Blood pressure							
Heart Rate and rhythm							
Pulse Bounding, thready							
Respirations Rate and rhythm							
Pupils Size, equality, reactivity							
Muscles Tense, flaccid, etc.							
Skin Color, moisture, temperature							
Movement Guarding, favoring, posture, alignment, other							

pects of the individual's life, a holistic approach to pain assessment is needed that incorporates physiologic, psychologic, and social components. Several pain assessment tools or components of pain assessment tools are available.[5,16,20,25]

The boxes on pp. 1977 to 1979 are one example of a pain assessment tool. This tool was developed and used in clinical practice. It is displayed in a flowsheet format with an accompanying key. Information derived from the individual will provide a basis for the development, implementation, evaluation, and revision of the care plan. Essential physiologic, psychologic, and social elements for assessment are stated on the flowsheet. The depth of assessment varies according to the individual's pain status, the situation, the setting, and the nurse's knowledge of pain assessment.

The flowsheet provides an area for time and date in the top of each column so that the frequency of assessment can be determined for each individual situation. The flowsheet is divided into three portions. The first part includes data necessary for the assessment of anyone

experiencing pain. The second part describes physiologic aspects of the pain experience. This information may be assessed more frequently with an individual in acute pain than with an individual in chronic pain. The third part assesses the impact of pain and general psychosocial areas to be assessed. A 1 to 5 subjective rating scale is used for the individual to answer these questions. We have found this scale easier to use than a scale with a larger selection of numbers. This area of assessment may be used more often for an individual with chronic pain. In an acute pain situation, such as in an emergency room setting or immediately after surgery, some of this information is not of high priority. The information is important to assess when the pain is at a controlled level, before an individual returns to a home or community setting.

The flowsheet provides essential parameters for assessment. Additional parameters can be added or deleted as necessary. This format is helpful because the data are displayed in a manner that enables the identification of trends. This helps evaluate the effectiveness of the

IMPACT OF PAIN*

Date and time

How much does the pain bother you?					
How much has the pain affected your ability to maintain your daily activities?					
What activities have been affected or eliminated because of pain? (list)					
How much as the pain affected the quality of your sleep?					
How much as the pain affected your energy level?					
How much has the pain affected your sexual activity?					
How much has the pain affected your ability to get along with others?					
How much as the pain affected your feelings of self-worth?					

*Use 0-5 scale for all questions: 0 = not at all; 5 = very much

nursing care to determine if expected patient outcomes are met.

If the individual is an outpatient, a daily log of activities that includes when the pain occurs or intensifies and the individual's subjective pain scale ratings identifies precipitating factors and monitors changes. In any setting, when an individual is starting a new pain intervention, it is beneficial to have the individual or the nurse graphically record the pain intensity using a subjective rating scale on the pain assessment flowsheet. This provides the nurse with information concerning the effectiveness of the intervention. In addition, for interventions such as analgesia administration, which is an interdependent function of nursing, the graphic display or flowsheet display documents for the physician the effectiveness of the analgesic.

The defining characteristics are divided into categories of acute and chronic pain. Individuals can reach a point of learning to live with chronic pain. In these situations defining characteristics of chronic pain may not be identified, since the self-care deficits encountered have been resolved and adaptation has occurred.

NURSING INTERVENTIONS

Patient Goal	Nursing Intervention
Identify measures that eliminate or control pain.	Explore measure that have been successful in the past. Identify measures that patient values as essential for pain reduction. Assess patient's willingness to incorporate nonpharmaceutical pain control measures. Instruct patient on pain-reduction strategies as pain experience dictates (for short attention span in acute pain give brief explanations; for chronic pain provide more detail). Administer medication per MD protocol: 1. Monitor effectiveness at frequent intervals.

Patient Goal	Nursing Intervention
	2. Graphically record pain assessment data.
	3. Provide physician with evidence of need to change medication.
	4. Provide or instruct the patient in the importance of regular doses.
	5. Intervene at the onset of pain.
	Implement several of the following strategies as indicated by patient condition and pain status:
	1. Position for comfort.
	2. Encourage attention to proper posture and alignment.
	3. Immobilize or rest affected area.
	4. Provide distraction.
	5. Suggest and instruct patient in relaxation techniques or imagery: short simple techniques with nurse directing for acute pain; more complex techniques for chronic pain.
	6. Provide music the patient finds relaxing.
	7. Provide massage, heat/cold applications if not contraindicated.
	8. Pace activities and plan activities ahead of time.
	9. Provide touch.
	10. Attempt interventions several times before judging success.
	11. Provide supportive environment.
	12. Determine realistic pain control goals with patient.
	13. Identify emotional responses from patient.
	14. Assess which pain reduction strategies patient finds helpful.
	15. Use several pain reduction strategies.
Identify and reduce activities that precipitate or enhance pain.	Help patient to identify activities that may enhance or precipitate the pain.
	Discuss measures to prevent or reduce the precipitation or enhancement of pain.
	Discuss measures to avoid these activities within the patient's life-style.
	Encourage family members to help the patient prevent the precipitation of a painful event.
	Encourage patient to keep a daily log to help identify other activities that precipitate or enhance pain.
Incorporate interventions to reduce or eliminate pain.	Assess patient's ability to implement interventions into present life-style.
	Discuss life-style modifications that may be necessary.
	Assess the patient's desire and ability to change these aspects of his life.
	Help patient to identify measures to implement life-style modifications.
	Provide referrals or information on community resources.
Set realistic goals.	Assess patient's ability to realistically project the impact of pain in all areas of life.
	Encourage patient to set priorities and plan ahead.
	Ask patient to identify one or two realistic goals to achieve each day.
	Discuss progress in goal attainment achieved.
	Teach the patient that realistic goal setting can aid in reducing fatigue, anxiety, and depression.
	Instruct patient in goal setting to normalize life-style and place pain on the periphery of life.
Verbalize positive feelings about self.	Assess patient's perception of his progress in goal attainment.
	If patient unable to return to work, help identify meaningful ways to fill time and promote positive feelings of self-worth during free hours.
	Provide patient with positive reinforcement for activities focused away from pain.
	Assist patient in developing normalizing strategies for activities encountered in daily life.
	Educate patient on community resources for prevention or reduction of problems related to job retraining, financial assistance, etc.
	Inform the patient of the importance of maintaining communication with all health professionals.
	Assess need for referrals for family or individual counseling, financial needs, sexual concerns.
	Encourage gradual reentry into family, society, and work activities; set realistic goals for reentry.
	Provide positive reinforcement for achievements.
	Discuss patient and family feelings regarding role changes.
	Assess patient's ability to identify strengths and weaknesses and to build on strengths.

Patient Goal	Nursing Intervention
	Encourage open communication between patient and family.
	Help patient and family understand the effects of the pain experience on each family member.
	Reinforce each person's role in helping the patient cope with the pain experience.
Avoid use of life-threatening, unproven remedies.	Inform patient and family about the identification of unproven remedies.
	Instruct patient in the dangers of unproven remedies: they can be life threatening; they may be expensive; they may serve as a substitute for ongoing health care.
	Assist patient in exploring feelings regarding unproven remedies.
	Assure patient of your willingness to discuss the desire to try unproven remedies.
	Assist patient in determining how to respond to individuals who suggest unproven remedies.
	Provide patient with community resources to assist in the identification of unproven remedies.
	Do not take unharmful unproven remedies from patient (patient may have faith in this remedy thus far not found in other treatments).
Maintain weight or move toward normal weight index for height and frame.	Instruct the patient on the effects of pain on nutrition and the influence of proper nutrition on their health status.
	Instruct the patient on the need for a balanced diet to maintain their ideal weight for their height and frame.
	Obtain a dietitian referral.
	Assess motivation toward obtaining proper nutrition and achievement of ideal weight.
	If underweight for height and frame, refer to nursing diagnosis nutrition, alteration in: less than body requirements.
	If overweight for height and frame, refer to nursing diagnosis nutrition, alteration in: more than body requirements.

The choice of nursing intervention for this diagnosis is derived from information elicited during the pain assessment. To determine which interventions should be incorporated into the nursing care plan, the nurse must first consider the pain assessment information and relate this to current knowledge derived from pain theories. The pain assessment information may or may not give clues to the source of pain. Knowing the etiology is helpful but not essential in selecting appropriate interventions. At times the nurse may be able to modify or act directly on the factors that cause pain. At other times, however, the etiology is unknown. The expected patient outcomes are appropriate for any individual in pain, but the emphasis may differ for patients in acute or chronic pain. The interventions are directed at achieving the expected patient outcomes and are not specific for either acute or chronic pain.

EVALUATION

Patient Outcome	Data Indicating That Outcome is Reached
Identifies strategies that eliminate or control pain.	Demonstrates ability to differentiate between strategies that are effective and ineffective.
	Applies previous strategies that have eliminated or controlled pain.
	Uses a variety of pain control strategies.
Incorporates interventions to reduce or eliminate pain.	Physiologic parameters move toward baseline.
	Fatigue controlled.
	Sleep pattern returns to normal or adapts to changes in sleep pattern.
	Activity returns to normal or activity is modified to control pain.
	Uses pain control strategies appropriately.
	Attention span returns to or moves toward prepain status.
	Reduction or absence of guarding, protective behavior.
	Verbalizes increased control over pain.
	Social and family interactions move toward prepain status.

Patient Outcome	Data Indicating That Outcome Is Reached
	Incorporates life-style modifications. Uses community resources or referrals appropriately.
Sets realistic goals.	Patient goals are realistic for the pain experience. Patient sets priorities for the achievement of goals. Identifies short-term achievable goals and progresses goals after accurate evaluation of previous goal attainment. Moves toward resumption of previous life-style or modifies life-style according to the limitations imposed by pain experience. Reduction in or ability to control fatigue, anxiety, and depression.
Verbalizes positive feelings about self.	Verbalizes positive statements about self. Identifies personal strengths and weaknesses. Builds on personal strengths. Sets realistic goals. Reenters family, society, and work activities at a level consistent with pain experience. Life no longer revolves around the pain experience. Verbalizes increased control over self. Incorporates effective coping strategies.
Avoids use of life-threatening, unproven remedies.	Identifies the dangers of life-threatening unproven remedies. Verbalizes knowledge of resources to assist in identification of unproven remedies. Seeks support to avoid using life-threatening unproven remedies. Maintains contact with health care system.
Weight remains at or moves toward normal weight index for patient height.	Incorporate strategies for weight gain or weight loss. Uses resources within family, community, health care agency as warranted. Weight moves toward identified goal.

References

1. Beland, I.L., and Passos, J.Y.: Clinical nursing: pathophysiology and psychosocial approaches, ed. 4, New York, 1981, Macmillan Publishing Co., Inc.
2. Bond, M.R.: Personality and pain. In Lipton, S., editor: Persistent pain: modern methods of treatment, New York, 1980, Grune & Stratton, Inc.
3. Bonica, J.J.: The need for a taxonomy of pain, Pain 6(3):247, June 1979.
4. Bonica, J.J., and Ventagridda, V., editors: Advances in pain research and therapy, vol. 2, New York, 1979, Raven Press.
5. Bourbonnais, F.: Pain assessment: development of a tool for the nurse and the patient, J. Adv. Nurs. 6(4):277, 1981.
6. Brand, K.P.: Alterations in comfort. In Snyder, M.: A guide to neurological and neurosurgical nursing, New York, 1983, John Wiley & Sons, Inc.
7. Curtis, S.M.: Mechanisms of pain. In Porth, C., editor: Pathophysiology: concepts of altered health states, Philadelphia, 1982, J.B. Lippincott Co.
8. Davis, G.C., Buchsbaum, M.S., and Bunney, W.E.: Pain and psychiatric illness. In Ng, L.K.Y., and Bonica, J.J., editors: Pain discomfort and humanitarian care: Proceedings of the National Conference, New York, 1980, Elsevier/North-Holland.
9. Feldman, H.R.: Psychological differentiation and the phenomenon of pain, Adv. Nurs. Sci. 50:50-57, Jan. 1984.
10. Fordyce, W.: Behavioral methods for chronic pain and illness, St. Louis, 1976, The C.V. Mosby Co.
11. Fordyce, W.E., and Steger, J.C.: Chronic pain in behavioral medicine: theory and practice. In Pomerleau, O.S., and Brady, J.P., editors: Baltimore, 1979, Williams & Wilkins Co.
12. Fortin, J.D.: A reformulation and methodologic approach to the diagnosis of chronic pain. In Kim, M.H., McFarland, G.K., and McLane, A.M. editors: Classification of nursing diagnoses: Proceedings of the Fifth National Conference, St. Louis, 1984, The C.V. Mosby Co.
13. Guyton, A.C.: Human physiology and mechanisms of disease, ed. 3, Philadelphia, 1982, W.B. Saunders Co.
14. Hendler, N.H.: The four stages of pain. In Hendler, N.H., Long, D.M., and Wise, T.N., editors: Diagnosis and treatment of chronic pain, Boston, 1982, John Wright, PSG Inc.
15. Huhman, M.: Endogenous opiates and pain, Adv. Nurs. Sci. 4:62, July 1982.
16. Jacox, A.: Pain: a source book for nurses and other health professionals, Boston, 1977, Little, Brown & Co.
17. Kim, M., McFarland, G., and McLane, A.: Pocket guide to nursing diagnosis, St. Louis, 1984, The C.V. Mosby Co.
18. Kim, M., and Mortiz, D.: Classification of nursing diagnosis: Proceedings of the Third and Fourth National Conferences, New York, 1982, McGraw-Hill Book Co.
19. Mastrovito, R.C.: Psychogenic pain, Am. J. Nurs. 74:514, March 1974.
20. McCaffery, M.: Nursing management of the patient with pain, Philadelphia, 1979, J.B. Lippincott Co.
21. Meinhart, N.T., and McCaffery, M.: Pain: a nursing approach to assessment and analysis, Norwalk, Conn., 1983, Appleton-Century-Crofts.
22. Melzack, R., and Wall, P.D.: Pain mechanisms: a new theory, Science 150:971, Nov. 1965.
23. Melzack, R.: Pain. In Sills, D.L., editor: International encyclopedia of the social sciences, vol. II, New York, 1968, Macmillan, Inc.

24. Melzack, R., and Wall, P.D.: Psychophysiology of pain, Int. Anesthesiol. Clin. **8**(1):3, 1970.
25. Wallace, K.G., and Hays, J.: Nursing management of chronic pain, J. Neurosurg. Nurs. **14**(4):185, Aug. 1982.
26. Zabrowski, M.: Cultural components in response to pain, J. Social Issues **8**:16, 1952.

Selected Readings

Beyerman, K.: Flawed perceptions about pain, Am. J. Nurs. **83**:302, Feb. 1982.

Check, W.: Results are better when patients control their own analgesia, J. Am. Med. Assoc. **247**:945, Feb. 19, 1982.

Cohen, F.L.: Postsurgical pain relief: patients' status and nurses' medication choices, Pain **9**:265, 1980.

Coyle, N.: Analgesia at the bedside, Am. J. Nurs. **79**:1554, Sept. 1979.

Davitz, L.J., Saneshima Y., and Davitz, J.: Suffering as viewed in six different cultures, Am. J. Nurs. **76**:1296, Aug. 1976.

Fagerhaugh, S.Y., and Strauss, A.: Politics of pain management staff-patient interaction, Palo Alto, Calif., 1977, Addison-Wesley Publishing Co.

Fordyce, W.: Behavioral methods for chronic pain and illness, St. Louis, 1976, The C.V. Mosby Co.

Gildea, J., and Quirk, T.R.: Assessing the pain experience in children, Nurs. Clin. North Am. **12**(14):631, Dec. 1977.

Heidrich, G., and Perry, S.: Helping the patient in pain, Am. J. Nurs. **83**:1828, 1982.

Kim, S.: Pain: theory, research and nursing practice, Adv. Nurs. Sci. **2**(2):43, Jan. 1980.

Maruta, T., and McHardy, M.J.: Sexual problems in patients with chronic pain, Medical Aspects Human Sexuality **17**:68J, Feb. 1983.

McCaffery, M.: Understanding your patient's pain, Nurs. 80 **10**:26, Sept. 1980.

McCaffery, M.: When your patient's still in pain don't just do something: sit there, Nurs. 81 **11**:58, June 1981.

McGuire, L., and Dizard, S.: Managing pain in the young patient, Nurs. 82 **12**:52, Aug. 1982.

Melzack, R., and Dennis, S.G.: Neurophysiological foundations of pain. In Sternbach, R.A., editor: The psychology of pain, New York, 1978, Raven Press.

Newman, R.G.: The need to redefine "addiction," N. Engl. J. Med. **308**(181):1096, 1983.

Schuster, G.D.: The effects of pain on the quality of life, Orthop. Rev. **12**(5):97, May 1983.

Sweeney, S.S.: OR Observations: key to post-op pain, J. Assoc. O.R. Nurses **32**(3):391, Sept. 1980.

Wallace, K.G., and Hays, J.: Nursing management of chronic pain, J. Neurosurg. Nurs. **14**:185, Aug. 1982.

Individual-Environment Interaction

INJURY, POTENTIAL FOR THEORY AND ETIOLOGY

Throughout the world, injuries are now the leading cause of death for persons under 40 years of age.[17] Injuries are the most serious public health problem facing developed societies, and in the United States injuries account for the majority of deaths among children and young adults.[3] The magnitude of the problem is sobering. Approximately 8 million people alive today in the United States can be expected to die from injuries.[16] This translates to one death in 12. Morbidity is far more difficult to estimate. The National Disease and Therapeutic Index estimates that in 1982 there were 1.1149 billion physician contacts as a result of injury.[5] Table 8 summarizes the current significance of the problem.

Injury has always been a significant problem. Industrialization brought new modes of injury as well as new therapeutic interventions. In early days the railroad was the predominant cause of injuries. More recently the automobile has become the leading cause of civilian injuries.

Injury will continue to be the leading cause of death for the young and the elderly until the problem is examined from a new perspective. Historically, injury control was thought to be impossible because accidents were believed to be the result of human action or error, luck, or acts of God.[14] This early conception of injury and the lack of control over its cause prohibited scientific injury into its causative mechanisms and preventive strategies.

During the past decade there have been initial efforts among research investigators to abandon the term *accident* and replace it with the term *injury*. An accident is an event or condition that occurs by chance or arises from unknown or remote causes.[6] The concept of chance implies the notion of randomness. Injury, on the other hand, is used interchangeably with trauma to refer to tissue damage caused by exchanges of environmental energy that are beyond the body's resilient capacity.[9] Differentiation of these two terms is important; the ability to separate and define the injury event correctly leads to prevention strategies and the ultimate systematic reduction of injuries. If we continue to view injury as an *accident,* the notions of chance, randomness, and victim will continue to dominate our thoughts and will interfere with injury investigation and prevention. If we redefine the problem as an *injury* that results from an inability to resist energy transfer, we are in a better position to precisely investigate the problem and to develop effective prevention methods.

Several injury models have been proposed. Benner[4] best summarizes these as (1) the single cause model, in which each injury event is the direct and total result of a single identifiable cause; (2) the random interaction model, in which multiple random factors result in the injury (not in common use); (3) the outcome model, in which the injury event is the outcome of specific human-environmental interactions during a preinjury phase that precedes the moment of energy release or mobilization; the injury phase is the transfer of released energy to people and property so that damage occurs; and (4) the systems analysis model, which attempts to identify all possible factors that can fail in the design, use, degradation, and destruction of a product or environmental situation. Waller[15] confirms that most multidisciplinary injury research is being conducted around the third model.

The preinjury, injury, postinjury model of human-environmental interaction was first defined by King in 1942 and Gibson in 1961. Both investigators identified injury as the result of a transfer of physical energy. Their work has more recently been expanded and redefined by Haddon.[8-10]

Haddon uses the epidemiologic characteristics of host (the human factors), agent (the energy sources), and environment (physical environment and social environment) to develop the framework. He further divides the injury into preevent (before the injury), event (the moment that energy is being transferred), and postevent (after the injury) stages. Fig. 8 depicts the injury model.

The injury process requires interaction of the human factors, the agents, and the environment. For the nursing diagnosis injury: potential for to be fully developed, all three factors must be considered. Injury researchers such

as Haddon,[8,9] Robertson,[13,14] and Baker[1-3] have consistently demonstrated that it is the interaction of these three variables that precipitates the injury. This approach alters the current North American Nursing Diagnoses Association's (NANDA) etiologies for the nursing diagnosis injury, potential for.[11] As proposed by NANDA, the etiology involves interactive conditions between the individual and the environment that impose a risk to the defensive and adaptive resources of the individual. The etiological factors as listed by NANDA include the following:

Internal factors, host
    Biologic
    Chemical
    Physiologic
    Psychologic perception
    Developmental
External environment
    Biologic
    Chemical
    Physiologic
    Psychologic
    People-provider

Although NANDA has provided many of the components of injury risk, the etiology as developed is disorganized and incomplete. The diagnosis is presented as being developed from an epidemiologic model, yet only two of the three epidemiologic variables (host and environment) are discussed. The agent variable is not developed. In the true epidemiologic sense it is the interaction of host, agent, and environment that leads to the potential of injury. In addition to the epidemiologic model components, the etiology as presented follows none of the previously researched models for injury as found in

Table 8

Injury Death Statistics Estimates: 1983*

	Birth-4 years		5-14 years		15-24 years		25-44 years		45-64 years	
	No.†	Rate‡	No.	Rate	No.	Rate	No.	Rate	No.	Rate
All injuries	4,000	22.4	4,700	13.9	19,800	48.4	24,600	35.4	15,300	34.3
Motor vehicle	1,200	6.7	2,500	7.4	14,700	36.0	14,400	20.7	6,500	14.6
Falls	250	1.4	100	0.3	450	1.1	1,000	1.4	1,900	4.3
Drownings	750	4.2	800	2.4	1,800	4.4	1,900	2.7	850	1.9
Fires, burns and deaths associated with fire	700	13.9	350	1.0	300	0 ˙	900	1.3	1,000	2.2
Suffocation (ingested object)	170	1.0	80	0.2	100	0.2	300	0.4	700	1.6
Poisoning (solids and liquids)	80	0.4	30	0.1	500	1.2	1,300	1.9	600	1.3
Firearms	60	0.3	200	0.6	600	1.5	550	0.8	350	0.8
Poisoning (gases and vapors)	40	0.2	40	0.1	300	0.7	450	0.6	300	0.7

Data from Accidents facts, 1984 Edition, Chicago, 1984, National Safety Council.
*All estimates based on 1983 population data.
†Actual number of deaths.
‡Rate per 100,000.

INJURY MODEL

	Human factors (host)	Energy-sources (agents)	Physical-sociocultural (environment)
Preevent phase			
Event phase			
Postevent phase			

Preevent Those events and factors before the injury. It is the interaction of these factors that leads to the injury.

Event During the injury process. It is the physical response, the intensity of the energy, and the environmental situation.

Postevent Following the injury. The body's response to the energy source, the final energy dose, and the emergency care provided by those in the environment.

Fig. 8

Injury model. Because of the nursing diagnosis "Injury: potential for," the major emphasis here is placed on the preevent phase.

the literature. It seems most appropriate that, as this diagnosis is further developed and clinically researched, it builds on the current research in the field of injury prevention. An important assumption of this approach is that the diagnosis must be narrowed to define injury to be congruent with the current injury literature. Specifically, this means that the nursing diagnosis injury, potential for as defined by NANDA should exclude some of the biologic defining characteristics, such as tissue hypoxia, malnutrition, immune-autoimmune factors, abnormal blood profiles, microorganisms, nutrients, and nosocomial agents. Although these factors certainly

may lead to an illness state, that state should not be confused with injury. To do so only burdens the investigator to clearly identify the true etiology and defining characteristics. It is recommended that new diagnoses be developed to consider many of the biologic defining characteristics as currently presented by NANDA. We have eliminated many of the biologic defining characteristics, which seem to confuse the clarity of the diagnosis.

Most familiar to nurses are the host and environmental characteristics. This is evidenced by the nursing diagnosis as it is currently developed. We must look to the research from other disciplines to identify the agent factors.

Host, or human, factors include variables that pertain specifically to the person being considered. Examples of this include the individual's age, physical condition, eyesight, muscle strength, mental ability, fatigue level, growth and development, personal habits and values, stress level, blood alcohol level, and dexterity. Also included is the individual's ability to cope with an unexpected energy source that may cause harm. These factors are essentially the individual's resistance characteristics.

Agent factors are the energy sources that challenge the individual's resistance characteristics and actually cause the injury. Haddon,[8,9] Robertson,[13] Baker,[1,2] and others have begun to isolate the energy sources that are known to be responsible for causing injury. These include mechanical/gravitational, thermal, radiant, chemical, and electrical sources, and lack of oxidation. Table 9 lists these energy sources. These are possible etiologies leading to the diagnosis injury, potential for.

Environmental factors may be divided into two sections—physical and sociocultural. Examples of physical

65-74 years		75 years and over		Totals	
No.	Rate	No.	Rate	No.	Rate
7,700	47.1	14,900	135.2	91,000	38.9
2,700	16.5	2,600	23.6	44,600	19.1
1,500	9.2	6,500	59.0	11,700	5.0
250	1.5	250	2.3	6,600	2.8
450	2.8	900	8.2	4,600	2.0
550	3.4	1,300	11.8	3,200	1.4
190	1.2	300	2.7	3,000	1.3
70	0.4	70	0.6	1,900	0.8
90	0.6	80	0.7	1,300	0.6

Table 9
Energy Sources: Agent Variables

Energy Source	Examples
Mechanical/gravitational	Motor vehicle crashes; falls; firearms; lacerations
Thermal	Heat exhaustion; burns
Radiant	Sunburn; radiation burns
Chemical	Poisoning: plant and animal toxins, drugs
Electrical	Electrical shock
Lack of oxidation	Drowning; suffocation

Table 10
Strategies and Countermeasures to Prevent Injury

Countermeasure	Examples
Prevent the creation of the hazard in the first place.	Raise driving age; outlaw fireworks; initiate handgun laws
Reduce the amount of the energy source brought into being.	Reduce auto speed; decrease temperature of hot water tank; decrease lead content in paint
Prevent the release of the energy source that already exists.	Self-extinguishing cigarettes; electrical outlets that break circuit if in contact with water source
Modify the rate or spatial distribution of the energy from its source.	Fixed-nozzle spray cans; modified brake design on automobiles; shut-off valves
Separate, in time or in space, the hazard or energy source and that which is to be protected.	Air bags and safety belts in automobiles; walkways around hazards
Separate the energy source by material barrier.	Flame-retardant clothing; childproof poison containers
Modify the basic qualities of the energy source.	Alter chemical agents to reduce poison content
Increase resistance to damage from energy source.	Athletic training; firewall
Counter damage already done by energy source.	CPR; emergency care
Repair and rehabilitate injured individual.	Trauma center; rehabilitation programs

Modified from Doenges, M., Jeffries, M., and Moorhouse, M.F.: Nursing care plans: nursing diagnosis in planning patient care, Philadelphia, 1980, F.A. Davis Co.

environmental factors are defective or unsafe equipment, hazardous road conditions, and exposure to solid, liquid, or gaseous poisons. Sociocultural environmental examples are unsupervised small children, lack of knowledge to establish a safe environment, family stress, and lack of knowledge regarding developmental ability.

Injury prevention strategies involve alteration or protection of the host and/or the environment against the agent. Ten strategies or countermeasures have been developed and refined by Haddon.[8-10] These strategies, as shown in Table 10, have been used as the basis for much injury prevention research and program development.

DEFINING CHARACTERISTICS[11]

Host Factors (Internal Factors)
Biologic and physiologic factors
    Age (under 40 years, over 60 years)
    Gender (males more than females)
    Chronic diseases
    Current disabilities, especially musculoskeletal, visual, hearing, and sensory
    Metabolism and nutritional status, especially calcium deficiency
    Fatigue
    High chemical substance or alcohol blood level
Mental/psychologic
    Mental disorders
    Orientation
    Temperament/mood
    Irritability, anger
    Emotional state/lability
    Personal stresses
    Social adjustment
    Altered levels of consciousness
    Aggressiveness/social deviance
Psychomotor
    Developmental level inappropriate for task or environment
    Skill/performance capabilities
    Muscle strength and coordination
Cognitive
    Experience
    Judgment
    Education (safety and general)
Behavioral
    Attitude
    Beliefs
    Habits
    Motivation
    Preoccupation

Environmental Factors (External Factors)
Physical factors
    Mechanical
        Defective or unsafe vehicle
        Excessive speeds
        Nonuse or misuse of safety belts
        Nonuse or misuse of headgear for bicycle or motorcycle riders
        Unsafe road or road-crossing conditions
        Play near vehicle pathways (driveways, laneways, railroad tracks)

Table 11
Injury, Potential for: Case Example for Football Player

Factor	Variable to Consider	High-Risk Indicators	Low-Risk Indicators
Host	Age Muscle development Bone maturity Hydration state	Young player with immature bone and muscle strength	Older player with mature bone and muscle strength
	Conditioning Muscle conditioning Use of warm-up Fatigue	Poor muscle conditioning and warm-up; fatigue	Good conditioning and warm-up; well rested
	Mental state Mood Stresses	Anxious, unprepared, stressed	Rested, prepared, low stress
	Psychomotor Skill performance Muscle coordination	Unable to perform skill demanded	Good coordination and able to perform required skill
	Cognitive Experience Judgment Education on football technique	Lack of experience and knowledge	Adequate experience and knowledge
Agent	Mechanical	Wet or rough playing surface Many unexpected or uncontrolled falls	Well maintained playing surface Dry surface Controlled falls
	Chemical	Environmental temperature hot, causing potential heat reaction	Environmental temperature cool
Environment	Physical Environmental temperature	Hot	Cool
	Playing surface	Rough and wet	Dry and smooth
	Equipment (padding quality, equipment quality, equipment fit)	Padding not adequate Shoes and equipment poor Equipment fits poorly	Adequate padding Good shoes and equipment Good equipment fit
	Social Coaches' attitude Coaches' knowledge about resources and hazards	Hard-driving coach unknowledgeable of injury potential or risk variables	Knowledgeable coach

Dangerous machinery and appliances
Sharp-edged toys
Slippery floors (wet or highly waxed)
Furniture with sharp edges, projections, or glass
Unanchored rugs
Bathtub without hand grip or antislip equipment
Unsteady furniture
Inadequately lit rooms
Unsturdy or absent stair rails
Unanchored electrical wires
Litter or liquid spills on floors or stairways
Unprotected open windows or stairs
Use of cracked dishes or glasses
Knives stored uncovered
Guns or ammunition stored unlocked
Fireworks or gunpowder
Absence of designated play areas
Shoes without traction

Thermal
 Playing with matches, candles, cigarettes
 Highly flammable children's toys or clothing
 Smoking in bed or near oxygen
 Grease waste collected on stoves
 Contact with intense cold
 Pot handles facing toward front of stove
 Hot water heater set higher than 130° F
 Lack of smoke detectors
 Potential igniting gas leaks
 Delayed lighting of gas burner or oven
 Experimenting with chemicals or gasoline
 Unscreened fires or heaters
 Improperly stored combustibles or corrosives (matches, oily rags, lye, gasoline)
Chemical
 Large supply of drugs in home
 Medicines stored in unlocked cabinets accessible to children

Hazardous products placed or stored within reach of young children
Lack of childproof caps
Products not stored in properly labeled storage container or space
Availability of illicit drugs potentially contaminated by poisonous additives
Flaking, peeling paint or plaster
Chemical contamination of food or water
Unprotected contact with heavy metals or chemicals
Paint, lacquer, etc. in poorly ventilated areas or without effective protection
Presence of poisonous vegetation
Presence of atmospheric pollutants
Contact with acids or alkalies
Radiant
Overexposure to sun, sunlamps, radiotherapy
Electrical
Overloaded fuse boxes
Lack of safety plugs or appliance outlets
Unused extension cords plugged in
Worn electrical cords
Electrical appliances and cords near water
Overloaded electrical outlets
Lack of oxidation
Household gas leaks
Fuel-burning heaters not vented to outside
Pacifier hung around infant's neck
Pools without structural barriers
Toys with cords
Pillow or plastic sheet placed in infant's crib
Propped bottle placed in an infant's crib
Vehicle running in closed garage
Children playing with plastic bags or inserting small objects into mouth or nose
Discarded or unused refrigerators or freezers without doors removed
Sociocultural factors
Lack of parental awareness of hazards
Lack of safety education
Fatalistic attitude about injuries
Lack of knowledge of developmental stages
Negligent, abusive, or overprotective child-rearing practices
Lack of parental supervision
Lack of resources to establish safe environment (knowledge, finances)
Presence of family stress (marital, financial, health)
Inadequate community emergency medical services response
Lack of public education (first aid and CPR)
Lack of community safety programs (water safety, lifeguards, crossing guards, building codes)

To establish the nursing diagnosis injury, potential for, one must reconsider the collective interrelationship of host, agent, and environmental factors. The diagnosis may then be defined as the interaction between the individual (the host), the energy source (the agent), and the environment (physical and sociocultural) that imposes a risk for physical harm to the individual. A working example of this definition is the case application to football players described in Table 11.

NURSING INTERVENTIONS

Patient Goal	Nursing Intervention
Host Factors	
Identify variables leading to increased susceptibility.	Inform that injury is more likely to occur in individuals under 40 years of age and over 60 years of age. Inform that injury is more likely to occur in males than in females.
Identify biologic and physiologic factors that increase risk of injury.	Perform assessment. Provide information regarding disease processes or physiologic conditions that increase risk of injury. Provide alteration strategies to adapt physical environment to the patient's physiologic state.
Identify psychomotor variables that increase risk of injury.	Conduct assessment of developmental level of individual. Provide educational information regarding safety strategies appropriate for individual. Assess skill competence and performance capabilities of individual. Assess muscle strength and coordination capabilities. Provide strategies to protect individual from potential injury. Assess and provide alteration strategies to increase self-protective capabilities for individual.
Identify mental and psychologic variables that may increase risk of injury.	Assess mental impairment or decision-making ability that may interfere with individual's ability to protect self from injury. Provide protective interventions that will protect individual from injury. Monitor mood and temperament, which may increase risk of injury. Assess individual's stress patterns, which may increase risk of injury. Assess personal and social adjustments, which may increase risk of injury. Provide protective interventions if necessary to prevent injury.

Patient Goal	Nursing Intervention
Identify behavioral factors that increase risk of injury.	Identify individual's habits or aggressive acts that place the individual at higher risk for injury. Assess social deviance or effect of TV violence, which may place individual at high risk for injury. Attempt to identify variables that affect individual behavior. Provide education and passive protection that will protect individual from injury. Assess for lack of motivation regarding injury protection. Where possible provide passive protection.
Evaluate cognitive ability to prevent injury.	Assess experience and judgment in individual's ability to determine and maintain adequate injury prevention strategies. Assess educational needs in area of safety education and injury prevention.
Agent Factors	
Use appropriate countermeasures to prevent injury from specific energy sources.	Provide education relevant to the 10 countermeasures (Table 10). Provide prevention strategies that will protect individual from injury.
Identify appropriate safety factors that protect the individual from injury.	Provide information regarding product design and characteristics: restraining devices, safety caps, barriers separating the individual from the hazard (stairs, windows, pools, streets).
Environmental Factors	
Identify physical environmental risks that increase potential of injury.	Assess physical risks in the environment. Provide education and structural recommendations to decrease injury risk. Assess task demand and provide protective intervention where necessary. Provide education regarding home hazards and methods to decrease injury potential.
Identify social environmental risks that increase potential of injury.	Assess parental expectations for child's behavior. Where appropriate, provide educational information congruent with growth and developmental level. Perform assessment of parental attitude toward injury prevention strategies. Where appropriate, provide information regarding injury potential and alternative prevention strategies. Assess components of family socioeconomic status that may place family in stress situation and thus increase injury risk. Assess child-rearing practices and provide alteration strategies to assist parents. Assess potential for family abusive behavior (see further intervention strategies under violence, potential for).
Identify family structure factors that may increase the potential of injury.	Assess family structure and potential family stresses such as income, physical, and emotional situation of family members that may increase family risk to injury.

The nursing care for this nursing diagnosis is directed toward the host, agent, and environmental factors that potentially lead to injury. The intent of the interventions is preventive and not curative. Because of this, many of the interventions are either educational or include strategies to alter the environment or the individual's position in the environment. Injury prevention is a very complex process that takes place in an equally complex environment. Attention to prevention requires careful evaluation of the individual, the environment, and the agents with which the individual may come in contact.

EVALUATION

Patient Outcome	Data Indicating That Outcome is Reached
Host Factors	
Accurate appraisal of susceptibility factors	Valid appraisal of age and gender factors that indicate increased risk of injury Appropriate steps to protect self or patients at high risk from injury
Appropriate recognition of biologic and physiologic factors that increase risk of injury	Identification of chronic diseases or physiologic conditions that increase risk of injury Protective strategies to alter risk potential Modification of environment to increase safety potential

Patient Outcome	Data Indicating That Outcome is Reached
Appropriate assessment of psychomotor variables that increase risk of injury	Appropriate assessment of developmental capabilities and recognition of injury risk Protective steps to prevent injury Accurate assessment of skill competence and performance ability Strategies to increase skill performance or to protect self from injury potential Exercise or training program to meet task demand Protective devices to separate self from potential injury source Accurate recognition of fatigue state, which may lead to potential injury Appropriate steps to prevent injury
Accurate assessment of mental and psychologic variables that increase risk of injury	Recognition of variables (mental, mood, temperament, stress, irritability, hostility) that may increase risk of injury Seeking new methods to express emotions that will not increase injury potential Demonstration of methods to decrease risk of injury
Appropriate behavioral response pattern to decrease risk of injury	Recognition of habits, aggressive behavior, and motivations that may increase injury potential Seeking new knowledge and skill to decrease potential risk Demonstration of methods that decrease risk of injury
Accurate assessment of cognitive ability to decrease risk of injury	Accurate assessment of own ability, experience, judgment, and education to reduce injury risk Seeking new information and skill to decrease deficit areas Use of new knowledge and skill to decrease injury risk

Agent Factors

Appropriate use of countermeasures to protect self from injury	Knowledge of countermeasures to reduce potential of injury (Table 10) Use of appropriate countermeasures Knowledge and use of safety devices and approved products that decrease risk of injury

Environmental Factors

Ability to reduce environmental physical risks of injury	Accurate assessment of exposure to environmental risks such as home products, hazardous materials, hazardous surfaces, and unprotected areas Knowledge to reduce environmental physical risk Altering physical environment to reduce risk of injury
Ability to reduce environmental social risks of injury	Recognition of social variables, such as child-rearing practices, child supervision, and discipline practices, that may increase risk of injury Seeking instruction to modify child-rearing practices where appropriate Seeking support to intervene when stress or knowledge limits adult's ability to provide safe environment for child-rearing Acknowledgment of own limitations regarding ability to cope with social environmental stress Seeking new knowledge and skill to cope with environmental social stress

References

1. Baker, S.: Medical data and injuries, Am. J. Public Health **73**(7):733-734, 1983.
2. Baker, S., and Dietz, P.: Injury prevention. In Healthy people: the Surgeon General's report on health promotion and disease prevention: background papers, DHEW-PHS Pub. No. 79-55071A, Washington, D.C., 1979, U.S. Government Printing Office.
3. Baker, S., O'Neill, B., and Karpf, R.: The injury fact book, Lexington, Mass., 1984, D.C. Heath & Co.
4. Benner, L., Jr.: Accident theory and accident investigators, Hazard Prevention **13**(4):18-21, March/April 1977.
5. Centers for Disease Control: Morbidity and Mortality Weekly Report, vol. 32, Dec. 1983.
6. Encyclopedia Britannica, Inc.: Webster's third new international dictionary, unabridged, Chicago, 1981, G. & C. Merriam Co.
7. Gordon, J.: The epidemiology of accidents, Am. J. Public Health **39**:504-515, April 1949.
8. Haddon, W.: On the escape of tigers: an ecological note, Am. J. Public Health **60**(12):2229-2234, 1970.
9. Haddon, W.: Advances in the epidemiology of injuries as a basis for public policy, Public Health Reports **95**(5):411-421, 1980.
10. Haddon, W., and Baker, S.: Injury control. In Clark, D., and MacMahon, B., editors: Preventive medicine, ed. 2, Boston, 1981, Little, Brown & Co.
11. Kim, M., McFarland, G., and McLane, A., editors: Pocket guide to nursing diagnosis, St. Louis, 1984, The C.V. Mosby Co.
12. National Safety Council: Accident facts, Chicago, 1983, National Safety Council.
13. Robertson, L.: Injuries: causes, control strategies, and public policy, Lexington, Mass., 1983, Lexington Books.
14. Robertson, L.: Injury epidemiology and the reduction of harm. In Mechanic, D.: Handbook of health, health care, and the health professions, New York, 1984, The Free Press.
15. Waller, J.: Injury as a public health problem. In Last, J., editor: Maxcy-Rosenau: public health and preventive medicine, ed. 11, New York, 1980, Appleton-Century-Crofts.
16. Whitefield, R., Zador, P., and Fife, D.: Expected mortality from injuries, Washington, D.C., 1984, Insurance Institute for Highway Safety.
17. Wintemute, G.: The size of the problem. In Wintemute, G., Mohan, D., and Teret, S., editors: Injury prevention in developing countries, Baltimore, 1984, The Johns Hopkins University.

HOME MAINTENANCE MANAGEMENT, IMPAIRED

THEORY AND ETIOLOGY

Social Influences on the Development of Home Health

Home is a very special place for Americans. We value personal privacy and personal property so much that they are protected by the constitution. Living in a private home is believed to provide a higher quality of life than institutional care because it supports independence and individuality. Private home life facilitates self-care, which is associated with self-esteem.[6] There currently is a trend to support community-based living for high-risk populations. This has led to an increase in home health care services.

The trend is an outgrowth of three separate social movements that have occurred since the 1960s. The first is the deprofessionalization of health care. In the 1950s Americans had come to expect the physician and other health care providers to cure their health problems through accurate diagnosis and intervention that included pharmacologic agents and high technology. Americans viewed the hospital as a place to go to be cured. By 1960 health professionals realized America's major health problems were long term and required active participation by the public for prevention and treatment. Disease was multicausal and related to life-style patterns. The patient and his family were recognized as important members of the health team.

Up to the 1960s home health care had been done by the family, physician, and nurse. Then home health care agencies began to employ licensed professional nurses, community aides, and trained homemakers to use a nursing team approach to provide home care. Agencies also began to hire professionals from other disciplines, such as social workers, physical therapists, speech therapists, and nutritionists to broaden the scope of home care. Home care then involved a multidisciplinary team with various levels of preparation that included family caregivers and the patient.[12]

The second social movement was the medical self-care or consumer movement. It is related to the deprofessionalization of health care. As Americans became more aware of having a role in health care, they also sought a more active role in planning, evaluating, and controlling care decisions. Health care knowledge no longer belonged exclusively to professionals such as physicians and nurses. New courses were developed in schools and the community in response to the public's interest in health promotion and the evaluation of professional health care. One example is the courses given by the Health Action Network in Reston, Virginia, sponsored by a health maintenance organization.[25]

The third social movement was deinstitutionalization.

Studies by Goffman[13] and others demonstrated the negative impact of institutionalization for the mentally ill, retarded, and the infirm. One result was legislation to ensure that people were placed in the least restrictive environment possible for both treatment and education. Judicial decisions upheld a handicapped person's right to education and treatment. Consequently, only people in need of asylum were not discharged to the community. This stimulated the development of community-based training and residential programs for these high-risk populations. State and federal funding was structured to provide incentives for the development of treatment programs. For instance, Medicare paid for skilled nursing care in the home but not custodial nursing care.[20,21]

Home health care is a traditional role for nurses. In fact, it was the original setting for nursing practice. The change from primarily home employment to hospital employment paralleled the post–World War I movement of acute care from the home to the hospital. Today home health care is a rapidly expanding field as acute care patients are discharged to the home needing complex, skilled care and long-term care patients are being maintained at home. The community health nurse provides home-based care for an identified patient by working with the family unit to (1) provide skilled nursing care, (2) coordinate care provided by the family, paraprofessionals, social agencies, and other health professionals, and (3) assist them in behavioral changes that will increase their level of self-care and home maintenance management.[1] In providing care the nurse, in cooperation with the patient, must assess not only the health care demands of the patient and family, but also the home and community environment. The nurse's documentation of services needs to include these activities. Mundinger[20] found that community health nurses do routinely provide both health promotion and maintenance services to the entire family unit. She also found nurses assessed and intervened at the environmental level, but they only recorded direct care to the identified patient. Documentation needs to reflect all nursing activities performed to ensure demonstration of the scope of nursing practice and justification of adequate compensation.

The National Conference on Nursing Diagnoses in 1978 recognized the legitimate concern of home health care nurses for the patient's environment by expansion of their nomenclature to include six diagnoses of the environment. The environment included both the physical and social surroundings of the individual. These diagnoses were refined in 1980 and plans were made for their further development. The refined diagnoses are parenting, alteration in: actual; parenting, alteration in: potential; home maintenance management, impaired; and injury, potential for.

This section focuses on impaired home maintenance management. When this diagnosis applies, the patient is unable to independently maintain a safe, growth-promoting immediate environment. The overall nursing goal is to enable the patient to continue living at home as long as it is safe and desirable.[15] Currently the literature on this subject is diffuse and poorly developed. We found only two references to this nursing diagnosis in the literature.[5,9] However, it is anticipated that it will increase in response to the current trend toward health promotion of the well population and home-based care of both the acutely ill and high-risk populations. High-risk populations include the physically and mentally handicapped, dependent children, frail elderly, and the chronically ill. Adaptation of the home for health care is also relevant to this diagnosis.

Self-Care Nursing Theory

This section uses Orem's self-care nursing theory as a framework for making the nursing diagnosis of home maintenance management, impaired. It is only one example of how a nursing theory may be used as a framework to develop a nursing diagnosis. Orem,[23] in her theory of nursing, identifies the patient as an individual, a family, a group, or a population. In home care there usually is an identified patient that is the source of referral for nursing care. However, the nurse assesses, plans, implements, and evaluates care for the entire family unit. The family is defined as the people living together in a dwelling who view themselves as a family unit. Community health nursing uses this inclusive view of the family as the patient to focus on prevention and health promotion. The health and welfare of any family member are intimately linked to the health and welfare of the other family members, who are also the primary source of care for the impaired patient. The dwelling and the community also interact with the patient and the family and may be a threat or a support of their health and welfare. Nursing assessment includes the identified patient, the family, the home environment, and the community.[4,18,27]

When a person becomes ill, he is socially released from his usual obligations. This includes caring for his immediate environment. The family is expected not only to assist in the treatment of the patient but also to do their usual tasks around the home. Thus the family is the patient's primary source of support. If the family lacks the physical, emotional, or developmental ability to assume these tasks, they need to seek assistance from the community. The home health nurse will include an assessment of the family's ability to compensate for the patient's usual roles in her assessment and care plan.[4]

Support for the identified patient and the family may also come from an extended family, neighbors, friends, or agencies. Their intermittent assistance with home adaptations or long-term maintenance needs is an important resource. They may also offer respite care so the family can get away to rejuvenate.[8] The patient with a wide network of affiliations and a decade or more of relationships within one community is in a very different position when he is unable to independently take care of his home than the isolated newcomer. The patient who lives alone needs to cultivate a network of social affiliations to supplement professional services.

Self-care theory of nursing speaks of assessing a patient's universal self-care requirements (USCR). One USCR is prevention of hazards to life and well-being.[23] The nursing diagnosis of home maintenance management, impaired is a therapeutic self-care deficit associated with this category. A number of excellent tools developed for the assessment of the family and the home environment are printed in the community health literature. Reutter[24] describes a tool that assesses the family using Orem's self-care nursing framework and also includes the collection of environmental data. Gordon[14] includes an assessment guide that addresses the nursing diagnosis of home maintenance management, impaired in her text. (See Suggested Readings for a listing of references pertaining to assessment of the household.)

For planning interventions, Orem identifies six nursing technologies. These are the nurse's specialized skills of practice. They include communicating, coordinating, assisting, creating a milieu for therapeutic practice, maintaining life processes, and promoting growth and development.[6,22,26] Nursing technologies are chosen based on assessment of the individual patient's degree of health deviation, state of growth and development, age, self-image, social roles, capacity for self-care, culturally derived goals, and his supports and home environment.[6,22] By means of the nursing process the plan is implemented and evaluated, with the nursing diagnoses as the organizing principles for care.

To facilitate discharge and effective long-term care, nurses in the hospital doing discharge planning also need to look beyond the identified patient to assess their family and home environment. Whether this is an acutely ill, chronically ill, newly disabled, or terminally ill person going home, the family will be the principal caregivers. Planning is ideally done before the patient is discharged to train the caregivers in the techniques of care of the patient and to adapt the home as a workplace to provide necessary nursing care.[11] The social roles of family members may also need to be permanently adapted to compensate for a patient handicap or susceptibility caused by the illness. Success or failure of home placement may also hinge on the structural characteristics of the dwelling and the supports available in the community both for family respite and professional services.[19] Training for self-care and adaptation, including home management, may be needed for the newly disabled or the person who becomes disabled over time with a chronic illness. A common example is the patient with severe arthritis who lives at home. The home care nurse works as a part of the multidisciplinary team to assist the family and patient to adapt their home and roles to allow maximum independence for the disabled member.[19] (See Suggested Readings for discharge planning for specific high-risk populations.)

Etiology

The diagnosis of home maintenance management, impaired is most common in cases where the family fails to adapt the home and family roles to care for a member who is disabled by disease, injury, maturational level, or congenital anomaly. However, it may occur in a well family or with a person living alone. The following are etiologies for impaired home maintenance management:

    Insufficient knowledge
        Lack of socialization (role model and/or emigration)
        Unfamiliarity with neighborhood resources
        Lack of training in adaptation of home maintenance skills
    Insufficient family organization and planning
    Insufficient finances
    Dysfunctional grieving
    Inadequate social support system
        Insufficient amount
        Insufficient quality
        Impaired family member
    Inadequate dwelling and/or furnishings
        Overcrowding
        Lack of adaptation of home structure or furnishings
        Structural defects
        Lack of equipment or aids for home care by disabled individual
    Inadequate community resources
        Insufficient community environmental sanitation or control of environmental contaminants or pollutants
        Lack of community professional and paraprofessional home care services

A safe, hygienic environment that offers social and physical stimulation for personal growth and development is the baseline sought for each identified patient. Failure to achieve this goal is associated with an imbalance in compensation by the patient, family, and/or community or a deficit in the dwelling and/or surrounding environment. The imbalance may be the result of lack of knowledge or insufficient support for the patient, family, and/or community. The dwelling may be unsuitable for the patient and family, in need of adaptation, or situated in a community that is unsafe or unhealthy for the patient.

Support may also be the home care nurse and other professionals in the community who provide social stimulation as well as refer the patient to appropriate resources. Citizens are often unaware of community services until they have a need for them. The consumer movement and health education campaigns by local, state, and federal governments and professional organizations have somewhat increased the public's knowledge of health practices and resources available in their communities. Many communities have homemaker services, extended payment plans for winter heating bills, institutional temporary respite care for the disabled, and other programs to help families maintain disabled members at home.

The community also contributes to the quality of life of its residents through its environmental health and sanitation programs. This support is especially important to community members who are disabled or sick. For instance, no matter how well the person maintains and adapts his home, if the building codes are not enforced and the pest control not done on a community-wide basis, the home will not be hygienic or safe. In addition, disabled people may be especially susceptible to pollutants that the general population can tolerate. An example is a person with emphysema living where there is smog.[2]

Lack of knowledge of community resources was mentioned previously. A person may also be unaware of how to maintain a safe, hygienic home or how to provide a growth-stimulating environment because of their developmental status, impaired cognitive functioning, or lack of role models. A very young person with few social supports may not have the necessary experience in caring for a dwelling to keep it clean or control pests. Or they may not know that a baby has poor internal temperature control and needs extra warmth in cold weather. Alternatively, an elderly person may not realize his declining ability to sense cold and fail to keep warm enough at night.

Impaired cognitive functioning is a problem both for mentally retarded adults and patients with organic brain dysfunctions. The health care trend of deinstitutionalization may have led to their placement in the community without the supports and training they need for home maintenance management. However, many programs do demonstrate how these patients can learn to care for themselves and their homes through training and continuing support in halfway houses, group homes, or foster homes.

Impaired home maintenance management is rarely the reason that a patient seeks nursing care in the home. However, in the nursing assessment of the patient, family, supports, dwelling, and community the nurse may identify current home maintenance management as a barrier to either healthful living or to providing nursing care. Necessary adaptations of the structure or furnishings for home care may be missing. Aids that could increase the patient's independence may be missing. Intervention for this diagnosis may take precedence over others to create a work place for safe care or to prevent injury of the patient and family. The home maintenance practices and facilities may be adequate for the family with healthy members but be hazardous for a patient.

Impaired home maintenance management may also be secondary to other nursing diagnoses or even a sign of their presence. For example, one objective sign of dysfunctional grieving is failing to participate in home maintenance tasks until the home is unsafe or unhygienic. Other diagnoses for which impaired home maintenance management may be a sign are alterations in parenting and ineffective coping by the individual or family. Impaired home maintenance may also be part of the etiology of another nursing diagnosis, such as potential injury, especially the subcategories of potential for poisoning (if garbage is not removed or food is stored under unsafe conditions) or potential for trauma (if necessary home repairs are not done).

DEFINING CHARACTERISTICS

The defining characteristics for this nursing diagnosis are listed under the headings of subjective (patient stated) and objective (nurse observed). Some examples are given to help clarify the characteristics. To establish the nursing diagnosis, any configuration of individual characteristics might be present. Any one critical defining characteristic is sufficient to form the diagnosis.

Subjective (patient stated)[15,17]; household member[15,17]:
  Express difficulty in maintaining their home in a comfortable, safe, and hygienic manner*
  Express difficulty in supporting personal growth of family members
  Request assistance with home maintenance management*
  Describe outstanding debts or financial crises that impede home maintenance management*
  Express ignorance of how to provide environment conducive for patient care
  Express exhaustion and/or inability to keep up the home
  Discuss dissatisfaction with dwelling because of overcrowding or lack of personal space
  Complain that furnishings are inadequate to maintain order or support healthful living patterns
  Show nurse defects in structure or utilities and express inability to have them repaired*
  Express lack of knowledge about community resources
  Express that environmental factors negatively affect their ability to maintain their home (for example, litter discarded in their yard every night makes it impossible for them to keep their yard maintained)

Express frustration that known resources are unavailable or insufficient in their community (for example, a patient may know that Meals on Wheels exists but is unavailable in their community)
Objective (nurse observed)[15,17]
  Presence of disease or disability necessitating adaptation of home maintenance
  Lack of knowledge of caregiver*
  Overtaxed family members (exhausted, anxious)*
  Inadequate support system
  Apparent lack of economic resources
  Disorganized home
  Knowledge of home maintenance inconsistent with current environment (for example, family moving from one country or culture to another may not know how to maintain a home in the new environment)
  Home lacks personal items and attempts at decoration
  Presence of indoor pets that are not housebroken
  Disorderly surroundings
  Unavailable cooking utensils, linen, or clothes because insufficient supply or unwashed*
  Accumulation of dirt, food waste, or hygienic waste*
  Offensive odors
  Inappropriate household temperature and/or insufficient ventilation
  Presence of vermin or rodents
  Repeated hygienic disorders, infestations, or infections*
  Lack of necessary equipment or aids
  Overcrowding for the available space
  Presence of structural barriers (for example, a family member must use wheelchair, but the home has thick carpeting and doorways are narrow)
  Unrepaired defects in structure or utilities*
  Characteristics of neighborhood make it difficult for effective home maintenance

Home maintenance management, impaired is defined as the state in which a patient is unable to or potentially unable to independently maintain a safe, growth-promoting home environment.[5,9,15,17] When assessing for this nursing diagnosis, the nurse must consider the individual, family, dwelling, and the community. The key observation is of the dwelling itself and its organization, cleanliness, and safety for both daily living and patient care. Observation for signs of provision for personal growth and individuality of family members is also necessary. The following parameters should be considered:

1. What is the individual patient's physical or mental status? Is there a disease or disability present that may impede home maintenance?
2. What is the home situation?
   a. Type of housing unit
   b. Location of housing unit
   c. Condition of housing unit
   d. Number of occupants in unit
3. What is patient's standard of home maintenance?
4. What is patient's perception of own ability to maintain the home?

---

*Critical defining characteristic.

*Critical defining characteristic.

5. What support system is available and what are its capabilities?
6. What community resources are available to enable patient to remain in the home situation?
7. Are financial resources adequate to maintain home?
8. What equipment is needed to facilitate adaptation?
9. Are there structural deficits and/or barriers that make home maintenance difficult?
10. What effect does the neighborhood or community have on the patient's ability to maintain the home?

NURSING INTERVENTIONS

Patient Goal	Nursing Intervention
Identify factors perceived as making it difficult to maintain the home.	Ask each member to identify how his home is different now and how long it has been unsatisfactory. Systematically identify factors that impede meeting the household standard. Have members state what factors in their home affect their health and how. Compare the patient's perceptions with nurse's observations. Share nurse's observations.
Recognize what daily maintenance can be realistically performed.	Discuss what each member now does and how often. Discuss possible role changes. Nurse differentiates hygienic factors that are esthetic from ones that negatively affect health.
Assess the current support system and develop a plan to supplement the family resources.	Identify members of current support system and assess their capabilities (assess daughter's contribution). Discuss community resources for daily home maintenance. Mutually develop a plan of care to increase supports.
Use community resources in an efficient, appropriate manner.	Initiate referrals for supplementation of daily home maintenance (homemaker service). Investigate community resources for long-term maintenance. Review with support system members how to use RN as continuing resource.
Adapt the home and/or life-style to promote maximum health and safety.	Discuss specific life-style and home changes that will promote health (consideration of adapting first floor rooms as bedrooms). Discuss rearranging furnishings for cleaning and safety. Reinforce changes by discussing positive impact; praise attempts at adaptation.
Repair structural defects.	Discuss relationship of defects to health (falling plaster to acute episodes of COPD). Discuss possible disease caused by defects (disease organisms in sewage from toilet). Investigate alternative ways to have repairs made within financial capabilities of family. Support attempts to obtain repairs.
Obtain and appropriately use equipment facilitating home maintenance.	Determine equipment and supplies needed, identify sources, obtain. Teach appropriate use and maintenance of equipment. Review means of maintaining sufficient supplies.
Manage home maintenance adequately.	Arrange for additional support on a regular basis. Have caregiver and family establish a mutually agreeable standard of cleanliness and order that is safe. Teach caregiver to support maximum independence of client. Observe couple for increased level of health secondary to cleaner home environment; when observed, compliment them on changes.
Increase awareness of the impact of neighborhood on home maintenance.	Identify factors in the community that negatively affect patient's ability to maintain home. Identify local resources that work to promote changes; encourage family participation. Assist family to assess safety of the neighborhood and periodically consider their housing options.

The following patient situation is presented here to illustrate the use of this nursing diagnosis.

Mrs. B. is a 73-year-old woman with a medical diagnosis of COPD. She has had repeated hospitalizations for acute episodes of this condition. Mrs. B. has recently been discharged and is undergoing steroid and oxygen therapy. The home health nurse has received a referral from the hospital to assess the home situation and identify home factors contributing to the frequency of the acute episodes.

On the first visit the nurse finds that Mrs. B. resides with her 76-year-old husband in a three-bedroom, two-story home in an older area of the city. All the bedrooms and the only full bathroom are on the second floor. The steps to the front of the house lead directly to the sidewalk along a busy thoroughfare. There is heavy truck traffic. The neighborhood appears to be declining. Litter has accumulated along the curbs, and many homes appear to need painting and general maintenance.

Mrs. B. greets the nurse by apologizing for "the mess." "I just don't have the energy to keep it up anymore," she states. The conversation and health history reveal that they own their home and have lived there for 41 years. They have many friends and a daughter who lives two blocks away. Mr. B. had a CVA 3 years ago. He has some slight weakness on the right side, but no paralysis. The nurse notes that he does not use a walker or cane to compensate for his unsteady gait. He uses furniture as a means to steady himself. Mr. B. contributes little help around the house. He also goes to a city hospital for his care. He takes hypertension medication regularly.

Mrs. B. has her medication and appears knowledgeable about dosage and possible side effects. Mrs. B. becomes very short of breath on exertion and especially when she must go upstairs. Arrangements have been made to deliver the oxygen tank the next day. It will be kept in the living room, where she spends most of the day watching television, sitting near an open window. The house has no air conditioning and it is summer. She is looking forward to the oxygen because it helped so much in the hospital. Neither of them smoke.

The house appears cluttered with furniture and memorabilia. It is dusty and some unwashed dishes are in the sink. There is a large, heavy, dusty upright vacuum cleaner in a corner of the living room. The walls are soiled, and paint is peeling off the kitchen walls. There is a hole in the ceiling near the peeling paint, and bits of plaster can be seen on the floor. Mr. B. explains there is a leaky toilet upstairs that occasionally overflows. It did so a few weeks ago and then the hole appeared in the ceiling below it. They would like to have it repaired, "but with Mary being sick, we cannot afford it." They live on a fixed income. Their only insurance coverage is Medicare.

Based on her observations and discussions, the nurse assesses the couple as her patient. She determines several nursing diagnoses, including home maintenance management, impaired. This care plan pertains only to this one diagnosis. Her notes state:

S: Mrs. B. stated lack of energy to maintain home.
   Mr. B. stated insufficient income to repair ceiling and toilet.
O: Insufficient support system to compensate for family disability related to disease (Mrs. B: COPD; Mr. B: CVA)
   Disorderly surroundings (crowded furniture and memorabilia)
   Lack of necessary aids or equipment (no dishwasher, quad cane, lightweight vacuum, or air conditioner)
   Insufficient family planning for adaptation to home care
   Accumulation of wastes (plaster and dust)
   Structural defects (unrepaired toilet and hole in ceiling)
   Structural barriers (stairs, bedrooms and bath upstairs)
   Characteristics of neighborhood make home maintenance difficult (litter, heavy road traffic polluting area)
Diagnosis: Home maintenance management, impaired

The above care plan is generalized to provide an example for any patient with this diagnosis. For illustration purposes, some examples from the case description of Mr. and Mrs. B. are given in parentheses. The overall goal is for the patient to remain in the home for as long as it is safe, feasible, and desirable.

EVALUATION

Patient Outcome	Data Indicating That Outcome is Reached
Accurate assessment of factors associated with home maintenance	Home maintenance defined as health problem. Each member states personal standard of home maintenance. Each member contributes in identification of factors that impede home maintenance. Nurse shares validation and discrepancies observed with family.
Realistic assessment of family members' capacity for daily maintenance	Current roles stated; possible role changes discussed. Hygienic factors differentiated.
Accurate assessment of support system and development of a realistic plan	Share perception of their support system, its strengths and weaknesses. Need for outside help defined. States what resources are available after the nurse shares her knowledge of available resources. Nurse and patient develop plan of care.

Patient Outcome	Data Indicating That Outcome is Reached
Appropriate and efficient use of community resources.	Contact with resources is initiated. Deficits in support are compensated. Support system members use RN appropriately.
Adaptation of home and/or life-style to promote health	Adaptation of home or life-style present. Expresses awareness of association of change with health.
Completion of repairs to structural defects	States relationship between defects and maintaining healthy, safe home. Sought help from community resources for repair of and financial help in eliminating structural defects. Observation of repairs.
Appropriate use of equipment and supplies	Equipment and supplies obtained. Equipment used appropriately. Verbalizes how to obtain future supplies and how to arrange for repair of equipment.
Adequate home maintenance management	Additional support obtained. Patient and household help mutually determine standard of cleanliness for home. Family maximally participates in own home maintenance. Family discusses own roles in maintaining a cleaner, safer environment.
Awareness of impact of neighborhood on home maintenance	Verbalizes factors negatively affecting home maintenance. Identifies neighborhood improvement resources; at least one member of the family participates. Verbalizes factors that would lead to changing residence.

References

1. American Nurses' Association: A conceptual model of community health nursing, Kansas City, 1980, American Nurses' Association.
2. Anderson, C.L., Morton, R.F., and Green, L.: Community health, St. Louis, 1978, The C.V. Mosby Co.
3. Burgess, W.: Community health nursing practice: a workbook in skill building modules, Norwalk, Conn., 1983, Appleton-Century-Crofts.
4. Burgess, W., and Ragland, E.: Community health nursing: philosophy, process, and practice, Norwalk, Conn., 1983, Appleton-Century-Crofts.
5. Carpenito, L.: Nursing diagnosis: application to practice, Philadelphia, 1983, J.B. Lippincott Co.
6. Coleman, L.J.: Orem's self-care concept of nursing. In Riehl, J.P., and Roy, C., editors: Conceptual models for nursing practice ed. 2, Norwalk, Conn., 1980, Appleton-Century-Crofts.
7. Coombs, E.M.: A conceptual framework for home nursing, J. Adv. Nurs. **9**:157-163, 1984.
8. Davis, A.J.: Disability, home care, and the caretaking role in family life, J. Adv. Nurs. **5**:475-484, 1980.
9. Doenges, M., Jeffries, M., and Moorhouse, M.F.: Nursing care plans: nursing diagnosis in planning patient care, Philadelphia, 1980, F.A. Davis Co.
10. Fortinsky, R., Granger, E., and Seltzer, G.B.: The use of functional assessment in understanding home care needs, Medical Care **19**:489-497, 1981.
11. Fralic, M.: Simultaneous imperatives (editorial), J. Nurs. Admin. **14**(9):9-10, 1984.
12. Gallager, B.: Nursing role in home health care. In Jarvis, L., editor: Community health nursing, Philadelphia, 1981, F.A. Davis Co.
13. Goffman, E.: Asylums, New York, 1961, Aldine Publishing Co.
14. Gordon, M.: Nursing diagnosis, New York, 1982, McGraw-Hill Book Co.
15. Jakob, D.: Home maintenance management impaired. In Kim, M.J., and Moritz, D.A., editors: Classification of nursing diagnoses, New York, 1982, McGraw-Hill Book Co.
16. Joseph, L.S.: Self-care and the nursing process, Nurs. Clin. North Am. **20**:131-143, 1980.
17. Kim, M.J., McFarland, G., and McLane, A.: Pocket guide to nursing diagnosis, St. Louis, 1984, The C.V. Mosby Co.
18. MacIvar, M., and Archoid, P.A.: A framework for family assessment in chronic illness, Nurs. Forum **15**:180-194, 1976.
19. Martin, N., Holt, N., and Hicks, D.: Comprehensive rehabilitation nursing, New York, 1981, McGraw-Hill Book Co.
20. Mundinger, M.: The relationship between policy and practice in the delivery of medicare home health services, Doctoral dissertation, 1981, Columbia University.
21. Mundinger, M.: Home care controversy, Rockville, Md., 1983, Aspen Systems Corporation.
22. Norris, C.M.: Self care, Am. J. Nurs. **79**:486-489, 1979.
23. Orem, D.: Nursing: concepts of practice, ed. 2, New York, 1980, McGraw-Hill Book Co.
24. Reutter, L.: Family health assessment: an integrated approach, J. Adv. Nurs. **9**:391-399, 1984.
25. Sehnert, K.: The medical care self care movement: past, present, and future. In Lorentz, N.G., and Davis, D., editors: Strategies for public health, New York, 1981, Van Nostrand Reinhold Co.
26. Smith, M.C.: Proposed metaparadigm for nursing research and development: an analysis of Orem's self care theory, Image **11**(3):75-79, 1979.
27. Williamson, J.A.: Mutual interaction: a model of nursing practice, Nurs. Outlook **29**:104-107, 1981.

Suggested Readings

Readings that include assessment tools of the home:

Block, G., Nolan, J., and Dempsey, M.: Health assessment for professional nursing, Norwalk, Conn., 1981, Appleton-Century-Crofts.

Fields, W., and McGinn, K.C.: Introduction to health assessment, Reston, Va., 1983, Reston Publishing Co., Inc.

Harnish, Y.: Patient care guides: practical information for public health nurses, New York, 1976, National League for Nursing, Pub. No. 21-1610.

Helvie, C.: Community health nursing, Philadelphia, 1981, Harper & Row, Publishers.

Stanhope, M., and Lancaster, J.: Community health nursing, St. Louis, 1984, The C.V. Mosby Co.

Young, R.: Community health nursing workbook: family as client, Norwalk, Conn., 1982, Appleton-Century-Crofts.

Readings pertaining to discharge planning:

Altman, H.: A collaborative approach to discharge planning for chronic mental patients, Hospital Community Psychiatry **34**(7):641-642, July 1983.

Bachman, C., and Preston, K.: Effective rehabilitation: reintegration into the community, Rehab. Nurs. **9**(1):14-16, Jan./Feb., 1984.

Cagan, J.: Evaluation of a discharge planning tool for use with families of high risk infants, Nurs. '83 **13**(8):65-67, Aug. 1983.

Chisholm, M.: Promises and pitfalls of discharge planning, Nurs. Manage. **14**(11):26-29, 1983.

Dwyer, J., and Heed, D.: Home management of the adult patient with leukemia, Nurs. Clin. North Am. **17**(4):665-676, Dec. 1982.

Marvin, J.A.: Planning home care for burn patients, Nurs. '83 **13**(8):65-67, Aug. 1983.

Shine, M.: Discharge planning of the elderly, Nurs. Clin. North Am. **18**(2):403-410, 1983.

Sexuality-Reproductive

SEXUAL DYSFUNCTION

Sexual dysfunction is a disruption of extreme variation of sexual behavior. It is defined further by an identifiable disturbance of a phase or phases of the sexual response pattern (orgasm phase disorders, excitement phase disorders, and desire phase disorders) and excessive pain and phobic avoidance of sex (both simple and panic). Sexual dysfunction as an extreme variation of sexual behavior is defined by the object, animate or inanimate, required for sexual arousal and release; its habitual use; and a disregard for the rights, damage, pain, fear, and sensitivities when the object is animate.

THEORY AND ETIOLOGY

Dysfunctional sexual response patterns can be primarily psychogenic, organic, or secondary to illness, psychologic disorders, or stress. The identification of disruption in one of the three phases is critical when considering focused sex therapy interventions. Self-report of sexual problems is insufficient evidence of actual dysfunctional sexual response patterns. When dysfunctional sexual response patterns are not in evidence, self-report of sexual problems and dissatisfaction most often have their etiological roots in psychiatric disorders or relationship problems rather than primary dysfunctional sexual responses.[2] Situational sexual response symptoms, avoidance and phobic responses, and situational inhibition are most often sexual problems not associated with medical problems.[2]

As a general rule, a primary sexual symptom that has "always" been present is more likely to be psychogenic than a secondary disorder that occurs after a period of good functioning, especially in the absence of trauma and stress.[2]

Organic causes should be suspected in a person whose sexual functioning has been normal for a significant period, especially when there is deterioration of ejaculatory functions or orgasm becomes delayed.[2,3] Precipitous impairment of erection, orgasm, or libido suggests that drugs with sexual side effects or injury to the genitals may be involved.[2] Estrogen deficiency in a woman is characterized by gradually increasing vaginal dryness.[2] Slowly diminished libido in a male can be associated with age-related diminution of testosterone or a slowly growing pituitary adenoma.[2,3]

Sexual disorders frequently associated with organic causes are as follows[2]:

Impotence
Dyspareunia
Vaginismus
Unconsummated marriage
Low or absent libido
Secondary anorgasmia in males and females
Secondary premature ejaculation
Secondary retarded ejaculation

In healthy medically asymptomatic individuals the following disorders are seldom associated with organic causes[2]:

    Primary premature ejaculation
    Primary impairment of female orgasm
    Retarded ejaculation

Sexual dysfunction as an extreme variation of sexual behavior, often called sexual deviations, by virtue of its long-standing and habitual characteristics is most often psychogenic with roots in psychic conflict and early conditioning. Even though there may be a disruption of the phases of the sexual response pattern in these individuals, more often the sexual response pattern is only invoked by the extremely variant object, animate or inanimate. The behavior (such as voyeurism, exhibitionism, pedophilia) often brings the individual in conflict with the law; or family members are implicated, as in incest, when the child comes to the attention of the health professional.

A framework of categorizing the broad nursing diagnoses of sexual dysfunction into subdiagnoses is used here. Each subdiagnostic category is described separately regarding the etiology and defining characteristics. Within this framework common organic causes and common psychosocial causes are identified.

The eight nursing subdiagnoses to be discussed include the following[1-3]:

1. Concern about sexual functioning without disruption of sexual patterns (secondary to organic and/ or psychosocial causes)
2. Disruption of sexual response pattern: orgasm/ejaculation phase
3. Disruption of sexual response pattern: excitement phase
4. Disruption of sexual response pattern: desire phase
5. Pain (pre- and post-orgasm/ejaculation phases)
6. Functional pain/disgust (dyspareunia)
7. Phobic avoidance of sexual experience (simple/complex)
8. Extreme variation of sexual behavior and object of sexual arousal without regard for the welfare of the object

Etiologies of Sexual Dysfunction[1-3]

Concern About Sexual Functioning Without Disruption of Sexual Response Pattern (Secondary to Organic and/or Psychosocial Causes)

Common organic causes
    Pregnancy, childbirth
    Mild infections of genitourinary tract and genitals (epididymitis, trichomoniasis)
    Disease states (heart attack, back surgery)
    Drugs or medication
Common psychosocial causes
    Unrealistic expectations of self and others
    Inadequate sexual techniques and poor communications
    Religious beliefs or cultural taboos
    Diminished interest and attachment to present sexual object
    Preoccupation with demanding and/or stressful activity
    Disruption and/or lack of comfort and privacy
    Lack of desired sex object (for example, isolation imposed because of travel, imprisonment)
    Age changes (such as in appearance, social functioning)
    More serious psychologic disorders (obsessional disorders, affective disorders, psychotic disorders)
    More serious, complex relationship issues (pathologic spouse, parental transference problems, incompatible marriage)

Disruption of Sexual Response Pattern: Orgasm/Ejaculation Phase

Common organic causes
    Male
        None for primary premature ejaculation
        Possible prostatism
        Secondary ejaculatory disorders due to organic factors (radical abdominal surgery and pelvic surgery, trauma or disease of lower spinal cord)
        Alpha-adrenergic blocking drugs; thioridazine
    Female
        None for primary anorgasmia
        Secondary anorgasmia disorders due to organic factors (advanced diabetes, MAO inhibitors, spinal cord injury, neurologic injury)
Psychosocial causes
    Obsessive self-observation during sex (critical appraisal, dissociated appraisal)
    Inability to "let go," (images and thoughts that distract, lower sexual responsiveness)
    For men: failure to perceive or register erotic sensations prior to orgasm (involved in self-observation, unaware of increasing penile sensations and mounting pleasure); for women: thoughts, images distracting from mounting pleasure
    Deeper intrapsychic and relationship problems (unconscious hostility toward men or women, unconscious guilt over pleasure, withholding, power struggle)

Disruption of Sexual Response Pattern: Excitement Phase

Common organic causes
    Men
        Diabetes
        Penile circulatory problems
        Endocrine problems
        Drugs: antihypertensive, beta-blockers, alcohol
        Radical pelvic surgery
        Spinal cord injuries
    Women
        Estrogen deficiency (menopause)
        Atropic vulvovaginitis
        Oophorectomy
        Radical pelvic surgery
        Vascular problems
        Endocrine: thyroid deficiency, Addison's disease, Cushing's syndrome
        Drugs, alcohol: antihistamines, anticholinergic drugs, psychotropic drugs
Psychosocial causes
    Performance anxiety

Partner pressure

Overconcern with pleasuring partner

Deeper psychologic causes

Not specific to sex; vary from minor to severe

Ambivalence about intercourse; minor to severe

Intrapsychic: oedipal problems; cultural guilt about sex; identity problems, seen more in males

Relationship: ambivalence toward partner, overconcern with pleasing, fear of rejection, inability to request desired sexual stimulation; partner "turn off"

Disruption of Sexual Responses Pattern: Desire Phase

Common organic causes

Disease state that reduces testosterone

Depression

Severe stress

Drugs (those which impair the sex circuits of the brain; beta-blockers, narcotics, alcohol)

Psychosocial causes

"Anti-fantasies"—focus on negative aspects of partner or sexual situations

Avoidance of erotic stimulation

Avoidance of erotic fantasies

Intrapsychic: fear of intimacy and commitment; complex dynamic connections to parental/sibling relationships

Psychiatric disorders

Relationship: anger, fear, out of love with partner

Pain (Pre- and Post-Orgasm/Ejaculatory Phase)

Organic causes

Genital muscle spasm

Infection in urinary tract (prostatitis, vesiculitis, herpes)

Painful gynecologic conditions (pelvic inflammatory disease, endometriosis, hymenal remnants, ovarian pathology, ectopic pregnancy, lower bowel disease, herpes)

Conditioned, voluntary painful spasm of perineal muscles of internal reproductive organs; secondary to psychologic problems, can range from minor to severe; neurosis and relationship problems

Functional Pain/Disgust (Dyspareunia)

Organic causes (Pain is more often organic than psychogenic; therefore, organic causes must be ruled out.)

Psychogenic causes (Usually complex and moderate to severe intrapsychic and relationship problems. Pain provides a defense against pleasure.)

Hyperchondriacal reaction to hormonal shifts

Pain: hysterical, depression syndrome

Intractable schizophrenia

Functional genital muscle spasm

Brutal sexual assault; intercourse; foreign object

Phobic Avoidance of Sexual Experience (Simple/Complex)

Associated with panic disorders (hypothesized to panic threshold, as if alarm is on; overreacts to hazards and separations)

Simple sexual phobia (conditioning and neurotic conflicts)

Sexual trauma (rape, sexual exploitation, sex stress situations [acute/chronic], delayed, "silent")

Extreme Variation of Sexual Behavior and Object of Sexual Arousal Without Regard for the Welfare of the Object

Object: pedophile: infant, child, adolescent

Etiology unknown (hypothesize that there is an excess or imbalance of endocrines, leading to hypersexuality)

Possible lowered hormonal functioning as a process of aging; compensating fear of failing sexual prowess

Transitory life experience (such as loss of spouse, loss of self-esteem)

Organic brain disease

Complex and severe psychological disorders with primary character disorder; disturbed social relations

Marked cognitive set justifying object choice and behavior; claiming it is nonharmful to immature individuals

History of victimization as a child (sexual or physical)

Primary social networks and family that overlooks, condones indirectly, and supports behavior

Sexual trauma: rape, sexual exploitation (chronic, delayed, silent)

Object: rapist

Organic causes

Never established (some hypotheses regarding endocrine and genetic considerations)

Severe psychologic and relationship issues

Antisocial traits, borderline, paraphiliac, paranoid, psychotic state

History of victimization

History of impulsivity and sadism toward animals

Shallow relationships; intimacy/commitment issues

History of witnessing violence, in particular in the family by father or male caretaker

DEFINING CHARACTERISTICS

Concern about sexual functioning without disruption of sexual response pattern (secondary to organic and/or psychosocial causes)

Concern over sexual functioning because of sudden minor alterations in responsiveness (such as time it takes to achieve sexual satisfaction)

Questions regarding sexual practices (such as amount, exertion, should erection be encouraged)

Confusion, anxiety toward expression of sexual drive

Confusion over intensity of response

Concern over adequacy in meeting sexual desire of partner

Confusion over object of sexual arousal (same for male and female)

Disruption of sexual response pattern: orgasm/ejaculation phase

Men

Premature ejaculation (inadequate control of ejaculation reflex)

Retarded ejaculation (delayed or absent)

Partial retarded ejaculation; inhibition of emission phase only; no pleasure

Retarded ejaculation

Premature ejaculation

Women

Inhibited orgasm (delayed or absent orgasm, missed orgasm)

Insufficient stimulation

Disruption of sexual response pattern: excitement phase

Men

Impotence

Disturbance of sexual pleasure

Diminished excitement

Women

Vaginal dryness

Painful coitus
Disturbance of sexual pleasure
Disruption of sexual response pattern: desire phase
  Total loss of desire
  Loss of desire in specific situations only
  Chronic, low sexual desire
Pain (pre- and post-orgasm/ejaculatory phase)
  Pain prior to sex (prevents entry or ejaculation)
  Perineal pain (muscle spasm)
  Vaginal spasms after penis has entered
  Postorgasmic uterine spasms
Functional pain (dyspareunia)
  Pain on entry (deep thrusting)
  Vaginismus
Phobic avoidance of sexual experience (simple/complex)
  Phobic avoidance of sexual experience and sexual arousal
Extreme variations of sexual behavior and object of sexual arousal without regard for the welfare of object
  Pedophile
    Expression of primary sexual interest in infant, child, and/or adolescent by an adult male or female
    Hypersexual activity with underaged persons
    Compulsion for involvement with immature sex object
    Focusing on one object at a time or on a group of children
    Involvement in pornography purchases and/or production
    Prefers to be alone (however, can be involved in work activities that either provide contact with immature individuals or time to pursue sexual activities with immature individuals or time to pursue sexual activities with one underaged person)
    Uses bribes, coercion, and intimidation with object
    Potentially violent; potentially homicidal
    Marriage of convenience (cover); or marriage to have access to child
    May be in clandestine social relationships with other pedophiles

More males than females as perpetrators
History of legal confrontation for involvement with immature individuals
Intelligence often average to above average
Rapist
  Requires absolute control of the object
  Uses force
  Inflicts physical abuse; can result in murder
  Justifies actions
  Blames victim
  Expresses high level of psychologic abuse (displays disqualifying degrading behavior)
  Requires power, control, and/or aggression for sexual arousal
  Experiences disruption of excitement phase with impotence and disruption frequently
  Experiences orgasm phase with partial ejaculation frequently

Assessment requires not only an awareness of defining characteristics but their relationship to organic or psychosocial etiologies and whether the behaviors are primary or secondary to the presumed etiologies. The first step in clustering behaviors is understanding that their etiologies can be either organic or psychosocial or a complex combination. As such, certain characteristics can be the same regardless of etiology. As such, the clusters of characteristics can lead to a process of differential diagnoses. Characteristics defined above are those major behaviors supporting the subdiagnoses, after a careful process of assessment.

NURSING INTERVENTIONS

Patient Goal	Nursing Intervention
Organic	
Understand organic issues or illness states' impact on sexual functioning.	Educate regarding physical illness, illness process, treatment interventions, such as drugs. Reframe distorted beliefs regarding sexual functioning given illness and treatment.
Reduce stress regarding sexual response disruption that is reversible and secondary to organic issues.	Provide accurate information regarding the temporary disruption caused by organic impairment. Instruct to modify attitudes to accommodate needed behavior change. Counsel the partner or couple.
Reduce stress and institute viable alternatives when disruption is not reversible because of organic problem	Counsel and educate client and sexual partner regarding prosthetics, implants, techniques, attitudes or beliefs regarding sexual expression.
Resolve past sexual trauma.	Focus counseling on reactions to sexual trauma.
Psychosocial	
Achieve more flexibility in attitudes regarding self and others around sexual functioning.	Counsel around expectations of self and others. Counsel around partnership issues. Educate about sexual techniques and interpersonal communication. Stress reduction instruction.
Reduce cognitive interference that distracts and lessens sexual responsiveness.	Use cognitive-behavioral approach to stop disruptive cognitive operations.

Patient Goal	Nursing Intervention
Reduce critical self-observations; reduce dissociation.	Alter beliefs regarding performance, adequacy. Provide training for moving into images of self, increasing awareness of kinesthetic responses, reducing self-imagery that dissociates feeling states.
Enhance kinesthetic, erotic experience.	Teach sensation-enhancing exercises with self and partner: increase awareness of mounting pleasure; explore means of intensifying sensations; block disruptive thoughts.
Reduce unconscious, intrapsychic conflicts with self and in relationships.	Counsel the individual or couple: work through unconscious hostility to opposite sex; work through guilt regarding pleasure; work through interpersonal problems, such as withholding and power plays.
Reduce chronic, delayed reactions to sexual trauma.	Focus counseling on chronic, delayed reactions to sexual trauma.
Reduce primary organic source of pain.	Educate in carrying out necessary medical interventions to reduce underlying disease process.
Reduce conditioned, painful voluntary muscle response (secondary to psychologic problems).	Refer to sex therapist for biofeedback and counseling for psychologic problems.
Reduce underlying psychologic conflicts.	Refer to counseling and sex therapy.
Reduce avoidance behavior.	Refer for differential diagnosis of simple/complex phobic response with drug therapy or sex therapy and desensitization.
Prevent further sexual assaults.	Report to authorities. Refer to experienced counselor: confront behavior and its impact on others; drug intervention; individual/family counseling; hypnotherapy, age regression; concerted efforts to have perpetrator identify with the victim; management of secondary psychiatric problems.

When a behavioral matrix such as sexual functioning becomes a problem, the characteristics of the problem must be understood by the objective evidence as well as the subjective data. The closer the objective evidence coincides with a definitive etiology, the more apt the specific intervention will be.

The following sequencing of data illustrates decisions in the evaluation of defining characteristics and in terms of broad etiologic considerations.

Does the patient have a disruption of sexual response patterns?

If normal functioning, then consider psychiatric diagnosis.

If no psychiatric problems, then provide education, reassurance.

If yes for psychiatric diagnosis, then differentiate problems, and provide appropriate psychiatric treatment (or refer).

If yes for abnormal functioning, then diagnosis: organic or psychogenic.

If organic then medical diagnosis. Is it a treatable medical problem that will result in correction or is it nontreatable? If yes, then sexual rehabilitation, counseling, penile implant.

If psychogenic, then check etiology. If it is a major psychologic cause, then long-term therapy. If it is a minor and moderate psychologic cause, then sex therapy.

If sexual problem is secondary to other psychiatric disorder, such as stress, depression, panic disorder, severe marital discord, substance abuse, major mental or emotional illness, then appropriate psychiatric treatment.

Sexual dysfunction as a diagnosis provides a broad spectrum of general data with a broad array of etiological factors. When these factors are considered, second and third order levels of assessment are required for specifying the particular type of sexual dysfunction and its relationship to important biopsychosocial parameters. In addition, particular types of intervention must be evaluated as to their impact physically, psychologically, and interpersonally. Assessment and differential diagnosis as well as specialized assessment diagnostic skill are necessary given the complexity of the functional disorder. Collaboration with other professionals as well as specialized expertise of the nurse are required both for differential diagnostic activities and particular intervention modes.

Concern about Sexual Functioning

When the etiological consideration is organic, nursing care focuses on educating the client and counseling about misconceptions that provoke anxiety and depression. Since sexual functioning most often involves a partner, nursing intervention is also directed at the appropriate partner.

For example, consider a husband recovering from a mild heart attack. The husband and wife are hesitant to resume their sexual relationship for fear the husband will have a heart attack. Sexual desire is present, as are sexual arousal and orgasmic experiences. For these people a causal connection between the energy expended in the sexual act and heart attack have been linked. Information and experience in monitoring exertion with concomitant signs such as pulse rate and chest pain become important for the husband. This is usually done through gradual increments in physical activity. Involvement of the wife provides experience for her as well as an opportunity for them to open up communication between them. Unrealistic expectations can be revealed and countered. In addition, the couple can become comfortable exploring, relaxing, and finding less strenuous methods for enjoying their sexual relationship. Steps in nursing care are as follows:

1. Assess and establish existence of sexual response patterns and that there is no extreme variation of sexual behavior.
2. Establish clear definition of primary organic problem.
3. Establish information relevant to the organic problem's influence on sexual behavior.
4. Clarify to patients and significant others any key perceptions regarding the relationship of the organic problem to sexual functioning.
5. Provide experiences necessary to enhance functioning, such as information, counseling, focused exercises.
6. Evaluate effectiveness of intervention.

When the etiological factors are psychologic and secondary to organic causes, education and counseling are the primary interventions. This is particularly true when the problems are minor. Severity of the primary psychologic and relationship problems is determined in part by assessment of the psychologic makeup of the person and/or couple and the critical interactional components of the relationship.

Some medical interventions greatly alter body structure as well as impinge on the physiology of penile erection and erotic responses; therefore special attention has to be paid to the process of the patient gaining acceptance of the body image changes. Partners need support and counseling during periods of adjustment.

When the etiological conditions have immediate psychologic causes, out of awareness cognitive patterns (images, internal dialogue, expectations), there can be interference with ejaculatory processes in the man and orgasm in the woman. Anorgasm and inhibited orgasm in the woman have recently been investigated for their or-

igins. There is debate as to whether orgasm is an essential feature of female sexuality. The purpose of the nursing care discussion is not to enter this disputed issue but rather to present some etiological factors and interventions that alter the dysfunctional response patterns in some women. When internal images and thoughts lead to habitual distraction and lessening of sexual pleasure, a variety of behavioral and cognitive approaches are used, such as thought stopping and reeducation. These are best accomplished when the patient's partner is also involved. Special knowledge, techniques, and counseling skills are necessary for identifying and changing these cognitive patterns. Some clinical specialists in psychiatric nursing do this type of sex therapy, as do nurse clinical specialists in the area of degenerative diseases or neurologic diseases and nurses who are primarily sex therapists.

Sex therapy provokes anxiety and requires patient motivation to carry through with exercises. People with problematic psychologic functioning and precarious relationships may not withstand the therapy and decompensate under its stress. On the other hand, a patient with a known psychiatric problem who has had periods of undisputed sexual functioning can be assisted with an approach that focuses directly on sexual functioning rather than deep psychotherapy. In these situations the disruption is not a defense against the underlying psychologic problem.

When there is a primary sexual response pattern dysfunction and a major psychologic problem, it is important to use long-term therapy prior to direct focus on the behavioral components of the sex pattern disruption. In summary, nursing care of orgasm disorders depends on their relation to minor and major psychologic and relationship causes. If minor, direct attention to the cognitive input of the patient and its interference with orgasm is the focus, with experiential tasks to alter the behavior. When there is a major psychologic problem, this is addressed first. When orgasm problems are secondary to other psychiatric disorders, appropriate intervention is to be established. This is usually by referral to specialists in these areas.

Nursing care of excitement phase disorders is similar to that for orgasmic disorders. First, when the excitement phase is disrupted secondarily to organic problems, appropriate medical attention is necessary. In males the impotence may or may not exclude erotic feelings and penile sensation. Penile implants have helped a great deal in reestablishing sexual relationships in otherwise irreversible organic conditions.

Vaginal dryness that impedes the enhancement of sexual excitement may be related to estrogen deficiency, most often associated with menopause. When hormonal replacement is contraindicated or not desired, lubricants can greatly reduce the problem.[2,3] Nursing care is influenced according to whether the medical problem is reversible. With reversible problems nursing care supports the patient and partner until the reestablishment of sexual functioning. If irreversible, rehabilitative efforts and counseling are the modes of intervention.

A general guide for simple nursing care follows:

1. Explain causal connection between attitudinal set and behavior and its relationship to sexual concern.
2. Gain cooperation and agreement to work toward change. Clarify that change is compatible and comfortable, acceptable to patient and partner.
3. Evaluate outcome. If unsatisfactory, reassess and if necessary refer for further evaluation or more specific psychiatric treatment of psychologic or relationship problem.

Removing a sexual complaint can escalate anxiety by exposing other human demands of relating, such as commitment and intimacy. Problems in these personal areas are masked through many symptoms of dysfunction. The symptoms may be viewed as defenses for the individual. At times in complex relationship problems the partner with the complaint may in fact be a foil for the more severe psychologic problems of the nonsymptomatic partner. When the symptom is removed, there is an imbalance in the relationship and the partner's underlying psychologic difficulties are revealed.

Disruption of Sexual Response Pattern

Orgasm/ejaculation phase. The orgasm/ejaculatory phase is quite susceptible to primary psychologic causes and secondary organic problems. This is true for both men and women. The effectiveness of nursing care depends on proper medical intervention and an understanding of the impact of the medical problem and treatment regimen. Since many of the medical interventions cause irreversible states or they are necessary for the total functioning of the individual, nursing care focuses on rehabilitative measures. If the medical problem is treatable, the nursing care is aimed at quelling the anxiety of the individual regarding sexual functioning during the treatment period as well as working with the partner. Education and counseling in conjunction with the medical regimen constitute primary nursing intervention.

Excitement phase. Immediate psychologic problems have been established in cases of male impotence. Nursing care, when organic cause is ruled out, focuses on counseling, which clarifies issues of performance, pressure to please the partner, or pressure from the partner. All these issues can affect the excitement phase.

Deeper psychologic problems and relationship problems require psychotherapy that focuses on the underlying issues. Referral and follow-through are often the primary nursing interventions.

Desire phase. Desire phase disorders have organic causes; included in the category are depression and severe stress. There is an established alteration in neural hormones that specifically mediate sexual desire. When the immediate psychologic causes are considered, they underscore behavior that avoids sexual involvement. The length of time without sexual desire becomes important in planning care. If it is chronic in a physically healthy, functioning individual without signs of severe mental illness, complex dynamic intrapsychic issues are usually considered. These require long-term psychotherapy with possible combined sex therapy. Nursing care most often involves referral.

When the response is more immediate and related to stress and depression, nursing care focuses on their reduction, making clear their causal link with low or absent sexual desire. If there is a pattern of avoidance of sexually stimulating experiences, this is to be explored with the client. This is particularly true in someone who has lost a spouse and is confused as to the meaning of continued sexual desire.

Pain: Pre- and Post-Orgasm/Ejaculation Phase

Pain associated with sex is more often than not based on organic causes. Nursing intervention is primarily directed toward making sure the client is thoroughly evaluated for underlying organic causes.

Functional Pain/Disgust (Dyspareunia)

When organic disease and physiologic issues are ruled out, psychogenic issues are addressed. Of particular importance is understanding whether the client has been the object of rape, incest, or a brutal sexual assault. Counseling around this issue is the primary intervention. Focused sex therapy may be required in conjunction with the resolution of the past event.

When counseling is addressed to underlying psychologic or relationship issues or past sexual trauma, it must be remembered that pain can be a defense against pleasure and until acceptance of pleasure has been established, removing the pain may provide intense anxiety and withdrawal from counseling.

Phobic Avoidance of Sexual Experience

Avoidance of sex and sexual arousal must be evaluated carefully for underlying panic disorder. In recent years it has been hypothesized that panic disorders are related to an underlying propensity to overreact physiologically to intense feeling states.[2] Some people speculate that there is a genetic precursor.[2] At any rate, experiments with drugs have demonstrated a reduction in the panic response. When the response is down and psychotherapy and sex therapy are combined, there have been favorable results. However, severe neurotic and borderline states can underlie the panic.

Simple phobic response with conditioning is usually amenable to psychotherapy or behavior therapy combined with instruction. When panic and phobic avoidance are evident, referral is the appropriate nursing intervention.

In general, the nurse should determine if the disorder has an organic or a psychogenic cause. If there is doubt, refer for more specialized evaluation. If organic and psychogenic causes are established, as well as their primary and secondary relationships, then use one of the following nursing interventions most appropriate to the causes and the level of sexual behavior issues: education, general counseling around personal and relationship issues, focused exercises to alter cognitive sets and physical behavior that impede sexual and erotic behaviors, and inclusion of the partner.

Extreme Variation of Sexual Behavior

Intervention for this disorder requires the efforts of a specialist. Unfortunately, the cause and effective interventions have not yet been established. Because of the degree of deviance and often the pain and exploitation of others, there are spotty efforts in developing consistent exploration into the management and cessation of the behaviors involved. The behavior is compulsive and often repeated.

Nurses are in contact with these people in many settings: the prison, the home, and areas of the health care system. In addition, nurses are often involved in providing services to the victims of people who fall under this category of sexual dysfunction.

When infants, children, and adolescents are the object, or when violence is engaged in with or without an age-appropriate partner, endocrine and genetic causes should be explored. With the pedophile, experiments are underway using hormonal therapy in conjunction with behavioral and psychotherapeutic efforts. This treatment group is a small population. For the most part pedophiles are released and reside in the general community without much offered either for their treatment or the treatment of their victims.

The following community nursing care is suggested. First, attempt to get some supervision from an interested mental health professional. Second, establish a contract with the individual to stop the behavior; make it clear that transgressions must be reported to the authorities; establish protection for potential victims and establish methods of stopping the behavior through substitution, diversion, distance, and attempts to help the perpetrator develop empathy for the victim. If the perpetrator has been sexually victimized during childhood, establish that the event has not been resolved and is being acted out. Also, help establish a positive social support system and review periodically the effectiveness of efforts to change behavior.

EVALUATION

Patient Outcome	Data Indicating That Outcome is Reached
Separation of attitudes toward sexual functioning that have been linked to organic illness	Sex not confused with organic issues; response to educative information and necessary medical regimen Concern over sexual functioning (self-report) diminishes
Cognitive shifts in restrictive expectations toward self and others.	No unrealistic expectations Relaxation Loss of concern over sexual functioning
Understanding of impact of medical treatment and illness on phases of sexual response	Acceptance of temporary problem or irreversibility with no evidence of depression, avoidance, self-recrimination
Participation in educational counseling programs for reduction of depression and anxieties surrounding illness and enhanced relationship with sexual partner	Techniques to compensate for restrictions Sense of pleasure and gratification in sexual response Physiologic measurements of increased penile circulation Disease process under control
Reduction of psychologic, behavioral patterns that affect phases of sexual response pattern	Alteration in beliefs and attitudes restrictive to sexual behavior and sense of pleasure Alteration in internal thought processes that restrict sexual behavior and sense of pleasure: reduction in disruptive imagery; reduction of negative internal dialogue; increased sense of erotic sensations and how one individual enhances and controls excitement and arousal

Patient Outcome	Data Indicating That Outcome is Reached
Resolution of intrapsychic conflicts	Self-report of more comfort, acceptance of self Increased positive experiences with opposite sex/sex partner
Resolution of conflicting interpersonal relationship with sexual partner	Increased sense of erotic sensations Divorces and leaves partner Working through role and dependency issues with partner Increased pointed conversations between partners Increased ease and flexibility in exploring reciprocal, sexually desirable experiences in one another

Evaluating nursing interventions depends on the specificity of etiology and the current level of the art of treatment. Dysfunctions associated with organic causes that are reversible either through specific medical intervention or the limited nature of the disorder, have a high probability of being offset. Simple psychosocially determined etiologies respond to education and constructive experiences.

Complex organic problems, reversible and irreversible, not only tax intervention techniques but also further compound predictable outcomes because of psychosocial responses to the illness phenomena with the medical regimen. This is further confounded by the social matrix of sexual behavior, that is, interventions and outcomes must frequently address the sexual partner of the patient. In these latter situations a process of constant evaluations and clarification of therapeutic goals is ensured so that changes can be made in strategies until maximum physical, psychologic, and social functioning returns or is established with regard to sexual functioning.

References

1. Hartman, C.R.: Sexual dysfunction. In Burgess, A.W., editor: Psychiatric nursing in the hospital and the community, ed. 4, Englewood Cliffs, N.J., 1985, Prentice-Hall, Inc.
2. Kaplan, H.S.: The evaluation of sexual disorders: psychological and medical aspects, New York, 1983, Brunner/Mazel.
3. Meyer, J., Schmidt, C., and Wise, T., editors: Clinical management of sexual disorders, Baltimore, 1983, Williams & Wilkins.

SEXUAL TRAUMA
THEORY AND ETIOLOGY

Rape Trauma Syndrome

Rape trauma syndrome is the acute and long-term psychosocial process of reintegration that occurs as an aftermath of forcible rape or attempted forcible rape.[1] The syndrome is influenced by the type of rape activity: forcible, nonconsenting, sexual exploitation, or sex-stress situation. The legal definition of rape varies from state to state; however, the issues generally addressed include lack of consent, force or threat of force, and sexual penetration. The clinical definition of rape trauma—the focus of this nursing diagnosis—is the stress response pattern of the victim following forced, nonconsenting sexual activity. The rape trauma syndrome of somatic, cognitive, psychologic, and behavioral symptoms is an active stress reaction to a life-threatening situation.[1]

The trauma to the victim results from that person being confronted with the life-threatening and highly stressful situation of rape and sexual abuse. The crisis or reaction that results is in the service of self-preservation. It is the nucleus around which an adaptive pattern may be noted.[1]

What is traumatizing to a rape victim (in all types of rape) is that her life is in jeopardy and she is helpless in the situation. Forcible rape—an act forced on a victim (usually female) by an assailant (usually male)—is viewed as an act of violence expressing power, aggression, conquest, degradation, anger, hatred, and contempt.[12] Hilberman[10] characterizes rape as the "ultimate violation of the self, short of homicide, with the invasion of one's inner and most private space, as well as loss of autonomy and control." Hilberman argues that it is the person's self, not an orifice, that has been invaded and that the core meaning of rape is the same for a virgin, a housewife, a lesbian, and a prostitute.[10]

A study of motivational intent of the offender indicates that rape behavior involves a hierarchy of life issues such as power, anger, and sexuality.[7] On the basis of clinical data on 133 convicted rapists and 92 adult victims, Groth, Burgess, and Holmstrom[7] viewed rape as complex and multidetermine, and they addressed issues of hostility (anger) and control (power) more than passion (sexuality). Subdivisions of these categories include the power-assertive rapist, who perceives rape as a means of expressing his virility and dominance; the power-reassurance rapist, who uses the act of rape to resolve doubts about his sexual adequacy; the anger-retaliation rapist who seeks revenge by degrading and humiliating women; and the anger-excitation rapist who derives sexual excitement from inflicting pain and punishing his victim.

In pair or group rape the motive of seeking male ca- maraderie has been suggested, and the motive of a sense of entitlement to sexual services has been observed in data on father-daughter incest,[9] wife rape,[13] and date situations.[4]

Analysis of the dynamics and method of operation of the rapist helps to explain what specific aspects have terrorized and victimized the person. Style of attack has been found to contain characteristics classified as blitz, in which the victim is quickly subdued and propelled into the assault[4]; con, in which the victim is approached ver- bally and then betrayed and assaulted[4]; and surprise, in which the rapist waits and targets a victim or sneaks up on and surprises her.[8]

Sexual Exploitation

Rape trauma syndrome falls within the general category of sexual traumas. Two additional sexual traumas were identified in the study in which rape trauma syndrome was reported.[11] A differential diagnosis needs to be made regarding the additional two sexual traumas.

A second group of sexual assault victims, most of whom were children and young adolescents, were cat- egorized as accessory-to-sex victims. In this type of sex- ual assault victims are pressured into sexual activity by a person or persons who stand in a power position over them through age or authority. Victims are unable to make a responsible decision of consent because of their level of personality or cognitive development or their learned rules of behavior. The emotional reaction of the victim results from being pressured into sexual activity and from the tension to keep the activity secret. The offender gains access to the victim in several ways: of- fering material rewards (candy, money); offering psy- chologic rewards (attention, interest, affection); or mis- representing moral standards (''It's okay to do this— your mother and I do it.'').[2]

This trauma syndrome is often characterized by a grad- ual social and psychologic withdrawal from usual life activities. This withdrawal is most apt to occur when the sexual activity is repeated with the same person over an extended time. Physical symptoms of trauma may be evidenced through changes in motor behavior and signs of infection. Such overall signs and symptoms are es- pecially prominent when the victim has been pressured into secrecy by the offender. The burden of carrying the secret creates considerable tension, and the victim feels constantly on guard to maintain the secret.[2]

Sex-Stress Situation

A third group of sexual trauma situations results from a sexual encounter in which both parties initially consent to sexual activity. The person for whom the sexual sit- uation produces the most anxiety usually brings the sit- uation to the attention of the nurse. The situation usually includes two consenting people for whom something ''goes wrong'' during the sexual activity; or there may be anxiety about the results of the sexual activity (preg- nancy, infection, disease).[4]

Etiologies for Sexual Trauma

Rape trauma: nonconsenting forcible rape
  Acute reactions
    A. Type of rape:
      1. Force/threat
      2. Damage/physical
    B. Age
    C. Demand for cognitive/behavioral assimilation of ex- perience (how the process proceeds):
      1. Surprise
      2. Death threat
      3. Physical penetration
      4. Physical injury
      5. Immobilization
      6. Attributions for cause of rape
      7. Self-appraisal of response to rapist or victim, mas- tery
      8. Stored sounds, smells, images, sensations
    D. Major coping behaviors employed to handle assault
    E. Demand for cognitive/behavioral assimilation of dis- closing experience to others:
      1. Response of judicial/police system
      2. Response of immediate social support system
    F. Prior psychosocial issues:
      1. Prior victimization
      2. Prior stress experiences
      3. Social network response
      4. Major coping behaviors
  Chronic reactions
    A through F of acute reactions plus particular emphasis on:
    Amount of physical violence
    Coping mechanisms employed to master rape
    Quality of support system
    Older age of victim
  Delayed reactions
    A through F with particular emphasis on dissociative de- fenses and avoidant coping behavior
Sexual exploitation (acute, chronic, delayed)
  Acute reactions
    A. Type of rape (particular attention to the threat/fear of violence used to control and the distortion of sense of self, sense of right, wrong, responsibility, perpetrated)
    B. Disclosure:
      1. Confrontation by self/others of the sexual exploi- tation
      2. Police/judicial proceedings
      3. Immediate social support system
      4. Peer and school reaction
    C. Demand for cognitive/behavioral assimilation of ex- perience (how the process proceeds):
      1. Betrayal
      2. Sorting out responsibility
      3. Dealing and subtle threats, coercion, distortion

4. Blurring of aggressive/sexual impulses
5. Stress reaction to disclosure
6. Stored sounds, smells, images, sensations
D. Major coping mechanisms employed to handle exploitation
E. Prior psychosocial issues; prior victimization

Chronic reactions

A through F of acute reactions with particular emphasis on:

Major defenses and coping mechanisms employed to handle the exploitation

Characteristics of the social support system:

1. Excessive blame
2. Excessive worry, reinforcement of victim role

Prior psychosocial issues

Chronic reactions

A through F of acute reactions plus:

Attachment to perpetrator

Degree of political, personal, and financial power of victimizer over victim

Chronic history of abuse, self-deprecation

Limited sense of alternatives

Limited psychologic capacities

Delayed reactions

A through F of acute reactions and 1 through 5 of chronic reactions, plus:

Socialization (delayed labeling of experience[s] as rape because of prevailing sense of social milieu holding victim responsible, deserving and provoking sexual abuse)

The primary use of dissociative and avoidant defenses and coping behaviors during time of sexual exploitation and through disclosure process, plus perception of self vis-à-vis social support system seem most important

Sex-stress situations

Acute reaction

Amount of violence

Betrayal

Self-blame, shame

Age

Sense of powerlessness

Demand for cognitive/behavioral assimilation of the experience (how the process proceeds)

Defensive and coping mechanisms employed to withstand assault

Prior psychosocial issues:

1. Prior abuse
2. Psychologic problems
3. Coping mechanisms

DEFINING CHARACTERISTICS

Somatic reactions

Physical trauma: cuts, bruises on neck, throat, breasts, thighs, legs, arms

Physical trauma to genitals

Gastrointestinal irritability

1. Stomach pains
2. Nausea
3. Change in appetite

Skeletal, muscle tension, headaches, fatigue

Sleep disturbance reactions

Genitourinary disturbances

1. Vaginal discharges
2. Rectal bleeding
3. Burning in urination
4. Itching

Psychologic/behavioral reactions

Disturbance of mood: depressed, anxious

Cognitive disruption: confusion, failure of memory, indecisiveness

Self-appraisal: fear, embarrassment, humiliation, self-blame

Fear of violence toward self and others

Desire for revenge

Intrusive thoughts, nightmares, daymares

1. Replication of the victimization
2. Thoughts of the rape
3. Mastery dreams of overcoming the assailant

Phobic reactions

1. Avoidance of sex
2. Avoidance of people
3. Avoidance of crowds
4. Avoidance of being alone

More severe psychologic reactions

1. Ideas of reference
2. Psychotic states
3. Severe acting out

Dysfunctional coping

1. Alcohol, drugs
2. Promiscuity, prostitution

Suicidal behavior, homicidal behavior

Self-blame, low self-esteem

Restrictive and avoidance behaviors

Fear that something is wrong with sexual organs

Social reactions

Dependence on others

Work or school failure, withdrawal

Avoidance of close or family relationships; social isolation

Disruption of couple's relationship

Social stigmatization

Constant moves to deal with anxiety and fear

Additional aspects

When a patient presents herself as psychotic or sexually promiscuous, has psychosomatic complaints, avoids sexual relationships, has sudden social withdrawal and alcohol and drug abuse, evaluation should be done to rule out the sexual trauma diagnoses. These major behavioral deviations often mask sexual trauma, either because prior psychiatric problems are exacerbated by the trauma or because these other syndromes defend against the sexual event.

There is also a group of victims who do not reveal to others the fact that they have been raped (silent reaction). This population appears different from the delayed reactions in that the total event is not dissociated and repressed, rather, there is memory of the event, but the emotional reaction and assimilation of the event are not addressed, nor is the event disclosed to others.

The following characteristics are associated with this later reaction:

Marked anxiety in personal interviews with long periods of silence, blocking of associations, minor stuttering, and physical distress

Reported marked irritability or actual avoidance of relationships with men

History of marked change in sexual behavior
History of sudden onset of phobic reactions; fear of being alone, going outside, being inside alone
Persistent loss of self-confidence and self-esteem; self blame
Suspiciousness
Frequent dreams of violence and nightmares

In the acute phase of rape trauma syndrome there is a great deal of disorganization in the victim's life-style. This disorganization is evidenced as follows.[1]

In *impact reactions* one of two styles of reaction is generally noted, either the expressed style, in which feelings of fear, anger, and anxiety are shown through behavior such as crying, sobbing, smiling, restlessness, and tenseness, or the controlled style, in which feelings are masked or hidden and a calm, composed, or subdued affect is noted.[3]

In the first several weeks after a rape the following acute *somatic manifestations* may be evident:

1. Physical trauma, which includes general soreness and bruising from the physical attack in various parts of the body such as the throat, neck, breasts, thighs, legs, and arms.
2. Skeletal muscle tension, which includes tension headaches and fatigue, as well as sleep pattern disturbances and complaints of hyperalertness, feeling edgy and nervous.
3. Gastrointestinal irritability, which includes stomach pains, appetite disruption, nausea.
4. Genitourinary disturbance, which includes gynecologic symptoms of vaginal discharge, itching, burning on urination, and generalized pain. Also symptoms from sexual penetration of the mouth and rectum are noted.

A wide gamut of *emotional reactions* may be expressed and include fear, humiliation, embarrassment, anger, revenge, and self-blame. Fear of physical violence and death is usually the primary affect experienced during the rape.

The long-term process of reorganization is the second phase of the rape trauma syndrome. Although the time of onset varies from victim to victim, this phase often begins several weeks after the assault or identification of the rape. Various factors affect the coping behavior of victims, for example, ego strength, social network support, and the way people treat them as victims.[3] The following characteristics are noted:

1. *Motor activity:* There generally is an increase in motor activity, especially changing residence and taking trips. Victims also turn for support to family members not necessarily seen daily as well as to friends, associates, and colleagues.
2. *Dreams and nightmares:* Intrusive thoughts of the rape break into the victim's conscious mind as well as during sleep (nightmares). Three types of nightmares may be reported: (1) replication of the state of victimization and helplessness; (2) symbolic dreams, which include a theme from the rape; and (3) mastery dreams in which the victim is powerful in assuming control. Nonmastery dreams dominate until the victim is recovered.
3. *Traumatophobia:* Fears and phobias are common characteristics following rape. The phobia develops as a defensive reaction to the circumstances of the rape. Some common phobias include fear of indoors, fear of outdoors, fear of being alone, fear of crowds, fear of people behind them, sexual fears.

NURSING INTERVENTIONS

Patient Goal	Nursing Intervention
Reduce the immediate negative reactions to the rape experience and disclosure.	Provide safety by: 1. Effective, considerate physical examination, necessary prescriptions, repair of injuries 2. Close relationship with safe person to provide for catharsis with attention to correction of distorted premises regarding self-blame 3. Establish self-control over person, decisions 4. Establish supportive social network 5. Counseling regarding stress response images, sounds, smells, sensations that provoke anxiety; relaxation exercises 6. Counseling for immediate family, spouse, partner
Gain support for the criminal judicial experience.	Careful preservation of evidence; reporting Assign to rape crisis Counsel regarding exacerbation of earlier crisis symptoms with prolonged investigative procedures and court appearances Continue counseling of important family member, spouse, partner

Patient Goal	Nursing Intervention
	With children particular photographic strategies can be used to provide evidence of physical injury from penetration (vaginal and anal)
Achieve reduction of any prolonged symptoms	Provide counseling and focused therapy for: 1. Prolonged anxiety reactions associated with specific flashback phenomena 2. Reframing of descriptive belief patterns Provide couples counseling where conflict, restriction in sexual activity occurs Careful examination and follow-up on physical injuries, symptoms

The nursing care of the rape trauma victim is based on four models of nursing intervention: the biological, the social, the cognitive-behavioral, and the psychologic.[5]

Biologic Model of Intervention

During the acute phase following the assault the nurse should carefully review any somatic alteration in the body system such as the following: circulatory system (flushing, perspiration, feeling hot or cold, headaches); respiratory system (breathing style, sighing respirations, rapid breathing, dizziness); gastrointestinal system (abdominal pain, nausea, lack of appetite, constipation); genitourinary system (urinary frequency, interference with sexual functioning).

On the follow-up it is essential for the nurse to document carefully the nature and intensity of the symptoms over a 24-hour period. The somatic side effects of any medication prescribed need to be distinguished from the somatic aftereffects of the assault. For example, the nausea and vomiting from antipregnancy medication should significantly decrease when the medicine is stopped. It is important to check if nausea is from an emotional reaction to thinking about the rape. Similarly, itching and vaginal discharge may be a result of the heavy dose of antibiotics and should decrease upon completion of the medication. A careful note should be made that the patient is taking the correct amount prescribed. Physical symptoms after 5 days should be carefully investigated, since the therapeutic regimen of medication is usually completed by then. Minor tranquilizers and sleeping medication should not be routinely prescribed without a careful assessment of the patient's needs.

The victim should have a gynecologic and medical follow-up appointment after she completes her first menstrual period following the assault. All victims, male and female, should have blood test for syphilis and a culture for sexually transmitted diseases taken during a 4- to 6-week follow-up visit. The referral and follow-up is a primary nursing intervention and may be made to either a nurse practitioner or physician.

Social Model of Intervention

This nursing intervention makes explicit use of the victim's social network. The goal of using family and friends of the victim is to strengthen the victim's self-confidence to help him or her resume a normal style of living. Whether or not the victim chooses to tell family and friends about the rape is not the point, but rather that the victim seeks support from the network.

The victim is encouraged to resume a normal style of activity according to her ability to pace the activities. The longer a victim avoids a normal activity such as school or work, the greater the difficulty in trying to return to it.

An important nursing intervention is to encourage the victim to seek out understanding people to talk to about any concerns. The victim often has specific decisions to make and seeks advice about issues such as whether to press charges against the rapist, whether to quit work, or how to tell people about the incident. It is important for the victim to have an active involvement with a social network and environment to resume a somewhat normal life-style. Repairing estranged family and social relationships is encouraged to provide the victim with additional emotional support during this time.

Cognitive-Behavioral Model of Intervention

The focus of this model is on the belief patterns the victim holds regarding rape and sexual assault as well as on desensitizing the person to the behavior that results from the assault—specifically the phobic reactions. Identifying the belief patterns (why the victim thinks the rape occurred) provides the nurse with a measurement of the victim's attribution of blame. For example, if the victim believes women are raped because of the way they dress, she will need to be educated as to the myths about rape. If the victim believes that rapists stalk victims and therefore anyone may become a victim, attention can be placed on increasing safety tactics for the prevention of invasion from predators.

One goal of this intervention is to deflate the fears, stresses, and anxieties the victim experiences after the assault and to help inflate the victim's own self-esteem and self-confidence in dealing with the world again. The victim has the potential to reach her previous level of adaptive functioning and to strengthen capabilities to feel secure again.

The nursing intervention is aimed at desensitizing the victim to the memory of the rape. Talking about the painful parts gives the victim psychologic control over the memory and strips it of its power to distress the victim. The victim is encouraged to master her fears, that is, to think back over the very frightening situation with support from the nurse and friends. Gradually, this method desensitizes the victim so that the thoughts can gradually enter the mind without the terrifying reactions. This technique may be used with the physical setting or other circumstances of the assault.

As the nurse talks with a victim, it is essential to help the victim make psychologic connections between the symptoms and the rape trauma. Although repression may be a protective process, it absorbs valuable psychic energy necessary for the victim to settle the crisis.

A common fear of victims and their families is that the offender will retaliate in some manner or that he will try to harm the victim in some other way. If concrete data exist that the offender is harassing the victim, the police can be notified to help in the matter. In some cases the victim is threatened by the defendant's family, and in such cases the judge may be explicit in condemning such behavior and in stating the sanctions for the assailant if such behavior continues. Retaliative behavior can be quite frightening to the victim.

Psychologic Model of Intervention

During the acute phase the nurse should carefully review (1) mental functioning in terms of impaired attention, poor concentration, poor memory, changes in outlook, and future planning, and (2) emotional reaction in terms of irritability, mood changes, dream disturbance, and changes in relationships with family and friends.

Talking with the victim during the impact phase, or as close as possible to the actual time of the rape, is essential to help repair the emotional damage inflicted on the victim. This intervention also attempts to minimize the psychologic aftereffects of the rape by providing emotional support of a nonjudgmental nature. Talking with the victim helps to establish an alliance and provides an opportunity for maximum assessment of the impact of the assault and the victim's reactions.

The overwhelming impulse of the victim is to avoid dealing with the experience. In such situations the nurse encourages the victim to talk about the rape and supports any fearful reaction by saying that the fear is a natural reaction to the danger to which the victim was exposed.

Talking about the assault and bearing the accompanying distressing feelings are essential steps in the total process of settling the crisis and mastering the experience. The treatment goals for the victim is to reestablish a normal style of living and to restore a sense of equilibrium. This means the victim must come to terms intellectually and viscerally by acknowledging the impact of the rape on her life and incorporating it as a stressful memory in the total life experience. The meaning of the assault must be talked about and thought about. The feelings, which may be accompanied by various physical and emotional manifestations, must be experienced. In this way the victim can diminish the painful impact of the experience.

EVALUATION

Patient Outcome	Data Indicating That Outcome is Reached

Absence of stress response symptoms	Self report:
	    Normal sleep patterns
	    Ability to think and talk of event without excessive signs of distress
	    Absence of flashbacks, intrusive thoughts

Return to physical functioning	Absence of physical symptoms; repair rehabilitation from physical injury
Return to psychologic functioning, balance, and flexibility	Memory intake Positive self-regard Absence of mood disturbance; no depression Physical energy for learning, solving problems
Return to social functioning	Return to critical role activities at work and as family member Comfortable in sex role Comfortable in social situations Reasonable sense of safety and caution in strange situation, at night, with people

The nurse can assume the victim has come to terms with the assault when she or he can honestly say that the memory is not as frequent, the physical distress is not as great, and the intensity of the memory has decreased. The victim will then have psychologically let go of the pain and fear and will feel a degree of calm that enables her to go about the business of living again. Two additional life areas must be assessed—the social and sexual—in terms of resuming precrisis levels of functioning. The social recovery depends greatly on who was told within the victim's social network and the reactions of the person. The nurse can make careful inquiry as to the level of resolution regarding social acknowledgment of the rape trauma.

In a 6-year follow-up study the effects of the rape on subsequent sexual functioning were analyzed in 81 adult rape victims.[6] Most victims who had been sexually active were found to experience changes in frequency of sexual activity and in sexual response. Six clinical issues were identified from the study, which deserve attention from nurses who evaluate the impact of rape on the sexual functioning of victims.

1. *Rape as a first sexual experience*. It is important to assess the value that the victim has placed on sexual activity to predict the magnitude of the sexuality issue following rape. For example, one woman who placed a high value on being a virgin when she married, indicated on follow-up that the issue was still very much present.

2. *Rape as an unresolved issue*. There can be complications with sexual recovery for the victim who has been previously raped or assaulted. Careful inquiry as to prior victimization history is crucial to determine if there has been resolution of the prior experiences.

3. *Victims not sexually active at the time of the rape*. Women who have been sexually active at some point in their lives may be inactive at the time they become rape victims. Many times these women decide to continue to abstain from sexual activity with a partner. However, when they do resume sexual relations, problems may arise. Thus it is important for the nurse to help victims anticipate some of the issues they may face when they resume sex, whether their resumption is immediate or comes weeks, months, or years later.

4. *Resuming sexual activity*. Victims may be helped to gain control over their sexual recovery by talking about their experiences. The nurse can help to monitor the victim's reactions to resuming sexual activity and can note the gradual decrease or increase in symptoms and problems. Problems identified by victims include sexual aversion, flashbacks to the rape during sexual activity, pain and discomfort during intercourse, vaginismus, orgasmic changes, and lack of libido. The victim may be overly concerned about resuming sexual relations and need reassurance that the experience went well.

5. *Partner counseling*. Both victim and partner have to readjust to the disruption caused by the rape. Counseling needs to be provided for both victim and partner. Individual as well as joint sessions will help to negotiate sexual activity as well as issues in other areas.

6. *Intensification of sexual problems*. Not all victims will recover their previous level of sexual functioning. For victims who have persistent difficulty in recovering their sexual equilibrium, additional referrals are indicated to clinicians trained in sex therapy and possessing a solid understanding of the physiologic and psychologic trauma of rape.

In summary, there are a number of evaluation methods used by various human service organizations for assessing relative attainment of individualized patient goals. Goal attainment scaling and self-report methods are highly recommended in the treatment of rape trauma syndrome.

References

1. Burgess, A.W., and Holmstrom, L.L.: Rape trauma syndrome, Am. J. Psychiatr. **131**:981-986, 1974.
2. Burgess, A.W., and Holmstrom, L.L.: Sexual trauma of children and adolescents: pressure, sex and secrecy, Nurs. Clin. North Am. **10**:551-563, 1975.
3. Burgess, A.W., and Holmstrom, L.L.: Coping behavior of the rape victim, Am. J. Psychiatr. **133**:413-418, 1976.
4. Burgess, A.W., and Holmstrom, L.L.: Rape: crisis and recovery, Bowie, Md., 1979, Brady Co.
5. Burgess, A.W., and Holmstrom, L.L.: Victims of sexual assault. In Lazare, A., editor: Outpatient psychiatry, Baltimore, 1979, Williams & Wilkins.
6. Burgess, A.W., and Holmstrom, L.L.: Rape: sexual disruption and recovery, Am. J. Orthopsychiatr. **49**:648-657, 1979.
7. Groth, A.N., Burgess, A.W., and Holmstrom, L.L.: Rape: power, anger and sexuality, Am. J. Psychiatr. **134**:1239-1243, 1977.
8. Hazelwood, R.R.: A behavioral interview of the rape victim, FBI Bulletin. (In press.)
9. Herman, J., and Hirschman, L.: Families at risk for father-daughter incest, Am. J. Psychiatr. **138**:967-970, 1981.
10. Hilberman, E.: The rape victim, Washington, D.C., 1976, American Psychiatric Association.
11. Holmstrom, L.L., and Burgess, A.W.: Assessing trauma in the rape victim, Am. J. Nurs. **75**:1288-1291, 1975.
12. Holmstrom, L.L., and Burgess, A.W.: Sexual behavior of assailants during reported rape, Arch. Sexual Behav. **9**:427-439, 1980.
13. Russell, D.E.H.: Rape in marriage, New York, 1982, Macmillan Co.

Suggested Readings

Bart, P.B.: Rape doesn't end with a kiss, Viva, June 1975.
Brownmiller, S.: Against our will: men, women and rape, New York, 1975, Simon & Schuster.
Burgess, A.W., editor: Rape and sexual assault: a research handbook, New York, Garland Publishing Co. (In press.)
Foley, T.S., and Davies, M.A.: Rape: nursing care of victims, St. Louis, 1983, The C.V. Mosby Co.
Ipena, D.K.: Rape: the process of recovery, Nurs. Res. **28**:272-275, 1979.
Katz, S., and Mazur, M.A.: Understanding the rape victim: a synthesis of research findings, New York, 1979, John Wiley & Sons, Inc.

McCahill, T.W., Meyer, C., and Fischman, A.M.: The aftermath of rape, Lexington, Mass., 1979, D.C. Heath Co.

McCombie, S.L., editor: The rape crisis intervention handbook, New York, 1980, Plenum Press.

President's Task Force on Victims: Final Report, Washington, D.C., 1982, Department of Justice.

Russell, D.E.H.: The politics of rape, New York, 1975, Stein & Day.

Silverman, D.: Sharing the crisis of rape: counseling the mates and families of victims, Am. J. Orthopsychiatr. **48:**166-173, 1978.

White, P.N., and others. Rape: a family crisis, Family Relations **39:**103-109, 1981.

Physiologic

SKIN INTEGRITY, IMPAIRMENT OF: ACTUAL

THEORY AND ETIOLOGY

Actual impairment of skin integrity is defined as the interruption of the intact covering of the body. In an average adult the skin covers 3000 square inches of surface area, weighs approximately 6 pounds, and receives about one third of the circulating blood volume. Skin is both elastic and self-regenerating.[9] Functions of the skin include sensation, protection, thermoregulation, secretions, and vitamin D production. Located in the skin are nerve receptors for pain, touch, temperature, and pressure. When stimulated, these afferent nerves send impulses through the spinal cord to the cerebral cortex, where messages are interpreted. Skin protects the body from physical and chemical agents and from loss of fluids and electrolytes. The skin surface is the first line of defense against bacteria. Thermoregulation is accomplished by conduction, convection, radiation, and evaporation, which are controlled by activation of sweat glands and by dilation and constriction of cutaneous blood vessels. Secretions of the skin include sebum from sebaceous glands, which lubricates the skin, and sweat from sweat glands, which cools the body. The skin synthesizes vitamin D by using ultraviolet rays from the sun.

Both external (environmental) and internal (somatic) factors that alter skin functions can impair skin integrity. External factors include hyperthermia and chemical substances that cause first-, second-, and third-degree burns. Prolonged hypothermia, as in frostbite, can damage local tissue as a result of ischemia. The earlobes, fingers, and toes are most commonly affected. When the temperature of tissues falls almost to freezing, the vascular smooth muscle becomes paralyzed. A sudden vasodilation to prevent frostbite circulates blood to the skin. This mechanism unfortunately is not well developed in humans.[5] Mechanical shearing forces caused by scratching damage the epidermis. The mechanical forces of pressure and restraint cause damage by impairing circulation. Radiation can cause a local inflammatory reaction of skin similar to that caused by a first-degree burn. Physical immobilization causes ischemia of the skin over the dependent parts of the body, especially over bony prominences. Prolonged exposure to moisture from humidity, secretions, or excretions alters skin turgor and the protective mechanism of the epidermis so that the skin is vulnerable to impairment and more susceptible to bacterial invasion.

Internal or somatic factors also impair skin integrity. Medications may produce the allergic reaction of urticaria (hives), which results in edema and disruption of blood vessel walls. This allergic reaction also can initiate the liberation of histamine, which causes itching. The person's scratching often is the direct cause of the skin impairment rather than the medication.

The altered nutritional state in cases of obesity contributes to skin integrity impairment because additional adipose tissue increases the chance of damage by pressure; for example, clothing may fit tighter and restrict circulation. Position changes might be required more often for the obese person. Obesity indirectly affects skin integrity, since obese persons have a higher incidence of diabetes mellitus, atherosclerosis, ischemic heart disease, and hypertension. The altered nutritional state in

2017

cases of emaciation contributes to skin integrity impairment because the protective function of the skin is compromised by poor turgor and inadequate protein intake for growth and repair. Altered metabolic states interfere with skin maintenance and regeneration. Protein, carbohydrates, iron, and vitamins A, B-complex, C, D, and E are needed. Altered circulation interrupts the blood flow to skin, preventing delivery of nutrients and oxygen. When circulation is altered for a prolonged period, tissue ischemia results, followed by skin ulceration. Alteration of sensation removes the protective mechanism of interpreting sensory (afferent) messages regarding heat, pain, or pressure. For example, a paraplegic can burn the foot but not feel the pain to move away from the heat source in time to minimize the damage. Pruritus (itching) occurs when mechanoreceptors or chemical stimuli are transmitted by unmyelinated nerve fibers.[5] Histamine is an example of a chemical stimulant that initiates itching. These nerve fibers become more sensitive during capillary dilation; thus vasoconstriction reduces the perception of pruritus. Tissue anoxia caused by venous stasis results in itching also.[14]

Alteration in pigmentation can impair skin integrity. Pigmentation depends on skin thickness and the amount of melanin present in the dermis. Decreased pigment accompanies hyperthyroidism, hypoparathyroidism, and pernicious anemia. Increased pigmentation is manifested in Addison's disease and lupus erythematosus. The skin of patients with these diseases becomes hypersensitive to sunlight; thus the danger of sunburn caused by chemical changes increases. Elderly persons normally lose subcutaneous fat, which makes their skin more susceptible to impairment by external factors. Individuals with altered skin turgor also are more susceptible to skin impairment. Infants and toddlers are susceptible to skin impairment through accidental injury.

An immunologic deficit including humoral and cellular elements alters the normal protective mechanism of the immune system. This might result in skin lesions and itching because of the lack of a normal immune response. The patient's protective function of the skin becomes more important because the immune system is not able to adequately protect the body if the skin is broken.[14]

Psychogenic reactions can initiate urticaria and itching. Edema can impair skin by exerting pressure from within via the interstitial spaces. This pressure thins the skin, making it more prone to injury. Edema also compromises blood supply to the skin.

In summary, the major etiological factors associated with impaired skin integrity include the following[13]:

External (environmental)
    Hyperthermia or hypothermia
    Chemical substance
    Mechanical factors
        Shearing forces
        Pressure
        Restraint
    Radiation
    Physical immobilization
    Excretion and secretions
    Humidity
Internal (somatic)
    Medication
    Altered nutritional state (obesity, emaciation)
    Altered metabolic state
    Altered circulation
    Altered sensation
    Altered pigmentation
    Skeletal prominence
    Developmental factors
    Immunologic deficit
    Alterations in skin turgor (change in elasticity)
    Excretions and secretions
    Psychogenic factors
    Edema

DEFINING CHARACTERISTICS[13]

Disruption of skin surface (pustule, papule, macule)
Destruction of skin layers (e.g., burns)
Invasion of body structures
Hemorrhage
Reports of pain from impaired area
Area of red skin

NURSING INTERVENTIONS

Patient Goal	Nursing Intervention
Regain skin integrity.	Assess vital signs.
	Position patient on an egg crate mattress or Clinitron bed.
	Change position frequently.
	Cover areas of impaired skin integrity as ordered with dressings, ointments, etc.
	Administer intravenous fluids as ordered.
	Administer antiinfectives as ordered.
	Maintain sterile technique when caring for wounds.

Patient Goal	Nursing Intervention
	Monitor leukocyte count.
	Provide balanced diet as ordered: high in protein, iron, and vitamins via oral, nasogastric tube, or total parenteral nutrition.
Achieve comfort.	Reduce itching sensation.
	Encourage patient to discuss feelings about impaired skin integrity and body image changes.
	Use distraction techniques for pain relief.
	Administer local and systemic analgesics as ordered.
	Evaluate the therapeutic, adverse, and toxic effects of drugs given.
Achieve awareness of learning needs.	Assess what patient and family need to learn
	Provide information concerning:
	1. Prevention of skin integrity alterations
	2. How to change dressing and apply topical medication
	3. Purpose, frequency of administration, and side effects of medication
	4. Dietary intake to promote wound healing
	5. How to achieve comfort and relieve pain

Three nursing goals emerge for the patient with actual impairment of skin integrity. In order of priority the goals are to repair skin integrity, to provide comfort, and to achieve awareness of learning needs. Skin integrity is regained by protecting the skin from further damage and by promoting wound healing. Because the protective function of the skin is lost where skin integrity is impaired, the patient requires artificial protection until the skin regenerates or new skin is grafted. The severity of this loss of protection varies with the amount of surface area involved as well as the layers of skin involved. A surgical incision requires a gauze dressing to provide protection from invading bacteria. A third-degree burn over a large area of the body might require opened and closed methods of treatment, according to protocol, to protect against bacteria and fluid and electrolyte loss. Healing is promoted by adequate oxygen and blood supply along with nutrients to support tissue growth. These nutrients include protein and carbohydrate to maintain a positive nitrogen balance. Iron and vitamins A, B-complex, C, D, and E are required also. The age of the patient is a factor in wound healing because children normally heal more rapidly than do adults. Elderly persons often heal more slowly because of decreased fibroblastic activity and impaired circulation. Patients receiving steroids have delayed wound healing because these drugs depress the inflammatory response, which occurs prior to wound healing. An infected wound heals more slowly because a greater inflammatory response is required to fight against bacteria.

Comfort is the next goal for the nurse and consists of relief of pain and itching. This itching sensation is felt at varying stages of tissue repair. The normal response, of course, is to scratch the area, but one gentle scratch can infect an area. Repeated scratching in one area can further damage the epidermis. Cold applied to the itch can anesthetize the area for a short time. The patient's nails must be clipped short and kept as clean as possible. The patient can be encouraged to press on the itching area rather than scratch. This pressing briefly interrupts the sensory (afferent) nerve impulse without damaging the epidermis. Distraction techniques may be effective to relieve itching perception.

Another aspect of comfort for some patients is psychologic. Impaired skin integrity can disfigure a person, resulting in a disturbance in self-concept (refer to Pattern 1). The patient should verbalize feelings about the body image change and consider how to cope with the reactions of others to this change.

EVALUATION

Patient Outcome	Data Indicating That Outcome is Reached
Regain skin integrity.	Skin intact
	Skin warm, dry, natural color
	No reports of pain or itching from involved area(s)
Demonstrate knowledge of self-care.	Patient/family can explain:
	1. Cause and prevention of altered skin integrity
	2. Medications and treatment for home use
	3. Dietary intake to promote wound healing
	4. Plan for follow-up care

SKIN INTEGRITY, IMPAIRMENT OF: POTENTIAL
THEORY AND ETIOLOGY

Etiological factors for the diagnosis of potential impaired skin integrity are actually risk factors, which follow under Defining Characteristics. If skin integrity impairment actually occurs, one or more of the risk factors become the etiology, and the nursing diagnosis changes.

DEFINING CHARACTERISTICS

External (environmental)
  Hyperthermia or hypothermia
  Chemical substance
  Mechanical factors
    Shearing forces
    Pressure
    Restraint
    Radiation
    Physical immobilization
    Excretions and secretions
    Humidity
Internal (somatic)
  Medication
  Altered nutritional state (obesity, emaciation)
  Altered metabolic state
  Altered circulation
  Altered sensation (anesthesia, paresthesia, pruritus)
  Altered pigmentation
  Skeletal prominence
  Developmental factors
  Alterations in skin turgor (change in elasticity)
  Psychogenic factors
  Immunologic deficit

NURSING INTERVENTIONS

Patient Goal	Nursing Intervention
Assess skin.	Assess skin integrity daily. Teach patient and family members to inspect skin daily for reddened areas, broken skin, and bruised areas, blisters, and swelling; include what healthy skin looks like and actions to take when abnormalities are found.
Identify diet needed to ensure tissue growth and repair.	Present information on correcting nutritional deficits by increasing intake of protein, carbohydrates, vitamins, and iron.
Maintain adequate circulation to the skin.	Facilitate circulation by changing positions frequently. Avoid use of tobacco because it constricts blood vessels. Keep warm with warm stockings and appropriate layers of clothing because cold constricts blood vessels. Avoid wearing clothing that restricts circulation, such as garters or constricting stockings. Massage feet gently to stimulate circulation; DO NOT MASSAGE LEGS. Regular exercise stimulates circulation; exercise ranges from ROM to aerobics and must be planned individually for each person. Swelling of feet and legs may indicate circulatory problem requiring use of support stockings and periodic leg elevation; could also indicate need to reduce sodium intake and restrict fluid intake.
Protect skin.	Present information about protecting skin when it is more sensitive than normal. Individuals with altered pigmentation must wear long sleeved shirts or blouses and hats to shield the skin. Children and adults playing and working in the sun need to wear clothes to protect their skin, to apply a sun screen lotion, or to limit exposure time. The skin needs to be clean and dry to prevent infection and skin breakdown; individuals receiving radiation need to blot dry their skin rather than rub. Dry skin needs to be lubricated with lotion or oil to prevent cracking. Blisters or redness may occur from ill-fitting clothes or shoes; skin should be padded with bandage and clothing or shoes changed until blister or redness subsides. When itching is a problem, the individual needs to be encouraged not to scratch; pressing the area or applying ice decreases the sensation and does not damage the skin. A cool environment is soothing as opposed to a warm environment, which tends to increase the perception of itching; lubricating the skin with oil or lotion may decrease itching sensation; tub bath containing oatmeal powder, potassium permanganate, or corn starch at 32° to 38° C (89.6° to 100.4° F) relieves itching; when other methods are unsuccessful, antihistamines are given as ordered by a physician.

The nursing care for patients with this nursing diagnosis is directed toward eliminating internal and external factors that might lead to impaired skin integrity. The intent of the diagnosis is preventive and not curative. As a result, many of the interventions are either educational or include strategies to alter the environment.

EVALUATION

Patient Outcome	Data Indicating That Outcome is Reached
Skin assessed	Skin assessed Skin warm, dry, natural color, moist, adequate turgor
Diet needs identified	Knowledge of foods that maintain nutritional balance; allowances for cultural and socioeconomic factors considered
Adequate circulation maintained	Describes actions to avoid pressure, avoid vasoconstriction, and stimulate circulation
Skin protected	Describes actions to protect the skin from sun, moisture, dryness, pressure, and scratching

TISSUE PERFUSION, ALTERATION IN: CEREBRAL, CARDIOPULMONARY, RENAL, GASTROINTESTINAL, PERIPHERAL
THEORY AND ETIOLOGY

Body cells depend on delivery of oxygen and nutrients and removal of metabolic waste products. Conditions that interrupt the pumping or transportation of blood systematically, regionally, compartmentally, or locally can precipitate decreased tissue perfusion. Ischemia refers to local, compartmental, and regional decreases in perfusion, whereas shock refers to rapid systemic decreases in tissue perfusion.[6] When tissue perfusion is decreased, cellular function and energy metabolism decrease. The effect of this decrease varies with the intensity of the ischemia, the rate of onset, and the metabolic demands of the particular tissue. For example, the degree of arterial occlusion is tolerated better when the metabolic demand is low and collateral circulation develops.

Cells require adenosine triphosphate (ATP) to perform their normal functions. About 90% of ATP is formed in the cell's mitochondria by oxidative phosphorylation, a complex process that involves the breakdown of glucose (glycolysis). During glycolysis adenosine diphosphate (ADP) combines with phosphate to become ATP. The availability of ADP becomes an important feedback mechanism to control the amount of ATP formed. Once the ADP in the cells has been converted to ATP, the glycolytic and oxidative processes stop. When ATP releases energy to perform cellular functions, a phosphoric acid radical is split away from ATP to form ADP, which automatically initiates the glycolytic process to form ATP again.[5]

Cells use ATP for three major functions. The first function is membrane transport, which includes movement of sodium and potassium ions and in certain cells calcium ions, phosphate ions, chloride ions, urate ions, and hydrogen ions. "Membrane transport is so important to cellular function that some cells, the renal tubular cells for instance, utilize as much as 80% of the ATP formed in the cells for this purpose alone."[5]

The second function is synthesis of chemical compounds such as protein by ribosomes, phospholipids, cholesterol, purines, and pyrimidine. The third function is supply of energy for special cells to perform mechanical work, such as smooth, skeletal, and cardiac muscle contractions, ciliary movement in the respiratory tract and fallopian tubes, and ameboid motion, which is movement of an entire cell, such as a white blood cell, through tissues.[5]

The usual oxidative phosphorylation process requires an adequate oxygen supply. (Normally 38 molecules of ATP are formed from one glucose molecule.) When oxygen is inadequate or unavailable, this process cannot take place. A small amount of ATP can be formed from anaerobic glycolysis (two ATP molecules formed from one glucose molecule).[22] End products of anaerobic glycolysis are pyruvic acid and hydrogen, which combine with nicotinamide adenine dinucleotide (NAD$^+$) to form NADH and H$^+$. Accumulation of either interrupts the glycolytic process to prevent further ATP formation. When accumulation does occur, NADH and H$^+$ react together to form lactic acid, which diffuses out of the cells into extracellular fluids. The diffusion of lactic acid allows the anaerobic glycolysis to continue for several minutes, providing ATP in the absence of oxygen.[5]

Decreased tissue perfusion interrupts the cellular supply of oxygen and nutrients for ATP formation and use. The ability of the tissue to survive depends on the severity and duration of the deficit. The reaction of the microcirculation is an important factor of tissue survival because when ischemic capillaries lose their integrity, tissue edema results.[6] The ATP-dependent functions (membrane transport, synthesis of chemical compounds, and energy supply for mechanical work) cannot occur efficiently. For example, sodium and calcium move into the cell while potassium and magnesium move out. Movement of sodium into the cell is followed by cellular swelling. This cellular swelling produces pressure against adjacent vessels to cause further ischemia.

Cellular hypoxia accompanies prolonged decreased tissue perfusion. The lactic acid waste products of anaerobic metabolism lower the cell's pH. An acidic condition can trigger release and activation of lysosomal enzymes, which destroy mitochondrial and plasma membranes and digest cell contents. When the integrity of the cell membrane is disrupted, intracellular enzymes leak out. These enzymes include lactic dehydrogenase (LDH), serum glutamic oxaloacetic transaminase (SGOT), and creatine phosphokinase (CPK).[6]

Cerebral

Altered cerebral tissue perfusion can be related to a change in blood vessels or compression from surrounding tissue. Cerebral infarction is significant because of the lack of tissue reserve and inability for tissue regeneration. Cerebral vascular accident (CVA) covers a wide range and gradation of symptoms from mild ischemic attack to major stroke. Causes of a CVA include thrombus, emboli, and hemorrhage, which interrupt blood flow to the areas of the brain supplied by the involved vessels. Thus the symptoms depend on which vessels are involved. Cerebral aneurysm is a round saccular dilation or ballooning of a weak arterial wall. Most patients are not symptomatic until the aneurysm ruptures and bleeds. Again, symptoms vary depending on the vessel involved. Arteriovenous malformation is an aggregation of abnormal veins and twisted, dilated arteries, each with deficient muscle coats. Head injury, both open and closed, can cause vascular rupture. Epidural hematoma results from a laceration of a vessel, most commonly the middle meningeal artery. Blood collects rapidly between the skull and dura. Subdural hematoma occurs when blood from a lacerated vessel, usually a vein, collects slowly between the dura and arachnoid.

Compression of cerebral vessels can be caused by tumors, benign or malignant, that exert pressure on adjacent arteries and veins to impede the blood flow. Hydrocephalus is another disorder that compresses cerebral vessels. Both communicating and noncommunicating hydrocephalus result from an excessive accumulation of cerebrospinal fluid that compresses vessels adjacent to the ventricles.

Cardiopulmonary

Altered cardiopulmonary tissue perfusion can result from faulty coronary artery perfusion or pulmonary capillary perfusion. Ischemic heart disease develops from atherosclerosis of the coronary arteries. Atherosclerosis refers to lesions of the intimal walls resulting from lipid deposits and fibrosis plaques. Endothelial cell injury, smooth muscle cell proliferation, and lipid and cell debris accumulation are among the factors that seem to contribute to lesion development. Narrowing or obstruction of these arteries by these lesions reduces the blood supply to the myocardium, resulting in angina and tachycardia. Severe reduction of the blood supply may lead to myocardial infarction with resulting reduction in cardiac output. Infarction causes significant damage in the heart because there is little reserve and no ability to regenerate damaged tissue.

Pulmonary infarct or emboli can interrupt the blood supply to the pulmonary capillaries, where gas exchange occurs in conjunction with the alveoli. Blood supply to the pulmonary capillaries can be interrupted by the same conditions as those which precipitate altered gas exchange due to perfusion alterations (high $\dot{V}/\dot{Q}$ ratio) (see box on p. 2034). These conditions include decreased cardiac output, circulatory collapse, blockage or compression of pulmonary capillaries, decrease in blood pH, and destruction of the capillary bed. Tissue necrosis produced by ischemia is accompanied by hemorrhage from damaged vessels at the edges of the infarcted area. In the lung this hemorrhage is extensive. A pulmonary infarct can be serious because it usually results from pulmonary emboli. There is concern that subsequent and larger emboli may originate from the source of the first embolus.[19]

Renal

Altered renal tissue perfusion can be related to any condition causing ischemia of the kidney. These include hypovolemia, blood loss following surgery or trauma, plasma loss due to burns, surgery, or acute pancreatitis, sodium and water loss, cardiac failure, myocardial infarction, cardiac arrhythmias, congestive heart failure, and septic shock. The kidney's normal response to ischemia is vasoconstriction to maintain flow through glomeruli; however this vasoconstriction increases ischemia. Prolonged ischemia results in tissue death and renal failure develops. A large renal infarct is not of particular concern because of the tissue reserve of the kidney.[17]

Gastrointestinal

Altered gastrointestinal tissue perfusion results from vascular disease and postoperative complications. Vascular disease precipitates occlusion of the superior mesenteric vessels to decrease the blood supply to the intestines.[17] Ischemic bowel disease can occur in the early postoperative period after kidney transplantation. Lack of perfusion results in decreased peristalsis. Since intestinal contents cannot move distally, the gastrointestinal tract attempts to get rid of its contents through vomiting. Infarcts of the bowel quickly become gangrenous.[19] During shock the liver is one of the first organs to deteriorate because of its rapid exposure to concentrated toxins and its high rate of metabolism. Ischemia of the liver results in elevation of serum enzymes (SGOT, SGPT, and LDH). As liver tissue damage continues, it becomes unable to detoxify materials. Decreased perfusion of the pancreas activates pancreatic enzymes and causes release of toxic factors into the blood. One of these, myocardial toxic factor, decreases myocardial contractility by 50% by interfering with the action of calcium ions.[6]

Peripheral

Altered peripheral tissue perfusion can be related to arteriosclerosis, atherosclerosis, inflammation, spasm, or obstruction of peripheral arteries and veins. Arteriosclerosis, hardening of the arteries, primarily affects the medial layers. It occurs with advancing age and calcification, and results in the loss of elastic properties of arteries. Cerebral and peripheral arteries are most commonly affected. Atherosclerosis is a form of arteriosclerosis that results from lesions of the intestinal wall. Endothelial cell injury, smooth muscle cell proliferation, and lipid and cell debris accumulation are among the factors that seem to contribute to lesion development. Thrombophlebitis, inflammation of the vein and clot formation, occurs in veins. Thromboangiitis obliterans (Buerger's disease) causes inflammation of vessel walls, thrombus formation, fibrosis thickening and scarring, and eventual occlusion of the vessel. Arteriolar spasm aggravates the fibrous constriction. Raynaud's disease also is characterized by arterial spasms, most often in the hands. Abnormal sympathetic innervation is thought to be a cause. Emboli are floating blood clots that can lodge in a bifurcation of arteries to narrow or occlude the vessel. Aneurysms occur in arteries of lower extremities, especially in the popliteal area in people over 60 years of age who have pronounced arteriosclerosis. Thrombi form at the aneurysm, and emboli may move to the distal part of the artery. On auscultation of the aneurysm, a bruit is heard that alternates with arterial pulsations. Arteriovenous fistulas occur in peripheral vessels as the result of congenital malformation or trauma. Because there is abnormal communication between the artery and the vein, the capillary is bypassed. A constant bruit is heard over the site of the fistula.[17]

Systemic ischemia, or shock, results from failure of one or all of the three physiologic mechanisms that support adequate circulation, that is, blood volume, cardiac output, and vascular tone. In hematogenic shock, perfusion is altered because of a marked reduction in blood volume. Examples include loss of whole blood in hemorrhagic shock, loss of plasma in burn shock, and severe dehydration and acidosis in diabetic shock. In cardiogenic shock, tissue perfusion alteration occurs because of failure of the heart to pump blood. In neurogenic shock, perfusion alteration occurs by interrupting the nerve supply to the blood vessels so that vascular tone is decreased. In anaphylactic shock, vasodilation occurs because an antigen-antibody reaction liberates histamine.[14]

• • •

The etiologies for altered tissue perfusion include the following:[13]
Interruption of arterial flow
Interruption of venous flow
Exchange problems
Hypervolemia
Hypovolemia

DEFINING CHARACTERISTICS[13]

Skin temperature: cold extremities
Skin color
  Dependent, blue or purple
  Pale on elevation, and color does not return on lowering
  Diminished arterial pulsation
Skin quality: shining
Lack of lanugo
Round scars covered with atrophied skin
Gangrene
Slow-growing, dry, thick brittle nails
Claudication

Blood pressure changes in extremities
Bruits
Slow healing of lesions
Cerebral
   Decrease in consciousness
   Restlessness
   Altered thought processes
   Memory loss
Cardiopulmonary
   Low systolic and diastolic blood pressure readings
   Cold clammy skin
   Slow capillary filling
   Tachycardia
   Angina
   Tachypnea

Renal
   Edema
   Decreased urinary output
   Hypertension
Gastrointestinal
   Abdominal distention
   Positive guaiac findings of stool
   Nausea or vomiting
   Thirst
Peripheral
   Edema
   Pain
   Numbness, tingling
   Muscle weakness
   Diminished sensitivity to pressure, temperature, tissue trauma

NURSING INTERVENTIONS

Patient Goal	Nursing Intervention
Maintain tissue perfusion and cellular oxygenation.	Assess vital signs and peripheral pulses. Assess skin color and temperature. Measure intake and output. Position extremities to facilitate circulation: elevation for venous problems, downward for arterial problems. Change position frequently. Regular active or passive exercise. Administer drugs as ordered to improve circulation: anticoagulants, vasodilators. Evaluate the therapeutic, adverse, and toxic effects of drugs given. Administer oxygen as ordered. Encourage balanced diet with adequate iron.
Reduce metabolic needs.	Encourage alternate periods of rest and activity. Protect extremities from extreme temperatures. Discuss stress reduction strategies.
Achieve awareness of learning needs.	Assess what patient and family need to know. Provide information concerning: 1. Changes required in activities of daily living 2. Maintaining reduction in metabolic needs 3. Assessing skin and peripheral circulation daily 4. Purpose, frequency of administration, and side effect of medication 5. Safety needs for patients taking anticoagulants 6. Providing balanced diet 7. Taking action to prevent recurrence of alteration in tissue perfusion 8. Plans for rehabilitation

Three nursing goals emerge for the patient with altered tissue perfusion. In order of priority the goals are to maintain tissue perfusion and cellular oxygenation, to reduce cellular needs, and to achieve awareness of learning needs.

Nursing actions to maintain tissue perfusion are based on the cause of the alteration. Elevation of the affected extremity is appropriate when venous circulation is altered, since this position uses gravity to facilitate return of blood toward the heart. Likewise, elevating both legs is helpful when the patient has hypovolemic shock to facilitate blood flow from the lower extremities to the trunk. Conversely, arterial circulation is hindered by prolonged elevation of lower extremities because the normal flow of arterial blood is downward. The flat position is best for long periods. The patient needs a firm bed to prevent hip flexion allowed on a soft mattress. Flexion of the hip may compromise circulation to the legs. The patient must also select chairs carefully. The knees must not be bent at more than a 90° angle, and the popliteal space must not press against the chair seat. Active and passive exercises as well as walking stimulate blood flow to the legs. External pressure on the legs is reduced by not crossing legs, not wearing tight clothing on the legs, and not sitting for prolonged periods. Drug administration may include heparin or dihydroxycoumarin as prophylaxis against blood clotting per physician order. Vasodilators are given, as ordered by physician, for arterial spasm and to improve general circulation. Cellular oxygenation is promoted by maintaining tissue perfusion. In acute conditions, however, supplemental oxygen may be ordered. Anemia needs to be treated per physician's orders to maximize oxygen transport.

Cellular metabolic needs are reduced by alternating periods of rest and activity. The patient needs to protect affected extremities from trauma and infection, which increase metabolic needs. Extremities need to be warm without becoming overheated. To accomplish this, heating pads, time spent in hot tubs, and exercise must be used in moderation. Fear, worry, and anxiety can increase the metabolic needs of tissue. To the extent possible, the patient needs to use stress reduction strategies to prevent detrimental physical effects of these psychologic states.

To achieve awareness of learning needs, the nurse discusses with the patient and family the actions needed to maintain tissue perfusion and decrease metabolic demands. Activities of daily living may need to be changed. The need for rehabilitation also will vary depending on the site and extent of altered perfusion. Safety needs to be emphasized for the patient taking anticoagulants. This includes watching for signs of bleeding from the gums, rectum, and skin. They should be informed about the anticoagulation properties of aspirin and cautioned against using it in combination with other anticoagulants. A well-balanced diet is important to provide sufficient glucose for ATP formation. Family members need to discuss action needed to prevent recurrence of this problem. This may include smoking cessation, dietary alterations, stress reduction strategies, and exercise programs.

EVALUATION

Patient Outcome	Data Indicating That Outcome is Reached
Adequate tissue perfusion	All pulses palpable Extremities warm and normal color Vital signs normal for patient
Urine output within normal limits	1500-3000 ml or equivalent to intake

Laboratory data within normal limits	LDH
	   0-2 yr: up to 450 IU/L
	   2-5 yr: up to 320 IU/L
	   5-8 yr: up to 270 IU/L
	   8-12 yr: up to 260 IU/L
	  12-14 yr: up to 260 IU/L
	  14-15 yr: up to 235 IU/L
	  15-18 yr: up to 225 IU/L
	  18-44 yr: 115-200 IU/L
	  44 yr and up: 115-225 IU/L
	SGOT: Levels in infancy are 2-3 times those found in adults; Ranges decrease during childhood; SMA method, 16 yr and up: 8-42 IU/L.
	CPK: Method dependent
	Hgb (g/dl)
	  1 day: 19.4 ± 2.1
	  11-13.5 mo: 11.9 ± 0.6
	  1.5-3 yr: 11.8 ± 0.5
	  5 yr: 12.7 ± 1.0
	  10 yr: 13.2 ± 1.2
	  Men: 15.5 ± 1.1
	  Women: 13.7 ± 1.0
	BUN
	  Birth-1 yr: 4-19 mg/dl
	  1-40 yr: 5-20 mg/dl
	  Gradual slight increase subsequently occurs.
	Serum creatinine
	  1-5 yr: 0.30-0.50 mg/dl
	  5-10 yr: 0.50-0.80 mg/dl
	  Men: up to 1.2 mg/dl

Patient Outcome	Data Indicating That Outcome is Reached
	Women: up to 1.1 mg/dl There are slight differences between the sexes with males higher, since the range relates to the amount of muscle mass present. PTT: 25-39 seconds (usually stated to be within 10 seconds of control) Arterial blood gases pH: 7.35-7.45 Po_2: 80-95 mm Hg Pco_2: 35-45 mm Hg O_2 sat: 95%-99%
Awareness of learning needs	Patient/family can explain: 1. Reasons for altered tissue perfusion 2. Medication and treatments for home use 3. Dietary and activity modification 4. Safety precautions 5. Follow-up treatment regimen

Oxygenation is a continuous process used to exchange gases between the body tissues and the atmosphere. This process involves four phases: ventilation, external respiration, transportation, and internal respiration. Alterations in ventilation can result from ineffective airway clearance or from ineffective breathing patterns, depending on the pathologic mechanism. When these two nursing diagnoses are not or cannot be resolved, they can precipitate a third nursing diagnosis of impaired gas exchange. This latter diagnosis can also be precipitated by alterations in external respiration and transportation.

AIRWAY CLEARANCE, INEFFECTIVE
THEORY AND ETIOLOGY

This diagnosis implies two problems: the upper and/or lower airways are not cleared and the normal mechanisms for clearance are not functioning. Clearance is required when narrowed airways alter the laminar airflow from the nose to the terminal bronchioles. This narrowing results from obstruction, such as excessive mucus production, or from restriction, such as bronchospasm.

Normal mechanisms for clearing airways include mucus production, ciliary function, cough reflex, and swallowing. Mucus is produced in response to irritants by surface goblet cells and serous glands in the tracheobronchial tree. Additionally, submucous glands continually produce 100 ml of mucus daily, which lies atop the pulmonary epithelium. Mucus forms an uninterrupted covering for the tracheobronchial tree and moves by the process of mucokinesis at a rate of 1 to 2 cm/minute to completely clean a normal adult lung in about 20 minutes.[20] The mucus blanket warms, filters, and humidifies air entering the nose. It contains immunoglobulins, polymorphonuclear neutrophils, interferon, and specific antibodies to defend the respiratory tract. The mucous blanket is interrupted by dehydration and by the inflammatory process and irritants, which produce excessive mucus to interfere with airflow.

Cilia are hairlike projections adjacent to the mucosal surface. They move mucus posteriorly in the nasal cavity and superiorly in the lower respiratory tract toward the pharynx to be swallowed or expectorated.[19] Factors altering cilia function include smoking, viral disease, chilling, and inhalation of irritating gases.[18] The cough reflex forcefully expels secretions from the airways to the pharynx for swallowing or expectorating. The cough reflex is diminished by depression of the medulla oblongata, as occurs after head injury and morphine administration. Also, the ability to remove secretions by coughing is impaired in chest trauma, debilitating diseases, and neuromuscular diseases such as multiple sclerosis, myasthenia gravis, cerebral palsy, and Guillain-Barré syndrome. This inability to cough occurs because intercostal and abdominal muscular contractions needed to expel secretions from airways are unattainable. Any condition that interrupts swallowing (dysphagia) causes potential threat of aspiration into lower airways. Swallowing can be interrupted by edema of the medulla, causing pressure on the glossopharyngeal, vagus, or hypoglossal cranial nerves. Dysphagia also is caused by congenital defects such as cleft palate and esophageal obstruction.

Upper Airway Obstruction

Upper airways, including the nose, pharynx, and larynx, are obstructed by six causes. First, the tongue occludes the airway when it falls on the posterior wall of the pharynx. This occurs during unconsciousness from a variety of causes, including grand mal seizures and cardiopulmonary arrest. Second, foreign objects obstruct the airway. These can include food, dentures, or a small toy. The object prevents movement of gases through the airways. Third is laryngeal spasm, which decreases the airway diameter. This may be caused by anaphylaxis, acute laryngitis, inflammation of the throat, and edema following extubation.[17] Fourth, nasal congestion or edema secondary to trauma or infection obstructs air flow. Congestion, the accumulation of blood in tissues, occurs in the nose secondary to fractures of the bones of the nose, including maxillary, nasal, vomer, palatine, ethmoid, and sphenoid. Damage to nasal cartilage also results in congestion. Edema of nasal mucosa is precipitated by the inflammatory process from rhinitis or acute sinusitis. Fifth, sinus congestion or edema obstructs upper airways as the result of allergic response, viral or bacterial infection, trauma, or inadequate drainage. Allergic responses, infection, and trauma cause obstruction by the processes of inflammation and edema. Inadequate drainage occurs when gravitational drainage is not possible, for example, a patient on a turning frame who lies in the prone position for a number of hours. Finally, polyps and tumors obstruct the nose and can be surgically removed.

Lower Airway Obstruction

Lower airways include the trachea, bronchi, and bronchioles. Obstruction occurs in these structures in four ways. First, constriction results from smooth muscle contraction initiated by parasympathetic (cholinergic) nerve stimulation or by the antibody-medicated immune response. This immune response takes place after the release of histamine and slow-reacting substance of anaphylaxis (SRS-A). For those with asthma, this narrowing occurs from partial blockage of beta-adrenergic receptors.[5] The second cause is congestion and edema. This results from the inflammatory response against microorganisms, as occurs in chronic bronchitis and tuberculosis. Edema of bronchial tissue also obstructs airways. The third cause of obstruction of the lower airway includes blockage by mucus plugs, mucus cohesion, tumors, or foreign bodies. Tenacity of mucus is greater when the patient is dehydrated. Tumors, whether malignant or benign, occlude airways. Bronchogenic carcinoma, which creates primary malignant tumors of the lower airways, is epithelial and arises from the mucosa of the bronchial tree. Smoking, industrial hazards, and air pollution increase the incidence. Bronchogenic carcinomas affecting airway clearance are divided into squamous cell or epidermoid, anaplastic or undifferentiated, and adenocarcinoma. Finally, the compression of lower airways by fibrosis impairs the flow of air and prevents expansion.

• • •

Etiologies for ineffective airway clearance include the following[13]:

Decreased energy and fatigue
Tracheobronchial
Infection
Obstruction
Secretion
Perceptual/cognitive impairment
Trauma

DEFINING CHARACTERISTICS[13]

Abnormal breathing sounds (rales, rhonchi)
Changes in rate or depth of respiration
Tachypnea
Cough, effective or ineffective, with or without sputum (indicates an irritant or secretion is stimulating the cough reflex; thus cough is both a sign of as well as a treatment for ineffective airway clearance)
Cyanosis (bluish discoloration of skin and mucous membranes; a late sign of hypoxia, not observed until O_2 saturation has fallen below 78%)
Dyspnea
Fever
Nasal bogginess (edema of the mucous membranes in the nasal cavity)
Altered speech (edematous sinuses cause nasal sounding speech; dyspnea may interrupt speech while patient catches breath; total airway obstruction causes inability to speak)
Increased anteroposterior diameter
Prolonged expiratory phase of respiration through pursed lip breathing
Use of accessory muscles for breathing
Choking or gasping
Noisy respirations
Nasal flaring
Anxiety
Fearfulness
Hemoptysis

NURSING INTERVENTIONS

Patient Goal	Nursing Intervention

Acute

Achieve airway patency.

Auscultate lungs.
Perform head tilt to remove tongue from obstructing the airway.
Perform the Heimlich maneuver to remove foreign object.
Prepare equipment for bronchoscopy if patient aspirated solid material.
Suction mucus and secretions from airways.
Administer medication as ordered: corticosteroids, antibiotics, bronchodilators, and decongestants.
Evaluate the therapeutic, adverse, and toxic effects of medications.
Provide humidification to airways as ordered.

Achieve adequate ventilation.

Administer oxygen as ordered.
Monitor arterial blood gases and hemoglobin.
Provide mechanical ventilation as ordered.

Achieve physical and psychologic comfort.

Provide oral care as needed for the patient who is coughing.
Plan rest periods of at least 1 hour during the day.
Assist in decreasing fear or anxiety.

Chronic

Maintain airway patency.

Encourage patient to breath deeply and cough each hour while awake.
Encourage fluid intake to thin secretions if patient is not fluid restricted.
Assist patient to the appropriate position for postural drainage.
Use percussion and vibration to dislodge pulmonary secretions.
Turn and position patient every 2 hours.
Administer medications as ordered: corticosteroids, bronchodilators, antiinfectives, and decongestants.
Evaluate the therapeutic, adverse, and toxic effects of medication given.
Discourage patient and family from smoking.

Achieve physical and psychologic comfort.

Place warm, moist compresses over painful sinuses.
Elevate head of bed to facilitate gravity drainage of sinus and reduce the work of breathing.
Provide oral care as needed for the patient who is coughing productively.
Plan rest periods of at least 1 hour during the day.
Assist in decreasing fear or anxiety.

Achieve awareness of learning needs.

Assess what patient and family need to learn.
Provide information concerning:
  1. How to prevent recurrence of airway obstruction
  2. How to perform diaphragmatic and pursed-lip breathing
  3. Purpose of drugs taken at home, the frequency of administration, and side effects
  4. Smoking cessation
  5. Eating balanced meals with adequate fluids
  6. Performing bronchial hygiene and productive coughing techniques
  7. Changing daily activities to decrease oxygen demands
  8. Plans for follow-up

Three nursing goals emerge for the patient with ineffective airway clearance. In order of priority the goals are to maintain oxygen to cells, to provide comfort, and to achieve awareness of learning needs. Nursing actions to attain goals is subdivided into upper and lower airway obstruction.

Upper Airway Obstruction

When the cause of upper airway obstruction is the tongue or a foreign object, the patient requires immediate care to clear the obstruction. When a foreign body is suspected, the nurse determines if the patient can speak to distinguish an occluded airway from another condition such as myocardial infarction. The person with an occluded airway will be unable to speak. To dislodge the obstruction, the nurse uses the Heimlich maneuver: four quick back blows to the victim between the scapula followed by abdominal thrusts. To deliver the abdominal thrusts, the nurse stands behind the patient and places both hands at the patient's diaphragm, grabs the right fist with the left hand, and gives a sudden, strong upward thrust against the abdomen. This pressure compresses the lungs, forcing the object into the mouth to clear the airway. This procedure can be done with the patient supine and the nurse kneeling astride and facing the patient. The nurse places the heel of one hand just above the umbilicus and places the other hand atop the first. A quick upward thrust is delivered against the abdomen to dislodge the object. The back blows and abdominal thrusts are continued until the obstruction is relieved or advanced life support is available. The airway is suctioned to remove excess secretions.

Ineffective airway clearance related to laryngospasm occurs most frequently in infants and children. It requires prompt care also but is placed in order of priority after obstruction by foreign object or tongue. Initially, the airway is opened using the head tilt with forward displacement of the mandible. An oropharyngeal airway is inserted followed by artificial ventilation by mouth-to-mouth means or inflation bag. A medical treatment of laryngospasm is administration of a paralytic drug followed by oral-tracheal intubation. If this action is not adequate and the patient is unconscious, the nurse, in collaboration with the physician, inserts an esophageal obturator airway. An emergency tracheostomy is performed by a physician as a last resort to open the airway. Once the airway is opened, the patient is placed in an upright position and encouraged to breathe deeply. Humidified oxygen is given as ordered.

Lower Airway Obstruction

When the cause of lower airway obstruction is edema or excessive mucus and secretion production, the airways are cleared by effective coughing. The patient is instructed to sit up as high as possible to facilitate chest expansion. Then the patient inhales slowly and deeply to dilate airways and force air behind the mucus and secretions. The patient exhales forcibly until the cough reflex is stimulated. Endotracheal stimulation is used to produce coughing when the patient is too weak to cough. Coughing is necessary but does require work that can fatigue the patient. The nurse determines the frequency of coughing needed by patients to clear the airways but not to tire them unnecessarily. Along with coughing, postural drainage is recommended to allow gravity to drain secretions from segmental bronchi. Percussion and vibration are used to dislodge pulmonary secretions. The patient who is obese, has unstable vital signs, or has extreme dyspnea may not be able to tolerate postural drainage.

To maintain comfort, the nurse encourages frequent oral and nasal hygiene for the patient who has a productive cough. The patient should blow his nose gently to remove mucus. Nostrils may be cleaned with moistened cotton-tipped applicators. Since coughing can cause fatigue and can interfere with sleep, the patient needs planned rest periods of at least 1 hour. After receiving treatments for airway clearance and medications, the patient can be encouraged to sleep. A dyspneic apprehensive patient may need to talk with the nurse about fears and anxieties related to breathing. The patient also may want to speak with a chaplain about these concerns.

EVALUATION

Patient Outcome	Data Indicating That Outcome is Reached
Acute	
Patent airway	Breath sounds clear bilaterally Normal respirations
Adequate ventilation	Arterial blood gases normal for patient Skin, nails, lips, and earlobes natural color
Chronic	
Patent airway	Breath sounds clear bilaterally Normal respirations Skin, nails, lips, and earlobes natural color
Knowledge of self-care	Patient and family can explain: 1. Reason for ineffective airway clearance 2. Actions to avoid it 3. Medications and treatments for home use 4. Plan for follow-up care

BREATHING PATTERN, INEFFECTIVE
THEORY AND ETIOLOGY

Breathing patterns provide the mechanism for ventilation, that is, the movement of air in and out of the lungs. These patterns depend on the integration of the nervous, muscular, and skeletal systems. The primary respiratory center located in the medulla oblongata contains mutually inhibiting inspiratory and expiratory centers in addition to chemoreceptors that are stimulated by arterial and cerebrospinal fluid, carbon dioxide tension, and hydrogen ion content. The pneumotaxic center in the pons provides the rhythmic quality of breathing. When the stimulus occurs, neurons transmit impulses down the spinal cord via the phrenic nerve, which innervates the diaphragm, to contract downward. Simultaneously, the thoracic intercostal nerves transmit impulses to the external intercostal muscles, which move the thorax up and out. The contraction of these muscle groups expands the thorax, which increases the volume within the lung. Movement of the thorax and lung occurs because the pleural fluid between the parietal and visceral pleura prevent their separation. Thus, as the thorax expands the lung volume increases, and as the thorax recoils the lung volume decreases. The amount of expansion or depth of respiration is controlled by the Hering-Breuer reflex. As the lungs inflate, the stretch receptors in the bronchi and bronchioles signal the respiratory center via the vagus nerve to stop sending impulses to breathe. The absence of these impulses is followed by passive recoil of the lungs. One voluntarily alters the breathing under the control of the cerebral cortex when talking, crying, or laughing.

The change in volume of the lung during contraction of respiratory muscles creates a negative pressure within the lungs that pulls in atmospheric air. When the lungs passively recoil, a more positive pressure is created that forces air out of the lungs.

When carbon dioxide is retained for a long time, CO_2 narcosis develops and the respiratory center becomes depressed and unable to initiate respiration. When this happens, the peripheral chemoreceptors in the carotid arch and aortic bodies stimulate the respiratory center. These chemoreceptors are sensitive to decreases in arterial oxygen tension.

Breathing patterns are interrupted by restrictive neuromuscular and respiratory disorders that (1) alter the synapses between nerves or between nerves and muscles, (2) alter the anatomic structure of the chest, or (3) cause pain. Central nervous system disorders altering synapses include general anesthesia, drug overdose, head injury, spinal cord injury, poliomyelitis, multiple sclerosis, amyotrophic lateral sclerosis, fatigue, and anxiety. General anesthesia and drug overdose depress the cerebral cortex and respiratory centers, preventing the receipt of incoming impulses from chemoreceptors stimulated by elevated arterial carbon dioxide or low arterial pH. Head injury also can depress the cerebral cortex or midbrain function, depending on the site and extent of injury, as well as cause direct anatomic damage to the medulla and pons.

Spinal cord injuries affect breathing patterns in quadriplegics as well as high paraplegics. The phrenic nerve travels through the third, fourth, and fifth cervical segments of the cord. In most cases individuals with an injury at C1 or C2 die of respiratory arrest because the muscles of respiration cannot receive impulses from the respiratory center. The intercostal nerves exit the spinal cord at the first and second thoracic levels. Individuals with spinal cord injuries at T2 and above would be expected to have altered breathing patterns.

Poliomyelitis is an acute viral infection that damages primarily the anterior horns of the spinal cord. Efferent fibers of the brainstem and brain also may be damaged in bulbar poliomyelitis. Since the anterior horns carry impulses to muscles, damage to those horns innervating muscles of respiration alter breathing patterns. Many poliomyelitis patients have respiratory deficits that result in ineffective breathing patterns.

Multiple sclerosis is an autoimmune disease that causes degenerative changes in the myelin of nerves. The signs and symptoms of this disease are varied and unpredictable; it can alter breathing patterns when the myelin of the spinal cord from T2 or above degenerates. Amyotrophic lateral sclerosis is a fatal motor neuron disease resulting from degeneration of anterior motor cells in the spinal cord; the motor nuclei of the hypoglossal (XII), vagus (X), spinal accessory (XI), facial (VII), and trigeminal (V) cranial nerves; and the corticobulbar and corticospinal tracts. Again, nerve damage prevents innervation of the muscles of respiration.

Fatigue, from multiple causes, can result in inadequate respiratory effort. One frequently overlooked cause of muscle fatigue is malnutrition in a patient who is intubated and given only intravenous dextrose. Since this patient cannot take oral fluids, he should receive total parenteral nutrition intravenously to supply adequate protein and carbohydrates. Characteristics of severe anxiety and panic include rapid and deep respirations resulting from sympathetic nervous system stimulation.

Peripheral neuromuscular disorders that alter breathing patterns include Guillain-Barré syndrome, myasthenia gravis, and muscular dystrophy. Guillain-Barré syndrome is a polyneuritis involving spinal roots, peripheral nerves, and occasionally cranial nerves. It is characterized by sudden, usually ascending, motor paralysis with loss of reflexes, paresthesia, and tender muscles. When the paralysis ascends to the level of the intercostal nerves and muscles, it alters breathing patterns.

Myasthenia gravis alters the breathing pattern because impulses from the phrenic and intercostal nerves to the diaphragm and anterior intercostal muscles are inconsistent. The number of acetylcholine receptor sites at the myoneural junction are inadequate. Muscle strength improves after rest and worsens after exertion.

Pseudohypertrophic (Duchenne) muscular dystrophy is a childhood disease. It is inherited as an X-linked recessive disorder affecting males primarily. Myofibrils in muscle fibers are destroyed, and increased fat cells are present in muscle tissue. Initially the gastrocnemius, deltoid, and quadricep muscles are involved. In the terminal stages the facial, oropharyngeal, and respiratory muscles are affected.[25]

Alterations of the anatomic structure of the chest include pneumothorax, hemothorax, paradoxic breathing, and kyphoscoliosis. The first three can follow blunt or penetrating chest injuries, but there are other causes. For example, pneumothorax occurs spontaneously in otherwise healthy individuals, but also after the rupture of an emphysematous bleb. Pneumothorax occurs when air separates the parietal from visceral pleura. The positive pressure of this air compresses the lung and may be severe enough to cause mediastinal shift. Hemothorax is the presence of blood in the pleural space. The effect of the blood is the same as that of the air—pressure on the lung and perhaps mediastinum. Paradoxic breathing occurs with rib fractures that interfere with the structure of the chest. The breathing pattern on the affected side is the opposite of that on the unaffected side. During inhalation the chest lowers, and during exhalation the chest rises. This problem leads to inadequate gas exchange. Breathing patterns are altered when extrapulmonary conditions limit chest expansion. One example is kyphoscoliosis, which results from curvature of the spine and deformity of the rib cage. This restricts the expansion of the chest.

Pain perception alters breathing patterns when it prevents one from inhaling or exhaling fully. This can accompany trauma, incisions, or disease processes of the chest or abdomen. Movement of chest muscles stimulate A-delta and C fibers. which carry pain impulses to the spinal cord.[5]

In summary, etiologies for ineffective breathing pattern include the following[13]:

Neuromuscular impairment
Pain
Musculoskeletal impairment
Anxiety
Decreased energy and fatigue
Inflammatory process
Decreased lung expansion
Tracheobronchial obstruction

DEFINING CHARACTERISTICS[13]

Dyspnea
Shortness of breath
Tachypnea
Fremitus
Abnormal arterial blood gases
Cyanosis
Cough
Nasal flaring
Respiratory depth changes
    Shallow respirations
    Cheyne-Stokes respirations
    Hyperventilation
Assumption of three-point position
Pursed-lip breathing or prolonged expiratory phase
Increased anteroposterior diameter
Use of accessory muscles
Altered chest excursion (paradoxic breathing or flail chest)
Orthopnea
Bradypnea
Tachycardia
Bounding pulse
Rising blood pressure
Reduced vital capacity

NURSING INTERVENTIONS

Patient Goal	Nursing Intervention
Acute	
Achieve full lung expansion with adequate ventilation.	Auscultate lungs.
	Administer humidified oxygen as ordered.
	Encourage patient to breathe deeply and cough; splint chest during coughing.
	Elevate head of bed unless contraindicated (as in spinal cord injury).
	Suction airway as needed using sterile technique.
	Turn the patient frequently.
	Monitor arterial blood gases.

Patient Goal	Nursing Intervention
	Measure total volume.
	Assist with procedures to achieve adequate ventilation: endotracheal intubation, tracheostomy, chest tube insertion.
	Maintain ventilator settings as ordered.
	Observe chest x-ray results.
	Monitor air bubbling down the chest tube into underwater seal chamber.
	Strip or milk chest tube as necessary.
Achieve comfort without depressing respiration.	Splint patient's chest during coughing.
	Use mild sedatives and small doses of meperidine (Demerol) or codeine to control pain as ordered by physician.
	Unless patient is intubated, encourage him to discuss fears of inadequate ventilation.
	Change patient's position frequently and position comfortably.
	Plan periods of rest for at least 1 hour.
	Achieve pain relief by distraction, mental imagery, meditation, physical pressure on the painful site, massage, and relaxation.
Chronic	
Maintain adequate ventilation.	Auscultate lungs.
	Assess skin and nail color.
	Observe chest x-ray results.
	Encourage patient to deep breathe and cough.
	Evaluate patient's ability to perform activities of daily living without experiencing shortness of breath.
Achieve awareness of learning needs.	Assess what patient and family need to know.
	Review reasons for ineffective breathing patterns.
	Make referral for ventilatory equipment to be used in the home.
	Review reason for medications and treatments ordered for home use.
	Review plan for follow-up care.

Three nursing goals emerge for the patient with ineffective breathing patterns. In order of priority the goals are to maintain oxygen delivery to cells, to achieve comfort, and to achieve awareness of needs.

To accomplish the first goal, the nurse assesses the respiratory system and maintains ventilation. The patient who has had trauma may have fractured ribs or penetrating chest wounds that can result in pneumothorax, hemothorax, or paradoxic breathing. The patient with pneumothorax is reassured and not left alone. The physician is summoned and performs a thoracentesis to remove the air and restore intrathoracic pressure. When the pneumothorax is caused by a sucking chest wound, it is covered with Vaseline gauze until it can be sutured by the physician. If air continues to flow into the pleural space, a chest tube is left in place and attached to water seal drainage.

Hemothorax is treated by the physician with thoracentesis followed by chest tube placement to remove blood. A central venous pressure line or pulmonary catheter is inserted by the physician when mediastinal shift or cardiac tamponade has occurred to monitor for signs of shock. When water seal drainage is used, the nurse maintains the seal in addition to measuring and describing the drainage.

When the patient's altered breathing pattern is related to rib fractures (flail chest), the ribs are treated by the physician by internal or external stabilization. Internal stabilization more commonly is obtained by intubating the patient and using a volume-controlled ventilator to maintain ventilation and expand the thorax. The ventilator is set to control the patient's breathing pattern. When breathing against the ventilator, the patient is sedated per physician order with narcotics, sedatives, or muscle relaxants to provide rest, decrease the work of breathing, and control ventilation until the ribs are stabilized. Patients who have had head injuries receive only muscle relaxants. External stabilization has not been used as often since the refinement of the volume ventilator. This stabilization is accomplished by attaching steel wire to the ribs or sternum or pull the chest wall outward. The wire is then attached to traction with a rope and pulley with 5 pounds of weight for 2 to 3 weeks until the ribs are stable.[17]

Altered breathing patterns related to neuromuscular disorders require prompt attention but are not the emergent conditions seen following trauma. The volume ventilator is used for patients with neuromuscular disorders to maintain breathing patterns via a tracheostomy or endotracheal tube.

Patients who cannot be weaned from the ventilator may use alternate forms of respiratory assistance. These patients include those with severe bulbar poliomyelitis, spinal cord injuries at C1 or C2, and amyotrophic lateral sclerosis. The iron lung can be used to maintain respirations by negative pressure, which acts like suction to pull the respiratory muscles outward and downward. This movement of the muscles allows air to move into the lungs. When the negative pressure is released, the muscles recoil passively for exhalation. For wheelchair-

bound patients, a pneumobelt can be used. It is a wide belt containing a rubber bladder that fits around the diaphragm. The belt is attached to a battery that produces alternating positive and negative pressure against the diaphragm.

EVALUATION

Patient Outcome	Data Indicating That Outcome is Reached

Maintain adequate ventilation.	Arterial blood gases:
	  pH: 7.35-7.45
	  Po_2: 80-95 mm Hg (lower for COPD patient)
	  Pco_2: 35-45 mm Hg (lower for COPD patient)
	  O_2 saturation: 95%-99%
	Chest rises symmetrically on inhalation and falls symmetrically on exhalation
	No use of accessory muscles
	Respiratory rate:
	  Adults: 12-20/min
	  Children:
	    Newborn: 30 to 50 resp/min
	    6 months: 20 to 40 resp/min
	    1 year: 20 to 40 resp/min
	    3 years: 20 to 30 resp/min
	    6 years: 16 to 22 resp/min
	    10 years: 16 to 20 resp/min
	    17 years: 14 to 20 resp/min

Knowledge of self-care.	Patient and family can explain: 1. Reasons for ineffective breathing 2. Medication and treatment for home use 3. Plan for follow-up care

GAS EXCHANGE, IMPAIRED
THEORY AND ETIOLOGY

The two nursing diagnoses discussed previously were related to conditions precipitated by alterations in ventilation, the first phase of oxygenation. If these diagnoses are not resolved, they can progress to impaired gas exchange. Airway patency and adequate breathing patterns are crucial to the maintenance of gas exchange. In addition to ventilation, alterations of two other phases of oxygenation (external respiration and transportation) can impair gas exchange.

External respiration is a process of oxygen diffusion across the alveolar capillary membrane into the blood. Diffusion depends on adequate distribution of air into the alveoli (ventilation) with adequate distribution of pulmonary capillary blood adjacent to the alveolus (perfusion). Also, alveolar surface area and integrity are required for diffusion. Adequate distribution of air is initiated by ventilation, the movement of air in and out of

the lungs. (The etiology and theory for ventilation are discussed under Ineffective Airway Clearance and Ineffective Breathing Patterns.) Oxygen diffusion across the alveolar wall varies with the thickness of the membrane, the surface area of the membrane, and the pressure difference between the two sides. The actual alveolar gas composition is determined by the ventilation/perfusion ratio ($\dot{V}/\dot{Q}$). $\dot{V}$ = gas volume per unit of time; $\dot{Q}$ = blood flow volume per unit of time.[5] Ideally, a perfect match between all alveoli and all pulmonary capillaries would yield a $\dot{V}/\dot{Q}$ ratio of 1.0. The normal $\dot{V}/\dot{Q}$ ratio is 0.8, however, because in the upright lung the gravity-dependent position receives more blood flow than airflow. Likewise, the apex of the lung receives more airflow than blood flow. A high $\dot{V}/\dot{Q}$ ratio occurs when ventilation (the numerator of the fraction) is greater than the perfusion of blood (the denominator of the fraction). Thus a high $\dot{V}/\dot{Q}$ ratio indicates inadequate perfusion around the alveolus with adequate ventilation. This condition has been called a *deadspace anatomic shunt*, that is, blood that flows from the right side of the heart to the left side of the heart without traversing pulmonary capillaries.[20] Hypoxia results because blood is unavailable to carry oxygen, and hypercapnia results because carbon dioxide cannot be eliminated. Causes of perfusion alterations are listed in the box below.

Causes of Hypoxia and Hypercapnia

Ventilation (Low $\dot{V}/\dot{Q}$ Ratio)
Inhibition of thorax or lung expansion (chest trauma, pneumothorax, hemothorax, fatigue, kyphoscoliosis, obesity, pulmonary fibrosis, pain)
Airway obstruction (bronchial asthma, chronic bronchitis, carcinoma)
Interference with respiratory center activity (drugs, central nervous system disturbances)
Decreases in elastic recoil (emphysema)
Low oxygen concentration at high altitude

Perfusion (High $\dot{V}/\dot{Q}$ Ratio)
Decreased cardiac output (myocardial infarction, cardiac arrhythmias, increased vascular resistance)
Circulatory collapse (shock)
Blockage of pulmonary capillaries (pulmonary embolus, pulmonary infarction)
Compression of pulmonary capillary bed (increase in alveolar pressure)
Decrease in blood pH
Destruction of capillary bed

Diffusion
Decrease in alveolar surface area; thickening of alveolar membrane (hyaline membrane disease, adult respiratory distress syndrome, extensive pulmonary resection)
Increase in fluid or secretions in interstitial space or alveoli (pulmonary edema, pneumonia)

Transportation
Inadequate hemoglobin (anemia, carbon monoxide poisoning)
Pump failure (congestive failure, aortic stenosis, aortic insufficiency, mitral stenosis, mitral regurgitation)
Inadequate vessel patency (arteriosclerosis, venous embolus, hemorrhage, peripheral edema)

Modified from Phipps, W.J., Long, B.C., and Woods, N.F.: Medical-surgical nursing: concepts and clinical practice, St. Louis, 1979, The C.V. Mosby Co.; and Wade, J.F.: Comprehensive respiratory care, ed. 3, St. Louis, 1982, The C.V. Mosby Co.

A low $\dot{V}/\dot{Q}$ ratio occurs when ventilation is lower than perfusion. Thus a low $\dot{V}/\dot{Q}$ ratio indicates inadequate ventilation with adequate perfusion. This condition has been called a *shunt unit*[22] and a capillary shunt, which indicates that blood flows through the pulmonary capillaries without participating in gas exchange.[20] Hypoxia results because oxygen is unavailable to the pulmonary capillaries, and hypercapnia results because carbon dioxide cannot be eliminated. When neither ventilation nor perfusion occurs, the condition is called a *silent unit*. Causes of ventilation alterations are listed in the box at left.

When ventilation and perfusion are adequate, gas exchange may be impaired by alterations of the alveoli that prevent adequate diffusion, the process by which oxygen and carbon dioxide are exchanged across the alveolar capillary membrane. Causes of diffusion alterations are listed in the box at left.

Transportation of oxygen is the third phase of the oxygenation process. After diffusing into the blood, oxygen combines with hemoglobin to form oxyhemoglobin. Hemoglobin has a greater affinity for oxygen when there is an increase in arterial pH or a decrease in P_{CO_2} or body temperature. This is a shift to the left of the oxyhemoglobin dissociation curve. Conversely, hemoglobin has less affinity for oxygen when there is a decrease in arterial pH or an increase in P_{CO_2} or body temperature. This is a shift to the right of the dissociation curve.[19] Circulation of oxyhemoglobin depends on an adequate pump to create pressure as well as patent vessels in which to flow. Causes of transportation alterations are listed in the box at left.

In summary, etiologies for impaired gas exchange are the following[13]:
    Altered oxygen supply
    Alveolar capillary membrane changes
    Altered blood flow
    Altered oxygen-carrying capacity of blood

DEFINING CHARACTERISTICS[13]

Confusion
Somnolence
Restlessness
Irritability
Inability to move secretions
Hypercapnia
Hypoxia
Polycythemia (a compensatory mechanism)
Increased anteroposterior diameter
Hyperresonance on chest percussion
Tachycardia/arrhythmias
Anxiety

Dyspnea
Cyanosis
Decreased mental acuity
Tachypnea

Widened A-a gradient
Three-point position
Pursed-lip breathing with prolonged expiratory phase

NURSING INTERVENTIONS

Patient Goal	Nursing Intervention

Acute Care

| Maintain adequate ventilation. | Ausculate lungs.
Measure vital signs.
Monitor cardiac rhythm.
Monitor arterial blood gases and hemoglobin.
Administer humidified oxygen as ordered.
Suction airway as needed using sterile technique.
Maintain ventilator settings as ordered.
Encourage patients to cough and deep breathe when not receiving mechanical ventilation.
Administer drugs as ordered: bronchodilators, antihistamines, antiinfectives, expectorants, and corticosteroids.
Evaluate the therapeutic, adverse, and toxic effects of drugs given.
Turn patient at least every 2 hours.
Elevate head of bed.
Administer packed cells or whole blood as ordered; observe for adverse reaction to blood administration. |
| Achieve physical and psychologic comfort. | Explain care being given and being planned.
If patient not intubated, encourage verbalization of feelings.
Provide back rub and position change frequently.
Provide oral hygiene.
Provide pain relief with independent nursing measures and with medications as ordered.
Provide planned periods of rest for at least 1 hour. |

Chronic Care

| Maintain adequate ventilation. | Ausculate lungs.
Measure blood pressure, pulse, and respiratory rate.
Monitor heart rhythm.
Administer oxygen as ordered.
Encourage patient to deep breathe and cough.
Administer drugs as ordered: bronchodilators, antiinfectives, corticosteroids.
Evaluate therapeutic, adverse, and toxic effects of drugs given.
Evaluate tolerance of patient while performing activities of daily living. |
| Achieve adequate knowledge level. | Assess what patient and family need to know.
Provide information about pursed-lip breathing and diaphragmatic breathing.
Discover reason for altered gas exchange and its prevention in the future.
Know actions, side effects, dosage, and frequency of administration for all medications ordered by the physician.
Plan a referral for ventilatory equipment to be used in the home.
Alter daily activities as necessary to decrease oxygen demand. |

There are three nursing goals for the patient with altered gas exchange. In order of priority the goals are to maintain oxygen delivery to cells, to achieve comfort, and to achieve awareness of needs.

A patent airway is needed for gas exchange. Patency is maintained by coughing or by suctioning. The patient's environment should have proper ventilation and humidity with an absence of cigarette smoke. Tracheostomy or endotracheal intubation with mechanical ventilation may be a necessary medical intervention to maintain gas exchange. Positive end expiratory pressure (PEEP) may be necessary to keep the alveoli open. Supplemental nutrition is needed for the intubated patient with sufficient calories to maintain a positive nitrogen balance. The hypoxic patient needs to reduce tissue oxygen demands. This is accomplished by performing activities of daily living for the patient and by spacing activities throughout the day. The risk of infection can be lessened by use of sterile technique when suctioning, hand washing by personnel, daily fluid intake of at least 3000 ml, adequate nutrition to maintain positive nitrogen balance, and prevention of exposure to others with infections.

EVALUATION

Patient Outcome	Data Indicating That Outcome is Reached
Adequate ventilation	Arterial blood gases (see Ineffective Breathing Patterns) Hemoglobin: 12-14 g/dl (women) 14-16 g/dl (men) Effortless breathing No use of accessory muscles Respiratory rate (see Ineffective Breathing Patterns) Perform activities of daily living without becoming short of breath
Knowledge of self-care	Patient and family can explain: 1. Reasons for altered gas exchange 2. Medication and treatment for home use 3. Plan for follow-up care

CARDIAC OUTPUT, ALTERATION IN: DECREASED

THEORY AND ETIOLOGY

Cardiac output is the amount of blood ejected from the left ventricle each minute and normally ranges from 4 to 8 L. Cardiac output is a function of the stroke volume (amount of blood ejected per contraction) and the heart rate (number of contractions per minute).

Stroke volume is determined by three factors: preload, contractility, and afterload. *Preload* refers to the blood volume in the ventricle at the end of diastole, the resting phase of the cardiac cycle, when ventricles fill with blood from the atria. Factors that determine blood flow from the atria to ventricle are the amount of venous return to the heart, the adequacy of atrial contraction, the functioning of cardiac valves (tricuspid, pulmonic, mitral, and aortic), and the stretch and contraction of the ventricles. As the ventricles fill, the muscle fibers in the ventricles stretch. Starling's law states that stretching the myocardial fibers during diastole increases the force of contraction during systole. The part of the muscle that stretches is the sarcomere, the basic functional unit of contraction. Myocardial sarcomeres normally stretch 2 μm during diastole, and the force of the contraction does not increase when the sarcomeres are stretched beyond this.[8] When the sarcomere is stretched beyond 2 μm, it does not generate adequate tension for muscle contraction.[5] When the muscle is overstretched, the force of systole is reduced and decreases ventricular emptying.[8]

Once the ventricle is filled with blood, the myocardial muscle contracts to eject the blood from the right ventricle into the pulmonary artery and the left ventricle into the aorta.

Contractility refers to the depolarization of the sarcomere of the myocardial cells. Each myocardial cell is composed of myocardial fibrils, a nucleus, and sarcoplasmic reticulum. The myocardial fibril is made up of sarcomeres. Sarcomeres comprise myosin and actin, which slide together during contraction. Stretching of the sarcomere increases the number of chemical interaction sites available for actin and myosin. The actions of myosin and actin require ATP, calcium, magnesium, potassium, and sodium. Physiologic and pharmacologic agents affect contractility at this level.[8]

The final determinant of stroke volume is *afterload*, which refers to the resistance to the flow of blood from the ventricle. This discussion is limited to the systemic vascular resistance because the pulmonary vascular system is a low-pressure system. When systemic vascular resistance is high, as in hypertension, the left ventricle must pump more forcefully to eject a normal cardiac output. Peripheral resistance is increased mainly by vasoconstriction or increased blood viscosity. Peripheral vascular resistance is decreased mainly by vasodilation. The box on the opposite page lists conditions that relate to a decrease in stroke volume.

Conditions That Decrease Stroke Volume

Conditions Affecting Preload

Diuresis
Hemorrhage
Third spacing
Burns   } Decrease venous return to the heart
Fever
Allergy (anaphylactic shock)
Atrial or ventricular septal defects

Atrial fibrillation   } Alter atrial contraction
Atrial flutter

Myocardial infarction
Ventricular dysrhythmia
Left ventricular hypertrophy   } Interfere with stretch and contraction of the myocardium
Cardiac tamponade
Mediastinal shift
Constrictive pericarditis

Conditions Affecting Contractility

Hypocalcemia, hypercalcemia
Hypokalemia, hyperkalemia
Myocardial infarction
Left ventricular hypertrophy
Mediastinal shift   } Interfere with sarcomere function
Hypoxemia
Hypercapnia
Metabolic acidosis

Conditions Affecting Afterload

Hypertension
Hypothermia (vasoconstriction)   } High systemic vascular resistance

Hemorrhage
Allergy
Diuresis   } Low systemic vascular resistance
Third spacing
Hyperthermia (vasodilation)

Heart rate is the second determinant of cardiac output. The beating of the heart depends on the conduction of impulses from the sinoatrial (SA) node to the bundle branches. The rate of the contraction is influenced by the sympathetic and parasympathetic nervous systems' stimulation of the SA and atrioventricular (AV) nodes. Epinephrine increases the rate and is supplied both by the sympathetic free nerve endings and the adrenal medulla. The vagus nerve from the parasympathetic nervous system affects the SA node to slow the rate. The body uses compensatory mechanisms to correct abnormal functions. For example, when hemorrhage occurs, the heart rate increases and vasoconstriction occurs to maintain an adequate blood pressure. Conversely, when fluid overload occurs, the body attempts to shift the fluid out of the intravascular space. The resulting signs of this compensation are dependent edema, ascites, and pulmonary and cerebral edema. Many of the defining characteristics reported are compensatory mechanisms.

Etiologies for decreased cardiac output include the following:[13]

Mechanical
    Alteration in preload
    Alteration in afterload
    Alteration in inotropic changes in heart
Electrical
    Alterations in rate
    Alterations in rhythm
    Alterations in conduction
Structural

DEFINING CHARACTERISTICS[13]

Variations in hemodynamic readings
Arrhythmias (ECG changes)
Fatigue
Jugular vein distention*
Cyanosis (pallor of skin and mucous membranes)
Oliguria
Anuria
Decreased peripheral pulses
Cold clammy skin
Rales†

Dyspnea†
Orthopnea†
Restlessness
Change in mental status†
Syncope†
Vertigo†
Edema, dependent*
Cough†
Frothy sputum†
Abnormal heart sounds (such as gallop rhythm)†
Weakness
Liver engorgement and tenderness*
Ascites*
Tachycardia
Angina

*Occurs with right ventricular failure.
†Occurs with left ventricular failure.

NURSING INTERVENTIONS

Patient Goal	Nursing Intervention
Acute Care	
Restore cardiac output.	Assess vital signs frequently according to patient's condition.
	Monitor cardiac rhythm continuously.
	Initiate prompt treatment of life-threatening arrhythmias per protocol:
	1. Cardiopulmonary resuscitation
	2. Appropriate drug therapy as ordered
	3. Prepare for insertion of pacemaker
	Monitor hemodynamic parameters:
	1. Pulmonary artery pressures
	2. Central venous pressures
	3. Cardiac output
	Monitor intravenous fluids with electrolytes as ordered
	Administer antiarrhythmic drugs as ordered.
	Administer inotropic drugs as ordered by physician.
	Observe cardiac enzyme values, electrolyte values (especially potassium), and arterial blood gases.
	Observe for therapeutic, adverse, and toxic effects of drugs given.
	When intraaortic balloon pump is inserted by physician, nurse assesses heart rate, mean arterial pressure, and pulmonary capillary wedge pressure, heart rhythm and regularity (especially R waves), urine output, skin color, peripheral perfusion, and mental status.
Reduce heart workload.	Assist patient to semi-Fowler's position.
	Maintain patient on complete bed rest according to policy.
	Perform activities of daily living for patient.
	When able to get out of bed, patient may use bedside commode.
	Assess hemodynamic parameters as ordered.
	Measure intake and output to monitor fluid balance.
	Administer stool softener as ordered.
	Administer diuretics as ordered.
	Administer oxygen as ordered.
	Encourage deep breathing and coughing.
	Administer nitrates as ordered.
	Administer hypnotics or analgesics as ordered to provide rest.
	Administer morphine as ordered.
	Observe for therapeutic, adverse, and toxic effects of drugs given.
	Provide a restful, quiet environment.
Chronic Care	
Ensure adequate cardiac output.	Assess blood pressure, apical pulse, and peripheral pulses.
	Assess cardiac rhythm.
	Measure intake and output.

Patient Goal	Nursing Intervention
	Evaluate patient's tolerance to activities of daily living; monitor for hypotension and arrhythmias.
	Administer drugs as ordered: antiarrhythmics, inotropics, diuretics, and potassium.
	Evaluate the therapeutic, adverse, and toxic effects of drugs given.
Achieve awareness of learning needs.	Assess patient's current knowledge and provide information as needed.
	Provide information concerning:
	1. Prevention of recurrence
	2. Risk factors to avoid
	3. Pathophysiology of illness
	4. Medication uses, side effects, and frequency of administration
	5. Stress management techniques
	6. Physical activity program
	7. Dietary alterations
	8. Guidelines for resuming sexual relations
	9. Guidelines for returning to work

The three nursing goals for the patient with decreased cardiac output, in order of priority, are to restore cardiac output, to reduce the workload of the heart, and to achieve awareness of learning needs. The goals of care vary with the acuity of the problem. To restore cardiac output, the causative condition must be corrected. Assessment data the nurse collects to meet this goal include the following:

Auscultating the heart

Measuring the heart rate and blood pressure

Palpating pulses

Identifying the rhythm of the heart via ECG pattern

Measuring the pressures of the right atria, pulmonary artery, and pulmonary capillary wedge via pulmonary artery catheter

Measuring cardiac output and urinary output

Measuring daily body weight

The nurse is aware of laboratory data, including electrolytes, cardiac enzymes, arterial blood gases, hemoglobin, and hematocrit. Under physician orders the nurse administers medications to maintain cardiac output and monitors the therapeutic effects and side effects of these drugs. When preload is reduced because of decreased volume, the nurse administers intravenous fluids as ordered. Per physician orders antiarrhythmic drugs are given to stabilize the rhythm, inotropic drugs are given to increase the force of contractility, and electrolytes are given to correct imbalances and facilitate contractility.[16] An intraaortic balloon is inserted by the physician to increase oxygen supply to the myocardium, decrease left ventricular work, and improve cardiac output. Assessment of the patient with balloon pump therapy includes monitoring heart rate, mean arterial pressure, pulmonary capillary wedge pressure, heart rhythm and regularity, urine output, skin color, peripheral perfusion, and mental status.[8]

To reduce the workload on the patient's heart, the nurse intervenes to meet physical and psychologic needs. Oxygen is provided as ordered to ensure an adequate supply for the myocardium. Pain medication is given based on protocol for comfort as needed. Morphine is a preferred drug because it not only relieves pain but also provides peripheral vasodilation to reduce venous return.[8] Diuretics and vasodilators are given to reduce systemic vascular resistance. The patient is asked to reduce physical activity by resting in bed in a semi-Fowler or Fowler position or in a chair. This position also reduces the patient's work of breathing, which reduces the workload of the heart. The patient's hygiene activities are performed for him. Specific times of rest are planned throughout the day. As the patient improves, a progressive activity schedule is implemented. The physician may prescribe stool softeners to prevent straining during defecation. The diet is changed as needed. Frequently caffeine and sodium are restricted. Small meals require less work by the heart.

To meet psychologic needs, the nurse attempts to reduce the patient's stress and anxiety. A quiet, pleasant environment relieves stress. The patient is encouraged to discuss feelings and is given as much information as possible. Relaxation techniques are taught to reduce tension (see Coping, ineffective individual).

To achieve awareness of learning needs, the nurse first assesses what the patient and family already know. They need to know what caused the decrease in cardiac output and how to avoid its recurrence. The patient and family will need to know actions and side effects of medications. Life-style changes will require regular exercise of at least 30 minutes three times a week. Dietary alterations are needed to restrict sodium or cholesterol. It is important to consider the patient's cultural food preferences when adapting dietary alterations to fit the life-style. When obesity is a problem, the patient needs to understand that extra weight increases the heart's workload. Smoking adds a burden to the heart by causing vasoconstriction.

EVALUATION

Patient Outcome	Data Indicating That Outcome is Reached

Cardiac output adequate	Normal sinus rhythm
	Heart rate within 20 beats of normal
	Blood pressure:
	  Adult upper limits:
	    140 mm Hg systolic
	    90 mm Hg diastolic
	    30 to 40 mm Hg pulse pressure
	  Children

	Mean systolic (±2 S.D.)	Mean diastolic (±2 S.D.)
Newborn	80 ± 16	46 ± 16
2 mo to 1 yr	89 ± 29	60 ± 10
1 yr	96 ± 30	66 ± 25
2 yr	99 ± 25	64 ± 25
3 yr	100 ± 25	67 ± 23
4 yr	99 ± 20	65 ± 20
5 to 6 yr	94 ± 14	55 ± 9
6 to 7 yr	100 ± 15	56 ± 8
7 to 8 yr	102 ± 15	56 ± 8
8 to 9 yr	105 ± 16	57 ± 9
9 to 10 yr	107 ± 17	57 ± 9
10 to 11 yr	111 ± 17	58 ± 10
11 to 12 yr	113 ± 18	59 ± 10
12 to 13 yr	115 ± 19	59 ± 10
13 to 14 yr	118 ± 19	60 ± 10

Patient Outcome	Data Indicating That Outcome is Reached
	Clear breath sounds bilaterally Alert, oriented Absence of angina Urinary output at least 30 ml/hr Skin warm, dry Peripheral pulses present and strong (normal for patient) Able to perform activities of daily living
Knowledge of self-care	Patient and family can explain: 1. Reasons for decreased cardiac output and how to prevent recurrence 2. Dietary alterations 3. Exercise program 4. Stress management activities 5. Medication uses and side effects 6. Plan for follow-up care

NUTRITION, ALTERATION IN: LESS THAN BODY REQUIREMENTS

THEORY AND ETIOLOGY

Nutrition is defined as the sum of all processes by which a living organism receives and uses nutrients for growth, maintenance, and repair of the body. Nutritional integrity requires the integration of multiple organs. The nervous system regulates food intake; the gastrointestinal system receives, digests, absorbs, metabolizes, and eliminates nutrients; the circulatory system transports nutrients; and the liver and adipose tissue regulate and store excess calories. Nutrients include proteins, carbohydrates, fats, vitamins, minerals, and water. The amount of nutrients one needs varies with the body's requirements. For example, during a growth period a child requires additional nutrients to meet growth needs. This same child who also has an infectious disease requires increased nutrients to meet repair needs. Since the body cannot manufacture or synthesize nutrients, it requires a regular supply from a balanced diet. Conditions that interrupt the supply or create an excessive demand contribute to an alteration in nutrition of less than body requirements.

Mineral ions in body fluids regulate metabolism of many enzymes, maintain acid-base balance and osmotic pressure, maintain nerve and muscle irritability, and in some cases are involved in tissue growth. Vitamins regulate metabolism, help convert fat and carbohydrate into energy, and assist in bone and tissue formation. Water functions in digestion, absorption, circulation, and excretion. Carbohydrates are converted to glucose, which is used by all body cells for energy. Some glucose is stored as glycogen in the liver and muscle while the remaining glucose is converted and stored as fat. Proteins are the fundamental structural component of cells, antibodies, enzymes, and many hormones. Protein is used also for energy but at a higher energy cost than carbohydrates, which burn completely to carbon dioxide and water. Proteins, on the other hand, have an end product of nitrogen, which requires energy to excrete. Fats function as a concentrated energy source. Use of fats for energy spares the use of protein for tissue building. Fats also insulate and protect the body as well as transport and absorb fat-soluble vitamins.

The etiology for the nursing diagnosis, defined by Kim, McFarland, and McLane,[13] is "inability to ingest or digest food or absorb nutrients because of biologic, psychologic, or economic factors." This definition is used as the organizing framework for the discussion of the diagnosis.

The following are etiologies for this diagnosis:
Lacks availability of food
   Socioeconomic factors
      Lack of transportation to obtain food
      Unable to speak language to request food
      Lacks money to buy food
      Lacks knowledge of what foods to obtain
Inadequate preparation of food
   Socioeconomic factors
      Different cultural/religious beliefs about what food may be eaten
      Lacks knowledge of how to prepare food
      Lacks refrigerator to store food
      Lacks cooking appliances to prepare food
   Psychologic factors
      Depression
      Anxiety
      Social isolation
      Anorexia
      Poor self-image or self-concept
   Biologic factors
      Nausea
      Absence of smell or taste
Inadequate digestion of food
   Biologic factors
      Chewing
         Pain
         Facial muscle weakness

         Malocclusion
         Broken or missing teeth
         Ill-fitting dentures
         Jaw wired closed
      Swallowing
         Muscle weakness
         Compression of hypoglossal cranial nerve (XII)
         Tracheal intubation
      Peristalsis through esophagus
         Stricture
         Obstruction
         Hiatal hernia
         Impaired peristalsis
      Peristalsis through stomach
         Pain
         Vomiting
         Gastritis
         Reduced stomach size
      Peristalsis through and absorption in small intestine
         Malabsorption
         Obstruction
         Construction
         Pain
         Hyperactive peristalsis
Increase in body's demand for nutrients
   Biologic factors
      Fever
      Chronic infection
      Rapid growth
      Excessive tissue repair (such as after multiple system trauma or burns)
      Cancer (disease-related problems include anemia, diarrhea, constipation, protein deficits, and fatigue; problems related to cancer therapy include nausea, vomiting, stomatitis, diarrhea, anorexia, and fatigue)

DEFINING CHARACTERISTICS[13]

Loss of weight with adequate food intake
Body weight 20% or more under ideal for height and frame
Reported inadequate food intake less than Recommended Daily Allowance (RDA)
Weakness of muscles required for swallowing or mastication
Reported or evidence of lack of food
Lack of interest in food
Perceived inability to ingest food
Aversion to eating
Reported altered taste sensation
Satiety immediately after ingesting food
Abdominal pain with or without pathology
Sore, inflamed buccal cavity
Capillary fragility
Abdominal cramping
Diarrhea and/or steatorrhea

Hyperactive bowel sounds
Pale conjunctiva and mucous membranes
Poor muscle tone
Excessive hair loss
Lack of information, misinformation
Misconceptions
Decreased triceps skinfold
Decreased midarm circumference
Decreased midarm muscle circumference

Decreased serum albumin
Decreased serum transferrin or iron-binding capacity
Decreased lymphocyte count
Anorexia
Dry, scaly, inelastic skin
Pallor of the oral mucosa
Edema
Absence of subcutaneous fat

NURSING INTERVENTIONS

Patient Goal	Nursing Intervention
Obtain nutrients to maintain body function.	Weigh patient daily. Medicate as ordered to reduce nausea and pain prior to eating. Assess ability to swallow and chew. Provide foods in the form appropriate for patient: general diet, mechanical soft, blenderized, formula via nasogastric or gastrostomy tube, or total parenteral nutrition as ordered by physician given via subclavian vein. Consider cultural and religious food preferences when patient has a choice. When patient feeds self, serve food at its appropriate temperature; ensure patient is comfortable and can reach necessary utensils for eating. When the patient is fed by mouth, serve food at its appropriate temperature; ensure patient is comfortable; allow patient sufficient time between bites; talk with the patient during the meal. When the patient is fed by nasogastric tube: 1. Ensure tube is in the stomach. 2. Aspirate gastric contents to determine the amount of the last feeding still in stomach. 3. If aspirated contents is less than 50 ml, proceed with the feeding. 4. Formula should be at room temperature and should flow in slowly. When the patient is fed by total parenteral nutrition: 1. Check infusion rate every hour or use infusion pump. 2. Monitor glucose daily. 3. Change dressing daily, using sterile technique; inspect insertion site.
Identify socioeconomic factors that contribute to inadequate nutritional intake.	Problem-solve with patient and family to identify socioeconomic factors contributing to inadequate nutrition. Determine with patient and family appropriate strategies to use to solve problems. Use referrals to other members of the health care team as needed (dietitian, social worker, community health nurse).
Identify psychologic and emotional factors.	Discuss with patient perceptions of factors interfering with ability or desire to eat. Discuss with the patient strategies useful to improve nutrition. Refer patients for additional therapy as needed.
Achieve adequate knowledge base.	Assess learning needs of the patient and family. Determine their understanding of the reason for altered nutrition. Teach types of menus to be used. Teach foods to avoid. Determine their understanding of the plan for follow-up treatment. Teach them reason for vitamin and mineral supplements to be taken. Provide them with names and phone numbers of personnel in community agencies.

There are three nursing goals for the patient with nutrition less than body requirements. In order of priority the goals are to supply nutrients to all cells, to eliminate the contributing factors, and to achieve an awareness of learning needs. Assessment data for the patient include skinfold measurements (anthropometric measurements), serum albumin, lymphocytes, and body weight. Triceps skinfold thickness gives data about fat stores, and arm circumference provides data about protein stores. The site measured for both the skinfold thickness and arm circumference is at the midpoint between the shoulder (acromial process) and the elbow (olecranon) of the nondominant arm. The average of three measurements is recorded. Measurement is made by pinching the skin and measuring its thickness with calipers. The arm circumference is measured at the same place on the arm (Fig. 9). Midarm muscle circumference (cm) = mean arm circumference (cm) − (0.314 × triceps skinfold thickness [mm]). The standards for these anthropometric measurements are in the evaluation section. Serum albumin values[11] are no longer useful after an infusion of albumin to maintain intravascular pressure. Visceral protein depletion is indicated when total lymphocyte count falls below 1500 (Table 12).

The patient's height and weight are compared with tables of ideal weight for the height. Regardless of the specific cause of the alteration in nutrition, the patient

Table 12

Serum Assessments in Malnutrition

	Serum albumin (g/dl)	Lymphocytes (per ml³)
Mild deficit	3.0-3.5	1500-1800
Modest deficit	2.1-3.0	900-1500
Severe deficit	2.1	900

requires a supply of nutrients to maintain body functions. Nutrients can be provided in a general diet or specialized diet taken by mouth, in a formula or blenderized general diet given through a nasogastric or gastrostomy tube, or in collaboration with the physician in the form of total parenteral nutrition through a subclavian vein. In each route proteins, carbohydrates, water, minerals, and vitamins are given. One form of fluid not recommended is intravenous dextrose in a peripheral vein because it provides minimal calories (400 calories in 1 L of 10% dextrose) and provides no protein.

For patients who eat a general diet the nurse considers cultural or religious food preferences. Offering patients some selection in the food gives them a feeling of control in their lives. When meals are served, patients need to feel as comfortable as possible, which may require oral hygiene, position change, or medication. They need to be able to reach their food, and some patients may require

Fig. 9
Triceps skinfold measurement.

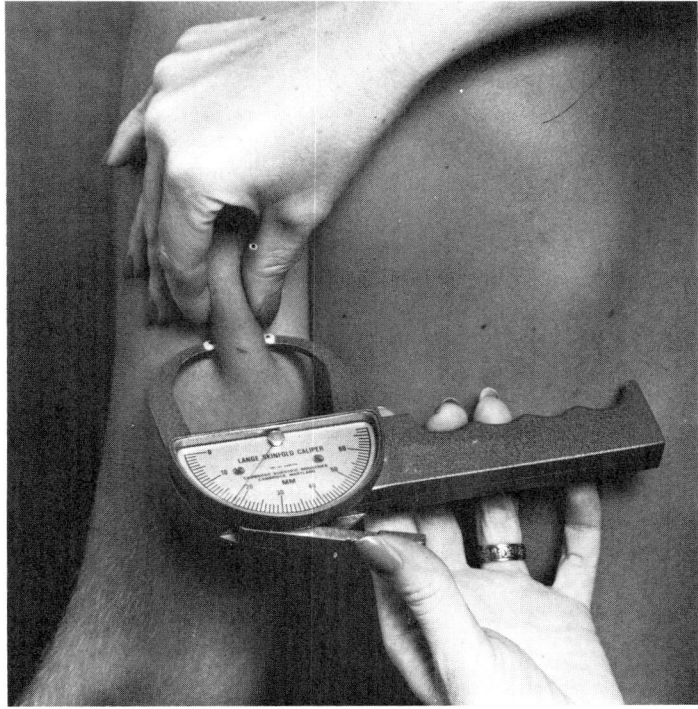

assistance with cutting food or opening containers. A pleasant eating environment free from unpleasant aromas enhances eating, as does an appropriate temperature for the food. Nasogastric tube feedings are continual via a pump or are intermittent. Placement of the tube needs to be checked each shift to ensure it is in the stomach. In collaboration with the physician, total parenteral nutrition is given continually through infusion into a subclavian vein. This solution comprises 50% dextrose, protein, electrolytes, vitamins, and trace elements.

The second goal is to eliminate the factors contributing to the alteration. When socioeconomic factors contribute to lack of food available, the nurse may need to make a referral to social agencies for assistance. The patient may be eligible for food stamps or other government-funded programs. The patient or family can shop in a cooperative, buy food on sale and freeze it for later use, or participate in a community garden. Cheaper forms of protein can be purchased, such as beans and legumes.

Psychologic factors need to be discussed with the patient to determine his perceptions. Referrals to appropriate specialists may be needed. The patient's social support system can be consulted for additional perceptions of the situation and possible solutions to the nutritional problems.

Chewing can be hampered by pain or muscle weakness. The patient with periodontal disease may need a referral to a dentist or oral surgeon. Patients with periodontal disease and those with dental caries need to receive oral hygiene and be encouraged to continue it after discharge. Aqueous lidocaine (Xylocaine) may be applied as ordered to painful areas in the mouth at mealtime. The patient who is physically able to brush and floss the teeth may need only a reminder. The patient with upper extremity muscle weakness may need to change to an electric toothbrush or to allow someone else to perform the brushing. The unconscious patient needs oral hygiene also. The mouth is inspected frequently to ensure that food is being swallowed rather than collected in the cheeks.

The patient with swallowing difficulties needs to be carefully assessed and advanced slowly. The patient's cough and gag reflexes must be present. The patient needs to be in a sitting position, and a suction machine should be ready at the bedside. First the nurse determines if the patient can swallow his own saliva. If this is successful, it is followed by about 1 teaspoon of water. This progression continues to semisolid food (applesauce), to pureed food, to soft diet, and to a regular diet. The person who has dysphagia due to a neuromuscular disorder may benefit from the food being placed on the back of the tongue. These patients are fed slowly and in an environment without distraction such as television, radio, or visitors. They need to concentrate on swallowing until the behavior is learned again. Tilting the head forward 45 degrees keeps the esophagus patent to facilitate swallowing. The mouth is inspected frequently to ensure food is being swallowed rather than collected in the cheeks.

Nausea and vomiting can be lessened with small amounts of cool liquids (cola, ginger ale, Jello water). Cleaning the mouth and blowing the nose after vomiting eliminates nauseous tastes and smells. Alteration of medicines should be considered to prevent nausea and vomiting. Rectal administration of medication rather than oral may help. The vomiting center stimulation is decreased by slow deep breathing through the mouth, removal of unpleasant sights and smells, and eating and drinking slowly.

The final goal is to achieve an awareness of learning needs. The patient and family need to understand the cause of inadequate nutrition and the actions to take to ensure adequate nutrition. The nurse needs to assess what the patient and family already know about nutrition. In many situations it may be appropriate to refer this family to a dietitian. Family members may need to learn how to prepare food in a specific manner. It is very important that the person who buys and prepares the food participate in the learning process.

EVALUATION

Patient Outcome	Data Indicating That Outcome is Reached
Adequate nutrition	Good bone and tooth development
	Erect body posture
	Good skin turgor
	Clear skin and eyes
	Firm muscles
	Triceps skinfold: men, 12.5 mm; women, 16.5 mm
	Midarm circumference: men, 29.3 cm; women, 28.5 cm
	Serum albumin: 3.5-5.0 g/dl or 53% of total protein
	Lymphocytes 2100 or 30% of leukocyte per ml^3 blood
	Midarm muscle circumference: men, 25.3; women 23.2

Patient Outcome	Data Indicating That Outcome is Reached
	Adequate elimination
	Prompt healing
	Weight at normal level for body build
	Growth of 3-5 inches annually for children
	Mental alertness
	Energy to perform activities of daily living
	Absence of malaise, fatigue, weakness
	Includes meats, milk, fruits, vegetables, breads in daily diet
Knowledge of self-care	Patient and family can explain:
	1. Reason for altered nutrition
	2. Actions to avoid it
	3. Types of menus to be used
	4. Any necessary dietary alterations (foods to include and avoid)
	5. Community agencies to be contacted for assistance
	6. Medication program to be followed: state dosage, action, and side effects of prescribed drugs; list over-the-counter drugs to avoid

NUTRITION, ALTERATION IN: POTENTIAL FOR MORE THAN BODY REQUIREMENTS

THEORY AND ETIOLOGY

Individuals who are at risk for more nutrition than the body requires benefit from primary prevention regarding overweight or obesity. Overweight is defined as 10% above the desirable weight for individuals according to their height and body build. Obesity is defined as 20% to 25% above the desirable weight according to height and body build. These two definitions assume a normal muscle/fat ratio. Athletes often do not fall within this assumption, since they exceed their ideal body weight because their developed muscle tissue weighs more than fat. Causes of this alteration of nutrition are the outcome of (1) excessive food intake with lack of physical activity, (2) hereditary predisposition, (3) dysfunctional psychologic conditioning in relation to food, (4) socioeconomic environment, (5) hormonal imbalances, and (6) disorders of the hypothalamus. When the body receives more calories than it can use, it stores the excess in the form of lipids in adipose tissue and muscle. Prolonged overeating without burning of calories leads to overweight and then obesity.

The adipose cell theory describes critical periods in the life span that determine the number and size of adipocytes (fat cells). These critical periods are the first half of pregnancy, birth to 2 years, childhood (7 to 11 years), and adolescence. If nutrition is provided beyond the need during these critical times, the number of adipocytes in adipose tissue increases (hyperplasia) or the existing adipocytes stretch (hypertrophy). Childhood or adolescent-onset obesity is characterized by adipocyte hyperplasia, whereas adult-onset obesity is characterized by adipocyte hypertrophy.[4] Other critical periods not specifically named in this theory are between 25 and 40 years of age, when activity declines, and after age 50 for both men and women because of a decrease in basal metabolic rate and activity.

Hereditary predisposition influences body build and rare genetic disorders. The influence of family members affects more often the psychologic and socioeconomic causes of altered nutrition. For example, individuals who perceive food as a reward or punishment or who did not experience gratification of oral needs might eat excessively. Eating behaviors demonstrated by parents influence their children. Thus some children learn overeating as a norm of their culture. Williams[24] reported research findings indicating that families of lower socioeconomic level tend to be overweight. With increasing upward mobility the incidence of obesity often declines.[24]

A relationship exists between psychologic components and obesity, but the exact cause and effect remain unclear. Body image problems relate to obesity when the onset occurs in childhood and adolescence, when emotional problems (depression, anxiety, and impulsiveness) are prevalent, and when disapproval of obesity is perceived by significant others.[23] Hormonal imbalances are identified as causes of overweight or obesity but are rarely the sole cause. Cushing's disease results from excessive secretion of glucocorticoids caused by (1) an adrenal tumor secreting cortisol, (2) a pituitary tumor secreting excessive adrenocorticotrophic hormone (ACTH), (3) an ectopic hypersecretion of ACTH from a tumor in another part of the body, such as a bronchogenic oat cell carcinoma, or (4) prolonged administration of synthetic glucocorticoids. Weight is gained because of sodium and water retention as well as an abnormal fat distribution. Myxedema (hypothyroidism) occurs when inadequate thyroid hormone is synthesized to metabolize fats and carbohydrates. Trauma, tumor, or other disorders to the ventromedial nucleus of the hypothalamus influence food intake because this nucleus contains the satiety center. When this center is destroyed or unable to function, the person has a voracious appetite. Hypothalamus disorders are a rare cause of obesity.

Etiologies for potential for more than nutritional body requirements include the following[13]:

Hereditary predisposition

Excessive energy intake (during late gestational life, early infancy, and adolescence)

Frequent, closely spaced pregnancies

Dysfunctional psychologic conditioning in relation to food

Membership in lower socioeconomic group

DEFINING CHARACTERISTICS[13]

Reported or observed obesity in one or both parents*

Rapid transition across growth percentiles in infants and children*

Reported use of solid food as major food source before 5 months of age

Observed use of food as reward or comfort measure

Reported or observed higher baseline weight at beginning of pregnancy

Dysfunctional eating patterns

Pairing foods with other activities; concentrating food intake at end of day

Eating in response to external cues, such as time of day, social situation

Eating in response to internal cues other than hunger, such as anxiety

Reported excessive appetite

Reported little or no physical exercise

Reported administration of glucocorticoids

*Critical defining characteristic.

NURSING INTERVENTIONS

Patient Goal	Nursing Intervention
Acknowledge the risk for obesity.	Discuss with patient the relationship between food intake, exercise, and obesity.
	Discuss risks of obesity: increased incidence for diabetes mellitus, hypertension, and atherosclerosis.
	Determine patient motivation for changing eating habits.
Achieve awareness of learning needs.	Design with the patient a diet and exercise plan for the family; consider the growth needs of each family member.
	Encourage patient to write down realistic weekly goals for food intake and exercise and to display them in a location where they can be reviewed daily.

Two nursing goals emerge for the patient with alteration in nutrition: potential for more than body requirements. The first goal is to acknowledge they are at risk, and the second is to achieve an awareness of learning needs to prevent obesity.

A person's acknowledgment of being at risk for obesity can occur at various times in the life span. A pregnant mother may need to know about food and exercise for her infant. A child or adolescent may want to prevent being overweight like a parent or older sibling. An adult may want to change behavior to avoid overweight in later years. The goal can be met through public education from agencies such as the American Heart Association and American Diabetes Association. Also, on an individual basis the nurse can give information to clients and family members when planning and implementing home care. Attaining and maintaining one's health includes weight control.

This first goal is the motivating factor for the second goal: achieving awareness of learning needs about the balance between food and fluid intake with regular physical exercise within the sociocultural environment of the client and family. The nurse first assesses the current knowledge of the patient and family. Considering the critical periods identified, one would initiate diet instruction during the antepartal period. The expectant mother needs a diet adequate in nutrients for herself and the fetus. For the breast-fed infant parents use weight gain as the criterion for adequacy of feeding. For the bottle-fed infant, parents use this same criterion rather than whether the infant finishes all feedings. Infants and children should not be forced to eat, since this may contribute to overeating. Children should be offered well-balanced meals in an environment free from distractions such as television and be encouraged to eat at their own pace. Food should not be used as reward or punishment for children because this practice may cause compulsive eating. While growing up, the child needs to learn the foods needed for a balanced diet as well as the importance of physical activity. When the child becomes an adolescent and begins taking responsibility for foods eaten, he will have a sufficient knowledge base about nutrition and exercise from which to make decisions. Adolescents and adults also need to balance food intake with physical activity. The hormonal change that occurs during puberty requires a change in eating and activity patterns. Likewise, after 50 years of age hormonal changes again necessitate reassessment of one's food intake and activity balance.

Instruction on how to prevent overweight and obesity is facilitated when all family members are present to discuss eating patterns and the meaning of food to them. If this is not possible, at least those individuals responsible for selecting food and preparing meals need to learn about overweight prevention practices. Sometimes this is the same person, but in some cultures one person selects food for another to prepare. Potential obesity caused by hormonal imbalances or hypothalamic disorders must be treated with specific medical or surgical regimens. This treatment protocol is carried out in conjunction with a balance between food intake and exercise.

EVALUATION

Patient Outcome	Data Indicating That Outcome is Reached
Acknowledges risk of obesity	Asks for help to revise own eating and exercising behaviors Knows consequences of obesity (diabetes mellitus, hypertension, atherosclosis) Does not want own children to be overweight
Knowledge of self-care	Patients can explain: 1. Dietary plan to maintain ideal body weight 2. Activity plan to maintain ideal body weight

NUTRITION, ALTERATION IN: MORE THAN BODY REQUIREMENTS

THEORY AND ETIOLOGY

Refer to the previous nursing diagnosis for the theory and etiology for this diagnosis. The adipose cell theory is important in helping to explain the difficulty in treating obesity. Most literature has concluded that the fat cell number alone does not account for obesity. The etiology is excessive intake in relation to metabolic need.[13]

DEFINING CHARACTERISTICS[13]

Weight 10% over ideal for height and frame
Weight 20% over ideal for height and frame*
Triceps skinfold greater than 15 mm in men and 25 mm in women*
Sedentary activity level
Reported or observed dysfunction eating patterns
    Pairing food with other activities
    Concentrating food intake at the end of the day
    Eating in response to external cues such as time of day, social situation
    Eating in response to internal cues other than hunger
Reported excess in food intake
Reported little or no physical exercise

*Critical defining characteristic.

NURSING INTERVENTIONS

Patient Goal	Nursing Intervention
Reduce body weight.	Weigh patient. Determine patient's desire to reduce body weight. Set a realistic plan with the patient; for example, plan to lose 1-2 pounds a week by walking a mile each day and reducing the caloric intake by 500 each day. The goal for weight loss should be posted in a strategic location. Discuss eating a balanced diet. Ask patient to keep a diary of what, when, and where he or she eats to evaluate changes that need to be made in life-style. Reward the patient for attaining goals and encourage the patient to use an internal reward system when goals are accomplished. Provide a list of support groups for weight loss: Overeaters Anonymous and TOPS (Taking Off Pounds Sensibly)

The one nursing goal for this diagnosis is to achieve and maintain reduction in body fat as well as body weight. The nurse's role may be to provide information to the patient about how to lose weight, or the role may include assisting with the weight reduction program. Motivation for weight reduction comes from within the person. The person must want to lose weight before a program can be successful. Learning the hazards of obesity may be a motivator. These hazards include atherosclerosis, hypertension, and diabetes mellitus. Realistic goals are written by the patient and posted at strategic places, such as on the refrigerator door, pantry door, or bathroom mirror. A goal of 1 to 2 pounds a week frequently is suggested as a starting point. This goal is based on the fact that 1 pound of adipose tissue has the energy potential of 3500 calories. Reducing one's caloric intake by 500 calories for 7 days theoretically yields a weight loss of 1 pound. In conjunction with decreased caloric intake, one needs to begin an exercise program and work toward a goal. The goal can be *minutes* of exercise or activity or *distance* (walking, jogging, swimming). These goals also should be written down and posted in strategic places.

Patients need to examine their eating patterns and behaviors. To assist them, they can keep a diary of what they eat, when they eat, where they eat, and the circumstances around which they eat. This activity will provide a data base for both the adequacy of nutrients eaten as well as the psychosocial conditions of eating. What one eats reveals how well balanced the diet is. Meats, fruits, vegetables, milk, cereals, and bread are needed daily for essential nutrients. To decrease food intake, a person can drink an 8-ounce glass of water before eating and use a smaller than usual plate so that the smaller serving will not look small. The person needs to eat slowly, chew thoroughly, and think about the taste and smell of the food. One needs to avoid doing any other activity while eating such as reading or watching television. Low-calorie snacks recommended are carrots, celery, and ap-

ples, which satisfy the oral need for chewing as well as provide needed vegetables and fruits. Low-calorie soft drinks are recommended also, along with water.

When one eats is important also. One person may skip breakfast, work through lunch, snack while preparing dinner, and eat dessert while watching television. The caloric intake needs to be subdivided throughout the waking hours. Instead of eating while watching television, perhaps the person can do something else with the hands and chew sugar-free gum. Where one eats includes the type of restaurant as well as which room of one's home. Fast-food restaurants often provide food quickly that is filling; however, it often is high in carbohydrates. Excessive consumption of foods from fast-food restaurants may contribute to obesity. The room where one chooses to eat is important when one is reducing caloric intake. Eating in only one place, such as the dining room table or kitchen, is helpful.

The circumstances around which one eats poses the most difficult data-collection problem. This includes the motivation for eating, those external and internal cues. Among the cues are anxiety, stress, fear, anger, peer pressure, loneliness, and depression. Some overeating problems are due to psychologic factors. Support groups or psychologic counseling may be needed to identify and deal with the problem. These include Overeaters Anonymous and TOPS (Take Off Pounds Sensibly). Behavior modification is another strategy used for reinforcement and cue elimination.

Surgical procedures may be considered for the obese person who is unsuccessful in repeated weight reduction attempts or whose health is jeopardized by the obese state. An intestinal bypass (jejunoileal bypass) is performed by the surgeon to decrease absorptive surfaces of the jejunum. Preoperatively the patient requires counseling about causes of the obese condition and the consequences of this kind of surgery. Postoperative care is similar to that for patients undergoing abdominal surgery.

EVALUATION

Patient Outcome	Data Indicating That Outcome is Reached
Weight reduced	Firm muscles Subcutaneous fat sufficient to pad bones and muscles; triceps skinfold within normal limits Daily weight stabilized at normal level for body build Diet includes meat, milk, fruits, vegetables, and breads
Aware of learning needs	The patient can explain: 1. Reason for obesity 2. Dietary plan for weight reduction 3. Exercise plan for weight reduction 4. Plans for follow-up care

FLUID VOLUME DEFICIT, POTENTIAL

THEORY AND ETIOLOGY

Fluid is present in cells, interstitial spaces, and intravascular spaces. The body has homeostatic mechanisms to regulate the intake and excretion of fluids. Water enters the body from fluids and foods consumed and is gained by the oxidation of foodstuffs and body tissue. Fluid intake is influenced by the thirst center located in the lateral hypothalamus, which is stimulated when the electrolytes inside its neurons become concentrated. Stimulation from the thirst center causes a person to sense thirst and drink fluids.

The excretion of fluid is influenced by the actions of antidiuretic hormone (ADH) and aldosterone. When body fluids become too concentrated, the neurons in the supraoptic nuclei of the hypothalamus stimulate the posterior pituitary to secrete ADH into the blood. Then ADH acts on the collecting ducts of the nephron to retain water. The action of aldosterone is to stimulate the retention of sodium and the excretion of potassium in both the distal tubules and collecting ducts. Three factors that stimulate aldosterone secretion are an increase in potassium ion concentration, an increase in angiotensin, and a decrease in sodium ion concentration.[5]

The potential for fluid volume deficit occurs after insufficient intake and excessive losses. Intake is insufficient when fluids are unavailable, either because of inadequate economic resources to purchase fluids or because of one's inability to independently drink as an infant, quadriplegic, or unconscious person. Inability to suck or swallow is another factor.

Fluid volume deficits occur from excessive losses of fluid. Excessive losses from the lungs take the forms of water from hyperventilation and secretions from a tracheostomy or endotracheal tube. Profuse diaphoresis causes fluid loss through the skin. Losses from the gastrointestinal tract include vomiting and drainage from a nasogastric tube, T-tube, or gastrostomy tube as well as from diarrhea. Finally, fluid losses occur as the result of medications, such as diuretics, given to decrease the body's fluid volume. When a person takes diuretics over time, there is a potential for fluid volume deficit.

When losses occur, regardless of the cause, the body tries to compensate by moving fluids from one space to another to maintain fluid balance within the body. For example, after excessive vomiting or diarrhea, the body tries to compensate for this loss of interstitial fluid by causing vasoconstriction, which in turn forces some intravascular fluid into the interstitial spaces. This compensatory action is followed by tachycardia to maintain systemic blood pressure and hemoconcentration due to the movement of fluid from the blood.

Etiologies for potential fluid volume deficit include the following[13]:

Extremes of age
Extremes of weight
Excessive losses through normal routes (diarrhea)
Loss of fluid through abnormal routes (indwelling tubes)
Deviations affecting access to, intake of, or absorption of fluids (physical immobility)
Factors influencing fluid needs (hypermetabolic states)
Knowledge deficiency related to fluid volume
Medications (diuretics)

DEFINING CHARACTERISTICS[13]

Increased fluid output
Urinary frequency
Thirst
Altered intake
Hyperventilation

NURSING INTERVENTIONS

Patient Goal	Nursing Intervention
Achieve fluid replacement.	Monitor vital signs.
	Weigh patient.
	Assess skin turgor.
	Measure intake and output.
	Maintain intravenous fluids and electrolytes as ordered.
	Observe electrolyte values.
	Maintain total parenteral nutrition as ordered.
	Administer medication as ordered to prevent fluid losses: antiemetics, antidiarrheals.
	Evaluate therapeutic, adverse, and toxic effects of medications given.
Achieve adequate knowledge base.	Assess what patient and family already know.
	Provide information concerning:
	1. Actions to prevent actual deficit
	2. Reasons for treatments
	3. What foods and fluids to consume
	4. What foods and fluids to avoid

The two nursing goals for the patient with potential fluid volume deficit are to prevent further deficit and to achieve awareness of learning needs.

The first goal is subdivided according to etiology into providing needed fluid and preventing further losses. The patient requires fluid by some route, usually intravenously, until the cause of the deficit can be found and corrected. Intravenous fluids can provide water, glucose, electrolytes, and vitamins. Albumin may be given intravenously, per physician order, to provide protein to maintain oncotic pressure. Total parenteral nutrition is frequently ordered by the physician when prolonged fluid therapy is required, since it supplies additional calories in the form of 50% dextrose as well as proteins, electrolytes, vitamins, and water. Nasogastric tube feeding is another means of providing fluids along with nutrients. Data on body weight and daily fluid balance must be obtained.

The second half of the goal deals with decreasing fluid loss. Loss from vomiting can be lessened by discontinuing oral intake of fluids and food, in addition to changing medications that cause vomiting as a side effect. When medications causing vomiting cannot be discontinued, then administration of antiemetics as ordered by the physician should be considered. Drainage from abnormal routes is difficult to stop. At times the drainage is necessary and must be replaced with fluids. Surgical intervention may be required to halt the drainage. Profuse diaphoresis requires fluid replacement also until the cause can be treated and fluid balance regained. Diarrhea is arrested by discontinuing oral intake and administering drugs as ordered to slow peristalsis.

The second goal is to achieve awareness of learning needs. Family members need to know the kinds of fluid replacements to use. For example, milk and milk products should not be withheld from individuals with diarrhea. Clear liquids are the fluids of choice, such as, ginger ale, apple juice, beef broth, popsicles. Family members need to know the purpose, frequency of administration and side effects of medications to be taken. They can keep a record of the intake and output to evaluate fluid balance.

EVALUATION

Patient Outcome	Data Indicating That Outcome is Reached
Fluid replaced	Vital signs within normal limits
	Good skin turgor
	Moist mucous membranes
	Absence of thirst
	Balanced intake and output
	Blood:
	Sodium: adult, 135-145 mEq/L
	Potassium: 3.5-5.0 mEq/L; add approximately 0.2 to normal range if serum is sampled rather than plasma; pediatric ranges are sometimes reported as slightly higher than adult levels

Patient Outcome	Data Indicating That Outcome is Reached
	Chloride (serum): full term, 96-106 mEq/L; children and adults, 97-107 mEq/L Urine specific gravity: range of 1.001-1.035; adult on normal fluid intake 1.016-1.022; specific gravity decreases with increasing age
Awareness of learning needs	Patient and family can explain: 1. Actions to prevent actual loss 2. Foods and fluids to consume 3. Foods and fluids to avoid 4. Medications and treatments for home use 5. Plan for follow-up care

FLUID VOLUME DEFICIT, ACTUAL
THEORY AND ETIOLOGY

Actual fluid volume deficit occurs when there is failure of regulatory mechanisms or when an active loss occurs. The ADH-thirst mechanisms are the primary regulating mechanisms of fluid volume. The aldosterone feedback system plays a small part in fluid regulation.

ADH is secreted by the supraoptic nuclei cells in the hypothalamus and stored in the posterior pituitary gland. The release of ADH is controlled by the neural impulses of the osmoreceptors cells in the hypothalamus by a negative feedback mechanism. The intake of fluid makes the extracellular fluid hypotonic. When this hypotonic fluid moves into the osmoreceptor cells, they swell and decrease neural impulses of the osmoreceptors. When impulses are decreased, there is less ADH released into the blood, which causes less water reabsorption from the renal tubules. Conversely, when the extracellular fluid is hypertonic, it causes the osmoreceptor cells to shrink, which stimulates neural stimulation of the hypothalamus to release the ADH from the posterior pituitary. The increased ADH causes water absorption from the renal tubules into the blood. The increased amount of water in the extracellular fluid reduces the tonicity of extracellular fluid, which decreases stimulation osmoreceptors. When the osmotic equilibrium is attained, the ADH secretion returns to its normal rate.[5]

Thirst is the primary regulator of fluid intake in the conscious person. Adjacent to the supraoptic nuclei is the lateral preoptic area of the hypothalamus, where the thirst center is located. The neuronal cells of the thirst center function almost identically as the osmoreceptors in the supraoptic nuclei. Any factor that will cause intracellular dehydration will cause the sensation of thirst. The most common cause of intracellular dehydration is an increased osmolar concentration of the extracellular fluid, such as increased sodium concentration, which causes osmosis of fluid from the neuronal cells of the thirst center. Excessive potassium loss also stimulates the

neuronal cells of the thirst center. Other factors that stimulate the thirst center are excessive angiotensin II, hemorrhage of up to 10% of the blood volume, low cardiac output, and dry mouth.[5]

Aldosterone is secreted by the adrenal cortex and regulates renal excretion of sodium. By controlling sodium ions, aldosterone also exerts control on potassium, chloride, and bicarbonate ions. For example, when sodium ions are retained, then potassium ions often are excreted to maintain the balance of cations. Likewise, chloride and bicarbonate often are attached to the sodium and potassium cations. A pathologic condition of the adrenal gland may not of itself cause fluid volume deficit, since the ADH-thirst mechanism is such a powerful controller of water and sodium concentration.[5]

Fluid volume deficit from active loss can be vascular fluid or gastrointestinal loss. Vascular fluid losses include hemorrhage and losses from profuse diaphoresis, burns, or wound drainage. When blood glucose levels are high, which occurs in uncontrolled diabetes mellitus, the glucose acts as an osmotic diuretic to cause fluid loss. Gastrointestinal losses may be from vomiting, diarrhea, fistula formation, gastric distention, or gastric suction. Third spacing, another cause of gastrointestinal fluid loss, occurs when fluid is trapped in a distended intestine due to intestinal obstruction, paralytic ileus, peritonitis, or ascites. Fluid is not lost from the body but is lost to the circulating blood volume.

Etiologies for actual fluid volume deficit include the following[13]:

Failure of regulatory mechanisms
Active loss

DEFINING CHARACTERISTICS[13]

Failure of regulatory mechanism
  Dilute urine

Increased urine output
Sudden weight loss
Possible weight gain
Hypotension
Decreased venous filling
Increased pulse rate
Decreased skin turgor
Decreased pulse volume and pressure
Increased body temperature
Dry skin
Dry mucous membranes
Hemoconcentration
Weakness
Edema
Thirst

Active loss
    Decreased urine output
    Concentrated urine
    Output greater than intake
    Sudden weight loss
    Decreased venous filling
    Increased serum sodium
    Hypotension
    Thirst
    Increased pulse rate
    Decreased skin turgor
    Decreased pulse volume and pressure
    Change in mental status
    Increased body temperature
    Dry skin
    Dry mucous membranes
    Weakness

NURSING INTERVENTIONS

Patient Goal	Nursing Intervention
Attain adequate fluid volume.	Measure vital signs. Measure intake and output. Weigh patient. Observe electrolyte values. Assess skin turgor. Administer intravenous and/or oral fluid as ordered by physician.
Reduce fluid volume deficit.	Measure vital signs. Measure intake and output. Observe electrolyte values. Measure fluid loss when possible. Measure abdominal girth when ascites and third spacing occur. Administer medications as ordered to prevent further fluid losses (antiemetics, antidiarrheals). Evaluate the therapeutic, adverse, and toxic effects of medications given. Cover wounds according to protocol.
Achieve awareness of learning needs.	Assess what patient and family already know. Provide information concerning: 1. Cause of this fluid deficit and how to prevent recurrence 2. Reasons for treatments 3. Foods and fluids to consume 4. The purpose, frequency of administration, and side effects of medications ordered by the physician for the patient to take at home When the patient is going home with total parenteral nutrition as ordered by the physician, the family needs to demonstrate how to change tubing and fluid bags as well as what to do when problems arise. Review the plan for follow-up.

Three nursing goals emerge for the patient with actual fluid volume deficit. These goals are to replace fluid loss, prevent further fluid losses, and achieve awareness of learning needs.

First, fluid is replaced in collaboration with the physician by an intravenous route in the form of blood or blood products, and/or glucose in water or saline with electrolytes. When long-term therapy is needed, total parenteral nutrition is used as ordered to provide concentrated glucose and proteins for calories and positive nitrogen balance, respectively.

Next, treatment is initiated to reduce and stop the fluid loss: stop hemorrhage, treat burns, give drugs as ordered to halt diarrhea or vomiting. This goal may be met quickly or require long-term therapy, depending on the cause (hemorrhage is stopped faster than ascites).

When excessive diaphoresis is caused by fever, it is treated with aspirin or acetaminophen as ordered by the physician and with tepid sponge baths.

The nurse assesses learning needs of the family to determine what content to provide. The patient and family may need instructions about nutrition. They will need to know the purpose, frequency of administration, and side effects of medications ordered by the physician to be taken at home. Return demonstration will be needed by the family who will care for a patient receiving intravenous fluids at home.

EVALUATION

Patient Outcome	Data Indicating That Outcome is Reached

Adequate fluid volume	Good skin turgor
	Moist mucous membranes
	Absence of thirst
	Balanced intake and output
	Clearing of mentation
	Blood pressure:
	  160/95 (over 65 years)
	  150/95 (45-65 years)
	  140/95 (18-44 years)
	  130/80 (11-17 years)
	  120/80 (7-10 years)
	  110/70 (3-6 years)
	  90/60 (infants)
	Pulse:
	  70-80/min (adults)
	  50-110/min (adolescents)
	  70-140/min (children)
	  80-180/min (infants)

Laboratory studies within normal limits

Blood (see Potential Fluid Volume Deficit)
Serum osmolality: 280-300 mOsm/kg water

Hemoglobin: (g/dl)	Birth (cord blood)	17.1 ± 1.8
	1 day	19.4 ± 2.1
	2-2.5 months	11.4 ± 1.1
	3-3.5 months	11.2 ± 0.8
	11-13.5 mo	11.9 ± 0.6
	1.5-3 yr	11.8 ± 0.5
	5 yr	12.7 ± 1.0
	10 yr	13.2 ± 1.2
	Men	15.5 ± 1.1
	Women	13.7 ± 1.0

Hematocrit: (%)	Birth (cord blood)	52.0 ± 5
	11-13.5 mo	39.0 ± 2
	1.5-3 yr	39.0 ± 2
	1.5-3 yr	39.0 ± 2
	5 yr	37.0 ± 3
	10 yr	39.0 ± 3
	Men	46.0 ± 3.1
	Women	40.9 ± 3

Urine
  Specific gravity: range of 1.001-1.035; adult on normal fluid intake, 1.016-1.022; specific gravity decreases with increasing age
  Osmolality: 250-900 mOsm/kg for random specimens

Adequate knowledge base

Patient and family are able to explain:
1. Reasons for fluid deficit
2. Foods and fluids to consume to prevent recurrence
3. Purpose, dosage, and side effects of medications ordered by physician
4. Plan for follow-up care

FLUID VOLUME EXCESS
THEORY AND ETIOLOGY

An excess in fluid volume occurs following (1) inadequate circulation of fluids, (2) retention of fluids, or (3) excessive intake of fluid or sodium. The body adapts to excessive fluid by redistributing it to potential spaces. Excessive fluid moves from intravascular to interstitial and potential spaces, resulting in edema of the cerebrum or joints, rales or pleural effusion, pericardial effusion, and ascites. When blood vessels cannot redistribute fluids sufficiently, they retain the fluid and the blood pressure rises due to excessive blood volume. Fluid accumulation in all body tissues results in anasarca (generalized edema).

Inadequate circulation of blood is one mechanism of fluid volume excess. Others are inadequate circulation of blood; inadequate cardiac output (ventricular hypertrophy, congestive heart failure); retention of fluid (renal failure, corticosteroid therapy, Cushing's syndrome); retention of aldosterone (primary aldosteronism, renal failure, cirrhosis); inadequate plasma protein (cirrhosis, malnutrition, hemorrhage, burns, draining wounds, fistulas, nephrosis); and excessive intake of fluids or sodium. The heart fails to pump fluid adequately due to left ventricular failure. Fluid backs up into the left atria and into the lungs, a low-pressure circulatory system. This extra fluid moves to the interstitial spaces of the alveoli, resulting in rales. This backup of fluid can continue to the right side of the heart and into the venous circulation. When the right side of the heart has excessive fluid to pump or the right ventricle has hypertrophied, then fluid backs up into the venous system. Dependent edema is observed most often in the ankles of ambulatory or sitting patients and in the sacrum of those confined to bed. Fluid accumulation may advance to ascites.

Retention of fluids is another cause of fluid volume excess. In renal failure the fluid to be excreted cannot be filtered through the nephrons and is therefore retained in the circulating blood volume. Increases in sodium retain fluid, since water goes where the salt is. Sodium is retained when cortisol levels rise, as during corticosteroid therapy or in Cushing's syndrome. Aldosterone's function is to retain sodium, so any retention of aldosterone will increase the serum sodium levels. Plasma proteins are needed in the circulatory system to bind with fluid to maintain oncotic pressure. Since proteins are supplied by dietary intake and synthesis in the liver, both malnutrition and cirrhosis interfere with the protein supply. Protein is lost by hemorrhage, burns, draining wounds, fistulas, and nephrosis.

Excessive intake of fluids (packed cells, IV fluids, plasma expanders) occurs most frequently as the result of rapid administration of the fluids. Sometimes this is initiated as treatment that continues beyond the point of therapeutic benefit.

Etiologies for fluid volume excess include the following[13]:

Compromised regulatory mechanism
Excess fluid intake
Excess sodium intake

DEFINING CHARACTERISTICS[13]

Edema
Effusion (pleural, pericardial)
Anasarca (generalized massive edema)
Weight gain
Shortness of breath, orthopnea
Intake greater than output
Third heart sound
Pulmonary congestion on x-ray film
Abnormal breath sounds: crackles (rales)
Change in respiratory pattern
Change in mental status
Decreased hemoglobin, hematocrit
Blood pressure changes
Central venous pressure changes
Pulmonary artery pressure changes
Jugular venous distention
Positive hepatojugular reflex
Oliguria
Specific gravity changes
Azoturia
Altered electrolytes
Restlessness and anxiety

NURSING INTERVENTIONS

Patient Goal	Nursing Intervention
Regain fluid balance.	Measure vital signs. Weigh patient. Measure intake and output. Restrict sodium and fluid as ordered. Observe electrolyte, albumin, urea nitrogen, creatinine, hemoglobin, and hematocrit values. Measure abdominal girth. Assess skin turgor and inspect skin for redness. Administer drugs as ordered: diuretics, albumin. Evaluate the therapeutic, adverse, and toxic effects of drugs given. Assist with thoracentesis and dialysis.
Avoid complications of fluid excess.	Inspect skin continuously for redness. Reposition patient frequently. Passive or active range of motion several times each day. Apply elastic stockings. Encourage the patient to cough and deep breathe.

Achieve awareness of learning needs.	Assess what the patient and family already know.
	Provide information concerning:
	  1. Reasons for fluid excess
	  2. Reasons for treatments
	  3. Dietary alterations required, such as low sodium diet
	  4. Purpose of drugs ordered for home use
	  5. Ways to support peripheral circulation
	  6. Plan for follow-up care

The three nursing goals for the patient with fluid volume excess are to regain fluid balance by removing excess fluid and treating the underlying cause, to prevent complications of fluid excess, and to achieve awareness of learning needs. Therapy to remove excessive fluid is based on the cause of the problem. In collaboration with physician orders diuretics are given for excessive fluid due to inadequate circulation, albumin is given to provide protein to pull fluid into the intravascular space so that it can be excreted by the kidneys, dialysis is used in renal failure when diuretics and albumin are inappropriate, thoracentesis is used to remove fluid from the pleural space, and paracentesis is used to remove fluid from the abdomen. In addition to removing fluid, treatment also includes restricting sodium and fluid intake to prevent further fluid excess.

While administering treatment for fluid excess, the nurse protects edematous parts of the body from prolonged pressure, injury, and extremes of hot and cold. Skin is inspected for redness and blanching. The patient's position is changed every 1 or 2 hours to prevent pressure on edematous areas. Active or passive range of motion is done to prevent contractures as well as to improve venous return. Application of elastic stockings provides support to veins and prevents venous stasis. Thirst becomes a problem because oral intake is limited but the patient is thirsty. Chewing gum or sucking hard candy may stimulate enough saliva to reduce the patient's thirst. There is a psychologic advantage for the patient when the nurse puts the small amount of oral fluid allowed in a small (medicine) cup rather than a standard size cup.

To plan learning needs, the nurse determines what the patient and family already know. They need to understand the cause of the fluid volume excess. Many patients will require dietary alterations of low sodium or altered protein intake. The person who buys the food and prepares the meals needs written information on appropriate menus. They need to read labels of food for sodium content. Information about medications to be taken includes the purpose, frequency of administration, and side effects. The patient needs to know how to support peripheral circulation. This includes applying elastic stockings before rising and avoiding crossed legs and standing for long periods. The feet and legs need to be inspected daily for edema and redness to prevent pressure sores.

EVALUATION

Patient Outcome	Data Indicating That Outcome is Reached
Fluid balance regained	Blood pressure (see Decreased Cardiac Output) Respiration (see Ineffective Breathing Patterns)
Laboratory studies within normal limits	Blood (see Potential Fluid Volume Deficit, Altered Tissue Perfusion)

Hemoglobin (g/dl)

Birth (cord blood)	17.1 ± 1.8
11-13.5 months	11.9 ± 0.6
1.5-3 years	11.8 ± 0.5
5 years	12.7 ± 1.0
10 years	13.2 ± 1.2
Men	15.5 ± 1.1
Women	13.7 ± 1.0

Hematocrit (%)   (see Actual Fluid Volume Deficit)
Albumin: 3.2-5.6 g/dl blood
Good skin turgor
Balanced intake and output
Clearing of mentation
Absence of edema

Patient Outcome	Data Indicating That Outcome is Reached
Awareness of learning needs	Patient and family can explain: 1. Reasons for fluid volume excess 2. Dietary alterations 3. Medication and treatments for home use 4. Plan for follow-up care

ORAL MUCOUS MEMBRANE, ALTERATION IN

THEORY AND ETIOLOGY

The oral mucous membrane is altered by pathologic conditions that damage tissue and by dehydration that dries the membrane. Tissue is damaged by chemical and mechanical trauma. Chemical trauma includes acidic foods and noxious agents. Mechanical trauma results from ill-fitting dentures, jagged teeth, braces, insertion of endotracheal tubes, and oral surgery. Some drugs cause mouth ulcers and stomatitis as delayed toxic effects. Infections in the oral mucosa result from microorganisms, mechanical trauma, vitamin deficiencies, liver and kidney diseases, and chemotherapy. Dryness of the mucous membrane results from dehydration, no oral intake for more than 24 hours, mouth breathing, lack of or decreased salivation, or side effects of medications (antihistamines, anticholinergics, phenothiazines, narcotics, and chemotherapy).

Etiologies for altered oral mucous membrane include the following[13]:

Pathologic conditions of oral cavity (radiation to head and/or neck)
Dehydration
Trauma
Chemical (acidic foods, drugs, noxious agents, alcohol)

Mechanical (ill-fitting dentures, braces, endotracheal, nasogastric, or surgery tubes)
NPO instructions for more than 24 hours
Ineffective oral hygiene
Mouth breathing
Malnutrition
Infection
Lack of or decreased salivation
Medication

DEFINING CHARACTERISTICS

Coated tongue
Xerostomia (dry mouth)
Stomatitis
Oral lesions or ulcers
Lack of or decreased salivation
Leukoplakia
Edema
Hyperemia
Oral plaque
Oral pain or discomfort
Desquamation
Vesicles
Hemorrhagic gingivitis
Carious teeth
Halitosis

NURSING INTERVENTIONS

Patient Goal	Nursing Intervention
Achieve nutrition and hydration.	Assess patient's teeth, gums, and oral mucosa.
	Measure intake and output.
	Provide oral hygiene (brushing, flossing, mouthwash).
	Lubricate lips.
	Administer local anesthetics as ordered prior to mealtime.
	Serve food and fluids at appropriate temperatures; avoid extreme temperatures (hot or cold) when they cause discomfort.
	Change texture of food to soft or puree when necessary.
	Maintain intravenous or oral fluids as ordered.
Achieve adequate knowledge base.	Assess what the patient and family already know.
	Provide information about:
	1. Reasons for alteration in oral mucous membrane
	2. Importance of dental hygiene for all family members
	3. Review medications and treatments ordered for home use
	4. Plan for follow-up care

Two nursing goals emerge for the patient with alteration in oral mucous membrane. These goals are to maintain nutrition and hydration and to achieve awareness of learning needs. The toothbrush used needs to have soft bristles of equal lengths. A commercial toothpaste or sodium bicarbonate may be used. The brushing motion is in small circles or sweeping motion moving downward from the gums. The tongue needs to be brushed also.

Oral care for the unconscious patient is performed with the patient in a side-lying position with the head of the bed elevated at least 30 degrees to prevent aspiration. The brushing procedure is the same for the alert patient. Rinsing is done using an a large syringe and oral suction. When the patient has an oral airway in place, it is changed or cleaned also. Dentures and bridges require soaking and brushing daily. After brushing, the mouth is rinsed. Commercial mouthwashes are not recommended because they contain alcohol, which is painful; instead, saline solution or water can be used. Hydrogen peroxide when used 1:2 or 1:4 with water acts well as a germicide to destroy bacteria chemically and clean mechanically. Its bubbling action removes film from tongue and teeth. Glycerin swabs tend to dry mucous membranes and are recommended only daily for clean, healthy mouths.[25]

Fluid and food intake decreases when it causes pain. Relief of the pain can be accomplished by changing the temperature of the fluid or food to tepid or to warm, or the texture of the food to soft or pureed. Foods to avoid include fried foods, spicy foods, citrus fruits, crusty foods, and foods of extreme temperatures. Local anesthetics, per physician's orders, are useful before mealtime to provide temporary pain relief to increase intake. These include lidocaine (Xylocaine) viscous 2%; 0.5 aqueous Benadryl solution and Maalox; or equal parts of 0.5 aqueous Benadryl solution and Kaopectate. The patient swishes the solution and then swallows or expectorates. When lidocaine is swallowed, however, it may affect the gag reflex.[3]

The nurse assesses the patient's and family's knowledge to determine what content to teach. Prevention of alteration of oral mucous membranes is very important. The patient and family need to review their dental hygiene practices. Children benefit from visits to the dentist every 6 months after the age of 2 years. Fluoride supplements are helpful for children. They will need help brushing their teeth until age 6, but it is important for children to develop the recommended dental hygiene practices. Infants who are put to bed with a bottle should receive a bottle of water rather than juice or milk. The infant who is teething needs safe objects to put in the mouth. Adults require annual visits to the dentist. Daily brushing and flossing with sufficient fluids and adequate nutrition will help prevent dental caries.

EVALUATION

Patient Outcome	Data Indicating That Outcome is Reached
Adequate nutrition and hydration	Moist oral mucous membranes, coral color Able to drink and chew without discomfort Lack of halitosis
Adequate knowledge base	Patient and family can explain: 1. Reasons for alteration in oral mucous membrane 2. Plan for dental hygiene for all family members 3. Medications and treatment for home use 4. Plan for follow-up care

References

1. Billings, D.M., and Stokes, L.G.: Medical-surgical nursing, St. Louis, 1982, The C.V. Mosby Co.
2. Campbell, C.: Nursing diagnosis and intervention in nursing practice, New York, 1978, John Wiley & Sons, Inc.
3. Carpenito, L.J.: Nursing diagnosis: application to clinical practice, Philadelphia, 1983, J.B. Lippincott Co.
4. Groer, M., and Shekleton, M.: Basic pathophysiology: a conceptual approach, ed. 2, St. Louis, 1983, The C.V. Mosby Co.
5. Guyton, A.C.: Textbook of medical physiology, ed. 6, Philadelphia, 1981, W.B. Saunders Co.
6. Hart, L.K., Reese, J.L., and Fearing, M.O., editors: Concepts common to acute illness: identification and management, St. Louis, 1981, The C.V. Mosby Co.
7. Hirsch, J., and Hannock, L., editors: Manual of clinical nursing procedures, St. Louis, 1981, The C.V. Mosby Co.
8. Hudak, C.M., Gallo, B.M., and Lohr, T., editors: Critical care nursing, ed. 3, Philadelphia, 1982, J.B. Lippincott Co.
9. Jacob, S.W., and Francone, C.A.: Structure and function in man, ed. 3, Philadelphia, 1974, W.B. Saunders Co.
10. Johanson, B.C., and others: Standards for critical care, St. Louis, 1981, The C.V. Mosby Co.
11. Kennan, R.A., and Blackburn, G.L.: Clinical nutritional assessment of the hospitalized patient, Surgical Rounds, Oct. 1981, pp. 34-44.
12. Kim, M.J., McFarland, G.K., and McLane. A., editors: Classification of nursing diagnosis, St. Louis, 1984, The C.V. Mosby Co.
13. Kim, M.J., McFarland, G.K., and McLane, A.: Pocket guide to nursing diagnosis, St. Louis, 1984, The C.V. Mosby. Co.
14. Luckmann, J., and Sorenson, K.: Medical-surgical nursing, ed. 2, Philadelphia, 1980, W.B. Saunders Co.
15. Malasanos, L., and others: Health assessment, ed. 2, St. Louis, 1981, The C.V. Mosby Co.
16. Palmer, P.: Advanced hemodynamic assessment, Dimensions Crit. Care 1:139-144, 1982.
17. Phipps, W.J., Long, B.C., and Woods, N.F.: Medical-surgical nursing: concepts and clinical practice, St. Louis, 1979, The C.V. Mosby Co.
18. Porth, C.: Pathophysiology: concepts of altered health states, Philadelphia, 1982, J.B. Lippincott Co.
19. Price, S.A., and Wilson, L.M.: Pathophysiology: clinical concepts of disease processes, ed. 2, New York, 1982, McGraw-Hill Book Co.
20. Shapiro, B.A., Harrison, R.A., and Trout, C.A.: Clinical application of respiratory care, ed. 3, Chicago, 1979, Year Book Medical Publishers, Inc.
21. Tucker, S.M., and others: Patient care standards, ed. 3, St. Louis, 1984, The C.V. Mosby Co.
22. Wade, J.F.: Comprehensive respiratory care, ed. 3, St. Louis, 1982, The C.V. Mosby Co.
23. White, J.W.: An overview of obesity: its significance to nursing, Nurs. Clin. North Am. 17:191-198, 1982.
24. Williams, S.R.: Nutrition and diet therapy, ed. 4, St. Louis, 1981, The C.V. Mosby Co.
25. Wilson, S.: Neuronursing, New York, 1979, Springer Publishing Co.

Elimination

BOWEL ELIMINATION, ALTERATION IN: CONSTIPATION

THEORY AND ETIOLOGY

A normal bowel movement is regular and easy and results in a complete passage of a formed stool. Although the range of normal bowel patterns is wide, a range between three bowel movements per week and three per day is frequently cited in the literature with no obvious difference between males and females.[6,11,28] In a more recent study of 789 students and hospital employees 94.2% reported stool frequencies between three per day and three per week, confirming the earlier studies of frequency in a healthy population.[13]

The relationship of bowel frequency with advancing age is unclear. The masking effect of laxative ingestion in older subjects may account for similarities in the distribution of bowel frequency across ages. However, taking laxatives for reasons unrelated to bowel frequency contributes to the ambiguity surrounding the age-frequency question.[11] Furthermore, there is some discrepancy between what persons say about their bowel habits during interviews and what they record in a bowel diary. Manning, Wyman, and Heaton[27] reported that one in six patients was wrong in predicting bowel frequency by as much as three bowel movements a week.[27]

The nature of true constipation is even more elusive than the nature of normal bowel function. Most definitions include the following characteristics: a decrease in frequency, the difficult passage of excessively hard stools, and a sense of incomplete evacuation. The failure of most people who claim to be constipated to satisfy any reasonable definition of the disorder creates problems for both clinicians and researchers.[37]

Since constipation may be a symptom of some underlying disease as well as a functional health problem, a medical evaluation, including abdominal and rectal examinations, should be done to exclude organic causes. "Constipation associated with weight loss, abdominal pain, or fresh rectal bleeding, particularly in the elderly, should alert the doctor to possible serious organic disease."[37] "Patients with constipation of recent onset, sudden aggravation of existing constipation with recent abdominal pain, or the passage of blood and mucus in the stools should always be subjected to sigmoidoscopy and barium enema examination."[2] Sklar[38] reviewed the records of 300 patients, age 65 or over, who were being seen in a large university gastrointestinal clinic. Only 44% had organic disease; 55% were considered to have a functional bowel disturbance, that is, symptoms of gastrointestinal distress (including constipation) without anatomic structural changes. Sklar pointed out that gastrointestinal problems of older persons did not differ greatly from those of the young: there is no wearing out of the digestive tract, mobility and absorption are not significantly impaired, there is no evidence that decreased gastric secretions induce symptoms, and digestive enzymes decrease, but sufficient quantities remain for normal digestion.

Numerous examples of variables believed to influence constipation have been identified. Diet, lack of exercise, ignoring the gastrocolic reflex, environmental factors, stress and tension, depression, and overuse of laxatives have been implicated as factors contributing to constipation. Lack of exercise has long been considered an important etiology, yet there are few data to support a relationship between exercise and elimination.

During the last decade researchers focused primarily on fiber and its effect on gut physiology. Most of the fiber-related studies concentrated on the effects of increased fiber on groups of institutionalized persons, such as nursing home residents.[40] Godding[14] cautioned health professionals not to regard edible fiber as something of a harmless cure-all: "The adsorptive and cation exchange properties of the fiber . . . do not always operate beneficially." For example, if nutritional levels are low, excess fiber intake further reduces availability of essential nutrients and threatens mineral malnutrition, especially zinc, calcium, and iron. Godding also suggested that major changes in diet, such as increasing the amount of edible fiber, require a period of adjustment, 3 weeks to a month before the body reaches a new steady state.

A review of a decade of research published in nursing journals from 1970 to 1980 was organized by Lindsey[26] under three major classifications in which the phenomenon of concern related (1) to the individual, (2) to the individual's environment, or (3) to some aspect of a therapy or procedure. No studies of bowel elimination were located in the first two categories and only two studies in the third. One[32] was a study of variables that account for proper bowel preparation for radiology, and the second[12] was a comparison of three methods for providing bowel control for spinal cord–injured patients.

As part of an ongoing effort to identify and validate the etiological factors and defining characteristics for this diagnosis two research instruments—*Nursing Practice and Constipation Tool: Nurse Perspective* and *Health Practices Tool, Elimination: Client Perspective*—were developed by McLane, McShane, and Sliefert.[29] To gain a better understanding of bowel elimination practices from the patient's perspective and to contribute to the establishment of construct validity for the latter instrument, the researchers interviewed 20 elderly persons living in a senior citizen residential community. Content analysis of data from the interviews was done to establish conceptual categories of diagnostic indicators for bowel elimination, alteration in: constipation. Five categories and eight subcategories with definitions were established.[29] The conceptual categories provide a beginning theoretical explanation for the diagnosis of constipation and also serve as a framework for assessment of bowel elimination practices of healthy adults from a nursing perspective.

I. Signs and symptoms
   A. Description of constipated stool
      1. Character: qualities of the stool, color, consistency
      2. Amount: amount of stool
      3. Frequency: lapse of time between stools
   B. Feelings and sensations: physical feelings and sensations associated with constipation, such as stomachache, bloating
II. Etiology: contributing factors, such as diet, fluids, inadequate exercise, medications, change in routine
III. Attending behaviors: consistent use of measures for the expressed purpose of alleviating or preventing constipation
   A. Treatment: measures taken to relieve constipation
   B. Prevention: measures taken to prevent constipation
IV. Health behaviors: health behavior influencing normal elimination, diet, fluid intake, exercise
V. Patterning: behaviors related to the production of a bowel movement, including toilet routine
   A. Expected frequency of bowel movement(s)
   B. Time of day of bowel movement(s)
   C. Stimulus behaviors
      1. Actions taken to stimulate a bowel movement, short term, within the hour, such as drinking hot water.
      2. Actions in daily routine that result in a bowel movement, such as eating breakfast
   D. Response to reflexes: behaviors in response to the urge to defecate

The five categories and eight subcategories of diagnostic indicators reflect the complexity of normal bowel elimination and constipation. Despite its complexity, constipation is usually diagnosed by patients themselves. However, their understanding of the phenomenon does not extend to analyzing the multiple factors that contribute to producing acute or chronic constipation. Nurses are similar to patients in their ability to diagnose an instance of altered bowel function, and like the patients they often fail to recognize or search for multiple etiological factors.

An analysis of the historical record of five National Conferences on the Classification of Nursing Diagnoses lends additional support to the preceding statements. No etiologies of constipation are identified in the proceedings of the first four conferences. At the Fifth National Conference, the following list of suggested etiologies was developed[21]:

Less than adequate fluid intake
Less than adequate dietary intake and bulk
Less than adequate physical activity or immobility
Personal habits
Chronic use of medication and enemas
Gastrointestinal obstructive lesions
Neuromuscular impairment

Musculoskeletal impairment
Pain on defecation
Diagnostic procedures
Lack of privacy
Weak abdominal musculature
Pregnancy
Emotional status

DEFINING CHARACTERISTICS

Decreased activity level (risk factor)
Frequency less than usual pattern
Hard formed stool
Palpable mass
Reported feeling of pressure in rectum
Reported feeling of rectal fullness
Straining at stool

Data supporting these defining characteristics, which are listed in the Proceedings of the Fifth National Conference on Classification of Nursing Diagnoses, were reported by McLane and McShane.[30]

Constipation has appeared as a diagnostic label on the list of "accepted diagnoses" of the National Group for Classification of Nursing Diagnoses (now known as NANDA) since the First National Conference in 1973.

The original label, Bowel function, irregular: constipation, was changed at the Second National Conference in 1975 and has remained unchanged since.[20-22]

Despite agreement of the participants of five national conferences that nurses diagnose and treat constipation, in the absence of a research base none of the defining characteristics has been upgraded to the category of critical defining characteristic, which Gordon[16] defines as "highly reliable, highly valid cues . . . which . . . increase confidence in diagnostic judgments." In addition, some of the so-called defining characteristics are risk factors, not indicators.

There is little agreement in the nursing diagnosis literature on a definition of constipation as evidenced by the absence of a definition in the publication of the national conferences.[20-22] Gordon[15] defined constipation as "periodic episodes of hard stools or absence of stools *not* associated with a pathological state." According to this definition all constipation that is associated with a pathologic state is outside the domain of nursing. The logical outcome of such reasoning would place constipation associated with such states as spinal cord injuries outside the realm of nursing practice. Clearly such a definition does not add to our understanding of the phenomenon nor does it provide the criteria by which to recognize an instance of the phenomenon. Carpenito's

Table 13

Historical Development of Consensual and Empirical Validation of Diagnostic Indicators: Constipation

First National Conference (1973)	Second National Conference (1975)	Third National Conference (1978)	Fourth National Conference (1980)	Fifth National Conference (1982)	Sixth National Conference (1984)
Infrequent stools Difficult evacuation of feces	Abdominal mass Decreasing appetite Hard, formed stool Frequency <3 times per week Headache Rectal fullness Rectal pressure Straining at stool	Abdominal mass Decreasing appetite Hard, formed stool Frequency <3 times per week Headache Rectal fullness Rectal pressure Straining at stool	Abdominal mass Abdominal pain Decreasing appetite Hard, formed stool Frequency <usual patterns Headache Rectal fullness Rectal pressure Straining at stool	Decreasing bowel sounds Abdominal mass Abdominal pain Increasing abdominal pressure Decreasing appetite Hard, formed stool Frequency <usual patterns Headache Nausea Rectal fullness Rectal pressure <usual amount of stool Straining at stool	Abdominal distention Change in abdominal growling Abdominal mass Abdominal pain Increasing abdominal pressure Change in abdominal size Decreasing appetite Blood with stool Dry, hard stool Change in flatus Change in frequency Headache Indigestion Mass in rectum Oozing liquid stool Rectal fullness Rectal pain with stool Rectal pressure Small volume of stool Straining at stool Swollen rectal veins Unable to pass stool

definition[7] further obscures the true nature of constipation: ''The state in which the individual experiences or is at high risk of experiencing stasis of the large intestine resulting in infrequent elimination and hard, dry feces.'' Inclusion in the definition of persons at risk of developing constipation reduces the conceptual clarity of the definition, and the term *infrequent* is conceptually ambiguous.

OTHER DEFINING CHARACTERISTICS

Other possible defining characteristics include those listed in the official publication of the conference,[22] defining characteristics identified in other nursing diagnosis literature, and indicators identified in a recent study of 300 subjects.[30] Also considered as other possible defining characteristics by participants of the Fifth National Conference were the following:

Abdominal pain
Appetite impairment
Back pain
Headache
Interference with daily living (consequence)
Use of laxatives (risk factor)

Data supporting abdominal pain, appetite impairment, and headache as other defining characteristics were reported by McLane and McShane.[29,30] No data were available to support back pain as a defining characteristic.

Interference with daily living is viewed as a consequence of constipation, and use of laxatives could be either a risk factor or an etiology. In addition to supporting the previously identified defining characteristics, McLane and McShane identified increased abdominal pressure, indigestion, increased size of the abdomen (distention, bloating), changes in abdominal growling, changes in amount of gas passed, swollen rectal veins, oozing liquid stool, and abdominal mass. Gordon[15] listed the same defining characteristics and other defining characteristics as listed in Kim and Moritz,[22] with the exception of abdominal pain, which she moved to the other defining characteristics category.

An analysis of the historical development of consensual and empirical validation of the diagnostic indicators for the category of constipation by the participants in six national conferences is presented in Table 13. The 22 defining characteristics listed in the last column of the table were supported by data from 300 healthy adults.[30]

NURSING INTERVENTIONS

Patient Goal	Nursing Intervention
Describe health behaviors that prevent constipation in relation to diet, fluid, exercise.	Provide instruction for: 1. Appropriate use of bulk in diet 2. Adequate daily fluid intake 3. Appropriate level of exercise for age and physiologic status 4. Recognition and attention to stimulus behaviors, for example, warm fluids on arising
Avoid habit-forming aids to defecation.	Assess and monitor laxative and enema use.
Take oral laxatives when other measures are ineffective.	Provide instruction for appropriate use of oral laxatives. Assess and monitor side effects of medication.
Establish a bowel repatterning program to establish normal bowel functioning.	Provide instruction for understanding: 1. Role of stimulus behaviors 2. Importance of immediate response to defecation urge Assist with implementation of new health behaviors relative to good bowel habits, including diet, fluids, exercise, and emotional equilibrium.

Attention to a learned function, such as elimination, occurs when there is a deviation from what is perceived by the patient as normal. Constipation has different meanings for different people. Some individuals consider not having a bowel movement every day as constipation; others perceive it as difficulty in passing feces. In a study done by McLane and McShane,[29] the majority of middle-aged and older adults defined constipation as not having a bowel movement every day.

The key to providing nursing care to patients lies in prevention of its occurrence. Because normal bowel functioning is a prerequisite for health, every person uses individual self-care practices for acquiring a regular pattern of elimination. There is seldom a single cause for constipation; rather it consists of a complex interaction of diet, fluid, exercise, patterning, attending behavior, and relief from emotional distress.

Health Behaviors

Diet. Health behaviors, such as a well-balanced diet, adequate fluid intake, and exercise are essential to the promotion of normal bowel functioning. A diet adequate in dietary fiber provides bulk and keeps the stool soft through the mechanism of water absorption. The fiber acts as a bulking agent through its water-binding properties. Kirwan[23] reported a direct relationship between the water-holding capacity of bran and the size of the bran particle. Pollmann and others[34] refer to dietary fiber as unavailable carbohydrates and lignin (noncarbohydrates) that originate from plant cell walls. The cell wall is composed of carbohydrates, cellulose, hemicellulose, and pectins as well as lignin. Unavailable carbohydrates are those which compose the cell wall and are not hydrolyzed by the human digestive tract.

It has been reported that the addition of natural fiber to the diet results in decreased extracolonic pressure and that this decrease has beneficial effects in conditions such as irritable colon and diverticular disease.[10] The mechanism increases the speed at which the stool passes through the intestines. The increased speed decreases the amount of water absorbed by the large intestine, and the stool remains soft and bulky.

Some high-fiber foods are whole-grain cereals and breads, leafy vegetables, and raw and cooked fruits. Fruits such as bananas, prunes, dates, figs, and rhubarb are good laxatives as well as being high in fiber.[42] The laxative substance found in prunes is dihydroxphenyl isatin. Other foods may have these same properties, but data on pharmacologic laxative properties of food are limited.[24] Unprocessed bran can also be used to increase fiber intake. Unprocessed bran is inexpensive and can be easily purchased in health food stores and many large supermarkets. It has been used successfully to treat constipation, diverticulosis, and irritable bowel syndrome.[19]

Bran is the end product of the milling of rice or wheat. Bran milled from wheat contains about 20% indigestible cellulose and is an excellent source of bulk. Unprocessed bran contains approximately 14% fiber, in contrast to the lesser fiber content of 100% Bran (7.5%), All Bran (7%), Bran Buds (7%), and Raisin Bran (3%). Since the fiber in unrefined bran is the important ingredient, Hui[19] recommends natural bran flakes or whole bran. For this reason products such as 40% Bran Flakes or compressed pellets such as All Bran are not recommended.

In health, body fluids (water and electrolytes) are constantly being metabolized and must be replaced to maintain normal processes. In health, normal fluid intake should be about 2500 ml per day. Of this amount approximately 1000 ml is obtained from water in food, 300 ml from oxidation, and 1200 ml as liquid.[33] These fluids enter the intestines each day, along with saliva, gastric secretions, pancreatic juices, and bile to comprise total body fluids of 9 to 10 L for absorption of nutrients and electrolytes. In health, most of this fluid is reabsorbed; only about 100 ml of water is excreted in feces.[31]

Insufficient fluids and fiber provide inadequate roughage, which slows the passage of food through intestines, permitting increased reabsorption of water and thereby causing a very hard constipated stool. Persons who are constipated can be helped by increasing their intake of both fiber and fluid.

Interventions include counseling the patient that good health does not depend on a daily bowel movement. However, if a problem exists, information about common conditions that cause constipation may be helpful. Among these are irregular or culture-bound dietary habits, a diet that does not contain the basic four food groups, omission of breakfast, very little activity or exercise, use of certain drugs or prolonged laxative use, pregnancy, and obesity. Helping the client change family food habits and plan meals is one intervention. Foods that are valuable sources of fiber and can be readily incorporated into the daily diet should be specified. The connection between constipation and ignoring the defecation urge should be explained. Various situations may be responsible for this inattention, such as change in home environment or job, working routines, inconvenience, travel, social activities, increased age, emotional disturbances and stress, and recuperating from an illness.

Older people with constipation have special needs. Their constipation problems may be directly related to loss of muscle strength, lack of exercise, or a dental handicap. A declining interest in food and its preparation because of living alone may be a significant factor. Older people may dislike high-fiber foods such as raw fruits and vegetables. McLane and McShane[30] found that cooked fruits and vegetables were preferred by healthy older persons. This population, because of living on fixed incomes, may also be unable to afford foods with high roughage content. It is necessary to emphasize the importance of avoiding laxatives and enemas on a routine basis because they contribute to loss of large bowel tone.

Exercise. Exercise in any form is essential for total body functioning and well-being. Normal defecation depends on adequate muscular strength in the abdominal and pelvic muscles. People who are sedentary, immobile, or debilitated from illness benefit from conditioning exercises to strengthen the muscles of the abdomen and pelvic floor. Lack of tone in abdominal muscles can be best corrected by doing situps. These should be done with knees bent and arms flexed behind the head, so as not to put undue strain on the back. Isometric contraction of perineal muscles and the pelvic tilt strengthen muscles of the pelvic floor. Walking briskly for at least 15 minutes a day is the easiest overall exercise.[8] McLane and McShane[30] found that exercise in the form of strenuous activity was related to preventing an incidence of constipation. There is highly suggestive evidence supporting exercise and conditioning not only as legitimate health behaviors in preventing constipation, but as self-esteem enhancers, stress reducers, and overall contributors to the quality of life.[5]

Patterning: stimulus behavior and response to reflex. Persons can be educated to use health behaviors for maintaining bowel function that are familiar and have proved helpful, such as a cup of hot liquid before breakfast, prune juice, or other measures. Many of these measures are based on stimulating physiologic processes and have sound bases for their effectiveness. The practice of drinking warm fluids on arising, for example, sets in motion the duodenocolic, gastrocolic, gastroileal, enterogastric, and defecation reflexes.

When feces are forced into the rectum, the process of defecation is normally initiated, including reflex contraction of the rectum and relaxation of anal sphincters.[17] The defecation reflex is described by Guyton as follows[17]:

When feces enter the rectum, the distended rectal wall initiates afferent nerve signals that spread through the myenteric plexus to initiate peristaltic waves in the descending colon, sigmoid, and rectum, forcing feces toward the anus. As the peristaltic waves move toward the anus, the internal anal sphincter is inhibited by "receptive relaxation" and if the external anal sphincter is relaxed, defecation will occur. This overall phenomenon is called the defecation reflex.

Because the defecation reflex is extremely weak, other reflexes intensify the peristaltic waves and convert the defecation reflex into a powerful process of defecation that is capable of emptying the large bowel from the splenic flexure to the anus. The reflexes enter the spinal cord and initiate other effects, such as deep inspiration, closure of the glottis, and contraction of the abdominal muscles to force fecal content downward. At the same time the pelvic floor muscles pull outward and upward on the anus to evaginate the feces downward. However, before actual defecation occurs, the conscious mind takes over voluntary control of the external sphincter and either inhibits it to allow the process to occur or further contracts it if the moment is not socially acceptable. When contraction of the external sphincter is maintained, the defecation reflex stops after several minutes and will not return until an additional amount of feces enters the rectum, which may not happen for several more hours.

When the time is more convenient for the person to defecate, defecation reflexes can usually be initiated by taking a deep breath to force the diaphragm downward and then contracting the abdominal muscles to increase abdominal pressure, thereby forcing feces into the rectum to initiate new reflexes. However, it should be noted that reflexes initiated this way are never as effective as those which arise naturally. For this reason people who inhibit their natural reflexes often become severely constipated.[17]

Stress and tension can interfere with normal bowel elimination, especially in an already stressful hospital environment. Stimulation of the sympathetic nervous system inhibits gastrointestinal activity, slowing the peristaltic waves yet innervating the internal anal sphincter at the same time. Therefore, during a time of stress, movement is delayed temporarily, but incontinence can occur. It follows that, in addition to including measures to decrease stress and ensuring adequate privacy, it is important to provide enough time for a bowel movement. In the acute care setting, treatments and tests are frequently scheduled so closely that the person has no relaxed uninterrupted time for a bowel movement.[31] This situation can be very serious for a person with constipation who has succeeded in developing a satisfactory schedule of elimination, only to have it thoughtlessly disrupted during a hospitalization.[30,31] This problem can be minimized by making sure that hospitalized patients participate in decision-making and planning related to their care.

The most physiologically effective position for defecation is a squatting position in which the pressure of the thighs increases the intraabdominal pressure and thus aids expulsion of the stool. Most adults can achieve this position by leaning forward while sitting on the toilet, but children and short people may find it comfortable to use a footstool to raise their thighs when using the toilet. Some elderly people who find it difficult to use a low seat use an elevated toilet seat to get off the toilet without assistance. A higher toilet seat often means that their feet barely touch the floor; they may therefore need a footstool to flex knees and hips for effective defecation.

Immobility

Constipation is perhaps the most frequent complication of immobility. Lack of activity, changes in eating habits and fluid intake, and the necessity of having to use the bedpan are contributing factors. Nursing management includes frequent toileting, active or passive exercises, good dietary intake with special attention to laxative foods and foods high in roughage, use of stool softeners, bulk-producing laxatives, intestinal wall–stimulating laxatives, or suppositories to which a patient is accustomed. Use of the commode, if possible, will also help to alleviate the problem.[33]

Table 14
Nonprescription and Prescription Drug Therapy to Relieve Constipation

Generic Name	Trade Name	Dosage and Administration	Comments
Bulk-Forming Agents			
Karaya gum		Oral: 5 to 10 g daily, taken with water	Nonprescription
Methylcellulose, car-boxymethylcellulose	Cologel Hydrolose	Oral: adults, 4 to 6 g daily; children over 6 yr, 1 to 1.5 g daily	Nonprescription
Mantago (psyllium) seed		Oral: adults 2-5 to 30 g daily; children over 6 yr, 1.25 to 15 g daily; add to water and drink rapidly	Nonprescription
Polycarbophil		Oral: adults, 4 to 6 g daily; children 6 to 12 yr, 1.5 to 3 g daily; 2 to 5 yr, 1 to 1.5 g daily; to 2 yr, 0.5 to 1 g daily	Nonprescription
Psyllium hydrocolloid Psyllium hydrophilic Pscilloid	Effersyllium Konsyl L A Formula Metamucil Modane Bulk	Oral: adults, 1 round teaspoon (7 g) or 1 packet; add to a glass of water and drink rapidly and then follow with a second glass of water; repeat 1 or 2 times daily if necessary	Nonprescription
Stimulant (Irritant) Cathartics			
Blacodyl	Biscolax Dulcolax Various others	Oral: adults, 10 mg, up to 30 mg may be given to clear gastrointestinal tract; children over 6 yr, 5 mg Rectal: adults and children over 2 yr, 10 mg; children under 2 yr, 5 mg	Initial response in 6 to 12 hr; nonprescription; do not take within 60 min of milk or antacids; rectal administration effective in 15 min
Cascara sagrada	Bileo-Secrin Cas-Evac	Oral: adults, 200 to 400 mg of extract; 0.5 to 1.5 ml of fluid extract or 5 ml of aromatic extract	Nonprescription; one of the mildest of the stimulant cathartics
Castor oil		Oral: adults, 15 to 60 ml; children over 2 yr, 5 to 15 ml; under 2 yr, 1 to 5 ml	Castor oil is degraded to ricinoleic acid, which is the active drug; nonprescription
Castor oil, emulsified	Neoloid	Oral: adults, 30 to 60 ml; children over 2 yr, 7.5 to 30 ml; under 2 yr, 2.5 to 7.5 ml	Nonprescription; mint flavored; turns alkaline urine pink
Damron	Anavac Danvac Dorbane Modane Weslax	Oral: adults, 75 to 150 mg; children 6 to 12 yr, 37 to 75 mg; 1 to 6 yr, 10 to 15 mg	Nonprescription; turns alkaline urine pink
Glycerine suppositories		Rectal: adults, 3 g; children under 6 yr, 1 to 1.5 g	Nonprescription; effective in 15 to 30 min
Phenolpthalein	Chocolax Exlax Feen-A-Mint	Oral: adults, 30 to 270 mg daily; children over 6 yr, 30 to 60 mg daily; 2 to 6 yr, 15 to 20 mg daily	Nonprescription; turns alkaline urine pink
Senna, whole leaf		Oral: adults, 0.5 to 2 g or 2 ml of senna fluid extract; children 6 to 12 yr, one-half adult dose; 2 to 5 yr, one-fourth adult dose; under 2 yr, one-eighth adult dose	Nonprescription
Sennosides A and B	Glysennid	Oral: adults, 12 to 24 mg at bedtime; children over 10 yr, same as adult; 6 to 10 yr, 12 mg at bedtime	Nonprescription
Saline Cathartics			
Magnesium hydroxide	Milk of magnesia	Oral: adult, 10 to 15 ml (concentrated) or 15 to 30 ml (regular)	Nonprescription
Magnesium sulfate	Epsom salt	Oral: adults, 15 g in a glass of water	Nonprescription

From Clark, J.B., Queener, S.F., and Burke-Karp, V.B.: Drugs affecting the gastrointestinal tract. In Clark, J., Queener, S., and Burke-Karp, V., editors: Pharmacological basis of nursing practice, St. Louis, 1982, The C.V. Mosby Co.   *Continued.*

Table 14, cont'd

Generic Name	Trade Name	Dosage and Administration	Comments
Monosodium phosphate	Sal Hepatica	Oral: adult, 5 to 20 ml with water	Nonprescription
Sodium phosphate		Oral: adults, 4 g in a glass of warm water	Nonprescription
Sodium phosphate with sodium biphosphate	Phospho-Soda	Oral: adults, 20 to 40 ml in a glass of cold water	Nonprescription
Lubricants			
Mineral oil	Agoral, Plain Kondremul, Plain Neo-Cultol Petrogalar, Plain	Oral: adults, 15 to 30 ml at bedtime; children, 5 to 15 ml at bedtime	Nonprescription; to ease strain of passing hard stools; should not be used regularly because the fat-soluble vitamins (A, D, E, and K) are not absorbed; response in 1 to 3 days
Fecal Softeners			
Dioctyl calcium sulfosuccinate	Surfak	Oral: adults, 50 to 360 mg daily; children, 50 to 150 mg daily	Nonprescription
Dioctyl sodium sulfosuccinate	Colace Comfolax D-D-S Various others	Oral: adults, 50 to 360 mg; children 6 to 12 yr, 40 to 120 mg; 3 to 6 yr, 20 to 60 mg; under 3 yr, 10 to 40 mg	Nonprescription

Attending Behaviors Treatment

Oral laxatives. The terms *laxative, cathartic,* and *purgative* all describe drugs that act on the large intestine. Their definitions reflect different degrees of action. A laxative is defined as a substance that promotes bowel evacuation by a mild action. It acts by increasing the bulk of feces, by softening the stool, or by lubricating the intestinal wall. On the other hand, a cathartic promotes bowel evacuation by stimulating peristalsis, increasing the fluidity or bulk of intestinal contents, softening the feces, or lubricating the intestinal wall. Cathartic means a fluid evacuation. Purgatives produce a watery stool and violent cramping, which can cause fluid and electrolyte depletion. For that reason they are no longer used in medical practice, and only stimulant cathartics are used.[9]

Clark and co-workers[9] classify laxatives as (1) bulk-forming, (2) stimulant (irritant) cathartic, (3) saline (osmotic cathartic), (4) wetting agent (softener), and (5) lubricant.

Bulk-forming laxatives. Bulk-forming laxatives provide what should be obtained through good dietary habits. Because of the increasing processing and refinement of fruits, vegetables, and grains, the American diet is very low in fiber. Laxatives in this class include bran, methylcellulose, polycarbophil, and psyllium hydrophilic mucilloid. Bulk-forming laxatives act by retaining water so that the stool increases in volume and remains soft.

An effect from bulk-forming laxatives is expected in 12 to 24 hours in a person who does not habitually use laxatives. An additional use of bulk-forming laxatives is to relieve a mild watery diarrhea by absorbing water to produce a soft stool.[9]

Stimulant-irritant cathartics. Stimulant cathartics stimulate peristalsis by irritating the mucosa, by stimulating the nerve plexus, or by direct action on smooth muscle. These drugs form a soft to fluid stool in 6 to 12 hours, depending on the dosage. Stimulant cathartics are the most abused group of laxatives because of their easy availability over the counter. When these drugs are used for more than a week, intestinal muscle tone is lost and becomes less responsive to any stimulation. Continued use can produce a diarrhea severe enough to induce dehydration through the loss of fluids and lower blood concentrations of sodium and potassium. In their discussion of stimulant cathartics Clark and associates[9] include cascara, danthron, senna, phenolphthalein, bisacodyl, castor oil, and glycerin.[9]

Table 14 describes the generic name, trade name, dosage, and administration and whether the laxative is nonprescription or prescription drug therapy.

Saline osmotic cathartics. The saline cathartics include several magnesium, sodium, and potassium salts. The most popular saline cathartics are magnesium citrate, sulfate, or hydroxide and sodium phosphate. Because these agents are incompletely absorbed, water is retained in the intestinal lumen, which leads to an increase in peristalsis. Transit time is reduced, and a semifluid stool is evacuated in 3 to 6 hours.[39]

Stool softeners (wetting agents). Stool softeners inhibit the absorption of water so that the fecal mass remains large and soft. Their advantage is that they can be used when straining at stool is to be avoided. Dioctyl calcium sulfosuccinate (Surfak) is the one most frequently used in this group. Although stool softeners are effective 24 to 48 hours after they are administered, dietary modalities may be just as effective, safer, and cheaper.

Lubricant. Mineral oil is the only laxative in this group that is used occasionally. It acts by softening stools and aids in easy passage of stools. Because the long-term effects of mineral oil interfere with the absorption of fat-soluble vitamins A, D, E, and K, it is inferior to the stool softeners, such as Surfak and Colace.[9]

Suppositories. Glycerin suppositories are a popular drug for relieving constipation in infants and adults. They act specifically on the lower bowel, but their efficacy is questionable when hard stool is present.

Bisacodyl (Dulcolax) 10 mg suppositories are frequently used in hospital settings. They are used to prepare the lower bowel for x-ray examination or surgery or to treat a single incidence of constipation.[39]

Enemas. Enemas are used when lower bowel and rectal evacuation are indicated in the management of a fecal impaction or to prepare a patient for endoscopic and radiographic tests and surgery. They should not be used regularly for the treatment of constipation. The normal saline enema is the safest, most effective, and best tolerated. Large volumes of normal saline solution, when correctly administered, cleanse the rectum and sigmoid colon with little mucosal irritation or disturbance in fluid and electrolyte balance. Disposable oil-retention enemas are frequently used in small volumes to soften a fecal impaction. Removal of the impaction is easily achieved if the oil-retention enema is followed by a normal saline enema after a period of 4 to 6 hours. Disposable hypertonic saline solution enemas (Fleet) are safe and frequently used. They contain a mixture of sodium phosphates and citrates. They are easy to self-administer and are disposable. They act by drawing water into the lumen from the body in significant quantities so that adequate fluid and electrolyte balance is maintained.[39]

EVALUATION

Patient Outcome	Data Indicating That Outcome is Reached
Describes health behaviors that prevent constipation in relation to diet, fluid, exercise	Explains the importance of a well-balanced diet, including the importance of eating breakfast Describes the importance of bulk in the diet through the ingestion of dietary fiber and bran Names 6 readily available foods high in fiber Discusses the importance of including 8-10 glasses of fluid in daily intake Recognizes and integrates daily exercise into life-style (15-minute walk/day minimum amount) Describes individual stimulus behaviors, such as warm fluids on arising or prune juice, that are helpful in initiating a bowel movement Expresses the importance of responding to the defecation urge when it arises naturally
Oral drug therapy produces a bowel movement within 12 to 24 hours	Takes oral laxative correctly Understands the desired effects of the medication Makes a correct decision if prescribed therapy is no longer effective
Bowel repatterning program to establish normal bowel functioning	Eliminates use of laxatives or enemas on a regular basis Attends to defecation urge when it arises naturally Consumes well-balanced diet, including sufficient fiber and laxative foods Relates the following process of bowel repatterning: 1. Eats large breakfast; sits on toilet 10 minutes 2. Relaxing environment; diversional activities, reading, listening to music 3. When defecation urge occurs, respond to it so it does not weaken

Patient Outcome	Data Indicating That Outcome is Reached
Describes contributing factors when known, methods to reduce contributing factors, and health behaviors to prevent constipation	Understands the physiology of defecation Names conditions that promote normal bowel functioning as well as those that contribute to the development of constipation

Constipation is a common problem encountered in all areas of nursing. Yet few nurses have a systematic approach to help people establish normal bowel functioning with minimal dependence on medication. The following section includes the overall goals, outcome criteria, and data indicating that criteria have been met for the prevention, treatment, education, and repatterning of this nursing diagnosis.

References

1. Aman, R.A.: Treating the patient, not the constipation, Am. J. Nurs. **80**(9):1634, 1980.
2. Banks, S., and Marks, I.N.: The aetiology, diagnosis and treatment of constipation and diarrhea in geriatric patients, South Afr. Med. J. **51**:409-414, 1977.
3. Bass, L.: More fiber, less constipation, Am. J. Nurs. **77**(2):254-255, 1977.
4. Battle, E.H., and Hanna, C.E.: Evaluation of a dietary regimen for chronic constipation: report of a pilot study, J. Gerontol. Nurs. **6**(9):527-532, 1980.
5. Blattner, B.: Lifestyling. In Blattner, B., editor: Holistic nursing, Englewood Cliffs, N.J., 1981, Prentice-Hall, Inc.
6. Brocklehurst, J.C.: How to define and treat constipation, Geriatrics June 1977, pp. 85-87.
7. Carpenito, L.J.: Nursing diagnosis: application to clinical practice, New York, 1983, J.B. Lippincott Co.
8. Clark, C.C.: Enhancing wellness: a guide for self-care, New York, 1981, Springer.
9. Clark, J.B., Queener, S.F., and Burke-Karp, V.B.: Drugs affecting the gastrointestinal tract. In Clark, J., Queener, S., and Burke-Karp, V., editors: Pharmacological basis of nursing practice, St. Louis, 1982, The C.V. Mosby Co.
10. Connell, A.: The effects of dietary fiber on gastrointestinal motor function, Am. J. Clin. Nutr. Oct. 1978, pp. 5152-5156.
11. Connell, A.M., and others: Variation of bowel habit in two population samples, Br. Med. J. **2**:1095-1099, 1965.
12. Cornell, S.A., and others: Comparison of three bowel management programs during rehabilitation of spinal cord injured patients, Nurs. Res. **22**:321-328, 1973.
13. Drossman, D.A., and others: Bowel patterns among subjects not seeking health care, Gastroenterology **83**:529-534, 1982.
14. Godding, E.W.: Physiological yardsticks for bowel function and the rehabilitation of the constipated bowel, Pharmacology **20**:88-103, 1980.
15. Gordon, M.: Manual of nursing diagnosis, New York, 1982, McGraw-Hill Book Co.
16. Gordon, M.: Nursing diagnosis: process and application, New York, 1982, McGraw-Hill Book Co.
17. Guyton, A.C.: Movement of food through the alimentary tract. In Guyton, A.C., editor: Textbook of medical physiology, Philadelphia, 1976, W.B. Saunders Co.
18. Hoopes, J.M., and Gunnett, A.E.: Constipation and diarrhea. In Wiener, M.B., and others, editors: Clinical pharmacology and therapeutics in nursing, New York, 1979, McGraw-Hill Book Co.
19. Hui, Y.H.: Diet and diseases of the gastrointestinal system. In Hui, Y.H., editor: Human nutrition and diet therapy, Belmont, Calif., 1983, Wadsworth.
20. Kim, M.J., McFarland, G., and McLane, A.M.: Classification of nursing diagnoses: Proceedings of the Fifth National Conference, St. Louis, 1984, The C.V. Mosby Co.
21. Kim, M.J., McFarland, G., and McLane, A.M.: Pocket guide to nursing diagnoses, St. Louis, 1984, The C.V. Mosby Co.
22. Kim, M.J., and Moritz, D.: Classification of nursing diagnoses: Proceedings of the Third and Fourth National Conferences, New York, 1982, McGraw-Hill Book Co.
23. Kirwan, W.O.: Actions of bran on colonic motility related to its physical properties, Gut **15**(10):829, 1974.
24. Krause, M.V., and Mahan, K.L.: Nutritional care in intestinal disease. In Krause, M.V., and Mahan, K.L., editors: Food, nutrition, and diet therapy, Philadelphia, 1984, W.B. Saunders Co.
25. Lindsey, A.M.: Phenomena and physiological variables of relevance to nursing: review of a decade of work. Part I, West. J. Nurs. Res. **4**:343-364, 1982.
26. Lindsey, A.M.: Phenomena and physiological variables of relevance to nursing: review of a decade of work. Part II, West. J. Nurs. Res. **5**:41-63, 1983.
27. Manning, A.P., Wyman, J.B., and Heaton, K.W.: How trustworthy are bowel histories? Comparison of recalled and recorded information, Br. Med. J. **2**:213-214, 1976.
28. Martelli, H., and others: Some parameters of large bowel motility in normal man, Gastroenterology **75**:612-618, 1978.
29. McLane, A.M., McShane, R., and Sliefert, M.: Constipation: conceptual categories of diagnostic indications. In Kim, M.J., McFarland, G., and McLane, A.M., editors: Classification of nursing diagnoses: Proceedings of the Fifth National Conference, St. Louis, 1984, The C.V. Mosby Co.
30. McLane, A.M., and McShane, R.: Bowel elimination practices of healthy adults, Unpublished manuscript.
31. Narrow, B.W., and Buschle, K.B.: Elimination. In Narrow, B.W., and Busehle, K.B., editors: Fundamentals of nursing practice, New York, 1982, John Wiley & Sons, Inc.
32. Padilla, G.V., and Baker, V.E.: Variables affecting the preparation of the bowel for radiologic examination, Nurs. Res. **21**:305-311, 1972.
33. Phipps, W.J., Long, B.C., and Woods, N.F.: Mechanisms for maintaining dynamic equilibrium. In Phipps W.J., Long B.C., and Woods N.F., editors: Medical-surgical nursing concepts and clinical practice, St. Louis, 1983, The C.V. Mosby Co.
34. Pollman, J.W., Morris, J.J., and Rose, P.: Is fiber the answer to constipation problems in the elderly? A review of literature, Int. J. Nurs. Studies **15**:107-114, 1978.
35. Rabb, R.R.: Constipation and laxative abuse, West. J. Med. **122**:93-96, 1975.
36. Roach, J.J. Constipation, J. Nat. Med. Assoc. **70**:591-596, 1978.
37. Rutter, K., and Maxwell, D.: Diseases of the alimentary system: constipation and laxative abuse, Br. Med. J. **2**:997-1000, 1976.
38. Sklar, M.: Functional bowel distress and constipation in the aged, Geriatrics Sept. 1972, pp. 79-85.
39. Weiner, M.B., and others, editors: Clinical pharmacology and therapeutics in nursing, New York, 1979, McGraw-Hill Book Co.
40. Wichita, C.: Treating and preventing constipation in nursing home residents, J. Gerontol. Nurs. **6**:35-39, 1977.
41. Wyman, J.B., and others: Variability of colonic function in healthy subjects, Gut **19**:146-150, 1978.
42. Zimring, J.G.: High-fiber diet versus laxatives in geriatric patients, N.Y. State J. Med. Dec. 1976, pp. 2223-2224.

BOWEL ELIMINATION, ALTERATION IN: DIARRHEA
THEORY AND ETIOLOGY

Diarrhea is the frequent passage of loose or watery stools. Consistency is a more reliable indicator of diarrhea than frequency, since there is general agreement that loose or watery stools are abnormal.[19] "Quantitatively, diarrhea is defined as the passage of over 200 g of stool per day containing 70% to 90% water. . . . Normal stool is 60%-80% water, and an increase in daily rectal water excretion of 100 to 200 ml will markedly alter the frequency and consistency of bowel movements."[2] Acute diarrhea is usually self-limiting, lasting 24 to 48 hours, whereas chronic diarrhea persists for several weeks or is intermittently present for several weeks.

The incidence of diarrhea in the general population is unknown. In a sample of 301 healthy volunteers 3.7% reported frequent runny stools and 26.7 reported occasional runny stools.[19] The 14 subjects comprising the frequent group reported loose or watery stools on more than 25% of occasions. They had 12.6 ± 1.8 bowel movements per week when compared with the 8.6 ± 0.2 in the remainder. The elderly are especially intolerant of diarrhea. In a retrospective study of 100 consecutive hospital admissions of the elderly for diarrhea, Pentland and Pennington[17] reported that 65 were admitted within 1 week of the onset of symptoms.

Common causes of acute diarrhea are infection, drug reactions, and major alterations in diet. The majority of cases of diarrhea occur secondary to infection or the ingestion of toxins. Although viral infections account for most cases of diarrhea, food poisoning caused by improper cooking or mishandling of food is frequently the offending agent. Bacteria implicated in food poisoning include *Staphylococcus aureus, Clostridium perfringens, Salmonella* organisms, *Campylobacter fetus,* and *Escherichia coli* (traveler's diarrhea). Traveler's diarrhea can also be caused by protozoan-infected drinking water *(Giardia lamblia).* Bloody diarrhea, usually of small volume, is associated with shigellosis, amoebic colitis, and ischemic colitis.[6]

Causes of chronic diarrhea include irritable bowel syndrome, lactase deficiency, cancer of the colon, inflammatory bowel disease, gastrointestinal surgery, radiation enterocolitis, malabsorption diseases, and laxative abuse. Functional diarrhea is a subset of irritable bowel syndrome and is characterized by alternating diarrhea and constipation with bloating and abdominal pain. Lactose intolerance produces symptoms similar to those of irritable bowel syndrome with cramping, flatulence, and diarrhea associated with ingestion of milk sugars. Another diet-induced type of diarrhea is produced by the sudden ingestion of fruits and vegetables containing large quantities of long-chain carbohydrates, which are incompletely digested in the small intestine.[2]

Persistent or chronic diarrhea is frequently thought to have a functional or psychogenic basis but may be the consequence of limited understanding of the mechanisms producing diarrhea. The diarrhea is often accompanied by fecal incontinence, a psychologically disabling symptom. In a study[14] of 76 consecutive patients with diarrhea, 39, or 51%, had incontinence. Only 19 of the 39 volunteered the information; the remaining admitted to incontinence only after careful questioning. Persons with a medical history of diabetes, anorectal surgery (hemorrhoidectomy), or trauma are more likely to experience fecal incontinence as a complication of diarrhea.[18]

In a prospective study of 100 consecutive patients with the dominant symptom of diarrhea, Bolin, Davis, and Duncombe[1] made a diagnosis of irritable bowel syndrome in 28 patients.[2] An etiological factor in 40% of the 28 patients was lactase deficiency. Organic causes for the persistent diarrhea were found in another 52 patients. Weight loss, rectal bleeding, and symptoms in childhood were historical factors that implicated an organic cause. Alcohol abuse or drug ingestion, including laxative abuse, was identified as the basis of symptoms in 10 subjects.

Compromised defense mechanisms, both nonimmune and immune factors, contribute to an increased incidence of diarrhea in the elderly. The nonimmune factors include a decline in stomach acid production, which permits substantial bacterial overgrowth; changes in intestinal microflora resulting from antibiotic therapy; changes in intestinal motility associated with diabetic neuropathy and regular use of drugs, especially anticholinergics, which alter intestinal clearance of bacteria; gastrointestinal surgery; travel; and institutionalization. Immune mechanisms include deficiencies in both cell-mediated immunity and antibody production.[17]

In two separate studies of 100 subjects, one prospective with an age range of 15 to 82 years[1] and one retrospective with a mean age of 80 years,[16] antibiotics were implicated as an etiological factor more frequently than any other single drug with the exception of laxatives. In the latter study five subjects developed diarrhea following courses of broad-spectrum antibiotic therapy, and two developed pseudomembranous colitis after treatment with clindamycin. Laxative abuse was implicated in 4 of 10 subjects, with drug use as a factor, in the first study and in 6 of 17 subjects in the second. A variety of other drugs fall into the miscellaneous category and include digitalis (toxicity), indomethacin, gold, guanethidine, and methyldopa.

Etiological factors were not identified for 28 subjects in the first study and for 34 in the second. Surreptitious laxative abuse has been reported in the literature and may account for some subjects in whom etiological factors were not identified. In a case report of a 54-year-old woman with a 6-month history of diarrhea, Morris and Turnberg[15] described the woman's denial when given the evidence of taking laxatives as not deliberate but as some form of internal block. "All the features of hysterical behavior, including the capacity for self-deception, lack of insight, and manipulation of relatives, friends and physicians, often in the absence of an obvious motive for gain, may be detected in surreptitious laxative abusers."

Etiologies for diarrhea are as follows:

Acute diarrhea
   Diet alteration
   Drug reactions
   Spoiled food
   Ingestion of toxins
   Infection
Chronic diarrhea
   Irritable bowel syndrome
   Lactase deficiency
   Cancer of the colon
   Inflammatory bowel disease
   Gastrointestinal surgery
   Radiation
   Malabsorption diseases
   Laxative abuse
   Chemotherapeutic agents

DEFINING CHARACTERISTICS

Abdominal pain
Cramping
Increased stool frequency
Increased frequency of bowel sounds
Loose, liquid stools
Urgency

Diarrhea has appeared as a diagnostic label on the list of accepted diagnoses of the National Group for classification of Nursing Diagnoses (NANDA) since the First National Conference in 1973. The original label—bowel function, irregular: diarrhea—was changed to bowel elimination, alteration in: diarrhea at the Second National Conference in 1975, and the label remained unchanged during succeeding conferences.[10-12] The conference participants did not submit an agreed on definition of diarrhea.

Several authors who contribute regularly to the nursing diagnosis literature formulated definitions of diarrhea, but there is no normative definition. Gordon[7] defines diarrhea as loose, fluid stools not associated with a pathologic state. She limits nurses to diagnosing and treating diarrhea that has food intolerance as the etiology. Carpenito[4] lists many etiologies but limits treatment to persons experiencing diarrhea caused by tube feedings, dietary indiscretions, or food allergies. In addition, she includes persons at high risk of experiencing frequent passage of liquid or unformed stool in her definition. The inclusion of at-risk statements in definitions serves to cloud rather than clarify the nature of the phenomenon.

OTHER DEFINING CHARACTERISTICS

The only other defining characteristic listed by Kim and Moritz[13] is changes in color. With some minor changes in wording, Gordon's defining characteristics[10-12] are identical with those listed in the official publications. Carpenito[4] includes weakness and observable signs of dehydration (under assessment data rather than defining characteristics) and also specifies that frequent stools means more than three times daily.

None of these nurse authors mentions the volume of diarrheal fluid, which Doe[6] considers an important indicator of the mechanism of the diarrhea. Stools of high volume, often exceeding 1 L a day, suggest a small intestinal origin for the diarrhea whereas a small stool volume suggests a colonic origin, as does the presence of bright blood and mucus. Doe associated tenesmus and urgency with rectal inflammation, periumbilical, colicky pain with small intestines, and lower abdominal pain on the left side as colonic in origin.[6]

NURSING INTERVENTIONS

Patient Goal	Nursing Intervention
Achieve relief of symptoms.	Provide instructions for: 1. Use of antidiarrhea medications 2. Modifications of diet 3. Perirectal skin care

Patient Goal	Nursing Intervention
	Assess/monitor hydration.
	Assess/monitor body weight.
Take prescribed medications.	Provide instructions for use of antidiarrhea medications.
	Assist with implementation of medication taking as part of activities of daily living.
	Assess/monitor side effects of medications.
Decrease number of episodes of diarrhea.	Provide instructions for:
	1. Use of food and elimination diary
	2. Personal hygiene measures, such as hand-washing techniques

The goals of nursing care include prevention, treatment, health teaching, and repatterning of bowel elimination. Although these categories are not mutually exclusive, they do provide a framework for considering various aspects of the problem that fall within the domain of nursing.

Prevention begins with a determination of the etiology or mechanism of the diarrhea, maintenance of fluid, electrolyte and nutritional status, and assessment of the need for health teaching. An accurate and detailed history must be taken, including assessment of usual and altered bowel elimination pattern, dietary habits, food intolerances and recent food ingestion, travel, symptoms, stool characteristics, including volume, color, and frequency, and the effect of diarrhea on the usual pattern of daily living. Stool cultures for organisms, cysts, and blood should be obtained if the diarrhea persists.

Treatment of acute diarrhea is focused on management of symptoms, elimination of the offending agent, and physician referral when indicated. Antidiarrheal drugs are not recommended for routine use in acute infectious diarrhea, since they may delay the natural eradication of the infection.[13] Physician referrals should be made when specific drug therapy is needed, when the diarrhea persists for more than 3 days, when the stool contains blood or has the appearance of steatorrhea, and when patients admit to fecal incontinence. Diarrhea associated with the use of antiinfective agents is normally alleviated when the offending agent is withdrawn. However, some persons continue to have diarrhea associated with cramps, tenderness, and fever because of an overgrowth of anaerobic organisms and/or the presence of their toxins. Physician consultation is suggested, since the individual may have developed pseudomembranous colitis. Tube feeding–induced diarrhea can be controlled by the use of Metamucil or by adjusting the type of tube feeding. Lactose-intolerant individuals will experience immediate relief when all lactose is removed from their diet. Although this may seem a simple solution, the actual implementation of a lactose-free diet is complicated by the presence of powdered whey and nonfat dry milk in many food products, including crackers, cookies, cereals, and sausages. Maintaining an adequate fluid and caloric intake may be difficult in more severe cases of diarrhea, and hospitalization for intravenous replacement of fluid and electrolytes might be required.

The type of health teaching required is unique to the situation and the patient. Initially, sufficient information should be given to the patient and family to help them understand the nature of the problem, treatment objectives, and rationale for laboratory studies, drugs, and supportive care. The patient's history and results of microbiologic studies provide a guide for other patient education programs designed to improve safe handling of food, hand-washing techniques, and understanding of the mechanisms of disease transmission at home and when traveling in foreign countries.

In developing countries diarrhea is a leading cause of morbidity and mortality among people who live with hunger and poverty. Social programs aimed at developing a safe supply of water and proper sewage disposal must accompany any personal or group health teaching. How to prepare and use an oral rehydration salt solution (ORS), such as the one recommended by the World Health Organization or the cheaper and more readily available labon-gur (brown sugar and salt) solutions,[9] should be incorporated in all teaching programs.

Repatterning of health practices related to bowel elimination that coincide with a patient's defined normal pattern usually occurs spontaneously, since the majority of cases of acute diarrhea are self-limiting. Those patients requiring drug therapy may expect to have relief of symptoms in 7 to 10 days. If the diarrhea is caused by an impaction, a common etiological factor in the elderly, attention must be given to all factors that influence bowel elimination, especially food and fluid intake, exercise, and the individual's response to the stimulus to have a bowel movement. Persons with chronic diarrhea associated with irritable bowel syndrome may benefit from individual and group counseling and from learning stress reduction techniques, such as systematic relaxation. It is important to remember that an individual's bowel elimination pattern is a reflection of the total life process and is not comprised of isolated physiologic events.

EVALUATION

Patient Outcome	Data Indicating That Outcome is Reached
Number and consistency of stools within normal limits	No more than three bowel movements per day Stool is formed and easy to pass
Adequate dietary intake	Skin well hydrated Urinary output maintained at 50 ml/hour Body weight stabilized within normal limits
Pain relief	No complaints of abdominal pain or discomfort
Decrease in episodes of fecal incontinence	Seeks medical consultation for evaluation of fecal incontinence Keeps a record of incontinent episodes
Perirectal skin normal in appearance	Absence of areas of redness, itching, and irritation in perirectal area
Plans to take medications	Schedules taking medications as part of daily activities
Reports side effect of medications to health professional	Verbalizes actions, dosages, and side effects of medications
Understands mechanism of diarrhea	Describes factors associated with diarrhea Lists two changes in health practices that will affect bowel elimination pattern, such as washing hands after use of toilet, reading labels on food products to avoid ingestion of lactose

References

1. Bolin, T.D., Davis, A.E., and Duncombe, V.M.: A prospective study of persistent diarrhea, Aust. N.Z. J. Med. **12**:22-26, 1982.
2. Bond, J.H.: Office-based management of diarrhea, Geriatrics **37**:52-64, Feb. 1982.
3. Burakoff, R.: An updated look at diverticular disease, Geratrics **36**:83-91, March 1981.
4. Carpenito, L.J.: Nursing diagnosis: application to clinical practice, New York, 1983, J.B. Lippincott Co.
5. Chernoff, R., and Dean, J.A.: Medical and nutritional aspects of intractable diarrhea, J. Am. Dietet. Assoc. **76**:161-169, 1980.
6. Doe, W.V., and Barr, G.D.: Acute diarrhea in adults, Austr. Family Physician **10**:438-446, June 1981.
7. Gordon, M.: Manual of nursing diagnosis, New York, 1982, McGraw-Hill Book Co.
8. Hobsley, M.: Dumping and diarrhea, Br. J. Surg. **68**:681-684, 1981.
9. International reflections, Health Values: Achieving High Level Wellness **7**:32, July/Aug. 1983.
10. Islam, M.R., and others: Labon-gur (common salt and brown sugar) oral rehydration solution in the treatment of diarrhea in adults, J. Trop. Med. Hygiene **83**:41-45, 1980.
11. Kim, M.J., McFarland, G.K., and McLane, A.M.: Pocket guide to nursing diagnoses, St. Louis, 1984, The C.V. Mosby Co.
12. Kim, M.J., McFarland, G.K., and McLane, A.M.: Classification of nursing diagnoses: Proceedings of the Fifth National Conference, St. Louis, 1984, The C.V. Mosby Co.
13. Kim, M.J., and Moritz, D.A.: Classification of nursing diagnoses: Proceedings of the Third and Fourth National Conferences, St. Louis, 1982, The C.V. Mosby Co.
14. Kronborg, I.J., and Wall, A.J.: Diagnosis and management of acute diarrhoea in adults, Austr. Family Physician **7**:1453-1460, Nov. 1978.
15. Leigh, R.J., and Turnberg, L.A.: Faecal incontinence: the unvoiced symptom, Lancet June 12, 1982. pp. 1349-1351.
16. Morris, A.I., and Turnberg, L.A.: Surreptitious laxative abuse, Gastroenterology **77**:780-786, 1979.
17. Pentland, B., and Pennington, C.R.: Acute diarrhoea in the elderly, Age and Aging **9**:90-92, 1980.
18. Ravdin, J.I., and Guerrant, R.L.: Infectious diarrhea in the elderly, Geratrics **38**:95-101, April 1983.
19. Read, N.W., and others: A clinical study of patients with fecal incontinence, Gastroenterology **76**:747-756, 1979.
20. Thompson, W.G., and Heaton, K.W.: Functional bowel disorders in apparently healthy people, Gastroenterology **79**:283-288, 1980.
21. Tilson, M.D.: Pathophysiology and treatment of short bowel syndrome, Surg. Clin. North Am. **69**:1273-1284, Oct. 1980.

BOWEL ELIMINATION, ALTERATION IN: INCONTINENCE
THEORY AND ETIOLOGY

Anal continence is maintained by the combined actions of the puborectalis muscle, the external and internal anal sphincters, and the rectum, although the mechanism is not clearly understood. According to Dickinson,[2] the puborectalis sling is the most important muscle in the system, and damage to it produces major defects of continence. Sensory pathways from the anorectal region that provide awareness of rectal filling and the urge to defecate are also of importance in the maintenance of continence. Persons at high risk for becoming incontinent are the elderly, persons with a low level of awareness, patients with a long-standing dependence on suppositories, individuals with neurologic abnormalities regardless of age, diabetic patients with neuropathy, patients with chronic diarrhea, persons with a history of rectal surgery, especially hemorrhoidectomy, and those with a history of trauma to the lumbosacral area.

Three abnormal patterns were found in a study of 24 women and 5 men, 19 to 74 years of age, with diarrhea and fecal incontinence.[11] Sphincter pressures, stool volume, and incontinence to rectally infused saline were used to differentiate the three patterns. The majority of the subjects were in a category characterized by low sphincter pressures, impaired continence to saline, and small stool volumes. The second pattern was characterized by normal sphincter pressures, low stool volume, and impaired incontinence to infused saline. Persons in the third category had normal sphincter pressures, good continence to infused saline, but very large amounts of daily stool. The authors recommend preoperative tests to predict susceptibility to fecal incontinence for liquids in persons undergoing elective surgery that could result in diarrhea, such as vagotomy and jejunoileal bypass. They also recommend avoidance of rectal surgery for persons with diarrhea and others at high risk.

Fecal incontinence with diarrhea was described as the "unvoiced symptom" by Leigh and Turnberg,[10] who studied 76 consecutive patients referred to a gastrointestinal clinic with a complaint of diarrhea. Thirty-nine (51%) had incontinence, but only 19 volunteered the information spontaneously. Reluctance to admit to fecal incontinence was probably associated with embarrassment.

Fecal incontinence is often functionally disabling.[10,11] Social isolation and depression may occur as individuals attempt to cope with odor and continence aids by remaining at home. Patients in long-term care agencies also tend to withdraw from social interaction as they attempt to deal not only with the incontinence but also with the reactions of personnel who continually face the unpleasant task of "cleaning up."

Despite the magnitude of the problem in terms of human suffering and the consumption of nursing and other health care resources needed to manage incontinent individuals, few clinical reports and empirical studies have appeared in the nursing literature. In a recent review of incontinence in the elderly, Wolanin[13] cited four studies of urinary incontinence and none of bowel incontinence.

Bowel management programs are designed to reduce the unpredictability of fecal incontinence and provide individuals with more security from episodes of incontinence. Sixty patients undergoing rehabilitation for spinal injuries (52 men and 8 women) were randomly assigned to one of three bowel training protocols: irritant contact bowel medications, bowel stimulant medications,

and a mechanical evacuation procedure.[1] Criteria used to determine the effectiveness of the bowel training protocol included the number of minutes from stimulation to evacuation, the number of times evacuation did not occur, and the number of accidental evacuations. The third method, mechanical evacuation, was found to be the most effective after the first week of the program. Habeeb and Kallstrom[7] used a nonresidue diet to reduce the number and unpredictability of incontinent episodes in nine men in a long-term care institution for the disabled. The diet plus vitamin and mineral supplements, daily doses of dioctyl sodium sulfosuccinate, and a weekly bisacodyl suppository to promote evacuation was successful in producing one predictable stool per week after 2 months of the program. Other benefits of the program included weight gain and elimination of episodes of fecal impaction. Staff reactions to the altered bowel routine and family reactions to the altered diet created unanticipated problems during implementation of the program. Nurses found it difficult to change ritualistic bowel routines, and families complained about food restrictions.

The following are etiologies for this diagnosis:
Autoimmune diseases such as myasthenia gravis
CNS disruptions such as stroke
Cogitive-perceptual impairment
Demyelinating diseases
Depression
Diarrhea
Fecal impaction
Loss of sphincter control
Musculoskeletal involvement
Neuromuscular involvement
Severe anxiety
Spinal cord injuries (transient or permanent)

DEFINING CHARACTERISTICS

Involuntary passage of stool
Embarrassed conduct
Fecal odor
Stained clothing
Stained bed linens
Decrease in social interaction
Washed underwear

Incontinence has appeared as a diagnostic label on the list of accepted diagnoses since the Second National Conference.[4] The label Bowel elimination, alteration in: incontinence has remained unchanged. Only one defining characteristic, involuntary passage of stool, was listed in the reports of the Second, Third, Fourth, and Fifth National Conferences[4,8,9] and in pocket guides by other authors.[3,6] Additional signs and symptoms identified by Wolanin[14] include stained clothing or beds, washed underwear, embarrassed conduct, refusal to participate in social activities or to leave the room, and withdrawal. Gettrust, Ryan, and Engelman[5] listed observed incontinence, states inability to be continent, and urgency as defining characteristics. Descriptive and validation studies are needed to refine both the etiologies and defining characteristics of the diagnosis of incontinence.

NURSING INTERVENTIONS

Patient Goal	Nursing Intervention
Elimination or reduction of episodes of incontinence.	Reduce or eliminate contributing factors when possible Teach alternate contraction and relaxation of pelvic floor muscles Ingest foods/fluids consistent with bowel elimination program
Prevention of skin breakdown.	Wash area, rinse, and dry after each incontinent episode
Repatterning	

Regular elimination of fecal contents (usually every other day).	Implement bowel retraining program:
	    Initiate when bowel sounds return and ileus is resolved
	    Establish evacuation schedule consistent with patient/family preferences
	    Teach patient/family use of laxatives and stool softeners to aid timing of defecation

Promotion of self-esteem, personal integrity, and social functioning.	Use incontinence aids temporarily until elimination pattern is established Changes clothes immediately after an incontinent episode

The psychologic responses of persons to fecal incontinence, embarrassment, social isolation, loss of self-esteem, and depression are similar to those discussed in the section on urinary incontinence (see p. 2075). Reestablishment of continence through a successful bowel training program and the assistance of supportive, understanding nurses who provide privacy and an unhurried atmosphere are the key elements in the treatment of incontinence. The type of bowel retraining program selected for a patient depends on the etiology of the incontinence and the preferences of the patient and family. Retraining a cord-injured patient is delayed until bowel sounds have returned and paralytic ileus is resolved.

EVALUATION

Patient Outcome	Data Indicating That Outcome is Reached
Amount and number of stools fall within normal limits	Regular evacuation of bowel contents Rare episodes of incontinence
Perirectal skin is normal in appearance	Absence of areas of redness, itching, and irritation in perirectal area
Reestablishes patterns of social interaction	Engages in social activities Engages in planning future goals Free of odor

References

1. Cornell, S.A., and others: Comparison of three bowel management programs during rehabilitation of spinal cord injured patients, Nurs. Res. **22**:321-328, 1973.
2. Dickinson, V.A.: Maintenance of anal continence: a review of pelvic floor physiology, Gut **19**:1163-1174, 1970.
3. Doenges, M., and Moorhouse, M.F.: Nurse's pocket guide: nursing diagnoses with interventions, Philadelphia, 1985, F.A. Davis.
4. Gebbie, K.M.: Summary of the Second National Conference: classification of nursing diagnoses, St. Louis, 1976, Clearinghouse–National Group for Classification of Nursing Diagnoses.
5. Gettrust, K.V., Ryan, S.C., and Engelman, D.S.: Applied nursing diagnoses: guides for comprehensive care planning, New York, 1985, John Wiley & Sons, Inc.
6. Gordon, M.: Manual of nursing diagnosis, New York, 1982, McGraw-Hill.
7. Habeeb, M.C., and Kallstrom, M.D.: Bowel program for institutionalized adults, Am. J. Nurs. **76**:606-608, 1976.
8. Kim, M.J., McFarland, G.K., and McLane, A.M.: Pocket guide to nursing diagnoses, St. Louis, 1984, The C.V. Mosby Co.
9. Kim, M.J., and Moritz, D.A.: Classification of nursing diagnoses:

proceedings of the Third and Fourth National Conferences, New York, 1982, McGraw-Hill.

10. Leigh, R.J., and Turnberg, L.A.: Faecal incontinence: the unvoiced symptom, Lancet, pp. 1349-1351, June 12, 1982.

11. Read, N.W., and others: A clinical study of patients with fecal incontinence, Gastroenterology **76**:747-756, 1979.

12. Rudy, E.B.: Advanced neurological and neurosurgical nursing, St. Louis, 1984, The C.V. Mosby Co.

13. Wolanin, M.D.: Confusion: prevention and care, St. Louis, 1981, The C.V. Mosby Co.

14. Wolanin, M.O.: Clinical geriatric nursing research. In Werley, H.H., and Fitzpatrick, J.J., editors: Annual review of nursing research, vol. 1, New York, 1983, Springer.

URINARY ELIMINATION, ALTERATION IN PATTERNS: INCONTINENCE

THEORY AND ETIOLOGY

Incontinence is a condition characterized by the involuntary escape of urine from the lower urinary tract to a degree that a social and hygienically unacceptable situation is imposed on the individual. It is a symptom of a number of underlying conditions that affect the anatomy and innervation of the lower urinary tract.[4] Many etiologies produce incontinence. It is important, when planning a successful program to reestablish continence and decrease the frequency of uncontrolled urinating, that the exact cause be established. However, the person is given help with the immediate problem first.[17]

Urinary incontinence is a common disorder, and various estimates have revealed that many more people experience the problem than was previously recognized. Incontinence of urine affects all age groups from infancy to old age. Feneley, Thomas, and Blannin[7] reported that normal healthy individuals may experience an occasional episode of urinary loss.[7] They reported a 58% incidence of stress incontinence among 1300 college women, including 5% who experienced the problem regularly. In addition, they reported a similar study of 4211 young, healthy nursing students who had never been pregnant. The results of this study showed that 50.7% had some degree of stress incontinence, and 16.7% cited a daily incidence. No one in the sample sought medical advice either because of embarrassment or because they did not think their problem was abnormal.

Control of urine is required for social survival, and it has been described as one of the essentials for survival in old age. The healthy older person tends to pass urine more frequently and will have a degree of urgency. Although two researchers reported that increasing age does not necessarily cause incontinence,[9,23] Shepard, Tribe, and Torrens[19] estimated that one in three women and one in 10 men over the age of 55 years suffer from urinary incontinence.[19] Some researchers contend that 10% to 15% of the adult population may have an unstable bladder, that is, one that contracts involuntarily in particular situations.[23]

Urinary problems are considered a very personal and private problem. If the problem cannot be managed, it can lead to isolation from family and friends. Every activity of daily living can be interrupted, and the problem can cause fear of the company of others at home, school, or work. In addition, urinary incontinence is one of the leading causes of admissions to nursing homes. Wells[23] reported that 55% of the total number of patients in skilled nursing facilities (long-term care facility improvement study) were described as being incontinent of urine.[23]

Cycle of Micturition

Urination (micturition) is the process by which the urinary bladder empties itself when it becomes filled. Basically, the bladder progressively fills, causing increased tension in the bladder walls.[13] When the tension in the walls rises above a threshold value, a nervous reflex, the micturition reflex causes micturition or at least a conscious desire to urinate. As the bladder approaches fullness, many superimposed micturition contractions begin to appear. These contractions are a result of a stretch reflex that is initiated by stretch receptors in the bladder wall and proximal urethra. Sensory signals are conducted to the sacral portion of the spinal cord through the pelvic nerves and then back again to the bladder through the parasympathetic fibers. The micturition reflex is self-regenerative, that is, initial bladder contraction further activates receptors to cause a still further increase in afferent impulses from the bladder, which causes increasing reflex contraction of the bladder. This cycle repeats itself again and again until the bladder has reached a strong degree of contraction. Then, within a few seconds to more than a minute, the reflex fatigues and the regenerative cycle of the micturition reflex stops, allowing rapid reduction in bladder contractions. In other words, the micturition reflex is a single complete cycle of (1) progressively rapid increase in pressure, (2) a period of sustained pressure, and (3) return to basal bladder tone pressure.

Once a micturition reflex occurs and does not succeed in emptying the bladder, the nervous elements generally remain in an inhibited state for several minutes or as long as an hour before another micturition reflex occurs. However, as the bladder becomes more distended, micturition reflexes occur more frequently and powerfully. The micturition reflex is a completely automatic spinal cord reflex, but it can be inhibited or facilitated by higher centers in the brain. For this reason, the higher centers partially inhibit micturition except when there is a desire to urinate, or to prevent urination by continual contraction of the external urinary sphincter until a convenient time. When the time arrives, the higher centers facilitate the sacral micturition centers to initiate a micturition reflex and inhibit the external urinary sphincter so that urination is possible.[13]

Guyton[13] defines abnormalities of micturition as the atonic bladder, the automatic bladder, and uninhibited bladder. The atonic bladder results from destruction of sensory nerve fibers from the bladder to the spinal cord. This prevents transmission of stretch signals from the bladder and prevents micturition reflex contractions. Consequently, the person loses all bladder control despite intact efferent fibers from the spinal cord to the bladder and regardless of intact neurogenic connections with the brain. The bladder then fills to capacity and overflows a few drops at a time through the urethra. Guyton calls this overflow dribbling. A common cause of this condition is crushing injuries to the sacral portion of the spinal cord. A less frequent occurrence is widespread syphilis.

The second abnormality defined by Guyton is the automatic bladder. This occurs if the spinal cord is damaged above the sacral region but the sacral segments are still intact. Typical micturition reflexes still occur, but they are no longer controllable by the brain. It is interesting that stimulating the skin in the genital area can sometimes elicit the micturition reflex when this condition occurs, thereby providing a means by which some patients still can control urination.

The uninhibited neurogenic bladder results in frequent uncontrollable urination. This condition is caused by damage to the spinal cord or brainstem that interrupts the inhibitory signals. Facilitory impulses passing continually down the cord keep the sacral centers so excitable that even very small amounts of urine will initiate an uncontrollable micturition reflex.

Classification of Causes

A classification of urinary incontinence that Willington[24,25] presented as a working concept divides incontinence into three broad etiological divisions: (1) central nervous system causes, including neurogenic and psychogenic causes; (2) genitourinary causes, including any organic lesion affecting the bladder, genitalia, and associated muscles; this group is the largest and includes stress incontinence; and (3) spurious causes, divided into iatrogenic (resulting from treatment) and associated factors that refer mainly to locomotor incompetence or loss of manual dexterity.

Central nervous system causes. Willington[24,25] further subdivides neurogenic causes into uninhibited, automatic, autonomous, and hypoesthetic. Unhibited causes refers to loss of conscious inhibition. Areas of the cerebrum associated with bladder activity are the cortex, basal ganglia, hypothalamus, and medulla. Characteristic patterns of bladder action in the elderly include a diminished ability to inhibit urination, resulting in precipitous voiding, and often a small contracted hyperactive bladder. In addition, poor neuromuscular action often produces incomplete emptying of the bladder. These effects are probably the result of impairment in the cerebral control of urination.[24,25]

Automatic causes mean uncontrolled voiding of large amounts infrequently due to reflex action of the spinal cord. This effect accompanies lesions of the spinal cord above the level of L2. Autonomous causes are related to a breakdown of the primary reflex arc. Defective automatic emptying occurs based on local connections of the vesical plexus in the bladder wall. Hypoesthetic causes are related to damaged sensory nerves from the bladder. The primary part of the reflex arc is damaged, and a large hypotonic bladder results. The motor fibers are intact. Sensations of fullness are impaired, which results in a large bladder with overflow incontinence.

Sutherland[22] and Bartol[2] described the psychologic mechanisms surrounding incontinence and categorized them as reactions of the person to the symptom and reactions of their caregivers.

Reactions of the person

1. *Regression.* Temper tantrums and emotional lability may occur in a hospitalized child or in an older person who is coping with sequential losses in life.
2. *Dependency.* A situation of role reversal can occur when older adults are put in dependent position, such as a bedfast state. Frequently, the caretaker assumes the role of surrogate mother, and dependency can develop.
3. *Rebellion.* This may occur as an expression of hostility against the system that places the person in the situation.
4. *Insecurity.* Insecurity can accompany a dramatic change of environment, such as admission to an acute or long-term care facility. The attendant anxieties and fears of old age may also be contributing factors.
5. *Attention-seeking.* This may be a response to the insecurity arising from feelings of rejection, abandonment, or neglect. It may also be a manipulative way of seeking attention.
6. *Disturbance of conditioned reflexes.* Performance

of the act of urination in an unaccustomed position with unfamiliar equipment and lack of privacy may contribute to incontinence.

7. *Sensory deprivation*. The frequent reduction in sensory stimulation in old age and the progressive lessening of a stimulating relationship in hospitalized persons may contribute to perceptual decrements.

8. *Symptom selection*. Emotional complications are more prevalent in older persons than in younger ones because the bladder in old age is more vulnerable. Cystometric studies in the aged, regardless of continence or incontinence, indicate a reduction in bladder capacity.

The psychologic reactions of the person to incontinence are uncertainty, insecurity, and perceived lack of support. Incontinent persons are filled with shame and guilt because of the burdens they are inflicting on others. In incontinent persons suffering from depression, self-punishing responses become more intense. They may feel their loss of urinary control is punishment for previous "bad" acts and that they are committing further offenses against society by the "filthy" behavior. Insecurity is further increased because of fear of damaging relationships that are already tenuous. This may lead to increased vulnerability and further social isolation and sensory deprivations. Tendency to develop apathy about their incontinence can easily be engendered by nurses who feel they are helping the person by dismissing the symptom completely. This may lessen the anxiety in a destructive way, since by implication they would be acknowledging the irreversibility of the symptom.[22]

Reactions of nurses and other caregivers. The person who is incontinent will be involved primarily with three groups of people: family members, friends, and nurses. The first automatic reaction to incontinence is one of aversion and revulsion. Healthy disgust is a normal reaction to the situation. A more serious problem is guilt feelings generated by the disgust.[2] Many nurses have allowed themselves to become thoroughly conditioned to avoid such feelings. If nurses do not feel free to discuss their reactions openly and honestly, it only adds to the intensity of the conflict situation. Where caregivers are family members, the situation is similar except that the unexpressed negative feelings are not the result of conditioning but grow out of respect and love for the parent or relative. The conflict becomes more intense if unconscious parent-child experiences are rekindled.[21] Bartol[2] warns of a repressive dependency developing if the caretaker compensates by reaction-formation. Guilt feelings are buried by overindulging, being ultrapermissive, and becoming excessively caring toward the incontinent individual. Other common reactions are that unexpressed negative feelings become displaced onto the incontinent person or buried at an unconscious level to lessen anxiety. Both reactions are likely to occur if there is no outlet for

caregivers to discuss their feelings in an honest and open way.[2]

Additional consequences of intractable incontinence described by Sutherland[21] and Bartol[2] that produce hostility and anger include the following:

1. Heavy expenses in terms of time, energy, resources, and supplies
2. Difficulty staffing units where there is a high level of incontinence
3. Treating the symptom of incontinence by concentrating on reduction of unpleasant effects rather than focusing on rehabilitating the whole person
4. Loss of sensitivity for a person's right to respect, privacy, care, and emotional support

Research and nursing diagnoses. Incontinence is an enormous concern for the incontinent individual, the family, and caregivers. In a critical review of nursing research on the topic, Wolonin[26] reported that several studies of incontinence and behavior modification or operant conditioning did not take the problem of organic dysfunction into account. The studies are 14 years old and have not been followed by any subsequent published work, although incontinence is a major problem in long-term care. Stevenson[21] reported a study conducted by Catanzaro of 126 persons with urinary bladder dysfunction secondary to multiple sclerosis. Nearly all of the respondents had stopped participating in community activities such as attending church and social functions. The result was an isolated life-style, lowered self-concept, and fixation on the urinary incontinence and its management aspects. Catanzaro concluded that these persons were delayed in completing normal adult developmental tasks and that their life-styles were "shamefully different."

Adams[1] found an 83% incidence of incontinence in patients who suffered a first cerebral vascular accident. "It was associated with age, inability to walk, speech pathology, dependence on others for care, and inability to perform simple commands." Other associated factors were hemiplegia and loss of proprioception.[26] The paucity of published nursing research is evident in Wolonin's review. However, gerontologic nursing journals and textbooks have begun to provide helpful information for this complex clinical problem.[23]

Genitourinary causes. A helpful way to classify these etiologies is to consider the cycle of micturition (filling, voluntary postponement, and emptying) and to divide the types of incontinence broadly into active and passive.[20,23,24] Active incontinence implies either failure of neurologic control in the voluntary postponement phase or defective outflow on micturition. The latter can occur with or without residual urine. On the other hand, passive incontinence means that muscles controlling continence are hypotonic, and the result is leakage during filling when the pressure is building up.[20,24,25]

Bladder outflow obstruction. Willington[24,25] reported an enlarged prostate gland as the most common cause of bladder outflow obstruction. In addition, he cited fibrous bladder neck obstruction, which can occur in both males and females, as another important cause. Other genitourinary causes affecting bladder outflow include defective neuromuscular relaxation, contraction of the bladder, and gynecologic causes.[3] Cystoceles and trigonitis associated with senile vaginitis may prevent effective emptying of the bladder.[3,24,25]

Loss of muscle tone. The decline in muscle tone in older adults is a cause of incontinence, particularly in females. The muscles and structures of the pelvic diaphragm are normally weaker in females than in males. In addition, as a result of the aging process, muscle tissue is decreased and replaced by adipose connective tissue, and pelvic support structures are weakened by a decline in estrogen.[8] When intraabdominal pressure is increased by sudden exertion such as sneezing, coughing, laughing, or standing, a small leakage of urine occurs. This condition is known as stress incontinence and is estimated to be present in 12% of older women.[8]

Urinary tract infections and fecal impactions. Urinary tract infection or irritation leads to increased bladder contractibility and may result in loss of urine control.[26] A bacterial count over 100,000/ml³ is usually considered indicative of infection.[24]

A common phenomenon on geriatric units is the occurrence of fecal impactions in patients admitted with urinary incontinence.[3] The hard stool puts pressure on the bladder and incontinence occurs. Removal of an impaction usually results in immediate resolution of the problem of incontinence.

Spurious incontinence. Spurious incontinence,[24] often seen in older adults, includes iatrogenic incontinence, incontinence caused by locomotor defects, and that caused by environmental factors. Iatrogenic incontinence is defined as a "treatment" that results in incontinence.[24] Drug therapy, as an iatrogenic cause, may take many forms. The most common is furosemide (Lasix), the diuretic action of which is so rapid that the person becomes incontinent. Hypnotics can cause a depth of sleep from which the person cannot be awakened by the customary bladder sensation. Sedation with diazepam (Valium) and the phenothiazines (for example, Sparine) is troublesome. Tricyclic antidepressants (Elavil) may also cause incontinence.[20,24]

Other etiologic factors that lead to loss of control of urine include locomotor defects, manual dexterity in manipulating clothing, distance to the bathroom, and environmental factors.[20,24]

Following are the etiologies for incontinence:

Central nervous system causes
  Neurogenic causes
    Uninhibited
    Automatic
    Autonomous
    Hypoesthetic
  Psychogenic causes
    Repression
    Dependency
    Rebellion
    Insecurity
    Attention seeking
    Disturbance of conditional reflexes
    Sensory deprivation
    Symptom selection
Genitourinary causes
  Bladder outflow obstruction
    Enlarged prostate gland
    Fibrous bladder neck obstruction
    Defective neuromuscular relaxation of the sphincter
    Contraction of the bladder
    Cystocele
    Trigonitis associated with senile vaginitis
  Loss of muscle tone
  Fecal impaction
Spurious incontinence
  Iatrogenic incontinence
  Locomotor defects
  Environmental factors
Other causes
  Dehydration[3]
  Sensory motor impairment[15]
  Neuromuscular impairment[15]
  Mechanical trauma[15]

DEFINING CHARACTERISTICS

Dysuria
Frequency
Hesitancy
Incontinence
Nocturia
Retention
Urgency

Incontinence has appeared as a diagnostic label on the list of accepted diagnoses of NANDA since the First National Conference in 1973.[11] The original label—urinary elimination, impairment of—was specified to include inability to control initiation, cessation, and generation of urine flow. The label was changed to urinary elimination, impairment of: alterations in patterns at the Second National Conference in 1975.[11] Three labels—urinary elimination, impairment of: alteration in patterns; urinary elimination, impairment of: incontinence; and urinary elimination, impairment of: retention—appeared on the list of nursing diagnoses accepted at the Third National Conference.[16] On the 1980 Fourth National Conference list of accepted diagnoses the label was changed and refined to urinary elimination, alterations in pattern and has remained unchanged during succeeding conferences in 1982 and 1984.[14,16]

In Gordon's *Manual of Nursing Diagnosis* the diagnostic category, urinary elimination, impairment of: incontinence appeared with the definition and defining characteristics as involuntary passage of urine. Gordon further ascertained that, if the etiology of incontinence is diagnosed, the patient should be referred for medical evaluation.[12]

Carpenito[5] lists three etiologies—enuresis, dysuria, and incontinence—and derives interventions specific to each cause. In addition, she notes that the diagnostic category pertains to alterations in urine elimination, not urine formation. It is within the domain of nursing to diagnose and treat an alteration in patterns of elimination, but nurses cannot alter polyuria, retention, anuria, and oliguria with independent nursing treatments.

It is interesting to note that incontinence has been included as a defining characteristic since the Fourth Conference. Carpenito[5] includes incontinence and enuresis as both etiologies and defining characteristics. In addition, Carpenito considers dribbling and bladder distention as defining characteristics in her classification system.

It can be said that incontinence is a symptom that may result from one or a combination of factors. Although increased attention has been given to various classification systems in the medical literature, no precise specification of the problem exists at this time in the nursing literature.

NURSING INTERVENTIONS

Patient Goal	Nursing Intervention
Eliminate or reduce the number of incontinent episodes.	Reduce or eliminate contributing physiologic, psychologic, and environmental factors when possible. Assess/monitor hydration. Assess/monitor nutrition. Assess/monitor voiding pattern. Promote micturition. Initiate bladder training or reconditioning. Establish a voiding schedule. Teach intermittent catheterization to person and family if indicated.
Increase self-esteem, personal integrity, and social functioning.	Encourage and assist with good grooming. Change clothes when wet immediately after incontinent episode. Uses incontinence aids temporarily until control is established.
Prevent skin breakdown.	Wash area, rinse, and dry well after incontinent episode.

The goals of nursing care include prevention, treatment, health teaching, and repatterning of urine elimination. Although these categories are not mutually exclusive, they do provide a framework for considering various aspects of the nature of incontinence that fall within the domain of nursing.

Prevention of incontinence depends on intelligent and thoughtful nursing care. Communication of the plan of care between all staff members, the individual, and the family is of utmost importance. Understanding and management of central nervous system causes, genitourinary causes, and spurious incontinence resulting from environmental factors depend on knowledge of the micturition cycle and the factors that can affect this cycle. An accurate and detailed assessment must be taken, including physiologic, psychosocial, and environmental factors. During assessment, information is gathered through observation, interview, physical examination, and consultation. Many of the physical causes of urinary incontinence require extensive evaluation by urologists and other specialists because of their complexity. However, some of the more common physical causes (for example, fecal impaction and stress incontinence), the psychologic causes, and spurious incontinence are frequently observed by nurses and respond to nursing interventions.

Nursing treatment of urinary incontinence should be aimed at careful elucidation of the underlying causes. Individuals who experience incontinence fall into three broad categories[6]:

1. Those with temporary loss of urine control due to reversible causes, such as inappropriate drug therapy, toxic confusional states, effects of translocation, and treatable medical conditions (cystoceles, prostatic hypertrophy, and cerebral vascular accidents)

2. Those who are ambulatory and incontinent and who may be mentally competent or incompetent
3. Those who are incontinent and bedfast

For individuals in all three groups an essential first step is to determine the present voiding pattern and compare it with the usual pattern or pattern elicited during the initial assessment. More detailed information can be included through the use of an incontinence chart that specifies intake and output data as well as circumstances related to incidences of urine control or loss.[6] Together these form the baseline for planning creative care that is sensitive to the attitudes of the individual and caregiver.

Measures to promote continence are essential to an individual's self-esteem. When specific treatment fails, external collecting devices may be helpful. Indwelling catheters may be used temporarily, intermittently, or as a last resort prior to an incontinent episode. Other measures include use of incontinence aids that are acceptable to the individual until control can be established; teaching intermittent self-catheterization if the person is functionally competent; and teaching a family member to do the procedure if indicated. Referrals to community nurses may be necessary if bladder reconditioning is called for.[5,19]

Repatterning of urine elimination can be attempted with persons complaining of urgency and frequency of micturition with incontinence. They can be trained to increase bladder capacity by increasing the time between voiding. The importance of keeping an accurate record of the amount of urine voided and time between voidings should be emphasized. A strict regimen enables the person to learn to inhibit bladder contractions with subsequent improvement in symptoms and urodynamics. The symptomatic cure rate for bladder retraining is reported consistently at over 80% after 3 to 6 months. The urodynamic improvement rate was reported to be about 30% in returning unstable bladders to normal.[19]

EVALUATION

Patient Outcome	Data Indicating That Outcome is Reached
Amount and number of voidings within normal limits	No more than eight voidings per day within range of 1000-1500 ml per day
Adequate dietary intake	Skin well hydrated Urinary output maintained at 50 ml/hour
Decrease in episodes of urinary incontinence	Seeks medical consultation for evaluation of urinary incontinence if indicated Keeps a record of incontinent episodes
Perineal skin normal in appearance	Absence of areas of redness, itching, and irritation in perineal area
Understands mechanisms of incontinence	Describes factors associated with incontinence Lists two changes in health practices that will affect urinary elimination pattern, such as strengthening pelvic floor muscles, holding urine until set voiding time, taking diuretics early in morning
Positive self-concept	Maintains interpersonal relationships Engages in social activities
Free from odor	Keeps skin clean and dry Wears protective clothing

References

1. Adams, M.: Urinary incontinence in the acute phase of cerebral vascular accident, Nurs. Res. 15:100-108, 1966.
2. Bartol, M.A.: Psychosocial aspects of incontinence in the aged person. In Mortenson-Burnside, I., editor: Psychosocial nursing care of the aged, New York, 1980, McGraw-Hill Book Co.
3. Brink, C.: Assessing the problem, Geriatric Nurs. 1:241-245, 1980.
4. Caldwell, K.P.S.: Urinary incontinence, New York, 1975, Grune & Stratton, Inc.
5. Carpenito, L.J.: Nursing diagnosis: application to clinical practice, New York, 1983, J.B. Lippincott Co.
6. Demmerle, B., and Bartol, M.A.: Nursing care for the incontinent person, Geriatric Nurs. Nov.-Dec. 1980, pp. 246-250.
7. Feneley, R.C.L., Thomas, D.G., and Blannin, J.B.: Urinary incontinence, J. Royal College Phys. Lond. 16:89-93, 1982.
8. Field, M.A.: Urinary incontinence in the elderly: an overview, J. Gerontol. Nurs. 5:12-19, 1979.
9. Freed, S.L.: Urinary incontinence in the elderly, Hosp. Pract. 17:81-94, March 1982.
10. Gebbie, K.M.: Summary of the Second National Conference, St. Louis, 1976, National Group for Classification of Nursing Diagnosis.

11. Gebbie, K.M., and Lavin, M.A.: Classification of nursing diagnoses: Proceedings of the First National Conference, St. Louis, 1975, The C.V. Mosby Co.

12. Gordon, M.: Manual of nursing diagnosis, New York, 1982, McGraw-Hill Book Co.

13. Guyton, A.C.: Micturition, renal disease, and diuresis. In Guyton, A.C., editor: Textbook of medical physiology, Philadelphia, 1976, W.B. Saunders Co.

14. Kim, M.J., McFarland, G.K., and McLane, A.M.: Classification of nursing diagnoses: Proceedings of the Fifth National Conference, St. Louis, 1984, The C.V. Mosby Co.

15. Kim, M.J., McFarland, G.K., and McLane, A.M.: Pocket guide to nursing diagnoses, St. Louis, 1984, The C.V. Mosby Co.

16. Kim, M.J., and Moritz, D.A.: Classification of nursing diagnoses: Proceedings of the Third and Fourth National Conferences, St. Louis, 1982, The C.V. Mosby Co.

17. Milne, J.S.: Prevalence of incontinence in the elderly age groups. In Willington, F.S., editor: Incontinence in the elderly, London, 1976, Academic Press, Inc.

18. Shepard, A.M., Blannin, J.P., and Feneley, R.C.L.: Changing attitudes in the management of urinary incontinence: the need for specialist nursing, Br. Med. J. 284:645-646, Feb. 1982.

19. Shepard, A., Tribe, E., and Tarrens, M.J.: Simple practical techniques in the management of urinary incontinence, Int. Rehab. Med. 4(1):15-19, 1982.

20. Spect, J., and Cordes, A.: Incontinence. In Carnevali, D.L., and Patrick, M., editors: Nursing management for the elderly, Philadelphia, 1979, J.B. Lippincott Co.

21. Stevenson, J.S.: Adulthood: a promising focus for future research. In Werley, H.H., and Fitzpatrick, J.J., editors: Annual review of nursing research, vol. 1, New York, 1984, Springer Publishing Co.

22. Sutherland, S.S.: The psychology of incontinence. In Willington, F.L., editor: Incontinence in the elderly, London, 1976, Academic Press, Inc.

23. Wells, T.: Promoting urine control in older adults, Geriatric Nurs. 1:236-269, 1980.

24. Willington, F.L.: Problems in the aetiology of urinary incontinence, Nurs. Times 71:379-381, 1975.

25. Willington, F.L.: Incontinence in the elderly, London, 1976, Academic Press, Inc.

26. Wolanin, M.D.: Clinical geriatric nursing research. In Werley, H.H., and Fitzpatrick, J.J., editors: Annual review of nursing research, vol. 1, New York, 1984, Springer Publishing Co.

Activity-Exercise

Activity can be defined as "an action which brings about a change in an existing situation by means of an expenditure of energy."[2] Exercise is an activity performed especially for the sake of training or improvement.[5] The immediate goal of activity may be to dress oneself; the immediate goal of exercise is more likely to be conditioning or physical fitness. In either case to be active provides one with a sense of control over the environment. Activity involves the expenditure of energy and necessitates mental and physical functioning. The pattern of behavior that individuals use to respond to the need for activity and exercise is influenced by physiologic, psychologic, cultural, social, and spiritual factors. Inherent within these factors are the developmental level and cognitive functioning ability of the individual.

Patterns of activity and exercise have evolved over the decades. Prior to the Industrial Revolution vigorous physical activity was required to meet survival needs. The advent of machines and the growth of technology introduced more sedentary habits and life-styles. Changes in activity altered expenditures of energy. Only 1% of the energy used on farms and in factories and workshops today is supplied by human labor; a century ago it comprised one third.[6] The work and school patterns of most adults and children do not provide adequate opportunities for exercise. Leisure time activities have not compensated for most of these losses.

Concerned about the loss of the benefits of exercise, President Eisenhower in 1956 created what is now the President's Council on Physical Fitness and Sports. The Kennedy administration emphasized youth and fitness.

The 1960s and the 1970s occasioned greater interest in exercise and fitness through the influence of the media, advertising, and the recreation industry. Title IX of the Educational Act Amendment of 1972 furthered women's involvement in exercise by encouraging more spending in schools for girls' athletics. The 1980s have seen continued emphasis on the need for physical exercise, but more rigorous study of how much and what types of activity and the specific benefits to be obtained are yet to be done. Reflecting on trends in the patterns of exercise in the United States as revealed in numerous investigations, including a Gallup poll in 1977 and a Harris poll in 1978, Thomas and co-workers[6] concluded:

1. The number of adults in the United States who report that they exercise regularly has increased significantly during the past 20 years.
2. The majority of adults, however, still do not exercise regularly, and only one in three children now participates in a daily program of school physical education.
3. The elderly, low-income populations, minorities, and women are underrepresented among the exercising population.
4. Many people who do exercise regularly probably do not achieve levels of activity that might promote physical fitness or condition the heart and lungs.

Exercise alters the chemistry and physiology of the body. It increases the maximal oxygen uptake, slows the resting heart rate, lowers elevated blood pressure, improves the efficiency of cardiac action, increases cardiac output, and enhances physical work activity.[6] It slows the loss of minerals from bones, which accompanies aging and may retard other age-related losses.[4] Carbohydrate metabolism is altered favorably; overweight and obesity decline. Exercise also contributes to improved sleep patterns, self-confidence, and a sense of well-being.

That exercise is beneficial is well documented. Public policy and plans of action to support further education of the population and to expand research in exercise and fitness have been promulgated.[1] Nurses have a role to play in both. One epidemiologic study[3] has provided some of the information for the nursing diagnoses described here.

References

1. Disease prevention and health promotion: federal programs on prevention, DHEW PHS pub. no. 79-55071B, Washington, D.C., 1978, U.S. Government Printing Office.
2. Fromm, E.: The art of loving, New York, 1956, Harper & Row Publishers.
3. Hoskins, L.M., and others: Nursing diagnoses in the chronically ill. Research in progress, The Catholic University of America, Washington, D.C.
4. Maranto, G.: Exercise: how much is too much? Discovery Oct. 1984, pp. 18-22.
5. Random house dictionary of the English language, New York, 1966, Random House.
6. Thomas, G.S., and others: Exercise and health: the evidence and the implications, Cambridge, Mass., 1981, Oelgeschlager, Gunn & Hain Publishers, Inc.

SELF-CARE DEFICIT: FEEDING, BATHING/HYGIENE, DRESSING/GROOMING, TOILETING

THEORY AND ETIOLOGY

The nursing diagnosis of self-care deficit: feeding, bathing/hygiene, dressing/grooming, toileting may be defined as the inability of the individual to adequately and capably perform these tasks for himself as a result of decreased motor function or cognitive function. The changes in function may be temporary or permanent and they result from physiologic or psychologic impairment or restraint. Performance of these activities is necessary for a healthy sense of self. Self-care theory emphasizes the importance of this diagnosis.

Self-care concerns activities that people perform for themselves in response to the needs and demands of daily living. Human needs must be fulfilled for gratification purposes and to make human survival and development possible. As stated by Orem[18]: "Self-care is the practice of activities that individuals initiate and perform on their own behalf in maintaining life, health, and well-being." We assume that adults have the right and responsibility for their own self-care. The ability to perform self-care provides them with a sense of control necessary for a healthy self-concept.

Self-care is deliberate and functional, that is, it serves a purpose, and it has a pattern or a sequence of behavior. Self-care is learned; it develops over time and therefore is influenced by teachers—the family and the sociocultural environment in which the individual lives and grows. Self-care to perform the activities of daily living becomes a habit about which there is little thought (until it is disrupted). Self-care has a value orientation with respect not only to what is done, but how it is done, when, and where.

The performance of self-care becomes a pattern of daily activity. Patterns of activity are affected by the functional health status of the individual, and this in turn is influenced by the individual's interaction with the environment and particularly the people therein. The functional health status must be assessed to determine the level of self-care ability of the patient and whether self-care deficits are present. The assessment of the patient-environment interaction identifies situational and social factors that may contribute either positively or negatively to the individual's ability to perform self-care and maintain independence.

The functional health status includes three components: (1) age-related biologic status, (2) developmental task status, and (3) disease (if present) and its treatment.[2] Age-related biologic status incorporates an assessment of the body systems and a comparison of that assessment with norms for that age. Changes in structure and function may occur during maturation that predispose the individual to self-care deficits. For example, musculoskeletal changes that normally accompany aging may lead to a slowing in movement that could create problems in self-care. The problem may be made more acute if those around the elderly individual are not tolerant of his need for more time to accomplish activities such as feeding, dressing, and bathing. This is an example of the interaction between patient-environment and functional health status in meeting the needs and demands of daily living. Other age-related changes that may affect basic self-care include decreased visual and hearing acuity, changes in dentition, and changes in strength and endurance.

The assessment of developmental task level enables comparison of the patient's age and stage of development to expected norms to identify differences that might affect self-care. The degree of independence or dependence and control is a factor. Infants, for example, are not expected to perform their own self-care, whereas the expectation is for adults to voluntarily perform their own feeding, bathing, dressing, and toileting. Maturation in terms of cognitive-perceptual abilities is also assessed. Knowledge, skill, and motivation are significant factors in self-care.[9]

Pathologic states caused by trauma or disease may alter structure and function and thus compromise self-care ability in all age groups. A young adult paralyzed in all extremities from a head injury is an extreme example. Severe coronary artery disease may decrease the middle-aged individual's tolerance to activity such that he cannot bathe and eat without assistance. Severe respiratory disease may have a similar effect. Mental confusion may develop in the elderly because of nutritional deficiencies or unknown causes and compromise the self-care ability. Also, the treatment regimen for a particular medical diagnosis may render the individual incapable of performing complete self-care. Surgically created diversions to normal activities, such as tracheotomies, colostomies, and gastrostomies, are examples. Pain may immobilize the individual and make self-care uncomfortable or impossible. Temporary deficits in self-care may also be encountered, such as being immobilized by intravenous tubing, splints and casts, and prescribed bed rest.

Lack of the ability to independently perform the necessary activities of daily living prolongs the length of stay of patients in acute care facilities.

The elements of the functional health status (age-related biologic status, developmental task level, and pathologic state) are interrelated, and all contribute directly to the level of self-care ability. This is best personified in the elderly, in whom pathologic changes can be superimposed on maturational changes, leading to self-care deficits.[5]

Eighty percent of the elderly population have chronic disease.[5] In this group physical immobility and mental confusion have been identified as the major causes of their "functional dependency" or their inability to tend to their own bodily needs, specifically ambulation, dressing, feeding, grooming, and toileting. Furthermore, 5% of the U.S. population ages 65 and over are in long-term care facilities, with the other 95% residing in the community. Of those in the community, by one estimate, about 15% are functionally disabled. "Another estimate is that 40% to 50% of the elderly in the community are limited in amount or kind of activity, with 18% having limited mobility (and 5% confined to home)."[5] About 25% to 41% are in need of home care services because of some impairment. It is obvious that as the number of elderly continues to grow, efforts to maintain their level of self-care ability and to promote independence will expand.

Changes in the functional health status have a direct effect on the ability to perform self-care: they are the basis for the formation of self-care deficits. However, independence in self-care can be influenced by factors and resources in the environment. If strength and endurance are limited, what is the household arrangement, how close is the bathroom, how many stairs must be climbed? In all situations of self-care deficit how accessible is transportation to professional services, to grocery stores, and shops? Is the neighborhood safe for walking? Is there a sense of security? The availability of home care services, nursing, cooking, and cleaning must be assessed as well as the individual's ability to afford them. Social support systems must be assessed; this includes family, friends, and neighbors. For some who are partially dependent in self-care, having someone come into the home to help them with the bath or to prepare food for future use may provide them with the necessary assistance to keep them living in their own home or apartment. The nurse should be aware that these same resources also generate demands.[2] This is the element of client-environment interaction in which the family that provides support also places demands on the individual, for example, when and where and how long it will take to eat, to bathe, to dress. The other environmental factors and resources must also be evaluated for the demands they make on the individual versus the strength they provide.

Functional Dependency: Quality of Life

Being functionally dependent, that is, requiring assistance from others in the activities of feeding, bathing/hygiene, dressing/grooming, and toileting, affects the individual's morale, self-esteem, and sense of dignity. These are human needs that contribute to the quality of life. Again, the elderly are the most rapidly growing population with the greatest number of dependency needs proportionally. Chang[3] found that elderly nursing home residents who had self-determined situational control over their own daily activities had higher morale than those elderly for whom others determined control of their daily activities. Chang also developed a tool to measure situational control of daily activities. Ryden[22] looked for patterns of causal relationships among the following variables: perception of situational control, health, socioeconomic status, functional dependency, length of stay, and morale in nursing home residents. She studied two groups of residents—those having skilled care and those having intermediate care. She found that "perception of situational control was a key variable, significantly related to the morale of residents on both levels of care."[22] For the skilled care group, perceived control was the only variable with a significant direct relationship to morale; for the intermediate care group, health, perceived control, functional dependency, and socioeconomic status, in that order, all had significant direct effects on morale. For the latter group, functional dependency influenced perceived control, making functional dependency the variable with the strongest effect on morale. "The greater the functional dependency, the less sense of control and the lower the morale score."[22]

The need for self-esteem is an integral part of the self-concept and closely related to one's body image; it is one's perception of self-worth.[4] Taylor[24] provided a theoretical framework for self-esteem using the four bases of self-esteem identified in the work of Coopersmith. These include the following:

1. Significance—the way a person feels he is loved and approved of by the people important to him
2. Competence—the way tasks which are considered important are performed
3. Virtue—the attainment of moral and ethical standards
4. Power—the extent to which a person influences his own and others' lives

The loss of the ability to perform a functional task and the loss of respect, threatened or real, that may accompany that loss may have a devastating effect on the sense of self of the individual. Rubin[21] stated that one expects to be in control of one's simplest functions and of the appropriateness of the time and place of their occurrence, and when this control is lost one is ashamed of oneself. A personal judgment of failure is made and the ego is threatened; it is even more telling when one's failure is witnessed by others. Miller[16] observed that lack of participation in activities of daily living and verbal responses indicating lack of control over activities and outcomes, associated with negative affective responses (withdrawal, pessimism, submissiveness, undifferentiated anger), indicate the diagnosis of powerlessness.

The interventions of the nurse or caregiver and their attitudes are essential in determining the responses and outcomes to self-care deficits in body functions. The outcome will also be affected by the specific nature of the deficit and whether it is temporary or long term. For example, individuals who are temporarily restrained by intravenous tubing and have to be fed by others may feel uncomfortable and prefer not to eat. On the other hand, the sudden traumatic deficits of accident-related quadriplegia and the progressive deficits that sometimes accompany growing older present more serious problems that may eventually threaten the ego.

Etiologies for self-care deficit may be any of the following:

Intolerance to activity, decreased strength and endurance
Pain, discomfort
Perceptual or cognitive impairment
Neuromuscular impairment
Musculoskeletal impairment
Depression, severe anxiety

DEFINING CHARACTERISTICS

Feeding
Inability to bring food from a receptacle to the mouth
Inability to cut food

Bathing/Hygiene
Inability to wash body or body parts*
Inability to obtain or get to water source
Inability to regulate temperature or flow

Dressing/Grooming
Impaired ability to put on or take off necessary items of clothing*
Impaired ability to obtain or replace articles of clothing
Impaired ability to fasten clothing
Inability to maintain appearance at a satisfactory level

Toileting
Unable to get to toilet or commode*
Unable to sit on or rise from toilet or commode*
Unable to manipulate clothing for toileting*
Unable to carry out proper toilet hygiene*
Unable to flush toilet or empty commode

*Critical defining characteristic.

The critical defining characteristics must be present for the diagnosis to be made; other characteristics may or may not be present.

The defining characteristics,[11,13] are observable signs and symptoms that are present when the particular self-care deficit is diagnosed. Functional levels indicating the degree of dependence or independence in performing the

Table 15
Classification of Functional Levels of
Self-Care*[1,6-8]

Level	Behavioral Indicator	Numeric Index
I	Independent; able to initiate and complete activity for self	0
II	Requires minimal assistance; may use equipment but manages it himself; does at least 75% of work	1
III	Requires moderate assistance, supervision, or teaching; does approximately 50% of work	2
IV	Requires extensive assistance from another person *and* equipment or devices; does less than 25% of work	3
V	Dependent on caregivers, total care; does not participate actively	4

*Self-care deficits exist for numeric indices 1 through 4.

task must also be included in any assessment of patient's abilities.

As stated previously, it is necessary in the assessment of self-care deficits to determine the functional level of ability. Commonly five levels of self-care are described on a continuum from independence, level I, to dependence, level V.[6] Table 15 describes the five functional levels and also contains a numeric code that can be used in a patient care classification system. By adding the numeric indices, a weighted value can be obtained to indicate the overall amount of nursing care required. Use of behavioral indicators makes it possible for the staff to identify and agree on consistent indicators of change, especially important in a progressive rehabilitation program. It should be noted that the client may be at different levels for different activities, for example, be able to eat but require help with dressing or with toileting at night.

In conjunction with the system in Table 15 an assessment sheet[10,14,15] reflecting specific areas of the body and specific activities is useful, especially in planning and evaluating the care of a patient requiring long-term care (Fig. 10). Functional levels or numeric indices can be coded for the appropriate date, and nursing interventions can be written to correspond to the respective code and deficit. A number of similar tools exist. For example, *feeds self* may have a numeric index of 3, indicating moderate assistance is required; in the nursing care plan the exact nature of the assistance would be indicated. In *dressing/grooming* the individual may be independent for upper extremities, indicated with a numeric index of 0, but dependent in lower extremities, indicated with a 4. The total score could be summed with the average determined (0 to 4), which would indicate the amount of assistance needed or the level of self-care ability. As rehabilitation takes place, improvement is indicated in specific areas with successive observations over time, and the flow sheet indicates this.

Fig. 10
Assessment sheet for self-care.

ACTIVITY

CODE AND DATES

Date						
FEEDING						
Diet: _____						
Moves to dining area						
Fixes own food						
Feeds self						
BATHING/HYGIENE						
Bath: upper extremities						
lower extremities						
Oral care						
Shampoo						
Shave						
DRESSING/GROOMING						
Upper extremities						
Lower extremities						
Shoes						
Buttons, zippers						
Make-up						
TOILETING						
Bathroom						
Bedside commode						
Bedpan						
Urinal						
Catheter care						
Incontinent of bladder						
Incontinent of bowel						

NURSING INTERVENTIONS

Patient Goal	Nursing Intervention
Achieve or maintain behavioral control.	Assess with patient his strengths and weaknesses; discuss what behavioral activities he can do for himself. Explore the use of assistive devices that can help the patient become more self-sufficient. Encourage or allow patient to do as much as possible for himself. Observe for evidence of readiness to increase amount of self-care. Provide help, supervision, and teaching as necessary to improve self-care. Act as patient advocate to increase sensitivity of others to effects of their actions on the patient.
Achieve or maintain cognitive control.	Plan care with patient; validate conclusions with him. Discuss any changes in his condition with him. Inform of anticipated effects of therapy. Assist in relating concerns to physician.
Achieve or maintain decisional control.	Discuss daily routines with patient; allow him a voice in scheduling functional activities. Consult with patient in making choices about his treatment; do not plan activities without his knowledge. Evaluate outcomes of care with patient.

Feeding

Achieve or maintain responsibility for feeding congruent with level of self-care ability (see Table 15).	Level I, independent: Praise and encourage to maintain independence. Level II, minimal assistance: Cut or prepare food as necessary. Level III, moderate assistance: Arrange tray, prepare food; encourage patient to eat and feed self. Level IV, extensive assistance: Feed patient as necessary (patient may have some difficulty with chewing or swallowing and require special diet); encourage patient to eat, allow adequate time, use pleasant manner. Level V, dependent, total care: Feed patient through manner prescribed (may be tube feeding or parenteral therapy); have equipment available for emergencies, such as suctioning.

Bathing/Hygiene

Achieve or maintain responsibility for bathing/hygiene congruent with level of self-care ability (see Table 15).	Level I, independent: Praise and encourage to maintain independence. Level II, minimal assistance: May provide care to one area, such as back. Level III, moderate assistance: Prepare bath, provide back, leg and foot care, comb hair. Level IV, extensive care: Provide majority of bath, hair care, and oral care. Level V, dependent, total care: Provide complete bath and hygiene care.

Dressing/Grooming

Achieve or maintain responsibility for dressing/grooming congruent with level of self-care ability (see Table 15).	Level I, independent: Praise and encourage to maintain independence. Level II, minimal assistance: Help with buttons, zippers, shoelaces. Level III, moderate assistance: Provide help with clothing on lower extremities, with shoes, with fasteners. Level IV, extensive assistance: Provide help with putting on all of clothing; do not hurry; allow patient to make choices in order of activity, makeup, etc., if able; comb hair, shave. Level V, dependent, total care: Dress/groom patient.

Toileting

Achieve or maintain responsibility for toileting congruent with level of self-care ability (see Table 15).	Level I, independent: Praise and encourage to maintain independence. Level II, minimal assistance: Provide needed support or equipment for patient to manage own toileting; be prompt in responding to patient's request. Level III, moderate assistance: Respond promptly to patient's request; assist with needed equipment. Level IV, extensive assistance: Provide and position toilet equipment; anticipate toileting needs; clean patient, rearrange clothing or bedding; be prompt, nonjudgmental. Level V, dependent, total care: If possible develop routine to stimulate or anticipate urination or defecation such that it may be controlled or expected at a certain time; promptly clean patient, rearrange clothing/bedding.

The primary goal of care is that the functional requirements, the basic human needs, be met.* At all levels of care the nurse must consider the patient's need for control. The patient who is independent in care, level I, has the ability to make choices about his own care, to carry out his self-care, and to be responsible for his own actions. He does not require help but should be praised and encouraged to maintain his independence. At the other extreme is the dependent patient, level V, who needs total care in the particular activity or activities affected. This level could include a patient in the intensive care setting who requires continuous monitoring and is unable to participate or to make decisions about any aspects of his care. Self-care levels II, III, and IV, requiring minimal, moderate, and extensive assistance, do require judgments concerning the patient's control and responsibility for his own care.

Miller[16] categorizes control as behavioral, cognitive, and decisional. Behavioral control refers to the "availability of a response," the capability of modifying an

*References 1, 8, 10, 14, 16, 18, 19, 23, 24.

event by direct action, such as turning off the television. Cognitive control means having knowledge of an event and interpreting it accurately, such as being informed of the exact nature of one's diagnosis and how it will be treated. Decisional control concerns being able to make choices from alternatives. Yura and Walsh[23] address the individual's need for self-control, self-determination, and responsibility: having command over resources and choosing and being accountable for one's self-care actions.

This section addresses general and specific care for each of the functional levels. Patients in acute care or long-term care settings are rarely independent in all areas of self-care; instead, there is a mix of self-care abilities, and the nursing assessment, interventions, and expected outcomes reflect this mix. The plan of care provides general guidelines; it must be individualized to the patient. At each level the nurse should specify what particular help or what assistive device is needed. The expected outcomes, or level of human need fulfillment that can be achieved by the patient, should be stated realistically by considering the reason for the alteration initially.

EVALUATION

Patient Outcome	Data Indicating That Outcome is Reached
Control over physical activities and environment in so far as capable	States realistic appraisal of own self-care ability Initiates and completes as much of care as physically possible
Knows and understands what is happening; maintains sense of self-esteem and self-worth	Takes active interest in own care; asks questions, shares own values, helps to prioritize care Verbalizes positive feelings about self; does not express feelings of insecurity, worthlessness
Makes choices concerning care; influences others	Sets reasonable goals for self; takes physical strength and endurance into account Sets specific time for performing activities but shows respect for goals and time constraints of nursing staff also; negotiates Takes active part in assessing activities and outcomes
Feeding	
Level I, independent	Initiates and completes feeding self; no help
Level II, minimal assistance needed	Completes feeding self; does approximately 75% of work
Level III, moderate assistance needed	Feeds self satisfactorily with supervision; does approximately 50% of work
Level IV, extensive assistance needed	Feeding completed with assistance; client does less than 25% of work
Level V, dependent, total care needed	Ingests diet when fed
Bathing/Hygiene	
Level I, independent	Initiates and completes own bath; clean body, hair, nails, teeth, no offensive odors (applies to all levels)
Level II, minimal assistance	Does approximately 75% of the work
Level III, moderate assistance	Does approximately 50% of the work

Patient Outcome	Data Indicating That Outcome is Reached
Level IV, extensive assistance	Does less than 25% of work; may perform light hygiene with some assistive devices, such as electric toothbrush
Level V, dependent, total care	No participation; bath and hygiene completed by caregivers
Dressing/Grooming	
Level I, independent	Initiates and completes own dressing/grooming appropriately
Level II, minimal assistance	Initiates dressing activity, dresses appropriately; does majority of work; pleased with appearance
Level III, moderate assistance	Does approximately 50% of the work
Level IV, extensive assistance	Does less than 25% of the work
Level V, dependent, total care	No active participation; dressed/groomed by caregivers
Toileting	
Level I, independent	Performs toileting activities for self; clean, no odors
Level II, minimal assistance	Goes to bathroom, cleans self; may need support getting to and from bathroom; may use bedpan or urinal by self at night if placed conveniently; continent
Level III, moderate assistance	Requests bedside commode, bedpan, or urinal when needed; able to transfer to same and to complete elimination; may need assistance with cleaning
Level IV, extensive assistance	Uses equipment provided; may have occasional episodes of incontinence
Level V, dependent, total care	Toileting care initiated and completed by caregivers

References

1. Baer, C.A., Delorey, M., and Fitzmaurice, J.B.: A study to evaluate the validity of the rating system for self-care deficit. In Kim, M.J., McFarland, G.K., and McLane, A.M., editors: Classification of nursing diagnoses: Proceedings of the Fifth National Conference, St. Louis, 1984, The C.V. Mosby Co.
2. Carnevali, D.L., and others: Diagnostic reasoning, Philadelphia, 1984, J.B. Lippincott Co.
3. Chang, B.L.: Generalized expectancy, situational perception, and morale among institutionalized aged, Nurs. Res. 27(5):316-324, 1978.
4. Driever, M.J.: Theory of self-concept. In Roy, Sr. C., editor: Introduction to nursing: an adaptation model, Englewood Cliffs, N.J., 1976, Prentice-Hall, Inc.
5. Filner, B., and Williams, T.F.: Health promotion for the elderly: reducing functional dependency. In Healthy people: The Surgeon General's Report on Health Promotion and Disease Prevention, DHEW PHS pub. no. 79-55071A, Washington, D.C., 1979, U.S. Government Printing Office.
6. Goldstein, N., and others: Self-care: a framework for the future. In Chinn, P.L., editor: Advances in nursing theory development, Rockville, Md., 1983, Aspen Systems Corp.
7. Gordon, M.: Manual of nursing diagnosis, New York, 1982, McGraw-Hill Book Co.
8. Johnson, K.: A practical approach to patient classification, Nurs. Management 15(6):39-46, 1984.
9. Joseph, L.S.: Self-care and the nursing process, Nurs. Clin. North Am. 15(1):131-143, 1980.
10. Katz, S.: Index of independence in activities of daily living (Index of ADL). In Instruments for measuring nursing practice and other health care variables, vol. 1, DHEW pub. no. HRA 78.53, Washington, D.C., 1981, U.S. Government Printing Office.
11. Kim, M.J., McFarland, G.K., and McLane, A.M.: Pocket guide to nursing diagnosis, St. Louis, 1980, The C.V. Mosby Co.
12. Kim, M.J., McFarland, G.K., and McLane, A.M.: Classification of nursing diagnoses: Proceedings of the Fifth National Conference, St. Louis, 1984, The C.V. Mosby Co.
13. Kim, M.J., and Moritz, D.: Classification of nursing diagnoses: Proceedings of the Third and Fourth National Conferences, New York, 1982, McGraw-Hill Book Co.
14. Loxley, C.M., and Cress, S.S.: The pocket guide to clinical nursing process for the adult medical-surgical client, New York, 1983, The Miller Press.
15. The Maryland Appraisal of Patient's Progress (M.A.P.P.): a patient care management system instructional manual, Department of Health and Mental Hygiene, Baltimore, Md., 1982.
16. Miller, J.M.: Coping with chronic illness: overcoming powerlessness, Philadelphia, 1983, F.A. Davis Co.
17. Mullin, V.I.: Implementing the self-care concept in the acute care setting, Nurs. Clin. North Am. 15(1):177-190, 1980.
18. Orem, D.: Nursing: concepts of practice, ed. 2, New York, 1980, McGraw-Hill Book Co.
19. Panicucci, C.L.: Functional assessment of the older adult in the acute care setting, Nurs. Clin. North Am. 18(2):355-363, 1983.
20. Power, D.J., and Craven, R.F.: ALS and aging: a case study in autonomy and control, Image: J. Nurs. Scholarship 15(1):22-25, 1983.
21. Rubin, R.: Body image and self-esteem, Nurs. Outlook June 1968, pp. 10-23.
22. Ryden, M.B.: Morale and perceived control in institutionalized elderly, Nurs. Res. 33(3):130-136, 1984.
23. Yura, H., and Walsh, M.: The nursing process, ed. 4, Norwalk, Conn., 1983, Appleton-Century-Crofts.
24. Taylor, Sr. M.C.: The need for self-esteem. In Yura, H., and Walsh, M., editors: Human needs and the nursing process, Norwalk, Conn., 1982, Appleton-Century-Crofts.

ACTIVITY INTOLERANCE
THEORY AND ETIOLOGY

Activity in which individuals engage reflects their physical capacity, structural and functional abilities, interests, and desires. Activity is a basic human need. It contributes to physical and emotional well-being. Activity is action; it requires intent and expenditure of energy. Activity is purposeful; it is required to maintain self-care, to accomplish occupational tasks, and to engage in physical exercise.

Unrestricted choice of activities contributes to one's sense of autonomy and independence. When an individual has no physiologic or psychologic constraints on the activities in which he chooses to engage, a sense of control is felt. But when limitations are imposed on an individual's usual activity pattern, this sense of control can be altered. White and co-workers,[19] in their discussion of the effects of the prolonged inactivity that was recommended for myocardial infarction patients in the 1950s, confirmed this effect. They stated: "The end of the ability to engage in constructive, purposeful activity is, for most persons, a tragedy—it symbolizes the end of independence and purpose in life."

The consequences of inactivity, imposed or assumed, affects the individual's total well being—physiologic, psychologic, social, cultural, and spiritual. Any alteration in an individual's activity pattern that occurs in response to a potential or actual health problem is of concern to professional nurses. When a potential or actual health problem affects the individual's ability to tolerate physical activity, the response is labeled activity intolerance.

The diagnosis of activity intolerance was accepted for clinical testing in 1982 at the Fifth National Conference on Nursing Diagnosis.[11] Although no definition of the diagnostic label was presented at the conference, various authors have provided relevant definitions. Campbell's definition[2] is presented in terms of the degree of activity that can be tolerated, that is, minimum, mild, and moderate activity tolerance. Her definitions are as follows:

Minimum activity tolerance: the inability to tolerate any physical activity without the presence of discomforts. . . . Mild activity tolerance: the ability to tolerate only a very limited amount of physical activity without the presence of discomforts. . . . Moderate activity tolerance: the ability to tolerate a moderate, but not a full day of physical activity without the presence of discomfort.

Campbell identified six possible etiologies of these three levels of altered activity tolerance: endocrine disturbances, tissue toxicity, inadequate tissue oxygenation, recovery from surgical procedures, poor nutrition, and depression.

Gordon[7] offered a similar diagnostic label—activity tolerance, decreased—that implies a change (decrease) in the level of tolerance for activity. It was defined as "insufficient energy to complete required or desired daily activities due to physiological or therapeutic limitations." Four levels are specified that, when used with the diagnostic label, describe an individual's response to specific activities. The physiologic and therapeutic limitations addressed by Gordon in her definition could be related to etiologies that are functional, structural, or situational in nature.

The label activity intolerance was used by Carpenito[4] as a descriptor of "a state in which the individual experiences an inability, physiologically or psychologically, to endure or tolerate an increase in activity." The definition implies that the response of activity intolerance would be identified as an individual increases activity. This increase of activity could occur as an ill individual attempts to resume usual activities or as a deconditioned individual attempts to increase the level of usual activity. In the first situation activity intolerance could be related to a pathophysiologic etiology; in the second, activity intolerance could be related to a situational etiology.

Drawing from these definitions, activity intolerance is defined as the inability to engage in and endure a required or desired physical activity as a result of functional, structural, or situational limitations. Physical activity encompasses all activity that requires the expenditure of energy. Self-care activities such as bathing, eating, and dressing as well as exercise and leisure activities are included when assessing an individual's ability to tolerate activity. The limitations that can contribute to an intolerance of such activity can be classified as functional, structural, or situational.

Functional limitations include those factors reflecting altered or impaired physiologic functioning. The required energy expenditure to perform the activity may be more than the individual has to expend. For an individual with cardiac disease the required myocardial oxygen consumption during various activities may exceed the amount of oxygen available.[14,17] Pulmonary diseases are often characterized by alterations of the oxygen and carbon dioxide transport process,[16] which compromises the supply of oxygen available to support the performance of activities.

Diseases causing endocrine disturbances (such as hypothyroidism), fluid-electrolyte imbalances (such as chronic renal disease), neurologic alterations (such as multiple sclerosis and Guillain-Barré syndrome), hepatic dysfunction (such as hepatitis), and circulatory and hematologic disorders (such as Raynaud's disease and anemia) also present functional limitations that can cause discomfort during activity. These disease-related functional limitations include generalized weakness, decreased mobility or immobility, and an imbalance between oxygen supply and demand.[2-4,9,11]

Structural limitations that can lead to activity intolerance are associated with an impairment or alteration of the anatomic structure. A structural impairment is related to a congenital or acquired anatomic deficit (for example, an individual whose right leg is shorter than the left leg) that limits mobility. A structural alteration can be caused by a therapeutic intervention (for example, a surgical incision that is painful or a cast applied to a leg rendering the leg immobile) or to the use of therapeutic equipment (such as a leg or back brace). The intervention or the use of equipment, although therapeutic in nature, can temporarily or permanently impose constraints (for example, the pain from an incision or fatigue from the weight of a cast or brace) that decrease an individual's willingness or ability to be mobile and active. The extent of the structural impairment or alteration influences the degree to which the individual's mobility is restricted and the consequent effect on his ability to tolerate activity.

Situational limitations that can alter an individual's tolerance for activity include factors relevant to the individual's cognitive and emotional status and environment. These limitations include lack of knowledge, lack of motivation, deconditioning, and lack of support. The individual may lack the knowledge necessary to engage in a particular activity in a manner that would provide for conservation of energy. An example of this is an individual with chronic obstructive pulmonary disease who avoids all activity to prevent shortness of breath.[5] The individual becomes more and more deconditioned and experiences an increasing resting oxygen consumption. Although the disease imposes functional constraints, the individual's avoidance of all activity because of a lack of knowledge imposes unnecessary restrictions on certain activities in which he could participate in a comfortable and safe manner. With proper instruction the individual can be made aware of the importance of specific conditioning exercises tailored to meet his physiologic needs.

Even though an individual may be knowledgeable of the importance of physical activity and how to engage in it so as to conserve energy, he may avoid activity because of depression.[2,4] Consequently the individual lacks the motivation required to endure physical activity. Even when the cognitive and emotional status of the individual is such that he is encouraged to participate in activity, the environment can contribute to his reluctance in becoming involved. A sedentary life-style that promotes deconditioning also promotes intolerance of activity.[4,11]

Support of the individual by significant others is another important factor in encouraging an individual's participation in and endurance of physical activity. Willingness of family members and friends to schedule meals, group activities, and time for personal activities in consideration of the individual's activity needs contributes to tolerance of and adherence to therapeutic activities. Encouragement and guidance from health care professionals can further enhance motivation and willingness to engage in activity.

The diagnosis of activity intolerance is made in relation to a specified etiology or causative factor. The etiology can be a functional, structural, or situational limitation that is experienced by an individual.

Possible etiologies for the nursing diagnosis of activity intolerance are listed below.[2,4,11]

Functional limitations
  Generalized weakness
  Decreased mobility or immobility
  Imbalance between oxygen supply and demand
Structural limitation
  Decreased mobility or immobility
Situational limitations
  Lack of knowledge
  Lack of motivation
  Deconditioning (related to life-style)
  Lack of support

DEFINING CHARACTERISTICS

Decrease in activity (self-care, exercise, leisure)
Avoidance of activity
Verbal report of fatigue or weakness*
Cardiovascular response to activity
  Bradycardia
  Inappropriate tachycardia
  Dysrhythmia
  Decrease in pulse strength
  Decrease in systolic pressure
  Excessive increase in systolic pressure
  Excessive increase in diastolic pressure
Respiratory response to activity
  Dyspnea
  Excessive increase in rate
  Decrease in rate
  Irregular rhythm
Skin in response to activity
  Pallor
  Cyanosis
  Excessive redness
  Cool
  Dry with strenuous activity
Posture
  Drooping of shoulders or head
  Decrease in muscle tone and strength

*Critical defining characteristic.

Equilibrium
    Ataxia
    Dizziness
Emotional status
    Lack of interest in activity
    Fearful of activity

The following parameters provide a guide for gathering data relative to assessing an individual's tolerance for or intolerance to activity.[1,4,6,10,18] The type, intensity, duration, and frequency of each activity in which an individual engages also must be considered when evaluating response to activity.

1. Activity pattern, past and present
   a. What activities (self-care, exercise, and leisure) were engaged in in the past? How were these activities tolerated?
   b. What activities are now engaged in? How are these activities tolerated?
2. Physical impediments
   a. Are there physical impediments that restrict participation in particular activities?
   b. Are there physical impediments that prevent active participation in activities?
3. Physiologic status
   a. Is there a change in physiologic status when engaging in activity?
   b. Cardiovascular response: note heart rate and rhythm; pulse strength; blood pressure.
   c. Respiratory response: note rate, depth, and rhythm of respirations.
   d. Skin: note color, signs, temperature, moisture.
   e. Posture: note signs of muscle fatigue.
   f. Equilibrium: note gait, fine and gross movements.
4. Emotional status
   a. Is there a change in emotional status prior to or upon engaging in activity?
   b. Is the individual fearful of harming himself?

In using this assessment guide, the presence of the defining characteristics can be determined. Presence of any or some of these characteristics may indicate that an individual is intolerant of engaging in particular activities.

NURSING INTERVENTIONS

Patient Goal	Nursing Intervention
Participate in activities that enhance physiologic well-being.	Provide patient information about activities in which to participate.
	Assist patient in interpretation of activity/exercise prescription.
	Seek consultation with physician, exercise physiologist, and occupational and physical therapists as necessary.
	Assist patient in identifying factors that reduce activity tolerance (inadequate sleep, medication, treatments, environmental conditions).
	Engage immobile patient in passive exercise regimen.
	Assist patient with structural limitations to adapt self-care, exercise, and leisure activities to meet needs.
	Provide assistance to patient as needed, encouraging independence in performing activities.
	Encourage patient to engage in self-care, exercise, and leisure activities that he can tolerate.
	Guide patient in increasing activity within therapeutic limits.
Develop activity/rest pattern supporting increased tolerance of activity.	Discuss with patient usual activity/rest pattern; suggest ways to modify an ineffective pattern.
	Discuss the importance of increasing activity tolerance.
	Encourage patient to participate in planning daily rest periods and activity periods.
	Adjust medication and treatment schedule to support adequate rest.
	Teach patient to monitor response to activity and to alter activity when signs and symptoms of anoxia or excessive fatigue are present.
	Encourage patient to gradually increase active participation in self-care, exercise, and leisure activities.
	Encourage patient to adhere to activity/rest schedule that best promotes increase in activity tolerance.
Use support of family, friends, and health care providers in adjusting activity/rest pattern to meet the need for activity.	Provide patient and significant others information about the importance of establishing a therapeutic activity/rest pattern.
	Review schedule of daily activities of significant others and identify with them how it can be altered to support fulfillment of the patient's needs.
	Encourage patient and significant others to participate in planning a mutually agreeable daily schedule of activity/rest periods.

Patient Goal	Nursing Intervention
	Facilitate expression of patient and significant others' concerns regarding proposed schedule. Identify support available from health care providers if need arises to revise or alter schedule. Encourage family and friends to support patient in efforts to meet need for activity.

The initial nursing assessment provides the opportunity to collect data relevant to an individual's ability to engage in activity and his response to activity. The identification of factors contributing to an inability to tolerate activities (the etiologies) and the presence of signs and symptoms that reflect this inability (the defining characteristics) lead to a nursing diagnosis of activity intolerance.

In the preceding section, goals and nursing interventions supporting goal achievement were specified.[2-4,13,15,18] Although the goals and interventions are presented in general terms, it is assumed that these will be adapted and expanded according to the needs of each individual. The general physiologic and emotional status of the individual, as well as the optimal therapeutic level of activity that should be attained, must be a primary consideration in planning nursing care.

Evaluation of the effectiveness of the nursing interventions is done in terms of whether the patient has achieved the expected outcomes. Each identified outcome reflects elimination or reduction of a specific etiology, thus enhancing the patient's tolerance to activity.

EVALUATION

Patient Outcome	Data Indicating That Outcome is Reached
Absence of weakness during or after engaging in activity	No verbal report of fatigue or weakness after engaging in activity Increased participation in self-care, exercise, and/or leisure activities Erect posture Desire to engage in activity
Optimal level of mobility	Active participation in self-care, exercise, and leisure activity Verbalizes need for active and/or passive exercise and participation as able Adapts activities to meet requirements
Evidence of balance between oxygen supply and demand	Heart rate, rhythm, and quality within therapeutic limits Blood pressure within therapeutic limits Respiratory rate, rhythm, and depth within therapeutic limits Skin color, temperature, and moistness appropriate for amount and intensity of activity Absence of ataxia, dizziness, and confusion
Knowledge of the importance of and the intensity, duration, and frequency of various activities	Describes the benefits of engaging in activity Specifies the recommended intensity, duration, and frequency of various activities Participation in activities in recommended manner
An appreciation of the need to participate in activities	Expresses desire to engage in activities Willing participation in self-care, exercise, and leisure activities
State of being physiologically conditioned to regularly participate in activities	Cardiovascular and respiratory status supports participation in activities Regularly engages in a variety of activities
Uses support of significant others to achieve and maintain therapeutic levels of activity	Identifies persons available to support efforts to enhance activity tolerance Plans activities with those persons who can assist in achieving optimal activity tolerance Seeks advice of health care providers as needed Maintains therapeutic activity schedule

References

1. American Heart Association, The Committee on Exercise: Exercise testing of individuals with heart disease or at high risk for its development, Dallas, 1975, American Heart Association, Inc.
2. Campbell, C.: Nursing diagnosis and intervention in nursing practice, New York, 1978, John Wiley & Sons, Inc.
3. Campbell, C.: Nursing diagnosis and intervention in nursing practice, ed. 2, New York, 1980, John Wiley & Sons, Inc.
4. Carpenito, L.J.: Nursing diagnosis: application to practice, Philadelphia, 1983, J.B. Lippincott Co.
5. Glass, L.B.: Exercise therapy for the patient with pulmonary dysfunction, Top. Clin. Nurs. **3**:87-93, 1981.
6. Gordon, M.: Assessing activity tolerance, Am. J. Nurs. **76**(1):72-75, 1976.
7. Gordon, M.: Manual of nursing diagnosis, New York, 1982, McGraw-Hill Book Co.
8. Gordon, M.: Nursing diagnosis: process and application, New York, 1982, McGraw-Hill Book Co.
9. Gould, M.T.: Nursing diagnoses concurrent with multiple sclerosis, J. Neurosurg. Nurs. **15**(6):339-345, 1983.
10. Halfman, M.A., and Hojnacki, L.H.: Exercise and maintenance of health, Top. Clin. Nurs. **3**:1-10, 1981.
11. Kim, M.J., McFarland, G.K., and McLane, A.M.: Classification of nursing diagnoses: Proceedings of the Fifth National Conference, St. Louis, 1984, The C.V. Mosby Co.
12. Kim, M.J., McFarland, G.K., and McLane, A.M.: Pocket guide to nursing diagnoses, St. Louis, 1984, The C.V. Mosby Co.
13. Miller, J.F.: Energy deficits in the chronically ill: the patient with arthritis. In Miller, J.F., editor: Coping with chronic illness: overcoming powerlessness, Philadelphia, 1983, F.A. Davis Co.
14. Muir, B.L.: Pathophysiology: an introduction to the mechanisms of disease, New York, 1980, John Wiley & Sons, Inc.
15. Orem, D.E.: Nursing concepts of practice, ed. 2, New York, 1980, McGraw-Hill Book Co.
16. Price, S.A., and Wilson, L.M.: Pathophysiology: clinical concepts of disease processes, ed. 2, New York, 1982, McGraw-Hill Book Co.
17. Sanderson, R.G., and Kurth, C.L.: The cardiac patient: a comprehensive approach, Philadelphia, 1983, W.B. Saunders Co.
18. Sculco, C.D.: The need for activity. In Yura, H., and Walsh, M., editors: Human needs and the nursing process, New York, 1978, Appleton-Century-Crofts.
19. White, P.D., and others: Rehabilitation of the cardiovascular patient, New York, 1958, McGraw-Hill Book Co.

DIVERSIONAL ACTIVITY, DEFICIT
THEORY AND ETIOLOGY

Philosopher Arthur Schopenhauer wrote that "the two foes of human happiness are pain and boredom."[1] Nursing has devoted much of its efforts to the treatment of pain but very little to the alleviation of boredom. A deficit in diversional activity often is manifested by reports of boredom by patients whose usual forms of activity are interrupted by illness, disability, or life changes. Boredom is especially prevalent in those persons whose illnesses extend for a long time, those who are hospitalized or otherwise institutionalized, or those who spend many hours in health treatment situations.

Integral to quality of life, diversion is a phenomenon that merits further study by nurses. Work on the nursing diagnosis of diversional activity deficit by the National Conference on the Classification of Nursing Diagnoses (now known as NANDA) has thus far resulted in no conclusive definition of the phenomenon. Gordon[3] has offered this definition: "decreased engagement in recreational or leisure activities." Although this definition provides a start in explaining a diversional deficit, the concept may be more complex than it appears. One of the issues raised at the Fifth National Conference was a need for careful definition of diversion.[4]

Webster's Dictionary offers one definition of diversion as "pastime or amusement" and two other definitions: "distraction of attention" and "anything that diverts or distracts the attention."[8] The second and third definitions imply a component of change, variety, or digression in one's focus of attention, but they do not qualify that state as being necessarily pleasurable or amusing. The first definition does not directly address change or variety of activity but focuses on the pleasurable quality.

Roget's Thesaurus offers several sets of synonyms for diversion that support this duality of definition. One set is oriented toward pleasure and amusement (recreation, relaxation, pastime, enjoyment, entertainment, and solace). Others are classified under change, deviation, and distraction (variety, transition, renewal, departure, digression, variation, and divided attention).[6]

From this study of words it appears that diversional activity could be defined with a focus on either the ideas of change and deviation or on the ideas of enjoyment and pleasure. Diversion as change simply could mean activities that are different from one's usual activities. There are many examples of this type of diversion. Persons who slow down to stare at accidents along the road as they are driving are experiencing a diversion from their usual driving pattern. The attention of a bedridden patient is diverted when a patient in the next bed cries out or when there is a commotion in the hallway. These types of diversions are not necessarily pleasurable or satisfying, but they do interrupt routines and often alleviate boredom.

Diversion as enjoyment or pleasure is more closely related to the concept of recreation and is the basis for Gordon's definition. Frye and Peters[2] offer a definition of recreation as "experience derived from participation in voluntarily chosen pursuits engaged in during unobligated time (leisure) primarily for purpose of personal satisfaction or enjoyment." This type of diversion focuses on the personal choice to do something one enjoys.

It connotes self-expression and self-development and usually is therapeutic.

The two defined aspects of diversion may be equally valid as nursing concerns. A need for diversion as change or variety in activities may be as important as a need for diversion as recreation or enjoyment. Variety of experience and recreation may be seen as subcategories of the broader concept of diversion. However, within the pattern of activity-exercise a recreational orientation may be more relevant.

Diversion as change or variety is closely related to sensory input and as such has many cognitive-perceptual elements that could be explored within that context. The optimal balance between stability in routines and variety or distraction from the routine largely depends on sensory intactness. Persons who suffer from dementia, such as Alzheimer's disease, function best with a minimum of diversions in a consistent routine; however, a young person immobilized with multiple fractures could benefit from a daily regimen that includes a high degree of variety.

There is a need to research the relevance of diversion within a cognitive-perceptual context. An exploration of relationships among sensory deprivation, sensory overload, and diversional activities might provide valuable insight into the study of diversion as change or variety.

For the purposes of this discussion the second focus, that of pleasurable or recreational activities, is explored. Therefore the following definition of diversion is offered: Diversion encompasses those activities which are recreational and are pursued during leisure time for the purpose of personal amusement or satisfaction. Leisure is that time which is free from obligations.

The amount of time that Americans leave free and unobligated is increasing steadily. It is projected that by the year 2000 about 39% of the nation's time will be spent at leisure; this is compared with figures of 25% in 1900 and 34% in 1950.[9] Americans engage in many diversional or recreational activities.

For many individuals their self-expression is linked closely to their leisure activities. Frye and Peters[2] see the "relaxed freedom of self chosen activity in unobligated time (as) . . . a good frame of reference for seeing oneself as one truly is." Obligated time (time "on the job" for most people) is spent doing things required by one's boss, one's need to earn money, one's own expectations of a job requirement, or the social norms of the work place. Unobligated time is spent in those activities one chooses. There is a freedom in making the choices of leisure activities that allow one to do what one wants to do rather than what one should do.

Those are personal choices and are largely dependent on a person's knowledge of various options. A person who has never seen snow is unlikely to be a skier. An activity that requires a large expenditure of money is unlikely to be chosen by a poor person. Persons who have never heard an opera would not consider opera a diversional option.

Because diversional activities have meaning, purpose, and value to the individual, the determination of a deficit in those activities is highly personal. The amount of time spent idly and the point at which boredom occurs vary greatly. Therefore to study diversion and diagnose a deficit in this area, a patient's own preillness or pre–life change schedule of activities must be a baseline for comparison with the postillness or post–life change schedule. A person who has a definite set of hobbies or recreational activities may experience more of a deficit than a person who normally engages in few activities when they become impossible.

Time perception is an important indicator of a person's diversional needs and is also a highly individual phenomenon. Smith[7] concluded that time perception may be related to the pace of one's geographic location. A city dweller who is accustomed to a rapid pace of living and constant sensory stimulation may be bored more quickly in a confined situation than a rural resident who has a slower life-style. This is a broad generalization, however, and needs to be validated in each situation rather than be assumed.

Time has another specific relationship to diversion, that is, the amount of unobligated time available. A person who has little or no unobligated time may have a diversional activity deficit because the time necessary to engage in such activities is unavailable. Likewise, a person who has more idle time than usual may have a deficit because there are not enough activities to fill the time.

A deficit of leisure time is more likely to occur for persons who are not confined to a treatment center and who have an excess of obligations in their lives. Such persons may be essentially healthy or suffering from chronic illnesses that do not interfere with their usual life-style. Their contact with nurses is frequently in an outpatient setting.

People with an excess of unobligated time are seen more frequently in an inpatient situation. Patients who are confined for extended periods have their usual obligated activities curtailed and have an increase in unobligated or leisure time. In addition, having an increase in leisure time with no diversions to fill that time may also be a problem to persons who retire from their jobs but have not planned activities for themselves.

Space is a factor that often limits the type of diversional activities. Patients who are hospitalized, especially those who are bedridden, live in a confined space where usually the only obvious diversion is television viewing. If a person does not enjoy television, problems arise. Patients may not be able to identify alternative diversions within their limited space. The confinement of space becomes even more of a problem to those whose usual diversions take place in large areas, for example, those whose leisure activities center around sports or total-body exercises. Space confinement is less of a problem for persons who enjoy reading or small crafts.

Although availability of time and space often limit the types of activities a person engages in, the desire to do something of a diversional nature is more closely related to personal energy levels. Given similar amounts of time and space, one person may have sufficient energy to engage in diversional activities and another may not. Of course, energy is linked to one's state of health, and nurses need to be aware of a person's capabilities before presuming a deficit exists. Persons who have little energy are content to spend time doing nothing, whereas those persons who have a higher energy level may be bored in the same circumstances.

In summary, the relationship among variables that determine diversional activities is more important than each variable alone. Available time and space allow for diversions, but energy level and desire of activities must be considered. What constitutes boredom for one person would not for another.

Some of the factors that contribute to the lack of fulfillment of the need for diversional activity have been defined at the Nursing Diagnosis Conferences.[5] They are environmental lack of diversional activity, long-term hospitalization, and frequent, lengthy treatments. Gordon adds the term *apathy* to long-term hospitalization.[3]

These etiologies are broad in scope and could be stated more explicitly. Environmental factors are different for a person who resides in a treatment center (hospital, nursing home) than for a person who lives at home and receives treatment as an outpatient. Persons who live at home may have problems such as limited finances, lack of transportation, social isolation, impaired mobility, impaired sensory functions (deafness, blindness), fear of neighborhood crime, or respiratory or cardiac difficulties with exertion, any of which would contribute to their being homebound or could limit diversional opportunities. Many of these factors are especially prevalent in elderly persons who have chronic illnesses or in people of any age who have severe handicaps.

At the other end of the continuum are persons who may not suffer from any overt altered health state but who have diversional activity deficits because they perceive that they have very little unobligated time. Etiologic factors causing these persons to have a deficit may be problematic time management, excessive job obligations, or fatigue. These persons may be seen in a health care situation because they have an excess of stress or have stress-related health problems. They feel caught in a cycle of their increased stress precluding leisure activities and the lack of diversional activities contributing to their stress.

Persons who are hospitalized, especially for lengthy periods, develop diversional activity deficits because their usual leisure habits frequently are impossible. Often they cannot think of alternative activities, nor do they consider the possibility of developing new methods of expression. The social structure of hospitals is such that patients have little say in establishing routines. Their world becomes small and detail oriented. Etiologies for diversional activity deficits in these patients may be lack of specification of alternative diversions, lack of accessibility of resources, lack of space, or lack of knowledge about activities that might be possible.

Mental state is an integral influence on participation in diversional activities and is important for patients who reside either in or outside of treatment centers. Depression or apathy may limit seriously a person's participation in activities that are possible and also may impede the imagination of new diversions.

In summary, the following list of possible etiologies for diversional activity deficit is offered:

Personal factors
    Problematic time management
    Lack of specification of desired diversions
    Depression
    Apathy
    Fatigue
    Impaired mobility
    Impaired sensory functions
    Impaired cardiopulmonary functions
    Lack of knowledge
    Lack of exposure/orientation to diversional activity
Environmental factors, home-based patients
    Limited finances
    Lack of transportation
    Social isolation
    Fear of neighborhood crime
Environmental factors, patients in treatment centers
    Lack of space
    Lack of resources
    Lack of knowledge of treatment center routines

DEFINING CHARACTERISTICS[3,5]

Little or no unobligated time or increase in amount of unobligated time
No pattern of leisure time activities*
Preillness leisure activities impossible since illness
No postillness substitute activities defined
Unavailability of resources for identified leisure activities
Confined space
Perception of impossibility of leisure activities

*Critical defining characteristic.

Perception of time passing slowly
Statement of desire for something to do*
Statement of boredom*
Daytime napping
Disinterest in television viewing
Energy level sufficient for recreational activities but no
    participation in such activities

Defining characteristics are raw data that together operationally define a deficit in diversional activities. Nurses collect data, first to determine if a problem exists; then they look at possible etiologies or contributing factors to the problem. Before care is planned, it is necessary to collect data to determine strengths that may be tapped by the patient to offset the problem. In most patient situations these three sets of information are collected and then sifted during the data analysis phase.

*Critical defining characteristic.

The following parameters are suggested as guidelines in collecting data to determine only if a diversional activity deficit exists. These parameters can be adapted for patients who are in treatment centers or are outpatients.
A. Usual activity routines before illness
    1. Amount of unobligated time
    2. Leisure activities, type and amount
        a. Resources used in leisure activities
    3. Knowledge of recreational options
B. Usual activity routines since illness or hospitalization
    1. Amount of unobligated time
    2. Leisure activities, type and amount
        a. Resources used in leisure activities
    3. Degree of confinement
C. Energy level (sufficient for diversional activities?)
D. Desire for activity
E. Mental status

NURSING INTERVENTIONS

Patient Goal	Nursing Intervention
Describe usual pattern of diversional activities.	Let patient know rationale for this—that usual pattern is a baseline for planning. Maintain nonjudgmental response to patient report. Elicit details of amount of time spent in diversional activity, location, resources.
Identify changes in ability to engage in usual diversional activities, or identify problems perceived with usual pattern of activities. (Consider etiology of problem to choose one outcome or the other.)	Ascertain patient's perceptions of present situation. Avoid leading questions. Encourage patient to consider changes in desire, available time, energy level, space, other constraints.
Choose one usual diversional activity to continue, and/or identify usual diversional activity that may be adapted to new constraints, and/or identify new diversional activity that may be started.	Whenever possible encourage patient to continue with those activities that were meaningful to him. Encourage creativity in choices. Encourage patient to identify activity; avoid suggestions unless patient unable to think of possibilities. Remember that diversional activities should be personally meaningful. Focus on the positive more than negative (''You can do this'' rather than ''You can't do that''). Orient patient to options available within the system, such as recreational therapy programs. After patient makes choice, if appropriate, validate with medical team patient capabilities to engage in chosen activity.
List resources needed for chosen activity.	Maintain emphasis on personal choice. Be careful not to assume what patient needs for chosen activity.
Identify means to obtain needed resources.	Consider what can be obtained within the system; what could be provided by family, friends; what are vital to activity; and what can be adapted from available options.
Engage in chosen diversional activity.	Support patient in chosen activity. Adapt environment as necessary. Provide positive feedback.
Express satisfaction with chosen activity.	Evaluate patient's perception of chosen activity. Allow for change of plans if activity unsatisfactory.

Once it has been established that a problem exists, it is necessary to determine the etiology for the deficit. In an actual clinical situation the etiology specifies the parameters of the problem more explicitly and allows for personalization of nursing care. Expected patient outcomes and nursing interventions presented in the preceding plan are general for most patients who have a diversional activity deficit. A key theme in this plan is a personal choice of activity by the patient. With such an approach the patient's diversional activity has meaning and purpose to that patient and is not just "something to do."

EVALUATION

Patient Outcome	Data Indicating That Outcome is Reached
Describe usual pattern of diversional activities	Indicates time free from obligations Lists activities that are self-chosen Relates the what, where, when, and how of diversional activities
Identify changes in ability to engage in usual diversional activities, *or* identify problems perceived with usual pattern of activities	Can realistically list changes in situation Compares present situation to past
Choose one usual activity to continue, *or* identify usual activity that may be adapted, *or* identify new diversional activity.	Makes a personal choice Sees possibilities of continuation of activity within constraints, *or* is able to see old activity in new light, *or* lists other interests that could be tried Can use a problem-solving approach to changed situation
List resources needed for chosen activity.	Gets involved in details of activity chosen Exhibits an action orientation
Identify means to obtain needed resources.	Takes responsibility for choice Uses problem-solving approach
Engage in chosen diversional activity.	Is seen actually doing something Fits activity into daily routine Makes choices as to when activity occurs Establishes new pattern that decreases idle time
Express satisfaction with chosen activity.	No reports of boredom Discusses activity Shows increase of interest in self

References

1. Bartlett, J.: Familiar quotations, ed. 14, Boston, 1968, Little, Brown & Co.
2. Frye, V., and Peters, M.: Therapeutic recreation: its theory, philosophy, and practice, Harrisburg, Pa., 1972, Stockpole Co.
3. Gordon, M.: Manual of nursing diagnosis, New York, 1982, McGraw-Hill Book Co.
4. Kim, M.J., McFarland, G.K., and McLane, A.M.: Classification of nursing diagnoses: Proceedings of the Fifth National Conference, St. Louis, 1984, The C.V. Mosby Co.
5. Kim, M.J., McFarland, G.K., and McLane, A.M.: Pocket guide to nursing diagnoses, St. Louis, 1984, The C.V. Mosby Co.
6. Roget's international thesaurus, ed. 4, New York, 1977, Thomas Y. Crowell, Publishers.
7. Smith, M.J.: Duration experience for bed-confined subjects: a replication and refinement, Nurs. Res. **28**(3):139-144, 1979.
8. Webster's new world dictionary of the American language, New York, 1972, The World Publishing Co.
9. The 1981 White House Conference on Aging: report of technical committee on the physical and social environment and quality of life, Washington, D.C., 1981, U.S. Government Printing Office.

SLEEP PATTERN DISTURBANCE

THEORY AND ETIOLOGY

Sleep is identified as a basic human need by Yura and Walsh.[15] Most individuals view sleep as a relatively passive state that is not a problem until it concerns amount. According to Steincrohn,[13] over 100 million Americans complain each year of some sleep problems, identified as insomnia, chronic fatigue, or listlessness. Nicholson and Marks[10] state that one out of every three adults suffers some difficulty sleeping some time each year. The difficulties may consist of delayed onset of sleep, early awakening, insufficient or broken sleep, or a combination of these problems. Sleep pattern disturbances are common among patients with medical or psychiatric illnesses and can sometimes compound the illness. Nurses can help patients meet their physiologic needs for sleep.

Before sleep pattern disturbances can be discussed, the minimum requirements for sleep and the function of sleep need to be described. There are wide variations in individuals' required sleep. Both the total sleep time and the total nightly amounts of sleep are age dependent. Mendelson and co-workers[9] report that in general total sleep time is greatest in infancy and gradually decreases in childhood. Total sleep time is stable in adulthood until old age, when it decreases.[11] In addition, the number of awakenings during sleep is highest in infancy and childhood. However, Mendelson[9] states that the number of awakenings per night also tends to increase after age 40. Normal amounts of sleeping time for adults have been described as anywhere from 6 to 9 hours. Nicholson and associates[10] described some variations from the ''normal'' adult that are not considered pathologic for these individuals. There are naturally short and naturally long sleepers. Short sleepers generally require less than 6 hours of sleep per night and show no signs of sleep deprivation when they achieve this amount. The naturally long sleepers seem to require 9 to 14 hours of sleep per night to show no signs of sleep deprivation. Mendelson[9] also describes individuals who have variations in their sleep phase cycle. Those individuals with an advanced sleep cycle tend to need to sleep early in the evening and then arise early in the morning. There are also individuals who could be described as ''late night owls,'' whose natural pattern is to stay up late into the early morning hours and then to arise in the late morning. These normal patterns sometimes result in difficulty because the individual's pattern is not in congruence with the rest of society. The ''late night owl'' may suffer from sleep deprivation because he or she goes to bed late and must arise early to go to work. Since there are such wide variations in the sleep requirements for individuals, the nurse and the patient must learn to assess the sleep requirements of and the natural pattern for the individual carefully so that sleep deprivation can be avoided or treated.

For a single individual, sleep needs vary at times during their life. Certain normal physiologic changes that occur during the lifespan can affect sleep needs. For example, Dement[2] states that a pregnant woman on the average needs 2 additional hours of sleep per night. Although there is not enough scientific evidence to document by what amount sleep needs vary during illness, experience seems to indicate that certain pathologic conditions alter the need for sleep. Many individuals sleep more hours when they have a cold or a fever, and with

more serious illnesses such as cancer individuals tend to spend more hours sleeping. Conversely, there may be times in an individual's life when less sleep is required. Recognition of these changing needs by the client may reduce the number of complaints of sleep difficulties.

Some complaints of sleep difficulties may be related to a discrepancy between individuals' expectations for sleep and their actual ability to sleep.[11] For instance, Mendelson[9] states that it is just as unrealistic for a 65-year-old person to expect to be able to sleep as well as he or she did at age 20 as to expect to be able to run as well as he or she did at age 20. In a study of elderly patients Hayter[5] found that many were dissatisfied with the amount of sleep that they were obtaining. Complaints of both too little and too much sleep were expressed by these clients. As age increases, Hayter[5] found that the amount of time spent in bed also increases. After age 85 there is a greater perceived need for something to promote sleep. With increasing amounts of time spent in bed and a decrease in the need for sleep, complaints of sleep difficulties are more likely. Anxiety about not meeting sleep expectations can actually lead to real long-term sleep difficulties.[9]

Sleep needs and the functions of sleep are little understood by medical science. In recent years there has been an increasing number of studies on sleep. Sleep is a behavioral state that can be defined as a ''recurrent, easily reversable condition characterized by a relative quiescence and by a greatly increased threshold for response to external stimulation.''[4] Common sense tells us that sleep and fatigue are related, but scientific evidence indicates that the relief of fatigue is not the sole function of sleep. Through studies of sleep deprivation some clues to the functions of sleep have been identified. Sleep is a restorative process in nature.[4] Physical restoration with RNA and protein synthesis occurs during sleep. Also, attentional ability, ability to learn, ego mechanisms, and sense of self apparently are restored by sleep.

Normal sleep patterns have definite cycles and rhythms. Two distinct types of sleep have been identified through the electroencephalogram, the electrooculogram, and the electromyogram. These are REM and nonREM sleep.[2] The initial sleep that the individual experiences is nonREM sleep, or quiet sleep.[2] NonREM sleep is characterized by slow regular breathing, absence of body movement, slow regular brain activity, and snoring. Four stages of nonREM sleep have been identified. During stages 1 through 4 the individual is said to descend into deep sleep. In stage 4, it is extremely difficult to waken an individual. Sleep-walking, night terrors, and bed-wetting usually occur during stage 4 sleep. REM sleep, or active sleep, is characterized by twitches of the face and fingertips, irregular breathing (very fast then slow), no snoring, and rapid eye movements. During REM sleep the large muscles of the body are completely paralyzed, and both cerebral blood flow and body temperature are increased. During sleep there is a regular pattern or cycle of nonREM and REM sleep. The sleep cycle lasts anywhere from 70 to 110 minutes with an average of 90 minutes. The percentage of time within the various stages of sleep varies over the life cycle.[2] Infants have the highest amount of stage 4 sleep. On the average, young adults spent 50% of sleep time in stage 2, 25% in REM, 10% in stage 3, 10% in stage 4, and 5% in stage 1.[9] Not only can the total sleep time be deprived, but also REM sleep deprivation can occur in the individual who is receiving enough sleep.[2] Symptoms of REM deprivation are impaired memory, psychologic problems, and difficulty in acquiring new data. Alcohol, hypnotics, stimulants, and antidepressants all can suppress REM sleep.[9] When the depriving factor is discontinued, a rebound in REM sleep occurs. During rebound REM sleep individuals experience vivid dreams. For some individuals their dreams prove frightening. Sometimes preknowledge that vivid dreams are likely to occur after a hypnotic is discontinued serves to reassure the patient.

There is much discussion in the literature of the consequences of sleep deprivation. However, when sleep deprivation has been studied, it has been in extreme cases. Individuals are deprived of sleep for several days while their physiologic and psychologic states are observed. Individuals who are deprived of sleep experience strong desires to fall asleep, especially during the night hours.[2] These individuals also experience difficulty in performing repetitive tasks without falling asleep, shortened attention spans, and sometimes paranoid psychoses.[4] For individuals to keep themselves awake, a great deal of physical effort is required. What is not clear from these studies of sleep deprivation is the consequence of shorter deprivations, such as only receiving 4 hours of sleep for several nights when 7 hours is the physiologic requirement. There is not enough scientific evidence in current sleep research to give us that answer. Anecdotally, people complain of fatigue, drowsiness, excessive daytime sleep, and sometimes personality changes. Whether the shorter deprivations have serious health consequences is unknown. Certainly, this is an important question, since so many individuals complain of the consequences of sleep difficulty. Productivity in society may be impaired because of these deprivations.

When discussing sleep pattern disturbances, it is important to identify the type of disturbance occurring. Sleep pattern disturbances could be divided into three types: (1) interrupted sleep, (2) difficulty in falling asleep, or (3) excessive daytime sleepiness. Individuals may complain of just one of these types or may have a combination. These sleep pattern disturbances can either be acute or chronic. Acute disturbances are quite normal reactions to grief and do not necessarily present a problem because of their short duration. However, sometimes disturbances that are expressions of normal grief may lead to chronic difficulties that require intervention.

Sleep interruption can be caused by external or internal factors. Excessive noise, bright lights, and children awakening during the night can all disturb sleep as well as uncomfortable or crowded beds.[13] Many individuals are sensitive to changes in their environment and have difficulty sleeping in hospitals or when they travel.[2,9] Internal states of the individual can also interrupt sleep. Pain, nocturia, hunger, coughing, difficulty breathing, ingested chemicals (such as caffeine, alcohol, and hypnotics) all can interrupt sleep.[2,9] Difficulty in falling asleep may be caused by the same factors.

Insomnia is a common term used to describe sleep pattern disturbances. It is usually defined as the subjective feeling that one is not getting enough sleep. One survey[14] found that the incidence of insomnia was about 14%. Insomnia is really difficulty in falling asleep either at bedtime or after awakening during the night. There may be a psychogenic cause such as anxiety, depression, sexual arousal, fear of some phenomenon associated with sleep (such as loss of consciousness, death, content of dreams), fear of not sleeping, or psychiatric disturbances. Furthermore, nightmares can cause insomnia. Pain or other discomforts such as asthma can prevent sleep. There is also evidence that lack of regular exercise can be related to sleep difficulties. However, any exercise that is done should be in the daytime or early evening. Exercise at bedtime can inhibit sleep.[9]

Excessive daytime sleepiness is most often related to two physiologic illnesses—sleep apnea and narcolepsy.[2,9-11] Sleep apnea can either be caused by an abnormality in the central nervous system or obstruction of the nasopharynx passages. Both sleep apnea and narcolepsy are conditions that require medical supervision. In assessing the client the nurse should try to rule out these conditions. It is most common for the sleep apnea client to have problems with snoring or sleeping in rather strange positions. One assessment technique is to tape record the client during sleep.[9] A client with a history of daytime sleepiness and snoring should be referred for further medical diagnosis.

Listed below are possible etiologies for the nursing diagnosis of sleep pattern disturbance[1-3,7,9-11,13,14]:

Noise
Excessive light
Uncomfortable surroundings (bed or bedclothing)
Excessive heat or cold
Crowded bed
Children disturbing sleep
Unfamiliar environment

Rapid time zone change, jet lag

Shift work or frequent changes in schedules

Physical discomfort (e.g., pain, asthma, nocturia, hunger)

Ingested chemicals (e.g., caffeine, hypnotics, antihistamines, alcohol, decongestants, stimulants)

Sleep apnea

Psychiatric disorders

Anxiety

Depression

Stress, personal or family

Inadequate physical activity

Excessive daytime sleep

Fear of some phenomenon associated with sleep

Fear of not sleeping

DEFINING CHARACTERISTICS

Verbal complaints of difficulty falling asleep

Early awakening

Interrupted sleep (list type of interruption)

Verbal complaint of not feeling well rested

Reduction in performance (work, school, or home)

Increasing irritability

Restlessness

Disorientation (progressive)

Lethargy

Listlessness

Mild fleeting nystagmus

Slight hand tremor

Ptosis of eyelids

Expressionless face

Thick speech with mispronunciation and incorrect words

Dark circles under eyes

Frequent yawning

Changes in posture

Naps during day

Excessive sleepiness during day

Less than 5 hours of sleep per night

In diagnosing sleep pattern disturbance, the nurse may find any number of defining characteristics in the patient.[3,7,8,15] However, the critical indicators of a diagnosis are complaints of difficulty falling asleep, interrupted sleep, and complaints of not feeling well rested. The other characteristics are consequences of sleep pattern disturbances or further specification of the extent of the disturbance.

The following parameters should be used to arrive at the diagnosis of sleep pattern disturbance:

A. Sleep initiation: How long does it take the patient to fall asleep?

B. Sleep interruptions
1. How many times per night is sleep interrupted?
2. What interrupts sleep?

C. Quality of sleep
1. How does patient feel in the morning?
2. How does patient describe his sleep?
3. Is the patient disturbed by long periods of wakefulness during the night?
4. Is the patient satisfied with his sleep?
5. Does the patient have complaints about his sleep? Specify.

D. Sleep habits
1. What is the patient's usual bedtime?
2. How many hours of sleep does the patient receive each night?
3. Does the patient snore?
4. What is the patient's usual awakening time?
5. How many hours of sleep does the patient feel he needs to be well rested and to function at optimal level?
6. What is the patient's usual bedtime routine?
7. What methods does the patient habitually use to fall asleep?
   a. Reading
   b. Prayer
   c. Meditation
   d. Relaxation
   e. Watching television
   f. Medication (name type)
   g. Beverage (name type)
8. How many individuals sleep in the same bedroom as the patient?
9. What type of bed does the patient prefer?
10. How many pillows does the patient use?
11. Does the patient prefer the window opened or closed?

E. Dreams
1. Does the patient have dreams?
2. How frequent are the patient's dreams?
3. How vivid are the patient's dreams?

F. Social habits
1. On the average, how many of the following beverages does the patient drink each day?
   a. Regular coffee
   b. Decaffeinated coffee
   c. Regular tea
   d. Herbal tea
   e. Cola drinks with caffeine
   f. Other carbonated drinks
   g. Alcoholic beverages
2. What are the patient's eating times during the day? Specifically examine the times that the patient eats in relation to bedtime and examine what types of food are eaten late at night.

NURSING INTERVENTIONS

Patient Goal	Nursing Intervention
Consume a diet and adhere to a medication schedule that is congruent with satisfactory sleep.	Instruct patient about relationship between sleep and diet. Teach patient to eliminate caffeine from diet. Instruct patient regarding relationship between alcohol intake and sleep. Teach patient to drink no more than one alcoholic beverage per day. Obtain daily medication schedule from patient and examine these medications for side effects of sleep disturbances; for prescribed medications, discuss the medications with the physician. Discourage the patient from taking sleeping medications, either prescribed or over the counter; explain that sleeping medications are only effective for a short-term disturbance and that sleeping medications on a long-term basis can induce sleep disturbances. Discuss with the patient the possibility that both hunger and spicy foods can interfere with sleep. Encourage the patient to eat a bedtime snack such as milk and crackers to prevent disturbance from hunger.
Establish a regular routine at bedtime.	Identify patient's sleep needs based on an assessment of patient's physiologic state, age, and previous sleep patterns. Instruct the patient about the internal and external factors that interfere with sleep. Assist the patient to identify those internal and/or external factors that interfere with sleep. Assist the patient to select one interfering factor to eliminate for 1 week. (After eliminating that factor, the patient selects another factor to eliminate. This pattern continues until all possible elimination is accomplished.) Instruct the patient about circadian rhythms and their importance to sleep. (If regular routines are established, sleep should become easier.) Establish a regular rising time and encourage patient to get up at that time no matter how well or how poorly he has slept. Instruct the patient that excessive time in bed tends to lead to lighter sleep and that time in bed worrying about getting to sleep tends to further exacerbate sleep difficulties. Encourage patient to go to bed only when sleepy. Establish a maximum time that the patient should spend in bed trying to fall asleep (between 15 and 30 minutes is usually a good amount). Encourage patient to get out of bed and engage in another activity if he has not fallen asleep in the established time period. (The same rule should be applied to those times that the patient awakes in the course of the night and is unable to fall asleep.)
Establish a program of regular activity and exercise during the day.	Instruct the patient about the relationship between sleep and regular exercise. (For satisfactory sleep, it is important that exercise is on a regular basis and that the exercise is during the day or early evening hours.) Assist patient in selecting an exercise activity that is enjoyable and appropriate for his physiologic condition. Encourage patient to begin exercise program. Instruct the patient about the relationship between napping and nighttime sleep. Encourage the patient to skip naps to maximize quality of nighttime sleep.
Develop a bedroom environment that is congruent with satisfactory sleep.	Instruct the patient about relationship between sleep environment and the quality of sleep. (When sleep difficulties occur, it is important that the bedroom is used solely for the purpose of sleep. When the bedroom is used for other activities, anxieties associated with these activities may become a problem when the patient is attempting to sleep.) Encourage patient to use the bedroom only for sleep. Alter lighting, temperature, and noise levels in bedroom so that sleep can be maximized.

As with most diagnoses, the preferable plan of care aims at the cause or the etiology of the disturbance. In the case of sleep pattern disturbances the nurse, after the assessment of the patient, should attempt to change the cause of the problem. If the etiology of the sleep pattern disturbance is pain, anxiety, spiritual distress, ineffective airway clearance, ineffective breathing pattern, alteration in urinary patterns, or abnormal grieving, the reader should refer to those sections in this text. In this care plan a behavioral approach to sleep pattern disturbances is taken. Regardless of the etiology of the sleep pattern disturbance, certain factors that are minor causes may need to be altered to minimize the problem. For example, alterations in the external environment may be necessary in any case to maximize the patient's ability to sleep undisturbed. Education with regard to normal require-ments of sleep should be discussed with all patients who have this diagnosis. The care plan should also focus on the elimination of internal states that may disturb sleep, such as hunger and ingested chemicals.

The nursing interventions given here assume that the patient is an outpatient. If the patient is in the hospital, the nurse has much more control over the environment and therefore more responsibility to examine and alter the environment to promote sleep. The nurse should determine the necessity of taking vital signs and other night-shift routines that may awaken the patient. The nurse should ensure that the hospital environment (especially the ICU) provides the patients with a clear differentiation between night and day. Sensitivity to the environmental factors that interfere with sleep may do much to promote satisfactory sleep within the hospital.

EVALUATION

Patient Outcome	Data Indicating That Outcome is Reached
Diet and medication intake congruent with satisfactory sleep	No caffeine consumption One or less alcoholic beverage consumed per day No sleeping medications Patient eats a bedtime snack Elimination of interfering factors
Regular bedtime routine conducive to satisfactory sleep	Patient arises at same time each day No more than 30 minutes spent in bed trying to get to sleep Patient goes to bed only when sleepy; bedtime approximately same time each night Patient gets out of bed when sleep does not occur within 30 minutes of bedtime
Regular exercise program implemented	Daily exercise routine No naps during the day
Bedroom conducive to sleep	Bedroom used for sleeping only External interferences in bedroom removed
Satisfactory sleep experienced	No or fewer than previous interruptions to sleep No symptoms of insufficient sleep Satisfaction with amount and quality of sleep

References

1. Carlson, J.H., Craft, C.A., and McGuire, A.D.: Nursing diagnosis, Philadelphia, 1982, W.B. Saunders Co.
2. Dement, W.C.: Some must watch while others sleep, San Francisco, 1974, W.H. Freeman Co.
3. Gordon, M.: Nursing diagnosis: process and application, New York, 1982, McGraw-Hill Book Co.
4. Hartmann, E.L.: The functions of sleep, New Haven, Conn., 1973, Yale University Press.
5. Hayter, J.: Sleep behaviors of older persons, Nurs. Res. 32(4):242-246, 1983.
6. Jovanovic, U.J.: Normal sleep in man, Stuttgart, 1971, Hippokrates Verlag.
7. Kim, M., McFarland, G., and McLane, A.: Pocket guide to nursing diagnosis, St. Louis, 1984, The C.V. Mosby Co.
8. Kim, M., and Moritz, D.: Classification of nursing diagnoses: Proceedings of the Third and Fourth National Conferences, New York, 1982, McGraw-Hill Book Co.
9. Mendelson, W.B., Gillin, J.C., and Wyatt, R.J.: Human sleep and its disorders, New York, 1977, Plenum Press.
10. Nicholson, A.N., and Marks, J.: Insomnia: a guide for medical practitioners, Boston, 1983, MTP Press Limited.
11. Orr, W.C., Altshuler, K.Z., and Stahl, M.L.: Managing sleep complaints, Chicago, 1982, Year-Book Medical Publishers, Inc.
12. Oswald, I.: Sleep, London, 1980, Penguin Books.
13. Steincrohn, P.J.: How to get a good night's sleep, Chicago, 1968, Henry Regnery Co.
14. Williams, R.L., and Karacan, I., editors: Sleep disorders: diagnosis and treatment, New York, 1978, John Wiley & Sons, Inc.
15. Yura, H., and Walsh, M.B.: Human needs and the nursing process, New York, 1978, Appleton-Century-Crofts.

MOBILITY, IMPAIRED PHYSICAL
THEORY AND ETIOLOGY

Mobility, the ability of an individual to move about freely, is a highly valued aspect of physical functioning. Through movement a person can perform an almost endless variety of physical actions, ranging from withdrawing from danger to seeking pleasurable experiences.[20] Mobility is also "one of the central attributes by which human beings define and express themselves and by which they measure their health and physical fitness."[21]

Recognizing the essential significance of mobility to both physical and psychologic well-being, it seems reasonable to assume that nurses are actively concerned with impairments in physical mobility. Indeed, "because mobility is so central to one's daily life, the problems associated with changes in mobility and the adaptation to these changes are among the most important problems with which nurses deal."[21]

The following definition of nursing is offered: "Nursing is the diagnosis and treatment of human responses to actual or potential health problems."[1] Impaired functioning in the area of activity is included in a listing of human responses that are the focus for nursing intervention.

In 1980 the National Conference Group for Classification of Nursing Diagnoses (NANDA) accepted mobility, impaired physical with defining characteristics as a diagnostic category label.[8,16] This action constitutes further evidence that the nursing profession recognizes the importance of physical mobility and accepts the problems associated with impaired physical mobility as being within the province of nursing.

Impaired physical mobility is defined as "the limitation of ability for independent movement within the environment."[8] It should be quite clear from this definition that the diagnosis of impaired physical mobility could be appropriately applied in a wide variety of situations. Indeed, the diagnosis could be made for the person who lies unconscious in a trauma unit after a motor vehicle accident, or for the person who is left with residual weakness of one side of the body following a stroke, or even for the person who has sustained an exercise-related injury of bone, joint, or muscle.

To further delineate how immobile a person is, four levels of impaired physical mobility have been identified. They are as follows[11]:

Level I: Requires use of equipment or device

Level II: Requires help from another person(s)—assistance, supervision(s), or teaching

Level III: Requires help from another person(s) and equipment or device

Level IV: Is dependent and does not participate in movement

In addition, to assist in determining more precisely just how impaired mobility will influence an individual, Milde[20] suggests that the following five parameters be considered: the duration or length of the event, the degree of restriction to movements, the amount of the body affected by the restrictions, the degree to which an upright position can be assumed, and the individual's control of both the quantity and quality of movements.

Most of the literature that serves as a theoretical base for the nursing diagnosis of impaired physical mobility relates to the concept of immobility. Immobility is defined as the state in which physical movement is decreased, restricted, or absent.[20] Even though immobility is a relative term, most of the documentation focuses on one of the most extreme forms of immobility—bed rest.

Immobility can affect all major body systems. The major possible consequences of immobility include effects on (1) the muscular system (decreased muscle mass, or atrophy, decreased muscle strength, decreased endurance, contractures), (2) the skeletal system (fibrosis and ankylosis of joints, osteoporosis), (3) the cardiovascular system (increased workload of the heart, decreased exercise tolerance, postural hypotension, venous stasis, thrombus and embolus formation), (4) the respiratory system (decreased respiratory rate, decreased chest expansion, decreased tidal volume, impairment of coughing mechanism, atelectasis, pneumonia, respiratory acidosis), (5) the nervous system (perceptual changes, altered sensation, autonomic lability, peripheral nerve palsy), (6) the digestive system (anorexia, constipation), (7) the integumentary system (decubitus ulcer, increased heat loss through skin), (8) the urinary system (urinary stasis, urinary retention, renal calculi, proteinuria), (9) metabolism (negative nitrogen balance, negative calcium balance, decreased metabolic rate), and (10) psychosocial functioning (sensory deprivation, role changes, decreased problem-solving ability, body-image distortions, changes in sleep patterns, mood changes).[2-4,13,18-24]

To help determine whether the nursing diagnosis of impaired physical mobility is appropriate for a given patient, the nurse needs to understand both the common etiologies and the defining characteristics for the diagnosis. The etiologies help the nurse identify populations of patients at high-risk for the diagnosis. Etiologies for impaired physical mobility include the following*:

Intolerance to activity

Decreased strength and endurance

Pain or discomfort

Perceptual or cognitive impairment

Certain physical disorders or states

*References 2, 5, 8, 14, 15, 20, 21.

Cranial lesion or disease
Central nervous system disorders
Muscular conditions
Neuromuscular junction disease
Connective tissue disorders
Peripheral neuropathies
Joint and bone disorders
Depression
Severe anxiety
Schizophrenic disorders
Paranoid disorders
Substance use disorders
Restrictive or suppressive therapeutic regimens
    External devices (casts, splints, traction, braces,
        IV tubing, cardiac monitors, ventilators)
    Pharmacologic agents (sedatives, anesthetics)
    Trauma or surgical procedure
    Bed rest

DEFINING CHARACTERISTICS[5,8,14-16]

Internal
    Inability to purposefully move within the physical environment, including bed mobility, transfer, and ambulation
    Reluctance or refusal to attempt movement
    Constancy of body posture in relation to gravity
    Decreased physical activity
    Limited range of motion
    Decreased muscle strength, control, and/or mass
    Impaired coordination
    Impaired perception of position or presence of body parts
    Perceived inability to move
External
    Imposed restrictions of movement (mechanical or medical protocol restrictions)

NURSING INTERVENTIONS*

Patient Goal	Nursing Intervention
Maintain normal musculoskeletal functioning during period of bed rest.	Teach and monitor active range-of-motion exercises for all joints should be performed at least two or three times daily (each movement should be performed at least twice during each exercise period).
	Perform passive range-of-motion exercises for patient if above intervention is not possible; same frequency as above.
	Teach and monitor isometric and isotonic exercises.
	Assist patient with position changes *at least* every 2 hours.
	Assist patient to maintain proper body alignment, using supportive devices as necessary.
	Encourage self-care activities.
	Consider referral to physical therapist.
Exhibit minimal cardiovascular alterations during period of bed rest.	Teach and monitor leg exercises.
	Teach patient to exhale through mouth when exercising or moving in bed.
	Teach patient to avoid straining while defecating.
	Assist patient with frequent position changes.
	Apply elastic stockings.
	Teach patient to avoid compression of veins.
Maintain normal respiratory functioning during period of bed rest.	Teach and monitor deep breathing and coughing regimen.
	Assist patient with frequent position changes.
	Teach and monitor use of incentive spirometer.
	Encourage increased activity level.
	Encourage increased fluid intake.
Maintain normal nervous system functioning during period of bed rest.	Assist patient to function at the highest possible cognitive level.
	Avoid use of positions that put prolonged pressure on nerves.
	Assist patient with frequent position changes.
Maintain normal digestive functioning during period of bed rest.	Provide small, frequent meals containing desired foods.
	Encourage increased activity level.
	Provide companionship during meals, if desired by patient.
	Encourage increased bulk and fluids in diet.
	Assist patient to assume a sitting position for defecation, if possible.
	Provide privacy for defecation.
	Offer bedpan after meals, especially after breakfast.

*References 4, 6, 7, 10, 12, 17, 20-23.

Patient Goal	Nursing Intervention
	Obtain order for stool softener, if indicated.
	Provide foods that are natural laxatives, such as prunes.
	Obtain order for laxative, suppository, or enema; give only if absolutely necessary.
Maintain a healthy integument during period of bed rest.	Assist patient with position changes *at least* every 2 hours.
	Inspect susceptible areas of skin (such as areas over bony prominences) for condition at time of each position change.
	Gently massage areas over bony prominences at time of each position change.
	Keep skin clean and dry but lubricated.
	Provide pressure-equalizing or pressure-reducing equipment, if indicated (such as alternating pressure mattress).
	Avoid shearing force when moving patient.
	Encourage well-balanced diet with adequate fluids, protein, and vitamin C.
Maintain normal urinary functioning during period of bed rest.	Encourage increased fluid intake.
	Provide foods and fluids that acidify urine (meats, fish, nuts, cereals, cranberry juice).
	Encourage increased activity level.
	Assist patient to assume a sitting position for urination, if possible.
	Provide privacy for urination.
	Assist patient with frequent position changes.
	Try nursing measures to relieve urinary retention, if it is present: sound of running water, pouring warm water over perineum (of females), having females contract and release perineal muscles.
	Perform catheterization as a last resort (per physician's order and using strict sterile technique).
Maintain normal psychosocial functioning during period of bed rest.	Provide meaningful interactions with patient.
	Encourage family and/or significant other(s) to visit patient.
	Provide meaningful sensory input.
	Encourage use of glasses and/or hearing aid if these devices are needed.
	Provide time-orienting devices (clocks, calendars, newspapers).
	Encourage self-care activities.
	Encourage responsibility for decision-making about own care.
	Encourage ventilation of feelings about illness and immobility.
	Provide meaningful diversions for patient.
	Provide uninterrupted periods for sleeping.
	Deliberate use of touch in providing nursing care.

The nursing management for a person with this nursing diagnosis differs according to the existing level of impairment. Recall the four levels of impaired physical mobility that have been identified. Level I reflects the least degree of impairment, and level IV reflects the greatest degree. The nursing care described assumes physical mobility at either level III or level IV. The nursing care is further based on the assumption that the patient is an adult. Not all the interventions listed are appropriate for every patient. In certain situations some of the interventions are contraindicated. The nursing care is presented as a general model for intervention. Specific nursing intervention strategies must be selected to meet the unique needs of the patient for whom the nurse is providing nursing care. Certain interventions may require a physician's order, depending on the practice setting.

EVALUATION*

Patient Outcome	Data Indicating That Outcome is Reached
Normal musculoskeletal function	Usual range of motion in all body joints maintained
	Usual muscle mass and strength maintained
	Participates actively in self-care activities
Minimal cardiovascular alterations	Normal heart rate (from 60 to 100 beats per minute) and blood pressure (from 100 to 140 mm Hg for systolic and from 70 to 90 mm Hg for diastolic)

*References 4, 6, 7, 10, 12, 17, 20-23.

Patient Outcome	Data Indicating That Outcome is Reached
	Maintains normal venous return
	No evidence of vein compression
	No evidence of thrombus or embolus
Normal respiratory function	Clear lungs on auscultation
	Normal tidal volume (approximately 500 ml)
	Normal chest expansion
	No evidence of atelectasis
	No evidence of pneumonia
	No evidence of respiratory acidosis
Normal nervous system function	Oriented to time, person, and place
	Normal peripheral nerve functioning (no abnormal pain or tingling present)
Normal digestive function	Maintains usual weight
	Maintains usual bowel elimination habits
	No evidence of fecal impaction
Normal integument	Intact skin
	No evidence of pressure (pallor, redness, increased warmth, or tenderness in involved area)
Normal urinary function	Adequate urine output (at least 1500 ml/day)
	No evidence of renal calculi
	No evidence of urinary retention
Normal psychosocial function	Relationships with family and/or significant other(s) maintained
	Participates actively in decisions about own care
	Verbalizes fears, concerns, and other feelings
	Accepts support from others
	Uses defense mechanisms constructively

References

1. American Nurses Association: Nursing: a social policy statement, Kansas City, 1980, American Nurses Association.
2. Aspinall, M.J., and Tanner, C.A.: Decision making for patient care: applying the nursing process, New York, 1981, Appleton-Century-Crofts.
3. Boland, M.: Relationship of mobility and body mechanics to maintenance of adaptation. In Murray, R.B., and Zentner, J.P., editors: Nursing concepts for health promotion, ed. 2, Englewood Cliffs, N.J., 1979, Prentice-Hall, Inc.
4. Brill, E.L., and Kilts, D.F.: Foundations for nursing, New York, 1980, Appleton-Century-Crofts.
5. Carpenito, L.J.: Nursing diagnosis: application to clinical practice, Philadelphia, 1983, J.B. Lippincott Co.
6. Ciuca, R., Bradish, J., and Trombly, S.M.: Active range-of-motion exercises: a handbook, Nursing 78 8(8):45-49, 1978.
7. Ciuca, R., Bradish, J., and Trombly, S.M.: Passive range-of-motion exercises: a handbook, Nursing 78 8(7):59-65, 1978.
8. Gordon, M.: Manual of nursing diagnosis, New York, 1982, McGraw-Hill Book Co.
9. Gordon, M.: Nursing diagnosis: process and application, New York, 1982, McGraw-Hill Book Co.
10. Hirschberg, G.G., Lewis, L., and Vaughan, P.: Promoting patient mobility and other ways to prevent secondary disabilities, Nursing 77 7(5):42-47, 1977.
11. Jones, E., and others: Patient classification for long term care: users manual, HEW pub. no. HRA-74-3107, Washington, D.C., Department of Health, Education, and Welfare, Health Resources Administration, Bureau of Health Services Research and Evaluation, Nov. 1974.
12. Jungreis, S.W.: Exercises for expediting mobility and decreasing disability in bedridden patients, Nursing 77 7(8):47-51, 1977.
13. Kavanagh, T.: General deconditioning. In Basmajian, J.V., and Kirby, R.L., editors: Medical rehabilitation, Baltimore, 1984, Williams & Wilkins.
14. Kim, M.J., McFarland, G.K., and McLane, A.M.: Classification of nursing diagnoses: Proceedings of the Fifth National Conference, St. Louis, 1984, The C.V. Mosby Co.
15. Kim, M.J., McFarland, G.K., and McLane, A.M.: Pocket guide to nursing diagnoses, St. Louis, 1984, The C.V. Mosby Co.
16. Kim, M.J., and Mortiz, D.A.: Classification of nursing diagnoses: Proceedings of the Third and Fourth National Conferences, New York, 1982, McGraw-Hill Book Co.
17. Kinney, A.B., and Blount, M.: Effect of cranberry juice on urinary pH, Nurs. Res. 28(5):287-290, 1979.
18. Lentz, M.: Selected aspects of deconditioning secondary to immobilization, Nurs. Clin. North Am. 16(4):729-737, 1981.
19. Mazess, R.B., and Whedon, G.D.: Immobilization and bone, Calcified Tissue Int. 35(3):265-267, 1983.
20. Milde, F.K.: Physiological immobilization. In Hart, L.K., Reese, J.L., and Fearing, M.O., editors: Concepts common to acute illness: identification and management, St. Louis, 1981, The C.V. Mosby Co.
21. Mitchell, P.H.: Motor status. In Mitchell, P.H., and Loustau, A., editors: Concepts basic to nursing, ed. 3, New York, 1981, McGraw-Hill Book Co.
22. Murray, R.B., Huelskoetter, M.M.W., and O'Driscoll, D.L.: The nursing process in later maturity, Englewood Cliffs, N.J., 1980, Prentice-Hall, Inc.
23. O'Neill, R.H.: Problems associated with disuse syndromes including the integument. In Beland, I.L., and Passos, J.Y., editors: Clinical nursing: pathophysiological and psychosocial approaches, ed. 4, New York, 1981, Macmillan Co.
24. Vallbona, C.: Bodily responses to immobilization. In Kottke, F.J., Stillwell, G.K., and Lehmann, J.F., editors: Krusen's handbook of physical medicine and rehabilitation, ed. 3, Philadelphia, 1982, W.B. Saunders Co.

Appendixes

Current Status and Historical Evolution of the North American Nursing Diagnoses Association

The North American Nursing Diagnoses Association (NANDA) officially came into being in April 1982 at the Fifth National Conference on Classification of Nursing Diagnoses in St. Louis. The purpose of NANDA is to develop, refine, and promote a taxonomy of nursing diagnostic terminology of general use to professional nurses. To achieve this NANDA conducts conferences, publishes documents, facilitates research, and serves as an information resource.

NANDA's roots may be traced to the 1973 First National Conference on the Classification of Nursing Diagnosis, which was conceived to clearly articulate the health problems that comprise the domain of nursing and to classify these health problems into a taxonomic system. The Second, Third, Fourth, Fifth, and Sixth National Conferences on Classification of Nursing Diagnoses followed in 1975, 1978, 1980, 1982, and 1984, respectively. All were held in St. Louis. The Seventh National Conference on Classification of Nursing Diagnoses is planned for March 9 to 12, 1986, in St. Louis.

The theme of the Seventh Conference is "Nursing Diagnosis: Gateway to Scientific Practice.

Before the official beginning of NANDA, work between national conferences was conducted by the National Conference Group for Classification of Nursing and in particular its Steering Committee. Membership of the Steering Committee in the most recent years included Dr. Marjory Gordon, Ann Becker, Dr. Mi Ja Kim, Dr. Gertrude K. McFarland, and Dr. Audrey M. McLane.

The evolution of nursing diagnoses and NANDA's foundations can be explored in depth through the official publications of the organization. These include:

Gebbie, K., editor: Summary of the Second National Conference: classification of nursing diagnoses, St. Louis, 1976, The Clearinghouse.

Gebbie, K., and Lavin, M., editors: Classification of nursing diagnoses: proceedings of the First National Conference, St. Louis, 1975, The C.V. Mosby Co.

Kim, M., McFarland, G., and McLane, A., editors: Classification of nursing diagnoses: proceedings of the Fifth National Conference, St. Louis, 1984, The C.V. Mosby Co.

Kim, M., McFarland, G., and McLane, A., editors: Pocket guide to nursing diagnoses, St. Louis, 1984, The C.V. Mosby Co.

Kim, M., and Mortiz, D., editors: Classification of nursing diagnoses: proceedings of the Third and Fourth National Conferences, New York, 1982, McGraw-Hill Book Co.

The current elected officers of NANDA are: President, Dr. Marjory Gordon, RN, Professor, Boston College, Boston; Vice President, Dr. Phyllis Kritek, RN, Associate Professor, University of Wisconsin, Milwaukee; Secretary, Jane Lancour, RN, MSN, Nurse Consultant, Lancour & Lancour Ltd., Wauwatosa, Wisconsin; Treasurer, Kristine Gebbie, RN, MN, Administrator, Oregon State Health Division, Portland; Board of Directors, Dr. Mi Ja Kim, RN, Professor, University of Illinois, Chicago, Lynda Carpenito, RN, MSN, Consultant, Mickleton, N.J.; Dr. Gertrude K. McFarland, RN, Nurse Consultant, Division of Nursing, Health Resources & Services Administration, U.S. Department of Health & Human Services, Rockville, Md.; Dr. Audrey McLane, RN, Professor, Marquette University, Milwaukee; Winnifred Mills, RN, MEd, Assistant Professor, University of British Columbia, Vancouver, British Columbia; Derry Mortiz, RN, MS, MEd, Staff Nurse, New Haven, Conn.; and Dr. Joyce Shoemaker, RN, Dean, University of Alabama, Huntsville.

NANDA's committees include Program, Publications, Membership, Diagnosis Review, Nominations, Research, Public Relations, and Taxonomy. Work on a nursing diagnoses label for acceptance by NANDA should be submitted to the Diagnostic Review Committee. This committee reviews proposed diagnoses, receives input from specialized clinical and technical review task forces, and recommends acceptance, modification, or rejection to the Board.

A registered nurse may become a member of NANDA by paying yearly dues of $20, provided that he or she has been granted a license to practice as a registered nurse and does not have a license under suspension or revocation. Information on becoming a member may be obtained from Karen K. Murphy, Executive Director, North American Nursing Diagnoses Association, St. Louis University, School of Nursing, 3525 Caroline St., St. Louis, Missouri 63104; phone: (314) 664-9800, ext. 675.

The current approved nursing diagnoses are the following:

Activity intolerance
Activity intolerance, potential
Airway clearance, ineffective
Anxiety
Bowel elimination, alteration in: constipation
Bowel elimination, alteration in: diarrhea
Bowel elimination, alteration in: incontinence
Breathing pattern, ineffective
Cardiac output, alteration in: decreased
Comfort, alteration in: pain
Communication, impaired: verbal
Coping, family: potential for growth
Coping, ineffective family: compromised
Coping, ineffective family: disabling
Coping, ineffective individual
Diversional activity, deficit
Family process, alteration in
Fear
Fluid volume, alteration in: excess
Fluid volume deficit, actual
Fluid volume deficit, potential
Gas exchange, impaired
Grieving, anticipatory
Grieving, dysfunctional
Health maintenance, alteration in
Home maintenance management, impaired
Injury, potential for
Knowledge deficit (specify)
Mobility, impaired physical
Noncompliance (specify)
Nutrition, alteration in: less than body requirements
Nutrition, alteration in: more than body requirements
Nutrition, alteration in: potential for more than body requirements
Oral mucous membrane, alteration in
Parenting, alteration in: actual or potential
Powerlessness
Rape trauma syndrome
Self-care deficit: feeding, bathing/hygiene, dressing/grooming, toileting
Self-concept, disturbance in: body image, self-esteem, role performance, personal identity
Sensory-perceptual alteration: visual, auditory, kinesthetic, gustatory, tactile, olfactory
Sexual dysfunction
Skin integrity, impairment of: actual
Skin integrity, impairment of: potential
Sleep pattern disturbance
Social isolation
Spiritual distress
Thought processes, alteration in
Tissue perfusion, alteration in: cerebral, cardiopulmonary, renal, gastrointestinal, peripheral
Urinary elimination, alteration in patterns
Violence, potential for

Conversion Factors to International System of Units (SI Units)

Conversion factors (SI Units)

Component	Normal Range in Units as Customarily Reported	Conversion Factor	Normal Range in SI Units, Molecular Units, International Units, or Decimal Fractions
Biochemical Components of Blood*			
Acetoacetic acid (S)	0.2-1.0 mg/dL	98	19.6-98.0 μmol/L
Acetone (S)	0.3-2.0 mg/dL	172	51.6-344.0 μmol/L
Albumin (S)	3.2-4.5 g/dL	10	32-45 g/L
Ammonia (P)	20-120 μg/dL	0.588	11.7-70.5 μmol/L
Amylase (S)	60-160 Somogyi units/dL	1.85	111-296 U/L
Base, total (S)	145-160 mEq/L	1	145-160 mmol/L
Bicarbonate (P)	21-28 mEq/L	1	21-28 mmol/L
Bile acids (S)	0.3-3.0 mg/dL	10	3-30 mg/L
		2.547	0.8-7.6 μmol/L
Bilirubin, direct (S)	Up to 0.3 mg/dL	17.1	Up to 5.1 μmol/L
Bilirubin, indirect (S)	0.1-1.0 mg/dL	17.1	1.7-17.1 μmol/L
Blood gases (B)			
Pco₂ arterial	35-40 mm Hg	0.133	4.66-5.32 kPa
Po₂ arterial	95-100 mm Hg	0.133	12.64-13.30 kPa
Calcium (S)	8.5-10.5 mg/dL	0.25	2.1-2.6 mmol/L
Chloride (S)	95-103 mEq/L	1	95-103 mmol/L
Creatine (S)	0.1-0.4 mg/dL	76.3	7.6-30.5 μmol/L
Creatinine (S)	0.6-1.2 mg/dL	88.4	53-106 μmol/L
Creatinine clearance (P)	107-139 mL/min	0.0167	1.78-2.32 mL/s
Fatty acids (total) (S)	8-20 mg/dL	0.01	0.08-2.00 mg/L
Fibrinogen (P)	200-400 mg/dL	0.01	2.00-4.00 g/L
Gamma globulin (S)	0.5-1.6 g/dL	10	5-16 g/L
Globulins (total) (S)	2.3-3.5 g/dL	10	23-35 g/L
Glucose (fasting) (S)	70-110 mg/dL	0.055	3.85-6.05 mmol/L
Insulin (radioimmunoassay) (P)	4-24 μIU/ml	0.0417	0.17-1.00 μg/L
	0.20-0.84 μg/L	172.2	35-145 pmol/L
Iodine, BEI (S)	3.5-6.5 μg/dL	0.079	0.28-0.51 μmol/L
Iodine, PBI (S)	4.0-8.0 μg/dL	0.079	0.32-0.63 μmol/L
Iron, total (S)	60-150 μg/dL	0.179	11-27 μmol/L
Iron-binding capacity (S)	300-360 μg/dL	0.179	54-64 μmol/L
17-Ketosteroids (P)	25-125 μg/dL	0.01	0.25-1.25 mg/L
Lactic dehydrogenase (S)	80-120 units at 30 °C	0.48	38-62 U/L at 30 °C
	Lactate → pyruvate		
	100-190 U/L at 37 °C	1	100-190 U/L at 37 °C
Lipase (S)	0-1.5 U/ml (Cherry-Crandall)	278	0-417 U/L

From Tilkian, S.M., Conover, M.B., and Tilkian, A.G.: Clinical implications of laboratory tests, ed. 3, St. Louis, 1983, The C.V. Mosby Co.
*This is a selected (not a complete) list of biochemical components. The ranges listed may differ from those accepted in some laboratories and are shown to illustrate the conversion factor and the method of expression in SI molecular units. For a more complete listing, see Henry, J.B., editor: Todd-Sanford-Davidsohn clinical diagnosis and management by laboratory methods, ed. 16, Philadelphia, W.B. Saunders Co.

Conversion factors (SI Units)

Component	Normal Range in Units as Customarily Reported	Conversion Factor	Normal Range in SI Units, Molecular Units, International Units, or Decimal Fractions
Lipids (total) (S)	400-800 mg/dL	0.01	4.00-8.00 g/L
Cholesterol	150-250 mg/dL	0.026	3.9-6.5 mmol/L
Triglycerides	75-165 mg/dL	0.0114	0.85-1.89 mmol/L
Phospholipids	150-380 mg/dL	0.01	1.50-380 g/L
Free fatty acids	9.0-15.0 mM/L	1	9.0-15.0 mmol/L
Nonprotein nitrogen (S)	20-35 mg/dL	0.714	14.3-25.0 mmol/L
Phosphatase (P)			
Acid (units/dL)	Cherry-Crandall	2.77	0-5.5 U/L
	King-Armstrong	1.77	0-5.5 U/L
	Bodansky	5.37	0-5.5 U/L
Alkaline (units/dL)	King-Armstrong	1.77	30-120 U/L
	Bodansky	5.37	30-120 U/L
	Bessey-Lowry-Brock	16.67	30-120 U/L
Phosphorus, inorganic (S)	3.0-4.5 mg/dL	0.323	0.97-1.45 mmol/L
Potassium (P)	3.8-5.0 mEq/L	1	3.8-5.0 mmol/L
Proteins, total (S)	6.0-7.8 g/dL	10	60-78 g/L
Albumin	3.2-4.5 g/dL	10	32-45 g/L
Globulin	2.3-3.5 g/dL	10	23-35 g/L
Sodium (P)	136-142 mEq/L	1	136-142 mmol/L
Testosterone: Male (S)	300-1,200 ng/dL	0.035	10.5-42.0 nmol/L
Female	30-95 ng/dL	0.035	1.0-3.3 nmol/L
Thyroid tests (S)			
Thyroxine (T_4)	4-11 μg/dL	12.87	51-142 nmol/L
T_4 expressed as iodine	3.2-7.2 μg/dL	79.0	253-569 nmol/L
T_3 resin uptake	25%-38% relative uptake	0.01	0.25%-0.38% relative uptake
TSH (S)	10 μU/mL	1	$<10^{-3}$ IU/L
Urea nitrogen (S)	8-23 mg/dL	0.357	2.9-8.2 mmol/L
Uric acid (S)	2-6 mg/dL	59.5	0.120-0.360 mmol/L
Vitamin B_{12} (S)	160-950 pg/mL	0.74	118-703 pmol/L
Hematology Values*			
Red cell volume (male)	25-35 mL/kg body weight	0.001	0.025-0.035 L/kg body weight
Hematocrit	40%-50%	0.01	0.40-0.50
Hemoglobin	13.5-18.0 g/dL	10	135-180 g/L
Hemoglobin	13.5-18.0 g/dL	0.155	2.09-2.79 mmol/L
RBC count	$4.5\text{-}6 \times 10^6/\mu L$	1	$4.6\text{-}6 \times 10^{12}/L$
WBC count	$4.5\text{-}10 \times 10^3/\mu L$	1	$4.5\text{-}10 \times 10^9/L$
Mean corpuscular volume	80-96 μm³	1	80-96 fL

*The International Committee for Standardization in Hematology recommends that the numbers remain the same but that the units change, so that hemoglobin is expressed as grams per deciliter (g/dL) even though other measurements are expressed as units per liter (U/L).

Chemotherapeutic Agents

This appendix has been developed primarily by abstracting the *American Hospital Formulary Service* (AHFS) information. Where necessary, the AHFS information has been supplemented by a variety of other references. Canadian trade names are taken from the *Compendium of Pharmaceuticals and Specialties*. The appendix was developed to coincide with the format of the AHFS and to include the chemotherapeutic agents referenced in this text. It is not intended to be an inclusive listing of all generic agents and their uses. The purpose of the appendix is to provide the reader with a quick reference regarding generic and trade names available both in the United States and Canada as well as to list the categories, actions, uses, side effects, adverse reactions, contraindications, and nursing considerations.

Reference

McEvoy, G.K., editor: American hospital formulary service: drug information 1985, Bethesda, Md., 1985, American Society of Hospital Pharmacists.

ADDITIONAL REFERENCES

Center For Disease Control: Morbidity and mortality weekly report: supplement on adult immunizations, Waltham, Mass., Sept. 28, 1984, Massachusetts Medical Society.

Clayton, B.D.: Mosby's handbook of pharmacology in nursing, ed. 3, St. Louis, 1984, The C.V. Mosby Co.

Compendium of pharmaceuticals and specialties, ed. 20, 1985, Canada.

Gahart, B.L.: Intravenous medications: a handbook for nurses and other allied health personnel, ed. 4, St. Louis, 1985, The C.V. Mosby Co.

Gilman, A.G., Goodman, L.S., and Gilman, A.: Goodman and Gilman's the pharmacological basis of therapeutics, ed. 6, New York, 1980, Macmillan Publishing Co., Inc.

Hahn, A.B., Barkin, R.L., and Oestreich, S.J.K.: Pharmacology in nursing, ed. 16, St. Louis, 1986, The C.V. Mosby Co.

Pagliaro, L.A., and Pagliaro, A.M.: Pharmacologic aspects of nursing care, St. Louis, 1986, The C.V. Mosby Co.

Rodman, M.J., et al.: Pharmacology and drug therapy in nursing, ed. 3, Philadelphia, 1985, J.B. Lippincott Co.

Scherer, J.C.: Lippincott's nurses' drug manual, Philadelphia, 1985, J.B. Lippincott Co.

ANTIHISTAMINE AGENTS

CATEGORY: ANTIHISTAMINES (AHFS 4:00*)

	Trade Names	
Generic Name	*U.S.*	*Canada*
Azatadine	Optimine	Optimine
Brompheniramine	Dimetane	Dimetane
Carbinoxamine	Clistin	—†
Chlorpheniramine	Chlor-Trimeton	—‡
Clemastine	Tavist	Tavist Fumarate
Cyproheptadine	Periactin	Periactin
Diphenhydramine	Benadryl	Benadryl
		Allerdryl
Doxylamine	Decapryn	—†
Methdilazine	Tacaryl	—†
Promethazine	Phenergan	Phenergan
Trimeprazine	Temaril	—†
Tripelennamine	Pyribenzamine	Pyribenzamine
Triprolidine	Actidil	Actidil

Actions: Competitively antagonize most of the smooth muscle–stimulating actions of histamine on the H_1 receptors of the gastrointestinal tract, uterus, large blood vessels, and bronchial muscles; specifically, by blocking H_1 receptor sites,

2117

thereby preventing the action of histamine on the cells; do not prevent the release of histamine.

Uses: Provide symptomatic relief of allergic symptoms caused by histamine release; not curative; some also useful in the prevention of motion sickness and the symptomatic treatment of vertigo associated with diseases affecting the vestibular system.

General side effects: Sedation, dizziness, lassitude, disturbed coordination, muscular weakness, anorexia, nausea, vomiting, diarrhea, and constipation.

Adverse reactions: Some patients, especially children and elderly persons, may experience paradoxical excitement characterized by restlessness, insomnia, tremors, euphoria, nervousness, delirium, palpitations, and convulsions; rarely, agranulocytosis, hemolytic anemia, leukopenia, thrombocytopenia, and pancytopenia.

Contraindications: Narrow-angle glaucoma or intraocular pressure from any cause, prostatic hypertrophy, stenosing peptic ulcer, and duodenal obstruction; history of asthma: cautious use.

Nursing considerations:
1. Advise patient of side effects leading to drowsiness, vertigo, and lightheadedness. Alcohol potentiates the drug effect.
2. Advise patient that the drug does not cure the problem but that it only provides symptomatic relief.
3. Alcohol and other CNS depressants have additive effects.
4. Long-term use requires periodic complete blood counts.

ANTI-INFECTIVE AGENTS (AHFS 8:00*)

Anti-infective agents are divided into nine major categories. Antibiotics are subdivided into eight subcategories.

CATEGORY: AMEBICIDES (AHFS 8:04)

Generic Name	Trade Names U.S.	Canada
Dehydroemetine	—§	—‡
Emetine	—§	—‡
Iodoquinol	Diiodohydroxyquin	Gynovules†
	Panaquin	
	Yodoxin	
Diloxanide furoate	Furamide	—‡

Actions: Amebicidal to motile intestinal protozoa. Some have amebicidal action against extraintestinal motile and cyst forms of protozoa.

Uses: Treatment of intestinal amebiasis such as intestinal *Entamoeba histolytica, Giardia lamblia,* and amebic hepa-

*American Hospital Formulary Service classification.
†Drug is not available in Canada although it is listed in 1985 *Compendium of Pharmaceuticals and Specialties.*
‡U.S. trade name (or sometimes generic name) not listed in 1985 *Compendium of Pharmaceuticals and Specialties.*
§Drug is known by generic name.

titis; usually involves the use of several drugs; may also be used to treat asymptomatic amoeba cyst carriers.

General side effects: Nausea, vomiting, diarrhea, intestinal distress or cramps, loss of appetite, headache, dizziness, and skin rash.

Adverse reactions: Cumulative toxicity is a risk with these agents; depending on the drug, there may be neural, cardiovascular, hepatic, thyroid, or cerebral toxicity. Consumption of alcoholic beverages while taking these drugs may cause flushing, vomiting, abdominal cramps, and headache.

Contraindications: Renal or liver disease, pregnancy, thyroid disease, organic heart disease, and bowel obstruction are contraindications for some agents.

Nursing considerations:
1. Patients being treated with amebicides may already have acute dysentery, dehydration, electrolyte imbalance, and malnutrition, all of which may be exacerbated with drug therapy.
2. Amebicides are administered for a given period of time. This is generally followed by a designated period of abstinence from drug therapy before therapy may be administered again.
3. The patient's activity should be curtailed during the acute disease and therapy period.
4. Amebicides must be discontinued if symptoms of toxicity develop. In some cases toxic symptoms will persist for variable periods after the drug is stopped.
5. Patients and carriers must return following therapy for stool examination. The time for reexamination depends on the drug and disease.

CATEGORY: ANTHELMINTICS (AHFS 8:08*)

Generic Name	Trade Names U.S.	Canada
Diethylcarbamazine	Hetrazan	Hetrazan
Mebendazole	Vermox	Vermox
		Pantelmin†
		Telmin†
Niclosamide	Niclocide	—‡
Piperazine citrate	Antepar	Entacyl
Pyrantel pamoate	Antiminth	Antiminth†
		Combantrin
Pyrvinium pamoate	Povan	Povan†
Quinacrine; mepacrine	Antabrine	Antabrine
		Tenicridine†
Thiabendazole	Mintezol	Mintezol
		Minzolum†

Actions: Individual drugs are toxic for specific helminths. Drug action causes paralysis or death to the intestinal helminths. Drugs also facilitate expulsion of the intestinal worms from the body. A few of the drugs are absorbed and immobilize or kill tissue helminths.

Uses: The most common intestinal infestations are with enterobiasis (pinworms), ascariasis (roundworms), and trichuriasis (whipworms). Less frequent are infections with strongyloidiasis (threadworms), ancylostomiasis (hookworms), and taeniasis (tapeworms).

General side effects: Nausea, vomiting, abdominal cramps, diarrhea, malaise, headache, and vertigo.

Adverse reactions: Individual drugs may elicit allergic reactions as a result of the death of the worms or stimulate elevations in SGOT levels. Toxic reactions include CNS disturbances, transient psychosis, skin rash, and photosensitivity or other visual disturbances.

Contraindications: Pregnancy and hepatic, renal, cardiac, or neurologic disease.

Nursing considerations:

1. Provide patient and family, who is to be treated on an outpatient basis, written instructions regarding premedication diet, manner of taking the medication, use of cathartics and enemas, and the need for follow-up stool examination. Retreatment may be necessary.

2. Teach hygiene measures to prevent the spread of the specific helminth. Suggestions include daily showers; clean underwear and bedclothes daily; short, clean fingernails; and frequent hand washing.

3. Fluid and nutritional therapy should accompany treatment for debilitating worm infections.

4. Advise patient that some agents cause discoloration of stool; for example, pyrvinium causes stools to become bright red in color.

CATEGORY: ANTIBIOTICS[1]
Class: Aminoglycosides (AHFS 8:12.02*)

	Trade Names	
Generic Name	U.S.	Canada
Gentamicin	Garamycin	Garamycin
		Cidomycin
Kanamycin	Kantrex	Kantrex
		Anamid
Neomycin	Mycifradin	Mycifradin
		Myciguent
Paromomycin	Humatin	Humatin†
		Humagel†
Streptomycin	—§	Streptolin†
		Streptosol 25%†
Tobramycin	Nebcin	Nebcin
		Tobrex

Actions: These antibiotics and semisynthetic antibiotic derivatives are bactericidal in action and are active against many aerobic gram-negative and some aerobic gram-positive bacteria: *Acinetobacter, Citrobacter, Enterobacter, E. coli, Klebsiella, Proteus, Providencia, Pseudomonas, Salmonella, Serratia, Shigella,* and most strains of *Staphylococcus aureus* and *S. epidermidis.* They are inactive against fungi, viruses, and most anaerobic bacteria.

Uses: Treatment of severe infections: nosocomial gram-negative sepsis, bone and joint infections, skin and soft-tissue infections, respiratory infections, and select urinary tract infections; oral kanamycin and neomycin for bowel sterilization before surgery; oral neomycin for patients with cirrhosis to prevent encephalopathy.

[1]For topical preparations see "Skin and Mucous Membrane Preparations (AFHS 84:04.04)."

General side effects: Headache, nausea, and diarrhea with oral use; tinnitus and dizziness with parenteral use; pain and irritation at injection site.

Adverse reactions: Ototoxicity and nephrotoxicity (particularly in the elderly and dehydrated patient with renal disease), hypersensitivity reactions, paralysis of skeletal muscles, hematologic changes, and changes in hepatic function.

Contraindications: Oral use in patients with bowel obstruction; concurrent administration with other nephrotoxic or ototoxic drugs; long-term use for patients with renal dysfunction.

Nursing considerations:

1. Monitor for signs of nephrotoxicity including decreased urinary output, decreased urinary creatinine levels, and increased BUN and serum creatinine. Risk increases with therapy beyond 7 to 10 days.

2. Monitor for signs of ototoxicity during and for 3 to 4 weeks following therapy. Signs of ototoxicity include dizziness, tinnitus, ataxia, nystagmus, and hearing loss at high frequencies. Risk increases with therapy extended beyond 7 to 10 days.

3. Keep patient well hydrated.

4. Monitor for signs of bacterial or fungal overgrowth.

5. Do not administer with other ototoxic or nephrotoxic drugs.

6. Inject deeply intramuscularly and rotate injection sites.

7. Advise patients using topical drugs to discontinue use during aminoglycoside therapy.

CATEGORY: ANTIBIOTICS
Class: Antifungal Antibiotics (AHFS 8:12.04*)

	Trade Names	
Generic Name	U.S.	Canada
Amphotericin B	Fungizone	Fungizone
Griseofulvin	Fulvicin-U/F	Fulvicin-U/F
	Grisactin	Fulvin P/G
		Grisovin-FP
Miconazole	Monistat	Monistat
	Declostatin	Micatin
Nystatin	Mycostatin	Mycostatin
	Nilstat	Nadostine
		Nilstat
		Nyaderm (K-Line)

Actions: Fungistatic and/or fungicidal against specific systemic and local fungi.

Uses: Systemic and local fungal infections; some agents sufficiently toxic to warrant use only for severe systemic infections. Other agents for cutaneous use only are discussed under the section on skin and mucous membrane preparations.

General side effects: Nausea, vomiting, and diarrhea.

Adverse reactions: Vary significantly with the drug and route of administration. Amphotericin B is extremely toxic with potential for allergic reactions; CNS, renal, hepatic, and cardiac toxicity; blood dyscrasias.

Contraindications: Drug dependent; in life-threatening systemic fungal disease, there may be no contraindications.

Nursing considerations: Drug dependent; refer to specific drugs.

Class: Cephalosporins (AHFS 8:12.06*)

Generic Name	U.S.	Canada
	Trade Names	
Cefamandole nafate	Mandol	Mandol
Cefazolin	Ancef	Ancef
	Kefzol	Kefzol
Cefotaxime	Claforan	Claforan
Cephalexin	Keflex	Keflex
		Ceporex
		Noralexin
Cephalothin	Keflin	Keflin
		Ceporicin

Actions: Bacteriostatic or bactericidal depending on the dose and tissue concentration of the drug, organism susceptibility, and rate of bacterial multiplication; interferes with mucopeptide synthesis in the bacterial cell wall, producing deficiencies in the cell wall that cause it to function as a semipermeable membrane; broad-spectrum effect against most gram-positive and some gram-negative bacteria; cephalosporins inactive against fungi and viruses.

Uses: Treatment of serious infections; usually not considered the drugs of choice for many infections unless alternate drugs are unsuitable because of toxicity, bacterial resistance, and patient hypersensitivity; may be preferred for infection caused by *Klebsiella;* used as prophylaxis for some surgery patients.

General side effects: Pain at IM site; thrombophlebitis following IV administration; diarrhea with oral administration.

Adverse reactions: Allergic reaction; potentially nephrotoxic; transient alteration in hepatic functions; Antabuse-like reactions; bleeding; ulcerative colitis; superinfections.

Contraindications: History of allergic reaction to cephalosporins or an anaphylactic reaction to penicillin; renal impairment.

Nursing considerations:
1. Obtain allergic or sensitivity history. If patient describes allergic history to cephalosporins or penicillin, do not administer.
2. Do not administer concurrently with nephrotoxic drugs. Monitor urinary output.
3. Cephalosporin administration is usually by intermittent IV infusion.
4. Monitor for signs of superinfection, particularly from fungi.
5. Oral cephalosporins should be taken 1 hour before or 2 hours after food intake. Add lactobacillus supplement (i.e., buttermilk, plain yogurt, or Lactinex) to the diet to replace normal gastrointestinal microbial flora.

*American Hospital Formulary Service classification.
†Drug is not available in Canada although it is listed in 1985 *Compendium of Pharmaceuticals and Specialties.*
‡U.S. trade name (or sometimes generic name) not listed in 1985 *Compendium of Pharmaceuticals and Specialties.*
§Drug is known by generic name.

Class: Miscellaneous β-Lactam Antibiotics (AHFS 8:12.07*)

Generic Name	U.S.	Canada
	Trade Names	
Cefoxitin	Mefoxin	Mefoxin

Nursing considerations: Similar in all respects to the cephalosporins.

Class: Chloramphenicol (AHFS 8:12.08*)

Generic Name	U.S.	Canada
	Trade Names	
Chloramphenicol	Chloromycetin	Chloromycetin
		Chloroptic
		Fenicol
		Isopto Fenicol

Actions: Bacteriostatic against a wide range of gram-positive and gram-negative bacteria, rickettsiae, and chlamydiae; acts to inhibit protein synthesis in susceptible bacteria.

Uses: Because of its toxic potential, this drug used primarily in severe systemic infections that do not respond to other anti-infection agents; commonly used for typhoid fever, influenzal meningitis, anaerobic infections, cholera, brucellosis, and rickettsial infections.

General side effects: Gastrointestinal distress.

Adverse reactions: Bone marrow depression: (1) dose related and reversible when drug is discontinued: reticulocytosis, leukopenia, vacuolation of erythroid cells, and thrombocytopenia; (2) non–dose related and irreversible: pancytopenia, agranulocytosis, and aplastic anemia; usually fatal; also hypersensitive reactions causing skin lesions, superinfections, optic neuritis, enterocolitis, and circulatory collapse and death in newborns (may be called the gray baby syndrome).

Contraindications: Infections for which other agents are effective; neonates, pregnant and nursing women, and patients with hepatic dysfunction.

Nursing considerations:
1. Screen patient for history of sensitivity to the drug or liver dysfunction.
2. Do not administer if the necessity for the use of this drug is questionable.
3. Verify that the patient has been informed of the risks associated with chloramphenicol.
4. Administer only to hospitalized patients.
5. Obtain baseline blood counts and monitor frequently (leukocytes, erythrocytes, and thrombocytes) during treatment. Discontinue drug therapy if decreases are detected.
6. Monitor also for weakness and tiredness, sore throat, easy bruising, and optic and peripheral neuritis. Discontinue therapy if any of these reactions are noted.
7. Irreversible bone marrow suppression may appear weeks or months after the drug has been discontinued. Patients should therefore continue to be monitored for sore throat, fever, fatigue, petechiae, and bleeding.

Class: Erythromycins (AHFS 8:12.12*)

Generic Name	Trade Names	
	U.S.	Canada
Erythromycin	E-Mycin	E-Mycin
	Erythrocin	Apo-Erythro-S
	Ilosone	Erythromid
		Ilosone Estolate

Action: Usually bacteriostatic but may be bactericidal in high concentrations or against highly susceptible organisms; inhibits protein synthesis in susceptible organisms, particularly gram-positive cocci (staphylococci, streptococci, enterococci, and pneumococci) and gram-positive bacilli (*Bacillus anthracis, Corynebacterium diphtheriae,* and *Clostridium*).

Uses: Mild to moderately severe infections of the upper and lower respiratory tract, skin, and soft tissue caused by *Streptococcus pyogenes;* pertussis; adjunct to diphtheria antitoxin; mycoplasma pneumonia; for penicillin-sensitive patients in the treatment of syphilis, gonorrhea, and other susceptible bacteria.

General side effects: Abdominal discomfort and cramping; nausea, vomiting, and diarrhea; irritation or phlebitis with IV administration.

Adverse reactions: Allergic reactions ranging from urticaria to anaphylaxis; superinfection; cholestatic hepatitis; and impaired hearing.

Contraindications: Hepatic disease associated with erythromycin estolate; history of hypersensitivity; safe use in pregnancy has not been established.

Nursing considerations:

1. Assess patient for history of liver disease or dysfunction. Do not administer erythromycin estolate if hepatic dysfunction is present. Administer other erythromycin preparations cautiously in patients with hepatic dysfunction.
2. Monitor patients for signs of gastrointestinal distress, skin rash, and liver impairment. Discontinue the drug if hypersensitivity or liver dysfunction develops.
3. Do not administer to persons with a history of hypersensitivity.
4. Administer oral drugs with a full glass of water on an empty stomach. Have patient avoid fruit juices or acidic beverages. Enteric coated tablets should be swallowed whole.
5. Monitor patient for signs of a superinfection.
6. Instruct ambulatory patients to report signs of persistent abdominal discomfort, jaundice, or skin rash to the physician. Changes in hearing should also be reported.
7. IM injections should be given deep into the muscle.

Class: Penicillins (AHFS 8:12.16*)

Generic Name	Trade Names	
	U.S.	Canada
Amoxicillin	Amoxil	Amoxil
	Larotid	Clavulin Trihydrate
Ampicillin	Amcill	Ampicin
	Omnipen	Ampilean
		Nova-Ampicillin
		Penbritin
Carbenicillin disodium	Geopen	Geopen Oral
	Pyopen	Pyopen Disodium
Carbenicillin indanyl	Geocillin	—§
Cloxacillin	Tegopen	Tegopen
		Bactopen
		Novocloxin
		Orbenin
Dicloxacillin	Dynapen	Dynapen
	Veracillin	Veracillin†
Methicillin; meta-cillin	Staphcillin	Staphcillin
Nafcillin	Unipen	Nafcillin
Oxacillin	Bactocill	Bristopen†
Penicillin G benzathine; benzethacil	Bicillin	Bicillin
		Megacillin
Penicillin G	Pentids	Crystapen
	Pfizerpen	
Penicillin G procaine	Wycillin	Wycillin
		Ayercillin
Penicillin V: phenoxymethyl penicillin	Pen-Vee-K	Pen-Vee K
	V-Cillin-K	Pen-Vee Potassium
Ticarcillin disodium	Ticar	Ticar

Actions: Bacteriostatic or bactericidal, depending on drug concentration; interfere with the formation of the bacterial cell wall and are therefore more effective against actively dividing organisms; effective against a broad spectrum of bacteria.

Uses: Pneumonia, meningitis, gonorrhea, urinary tract infections, upper respiratory infections, syphilis, diphtheria, beta-hemolytic streptococcus, anthrax, and as a prophylaxis for patients with rheumatic fever.

General side effects: Allergic skin rash, pain at the injection site, phlebitis, nausea, vomiting, and diarrhea.

Adverse reactions: Anaphylaxis and other hypersensitivity reactions (may be immediate or delayed); gastrointestinal upset; renal and hepatic toxicity and neurotoxicity; blood dyscrasias.

Contraindications: History of allergic reaction to a penicillin or cephalosporin; use with caution in patients with a history of asthma, urticaria, or hay fever.

Nursing considerations:

1. Take a careful drug history. Do not administer to anyone with a history of hypersensitivity to penicillin or cephalosporin. Observe patient for adverse reaction for 30 minutes following parenteral administration. Have emergency response drugs and equipment available.
2. Obtain cultures for sensitivity tests before first dose.
3. Monitor patient for gastrointestinal, oral, or vaginal superinfections.
4. Oral penicillin should be taken 1 hour before or 2 hours after meals. (Antacids should not be used.) An around-the-clock dosing schedule is necessary to maintain constant therapeutic levels. Oral suspensions should be refrigerated.
5. Instruct patient to complete the entire course of prescribed therapy, to refrain from self-medication with leftover antibiotics, and to report treatment failures to the physician.

6. Do not administer long-acting penicillins IV (penicillin G benzathine, penicillin G procaine, and others). Inject drugs deeply IM, and do not massage IM site or apply heat after administering long-acting penicillins.

7. Serum electrolyte monitoring is necessary during prolonged use with sodium or potassium penicillins.

Class: Tetracyclines (AHFS 8:12.24*)

	Trade Names	
Generic Name	U.S.	Canada
Doxycycline	Vibramycin	Vibramycin
Tetracycline	Achromycin V	Achromycin V
	Sumycin	Cefracycline
		Tetracyn

Actions: Usually bacteriostatic but may be bactericidal in high concentrations or against some susceptible organisms; alter protein synthesis in microorganisms and in mammalian cells if used in high concentrations; effective against a broad spectrum of organisms particularly *Rickettsia,* chlamydia, mycoplasma, spirochetes, and many gram-negative and gram-positive bacteria. Resistance to one drug in the group is accompanied by cross-resistance to the whole group.

Uses: Rickettsial diseases such as Rocky Mountain spotted fever, pneumococcal pneumonia, brucellosis, some *Haemophilus influenzae* infections, meningococcemia, lymphogranuloma venereum, gonococcemia, amebiasis, and inflammatory acne vulgaris; not used for common gram-positive or gram-negative bacteria for which there are other effective drugs.

General side effects: Diarrhea, gastrointestinal distress, and ulcers from oral administration; photosensitivity (from select agents); pain from IM injection.

Adverse reactions: Reversible renal tubular dysfunction when outdated drugs have been used (Fanconi's syndrome), abrupt rise in BUN, permanent discoloration of teeth and bone deformities if administered during the time of tooth and bone formation, hypersensitivity reactions, blood dyscrasias, superinfections with severe enteritis, hepatic damage, and vestibular dysfunction.

Contraindications: Renal or liver impairment, pregnancy (after first trimester), children from birth to 8 years of age, nursing mothers, and any person with a history of a hypersensitive reaction to any tetracycline.

Nursing considerations:

1. Do not administer to pregnant or lactating women, persons with a history of a hypersensitive reaction to any tetracycline, or patients with renal or hepatic dysfunction.

2. Administer oral tetracyclines with ample fluids, preferably on an empty stomach. They may be taken with food, if necessary, provided that no milk or milk products or drugs containing magnesium, calcium, aluminum, or iron are given.

*American Hospital Formulary Service classification.
†Drug is not available in Canada although it is listed in 1985 *Compendium of Pharmaceuticals and Specialties.*
‡U.S. trade name (or sometimes generic name) not listed in 1985 *Compendium of Pharmaceuticals and Specialties.*
§Drug is known by generic name.

3. Never administer outdated parenteral preparations. Promptly use powders after reconstitution.

4. Dilute IV solutions well and administer by slow drip. Monitor for phlebitis.

5. IM administration is not recommended. If tetracycline must be given by this route, inject deep into a large muscle and apply ice pack to relieve pain.

6. Monitor for signs of hepatic or renal dysfunction, bone marrow depression, superinfection, and enteritis. Instruct patient to report any untoward symptoms to physician, particularly acute-onset diarrhea different from the diarrhea associated with onset of the drug regimen.

7. Instruct patient on long-term therapy of the need for periodic laboratory analysis of blood components.

8. Instruct patient to destroy unused tetracyclines and to never share these drugs with others.

9. Advise patient to avoid prolonged exposure to direct sunlight or ultraviolet light during therapy to prevent photosensitization. Drug may need to be discontinued if skin irritation develops.

10. Do not expose drug to heat or light. Protect from sunlight during infusion.

Class: Miscellaneous Antibiotics (AHFS 8:12.28*)

	Trade Names	
Generic Name	U.S.	Canada
Clindamycin	Cleocin	Cleocin†
		Dalacin
Polymyxin B	Aerosporin	Aerosporin
Spectinomycin	Trobicin	Trobicin

Nursing considerations: These antibiotics have structural and action characteristics that are agent specific. The nurse should refer to the *Physicians' Desk Reference (PDR)* or to the *American Hospital Formulary Service* for information on each of these drugs; in Canada the nurse should consult the *Compendium of Pharmaceuticals and Specialties.*

CATEGORY: ANTITUBERCULOSIS AGENTS (AHFS 8:16*)

	Trade Names	
Generic Name	U.S.	Canada
Aminosalicylic acid	PAS	PAS
		Nemasol
Capreomycin sulfate	Capastat	Capastat
Cycloserine	Seromycin	Seromycin†
		Closina†
Ethambutol	Myambutol	Myambutol
		Etibi
Ethionamide	Trecator	Trecaton†
		Trescatyl†
Isoniazid; isonicotinic acid hydrazide (INH)	Niconyl	Isotamine
	Nydrazid	PMS Isoniazid
		Rimifon
Pyrazinamide	Aldinamide	Aldinamide†
		Tebrazid
Rifampin	Rifadin	Rifadin
	Rifamycin	
Viomycin	Viocin	Viocin†
		Vinactane-P†

Actions: The antituberculosis agents used in clinical practice vary as to their action, effectiveness, and toxicity.

Uses: The primary agents used in the treatment of tuberculosis include ethambutol, isoniazid, rifampin, and streptomycin (an aminoglycoside). The other antituberculosis agents are generally less effective and more toxic; these secondary agents are reserved for use when there is bacterial resistance to the primary drugs. Antituberculosis agents are generally administered as combinations of two or three drugs, one of which is isoniazid.

General side effects: Vary with the individual agent.

Adverse reactions: Ototoxicity, nephrotoxicity, hepatotoxicity; some cause CNS stimulation; peripheral neuropathy with isoniazid.

Contraindications: Vary with the individual agent.

Nursing considerations:

1. Treatment for tuberculosis is lengthy (1 to 2 years) in order to be effective. Education of the patient regarding the medication regimen and side effects is necessary to ensure compliance with treatment.
2. Monitor for toxic manifestations of specific agents.
3. Encourage patient to report symptoms of toxicity to physician. Provide mechanism for patient to receive assurance or answers to questions between physician visits.
4. Administer vitamin B$_6$ with isoniazid to prevent neurotoxic effects.

CATEGORY: ANTIVIRALS (AHFS 8:18*)

Generic Name	Trade Names	
	U.S.	Canada
Acyclovir	Zovirax	Zovirax
Amantadine	Symmetrel	Symmetrel
		Solu-Contentun†
Vidarabine	Vira-A	Vira-A

Actions: Inhibition of intracellular viral replication (also block normal human cell response); prevention of viral penetration into host cell (amantadine only).

Uses: Clinically limited because of the thin margin between effectiveness and damage to host cells; influenza prophylaxis (amantadine); herpes simplex and keratoconjunctivitis (topical ophthalmic vidarabine); genital herpes (acyclovir); systemic herpes encephalitis (vidarabine).

General side effects: Ophthalmic preparations: tearing, irritation, and photophobia; systemic preparations may cause CNS reactions, nausea and vomiting, and phlebitis at infusion site; topical ointments may cause burning, stinging, and pruritus.

Adverse reactions: Allergic reactions to topical preparations, hepatic and bone marrow toxicity, orthostatic hypotension and congestive heart failure with amantadine, and severe CNS reactions.

Contraindications: Pregnant and nursing women should not receive amantadine.

Nursing considerations:

1. Apply topical preparations with a finger cot.
2. Caution patient to use only ophthalmic preparations in the eye. Advise that they may cause temporary clouding of vision. Instruct patient regarding the use and storage of ophthalmic preparations.
3. Systemic antivirals should not be used for trivial infections.
4. Monitor for toxicity to systemic antivirals. Prepare patient for hypotensive reaction to amantadine, advising patient to rise slowly from sitting or lying position.

CATEGORY: ANTIMALARIAL AGENTS (AHFS 8:20*)

Generic Name	Trade Names	
	U.S.	Canada
Chloroquine	Aralen	Aralen
		Avloclor†
		Quinachlor†
Hydroxychloroquine	Plaquenil	Plaquenil
Pyrimethamine	Daraprim	Daraprim
Quinine sulfate	—§	Novoquinine
Sulfadoxine-pyrimethamine	Fansidar	—‡

Actions: Vary with the drug and the life cycle of the *Plasmodium* in humans; agents effective against the erythrocytic phase of the *Plasmodium* include chloroquine, quinine, quinacrine (an anthelmintic); agents effective against the fixed tissue phases of the pathogen include pyrimethamine and sulfadoxine-pyrimethamine.

Uses: Malaria; drug choice depends on the type of *Plasmodium* (*P. vivax, P. ovale, P. malariae, P. falciparum*) and the stage in the organism's life cycle. Agents effective against the erythrocytic phase are used for treatment during an acute attack. They have no effects on the tissue stage of the organism and therefore do not prevent relapses. Primaquine is used to prevent relapses. Pyrimethamine is used for prophylaxis. Drugs are frequently used in combination.

General side effects: Gastrointestinal distress; other effects are agent specific.

Adverse reactions: CNS stimulation, visual disturbances (nonreversible retinopathy with chloroquine and hydroxychloroquine), hypotension, cardiotoxicity, skin eruptions, blood dyscrasias, and hepatotoxicity.

Contraindications: Vary with the drug and its toxic potential.

Nursing considerations:

1. These are toxic drugs with potential for causing irreversible reactions, particularly with prolonged therapy. Patients receiving outpatient therapy should be informed as to reactions to observe and report to their physician. Hospitalized patients should be monitored for reactions according to the agent being administered.
2. Complete cure for malaria may require prolonged therapy with more than one drug. Instruct patient to report relapses, to return for reexamination, and to comply with regimen.

CATEGORY: SULFONAMIDES (AHFS 8:24*)

Generic Name	Trade Names	
	U.S.	Canada
Co-trimoxazole	Bactrim	Bactrim
	Septra	Septra
Sulfacetamide	Sulamyd	Sodium Sulamyd
		Sulfex
Sulfadiazine	Suladyne	Solu-Diazine Sodium†
		Sulfadets†
Sulfamethoxazole	Gantanol	Gantanol
		Apo-Sulfamethoxazole

| Generic Name | Trade Names | |
	U.S.	Canada
Sulfapyridine	—§	Dagenan
Sulfisoxazole	Gantrisin	Gantrisin
		Apo-Sulfisoxazole
Trisulfapyrimidine	Trisulfazine	—‡

Actions: Bacteriostatic against a broad spectrum of gram-positive and gram-negative bacteria; interfere with folic acid synthesis, which inhibits bacterial cell replication and thus the bacteria are starved.

Uses: Clinical use limited because of the development of many bacterial strains resistant to the drugs; may be used for urinary tract infections, otitis media, chancroid, trachoma, inclusion conjunctivitis, and norcardiosis and as an adjunct therapy for select infections.

General side effects: Nausea, vomiting, and diarrhea.

Adverse reactions: Hypersensitivity, dermatologic reactions, photosensitivity, fever and serum-sickness–type reactions, blood dyscrasias, hepatic and renal damage, crystalluria, CNS symptoms, Stevens-Johnson syndrome, and decreased synthesis of vitamin K.

Contraindications: Hypersensitivity to any sulfonamides, renal or hepatic impairment, infants younger than 2 months, patients with bowel obstruction, group A beta-hemolytic streptococcal infections, and pregnant women at term.

Nursing considerations:

1. The patient's fluid intake should be sufficient (3000 ml/d) to produce a urinary output of 1200 to 1500 ml/d. Maintain sufficient fluid intake and output for 48 hours after discontinuation of long-acting sulfonamides.
2. Patients being given prolonged therapy should be directed to return for blood counts and urinalyses at 2-week intervals.
3. Seven to ten days after initiation of therapy monitor for skin rash, blood dyscrasias, sore throat, fever, pallor, purpura, jaundice, weakness, serum sickness, renal involvement (oliguria, anuria, hematuria, proteinuria, colic), ecchymosis and hemorrhage associated with decreased synthesis of vitamin K, and symptoms of Stevens-Johnson syndrome (high fever, severe headache, and mucous membrane inflammation).
4. Caution patient to avoid direct sunlight.
5. Do not administer sulfonamides to patients with beta-hemolytic streptococcal infections.
6. During drug therapy as a precautionary measure, avoid juices or vitamin C to avoid acidifying the urine pH.

CATEGORY: SULFONES (AHFS 8:26*)

| Generic Name | Trade Names | |
	U.S.	Canada
Dapsone; diaphenyl-sulfone	Avlosulfon DDS	Avlosulfon DDS

*American Hospital Formulary Service classification.
†Drug is not available in Canada although it is listed in 1985 *Compendium of Pharmaceuticals and Specialties.*
‡U.S. trade name (or sometimes generic name) not listed in 1985 *Compendium of Pharmaceuticals and Specialties.*
§Drug is known by generic name.

Actions: Bacteriostatic against *Mycobacterium leprae* by interfering with bacterial metabolism; drug accumulates in body tissues.

Uses: Lepromatous and tuberculoid types of leprosy until lesions are bacteriologically negative (1½ to 5 years).

General side effects: Decrease in hemoglobin during first weeks of therapy followed by stabilization at pretreatment levels; gastrointestinal and neurologic disturbances.

Adverse reactions: Persistent anemia, other blood dyscrasias, allergic dermatitis, hepatitis, drug fever, rhinitis, hepatotoxicity, psychosis, and erythema nodosum as a reaction to circulating dead bacterial antigens.

Contraindications: Amyloidosis of the kidneys.

Nursing considerations:

1. Patients will be required to take these drugs for years and may need assistance with compliance.
2. Administer with food. Dosage is increased slowly at first.
3. Instruct patient to return for periodic liver function and blood studies.
4. After several weeks of therapy, monitor for allergic dermatitis. Reaction may be temporary.
5. Monitor for anemia and cyanosis. Both should be temporary.

CATEGORY: URINARY ANTI-INFECTIVES (AHFS 8:36*)

| Generic Name | Trade Names | |
	U.S.	Canada
Methenamine mandelate	Mandelamine	Mandelamine Sterine
Nitrofurantoin	Macrodantin	Macrodantin Apo-Nitrofurantoin

Actions: Agent specific.

Uses: Initial or recurrent urinary tract infection; treatment of acute and chronic urinary tract infections when other agents are not effective; prophylaxis or suppression of chronic urinary tract infections requiring long-term therapy.

General side effects: Gastrointestinal disturbances, nausea, and vomiting.

Adverse reactions: Agent-specific reactions; examples include allergy to dye, dysuria with large doses, headache, dyspnea, edema, tinnitus, hepatic malfunction, and crystalluria; CNS and visual disturbances, photosensitivity, and toxic psychoses, convulsions, increased intracranial pressure, and metabolic acidosis; and peripheral polyneuropathy, pulmonary hypersensitivity, and hemolytic anemia.

Contraindications: Renal insufficiency, hepatic dysfunction, epilepsy, pregnant or nursing women, and infants under 1 month of age.

Nursing considerations:

1. Encourage large amounts of fluids during drug course. Intake should be at least 2000 ml/d. Monitor intake and output.
2. Teach patient to check urine pH with Labstix or Nitrazine paper (desired is pH less than 5.5). Ascorbic acid and acid-ash foods or juices such as cranberries, plums, and prunes assist to acidify the urine (for methenamine mandelate only).
3. Discontinue drug if CNS reactions such as irritability, headache, excitement, numbness, paresthesias, or vertigo appear.

4. Caution patients to avoid prolonged direct sunlight.
5. Patients being given prolonged therapy should return every 6 months for periodic hematologic examinations to detect hemolytic anemia and to have hepatic function studies, urinalysis, and culture and sensitivity tests done.

CATEGORY: MISCELLANEOUS ANTI-INFECTIVES (AHFS 8:40*)

	Trade Names	
Generic Name	U.S.	Canada
Furazolidone	Furoxone	Furoxone
Metronidazole	Flagyl	Flagyl
		Apo-Metronidazole

Nursing considerations: These anti-infective agents have structural and action characteristics different from other anti-infective categories. The nurse should refer to the *Physicians' Desk Reference (PDR)* or the *American Hospital Formulary Service* for information on each of these drugs; in Canada the nurse should refer to the *Compendium of Pharmaceuticals and Specialties.*

CATEGORY: ANTINEOPLASTIC AGENTS (AHFS 10:00*)

	Trade Names	
Generic Name	U.S.	Canada
Asparaginase	Elspar	Kidrolase
Azathioprine	Imuran	Imuran
Bleomycin	Blenoxane	Blenoxane
Busulfan	Myleran	Myleran
Carmustine (BCNU)	BiCNU	BiCNU
Chlorambucil	Leukeran	Leukeran
Cisplatin	Platinol	Platinol
Cyclophosphamide (CTX)	Cytoxan	Cytoxan
		Procytoc
Cytarabine; Ara-C	Cytosar-U	Cytosar-U
Dacarbazine	DTIC	DTIC
Dactinomycin; actinomycin D	Cosmegen	Cosmegen
Dibromomannitol	Mitrobronitol	—‡
Doxorubicin	Adriamycin	Adriamycin
Fluorouracil (5 FU)	Adrucil	Adrucil
		Etudex
Hydroxyurea	Hydrea	Hydrea
Mechlorethamine; nitrogen mustard	Mustargen	Mustargen
Melphalan	Alkeran	Alkeran
Mercaptopurine (6-MP)	Purinethol	Purinethol
Methotrexate (MTX); amethopterin	Mexate	Methotrexate
Mitomycin	Mutamycin	Mutamycin
Mitotane	Lysodren	Lysodren
Procarbazine	Matulane	Natulan
Tamoxifen	Nolvadex	Nolvadex
Thioguanine (6-TG)	—§	Lavis
Thiotepa	—§	—§
Triethylene melamine (TEM)	—§	Tretamine
Vinblastine (VLB)	Velban	Velbe
Vincristine (VCR)	Oncovin	Oncovin

Actions: These complex agents most generally exert their effects during the mitotic cycle (or proliferating stage) of malignant cells. The agents are cytotoxic and act on certain biochemical pathways of the rapidly proliferating malignant cells. Other rapidly proliferating tissues such as bone marrow, gastrointestinal epithelium, skin, hair follicles, germinal epithelium of gonads, and embryonic tissue may also be affected.

In addition to their cytotoxic properties, these agents are immunosuppressive. This immunosuppression increases the susceptibility of the patient to opportunistic infections.

Antineoplastic agents are divided into two groups: those that are most effective against dividing cells (cell cycle specific agents) and those that are effective against nondividing cells (cell cycle nonspecific agents). Most of the agents fall in the former group. Only two agents, carmustine and a related compound lomustine, are classified as cell cycle nonspecific agents. Use of cell cycle nonspecific agents is indicated for those tumors that are slow growing. There are still other antineoplastic agents that may not be classified by means of their effect on the cell life cycle. These agents act by methods other than cytotoxicity, or their precise action method has not been exactly determined.

Uses: Neoplastic disease.

General side effects: Nausea and vomiting, stomatitis, diarrhea that may lead to fluid and electrolyte imbalance, alopecia, anorexia, fever, fluid retention, masculinization by some agents, and amenorrhea or reduced spermatogenesis.

Adverse reactions: Bone marrow depression resulting in WBC counts less than 3000/ml or platelet counts below 100,000 cells/ml, hepatic or renal toxicity, ototoxicity, pulmonary fibrosis, hemorrhagic cystitis, cardiotoxicity, and pain or skin reaction along injection site.

Contraindications: All of these agents are extremely toxic and should be used only with extreme caution and careful monitoring; contraindications or reasons to discontinue or reduce the dosage of the agent depend on the toxic or adverse reactions exhibited by the patient.

Nursing considerations:

1. Administer antiemetics as necessary for nausea and vomiting. Carefully monitor intake and output, weight, and electrolytes.
2. Monitor for diarrhea, and if necessary administer antidiarrheal agents per physician order. Observe stool number and consistency. Test for occult blood.
3. Observe condition of oral mucous membrane. Encourage good oral hygiene and if necessary nystatin oral suspension.
4. Carefully observe for agent-specific toxic reactions as described above. Monitor laboratory values as indicated.
5. Observe and care for skin integrity disturbances such as alopecia, dermatitis, jaundice, and changes in the color of skin or nail beds.
6. Protect patient from infection or secondary disease. Use reverse isolation as indicated. Monitor temperature and leukocyte count. If possible avoid invasive procedures such as indwelling catheters and IM injections.
7. Assess patient's coping ability. Reassure patient that mood changes are temporary.
8. Health care provider handling, mixing, and administering cytoxic agents should follow recommendations as distrib-

RECOMMENDATIONS FOR HANDLING CYTOTOXIC AGENTS

Preamble: The increasing use of cytotoxic agents and the growing awareness of potential hazards require special attention to the procedures utilized in the handling, preparation and administration of these drugs. Equally important is the proper disposal of chemical residues and wastes. These recommendations are intended to provide information for the protection of personnel participating in the clinical process of chemotherapy. The mutagenic and carcinogenic potential of many cytotoxic agents is well established and is a possible hazard to the health of exposed individuals. It is the responsibility of institutional and private health care providers to adopt and use appropriate procedures for protection and safety.

I. Environmental protection
1. All mixing of cytotoxic agents should be performed in a Class II, biological safety cabinet. Type A cabinets are the minimal requirement. Type A cabinets which are vented (some now classified as Type B3) are preferred.
2. Special techniques and precautions must be utilized because of the vertical (downward) laminar airflow (see Supplement I).
3. The biological safety cabinet must be certified by qualified personnel annually or any time the cabinet is physically moved.
4. The biological safety cabinet should be operated with the blower on, 24 hours per day—seven days per week.
5. Drug preparations must be performed only with the view screen at the recommended access opening. Professionally accepted practices concerning the aseptic preparation of injectable products should be followed.

From National Study Commission on Cytotoxic Exposure. Copyright 1984.

---

uted by the National Study Commission on Cytotoxic Exposure (see box above).

9. Discuss sperm banking with male patients who plan to have children.

AUTONOMIC AGENTS (AHFS 12:00*)

Autonomic agents are divided into five major categories.[2]

CATEGORY: PARASYMPATHOMIMETIC (CHOLINERGIC) AGENTS (AHFS 12:04*)

Generic Name	Trade Names	
	U.S.	Canada
Ambenonium	Mytelase	Mytelase
Bethanechol	Urecholine	Urecholine
Neostigmine	Prostigmin	Prostigmin Methylsulfate
Pyridostigmine	Mestinon	Mestinon

Actions: There are two types of cholinergic agents: parasympathomimetic agents act on the receptors of the effector cells

*American Hospital Formulary Service classification.
†Drug is not available in Canada although it is listed in 1985 *Compendium of Pharmaceuticals and Specialties.*
‡U.S. trade name (or sometimes generic name) not listed in 1985 *Compendium of Pharmaceuticals and Specialties.*
§Drug is known by generic name.
[2]Beta blockers are discussed in the cardiovascular drug section (AHFS 24:00).

that receive postganglionic nerve fibers from the autonomic nervous system; and anticholinesterase agents act to inhibit the enzyme cholinesterase, which is responsible for degrading acetylcholine.

Uses: Many potential therapeutic uses; gastrointestinal tract: used postoperatively for gastric atony and paralytic ileus; postpartum or postoperatively: used to stimulate bladder contraction and thus micturition; cardiovascular system: may be used to treat paroxysmal atrial tachycardia; peripheral vascular system (Raynaud's disease): causes vasodilation; ocular: reduces intraocular pressure in chronic simple wide-angle glaucoma; skeletal muscles (myasthenia gravis): causes stimulation and improvement of abnormally weak muscle fibers.

General side effects: The clinical usefulness of these agents may be limited because of their many side effects: intestinal cramps, diarrhea, increased heartburn and belching, nausea, vomiting, involuntary micturition, bradycardia and hypotension, blurring of vision, muscle twitching and cramps, anxiety, confusion, and restlessness.

Adverse reactions: Some compounds may cause bronchospasms, ataxia, depression of respiration, cyanosis, coma, cardiovascular collapse, respiratory failure, and death.

Contraindications: Hyperthyroidism, peptic ulcer or spastic or obstructive gastrointestinal disturbances, narrow-angle glaucoma, bronchial asthma, renal failure, and patients in cholinergic crisis.

Nursing considerations:
1. For many agents, there is a narrow index between therapeutic effect and adverse or side effects.
2. Side effects should be monitored closely and reported to the physician.

RECOMMENDATIONS FOR HANDLING CYTOTOXIC AGENTS, cont'd

II. Operator protection
1. Disposable surgical latex gloves are recommended for all procedures involving cytotoxic drugs. Polyvinyl chloride (PVC) gloves should not be worn while handling cytotoxic agents. Several types of PVC gloves are permeable to a variety of drugs.
2. Gloves should routinely be changed approximately every 30 minutes when working steadily with cytotoxic agents. Gloves should be removed immediately after overt contamination.
3. Double gloving is recommended for cleaning up of spills.
4. Protective barrier garments should be worn for all procedures involving the preparation and disposal of cytotoxic agents. These garments should have a closed front, long sleeves and closed cuff (either elastic or knit).
5. All potentially contaminated garments must not be worn outside the work area.

III. Compounding procedures and techniques
1. Hands must be washed thoroughly before gloving and after gloves are removed.
2. Care must be taken to avoid puncturing of gloves and possible self-inoculation.
3. Syringes and I.V. sets with Luer-lock fittings should be used whenever possible.
4. Vials should be vented with a hydrophobic filter to eliminate internal pressure or vacuum.
5. Before opening ampules, care should be taken to insure that no liquid remains in the tip of the ampule. A sterile, disposable alcohol dampened gauze sponge should be wrapped around the neck of the ampule to reduce aerosolization.
6. For sealed vials, final drug measurement should be performed prior to removing the needle from the stopper of the vial and after the pressure has been equalized.
7. A closed collection vessel should be available in the biological safety cabinet or the original vial may be used to hold discarded excess drug solutions.
8. Special procedures should be followed for acute exposure or spills (Supplement II).
9. Cytotoxic agents which are handled within the treatment area should be properly labeled (e.g., "Chemotherapy: Dispose of Properly").

IV. Precautions for medication administration
1. Disposable surgical latex gloves should be worn during all cytotoxic drug administration activities.
2. Syringes and I.V. sets with Luer-lock fittings should be used whenever possible.
3. Special care must be taken in priming I.V. sets. The distal tip cover must be removed before priming. Priming should be performed into a sterile, alcohol-dampened gauze sponge, which then is disposed of appropriately.

V. Disposal procedures
1. Place contaminated materials in a leakproof, puncture-proof container appropriately marked as hazardous waste.
2. Cytotoxic drug waste should be transported according to the institutional procedures for contaminated material.
3. There is insufficient information to recommend any single preferred method for disposal of cytotoxic drug waste.
    3.1 One method for disposal of hazardous waste is by incineration at a temperature considered sufficient by the Environmental Protection Agency (EPA) to destroy organic compounds. Incineration should be done in an EPA permitted hazardous waste incinerator.
    3.2 Another method of disposal is by burial at an EPA permitted hazardous waste site.
    3.3 A licensed hazardous waste disposal company may be consulted for information concerning available methods of disposal in the local area.

VI. Personnel policy recommendations
1. All personnel working with cytotoxic agents must receive special training.
2. Access to the compounding area must be limited to only necessary authorized personnel.
3. The personnel working with these agents should be observed regularly by supervisory personnel to insure compliance with procedures.
4. Acute exposure episodes must be documented. The employee must be referred for professional medical examination.

VII. Monitoring procedures
1. Procedures to monitor the equipment and operating techniques of the personnel should be performed on a regular basis and documented. Specific methods of monitoring should be developed to meet the complexities of the function.
2. It is recommended that personnel involved in the preparation of cytotoxic agents on a full time basis be given periodic health examinations in accordance with institutional policy.

RECOMMENDATIONS FOR HANDLING CYTOTOXIC AGENTS, cont'd

Special Techniques and Precautions for Use in the Class II Biological Safety Cabinet Supplement I

1. All equipment needed to complete the procedure in the Class II Biological Safety Cabinet should be placed into the cabinet before beginning and the view screen should be placed at the recommended operating position. A wait of at least two to three minutes before beginning work to allow the unit time to purge itself of airborne contaminants is recommended.

2. The proper procedures for use in the Biological Safety Cabinet are not the same as those used in the horizontal laminar hood. In many cases they seem contradictory, although in theory they are not. This is because of the nature of the airflow pattern in the Biological Safety Cabinet. Clean air descends through the work zone from the top of the cabinet toward the work surface. As it descends, the air is split, with some leaving through the rear perforation and some leaving through the front perforation. The region where the airflow splits is known as the "smoke split" because smoke introduced into this area appears to split into two directions.

3. It is recommended that the smoke split be determined and marked on each cabinet after it is purchased even if the manufacturer states its location. This can be easily done by using an incense stick to generate smoke and moving it gently from front to rear laterally along the work surface of the cabinet near the center.

4. Routinely used large equipment should be placed in the cabinet in its normal position when the determination of the smoke split is made. The equipment should then be placed in the same position every time the cabinet is used.

5. Personnel should refrain from applying any face powder, eye make-up, rouge, fingernail polish, hairspray or other cosmetics in the work area. These cosmetics may provide a source of prolonged exposure if contaminated.

6. Eating, drinking, chewing of gum, storage of food or smoking in, around or near the Biological Safety Cabinet should be prohibited. Each of these are sources of ingestion if they are accidentally contaminated by the cytotoxic agent or other hazardous products.

7. Sterile products should be arranged in the cabinet so as to minimize the possibility of contamination. This may mean locating them in the immediate vicinity of the smoke split. If appropriate, due to quantity or configuration, the sterile items should be kept only in the center and nonsterile items on either side.

8. For additional operator protection, it is recommended that the area behind the smoke split be used whenever possible since the airflow direction in that area is away from the operator, lessening the chance of accidental exposure.

9. The least efficient area of the cabinet in terms of product and personnel protection is within three inches of the sides near the front opening. Therefore, you should not work within three inches of the sides of the cabinet.

10. Periodic evaluation of the smoke split should be performed on a routine basis. A constantly changing smoke split location may be indicative of problems with the operation of the cabinet.

11. Entry into and exit from the cabinet should be in a direct manner perpendicular to the face of the cabinet. Rapid movements of the hands in the cabinet and laterally through the protective air barrier should be avoided.

Special Procedures for Acute Exposure or Spills Supplement II

1.0 Acute exposure

  1.1 Overtly contaminated gloves or outer garments should be removed and replaced immediately after an exposure.

  1.2 Hands should be washed after removing gloves. Gloves are not a substitute for handwashing.

  1.3 In case of skin contact with a cytotoxic drug product, the affected area should be washed thoroughly with soap and water as soon as possible. Refer to professional medical attention as soon as possible.

  1.4 For eye exposure, flush affected eye with copious amounts of water. Refer to professional medical attention immediately.

2.0 Spills

  2.1 All personnel involved in the clean-up of a spill should wear protective clothing (e.g. gloves, gowns, etc.). All clothes and other material used in the process should be treated or disposed of properly.

  2.2 Double gloving should be used in the cleaning up of spills.

3. If agents are being used to force urination postpartum or postoperatively, must make sure patient does not have bladder obstruction.
4. Atropine should be available to counteract cholinergic side effects.
5. These agents may slow heart rate, dilate vessels, and lower blood pressure. Therefore the nurse must be aware of potential orthostatic hypotension and patient advised accordingly.
6. For patients with myasthenia gravis, regular timing of taking medication is vitally important.

CATEGORY: ANTICHOLINERGIC AGENTS (AHFS 12:08*)

| Generic Name | Trade Names | |
	U.S.	Canada
Atropine	—§	Isopto Atropine Sulfate SMP Atropine
Benztropine	Cogentin	Cogentin
Dicyclomine	Bentyl	Bentyl
Ethopropazine	Parsidol	Parsidol†
Orphenadrine	Disipal	Disipal
Propantheline	Pro-Banthine	Pro-Banthine
Scopolamine; methscopol-amine	Transderm-V	Transderm-V
Trihexyphenidyl	Artane	Artane

Actions: Interfere with the transmission of nerve impulses from cholinergic nerves to postganglionic nerves in various structures and organs; specifically act to block acetylcholine from interacting with its receptors, thus inhibiting organ response.
Uses: Antisecretory and antispasm effect of the gastrointestinal tract: used in peptic ulcer disease, preoperatively as an antisecretory agent, urologic disorders to reduce reflex spasms or feelings of urgency, and to increase bladder capacity in children with nocturnal enuresis; atropine used as cardiac agent to increase heart rate in sinus bradycardia and partial heart block; used in ophthalmologic examinations to dilate the pupil and paralyze muscles of accommodation. The belladonna alkaloids have central effects and may be used to treat motion sickness or in anesthesia; overall, their use has decreased; they are no longer used to treat parkinsonism.
General side effects: Dryness of mouth; mydriasis, which causes possible photophobia or blurred vision; heart palpitations and tachycardia; and constipation.
Adverse reactions: Skin dry and hot, fever, urinary retention, impotence, coronary insufficiency or chest pain, restlessness, confusion, hallucinations, and delirium.
Contraindications: Narrow-angle glaucoma, prostatic hypertrophy, angina, and gastrointestinal obstruction from causes such as pyloric stenosis.

*American Hospital Formulary Service classification.
†Drug is not available in Canada although it is listed in 1985 *Compendium of Pharmaceuticals and Specialties.*
‡U.S. trade name (or sometimes generic name) not listed in 1985 *Compendium of Pharmaceuticals and Specialties.*
§Drug is known by generic name.

Nursing considerations:
1. Carefully monitor desired effects vs. potential side effects.
2. Be alert for contraindications of the use of these agents and advise the physician accordingly.
3. Explain the effect of the select agent to the patient so that the patient can expect a therapeutic response.

CATEGORY: SYMPATHOMIMETIC (ADRENERGIC) AGENTS (AHFS 12:12*)

| Generic Name | Trade Names | |
	U.S.	Canada
Albuterol; salbutamol	Proventil	Albuterol† Ventolin
Dobutamine	Dobutrex	Dobutrex
Dopamine	Intropin	Intropin Revimine
Epinephrine	Adrenalin	Adrenalin
Isoetharine	Bronkosol	—‡
Isoproterenol	Isuprel	Isuprel
Levarterenol	Levophed	Levophed
Metaproterenol; orciprenaline	Alupent	Alupent
Metaraminol	Aramine	Pressonex† Pressorol†
Pseudoephedrine	Sudafed	Afrinol†
Ritodrine	Yutopar	Yutopar
Terbutaline	Bricanyl Brethine	Bricanyl

Actions: Act on either alpha- or beta-adrenergic receptors of the sympathetic nervous system; those drugs that affect the beta receptors act to stimulate the heart rate and dilate the bronchioles and blood vessels; those drugs that affect the alpha receptors act primarily to cause peripheral vasoconstriction; some agents may interact with both alpha and beta receptors.
Uses: Primary use: shock and acute hypotension to increase the rate and strength of systole; additional areas of use: severe bradycardia or heart block, bronchodilation such as in acute asthma or allergic reaction, paroxysmal atrial tachycardia, and local or systemic vasoconstriction.
General side effects: Tachycardia or palpitations, headache, anxiety, nervousness, nausea or vomiting, restlessness, dysuria, and tremors.
Adverse reactions: Cardiac arrhythmias, severe hypertension, cardiac dilation, and pulmonary edema.
Contraindications: Agents should be used with caution in patients with aortic stenosis, enlarged prostate glands, diabetes, hypertension, hyperthyroidism, and coronary insufficiency or other heart disease.
Nursing considerations:
1. When agents are administered intravenously, monitor patient's blood pressure, pulse, and respirations at least every 5 minutes.
2. These agents are toxic to the tissues. Should the IV needle or cannula become dislodged from the vessel, stop IV solution immediately if infiltration into the tissue is noted.

CATEGORY: SYMPATHOLYTIC (ADRENERGIC BLOCKING) AGENTS (AHFS 12:16*)

Generic Name	Trade Names	
	U.S.	Canada
Dihydroergotamine; ergometrine	DHE 45	Dihydroergotamine
Ergoloid mesylates; ergonovine	Hydergine	Hydergine
		Ergotrate Maleate
		Ergobasine†
		Ergoklinine†
	Cafergot	—‡
Ergotamine	Gynergen	Gynergen
		Ergomor
		Medihaler-Ergotamine
Methysergide	Sansert	Sansert
		Deseril†
Phenoxybenzamine	Dibenzyline	Dibenzyline
Phentolamine	Regitine	Rogitine

Actions: Interference with the transmission of sympathetic nerve impulses to adrenergic receptor sites on the neuroeffectors; act primarily on smooth muscles to block alpha-stimulated vasoconstriction.

Uses: Phenoxybenzamine used to control or prevent paroxysmal hypertension and sweating in patients with pheochromocytoma; in addition, may be used to treat vasospastic peripheral vascular disorders such as Raynaud's syndrome. Phentolamine used in the diagnosis of pheochromocytoma and in the control of hypertensive episodes before and during surgical removal of pheochromocytoma; in addition, used to prevent and treat tissue necorsis that can occur if either levarterenol or dopamine extravasate during IV infusion. These agents (phentolamine and phenoxybenzamine) are no longer used for essential hypertension.

General side effects: Nasal congestion, postural hypotension with dizziness and reflex tachycardia, tiredness, weakness, malaise, headache, and dry mouth.

Adverse reactions: Severe postural hypotension, which may lead to heart attack, congestive heart failure, stroke, or kidney failure.

Contraindications: Coronary artery disease or angina pectoris, renal damage, severe cerebral atherosclerosis, gastritis, or peptic ulcer.

Nursing considerations:
1. Carefully observe patient for side effects.
2. Inform patient of possible side effects such as syncopy or postural hypotension so that they may be identified early and reported.
3. When phentolamine is used to prevent tissue necrosis and sloughing following IV administration or extravasation of levarterenol (Levophed), 5 to 10 mg of phentolamine in 10 ml of 0.9% sodium chloride injection should be infiltrated into the affected area.

---

*American Hospital Formulary Service classification.
†Drug is not available in Canada although it is listed in 1985 *Compendium of Pharmaceuticals and Specialties.*
‡U.S. trade name (or sometimes generic name) not listed in 1985 *Compendium of Pharmaceuticals and Specialties.*
§Drug is known by generic name.

SKELETAL MUSCLE RELAXANTS (AHFS 12:20*)

Generic Name	Trade Names	
	U.S.	Canada
Baclofen	Lioresal	Lioresal
Cyclobenzaprine	Flexeril	Flexeril
Dantrolene	Dantrium	Dantrium
Mephenesin	Tolserol	Tolserol†
Methocarbamol; glyceryl guaiacolate carbamate	Robaxin	Robaxin
		Tresortil†
Pancuronium bromide	Pavulon	Pavulon
Succinylcholine; suxamethonium	Anectine	Anectine
		Quelicin Chloride

Actions: Act selectively to decrease the tone of skeletal muscles; specifically, these neuromuscular blocking agents interrupt the transmission of impulses from motor neurons at the skeletal-neuromuscular junction; have no central nervous system effect in that they do not alter the patient's memory, level of consciousness, or pain threshold.

Uses: Muscle spasticity that may result from acute injury or spasm or from chronic neurologic disorders such as cerebral palsy, multiple sclerosis, hemiplegia, spinal tumors, and tetanus; pancuronium used to facilitate mechanical respiration in patients with status asthmaticus who have failed to respond to conventional measures; succinylcholine usually administered before pancuronium to facilitate endotracheal intubation.

General side effects: Transient drowsiness, dizziness and vertigo, lethargy, nausea, vomiting, dry mouth, blurred vision, and postural hypotension with feelings of weakness.

Adverse reactions: Mental depression, hallucinations, seizure, gastrointestinal bleeding, extreme muscle weakness, loss of peripheral vision, hematuria resulting from red cell hemolysis, and dependency on agent.

Contraindications: Cardiac arrhythmias, heart block, congestive heart failure or a recent myocardial infarction, liver disease, and kidney disease; succinylcholine causes an abrupt change in intraocular pressure that may be hazardous to patients with glaucoma or penetrating wounds of the eye.

Nursing considerations:
1. Use these agents in conjunction with programs of rest, physical therapy, and analgesics.
2. Perform baseline clinical assessments before initiating these agents so that the benefits from the specific drugs may be measured. Use of test dose is advised, especially with succinylcholine.
3. Use with caution in patients with seizure disorders. These agents may cause a deterioration in the patient's seizure control.
4. Advise patient that these agents may cause drowsiness. Warn patient to evaluate how the agents affect his performance before operating an automobile or machinery.

BLOOD DERIVATIVES

CATEGORY: BLOOD DERIVATIVES (AHFS: 16:00*)

Generic Name	Trade Names	
	U.S.	Canada
Albumin, human	Albumisol	Normal Serum Album
	Albutein	—‡
Plasma protein fraction, human (PPF)	Plasmanate	Plasmanate
	Plasmatein	—‡

Actions: Important factors in the regulation of plasma volume and tissue fluid balance through their contribution of the colloid oncotic pressure of plasma; when administered intravenously, they cause a shift of fluid from the interstitial spaces into the circulation; also cause a slight increase in the concentration of plasma proteins.

Uses: Plasma volume expansion and maintenance of cardiac output in the treatment of trauma, burns, hemorrhage, or other conditions where there is a circulating volume deficit; may also be used for short-term treatment of hypoproteinemia; administered in conjunction with or combined with whole blood, plasma, or crystalloid IV solutions.

General side effects: Infrequently occur.

Adverse reactions: May occur because of allergy or protein overload resulting from high dosage or repeated administration; include chills, nausea, fever, urticaria, hypotension, flushing, erythema, headache, and backache; rapid infusion may cause fluid volume overload.

Contraindications: Patients undergoing cardiopulmonary bypass procedures and patients with severe asthma.

Nursing considerations:

1. Monitor patient for signs of fluid overload or for adverse reactions.
2. The rate of administration should be related to the patient's clinical response.

BLOOD FORMATION AND COAGULATION (AHFS 20:00*)

CATEGORY: ANTIANEMIA DRUGS
Class: Iron preparations (AHFS 20:04.04*)

Generic Name	Trade Names	
	U.S.	Canada
Ferrous gluconate	Fergon	Fergon
		Fertinic
Ferrous sulfate	Feosol	Fesofor
		Slow-Fe
Iron dextran	Imferon	Imferon

Actions: Help to correct erythropoietic abnormalities from deficiency of iron.

Uses: Prevention and treatment of iron-deficient anemia and relief of symptoms caused by iron deficiency, such as tongue sores, fissures of the angles of the lips, dysphagia, and dystrophy of the nails and skin.

General side effects: Constipation, diarrhea, dark stools, nausea or epigastric pain, headache, arthralgia, hypotension, diz-ziness, and metallic taste in mouth; most usually subside within a few days.

Adverse reactions: Anaphylactoid reaction following rapid IV administration; acute toxicity by overdose may occur with as small ingestion as 1 g; signs of acute iron poisoning occur in stages:

Stage one (6 to 8 hours after ingestion): gastrointestinal irritation, epigastric pain, nausea, vomiting, diarrhea, green and tarry stools, hematemesis, drowsiness, pallor, cyanosis, and coma

Stage two (8 to 24 hours): local erosion of stomach and small intestine from increased iron absorption

Stage three (over 24 hours): CNS abnormalities, metabolic acidosis, hepatic dysfunction, and progressive circulatory collapse, coma, and death

Contraindications: Use with extreme caution in patients with impaired hepatic function; should not be used in patients with primary hemochromatosis, peptic ulcers, regional enteritis, and ulcerative colitis.

Nursing considerations:

1. Do not administer oral and parenteral iron preparations concomitantly.
2. Blood hemoglobin and hematocrit levels should be monitored periodically during administration period.
3. Patient should be advised that stools will turn dark in color.
4. Use the Z-track method of IM injection to administer iron dextran. If it is not used, staining of the skin may result from the medication.
5. Oral dosages may need to be taken with food or milk to decrease epigastric distress.

CATEGORY: COAGULANTS AND ANTICOAGULANTS
Class: Anticoagulants (AHFS 20:12.04*)

Generic Name	Trade Names	
	U.S.	Canada
Dicoumarol; bishydroxy-coumarin	—§	—‡
Heparin sodium	Heprinar	Hepalean
		Minihep
Warfarin	Coumadin	Coumadin Sodium
		Warfilone Sodium

Actions: Alteration of synthesis of blood coagulation factors II (prothrombin), VII (proconvertin), IX (Christmas factor), and X (Stuart-Prower factor) in the liver; specifically, they interfere with the action of vitamin K. Coumadin indirectly interferes with blood clotting by suppressing hepatic synthesis of vitamin K–dependent clotting factors: II, VII, IX, and X. Heparin exerts a direct effect on blood coagulation by enhancing the inhibitory actions of antithrombin III or several factors essential to normal blood clotting. This then blocks the conversion of prothrombin to thrombin and fibrinogen to fibrin.

Uses: Anticoagulant therapy as indicated in the treatment of pulmonary embolism, deep venous thrombosis, coronary occlusion, cerebral embolism, heart valve prosthesis, and acute peripheral arterial embolism; may also be used prophylactically before and during cardiovascular surgery and hemodialysis procedures.

General side effects: Coumadin: anorexia, nausea, vomiting, diarrhea, abdominal cramps, dermatitis, and urticaria; heparin: diarrhea and reversible transient alopecia.

Adverse reactions: Hemorrhage, thrombocytopenia, and hypersensitivity as evidenced by fever, chills, urticaria, asthma, and cardiovascular collapse.

Contraindications: Patients without coagulation test information or patients with uncontrolled bleeding; patients with thrombocytopenia and other blood dyscrasias, bacterial endocarditis, and gastrointestinal ulcers.

Nursing considerations:
1. The antidote to warfarin sodium overdosage is vitamin K given 5 to 25 mg IM or IV. Bleeding is usually brought under control within 6 hours.
2. PTT and Lee-White whole blood clotting time (WBCT) should be performed periodically for patients taking heparin.
3. Prothrombin time (PT) should be performed periodically for patients taking warfarin.
4. Watch for signs of excess bleeding of injection sites, gums, palate, nose, stool, and urine.
5. Be alert to complaints of backaches, abdominal discomfort, and flank pain, which may indicate retroperitoneal or intestinal bleeding.
6. Administer heparin by deep subcutaneous injection rotating sites so as to avoid hematoma development. Heparin is not recommended for IM injections.
7. Heparin antidote is protamine sulfate.
8. Advise female patients that menstrual bleeding may be increased and prolonged.
9. Avoid any medications containing aspirin.

Class: Antiheparin Agents (AHFS 20:12.08*)

| Generic Name | Trade Names | |
	U.S.	Canada
Protamine sulfate	—§	—§

Actions: Acts as a heparin antagonist by complexing with heparin to neutralize the heparin effect.

Uses: Antidote to heparin is protamine sulfate; 1 mg will neutralize approximately 120 units of heparin. Its use should be reserved for major bleeding problems. Although not clinically significant, protamine sulfate is also a weak anticoagulant.

General side effects: Rapid IV administration may cause acute hypotension, dyspnea, bradycardia, transient flushing, and a feeling of warmth.

Adverse reactions: Allergic reactions resulting in urticaria and angioneurotic edema; heparin rebound reaction with anticoagulation and bleeding.

Contraindications: Hemorrhage not caused by heparin overdose; cautious use if allergic to fish.

*American Hospital Formulary Service classification.
†Drug is not available in Canada although it is listed in 1985 *Compendium of Pharmaceuticals and Specialties.*
‡U.S. trade name (or sometimes generic name) not listed in 1985 *Compendium of Pharmaceuticals and Specialties.*
§Drug is known by generic name.

Nursing considerations:
1. Perform coagulation tests 5 to 15 minutes after administration of protamine sulfate.
2. Observe patient for heparin rebound reaction 2 to 8 hours after agent administration.
3. Monitor blood pressure.

Class: Hemostatics (AHFS 20:12.16*)

| Generic Name | Trade Names | |
	U.S.	Canada
Aminocaproic acid	Amicar	Amicar
Antihemophilic factor	Factor VIII	—§
Factor IX complex	Konyne	—§

Actions: Artificial replacement of the missing clotting factor so that the patient's blood may clot.

Uses: For patients who are lacking one or more natural clotting components. Aminocaproic acid used to treat disorders in which there is insufficient fibrinogen (factor I); specifically, acts as an antifibrinolytic agent. Antihemophilic factor used to treat the classic form of hemophilia (hemophilia A) where there is a congenital lack of functional factor VIII. Factor IX complex (containing factor IX along with other vitamin K–dependent factors [II, VII, and X]) used to treat Christmas disease (hemophilia B) that occurs as a result of factor IX deficiency.

General side effects: Nausea, cramping, diarrhea, dizziness, tinnitus, malaise, headache, tachycardia, hypotension, clouding of consciousness, chills, and fever; most directly related to the rapidness of infusion; likewise, they quickly disappear when agent administration is stopped.

Adverse reactions: Viral hepatitis, cyanosis, hypotension, bradycardia, and arrhythmias.

Contraindications: Known liver disease, kidney disease, uremia, or cardiac disease.

Nursing considerations:
1. Monitor patient for blood clotting time and monitor vital signs.
2. Observe for signs of thrombosis (leg pain or tenderness).

CATEGORY: THROMBOLYTIC AGENTS (AHFS 20:40*)

| Generic Name | Trade Names | |
	U.S.	Canada
Streptokinase	Kabikinase	—†
	Streptase	Streptase
Urokinase	Abbokinase	—‡

Actions: Promotion of thrombolysis by speeding up the natural clot-resolving process; both are proteolytic enzymes capable of rapidly dissolving vessel-occluding blood clots.

Uses: Treatment of acute massive pulmonary embolism, acute deep vein thrombosis, and some cases of acute myocardial infarction caused by coronary thrombosis.

General side effects: Fever.

Adverse reactions: Massive bleeding, urticarial skin eruptions, bronchospasms, and angioneurotic edema.

Contraindications: Patients with preexisting hemostatic defects, recent surgery, ulcerative wounds, massive trauma, ulcerative colitis, diverticulitis, hepatic or renal disease, thrombocytopenia, chronic lung disease with cavitation, rheumatic valvular disease, and subacute bacterial endocarditis; have not been established as safe for pregnant women or children.

Nursing considerations:

1. Before beginning treatment, obtain a thrombin time.
2. Carefully observe patient for signs of bleeding, either external or internal.
3. If heparin therapy has been used before the use of these agents, stop the heparin therapy.
4. Avoid unnecessary handling of patients while thrombolytic agent therapy is being used. This will help avoid damage and potential bleeding.

CARDIOVASCULAR AGENTS (AHFS 24:00*)

CATEGORY: CARDIAC DRUGS (AHFS 24:04*)

Generic Name	Trade Names	
	U.S.	Canada
Amiodorone (investigational)	—§	—‡
Amrinone	Inocor	Inocor
Aprindine (investigational)	—§	—‡
Atenolol	Tenormin	Tenormin
Bretylium	Bretylol	Bretylate
Digitalis	Digifortis	—†
Digitoxin	Crystodigin	—†
Digoxin	Lanoxin	Lanoxin Novodigoxin
Disopyramide	Norpace	Norpace Rythmodan
Lidocaine	Xylocaine	Xylocaine Xylocard
Mexiletine (investigational)	—§	—†
Nadolol	Corgard	Corgard
Pindolol	Visken	Visken
Procainamide	Pronestyl	Pronestyl
Propranolol	Inderal	Inderal Detensol
Quinidine gluconate	Quinaglute	Quinate
Quinidine polygalacturonate	Cardioquin	Cardioquin
Quinidine sulfate	Cin-Quin	Quinicardine
Timolol	Blocadren	Blocadren
Tocainide	Tonocard	Tonocard
Verapamil	Calan Isoptin	Isoptin

Actions: There are two types of agents in this category. The cardiac glycosides, which include digitalis, digitoxin, and digoxin, act by increasing the strength of the heartbeat (positive inotropic effect) and by altering the electrophysiologic properties of the heart; both actions affect the rate and quality of contractility and rhythm. All of the remaining agents in the category are antiarrhythmics; although these agents are all similar, each has a unique electrophysiologic action in its ability to alter conduction and influence the initiation of membrane response.

Uses: Digitalis preparations used to treat heart failure and certain supraventricular arrhythmias; specifically they are used to assist the heart to increase stroke volume and thus improve cardiac output. Antiarrhythmic agents used to treat specific ventricular or supraventricular arrhythmias; also may be used to treat premature atrial and ventricular contractions, tachycardia, and atrial flutter and fibrillation.

General side effects: Antiarrhythmia agents may cause drowsiness; anticholinergic effects; gastrointestinal upset; metallic or bitter taste in the mouth; diarrhea; visual disturbances; and CNS side effects such as dizziness, headache, slurred speech, and in rare cases coma.

Adverse reactions: Digitalis toxicity evidenced by anorexia, nausea, vomiting, excessive slowing of the pulse (well below 60/min), visual disturbances, cardiac arrhythmias, dizziness, lethargy, insomnia, irritability, restlessness, and headache. Antiarrhythmic agent toxicity causes various degrees of heart block, acute hypotension, widening of QRS complex on electrocardiogram, chest pain, difficulty in breathing, fluid retention, tachycardia or bradycardia, and additional arrhythmias. In addition to these general signs, each agent has numerous specific toxicity signs.

Contraindications: Digitalis preparations contraindicated for persons with heart block or those prone to suffer Stokes-Adams attacks; caution must be used when the patient has congestive heart failure because quinidine, propranolol, procainamide, and disopyramide cause decreased contractility; contraindications for the arrhythmic agents are agent specific.

Nursing considerations:

1. Closely monitor patients receiving these agents for signs of toxic response. Be familiar with the toxic signs of the specific agent prescribed.
2. Before each dose of a digitalis preparation, carefully assess the patient. This includes full minute apical pulse evaluation noting rate, rhythm, and presence of extra sounds (S_3) and history of adverse effects.
3. If toxic signs are suspected for the digitalis preparations, obtain a serum digitalis level. Also periodically monitor the potassium level.
4. Therapeutic effects of digitalis preparations include improvement in patient's condition including a loss of weight, decreased peripheral edema, relief of dyspnea, increased urine output, and reduced restlessness and anxiety.
5. Follow specific instructions for antiarrhythmic agents: procainamide should be taken around the clock; quinidine and disopyramide may be taken with food if gastrointestinal upset occurs (avoid citrus foods that will make the urine alkaline); verapamil should be taken on an empty stomach, 1 hour before or 2 hours after a meal.

CATEGORY: ANTILIPEMIC AGENTS (AHFS 24:06*)

	Trade Names	
Generic Name	U.S.	Canada
Cholestyramine	Questran	Questran
Clofibrate	Atromid-S	Atromid-S
Gemfibrozil	Lopid	Lopid
Niacin	Nicobid	Novoniacin
Probucol	Lorelco	Lorelco
Sitosterols	Cytellin	—‡

Actions: Reduction of serum low-density (prebeta) lipoprotein (VLDL) and low-density (beta) lipoprotein (LDL) levels in the blood; exact mechanism by which they reduce cholesterol and triglycerides is unknown; as the low-density lipoproteins are reduced, the high-density (alpha) lipoprotein levels may increase.

Uses: Adjuncts to dietary therapy to decrease elevated serum triglyceride and cholesterol levels in patients with significant hyperlipidemia and a high risk of coronary artery disease; select agents such as niacin may be used in the treatment of type II, III, IV, or V hyperlipoproteinemia.

General side effects: Nausea, constipation or diarrhea, abdominal pain, flulike muscle aches, headache or dizziness, flushing of the face and neck, pruritus, and burning or stinging of the skin; generally last less than 2 weeks.

Adverse reactions: Thromboembolism and ischemic disorders, chest pains, palpitations, syncope, extrasystoles, anemia, liver function changes, and glycosuria and abnormal glucose tolerance.

Contraindications: Patients with gallbladder disease or a history of liver disease, diabetes, gout, and peptic ulcer should be carefully evaluated before the use of these agents.

Nursing considerations:
1. Give agents just before or with meals.
2. Advise patient to always take agent with something; it may be mixed thoroughly with soup, cereal, or juices.
3. Patients taking these agents for a prolonged period are at risk for developing vitamin A, D, and K deficiencies.
4. Monitor for the effectiveness of the agents as evidenced by decreased serum lipid levels and decreased skin lesions.

CATEGORY: HYPOTENSIVE AGENTS (AHFS 24:08*)

	Trade Names	
Generic Name	U.S.	Canada
Captopril	Capoten	Capoten
Clonidine	Catapres	Catapres
		Dixarit
Diazoxide	Hyperstat	Hyperstat
Guanethidine	Ismelin	Ismelin
		Apo-Gua-nethi-dine

*American Hospital Formulary Service classification.
†Drug is not available in Canada although it is listed in 1985 *Compendium of Pharmaceuticals and Specialties.*
‡U.S. trade name (or sometimes generic name) not listed in 1985 *Compendium of Pharmaceuticals and Specialties.*
§Drug is known by generic name.

	Trade Names	
Generic Name	U.S.	Canada
Hydralazine	Apresoline	Apresoline
Methyldopa	Aldomet	Aldomet
		Dupamet
Metoprolol	Lopressor	Betaloc
Minoxidil	Loniten	Loniten
Prazosin	Minipress	Minipress
Reserpine	Serpasil	Serpasil
		Reserfia
Sodium nitroprusside	Nipride	Nipride

Actions: Act in a variety of ways. Prazosin is an alpha-adrenergic receptor blocker that acts by blocking the alpha receptors in the vasculature that mediate sympathetic vasoconstrictor tone. Metoprolol is thought to act by its ability to suppress renin release and to block beta receptors which in turn reduces blood pressure. Captopril is a renin-angiotensin system inhibitor that acts to block the conversion of angiotensin I to angiotensin II, thus reducing blood pressure. Clonidine has a central effect that depresses the cardiovascular control center. Guanethidine sulfate depletes and then blocks norepinephrine release from the sympathetic nerve fibers. Reserpine acts as an adrenergic neuron blocking agent that interferes with the synthesis, storage, and release of norepinephrine by the sympathetic nervous system. Clonidine and methyldopa act on both the central and peripheral nervous systems to reduce blood pressure. Hydralazine and minoxidil both act directly on the arteriolar smooth muscles to vasodilate. Reserpine acts on the central and peripheral nervous systems to deplete and then occupy the storage granules; this interferes with the synthesis of norepinephrine.

Uses: Treatment of hypertension.

General side effects: Dizziness, postural hypotension, diarrhea, impotence or interference with normal ejaculation in males, amenorrhea and inability to conceive in females, drowsiness and dry mouth, rash, pruritus, eosinophilia, and vivid dreams or nightmares.

Adverse reactions: Proteinuria that may exceed 1 g/d; weight gain from fluid; profound hypotension with weakness, vomiting, skin pallor, and weak irregular heartbeat (if medication is abruptly discontinued); Raynaud's disease; lupuslike reaction; rebound hypertension; and blood dyscrasias. Minoxidil may cause hypertrichosis.

Contraindications: Patients with asthma and heart failure, advanced degrees of heart block, emotional depression, liver disease, and active peptic ulcers or ulcerative colitis.

Nursing considerations:
1. Many of these agents are given in conjunction with diuretics and diet and exercise programs.
2. Abrupt withdrawal of these agents may cause a rebound hypertensive reaction, angina, or even sudden death.
3. Warm or hot climates may affect the patient's response to the drugs. Patients may need drug dosages readjusted.
4. Teach patient to monitor his own blood pressure and pulse before taking each dose of the medication.
5. No improvement in the patient's blood pressure may indicate poor compliance by the patient.
6. Many of these agents may cause drowsiness. It may be advisable to instruct patient to take them at bedtime.

7. Inform the patient of the first dose effect of prazosin, which may be characterized by signs of weakness progressing to syncope.

CATEGORY: VASODILATING AGENTS (AHFS 24:12*)

Generic Name	Trade Names	
	U.S.	*Canada*
Amyl nitrite	—§	Isoamyl Nitrite
Dipyridamole	Persantine	Persantine
		Apo-Dipyri-
		damole
Isosorbide dinitrate	Isordil	Isordil
	Sorbitrate	Coronex
Nicotinyl alcohol	Roniacol	Roniacol
Nifedipine	Procardia	Adalat
Nitroglycerin	Nitro-Bid	Nitro-Bid
	Transderm-Nitro	Tridil
Tolazoline	Priscoline	Priscoline

Actions: Vasodilation of healthy cardiac vasculature and thus increase in coronary blood flow.

Uses: Acute relief of angina pectoris and other peripheral vasospastic disorders.

General side effects: Throbbing headache, flushing of face and neck, postural hypotension with dizziness, and gastrointestinal upset.

Adverse reactions: Persistent headache, increased severity or frequency of angina, and severe hypotensive response with cardiovascular collapse.

Contraindications: Narrow-angle glaucoma and recent cerebral hemorrhage or head trauma.

Nursing considerations:

1. Patients taking nitrates should not use alcohol. A hypotensive response may result.
2. For patients taking nitroglycerin tablets, the number of tablets and time of relief from angina should be recorded.
3. Nitroglycerin sublingual tablets will lose potency if exposed to air and light. They should therefore be left in the original container, tightly closed, and stored in a cool location. The patient should be instructed to obtain a new and fresh supply of nitroglycerin every 6 months.
4. Nitroglycerin dermal patches should be rotated on areas of the chest, upper arm, upper thigh, and back. The area should be free from hair (do not shave the area, use an electric razor).
5. Amyl nitrite is administered by nasal inhalation. The patient should be sitting during and immediately following inhaling amyl nitrite. The ampule, wrapped in a woven absorbent covering, is crushed between the fingers and held to the nostrils for inhalation.

CATEGORY: SCLEROSING AGENTS (AHFS 24:16*)

Generic Name	Trade Names	
	U.S.	*Canada*
Morrhuate sodium	—§	—‡
Sodium tetradecyl sulfate	Sotradecol	Trombovar

Actions: When injected into a vein, these agents cause inflammation of the vein and formation of a thrombus. The blood clot occludes the injected vein and fibrous tissue develops, resulting in obliteration of the vein.

Uses: Obliteration of primary varicose veins that consist of simple dilation with competent valves.

General side effects: Burning, cramping, or itching at the injection sites.

Adverse reactions: Sloughing or necrosis of tissue if the agents are administered incorrectly; hypersensitivity to the agents resulting in dizziness, weakness, asthma, vascular collapse, and respiratory depression.

Contraindications: Should not be used when the patient has significant valvular or deep vein incompetence; also contraindicated in patients with thrombophlebitis, underlying arterial disease, uncontrolled diabetes, neoplasms, sepsis, blood dyscrasias, and acute respiratory or skin diseases.

Nursing considerations:

1. These agents should be used in conjunction with the use of support elastic stockings.
2. Specifically, the area to be injected is closed off and isolated from general circulation by the use of compression bandages. These bandages are left in place for several weeks following agent injection. They are removed when it is felt that the sclerosing process is complete.

CENTRAL NERVOUS SYSTEM AGENTS (AHFS 28:00*)

CATEGORY: ANALGESICS AND ANTIPYRETICS (AHFS 28:08*)

Generic Name	Trade Names	
	U.S.	*Canada*
Acetaminophen	Tylenol	Tylenol
Butorphanol	Stadol	—†
Codeine	—§	Paveral
Meperidine	Demerol	Demerol
Methadone	Dolophine	—†
Morphine	—§	Epimorph
Oxycodone	Percodan	Percodan
		Supeudol
Pentazocine	Talwin	Talwin
Phenacetin	Acetophenetidin	—‡
Sulfinpyrazone	Anturane	Anturane
		Antazone

Actions: Four types of agents are found in this category. First, the opioid analgesics, consisting of codeine, meperidine, methadone, morphine, and oxycodone, act on the central nervous system to interfere with pain conduction or the central response to pain; in addition, opioid analgesics act on the central nervous system to cause suppression of the cough reflex. Second, the mixed agonist/antagonist agents include butorphanol and pentazocine; they act by an unknown mechanism to cause potent analgesia; they also increase arterial resistance, thus increasing myocardial work and oxygen demand. Third, sulfinpyrazone is a potent uricosuric agent that also has antithrombotic and platelet inhibitory effects; this agent has minimal anti-inflammatory and analgesic activity. Fourth are the para-aminophenol derivatives consisting of acetaminophen and phenacetin; these nonsalicylate analgesics produce analgesia and antipyresis by a mechanism similar to the salicylates, but they do not have the anti-inflammatory activity of the salicylates.

Uses: Opioid analgesics and opioid agonists/antagonist agents: temporary analgesia in the treatment of moderate to severe pain; sulinpyrazone: chronic gouty arthritis and intermittent gouty arthritis; para-aminophenol derivatives: temporary analgesia in the treatment of mild to moderate pain; most effective in relieving low intensity pain of nonvisceral origin.

General side effects: Opioid analgesics and agonist/antagonist agents tend to cause respiratory depression, drowsiness, sedation, change in mood, euphoria, mental clouding, nausea and vomiting, dizziness, restlessness, faintness and weakness, and decreased peristalsis; sulfinpyrazone may cause gastrointestinal disturbances or may aggravate or reactivate peptic ulcers.

Adverse reactions: Opioid analgesics and agonist/antagonists may cause respiratory arrest, shock, and cardiac arrest. Sulfinpyrazone should not be used in patients who have diminished renal function. Toxic doses of the para-aminophenol derivatives may cause nausea, vomiting, circulatory failure, rapid shallow breathing, methemoglobinemia, hemolytic anemia, hepatotoxicity, and nephrotoxicity. On rare occasions, phenacetin has been reported to increase occult blood loss. Hepatic necrosis and coma may occur with the use of acetaminophen in overdose amounts when the half-life of the agent exceeds 4 hours.

Contraindications: Increased intracranial pressure or head injury, chronic obstructive pulmonary disease (COPD), hypotension, hepatic failure, renal failure, severe gallbladder disease, thyroid disease, and pregnancy.

Nursing considerations:

1. If gastrointestinal upset occurs, advise patient to take these agents with food or milk.
2. Opioid analgesics and opioid agonist/antagonists may cause drowsiness, dizziness, or visual changes. Advise patient not to operate machinery or drive.
3. Adequate fluid intake and alkalinization of the urine are recommended for sulfinpyrazone.
4. The para-aminophenol derivatives produce a lower incidence of gastric irritation, ulceration, and bleeding than do salicylates.
5. The opioid agents and pentazocine are all controlled substances.

*American Hospital Formulary Service classification.
†Drug is not available in Canada although it is listed in 1985 *Compendium of Pharmaceuticals and Specialties.*
‡U.S. trade name (or sometimes generic name) not listed in 1985 *Compendium of Pharmaceuticals and Specialties.*
§Drug is known by generic name.

CATEGORY: NONSTEROIDAL ANTI-INFLAMMATORY AGENTS (AHFS 28:08.04*)

Generic Name	Trade Names U.S.	Canada
Aspirin	ASA Enseals Bayer Zorprin	Entrophen
Fenoprofen	Nalfon	Nalfon
Ibuprofen	Motrin	Motrin Amersol
Indomethacin	Indocin	Indocin Novomethacin
Meclofenamate	Meclomen	—†
Naproxen	Naprosyn	Naprosyn Naxen
Oxyphenbutazone	Tandearil	Tandearil Oxybutazone
Phenylbutazone	Butazolidin	Butazolidin Algoverine
Salicylate	—§	—‡
Sulindac	Clinoril	Clinoril
Tolmetin	Tolectin	Tolectin

Actions: Aspirin is a nonsteroidal anti-inflammatory and analgesic agent that acts at all sites within the central nervous system. The exact action of the other nonsteroidal anti-inflammatory agents is unknown. They are thought to initiate anti-inflammatory action by inhibiting the synthesis or release of prostaglandins.

Uses: Aspirin is used in the treatment of moderate to mild pain, fever, and inflammatory diseases; it may also be used in the prevention of arterial and possibly venous thrombosis. The nonsteroidal anti-inflammatory drugs (NSAIDs) are used primarily to reduce acute inflammatory reactions as seen in rheumatoid and other forms of arthritis, including gout. They have also been used most recently to treat inflammation and discomfort associated with bursitis, tendinitis, and dysmenorrhea.

General side effects: Although aspirin is tolerated well by most people, some individuals may experience ringing in the ears, increased respirations, and gastrointestinal disturbances. The newer NSAIDs result in fewer complaints of gastrointestinal upset than aspirin. In general they are well tolerated with few side effects. Fenoprofen and naproxen may both cause drowsiness severe enough to make driving hazardous. Blurring of vision may also occur with long-term use.

Adverse reactions: Aspirin may induce prolonged bleeding times in some patients, nausea, and vomiting. Salicylate poisoning may occur, resulting in tinnitus, dizziness, blurred vision, hemorrhaging, and acid-base imbalances. Adverse reactions to the NSAIDs include gastrointestinal hemorrhage and peptic ulcer disease. Uncommon but more severe adverse reactions to the newer NSAIDs include changes in liver function studies, sodium retention, and blood dyscrasias.

Contraindications: Active ulcer diseases, blood dyscrasias, hypertension, and cardiovascular, renal, or liver diseases.

Nursing considerations:

1. To minimize gastric irritation, advise patient to take aspirin with large quantities of water or milk or with food.

2. To minimize the risk of aspirin overdosage, advise patient to take no more than five doses of aspirin during a 24-hour period.
3. Because of evidence showing a potential relationship between the use of aspirin and Reye's syndrome, aspirin should be used with caution in young children. Many advocates are recommending that children under the age of 12 years take acetaminophen. If aspirin must be used, the recommended dosage schedule is as follows:

   Children under 2 years: individualized
   Children 2 to 11 years: 65 mg/kg daily administered in four to six divided doses
   Individuals over 11 years of age: 454 mg, repeated as necessary; daily dose should not exceed 3.63 g.

4. Many of the nonsteroidal anti-inflammatory agents are started in low doses and slowly increased as the patient's tolerance to the agents increases.
5. Patients receiving long-term therapy with agents such as phenylbutazone and indomethacin should have regularly scheduled blood studies to monitor for blood dyscrasias.
6. If the patient is allergic to aspirin, there may also be an increased sensitivity to the other NSAIDs. These agents should be used with extreme caution and with close observation for allergic or sensitivity response.
7. Aspirin should be used cautiously in those patients with asthma, hay fever, and nasal polyps. This triad of clinical signs is known as the ASA triad.

CATEGORY: OPIATE ANTAGONISTS (AHFS 28:10*)

	Trade Names	
Generic Name	U.S.	Canada
Levallorphan	Lorfan	Lorfan
Naloxone	Narcan	Narcan

Actions: Naloxone is an opioid antagonist agent that acts to stimulate respiratory rate and minute volume, arterial P_{CO_2}, and blood pressure. Levallorphan is a narcotic antagonist that also possesses agonistic activities. The precise mechanism of action of these agents is unknown.

Uses: Naloxone effective only as a pure opioid antagonist; used in the treatment of respiratory depression induced by natural and synthetic opioids such as morphine, methadone, and heroin. These agents generally ineffective in the treatment of respiratory depression caused by barbiturates or other sedatives and hypnotics, anesthetics, or other nonnarcotic CNS depressants. Naloxone now being used investigationally as an agent to block the endorphin response following severe trauma.

General side effects: Levallorphan may also produce unpleasant side effects such as transient dysphoria or hallucinations.

Adverse reactions: Naloxone is very short acting and must be closely monitored and readministered if necessary. Patients must be carefully monitored and supported with artificial ventilation if necessary.

Contraindications: Known sensitivity.

Nursing considerations:
1. Naloxone is the preferred agent to levallorphan because of its pure antagonist quality.
2. Use these agents in conjunction with the administration of oxygen and mechanical ventilation.
3. Carefully monitor the patient for the wearing off of the opioid antagonist agent and the patient's deteriorating respiratory state.

CATEGORY: ANTICONVULSANTS (AHFS 28:12*)

	Trade Names	
Generic Name	U.S.	Canada
Carbamazepine	Tegretol	Tegretol
		Mazepine
Ethosuximide	Zarontin	Zarontin
Phenobarbital	Luminal	Luminal
		Gardenal
Phenytoin	Dilantin	Dilantin
		Novophenytoin
Primidone	Mysoline	Mysoline
		Sertan

Actions: Increase in the convulsive threshold of the motor cortex to chemical or electrical stimulation. Although the precise mechanism or mechanisms of action of the agents have not been confirmed at the molecular level, they are thought to probably stabilize the cell membrane due to modification of calcium, sodium, and potassium transport either by increasing sodium efflux or inhibiting sodium influx.

Uses: Treatment and prevention of seizure activity. The agents are selective regarding the types of seizures best treated. Although intravenous administration of diazepam (Valium) is the agent of choice for status epilepticus, the agents listed above are those most commonly used to treat chronic seizure disorders.

General side effects: Most common: drowsiness, vertigo, ataxia, irritability, headache, restless, and nystagmus; generally more pronounced when therapy is initiated; may subside with continued therapy or may be reduced by initiating therapy at a lower dosage; in addition, signs of nausea, vomiting, dysphagia, constipation, diarrhea, and anorexia may be seen.

Adverse reactions: Severe and uncommon adverse reactions include high fever, severe headache, conjunctivitis, alopecia and chloasma-like hyperpigmentation, lymphadenopathy, eosinophilia, jaundice, and blood dyscrasias.

Contraindications: Renal or liver disease or insufficiency.

Nursing considerations:
1. Start at low doses and increase as the patient's tolerance adjusts to the common side effects. By the end of a 1-week period, the maximal dosage level should be reached.
2. Withdraw agents very gradually because of the potential of precipitating seizure activity.
3. Laboratory blood level monitoring as well as a patient log recording the patient's response to the designated agent may assist to determine the therapeutic dosages to be maintained by the patient.
4. Because many of these agents may cause blood dyscrasias, laboratory complete blood counts should be performed on a regular periodic schedule.

5. Patient education regarding compliance and the recognition of side and adverse effects is extremely important.
6. Safe use of these agents during pregnancy has not been established. Dilantin is known to be associated with a higher than normal incidence of fetal malformations.

CATEGORY: PSYCHOTHERAPEUTIC AGENTS (AHFS 28:16*)
Class: Antidepressants (AHFS 28:16.04*)

	Trade Names	
Generic Name	*U.S.*	*Canada*
Amitriptyline	Elavil	Elavil
		Levate
Amoxapine	Asendin	Asendin
Desipramine	Norpramin	Norpramin
Doxepin	Sinequan	Sinequan
Imipramine	Tofranil	Tofranil
		Novopramine
Isocarboxazid	Marplan	Marplan
Nortriptyline	Aventyl	Aventyl
Phenelzine	Nardil	Nardil
Protriptyline	Vivactil	Triptil
Tranylcypromine	Parnate	Parnate
Trazodone	Desyrel	Desyrel

Actions: The two types of antidepressant agents discussed in this section include the tricyclic agents and the monoamine oxidase (MAO) inhibitors. The tricyclic agents include amitriptyline, amoxapine, desipramine, doxepin, imipramine, nortriptyline, protriptyline, and trazodone; these agents act by increasing the amount of norepinephrine and serotonin neurotransmissions at the synaptic cleft. The MAO inhibitors include isocarboxazid, phenelzine, and tranylcypromine; they act by inhibiting the enzyme monamine oxidase and thereby increasing the concentration of norepinephrine and serotonin.

Uses: Tricyclic agents used for treating all categories of depression; imipramine also used to help prevent enuresis in children over 6 years of age. MAO inhibitors are second-line agents and are used primarily when the tricyclic agents have failed; patients thought to respond best to MAO agents are those who are suffering severe neurotic or atypical depression.

General side effects: Most of the tricyclic agents exert a sedative effect during the first few days of their use. After several weeks of treatment, however, most patients respond with a decrease of their target symptoms. Common side effects for both the tricyclic and MAO agents include dry mouth, blurred vision, difficulty with micturition and in males with impotence or delayed ejaculation. CNS side effects felt with both agents include feelings of euphoria or feelings of hyperactivity, hyperreflexia, restlessness, and jitteriness or agitation. Some patients may show overt motor stimulation in the form

*American Hospital Formulary Service classification.
†Drug is not available in Canada although it is listed in 1985 *Compendium of Pharmaceuticals and Specialties.*
‡U.S. trade name (or sometimes generic name) not listed in 1985 *Compendium of Pharmaceuticals and Specialties.*
§Drug is known by generic name.

of paresthesia or tinnitus. The more serious side effects, especially in elderly persons taking MAO agents, are a potential sudden rise or fall in blood pressure.

Adverse reactions: CNS effects of the tricyclic agents include drowsiness or restlessness along with confusion, dizziness, and headaches. Cardiovascular adverse reactions include arrhythmias, tachycardia, and A-V block defects. The MAO inhibitors have been known to cause hypertensive crisis, severe headache, neck ache, sweating, nausea, and vomiting. Other adverse reactions may be noted by patients taking other agents such as narcotic analgesics, other CNS depressants, adrenergic agents, insulin or hypoglycemic agents, antihypertensive or antiparkinsonism agents, or other agents that affect catecholamine metabolism. Each of these combinations should be individually investigated.

Contraindications: MAO inhibitors: cerebrovascular or cardiovascular disease, hypertension, severe headaches, or congestive heart failure.

Nursing considerations:
1. Oral contraceptives may inhibit the effect of tricyclic antidepressents.
2. Alcohol, CNS depressants, and barbiturates may enhance the effects of these agents and may lead to toxicity.
3. Certain agents may cause increased sensitivity to the sun.
4. Because many of these agents cause drowsiness or visual changes, especially early in the course of treatment, advise patients to use extreme care when driving or operating heavy machinery.
5. Tricyclic antidepressants should be used cautiously in patients with benign prostatic hypertrophy and angle-closure glaucoma.
6. Patients taking MAO inhibitors should be cautioned to avoid foods and beverages that are high in tyramine, an amino acid found in many "aged" foods, such as cheeses, yogurt, sour cream, fermented sausages, figs, raisins, chocolate, yeast extract, beer, and wine.

Class: Tranquilizers (AHFS 28:16.08*)

	Trade Names	
Generic Name	*U.S.*	*Canada*
Chlorpromazine	Thorazine	Largactil
		Chlorpromanyl
Haloperidol	Haldol	Haldol
Prochlorperazine	Compazine	Stemetil

Actions: Antagonists of dopamine receptors in the central nervous system; which thus act to decrease transmission; tend to depress the central nervous system at the subcortical, midbrain, and brainstem levels; schizophrenia thought to be caused by "excessive" dopaminergic transmission; phenothiazines exert actions in the central nervous system that produce sedation without hypnosis or anesthesia, block avoidance behavior, have an antiemetic effect, alter temperature regulation, exert an antipruritic effect, produce analgesia, alter seizure threshold, and produce endocrine alterations.

Uses: Treatment of psychomotor agitation associated with various acute and chronic psychoses including schizophrenia, manic phase, and alcohol withdrawal; also may be used to control or prevent nausea and vomiting and in the control of hiccups. Hydroxyzine may be useful as a mild calming agent in the symptomatic treatment of emotional or psychoneurotic states characterized by anxiety, tension, and agitation; also useful in the treatment of chronic urticaria, but the agent should not be used alone in the treatment of psychoses or depression.

General side effects: Numerous; may involve almost every organ system (the reader is referred to further information on each specific agent for possible effects); common side effects include dizziness, drowsiness, sensitivity to sunlight, pink or reddish urine, sensitivity to heat, and constipation.

Adverse reactions: Agranulocytosis, eosinophilia, thrombocytopenia, aplastic anemia, photosensitivity, dermatoses or melanosis, and extrapyramidal symptoms (again the reader must be aware of the adverse effects of the specific agent being used).

Contraindications: Administer with great caution to patients with renal or hepatic disease.

Nursing considerations:
1. These agents may cause increased patient drowsiness. Therefore warn patient about operating equipment or driving.
2. Carefully observe patient for agent-specific side and adverse reactions.
3. Avoid alcohol or other depressants while these agents are being taken.
4. While patient is taking these agents, monitor blood pressure on a regular basis.
5. These agents may cause patients to become hypothermic. Closely monitor elderly persons for temperature control and potential for burning during bathing.

Class: Miscellaneous Psychotherapeutic Agents (AHFS 28:16.12*)

| Generic Name | Trade Names | |
	U.S.	Canada
Lithium	Lithane	Lithane
		Carbolith

Actions: Unknown; thought to alter the metabolism of norepinephrine in the brain and thus limit the availability of the neurotransmitter at receptor sites; the full and maximal effect is reached within 6 to 10 days after beginning treatment.

Uses: Control of manic episodes in patients with manic-depressive psychoses; has no apparent effect in the treatment of schizophrenia.

General side effects: Serious side effects uncommon for serum levels below 2.0 mEq/L; if seen, these generally consist of fine motor tremor, polyuria, mild thirst, diarrhea, vomiting, drowsiness, muscular weakness, and lack of coordination.

Adverse reactions: Toxic reactions occur when the serum level exceeds 2.0 to 3.0 mEq/L; signs include ataxia, tremor, muscle hyperexcitability, muscle twitching of the limbs, seizures, slurred speech, restlessness, stupor, and coma; in addition, the patient may have cardiovascular irregularities and circulatory failure.

Contraindications: Extreme caution must be used when using lithium in elderly persons or in any patient with impaired renal function.

Nursing considerations:
1. All patients taking lithium should have routine serum lithium levels drawn on a routine basis. This means that during the first month of therapy levels should be drawn once or twice a week using samples drawn 8 to 12 hours after the previous dose. Once the patient is on maintenance therapy, serum levels should be drawn at least once each month. The serum lithium levels should not be permitted to exceed 2 mEq/L during the acute treatment phase or 1.5 mEq/L during maintenance therapy.
2. Encourage patient to maintain adequate fluid intake.
3. Because lithium may cause drowsiness, caution regarding the operation of automobiles and heavy equipment.
4. Because restricted sodium intake may potentiate lithium toxicity by facilitating lithium reabsorption, it is essential that patients receive a diet containing the normal amounts of sodium chloride. In addition, sodium-depleting diuretics such as thiazides should be avoided.
5. If drug toxicity signs are noted, lithium is generally withheld for 24 hours and is then restarted at a lower dose.

CATEGORY: RESPIRATORY AND CEREBRAL STIMULANTS (AHFS 28:20*)

| Generic Name | Trade Names | |
	U.S.	Canada
Diethylpropion	Tenuate	Tenuate
		Dietic
Phentermine	Fastin	Fastin
	Ionamin	Ionamin

Actions: Anorexigenic effect and loss of weight.

Uses: Adjunct therapy in the treatment of obesity.

General side effects: May cause headache, nervousness, dizziness, insomnia, dryness of the mouth, blurred vision, and urticaria.

Adverse reactions: May cause tachycardia, palpitations, and gastrointestinal upset.

Contraindications: Use with extreme caution in patients with hyperthyroidism, hypertension, angina pectoris, and other severe cardiac diseases; contraindicated in patients taking MOA inhibitors and patients with narrow-angle glaucoma.

Nursing considerations:
1. Diethylpropion is only an adjunct therapy that helps to bring about weight loss. This agent must be supplemented with a program to curtail overeating and a suitable diet.
2. Habituation or addiction is possible with both of these agents.

CATEGORY: ANXIOLYTICS, SEDATIVES, AND HYPNOTICS (AHFS 28:24*)

| Generic Name | Trade Names | |
	U.S.	Canada
Alprazolam	Xanax	Xanax
Amobarbital	Amytal	Amytal
		Isobec
Chlordiazepoxide	Librium	Librium
		Medilium
Diazepam	Valium	Valium
		Vivol

	Trade Names	
Generic Name	*U.S.*	*Canada*
Flurazepam	Dalmane	Dalmane
		Novoflupam
Glutethimide	Doriden	Doriden
Hydroxyzine HCl	Atarax	Atarax
		Multipax
Hydroxyzine pamoate	Vistaril	—‡
Meprobamate	Equanil	Equanil
		Meditran
Oxazepam	Serax	Serax
		Zapex
Pentobarbital	Nembutal	Nembutal
Phenobarbital	Luminal	Luminal
		Gardenal
Secobarbital	Seconal	Seconal
		Novosecobarb

Actions: The three groups of agents in this category include the barbiturates, the nonbarbiturates, and the antianxiety agents. The barbiturates include amobarbital, pentobarbital, phenobarbital, and secobarbital. Although their mechanism of action is not completely understood, they are thought to act throughout the central nervous system to produce sedation from mild forms to deep coma. The nonbarbiturates include glutethimide and flurazepam; they are very similar to the barbiturates; although they were developed to be more effective and safer than the barbiturates, little research verifies their advantage. In fact, in the case of overdose, they may be more difficult to treat. The antianxiety agents or minor tranquilizers are mostly benzodiazepines; these agents include alprazolam, chlordiazepoxide, diazepam, meprobamate, and oxazepam; they act on the subcortical levels of the central nervous system; although their full action mechanism is not fully understood, they have a general benefit over the other agents in this category because of their wide margin of safety. Hydroxyzine has antihistaminic effects in addition to its sedative and antiemetic activity.

Uses: Barbiturates and nonbarbiturates are used primarily as hypnotic agents in the treatment of simple insomnia. The barbiturates are also used preoperatively to relieve anxiety and to provide sedation. Amobarbital, pentobarbital, and phenobarbital are useful seizure control agents. Amobarbital may also be used as a diagnostic aid in schizophrenia. The antianxiety agents are used for anxiety disorders. They are not intended for use in patients with a primary depressive disorder or psychosis or for those psychiatric disorders in which anxiety is not a prominent feature. The use of meprobamate has declined because of its high addiction potential.

General side effects: Barbiturates and nonbarbiturates may cause drowsiness, a feeling of hangover, lethargy, vertigo, headache, heartburn, nausea, vomiting, and CNS depression. The antianxiety agents may cause a transient mild drowsiness during the first few days of therapy; other side effects are similar to those of the barbiturates and nonbarbiturates.

*American Hospital Formulary Service classification.
†Drug is not available in Canada although it is listed in 1985 *Compendium of Pharmaceuticals and Specialties.*
‡U.S. trade name (or sometimes generic name) not listed in 1985 *Compendium of Pharmaceuticals and Specialties.*
§Drug is known by generic name.

Adverse reactions: Hypersensitivity reactions to barbiturates and nonbarbiturates include angioneurotic edema, fever, serum sickness, urticaria, erythema multiforme, blood dyscrasias, and Stevens-Johnson syndrome. In children, phenobarbital may produce a paradoxical excitement and hyperactivity. Elderly persons may react to usual doses of barbiturates with excitement, confusion, or depression. IV administration of barbiturates may produce severe respiratory depression, apnea, laryngospasm, bronchospasm, coughing, vasodilation, and hypotension. Antianxiety agents may cause changes in libido, urinary retention, menstrual irregularities, bradycardia, tachycardia, peripheral edema, and visual disturbances.

Contraindications: Barbiturates are to be administered cautiously in patients with mental depression or a history of drug abuse. In addition, extreme caution should be used when administering any of these agents to pregnant patients (first-trimester administration should be avoided) or patients with renal or hepatic disease or dysfunction or pulmonary insufficiency.

Nursing considerations:

1. If barbiturates are to be administered by IV route, carefully read the potential adverse effects listed above.
2. Forgetfulness sometimes follows the use of moderate doses of barbiturates. This may lead to potential injury or to unintentional overdose or acute intoxication.
3. When these agents (especially high doses of barbiturates) are to be discontinued, the dosage should be gradually decreased to avoid withdrawal symptoms.
4. Avoid the use of these agents with other CNS depressants or with alcohol.
5. Cigarette smoking may alter the clinical effects of the antianxiety agents.
6. All of these agents, except hydroxyzine, are controlled substances.
7. Caution should be used when these agents are used in elderly persons; they may accumulate because of decreased liver function.

DIAGNOSTIC AGENTS (AHFS 36:00*)

These agents are discussed where appropriate in each chapter throughout the text. The reader is referred to the index for page references.

ELECTROLYTIC, CALORIC, AND WATER BALANCE (AHFS 40:00*)

CATEGORY: ACIDIFYING AGENTS (AHFS 40:04*)

	Trade Names	
Generic Name	*U.S.*	*Canada*
Ammonium chloride	—§	Ammonium Muriate

Actions: An acid-forming salt that is rapidly absorbed from the gastrointestinal system.

Uses: Systemic acidifier in patients with metabolic alkalosis resulting from chloride loss following vomiting or gastric suction; may also be used to correct hypochloremia from depletion following diuretic therapy and a decrease of pH in the urine.

General side effects: May cause skin rash, headache, hyperventilation, bradycardia, drowsiness, and mental confusion.

Adverse reactions: When used in large doses, may irritate the gastric mucosa and may cause gastric distress, anorexia, and vomiting, large doses may also cause metabolic acidosis; in patients with hepatic disease, the ammonia may have a toxic response causing calcium-deficient tetany, hyperglycemia, glycosuria, and twitching; due to inability of diseased liver to convert ammonium ion to urea.

Contraindications: Should be administered with caution in patients with pulmonary insufficiency, hepatic disease, or cardiac disease.

Nursing considerations:

1. Monitor patient's acid-base balance periodically. Report clinical signs of acidosis or alkalosis.
2. Closely monitor signs of gastric irritation.
3. Give this agent with food to decrease the gastrointestinal side effects.
4. Monitor the rate and depth of respirations. Shortness of breath and increased ventilatory rate are signs of acidosis.
5. Monitor diabetic patients closely. This agent may lead to hyperglycemia.
6. Rapid IV administration may lead to ammonia toxicity. Signs include vomiting, pallor, diaphoresis, irregular breathing, arrhythmias, convulsions, and coma.

CATEGORY: ALKALINIZING AGENTS (AHFS 40:08*)

Generic Name	Trade Names	
	U.S.	*Canada*
Sodium bicarbonate (IV and oral)	—§	—§
Sodium citrate (oral)	—§	—§

Actions: Systemic alkalizers with systemic antacid effects that neutralize hydrochloric acid.

Uses: Sodium bicarbonate used to treat metabolic acidosis; may be administered with gastric irritant agents to counteract the hyperacidity of the stomach; may also be used to minimize uric acid crystallization associated with uricosuric agents and certain chemotherapy protocols. Sodium citrate used as an alkalinizing agent in those patients with conditions that require long-term maintenance of alkaline pH urine or in those patients with chronic metabolic acidosis associated with chronic renal insufficiency or renal tubular acidosis; used to alkalinize the urine or to restore the bicarbonate reserve in acidosis; used also as an anticoagulant in the collection of blood and as an agent to prevent the curdling of milk.

General side effects: May cause increased gastrointestinal distress by causing gastric distention, belching, and flatulence; may also cause sodium overload, hypocalcemia, and hypokalemia. Chronic use of oral preparations taken with milk may cause milk alkali syndrome, consisting of anorexia, nausea, vomiting, and metabolic alkalosis.

Adverse reactions: Large doses of sodium bicarbonate may lead to alkalosis. Large doses of sodium citrate may depress cardiac contractility and cause tetany be decreasing blood calcium levels.

Contraindications: Hypertension, congestive heart failure, renal insufficiency, or fluid retention; should be used with extreme caution in elderly persons and patients with decreased chloride levels secondary to vomiting, diuresis, and suctioning.

Nursing considerations:

1. Rapid administration of sodium bicarbonate is dangerous and may cause death. The agent is to be injected slowly.
2. Closely monitor electrolyte, acid-base, and fluid balance.
3. Because sodium citrate may have a laxative effect, give after meals to help decrease this unwanted effect.
4. For urinary alkalinization, carefully monitor the urine pH.
5. Sodium bicarbonate when injected into the tissues may cause severe tissue damage. Stop dislodged IV lines immediately.
6. Sodium bicarbonate is not compatible with all IV solutions. Compatibility should be evaluated before IV administration.

CATEGORY: AMMONIA DETOXICANTS (AHFS 40:10*)

Generic Name	Trade Names	
	U.S.	*Canada*
Lactulose	Cephulac	Cephulac

Actions: Synthetic derivative of lactose; acts to reduce blood levels of ammonia; although the exact mechanism of action has not been determined it is associated with the conversion of ammonia (NH_3) in the colon to ammonium (NH_4), which cannot be absorbed into the bloodstream.

Uses: Reduction of blood ammonia concentration in patients with portal-systemic encephalopathy (PSE); by doing this, it reduces severity of PSE during both hepatic coma and precoma states. Used as adjunct therapy to the restriction of protein; may also be used to treat PSE resulting from surgical portacaval shunts or chronic hepatic diseases such as cirrhosis; investigationally, this agent has been successfully used as a laxative in the treatment of chronic constipation in both children and adults.

General side effects: Diarrhea is the most common side effect, especially during the first few days of therapy; other side effects include abdominal cramping and flatulence; all of these signs usually subside with continued therapy; if not, dosage may need to be lowered.

Adverse reactions: Overdose of this agent leads to diarrhea and severe fluid and electrolyte depletion.

Contraindications: Not helpful in treatment of infectious hepatitis or other acute liver disorders.

Nursing considerations:

1. Initial large doses of the agent help to lower hyperammonemia by 25% to 50% and thus help to increase patient's ability to tolerate larger amounts of dietary protein.
2. If the side effect of diarrhea is seen, dosage should be decreased until the patient adjusts to the medication.
3. The sweet taste of the agent may be decreased by mixing it with water or fruit juice or by administering it in a food such as dessert.

Electrolyte Concentrations of Several Commonly Used Parenteral Solutions

Solution	g/L	Cations (mEq/L)	Anions (mEq/L)
Ammonium chloride 0.9%	9.0	167 NH₄	167 Cl
Ammonium chloride 2.14%	21.4	400 NH₄	400 Cl
Potassium chloride 0.3%	3.0	40 K	40 Cl
Sodium bicarbonate 1.5%	15.0	178 Na	178 mM Bicarbonate
Sodium chloride 0.45%	4.5	77 Na	77 Cl
Sodium chloride 0.9%	9.0	154 Na	154 Cl
Sodium chloride 5.0%	50.0	850 Na	850 Cl
Sodium lactate ⅙ molar	19.0	167 Na	167 mM Lactate
Ringer's USP	8.6 NaCl	147 Na	155.5 Cl
	0.3 KCl	4 K	
	0.33 CaCl₂ (2 H₂O)	4.5 Ca	
Lactated Ringer's USP (Hartmann's)	6.0 NaCl	130 Na	109.7 Cl
	0.3 KCl	4 K	
	0.2 CaCl₂ (2 H₂O)	2.7 Ca	
	3.1 Na Lactate		27 mM Lactate
Lactated potassic saline NF (Darrow's)	4.0 NaCl	122 Na	104 Cl
	2.6 KCl	35 K	
	5.9 Na Lactate		50 mM Lactate
Duodenal	5.1 NaCl	138 Na	100 Cl
	0.9 KCl	12 K	
	5.6 Na Lactate		53 mM Lactate
Gastric	3.7 NaCl	63 Na	150 Cl
	1.3 KCl	17 K	
	3.74 NH₄Cl	70 NH₄	

From American hospital formulary service, Bethesda, Md., 1983, American Society of Hospital Pharmacists.

CATEGORY: REPLACEMENT SOLUTIONS (AHFS 40:12*)

For the purposes of discussion, this category has been broken down into five class units, each discussed separately: calcium salts, dextran solutions, potassium supplements, Ringer's solutions, and sodium supplements (see table above).

Class: Calcium Salts

Generic Name	Trade Names U.S.	Canada
Calcium carbonate	Titralac	Biocat Caltrate
Calcium chloride	—§	—§
Calcium glubionate	Neo-Calglucon	—‡
Calcium gluconate	Kalcinate	—§
Calcium lactate	—§	—§

*American Hospital Formulary Service classification.
†Drug is not available in Canada although it is listed in 1985 Compendium of Pharmaceuticals and Specialties.
‡U.S. trade name (or sometimes generic name) not listed in 1985 Compendium of Pharmaceuticals and Specialties.
§Drug is known by generic name.

Actions: Calcium acts as an important activator in the transmission of nerve impulses for both smooth and skeletal muscles and plays an important part in the contraction of the cardiac muscle as well as in proper renal function, respiration, and blood coagulation.

Uses: Source of calcium cation in treatment of calcium depletion; may be administered intravenously during acute periods such as cardiac resuscitation when epinephrine has failed to improve weak or ineffective myocardial contraction; hypocalcemic tetany secondary to renal failure and numerous poisoning agents; hypoparathyroidism, premature delivery, or maternal diabetes in infant; severe muscle cramps; and numerous other case-specific situations; available for oral administration, including carbonate, glubionate, gluconate, and lactate; calcium gluconate and lactate available in injectable forms.

General side effects: Gastrointestinal irritation, constipation, and alterations in urinary output.

Adverse reactions: Cardiac arrhythmias; hypercalcemia with chronic administration.

Contraindications: Cautious use of calcium salts with renal or cardiac disease, sarcoidosis, respiratory disease, or patients who are receiving digitalis; contraindicated in patients with active ventricular fibrillation or high serum calcium levels, should not be given if bone metastases caused by cancer are present.

Nursing considerations:

1. Calcium salts are irritating to the tissues and may cause tissue reactions or damage.
2. IV calcium should be administered very slowly. Rapid administration may precipitate complaints of tingling sensations, heat wave feelings, and a chalky taste in the mouth.
3. Frequent serum calcium and phosphorus levels should be monitored and should be maintained at 4.3 to 5.3 mEq/L (calcium) and 1.8 to 2.6 mEq/L (phosphorus).
4. Arrhythmias may develop if calcium salts are administered in patients who are also receiving cardiac glycosides.
5. If the agent is administered intravenously, the compatibility of the agent with the IV solution must be evaluated before administration.

Class: Dextran Agents

Generic Name	Trade Names	
	U.S.	Canada
Dextran 40	Gentran	—‡
Dextran 70	Macrodex	Macrodex
Dextran 75	Gentran 75	Dextran 75

Actions: Act with a colloidal osmotic effect to draw fluid from the interstitial spaces into the intravascular spaces; accompanying an increase in intravascular volume is an increase in central venous pressure, cardiac output, blood pressure, urinary output, capillary perfusion, and pulse pressure; conversely there is a decrease in heart rate, peripheral resistance, and blood viscosity; dextrans 70 and 75 produce a plasma volume expansion slightly in excess of the volume of the dextran solution infused.

Uses: Although the agents dextran 40, 70, and 75 are different, all are used as early fluid replacement for plasma volume during a shock episode when whole blood or blood products are not yet available. Dextran 40 has a low molecular weight and is more readily available, is excreted more readily, has a shorter action, and effectively improves microcirculation. Maximal plasma volume expansion is reached several minutes after the end of infusion. Dextran 40 is short acting, and the drug level falls rapidly during the first hour following administration; one advantage of dextran 40 over the higher-molecular weight dextrans is that it minimizes the sludging of blood as a result of its effects on microcirculation; dextran 40 has also been used investigationally to improve circulation in conditions such as myocardial infarction and sickle cell crisis. Dextrans 70 and 75 are helpful in the treatment of burns and hypovolemic shock; they should not be used if hypovolemia is not present; they have molecular weights more similar to that of serum albumin and reach peak action approximately 1 hour after infusion.

General side effects: Mild development of metabolic acidosis following administration; may cause urticaria, nasal congestion, wheezing, tightness of the chest, and mild hypotension; seems to be transient and the exact cause is not well understood.

Adverse reactions: Allergic reactions as evidenced by mild urticarial reactions to severe anaphylactoid reactions; severely injured patient who has decreased urinary output following the administration of dextran; less common: gastrointestinal disturbances including diarrhea, vomiting, and involuntary defecation in unconscious patients.

Contraindications: Allergic history to dextrans; history of renal disease; patients with congestive heart failure who may already have fluid overload. Patients with active hypovolemic hemorrhage may have increased bleeding following the administration of dextran 40; caused by improved microcirculation and tissue perfusion. Dextran 40 contraindicated in patients with thrombocytopenia or hypofibrinogenemia.

Nursing considerations:

1. Because of potential allergic reactions, make special patient observation and assessments during the first 10 to 15 minutes of IV administration.
2. Because of the rapid excretion of dextran 40, urine specific gravity and viscosity should be expected to increase.
3. Careful monitoring of urinary output should be done while the patient is receiving dextran. If oliguria or anuria occurs, physician consultation should be sought, the infusion should be terminated, and the administration of mannitol should be considered. In the case of severe injury, it may be very difficult to determine if the oliguria or anuria is caused by the use of dextran or acute renal failure.
4. During the first 24 hours of therapy, the total dosage of dextran 40 in a 10% solution should not exceed 2 g/kg body weight. In cases of severe shock, the first 500 ml of the solution may be administered rapidly providing that the patient's central venous pressure is carefully monitored.
5. During the first 24 hours of therapy, the total dosage of dextran 70 or 75 in a 6% solution should not exceed 1.2 g/kg body weight. In emergency situations, dextran 70 or 75 may be given to adults at a rate of 1.2 to 2.4 g/min.

Class: Potassium Supplements

Generic Name	Trade Names	
	U.S.	Canada
Potassium chloride	K-Lyte/CL	K-Lor
	K-Lor	Kalium Durules
Potassium citrate	—§	—†
Potassium gluconate	Kaon	Kaon

Actions: Potassium is the major cation of intracellular fluid and is essential for the maintenance of acid-base balance; essential for the transmission of nerve impulses, cardiac contraction, renal function, smooth and striated muscle contraction, tissue synthesis, and carbohydrate metabolism.

Uses: Prevention or treatment of potassium depletion as caused by inadequate diet or the use of diuretics.

General side effects: May cause nausea, vomiting, diarrhea, and abdominal cramping.

Adverse reactions: Hyperkalemia is the most serious adverse reaction.

Contraindications: Should be administered with caution in patients with renal or cardiovascular disease or untreated Addison's disease; should not be administered to patients receiving potassium-sparing agents such as spironolactone and triamterene.

Nursing considerations:

1. Determine the patient's renal status before beginning potassium therapy.

2. Periodically monitor serum potassium levels.

3. Perform electrocardiac evaluation periodically to evaluate for potassium toxicity. The clinical signs include peaked T waves, depression of the S-T segment, disappearance of the P wave, prolongation of the Q-T interval, and widening and slurring of the QRS complex.

4. Clinical signs of potassium toxicity include extremity paresthesia or feelings of weakness or heaviness, mental confusion, gray pallor, and peripheral vascular collapse with decreased blood pressure and cardiac arrhythmias.

5. Potassium administered by IV solution must be dilute and administered slowly. The concentration of potassium should not exceed 40 mEq/L of fluid. The rate of a solution containing potassium should not exceed 20 mEq/h. If the patient is receiving potassium supplements intravenously, there may be pain at the infusion site if the potassium concentration is greater than 30 mEq/L.

6. Oral administration of potassium agents should be as a liquid with or after meals. Adverse agent taste and gastrointestinal irritation will be decreased if the potassium is mixed with or followed by a full glass of fruit juice or water.

Class: Ringer's Solutions

Generic Name	Trade Names	
	U.S.	Canada
Ringer's injection	—§	—§
Ringer's injection, lactated	—§	—§

Actions: These two agents are quite different. The Ringer's injection is a well-balanced electrolyte solution that is better than isotonic sodium chloride. It contains sodium chloride (147 mEq/L), potassium chloride (4 mEq/L), and calcium chloride (4.5 mEq/L); in action the Ringer's injection approximates isotonic sodium chloride solution. Ringer's injection, lactated, is a well-balanced electrolyte solution that is a modification of Hartmann's solution containing sodium (130 mEq/L), potassium chloride (4 mEq/L), calcium chloride (2.7 mEq/L), and sodium lactate (27 mEq/L). In action, it closely approximates the electrolyte concentrations in blood plasma; thus its primary use is as a simple plasma volume expander as well as a product that promotes hemodynamic physiologic activity.

Uses: Ringer's injection used primarily for the same indications as isotonic sodium chloride; has less tendency to produce abnormal sodium retention and edema in hypoproteinemic patients than does sodium chloride solution. Ringer's injection, lactated, used primarily in dehydration or other fluid volume deficit situations such as hypovolemic-induced trauma, burns, and severe diarrhea.

General side effects: None known.

Adverse reactions: The major adverse reactions relate to fluid overload and fluid dilution of actual blood components; ex-

*American Hospital Formulary Service classification.
†Drug is not available in Canada although it is listed in 1985 *Compendium of Pharmaceuticals and Specialties.*
‡U.S. trade name (or sometimes generic name) not listed in 1985 *Compendium of Pharmaceuticals and Specialties.*
§Drug is known by generic name.

cess administration may cause metabolic alkalosis; local injection site reaction, infection, or thrombosis may occur.

Contraindications: None known; not intended to replace blood or plasma expanders.

Nursing considerations:

1. Carefully monitor patients receiving large quantities of Ringer's injection, lactated, for treatment of hypovolemia or dehydration for signs of fluid overload. This is most frequently done by central venous pressure (greater than 12 indicates potential hypervolemia) or wedge pressure monitoring (greater than 15 indicates potential hypervolemia).

2. Patients should also have frequent laboratory monitoring for blood component dilution. Most frequently Ringer's injection, lactated, is given in conjunction with units of whole blood or packed cells.

Class: Sodium Agents

Generic Name	Trade Names	
	U.S.	Canada
Sodium chloride	—§	Urogate
Sodium-potassium-ammonium chloride	—§	—‡
Sodium-potassium chloride and sodium lactate	—§	—‡

Actions: Sodium chloride is a natural ion of the body. Isotonic sodium chloride is 0.9% solution containing approximately 154 mEq/L of both sodium and chloride. A liter of blood plasma or serum contains approximately 140 mEq sodium and 102 mEq chloride. Thus solutions of isotonic sodium chloride have slightly greater concentrations of both sodium and chloride than the actual blood serum or plasma. Sodium-potassium-ammonium contains sodium chloride (63 mEq/L), potassium chloride (17 mEq/L), and ammonium chloride (70 mEq/L). Sodium-potassium chlorides and sodium lactate contains sodium chloride (138 mEq/L), potassium chloride (12 mEq/L), and sodium lactate (100 mEq/L).

Uses: Isotonic (0.9%) solutions of sodium chloride (normal saline) primarily used in situations where the chloride loss is greater than the sodium loss, such as in vomiting, diarrhea, or nasogastric irrigation. Hypotonic (0.45%) solutions of sodium chloride used for the initial treatment of conditions in which the immediate need is water replacement without increasing osmotic pressure or serum sodium levels. Hypertonic (3% or 5%) solutions of sodium chloride used rarely to increase the sodium levels of seriously ill patients or patients in addisonian crisis and diabetic coma. Sodium-potassium-ammonium chloride solutions used to replace electrolytes lost in gastric fluid secondary to suction drainage. Sodium-potassium chloride solution used for replacement of electrolytes lost in duodenal fluid through intestinal suction or biliary or pancreatic drainage.

General side effects: None known.

Adverse reactions: Fluid overload or abnormalities of electrolyte values; reactions that may occur because of the solution or because of the technique of administration include febrile response, infection at the site of administration, venous thrombosis, or phlebitis extending from the site of injection.

Contraindications: Should be used with caution in patients with congestive heart failure, circulatory insufficiency, or signs of postoperative sodium intolerance; because of the high fatty concentration of the sodium-potassium-ammonium chloride solution, agent should be used with extreme caution in patients with renal or hepatic disease.

Nursing considerations:

1. Administration of too much sodium chloride may result in electrolyte imbalances leading to water retention, edema, potassium depletion, and aggravation of existing acidosis.
2. Sodium-potassium-ammonium chloride solution may be administered slowly subcutaneously or intravenously. The IV rate should not exceed 500 ml/h.
3. Sodium-potassium chloride solution fluid replacement must be based on the amount of duodenal fluid lost. The solution should not be administered at an IV rate to exceed 500 ml/h.

CATEGORY: CALORIC AGENTS (AHFS 40:20*)

| | Trade Names | |
Generic Name	U.S.	Canada
Dextrose	—§	—§
Dextrose and sodium chloride	—§	—§
Fructose	Levugen	—‡
Protein hydrolysate	Amigen	Amigen†

Actions: Provision of calories required for metabolic needs and supplying the body with needed fluids; fructose more easily and quickly metabolized than dextrose and therefore more rapidly available to act; an advantage of the fructose injection is that insulin is not necessary for conversion of fructose to glycogen. Protein hydrolysates are artificial digests of protein.

Uses: Low concentrations of dextrose solutions (e.g., 5% and 10%) used for both caloric supplements with different amounts of fluid supplementation; 20% dextrose solutions used for a diuretic effect to aid in tissue dehydration as seen in pregnancy toxemia; 50% dextrose solutions used in shock situations to rapidly increase blood glucose levels; dextrose may also be used orally via feeding tubes as a dietary supplement. Ten percent solutions of fructose used as fluid and dietary supplements. Protein hydrolysates used as nutritional protein supplements in patients with special protein needs and infants who are allergic to milk.

General side effects: Intravenous administration of protein hydrolysates may cause nausea, vomiting, and increased body temperature.

Adverse reactions: Prolonged administration of protein hydrolysates may cause vasodilation, abdominal pain, convulsions, and thrombosis.

Contraindications: Protein hydrolysates should be given with extreme caution in acidotic patients and patients with hepatic or renal disease.

Nursing considerations:

1. Routinely monitor blood sugar values in diabetic patients receiving dextrose solutions.
2. Administer protein supplements with adequate amounts of carbohydrates. If not, the protein will be used for the body's caloric needs rather than for tissue repair.

CATEGORY: DIURETICS (AHFS 40:28*)

| | Trade Names | |
Generic Name	U.S.	Canada
Amiloride	Madamor	Madamor
Bendroflumethiazide	Naturetin	Naturetin
Chlorothiazide	Diuril	Diuril
Ethacrynic acid	Edecrin	Edecrin
Furosemide	Lasix	Lasix
		Foroside
Hydrochlorothiazide	Hydro-Diuril	Hydro-Diuril
	Esidrix	Esidrix
	Oretic	Oretic
Mannitol	Osmitrol	Osmitrol
Spironolactone	Aldactone	Aldactone
		Sincomen
Triamterene	Dyrenium	Dyrenium

Actions: Of the agents listed above, there are four types: thiazide (sulfonamide-type) diuretics, high-ceiling (loop-type) diuretics, osmotic diuretics, and potassium-sparing diuretics. The thiazide-type diuretics (bendroflumethiazide, chlorothiazide, and hydrochlorothiazide) act at the distal tubule to block the chloride pump, which in turn prevents reabsorption of both chloride and sodium. The loop-type diuretics (ethacrynic acid and furosemide) act at the loop of Henle to block the chloride pump, which again decreases the reabsorption of both sodium and chloride. The osmotic diuretics (mannitol) act to increase the volume of urine that the kidney produces; more specifically the osmotic action of the agent molecules draws fluid into the plasma from the extravascular spaces; this helps to decrease excess fluids elsewhere in the body, such as to reduce cerebral edema secondary to surgery or trauma. The potassium-sparing diuretic (spironolactone) acts as a competitive antagonist of aldosterone to inhibit the reabsorption of sodium in the distal tubule without causing a loss of potassium. Triamterene and amiloride both act at the distal renal tubule to inhibit sodium-potassium ion exchange.

Uses: The thiazides are moderate diuretics that are relatively safe to use as a first-level diuretic agent, particularly in the treatment of hypertension. Loop diuretics are most commonly used as the agent of choice for reducing edema associated with renal disease, congestive heart failure, and hepatic cirrhosis. These agents tend to be effective even if there is a drug-induced electrolyte or acid-base imbalance. Osmotic diuretics are most commonly used to keep the kidneys producing urine when they would normally shut down, such as in times of severe hypovolemia secondary to trauma or severe burns. Potassium-sparing agents are weak diuretics and are most commonly used in combination with other diuretic agents. Spironolactone is specifically useful in the treatment of liver and nephrotic disorders that lead to hyperaldosteronism.

General side effects: Hypokalemia is the most common problem encountered and may first appear as complaints of weakness, muscle cramps, and cardiac irregularities. Signs of hypovolemia may appear as weakness, tachycardia, light-headedness, confusion, headache, and nausea and vomiting.

Adverse reactions: Dehydration or sudden hypovolemia leading to hypotension and severe electrolyte imbalances are the most common serious adverse reaction. The loop agents have been shown to interact with aminoglycoside antibiotics to potentially cause ototoxicity resulting in ringing in the ears or reversible deafness. Furosemide may also potentiate the effect of succinylcholine, thus leading to prolonged paralysis following surgery. Furosemide may also block the excretion of salicylates, thus leading to salicylate toxicity. The loop agents may also lower calcium levels and thus in rare occasions cause tetany. Potassium-sparing agents may cause hyperkalemia, signs of which include muscle cramps, lethargy, confusion, ataxia, and cardiac arrhythmias. Spironolactone may specifically cause gynecomastia, impotence, and menstrual abnormalities. Thiazides must be used with extreme caution in patients with hyperglycemia, hyperuricemia, and hyperlipidemia.

Contraindications: Must be used with extreme caution in patients with electrolyte disturbances or renal or urinary tract dysfunction; contraindicated in patients with hypersensitivities to sulfonamides or thiazides, pregnant or lactating women, or patients taking digitalis preparations; also contraindicated for any patient with increased serum potassium levels or renal insufficiency or dysfunction.

Nursing considerations:

1. In addition to increasing sodium and chloride excretion, these agents also cause excretion of other electrolytes. Periodic electrolyte evaluations must be monitored for all patients on diuretic agents. This is especially important for patients receiving loop diuretics.
2. Thiazide diuretics are more efficiently absorbed when taken with food. Instruct patients to take these agents with meals.
3. Accurate daily weights and intake and output should be monitored for patients taking potent diuretics such as the loop diuretics. The recommended daily fluid weight reduction is 1 to 2 pounds per day.
4. Osmotic diuretics such as mannitol should be given only in emergency situations where the patient may be closely monitored for sudden hypovolemia, hypotension, and related cardiac arrhythmias.
5. If a patient is taking a diuretic with a potassium supplement and the physician wishes to add a potassium-sparing diuretic agent, the potassium supplement should be terminated. Close electrolyte evaluation by laboratory studies is still required.
6. Patients taking potassium-sparing agents should be advised to avoid excessive consumption of foods high in potassium.

*American Hospital Formulary Service classification.
†Drug is not available in Canada although it is listed in 1985 *Compendium of Pharmaceuticals and Specialties.*
‡U.S. trade name (or sometimes generic name) not listed in 1985 *Compendium of Pharmaceuticals and Specialties.*
§Drug is known by generic name.

CATEGORY: URICOSURIC AGENTS (AHFS 40:40*)

	Trade Names	
Generic Name	*U.S.*	*Canada*
Probenecid	Benemid	Benemid
		Benoryl
	Probalan	—‡
	Probenimead	—‡
Sulfinpyrazone	Anturane	Anturane
		Antazone

Actions: Inhibition of renal tubular reabsorption or uric acid; increased plasma levels of penicillins and cephalosporins occur because the uricosuric agents inhibit their renal tubular excretion.

Uses: Lowering of serum urate levels in the treatment of chronic gouty arthritis and tophaceous gout; probenecid also used as adjunct therapy to elevate and prolong the plasma levels of penicillin agents: common practice when penicillin is used in the parenteral or oral treatment of venereal diseases.

General side effects: Although not commonly seen, the side effects for these agents include headache, anorexia, nausea, vomiting, dyspepsia, abdominal pain, and aggravation of peptic ulcers; hypersensitivity reactions include skin rash, dizziness, vertigo, and tinnitus.

Adverse reactions: Rarely, probenecid may cause nephrotic syndrome, hepatic necrosis, and aplastic anemia; because probenecid increases the concentration of uric acid in the renal tubules, rarely patients with gout may develop uric acid deposits that may cause renal colic, hematuria, and costovertebral pain. Acute toxicity of sulfinpyrazone evidenced by ataxia, labored breathing, convulsions, and coma; has been reported that sulfinpyrazone may rarely cause blood dyscrasias.

Contraindications: Both agents should be used cautiously in patients with peptic ulcer history or known renal calculi or renal disease; sulfinpyrazone contraindicated in patients with allergic reactions to pyrazolone derivatives such as oxyphenbutazone or phenylbutazone; also contraindicated in patients with a creatinine clearance of less than 50 ml/min.

Nursing considerations:

1. Because these agents have no analgesic or anti-inflammatory effect, they are of no value during an acute gout attack. They may exacerbate and prolong inflammation during the acute phase and should therefore not be started until 2 or 3 weeks after an acute gout attack.
2. The uricosuric actions of probenecid and salicylates are mutually antagonistic. Salicylates are contraindicated during probenecid therapy. If an analgesic is required, acetaminophen should be recommended.
3. Probenecid produces maximal renal clearance of uric acid within 30 minutes after being administered. It also exerts its effect on penicillin plasma levels for approximately 2 hours. The administration of penicillin should therefore be withheld for at least 30 minutes after the administration of probenecid.
4. Once uricosuric therapy is initiated for chronic gout, it should be continued indefinitely. Irregular dosage schedules may actually increase the serum urate concentrations. Pa-

tients should be periodically scheduled for blood testing to evaluate serum urate levels and blood dyscrasias.

5. Because of the gastrointestinal sensitivity to sulfinpyrazone, the patient should be advised to take the agent with meals, milk, or antacids. Fluids should be encouraged, and the urinary output should be at least 2 to 3 L/d.

6. Urinary alkalinizers may be used to prevent the formation of uric acid kidney stones.

ANTITUSSIVES, EXPECTORANTS, AND MUCOLYTIC AGENTS (AHFS 48:00*)

CATEGORY: EXPECTORANTS AND COUGH PREPARATIONS

Generic Name	Trade Names U.S.	Canada
Acetylcysteine	Mucomyst	Mucomyst Airbron
Codeine; methylmorphine (many combination products)	Phenergan with Codeine Actifed-C Novahistine Nucofed	Phenergan with Codeine —‡ Novahistex-C —‡
Dextromethorphan (many combination products)	Romilar Benylin DM	Balminil DM Syrup Robidey
Diphenhydramine	Benylin Cough Syrup Benadryl Elixir Nordryl	Allerdryl Benadryl Elixir Insumnal —‡
Glyceryl guaiacolate; guaifenesin		
With theophylline	Quibron	Quibron-T/SR
Plain	Robitussin 2/G Glycotuss	Robitussin —‡ —‡
With other combined products	Robitussin AC Dimetane Dimetane-DC Actifed C Expectorant Novahistine Cough Formula Robitussin DM	Robitussin AC Dimetane Dimetane-DC —‡ Novahistine DH Robitussin DM
Hydrocodone; dihydrocodeinone	Dicodid Codone	Robidone
Iodinated glycerol	Organidin Ipsatol	Organidin —‡
Levopropoxyphene	Novrad	—†
Noscapine	Tusscapine	—†
Potassium iodide	Pima Syrup SSKI	KI Thyro-Block
Terpin hydrate	Terp Liquid	—‡

Actions: This category includes various types of agents: mucolytic, opioid, and nonopioid antitussives and peripheral-acting expectorants. The mucolytic agent (acetylcysteine) acts by reducing the viscosity of purulent and nonpurulent pulmonary secretions. Opioid antitussive-analgesic agents (codeine, hydrocodone, and noscapine) and the nonopioid antitussive agents (dextromethorphan, diphenhydramine, and levopropoxyphene) both act centrally to depress the medullary cough center and thus to reduce its sensitivity to nerve irritations from the respiratory tract. The opioid derivatives also exert a drying effect on the respiratory tract mucosa that leads to an increase in the viscosity of bronchial secretions. The expectorants (glyceryl guaiacolate, iodinated glycerol, potassium iodide, and terpin hydrate) act by increasing respiratory tract fluid. Once the secretions are liquefied, they may be expectorated.

Uses: Acetylcysteine: adjunct therapy in treatment of pulmonary diseases with mucous obstruction (i.e., cystic fibrosis). Nonopioid antitussive and opioid antitussive-analgesic agents: used alone or in combination with other agents in the symptomatic relief of a nonproductive cough. Dextromethorphan: only morphine-derivative antitussive agent that is not included under federal narcotic law; about equal to codeine in depressing the cough reflex and has no expectorant action. Expectorant agents: liquefy bronchial secretions and thus make a productive cough more likely; may be used as adjunctive therapy in treatment of bronchial asthma, bronchitis, emphysema, and other respiratory conditions in which expectorant action is desirable. Glyceryl guaiacolate: usually used in combination with bronchodilators, decongestants, antihistamines, or cough suppressants. The reader is advised to review a more specific reference for the exact agent being used.

General side effects: Acetylcysteine may cause stomatitis, hemoptysis, nausea, and rarely fever and chills. Opioid antitussive agents may cause nausea, vomiting, dizziness, drowsiness, palpitations, excessive perspiration, agitation, and constipation. Although uncommonly seen, side effects for the nonopioid antitussive agents include nausea, dizziness, drowsiness, and jitteriness. Expectorant agents containing iodine may cause skin eruptions, eye and throat irritation, headache, and inflammation of the pharynx and larynx.

Adverse reactions: Acetylcysteine has been reported to cause bronchospasm in patients with asthma. Opioid antitussive agents used in excess may cause respiratory depression. Toxic doses of codeine may produce exhilaration, excitement, convulsions, delirium, hypotension, tachycardia, muscular weakness, circulatory collapse, and respiratory paralysis.

Contraindications: Opioid antitussive agents should be used with caution in patients who have just undergone thoracic surgery or who should not have the cough center suppressed such as patients with atelectasis. Dextromethorphan is incompatible with penicillins, the tetracyclines, salicylates, phenobarbital sodium, hydriodic acid, and high concentrations of sodium or potassium iodide.

Nursing considerations:

1. The above agents should not be used alone in the treatment of coughs. In addition, the patient should be advised to

consume large quantities of fluids to liquefy secretions and to avoid those products that may increase mucous production. Humidification with a vaporizer may be used.

2. Acetylcysteine is most commonly administered by nebulization. All precautions regarding nebulization procedures should be followed.

3. Opioid antitussives may potentiate the effect of other narcotic or sedative agents or alcohol. Advise patients accordingly.

4. Carefully monitor patients for addiction to opioid-type agents such as codeine and hydrocodone.

EYE, EAR, NOSE, AND THROAT PREPARATIONS (AHFS 52:00*)

Many of the agents that are used for the eye, ear, nose, and throat are discussed elsewhere in this appendix. Only those agents with special properties specifically related to the eye, ear, nose, and throat are discussed here. Refer to the index for further agent information if not found in this section.

CATEGORY: ANTI-INFECTIVES (AHFS 52:04*)
Class: Sulfonamides (AHFS 52:04.08*)

	Trade Names	
Generic Name	*U.S.*	*Canada*
Sulfacetamide sodium (ophthalmic)	Bleph-10 Bleph-30 Liquifilm Cetamide Sulf-10 Sulamyd	Bleph-10 Bleph-30 Liquifilm Cetamide Sulfex 10% Sodium Sulamyd
Sulfisoxazole diolamine (ophthalmic)	Gantrisin Sulfium	—‡ —‡

Actions: Bacteriostatic against a broad spectrum of gram-positive and gram-negative bacteria; interfere with folic acid synthesis, which inhibits nucleic acid synthesis and thus bacterial cell replication.

Uses: Used topically on the eye to treat conjunctivitis, corneal ulcers, and other superficial eye infections; sulfacetamide has also been used to prevent infection following foreign body removal from the eye; except in the treatment of very superficial infections, systemic anti-infective therapy may also be necessary.

General side effects: See section AHFS 8:24 in this appendix.

Adverse reactions: See section AHFS 8:24 in this appendix. Use of sulfonamides may result in overgrowth of nonsusceptible organisms such as fungi; these ophthalmic agents like others may retard corneal healing.

*American Hospital Formulary Service classification.
†Drug is not available in Canada although it is listed in 1985 *Compendium of Pharmaceuticals and Specialties.*
‡U.S. trade name (or sometimes generic name) not listed in 1985 *Compendium of Pharmaceuticals and Specialties.*
§Drug is known by generic name.

Contraindications: See section AHFS 8:24 in this appendix.

Nursing considerations:

1. The concentration of the solution or ointment will dictate frequency and methods for application. In all cases, these agents are applied topically.

2. Care must be taken to avoid contamination of the tip of the dropper or the ointment tube.

3. To instill eye drops, the patient should tilt the head backward. The health care provider then exposes the lower conjunctival sac by applying gentle downward pressure. The drops are instilled into the area between the eyeball and the lower lid. The patient is then instructed to gently close the eyes. Ophthalmic ointments are applied in a similar manner except that once the conjunctival sac is exposed, a thin line of ointment is placed along the inner lid.

CATEGORY: ANTI-INFLAMMATORY AGENTS (AHFS 52:08*)

	Trade Names	
Generic Name	*U.S.*	*Canada*
Dexamethasone Ophthalmic	Maxidex Decadron	Maxidex Decadron
Nasal	Decadron	—‡
Fluorometholone (ophthalmic)	FML Liquifilm	—‡
Hydrocortisone (ophthalmic)	Optef	—§
Hydrocortisone acetate (ophthalmic)	Hydrocortone	—§
Medrysone (ophthalmic)	HMS Liquifilm	—‡
Prednisolone acetate (ophthalmic)	Pred Mild Predulose Pred Forte	Pred Mild —‡ Pred Forte
Prednisolone sodium phosphate (ophthalmic)	Hydeltrasol Inflamase	—‡ Inflamase

Actions: Inhibition of the inflammatory response to the topical area on which they are applied; when used in high doses, may delay tissue healing.

Uses: Ophthalmic corticosteroids used for the symptomatic relief of inflammatory conditions of the conjunctiva, cornea, and anterior globe; may also help treat chemical or thermal injuries to the eye by preventing fibrosis and scarring of the injured tissue; may be used in combination agents to treat some ocular bacterial infections (see "Adverse Reactions"); not curative and should be discontinued as quickly as possible. Corticosteroids applied to the nasal mucosa help reduce inflammation of nasal congestion and nasal polyps.

General side effects: Rarely, topical burning or stinging may occur following application; nasal application of corticosteroids may cause nasal irritation and dryness, headache, rebound congestion, and rarely insomnia.

Adverse reactions: Topical steroids applied to the eye may reduce the facility of aqueous outflow and therefore increase intraocular pressure; likewise, these steroids may aggravate open-angle (simple) glaucoma. Combination ophthalmic corticosteroids with anti-infective properties may reduce the body's resistance to the infective agent. Prolonged use (usually longer than 2 years) of topical ophthalmic corticosteroids may cause posterior subcapsular cataracts that do not regress when the agent is discontinued.

Contraindications: Ophthalmic corticosteroids should not be used to treat minor abrasions or injuries; also not indicated in the treatment of patients with acute, untreated purulent bacterial, viral, or fungal ocular or otic infections. Topical otic solutions should not be used if the patient has a perforation of the tympanic membrane.

Nursing considerations:

1. If intraocular pressure is increased because of the use of corticosteroids applied to the eye, the pressure may stay elevated for 1 to 6 weeks following termination of therapy. The problem is reversible, and the pressure should return to normal following termination of therapy.

2. Chronic topical ophthalmic corticosteroid therapy should be used only if the patient is under close observation of an ophthalmologist. The patient's intraocular pressure should be monitored during physician visits.

3. As with all ophthalmic solutions, care should be taken to avoid contamination of the tip of the applicator.

4. All of the above listed agents differ in concentration. The health care provider should be aware of the strength of medication ordered and the care considerations of the specific agent.

CATEGORY: CARBONIC ANHYDRASE INHIBITORS (AHFS 52:10*)

	Trade Names	
Generic Name	U.S.	Canada
Acetazolamide	Acetazide	Acetazolam
		Apo-Acetazolamide
	Diamox	Diamox
	Hydrazol	—‡
Dichlorphenamide	Daranide	—‡
	Oratrol	—‡

Actions: Reduction of formation of hydrogen and bicarbonate ions by inhibiting the enzyme carbonic anhydrase; because of this, the ions are not available for transport into secretions. Specifically, these agents decrease the formation of aqueous humor, thereby lowering intraocular pressure in individuals with glaucoma.

Uses: Prolonged therapy in patients with open-angle (noncongestive, chronic, simple) glaucoma that is not controlled by miotics alone; may also be used to treat secondary glaucoma and for short-term preoperative therapy in narrow-angle (obstructive, closed-angle) glaucoma when delay of surgery is desired in order to lower intraocular pressure; acetazolamide has other uses, including treatment of edema secondary to congestive heart failure and use as an anti-epilepsy agent in the prophylactic management of petit mal epilepsy.

General side effects: Most reactions are dose related and respond well to lower doses of the medications; common side effects include malaise, nausea, vomiting, diarrhea or con-stipation, weight loss, altered taste and smell, abdominal distention, drowsiness, confusion, depression, excitement, nervousness, dizziness, fatigue, and irritability; in some instances the diuresis would be considered a side effect if not the primary purpose of use.

Adverse reactions: Paresthesia or tingling sensations of the extremities, tongue, lips, or anus; more serious adverse reactions: bone marrow depression, hypokalemia, hyperbili-rubinemia, renal colic, renal calculi, and dysuria.

Contraindications: Should be used with caution in patients with respiratory acidosis or decreased respiratory function; also contraindicated in patients with hepatic or renal disease or depressed adrenocortical insufficiency or hyperchloremic acidosis.

Nursing considerations:

1. These agents should be used in conjunction with topical epinephrine-miotics which facilitate the aqueous outflow.

2. Because some of the side effects of these agents are sedative, patients should be warned that mental alertness and physical coordination may be impaired.

3. Because bone marrow depression is an adverse reaction, patients should have periodic monitoring of laboratory values. If blood dyscrasias occur, the agent should be discontinued and appropriate therapy instituted. Serum bilirubin and electrolytes should also be monitored.

4. These agents increase excretion of lithium. Patients taking lithium should have serum levels closely monitored.

CATEGORY: LOCAL ANESTHETICS (AHFS 52:16*)

	Trade Names	
Generic Name	U.S.	Canada
Proparacaine (ophthal-mic)	Ophthaine	Ophthaine
		Alcaine
	Ophthetic	Ophthetic
Tetracaine (ophthal-mic, nasal, or oral)	Pontocaine	Pontocaine

Actions: Act on the surface of the eye by temporarily interrupting the production and conduction of nerve impulses; anesthetic potency of proparacaine is about equal to that of tetracaine.

Uses: Topical anesthetic agent used for the surface of the eye.

General side effects: Instillation of these agents at recommended doses should not cause local irritation; if side effects are seen, they commonly include initial irritation, stinging or burning, and increased lacrimation.

Adverse reactions: Although rare, systemic toxicity may include CNS stimulation followed by depression.

Contraindications: Should be used cautiously in patients with known allergies to local anesthetics, cardiac disease, and hyperthyroidism.

Nursing considerations:

1. Installation of a 0.5% solution in the eye produces local anesthesia within 20 seconds. The duration of action is about 15 minutes.

2. Refrigeration of solutions previously used helps to retard color changes. Discolored solutions should not be used.

3. Patients who have received treatments requiring the use of local ophthalmic anesthetics should have the treated eye patched until the anesthesia wears off. If not, foreign bodies or injury to the eye could occur without the patient's awareness.

CATEGORY: MIOTICS (AHFS 52:20*)

Generic Name	Trade Names	
	U.S.	*Canada*
Echothiophate	Echodide	—‡
	Phospholine	Phospholine Iodide
Isoflurophate	Floropryl	—†
Physostigmine	Isopto Eserine	—‡
Pilocarpine	Almocarpine	—†
	Isopto Carpine	Miocarpine Hydrochloride
	Pilocel	Ocusert Pilo-20 and 40
	Pilocar	P.V. Carpine Nitrate
	Piloptic	Isopto Carpine
	M-Pilo	

Actions: Primarily topical cholinergic agents that directly cause the sphincter muscles of the iris and ciliary body of the eye to contract; by this mechanism, they reduce intraocular pressure in the eye. Precise mechanism of action has not been determined; it is thought that in the treatment of open-angle glaucoma these agents reduce the intraocular pressure by causing contraction of the ciliary muscle and thus permit a widening of the trabecular meshwork; in narrow-angle (closed-angle) glaucoma it is thought that these agents reduce intraocular pressure by constricting the pupil and stretching the iris. Echothiophate is a long-acting indirect cholinergic agent.

Uses: Used topically in the eye for the medical treatment of open-angle (or chronic, simple) glaucoma; in some cases, may also be used for acute narrow-angle (closed-angle) glaucoma. The long-acting agent echothiophate is not ordinarily administered for narrow-angle glaucoma; instead, it is used in the treatment of open-angle glaucoma and in diagnostic studies and initial treatment management of convergent strabismus. Physostigmine is not as well tolerated as pilocarpine and is not recommended for long-term therapy. In the treatment of open-angle glaucoma, a miotic is often used in conjunction with a carbonic anhydrase inhibitor, epinephrine, or timolol. Pilocarpine may be used in emergency situations of acute narrow-angle glaucoma to lower the intraocular pressure before surgery. Because the pigment of the iris absorbs these agents, the agents are less effective in patients with dark-colored pigments (e.g., black, brown, or hazel) than those with light-colored pigments.

General side effects: Side effects reduced if the agents are started at low doses and gradually increased. Common effects include painful ciliary or accommodation spasm, blurred vision or myopia, poor vision in dim light, ciliary or con-

*American Hospital Formulary Service classification.
†Drug is not available in Canada although it is listed in 1985 *Compendium of Pharmaceuticals and Specialties.*
‡U.S. trade name (or sometimes generic name) not listed in 1985 *Compendium of Pharmaceuticals and Specialties.*
§Drug is known by generic name.

junctival congestion, twitching of the eyelids, burning or stinging sensation of the eyes, ocular or brow pain, headache, photophobia, and increased visibility of floaters.

Adverse reactions: The long-acting agents (e.g., echothiophate) may also cause vasodilation of blood vessels of the conjunctiva, iris, and ciliary body. This vasodilation may lead to vascular congestion and ocular inflammation. Systemic adverse reactions, which occur most commonly in children, include nausea, vomiting, diarrhea, abdominal pain, and intestinal cramping. More serious adverse reactions include cardiac arrhythmias and CNS excitement followed by confusion, convulsions, and coma.

Contraindications: Long-acting agents such as echothiophate should not be used in patients before surgery because of the risk of further angle narrowing; use with extreme caution in patients with a history of previous retinal detachment of who are at high risk for retinal detachment; also contraindicated for any patient in whom pupillary constriction is undesirable or patients with history of bronchial asthma, vascular hypertension, hyperthyroidism, epilepsy, or other CNS or cardiovascular disorders.

Nursing considerations:

1. Because of the potential side effect of poor vision in dim light and because of the potential spasm of accommodation, advise patients to avoid driving at night.
2. Alcohol consumption may increase the incidence of adverse reactions.
3. Initial side effects felt by the patient may be reduced by administering (physician ordered) a diluted solution of the medication.
4. Because of the potential for these agents to be systemically absorbed, carefully monitor the patient for signs of systemic adverse reactions.
5. Take care to keep medication tubes and containers free from contamination. Select agents such as isoflurophate may also hydrolyze if permitted to come in contact with a moist surface.
6. These agents may be irritating to the hands and eyelids. Any excessive ointment or solution should be wiped away immediately following application. The patient should also be instructed to carefully wash the hands.
7. Following topical administration of select agents, finger pressure should be applied on the lacrimal sac for 1 or 2 minutes to minimize drainage into the nose and throat and to reduce the risk of systemic absorption. Specific instructions regarding individual agents should be verified before administration.

CATEGORY: MYDRIATICS (AHFS 52:24*)

Generic Name	Trade Names	
	U.S.	*Canada*
Atropine	—§	Isopto Atropine
Cyclopentolate	Cyclogyl	Cyclogyl
		Noa-Cyclo
Phenylephrine	Neo-Synephrine	Neo-Synephrine
		Mydfrin
Tropicamide	Mydriacyl	Mydriacyl
Combination	Alconefrin	—‡
agents	Prefrin Liquifilm	Prefrin Liquifilm

Actions: Mydriatics (pupil-dilating) and cycloplegics (responsible for the paralysis of the ciliary muscles of the eyes) are basically anticholinergic topical agents; primary actions of these agents are the same as those described in section AHFS 12:08 in this appendix.

Uses: Mainly dilation and paralysis of the ciliary muscles of the eye to facilitate examination of the internal eye structure and function during diagnostic and refractory eye examinations. Atropine is the most potent of the category (its mydriatic action may persist for as long as 10 days while the cycloplegic action may last for 5 days); major advantage of the other agents over atropine is the short-term action (maximal effect within 15 minutes to 1 hour, complete recovery within 3 to 24 hours). Mydriatics such as cyclopentolate and phenylephrine may also be used to evaluate for glaucoma (see "Nursing Considerations"). Phenylephrine used to produce mydriasis without cycloplegia and is especially helpful during select diagnostic procedures; may also be used to decrease intraocular pressure in normal eyes or in patients with open-angle (chronic, simple) glaucoma; may also be used in the diagnosis and treatment of Horner's or Raeder's syndrome. Because the pigment of the iris absorbs all of these agents, they may be less effective in dark-colored eyes than in light-colored eyes.

General side effects: The normal action of the agent, which may be perceived as a side effect by the patient, is blurred vision and increased sensitivity to light. Phenylephrine may also cause transient burning or stinging, hyperemia, keratitis, and headache.

Adverse reactions: Rarely, systemic effects may be seen (especially in children); refer to the discussion of adverse reactions of atropine and other parasympatholytic agents listed under AHFS 12:00. Local adverse reactions include allergic conjunctivitis. Rarely systemic reactions may occur to phenylephrine: palpitations, tachycardia, premature ventricular contractions, tremors, diaphoresis, and hypertension.

Contraindications: Glaucoma; if used with these patients, an angle-closure attack may be precipitated.

Nursing considerations:

1. Because of the blurred and hypersensitive light effect of these agents, advise the patient to wear sunglasses and not drive until normal accommodation is achieved.

2. To use these agents to test for possibility of narrow-angle glaucoma, a baseline intraocular pressure is measured and the drops are instilled in one eye. In 1 hour, a second intraocular pressure reading is measured. If a pressure increase of 8 mm or more is observed, the test is considered positive. A miotic agent such as pilocarpine is then administered to reduce the increased pressure. There are other darkroom physiologic tests that may be safer for the patient than the above described pharmacologic test.

3. Because phenylephrine may lower intraocular pressure in the eye, baseline tonometry should be performed before the agent is administered.

CATEGORY: VASOCONSTRICTORS (AHFS 52:32*)

Generic Name	Trade Names	
	U.S.	*Canada*
Epinephrine	Adrenalin	Adrenalin
		Glaucon
Oxymeta-	Afrin	—†
zoline	Duration	—‡
Phenylephrine	Neo-Synephrine	Neo-Synephrine
Nasal		Mydrin
	Biomydrin	—‡
	Isophrin	—‡
	Rhinall	—‡
Ophthalmic	Mistura	—‡
	Prefrin Liquifilm	Prefrin Liquifilm

Actions: Sympathomimetic agents that reduce edema of the skin and mucous membranes by their effect on the alpha-adrenergic receptors, which in turn causes vasoconstriction; a more detailed discussion of their action is found in the autonomic agent section of this appendix under AHFS 12:12.

Uses: Epinephrine used to produce local vasoconstriction and hemostasis in bleeding from small surface vessels such as those of the skin and mucous membranes of the eye, mouth, throat, nose, and larynx (effect begins within 5 minutes and lasts less than 1 hour); may also be used to produce effective mydriasis when the permeability of the eye increases following trauma or surgery. Oxymetazoline and phenylephrine may be applied topically to relieve nasal congestion with acute rhinitis, colds, sinusitis, hay fever, and other similar conditions. Phenylephrine also applied topically to the conjunctiva to temporarily relieve allergic atopic conjunctivitis, congestion, itching, and minor irritation from mechanical and chemical sources; may also be used during select ocular diagnostic procedures and applied topically before ocular surgery to aid in the control of bleeding.

General side effects: See AHFS 12:12 in this appendix. CNS side effects include nervousness and restlessness; tricyclic antidepressants and thyroid hormones may potentiate effects of epinephrine; oxymetazoline and phenylephrine, especially in children, may cause transient burning, stinging, and dryness of the mucosa.

Adverse reactions: Epinephrine and oxymetazoline may cause a rebound vasodilation effect when use is discontinued. Ophthalmic use of epinephrine may cause allergic reactions as noted by diffuse vascular engorgement, conjunctivitis, and iritis; prolonged ophthalmic use of epinephrine may cause localized melanin-like pigmentary deposits in the conjunctiva, cornea, and eyelids. Oxymetazoline and phenylephrine may also cause systemic sympathomimetic effects as described in section AHFS 12:12 in this appendix.

Contraindications: Before these agents are used, the cardiovascular status of the patient must be assessed; epinephrine and phenylephrine contraindicated as any type of local anesthesia for use in ears, nose, fingers, toes, or genitalia.

Nursing considerations:

1. These agents are all applied topically. Care must be taken to prevent contamination of the container dropper or spray dispenser.

2. If the agent is administered by drops, the patient should lie

in a supine, head-low position for at least 5 minutes after agent administration.
3. If the agent is administered by nasal spray, the patient should be in an erect position. Three to five minutes after agent administration, the nose should be blown.
4. Some manufacturers state that the ophthalmic solutions of phenylephrine should not be used in patients who wear soft contact lenses.

CATEGORY: MISCELLANEOUS EENT DRUGS (AHFS 52:36*)

	Trade Names	
Generic Name	U.S.	Canada
Glycerin		
Oral	Osmoglyn	—†
	Glyrol	—†
Ophthalmic	Ophthalgan	—‡
Timolol		
Ophthalmic	Timoptic	Timoptic
		Blocadren

Actions: Glycerin acts to elevate the osmotic pressure of the plasma to such an extent that water is drawn from the extravascular spaces into the blood. Timolol is a beta-adrenergic blocking agent; exact mechanism by which it acts is unclear; does not have significant intrinsic local anesthetic, sympathomimetic, or parasympathomimetic actions.
Uses: Glycerin is an alcohol-type agent used orally as an osmotic agent to lower intraocular pressure or topically to reduce superficial corneal edema (a reduction in intraocular pressure may be seen within 10 minutes following oral agent administration, peak is reached in 30 to 90 minutes, and agent duration is 4 to 8 hours); used clinically before surgery and along with other agents to reduce the intraocular pressure in patients with acute narrow-angle glaucoma; sterile glycerin may be used topically to reduce trauma-caused superficial corneal edema. Timolol used topically to lower the intraocular pressure in patients with open-angle (chronic, simple) glaucoma as well as ocular hypertension and other types of glaucoma.
General side effects: Oral administration of glycerin may cause mild headache, dizziness, nausea, vomiting, thirst, and diarrhea. Timolol has been reported to cause mild ocular irritation and local hypersensitivity.
Adverse reactions: Rarely, glycerin has been reported to cause convulsion and seizure disorders.
Contraindications: Glycerin should be administered with caution to patients with a history of cardiac, renal, or hepatic disease. Before using timolol, the contraindications should be reviewed for administering other beta-adrenergic blocking agents; specifically, the reader is referred to section AHFS 12:00 in this appendix; safe use of timolol during pregnancy and with children has not been established.

*American Hospital Formulary Service classification.
†Drug is not available in Canada although it is listed in 1985 *Compendium of Pharmaceuticals and Specialties.*
‡U.S. trade name (or sometimes generic name) not listed in 1985 *Compendium of Pharmaceuticals and Specialties.*
§Drug is known by generic name.

Nursing considerations:
1. Lying down after administration of oral doses of glycerin may assist to reduce the side effects of the agent.
2. Although dehydration is unlikely, patients (especially elderly ones) taking glycerin should be monitored for signs of dehydration. Likewise, diabetic patients should be monitored for blood sugar levels.

GASTROINTESTINAL AGENTS (AHFS 56:00*)

CATEGORY: ANTACIDS AND ADSORBENTS (AHFS 56:04*)

	Trade Names[3]	
Generic Name	U.S.	Canada
Aluminum carbonate	Basalgel	Basalgel
Aluminum hydroxide	Alu-Cap	Alu-Tab
	Dialume	—‡
	Amphojel	Amphojel
Calcium carbonate	Titralac	Biocal
	Tums	Caltrate Os-Cal
		Tums
Charcoal, activated (universal poison antidote)	Charcocaps	—‡
	Charcotabs	—‡
Dihydroxyaluminum sodium	Rolaids	Rolaids
Magaldrate	Riopan	Riopan
Magnesium hydroxide	Phillips' Milk of Magnesia	Phillips' Milk of Magnesia
Sodium bicarbonate; baking soda	Alka-Seltzer	Alka-Seltzer

Actions: Antacids are inorganic salts that dissolve in acid gastric secretions; once dissolved, they release anions that partially neutralize gastric hydrochloric acid. Sodium bicarbonate rapidly reacts with hydrochloric acid to form sodium chloride, carbon dioxide, and water. Excess bicarbonate empties into the small intestine and is systemically absorbed. The result may be mild metabolic alkalosis. The antacids other than sodium bicarbonate generally do not cause metabolic alkalosis. Activated charcoal is a nonspecific adsorbent that acts to adsorb a wide variety of drugs and chemicals; this adsorbent quality prevents the drug or chemical from being systemically adsorbed from the gastrointestinal tract. The charcoal is neither adsorbed nor metabolized but is excreted unchanged in the feces.
Uses: Clinical use of antacids is based on their ability to increase the pH of gastric secretions; routinely used to increase gastric pH to facilitate healing of peptic ulcers. Although studies are not available on the efficacy of antacids for the relief of acid indigestion, heartburn, and sour stomachs, most practitioners advocate their use to reduce gastric acidity, which in turn may decrease clinical distress; may also be useful in the management of esophageal reflux by increasing gastric

[3]There are many other products, such as Citrocarbonate, that are mixtures of the listed generic agents.

pH, which increases the lower esophageal sphincter pressure. Activated charcoal is most commonly used during emergency situations as a general purpose poisoning antidote since it will not adsorb cyanide, ethanol, methanol, ferrous sulfate, caustic alkalies, and mineral acids.

General side effects: Side effects for antacids are agent specific: magnesium antacids have a laxative effect, calcium and aluminum antacids have a constipating effect, and calcium and sodium bicarbonate antacids may cause increased flatulence. No side effects of activated charcoal are known.

Adverse reactions: Metabolic alkalosis may result from systemically absorbed antacids such as sodium bicarbonate and rarely calcium carbonate; signs are vague and include a loss of taste for food and malaise, which may be followed by nausea, vomiting, stomach pain, and later irritability, dizziness, muscle twitching, and finally severe metabolic response; extremity edema and fluid retention may occur secondary to electrolyte imbalances. Some agents such as calcium may cause a rebound of gastric hypersecretion.

Contraindications: Most antacids contain sodium to some degree; product must be labeled as such if the level of sodium is greater than 0.2 mEq per dose. Agents containing high levels of sodium are contraindicated for those patients on low-sodium diets and those with renal, cardiovascular, and hepatic disease. Antacids containing more than 25 mEq per dose should be used very cautiously in patients with renal disease.

Nursing considerations:

1. With normal doses of antacids, the gastric pH is generally not increased above 4 or 5.
2. The following antacids are listed in decreasing order of their ability to neutralize a given amount of gastric acid: calcium carbonate, sodium bicarbonate, magnesium salts, and aluminum salts.
3. Following are pros and cons for the use of select agents:
   a. Sodium bicarbonate: because of high sodium content, use only for occasional heartburn or indigestion; because it is systemically absorbed, it is not used for long-term, high-dose management of peptic ulcer disease
   b. Magnesium antacids and aluminum antacids: Because these agents are not systemically absorbed, they are safe for long-term therapy; main disadvantage is potential side effects stated above
   c. Calcium carbonate: an inexpensive substance that is not systemically absorbed; a portion of the compound may react with calcium chloride and rarely lead to systemic hypercalcemia (may be especially true for patient also taking lots of milk and cream products); therefore not recommended for use in long-term ulcer therapy; may also cause a rebound hyperacidic gastric response
4. Carefully monitor patients receiving sodium bicarbonate for signs of metabolic alkalosis.
5. Use antacids only as adjunct therapy for patients with peptic ulcers and gastric distress. In addition, physical and emotional rest must be encouraged.
6. In patients with uncomplicated ulcers, an antacid may be administered 1 and 3 hours postprandially and at bedtime. The duration of treatment should be no longer than 4 to 6 weeks.
7. For the management of acute esophageal reflux, antacids may be administered as frequently as every 30 minutes to 1 hour.
8. Activated charcoal is most effective when used in the powder form. Depending on the patient's weight, 5 to 50 g of the agent may be mixed with water, to make a thick solution. This solution may be inserted via a nasogastric tube or taken orally. If taken orally, a flavoring agent such as fruit juice may be added. The use of activated charcoal is generally a second-level intervention following the use of ipecac or gastric lavage.
9. Activated charcoal will make the patient's feces black.

CATEGORY: ANTIDIARRHEAL AGENTS (AHFS 56:08*)

	Trade Names	
Generic Name	U.S.	Canada
Bismuth	Pepto-Bismol	Pepto-Bismol
Diphenoxylate with atropine sulfate	Lomotil	Lomotil
Kaolin and pectin	Kaopectate	Keopectate
Loperamide	Imodium	Imodium
Paregoric	—§	—§

Actions: Agents such as bismuth and kaolin and pectin are not systemically absorbed but act locally to coat the intestinal mucosa. This coating protects against irritation and thus helps to reduce inflammation. In addition, they may help to filter out toxins and bacteria that may be in the gastrointestinal tract. The other antidiarrheal agents (diphenoxylate, loperamide, and paregoric) are opiate agents that act systemically on the smooth muscle of the intestine to decrease hyperperistaltic activity.

Uses: Treatment of diarrhea; loperamide may specifically be used to treat chronic diarrhea associated with inflammatory bowel disease or to reduce the volume of discharge from ileostomies.

General side effects: Opiate-type agents may cause nausea, vomiting, dry mouth, abdominal discomfort, blurred vision, paralytic ileus, malaise, lethargy, and restlessness.

Adverse reactions: Diphenoxylate in rare occasions may cause tachycardia, miosis, numbness of the extremities, swelling of the gums, mental depression, loss of tendon reflexes, and coma and respiratory arrest; it is thought that these reactions may be caused by the atropine sulfate in the preparation.

Contraindications: Opiate-type antidiarrheal agents should not be used in cases of acute poisoning until the toxic poisons have been eliminated from the gastrointestinal tract; should also be avoided in patients in whom constipation must be avoided; should be used with extreme caution in patients with asthma, severe prostatic hypertrophy, hepatic disease, or narcotic dependency. Diphenoxylate should not be administered to children under the age of 2 years because of the narrow range between therapeutic and toxic dosages. Lomotil contraindicated for those patients known to be allergic to atropine.

Nursing considerations:

1. Be aware of the possibility of chemical dependence of these agents, especially those opiate-type preparations that are systemically adsorbed.
2. Diphenoxylate may potentiate the effect of other CNS depressants and should therefore be carefully monitored. The patient should also be advised.
3. All patients with diarrhea should be carefully monitored for fluid, electrolyte, and acid-base balance.

CATEGORY: CATHARTICS AND LAXATIVES (AHFS 56:12*)

	Trade Names	
Generic Name[4]	U.S.	Canada
Bisacodyl	Biscolax	Biscolax
		Apo-Bisa-codyl
	Dulcolax	Dulcolax
Cascara sagrada	Cas-Evac	Cascara
Castor oil	—§	—§
Danthron	Anavac	Anavac
	Danvac	Danvac
	Dorbane	Dorbane
	Modane	Modane
Dioctyl calcium sulfosuccinate	Surfak	Surfak
Dioctyl sodium sulfosuccinate	Colace	Colace
	Comfolax	—‡
	D-S-S	—‡
Glycerin	Glycerol	Glycerol
Karaya	—§	—‡
Magnesium citrate	—§	Citro-Mag
		National Laxative
Magnesium hydroxide	Milk of Magnesia	Milk of Magnesia
Magnesium sulfate	Epsom Salt	Epsom Salt
Malt soup extract	Maltsupex	—†
Methylcellulose	Cologel	Gonio-Gel
	Hydrolose	Lacril
	Cellothyl	Murocel
Mineral oil	Fleet Mineral Oil	Fleet Mineral Oil
	Agoral Plain	Agoral Plain
	Neo-Cultol	—‡
	Petrogalar Plain	—‡
Monosodium phosphate	Sal Hepatica	—‡
Phenolphalein	Chocolax	Fructines-Vichy
	Ex-Lax	—‡
	Feen-A-Mint	—†
Psyllium	Effersyllium	—†
	Konsyl	—†
	L.A. Formula	—†
	Metamucil	Metamucil
	Modane Bulk	—‡

	Trade Names	
Generic Name[4]	U.S.	Canada
Sodium phosphate with sodium biphosphate	Phospho-Soda	—‡
Sorbitol	—§	

[4]Many other combination agents exist beyond those listed.

*American Hospital Formulary Service classification.
†Drug is not available in Canada although it is listed in 1985 *Compendium of Pharmaceuticals and Specialties.*
‡U.S. trade name (or sometimes generic name) not listed in 1985 *Compendium of Pharmaceuticals and Specialties.*
§Drug is known by generic name.

Actions: These agents may be divided into six groups: bulk forming, hyperosmotic, stimulant (anthraquinone), saline, mineral oil, and stool softeners. The bulk-forming laxatives (karaya, malt soup extract, methylcellulose, and psyllium) swell in water to form an emollient, gel-type solution; it is thought that when the agent is taken orally, it results in providing bulk to the feces and promotes peristalsis. Hyperosmotic laxatives (glycerin and sorbitol) are administered rectally to promote local irritation and the drawing of water from the tissues into the feces; reflex evacuation is therefore stimulated. Stimulant laxatives (bisacodyl, cascara sagrada, castor oil, danthron, and phenolphalein) induce defecation by stimulating peristaltic activity of the intestine through local irritation of the mucosa. Saline laxatives (magnesium citrate, magnesium hydroxide, magnesium sulfate, monosodium phosphate, and sodium phosphate with sodium biphosphate) are orally administered agents that act to draw water into the small intestine; it is the fluid that causes stretching of the intestine and stimulates peristalsis. Select saline agents may be administered rectally; their action is slightly different and agent specific. Mineral oil acts by lubricating fecal material and the intestinal mucosa. When these agents are used in enema form, it is the lubrication and extra fluid bulk that stimulates evacuation. Stool softeners (dioctyl calcium sulfosuccinate and dioctyl sodium sulfosuccinate) soften fecal material by lowering surface tension at the oil-water interface of the fecal material; thus the fecal material is softened and easier to defecate.

Uses: Cathartics are agents used to promote rapid evacuation of the intestine. Laxatives are used basically for the same purpose, but the evacuation action may be less pronounced. Both of these agents are used to alter stool consistency and to relieve constipation or to empty the lower intestine. Although most agents work only on the lower colon, select agents such as castor oil, phenolphthalein, and magnesium citrate also increase activity of the small intestine.

General side effects: Abdominal cramping and generalized discomfort most commonly seen; suppositories may cause a localized burning sensation.

Adverse reactions: Prolonged use of these agents may cause dehydration and electrolyte imbalances; agent dependency should also be considered an adverse reaction; depletion of oil-soluble vitamins (A, D, K, and E) may occur with excessive use of mineral oil and castor oil.

Contraindications: Should not be used habitually as a routine measure for inducing stool evacuation; before agents are administered for complaints of abdominal pain and cramping, medical pathologic conditions such as appendicitis, diverticulitis, and ulcerative colitis must be ruled out.

Nursing considerations:

1. Stimulant laxatives may alter fluid and electrolyte absorption. The patient, especially young children and elderly persons, should be monitored closely.

2. Because many of these agents are available over the counter, they are generally self-prescribed and overused. Constipation is best avoided or relieved by a diet high in fiber, adequate fluid intake, prompt response to defecation reflex, and exercise.
3. Fat-soluble vitamins (A, D, E, and K) may not be adequately absorbed if a patient is taking mineral oil.
4. Laxatives, especially castor oil and mineral oil, should not be used during pregnancy and should be used cautiously postpartum if the mother is breast feeding.

CATEGORY: DIGESTANTS (AHFS 56:16*)

	Trade Names	
Generic Name	*U.S.*	*Canada*
Pancreatin	Panteric	—‡
Pancrelipase	Cotazym	Cotazym
	Viokase	Pancrease
		Viokase

Actions: Both of these agents, obtained from hog or cattle pancreases, contain enzymes that break down starches (amylases) and fats (lipases) as well as the enzymes trypsin and chymotrypsin, which are necessary for proper digestion.

Uses: Pancreatin used for preparation of partially or completely predigested foods for administration to invalids and persons with poor digestion caused by pancreatic hypofunction. Pancrelipase is a more concentrated mixture of pancreatic enzymes and is recommended as replacement therapy for patients with cystic fibrosis of the pancreas, chronic pancreatitis, and cancer of the pancreas and patients who have had their pancreas surgically removed.

General side effects: In the recommended doses, no known side effects.

Adverse reactions: None known.

Contraindications: None indicated.

Nursing considerations:

1. These agents are normally taken orally with meals. For small children the tablet may be crushed or the capsule opened and the agent sprinkled on the food.

CATEGORY: EMETICS AND ANTIEMETICS (AHFS 56:20 and 56:22*⁵)

	Trade Names	
Generic Name	*U.S.*	*Canada*
Ipecac syrup	—§	—§
Meclizine	Antivert	Bonamine
	Roclizine	
Metoclopramide	Reglan	Maxeran
		Reglan
Prochlorperazine	Compazine	Stemetil
	Combid	
Thiethylperazine	Torecan	Torecan Maleate
Trimethobenzamide	Tigan	—‡

⁵Also refer to appendix section AHFS 28:24 for discussion of promethazine (Phenergan).

Actions: These agents may easily be divided into two groups, those that promote emesis (ipecac) and those that are antiemetic (meclizine, metoclopramide, prochlorperazine, and trimethobenzamide). Ipecac syrup acts centrally by stimulating the chemoreceptor trigger zone of the medulla and locally to produce emesis; it also causes localized gastric irritation. Antiemetic agents act in one of two ways, either by depressing the chemoreceptor emesis trigger zones along the vestibular-cerebellar pathways or by acting directly on the vomiting center in the medulla; some agents act only by one action, and other agents act in both ways.

Uses: Ipecac syrup used to induce vomiting in the early management of acute oral poisonings. Meclizine used primarily in the prevention and treatment of motion sickness; may also be used in the symptomatic treatment of diseases such as labyrinthitis that affect the vestibular system. Prochlorperazine and thiethylperazine are phenothiazine agents used in the general treatment of nausea and vomiting in adults (these agents are discussed in greater detail in section AHFS 28:16.08 of this appendix). Thiethylperazine recommended to be used only as an antiemetic agent. Metoclopropamide used most commonly as an IV antiemetic agent approximately ½ hour before cisplatin cancer chemotherapy. Trimethobenzamide may be useful for nausea and vomiting associated with surgery, the treatment of radiation therapy, labyrinthitis, and motion sickness; may be less effective than the phenothiazines when used on a short-term basis but may be more effective when long-term therapy is needed.

General side effects: Antiemetic agents may cause drowsiness, fatigue, dry mouth, and blurred vision; depression or restlessness may occur if phenothiazine agents are used postoperatively.

Adverse reactions: Ipecac in doses of 30 ml or less should have no adverse reaction. If prochlorperazine is used over several days, patient may show significant adverse reactions, including severe muscle spasms, motor restlessness, and other extrapyramidal motor system reactions. Although rare, trimethobenzamide may cause parkinson-like symptoms, hypotension, and extrapyramidal symptoms.

Contraindications: Ipecac should not be administered if the patient's consciousness level is decreasing, the patient is unconscious, or the patient was known to have ingested a caustic or corrosive substance. The safety of most of the antiemetics during pregnancy has not been established. Phenothiazines and specifically prochlorperazine are not indicated for the treatment of nausea and vomiting in children and should not be used in young children under the age of 2 years. Thiethylperazine should not be used if the patient is comatose or has a depressed CNS status.

Nursing considerations:

1. If administered correctly, ipecac will produce emesis in almost all patients treated. The proper oral administration of ipecac is as follows:
   a. Under 1 year of age: 5 to 10 ml
   b. 1 to 5 years of age: 10 to 15 ml
   c. Over 5 years: 15 to 30 ml
2. Following oral administration, the patient should immediately consume 200 to 300 ml (less for small children) of milk (evaporated is preferred). The use of water following

oral ipecac administration may increase poison agent absorption. Patient ambulation after taking the ipecac and milk seems to facilitate an emesis response. If emesis does not occur within 20 minutes, the ipecac dose should be repeated.

3. Because the emesis may not evacuate all of the toxic substance, activated charcoal may be administered after vomiting from the ipecac has stopped.

4. Patients taking antiemetic agents should be warned about the potential sedative-type side effects and warned not to drive or operate machinery until the extent of individual side effects may be evaluated. In addition, CNS depressants and alcohol may potentiate the agent's sedative effects.

5. Many of these agents when administered intramuscularly may cause localized pain, stinging, burning, redness, and swelling at the injection site.

CATEGORY: MISCELLANEOUS GASTROINTESTINAL AGENTS (AHFS 56:40*)

	Trade Names	
Generic Name	U.S.	Canada
Cimetidine	Tagamet	Tagemet
		Novo-Cimetine
Ranitidine	Zantac	Zantac

Actions: These agents are histamine H$_2$ receptor antagonists; they specifically inhibit the action of histamine on the H$_2$ receptors of the parietal cells, which in turn reduces gastric acid output and concentration.

Uses: Treatment of patients with peptic ulcer disease and Zollinger-Ellison syndrome by inhibition of gastric acid secretion; reduce diarrhea, anorexia, and pain and promote healing of peptic ulcers; cimetidine also being used investigationally in the treatment of urticaria.

General side effects: Mild and usually transient; include mild diarrhea, dizziness, rash, and muscle pains.

Adverse reactions: High doses may cause impotence; when dose is reduced, problem subsides.

Contraindications: Used with caution in patients (especially elderly persons) with organic brain syndrome or impaired cardiovascular, hepatic, or renal function.

Nursing considerations:

1. When these agents are used for the treatment of peptic ulcer disease, antacids are concomitantly used to relieve gastric pain.

2. When taken with meals, cimetidine reduces meal-stimulated acid secretion by about two thirds during peak secretion times.

3. When these agents have been administered by IV bolus to control gastrointestinal bleeding, episodes of bradycardia and hypotension have resulted. To avoid such adverse reaction, dilute the drug agent in 100 ml of sodium chloride, Ringer's lactate, or dextrose solution and administer over 15 to 20 minutes.

*American Hospital Formulary Service classification.
†Drug is not available in Canada although it is listed in 1985 *Compendium of Pharmaceuticals and Specialties.*
‡U.S. trade name (or sometimes generic name) not listed in 1985 *Compendium of Pharmaceuticals and Specialties.*
§Drug is known by generic name.

GOLD COMPOUND AGENTS (AHFS 60:00*)

CATEGORY: GOLD COMPOUNDS

	Trade Names	
Generic Name	U.S.	Canada
Aurothioglucose	Solganal	—†
Gold sodium thiomalate	Myochrysine	Myochrysine

Actions: Production of anti-inflammatory effects during active stage of rheumatoid arthritis; although the precise method of action is unknown, gold salts have a strong affinity for sulfur and therefore provide an inhibitory effect on pyruvic dehydrogenase, which in turn alters cellular metabolism.

Uses: Treatment of rheumatoid arthritis; of less value in advanced cases and in the presence of extensive deformities and not indicated for old, burned-out, or arrested cases of rheumatoid arthritis; use in treatment of juvenile rheumatoid arthritis still considered investigational.

General side effects: Most common side effects occur to skin and mucous membrane and include erythema, urticaria, and papular or vesicular lesions on the skin, or stomatitis, gingivitis, pharyngitis, colitis, proctitis, and vaginitis of the mucous membranes. A metallic taste in the mouth may precede oral mucous membrane reactions. Other side effects include nausea, vomiting, anorexia, diarrhea, abdominal cramps, headache, conjunctivitis, iritis, and corneal ulcers.

Adverse reactions: Most adverse reactions occur following 2 or 3 months of treatment. More severe adverse reactions include severe exfoliative dermatitis that may lead to alopecia, chrysiasis (gray-to-blue pigmentation), or lichenoid lesions on the skin or mucous membrane. Although rare, the most toxic reaction of gold salts is the occurrence of a variety of blood dyscrasias; if these occur, they are serious and may be fatal. Gold salts may be nephrotoxic and hepatotoxic and may produce a nephrotic syndrome, glomerulitis with hematuria, and toxic hepatitis with jaundice. Transient proteinuria may also occur in patients receiving treatment. If adverse reactions occur, recovery may be facilitated by the use of corticosteroids or penicillamine.

Contraindications: Hypertension and renal or hepatic disease or dysfunction; should be administered only with extreme caution in patients with a history of blood dyscrasias; safe use of gold salts during pregnancy has not been established.

Nursing considerations:

1. The use of gold salts in the treatment of the active stage of rheumatoid arthritis is in addition to a regimen of salicylates, rest, and physical therapy.

2. The oral metallic taste of the agent in the mouth should be considered a warning sigh of impending gold toxicity.

3. Before therapy is begun, patients should have baseline hematologic evaluation. Patients taking gold salts should be monitored on a regular basis for the presence of blood dyscrasias. Eosinophilia frequently precedes or accompanies severe gold toxicity and may be a useful laboratory parameter.

4. Patients should also be monitored for renal and hepatic function before and during treatment with gold salts. If

albumin is seen in the urine after initiation of therapy, treatment should be discontinued until the symptom cause is verified.

5. The patient should be informed about the possible toxic and adverse reactions and should report to the health care provider any signs of pruritus, rash, mouth sores, or a metallic taste in the mouth.

6. Patients should also be warned about the possibility of photosensitivity reactions after exposure to sunlight or artificial ultraviolet light.

7. Because the possibility of anaphylactic reaction may occur following IM injection, the patient should be observed for 30 minutes after the injection.

HEAVY METAL ANTAGONISTS (AHFS 64:00*)

	Trade Names	
Generic Name	*U.S.*	*Canada*
Deferoxamine mesylate	Desferal	Desferal
Edetate calcium disodium	Calcium Disodium Versenate	Calcium Disodium Versenate
Penicillamine	Cuprimine Depen Titratabs	Cuprimine Depen

Actions: Deferoxamine mesylate and edetate calcium disodium bind iron and keep it from entering into chemical reactions. Penicillamine is a synthetic sulfhydryl compound that is an inactive degradation product of penicillin; combines with copper, iron, mercury, lead, gold, and arsenic to form soluble complexes that are readily excreted by the kidneys.

Uses: Deferoxamine mesylate and edetate calcium disodium used in acute and chronic iron intoxication poisoning as well as in the long-term management of iron storage diseases or iron overload as may occur with multiple transfusions. Parenteral administration of edetate calcium disodium may be useful in the treatment of poisoning by other heavy metals such as chromium, manganese, nickel, zinc, and possibly vanadium. Penicillamine used in treatment of rheumatoid arthritis (restricted to those patients with severe and active disease who have not responded to other therapy); also used to treat Wilson's disease (hepatolenticular degeneration) to promote excretion of copper deposited into the tissues, cystinuria to prevent renal calculi development, some cases of lead poisoning, and rheumatoid arthritis; effective orally and is also given to selected patients with severe acute arthritis that is unresponsive to conventional therapy.

General side effects: Deferoxamine mesylate and edetate calcium disodium may cause allergic reactions, blurred vision, abdominal discomfort, diarrhea, leg cramps, and fever. Penicillamine reactions of some type occur in approximately one third of all patients taking the agent; most common are mild allergic sensitivities such as generalized pruritus and erythematous rash, increased friability of skin, anorexia, nausea, epigastric pain, vomiting, and diarrhea. Slight to moderate proteinuria (less than 2/24 h) may occur in some patients; generally improves with continued drug use.

Adverse reactions: Although deferoxamine mesylate is relatively nontoxic, pain and induration at the site of injection may occur; rapid IV injection may cause generalized erythema, hypotension, and shock; prolonged therapy with deferoxamine mesylate has been reported to cause cataracts. One of the most serious adverse reactions of these agents is renal damage such as renal tubular necrosis. Penicillamine may cause severe adverse reactions such as leukopenia, thrombocytopenia, bone marrow depression, hemolytic anemia, monocytosis, and thrombocytosis. Fatalities have been reported.

Contraindications: Renal disease or dysfunction; not effective in treatment of mercury, gold, or arsenic poisoning. Deferoxamine mesylate not indicated for children under 3 years of age. Penicillamine has numerous agent-specific contraindications; the reader should investigate these in detail before agent administration.

Nursing considerations:

1. The use of deferoxamine mesylate for acute iron poisoning should not preclude the use of other emergency measures such as induction of emesis, gastric lavage, and correction of acidosis.

2. Signs of acute lead poisoning include vomiting, diarrhea, abdominal pain, tarry or bloody stools, metallic breath or taste in the mouth, and coma. Signs of chronic lead poisoning include anorexia, weight loss, gingival margin blueblack lines, metallic taste in the mouth, nausea and vomiting, vague leg and arm pains, sensory disturbances, and finally convulsions and coma.

3. IM injection of these agents may cause localized discomfort and tissue induration. Injection site observation and rotation of sites are very important.

4. If these agents are administered by IV route, the patient should be very carefully monitored and signs of cardiac changes, decrease in urinary output, or changes in the CNS status should be reported immediately. Cardiac monitoring by ECG is recommended during agent administration.

5. While these agents are administered, periodic renal function tests should be performed. The BUN should also be monitored. If urinary output is decreased after administration, the agent should be withheld until the cause of the decrease is evaluated.

6. Because of the serious adverse reactions such as renal damage, the recommended dosages should not be exceeded.

7. The use of penicillamine is very disease specific and generally accompanies many other care considerations such as other drug agents, diet, and avoidance of certain therapies. Because of the serious potential adverse reactions and the specific considerations for beneficial effect, the health care provider should read extensively about this drug and the special disease care considerations before beginning therapeutic use.

8. It is very important to perform baseline and periodic hematologic, urologic, and hepatic studies on all patients receiving penicillamine therapy.

HORMONE AND SYNTHETIC SUBSTITUTES (AHFS 68:00*)

CATEGORY: ADRENALS (AHFS 68:04*)

	Trade Names	
Generic Name	U.S.	Canada
Beclomethasone	Beclovent	Beclovent Inhaler
	Vanceril	Vanceril Inhaler
Betamethasone	Celestone	Celestone
Cortisone	Cortistan	—‡
	Cortone	Cortone
	Pantisone	—‡
Dexamethasone	Decadron	Decadron
	Hexadrol	Hexadrol
	Maxidex	Maxidex
Fludrocortisone	Florinef	Florinef Acetate
Fluprednisolone	Alphadrol	—†
Hydrocortisone	Cortef	Cortef
	Hydrocortone	—‡
	Hytone	—‡
	Solu-Cortef	Solu-Cortef
		Unicort
Methylprednisolone	Medrol	Medrol
	Depo-Medrol	Depo-Medrol
	Solu-Medrol	Solu-Medrol
Prednisolone	Delta-Cortef	Pred Forte
		Pred Mild
	Panisolone	Inflamase
Prednisone	Deltasone	Deltasone
		Winpred
	Orasone	—†
	Ropred	—‡
Triamcinolone	Aristocort	Aristocort
	Kenacort	Kenacort
	Kenalog	Kenalog-E Acetonide

Actions: This group of agents may be divided into two groups: the mineralocorticoids (fludrocortisone) and the glucocorticosteroids (the rest of the list). Effects of the glucocorticosteroids on the body are complex and affect almost every body system; in addition to regulating carbohydrate metabolism, they also regulate metabolism of proteins and fats. Primary function of the mineralocorticoids is to maintain proper fluid and electrolyte balance in the body.

Uses: Generally administered not as curative but as palliative treatment for inflammatory, allergic, and stress reactions; in specific diseases, also used to replace deficient endogenous hormones. For primary adrenal insufficiency, steroid replacement therapy is considered a primary life-sustaining therapy; corticosteroids also have both therapeutic and diagnostic applications because of their ability to suppress secretions of normal adrenal hormones. With the exception of the use of IV glucocorticoids during shock caused by adrenocortical insufficiency, the value of these agents during other types of shock is controversial. Goal of treatment therapy with corticosteroids is to administer the lowest daily dose of the agent

*American Hospital Formulary Service classification.

†Drug is not available in Canada although it is listed in 1985 *Compendium of Pharmaceuticals and Specialties.*

‡U.S. trade name (or sometimes generic name) not listed in 1985 *Compendium of Pharmaceuticals and Specialties.*

§Drug is known by generic name.

possible for the shortest period of time and still receive beneficial results.

General side effects: Short-term (1 to 2 weeks) administration of these agents very unlikely to cause side effects; if seen, they may include such signs as headache, fatigue, absence of signs of infection (even when the infection is present), flushing of face, and increased diaphoresis. Side effects of long-term therapy are significant and include Cushing-like syndrome ("moon" face, hump back, redistribution of fat), hirsutism, thinning of scalp hair, abdominal distention, weight gain, psychic disturbances, increased intracranial pressure, convulsions, increased intraocular pressure, posterior subcapsular cataracts, hypertension, gastrointestinal ulcers, protein depletion, osteoporosis, suppression of growth in children, diabetes, and amenorrhea.

Adverse reactions: May be adrenal suppression seen as actual adrenal atrophy "turn off" or an extension of the side effects listed above. The turn off is caused by an inhibition of hypothalamic-pituitary adrenal function; some degree of adrenal suppression may persist for up to 12 months in patients who have received large doses of corticosteroids for extended periods of time (see nursing consideration 3 below). Additional adverse reactions of these agents may include suppressed growth in children, suppression of the inflammatory response, and immunosuppressive effect and may cause sodium and water retention. Large doses may precipitate signs of psychosis, depression, euphoria, or disorientation.

Contraindications: Should be used with extreme caution in patients with active or healed tuberculosis; topical use contraindicated for fungal infections; allergic reaction or infections may be masked because of these agents; should be used very cautiously in patients with diabetes mellitus (may cause hyperglycemia), peptic ulcer, or cardiovascular disease.

Nursing considerations:

1. The effect of these agents may not be evident for several hours, so the agent should not be used as the only treatment during the time of an emergency. It is generally administered as a secondary agent.
2. For patients who have been receiving these agents for extended periods of time, withdrawal of the agents should be tapered because of suppression. Encourage the patient not to discontinue the medication even if symptoms improve. The patient should be evaluated for withdrawal effects, which may include fatigue, nausea or vomiting, diarrhea, weight loss, and dizziness.
3. Patients who have been taking these agents for long periods of time and then stop them will have reduced adrenal function for up to 12 months. These patients should be advised to notify the physician of previous therapy before any surgery or in case of any signs of infection or injury so that the patient may be evaluated for the necessity to provide supplemental corticosteroid therapy.
4. Important nursing considerations for patients taking these agents includes awareness of the many side effects of these agents. Specifically, the nurse should be aware of potential unnoticed patient infections and take extra precautions to prevent infection. Also, the nurse should assess for increased bleeding tendencies, fluid volume increase, changes in self-concept, or other signs listed above.

CATEGORY: ANDROGENS (AHFS 68:08*)

Generic Name	Trade Names	
	U.S.	Canada
Danazol	Danocrine	Cyclomen
Fluoxymesterone	Halotestin	Halotestin
	Ultandren	—†
Testosterone	Android-T	Delatestyl
	Depotest	Malogex
	Perandren	
	Tesone	

Actions: Two effects: an androgenic activity and an anabolic activity. Androgenic activity associated with development and maintenance of secondary male sex characteristics. Anabolic function of androgenic hormones maintains a positive nitrogen balance, stimulates growth of skeletal muscles, bones, skin, and hair, accelerates epiphyseal closure, and stimulates erythropoiesis. Derivatives of androgens have been synthesized that possess either predominately an androgenic activity or an anabolic activity. Large doses of androgens will suppress gonadotropic secretions in males, which in turn will lead to testicular atrophy.

Uses: Replacement therapy in various states of male sex hormone deficiencies: hypogonadism, male climacteric, cryptorchidism, and some cases of impotence. In females, used for postpartum breast pain, breast engorgement, and palliative treatment of breast cancer diagnosed as responsive to androgen therapy. May also be used in treatment of refractory anemias and osteoporosis to reverse protein loss after trauma, burns, debilitating diseases and growth stimulation in preadolescent males.

General side effects: Agent specific but general categories include dizziness, headache, fatigue, irritability, depression, decreased ejaculatory volume, appetite changes, and gastrointestinal distress.

Adverse reactions: Agent specific; serious reaction categories include such things as hypercalcemia, suppression of clotting factors, increased serum chloesterol levels, abnormal liver function studies, and cholestatic hepatitis; in men: prostatic hypertrophy, increased frequency and duration of penile erections, increased libido, impotence, epididymitis, bladder irritability, and gynecomastia; in women: hirsutism, amenorrhea and irregular menses, clitoral enlargement, and voice deepening.

Contraindications: Fluoxymesterone should be discontinued if priapism occurs or if the patient has prostatic carcinoma; should also be given with extreme caution in young boys to avoid premature epiphyseal closure or precocious sexual development.

Nursing considerations:
1. Close monitoring of all patients receiving these agents is necessary. Any signs of side or adverse reactions should be reported immediately.
2. Patients receiving these therapeutic agents should have periodic laboratory evaluations. The specific tests required will be agent specific. In summary most tests should include monitoring of serum calcium levels, complete blood counts, serum cholesterol levels, and blood clotting times.

4. Prepubertal males receiving treatment should have x-ray evaluation of bone age approximately every 6 months.
5. Monitor closely for cardiovascular problems.
6. Liver function tests should be performed as pretreatment baseline data and periodically repeated during therapy.

CATEGORY: CONTRACEPTIVES (AHFS 68:12*)

Generic Name	Trade Names	
	U.S.	Canada
Estrogen-progestogen combinations	(see tables, p. 2160)	
Progestogens, oral		
Norethindrone	Micronor	
Norgestrel	Ovrette	
	(see tables, p. 2160)	

Actions: Suppression of ovulation by inhibition of release of pituitary gonadotropins that regulate ovulation; also thicken cervical mucus, which inhibits penetration of sperm; other agent effects include changes in endometrium that make environment unfavorable for implantation; in addition, tubal transport of ovum may be affected.

Uses: Primary purpose: prevention of conception; Also treatment of endometriosis and regulation of menstrual cycles. Although most products are available and used in combination (estrogen-progestin products), there are a few products (called minipills) that are progestin-only products and are less likely to cause adverse effects; progestin-only products may also be somewhat less reliable than combination products.

General side effects: Minor side effects of most of these products are similar to those of early pregnancy, including nausea and vomiting, dizziness and headache, weight gain, breast fullness, and increased skin pigmentation. Some women may experience breakthrough bleeding or spotting. Other women may miss a period after termination of the agents.

Adverse reactions: Women using oral contraceptives may be at higher risk than other women for developing thromboembolic disorders, hypertension, and delayed ovulation following termination of the agent.

Contraindications: Family or personal history of breast cancer, genital cancer, coronary disease, hepatic or renal disease, thromboembolic disorders, permanent sterility, or diabetes.

Nursing considerations:
1. Advise patient taking oral contraceptives to notify the health care provider if she has any signs of calf, chest, or groin pain; increased lumps in the breast; severe headache, dizziness, or visual disturbances; severe abdominal pain, breakthrough bleeding, or suspected pregnancy.
2. Patient instructions regarding regularity of taking this medication are very important. If pills are missed, the patient should be advised to use a secondary protection source. Agent-specific package inserts provide more specific information.
3. The patient should be encouraged to report any other medications being taken. There is evidence to support the theory

Composition and Doses of Some Oral Contraceptives

Estrogen (mg)	Progestin (mg)	Trade Name
Combinations*		
Ethinyl estradiol (0.02)	Norethindrone (1)	Loestrin 1/20; Zorane 1/20
Ethinyl estradiol (0.03)	Norgestrel (0.3)	Lo/Ovral
Ethinyl estradiol (0.03)	Norethindrone (1.5)	Loestrin 1.5/30; Zorane 1.5/30
Ethinyl estradiol (0.035)	Norethindrone (0.4)	Ovcon-35
Ethinyl estradiol (0.035)	Norethindrone (0.5)	Brevicon; Modicon
Mestranol (0.05)	Norethindrone (1)	Norinyl 1 + 50; Ortho-Novum 1/50
Ethinyl estradiol (0.05)	Norgestrel (0.5)	Ovral
Ethinyl estradiol (0.05)	Ethynodiol diacetate (1)	Demulen
Ethinyl estradiol (0.05)	Norethindrone (1)	Ovcon-50; Zorane 1/50
Ethinyl estradiol (0.05)	Norethindrone acetate (1)	Norlestrin, 1
Ethinyl estradiol (0.05)	Norethindrone acetate (2.5)	Norlestrin, 2.5
Mestranol (0.06)	Norethindrone (10)	Ortho-Novum, 10 mg
Mestranol (0.075)	Norethynodrel (5)	Enovid, 5 mg
Mestranol (0.08)	Norethindrone (1)	Norinyl 1 + 80; Ortho-Novum 1/80
Mestranol (0.10)	Ethynodiol diacetate (1)	Ovulen
Mestranol (0.10)	Norethindrone (2)	Norinyl, 2 mg; Ortho-Novum, 2 mg
Mestranol (0.10)	Norethynodrel (2.5)	Enovid-E
Mestranol (0.15)	Norethynodrel (9.85)	Enovid, 10 mg
"Minipills"†		
—	Norethindrone (0.35)	Micronor; Nor-Q.D.
—	Norgestrel (0.075)	Ovrette

From Gilman, A.G., Goodman, L.S., and Gilman, A: Goodman and Gilman's the pharmacological basis of therapeutics, ed. 6, New York, 1980, Macmillan Publishing Co., Inc.
*Combination tablets are taken for 20 or 21 days and off for 7 or 8 days. These preparations are listed in order of increasing content of estrogen.
†"Minipills" are taken daily continually.

Canadian Oral Contraceptive Products

Progestin Component	Phasic Formation	<50 µg Estrogen	50 µg Estrogen	>50 µg Estrogen	Progestin Only
Norethindrone	Ortho 7/7/7 (tabs)	Ortho 1/35 (tabs)	Ortho-Novum 1/50 (tabs)	Ortho-Novum 1/80 (tabs)	Micronor (tabs)
	Ortho 10/11 (tabs)	Ortho 0.5/35 (tabs)	Norinyl 1 + 50	Ortho-Novum 0.5 mg (tabs)	
		Brevicon 1/35		Ortho-Novum 2 mg (tabs)	
		Brevicon		Ortho-Novum 5 mg (tabs)	
				Norinyl 1 + 80	
				Norinyl 2 mg	
Norethindrone Acetate		Minestrin 1/20	Norlestrin 1/50	Norlestrin 2.5	
		Loestrin 1/30			
Ethynodiol Diacetate		Demulen 30	Demulen 50	Ovulen 0.5 mg	
				Ovulen 1 mg	
d-Norgestrel	Triphasil	Min-Ovral	Ovral		

Data from Ortho Pharmaceutical, Canada.

that oral contraceptives may have reduced effectiveness with certain other prescribed medications. Specific agents should be investigated.

4. While women are taking oral contraceptives, they should be encouraged to have regularly scheduled physical examinations including breast examination, Pap tests, and periodic laboratory studies.

5. Some health care providers advise women to terminate oral contraceptive therapy at least 3 months before trying for conception. Other contraceptive measures should be used during this time. It may take other women at least 3 months to begin to ovulate and have menstrual periods after termination of the contraceptive agent.

CATEGORY: ESTROGENS (AHFS 68:16)

	Trade Names	
Generic Name	U.S.	Canada
Diethylstil-bestrol (DES)	Stilbestrol	Itonvol
Estradiol	Aquadiol	—‡
	Aquagen	—‡
	Estrace	—†
	Progynon	Progynon
Estrogens, con-jugated	Menogen	—‡
	Premarin	Premarin
Estrone	Estronol	Femogen
	Theelin	—†

Actions: Female hormones secreted primarily by the ovarian follicles. Associated with development and maintenance of female secondary sex characteristics. At menopause, ovarian secretion of estrogens declines at various rates. The estrogen preparations are divided into two groups according to structure: steroidal and nonsteroidal. The natural steroidal agents include estradiol, estrone, and their conjugated forms; DES is classed as a nonsteroidal derivative.

Uses: Used most frequently in treatment of a variety of conditions associated with estrogen hormone deficiencies, such as natural or surgical menopausal symptoms, suppression of lactation, prevention or treatment of postmenopausal osteoporosis, palliative treatment of advanced prostatic cancer in men, and inoperable breast cancer in women at least 5 years after menopause; DES also used following sexual assault to prevent postcoital contraception.

General side effects: Most common side effect of these agents is a transient nausea when therapy is begun; other side effects include gastrointestinal upset and abdominal cramps, anorexia, diarrhea, headache, breakthrough bleeding, and breast engorgement.

Adverse reactions: Generally only high-dose long-term therapy leads to adverse reactions, which may include endometrial cancer when agents are taken by postmenopausal women; other cancers under current evaluation are breast, cervix,

*American Hospital Formulary Service classification.
†Drug is not available in Canada although it is listed in 1985 *Compendium of Pharmaceuticals and Specialties.*
‡U.S. trade name (or sometimes generic name) not listed in 1985 *Compendium of Pharmaceuticals and Specialties.*
§Drug is known by generic name.

vaginal, liver, and kidney. Patients should also be observed for an increased incidence of gallbladder disease, thromboembolic disorders, or severe visual disorders.

Contraindications: Should be used with extreme caution in patients with the following conditions: asthma, epilepsy, cardiac or renal disease, migraine or other serious headaches, epilepsy, and history of thrombophlebitis.

Nursing considerations:

1. Signs of estrogen deficiency include hot flashes, chills, muscle cramps, myalgia, arthralgia, and paresthesia.

2. Caution patients to avoid exposure to ultraviolet light and prolonged exposure to sunlight while taking estrogens.

3. Instruct patient to report any signs of side effects or adverse reactions immediately.

4. Postmenopausal use requires regular checks for endometrial cancer.

5. Closely monitor the diabetic patient for potential medication adjustment.

6. Patients taking these agents should have blood pressure routinely screened for potential cardiovascular adverse reactions.

CATEGORY: GONADOTROPINS (AHFS 68:18*)

	Trade Names	
Generic Name	U.S.	Canada
Chorionic gonadotropin (HCG)	Antuitrin	Antuitrin, A.P.L.
	Chorex	
	Follutein	
Clomiphene citrate	Clomid	Clomid
Menotropins (HMG)	Pergonal	Pergonal
		Profasi HP

Actions: Chorionic gonadotropin (HCG) is a polypeptide hormone produced by human placenta during pregnancy; its purpose is to stimulate production of gonadal steroid hormones by stimulating the cells of the testes to produce androgens and the corpus luteum of the ovary to produce progesterone. In women the agents are thought to act by increasing secretion of luteinizing hormones (LHs), follicle-stimulating hormones (FSHs), and gonadotropins; this in turn acts to induce the ovulatory response in anovulatory women. Menotropins are a purified preparation of FSH and LH. Clomiphene is structurally a nonsteroidal-agent, synthetic derivative that increases output of pituitary gonadotropins; this in turn stimulates maturation and endocrine activity of ovulation and development of a functional corpus luteum.

Uses: Used only after careful and complete endocrinologic patient assessment. Chorionic gonadotropin used for two major purposes: in boys, for treatment of cryptorchidism and to assist in decision if an orchiopexy will be needed (it is hoped that following the administration of HCG the testes will descend); in females chorionic gonadotropin, clomiphene citrate, and menotropins are given sequentially and in combinations for induction of ovulation and pregnancy. Chorionic gonadotropin along with menotropins has been used investigationally in male infertility.

General side effects: May cause dose-related side effects including headache, irritability, fatigue, nausea and vomiting, vasomotor flushes, abdominal discomfort, and pain at injection site; should only be used when careful patient monitoring can be maintained; multiple births are also considered a side effect.

Adverse reactions: May cause weight gain, urticaria, and allergic dermatitis. In addition, HCG and menotropins may cause precocious puberty or gynecomastia; if noted, agent should be stopped. Chorionic gonadotropin may also cause fluid retention and should therefore be used with caution in patients with epilepsy, migraine, and cardiac or renal diseases. Clomiphene citrate reported to cause blurring of vision or decreased vision; symptoms disappear once agent is stopped. Birth defects have occurred while women have taken these agents.

Contraindications: History of liver disease or dysfunction, high urinary gonadotropin levels that may indicate primary ovarian failure, abnormal thyroid function, adrenal dysfunction, abnormal bleeding of undetermined origin, ovarian cysts, and pregnancy.

Nursing considerations:

1. The patient's weight and evidence of edema should be monitored during outpatient administration of these agents.
2. It is recommended that the patient undergo hepatic function studies before beginning therapy with these agents.
3. When clomiphene citrate is used for women who wish to become pregnant, the agent is taken for 5 days. The physician will discuss the timing of sexual intercourse. If side effects or adverse reactions are noted while the patient is taking the agent, these should be reported immediately.
4. Men taking these agents to produce increased spermatogenesis must undergo treatment for at least 3 months.
5. The close and careful monitoring of all patients taking these agents must be maintained. This monitoring includes clinical evaluation, observation of side and adverse reactions, and laboratory test monitoring.
6. Multiple pregnancies have been reported to occur in about 20% of pregnancies when conception has occurred following therapy by these agents; therefore before treatment, the patient and male partner must be informed of the possibility and potential hazards of multiple pregnancy.
7. Pregnancy should be monitored with ultrasound to determine the number of fetuses.

CATEGORY: ANTIDIABETIC AGENTS (AHFS 68:20*)
Class: Insulins (AHFS 68:20.08*)

| Generic Name | Trade Names | |
	U.S.	Canada
Rapid-acting		
Insulin injection (regular)	Regular Insulin	Insulin Toronto
	Regular Iletin I	Eletin Regular
	Velosulin	Velosulin

*American Hospital Formulary Service classification.
†Drug is not available in Canada although it is listed in 1985 *Compendium of Pharmaceuticals and Specialties.*
‡U.S. trade name (or sometimes generic name) not listed in 1985 *Compendium of Pharmaceuticals and Specialties.*
§Drug is known by generic name.

| Generic Name | Trade Names | |
	U.S.	Canada
Insulin injection (regular, recombinant DNA origin)	Novolin R	Actrapid Human
	Humulin R	Humulin R
Prompt insulin zinc suspension (semilente)	Semilente	Semilente
	Semilente Iletin I	Iletin-Semilente
	Semilente	—‡
Intermediate-acting		
Isophane insulin suspension (NPH)	NPH Iletin	Iletin-NPH
	NPH Insulin	NPH Insulin
	Humulin N	
Insulin zinc suspension (Lente)	Lente Iletin I	Iletin Lente
	Lente Insulin	Iletin Pork Lente
	Lentard	—‡
Isophane human insulin suspension (recombinant DNA origin)	Humulin N	Humulin N
	Novolin L	Monotard Human
Long-acting		
Extended insulin zinc suspension (ultralente)	Ultralente Insulin	Ultralente Insulin
	Ultralente Iletin	Iletin Ultralente
	Ultralente	—‡
Protamine zinc insulin (PZI)	Protamine Zinc and Iletin I or II	Iletin PZI

Actions: Insulin, which is normally derived from the beta cells of the pancreas, is the principal hormone required for proper glucose utilization in the metabolism process. Insulin preparations are currently available as porcine insulin, as bovine insulin, or by genetic engineering (recombinant DNA origin); because insulin from the porcine pancreas is considered to be more similar to that of human insulin, it is less likely to be antigenic.

Uses: Available in different types of preparations because of different patient needs; summary information described below under "Nursing Considerations"; dosages are highly individualized and may differ from one dose to the next based only on patient's blood glucose or ketone testing.

General side effects: Most commonly seen as localized reactions such as burning at the injection site; in addition, and especially if the injection sites are not rotated, patient may have hypertrophied or atrophied subcutaneous areas secondary to repeated injections.

Adverse reactions: See specific hypoglycemia and hyperglycemia signs listed below under "Nursing Considerations"; in addition, there may be local or systemic allergic reactions and insulin resistance.

Contraindications: Inadequate control of blood sugar by diet, coma related to hypoglycemia, lipodystrophy, insulin allergy, hypoglycemia, and insulin resistance.

Nursing considerations:

1. The table on the opposite page summarizes the onset, peak, and duration of the various preparations.

Agent Type	Onset of Action (h)	Peak Effect (h)	Duration of Action (h)
Rapid-Acting			
Insulin injection (regular)	½-1	2-3	5-7
Prompt insulin zinc suspension (semi-lente)	½-1	4-7	12-16
Intermediate-Acting			
Isophane insulin suspension (NPH)	1-2	8-12	18-24
Insulin zinc suspension (lente)	1-2	8-12	18-24
Isophane human suspension (recombinant DNA origin)	>1.5	>8	>24
Long-Acting			
Extended insulin zinc suspension (ultra-lente)	4-8	16-18	36
Protamine zinc insulin (PZI)	4-8	14-20	36

2. *Diabetic ketoacidosis* may be present before the administration of insulin. Signs include drowsiness, dim vision, thirst, Kussmaul breathing, air hunger, dry mouth, fruity breath odor, nausea, vomiting, abdominal pain, flushed skin, and rapid pulse.

3. *Signs of hyperglycemia* include polyphagia, polyuria, polydipsia, dehydration, glucosuria, ketonuria, blurred vision, weight loss, hypovolemia, recurrent or persistent infections, weakness, fatigue, muscle wasting, and muscle fatigue.

4. *Signs of hypoglycemia* (hyperinsulinism) include fatigue, weakness, confusion, headache, diplopia, psychosis, personality changes, rapid shallow respirations, peripheral limb tingling, slurred speech, staggering gait, tremors, diaphoresis, slow coordination, slow cerebration, dizziness, convulsions, and coma.

5. There are many nursing considerations for patients taking insulin. The reader is referred to Chapter 8 for more specific information.

Class: Sulfonylureas (AHFS 68:20.20*)
Class: Miscellaneous Antidiabetic Agents (AHFS 68:20.92*)

Generic Name	Trade Names	
	U.S.	*Canada*
Acetohexamide	Dymelor	Dimelor
Chlorpropamide	Diabinese	Diabenese
		Chloronase
Glucagon	—§	—§
Tolazamide	Tolinase	—†
Tolbutamide	Orinase	Orinase
		Mobenol

Actions: Useful in management of select cases of diabetes mellitus. Sulfonylurea acts on blood sugar level by stimulating insulin secretion from beta cells of pancreatic islets; ineffective in the absence of functioning beta cells and therefore not appropriate therapy for absolute insulin deficiencies. Agents are also not oral insulin or a substitute for insulin.

Glucagon is a hyperglycemic glycogenolytic agent that has no structural resemblance to insulin and that elevates blood sugar by stimulating hepatic gluconeogenesis through activation of cyclic adenosine monophosphate and phosphorylase activity.

Uses: Most effective in treatment of maturity-onset diabetes when patient has little or no tendency toward ketoacidosis; most frequently instituted when hypoglycemia cannot be controlled by diet alone; patients most likely to respond are those with adult-onset diabetes. Glucagon used in emergency situations to treat severe hypoglycemic reactions in diabetic patients receiving insulin and in psychiatric patients during insulin shock therapy. If patient has adrenal insufficiency, starvation, or chronic hypoglycemia, agent may not be helpful.

General side effects: Side effects similar to other sulfonylurea agents, including gastrointestinal upset, diarrhea, weakness, fatigue, tachycardia, sweating, tremor, and rarely skin eruptions. Chlorpropamide may have more serious side effects, including dose-related manifestations of gastrointestinal upset, severe diarrhea, and lower gastrointestinal bleeding. Rarely, photosensitivity has been reported to occur.

Adverse reactions: Transient leukopenia, thrombocytopenia, and mild anemia have been reported; in addition, other potential adverse reactions include severe hypoglycemia (see signs below). Adverse reactions, collapse, and hypotension have been reported with IV administration of glucagon of 2 mg or less over a 45-minute period. Tolbutamide has been reported to rarely cause blood dyscrasias, including thrombocytopenia, hemolytic anemia, leukopenia, agranulocytosis, aplastic anemia, and pancytopenia.

Contraindications: Should be administered with caution to patients who are debilitated or malnourished because of increased risk of hypoglycemia. Because these agents have no blood glucose–lowering effects in absence of pancreatic beta cells, they should not be used as therapy in type I (juvenile) diabetes; also contraindicated in cases of brittle or unstable types of diabetes, or diabetes associated with ketosis, diabetic coma, major surgery, or renal, thyroid, or hepatic dysfunction; should be avoided during pregnancy. Safety and efficacy in children have not been established.

Nursing considerations:

1. Advise patients regarding signs of hyperglycemia and hypoglycemia (listed below under "Nursing Considerations"). Patients are usually started on a 7-day supply of the agent and then are clinically reevaluated to assess agent effect. Severe hypoglycemia may be a serious problem.

2. In order for therapy from these agents to be successful, the patient must be carefully chosen for compliance potential and instructed as to the nature of adult-onset diabetes. Patients must be under close medical supervision (for at least 6 consecutive weeks) and instructed to notify the physician immediately if any adverse or side reactions occur. In addition, the patient must fully understand the medication therapy recommendations (when to take the agent), the dietary instructions, and other instructions related to body weight, personal hygiene, and other case-related points.

3. Elderly patients may be hyperresponsive to these agents when first administered; it may be helpful to start with a low dose, evaluate for side effects, and then increase the dose over several days.

4. Patients must be taught how and when to test for glucosuria and ketonuria.

5. Significant drug interactions occur between these agents and other agents such as barbiturates, hypnotics, sedatives, sulfonamides, salicylates, probenecid, and monoamine oxidase inhibitors. Carefully review the specific agent prescribed and the possible interactions that may occur.

CATEGORY: PITUITARY (AHFS 68:28*)

Generic Name	Trade Names	
	U.S.	Canada
		Acthar
Corticotropin (ACTH)	Acthar	Duraton
Desmopressin	DDAVP	DDAVP
Lypressin	Diapid	—‡
Somatropin (human growth hormone)	Asellacrin	—‡
	Crescormon	Crescormon
		Pitressin
Vasopressin (ADH)	Pitressin	Pitressin Tannate

Actions: There are two primary types of pituitary hormones: the anterior hormones (follicle-stimulating hormone, luteinizing hormone, human chorionic gonadotropin, somatotropin, and prolactin) and the posterior hormones (antidiuretic hormone and oxytocin). For the anterior pituitary hormones the main action is either hormone secreting or hormone producing. The regulation of most anterior hormones is done primarily via a negative-feedback mechanism to stop or slow down the production or excretion of a hormone. Somatropin, for example, increases the renal tubular reabsorption of phos-

*American Hospital Formulary Service classification.

†Drug is not available in Canada although it is listed in 1985 *Compendium of Pharmaceuticals and Specialties.*

‡U.S. trade name (or sometimes generic name) not listed in 1985 *Compendium of Pharmaceuticals and Specialties.*

§Drug is known by generic name.

phorus and decreases that of calcium; intestinal absorption of calcium is increased. This may then be secondary to somatropin's stimulation of skeletal growth at the epiphyses and to stimulation of soft-tissue growth. The posterior pituitary hormones affect the functioning of peripheral target tissue by either an oxytocin or antidiuretic vasopressin activity.

Uses: Use of the anterior pituitary hormones is primarily agent specific. Bromocriptine used in the short-term management of amenorrhea associated with hyperprolactinemia; may also be used to treat postpartum breast engorgement and to treat investigationally the symptoms of idiopathic or postencephalitic Parkinson's disease. Corticotropin used primarily as an aid in the diagnosis of adrenocortical insufficiency; has also been used effectively to increase muscle strength in patients with severe myasthenia gravis; is not curative and is indicated only as supportive therapy. Somatropin used to promote linear growth in patients with growth failure caused by a deficiency of endogenous growth hormone; should be used only by those physicians experienced in diagnosis and management of pituitary growth hormone deficiency. Posterior pituitary agents used both as vasopressive agents and antidiuretic agents to prevent or control polydipsia, polyuria, and dehydration in patients with diabetes insipidus. Desmopressin has been used throughout pregnancy and lactation without adverse effects on the mother or fetus.

General side effects: Potential side effects of anterior pituitary hormones involve almost every body system: cardiovascular signs include, for example, fluid retention; gastrointestinal signs may be abdominal discomfort, nausea and vomiting, and ulcerative esophagitis; CNS signs include fever, headache, dizziness, depression, mood swings, personality changes, and even convulsions. If anterior agents are injected, there may be local discomfort at the injection site. Posterior hormones cause infrequent and mild side effects, including rhinorrhea, nasal congestion, irritation with burning sensation, and pruritus of the nasal passages; infrequently, patient may experience nasal ulceration, headache, abdominal cramps, and increased bowel movements.

Adverse reactions: Short-term use of corticotropin unlikely to cause any adverse reactions; long-term use may cause skin atrophy, fluid retention, hyperpigmentation, and adverse androgenic effects such as amenorrhea, postsubcapsular cataracts, exophthalmos, increased intraocular pressure, acne, and hirsutism; when used for prolonged periods, may suppress pituitary release of corticotropin and cause agent-induced hypothalamic insufficiency; severe reactions such as anaphylactic shock, wheezing, and circulatory failure have been reported.

Contraindications: Before these agents are used for the treatment of amenorrhea and infertility, patient must be carefully screened for pituitary dysfunction and tumor. Corticotropin ineffective in treatment of primary adrenocortical insufficiency and congenital adrenogenital syndrome; should also be used with caution in patients with hypothyroidism, cirrhosis, peptic ulcer disease, hepatic disease, congestive heart failure, scleroderma, or recent surgery; long-term use in children should be avoided because the agent may retard bone growth. Posterior pituitary agents should be used with caution in patients who have coronary vasospasm or elevated blood pressure.

Nursing considerations:

1. Vaccines and immunizations should not be administered to patients receiving corticotropin because of potential neurologic reactions and because corticotropin may inhibit the antibody response.
2. Before patients begin treatment with the anterior pituitary agents the adrenal responsiveness to the agent should be verified.
3. These agents have multiple interactions, especially the anterior agents with other agents. The nurse should be aware of the agent-specific interactions before administration.
4. If the patient is taking any of the anterior agents and also becomes pregnant, the physician should be notified as soon as possible.
5. The posterior pituitary agents are administered intranasally according to the manufacturer's instructions to ensure that the agent is deposited high in the nasal cavity and does not pass down the throat. The package insert should be carefully read.

CATEGORY: PROGESTINS (AHFS 68:32*)

Generic Name	Trade Names	
	U.S.	Canada
Hydroxyprogesterone	Delalutin	Delalutin
	Duralutin	—‡
Medroxyprogesterone	Provera	Provera
	Depo-Provera	Depo-Provera
	Amen	—‡
Norethynodrel	Enovid	Enovid
Progesterone	Gesterol	Gesterol
	Lipo-Lutin	Progestasert
	Prorone	—‡

Actions: Production of a pharmacologic response usually produced by progesterone; includes induction of secretory changes in the endometrium, an increase in basal body temperature, production of histologic changes in vaginal epithelium, relaxation of uterine smooth muscle, stimulation of mammary alveolar tissue growth, pituitary inhibition, and production of withdrawal bleeding in the presence of estrogen.

Uses: Treatment of functional uterine bleeding, premenstrual tension, dysmenorrhea, threatened and habitual abortion, primary amenorrhea, and toxemia of pregnancy; norethynodrel suppresses ovulation and has therefore also been used for prevention of conception; duration and method of agent administration vary with the purpose for which the agent is being used.

General side effects: At usual doses and for short periods, most agents produce only minor side effects including spotting, irregular bleeding, nausea, and lethargy. High dosages may cause gastrointestinal upset, extremity edema and weight gain, headache and dizziness, oligomenorrhea, amenorrhea, breast congestion, and decreased libido. Parenteral administration of progesterone may result in pain and swelling at the injection site.

Adverse reactions: Jaundice has been reported with the use of select agents as well as androgenic effects and masculinization of the female fetus; patients receiving prolonged therapy should be carefully monitored for androgenic effects.

Contraindications: Some progestogens may aggravate asthma, epilepsy, and migraine headaches; should be used with extreme caution in patients with liver disease.

Nursing considerations:

1. There is no evidence to indicate that patients discontinuing the medications will have subsequent difficulty in achieving conception.
2. If a patient misses two consecutive menstrual periods while taking medroxyprogesterone, treatment should be discontinued and pregnancy ruled out before continuing therapy.

CATEGORY: THYROID AND ANTITHYROID AGENTS (AHFS 68:36*)

Generic Name	Trade Names	
	U.S.	Canada
Calcitonin	Calcimar	Calcimar
Iodine	—§	—‡
Levothyroxine	Levoid	—‡
	Levothroid	—‡
	Synthroid	Synthroid
Liothyronine	Cytomel	Cytomel
Liotrix	Euthroid	—‡
	Thyrolar	—‡
Methimazole	Tapazole	Tapazole
	Thiamazole	—‡
Propylthiouracil	Propacil	Propyl-Thyracil
Thyroglobulin	Proloid	Proloid
Thyroid	S-P-T	—‡
	Thyrar	—‡

Actions: These agents may be divided into the antithyroid agents and the thyroid agents. The antithyroid agents (calcitonin, iodine, methimazole, and propylthiouracil) act to inhibit one or more steps in hormone synthesis; the precise physiologic role of the agents is not known. The thyroid agents (levothyroxine, liothyronine, liotrix, thyroglobulin, and thyroid) are either natural hormones of animal origin (called desiccated thyroid extract) or synthetic replacement hormones; these agents are composed of T_3, T_4, or a combination of both hormones; natural hormones have been largely replaced by synthetic hormones.

Uses: With the exception of calcitonin, the antithyroid agents are used to treat hyperthyroidism. Calcitonin used to reduce high blood calcium levels and may be used as an emergency hormone to lower serum calcium in patients with hypercalcemia; also used in patients with Paget's disease of the bone to decrease the rate of bone turnover with a resultant decrease in elevated serum alkaline phosphatase level and urinary hydroxyproline excretion. Patients treated frequently show steady improvement with a plateau after 6 to 9 months and a relapse toward pretreatment levels after 1 to 2 years of therapy. Iodine used to treat simple and colloid goiter and may be used alone as preoperative preparation or more commonly with other antithyroid agents. Thyroid preparations used as replacement therapy to treat primary and secondary myxedema, myxedemic coma, cretinism, and simple non-toxic goiter.

General side effects: Side effects of antithyroid agents have been infrequent and mild; they include fever, chills, decreased hair growth, pigmentation changes, nausea, vomiting, paresthesias, and confusion. Side effects of thyroid preparations may be indicative of overdosage and may include palpitations, angina, dyspnea, headache, excessive warmth, diarrhea, nervousness, and mental agitation.

Adverse reactions: All antithyroid agents given in excessive quantities over prolonged periods may induce hypothyroidism; the most serious adverse reactions to methimazole therapy are agranulocytosis, leukopenia, and thrombocytopenia. Adverse reactions indicating overdose of thyroid agents may not appear for 1 to 3 weeks after initiation of therapy; signs include diarrhea, cramps, vomiting, continued weight loss, hyperhidrosis, intolerance to heat, hyperirritability, nervousness, insomnia, increased cardiac output, tachycardia, and arrhythmias; these patients should be carefully watched for signs of thyrotoxicosis.

Contraindications: Propylthiouracil and methimazole both cross the placenta, are excreted in milk, and are therefore contraindicated for use in nursing mothers. Because the effects of calcitonin in pregnant women are unknown, the agent should not be administered to women who are pregnant or women who want to become pregnant; calcitonin may cause hypersensitivity reactions to fish. Iodine contraindicated in patients with tuberculosis, iododerma, laryngeal edema, and swelling of the salivary glands or increased salivation on previous exposure to iodides; not effective in treatment of postoperative thyroid crisis. Thyroid preparations should not be used in treatment of metabolic insufficiency not associated with thyroid deficiency; should be used with extreme caution in patients with coronary artery disease; contraindicated in patients with myocardial infarction or thyrotoxicosis.

Nursing considerations:
1. Patient education regarding the use of these agents for long-term therapy is important.
2. Patients receiving long-term calcitonin therapy should have periodic examinations of urine sediment for observation of coarse granular casts.
3. For calcitonin, skin testing is recommended before subcutaneous or intramuscular injection. The appearance of a small wheal or erythema within 15 minutes is a positive reaction, and the agent should not be administered.
4. Patients may be taught to self-inject calcitonin. When this is done, all precautions such as site rotation and aseptic techniques must be taught.
5. Because of the potential adverse reaction with several of the antithyroid agents, patients should be advised to report symptoms of sore throat.

*American Hospital Formulary Service classification.
†Drug is not available in Canada although it is listed in 1985 *Compendium of Pharmaceuticals and Specialties.*
‡U.S. trade name (or sometimes generic name) not listed in 1985 *Compendium of Pharmaceuticals and Specialties.*
§Drug is known by generic name.

OXYTOCIC AGENTS (AHFS 76:00*)

CATEGORY: OXYTOCICS

| Generic Name | Trade Names | |
	U.S.	Canada
Ergonovine maleate	Ergotrate Maleate	Ergotrate Maleate
Methylergonovine maleate	Methergine	Methylergobasine-Sandoz
Oxytocin	Pitocin	—‡
	Syntocinon	Syntocinin

Actions: Ergonovine and methylergonovine act to intensify uterine and cervical contractions. Oxytocin is an endogenous hormone produced by the posterior pituitary that indirectly stimulates uterine contraction by increasing the sodium permeability of uterine myofibrils; also has a vasopressive and antidiuretic effect.

Uses: Ergonovine and methylergonovine used by IM or IV injection for prevention and treatment of postpartum and postabortion hemorrhage (IV injection only for severe postpartum hemorrhage). Oxytocin used by IV infusion to induce labor at term by stimulating uterus to contract during first and second stages of labor; frequently used postpartum or following cesarean delivery to stimulate immediate contractions of uterus and to control uterine bleeding. Because ergonovine and methylergonovine produce more sustained contractions and higher uterine tone, most physicians prefer their use over oxytocin for management of postpartum hemorrhage.

General side effects: Nausea and vomiting are the most common side effects; others include dizziness and headache. Large and rapid doses of oxytocin may cause severe decreases in maternal systolic and diastolic blood pressure and increase in heart rate and systemic venous return and cardiac output, and arrhythmias may result; postpartum bleeding may increase with administration of oxytocin.

Adverse reactions: IV administration of these agents not adequately diluted may cause serious adverse reactions including hypertension, generalized headache, arrhythmias, tinnitus, diaphoresis, palpitations, temporary chest pains, dyspnea, and allergic reactions. Especially when oxytocin is administered in excessive dosage, tetanic contractions with risk of uterine rupture or injury to fetus may occur.

Contraindications: Ergonovine and methylergonovine should not be used for induction or augmentation of labor; if these agents are administered during the third stage of labor before delivery of the placenta, complications such as captivation of the placenta may occur; should be used with extreme caution in patients with sepsis or renal or hepatic dysfunction. Oxytocin contraindicated as a method to stimulate term pregnancy until maternal and fetal adequacy has been evaluated.

Nursing considerations:
1. Usual doses of ergonovine and methylergonovine intensify uterine contractions and then provide periods of relaxation. Larger doses of the agents produce forceful contractions with shorter or no periods of relaxation.
2. These agents administered intravenously should be adequately diluted according to the agent directions and ad-

ministered slowly and precisely by use of an infusion pump or other type of microdrip unit. Nausea and vomiting and other signs of maternal or fetal distress may result from rapid infusion.

3. Before oxytocin is used for the function of labor at term, pelvic adequacy and other maternal and fetal conditions must be carefully evaluated and monitored. During the administration of oxytocin, maternal and fetal monitoring should be maintained. The physician should be notified immediately of any signs of fetal distress such as decreased fetal heart rate or any signs of maternal distress such as increased vaginal bleeding or a rapid change in vital signs or discomfort. The duration and status of contractions should also be monitored. Discontinue infusion immediately if any signs of distress are noted.

4. Buccal or parenteral oxytocin administration should be used only by hospital professionals where intensive care and surgical facilities are immediately available.

RADIOACTIVE AGENTS (AHFS 78:00*)[6]

CATEGORY: RADIOACTIVE AGENTS

	Trade Names	
Generic Name	*U.S.*	*Canada*
Iodinated ^{125}I serum albumin	Albumotope I-125 Risa-125	—§
Iodinated ^{131}I serum albumin	Albumotope I-131 Risa-131	—§
Iodinated ^{131}I serum albumin (macroaggregated)	Albumotope-LS Macroscan-131	—§
Sodium iodide ^{125}I	Iodotope I-125	—§
Sodium iodide ^{131}I	Iodotope I-131	—§
Sodium phosphate ^{32}P	Phosphotope	—§

Actions: Can be used in two ways (therapeutic and diagnostic); act selectively as tracer components to monitor or modify specific physiologic activity within the body. ^{131}I used for both diagnostic testing of thyroid function and therapeutically as a source of radioactivity to selectively destroy thyroid function. ^{32}P used only as a source of radioactivity to selectively destroy cells with a high phosphate turnover (e.g., neoplastic bone marrow cells).

Uses: May either be used diagnostically as radioactive tracers or therapeutically as radioactive sources in pathologic conditions in which there is significant metabolic malfunction or in which an organ or tissue produces physiologic harm through overactivity. There are three types of agents discussed in this section: the iodinated serum albumin agents (iodinated ^{125}I, iodinated ^{131}I, and iodinated ^{131}I [macroaggregated]) are used primarily as diagnostic agents to evaluate blood and plasma volume (iodinated ^{125}I and iodinated ^{131}I tag onto plasma albumin and are therefore used primarily as

[6] Not listed in 1985 edition of AHFS.

diagnostic agents to determine blood or plasma volume); the sodium iodide agents (sodium iodide ^{125}I and sodium iodide ^{131}I) are used either for diagnostic testing of thyroid disorders or for therapeutic intervention of thyroid disease or cancer; and sodium phosphate (sodium phosphate ^{32}P) is used for both diagnostic evaluation and therapeutic intervention of intraocular and cerebral tumors and in the treatment of certain types of leukemia. In addition, iodinated ^{131}I used to determine placenta localization and to diagnose placenta previa. Macroaggregated iodinated ^{131}I prepared by heating iodinated ^{131}I to produce aggregated albumin particles; the macroaggregated agent is used as a diagnostic aid in conjunction with lung imaging procedures (see Chapter 2) to evaluate total, unilateral, and regional arterial perfusion of lungs. This diagnostic procedure is used with others to evaluate pulmonary embolism, pulmonary arterial thrombosis, regional pulmonary hypoxia, pulmonary hypertension, pulmonary vascular bed compression, malignant bronchogenic carcinoma, lung abscesses, and tuberculosis. Sodium iodide ^{125}I and ^{131}I preparations used in low doses as diagnostic aids to estimate functional status of the thyroid gland, to study the morphology of the thyroid, to locate substernal and lingual thyroid tissue, and to locate thyroid tumors; thyroid function studies may be made by measuring the percentage of specific tracer doses or by using scintillation scanning techniques. Use and value of the iodide for thyroid uptake tests depend on several factors, including techniques employed and patient's level of dietary iodide. When radioactive iodide is used for therapy, goal is to destroy or reduce amount of functioning thyroid tissue in select cases of hyperthyroidism and thyroid carcinoma. Radiation by use of iodide ^{125}I and iodide ^{131}I is most often chosen because it is less expensive and less disfiguring than surgery. Radioactive iodide is treatment of choice for patients with Graves' disease who are unable to tolerate antithyroid agents and for patients who experience a recurrence of Graves' disease following thyroid surgery. Sodium phosphate ^{32}P infrequently used diagnostically to aid in location of certain ocular and cerebral tumors; more commonly used to reduce number of red blood cells in palliative treatment of polycythemia vera and in treatment of chronic myelocytic (granulocytic) leukemia.

General side effects: Although side effects are uncommon with the iodinated diagnostic agents, fever, aseptic (chemical) meningitis, and allergic reactions have been reported; other side effects are agent specific; review of these effects should be made before agent administration.

Adverse reactions: In large doses, the sodium iodide agents may cause thyroiditis manifested by hyperthyroidism, swelling and tenderness of the neck, and sore throat, as well as transient aggravation of symptoms of thyrotoxicosis. These signs of thyroiditis may develop 1 or 2 weeks following therapy. The major disadvantage of use of radioactive iodides ^{131}I and ^{125}I for treatment of hyperthyroidism or thyroid cancer is the long period of time that may be necessary to see results; a second disadvantage is that hypothyroidism may develop; in addition, there may be systemic radiation effects. Radiation sickness may occur following therapeutic doses of sodium phosphate ^{32}P.

Contraindications: Although in low doses there is no evidence that patients incur measurable doses of radiation from any of these agents used for diagnostic procedures, for all agents described above, unnecessary radiation exposure should be avoided, especially in pregnant women and young children. Because these agents are primarily excreted by the urine, they should be used with caution in patients with renal dysfunction. Sodium iodide ^{131}I contraindicated in nursing mothers; when used in larger therapeutic doses, sodium iodide agents are carried across the placenta and may destroy fetal development.

Nursing considerations:

1. Health care professionals using radioactive agents should be aware of the Atomic Energy Commission (AEC) and utilize the recommended precautions such as wearing monitoring badges. Other precautions include adequate shielding to protect personnel and patients from unnecessary radiation, disposal of used radioactive materials in a standard procedural manner congruent with the AEC recommendations, frequent washing of hands, and frequent monitoring of the physical environment for radiation levels.

2. After patients receive therapeutic treatment with radioactive agents, the patient's saliva, perspiration, urine, feces, vomitus, wound drainage, and breast milk should be considered as radioactive for a dose- and agent-related period of time.

3. To minimize thyroidal uptake of the radioactive iodide agents, a thyroid-blocking agent such as strong iodine solution (Lugol's solution) should be administered before and for 3 to 5 days following administration of the radioactive agent.

4. Because the iodide agents are excreted primarily in the urine, the possibility of increased radiation effects from accumulation should be considered in patients with renal compromise.

5. Thyroid uptake may be decreased in the diagnostic use of sodium iodide ^{131}I in patients with congestive heart failure; it may also be increased in patients with congestive heart failure who are on low-sodium diets and in patients with chronic cirrhosis.

6. Iodine-containing preparations such as strong iodine solution (Lugol's solution), iodides, white bread, antitussives, iodine-containing suppositories, and radiographic contrast media may decrease thyroidal uptake of iodide for up to 1 month.

7. Antithyroid agents may be given before radiation therapy. When this is done, the drugs should be discontinued 48 to 72 hours before the administration of ^{125}I or ^{131}I. Iodide-containing agents should not be administered before therapy.

8. When patients are receiving large doses of radioactive iodine as a therapeutic treatment, they require hospitalization and isolation. Isolation should consist of a private room at least 6 feet away from other patients and traffic flow; special protective measures for care givers, including gowns, gloves, booties, special method by which to dispose of body wastes, dosimeter and radiation badges, and consultation by the radiation safety branch of the hospital; and special precautions regarding visitors, such as no children and no pregnant women.

9. For patients receiving any of these agents as cancer therapy, careful blood studies including hemoglobin, leukocyte, erythrocyte, and platelet counts should be conducted as baseline information before beginning therapy as well as at monthly intervals during treatment. Some sources recommend reevaluation of these parameters throughout life even after therapy is terminated.

SERUM, TOXOID, AND VACCINE AGENTS (AHFS 80:00*)

CATEGORY: SERUMS (IMMUNE GLOBULINS) (AHFS 80:04*)

	Trade Names	
Generic Name	U.S.	Canada
Hepatitis B immune globulin	H-BIG	Heptavax-B
	Hep-B-Gammagee	—‡
	HyperHep	—‡
Immune serum globulin; gamma globulin	Gamastam	Immune Serum
	Gammagee	Globulin-Gamma
	Immuneglobulin	Globulin
	Gamastan	—‡
Human rabies immune globulin	Hyperab	Globulin (Human)
Rho(D) immune globulin	RhoGAM	Rh₀ (D) Immune Globulin
	Hyper Rho-D	Win-Rho
	Gamulin Rh	—‡
Tetanus immune globulin	Hyper-Tet	Tetanus Immune Globulin
	Immu-Tetanus	—‡
	Pro-Tet	—‡
Varicella-zoster immune globulin (investigational)	—§	—§

Actions: Prevention or modification of certain diseases in specific circumstances; most often given as postexposure prophylaxis following either parenteral (needle stick, laceration, or bite), direct mucous membrane (cough), or oral ingestion (pipetting) exposure.

Uses: Each agent is disease or exposure specific; most common method of agent administration is by IM injection. Hepatitis B immune globulin (H-BIG) used alone or in combination as postexposure prophylaxis against known exposure to hepatitis B virus. Immune serum globulin (IG) given as preexposure prophylaxis against hepatitis A to travelers in areas of high potential contact with the virus; also indicated for postexposure prophylaxis for close household and sexual contacts of persons with hepatitis A or for staff or professional members of health care institutions in which hepatitis A has been identified; to be most effective, it should be given within 2 weeks of known contact. Human rabies immune globulin (HRIG) indicated as postexposure prophylaxis for

---

*American Hospital Formulary Service classification.
†Drug is not available in Canada although it is listed in 1985 *Compendium of Pharmaceuticals and Specialties.*
‡U.S. trade name (or sometimes generic name) not listed in 1985 *Compendium of Pharmaceuticals and Specialties.*
§Drug is known by generic name.

rabies unless contraindicated as listed below. Rho(D) immune globulin used in Rh-negative women to prevent sensitization to the Rho(D) factor and to prevent hemolytic disease of the newborn in subsequent pregnancies. Tetanus immune globulin used for those patients with clean and minor wounds who (1) have unknown or uncertain previous tetanus toxoid immunization status, (2) have received fewer than two previous tetanus toxoid doses, or (3) have received only two previous tetanus toxoid doses and whose wound is more than 24 hours old. Varicella-zoster immune globulin should be administered to immunosuppressed or compromised patients who have contracted varicella or who are known to have been exposed to varicella; may be used on an individual basis with other noncompromised adults if risk of contracting disease is greater than immunization risk.

General side effects: Local injection site soreness or redness has been reported.

Adverse reactions: If agents are administered in accord with agent-specific technique, serious adverse reactions are rare.

Contraindications: Human rabies immune globulin (HRIG) contraindicated for persons who have been previously immunized with recommended therapy or for those individuals with an adequate rabies antibody titer. Other individuals with special health states such as pregnancy, conditions that compromise the immune system, hemodialysis, splenic dysfunction or anatomic asplenia, factor VIII or IX deficiencies, chronic alcoholism, or other high-risk diseases should receive these agents only after complete investigation of the agent's risks and benefits as described on package inserts.

Nursing considerations:

1. If more than one injection is given, use different injection sites. Carefully document the agent and the site. If a reaction occurs, it is important to identify the agent of cause.

2. Give parenterally administered live-virus vaccines at least 14 days before or at least 6 weeks (preferably 3 months) after administration of immune globulins.

CATEGORY: TOXOIDS (AHFS 80:08*)

Generic Name	Trade Names	
	U.S.	Canada
Diphtheria toxoid	—§	—§
Diphtheria and tetanus toxoids, adsorbed (DT)	—§	—§
Tetanus and diphtheria toxoids, adsorbed, for adult use (Td)	—§	—§
Diphtheria and tetanus toxoids and pertussis vaccine, adsorbed (DPT, DTP)	—§	—§
Tetanus toxoid (TT)	—§	—§

Actions: Provision of active immunity by inducing production of injected antitoxin. Single injections do not provide adequate immunity; the body requires three primary immunizations at scheduled intervals and then periodic reimmunization to provide continued disease protection.

Uses: Three toxoids currently available for active immunity (tetanus, diphtheria, and pertussis). All vaccines administered by IM injection and available in the agents listed above to provide single or combination ingredients. Diphtheria toxoid is an active immunization against diphtheria for children under the age of 6 years. Diphtheria and tetanus toxoids, adsorbed, provide active immunity against diphtheria and tetanus for children 6 weeks through 6 years of age. Tetanus and diphtheria toxoids, adsorbed, are for adult use in providing active immunity against tetanus and diphtheria. Diphtheria and tetanus toxoids and pertussis vaccine, adsorbed, used to provide active immunity to diphtheria, tetanus, and pertussis in children 6 weeks through 6 years of age. Tetanus toxoid and tetanus toxoid, adsorbed, used to provide active immunity to tetanus in adults and children over 6 weeks of age (it is recommended, however, that children less than 7 years of age receive DPT and that adults receive Td). The recommended schedule for immunizations is listed in Chapter 15.

General side effects: Local injection site reactions with signs of redness and slight swelling are most common; infrequently, the patient may have a low-grade fever.

Adverse reactions: Although rare, diphtheria and tetanus toxoid has been reported to cause systemic reactions including high fever, malaise, generalized aches and pains, flushing, generalized urticaria or pruritus, tachycardia, and hypotension.

Contraindications: Acute or active infection. Other individuals with special health states such as pregnancy, conditions that compromise the immune system, hemodialysis, splenic dysfunction or anatomic asplenia, factor VIII or IX deficiencies, chronic alcoholism, or other high-risk diseases should receive these agents only after complete investigation of the agent's risks and benefits as described on the package inserts. It has been recommended that children with history of CNS damage or convulsions should have their primary immunizations postponed until they are at least 2 years of age.

Nursing consideration:

1. If passive tetanus immunization is needed, human immune globulin is the agent of choice (see discussion in section on serums above). The adsorbed tetanus toxoid preparation should be used for the tetanus toxoid injection when both passive and active immunizations are given during the same clinical situation. Separate syringes and separate body locations should be used for the two preparations. Careful documentation of the agent and site should be made.

CATEGORY: VACCINES (AHFS 80:12*)

Generic Name	Trade Names	
	U.S.	Canada
BCG vaccine	—§	—§
Cholera vaccine	—§	—§
Hepatitis B vaccine	Heptavax-B	Heptavax-B
Influenza vaccine, polyvalent	—§	Influenza Vaccine Whole Virion, Subvirion
Measles virus vaccine	Attenuvax M-Vac	Measles Vaccine —‡
Measles, mumps, and rubella virus	M-M-R II	M-M-R II
Mumps virus vaccine	Mumpsvax	Mumpsvax
Pneumococcal vaccine, polyvalent	Pneumovax Pnu-Immune	Pneumovax Pneumovax 23
Poliovirus vaccine, inactivated (Salk)	—§	—§

	Trade Names	
Generic Name	*U.S.*	*Canada*
Poliovirus vaccine, live oral (Sabin)	Orimune	Poliovirus Vaccine (Sabin)
Rabies vaccine	—§	—§
Rubella virus vaccine	Meruvax II	Meruvax II
Rubella and mumps vaccine	Biavax II	—‡
Typhoid vaccine	—§	—§

Actions: Vaccines may be divided into four types. The *live-virus vaccines* (measles, mumps, and rubella virus vaccines both individually and in combination [M-M-R II]; poliovirus, live oral) are live virus vaccines that promote active immunity by inducing the production of specific antibodies. The *inactivated-virus vaccines* (hepatitis B vaccine; poliovirus vaccine, inactivated; influenza vaccine; and rabies vaccine) are killed viruses used to induce active immunization against the stated select agent. The *live-bacterial vaccine* (tuberculosis BCG vaccine) is used to produce active immunity to tuberculosis. The *inactivated-bacterial vaccines* (cholera, pneumococcal polysaccharide vaccine, and typhoid vaccine) are killed bacterial agent vaccines that promote active immunity by inducing production of specific antibodies.

Uses: Primary vaccines required of all children in the United States: measles; rubella; mumps; and trivalent polio virus, live oral. In Canada, measles, mumps, rubella, polio adsorbed, and DPT required. BCG vaccine recommended for administration to children and health care professionals who live in areas of the world where there is a high prevalence of tuberculosis. Other vaccines used on a case-by-case basis for individuals with known or potential exposures or for individuals who would be highly compromised if they should contract the disease; for example, mumps vaccination may be of particular value in boys nearing puberty and in men who have not had mumps. Primary purpose of rubella immunization: prevention of infection of fetus and congenital rubella syndrome; rubella vaccine therefore indicated as a single subcutaneous dose for adults, particularly women, unless proof of immunity is available by childhood record or by titer evaluation. Hepatitis B vaccine specifically recommended for adults at increased risk of occupational, social, family, environmental, or illness-related exposure to hepatitis B; high-risk group includes homosexual males, users of illicit injectable drugs, household or sexual contacts of hepatitis B carriers, and health care professionals with high exposure risk. Typhoid and cholera vaccines only recommended for overseas travelers. Immunity of cholera vaccine is short duration, not exceeding 4 to 6 months. Because all of these vaccines are disease specific and require different administration techniques and frequencies, the reader is also referred to the implied disease for further discussion of their use.

General side effects: For those agents that are injected, the side effects are most commonly localized redness and discomfort around the injection site as well as malaise, fever, and chills. Rubella vaccine may cause joint pain or peripheral aching.

Adverse reactions: Measles vaccine may cause fever for 1 or 2 days beginning between 5 to 12 days after administration. Parotitis following mumps vaccination has been reported. BCG vaccine may cause local adverse reactions including streaking from the injection site toward regional lymph nodes and localized abscess or ulceration around the injection site.

Contraindications: Each agent has specific contraindications for administration; the health care provider should carefully read the package inserts before agent administration. Individuals with special health states such as pregnancy, conditions that compromise the immune system, hemodialysis, splenic dysfunction or anatomic asplenia, factor VIII or IX deficiencies, chronic alcoholism, or other high-risk diseases should receive these agents only after complete investigation of the agent's risks and benefits as described on the package inserts.

Nursing considerations:

1. Individuals born since 1957 should be considered immune to rubella, measles, and mumps only if there is documentation of adequate immunization with live virus or if there is serologic evidence of measles immunity. The measles, mumps, and rubella virus vaccine should not be administered until the child is approximately 15 months of age. Protection requires a single dose of the live virus.

2. The live oral trivalent polio virus vaccine is administered orally to the child at four times: approximately 2 months, 4 months, 18 months, and 4 to 6 years. Routine immunization of adults is not necessary unless the adult is at professional or personal high risk for contracting polio.

3. Hepatitis B virus vaccine is intended for primary preexposure prophylaxis. Recently, however, it has also been recommended as a postexposure treatment for high-risk groups. More commonly recommended for postexposure protection, however, is the hepatitis B immune globulin.

4. BCG vaccine offers no protection to individuals who are already tuberculin positive. Also, following BCG administration, the individual will always elicit a positive TB skin test.

5. New data available regarding the vaccine efficacy using pneumococcal polysaccharide vaccines recommend that these agents be administered for the following persons: (a) adults with chronic illness, especially those with cardiovascular disease and chronic pulmonary disease, who sustain increased morbidity with respiratory infections; (b) adults with chronic illnesses specifically associated with increased risk of pneumococcal disease or its complications; these include splenic dysfunction or anatomic asplenia, Hodgkins' disease, multiple myeloma, cirrhosis, alcoholism, renal failure, cerebrospinal-fluid leaks, and conditions associated with immunosuppression; and (c) older adults, especially those over age 65, who are in good health. Because of the marked increase in possible adverse reactions, a booster dose of this agent should not be given.

*American Hospital Formulary Service classification.
†Drug is not available in Canada although it is listed in 1985 *Compendium of Pharmaceuticals and Specialties.*
‡U.S. trade name (or sometimes generic name) not listed in 1985 *Compendium of Pharmaceuticals and Specialties.*
§Drug is known by generic name.

SKIN AND MUCOUS MEMBRANE AGENTS (AHFS 84:00*)

Almost all of the agents of the following categories and classes are available in a variety of product forms including lotions, ointments, creams, suppositories, and liquids. Many of the trade names are specific to the form of the agent's preparation. Also, although not elaborated in this appendix, most of these agents are also available in combination products. The health care provider must carefully investigate the exact ingredients of prescribed agents.

CATEGORY: ANTI-INFECTIVES (AHFS 84:04*)
Class: Antibiotics (AHFS 84:04.04*)[7]

Generic Name	Trade Names	
	U.S.	*Canada*
Bacitracin	Baciguent	Baciguent
Gentamicin	Garamycin	Garamycin
Neomycin	Myciguent	Myciguent

Actions: Topical agents; bactericidal or bacteriostatic in action depending on the concentration of the agent attained at the site of infection and the susceptibility of the infecting organism; generally inactive against fungi and viruses.

Uses: Alone or in combination with other anti-infectives or corticosteroids in treatment of superficial skin infections; agents listed are active against many gram-positive and gram-negative organisms; there is some controversy regarding when they are really needed vs. when the lesion kept clean and dry would heal adequately on its own.

General side effects: Applied topically, these agents have a low order of reaction; when seen, it generally appears as a localized allergic reaction including erythema and pruritus.

Adverse reactions: Rarely, topical use of these agents may cause systemic reactions ranging from generalized itching to hypotension and cardiac arrest. Occasionally, overgrowth of nonsusceptible organisms such as fungi occurs; if this type of superinfection is noted, agent should be discontinued and infection reevaluated.

Contraindications: Known allergic reactions; discontinue use if any allergic reactions appear.

Nursing considerations:
1. The concomitant use of topical steroids may mask the clinical signs of bacterial, fungal, or viral infections.
2. These agents should be applied topically two or three times each day. Before a new application, the old ointment as well as any wound crusting or blood should be cleansed off. Care should also be taken to avoid further contamination of infected skin.
3. These agents are not usually absorbed following topical application to intact skin. They (especially gentamicin and neomycin) may, however, be readily absorbed through skin that is denuded or that has lost the keratin layer, such as in

---

[7]Many of the topical antibiotics are mixed combinations.

---

wounds, burns, and ulcers. Because of this increased absorption potential, the reader is referred to the cautions of side effects and adverse reactions that may be seen in the systemic ingestion of these agents (see section AHFS 8:12.02).

Class: Antivirals (AHFS 84:04.06*)

Generic Name	Trade Names	
	U.S.	*Canada*
Acyclovir	Zovirax	Zovirax

Actions: A synthetic acyclic purine nucleoside analogue that is active against varicella zoster.

Uses: Management of initial herpes genitalis and mucocutaneous herpes simplex virus types 1 and 2 infections in immunocompromised patients. On clinical trials and during the first episode of the disease, agent tends to decrease healing time and decrease discomfort; during subsequent episodes of herpes, agent has shown no clinical benefit.

General side effects: Topical application may cause localized irritation and discomfort.

Adverse reactions: IV administration may cause renal compromise, irritation at IV site, transient elevations of serum creatinine, rash, and hives.

Contraindications: Should not be applied near the eye; effects during pregnancy and for nursing mothers are not known.

Nursing considerations:
1. For use in the management of genital herpes, the agent is applied by ointment. The recommended dosage should not be exceeded. Treatment consists of application six times per day for a duration of 7 days. The old ointment should be removed before applying new ointment.
2. For use in the treatment of mucosal or cutaneous herpes in immunocompromised patients, the agent is administered intravenously and slowly and should be considered very potent. The health care provider should be aware of systemic absorption and adverse reactions before its administration. Renal function studies and a baseline creatinine level should be done before agent administration.

Class: Antifungals (AHFS 84:04.08*)

Generic Name	Trade Names	
	U.S.	*Canada*
Clotrimazole	Lotrimin	Canesten
	Mycelex	Myclo
	Gyne-Lotrimin	—‡
Gentian violet	GVS Vaginal Cream/Inserts	—‡
Haloprogin	Halotex	Halotex
Miconazole nitrate	MicaTin	MicaTin
	Monistat	Monistat
Nystatin	Mycostatin	Mycostatin
	Nilstat	Nilstat
Tolnaftate	Tinactin	Tinactin

Actions: Alteration of cell membrane permeability and binding with the phospholipids in the fungal cell membrane; most agents not absorbed from healthy intact skin.

Uses: Most agents used in topical treatment of tinea pedis, tinea cruris, tinea corporis, and tinea manuum. Nystatin used to treat monilia infections, vulvovaginal candidiasis, and diaper rash. Clotrimazole also used intravaginally347o treat candidiasis. Gentian violet inhibits growth of many types of fungi including yeasts and dermatophytes; also used to treat staphylococcal gram-positive bacteria infections.

General side effects: If side effects are seen, they are generally localized irritation, burning, and vesicle formation. If reaction is more than this, agent should be stopped.

Adverse reactions: Occasionally, clotrimazole may cause blistering, erythema, edema, pruritus, burning, stinging, skin peeling, and fissures. Esophageal irritation and obstruction have been reported from swallowing gentian violet.

Contraindications: Not intended for ophthalmic use. Use of these agents for pregnant women varies from agent to agent; specific agent should be investigated before beginning its use.

Nursing considerations:

1. Clinical use of these agents may take from 1 to 8 weeks depending on the agent and its strength and the organism. Most vaginal fungal infections should be treated for 2 weeks while topical infections may take at least 8 weeks of treatment. If after 8 weeks of therapy, the patient is not significantly improved, the clinical status must be reevaluated.

2. Gentian violet is applied as a solution by painting the area to be treated or intravaginally. It should not be swallowed. Applied topically, the agent has both local irritant as well as staining properties. A purple stain will occur on all skin and clothing that comes in contact with the agent. Concomitant therapy of adequate hygiene should be initiated to prevent the spread of infection or reinfection.

Class: Scabicides and Pediculicides (AHFS 84:04.12*)

Generic Name	Trade Names	
	U.S.	Canada
Benzyl benzoate	—§	Scabanca
Crotamiton	Eurax	Eurax
Lidane (gamma benzene hexachloride)	Kwell	—‡
Pyrethrins with piperonyl butoxide	RID A-200 Pyrinate Vonce	—‡

Actions: Toxic to parasitic arthropods.

Uses: Topical treatment of scabies, head lice, body lice, crab lice, and possibly their respective nits. Some agents such as gamma benzene hexachloride are the usual treatment of choice for either scabies or lice, while other agents are arthropod specific. For infants and young children, agents other than gamma benzene hexachloride are preferred. Crotamiton indicated only for treatment of scabies. Pyrethrins with pi-

*American Hospital Formulary Service classification.
†Drug is not available in Canada although it is listed in 1985 *Compendium of Pharmaceuticals and Specialties.*
‡U.S. trade name (or sometimes generic name) not listed in 1985 *Compendium of Pharmaceuticals and Specialties.*
§Drug is known by generic name.

peronyl butoxide used only for treatment of head lice, body lice, crab lice, and their nits.

General side effects: When used according to directions, topical application of these agents has few side effects; may be slight local irritation if agents come in contact with face, eyes, mucous membranes, and urethral meatus.

Adverse reactions: Inhalation of agents may cause headache, nausea, vomiting, and irritation of eyes, nose, and throat. Gamma benzene hexachloride may cause acute toxicity evidenced by serious CNS seizures and hepatic and renal toxicity.

Contraindications: Should not be applied to acutely inflamed or raw, weeping skin. Gamma benzene hexachloride should be used very cautiously in infants and small children; long-term exposure to vapors has caused fatal aplastic anemia and other hematologic disorders.

Nursing considerations:

1. Do not administer orally. Treatment is by topical application.

2. Before applying the drugs topically, instruct the patient to bathe in soap and water and scrub the body to remove scaling or crusted detritus and then towel dry.

3. The specific treatment protocol will differ with treatment of scabies and lice. Refer to Chapter 5 for a detailed discussion of agent application and care.

Class: Miscellaneous Local Anti-Infectives (AHFS 84:04.16*)

Generic Name	Trade Names	
	U.S.	Canada
Hexachlorophene	pHisoHex	pHisoHex
Mafenide	Sulfamylon	Sulfamylon
Nitrofurazone	Furacin	Furacin
	Nisept	—‡
Povidone-iodine	Betadine	Betadine
	ACU-dyne	—‡
	Povadyne	Proviodine
Silver sulfadiazine	Silvadene	Flamazine

Actions: Topical agents; act in individual ways as topical germicides and as bacteriostatic agents against many gram-negative and gram-positive organisms and several strains of anaerobes.

Uses: Hexachlorophene and povidone-iodine act primarily as postwound or preoperative bacteriostatic skin cleansers (see caution below). Povidone-iodine is not absorbed. Mafenide used in treatment of primary and secondary infection of skin and mucous membranes. Commonly, mafenide, nitrofurazone, and silver sulfadiazine used in topical treatment of second- and third-degree burns. Nitrofurazone may also be used to prevent infection of skin grafts and donor sites and in prevention and treatment of nonspecific bacterial urethritis and bacterial vaginitis and cervicitis.

General side effects: Localized redness or irritation, especially if povidone-iodine is used and patient is allergic to iodine. Pain or burning following application of mafenide and nitrofurazone are commonly reported. Most frequently reported side effect of these agents is some type of topical allergic sensitization; most common signs of sensitization include rash, facial edema, blisters, urticaria, and dermatitis around area of application.

Adverse reactions: If hexachlorophene is not thoroughly rinsed from sensitive areas of skin after use, it may be rapidly absorbed and may lead to toxic blood levels; adverse CNS signs include irritability. Adverse reactions for mafenide include systemic acidosis, hyperventilation, and increased serum chloride and decreased carbon dioxide levels. Silver sulfadiazine may accumulate in patients with impaired hepatic or renal function; risk-to-benefit ratio must be carefully evaluated.

Contraindications: Hexachlorophene contraindicated on burned or denuded skin; has been reported to be absorbed in young premature infants. Sulfonamide therapy and silver sulfadiazine contraindicated in pregnant women at term and premature or newborn infants.

Nursing considerations:

1. Povidone-iodine does not permanently stain the skin or clothing. The agent may be washed away with soap and water.
2. Mafenide acetate cream for the management of burn treatment is reported to be more painful than silver nitrate or silver sulfadiazine.
3. For application and management of these agents in the care of the burned patient, see Chapter 5.

CATEGORY: ANTI-INFLAMMATORY AGENTS (AHFS 84:06*)

The corticosteroids discussed here are single-agent products. Many times these products are used in combination with other products. Additional information may be located on the use of corticosteroids in sections AHFS 52:08 and 68:04.

	Trade Names	
Generic Name	U.S.	Canada
Group 1		
Betamethasone dipropionate ointment, 0.05%	Diprosone	Diprosone
Desoximethasone cream, 0.25%	Topicort	—‡
Fluocinonide jelly, 0.05%	Topsyn	Topsyn Gel
Halcinonide cream, 0.1%	Halog	Halog
Group 2		
Betamethasone benzoate jelly, 0.025%	Benisone	—‡
Betamethasone valerate ointment, 0.1%	Valisone	Valisone
Triamcinolone acetonide cream, 0.5%	Aristocort HP	Aristocort Acetonide Topicals
Group 3		
Betamethasone valerate lotion, 0.1%	Valisone	Valisone
Fluocinolone acetonide cream, 0.025%	Sunalar	Synalar
Flurandrenolide ointment, 0.05%	Cordran	Cordran
Triamcinolone acetonide ointment, 0.1%	Aristocort R Kenalog	Aristocort R Kenalog

	Trade Names	
Generic Name	U.S.	Canada
Group 4		
Betamethasone valerate cream, 0.1%	Valisone	Valisone
Cortisol valerate cream, 0.2%	Westcort	Westcort
Fluocinolone acetonide cream, 0.025%	Synalar	Synalar
Triamcinolone acetonide cream, 0.1%; lotion, 0.025%	Kenalog	Kenalog
Group 5		
Desonide cream, 0.05%	Tridesilon	Tridesilon
Flumethasone pivalate cream, 0.03%	Lotcorten	Locorten

Action: Hydrocortisone or synthetic derivatives of hydrocortisone used topically as anti-inflammatory agents.

Uses: Used alone or in combination with other skin preparations discussed elsewhere to treat dermatosis and to produce anti-inflammatory, antipruritic, and vasoconstrictive actions. Although absorption is minimal over most body surface areas such as the knees, palms of the hands, soles of the feet, forearms, and elbows, agents are readily absorbed along the scrotum, axilla, eyelids, face, and scalp. Agents listed above by group indicate relative activity of the corticosteroid preparation: group 1 has a high degree of relative activity while group 5 has a much lesser degree of activity.

Adverse reactions: Topical application generally does not elicit any adverse reactions; combination products may cause adverse reactions. Long-term use of topical corticosteroids may cause atrophy of the epidermis and dermal collagen and drying of the skin. Epidermal thinning, telangiectasis, increased fragility of cutaneous blood vessels, purpura, and atropic striae possible. Significant systemic absorption and rebound responses possible if agents are used for longer than 2 months.

Contraindications: Fungal infection.

Nursing considerations:

1. The percutaneous penetration of corticosteroids may be increased by the use of an occlusive dressing over the treated area. Use of an occlusive dressing should be evaluated on an individual-case basis determined by the reason for treatment and the appearance of the lesion being treated.
2. The type of agent substance (cream, lotion, jelly, etc.) that is chosen depends on the location of the lesion and the condition being treated. Lotions may be best for weeping, erupting lesions. Lotions, gels, and aerosols are best for hairy areas. Creams are best for dermatoses; and ointments may be best for treatment of dry, scaly lesions.
3. See Chapter 5 for details of agent application, skin-cleansing procedure, and use of occlusive dressings.

CATEGORY: ASTRINGENTS (AHFS 84:12*)

	Trade Names	
Generic Name	U.S.	Canada
Aluminum acetate	Burow's Solution	Burow's Solution
Silver nitrate	—§	—§
Tannic acid	—§	—§

Actions: Germicides and astringents to treat tissue and mucous membrane.

Uses: Aluminum acetate used topically to treat acute and subacute inflammatory conditions; in ointment form, used to treat ulcerative conditions of skin. Silver nitrate used as a topical germicide agent or as an astringent to mouth, bladder, or urethral membranes; in stronger solutions, used for chemical cauterization to remove excess granulation tissue or warts; 1% solution of silver nitrate used in eyes of newborns for prophylaxis against ophthalmia neonatorum. Tannic acid used to treat hyperhidrosis, to toughen tender skin, and in management of intertrigo, receding gums, and sore throat; may also be used internally to treat bleeding hemorrhoids and to control bleeding and diarrhea.

General side effects: Local reactions include increased irritation, redness, or slight discomfort.

Adverse reactions: Use of large amounts of tannic acid applied topically in treatment of burns may lead to liver failure.

Contraindications: With exception of tannic acid, agents should not be swallowed; silver nitrate is highly toxic to gastrointestinal tract and central nervous system.

Nursing considerations:

1. Aluminum acetate is used generally as a wet dressing or as a gargle. The agent must be mixed and diluted according to package instruction before use. (More discussion is found in Chapter 5).
2. Silver nitrate must be handled carefully since it will leave a gray or black stain on skin or utensils. Silver nitrate may be removed from linen by an application of iodine tincture followed by sodium thiosulfate solution.
3. Aqueous solutions of tannic acid should be freshly prepared before use because they are unstable in the presence of light and oxygen. Glycerin solutions of tannic acid are relatively stable.

CATEGORY: CELL STIMULANTS AND PROLIFERANTS (AHFS 84:16*)

Generic Name	Trade Names	
	U.S.	Canada
Isotretinoin	Accutane	Accutane
Tretinoin	Retin-A	Stie VAA
		Vitamin A Acid

Actions: Both agents related to retinoic acid and vitamin A; precise action of topical (tretinoin) or capsule (isotretinoin) use is not yet determined; it is believed that these agents inhibit keratinization.

Uses: Isotretinoin used in treatment of severe recalcitrant cystic acne; single course of therapy may result in complete and prolonged remission. Tretinoin used topically in treatment of acne vulgaris, primarily grades I to III, in which comedones, papules, and pustules predominate. Tretinoin therapy is not curative, and relapses generally occur between 3 and 6 weeks from drug withdrawal.

*American Hospital Formulary Service classification.
†Drug is not available in Canada although it is listed in 1985 *Compendium of Pharmaceuticals and Specialties*.
‡U.S. trade name (or sometimes generic name) not listed in 1985 *Compendium of Pharmaceuticals and Specialties*.
§Drug is known by generic name.

General side effects: Side effects associated with isotretinoin are usually dose related and include such things as eye irritation; dry, itching skin; dry mouth; nausea and vomiting; insomnia or lethargy and fatigue; and elevated laboratory values of sedimentation rate, triglyceride level, and increased lipoproteins. Side effects of topical tretinoin therapy are local inflammatory reactions that reverse after therapy has been terminated; skin may show increased redness, scaling, blistering, or crusting; if these are seen, patient should be advised to use the agent less often or to discontinue therapy for a few days.

Adverse reactions: Isotretinoin: hypertriglyceridemia, musculoskeletal aches and pains, and corneal opacities.

Contraindications: Isotretinoin should not be given to women of child-bearing potential; fetal abnormalities have been reported. Concomitant use of tretinoin with other topical medications should be avoided.

Nursing considerations:

1. Patients may experience a prolonged healing response while taking these agents.
2. Because of the numerous side effects, adverse reactions, and contraindications, the risk-to-benefit ratio must be discussed with the patient before use.
3. While patients are using these agents, vitamin A supplements should not be used. An additive toxic reaction may result.
4. Sun or ultraviolet light may cause an increased sensitivity to sunburn while the patient is taking these agents.
5. Pregnancy should not be attempted until 1 month has passed since the termination of these agents and until one menstrual cycle has occurred.

CATEGORY: KERATOLYTIC AGENTS (AHFS 84:28*)

Generic Name	Trade Names	
	U.S.	Canada
Anthralin	Anthra-Derm	Anthraforte
		Anthranol
		Lasan
Benzoyl peroxide	Desquam-X	—‡
	Benoxyl-5	—‡
	PanOxyl-5	—‡
Podophyllium resin	—§	Podofilm
Salicylic acid	Calicylic	Keralyt
	Salacid	Gel
		Saligel
Silver nitrate	—§	—§

Actions: Chemical action rather than physical abrasive action.

Uses: Anthralin and benzoyl peroxide used in treatment of psoriasis to actually loosen comedones and to exert a peeling, or desquamating, effect; anthralin preferred because it has less tendency to produce conjunctivitis when used about the face and scalp and is less likely to cause dermatitis or discoloration of skin. Some agents such as benzoyl peroxide may also provide a desquamating, drying, and antibacterial effect. Podophyllium resin used in the treatment of venereal warts (condylomata acuminata) and granuloma inguinale. Salicylic acid used in treatment of localized hyperkeratosis and for removal of plantar warts and calluses.

General side effects: Some agents when used around face and eyes may cause conjunctivitis.

Adverse reactions: Resin in podophyllium is cytotoxic and irritating; skin adjacent to treatment area must be protected.

Contraindications: Acute inflammation of skin; likewise, they should be discontinued if irritation appears.

Nursing considerations:

1. Podophyllum should be applied to the affected area and covered for 12 to 24 hours. At that time, the agent should be washed off. Timed treatments should occur weekly until the lesions regress. Within a few hours, the lesions become blanched and in 24 to 48 hours they become necrotic. On about the third day they begin to slough and gradually disappear without scarring.
2. See Chapter 5 for the procedures to use salicylic acid in the removal of plantar warts and calluses.

CATEGORY: KERATOPLASTIC AGENTS (AHFS 84:32*)

	Trade Names	
Generic Name	*U.S.*	*Canada*
Coal tar	Cotasol	Estar
	Estar	Bainetar
	Psorigel	Zetar

Actions: Coal tar by-product that has keratoplastic, stimulating, and antipruritic properties.

Uses: Treatment of psoriasis and other eczematous dermatoses such as atopic dermatitis, seborrheic dermatitis, lichen simplex chronicus, and chronic eczematous dermatitis; often used in combination with other topical agents.

General side effects: May cause severe dermatitis when used for extended periods of time; irritation is dose related.

Adverse reactions: Severe skin irritation leading to blister formation and localized tissue damage.

Contraindications: Infected lesions.

Nursing considerations:

1. Refer to Chapter 5 for coal tar application procedures.
2. Because of a potential dermatitis reaction, coal tar should not be applied to more than one fourth of the body at any one time.

CATEGORY: PIGMENTING AND DEPIGMENTING AGENTS
Class: Depigmenting Agents (AHFS 84:50.04*)

	Trade Names	
Generic Name	*U.S.*	*Canada*
Hydroquinone	Artra	—‡
	Eldopaque	—‡
	Eldoquin	—‡
Monobenzone	Benoquin	—†

Actions: Inhibition of tyrosinase in the melanocytes to decrease production; there is also thought to be some direct toxicity to the melanocytes themselves.

Uses: Hydroquinone used topically to reduce hyperpigmentation in conditions such as freckling, inactive chloasma, generalized and senile lentigo, and photosensitization associated with inflammation or use of certain perfumes; depigmentation may take 1 to 4 months and may persist for 2 to 6 months following termination of treatment. Monobenzone applied topically to permanently depigmented normal skin surrounding vitiliginous lesions in patients with disseminated idiopathic vitiligo.

General side effects: May cause mild skin irritation including burning, stinging, and allergic dermatitis.

Adverse reactions: Repeated use of monobenzone causes destruction of melanocytes, or permanent depigmentation. An acute toxic overdose reaction may cause signs similar to a phenol overdose including tremors, convulsions, and severe hemolytic anemia.

Contraindications: Do not apply these agents near the eyes or mouth; monobenzone contraindicated for any condition other than disseminated vitiligo.

Nursing consideration:

1. Topical application of these agents is disease specific. See Chapter 5 for further information.

Class: Pigmenting Agents (Psoralens) (AHFS 84:50.06*)

	Trade Names	
Generic Name	*U.S.*	*Canada*
Methoxsalen	Oxsoralen	—†
Trioxsalen	Trisoralen	—‡

Actions: When exposed to long-wavelength ultraviolet light, these agents tend to increase melanin-producing cells.

Uses: Used in conjunction with ultraviolet light treatments to repigment vitiliginous skin in patients with idiopathic vitiligo. Topical application of these agents produces a more intense photosensitizing response than does oral agent ingestion. Topical application should only be used when the area is small and well defined (less than 10 sq cm).

General side effects: Side effects most commonly follow oral agent administration and include nausea, vomiting, nervousness, vertigo, insomnia, and mental depression.

Adverse reactions: These agents are strong photosensitizers and capable of producing severe burns if improperly used. The ultraviolet light exposure must be controlled (310 to 365 nm). Phototoxic reactions include severe blistering, edema, erythema, and peeling of the skin. If severe reactions occur, the agents should be discontinued.

Contraindications: Should not be administered concomitantly with other local or systemic photosensitizing agents; also contraindicated in patients with gastrointestinal diseases, chronic infections, or diseases associated with photosensitivity such as porphyrias, acute lupus erythematosus, or leukoderma; have not been established as safe for young children or pregnant women.

Nursing considerations:

1. Complete cures following therapy are infrequent. About one third of the patients treated have significant amounts of pigmentation restored.
2. The patient's skin should be protected from sunlight for at least 8 hours if the agents are orally administered and for 12 to 48 hours following topical administration.
3. Side effects from oral administration of these agents may

be reduced by administering the agent with milk or at mealtime.

4. These are complex agents. Before assisting with administration, the nurse should be very familiar with all implications, adverse reactions, and complications. Refer to the package insert.

5. For psoralen therapy in combination with ultraviolet light, see also Chapter 5.

CATEGORY: SUNSCREEN AGENTS (AHFS 84:80*)

	Trade Names	
Generic Name	U.S.	Canada
Para-aminobenzoic acid (PABA)	PreSun	PreSun 4
	Pabanol (many others)	PreSun 8
Glyceryl para-aminobenzoate	Sea and Ski	
Homosalate	Coppertone	
Padimate O	Protan	
	Sundown	
	Sea and Ski	
Zinc oxide[x]	—§	Herisan
		Zincoflax

Actions: Act in varying degrees to decrease amount of radiant energy that the body's skin absorbs; the wavelength to which skin is maximally sensitive is 296.7 nm; the sun provides wavelengths that reach the earth's surface at approximately 310 nm; sunscreens to varying degrees block excess radiant energy to which the body is exposed.

Uses: Effectiveness depends on amount of radiant energy that the sunscreen is able to absorb; most now have a rating factor indicating the amount of sun protection factor (SPF) available in the agent. The rating scale goes from 2 (least protection against burning) to 15 (maximal protection against burning). Products containing para-aminobenzoic acid (PABA) considered best for prevention of burning.

SMOOTH MUSCLE RELAXANTS (AHFS 86:00*)

CATEGORY: SPASMOLYTIC AGENTS

	Trade Names	
Generic Name	U.S.	Canada
Oxybutynin	Ditropan	Ditropan
Papaverine	Cerespan	—§

*American Hospital Formulary Service classification.
†Drug is not available in Canada although it is listed in 1985 *Compendium of Pharmaceuticals and Specialties.*
‡U.S. trade name (or sometimes generic name) not listed in 1985 *Compendium of Pharmaceuticals and Specialties.*
§Drug is known by generic name.
[x]There are many more agents that contain combination ingredients, for example, oxyhenrone (combination of octyl salicylate and padimate O), marketed in the United States under the trade names of Solbar, Pre Sun 15 Lip Protection, Pre Sun 15, and Total Eclipse.

	Trade Names	
Generic Name	U.S.	Canada
	Pavacap	—‡
	Pavabid	—‡
Theophyllines[9]		
Aminophylline; theophylline ethylene	Somophyllin	Somophyllin
Dyphylline	Dilor	—†
	Airet	—‡
Theophylline	Bronkodyl	—‡
	Slo-Phyllin	—‡
	Theo-Dur	Theo-Dur
		Elixophyllin

Actions: Theophyllines (aminophylline, dyphylline, and theophylline) dominate this major grouping; major difference in these agents is their method of administration; act directly on smooth muscles of respiratory tract to produce relief of bronchospasm and increase flow rates and vital capacity; also dilate pulmonary arterioles, reduce pulmonary hypertension and alveolar carbon dioxide tension, increase pulmonary blood flow, and lower threshold of respiratory center to carbon dioxide. Oxybutynin and papaverine both exert a direct spasmolytic action on other smooth muscles throughout the body.

Uses: Theophyllines used as bronchodilators in symptomatic treatment of mild bronchial asthma and reversible bronchospasm that may occur in association with chronic bronchitis, emphysema, and other obstructive pulmonary diseases. Each of the theophylline agents have slightly different implications for use and should be investigated individually by the nurse before use. Oxybutynin used primarily as an antispasmotic in patients with uninhibited neurogenic or reflex neurogenic bladders for relief of symptoms associated with voiding, such as urgency, urge incontinence, frequency, nocturia, and incontinence. Papaverine used for cardiovascular system diseases in which there is spasm of blood vessels resulting in myocardial, cerebral, or peripheral ischemia.

General side effects: Theophyllines stimulate all levels of the central nervous system promoting headache, nervousness, irritability, restlessness, dizziness, peripheral vasoconstriction, and tachycardia; also irritating to gastrointestinal tract and may cause nausea, vomiting, epigastric pain, abdominal cramps, anorexia, and sometimes diarrhea; most of these side effects are transient and mild. Other side effects are similar to those of anticholinergic agents such as dry mouth, decreased sweating, urinary hesitancy, tachycardia, palpitations, blurred vision, and cycloplegia. Side effects from papaverine include general discomfort, flushing of face, sweating, dryness of mouth or throat, hypotension, gastrointestinal upset, drowsiness, dehydration, malaise, dizziness, and headache.

Adverse reactions: High plasma levels of theophyllines may increase sinus rate, tachycardia, acute hypotension, extrasystole, or ventricular arrhythmias; other more serious and rare adverse reactions of theophyllines include suppression

[9]Also available in combination with numerous other agents.

of bone marrow, leukopenia, and thrombocytopenia. Acute toxicity resulting from oxybutynin ingestion includes CNS excitability, fever, flushing, cardiovascular stimulation, and later hypotension and circulatory and respiratory collapse. IV administration of papaverine should be done only under direct physician supervision; fatal arrhythmias and apnea have resulted following rapid injection.

Contraindications: Should be used with caution in young children, elderly persons, and patients with angina pectoris, history of recent myocardial infarction, congestive heart failure, cor pulmonale, or renal or hepatic disease. Oxybutynin should be used with caution in patients with hepatic, renal, cardiovascular, or CNS dysfunction or ulcerative colitis; may also aggravate symptoms of reflux esophagitis. Papaverine contraindicated for patients with atrioventricular heart block and should be administered with extreme caution in patients with cardiac arrhythmias and glaucoma.

Nursing considerations:

1. Theophylline plasma or serum levels of about 10 to 20 μg/ml are required to produce optimal bronchodilator response. This may be reached by a single diluted IV dose of aminophylline (5 mg/kg) administered over a 30-minute period. Adverse reactions from the theophyllines should be anticipated if the plasma level exceeds 20 μg/ml.
2. Patients should be closely monitored while receiving IV theophylline agents. Rapid IV injection may cause dizziness, faintness, light-headedness, palpitations, syncope, precordial pain, premature ventricular contractions, severe hypotension, and cardiac arrest.
3. Successful therapy by the theophyllines includes a decrease in shortness of breath, wheezing, dyspnea, and improved pulmonary function studies.
4. These agents interact specifically with numerous other drugs. The health care provider should become familiar with the interactions of all agents being taken by the patient.
5. The theophyllines have low therapeutic indexes. Cautious dosage determinations are essential.
6. Patients taking oxybutynin should be cautioned of potential drowsiness and weakness while taking the agent. Precautionary measures should be taken until the effect of the agent may be evaluated.
7. IV administration of papaverine should only be done under direct physician supervision. When administered intravenously, the administration should be very slow (over a 1- to 2-minute period).
8. Papaverine is not compatible with Ringer's lactate IV solution.

VITAMINS (AHFS 88:00*)

The table on pp. 2178 and 2179 provides a summary of the recommended daily dietary allowances of fat- and water-soluble vitamins as well as minerals.

Many of the following vitamins are also available in combination with other vitamins, minerals, laxatives, hormones, enzymes, amino acids, and protein supplements. Many of the trade names listed below are different because of the strength of vitamin in the product. Others are different because of the extended-release component. Because the side effects, adverse reactions, contraindications, and nursing considerations are agent specific and differ depending on whether the vitamin is water soluble or fat soluble or the combination of the agent, these discussions have not been included. Vitamins A, D, E, and K have been discussed in greater detail. Because these are fat-soluble vitamins, they may be stored in the body, accumulate, and cause toxicity and overdosage. The remaining vitamins, because they are water soluble and are readily excreted in the urine, are thought not to be toxic. There is some beginning investigational concern that prolonged intake of excessive amounts of pyridoxine, niacin, and ascorbic acid may cause some adverse effects. The reader should thoroughly investigate the specific agent prescribed before its administration and should always consider the potential of adverse or accumulative reactions.

CATEGORY: VITAMIN A (AHFS 88:04*)

Generic Name	Trade Names	
	U.S.	Canada
Vitamin A	Alphalin	—÷
	A-Cap	—÷
	Aquasol A	Aquasol A

Actions: A fat-soluble dietary substance found in the fat of milk, egg yolks, liver, meat, and oily saltwater fish; available as retinol formed from edible fatty acids.

Uses: Required for growth and bone development, vision, reproduction, and integrity of mucosal tissue; used to prevent and treat symptoms of agent deficiency such as xerophthalmia and night blindness; may be used as a screening test for fat malabsorption; may also be used in Darier's disease and other skin disorders such as ichthyosis and psoriasis.

Adverse reactions: Absorption is incomplete in larger doses or in patients with fat malabsorption, low protein intake, hepatic disease, or pancreatic disease. Patients with glomerulonephritis or lipoid nephrosis may have increased serum levels of vitamin A because of storage abnormalities. If large doses of fat-soluble vitamin A are administered after saturation storage sites have been exceeded, unbound retinol may carry lipoproteins into circulation and may lead to toxic effects on cellular membranes that lead to hypervitaminosis. Acute toxicity (more common in young children than adults) may be seen if greater than 25,000 units of vitamin A per kilogram of body weight is ingested; signs include drowsiness, vertigo, coma, vomiting, diarrhea, papilledema, increased intracranial pressure, and visual disturbances. Erythema and generalized peeling of the skin occur a few days later and may persist for several weeks.

Contraindications: Hypervitaminosis and sensitivity to vitamin A; malabsorption syndromes.

Food and Nutrition Board, National Academy of Sciences–National Research Council Recommended Daily Dietary Allowances*

	Age (yr)	Weight (kg)	Weight (lb)	Height (cm)	Height (in)	Protein (g)	Fat-soluble vitamins			
							Vitamin A (μg_{RE})†	Vitamin D (μg)‡	Vitamin E (mg $_{\alpha\text{-TE}}$)§	Vitamin C (mg)
Infants	0.0-0.5	6	13	60	24	kg × 2.2	420	10	3	35
	0.5-1.0	9	20	71	28	kg × 2.0	400	10	4	35
Children	1-3	13	29	90	35	23	400	10	5	45
	4-6	20	44	112	44	30	500	10	6	45
	7-10	28	62	132	52	34	700	10	7	45
Males	11-14	45	99	157	62	45	1000	10	8	50
	15-18	66	145	176	69	56	1000	10	10	60
	19-22	70	154	177	70	56	1000	7.5	10	60
	23-50	70	154	178	70	56	1000	5	10	60
	51+	70	154	178	70	56	1000	5	10	60
Females	11-14	46	101	157	62	46	800	10	8	50
	15-18	55	120	163	64	46	800	10	8	60
	19-22	55	120	163	64	44	800	7.5	8	60
	23-50	55	120	163	64	44	800	5	8	60
	51+	55	120	163	64	44	800	5	8	60
Pregnant						+30	+200	+5	+2	+20
Lactating						+20	+400	+5	+3	+40

Reproduced from Recommended Dietary Allowances, ed. 9 (1980), with the permission of the National Academy of Sciences, Washington, D.C.
*Designed for the maintenance of good nutrition of practically all healthy people in the United States. The allowances are intended to provide for variety of common foods in order to provide other nutrients for which human requirements have been less well defined.
†Retinol equivalents. 1 retinol equivalent = 1 μg retinol or 6 μg β-carotene.
‡As cholecaliferol. 10 μg cholecalciferol = 400 IU vitamin D.
§α-Tocopherol equivalents. 1 mg d-α tocopherol = 1 $_{\alpha\text{-TE}}$.
‖1 NE (niacin equivalent) is equal to 1 mg of niacin or 60 mg of dietary tryptophan.
¶The folacin allowances refer to dietary sources as determined by *Lactobacillus casei* assay after treatment with enzymes (conjugases) to make
**The recommended daily allowance for vitamin B$_{12}$ in infants is based on average concentration of the vitamin in human milk. The allowances intestinal absorption.
††The increased requirement during pregnancy cannot be met by the iron content of habitual American diets nor by the existing iron stores of many those of nonpregnant women, but continued supplementation of the mother for 2 to 3 months after parturition is advisable in order to replenish

CATEGORY: VITAMIN B COMPLEX (AHFS 88:08*)

	Trade Names				Trade Names	
Generic Name	U.S.	Canada	*Generic Name*	U.S.	Canada
Folic acid; folate	Folvite	Folvite	Riboflavin	—§	—§
Niacin; niacinamide	Wampocap	Niacinamide	Vitamin B$_2$		
	Nicobid	Novoniacin	Vitamin G		
	Niac	—‡	Thiamin	Betalin S	—‡
	Nicotinex	—‡	Vitamin B$_1$	Thia	—‡
	Vasotherm	—‡		Bewon	Bewon
	Pan-B-3	—‡	Vitamin B$_{12}$		
Pyridoxine; vitamin B$_6$	TexSix T.R.	—‡	Cyanocobalamin	Betalin 12	—§
	Hexa-Betalin	Hexa-Betalin		Redisol	
	Hexacrest	—‡		Rubramin	—‡
	Pan-B-6	—‡		Stytobex	—‡
					—‡
			Hydroxocobalamin	AlphaREDISOL	Acti-B$_{12}$
				Alpha-Ruvite	—‡
				Codroxomin	—‡
			Liver extract	Pernaemon	—‡

*American Hospital Formulary Service classification.
†Drug is not available in Canada although it is listed in 1985 *Compendium of Pharmaceuticals and Specialties.*
‡U.S. trade name (or sometimes generic name) not listed in 1985 *Compendium of Pharmaceuticals and Specialties.*
§Drug is known by generic name.

Water-soluble vitamins						Minerals					
Thia-min (mg)	Ribo-flavin (mg)	Niacin (mg NE)‖	Vita-min B$_6$ (mg)	Fola-cin¶ (µg)	Vita-min B$_{12}$ (µg)	Cal-cium (mg)	Phos-phorus (mg)	Mag-nesium (mg)	Iron (mg)	Zinc (mg)	Iodine (µg)
0.3	0.4	6	0.3	30	0.5**	360	240	50	10	3	40
0.5	0.6	8	0.6	45	1.5	540	360	70	15	5	50
0.7	0.8	9	0.9	100	2.0	800	800	150	15	10	70
0.9	1.0	11	1.3	200	2.5	800	800	200	10	10	90
1.2	1.4	16	1.6	300	3.0	800	800	250	10	10	120
1.4	1.6	18	1.8	400	3.0	1200	1200	350	18	15	150
1.4	1.7	18	2.0	400	3.0	1200	1200	400	18	15	150
1.5	1.7	19	2.2	400	3.0	800	800	350	10	15	150
1.4	1.6	18	2.2	400	3.0	800	800	350	10	15	150
1.2	1.4	16	2.2	400	3.0	800	800	350	10	15	150
1.1	1.3	15	1.8	400	3.0	1200	1200	300	18	15	150
1.1	1.3	14	2.0	400	3.0	1200	1200	300	18	15	150
1.1	1.3	14	2.0	400	3.0	800	800	300	18	15	150
1.0	1.2	13	2.0	400	3.0	800	800	300	18	15	150
1.0	1.2	13	2.0	400	3.0	800	800	300	10	15	150
+0.4	+0.3	+2	+0.6	+400	+1.0	+400	+400	+150	††	+5	+25
+0.5	+0.5	+5	+0.5	+100	+1.0	+400	+400	+150	††	+10	+50

individual variations among most normal persons as they live in the United States under usual environmental stresses. Diets should be based on a

polyglutamyl forms of the vitamin available to the test organism.
after weaning are based on energy intake (as recommended by the American Academy of Pediatrics) and consideration of other factors such as

women; therefore the use of 30 to 60 mg of supplemental iron is recommended. Iron needs during lactation are not substantially different from stores depleted by pregnancy.

Actions: These agents are water soluble and are all found in the same types of food, including meat, eggs, milk, yeast, leafy green vegetables, and cereal grains. Folic acid required for nucleoprotein synthesis and maintenance of normal erythropoiesis. Niacin required for lipid metabolism. Pyridoxine required for amino acid metabolism. Riboflavin required for tissue respiration. Thiamin required for carbohydrate metabolism. Vitamin B$_{12}$ required for nucleoprotein and myelin synthesis, cell reproduction, normal growth, and maintenance of normal erythropoiesis.

Uses: Folic acid used in treatment of megaloblastic and macrocytic anemias resulting from folate deficiency. Niacin used in treatment of niacin deficiency and pellagra. Pyridoxine used to prevent and to treat vitamin B$_6$ deficiency, which is rarely identified in humans except in conjunction with other vitamin deficiencies or in relation to drug induction; there is some indication that pyridoxine needs during pregnancy may increase; patients with hereditary sideroblastic anemia should be treated with daily oral doses of pyridoxine. Riboflavin as a drug agent is used to prevent riboflavin deficiency and to treat ariboflavinosis and micro-

cytic anemia. Although adequate amounts of riboflavin are obtained from dietary sources, patients with liver disease, alcoholism, malignancy, and long-standing infections may require supplemental amounts. Thiamin used to treat thiamin deficiency syndromes as seen in alcoholic patients, such as beriberi, Wernicke's encephalopathy syndrome, and peripheral neuritis associated with pellagra; may be used as an emergency IM or IV dose to treat the high-output heart failure caused by beriberi and Wernicke's encephalopathy; may also be used in the treatment of select metabolic disorders. Vitamin B$_{12}$ used in treatment of pernicious anemia and other vitamin B$_{12}$ deficiency states.

Adverse reactions: Becuase the B vitamins are water soluble, they are relatively nontoxic; if adverse reactions are seen, they are most commonly manifested as allergic skin reactions, general malaise, or gastrointestinal upset. Niacin releases histamine and may cause flushing of the skin; orthostatic hypotension may follow administration; large doses may cause exacerbation of asthma, uricosuria, or precipitated gouty arthritis. Pyridoxine interferes with therapeutic effect of levodopa; continued high-level doses have been reported to lead to severe peripheral neuropathies. Although vitamin B$_{12}$ is usually nontoxic, there may be mild transient diarrhea, peripheral vascular thrombosis, itching, and a feeling of generalized body swelling.

Contraindications: Folic acid: undiagnosed anemia. Vitamin B$_{12}$: undiagnosed anemia, heart disease, known reactions to cobalt, or Lever's disease.

CATEGORY: VITAMIN C (AHFS 88:12*)

	Trade Names	
Generic Name	U.S.	Canada
Ascorbic acid	Ascor	Apo-C
	Ascorspan	Ce-Vi-Sol
	Cebid	Reduxon
	Cevalin	
	Ceeject	
	Ce-Vi-Sol Drops	
	Cecon Drops	
	Vitacee	
	Vitamin C Neo-Vadrin	
	Cemill	

Actions: A water-soluble vitamin found in citrus fruits, other fresh fruits, and vegetables; required for oxidation-reduction reactions and for collagen formation and tissue repair; deficiencies lead to disruption of connective tissue integrity.

Uses: Prevention and treatment of scurvy; also in large doses, it has been advocated for lessening the severity of and preventing the common cold. Vitamin C is also used as a urinary acidifier.

Adverse reactions: Large ingestion of vitamin C may lead to diarrhea and uricosuria; high doses may also predispose patient to decreased efficacy of oral anticoagulants and increased estrogen levels; because each gram of ascorbic acid contains 5 mEq of sodium, this agent should be used with caution in patients with sodium intake restrictions.

CATEGORY: VITAMIN D (AHFS 88:16*)

	Trade Names	
Generic Name	U.S.	Canada
Dihydrotachysterol	Hytakerol	Hytakerol
Ergocalciferol	Deltalin	—‡
	Drisdol	Drisdol
		Ostoforte
		Radiostol

Actions: A fat-soluble vitamin not readily available in natural dietary sources; main source in the United States is by the addition of vitamin D concentrates to milk products. Main action of vitamin D after being metabolically activated is to aid in absorption of ingested calcium from the gastrointestinal tract so that the calcium may act on the bones throughout the body.

Uses: Primarily administered to prevent or treat rickets or osteomalacia and to manage hypocalcemia associated with hypoparathyroidism or pseudohypoparathyroidism.

Adverse reactions: Because vitamin D is a fat-soluble vitamin, it is very important that the patient be monitored for evidence of hypercalcemia. Although adverse reactions are not common, infants and patients with sarcoidosis or hypoparathyroidism may have increased sensitivity to vitamin D. Toxicity is most commonly seen when the agent is taken for several months. Hypervitaminosis D results from the movement of calcium from the bones into the blood. Clinical signs include symptoms of headache, anorexia, nausea, vomiting, abdominal cramps, diarrhea or constipation, irritability, vertigo, and ataxia or hypotonia. Laboratory values show increased evidence of calcium in kidney, heart, and blood samples. Fatalities may result from renal dysfunction.

CATEGORY: VITAMIN E (AHFS 88:20*)

	Trade Names	
Generic Name	U.S.	Canada
Vitamin E	E-Ferol Acetate	Aquasol E
	Eprolin	
	Alpha-E 100	
	Alpha-E 300	
	Maxi-E	
Water miscible	Aquasol E	
	Solucap E	

Actions: A fat-soluble vitamin that is available in wheat germ oil, fresh lettuce leaves, and the fat of eggs aned milk; may increase the absorption, utilization, and storage of vitamin A and may protect against hypervitaminosis; effects are controversial.

Uses: Low–birth weight infants to treat hemolytic anemia caused by vitamin E deficiency; abundant in normal diets; deficiency does not occur in normal adults. There is no evidence to support that vitamin E therapy cures sterility, strengthens muscles in dystrophic patients, or is beneficial in cardiovascular disorders.

Adverse reactions: Doses of more than 300 units of vitamin E per day may cause diarrhea, intestinal cramps, nausea, fatigue, headache, blurred vision, increased serum creatine kinase, increased cholesterol and triglycerides, and increased urinary estrogens and androgens; may also cause decreased serum thyroxine and triiodothyronine; injections of vitamin E have on rare occasions caused a sterile abscess; topical application may cause dermatitis.

CATEGORY: VITAMIN K (AHFS 88:24*)

	Trade Names	
Generic Name	U.S.	Canada
Menadione; vitamin K$_3$	—§	—§
Menadiol sodium diphosphate; vitamin K$_4$	Synkayvite	Synkavite
	Kappadione	—†
Phytonadione; vitamin K$_1$	Aqua-MEPHYTON	Aqua-MEPHYTON
	Konakion	Konakion
	Mephyton	—‡

*American Hospital Formulary Service classification.
†Drug is not available in Canada although it is listed in 1985 *Compendium of Pharmaceuticals and Specialties*.
‡U.S. trade name (or sometimes generic name) not listed in 1985 *Compendium of Pharmaceuticals and Specialties*.
§Drug is known by generic name.

Actions: A fat-soluble vitamin required for synthesis of blood coagulation factors II (prothrombin), VII (proconvertin), IX (Christmas factor), and X (Stuart-Power factor) in the liver; so abundant in foods, including plant leaves and vegetable oils, that deficiency is rarely the result of poor diet; deficiency comes from inability of the body to absorb the vitamin because of an intestinal disorder or because of the presence of antagonists (coumarin and indanedione agents).

Uses: Antidote to overdosage with oral anticoagulants as well as in the prevention and treatment of hypoprothrombinemia caused by vitamin K deficiency. Although the dietary source of vitamin K is usually adequate, malabsorption syndromes such as sprue, celiac disease, ulcerative colitis, cystic fibrosis, prolonged diarrhea, and obstructive jaundice may cause deficiencies. Phytonadione (vitamin K_1) and menadione (vitamin K_3) require bile salts for absorption from the gastrointestinal tract; menadiol sodium (vitamin K_4) does not. Phytonadione (vitamin K_1) is the agent of choice for treatment of hemorrhage induced by coumarin; it will not, however, antagonize the anticoagulant action of heparin; is used in the prophylaxis and treatment of hemorrhagic disease of the newborn and is effective in the prevention of neonatal hemorrhage resulting from anticonvulsant therapy during therapy. Menadione (vitamin K_3) and menadiol sodium diphosphate (vitamin K_4) ineffective and should not be used in the treatment of oral anticoagulant–induced hypoprothrombinemia.

Adverse reactions: Menadione (vitamin K_3) and menadiol sodium (vitamin K_4) may produce severe hemolytic anemia, hyperbilirubinemia, hemoglobinuria, kernicterus, brain damage, and death in newborn infants, particularly premature infants. If these agents are administered to the mothers during the last few weeks of pregnancy, the agents may also induce an adverse reaction. Less severe adverse reactions include nausea, vomiting, headache, and hypersensitivity allergic reactions. Phytonadione (vitamin K_1) is relatively nontoxic; however, severe reactions have occurred rarely during or immediately following IV administration; signs include cramping pains, convulsions, cardiac irregularities, chest pain, cyanosis, dulled consciousness, sense of chest constriction, hypotension, and circulatory collapse.

UNCLASSIFIED THERAPEUTIC AGENTS (AHFS 92:00*)

Because of the nature of this section, each of the following agents will be treated as a separate class.

Class: Allopurinol

Generic Name	Trade Names	
	U.S.	Canada
Allopurinol	Lopurin	Purinol
	Zyloprim	Zyloprim

Actions: Inhibition of xanthine oxidase, the enzyme that catalyzes the conversion of hypoxanthine to xanthine and of xanthine to uric acid; uric acid level is therefore reduced.

Uses: Lower serum and urinary uric acid levels in treatment of primary gout and in treatment of primary or secondary gouty nephropathy with or without secondary oliguria; most helpful for patients with frequent and disabling attacks of gout. Some physicians believe that therapy should be initiated when serum urate levels exceed 9 mg/dl. Considered the treatment of choice for gout when uricosurics cannot be used; goal of therapy is to lower serum urate levels to about 6 mg/dl.

General side effects: Although incidence is low, the most common side effect is a pruritic maculopapular skin rash, fever, nausea, vomiting, chills, alopecia, and malaise.

Adverse reactions: Rarely, severe furunculoses of the nose, Stevens-Johnson syndrome, leukopenia, leukocytosis, eosinophilia, and arthralgia have been reported; transient alterations in liver function tests have been reported.

Contraindications: Because this agent has no analgesic or antiinflammatory activity, its use during acute gout attacks may actually prolong or exacerbate the inflammation; should be used cautiously in patients with renal or liver disease; effects of this agent on pregnant women are unknown; should also not be administered to nursing mothers or young children.

Nursing considerations:

1. Allopurinol may increase the frequency of acute gouty attacks during the first 6 to 12 months of therapy.
2. Patients taking long-term allopurinol treatment should have periodic liver function and renal function studies performed.

Class: Bromocriptine

Generic Name	Trade Names	
	U.S.	Canada
Bromocriptine	Parlodel	Parlodel

Actions: A dopamine agonist that reduces serum prolactin levels by inhibiting the release of prolactin from the anterior pituitary gland and thus restoring ovulation and ovarian function in amenorrheic women and suppressing puerperal or nonpuerperal lactation in women with adequate gonadotropin levels and ovarian function.

Uses: Approved only for short-term use in treatment of amenorrhea or galactorrhea associated with hyperprolactinemia of various etiologies, excluding pituitary tumors; restores ovulation without ovarian hyperstimulation and risk of multiple pregnancy; has also been used to restore fertility in oligospermic men without pituitary tumors; has been used investigationally for treatment of several other diseases such as Parkinson's disease, acromegaly, Cushing's disease, and chronic hepatic encephalopathy.

General side effects: Side effects include nausea, vomiting, anorexia, abdominal or leg cramps, metallic taste in the mouth, burning discomfort of the eyes, epigastric pain, dyspepsia, and constipation or diarrhea; CNS effects include headache, dizziness, fatigue, light-headedeness, and sedation.

Adverse reactions: Rarely, the increased gastrointestinal acid production by the agent may cause a peptic ulcer or gastrointestinal bleeding. Confusion, hallucinations, delusions, headaches, nasal congestion, and nightmares are related to high doses over long periods of time.

Contraindications: Pregnancy; not recommended for children under 15 years of age.

Nursing considerations:

1. When therapy is begun with doses greater than 20 mg/d, the incidence of side effects is high. If noted, reduce the dosage and increase it slowly.
2. If side effects are noted, they may be decreased by administering the agent with food, using antacids, or if necessary antiemetics as ordered.
3. It is recommended that a pregnancy test be performed every 4 weeks in amenorrheic women, and once menses are reinstated, whenever a menstrual period is missed. If pregnancy is suspected, the agent should be terminated at once.
4. Orthostatic hypotension or dizziness may result secondary to agent administration. Proper education and precautions should be utilized.

Class: Cromolyn

	Trade Names	
Generic Name	U.S.	Canada
Cromolyn		
Ophthalmic	Opticrom	Opticrom
Nasal	Nasalcrom	Rynacrom
Tracheobronchial inhalation	Intal	Intal

Actions: Acts primarily through a local effect on the mucosa; prevents release of mediators of type I allergic reactions, including histamine and slow-reacting substances of anaphylaxis from sensitized mast cells after an antigen-antibody reaction has taken place; have no bronchodilator, antihistamine, or corticosteroid-like properties.

Uses: Capsule powder inhalation directly into tracheobronchial tree or by nasal spray solution for management of severe bronchial asthma; prophylactic in nature and has no value in treatment of acute asthma attacks; ophthalmologic cromolyn used investigationally in treatment of vernal keratoconjunctivitis.

General side effects: Local mucous irritation is most common side effect.

Adverse reactions: Inhalation of powder may cause bronchospasm, cough, laryngeal edema, and wheezing; other adverse reactions to these agents include angioedema, joint swelling, dysuria, nausea, headache, and urticaria.

Contraindications: Children under 5 years of age or any individual showing an allergic response to the agent.

Nursing considerations:

1. The dosage of these agents should be reduced very slowly so as not to precipitate a disease response.
2. This agent is administered by inhalation or by ophthalmic solution. It is not effective when administered orally. Carefully read the package insert for specific directions before attempting agent administration.

*American Hospital Formulary Service classification.
†Drug is not available in Canada although it is listed in 1985 *Compendium of Pharmaceuticals and Specialties.*
‡U.S. trade name (or sometimes generic name) not listed in 1985 *Compendium of Pharmaceuticals and Specialties.*
§Drug is known by generic name.

Class: Levodopa

	Trade Names	
Generic Name	U.S.	Canada
Levodopa	Bio-Dopa	—†
	Dopar	—†
	Larodopa	Larodopa

Actions: Not completely known; penetrates the central nervous system and increases the dopamine concentration in the brain.

Uses: Symptomatic treatment of idiopathic parkinsonism and parkinsonian syndrome resulting from lethargica encephalitis, carbon monoxide intoxication, chronic manganese intoxication, or cerebral arteriosclerosis; although the agent may alter the symptoms of parkinsonism, it does not alter the course of the disease.

General side effects: Side effects are common and include signs from almost every body system. Gastrointestinal signs include nausea, vomiting, anorexia, constipation, and abdominal or epigastric distress. CNS signs include decreased attention span, nervousness, increased anxiety, vivid dreams, nightmares, and feelings of euphoria, malaise, and fatigue. Respiratory signs may include bizarre breathing patterns or episodic hyperventilation. Urinary tract signs include urinary frequency, incontinence, and dark urine. Ocular signs include blurred vision, diplopia, mydriasis, or miosis. In addition, renal and hepatic laboratory values may be elevated.

Adverse reactions: More serious reactions include duodenal ulcers or gastrointestinal bleeding and choreiform, dystonic, dyskinetic, and other adventitious movements; approximately 50% of patients receiving long-term therapy have some type of rhythmic or jerky movement secondary to the agent.

Contraindications: Severe cardiovascular, pulmonary, renal, hepatic, or endocrine disease; because of the potential psychiatric side effects it should also be used with extreme caution if the patient is depressed or has other psychiatric distress; contraindicated in patients taking monoamine oxidase inhibitors; safety during pregnancy has not been established.

Nursing considerations:

1. The patient should be warned that orthostatic episodes may follow therapeutic doses of levodopa as well as about the many common side effects and adverse reactions. Any agent-related symptom should be reported and evaluated.
2. If signs indicating potential psychiatric disturbance are noted, they must be evaluated to determine if they are levodopa dependent.
3. Hepatic, hematopoietic, cardiovascular, and renal function studies should be performed as a baseline before beginning therapy as well as periodically while the patient is taking levodopa.

Drug Index

2183

Sodium sulamyd, 2123, 2148
Sodium tetradecyl sulfate, 2135
Sodium-potassium chloride and sodium lactate, 2144
Sodium-potassium-ammonium chloride, 2144
Solganal, 2156
Solu-Contentun, 2123
Solu-Cortef, 2158
Solu-Diazine Sodium, 2123
Solu-Medrol, 2158
Solucap E, 2180
Somatropin (human growth hormone), 2164 spelling?
Somophyllin, 2176
Sorbitol, 2154
Sorbitrate, 2135
Sotradecol, 2135
Spasmolytic agents, 2176
Spectinomycin, 2122
Spironolactone, 2145
S-P-T, 2165
SSKI, 2147
Stadol, 2135
Staphcillin, 2121
Stemetil, 2138, 2155
Sterine, 2124
Stie VAA, 2174
Stilbestrol, 2161
Streptase, 2132
Streptokinase, 2132
Streptolin, 2119
Streptomycin, 2119
Streptosol 25%, 2119
Stytobex, 2178
Succinylcholine, 2130
Sudafed, 2129
Suladyne, 2123
Sulamyd, 2123, 2148
Sulf-10, 2148
Sulfacetamide, 2123
Sulfacetamide sodium (ophthalmic), 2148
Sulfadets, 2123
Sulfadiazine, 2123
Sulfadoxine-pyrimethamine, 2123
Sulfamethoxazole, 2123
Sulfamylon, 2172
Sulfapyridine, 2124
Sulfex, 2123, 2148
Sulfinpyrazone, 2135, 2146
Sulfisoxazole, 2124
Sulfisoxazole diolamine (ophthalmic), 2148
Sulfium, 2148
Sulfonamides, 2123, 2148
Sulfones, 2124
Sulfonylureas, 2163
Sulindac, 2136
Sumycin, 2122
Sunalar, 2173
Sundown, 2176
Sunscreen agents, 2176
Supeudol, 2135
Surfak, 2154
Suxamethonium, 2130
Symmetrel, 2123

Sympatholytic agents, 2130
Sympathomimetic agents, 2129
Synalar, 2173
Synkayvite, 2180
Synthroid, 2165
Syntocinon, 2166

T

Tacaryl, 2117
Tagamet, 2156
Talwin, 2135
Tamoxifen, 2125
Tandearil, 2136
Tannic acid, 2173
Tapazole, 2165
Tavist Fumarate, 2117
Tavist, 2117
Tebrazid, 2122
Tegopen, 2121
Tegretol, 2137
Telmin, 2118
Temaril, 2117
Tenicridine, 2118
Tenormin, 2133
Tenuate, 2139
Terbutaline, 2129
Terp liquid, 2147
Terpin hydrate, 2147
Tesone, 2159
Testosterone, 2159
Tetanus and diphtheria toxoids, adsorbed, for adult use (Td), 2169
Tetanus immune globulin, 2168
Tetanus Immune Globulin, 2168
Tetanus toxoid (TT), 2169
Tetracaine (ophthalmic, nasal, or oral), 2149
Tetracyclines, 2122
Tetracyn, 2122
TexSix T.R., 2178
Theelin, 2161
Theo-Dur, 2176
Theophylline, 2176
Theophylline ethylene, 2176
Thia, 2178
Thiabendazole, 2118
Thiamazole, 2165
Thiamin, 2178, 2179
Thiethylperazine, 2155
Thioguanine (6-TG), 2125
Thiotepa, 2125
Thorazine, 2138
Throat preparations, 2148
Thrombolytic agents, 2132
Thyrar, 2165
Thyro-Block, 2147
Thyroglobulin, 2165
Thyroid, 2165
Thyroid agents, 2165
Thyrolar, 2165
Ticar, 2121
Ticarcillin disodium, 2121
Tigan, 2155
Timolol, 2133
Timolol (ophthalmic), 2152

Timoptic, 2152
Tinactin, 2171
Titralac, 2152
Tobramycin, 2119
Tobrex, 2119
Tocainide, 2133
Tofranil, 2138
Tolazamide, 2163
Tolazoline, 2135
Tolbutamide, 2163
Tolectin, 2136
Tolinase, 2163
Tolmetin, 2136
Tolnaftate, 2171
Tolserol, 2130
Tonocard, 2133
Topicort, 2173
Topsyn Gel, 2173
Topsyn, 2173
Torecan, 2155
Torecan maleate, 2155
Toxoid agents, 2168
Toxoids, 2169
Tranquilizers, 2138
Transderm-Nitro, 2135
Transderm-V, 2129
Tranylcypromine, 2138
Trazodone, 2138
Trecator, 2122
Trescatyl, 2122
Tresortil, 2130
Tretamine, 2125
Tretinoin, 2174
Triamcinolone, 2158
Triamcinolone acetonide cream, 2173
Triamcinolone acetonide ointment, 2173
Triamterene, 2145
Tridesilon, 2173
Tridel, 2135
Triethylene melamine (TEM), 2125
Trihexyphenidyl, 2129
Trimeprazine, 2117
Trimethobenzamide, 2155
Trioxsalen, 2175
Tripelennamine, 2117
Triphasil, 2160
Triprolidine, 2117
Triptil, 2138
Trisoralen, 2175
Trisulfapyrimidine, 2124
Trisulfazine, 2124
Tritalac, 2142
Trobicin, 2122
Trombovar, 2135
Tropicamide, 2150
Tums, 2152
Tusscapine, 2147
Tylenol, 2135
Typhoid vaccine, 2170

U

Ultandren, 2159
Ultralente, 2162
Ultralente Iletin, 2162
Ultralente Insulin, 2162

Index